# Avery's
# Drug Treatment

## 4TH EDITION

Edited by

**Trevor M. Speight**

Senior Editor
Adis International Limited
Auckland

and

**Nicholas H.G. Holford**

Associate Professor
Department of Pharmacology & Clinical Pharmacology
University of Auckland School of Medicine
Auckland

A guide to the properties, choice, therapeutic use and economic value of drugs in disease management

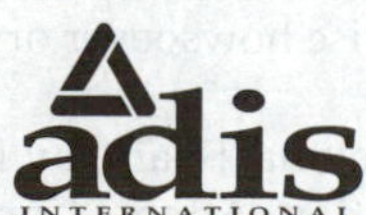


**Adis International**

Auckland Chester Frankfurt Hong Kong Madrid Milan Osaka Paris Philadelphia Sydney

# Avery's
# Drug Treatment
## 4TH EDITION

ISBN 0-86471-036-4

1ST edition 1976
2ND edition 1980
3RD edition 1987

**Adis International Limited**
**41 Centorian Drive, Mairangi Bay, Auckland 10, New Zealand**



Printed in Barcelona, Spain, by Ingoprint S.A.
Technical collaboration, Adonis Communications S.L.

## Preface to Fourth Edition

The first edition of this textbook published some 20 years ago sought to bridge the gap between standard texts on pharmacology on the one hand, and medicine on the other, by discussing the uses and effects of drugs in a disease-oriented context. The preface to the First Edition is again reprinted in this edition to restate the rationale for the structure of ***Drug Treatment***, and to emphasise that the book's original aims and objectives have been retained, i.e. to assist clinicians in gaining an understanding of drug responses in disease states and in selecting the most appropriate drug for a particular patient. Precisely what drugs can and cannot achieve and, when they are clearly indicated, their optimum clinical use, remains a primary focus of this book.

As with earlier editions, the Fourth Edition of ***Drug Treatment*** covers the clinical pharmacological basis of therapeutics and emphasises the importance of the pharmacodynamic and pharmacokinetic properties of drugs in their selection and rational usage in disease management. The Fourth Edition is, however, largely a 'new' one (rather than simply an 'update') written to a new/revised format. In doing so, an attempt has been made to apply a consistent set of clinical pharmacological principles throughout all chapters. Tabular compilations of the clinical pharmacological properties of drugs of various therapeutic classes have been included to assist in an understanding of the differences and similarities of the various agents that may be prescribed for the treatment of a diseased patient. At the same time, the influence of intercurrent diseases on the pharmacokinetics and clinical responses to drugs is emphasised so that the changes in drug therapy that need to be undertaken, either in the initial selection of a therapeutic agent or in the dosage given, are made clear.

The new edition of ***Drug Treatment*** contains more information on therapeutics than earlier editions, and the 'optimum treatment' section for each disease state has been extensively rewritten to provide current evidence-based guidelines on management. As part of this process, a number of *clinical algorithms* have been included to assist in an understanding of the often complex considerations in managing important disease states. Additionally, the new edition provides information on the relevant *economic considerations* that should be taken into account when undertaking treatment of a diseased patient. Where data are available, a new section 'Clinical Outcome and Economic Considerations' has been included as part of the disease treatment discussion to provide information on: (a) the economic costs of the illness; and (b) the desirable objectives of treatment in relation to the costs of achieving these objectives. A new chapter on 'Pharmacoeconomics and Drug Prescribing' discusses the principles of pharmacoeconomic evaluation of drugs and emphasises that drugs should be appreciated for the value they contribute rather than the costs they generate.

In addition to the chapter on pharmacoeconomics, the Fourth Edition of ***Drug Treatment*** contains a number of other important new contributions including chapters on 'Maternal and Fetal Clinical Pharmacology'; 'Principles of Pharmacoepidemiology'; 'Drug Development and Approval Processes' and 'Immune System Disorders' *plus* new appendices providing a 'Guide to Safety of Drugs in Breast Feeding' and the 'Clearance and Volume Method of Dose Prediction'. These new contributions enhance the book's coverage of important concepts in clinical pharmacology and therapeutics, and its overall value as a guide to disease management.

The editing of this book has been a massive but very rewarding task, and we trust that it will assist in meeting information requirements in the new environment that is medicine in the 1990s. We would like to record our thanks to the international panel of experts who contributed the various chapters and appendices for their cooperation and enthusiasm. We would also like to thank our colleagues at Adis International who assisted in the production of this new edition, particularly Cushla Goode, Heather Langtry and Lisa Aalbers (who had the unenviable task of keying the entire book), as well as David Britten, Joy Robinson and Lisa O'Carroll. Last, but by no means least, the input and encouragement of the book's founding editor Graeme Avery is gratefully acknowledged.

*Trevor M. Speight*
*Nicholas H.G. Holford*
Auckland, December 1996

## Preface to First Edition

The aim of this book is to discuss the use and effects of drugs within a disease orientated context and so assist clinicians in an understanding of drug response in disease states and in the selection of the most appropriate drug and dosage for a particular patient. The book has been highly structured to achieve this purpose and covers: (1) the clinical pharmacological basis of therapeutics, with particular emphasis on pharmacokinetics; (2) rational selection and individualised use of drugs; (3) the influence of associated disease or intercurrent illness on drug response; (4) diseases caused by drugs; and (5) summary tables and appendices to enable quick reference and correlation of data on individual drugs and classes of drugs. Such a wide scope has never before been attempted in a single book. It was felt, however, that an integrated format describing the effects and response to drugs within the context of their clinical use was essential for a proper understanding of clinical pharmacology and therapeutics. Knowledge of what drugs can and can not achieve in a particular disease and how that disease can modify the response to a drug are a prerequisite to safe and effective drug therapy.

A discussion of pathophysiological principles and the mode of action of drugs has only been included where these are of particular importance in the selection of a drug or dose regimen. This is not to say that an understanding of these aspects is not important generally - *it is,* but the central aim of this book is to show that before selecting a drug or dose regimen, the clinician should think first about the patient and his/her disease(s) and how this might modify drug response. In this way it is hoped that the desired therapeutic effect with minimum adverse effects may be more easily attained. A number of standard texts are available which discuss the pathophysiological and pharmacological basis of therapeutics. Such texts, although extremely valuable and important, describe drugs from the viewpoint of their actions and various uses, which is not ideal for the prescribing clinician whose special primary need is to know how to select and use a drug for an individual patient with a particular disease. The starting point in the therapeutic decision-making process is the patient and his/her disease or pathophysiological condition and how this relates to the pharmacodynamic actions and characteristic pharmacokinetic properties of individual drugs. The purpose of the book is therefore to complement standard texts in pharmacology on the one hand, and medicine on the other - a kind of 'bridge text'.

The teaching of therapeutics is difficult. Traditional teaching of medicine places an excessive emphasis on proficiency in diagnosis while teaching in pharmacology has until recently placed too much emphasis on the pharmacological action of drugs and too little emphasis on how they behave and what they achieve in sick patients. This book aims to bridge this gap by defining clinical pharmacological principles of therapy within a disease orientated context and by describing established approaches to therapy on the basis of drug availability and specialist clinical experience with drugs on a worldwide basis. (Certain indications given in the book for use of some drugs may not be those at present 'approved' for general use in some countries.) A synopsis of important principles appears at the head of each chapter. These synopses might help in defining learning objectives by itemising that material which is of most general significance and importance, which should be read during skimming for high points and for review, and also that material which most students should master. The relatively young discipline of clinical pharmacology is an essential component of modern medical practice. Already, it has made a very important contribution to improvement in teaching of therapeutics, but academic clinical pharmacology is developing so rapidly that if not careful, it runs the risk of moving away from the present level of understanding of the clinicians whom it is trying to serve. Perhaps also, too much effort in clinical pharmacology has been placed on the valuation of new drugs rather than on the better utilisation and understanding of existing drugs.

Clinicians use drugs to achieve a preconceived clinical endpoint. This having been decided upon, it remains to select the most appropriate drug and dose regimen for a particular patient. Since clinical drug effects are the result of complex interaction between the drug, the patient and his/her disease, much emphasis in this book has therefore been placed on individualisation of therapy - both in terms of the characteristic pharmacokinetic properties of individual drugs and the response to a particular drug in an individual patient with a particular disease. Individualised dosage is the heart of therapeutics. Doses discussed in this book are not necessarily those 'approved by a regulatory body' but rather those which competent clinicians have by experience found to be both effective and safe. There is no such thing as a standard dose for all patients, nor a maximum dose for all patients. Therapeutics deals with individuals, not groups of patients.

***Drug Treatment*** is primarily aimed at the student and the clinician in practice, but it should also be of use as a starting point for those studying for higher exams. It is hoped too that the wide scope of information, particularly the many reference tables of drug data, will provide something of value for everyone involved in the study, use and provision of information on drugs. For the prescribing clinician, information on drugs needs to be practical and authoritative. Great care has been placed in the writing and editing to achieve this purpose, all the time keeping the scope of the book within the bounds of understanding of its intended primary audience. It is a book for those who wish to prescribe drugs rationally and with confidence that therapy will be likely to be both effective and safe. The various discussions have been kept as concise as possible with emphasis placed on principles and major aspects of therapy and drug related effects. Those diseases which are most common and those drugs which are most often used have received the greatest attention, as have common therapeutic dilemmas and areas which illustrate clinical pharmacological principles of therapy. The planning of the book coincided with the rapid development of research interest in the study of pharmacokinetics of drugs in sick patients. Much of this information is still poorly defined, particularly its application to therapeutics. Interpretation of these data and the implications to therapy was one of the most difficult tasks in writing and editing the material in the book. Further study will no doubt elucidate many of the uncertain areas. In the meantime, the material pertaining to pharmacokinetic concepts in sick patients therefore relates to the better established principles and those findings of most practical application to therapeutics.

References have been selected both for the purpose of supporting statements made in the text and also to act as a starting point for those who wish to study a particular aspect in more depth. Major review articles and specific text books have been included for this purpose. Source data given in tables and figures are acknowledged separately at the beginning of the book, rather than in the text itself.

Therapeutics can and should be an enjoyable experience and I can only hope that this book gives readers as much pleasure (and assistance) as I have had in compiling and editing it.

*Graeme S. Avery*
Auckland, January 1976

# Contributors

*Abel, A.D.*
Jefferson Medical College, Thomas Jefferson University, Philadelphia, Pennsylvania, USA

*Abel Jr, R.S.*
Clinical Professor of Ophthalmology, Thomas Jefferson University, Philadelphia, Pennsylvania, USA

*Atkinson, H.C.*
Medical Director, Roche Products (New Zealand) Ltd, Penrose, Auckland, New Zealand

*Begg, E.J.*
Associate Professor, Department of Medicine, Christchurch School of Medicine, Christchurch Hospital, Christchurch, New Zealand

*Bennett, W.M.*
Professor of Medicine and Pharmacology, Department of Medicine, Division of Nephrology, Hypertension and Clinical Pharmacology, Oregon Health Sciences Center, Portland, Oregon, USA

*Benowitz, N.L.*
Professor of Medicine and Chief, Division of Clinical Pharmacology and Experimental Therapeutics, University of California at San Francisco, San Francisco General Hospital Medical Center, San Francisco, California, USA

*Bergman, U.*
Associate Professor of Clinical Pharmacology, Department of Medical Laboratory Sciences and Technology, Division of Clinical Pharmacology, Karolinska Institute, Huddinge University Hospital, Huddinge, Sweden

*Boogaerts, M.A.*
Professor of Internal Medicine and Chairman, Research Department of Pathophysiology, University of Leuven, Leuven, Belgium

*Borgå, O.*
Scientific Adviser and Pharmacokineticist, Astra Pharmaceuticals Ltd, Lund, Sweden. Formerly Pharmacokineticist, Office of Clinical Pharmacology and Biopharmaceutics, US Food and Drug Administration, Washington DC, USA

*Bowie, W.R.*
Professor, Department of Medicine, Division of Infectious Diseases, The University of British Columbia, Vancouver, British Columbia, Canada

*Boyages, S.C.*
Clinical Associate Professor and Head of Diabetes and Endocrinology, Westmead Hospital, Westmead, NSW, Australia

*Brooks, B.A.*
Nurse Consultant, Diabetes Centre, Endocrinology Institute, Royal Prince Alfred Hospital and the University of Sydney, Sydney, NSW, Australia

*Brooks, P.M.*
Professor of Medicine and Head, Medical Professorial Unit, St Vincent's Hospital, University of New South Wales, Sydney, Australia

*Bulpitt, C.J.*
Professor, Division of Geriatric Medicine, Hammersmith Hospital, London, England

*Capstick, F.*
Nurse Specialist, Diabetes Centre, Endocrinology Institute, Royal Prince Alfred Hospital and the University of Sydney, Sydney, NSW, Australia

*Caterson, I.D.*
Clinical Associate Professor and Director of Clinical Endocrinology, Endocrinology Institute, Royal Prince Alfred Hospital and the University of Sydney, Sydney, NSW, Australia

*Chan, T.Y.K.*
Associate Professor, Department of Clinical Pharmacology, The Chinese University of Hong Kong, Prince of Wales Hospital, Shatin, N.T., Hong Kong

*Cormican, M.G.*
Department of Immunology, University College Hospital, Galway, Ireland

*Crawford, D.H.G.*
Joint Liver Program, Department of Medicine, Queensland Institute of Medical Research, Brisbane, Queensland, Australia

*Critchley, Julian A.J.H.*
Professor of Clinical Pharmacology, Chairman, Department of Clinical Pharmacology, The Chinese University of Hong Kong, Prince of Wales Hospital, Shatin, N.T., Hong Kong

*Cumming, A.D.*
Senior Lecturer, Department of Medicine, University of Edinburgh, and Consultant, Department of Renal Medicine, Royal Infirmary Trust, Edinburgh, Scotland

*Cusack, B.J.*
Chief, Geriatrics Section, Department of Veterans Affairs Medical Center, Boise, Idaho, and Associate Professor of Medicine, Division of Gerontology and Geriatric Medicine, University of Washington, Seattle, Washington, USA

*Dahl, M.-L.*
Associate Professor of Clinical Pharmacology, Karolinska Institute, Department of Medical Laboratory Sciences and Technology, Division of Clinical Pharmacology, Huddinge University Hospital, Huddinge, Sweden

*Darlow, B.A.*
Senior Lecturer, Department of Paediatrics, Christchurch School of Medicine, Christchurch Hospital, Christchurch, New Zealand

*Davey, P.G.*
Reader in Clinical Pharmacology and Infectious Diseases, Pharmacoeconomics Research Centre, Department of Clinical Pharmacology, University of Dundee, Ninewells Hospital and Medical School, Dundee, Scotland

*Day, R.O.*
Professor of Clinical Pharmacology, St Vincent's Hospital, School of Physiology and Pharmacology, University of New South Wales, Sydney, Australia

*de Carle, D.J.*
Associate Professor of Medicine, The University of New South Wales, Sydney, and Consultant Gastroenterologist, The St George Hospital, Kogarah, NSW, Australia

*deShazo, R.D.*
Professor of Medicine and Pediatrics, and Chairman of the Department of Internal Medicine, College of Medicine, University of South Alabama, Mobile, Alabama, USA

*Dettli, L.*
Professor Emeritus, Department of Internal Medicine, University Hospital, Basel, Switzerland

*Dodd, T.*
Director of Pharmacy, Manchester Royal Infirmary, Manchester, England

*Donnelly, R.*
Senior Lecturer, Department of Clinical Pharmacology, and Endocrinology Institute, Royal Prince Alfred Hospital and the University of Sydney, Sydney, NSW, Australia

*Douglas, J.G.*
Consultant Physician in Respiratory Medicine and Infection, Aberdeen Royal Hospitals NHS Trust, Aberdeen Royal Infirmary, Foresterhill, Aberdeen, Scotland

*Eadie, M.J.*
Professor of Clinical Neurology and Neuropharmacology, Department of Medicine, The University of Queensland, Royal Brisbane Hospital, Brisbane, Queensland, Australia

*Edwards, I.R.*
Professor and Director, WHO Collaborating Centre for International Drug Monitoring, Uppsala, Sweden

*Einarson, T.R.*
Associate Professor, Faculty of Pharmacy, and Department of Health Administration, Faculty of Medicine, University of Toronto, and Department of Clinical Pharmacology, Hospital for Sick Children, Toronto, Ontario, Canada

*Feely, J.*
Professor, Department of Pharmacology and Therapeutics, Trinity College, Dublin, Ireland

*Friend, J.A.R.*
Consultant Physician in Thoracic Medicine, Aberdeen Royal Hospitals NHS Trust, Aberdeen Royal Infirmary, Foresterhill, and Clinical Reader in Medicine, University of Aberdeen, Aberdeen, Scotland

*Gallagher, N.D.*
Clinical Professor of Gastroenterology, University of Sydney, The A.W. Morrow Gastroenterology and Liver Centre, Royal Prince Alfred Hospital, Camperdown, NSW, Australia

*Gazzard, B.G.*
Consultant and HIV/GUM Clinical Director, Chelsea and Westminster Hospital, London, England

*Gibson, P.R.*
Associate Professor of Medicine, University of Melbourne Department of Medicine, and Gastroenterologist, The Royal Melbourne Hospital, Melbourne, Victoria, Australia

*Hall, M.H.*
Consultant Obstetrician/Gynaecologist, Aberdeen Maternity Hospital, Foresterhill, Aberdeen, Scotland

*Handelsman, D.J.*
Associate Professor and Director of Andrology Unit, Endocrinology Institute, Royal Prince Alfred Hospital and the University of Sydney, Sydney, NSW, Australia

*Hebert, M.F.*
Associate Professor of Pharmacy, Department of Pharmacy, University of Washington, Seattle, Washington, USA

*Holford, N.H.G.*
Associate Professor, Department of Pharmacology and Clinical Pharmacology, University of Auckland School of Medicine, Auckland, New Zealand

*Jackson, R.T.*
Professor of Otolaryngology, Emory University School of Medicine, Atlanta, Georgia, USA

*Jones, R.N.*
Professor and Director of the Medical Microbiology Division and Anti-Infectives Research Center, Department of Pathology, University of Iowa College of Medicine, Iowa City, Iowa, USA

*Kellow, J.E.*
Associate Professor of Medicine and Gastroenterologist, University of Sydney Department of Medicine, The Royal North Shore Hospital, St Leonards, NSW, Australia

*Koren, G.*
Director, Division of Clinical Pharmacology and Toxicology, and Professor of Pediatrics, Pharmacology, Pharmacy and Medicine, University of Toronto, The Hospital for Sick Children, Toronto, Ontario, Canada

*Krishnaswamy, K.*
Deputy Director, National Institute of Nutrition, Jamai-Osmania, Hyderabad, India

*Krum, H.*
Senior Lecturer in Clinical Pharmacology, Department of Epidemiology and Preventive Medicine, and Department of Medicine, Monash University Medical School, Alfred Hospital, Prahran, Victoria, Australia

*Lader, M.*
Professor of Clinical Psychopharmacology, Institute of Psychiatry, De Crespigny Park, Denmark Hill, London, England

*Leatherman, J.*
Assistant Professor of Medicine, University of Minnesota Medical School, Division of Pulmonary and Critical Care Medicine, Hennepin County Medical Center, Minneapolis, Minnesota, USA

*Legge, J.S.*
Consultant Physician in Thoracic Medicine, Aberdeen Royal Infirmary, Foresterhill, Aberdeen, Scotland

*Lewitt, M.*
Staff Specialist and Senior Lecturer, and Director of Diagnostic Endocrinology, Endocrinology Institute, Royal Prince Alfred Hospital and the University of Sydney, Sydney, NSW, Australia

*MacDonald, T.*
Senior Lecturer in Clinical Pharmacology, University of Dundee, Ninewells Hospital and Medical School, Dundee, Scotland

*Maibach, H.I.*
Professor, Department of Dermatology, School of Medicine, University of California, San Francisco, California, USA

*Malek, M.*
Professor in Health Policy, Planning and Management, Department of Management, The University of St Andrews, Fife, Scotland

*McCaughey, W.*
Lecturer, Department of Anaesthetics, The Queen's University of Belfast, Whitla Medical Building, Lisburn Road, Belfast, Northern Ireland

*McCombs, C.C.*
Professor of Medicine and Director of the Division of Experimental Medicine, College of Medicine, University of South Alabama, Mobile, Alabama, USA

*McNeil, J.J.*
Professor and Head, Department of Epidemiology and Preventive Medicine, Monash University Medical School, Alfred Hospital, Prahran, Victoria, Australia

*Mirakhur, R.K.*
Senior Lecturer, Department of Anaesthetics, The Queen's University of Belfast, Whitla Medical Building, Lisburn Road, Belfast, Northern Ireland

*Muggia, F.M.*
Professor of Medicine, University of Southern California School of Medicine, and Director, Medical Oncology and Clinical Investigations, University of Southern California, Kenneth Norris Jr. Comprehensive Cancer Center and Hospital, Los Angeles, California, USA

*Nielson, C.P.*
Co-Director, Critical Care, Department of Veterans' Affairs Medical Center, Boise, Idaho, and Associate Professor of Medicine, Division of Gerontology and Geriatric Medicine, University of Washington, Seattle, Washington, USA

*O'Brien, A.A.J.*
Consultant Physician, Department of Medicine for the Elderly, Southend General Hospital, Prittlewell Chase, Westcliffe on Sea, Essex, England

*Orme, M.L'E.*
Professor of Pharmacology and Therapeutics, University of Liverpool, and Director of Education and Training, NW Regional Office of the NHS Executive, Warrington, England

*Peerlinck, K.*
Assistant Professor, Center for Molecular and Vascular Biology, University of Leuven, Leuven, Belgium

*Pentel, P.*
Professor of Medicine and Pharmacology, University of Minnesota Medical School, Division of Clinical Pharmacology and Toxicology, Hennepin County Medical Center, Minneapolis, Minnesota, USA

*Petrie, J.C.*
Professor of Clinical Pharmacology, Head, Department of Medicine and Therapeutics, University of Aberdeen, Foresterhill, Aberdeen, Scotland

*Pfaller, M.A.*
Professor and Co-Director, Clinical Microbiology and Molecular Pathology Laboratories, Department of Pathology, University of Iowa College of Medicine, Iowa City, Iowa, USA

*Piper, D.W.*
Professor Emeritus, University of Sydney Department of Medicine, The Royal North Shore Hospital, Sydney, NSW, Australia

*Powell, L.W.*
Professor of Medicine, University of Queensland, Director, Queensland Institute of Medical Research, Brisbane, Queensland, Australia

*Proudfoot, A.*
Director, Scottish Poisons Information Bureau, Royal Infirmary, Edinburgh, Scotland

*Qu, X.*
Research Fellow, Department of Clinical Pharmacology, University of Sydney, Sydney, NSW, Australia

*Quinn, D.I.*
NHMRC Research Scholar, Garvan Institute of Medical Research, and Clinical Lecturer, Department of Clinical Pharmacology and Toxicology, St Vincent's Hospital, The University of New South Wales, Sydney, Australia

*Roberts, R.K.*
Consultant Gastroenterologist, Royal Brisbane Hospital, Brisbane, Queensland, Australia

*Sjöqvist, F.*
Professor of Clinical Pharmacology, Department of Medical Laboratory Sciences and Technology, Division of Clinical Pharmacology, Karolinska Institute, Huddinge University Hospital, Huddinge, Sweden

*Sorrell, T.C.*
Professor and Director, Centre for Infectious Diseases and Microbiology, University of Sydney, Westmead Hospital, Westmead, NSW, Australia

*Spilker, B.*
Executive Director, Orphan Medical, Minnetonka, Minnesota, USA

*Steinbeck, K.S.*
Staff Specialist and Director of Metabolism and Obesity Services, Endocrinology Institute, Royal Prince Alfred Hospital and the University of Sydney, Sydney, NSW, Australia

*Swaraj, S.*
Research Fellow, Andrology Unit, Endocrinology Institute, Royal Prince Alfred Hospital and the University of Sydney, Sydney, NSW, Australia

*Taeschner, W.*
Frosch-Apotheke, Lörrach, Germany

*Talley, N.J.*
Professor of Medicine, Department of Medicine, University of Sydney, Nepean Hospital, Penrith, NSW, Australia

*Tett, S.*
Associate Professor and Head, School of Pharmacy, University of Queensland, Brisbane, Queensland, Australia

*Theis, J.G.W.*
Clinical and Research Fellow, Clinical Pharmacology, Division of Clinical Pharmacology and Toxicology, Department of Paediatrics, University of Toronto, The Hospital for Sick Children, Toronto, Ontario, Canada

*Todd, N.W.*
Professor of Otolaryngology and Pediatrics, Emory University School of Medicine, and Chief of Otorhinolaryngology, Egleston Children's Hospital, Atlanta, Georgia, USA

*Turner Jr, J.S.*
Emeritus Professor and Chief of Otolaryngology, Emory University School of Medicine, Atlanta, Georgia, USA

*Turtle, J.R.*
Professor of Medicine and Head, Endocrinology Institute, Royal Prince Alfred Hospital and the University of Sydney, Sydney, NSW, Australia

*Vale, J.A.*
Director, West Midlands Poisons Unit, City Hospital, Birmingham, England

*Verhaeghe, R.*
Associate Professor of Medicine, Center for Molecular and Vascular Biology, University of Leuven, Leuven, Belgium

*Verstraete, M.*
Professor of Medicine (Emeritus), Center for Molecular and Vascular Biology, University of Leuven, Leuven, Belgium

*Vestal, R.E.*
Chief of Clinical Pharmacology and Gerontology Research Unit, Associate Chief of Staff for Research and Development, Department of Veterans' Affairs Medical Center, Boise, Idaho, USA, and also Professor of Medicine, Adjunct Professor of Pharmacology, Division of Gerontology and Geriatric Medicine, University of Washington, Seattle, Washington, USA

*Von Hoff, D.D.*
Director, Institute of Drug Development, Cancer Therapy and Research Center, San Antonio, and Department of Medicine, University of Texas Health Science Center at San Antonio, Texas, USA

*Vozeh, S.*
Professor, Medical Division, Intercantonal Office for the Control of Medicines, Berne, Switzerland

*Walson, P.D.*
Division Head, Clinical Pharmacology/Toxicology, Children's Hospital, and Professor, Pediatrics, Pharmacology, Pharmacy and Allied Health Services, The Ohio State University, Columbus, Ohio, USA

*Webster, J.*
Consultant Physician, Aberdeen Royal Infirmary, Foresterhill, Aberdeen, Scotland

*Weltfriend, S.*
Department of Dermatology, Rambam Medical Center, and Faculty of Medicine, Technion, Israel Institute of Technology, Haifa, Israel

*Wiholm, B.-E.*
Head, Section of Pharmacoepidemiology, Medical Products Agency, Uppsala, Sweden, and Associate Professor of Clinical Pharmacology, Department of Clinical Pharmacology, Karolinska Institute, Huddinge University Hospital, Huddinge, Sweden

*Wilson, J.S.*
Senior Staff Specialist, Gastrointestinal Unit, The Prince of Wales Hospital, Randwick, NSW, Australia

*Yue, D.K.*
Professor and Director of Diabetes Services, Endocrinology Institute, Royal Prince Alfred Hospital and the University of Sydney, Sydney, NSW, Australia

*Zegarelli, D.J.*
Professor, Columbia University School of Dental and Oral Surgery (in Stomatology) and College of Physicians and Surgeons (in Pathology), Columbia Presbyterian Medical Center, New York, NY, USA

# Contents

Chapter 1

# Fundamentals of Clinical Pharmacology

*F. Sjöqvist, O. Borgå, M.-L. Dahl* and *M.L'E. Orme*

## Synopsis of Important Principles

1) Drugs act by affecting biochemical or physiological processes in the body. Most drugs act at specific receptors. The action of a drug is characterised by two variables: the magnitude of the response and the concentration required to produce the response.

2) A specific drug acts only at one receptor but may produce multiple effects due to the location of the receptor in various organs. A selective drug acts on one receptor in a particular tissue at concentrations that produce little effect on the receptor in other organs. Most drugs have multiple actions and it is usually preferable to use more specific or more selective agents.

3) Drugs are molecules with characteristic physicochemical and pharmacokinetic properties. Knowledge of these properties helps to predict the behaviour of a drug in the body and is an important guide in the selection of appropriate doses and dosage intervals.

4) The special and simultaneously operating processes in pharmacokinetics are drug absorption, distribution, metabolism (biotransformation) and excretion. The rate at which these processes proceed and consequently the concentration of drug in the body, is influenced by many factors pertaining to the drug and its dosage form, to pathophysiological or genetic variables of the individual patient, and to effects of other drugs taken concurrently.

5) Many drugs are bound to plasma proteins. Changes in the binding of a drug due to diseases such as uraemia or chronic inflammation affect its distribution and elimination in the body in a way which is predictable from its kinetic properties. However, for most drugs, changes in protein binding are of little clinical significance since for low clearance agents at least, the unbound (pharmacologically active) drug concentration will be unaltered, and only the total drug concentration (bound plus unbound) will be changed.

6) For many drugs, individual patients show a wide variation in response to the same dose. Much of this variability in drug response between patients can be explained by individual kinetic factors, particularly genetically-determined differences in drug metabolism, and by the effects of environmental factors, intercurrent illness or disease states on pharmacokinetics or tissue response.

7) Drug dosages must be individualised if the desired therapeutic response with minimal adverse effects is to be obtained. The response to some drugs is better correlated with plasma concentrations than with dosage. Increasing knowledge on the role of individual enzymes in drug metabolism, and the regulation thereof, provides new possibilities for individualised drug dosages based on prediction of an individual's metabolic capacity by the use of enzyme-specific probe drugs and/or genotyping.

8) Rational drug prescribing involves a decision on whether to use a drug, and if so, selection of a suitable drug and regimen, consideration of compatibility between the drug and patient or any other drugs being given, a legibly written prescription, and appropriate instruction of the patient about use of the drug and expectations from treatment and follow-up.

The rational pharmacological treatment of any patient requires adequate knowledge about the disease process, the pharmacodynamic properties of the drug(s) selected, and the individual's handling of the drug(s) [pharmacokinetics]. This chapter discusses clinical pharmacological principles which can be applied in any therapeutic situation, particularly as they relate to dose and dose interval. Assuming that the diagnosis and the selection of the drug are appropriate, the remaining problem for the clinician is to find a dosage schedule which gives an optimum drug concentration in the diseased organ. The concentration must not be too low, nor too high. In the former case, therapeutic failure may occur, while in the latter, adverse effects may prove troublesome to the patient.

General principles in drug therapy should be based on the concept that drugs, besides being remedies for a particular disease, are molecules with characteristic physicochemical and pharmacokinetic properties. Many of these properties are not readily available in usual reference sources; however, appendix A to this book presents a useful compilation of pharmacokinetic parameters for commonly used drugs. It is our hope that clinicians reading this chapter will become motivated to make use of such information and when it cannot be located, to request it from representatives of pharmaceutical firms, members of hospital formulary committees, drug information centres or regulatory agencies.

## 1. Basic Concepts of Drug Action

Drug action is determined by a physicochemical interaction between the drug and functionally important molecules (usually a 'receptor') in the body. The magnitude of the response is related to the concentration of the drug at the appropriate site of action, which in turn, depends on the dosage and the time-course of the drug in the body. Knowledge of the physicochemical and pharmacokinetic properties of drugs and how they act can help greatly in understanding why individual drugs produce particular effects.

### 1.1 Physicochemical Characteristics of Drugs

There are three important physicochemical properties of a drug molecule – its lipid solubility, the extent to which it is ionised, and its molecular size.[1,2] Many therapeutic agents are highly soluble in lipids and this property allows them to cross the gastrointestinal wall, the placenta, blood-brain 'barrier' and cell membranes. Having been filtered through the glomerulus, lipid soluble drugs will be almost completely reabsorbed during their passage through the nephron. Such drugs would remain in the body for an indefinite period unless they are metabolised to more water soluble metabolites, which can then be excreted in the urine.

To gain access to their site of action, drugs must cross one or more barriers – the surface and capillary endothelia, the plasma membranes of the cell, and the intracellular membranes. This transfer is usually accomplished by passive diffusion, although other processes such as active transport may occur.

The process of *passive diffusion* is characterised by the movement of drug molecules down a concentration gradient with no expenditure of energy. The rate of diffusion depends on the physicochemical properties of the drug. Many drugs can be considered as weak electrolytes and exist in two forms – ionised and nonionised – depending on the pH of the medium (fig. 1). It is usually assumed that only the nonionised drug is sufficiently lipid soluble to diffuse through biological membranes, and that a highly ionised water soluble drug will only cross biological membranes if it is of small molecular size. Thus, the passage of water soluble ions through the pores of the plasma membrane

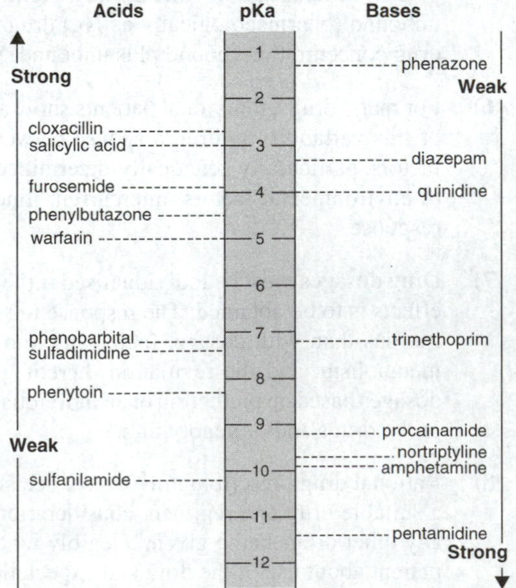

**Fig. 1.** pKa values for some representative acidic and basic drugs (see also appendix A).

is sharply limited when the molecular weight is above 100D (dalton), a notable exception being hepatic parenchymal cells. Almost all drugs have molecular weights well above 100D and thus cannot pass through these pores, one exception being lithium ion which has a molecular weight of 7D.

In describing the lipid solubility of a drug, it is understood that the various lipid : water partition coefficients used are crude indices of the diffusion process *in vivo*. Nevertheless, it has been shown that within the group of thiazide diuretics, there is a close relationship between the chloroform : water partition coefficient, the uptake in renal tubular cells, and the natriuretic activity.[3]

The extent to which ionisation takes place is dependent on the pKa of the drug and the pH of the solution in which the drug is dissolved. The ionisation of a weak *acidic* drug (e.g. phenobarbital) is an equilibrium reaction:

$$HA \Leftrightarrow H^+ + A^-$$

The following mathematical relationship exists:

$$Ka = \frac{[H^+] \cdot [A^-]}{[HA]}$$

where [HA] is the concentration of the non-ionised acidic drug, and [H+] and [A⁻] represent the concentrations of the hydrogen ions and ionised drug, respectively. The relationship between the ionisation of a weak acidic drug, its pKa and the pH of the solution is given by the Henderson-Hasselbach equation, which is obtained by logarithmic expression of the above equation:

$$pH = pKa + \log\frac{[A^-]}{[HA]}$$

The pKa of a drug is defined as the pH at which the drug is 50% ionised, and if the above equation is rearranged such that:

$$\log\frac{[A^-]}{[HA]} = pH - pKa$$

it can be seen that small changes of pH near the pKa of a weak acidic drug will markedly affect its degree of ionisation and, under certain conditions, its distribution in the body.

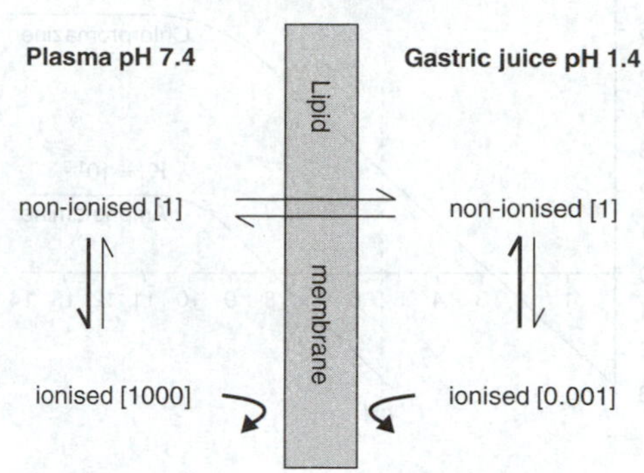


**Fig. 2.** The distribution of a weak acid (e.g. warfarin pKa 5) between plasma and gastric juice separated by a lipid membrane permeable only to the non-ionised form of a drug. The figures in square brackets refer to the approximate, relative concentrations of drug in arbitrary units (after Brodie[4]).

For a *base*, the constants Ka and pKa can be used, remembering that these terms now refer to the reaction:

$$BH^+ \Leftrightarrow B + H^+$$

The same equations thus apply if [B] and [BH⁺] are exchanged for [A⁻] and [HA], respectively.

Knowledge of the pKa of a drug is useful in predicting its behaviour in various body fluids. Phenobarbital, with a pKa of 7.2, is largely non-ionised at acid pH and will be about 40% non-ionised in plasma.

$$\log\frac{[A^-]}{[HA]} = 7.4 - 7.2 = 0.2$$

$$\frac{[A^-]}{[HA]} = 1.58$$

On the other hand, phenobarbital can be trapped in ionised form in alkalinised urine. The principle is illustrated in figure 2 with warfarin, which has a pKa of 5 and will thus be non-ionised in gastric fluid (pH 1.4), which will aid its absorption. The situation is reversed for basic drugs, such as amphetamine, which will be more ionised at an acidic pH. Such drugs will in fact diffuse from plasma into gastric fluid upon parenteral administration. Drugs with a similar pKa may, nevertheless, be differently affected by changes in pH of body fluids. This is due to their different lipophilicities. For example, the urinary excretion of amphetamine, but not that of chlorpromazine, is markedly

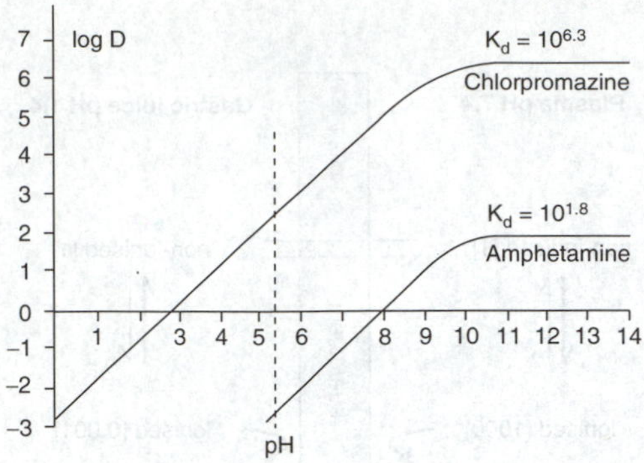


**Fig. 3.** Logarithmic representation of the partition ratio (D) between dichloromethane and water at different pH values for two different basic drugs with similar pKa values, chlorpromazine (pKa 9.3) and amphetamine (pKa 9.9). Although both drugs are almost completely ionised at pH 5.5 (indicated by the broken line), the partition ratio of chlorpromazine is $10^{2.5} = 316$ but only $10^{-2.5} = 0.00316$ for amphetamine. This is due to the great difference in lipophilic properties of the drugs in non-ionised form. Thus, the partition coefficient ($K_d$) of non-ionised chlorpromazine is more than 30,000 × higher than that of amphetamine.

enhanced by acidifying the urine. This is explained by a much more effective tubular reabsorption of chlorpromazine, which in turn is due to its much higher lipophilicity (fig. 3).

## 1.2 Receptors and Drug Response

Drugs act by affecting normal physiological or biochemical processes in the body, or by controlling changes in these processes brought about by disease. Whatever effects a drug produces, they are a consequence of physicochemical interactions between the drug and functionally important molecules in the body. Some drugs act by combining with a small molecule or ion (e.g. neutralisation of gastric acid by antacids or chelation of ferrous ion by deferoxamine in treatment of iron poisoning), or by a nonspecific effect on membrane function (e.g. local anaesthetics). However, in the majority of cases, drugs are presumed to interact with macromolecular components of tissues. Such elements with which a drug combines to produce its characteristic effects are called *receptors*.

A receptor is not a readily identifiable physical entity. In many cases, receptors are areas of cell membranes with special structural features that result in the binding of endogenous compounds such as adrenaline (epinephrine), noradrenaline (norepinephrine), histamine, acetylcholine, etc. In other cases, the functioning macromolecule may be an enzyme which is inhibited by a drug, or a nucleic acid molecule to which the drug binds. If the drug has an appropriate chemical structure, it will also bind to these receptors and may produce a similar response to the endogenous transmitter, or it may block the response to the transmitter. The structural requirements for combining with a receptor site are specific, both molecular structure and stereochemistry playing important roles in determining the 'fit' of the drug to the receptor; for example, the *l*-form of a stereoisomer pair may be pharmacologically active while the *d*-form is less active (e.g. β-adrenoceptor blocking action of propranolol) or inactive (e.g. opioid analgesics).

The advent of modern molecular biology techniques has allowed more detailed investigation of the nature of some receptors. It is clear that there is a family of receptors which binds to GPT-activated proteins (G-proteins) to initiate a response. The receptor protein recognises and then responds to agonists and is thereby altered. The genes for some receptors (e.g. muscarinic, serotonergic) have been cloned and as a result, structural analysis has been performed. A general pattern emerges for these G-protein linked receptors of an *N*-terminus in the extracellular space with 7 transmembrane spanning regions, 3 extracellular and 3 cytoplasmic loops, and an intracellular C terminus. How widely this model is representative is unknown.[5]

This section is intended as a very brief overview of how drugs act in normally responding tissues. It should be noted that receptor changes can play a part in altered sensitivity to some drugs (for a review, see Snyder[6]).

### *1.2.1 Drug-Receptor Interactions*

A drug response is usually the result of a reversible combination between a drug and receptor to form a drug-receptor complex – the response being assumed to be directly proportional to the amount of drug-receptor complex formed. A drug which 'fits' the receptor well, will bind strongly and is said to have a high affinity for the receptor. The graded dose-response relationship seen with most drugs (usually shown graphically as a plot of the logarithm of the drug concentration *versus* the response) is partially a reflection of the extent of occupancy of receptor sites by that drug, in which case the maximal response should correspond to occupancy of all receptor sites. However, this is an oversimplification since other steps involved between the interaction of a drug and receptor and the subsequent biological effect (e.g. 'second messenger' steps involving such agents as cyclic-AMP) may be the limiting factors in production of the maximal response. The relative affinity of a drug for the receptor can be defined as the concentration ($C_{50}$) required to produce half the maximal response (fig. 4).

To explain the different magnitude of response which may be seen between drugs that act on the same receptor site, and apparently have a similar affinity for the receptor, the property of intrinsic activity has been postulated. The intrinsic activity of a drug is a measure of the maximal response that the drug can produce when given in very high concentrations. Thus, two similarly acting drugs with the same affinity but differing intrinsic activities will require a different extent of receptor occupation to produce the same response. The drug with lower intrinsic activity will require a greater extent of receptor occupation, and so a larger dose. A drug with high affinity and high intrinsic activity is termed an *agonist*, while an agent with high affinity but no intrinsic activity is termed an *antagonist* since it prevents or tends to prevent a drug that does possess intrinsic activity from interacting with the receptor site. Falling between these two extremes are *partial agonists* (see further below), drugs which no matter how high their concentration will not produce the full response of which the tissue is capable (fig. 4).

Antagonists are of two main types. An antagonist is said to be *competitive* if it combines reversibly with the same receptor site as the agonist. Since the antagonist-receptor complex can be reversed, the maximum response to the agonist can still be obtained provided the concentration of agonist is high enough – i.e. the dose-response curve shifts to the right (fig. 5). An antagonist is said to be *non-competitive* if it 'inactivates' the receptor so that an effective agonist-receptor complex cannot be formed. In this case, the effect of the antagonist on the receptor may be reversible or irreversible; the result is to reduce the intrinsic activity of the agonist without changing its affinity, so that a maximal response cannot be obtained by increasing the concentration of the agonist (fig. 6).

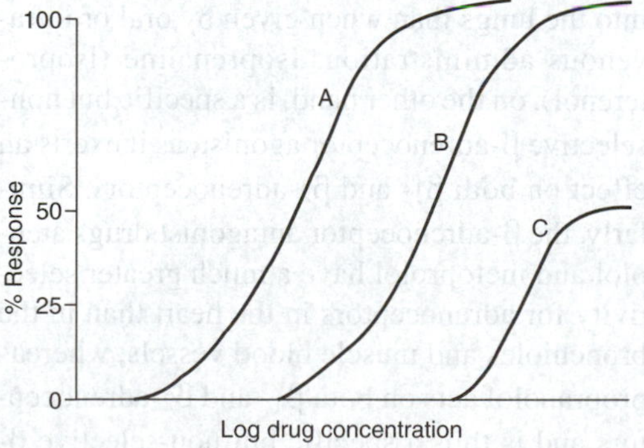


**Fig. 4.** Log concentration-response curves for two full agonist drugs which produce the maximum response at high concentrations. Drug A has a higher affinity than drug B, as lower concentrations of drug A than B are required to produce the same degree of response. Drug C is a partial agonist. Very high concentrations of drug C produce a maximum response less than that produced by the two full agonist drugs A and B (after Meffin et al.[7]).

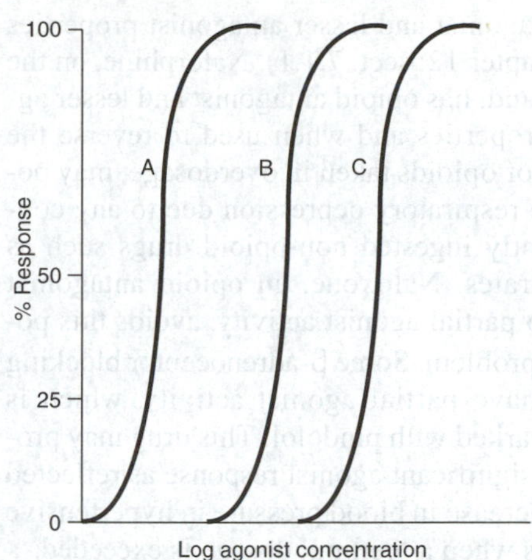


**Fig. 5.** Log concentration-response curves for an agonist in the presence of a competitive antagonist. Curve A shows the response of the agonist alone and curves B and C in the presence of increasing concentrations (C > B) of a competitive antagonist (after Meffin et al.[7]).

Partial agonists also have antagonist properties, since they occupy receptor sites, preventing access of full agonists to the receptor, but possess only relatively weak intrinsic activity of their own and do not elicit a maximal response of the tissue involved, even at very high concentrations. The net effect of a combination of a partial agonist and a full agonist is dependent upon the concentrations present. At low agonist concentrations, addition of a partial agonist will increase the response by occupying previously empty receptor sites, while at higher agonist concentrations, the response may be decreased on addition of a partial agonist since receptor sites previously occupied by the full agonist may now become occupied by the less active (intrinsic activity) partial agonist (fig. 7).

Some drugs used therapeutically have this dual action. Strong analgesics such as pentazocine, butorphanol and buprenorphine have both opioid agonist and lesser antagonist properties (see chapter 12; sect. 7.1.1). Nalorphine, on the other hand, has opioid antagonist and lesser agonist properties and when used to reverse the effects of opioids taken in overdosage, may potentiate respiratory depression due to any concomitantly ingested non-opioid drugs such as barbiturates. Naloxone, an opioid antagonist with no partial agonist activity, avoids this potential problem. Some β-adrenoceptor blocking drugs have partial agonist activity, which is most marked with pindolol. This drug may produce a significant agonist response as reflected in an increase in blood pressure in hypertensive patients when a 'ceiling' dosage is exceeded.

### *1.2.2 Specificity and Selectivity of Drug Action*

Most drugs have multiple effects, some of which in varying degree may be undesirable, rather than a single one thought to be most important. It is therefore usually preferable to give more specific or more selective drugs. The phenothiazines as a class, are relatively nonspecific drugs because they act on a variety of different receptors (see chapter 30; sect. 3.1). Drugs may still act on a particular receptor but produce a number of pharmacological responses because of a wide distribution of this receptor in body tissues (e.g. atropine action on muscarinic receptors).

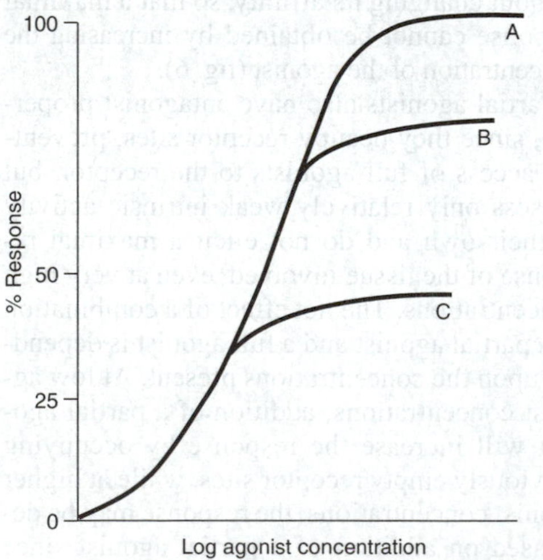


**Fig. 6.** Log concentration-response curves for an agonist in the presence of a non-competitive antagonist. Increasing concentrations of the antagonist (C > B) produce a reduced maximum effect with respect to that obtained with the agonist alone (A). In contrast to competitive antagonism (fig. 5), increasing the concentration of the agonist fails to restore the maximum response (after Meffin et al.[7]).

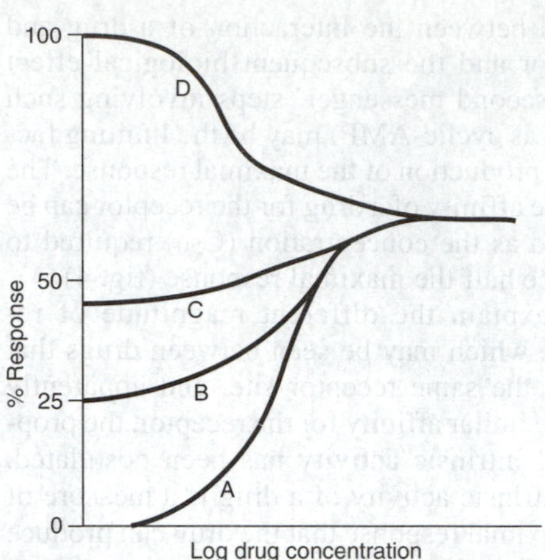


**Fig. 7.** Log concentration-response curves for a partial agonist in the presence of a full agonist. Curve A: partial agonist only. The relative concentrations of full agonist are B < C < D. In curves B and C, the concentrations of full agonist are less than that which will produce the maximum response of the partial agonist, and so the agonist effects are additive. In curve D, the response due to the full agonist exceeds that of the partial agonist, and the response is antagonised to the maximum response of the partial agonist (after Meffin et al.[7]).

Some drugs can be both specific and selective, as is well illustrated by drugs acting on β-adrenoceptors. Selectivity however, is not absolute. Thus, β-adrenoceptor agonist bronchodilators such as salbutamol (albuterol) and terbutaline show relative selectivity for the $\beta_2$-adrenoceptors in bronchial smooth muscle at doses which cause little stimulation of the $\beta_1$-adrenoceptors in the heart. Such relative selectivity is greater when these drugs are inhaled into the lungs than when given by oral or intravenous administration. Isoprenaline (isoproterenol), on the other hand, is a specific but nonselective β-adrenoceptor agonist, as it exerts an effect on both $\beta_1$- and $\beta_2$-adrenoceptors. Similarly, the β-adrenoceptor antagonist drugs atenolol and metoprolol have a much greater selectivity for adrenoceptors in the heart than in the bronchioles and muscle blood vessels, whereas propranolol acts on both $\beta_1$- and $\beta_2$-adrenoceptors and is thus a specific but non-selective β-blocker (see chapter 21; sect. 3.2).

In clinical terms, it is important to remember that the selective nature of β-adrenoceptor antagonists such as atenolol and metoprolol is not absolute and thus these drugs should never be regarded as 'cardiospecific'. It is still possible to precipitate an attack of asthma in a sensitive patient by the use of atenolol or metoprolol.

### 1.3 Potency and Drug Effect

Potency must not be confused with specificity and selectivity, nor used to indicate clinical efficacy. Furosemide and other loop diuretics produce a greater diuresis (i.e. have greater efficacy) in renal failure than that from any dose of a thiazide diuretic. On the other hand, the different mg dose equivalents of the individual thiazides do not have clinical relevance, since the maximum diuretic effect produced by each is the same when used at adequate dosage.

## 2. Basic Concepts of Pharmacokinetics

### 2.1 Plasma Concentration-Time Curves

Pharmacokinetics deals with the time course of the drug in the body. It requires assay methods for the determination of drug in tissues and body fluids, e.g. plasma and urine. The blood is a unique body fluid in that it stays in intimate contact with all tissues. Hence the drug concentration in blood plasma continuously mirrors the fate of the drug in various tissues and organs. Additional information on what has happened to the drug can be obtained by measuring the drug and its metabolites in the urine and faeces. In animals, powerful methods such as the administration of radiolabelled drugs followed by autoradiography or direct sampling of various tissues of the sacrificed animal may provide deeper insight into the fate of the drug than can usually be obtained in humans.

In humans, mathematical models may be useful in describing the time-course of the various events that a drug dose may undergo: absorption, distribution, metabolism and excretion. However, a simple first approach is to plot the experimentally determined drug concentrations in, for example, plasma *versus* time. The maximum plasma concentration ($C_{max}$) and the corresponding time ($t_{max}$) after an oral dose are important values that are then readily apparent. The time period at which plasma concentrations stay above a certain limit, e.g. the lowest concentration for a certain pharmacological response, will also be apparent from the graph. However, the use of simple pharmacokinetic concepts may reveal many more details of importance as will be described below.

### 2.2 Simple Pharmacokinetic Characterisation of Drugs

Pharmacokinetics deals with the mathematical description of the biological processes which affect the time-course of the absorption and fate of drugs, and which are themselves affected by drugs.[8] The description of the fate of drugs in the body can be simplified by the introduction of certain models. The mathematical formulae derived from these models make it possible to determine appropriate dosage regimens. The relevance of both the formulae and the derived dosage regimens can be tested by direct measurement of drug plasma concentrations. Usually, the body is depicted as a system of compartments, even though these lack physiological or anatomical reality. The one-compartment model (fig. 8) depicts the body as a single homogeneous unit (see further section 2.2.4). The two-compartment open model consists of a so-called central compartment (which includes plasma) and a peripheral or 'tissue'

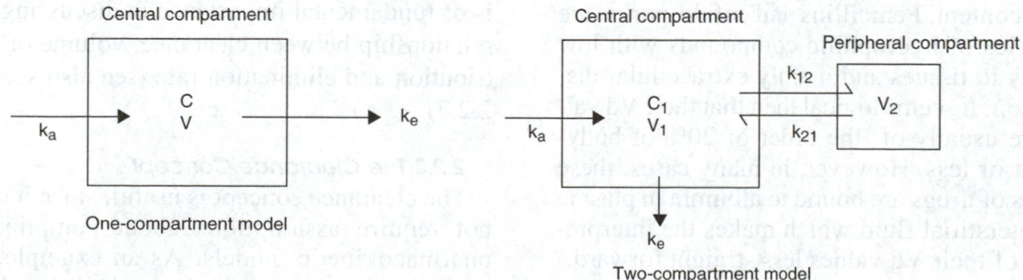


**Fig. 8.** Schematic diagram of the body (left) as a one-compartment model, and (right) as a two-compartment open model. $k_a$ is the rate constant of absorption and $k_e$ the rate constant of elimination (including both metabolism and excretion). $k_{12}$ and $k_{21}$ are transfer rate constants between the two compartments (i.e. from compartment one to compartment two and *vice versa*). The amount of drug in the body is given by the concentration of drug (C) times the apparent volume of distribution (V). In the two-compartment model, $V_1$ and $V_2$ are the apparent volumes of distribution and $C_1$ the concentration of drug in the central compartment (see text). C and $C_1$ are assumed to be the concentration of drug in plasma.

compartment. It is assumed that absorption to and elimination from the system involve only the central compartment (fig. 8). Sometimes more complicated models are used.

#### *2.2.1 Linear Kinetics*

In linear or first-order kinetics, rates of transport or elimination are proportional to drug concentrations in the compartments. If, on the other hand, the elimination rate has a maximum value, as for instance the rate of ethanol metabolism, then we are dealing with a nonlinear or *capacity-limited* process. As a first approach, the simple pharmacokinetic models usually assume linear kinetics, but capacity-limited processes can usually be dealt with by incorporation of Michaelis-Menten expressions for the critical step (see section 2.2.8).

#### *2.2.2 Apparent Volume of Distribution*

The apparent volume of distribution (Vd) relates the amount of drug in the total body relative to that in plasma at any one time. In the phenazone (antipyrine) example in figure 9, the oral dose given was 10 mg/kg and $C_0$ was 19.1 mg/L (where $C_0$ is the fictitious plasma concentration at time zero; see further section 2.2.4). The Vd of the system that would tally with these figures can be calculated from the equation:

$$Vd = Dose/C_0 = (10\ mg/kg)/(19.1\ mg/L) = 0.52\ L/kg$$

This Vd value of 0.52 L/kg of bodyweight seems to indicate that phenazone distributes in a volume corresponding to about 52% of the bodyweight. The figure is in agreement with the fact that phenazone, which is not bound to plasma proteins, distributes in the body water (intra- and extracellular). Because of this feature, phenazone has been used to measure body water content. Penicillins and cefalosporins are examples of hydrophilic compounds with low affinity to tissues and mainly extracellular distribution. It seems logical then that their Vd values are usually of the order of 20% of bodyweight or less. However, in many cases, these classes of drugs are bound to albumin in plasma and interstitial fluid which makes the interpretation of their Vd values less straight forward.

The body is obviously not homogeneous, even if it can be treated as such in a mathematical model. Drug concentrations in the liver, kidneys, muscle, fat and other tissues will therefore differ from one another as well as from the concentration in the plasma. The apparent volume of distribution of a drug should therefore be interpreted with caution. Vd values of several L/kg, while being seemingly impossible to explain, are often seen with lipophilic drugs. However, these values simply indicate that the drug is bound to solid constituents of the body. In other words, the drugs preferentially distribute to tissues relative to plasma. Small Vd values (0.2 L/kg or less) for lipophilic drugs that in animals have been shown to gain access to all sorts of tissues, may often be explained by a high affinity for plasma proteins, as is discussed below (see section 2.2.6). The volume of distribution calculated from the unbound plasma drug concentration ($Vd_u$) will then be much higher and will reveal the true distribution.

From a practical mathematical standpoint, Vd can be looked upon as a proportionality constant, which will allow the calculation of the amount of drug in the body at any time from the known plasma concentration (C):

$$\text{Amount in the body} = Vd \cdot C$$

In the simple one-compartment model (fig. 8), Vd is calculated as Dose/$C_0$. However, there are several other ways of defining and calculating the volume of distribution in more complicated models, as will be described below. One method makes use of the total plasma clearance (CL) of the drug (see section 2.2.3). Vd may then be calculated as CL divided by the appropriate rate constant. If applied to the one-compartment model, this gives:

$$Vd = CL/k_e$$

This expression, which may be rewritten as:

$$k_e = CL/Vd$$

is of fundamental importance in discussing the relationship between clearance, volume of distribution and elimination rate (see also section 2.2.7).

#### *2.2.3 The Clearance Concept*

The clearance concept is useful, since it does not require assumptions about complicated pharmacokinetic models. As an example, all that is needed to calculate the total plasma clearance of a drug after a single intravenous dose is an estimate of the total area under the plasma concentration-time curve from time zero to infinite time, $AUC_{(0-\infty)}$. At this time, all of the dose (D) has been eliminated and the total plasma clearance (CL) is calculated as $D/AUC_{(0-\infty)}$.

Clearance reflects the relationship between the elimination rate and concentration of a drug, i.e.:

Rate of elimination = Concentration (C) · Clearance (CL)

The units of clearance are L/h, ml/min or any other unit of volume per time, but are most conveniently expressed as L/h (see further chapter 5; sect. 1.6.7 and appendix G). The straightforward interpretation of CL is the number of litres of plasma that are cleared of drug (i.e. completely freed of drug) per hour by the eliminating organs of the body (liver, kidneys and others). In an analogous manner, the total blood clearance ($CL_b$) may be defined from the blood concentration data. Total blood clearance can often be directly interpreted physiologically. If, for instance, the drug is known to be exclusively eliminated by hepatic metabolism in man, and $CL_b$ is found to be 90 L/h, one knows that the blood reaching the liver is completely cleared of drug by this organ in one single passage. This conclusion is based upon the fact that the blood flow to the liver in man is approximately 90 L/h (1.5 L/min).

In general, drugs are eliminated by both renal ($CL_R$) and hepatic clearance ($CL_H$) so that:

$$CL = CL_R + CL_H$$

If urine is completely collected from time zero to time infinity (usually approximated to 7 half-lives), $CL_R$ may be directly measured from the total amount of unchanged drug excreted in the urine, $A_{e(0-\infty)}$:

$$CL_R = A_{e(0-\infty)}/AUC_{(0-\infty)}$$

The analogy with the definition of CL is apparent. Renal clearance may also be estimated as $A_e/AUC$ for a short period of time in a single or repetitive dose experiment. This requires accurate urine collection and plasma sampling during the same period. From the magnitude of the renal clearance figures, one may sometimes draw direct conclusions. For a compound that is not bound to plasma proteins and undergoes no active tubular secretion, a $CL_R$ value similar to that of inulin is to be expected, i.e. 7.2 to 7.8 L/h (120 to 130 ml/min) in normal healthy individuals. If, in this example, $CL_R$ is calculated to be 0.6 L/h, this then indicates tubular reabsorption of the drug by active or passive processes.

The main advantage in using clearance values in characterising elimination processes lies in the fact that CL, $CL_R$ and $CL_H$ may all be given some physiological interpretation. This is in contrast to $k_e$ or $t^{1/2}$ values as will be discussed below (section 2.2.7). To be allowed to use a constant value of clearance, one has to know that there are no capacity-limited processes involved, i.e. one is dealing with a system that is linear or dose-independent. If the elimination is capacity-limited, CL will not be a constant but will decrease with increasing doses. Of course, many of the processes that we consider dose-independent are in fact capacity-limited at drug doses higher than those normally used in therapy. This may become apparent in cases of overdosage.

In calculating clearance by the relationship $D/AUC_{(0-\infty)}$, $AUC_{(0-\infty)}$ needs to be determined. This calculation is usually done by the trapezoidal rule which approximates the area under the experimentally found curve as the sum of trapezoids defined by straight lines connecting the experimental points. The area from the last experimental point ($t_n$, $C_n$) to infinity is estimated as $C_n/\beta$ where β is the slope of the last part of the curve in a log concentration *versus* time plot. Thus:

$$AUC_{(0-\infty)} = \text{Sum of trapezoids} + C_n/\beta$$

The shape of the curve is not critical and it may contain any number of exponential components, as long as it is possible to estimate the final log-linear part with some accuracy.

Thus, CL can be calculated by non-compartmental methods. One of the main advantages of the clearance concept is therefore that no assumption has to be made except that we are dealing with a linear system, i.e. all concentrations that we measure are proportional to the dose.

### 2.2.4 The One-Compartment Model

This is the simplest and most widely used of the pharmacokinetic compartmental models. In this model (fig. 8), the body is depicted as one vessel with an apparent volume, V and the drug concentration therein is equal to the plasma concentration, C. The elimination from the body is controlled by the first-order rate constant $k_e$, which as shown in section 2.2.2 above, is equal to the total plasma clearance (CL) divided by the volume of distribution. The model can be applied on the post-absorption plasma concentration-time data obtained after an oral dose of phenazone (antipyrine) [fig. 9], a drug that has virtually complete absorption. The concentrations can be reasonably well described by the following mathematical expression for the one-compartment model:

$$C = C_0 \cdot e^{-k_e \cdot t} = C_0 \cdot e^{-CL/V \cdot t}$$

in which C is the plasma concentration at time t after administration; $C_0$ is the fictitious concentration at time zero which may be calculated by back-extrapolation of the curve (fig. 9); and e is the base for the natural logarithms (ln). The monoexponential behaviour of the plasma data are best revealed by plotting them in a logarithmic scale *versus* a linear time scale as shown in figure 9. The corresponding equation is then:

$$\ln C = \ln C_0 - CL/V \cdot t$$

and the negative of the slope of the curve is identified as CL/V or $k_e$. The ordinate intercept is $C_0$. The elimination or plasma half-life ($t_{1/2}$) of the drug, i.e. the time for halving any given plasma concentration, is calculated as:

$$\ln 2 \cdot V/CL \textit{ or } 0.7 \cdot V/CL$$

In the example in figure 9, the post-absorption plasma concentration data can be described by the equation:

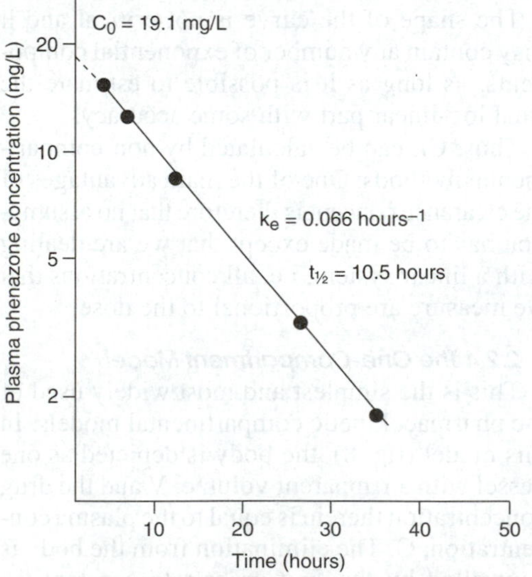


**Fig. 9.** An application of the one-compartment model. Plasma concentration-time curve of phenazone (antipyrine) after a single oral dose (10 mg/kg) given to a healthy volunteer. The drug is eliminated by an overall first-order process, and thus the disappearance curve becomes linear if plotted on log-linear paper.

$$C = 19.1 \cdot e^{-0.066 \cdot t}$$

and the half-life can be calculated as 10.5 hours. This semilogarithmic-type plot may be very useful even with data that are best described as the sum of two or more exponential functions. The number of straight phases of the plasma concentration *versus* time decay then indicates the minimum number of exponential terms required to describe the data.

### 2.2.5 Multiexponential Curves

As mentioned above (section 2.2.4), the plot of log concentration *versus* time often yields more than one linear phase. If two phases are seen (fig. 10), the drug may be described by a two-compartment model. In contrast to CL and Vd, the constants of such a model (see fig. 8) usually have no direct physiological counterparts and differences between individuals in the actual values are difficult to interpret. However, the model may be useful for descriptive and predictive purposes, e.g. to predict the effect of changing from one dosage regimen to another. In fact, the shape of the plasma concentration-time curve can easily be simulated for any dosage regimen, even a complicated combination of oral and intravenous doses or infusions, if the constants in the model are known.

The first steeper part of the curve is often considered to represent mainly distribution of the drug into the tissues of the body and is therefore referred to as the *distribution phase* (or α-phase). The latter part is referred to as the *elimination phase* (or β-phase) since the decline obviously represents elimination. This terminology may be adequate for drugs with short α-phases of up to 15 minutes, but may be very misleading when it comes to drugs with α-phases of several hours. If the AUC associated with the α-phase is much higher than that associated with the β-phase, it is clear from clearance considerations that most of the elimination actually occurs during the α-phase. This is so because the rate of elimination is $CL \cdot C$, and the amount eliminated during a time period (0-t) is $CL \cdot AUC_{(0\text{-}t)}$, where $AUC_{(0\text{-}t)}$ is the area under the curve for the actual time period. The β-phase is then best referred to as the redistribution phase, since using the two-compartment terminology, the drug is returning or redistributing from the peripheral (or tissue) compartment to the central (or plasma) compartment from which it is sub-

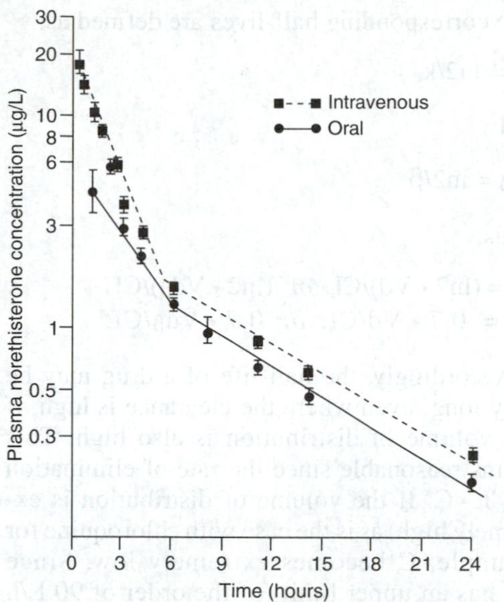


**Fig. 10.** Biphasic disappearance of the plasma concentrations of the contraceptive steroid norethisterone (norethindrone) after oral and intravenous administration of 1mg to 6 individuals (mean values ± SE) [after Back et al.[9]].

sequently eliminated (assuming a two-compartment open model; see fig. 8).

Well perfused organs such as the liver and kidney are usually thought to belong to the central compartment. For some drugs such as chlorthalidone, the half-life defined by the slope of the β-phase ($t_{½β}$) may be very long, because of high affinity binding within the tissue. The long $t_{½β}$ of chlorthalidone (30 to 60h) is due to drug dissociation from the enzyme carbonic anhydrase present in red blood cells, which in this case represent the tissue compartment. Acetazolamide, another drug with carbonic anhydrase affinity, is able to displace chlorthalidone from carbonic anhydrase, thereby decreasing its volume of distribution considerably. This results in a much shorter half-life of chlorthalidone, of the order of 15 hours, in the presence of acetazolamide.[10] This exemplifies the fact that the elimination rate constant is the ratio of clearance and volume of distribution (i.e. $k_e$ = CL/Vd). An increased elimination rate, as in this example, is therefore not necessarily a reflection of an increased clearance. For further discussion of this point, see section 2.2.7.

It is very important in studies of drug elimination to extend the period of blood sampling enough to be able to estimate the $AUC_{(0-\infty)}$ accurately. Theoretically, it is necessary to follow the plasma curve until all drug has been eliminated. In practice, this can only be done by use of radioisotopes where one may sometimes follow the fate of the drug until 97% or so of the label has been recovered in urine, faeces, and expired air. In other cases, one has to assume that the β-phase is not followed by another more long-lasting phase.

In general, the plasma concentration curve for any compartmental model can be described as a sum of exponential terms:

$$C = A \cdot e^{-\alpha t} + B \cdot e^{-\beta t} + \ldots N \cdot e^{-\omega t}$$

In this general case, $AUC_{(0-\infty)}$ is described by the equation:

$$AUC_{(0-\infty)} = A/\alpha + B/\beta + \ldots N/\omega$$

When the constants (i.e. A, α, B, β etc.) have been determined, e.g. by use of a least-squares fitting program, it is possible to assess the relative importance of the various half-lives ($t_{½α}$, $t_{½β}$, etc.) associated with the different rate constants on the accumulation of the drug with repeated administration. If, for example, the term A/α accounts for 95% of $AUC_{(0-\infty)}$, and $t_{½α}$ is 3 hours, one can predict that repeated doses given every 12 or 24 hours will produce virtually no accumulation. This will be so even if the terminal half-life is, e.g. 80 hours. The rule of thumb that 3 half-lives are required to approximately reach steady-state does not seem to apply here, since the dose given at 240 hours and the first dose will look virtually identical. In fact, the rule does apply, at least approximately, if only the dominant half-life (in this case the 3-hour $t_{½α}$) is considered. Thus, in a multicompartment model, the contribution of the terminal half-life (often misleadingly called the biological half-life) to the accumulation of the drug is not related to the magnitude of the half-life alone, but rather to the ratio of N/ω (the AUC associated with the terminal phase according to the expression shown above) to the total $AUC_{(0-\infty)}$.

#### *2.2.6 Volume of Distribution for Multiexponential Systems*

The simple one-compartment definition of Vd cannot be applied in these systems. Two other Vd terms, $Vd_β$ (often called $Vd_{area}$ or $V_z$) and $Vd_{ss}$ have proved very useful. $Vd_β$ is defined as the volume of distribution during the last log-linear phase (β-phase). Thus, the amount of drug in the body at any time t during this phase is Vdβ • C, where C is the plasma concentration at time t. Vdβ is calculated as CL/β, where β is the slope of the β-phase in the ln C *versus* time plot (see fig. 10).

$Vd_{ss}$ relates drug concentration to the total amount of drug in the body at steady-state, i.e. $Vd_{ss} \cdot C^{ss}$ is the amount of drug in the body at steady-state. A simple non-compartmental method to calculate $Vd_{ss}$ from plasma data after a single intravenous dose (D) has been described.[11] The assumptions that have to be made for this calculation, such as linear kinetics and elimination from the central (i.e. plasma) compartment, seem to be reasonably justified with most drugs. After an intravenous bolus dose, $Vd_{ss}$ is calculated from:

$$Vd_{ss} = \frac{D \cdot AUMC_{(0-\infty)}}{[AUC_{(0-\infty)}]^2}$$

where $AUMC_{(0\text{-}\infty)}$ is defined as the area under the 'first moment' of the plasma concentration-time curve, i.e. the area under the curve of the product of time, t, and plasma concentration, C, over the time span zero to infinity.

The main use of $Vd_{ss}$ values, apart from calculating the amount of drug in the body at steady-state, is for comparative purposes. Since they are valid during equilibrium conditions, they indicate the relative affinity of the drug for tissues as compared with plasma. Vdβ values, on the other hand, may be risky to use in this manner, since Vdβ is highly dependent on the rate of elimination, the value increasing with increasing rates of elimination. However, for drugs with a kinetic behaviour not deviating very much from the one-compartment model, Vdβ is not significantly larger than $Vd_{ss}$, and in this instance, Vdβ gives a fair estimate of the relative tissue/plasma affinities.

### *2.2.7 The Half-Life Concept*

The rate at which a drug leaves the body is dependent on CL and Vd. In the one-compartment model:

$$k_e = CL/Vd$$

In two- or multicompartment models where β is defined as the slope of the β-phase of the log concentration *versus* time curve:

$$\beta = CL/Vd\beta$$

The corresponding half-lives are defined as:

$$t\tfrac{1}{2} = \ln 2/k_e$$

and

$$t\tfrac{1}{2}\beta = \ln 2/\beta$$

Thus,

$$t\tfrac{1}{2} = (\ln 2 \cdot Vd)/CL \text{ or } (\ln 2 \cdot Vd\beta)/CL$$
$$= 0.7 \cdot Vd/CL \text{ or } 0.7 \cdot Vd\beta/CL$$

Accordingly, the half-life of a drug may be very long, even where the clearance is high, if the volume of distribution is also high. This seems reasonable since the rate of elimination is CL • C. If the volume of distribution is extremely high, as is the case with chloroquine for example, C becomes extremely low. Since CL has an upper limit (of the order of 90 L/h for drugs metabolised in the liver), the product CL • C may be very low, even for so-called high clearance drugs. Thus, the half-life of a drug may be a very poor indicator of the actual capacity for elimination, especially for drugs with Vd values that are large and vary between individuals. However, the use of half-life as an in-

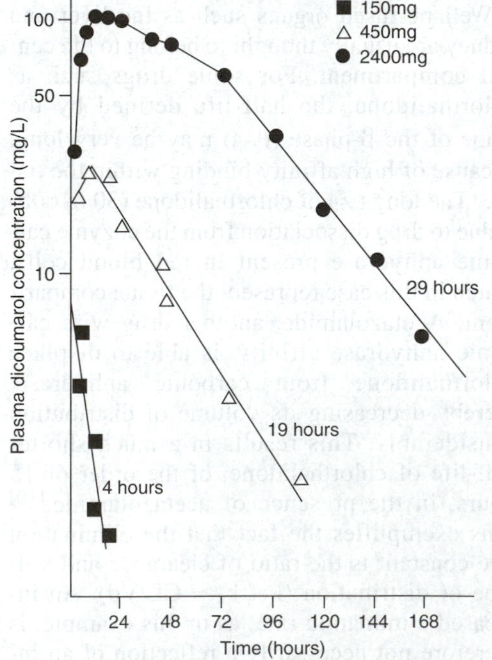


**Fig. 11.** Log plasma concentrations of dicoumarol (in mg/L) *versus* time after varying oral doses of dicoumarol in humans. The plasma half-life is prolonged from 4 hours to 29 hours when the dose is increased. An example of dose-dependent kinetics (after O'Reilly et al.[12]).

dicator of interindividual variability in metabolism of a drug may sometimes be justified, e.g. for phenazone, for which the variability in Vd is fairly small. For some high clearance drugs, CL varies little between individuals while the variation in Vd may be quite considerable. Variations in half-life then mirror the variability in Vd rather than hepatic activity.

*In summary*, the half-life is a measure of how the body as a whole handles the drug, but it is a poor indicator of the capacity for elimination at the cellular or organ level.

### 2.2.8 Michaelis-Menten Kinetics

Alcohol metabolism in a person who has imbibed several drinks will proceed at a rate that is essentially constant in terms of amount per unit of time, i.e. by *zero-order kinetics*. The rate of metabolism is largely independent of the concentration of alcohol in the body. This is so because the metabolic process proceeds at its maximum capacity, e.g. 10g alcohol/hour. When blood concentrations have declined enough, an intermediate phase is reached where Michaelis-Menten kinetics are applicable. The enzymatic process no longer occurs at its maximum rate ($V_{max}$) but at a rate that is dependent on (but not proportional to) the plasma concentration. Finally, as concentrations drop far below the Km value (the plasma concentration at which the rate of metabolism proceeds at a rate equal to $V_{max}/2$), first-order kinetics will prevail.

If Michaelis-Menten kinetics apply, then the rate of elimination will increase with increasing dose, but the increase will be less than proportional to the increase in dose. With increasing doses, zero-order kinetics will be approached asymptotically. In such cases, the half-life concept will lack any relevance since $t_{1/2}$ will vary with drug concentration (fig. 11).

Michaelis-Menten or capacity-limited elimination has been documented for salicylic acid, dicoumarol (bishydroxycoumarin) and phenytoin (diphenylhydantoin), drugs that are all mainly metabolised. If the dose-dependent kinetics occur with clinically used doses, their clinical use is made more difficult because small increments in dosage may result in large increases of the plasma concentrations, thereby resulting in toxicity.

### 2.2.9 Bioavailability

An important application of pharmacokinetics is in the determination of the proportion (fraction) of unchanged drug that reaches the systemic circulation – known as the bioavailability. This can be determined from plasma concentration (or urinary excretion) data. The bioavailability of an orally administered drug is often calculated by comparing the $AUC_{(0-\infty)}$ after oral and intravenous (IV) administration. The bioavailable fraction F of an oral dose is then simply expressed as:

$$F = \frac{AUC_{(0-\infty)} \text{ after oral dose}}{AUC_{(0-\infty)} \text{ after IV dose}}$$

Low oral bioavailability may not necessarily mean poor absorption but can be caused by metabolism of the drug in the gut wall, or in particular by rapid uptake and metabolism in the liver during the first circulation through this organ (see section 3.3.3), such that only a small fraction of the drug absorbed from the gastrointestinal tract actually reaches the systemic circulation.

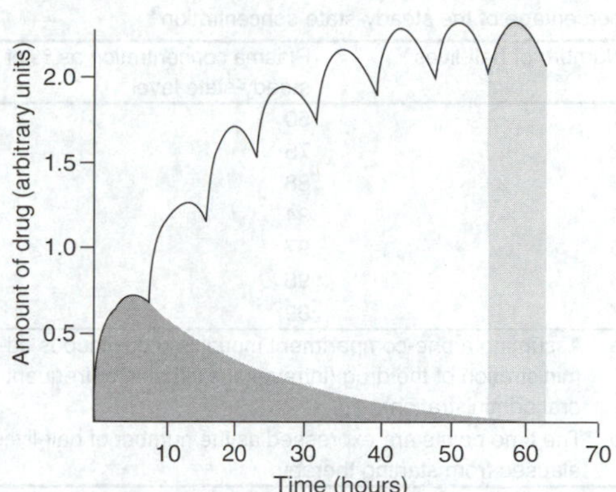


**Fig. 12.** Schematic representation of the accumulation of drug in the body (or plasma) after oral administration. The drug is given every 8 hours and has a half-life of 12 hours. The area under the plasma concentration-time curve after the first dose is equal to the area under the curve during the dosage interval, provided that plateau concentrations (steady-state) have been reached (after Rowland[13]).

## 2.3 Steady-State Plasma Concentration

Thus far, we have considered only the administration of a single dose of a drug. While a number of drugs such as analgesics or hypnotics may be given in this way, it is more common to give drugs on a regular basis. As an example, consider digoxin, given without a loading dose, twice a day.

Digoxin has a half-life of about 40 hours (assuming normal renal function) and by the time the second dose of digoxin is given at 12 hours, the plasma concentration will still be more than

**Table I.** The plasma concentration at different time points as a percentage of the steady-state concentration[a]

| Number of half-lives[b] | Plasma concentration as % of steady-state level |
|---|---|
| 1 | 50 |
| 2 | 75 |
| 3 | 88 |
| 4 | 94 |
| 5 | 97 |
| 6 | 98 |
| 7 | 99 |

a Assuming a one-compartment model and continuous administration of the drug (intravenous infusion or frequent oral administration).

b The time points are expressed as the number of half-lives elapsed from starting therapy.

half its peak value and thus the concentration of the second dose of digoxin will rise to higher levels than after the first dose. With each succeeding dose, this pattern will be repeated until a steady-state concentration is reached. The elimination of digoxin from the plasma obeys first-order kinetics so that as the concentration of drug in plasma increases, the amount of drug eliminated per unit of time increases.

The tendency for a drug to accumulate will therefore be balanced by the increased amount of drug being eliminated. As a result, a steady-state will be reached during which the amount of drug absorbed will equal the amount of drug being eliminated. The plasma concentration will then fluctuate around a mean or plateau concentration (fig. 12).

Assuming that a one-compartment model can be applied, the rate at which the plateau or steady-state plasma concentration ($C^{ss}$) will be reached can be calculated (table I). Thus, 50% of the $C^{ss}$ will be reached in one half-life, 75% in two half-lives, 87.5% in three half-lives, etc. Consequently, during oral administration of digoxin once daily, it will take 200 hours ($5 \times t_{1/2}$) to reach 97% of the steady-state concentration. This can be exemplified further (fig. 13) with data on nortriptyline and desipramine (desmethylimipramine). The time taken to reach the steady-state concentration is well illustrated and corresponds to about 4 to 5 half-lives. Clinically, a drug intended for maintenance therapy can be expected to have its full benefit when a therapeutic steady-state plasma concentration has been reached. A number of concepts follow from these observations:

1) The shorter the elimination half-life of a drug, the sooner the $C^{ss}$ will be reached. (A drug with a half-life of 8 hours, given every 8 hours, will reach 90% of the $C^{ss}$ in 26 hours.)

2) The shorter the elimination half-life of a drug, the more the plasma concentration will fluctuate between doses and it is difficult in practice to dose more often than 4 times daily. Thus, drugs like alprenolol and procainamide with half-lives between 2 to 3 hours will show marked variations in plasma concentrations between doses when given every 6 hours. One way to avoid drastic fluctuations is to prepare such drugs in sustained-release forms. As an example, procainamide as sustained-release tablets can be given twice daily while ordinary tablets have to be given every 3 hours to avoid marked fluctuation in plasma concentrations.[15]

3) If the elimination half-life of a drug is prolonged above the normal value, as will happen with digoxin and aminoglycoside antibiotics (e.g. gentamicin, kanamycin) in patients with renal failure, the time taken to reach a steady-state will be longer than before, and concentrations reached will be considerably higher than under normal conditions. The dose must therefore be decreased and the dosage interval prolonged (see chapter 24; sect. 11.1 and appendix D). On the other hand, if a clinical effect is required quickly, it is possible to shorten the time taken to reach the steady-state concentration by giving a loading dose at the beginning, as is

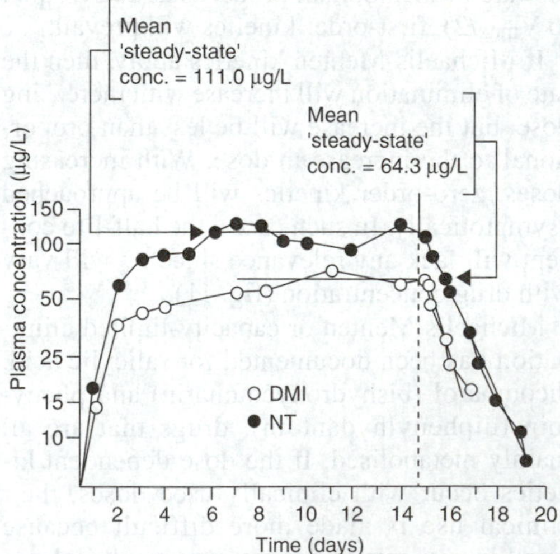


**Fig. 13.** Log plasma concentrations of desipramine (desmethylimipramine; DMI) and nortriptyline (NT) *versus* time during repetitive oral administration. The drugs were given to the same volunteer several weeks apart in a daily dose of 0.4 mg/kg administered every 8 hours for 15 days. Steady-state concentrations are reached within 4 to 5 days. When medication is stopped, plasma concentrations decline monophasically with half-lives of 25 (NT) and 21 hours (DMI), respectively (after Alexanderson[14]).

sometimes used for digoxin. The loading dose ($L_D$) can be calculated as:

$$L_D = C^{ss} \cdot Vd$$

where $C^{ss}$ is the required plasma concentration and Vd the apparent volume of distribution.

In practice, particularly with a drug which has a long elimination half-life, it is usually better to allow gradual accumulation following the usual maintenance dose and dosage interval. The patient will reach his or her individual steady-state concentration in due course.

4) It is possible to predict the steady-state concentrations of a drug in plasma after multiple doses from the kinetic behaviour of a single dose. This requires information about the clearance (CL) and the bioavailability (F). The formula used is:

$$C^{ss} = (F \cdot D)/(CL \cdot \tau)$$

where D is the dose and $\tau$ the dosage interval. As pointed out in section 2.2.9, bioavailability (F) is dependent on both the fraction absorbed and the degree of metabolism during the first passage of the drug through the gut wall and/or liver. The above formula implies linear kinetics. If the prediction does not hold, induction or inhibition of drug metabolism or capacity-limited elimination may operate. For example, actual steady-state plasma concentrations of carbamazepine are always lower than those predicted since autoinduction of its metabolism occurs after a few doses.[16]

The steady-state concentration, $C^{ss}$ may be calculated from the $AUC_{(0\text{-}\tau)}$ during the dosage interval divided by the length of the dosage interval ($\tau$). As shown below, $C^{ss}$ can also be predicted from the area under curve after a single dose [$AUC_{(0\text{-}\infty)}$] as $C^{ss} = AUC_{(0\text{-}\infty)}/\tau$:

$$C^{ss} = \text{Dose rate}/CL$$

$$\text{Dose rate} = \text{Dose}/\tau$$

$$CL = \text{Dose}/AUC_{(0\text{-}\infty)}$$

Thus,

$$C^{ss} = (\text{Dose}/\tau)/[\text{Dose}/AUC_{(0\text{-}\infty)}] = AUC_{(0\text{-}\infty)}/\tau$$

Hence $AUC_{(0\text{-}\infty)}$ and $AUC_{(0\text{-}\tau)}$ are equal (fig. 12). This illustrates an important characteristic of a linear system, namely that a particular dose gives rise to a certain AUC independent of whether it is after a single dose or after a maintenance dose at steady-state. However, the fact that a $C^{ss}$ can be calculated does not imply that the levels are 'steady'. To indicate variations within a dosage interval, it is customary to use peak-trough ratios. The maximum plasma concentration, $C_{max}$, and the time to reach this, $t_{max}$, both give valuable additional information.

### 2.4 Drugs as Chemical Individuals: Conclusions

Any drug can be characterised by several variables which will help to predict its behaviour in the body, as well as guide the clinician in selecting appropriate doses and dosage intervals. These variables include:

a) Bioavailability
b) Plasma clearance
c) Apparent volume of distribution
d) Elimination half-life
e) The pKa value
f) Lipophilicity as measured, for example, by the octanol : water partition coefficient.

We have also seen that the steady-state plasma concentration ($C^{ss}$) can be predicted from the bioavailability and clearance. Both variables may vary widely between individuals and this is the pharmacokinetic basis for individualised dosage regimens (see also chapter 5 and appendix G).

## 3. Special Processes in Pharmacokinetics

### 3.1 Drug Absorption

#### *3.1.1 Drug Absorption After Oral Administration*

Before a drug can be absorbed after oral ingestion, a drug tablet or capsule must disintegrate and the drug must dissolve in the gastrointestinal fluids. Most studies of the process of absorption have been performed with the drug in solution. This has tended to emphasise the importance of factors such as lipid solubility for drug absorption and de-emphasise the many factors that can interfere with the dissolution of the drug product in the gastrointestinal tract.

There are four possible mechanisms of absorption:

1) Passive diffusion.
2) Active transport.
3) Filtration through pores.
4) Pinocytosis.

#### Passive Diffusion

This is by far the most important process. No energy is required for the absorption of the drug and the net transfer of the drug is directly proportional to the concentration gradient and to the lipid : water partition coefficient of the drug. Lipid soluble drugs are absorbed more rapidly than water soluble drugs and no competition for absorption will be seen between two drugs of similar chemical composition. The drug must initially be present in aqueous solution at the surface of the cell membrane, then dissolve in the lipid membrane and finally pass into the aqueous phase on the other side of the membrane. Drug absorption will depend on the physicochemical properties of the compound as illustrated in section 1.1, especially its degree of ionisation in the gastrointestinal lumen. The ionised forms of drugs are not appreciably lipid soluble and thus in theory, acids should be better absorbed at acid pH (when they are relatively non-ionised) in the stomach than at the higher pH in the intestine. However, the short sojourn of the drug in the stomach and its limited surface area compared with that of the intestine outbalance the importance of this pH factor.

It is worth noting that drugs absorbed by passive diffusion are well absorbed not only in the small intestine, but also in the large intestine and the rectum. This is the basis for development of many sustained-release (SR) formulations and rectal administration forms.

#### Active Transport

This term implies the utilisation of energy to convey a drug across a cell, often against a concentration gradient. This mechanism is highly specific and is used for the transport of naturally occurring substances, such as amino acids, sugars and some vitamins, but rarely for drugs unless they have close structural similarity to a naturally occurring compound. Methyldopa and levodopa are both absorbed by active transport via an amino acid transport mechanism. The extent of absorption of actively transported drugs may be dependent upon the dose given because of saturation of the carrier mechanisms involved.

#### Filtration Through Pores

It has long been believed that the pores between cells are so small that only compounds with a molecular weight of less than 100D can be absorbed in this way. However, newer research indicates that the paracellular route is of great significance.[17] Drugs utilising this route often have an absorption window in the small intestine. Once past that window, the absorption rate drops dramatically, leading to incomplete absorption. Examples of such drugs are furosemide and atenolol; these drugs are unsuitable for sustained-release formulation.

#### Pinocytosis

This mechanism of absorption, whereby microscopic particles are engulfed by the cell membrane, is not of major importance for the absorption of drugs, although it may have some relevance to the uptake of macromolecules.

**Table II.** Factors affecting drug absorption from the gastrointestinal tract

| |
|---|
| **1. Formulation and characteristics of drug product:** |
| a) Tablet disintegration time |
| b) Dissolution time |
| c) Presence of excipients in tablet or capsule formulation |
| d) Stability in gastrointestinal tract |
| **2. Patient characteristics:** |
| a) pH of lumen |
| b) Gastric emptying time |
| c) Intestinal transit time |
| d) Surface area of gastrointestinal tract |
| e) Gastrointestinal disease |
| f) Mesenteric blood flow |
| **3. Presence of other substances in the gastrointestinal tract:** |
| a) Interaction with other drugs, ions |
| b) Food |
| **4. Pharmacokinetic characteristics of drug:** |
| a) Drug metabolism by gut bacteria |
| b) Drug metabolism in gut wall |

### *3.1.2 Factors Affecting Oral Absorption*

Table II lists some of the factors known to affect the absorption of drugs.

The formulation of the drug product may have dramatic effects on its solubility and hence absorption. Thus, the acid form of phenytoin is absorbed at rates which depend on its crystal size. An epidemic of phenytoin intoxication occurred in Australasia when the excipient was changed in the most commonly used product.[18] In Sweden, the most commonly used phenytoin product was shown to have less than 50% bioavailability and instances of severe intoxication have occurred when patients were changed to other brands of phenytoin, which were subsequently found to have much higher bioavailability.[19]

The presence of other drugs or even excipients believed to be inert may also modify drug absorption. The absorption of tetracyclines and fluoroquinolone derivatives is reduced by cations such as iron or calcium which produce insoluble chelates.[20] Bentonite, a constituent in, for example, some *p*-aminosalicylic acid (PAS) granules, is responsible for a marked impairment of the absorption of rifampicin when given together with some PAS products. This is due to adsorption of rifampicin onto bentonite.[21] Drugs that are well absorbed are probably less affected by the presence of other drugs in the gut, compared with poorly absorbed drugs (see further chapter 7).

Gastric emptying and motility determine the rate of delivery of a drug to the small intestine where absorption of most drugs occurs. As a general rule, factors slowing gastric emptying will decrease the rate of absorption of most drugs (and *vice versa*) but for some drugs, such as those that are poorly soluble, erratically absorbed, or metabolised in the gut, the amount of drug absorbed may be increased when gastric emptying or intestinal motility is slowed (see section 5.4.1).

#### Influence of Food

The presence of food might be expected to interfere with drug absorption by slowing gastric emptying, or by altering the degree of ionisation of the drug in the stomach. In the past, it has been assumed that food will in general delay drug absorption without affecting the total amount of drug absorbed, but this is an oversimplification.[22] Food intake may actually influence absorption of drugs in different ways – increasing, decreasing or having no consistent effect on the amount absorbed. The rate of absorption of some drugs will be decreased by the presence of food in the stomach. Thus, the absorption of digoxin is delayed by the presence of food. Conversely, concurrent food intake may enhance the rate of absorption of some drugs such as phenytoin.

The direction of this interaction is not only dependent on the physicochemical characteristics of the drug itself, but is also largely influenced by the drug formulation. Thus, one sustained-release formulation of theophylline was shown to release a large fraction of its contents (so-called 'dose-dumping') when given together with a high-fat, high-calorie meal,[23] producing intolerable adverse effects. Other sustained-release formulations (of theophylline as well as many other drugs) are insignificantly affected by a meal. The magnitude of the effect of the meal on a particular drug formulation, if any, is difficult to predict. Food studies are part of the regulatory requirements for new sustained-release formulations required by many regulatory authorities, and are an important part of the product's labelling.

The *extent* of absorption of some drugs is now known to be affected by the presence of food in the stomach. For most drugs, the effect, if any, is clinically insignificant; however, food enhances the absorption of hydrochlorothiazide, phenytoin, nitrofurantoin, and the anthelmintic drugs thiabendazole, mebendazole and albendazole. The latter were designed to be poorly absorbed and to kill intestinal helminths. They are now known to be effective against hydatid disease and food, particularly fatty food, markedly enhances the extent of their absorption. The antimalarial drug halofantrine is also more extensively absorbed if taken with food.[24]

In contrast, some antibiotics such as penicillin, rifampicin and isoniazid are comparatively poorly absorbed if taken with food. Tetracycline is a chelating agent and ions such as calcium and magnesium in food will bind to, and inactivate tetracyclines thereby preventing their absorption. The same applies to the fluoroquinolone derivative ciprofloxacin. As a generalisation, it is better to take such drugs a couple of hours before food to avoid these problems.[20]

The bioavailability of some drugs may be low because of first-pass metabolism in the gut wall or liver. Concurrent food intake may reduce this presystemic clearance and thus increase the bioavailability of lipophilic bases such as propranolol, metoprolol and hydralazine, but only when the drugs are given as conventional immediate-release preparations. The mechanisms of these food-induced changes in bioavailability remain to be fully explained, but competitive inhibition of drug metabolising enzymes and effects on splanchnic blood flow have been proposed. Unlike the above drugs, however, bases which undergo presystemic dealkylation such as codeine, amitriptyline and prazosin do not have their bioavailability affected by food intake.

### *3.1.3 Alternative Sites of Drug Absorption*

Although drugs are usually administered by mouth, they may be given by a variety of other routes as well.

#### Intramuscular Absorption

Drugs may be administered by the parenteral route:

- Because they are destroyed in the stomach (e.g. benzylpenicillin).
- Because they are subject to extensive and rapid hepatic first-pass metabolism (e.g. lidocaine).
- To ensure compliance with therapy.
- To ensure a more rapid onset of action.

However, intramuscular administration of some drugs does not always assure rapid or complete absorption, and some degree of local discomfort is probably inevitable with any intramuscular injection.

Although lipid solubility favours absorption of drugs from an intramuscular injection, the water solubility of a drug is a major determinant of the rate and completeness of absorption. The drug must be sufficiently water soluble at physiological pH to remain in solution in the interstitial fluid of muscle tissue until absorption occurs. Drugs that are poorly soluble in water (e.g. diazepam) or soluble in water only at non-physiological pH (e.g. phenytoin, chlordiazepoxide) are most likely to have bioavailability problems after intramuscular injection. Such drugs precipitate at the injection site once the non-aqueous solvent diffuses away or buffering occurs. Absorption of phenytoin and digoxin can be very slow and erratic. Intramuscular injection is therefore not a reliable means of administration of these drugs and should be avoided. Chlordiazepoxide and diazepam are slowly absorbed after intramuscular injection and diazepam may be incompletely absorbed. More rapid and reliable effects can be obtained by oral or intravenous administration of these drugs.

Absorption after intramuscular injection is also influenced by local blood flow. Thus, blood flow to skeletal muscle may be decreased by circulatory disturbances associated with reduced cardiac output. Morphine, for example, may be slowly absorbed after intramuscular injection in acute myocardial infarction. Differences in blood flow to specific muscle groups may also explain different rates of absorption. Lidocaine absorption, for example, is more rapid after injection into the deltoid muscle than into the vastus lateralis and gluteus maximus.

#### Rectal Absorption

The rectal route may be chosen to avoid direct gastric irritation or because of therapeutic customs in different countries. Absorption from the rectum is governed by the same processes which operate in other parts of the gastrointestinal tract. The surface area of the mucosa is less and thus in general, absorption is not as rapid or as complete as after oral administration. Rectal administration offers an alternative to parenteral administration where nausea and vomiting are a problem, and some drugs (e.g. metronidazole) are absorbed almost as well from the rectum as by parenteral administration. Speed of absorption can be impressive; the use of rectal diazepam in children with febrile convulsions has been a major therapeutic advance for these children, and has obviated the need for intravenous administration.

There may be partial avoidance of hepatic first-pass metabolism when the drug is given rectally and this can explain the better bioavailability (compared with oral administration) of drugs such as propranolol, metoclopramide and morphine. However, it is rare to avoid all first-pass metabolism in this way. The composition of the rectal preparation is particularly important for drugs given rectally, and this explains the poor absorption from the rectum of certain preparations of diazepam, indomethacin, paracetamol and diflunisal.[25]

#### Pulmonary Absorption

Many drugs can be readily absorbed from the lungs by passive diffusion. This applies particularly to inhaled anaesthetic gases but also to drugs delivered either as aerosols or as particulate inhalations. Most drugs, initially produced in aerosol form to allow direct medication to the lung, are in fact absorbed into the body via this route. Dosage levels are usually small and thus little therapeutic effect is seen outside the lungs, but repetitive inhalation of isoprenaline (isoproterenol) aerosols was probably responsible for a number of deaths from cardiac arrhythmias in the 1960s. The smaller the particle size, the more likely the drug is to be absorbed. Particles greater than 20μm in size are likely to be deposited on the bronchiolar epithelium and then the respiratory cilia will sweep the particles back to the larynx where they will be swallowed. Particles of 2μm in size are likely to reach the smallest bronchioles.

#### Local Absorption from the Mouth and Nose

Local delivery of drugs to these sites is increasingly used for therapeutic purposes. Although there are a number of potential advantages with these routes of administration, there are also some disadvantages. Buccal and sublingual administration allows rapid absorption of a drug and avoids the first-pass metabolism that may follow absorption from the small intestine. In addition, the drug formulation can be spat out by the patient if the therapeutic effect becomes too marked. Disadvantages include problems with the taste of the preparation and the need to keep it in place for a period of time and not chew or swallow it. This route is often used for administration of nitrates but is increasingly used for drugs such as captopril, prochlorperazine and pentazocine. Sublingual buprenorphine and morphine may allow more rapid pain relief that the corresponding oral dose.[26]

The intranasal route of drug delivery has been conventionally used for the administration of peptides such as desmopressin, gonadotrophin-releasing hormone (GnRH) and its analogues (e.g. buserelin). Although less than 1% of the dose may be absorbed, it is still considered an effective method of drug administration, and avoids the problems of compliance seen with injection methods. Recently, other peptides have been given by the nasal route, e.g. calcitonin and somatorelin (growth hormone-releasing hormone; GHRH), and studies are in progress with other drugs such as propranolol and contraceptive steroids. In general, a nasal spray is more effective than nasal drops, and many peptides are better absorbed if 'promoters' are included in formulation; these agents may alter the mucous covering of the nasal mucosa or open up the tight junctions of the epithelial cells. However, there are some concerns over local toxic effects to the mucosa with long term use.[27]

### Percutaneous Absorption

Is it now known that human skin is a very effective way of delivering drugs to the body as a whole, and the science involved has revealed much more information about the skin. Most drugs are absorbed across the skin to a certain extent, and this absorption is increased if the skin surface is occluded with polythene. In humans, many factors will affect the absorption of drugs across the skin. For example, the thickness of the skin and its regular exposure to the atmosphere are important. In general, drug absorption is better across thin skin (e.g. behind the ear) or across skin not regularly exposed to the environment. There are also important racial differences in skin composition and in the response of different skin types to various chemical stimuli. Drugs are absorbed slightly better across White skin than across Black skin, although it is doubtful if this is of clinical significance. It has been assumed that drug absorption would be more rapid across diseased skin than across normal skin but this is not necessarily true.[28]

**Table III.** Some advantages of transdermal drug delivery compared with conventional oral therapy (after Ridout et al.[29])

- Avoidance of gastrointestinal or hepatic first-pass metabolism
- Avoidance of 'peaks' and 'troughs' in plasma concentration *versus* time curves
- Rapid termination of drug input
- Reduction in interindividual variability in absorption seen usually with oral administration
- Prolonged duration of action
- Improved patient compliance

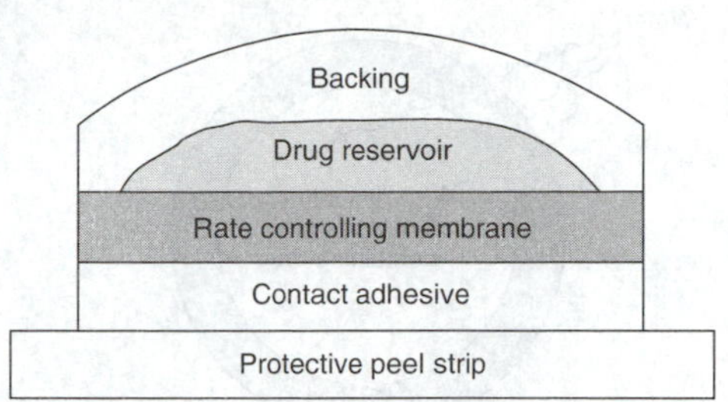


**Fig. 14.** Schematic cross-section of a typical transdermal drug delivery system.

Drugs may be used in transdermal formulations for single-dose use or for multiple-dose therapy. Some of the advantages of transdermal drug delivery compared with conventional oral therapy are listed in table III. Single-dose therapy is exemplified by scopolamine (hyoscine) which was the first transdermal drug delivery system to be developed; this has been shown to be effective for the treatment of both motion sickness and postoperative nausea. Other drugs for single-dose use include azatidine and fentanyl.

A number of drugs are now given as transdermal formulations for multiple-dose therapy, including clonidine, estradiol, nitroglycerin (glyceryl trinitrate), timolol, nicotine and testosterone. The development of rate-controlling has helped greatly in this and a typical example is shown in figure 14. A number of technical devices have been produced and these are discussed in detail elsewhere (see review by Ridout et al.[29]). These devices all aim to produce a standard delivery of drug across the skin from a reservoir which is progressively depleted of its drug content. The systems now in

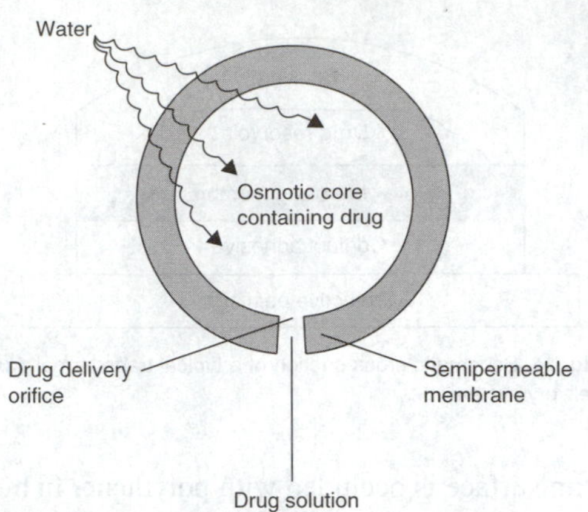


**Fig. 15.** Schematic cross-section of a typical osmotic drug delivery system.

use are mostly very effective but do not solve all problems of therapy. Thus, the tolerance that develops to oral nitrate therapy still occurs with the transdermal formulation and can only be relieved by taking the delivery system (patch) off the skin for a defined period every day.

**Conjunctival Absorption**

The conjunctiva functions as a specialised skin surface, and drugs can be administered into the conjunctiva for local therapy to the eye or for more general therapy. Some success has been achieved with locally inserted sustained-release preparations of drugs such as pilocarpine 'Ocusert' (see chapter 15; sect. 5.1.4).

### *3.1.4 Rate-Controlled Oral Drug Delivery Systems*

Although oral administration is the most common way of giving drugs, standard formulations may cause problems. In some cases, the drug in question may have a very short half-life and thus has to be given very frequently to maintain steady-state concentrations (e.g. procainamide). In other cases, adverse effects may be caused by high peak plasma concentrations following rapid release of the drug from a standard oral formulation (e.g. indomethacin, carbamazepine). The initial approach to these problems was to produce a variety of sustained-release preparations to slow down the rate of absorption. Modern technology has now developed a number of different approaches to the problem and pharmacokinetic techniques have been developed to evaluate the data produced.[30]

Some of the available rate-controlled systems depend upon osmosis for their effect (fig. 15). The principle of this system is a semipermeable membrane surrounding an osmotically active core of drug. A single hole is drilled very accurately into each capsule using laser technology. When the capsule/device is swallowed, water from the intestine enters the core of the capsule through the semipermeable membrane, dissolving the drug on the surface of the core. A steady osmotic pressure is thus developed inside the device which pushes the drug solution out through the opening. The drug is therefore delivered in a zero-order fashion. The rate of drug delivery is primarily regulated by the size of the hole drilled into the device. The release rate will stay constant until the contents of the capsule/device are all dissolved and progressive dilution then leads to a gradual slowing of the delivery of the drug. Such a system was first used extensively for indomethacin but has been extended to other drugs such as β-adrenoceptor blockers.[31] The indomethacin delivery system initially produced problems due to local intestinal ulceration; it is not clear whether this was due to high local concentrations of indomethacin or to high local concentrations of potassium.

A number of different rate-controlled systems have been developed. These systems have two principal aims:

1) To supply pharmacological amounts of a drug to the patient but without exposing him/her to subtherapeutic or supratherapeutic concentrations.

2) To provide good control of drug therapy but without incurring additional costs.

In mechanical terms, the devices may be very complicated but the main ones in use are relatively simple. In some areas of therapy, e.g. contraceptive steroid therapy, devices are being developed which can be implanted under the skin through a needle and which can deliver the drug at the required rate for several years. In other cases, newer oral formulations have been developed (e.g. 'Oros' systems). The systems continue to advance in technological terms and it is now necessary to tie the technology in with the goals of improved drug therapy.

### *3.1.5 Other Drug Delivery Systems*

Other methods of delivering drugs to their site of action are being actively investigated. The use of *monoclonal antibodies* and *liposomes* has been under investigation for the last decade but progress has not been as rapid as expected. Liposomes have the potential to carry a wide range of drugs to their site of action and in the process, reduce the risk of toxicity to specific organs that are not the intended site of therapeutic action. Studies with liposome formulations are in progress with drugs such as amphotericin B, doxorubicin and gentamicin. The last decade has seen greatly improved technology in terms of drug capture and liposome stability, and liposomal systems are likely to have a significant clinical impact in the near future.[32]

Studies are also in progress with the *intrathecal delivery* of drugs. Here drugs such as the opioids are delivered via a fine catheter into the subarachnoid space in the cauda equina. Although this is an invasive method of drug delivery, there are advantages for some conditions. Thus, the dose of baclofen given orally for spinal cord spasticity is 60 mg/day but an intrathecal dose of 600 μg/day has an even more pronounced effect.[33]

## 3.2 Binding and Distribution of Drugs

After absorption, a number of factors influence the subsequent fate of a drug. Thus, it will be distributed to receptors at its site of action, to silent or inactive receptors in other tissues, and to sites of metabolism and excretion (fig. 16). The process of distribution largely depends on the physicochemical properties of the drug such as lipid solubility and binding to macromolecules, but is also affected by factors such as blood flow to various organs.

Drugs are transported from the site of administration to receptor sites by plasma proteins and red blood cells. Serum albumin can carry many types of drugs, but haemoglobin, lipoproteins, $\alpha_1$-acid glycoprotein and certain other globulins are also important. The processes of distribution, metabolism and excretion operate simultaneously and thus a change in protein binding of a drug will affect its distribution and elimination, and hence steady-state plasma concentration, in the body in a way which is predictable from its pharmacokinetic properties.[34,35]

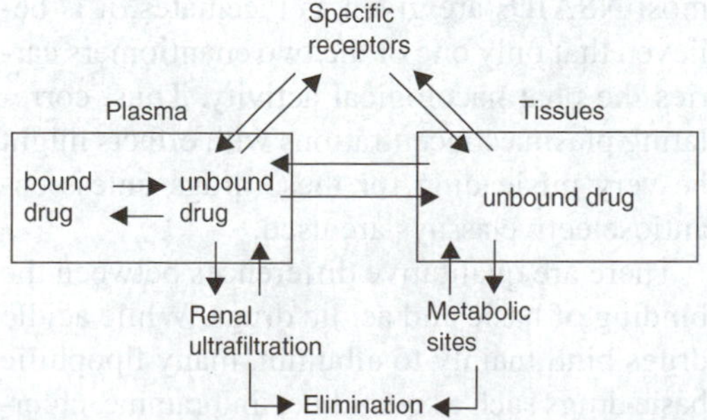


**Fig. 16.** Schematic representation of the fate of a drug in the body. During distribution equilibrium, the unbound concentration of drug is assumed to be the same in various parts of the body.

### *3.2.1 Protein Binding of Drugs*

The exterior surface of a protein is composed principally of polar amino acids with the side chains projecting into the surrounding environment. A given protein, e.g. serum albumin, may have several specific structures and reactive groups, permitting reversible binding of many structurally diverse small molecules. The forces involved in binding include ionic, hydrogen and hydrophilic bonds and weaker bonds called van der Waal forces.

Proteins are structures with clefts and holes that can also allow entry of small molecules into their interior areas. Once a small molecule is attached to a protein, it travels in the bloodstream until it dissociates from the protein and attaches to another macromolecule. Thiopental, for example, is highly bound (75%) to plasma proteins but when the blood reaches the brain or fat tissue, the drug rapidly dissociates from the protein in blood and binds to lipids in the tissue.

Serum albumin (MW 66,400D) probably exists in several closely related conformations, and the location and number of binding sites may differ for different drugs. Albumin has a particularly high affinity for acidic drugs, such as warfarin, nonsteroidal anti-inflammatory drugs (NSAIDs), penicillins, sulfonamides and salicylic acid.

Two independent binding sites (I and II) for acidic drugs have been particularly well characterised on human serum albumin.[36,37] Site I, the less specific of the two sites, binds a variety of structurally diverse drugs such as warfarin, phenylbutazone, the antiepileptic drugs phenytoin and valproic acid (sodium valproate), and various sulfonamides (table IV).

Warfarin is bound specifically to this site, and the ability of various drugs to displace warfarin has been used as a criterion of site I binding. Similarly, diazepam has been used as a marker for the more specific site II. With the exception of the benzodiazepines, site II drugs are generally carboxylic acids (table IV), among them the extremely strongly bound anti-inflammatory analgesic drugs naproxen and ibuprofen and their analogues. The latter drugs are also bound to site I, but in general with lower relative affinity. This means that they are less efficient in displacing type I drugs, unless in very high concentration, when binding to the less specific secondary site occurs.

Among endogenous compounds, it may be noted that tryptophan is bound to site II, while bilirubin is primarily bound to site I. This explains why bilirubin may be displaced by several sulfonamides (site I drugs) and salicylic acid (bound equally strongly to sites I and II). It is a widespread misconception that compounds bound with very high affinity, such as bilirubin, cannot be displaced by compounds with lower affinity for the protein (e.g. sulfonamides). According to accepted theory, competitive displacement occurs when the product of the *free* concentration of displacer and its binding constant is high enough. This implies that important displacement will be caused by drugs that have unbound concentrations high enough to exceed the binding capacity of their own primary binding sites on albumin. In other words,

**Table IV.** Binding sites of highly bound acidic drugs on human serum albumin (after Sjöholm et al.;[36] Sudlow[37])

| Site I (warfarin site) | Site II (diazepam site) |
|---|---|
| Warfarin | Benzodiazepines |
| Ethylbiscoumacetate | |
| Acenocoumarol | Ibuprofen |
| (nicoumalone) | Flurbiprofen |
| Phenprocoumon | Ketoprofen |
| Dicoumarol | Naproxen |
| | Indomethacin |
| Chlorothiazide | Salicylic acid |
| Furosemide (frusemide) | Diflunisal |
| Bumetanide | Flufenamic acid |
| Several sulfonamides | Ethacrynic acid |
| Azidocillin | |
| Nalidixic acid | Clofibric acid[a] |
| Phenytoin | Cloxacillin |
| Valproic acid | Dicloxacillin |
| Salicylamide | Probenecid |
| Salicylic acid | |
| Diflunisal | Sulfobromophthalein |
| Phenylbutazone | |
| Oxyphenbutazone | Tolazamide |
| Azapropazone | Glibenclamide (glyburide) |
| Sulfinpyrazone | Tolbutamide |
| Indomethacin | |
| Naproxen | Tryptophan |
| Chlorpropramide | |
| Glibenclamide (glyburide) | |
| Tolbutamide | |
| Bilirubin | |

a Active metabolite of clofibrate.

drugs that exhibit concentration-dependent binding at therapeutic doses are the only drugs that may be potential displacers of other drugs. This prerequisite makes salicylate, phenylbutazone, valproic acid, naproxen, dicloxacillin and several sulfonamides likely candidates for displacement of other drugs bound to the same site, but rules out warfarin, diazepam, indomethacin and phenytoin. This is because therapeutic plasma concentrations of the latter drugs are much below the saturation concentration of their albumin binding.

Fatty acids have their own specific primary binding sites on albumin. By inducing conformational changes in the albumin molecule, fatty acids can affect the binding of other compounds to separate sites on albumin. Thus, high serum concentrations of free fatty acids released by heparin injection, may cause either decreased or increased binding of drugs, as shown with digitoxin[38] and warfarin,[39] respectively. Normal physiological fluctuations in free fatty acid levels usually have little effect on drug binding.

Many drugs, among them the NSAIDs, occur in two different enantiomeric forms. Since proteins are chiral compounds, they have the potential to distinguish between these two forms. As an example, the binding of *S*-flurbiprofen and *S*-carprofen to plasma proteins is greater than that of the *R*-enantiomers of these drugs, but the opposite is true for *S*-etodolac and *S*-pirprofen.[40] Since NSAIDs are, in general, low clearance drugs with low volumes of distribution, their clearances will be directly proportional to the unbound fraction of drug. The main implication of the enantioselective binding is that it will translate into different pharmacokinetic properties of the two enantiomers. While most NSAIDs are given as racemates, it is believed that only one of the two enantiomers carries the pharmacological activity. Thus, correlating plasma concentrations with effects might be very misleading for these drugs unless enantioselective assays are used.

There are qualitative differences between the binding of basic and acidic drugs. While acidic drugs bind mainly to albumin, many lipophilic basic drugs such as quinidine, imipramine, chlorpromazine, alprenolol and propranolol bind more avidly to other proteins in the plasma such as $\alpha_1$-acid glycoproteins and lipoproteins.[41,42]

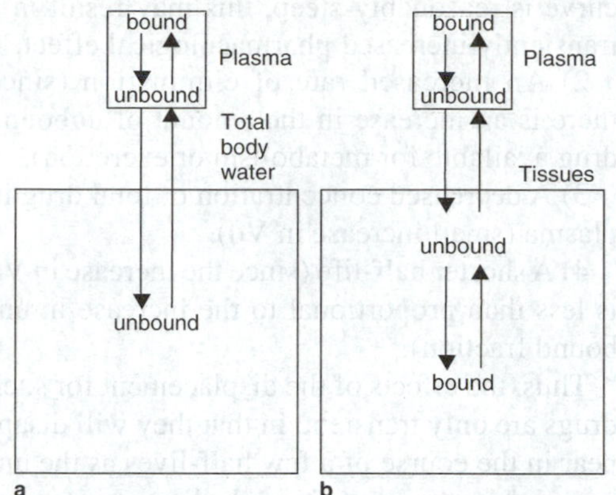


**Fig. 17. (a)** Schematic representation of the partitioning of a non-tissue bound drug between the plasma pool and total body water. **(b)** Schematic representation of the partitioning of a tissue and plasma bound drug between plasma and other tissues.

### *3.2.2 Pharmacological Implications of Protein Binding*

The interaction between a protein and a drug is reversible and obeys the law of mass action:

Drug + Protein ⇔ Drug-protein complex

The rate at which a drug-protein complex can dissociate is very rapid (with a half-life of about 20 milliseconds) so this is probably not a rate-limiting factor in the removal of drug from plasma. Only unbound drug can diffuse into tissues because the drug-protein complex is unable to cross cell membranes. The drug-protein complex therefore acts as a store of drug and as unbound drug is removed from plasma, more of the complex dissociates.

The consequences of protein binding are quite different for drugs that are extensively bound in tissues compared with those that are not bound in the tissues. Much of the discussion in the literature concerning the importance of plasma protein binding has not taken this into account. It is also important to consider that the consequences of protein binding are different during the distributive phase after drug administration, compared with the distribution equilibrium that may occur during steady-state conditions. Also, in other non-equilibrium situations, plasma protein binding can have unexpected effects, as illustrated by the following examples.

For tissue bound drugs, the plasma can be completely cleared of drug during a single passage through an organ such as the brain (e.g. thiopental), the kidney or the liver, irrespective of the extent of plasma protein binding. In such cases, the protein binding actually increases the concentration of drug available for diffusion into the tissues or the sites of elimination. For example, with some drugs that have a high hepatic clearance, such as alprenolol, propranolol and hydralazine, virtually all drug in blood, unbound and bound, is cleared during one passage through the liver. For these drugs, with a high 'hepatic extraction ratio' (see sections 3.3.3 and 5.4.3), increased protein binding may increase rather than decrease the amount metabolised per unit of time, simply because increased binding to plasma protein results in elevated total drug concentrations in blood and thus a higher drug delivery rate at any given blood flow.

While the above examples relate to non-equilibrium situations, the following discussion relates to *low clearance* drugs only, and is based on the assumption that distribution equilibrium has been obtained, i.e. a plateau concentration at steady-state. Under these circumstances, the unbound concentration of a drug should be equal in the plasma and tissues, and at receptor and metabolic (excretory) sites. For example, during long term treatment with phenytoin, the concentration of unbound drug in plasma during steady-state conditions is the same as the concentration in cerebrospinal fluid (CSF) and saliva, which essentially can be considered as protein-free solutions. Thus, CSF and saliva concentrations are about 10% of the total steady-state plasma concentration, corresponding to 90% binding of phenytoin in plasma.

### *3.2.3 Displacement of Protein Bound Drugs*

For a drug with negligible binding to tissues other than plasma, the model depicted in figure 17a can be used to describe some pharmacological consequences of a displacement interaction. Unbound drug in the plasma pool (4% of

**Table V.** Relationship between degree of binding to plasma proteins and total amount of drug in plasma (after Martin[43])

| Binding to plasma proteins (%) | Drug in plasma as % of total amount in the body |
|---|---|
| 0 | 6.7 |
| 50 | 12 |
| 60 | 15 |
| 70 | 19 |
| 80 | 26 |
| 90 | 42 |
| 95 | 59 |
| 98 | 78 |
| 99 | 88 |
| 100 | 100 |

**Table VI.** Predicted increase in concentration of unbound drug *in vivo* resulting from drug displacement found *in vitro* (chosen as a doubling of the unbound percentage)

| Displacement observed *in vitro* | | | | Predicted[a] increase of unbound concentration *in vivo* by a factor of: |
|---|---|---|---|---|
| % bound | | % unbound | | |
| before | after | before | after | |
| 99 | 98 | 1 | 2 | 1.8 |
| 95 | 90 | 5 | 10 | 1.4 |
| 90 | 80 | 10 | 20 | 1.3 |
| 80 | 60 | 20 | 40 | 1.14 |
| 70 | 40 | 30 | 60 | 1.11 |
| 50 | 0 | 50 | 100 | 1.06 |

a Based on the calculated total amount of drug in the plasma for a given degree of protein binding (see table V). For example, displacement of a drug which is 90% protein bound to 80% *in vivo* results in a decrease in the total amount of drug in the plasma from 42 to 26% so that the concentration of unbound drug is increased, albeit transiently (see section 3.2.3), by a factor of 1.3 [i.e. (100 – 26)/(100 – 42) = 1.3], rather than a factor of 2 as observed *in vitro*. Protein binding displacement leading to increases in the fraction of unbound drug becomes unimportant at binding degrees below 80%.

bodyweight) is in equilibrium with unbound drug in the 15 times bigger pool consisting of total body water (60% of bodyweight). Table V shows that most of the total amount of drug (bound + unbound) in the body occurs in plasma at binding degrees above 90%. Table VI shows the consequences *in vivo* of a displacement interaction observed *in vitro*. This model helps to show that the rise in unbound concentration as found *in vitro* never occurs to the same extent *in vivo*. In fact, protein binding displacement will affect the unbound concentration of drug in the body only at binding degrees above 80%. The model does not take extravascular albumin into account which might increase the quantitative importance of displacement.[44]

Model 1 (fig. 17a) can be used to discuss the possible consequences of a displacement interaction. A basic assumption here is that the displaced drug is a low clearance one; high clearance drugs invariably seem to have high tissue binding and thus do not conform with model 1. Another assumption is that the displaced drug had been administered until steady-state has been reached. If the displaced drug has high initial binding of 80% or more, the following events may result from a displacement interaction:

1) A *transiently* increased unbound drug concentration in plasma; if the concentration-effect curve is reasonably steep, this may result in a transiently increased pharmacological effect.

2) An increased rate of elimination (since there is an increase in the amount of unbound drug available for metabolism or excretion).

3) A decreased concentration of total drug in plasma (small increase in Vd).

4) A shorter half-life (since the increase in Vd is less than proportional to the increase in unbound fraction).

Thus, the effects of the displacement for such drugs are only transient, in that they will disappear in the course of a few half-lives as the unbound drug concentration declines to its pre-displacement steady-state value. As already pointed out, this sequence of events will only occur for drugs with high initial binding; the unbound drug concentration will not be significantly affected in the case of drugs with lower degrees of protein binding (< 80%).

In model 2 (fig. 17b), which is generally applicable, the prerequisites are the same as in model 1, with the exception that the drug now may bind considerably to tissue components as well. Table VII shows that with an increasing volume of distribution, less and less drug occurs in plasma compared with tissues. One consequence of this is that induced changes in plasma protein binding (see also section 5.4.2) will be potentially important clinically only at small Vd values of the order of 0.15 L/kg or less. At Vd values above this, less than 27% of the total drug in the body occurs in plasma.

The consequences of a displacement interaction for highly bound drugs with a large Vd value can be discussed using model 2 (fig. 17b). If the drug is a low clearance one and has been administered until steady-state has been reached, a displacement interaction at protein binding sites will lead to:

1) A negligible increase in the unbound concentration in plasma.

**Table VII.** Relationship between apparent volume of distribution (Vd) and amount of drug in plasma (assuming a plasma volume equal to 4% of bodyweight)

| Vd (L/kg) | % Drug in plasma of total amount in body |
|---|---|
| 0.045 | 89 |
| 0.10 | 40 |
| 0.15 | 27 |
| 0.6 | 6.7 |
| 1.0 | 4.0 |
| 10 | 0.40 |

**Table VIII.** Apparent volumes of distribution[a] of various drugs (approximate average values in healthy individuals)

| Drug | Vd (L/kg) |
|---|---|
| Furosemide (frusemide) | 0.1 |
| Phenylbutazone | 0.1 |
| Warfarin | 0.1 |
| Naproxen | 0.1 |
| Sulfamethoxazole | 0.1 |
| Ibuprofen | 0.14 |
| Tolbutamide | 0.14 |
| Valproic acid | 0.15 |
| Sulfafurazole (sulfisoxazole) | 0.2 |
| Dicloxacillin | 0.2 |
| Glibenclamide (glyburide) | 0.3 |
| Nalidixic acid | 0.3 |
| Benzylpenicillin (penicillin G) | 0.3 |
| Phenazone (antipyrine) | 0.6 |
| Phenytoin (diphenylhydantoin) | 0.6 |
| Diazepam | 0.7 |
| Pentobarbital | 0.7 |
| Indomethacin | 0.9 |
| Carbamazepine | 1 |
| Lidocaine (lignocaine) | 1.3 |
| Procainamide | 2 |
| Pentazocine | 3 |
| Digoxin | 6 |
| Chlorpromazine | 20 |
| Nortriptyline | 20 |

a It should be noted that the Vd term is not unequivocally defined unless the pharmacokinetic model is defined. Even then, there are several volume terms, e.g. $Vd_\beta$, $Vd_{area}$, $Vd_{ss}$ (see sections 2.2.2 and 2.2.6). For this table, Vd (= $Vd_{extrap}$) has been used where the log plasma concentration-time curve was essentially monoexponential, and $Vd_\beta$ (= $Vd_{area}$) where there was a biphasic decline of plasma concentrations with time.

2) A decreased concentration of total drug in plasma (increased Vd).

3) Little or no pharmacological consequences.

4) A changed relationship between total drug concentration and clinical effects (i.e. effects will occur at a lower concentration of *total* drug).

A discussion of the consequences of displacement of a *high clearance drug* requires introduction of a number of new concepts and is beyond the scope of this chapter. For further discussion of this topic, see Rowland & Tozer.[45]

While the predictions using model 1 are mainly theoretical with little clinical support, the predictions using model 2 have been validated by clinical studies. After adding the displacer valproic acid to maintenance therapy with phenytoin, the unbound *fraction* of phenytoin in plasma increased, the total plasma concentration decreased, while the unbound concentration remained relatively stable.[46] The same phenomenon occurs with phenytoin in uraemia as a consequence of decreased protein binding.[47] In both cases, the therapeutic plasma concentration range of phenytoin (measured as bound plus unbound drug) was lowered (see also sections 5.4.2, 6.1; and chapter 5; sect. 1.6.3).

Hence by knowing the Vd of a drug and its degree of plasma protein binding, we can predict the possible importance of a protein binding displacement interaction. Vd values for some drugs are listed in table VIII and for many others in appendix A.

As discussed in section 3.2.1, displacement will only occur if the two drugs are bound to the same site on albumin. Ibuprofen has a low Vd value (table VIII) and is highly protein bound (99%) but binds to a different primary site on albumin than, for example, warfarin or tolbutamide (table IV). Also, plasma concentrations of ibuprofen obtained with normal therapeutic doses are relatively low. This explains why ibuprofen does not displace warfarin.[48] Phenylbutazone, on the other hand, is bound to the same site on albumin as warfarin and tolbutamide and is a predictable cause of interaction with these drugs. However, this is because phenylbutazone not only displaces warfarin and tolbutamide, but also inhibits the metabolism of these drugs.[49] In fact, inhibition of metabolism appears to be the more important mechanism. Most clinically important interactions that were formerly thought to be due to protein binding displacement usually have another interaction mechanism involved as well, commonly decreased metabolism or renal excretion (see also chapter 7; sect. 2.3.2).

To summarise the pharmacokinetic importance of drug protein binding, the rate-limiting factor for entry of a drug into tissue fluid appears to be diffusion of unbound drug and not the rate of dissociation of the drug-albumin complex. The best available indication of the concentration of unbound drug in tissue fluids is the unbound drug concentration in plasma. Displacement interactions are only likely to be of clinical importance for highly albumin bound acidic drugs which are bound to the same site on the albumin molecule and which have small apparent volumes of distribution of the order of 0.15 L/kg or less (for a list of Vd values, see appendix A).

As discussed in section 3.2.1, a prerequisite for a displacer is that its concentration is high enough to begin saturating (complete saturation can never be achieved at any concentration) its own binding sites. Very few drugs meet this criterion. Some acidic drugs that have been identified as displacers for albumin binding are clofibric acid, phenylbutazone, salicylic acid, sulfamethoxazole, and valproic acid. Erythromycin appears to be a potential displacer for $\alpha_1$-acid glycoprotein binding.[50]

## 3.3 Drug Metabolism

### *3.3.1 General Principles*

In general, drugs can be divided into water soluble (polar) and lipid soluble compounds. Water soluble drugs are mainly excreted unchanged through the kidneys and will reach toxic concentrations in the body when kidney function deteriorates, unless the dose is reduced. Lipid soluble drugs are initially filtered in the glomeruli but may be fully reabsorbed further on in the distal portion of the nephron. Such drugs therefore have to be metabolised to more polar compounds before they can be excreted in the urine. Their rate of metabolism will determine the duration of action of single doses and the intensity of action of multiple doses. This is because the steady-state concentration largely depends on the elimination rate constant (see section 2.2.4).

The metabolites formed are usually, but not always, less active than the parent compound (bioinactivation). Exceptions to this rule are drugs like many of the ACE inhibitors which are hydrolysed to their active forms following oral administration, and the cytotoxic drug cyclophosphamide which has to be bioactivated by enzymatic hydroxylation (see chapter 27; sect. 1). Many other drugs like imipramine, alprenolol, propranolol, procainamide, diazepam and phenylbutazone are active *per se,* but also have active metabolites whose pharmacokinetic or pharmacodynamic profiles differ to some extent from that of the parent drug. The contribution of active metabolites to the therapeutic and/or toxic effects of a drug is determined by their relative activity and quantitative importance (e.g. hydroxyhexamide, a major metabolite of acetohexamide, has 2.5 times the antihyperglycaemic activity of acetohexamide but is present in plasma in only small amounts in patients with normal renal function), and whether they accumulate with repeated administration (e.g. nordazepam in the elderly) or in patients with impaired renal function (e.g. procainamide).

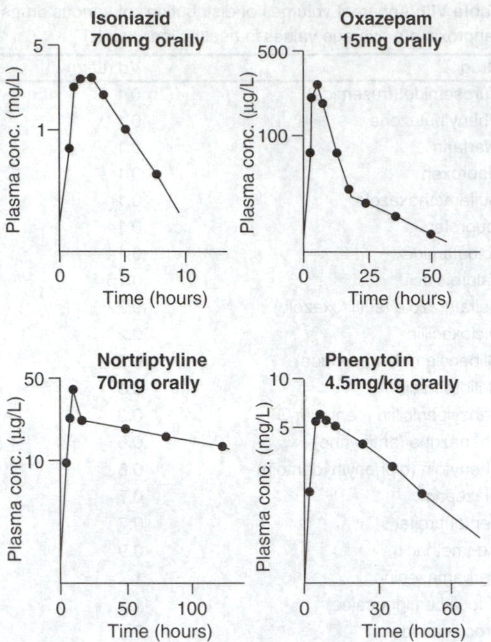


**Fig. 18.** Plasma concentration-time curves after oral administration of single doses of isoniazid, oxazepam, nortriptyline and phenytoin, which are all metabolised by different pathways.

Figure 18 shows the plasma pharmacokinetics of a single oral dose of four drugs – isoniazid, oxazepam, nortriptyline and phenytoin. They have in common that they are extensively metabolised in the body and that the metabolites have weaker or no pharmacodynamic activity compared with the parent compound.

Isoniazid is rapidly absorbed and then disappears monophasically from plasma with a half-life of a few hours due to acetylation by a mitochondrial hepatic enzyme *N*-acetyltransferase (see section 5.2.1). Oxazepam and nortriptyline are much more slowly absorbed and their disappearance from plasma is biexponential. The first part of the plasma disappearance curve ($\alpha$-slope) reflects the distribution of the drug in the body, while the second part ($\beta$-slope) reflects elimination from the body.

Oxazepam has a plasma half-life of the order of 12 hours (range 6 to 25 hours) and is conjugated directly with glucuronic acid to an inactive metabolite. Oxazepam, being itself an end metabolite of diazepam, thus has a much simpler metabolism than many other benzodiazepines. Lorazepam is also eliminated by conjugation with glucuronic acid (see chapter 30; sect. 6.1.2).

Nortriptyline is an example of a drug which is metabolised in a more complicated way. Two main metabolic reactions occur: an initial hydroxylation followed by conjugation. Demethylation is also involved. The plasma half-life of nortriptyline varies greatly between individuals (range 15 to 90 hours), depending on the genetically determined capacity to metabolise the drug via the hepatic CYP2D6 enzyme (see section 5.2.2). The main metabolite E10-hydroxynortriptyline may also contribute to the antidepressant activity of nortriptyline.[51]

Phenytoin has a slow absorption and its disappearance from plasma is slower at high than at low plasma concentrations (i.e. concentration-dependent metabolism). Its elimination half-life therefore varies over the concentration range. Phenytoin is initially hydroxylated in one of the benzene rings and then conjugated with glucuronic acid. Both metabolites are inactive.

Many drugs are racemic mixtures of two optical isomers (enantiomers). Both the pharmacokinetics and pharmacodynamics of the enantiomers of a drug may differ markedly and they should thus be considered as two separate compounds.[52,53] For example, in terms of clearance, *R*-metoprolol is cleared more rapidly than *S*-metoprolol and this is particularly obvious in individuals who are extensive metabolisers of debrisoquine (see section 5.2.2). In qualitative terms, *S*-warfarin is primarily metabolised to hydroxylated derivatives while *R*-warfarin is metabolised to warfarin alcohols. Differences in metabolism may also explain some drug interactions which have been misunderstood until the enantiomers were examined. Thus, phenylbutazone inhibits the metabolism of *S*-warfarin (the more potent enantiomer) while inducing the metabolism of *R*-warfarin. This explains the important interaction between these two drugs which has, in the past, been wrongly ascribed only to a displacement from protein binding sites.

The metabolism of a drug may also lead to the formation of several possible isomers. For example, the 10-hydroxylation of nortriptyline is stereospecific in that mainly E10-hydroxynortriptyline is formed, Z10-hydroxynortriptyline being only a minor metabolite. The formation of E10-hydroxynortriptyline, but not that of Z10-hydroxynortriptyline, is related to the activity of the polymorphic cytochrome P450 isoenzyme CYP2D6,[54] indicating that different enzymes catalyse the formation of the two isomers.

#### *3.3.2 Sites of Drug Metabolism*

The main site of drug metabolism is the liver but other tissues may also metabolise drugs, such as the lung, kidneys, blood, brain, skin and intestine (extrahepatic metabolism). For example, isoprenaline (isoproterenol) is metabolised in the gut wall to inactive conjugates.[55] Metabolism in the gut wall contributes to the first-pass metabolism of the drug and thus reduces its bioavailability. The gut bacterial flora may also metabolise certain drugs.

#### *3.3.3 First-Pass Metabolism*

Orally administered drugs will traverse the gut wall, the hepatic portal system, and the liver before reaching the systemic circulation. If a drug is extensively cleared by the liver, only a small fraction of the administered unchanged drug will reach the systemic circulation and exert its pharmacodynamic effects. This so-called 'first-pass metabolism' is seen for a number of drugs in common use. The fraction of drug removed from the blood during a single transit through the liver is referred to as the *extraction ratio* and drugs subject to extensive first-pass elimination in the liver therefore have a high hepatic extraction ratio (i.e. >0.7).

Significant first-pass metabolism is one explanation of why an intravenous dose of certain drugs is much smaller than an equipotent oral dose. For example, the β-adrenoceptor blocking drugs propranolol and alprenolol are extensively metabolised in the liver on their first passage through the organ. This explains why their oral bioavailabilities are around 10 to 30% (see appendix A), despite complete absorption. For alprenolol, the pharmacodynamic consequences of this kinetic behaviour after oral administration are diminished by the formation of an hydroxylated metabolite with β-blocking properties.[56]

Some drugs (e.g. lidocaine) have such extensive and rapid first-pass metabolism that they cannot be used orally. Use of high lidocaine doses orally is further hampered by toxicity due to a metabolite formed during first-pass metabolism.[57] Morphine also has extensive first-pass metabolism (oral bioavailability in the range 15 to 65%) and has traditionally been used only by the parenteral route. In the last decade, however, it has become available as oral preparations in dosages which are up to 10 times higher than those used parenterally.

Although first-pass metabolism in the liver is quantitatively more important, several drugs undergo extensive metabolism in the gut wall.

**Table IX.** Examples of important drug metabolic reactions

| Reaction | Substrates |
|---|---|
| 1. Cytochrome P450 mediated oxidation | Many drugs, carcinogens, insecticides, endogenous steroids and fatty acids |
| 2. Oxidation of alcohols and aldehydes (dehydrogenases) | Chloral hydrate, ethanol |
| 3. Oxidation of purines (xanthine oxidase) | Mercaptopurine and azathioprine |
| 4. Oxidation by monoamine oxidase (MAO) | Tyramine, catechol- and indolamines |
| 5. Hydrolysis (serum cholinesterase) | Suxamethonium (succinylcholine) |
| 6. Glucuronidation | Phenols, carboxylic acids, oxazepam, morphine |
| 7. Acetylation | Isoniazid, hydralazine, procainamide, dapsone, sulfonamides |

Such drugs include isoprenaline, paracetamol, ethinylestradiol, cyclosporin, and ascorbic acid. The metabolic steps most commonly involved are conjugation processes to form either glucuronide or sulfate, and the metabolites produced are usually inactive. However, one of the main metabolites of morphine, morphine 6-glucuronide, has been shown to have analgesic activity *per se*.[58]

The presence of cytochrome P450 3A (CYP3A) in the gut wall is probably the main reason for the extensive first-pass metabolism of cyclosporin.[59] Studies of cyclosporin, before and after induction of oxidative drug metabolism by treatment with rifampicin 600mg daily for 11 days, showed a marked increase in first-pass metabolism, although the total systemic clearance of cyclosporin was only moderately increased.[60] This indicates that gut wall metabolism by CYP3A (possibly CYP3A4) is inducible in a similar manner as hepatic metabolism. The potential for important drug-drug interactions at this level is indicated by the finding that concomitant administration of cyclosporin and erythromycin leads to an increased AUC of cyclosporin when erythromycin is given orally but no increase when erythromycin is given intravenously.[61]

### 3.3.4 Pathways of Drug Metabolism

A wide variety of biochemical reactions can take place during the metabolism of a drug to more water soluble compounds (table IX). Traditionally, metabolic reactions have been divided into two basic types. In phase I reactions, polar groups are introduced into the drug molecule by, for example, oxidation, reduction, or hydrolysis. Oxidation is by far the most common pathway and is considered in more detail below. Phase II reactions are synthetic and involve conjugation with glucuronic acid, sulfate, glycine, acetyl or other groups. Some drugs may undergo metabolism by both phase I and phase II reactions, while others only pass through phase I and yet others are directly conjugated (fig. 19). The metabolites formed are generally more water soluble than the parent compound, and are excreted in the urine or in the bile.

As pointed out in section 3.3.1, metabolites are by no means always pharmacologically inactive but may contribute to the therapeutic or adverse effects of the parent drug (e.g. the metabolites of many antipsychotic and antidepressant drugs). Others, for example the antiarrhythmic drug encainide, are inactive as such and need to be metabolised to the active compound (*O*-demethylencainide). Glucuronide conjugates have until recently been assumed to be pharmacologically inactive. However, several lines of evidence indicate that glucuronides may contribute to drug effects. For example, as pointed out above (section 3.3.3), morphine 6-glucuronide seems to have analgesic activity *per se*. Also, the active parent compound may be released by enzymatic cleavage from the already formed glucuronide. Such systemic cycling has also been demonstrated for clofibric acid.[58]

#### The Cytochrome P450 System

Cytochrome P450 is the collective term for a group of related enzymes or isozymes located in the membranes of the endoplasmic reticulum. It is responsible for the oxidative metabolism of numerous drugs and other foreign compounds, as well as many endogenous substrates including prostaglandins, fatty acids and steroids. Each P450 enzyme consists of a single protein and one haeme group as the prosthetic group. Assisted by the reduced form of nicotinamide adenine dinucleotide phosphate (NADPH), each P450 enzyme has the unique ability to incorporate one atom of molecular oxygen into the substrate. The cytochrome P450 superfamily is divided into families and subfamilies of enzymes that are defined on the basis of their amino acid sequence similarities.[63] With a few exceptions, enzymes that share more than 40% of their amino acid sequence belong to the same family, while P450s in a single subfamily share greater than 55% sequence homology. P450s are named with the root CYP, followed by an arabic numeral designating the family, a capital letter for the subfamily and, finally, another arabic numeral denoting the individual enzyme. The same code is used for the genes that code for proteins. Currently, twelve families of P450s have been described in mammals, and in humans, over 30 P450 genes have been cloned. Four of the families (CYP1-CYP4) have been found to be involved in drug metabolism, while the other families are of importance for the synthesis and metabolism of endogenous compounds.[64]

Drug-metabolising P450s have a distinct but overlapping substrate specificity. However, a drug may, in certain cases, have a high affinity for a particular P450, which will in practise almost completely catalyse a certain oxidative reaction (e.g. 4-hydroxylation of debrisoquine by CYP2D6, see section 5.2.2). Depending on the chemical structure of the substrate, the initial reaction may involve hydroxylation of an aromatic ring (e.g. phenytoin, imipramine) or of a hydrocarbon side chain (e.g. barbiturates), dealkylation (e.g. demethylation of a number of psychotropic drugs), or sulfoxidation (e.g. chlorpromazine). Another characteristic of P450s is a large intra- and interspecies variability in regulation and in catalytic activity. Knowledge of the role of specific P450s in drug metabolism and the factors influencing their activity has increased enormously during the last years by studies in human liver microsomes, studies with purified enzymes, use of specific inducers and inhibitors, and the expression of specific P450 cDNAs in *in vitro* systems.

Table X shows the main human P450 isoenzymes involved in drug metabolism, with examples of known drug substrates, model substances (marker drugs) used to characterise the catalytic activity, selective inhibitors and important inducers of individual P450s. More than one P450 isoenzyme is often involved in the metabolism of a drug. Thus, for example, the hydroxylation of imipramine is catalysed by CYP2D6 while its demethylation is catalysed by CYP1A2, CYP2C19, and, possibly, CYP3A4. Two of the enzymes, CYP2D6 and CYP2C19, exhibit genetic polymorphism in catalytic activity, and will be discussed in more detail in section 5.2 (below). On the basis of expression in the liver, it appears that enzymes belonging to the CYP3A (about 30% of total hepatic P450) and CYP2C (about 20%) subfamilies are the most abundant forms, followed by CYP1A2 (13%), CYP2E1 (7%), CYP2A6 (4%), and CYP2D6 (2%), and that these P450s

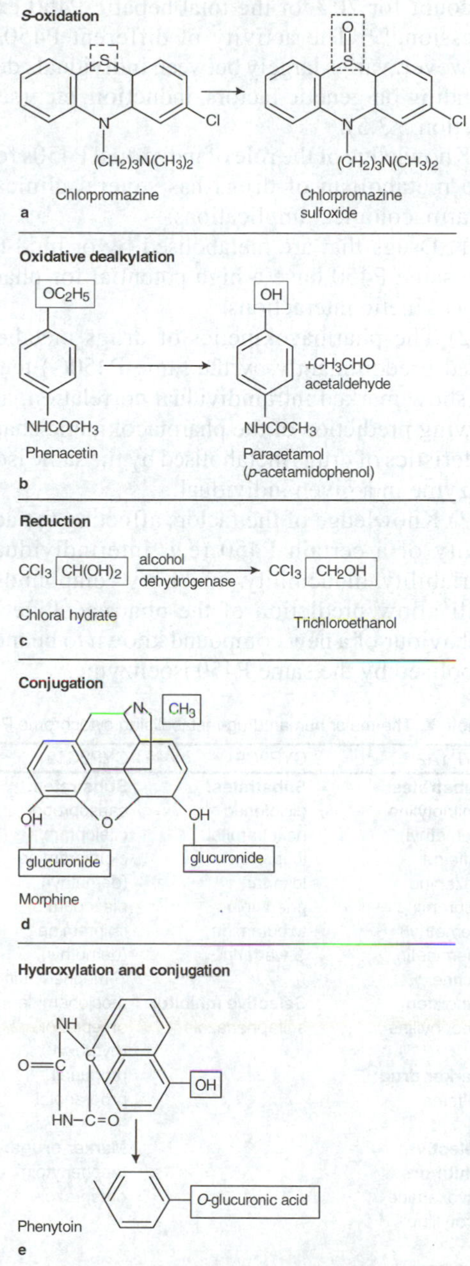


**Fig. 19.** Some examples of the metabolic transformation of drugs. (a) Cytochrome P450 catalysed metabolism of chlorpromazine by *S*-oxidation (i.e. introduction of an oxygen group); one of the many metabolic pathways of chlorpromazine. (b) Cytochrome P450 catalysed metabolism of phenacetin by oxidative dealkylation (i.e. removal of an alkyl group). (c) Metabolism of chloral hydrate to an alcohol by the non-microsomal enzyme alcohol dehydrogenase (i.e. a reduction reaction). (d) Microsomal enzyme catalysed (transferase) metabolism of morphine by union of the endogenous substance glucuronic acid with the hydroxyl group of the molecule (i.e. conjugation by glucuronidation). A metabolic side reaction, oxidative demethylation, also occurs. (e) Phenytoin is initially hydroxylated and then conjugated with glucuronic acid (after Crossland[62]).

account for 70% of the total hepatic P450 expression.[65] The activity of different P450s, however, varies largely between individuals depending on genetic factors, induction, etc. (see section 3.3.5).

Knowledge of the role of individual P450s for the metabolism of drugs has several clinical pharmacological implications:

1) Drugs that are metabolised by or bind to the same P450 have a high potential for pharmacokinetic interactions.

2) The pharmacokinetics of drugs metabolised predominantly by the same P450(s) tend to show marked intraindividual correlation, allowing prediction of the pharmacokinetic characteristics of drugs metabolised by the same isoenzyme in a given individual.

3) Knowledge of the factors affecting the activity of a certain P450 (e.g. interindividual variability, inducibility, inhibitory compounds) will allow prediction of the pharmacokinetic behaviour of a new compound known to be metabolised by the same P450 isoenzyme.

**Conjugation Reactions**

Glucuronidation is another major reaction in the metabolism of xenobiotics and endogenous compounds to more water soluble substances. This reaction is catalysed by uridine diphosphoglucuronosyltransferases (UDPGTs) located in the endoplasmic reticulum of the cells. The highest activity is found in the liver, but a variety of organs such as the skin, lung, kidneys and small intestine also express the enzymes (extrahepatic glucuronidation). There is accumulating evidence that, homologous to the cytochrome P450 family, UDPGTs exist in multiple forms in most species.[66] Usually, many UDPGTs are capable of reacting with different classes of xenobiotics or drugs. Also, many drugs react with more than one isoform of UDPGT. A 10-fold variation in the rate of glucuronidation is not uncommon in healthy human populations. The role of genetic factors, environmental factors and host-dependent factors in the regulation of this variability remains to be determined.[58]

**Table X.** The major human drug-metabolising cytochrome P450 isoenzymes

| CYP1A2 | CYP2C9 | CYP2C19 | CYP2D6 | CYP2E1 | CYP3A4 |
|---|---|---|---|---|---|
| **Substrates:** | **Substrates:** | **Substrates:** | **Substrates:** | **Substrates:** | **Substrates:** |
| amitriptyline | diclofenac | carisoprodol | amitriptyline | chlorzoxazone | codeine (*N*-demethyl) |
| (demethyl) | hexobarbital | citalopram | (hydroxyl) | enflurane | cyclophosphamide |
| caffeine | ibuprofen | clomipramine | codeine (*O*-demethyl) | ethanol | cyclosporin |
| clozapine | losartan | (demethyl) | clomipramine | halothane | dapsone |
| imipramine | phenytoin | diazepam | (hydroxyl) | paracetamol | diltiazem |
| (demethyl) | tolbutamide | imipramine | debrisoquine | | erythromycin |
| phenacetin | *S*-warfarin | (demethyl) | desipramine | **Marker drug:** | estradiol |
| tacrine | | *S*-mephenytoin | dextromethorphan | chlorzoxazone | granisetron |
| tamoxifen | **Selective Inhibitor:** | moclobemide | encainide | | lidocaine |
| theophylline | sulfaphenazole | omeprazole | ethylmorphine | **Inducer:** | midazolam |
| | | (hydroxyl) | flecainide | ethanol | nifedipine |
| **Marker drug:** | | proguanil | haloperidol | | omeprazole (sulfone |
| caffeine | | propranolol | imipramine (hydroxyl) | | formation) |
| | | | metoprolol | | protease inhibitors |
| **Selective** | | **Marker drugs:** | mianserin | | (ritonavir, saquinavir, |
| **inhibitors:** | | mephenytoin | nicotine | | indinavir) |
| fluvoxamine | | omeprazole | nortriptyline | | quinidine |
| furafylline | | | paroxetine | | tamoxifen |
| | | | perphenazine | | terfenadine |
| **Inducer:** | | | propafenone | | triazolam |
| smoking | | | thioridazine | | verapamil |
| | | | tropisetron | | |
| | | | zuclopenthixol | | **Marker drugs:** |
| | | | | | 6β-hydroxycortisol? |
| | | | **Marker drugs:** | | midazolam? |
| | | | debrisoquine | | $^{14}$C-erythromycin? |
| | | | dextromethorphan | | |
| | | | sparteine | | **Selective inhibitor:** |
| | | | | | ketoconazole |
| | | | **Selective inhibitor:** | | |
| | | | quinidine | | **Inducers:** |
| | | | | | glucocorticoids |
| | | | | | antiepileptics |
| | | | | | rifampicin |

Other enzyme systems mediating conjugation reactions such as *N*-acetyltransferases, glutathione transferases, and sulfotransferases also exist as gene superfamilies. However, the development of isoform-specific substrate and inhibitor probes is currently less advanced than with the cytochrome P450s. *N*-Acetyltransferases are discussed in more detail below due to the existence of genetic polymorphism (see section 5.2.1).

### *3.3.5 Factors Affecting Drug Metabolism*

Large interindividual variability in drug metabolism is more a rule than an exception. Many factors contribute to this variability and some are listed in table XI. The activity of many drug-metabolising enzymes is under genetic control and may vary between different ethnic groups. These aspects are discussed in more detail in sections 5.2 and 5.3.

**Table XI.** Factors affecting drug metabolism

| Factor | Response |
|---|---|
| Genetic influences | See section 5.2 |
| Interethnic differences | See section 5.3 |
| Age | |
| neonates | Reduced rate of drug metabolism |
| elderly | may occur (see also chapters 3 and 4) |
| Gender | Reduced rate of drug metabolism |
| Pregnancy | may be present in females,[a] and an increased rate during pregnancy (see chapters 2 and 18) |
| Liver disease | Reduced rate of elimination of some drugs (depends on pharmacokinetic characteristics of drug and type and stage of liver disease); increased bioavailability and reduced elimination of orally administered high clearance drugs in cirrhosis (see section 5.4.3) |
| Time of day | See section 3.3.5 |
| Environmental | Enhanced rate of metabolism with occupational exposure to chlorinated insecticides and benzo(a)pyrene (cigarette smoking, charcoal broiling) |
| Diet | Enhanced rate of metabolism (of certain drugs) by high protein/carbohydrate ratio and cruciferous vegetables (therapeutic implications not clear) Inhibition of metabolism (e.g. bioflavonoids in grapefruit juice) |
| Malnutrition | Reduced rate of drug metabolism probable in severe malnutrition[a] (see chapter 34) |
| Alcohol | |
| acute ingestion | Inhibition of certain drug metabolising enzymes |
| chronic long term intake | Induction of certain drug metabolising enzymes |
| Other drugs | Inhibition or induction of metabolism (see chapter 7) |

a Mainly based on studies in animals. More data therefore needed in humans.

#### Age

There is clear evidence that age does affect the pharmacokinetics of drugs. In the *neonate*, the ability to metabolise drugs may be reduced and there are often changes in the volume of distribution and protein binding of drugs as well (see also chapter 3). Different enzymatic processes develop at different phases of fetal and neonatal life. Sulfate conjugation is rather well developed in the newborn, while other reactions such as glucuronide conjugation and oxidation occur at a lower rate in the newborn than in adults.[67,68] Consequently, there are not only quantitative but also qualitative differences in the metabolic pattern between newborns and adults. A well known example is paracetamol, which is metabolised in the newborn mainly by sulfate conjugation and in adults by glucuronide conjugation. Newborn babies are able to metabolise some transplacentally transferred drugs (phenytoin, carbamazepine) at adult rates. This may be due partly to transplacental induction of the cytochrome P450 system.

The development of enzymatic capacity is highest during the first weeks or months of life. The oxidative metabolic capacity for certain drugs, e.g. phenytoin, carbamazepine and theophylline is highest in children at the age of 1 to 5 years. At this time, the clearance of theophylline is 1.5 to 2 times higher than in adults. This may be due to the large relative size of the liver (and thus enzyme amount) or higher enzyme activity in children. The metabolic rates decrease to the adult level at puberty.

In the *elderly,* there are a number of factors that may affect pharmacokinetics. Renal function declines with age and this will cause the accumulation in plasma of drugs (or their active metabolites) that are cleared by the kidney. The volume of distribution of lipophilic drugs is increased due to the increased fat content of the body. Plasma protein binding of acidic drugs (e.g. phenytoin) is often reduced due to lower albumin concentrations in plasma. This may lead to decreased total drug concentrations in the plasma, although the concentration of free drug is unchanged provided that drug elimination is not impaired. On the other hand, the concentration of $\alpha_1$-acid glycoprotein which binds many basic drugs, is often increased in the elderly, leading to higher total drug concentrations with unchanged free drug concentrations.

The metabolism of some drugs is affected in the elderly, leading to accumulation of the drug in plasma. However, the decrease in metabolism with increasing age is usually minor in relation to the large interindividual variability in drug metabolism due to other reasons. Based on presently available biochemical data, the intrinsic hepatic drug-metabolising activity does not decrease significantly with increasing age in humans. The observed age-related differences in drug clearance[69] appear to be mainly accounted for by an age-related decrease in liver size (for low intrinsic clearance drugs) or in liver blood flow (for high intrinsic clearance drugs) [see also section 5.4.2]. The liver weight decreases about 18 to 25% between the ages of 20 and 80 years as indicated by autopsy studies. Similarly, the liver blood flow is reduced by 25 to 35% between the ages of 30 and 75 years. Consequently, the first-pass metabolism of high clearance drugs such as propranolol and labetalol is reduced in old age, leading to an increased oral bioavailability of these agents. In this respect, it should be noted that many studies in the elderly are performed in very fit, drug-free individuals and the findings may not be appropriate for many elderly patients who are infirm and taking other drugs (see also chapter 4).

#### Gender and Pregnancy

Sex-related differences in the metabolism of some drugs, e.g. certain anxiolytics and hypnotics, have been observed.[70] This may be due to gender-related differences in the activity of specific drug metabolising enzymes (for a review, see Harris et al.[71]). However, these variations are in general small and do not necessitate any adjustment in drug dosage. Some changes may in fact be due to concomitant administration of combined (estrogen-progestagen) oral contraceptives. It is now clear that the pill does inhibit the oxidative metabolism of certain drugs while inducing the glucuronide conjugation process.[72]

Pregnancy is associated with an increased clearance of some drugs that are oxidised. A striking example is the manifold increase in hepatic metabolism of metoprolol during pregnancy.[73] The mechanism for this still remains to be clarified.

#### Foreign Compounds and Environmental Factors

A large variety of foreign compounds have the ability to increase the rate of drug metabolism (in particular oxidation but also glucuronidation) by enzyme induction. The induction process involves increased synthesis of the enzyme involved and increased formation of liver cell membranes containing this enzyme, and therefore becomes apparent only after a certain period of time. The molecular mechanisms by which P450 genes are regulated are beginning to be unravelled.[74]

Environmental factors such as heavy cigarette smoking [benzo(a)pyrene] and occupational exposure to chlorinated hydrocarbon insecticides may induce certain metabolic pathways and thereby modify the response to drugs.[75,76] The metabolism of theophylline in particular is enhanced in heavy smokers who therefore may need higher average doses than non-smokers.[77] Theophylline is metabolised by the cytochrome P450 enzyme CYP1A2, the inducibility of which by smoking has been documented using caffeine as a probe drug. Another substrate for CYP1A2 is the antipsychotic drug clozapine.[78] Lower plasma concentrations of clozapine in smokers than in non-smokers for a given dose are consistent with the induction of CYP1A2 by smoking.[79] Similarly, the effectiveness of usual doses of analgesics such as pentazocine and dextropropoxyphene may be decreased in heavy cigarette smokers. A case of lack of response to usual dosages of warfarin has been observed following temporary intensive occupational exposure to chlorinated insecticides.[80]

#### Diet and Alcohol

An extreme example of environmental influence on drug metabolism is the effect of charcoal broiled beef on the oral bioavailability of phenacetin (fig. 20).[81] Probably, benzo(a)pyrene and other polycyclic aromatic hydrocarbons contaminating the beef during broiling induce the first-pass dealkylation of phenacetin, resulting in lowered AUCs of the parent drug. A marked interindividual variation is seen in the induction. The ratio between the concentrations of the active metabolite paracetamol (acetaminophen) and phenacetin is increased markedly. A similar effect of charcoal broiled beef has been observed on the metabolism of theophylline and phenazone. Presumably, other drugs which are metabolised by the 'benzo(a)pyrene inducible'

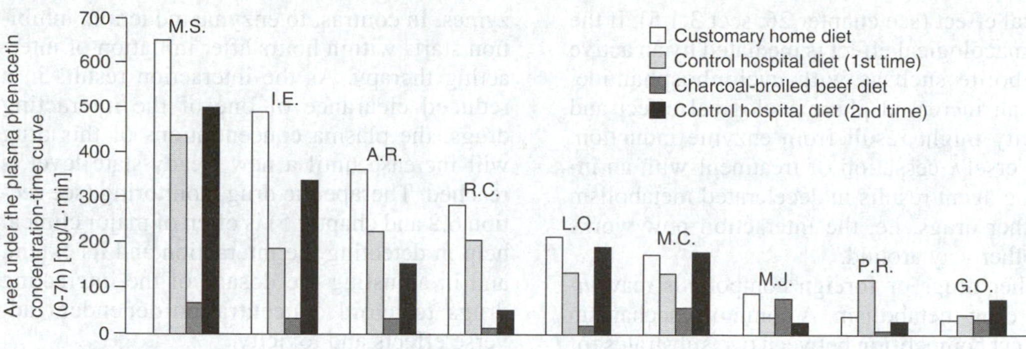


**Fig. 20.** Effect of a charcoal-broiled beef diet on the area under the plasma concentration-time curve of orally administered phenacetin. Note the marked interindividual variation in the inducing effect on phenacetin metabolism (after Conney et al.[81]).

forms of cytochrome P450 will also be affected.[75]

More modest manipulation of the diet has also been found to affect the metabolism of a few drugs (theophylline, phenazone, phenacetin), as evidenced by an increased rate of metabolism of these drugs the higher the protein : carbohydrate ratio in the diet.[75,82,83] Dietary intake of cruciferous vegetables such as brussels sprouts and cabbage can also increase the rate of metabolism of phenazone and phenacetin.[84] These effects of diet clearly add to the variability of drug metabolism in different individuals, but the clinical significance is not clear. On the other hand, severe malnutrition states may have a profound influence on drug metabolism and disposition (see chapter 34; sect. 2.1.3, 2.2).[85]

Food constituents may also inhibit drug metabolism. An interesting example is the strong inhibitory effect of *bioflavonoids* present in grapefruit juice (but not orange juice), on the first-pass metabolism of calcium antagonists. A 2- to 3-fold increase in the area under the plasma concentration-time curve (AUC) of orally administered nifedipine and felodipine is seen when these drugs are taken together with grapefruit juice. A similar effect on the concentrations of cyclosporin has also been documented. Calcium antagonists and cyclosporin are metabolised by the cytochrome P450 isoenzyme CYP3A4 which is present in the gut wall and in the liver, and the bioflavonoids inhibit this enzyme activity.[86]

The effect of *alcohol* on drug metabolism depends on the amount of alcohol consumed, as well as the duration and regularity of alcohol intake. Even a few days' intake of relatively high doses of alcohol may cause a non-specific inhibition of various cytochrome P450 enzymes, leading to increased plasma concentrations of drugs and an increased risk of adverse effects. This type of interaction with alcohol intake has been documented for warfarin, amitriptyline and diazepam. On the other hand, regular long term intake (weeks to months) of relatively high doses of alcohol (50 g/day) may cause the opposite phenomenon, i.e. induction of drug metabolism via the cytochrome P450 system. Drugs whose metabolism may be induced by long term alcohol intake are phenytoin and warfarin; this may lead to difficulties in adjusting the dosage of these drugs due to their narrow therapeutic ranges. Another example of toxicological significance is the increased liver toxicity of paracetamol in alcoholic individuals. Paracetamol is converted to a hepatotoxic metabolite by the cytochrome P450 isoenzyme CYP2E1, the activity of which is induced by alcohol. Even low doses of drugs containing paracetamol may therefore be hepatotoxic in individuals with regular high alcohol consumption.

#### Other Drugs

Many barbiturates, the antiepileptics phenytoin and carbamazepine, and the antituberculosis drug rifampicin (rifampin) increase the rate of metabolism of other drugs through *induction* of mainly cytochrome P450 enzymes (particularly CYP3A4) but also other enzymes, e.g. glucuronosyltransferases.[87-89] A large number of clinically important drug interactions due to enzyme induction have been documented. Thus, the rate of metabolism of coumarin derivatives (e.g. warfarin) is enhanced by phenobarbital, rifampicin and carbamazepine, causing a decrease in the steady-state plasma concentration of warfarin and a decrease in its pharmacological effect (see chapter 26; sect 3.1.5). If the pharmacological effect is mediated by an active metabolite such as with cyclophosphamide, then an increased pharmacological effect and toxicity might result from enzyme induction. Conversely, cessation of treatment with an inducing agent results in decelerated metabolism of other drugs, i.e. the interaction now works the other way around.

Other drugs or foreign compounds may *inhibit* drug metabolism. A common mechanism is direct competition between two substrates for the metabolic site on the same enzyme, e.g. the same cytochrome P450. Thus, all drugs metabolised by the same enzyme may potentially interact with each other, leading to increased plasma concentrations of the drug(s). The extent of the inhibition depends on the affinities of the interacting drugs for the enzyme involved, as well as on the concentrations of the individual drugs. The clinical consequences also depend on the pharmacodynamic properties of the parent compounds and their metabolites. Common clinical examples of interactions between drugs metabolised by the same enzyme are those between antidepressants, antipsychotics and antiarrhythmics involving CYP2D6.[90] Many phenothiazine antipsychotics have a high affinity to CYP2D6 and inhibit the metabolism of, for example, tricyclic antidepressants. Erythromycin, verapamil and cyclosporin are metabolised by CYP3A4, and the elimination of cyclosporin is inhibited by the other two drugs. Ketoconazole and itraconazole are also very potent inhibitors of CYP3A4 and thus of the metabolism of the antihistamine drug terfenadine. Cases of terfenadine-induced torsades de pointes have been documented in patients treated simultaneously with terfenadine and ketoconazole, and the same interaction also occurs between terfenadine and erythromycin, another inhibitor of CYP3A4. These combinations should therefore be avoided.

A drug may also be a potent inhibitor of a certain cytochrome P450 without being a substrate for it. Thus, quinidine selectively inhibits CYP2D6 at low concentrations. The antidepressant drug fluvoxamine is a potent inhibitor of CYP1A2, and up to 10-fold increased steady-state plasma concentrations of clozapine (a CYP1A2 substrate) have been reported in patients treated with these two drugs.[91] Cimetidine, on the other hand, inhibits a number of different cytochrome P450s and thus interacts with many drugs metabolised by different enzymes. In contrast to enzyme induction, inhibition starts within hours after initiation of interacting therapy. As the interaction results in a reduced clearance of one of the interacting drugs, the plasma concentrations of this drug will increase until a new steady-state level is reached. Therapeutic drug monitoring (see section 6.2 and chapter 5) is often of major clinical help in detecting the interaction and its extent, and in adjusting the dosage of the interacting drugs to avoid concentration-dependent adverse effects and toxicity.

#### Time of Day (Chronopharmacology)

Recent studies have demonstrated that the therapeutic response to a drug and its adverse effects may depend on the time of day when the drug is administered. We are used to the idea of diurnal rhythm in terms of hormonal release so it should be no surprise that some of the control processes of the pharmacodynamics and pharmacokinetics of drugs may be time-of-day dependent.[92] Drugs for which chronopharmacological changes have been reported include ampicillin, carbamazepine, corticosteroids, cyclosporin, digoxin, indomethacin, lithium and theophylline. In the case of cyclosporin, a 23% increase in the area under the plasma concentration *versus* time curve has been demonstrated when the drug was given at 9.00pm compared with the same dose given at 9.00am.[93]

Although studies in this area have been performed for some years, it is still not possible to know what the clinical impact in an individual patient will be. It is known that the timing of administration of some cytotoxic drugs affects both the therapeutic response and the adverse effects.[94]

### 3.4 Renal Excretion of Drugs

Comparatively few drugs are excreted unchanged by the kidney because of tubular reabsorption of lipid soluble drug. However, a number of important drugs are primarily excreted unchanged or as active metabolites by glomerular filtration and if renal function is impaired, this will have important consequences for drug therapy. If the usual dosage is not modified, the plasma concentration of such drugs or their active metabolites will rise producing toxic symptoms (see section 5.4.4).

Active tubular secretion occurs for a few organic bases such as chloroquine and for organic acids such as penicillin, probenecid and salicylates. It is envisaged that the organic acid is carried across the tubular cell by a carrier which liberates the drug into the tubule and returns to carry more drug.[95] Competition for this carrier may occur and, in this way, probenecid impairs the excretion of penicillin by the kidney leading to higher plasma concentrations of penicillin. Digoxin is another drug that is actively secreted in the kidney. A number of drugs (quinidine and spironolactone are particularly well studied) decrease the renal excretion of digoxin, leading to higher plasma concentrations of the drug. For some drugs (e.g. the cefalosporins), saturable renal reabsorption has been described.[96]

The renal clearance of many acidic and basic drugs varies over the urinary pH range (4.8 to 7.5) in accordance with the pH partition hypothesis. Strong acids (pKa less than 2) and strong bases (pKa greater than 12) are virtually completely ionised over the physiological range of urinary pH and their clearances are therefore unaffected by pH changes in urine. Weak organic bases (pKa 7.5 to 10) and acids (pKa 3.0 to 7.5) however, may be affected by urinary pH. Amphetamine, a weak organic base, is excreted unchanged and is more ionised at acidic pH. Its rate of excretion may therefore be increased by acidifying the urine with ammonium chloride. Phenobarbital and salicylates are excreted in part in the unchanged form and, being weak organic acids, are ionised at alkaline pH. Their excretion rates may therefore be increased by the use of sodium bicarbonate to make the urine alkaline (see also section 1.1).

Renal excretion of drugs and modification of dosages in renal disease is discussed in more detail in section 5.4.4 and in chapter 24 (sect. 11) and appendix D.

### 3.5 Biliary Excretion of Drugs

Many drugs are actively transported by hepatic cells from blood to bile. Drugs and drug metabolites (particularly glucuronide conjugates) are likely to be excreted in bile if they are polar and if their molecular weight exceeds 400D. Ampicillin and rifampicin for example, are excreted in high concentration in the bile and good use may be made of this characteristic in the treatment of infections of the biliary tract.

Some drugs undergo an 'enterohepatic' circulation (e.g. digitoxin, estrogens, indomethacin). A drug, or more usually a drug conjugate, is excreted into the bile and enters the gastrointestinal tract where, in the case of the metabolite, it may be broken down by enzymes in gut bacteria to liberate the unchanged drug. Any drug appearing in this way may then be reabsorbed into the body along with any drug that may have appeared in the gut from a recently taken oral dose. Theoretically, the enterohepatic circulation may be interfered with by drugs such as broad-spectrum antibiotics which will destroy any gut bacteria, and any drug conjugate then entering the gut from the bile will be excreted in the faeces. This would lead to a lowering of plasma concentrations of the drug in question and could be a possible cause of adverse drug interactions in certain situations. It has been suggested that the effectiveness of combined oral contraceptive steroids is reduced because of such an interaction with antibiotics like ampicillin, but the evidence that this interaction is clinically important is slim.[97]

Biliary excretion may serve as an alternative route of elimination of some polar drugs in patients with renal impairment, but for drugs such as digoxin, the reduction in the rate of renal elimination is only partially compensated by biliary excretion.[98] Oxazepam seems to have a more pronounced enterohepatic circulation in uraemic patients compared with individuals with normal renal function.[99] Drugs may also interact at the level of biliary excretion. Thus, quinidine decreases not only the renal but also the biliary excretion of digoxin (see further chapter 7, sect. 2.3.6 and 2.3.8). Verapamil appears to inhibit mainly the biliary excretion of digoxin.[100]

## 4. The Time-Course of Drug Effects

Understanding the time-course of drug effects is based on knowledge of the relationship between drug concentration and effect. This is determined by the pharmacodynamic properties of the drug which can usually be described in terms of the maximum drug effect, $E_{max}$, and the concentration producing 50% of $E_{max}$, the $EC_{50}$. The time-course of drug concentrations, i.e. its pharmacokinetics, then provides the means to predict the time-course of drug effects. Thus, pharmacokinetics is a necessary prerequisite for predicting drug effects *in vivo*.

In general, drug effects will be delayed in relation to changes in drug concentration at easily measured sites, e.g. in plasma. This delay may be accounted for in terms of:

1) The distribution kinetics of the drug to its site of action; and

2) Subsequent changes in physiological mediators of the effect.

The clinical effects of drugs may frequently reflect the cumulative action of a drug and the time-course of this cumulative effect may be dependent on the pattern of concentrations after each dose.

### 4.1 Immediate Drug Effects

If plasma drug concentrations are not changing rapidly, the drug effect may be predicted quite well from the plasma concentration because the distributional and physiological delays are short. This is often assumed when drug concentrations are measured as part of a therapeutic drug monitoring strategy (see section 6 and also chapter 5) and the measured concentration is then used to assess an individual's pharmacodynamics, e.g. in the use of theophylline. For practical purposes, the drug effects can be considered as immediately related to the plasma concentration.

### 4.2 Delayed Drug Effects

#### *4.2.1 Distributional Delay*

Drugs which are administered by rapid intravenous injection or infusion, as is commonly the case in anaesthetic practice, will frequently show some delay of effect in relation to concentration. One of the first well described examples of this phenomenon was the neuromuscular blocking effect of tubocurarine[101] for which the concept of an *effect compartment* was introduced to account for the delay in equilibration of drug between the plasma and the site of action. The equilibration delay is characterised by the *equilibration half-time*. If the plasma concentration changes suddenly from zero to a new value and then remains constant, the time-course of drug at its site of action can be predicted via the *effect compartment* model to increase and eventually equilibrate with the plasma concentration. The concentration increases in an exponential fashion such that 50% of the eventual equilibrated value is achieved after one equilibration half-time, 75% after 2 equilibration half-times, etc. Equilibration half-times are usually of the order of a few minutes and are largely determined by perfusion of the target organ and its size (the apparent volume of distribution).

#### *4.2.2 Physiological Delay*

All drug action starts with an interaction of the agent with its site of action, e.g. a receptor binding site, followed by a chain of events which lead to expression of the drug effect. The intermediate links in the chain may be relatively rapid in relation to the time-course of drug concentration changes, in which case effects may appear to be immediately related to drug concentration. Many drug actions are known to change the rate of production or elimination of a physiological mediator which itself leads to the drug effect that is observed. The kinetics of such a physiological mediator can be the rate-limiting factor in the appearance of a drug effect. If production of the mediator is decreased or increased, the half-life of the mediator is not changed and the time-course of expression of the drug effect will have a similar delay when drug concentrations increase and when they decrease.

On the other hand, if the action of the drug decreases mediator elimination, then the half-life of the mediator will become longer and the delay in onset of drug effect will be slower when drug concentrations are increasing than the disappearance of drug effect when drug concentrations are falling. The converse will apply if the drug action enhances elimination of the mediator. The anticoagulant effect of warfarin is a clear example of physiological delay in expression of a drug action. Warfarin inhibits the recycling of vitamin K which is a cofactor in the synthesis of clotting factors. This inhibition appears to be quite rapid and closely related to warfarin concentration. The clotting factors themselves have relatively long half-lives with a typical overall value of about 14 hours. The anticoagulant effect of warfarin takes over 2 days (4 half-lives) before it reflects the warfarin concentration because of the time taken to reach a new steady-state concentration of clotting factors.

The time-course of physiological intermediates is probably a better explanation for most delayed drug effects than the *effect compartment* model, especially when the delays are more than a few minutes.

### 4.3 Cumulative Drug Effects

The time-course of some drug effects can be explained readily by the pattern of drug concentrations but the clinical effect of interest may be essentially independent of the fluctuation of concentrations after each dose. The effects of diuretics on sodium and water excretion by the kidney are clearly linked to the time-course of the diuretic in plasma and its excretion in the renal tubule. The clinical benefit of diuresis is not directly related to the increase in sodium or water excretion rate, but rather to the cumulative loss of sodium and water. The cumulative effect of a diuretic can be predicted by integrating the instantaneous concentration-effect relationship so that even though the time-course of drug concentration after a single dose is not directly related to clinical benefit, the pattern of concentrations after several doses will determine the therapeutic outcome.

Other classes of drug, e.g. anticancer agents and antibiotics have clinical outcomes that represent the cumulative effect of preceding doses. These drugs may be sensitive to the profile of drug concentrations such that greater benefits may be obtained by giving drug more continuously than by intermittent use. Alternatively, the clinical benefit may be the same but toxicity is reduced with intermittent administration, e.g. once-daily aminoglycoside use compared with three-times-daily use. This phenomenon is know as schedule dependence and is a reflection of a non-linear concentration-effect relationship and the expression of a cumulative drug effect.

## 5. Interindividual Differences in Pharmacokinetics

### 5.1 General and Methodological Aspects

Kinetic processes such as passive diffusion which are rate-limited by the physicochemical characteristics of the drug, are not likely to vary significantly among patients unless pathophysiological factors exert an influence (see section 5.4). For example, buccal absorption of drugs seems to proceed at rates that differ markedly between drugs but not between individuals. In contrast, whenever enzymatic processes are involved in the fate of drugs in the body, biochemical individuality is to be expected. The extent of this variability has not been appreciated until relatively recently.

Although active transport of drugs through biological membranes occurs and some interindividual variability has been documented in the binding and distribution of drugs, the quantitatively most important determinant of pharmacokinetic individuality is in the rate of drug metabolism.[102] For example, steady-state plasma concentrations of tricyclic antidepressants vary 20- to 30-fold on a fixed maintenance dose, and most of this variability can be accounted for by differences in the rate of hydroxylation, while interindividual differences in binding and distribution are approximately 2-fold.[103]

It is important to use appropriate methods in assessing interindividual differences in drug metabolism. The clinically used laboratory procedures for liver function are of very little, if any, predictive value for the ability of an individual to metabolise a drug. Measurements of D-glucaric acid and 6β-hydroxycortisol in urine may give an idea about the degree of induction of a patient's microsomal enzyme system. The correlation coefficients obtained between the extent of excretion of these two compounds in urine and the rate of metabolism of various drugs are, however, far too weak to have any clinical significance for a particular patient. The same holds true for the phenazone (antipyrine) half-life as a predictor of the rate of oxidation of another drug.[104]

For drugs whose elimination is to a major extent catalysed by a specific cytochrome P450 enzyme, the pharmacokinetics may to a certain extent be predicted by the use of a marker drug for this enzyme (table X). For example, the debrisoquine metabolic ratio, a measure of the catalytic activity of the polymorphic CYP2D6, predicts the steady-state plasma concentrations of desipramine, a tricyclic antidepressant metabolised predominantly by CYP2D6.[105] Similarly, caffeine may be used as a marker drug for CYP1A2, and may be of value for the prediction of the pharmacokinetics of drugs metabolised by this enzyme, e.g. clozapine. The use of marker drugs for these and other cytochrome P450 isoenzymes may be especially useful to identify individuals with an exceptionally high or low metabolic capacity, thus requiring higher or lower doses than those generally recommended.

The elimination of many drugs is, however, influenced by several factors and therefore the only accurate way to assess the rate of metabolism of a particular drug is to study it with appropriate chemical and kinetic methodology. Depending on the drug, different pharmacokinetic variables have to be used to assess rates of metabolism:

1) A drug which rapidly equilibrates between the plasma and tissues after intravenous administration and does not have substantial first-pass elimination can usually be adequately described from the pharmacokinetic point of view by a one-compartment model (see section 2.2.4). For such drugs, e.g. phenazone (antipyrine), the

**Table XII.** Genetically determined abnormal drug responses

| Condition | Response | Drugs involved | Mechanism | Inheritance | Frequency |
|---|---|---|---|---|---|
| Slow and rapid acetylators | Rapid acetylators may respond poorly<br>Slow acetylators more likely to show toxicity | Isoniazid<br>Hydralazine<br>Procainamide<br>Some sulfonamides<br>Dapsone | Polymorphic *N*-acetyltransferase in liver | Autosomal recessive | 40% of Caucasians are rapid; 80 to 90% of Asians are rapid |
| Slow (poor) drug oxidation | Concentration-dependent adverse effects | Debrisoquine<br>Tricyclic antidepressants<br>Antipsychotics<br>Lipophilic β-blockers (see section 5.2.2) | Deficient CYP2D6 in liver | Autosomal recessive | 7% of Caucasians; 1% of Asians |
| | | Diazepam<br>Omeprazole<br>*S*-Mephenytoin | Deficient CYP2C19 in liver | Autosomal recessive | 3% of Caucasians; 15% of Asians |
| | | Phenytoin | See text (sect. 5.2) | See text | Rare |
| Suxamethonium sensitivity | Prolonged apnoea | Suxamethonium (succinylcholine) | Abnormal plasma cholinesterase | Autosomal recessive | 1 in 2500 commonest type of allele |
| Porphyria | Abdominal pain<br>Paralysis | Barbiturates | Abnormal inducibility of δ-amino laevulinic acid synthetase | Autosomal dominant | |
| Warfarin resistance | Resistance to anticoagulation | Warfarin | Increased sensitivity to vitamin K in liver | Autosomal dominant | 2 large pedigrees described |
| Favism, drug-induced haemolysis | Haemolysis on exposure to certain drugs or chemicals | Many drugs, e.g:<br>Primaquine<br>Nitrofurantoin<br>Aminophenazone (amidopyrine)<br>Sulfonamides | Deficient glucose-6-phosphate dehydrogenase (G6PD) | Sex-linked incomplete dominant | Approx. 100 million affected worldwide |
| Malignant hyperpyrexia | Uncontrolled rise in body temperature, muscular rigidity | Certain drugs used in anaesthesia, especially halothane and suxamethonium | Unknown | Autosomal dominant | 1 in 20,000 |
| Glaucoma | Glaucoma due to abnormal response to intraocular corticosteroids | Topical corticosteroids<br>Systemic corticosteroids (long term) | Unknown | Autosomal recessive | 5% of US population |
| Chlorpropamide alcohol flushing | Facial flushing after alcohol (non-insulin dependent diabetes) | Chlorpropamide | Unknown | Autosomal dominant | 30% of Caucasians |

elimination half-life is a good estimate of the rate of metabolism.

2) A large number of drugs confer on the body the characteristics of a two or multicompartment system. In the former situation, the liver is part of the central compartment, from where elimination occurs (see section 2.2.5). For such drugs, the elimination half-life will depend on metabolism and distribution, and therefore plasma clearance (see section 2.2.3) should be used to assess rates of elimination.

3) For drugs undergoing substantial first-pass elimination in the liver (see section 3.3.3), pharmacokinetic models have been developed where the hepatoportal system is added as a separate compartment. For such high clearance drugs, the elimination half-life is a poor index of rates of metabolism and changes thereof (e.g. enzyme induction), and the most accurate term to use is clearance or the area under the plasma concentration-time curve (AUC) after oral administration.

As an example, treatment with pentobarbital lowers the AUC (increases the first-pass metabolism) of orally administered alprenolol due to induction of cytochrome P450,[106] but has little effect on the half-life of alprenolol. The latter will be determined mainly by distribution factors, particularly the rate at which the drug is delivered to the liver, which is determined by liver blood flow. Following intravenous doses of alprenolol, there is little effect of pentobarbital on its plasma concentration-time curve.[107] This is because after intravenous administration, the drug is distributed in the body before passing through the liver. Since virtually the whole amount of drug presented to the liver per unit of time will be metabolised in any case, induction of drug metabolising enzymes cannot be expected to enhance hepatic clearance more than marginally. After oral administration, only a small part of the drug will pass the liver without undergoing metabolic degradation. If the liver enzymes are induced, this fraction will then be further substantially reduced. Thus, the amount of drug actually reaching the circulation will be relatively more affected after oral than after intravenous administration. These concepts have been elegantly described in mathematical terms by several authors.[108,109] An important consequence is that drug metabolism interactions between high clearance drugs should be studied after oral administration.

4) In clinical practice, drug metabolism usually has to be evaluated during continued therapy (items 1 to 3 above refer to single-dose studies), and then the measurement of plasma clearance or steady-state plasma concentrations (section 2.3) as related to dose gives an accurate index of drug metabolism. With the use of tracer doses of stable radioisotopes, the pharmacokinetic variables in 1 to 3 above may be assessed without interrupting therapy.

## 5.2 Pharmacogenetics

Pharmacogenetics deals with the study of genetically-determined variations in drug response. The observation that certain adverse reactions to drugs are due to genetically-determined variations in drug metabolising enzymes was first made by Motulsky[110] and Kalow.[111] Examples are plasma cholinesterase variants associated with suxamethonium (succinylcholine) sensitivity, and inherited abnormalities of red cell glutathione metabolism as a cause of primaquine sensitivity. At about the same time, genetic differences in the capacity to acetylate isoniazid were discovered.[112] Table XII shows some examples of abnormal drug responses due to inherited individual traits. Although not all the variations in drug response involve drug metabolism, pharmacogenetic research has since the 1970s and the discovery of the debrisoquine/sparteine hydroxylation polymorphism (see section 5.2.2), expanded vigorously in the study of the interplay between environmental influences and genetic factors controlling the rate of drug metabolism. More recently, interethnic differences in drug metabolism and response have gained increasing interest and will be discussed below (section 5.3). In general, the objectives of pharmacogenetic research may be defined as:

1) Identification of genetically-controlled variations in drug metabolism and response.

2) The study of the molecular mechanisms causing these variations.

3) Evaluation of the clinical implications and relevance of these variations.

4) The development of methods to identify susceptible individuals in order to prospectively avoid undesirable drug responses.

As discussed in section 5.1, there are large interindividual differences in the capacity to metabolise drugs and other xenobiotics. This variability can be due to genetic factors, non-genetic constitutional factors such as age and disease, or environmental influences.[113] Genetic factors can be either polygenic or monogenic. Monogenic traits are inherited in a Mendelian fashion and present themselves as either polymorphisms or rare phenotypes. The term genetic polymorphism defines monogenic traits that exist in the population in at least two phe-

**Table XIII.** Genetic polymorphisms of drug metabolism

| Pathway | Marker drugs | Enzyme | Drug substrates | Incidence of deficiency (%) | |
|---|---|---|---|---|---|
| | | | | Caucasians | Asians |
| Acetylation | Isoniazid<br>Caffeine | NAT2 | Certain sulfonamides<br>Hydralazine<br>Dapsone<br>Procainamide | 50-70 | 10-15 |
| Oxidation | Debrisoquine<br>Dextromethorphan<br>Sparteine<br>Desipramine | CYP2D6 | Antidepressants<br>Antipsychotics<br>β-Blockers<br>Antiarrhythmics | 5-10 | 1 |
| | Mephenytoin<br>Omeprazole | CYP2C19 | Clomipramine<br>Imipramine<br>Citalopram<br>Omeprazole<br>Proguanil | 3 | 15-25 |

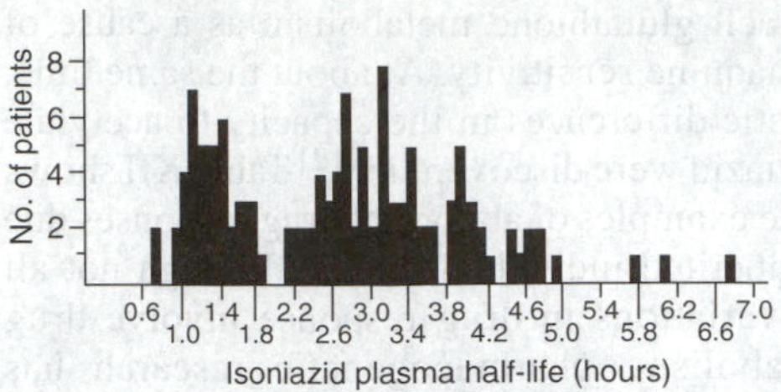


**Fig. 21.** Bimodal distribution of the plasma half-lives of isoniazid in Swedish patients with tuberculosis. The antimode is at 2.1 hours (after Hanngren et al.[117]).

notypes, the rarest phenotypes occurring at a frequency of more than 1% (those with a lower frequency are defined as rare phenotypes).

In drug metabolism, three polymorphisms (table XIII) have currently been well characterised and these will be discussed in detail below. In addition to these, a number of rare phenotypes are known. A case of deficiency of *amobarbital* (amylobarbitone) metabolism has been described,[114] although this was later found to be an inability to *N*-glucosidate amobarbital.[115] Unusually slow metabolism of *phenytoin*, leading to excessive steady-state plasma concentrations and toxicity has been described in rare individuals.[116] Family studies of the propositi are compatible with the assumption of dominant inheritance, but it still remains an open question whether this rare phenotype with abnormally slow phenytoin metabolism exists. Genetic polymorphism has also been suggested for the oxidative metabolism of drugs such as theophylline, tolbutamide and nifedipine, the sulfoxidation of carbocisteine (*S*-carboxymethyl-L-cysteine), and the *N*-oxidation of trimethylamine. However, the presence of a classical genetic polymorphism has not been confirmed in these cases.

### 5.2.1 Acetylation Polymorphism

The classic example of genetic defect in drug metabolism is the acetylation polymorphism, first described more than 30 years ago.[112] The polymorphism was initially discovered from observations of a bimodal distribution of the plasma concentrations of isoniazid, a first-line drug in the treatment of tuberculosis. Isoniazid is mainly eliminated by *N*-acetylation in the liver. Individuals can be classified as either rapid or slow acetylators of the drug, either using the isoniazid plasma half-life (antimode around 2 hours; fig. 21) or by measuring the ratio between acetylated and unchanged isoniazid in plasma or urine. Family studies confirmed that the capacity to acetylate isoniazid is genetically controlled, slow acetylators being homozygous for a recessive allele at a single autosomal gene locus.[118]

The proportion of rapid and slow acetylators varies markedly (from 5 to 90%) in populations of different ethnic and geographic origin.[119] Thus, in Caucasian populations of Europe and North America, approximately 50% are rapid acetylators, while 80 to 90% of Asians and nearly 100% of Canadian Eskimos are rapid acetylators. Recently, the polymorphic enzyme has been identified as the cytosolic arylamine *N*-acetyltransferase NAT2.[120] A number of mutated alleles of the *NAT2* gene locus causing deficient acetyltransferase activity have been identified, with marked allelic variation between Caucasian and Asian populations (see also section 5.3).

The acetylation polymorphism affects the metabolism of a number of drugs including sulfadimidine (sulfamethazine), sulfapyridine and several other sulfonamides, hydralazine, procainamide, dapsone, phenelzine, clonazepam, nitrazepam, aminoglutethimide and caffeine. In addition to isoniazid, sulfadimidine and sulfapyridine and, more recently, caffeine have been used for phenotyping purposes.[119]

A number of clinical implications of polymorphic acetylation have been documented,

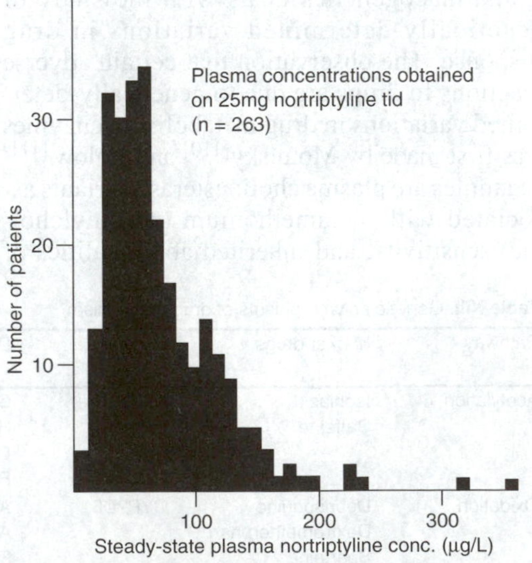


**Fig. 22.** The skewed distribution of steady-state plasma concentrations of nortriptyline in 263 patients treated with 25mg 3 times daily (tid). Note that the interindividual variability in plasma concentration is of a similar order of magnitude even if the dose is adjusted according to bodyweight.

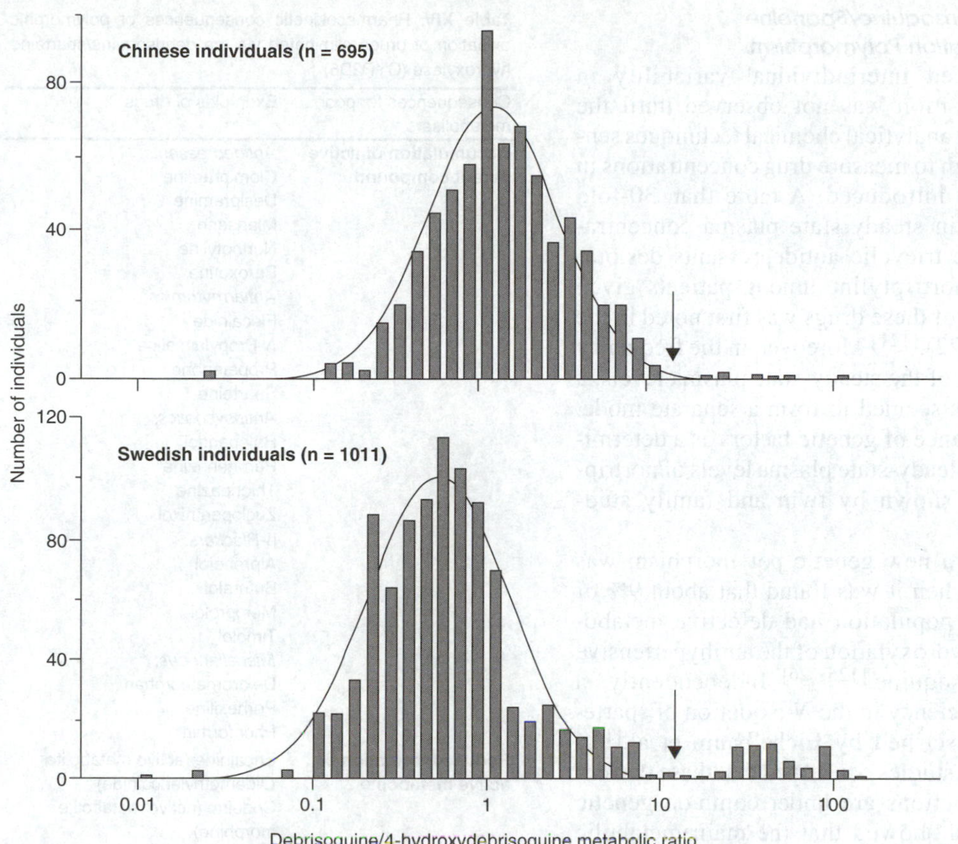


**Fig. 23.** Distribution of the urinary debrisoquine/4-hydroxydebrisoquine metabolic ratios among Chinese and Swedish individuals. The arrows indicate the metabolic ratio of 12.6, the antimode between extensive and poor metabolisers of debrisoquine established in Caucasian populations (after Bertilsson et al.[129]).

both with respect to drug therapy and toxicity.[119] The effective antihypertensive dose of hydralazine is lower in slow than in rapid acetylators. Administration of doses higher than 200mg hydralazine per day to a slow acetylator usually results in excessive plasma concentrations. The lupus-like syndrome, a severe adverse effect of hydralazine treatment, is more likely to develop in slow than in rapid acetylators. A similar syndrome may be provoked by procainamide, with earlier onset in slow acetylators. Some cases of dapsone-resistant leprosy seem to be associated with the rapid acetylator phenotype, while in ulcerative colitis, slow acetylators require a lower daily dose of the sulfapyridine analogue sulfasalazine to maintain remission without causing haemolysis, nausea or headache. Slow acetylators are also at increased risk of isoniazid-induced peripheral neuropathy, which can, however, be prevented by daily administration of pyridoxine. A phenotype-dependent drug interaction has been described between isoniazid and phenytoin. Serum phenytoin concentrations may be increased in slow acetylators during concomitant treatment with isoniazid due to higher isoniazid concentrations causing inhibition of phenytoin metabolism.

In addition to drug-induced toxicity, a number of disease states have been found to be associated with either acetylator phenotype. For example, the slow acetylator phenotype has been associated with bladder cancer, while rapid acetylators may be at a higher risk of developing cancer of the colon. The polymorphic *N*-acetyltransferase catalyses the metabolism of a number of arylamine carcinogens and might thus play a role in the metabolic activation or detoxification of these exogenous compounds. Other examples are the association, albeit weak, between the rapid acetylator phenotype and diabetes as well as breast cancer, and between the slow acetylator status and leprosy. These associations remain unexplained.

### 5.2.2 Debrisoquine/Sparteine Hydroxylation Polymorphism

Pronounced interindividual variability in drug disposition was not observed until the 1960s when analytical chemical techniques sensitive enough to measure drug concentrations in blood were introduced. A more than 30-fold variability in steady-state plasma concentrations of the tricyclic antidepressants desipramine and nortriptyline among patients given fixed doses of these drugs was first noted in the 1960s (fig. 22).[121] Moreover, in the frequency distribution of the steady-state plasma levels, a few patients seemed to form a separate mode. The importance of genetic factors as a determinant of the steady-state plasma levels of nortriptyline was shown by twin and family studies.[122-124]

In 1977, a new genetic polymorphism was identified when it was found that about 9% of the British population had defective metabolism by 4-hydroxylation of the antihypertensive drug debrisoquine.[125,126] Independently, a similar deficiency in the *N*-oxidation of sparteine was described by Eichelbaum et al.[127] Subsequent studies confirmed that these two enzymatic reactions are under common genetic control, and showed that the main metabolic pathways of the tricyclic antidepressants nortriptyline and desipramine (10-hydroxylation and 2-hydroxylation, respectively) cosegregated with it.[54,128] It has since been shown in a number of studies that the capacity to 4-hydroxylate debrisoquine, measured as the ratio between the urinary recovery of debrisoquine and that of 4-hydroxydebrisoquine after a single oral dose of the drug (i.e. the metabolic ratio), varies greatly between individuals and is bimodally distributed in Caucasian populations (fig. 23). About 7% have a deficient metabolism and are classified as poor metabolisers, while the rest are extensive metabolisers.[130,131] Family studies have clearly shown that poor metabolisers are homozygous for a recessive gene, while extensive metabolisers are either homozygous or heterozygous for the dominant gene [autosomal recessive inheritance of the poor metaboliser (PM) phenotype].[130,132] The enzyme responsible for the 4-hydroxylation of debrisoquine and the *N*-oxidation of sparteine has been shown to be the hepatic cytochrome P450 enzyme CYP2D6, which exhibits large interindividual variability in activity and is deficient in poor metabolisers.

**Table XIV.** Pharmacokinetic consequences of polymorphic oxidation of drugs eliminated via the debrisoquine/sparteine hydroxylase (CYP2D6)

| Consequences for poor metabolisers | Examples of drugs |
|---|---|
| **Accumulation of active parent compound** | *Antidepressants:*<br>Clomipramine<br>Desipramine<br>Mianserin<br>Nortriptyline<br>Paroxetine<br>*Antiarrhythmics:*<br>Flecainide<br>*N*-Propylajmaline<br>Propafenone<br>Sparteine<br>*Antipsychotics:*<br>Haloperidol<br>Perphenazine<br>Thioridazine<br>Zuclopenthixol<br>β-*Blockers:*<br>Alprenolol<br>Bufuralol<br>Metoprolol<br>Timolol<br>*Miscellaneous:*<br>Dextromethorphan<br>Perhexiline<br>Phenformin |
| **Reduced formation of active metabolite** | Encainide (active metabolite *O*-demethylencainide)<br>Codeine (active metabolite morphine) |
| **Accumulation of active parent compound and metabolite** | Amitriptyline (active metabolite nortriptyline)<br>Thioridazine (active metabolite sulforidazine) |

The molecular genetic basis of the polymorphic hydroxylation of debrisoquine and sparteine has been characterised.[133,134] Several mutated alleles of the *CYP2D* locus causing deficient enzyme have been described, allowing genotyping of individuals (e.g. from leucocyte DNA) with prediction of the phenotype (poor metaboliser *vs* extensive metaboliser) with high accuracy in Caucasian populations. More recently, new variants of the *CYP2D* locus with duplication or amplification of the active *CYP2D6* gene and associated with ultrarapid metabolic capacity have been identified.[135,136] As discussed in section 5.3.1, pronounced interethnic differences exist both with respect to the metabolic capacity as well as the allelic distribution at the *CYP2D* locus.

The polymorphic CYP2D6 metabolises a large number of important drugs such as tricyclic and newer antidepressants, antipsychotics, many antiarrhythmics, lipophilic β-blockers and opioids. Table XIV shows examples of the principal pharmacokinetic consequences of the polymorphism for drugs eliminated by CYP2D6, depending on which metabolic step is CYP2D6-dependent, and the pharmacodynamic properties of the parent compound and metabolites. If the elimination of the active principle (parent compound and/or metabolite) is dependent on CYP2D6, this will accumulate in poor metabolisers as compared with extensive metabolisers, leading to higher steady-state plasma concentrations per given dose in the former. This is of potential clinical importance, especially for drugs with a narrow therapeutic range. Thus, poor metabolisers will be at a risk of developing concentration-dependent adverse effects when given ordinary doses of the drug. Examples of this are cardiotoxicity with tricyclic antidepressants, extrapyramidal effects with antipsychotics (see fig. 24), or peripheral neuropathy with perhexiline.[90,134,138,139]

On the other hand, an inadequate therapeutic effect due to subtherapeutic plasma concentrations may be obtained at ordinary doses in patients who are extremely rapid metabolisers, as seen for example with some tricyclic antidepressants. For drugs with a narrow therapeutic range and large interindividual variability, the dosage will need to be adjusted individually according to the clinical response, aided by therapeutic drug monitoring and/or determination of the patient's metabolic capacity by phenotyping or genotyping. However, the very broad therapeutic range of the β-blockers seems to balance the potential clinical consequences of polymorphic metabolism for these drugs. CYP2D6 also shows marked stereospecificity with some drugs, e.g. metoprolol.[140,141] It must be emphasised that drugs whose metabolism cosegregates with the polymorphic CYP2D6 will exhibit a varying degree of selectivity for this enzyme, and the pathway catalysed by it is of varying importance for the overall metabolism and elimination of the drug in question. Thus, the clinical implications of polymorphic metabolism need to be evaluated separately for each drug.

#### 5.2.3 S-Mephenytoin Hydroxylation Polymorphism

*S*-Mephenytoin hydroxylation polymorphism is another autosomal recessive trait affecting oxidative drug metabolism.[142] About 3% of Caucasians and 15 to 25% of Asians have a deficient capacity to 4-hydroxylate the *S*-enantiomer of the antiepileptic drug mephenytoin (methoin). The polymorphic enzyme, recently identified as CYP2C19,[143] also catalyses the metabolism of other drugs such as diazepam and its metabolite nordazepam (*N*-desmethyldiazepam), the acid (proton) pump inhibitor omeprazole, propranolol, and some antidepressant drugs (e.g. imipramine, clomipramine, citalopram, moclobemide) [table X].[134,144] The clinical significance of the polymorphic metabolism of these compounds remains to be established but it undoubtedly contributes to variability in the disposition of these drugs. Interestingly, the bioactivation of the antimalarial drug proguanil to the active moiety cycloguanil cosegregates with the *S*-mephenytoin hydroxylase activity,[145] and plasma cycloguanil concentrations are 3 times lower in poor metabolisers than in extensive metabolisers. It remains to be established whether concentrations of this active metabolite are sufficient to exert an antimalarial effect following the standard dosage in poor metabolisers.

Genetically determined variability in drug metabolism seriously questions the therapeutic tradition of giving similar doses to all patients. Clearly, whenever drug response is abnormal (poor response, severe adverse effects) follow-

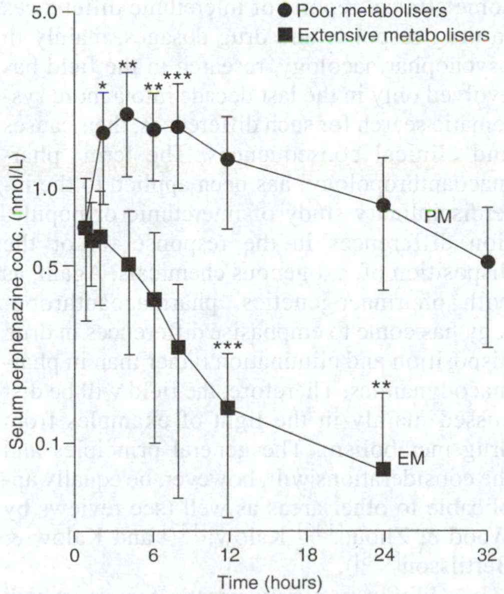


**Fig. 24.** Serum concentration of perphenazine (mean ± SD) in 6 poor metabolisers and 6 extensive metabolisers of debrisoquine after a single oral dose of 6mg perphenazine. Significant differences in serum concentration between extensive and poor metabolisers are indicated: *$p < 0.05$; **$p < 0.01$; ***$p < 0.001$ (after Dahl-Puustinen et al.[137]).

ing an apparently normal therapeutic dose, an explanation should be sought in pharmacokinetic terms. Studies are now in progress in many laboratories on the possible interindividual variations in receptor response at a constant concentration of drug in the biophase surrounding tissue receptor sites. If significant differences are revealed, it will be even more important in the future to develop accurate and clinically applicable methods for measuring drug responses (see also sections 6.1, 8).

### 5.3 Interethnic Differences in Drug Metabolism and Response

Interethnic or interracial differences in drug metabolism and response (table XII) have been increasingly recognised in parallel with new findings in pharmacogenetic research. An early observation during the second world war was that primaquine-induced haemolysis occurred mostly in Black US army soldiers. Later, the association was found to be due to a genetic deficiency of glucose-6-phosphate dehydrogenase (G6PD) which is more common in populations from malaria-infected regions. Also, the large interethnic variations in the proportions of slow acetylators between different populations were soon discovered (see above). Despite some clinical reports of interethnic differences in drug response and drug dosages, mainly in psychopharmacology, research in the field has evolved only in the last decade into a more systematic search for such differences, their causes and clinical consequences. The term 'pharmacoanthropology' has been applied to the interdisciplinary study of interethnic or population differences in the response to, or the disposition of, exogenous chemicals. Again, as with pharmacogenetics, pharmacoanthropology has come to emphasise differences in drug disposition and elimination rather than in pharmacodynamics. Therefore, the field will be discussed mainly in the light of examples from drug metabolism. The general principles and the considerations will, however, be equally applicable to other areas as well (see reviews by Wood & Zhou;[146] Kalow;[147] and Kalow & Bertilsson[148]).

In addition to purely genetic factors, which are especially easy to observe for polymorphic traits, other fundamental factors that may create interethnic differences in drug disposition and response include environmental factors such as climate, nutritional state, diet, life-style, health, cultural factors, or differences in the pathophysiology of the underlying disease.

#### *5.3.1 The CYP2D6 Polymorphism*

Numerous studies in Caucasian populations of Europe and North America have shown very similar frequency distribution curves for the debrisoquine/sparteine metabolic ratio, with a rather consistent incidence of the poor metaboliser phenotype (5 to 10%). Asian populations, however, differ from the Caucasian ones in two respects. Firstly, no clear bimodality of the distribution of the debrisoquine metabolic ratio can be observed in Chinese populations, and using the antimode defined in Caucasians, only about 1% of Chinese can be classified as poor metabolisers (fig. 23; table XIII).[105] Secondly, the distribution of the metabolic ratios is shifted to the right towards higher values in Chinese extensive metabolisers compared with Caucasian extensive metabolisers (fig. 23), indicating lower average CYP2D6 activity in Chinese. Similar results have been obtained comparing other Asian (Japanese and Korean) and Caucasian populations.

The reasons for these differences remained unexplained until the CYP2D6 gene was cloned and the molecular genetic basis of the polymorphism could be explored. Comparative studies subsequently showed that the differences in *CYP2D6* activity between Asian and Caucasian extensive metabolisers are due to a high frequency (about 50%) in the Asian population of an allele giving rise to an unstable gene product (CYP2D6 enzyme) with decreased enzymatic activity (for a review, see Bertilsson et al.[134]). This allele is practically absent in Caucasian populations. On the other hand, the low frequency of true poor metaboliser phenotype in Chinese is inherent in the low frequency of two of the most common mutated alleles of the *CYP2D* locus, *CYP2D6A* and *CYP2D6B*, causing absent CYP2D6 activity among Caucasians. Recent data indicate that Black populations differ markedly from both Asians and Caucasians in this respect.[149] The experience from the CYP2D6 research highlights the fundamental importance of solid pharmacological data on the phenotypic expression of a gene in order to evaluate the functional consequences of the allelic variation observed at DNA level. Also, a genotyping method based on the screening for the most common mutations in one population cannot be applied directly to another population without data on its validity.

The clinical importance of the interethnic differences in *CYP2D6* gene structure and expression lies in the large number of drugs whose elimination covaries with this enzyme activity (table X). Examples of drugs for which interethnic differences in pharmacokinetics have been documented include the tricyclic antidepressants and antipsychotics, both drug groups being metabolised by CYP2D6 (for reviews, see Wood & Zhou;[146] Kalow & Bertilsson[148]). The oral plasma clearance of desipramine and haloperidol, for example, is significantly lower in Chinese compared with Caucasian individuals, the difference remaining significant even if gender and bodyweight are taken into account. There is a clinical impression that individuals of Asian origin are less tolerant to the adverse effects of tricyclic antidepressants than Caucasians and that they also develop extrapyramidal effects on significantly lower doses of antipsychotic compounds. These observations could be explained by the lower average CYP2D6 activity in Chinese compared with Caucasian extensive metabolisers of debrisoquine, constituting 99% and 93% of the populations, respectively.

Moreover, a more pronounced serum prolactin response to haloperidol has been observed in Chinese compared with sex and bodyweight matched Caucasian individuals. These differences could not be fully accounted for by pharmacokinetic variability, suggesting that pharmacodynamic differences may also exist between the two populations.

#### 5.3.2 The CYP2C19 Polymorphism

This polymorphism also shows marked interethnic differences. Thus, the incidence of poor metabolisers is only about 3% in Caucasian populations, but as high as 15 to 25% in Chinese, Japanese and Koreans.[134] In a Black Zimbabwean population, 4% were poor metabolisers of mephenytoin.[149]

The pharmacokinetics of two substrates of the polymorphic *S*-mephenytoin hydroxylase, diazepam and omeprazole, have been compared between Swedish, Chinese and Korean healthy volunteers.[134] While the plasma half-life of diazepam was twice as long in Swedish poor metabolisers of *S*-mephenytoin compared with extensive metabolisers, no interphenotypic difference in diazepam pharmacokinetics was found in Chinese individuals. The mean half-lives in Chinese extensive and poor metabolisers were long and similar to those in Caucasian poor metabolisers. Similarly, the clearance of omeprazole was also significantly lower in Asian extensive metabolisers compared with Caucasian extensive metabolisers. A possible explanation for these differences in the elimination of omeprazole and diazepam between the two ethnic groups is that a higher proportion of Asian extensive metabolisers are heterozygous carriers of a defect allele coding for the *S*-mephenytoin hydroxylase activity, and might thus have lower enzymatic capacity compared with Caucasian extensive metabolisers.

#### 5.3.3 Acetylation Polymorphism

The percentage of slow acetylators varies largely between different populations, being around 60% in Europe, 50% in Africa, 15% in Japan and China, close to 12% in the South Pacific, and as low as 5% among Canadian Inuit (Eskimos). It also follows that about 60% of the Inuit but only 5% of Europeans are homozygous rapid acetylators. This high acetylation activity in a large proportion of the Inuit population calls for the use of high doses of isoniazid in a slow-release formulation for the treatment of tuberculosis.[148,150]

Eight structural variants of the polymorphic *NAT2* gene have been described, six of which are associated with the slow acetylator phenotype. Four of the variants occur frequently enough to explain about 95% of the acetylation polymorphism in different populations. It appears that the low frequency of slow acetylators in East Asian populations can be explained by the relative lack of one of the mutated alleles in this population.[120]

#### 5.3.4 Other Metabolic Differences

The CYP3A subfamily is the most abundantly expressed cytochrome P450 in the human liver, and CYP3A4 seems to be the major form. This enzyme metabolises a number of important drugs such as cyclosporin, erythromycin, nifedipine and other dihydropyridine calcium antagonists, and lidocaine (table X). The AUC of nifedipine has been shown to be higher in South Asians than in Caucasians,[151] indicating that South Asians might have lower CYP3A activity compared with Caucasians. Similarly, the elimination of codeine by *N*-demethylation, a metabolic pathway catalysed by CYP3A4, is lower in Chinese compared with Swedes.[152] The CYP3A subfamily is readily inducible, and it is therefore unclear whether the possible interethnic differences in this enzyme activity are of genetic or environmental origin.

Other enzyme systems for which interethnic differences have been documented include glucuronidation, esterases, and alcohol-metabolising enzymes. The elimination of codeine by glucuronidation shows marked normal distribution in both Chinese and Swedish individuals, but the average activity is significantly lower in Chinese.[152] Both the cause and the relevance of this finding remain unclear.

A genetic variant of butyrylcholinesterase, designated atypical cholinesterase, was one of the first examples of genetically determined abnormal drug responses (table XII; see also chapter 6; sect. 4.2.1). Several other variants of the enzyme have later been identified and the molecular basis of most of them elucidated.[148] Large interethnic differences in the activity of paraoxonase, a polymorphic enzyme capable of hydrolysing several organophosphate esters, are known (for a review, see La Du[153]). The clinical significance of these differences remains speculative.

The mitochondrial enzyme aldehyde dehydrogenase ALDH2 metabolises acetaldehyde derived from ethanol. Deficiency of this enzyme activity is a dominant trait causing accumulation of acetaldehyde after ethanol intake, with resultant unpleasant symptoms such as facial flushing, decrease in blood pressure, and tachycardia. This deficiency does not occur in Caucasian populations but is very common in Asians.[154] Interestingly, disulfiram used to treat alcohol-dependent patients acts by blocking ALDH2.

#### *5.3.5 Interethnic Differences in Drug Responses*

In comparison with the numerous examples of interethnic differences in drug metabolism, the literature on differences in drug response, not due to pharmacokinetic reasons, is meagre. However, it has been reported that Black individuals may show less pronounced reduction of exercise-induced increases in heart rate in response to propranolol.[146] This difference could not be accounted for by differences in the pharmacokinetics of propranolol, and was later suggested to be due to a greater parasympathetic tone in Black individuals. The pharmacokinetics and effects of propranolol were later studied in Chinese and Caucasian individuals. It was found that the concentration-response curves relating reduction in heart rate and propranolol concentration were shifted to the left in Chinese compared with Caucasians. Chinese were also more sensitive to the antihypertensive effects of propranolol. Extensive studies have failed to explain the observed pharmacodynamic differences in pharmacokinetic terms. It has furthermore been shown that Chinese also have an increased sensitivity to β-receptor-mediated effects on renin activity. This may partially explain the increased sensitivity to the antihypertensive effects of propranolol in Chinese individuals.[146]

Black individuals have been found to be resistant to the initial bradycardia caused by atropine, but more susceptible to the late effects of this drug than Caucasians. Chinese individuals have also been found to react with a higher increase in heart rate after repeated doses of atropine compared with Caucasians.

### 5.4 Effects of Disease States

Most pharmacokinetic drug studies are initially performed in volunteers and the drug is then used in patients who may have a variety of diseases apart from the one for which the drug is given. Thus, attention has been paid to the effects that various disease states may have on the absorption, distribution, metabolism and excretion of drugs. In addition to altering the pharmacokinetics of drugs, certain disease states may alter their pharmacodynamic properties through an effect on the intrinsic sensitivity of receptors.[155] Thus, hypokalaemia enhances the toxicity of digitalis as well as potentiating the action of non-depolarising skeletal muscle relaxants.

#### *5.4.1 Absorption in Disease*

Gastrointestinal disease may alter both the rate of absorption of an orally administered drug, as well as the amount of drug that may be absorbed (see chapter 22; sect. 1.1). Further information is required before all the possible variations with particular drugs can be elucidated but some important concepts have emerged.

The gastric emptying rate is an important factor in drug absorption, since this influences the rate of delivery of a drug from the stomach to the small intestine where most drugs are absorbed. In general, an increase in the rate of gastric emptying or in gastrointestinal motility increases the rate of drug absorption (and *vice versa*), but for poorly soluble drugs such as digoxin, the opposite holds (see further chapter 7, sect. 2.3.1). A change in the *rate* of absorption however, does not necessarily result in alteration of the *amount* of drug absorbed and depends on the clinical circumstances, the physicochemical and pharmacokinetic characteristics of the particular drug, and on formulation factors of the drug product (see chapter 22; sect. 1.1). If the drug is in solution by the time it reaches the small intestine, absorption will be rapid and may be complete, but if the drug dissolves relatively slowly, delayed intestinal transit may increase the amount absorbed. This is particularly the case for drugs with an 'absorption window' in the small intestine.

Delayed drug absorption due to slowed gastric emptying is most likely to be important when a rapid onset of effect is required, particularly if the drug has a short elimination half-life (e.g. paracetamol), since therapeutic plasma concentrations may never be attained; or if the drug is metabolised in the stomach or gut wall. Therapeutic failure with levodopa may occur in patients with delayed gastric emptying, partly because it is metabolised (decarboxylated) in the stomach wall, and partly because the drug is absorbed in the small intestine (by active transport), the amount of unchanged drug available for absorption thereby being reduced.

Studies of drug absorption in malabsorption syndromes have yielded conflicting information. However, for most drugs there is little evidence that absorption is significantly altered. Where incomplete absorption of drugs has occurred (e.g. penicillin in coeliac disease), treatment of the condition has restored absorption to normal. In some situations, bioavailability may actually be increased by a malabsorption state. The oral contraceptive steroid ethinylestradiol is normally extensively metabolised in the gut wall by conjugation with sulfate and this process is markedly impaired in patients with coeliac disease (mean 75%) but returns to its more usual lower level (mean 40%) when the disease is successfully treated.[156]

Other diseases or pathophysiological conditions may alter the absorption of some drugs, particularly as a result of altered gastric emptying (e.g. acute myocardial infarction, acute migraine, labour). Renal disease can also affect the bioavailability of certain drugs. These and other examples are discussed in the relevant chapters. Low cardiac output states might impair the absorption of some drugs after intramuscular injection (see section 3.1.3).

#### *5.4.2 Drug Distribution in Disease*

The onset and duration of action of a drug is dependent on its rate of distribution, which in turn depends on factors such as cardiac output, blood flow through tissues, and cell membrane permeability. For drugs with pKa values close to 7.4 (see appendix A), it has been shown that small changes in acid-base balance have a disproportionate effect on ionisation of weak organic acids and bases and may affect their uptake in tissues; for example, the myocardial uptake and efficacy of lidocaine (pKa 7.86) may be reduced by severe acidosis.[157] In myocardial infarction, particularly that complicated by shock, or in heart failure, the apparent volumes of distribution of lidocaine and procainamide are reduced from normal – probably due to the reduced blood supply to peripheral tissues. This results in higher blood concentrations than expected and undue toxicity from rapidly administered doses. Clearance is also reduced, necessitating a decrease in maintenance intravenous doses of lidocaine and procainamide (see further chapter 20).

Protein binding too is affected by disease.[158] In severe hypoalbuminaemia, such as in the nephrotic syndrome or severe protein malnutrition (kwashiorkor in children), and in severe hepatic disease (both cirrhosis and hepatitis), the protein binding of drugs may be reduced. Thus, the binding of drugs such as diazepam, naproxen, tolbutamide, valproic acid and verapamil has been shown to be decreased in patients with hepatic disease. In general, binding is only reduced when the liver disease is

**Table XV.** Binding of drugs to plasma proteins in patients with reduced renal function (after Zini et al.[158])

| Drug | Acid (A) or base (B) | Binding |
|---|---|---|
| Azapropazone | A | Decreased |
| Azlocillin | A | Slightly decreased |
| Furosemide | A | Decreased |
| Indomethacin | A | Decreased |
| Naproxen | A | Decreased |
| Phenytoin | A | Decreased |
| Sulfonamides | A | Decreased |
| Theophylline | A | Decreased |
| Valproic Acid | A | Decreased |
| Warfarin | A | Decreased |
| Dapsone | B | No change |
| Diazepam | B | Decreased |
| Disopyramide | B | Increased |
| Maprotiline | B | No change |
| Morphine | B | Increased |
| Pindolol | B | No change |
| Propafenone | B | Increased |
| Triamterene | B | Decreased |
| Verapamil | B | No change |

associated with hypoalbuminaemia (or occasionally hyperbilirubinaemia) and is associated with a lower concentration of albumin in plasma. There is no evidence of a conformational change in the albumin molecule in patients with cirrhosis. Bilirubin is bound with high affinity to albumin and can be displaced from its primary binding site by drugs such as the sulfonamides, cefalosporins, and nonsteroidal anti-inflammatory drugs.[159] The resulting rise in free bilirubin concentration in neonates may produce kernicterus.

Binding of drugs to plasma proteins is well known to be affected in renal disease.[160] The binding of most acidic drugs to albumin is reduced but the binding of basic drugs – usually to $\alpha_1$-acid glycoprotein, is less uniformly affected (table XV). The cause of reduced binding is less clear than in hepatic disease since binding may be decreased even in the presence of normal albumin levels. There is good evidence for the accumulation of endogenous substances in the plasma of patients with renal failure which can interfere with binding to albumin.[161] A number of endogenous substances have been identified such as free fatty acids (FFA), hippuric acid, indoxyl sulfate and various furan carboxylic acids, and many of these bind to site I or site II on the human serum albumin molecule. Normal binding can be restored by dialysis or by acidification of albumin (to pH 3) and extraction with activated charcoal. It is also partly restored a few days after kidney transplantation.[99]

There is also some evidence for a change in the conformational structure of albumin in patients with renal disease. Thus, carbamylation of albumin is known to occur and can affect the protein binding of drugs, particularly those that bind to site I on the albumin molecule. In the nephrotic syndrome, the reduced binding of drugs to albumin is due primarily to the low albumin levels in plasma.

Many basic drugs bind to acute phase proteins, particularly $\alpha_1$-acid glycoprotein.[41] The rise of $\alpha_1$-acid glycoprotein levels in some renal diseases may explain the increased binding of various drugs noted in table XV. $\alpha_1$-Acid glycoprotein levels are increased in many disease processes, especially inflammatory diseases and following trauma such as surgery. Thus, the binding of basic drugs may be increased in patients following a myocardial infarction or severe burns, as well as in patients with rheumatoid arthritis or infections (fig. 25). In patients with malaria, the binding of quinine is increased due to the higher concentrations of $\alpha_1$-acid glycoprotein and this may explain the reduced likelihood of eye and ear toxicity in such patients despite high total plasma concentrations of quinine (since the increased binding may not have had any clinically relevant effect on the unbound drug concentration).

While the free fraction ($f_u$) of a drug may be changed in patients with disease, this does not imply a corresponding change in the free concentration of the drug in question. The volume of distribution may be affected but the clearance of the drug will depend on other factors, particularly the hepatic extraction ratio (see also section 3.3.3).

Drugs metabolised by the liver can be divided into two main types with respect to their hepatic clearance – *high clearance* (flow-dependent) and *low clearance*.[34] For the former (e.g. propranolol, lidocaine), the extraction ratio in the liver is high and the liver's ability to metabolise them is dependent upon the activity of drug metabolising enzymes and on the rate of transport of the drug (bound and unbound) to the organ, i.e. hepatic blood flow and plasma protein bind-

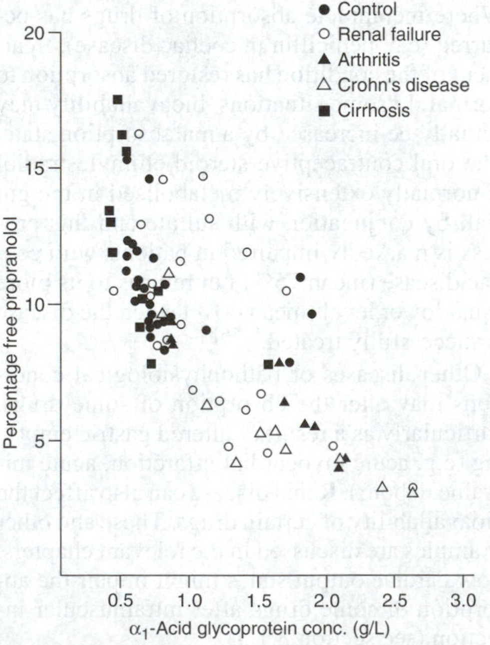


**Fig. 25.** Relationship between the binding of propranolol and the plasma concentration of $\alpha_1$-acid glycoprotein. Note the decrease in free fraction of propranolol in arthritis and Crohn's disease (after Piafsky et al.[162]).

**Table XVI.** Potential mechanisms of altered drug disposition in liver disease (after McLean & Morgan[163])

1. Reduction in total cell mass
2. Reduction in portal venous perfusion due to:
   a) Extrahepatic shunting of portal blood
   b) Intrahepatic shunting of portal blood
   c) Reduction in portal flow following increased vascular resistance
   d) Altered access from axial flow to sinusoid
3. Increase in arterial perfusion of liver due to:
   a) Preferential perfusion of sinusoid mid-zone and terminal zones by arterioles
   b) Higher arterial inflow into sinusoids
   c) Direct proximity of arterial blood to sinusoidal plates
4. Reduced exchange of water and small molecules across the endothelial lining
5. Impaired diffusion of substates within space of Disse

ing. The pharmacokinetics of such drugs will thus be affected by processes that lower the capacity of the liver to metabolise drugs and change hepatic blood flow and/or protein binding. For low clearance drugs, hepatic elimination is dependent solely upon the concentration of unbound drug presented to the liver.

### *5.4.3 Drug Metabolism in Disease*

A number of diseases and pathophysiological states are capable of altering the rate of drug metabolism as a consequence of changes in hepatic blood flow or hepatic microsomal drug metabolising enzyme activity.

#### Liver Disease

The liver is the main organ of metabolism for many drugs and it would not be surprising if liver disease were to lead to impaired drug metabolism and thus to altered pharmacokinetics. In health, the liver has a mass of 0.015 to 0.02 kg/kg bodyweight. There is a dual blood supply providing on average 1.2 to 1.5L blood per minute. Normally 80% of the blood comes via the hepatic portal vein from the splanchnic circulation while the remaining 20% arrives at the liver from the hepatic artery. Vascular exchange takes place in the liver sinusoids which are modified capillaries. These are low pressure systems and in health, the hepatic venous pressure is 1 to 2mm Hg while the hepatic portal venous pressure is 8 to 10mm Hg. The high blood flows of 1.0 to 1.5 ml/kg/min are needed since the hepatic portal blood is partly desaturated with oxygen (normally 70 to 80% saturated with oxygen compared with 100% for the hepatic artery).

In liver disease, there are a number of variables that can affect the pharmacokinetics of a drug (table XVI), including hepatic blood flow, reduction in hepatic cell mass, portal-systemic shunting of blood, cholestasis, and changes (usually a decrease) in drug protein binding. The latter is discussed in more detail in section 5.4.2. Clearance (CL) can be defined in terms of the extraction of the drug by the liver (E) and hepatic blood flow (Q). Hepatic extraction is defined as the fraction of drug that is extracted as it passes through the liver, i.e.:

$$E = (C_i - C_o)/C_i$$

where $C_i$ is the input concentration presented to the liver and $C_o$ is the output concentration that exits from it. Hepatic clearance ($CL_H$) is then defined by:

$$CL_H = Q \cdot E$$

As the ability of the liver to extract a drug from the circulation increases, $C_o$ approaches zero and the extraction ratio approaches unity. The extraction ratio is also the extent to which a drug is cleared from the blood on a single pass through the liver.

The effect of liver disease on drug kinetics has been examined for different categories of drugs, depending on their hepatic clearances (table XVII; see also appendix F), i.e. whether they are low clearance drugs or high clearance drugs:

*Low clearance, high degree of protein binding drugs:* the situation with drugs of this type

**Table XVII.** Percentage changes in total systemic clearance of drugs in patients with severe liver disease (after Bass & Williams[164])

| | |
|---|---|
| **High clearance drugs:** | |
| Morphine | –7 |
| Metoprolol | –25 |
| Lidocaine | –40 |
| Pentazocine | –46 |
| Verapamil | –50 |
| Pethidine | –50 |
| Propranolol | –62 |
| **Low clearance drugs:** | |
| Ampicillin | –16 |
| Atenolol | +23 |
| Chloramphenicol | –65 |
| Diazepam | –53 |
| Furosemide | –15 |
| Lorazepam | +8 |
| Oxazepam | +14 |
| Tolbutamide | +44 |
| Warfarin | No change |

**Table XVIII.** Changes in bioavailability and clearance of high clearance drugs in patients with liver disease

| Drug | Hepatic extraction ratio | Clearance | Bioavailability |
|---|---|---|---|
| Clomethiazole (chlormethiazole) | 0.9 | Reduced | Much increased |
| Labetalol | 0.7 | Reduced | Increased |
| Lidocaine | 0.7 | Reduced | |
| Pentazocine | 0.8 | Reduced | Much increased |
| Pethidine (meperidine) | 0.5 | Reduced | Increased |
| Propranolol | 0.6 | Slightly reduced | Slightly increased |

is a specialised one and few examples exist. Where examples do exist, the final result will depend on the balance between changes in intrinsic clearance and changes in the unbound fraction. Thus, for mexiletine, the unbound fraction is unchanged in patients with liver disease, while intrinsic clearance is reduced leading to an overall reduction in hepatic clearance of 75%.[165] In contrast, for tolbutamide, the reverse is seen in patients with acute viral hepatitis[166] – no change in intrinsic clearance and an increase in the unbound fraction of tolbutamide, leading to an apparent 44% increase in the hepatic clearance of the drug (based on total drug concentrations). Studies with naproxen have revealed an intermediate position with no net change in hepatic clearance of this drug in patients with cirrhosis of the liver.[167]

*Low clearance, low degree of protein binding drugs:* there have been many studies with drugs of this type in patients with both acute hepatitis and cirrhosis of the liver.[163] In general, oxidative drug metabolism is impaired in liver disease and the degree of impairment correlates best with the degree of access of the drug from the sinusoid to the hepatocyte. This may in part be linked with the degree of access of oxygen to the hepatocytes. The clearance of phenazone (antipyrine), a typical marker drug that has been frequently studied, is reduced by 50 to 70% in patients with severe liver disease[163] but in mild to moderate disease, no change is seen. Although hepatocyte cell mass is reduced in severe liver disease, there is evidence that the activity of cytochrome P450 isozymes is variably affected by liver disease and this may explain the variable results of human studies in this field.[168]

Conjugation processes are less uniformly affected by liver disease. Thus, for many drugs that are metabolised to a glucuronide conjugate (e.g. oxazepam, furosemide, lorazepam), there is no impairment in liver disease, while for others (e.g. chloramphenicol and paracetamol), there is evidence of reduced conjugation in liver disease.[163] On balance, it seems that conjugation processes are relatively little affected by liver disease.

*High clearance drugs:* examples of changes in bioavailability and clearance with these drugs in patients with liver disease are shown in table XVIII. In early studies with drugs of this type, e.g. propranolol, lidocaine, good correlations were found between the changes in pharmacokinetics in liver disease and alterations in blood flow. However, as the studies became more sophisticated, it proved increasingly difficult to attribute changes in pharmacokinetics to intra- or extrahepatic shunting of blood. In general, while there is good evidence for a reduced clearance of these drugs in patients with severe liver disease, this is more to do with access of the drugs from the sinusoid to the hepatocyte than to changes in hepatic blood flow.[163]

***Pharmacodynamic changes in liver disease:*** in addition to the well recognised pharmacokinetic changes in patients with severe liver disease, the altered drug response that is sometimes seen in such patients may be due to pharmacodynamic changes. Thus, there appears to be a reduced sensitivity of the kidney to diuretics and an increased sensitivity of the brain to sedatives and antianxiety agents. The reduced sensitivity of the kidney to diuretics is not due to a reduced sensitivity of a nephron but rather to a reduced number of functioning nephrons.[169] However, the increased sensitivity of the brain to drugs such as the benzodiazepines is an area that has generated intense debate and confusion. While early studies appeared to show such increased sensitivity, apparently due to an increased number of benzodiazepine binding sites in the brain,[170] more recent studies have not confirmed this.[171]

### Thyroid Disease

The influence of thyroid disease on drug metabolism has been studied intensively in recent years, and controlled studies are relatively easy to perform since the patient can be restudied when the thyroid status is restored to normal. In general, drug metabolism is accelerated in hyperthyroidism and reduced in hypothyroid states (see further chapter 19; sect. 1.3).[172]

#### Renal Disease

It has generally been assumed that the rate of metabolism of a drug will not be altered in patients with renal impairment, but this is not necessarily true. Thus, oxidation of some drugs may be enhanced, leading to a more rapid rate of drug metabolism, while for others, oxidation may be decreased. Most glucuronide conjugation reactions are unaltered by renal disease but hydrolytic reactions may be slowed, as is seen with the hydrolysis of insulin, procaine and cefalothin. Reduction may also be slowed, e.g. with cortisol (see further chapter 24; sect. 1.3).

#### Surgery and Trauma

Many factors that can alter the disposition of drugs exist after surgery.[173] Apart from slowed gastric emptying and altered protein binding (see section 5.4.2), liver blood flow increases and hepatic microsomal drug metabolising enzyme activity increases. The increase in drug metabolic capacity, as reflected in an enhanced rate of elimination of phenazone (antipyrine), may be due to altered secretion of hormones or concomitant use of enzyme-inducing drugs. Impaired renal function is only likely after severe trauma with hypotension.

The possible adverse effects of general anaesthetics on liver and kidney function must also be considered (see chapter 12; sect. 2.1). This area requires further study with drugs with different pharmacokinetic characteristics before the clinical implications are clear.

**Table XIX.** Elimination half-lives of some drugs in patients with normal renal function and in patients with impaired renal function (after Fillastre & Singlas;[174] Peter et al.;[175] Singlas & Fillastre[176])

| Drug | Half-life (hours) | |
|---|---|---|
| | normal renal function | end-stage renal disease[a] |
| Amoxicillin | 1.0 | 12.5 |
| Benzylpenicillin (penicillin G) | 0.5 | 5 |
| Cefuroxime | 1.6 | 14 |
| Cefixime | 3 | 12 |
| Gentamicin | 2.7 | 42 |
| Erythromycin | 1.8 | 3.2 |
| Tetracycline | 6 | 65 |
| Doxycycline | 17.5 | 23 |
| Trimethoprim | 12.5 | 27 |
| Ciprofloxacin | 4.6 | 8.0 |
| Ofloxacin | 5.5 | 32.5 |
| Ethambutol | 11 | 11 |
| Fluconazole | 25 | 125 |
| Digoxin | 30 | 85 |
| Omeprazole | 1.5 | 1 |
| Zidovudine | 1 | 1.4 |
| Nabumetone | 20 | 40 |

a End-stage renal disease is defined as a creatinine clearance of less than 2 ml/min.

### 5.4.4 Drug Excretion in Disease

Drugs that are largely eliminated by renal excretion show a decreased clearance in patients with age-dependent (elderly and newborn) or pathological impairment of renal function. Thus, accumulation of the drug will occur on normal doses and toxicity may ensue. Table XIX shows the expected elimination half-lives of some drugs in both healthy individuals and in patients with end-stage renal disease (creatinine clearance <2 ml/min). In many cases, the half-lives are greatly prolonged in end-stage renal disease (e.g. gentamicin, tetracycline, ofloxacin, fluconazole) but in other cases, there is little change in half-life. Examples of the latter include erythromycin, doxycycline, ethambutol and zidovudine. With these drugs, the main route of elimination is metabolism.

It is generally assumed that drugs that are metabolised can be safely given in normal doses to patients with renal function impairment. This assumption is only true if the polar metabolites, which will accumulate in the plasma of such patients, are biologically inert. It is now well established that many drugs have active metabolites and these, if not further metabolised, will accumulate in the plasma of patients with renal failure.[177] This may lead to enhanced therapeutic efficacy, adverse effects or both. Thus, the main active metabolite of procainamide, *N*-acetylprocainamide (acecainide) accumulates in the plasma of patients with impaired renal function and has been associated with the causation of cardiac arrhythmias. Norpethidine (normeperidine) is an active metabolite of pethidine, the plasma concentration of which increases in renal impairment. The metabolite is less active as an analgesic than the parent drug but is more active as a convulsive agent, and this leads to muscle irritability and twitching in some patients. The toxicities associated with nitrofurantoin (peripheral neuropathy) and allopurinol (skin rash) are at least partly due to the metabolites of these drugs which accumulate to high concentrations in the plasma of patients with impaired renal function.

It is therefore a *sine qua non* for scientifically sound drug therapy in uraemia to know the fate and likely plasma concentrations of such metabolites, and to adjust the dose in accordance with the known pharmacokinetics of pharmacologically active compounds.

In general, haemodialysis will remove drugs and their metabolites, that have accumulated in the plasma of patients with renal failure (see further chapter 8; sect. 6.5). However, there are many factors that affect drug removal by dialysis. Some of these are drug-specific (e.g. molecular size, lipid solubility), others are patient-specific (e.g. type of vascular access), while sometimes dialysis-specific factors may be important. These include the dialyser flow rate, and the intrinsic properties of the dialyser membrane. Thus, drug dosage regimens in patients undergoing haemodialysis may not be simply a matter of using routine doses as applied to patients with normal renal function.[175]

In order to achieve a required steady-state plasma concentration when the clearance of a drug is decreased in renal failure, the following three facts should be understood:

1) The priming or loading dose will not need to be changed.

2) A smaller maintenance dose of the drug will be needed and/or that dose should be given less frequently than before.

3) The time taken to achieve the steady-state plasma concentration will be longer – since to achieve 90% of that concentration will take 3 times the half-life (see section 2.3; table I).

During recent years, a number of nomograms have been published to guide the clinician in the dosage of drugs in renal insufficiency, particularly those with a narrow therapeutic range such as gentamicin, kanamycin and digoxin (see also appendix E). These nomograms take into account creatinine clearance (or serum creatinine), bodyweight and age of the patient. When using such nomograms, it must be remembered that the determination of creatinine may be inaccurate, that compensatory excretory routes such as faecal excretion may vary among individuals, and that kidney function may change quickly. Such nomograms are thus poor replacements for longitudinal monitoring of steady-state plasma concentrations, which should be performed liberally when toxic drugs are used. This is particularly true in elderly patients, where kidney function may be impaired despite normal serum creatinine. Drug disposition and response and the principles of use of drugs in renal disease are discussed further in chapter 24 (sections 1 and 11).

### 5.5 Multiple Drug Therapy: Drug Interactions

Drugs are often used in combination and it may be necessary to prescribe several potent drugs for the same individual. It then becomes important to recognise *potential* possibilities for drug interactions and to plan the treatment of the patient accordingly. In general, most problems can be avoided by adjustment of the dosage or dosage interval of the interacting drugs but in rare instances, a particular drug combination may be contraindicated.

Knowledge of the mechanisms involved in drug interactions is crucial in trying to predict drug interaction possibilities. As an example, new insight into the genetics and substrate specificity of the cytochrome P450s is a rational basis for predicting the many possibilities of clinically important drug metabolic interactions. On the other hand, understanding the basic concepts regarding protein binding and distribution of drugs leads to the unequivocal conclusion that interactions between drugs at plasma protein binding sites have little clinical importance (see section 3.2.2). Drug interactions are discussed further in the clinical context in chapter 7 and appendix B.

In order to clarify both the mechanisms of interactions and their clinical importance, several fundamental points need to be taken into consideration:

1) Specific drug analytical techniques must be used. This includes enantioselective methods in the case of racemic drugs.

2) Pharmacokinetic data obtained must be correctly interpreted. Drug-induced changes in measurements such as the elimination half-life of a drug may have several explanations, e.g. either the clearance or volume of distribution may have changed. To distinguish between these, it may be necessary to measure drug metabolites in body fluids, binding to plasma proteins, etc.

3) Animal data can seldom be extrapolated to man. Some tabulations of drug interactions contain both human and animal data. This may confuse the clinician when using the information in clinical practice.

4) *In vitro* data on, for example, synergism or antagonism between antibiotics and *in vitro* observations on drug binding displacement inter-

actions are not necessarily applicable to the conditions *in vivo* (see section 3.2.2). In fact, there are very few known examples of drug-drug displacement interactions that have been demonstrated to be of clinical importance.

5) The results of drug interaction experiments in healthy volunteers (often single-dose experiments) may not be relevant for patients who are treated long term with drugs.

6) Many interaction studies are based on rather small patient or volunteer samples and some are even 'case reports'. There are relatively few prospective studies aimed at documenting the prevalence of clinically important drug interactions (see further chapter 7).

7) There is interindividual variability in the intensity of drug metabolic interactions.

8) Ultimately, the clinical importance of a particular interaction has to be assessed in controlled clinical investigations.

9) As a rule of thumb, drug interactions are particularly important for drugs with a narrow therapeutic range (steep concentration-effect curve) when the effects are difficult to assess.

10) The best method of discovering pharmacokinetic drug interactions is monitoring of drug concentrations in plasma.

## 6. The Role of the Clinical Pharmacological Laboratory in Improving Drug Therapy

It is now realised that it may be clinically useful to monitor plasma concentrations of certain drugs in patients for whom therapy is essential (e.g. see Richens;[178] Sjöqvist[179]). For example, the effect of phenytoin (diphenylhydantoin) is much better correlated in patient populations to its steady-state plasma concentration than to dosage.[180] This may also be true for many other drugs that are extensively metabolised. As discussed in section 5, a fixed dose of such a drug may produce a 10-fold interindividual range in steady-state plasma concentrations due to the combined influence of genetic and environmental factors on drug metabolism.

There is no general biochemical test available to detect patients with extreme rates of drug metabolism. However, developments in pharmacogenetics promise to provide the clinician with reliable phenotyping and genotyping tests for assessing the function of individual drug metabolising enzymes (see table X). In assessing drug metabolism, the best method is still to study each compound separately, e.g. by measuring the steady-state plasma concentration. This is not only practical (in that it avoids stopping treatment and manipulation of dosage for clearance measurements), but also reveals important drug metabolic and psychological (i.e. drug compliance; see section 6.2.2) information about the patient.

The position with drugs that are excreted *unchanged* by the kidney is better, because laboratory tests such as serum creatinine or creatinine clearance are reasonable guidelines for the modification of dosage when there is impairment of renal function (see further section 5.4.4).

### 6.1 Correlation Between Drug Plasma Concentrations and Clinical Effects

The idea of using the plasma concentration of a drug as an objective means towards safer and more rational therapy in an individual patient is based on several prerequisites which are summarised in table XX and discussed below.

#### *6.1.1 Action at Receptor Sites*

The drug should have a reversible action. For 'hit and run' drugs like irreversible monoamine oxidase inhibitors, the action may persist even though the drug is no longer measurable in plasma. Most drugs in common use exert a reversible, concentration-dependent interaction with receptor sites (see section 1.2).

The development of tolerance at receptor sites should not be an important problem, as it is for example with barbiturates, ethanol and morphine.[6]

**Table XX.** A correlation between the steady-state plasma concentration of a drug and clinical effect can be expected when the following criteria are fulfilled

1. The drug has a reversible action and acts *per se* (not through metabolites)
2. Development of tolerance at receptor sites does not occur
3. The concentration of unbound drug in plasma is equal to the concentration of unbound drug at receptor sites – i.e. plasma and tissue concentrations of unbound drug should be in equilibrium after some period of continued treatment
4. The clinical effects of the drug are measured accurately
5. Factors that modify the plasma concentration-clinical effect relationship are taken into account, e.g. other drugs, abnormal protein binding, stage of disease
6. The pharmacokinetic properties of the drug are taken into account, e.g. time of sampling plasma, when to measure area under plasma concentration-time curve, etc.
7. The chemical analytical method must be both sensitive and selective and sometimes even enantioselective

### 6.1.2 Distribution Equilibrium

At distribution equilibrium, the concentration of unbound drug in plasma should be equal to the concentration of unbound drug at receptor sites. This equilibrium will occur after a period of continued treatment, the length of which will vary considerably between drugs.

There is little reason to believe that the ratio between the concentration of unbound drug in plasma and in the biophase surrounding tissue receptor sites should differ markedly between patients, as long as we consider drug distribution as a passive process depending upon the physicochemical properties of the drug rather than upon the genetic constitution of the individual.

An important question is whether total or unbound plasma concentrations should be measured or both. From a theoretical standpoint, it is clear that measurement of the unbound concentration is preferable. However, it is impractical, since present methodology to measure protein binding (equilibrium dialysis and ultrafiltration) is time consuming and labour intensive. Experience with a number of drugs indicates that, under normal circumstances, interindividual differences in protein binding are small, at least in comparison with the marked interindividual differences in metabolism (see section 5). This suggests that the present practice of monitoring total plasma concentrations is, in most cases, acceptable. However, when the patient is treated simultaneously with two or more highly bound acidic drugs with a small apparent volume of distribution and which bind to the same site on albumin (e.g. warfarin and phenylbutazone), the fraction of the displaced drug (warfarin) that is unbound increases and while (as pointed out in section 3.2.3) the unbound drug concentration rapidly returns to its original predisplacement level, the total drug concentration is decreased.

The fraction of unbound drug may also be increased in certain diseases and decreased in others (see section 5.4.2). For example, the unbound fraction of phenytoin is increased markedly in patients with uraemia. These patients can therefore be expected to respond therapeutically or with adverse effects at much lower *total* plasma concentrations than epileptics with normal renal function.

Hence monitoring of the *unbound* drug concentration is important in this and similar situations. Methods now exist for the measurement of unbound plasma concentrations of drugs, usually by ultrafiltration devices which are relatively simple to use. Studies suggest that in selected patients, measurement of unbound concentrations may be useful and may give a truer account of the pharmacokinetic situation, particularly for phenytoin (see also chapter 5; sect. 1.6.3, 1.6.9, 4).[181,182]

### 6.1.3 Measurement of Clinical Effects

In many areas of pharmacology, the ability to measure minute concentrations of drugs in biological fluids has become satisfactory. Drug analytical methods allow accurate measurement of concentrations down to 1 μg/L or lower. Attempts to correlate plasma concentrations of drugs with their clinical effect are therefore dependent upon the ability to accurately detect and quantify the latter. In some areas of therapeutics, this is relatively easy (e.g. for cardiovascular drugs) but in others more difficult (e.g. CNS active drugs), as discussed in section 8.

It is important that the variable being measured is related to the pharmacodynamic effect of the drug, otherwise no single relationship to drug plasma concentration can be expected. Even measuring such an apparently simple parameter as systemic arterial blood pressure imposes a number of questions: should it be measured continuously or on a few occasions every day, in the sitting, standing or lying position, at rest or after exercise or both, in the clinic or at home?

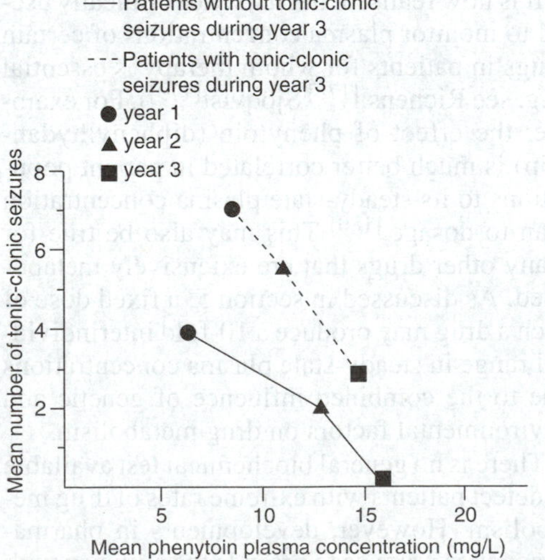


**Fig. 26.** The relationship between the annual mean number of tonic-clonic (grand mal) seizures and the mean concentration of phenytoin in two groups consisting of patients with or without seizures during the third year of a prospective study (after Lund[180]).

#### 6.1.4 Factors that Modify the Plasma Concentration-Effect Relationship

A number of factors may modify the plasma concentration-clinical effect relationship in an individual patient. Intercurrent illness, surgery or a change in environmental and dietary factors may alter the usual absorption and disposition of a drug, as considered in sections 3.3.5 and 5.4. Concomitant drug therapy (section 5.5) is probably the most important factor and often impossible to control. The stage of the disease is also important, amply illustrated in the case of phenytoin and tonic-clonic (grand mal) epilepsy. With increasing severity of seizures, the plasma concentration needed for seizure control rises (fig. 26).

#### 6.1.5 The Drug and its Chemical Assay

There are a number of points to take into consideration regarding the drug and its chemical assay. Ideally, the drug is characterised by slow absorption and a long elimination half-life relative to the dosage interval such that only minor fluctuations of drug plasma concentrations occur during the day. In this case, the time for sampling plasma may be of little importance (e.g. phenytoin). For other drugs, very strict protocols have to be set up, with plasma concentrations measured at a specific time point in relation to dosage, e.g. 12 hours after the last dose with lithium and at least 6 to 8 hours with digoxin (see further chapter 5; sect. 2.2, 4). For drugs with short half-lives (a few hours) and hence major fluctuations of plasma concentrations at conventional dosage intervals, the trough concentration obtained just before the next dose is to be administered, and the peak concentration obtained 1 to 2 hours after a dose, are appropriate times to obtain samples for evaluation (e.g. aminoglycoside antibiotics). Sometimes it may be desirable to measure the area under the plasma concentration-time curve (AUC) during the dosage interval.

In plasma concentration estimations, it is an advantage if the drug is active *per se*. However, with many drugs used in clinical practice, the pharmacological effects of the metabolites are often unknown and the main metabolites may not even be identified. It becomes more complicated to measure several compounds in plasma.

#### 6.1.6 Drug Analytical Methods

The chemical analytical methods must be both sensitive and selective. In some conventional analytical methods, the drug history of the patient has importance for the choice of the procedure but with modern techniques, this problem is minimised. The development of drug analysis has been particularly rapid during the last 20 years with methods such as conventional gas chromatography, gas chromatography-mass spectrometry (GC-MS), radioimmunoassays, and high-performance liquid chromatography (HPLC). The latter technique allows many different methods of detection, e.g. based on ultraviolet absorption, fluorescence, or electrochemical reduction or oxidation reactions. The recent marriage of HPLC to mass spectrometry (LC-MS) has extended the latter highly sensitive and specific detection technique to compounds too polar to analyse by GC-MS, e.g. various conjugated metabolites.

How then can advancements in clinical pharmacokinetics be utilised in patient care when the research requires a team of professionals and sophisticated analytical methods? Two ways of utilising this knowledge are apparent:

1) To refer selected patients to regional centres for pharmacokinetic or drug metabolic work-ups in analogy with what is now done in cases of inborn errors of endogenous metabolism; and

2) To develop simpler analytical methods that can be applied in routine laboratories.

It is important that a pharmacokinetic service laboratory participates in quality control programmes and adheres to the principles of good laboratory practice (GLP).

### 6.2 Main Indications for Measuring Drugs in Plasma (or Other Body Fluids)

#### 6.2.1 Therapeutic Drug Monitoring

For the drugs listed in table XXI, the relationship between plasma concentration and clinical effects has been studied under relatively satisfactory conditions. Many of these drugs have a narrow therapeutic ratio (digoxin, lithium), while others have dose-dependent elimination kinetics (phenytoin) and others show marked interindividual variability in elimination kinetics (nortriptyline). These factors strengthen the need to monitor plasma concentrations, but the prime reason for doing this should be that it is difficult to reach an optimum dosage schedule solely on the basis of a clinical evaluation of drug response.

With this philosophy, the monitoring of plasma concentrations of antidiabetic, antihypertensive and anticoagulant drugs is not justified, but an open mind according to individual circumstances has to be kept in relation to drugs

**Table XXI.** Examples of drugs for which therapeutic and toxic ranges of plasma concentrations have been defined or proposed[a] (see also chapter 5; sect. 4)

| Drug | Therapeutic range | Toxicity | References |
|---|---|---|---|
| **Antiepileptic drugs** | | | |
| Phenytoin | 10-20 mg/L (40-80 μmol/L) | >25 mg/L (>100 μmol/L) | Kutt;[183] Lund;[180] Hvidberg & Dam[184] |
| Phenobarbital | 10-30 mg/L (45-130 μmol/L) | >35 mg/L (>150 μmol/L) | Buchtal & Lennox-Buchtal;[185] Hvidberg & Dam[184] |
| Carbamazepine[b,d] | 5-10 mg/L (20-40 μmol/L) | >12 mg/L (>50 μmol/L) | Bertilsson & Tomson;[186] Hvidberg & Dam[184] |
| Ethosuximide[b] | 40-100 mg/L (300-700 μmol/L) | >100 mg/L (>700 μmol/L) | Penry[187] |
| Valproic acid[b] | 50-100 mg/L (350-700 μmol/L) | >100 mg/L (>700 μmol/L) | Richens & Warrington[188] |
| **Cardiovascular drugs** | | | |
| Digoxin | <2 μg/L (<2.6 nmol/L) | >3 μg/L (>4 nmol/L) | Smith et al.;[189] Iisalo;[190] Weintraub[191] |
| Digitoxin[b] | 10-25 μg/L (13-33 nmol/L) | >38 μg/L (>50 nmol/L) | Perrier et al.[192] |
| Quinidine | 1.3-4 mg/L (4-12 μmol/L) | >4 mg/L[c] (>12 μmol/L) | Sokolow & Ball;[193] Koch-Weser[194] |
| Procainamide[d] | 3-10 mg/L (10-35 μmol/L) | >10 mg/L (>35 μmol/L) | Koch-Weser;[195] Karlsson[15] |
| **Psychotherapeutic drugs** | | | |
| Lithium | 0.5-1.0 mmol/L | >1.5 mmol/L | Amdisen[196] |
| Nortriptyline[e] | 50-160 μg/L (200-600 nmol/L) | >210 μg/L (>800 nmol/L) | Kragh-Sorensen;[197] Åsberg & Sjöqvist[198] |
| Imipramine[e] | 150-270 μg/L[f] (540-960 nmol/L) | | Gram;[199] Perrel et al.[200] |
| Perphenazine | 0.8-2.4 μg/L (2-6 nmol/L) | >2.4 μg/L (>6 nmol/L) | Hansen et al;[201] Hansen & Larsen[202] |
| **Miscellaneous** | | | |
| Theophylline | 7-20 mg/L (40-110 μmol/L) | >20 mg/L (>110 μmol/L) | Ogilvie[77] |
| Cyclosporin[g] | 60-240 μg/L[h] | | Lindholm[203] |

a Excluding antibiotics.
b More clinical data needed.
c Varies with assay method.
d Has an active metabolite (see text).
e Data relate to endogenous depression.
f Sum of imipramine and desipramine.
g Data relate to renal transplantation.
h Data relate to specific analysis in whole blood.

affecting subjective variables such as mood and pain and drugs used prophylactically such as antiarrhythmics. Only for a few drugs is routine monitoring justified.[188] Monitoring the plasma concentrations of antiepileptic drugs has increased the effectiveness and safety of drug therapy in epilepsy (see chapter 5, sect. 4.3 and chapter 29, sect. 4.1.3), while monitoring of plasma lithium is necessary to avoid toxicity in long term prophylaxis of bipolar disorder (see chapter 30; sect. 4.1.1). Monitoring of tricyclic antidepressants has become more important in the light of new knowledge about their pharmacogenetics (see section 5.2). The list of drugs for which a desirable therapeutic plasma concentration 'range' has been defined is short but in some countries, drug regulatory agencies now require that new drugs are introduced to the market with this knowledge in the documentation file. Cyclosporin is an example of a drug where the manufacturer requests clinicians to monitor plasma (whole blood) concentrations to avoid toxicity. Antipsychotic drugs are now increasingly monitored in sophisticated psychiatric clinics after the discovery that most of them are metabolised by the polymorphic CYP2D6 (see further sections 5.2 and 5.3.1).

The measurement of drugs in plasma does not replace sound clinical judgement. On the contrary, this is a prerequisite for proper utilisation of the service, which should be part of a consultation in clinical pharmacology used mainly when patients are responding abnormally to a drug or when routine monitoring is justified to guide safe and effective use of a drug. It should also be appreciated that estimation of drug concentrations from a given plasma sample (as with antibacterial sensitivity testing) can vary between laboratories, as shown with antiepileptic drugs.[178,204] This fact must always be borne in mind when plasma concentration estimations are requested. Contrary to the general belief, many more patients are under-medicated than over-treated to judge from drug concentrations obtained in plasma.

A further consideration is the phenomenon of stereoisomerism (see also chapter 5; sect. 1.6.5). For some drugs that are administered as a racemic mixture of two enantiomers, one is frequently more potent than the other and they may be subject to stereoselective metabolism. As an example, with verapamil, the *S*(–) enantiomer is mainly responsible for the drug's negative dromotropic activity, and due to stereoselective first-pass metabolism, the same plasma concentration of total verapamil consists of a 2- to 3-times smaller proportion of the *S*(–) enantiomer after oral administration in comparison with intravenous administration. Measurements of the sum of the two enantiomers (*S* plus *R*) is therefore less meaningful, as the target concentration after intravenous administration will be much lower than after oral administration. Thus, the use of enantioselective assays, e.g. by use of chiral HPLC columns, is highly recommended in cases where the two enantiomers have different pharmacodynamic and pharmacokinetic properties (for a review on drug enantiomers, see Williams & Lee[52]).

### 6.2.2 Checking Drug Compliance

It is often justified to question whether the patient is complying with the prescription or not.[205-207] Experience with many years' monitoring of phenytoin in plasma shows that many epileptic patients forget to take their medication. This is not only due to kinetically inappropriate dosage schedules, such as 3 to 4 times daily when once or twice daily will suffice, but is probably also due to the failure of the clinician to explain the benefit : risk equation to the patient (fig. 27).

It is possible to distinguish between poor drug compliance and rapid metabolism of drugs known to be completely absorbed. If the patient is at steady-state, then one should be able to account for a defined amount of the drug in a 24-hour urinary specimen as the main metabolite. For example, *p*-hydroxyphenytoin in conjugated and unconjugated form should amount to 80% of the daily ingested dose of phenytoin. Therefore, a pharmacokinetic service laboratory should have methods available for the main metabolite(s) of drugs.

### 6.2.3 At-Risk Patients and Special Situations

These include patients with poor and rapidly changing kidney function, where even short term treatment with ordinary doses of drugs such as digoxin or aminoglycoside antibiotics may result in toxic concentrations and, in the latter case, irreversible damage of the inner ear (see chapter 14; sect. 8.1). Other patients in whom drug monitoring may be valuable include those with compromised cardiovascular functions (to adapt the dosage according to disease-mediated changes in clearance), and those on complex combination therapy (to control drug interactions). Other indications may include suspicion of malabsorption.

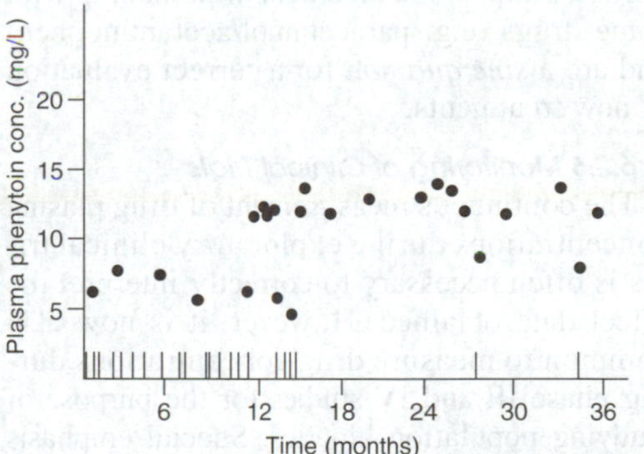


**Fig. 27.** Plasma concentrations of phenytoin and seizure frequency in long term therapy. The patient was a 44-year-old woman with generalised epileptic seizures of unknown aetiology of 15 years duration. A constant dose of phenytoin (6.8 mg/kg/day) was prescribed over a 3-year period. Too little attention was paid to the low plasma concentrations during the first year, and other antiepileptic drugs were tried with unsatisfactory results. During hospitalisation in month 12, plasma concentrations rose (unreliable drug intake). Following a 'pedagogic' intervention, plasma concentrations remained between 12 and 15 mg/L, and the number of seizures diminished markedly. Only two seizures occurred during the last 2 years; on both occasions, the plasma concentration had dropped because of interruptions in drug intake. Seizures are shown by the event markers on the abscissa (after Lund[208]).

#### 6.2.4 Diagnosis of Extreme Rates of Drug Metabolism (Pharmacogenetics)

As discussed in detail in section 5.2, mutations of the genes regulating the activity of different cytochrome P450 enzymes will lead to extremely slow metabolism of a vast number of drugs. The poor metaboliser phenotype can be tentatively diagnosed by simple measurements of drug plasma concentrations (i.e. very high plasma concentration relative to dose). A confirmation can later be made with a phenotyping test or, under ideal circumstances, a genotyping test. It may be vital for certain patients (and their clinicians) to know their phenotype in order to benefit from an individually tailored dosage regimen.

The other extreme, ultrarapid metabolism, caused by duplication or amplification of the *CYP2D6* gene, may be diagnosed accordingly. The combination of conventional therapeutic drug monitoring and modern pharmacogenetic techniques has great potential in the monitoring of sophisticated drug therapy.

#### 6.2.5 Management of Certain Drug Intoxications

Since most treatment of drug overdosage and poisoning is symptomatic and unspecific, there is usually no urgency in these measurements (see also chapter 8). They are, however, an important guide to management of poisoning with some drugs (e.g. paracetamol/acetaminophen) and are a *sine qua non* for a correct evaluation of new treatments.

#### 6.2.6 Monitoring of Clinical Trials

The continuous measurement of drug plasma concentrations during exploratory clinical trials is often necessary to correctly interpret the effect data obtained. However, it is now also common to measure drug concentrations during phase III and IV studies for the purpose of studying population kinetics. Special emphasis should be put on the occurrence of kinetic (metabolic) outliers. Clinicians involved in clinical trials should request such determinations to be made.

## 7. Pharmacokinetics in Drug Selection

It is useful to consider whether the various theoretical factors discussed in the preceding sections can assist in drug selection. This can be best illustrated by thinking about a therapeutic situation and considering what the clinician should ask him/herself about the drug when selecting the best agent of a particular drug class. Table XXII shows a check list for the pharmacokinetic and clinical documentation of drugs which may be used for this purpose.

**Table XXII.** Checklist on clinical documentation of drugs

1. Structural formula – relationship to other drugs on the market
2. Mechanism(s) of action
3. Indications based on acceptable evidence of therapeutic efficacy in controlled clinical trials (see also section 9; 10.2)
4. Pharmacokinetics:
   a) Pharmaceutical aspects
   b) Bioavailability
   c) Binding and distribution
   d) Metabolism (pathways, rates, active metabolites, interindividual variations)
   e) Excretion
   f) Pharmacokinetic and/or pharmacodynamic rationale for dosage regimens
   g) Pharmacogenetic phenotypes needing special dosages
   h) Effects of disease on pharmacokinetics
   i) Anticipated or documented drug interactions
5. Contraindications and adverse effects (pharmacokinetic basis). Care with which adverse effects have been sought
6. Comparative clinical pharmacology and therapeutic efficacy in relation to other drugs used for the same indication
7. Comparative drug price (see also chapter 10)

To the academic clinical pharmacologist, an overwhelming therapeutic problem is the inappropriate or suboptimal use of drugs that are already on the market. Studies of the mechanisms involved in interindividual variations in pharmacokinetics and pharmacodynamics will, in the long term, help to define the properties of ideal drugs. This research will provide an important feedback to the chemists in the pharmaceutical industry concerned with drug design. Any new, highly effective and non-toxic drug which represents a novel pharmacodynamic principle will be welcomed in clinical medicine. However, many drugs that are offered to the clinical academic community for trials are not in this category but are rather modifications of existing drugs. Nevertheless, for such drugs, the following characteristics may represent improvements:

1) The drug is not a racemate.

2) The drug acts *per se* rather than through metabolites (simplified monitoring of plasma concentration when necessary).

3) The drug does not have dose-dependent elimination kinetics (upon 'saturation' of the metabolic pathways, disproportionate increases in plasma concentrations may occur after small dose increases).

4) The drug does not have variable absorption or different bioavailability when given with a meal.

5) Dose-response studies have been performed.

6) The relationships between steady-state plasma concentration and the clinical effects (including adverse effects) have been explored.

7) An analytical method should be available for specific measurement of the drug in plasma.

The best way for clinicians to cope with interindividual variations in kinetics may be to use drugs whose pharmacological effects are easy to measure or which have such a large therapeutic ratio that fixed doses can be used without complications.

## 8. Clinical Assessment of Drug Effects

Reliable and accurate methods of assessing the clinical response to drugs are essential, not only to determine if the desired therapeutic goal has been achieved but also to control measurements of drug response in therapeutic trials and to study the correlation between plasma concentrations of drugs and their pharmacodynamic effects.

### 8.1 Cardiovascular Drugs

Much clinical pharmacological information arose initially in the field of cardiovascular medicine since it is easy to measure the blood pressure and pulse rate and to relate changes to the drugs given. Use of simple apparatus, such as the muddled zero sphygmomanometer, enables the blood pressure to be measured relatively free of observer bias. The therapeutic effect can be measured in more sophisticated ways and the effect of β-adrenoceptor blocking drugs is commonly measured by the effect on submaximal exercise-induced heart rate. The exercise needs to be submaximal to eliminate as far as possible the effects of vagal activity on the heart rate. Without resorting to invasive methods, other cardiac drugs can be monitored fairly accurately, either for therapeutic benefit to the patient or for use in clinical trials. Thus, an antianginal drug may be monitored in the laboratory by assessing the work done by the patient (e.g. on a treadmill or bicycle ergometer) before the onset of chest pain. More simply, the patient can keep a diary card, recording every anginal attack and then relate these to the use or dosage of the drug concerned.

There are now a number of new methods which allow accurate measurement of cardiovascular function in a non-invasive way. Such methods include Colour-Doppler studies for measurement of blood flow, and impedance methodology for measurement of cardiac output.

Antiarrhythmic drugs can be monitored by the use of a Holter electrocardiogram.[209] An electrocardiogram (ECG) lead is attached to the chest wall, and is connected to a small transmitter powered by a battery, which can be easily carried by the patient for days on end if necessary. The ECG is transmitted to a tape recording device which can be several miles away and the tape can be rapidly analysed by computer for the presence of cardiac arrhythmias and related to the drug used. This is often used in clinical trial work.

### 8.2 Antiasthmatic and Antidiabetic Drugs

In asthmatic patients, it is common practice to measure the vital capacity (VC) and forced expiratory volume in one second ($FEV_1$) in the clinic, while airways resistance can be measured more specifically by non-invasive methods. This is useful to assess the response of patients to their drugs (see chapter 23; sect. 3.2). It is now possible to equip patients with a simple device for use at home to measure their peak expiratory flow rate (PEFR). This will enable day-to-day or even hour-to-hour changes to be quantified and there is some evidence that the peak expiratory flow rate starts to fall some time before the patient experiences wheezing, thus enabling changes in drug therapy to be made before an asthma attack develops.[210]

In diabetes mellitus, it has been common practice to monitor therapeutic progress and drug effect by the measurement of urinary glucose. It has however, been recognised for some time that this method is insensitive and changes seen in urinary glucose occur too late for any effective preventive measures to be taken with the drug therapy.[211] Until recently, monitoring of blood glucose has not been practicable because of the apparatus required. However, there are now available simple and relatively cheap devices that, working on the reflectance principle, can accurately and reliably measure the concentration of glucose in a finger prick sample of blood. Long term measurement of the efficacy of blood glucose control can be best performed by monitoring glycosylated haemoglobin concentrations (HbA1C).

### 8.3 Analgesics and Other CNS Active Drugs

It is in the field of pain states and psychiatric or neurological disease that it is most difficult to measure the clinical effect of drugs with any accuracy. Even in diseases such as rheumatoid arthritis, where the appreciation of pain and discomfort is dependent on the central nervous system, accurate quantification is difficult. Objective measures such as the measurement of digital joint size exist, but are not very sensitive to anti-inflammatory drugs. Appreciation of pain is revealed by such tests as the duration of morning stiffness, and the articular index of joint tenderness but undoubtedly the development of analogue pain scores has helped considerably in the quantification of drug action in this area of therapeutics.[212] In this test, the patient is confronted with a line of fixed length and marks on it with a pen how severe the pain has been using the two indicators – one at each end of the line – as a reference (fig. 28). No other helping marks should be used. The patient's pain is then quantified by measurement (in cms) from the 'no pain' end of the line and the scale can be made as large as is needed. This test is remarkably sensitive to changes in pain and is also repeatable with little variation by the patient. Such scales can be extended to quantify other subjective phenomena such as sedation, or severity of dry mouth with an anticholinergic drug.

In epilepsy, it is conventional to rely on the patient's own assessment of his or her fit frequency to determine the effectiveness of drug therapy. This is unreliable since most patients have no warning of a fit, and some have no knowledge that a fit has taken place, particularly if fits occur only at night. Epileptic fits can be monitored by closed circuit television and

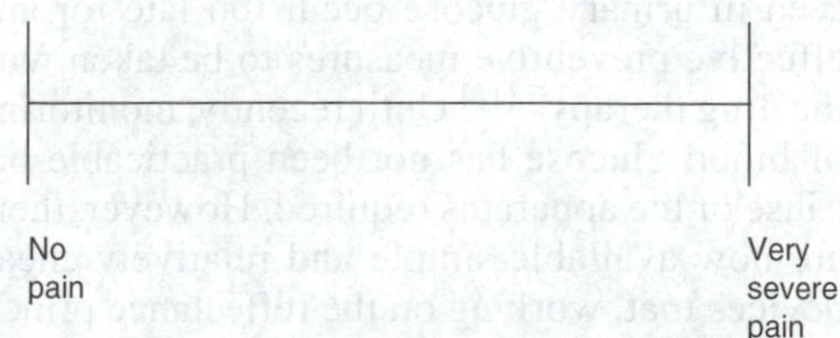


**Fig. 28.** Line of fixed length (no more than 10cm) for a patient to mark the severity of pain (see text).

electroencephalogram (EEG) records but this is only practicable in a few specialised units. The EEG can be recorded in the same way as the ECG, using a few leads only and a portable transmitter. However, analysis of the spike and wave activity has to be done by hand. There is promise for computer-based analysis and within a few years, a readily usable method should be available for monitoring the response to antiepileptic drugs.

Hypnotics, antipsychotic, antianxiety and antidepressant drugs are probably the most difficult group of drugs to assess clinically in patients. A variety of different methods has been evolved, some objective and some subjective. With sedative drugs, tests of mental concentration have been devised, particularly as related to driving automobiles, and performance in such tests can be related to the plasma concentration of the drug in question. A variety of rating scales have been proposed for the quantification of the degree of anxiety or depression, but most are complicated and require skilled persons to undertake them.[213] Certainly, in these fields, reliable and accurate methods of assessing drug action are badly needed. Considerable sophistication now exists in using rating scales in psychiatry but most of these were not developed for measuring drug effects.

In phase I trials of antipsychotic and antidepressant drugs, biochemical assessment of drug effects is possible by measuring changes in transmitters and their metabolites in cerebrospinal fluid.

Recent advances in technology are beginning to allow more routine studies into the biochemistry and cellular function of tissues without invasive procedures. Nuclear magnetic resonance (NMR) imaging, acting in a spectroscopy mode, can examine biochemical function in tissues. For example, changes in skeletal muscle metabolism can be examined by changes in $P^{31}$ NMR spectra and this is sensitive to small changes in concentration of compounds such as adenosine triphosphate.[214] Positron emission tomography (PET) is able to provide a 3-dimensional picture of the biochemistry and physiology of human tissues.[215] In the CNS, PET can provide data on receptor status in various tissues and has been used to examine serotonin and dopamine receptors in localised areas such as the striatum. An alternative to PET is single-photon emission computed tomography (SPECT) which examines the computerised image of a tissue after a dose of a radiopharmaceutical.

**Table XXIII.** Factors affecting drug response in patients (after Lawrence[217])

| | |
|---|---|
| 1. | Pharmacodynamics of the drug |
| 2. | Pharmacokinetics of the drug |
| 3. | Potential drug interactions |
| 4. | Receptor sensitivity |
| 5. | Mood, personality and attitude of the patient |
| 6. | Mood, personality and attitude of the doctor |
| 7. | Doctor's explanation to the patient |
| 8. | Patient's prior experience of doctors and drugs |
| 9. | Patient's estimate of what ought to happen |
| 10. | Social environment of the patient |

This technique is less sensitive than PET but is more routinely available since a cyclotron is not needed. These new techniques have been successfully used to study the binding of antipsychotic drugs at different dose levels to dopamine receptors. Haloperidol, for example, has been found to saturate its binding sites at commonly used dosages.[216]

### 8.4 Adverse Effects

It is important to realise that not only the benefits of drug therapy, but also its adverse effects should be closely assessed, particularly in clinical trials. It is no longer acceptable to ask the patients if the tablets are upsetting them or if they have had any ill effects they attribute to the drug. Such non-specific questions should be accompanied by a self-administered questionnaire which can be completed by the patient. Such a questionnaire will list most of the adverse effects that have been linked with the particular drug under study and the patient will be asked to indicate their presence or absence. Such an approach reveals a much higher incidence of ill effects than traditional methods, not all of which will be associated with the drug. However, by comparison with a placebo or other treatment group, it will be much easier when studying numbers of patients to see which adverse effects are, and which are not, associated with the use of a particular drug.

## 9. Principles of Controlled Clinical Trials

There is no doubt that in good hands, the controlled clinical trial is a very powerful tool for the investigation of both new and old drugs. When a drug is administered to a patient, the response to it is dependent on a number of variable factors (table XXIII). The aims of a controlled clinical (therapeutic) trial are to standardise or minimise those factors as far as possible. Many considerations and much careful planning are necessary for the successful conduct of a clinical trial. This section is only intended as a very brief overview of some important general principles. For more detailed discussion, see chapter 11 and reviews by Good;[218] Harris & Fitzgerald;[219] and WHO.[220]

### 9.1 Initial Clinical Trials

When a new drug is first tested in humans, it is likely that the study will in fact be an open one, with little attempt to overcome bias. In some cases, the drug will be given to a healthy volunteer and the pharmacological response assessed by appropriate tests. In other cases, the drug will be given first to patients with the disease for which the drug has been developed. This is especially the case with new cytotoxic drugs. The drug is likely to be given to a very few individuals, perhaps 6 to 10, under closely supervised conditions. The main aim is to see if the pharmacodynamics and pharmacokinetics of the drug are similar to what has been predicted from preclinical studies. To this end, it is very useful if a method is already available for measuring plasma concentrations of the drug and its metabolites. This will help in achieving another goal of phase I studies, i.e. to get a preliminary idea about dose-response and concentration-effect relationships.

It is not a main aim at this stage to look for toxic effects, although comprehensive adverse effect and biochemical screening will be undertaken. The clinician has to satisfy him/herself that the animal toxicity studies are adequate to justify the risk of administering the drug for the first time to humans. However, there is no doubt that it is possible to waste too much time in testing a drug in animals before studying it in humans. The correct balance of information is difficult to achieve.[221]

### 9.2 Design of Clinical Trials

Much has been written about the need for clinical trials to be randomised and double-blind for reliable evaluation of the efficacy of treatments.[222] It is probably in the field of cancer that the randomised trial has attained its most sophisticated and rigid form.[223,224] In some situations, this design is unnecessary and unsuitable. Thus, in early drug studies in humans, the double-blind technique is not appropriate and in specialised techniques, where perhaps the rate of onset of a drug's action is being studied, the open study may be more appropriate, provided the observations are made as bias-free as possible. The requirements for adequate design of a trial depend on the disease and drug effect being investigated.

The aims of a clinical trial may vary from trial to trial but must always be very carefully formulated before the start of the study. The aim should be to answer *one* precisely framed question – with perhaps one or two subsidiary questions. The more questions that are posed initially, the more complicated the trial becomes, and the more likely is it that the trial will break down in practice. Questions that may be asked include: 'is this drug effective?'; 'how does it compare with other drugs?'; 'in what patients is it of value?'; and 'what is the most appropriate dosage?'

The clinical trial should be carried out in like or equivalent (homogeneous) groups of patients, so that the patients in each treatment group are as closely matched as possible for all known variables – such as age, sex, race, duration and severity of disease, etc. The best way of achieving homogeneous groups of patients is by random allocation – it is not acceptable to allot patients alternatively to the two treatments under test as the clinician will almost certainly become biased in his/her allocation of patients to the regimens. Once the decision to enter the patient into the trial is taken, the individual is allotted treatment A or B depending on an agreed randomisation schedule – such as the use of random number tables.

In some trials, it is important to stratify patients at random into evenly divided subgroups according to defined criteria that may affect outcome – such as trials in acute myocardial infarction in which patients are stratified according to the factors known to influence prognosis. Such stratification produces more homogeneous subgroups in which significant results may be obtained, that would otherwise be less apparent if only the group as a whole was considered. However, random allocation does not guarantee like groups and it is still necessary to show that the treatment groups are comparable. The larger the number of patients in each group or subgroup, the greater the chance that they will be reasonably well matched.

Treatments should ideally be carried out *concurrently* because diseases may vary in severity with time. However, consecutive or crossover studies are acceptable in some diseases where the severity of the disease is known to be relatively stable (e.g. hypertension).

Any ancillary treatments should be the same for each study group and should also be defined, since they may influence the outcome. This requires much coordination of treatments in multicentre (multiclinic) trials, in which it is also particularly important to achieve comparable groups both within and between centres.

The methods of assessment of the response should obviously be relevant to the aim of the trial and the drug effect being studied. The person who is to make the assessments (patient, clinician, auxiliary), their nature (subjective and/or objective), type (particularly in relation to statistical considerations), and timing (daily, weekly, etc. or before and after) require much consideration prior to commencing the trial.

Before the start of the trial, it is important to formulate as simple an aim as possible, to write out a detailed protocol, and to adhere to the protocol throughout the study. This latter requirement may seem trite but it is surprising how often the design of a trial is altered half way through because of an observation in an early patient. This may well destroy the results of the whole trial.

### 9.3 Use of Controls

Although in early clinical trials, controls may not be needed, it is vital to introduce control observations as soon as possible.[225] Controls may consist of patients receiving no treatment, a different treatment (active or inactive pharmacologically), or patients receiving the same treatment but at a different dose or according to a different schedule.

Whichever control method is used, it must be both valid and suitable in relation to the aim of the trial. Historical controls in most cases are not satisfactory, since with the passage of time, many variables may have changed the course of the disease or influenced outcome. Usually, the treatments are studied in comparable groups of patients over the same period of time. It is hoped that the groups will be large enough to minimise any interpatient variability. When the variability of disease between individuals is a cause for concern, it is sometimes useful to use a patient as his or her own control, provided the disease process is stable. Here each patient is exposed to every available treatment having first one and then the other. In such a crossover design, it is then important to ensure that each treatment

| | Treatment periods | | | |
|---|---|---|---|---|
| | 1 | 2 | 3 | 4 |
| Patient No. 1 | A | B | D | C |
| Patient No. 2 | B | C | A | D |
| Patient No. 3 | C | D | B | A |
| Patient No. 4 | D | A | C | B |

**Fig. 29.** 'Latin square' design to assign patients to treatments (*viz* A, B, C, D) so that each is as likely to precede as to follow each other.

both precedes and follows each other treatment the same number of times to avoid the risk of systematic bias or 'carry over' effect. It is sometimes necessary to include a control 'washout' period of adequate duration between active treatment periods. The most usual way to arrange this is the use of a 'latin square' design (fig. 29), where each treatment is as likely to precede as to follow each other.

Having decided to include a control, should a placebo or pharmacologically active medication be used? In some circumstances, it may be unethical to give a placebo medication (e.g. in epilepsy or tuberculosis) and thus comparison of the active drug is made not with a pharmacologically inert placebo preparation but with the best available therapy. If a placebo is used, it should match the active drug as closely as possible in colour, texture, shape and taste, as this will help to distinguish between the pharmacological effects of the drug and the psychological effects associated with the trial (e.g. more clinician interest, more frequent visits, etc.). It will also help to avoid false-positive and false-negative conclusions. It is important to realise that in clinical trials, an inert placebo will produce benefit in a certain proportion of patients and will produce adverse effects in some patients.[226,227] Placebos are not totally inactive; rather they are pharmacologically inactive.

### 9.4 Double-Blind Technique

Since both clinicians and patients are capable of bias due to previously held beliefs, the double-blind technique is used as a control device to prevent this bias from influencing the results. However, the use of a double-blind technique does not guarantee that the results of the trial will be either the whole truth or beyond reproach. Many factors other than the design of the trial influence the adequacy and interpretation of the results (see section 10.2). However, if a double-blind technique is used properly, it is a most useful way of assessing the therapeutic efficacy of a drug, since neither the patient nor the clinician will know the true nature of the medication that is taken until the end of the trial. The temptation to break open a code half way through a trial should be resisted, even with drop-outs, since it makes it more likely that the true nature of the other treatments will be discovered.

When two active drug treatments are compared, it is often difficult to arrange a double-blind study. It is tempting to arrange for drug A to be reformulated to make it appear to be identical to drug B. This, however, will mean that the bioavailability of drug A might be different from the original formulation and tests to ensure that this is not so, are necessary. It is easier to use a 'double dummy' technique where active drug A plus placebo drug B is compared with placebo drug A plus active drug B.

### 9.5 Statistical Considerations

It is possible only to consider this, as with many other aspects of controlled trials, in brief in this section. In designing a clinical trial, the initial hypothesis is usually that of 'no difference', i.e. that there is no difference between treatment A and treatment B. It then has to be decided if the results obtained could be due to chance or if there is a real probability of difference between the two treatments. In most cases, it can be assumed that the data are normally distributed and relatively simple statistical tests can be used. However, in some cases, the normal distribution does not apply and then more sophisticated statistics are necessary.

Before the start of a trial, it is usual to assume that a given level of probability (p) will be accepted. If p is less than 0.05, a difference would be found by chance only 5 times in every 100 studies. Thus, by implication, the null hypothesis would be considered wrong and the conclusion would be that a statistical difference existed between the treatments. In some cases, it may be preferred only to accept a result if p is less than 0.01. It is important to realise however, that even here, there is a 1 in 100 risk of the treatments being different by chance alone. Thus, it is not surprising that, with many similar trials being performed with a drug in different population groups and with a different design, results sometimes appear to be conflicting.

Sometimes too, results may be found that suggest that treatment A tends to be better than treatment B, but in statistical terms there is no

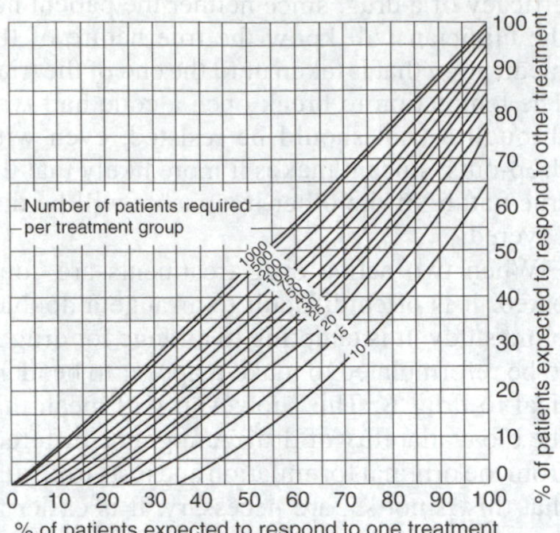


**Fig. 30.** Number of patients required for a clinical trial – assuming a minimum chance (50%) of successful conclusion at 5% level of significance ($p < 0.05$) [after Clark & Downie[229]]. The treatment with the greater response is plotted on the horizontal scale. The graph can be used as a guide to: (a) Indicate the smallest number of patients likely to provide results from which significant conclusions can be drawn; (b) Determine from the actual number of patients studied, whether the observed difference in response is large enough to be significant at the 5% level.

significant difference between them. This may be seen with small patient numbers. It should be noted that failure to find a difference between two treatments does not necessarily mean that they are equal, but rather that any difference which might exist could not be detected with the number of patients studied. It may sometimes mean (e.g. where the response rate is high with both treatments) that any difference is not of much clinical importance. On the other hand, a statistically significant difference between two treatments may not be *clinically* important (i.e. if the magnitude of the difference is not worthwhile), such as on average an extra 15 minutes duration of sleep between two hypnotics.[228] Similar considerations apply in bioavailability studies.

It must be emphasised that statistical analysis, however good, will not salvage a trial that is poorly designed or poorly conducted and based on insensitive methods for assessing the clinical effects.

## 9.6 Patient Numbers

It is often very difficult to know how many patients will be needed in a clinical trial in order that the result will be meaningful. In general, the mistake is to use too few patients. The smaller the expected difference between two treatments, the greater the number of patients required to achieve a significant result (fig. 30). The clinical investigator is best advised to consult with a statistician at the design stage of a trial. The statistician will need to know what magnitude of difference the clinician is interested in detecting (e.g. halving the death rate) and what risks he or she will tolerate of missing a difference that does genuinely exist. It is particularly difficult to obtain adequate numbers of patients in long term studies; for example, in the assessment of whether long term β-adrenoceptor blockade will reduce the death rate from myocardial infarction. The study of a few dozen patients can, in most cases, detect an ideal treat-

**Table XXIV.** Rational drug prescribing – decisions and considerations

**Decisions**

1. Diagnosis
   a) Accurate, or
   b) At least probable
2. Disease understanding
   a) Pathophysiology
   b) Natural history
3. To treat or not
   a) Is a drug necessary at all?
      i) no need to treat?
      ii) other form of treatment more appropriate?
   b) If a drug is necessary:
      i) what benefit is expected?
      ii) what harm may result from a drug?
      iii) what harm will result if a drug is not used?
4. Drug and regimen
   a) Choice of drug, preparation, route of administration
   b) Selection of an appropriate dosage and dose schedule (patient factors)
   c) Duration of treatment (nature of disease)

**Considerations**

1. Compatibility between drug and patient (adverse effects)
2. Compatibility between drugs (interactions)
3. Review decision in 4a, b above if necessary

**Action**

1. Write prescription (legibly)
2. Instruct the patient about:
   a) The therapeutic aim and that the potential benefit is expected to outweigh the risk of adverse effects
   b) Reporting and action to take on any important adverse effects
   c) How to take or use the medication (e.g. oral dose in relation to food, need to complete prescribed course, correct use of an asthma aerosol inhaler, etc.)
3. Follow-up
   a) Of symptoms; titration of dose
   b) Check compliance with medication instructions

ment which prevents more than two-thirds of the deaths. However, in cases like the example quoted, where the death rate is small, and the interest is in detecting a small reduction in the death rate, it will be necessary to follow several hundred patients over a number of years.

### 9.7 Sequential Analysis

This sophisticated technique has been widely used for trials in acute diseases and allows a trial to be continually monitored and to be stopped when a significant result is achieved. In this way, the numbers of patients involved can be kept to a minimum, and ethical objections can be best resolved. The most familiar of these procedures requires allocation of the study participants in pairs to two treatments.[230] Other designs have been developed which do not involve pairwise allocation.[231]

### 9.8 Ethical Considerations

In the conduct of a controlled clinical trial, whether in normal volunteers or patients, it is important to consider the ethical aspects of the study and nowadays, all protocols have to be vetted by an independent ethical review body. In addition, each participant in the study should give their informed consent to the study. Some of the important and vexed ethical aspects which can arise are considered in chapter 11. Scientific medical ethics are founded on the moral principles and standards of reason that are a part of ethics generally, and on the cumulative wisdom and experience of scientific knowledge and practice.[232]

### 9.9 Good Clinical Practice (GCP)

Compared with all other clinical research, clinical drug evaluation is heavily regulated by national health authorities. For a number of years, the World Health Organization and individual countries have developed guidelines for so-called good clinical practice (GCP) for trials on pharmaceutical products. The guidelines define the terminology used in clinical trials and lay down the responsibilities of the investigator and the sponsor. They also define the concept of monitoring clinical trials, as well as methods for quality assurance for conduct of clinical trials. These documents are in fact recommended reading for any physician involved in clinical drug evaluation and can be obtained from most national drug control agencies.

**Table XXV.** Principles of assessing reports of therapeutic trials

**1. Basic principles**

a) Any individual trial provides limited information – what happens in a selected group of patients under defined conditions

b) One study cannot provide all evidence – the answers to the many questions that may need to be considered in evaluating a drug cannot be provided by any one study

c) Statements made must be critically evaluated – statements made and conclusions drawn by authors cannot necessarily be accepted as read. Critical faculties must be maintained at all times

**2. Important general requirements**

a) Appropriate controls – were controls adequate (or not necessary) to avoid bias or reduce variation which might influence the results?

b) Appropriate and adequate methods of assessing therapeutic effects – were the methods fully defined, relevant to the aims and reproducible?

c) Adequate number of subjects – the smaller the difference between two drugs, the greater the number of patients required to achieve a significant result (failure to find a difference between two drugs does not necessarily mean that they are equal, but rather that any difference which might exist could not be detected with the number of patients used)

d) Homogeneous population – when two or more treatments are compared, were the groups sufficiently well matched? (*NB.* allocation of patients at random to treatment does not guarantee like groups)

e) Appropriate duration of treatment – was therapy sufficiently long for an optimum drug effect and for the nature of the disease?

f) Appropriate dosage – were dosages chosen adequate (if a dose-effect study) or comparable (if two drugs being compared)?

g) Measurement of adverse effects – were the methods of assessment adequate and with a defined protocol (the incidence of adverse effects depends on the care with which they are sought and how and by whom patients are interrogated)?

h) Appropriate statistical validation – where necessary (most trials fall down before this point is reached). *NB.* Elaborate statistics cannot validate a poorly designed or executed trial, make unlike treatment groups equal, or be used to extend the results obtained in a selected group of patients under defined conditions to individualised use of a drug in actual clinical practice

**3. Interpretation of results and conclusions**

a) Is the result clinically significant (would the patient benefit) or acceptable (does it satisfy *current* desirable criteria)?

b) Are comparisons with other drug trials (e.g. in the discussion) valid? – was a comparison made with the *currently* accepted treatment of choice? If so, was the comparison valid? If not, was such a comparison unnecessary or was a comparison made against a superseded treatment of choice? Is the discussion a fair review of reliable results?

c) Are the author's conclusions justified? – conclusions must be made on the basis of what has been established in the trial and not extended beyond these findings

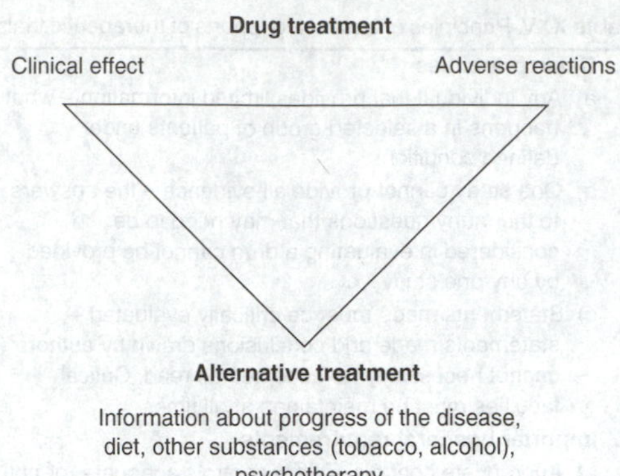


**Fig. 31.** The therapeutic triangle.

## 10. Clinical Pharmacological Principles in Drug Prescribing

### 10.1 The Drug Prescription

The decisions and considerations to be made in connection with the prescribing of modern drugs involve the same analytical principles as does sophisticated differential diagnosis (see table XXIV).[233-235] Yet, the prescription is traditionally made in a hurry at the very last moment of the consultation or at the crowded time of discharge from hospital, with insufficient time left for informing the patient about the therapeutic aims or for providing appropriate instructions in use of the medication.[236,237] Worse than this, the illegibility of prescriptions is a well known joke, even within the medical profession. It is high time to change these poor habits.

The causes of unnecessary, unsuitable or ineffective therapy include inadequacy of time and facilities available for proper diagnosis, ignorance of the cause and natural history of disease, inadequacies of teaching in clinical pharmacology and drug evaluation, ineffectiveness of official advice about drug usage relative to that given by the industry, and pressures exerted by patients and colleagues.[238,239] Many patients expect a remedy for any symptom and it is the clinician's duty to explain to them that drugs are not needed for self-limiting diseases or short-lasting minor symptoms of unknown nature. It is a regrettable fact that many prescriptions in these situations come to resemble conditioned reflexes. It is even more regrettable that many drugs are used in a stereotyped manner, in fixed, often too low dosage schedules, and with little regard for the basic principles of pharmacokinetics and drug response. It is also important to realise that in several instances, alternative treatment may be the correct therapeutic choice. Drug treatment with its benefits and risks should always be compared with the outcome of alternative treatment (fig. 31).

### 10.2 Assessing Reports of Therapeutic Trials

New drugs are not necessarily better than older ones, but they are almost always more expensive. Unexpected and important adverse effects can still occur after marketing of a new drug, even though it has complied with all the required tests. Familiarity with the use of a particular drug is a valid reason for continuing to use it until adequate and convincing reasons for change are apparent. Such evidence is generally

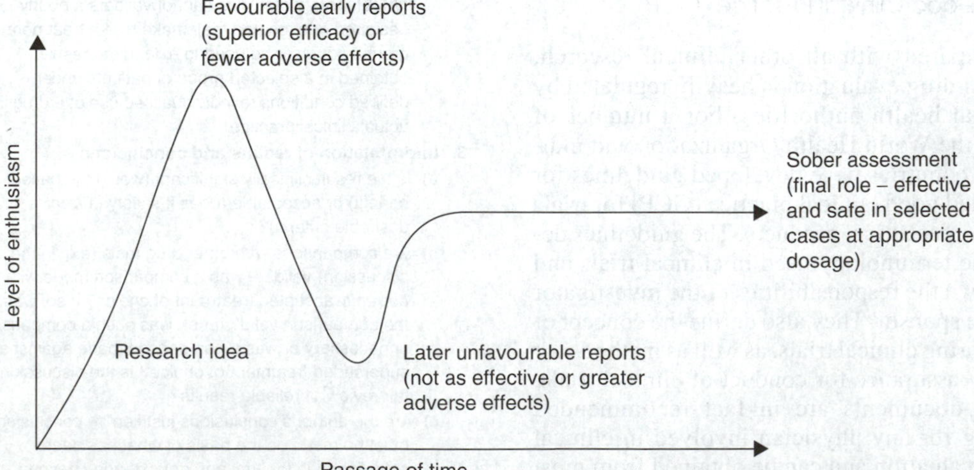


**Fig. 32.** Enthusiasm and therapeutic role for a new drug with the passage of time.

based on the results of therapeutic trials, but these must be evaluated critically (table XXV) because clinical trials vary greatly in quality and value.[240] Statements made cannot necessarily be accepted as read.

The fundamental problem with assessment of drug literature lies in the varying acceptability of published reports and in the subsequent interpretation and use of the data. Many factors, apart from study design (see section 9), may influence data in therapeutic trials. For example, even if randomisation was made, were the treatment groups reasonably well matched?; were doses of the drugs under study equivalent?; were patient numbers large enough to detect any differences?; was the drug taken as intended?; who made the observations and how were they made, etc.?[240] Also, it should be borne in mind that the enthusiasm for a new drug generally changes with the passage of time, and thus the nature and quality of evidence depends on the adequacy of studies and extent of actual clinical experience at any given time of publication (fig. 32).

As discussed in section 8, in its most rigorous form, a therapeutic trial to establish the efficacy of a new drug demands homogeneous groups of patients, concurrently treated in different ways (i.e. other standard drug or treatment). The less the differences within the groups and between them (apart from the treatment), the better the design of the trial. What constitutes an adequately designed trial necessarily varies, depending on the disease and drug effect being evaluated. Each trial however, affords precise and limited information and can only show what on average is likely to happen to a selected group of patients under defined conditions. Indeed, the more rigid the methodology of the trial, the more artificial the conditions are likely to be and the narrower the general applicability of the results.

These limitations must be borne in mind when extending the results (efficacy or adverse effects) of a particular therapeutic trial to clinical practice. Thus, many trials are conducted under conditions that are far removed from those in which drugs are ultimately used, and it is a major objective for the future to evaluate drugs and monitor drug use under actual conditions of practice.[241] There is an important balance between clinical sense and clinical science.[242]

### 10.3 Utilisation of Existing Drugs and Individualisation of Therapy

Better utilisation of existing drugs and individualisation of drug therapy have increased in importance for three reasons:

1) The development of new, effective drugs is becoming more difficult, because the pharmaceutical industry is facing complex and far reaching demands from governmental health authorities regarding the documentation of drug safety and efficacy.

2) There is a tendency among patients and pressure groups to be sceptical about drugs and their usage by clinicians, particularly the use of unnecessarily expensive drugs.

3) As outlined in this chapter, clinical pharmacological research has shown that much of the variability in drug response between patients can be explained by individual pharmacodynamic and pharmacokinetic factors.

## Further Reading

Gibaldi M. Biopharmaceutics and clinical pharmacokinetics. 4th ed. Philadelphia: Lea and Febiger, 1991

Grahame-Smith DG, Aronson JK. Oxford textbook of clinical pharmacology and drug therapy. 2nd edition. Oxford: Oxford University Press, 1992

Pratt WB, Taylor P. Principles of drug action: the basis of pharmacology. 3rd ed. New York: Churchill Livingstone, 1990

Hardman JGG, Gilman A, et al. editors. Goodman and Gilman's The pharmacological basis of therapeutics. 9th ed. New York: McGraw Hill, 1995

Laurence DR, Bennett PN. Clinical pharmacology. 7th ed. Edinburgh: Churchill Livingstone, 1992

Melmon KL, Morrelli HF. Clinical pharmacology: basic principles in therapeutics. 3rd ed. New York: McMillan, 1991

## References

1. Garrett ER. The physico-chemical and pharmacokinetic basis for the biopharmaceutical evaluation of drug biological availability in pharmaceutical formulations. Acta Pharmacologica et Toxicologica 1971; 29 Suppl. 3: 1
2. Keberle H. Physico-chemical factors of drugs affecting absorption, distribution, and excretion. Acta Pharmacologica et Toxicologica 1971; 29 Suppl. 3: 30
3. Duggan DE. The accumulation of chlorothiazide and related saluretic agents by isolated renal tubules. Journal of Pharmacology and Experimental Therapeutics 1966; 152: 122
4. Brodie BB, Binns, editors. Absorption and distribution of drugs. London: Livingstone, 1964
5. Kenskin T. Drugs and receptors: an overview of the current state of knowledge. Drugs 1990; 40: 666
6. Snyder S. Receptors, neurotransmitters and drug responses. New England Journal of Medicine 1979; 300: 465

7. Meffin PJ, Birkett DJ, Wing LMH. Fundamentals of clinical pharmacology. 2: how drugs act. Current Therapeutics 1979; 20: 87
8. Gibaldi M. Biopharmaceutics and clinical pharmacokinetics. 2nd ed. Philadelphia: Lea and Febiger, 1977
9. Back DJ, Breckenridge AM, Crawford FE, et al. Kinetics of norethindrone in women: II. Single-dose kinetics. Clinical Pharmacology and Therapeutics 1978; 24: 448
10. Beermann B, Hellström K, Lindström B, et al. Binding site interaction of chlorthalidone and acetazolamide, two drugs transported by red cells. Clinical Pharmacology and Therapeutics 1974; 17: 424
11. Benet LZ, Galeazzi RL. Non-concentrated determination of the steady-state volume of distribution. Journal of Pharmaceutical Sciences 1979; 68: 1071
12. O'Reilly RA, Ageler PM, Leong LS. Studies on the coumarin anticoagulant drugs: a comparison of the pharmacodynamics of dicoumarol and warfarin in man. Thrombosis et Diathesis Haemorrhagica 1964; 11: 1
13. Rowland M. Drug administration and regimens. In: Melmon & Morrelli, editors. Clinical pharmacology, basic principles in therapeutics. 1st ed. New York: Macmillan, 1972: 21
14. Alexanderson B. Pharmacokinetics of desmethylimipramine and nortriptyline in man after single and multiple oral doses – a crossover study. European Journal of Clinical Pharmacology 1972; 5: 1
15. Karlsson E. Clinical pharmacokinetics of procainamide. Clinical Pharmacokinetics 1978; 3: 97
16. Bertilsson L. Clinical pharmacokinetics of carbamazepine. Clinical Pharmacokinetics 1978; 3: 128
17. Lennernäs H, Ahrenstedt O, Ungell AL. Intestinal drug absorption during induced net water absorption in man: a mechanistic study using antipyrine, atenolol and enalaprilat. British Journal of Clinical Pharmacology 1994; 37: 589
18. Bochner F, Hooper WD, Tyrer JH, et al. Factors involved in an outbreak of phenytoin intoxication. Journal of the Neurological Sciences 1972; 16: 481
19. Neuvonen PJ. Bioavailability of phenytoin: clinical pharmacokinetic and therapeutic implications. Clinical Pharmacokinetics 1979; 4: 91
20. Neuvonen PJ, Kivistö KT, Lehto P. Interference of dairy products with the absorption of ciprofloxacin. Clinical Pharmacology and Therapeutics 1991; 50: 498
21. Boman G, Lundgren P, Stjernström G. Mechanism of the inhibitory effect of PAS granules on the absorption of rifampicin: adsorption of rifampicin by an excipient, bentonite. European Journal of Clinical Pharmacology 1975; 8: 293
22. Melander A. Influence of food on the bioavailability of drugs. Clinical Pharmacokinetics 1978; 3: 337
23. Hendeles L, Weinberger M, Milaretz G, et al. Food-induced 'dose dumping' from a once a day theophylline product as a cause of theophylline toxicity. Chest 1985; 87: 758
24. Milton KA, Edwards G, Ward SA, et al. Pharmacokinetics of halofantrine in man – effects of food and dose size. British Journal of Clinical Pharmacology 1989; 28: 71-7
25. Van Hoogdalem EJ, de Boer AG, Breimer DD. Pharmacokinetics of rectal drug administration (Pts I and II). Clinical Pharmacokinetics 1991; 21: 11 and 110
26. Motwani JG, Lipworth BJ. Clinical pharmacokinetics of drugs administered buccally and sublingually. Clinical Pharmacokinetics 1991; 21: 83
27. Pontiroli AE, Calderara A, Pozza G. Intranasal drug delivery – potential advantages and limitations from a clinical pharmacokinetic perspective. Clinical Pharmacokinetics 1989; 17: 299
28. Wester RC, Maibach HI. Percutaneous absorption of drugs. Clinical Pharmacokinetics 1992; 23: 253
29. Ridout G, Santus GC, Guy RH. Pharmacokinetic considerations in the use of newer transdermal formulations. Clinical Pharmacokinetics 1988; 15: 114
30. Banerjee PS, Robinson JR. Novel drug delivery systems: an overview of their impact on clinical pharmacokinetic studies. Clinical Pharmacokinetics 1991; 20: 1
31. Theeuwes F, Swanson DR, Guittard G, et al. Osmotic delivery systems for the β-adrenoceptor antagonists metoprolol and oxprenolol: design and evaluation of systems for once-daily administration. British Journal of Clinical Pharmacology 1985; 19: 69S
32. Gregoriadis G, Florence AT. Liposomes in drug delivery: clinical diagnostic and ophthalmic potential. Drugs 1993; 45: 15
33. Kroin JS. Intrathecal drug administration: present use and future trends. Clinical Pharmacokinetics 1992; 22: 319
34. Blaschke TF. Protein binding and kinetics of drugs in liver disease. Clinical Pharmacokinetics 1977; 2: 32
35. Jusko WJ, Gretch M. Plasma and tissue protein binding of drugs in pharmacokinetics. Drug Metabolism Reviews 1976; 5: 43
36. Sjöholm I, Ekman B, Kober A, et al. Binding of drugs to human serum albumin: XI. The specificity of three binding sites as studied with albumin immobilized in microparticles. Molecular Pharmacology 1979; 16: 767
37. Sudlow G. The specificity of binding sites on serum albumin. Proceedings of the 7th International Congress on Pharmacology, Paris, 1978. Oxford: Pergamon, 1979
38. Storstein L. The effect of heparin on serum protein binding of digitoxin and digoxin. Clinical Pharmacology and Therapeutics 1976; 20: 15
39. Nilsen OG, Storstein L, Jacobsen S. Effect of heparin and fatty acids on the binding of quinidine and warfarin in plasma. Biochemical Pharmacology 1977; 26: 229
40. Lapicque F, Muller N, Payan E, et al. Protein binding and stereoselectivity of non-steroidal anti-inflammatory drugs. Clinical Pharmacokinetics 1993; 25: 115
41. Borgå O, Piafsky KM, Nilsen OG. Plasma protein binding of basic drugs: I. Selective displacement from $\alpha_1$-acid glycoprotein by tris(2-butoxyethyl) phosphate. Clinical Pharmacology and Therapeutics 1977; 22: 539
42. Fremstad D, Bergerud K, Haffner JFW, et al. Increased protein binding of quinidine after surgery: a preliminary report. European Journal of Clinical Pharmacology 1976; 10: 441
43. Martin BK. Potential effect of the plasma proteins on drug distribution. Nature 1965; 207: 274
44. Øie S, Tozer TN. Effect of altered plasma protein binding on apparent volume of distribution. Journal of Pharmaceutical Sciences 1979; 68: 1203
45. Rowland M, Tozer TN. Clinical pharmacokinetics: concepts and application, 3rd ed. Baltimore: Williams & Wilkins, 1995: 166
46. Mattson RH, Cramer JA, Williamson PD, et al. Valproic acid in epilepsy: clinical and pharmacological effects. Annals of Neurology 1978; 3: 20
47. Odar-Cederlöf I, Borgå O. Kinetics of diphenylhydantoin in uraemic patients: consequences of decreased

plasma protein binding. European Journal of Clinical Pharmacology 1974; 7: 31
48. Penner JA, Abbrecht PH. Lack of interaction between ibuprofen and warfarin. Current Therapeutic Research 1975; 18: 862
49. Hansen JM, Christensen LK. Drug interactions with oral sulphonylurea hypoglycaemic drugs. Drugs 1977; 13: 24
50. Barre J, Riant P, Tillement JP. Measurement of free drug in phase I: is it useful? Fundamental and Clinical Pharmacology 1990; 4 Suppl. 2: 141s
51. Nordin C, Bertilsson L, Siwers B. Clinical and biochemical effects during treatment of depression with nortriptyline: the role of 10-hydroxynortriptyline. Clinical Pharmacology and Therapeutics 1987; 42: 10
52. Williams K, Lee E. Importance of drug enantiomers in clinical pharmacology. Drugs 1985; 30: 333
53. Drayer DE. Pharmacodynamic and pharmacokinetic differences between drug enantiomers in humans: an overview. Clinical Pharmacology and Therapeutics 1986; 40: 125
54. Mellström B, Bertilsson L, Säwe J, et al. E- and Z-hydroxylation of nortriptyline in man – relationship to polymorphic hydroxylation of debrisoquine. Clinical Pharmacology and Therapeutics 1981; 30: 190
55. Connolly EM, Davies DS, Dollery CT, et al. Metabolism of isoprenaline in dog and man. British Journal of Pharmacology 1972; 46: 458-72
56. Johnsson G, Regårdh C-G. Clinical pharmacokinetics of β-adrenoceptor blocking drugs. Clinical Pharmacokinetics 1976; 1: 233
57. Bennett PN, Aarons LJ, Bending MR, et al. Pharmacokinetics of lidocaine and its deethylated metabolite: dose and time dependency studies in man. Journal of Pharmacokinetics and Biopharmaceutics 1982; 10: 265-81
58. Kroemer HK, Klotz U. Glucuronidation of drugs: a reevaluation of the pharmacological significance of the conjugates and modulating factors. Clinical Pharmacokinetics 1992; 23: 292
59. Kolars JC, Awni WM, Merion RM, et al. First-pass metabolism of cyclosporin by the gut. Lancet 1991; 338: 1488
60. Hebert MF, Roberts JP, Prueksaritanont T, et al. Bioavailability of cyclosporine with concomitant rifampin administration is markedly less than predicted by hepatic enzyme induction. Clinical Pharmacology and Therapeutics 1992; 52: 453
61. Gupta SK, Bakran A, Johnson RWG, et al. Cyclosporin-erythromycin interaction in renal transplant patients. British Journal of Clinical Pharmacology 1989; 27: 475
62. Crossland J. Modern views on pharmacology. II. Drug metabolism. Practitioner 1971; 206: 293
63. Nelson DR, Kamataki T, Waxman DJ, et al. The P450 superfamily – update on new sequences, gene mapping, accession numbers, early trivial names of enzymes, and nomenclature. DNA and Cell Biology 1993; 12: 1
64. Gonzalez FJ. Human cytochromes P450: problems and prospects. Trends in Pharmacological Sciences 1992; 13: 346
65. Shimada T, Yamazaki H, Mimura M, et al. Interindividual variations in human liver cytochrome P450 enzymes involved in the oxidation of drugs, carcinogens and toxic chemicals: studies with liver microsomes of 30 Japanese and 30 Caucasians. Journal of Pharmacology and Experimental Therapeutics 1994; 270: 414
66. Tephly TR, Burchell B. UDP-glucuronosyltransferases: a family of detoxifying enzymes. Trends in Pharmacological Sciences 1990; 11: 276
67. Pelkonen O. Prenatal and neonatal development of drug and carcinogen metabolism. In: Estabrook & Lindenlaub, editors. The induction of drug metabolism. Symposia Medica Hoechst 14. Stuttgart: Schattauer Verlag, 1979: 507
68. Rane A, Sjöqvist F, Orrenius S. Drugs and fetal metabolism. Clinical Pharmacology and Therapeutics 1973; 14: 666
69. Woodhouse KW, Wynne HA. Age-related changes in liver size and hepatic blood flow: the influence of drug metabolism in the elderly. Clinical Pharmacokinetics 1988; 15: 287
70. Wilson K. Sex-related differences in drug disposition in man. Clinical Pharmacokinetics 1984; 9: 189
71. Harris RZ, Benet LZ, Schwartz JB. Gender effects in pharmacokinetics and pharmacodynamics. Drugs 1995; 50: 222-39
72. Stoehr GR, Kroboth PD, Juhl RP, et al. Effect of oral contraceptives on triazolam, temazepam, alprazolam and lorazepam kinetics. Clinical Pharmacology and Therapeutics 1984; 36: 683
73. Högstedt S, Lindberg B, Peng DR, et al. Pregnancy-induced increase in metoprolol metabolism. Clinical Pharmacology and Therapeutics 1985; 37: 688
74. Gonzalez FJ, Liu SY, Yano M. Regulation of cytochrome P450 genes: molecular mechanisms. Pharmacogenetics 1993; 3: 51
75. Alvares AP. Interactions between environmental chemicals and drug biotransformation in man. Clinical Pharmacokinetics 1978; 3: 462
76. Jusko WJ. Role of tobacco smoking in pharmacokinetics. Journal of Pharmacokinetics and Biopharmaceutics 1978; 6: 7
77. Ogilvie RI. Clinical pharmacokinetics of theophylline. Clinical Pharmacokinetics 1978; 3: 267
78. Bertilsson L, Carrillo JA, Dahl ML, et al. Clozapine disposition covaries with CYP1A2 activity determined by a caffeine test. British Journal of Clinical Pharmacology 1994; 38: 471-3
79. Haring C, Meise U, Humpel C, et al. Dose-related plasma levels of clozapine: influence of smoking behaviour, sex and age. Psychopharmacology 1989; 99: S38
80. Jeffery WH, Ahlin TA, Goren C, et al. Loss of warfarin effect after occupational insecticide exposure. Journal of the American Medical Association 1976; 236: 2881
81. Conney AH, Pantuck EJ, Hsiao KC, et al. Enhanced phenacetin metabolism in humans fed charcoal broiled beef. Clinical Pharmacology and Therapeutics 1976; 20: 633
82. Conney AH, Pantuck EJ, Pantuck CB, et al. Role of environment and diet in the regulation of human drug metabolism. In: Estrabrook & Lindenlaub, editors. The induction of drug metabolism. Stuttgart: Schattauer Verlag, 1979
83. Anderson KE, Kappas A. Dietary regulation of cytochrome P450. Annual Review of Nutrition 1991; 11: 141
84. Pantuck EJ, Pantuck CB, Garland WA, et al. Stimulatory effect of brussels sprouts and cabbage on human drug metabolism. Clinical Pharmacology and Therapeutics 1979; 25: 88
85. Krishnaswamy K. Drug metabolism and pharmacokinetics in malnutrition. Clinical Pharmacokinetics 1978; 3: 216

86. Bailey DG, Arnold JMO, Spence JD. Grape fruit juice and drugs: how significant is the interaction? Clinical Pharmacokinetics 1994; 26: 91
87. Park BK, Breckenridge AM. Clinical implications of enzyme induction and enzyme inhibition. Clinical Pharmacokinetics 1981; 6: 1
88. Zilly W, Breimer DD, Richter E. Pharmacokinetic interactions with rifampicin. Clinical Pharmacokinetics 1977; 2: 61
89. Bock KW, Bock-Hennig BS. Differential induction of human liver UDP-glucuronosyltransferase activities by phenobarbital-type inducers. Biochemical Pharmacology 1987; 36: 4137
90. Lennard MS. Genetically determined adverse drug reactions involving metabolism. Drug Safety 1993; 9: 60
91. Jerling M, Lindström L, Bondesson U, et al. Fluvoxamine inhibition and carbamazepine induction of the metabolism of clozapine: evidence from a therapeutic drug monitoring service. Therapeutic Drug Monitoring 1994; 16: 368
92. Reinberg A, Smolensky MH. Circadian changes of drug disposition in man. Clinical Pharmacokinetics 1982; 7: 401
93. Cipolle RJ, Canafax DM, Rabatin J, et al. Time dependent disposition of cyclosporine after pancreas transplantation and application of chronopharmacokinetics to improve immunosuppression. Pharmacotherapy 1988; 8: 47
94. Hrushesky WJ, Von Roemeling R, Fraley EE, et al. Circadian-based infusion chronochemotherapy controls progressive metastatic renal cell carcinoma. Seminars in Surgical Oncology 1988; 4: 110
95. Caffruny EL. Renal tubular handling of drugs. American Journal of Medicine 1977; 62: 491
96. Arvidsson A, Borgå O, Alván G. Renal excretion of cephapirin and cephaloridine: evidence for saturable tubular reabsorption. Clinical Pharmacology and Therapeutics 1979; 25: 870
97. Orme ML'E, Back DJ, Breckenridge AM. Clinical pharmacokinetics of oral contraceptive steroids. Clinical Pharmacokinetics 1983; 8: 95
98. Bloom PM, Nelp WP. Relationship of the excretion of tritiated digoxin to renal function. American Journal of the Medical Sciences 1966; 251: 133
99. Odar-Cederlöf I, Vessman J, Alvan G, et al. Oxazepam disposition in uremic patients. Acta Pharmacologica et Toxicologica 1977; 40 (Suppl. 1): 52-62
100. Hedman A, Angelin B, Arvidsson A, et al. Digoxin-verapamil interaction: reduction of biliary but not of renal digoxin clearance in humans. Clinical Pharmacology and Therapeutics 1991; 49: 256
101. Sheiner LB, Stanski DR, Vozeh S, et al. Simultaneous modeling of pharmacokinetics and pharmacodynamics: application to d-tubocurarine. Clinical Pharmacology and Therapeutics 1979; 25: 358-71
102. Alván G. Individual differences in the disposition of drugs metabolised in the body. Clinical Pharmacokinetics 1978; 3: 155
103. Alexanderson B, Sjöqvist G. Individual differences in the pharmacokinetics of monomethylated tricyclic antidepressants: role of genetic and environmental factors and clinical importance. Annals of the New York Academy of Sciences 1971; 179: 739
104. Sjöqvist F, von Bahr C. Interindividual differences in drug oxidation: clinical importance. Drug Metabolism and Disposition: The Biological Fate of Chemicals 1973; 1: 469
105. Bertilsson L, Åberg-Wistedt A. The debrisoquine hydroxylation test predicts steady state plasma levels of desipramine. British Journal of Clinical Pharmacology 1983; 15: 388
106. Grundin R, Moldeus P, Orrenius S, et al. The possible role of cytochrome P-450 in the liver 'first pass elimination' of a β-receptor blocking drug. Acta Pharmacologica et Toxicologica 1974; 35: 242
107. Alván G, Piafsky K, Lind M, et al. Effect of pentobarbital on the disposition of alprenolol. Clinical Pharmacology and Therapeutics 1977; 22: 316
108. Wilkinson GR, Shand DG. A physiological approach to hepatic drug clearance. Clinical Pharmacology and Therapeutics 1975; 18: 377
109. Nies AS, Shand DG, Wilkinson GR. Altered hepatic blood flow and drug disposition. Clinical Pharmacokinetics 1976; 1: 135
110. Motulsky A. Drug reactions, enzymes and biochemical genetics. Journal of the American Medical Association 1957; 165: 835
111. Kalow W. Pharmacogenetics: heredity and the response to drugs. Philadelphia: WB Saunders, 1962
112. Evans DAP, Manley GA, McKusick VA. Genetic control of isoniazid metabolism in man. British Medical Journal 1960; 2: 485
113. Vesell ES. Pharmacogenetics: multiple interactions between genes and environment as determinants of drug response. American Journal of Medicine 1979; 66: 183
114. Kalow W, Kadar D, Inaba T, et al. A case of deficiency of N-hydroxylation of amobarbital. Clinical Pharmacology and Therapeutics 1977; 21: 530
115. Tang BK, Kalow W, Inaba T, et al. Variation in amobarbital metabolism: evaluation of a simplified population study. Clinical Pharmacology and Therapeutics 1983; 34: 202
116. Kutt H, Wolk M, Scherman R, et al. Insufficient parahydroxylation as a cause of diphenylhydantoin toxicity. Neurology 1964; 14: 542
117. Hanngren A, Borgå O, Sjöqvist F. Inactivation of isoniazid (INH) in Swedish tuberculous patients before and during treatment with para-aminosaalicylic acid (PAS). Scandinavian Journal of Respiratory Diseases 1970; 51: 61
118. Iselius L, Evans DAP. Formal genetics of isoniazid metabolism in man. Clinical Pharmacokinetics 1983; 8: 541
119. Weber WW, Hein DW. N-Acetylation pharmacogenetics. Pharmacological Reviews 1985; 37: 25
120. Grant DM. Molecular genetics of the N-acetyltransferases. Pharmacogenetics 1993; 3: 45
121. Hammer W, Sjöqvist F. Plasma levels of monoethylated tricyclic antidepressants during treatment with imipramine like compounds. Life Sciences 1967; 6: 1895
122. Alexanderson B, Evans DA, Sjöqvist G. Steady-state plasma levels of nortriptyline in twins: influence of genetic factors and drug therapy. British Medical Journal 1969; 4: 764
123. Alexanderson B. Prediction of steady-state plasma levels of nortriptyline from single oral dose kinetics: a study in twins. European Journal of Clinical Pharmacology 1973; 6: 44
124. Alexanderson B, Sjöqvist G. Pharmacokinetic and genetic studies of nortriptyline and desmethylimipramine in man: the predictability of therapeutic plasma levels from single-dose plasma concentration data. In: Okita & Acheson, editors. Pharmacology and the future of man. Proceedings of the 5th International Congress of Pharmacology, Vol. 3. Basel: Karger, 1973: 150

125. Mahgoub A, Idel JR, Dring LG, et al. Polymorphic hydroxylation of debrisoquine in man. Lancet 1977; 2: 584
126. Tucker GT, Silas JH, Iyn AO, et al. Polymorphic hydroxylation of debrisoquine in man [letter]. Lancet 1977; 2: 718
127. Eichelbaum M, Spannbrucker N, Dengler HJ. A probably genetic defect of the metabolism of sparteine. In: Gorrod, editor. Biological oxidation of nitrogen. Amsterdam: Elsevier/North Holland Biomedical Press, 1978: 113
128. Spina E, Birgersson C, von Bahr C, et al. Phenotypic consistency in the hydroxylation of desmethylimipramine and debrisoquine in healthy subjects and in human liver microsomes. Clinical Pharmacology and Therapeutics 1984; 36: 677
129. Bertilsson L, Lou YQ, Du YL, et al. Pronounced differences between native Chinese and Swedish populations in the polymorphic hydroxylations of debrisoquine and S-mephenytoin. Clinical Pharmacology and Therapeutics 1992; 51: 388
130. Price Evans DA, Mahgoub A, Sloan TP, et al. A family and population study of the genetic polymorphism of debrisoquine oxidation in a white British population. Journal of Medical Genetics 1980; 17: 102
131. Alván G, Bechtel P, Iselius L, et al. Hydroxylation polymorphisms of debrisoquine and mephenytoin in European populations. European Journal of Clinical Pharmacology 1990; 39: 533
132. Steiner E, Iselius L, Alván G, et al. A family study of genetic and environmental factors determining polymorphic hydroxylation of debrisoquine in man. Clinical Pharmacology and Therapeutics 1985; 38: 394
133. Meyer UA, Skoda RC, Zanger UM, et al. The genetic polymorphism of debrisoquine/sparteine metabolism. Molecular mechanisms. In: Kalow W, editor. Pharmacogenetics of drug metabolism. New York: Pergamon Press, 1992: 609-23
134. Bertilsson L, Dahl ML, Ingelman-Sundberg M, et al. Interindividual and interethnic differences in polymorphic drug oxidation – implications for drug therapy with focus on psychoactive drugs. In: Pacifici GM, Fracchia GN, editors. Advances in drug metabolism in man. Luxembourg: European Commission, 1995: 85-136
135. Johansson I, Lundqvist E, Bertilsson L, et al. Inherited amplification of an active gene in the cytochrome P450 *CYP2D* locus as a cause of ultrarapid metabolism of debrisoquine. Proceedings of the National Academy of Sciences of the United States of America 1993; 90: 11825
136. Dahl M-L, Johansson I, Bertilsson L, et al. Ultrarapid hydroxylation of debrisoquine in a Swedish population: analysis of the molecular genetic basis. Journal of Pharmacology and Experimental Therapeutics 1995; 274: 516
137. Dahl-Puustinen ML, Liden A, Alm C, et al. Disposition of perphenazine is related to polymorphic debrisoquine hydroxylation in human beings. Clinical Pharmacology and Therapeutics 1989; 46: 78-81
138. Eichelbaum M, Gross AS. The genetic polymorphism of debrisoquine/sparteine metabolism – clinical aspects. Pharmacology and Therapeutics 1990; 46: 377
139. Dahl ML, Bertilsson L. Genetically variable metabolism of antidepressants and neuroleptic drugs in man. Pharmacogenetics 1993; 3: 61
140. Lennard MS, Tucker GT, Silas JH, et al. Differential steroselective metabolism of metoprolol in extensive and poor debrisoquine metabolisers. Clinical Pharmacology and Therapeutics 1983; 34: 732
141. Lennard MS, Tucker GT, Woods HF. The polymorphic oxidation of β-adrenoceptor antagonists: clinical pharmacokinetic considerations. Clinical Pharmacokinetics 1986; 11:
142. Küpfer A, Preisig R. Pharmacogenetics of mephenytoin: a new drug hydroxylation polymorphism in man. European Journal of Clinical Pharmacology 1984; 26: 753
143. Goldstein JA, Faletto MB, Romkes-Sparkes M, et al. Evidence that CYP2C19 is the major (S)-mephenytoin 4'-hydroxylase in humans. Biochemistry 1994; 33: 1743
144. Wilkinson GR, Guengerich FP, Branch RA. Genetic polymorphism of S-mephenytoin hydroxylation. Pharmacology and Therapeutics 1989; 43: 53
145. Ward SA, Helsby NA, Skjelbo E, et al. The activation of the biguanide antimalarial proguanil co-segregates with the mephenytoin oxidation polymorphism: a panel study. British Journal of Clinical Pharmacology 1991; 31: 689
146. Wood AJJ, Zhou HH. Ethnic differences in drug disposition and responsiveness. Clinical Pharmacokinetics 1991; 20: 350
147. Kalow W. Interethnic variation of drug metabolism. Trends in Pharmacological Sciences 1991; 12: 102
148. Kalow W, Bertilsson L. Interethnic factors affecting drug response. Advances in Drug Research 1994; 25: 1
149. Masimirembwa CM. Pharmacogenetics of drug metabolizing enzymes in a black African population. MD Thesis. Stockholm: Karolinska Institute, 1995
150. Jeanes CWL, Schaefer O, Eidus L. Inactivation of isoniazid by Canadian Eskimos and Indians. Canadian Medical Association Journal 1972; 106: 331
151. Ahsan CH, Renwick AG, Macklin B, et al. Ethnic differences in the pharmacokinetics of oral nifedipine. British Journal of Clinical Pharmacology 1991; 31: 399
152. Yue QY, Svensson J-O, Alm C, et al. Interindividual and interethnic differences in the demethylation and glucuronidation of codeine. British Journal of Clinical Pharmacology 1989; 28: 627
153. La Du BN. Human serum paraoxonase/arylesterase. In: Kalow W, editor. Pharmacogenetics of drug metabolism. New York: Pergamon Press, 1992: 51-91
154. Agarwal DP, Goedde HW. Pharmacogenetics of alcohol dehydrogenase. In: Kalow W, editor. Pharmacogenetics of drug metabolism. New York: Pergamon Press, 1992: 263-80
155. Prescott LF. Pathological and physiological factors affecting drug absorption, distribution, elimination and response in man. In: Gillette & Mitchell, editors. Handbook of experimental pharmacology: concepts in biochemical pharmacology, part 3. Berlin: Springer-Verlag, 1975: 234
156. Grimmer SFM, Back DJ, Orme ML'E, et al. The in-vitro mucosal conjugation of ethinyloestradiol and the bioavailability of oral contraceptive steroids in patients with treated and untreated coeliac disease. Alimentary Pharmacology and Therapeutics 1992; 6: 79-85
157. Hayes AH. Intravenous infusion of lidocaine in the control of ventricular arrhythmias. In: Scott & Julian, editors. Lidocaine in the treatment of ventricular arrhythmias. Edinburgh: Livingstone, 1971: 189
158. Zini R, Riant P, Barre J, et al. Disease induced variations in plasma protein levels: implications for drug dosage regimens (Pts I and II). Clinical Pharmacokinetics 1990; 19: 147 and 218

159. Walker PC. Neonatal bilirubin toxicity: a review of kernicterus and the implications of drug induced bilirubin displacement. Clinical Pharmacokinetics 1987; 13: 26
160. Reidenberg MM, Drayer DE. Alterations of drug-protein binding in renal disease. Clinical Pharmacokinetics 1984; 9 Suppl. 1: 18
161. Sjöholm I, Kober A, Odar-Cederlöf I, et al. Protein binding of drugs in uraemic and normal serum: the role of endogenous binding inhibitors. Biochemical Pharmacology 1976; 25: 1205
162. Piafsky KM, Borgå O, Odar-Cederlöf I, et al. Increased plasma protein binding of propranolol and chlorpromazine mediated by disease-induced elevations of plasma $\alpha_1$-acid glycoprotein. New England Journal of Medicine 1978; 299: 1435
163. McLean AJ, Morgan DJ. Clinical pharmacokinetics in patients with liver disease. Clinical Pharmacokinetics 1991; 21: 42
164. Bass NM, Williams RL. Guide to drug dosage in hepatic disease. Clinical Pharmacokinetics 1988; 15: 396
165. Pentikäinen PJ, Hietakorpi S, Halinen MO, et al. Cirrhosis of the liver markedly impairs the elimination of mexiletine. European Journal of Clinical Pharmacology 1986; 30: 83
166. Williams RL, Blaschke T, Meffin PJ, et al. Influence of acute viral hepatitis on disposition and plasma binding of tolbutamide. Clinical Pharmacology and Therapeutics 1977; 21: 301
167. Williams RL, Upton RA, Cello JP, et al. Naproxen disposition in patients with alcoholic cirrhosis. European Journal of Clinical Pharmacology 1984; 27: 291
168. Murray M, Zaluzny L, Farrell GC. Drug metabolism in cirrhosis: selective changes in cytochrome P450 isozymes in the choline deficient rat model. Biochemical Pharmacology 1986; 35: 1817
169. Villeneuve JP, Verbeeck RK, Wilkinson GR, et al. Furosemide kinetics and dynamics in patients with cirrhosis. Clinical Pharmacology and Therapeutics 1986; 40: 14
170. Bakti G, Fisch HU, Karlaganis G, et al. Mechanism of the excessive sedative response of cirrhotics to benzodiazepines: model experiments with triazolam. Hepatology 1987; 7: 629
171. Butterworth RF, Lavoie J, Giguere JF, et al. Affinities and densities of high affinity ($^3$H) muscimol (GABA-A) binding sites of central benzodiazepine receptors are unchanged in autopsied brain tissue from cirrhotic patients with hepatic encephalopathy. Hepatology 1988; 8: 1084
172. Eichelbaum M. Drug metabolism in thyroid disease. Clinical Pharmacokinetics 1976; 1: 339
173. Elfström J. Drug pharmacokinetics in the postoperative period. Clinical Pharmacokinetics 1979; 4: 16
174. Fillastre J-P, Singlas E. Pharmacokinetics of newer drugs in patients with renal impairment (Pt 1). Clinical Pharmacokinetics 1991; 20: 293
175. Peter WL, Redic-Kill KA, Halstenson CE. Clinical pharmacokinetics of antibiotics in patients with impaired renal function. Clinical Pharmacokinetics 1992; 22: 169
176. Singlas E, Fillastre J-P. Pharmacokinetics of new drugs in patients with renal impairment (Pt II). Clinical Pharmacokinetics 1991; 20: 389
177. Drayer D. Active drug metabolites and renal failure. American Journal of Medicine 1977; 62: 486
178. Richens A. Drug level monitoring – quality and quantity. British Journal of Clinical Pharmacology 1978; 5: 285
179. Sjöqvist F. Therapeutic drug monitoring – twenty years experience. In: Lemberger & Reidenberg, editors. Proceedings of the Second World Conference on Clinical Pharmacology and Therapeutics. Washington DC: American Society for Pharmacology and Experimental Therapeutics, 1984: 38
180. Lund L. Anticonvulsant effect of diphenylhydantoin relative to plasma levels: a prospective three-year study in ambulant patients with generalised epileptic seizures. Archives of Neurology 1974; 31: 289
181. Perruca E. Free level monitoring of antiepileptic drugs: clinical usefulness and case studies. Clinical Pharmacokinetics 1984; 9 Suppl. 1: 71
182. Peterson BM, McLean S, Von Witt RJ, et al. Audit of a monitoring service for free phenytoin. British Journal of Clinical Pharmacology 1985; 19: 693
183. Kutt H. Pharmacodynamic and pharmacokinetic measurements of antiepileptic drugs. Clinical Pharmacology and Therapeutics 1974; 16: 243
184. Hvidberg E, Dam M. Clinical pharmacokinetics of anticonvulsants. Clinical Pharmacokinetics 1976; 1: 161
185. Buchtal F, Lennox-Buchtal MA. Phenobarbital relation of serum concentration to control of seizures. In: Woodbury et al., editors. Antiepileptic drugs. New York: Raven Press, 1972: 335
186. Bertilsson L, Tomson T. Clinical pharmacokinetics and pharmacological effects of carbamazepine and carbamazepine-10, 11-epoxide. Clinical Pharmacokinetics 1986; 11: 177
187. Penry JK. Correlation of serum ethosuximide levels with clinical effect. In: Schneider et al., editors. Clinical pharmacology of antiepileptic drugs. Berlin: Springer-Verlag, 1975: 217
188. Richens A, Warrington S. When should plasma drug levels be monitored? Drugs 1979; 17: 488
189. Smith RW, Butler VP, Haber E. Determination of therapeutic and toxic serum digoxin concentrations by radioimmunoassay. New England Journal of Medicine 1969; 281: 1212
190. Iisalo E. Clinical pharmacokinetics of digoxin. Clinical Pharmacokinetics 1977; 2: 1
191. Weintraub M. Interpretation of the serum digoxin concentration. Clinical Pharmacokinetics 1977; 2: 205
192. Perrier D, Mayersohn M, Marcus FI. Clinical pharmacokinetics of digitoxin. Clinical Pharmacokinetics 1977; 2: 292
193. Sokolow M, Ball RE. Factors influencing conversion of chronic atrial fibrillation with special reference to serum quinidine concentration. Circulation 1956; 14: 568
194. Koch-Weser J. Correlation of serum concentrations and pharmacological effects on antiarrhythmic drugs. Proceedings of the 5th International Congress on Pharmacology, San Francisco 1972. Basel: Karger, 1973; 3: 69
195. Koch-Weser J. Serum procainamide levels as therapeutic guides. Clinical Pharmacokinetics 1977; 2: 389
196. Amdisen A. Serum level monitoring and clinical pharmacokinetics of lithium. Clinical Pharmacokinetics 1977; 2: 73
197. Kragh-Sorenson PW. Correlation between plasma levels of nortriptyline and clinical effects. Communications in Psychopharmacology 1978; 2: 451
198. Åsberg M, Sjöqvist F. On the role of plasma level monitoring of tricyclic antidepressants in clinical practice. Communications in Psychopharmacology 1978; 2: 381

199. Gram L. Plasma level monitoring of tricyclic antidepressant therapy. Clinical Pharmacokinetics 1977; 2: 237
200. Perrel JM, Stiller RL, Glassman AH. Studies on plasma level/effect relationships in imipramine therapy. Communications in Psychopharmacology 1978; 2: 429
201. Hansen LB, Larsen N-E, Vestergård P. Plasma levels of perphenazine (Trilafon) related to development of extrapyramidal side effects. Psychopharmacology 1981; 74: 306
202. Hansen LB, Larsen N-E. Therapeutic advantages of monitoring plasma concentrations of perphenazine in clinical practice. Psychopharmacology 1985; 87: 16
203. Lindholm A. Therapeutic drug monitoring of cyclosporin – an update. European Journal of Clinical Pharmacology 1991; 41: 273
204. Pippenger C, Penry JK, White BG, et al. Interlaboratory variability in determination of plasma antiepileptic drug concentrations. Archives of Neurology 1976; 33: 351
205. Blackwell B. Patient compliance. New England Journal of Medicine 1973; 289: 249
206. Blackwell B. Treatment adherence. British Journal of Psychiatry 1976; 129: 513
207. Mazullo JM. The non-pharmacologic basis of therapeutics. Clinical Pharmacology and Therapeutics 1972; 13: 157
208. Lund L. Bestämning av fenytoin i plasma – kliniska erfarenheter. Läkartidningen 1971; 68: 73
209. Clarke JM, Hamer J, Skeleton JR, et al. The rhythm of the normal human heart. Lancet 1976; 2: 508
210. Clark TJH, Hetzel MR. Diurnal variation of asthma. British Journal of Diseases of the Chest 1977; 71: 87
211. Holman RR, Turner RC. Basal normoglycaemia attained with chlorpropamide in mild diabetes. Metabolism: Clinical and Experimental 1978; 27: 539
212. Revill S, Robinson JO, Rosen M, et al. The reliability of a linear analogue for evaluating pain. Anaesthesia 1976; 31: 1191
213. Hamilton M. Comparative value of rating scales. British Journal of Clinical Pharmacology 1976; 3 Suppl. 1: 58
214. Radda GK. The use of NMR spectroscopy for the understanding of disease. Science 1986; 233: 640
215. Forstrom LA. Positron emission tomography – the promise of metabolic imaging. Mayo Clinic Proceedings 1989; 64: 720
216. Farde L, Nordström A-L, Wiesel F-A, et al. Positron emission tomographic analysis of central D1 and D2 dopamine receptor occupancy in patients treated with classical neuroleptics and clozapine. Archives of General Psychiatry 1992; 49: 538
217. Lawrence D. Clinical pharmacology. London: Churchill Livingstone, 1973
218. Good CS. The principles and practice of clinical trials. Edinburgh: Churchill Livingstone, 1976
219. Harris EL, Fitzgerald JD. The principles and practice of clinical trials. Edinburgh: Livingstone, 1970
220. World Health Organization. Guidelines for evaluation of drugs for use in man. Technical Report Series No. 563. Geneva: World Health Organization, 1975
221. Dollery CT, Davies DS. The conduct of initial drug studies in man. British Medical Bulletin 1970; 26: 233
222. Byar DP, Simon RM, Friedewald WT, et al. Randomized clinical trials. New England Journal of Medicine 1976; 295: 74
223. Peto R, Pike MC, Armitage P, et al. Design and analysis of randomized clinical trials requiring prolonged observation of each patient: I. Introduction and design. British Journal of Cancer 1976; 34: 485
224. Peto R, Pike MC, Armitage P, et al. Design and analysis of randomized clinical trials requiring prolonged observation of each patient: II. Analysis and examples. British Journal of Cancer 1977; 35: 1
225. Hill AB. Controlled clinical trials. Oxford: Blackwell, 1960
226. Blackwell B, Bloomfield SS, Buncher CR. Demonstration to medical students of placebo-responses and non-drug factors. Lancet 1972; 1: 1279
227. Lasagna L, Laties VG, Dihan JL. Further studies on the pharmacology of placebo administration. Journal of Clinical Investigation 1958; 37: 533
228. Wade OL, Waterhouse JAH. Significant or important? British Journal of Clinical Pharmacology 1977; 4: 411
229. Clark CJ, Downie CC. A method for the rapid determination of the number of patients to include in a controlled clinical trial. Lancet 1966; 2: 1357
230. Armitage P. Sequential medical trials. Oxford: Blackwell, 1960
231. Day NE. Two-stage designs for clinical trials. Biometrics 1969; 25: 111
232. Reiser SJ, Dyck AJ, Curran WJ. Ethics in medicine. Cambridge, Mass: MIT Press, 1977
233. Binns TB. Sensible prescribing: I – the context of prescribing. Practitioner 1975; 214: 118
234. Smithells RW. Iatrogenic hazards and their effects. Postgraduate Medical Journal 1975; 51 Suppl. 2: 39
235. World Health Organization. Guide to good prescribing. Division of drug management and policies. Geneva: World Health Organization, 1994
236. Kellaway GSM, McCrae E. Non-compliance and errors of drug administration in patients discharged from acute general medical wards. New Zealand Medical Journal 1975; 81: 508
237. Kellaway GSM, McCrae E. The effect of counselling on compliance-failure in patient drug therapy. New Zealand Medical Journal 1979; 89: 161
238. Hemminki E. Review of literature on the factors affecting drug prescribing. Social Science and Medicine 1975; 9: 111
239. Modell W, Houde RW. Factors influencing clinical evaluation of drugs. Journal of the American Medical Association 1958; 167: 2190
240. Lionel NDW, Herxheimer A. Assessing reports of therapeutic trials. British Medical Journal 1970; 3: 637
241. Lasagna L. A plea for 'naturalistic' study of medicines. European Journal of Clinical Pharmacology 1974; 7: 1
242. Armstrong D. Clinical sense and clinical science. Social Science and Medicine 1977; 11: 599

Chapter 2

# Maternal and Fetal Clinical Pharmacology

*J.G.W. Theis* and *G. Koren*

## Synopsis of Important Principles

**1)** During pregnancy, the mother and the fetus represent a non-separable unity, the maternal-fetal unit. Maternal well-being is an absolute prerequisite for the optimal functioning and development of both parts of this unit. Consequently, it is important to treat the mother whenever needed while protecting the unborn fetus to the greatest possible extent.

**2)** Major congenital malformations occur in 2 to 4% of all live births; up to 15% of all diagnosed pregnancies will result in fetal loss. The cause of these adverse pregnancy outcomes is understood in only a minority of the incidents. It is important to acknowledge this 'background risk' in the context of the prevalence of drug-induced adverse pregnancy outcomes.

**3)** Associations of malformations with drugs have been described in case reports and case series. While these are important in drawing attention to a suspected teratogen, they cannot prove teratogenicity. Epidemiological studies are powerful tools to detect associations between exogenous factors and adverse pregnancy outcomes. These studies require that confounding factors are identified and corrected for, statistical analysis is performed appropriately, and investigators remain unbiased.

**4)** Malformations are not induced during the first 2 weeks after conception, the 'none or all' period. Embryogenesis (weeks 4 to 10 of gestation) is the period of greatest susceptibility to malformations, a period during which many women do not know they are pregnant. During the later fetogenesis stage (after week 10 of gestation), the major risk is to the development of the CNS.

**5)** Factors affecting the occurrence of malformations include the dose of the teratogen, timing of exposure, and susceptibility of the developing organism. Mechanisms of teratogenicity are still poorly understood. They may include direct effects on the embryo, multifactorial effects, and effects on the placenta or the maternal part of the maternal-fetal unit.

**6)** Both maternal and fetal pharmacokinetics may need consideration in drug selection. Maternal pharmacokinetics may be altered due to the physiological changes during pregnancy, necessitating dosage adjustment of a number of drugs.

**7)** Except for drugs with very high molecular weights (e.g. heparin), almost all drugs pass the placenta. The degree of transfer depends on physicochemical properties of the drug and properties of the placenta such as expression of carrier mechanisms or metabolising enzymes.

**8)** Counselling of women before a planned pregnancy should include discussion of a variety of factors that may affect the offspring. These include risks associated with specific therapeutic agents and the abuse of substances such as smoking and alcohol, and pre-existing risks such as genetic factors or maternal age. Folic acid should be supplemented during pregnancy planning, as folic acid taken periconceptually can reduce neural tube defects.

**9)** During pregnancy, women needing drug treatment should be informed about the associated risks and benefits in an unbiased fashion. Irrational maternal fears based on poor or false information may lead to a lack of compliance, which may endanger both the mother and the unborn child, and in the worst cases, may even lead to termination of otherwise wanted pregnancies.

**10)** The most common causes of poisoning during pregnancy are iron, aspirin, and paracetamol (acetaminophen). The usual treatment of the mother for overdose must not be withheld because of the pregnant state. Fetal and maternal risks are not necessarily equal and may be dependent on placental transfer and different expressions of maternal and fetal metabolic pathways.

During the history of modern medicine, the focus of embryonal, fetal and maternal medicine has dramatically shifted. Until the middle of the 20th century, infections were the leading cause of morbidity and mortality of both pregnant mothers and their infants, and thus were the main focus of attention and treatment. Congenital malformations had been described but were felt to be unpreventable and untreatable.

Since the middle of this century, this concept has been challenged. The first reports appeared showing associations of congenital malformations with exogenous factors during pregnancy, such as rubella.[1] The thalidomide disaster[2-4] and its worldwide publicity caused a revolution in the way pharmacotherapy is used during pregnancy. Soon after this, many drugs and chemicals and a multitude of environmental factors were accused of being human teratogens, although only a very limited group of drugs and chemicals have proven to be teratogenic (table I) and many others are now considered 'safe', i.e. not associated with an increase in adverse pregnancy outcomes (table II).

Irrational fear on the part of patients and practitioners, augmented by misinformed media reports, result in unfortunate and tragic events. Irrational fears of the pregnant patient may lead to impaired compliance with therapy. Insufficient information to practising physicians may lead to suboptimal treatment either via avoidance of necessary drug treatment or selection of suboptimal regimens. Such approaches may impose a risk to maternal well-being, and may also affect the unborn child.

Programmes aimed at informing, counselling and following up pregnant women exposed to drugs, chemicals, or radiation during pregnancy are useful sources of data on maternal concerns over exposure. Experience with women counselled at the Motherisk Clinic in Toronto demonstrates that pregnant women tend to assign the risks associated with their own intake of medications at unrealistically high values.[7] This misperception of risks may lead to the unwarranted termination of otherwise wanted pregnancies.[7] Such behaviour has been documented by the Greek experience after the Chernobyl catastrophe, where a large number of desired pregnancies were terminated because of unrealistic fears of congenital malformations.[7,8]

**Table I.** Drugs and chemicals proven to be teratogenic in humans (after Koren & Nulman;[5] reproduced with permission of the publisher)

| Drug/chemical | Fetal adverse effects | Relative risk for teratogenicity | Clinical intervention |
|---|---|---|---|
| Alcohol (ethanol) | *Fetal alcohol syndrome*: mental retardation, microcephaly, poor coordination, hypotonia, hyperactivity, short upturned nose, micrognathia or retrognathia (infancy) or prognathia (adolescence), short palpebral fissures, hypoplastic philtrum, thinned upper lips, microphthalmia, antenatal/postnatal growth retardation, occasional pathologies of eyes, mouth, heart, kidneys, gonads, skin, muscle and skeleton | In alcoholic women consuming over 2 g/kg/day ethanol during the first trimester: 2- to 3-fold higher risk for congenital malformations (about 10%) | Calculate accurate dosage of alcohol. *Prospective*: discontinue exposure; if woman is alcoholic, refer to addiction centre *During pregnancy*: alleviate fears in mild or occasional drinkers who may terminate pregnancy based on unrealistic perception of risk; level 2 ultrasound to rule out visible malformation |
| Alkylating agents (busulfan, chlorambucil, cyclophosphamide, chlormethine) | Growth retardation, cleft palate, microphthalmia, hypoplastic ovaries, cloudy corneas, agenesis of kidney, malformations of digits, cardiac defects, multiple other anomalies | Case reports show 10-50% of cases were malformed, depending on the drug. Adverse outcome may have been over-represented | Level 2 ultrasound to rule out visible malformations |
| Antimetabolite agents (aminopterin sodium, azauridine, cytarabine, fluorouracil, mercaptopurine, methotrexate) | Hydrocephalus, meningoencephalocele, anencephaly, malformed skull, cerebral hypoplasia, growth retardation, eye and ear malformations, malformed nose and cleft palate, malformed extremities and fingers *Aminopterin syndrome*: cranial dysostosis, hydrocephalus, hypertelorism, anomalies of external ear, micrognathia, posterior cleft palate | Case reports show 7-75% of cases were malformed. Adverse outcome may have been over-represented | Level 2 ultrasound to rule out visible malformations. Supplement folic acid in women receiving antifolates (e.g. methotrexate) |

**Table I.** *(Continued)*

| Drug/chemical | Fetal adverse effects | Relative risk for teratogenicity | Clinical intervention |
|---|---|---|---|
| Carbamazepine | Increased risk of NTDs | NTDs estimated at 1% with carbamazepine | Periconceptional folic acid; maternal and/or amniotic α-fetoprotein; ultrasound to rule out NTDs |
| Carbon monoxide | Cerebral atrophy, mental retardation, microcephaly, convulsions, spastic disorders, intrauterine or postnatal death | Case reports show high risk for neurological sequelae when mother is severely poisoned; no increased risk in mild accidental exposures | Measure maternal carboxyhaemoglobin levels; use 100% oxygen for 5h after maternal carboxyhaemoglobin returns to normal (fetal equilibration takes longer); use hyperbaric chamber if available, as elimination $t_{½}$ of CO is more rapid; fetal monitoring by an obstetrician; sonographic follow-up |
| Coumarin anticoagulants | *Fetal warfarin syndrome*: nasal hypoplasia, chondrodysplasia punctata, brachydactyly, skull defects, abnormal ears, malformed eyes, CNS malformations, microcephaly, hydrocephalus, skeletal deformities, mental retardation, optic atrophy, spasticity, Dandy Walker malformations | 16% of exposed fetuses have malformations; 3% haemorrhages; 8% stillbirths | *Prospective*: switch to heparin for the first trimester; deliver by a caesarean section; follow-up mothers in a high-risk perinatal unit |
| Stilbestrol (diethylstilbestrol, DES) | *Female offspring*: clear cell vaginal or cervical adenocarcinoma in young female adults exposed *in utero* (before 18th week); irregular menses (oligomenorrhoea), reduced pregnancy rates, increased rate of preterm deliveries, increased perinatal mortality and spontaneous abortion<br>*Male offspring*: cysts of epididymis, cryptorchidism, hypogonadism, diminished spermatogenesis | Exposure before 18 weeks of gestation: ≤1.4 per 1000 exposed females with carcinoma. Congenital morphological changes in vaginal epithelium in 39% of exposures | *Diagnosis*: direct observation of mucosa and Shiller's test<br>*Treatment*: mechanical excision or destruction in relatively confined area; surgery/radiotherapy for diffused tumour |
| Lead | Lower scores in developmental tests | Higher risk when maternal lead concentration is >10 μg/dl | *Maternal lead concentrations >10 μg/dl:* investigate for possible source of contamination<br>*Concentrations >25 μg/dl:* consider chelation |
| Lithium | Possibly higher risk for Ebstein's anomaly; no detectable higher risk for other malformations | | Women who need lithium should continue therapy, with sonographic follow-up; patients may need higher doses because of increased clearance |
| Methyl mercury, mercuric sulfide | Microcephaly, eye malformations, cerebral palsy, mental retardation, malocclusion of teeth | Women with affected offspring consumed Hg 9-27 ppm; greater risk at 6-8 gestational months; relative risk not known, but severe disease seen in 13 of 220 neonates born after contamination in Minamata, Japan | Good correlation between Hg levels in maternal hair follicles and fetal neurological outcome; hair Hg content >50 ppm used successfully as threshold for termination of pregnancy; in acute poisoning, fetus is 4-10 times more sensitive than adults to methyl-Hg toxicity |

*[Continued over]*

**Table I.** *(Continued)*

| Drug/chemical | Fetal adverse effects | Relative risk for teratogenicity | Clinical intervention |
|---|---|---|---|
| Polychlorinated biphenyls (PCBs) | Stillbirth<br>Signs at birth: white eye discharge, 30% (32/108); teeth present, 8.7% (11/127); irritated/swollen gums, 11% (11/99); hyperpigmentation ('cola' staining), 42.5% (54/127); deformed/small nails, 24.6% (30/122); acne, 12.8% (16/125)<br>*Subsequent history*: bronchitis or pneumonia, 27.2% (30/124); chipped or broken teeth, 35.5% (38/107); hair loss, 12.2% (14/115); acne scars, 9.6% (11/115); generalised itching, 27.8% (32/1150)<br>*Developmental*: do not meet milestones, lower scores than unexposed controls, evidence of CNS damage | 4% (6/159) to 20% (8/39) | These figures from cases poisoned by high consumption of PCB-contaminated rice oil cannot be extrapolated to cases in which maternal poisoning is not verified. Women working near PCBs (e.g. hydroelectric facilities) should use effective protection |
| Penicillamine | Skin hyperelastosis | Few case reports; risk unknown | |
| Phenytoin | *Fetal hydantoin syndrome*: low nasal bridge, inner epicanthal folds, ptosis, strabismus, hypertelorism, low set or abnormal ears, wide mouth, large fontanelles, anomalies and hypoplasia of distal phalanges and nails, skeletal abnormalities, microcephaly and mental retardation, growth deficiency, neuroblastoma, cardiac defects, cleft palate/lip | 5-10% of typical syndrome; about 30% of partial picture; relative risk of 7 for offspring with IQ ≤84 | Consider changing to other medications and/or keep phenytoin concentrations at lower effective levels; level 2 ultrasound to rule out visible malformations; vitamin K to neonate; epilepsy itself increases teratogenic risk |
| Systemic retinoids (isotretinoin, etretinate) | Spontaneous abortions; deformities of cranium, ears, face, heart, limbs, liver; hydrocephalus, microcephalus, heart defects; cognitive defects even without dysmorphology | For isotretinoin: 38% risk; 80% of malformations are CNS | Treated women should have an effective method of contraception; terminate pregnancy if possible; if diagnosed too late, sonographic follow-up to rule out confirmed malformations |
| Trimethadione (troxidone) | *Fetal trimethadione syndrome*: intrauterine growth retardation, cardiac anomalies, microcephaly, cleft palate and lip, abnormal ears, dysmorphic face, mental retardation, tracheo-oesophageal fistula, postnatal death | Based on case reports: 83% risk; 32% infantile or neonatal death | No need for this antiepileptic because other alternatives are available |
| Thalidomide | Limb phocomelia, amelia, hypoplasia, congenital heart defects, renal malformations, cryptorchidism, abducens paralysis, deafness, microtia, anotia | About 20% risk when exposure to drug occurs in days 34-50 of gestation | Thalidomide is effective for some forms of leprosy; treated women should have an effective mode of contraception |
| Tetracycline | Yellow, grey-brown or brown staining of deciduous teeth, destruction of enamel | From 4 months of gestation and on, occurs in 50% of fetuses exposed to tetracycline, 12.5% to oxytetracycline | If exposure before 14-16 weeks of gestation, no known risk |
| Valproic acid | Lumbosacral spina bifida with meningomyelocele; CNS defects, microcephaly, cardiac defects | 1.2% risk of NTDs | Level 2 ultrasound and maternal $\alpha$-fetoprotein or amniocentesis to rule out NTDs; epilepsy itself increases teratogenic risk |

*Abbreviations and symbols:* NTDs = neural tube defects; $t_{1/2}$ = half-life; CNS = central nervous system; CO = carbon monoxide; ppm = parts per million; Hg = mercury; IQ = intelligence quotient.

**Table II.** Drugs of choice in pregnancy (after Smith et al.;[6] reproduced with permission of the publisher)

| Condition | Drug(s) of choice | Alternative(s) | Comments |
|---|---|---|---|
| Acne | *Topical:*<br>Erythromycin<br>Clindamycin<br>Benzoyl peroxide | *Systemic:*<br>Erythromycin<br>*Topical:*<br>Tretinoin (vitamin A acid) | Isotretinoin is contraindicated in pregnancy |
| Allergic rhinitis | *Topical:*<br>Corticosteroids<br>Sodium cromoglycate (cromolyn sodium)<br>Decongestants (*NB.* use sparingly):<br>• xylometazoline<br>• oxymetazoline<br>• naphazoline<br>• phenylephrine<br>*Systemic:*<br>Diphenhydramine<br>Dimenhydrinate<br>Tripelennamine | Immunotherapy | Limited experience with terfenadine and astemizole has not revealed a substantial teratogenic risk |
| *Anaemias:* | | | |
| Iron deficiency anaemia | Iron supplements | | |
| Folic acid deficiency | Folic acid | | Folic acid recommended for all pregnant women commencing before conception |
| Cyanocobalamin (vitamin $B_{12}$) deficiency | Cyanocobalamin PO/IM, multivitamins | | |
| Pernicious anaemia | Cyanocobalamin IM or PO + intrinsic factor PO | | |
| Haemolytic anaemia | Corticosteroids<br>Iron supplements<br>Blood transfusion | | |
| Sickle cell anaemia | *Prophylaxis:*<br>Penicillin<br>Folic acid supplement<br>Iron supplement<br>Blood transfusion<br>*Crisis:*<br>Morphine<br>Pethidine (meperidine)<br>Sodium bicarbonate, $O_2$ | | Vaccinate with pneumococcal vaccine before pregnancy; vaccinate during pregnancy only if patient at risk of contracting disease |
| Anticoagulation (after prosthetic valve replacement) | Heparin<br>Aspirin | Warfarin (trimesters 2 + 3; avoid at term; see text, sect. 7.2.3)<br>Dipyridamole<br>Streptokinase (use for pulmonary embolism if heparin fails) | Avoid aspirin in 3rd trimester; risk of bleeding with streptokinase (if used at term, deliver by caesarean section) |
| Anxiety disorders | Benzodiazepines | | |
| Arrhythmias | Quinidine<br>Digoxin | Procainamide<br>Propranolol<br>Lidocaine (late in pregnancy, short term)<br>Verapamil (late in pregnancy, short term) | Amiodarone has been associated with adverse thyroid effects in neonates |
| Asthma | *Inhalational:*<br>$\beta_2$-adrenoceptor agonists (e.g. salbutamol)<br>Corticosteroids<br>Sodium cromoglycate<br>Ipratropium bromide<br>*Systemic:*<br>Theophylline<br>Corticosteroids | | *Emergency treatment:*<br>Adrenaline (epinephrine) SC, IV |

[Continued over]

**Table II.** [*Continued*]

| Condition | Drug(s) of choice | Alternative(s) | Comments |
|---|---|---|---|
| Constipation | *Bulk-forming agents:*<br>Psyllium mucilloid<br>Bran<br>*Stool softeners/osmotic agents:*<br>Docusate sodium/calcium<br>Glycerin<br>Sorbitol<br>Lactulose<br>Mineral oil<br>Magnesium hydroxide | *Saline laxatives:*<br>Magnesium citrate<br>Sodium phosphate/ biphosphate enena<br>*Gastrointestinal stimulants:*<br>Bisacodyl<br>Phenolphthalein | Avoid gastrointestinal stimulants if possible |
| Cough | Candy cough lozenges<br>Diphenhydramine<br>Codeine | Dextromethorphan | |
| Depression | Tricyclic antidepressants<br>Fluoxetine | Lithium | When lithium is used in 1st trimester, fetal echocardiogram and level 2 ultrasound recommended owing to small risk of Ebstein's anomaly |
| Diabetes mellitus | Human insulin | Beef or pork insulin | Avoid oral antidiabetic agents if possible |
| Diarrhoea | Oral rehydration solution<br>Attapulgite (kaolin + pectin)<br>Bulk-forming agents (methylcellulose, psyllium mucilloid) | | |
| Dyspepsia, heartburn | *Antireflux:*<br>Alginic acid + antacids<br>*Antacids:*<br>Magnesium hydroxide<br>Aluminium hydroxide<br>Magaldrate<br>Calcium carbonate<br>*Antiflatulants:*<br>Simethicone | $H_2$-Blockers (e.g. ranitidine, cimetidine) | Limited experience with $H_2$-blockers suggests that they are not human teratogens |
| Fever | Paracetamol (acetaminophen) | Aspirin<br>Ibuprofen | Avoid aspirin and ibuprofen in 3rd trimester |
| *Headache:* | | | |
| Tension headache | Paracetamol | Aspirin/nonsteroidal anti-inflammatory drugs (NSAIDs)<br>Benzodiazepines | Avoid aspirin and NSAIDs in 3rd trimester |
| Migraine headache | *Treatment:*<br>Paracetamol<br>Codeine<br>Morphine<br>Pethidine<br>Dimenhydrinate | *Prophylaxis:*<br>β-Adrenoceptor blockers<br>Tricyclic antidepressants<br>*Treatment:*<br>Butalbital/aspirin/codeine | Limited experience with ergotamine shows no evidence of teratogenicity, but concerns of potent vasoconstriction remain |
| Cluster headache | *Prophylaxis:*<br>Corticosteroids<br>Amitriptyline<br>Propranolol<br>*Treatment:*<br>Corticosteroids | | |
| Hypertension | Methyldopa<br>Hydralazine | β-Adrenoceptor blockers (e.g propranolol, labetalol)<br>Prazosin<br>Nifedipine (in later stages of pregnancy) | ACE inhibitors should be avoided |

**Table II.** *[Continued]*

| Condition | Drug(s) of choice | Alternative(s) | Comments |
|---|---|---|---|
| Hyperthyroidism | Propylthiouracil<br>Thiamazole (methimazole) | *Symptomatic:*<br>β-Adrenoceptor blockers (e.g. propranolol) | Surgery may be needed if illness not controlled with drugs; maternal propylthiouracil doses >200mg may affect fetal thyroid |
| Hypothyroidism | Levothyroxine<br>Liothyronine | Desiccated thyroid | |
| Idiopathic thrombocytopenic purpura | Corticosteroids<br>IV immunoglobulins<br>Blood transfusions | | |
| *Infections:* | | | |
| Bacterial infections | *Systemic:*<br>Penicillins<br>Cefalosporins<br>Cotrimoxazole<br>Erythromycin<br>Clindamycin<br>Nitrofurantoin<br>*Topical:*<br>Polymixin B/bacitracin | Aminoglycosides<br>Metronidazole<br>Trimethoprim<br>Nalidixic acid | Try to avoid sulfonamides in late pregnancy<br>Avoid tetracycline during pregnancy |
| Viral infections | Aciclovir<br>Zidovudine | Amantadine<br>Idoxuridine<br>Trifluridine<br>Vidarabine | |
| Tuberculosis | Isoniazid<br>Ethambutol | Rifampicin<br>Streptomycin | |
| Fungal infections | Nystatin: oral, topical, vaginal<br>Miconazole: topical, vaginal<br>Clotrimazole: topical, vaginal<br>Econazole: vaginal<br>Ketoconazole: topical | Ketoconazole PO: use only if absolutely necessary | |
| Toxoplasmosis | Pyrimethamine/sulfadiazine<br>Spiramycin | | |
| Malaria | *Prophylaxis:*<br>Chloroquine<br>*Treatment:*<br>Chloroquine<br>Quinine/quinidine<br>Quinine + clindamycin | Pyrimethamine + dapsone/sulfadoxine | |
| Trichomoniasis | Metronidazole | | |
| Inflammatory bowel disease (ulcerative colitis and Crohn's disease) | Mesalazine (5-aminosalicylic acid; mesalamine)<br>Olsalazine<br>Sulfasalazine<br>Corticosteroid (PO, rectal, IV)<br>Antibiotics (see bacterial infections above)<br>Vitamin supplements<br>Calcium carbonate | Metronidazole<br>Codeine<br>Loperamide (for severe diarrhoea) | |
| Insomnia | Diphenhydramine<br>Dimenhydrinate<br>Benzodiazepines | | |
| Lice | Pyrethrins<br>Permethrins<br>Petrolatum ointment to eyelashes | Lindane (gamma-benzene hexachloride) | |
| Lichen planus | Topical corticosteroids<br>Intralesional corticosteroids<br>Systemic hydroxyzine (for itching), corticosteroids | | |

*[Continued over]*

**Table II.** [*Continued*]

| Condition | Drug(s) of choice | Alternative(s) | Comments |
|---|---|---|---|
| Mania (and bipolar affective disorder) | Lithium<br>Antipsychotics (chlorpromazine, haloperidol) | *Depressive episodes:*<br>Tricyclic antidepressants<br>Fluoxetine | If lithium is used in 1st trimester, fetal echocardiogram and level 2 ultrasound recommended owing to small risk of Ebstein's anomaly |
| Myasthenia gravis | Pyridostigmine<br>Prednisone | | |
| Nasal congestion | *Nasal drops/spray:*<br>Normal saline<br>Xylometazoline<br>Oxymetazoline<br>Phenylephrine<br>Naphazoline | Pseudoephedrine | |
| Nausea, vomiting, motion sickness | *Antihistamines:*<br>Doxylamine + pyridoxine<br>Diphenhydramine<br>Dimenhydrinate<br>Meclozine<br>Cyclizine | Chlorpromazine<br>Metoclopramide (used safely in 3rd trimester) | |
| Pain | *Systemic:*<br>Paracetamol<br>Morphine<br>Codeine<br>Pethidine<br>*Topical:*<br>Capsaicin<br>Local anaesthetics<br>Salicylates | Aspirin<br>NSAIDs | Avoid aspirin, salicylates and NSAIDs in 3rd trimester; opioids (e.g morphine, pethidine, codeine) may cause neonatal withdrawal syndrome |
| Peptic ulcer disease | *Antacids:*<br>Magnesium hydroxide<br>Aluminium hydroxide<br>Magaldrate<br>Calcium carbonate | Sucralfate<br>$H_2$-Blockers<br>Bismuth subsalicylate/ subcitrate | Avoid salicylates in 3rd trimester |
| Pinworms | Piperazine citrate/adipate | Pyrantel pamoate<br>Pyrvinium pamoate | |
| Pruritus | *Topical:*<br>Moisturising creams/lotions<br>Wet dressings:<br>• Aluminium acetate<br>• Oatmeal bath<br>Zinc oxide cream/ointment<br>Calamine lotion<br>Corticosteroids<br>*Systemic:*<br>Hydroxyzine<br>Diphenhydramine<br>Corticosteroids | Topical local anaesthetics | |
| Psoriasis | *Topical:*<br>Corticosteroids<br>Salicylic acid<br>Emollient ointments<br>Calamine lotion (acute lesions) | | Avoid salicylates in 3rd trimester; etretinate contraindicated in pregnancy |
| Reflux oesophagitis | Alginic acid + antacids<br>*Antacids:*<br>Magnesium hydroxide<br>Aluminium hydroxide<br>Magaldrate<br>Calcium carbonate | | Sitting and sleeping posture is important; frequent, small meals may help |

**Table II.** *[Continued]*

| Condition | Drug(s) of choice | Alternative(s) | Comments |
|---|---|---|---|
| Rheumatoid arthritis | Aspirin<br>NSAIDs<br>Corticosteroids (systemic, intra-articular) | Gold<br>Chloroquine<br>Hydroxychloroquine<br>Azathioprine (after 1st trimester if necessary) | Avoid aspirin and NSAIDs in 3rd trimester<br>Avoid cancer chemotherapeutic agents as much as possible |
| Rosacea | *Topical:*<br>Erythromycin<br>Benzoyl peroxide<br>Metronidazole | Systemic corticosteroids | |
| Scabies | Permethrins<br>Pyrethrins + piperonyl butoxide | Crotamiton<br>Lindane<br>Benzyl benzoate<br>Sulfur 5% in petrolatum | |
| Schizophrenia | Phenothiazines | | |
| Seborrhoeic dermatitis | Salicylic acid shampoo | | Avoid salicylates in 3rd trimester |
| Seizures | Benzodiazepines<br>Carbamazepine<br>Ethosuximide | Valproic acid<br>Phenobarbital<br>Primidone<br>Phenytoin | Folic acid supplementation recommended; carbamazepine and valproic acid associated with small risk of neural tube defects; level 2 ultrasound and α-fetoprotein monitoring recommended; phenytoin causes fetal hydantoin syndrome |
| Systemic lupus erythematosus | Corticosteroids | Azathioprine (after 1st trimester if necessary)<br>Chloroquine<br>Hydroxychloroquine | Avoid cancer chemotherapeutic agents as much as possible |
| Superficial vein thrombosis | Warm compresses<br>Aspirin/NSAIDs | | Avoid aspirin and NSAIDs in 3rd trimester |
| Thrombophlebitis, deep vein thrombosis | *Anticoagulants:*<br>Heparin<br>Warfarin (2nd + 3rd trimester; avoid at term)<br>*Thrombolytics:*<br>Streptokinase | | Risk of bleeding with streptokinase; if used at term, deliver by caesarean section |
| Trigeminal neuralgia | | Carbamazepine<br>Tricyclic antidepressants<br>Phenothiazines | Carbamazepine associated with small risk of neural tube defects; level 2 ultrasound and α-fetoprotein monitoring recommended |

*Abbreviations:* IM = intramuscular; IV = intravenous; PO = oral; SC = subcutaneous; NSAID = nonsteroidal anti-inflammatory drug; ACE = angiotensin-converting enzyme.

Another painful example of misinformation and misperceptions falsely associating a drug with congenital malformations is highlighted by the 'Bendectin' story. This combination of doxylamine with pyridoxine was used and studied most widely as a treatment for morning sickness during pregnancy.[9] However, it was removed from the market by its manufacturer in 1983 despite strong scientific evidence showing its reproductive safety. This decision was based on negative publicity, numerous lawsuits and the resulting increase in insurance premiums. Many pregnant women were thus deprived of the only approved therapy for morning sickness that was known to be safe.[10-12] Recently, the negative effect of this decision on public health was documented by demonstrating an increase in hospital admissions for hyperemesis during pregnancy after 'Bendectin' was no longer available.[13] At present, the drug is available in only a few countries. In Canada, the local brand ('Diclectine') has been labelled by the government as the drug of choice for morning sickness.

Despite the necessity of adequate treatment of pregnant women, protection of the developing fetus from teratogenic effects must be equally considered. Since most adverse drug effects observed in the fetus are irreversible, extreme care is needed when exposing the maternal-fetal unit to drugs. Balancing the risks and benefits of therapy during pregnancy on evidence-based data presents an important challenge for every clinician involved in the care of women during pregnancy.

The aim of this chapter is to provide the clinician with the tools to meet this challenge. These include a basic understanding of the unique pharmacokinetics of the maternal-fetal unit, the effect of drugs during different developmental stages, and a brief review of the effects on the unborn child of a number of commonly used or abused drugs.

## 1. General Considerations

### 1.1 Definitions

*Congenital malformations* are defined as nonreversible functional or morphological defects present at birth. The underlying cause can be genetic, environmental (drugs, chemicals, radiation, pathogens and maternal illnesses), or multifactorial. The cause of most anomalies remains unknown. Congenital malformations, although sometimes not detectable at birth, may lead to functional impairment that becomes evident later in life. Thus, it is important not to restrict the term to macroscopically detectable morphological abnormalities.

**Table III.** Amalgamation of criteria for proof of human teratogenicity. Items 1 to 3 or 1, 3, and 4 are essential criteria; 5 to 7 are helpful but not essential (after Shepard,[17] reproduced with permission)

| | |
|---|---|
| 1. | Proven exposure to agent at critical time(s) in prenatal development (prescriptions, physicians' records, dates) |
| 2. | Consistent findings by 2 or more epidemiological studies of high quality with:<br>a) control of confounding factors<br>b) sufficient numbers<br>c) exclusion of positive and negative bias factors<br>d) prospective design, if possible, and<br>e) relative risk of 6 or more (?) |
| 3. | Careful delineation of the clinical cases. A specific defect or syndrome, if present, is very helpful |
| 4. | Rare environmental exposure associated with rare defect. Probably 3 or more cases [e.g. oral anticoagulants and nasal hypoplasia; thiamazole (methimazole) and scalp defects (?), and heart block and maternal rheumatism] |
| 5. | Teratogenicity in experimental animals is important but not essential |
| 6. | The association should make biological sense |
| 7. | Proof in an experimental system that the agent acts in an unaltered state. Important information for prevention |

Congenital malformations are usually divided into major and minor, although neither term has been well defined. A *major malformation* has been described as being either life-threatening, requiring major surgery, or having serious cosmetic effects.[14] Any structural and functional conditions that impair quality of life, such as reduced intelligence quotient (IQ), should be included into this definition. *Minor malformations or minor anomalies* are less well defined. The term incorporates unusual morphological features that are of no serious medical or cosmetic consequence to the affected individual.[15]

A *teratogen* is generally defined as an exogenous agent that has the ability to produce congenital malformations or functional defects during embryonic or fetal development.[16] Despite this definition, it often remains difficult to decide whether an individual substance is a teratogen or not, for reasons described in sections 3 and 1.3 of this chapter. A current attempt to outline criteria for proof of human teratogenicity is depicted in table III.

### 1.2 Epidemiology of Congenital Malformations and Other Adverse Pregnancy Outcomes

The prevalence of major congenital malformations has been reported to be in the range of 2 to 4% of all live births, depending on the methods and sources used.[14,18-22] On the basis of the defects that are detectable at birth or in the immediate neonatal period, a 2 to 3% risk is usually quoted for malformations in the normal population. While these numbers may be useful for counselling and other clinical or epidemiological purposes, they underestimate the true figure of malformations, since an equally high number of birth defects becomes apparent throughout the first 5 years of life (e.g. some cardiac abnormalities, absent kidney).[23,24]

The true incidence of fetal defects throughout pregnancy is much higher, but the majority of these result in fetal loss and, thus, are not counted as congenital malformations.[25] It has been estimated that up to 15% of diagnosed pregnancies result in fetal losses, most of them

**Table IV.** Timetable of pregnancy: pharmacological considerations (after Moore;[27] Kline et al.;[25] Tuchmann-Duplessis;[28] Chitayat et al.[29])

| Gestational age (weeks after last menstrual period) | Embryonic age (days after conception) | Number of surviving conceptuses (% of conceived) | Likelihood to survive until live birth | Important developmental steps | Maternal perception | Diagnostic or preventive procedures |
|---|---|---|---|---|---|---|
| Planning period | | | | | | Folate supplementation recommended; if chronic conditions exist, optimise therapy for pregnancy |
| 0 | | | | | Last menstrual period | |
| 2 | 0-6 | 100% | 50% | Conception<br>Forming of blastocyst | | |
| 3 | | | | Start of implantation | | |
| 4 | 7-13 | | | Formation of bilaminar embryo<br>Differentiation of trophoblast | | |
| 5 | 14-20 | 71% | 70% | Formation of 3 germ layers<br>Start of organogenesis<br>Day 17-27: neural tube | First missed menstrual period | |
| 6-7 | 21-35 | 57-63% | 79-88% | Day 26-37: formation of limbs<br>Day 28: neural tube closed; brain development continues<br>Day 20-40: heart | Pregnancy usually clinically recognised; maternal morning sickness | |
| 8-9 | 36-49 | 55% | 90% | *Until early fetal stage:*<br>• formation of lip and palate<br>*Throughout fetal period:*<br>• development of external genitalia<br>• development of teeth | | |
| 10 | 50-56 | 51% | 98% | | | Chorionic villus sampling at 9-12 weeks gestational age |
| 11-14 | | | | Begin fetal stage<br>Palate closed | | Early amniocentesis |
| 15-17 | | | | | | Ultrasound for detection of malformations<br>Amniocentesis<br>Maternal $\alpha$-fetoprotein measurement |
| 18-20 | | | | | Maternal perception of fetal movements | |
| 24 | | | | Fetus starts to be viable if born prematurely | | |
| 34 | | 50% | | Neonatal mortality not significantly higher than at 40 weeks | | |
| 40 | | 50% | | | Live birth | |

occurring during early gestation.[26] However, this number varies between studies[25] and tends to decrease when pregnancy is diagnosed later in its course (table IV).

It has been estimated that only 5% of all congenital malformations are caused by environmental factors, including drugs and chemicals, infectious agents, and maternal illness.[30] The causes of a further 25% are considered to be multifactorial and may extend the number of congenital malformations co-induced by environmental factors. These numbers are rough estimates, since there is no proven cause for most congenital malformations.

The prevalence of congenital malformations induced by environmental factors, at 0.1 to 0.2% of all live births, may appear to be low. However, this is a very significant number, considering the effect of congenital malformations on the future of the individual child, the child's family, and the community. In the US in 1986, congenital birth defects were the leading cause of infant mortality, responsible for more than one-fifth of all infant deaths.[31] Since congenital malformations are usually irreversible, the morbidity and disability experienced by those children who survive is equally important.

The effect of a congenital malformation on the child's life depends on the type and severity of malformation, and may be substantial. In addition, the effects on the family cannot be underestimated. From the rates in the previous paragraph, 1 to 2 in 1000 families are directly affected by the birth of a child born with congenital malformations caused by environmental factors. The health costs are significant: the financial burden of having a child survive with major malformations has been estimated to range between $1.5 million and $4.5 million throughout life.[32]

## 1.3 Identification of Drugs or Chemicals as Teratogens

The identification of a drug, chemical, or environmental factor as a teratogen is hampered by a variety of factors. No known teratogens cause congenital malformations in all exposed conceptuses. Even substances with an extremely high teratogenic potential such as thalidomide or the retinoids cause malformations in only 20% and 38% of the prenatal exposures, respectively.[5] Other substances with lower teratogenic potential such as valproic acid and carbamazepine, cause major malformations in only about 1 to 2% of all prenatal exposures.[5] Hence, a high number of incidences must be recorded before a statistically valid association can be proven.

Unfortunately, animal models have only a limited value. While all drugs which to date are known to be teratogens have expressed teratogenicity in at least one animal species, they have often failed to do so in other species. Moreover, drugs considered to be safe during human pregnancy have shown teratogenic effects in some animal species. For ethical reasons, it is impossible to test most new drugs in pregnant women. Therefore, a delay in detection of human teratogenicity is unavoidable, although attempts should be made to shorten this delay as much as possible by having reporting and data collection systems for pregnancy exposure and outcome in place and functional.

Given the expected rate of malformations in children, if a non-teratogenic drug is widely used during pregnancy, on average 2 to 4% of the exposed offspring will spontaneously be born with a congenital malformation. These may be reported as single cases stating the antenatal exposure and speculating on a causative association, as occurred with 'Bendectin'.[11] Thus, a drug widely used during pregnancy may be falsely associated with malformations. This demonstrates the necessity for carefully designed epidemiological studies.

New data on the teratogenic risk of a variety of drugs are constantly arising. Unfortunately, studies often provide as much misinformation as information. To provide optimal patient care, clinicians need to evaluate the current literature critically. It is, thus, important to understand the epidemiological methods typically employed in the reports and studies dealing with the causes of congenital malformations and their association with environmental factors. For a further discussion of these methods, see chapter 9.

### *1.3.1 Case Reports*

The common practice of reporting single cases of malformation as they arise may raise suspicions and lead to a hypothesis. However, by themselves, single cases are generally not sufficient to prove an association. An association between an environmental factor and malformations can be suspected when a number of cases is described in a case series. The homogeneous pattern of rare malformations produced by isotretinoin may serve as an example of such series proving causation long before large cohorts were collected.

#### Lithium

Lithium, a drug used to treat bipolar mood disorders, is used by approximately 0.1% of pregnant women.[33] Fetal effects of lithium have frequently been described, mostly by the Lithium Baby Register. This effort, founded in 1968 in Denmark and later expanded internationally, was a voluntary reporting system that collected information about children who were exposed to lithium during the first trimester of pregnancy. By 1983, the register listed 225 cases, including 25 (11%) with major malformations. 18 of these patients had cardiac malformations, one-third of them being the rare Ebstein's anomaly. On the basis of this information, lithium has widely been regarded as a human teratogen.[32,34]

Recently, the association between lithium and cardiac malformations was the topic of several retrospective case control studies and 2 prospective studies which became the basis for a meta-analysis.[35] This meta-analysis calculated risk ratios for cardiac malformations of 7.7 (95% confidence interval, 1.5 to 41.2) in the case control studies and 1.2 (95% confidence interval, 0.1 to 18.3) in the prospective cohorts. It was concluded that epidemiological data indicate that the teratogenic risk of first-trimester lithium exposure is substantially lower than previously suggested.

The comparison between case series based on a voluntary register and epidemiological evidence with a known denominator highlights the shortcomings of anecdotal reporting. Without a knowledge of the total number of exposures, an increased risk cannot be accurately defined. It is more likely that adverse pregnancy outcomes are voluntarily reported to a register than normal outcomes. Since the denominator of exposures remains unknown, registers of case reports and case series do not allow for risk estimates. If risk estimates are, nevertheless, calculated they are likely to produce overestimates.

Case reports or case series have been the basis for the detection of most known teratogens. While they can serve to draw attention to a suspected association, suspected associations must be subsequently supported by carefully designed epidemiological studies.

### *1.3.2 Case Control Studies*

Case control studies begin with a particular outcome and compare retrospectively the pregnancies of mothers with offspring presenting certain conditions or malformations with a control group consisting of the pregnancies of mothers with offspring not presenting the studied malformation.

#### Aspirin

The relationship between aspirin (acetylsalicylic acid) and congenital defects is controversial,[34] as shown by the results of a number of studies with different designs: 4 retrospective case control studies and 2 cohort studies. Three of the case control studies involved the pregnancies of 833 mothers in Wales[36] and 458 mothers in Scotland[37] resulting in birth of malformed children, and the pregnancies of 599 mothers in Finland[38] resulting in birth of children with cleft palates. The exposures of these index pregnancies were compared with controls consisting of the pregnancies resulting in the delivery of normal children. In each study, intake of aspirin during pregnancy was more often reported by mothers who had given birth to malformed children. Consequently, it was suggested that aspirin may be teratogenic. However, an association was not found between aspirin and cardiac malformations in another case control study, the Slone Epidemiology Unit Birth Defects Study,[39] involving 1381 infants with structural cardiac defects. The main difference between this study and the previous 3 was the assessment of 6966 infants with other malformations as controls instead of normal infants, and careful adjustments for potential confounding factors. This study found no differences in the maternal intake of aspirin between the cases and controls during the period critical for cardiac development.

Two cohort studies (see section 1.3.3) of gestational exposure to aspirin have been undertaken: an FDA surveillance study of Michigan Medicaid recipients involving 1709 completed pregnancies in which mothers were exposed to aspirin during the first trimester,[34] and the Collaborative Perinatal Project involving 14,864 pregnancies with mothers exposed to aspirin during the first trimester.[40] They did not result in a statistical association between aspirin exposure and congenital malformations. It appears that the epidemiological association between aspirin and congenital malformation is only based on early studies performed without appropriate measures now used to remedy typical pitfalls of the case control approach. Hence, aspirin use in recommended dosages during the first trimester of pregnancy is regarded today to be safe to the fetus.

#### Stilbestrol

The best example of the retrospective case control approach is probably the epidemiological investigation into the adverse effects of stilbestrol (diethylstilbestrol) on pregnancy outcome. The first epidemiological association between adenocarcinoma of the vagina in young women and their prenatal exposure to stilbestrol was made in a case control study involving 8 cases and 8 matched controls.[41] Because of the rarity (0.014 to 0.14% risk up to the age of 24 years) of this specific outcome, early cohort studies failed to confirm this association.[42] However, the frequency of dysplasia and carcinoma *in situ* of the cervix and vagina was significantly increased over controls with a relative risk of 2- to 4-fold in a cohort study involving 3980 Diethylstilbestrol Adenosis (DESAD) Project patients.[43] Moreover, the high incidence of cervical or vaginal structural changes in women following antenatal stilbestrol exposure, reported to be approximately 25% by the DESAD Project,[44] and the relationship between such changes and adenocarcinoma of the vagina underline the association seen in the case control studies.

#### Advantages of Case Control Studies

Case control studies are often used to acquire further and better evidence about whether congenital malformations or specific malformations are associated with a certain risk factor. The major advantage of retrospective case control studies is that they can be performed within a short time frame at a tolerable expense. Moreover, they allow for epidemiological investigation of exposures that only rarely result in specific adverse pregnancy outcomes. This avoids the necessity of screening hundreds or thousands of pregnancies with a certain exposure to find a significantly different rate of outcomes.

#### Disadvantages of Case Control Studies

Case control studies may have important disadvantages, including their vulnerability to selection or recall bias. This may be the reason for the significant outcome of the 3 aspirin studies cited above. Aspirin is a drug taken by large numbers of pregnant women. When a pregnancy results in an adverse outcome, it is likely that the woman reflects about the pregnancy and remembers each exposure. In contrast, when a pregnancy does not result in any problems, minor events including the intake of aspirin might be easily forgotten. Such behaviour can result in recall bias, which may falsely associate a frequently taken drug with congenital malformations. The Slone Epidemiology Unit Birth Defects Study[39] recruited infants with other malformations instead of normal infants as controls. By this means, recall bias was likely to be greatly reduced.

### *1.3.3 Cohort Studies*

Prospective cohort studies represent the gold standard of epidemiological research. They involve recruitment and follow-up of individuals who were exposed or not exposed to a certain potential risk factor. Outcomes are then collected prospectively and analysed statistically.

#### Fluoxetine

In a study comparing 128 pregnancies in women exposed to fluoxetine during the first trimester with a control group of 128 pregnant women with no exposure,[45] two women in each group had offspring with major malformations, a nonsignificant difference. There was a tendency for a higher rate of spontaneous abortions in the fluoxetine-exposed group (14.8 *vs* 7.8%), but this was not statistically significant. In addition, 74 fluoxetine-exposed pregnancies were compared with 74 control pregnancies during which the women were exposed to tricyclic antidepressants and 74 in which women were exposed to non-teratogenic drugs. Here too, there was no statistical difference between the groups with regard to pregnancy outcome. There was a nonsignificant tendency towards a higher rate of spontaneous abortions compared with that in pregnancies involving no exposure to antidepressant drugs (13.5 *vs* 6.8%); however, this tendency was not seen when compared with pregnancies in women exposed to tricyclic antidepressants (13.5 *vs* 12.2%). It was concluded that fluoxetine is very unlikely to be a major human teratogen, although it was acknowledged that the power of the study was insufficient to rule out minimal risk above the baseline.

Disregarding the statistical power issue of sample size, the study of Pastuszak et al.[45] demonstrates the state of the art in prospective cohort studies investigating the human teratogenicity of xenobiotics. Selection bias was minimised by choosing a control group of women who called the teratogen information service about exposure to non-teratogens. These women are likely to be equally concerned about the effect of an exposure to drugs during their pregnancy as are the mothers exposed to the studied drug, and this should lead to similar recall patterns. A second control group of women taking tricyclic antidepressants for their depression was aimed at separating the effects of the psychiatric condition from drug intake. The potential confounding factor of maternal age was minimised by matching controls on this variable. Other possible confounders such as obstetric history, alcohol (ethanol) and cigarette use were also compared and would have been adjusted for if they were different.

Prospective cohort studies have a number of advantages when compared with case control studies. Data are prospectively collected at a time when outcome is not yet known, thus defining a true denominator for later calculation of risk. The exposure is well defined, and sensitivity to a specific outcome is increased by careful prospective collection of outcome data. Prospective cohort studies are not free of pitfalls. However, the fluoxetine study demonstrates how some of these shortcomings can be obviated by careful selection of controls and by addressing possible confounding factors.

The prospective cohort approach is extremely powerful in elucidating the reproductive effects of xenobiotics with special focus on the prevalence of congenital malformations. A major drawback, however, is that to have sufficient power to rule out major teratogenic effects, there is a need to collect a large number of cases exposed to the xenobiotic in question.

### 1.3.4 Studies of Birth Prevalence or Incidence

Birth registries exist in a number of countries to monitor several neonatal characteristics and may, thus, be employed to draw useful conclusions. Although, to date, no human teratogens have been detected through the use of birth registries, this detection may not be impossible.

#### Thalidomide

Phocomelia, the main malformation typically induced by thalidomide during postconceptional days 22 to 36, is a very rare malformation, with an incidence of about 3.1 to 3.4 in 10,000 live births.[46] In October 1960, 2 cases of phocomelia were reported at a meeting in Germany[47] and other reports followed.[48] By this time, hundreds of babies were born with thalidomide embryopathy. The association between these defects and thalidomide was not made until late 1961 when Lenz[49] in Germany and McBride[4] in Australia suspected thalidomide to be the cause of these new cases.

Retrospectively, it was later noted that, had the Swedish monitoring system been in place at the time, the epidemic would have been signalled in Sweden after the birth of only 7 affected infants in a 4-month period.[50] In fact, at least 147 malformed infants were born in Sweden between 1960 and 1962.[2] However, it needs to be noted that the presentation of the thalidomide embryopathy was very unusual, being characterised typically by symptomatology which is extremely rare in unexposed newborns. In contrast, a teratogen that increases frequent malformations such as cardiac or neural tube defects by a small margin will need many more cases to be detectable by birth registries.

### 1.3.5 Experimental/Interventional Studies

For ethical and common sense reasons, pregnant women should only be exposed to interventions that are beneficial, or that have at least the potential of leading to benefits that may outweigh the involved risks. This is rarely the case when pregnant women are exposed to agents with questionable teratogenic potential. However, interventional studies can be used to determine whether a modality will reduce the risk of adverse pregnancy outcome. This approach has been used to investigate whether periconceptional folic acid reduces the incidence of neural tube defects.

#### Folic Acid and Neural Tube Defects

Evidence had been accumulating that low intake of folic acid may be associated with neural tube defects. However, it remained unclear whether confounding factors such as socioeconomic class or low intake of other vitamins may be responsible for these observations. This question was answered only through a large, British Medical Council-sponsored, international study in women who had had a previous child with neural tube defects. This randomised, double-blind, placebo-controlled study clearly demonstrated that folic acid reduced the risk of recurrence of neural tube defects and that other vitamins (without folic acid) failed to do so.[51] The validity of these data in a normal population was demonstrated by another randomised, double-blind, placebo-controlled study from Hungary involving pregnant women not having other risk factors. This study clearly showed the protective effect of folic acid 0.8 mg/day plus vitamins when compared with placebo.[52]

It is not clear whether 0.8 mg folic acid daily, as given in the Hungarian study, is superior to slightly smaller doses. However, it is likely that a dietary intake of 0.2 mg/day or less, which is characteristic of most Western women, is insufficient. Hence, the results of the two interventional studies have led to new recommendations for periconceptional supplementation of folic acid (see further section 5.1).

#### 1.3.6 Meta-Analysis

Meta-analysis is a method of analysing data combined from a number of separately performed epidemiological studies. The result is an overall odds ratio (see further chapter 9; sect. 4.2.5) that describes the association between an exposure and outcome. The strength of this method is its ability to increase sample size and consequent statistical power.

##### Metronidazole

Metronidazole is a first-line drug in the treatment of trichomoniasis[53] and has been commonly used by women during their reproductive years. It easily crosses the placenta to achieve a similar concentration in fetal and maternal blood.[54] Metronidazole has been in use for over 30 years and during this time it has never been reported to be teratogenic. Human and animal studies failed to document any harm to the offspring associated with its use during pregnancy.

While metronidazole is mutagenic in bacteria and carcinogenic in rodents, similar effects have never been documented in humans.[55] Nevertheless, these findings have been a major drawback when evaluating its safety during early human pregnancy.[34,54] The manufacturer and the US Centers for Disease Control consider metronidazole to be contraindicated during the first trimester in patients with trichomoniasis.[34] Since there have been a number of well controlled epidemiological studies investigating the association between metronidazole use in the first trimester and teratogenic effects, a meta-analysis was performed.

The meta-analysis used data from published studies including a total of 1336 women exposed to the drug. The result yielded an odds ratio for congenital malformations of 0.93 (95% confidence interval, 0.73 to 1.18). The result was supported by each of the studies. It was stated that metronidazole should consequently be considered non-teratogenic and its use should be encouraged in pregnant women who need the drug during the first trimester of pregnancy.[56]

Prospective human studies with a typical sample size of around 100 exposed pregnant women, like the fluoxetine study described in section 1.3.3, may be able to prove an association between a certain chemical exposure and an outcome, if the result yields a significant odds ratio. It is much more difficult to prove *safety* of a drug, because very large cohorts (i.e. in thousands) are needed to prove, for example, a relative risk of less than 2-fold. Yet, if smaller but well performed studies are available, these can be jointly analysed using meta-analysis to lead to risk estimation with much greater power.

## 2. Embryonic and Fetal Development

Antenatal human development can be divided into 3 major periods: blastogenesis, embryogenesis, and fetogenesis (table IV). Since the damage caused by xenobiotics avidly depends on the time of exposure, it is essential to review the characteristics of these developmental periods.

### 2.1 Blastogenesis

During the first week after conception, the conceptus develops from one cell to a bilaminar embryo surrounded by the trophoblast. At the same time, the conceptus travels via the fallopian tube to the uterine cavity to begin implantation at the end of the first week. At the end of the second week, implantation has progressed, with formation of lacunae that connect to maternal capillaries resulting in the first uteroplacental perfusion. Meanwhile, the inner cell mass has developed into a trilaminar leaf-shaped embryo, the cells of which are differentiating into ectodermal, mesodermal and entodermal cells with distinct destinies.

Congenital malformations due to exposure to toxins are usually not observed during this stage.[27] Damage may be inflicted on the developing organism if toxins achieve sufficient concentrations in the fallopian tube or at the site of implantation *in utero*. Such damage is most likely to lead to death of the organism, followed by an early abortion, which may not be noticed by the woman. If the organism survives, it is most likely to develop into a healthy embryo and fetus because of the still existing totipotency of its cells. Although animal experiments have shown that congenital malformations can be induced during this period,[57] clinical experience points towards the validity of this concept in humans. This period has, thus, been named as the ‘none or all’ period.

### 2.2 Embryogenesis

The embryonal period covers the time up to and including the 8th week after conception, or up to and including the 10th gestational week, and is characterised by the rapid development of almost all major organs. During the third week after conception, the neural groove appears and the future heart becomes visible. Thereafter, the neuropores close and the optic vessels become discernible during the fourth week. Simultaneously, the digestive system differentiates, the foregut and hindgut appear, the buccopharyngeal membrane ruptures, and the primordia of the liver and pancreas become visible.

At the end of the 4th week, at the 26th to 28th days, the arm and leg buds are noticed as mesodermal thickenings. During the 5th week, the olfactory pits appear, the superficial ectoderm of the optic vesicle forms the lens primordium, and in the heart the interatrial septum divides the atrial cavity into right and left sides. From this moment, the growth of the embryo is accelerated: the cardiac structures and the limb buds differentiate and the Mullerian ducts appear in the 6th week. During the next 2 weeks, the atrial and interventricular septa are completed, the primary ossification centres appear, the anal membrane ruptures and the gender of the embryo becomes well determined.

In this rapid development period, the embryo is most susceptible to the induction of malformations by teratogens. Unfortunately, at this early stage of pregnancy the woman is often unaware of her pregnancy and, thus, she may unknowingly use xenobiotics that are potentially hazardous to the embryo.

### 2.3 Fetogenesis

The fetal period begins at the end of the 8th week after conception, when little further differentiation of organs remains to be completed. The period is characterised by rapid growth and differentiation of organ systems.

Important events during the early fetal period include the complete closure of the palate, the reduction of the umbilical hernia, the differentiation of the external genitalia, as well as the histogenesis of the central nervous system. The latter process lasts for the entire fetal period and is completed only several months after birth. This explains the vulnerability of the brain to fetotoxic agents throughout the entire pregnancy. Interference with the development of the central nervous system can lead to various types of impairment of mental development such as reduced IQ, specific learning difficulties, or behavioural changes in postnatal life.

**Table V.** Basic principles of abnormal development (after Wilson[58])

| | |
|---|---|
| 1. | Susceptibility to abnormal development depends on the genotype of the conceptus and on the manner in which this genetic composition interacts with the environment |
| 2. | Agents that cause abnormal development vary with the developmental stage at the time of exposure |
| 3. | Teratogenic agents act in specific ways (mechanisms) on developing cells and tissues to initiate abnormal embryogenesis (pathogenesis) |
| 4. | The final manifestations of abnormal development are death, malformation, growth retardation, and functional disorders |
| 5. | The access of adverse environmental influences to developing tissues depends on the nature of the influences (agents) |
| 6. | Manifestations of deviant development increase in degree as dosage increases, from no effect to totally lethal effect |

## 3. Basic Principles of Teratogenicity

None of the presently known teratogens causes malformations in all exposures. The specific malformations induced by a given teratogen are often similar, but represent a spectrum of related malformations. This illustrates that the induction of malformations by a specific teratogen is influenced and dependent on a number of contributing factors, mainly genetic susceptibility, the developmental stage, and the dose of the exposure. Five principles of abnormal development were laid out as early as 1959 (before the thalidomide tragedy), and with minor modifications they still hold true today (table V).[58]

### 3.1 Time of Exposure to Toxins or 'Window of Opportunity'

Some teratogens (e.g. thalidomide) cause malformations only during a specific period of development. The 'window of opportunity' for thalidomide is between the postconceptional days 22 to 36.[46] Knowing when this period exists may allow the use of teratogenic drugs outside these periods in cases when therapy is essential. For example, coumarin anticoagulants are known to induce specific malformations during the 6th to 9th gestational weeks. None of 19 fetuses exposed to maternal treatment with warfarin after the 12th postconceptional week showed any signs of malformations associated with oral anticoagulants.[59] Yet, it should be remembered that there is a small risk of cerebral pathology and a risk of bleeding if coumarins are given during the fetal period.

The damage caused by a single exposure to an embryotoxin depends highly on the exact time of the exposure. The target organ system is usually either developing at this time or is about to develop. This has clearly been demonstrated with thalidomide, which has the potential for inducing a spectrum of malformations. If exposure occurred during postconceptional days 20 to 22, ear malformations resulted sometimes even without limb defects. In contrast, exposure during days 28 to 33 was likely to cause defects of the lower limbs. These days coincide with ear and lower limb development.

Knowledge of fetal developmental milestones is, thus, clinically important. For example, carbamazepine will only cause open neural tube defects during the first postconceptional weeks. On the other hand, folic acid will not prevent neural tube defects if given after the fourth week of conception.

Exposure to fetotoxic xenobiotics after the 10th postconceptional week does not lead to major malformations, except those associated with brain development. Exposure to xenobiotics during the fetal stage may lead to growth arrest, cell depletion, or functional anomalies, which are often difficult to detect at birth. Deformations caused by mechanical forces during the fetal period may mimic malformations, but should be distinguished. For instance, intrauterine compression associated with oligohydramnios can produce alterations in the shapes of the legs and feet.

During the fetal period, functional mechanisms of fetal toxicity become more apparent. Angiotensin-converting enzyme (ACE) inhibitors, for instance, may interfere with fetal cardiovascular and renal function and lead to oligohydramnios and fetal hypotension.[34] Exposure to cigarette smoking may inhibit fetal growth, partially because of decreased oxygen delivery to fetal tissues.[60,61]

### 3.2 Dose Dependency

Teratogenic effects are typically dependent on the dose of teratogen exposure to the pregnant woman, ranging from no effect to death at high doses. This dose dependency may have a clear threshold, often followed by a steep increase in the dose-response curve. The dose required to induce teratogenicity often differs widely between species and even between individuals. This is because of differences in placental morphology and physiology, genetic and environmental differences altering the susceptibility of the target organs, and differences in the fetal and maternal metabolism of xenobiotics leading to detoxification or toxification of a substance. Metabolic variability can be of particular importance if the teratogen is not the parent drug of exposure but one of its metabolites. A typical example for the importance of metabolic toxification is cyclophosphamide, which is converted to the cytotoxic and embryotoxic metabolites phosphoramide and acrolein.[62]

### 3.3 Species Differences

A complicating factor in teratology is the large difference between species regarding the adverse fetal effects of xenobiotics. While all known human teratogens have been found to be teratogenic in at least one animal species, there have been large interspecies differences. Coumarins, for instance, are teratogenic in humans, whereas until recently no other species was known to be susceptible to this class of agents. Conversely, drugs that are not teratogenic in humans (e.g. aspirin) may induce teratogenicity in a number of animal species. Furthermore, the type of malformations produced by a specific teratogen may be different among species. For example, carbutamide produces eye anomalies in rats and in mice while, in the rabbit, facial and visceral malformations have been observed.[28]

### 3.4 Mechanisms of Teratogenicity

The mechanisms leading to the induction of malformation by xenobiotics are still poorly understood. For example, more than 25 years after the discovery of the teratogenic potential of thalidomide, 24 proposed mechanisms are still considered, with no single one being particularly attractive.[63] That corticosteroids induce oral clefts in animals, but not in humans, has been linked to localisation of glucocorticoid receptors in this area in animals but not humans.

#### *3.4.1 Direct Fetal Toxicity*

During embryonal development, the organism is undergoing rapid growth, with a degree of cell and organ differentiation never to be experienced again later in life. This rapid development involves cell division and growth, cell and cell-layer migration, cell and tissue differentiation, fusion of cell layers, growth arrest, and programmed cell death.[64]

Coordination and regulation of cell growth and specialisation requires a complex system of interactions and regulations at intracellular levels in conjunction with various inter- and extracellular factors. Intracellularly, the expression of specific genes is regulated, with the resulting messenger RNA post-transcriptionally modified and translated into specific proteins. The intracellular transport and compartmentation appear to be essential for the development of specialised structures. Expression of specific adhesion molecules allows communication with neighbouring cells, the release of signal molecules and the expression of corresponding receptors coupled to specific second messenger mechanisms that enable interactions with more distant cells.

This short and incomplete list of mechanisms necessary for embryonic development contains a number of possible targets for xenobiotics. It is well known that DNA and RNA synthesis can be affected by chemotherapeutic agents and radiation. However, the mechanisms leading to the teratogenicity of such diverse substances as antiepileptic drugs (trimethadione, phenytoin, valproic acid and carbamazepine), heavy metals (mercury and lead), anticoagulants (coumarins), and others (e.g. thalidomide, stilbestrol, alcohol, etc.) are still poorly understood.

#### *3.4.2 Genetic Susceptibility to Teratogens*

The variability in susceptibility to teratogens by different species has been discussed in section 3.3. Similarly, interindividual differences in susceptibility are observed within species. In humans, such genetic susceptibility has been documented for phenytoin. Only a small percentage of offspring of women who have taken phenytoin during the first trimester exhibit the fetal hydantoin syndrome (for clinical signs, see table I). The occurrence of this syndrome has been shown[65] to be associated with the expression and activity of an epoxide hydrolase that is genetically controlled. Fetuses with low activity of this enzyme are believed to be unable to inactivate the teratogenic epoxide metabolite of phenytoin with the result that they experience fetal hydantoin syndrome.[65] Subsequent animal studies support these findings. The incidence of phenytoin-induced congenital malformations was significantly lowered by coadministration of the cytochrome P450–inhibiting antiepileptic drug stiripentol by reducing the level of fetal exposure to oxidative metabolites of phenytoin.[66]

#### *3.4.3 Mechanisms Involving the Placental-Maternal Unit*

The mammalian embryo is fully dependent on its mother to maintain homeostasis by providing nutrients and oxygen, and removing metabolic waste. Disruption of these functions at the maternal or placental level may impair embryonic development and may lead to adverse pregnancy outcomes. The importance of maternal well-being for fetal outcome has been realised by clinicians for generations. Fetal damage caused by maternal-placental mechanisms has been demonstrated in animal experiments. For example, cadmium (Cd) 40 μmol/kg injected into rats on gestation day 18 caused a 75% incidence of fetal death, even though the fetal Cd burden was low. Direct intraperitoneal injection into the fetus, producing a 10-fold greater body burden of Cd, caused only an 8% increase in fetal death. It has been speculated that the mechanism leading to this toxicity could be fetal zinc deficiency caused by Cd-dependent interference with placental zinc transport.[67]

#### *3.4.4 Multifactorial Effects*

All of the effects described in this section may interact and complicate the understanding of fetal outcome. However, multifactorial effects may be more the rule than the exception. An illustrative example is the fetal alcohol syndrome in which several factors are likely to affect fetal outcome: the dosage and rate of ethanol intake, maternal metabolism, and finally, the genetics of the fetus. The latter is indicated by the concordance of effect in monozygous twins and discordance in dizygous twins.[68]

## 4. Pharmacokinetic Considerations

### 4.1 Maternal Pharmacokinetics During Pregnancy

Pregnancy is accompanied by a multitude of changes in maternal physiology (table VI). These alterations may have significant effects on many aspects of maternal drug handling and need to be taken into account when treating pregnant women. However, because of many discrepancies between the handling of different drugs, high inter- and intraindividual variability, and the progressive nature of these changes, it is impossible to arrive at a general and consistent pharmacokinetic paradigm in pregnancy.[70] Hence, predictions of maternal pharmacokinet-

**Table VI.** Maternal physiological changes during pregnancy possibly affecting maternal pharmacokinetics (after Hytten & Chamberlain[69])

| Body system/ function | Physiological changes | Extent of change |
|---|---|---|
| Cardiovascular system | Cardiac output | ↑ 30-35% |
| | Heart rate | ↑ 20% |
| | Stroke volume | ↑ 10% |
| | Arterial blood pressure | ↔ |
| | *Blood flow:* | |
| | uterus | ↑ 950% to 500ml |
| | kidneys | ↑ 60-80% |
| | liver | ↔ or ↑ 75%? |
| | skin (hands) | ↑ 600-700% |
| Haematological system | Plasma volume | ↑ 50% |
| | Red cell mass | ↑ 18-30% |
| | Plasma albumin concentration | ↓ 30% |
| | Serum lipids | ↑ 66% |
| Respiratory system | Tidal volume | ↑ 40% |
| | Respiratory rate | ↔ |
| Gastrointestinal system | Gastric tone/mobility | ↓ |
| | Intestinal mobility | ↓ |
| Kidney function | GFR | ↑ 50% |
| Body composition | Water | ↑ |
| | Fat | ↑ |

*Abbreviations & symbols:* GFR = glomerular filtration rate; ↑ = increased; ↓ = decreased; ↔ = unchanged.

ics at different stages of pregnancy are bound to be inaccurate. When there are doubts about the clinical effectiveness or important dose-dependent adverse effects, especially for drugs with narrow therapeutic ranges, then plasma drug concentrations should be monitored (see further chapter 5).

The effects of the physiological changes during pregnancy on the principal determinants of maternal pharmacokinetics (absorption, distribution, metabolism and excretion) are discussed in sections 4.1.1, 4.1.2, and 4.1.3. For the sake of simplicity, the contributions of the fetus, placenta, uterus and amniotic fluid, as an additional compartment having a possible effect on maternal pharmacokinetics, are not discussed.

#### 4.1.1 Absorption

Absorption of enterally-administered drugs may be delayed in pregnancy, resulting in delayed and lower peak plasma concentrations because of slow gastric and intestine motility. The total amount absorbed may increase if absorption of a particular drug is slow and depends on the time the drug remains in the intestine. It may decrease if emesis and oesophageal reflux, which occur frequently during pregnancy, interfere with proper absorption.

As tidal volume and pulmonary blood flow are increased, gaseous xenobiotics that enter the circulation via the lung may equilibrate faster with blood concentrations, resulting in increased total absorption. Transdermal absorption may be altered by a variety of factors, including increases in cutaneous blood flow, extracellular water, and in amounts of subcutaneous fat tissue.

Despite absorption being significant in delineating maternal plasma concentrations and consequent fetal exposure to xenobiotics, there are very few data evaluating changes in absorption of drugs during pregnancy.

#### 4.1.2 Distribution

Total body water increases during the course of pregnancy by about 8L. However, this value may vary considerably between individuals and is also dependent on the method of determination.[71] 60% of the increase is distributed to the placenta, fetus, and amniotic fluid, while another 40% is distributed to maternal tissues, resulting in maternal plasma volume increasing by 50% during pregnancy. These changes mainly affect the volume of distribution of polar drugs, which have a relatively low volume of distribution that corresponds to water compartments.

The 25% average increase in body fat during pregnancy[72] leads to increased volumes of distribution of drugs that are predominantly deposited in fatty tissues, often resulting in a decrease in their plasma concentration.

The tendency towards lower plasma concentrations of drugs is complicated by a decrease in protein binding and, hence, an increase in the fraction of the unbound (free) drug present. Serum albumin concentrations are decreased during pregnancy and, in addition, drugs may be displaced from their plasma proteins by the increased amount of circulating free fatty acids and other endogenous substances.[73] As discussed in chapter 1, section 3.2.3, changes in the free fraction of drugs are of no clinical relevance unless they are rapid or accompanied by changes in absorption or elimination capacity. However, pregnancy is accompanied by a number of physiological changes that may concomitantly affect other pharmacokinetic parameters.

#### 4.1.3 Metabolism and Excretion

Both induction and inhibition of enzymes have been reported during pregnancy, depending on the metabolising system.[74] For example, while the cytochrome P450 enzyme metabolising caffeine is less active,[75,76] there is an increase in liver metabolism of phenytoin during gestation.[77,78]

A gradual increase in renal function will generally result in an augmented elimination rate of xenobiotics that are excreted by the kidneys, including penicillins, aminoglycosides, digoxin and many others. To ensure sufficient therapeutic drug concentrations at the site of action, an increase in dose of these drugs needs to be considered.

## 4.2 Placental Function

The human placenta is derived mainly from embryonic tissue except for one basal cell layer on the uterine side, the decidua basalis. During the first week of conception the conceptus differentiates into 2 parts, the outer trophoblast and the inner cell mass. Growth of the trophoblast, which will form the placenta, initially exceeds the growth of the inner cell mass, which will eventually form the embryo. At the end of the first week, the trophoblast is superficially implanted whereas, during the second week, uteroplacental perfusion is established by formation of lacunae through which maternal blood circulates. During the third week, fetal capillaries are formed in the chorionic villae and perfused by fetal blood cells. The essential dual perfusion of the mammalian placenta is established.

During the following months until birth the surface area for maternal-fetal exchange increases proportionally to the weight of the fetus.[79,80] The fetal capillaries are arranged in direct proximity to the trophoblast syncytium, allowing close contact between the two circulation systems. The syncytial trophoblast is a highly specialised tissue that consists of a single layer of fused cells; it is the only continuous barrier between the maternal and fetal circulation. The transfer across this barrier regulates and limits the maternal-fetal exchange of xenobiotics in both directions. This arrangement differs from that seen in many animals, which limits the validity of extrapolation of data derived from animal experiments to the understanding of human placental physiology and pathophysiology.

### *4.2.1 Placental Transfer of Drugs*

Little is known about placental transfer during early pregnancy, the period of the greatest teratogenic vulnerability. All present knowledge has been derived from placentas at term. Generalisation to earlier periods must be made with caution.

#### Diffusion

Diffusion is the most important mode of xenobiotic distribution in tissues; this is likely to be true also for the placental tissue. Passive diffusion is defined by the passage of molecules across a barrier without the input of energy, and can be described by Fick's equation:

$$\Delta q/\Delta t = KA(C_m - C_f)/d$$

where $\Delta q/\Delta t$ is the rate of transfer of a substance, K is the diffusion constant of the drug in question, A the surface area of the membrane, $C_m$ is the maternal free blood concentration, $C_f$ is the fetal free blood concentration, and d is the thickness of the membrane. According to this equation, the rate of net transfer is dependent on the physicochemical characteristics of the transferred substance, the area available for diffusion, the concentration gradient of free (i.e. not protein bound) substance between the maternal and fetal sides, and is inversely correlated to the thickness of the membrane. Since surface area and thickness of the membrane are constants at a given developmental period, transfer depends mainly on the concentration gradient and the physicochemical properties of the transported substance.

#### Influence of Physicochemical Properties

Physicochemical properties of xenobiotics with importance for placental transfer are molecular weight, water/lipid solubility, and ionisation of the substance. Drugs with a molecular weight of less than 500D tend to easily cross the human placenta, while drugs with a higher molecular weight might only achieve incomplete transfer, thus reaching lower concentrations in the fetal circulation. Heparin, for example, which has a molecular weight of more than 5000D, is not transported to the fetus at all.

Lipid solubility favours transfer across the placenta in comparison with water solubility. Most molecules of acidic drugs with a low pKa and of basic drugs with a high pKa are charged at physiological pH values. This complicates transport or diffusion across biological membranes and, thus, transplacental transport of these agents tends to be incomplete.

#### Influence of pH Differences

Fetal blood pH is slightly lower than the maternal value. Weak bases with a pKa close to the blood pH are predominantly non-ionised on the maternal side of the placenta and easily cross into fetal blood. On the fetal side, these molecules become ionised because of the more acidic environment. This results in a lower concentration of non-ionised drug and leads to further diffusion of non-ionised drugs across the placenta, leading to a net movement from maternal to fetal systems ('ion trapping'). The same mechanism may cause weak acids to be less concentrated on the fetal side of the placenta.[81]

#### Facilitated Transfusion and Active Transport

In addition to passive diffusion, xenobiotics can be transported across the placenta by facilitated transfusion and active transport. Facilitated transfusion involves mediation by a carrier, but is not energy dependent. While facilitated transfusion is an important mode for endogenous compounds such as glucose, drugs may also be transported by such carriers, an example being cefalexin. Facilitated transfusion allows a drug to reach higher peak concentrations, but does not alter the concentration at equilibrium.

In contrast, active transport allows the transport of molecules against an existing concentration gradient through the expenditure of energy. Substrates for active transport are usually molecules essential for the growth of the embryo (i.e. amino acids). Most drugs are not actively transported unless they are analogues of endogenous compounds; examples are methyldopa and fluorouracil.[82]

#### Influence of Uterine Blood Flow and Fetal Tissue Distribution

If a drug is rapidly transported across the placenta, its availability at the site of exchange becomes a rate-limiting factor for maternal-fetal transfer. Uterine blood flow determines the rate of presentation of a drug and, thus, may determine the rate of transport. On the fetal side, placental blood flow and tissue distribution become rate-limiting factors, because they determine the fetal contribution to the concentration gradient.

#### Influence of Protein Binding

Fetal albumin concentrations increase during pregnancy from very low levels during the first trimester to levels exceeding adult values during late pregnancy. Conversely, maternal albumin concentrations progressively decrease throughout gestation so that they are higher than fetal concentrations during early gestation, achieve equivalency at around week 30 of gestation, and are lower than fetal levels later in the late third trimester.[83] In contrast, fetal concentrations of

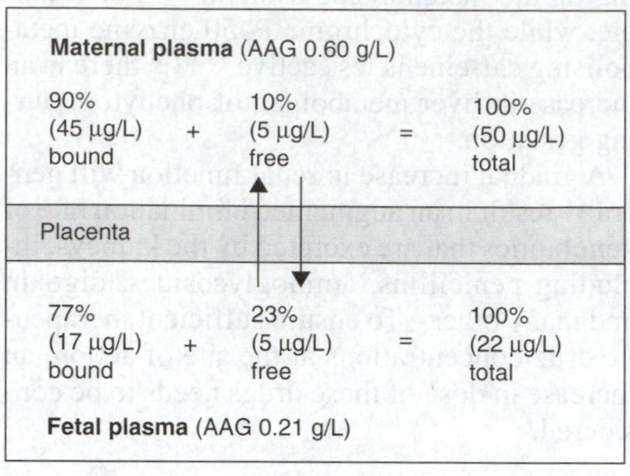


F/M = 22 μg/L ÷ 50 μg/L = 0.44

**Fig. 1.** Equilibrium concentrations of a drug across the placenta is determined by the percentage of the drug bound to its binding protein, as established by the transplacental plasma protein concentration ratio. A drug (total concentration 50 μg/L) is 90% bound to maternal plasma $\alpha_1$-acid glycoprotein (AAG), producing a bound to free (B/F) ratio of 9.0. Fetal plasma contains only 37% of the maternal AAG concentration, and the B/F ratio is reduced to 3.4 [$B/F_{maternal} \times 0.37 = B/F_{fetal}$ ($9.0 \times 0.37 = 3.4$)]. Unbound drug freely equilibrates between maternal and fetal compartments (↓↑). The resulting fetal/maternal concentration ratio (F/M) is the sum of the bound and free concentrations in fetal plasma divided by the total concentration in maternal plasma (F/M = 0.44) [after Hill & Abramson;[85] with permission].

$\alpha_1$-acid glycoprotein remain low throughout pregnancy.[83] These differences have distinct effects on the fetal/maternal ratio of total (bound and free) concentrations of drugs that bind to these proteins.

Xenobiotics cross the placenta as free, unbound molecules. Dissociation from plasma proteins occurs almost instantaneously and, thus, this process should not affect the diffusion across the placenta.[84] Consequently, the concentration driving diffusion and eventually equilibrating across the placenta is the level of free drug. Once it arrives on the other side, some free drug will again become protein bound. Since protein concentrations differ between maternal and fetal plasma, this may result in different concentrations of total drug despite similar concentrations of free drug.

Thus, in the case of albumin-bound acid drugs, the ratio of maternal to fetal drug concentration (when measured as total drug concentration) changes throughout pregnancy due to changes in maternal and fetal albumin concentrations. In the case of basic a1-acid glycoprotein–bound drugs, maternal total drug concentrations will exceed fetal total drug concentrations

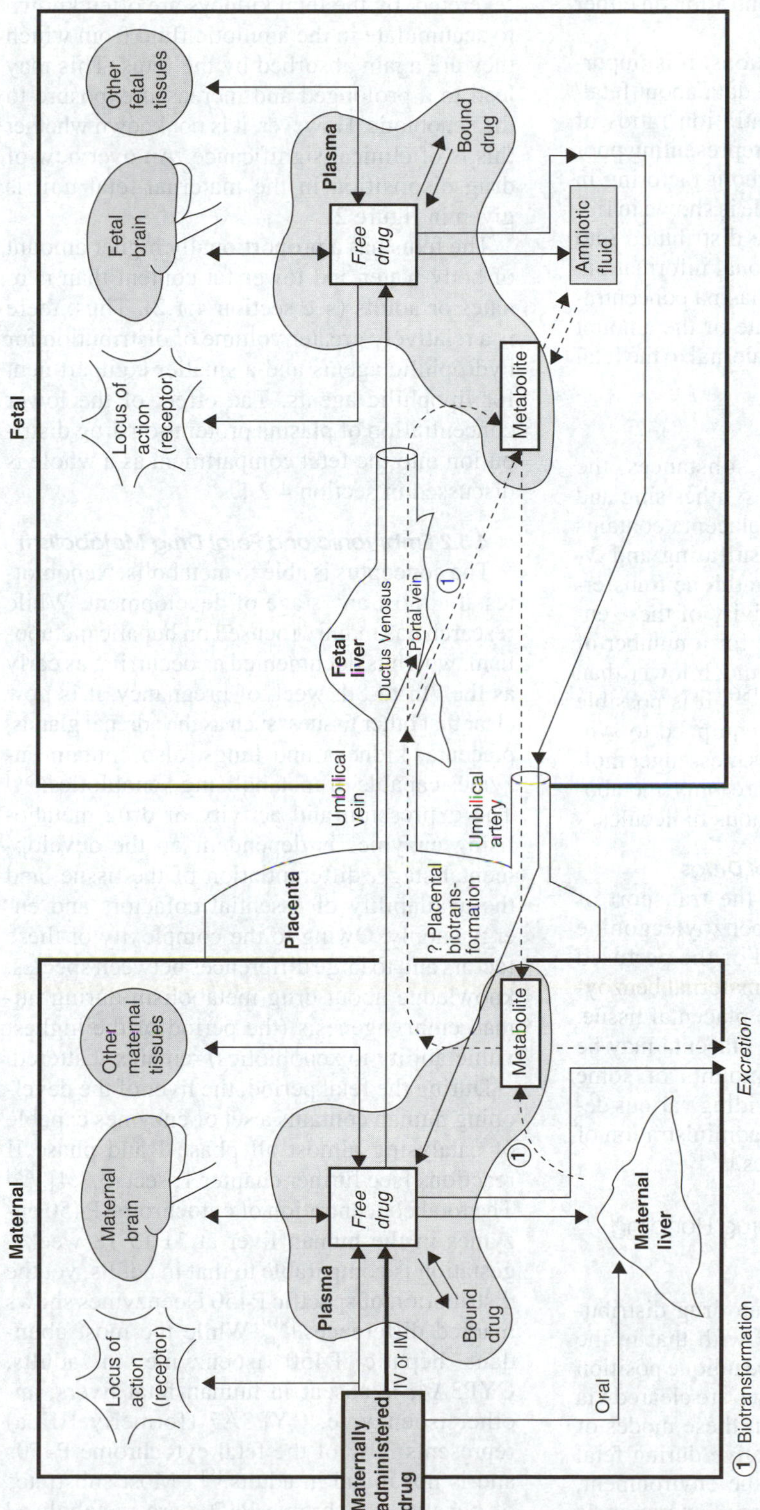


**Fig. 2.** Drug disposition in a model of the maternal-placenta-fetal unit (after Mirkin;[87] with permission).

throughout the entire pregnancy, although free drug may have the same concentration on either side of the placenta.

Because of these considerations, it is important not to interpret published data about fetal/maternal total plasma concentration ratios of highly protein bound drugs as representing poor or good placental transfer without factoring in protein binding.[85] An example is shown in figure 1. Finally, since drugs are distributed into various tissues, without additional information, neither the total nor the free plasma concentration allows a complete estimate of the amount of drug transferred from the maternal to the fetal compartment.

#### 4.2.2 Placental Metabolism

In addition to transferring substances, the placenta has the capability of synthesising and metabolising molecules. The placenta contains cytochrome P450 enzymes, sulfating and *N*-acetylation enzymes, and glutathione transferase activity. However, the activity of these enzymes appears to be selective for a number of substances and the activity is much lower than that of fetal hepatic enzymes.[86] It is possible that the placenta is primarily equipped to synthesise and modify endogenous messenger molecules and that xenobiotics are only metabolised if they resemble endogenous molecules.

#### 4.2.3 Placental Absorption of Drugs

A recent study evaluating the transport of cocaine and its metabolite benzoylecgonine revealed that about one-third of the perfused cocaine and one-eighth of the maternal benzoylecgonine was retained by the placental tissue. These results suggest that the placenta may be able to retain significant amounts of some xenobiotics, thus perhaps providing various degrees of fetal protection after administration of potentially harmful xenobiotics.[86]

### 4.3 Embryonic and Fetal Drug Handling

#### 4.3.1 Fetal Drug Distribution

The main difference between drug distribution in the fetus as compared with that in the neonate or adult is related to the unique position *in utero*. After birth, xenobiotics are cleared via the liver, kidney, and lung, but these modes of excretion are minimally operative during fetal life. The only connection to the environment, and consequently the only route of excretion, is via the placenta. The fetal 'extracorporeal' environment, the amniotic fluid, is a fetal compartment on its own. For example, drugs that are 'excreted' by the fetal kidneys are often known to accumulate in the amniotic fluid from which they are again absorbed by the fetus. This may lead to a prolonged and increased exposure to the xenobiotic. However, it is not known whether this is of clinical significance. An overview of drug disposition in the maternal-fetal unit is given in figure 2.

The fetus has a proportionally higher amount of body water and lower fat content than neonates or adults (see section 4.1.2). Thus, there is a relatively greater volume of distribution for hydrophilic agents and a smaller compartment for lipophilic agents. The effect of the lower concentration of plasma proteins on drug distribution into the fetal compartment as a whole is discussed in section 4.2.1.

#### 4.3.2 Embryonic and Fetal Drug Metabolism

The conceptus is able to metabolise xenobiotics at almost any stage of development. While research has mainly focused on hepatic metabolism, which is documented as occurring as early as the 7th to 8th week of pregnancy, it is now clear that other tissues, such as the adrenal glands, placenta, kidneys and lungs, also contain enzymes capable of metabolising xenobiotics.[88] The expression and activity of drug-metabolising enzymes is dependent on the developmental stage, differentiation of the tissue, and the availability of essential cofactors and energy supply. Owing to the complexity of these factors and to large differences between species, knowledge about drug metabolism during human embryogenesis (the period of the highest vulnerability to xenobiotics) remains scattered.

During the fetal period, the liver of the developing human contains a set of enzymes capable of catalysing almost all phase I and phase II reactions [see further chapter 1; sect. 3.3.4].[88] The total concentration of cytochrome P450 enzymes in the human liver at 11 to 18 weeks' gestation is comparable to that in adults, yet the distribution of specific P450 isoenzymes shows marked differences.[89] While the most abundant hepatic P450 isoenzyme in adults, CYP3A4, is absent in human fetal livers, another isoenzyme, CYP3A7 (formerly HFLa) represents 30% of the fetal cytochrome P450s and is not found in adults.[90] Most substrates of hepatic cytochrome P450s are metabolised with a significantly lower activity compared with adults.[88]

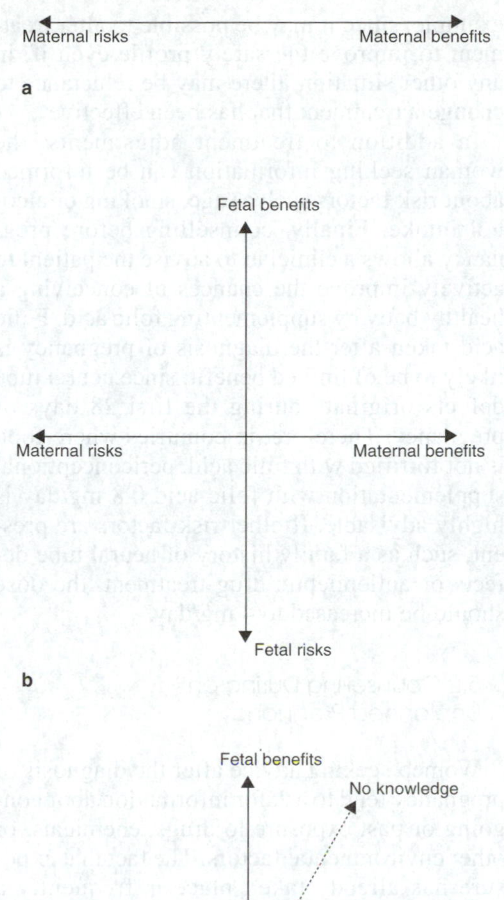


**Fig. 3.** Factors in the process of deciding whether to use a drug in a female patient. (a) Non-pregnant patient; (b) pregnant patient; (c) pregnant patient with analysis of evidence.

Information about other phase I reactions is relatively scarce. Activities of monoamine oxidase, alcohol dehydrogenase, aldehyde dehydrogenase, nitroreduction and epoxide hydrolase have all been detected in the human fetal liver; however, these activities were usually lower than in adults.[74,89]

Glucuronidation, quantitatively the most important phase II reaction in adults, is substantially reduced or even absent in the human fetal liver, with the exception of one isoenzyme that metabolises 5-hydroxytryptamine. The activity of this enzyme almost reaches adult levels.[91] In contrast, sulfation is well developed in the human fetus. This constellation leads to a shift in metabolic pathways for drugs that can be both glucuronidated and sulfated. Whereas in adults, paracetamol (acetaminophen), salicylamide, and ritodrine are usually glucuronidated, they are usually sulfated in human fetuses.[89]

*N*-Acetyltransferase (NAT), in particular NAT1 activity, has been detected in human fetal liver[92] and placenta.[93,94] The activity reaches about 60% of adult levels in human liver.[92]

The human fetus is able to metabolise xenobiotics by glutathione conjugation. Similar to the situation with cytochrome P450 isoenzymes, the expression of isoenzymes appears to differ significantly between intra- and extrauterine life.

*In summary*, the human fetus is equipped with an array of mechanisms to metabolise xenobiotics. Several isoenzymes are uniquely expressed during fetal life. The mechanisms leading to differential expression before and after birth remain unknown, as does their potential benefit to the fetus. In general, the activities of enzymes capable of metabolising xenobiotics appear to be lower during fetal than during later life. This may prevent rapid metabolism to more polar molecules that may not be able to freely cross the placenta and may accumulate in the fetal circulation. Metabolism of xenobiotics can lead to either detoxification or toxification. The large differences between the enzymes expressed in fetuses of different species compared with humans may account for many of the observed interspecies differences in teratogenicity.

## 5. General Principles of Counselling and Drug Therapy in Pregnancy

In general, the decision to employ a certain drug for treatment is made by evaluating benefits *versus* risks to the patient (fig. 3a). This situation is complicated during pregnancy since, in essence, this evaluation must be made for two patients, the mother and the unborn child. In addition, a different quality of risk must be considered because adverse effects in the offspring may often be irreversible. While the physician must select a treatment with the lowest possible risk to the unborn child, the risks and benefits for the mother must not be neglected. This concept may be visualised by the 2-dimensional graph depicted in figure 3b.

Unfortunately, the evaluation of risks *versus* benefits is often hampered by the fact that the risks to the conceptus imposed by maternal use of many new prescription drugs are not yet known. This further complicates the decision process, as depicted in figure 3c. However, in most instances, it may be possible to replace a novel drug with an older, more established agent for which sufficient data are available to allow an informed decision. Sacrifices made, such as the potential for increased adverse effects in the pregnant women or slightly decreased efficacy, may be outweighed by the known safety for the offspring.

To shorten the process of information gathering for the clinician, table II presents an extensive list of drugs that have shown no increased risk for the fetus during pregnancy or that will involve the least fetal risk if maternal treatment is essential.[6] It should not be inferred that drugs not included in this table may be teratogens or may have adverse effects on the offspring, but rather that there are insufficient good studies to indicate with a high degree of likelihood that the particular drug can be adequately defined as 'safe'. The data presented in table II are valid at present but will need to be re-evaluated as additional information becomes available.

When risks to the fetus are estimated or when women are counselled, it should be kept in mind that there is no guarantee of an uncomplicated pregnancy outcome. A 2 to 3% baseline risk of major congenital malformation cannot be circumvented with our present knowledge. The increase in risk by 1%, as for instance estimated to be induced by therapy with carbamazepine, may appear high but must be viewed in relation to this baseline risk.

It is beneficial to inform pregnant women of the facts leading to the choice of a specific treatment. Accurate information will alleviate fears, improve patient compliance and, thus, eventually lead to better treatment.

### 5.1 Counselling For a Planned Pregnancy

Counselling of women who are planning pregnancy is an ideal situation. If chronic conditions are present, adjustments of treatment can be made to account for any risks to the conceptus. The therapy of seizure disorders serves as a good example, since it may be possible to alter treatment to improve the safety profile even if, in any other situation, there may be reluctance to change a treatment that has been effective.

In addition to treatment adjustments, the woman seeking information can be informed about risk factors such as age, smoking or alcohol intake. Finally, counselling before pregnancy allows a clinician to advise the patient to actively improve the chances of conceiving a healthy baby by supplementing folic acid. Folic acid taken after the diagnosis of pregnancy is likely to be of limited benefit, since neural tube defects originate during the first 28 days of pregnancy. Therefore, in countries where food is not fortified with folic acid, periconceptional supplementation with folic acid 0.8 mg/day is highly advisable. If other risk factors are present, such as a family history of neural tube defects or antiepileptic drug treatment, the dose should be increased to 4 mg/day.

### 5.2 Counselling During an Unplanned Pregnancy

Women seeking advice after the diagnosis of pregnancy tend to ask for information about ongoing or past exposure to drugs, chemicals, or other environmental factors. The fact that exposure has already taken place is frequently a cause of a high degree of anxiety. Since the information given may have a significant effect on the decision to terminate pregnancy, it is important to inform the patient accurately about the possible risks or to emphasise that there is no increased risk if the exposure was to drugs or chemicals that are considered safe. It is not enough to tell the patient that a drug may be teratogenic; a quantitative assessment of the risk should be given (see table I), since women tend to overestimate the incidence of adverse pregnancy outcomes after exposure to any teratogen.[95]

Proper information can only be given after having taken a thorough history, including time of conception (based on last menstrual period), exact time of the exposure and dosage of the xenobiotic, indications for any drugs taken, and other maternal medical conditions possibly posing risks, such as age or chronic diseases. It may be appropriate to confirm this information by physical examination and comparison with previous medical records. Ultrasound examination may be beneficial to determine the exact stage of the pregnancy and at a later stage of pregnancy to screen for visual fetal defects. Amniocentesis and measurement of α-fetoprotein should be offered if indicated, when chromosomal abnormalities or neural tube defects need to be ruled out.

In addition to giving an estimate of the possible risk to the conceptus, advice should be given about possible future avoidance of exposure if a xenobiotic is thought to bear a risk to the pregnant woman or her unborn child.

### 5.3 Retrospective Evaluation of the Role of Teratogens in Adverse Pregnancy Outcomes

Retrospective evaluation after an adverse pregnancy outcome leads to a different kind of risk assessment. As with prospective risk estimation, this assessment relies on a thorough history, elucidating exact exposure dates and dosages, a thorough medical history and physical examination of mother and offspring. The medical history should be verified by past medical records whenever possible. Xenobiotic exposures during pregnancy as well as all possible confounding factors must then be compared with the current knowledge about their effects during pregnancy. If an association between the xenobiotic(s) in question and symptomatology of the offspring appears plausible, it is important to search for other likely causes of the malformation. A genetic consultation must be incorporated to exclude or include genetic causes of the adverse pregnancy outcome, since far more malformations occur due to genetic causes than to exposure to xenobiotics.

Finally, careful wording of the medical opinion rendered is extremely important since it is almost never possible to pinpoint a causal relationship with absolute certainty, and retrospective assessments may be used in later litigation.

## 6. Known Human Teratogens

A limited number of drugs and commonly used chemicals have been proven to be human teratogens. These are listed in table I in conjunction with the fetal adverse effects caused by each molecule, the relative risks that these effects will occur after exposure, and clinical interventions that should be undertaken. The table focuses on drugs and chemicals as teratogens, but viruses, such as rubella or varicella, and pathological maternal conditions, such as diabetes mellitus, may also act as 'environmental' teratogens.

## 7. Effects of Commonly Used Therapeutic Agents on the Embryo and Fetus

The literature about the risks and benefits of drug treatment during pregnancy is continuously expanding. While there is almost no drug that has not been rightly or wrongly associated with some adverse pregnancy outcome in at least one case report, many drugs are now considered safe during pregnancy. Other drugs, such as antiepileptics, may impose fetal risks, but are nevertheless necessary for a pregnant woman with serious or chronic disease.

It is no longer possible to summarise in a single chapter the complete knowledge about drug treatment in pregnancy. For detailed information, large collections of references are available, e.g. Briggs et al.;[34] Koren;[96] Shepard;[16] Gilstrap and Little;[97] Petrie;[98] Schardein;[99] and Heinonen et al.[14]

With the needs of the clinical pharmacologist and practising physician in mind, a 2-tiered approach has been taken to extract the relevant essentials from the literature and present them here. The first consists of a list of drugs for which there is sufficient evidence to consider them safe during pregnancy if used in therapeutic dosages (table II). This information can, of course, only serve as a rough guideline. Treatment must be oriented primarily to maternal pathology and needs to be individualised for each patient.

The second part discusses in more detail the effects of a selected group of important or frequently used drugs on the developing offspring. Since maternal, fetal or embryonic effects of drugs may differ widely between humans and many animal species, animal experiments remain of limited value and great caution must be exercised when extrapolating the results to human drug use. Therefore, this discussion of drug effects during pregnancy focuses on available human data and uses animal data only where absolutely necessary.

New agents are constantly being developed for therapeutic use in humans. Since human data about their use in pregnancy may be unavailable, many newer drugs are not included in this discussion. Many of these agents are similar to existing drugs used for the same indications. However, for use in pregnancy, it is often advisable to replace newer drugs with others for which more safety information is available.

7.1 Drugs Acting on the Nervous System

#### *7.1.1 Opioid Analgesics*

All of the centrally-acting analgesics readily cross the placenta.[97] *Pethidine* (meperidine), the opioid analgesic most frequently used during delivery, appears in the fetal blood 2 minutes after intravenous administration to the mother, and equilibrium between maternal and fetal circulation occurs after 6 minutes.[100] Since *methadone* has a longer elimination half-life in the fetus (23h) than in the mother (3h),[101] fetal drug concentrations may exceed maternal concentrations during elimination.

Despite the use of opioids over many decades, no reports have linked them to congenital malformations when used for medical purposes. However, concern exists about the respiratory depression in neonates exposed *in utero* to morphine given to alleviate pain during the course of delivery.[102] While early reports have stated that morphine causes more pronounced respiratory depression than pethidine in the neonate, others have found no differences if the analgesics were used in equipotent doses.

The concern over neonatal respiratory depression first led to replacement of morphine by pethidine and later to a general decrease in systemic use of all opioid analgesics.[100,102] More recently, the employment of opioids has resurged with the development of intrathecal methods of administration, often in combination with local anaesthetics.[102,103] The lower systemic doses given with this technique results in smaller effects on the fetus or neonate.

Hypertonic uterine contractions are a possible adverse effect of pethidine when used during labour[100] and these contractions have not been described during morphine use. When used for prolonged periods (i.e. illicit use, see section 8), all opioid agonists can produce varying degrees of maternal and fetal addiction, followed by withdrawal symptoms in the neonate after birth. However, when opioids are used only during labour, this is of no concern.

In the search for opioid analgesics that are potent, but have fewer adverse effects and cause no dependence, a large number of agents have been developed and are currently used for various indications. Advantages of some of these agents may be the absence of active metabolites, a more selective effect on subgroups of opioid receptors, or partial opioid antagonist activity. In the neonate, adverse effects similar to those described above for morphine and pethidine should be expected after administration of these agents to a woman in labour. When evaluating the safety of these agents, it should be remembered that there is very little experience with their use in the first trimester of pregnancy and that there is much less experience during late pregnancy than with morphine and pethidine. Nevertheless, the following analgesics appear to be safe when used in pharmacological doses during late pregnancy:[34] alfentanil, alphaprodine, anileridine, butorphanol, fentanyl, levorphanol, nalbuphine, oxymorphone, pentazocine, phenazocine and sufentanil.

*Codeine* is a widely used analgesic and antitussive agent, and embryonic or fetal exposure is common. Several cohort studies (summarised in the review by Briggs et al.[34]) have associated the agent with a number of congenital malformations. However, it appears unlikely that these are of any statistical significance especially since there is no single defect observed in all or most of the studies. Codeine appears to be safe when used in pharmacological doses during pregnancy, and this appears also to be true for *oxycodone* and *hydromorphone*.

*Naloxone* is an opioid antagonist with no agonist properties. It is frequently used in neonates to counteract respiratory depression caused by opioid agonists given in the immediate antenatal period. No adverse effects are known when appropriate neonatal doses are used, unless it is administered to a neonate of an addicted mother. In this case, acute neonatal withdrawal symptoms can be induced. After administration, the neonate should be carefully observed, since the effects of the opioid agonist may outlast the effects of the antagonist, resulting in recurrent neonatal respiratory depression.

Analgesics or local anaesthetics given during labour may have an effect on the neonate. It remains unknown whether this effect may be sustained over the first days of life. On the other hand, management of pain associated with labour is an extremely sensitive issue for the mother. Management that is perceived by the mother as inappropriate may arouse feelings of anger or even guilt over having exposed their offspring to potentially harmful drugs. This may affect the process of maternal bonding. It is, thus, extremely important to discuss treatment options and their potential benefits and risks with the pregnant woman during the early stages of labour.

#### 7.1.2 Non-Opioid Analgesics

*Paracetamol* (acetaminophen) is commonly used throughout all stages of pregnancy to treat pain or fever. When used in appropriate doses, no teratogenic or adverse fetal effects have been observed in a number of cohort studies.[34] The implications of overdosage are discussed in section 9.2.

*Aspirin* (acetylsalicylic acid) has been used for a number of conditions during pregnancy including pain, inflammation, pregnancy-induced hypertension, pre-eclampsia and eclampsia, and tocolysis. Salicylates easily cross the placenta and reach a total fetal plasma concentration higher than the maternal level, a difference that has been attributed to the greater binding of salicylates to fetal proteins.[104] The difference between maternal and fetal total plasma concentrations is therefore unlikely to be of any clinical significance.

As discussed in detail in section 1.3.2, aspirin is not associated with teratogenic effects during the first trimester of pregnancy. Yet, caution with the use of aspirin is warranted during the third trimester, especially in the immediate prepartum period. Aspirin interferes with the thromboxane $A_2$ synthesis of maternal platelets and may, if given in high enough doses, also interfere with fetal prostaglandin synthesis, which can result in peripartum bleeding and central nervous system haemorrhages.[105] Low-dose aspirin (e.g. 40 to 150 mg/day) has been given for the prevention of pregnancy-induced hypertension, eclampsia, and pre-eclampsia. Although no adverse fetal effects were noted in a number of studies,[106-108] whether it has beneficial maternal effects is still debated (see further chapter 18; sect. 3.3).

Nonsteroidal anti-inflammatory drugs (NSAIDs) have not been associated with malformations. However, NSAIDs cross the placenta and have the potential of inhibiting fetal cyclo-oxygenases. During late pregnancy, this has been described in various reports as being associated with functional adverse effects such as constriction of the ductus arteriosus, oligohydramnios, and after birth with primary pulmonary hypertension, patent ductus arteriosus, and necrotising enterocolitis.[34] Nevertheless, both intrauterine ductal contraction and oligohydramnios are usually only observed after prolonged treatment and have been reversible on discontinuation of the NSAIDs. Prospective studies of indomethacin employed as a tocolytic agent have failed to confirm the association of indomethacin with adverse neonatal effects.

*In summary,* other agents such as paracetamol appear to have a better safety profile than NSAIDs in the treatment of pain during pregnancy. For other indications (i.e. tocolysis, polyhydramnios), NSAIDs should be used with caution until the results of further necessary prospective studies are available (see section 7.4).

#### 7.1.3 Drugs Used in Anaesthesia

Exposure to general anaesthetics during pregnancy is common, with up to 2% of women requiring surgery during pregnancy.[109] Moreover, anaesthetics may represent an occupational hazard to pregnant women working in operating rooms. Intravenous anaesthetics are lipophilic molecules that freely cross the placenta and result in fetal plasma concentrations similar to maternal levels.[110] In contrast, neuromuscular blocking agents such as *atracurium* and *vecuronium* are large charged molecules that result in a fetal plasma concentration of only about 10% of the maternal concentration.

##### Use During Early Pregnancy

There is no evidence to date that a single course of anaesthesia during early pregnancy can induce malformations in the conceptus.[111] Safety has been demonstrated for *nitrous oxide* gas,[112] while the volatile liquids *enflurane* and *halothane* were not associated with any adverse embryonic and fetal effects in the patients included in the Collaborative Perinatal Project.[14] In the same study, the intravenous anaesthetics *thiopental*, *methohexital* and *thiamylal* were also not associated with increased risks to the offspring.

A recent retrospective case control study has, however, suggested an association between first-trimester exposure to general anaesthesia and hydrocephalus in combination with another major defect.[113] No significant association was found between first-trimester exposure to general anaesthesia and isolated hydrocephalus (i.e. no other birth defects) or all central nervous system defects. This study has several significant limitations: gross details of the surgery were not known, correlation with hospital record was not consistently possible, and recall bias could not be excluded. Consequently, the results have to be interpreted with great caution. At present, it appears to be justified to regard first-trimester anaesthesia as non-teratogenic.

##### Use During Delivery

The use of general anaesthetics during delivery requires different considerations, since fetal exposure may lead not to malformations but to neonatal depression with possible sequelae. General anaesthesia is typically initiated with intravenous fast-acting agents such as *thiopental* and *methohexital*. These are quickly transferred to the fetus; peak fetal concentrations of thiopental and methohexital have occurred within 2 to 3 minutes of intravenous injection.[110] However, the fetal brain is not exposed to high concentrations of drug because peak concentrations necessary for high initial brain concentrations do not occur in the fetus.[114]

Fetal concentrations of *nitrous oxide* increase over time with continuous exposure. Therefore, it is beneficial to keep the duration of anaesthesia before delivery as short as possible. Although the volatile fluids *halothane, enflurane,* and *isoflurane* used in combination with nitrous oxide to maintain anaesthesia are known to decrease uterine tone and contractility, maternal blood loss is not increased by their use.

**Occupational Exposure to Anaesthetics**

A large number of studies dealing with the occupational exposure to anaesthetic agents during pregnancy has been published. Interpretation of the results is hampered by study design problems.[115] All but one[116] of these investigations are retrospective cohort studies which are subject to biases in sample selection and responses. Confounding factors have not been adequately addressed, and response rates were often low. When summarised, these studies did not show any increase in congenital malformations, but a 1.5- to 2-fold higher risk of spontaneous abortion occurred. Whether this result represents a true increase in the risks of pregnancy loss is still not known in view of the limitations of the studies.

#### 7.1.4 Anticholinergics

*Atropine* readily crosses the placenta. While an effect on fetal breathing movements was noted in one study,[117] no effect on fetal heart rate was observed.[117,118] Congenital malformations have not been associated with the use of atropine.[34]

#### 7.1.5 Antiepileptic Drugs

Seizures occurring during pregnancy endanger both the mother and her offspring. Thus, it is generally agreed that seizure disorders require appropriate treatment during pregnancy.[119] Maternal seizure disorders were associated with an increased frequency of stillbirth, microcephaly, mental retardation and nonfebrile seizure disorders in the Collaborative Perinatal Project of the National Institute of Neurological and Communicative Disorders and Stroke; the overall risk of any unfavourable pregnancy outcome was double when compared with controls.[120]

Almost all of the antiepileptic drugs commonly used today (carbamazepine, phenobarbital, phenytoin, primidone, and valproic acid) have been associated with congenital malformations. For a discussion of the benzodiazepines, see section 7.1.7. To date, there are insufficient human data available to draw conclusions about the gestational use of the newer agents, such as gabapentin, lamotrigine, and vigabatrin. The manufacturers of these drugs have established a prospective registry in 1995 to address their reproductive safety.

As is to be expected for centrally-acting drugs that are able to easily penetrate the blood-brain barrier, all antiepileptic agents readily cross the placenta and appear in the fetal blood in therapeutic concentrations. The cord blood concentrations of *valproic acid* were determined to be even greater than maternal levels.[121]

The pharmacokinetics of most antiepileptic drugs undergo major changes during pregnancy. Maternal plasma concentrations of *phenytoin, phenobarbital, primidone* and *valproic acid* tend to decrease during pregnancy while those of *carbamazepine* and *ethosuximide* remain fairly stable. Factors that may reduce maternal plasma concentrations of antiepileptic drugs include increased renal and hepatic function, a higher volume of distribution, decreased protein binding, and lack of patient compliance. As was recently demonstrated for phenytoin, the reduction of total drug concentrations can be explained by reduced protein binding, resulting in plasma concentrations of the active free drug that are close to concentrations seen in the nonpregnant state.[122,123] Therapeutic monitoring of the antiepileptic drugs may be of benefit in late pregnancy because the changes in plasma concentrations can considerably vary between and even within patients (see chapter 5; sect. 2.3). If concentrations are monitored, it is useful to measure free drug.

Several risk factors for congenital malformations after exposure to antiepileptic drugs can be reduced by proper management. Polytherapy should be avoided whenever possible, antiepileptic treatment should only be given when considered necessary, seizures should be controlled as well as possible, and adequate folic acid levels should be achieved by periconceptional supplementation with folic acid 4 mg/day.

Antiepileptic drug treatment during pregnancy has been associated with fetal haemorrhages.[124] Recently, Cornelissen et al.[125] showed that the incidence of vitamin K deficiency is increased in neonates prenatally exposed to enzyme-inducing antiepileptic drugs. This deficiency can be prevented by administration of vitamin K to the mother starting at the 36th gestational week.[126] Maternal oral vitamin K supplementation during the last week(s) of pregnancy should be recommended.

The choice of antiepileptic drugs to use during pregnancy depends on a number of factors. While polytherapy should be avoided whenever possible, the chosen antiepileptic drug should render optimal seizure control. Carbamazepine and benzodiazepines have been considered the drugs of choice.[6,119] Use of *carbamazepine* increases the risk of neural tube defects to about 1%.[127] Neural tube defects are detectable *in utero* by measurement of α-fetoprotein and fetal ultrasound during the 18th week of pregnancy, thus allowing for secondary prevention by elective abortion if chosen by the family. A clinical presentation similar to the fetal hydantoin syndrome has also been described for carbamazepine;[128] however, its prevalence appears to be extremely low.

Similarly, *valproic acid* also increases the incidence of neural tube defects. In addition, a multitude of other congenital malformations and, as well, intrauterine growth retardation, fetal hepatotoxicity and neonatal withdrawal symptoms have been described as occurring after administration of this drug.[34,129] The prevalence of neural tube defects after valproic acid exposure during early pregnancy is 1 to 2%.[127] The exact prevalence of the other malformations remains unknown.

*Phenytoin* treatment during pregnancy has been associated with a constellation of malformations collectively known as the fetal hydantoin syndrome. Abnormalities include craniofacial malformations, hypoplasia of the distal phalanges and nails, growth deficiency, mental retardation, and cardiac defects (for more details, see table I). Children exposed *in utero* to phenytoin monotherapy had a mean global IQ that was 10 points lower than in matched control individuals.[119]

Children born to mothers treated with *phenobarbital* and *primidone* have a 2- to 3-fold risk for malformation compared with the normal population. While a specific constellation of abnormalities has not been described for these drugs, rates of microcephaly and cardiovascular effects have been reported to be increased. In addition, it has been suggested that the cognitive development of the exposed offspring may be impaired.[130]

For petit mal epilepsy, the succinimides are considered to be the drugs of choice during the first trimester of pregnancy.[34] The succinimides are presently thought to have a low or no teratogenic potential; however, very few epidemiological data are available in humans.

#### *7.1.6 Barbiturates*

Data about the possible teratogenicity of barbiturates are inconclusive. *Phenobarbital* has been associated with an increased risk of major malformations in the offspring of epileptic mothers. However, this association may be more related to the maternal condition than to the drug. A typical constellation of symptoms as described for a number of teratogens does not occur with barbiturates.[34]

A clinical condition compatible with neonatal withdrawal syndrome has been described in infants antenatally exposed to barbiturates. Symptoms include tremor, hyperactivity, restlessness, hyperreflexia, disturbed sleep and excessive crying. Due to the long half-lives of these drugs, onset of these symptoms may occur as late as 2 weeks postpartum. Infants demonstrating signs and symptoms of barbiturate withdrawal consistent with a positive maternal history may be effectively treated with phenobarbital.[131]

#### *7.1.7 Benzodiazepines*

Impaired neurodevelopment at 10 months of age has been reported in infants exposed to benzodiazepines throughout pregnancy.[132] In this study, 17 infants born to mothers who used benzodiazepines throughout pregnancy for psychiatric disorders were compared with 29 infants of healthy mothers who did not take benzodiazepines during pregnancy. Unfortunately, this study had no means of controlling for a number of confounding factors. Mothers in the benzodiazepine group smoked more frequently, lived in stable relationships less frequently, and had more psychiatric diagnoses, mostly panic disorder. These differences may well have an influence on postnatal development and appear more likely to be responsible for the differences than is the antenatal benzodiazepine use. The results of this study must therefore be interpreted with extreme caution.

Benzodiazepines have repeatedly been associated with an increased incidence of cleft lip and or cleft palate. However, a number of epidemiological studies failed to confirm this association.[34] A recently performed prospective cohort study involving 137 benzodiazepine-exposed pregnancies and an equal number of controls failed to show an increased risk of malformations.[133] While larger prospective cohort studies are needed to settle the remaining uncertainties, it can be concluded that exposure to benzodiazepines during pregnancy is not associated with a clinically significant increase in major malformations.

## 7.2 Drugs Acting on the Cardiovascular System

### *7.2.1 Antihypertensive Drugs*

Maternal hypertension or the presence of pre-eclampsia or eclampsia complicates 5 to 10% of all pregnancies, is associated with increased fetal loss, and is responsible for approximately 12% of all perinatal death as a consequence of preterm births.[134] These facts underline the need for appropriate treatment of these conditions. Yet they also complicate the interpretation of data available on the safety of drugs employed to treat hypertension. For example, drugs that are usually used only for severe hypertension may be associated with an increased risk of adverse fetal effects, when these effects are actually caused by the severe disease necessitating the aggressive treatment.

#### α-Adrenoceptor Blocking Drugs

There are few reports of the efficacy and fetal risks of α-adrenoceptor blocking agents during pregnancy. Treatment with *prazosin* has been evaluated in only small studies during pregnancy, mostly in combination with a β-blocker. Prazosin combined with oxprenolol was effective in pregnant women with essential hypertension,[135,136] while prazosin given in combination with atenolol for pregnancy-induced hypertension appeared to be less effective.[137] Fetal losses occurred, but were attributed to the severity of the underlying disease. Adverse neonatal effects were not observed. Prazosin crosses the placenta, but is found in fetal serum only at a concentration of 10 to 20% of maternal levels when given orally in a sustained release formulation.[138]

#### β-Adrenoceptor Blocking Drugs

β-Adrenoceptor blocking drugs are widely used during pregnancy. Indications have included hypertension, hyperthyroidism, and tachyarrhythmias of the mother and tachyarrhythmias of the fetus. All β-blocking drugs readily cross the placenta and reach fetal blood concentrations that are either below corresponding maternal values or similar to maternal levels. However, direct fetal effects such as bradycardia have only rarely been observed. There are sufficient data to conclude that the β-adrenoceptor blocking agents *acebutolol, atenolol, labetalol* (an α- and β-blocking agent), *metoprolol, oxprenolol, pindolol,* and *propranolol* have no teratogenic effects in humans and that they can be considered to be safe during pregnancy.[6,34,139]

A number of possible adverse perinatal effects have, however, been reported. Among these are intrauterine growth retardation, decreased fetal heart rate, and bradycardia and hyperglycaemia occurring shortly after birth. In one report, intrauterine growth retardation in neonates was most severe after antenatal exposure to atenolol (mean birthweight 2745g) and less severe after exposure to acebutolol (3160g) or pindolol (3375g).[140] A similar study comparing the birthweights of neonates born to mothers treated with atenolol *vs* labetalol also found a significant difference (2750 *vs* 3280g).[141] In contrast, a randomised, double-blind study involving 120 pregnant women with mild to moderate hypertension treated with either atenolol or placebo found no differences in neonatal birthweight (2961 *vs* 3017g).[142] Thus, intrauterine growth retardation may not be caused by the β-blocking drugs, but by the underlying disease. Differences in disease severity may also account for the differences in outcome of the studies.

In theory, non-selective β-blockers may increase uterine tonus but clinically, this is not a problem. It remains unclear whether β-blocking drugs have an effect on fetal heart rate. Attempts to treat fetal tachyarrhythmias using propranolol have, in most cases, not been successful. It has been speculated that this nonresponsiveness may either be due to dosages too low to achieve an effect or to a possible immaturity of fetal β-adrenoceptors.[143]

Pharmacokinetics in pregnancy have been described for propranolol[144] and labetalol,[145] and remain similar to those in the non-pregnant state so that no dosage adjustments are needed. Metoprolol pharmacokinetics have been determined in 5 women during the third trimester of pregnancy and repeated 3 to 5 months after delivery. While serum half-lives were similar (1.3

*vs* 1.7h), peak concentrations during pregnancy were only 20 to 40% of those measured after delivery, which may signal a need for dosage adjustment.[146]

*In summary,* β-adrenoceptor blocking drugs appear to be safe and efficacious for maternal treatment during pregnancy. Although most neonates have not shown any adverse clinical signs, it is advisable to closely observe neonates exposed *in utero* to β-blocking agents for any signs of β-blockade such as bradycardia or hypoglycaemia.

#### Centrally-Acting Antihypertensives

*Methyldopa,* a drug widely used to treat hypertension during pregnancy, readily crosses the placenta and achieves fetal concentrations similar to maternal levels.[147] A review of 1157 pregnancies in hypertensive women exposed to methyldopa demonstrated no adverse fetal effects.[34] A reduction in systolic blood pressure by 4 to 5mm Hg was seen during the first 2 days of life in a cohort of neonates exposed to methyldopa *in utero*.[148] However, the mild reduction in blood pressure did not seriously compromise the neonates. Due to its safety profile, methyldopa is considered to be one of the drugs of choice for the treatment of maternal hypertension during pregnancy.[6]

*Clonidine* has also not been associated with adverse fetal effects. However, there are considerably fewer studies presenting experiences with the use of clonidine during pregnancy than with methyldopa. Clonidine crosses the placenta and achieves fetal serum concentrations close to maternal levels.[149] No neonatal hypotension was observed.

#### Direct-Acting Vasodilators

*Hydralazine* is frequently used during pregnancy. In fact, in 1985, it was reported to be the most common antihypertensive agent used by pregnant women in England.[150] Like most other antihypertensives, hydralazine readily crosses the placenta and achieves fetal serum concentrations equal to or greater than maternal levels.[151] Numerous reports have confirmed the safety of hydralazine use during pregnancy either as monotherapy or in combination with other antihypertensive agents.[34]

Nevertheless, several case reports have linked hydralazine to a variety of adverse fetal or maternal effects: fetal premature atrial contractions in a fetus at 35 weeks' gestation that resolved after discontinuation of hydralazine therapy,[152] fatal maternal hypotension in a pregnant woman after combined therapy with hydralazine and diazoxide,[153] a lupus erythematosus-like syndrome in both a mother and her growth-retarded offspring delivered after 6 days of hydralazine treatment during the 28th gestational week, and neonatal thrombocytopenia and bleeding in a case series of 3 infants after maternal hydralazine treatment throughout the third trimester.[63] However, the latter has been shown to be also associated with the maternal condition independent of hydralazine therapy.[154]

Considering the large number of pregnant women treated with hydralazine, the low number of reports of adverse effects, and the safety and efficacy demonstrated by a number of clinical studies, this drug must still be considered a first-line agent for antihypertensive therapy in pregnancy.[6]

*Diazoxide* has been used by a number of groups during pregnancy. It crosses the placenta to reach fetal blood concentrations close to the maternal levels.[155] Diazoxide has been associated with alopecia and hypertrichiosis lanuginosa in a case series.[155] However, this study has not been confirmed by subsequent reports. Another concern is neonatal hyperglycaemia.[34] Since other potent alternatives to diazoxide are available, the use of this drug should be considered only for very special indications, i.e. if other therapies have failed.

*Sodium nitroprusside* and *nitroglycerin* have not been linked to congenital malformations.[34] On the basis of animal experiments, concern had been raised about possible fetal toxicity of cyanide released from sodium nitroprusside.[156,157] However, if prolonged use is avoided, this is not thought to pose a major risk to the human fetus.[158,159] Very few data about use of these drugs in pregnancy are available, which renders it currently impossible to conclude that either drug can be regarded as safe for the fetus.

#### Dihydropyridine Calcium Antagonists

*Nifedipine* and other dihydropyridines have been used to treat hypertension during pregnancy and to inhibit premature labour. Nifedipine crosses the placenta.[160] In a recent review, the dihydropyridines, and particularly nifedipine, were considered safe for both the mother and the fetus.[161] While the effectiveness of nifedipine as an antihypertensive agent has been demonstrated in several studies, controlled studies proving the efficacy of its use as a tocolytic are still lacking.

Experience with dihydropyridines during the embryonic period of pregnancy is limited and embryotoxicity has been demonstrated in animal studies.[162,163] The relevance of these results to human use of the drugs are unknown and further human data are awaited. Thus, the use of dihydropyridines should be limited to the second and third trimester of pregnancy.

#### Diuretics

Pregnancy is physiologically accompanied by an expansion of the plasma volume. Since diuretics may reduce intravascular volume and decrease placental perfusion, several authors have cautioned against the use of diuretics during pregnancy. However, a review summarising the results of 9 randomised trials of diuretics in pregnancy involving nearly 7000 patients has shown that diuretics are effective in reducing pre-eclampsia. Moreover, perinatal mortality was not increased when diuretics were used. Except for maternal hypokalaemia in patients not receiving potassium supplements, no significant maternal side effects were observed.[164]

*Furosemide* (frusemide) crosses the placenta[165] and appears to have a diuretic effect on the fetus *in utero*.[166,167] Nevertheless, an alteration of amniotic fluid volume has not been observed.[168] Neonates exposed to the drug shortly before birth voided urine more often after birth than non-exposed newborns. In addition, the urine of the exposed newborns had higher sodium and potassium concentrations.[169]

Thiazides have not been associated with malformations in humans. *Chlorothiazide* and *chlorthalidone* (a thiazide-like agent) cross the placenta, which is also assumed to occur with other clinically used thiazides. Adverse fetal effects are rare. Neonatal thrombocytopenia, hyponatraemia and hypotonia have been described in case reports.[34]

Although human data about the safety and benefits of *potassium-sparing* and *osmotic diuretics* are limited, it appears unlikely that any of these drugs are associated with human malformations.[34] However, use of these diuretics during pregnancy should only be considered if other means of treatment fail.

#### ACE Inhibitors

Exposure to ACE inhibitors during the second and third trimesters of pregnancy is associated with a certain combination of sequelae.[170] These consist of intrauterine growth retardation, oligohydramnios due to fetal renal failure, and hypoplasia of the membranous bones of the skull, and, during the neonatal period, hypotension, anuria or oliguria, and persistent ductus arteriosus.[171] ACE inhibitors inhibit the conversion of angiotensin I to angiotensin II, and the metabolism of bradykinin. These inhibitory effects lead to fetal vasodilatation, reducing blood pressure and impairing fetal circulation. In addition, bradykinin appears to release vasoconstrictive prostaglandins in the human fetal placenta. Enhanced vasoconstriction may reduce placental blood flow and thereby cause fetal damage.[172]

Neither animal nor human reports associate ACE inhibitors taken only during the first trimester of pregnancy with malformations or embryonic loss. ACE inhibitors, thus, appear not to interfere with embryonic development and are consistent with being *functional* teratogens. Functional teratogens are exogenous factors that do not directly interfere with embryonic development but may have a toxic effect on the function of a developed organ, possibly leading to subsequent damage of the organ or the fetus.

ACE inhibitors are however, contraindicated during the second and third trimester of pregnancy. Inadvertent use during the first trimester should not be considered an indication for terminating pregnancy, but an alternative treatment should be substituted for the remainder of the pregnancy. Children born to mothers who have been taking ACE inhibitors during pregnancy should be carefully monitored for renal function and blood pressure.

#### Other Antihypertensives

Concern about the use of *reserpine* during pregnancy has arisen since neonates exposed to maternal reserpine treatment near term were reported to experience nasal discharge, respiratory distress, lethargy, and poor appetite.[173] An incidence of 8% (4 in 48 exposed mother-child pairs) malformations has been recorded by the Collaborative Perinatal Project.[14] However, no major category of malformations was identified.

### *7.2.2 Antiarrhythmic Drugs and Cardiac Glycosides*

#### Digoxin

After many years of relatively safe human experience, digoxin has been considered the drug of choice for the appropriate cardiac arrhythmias during pregnancy.[6] Digoxin readily crosses the placenta and reaches, under controlled *in vitro* conditions, about 40% of the maternal levels.[174,175] Neither malformations nor fetotoxicity have been associated with pharmacological maternal doses of digoxin.[34] When monitoring maternal, fetal, or neonatal plasma concentrations, it is important to realise that an endogenous immunoreactive digoxin-like substance can interfere with the digoxin assay and cause falsely elevated results.[176]

#### Quinidine

Quinidine easily crosses the placenta, achieves fetal serum concentrations similar to maternal levels, and over time accumulates in the amniotic fluid.[175] Despite its frequent use, no associated congenital malformations have been reported.[177]

#### Procainamide

Procainamide is a weak base with low protein binding. Thus, placental transfer and ion trapping are to be expected.[175,178,179]

#### Lidocaine (Lignocaine)

Most information about lidocaine derives from its use as a local anaesthetic. No association between the exposure to lidocaine and major congenital malformations was found in 947 exposures recorded by Heinonen et al.[14]

Lidocaine readily crosses the placenta and may have a central depressant effect on the neonate if high serum concentrations are achieved. However, a number of studies failed to detect adverse effects on neonatal neurobehaviour following lidocaine epidural administration.[34]

#### Verapamil

There is no evidence for any teratogenic effects of verapamil in humans.[34] Verapamil crosses the placenta as documented by reports of successful cardioversion of fetal arrhythmias after administration of the drug to the mother.[175] However, caution in the use of verapamil has been recommended since it may, theoretically, impair uterine blood flow in humans, as has been documented in pregnant ewes.[97]

#### Amiodarone

Amiodarone is used in the treatment of ventricular cardiac arrhythmias. The drug structurally resembles tri-iodothyronine and can change thyroid function either directly or by releasing iodine. Amiodarone and its major active metabolite mono-*N*-desethyl-amiodarone cross the placenta and reach fetal serum concentrations of approximately 10 to 25% of maternal values. Iodine also crosses the placenta. Concerns about amiodarone treatment during pregnancy are, thus, focused around fetal or neonatal cardiac effects and thyroid function.

Neonatal outcome in 17 pregnant patients who received amiodarone for maternal indications and 4 neonates who had received amiodarone for fetal arrhythmias during gestation have been described.[34] Congenital goitre and hypothyroidism was seen in 2 neonates, 1 exposed due to maternal treatment and the other due to fetal treatment. A third child had transient biochemical changes typical of hypothyroidism, but exhibited no clinical signs. Bradycardia was seen in 3 neonates born to treated mothers.

Twelve additional cases of maternal amiodarone treatment during pregnancy were recently reported from Canada.[180] One child was born with congenital hypothyroidism and 1 had transitional neonatal hypothyroidism. This report confirms that gestational exposure to amiodarone may be complicated by perinatal hypothyroidism. Fetuses and neonates exposed to amiodarone *in utero* should be carefully monitored for bradycardia, alterations of thyroid function, and neurodevelopment.

### *7.2.3 Anticoagulants, Antithrombotics and Thrombolytics*

Pregnancy is considered a hypercoaguable state. Venous thromboembolism is a major complication, with an incidence of approximately 1 in 1000, and pulmonary embolism is the most common cause of maternal death in the UK.[181] Anticoagulants are often used to prevent the occurrence of thromboembolic events in women with a history of such events and, thus, the use of these drugs is not unusual during pregnancy.

#### Coumarins

Use of coumarins during the first trimester may result in the fetal warfarin syndrome. Most clinical stigmata are nasal hypoplasia, which may result in neonatal respiratory distress due to upper airway obstruction and stippled epiphyses seen on x-rays (table I). In about 50% of cases with fetal warfarin syndrome, hypoplasia of the extremities with shortening of the fingers may result. The critical period for fetal exposure appears to be between 6 to 9 weeks of gestation.[59] None of 19 infants born to mothers treated with warfarin during the second and third trimester of pregnancy had fetal warfarin syndrome.[182]

Coumarin derivatives used during the second and third trimester have been associated with CNS defects, microcephaly, hydrocephalus, mental retardation and optic atrophy, among other rarely described problems. These defects are thought to be caused by fetal bleeding and subsequent scarring.[183] The incidence of adverse fetal effects associated with warfarin use during the second and third trimester has not been established, but appears to be very low.

It is recommended that coumarin derivatives be avoided during the 6th to 12th week of pregnancy and discontinued 2 to 3 weeks before delivery to prevent fetal or maternal bleeding during labour. During these times, heparin should be substituted.

#### Heparins

Heparin is one of the few drugs that, due to its size, does not cross the placenta.[184] Nevertheless, it was thought to be associated with a high incidence of fetal loss and prematurity,[59] although it is probable that this higher risk may in fact be caused by the underlying diseases. The fetal safety of heparin was demonstrated in a retrospective study involving 100 pregnancies in which the mothers were exposed to heparin. No heparin-associated adverse pregnancy outcomes resulted.[185]

The main untoward effects of long term heparin treatment during pregnancy are maternal osteopenia and thrombocytopenia. However, the incidence of severe manifestations of either appears to be relatively low.[181] On the day of delivery, the dosage should be reduced to 7500U or less every 12 hours to reduce the danger of excessive bleeding. The activated partial thromboplastin time (APTT) should be monitored and administration of protamine sulfate should be considered if prolongation indicates a danger of bleeding complications.

Low molecular weight (LMW) heparins also do not undergo placental transfer.[186] Positive experience with low molecular weight heparins in a limited number of pregnancies has been reported.[187]

#### Antiplatelet Agents

The safety of the most frequently employed antiplatelet agent *aspirin* is discussed in section 7.1.2, and has been documented by a number of studies. However, its efficacy for the prevention of maternal thromboembolic events in pregnancy needs further study. Thus, it cannot be recommended for this indication in pregnancy, due to lack of evidence of effectiveness.

### 7.3 Antihistamines

*Brompheniramine* was the only antihistamine significantly associated with congenital malformations in the Collaborative Perinatal Project.[14] Ten of 65 pregnancies exposed to brompheniramine during the first trimester resulted in a malformed neonate, but when used anytime during pregnancy, this association was not found (i.e. 6 malformations in 412 pregnancies).[14] In contrast, another report found no significant association between brompheniramine and major congenital malformations.[188] Similarly, a small prospective controlled cohort study also found no significant association between brompheniramine and major malformations.[189] A meta-analysis that followed this study confirmed the lack of association.

*Doxylamine,* being one of the active ingredients of 'Bendectin' or 'Debendox', has been widely studied. No association with congenital malformations has been found.[9,190]

*Diphenhydramine* has been reported to be associated with an increased risk of cleft palate. However, this association was not confirmed in any of the studies covered in a major review of the subject.[34]

In general, histamine $H_1$-receptor blockers appear not to be associated with major congenital malformations, although to date, no study has confirmed this trend with the newer non-sedating antihistamines.

### 7.4 Tocolytic Agents

The initial stimulus leading to the induction of premature labour remains unknown. Once uterine contractions have commenced, they are modulated by a number of agents. Enhancers of contractions are prostaglandin $F_{2\alpha}$, oxytocin, and increased intracellular calcium concentrations. Inhibitors of contractions are intracellular cyclic-AMP, which can be pharmacologically induced by activation of $\beta_2$-adrenoceptors, and intracellular cyclic-GMP, which is increased by nitric oxide and pharmacologically by its donors, e.g. sodium nitroprusside. These mechanisms, most of which are non-specific for the uterine smooth muscle cell, are, thus, the targets of tocolytic therapy.

*Ritodrine,* a $\beta_2$-adrenoceptor agonist, is presently the best studied agent employed to treat premature labour. A recent meta-analysis, summarising 16 randomised controlled studies of good quality including more than 1600 pregnant women, has shown that ritodrine is effective in prolonging labour for 48 hours[191] with no significant decrease in perinatal morbidity and mortality. Unfortunately, the use of ritodrine is often accompanied by a multitude of maternal adverse effects resulting from activation of non-uterine $\beta_2$- and $\beta_1$-receptors.[192]

*Indomethacin*, a non-selective inhibitor of cyclo-oxygenases, has also been effective in prolonging pregnancy for 7 to 10 days, as demonstrated by a meta-analysis of 5 randomised controlled trials involving approximately 500 mothers.[193] A significantly reduced risk of perinatal morbidity and mortality could not be demonstrated. Although adverse fetal or neonatal effects were not found in randomised controlled studies of tocolysis with indomethacin, theoretical considerations and case reports warrant caution when this drug is administered to pregnant women. In a prospective case series, the incidence of fetal ductal constrictions was reported to be 50% (7 of 14 fetuses at their gestational age of 26.5 to 31 weeks).[194] These constrictions were fully reversible within 24 to 48 hours after cessation of short term treatment (<72h). Indomethacin has also been associated with a decrease in fetal urine output that appears to be reversible on discontinuation of treatment.[195] Other potential neonatal adverse effects include persistent pulmonary hypertension and necrotising enterocolitis.[196]

Other agents employed in the treatment of preterm labour are magnesium sulfate, atosiban (an oxytocin receptor antagonist), and nifedipine. To date, the efficacy of these drugs in terms of prolonging labour or reducing neonatal morbidity and mortality has not been clearly shown.[197]

## 7.5 Antimicrobial Agents

Antibiotics are among the drugs most commonly used during pregnancy. This is reflected by the fact that concerns about the use of antibiotics during pregnancy are the leading cause for women and healthcare professionals to call Motherisk, the teratogen information centre in Toronto.[198]

Treatment of maternal infections during pregnancy should follow the general principles outlined in section 5 for any pharmacotherapy. While the safety to the embryo or fetus is an important concern, efficacy of maternal treatment should be as important for selection of therapy. Hence, an antibiotic should be chosen in the same way as in non-pregnant patients, either by susceptibility studies, or by empirical evaluation of the most likely group of pathogens and their most likely antibiotic susceptibility. These considerations will usually result in a number of antibiotics that are likely to be effective in the treatment of the infection. Selection from this group of drugs should then be guided by embryonic or fetal safety concerns.

To ensure efficacy of antibiotic treatment, adequate drug concentrations have to be achieved at the location of infection. As a result of alterations in volume of distribution, protein binding, renal and hepatic clearance during pregnancy, serum concentrations of a number of antibiotics tend to be lower than during the non-pregnant state.[7] This is particularly true for penicillins, cefalosporins, erythromycin, and aminoglycosides. The dosage of antibiotics possessing a wide therapeutic index should be adjusted empirically. Penicillins and cefalosporins, for instance, tend to achieve lower serum concentrations during pregnancy, and thus an increase of the dose should be considered.

Treatment of fetal and intrauterine infections present particular pharmacological challenges. Direct treatment is not feasible in most cases; hence drug delivery must be via the maternal circulation. The placenta is permeable to virtually every antibiotic. However, fetal peak concentrations will be reached at a later time, typically 1 to 3 hours after the maternal peak,[199] and will usually be lower than the maternal peak concentration. Fetal concentrations at steady-state may be similar to or significantly lower than maternal concentrations, depending on the characteristics of the antibiotic. This can be due to a relative barrier function of the placenta or to different protein binding on the fetal side. Unfortunately, most published fetal serum concentrations are total serum concentrations. As a result, free (active) fetal drug concentrations are poorly known for drugs with high protein binding.

The intrauterine compartment most difficult to reach is the amniotic fluid. To get there, a drug must be transferred to the fetus and subsequently excreted by the fetal kidneys into the amniotic fluid. With these obstacles to treatment, intrauterine infections have been compared with deeply located abscesses.[199] Accordingly, high intravenous doses of antibiotics must be given. Consequently, delivery of a viable fetus has to be considered as part of the treatment,[200] thus allowing for direct therapy of the newborn.

### 7.5.1 Antibacterial Agents Considered Safe During Pregnancy

Most *penicillins* cross the placenta well, exceptions being piperacillin and sulbenicillin.

Agents with low protein binding, ampicillin, amoxicillin and methicillin penetrate well and achieve concentrations in the amniotic fluid 0.5 to 1 times that of the maternal plasma concentration.[121] The penicillins are safe antibiotics during pregnancy, with no embryo- or fetotoxic effects having been described in large studies.[201] Since maternal serum concentrations tend to be lower during pregnancy because of increased renal clearance, a moderate increase in the dosage should be considered.

The first-generation *cefalosporins* cross the placenta poorly and achieve fetal serum concentrations approximately 10% of maternal concentrations.[202] The second- and third-generation cefalosporins also achieve fetal serum concentrations significantly below maternal levels. An exception to this rule may be ceftizoxime. Maternal, fetal and amniotic levels measured at delivery after at least 3 doses of ceftizoxime 2g at 8-hour intervals were 12, 24.5, and 43.5 μg/L, respectively.[203] Other studies have reported cord blood levels between 12 and 30 μg/L and amniotic fluid concentrations of 10 to 20 μg/L, while another study found a mean fetal/maternal ratio of only 0.28 after a 2g intravenous dose.[34] Maternal serum concentrations of all cefalosporins are reduced during pregnancy because of increased renal clearance; thus, an increase in dosage should be considered.[201] This is of particular importance if bactericidal concentrations are desirable in fetal blood.

*Erythromycin* does not have adverse effects on the unborn offspring but crosses the placenta in concentrations too low to be therapeutic on the fetal side. However, erythromycin treatment of maternal Mycoplasma infections results in a reduction of pregnancy loss and fewer low birthweight infants, underlining the importance of adequate treatment of such infections during pregnancy.[34,201] Erythromycin estolate is contraindicated during pregnancy because the risk of hepatotoxicity is increased in pregnant women.[204]

*Clindamycin* is frequently used for the treatment of drug-resistant anaerobic infections during the peripartum period, particularly intraamniotic and postpartum infections. It crosses the placenta and reaches fetal tissue concentrations that are considered therapeutic.[201]

*Nitrofurantoin* has not been associated with adverse fetal effects. Since it does cross the placenta, fetal haemolytic anaemia may be possible in glucose-6-phosphate dehydrogenase (G6PD) deficient fetuses, but this has not been reported. It appears safe for the treatment of maternal urinary tract infections.[34,54] A recent meta-analysis performed by Motherisk in Toronto confirmed the fetal safety of the drug.[205]

The safety of *metronidazole* is discussed in section 1.3.6. As pointed out in this section, metronidazole can be considered safe for the offspring during pregnancy.

The antituberculosis agents *ethambutol, isoniazid* and *rifampicin* (rifampin) all cross the placenta, achieving considerable concentrations in fetal plasma. None of these agents has been associated with major congenital malformation. The risk associated with treatment of tuberculosis during pregnancy is considerably lower than the risks associated with untreated disease.[34]

#### 7.5.2 Antibacterial Agents to be Used With Caution During Pregnancy

The *aminoglycosides* cross the placenta and achieve fetal plasma concentrations lower than those in the mother. The penetration of gentamicin and streptomycin into the amniotic fluid has been described as being very low (30 to 50% of those in the maternal serum), which contrasts with their renal excretion *ex utero*.[121] Marked concentration of aminoglycoside in fetal renal tissue has been noted.[201] While there has been concern about aminoglycoside-associated fetal ototoxicity, in fact, minimally increased frequencies of this complication have only been reported with the older agents streptomycin and kanamycin.[34] Since maternal plasma concentrations may be lower during pregnancy (because of increased renal clearance) compared with the non-pregnant state, therapeutic monitoring of these concentrations may be advisable during pregnancy (see further chapter 5).

Studies investigating the use of *vancomycin* during pregnancy are scarce, and none have associated the drug with congenital malformations. This agent crosses the placenta and has in one case achieved sufficient levels to treat chorioamnionitis during the second trimester.[206] One report investigated possible associations between vancomycin, sensory hearing loss and renal function; the study was complicated by methodological issues, but did not find adverse associations.[34]

*Fluoroquinolones* are neither embryotoxic nor teratogenic in animals. However, their manufacturers have labelled them as contraindicated during pregnancy because arthropathies of weight-bearing joints have occurred in immature animals.[34] No such reports have been published in humans. In Michigan Medicaid files, among 132 neonates exposed to ciprofloxacin, only 2 major birth defects were observed, which is less than expected from the baseline risk of 2 to 3%. Ciprofloxacin crosses the placenta slowly, but amniotic fluid concentrations exceed maternal serum concentrations by 10-fold after 12 hours.[34] Recently, the experience with 35 pregnant women treated with norfloxacin or ciprofloxacin mainly for urinary tract infections during the first trimester of pregnancy was reported. All gave birth to healthy neonates without indications of malformations or clinically detectable joint abnormalities. These data suggest that in humans, there may be no association between fluoroquinolones and musculoskeletal problems.[207]

*Sulfonamides* are commonly used to treat asymptomatic bacteriuria and cystourethritis in pregnancy.[121] Although the sulfonamides are teratogenic in some animal species, it is highly unlikely that they have high teratogenic potential in humans. Most human studies have found no association between sulfonamides and congenital malformations.[34]

Concerns about the use of sulfonamides during pregnancy have been expressed because of their ability to displace bilirubin from its binding sites on plasma albumin after transplacental passage. However, the amount of bilirubin that could be displaced by therapeutic sulfonamide concentrations would only cause a negligible change in unbound bilirubin. The possible mechanism is more likely to be due to inhibition of bilirubin clearance by sulfonamides. The fact that no cases in which the use of sulfonamides might have caused kernicterus have been described points towards the purely theoretical grounds of this discussion. Nevertheless, currently the sulfonamides are not commonly used during the last 2 weeks of pregnancy.

*Trimethoprim* is a folic acid antagonist either used alone or typically in combination with *sulfamethoxazole* (i.e. as cotrimoxazole). Both substances cross the placenta and achieve concentrations in fetal plasma and amniotic fluid similar to maternal plasma levels.[208] Concern has arisen about the use of cotrimoxazole because folic acid antagonists are known teratogens in animals. Until recently, no teratogenic effects of cotrimoxazole have been reported.[34,201] However, in a surveillance study of Michigan Medicaid recipients, 2296 neonates had been exposed to cotrimoxazole during the first trimester. 126 major birth defects were noted in this cohort where 98 would have been expected. 37 of the malformations were cardiovascular defects where 23 would have been expected.[34] Although these data may be suggestive of causation between cotrimoxazole and congenital defects, such an association will have to be confirmed by studies specifically investigating this issue.

#### 7.5.3 Antibacterial Agents Contraindicated During Pregnancy

The *tetracyclines* are the only group of antibacterials that have unequivocally been associated with adverse fetal effects. When given during the period of bone and teeth development after the fourth to fifth month of gestation, tetracyclines cause yellow discolouration by deposition of the antibiotic into the calcifying bones or teeth.[209] Because of this effect and because other alternative drugs are available, the tetracyclines are contraindicated during pregnancy.

#### 7.5.4 Antiviral Drugs

Remarkable progress has been made in the use of antiviral agents during pregnancy. A decade ago, a review on antimicrobials during pregnancy stated that systemic antivirals should be avoided during pregnancy.[201] Today, the systemic antivirals *aciclovir* and *zidovudine* are considered safe during pregnancy and the use of zidovudine in pregnant women infected with human immunodeficiency virus (HIV) is strongly indicated.

Much research has focused on the use of zidovudine in the acquired immunodeficiency syndrome (AIDS). Clear benefits have recently been shown in a group of pregnant HIV-infected women who had CD4+ T cell counts of more than 200 cells/μl and who had not been previously treated with zidovudine. The study regimen consisted of zidovudine 100mg 5 times daily started during weeks 14 to 34 of gestation and continued for the remainder of pregnancy. During labour, a loading dose of 2 mg/kg bodyweight was given over 1 hour followed by continuous infusion of 1 mg/kg bodyweight until delivery. The neonate received zidovudine syrup 2 mg/kg bodyweight every 6 hours for the first 6 weeks of life. A 67.5% reduction in HIV transmission to the child was seen in the treatment group when compared with a group receiving placebo. While the benefits are obvious, the long term effects of this treatment are not known and it remains unclear whether similar benefit would also be seen in women with lower CD4+ counts.[210]

The safety of zidovudine treatment during pregnancy is being evaluated by the Antiretroviral Pregnancy Registry, which was established in 1989. From the data prospectively collected in this registry it can be concluded that zidovudine treatment during pregnancy, including use in the first trimester, is not associated with an increased risk of congenital malformations.[211]

The pregnancy outcome data following exposures to aciclovir are similarly collected in a registry which was founded in 1984. Most patients in this registry were treated for herpes simplex and varicella zoster virus. Of the 311 live births following aciclovir treatment in the first trimester, 4% of infants had birth defects, which is not different from the general population, indicating no apparent increase in risk of congenital malformations.[212]

## 7.6 Antineoplastic Drugs

Cancer is a rare but serious event during pregnancy. Although different groups of chemotherapeutic agents are available, all are active in inhibiting growth and cell division, processes that are absolutely essential to the embryo or fetus. Virtually every chemotherapeutic agent crosses the placenta in considerable concentrations, thus reaching the embryo or fetus. Hence, therapy poses the dilemma that optimal maternal treatment may impair fetal well-being.[213]

Fortunately, the incidence of serious fetal adverse effects is much lower than would be expected on the basis of the mechanisms of actions of these drugs. Approximately 10 to 17% of fetuses exposed to cytotoxic drugs during the first trimester exhibit major malformations.[213] Major structural defects have not been detected when chemotherapy commenced after the end of the first trimester (i.e. when organogenesis is completed). However, continuous brain development may be adversely affected. Other possible adverse effects of chemotherapy during pregnancy include spontaneous abortion, organ toxicity, premature birth and growth retardation.[66]

## 7.7 Immunosuppressive Drugs

*Azathioprine* crosses the placenta and traces of its metabolite mercaptopurine have been detected in fetal blood. Exposure during the first trimester appears not to be associated with an increase in major congenital malformations. However, it has been associated with a higher risk of prematurity and growth retardation. Due to a lack of controlled studies and the presence of serious underlying pathology leading to azathioprine use, it is impossible to ascertain this risk.[34,214]

Despite its considerable molecular size, *cyclosporin* readily crosses the placenta and achieves fetal plasma concentrations about half those seen in the maternal circulation. Knowledge of risk to the exposed unborn child is based on a small number of known cases. Cyclosporin is unlikely to be a major human teratogen.[34] In a series of patients with renal transplants, 66% of fetuses exposed to cyclosporin were delivered prematurely and 56% were small for their gestational age. Due to underlying maternal condition, it is unlikely that this high incidence is caused solely by cyclosporin.

*Thalidomide* (see also section 1.3.4): in contrast to common belief, thalidomide is still in clinical use. The drug is used in the treatment of leprosy and it is being investigated as an immunosuppressive agent (e.g. in Behçet's disease). The benefits of thalidomide for these indications raises important ethical questions:

- Does a proven teratogenic drug have to be removed off the market?
- Should we withhold uniquely efficacious treatment from the general population because it may have detrimental effects if used against advice during pregnancy?
- Is it appropriate to educate, and to enforce effective contraception in women of childbearing age if they are treated with potent teratogens?

With regard to the last question, in South America, thalidomide embryopathy is thought to be prevented by injecting contraceptive steroid hormones in women treated with thalidomide for leprosy. Despite this effort, some women have used the drug after effective contraception had ceased.

## 7.8 Miscellaneous Drugs

A large number of medicinal agents are available to pregnant women over-the-counter (OTC) without prescription. In fact, OTC drugs are taken more commonly during pregnancy than prescription drugs. Requests for OTC drugs may increase during pregnancy because of the increase in symptoms such as nausea, backache, constipation and nasal congestion.[215] While most of these drugs are now considered safe, this is only true when they are administered in recommended dosages. During the last trimester, OTC drugs may affect the fetus or the maternal circulation, thus indirectly affecting the fetus. In general, OTC agents should be regarded as drugs by both pregnant women and clinicians. Inquiry about their use should be part of taking the obstetric history and appropriate counselling should be given, with recommendations for taking products with safe ingredients.[215]

## 8. Drugs of Abuse in Pregnancy

Drugs of abuse are frequently consumed among women of childbearing age. Because half of all pregnancies are not planned and because pregnancy is usually diagnosed 6 to 8 weeks after the last menstrual period, inadvertent embryonic exposure to drugs is common. While recreational drug users or drug-addicted women might appear unconcerned about the risks to themselves, they usually wish to spare their unborn children from risks associated with drug use.[216] Proper and unbiased information regarding the risks to the embryo is therefore very important at this time.

The potential fetal risks associated with drug abuse must be explained, but they must not be overblown, since perception of this information may have significant influence on maternal decision-making. This decision can range from reduction, alteration or discontinuation of drug use to the decision to abort an otherwise wanted pregnancy. Discontinuation of drug use should be advised. At the same time, the woman should be offered assistance and referral to professional services able to provide necessary addiction counselling. After the initial approach, the woman ideally should enter a follow-up programme that continues beyond childbirth.

### 8.1 Alcohol

Without doubt, alcohol is the teratogen most commonly used during pregnancy. Its teratogenic effects have been described since antiquity. The first reports in modern medicine appeared 1968 in France[217] and about 5 years later in the US.[218,219] The fetal alcohol syndrome (FAS) has been well described and includes central nervous system dysfunction (mental retardation with hypotonia and hyperactivity), craniofacial dysmorphology (microcephaly, microphthalmia, short palpebral fissures, short upturned nose, hypoplastic philtrum, thinned upper vermilion, retrognathia or micrognathia), antenatal and postnatal growth retardation, and a number of inconsistent other anomalies.

The prevalence of fetal alcohol syndrome varies between countries and is estimated to be 1 per 100 live births in Northern France, 1 per 600 in Sweden, 1 per 750 in Seattle, and from 1 to 3 per 1000 in the US; it averages 1.9 per 1000 worldwide.[220] The occurrence of FAS is clearly related to the amount of alcohol consumed during pregnancy, but appears to be multifactorial, since even heavy use of alcohol leads to full blown FAS in only 30 to 40% of the offspring of alcoholic women.[221] The rate of malformations appears not to increase unless the ingested amount of alcohol exceeds 6 drinks per day;[222] however, fetal alcohol effects (i.e. low birthweight) have been observed after maternal consumption of only 2 drinks (i.e. total 30ml) of alcohol per day.[34] The mechanisms leading to the teratogenic effects of alcohol are not yet understood.

### 8.2 Tobacco

Although maternal smoking has decreased, 25% of pregnant women in North America still smoke.[223] Cigarette smoke contains an array of toxins including nicotine, carbon monoxide, cyanide, sulfide, and carcinogenic hydrocarbons. Fetal adverse effects of cigarette smoke have mainly been attributed to nicotine and carbon monoxide.[60] Smoking is not associated with congenital malformations, but increases the risks for prematurity, spontaneous abortions, perinatal mortality and the sudden infant death syndrome.[224] It is long established that maternal smoking leads to impaired fetal growth, with birthweight on average 200g lower than in the offspring of nonsmokers.[225]

Recently, it has been shown that only women who smoked during the last trimester were at higher risk of having children who were small for their gestational age compared with offspring of nonsmoking mothers. Whether a mother had smoked during the first trimester was of no difference. The risk increased with the number of cigarettes smoked during the third trimester.[61]

### 8.3 Caffeine

Caffeine has not been associated with congenital malformations in humans.[34] Early reports linked high caffeine consumption with increased incidence of spontaneous abortion and low birthweight. Unfortunately, these studies were not corrected for cigarette smoking and alcohol consumption. A large number of more recent, better controlled studies were not able to confirm the link between caffeine and spontaneous abortions. Whether high amounts of caffeine during pregnancy increase the likelihood of fetal growth retardation is still being disputed.[226-229] If it does have an effect, this effect is negligible compared with the effect of smoking and there may be an additive effect with smoking.[229]

Caffeine should only be used in moderate amounts during pregnancy. In fact, caffeine clearance decreases as pregnancy proceeds. At the end of pregnancy, clearance is only 30% of that seen in the prepregnant state.[76] Thus, lower intake during pregnancy should still achieve the desired effects sought by coffee drinkers.

### 8.4 Cocaine

The high prevalence of cocaine use has become a major health concern during pregnancy. Hundreds of reports dealing with cocaine use during pregnancy have emerged in the medical literature. Cocaine crosses the human placenta, with varying proportions absorbed by placental tissues, suggesting that the placenta may offer some degree of fetal protection after bolus administration.[230] Moreover, the placenta expresses acetylcholinesterase and butyrylcholinesterase activity, and, thus, can metabolise cocaine.[86] Existing variability in placental handling of cocaine may determine fetal exposure and contribute to variability in fetal effects.

Cocaine is a CNS stimulant with effects thought to be due to sympathomimetic-driven fetal, uterine or maternal vasoconstriction and hypertension leading to infarcts or haemorrhages at any time during gestation and in any structure. This may explain the variability of clinical effects attributed to cocaine use. A typical well-defined 'fetal cocaine syndrome' does not exist.[231] Cocaine use during pregnancy has been associated with shorter gestation, premature delivery, spontaneous abortion, abruptio placentae and fetal death. Congenital malformations of almost every system have been reported and it has been stated that cocaine should be considered teratogenic.[34]

Reports about cocaine effects on pregnancy have often been controversial and it is difficult to extract a clear tendency. Interpretation of the results is hampered by the fact that cocaine use is commonly accompanied by confounding factors such as concomitant use of other recreational or addictive drugs, including tobacco, alcohol, cannabis, etc, which may affect pregnancy outcome by themselves. In addition, cocaine addicts often cluster in low socioeconomic groups, receive poor prenatal care and may carry sexually transmissible diseases.[232,233] In epidemiological studies, it is difficult to separate the effects of cocaine from effects of these confounding variables. Since it is an illicit drug, documentation of pregnancy exposure by history alone is prone to errors. This is likely to improve, as techniques such as hair analysis are emerging that allow cocaine use and fetal exposure to be traced back in time.[234] Finally, there seems have been some publication bias, with studies of 'positive' (i.e. adverse fetal) outcomes about the reproductive risks of cocaine having been more likely to be accepted for publication than studies with 'negative' results.[235]

Cocaine users form a heterogeneous group, consisting of social cocaine users who tend to stop use once pregnancy is detected, and cocaine-addicted women who tend to continue cocaine use throughout pregnancy. Recently, the risks of social cocaine use during the first trimester on pregnancy outcome have been studied. Women who stopped cocaine use after diagnosis of pregnancy were compared with drug-free women and cannabis users (to control for this confounding factor). No significant differences in pregnancy outcome and infant development were detected during the first and second years of life, indicating that cocaine is not a teratogen. Its use in early pregnancy does not provide an indication for elective abortion.[236]

A meta-analysis of the studies of outcomes of gestational cocaine exposure published between 1975 and 1989 found genitourinary malformations and spontaneous abortions significantly increased in offspring of cocaine users compared with drug-free women. When cocaine polydrug users were compared with polydrug users not using cocaine (to control for confounding factors), only genitourinary malformations remained significantly different. Thus, very few adverse reproductive effects can be associated with cocaine abuse and a variety of effects commonly associated with cocaine may in fact be caused by confounding factors.[237]

Cocaine probably does not cause withdrawal symptoms in the neonate. Due to the long half-life in neonates (noted by the presence of cocaine in urine for at least 4 days after exposure) it is possible that apparent withdrawal symptoms represent in fact cocaine intoxication. Marked symptoms of central nervous system hyperexcitability can be treated with benzodiazepines. Withdrawal symptoms should be managed supportively. It has been reported that infants of cocaine-abusing mothers are at a higher risk of sudden infant death syndrome,[131] but this effect may be caused by concomitant smoking.

Children exposed to cocaine throughout pregnancy may exhibit lasting neurodevelopmental effects, even after poverty and postnatal deprivation are excluded as causes. Exposed children had an 8-fold greater risk of microcephaly than a healthy control group, and this was not compensated for during extrauterine life, resulting in a lower mean head circumference. Cocaine-exposed children scored significantly lower on a language development test. However, since mothers who use cocaine during pregnancy almost inevitably smoke cigarettes and often use alcohol, it is impossible to attribute the measured toxic effects to cocaine alone.[238]

*In summary,* cocaine is transported across the placenta and acts as a vasoconstrictor in a variety of vascular beds. It does not appear to cause typical malformations when used during the first trimester. Cocaine use during the fetal period may be weakly associated with effects leading to a variety of adverse outcomes such as prematurity, reduced birthweight, abruptio placentae, spontaneous abortion, intrauterine death and genitourinary malformations. Its use during the fetal period is associated with many confounding variables that may be responsible for the adverse pregnancy outcomes attributed to the drug.

## 8.5 Opioids

The effects of medical use of opioids are discussed in section 7.1.1.

The use of heroin during pregnancy has been associated with a high incidence of premature birth, decreased birthweight and a higher incidence of medical and obstetric complications. However, since heroin abuse is commonly accompanied by cigarette smoking, alcohol consumption, low socioeconomic class, and poor prenatal care, it is difficult to attribute these problems solely to heroin. Methadone maintenance has been the treatment of choice for heroin addicts. Advantages of such treatment are suppression of maternal withdrawal symptoms, a more constant drug level compared with the fluctuations typically seen in illicit intravenous heroin use, and avoidance of medical problems associated with contaminated street drugs or needle sharing. Moreover, methadone treatment should provide a basis for counselling and social care.[216]

Neonatal problems are frequently observed in offspring of opioid-abusing mothers. A high incidence of low Apgar scores has been reported.[239] If naloxone is used during neonatal resuscitation, early and severe withdrawal symptoms may result. Neonatal opioid withdrawal is detected in 67 to 90% of neonates of opioid-using mothers and appears to be related to the maternal dosage of methadone but not of heroin.[131] It is thought to result at least in part from $\alpha_2$-adrenoceptor supersensitivity in the locus ceruleus.[240] Symptoms include, in order of frequency, irritability, tremor, hypertonicity, high pitched cry, respiratory distress, sneezing, and convulsions.

The onset of symptoms may be shortly after birth in offspring of heroin abusers and is usually delayed by 1 to 3 days in neonates of methadone-using mothers due to its longer half-life. Treatment is mainly symptomatic and should include conservative comfort measures such as holding, swaddling, and minimal stimulation. Pharmacotherapy is frequently necessary and many drugs including paregoric (a camphorated opium tincture containing anhydrous morphine 0.4 mg/ml), tincture of opium, morphine, methadone, diazepam, chlorpromazine, phenobarbital, and clonidine have been used to treat severe neonatal opioid withdrawal.[131] Controlled comparative clinical studies investigating the efficacy of these drugs are rare. Two studies have compared the efficacy of treatment with paregoric *versus* phenobarbital and found paregoric to be more efficacious.[241,242] Further studies to evaluate treatment are necessary.

Follow-up studies investigating the effects of maternal opioid use during pregnancy and neonatal withdrawal symptoms on infant development have yielded controversial results.[131] Environmental factors may be more important for infant development than prenatal opioid exposure.

## 8.6 Cannabinoids

Marijuana or hashish have not been associated with congenital malformations. Adverse pregnancy outcomes reported after the use of cannabinoids are most likely attributable to concomitant factors such as tobacco smoking.[216,220]

### 8.7 Hallucinogens

Lysergic acid diethylamide (LSD) was used by millions of women in the 1960s. Although sporadic case reports have appeared of infants with various malformations, no specific pattern or clear evidence of teratogenicity has been produced.[16]

## 9. Poisoning in Pregnancy

Many of the drugs discussed above are considered to be safe during pregnancy. This, of course, may only be true for therapeutic dosages. Overdoses and poisonings are a serious threat to both the mother and her offspring. However, the fetal and maternal risks are not necessarily equal. The extent of toxin exposure may be modified by its ability to cross the placenta and the effect of the toxin may depend on the different expression of metabolic pathways in the mother and the fetus. For a review of poisoning in pregnancy, see Tenenbein et al.[243]

The general approach to the poisoned pregnant patient should not differ from that for the non-pregnant patient (see further chapter 8). It is important not to endanger the mother (and thus also the fetus) by omitting necessary interventions out of fear that these may endanger the fetus.

The most common poisonings in pregnancy are due to paracetamol, aspirin, and iron.[244] These exposures are discussed here to serve as examples for the complex problem of poisonings in pregnancy.

### 9.1 Paracetamol Poisoning

Paracetamol (acetaminophen) becomes toxic only after oxygenation by hepatic cytochrome P450 enzymes. The resulting highly reactive metabolite ultimately causes hepatotoxicity by binding to hepatic macromolecules. This pathway becomes important once hepatic glutathione is depleted by metabolism of an excessive dose of paracetamol. Thus, treatment consists of substitution of glutathione by administration of *acetylcysteine* (*N*-acetylcysteine) [see also chapter 8; sect. 4.3.1].

Paracetamol crosses the placenta, as documented by measurements in cord blood of neonates delivered shortly after maternal doses. However, for fetal toxicity to occur, paracetamol must be metabolised by an active cytochrome P450 enzyme in the liver of the fetus. As discussed in section 4.3.2, cytochrome P450 activity is present in the fetal liver. However, at weeks 18 to 23 of gestation, the mean activity for paracetamol is only 10% of adult values, with a linear increase with gestational age. This implies that the potential for fetal toxicity of paracetamol increases with fetal age.

Management of paracetamol overdoses during pregnancy should thus be similar to their management in non-pregnant patients. Acetylcysteine has been shown to undergo negligible transplacental transfer in sheep and humans, and appears to be non-teratogenic in humans. Since the fetal prognosis may worsen with gestational age, delivery of the mature fetus may be considered during the third trimester of pregnancy to allow for direct extrauterine acetylcysteine therapy if maternal paracetamol concentrations are in the toxic range.[243]

### 9.2 Aspirin Poisoning

In contrast to paracetamol, the salicylates do not need to be metabolised to exert toxicity. Salicylates readily cross the placenta and reach concentrations in fetal plasma slightly higher than maternal levels. Due to the lower pH of fetal blood, less drug is ionised, which favours transport across cell membranes and into the brain. Central nervous system toxicity due to uncoupling of oxidative phosphorylation is thought to be the major cause of fetal death.

A recent review has summarised 5 reports of *in utero* salicylate intoxication, 3 of which were after acute maternal ingestion and 2 were after subacute or chronic ingestion.[243] In 2 of the acute ingestion cases, the fetus died. It is suggested that salicylate poisoning be treated during pregnancy in a manner similar to that recommended for non-pregnant patients (see chapter 8; sect. 6.4.1), with the hope that the treatment will have transplacental effects. If the fetus is viable, delivery and direct care *ex utero* should be considered during late pregnancy.[243]

### 9.3 Iron Poisoning

Prenatal vitamins and iron are the second most common overdose situations during pregnancy. In contrast to poisoning with salicylates, the fetus appears to do much better than the mother. In its physiological ferric state, iron is insoluble and is transported by transferrin. Its transport across membranes is a complicated process involving binding to a receptor and subsequent endocytosis. In the case of hyperferraemia, only a negligible amount of iron is transported across the placenta. Fetal damage, thus, can only be due to maternal toxicity.

Treatment should not differ from treatment of non-pregnant patients (see chapter 8; sect. 4.4.1). A complicating factor is that *deferoxamine* (desferrioxamine) is stated to be an animal teratogen. However, deferoxamine is a charged large molecule and is not thought to cross the placenta. Thus, toxicity in animals must be due to chelation of essential nutrients; this is much less likely to occur when the animal is in the hyperferric state. In the few reports of pregnant women exposed during the first trimester to deferoxamine as part of the management of thalassaemia, no embryotoxicity was observed. It is important not to endanger the mother by withholding necessary treatment because of concerns about fetal effects of deferoxamine.[243]

## 10. Fetal Therapy

In general, a proper and well documented diagnosis is an absolute prerequisite for effective treatment. Fetal therapy is not exempt from this principle. New technologies such as ultrasonographic imaging, fibre optics, and new biochemical and molecular biology assay systems have rapidly increased the likelihood of diagnosing fetal pathology well before delivery.[245,246] Surgical and pharmacological attempts to antenatally correct a number of these conditions have followed. While surgical interventions such as early corrections of diaphragmatic hernias[247] and obstructive uropathies[248] have received much attention, less dramatic drug interventions have become routine therapy.

Recently, a US National Institutes of Health consensus conference recommended administration of *betamethasone* or *dexamethasone* (intramuscularly to the mother) for all fetuses from weeks 24 to 34 of gestation who are at risk of preterm delivery.[249] This followed the finding of several studies that corticosteroids significantly decrease neonatal morbidity and mortality when given 24 hours to 7 days before preterm delivery. Additive effectiveness for neonates who postnatally receive pulmonary surfactant therapy and prenatal steroids has been demonstrated by a Finnish multicentre study.[250]

Fetal cardiac arrhythmias are another target for antenatal treatment. A number of agents has been used to treat fetal tachyarrhythmias.[143] The experience with various drugs with different mechanisms of action, different maternal kinetics, and different transplacental distributions illustrates the large number of factors that need to be considered when opting for fetal drug therapy.

Other examples for fetal drug therapy include the treatment of polyhydramnios with *indomethacin*,[251] of immune thrombocytopenia with *platelet transfusions* to the fetus or *corticosteroids* and/or IgG to the mother, and, if diagnosed early enough, the treatment of congenital adrenal hypoplasia with *dexamethasone*.[252] These examples illustrate the wide variety of indications for fetal drug treatment. However, they also illustrate the complexity of this approach. Therapy may be possible by direct injection to the fetus either into the umbilical vein under sonographic guidance or by administration to the mother and transplacental passage. While direct injection to the fetus is an invasive option, administration via the mother may be associated with maternal adverse effects and is dependent on placental function.[253]

Fetal therapy is a rapidly developing field with unforeseeable potential for fetal benefit. New therapeutic options are on the horizon, such as fetal gene therapy[254] and transplantation of fetal cells,[255] which have the potential to push boundaries far beyond what is currently thinkable.

### Further Reading

Briggs GG, Freeman RK, Yaffe SJ. Drugs in pregnancy and lactation. 4th ed. Baltimore: Williams & Wilkins, 1994

Gilstrap III LC, Little BB, editors. Drugs and pregnancy. New York: Elsevier, 1992

Heinonen OP, Slone D, Shapiro S. Birth defects and drugs in pregnancy. Littleton, Massechusetts: PSG Publishing Company, 1977

Koren G, editor. Maternal-fetal toxicology: a clinician's guide. 2nd ed. New York: Marcel Dekker, 1994

Petrie RH, editor. Perinatal pharmacology. Oradell: Medical Economics Books, 1989

Schardein JL. Chemically induced birth defects. New York: Marcel Dekker, 1985

Shepard TH. Teratogenic agents. 7th ed. Baltimore and London: The Johns Hopkins Press, Ltd, 1992

## References


1. Gregg NM. Congenital cataract following German measles in the mother. Transactions of the Ophthalmological Society of Australia 1941; 3: 35-46
2. Lenz W. A short history of thalidomide embryopathy. Teratology 1988; 38: 203-15
3. Newman CGH. Clinical aspects of thalidomide embryopathy: a continuing preoccupation. Teratology 1985; 32: 133-44
4. McBride WG. Thalidomide and congenital abnormalities (letter). Lancet 1961; 2: 1358
5. Koren G, Nulman I. Teratogenic drugs and chemicals in humans. In: Koren G, editor. Maternal-fetal toxicology: a clinician's guide. 2nd ed. New York: Marcel Dekker, 1994: 33-48
6. Smith J, Taddio A, Koren G. Drugs of choice for pregnant women. In: Koren G, editor. Maternal-fetal toxicology: a clinician's guide. 2nd ed. New York: Marcel Dekker, 1994: 115-28
7. Koren G, Bologa M, Pastuszak A. The way women perceive teratogenic risk. In: Koren G, editor. Maternal-fetal toxicology: a clinician's guide. 2nd ed. New York: Marcel Dekker, 1994: 727-36
8. Trichopoulos D, Zavitsanos X, Koutis C, et al. The victims of Chernobyl in Greece: induced abortions after the accident. British Medical Journal 1987; 295: 1100
9. McKeigue PM, Lamm SH, Linn S, et al. Bendectin and birth defects: I. A meta analysis of the epidemiologic studies. Teratology 1994; 50: 27-37
10. Ornstein M, Einarson A, Koren G. Bendectin/Diclectin for morning sickness: a Canadian follow-up of an American tragedy. Reproductive Toxicology 1995; 9: 1-6
11. Leeder JS, Spielberg S. Teratogenicity and litigation. In: Koren G, editor. Maternal-fetal toxicology: a clinician's guide. 2nd ed. New York: Marcel Dekker, 1994: 771-82
12. Orme MLE. Debendox saga. British Medical Journal 1985; 291: 918-9
13. Neutel CI, Johnansen HL. Measuring drug effectiveness by default: the case of Bendectin. Canadian Journal of Public Health 1995; 86: 66-70
14. Heinonen OP, Slone D, Shapiro S. Birth defects and drugs in pregnancy. Littleton, Massachussetts: PSG Publishing Company, 1977
15. Smith DW, Jones KL. Recognizable patterns of human malformations. 3rd ed. Philadelphia: WB Saunders Co, 1982
16. Shepard TH. Teratogenic agents. 7th ed. Baltimore and London: The Johns Hopkins Press Ltd, 1992
17. Shepard TH. 'Proof' of human teratogenicity [letter]. Teratology 1994; 50: 97-8
18. Knox EG, Lancashire RJ. Epidemiology of congenital malformations. London: HMSO Publications, 1991
19. Leppig KA, Werler MM, Cann CI, et al. Predictive value of minor anomalies I: association with major malformations. Journal of Paediatrics and Child Health 1987; 110: 531
20. van Regemorter N, Dodion J, Druart C, et al. Congenital malformations in 10,000 consecutive births in a university hospital: need for genetic counselling and prenatal diagnosis. Journal of Pediatrics 1984; 104: 386-90
21. Mehes K. Minor malformations in the neonate. Budapest: Akademiai Kiaddo, 1983
22. Marden PM, Smith DW, McDonald MJ. Congenital anomalies in the newborn infant, including minor variations. Journal of Pediatrics 1964; 64: 357
23. Stevenson RE, Hall JG. Terminology. In: Stevenson R, Hall J, Goodman R, editors. Human malformations and related anomalies. New York: Oxford University Press, 1993: 21-30
24. Lock FR, Gratling HB, Wells HB. Difficulties in the diagnosis of congenital abnormalities: experience in a study of the effect of rubella on pregnancy. Journal of the American Medical Association 1961; 178: 711-4
25. Kline J, Stein Z, Susser M. Developmental abnormalities; I: measuring frequencies. In: Conception to birth: epidemiology of prenatal development. New York: Oxford University, 1989
26. Wilcox AJ. Early pregnancy. In: Kiely M, editor. Reproductive and perinatal epidemiology. Boca Raton: CRC Press, 1991
27. Moore KL. The developing human - clinically oriented embryology. Philadelphia: WB Saunders Company, 1988
28. Tuchmann-Duplessis H. Embryonic clinical pharmacology. In: Speight TM, editor. Avery's drug treatment: principles and practice of clinical pharmacology and therapeutics. 3rd ed. Auckland: Adis Press, 1987: 65-78
29. Chitayat D, Hodgkinson KA, Wyatt PR. Prenatal diagnosis in clinical practice. In: Koren G, editor. Maternal-fetal toxicology: a clinician's guide. 2nd ed. New York: Marcel Dekker, 1994: 601-25
30. Kalter H, Warkany J. Congenital malformations: etiologic factors and their role in prevention. New England Journal of Medicine 1983; 308: 424-31, 491-7
31. Centers for Disease Control. Contribution of birth defects to infant mortality - United States, 1986. MMWR Morbidity and Mortality Weekly Report 1989; 38: 633
32. Koren G, Pastuszak A. Teratogen information services. In: Koren G, editor. Maternal-fetal toxicology: a clinician's guide. 2nd ed. New York: Marcel Dekker, 1994: 683-705
33. Zalzstein E, Koren G, Einarson T, et al. A case-control study on the association between first trimester exposure to lithium and Ebstein's anomaly. American Journal of Cardiology 1990; 65: 817-8
34. Briggs GG, Freeman RK, Yaffe SJ. Drugs in pregnancy and lactation. 4th ed. Baltimore: Williams & Wilkins, 1994
35. Cohen LS, Friedman JM, Jefferson JW, et al. A reevaluation of risk of in utero exposure to lithium. Journal of the American Medical Association 1994; 271: 146-50
36. Richards ID. Congenital malformations and environmental influences in pregnancy. British Journal of Preventive and Social Medicine 1969; 23: 218-25
37. Nelson MM, Forfar JO. Associations between drugs administered during pregnancy and congenital malformations of the fetus. British Medical Journal 1971; 1: 523-7
38. Saxen I. Associations between oral clefts and drugs taken during pregnancy. International Journal of Epidemiology 1975; 4: 37-44
39. Werler MM, Mitchell AA, Sharpiro S. The relation of aspirin use during the first trimester of pregnancy to congenital cardiac defects. New England Journal of Medicine 1989; 321: 1639-42
40. Slone D, Heinonen OP, Kaufman DW, et al. Aspirin and congenital malformations. Lancet 1976; 1: 1373-5
41. Herbst AL, Ulfelder H, Poskanzer DC. Adenocarcinoma of the vagina. New England Journal of Medicine 1971; 284: 878-81
42. Herbst AL. The epidemiology of vaginal and cervical clear cell adenocarcinoma. In: Herbst AL, Bern HA, editors. Developmental effects of diethylstilbestrol

(DES) in pregnancy. New York: Thieme-Stratton Inc., 1981: 63-80
43. Robboy SJ, Noller KL, O'Brian P, et al. Increased incidence of cervical and vaginal dysplasia in 3,980 diethylstilbestrol-exposed young women: experience of the National Collaborative Diethylstilbestrol Adenosis (DESAD) Project. Journal of the American Medical Association 1984; 252: 2979-83
44. Jefferies JA, Robboy SJ, O'Brian PC, et al. Structural anomalies of the cervix and vagina in women enrolled in the Diethylstilbestrol Adenosis (DESAD) Project. American Journal of Obstetrics and Gynecology 1984; 148: 59-66
45. Pastuszak A, Schick-Boschetto B, Zuber C, et al. Pregnancy outcome following first-trimester exposure to fluoxetine (Prozac). Journal of the American Medical Association 1993; 269: 2246-8
46. Brent RL, Holmes LB. Clinical and basic science lessons from the thalidomide tragedy: what have we learned about the causes of limb defects? Teratology 1988; 38: 241-51
47. Kosenow W, Pfeiffer RA. Micromelie, Haemangiom an Duodenalstenose. Wissenschaftlishe Ausstellung Nr. 39, 59. Kassel: Tagung der Deutschen Gesellschaft der Kinderheilkunde, 1960
48. Wiedemann HR. Hinweis auf eine derzeitige Haeufung hypo- und aplastischer Fehlbildungen der Gliedmaassen. Medizinische Welt 1961; 37: 1884-7
49. Lenz W. Thalidomide and congenital abnormalities. Lancet 1962; 2: 45
50. Kallen B, Winberg J. A Swedish register of congenital malformations. Paediatrics 1968; 41: 765-76
51. MRC Vitamin Study Research Group. Prevention of neural tube defects: results of the Medical Research Council Vitamin Study. Lancet 1991; 338: 131-7
52. Czeizel A. Controlled studies of multivitamin supplementation on pregnancy outcome. In: Keen CL, Bendich A, Willhite CC, editors. Maternal nutrition and pregnancy outcome. San Diego, CA: New York Academy of Sciences, 1992: 17-20
53. Lossick JG, Kent HL. Trichomoniasis: trends in diagnosis and management. American Journal of Obstetrics and Gynecology 1991; 165: 1217-22
54. Gilstrap III LC, Little BB. Antimicrobial agents during pregnancy. In: Little BB, Gilstrap III LC, editors. Drugs and pregnancy. New York: Elsevier, 1992: 39-67
55. Dobias L, Cerna M, Rosessner P, et al. Genotoxicity and carcinogenicity of metronidazole. Mutation Research 1994; 317: 177-94
56. Burtin P, Taddio A, Aribumu O, et al. Safety of metronidazole in pregnancy: a meta-analysis. American Journal of Obstetrics and Gynecology 1995; 172: 525-9
57. Pampfer S, Streffer C. Prenatal death and malformations after irradiation of mouse zygotes with neutrons or x-rays. Teratology 1988; 37: 599
58. Wilson JG. Experimental studies on congenital malformations. Journal of Chronic Diseases 1959; 10: 11-130
59. Hall JG, Pauli RM, Wilson KM. Maternal and fetal sequelae of anticoagulation during pregnancy. American Journal of Medicine 1980; 68: 122-40
60. Koren G. Fetal toxicology of environmental tobacco smoke. Current Opinion in Pediatrics 1995; 7: 128-31
61. Lieberman E, Gremy I, Lang JM, et al. Low birthweight at term and the timing of fetal exposure to maternal smoking. American Journal of Public Health 1994; 84: 1127-31
62. Mirkes PE. Cyclophosphamide teratogenesis: a review. Teratogenesis Carcinogenesis and Mutagenesis 1985; 5: 75
63. Stephens TD. Proposed mechanisms of action in thalidomide embryopathy. Teratology 1988; 38: 229-39
64. England MA. Cellular processes and tissue interactions in developmental pathology. In: Harrison MR, Golbus MS, Filly RA, editors. The unborn patient: prenatal diagnosis and treatment. 2nd ed. Philadelphia: WB Saunders Company, 1990: 43-52
65. Buehler BA, Delimont D, van Waes M, et al. Prenatal prediction of risk of the fetal hydantoin syndrome. New England Journal of Medicine 1990; 322: 1567-72
66. Doll DC, Ringenberg S, Yarbro JW. Antineoplastic agents and pregnancy. Seminars in Oncology 1989; 16: 337
67. Daston GP. Relationships between maternal and developmental toxicity. In: Kimmel CA, Buelke-Sam J, editors. Developmental toxicology. 2nd ed. New York: Raven Press, 1994: 189-212
68. Rutledge JC. Genetic factors in clinical development physiology. In: Kimmel CA, Buelke-Sam J, editors. Developmental toxicology. 2nd ed. New York: Raven Press, 1994: 333-45
69. Hytten F, Chamberlain G, editors. Clinical physiology in obstetrics. 2nd ed. Oxford: Blackwell, 1991
70. Cummings AJ. A survey of pharmacokinetic data from pregnant women. Clinical Pharmacokinetics 1983; 8: 344-54
71. Hytten FE. Weight gain in pregnancy. In: Hytten FE, Chamberlain G, editors. Clinical physiology in obstetrics. 2nd ed. Oxford: Blackwell, 1991: 173-203
72. Hytten FE. Weight gain in pregnancy. In: Hytten FE, Chamberlain G, editors. Clinical physiology in obstetrics. Oxford: Blackwell, 1980: 193-233
73. Notarianni LJ. Plasma protein binding of drugs in pregnancy and in neonates. Clinical Pharmacokinetics 1990; 18: 20-36
74. Perucca E. Drug metabolism in pregnancy, infancy and childhood. Pharmacology and Therapeutics 1987; 34: 129-43
75. Ortweiler W, Simon HU, Splinter FK, et al. Bestimmung der elimination von Koffein und Metamizol in der Schwangerschaft und im Wochenbett als in vivomethode zur Charakterisierung verschiedener Zytochrom P-450 abhängiger biotranformationsreaktionen. Biomedica Biochimica Acta 1985; 44: 1189-99
76. Aldridge A, Bailey J, Neims AG. The disposition of caffeine during and after pregnancy. Seminars in Perinatology 1981; 5: 310-4
77. Dickinson RG, Hooper WD, Wood B, et al. The effect of pregnancy in humans on the pharmacokinetics of stable isotope labelled phenytoin. British Journal of Clinical Pharmacology 1989; 28: 17-27
78. Dam K, Christiansen J, Munok O, et al. Antiepileptic drugs: metabolism in pregnancy. Clinical Pharmacokinetics 1979; 4: 53-62
79. Aherne W, Dunnil MS. Quantitative aspects of placental structure. Journal of Pathology Bacteriology 1966; 91: 123-39
80. Aherne W, Dunnil MS. Morphometry of the human placenta. British Medical Bulletin 1966; 22: 5-8
81. Koren G. Changes in drug disposition in pregnancy and their clinical implications. In: Koren G, editor. Maternal-fetal toxicology: a clinician's guide. 2nd ed. New York: Marcel Dekker, 1994: 3-13

82. Simone C, Derewlany LO, Koren G. Drug transfer across the placenta: considerations in treatment and research. Clinics in Perinatology 1994; 21: 463-81
83. Krauer B, Dayer P, Anner R. Changes in serum albumin and $\alpha_1$-acid glycoprotein concentrations during pregnancy: an analysis of fetal-maternal pairs. British Journal of Obstetrics and Gynaecology 1984; 91: 875-81
84. Tucker GT. Plasma binding and disposition of local anaesthetics. International Anesthesiology Clinics 1975; 13: 33-59
85. Hill MD, Abramson FP. The significance of plasma protein binding on the fetal/maternal distribution of drugs at steady-state. Clinical Pharmacokinetics 1988; 14: 156-70
86. Simone C, Derewlany LO, Oskamp M, et al. Acetylcholinesterase and butyrylcholinesterase activity in the human term placenta: implications for fetal cocaine exposure. Journal of Laboratory and Clinical Medicine 1994; 123: 400-6
87. Mirkin BL. Perinatal pharmacology and therapeutics. New York: Academic Press, 1976
88. Juchau MR, Chao ST, Omiecinski CJ. Drug metabolism by the human fetus. In: Gilbaldi M, Prescott L, editors. Handbook of clinical pharmacokinetics. Auckland: Adis, 1983: 58-78
89. Gregus Z, Klaassen CD. Hepatic disposition of xenobiotic during prenatal and early postnatal development. In: Polin RA, Fox W, editors. Fetal and neonatal physiology. Philadelphia: Saunders, 1992: 1103-22
90. Kitada M, Kamataki T. Cytochrome P450 in human fetal liver: significance and fetal specific expression. Drug Metabolism Reviews 1994; 26: 305-23
91. Leakey JEA, Hume R, Burchell B. Development of multiple activities of UDP-glucuronyltransferase in human liver. Biochemical Journal 1987; 243: 859-61
92. Pacifici GM, Bencini C, Rane A. Acetyltransferases in humans: development and tissue distribution. Pharmacology 1986; 32: 283-391
93. Derewlany LO, Knie B, Koren G. Arylamine N-acetyltransferase activity of the human placenta. Journal of Pharmacology and Experimental Therapeutics 1994; 269: 756-60
94. Derewlany LO, Knie B, Koren G. Human placental transfer and metabolism of p-aminobenzoic acid. Journal of Pharmacology and Experimental Therapeutics 1994; 269: 761-5
95. Koren G, Feldman Y, MacLeod SM. Motherisk II. In: Koren G, editor. Maternal-fetal toxicology: a clinician's guide. 2nd ed. New York: Marcel Dekker, 1994: 737-56
96. Koren G, editor. Maternal-fetal toxicology: a clinician's guide. 2nd ed. New York: Marcel Dekker, 1994
97. Gilstrap III LC, Little BB, editors. Drugs and pregnancy. New York: Elsevier, 1992
98. Petrie RH, editor. Perinatal pharmacology. Oradell: Medical Economics Books, 1989
99. Schardein JL. Chemically induced birth defects. New York: Marcel Dekker, 1985
100. Roberts WE, Norman PF, Morrison J. Meperidine for intrapartum analgesia. In: Petrie RH, editor. Perinatal pharmacology. Oradell: Medical Economics Books, 1989: 353-60
101. Caldwell J, Walkie LA, Notarianni LJ, et al. Transplacental passage and neonatal elimination of pethidine given to mothers in childbirth. British Journal of Clinical Pharmacology 1977; 4: 715
102. Lavery JP. Morphine for obstetric analgesia. In: Petrie RH, editor. Perinatal pharmacology. Oradell, NJ: Medical Economics Books, 1989: 345-52
103. Shnider SM, Levinson G. Anesthesia for obstetrics. In: Miller RD, editor. Anesthesia. 4th ed. New York: Churchill Livingstone, 1994: 2031-76
104. Hamar C, Levy G. Factors affecting the serum protein binding of salicylic acid in newborn infants and their mothers. Pediatric Pharmacology 1980; 1: 31-43
105. Stuart MJ, Gross SJ, Elrad H, et al. Effects of acetylsalicylic-acid ingestion on maternal and neonatal hemostasis. New England Journal of Medicine 1982; 307: 909-12
106. CLASP Collaborative Group. CLASP: a randomised trial of low dose aspirin for the prevention and treatment of pre-eclampsia among 9364 pregnant women. Lancet 1994; 343: 619-29
107. Sibai BM, Caritis SN, Thom E, et al. Prevention of pre-eclampsia with low-dose aspirin in healthy, nulliparous pregnant women. New England Journal of Medicine 1993; 329: 1213-8
108. Schiff E, Peleg E, Goldenberg M, et al. The use of aspirin to prevent pregnancy-induced hypertension and lower the ratio of thromboxane $A_2$ to prostacyclin in relatively high risk pregnancies. New England Journal of Medicine 1989; 321: 351-6
109. Finster M. Surgical anaesthesia for the pregnant patient. Canadian Journal of Anaesthesia 1988; 35: S14-7
110. Gin T. Pharmacokinetic optimisation of general anaesthesia in pregnancy. Clinical Pharmacokinetics 1993; 25: 59-70
111. Bentur Y, Zalzstein E, Koren G. Occupational exposures known to be human reproductive toxins. In: Koren G, editor. Maternal-fetal toxicology: a clinician's guide. 2nd ed. New York: Marcel Dekker, 1994: 399-424
112. Crawford JS, Lewis M. Nitrous oxide in early human pregnancy. Anaesthesia 1986; 41: 900-5
113. Sylvester GC, Khoury MJ, Lu X, et al. First-trimester anesthesia exposure and the risk of central nervous system defects: a population-based case-control study. American Journal of Public Health 1994; 84: 1757-60
114. Kosaka Y, Takahashi T, Mark LC. Intravenous thiobarbiturate anaesthesia for cesarian section. Anaesthesiology 1969; 31: 489-506
115. Tannenbaum TN, Goldberg RJ. Exposure to anesthetic gases and reproductive outcome: a review of the epidemiologic literature. Journal of Occupational Medicine 1985; 27: 659-68
116. Ericson A, Källén B. Survey of infants born in 1973 or 1975 to Swedish women working in operating rooms during their pregnancies. Anesthesia and Analgesia 1979; 58: 302-5
117. Roodenburg PJ, Wladimiroff JW, Van Weering HK. Effect of maternal intravenous administration of atropine (0.5mg) on fetal breathing and heart pattern. Contribution to Gynecology and Obstetrics 1979; 6: 92-7
118. Abboud T, Raya J, Sadri S, et al. Fetal and maternal cardiovascular effects of atropine and glycopyrrolate. Anesthesia and Analgesia 1983; 62: 426-30
119. Scolnic D, Nulman I, Rovet J, et al. Neurodevelopment of children exposed in utero to phenytoin and carbamazepine monotherapy. Journal of the American Medical Association 1994; 271: 767-70

120. Dalessio DJ. Current concepts: seizure disorders and pregnancy. New England Journal of Medicine 1985; 312: 559-63
121. Pacifici GM, Nottoli R. Placental transfer of drugs administered to the mother. Clinical Pharmacokinetics 1995; 28: 235-69
122. Tomson T, Lindborn U, Ekqvist B, et al. Epilepsy and pregnancy: a prospective study of seizure control in relation to free and total plasma concentrations of carbamazepine and phenytoin. Epilepsia 1994; 35: 122-30
123. Tomson T, Lindbom U, Ekqvist B, et al. Disposition of carbamazepine and phenytoin in pregnancy. Epilepsia 1994; 35: 131-5
124. Moslet U, Hansen ES. A review of vitamin K, epilepsy and pregnancy. Acta Neurologica Scandinavica 1992; 85: 39-43
125. Cornelissen M, Steegers-Theunissen R, Kollee L, et al. Increased incidence of neonatal vitamin K deficiency resulting from maternal anticonvulsant therapy. American Journal of Obstetrics and Gynecology 1993; 168: 923-8
126. Cornelissen M, Steegers-Theunissen R, Kollee L, et al. Supplementation of vitamin K in pregnant women receiving anticonvulsant therapy prevents neonatal vitamin K deficiency. American Journal of Obstetrics and Gynecology 1993; 168: 884-8
127. Rosa FW. Spina bifida in infants of women treated with carbamazepine during pregnancy. New England Journal of Medicine 1991; 324: 674-7
128. Jones KL, Lacro RV, Johnson KA, et al. Pattern of malformations in the children of women treated with carbamazepine during pregnancy. New England Journal of Medicine 1989; 320: 1661-6
129. Thisted E, Ebbesen F. Malformations, withdrawal manifestations, and hypoglycaemia after exposure to valproate in utero. Archives of Disease in Childhood 1993; 69: 288-91
130. van der Pol MC, Hadders-Algra M, Huisjes HJ, et al. Antiepileptic medication in pregnancy: late effects on the children's central nervous system development. American Journal of Obstetrics and Gynecology 1991; 154: 121-8
131. Besunder JB, Blumer JL. Neonatal drug withdrawal syndromes. In: Koren G, editor. Maternal-fetal toxicology: a clinician's guide. 2nd ed. New York: Marcel Dekker, 1994: 321-52
132. Viggedal G, Hagberg BS, Laegreid L, et al. Mental development in late infancy after prenatal exposure to benzodiazepines - a prospective study. Journal of Child Psychology and Psychiatry 1993; 34: 295-305
133. Pastuszak A, Koren G, Milich V, et al. Prospective assessment of pregnancy outcome following first-trimester exposure to benzodiazepines. In: Koren G, editor. Maternal-fetal toxicology: a clinician's guide. 2nd ed. New York: Marcel Dekker, 1994: 77-88
134. Martin Jr JN, Perry Jr KG. Hypertension and preeclampsia. In: Sweet AY, Brown EG, editors. Fetal and neonatal effects of maternal disease. St Louis: Mosby Year Book, 1991: 224-40
135. Dommissee J, Davey DA, Roos PJ. Prazosin and oxprenolol therapy in pregnancy hypertension. South African Medical Journal 1983; 64: 231-3
136. Lubbe WF, Hodge JV. Combined α- and β-adrenoceptor antagonism with prazosin and oxprenolol in control of severe hypertension in pregnancy. New Zealand Medical Journal 1981; 94: 169-72
137. Lubbe WF. β-blockers in pregnancy. New England Journal of Medicine 1982; 307: 753
138. Bourget P, Fernandez H, Ribou F, et al. Faible passage transplacentaire de la prazosine (Alpress) au cours du troisieme trimestre de la grossesse: a propos de trois cas. Journal de Gynecologie, Obstetrique et Biologie de la Reproduction 1993; 22: 871-4
139. Frishman WH, Chesner M. Beta adrenergic blockers in pregnancy. American Heart Journal 1988; 115: 147-52
140. Dubois D, Petitcolas J, Temperville B, et al. Treatment of hypertension in pregnancy with β-adrenoceptor antagonists. British Journal of Clinical Pharmacology 1982; 13 Suppl.: 375S-8S
141. Lardoux H, Gerard J, Blazquez G, et al. Hypertension in pregnancy: evaluation of two beta-blockers atenolol and labetalol. European Heart Journal 1983; 4 (Suppl. G): 35-40
142. Rubin PC, Butters L, Clark DM, et al. Placebo-controlled trial of atenolol in treatment of pregnancy-associated hypertension. Lancet 1983; 1: 431-4
143. Ito S, Magee L, Smallhorn J. Drug therapy for fetal arrhythmias. Clinics in Perinatology 1994; 21: 543-72
144. Smith MT, Livingstone I, Eadie MJ, et al. Chronic propranolol administration during pregnancy: maternal pharmacokinetics. European Journal of Clinical Pharmacology 1983; 25: 481-90
145. Rubin PC, Butters L, Kelman AW, et al. Labetalol disposition and concentration-effect relationships during pregnancy. British Journal of Clinical Pharmacology 1983; 15: 465-70
146. Hogstedt S, Lindberg B, Rane A. Increased oral clearance of metoprolol in pregnancy. European Journal of Clinical Pharmacology 1983; 24: 217-20
147. Jones HMR, Cummings AJ. A study of the transfer of α-methyldopa to the human foetus and newborn infant. British Journal of Clinical Pharmacology 1978; 6: 432-4
148. Whitelaw A. Maternal methyldopa treatment and neonatal blood pressure. British Medical Journal 1981; 283: 471
149. Hartikainen-Sorri A-L, Heikkinen JE, Koivisto M. Pharmacokinetics of clonidine during pregnancy and nursing. Obstetrics and Gynecology 1987; 69: 598-600
150. de Swiet M. Antihypertensive drugs in pregnancy. British Medical Journal 1985; 291: 365-6
151. Liedholm H, Wahlin-Boll E, Ingemarsson I, et al. Transplacental passage and breast milk concentrations of hydralazine. European Journal of Clinical Pharmacology 1982; 21: 417-9
152. Lodeiro JG, Feinstein SJ, Lodeiro SB. Fetal premature atrial contractions associated with hydralazine. American Journal of Obstetrics and Gynecology 1989; 160: 105-7
153. Heinrich WL, Cronin R, Miller PD, et al. Hypotensive sequelae of diazoxide and hydralazine therapy. Journal of the American Medical Association 1977; 237: 264-5
154. Brazy JE, Grimm JK, Little VA. Neonatal manifestations of severe maternal hypertension occurring before the thirty-sixth week of pregnancy. Journal of Pediatrics 1982; 100: 265-71
155. Milner RDG, Chouksey SK. Effects of fetal exposures to diazoxide in man. Archives of Disease in Childhood 1972; 47: 537-43
156. Naulty J, Cefalo RC, Lewis PE. Fetal toxicity of nitroprusside in the pregnant ewe. American Journal of Obstetrics and Gynecology 1981; 139: 708-11

157. Lewis PE, Cefalo RC, Naulty JS, et al. Placental transfer and fetal toxicity of sodium nitroprusside. Gynecologic and Obstetric Investigation 1977; 8: 46
158. Shoemaker CT, Meyers M. Sodium nitroprusside for control of severe hypertensive disease in pregnancy: a case reported and discussion of potential toxicity. American Journal of Obstetrics and Gynecology 1984; 149: 171-3
159. Stempel JE, O'Grady JP, Morton MJ, et al. Use of sodium nitroprusside in complications of gestational hypertension. Obstetrics and Gynecology 1982; 60: 533-8
160. Manninen AK, Johakoski A. Nifedipine concentrations in maternal and umbilical serum, amniotic fluid, breast milk and urine of mothers and offspring. International Journal of Clinical Pharmacology Research 1991; 11: 231-6
161. Childress CH, Katz VL. Nifedipine and its indications in obstetrics and gynecology. Obstetrics and Gynecology 1994; 83: 616-24
162. Danielsson BR, Danielson M, Danielson M, et al. Identical phalangeal defects induced by phenytoin and nifedipine suggest fetal hypoxia and vascular disruption behind phenytoin teratogenicity. Teratology 1992; 45: 247-58
163. Yoshida T, Kanamori S, Hasegawa Y. Hyperphalangeal bones induced in rat pups by maternal treatment with nifedipine. Toxicology Letters 1988; 40: 127-32
164. Collins R, Yusuf S, Peto R. Overview of randomised trials of diuretics in pregnancy. British Medical Journal 1985; 290: 17-23
165. Beermann B, Groschinsky-Grind M, Fahraeus L, et al. Placental transfer of furosemide. Clinical Pharmacology and Therapeutics 1978; 24: 560-2
166. Stein WW, Halberstadt E, Gerner R, et al. Effect of furosemide on fetal kidney function. Archiv fuer Gynecology 1977; 224: 114-5
167. Wladimiroff JW. Effect of furosemide on fetal urine production. British Journal of Obstetrics and Gynaecology 1975; 82: 221-4
168. Votta RA, Parada OH, Windgrad RH, et al. Furosemide action on the creatinine concentration of amniotic fluid. American Journal of Obstetrics and Gynecology 1975; 123: 621-4
169. Pecorari D, Ragni D, Autera C. Administration of furosemide to women during confinement, and its action on newborn infants. Acta Biomed (Italy) 1969; 40: 2-11
170. Pryde PG, Sedman AB, Nugent CE, et al. Angiotensin-converting enzyme inhibitor fetopathy. Journal of the American Society of Nephrology 1993; 3: 1575-82
171. Teratogen Update. Angiotensin-converting enzyme inhibitors. Teratology 1994; 50: 399-409
172. Soares de Moura R, Cerqueira Lopes MA. Effects of captopril on the human foetal placental circulation: an interaction with bradykinin and angiotensin I. British Journal of Clinical Pharmacology 1995; 39: 497-501
173. Budnik IS, Leikin S, Hoeck LE. Effect in the newborn infant of reserpine administration ante partum. American Journal of Diseases of Children 1955; 90: 286-9
174. Derewlany LO, Leeder JS, Kumar R, et al. The transport of digoxin across the perfused human placental lobule. Journal of Pharmacology and Experimental Therapeutics 1991; 256: 1107-111
175. Mitani GM, Steinberg I, Lien EJ, et al. The pharmacokinetics of antiarrhythmic drugs in pregnancy and lactation. Clinical Pharmacokinetics 1987; 12: 253-91
176. Koren G, Farine D, Maresky D, et al. Significance of the endogenous digoxin-like substance in infants and mothers. Clinical Pharmacology and Therapeutics 1984; 36: 759-64
177. Rotmensch HH, Rotmensch S, Elkayam U. Management of cardiac arrhythmias during pregnancy: current concepts. Drugs 1987; 33: 623-33
178. Allen NM, Page RL. Procainamide administration during pregnancy. Clinical Pharmacy 1993; 12: 58-60
179. Weiner CP, Thompson MIB. Direct treatment of fetal supraventricular tachycardia after failed transplacental therapy. American Journal of Obstetrics and Gynecology 1988; 158: 570-3
180. Magee LA, Downar E, Sermer M, et al. Pregnancy outcome after gestational exposure to amiodarone in Canada. American Journal of Obstetrics and Gynecology 1995; 172: 1307-11
181. Graeves M. Anticoagulants in pregnancy. Pharmacology and Therapeutics 1993; 59: 311-27
182. Iturbe-Alessio I, Fonseca MDC, Mutchinik O, et al. Risks of anticoagulant therapy in pregnant women with artificial heart valves. New England Journal of Medicine 1986; 315: 1390-3
183. Shoul WL, Hall JG. Multiple congenital abnormalities associated with oral anticoagulants. American Journal of Obstetrics and Gynecology 1977; 127: 191-8
184. Flessa HC, Kapstrom AB, Glueck HI, et al. Placental transfer of heparin. American Journal of Obstetrics and Gynecology 1965; 93: 570-3
185. Ginsberg JS, Kowalchuk G, Hirsh J, et al. Heparin therapy during pregnancy: risks to the fetus and to the mother. Archives of Internal Medicine 1989; 149: 2233-6
186. Forestier F, Daffos F, Rainaut M, et al. Low molecular weight heparin (CY 216) does not cross the placenta during the third trimester of pregnancy. Thrombosis and Haemostasis 1987; 57: 234
187. Melissari E, Parker CJ, Wilson NV, et al. Use of low molecular weight heparin in pregnancy. Thrombosis and Haemostasis 1992; 68: 652-6
188. Aselton P, Jick H, Milkunsky A, et al. First-trimester brompheniramine use and congenital disorders. Obstetrics and Gynecology 1985; 65: 451-5
189. Seto A, Einarson T, Koren G. Evaluation of brompheniramine safety in pregnancy. Reproductive Toxicology 1993; 7: 393-5
190. Einarson TR, Leeder JS, Koren G. A method for meta-analysis of epidemiologic studies. Drug Intelligence and Clinical Pharmacy 1988; 22: 813-82
191. Keirse MJNC. Betamimetic tocolysis in preterm labour. In: Enkin MW, Keirse MJNC, Renfrew MJ, et al., editors. Pregnancy and childbirth module ('Cochrane Database of Systematic Reviews': Review No. 03237, 17 Feb 1995). Oxford: Update Software ('Cochrane updates on disk'), 1994: Disk Issue 1
192. Canadian Preterm Labor Investigation Group. Treatment of preterm labor with the beta adrenergic agonist ritodrine. New England Journal of Medicine 1992; 327: 308-12
193. Keirse MJNC. Indomethacin tocolysis in preterm labour. In: Enkin MW, Keirse MJNC, Renfrew MJ, et al., editors. Pregnancy and childbirth module ('Cockrane Database of Systematic Reviews': Review No. 04383, 17 Feb 1995). Oxford: Update Software ('Cochrane updates on disk'), 1994: Disk Issue 1
194. Moise KJ, Huhta JC, Sharif DS, et al. Indomethacin in the treatment of premature labor. New England Journal of Medicine 1988; 319: 327-31

195. Kirshon B, Moise KJ, Wasserstrum N, et al. Influence of short term indomethacin therapy on fetal urine output. Obstetrics and Gynecology 1988; 72: 51-3
196. Norton ME, Merrill J, Cooper BAB, et al. Neonatal complications after the administration of indomethacin for preterm labour. New England Journal of Medicine 1993; 329: 1602-7
197. Hannah ME, et al. The Canadian consensus on the use of tocolytics for preterm labour. Journal of the Society of Obstetricians and Gynecologists of Canada 1995; 17: 1089-138
198. Bologa M. Direct drug toxicity to the fetus. In: Koren G, editor. Maternal-fetal toxicology: a clinician's guide. 2nd ed. New York: Marcel Dekker, 1994: 267-99
199. Philipson A. Principles and possibilities of antibiotic treatment of intrauterine infections. In: Krauer B, Krauer F, Hytten FE, et al., editors. Drugs and pregnancy. London: Academic Press, 1984: 177-89
200. Blanco JB. Intra-amniotic infections. In: Gleicher N, editor. Principles and practice of medical therapy in pregnancy. 2nd ed. Norwalk: Appleton & Lange, 1992: 712-6
201. Chow AW, Jewesson PJ. Pharmacokinetics and safety of antimicrobial agents during pregnancy. Reviews of Infectious Diseases 1985; 7: 287-313
202. Graham JM, Oshiro BT, Blanco JD. Limited spectrum (first-generation) cephalosporins. Obstetrics and Gynecology Clinics of North America 1992; 19: 449-59
203. Eriksen NL, Blanco JD. Extended-spectrum (second- and third-generation) cephalosporins. Obstetrics and Gynecology Clinics of North America 1992; 19: 461-74
204. McCormack WM, George H, Donner A, et al. Hepatotoxicity of erythromycin estolate during pregnancy. Antimicrobial Agents and Chemotherapy 1977; 12: 630-5
205. Motherisk Newsletter No. 3, Jan 1995. The Motherisk Program, The Hospital for Sick Children. Toronto, 1995
206. Bourget P, Fernandez H, Delouis C, et al. Transplacental passage of vancomycin during the second trimester of pregnancy. Obstetrics and Gynecology 1991; 78: 908-11
207. Berkovitch M, Pastuszak A, Gazarian M, et al. Safety of the new quinolones in pregnancy. Obstetrics and Gynecology 1994; 84: 535-8
208. Reid DWJ, Caille G, Kaufmann NR. Maternal and transplacental kinetics of trimethoprim and sulfamethoxazole, separately and in combination. Canadian Medical Association Journal 1975 Suppl. 112: 67S-72S
209. Cohlan SQ. Tetracycline staining of teeth. Teratology 1977; 15: 127-30
210. Centers for Disease Control. Zidovudine for the prevention of HIV transmission from mother to infant. MMWR Morbidity and Mortality Weekly Report 1994; 43: 285-7
211. Centers for Disease Control. Birth outcomes following zidovudine therapy in pregnant women. MMWR Morbidity and Mortality Weekly Report 1994; 43: 409, 415-6
212. Centers for Disease Control. Pregnancy outcomes following systemic prenatal acyclovir exposure - June 1, 1984 - June 30, 1993. MMWR Morbidity and Mortality Weekly Report 1993; 41: 806-9
213. Koren G, Weinewr L, Lishner M, et al. Cancer in pregnancy: identification of unanswered questions on maternal and fetal risks. Obstetrics and Gynecology Survey 1990; 45: 509-14
214. Gilstrap III LC, Little BB. Immunosuppressant during pregnancy. In: Little BB, Gilstrap III LC, editors. Drugs and pregnancy. New York: Elsevier, 1992: 199-207
215. Conover EA, Rayburn WF. Over-the-counter drugs during pregnancy. In: Rayburn WF, Zuspan FP, editors. Drug therapy in obstetrics and gynecology. 3rd ed. St Louis: Mosby Year Book, 1992
216. Schneiderman JF. Nonmedical drug and chemical use during pregnancy. In: Koren G, editor. Maternal-fetal toxicology: a clinician's guide. 2nd ed. New York: Marcel Dekker, 1994: 301-19
217. Lemoine P, Harroussean H, Borteym JP. Les enfants de parents alcooliques: anomalies observees: a propos de 127 cas. Questions in Medicine 1968; 25: 477-82
218. Ulleland CN. The offspring of alcoholic mothers. Annals of the New York Academy of Sciences 1972; 197: 167-9
219. Jones KL, Smith DW, Ulleland CN. Pattern of malformations in offspring of chronic alcoholic mothers. Lancet 1973; 1: 1267-71
220. Little BB, Snell LM, Gilstrap LC. Alcohol use during pregnancy and maternal alcoholism. In: Little BB, Gilstrap LC, editors. Drugs and pregnancy. New York: Elsevier, 1992: 367-85
221. Council on Scientific Affairs, American Medical Association. Fetal effects of maternal alcohol use. Journal of the American Medical Association 1983; 249: 2517-21
222. Mills JL, Graubard BI. Is moderate drinking during pregnancy associated with an increased risk for malformations? Pediatrics 1987; 80: 309-14
223. Kleinman JC, Kopstein A. Smoking during pregnancy, 1967-80. American Journal of Public Health 1987; 77: 823-5
224. Koren G, Klein J, Forman R, et al. Biological markers of intrauterine exposure to cocaine and cigarette smoking. In: Koren G, editor. Maternal-fetal toxicology: a clinician's guide. 2nd ed. New York: Marcel Dekker, 1994: 387-97
225. Longo LD. The biological effects of carbon monoxide on the pregnant woman, fetus and newborn infant. American Journal of Obstetrics and Gynecology 1977; 129: 69-103
226. Fortier I, Marcoux S, Beaulac-Baillargeon L. Relation of caffeine intake during pregnancy to intrauterine growth retardation and preterm birth. American Journal of Epidemiology 1993; 137: 931-40
227. Larroque B, Kaminski M, Lelong N, et al. Effects on birth weight of alcohol and caffeine consumption during pregnancy. American Journal of Epidemiology 1993; 137: 941-50
228. Narod SA, De Sanjose S, Victoria C. Coffee during pregnancy: a reproductive hazard? American Journal of Obstetrics and Gynecology 1991; 164: 1109-14
229. Peacock JL, Bland JM, Anderson HR. Effects on birthweight of alcohol and caffeine consumption in smoking women. Journal of Epidemiology and Community Health 1991; 45: 159-63
230. Simone C, Derewlany LO, Oskamp M, et al. Transfer of cocaine and benzoylecgonine across the perfused human placental cotyledon. American Journal of Obstetrics and Gynecology 1994; 170: 1404-10
231. Plessinger MA, Woods Jr JR. Maternal, placental, and fetal pathophysiology of cocaine exposure during pregnancy. Clinical Obstetrics and Gynecology 1993; 36: 267-78

232. Snodgrass SR. Cocaine babies: a result of multiple teratogenic influences. Journal of Child Neurology 1994; 9: 227-33
233. Forman R, Klein J, Meta D, et al. Maternal and neonatal characteristics following exposure to cocaine in Toronto. Reproductive Toxicology 1993; 7: 619-22
234. Koren G, Klein J, Forman R, et al. Biological markers of intrauterine exposure to cocaine and cigarette smoking. Developmental Pharmacology and Therapeutics 1992; 18: 228-36
235. Koren G, Graham K, Shear N, et al. Bias against the null hypothesis: the reproductive risks of cocaine. Lancet 1989; 335: 415
236. Graham K, Feigenbaum A, Nulman I, et al. Pregnancy outcome and infant development following gestational cocaine use by social cocaine users in Toronto, Canada. In: Koren G, editor. Maternal-fetal toxicology: a clinician's guide. 2nd ed. New York: Marcel Dekker, 1994: 371-86
237. Lutiger B, Einarson TR, Koren G, et al. Relationship between gestational cocaine use and pregnancy outcome: a meta-analysis. In: Koren G, editor. Maternal-fetal toxicology: a clinician's guide. 2nd ed. New York: Marcel Dekker, 1994: 353-69
238. Nulman I, Rovet J, Altmann D, et al. Neurodevelopment of adopted children exposed in utero to cocaine. Canadian Medical Association Journal 1994; 151: 1591-7
239. Lifschitz MH, Wilson GS, O'Brian-Smith, et al. Factors affecting head growth and intellectual function in children and drug addicts. Pediatrics 1985; 75: 269-74
240. Rivers RPA. Neonatal opiate withdrawal. Archives of Disease in Childhood 1986; 61: 1236-9
241. Kandall SR, Koberczak TM, Mauer KR, et al. Opiate v. CNS depressant therapy in neonatal drug abstinence syndrome. American Journal of Diseases of Children 1983; 137: 378-82
242. Carin I, Glass L, Parekh A, et al. Neonatal methadone withdrawal: effect of two therapy regimens. American Journal of Diseases of Children 1983; 137: 1166-9
243. Tenenbein M. Poisoning in pregnancy. In: Koren G, editor. Maternal-fetal toxicology: a clinician's guide. 2nd ed. New York: Marcel Dekker, 1994: 223-52
244. Rayburn W, Aronow R, Delancy B, et al. Drug overdose during pregnancy: an overview from a metropolitan poison control center. Obstetrics and Gynecology 1984; 64: 611-4
245. Plouffe Jr L, Donahue J. Techniques for early diagnosis of the abnormal fetus. Clinics in Perinatology 1994; 21: 723-41
246. Harrison MR, Golbus MS, Filly RA, editors. The unborn patient: prenatal diagnosis and treatment. 2nd ed. Philadelphia: W.B. Saunders Company, 1991
247. Harrison MR. The fetus with a diaphragmatic hernia: pathophysiology, natural history, and surgical management. In: Harrison MR, Golbus MS, Filly RA, editors. The unborn patient: prenatal diagnosis and treatment. 2nd ed. Philadelphia: WB Saunders Company, 1991: 295-313
248. Harrison MR, Filly RA. The fetus with obstructive uropathy: pathophysiology, natural history, selection and treatment. In: Harrison MR, Golbus MS, Filly RA, editors. The unborn patient: prenatal diagnosis and treatment. 2nd ed. Philadelphia: WB Saunders Company, 1991: 328-93
249. NIH Consensus Conference Panel of the Effect of Corticosteroids for Fetal Maturation on Perinatal Outcomes. Effect of corticosteroids for fetal maturation on perinatal outcomes. Journal of the American Medical Association 1995; 273: 413-7
250. Kari MA, Hallman M, Eronen M, et al. Prenatal dexamethasone treatment in conjunction with rescue therapy of human surfactant: a randomized placebo-controlled multicentre study. Pediatrics 1994; 93: 730-6
251. Kramer WB, Van den Veyver IB, Kirshon B. Treatment of polyhydramnios with indomethacin. Clinics in Perinatology 1994; 21: 615-30
252. Speiser PW, New MI. Prenatal diagnosis and management of congenital adrenal hyperplasia. Clinics in Perinatology 1994; 21: 631-45
253. Evans MI, Pryde PG, Reichler A, et al. Fetal drug therapy. In: Fetal medicine (special issue). Western Journal of Medicine 1993; 159: 325-32
254. Karson EM, Anderson WF. Prospects for gene therapy. In: Harrison ML, Golbus MS, Filly RA, editors. The unborn patient: prenatal diagnosis and treatment. 2nd ed. Philadelphia: WB Saunders Company, 1991: 481-94
255. Crombleholme TM, Zanjani ED, Langer JC, et al., editors. The unborn patient: prenatal diagnosis and treatment. 2nd ed. Philadelphia: WB Saunders Company, 1991: 495-507

Chapter 3

# Paediatric Clinical Pharmacology and Therapeutics

*P.D. Walson*

## Synopsis of Important Principles

1) Drug administration and the response to drugs in children is affected by a number of factors including age and growth. This is of particular importance in the neonatal period and when physiological variables are changing rapidly.

2) There may be major differences in the response to drugs in neonates, infants and children in comparison with adults. These differences are due more to altered pharmacokinetics and the difficulty of recognising effects in children than to altered tissue responsiveness.

3) With a few specific exceptions, drug absorption by either oral or parenteral routes is similar in children to that in adults but practical problems and a lack of appropriate pharmaceutical formulations can create major problems.

4) Drug distribution is affected by a number of factors including protein binding, body compartment size and composition, blood flow, rates of metabolism and excretion, and membrane permeability, all of which can be different in children.

5) Rates of drug metabolism and excretion are generally diminished in the neonatal period, especially in the premature infant, but increase to normal adult values in the first few months of life. Later in childhood, as well as in specific disease states (e.g. cystic fibrosis), rates of drug metabolism or excretion may exceed adult values.

6) Safe and effective drug therapy in the neonatal period is complicated by a paucity of acute dosage regimen data (although this situation is improving rapidly), by the lack of appropriate formulations which allow accurate dosage or delivery, and by the difficulty in detecting adverse drug reactions in this age group.

7) In the immediate postnatal period, problems may arise from medications given to the mother and transferred transplacentally to the infant. In addition, breast fed infants can be affected by their mother's medication, although this is of consequence for only a few drugs.

8) When prescribing drugs for children, the simplest possible dosage regimen should be used with attention paid to the dose, route of administration, formulation, and duration of therapy.

9) Provision of information to the parents and, if appropriate, the child, concerning the disease and its treatment, can be as important as the regimen. Attention needs to be given to whether therapy is indeed required, what can realistically be expected from the drug given, the duration of therapy, monitoring parameters, and possible adverse effects. The problems of noncompliance may be made worse if this sort of explanation is not provided.

Paediatric medicine differs from adult medicine in many ways, mostly because of the more rapid growth and development of the child. The child is not a 'little adult' and should not be regarded as such in psychological, medical or pharmacological terms. Paediatric pharmacology can be broadly subdivided into two major periods relevant to drug action: intrauterine and extrauterine life. The intrauterine period can be further divided into the periods of:

1) Embryogenesis and organogenesis – essentially the first trimester of pregnancy (see further chapter 2).

2) Fetal maturation – the second trimester to labour (see further chapters 2 and 18).

3) The period just before birth and during labour – drugs that the baby is born with (see further chapters 2 and 18).

This chapter deals with drug therapy in extrauterine life, which can be divided into a number of distinct, *albeit* somewhat arbitrary, stages:

*The early postnatal period:* this is a phase of physiological immaturity during which there is rapid growth and highly variable alterations in drug metabolism and elimination, especially in premature infants. This period is also associated with a greater need for individualised therapy, a lower tolerance for adverse effects, a higher incidence of therapeutic errors, and greater difficulty identifying efficacy or toxicity. Yet there is a lack of both data on which to base therapeutic decisions and formulations that allow safe and effective administration.

*Infancy:* this represents an extension of the first stage, but the type and severity of disorders being treated are different and require a modified approach. Bodyweight gain and body water composition change rapidly as does the ratio of bodyweight or surface area to organ size and function.

*The 'toddler':* this stage is mainly associated with recurrent minor illnesses, often leading to multiple short courses of therapy. There are problems actually getting the child to take the medication as prescribed and these children's motor skills and curiosity develop faster than their intellectual ability to understand risks. They become progressively more adventurous and are the most likely to be accidentally poisoned.

*The young child:* the difficulties of drug administration seen in the 'toddler' are less common in this age group. There is, however, enhanced metabolism (e.g. antiepileptic agents and theophylline) and excretion (e.g. aminoglycosides) of a number of drugs (in mg/kg or mg/m$^2$) in this age group when either dose or clearance per unit of bodyweight is considered. Clearance can change rapidly in children even during a single regimen, making dosage much more problematic than in adult medicine.

*Adolescence:* while significant pharmacokinetic alterations have not been described at this stage of development, sexual development produces major changes in body size and composition and may affect drug metabolism. Psychological changes and peer pressure result in behaviours, many of them hidden, that can alter drug metabolism (e.g. smoking) or lead to drug interactions (e.g. ethanol consumption or illicit drug use). While poorly studied, psychiatric disorders (e.g. bulimia or anorexia) can be associated with body composition changes or behaviours that alter drug distribution or metabolism and therefore the required dosage. Finally, the problem of compliance (under-, over- or erratic use) becomes a major issue.

## 1. General Considerations

Paediatric pharmacology developed from therapeutic practice in adults with children receiving 'scaled down' adult doses. Although clearly unsatisfactory, this approach has been used for a long time with considerable clinical success. Much has been written in the literature about the need for more precise dosage regimens, and dosage based on age, surface area or bodyweight has become common practice. The scientific evidence supporting these dosage methods is sparse. Nevertheless, results are usually satisfactory for the medications used in daily paediatric practice which are relatively non-toxic and have a wide therapeutic margin. The use of such drugs, even with relative dosage inaccuracy, will be satisfactory if the desired therapeutic result is obtained with minimal adverse effects. Such practice, however, may be unnecessarily costly.

The situation is quite different for drugs with a narrow therapeutic margin, where there is only a small difference in dosage between efficacy and toxicity. Consequently, for agents such as digoxin, aminoglycoside antibiotics, or cytotoxic drugs, much more specific dosage information is needed. This can be derived from well-conducted pharmacokinetic studies which allow the precise definition of dosage relative to age, bodyweight, renal and hepatic function, concomitant disease states, and so on. Such studies are now being performed by a number of paediatric pharmacology units worldwide, and these have been given impetus by the requirements of drug regulatory authorities for such information, as well as technical advances such as optimal sampling theory, small volume assay techniques, stable isotopes, and computer modelling programs.[1] However, these studies can be used only to define 'best guess' initial dosage guidelines for a population. Individual doses may still need to be adjusted on the basis of clinical observations and plasma concentration monitoring results (see chapter 5). Drug effectiveness can be seriously compromised or toxicity promoted by assuming that 'therapeutic ranges' established in adults are applicable to children.[2] For example, such extrapolation has resulted in overdosage of infants with theophylline for both asthma and apnoea, underdosage with phenobarbital for seizures, and a total lack of useful information for indomethacin for patent ductus arteriosus.

Clearly, more paediatric pharmacodynamic and pharmacokinetic studies are needed, but the priorities for paediatric pharmacology studies should be based on resources, need and drug utilisation. In this respect, there is obviously a very considerable difference between what is prescribed in a teaching hospital, a district hospital, and in general practice. There are even greater differences when over-the-counter drug use is considered, especially in countries where there is uncontrolled access to all drugs. Currently, the majority of children even in developed countries are treated as outpatients whenever possible, often without a clinician or any medical advice. In addition, with the improvement in their general standard of health, most children have only brief episodes of relatively mild acute illnesses. Treatment for these episodes, be it symptomatic or curative, requires medications that have a fairly wide therapeutic margin. This situation is obviously quite different from that of the sick child in a hospital or the child with a serious chronic disease (e.g. cystic fibrosis) being treated as an outpatient.

The differentiation between these broad groups of patients is important, as it lends perspective to the appropriate development of paediatric pharmacology. It is easy for academic disciplines to get lost in the minutiae of a particular teaching hospital problem and lose sight of the realities of the community at large. The treatment of many minor illnesses, which represent a considerable amount of the day-to-day workload of general practitioners and paediatricians, can be dealt with effectively using tried and trusted medications for which scientifically calculated dosage regimens are not available. In a child with pharyngitis, whether amoxicillin is given as 125mg 3 times daily or 250mg every 8 hours is probably of little importance, in terms of reality, efficacy or toxicity. It may not even matter whether the drug is given for 3, 7 or 10 days. However, treatment of sepsis in a 500g premature neonate is quite different.

In an attempt to protect children, a number of countries have introduced legislation which has prohibited the promotion or labelling of certain drugs for use in children. While such legislation has indeed been protective, it has also led to many children being denied the benefit of potentially useful drugs. The result has been the development of the so-called 'therapeutic orphan' situation.[3] All drugs used in children should have been studied in children. However, there will be certain situations where this is very difficult to do in a systematic way. For example, arrhythmias are much less common in children than adults; thus, new antiarrhythmics would be expected to be developed using only adult patients. Such compounds may infrequently be considered of potential use in children. Provided the adverse effects described in adults are acceptable, legislation should allow the use of this medication in selected children, initially using an extrapolated dosage. Individual pharmacokinetic and pharmacodynamic studies could be carried out while treating individual patients. An accumulation of such individual experiences would, in time, allow suitable paediatric data to be collected. At present, the performance of these and other paediatric drug trials has been limited, but this situation is improving.

## 2. Determinants of Altered Drug Responsiveness in Infants and Children

A number of factors determine drug dosage and response in infants and children.

### 2.1 Drug Absorption and Bioavailability

Drugs may be administered by a number of routes, including orally, parenterally, intraosseously, topically, and rectally. Other, less common routes such as by inhalation, sublingually, intravaginally, and by implantation will not be discussed, but all have unique paediatric considerations.

### 2.1.1 Oral Absorption

Physiologically, it has been shown that neonates, especially the premature, have greatly reduced gastric acid secretion with relative achlorhydria. Adult values are not achieved until about 3 years of age. In addition, gastric emptying, which has an influence on subsequent absorption, is prolonged. Absorption approaches adult values by 6 to 8 months of age and is altered by position, feeding, gestational and postnatal age. The importance of delayed gastric emptying is probably not as great as previously believed, except during the first few weeks of life, and the clinical importance of this is limited because sick neonates receive most of their medications parenterally. Because of relative achlorhydria, absorption of orally administered penicillins is enhanced in neonates. On the other hand, the absorption of some other drugs (e.g. phenobarbital, phenytoin and rifampicin) is reduced. Orally administered carbamazepine suspension is well absorbed, as are digoxin and diazepam.

Other than in the neonatal period, significant differences in the gastrointestinal absorption of drugs have not been well demonstrated except in children with gastrointestinal problems, such as coeliac disease. Bioavailability of orally administered drugs with a high hepatic clearance and first-pass elimination (e.g. propranolol and dextropropoxyphene) may, however, be low and show greater interindividual variability in children than in adults. Drugs such as cyclosporin, whose absorption depends on bile flow, diet, and intestinal transit, may also show greater inter- and intrapatient variability in children than in adults. Prolonged-release preparations such as those designed to release a drug over 24 hours are unlikely to produce reliable absorption in children, as both highly variable and much more rapid intestinal transit times than in adults are seen. And of course it is the actual amount of drug retained that determines the effects seen, not the amount measured since some may be spilled, or spat out.

Of considerable practical importance is the question of drug absorption relative to meals. There is a large, often conflicting, literature on this subject. The absorption of a few drugs [e.g. isoniazid, rifampicin, tetracyclines except doxycycline and minocycline, narrow-spectrum penicillins, and the antidiabetic drugs glibenclamide (glyburide) and glipizide] is clearly reduced by food. However, all other medications should be given with meals, even if only for simplicity and to enhance compliance. This is obviously problematic in severely ill, hospitalised children who are unable or unwilling to eat.

### 2.1.2 Absorption After Parenteral Administration

Rapid and complete absorption after *intramuscular* administration cannot be automatically assumed. In adults, resting muscle blood flow has been shown to be greatest in the deltoid, intermediate in the thigh, and least in the buttock. In neonates, muscle blood flow varies quite considerably over the first 2 to 3 weeks of life. In disease states where there is gross oedema (about 30% of bodyweight), such as the nephrotic syndrome or kwashiorkor, intramuscular bioavailability may be reduced. Also, muscle blood flow is dependent on activity, which is decreased in paralysed or sick children. Certain drugs (e.g. phenytoin, digoxin and diazepam) are poorly absorbed from any site and should not be administered intramuscularly, even to healthy children.

*Intraosseous* drug administration is a major, rediscovered advance in the emergency treatment of children, especially those in whom any delay in receiving drug or fluids could be life-threatening (e.g. those with septic shock). More studies are needed, but the intraosseous route appears to be a reliable, safe way to administer medications, even those such as adenosine which require rapid circulatory access.

### 2.1.3 Percutaneous Absorption

Percutaneous absorption of drugs is enhanced in infants, and to a lesser extent in children, especially in the presence of damaged skin or under an occlusive covering (e.g. plastic pants). In part, this is because children have a much larger surface area to bodyweight ratio. Significant absorption has been documented with continued use of strong topical corticosteroids in infants with moderately severe to severe eczema and nappy (diaper) rash. Boric acid may be absorbed, resulting in systemic toxicity, when certain dusting powders (which are also both ineffective and toxic) are used on damaged skin. Also, aniline dyes can be absorbed through unbroken skin and produce methaemoglobinaemia.

Problems with dermal absorption have also been documented with extensive topical use of the sulfonamide mafenide, and with povidone iodine or aminoglycoside-polymixin sprays for burns. Storage of clothes in naphthalene mothballs can potentially lead to haemolytic anaemia

**Table I.** Effect of site of injection and intravenous (IV) flow rate on the time to deliver 95% of an intravenously-administered dose (after Gould & Roberts[6])

| IV flow rate (ml/min) | **Approximate time to deliver 95% of an administered dose (min)** | | | |
|---|---|---|---|---|
| | Distance of injection site from patient (ml)[a]: | | | |
| | 0.15 | 8.15 | 12.15 | 17.75 |
| 3 | <10 | 190 | 200 | |
| 10 | <10 | 90 | 80 | |
| 25 | <10 | 70 | 70 | 130 |
| 100 | <5 | 15 | 30 | 70 |

a Distance in ml of volume in intravenous tubing.

and jaundice in infants with glucose-6-phosphate dehydrogenase (G6PD) deficiency. Hexachlorophene emulsion or powder, used in neonatal nurseries to prevent staphylococcal sepsis, may be associated with neurotoxicity or death as a result of percutaneous absorption. Use of hexachlorophene preparations should therefore be avoided in children, especially neonates.[4]

Neonatal skin is so permeable that it has been used to administer both theophylline and fatty acids and to non-invasively (i.e. transcutaneously) monitor theophylline drug concentrations.

#### *2.1.4 Rectal Absorption*

The rectal route is generally less favoured in Anglo-Saxon countries than in continental Europe. The attractions of rectal administration are that it can be useful in patients who are vomiting and in infants and young children who are reluctant to take oral medication, and that it might partially avoid hepatic first-pass metabolism to which a number of orally administered drugs are susceptible. However, in practice, the rectal route is not ideal because of considerable interindividual variation in both retention and rectal venous drainage and hence, in the rate and extent to which drugs are absorbed. Lack of suitable preparations, trauma from insertion, and irritation from excipients also limit use of this route. However, antiemetics (which are otherwise seldom indicated), antipyretics (e.g. paracetamol), hypnosedatives (e.g. chloral hydrate), opioids (e.g. hydromorphone) and anticonvulsants (e.g. diazepam) are commonly given rectally.

### 2.2 Factors Influencing Drug Availability After Intravenous Administration

Intravenous administration is usually assumed to deliver drugs into the circulation reliably and rapidly. In fact, intravenous administration can be associated with delayed or uncertain delivery. The amount of delay is determined by the site of administration, the intravenous flow rate, fluid and drug viscosity, and the length, dimensions, composition and even location of the line with respect to the patient (table I).[5] Dosage uncertainty can be caused by measurement or calculation errors as well as adsorption or absorption of the drug by the intravenous line (e.g. diazepam), photodecomposition (e.g. methotrexate), or deposition of precipitates (e.g. calcium phosphate in total parenteral nutrition solutions) on in-line filters. Complex problems can also be created by formulations such as chloral hydrate or cyclosporin preparations which can dissolve plastic or plasticisers, and opaque solutions (e.g. total parenteral nutrition solutions or propofol) can make particulate material difficult to see.

### 2.3 Drug Distribution

Numerous factors influence paediatric drug distribution, particularly body composition, plasma protein binding, and blood-brain barrier development. The influence of regional circulation or of drug specificity for tissue receptor sites is less clear.

#### *2.3.1 Body Composition*

Newborn infants have a much higher extracellular fluid volume – especially prematures (in whom it constitutes 50% of bodyweight) – than full term infants (45%), older infants (25% at 1 year of age), or adults (20 to 25%). Total body water is also much greater in neonates, varying from 92% in premature infants to about 75% in full term infants, compared with about 50 to 60% in adults. On the other hand, fat content is lowered, being about 3% in premature infants, 12% in full term neonates, 30% at 1 year of age, and about 18% in the average adult. As drugs are distributed between extracellular water and depot fat according to their lipid : water partition coefficient, these changes can have considerable significance for altered drug distribution, particularly in the neonatal period, but also in diseases associated with fluid excess.

In terms of drug dosage, especially with water soluble drugs, which are by far the most commonly used in paediatric practice, this implies that larger initial doses on a mg/kg bodyweight basis need to be given to achieve plasma concentrations similar to those seen in adults. However, after the initial or loading dose, the dosage interval may need to be increased or the amount per day decreased to compensate for diminished hepatic function and renal excretion (see section 2.4). Both drug distribution and clearance must be considered when selecting a dosage regimen. For example, a premature infant or anephric child with sepsis may need a larger than usual (i.e. 4 mg/kg) initial gentamicin dose to achieve an effective concentration, yet subsequent doses may be only 1 mg/kg given every 24 to 36 hours.

#### 2.3.2 Plasma Protein Binding

Plasma protein binding in the neonatal period, and especially in the premature infant, is less than in adults. This results in a higher free *fraction* of unbound drug, but this change considered in isolation (i.e. in the absence of concomitant changes in drug elimination capacity) would not be expected to result in increased pharmacological effects since the unbound drug concentration is unchanged and only the total (bound plus unbound) concentration will be affected. In part, reduced protein binding is due to lower plasma protein concentrations in neonates, especially plasma albumin, which is low until age 10 to 12 months. In addition, $\alpha_1$-acid glycoprotein levels are also low. There also appear to be differences in binding capacity, although changes in binding affinity have not been well described.

One consequence of a higher free fraction of a drug in the plasma is a larger apparent volume of distribution in neonates than in adults. Thus, a given plasma concentration of a drug in neonates may reflect a higher amount of drug in the body because of the larger plasma : tissue concentration ratio than in adults. This is a corollary to the comments made about body water (section 2.3.1).

In older children, there are a number of disease states that may affect drug protein binding including hepatic disease, the nephrotic syndrome, chronic renal failure, cardiac failure, and malnutrition (especially kwashiorkor, where hypoalbuminaemia is severe). The clinical significance of altered binding *per se* in these conditions is minimal, but may be of importance for some drugs such as salicylate for which higher penetration into the cerebrospinal fluid (CSF) and brain may result, especially in children with metabolic acidosis from salicylate intoxication.

Changes in protein binding must be considered when total rather than unbound drug concentrations are used to adjust dosage regimens (see further chapter 5; sect. 1.6.3).

#### 2.3.3 The Blood-Brain Barrier

The 'blood-brain barrier', a permeability barrier between the circulation and the brain parenchyma composed of endothelial cells as well as the adjacent astrocytic foot processes, is functionally incomplete in neonates. Except for drugs handled by active transport processes, the two most important factors that determine the rate of transport of drugs across the blood-brain barrier are lipid solubility and the degree of ionisation of the drug. Drugs that are predominantly non-ionised at physiological pH are much more lipid soluble than mostly ionised drugs and are therefore likely to achieve higher concentrations in the brain and cerebrospinal fluid (CSF).

Entry of drugs into the CSF occurs largely through the choroid plexus, where the capillaries have large fenestrations and are thus highly permeable. Secretion of CSF is an active process. CSF has a low protein concentration and an acid-base profile similar to venous blood. Thus, the non-ionised drug concentration and the proportion of drug molecules that are ionised are similar in CSF and plasma water. Drugs leave the brain by reverse passage through the blood-brain barrier (for lipid soluble drugs) or by clearance into the CSF and eventually into the general circulation *via* the arachnoid villi.

A number of factors, in addition to those already mentioned, influence drug passage into the CSF and, thus, by assumption, the brain. There is greater penetration of certain substances into the child's brain; the amount is determined by the degree of immaturity, acidosis, hypoxia, hypothermia and infection, and the sparseness of myelination.

The permeability of antibiotics into the CSF in children with meningitis is an important consideration. Although some agents penetrate poorly under normal circumstances, in the presence of meningeal inflammation, penetration may be considerably enhanced. Drugs in this category include penicillins such as benzylpenicillin (penicillin G), ampicillin, ticarcillin, azlocillin, mezlocillin and piperacillin; cefalosporins such as cefotaxime, ceftriaxone, ceftizoxime, ceftazidime and cefuroxime; and also rifampicin and vancomycin. Drugs which have good penetration into the CSF, even in the absence of meningeal inflammation, include chloramphenicol and cotrimoxazole (trimethoprim/sulfamethoxazole). Despite the development of drug resistance and the advent of effective cefalosporins which penetrate well, chloramphenicol still has a place in therapy, especially in developing countries, because of its low cost, excellent oral bioavailability, and good CNS penetration. Its dose-dependent toxicity can be minimised by appropriate dosage and plasma concentration monitoring. Dose-independent, lethal, idiosyncratic haematological toxicity is rare (1 in 10,000 to 50,000) and may occur as often with newer, much more expensive drugs.

Drugs that penetrate the CSF poorly regardless of inflammation include the aminoglycosides, clindamycin, erythromycin, fusidic acid and tetracycline. Although the aminoglycosides continue to be used for Gram-negative meningitis, the CSF concentrations achieved are generally low and inconsistent; higher concentrations have been obtained by direct intrathecal or intraventricular administration but the efficacy of such routes of administration is unproven. The newer cefalosporins appear more appropriate agents.

The use of corticosteroids in the management of meningitis is worthy of mention. Although becoming common, this practice has been shown to be effective only for *Haemophilus influenzae* meningitis, the management of adrenal insufficiency associated with meningococcal meningitis, and possibly tuberculous meningitis. Corticosteroid use in other forms of meningitis is of unproven clinical benefit and could be detrimental, since steroids reintegrate the blood-brain barrier and could inhibit drug penetration.

### 2.4 Drug Elimination

There are significant differences in drug elimination in neonates, infants and children which relate to the developmental physiological states of the various age groups. Sufficient information is now available to prove that in the neonatal period, there is a physiological immaturity in the capacity of the liver to metabolise a large number of drugs. For drugs that are mainly eliminated by hepatic metabolism, this leads to a longer plasma half-life, which results in a longer time to reach steady-state, a potential increase in the eventual steady-state concentration of the unchanged drug, and an associated decrease in, or absence of, metabolites. In general, the more premature the infant, the greater the degree of depression of hepatic metabolism (table II).

The same principle applies to drugs that are mainly eliminated unchanged by renal excretion. The glomerular filtration rate is very low prior to 34 weeks of gestation and does not reach adult levels until 2.5 to 5 months of age, after which it may exceed adult values until adolescence. Tubular secretion is also lower and does not reach adult levels until 7 months. The more premature the infant, the less the ability of the kidneys to excrete drugs and thus the longer the plasma half-life. Some examples are shown in table II.

#### 2.4.1 Hepatic Metabolism

**The Perinatal Period**

Hepatic drug metabolism, especially in the neonatal period, has been a subject of intense interest to paediatric pharmacologists for the past three decades. Not surprisingly, this has produced a wealth of information, from which certain general principles can be discerned:

1) Hepatic metabolism of many drugs is slow in the neonatal period compared with that in older children or adults.

2) In part, this is related to immaturity of hepatic drug metabolising enzyme systems in neonates.

3) Oxidation and glucuronidation processes (see chapter 1; sect. 3.3) are generally decreased more in neonates than demethylation or sulfation.

4) The maturation of hepatic metabolic rate or even a specific metabolic pathway (e.g. methylation of theophylline to caffeine) is determined by both postnatal and postgestational age.

5) Interindividual, pharmacogenetically determined differences in the rate of hepatic metabolism seen in adults are also seen in neonates, but neonates have additional, large intraindividual differences as a result of dosage problems and rapid changes in clinical condition, growth, and maturation.

6) Studies in animals may not accurately predict clinical effects. Studies using isolated human fetal hepatocytes have indicated that the human fetus is better equipped with hepatic drug metabolising enzymes, at least of the

**Table II.** Plasma half-lives (hours) of different drugs in neonates, infants, children and adults[a] (after Morselli;[7,8] Morselli & Baruzzi;[9] Besunder[10])

| Drug | Neonates (<7 days) | Infants (>1 month) | Children (1-15 years) | Adults[b] |
|---|---|---|---|---|
| **Drugs mainly eliminated by hepatic metabolism** | | | | |
| Carbamazepine | 8-28 | | 14; 19 | 16-36 |
| Diazepam | 22-46<br>38-120 (prematures) | 10-12 | 15-21 | 24-48 |
| Ethosuximide | | | 24-41 | 40-60 |
| Indomethacin | ≈15<br>13-24 (prematures) | | | 4-11 |
| Lidocaine[d] (lignocaine) | ≈3 | | | 1-2 |
| Mepivacaine | ≈9 | | | ≈2 |
| Nalidixic acid | ≈4 | ≈3 | ≈2 | 1.5-2.5 |
| Nortriptyline | ≈56 | | | 18-28 |
| Paracetamol (acetaminophen) | 2-5<br>≈5[c] | | ≈4.5[c] | ≈2<br>≈4[c] |
| Pethidine (meperidine) | ≈23 | | | ≈6 |
| Phenobarbital | 70-500 | 20-70 | 20-80 | 60-180 |
| Phenylbutazone | ≈27 | ≈18 | ≈18; 23[e] | ≈70 |
| Phenytoin[d] | 30-60 | 2-7 | 2-20 | 20-30 |
| Salicylate[d] | 4.5-11[c] | | 2-4[c] | 2-4[c] |
| Theophylline | 20-35<br>14-58 (prematures) | ≈5.6 | 1.4-8 | 3.5-8 |
| Tolbutamide | 10-40 | | | 4-10 |
| **Drugs mainly eliminated by renal excretion** | | | | |
| Digoxin | 26-170<br>90 (prematures) | 11-37 | 19-50 | 30-60 |
| Furosemide (frusemide) | 2.4-29.4<br>(8.6 term mean)<br>8.4-44 (26.8 premature mean) | | | 0.5 |

a Mean values or ranges shown are only intended to show trends in elimination with postnatal development. Some values in children and adults are not from the same laboratory as those for neonates and infants.

b Younger adults. Values can vary widely among individuals but those indicated are the usual mean values.

c Based on urinary excretion, rather than plasma concentration.

d Dose-dependent elimination. Values given are those at or around therapeutic concentrations.

e Value of ≈18h in children aged 2 to 7 years; ≈23h for older children.

mono-oxygenase system, than are animal fetuses.

As shown in table II, the plasma half-life of most drugs that are eliminated mainly by hepatic metabolism is prolonged, because of the immaturity of hepatic drug metabolising systems. However, the clinical effects of altered hepatic metabolism can be difficult to predict because these effects depend on the drug's chemistry – whether it is deactivated or activated, or has active or toxic metabolites – and on maternal drug exposure, gestational and postnatal age, whether the drug has a high or low hepatic extraction ratio (i.e. whether its metabolism is flow- or capacity-limited), and the specific metabolic pathway(s) involved.

Concentrations of ligandin (the Y protein that binds organic ions including certain drugs) are low in the fetus and neonate until 5 to 10 days after birth; this leads to lower clearance of ionic, low hepatic extraction ratio drugs. Drugs that are detoxified may therefore be more active, while prodrugs (e.g. chloramphenicol succinate) or drugs with active or toxic metabolites (e.g. propranolol, diazepam, methyldopa, paracetamol, pethidine, procainamide, and lidocaine) may be less active or less toxic. The immature liver is proportionally larger than at any other age and thus may have considerable metabolising potential despite low enzyme concentrations, if only on a relative mass basis. High hepatic extraction ratio (flow-limited) drugs may be less affected than low hepatic extraction ratio agents.

In fetal life, this metabolic capability may not be of great importance, since it is the maternal liver that largely carries out these functions. However, where the mother receives medication on a regular basis, or receives a drug which is slowly eliminated, fetal metabolism has a role to play and such exposure may induce neonatal metabolism. Both gestational and postnatal age determine the rate of metabolism. For example, with chloramphenicol and theophylline, it is the postconceptual rather than postnatal age that determines the metabolic rates in neonates.[11] While *N*-demethylation of pethidine and aromatic hydroxylation of chlorpromazine take place in the neonate, conjugated chlorpromazine metabolites are found in the urine only if the drug was administered to the mother before birth. This implies that the fetus is capable of hydroxylating chlorpromazine, but not of conjugating the metabolite. Similarly, diazepam has been shown to be reasonably well *N*-demethylated, but poorly hydroxylated and conjugated in preterm infants, when compared with full-term infants or older children.

The effects of deficient glucuronidation are best illustrated by chloramphenicol. When chloramphenicol is given in 'usual' mg/kg doses to neonates or young children, accumulation of unchanged drug can lead to high concentrations with consequent serious toxicity (circulatory collapse or death; the 'grey baby' or 'grey toddler' syndromes) – a result of the low concentrations of glucuronyl transferase and uridine diphosphate glucuronic dehydrogenase. Numerous pharmacokinetic studies carried out with chloramphenicol in the neonatal period have led to more precise dosage recommendations based on factors such as bodyweight and gestational or neonatal age. Problems remain, however, with the administration of chloramphenicol to newborn infants because of the considerable interindividual variation in metabolism, extent of illness, renal function and acidosis. Despite more precise dosage recommendations, limiting the dose to 25 mg/kg/day in neonates in the first week of life, and ensuring that serum chloramphenicol concentrations are maintained in the range of 15 to 25 mg/L using blood level monitoring, toxicity still occurs. This is also true for theophylline when used for treatment of apnoea and respiratory diseases. Neonates are capable of metabolising theophylline to 1,7-methyluric acid and 1,3-dimethyluric acid, but not to 3-methylxanthine; the latter is, however, produced by older infants and young children. The 'therapeutic range' for apnoea (7 to 12 mg/L) in neonates is also different from that for asthma (5 to 15 mg/L). Target ranges for asthma/wheezing are different for neonates (5 to 12 mg/L), children (5 to 15 mg/L) and adults (10 to 20 mg/L).

Finally, metabolism is susceptible to induction, as is the case in older children and adults. Phenobarbital is a well known inducer of hepatic metabolising enzymes, but other inducing agents such as tobacco or betamethasone (given to prevent the development of hyaline membrane disease) can have marked effects. In a study in premature infants who received theophylline for therapeutic purposes, parenteral administration of betamethasone in 4 cases induced hepatic microsomal function, such that these infants (with the exception of one) were capable of producing 6 metabolites of theophylline in the first week of life. This finding was in sharp contrast to 5 control infants who were not exposed to betamethasone *in utero* and in whom this enzymatic feat took much longer to achieve.[12] However, betamethasone-induced enzyme induction did not influence the initial plasma half-life of theophylline, which was not greatly different in the two groups, pointing to the overriding importance of renal function in this age group.[13] In a study in infants aged 3 weeks to 6.5 months, the mean renal clearance of theophylline was 27% of total clearance, and in some individuals it was as high as 43 and 45% of total clearance.[14] Similar observations have been made with metronidazole.[15]

*In summary*, a number of important changes occur in neonatal hepatic drug metabolism during the first few weeks of life. Most of these changes occur spontaneously as part of maturation and development; some may be induced by agents given to the infant or mother. In general, while these changes are important, their clinical effects can be difficult to predict and they do not influence dosage regimens as much as does renal function.

#### The Older Child

Because of the significance of the changes that occur in neonatal hepatic drug metabolism, less attention has been paid to the older child in this regard. It has long been known that dosage requirements of some drugs (e.g. antiepileptics and theophylline) to achieve similar plasma concentration are greater on a mg/kg bodyweight basis in the 1- to 8-year-old age group than in adults. This is because the rate of metabolism of these drugs is more rapid in the younger age group, such that their clearance is greater and half-life shorter. This necessitates the use of larger daily doses, given at more fre-

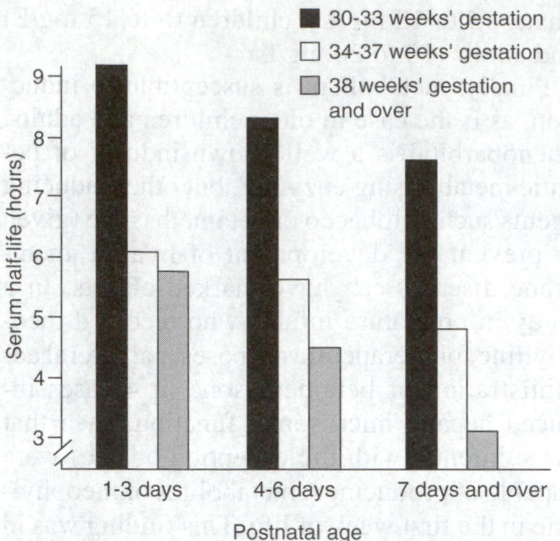


**Fig. 1.** Relationship between kanamycin half-lives and gestational and postnatal ages (after Howard & McCracken;[16] with permission).

quent intervals or as sustained-release preparations, to achieve therapeutic blood concentrations with acceptable peak to trough variation in this age group. This more rapid metabolism is almost certainly due to the fact that in children, the liver is larger relative to bodyweight than in adults. These proportions change to the usual adult pattern at puberty, at which time daily drug dosage requirements lessen and dosage intervals can be increased.

### *2.4.2 Renal Excretion*

Renal excretory capacity is decreased in neonates and shows progressive maturation with gestational and postnatal age. Adult values for glomerular filtration rate are reached after about 3 to 6 months of age, while tubular function matures at about 12 months. The differences in renal function demonstrated between premature infants born before 34 weeks of gestation and full-term infants persist for the first month of life. It would appear that the functional development of the glomerulus precedes that of the proximal tubule until at least the 36th to 39th week of gestation. In addition, it seems likely that there is active renal vasoconstriction around term. This maintains the glomerular filtration rate at a low level in the perinatal period, which may protect the proximal tubules from a relative overload of electrolytes, peptides, glucose and amino acids, and subsequent spillage of the compounds into the urine. The magnitude of the change is great; tubular secretion of para-aminohippuric acid (PAH), for example, can increase 10-fold in the first year of life.

Numerous studies have assessed the influence of altered renal function on drug elimination in neonates. Renal function is of particular importance to drug disposition in the neonatal period, as most sick neonates receive antibiotics for suspected, or proven, infection and most of these agents are water soluble. The example of kanamycin presented in figure 1 illustrates the fact that the less mature the infant, whether in terms of gestational or postnatal age, the lower is renal drug clearance and the longer the half-life of the drug. Further examples are given in table III, which lists plasma half-life values for some commonly used antibacterial drugs. Such data have led to the development of age- and bodyweight-related dosage regimens for some antimicrobial agents used in the neonatal period (tables IV and V).

For most agents excreted predominantly by the kidney, the plasma half-life is prolonged in the first week of life. The rate of elimination then increases rapidly during the ensuing weeks until shorter adult half-life values are seen, usually by the end of the first month of life. Later in childhood, renal function can exceed adult values and result in underdosage if not recognised. The implications of these changes are not always incorporated into therapy. For example, aminoglycoside dosages or dose intervals are adjusted to account for renal dysfunction based on plasma concentration monitoring results, but doses of concomitant penicillin or cefalosporin drugs (which are renally excreted

**Table III.** Plasma half-lives (mean or range in hours) of some antibacterial drugs in premature and term neonates and young infants (after McCracken;[17] Tognoni;[18] Paap & Nahata[19])

| Drug | Prematures (≤7 days) | Neonates (≤7 days) | Infants (7-14 days) | Infants (>14 days) | Adults |
|---|---|---|---|---|---|
| Ampicillin | ≈4-6 | 4 | 2.8 | 1.7 | 1-1.5 |
| Benzylpenicillin (penicillin G) | 3.8 | 2.6-4.9 | 1.7-2.6 | 1.4-3.8 | 0.7 |
| Carbenicillin | ≈5-6 | 3-5.7 | 2.1-3.6 | ≈1.5 | 1-1.5 |
| Gentamicin | 4.1-13.8 | 3.4-6.5 | 3-5.6 | 3-5 | 2-3 |
| Methicillin | 2.4-3.3 | 1.3-3.3 | 0.9-3.1 | 0.8-1.8 | 0.5 |
| Tobramycin | 5.6-11.3 | 4.6 | 3.9 | | 1-2 |

**Table IV.** Neonatal antibiotic dosage guidelines (after St Geme & Polin;[20] Paap & Bosso[21])

| Antibiotic (route) | Postnatal age | Bodyweight (g) | Dose (mg/kg) and interval |
|---|---|---|---|
| Amikacin/kanamycin | ≤1wk | <800 | 10 q36h |
| (IM or IV) | | 800-1500 | 10 q24h |
| | | 1500-2000 | 7.5 q18h |
| | | >2000 | 7.5 q12h |
| | >1 wk | Any weight | 7.5 q8-36h[a] |
| Ampicillin | <1wk | <2000 | 25 q12h |
| (PO, IM, IV) | | >2000 | 50 q12h |
| | >1wk | Any weight | 75 q6h |
| Benzylpenicillin (penicillin G) | | Any weight | 15 q12h |
| (IM, IV) | | | |
| Carbenicillin | | <2000 | 75 q8h |
| (IV) | | >2000 | 75 q6h |
| Cefazolin | | <2000 | 20 q12h |
| (IM/IV) | | >2000 | 20 q8-12h |
| Cefotaxime | <1wk | Any weight | 50 q12h |
| (IV) | >1wk | Any weight | 50 q8h |
| Chloramphenicol | <1wk | Any weight | 25 q24h |
| (PO, IM, IV) | >1wk | Any weight | 25 q12h |
| Clindamycin | | <2000 | 2.5-5 q8h |
| (PO, IM, IV) | | >2000 | 2.5-5 q6h |
| Gentamicin/tobramycin/netilmicin | ≤1wk | <800 | 3.5 q36h |
| (IM, IV) | | 800-1500 | 3.0 q24h |
| | | 1500-2000 | 2.5 q18h |
| | | >2000 | 2.5 q12h |
| | >1wk | Any weight | 2.5-3 q8-36h[a] |
| Oxacillin | | <2000 | 25 q12h |
| (PO, IM, IV) | | >2000 | 50 q12h |
| Piperacillin | | <2000 | 50 q8-12h |
| (IV) | | >2000 | 50 q6-8h |
| Polymixin B | | Any weight | 2 q12h |
| (IM, IV) | | | |
| Ticarcillin | | <2000 | 75 q8-12h |
| (IV) | | >2000 | 75 q6-8h |
| Vancomycin | ≤1wk | <800 | 20 q36h |
| (IV) | | 800-1500 | 20 q24h |
| | | 1500-2000 | 20 q18h |
| | | >2000 | 15 q12h |
| | >1wk | Any weight | 15-20 q8-36h[a] |

a See table V.

*Abbreviations:* IM = intramuscular; IV = intravenous; PO = oral.

but not monitored) are often left unchanged. This results in unnecessary dosages, expense and risk of toxicity (e.g. penicillin- or cefalosporin-induced seizures). Also, if doses of drugs which depend on renal excretion for activity (e.g. furosemide) are not increased, underdosage results.

In both physiological immaturity and renal failure in childhood, maintenance drug doses should be modified on the same basis as in adults (see chapter 24 and appendices D & E), i.e. by either maintaining the same amount of drug per dose but increasing the dose interval, maintaining the same dose interval and decreasing the amount of drug per dose, or a combination based on dosage practicalities. However, initial ('loading') doses may need to be increased because of distribution differences. Patients with cystic fibrosis exhibit a different pattern. It has been shown that penicillins, cefalosporins and aminoglycosides are renally cleared much more rapidly in children with cystic fibrosis than in healthy children (because of enhanced tubular secretion), and also have increased volumes of distribution. In the case of gentamicin, an increase in the volume of distribution has been observed in patients with cystic fibrosis when compared with controls (0.34 *vs* 0.24 L/kg), and plasma clearance was also increased (10.5 *vs* 5.7 L/h).[23] Some of these differences may be the result of changes in body composition. The underlying mechanisms, although not fully elu-

**Table V.** Antibacterial drug regimens for neonatal septicaemia and meningitis (modified from McCracken & Eichenwald;[22] St Geme & Polin;[20] Paap & Bosso[21]) [See text for dosage rationale]

| Clinical condition/cause | Initial therapy | Dose (mg/kg) and interval | | | | Duration (days)[a] |
|---|---|---|---|---|---|---|
| **1. Septicaemia** | | | | | | |
| a) Unknown cause[b] | Ampicillin[c] + aminoglycoside ± vancomycin | *Ampicillin* (IV): | *Amikacin/ kanamycin* (IM/IV): | *Gentamicin/ tobramycin/ netilmicin* (IM/IV): | *Vancomycin* (IV): | 3-14 |
| | i) *≤7 days postnatal age:* | | | | | |
| | <800g | 25 q12h | 10 q36h | 3.5 q36h | 20 q36h | |
| | 800-1500g | 25 q12h | 10 q24h | 3.0 q24h | 20 q24h | |
| | 1500-2000g | 25 q12h | 7.5 q18h | 2.5 q18h | 20 q18h | |
| | >2000g | 50 q12h | 7.5 q12h | 2.5 q12h | 15 q12h | |
| | ii) *>7 days postnatal age* (any weight): | | | | | |
| | <27 wks PCA | 75 q12h | 7.5 q36h | 3.0 q36h | 20 q36h | |
| | 27-30 wks PCA | 75 q12-24h | 7.5 q24h | 2.5 q24h | 20 q24h | |
| | 30-34 wks PCA | 75 q12-18h | 7.5 q18h | 2.5 q18h | 20 q18h | |
| | 34-38 wks PCA | 75 q12h | 7.5 q12h | 2.5 q12h | 15 q12h | |
| | >38 wks PCA | 75 q12h | 7.5 q8h | 2.5 q8h | 15 q8h | |
| | Cefotaxime or ceftazidime ± ampicillin | *Cefotaxime/ ceftazidime* (IV): | *Ampicillin:* as above | | | 3-14 |
| | i) *≤7 days postnatal age* (any weight) | 50 q12h | | | | |
| | ii) *>7 days postnatal age:* | | | | | |
| | <2000g | 50 q12h | | | | |
| | >2000g | 75 q8-12h | | | | |
| b) Group B streptococci | Benzylpenicillin (penicillin G)[c] ± aminoglycoside | *Benzylpenicillin* (IM/IV) [any postnatal age or weight]: 15-30 q12h | *Aminoglycosides as above* | | | 10-14 |
| c) *Escherichia coli, Klebsiella* spp., coliforms | Cefotaxime or ampicillin[c] + aminoglycoside | *Cefotaxime:* as above | *Ampicillin:* as above | *Aminoglycosides:* as above | | 14-21 |
| d) *Listeria monocytogenes, Proteus mirabilis, Streptococcus faecalis* | Ampicillin[d] ± aminoglycoside | *Ampicillin:* as above | *Aminoglycosides as above* | | | 14 |
| e) *Pseudomonas aeruginosa* | Ceftazidime + aminoglycoside | *Ceftazidime* (IV): | *Aminoglycosides:* as above | | | 14-21 |
| | i) *≤7 days postnatal age* (any weight) | 50 q12h | | | | |
| | ii) *>7 days postnatal age:* | | | | | |
| | <2000g | 50 q12h | | | | |
| | >2000g | 75 q12h | | | | |
| **2. Meningitis** | | | | | | |
| a) Unknown cause[b] [maternal- or community-acquired] | Ampicillin[c] + aminoglycoside[e] | *Ampicillin:* as above | *Aminoglycosides:* as above | | | 10-21 |
| | Ampicillin[c] + chloramphenicol | *Chloramphenicol* (IV/PO): | *Ampicillin:* as above | | | 10-21 |
| | i) *≤7 days postnatal age* | 25 q24h | | | | |
| | ii) *>7 days postnatal age* | 25 q12h | | | | |
| | Ampicillin[c] + cefotaxime | *Ampicillin:* as above | *Cefotaxime:* as above | | | 10-21 |
| | Benzylpenicillin[c] + aminoglycoside[e] | *Benzylpenicillin:* as above | *Aminoglycosides as above* | | | 10-21 |

**Table V.** *[Continued]*

| Clinical condition/cause | Initial therapy | Dose (mg/kg) and interval | | Duration (days)[a] |
|---|---|---|---|---|
| **Meningitis** *[continued]* | | | | |
| b) Nosocomial | Methicillin[c] + aminoglycoside[e] | *Methicillin* (IM/IV): | *Aminoglycosides:* as above | 10-21 |
| | i) *≤7 days postnatal age:* | | | |
| | <2000g | 25-50 q12h | | |
| | >2000g | 50 q8h | | |
| | ii) *>7 days postnatal age:* | | | |
| | <2000g | 50 q8h | | |
| | >2000g | 50 q6h | | |
| | Vancomycin + aminoglycoside[e] | *Vancomycin:* as above | *Aminoglycosides:* as above | 10-21 |
| | Vancomycin + cefotaxime | *Vancomycin:* as above | *Cefotaxime:* as above | 10-21 |
| c) *Bacteroides fragilis* | Metronidazole | 7.5 q12h (IV) | | |
| d) *Campylobacter fetus* | Chloramphenicol | As above (IV/PO) | | 14 |
| e) *Citrobacter freundii* or *Enterobacter* spp. | Cefotaxime + aminoglycoside[e] | *Cefotaxime:* as above | *Aminoglycosides:* as above | 14-21 |
| f) *Flavobacterium meningosepticum* | Vancomycin[e] | As above (IV) | | 14 |
| g) Group A streptococci | Benzylpenicillin[c] | As above (IV) | | 14 |
| h) Group D streptococci: | | | | |
| i] enterococcal | Ampicillin[c] + aminoglycoside[e] | *Ampicillin:* as above | *Aminoglycosides:* as above | 14 |
| ii] non-enterococcal | Benzylpenicillin[c] | As above (IV) | | 14 |
| i) *Haemophilus influenzae* | Ampicillin (if sensitive)[c] | As above (IV) | | 14 |
| j) *Staphylococcus epidermidis* or | Methicillin[c] | As above (IM) | | 10 |
| *Staphylococcus aureus* (methicillin-sensitive) | Nafcillin[c] | As for methicillin (see above) [IV] | | 14 |
| k) *Streptococcus pneumoniae* or *Treponema pallidum* | Benzylpenicillin[c] | As above (IV) | | 10 |
| l) *Pseudomonas* spp. | Carbenicillin[c] | | | 14-21 |
| | <2000g | 75 q8h (IV) | | |
| | >2000g | 75 q6h (IV) | | |

a Depending on culture results and clinical course.

b Once the organism is identified and susceptibilities are known, the most appropriate drug(s) and dosages should be used, added or substituted.

c A cefalosporin can be used in place of a penicillin in most penicillin-allergic patients, although rare patients will be allergic to both. If substituting a cefalosporin is considered unwise, chloramphenicol, vancomycin, or vancomycin + rifampicin are acceptable replacements.

d Cotrimoxazole (trimethoprim/sulfamethoxazole) can be used in penicillin-allergic patients.

e It is advisable to adjust doses based on measured blood concentrations (see further chapter 5).

f Vancomycin should be added if penicillin-resistant organisms likely.

**NB.** Dosages should be guided by serum drug concentrations for chloramphenicol, aminoglycosides and vancomycin. Clearances of aminoglycosides can be used to adjust dosages of penicillin (and its synthetic derivatives).

*Abbreviations:* IM = intramuscular; IV = intravenous; PO = oral; PCA = postconceptual age.

cidated, must be different for penicillins, since gentamicin is not actively secreted by the renal tubules. The clinical implication of these findings is that children with cystic fibrosis will frequently require higher initial and maintenance dosages and shorter dose intervals of antimicrobial drugs.

### 2.5 Metabolic Disturbances

Sensitivity to drugs in childhood may be affected by factors such as dehydration, fever and acidosis. Metabolic acidosis is quite common in sick children, especially the very young, and can alter drug penetration into cells. The tissue uptake of acidic drugs may be enhanced by acidosis whereas that of basic drugs is decreased. This is best demonstrated in salicylate poisoning where a decreased pH markedly affects the degree of ionisation of salicylate (pKa 3) which leads to enhanced salicylate penetration into the brain and other tissues. Control of acidosis by administration of alkali (sodium bicarbonate) is therefore a primary therapeutic goal in these children, as this leads to a reduction in salicylate concentrations in the brain and CSF and also enhances renal excretion of the drug. Acidosis has similar effects on phenobarbital distribution.

The state of hydration can also be of major importance, and severe dehydration is common in infancy. In diabetic acidosis, a larger dose of insulin is required if it is given to the child before rehydration. Fever readily occurs in older infants, especially in an underhydrated infant, and may also modify the response to some drugs. Underhydration may tend to increase the effect of many drugs with small volumes of distribution, such as nonsteroidal anti-inflammatory drugs (NSAIDs), aminoglycosides, antiepileptic agents, and theophylline, since most of these drugs are distributed into body fluid.

### 2.6 Genetically Determined Abnormal Drug Responses

Most studies of genetically determined abnormal responses to drugs have involved adults. However, such responses also occur in children. Indeed, some genetically determined abnormalities in drug response were first noted in children, e.g. glucose-6-phosphate dehydrogenase (G6PD) deficiency (see further chapter 26), and in some situations children seem to react more frequently than do adults, e.g. general anaesthesia and malignant hyperpyrexia (see further chapter 12; sect. 5.5). Patients with G6PD deficiency are extremely sensitive to a number of drugs. This is particularly important in the neonatal period, as the resulting haemolysis exacerbates already existing jaundice. Families with children known to have G6PD deficiency should be informed of the hazards of drugs that can precipitate episodes of haemolytic anaemia, and should be provided with a list of compounds that should be avoided (see chapter 26; sect. 5.2, table XVIII).

Many interindividual differences in pharmacokinetics and pharmacodynamics have been proven to be genetically determined. One area of special interest concerns the effect of genetic constitution on the development of drug-induced fetal abnormalities.[24] Pharmacogenetic differences explain – at least in part – why some, but not all, fetuses develop congenital abnormalities when exposed to a drug *in utero*. Importantly, recent work in this area has highlighted the risks of using the wrong animal models in this situation. For example, thalidomide, despite its devastating effect on the human fetus, has no teratogenic effect in the rat, but does have an effect in the monkey and rabbit (see also chapter 2; sect. 1.3.4). It is also possible that genetic susceptibility may be acquired, as is postulated for sulfonamide sensitivity in patients with human immunodeficiency virus (HIV) infection.

## 3. Problems with Drugs and Drug Therapy in Children

Because of growth and maturation, drug therapy needs to be considered somewhat differently in the various periods of childhood and adolescence.

### 3.1 Early Postnatal Period

As discussed in section 2, the early postnatal period is associated with the most significant and rapidly changing differences in drug handling as well as response. In addition to the general problems already discussed, there are particular problems associated with drug administration, dosage regimen selection, and exposure to maternal medication, either prenatally or via breast milk.

#### *3.1.1 Problems with Drug Administration*

Oral administration of drugs to neonates may result in aspiration or poor absorption (section 2.1.1), especially in the first few weeks of life. Intramuscular drug administration can be hazardous in infants as there is little muscle mass. The practice of using the buttocks as a site for intramuscular injections should be especially avoided because of the risk of damaging the sciatic nerve. The preferred site is the lateral aspect of the thigh, although gangrene of the foot has followed injection even in this area.

Intravenous drug administration is also not without hazard in the neonate, as problems of drug and fluid extravasation may lead to local tissue necrosis. In addition, intravenous drug administration is not as reliable as is often assumed. With the slow infusion rates used in neonates, the site of injection into the intravenous tubing can be particularly important. Much lower serum concentrations may be achieved with distal injections, as opposed to more proximal sites of administration, and there can be hours of delay in delivery of drug to the circulation (see table I).[6] This is especially critical for severely ill children, in whom such delay in drug delivery can be fatal (e.g. antibiotics for sepsis or vasopressor agents for shock). This fact has practical applications for hospital units which change tubing frequently, resulting in the discarding of a major portion of a daily dose. In transported neonates, this may result in the discarding of the critical first dose(s) and delay in giving the next (actually the first) dose. In our institution for example, in the past more than 25% of transported neonates had not received any antibiotics until the first dose given after arrival. This was because their first dose was administered into slow-running infusion lines, which were discarded on arrival.

### 3.1.2 Problems with Therapy, Dosage and Plasma Concentration Monitoring

As discussed in sections 2.4.1 and 2.4.2, hepatic and renal immaturity, particularly in the neonatal period, are important factors in determining drug dosage regimens. In older children, growth, formulations, behaviour, and certain diseases (e.g. cystic fibrosis) are more important. Plasma concentration monitoring (therapeutic drug monitoring) has a definite role to play in paediatric dosage selection, especially using the microimmunoassays available for the most commonly monitored drugs. Plasma concentration monitoring is discussed in detail in chapter 5. The main indications for its use in childhood include:

1) Use of drugs with saturable metabolism (e.g. phenytoin, theophylline and salicylates).

2) Use of drugs with narrow therapeutic indices and wide interindividual variations in clearance (e.g. digoxin).

3) Suspected noncompliance with drugs for which poor compliance (either under- or overdosage) can have major clinical consequences (e.g. cyclosporin).

4) Adjustment of drug doses for growth and development, especially for drugs for which this cannot be done simply on a bodyweight basis (e.g. antiepileptics or aminoglycosides).

5) Cases of therapeutic failure: either lack of effect or symptoms of toxicity.

6) Prevention of adverse drug reactions (e.g. with methotrexate).

7) Presence of major organ (renal, hepatic or cardiac) failure or dysfunction, altered organ blood flow or protein binding.

8) Drugs with variable absorption (e.g. cyclosporin).

Unique non-pharmacokinetic problems in therapeutic drug monitoring include interference from both maternal and endogenous substances [e.g. digitalis-like immunoreactive substance (DLIS) with digoxin], different 'therapeutic' ranges (e.g. adult asthma *vs* neonatal apnoea), and drug contamination of skin puncture samples.[25]

### 3.1.3 Maternal Drug Therapy

Administration of a drug to the mother exposes her infant to the effects of the drug (see further chapter 2). Drugs taken by the mother prior to or during delivery, including cigarettes and alcohol, can alter organ development, function and metabolism. Unfortunately, few objective data are available, partly because it is often difficult or impossible to assess maternal drug exposure. Even in many tertiary care centres, maternal medications are not recorded in a useful way. For example, recording only that the mother received '2% lidocaine' (lignocaine) for an episiotomy makes it impossible to calculate the dose given to the mother let alone to the child, yet local anaesthetics, even if not administered directly into the child accidentally, can produce seizures and cardiovascular instability, and many other maternal medications can affect neonates. Opioids given for pain control can result in significant neonatal respiratory depression. Liver enzyme-inducing drugs can alter the way drugs are handled by the neonate. Indomethacin or other NSAIDs given to the mother can alter renal function in the neonate.

Drugs administered to the mother can also confuse the results of plasma concentration monitoring. Aminoglycosides given to the mother for infection alter neonate drug concentration interpretations. Gentamicin concentrations in placental blood can be 40 to 70% of maternal concentrations or higher within 1 to 2 hours of maternal administration.[26,27] A complete discussion of this issue is beyond the scope of this chapter, but it is important that clinicians treating mothers and children realise that medication administered to the mother may affect the neonate or breast-feeding child.

#### 3.1.4 Drug Excretion in Breast Milk

Most drugs taken by a nursing mother are excreted to some extent in her milk. However, for most drugs, the amount ingested by the infant will be extremely small (only 1% or less of the maternal dose) and/or will not be harmful to the infant (see further appendix C). The decision to breast feed while taking a drug needs to be made carefully by weighing the benefits of breast feeding against the possible adverse effects in the infant. Unfortunately, individual decisions are rendered complex by a paucity of reliable information. Most of the literature on this subject consists of isolated case reports without adequate data on:

- Maternal drug dosage
- Maternal blood and concomitant breast milk concentrations
- Concentrations in the infant
- Complete dosage information and timing of the sampling in relation to administration and feeding
- Duration of maternal treatment
- Any observed adverse effects in the infant.

Fortunately, adverse clinical effects in the infant are rare, even for the few drugs (e.g. some antiepileptics) for which relatively large amounts of drug and/or its metabolites may be transferred to the infant and produce measurable concentrations in plasma. The presence of a drug in breast milk need not be a contraindication to breast feeding, except for toxic agents, drugs which suppress lactation (e.g. estrogens, thiazides or pyridoxine), or when infants have unique sensitivity (e.g. G6PD deficiency or allergy).

Breast feeding should be avoided with especially toxic drugs such as immunosuppressive, anticancer or radiolabelled drugs but, with these rare exceptions, it is generally appropriate to encourage all mothers to breast feed. However, infants should always be closely observed for any adverse effects, which, if they occur, should be reported [see further appendix C for data on the safety of drugs during breast feeding].

### 3.2 Second to Twelfth Months of Life

The physiological immaturity of the liver and kidneys lessens during this period and, after the first month of life, less detailed attention is needed to individualising drug dosages in all but the extremely premature infant. In children without organ dysfunction, drugs may be administered on a mg/kg or mg/m$^2$ basis without the need for issues of prematurity and gestational age to be taken into account.

### 3.3 The 'Toddler' and Early School Age Child

There are no particular pharmacokinetic problems in this age group, except that young children about 1 to 10 years of age generally eliminate (metabolise or excrete) drugs more rapidly than adults (see sections 2.4.1 and 2.4.2). This is particularly important for drugs that are metabolised by oxidation or hydroxylation such as phenobarbital, phenytoin and theophylline. It has been clinically appreciated for many years that children of this age require both larger daily doses of these drugs on a mg/kg bodyweight basis and more frequent administration than adults to achieve equivalent concentrations. Until about 10 to 12 years of age, children probably metabolise drugs more rapidly than adults, because they have larger liver volumes per kilogram of bodyweight. The main issues confronting clinicians who prescribe drugs for children in this age group include the following:

1) *Compliance:* the use of pleasant-tasting syrups and suspensions has made it easier to persuade children to take oral medication. However, these preparations can cause significant tooth decay from sucrose, or diarrhoea from sorbitol, in children who receive multiple courses of liquid medications containing sweeteners; and, unfortunately, not all useful medicines come in formulations that are easy to administer to children. Succimer (DMSA – an oral lead-chelating drug), for example, is available only in 100mg capsules which have an extremely unpleasant smell and taste. Effective dosage can be a formidable task, especially because efficacy was established using mg/m$^2$ dosages, yet package labelling contains a mg/kg

dosage table,[28] which if used, provides toddlers with 40 to 50% less drug than the mg/m$^2$ dose.

It is important, in the context of compliance, to realise that very few drugs need to be given more than 3 times daily, and some can be given once daily. Most parents will develop their own ways of getting their children to take medication; the need to monitor their success depends on the clinical situation. Recently, electronic monitoring devices have become commercially available to monitor how many times medication vials are opened (and soon will record how much is actually dispensed). Data from trials using these devices illustrate how difficult it is for patients to follow dosage regimens. Without such devices, clinicians cannot predict or detect noncompliant behaviour but can use data collected by these devices to alter compliance.[29,30]

2) *Normal childhood curiosity:* toddlers are in an exploratory phase of their lives and are naturally very inquisitive. For this reason, it is important that all medications and household products be safely stored in the home. At about the age of 6 years, a normal child understands the concept of cause and effect. Nonretarded children over the age of 6 who are poisoned should therefore be evaluated for underprotection and self-destructive behaviour.

3) *Recurrent infections:* young children, especially when they first go to school or preschool and are exposed to large numbers of other children, get what seems to be more than their share of coughs, colds, sore throats and ear infections. In fact, this is quite normal. It has been estimated that during the first 6 years of life, the average child can expect to have 17 minor colds, 7 severe colds, 3 ear infections, 6 other respiratory tract infections, 2 episodes of diarrhoea, and 2 skin infections. Most of these infections will be viral but this is difficult to prove clinically. Therefore, young children often receive recurrent courses of broad-spectrum antibiotics, the disadvantages of which are contentious.

4) *Growth:* the effects of normal growth mean that children receiving medication for chronic disorders such as epilepsy, asthma, etc. need their drug doses reviewed from time to time, with plasma concentration monitoring where appropriate.

### 3.4 Adolescence

Adolescence is associated with major changes in hormone secretion, growth and behaviour. Although the hormonal changes associated with puberty might be expected to produce alterations in drug disposition, there is little evidence that this constitutes a major problem for the prescriber. Problems that do occur involve the following:

1) *Growth:* major changes in bodyweight must be considered for long term medications, although the relative decrease in drug metabolism after childhood tends to compensate for greater size.

2) *Noncompliance:* adolescents may be very resistant to taking medication. While this may not be of much importance for acute self-limiting illnesses such as sore throats or tonsillitis, it can present difficulties in management of chronic disorders such as diabetes mellitus, asthma, epilepsy, juvenile rheumatoid arthritis and cystic fibrosis.

3) *Suicide attempts:* self-poisoning in this age group, unlike the inquisitive toddler, has a more sinister connotation. Suicidal gestures and attempts are common in adolescence. This is a further reason for medication in the home to be securely stored.

4) *Illicit drugs:* the use of such agents begins to appear in early adolescence. This possibility should always be borne in mind by the clinician.

5. *'Legal' drugs:* many potentially dangerous chemicals are readily available to adolescents. Steroid hormones (both anabolic and contraceptive) are widely abused. More than 50% of smokers begin smoking before adolescence. A large number of even very young children experiment with alcohol or organic solvents. Caffeine or caffeine/sympathomimetic combination dietary products are widely used. These substances can have a greater influence on prescription drug effects than most illicit drugs.

### 3.5 Poisoning in Children

Poisoning in childhood remains a common problem and can be divided into accidental, therapeutic, child abuse or neglect, and suicidal attempts. Accidental poisoning occurs often in toddlers but can also occur in older children, such as when substances are put in inappropriate containers (e.g. gasoline in soft drink/soda bottles) or medications are taken in the dark. Therapeutic poisonings, where excess medication is given by a clinician, nurse, pharmacist, parents, or other caregiver are not rare and can be lethal. Medication errors, especially 10-fold dosage errors, account for significant morbidity and mortality.[31] Child abuse or neglect includes cases where a caregiver deliberately gives excess drug or other toxic substance to a child,[32] or where poisoning occurs as the result of underprotection. Suicidal gestures or attempts can occur throughout childhood.

The nature of poisons taken by children varies temporally and geographically. Whereas salicylate poisoning was very common 20 years ago, this has now been largely replaced by overdosage with other drugs such as paracetamol and ibuprofen. In a study from Brisbane, Australia, the most commonly implicated substances causing hospital admission and death were petroleum distillates (13%), antihistamines (9%), benzodiazepines (9%), bleaches and detergents (7%), and aspirin (6%). Fatalities were most common with cardiotoxic drugs, followed by tricyclic antidepressants, sympathomimetic agents, caustic soda and aspirin. However, cases of accidental poisoning leading to death have decreased over the past decades in association with altered prescribing habits, safer packaging, the colouring of toxic substances (e.g. kerosene and antifreeze), the development of regional poison control centres, improved transport and supportive care, as well as the availability of specialists in medical toxicology and critical care.

The management of drug overdosage and poisoning is discussed in greater detail in chapter 8 (for reviews, see also Henry & Volans;[33] Prescott;[34] Olsen[35]). However, a number of general points concerning childhood poisoning warrant special consideration.

Children who have ingested, or are suspected of having ingested, a drug or poison should be considered for hospital admission. Often, caretaker anger and guilt interfere with family relations and make histories inaccurate. Admission for even 24 hours of observation can allay guilt, allow symptoms and signs to develop, permit discovery of underprotection, abuse or self-destructive behaviour, and provide a measure of safety.

With most drugs and poisons, absorption occurs rapidly. Gastric emptying is unlikely to be of value if undertaken more than 4 hours after the ingestion took place unless there is an intestinal concretion (i.e. bezoar) present, or gastric emptying has been delayed (e.g. by opioid analgesics, anticholinergic agents, CNS depressants, etc.).

Oral activated charcoal absorbs most toxins in the bowel, and for some agents will assist in drug elimination as well (see further chapter 8; sect. 6.2).

Toxicological analyses are indicated less often in children than in adults. They are most useful in cases of suspected poisoning due to salicylates, paracetamol, methanol, ethylene glycol, iron, xanthines, and heavy metals.

Poisoning should also be considered whenever there is an exaggerated or unexpected effect seen in a child receiving a therapeutic drug. Clinicians should examine actual prescription containers and compare them and their contents to what was prescribed. In the hospitalised child, all medications and syringes should be collected, and intravenous lines and tubing replaced and examined.

## 4. Drug Treatment in Infants and Children

### 4.1 General Principles

While many of the principles of good drug prescribing are the same in adults as in infants and children, some are qualitatively or quantitatively different. This review will discuss aspects of drug prescribing that require special consideration in infants and children (table VI).

#### *4.1.1 Is Drug Treatment Really Needed?*

Drug treatment is not always required. While some parents demand treatment, not all do. In fact, as many as 25% of prescriptions are never filled. There is growing interest in natural remedies (naturopathy) and non-medical treatments such as acupuncture, iridology, etc. This interest probably reflects the bad publicity received by a number of medications in the lay press and a general trend to get back to a more 'natural' lifestyle. This allows the clinician more chance of avoiding the common 'pressure to prescribe' but can also cause serious or lethal poisoning from home cures.

The decision to treat must be dictated by data (if available) or by common sense. Antibacterial drugs are overprescribed for viral sore throats and ear infections. A risk : benefit analysis may well favour prescribing, depending on the clinical situation. Otherwise-healthy children with a cough and a sore throat probably do not need anything but an examination, explanation and reassurance. However, a child with pus on the tonsils may be treated more inexpensively and effectively by giving penicillin than by doing a throat culture. And while antibiotics have been shown to have minimal effect on the course of

**Table VI.** Some principles of paediatric drug prescribing (after Buchanan;[36] Walson et al.[37])

**1. Is drug treatment needed?**

a) The decision to treat requires an accurate diagnosis and risk-benefit analysis.

b) Many acute childhood illnesses are self-limiting and need no treatment.

c) Well children with cough and a sore throat may not need anything but an examination, explanation and reassurance. However, a child with pus on the tonsils may be treated more inexpensively and effectively by giving penicillin than by doing a throat culture.

d) Although antibiotics have been shown to have minimal effect on the course of otitis media, the child with a bulging, red ear drum should sensibly still receive them.

e) In the case of fever, antipyretic drugs are not always necessary. While febrile convulsions are a matter for concern, fever *per se* is not a significant danger.

f) Avoid 'treating the caretaker'. Growing parental concern about the 'overuse' of drugs, especially antibacterial drugs, can be judiciously used to advantage to resist prescribing in a particular clinical situation.

g) When prescribing a drug for an acute illness, the reason for giving the drug should be explained. The parent who thinks that their child received an antibiotic for a 'cold' will be more likely to expect such treatment for the next illness than the parent who understands that it was the exudative pharyngitis or otitis, and not the cold, that prompted treatment.

h) Lack of paediatric trials and information about delayed effects create special problems.

**2. Choice of drug, formulation and brand**

a) Certain drugs should be avoided in children except in special circumstances (e.g. chloramphenicol and tetracyclines).

b) The most suitable preparation should be considered before prescribing. Ease of administration, available formulations, size, concentration, taste, excipients are all important in cost, acceptability and even safety considerations.

c) The dose, concentration, and excipients in preparations used must be considered to safely treat very small children.

**3. Dosage regimens**

a) In neonates, drugs that have been well studied, and have pharmacokinetically derived dosage schedules, are preferred.

b) It is important to individualise dosages as much as possible, especially for drugs with narrow therapeutic margins such as digoxin, theophylline, aminoglycosides and antiepileptic drugs.

c) The daily dose, loading doses, formulation, route, frequency and duration of therapy must all be considered.

d) Therapeutic drug monitoring, if correctly used, may be of value.

e) Proper prescribing, dispensing, communication and monitoring of response are important, often neglected aspects of treatment.

**4. Drug compliance**

a) Be realistic about what the patient or parents are being asked to do. Always consider noncompliance as a cause of unexpected results.

b) Keep the regimen as simple as possible. Whenever, possible prescribe once- or twice-daily doses.

c) The most important factor in enhancing compliance is a satisfactory relationship between the clinician and the patient (or parents). Provide a full explanation of the illness, aims and possible adverse effects of therapy.

d) Give responsibility for compliance to parents or older children, especially those with chronic disease.

e) Provide positive follow-up. Compliance decreases with time. Encouragement and explanation of the need for therapy given at each visit may help.

f) Give sensible instructions. Do not expect patients to do things you would not do yourself.

g) Consider the selected use of compliance aids and monitoring techniques.

**5. Duration of therapy**

a) Decisions must be dictated by available data or by common sense if data are unavailable.

b) For most illnesses, the duration of treatment depends on the nature of the illness (i.e. whether acute/self-limiting or chronic) and the drugs used.

otitis media, the child with a bulging, red ear drum should sensibly still receive them. Perhaps most importantly, when prescribing a drug for an acute illness, the reason for giving the drug should be explained. The parent who thinks that their child received an antibiotic for a 'cold' will be more likely to expect such treatment for the next illness than the parent who understands that it was the exudative pharyngitis or otitis, and not the cold, that prompted treatment.

#### *4.1.2 If Treatment Is Needed, Which Drug Is Appropriate?*

Wherever possible, drug selection should be based on pathophysiology. For example, the choice of an antibacterial agent should ideally be guided by a knowledge of the causative organism. In practice, this is often not possible. Treatment may need to be empirical, based on the likely causative agents and the fact that certain antibacterial drugs are less suitable for children.

Drug selection is also based on relative risk and clinical considerations. The risk of chloramphenicol toxicity is relatively high, especially in the neonatal period. In general, this drug should be used in children only in certain specific circumstances, including acute epiglottitis, *Haemophilus influenzae* meningitis, and typhoid fever, especially in some developing countries. Sulfonamides, including cotrimoxazole, should be avoided in neonates because of the possibility of kernicterus. Tetracyclines should not be used in childhood because of the risk of tooth staining and damage.

Drug selection can be quite complicated, even for minor conditions such as the choice of antipyretic for fever. The use of aspirin in young children is best avoided because of its possible, but still unproven, relationship to Reye's syndrome[38] and the availability of safer alternatives. Paracetamol (acetaminophen) is effective, has less gastrointestinal toxicity and fewer antiplatelet effects, and is available in liquid and rectal forms. Ibuprofen, while a longer-acting antipyretic (especially for higher temperatures)[39] and more effective analgesic, is more expensive and produces more mild toxicity than paracetamol when used therapeutically. It can also cause serious toxicity in children with renal diseases. However, ibuprofen appears to be much safer in accidental or intentional overdose than paracetamol.

Even topical medications require special consideration. Potent topical corticosteroids are unsuitable for routine use in neonates and young children because of the risk of significant systemic absorption, with consequent adrenal suppression and growth retardation.

#### *4.1.3 Which Preparation and Route of Administration?*

For paediatric patients, the choice of formulation can be more important than the choice of drug or brand. Lack of appropriate paediatric intravenous preparations is directly or indirectly responsible for a number of serious, occasionally fatal, medication errors.[31] Ease of administration, routes available, size, taste and the excipient ('inert' vehicle) can all be important considerations in the cost, acceptability and even safety of many non-parenteral formulations.

Clinicians should be aware of available formulations and their advantages and disadvantages, as well as local laws governing the ability of pharmacies to substitute one preparation for another. For example, I have treated a child who developed signs of toxicity when a rapidly absorbed preparation of theophylline was substituted for a sustained-release preparation by a pharmacy which was exempt from state substitution regulations. Similarly, children may have allergic reactions to an excipient present in one but not another preparation.

There are also non-allergic paediatric diseases which require special care in formulation selection. For example, patients with fructose intolerance can have lethal reactions to sorbitol-containing oral medications. A number of children have been poisoned by the use, usually inappropriate, of 2% viscous lidocaine (lignocaine) solution because of the mistaken perception that this low percentage equals a low dose, when in fact, this preparation contains 20 mg/ml lidocaine. Thus, a 10kg toddler who ingests 10ml of this medication ingests 200mg lidocaine (20 mg/kg), a dose which is likely to result in seizures from either the well-absorbed lidocaine or the metabolite formed by first-pass metabolism of the absorbed parent drug.[40]

Concentration and site-specific toxicity are also problems. When gentamicin 1% eye drops are used in the ear, this solution, which contains 1000 μg/ml of gentamicin, can be toxic to the middle ear if the tympanic membrane is not intact. Use of long-acting (depot) intramuscular penicillin injections (e.g. benzathine benzylpenicillin) can result in inadvertent intravascular injection, which is difficult to detect. Many clinicians are unaware that aspiration of these viscous preparations is unlikely to reveal blood in the syringe, even when the needle tip is in a vessel.[41]

Excipients are often considered unimportant, inactive components of medications, yet they can be responsible for a number of clinically significant allergic reactions.[42] These include anaphylaxis from gelatin or egg proteins in measles-mumps-rubella (MMR) vaccine, toxic effects such as potentially lethal benzyl alcohol-induced metabolic acidosis,[43] or mercury poisoning from thiomersal used as a preservative.[44]

Once a drug is selected, the clinician must decide on a dosage regimen – the dose, formulation, route of administration, frequency and duration of therapy. Paediatric drug administration is much more complicated than the 'one dose fits all' approach so common in adults. Dosage selection may be quite simple for a minority of drugs, but for the majority, the dosage must be calculated on the basis of bodyweight, surface area, developmental stage, metabolic rates, concomitant medication, and physiological function. All of these variables may be both more difficult to assess and quantitatively more important in children. Even something so apparently simple as bodyweight can be problematic in paediatric patients because of potentially major fluctuations in this variable (e.g. a 600g baby can be 720g a few days later, producing a major change in dosage requirements even if significant changes in metabolic and excretory functions are ignored). Accurate measurement of bodyweight is not trivial, especially in critically ill infants. Body surface area is superior to bodyweight for estimating the dosage of many drugs, but this also requires accurate bodyweight measurements if $(\text{bodyweight})^{0.67}$ is used to calculate surface area. This method of assessing surface area has been shown to be as good or better than nomograms based on height and bodyweight. Height measurements are even more difficult to obtain than bodyweight alone.

The rapidly changing size, bodyweight and physiological function present in children who are growing and recovering from illness make it necessary to adjust drug dosages constantly, even during the same hospitalisation. This is seldom necessary in older children or adults.

Specific paediatric concerns such as slow intravenous infusion rates, low muscle mass, skin absorption, lack of anal sphincter control, rapid gastrointestinal transit and poor compliance with administration necessitate familiarity with multiple routes of administration. For example, for drugs administered into an intravenous line running at 3 ml/h, it can take 6 to 8 hours before a detectable concentration begins to appear in the plasma,[6] a potentially lethal delay in certain critically ill patients (table I). If a life-saving drug is administered into a slowly running intravenous line, this delay in reaching the infant can cause significant problems. In our institution, we have found that discarding intravenous lines in transported infants can result in many infants not receiving aminoglycosides until their ‘2nd’ intravenous dose: their first dose was in the discarded transport intravenous tubing.

Rectal suppositories cannot be reliably absorbed unless they are retained, a difficult requirement in children. Additionally, not all suppositories contain evenly dispersed drug, making the practice of giving portions of a dose problematic. Rapid gastrointestinal transit present in most children makes absorption of slowly absorbed orally administered drugs or dosage forms unreliable (e.g. sustained-release preparations formulated to release drug over 12 to 24 hours cannot be expected to deliver their dose reliably if they are passed from the body in 2 to 4 hours).

Whenever possible, the oral route should be used, although in the critically ill child or the child with vomiting or significant diarrhoea, it may be more appropriate to administer the medication parenterally. Rectal drug administration is rarely indicated but can be useful, as in the case of diazepam for convulsions, glycerin for constipation, or paracetamol for fever with vomiting. For oral administration, liquid preparations are the most suitable for children under 5 years of age. Capsules that can be emptied and disguised in jam or honey are also used. Tablets are often difficult to break and then crush. The decision as to which oral preparation to use is based on a number of factors that include bioavailability, palatability, convenience, availability of various dosage forms, cost, stability and toxicity. Drug concentrations in many preparations make accurate dosage of small children impossible. For example, consider the volume needed to treat a 1kg baby when aminophylline (25 mg/ml) or morphine (50 mg/ml) solutions are used. Serious toxicity can occur if concentrated preparations such as these are not diluted before use. There are also problems when only fixed-dose preparations designed for use in adults are available and must be reformulated for use in children.[45] Unfortunately, there are scant data available on the methods or efficacy of such reformulation practices.

The inhaler is an important method of drug delivery in the management of respiratory diseases. However, this is an excellent example of the problems caused by using adult drug delivery methods in children. Young children may not be able to use standard inhalers efficiently. Such children may benefit from the use of a nebuliser, where the medication is made available in fine spray form without requiring the child’s active participation. Spacers, which are easier for the young child to use, have also been introduced.

#### *4.1.4 Estimation of Drug Dosage*

Many formulae have been used to derive total daily drug dosage in children, but none is of any particular value or use in deciding the dosage interval. In practical terms, most drugs commonly prescribed for children have a wide therapeutic margin, and thus an accurately in-

**Table VII.** Usually recommended doses for older infants and children of some commonly used drugs (normal renal and hepatic function)

| Drug | Dosage[a] | Notes[b] |
|---|---|---|
| **Analgesics/antipyretics** | | |
| Aspirin | 10 mg/kg/day (q4-8h) PO | Antipyretic/analgesic dose (avoid in young children) |
| | 90-120 mg/kg/day PO (divided q4-8h) | Anti-inflammatory dose |
| | | Avoid use under the age of 1 year |
| Paracetamol (acetaminophen) | 60 mg/kg/day PO (divided q4-6h) | Paracetamol has a wide therapeutic margin and is relatively safe in children (*NB.* accidental overdosage may cause hepatic or renal damage) |
| **Strong (opioid) analgesics** | | |
| Morphine | 0.1-0.2 mg/kg/dose SC (q3-4h)<br>0.05-0.1 mg/kg/dose IV or IM (q3-6h)<br>0.01-0.04 mg/kg/hr by IV infusion | Opioid doses depend on the stimulus, other drugs, and previous exposure to opioids |
| Pethidine (meperidine) | 1.0-2.0 mg/kg/dose PO or IM (q3-4h)<br>0.1-0.5 mg/kg/dose IV (q1-3h) | Avoid continuous use (especially in patients with renal dysfunction or seizure disorders) and avoid in patients receiving drugs with MAO inhibitory activity |
| **Anthelmintics** | | |
| Mebendazole | 100mg (1-2 doses)/day PO | Pinworms x 1 day, others x 3 days. May repeat after 2-3 weeks |
| Pyrantel pamoate | 11 mg/kg (single dose) PO (up to 1g maximum) | Threadworm, roundworm; repeat after 2-3 weeks. Give 3 daily doses for hookworm |
| Thiabendazole | 25-75 mg/kg/day PO divided q8-12h (up to 3g/day maximum) | 2-day course for threadworm, roundworm and intestinal Strongyloides; 5-day course for disseminated Strongyloides or visceral larva migrans; 3-day course for drancunculiasis or angiostrongyliasis |
| **Antibacterial agents** (see also table IV for important neonatal doses. In general, oral doses should be given for mild to moderate infections and parenteral doses for moderate to severe infections) | | |
| Amikacin | 15-30 mg/kg/day (q8-12h) IM/IV | Monitor serum concentrations, especially in renal failure |
| Amoxicillin | 20-50 mg/kg/day (q6-8h) PO/IM/IV | Better absorbed orally than ampicillin; modify dose in renal failure to avoid seizures |
| Ampicillin | 50-300 mg/kg/day (q6-8h) PO/IM/IV | High doses can cause seizures, especially in renal failure |
| Azithromycin[c] | 10 mg/kg PO on day 1, then 5 mg/kg PO days 2-5 | |
| Benzylpenicillin (penicillin G) | 25,000-90,000 U/kg/day [15-54 mg/kg/day] | High-dose penicillin can cause seizures, especially in renal failure |
| Carbenicillin | 30-50 mg/kg/day (q6h) IV | Modify dose in renal failure |
| Cefadroxil | 30 mg/kg/day (as 2 PO doses) | Modify dose in renal failure |
| Cefalexin | 25-100 mg/kg/day (q6-8h) PO | Modify dose in renal failure |
| Cefalothin | 75-150 mg/kg/day (q4-6h) IM/IV | Modify dose in renal failure |
| Cefamandole | 50-150 mg/kg/day (q4-8h) IM/IV | Modify dose in renal failure |
| Cefazolin | 50-150 mg/kg/day (q6-8h) IM/IV | Modify dose in renal failure |
| Cefixime | 8 mg/kg/day (as 1 or 2 PO doses) | Modify dose in renal failure |
| Cefotaxime | 100-200 mg/kg/day (q4-6h) IM/IV | Modify dose in renal failure |
| Cefoxitin | 80-160 mg/kg/day (q4-6h) | Modify dose in renal failure |
| Cefradine | 25-100 mg/kg/day (q6-12h) PO/IM | Modify dose in renal failure |
| Cefuroxime | 30-150 mg/kg/day (q8-24h) | Modify dose in renal failure |
| Chloramphenicol | *1 month-1 year:* 50 mg/kg/day (q8-12h) PO/IM/IV<br>*>1 year:* 50-100 mg/kg/day (q8-12h) PO/IM/IV | Should only be used to treat *Haemophilus influenzae* meningitis, acute epiglottitis, typhoid fever, or organisms resistant to other less toxic antibiotics. Monitor predose serum concentrations |
| Clarithromycin | 15 mg/kg/day (as 2 PO doses) | Decreases hepatic metabolism of some other drugs |
| Cloxacillin | 50-200 mg/kg/day (q8h) PO/IM/IV | Modify dose in renal failure |
| Cotrimoxazole (trimethoprim/sulfamethoxazole) | 2-20 mg/kg/day of trimethoprim (approx 5ml suspension per 18-22 lbs) in 2-4 divided doses PO.<br>Use lower doses for children <6mo | Suspension contains 40mg trimethoprim + 200mg sulfamethoxazole/5ml<br>Much higher doses for *Pneumocystis carinii* infection (trimethoprim 150mg + sulfamethoxazole 750mg per $m^2$/day given 3 times per week) |
| Erythromycin | 20-50 mg/kg/day (q6-12h) IM/IV | Avoid use with theophylline, terfenadine, astemizole, cisapride and carbamazepine (metabolism inhibited by erythromycin) |
| Gentamicin | 2-7.5 mg/kg/day (q8-24h) IM/IV | Monitor serum concentrations, especially in renal failure |
| Methicillin | 100-200 mg/kg/day (q6h) IM | Modify dose in renal failure |

**Table VII.** *[Continued]*

| Drug | Dosage[a] | Notes[b] |
|---|---|---|
| Phenoxymethylpenicillin (penicillin V) | 12.5-50 mg/kg/day (q4-8h) PO | Modify dose in renal failure |
| Ticarcillin | 150-300 mg/kg/day (q4-6h) IV/IM | Modify dose in renal failure |
| Tobramycin | 2-7.5 mg/kg/day (q8-24h) IM/IV | Monitor serum concentrations, especially in renal failure |
| **Antidepressants/antipsychotics** | | |
| Chlorpromazine | 1-4 mg/kg/day (q8-24h) IV/IM/PO | Also used as an antiemetic (see notes below under this heading) |
| Haloperidol | 0.025-0.15 mg/kg/day (q12h) PO | Can be given once per month IM once stabilised. May cause extrapyramidal symptoms |
| Imipramine | *Enuresis:* 6 years and older, initially 10-25mg PO at bedtime. If necessary, increase to 50mg in children <12 years, or to 75mg in children >12 years | Gradually taper dose when discontinuing. Monitoring of serum concentrations may be useful. Active metabolite (desipramine) present |
| **Antidiarrhoeal agents** (NB. seldom recommended) | | |
| Loperamide | *>8 years:* 2mg, repeated as needed up to a maximum of 8 mg/day (q6-8h) PO | Oral rehydration preferred. Avoid use in bacterial diarrhoea |
| **Antiemetics** (NB. antiemetics should not be used in the management of vomiting associated with gastroenteritis) | | |
| Ondansetron | *4 to 12 years:* 4 mg tid PO; *or* 0.15 mg/kg/dose IV for 1 to 3 doses (q4h) | For chemotherapy-induced vomiting, give 30 minutes before and 4 and 8 hours after chemotherapy |
| Prochlorperazine | *>2 years:* 0.1-0.2 mg/kg/day q8-24h PO or IM | Avoid in children weighing less than 10kg. Extrapyramidal symptoms common, especially with overdosage |
| Promethazine | 1-2 mg/kg/day (q8h) PO/IM/IV | Extrapyramidal symptoms common, especially with overdosage |
| **Antifungal agents** | | |
| Amphotericin B | *Test dose:* 0.1 mg/kg IV over 6 hours. Increase to 0.25 mg/kg/day initially, and as tolerance allows, to 1 mg/kg/day | Test dose recommended (0.1 mg/kg) Used for life-threatening infections. Total daily dose must not exceed 1.5 mg/kg |
| Griseofulvin | 10-20 mg/kg/day (q8h) PO [microsize] | Administer with fatty food. Dose of ultramicrosize form is about one-half of microsize dose |
| Ketoconazole | *>2 years:* 5-10 mg/kg/day (as 1 or 2 PO doses) | Clinically significant inhibition of hepatic metabolism of other drugs (e.g. terfenadine, theophylline, carbamazepine). Monitor hepatic function. Absorption decreased at high pH (avoid giving with antacids) |
| Miconazole | 20-40 mg/kg/day IV (q8h) | Infuse slowly (over 30 to 60 minutes) |
| Nystatin | 0.4-2.4 MU/day (q8h) PO | Retain oral suspension in mouth as long as possible |
| **Antihistamines** | | |
| Astemizole | *<6 years:* 0.2 mg/kg/day PO<br>*6-12 years:* 5 mg/day PO<br>*>12 years:* 10 mg/day PO | Give single daily dose on an empty stomach |
| Chlorpheniramine | 0.35 mg/kg/day (q6-12h) PO | Give with food or milk |
| Clemastine | *>6 years:* 0.67-4.02 mg/day | Give with food or milk |
| Cyproheptadine | *2 to 6 years:* 2mg bid/tid PO<br>*>6 to 14 years:* 4mg bid/tid PO<br>*>14 years:* 4mg tid PO or 0.25 mg/kg/day (up to 32 mg/day) | Commonly causes anticholinergic adverse effects |
| Diphenhydramine | 1.25 mg/kg (q4-6h) PO, IM or IV | Give higher doses (1-2 mg/kg IV) for anaphylaxis |
| Terfenadine | *3-6 years:* 15mg q12h PO<br>*7-12 years:* 20mg q12h PO<br>*>12 years:* 60 mg q12h PO | Avoid in patients receiving erythromycin, clarithromycin or ketoconazole |
| **Antituberculosis drugs** | | |
| Isoniazid | *Active disease:* 10-40 mg/kg/day (q24h) PO<br>*Prophylaxis:* 10 mg/kg/day (q24h) PO | Potentially hepatotoxic. Pyridoxine supplements recommended for breast fed babies and malnourished children |
| Rifampicin (rifampin) | 10-20 mg/kg/day (q12-24h) PO | Induces hepatic metabolism of many other drugs (see appendix B). Potentially hepatotoxic when used with other antituberculosis drugs. Colours urine, faeces, saliva, tears, etc. red-orange |
| Streptomycin | 20-40 mg/kg/day (q24h) IM | Use with caution in impaired renal function. Baseline audiological evaluation may assist in toxicity assessment |

**Table VII.** *[Continued]*

| Drug | Dosage[a] | Notes[b] |
|---|---|---|
| **Antitussives** | | |
| Dextromethorphan | 1 mg/kg/day (q8h) PO | Avoid in patients receiving drugs with MAO inhibitory activity |
| **Cardiac glycosides** | | |
| Digoxin | *Digitalising dose:* 1mo-2y, 35-60 μg/kg<br>2-5 years, 30-40 μg/kg<br>5-10 years, 20-35 μg/kg<br>>10 years, 10-15 μg/kg<br>Divide initial digitalising dose into 3 administrations (q8h)<br>*Maintenance dose:* 1/5 to 1/3 of the oral digitalising dose/day | Begin maintenance dose 24 hours after digitalising dose. Monitoring of serum concentrations may be useful to guide dosage, especially in patients with renal dysfunction, but presence of digitalis-like immunoreactive substance (DLIS) may give rise to spuriously high concentrations. Predose concentrations are most useful to monitor |
| **Central stimulants** | | |
| Methylphenidate | 5mg morning and noon in attention deficit disorder. If necessary, increase by 5-10 mg/week to maximum 60 mg/day or 2 mg/kg/day | Avoid in children under 4 years of age; monitor blood pressure and bodyweight.<br>Can precipitate Tourette's syndrome or sleep disturbance |
| **Corticosteroids** | | |
| Hydrocortisone | *Status asthmaticus:* 4-10 mg/kg/day (q3-6h) IV | |
| Prednisone/prednisolone | 0.5-2 mg/kg/day (q12h) PO initially, with incremental reductions relative to progress | Giving entire dose in the morning, or perhaps on alternate days, may lessen adrenal suppression |
| **Haematinics** | | |
| Iron (elemental) | *Prophylaxis:* 1-2 mg/kg/day (q24h) PO<br>*Treatment:* 6 mg/kg/day (q24h) PO | Dilute before administration and give 1 hour before or 2 hours after a meal |
| **Hypnosedatives** | | |
| Chloral hydrate | 25-50 mg/kg/dose PO<br>(100 mg/kg/day maximum) | Not recommended for long term use |
| Diazepam | 0.1-0.8 mg/kg/day (q8h) PO, IV or rectally | Both oral and rectal routes produce higher serum concentrations than IM administration (which is not recommended) |
| **Laxatives** | | |
| Bisacodyl | 0.3 mg/kg/day PO or rectally | Tablets should be swallowed whole and not chewed or crushed. Do not give within 1 hour of antacids or milk |
| Senna | *Powder:* sennosides 0.46-0.92 mg/kg/day PO | Long term use may result in dependence. Ensure good fluid intake |
| **Vitamins** | | |
| Vitamin $D_2$ (ergocalciferol) | *Prophylaxis:* 400-1000 IU/day<br>*Treatment:* 2000-4000 IU/day | Monitor serum calcium |
| Vitamin $K_1$ (phytomenadione) | *Haemorrhagic disease of the newborn:*<br>*Prophylaxis:* 1mg IM/IV<br>*Treatment:* 5-10mg IM/IV/SC/PO<br>*Other prothrombin deficiencies:*<br>Older children: 5-10mg IV/IM | Overdosage may cause kernicterus in premature infants. Monitor prothrombin time. Rapid IV injection can cause hypotension or anaphylaxis; other routes preferred. Oral absorption requires bile salts |

a Doses listed are average doses and are approximate. Variability of response may require alteration of dosage (see section 2).

b See also relevant discussion in this and other chapters.

c Not yet FDA approved for use in children in the US.

*Abbreviations:* IM = intramuscular; IV = intravenous; PO = oral; SC = subcutaneous; MAO = monoamine oxidase; tid = 3 times daily; bid = twice daily.

dividualised dosage regimen may not always be very important. In a child with tonsillitis, it probably does not matter greatly if phenoxymethylpenicillin (penicillin V) is given as 250mg 3 times daily, 250mg every 8 hours, or 500mg twice daily; a suitable therapeutic response is likely. However, for children with complex or chronic disorders treated at a tertiary referral level, drugs with a narrow therapeutic margin are often used and more specific dosage information is required. Such information is obtained from pharmacokinetic studies which allow the determination of dosage and dosage interval relative to age, bodyweight, maturity and so on. Most studies of this type relate dosage to bodyweight, a convenient variable which is almost always measured when children visit a doctor.

As has been mentioned, there are some advantages to dosages based on body surface area, but this requires first the calculation of surface area. Except for drugs for which efficacy data are based on surface area (e.g. cytotoxics and antivirals), dosage can be based on bodyweight alone (see table VII for examples of typical dosage recommendations for some commonly used drugs). However, not all hospitalised children have accurate bodyweights taken, and others (especially those in intensive care and premature neonates) have rapid, large bodyweight changes during a single illness.

#### 4.1.5 Dose Frequency

The frequency of administration is an important part of a dosage regimen and can have a major effect on compliance. Cost and other variables, such as fraction absorbed, peak to trough variation in plasma drug concentrations, gastrointestinal intolerance, and compliance, are all critical to efficacy. This aspect of drug administration often does not get the attention it deserves. Knowledge of pharmacokinetics and pharmaceutics is required to decide on the optimal dose frequency.

As a first step, clinicians need to be aware of the potentially major differences in response to administration every 6 hours *vs* 4 times daily,[46] especially for rapidly absorbed and rapidly cleared drugs (e.g. rapidly absorbed theophylline preparations). They also need to be aware that a more rapid elimination rate in younger children often equates with the need for more frequent, as well as higher, daily dosages of many drugs in this population (e.g. phenytoin 10 to 15 mg/kg/day given in 3 or 4 evenly divided doses may be required in a 6-year-old, whereas adolescents and adults seldom tolerate dosages >5 mg/kg/day given once daily or, at most, in 2 equally divided doses).[47] This is different again in infants, who often require rather large loading doses followed by infrequent and small maintenance doses. For example, a premature infant may need 20 to 30 mg/kg phenobarbital followed by a maintenance dosage of 3 to 4 mg/kg/day which need not be given twice or more often daily, as it often is.[48]

#### 4.1.6 Duration of Treatment

The duration of treatment is dictated by the nature of the illness. In the community at large, most children have recurrent episodes of acute, self-limiting illnesses. On the other hand, children attending hospitals or paediatric clinics on a regular basis may well have a much higher proportion of chronic disorders. Thus, general practice clinicians will be mainly involved in short term therapy, while tertiary referral paediatricians will be more involved in long term therapy.

For certain conditions (e.g. epilepsy, diabetes and cystic fibrosis), therapy will be prolonged and may be life-long. For other diseases such as tuberculosis, a defined course of therapy may be prescribed for 6, 9 or 12 months, depending on the regimen being used. In most illnesses, however, the duration of therapy depends on the drugs and nature of the illness and is largely empirical.

New, longer-acting medications have been shown to be effective when used for shorter periods than older drugs (e.g. azithromycin for 5 days rather than penicillin for 10 days for streptococcal pharyngitis), but shorter term use of older drugs may also be effective. For example, there is little difference in outcome between short and long term antibiotics (or indeed no antibiotics) for the treatment of otitis media, and even single-dose therapy of sexually transmitted diseases and urinary tract infections may be as effective as weeks of therapy. Obviously, much remains to be learned about the optimum duration of therapy.

#### 4.1.7 Economic Considerations

The cost of prescribing is a special problem in children, not only because many young families have limited funds, limited insurance coverage or both, but because there are ways the clinician can keep down the cost of treatment.

Use of older, less expensive drugs (e.g. amoxicillin for non-drug-resistant otitis media), generic prescribing, and use of commercially available packs rather than ones that require repackaging are all examples of cost-conscious prescribing, each of which can be considered in the appropriate clinical situation. Unfortunately, there are situations when each is not cost effective. Clinicians should establish a relationship with an unbiased source of pharmaceutical information and knowledge (written, electronic or human) in order to practice cost-effective prescribing. It is hoped, but not yet proven, that such action will decrease both the unnecessary cost of care and the large percentage of prescriptions that are never filled; this was estimated to be as high as 23% in a study of patients leaving an emergency department.[49]

#### *4.1.8 Prescription Writing*

The writing of a prescription can be considered the first step in drug administration. While good prescription writing practices are also needed for adults, the adverse effects of bad practices are more dangerous in children. For example, illegibility of prescriptions can prove fatal to children and adults alike, especially with drugs that have similar names or look alike, and must be avoided.[50] Furthermore, it is seldom critical for an adult's bodyweight to be included on a prescription, yet this omission can have devastating consequences for a neonate or small child. Other examples of poor prescription writing which are especially important in children include:

- Leaving off important instructions (e.g. an oral antibiotic prescribed for otitis media can be instilled in the ear canal)
- Using potentially confusing abbreviations (e.g. 'qd' which may be mistaken for 'qid' or 'AZT' being used for azathioprine, aztreonam or zidovudine (azidothymidine)[46]
- Not indicating the duration of use (e.g. repeated doses of colchicine).

These can all be dangerous.

Ten-fold dosage errors are an especially important paediatric problem. This can be the result of calculation errors, misplaced decimal point errors, or unit confusion. Such errors result in a disproportionate percentage of serious medication errors in children; almost all are preventable.[31]

#### *4.1.9 Dispensing and Medication Errors*

Once a drug is prescribed, it still must be obtained and given correctly. It is important to realise that, while uncommon, it is possible for a patient to get the wrong drug, dose or formulation from the pharmacy or the caregiver. It is even possible for the manufacturer to provide mislabelled or mispackaged drug. Whenever possible, patients should be made aware of what to expect (e.g. tablets or caplets, colour, consistency, etc.) so that they will have a greater chance of detecting dispensing errors.

It is also important for the prescriber to make clear when treatment should be started, and whether it is safe to wait to fill the prescription. Other items in the discussion should include whether a loading dose should be used, specific cautions (e.g. whether to take with meals), whether there is a major therapeutic difference between 4 times a day and every 6 hours, as well as advice as to the best way to increase compliance.

Special care is necessary when multiple prescriptions are given because the chance of confusion is increased. Some errors are minor, such as mistakenly using an antibiotic 3 times daily and a decongestant 4 times daily, rather than *vice versa*. However, others can be potentially lethal such as taking lindane lotion orally for scabies, and applying the similar-looking and coprescribed diphenhydramine syrup topically[51] – a totally preventable error since lindane has been replaced by equally efficacious, less toxic alternatives. Medication errors can also occur as a result of the difficulty in accurately measuring paediatric doses, or the use of inaccurate or incorrect measuring devices. Household teaspoons, for example, can contain between 2.5 and 7.5ml. They can also be confused with tablespoons, especially when abbreviations are used on prescriptions. Use of measuring devices such as oral syringes or cups can eliminate some errors, but create their own problems. There are examples of parents who have mistakenly thought that they should fill the cup for every dose or were unable to read or understand cup markings.[52]

Accurate measurement can be especially problematic with highly concentrated solutions and commercially available administration devices. Two drugs that have caused lethal overdosage are intravenous morphine and digoxin because both drugs are available as highly concentrated solutions.[31] Doses for neonates require the use of very small (i.e. <0.1ml) volumes if commercially available solutions are used without dilution. This can be lethal if done improperly. For example, if a 1ml syringe is used, the syringe may have as much as 0.2 to 0.3ml of 'dead space'. If the syringe is 'rinsed out' with intravenous fluid after a 0.1ml dose, the patient can receive up to a 2- to 3-fold overdose.[40]

#### *4.1.10 Medication Compliance and Patient/Parent Education*

The failure of patients to take medication as prescribed is well known. While most of the literature pertains to adults, there is a growing awareness of this problem among children and adolescents as well.

Noncompliance may take a number of forms: not filling the prescription, omission of doses, excessive dosages, taking medication at incorrect times, poor clinic attendance, and discontinuation of therapy prematurely. For example, noncompliance, especially with duration of therapy, occurs in 25 to 75% of children receiving oral penicillin for an acute illness. In patients with a chronic illness, whether adults or children, it is known that compliance decreases the longer the duration of therapy. Studies of children receiving medication for asthma, juvenile rheumatoid arthritis, diabetes, epilepsy, hyperactivity, organ rejection after renal transplantation, or cancer have all shown noncompliance to be a reality. Adolescents are generally recognised as showing poorer compliance than younger children, largely because only the latter receive medication under parental supervision.

It is appropriate to ask whether it really matters if patients are noncompliant. Patients may have the right to decide whether to take medication. However, failure to take medication does have both economic and therapeutic implications which extend beyond the noncompliance of the patient. Where a treatment is unsuccessful because of unrecognised noncompliance, the patient, apart from suffering poor health, may be subjected to unnecessary diagnostic tests, the administration of alternative and often inappropriate medications and, at times, repeated admissions to hospital. Early discontinuation of antibacterial therapy may lead to the emergence of resistant bacterial strains, while with some drugs, cessation of therapy may have life-threatening consequences. In addition, the accumulation of unused medications in a household may increase the risk of poisoning. However, since overprescribing is depressingly common, some noncompliance could well be advantageous. Many adult admissions to hospital result from adverse drug reactions, and 10 to 20% of patients experience an adverse drug reaction while in hospital.

Efforts to encourage compliance may be best directed at patients in whom noncompliance is mostly likely to have a deleterious effect. Patients taking drugs such as theophylline or phenytoin, which have a narrow therapeutic margin, deserve special consideration. In these patients, noncompliance may lead to an increase in dosage, which, if compliance suddenly improves, may result in intoxication.

#### Factors Leading to Noncompliance

Extensive efforts have been made to identify the most important factors in determining which patients will be compliant, but noncompliance remains unpredictable. A number of the factors that can affect compliance include the medication, dosage regimen, illness being treated, patient, caretaker, prescriber, treatment environment and monitoring. Adverse drug effects are often cited as a cause of noncompliance, but are in fact not a very common occurrence, especially in children. The medication itself is of special importance in paediatric practice, where appearance and taste are more likely to alter compliance. This is one reason sweetened liquid preparations are used for most children.

The frequency and complexity of the therapeutic regimen influences compliance in both adults and children. A clear correlation between the number of doses per day and compliance has been demonstrated; drugs administered once or twice a day had about 75% compliance, whereas those administered four times a day were associated with only 25% compliance. However, there is little to be gained from once- *vs* twice-daily administration[53] and there are risks associated with less frequent administration[54] such as the exaggerated effects of a missed dose. The choice of frequency of administration is a complex clinical decision based on the patient, disease, drug pharmacokinetics and formulations available. Many children are poor compliers if a dose needs to be taken at school, as are adolescents or adults at work. Whenever possible, therefore, dosage regimens should be tailored to the routine of the patient and his or her family. Meal times are the most obvious times to take medication (see section 2.1.1). Where possible, equal doses given at convenient times are preferred. Confusing dosage schedules should be avoided.

#### Measures to Improve Compliance

While little can be done to alter the nature of the illness, a great deal can be done to improve the patient's and parents' understanding of the illness and the need to take medication. Where the patient or the parents perceive the illness to be serious, compliance is likely to be better. Symptom-free periods are likely to be associated with lapses in compliance, no matter how serious the disease. Noncompliance is one of the leading problems in transplant rejection. It is not known whether this is the result of denial, misunderstanding or psychopathology.

The patient and caretaker, as well as their relationship, are other important determinants of compliance which must be considered and if possible altered by the prescriber.

The prescriber probably has the greatest influence in ensuring compliance. The clinician's ability to have the child and caretaker trust and like him/her, to be comfortable and friendly, to relate in a strong positive fashion, and other aspects of the prescriber and patient/parent interaction are important determinants of compliance. The doctor who is interested in the child and the family, who spends time discussing the illness and the medication, and who is welcoming and remains interested at follow-up consultations may be more likely to have compliant patients. Also, clinicians who encourage patients and parents to ask questions and not be reluctant to admit incomplete compliance will be less likely to be surprised.

The treatment environment influences compliance. If a patient waits several hours in a hospital outpatient clinic, is seen by the doctor perhaps briefly, and then waits another hour for medication at the pharmacy, it can be imagined that their enthusiasm for the medication, let alone the entire healthcare system, may be less than is desirable. Use of facilities which have efficient and experienced personnel and are reasonably priced is preferred.

Follow-ups and monitoring can improve compliance. Plasma concentration monitoring can be useful to identify noncompliance as can the use of electronic or even paper and pencil medication event recording systems. What the clinician must not do is assume that noncompliant patients can be easily identified. Numerous studies have demonstrated that clinicians do no better than chance at guessing which patients or parents are compliant.

*In summary*, noncompliance can be expected as a behavioural pattern in many situations where medication is being taken. Efforts to overcome this are time-consuming and therefore should be concentrated on those patients in whom compliance with therapy is most important.

## 4.2 Treatment of Infectious Diseases

Infections are the most common cause of illness in childhood. Many are self-limiting and of short duration; some are life-threatening or chronic. Many diseases of unknown origin are suspected of being infectious (e.g. inflammatory bowel disease and arthritic diseases) but causative agents have not been identified. However, once an infectious agent is identified, drug treatment may change drastically, such as occurred with antibacterial treatment of *Helicobacter pylori* infection in gastric and duodenal ulcers. Specific information on the management of many infectious diseases is given in other chapters. Some general principles and paediatric aspects of a few selected diseases will be briefly discussed here.

### *4.2.1 Fever*

Fever is the most common symptom treated in paediatric practice. While usually the result of an infection, fever may be the sign of many non-infectious systemic illnesses. Large quantities of antipyretics are ingested by children annually, but in an otherwise-healthy child, this is seldom necessary. Even fevers up to 40°C are unlikely to be harmful, and treatment can delay proper diagnosis or cause toxicity. Prevention is also important. Parents should be cautioned to prevent overheating by avoiding excessive clothing or bedding and by the liberal administration of fluids. However, in the young child (aged 3 to 36 months) fever may be the only sign of bacteraemia, prompting many clinicians to consider the use of empirical antibacterial therapy,[55] although the choice of antibacterial drug remains uncertain.[56]

Whether or not other therapy is given, when lowering of temperature is indicated, excessive clothing should be removed and perspiration allowed to evaporate. Tepid sponging is of value, but cold sponging or baths which induce peripheral vasoconstriction should be avoided, especially sponging with isopropanol (rubbing alcohol), since this both produces vasoconstriction and is associated with the additional toxicity of inhalation and dermal absorption of volatilised alcohols. This can lead to a chemical pneumonitis as well as metabolic problems (e.g. acetonaemia from the metabolism of isopropanol). When an antipyretic is required, the traditional agents have been aspirin or paracetamol, but aspirin has now been largely replaced by ibuprofen in many countries; these drugs are of equal efficacy as antipyretics. In the young child, paracetamol is preferred because of its greater safety with therapeutic doses and its availability in liquid and rectal preparations. Although the relationship between salicylate ingestion and Reye's syndrome is still unproven, the association is strong enough that in a number of countries, it is recommended that aspirin should not be given to children with fever due to viral infections.[38]

Use of ibuprofen is increasing in some countries. It is an effective antipyretic and analgesic but has potential renal and gastrointestinal toxicity in selected patient populations, though a superior safety record in overdose. While paracetamol cannot be administered to children with impunity, it does have a very wide therapeutic margin. Acute, therapeutic use of paracetamol causes less toxicity (mainly gastrointestinal upset) but, while rare in childhood, paracetamol poisoning with subsequent hepatic failure is well documented.[57,58] If paracetamol poisoning does occur, it should be treated as described in chapter 8 (sect. 4.3.1).

#### 4.2.2 Principles of Antimicrobial Drug Use in Children

The general principles of antimicrobial drug use are similar in children and adults. Decisions involve whether to treat, what to use, how much and for how long agents should be given. Details of these decisions are given in other chapters.

Ideally, the offending agent and drug sensitivities would be known before instituting therapy. While newer molecular biological techniques (e.g. polymerase chain reaction technology) promise to revolutionise infectious disease diagnosis and eventually drug therapy, for some time to come clinical diagnoses will be made and therapy chosen on the basis of clinical experience and a knowledge of the environment in which the patient is treated. This type of 'informed guesswork' usually produces quite acceptable results.

In the individual patient, the decision to treat or not is based on a risk-benefit analysis for patient and environment. Therapy is selected on the basis of a combination of clinical, laboratory, financial and societal factors. For example, while single-drug treatment is preferred, combination therapies may be sometimes given. Also, the drug or drugs used can differ greatly. A child with potential sepsis may receive an aminoglycoside, a cefalosporin and a penicillin in an industrialised nation, whereas in a developing county a similar child may receive only chloramphenicol.

Once a decision to treat is made and an agent(s) selected, the dose(s) must be chosen. This is clearly more complicated in children than adults: one dose doesn't 'fit all'. Dosages are also based on a combination of considerations including the disease, and its severity or duration, the clinical setting, economic considerations, and patient characteristics. Nutritional and physiological status, other diseases, the likelihood of compliance with therapy, age and developmental status all influence dosage regimens. Guidelines (table V) are based on a combination of empirical and scientific observations.

The duration of therapy is determined by whether a cure or only control of the disease is required, the cost of therapy, the likelihood of resistance, culture results, clinical course and patient- or drug-specific monitoring parameters (including blood drug concentrations, white cell counts, etc.).

Each decision – whether to treat, what to use, how much and for how long – can be altered by local and individual realities, and it is difficult to make dogmatic recommendations about therapy. Decisions concerning a 500g infant of a mother with human immunodeficiency virus (HIV) infection are quite different even for the same disease in a 3kg healthy neonate or a healthy 5-year-old. These decisions are also quite different in an industrialised *vs* a developing country.

#### 4.2.3 Common Neonatal Infections

Neonates, particularly premature and small-for-gestational-age infants, have diminished intrinsic defence mechanisms and are particularly susceptible to infection. This is especially hazardous for the infant with, for example, hyaline membrane disease with several intravenous lines who is being ventilated in an intensive care unit, with several potential entry points for bacteria. Improvements in neonatal care, including the use of surfactant preparations, have resulted in the survival of progressively more immature neonates with a greater number of invasive procedures (e.g. extracorporeal membrane oxygenation) and longer duration of indwelling lines. In addition to being unduly susceptible to infection, neonates are likely to be infected with different organisms, which are sometimes more difficult to treat than in older children. Also, clinical signs may be subtle in these infants and may include nonspecific features such as poor feeding or changes in temperature. For these reasons, many infants are treated with antibacterial drugs, after appropriate cultures have been taken, on the suspicion of being infected rather than waiting for conclusive proof. While there is a greater number of infants susceptible to overwhelming infection, more infected infants survive even the most fulminating infections such as septicaemia, pneumonia and meningitis.

#### Septicaemia

While rare in developed countries (1 to 5 per 1000 live births), septicaemia continues to have a 30 to 50% mortality[20] and significant morbidity in survivors. It should always be suspected in infants, especially the premature, who are in any way ill in the first few weeks of life. Such infants should have blood cultures taken, and urine, spinal fluid and skin sites cultured. While awaiting the results, therapy should be commenced. Therapy will depend on the most likely source and the bacteriological milieu of the intensive care unit in question, but as a generalisation, most units would start with a penicillin (or a cefalosporin) and an aminoglycoside, e.g. ampicillin and gentamicin. Others might consider the use of a single agent such as a newer broad-spectrum cefalosporin (e.g. cefotaxime or ceftazidime). Guidelines for therapy are shown in table V. The predominant pathogens are *Escherichia coli* and group B β-haemolytic streptococci, while *Staphylococcus aureus, Klebsiella* spp., *Enterobacter* spp., *Serratia* spp., *Pseudomonas aeruginosa*, *Proteus* spp., *Listeria* spp. and fungi are also potential problems. In the early period after birth, infections are usually the result of intrauterine or perinatal (especially ascending amniotic fluid) infections, while later, nosocomial sources predominate. In addition to antibacterial therapy, these infants also need general supportive care with attention to body temperature, and intravenous fluids with adequate calories. There is also a role for monitoring of plasma drug concentrations, especially with the aminoglycosides (see section 3.1.2).

#### Pneumonia

Neonatal pneumonia may be part of a generalised viral infection (e.g. herpes, cytomegalovirus, rubella) or may be due to organisms such as *Toxoplasma gondii, Listeria* spp., *Chlamydia* spp., or other organisms acquired during the perinatal period. Aspiration pneumonia may occur in infants who have suffered fetal distress, or in babies with tracheo-oesophageal fistulae or gastrointestinal obstruction. Acquired pneumonias are usually due to organisms present in the hospital, staphylococci and coliforms being especially common in the neonatal period. For these infections, antistaphylococcal penicillins such as methicillin, or – in the case of coliform organisms – gentamicin are appropriate choices (see table V for dosages).

The occurrence of multiresistant strains of *S. aureus* in many neonatal nurseries is of concern at present. In such cases, treatment with vancomycin is appropriate. There is a large and growing body of knowledge of antibiotic pharmacokinetics in neonates (see reviews by St Geme & Polin;[20] Paap & Nahata;[19] Paap & Bosso[21]).

#### Meningitis

Neonatal meningitis is a particularly distressing condition. Despite adequate antibacterial therapy, the mortality and morbidity remain very high.[21] The accepted signs of meningitis are not seen in neonates. The presenting features are often very nonspecific, causing late diagnosis. As with older children and adults, the later the presentation, the worse the outcome.

Initial therapy is aimed at the most likely organisms, followed by more specific therapy based on the results of Gram staining and, subsequently, cultures. A regimen of ampicillin and gentamicin is effective against both the major pathogens in this age group (group B streptococci, *E. coli* and other coliforms) and is also appropriate for infections caused by *Listeria monocytogenes, P. aeruginosa* and *Streptococcus pneumoniae*. Alternatively, a cefalosporin such as cefotaxime or ceftazidime may be selected. The newer cefalosporins penetrate the cerebrospinal fluid particularly well and are active against most of the likely organisms, with the exception of *L. monocytogenes*, the presence of which requires the addition of ampicillin. In comparison, the aminoglycosides penetrate the cerebrospinal fluid poorly even if given intraventricularly, and do not improve outcome.

### 4.2.4 Septicaemia and Meningitis Beyond the Neonatal Period

The pathogens most commonly causing sepsis after the neonatal period are *H. influenzae, S. pneumoniae* and *Neisseria meningitidis*. Staphylococcal septicaemia is also not uncommon and is usually associated with osteomyelitis or a tissue infection such as a psoas abscess (pyomyositis tropicans). In this age group, blood cultures are very useful with a reasonably high return (about 50% positivity). In immunocompromised children, ubiquitous organisms are common, as are infections with fungi, protozoa, and viruses such as varicella. In patients with sickle cell disease, both pneumococcal and *Salmonella* infections are possible.

When the bacteriological diagnosis is uncertain, therapy may be started with a broad-spectrum approach using a combination of ampicillin and gentamicin or a single cefalosporin such as cefotaxime or ceftazidime. Once the pathogen has been identified, a change in therapy may be indicated, especially in the case of staphylococcal infections, for which vancomycin may be needed. Previously, bacterial meningitis beyond the neonatal period was predominantly due to *H. influenzae*, which was treated with either ampicillin, a cefalosporin, or chloramphenicol, but there have been a growing number of ampicillin- and even chloramphenicol-resistant *H. influenzae* type b strains appearing. It is hoped that the success of *H. influenzae* immunisation in dramatically reducing the incidence of this disease in developed countries will be repeated in other countries where the disease remains common. There is also at least a theoretical concern that the disease will return as a problem in older children or adults who outgrow their vaccine-induced immunity.

#### *4.2.5 Respiratory Infections*

Most respiratory infections are viral in origin and do not require antibacterial therapy. Conditions and symptoms commonly treated include respiratory tract infections, cough, pharyngitis, tonsillitis, otitis media, croup and bronchitis.

Although most acute upper respiratory tract infections are of viral origin (colds), antibacterial, antihistamine, antipyretic and decongestant drugs are often prescribed.[59,60] There have been many controversial studies of therapy in this situation, but decisions are not clear-cut and practice is dictated by the individual clinician. Antibacterial drugs may help the child with sinusitis, otitis media, streptococcal pharyngitis, pneumonia or any of a number of bacterial infections, but will do no good for the child with a pure viral infection and will be associated with both cost and risk. Likewise, antihistamines can help control certain allergic symptoms and produce sedation, antipyretics can relieve discomfort (the primary reason they are taken by adults), and decongestants can produce temporary relief of congestion, but all increase costs and can cause adverse effects.

*Cough* is one of the most common reasons for a physician visit.[61] The decision to treat or not is difficult and is based on the severity, chronicity, and cause. Chronic cough is a symptom of many different, often treatable diseases (table VIII).[62] If the cough is the result of an underlying condition, treatment is designed to stop the cough with antitussives and treat the underlying condition (e.g. asthma, allergic rhinitis, gastro-oesophageal reflux, etc.). When the cough is part of a defensive reaction, therapy is selected to make it more effective using protussives.[61] Many antitussives have been demonstrated to have efficacy but the efficacy of protussives has not been as well demonstrated.

#### Pharyngitis and Tonsillitis

Many children with infections of the upper respiratory tract have pharyngitis or tonsillitis. Ideally, throat swabs should be performed and the results awaited before starting treatment. However, throat swabs are not very reliable in identifying pathogens and therapy usually needs to be started at the time of presentation. A pragmatic approach is to explain the clinical findings to the parent, emphasising that the majority (about 90%) of sore throats are due to viruses, which do not respond to antibacterial drugs, and begin an antipyretic/analgesic drug for symptomatic treatment. If the throat is particularly inflamed or if there is visible pus on the tonsils or elsewhere, then clinicians either take a throat swab and await the result before starting antibacterial drugs or start treatment empirically to cover group A β-haemolytic streptococci. Phenoxymethylpenicillin (penicillin V) or erythromycin should be given for 10 days, bearing in mind that most children will be better in 3 or 4 days and may well cease to take the medication. While streptococci resistant to penicillin, erythromycin or other common antibiotics have been reported in most situations, they are too uncommon a cause of pharyngitis to justify the use of newer, more convenient but much more expensive cefalosporins or macrolides (e.g. clarithromycin or azithromycin).

#### Otitis Media

Inflammation of the middle ear is a common problem in infancy and childhood; middle ear disease represents a very common cause of medical consultation in the first 5 years of life. While it might be expected that treatment of so common a condition would be clearly defined, this is not the case. Studies have found no difference in the end result between treatment groups receiving either antibiotics only, myringotomy only, or myringotomy and any of a number of antibiotics. This is mentioned only to emphasise the fact that there remains quite considerable controversy about the management of this condition. Currently, the accepted

**Table VIII.** Causes of chronic cough in children

| Condition | Clinical features |
|---|---|
| Allergic rhinitis | Usually clear, itchy nasal discharge. Symptoms can often be linked to allergen exposure. Family history usually positive. Nasal smear usually shows eosinophils |
| Asthma | Cough often worse with cold air, exercise and at night. May be initiated by a viral infection. Family history is usually positive. Pulmonary function tests and methacholine challenge are usually abnormal, but cough may be the only manifestation of asthma |
| Congenital anomalies | Congenital heart defects, tracheo-oesophageal fistulas, laryngotracheomalacia. Symptoms usually appear shortly after birth. There is often associated clubbing, cyanosis or failure to thrive |
| Cystic fibrosis | Family history often positive. Failure to thrive, meconium ileus, malabsorption, barrel chest, digital clubbing may be associated. May present as late as young adulthood |
| Drugs | ACE inhibitors can cause cough. β-Blockers can exacerbate asthma |
| Environmental exposure | Exposure to cigarette or wood smoke. Eyes and nasal mucosa usually red and irritated |
| Foreign body | History of sudden coughing and choking can usually be obtained. Toddler age group most likely, but can occur at any age. Foreign bodies in oesophagus, stomach and external ear canal can also cause cough |
| Gastro-oesophageal reflux | May cause aspiration in infants. There is often dyspepsia, but cough may be only feature. May worsen asthmatic cough |
| Immunodeficiency | Hypogammaglobulinaemia, immotile cilia syndrome, human immunodeficiency virus (HIV) disease, severe combined immunodeficiency. These children can present at any age and have histories of recurrent infections |
| Pneumonia | Viral or *Mycoplasma* pneumonia commonly cause prolonged cough. In infants, *Chlamydia*, *Ureaplasma*[a] infection likely. Tuberculosis should be considered especially when there is history of exposure |
| Psychogenic | Cough is loud and honking. Resolves during sleep. Child generally not concerned with cough |
| Sinusitis | Nasal congestion and discharge, postnasal drip, headaches, halitosis may be present. However, cough may be the only feature. Sinusitis may exacerbate asthmatic cough |
| Upper respiratory tract infection | Usually the result of consecutive infections. However, coughs from adenoviral, influenza, or pertussis infection can persist up to 8-12 weeks |
| Vasomotor rhinitis | Symptoms generally not associated with allergen exposure. Nasal smear usually normal |

a Ureaplasma refers to *Ureaplasma urealyticum*, a micro-organism similar in morphology to *Mycoplasma pneumoniae*.

view is that children diagnosed with otitis media using a pneumatic otoscope should be treated with an appropriate antibacterial drug (e.g. amoxicillin, erythromycin, cotrimoxazole or cefaclor) but antihistamines or nasal decongestants are of no value and may be counterproductive. Analgesic/antipyretic drugs are recommended as part of symptomatic treatment.

There is no doubt that the major complications of otitis media (mastoiditis, meningitis, etc.) which were common in the preantibiotic era are now very uncommon. On the other hand, serous otitis media ('glue ear') has become a frequent problem; whether this is in any way related to the extensive use of antibacterial drugs is unknown.

#### Croup

The term 'croup' is perhaps best regarded as a descriptive one – describing the noise made by a child with upper airway obstruction from whatever cause. The two most important causes are laryngotracheobronchitis and epiglottitis. Other causes may include laryngeal oedema, laryngeal foreign body, papillomas, vocal cord paresis, congenital abnormalities of the larynx, retropharyngeal abscess and diphtheria.

Laryngotracheobronchitis is the most common cause of croup. It is viral in origin, usually due to one of the parainfluenza viruses. Usually there is a prodromal upper respiratory tract infection followed by inspiratory stridor (croup). This is often frightening for both the child and the parents and always seems worse at night. It may be advisable to admit these children to hospital for observation and to allay parental anxiety. It is traditional for the child to be nursed in a humidified atmosphere, although there is no scientific evidence that this is of any value. Antibacterial drugs are necessary only if there is concomitant pneumonia. This is rare in developed countries but common in the developing world.

For most children, croup is a self-limiting illness of 2 to 4 days' duration. Corticosteroid use is controversial and is reserved for the most serious cases requiring intubation.

#### Acute Epiglottitis

Acute epiglottitis has a much more rapid onset, usually 12 to 24 hours, and is not usually preceded by any prodromal illness. These children appear acutely ill, are usually sitting up with their mouths open, and are drooling saliva.

They should be taken directly to the operating theatre for intubation or tracheostomy. If the disease is suspected, preparation for laryngeal intubation or tracheostomy should precede any examination of the throat. Depression of the posterior portion of the tongue has been the terminal event in precipitating complete respiratory obstruction.

Acute epiglottitis is caused by *H. influenzae* and is a septicaemic illness. Antibacterial therapy should be administered: either ampicillin, a cefalosporin or chloramphenicol. The epiglottic swelling usually recedes very rapidly and nearly all children can be extubated within 24 hours. Antibacterial drugs should be continued for 7 to 10 days.

#### Bronchitis

Acute bronchitis in childhood is usually viral in origin and thus does not require the use of antibacterial drugs. Most children recover in a few days, with recovery perhaps being assisted by the use of bronchodilators, preferably by inhalation. Antibacterial therapy should be reserved for the child who is still not well after 4 or 5 days when secondary bacterial infection may have occurred. In this situation, a penicillin drug is indicated, since the most likely causative bacterial organism is *Streptococcus pneumoniae*. It is important to remember that the child with 'recurrent bronchitis' or 'wheezy bronchitis' is likely to have underlying asthma and should be treated accordingly – not with repeated antibacterial drugs.

#### Pertussis

Pertussis is a preventable disease which has once again become a major problem in developed nations. This recrudescence is due to a multifactorial decrease in immunisation compliance, which is the result of adverse publicity concerning possible (but unproven) neurological damage associated with pertussis vaccination and failure of younger parents to see pertussis as a disease of any significance. The increase in cases and deaths has occurred in countries where medical resistance to immunisation was prominent (e.g. Japan, the UK and Australia), in countries where patient compliance with immunisation was poor (e.g. the US), and in developing countries with inadequate finances or delivery systems. Vaccination is clearly cost effective[63] but this fact has not been enough to guarantee compliance, even in developed countries, without resistance from the medical community. An epidemic occurred in the US in 1993, for example. It is hoped that the recent introduction of an acellular vaccine which produces effective immunity but fewer local reactions and less fever[64] will result in greater acceptance and use.

There is no specific therapy for pertussis, although the administration of erythromycin or other macrolide agents will reduce the infectivity of the patient to others. The basic treatment is good supportive care. Before the advent of modern intensive care, and today in areas where it is not available, pertussis can cause widespread morbidity and mortality, especially in children under the age of 6 months.

#### Acute Bronchiolitis

This condition, which is due to infection with respiratory syncytial virus (RSV), affects mainly young children and is rare over the age of 2 years. In most children, it is a mild illness with significant wheeze but not much distress, which lasts 2 to 4 days. In some infants, it may be considerably more severe, occasionally requiring artificial ventilation. Treatment consists of humidified oxygen and adequate hydration. Although widely used, *ribavirin* treatment is controversial and should be restricted to certain high risk populations (e.g. patients with congenital heart disease) where benefits may outweigh risks. More recently, RSV immune globulin has been proposed, but is unproven as a therapy. There is no role for the routine use of corticosteroids[65] or for antibacterial drugs.

#### Pneumonia

The management of pneumonia in children depends on the severity of the illness. In the mildly ill child, oral treatment with erythromycin, penicillin or a broader-spectrum antibacterial drug such as amoxicillin may well be sufficient. In the severely ill child, making an aetiological diagnosis is difficult. Sputum is often difficult to obtain and of limited value. Blood cultures are most useful. Occasionally in the very ill child, or those who are immunocompromised and in whom unusual organisms are suspected, it may be necessary to perform tracheal aspirates, direct lung punctures, thoracentesis or bronchopulmonary lavage. Throat swabs are of no value.

*Lobar pneumonia* is most often caused by *S. pneumoniae* and should be treated with benzylpenicillin (50,000 U/kg/day in 4 divided doses) parenterally for a few days, followed by oral phenoxymethylpenicillin for a total of 7 to 10 days. Other agents are used as appropriate for specific infections, e.g. flucloxacillin for *S. aureus*; gentamicin, cefotaxime or ceftazidime for *Klebsiella pneumoniae*; carbenicillin or ticarcillin for *P. aeruginosa*; and erythromycin for *Legionella pneumophila* (see further chapter 23; sect 6.2).

*Bronchopneumonia* is often viral, but of course this is difficult to demonstrate acutely and thus it may be appropriate to treat with antibacterial drugs on clinical grounds. *Mycoplasma pneumoniae* commonly causes bronchopneumonia and is best treated with erythromycin (30 to 50 mg/kg/day in divided doses).

*Empyema* may occur both in infants and in older children. This is usually due to *S. aureus*, but may also be due to *H. influenzae* or *S. pneumoniae*. An aetiological diagnosis is important and can usually be obtained by culturing the empyema fluid. Treatment should be directed at the specific organism. *Mycobacterium* spp. are an increasingly common cause, especially in malnourished or immunocompromised children.

Supportive treatment for pneumonia is important and includes adequate hydration, supplementary oxygen, analgesics/antipyretics and bronchodilators where necessary. Chest physiotherapy for patients with pneumonia is traditional but unproven.[66]

#### 4.2.6 Gastrointestinal Infections

Gastroenteritis remains one of the most common major disorders of early childhood, in both developed and developing countries. In the latter, it remains a major cause of mortality and morbidity. It is most common under the age of 2 years and is less frequent in breast-fed than bottle-fed babies.

*Diarrhoea and vomiting* in the young child is usually due to an acute infective enteritis (viral, bacterial or protozoal). However, other diseases can masquerade as gastroenteritis and need to be borne in mind. These include urinary tract infection, appendicitis, intussusception, Hirschsprung disease and other systemic disorders. Viruses account for 60 to 80% of cases of acute infantile diarrhoea in developed countries and about half that number in developing countries. The most common viral pathogen is the human rotavirus. Bacteria account for about 10 to 20% of cases in developed countries and considerably more than this in developing countries. *E. coli* is probably the most common bacterial pathogen, while *Shigella* spp. can cause an invasive enterocolitis with blood, mucus and pus in the stools. *Salmonella* enteritis often arises from a food-borne source and can cause severe bloody diarrhoea and a systemic illness. Other organisms to be considered include *Campylobacter* and *Yersinia* spp., while toxin-producing staphylococci and *Clostridium* spp. may also cause a severe diarrhoea. The most common protozoa responsible for diarrhoea is *Giardia lamblia*. Unusual organisms (e.g. *Cryptococcus* spp.) can cause disease in immune-deficient patients.

Treatment depends on the patient and degree of dehydration. Hospital admission is undesirable for the majority of patients with gastroenteritis; most parents can manage the child who is able to take adequate oral fluids at home. The disease is usually mild. In well-nourished children without dehydration, gastroenteritis is usually a short-lived, self-limiting condition lasting only a few days. However, hospital admission is warranted when:

- Parenteral therapy is necessary for rehydration
- Outpatient management has failed
- Uncertainty exists about the state of hydration or the diagnosis
- Gastroenteritis occurs in the first 1 to 2 months of life when septicaemia is a real risk
- Intractable vomiting is present
- There is pre-existing malnutrition or other debilitating illness.

Stool cultures are usually unnecessary, except if a bacterial or protozoal diarrhoea is suspected (i.e. blood and mucus are present in the stools). Plasma electrolytes, while not required routinely, should be determined in children in whom dehydration is severe, hypernatraemic dehydration is suspected on clinical grounds, or urine is not passed once the child has been rehydrated. The major advance in the management of gastroenteritis over the past decade has been the introduction of *oral rehydration therapy*. This unfortunately continues to be neglected[67,68] even when knowledge about its proper use is not an issue. A number of oral rehydration solutions are available, all based on the World Health Organization solution which contains sodium 90 mmol/L, potassium 20 mmol/L, bicarbonate 30 mmol/L, chloride 80 mmol/L, and glucose 111 mmol/L. This can be made up very simply by adding 3.5g sodium chloride, 2.5g sodium bicarbonate, 1.5g potassium chloride, and 20g glucose (or 40g sucrose) to 1L of water. In developed countries, the sodium concentration of this solution might lead to hypernatraemia in the well-nourished child.

Studies have shown that a sodium content of 50 mmol/L is as effective as 90 mmol/L both in the well-nourished and malnourished child.[69] Oral fluids such as flat lemonade, which has a high osmolality and no electrolytes, or the currently fashionable electrolyte solutions for sports people are not appropriate in the management of fluid loss associated with diarrhoea.

Oral rehydration can be successfully used in the majority of cases of gastroenteritis. In the recovery phase, usually within 24 hours of the commencement of oral fluids, full nutrient intake should be reinstated. There is no role for the use of graduated feeds as it has been shown that the reintroduction of a full feed is not detrimental to the child. Most children will recover within 2 to 5 days. Lactose-free foods should be considered only if lactose intolerance is proven, using simple tests such as stool 'Clinitest' tablets.

There is no role for antidiarrhoeal, antibiotic or antiemetic drugs in the routine management of gastroenteritis in children.[67] Although loperamide, when given in high doses, has been shown to reduce fluid and electrolyte secretion caused by various toxigenic bacteria, and to be effective in reducing symptoms of both chronic secretory diarrhoea and acute diarrhoea in childhood (in conjunction with oral rehydration therapy), its use is potentially hazardous in children because of possible CNS effects with large doses. Loperamide should not be regarded as a substitute for oral rehydration therapy, nor as a routine adjunct to such treatment. Oral bismuth subsalicylate has been shown to have additive effects to oral rehydration therapy, and may have a role in selected situations where the risk of salicylate and bismuth use is justified. The use of other, more absorbable bismuth preparations has no place in therapy, because of lack of evidence of efficacy and the proven neurotoxic risks of bismuth absorption.

*Antibacterial drugs* should be used only in certain specific circumstances such as:

1) *Shigellosis:* ampicillin (but not amoxicillin) or cotrimoxazole, given either orally or parenterally, are useful in shortening the duration of symptoms and the duration of faecal excretion of the organism.

2) *Salmonellosis:* treatment with ampicillin, cotrimoxazole or chloramphenicol is indicated if the child has a significant systemic illness. In children with diarrhoea alone, antibiotics do not shorten the course of the illness and may in fact prolong the carrier state.

3) *Campylobacter enteritis:* erythromycin (orally) is recommended in severe cases. This does not shorten the duration of the illness but markedly reduces the duration of bacterial shedding and reduces the incidence of relapse.[70]

4) *Enteropathogenic E. coli enteritis in infancy:* oral neomycin (100 mg/kg/day in 4 divided doses) or colistin (20 mg/kg/day in 4 divided doses) may be beneficial in patients with protracted symptoms.

5) *Gastritis caused by H. pylori:* this organism is increasingly reported to be the cause of symptoms as well as eventual gastric (and perhaps duodenal) ulcer disease and possibly even gastric carcinoma in adulthood. While knowledge is still evolving, it appears that aggressive combination therapies are indicated, many of which include nonabsorbable forms of bismuth (e.g. bismuth subcitrate or subsalicylate) [see further chapter 22; sect. 4.3].

Management of other gastrointestinal infections, including parasitic infections, is discussed in chapter 22 (section 10).

#### 4.2.7 Urinary Tract Infections

Urinary tract infection in children can be a potential marker of an underlying anatomical abnormality of the genitourinary tract. Thus prompt diagnosis, investigation and appropriate treatment are important but diagnosis is difficult. Symptoms of a urinary tract infection in older children are similar to those seen in adults, but in infants and young children, symptomatology may be nonspecific and includes irritability, lethargy, poor feeding, failure to thrive, or even unexplained jaundice in the neonate.

Collection of uncontaminated urine samples is difficult, especially in very young children. In the neonate, the confidence limits of a single voided specimen obtained by bag collection are only 20%, rising to 50% in infants and toddlers. In older, continent children, this rises to the adult value of 80%, which can be enhanced to 90% by duplicate collection. In some children, it may not be possible to obtain a clean bag specimen. Results may be suggestive, but not conclusive, of a urinary tract infection. This is an indication for suprapubic bladder aspiration. The presence of any pyuria or bacteriuria in a suprapubic specimen is significant.

If a urinary tract infection is diagnosed, treatment with antibacterial drugs should be started. Most children can be treated with short-acting sulfonamides (e.g. sulfafurazole/sulfisoxazole), cotrimoxazole, amoxicillin, a cefalosporin, or nitrofurantoin administered orally at home. Children who are vomiting or are quite ill should be admitted to hospital and given a parenteral antibacterial agent. Treatment should generally be continued for 5 to 7 days. In uncomplicated cases, single-dose therapy, e.g. with amoxicillin (100 mg/kg orally) or cotrimoxazole (0.72 to 1.44g orally) may produce comparable results to 5- or 7-day treatment courses (see also chapter 24; sect. 3.1).[71]

A urine specimen should be obtained for culture after the infection has been treated. Culture should be repeated if the child again becomes symptomatic. All children, both boys and girls, who have had a urinary tract infection should undergo intravenous urography. Children under 2 to 3 years of age, or older children who have an abnormal intravenous urogram, should have a micturating cystourethrogram. The role of renal ultrasound or renal scanning using technesium succimer (DMSA) is still controversial. In about 30% of children with a proven urinary tract infection, an anatomical abnormality of the urinary tract, especially some form of obstructive uropathy, will be demonstrated. Approximately 30 to 50% of infants with urinary tract infection will have vesicoureteric reflux, usually of a mild to moderate degree, which ceases spontaneously when the infection has been treated. These children, if they have recurrent infections, should receive 6 to 12 months of prophylactic therapy (e.g. nitrofurantoin 1 to 2 mg/kg/day or cotrimoxazole at half the normal recommended daily dose). In patients with severe reflux, development of renal scarring is a concern. Management of this group of patients remains controversial and consists of antibacterial therapy, surgical correction or both.

In all children, blood pressure should be measured from time to time and compared to age-appropriate normals as well as previous readings. In children who have had a urinary tract infection and especially in those with recurrent infections or significant reflux, blood pressure should be measured at each visit. Hypertension is a major problem in patients with reflux nephropathy and is usually seen from the second decade onwards. Persistent proteinuria is an ominous sign and in combination with hypertension, usually heralds deterioration in renal function.

#### *4.2.8 Tetanus*

Tetanus remains a major global disease. Neonatal tetanus is depressingly common in developing countries where the umbilical cord may be cut with a dirty implement (razor blade, knife, etc.) and subsequently covered with soil or dung. In general, where tetanus occurs commonly, intensive care facilities are limited. Most of the literature on the management of tetanus comes from the developed world, where the condition is uncommon and usually, patients present early. Thus, on a global scale there is a gulf between what might be regarded as appropriate treatment and that which is actually available for the vast majority of patients.

Treatment of tetanus requires maintenance of an airway, wound care, antitetanus serum, sedation, prevention of complications, nutritional support, tetanus toxoid, and follow-up.[36]

#### *4.2.9 Immunisations Against Infectious Diseases*

The development of effective vaccinations is a major, if not the major, advance in paediatric care. Unfortunately, the percentage of children who are fully immunised is low, even when cost is not an issue. Adequate treatment of children requires proper administration of a number of vaccines.

A discussion of all aspects of modern immunisation practice, including the fact that improperly stored vaccines are ineffective, is beyond the scope of this chapter. Both the incidence and adverse sequelae of viral (e.g. polio, rubella, rubeola, hepatitis B, and varicella) and bacterial diseases (e.g. diphtheria, pertussis, and *H. influenzae* meningitis) can be decreased significantly. The total elimination of variola (smallpox) as a disease of mankind is an example of what is possible. Even parasitic and protozoan diseases may eventually be controllable with immunisation. The dramatic reduction in *H. influenzae* meningitis following *H. influenzae* B (HIB) vaccines is another example of the potential impact of a successful vaccination programme. In contrast, the practical limitations of these possibilities are best illustrated by tetanus and pertussis.

### 4.3 Treatment of Other Common Disorders in Children

Treatment of diseases that can affect children is discussed in other chapters. A few are discussed here to illustrate paediatric aspects of disease therapy.

#### *4.3.1 Cystic Fibrosis*

Cystic fibrosis, an hereditary disease of exocrine gland secretion, is characterised by recurrent pulmonary infections, pancreatic insufficiency with maldigestion, malabsorption and an excessive loss of sweat and electrolytes. This condition is of growing importance in paediatric and adolescent practice and is now impinging upon adult respiratory medicine. It is the most common lethal genetic defect in Caucasian populations. However, the prognosis has improved greatly over the past 2 decades such that most patients now survive childhood and progress to adulthood if treated at a major centre. Cystic fibrosis is an important 'pharmacological condition'. These patients eliminate a number of drugs, especially penicillins, cefalosporins, aminoglycosides and antimicrobials, much faster than persons without the disease (see section 2.4.2). They also need numerous medications, and their treatment requires pharmacological knowledge of a number of new antibiotics, nutritional therapies, and established drugs given by novel routes (e.g. inhaled aminoglycosides and amiloride),[72] completely new drug classes [e.g. dornase-alfa (DNase) and uridine triphosphate (UTP)], and also the evolving principles of gene therapy.

The reasons for the enhanced clearance of many drugs in cystic fibrosis patients is unclear, but the clinical implication of these findings is that higher doses than are commonly recommended will be needed to achieve what would normally be regarded as 'therapeutic' serum concentrations. This is rendered more complex by the variable penetration of antimicrobial agents into the bronchial tree and sputum.

The management of cystic fibrosis has become a specialised, team approach, with two main aims:

a) Preventing progression of the pulmonary disease; and

b) Maintaining normal nutrition and growth.

**Prevention of Progression of Pulmonary Disease**

The most common pulmonary pathogens in cystic fibrosis are *S. aureus* and *P. aeruginosa*. Therapy consists of continuous prophylactic antibacterial drugs, often in combination. Acute pulmonary infective exacerbations, often due to *Pseudomonas* spp., require intravenous treatment with appropriate antibacterials as well as vigorous physiotherapy. The latter is an important part of both acute and prophylactic management, with most patients requiring one or two sessions of percussion and drainage daily. This should be done at home and combined with regular physical exercise.

Inhaled therapy is often given before physiotherapy in an attempt to loosen secretions; a bronchodilator such as salbutamol (albuterol) may be beneficial as about 50% of cystic fibrosis patients have underlying bronchial hyper-reactivity. However, there is no good evidence that mucolytics are of value. Regular treatment with inhaled antibiotics is controversial. Recently, nebulised *dornase-alfa* (DNase), which is designed to improve function by destroying the DNA of inflammatory cells and thereby decreasing the viscosity of secretions, has been shown to be effective in patients with less severe pulmonary compromise. However, it has not yet been shown to be effective in more severely compromised patients. Lung function rapidly returns to normal when dornase-alfa (DNase) treatment is stopped, and the therapy is very expensive. Inhaled amiloride, a potassium-sparing diuretic, has also been used on the basis of its effect on the chloride channel.

Inhaled uridine triphosphate (UTP) may also be useful. The recently discovered genetic cause of the abnormal pathophysiology in cystic fibrosis promises to provide molecular genetic methods to treat or even cure the disease.

**Maintenance of Normal Nutrition and Growth**

An important observation of the past decades has been that ensuring the best possible nutrition in cystic fibrosis patients increases survival and decreases the number of pulmonary infections. The diet should provide 150% of the recommended caloric intake, contain a moderate amount of fat, and be high in protein. For patients whose weight is less than ideal, high calorie oral supplements are recommended and in severely malnourished patients, either enteral (gastrotomy or nasogastric feeding) or parenteral therapy should be instituted. Pancreatic insufficiency requires replacement with pancreatic enzymes to prevent malabsorption and ensure normal growth. Infants are usually started on powdered preparations while older children are given capsules. Pancreatic enzymes should be taken with all meals containing fat or protein. Preparations are available in enteric-coated microspheres, which are less susceptible to acid degradation and can thus be taken in smaller dosages.

Longer survival of cystic fibrosis patients is unfortunately associated with a number of problems related to liver disease, diabetes and sterility.

### *4.3.2 Convulsive Disorders*

Neurological diseases are discussed in chapter 29, but seizures are dealt with here as largely a paediatric disease, both because of the high incidence of febrile convulsions and because about 80% of epilepsy begins in childhood and about 90% prior to adult life.

#### Febrile Convulsions

Febrile seizures are seizures occurring between the age of 3 months and 5 years associated with fever but without evidence of intracranial infection or a metabolic cause.[73] They are common: about 4% of children have at least one febrile convulsion, usually associated with respiratory infections, otitis media or tonsillitis. They can be prolonged (>30 minutes), unilateral (i.e. focal) or generalised, single or multiple (>2 in a day) and are frightening for the parents, who may think that the child is dying. Usually the seizures are brief and not even seen by the clinician; it is thus important to obtain a good history from the parents, paying particular attention to the duration of the seizure and the presence of any early focal component.

Nothing can be done to prevent the first febrile convulsion. Parents who are obviously not expecting it to occur will call or visit their doctor, call an ambulance or go to a hospital. In any of these situations, if the child is still convulsing when medical contact is made, the seizures should be controlled by administering *diazepam* (up to 0.25 mg/kg intravenously or 0.5 mg/kg rectally). There is little risk of long term neurological deficits, epilepsy, behavioural changes or any other sequelae despite the fact that seizures will recur once in about 32% of patients, twice in 15%, and three times in only 7%, most commonly between the ages of 12 and 24 months.[74] In 75%, this recurrence is within 12 months of the first seizure and in 92% within 24 months. The risk of recurrences is increased with:

- A prolonged seizure (more than 15 to 20 minutes)
- A neurological or developmental abnormality either present before or found after the seizure
- A focal seizure
- More than one seizure on the same day
- Previous non-febrile seizures
- A family history of febrile convulsions or epilepsy in a parent or sibling.

Long term therapy is controversial. There is no evidence that maintenance prophylaxis reduces the subsequent development of epilepsy in children with complex, as opposed to simple, febrile seizures, and febrile convulsions do not in themselves lead to epilepsy. However, it may be argued that features 2, 5 and 6 are indicators of epilepsy. Children with these features are more likely to have or develop epilepsy and their febrile seizures may be just the start of this. These children, if given antiepileptic drugs, are not receiving prophylaxis for febrile convulsions but rather treatment for epilepsy.

Until a diagnosis of epilepsy is made, however, continuous treatment is optional, since the great majority of children who have febrile seizures will not develop epilepsy, suffer harm, or be candidates for long term prophylaxis. Previously healthy children with normal development and neurological examinations are especially unlikely to have recurrent seizures. Their parents should be advised to use antipyretics alone or with tepid water sponging when their child develops a fever. To avoid unnecessary parental guilt, they should be informed that there is no way to predict or avoid a recurrence and that antipyretics can take hours to lower temperature.[59] For those requiring more definitive prophylaxis, there are 2 options:

- Intermittent therapy using rectal diazepam (up to 0.5 mg/kg) administered whenever the child has a fever and prior to immunisations
- Maintenance prophylaxis with either phenobarbital or valproic acid/sodium valproate.

For most children, intermittent diazepam is preferred because of the low risk of recurrence, benign natural history, and the risks of long term antiepileptic drug use (see further chapter 29; sect. 4). Intermittent use of phenobarbital, valproic acid, or any other non-benzodiazepine is ineffective, unproven or pharmacologically irrational. Once started, therapy should be continued until 5 years of age or for 1 year seizure-free (whichever occurs later) and then tapered over at least a month.

#### Epilepsy

The treatment of epilepsy is discussed in detail in chapter 29 (section 4). Only some issues particularly pertinent to children will be discussed here including growth, metabolism, compliance with therapy, adverse effects and duration of treatment, lifestyle changes, and use of newly introduced drugs.

***Growth and metabolism:*** because children are growing continuously, there is a need for regular dosage review, which may be assisted by plasma concentration monitoring, especially for phenytoin. As discussed earlier (section 2.4.1), drug metabolism in the child aged 1 to about 8 or 10 years is more rapid than in adults. Children in this age range require both higher doses on a mg/kg bodyweight basis and more frequent administration than do adults to achieve similar plasma concentrations.

***Compliance difficulties:*** it is often assumed that because children are, in the main, looked after by their parents, compliance is assured, but this is not always the case. It is necessary to obtain parental cooperation to achieve compliance. This, in turn, depends largely upon parents understanding the underlying condition and the treatment, and having a good rapport with the clinician. As the child gets older, responsibility for therapy should be progressively handed over to the child. It is also important for parents to understand the concept of the therapeutic range and the effects of missed doses. Once-daily administration of phenobarbital and twice- or thrice-daily administration of others is recommended wherever possible so that children do not have to take medication to school. Even on an 8-hourly schedule, it should be possible for a child to avoid taking a dose at school. As part of normal development, compliance may diminish during adolescence. However, seizure control may deteriorate in association with the onset of puberty. It has been suggested that this is due to metabolic changes but the evidence for this is somewhat anecdotal. In general, noncompliance is a much more common cause of poor seizure control.

***Adverse drug effects:*** phenobarbital is now seldom favoured as an antiepileptic drug because of the hyperactivity that it can produce in 20 to 40% of children. Phenytoin is less used in paediatric practice than in adults, largely because of its adverse effects of acne, gum hypertrophy and hirsutism. Sodium valproate/valproic acid is commonly used but can induce considerable weight gain which may be of concern, especially to girls.

The cognitive adverse effects of antiepileptic drugs are particularly disruptive in the school-age child. Carbamazepine is perhaps the least likely to produce cognitive dysfunction; nevertheless, it can occur.[75]

***Duration of treatment:*** as a matter of principle, in a child who has been free of seizures for about 2 years while taking antiepileptic drug therapy, cessation of therapy should be considered. Some specialists use 1 year seizure-free as a criterion, and others use 3 years seizure-free; most consider 2 years to be appropriate. While it cannot be predicted accurately which patients will have recurrences, certain generalisations can be made. Relapse is more likely in children whose seizures have been very difficult to control, those with established neurological problems, children who have had focal or mixed seizures, and those who have their medication withdrawn rapidly. Medication should therefore be withdrawn slowly, over 1 to 3 months. The role of the electroencephalogram in predicting relapse is limited and controversial.

It is extremely important that children with epilepsy lead as normal a life as possible. Obviously this has different implications for the child whose seizures are so severe that he or she has to wear a protective helmet as opposed to the youngster who has rare seizures. Children with epilepsy should be encouraged to participate in the normal activities of childhood; however, certain precautions should be taken:

- They should never be allowed to swim unsupervised.
- Rock or tree climbing should be discouraged.
- Showering is to be preferred to bathing; if a bath is taken, the water should be shallow and the bathroom door left unlocked, preferably ajar.

***Use of newer antiepileptic drugs:*** a number of newer agents (e.g. lamotrigine, felbamate and gabapentin) have been introduced (see further chapter 29; sect. 4). Unfortunately, repeating an old pattern, few studies have been carried out with these drugs in children. The data necessary to make recommendations for their use in children (both the largest population of patients and those most affected by the adverse effects of older antiepileptic drugs) should soon be available. Until then, these drugs will be used mainly in children with the most severe and least responsive seizures and syndromes.

#### 4.3.3 Corticosteroid Therapy in Children

Corticosteroids are valuable agents in a number of conditions seen in childhood such as asthma, atopic eczema, acute leukaemia, the nephrotic syndrome, chronic inflammatory bowel disease, rheumatic carditis, idiopathic thrombocytopenia purpura, and the adrenogenital syndrome.

Corticosteroids should not be withheld if they are genuinely required, but should be used with caution in children. Dosage depends on the disease being treated, the degree of control required, and the extent to which adverse effects can be accepted. For prednisone, a dose of 10mg in adults is equivalent to 0.2 mg/kg in children or 6 mg/$m^2$. This relationship can be used for approximate conversion purposes where only adult doses are quoted. All the adverse effects of corticosteroids seen in adults (see chapter 19; sect. 7.1.1) occur in children, although peptic ulceration and osteoporosis are rare. Psychiatric dysfunction is common but under-recognised. Growth retardation is by far the most important problem in children who receive these drugs on a long term basis. To minimise this, the smallest dose possible should be used. For some conditions (e.g. asthma), it may be worth administering the corticosteroid on an alternate-day basis. Alternate-day regimens have been shown to minimise (but not eliminate) adverse effects on growth, but are not always effective (e.g. for arthritis) and have not been proven to prevent the other adverse effects of long term corticosteroid use.

The use of inhaled corticosteroids in the treatment of asthma appears to produce minimal adrenal suppression and effects on growth.[76] The use of spacer devices also decreases the risk of both topical and systemic effects.

Some viral diseases, especially varicella, may be fulminating in children receiving corticosteroids. If these occur, the corticosteroid dosage should be reduced, although this may well produce relapse of the disease under treatment.

#### 4.3.4 Iron Deficiency Anaemia

Haematological disorders are discussed in greater detail in chapter 26. In children, iron deficiency is the most common cause of anaemia. It is usually due to nutritional iron deficiency in children from 3 months to 3 years of age and may be related to maternal iron deficiency, blood loss, or the excessive ingestion of cows' milk in infancy. Prevention is best achieved by identifying infants at risk: babies of anaemic mothers, premature and small-for-gestational-age infants, multiple-birth infants, and those who have suffered perinatal blood loss. In such infants, oral iron (2 mg/kg/day elemental iron given in a suitable liquid preparation) should be administered for a period of about 3 months.

In documented iron deficiency anaemia, 6 mg/kg/day of elemental iron should be given for 2 to 3 months. Parents should be advised that the iron will darken the stools and that the deciduous teeth may be slightly stained. This does not occur, however, with permanent teeth and the effect on deciduous teeth may be decreased by rinsing the mouth out after administration.

#### 4.3.5 Protein-Energy Malnutrition

Protein-energy malnutrition is the most common paediatric condition globally. It affects children who are either chronically ill or living in areas of poverty, crop failure, or armed conflicts, whether in developed or underdeveloped countries. It has been estimated that 100 million children less than 4 years of age were affected in 1974.[77] The condition is due to either protein or energy deficiency, usually the result of insufficient food intake. The clinical manifestations vary around the world, the most common manifestation being an underweight child, marasmus or kwashiorkor. Treatment consists of:

1) *Nutritional rehabilitation:* the reintroduction of a normal diet for age will allow nutritional recovery in a period of about 3 weeks if the problems which produced the malnutrition can be corrected.

2) *Vitamin supplementation:* this varies greatly; however, retinol (vitamin A) deficiency is fairly universal, leading to xerophthalmia and eventual blindness. Retinol 100,000U intramuscularly is also useful to decrease the complications of rubeola. Folic acid is given for megaloblastic anaemia due to folate deficiency and to all pregnant women (who are often 'children') to decrease the risks of birth defects.

3) *Electrolyte therapy:* these children, many of whom are potassium deficient from recurrent episodes of gastroenteritis, should all receive an oral potassium supplement.

4) *Antimicrobial therapy:* children with protein-energy malnutrition, especially kwashiorkor, are susceptible to recurrent and severe infections because of a quite profound depression of cell-mediated immunity, which recovers with refeeding. In addition, children with kwashiorkor exhibit abnormalities of drug metabolism, which although pharmacologically interesting, probably do not account for their poor response to standard antimicrobial therapy. In developed countries, undernutrition is less common, but not unknown, and obesity is a much more common form of malnutrition.

#### 4.3.6 Pain

Management of pain in children is changing rapidly as a result of improvements in the appreciation of paediatric pain, pharmacological knowledge, and drug delivery technology.[78-80] Numerous studies have shown that pain is under-recognised and often inappropriately treated in children, largely as a result of misperceptions of clinicians and allied health professionals concerning the ability of children to experience pain, as well as the inability or unwillingness of children to report pain. The important principles of pain management in children include the following:

1) Unrelieved pain causes significant physical and psychological harm in both the short and the long term.

2) It is easier to treat pain before it is established than after. Sufficient time must elapse between the administration of a drug and its effect to be maximal. With nonsteroidal anti-inflammatory drugs (NSAIDs), for example, it can take 1 to 2 hours before the maximal effect is seen.

3) Control and evaluation of pain requires communication between caregivers, parents and patients.

4) Although it may not be possible for all pain to be eliminated, pain is controllable in the vast majority of situations.

5) Children and caregivers must become actively involved in both the assessment and management of pain. While assessment can be difficult, especially in preverbal, unconscious or paralysed children, a number of assessment techniques (e.g. visual analogue scales, pictures of faces, poker chips, and behavioural scales) can be used to monitor both the need for and response to treatment.

6) Pain can be divided into acute, disease-related, and chronic non-disease-related pain, each of which may require somewhat different management but most principles are the same.

7) Continued use of medication can produce tolerance or even withdrawal but this must not be equated with 'addiction'. True addiction following the medical use of analgesics is extremely uncommon and should not be used as an excuse to undertreat pain. Also, normal coping behaviours (e.g. watching television or combing one's hair) must not be used as 'evidence' of lack of pain or an excuse to withhold treatment.

8) Whenever possible, the cause of the pain should be identified and treated specifically. It must be appreciated that when the source of pain is removed (e.g. when an abscess is drained), the sedative or respiratory depressant effects of administered drugs may be uncovered.

Analgesics and anaesthetics (local, regional and systemic) are the major drugs used for relief of pain, supplemented with anxiolytics, sedatives, antidepressants, and disease-specific treatments as appropriate. Irrational, dangerous combinations (e.g. pethidine/promethazine/ chlorpromazine) should be avoided. For adequate patient monitoring, skills in paediatric assessment, airway management and resuscitation are perhaps even more important than knowledge of the pharmacology of the drugs used.

*Local anaesthetics* may be injected or applied to reduce pain sensation. Individually titrated doses of oral, intravenous, intramuscular, rectal, transmucosal or topical *opioids* may be given until the desired analgesia is obtained or toxicity occurs. Incremental doses of *benzodiazepines* produce anxiolysis but not anaesthesia, while barbiturates are antianalgesic (i.e. can increase pain response). *Anaesthetics*, either inhaled (e.g. nitrous oxide) or systemic (e.g. ketamine), should be used only when experienced personnel and monitoring equipment are available.

Nonpharmacological management techniques (e.g. distraction, imagery, self hypnosis, etc.) should always be combined with or even substituted for drugs where possible, especially for chronic pain. Many sedative/hypnotic preparations can produce 'paradoxical' excitement in children, especially in overdose; too much of the sedative/hypnotic can produce as great a problem as too little.

*Nonsteroidal anti-inflammatory drugs* (especially injectable preparations such as ketorolac) are useful adjuncts for procedural pain, especially for inflammatory, periosteal, or bone pain.

*Morphine* is the standard by which other opioids are judged. *Pethidine* (meperidine) may be used, but only short term, in patients unable to tolerate morphine or hydromorphone. Pethidine is contraindicated in patients receiving drugs with monoamine oxidase inhibitory activity. Its major metabolite, norpethidine (normeperidine), is associated with significant potential to cause seizures and dysphoria, especially in patients with renal dysfunction.

Opioids should be given around the clock in a fixed dosage rather than 'prn', especially for chronic pain, and the intramuscular route should be avoided if possible.

*Patient-controlled analgesia* (PCA), where the patient controls how much drug is given (within certain preset maxima) with or without a background infusion dose, should be considered even in very young children if they can master the simple concept of pushing a button when their pain is getting worse. Rescue doses must be available during the dose-finding phase. Topical (e.g. fentanyl patch), mucosal (e.g. fentanyl 'lollipops'), rectal (e.g. hydromorphone suppositories) and oral routes can be used as substitutes for, or in addition to, intravenous administration. The proper dose must be individualised and repeatedly reassessed.[81]

#### 4.3.7 Respiratory Distress Syndrome, Bronchopulmonary Dysplasia, and Patent Ductus Arteriosus

Developments in obstetric and neonatal care have made possible the survival of progressively smaller, more immature infants but many still die and as many as 10% develop bronchopulmonary dysplasia. The major drug advances which have improved this have been the use of maternal corticosteroids (see further chapters 2 and 18) and exogenous surfactants.[82,83] Surfactants, either natural (extracted from human or animal amniotic fluid or lungs) or synthetic (*colfosceril palmitate*; the major component of natural surfactant) have been shown to improve survival and decrease the number of premature infants who develop bronchopulmonary dysplasia in a highly cost-effective way.[84] Their use is associated with no obvious long term toxicity but a higher incidence of apnoea of prematurity and of lung haemorrhage have been observed, possibly because of the survival of children who would otherwise die. Surfactants are being increasingly used for the treatment of infants and adults with other forms of lung damage leading to respiratory distress. Administration is by direct endotracheal instillation either before (prophylactic) and/or after the onset of distress (rescue). The ideal agent, dose, frequency and timing of administration are still the subject of active investigation. Surfactant use has decreased the incidence of bronchopulmonary dysplasia. Other treatments, especially prenatal and neonatal corticosteroids, are also being used.

The ability to pharmacologically manipulate the *patent ductus arteriosus* has also been a major advance. High-output cardiac failure has been treated successfully by closing the ductus with the cyclo-oxygenase inhibitor indomethacin (0.2 mg/kg dose followed by up to 2 additional 0.1 mg/kg doses in children >48 hours old and up to 0.25 mg/kg additional doses in older children depending on gestational and postnatal age), with or without plasma concentration monitoring. Conversely, children with patent ductus arteriosus-dependent cardiac lesions can be maintained with short term intravenous *alprostadil* (prostaglandin $E_1$; 0.002 to 0.5 μg/kg/min) or even long term (months) oral *dinoprostone* (prostaglandin $E_2$) therapy. Although life-saving, these treatments can cause serious toxicity and should be reserved for use by cardiac specialists in tertiary care centres.

#### 4.3.8 Hyperbilirubinaemia and Kernicterus

Hyperbilirubinaemia continues as a common, important condition of the newborn.[85] Kernicterus, a severe neurodevelopmental condition associated with hyperbilirubinaemia, remains a threat. Although levels of bilirubin and the use of methods to prevent kernicterus are associated, their cause and effect relationship remains unclear.[86] These methods include:

1) Avoiding drugs (such as the sulfonamides and salicylates), which are capable of raising bilirubin levels at clinically used concentrations.

2) Using drugs such as phenobarbital to stimulate hepatic conjugation [along with supplemental phytomenadione (vitamin $K_1$)].

3) Using phototherapy to degrade bilirubin into less toxic and more easily excreted products.

4) Performing exchange transfusions to rapidly lower bilirubin levels.

5) Experimental attempts either to prevent bilirubin production by blocking haemoxygenase (e.g. tin protoporphyrin) or blocking its intestinal reabsorption (e.g. using exogenous bilirubin oxidase or bilirubin binding agents such as charcoal).

#### 4.3.9 Growth Abnormalities: Use of Growth Hormone in Children

The use of human growth hormone (hGH) is an excellent example of the success of molecular biology as well as the ability of natural products to treat both primary deficiency states and related diseases. It is also an example of how long it takes to clarify the risks and benefits of any therapy. The primary use of hGH is to treat primary or secondary causes of growth hormone deficiency. Though still non-conventional or even experimental, the use of hGH has also gained favour in the treatment of other causes of short stature, most notably Turner's syndrome, certain chronic diseases (e.g. juvenile rheumatoid arthritis, Crohn's disease, or renal insufficiency), intrauterine growth retardation, skeletal dysplasias, uraemia, or even obesity.

The use of natural hGH also provides an excellent example of serious, unexpected and delayed toxicity. The initial source of hGH, human cadaver pituitaries, resulted in some instances of transmission of Creutzfeldt-Jakob disease. Although this has only occurred in isolated cases, the use of any animal source is associated with risk of transmission of infectious agents. Synthetically produced hGH differs by only one amino acid from natural hGH, but its use may be associated with the development of an antibody response or lack of activity, whether the alteration was planned (e.g. methionyl-hGH) or the result of misincorporation (e.g. *E. coli*-synthesised norleucine). Thyroid and carbohydrate metabolism and salt and water balance may also be affected. There is also concern about the effect of hGH on neoplastic transformation. Finally, it is possible that the pace of renal functional deterioration is hastened by the use of hGH in patients with renal failure.

## Acknowledgement

Supported by NICHD Pediatric Pharmacology Research Unit HD31316.

## Further Reading

Benet LZ, Massoud N, Gambertoglio JG. Pharmacokinetic basis for drug treatment. New York: Raven Press, 1984

Briggs GG, Bodendorfer TW, Freeman RK, et al. Drugs in pregnancy and lactation. A reference guide to fetal and neonatal risk. Baltimore: Williams and Wilkins, 1983

MacLeod SM, Radde IC. Textbook of paediatric clinical pharmacology. Littleton: PSG Publishing, 1985

Pagliaro LA, Pagliaro A-M, editors. Problems in pediatric drug therapy. 3rd edition. Hamilton, IL: Drug Intelligence Publications, 1995

Yaffe SJ, editor. Paediatric pharmacology: therapeutic principles in practice. New York: Grune and Stratton, 1980

## References

1. Kauffman RE, Kearns GL. Pharmacokinetic studies in paediatric patients. Clinical Pharmacokinetics 1992; 23: 10-29
2. Gilman JT, Gal P. Pharmacokinetic and pharmacodynamic data collection in children and neonates. Clinical Pharmacokinetics 1992; 23: 1-9
3. Shirkey HC. Therapeutic orphans. Journal of Pediatrics 1968; 72: 119
4. Walson PD, Bressler R, Fulginiti VA. The routine use of hexachlorophene (HCP) in the newborn nursery should be banned. In: Lasagna L, editor. Current controversies in therapeutics. Philadelphia: WB Saunders, 1980: 419-26
5. Roberts RJ. Drug therapy in infants: pharmacologic principles and clinical experience. Philadelphia: WB Saunders, 1984
6. Gould T, Roberts RJ. Therapeutic problems arising from the use of the intravenous route for drug administration. Journal of Pediatrics 1979; 95: 465
7. Morselli PL. Clinical pharmacokinetics in neonates. Clinical Pharmacokinetics 1976; 1: 81
8. Morselli PL. Drug disposition during development. New York: Spectrum, 1977
9. Morselli PL, Baruzzi A. Serum levels and pharmacokinetics of anticonvulsants in the management of seizure disorders. In: Mirkin BL, editor. Clinical pharmacology and therapeutics. A pediatric perspective. Chicago: Year Book Publishers, 1978: 89
10. Besunder JB, Reed MD, Blumer JL. Principles of drug biodisposition in the neonate. A critical evaluation of the pharmacokinetic-pharmacodynamic interface (Part I and II). Clinical Pharmacokinetics 1988; 14: 189-216
11. Kraus DM, Fischer JH, Reitz SJ, et al. Alterations in theophylline metabolism during the first year of life. Clinical Pharmacology and Therapeutics 1993; 54: 351-9
12. Jager-Roman E, Doyle PE, Thomas D, et al. Increased theophylline metabolism in premature infants after prenatal betamethasone administration. Developmental Pharmacology and Therapeutics 1982; 5: 127
13. Baird-Lambert J, Doyle PE, Thomas D, et al. Theophylline metabolism in preterm infants during the first week of life. Developmental Pharmacology and Therapeutics 1984; 7: 239
14. Franko TG, Powell DA, Nahata MC. Pharmacokinetics of theophylline in infants with bronchiolitis. European Journal of Clinical Pharmacology 1982; 23: 123-7
15. Doyle PE, Jager-Roman E, Baird-Lambert J, et al. Effect of prenatal exposure to betamethasone on metronidazole elimination in the premature infant. Journal of Pediatrics 1982; 101: 647
16. Howard JB, McCracken GH. Reappraisal of kanamycin usage in neonates. Journal of Pediatrics 1975; 86: 949
17. McCracken GH. Pharmacological basis for antimicrobial therapy in newborn infants. American Journal of Diseases of Children 1974; 128: 407
18. Tognoni G. Antibiotics. In: Morselli PL, editor. Drug disposition during development. New York: Spectrum, 1977: 123
19. Paap CM, Nahata MC. Clinical pharmacokinetics of antibacterial drugs in neonates. Clinical Pharmacokinetics 1990; 19: 280-318
20. St Geme III JW, Polin RA. Neonatal sepsis: progress in diagnosis and management. Drugs 1988; 36: 784-800
21. Paap CM, Bosso JA. Treatment options for the pharmacological therapy of neonatal meningitis. Drugs 1992; 43: 700-12
22. McCracken GH, Eichenwald HF. Antimicrobial therapy in infants and children. Part II. Therapy of infectious conditions. Journal of Pediatrics 1978; 93: 357
23. Kearns GL, Hilman BD, Wilson JT. Dosing implications of altered gentamicin disposition in patients with cystic fibrosis. Journal of Pediatrics 1982; 100: 312-8
24. Spielberg SP. Pharmacogenetics and the fetus. New England Journal of Medicine 1982; 307: 115
25. Walson PD. Pediatric TDM. Clinical Chemistry News 1992: 13-19

26. Weinstein AJ, Gibbs RS, Gallagher M. Placental transfer of clindamycin and gentamicin in term pregnancy. American Journal of Obstetrics and Gynecology 1976; 124: 688-91
27. Nichoga A, Skosyeva AM, Voropaeva SD. Transplacental passage of gentamicin and its effect on the fetus. (Russian). Antibiotiki Khiomioter 1982; 27: 46-50
28. Mortensen ME. Succimer chelation: what is known? Journal of Pediatrics 1994; 124: 313-7
29. Olivieri NF, Matsui D, Hermann C, et al. Compliance assessed by the medication event monitoring system. Archives of Disease in Childhood 1991; 66: 1399-402
30. Matsui D, Hermann C, Braudo M, et al. Clinical use of the medication event monitoring system: a new window into pediatric compliance. Clinical Pharmacology and Therapeutics 1992; 52: 102-3
31. Koren G, Barzilay Z, Greenwald M. Tenfold errors in administration of drug doses: a neglected iatrogenic disease in pediatrics. Pediatrics 1986; 77: 848-9
32. Dine MS, McGovern ME. Intentional poisoning of children - an overlooked category of child abuse: response of seven cases and review of the literature. Pediatrics 1982; 70: 32
33. Henry J, Volans G. ABC of poisoning. Problems in children. British Medical Journal 1983; 289: 486
34. Prescott LF. New approaches to managing drug overdosage and poisoning. British Medical Journal 1983; 287: 274
35. Olsen K, et al., editors. Poisoning and drug overdose. Norwalk: Appleton & Lange, 1990
36. Buchanan N. Paediatric clinical pharmacology and therapeutics. In: Speight TM, editor. Avery's drug treatment: principles and practice of clinical pharmacology and therapeutics. 3rd ed. Auckland: Adis Press, 1987: 119-59
37. Walson PD, Getschman S, Koren G. Principles of drug prescribing in infants and children: a practical guide. Drugs 1993; 46: 281-8
38. Glen-Bott AM. Aspirin and Reye's syndrome: a reappraisal. Medical Toxicology and Adverse Drug Experience 1987; 2: 161-5
39. Walson PD, Galletta G, Chomilo F, et al. Comparison of multidose ibuprofen and acetaminophen therapy in febrile children. American Journal of Diseases of Children 1992; 146: 626-32
40. Braden NJ, Walson PD. Drug reactions and interactions in pediatric practice. Pediatrics in Review 1985; 6: 297-303
41. Walson PD, Galletta G. Intravascular injection of long-acting penicillin [letter]. Pediatrics 1987; 79: 165
42. Kumar A, Rawlings RD, Beaman DC. The mystery ingredients: sweeteners, flavorings, dyes and preservatives in analgesic/antipyretic, antihistamine/decongestant, cough and cold, antidiarrheal, and liquid theophylline preparations. Pediatrics 1993; 91: 927-33
43. American Academy of Pediatrics: Committee on Fetus and Newborn and Committee on Drugs. Benzyl alcohol: toxic agent in neonatal units. Pediatrics 1983; 72: 356-8
44. Rohyans J, Walson PD, Wood GA, et al. Mercury toxicity following merthiolate ear irrigations. Journal of Pediatrics 1984; 104: 311
45. Nahata MC, Hipple TF, editors. Pediatric drug formulations. Ohio: Harvey Whitney Books, 1992
46. American Society of Hospital Pharmacists Scientific Affairs Department. Draft guidelines on preventable medication errors. American Journal of Hospital Pharmacists 1992; 49: 640-8
47. Curless RG, Walson PD, Carter DE. Phenytoin kinetics in children. Neurology 1976; 26: 715-20
48. Fischer JH, Lockman LA, Zaske D, et al. Phenobarbital maintenance dose requirements in treating neonatal seizures. Neurology 1981; 31: 1042-4
49. Saunders CE. Patient compliance in filing prescriptions after discharge from the emergency department. American Journal of Emergency Medicine 1987; 5: 283-6
50. Pincus JM, Ike RW. Norflux or Norflex? [letter]. New England Journal of Medicine 1992; 326: 1030
51. Lee B, Groth P, Turner W. Suspected reactions to gamma benzene hexachloride. Journal of the American Medical Association 1976; 236: 2846
52. Litovitz T. Implication of dispensing cups in dosing errors and pediatric poisonings: a report from the American Association of Poison Control Centers. Annals of Pharmacotherapy 1992; 26: 917-8
53. Greenberg RN. Overview of patient compliance with medication dosing: a literature review. Clinical Therapeutics 1984; 6: 592-9
54. Levy G. A pharmacokinetic perspective on medicament noncompliance. Clinical Pharmacology and Therapeutics 1993; 54: 242-4
55. Fleisher GR, Rosenberg N, Vinci R, et al. Intramuscular versus oral antibiotic therapy for the prevention of meningitis and other bacterial sequelae in young, febrile children at risk for occult bacteremia. Journal of Pediatrics 1994; 124: 505-12
56. Long SS. Antibiotic therapy in febrile children: 'best-laid schemes..'. Journal of Pediatrics 1994; 124: 585-8
57. Fowler PD. Aspirin, paracetamol and non-steroidal anti-inflammatory drugs: a comparative review of side effects. Medical Toxicology and Adverse Drug Experience 1987; 2: 338-66
58. Kelley MT, Walson PD, Hayes JR, et al. Safety of paracetamol and ibuprofen in febrile children. Drug Investigation 1993; 6: 48-56
59. Walson PD, Mortensen ME. Pharmacokinetics of common analgesics, anti-inflammatories and antipyretics in children. Clinical Pharmacokinetics 1989; 17: 116-37
60. Addy DP. Does treating common viral upper respiratory tract infections with antibiotics have any value such as shortening the illness or reducing morbidity or even mortality? British Medical Journal 1983; 287: 341
61. Irwin RS, Curley FJ, Bennett FM. Appropriate use of antitussives and protussives: a practical review. Drugs 1993; 46: 80-91
62. Hatch RT, Carpenter GB, Smith LJ. Treatment options in the child with a chronic cough. Drugs 1993; 45: 367-73
63. Conway SP, Leese B. Routine childhood immunization: is it worth it? PharmacoEconomics 1993; 3: 183-91
64. Blumberg DA, Mink C, Cherry JD, et al. Comparison of acellular and whole-cell pertussis component diphtheria-tetanus-pertussis vaccines in infants. Journal of Pediatrics 1991; 119: 194-204
65. Leer JA, Green JL, Heimlich EM, et al. Corticosteroid treatment in bronchiolitis: a controlled, collaborative study in 297 infants and children. American Journal of Diseases of Children 1969; 117: 495
66. Britton S, Bejstedt M, Vedin L. Chest physiotherapy in primary pneumonia. British Medical Journal 1985; 290: 1703
67. Davies A, Jenkins HR. Management of gastroenteritis in early childhood. Drugs 1992; 44: 57-64
68. Reis EC, Goepp JG, Katz S, et al. Barriers to use of oral rehydration therapy. Pediatrics 1994; 93: 708-11

69. Gracey M. Oral therapy for acute diarrhoea. Medical Journal of Australia 1984; 40: 348
70. Pai CH, Gillis F, Tuomanen E, et al. Erythromycin treatment of Campylobacter enteritis in children. American Journal of Diseases of Children 1983; 137: 286
71. Bailey RR. Single dose therapy of urinary tract infection. Sydney: Adis Health Science Press, 1983: 53
72. App EM, King M, Helfesrieder R, et al. Acute and long-term amiloride inhalation in cystic fibrosis lung disease: a rational approach to cystic fibrosis therapy. American Review of Respiratory Disease 1990; 141: 605-12
73. Knudsen FU. Optimum management of febrile seizures in childhood. Drugs 1988; 36: 111-20
74. Offringa M, Bossuyt PM, Lubsen J, et al. Risk factors for seizures recurrence in children with febrile seizures: a pooled analysis of individual patient data from five studies. Journal of Pediatrics 1994; 124: 574-84
75. O'Dougherty M, Wright FS, Cox S, et al. Carbamazepine plasma concentration: relationship to cognitive impairment. Archives of Neurology 1987; 44: 863-7
76. Boner AL, Piacentini GL. Inhaled corticosteroids in children: is there a 'safe' dosage? Drug Safety 1993; 9: 9-20
77. Bengoa JM. The problem of malnutrition. World Health Organization Chronicle 1974; 28: 3
78. Gaukroger PB. Paediatric analgesia. Drugs 1991; 41: 52-9
79. Steward DJ, editor. Management of childhood pain: new approaches to procedure-related pain. Journal of Pediatrics 1993; 122 Suppl. 5
80. Walson PD, Graves PS, Mortensen ME, et al. Patient-controlled versus conventional analgesia for postsurgical pain relief in adolescents. Developmental Pharmacology and Therapeutics 1992; 19: 32-9
81. US Department of Health and Human Services. Acute pain management: clinical practice guideline. US Government Printing Office: 312-092/73727, 1992
82. Dechant KL, Faulds D. Colfosceril palmitate: a review of the therapeutic efficacy and clinical tolerability of a synthetic surfactant preparation (Exosurf$^{R}$ Neonatal) in neonatal respiratory distress syndrome. Drugs 1991; 42: 877-94
83. Merritt TA, Hallman M, Spragg R, et al. Exogenous surfactant treatments for neonatal respiratory distress syndrome and their potential role in the adult respiratory distress syndrome. Drugs 1989; 38: 591-611
84. Mugford M, Howard S. Cost effectiveness of surfactant replacement in preterm babies. PharmacoEcononics 1993; 3: 362-73
85. Rubaltelli FF, Griffith PF. Management of neonatal hyperbilirubinaemia and prevention of kernicterus. Drugs 1992; 43: 864-72
86. Walker PC. Neonatal bilirubin toxicity: a review of kernicterus and the implications of drug-induced bilirubin displacement. Clinical Pharmacokinetics 1987; 13: 26-50

Chapter 4

# Geriatric Clinical Pharmacology and Therapeutics

***B.J. Cusack, C.P. Nielson*** and ***R.E. Vestal***

## Synopsis of Important Principles

1) In elderly patients, the decreased renal and hepatic clearance of some drugs increases the risk of adverse drug reactions.

2) Drug concentrations achieved for a given dose, the duration of drug activity, and the organ response to a given drug concentration may be altered in elderly patients.

3) Normal homeostatic responses to drug-induced perturbations are impaired with aging.

4) Elderly patients frequently experience multiple illnesses and take many drugs concurrently.

5) The combination of altered drug activity, impaired homeostasis, and the use of multiple drugs by elderly patients results in frequent adverse drug reactions.

6) Although they can be difficult to recognise in elderly patients, adverse drug reactions are a frequent cause of morbidity and may precipitate hospitalisation.

7) Because the risk of adverse drug reactions increases with the number of drugs taken, it is important to discontinue any treatment that is not efficacious.

8) Because of neurological, visual and auditory disabilities, elderly patients may have difficulty complying with complicated drug regimens.

9) Some chronic diseases in elderly patients cannot be effectively treated with drugs.

10) The importance of a critical and conservative approach to drug therapy in elderly patients cannot be overemphasised.

Pharmacological responses are altered with age and adverse drug reactions occur frequently in elderly patients. Older patients often have multiple chronic diseases that require concurrent medications. Because organ function and pharmacological responses are more variable among individuals as age increases the effects of standard doses are difficult to predict. Increased drug use, decreased predictability of response, and increased susceptibility to adverse reactions are among the factors that complicate effective therapeutic intervention in elderly patients. This chapter discusses the mechanisms of altered pharmacological responses and outlines a general approach to therapeutic management. Examples are given of disease entities in which pharmacological intervention is altered in elderly patients. For more detailed reviews on geriatric clinical pharmacology, see Bressler and Katz;[1] Montamat et al.;[2] Vestal and Cusack;[3] Durnas et al.;[4] and Vestal et al.[5]

## 1. General Considerations

The number and proportion of elderly people in the population are increasing as a result of decreasing birth rates and medical and economic factors that favour a longer life expectancy. 100 years ago, only 2% of the population was over 65 years of age. In 1990, 12.6%, or more than 31 million people, in the US were over 65 years of age and by 2050 the proportion may increase to 20%. While the elderly population as a whole grew 22% from 1980 to 1990, the number of individuals aged over 85 years increased by 38% during the same 10-year period and will nearly double by the 21st century. These demographic considerations have important ramifications both economically and for the practice of medicine.

In 1988, Americans spent $27.1 billion on prescription medications and $14.8 billion on nonprescription medications and other nondurable medical products. Elderly patients, who constituted 12% of the population in 1988, accounted for 35% of prescription drug expenditures in that year.[6] Similarly, in the UK, where elderly patients represent a similar percentage of the population, they are responsible for about 30% of drug costs.[7] With increasing medical knowledge, advances in technology and a greater variety of expensive therapeutic agents, the cost will continue to increase.

### 1.1 Drug Usage and Frequency of Adverse Reactions in Elderly Patients

Adverse drug reactions are an important cause of morbidity and hospital admission.[8] Risk factors include the number of diseases prior to admission and the number of drugs used.[9] 85 to 95% of ambulatory elderly take at least 1 medication, with an average of 3 to 4.[10,11] In a large, multicentre study, adverse reactions were a contributing cause in 10.5% of consecutive geriatric admissions.[12] Common adverse drug effects include confusion, ataxia, falls, postural hypotension, urinary retention, and constipation. Antihypertensives, anti-Parkinsonian agents, antipsychotic drugs and sedatives were the most common causes of significant adverse reactions. Thus, a careful drug history which includes over-the-counter medications is particularly important in elderly patients.

Although some studies have shown that the incidence of adverse drug reactions increases with age and may be as high as 10 to 25%, a rate that is 2- or 3-fold higher than in younger patients, the notion that age is a critical predisposing determinant of adverse reactions is controversial.[13,14] In fact, the incidence of adverse drug reactions increased with age in only 5 of 12 studies that evaluated age as a variable.[13] Of 5 studies in outpatients, only 2 showed an increased incidence with age. Two showed no effect, and 1 showed a U-shaped relationship between adverse drug reactions and age. Among 4 studies of hospital admission due to adverse drug reactions, 2 showed an increase with age and 2 showed no effect.[13] Many studies do not control adequately for disease severity, prevalence of drug use and type of drug taken. When prevalence of diseases and drug use has been considered, the numbers of diseases and drugs used, rather than age *per se*, are determinants of the frequency of adverse drug reactions.[9,15] Under-recognition of adverse effects in and by geriatric patients is also a factor to be considered.[16]

### 1.2 Importance of a Critical and Conservative Approach to Drug Therapy

Treatment of elderly patients requires careful consideration of whether the therapeutic objectives are symptomatic relief, disease suppression or cure. In the US, using a discrete state model, at the age of 65 years, a male has a life expectancy of 15.4 years, and a female of 20.9

**Table I.** Factors affecting drug disposition in the geriatric patients (adapted from Vestal & Dawson;[18] reproduced with permission)

| Pharmacokinetic variable affected | Age-related physiological changes | Pathological conditions | Therapeutic and environmental factors |
|---|---|---|---|
| Absorption | Increased gastric pH<br>Decreased absorptive surface<br>Decreased splanchnic blood flow<br>Decreased gastrointestinal motility | Achlorhydria<br>Diarrhoea<br>Postgastrectomy<br>Malabsorption syndromes<br>Pancreatitis | Drug interactions (e.g. antacids, anticholinergics, cholestyramine)<br>Food/meals |
| Distribution | Decreased cardiac output<br>Decreased total body water<br>Decreased lean body mass<br>Decreased serum albumin concentration<br>Increased $\alpha_1$-acid glycoprotein concentration<br>Increased proportion of body fat | Congestive heart failure<br>Dehydration<br>Oedema or ascites<br>Hepatic failure<br>Malnutrition<br>Renal failure | |
| Metabolism | Decreased hepatic mass<br>Decreased hepatic blood flow | Congestive heart failure<br>Fever<br>Hepatic insufficiency<br>Malignancy<br>Malnutrition<br>Thyroid disease<br>Viral infection or immunisation | Dietary composition<br>Drug interactions<br>Insecticides<br>Tobacco (smoking) |
| Excretion | Decreased renal blood flow<br>Decreased glomerular filtration rate<br>Decreased tubular secretion | Hypovolaemia<br>Renal failure | Drug interactions |

years. At age 75, this decreases to 9.8 years for a male and 14 years for a female.[17] Because life expectancy remains over 5 years even at age 85, definitive, curative intervention is often preferable to long term symptomatic treatment. The ability of elderly patients to tolerate surgery or toxic drug therapy is highly variable and an individual's mental status, cardiorespiratory condition, and quality of life are only a few of the factors that must be considered. Appropriate decisions require physician judgement and participation of the patient and his or her family.

Many disease states in elderly patients are chronic and symptoms are not always effectively treated with medications. Because of the increased frequency of adverse drug reactions and interactions with multiple medications, it is important that therapeutic effectiveness be continually re-evaluated and unnecessary agents discontinued. The need for a critical and conservative approach to drug therapy in elderly patients cannot be overemphasised.

## 2. Determinants of Altered Drug Responsiveness in Elderly Patients

Cross-sectional analysis demonstrates that a progressive decline in many parameters of physiological function occurs with aging and may influence the disposition of drugs in geriatric patients (table I). Impaired organ function, which may result from prior disease as well as from aging, alters drug kinetics, organ response and homeostatic counter-regulation to drug effect. The intensity and duration of drug action is determined mainly by the concentration of unbound drug at the site of action (see chapter 1; sect. 1.2), which in turn is related to drug absorption, distribution and elimination. Although absorption does not change with age for most drugs, distribution and metabolism or excretion may be altered and thus the dosage of some drugs must be adjusted. In addition, the physiological response to a standard drug concentration and the homeostatic response to a pharmacologically-induced stress may be altered in elderly patients. Thus changes in pharmacokinetics, end-organ response, and homeostatic regulation alter the pharmacological response and may predispose elderly patients to adverse drug reactions (fig. 1). It must be recognised that variability between individuals increases with age and generalisations concerning drug response in elderly patients are not equally applicable to all patients. Drug therapy must be individualised in each patient with careful monitoring of therapeutic effectiveness and attention to the development of adverse effects.

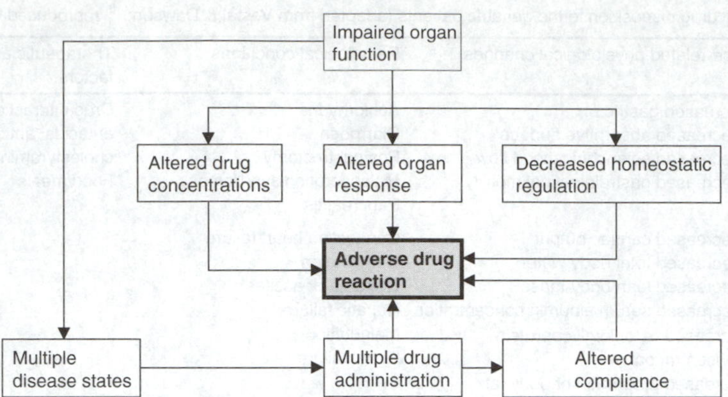


**Fig. 1.** Factors contributing to adverse drug reactions in elderly patients.

## 2.1 Pharmacokinetic Factors

### *2.1.1 Drug Absorption and Bioavailability*

The amount of drug that reaches the systemic circulation (bioavailability) following oral drug administration depends on gastrointestinal absorption and presystemic metabolism during its first passage through the gastrointestinal mucosa and the liver. Changes in gastrointestinal function with aging include an increase in gastric pH,[19] delayed gastric emptying, decreased motility, and decreased intestinal blood flow.[20] The absorption of substances that are actively transported from the intestinal lumen including some sugars, minerals and vitamins may therefore be decreased in elderly patients. However, most drugs are passively absorbed and, although the rate of absorption may be slightly decreased, major alterations with aging have not been identified.[3]

In contrast, pathological or surgical alterations in gastrointestinal function and concurrent administration of other drugs may cause significant changes in drug absorption. Specific examples of the former include gastrectomy, pyloric stenosis, pancreatitis, regional enteritis, and malabsorption syndromes.[21] Concurrently administered cholestyramine binds and decreases the absorption of many drugs including thiazides, phenobarbital, anticoagulants, thyroxine, digitalis glycosides, aspirin (acetylsalicylic acid), paracetamol (acetaminophen) and penicillin, while antacids decrease the absorption of drugs such as chlorpromazine, tetracycline, cimetidine, isoniazid and penicillamine. Drugs with anticholinergic activity such as propantheline decrease motility and delay (but do not necessarily decrease) the absorption of various other drugs.[22] Thus, although major changes in drug absorption from age alone have not been identified, the effects of disease and concurrent drug therapy may be important.

Following absorption, drugs pass through the portal system to the liver. Agents such as propranolol and the nitrates are subject to significant first-pass hepatic extraction which reduces their bioavailability. With aging, such hepatic extraction may be altered. For example, increased plasma concentrations of propranolol following oral administration in elderly patients may be related to decreased hepatic extraction.[23]

### *2.1.2 Drug Distribution*

Drug distribution is determined by body composition, plasma protein binding, and organ blood flow. Total body water and lean body mass decrease with age. As a result of these changes in body composition, use of standardised drug dosages in elderly patients may be expected to produce higher drug concentrations in the blood. Drugs that distribute primarily in body water may exhibit increased blood concentrations if a dose calculated on the basis of total bodyweight or surface area is given. This has been demonstrated for ethanol. Ethanol distributes in body water but its metabolism is not altered in elderly patients.[24] Body fat as a percentage of bodyweight increases with aging until the age of 85 years and then decreases. Increased body fat will increase the volume of distribution of fat-soluble drugs such as the benzodiazepines with a resultant decrease in the concentration and a more prolonged drug effect. Thus, it was demonstrated[25] that the elimination half-life of diazepam was prolonged with age despite the fact that systemic clearance was

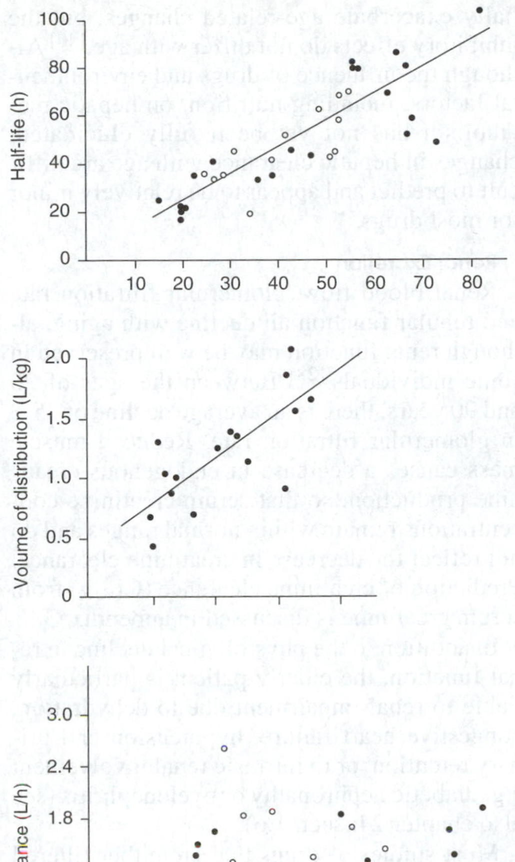


**Fig. 2.** Relationship between age and diazepam elimination half-life (upper panel), volume of distribution (middle panel), and total plasma clearance (lower panel) in health volunteers (after Klotz et al.,[25] with permission).

unaltered (fig. 2). The prolonged half-life was related to the increased volume of distribution with age. However, despite theoretical considerations, many drugs do not exhibit the expected change in volume of distribution with aging.

Change in organ blood flow with aging may also affect the rate of drug distribution. Some cross-sectional studies indicate that cardiac output decreases and peripheral vascular resistance increases with age.[26] Hepatic and renal blood flow are decreased[27,28] and an increased fraction of cardiac output is distributed to the brain, heart and skeletal muscle.[29] Although many of these changes are at least partly a result of prior illness, the average elderly patient will probably have altered blood flow compared with younger patients.

Plasma protein concentrations may also be altered in elderly patients, although the significance of this in terms of altered drug effects is negligible if there is no concomitant alteration in elimination capacity (metabolism or excretion) – which of course there may be in this age group (see section 2.1.3 below), and indeed it is the possible change in drug elimination capacity that is of most importance in this context. In 80-year-old individuals, some studies have shown that plasma albumin concentrations are approximately 20% less than in 20-year-olds, and the binding of many drugs predominantly bound to this protein may therefore be decreased. In contrast, the concentration of $\alpha_1$-acid glycoprotein may be increased in the presence of chronic diseases that frequently occur in the elderly population,[30] potentially increasing the binding of drugs such as antidepressants, antipsychotic drugs and β-blockers which are mainly bound to this protein. However, there is no known clinical relevance of these changes in plasma protein binding, except for the interpretation of measured drug concentrations (see chapter 5, sect. 1.6.3).

### 2.1.3 Drug Elimination

The principal mechanisms of drug elimination are hepatic metabolism and renal excretion. If drug elimination is decreased, the effects of a single dose are prolonged and the steady-state concentration is increased if the dosage is not adjusted.

#### Hepatic Metabolism

Although *in vitro* studies in animals suggest that both basal activity and inducibility of the hepatic microsomal mixed-function oxidase enzymes may be reduced with age, these alterations have not been demonstrated clearly in humans.[31,32] Hepatic blood flow and liver mass change in proportion to bodyweight and decrease with aging.[27]

Because phenazone (antipyrine) is minimally protein bound and is almost completely metabolised by the hepatic cytochrome P450 enzyme system prior to excretion, it is used as an index of hepatic metabolism. Although studies are not entirely in agreement, most data indicate a prolonged phenazone half-life and reduced metabolic clearance in elderly individuals. The clinical significance of any decrease is unclear since interindividual variation (6-fold) greatly exceeds the effect of age, which accounts for only 3% of the variance.[33]

The rate of metabolism of many drugs by the cytochrome P450 enzyme system is decreased by 20 to 40% with aging.[4] Examples include theophylline, propranolol, nortriptyline, alfentanil, fentanyl, trazodone, alprazolam, triazolam, diltiazem, verapamil, and levodopa.[4] Many benzodiazepines are metabolised by microsomal enzymes to active metabolites which are also eliminated by hepatic metabolism. Chlordiazepoxide, diazepam, clorazepate and prazepam are all converted to nordazepam (*N*-desmethyldiazepam), which has an elimination half-life as long as 220 hours in elderly patients. The age-related decline in clearance of some benzodiazepines has been shown to be more pronounced in males than females,[34,35] although reduced metabolism is a potential clinical problem in either sex. Non-microsomal enzyme pathways may be less affected by age. Thus, there is little effect of aging on the elimination of isoniazid, rifampicin, paracetamol (acetaminophen), valproic acid, salicylate, indomethacin and oxprenolol.[4] However, other studies have shown that the elimination of paracetamol, ketoprofen, salicylate, naproxen and morphine is reduced in elderly patients.[4]

Benzodiazepines that primarily undergo conjugation in the liver and are without active metabolites include oxazepam, lorazepam and temazepam (although oxazepam is a minor metabolite of temazepam). Cumulative or prolonged sedative effects may be less likely with these compounds because they have shorter half-lives and their elimination may be unaltered with aging.[4] Ethanol metabolism by alcohol dehydrogenase[24] and isoniazid elimination by acetylation[36] are unchanged in elderly patients. Although it is controversial whether drug acetylation (see chapter 1; sect. 3.3) is altered with age, a large study in healthy volunteers did not demonstrate a clinically important effect of age or gender.[37]

Concurrent drug administration, illness, genetics and environmental factors including smoking may have more important effects on hepatic drug metabolism than age. Although the data are not entirely consistent,[38] causes of enzyme induction such as smoking may have less effect in elderly than in young patients.[39] In contrast, drugs that decrease microsomal enzyme activity (such as cimetidine) may potentially exacerbate age-related changes, but the inhibitory effects do not differ with age.[40] Although the influence of drugs and environmental factors, including nutrition, on hepatic metabolism has not yet been fully elucidated, changes in hepatic clearance with age are difficult to predict and appear to be relatively minor for most drugs.

#### Renal Excretion

Renal blood flow, glomerular filtration rate and tubular function all decline with aging, although renal function may be well preserved in some individuals.[28] Between the ages of 20 and 90 years, there is an average decline of 35% in glomerular filtration rate. Reduced muscle mass causes a decrease in endogenous creatinine production, so that serum creatinine concentrations remain within normal ranges and do not reflect the decrease in creatinine clearance. Prediction of creatinine clearance ($CL_{CR}$) from serum creatinine is discussed in appendix G.

In addition to the physiological decline in renal function, the elderly patient is particularly liable to renal impairment due to dehydration, congestive heart failure, hypotension and urinary retention, or to intrinsic renal involvement e.g. diabetic nephropathy or pyelonephritis (see also chapter 24; sect. 1.6).

Most studies of drugs that are either filtered or secreted have identified an age-related decrease in excretion that correlates with altered renal function. Altered drug excretion generally parallels decreases in glomerular filtration. Drugs with significant toxicity that have diminished renal excretion with age include allopurinol, aminoglycosides, amantadine, lithium, digoxin, procainamide, chlorpropamide and cimetidine. These agents may have reduced clearance, prolonged half-lives and increased steady-state concentrations if dosages are not adjusted for renal function (see also chapter 24, sect. 11 and appendix D).

### 2.2 Pharmacodynamic Factors

In addition to changes in absorption, distribution, metabolism or excretion that may alter unbound drug concentrations, organ response and homeostatic counter-regulation may be altered with aging. Sites of drug action include cell surface receptors, intracellular receptors, enzymes and membrane ion channels. In the case of receptor agonists, tissue response is dependent on receptor binding, intracellular stimulus re-

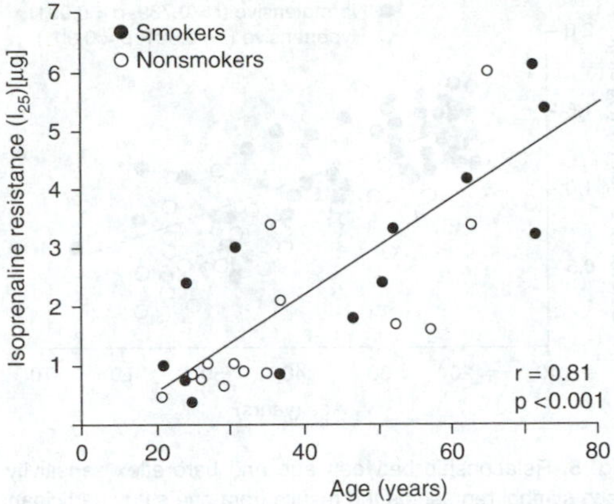


**Fig. 3.** Relationship between age and isoprenaline (isoproterenol) sensitivity (as determined by the dose of isoprenaline required to increase heart rate by 25 beats/min) in 27 healthy male volunteers, aged 21 to 73 years (after Vestal et al.[41]).

sponse coupling, and activation of effector mechanisms. The physiological response includes both the direct drug effect and the homeostatic responses to that pharmacological effect. Decreased homeostatic counter-regulation with aging may be a significant cause of adverse drug reactions.

### 2.2.1 Receptor Sensitivity

β-Adrenoceptor function in elderly patients has been more extensively studied than other receptor responses. Because the intravenous dose of isoprenaline (isoproterenol) that produces an increase in the heart rate of 25 beats/min is increased in elderly individuals compared with that in the young (fig. 3),[41] it appears that the β-adrenoceptor response is decreased with aging.

In rats, β-adrenoceptor density decreases with age in adipose tissue and in most brain areas, but the density is unchanged in lymphocytes, heart and lung and it increases in liver. In humans, there are no receptor density changes in either lymphocytes or brain.[42] However, the number of high-affinity receptors, which are coupled to adenylate cyclase, decreases with age in most tissues.

There is also a decrease in membrane adenylate cyclase activity with an associated decrease in the production of cyclic-AMP in response to stimulation with isoprenaline in a variety of tissues. It has been suggested that β-adrenoceptor agonist affinity is decreased with aging, perhaps secondary to elevated plasma catecholamine concentrations.[43]

Evidence that receptors other than β-adrenoceptors are altered with aging is not well established. However, elderly patients are known to be more sensitive to psychotherapeutic drugs. Impairment of psychomotor function by benzodiazepines, for example, occurs at lower concentrations in elderly than in young patients; altered responses have been demonstrated with nitrazepam[44] and diazepam.[45] Elderly patients appear to be more sensitive to the effects of morphine, warfarin, diltiazem, verapamil, enalapril and levodopa.[46] Also, adverse effects may be more frequent in elderly patients even when unbound drug concentrations are similar to those in the young. Increased receptor sensitivity has not been established, and these changes are likely due to a combination of increased tissue sensitivity, decreased ability to compensate for altered CNS function, and altered pharmacokinetic characteristics causing increased or prolonged tissue exposure. For example, the effect of triazolam on sedation is increased in elderly patients due to altered pharmacokinetics rather than to changes in sensitivity.[47] Interindividual variation in most physiological parameters also increases with age and drug effects may be difficult to predict in any one patient. Because sensitivity to drug effects is often increased and adverse reactions are common, initial doses should be low and the final dose adjusted according to individual tolerability.

There is also strong evidence that benzodiazepines contribute to falls in elderly patients.[35] Central nervous system (CNS) adverse effects including confusion, disorientation, agitation or sedation are more common in elderly patients with tricyclic antidepressants, phenothiazines, anticholinergic drugs, barbiturates, levodopa, and cimetidine.

### 2.2.2 Impaired Homeostasis

Homeostatic regulation requires appropriate sensing of an altered physiological state (whether due to disease or therapeutic intervention), endocrine or neurological transmission of sensory and regulatory signals, and appropriate organ compensatory responses. Impaired homeostasis is a frequent cause of adverse drug reactions as well as increased sensitivity to drug effects. For example, older individuals have an impaired ability to excrete free water load. Addition of hydrochlorothiazide further impairs free water excretion in elderly patients, placing the patient at risk of dilutional hyponatraemia (fig. 4).[48] The ability of younger individuals to excrete free water, when given ibuprofen, approaches that in elderly study participants. This suggests that the defect in elderly patients may be due to lower renal prostaglandin production.

Most clinicians recognise the susceptibility of elderly patients to congestive heart failure from the rapid infusion of saline. Cardiac output, renal function and possibly endocrine response to volume overload are all decreased with age. Although adequate to maintain homeostasis under normal circumstances, decreased glomerular filtration prevents the rapid excretion of a saline excess.

Volume depletion is also a risk. While the senescent kidney is able to decrease urinary sodium to low concentrations, the adaptive response is delayed and extracellular fluid loss may be significant during this period.[49] Volume depletion is further exacerbated by diminished plasma renin activity, the basal level of which is decreased by 30 to 50% in elderly patients. The relative decrease with age becomes greater following salt restriction, diuretic therapy, or upright posture.[50] Decreased renin may not only exacerbate the hypotensive effects of volume depletion, but is also associated with reduced aldosterone which impairs renal sodium conservation.

Postural hypotension is frequent in elderly individuals and may be exacerbated by many

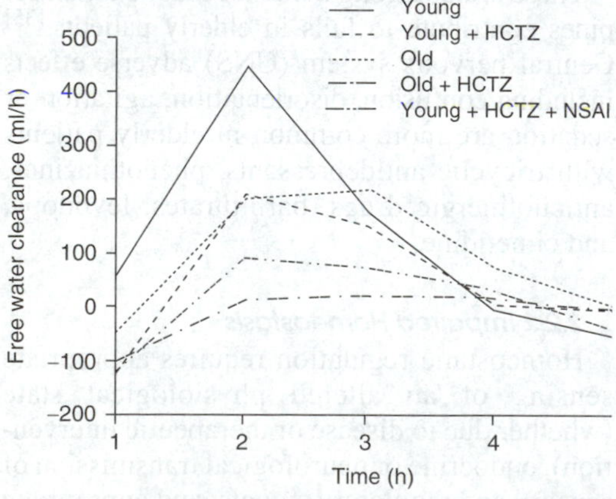


**Fig. 4.** The effect of age, hydrochlorothiazide (HCTZ) and ibuprofen (NSAI) on free water clearance after ingesting 20 ml/kg water load over 30 minutes. Free water clearance values are lower in elderly patients and the difference is increased following hydrochlorothiazide (100 mg/day for 3 days). When young volunteers were given both HCTZ and ibuprofen, their free water clearance became similar to that in the elderly individuals pretreated with HCTZ alone (after Clark et al.;[48] with permission).

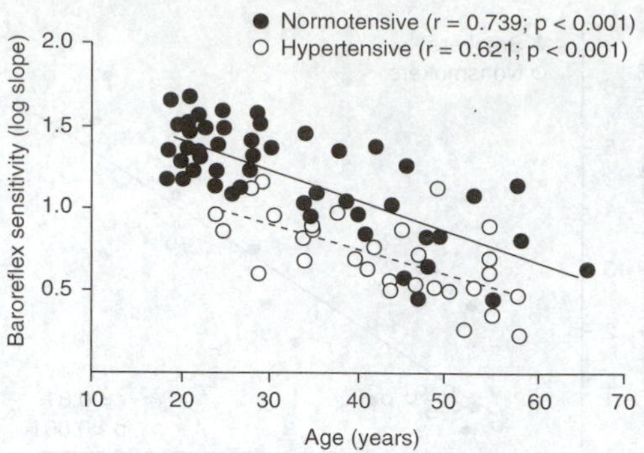


**Fig. 5.** Relationship between age and baroreflex sensitivity. Each symbol represents the results from one study participant (after Gribben et al.[51]).

drugs. The pathogenesis is probably multifactorial and includes decreased baroreceptor response, altered sympathetic activity and responsiveness, impaired vasomotor response in both arterioles and veins, and altered volume regulation. The baroreceptor response to changes in blood pressure is decreased and slower in elderly patients (fig. 5). However, sympathetic nervous system activity, as reflected by the plasma noradrenaline concentration, is increased;[52] basal noradrenaline concentrations and the increment with standing, cold pressor testing, and exercise are equal or increased in elderly as compared with young patients.

Although multifactorial in aetiology, decreased vasomotor response and increased venous capacitance may be the most important mechanisms of postural hypotension in elderly patients. Drugs that alter CNS function, sympathetic activity, vasomotor response, cardiac function, or volume regulation may exacerbate postural changes in blood pressure. Phenothiazines, tricyclic antidepressants, levodopa, antihypertensive drugs and diuretics are frequent causes of postural hypotension seen in clinical practice. Elderly patients who are at risk of fracture from falls must be observed carefully and have medication dosages adjusted slowly.

## 3. Principles of Prescribing Drugs for Elderly Patients

Elderly patients may have multiple disease states and may use a wide variety of drugs, increasing the potential for altered responsiveness to drugs and a higher incidence of adverse effects compared with the younger patient.[2,5] Thus, it is important to define certain basic principles of prescribing for the older patient before initiating therapy.

1) *Is drug therapy required?*

Many of the diseases which elderly patients experience either do not require treatment or are not effectively treated with available medications. Certainly, identification of a pathological process does not invariably require institution of drug therapy. Indeed, it is surprising how often elderly patients are better off without some drugs. Many old people admitted to hospital or reviewed during long term hospitalisation improve greatly when the regimen of drugs that they have been taking is stopped.[53,54] This also means that a drug should not be used for longer than necessary; the need for repeat prescriptions should be reviewed at periodic intervals.

These edicts do not mean, however, that drugs should be withheld on account of old age, particularly when appropriate drug treatment can improve the elderly person's quality of life.

2) *If drug treatment is required, which drug is appropriate?*

The margin between therapeutic effect and toxicity is so small in many cases that a drug which is indicated for a particular condition in younger patients may be unsuitable in elderly patients with the same condition. For example, the age-related toxicity of benzodiazepines with long half-lives has made the use of these drugs undesirable in elderly patients. Other types of hypnotics may be more appropriate (see section 4.8.3). Other drugs considered by some experts as inappropriate for use in elderly patients, at least in nursing homes, include amitriptyline, barbiturates, reserpine, indomethacin, chlorpromamide, dextropropoxyphene, pentazocine, cyclandelate, isoxuprine and dipyridamole.[55] The possibility of enabling drug abuse and dependence by inappropriate prescribing must also be considered when treating older patients.[56]

3) *Is the patient being asked to take more drugs than are tolerable or manageable?*

The smallest number drugs that the patient actually needs should always be used. The greater the number of drugs prescribed the greater the chance of adverse drug reactions (see also chapter 6) or drug interactions (see chapter 7). The likelihood of toxicity increases as the number of drugs prescribed rises.

In addition, there is an increased likelihood of errors by the patient in taking the medication, leading to a possible lack of efficacy or an increase in toxicity. Although most studies have failed to show a relationship between age and compliance, it still represents an important problem.[57] Noncompliance with medication regimens has been implicated as leading to hospitalisation in over 10% of hospitalised older patients.[58] Medication errors, especially errors of omission, noncomprehension and noncompliance with medication instructions, have long been recognised as occurring in elderly patients.[59,60] Slowness of comprehension and lapses of memory, particularly short term memory, which deteriorates with age, make it difficult for elderly patients to manage complex drug regimens.

4) *Which type of preparation should be used?*

The dosage form and the size, shape and colour of tablets and capsules, and their similarity to one another are all important considerations in prescribing drugs for elderly patients.[61] Many older people have difficulty in swallowing; consequently, large tablets and capsules should be avoided. There is a good case for the use of liquid preparations such as syrups for many patients, or of effervescent tablets. On occasion, suppositories may be the most suitable method of administration.

Many tablets and capsules with widely differing pharmacological actions are of similar size, shape and colour. This causes confusion for the patient. In particular, loss of vision in elderly patients makes it difficult for them to determine which preparation they are taking. Touch and colour vision, however, are well preserved in this patient population. Thus preparations to be used together should have distinctive colour and shape.

The more distinctive the pill is, the easier and safer it is to use.

5) *Should the standard dosage or dosage schedule be modified?*

As a rule, the elderly patient requires smaller doses of drugs than are customarily given to the young adult. Examples are the starting dose of thyroxine, due to increased risk of cardiac ischaemia, and the maintenance dose of digoxin, which is reduced because of decreased renal clearance (see also section 4.1.6). Drugs usually given in reduced dosage in elderly patients are shown in table II.

Whenever possible, intermittent schedules such as drugs given on alternate days or 5 days a week, should be avoided, since they are rarely followed accurately. Once-daily dosage ensures better compliance than more frequent regimens.[64] Apart from convenience to the pa-

**Table II.** Summary of important pharmacokinetic and pharmacodynamic changes in the elderly, guidelines for dosage adjustment, and common adverse effects in this age group[a]

| Drug | Pharmacokinetic changes | | | | Sensitivity | Dosage adjustment | Common adverse effects |
|---|---|---|---|---|---|---|---|
| | absorption or bioavailability | volume of distribution | clearance | half-life | | | |
| **Lipid-lowering drugs** | | | | | | | |
| Cholestyramine | | | | | | Indications unclear | Nausea, constipation |
| Clofibrate | | | | | | Indications unclear | Nausea, gallstones |
| Nicotinic acid | | | | | | Indications unclear | Flushing, glucose intolerance |
| Pravastatin | | | | | ↔ | None | |
| Simvastatin | | | | | ↔ | None | |
| **Antihypertensive drugs** | | | | | | | |
| β-*Adrenoceptor antagonists:* | | | | | | None | Increased with age: bronchospasm, congestive heart failure, peripheral vascular insufficiency |
| Atenolol | ↑ or ↔ | ↔ | ↔ | ↔ | | | |
| Metoprolol | ↓ or ↔ | | | ↓ or ↔ | | | |
| Pindolol | | | | ↔ | | | |
| Propranolol | ↑ or ↔ | ↔ | ↓ or ↔ | ↑ or ↔ | ↓ | | |
| Labetalol | ↑ | ↔ | ↔ | | | | |
| $\alpha_1$-*Adrenoceptor antagonists:* | | | | | | | |
| Doxazosin/terazosin | | | | | | None | Dizziness, headache |
| Prazosin | ↓ | ↑ | ↓ | | | Initial decrease | Orthostatic hypotension |
| *Calcium antagonists:* | | | | | | | |
| Dihydropyridines (e.g. nifedipine, amlodipine, felodipine) | | | | | ↔ | Initial decrease | |
| *ACE Inhibitors* | | | ↓ | ↔ | ↔ | Decrease | |
| *Centrally-acting drugs:* | | | | | | | |
| Methyldopa, clonidine | | | | | | None | Sedation, depression, impotence |
| **Diuretics** | | | | | | None | Orthostatic hypotension, hypokalaemia, hyponatraemia, glucose intolerance |
| Bumetanide | | | ↓ | | ↓ | | |
| Chlorthalidone | ↔ | | | ↑ | | | |
| Furosemide (frusemide) | | ↑ | ↓ | ↑ | Slow response | | |
| **Antianginal drugs** | | | | | | | |
| Nitrates | | | | | | | Hypotension |
| Verapamil | | | | ↑ | ↑ | | Conduction abnormalities |
| **Antiarrhythmic drugs** | | | | | | | |
| Amiodarone | | | | | | Decrease; monitor | |
| Sotalol | | | ↓ | ↑ | | Decrease; monitor | |
| Quinidine | | ↔ | ↓ | ↑ | | Decrease; monitor | Nausea, diarrhoea, arrhythmia |
| Procainamide | | | ↓ | | | Decrease; monitor | Nausea, lupus syndrome, arrhythmia |
| Disopyramide | | ↑ | ↓ | ↑ | | Avoid | Congestive heart failure, anticholinergic effects[b] |
| Lidocaine (lignocaine) | ↑ | ↑ or ↔ | ↔ or ↓ | ↑ | | Decrease; careful monitoring | Confusion |

**Table II.** *[Continued]*

| Drug | Pharmacokinetic changes | | | | Sensitivity | Dosage adjustment | Common adverse effects |
|---|---|---|---|---|---|---|---|
| | absorption or bioavailability | volume of distribution | clearance | half-life | | | |
| Digoxin | ↑ or ↔ | ↓ | ↓ | ↑ | | Decrease; monitor | Nausea, confusion, arrhythmia, vasoconstriction |
| **Anticoagulant, antiplatelet and antithrombotic drugs** | | | | | | | |
| Streptokinase | | | | | | | Increased risk of stroke in elderly |
| Alteplase (rt-PA) | | | | | | | Increased risk of stroke in elderly |
| Heparin | | ↔ | ↔ | ↔ | ↔ | None | Possible increased haemorrhage |
| Warfarin | | ↔ | ↔ | ↔ | ↑ or ↔ | Decrease initially | Possible increased haemorrhage |
| Ticlopidine | | | ↓ | ↑ | | Possible decrease in renal failure | Reversible neutropenia, diarrhoea, skin rash |
| Pentoxifylline | | | | | | Decrease in renal or hepatic failure | GI disturbance, dizziness, headache |
| Dextran | | | | | | None | Volume overload |
| **Pulmonary drugs** | | | | | | | |
| Theophylline | ↔ | ↑ or ↔ | ↓ or ↔ | ↔ or ↑ | | Decrease | Nausea, tremor, arrhythmia |
| $\beta_2$-Adrenoceptor agonists | | | | | ↓ | None | Tremor, arrhythmia |
| Beclomethasone dipropionate | | | | | | | Oropharyngeal candidiasis |
| Isoniazid | | | | ↔ | | None | Hepatitis |
| **Antibacterial drugs** | | | | | | | |
| Aminoglycosides | | ↑ or ↔ | ↓ or ↔ | ↑ or ↔ | | Decrease; monitor | Ototoxic, nephrotoxic |
| Cefalosporins | | | | ↑ | | Decrease | |
| Penicillins | | ↔ | | ↑ | | Decrease | Seizures |
| Nitrofurantoin | | | ↓ | | | Avoid if impaired renal function | |
| **Endocrine drugs** | | | | | | | |
| Estrogens | | | | | | | Gallbladder disease, possible endometrial carcinoma, exacerbation of breast cancer |
| Propylthiouracil | ↔ | ↔ | ↔ | | | None | |
| Thyroxine | | | ↓ | | | Initial very low dose | Angina, arrhythmia |
| Corticosteroids | | | | | | | Osteoporosis |
| Chlorpropamide | | | ↓ or ↔ | ↔ | | Decrease | Hypoglycaemia, hyponatraemia |
| Tolbutamide | | | ↔ | ↔ | ↓ or ↔ | | Hypoglycaemia |
| Sulphonylureas | | | | | | | Hypoglycaemia |
| Metformin | | | ↓ | | | Decrease; monitor blood glucose and renal function | Lactic acidosis |
| Insulin | ↔ | | ↓ | ↑ | | None | Hypoglycaemia |
| Calcium carbonate | ↓ | | | | | Give with meal | |

*[continued over]*

**Table II.** *[Continued]*

| Drug | Pharmacokinetic changes | | | | Sensitivity | Dosage adjustment | Common adverse effects |
|---|---|---|---|---|---|---|---|
| | absorption or bioavailability | volume of distribution | clearance | half-life | | | |
| **Antirheumatic drugs** | | | | | | | |
| Aspirin | ↔ | ↑ or ↔ | ↓ or ↔ | ↑ | | None | GI bleeding |
| Indomethacin | | | ↓ or ↔ | | | None | GI bleeding, renal dysfunction |
| **Gastrointestinal drugs** | | | | | | | |
| Cimetidine | ↑ or ↔ | ↓ | ↓ | ↔ | | Decrease | Confusion |
| Ranitidine | ↔ | | ↔ | | | None | |
| Omeprazole | ↑ | | ↓ | ↑ | | None | |
| Cisapride | | | | | | Decrease in renal or hepatic failure | GI disturbance |
| Metoclopramide | | | | | | None | Confusion, extrapyramidal symptoms (rare) |
| **Incontinence drugs** | | | | | | | |
| Oxybutynin | | | | | | Decrease, titrate slowly | Dry mouth, confusion, nausea, constipation, mydriasis and tachycardia |
| **Neurological drugs** | | | | | | | |
| Tacrine | | | | | | Increase slowly; monitor LFTs | Liver toxicity, GI disturbance |
| Levodopa | ↑ or ↔ | | | | ↑ or ↔ | Decrease | Hypotension, confusion |
| Phenytoin | | | ↓ or ↔ | | | Decrease; monitor | Ataxia |
| Carbamazepine | | | | | | Decrease; monitor | Ataxia, sedation |
| Phenobarbital | | | ↓ | | | Decrease; monitor | Confusion |
| **Psychotherapeutic drugs** | | | | | | | |
| Phenothiazines | | | | | | Decrease | Hypotension, anticholinergic effects[b], tardive dyskinesia, extrapyramidal symptoms |
| Risperidone | | | | | | Decrease | Sedation, insomnia |
| *Tricyclic antidepressants:* | | | | | | Decrease | Hypotension, anticholinergic effects[b] |
| Imipramine | | | ↓ or ↔ | ↑ or ↔ | | | |
| Desipramine | | | ↓ or ↔ | ↑ or ↔ | | | |
| *Other antidepressants:* | | | | | | | |
| Nefazodone | | | ↓ | | | Initial dosage decreased | |
| Venlafaxine | | | | | | Decrease in renal or hepatic failure | |
| *Mood-stabilising drugs:* | | | | | | | |
| Lithium | | | ↓ | | | Decrease | |
| *Benzodiazepines:* | | | | | ↑ | Decrease | Sedation, psychomotor impairment |
| Chlordiazepoxide | ↔ | ↑ | ↓ | ↑ | | | |
| Diazepam | | ↑ | ↓ or ↔ | ↑ | | | |
| Lorazepam | | ↔ | ↓ or ↔ | ↔ | | | |

**Table II.** *[Continued]*

| Drug | Pharmacokinetic changes | | | | Sensitivity | Dosage adjustment | Common adverse effects |
|---|---|---|---|---|---|---|---|
| | absorption or bioavailability | volume of distribution | clearance | half-life | | | |
| Oxazepam | ↔ | ↔ | ↔ | ↔ | | | |
| *Non-benzodiazepine hypnosedatives:* | | | | | | | |
| Zopiclone | | | | ↑ | | None | |
| Zolpidem | | | | ↑ | | Decrease | |
| *Analgesics and anaesthetics/skeletal muscle relaxants:* | | | | | | | |
| Paracetamol (acetaminophen) | ↔ | ↓ or ↔ | ↓ or ↔ | ↑ or ↔ | | None | |
| Pethidine (meperidine) | | ↔ | ↓ | ↑ | | Decrease | Confusion, seizures |
| Morphine | | | | ↑ or ↔ | ↑ or ↔ | Decrease | Confusion, respiratory depression |
| Halothane | | | | | ↑ | Decrease | |
| Pancuronium bromide | | ↔ | ↓ | ↑ | | Decrease | Delayed recovery |
| Thiopental | | ↑ | ↑ or ↔ | ↑ | | Decrease | |
| Tramadol | | | | ↑ | | Daily dosage not exceeding 300mg | Constipation, nausea, dizziness |

a Many studies have reached conflicting conclusions and data given here represent recent or most probable results. Discussion and references are included in the text as well as in reviews by Durnas et al.,[4] Plein & Plein,[62] Ouslander,[63] Vestal & Dawson.[18]

b Anticholinergic effects include confusion, blurred vision, tachycardia, increased intraocular pressure, dry mouth, urinary hesitancy or retention, constipation.

*Abbreviations:* ↑ = increased; ↓ = decreased; ↔ = unchanged; GI = gastrointestinal; SSRIs = selective serotonin reuptake inhibitors; LFTs = liver function tests; ACE = angiotensin-converting enzyme.

tient and thereby better patient compliance, once-daily dosage at night, for example of psychotherapeutic drugs,[65,66] may decrease troublesome adverse reactions since the patient would be asleep when these effects would be most annoying (see also sect. 4.7). Other drugs may be best given as a single dose in the morning, for example diuretics.

6) *Which adverse effects are likely to occur and which drugs should be avoided if possible?*

The elderly population differs from the young in that drugs more frequently lead to confusion and vague ill health. Drugs which act on various systems such as the gastrointestinal tract, for example, are more apt to produce gastrointestinal upset in the aged. Similarly, psychotherapeutic drugs may frequently induce markedly abnormal behavioural responses in older patients, while in younger patients these are much less common (see section 4.8).[67]

7) *Should the drug be specially packaged and labelled?*

Where possible, drugs prescribed for elderly patients living at home should be packaged in readily opened containers so that disabled patients in particular are able to use them.[68] Clear labelling in large print is also very important.[69] Blister packaging or unit dose packaging can reduce noncompliance significantly.[70,71] Elderly patients prefer medication organiser boxes to other compliance enhancers.[72]

8) *Can the patient living at home manage self medication?*

Elderly patients should be taught to understand the drugs they must take, particularly the relative importance of drugs to their well-being. Time should be spent to educate the patient in the use and administration of their regimen. Sometimes it may be necessary to provide clear instructions in writing about the manner in which a drug should be taken or to suggest the use of a diary or calendar to record daily drug administration.[73]

Collaboration with a responsible and interested relative, neighbour or friend can be helpful. Even with these and other considerations, discussed above, some drugs are best kept in the custody of others. Surveys have shown that many elderly patients living at home have potent drugs prescribed for them when they are mentally unfit to be responsible for their use.[74] It is imperative in such cases that a responsible relative should have charge of drug treatment. If there are no responsible relatives, it may be necessary to ask the community nurse to administer drug therapy. Sometimes these arrangements are necessary for physical reasons; for example, an elderly diabetic patient with impaired vision cannot be expected to measure out an injection of insulin with safety.

9) *Is there a need for continued medication?* When a drug such as digoxin has been prescribed in an acute episode (e.g. atrial fibrillation complicating pneumonia) there may be no reason for its continued use once the acute episode is satisfactorily treated. The same is true of many drugs commonly prescribed. It is useful to review treatment regularly and discontinue drugs that are no longer needed.[53]

Elderly patients tend to hoard drugs.[68] Accumulation of medication will only serve to confuse the patient and encourage use of drugs from prior treatment programmes. To aid in the review of old and current medication, patients should be encouraged to bring their containers to consultations in private practice and also in hospital outpatient departments. If their medications are outdated or clearly will not be required in the future, then this can be explained to the patient and the drugs discarded.

## 4. Optimum Drug Treatment in Elderly Patients

The principles of drug treatment which pertain to older patients are illustrated in this section by a discussion of certain clinical syndromes and symptoms that are frequently encountered in the care of elderly patients. Further discussion on these and other conditions occurring in elderly patients can be found in other chapters in this book. Guidelines for dosage adjustment of drugs commonly used in elderly patients are summarised in table II.

### 4.1 Disorders of the Cardiovascular System

The major cause of death in elderly patients is atherosclerotic disease; over 50% of deaths are due to coronary or cerebral infarction. The prevalence of significant coronary disease may be as high as 60% in men at the age of 60 years, although symptomatic disease is much less common.[75]

#### *4.1.1 Atherosclerosis*

*Hyperlipidaemia* is associated with an increased risk of ischaemic heart disease (IHD) and stroke in older persons. However, the relative risk of coronary disease in those over 65 years of age with high total cholesterol concentrations is less than in persons of younger age,[76] suggesting that high cholesterol loses power as a predictor of IHD. Nevertheless, since the absolute risk of coronary disease increases significantly with age, the total attributable risk of high cholesterol concentrations in fact increases with age.[77] Thus, lowering cholesterol concentrations theoretically may benefit more people of advanced age than those of middle age.

Using US National Cholesterol Education Program guidelines (which combine plasma cholesterol concentrations with other risk factors for IHD), one study performed in community-dwelling elderly people found that 36% of participants were eligible for treatment using a single cholesterol measurement.[78] This suggests that a substantial number of older persons are, in theory, candidates for lipid-lowering interventions. As yet, however, no studies have been performed to show the efficacy of cholesterol lowering in prevention of IHD in older people.

Similarly, the effects of drug therapy on non-IHD related mortality in older persons are unknown but their potential importance cannot be dismissed. Therefore, individualised clinical judgement is required in deciding whether to lower plasma cholesterol, with the patient's full understanding of the illness and its consequences. This should be based on an estimate of cardiovascular risk and on life expectancy. Primary prevention in the absence of other risk factors is likely to be of little benefit. The presence of other risk factors for IHD (e.g. hypertension, diabetes, obesity and left ventricular hypertrophy) may weight the decision in favour of initiating therapy. Secondary prevention is more justified, although it is not well documented in heart disease patients over 70 years of age. Frail patients with chronic disease or potentially fatal disease should not be subjected to the rigours of lipid-lowering therapy, since benefit is unlikely to be realised.

A low-fat, low-cholesterol diet is reasonable in older patients, provided that it does not jeopardise nutritional status. Many older patients may have difficulty in complying with a cholesterol-lowering diet. Patients should be advised to exercise as regularly as is tolerated. In those with higher LDL-cholesterol concentrations (>4.15 mmol/L; >160 mg/dl) despite these measures, many experts consider that drug therapy may be entertained in healthy, active persons, realising that the benefit is possible but not established.[77] Bile acid binding resins (e.g. cholestyramine, colestipol), nicotinic acid, clofibrate, and gemfibrozil have significant adverse effects that may be increased in elderly patients (see further chapter 20). However, HMG-CoA reductase inhibitors such as pravastatin and simvastatin appear well tolerated in the elderly population.[79,80]

### *4.1.2 Hypertension*

The prevalence of systolic and diastolic hypertension is high in elderly persons. Estimates in some studies show that in people over 65 years of age, less than 30% have diastolic blood pressure over 90mm Hg and more than 10% have isolated systolic hypertension over 160mm Hg.[81] Hypertension increases the risk of stroke, multi-infarct dementia, coronary heart disease, peripheral vascular disease, aortic aneurysms, and renal failure. In elderly patients, systolic pressure is a stronger predictor of complications than diastolic pressure. Treatment of systolic or diastolic hypertension improves outcomes in older patients.

Earlier studies conducted in young elderly (60 to 69 years) patients with diastolic hypertension showed that a 16 to 39% reduction in cardiovascular morbidity or mortality accompanies antihypertensive therapy.[81] More recent studies specifically included older patients (over 60 years). The European Working Party on Hypertension in the Elderly,[82] the British general practitioner study,[83] and the STOP study[84] demonstrated significant decreases in cardiovascular mortality, ranging from 22 to 38%. In general, these data support treatment of diastolic blood pressures of 90mm Hg or above in patients aged 60 to 75 years, and of 105mm Hg or more in those aged 70 to 84 years. Treatment of isolated systolic hypertension (>160mm Hg with diastolic pressure <90mm Hg) in patients 60 years or older has been shown to reduce stroke by 36% and coronary heart disease by 25%.[85] Adverse effects of antihypertensive therapy in studies specifically including older patient were minor and caused minimal withdrawals.

Thus, treatment of hypertension is effective and has a low risk in older patents aged at least up to 84 years. Drugs used in these studies included thiazide diuretics, β-blockers (metoprolol, atenolol and pindolol), methyldopa and reserpine. It should be remembered that most of the patients studied were relatively well and results might be different in medically frail elderly patients. The value of antihypertensive intervention in patients over 85 years remains unproven, but may be the same as in younger patients.

Initial therapy of mild hypertension with weight loss, exercise, salt restriction and discontinuation of smoking should be attempted. If ineffective, then an increasing array of antihypertensive agents is available. The choice of therapy involves the consideration of efficacy, medication cost, concurrent therapy, associated illness, and patient compliance (see also chapter 21; sect. 3, 4.2). Patients with severe or intractable hypertension despite multidrug therapy, or worsening azotaemia[86] should be evaluated for renal artery stenosis that may be managed with surgery or transluminal angioplasty.

#### Diuretics

Elderly patients are more likely than younger patients to have low plasma renin activity in association with elevated blood pressure.[87] Because diuretics may be most effective in patients with low renin hypertension,[87] these drugs are a logical initial choice for therapy. This prediction is borne out by recent trials discussed above. To minimise adverse effects, dosages should be low, equivalent to 12.5 to 25mg hydrochlorothiazide per day. However, it may be prudent to avoid diuretics in elderly men with electrocardiographic abnormalities, because of the potential for ventricular arrhythmias.

Hypokalaemia has an increased prevalence in elderly patients[88] and may be exacerbated by diuretic therapy. Although routine potassium supplementation is not indicated,[89] serum potassium concentrations must be monitored. Since potassium deficiency increases the risk of digitalis toxicity, monitoring of serum potassium concentrations is particularly important in patients receiving concurrent digoxin and diuretic therapy. The addition of potassium-sparing diuretics such as triamterene, amiloride or spironolactone may be effective in avoiding hypokalaemia, although these agents can cause hyperkalaemia and must be used with caution. However, they have the advantage of also exerting a magnesium-sparing effect. Patients with diabetes, on nonsteroidal anti-inflammatory drugs (NSAIDs) or with high potassium intake (such as some salt substitutes) are at particular risk of hyperkalaemia.

Hyponatraemia, which may be related to increased antidiuretic hormone concentrations with age,[90] may be induced by diuretics. This tends to occur most often in older female patients and happens early in the course of therapy.[91] Elderly patients must be observed for dehydration and postural hypotension after the start of therapy. Orthostatic hypotension is common in elderly patients,[92] and although not all studies have demonstrated that diuretics can exacerbate this condition,[93] cautious management is prudent.

#### Adrenoceptor Antagonists and Vasodilators

***β-Adrenoceptor antagonists (β-blockers)*** are widely used in older patients, although whether their antihypertensive efficacy is reduced in elderly patients remains controversial. The British general practitioner trial and the Swedish STOP trial attest to the benefits of both atenolol and metoprolol in older hypertensive patients.[83,84] However, another British study did not show a benefit of β-blockers in reducing mortality from stroke or all cardiovascular causes.[94]

If patients also have angina or certain types of arrhythmia, β-blockers may offer the advantage of treating multiple diseases with a single agent. However, they may worsen congestive heart failure, cardiac conduction abnormalities, bronchospasm, or peripheral vascular disease. Relatively $\beta_1$-specific ('cardioselective') drugs (see chapter 21; sect. 3.2) and those with significant partial agonist activity (e.g. pindolol) may be tolerated by patients with mild pulmonary disease or peripheral vascular disease, but must be used very cautiously in these populations. Some reports suggest that adverse reactions to β-blockers are increased in elderly patients.[95]

Because hepatic first-pass metabolism decreases, plasma concentrations of propranolol are increased with age.[23] However, changes in clearance with age may be less significant at high doses; in one study, elderly patients had a 50% lower clearance of propranolol after a 20mg dose, but there was no significant age-related difference after 40 or 160mg doses.[96] Because the pharmacological response may diminish in elderly patients[41] and there is marked variation between individuals, dosage adjustment for age cannot be reliably predicted. This concern is not critical, since the dose is adjusted according to blood pressure and heart rate response.

Other β-blockers have not been as extensively studied in elderly patients. Although metoprolol plasma concentrations are not altered, elevated concentrations of an active metabolite have been identified in elderly patients.[97] Although the clearance of atenolol, which is eliminated predominantly by the kidney, was not significantly reduced in a small group of healthy elderly individuals, dose requirements will likely be less in those with impaired renal function.[98] The bioavailability of labetalol, a combined α- and β-adrenoceptor blocker, is increased, but the clearance of labetalol is not changed with age.[99] Relatively $\beta_1$-selective agents such as metoprolol or atenolol are a reasonable choice for most patients who do not have contraindications to β-blocker therapy. Initial dosages should be conservative and the maintenance dose must be adjusted cautiously according to individual tolerability and response.

***$\alpha_1$-Adrenoceptor antagonists*** such as prazosin, doxazosin and terazosin, and ***peripheral vasodilators*** such as hydralazine and minoxidil are usually tolerated by elderly patients, although patients must be carefully followed for orthostatic hypotension. In particular, a small subset of elderly hypertensive patients who have concentric left ventricular hypertrophy may be at risk of severe hypotension.[100] Many of these patients have signs of pulmonary congestion related to diastolic dysfunction. Reflex tachycardia with hydralazine may be less significant in elderly patients because of impaired baroreceptor responses compared with those in younger adults.[101] A minor increase in plasma hydralazine concentrations with age is less significant than the genetic variability in its rate of metabolism.[102]

The bioavailability of prazosin is moderately decreased in elderly patients,[103] but total plasma clearance of the drug is unaltered. The initial dosage of prazosin should be conservative, given at night, and patients should be warned about possible first-dose hypotensive reactions. Other longer acting $\alpha_1$-blockers such as terazosin and doxazosin may be less likely to cause hypotension and have more convenient dosage schedules.

***Calcium antagonists*** such as verapamil, diltiazem and the dihydropyridines (e.g. nifedipine, amlodipine and felodipine) are widely used in older patients. These drugs are metabolised extensively in the liver (see also chapter

21; sect. 3.4). The plasma concentrations of calcium antagonists tend to increase with age, and the antihypertensive response appears unchanged, suggesting that dosage requirements may be reduced in older patients.[104] Although some authorities have proposed that these agents may be relatively more effective in elderly than in younger patients,[105] they are more expensive, and have not been as well studied as other available agents. They have no significant metabolic adverse effects, have potent antianginal properties, and can be used in patients with diabetes mellitus, obstructive lung disease, peripheral vascular disease and cerebrovascular disease. Thus, they have wide application in older patients. Recent data suggest that short-acting agents such as nifedipine may cause a dose-related increase in cardiovascular mortality.[106] This needs further corroboration before any definitive recommendation can be made about their use in elderly patients.

***Angiotensin-converting enzyme (ACE) inhibitors*** are effective in old age despite the fact that older patients tend to have low renin hypertension. Their effectiveness is equivalent to that of the calcium antagonists or β-blockers, as has been shown in a study in female patients.[107] Most of these drugs are eliminated by the kidney and their dosages must be reduced in old age. Elderly patients should be followed carefully for further deterioration in renal function after initiation of therapy with ACE inhibitors.

***Centrally-acting $\alpha_2$-adrenoceptor agonists*** such as methyldopa and clonidine decrease central sympathetic nervous system activity and may cause drowsiness, depression and impotence. Because these symptoms may be attributed to age, patients as well as relatives must be carefully questioned to determine the consequences of therapy. These are second-line drugs in older patients. Sudden interruption of clonidine therapy, particularly at high doses, may be complicated by rebound hypertension. Therefore, clonidine should not be given to unreliable or noncompliant patients. In the EWPHE study, methyldopa was associated with beneficial outcomes.[82]

***Adrenergic neuron blocking drugs*** such as bethanidine may cause severe orthostatic hypotension and should be avoided in elderly patients.

#### Quality of Life Considerations

Recent studies have investigated the relative therapeutic efficacy and the effects of different antihypertensive agents on quality of life in older patients. A randomised, controlled study comparing atenolol, enalapril and sustained-release diltiazem in older women found no differences in rates of adverse drug reactions or in measures of quality of life.[107] A US Veterans Affairs study of hydrochlorothiazide for systolic hypertension in men aged 60 years or over showed that cognitive-behavioural function 'was well preserved' without dose-related effects.[108] Data regarding effects of antihypertensive agents on quality of life in elderly patients are to date not definitive. Further studies, incorporating methodology designed to assess this feature in elderly patients, are awaited.

#### Choice of Drug

Although hypertension in old age is characterised by high peripheral vascular resistance, low renin concentrations, and decreased cardiac output, it does not follow that only drugs that are theoretically useful in such physiological conditions (e.g. diuretics, vasodilators and calcium antagonists) should be used in older patients. Drugs found efficacious in reducing complications of hypertension in older patients include diuretics and β-adrenoceptor blockers. However, many patients cannot tolerate these medications because of adverse effects or underlying interacting disease states (e.g. patients with asthma who cannot take β-blockers). The choice depends on cost, effectiveness and the adverse effect profile.

Some studies help to point the way for patients in certain groups. In elderly females (mean age 70 years), diltiazem was found to have a clinically unimportant but statistically greater effect compared with atenolol or enalapril.[107] A study in male patients, including a subset of older (>60 years) men, found that there was no difference in antihypertensive effectiveness between 6 drugs studied (hydrochlorothiazide, atenolol, captopril, clonidine, prazosin and sustained-release diltiazem) in White patients.[109] However, in Black patients, diltiazem, clonidine and hydrochlorothiazide were most effective, whereas captopril and atenolol were less effective. These observations require further study.

### 4.1.3 Orthostatic Hypotension

Postural hypotension (reduction in systolic blood pressure of ≥20mm Hg) is a common problem in older persons, with a prevalence as high as 20% in those over 65 years and up to 30% in persons over 75 years of age.[92] Postural hypotension is important because of the risk of complications including syncope, falls and fractures. In carefully selected individuals without risk factors, the prevalence was less than 7%,[110] suggesting that risk factors rather than aging are important in the pathogenesis of this condition. The most important risk factors include drugs, supine systolic hypertension, and cardiac impairment.

In addition to drugs and age-associated diseases, there are physiological changes that contribute to orthostatic hypotension. Elderly patients have impaired baroreceptor-mediated heart rate responses, decreased cardiac responses to sympathetic stimulation, and impaired ventricular compliance.[111] Thus, in the face of a decrease in venous return on assuming upright posture, the older adult can have a reduction in blood pressure because of altered heart rate responses, decreased cardiac inotropic responses, and stroke output reductions due to impaired ventricular filling.

If homeostatic responses are impaired, symptomatic orthostatic hypotension occurs after even minor provocation. Volume depletion associated with vomiting, diarrhoea, diuretic therapy, Addison's disease, or renal tubular sodium wasting may precipitate significant symptoms. Autonomic dysfunction, either peripheral (e.g. due to diabetes, alcohol, cancer, amyloidosis or of idiopathic origin) or central (e.g. Shy-Drager syndrome), is the most frequent cause of severe postural hypotension.

Iatrogenic causes of postural hypotension include many drugs (e.g. phenothiazines, tricyclic antidepressants, antihypertensives, diuretics, levodopa and nitrates) and prolonged bedrest. One of the most important dicta of therapeutics in elderly patients is to check for postural hypotension before using one of these drugs. If postural hypotension is found, the prescriber should use a more suitable alternative, if possible.

Orthostatic hypotension is detected by measuring blood pressure immediately on standing and 2 minutes after standing. In elderly patients with orthostasis, it is important to emphasise nondrug therapy with support stockings (thigh high), increased sodium intake, elevation of the head of the bed, foot dorsiflexion exercises, and instruction to avoid hot baths and standing too quickly. Lifting heavy weights, hot weather and hyperventilation can worsen orthostasis.[112]

If drug intervention is necessary, *fludrocortisone* is the usual first-line agent, although high dosages (up to 1 mg/day) may be necessary. Adverse effects including hypokalaemia are common, and the dose is often limited by the onset of congestive heart failure or severe supine hypertension. Other potentially useful drugs include caffeine (given with meals), α-adrenoceptor agonists (e.g. phenylpropanolamine, midodrine), and NSAIDs.[111] In some cases, epoetin may help ameliorate symptoms by its effects of reducing orthostatic hypotension and correcting anaemia that can occur in this condition.[113] Frequently, a combination of drugs is required to control symptoms. Severe nocturnal supine hypertension may be treatable with short-acting nifedipine.

#### 4.1.4 Angina Pectoris

Drug therapy of chronic stable angina generally is similar in all age groups (see chapter 20 for further discussion on management).

*Nitrates* are commonly administered for this condition. Although the effects of age on nitrate metabolism are unknown, the vascular effects of nitrates do not appear to change with age. The problem of tolerance to nitrates (probably unaffected by age) dictates that nitrate-free intervals be scheduled in the regimen, and these drugs often require cotherapy with other antianginal agents. Since older patients are at particular risk of cerebral hypoperfusion and falls, they should be instructed to take sublingual nitroglycerin (glyceryl trinitrate) only when sitting or lying down.

Other agents such as *β-blockers* and *calcium antagonists* may also be used. Important considerations in the use of β-blockers in elderly patients are discussed in section 4.1.2 above. Verapamil and diltiazem should be used cautiously in patients with pre-existing disease of the conducting system. As the elimination half-life of verapamil is longer in older patients than in younger adults,[114] elderly patients may, therefore, require lower dosages when they receive this agent long term. In using verapamil or diltiazem in elderly patients, care is required to monitor for conduction disturbance, especially if these drugs are given in conjunction with β-blockers. Low-dose *aspirin* (325mg on alternate days) is also of long term benefit in chronic stable angina in men (mean age 64 ± 9 years) in reducing the risk of myocardial infarction from 13% to 4% over an average of 60 months.[115] No women were included in this study.

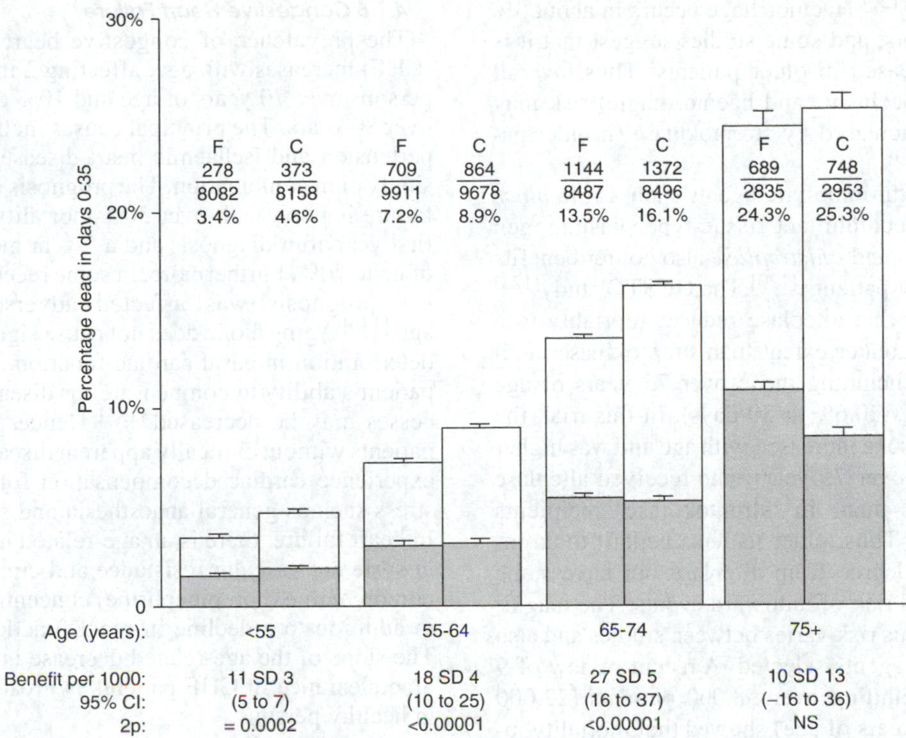


**Fig. 6.** Absolute effects of fibrinolytic therapy on mortality during days zero to 35 after myocardial infarction in different age groups. Unstratified percentages dead in days zero to 35 among all those allocated fibrinolytic therapy (F) and control patients (C) in these trials are plotted, subdivided according to age. The shaded portion of each column represents deaths during days zero to 1 and the unshaded portions represent deaths during days 2 to 35 (after The FTT Group,[124] with permission). *Abbreviations:* CI = confidence interval; SD = standard deviation; NS = not statistically significant.

Some studies have indicated that older patients (>60 and <80 years) with significant disease gain a greater survival benefit from coronary artery bypass grafting than with medical therapy of angina.[116]

In unstable angina, *aspirin* 80 to 325 mg/day (chew and swallow initially) should be given in the absence of absolute contraindications (e.g. allergy). It reduces the risk of subsequent myocardial infarction and cardiac death by 50 to 70% (from 10 to 18% down to 5 to 7%) over follow-up periods up to 24 months.[117] *Heparin* alone may be more efficacious, at least in patients under 75 years of age, reducing the risk of myocardial infarction from 12 to 0.8%, compared with 3% for aspirin.[118]

#### 4.1.5 Myocardial Infarction

Age is a major prognostic factor for death following myocardial infarction.[119] While the beneficial effects of thrombolytic therapy on morbidity and mortality have led to an increase in their use in younger patients, there is still some reluctance among clinicians to use them in older patients. However, data from large trials that included older patients with suspected acute myocardial infarction have indicated the benefits of thrombolytic therapy in patients over 65 and indeed over 75 years of age.[120] Results from the ISIS–2 study[121] showed that *streptokinase* reduced 5-week mortality, with an absolute reduction of 38 deaths per 1000 patients treated in those aged 60 to 69 years and 34 per 1000 patients treated in those over 70 years. The addition of aspirin further reduced mortality in older patients; absolute reductions in mortality were 25, 70, and 80 deaths per 1000 patients treated in those aged less than 60 years, 60 to 69 years and 70 years or over, respectively. Thus, because of the increased mortality rate, absolute benefit increased with age in that study.

Using a predictive model based on these and other earlier data, it has been determined that streptokinase is cost-effective in selected older patients.[122] Haemorrhage occurs in about 3% of patients, and some studies suggest that it is not increased in older patients. Thus, overall stroke (occlusive and haemorrhagic) risk may not be increased by streptokinase in older patients.[120]

Other thrombolytic agents such as *alteplase* (rt-PA, recombinant tissue-type plasminogen activator) and *anistreplase* also confer benefits in elderly patients.[120] The GUSTO study[123] indicates that alteplase reduces mortality to a slightly greater extent than streptokinase in all groups, including those over 75 years of age (19.3% *vs* 20.6% at 30 days). In this trial, the risk of stroke increased with age and was higher in those over 75 years who received alteplase (3.93%) than in streptokinase recipients (3.05%). Thus, older patients benefit to an increased degree from alteplase but have some increased risk of untoward events. The magnitude of this risk varies between studies and also between agents selected. A recent review of 9 trials including over 58,000 patients (22,000 over 65 years of age) showed that mortality increased with age and although the relative risk reduction decreased with age, the number of lives saved per 1000 patients treated was much the same in all age groups (fig. 6).[124] The difficulty in older patients is in quantifying the risk in individual patients, and selecting those whose risk does not outweigh the benefit. Because of concomitant disorders, delays in presentation, and absence of chest pain, the number of patients who do not qualify for therapy increases with age.[125] Also, allowing for conventional exclusion criteria, the number of elderly patients who do not receive thrombolytic therapy increases with age.[126]

Recent studies suggest that ACE inhibitors decrease mortality post-myocardial infarction. About 5 lives are saved per 1000 treated in the first month and this is likely also true in patients over 70 years.[127,128]

The use of other drugs of importance in management of myocardial infarction in older patients, such as aspirin, heparin, nitrates and β-blockers, is similar to that in other adult age groups. Although aspirin use was associated with decreased 6-month mortality in patients at least 65 years old (8.4 *vs* 17%), about 25% of eligible elderly patients did not receive the drug.[129]

#### *4.1.6 Congestive Heart Failure*

The prevalence of congestive heart failure (CHF) increases with age, affecting 2 to 3% of persons over 70 years of age and 10% of those over 80 years. The principal causes include hypertension and ischaemic heart disease, either singly or in combination. The prognosis of heart failure is poor, with over 30% mortality in the first year after diagnosis and a 5-year mortality of up to 70%. Furthermore, in some recent studies, prognosis was affected adversely by age.[130] Aging alone does not cause significant deterioration in basal cardiac function, but the patient's ability to compensate for disease processes may be decreased.[131] Hence, elderly patients without clinically apparent disease may experience cardiac decompensation following stress such as general anaesthesia and surgery. In heart failure, there is an age-related increase in systemic vascular resistance and circulating noradrenaline (norepinephrine) concentrations, in addition to a decline in renal function.[132] The slope of the age-related decrease in creatinine clearance in CHF patients is greater than in healthy persons.

Drugs such as the β-blockers and calcium antagonists can exacerbate congestive heart failure. Elderly patients with glaucoma frequently use eye drops containing a β-blocker (e.g. timolol) and this may be associated with significant systemic adverse effects, including precipitation of congestive heart failure.[133,134]

Drug therapy of congestive heart failure in elderly patients is the same as in younger adults (see further chapter 20), but with some notes of caution. *Digoxin* improves symptoms in older patients with heart failure with sinus rhythm as well as with atrial fibrillation. However, because of their decreased renal function, digoxin maintenance dosage requirements are decreased in elderly patients.[135] Diuretics remain a mainstay of therapy in older patients to reduce oedema and pulmonary congestion, but the peak effect of furosemide (frusemide) is reduced with age. Because of altered homeostasis, diuretic dosages should be adjusted cautiously in older patients to prevent volume depletion and electrolyte imbalance.

*ACE inhibitors* improve symptoms and reduce mortality in heart failure. However, more study is needed to show that these benefits extend to patients over 75 years of age. Since most ACE inhibitors are excreted by the kidney, maintenance dosages should be reduced in elderly patients. Where possible, target dosages of captopril should be 75 mg/day and of enalapril 20 mg/day, since these dosages are associated with improved outcomes. Many frail elderly patients cannot tolerate these doses, however, due to development of hypotension and azotaemia. In very elderly patients, initial dosages should be very low (e.g. captopril 6.25 mg/day or enalapril 1.25 to 2.5 mg/day) to avoid hypotension.

The role of promising new drug treatments, such as β-blockers, amiodarone or phosphodiesterase inhibitors (e.g. vesnarinone), is not yet established in older patients.

#### *4.1.7 Cardiac Arrhythmias*

Sinus node dysfunction and conducting system disease occur frequently in elderly patients. Symptoms of dizziness, palpitations, near syncope or syncope may warrant evaluation for arrhythmias. Bradyarrhythmias are identified in approximately 12% of elderly patients referred for Holter monitoring;[136] sinus node dysfunction occurs in 60% and atrioventricular conduction abnormalities in 40% of these patients. While most patients are asymptomatic and do not require therapy, use of β-blockers, digoxin, verapamil, diltiazem, amiodarone and other antiarrhythmic drugs can exacerbate underlying conduction disease.

Supraventricular ectopy is also common in old age. Supraventricular tachyarrhythmias include atrial fibrillation, flutter and atrioventricular nodal re-entrant tachycardias. Supraventricular tachyarrhythmias associated with a rapid ventricular response may be controlled with digoxin, verapamil, diltiazem, β-blockers or adenosine, as in younger patients (see further chapter 20). Causes of atrial fibrillation are similar to those in young adults. Hyperthyroidism with otherwise subtle clinical features is a more frequent cause of atrial fibrillation in older than in young patients,[137] and may be missed as a cause unless thyroid function is checked.

Ventricular arrhythmias are also common in elderly patients. A Holter monitor study of healthy, active elderly individuals demonstrated a 69% prevalence of this type of arrhythmia.[138] Among study participants with ventricular arrhythmias, 31% had complex premature ventricular contractions (PVCs) and 6% had ventricular tachyarrhythmia. A study which included many hospitalised patients demonstrated that multiform PVCs occurred in 85% and ventricular tachycardia in 22% of elderly patients.[136] However, these arrhythmias are frequently asymptomatic and the indications for treatment in elderly patients are not well established.

Therapy of ventricular arrhythmias should be restricted to symptom control or to prevention of sudden death. Antiarrhythmic drugs may not be well tolerated, and drugs of class I of the Vaughan-Williams classification in particular can aggravate rhythm disturbances (i.e. have proarrhythmic effects) in some patients. In this respect, it should be noted that antiarrhythmics can increase the risk of sudden death, as seen in the CAST study with encainide and flecainide (see further chapter 20).[139]

For drug therapy of troublesome palpitations due to ventricular ectopy, the clinician could reasonably use β-blockers or class IA or IB antiarrhythmics (see further chapter 20) if β-blockers are not successful or are contraindicated (e.g. due to chronic obstructive pulmonary disease). The end-point should be relief of symptoms. For treatment of life-threatening arrhythmias (e.g. symptomatic ventricular tachycardia), empirical drugs of choice include sotalol and amiodarone. In one study of 296 patients with a mean age of 65 years with ventricular tachyarrhythmias, sotalol was found to be more effective in preventing death and recurrence of arrhythmia than 6 other drugs (imipramine, mexiletine, pirmenol, procainamide, propafenone and quinidine).[140] Smaller studies suggest that amiodarone may also help reduce the risk of death, although this needs further evaluation.

Treatment is best guided by electrophysiological or Holter studies when possible. Patients should be evaluated carefully, since impairment of ventricular function (more common in older patients) carries a high risk of lethal arrhythmias. Patients should be managed urgently, with treatment directed towards control of the underlying heart disease as well as treatment of the ventricular arrhythmia.

##### Digoxin

Digitalis glycosides are effective for control of ventricular rate in atrial tachyarrhythmias. If a patient has a rapid ventricular response and is haemodynamically stable, digoxin loading with electrocardiographic monitoring may be performed. The total loading dose is calculated according to the patient's weight (8 to 12 μg/kg intravenously or 10 to 15 μg/kg orally). Treatment can often be titrated to achieve a decrease in ventricular response while observing the patient for indications of toxicity (e.g. accelerated junctional tachycardia). Because digoxin is mainly eliminated by the kidney, its systemic clearance is reduced[135] and the maintenance dosage required is decreased in elderly patients (sometimes to as low as 0.0625 mg/day) when the glomerular filtration rate is impaired.[141] Serum creatinine, as noted previously (see section 2.1.3), may not reflect this alteration in renal function (see appendix G for calculation of creatinine clearance from serum creatinine concentrations).

Toxic reactions to digoxin occur in up to 20% of elderly patients.[142] Over a 6-year period, 4.2% of older community patients in one study were hospitalised for digitalis toxicity; quinidine cotherapy and renal impairment appeared as risk factors for toxicity.[143] Renal impairment and advanced heart disease, which are more common in older patients, significantly increase the risk of digoxin toxicity. Extracardiac manifestations include anorexia, nausea, vomiting, disorientation, visual disturbances and hallucinations. Cardiac toxicity is characterised by increased automaticity and conduction block (supraventricular tachycardia with block and junctional tachycardia are typical arrhythmias). Other risk factors for cardiotoxicity include electrolyte abnormalities (hypokalaemia, hypomagnesaemia), hypothyroidism, advanced pulmonary disease and drug interactions. Quinidine, verapamil and amiodarone increase plasma digoxin concentrations and the dosage of digoxin may need to be reduced by up to 50% if any of these other agents are instituted (see further chapter 20 and also appendix B).[142]

#### Calcium Antagonists

Calcium antagonists such as verapamil and diltiazem have advantages over digoxin in patients with supraventricular tachyarrythmias. Rapid ventricular response to acute atrial fibrillation is more quickly and effectively controlled with intravenous verapamil or diltiazem than with digoxin. However, the blood pressure must be monitored carefully. Significant negative inotropic effects can be a problem when treating patients with cardiac impairment. Verapamil is a favourable alternative to digoxin for long term treatment of atrial fibrillation,[144] and has a beneficial effect on exercise tolerance. Diltiazem also helps control the ventricular rate and has less negative inotropic effect than verapamil.

Digoxin, verapamil and diltiazem must be used very cautiously, if at all, in elderly patients with conducting system disease in whom atrioventricular block may be exacerbated.

#### Other Antiarrhythmic Drugs

***Class I antiarrhythmics*** include quinidine, procainamide, disopyramide, lidocaine, mexiletine and tocainide. Quinidine is primarily metabolised by the liver, although around 20% is excreted by the kidney unchanged. Clearance is reduced and the half-life prolonged in elderly patients.[145,146] The adverse effects of quinidine, which may be more frequent in elderly patients, include nausea, diarrhoea, tinnitus, altered hearing, confusion, syncope and hypotension (see also chapter 20). Although moderately effective in the prevention of atrial fibrillation, quinidine, according to one report, may increase the risk of death.[147]

Procainamide is metabolised in the liver to an active metabolite, acecainide (*N*-acetylprocainamide; see also chapter 20). Both procainamide and acecainide undergo renal elimination. Because of decreased renal function in elderly patients, dosages of both quinidine and procainamide should be decreased initially and serum concentrations monitored during dosage adjustment.[145,148] Procainamide can induce a systemic lupus erythematosus-like syndrome, which is not infrequent after high-dose or prolonged therapy. Symptoms, including arthralgias, malaise, pleurisy and abdominal distress, may not be recognised immediately in some elderly patients.

Disopyramide has anticholinergic activity that may cause urinary hesitancy or retention in elderly men, in addition to confusion, constipation, and worsening of glaucoma in people of either gender. It also has greater negative inotropic effects than either quinidine or procainamide, and may cause significant cardiac depression in predisposed individuals. The elimination of disopyramide is decreased because of decreased renal function in older persons, mandating lower maintenance dosages.[149]

Lidocaine, a class IB agent, is effective for the acute treatment of ventricular arrhythmias. Clearance by the liver is decreased in the presence of congestive heart failure, myocardial infarction, or hepatic disease. Although some studies show that the clearance of lidocaine is not altered with age, the plasma half-life of the drug is increased in elderly patients.[150,151]

CNS adverse effects, including confusion, drowsiness, dizziness and convulsions, are more frequent in elderly patients.[152] About 8% of patients over 70 years of age experience adverse reactions, compared with 4% under the age of 50.[153] The dosage of lidocaine should be decreased by 50% in elderly patients and subsequently adjusted on the basis of measurement of lidocaine concentration.

Mexiletine and tocainide are other class IB agents in common usage. The pharmacokinetics of mexiletine appear unaltered with age;[154] however, the rate of metabolism of tocainide is reduced with age.

***Class II antiarrhythmics,*** i.e. β-blockers, are associated unequivocally with a reduction of sudden death (presumed due to cardiac arrhythmia) in post-myocardial infarction patients. This benefit is found with nonselective blockers (e.g. propranolol), relatively $\beta_1$-selective agents (e.g. metoprolol), and drugs with partial agonist activity (e.g. pindolol), and is most obvious in patients with impaired ventricular function.[155]

***Class III antiarrhythmics*** include sotalol and amiodarone. Sotalol is a β-blocker with class III antiarrhythmic properties at higher doses (see further chapter 20) and is beneficial in the treatment of ventricular arrhythmias. Sotalol is eliminated partly by the kidney and its systemic clearance is significantly reduced in older persons.[156] Amiodarone, which is effective in the treatment of both atrial fibrillation and ventricular arrhythmias, should be used with caution in older patients. Little is known of its pharmacokinetics in relation to age. Amiodarone can aggravate sinus node dysfunction and less frequently may cause atrioventricular block, complications that are likely to be more common in older patients. Hypothyroidism is another adverse effect and this may also be more common in elderly patients.[157] On the basis of limited adverse reaction data, some authors suggest that amiodarone dosages should be limited to 100 to 200 mg/day in older patients.[158]

#### 4.1.8 Cerebrovascular Disease

Approximately 80% of *strokes* occur in individuals over 55 years of age. The most important risk factor for stroke in any age group is hypertension. Myocardial infarction, valvular and other structural heart disease, diabetes mellitus and atrial fibrillation are also among the more important risk factors in the elderly population. These factors in combination produce a cumulative increase in risk. Modification of these risk factors (including systolic hypertension) remains important in older adults.

Although *carotid artery disease* is a frequent source of embolisation, asymptomatic carotid artery bruits are also common, but are not an indication for surgical intervention. *Transient ischaemic attacks* (TIAs) are a clear indication of cerebrovascular disease and are frequently caused by platelet or atheromatous emboli from the carotid bifurcation. Elderly patients with transient ischaemic attacks merit careful treatment because of an increased risk of stroke, myocardial infarction and death. If a high grade stenosis (>70%) is identified, endarterectomy should be considered, as it has an acceptably low risk in selected elderly patients. Myocardial infarction is a common complication of endarterectomy, and careful evaluation and management of coronary disease is important prior to surgery. Those with minimal (<33%) stenosis should receive medical rather than surgical care. Management of moderate disease (33 to 70% stenosis), until definitively established, should be medical in most elderly patients.

***Aspirin*** decreases the rate of fatal and nonfatal stroke and myocardial infarction by 20 to 25% in patients (mean age 60 to 70 years) with prior anterior circulation TIAs or small strokes.[159] A recent review of 8 randomised placebo-controlled trials of aspirin in patients with TIA or small strokes suggested that aspirin may be expected to reduce the number of strokes by 6 to 11 and non-stroke deaths by 5 to 9 per 1000 patient-years of treatment.[160] Dosages used have ranged from 75 to 1500 mg/day. Females benefit as well as males, according to recent studies. The recent European Stroke Prevention Study,[161] which used aspirin 330mg and dipyridamole 75mg 3 times daily, demonstrated by a subset analysis a similar benefit in stroke reduction in patients over 65 years of age (in whom the risk is increased) to that in younger patients.

The available data suggest that lower doses of aspirin (30 to 300mg daily) are no less beneficial than higher doses, with some reduction in adverse reactions. Nonetheless, even at low doses, there is an appreciable risk of bleeding; among 1555 patients (55% over 65 years of age) taking a dose of 30 mg/day, with a mean follow-up of 2.6 years, there were 40 major and 49 minor bleeding complications.[162]

Thus, treatment with aspirin should be considered carefully, especially in very elderly patients in whom the benefit is not well established. The dosage should be kept to a minimum, in the range of 80 to 325 mg/day.

***Ticlopidine*** is an effective alternative antiplatelet agent in patients who do not respond to or who cannot tolerate aspirin. Its cost and adverse effects including reversible neutropenia (<1%), diarrhoea and skin rash are the main drawbacks of this agent.[163]

***Oral anticoagulants*** are also used in the prevention of systemic thromboembolism (including stroke) in patients with non-valvular atrial fibrillation, rheumatic heart disease, prosthetic heart valves, mural thrombus and dilated cardiomyopathy. Atrial fibrillation, numerically the most important of these disorders in elderly patients (affecting about 5% of those over 65 years of age), carries an annual risk of stroke of about 5%. Furthermore, the risk of stroke increases with age.

Several studies have demonstrated that low-dose warfarin reduces the risk of stroke in persons with non-valvular atrial fibrillation by 42 to 86%, with an acceptably low risk of haemorrhagic complications.[164] Aspirin 325 mg/day has a similar benefit to warfarin in patients under 75 years of age, particularly those with a low risk of stroke (no hypertension, recent heart failure, previous thromboembolism, or mitral annular calcification). In older patients (>75 years), in whom the risk of thromboembolism is higher, aspirin is less efficacious than warfarin, but the benefits of warfarin are offset to some extent by the risk of intracranial haemorrhage.[165]

Aspirin may be adequate for patients under 75 years of age who are at a low risk and have unremarkable echocardiogram results. Warfarin is likely preferred for patients under 75 years of age who have a high risk and for carefully selected patients over 75 years, realising that even with treatment, the stroke risk remains significant. Anticoagulants should be used, if possible, for secondary prevention in patients with prior events.[166]

The international normalised ratio (INR) [see further chapter 26; sect. 3.1.5] may be used to help monitor warfarin dosage, the INR being kept between 2.0 and 3.0. Obvious contraindications to the use of warfarin include uncontrolled hypertension, previous intracranial bleeding, bleeding diathesis, peptic ulcer disease, falls, and poor compliance (see also chapter 26; sect. 3.1.5). Treatment of polycythaemia or other hyperviscosity syndromes is important in any patient with cerebrovascular disease.

Following a completed stroke, anticoagulant therapy is of no proven value for secondary prevention unless the stroke is considered embolic in origin. Low-dose subcutaneous ***heparin*** (e.g. 5000U twice daily) should be given for prophylaxis of deep venous thrombosis (see also section 4.1.10). Use of hypnosedatives and antipsychotic drugs should be minimised. Depression is a common complication and responds to antidepressant therapy.[167] Agents used to advantage have included tricyclics such as nortriptyline, while methylphenidate can be useful in some patients with significant psychomotor retardation.

The role of thrombolytic agents is not established in acute stroke in older persons and should be regarded as experimental at this stage.

#### *4.1.9 Peripheral Vascular Disease*

*Claudication* is a very common symptom in elderly patients. When it is severe, surgical revascularisation may be the only effective treatment. Acute thrombosis or embolic events may respond to local streptokinase infusion (see also chapter 26; sect. 3.2.2). Isolated stenotic lesions may be managed with transluminal angioplasty. Discontinuation of smoking and initiation or maintenance of a regular exercise programme often improve or decrease the progression of symptoms.

*Pentoxifylline (oxypentoxifylline)* increases exercise tolerance to a moderate degree in patients with intermittent claudication by reducing blood viscosity,[168,169] but the clinical significance of this effect is doubtful in most patients. Most vasodilators are not efficacious and may exacerbate symptoms by impairing local vasoregulation. Nonselective β-blockers inhibit peripheral vasodilatation through blockade of $\beta_2$-receptors and should be avoided. However, a relatively $\beta_1$-selective agent in a low dose (e.g. metoprolol) or a drug with partial agonist activity (e.g. pindolol) may be better tolerated.

#### *4.1.10 Thromboembolic Disease*

Thromboembolic disease is common in elderly patients. Two-thirds of hospitalised patients over 70 years of age develop calf vein thrombosis.[170] Although the reasons for this increased risk with age are not entirely established, stasis from venous dilatation, hypercoagulability, and reduced fibrinolysis may be contributory. Hypercoagulability is associated with malignancy, infection, surgery, and decreased reticuloendothelial clearance of activated coagulation factors. Risk factors for mortality associated with pulmonary embolism include age over 60 years, cancer, congestive heart failure and chronic lung disease.[171]

Since *deep venous thrombosis* (DVT) leading to fatal pulmonary emboli is frequently asymptomatic, prophylaxis is important in all high-risk patients. Conditions that predispose to thrombosis include congestive heart failure, stroke, malignancy, hip fracture, and immobility. Although hip and knee surgery are very high-risk procedures, most surgery is associated with thromboembolic disease.

Prophylaxis of DVT should be considered for elderly patients immobilised by acute illness. Graduated pressure elastic stockings and early ambulation may be helpful, but are not adequate in higher risk patients. Low-dose subcutaneous heparin 5000U every 8 to 12 hours provides effective prophylaxis against DVT and pulmonary embolism for most patients (see also chapter 26; sect. 3.2.1). Intermittent pneumatic compression and oral anticoagulants (INR maintained in the range 2 to 3) may be used if heparin is impractical. Low-dose heparin is less effective in patients undergoing hip or knee surgery and is of questionable value in retropubic prostatectomy. In patients undergoing total hip replacement, oral anticoagulation (INR 2 to 3) is one recommended choice.[172]

Although dextran may provide effective prophylaxis in hip surgery,[173] elderly patients often do not tolerate the associated volume expansion. Adjusted dosages of subcutaneous heparin to prolong the partial thromboplastin time to 31.5 to 36 seconds[174] may be useful in hip surgery (see chapter 26; sect. 3.1.4). Low molecular weight (LMW) heparin, which is associated with a lower risk of haemorrhage than standard heparin, lowers the risk of proximal DVT to 7.5% or less following hip surgery,[175] and is recommended for prophylaxis of DVT following total knee replacement.[172] Intermittent pneumatic compression is an effective measure in genitourinary surgery,[176] knee[177] and hip surgery and in current practice is used in combination with other methods.[178]

Some early studies have suggested that patients over 65 years probably have an increased frequency of bleeding after receiving anticoagulants.[179,180] This may occur particularly in the presence of other risk factors including prior stroke, heart failure, renal insufficiency, liver disease and concomitant NSAID therapy.[181] The possible mechanisms of altered anticoagulant effect with aging include increased drug sensitivity, decreased drug elimination, and increased vascular fragility predisposing to haemorrhage.

Although controversial,[182] it has been suggested that warfarin causes greater inhibition of vitamin K-dependent coagulation factor synthesis for a given plasma concentration in elderly patients than in younger adults.[183] The increased warfarin effect may be due to a combination of changes in vitamin K response with age. Elderly patients have decreased synthesis of clotting factors, increased clearance of vitamin K, greater accumulation of vitamin K oxide after warfarin administration, and reduced receptor sensitivity to vitamin K.[184] However, there do not appear to be significant age-related changes in warfarin pharmacokinetics that would increase unbound warfarin concentrations in elderly patients.[183] The increased sensitivity to warfarin may result in a 40% decrease in the required dosage for elderly patients,[185] although not all studies are in agreement on this point.[182] Anticoagulant treatment of patients with dementia, gait disorders or other illnesses predisposing to trauma must be undertaken very cautiously.

The response to heparin has not been well studied in elderly patients. No major changes in pharmacokinetics have been shown to occur with aging,[186] but most studies suggest that the risk of bleeding is increased in older persons.[181] Although specific data are not available, initial conservative dosage of heparin (guided by bodyweight and nomogram) together with careful monitoring may help reduce the risk of inadequate therapy or bleeding.[187] Though expensive, low molecular weight (LMW) heparins may be a useful alternative to standard heparin in elderly patients with a high risk of bleeding (see also chapter 26; sect. 3.1.4). Prolonged heparin administration (over 10,000 U/day for over 3 months) may cause osteoporosis.

## 4.2 Obstructive Airways Disease

### *4.2.1 Asthma*

Late-onset asthma in elderly patients is seldom associated with allergic manifestations.[188] Chronic cough, intermittent wheezing and often nocturnal dyspnoea or cough are predominant features. Asthma is underdiagnosed in older adults, with symptoms often being attributed to age, heart disease or chronic obstructive pulmonary disease. The age-adjusted death rate for asthma is increased in older patients, and the asthma-related mortality rate in this age group is increasing.[189] Elderly patients frequently take drugs such as aspirin, other NSAIDs, and β-blockers for heart disease or glaucoma, and these may aggravate bronchospasm. In confusing cases, measurement of non-specific bronchial reactivity with agents such as methacholine can be a safe, reproducible and efficient test for asthma in older patients.[190] By comparison, estimation of diurnal variation in peak expiratory flow rate may be less efficient.

Management of asthma in elderly patients is frequently complicated by concomitant cardiac disease. Bronchodilators including sympathomimetics and theophylline increase myocardial oxygen demand and exacerbate atrial and ventricular arrhythmias. Oral and parenteral sympathomimetics have greater cardiac adverse effects (including arrhythmias and angina) than inhaled medications, and should be avoided in elderly patients. Treatment of asthma in older patients, as in other age groups, consists of bronchodilators and corticosteroids.

#### Bronchodilators

***Inhaled $\beta_2$-adrenoceptor agonists*** such as salbutamol (albuterol), orciprenaline (metaproterenol), terbutaline, fenoterol and rimiterol are the agents of choice for bronchospasm in elderly patients. While $\beta_2$-selective agents have a relatively greater effect on bronchial smooth muscle than on the myocardium, higher inhaled doses may cause cardiac stimulation. Although it appears that the $\beta_2$-adrenoceptor response of the airways is reduced with aging,[191,192] most patients have a reasonable clinical response to usual doses of $\beta_2$-agonists. In apparently resistant cases, the response is best guided, if possible, by pulmonary function testing. Systemic adverse effects of these agents include tremor, tachycardia and hypokalaemia.

***Ipratropium bromide***, an anticholinergic agent, appears to exert a bronchodilator response in asthma patients that is unaffected by age.[192] The use of inhaled ipratropium as a first-line agent in asthma remains controversial, but it may be more justified in older patients. In the treatment of asthma, it may be best to use bronchodilators on an 'as needed' basis, rather than regularly.

Elderly patients frequently cannot use standard multidose inhalers effectively,[193] and other devices should be used to enhance drug delivery. Breath-activated autoinhalers,[193] spacer inhalers or portable electric nebulisers are useful alternatives.

The pharmacokinetic properties of ***theophylline*** and factors that alter its elimination are discussed in chapter 23 (sect. 3.1.1). Although absorption following oral administration is not altered with age,[194] most studies indicate that the elimination of theophylline is decreased in old age by approximately 30%.[4] Plasma concentrations of theophylline may be increased by other drugs such as cimetidine, erythromycin, troleandomycin, ciprofloxacin, allopurinol, and some influenza vaccines. The inhibition of theophylline metabolism by cimetidine or ciprofloxacin is not age-dependent.[195] Intravenous infusion of theophylline (as aminophylline) is seldom required since its bronchodilator effects may not add to the efficacy of $\beta_2$-adrenoceptor agonists and corticosteroid therapy.

Cigarette smoking or phenytoin cause induction of hepatic drug metabolising enzymes with a resultant increase in the maintenance dosage requirements of theophylline, even in older patients.[196] As well as causing bronchial smooth muscle relaxation, theophylline and other methylxanthines may also cause CNS stimula-

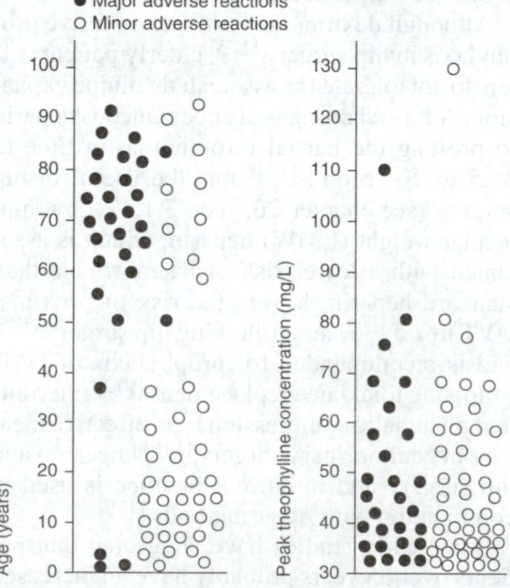


**Fig. 7.** Relationship between peak plasma theophylline concentrations and occurrence of major and minor adverse reactions to theophylline (after Shannon & Lovejoy,[199] with permission).

tion, diuresis and cardiac stimulation. Adverse reactions including nausea, cardiac arrhythmias and convulsions are frequent at serum concentrations over 20 mg/L and it is best to keep the theophylline concentration between 5 and 15 mg/L. Older patients are more likely to experience serious or fatal consequences of toxicity as a result of chronic theophylline use than younger patients (fig. 7).[197,198] For this reason, long term use of theophylline should be restricted in the treatment of asthma in elderly patients. Theophylline should be used mainly to help control nocturnal asthma.

#### Corticosteroids

Corticosteroids administered by inhalation such as beclomethasone dipropionate or budesonide are preferable to oral preparations for long term therapy. Long term, regular use of inhaled corticosteroids improves airway hyperresponsiveness, decreases the use of bronchodilators and improves the severity of symptoms.[200] Adverse effects are minimal, and the occurrence of oropharyngeal candidiasis can be reduced by oral rinsing after each use. If acute exacerbations do not respond to maximal doses of inhaled corticosteroids (e.g. beclomethasone dipropionate 1500 to 2000 μg/day) early systemic therapy is recommended. Although systemic corticosteroids are effective in the treatment of obstructive airway disease, their long term administration is associated with many adverse effects. Inhibition of calcium absorption and osteoblast activity with exacerbation of osteoporosis may be a particular risk. A combination of calcium and calcitriol reduces bone loss in patients receiving corticosteroids.[201] Alendronate may also be used to reduce bone loss.[202]

Patients with chronic positive tuberculin reactions who have not been treated for tuberculosis should be followed up closely or treated prophylactically when corticosteroid therapy is initiated.

### *4.2.2 Chronic Obstructive Pulmonary Disease*

Chronic obstructive pulmonary disease often overlaps significantly with asthma in older patients, especially in smokers. Smoking cessation is a primary requirement in patients of any age who have chronic obstructive pulmonary disease. Nicotine skin patches are useful in helping to stop smoking and long term success occurs in 20 to 40% of cases. Inhaled ipratropium generally has greater efficacy as a bronchodilator in chronic obstructive pulmonary disease than in asthma,[203] and has a similar effect to maximal doses of $\beta_2$-adrenoceptor agonists. Some clinicians prefer using ipratropium to $\beta_2$-agonists in chronic obstructive pulmonary disease. Combination of anticholinergic and $\beta_2$-agonist drugs may be helpful, blending the rapidity of action of the latter with the long duration of action of the former, while reducing the risk of dose-related adverse effects.

Although the benefits of corticosteroids remain controversial, recent evidence has suggested that long term inhaled corticosteroids improve expiratory flow rate, decrease symptoms, and slow deterioration in chronic obstructive pulmonary disease patients with a mean age of 52 years.[204] Long term oral corticosteroid therapy should be used only as a last resort, particularly in very old patients, because of its increased risks and undocumented benefits at that age.

It is wise to offer influenza and pneumonia vaccines to older patients with chronic lung disease, although the benefit of the latter in this population remains controversial. Influenza vaccine has been reported to decrease morbidity and mortality from influenza-related diseases including pneumonia, bronchitis and heart attack in a cost-effective fashion and should be strongly endorsed for use in older persons.[205]

## 4.3 Endocrine and Metabolic Disorders

### *4.3.1 Thyroid Disease*

Both hyperthyroid and hypothyroid states increase in frequency with age. The prevalence of hyperthyroidism in elderly patients ranges from 0.5 to 2.3%, depending on the population studied and the criteria used for diagnosis.[206] Approximately 15% of all thyrotoxic patients are over the age of 60 years.[207] Estimates of the prevalence of hypothyroidism range from 0.9 to 17.5%.[206]

Despite the frequency of thyroid disease, clinical recognition of altered thyroid function in elderly patients is often difficult. The diagnosis is easily overlooked because of subtle clinical manifestations, concurrent illness, and medications that modify the signs and symptoms of thyroid disease in older patients. Second-generation thyroid-stimulating hormone (TSH) tests are useful in determining hypothyroidism (raised TSH) and are sensitive but not as specific in diagnosing hyperthyroidism (decreased TSH).

#### Hyperthyroidism

Although the aetiologies of hyperthyroidism do not change greatly with age, Graves' disease is the most common cause of hyperthyroidism in elderly patients.[208] Thyrotoxicosis may be precipitated by a large iodide load (e.g. radiographic contrast media or drugs such as amiodarone) and 'natural' desiccated thyroid as a 'health food.'

Treatment of hyperthyroidism should be limited initially to the control of symptoms. In any form of hyperthyroidism, symptomatic relief of tachycardia, tremor and anxiety may be achieved with a nonselective β-blocker such as propranolol in carefully monitored doses.

Elderly patients frequently do not tolerate prolonged hyperthyroidism, and congestive heart failure occurs in over 50% of patients. Radioactive iodine is the preferred definitive treatment.[206] Because treatment is more urgent in elderly than in younger patients, prolonged therapy with multiple small doses of radioiodine is undesirable. Consequently, a relatively large dose of radioiodine (15 to 30 mCi) with the objective of thyroid ablation should be considered.[209] The notion that elderly patients may be at risk of exaggerated thyrotoxicosis following treatment with radioiodine[210] appears to be mostly anecdotal.[209]

Following initial radioiodine therapy, rapid restoration of the euthyroid state can be achieved with antithyroid drugs such as propylthiouracil, carbimazole or thiamazole (methimazole) [see also chapter 19; sect. 5.2].

#### Hypothyroidism

The most common cause of hypothyroidism is autoimmune thyroiditis, but iodine-containing drugs (e.g. amiodarone) and long term lithium therapy can induce overt disease.

Elderly patients should receive very low doses of thyroxine when replacement therapy is initiated to prevent precipitation of cardiac ischaemia or arrhythmia. An initial dose of 0.025 mg/day with increases at intervals of 4 to 6 weeks by increments of 0.025mg is usually safe. Maintenance dosages are usually decreased with age and 0.05 to 0.1 mg/day may be adequate.[211] The goal should ideally be restoration of a euthyroid state (normal TSH), but at least elimination of symptoms.

TSH concentrations may sometimes be spuriously elevated in elderly patients as a result of antibodies that cross-react in the radioimmunoassay.

### 4.3.2 Non-Insulin Dependent Diabetes Mellitus

Non-insulin dependent diabetes mellitus (NIDDM or type II diabetes mellitus) is principally a disorder of middle and old age and its prevalence increases with age. In the UK, approximately 50% of NIDDM patients are over 65 years of age,[212] which is similar to the demography in the US.[213]

Patients with fasting plasma glucose concentrations over 7.8 mmol/L (140 mg/dl) or over 11.1 mmol/L (200 mg/dl) at 2 hours following a glucose load are diabetic by the criteria of the US National Diabetes Data Group. However, not all elderly patients who are diabetic require drug treatment. Patients who are asymptomatic and do not have evidence of ketosis should be treated initially with dietary management and exercise if possible. Attainment and maintenance of ideal bodyweight is important and may be feasible in some patients. Even moderate bodyweight loss increases insulin sensitivity and may normalise glycaemic control.[214] Caloric restriction, with decreased saturated fat and cholesterol, and increased complex carbohydrate and fibre should be carefully supervised, with reminders and weight checks to help promote compliance and avoid undernutrition. There are few data, however, on the specific benefits of dietary intervention in elderly patients with diabetes. If possible, clinicians should avoid prescribing drugs that may exacerbate hyperglycaemia, including thiazide diuretics, estrogens, sympathomimetics and corticosteroids.

Symptoms of hyperglycaemia include polyuria, polydipsia, weight loss, fatigue and recurrent candidiasis. Significant symptoms, ketoacidosis or hyperglycaemic hyperosmolar coma are indications for pharmacological intervention (see further chapter 19; sect. 3). Short term symptoms due to hyperglycaemia respond to drug therapy.

Elderly patients are frequently affected by the long term complications of diabetes including cataracts, retinopathy, neuropathy, renal disease and vascular disease. These typically develop after 10 to 20 years. Some data suggest that the risks of coronary artery disease and retinopathy are increased in those with poorer blood sugar control.[215] It is not known, however, whether these long term complications occur less frequently or develop more slowly in patients treated with vigorous antidiabetic therapy. Such treatment has risks in elderly patients and therapy must be individualised with consideration of each patient's life expectancy, severity of disease, and ability to tolerate therapy. As in diabetic patients in any age group, hypertension control is very important; calcium antagonists and ACE inhibitors are the antihypertensive drugs of choice.

#### Oral Antidiabetic Agents

If diet alone does not provide adequate control of diabetes, an oral antidiabetic agent usually is added next. These agents are of major importance in the management of NIDDM[216] since they address the metabolic abnormalities of type II diabetes (e.g. peripheral insulin resistance) and are easy to take compared with insulin.

The sulphonylureas are well absorbed and are all at least partially metabolised by the liver, in some cases with the generation of active metabolites (see chapter 19; sect. 3.2.1). Although the pharmacokinetic behaviour of the short-acting sulphonylureas is very similar in young and old patients, decreased renal function may be associated with increased half-life and greater steady-state concentrations of renally excreted agents [e.g. chlorpropamide or the active metabolites of acetohexamide, glibenclamide (glyburide) and tolazamide]. Chlorpropamide has a half-life of 35 to 40 hours in older patients with normal renal function, and a steady-state plasma concentration may take more than a week to be achieved in elderly patients. Because plasma concentrations are highly variable between individuals following a standard dose,[217] the drug effect must be monitored carefully. The pharmacodynamic properties and efficacy of the sulphonylureas are not altered in elderly patients to a clinically important extent.[216]

Older patients are particularly susceptible to hypoglycaemic reactions due to sulphonylureas.[218] Probably because of its prolonged duration of action, adverse effects are most frequent with chlorpropamide,[219] but also occur with the newer, second-generation agents such as glibenclamide (glyburide) or glipizide.[220] Periods of decreased carbohydrate intake may be a significant risk factor. Potentially clinically important drug interactions that may result in hypoglycaemic reactions or decreased sulphonylurea dose requirements are listed in appendix B. Hypoglycaemic symptoms are variable in elderly patients. Insidious onset of impaired judgement, altered speech, decreased motor function or intermittent confusion may not be recognised as manifestations of hypoglycaemia; focal neurological deficits and Parkinsonian symptoms have also been reported. Recurrent hypoglycaemia may cause irreversible neurological deficits,[221] and fatal hypoglycaemic coma has been reported in elderly patients with blood glucose concentrations of 3.3 and 3.5 mmol/L (60 and 63 mg/dl).[222]

Chlorpropamide and, to a lesser degree, tolbutamide also increase renal tubular water resorption and may cause hyponatraemia. Because of its prolonged half-life and the risk of hyponatraemia, chlorpropamide is an undesirable agent in older individuals. Glipizide is a preferred agent in elderly patients because of a reduced risk of dilutional hyponatraemia or drug interactions and unaltered elimination in the presence of renal impairment.

In patients who remain hyperglycaemic on diet and sulphonylurea therapy, addition of metformin to the regimen is reasonable, especially in those with obesity and hyperlipidaemia. It helps improve glycaemic control by reducing hepatic glucose production and tissue glucose uptake. It also has a beneficial effect on hyperlipidaemia.[223] Metformin should be avoided in patients with serum creatinine >1.4 mg/dl or estimated creatinine clearance <60 ml/min (3.6 L/h). Very elderly patients may be at particular risk of lactic acidosis.[215]

All oral antidiabetic drugs should be initiated at low doses in elderly patients and then increased carefully.

#### Insulin

Although other studies are conflicting, an increase in insulin half-life[224] and a decrease in its clearance[225] probably occur with aging. Insulin absorption and time to peak effect vary between patients, but are not known to be significantly altered in elderly patients. Arthritis and visual impairment often cause practical difficulties with drug administration, but the use of premixed insulin has been shown to be associated with a reduction in dosage errors.[226]

Because hypoglycaemia may be difficult to recognise and may have severe consequences in elderly patients, therapy should be directed toward the elimination of symptoms but not necessarily normalisation of blood glucose. The target of insulin treatment should be discussed carefully with the patient and family with the goal of correcting hyperglycaemia as much as possible without raising the risk of hypoglycaemia. This typically results in more conservative target plasma glucose concentrations in the older patient, but some high-risk patients can cooperate well with standard adult goals.

#### *4.3.3 Osteoporosis*

Approximately 25% of women and 10% of men experience at least one spinal or hip fracture after the age of 60 years,[227] and more than 1.5 million Americans have osteoporosis-related fractures each year. Decreases in intestinal absorption of calcium, changes in serum 1α,25-dihydroxycholecalciferol, increased parathyroid secretion, and altered calcitonin and estrogen metabolism may all contribute to bone loss with age.[228] Reduced total bone mass in the third or fourth decades of life before bone loss begins may be a primary risk factor for significant osteoporosis and fractures in old age.[229] Subsequent postmenopausal and age-related bone loss can reach 30 to 40% of peak bone mass.[230] The further decrease in bone mass is associated with an increase in the risk of fractures. However, osteomalacia, hyperparathyroidism, multiple myeloma, metastatic disease and corticosteroid excess should all be considered in the differential diagnosis of pathological fracture in elderly patients.

In the management of osteoporosis, the emphasis must be on prevention, with intervention in young or middle-aged adult life, emphasising regular exercise, discontinuation of smoking or heavy alcohol intake, and adequate calcium diet. Postmenopausal women should take elemental calcium 1.0 to 1.5 g/day. Weight-bearing exercise increases bone mass. Elderly patients should receive 800U of vitamin $D_3$ (cholecalciferol) daily. Low-dose estrogen replacement therapy reduces the risk of fracture after the menopause from 7 to 5 per 1000 patients,[231] and should be strongly considered in patients at high risk, especially those with documented low bone mass. The duration of therapy should be at least 5 years, but longer periods of up to 20 years may be required to reduce hip fractures in patients over 75 years of age who are at highest risk of fracture. The optimum duration of treatment is not established. Benefit is best in current elderly users who started estrogen therapy within 5 years of menopause.[232]

Treatment of established osteoporosis is primarily concerned with the prevention of further bone loss and symptomatic treatment of pain. Regular weight-bearing exercise such as walking should be incorporated into every treatment regimen. Vitamin D supplementation (vitamin $D_3$ 800 U/day) and calcium supplementation (1.2 g/day) are safe and have been shown to reduce the risk of hip fractures in elderly (84 ± 6 years) female residents of nursing homes from 7.8 to 5.8% over 18 months, preventing 2 fractures per 100 persons treated.[233] Because calcium carbonate may not be well absorbed in elderly patients with achlorhydria,[234] administration with meals or the use of calcium citrate should be considered.

Vitamin D deficiency with osteomalacia has been noted in some elderly people with osteoporosis[235] and in 10 to 20% of those with hip fracture. This requires vitamin D supplementation (400 to 1000 U/day). Urinary calcium should be at least 100 mg/day in those with adequate calcium absorption. There is no convincing evidence as yet that treatment with estrogens or calcitonin is beneficial in those over 75 years of age with established osteoporosis (see also chapter 25; sect. 12.2).

***Estrogen therapy*** decreases postmenopausal bone resorption, possibly by decreasing parathyroid hormone activity.[236,237] Conjugated estrogens 0.625 mg/day are efficacious.[238] However, estrogen therapy is complicated by an increased risk of gallbladder disease and endometrial carcinoma.[239,240] Endometrial carcinomas are usually low grade, however, and increased mortality from endometrial disease has not been clearly established.[241] The risk of endometrial carcinoma is reduced if estrogens are combined with a progestagen (e.g. medroxyprogesterone). Resumption of menstrual bleeding, often unacceptable to older women, can be avoided by a continuous estrogen/progestagen regimen (see also chapter 18; sect. 11.4).

Estrogens may also exacerbate benign or malignant breast disease. Although hypertension and thrombotic disease are associated with the use of estrogens for contraception, the risk of these complications is low in regimens used to prevent or treat osteoporosis and is least with transdermal estrogen. Health screening for breast and uterine complications is advisable.

***Calcitonin*** inhibits osteoclastic activity. Although serum calcitonin appears to be elevated in some postmenopausal women with osteoporosis, intranasal calcitonin administration (100 U/day) decreases the rate of trabecular bone loss in this population and higher doses increase spinal mineral content.[242] Calcitonin reduces the incidence of hip, vertebral and forearm fractures and benefit has been shown in women over

65 years of age for hip and forearm fractures.[242] Calcitonin also has a useful analgesic effect on spinal pain, possibly due to endorphin secretion. The average dosage is 50 to 100 U/day of intranasal calcitonin given with calcium supplements.

***Bisphosphonates*** such as etidronate are taken up preferentially by the skeleton and suppress osteoclastic activity. They can increase spinal mineralisation modestly when given over a 2- to 4-year period. Some[243] but not all[244] studies have shown that etidronate can reduce the rate of vertebral fractures in postmenopausal osteoporosis. Effects on hip fracture are unknown. Alendronate, in women aged 45 to 80 years with osteoporosis, reduced vertebral fractures from 6.2 to 3.2% over 3 years.[202] The decreased risk was similar in patients <65 years of age and those 65 years of age or older.

***Fluoride*** has a strong, but variable anabolic effect on bone. Its use is frequently complicated by gastritis, tendinitis and possibly arthritis. There is no good evidence to date that fluoride is beneficial in older persons.

Acute spinal compression fractures are unfortunately a common complication of osteoporosis. Treatment is symptomatic, with a short period of bed rest. Pain from vertebral crush fractures should be managed aggressively with opioid analgesics if necessary. Physical therapy is important, if it can be tolerated, to improve paraspinal muscle strength and reduce the risk of further fracture. Temporary use of a brace can help reduce pain. It should be noted that prolonged immobilisation through either bed rest or a back brace can aggravate osteoporosis by increasing the rate of bone loss.

## 4.4 Rheumatic Diseases

Rheumatic diseases are a common and disabling problem in elderly patients. More than 85% of patients over the age of 65 are afflicted by osteoarthritis. Although osteoarthritis is the most common cause of joint pain, polymyalgia rheumatica and pseudogout are also primarily diseases of older patients. Treatment of these diseases is discussed in detail in chapter 25 (sect. 3, 4, 6 and 13.2.4).

### 4.4.1 Osteoarthritis

Osteoarthritis is characterised by cartilage deterioration and calcium deposition at joint margins. Although inflammation is less than that of rheumatoid and other inflammatory arthritides, pain is often partially responsive to salicylates, NSAIDs, or local injection of corticosteroids (see also chapter 25; sect. 4.1).

In elderly patients, the elimination half-life of salicylate is increased,[245] as are serum concentrations of its metabolites salicyluric and gentisic acids.[246] However, no increase in adverse effects with age has been identified. Plasma concentrations of indomethacin for a given dose are increased in elderly patients;[247] over 50% of elderly patients experience adverse effects with this drug and 20% have to discontinue treatment.[248] Salicylates and NSAIDs may cause gastrointestinal distress or bleeding in elderly patients, as in younger patients. Since iron intake is often decreased in elderly patients, an increased incidence of iron deficiency anaemia may occur with occult blood loss.[249]

Decreased renal blood flow, decreased glomerular filtration rate, oedema, or proteinuria may also result from NSAID administration.[250] Because complications may be more frequent in elderly patients,[251] renal function should be monitored carefully when these agents are prescribed. For further discussion of the use of NSAIDs, see section 4.10.

### 4.4.2 Rheumatoid Arthritis

Although rheumatoid arthritis usually beings in younger patients, and is more common in women, up to one-third of patients first present for treatment after the age of 60 years.[252] Therapy with NSAIDs, corticosteroids, and disease-modifying agents (e.g. gold, methotrexate, penicillamine, sulfasalazine, chloroquine derivatives) is similar in all age groups (see chapter 25; sect. 3.2), although the indications for disease-modifying agents in elderly patients are not well established.

The therapeutic efficacy of gold[253] and penicillamine[254] is not altered by age. However, elderly patients with rheumatoid arthritis may be more sensitive to the toxicity of azathioprine and methotrexate. In addition to drug therapy, the value of physical therapy in improving the functional quality of life for rheumatoid arthritis patients cannot be overemphasised.[252] Some patients may benefit from surgical intervention such as arthroplasty.

## 4.5 Gastrointestinal Disorders

### 4.5.1 Acid-Related Upper Gastrointestinal Disease

Acid-related upper gastrointestinal tract diseases such as gastro-oesophageal reflux and peptic ulcer disease are much more frequent in older patients than in younger adults. Older patients may present with atypical signs and symptoms (e.g. cough with gastro-oesophageal reflux or weight loss with peptic ulcer disease).

The increase in the frequency of peptic ulcer disease in elderly patients is in part related to the high use of NSAIDs by this age group.[255] The available evidence suggests that NSAIDs cause gastric ulcer and also probably duodenal ulcer, and that they increase the risk of bleeding or perforation by between 50 and 500%.[256] This effect is dose-related in elderly persons.[257] It therefore behoves clinicians to limit NSAID use and dosages in older persons and advise patients carefully of the risks of these agents.

There is little prospective information available to indicate whether aging affects the response to treatment of peptic ulcer disease. However, response rates to *$H_2$-receptor blockers*, including cimetidine, ranitidine and famotidine, appear similar in older patients to younger persons, with 75 to 100% healing at 8 weeks with full-dose therapy.[255] The response to *omeprazole* is satisfactory in elderly patients, perhaps in part because higher plasma concentrations[255] and efficient reduction of peak acid output occur at dosages of 20 mg/day.[258]

At standard dosages, blood concentrations of cimetidine[146] and other $H_2$-blockers[255] are increased, due to reduced clearance in elderly patients. Adverse reactions to cimetidine including confusion, hallucinations and psychotic reactions have been noted in up to 17% of nursing home residents receiving 'usual' doses of this drug.[259] Other $H_2$-blockers may also cause mental confusion, especially in the presence of renal impairment, since these drugs are excreted via the kidney. In most older patients, the $H_2$-blockers are well tolerated: a recent meta-analysis showed similar rates of adverse reactions (2%) in patients above and below 65 years of age.[260] Sucralfate can be given with success for treatment of duodenal and gastric ulcer disease, but should not be given with a $H_2$-blocker.

For maintenance treatment of peptic ulcer disease, ranitidine is perhaps the $H_2$-blocker of choice in elderly patients, as it has a simple dosage regimen, low risk of drug interactions, and proven benefit in this situation, including prevention of recurrent bleeding from duodenal ulcer.[261] On the basis of observations that eradication of *H. pylori* infection in patients with duodenal or gastric ulcer can markedly reduce the rate of recurrence in patients of all ages,[262] it is judicious to treat older patients with peptic ulcer disease and evidence of *H. pylori* infection with an antibacterial regimen such as either colloidal bismuth subcitrate (tripotassium dicitrato bismuthate) or bismuth subsalicylate, plus amoxicillin and metronidazole (see also chapter 22; sect. 4.3).

Agents used in treatment of gastro-oesophageal reflux disease include the *prokinetic agents* metoclopramide, cisapride and domperidone (see also chapter 22; sect. 3.1). Metoclopramide is a dopamine antagonist which can cause confusion, drowsiness, extrapyramidal symptoms, including tardive dyskinesia, and exacerbation of Parkinson's disease. Cisapride and domperidone cross the blood-brain barrier in lower amounts and are advantageous in patients who experience CNS effects from metoclopramide.

#### 4.5.2 Constipation

Constipation is a frequent problem in elderly patients and the use of laxatives rises dramatically with age; up to 30% of elderly community dwellers and over 70% of nursing home residents use laxatives regularly.[263] Although in healthy active adults, stool frequency and bowel transit are minimally changed with age, prolonged transit occurs in those with constipation and in frail elderly persons.[264] Decreased motility and constipation are exacerbated by drugs such as opioid analgesics, anticholinergics, tricyclic antidepressants, antipsychotics, antihypertensives, iron, and aluminium-containing antacids (see also chapter 22; sect. 11.2.4). Frail elderly people have decreased rectal tone and perception of rectal distension and may develop constipation or impaction through failure of defaecation.[265]

Because definitions of constipation vary (small hard stools, difficulty with passage, infrequency, incomplete evacuation), the character of a patient's complaint must be identified before initiating therapy. The differential diagnosis of severe constipation includes neoplastic disease, diverticulitis, diabetic or other autonomic neuropathy, hypercalcaemia, hypothyroidism, and depression. Factors that increase the risk of constipation include immobility, polypharmacy, dementia, and Parkinsonism.

Faecal impaction (best shown on abdominal x-ray) can be treated with a mineral oil retention enema (100 to 200ml), although manual fragmentation is often also required. Repeated enemas or suppositories (e.g. bisacodyl) may be required daily until the bowel is cleared and then treatment with oral agents can commence.

Debilitated patients with chronically infrequent, hard stools may require regular laxative treatment. Bulk laxatives such as psyllium should be used only if fluid intake is adequate. An osmotic laxative such as sorbitol or lactulose can be used if necessary. Saline laxatives such as magnesium hydroxide (milk of magnesia) can be effective, but the patient must be monitored for signs of dehydration and hypermagnesaemia. In resistant cases with poor bowel motility, oral senna preparations or bisacodyl taken initially at half the usual adult dose 3 times per week are often effective, with the goal of discontinuing this treatment when possible, and maintaining bowel control with bulk laxatives or osmotic agents.

In active elderly patients, constipation can usually be managed with a bowel training programme, which should allow laxatives to eventually be discontinued. A high fibre diet with added bran or the use of bulk laxatives [e.g. 15ml (1 tablespoon) of psyllium in 240ml liquid daily] should be used initially. Regular use of the toilet should be encouraged at fixed times for a standard period of time (e.g. 10 minutes, whether the patient feels an urge to defaecate or not) as this helps promote a consistent bowel habit. If after 4 or 5 days the patient has not had a bowel movement or if marked discomfort develops, a hypertonic phosphate enema or suppository is used and the process restarted. If this programme is unsuccessful, laxatives are instituted, as in debilitated patients.

Laxatives in either active or debilitated patients should be initiated at low doses, with repeated attempts to decrease or discontinue therapy. A number of hazards can result from inappropriate choice and use of laxatives in elderly patients (see further chapter 22; sect. 11.1.3).

#### 4.5.3 Faecal Incontinence

Faecal incontinence is extremely disabling. Intractable incontinence causes social isolation and frequently leads to institutionalisation. Transient, mild symptoms associated with diarrhoea may resolve if stools regain normal consistency. The principal causes include functional incontinence, faecal impaction, loss of normal defaecation control mechanisms, and psychological/mental causes.

Functional faecal incontinence occurs in patients with debilitation or diarrhoea who are unable to get to the toilet in time. These patients often have no abnormality of the bowel and sphincter. Treatment is that of the underlying debilitation or diarrhoea.

Faecal impaction, with holdup in the colon or rectum, can give rise to incontinence, often with leakage of soft stool. Incontinence usually resolves with elimination of the impaction and adequate management of constipation and underlying cause. However, elderly patients with impaction may have poor rectal sensation and hypotonic rectal function[266] which may give rise to recurrence of impaction.

Disturbance of control of defaecation and sphincter control can occur as a result of local causes such as rectal tumour, long term laxative abuse (with stimulant cathartics, e.g. bisacodyl), pelvic surgery, and local neurological disorders (e.g. autonomic or peripheral neuropathy). Diagnostic evaluation of neurological function and sphincter response should be considered in patients with significant, persistent symptoms. Central disorders causing disordered rectal function and incontinence include dementia, Parkinsonism and stroke. Such patients experience incontinence with passage of formed stool. This is usually associated with urinary incontinence.

Symptomatic control of faecal incontinence due to sphincter or bowel dysfunction can often be achieved. Antidiarrhoeal agents such as diphenoxylate/atropine or loperamide may be administered at minimum dosage to control stool frequency and then interrupted with a stimulant laxative (e.g. senna or bisacodyl) to produce a bowel movement 2 to 3 times per week. An increased time between bowel movements can sometimes be achieved with periodic enemas. Biofeedback training to increase recognition of rectal distension may be of value in competent patients.[267,268]

### 4.6 Urinary Incontinence

Urinary incontinence occurs in 15% of community-dwelling elderly persons and up to 50% of elderly patients in short or long term care institutions.[269]

***Acute incontinence*** associated with medical illness is often functional and results from confusion, immobility, cystitis, faecal impaction, or polyuria from diabetes, congestive heart failure or diuretic administration.[270] Hypnosedatives and drugs with anticholinergic effects (e.g. tri-

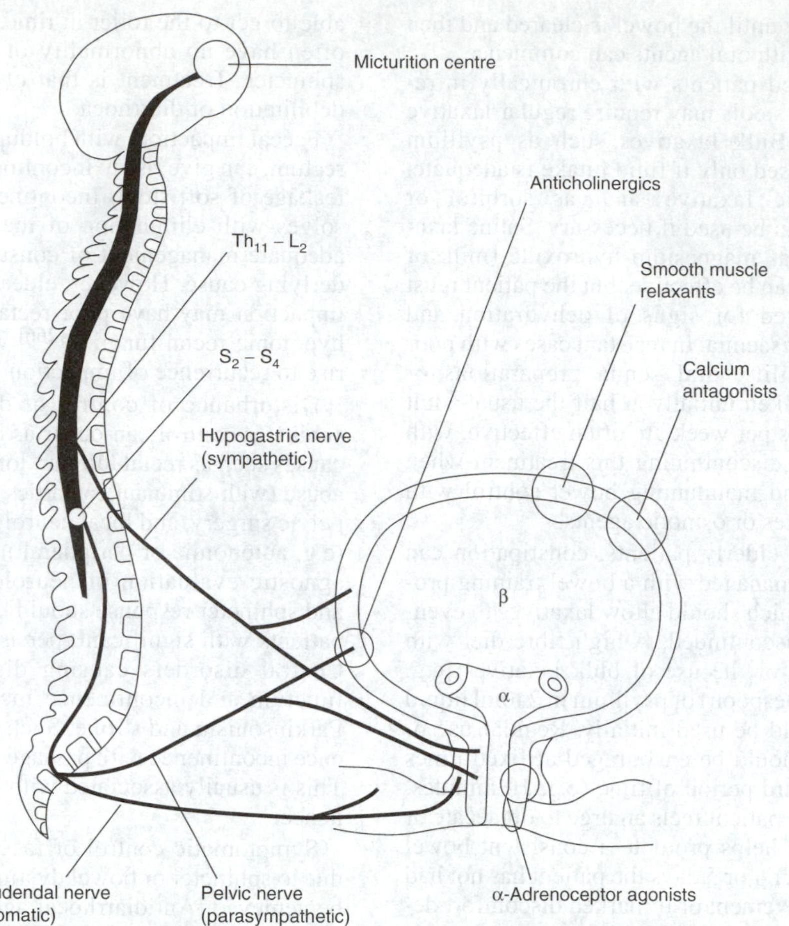


**Fig. 8.** Innervation of the bladder, internal and external sphincters, and sites of action of drugs used to help control urinary incontinence in elderly patients (after Sourander,[272] with permission).

cyclic antidepressants, disopyramide) frequently alter bladder control.

***Chronic incontinence*** can generally be categorised as being due to detrusor instability (uninhibited detrusor), overflow incontinence, or sphincter insufficiency.[271] If the cause of incontinence is unclear after history-taking, physical examination, and routine laboratory tests including urinalysis, then catheterisation for determination of postvoidal residual urine volume and cystometrography may be of diagnostic value. However, the precise role of invasive tests in the assessment of incontinence in geriatric patients has not been well established.

***Detrusor instability (uninhibited bladder)*** is the most frequent cause of incontinence in elderly patients. It results from the loss of cortical inhibition, increased afferent activity from the bladder, deconditioning from prolonged periods of low bladder volume, or spinal cord transection above vertebra T-7. Decreased cortical inhibition can result from cerebrovascular disease, Alzheimer's disease, Parkinson's disease, multiple sclerosis, normal pressure hydrocephalus, and intracranial neoplasm. Increased afferent activity may be associated with bladder infection, faecal impaction, and bladder neoplasm. Detrusor instability also commonly occurs in the absence of any of the above conditions.

The patient usually presents with urge incontinence, frequency, and nocturia. The bladder detrusor muscle characteristically contracts involuntarily at low bladder volumes. Because detrusor innervation is primarily parasympathetic (fig. 8), *anticholinergic drugs* including emepronium bromide, dicyclomine, flavoxate, oxybutynin, and propantheline may decrease detrusor contractions and increase bladder capacity. Of these, oxybutynin is probably the most commonly used drug.[273] Unfortunately, adverse effects including confusion, dry mouth, nausea, constipation, mydriasis and tachycardia limit the use of these drugs in elderly patients.[274]

*Imipramine* has anticholinergic properties and some authors also consider that it exerts an α-sympathomimetic effect due to reuptake antagonism. It also may have a direct inhibitory effect on bladder tone.[275] A starting dose of imipramine 25mg given at bedtime is often well tolerated and effective in elderly patients.[276]

Some *calcium antagonists* (e.g. flunarizine) decrease bladder tone and have been shown to decrease incontinence (fig. 8).[277] Because these agents are better tolerated than other alternatives, a therapeutic trial may be of value. A useful newer agent, with both calcium antagonist and anticholinergic activities was *terodiline.*[272,278] However, this drug was withdrawn from the market because of its proarrhythmic effects.

***Overflow incontinence*** is caused by bladder outlet obstruction such as prostatic enlargement or by peripheral motor or sensory neuropathy (frequently due to diabetes mellitus) which interrupts the sacral reflex arc and thus impairs bladder emptying. Post-voiding residual volume is elevated. Most cases of outflow obstruction require surgical intervention or, if surgery is not feasible, intermittent or continuous catheter drainage. Occasionally, retention due to a neuropathic bladder may be improved by decreasing the sphincter tone with an *α-adrenoceptor blocker* such as terazosin, doxazosin, prazosin or phenoxybenzamine.

In the absence of obvious outlet obstruction, *cholinergic agents* (e.g. bethanechol) increase bladder contraction but are frequently ineffective. Their use is also complicated by many muscarinic agonist adverse effects including nausea, diarrhoea, diaphoresis, bronchospasm and bradycardia.

***Stress incontinence*** is the loss of small volumes of urine associated with abrupt increases in intra-abdominal pressure. Tissue atrophy and changes in muscle tone with aging may lead to an alteration of the posterior urethrovesical angle and cause stress incontinence. Sphincter weakness associated with local neurological deficits or local urethral inflammation or tissue atrophy may also contribute to or independently cause symptoms.

Treatment with *estrogens* is often helpful in reversing tissue atrophy[279] and also increasing the response to *α-adrenoceptor agonists* such as phenylpropanolamine or ephedrine[280,281] used to augment sphincter tone (fig. 8). Although topical vaginal estrogens (e.g. conjugated estrogens cream 0.5 to 1.0g several times per week) may be used, significant systemic absorption should be expected. Systemic estrogen therapy may be complicated by an increased risk of gallbladder disease and endometrial carcinoma, as discussed in section 4.3.3.

## 4.7 Impotence

About 1 in 5 males between the ages of 50 and 70 years are unable to have intercourse because of impotence.[282] The cause is multifactorial in up to 65% of cases. Causes include vascular (arterial insufficiency, venous leakage), neurological (e.g. stroke, multiple sclerosis, spinal cord damage, peripheral sensory or autonomic neuropathy), endocrine disorders (e.g. diabetes, hypothyroidism, hypogonadism), psychiatric disorders such as depression, and performance anxiety. Drugs stated to cause impotence are numerous. They include diuretics (thiazides, spironolactone), centrally-acting antihypertensives (methyldopa, clonidine), β-blockers, verapamil, tricyclic antidepressants, antipsychotics, antiepileptic drugs, estrogens and corticosteroids.[282]

Treatment is directed at the cause if possible. Avoiding cigarette smoking and alcohol abuse should be emphasised. Careful review of medication and stopping possibly offending agents is important. Drug-induced impotence is usually closely temporally related to institution of a particular medication whereas other organic causes develop slowly. *Yohimbine*, an $\alpha_2$-adrenoceptor agonist, is most effective in patients with psychological (60% response) rather than organic (43% response) impotence.[283] Testosterone deficiency occurs in up to 50% of elderly men, many of whom do not experience impotence. The benefit of *testosterone* in those with impotence is unpredictable and sometimes short lived.[282] Testosterone should not be given to patients with symptomatic prostatic enlargement or prostate cancer. Haematocrit, prostatic specific antigen (PSA) concentrations, and digital prostate examination should be performed regularly.

Competent, cooperative older patients may be able to use *intracavernosal injections of va-*

*sodilators* such as papaverine, phentolamine, or, in particular, alprostadil (prostaglandin $E_1$) with a good degree of success (see also chapter 19; sect. 8.2.5, 8.3.6).[284] Careful instruction and initial trial of the minimal successful dosage is required to avoid overdose and risk of damaging priapism. Vacuum tumescence devices are very useful in older males and have a high satisfaction rate, especially in couples with a close relationship.[285] Failure to ejaculate, local pain or occasional bruising can occur.

If the above methods are unsuccessful or unsuitable, a penile prosthesis can be tried. These give over 80% satisfaction if used properly and with prior education. There are 3 kinds: semirigid rods, fully inflatable hydraulic devices, and self-contained hydraulic implants.[286] The semirigid device is the simplest, cheapest and safest choice. The applicability of vascular surgery for impotence in the older population is unknown.

## 4.8 Neurological and Psychiatric Disorders

### 4.8.1 Dementia

Dementia affects 5 to 10% of elderly people in the community and over 50% of patients in long term care institutions. Although Alzheimer's disease, multi-infarct dementia, and alcoholism are among the most frequent causes, evaluation for reversible causes of cognitive impairment including depression, normal pressure hydrocephalus, hypothyroidism, and vitamin $B_{12}$ deficiency is important. A history of brisk deterioration or delirium suggests metabolic abnormality, infection or adverse drug effect (table III). Thus, it is important to ensure that patients with dementia, in particular, remain in good physical health and receive only necessary medications. Patients should be routinely evaluated for depression, which is common in the earlier stages of dementia and can worsen cognitive function, but may respond to specific antidepressant therapy.

#### Antipsychotic Drugs

Antipsychotic drugs (see also chapter 30; sect. 3.1) are frequently and probably excessively prescribed, but these agents can be of some value in ameliorating psychotic complications when used cautiously.[287] Antipsychotics are of benefit in treating agitation, paranoia, restlessness and hostility. A review of over 60 studies suggested that a therapeutic response can be obtained in up to 70% of cases.[288] There is no single best agent, and it is important to recognise that although antipsychotics may relieve behavioural symptoms, multiple adverse effects including worsening of confusion can accelerate the progression of disability. Because behavioural disturbances are often transient, antipsychotics should not be prescribed indefinitely.

When antipsychotics are used, small initial doses should be administered. Although most antipsychotic drugs are tolerated at low doses, butyrophenones such as haloperidol (0.5mg 2 or 3 times daily) may have fewer cardiovascular and anticholinergic adverse effects than others. Informed consent is required in some countries when using antipsychotic drugs in view of their potential to cause tardive dyskinesia (most common in diabetic and elderly patients), which is often irreversible in elderly patients.[289] In addition, the abnormal involuntary movement scale (AIMS) test should be performed every 6 months.

Other adverse reactions to antipsychotic drugs are common (see table IV), and may not be easily recognised in a demented patient. Effects such as impairment of cognitive function, akathisia and blurred vision may paradoxically increase anxiety and agitation. Extrapyramidal effects appear most severe with haloperidol, thiothixene, and the piperazine phenothiazines including fluphenazine, perphenazine and trifluoperazine. Choreiform movements may oc-

**Table III.** Common causes of altered mental status in the elderly

**Infections:**
Urinary tract, pneumonia, meningitis

**Endocrine disorders:**
Hypothyroidism, hyperthyroidism
Addison's disease, Cushing's syndrome

**Metabolic disorders:**
Hypoxaemia, hepatic failure, renal failure
Thiamine deficiency, vitamin $B_{12}$ deficiency
Hypercalcaemia, hyponatraemia
Hypoglycaemia, hyperglycaemic hyperosmolar coma

**Neurological disturbances:**
Alzheimer's disease, multi-infarct dementia
Normal pressure hydrocephalus
Alcoholism
Subdural haematoma, intracranial neoplasm
Depression

**Iatrogenic causes:**
Altered environment
Sleep deprivation
Drugs (e.g. hypnosedatives, antipsychotics, tricyclic antidepressants, corticosteroids, levodopa, bromocriptine, NSAIDs, anticholinergics, antihistamines, $H_2$-receptor blockers)

cur more frequently in elderly patients than in younger adults.[290]

Newer antipsychotic agents such as *risperidone* may have advantages because of fewer extrapyramidal adverse effects. Sleep disturbances in association with dementia are treatable with the more sedating antipsychotics such as *thioridazine* (10 to 100mg) in those with psychotic disturbance. For more routine use, sedative antidepressant agents with little anticholinergic effect such as *trazodone* (25 to 75mg) are useful. *Carbamazepine* has helped control agitated behaviour in demented patients in some studies.[291]

Withdrawal of antipsychotic agents should be considered continuously. In a study conducted in nursing homes, residents whose antipsychotics were withdrawn were found to have significantly improved affect, with no discernible adverse effects resulting from withdrawal.[292]

**Tacrine**

A characteristic of Alzheimer's dementia is reduced cholinergic neuronal activity (see further chapter 30, sect. 11.1). Tacrine, a centrally acting, noncompetitive cholinesterase inhibitor, is of modest, but significant benefit in some patients with Alzheimer's dementia. In a review of 15 double-blind, placebo-controlled studies, cognitive improvement was seen in 10 and behavioural/functional improvement in 7.[293] Test items shown to improve included recall, naming, language, and word finding. Function becomes recognisably better in some cases. However, this modest, dose-related success is marred by liver toxicity and gastrointestinal disturbance. Liver toxicity (>3 times elevation of alanine aminotransferase, ALT) requiring cessation of therapy occurs in about 25% of cases, although many patients can tolerate tacrine on rechallenge. Many patients experience dose-related autonomic adverse effects such as nausea, vomiting, abdominal discomfort or diarrhoea. Benefit is dose-related and best seen at 160 mg/day. Less than one-third of patients will be able to tolerate that dose.[294]

**Table IV.** Adverse effects of antipsychotic medications

| |
|---|
| **Anticholinergic effects:** dry mouth, blurred vision, constipation, urinary retention, delirium |
| **Extrapyramidal effects:** stiffness, rigidity, drooling, tremor, akathisia, tardive dyskinesia |
| **Orthostatic hypotension** |
| **Sedation** |

### *4.8.2 Depression*

About 2% of older persons have major clinical depression and a further 2% experience dysthymic reactions. Depression is more common in those over 80 years of age and affects up to 20% of patients in extended care institutions.[295] The risk of suicide is increased 2 to 4 times in patients over 65 years of age when compared with that in younger adults. Depression often accompanies medical illness in hospitalised patients and occurs in 30 to 60% of post-stroke patients. Complaints of dysphoric mood are less common and weight loss or somatic symptoms are more frequent in elderly than in younger patients. Intervention to improve living conditions, minimise financial stress, and increase social activity is difficult but may be rewarding. Pharmacological treatment can be effective, and the choice of drug should be based on known efficacy, pharmacokinetic profile and risk of causing adverse effects in this age group.[1]

**Tricyclic Antidepressants**

Treatment with tricyclic antidepressants can be effective, but adverse effects are more frequent than in younger patients. Although the evidence is conflicting, most data indicate that plasma concentrations of many tricyclic and newer antidepressants are increased with age,[296] probably because of a decreased clearance of some of these drugs in elderly patients. One study demonstrated a decrease in the clearance of imipramine, but not desipramine, with age.[297] This suggested that tricyclic antidepressants that are eliminated by demethylation, such as imipramine, may be affected by age to a greater extent than agents eliminated by hydroxylation, such as desipramine. Although plasma concentrations may provide an index of drug absorption and elimination, correlations with therapeutic efficacy are not well established for many antidepressants (see also chapter 30; sect. 5.1.3). Therapeutic monitoring may be useful for imipramine and nortriptyline.

Since elderly patients may be more susceptible to adverse effects, dosages of tricyclic antidepressants should be conservative. The initial dosage should be on average 50% lower than in younger patients, and the patient carefully monitored during dosage adjustment for adverse anticholinergic, cardiovascular and sedative effects. Amitriptyline, doxepin and imipramine (25 to 150 mg/day) have the greatest sedative and anticholinergic properties, while nortriptyline (10 to 60 mg/day) and desipramine (25 to

150 mg/day) have fewer anticholinergic and also fewer sedative effects. Orthostatic hypotension is a frequent and potentially serious adverse effect of tricyclic antidepressants in elderly patients but is less of a problem with nortriptyline. Thus, selection of a tricyclic antidepressant is made on the basis of adverse effect profile (see further chapter 30, table VIII) rather than differences in efficacy, and consequently desipramine or nortriptyline are preferred drugs in elderly patients.

**Newer Antidepressants**

Newer agents used in older patients to treat depression include trazodone, amfebutamone (bupropion), selective serotonin reuptake inhibitors (SSRIs), and methylphenidate. *Trazodone* has proved effective in most studies, has little anticholinergic effect, and is purported to be less cardiotoxic than tricyclic agents. Its sedating effect, if tolerated, can benefit those with sleep disturbance. *Amfebutamone (bupropion)* has no anticholinergic or cardiovascular adverse effects, but can lower the seizure threshold and impair appetite. It is useful in those with significant cardiovascular disease or orthostatic hypotension.

The *SSRIs* (e.g. fluoxetine, sertraline, and paroxetine) are being used increasingly in frail elderly patients because of their relative safety and apparent efficacy in this population in initial clinical trials.[298] They do not cause anticholinergic effects and sedation is less common than with tricyclics. Both fluoxetine and sertraline have metabolites with long half-lives (7 to 14 days for norfluoxetine) and the relatively shorter-acting paroxetine may have some advantage in older persons. Some studies suggest that plasma concentrations of fluoxetine and paroxetine, but not sertraline, are increased with age.[299] Adverse reactions include nausea, anorexia, diarrhoea, insomnia and headache. Paroxetine and fluoxetine, but not sertraline, are potent inhibitors of the metabolism of tricyclic antidepressants, phenothiazines, class IC antiarrhythmic agents (e.g. flecainide, encainide and propafenone), and quinidine. Thus, sertraline appears the least complicated choice in elderly patients.

The recently introduced atypical antidepressants nefazodone and venlafaxine have a good safety profile suitable for elderly patients, but likely should be reserved for patients at risk from other, better established agents.[300,301] They require frequent administration, which may be a disadvantage in less motivated and reliable persons.

**Other Agents**

*Methylphenidate* can be a useful second-line antidepressant in patients with significant retarded depression, often associated with medical illness such as stroke. The efficacy of this drug is not affected by age. Its onset of action (2 to 4 days) is more rapid than other antidepressants.[302] Small studies suggest that it is well tolerated in older persons, with infrequent adverse effects including hypertension, anorexia, anxiety, tremor, tachycardia and psychosis.

*Lithium*, which is used for recurrent depression and bipolar (manic-depressive) illness, has decreased clearance in old age.[303] Doses should therefore be reduced in line with renal function, guided by plasma concentration monitoring, and should be adjusted when diuretics or NSAIDs are also used. Other mood stabilisers, including *carbamazepine* and *valproic acid*, may be used in patients who cannot tolerate lithium.

*Electroconvulsive treatment (ECT)* is well tolerated, even by patients over 80 years of age with a good but variable response rate. It does affect memory and its use should be restricted to cases of drug-resistant depression, potential suicide and antidepressant drug intolerance.

The prognosis of depression is relatively good, with over 60% of patients becoming well or having relapses that respond readily to treatment.[304] However, the prognosis is less favourable in those with significant medical illness, many of whom have contraindications to the use of tricyclic antidepressants. Some authors suggest that full dosage maintenance therapy is reasonable in older patients to help prevent recurrence. The duration of maintenance therapy is not known, but some experts suggest treatment for 4 to 5 years.

#### *4.8.3 Sleep Disturbances*

Changes in sleep occur with aging. Stage 4 and REM (rapid eye movement) periods of sleep decrease, and the frequency and length of awakenings increase. Sleep disorder is common in many diseases of elderly patients, including congestive heart failure, chronic obstructive pulmonary disease, Parkinsonism, dementia, arthritis, and prostatism. Reversible causes of sleep disruption should be considered and include sleep apnoea, nocturnal urinary frequency, leg cramps, and depression. Nocturnal urinary frequency may be decreased by avoiding diuretics and methylxanthines (e.g. theophylline, caffeine) in the evening. Leg cramps may be caused by electrolyte abnormalities (e.g. potassium and magnesium depletion induced by diuretic therapy), which may be treated by correction of the abnormality. For symptomatic treatment, quinine (300mg at bedtime) can decrease the frequency of leg cramps,[305] but the risk of adverse reactions, including marrow dysplasia has led to the withdrawal of the drug for this indication in the US by the FDA.

Antidepressants with sedative properties (e.g. amitriptyline, trazodone, doxepin) should be considered in patients with depressive symptoms. Many patients improve when told that their symptoms are not pathological.

Symptomatic treatment of insomnia requires advice about expected changes in sleep with aging, and advice about good sleep habits.[306] These include daily exercise, avoidance of catnaps, a fixed time for retiring and rising, and abstinence from alcohol, caffeine, and other liquids near bedtime. Drug treatment may be required in cases resistant to these measures.

#### Rational Use of Hypnotics

Hypnotics should be given for only a few weeks and then tapered off, since rebound disturbances in sleep may occur. The best agents for use in elderly patients are the medium and short-acting *benzodiazepines* (see chapter 30; sect. 6.1.1). Barbiturates have a prolonged duration of activity,[307] increased adverse effects[20] and should not be used as hypnotics in elderly patients.[308]

Some benzodiazepines (e.g. chlordiazepoxide, diazepam, clorazepate) are metabolised to nordazepam (*N*-desmethyldiazepam), which is pharmacologically active and has a half-life as long as 220 hours in elderly patients, whereas others such as oxazepam, lorazepam and temazepam do not have active metabolites and may be safer agents in older patients. However, drug accumulation and progressive deterioration of mental performance can occur in elderly patients, even with shorter-acting agents.[309]

Since elderly patients have an increased sensitivity to some benzodiazepines (see also section 2.2.1),[44,45] and an increased frequency of adverse effects (fig. 9), treatment should be initiated at lower doses than in younger patients. Although patients often obtain symptomatic benefit, sleep disturbances (decreased stage 4 and REM sleep) may be exacerbated and tolerance may occur with repeated use. Withdrawal symptoms including increased anxiety and insomnia may occur following long term use of benzodiazepines at higher dosages.

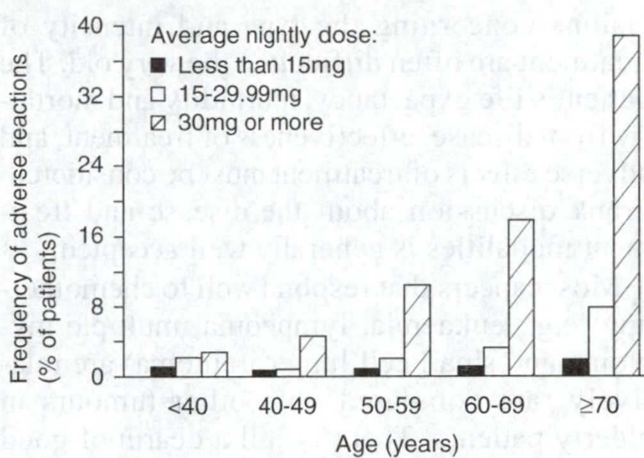


**Fig. 9.** Effect of age and average daily dose on the frequency of adverse reactions to flurazepam (after Greenblatt et al.[310]).

Benzodiazepines are associated with an increased risk of falls and trauma, including hip fracture.[311,312] Because long term administration may be associated with tolerance, dependence or possible drug accumulation and associated impaired mental function, benzodiazepine administration should only be intermittent. It is recommended to use an hypnotic for 3 weeks and observe sleep progress after withdrawal.

Other hypnotics used in older persons include *chloral hydrate* (0.5g nightly), which is relatively safe and effective but can cause gastric irritation. *Zopiclone* is a newer agent with a low potential for rebound insomnia or dependence, and a short half-life of 3 to 6 hours. This drug may be preferable to benzodiazepines in some older persons.[313] *Zolpidem*, a nonbenzodiazepine agent that binds to the type I benzodiazepine subtype of the benzodiazepine receptors,[314] does not alter the relative durations of sleep stages and may also be beneficial in older patients in reduced doses (usual dose, 5mg at night). It should be noted that, although hypnotics are widely used to treat sleep disturbances in nursing home patients, there is no clear relationship between patterns of sedative-hypnotic use and the presence, absence, or change in sleep complaints.[315]

### 4.9 Neoplastic Diseases

The incidence of neoplastic disease increases several-fold in elderly patients over that in younger patients. Because cancer treatment is often associated with significant morbidity, decisions concerning the type and intensity of treatment are often difficult in the very old. The patient's life expectancy, morbidity and mortality from disease, effectiveness of treatment, and adverse effects of treatment must be considered. Frank discussion about the disease and treatment modalities is generally well accepted.

Most cancers that respond well to chemotherapy (e.g. leukaemia, lymphoma, multiple myeloma and small cell lung carcinoma) are relatively rare compared with other tumours in elderly patients. There is still a dearth of good information to guide effective chemotherapy in patients over 65 years of age.

*Antineoplastic agents* have a narrow therapeutic index with typically severe toxicity. Adverse effects of many antineoplastic drugs are more frequent or more severe than in younger patients. For example, the risk of cardiomyopathy with the anthracycline agent doxorubicin may be increased in elderly patients.[316] Bone marrow reserve may be reduced with age, leading to an increased risk of neutropenia following more aggressive chemotherapeutic regimens such as in the treatment of lymphomas or acute leukaemias.[317] This may be part of the reason why treatment of these disorders is less successful in older patients. Chemotherapy of solid tumours (e.g. lung, breast and colorectal carcinomas) appears not to be associated with an increased risk of toxicity in otherwise healthy patients over 65 years of age.[318]

To minimise the risk of toxicity, treatment should be individualised carefully in elderly patients with clearly defined goals.[319] Dosages of drugs such as methotrexate, cyclophosphamide, mithramycin, bleomycin, streptozocin, cisplatin and etoposide are adjusted according to creatinine clearance in elderly patients, bearing in mind that these adjustments have not been validated.

Some hormonal agents are very useful in older patients. Tamoxifen, a nonsteroidal antiestrogenic agent is very useful for treatment of estrogen receptor positive breast cancer. It is a useful choice as primary treatment in frail elderly patients with breast cancer or as initial therapy for metastatic disease. Stilbestrol remains a drug to consider for treatment of symptomatic metastatic prostate cancer in older men, although it carries the risk of deep venous thrombosis.

Older patients tolerate radiation therapy of tumours quite well[320] and this should always be considered when appropriate, especially for palliation. Surgical morbidity and mortality are increased with age for nearly all surgical procedures.[321] Decreased respiratory, myocardial and renal function as well as atherosclerotic diseases that predispose to stroke and myocardial infarction are primary factors in the increased surgical risk.

## 4.10 Pain Management and Anaesthesia

### *4.10.1 Pain Management*

Many common diseases in elderly patients, such as degenerative joint disease, cancer and neuropathy, are associated with chronic pain. Thus, chronic pain is one of the most frequent symptoms in old age. Although the general principles of pain management are the same as in younger patients (see chapter 12; sect. 7.2), elderly patients require some differences in approach to therapy. Careful diagnosis of the cause, with consideration of depression, and attention to secondary functional impairment are of particular importance in older persons. A strategy for management is shown in table V.

Chronic benign pain (e.g. due to arthritis) is typically mild to moderate in degree and is treated with paracetamol (acetaminophen) or NSAIDs. Some studies indicate that clearance of paracetamol is reduced with age,[4] but there is no evidence to date that older patients are more susceptible to acute or chronic liver toxicity or to renal toxicity. Nevertheless, clinicians should advise patients that the dosage of paracetamol in humans should be less than 4g per day to avoid increased risk of chronic hepatotoxicity.

Aspirin and other NSAIDs are mainly eliminated by hepatic metabolism. Although age-related differences in these parameters may not be very important clinically, it remains wise to start with lower doses of NSAIDs in older patients. Salicylate toxicity most often occurs in older patients, especially in the presence of renal impairment.[323] Endoscopic studies have indicated that 14 to 30% of long term users of NSAIDs experience peptic ulceration.[324] Upper gastrointestinal haemorrhage is increased 4- to 5-fold and is dose-related; risk factors include age, among other factors such as smoking, prior peptic ulcer disease, and concomitant use of corticosteroids or anticoagulants.[325,326] Furthermore, older persons are at increased risk of dying from peptic ulcer complications. Prophylactic treatment with *misoprostol* appears effective[327] and should be considered in older

**Table V.** Suggested initial pain therapies in the elderly

| Pain type | Musculoskeletal | Neuropathic | Malignant |
|---|---|---|---|
| Mild | Aspirin/paracetamol<br>NSAID<br>Heat/cold<br>Physical therapy<br>Local injection<br>Cognitive therapy[a] | Aspirin/NSAID<br>Local anaesthetic injection or epidural corticosteroid | Aspirin/paracetamol<br>NSAID<br>Cognitive therapy[a] |
| Moderate | TENS<br>Acupuncture<br>Codeine/oxycodone<br>Combinations[b] | Antidepressant<br>Anticonvulsant (e.g. phenytoin, carbamazepine)<br>Codeine/oxycodone<br>Combinations[b] | Codeine<br>Oxycodone<br>Combinations[b] |
| Severe | Strong (opioid) analgesic | Neuroablation<br>Epidural opioid | Strong (opioid) analgesic |

a Relaxation, distraction, biofeedback, etc.

b Combination of a strong (opioid) analgesic and an NSAID or paracetamol.[322]

*Abbreviations:* NSAID = nonsteroidal anti-inflammatory drug; TENS = transcutaneous electrical nerve stimulation.

patients with other risk factors if NSAID use cannot be avoided.

Chronic renal disease is increased in men over 65 years[328] and reversible mild azotaemia is common in nursing home patients of advanced age who take NSAIDs.[329] The NSAIDs have a ceiling effect (i.e. the dose/analgesic effect plateaus at therapeutic concentrations) and in view of the added risk of toxicity in elderly patients, it is unwise to push the dosage to maximum recommended adult levels.

If paracetamol or NSAID treatment is ineffective, the addition of opioid analgesics should be considered. Some experts consider that dextropropoxyphene is not a good choice in older patients because, compared with other agents for mild pain, it is more toxic and not more efficacious.[55] In addition, the elimination of dextropropoxyphene and its metabolite norpropoxyphene is significantly delayed in elderly patients, increasing the risk of accumulation and dose-related toxicity.[330]

*Morphine* is the opioid of choice for severe pain. The risk of opioid addiction is low in older patients with pain. Clearance of morphine is decreased by 30% with age and elimination of the active metabolite morphine-6-glucuronide (renally excreted) is also age-dependent, resulting in an increased half-life.[4] This may largely explain the increased analgesic effect and prolonged duration of action in elderly compared with younger patients (fig. 10).[331] Plasma concentrations of pethidine (meperidine) are also increased with age following intramuscular administration.[333] Initial doses of opioid analgesics should therefore be conservative in elderly patients. Doses should be increased as needed according to progression of pain or as tolerance develops. Adverse effects, particularly nausea and constipation, should be anticipated.

Epidural and intrathecal morphine appear to be safe and effective in older people. This route may help to reduce systemic toxicity such as nausea and depression of sensorium. Lower starting and maintenance doses are required in the acute post-operative setting, but not necessarily for repeated administration.[334]

In the treatment of severe pain, particularly if there is a neuropathic component (neuropathy or radiculopathy), anticonvulsants (phenytoin or carbamazepine) are useful adjuvants. Antidepressants such as desipramine are also useful adjuvants for pain control and at the same time relieve depression, which is a common occurrence. Corticosteroids are useful for reflex sympathetic dystrophy and pain due to tumour invasion of bone or nerve roots. Local myofascial injection of painful trigger points with local anaesthetic sometimes is helpful. Epidural steroid injection for low back radicular pain can be helpful in relieving pain and promoting mobility in elderly patients.

#### *4.10.2 Anaesthesia*

Surgical morbidity and mortality are increased with age for nearly all surgical procedures.[335] Decreased respiratory, myocardial and renal function as well as atherosclerotic diseases that predispose patients to stroke and myocardial infarction are primary factors in the increased surgical risk. Changes in the CNS with aging, including decreased neurotransmitter synthesis and increased degradation,[336] alter anaesthetic and opioid analgesic responses. Older patients tend to have greater sensitivity

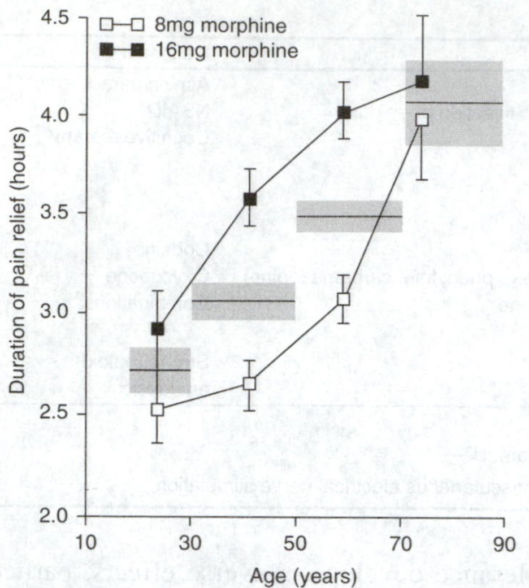


**Fig. 10.** Duration of pain relief in relation to age after either 8mg or 16mg doses of morphine. The vertical bars represent ± SEM and the shaded areas represent comparable data for the combined doses for each age group (after Kaiko[332]).

but less predictable responses than younger patients.

Interestingly, in the case of thiopental, the required dose for induction of anaesthesia is reduced by 50% in elderly patients. This appears to be due to impairment of rapid clearance from the central compartment, rather than altered sensitivity.[337] The minimum alveolar concentration (a measure of potency; see chapter 12, sect. 2.1.1) of inhalational anaesthetics decreases with age.[338] The concentration of halothane decreases by 25% and that of isoflurane by 18% from age 20 years to over 65 years.[339] Alveolar concentrations of sevoflurane and isoflurane on wakening decrease with age.[340]

Although recovery following neuromuscular blockade by tubocurarine and reversal by neostigmine is unchanged with age, pancuronium elimination is decreased and recovery is slower in older patients.[341] Increasing age is associated with slower onset of neuromuscular blockade due to suxamethonium (succinylcholine) and vecuronium.[342] The effects of rocuronium[343] and of vecuronium[344] are prolonged in older patients due to reduced drug clearance.

Epidural dosage requirements of local anaesthetics are decreased above the age of 40 years, but may not be altered further in old age.[345] Regional anaesthesia is well tolerated[346] and is the treatment of choice in elderly patients whenever possible.

## Further Reading


Bressler R, Katz MD, eds. Geriatric pharmacology. New York: McGraw-Hill, 1993

Chutka DS, Evans JM, Fleming KC, et al. Drug prescribing for elderly patients. Mayo Clinic Proceedings 1995; 70: 685

Durnas C, Loi CM, Cusack BJ. Hepatic drug metabolism and aging. Clinical Pharmacokinetics 1990; 19: 359

Gurwitz JH, Avorn J. The ambiguous relation between aging and adverse drug reactions. Annals of Internal Medicine 1991; 114: 956

Lamy PP, editor. Clinical pharmacology. Clinics in Geriatric Medicine. Philadelphia: WB Saunders, 1990; 6: 229

Montamat SC, Cusack BJ, Vestal RE. Management of drug therapy in the elderly. New England Journal of Medicine 1989; 321: 303

Rochon PA, Gurwitz JH. Geriatrics septet: drug therapy. Lancet 1995; 436: 32

Stewart RB, Cooper JW. Polypharmacy in the aged: practical solutions. Drugs & Aging 1994; 4: 449

Vestal RE, Cusack BJ. Pharmacology and aging. In: Schneider and Rowe, editors. Handbook of the biology of aging, 3rd ed. San Diego: Academic Press, 1990: 349

Vestal RE, Montamat SC, Nielson CP. Drugs in special patient groups: the elderly. In: Melmon, Morrelli, Hoffman et al. editors. Clinical pharmacology: basic principles in therapeutics, 3rd ed. New York: McGraw-Hill, 1992: 851

Walker J, Wynne H. Review: the frequency and severity of adverse drug reactions in elderly people. Age and Ageing 1994; 23: 225


## References


1. Bressler R, Katz MD. Drug therapy for geriatric depression. Drugs & Aging 1993; 3: 195
2. Montamat SC, Cusack BJ, Vestal RE. Management of drug therapy in the elderly. New England Journal of Medicine 1989; 321: 303
3. Vestal RE, Cusack BJ. Pharmacology and aging. In: Schneider & Rowe, editors. Handbook of the biology of aging. 3rd ed. San Diego: Academic Press, 1990: 349.
4. Durnas C, Loi C-M, Cusack BJ. Hepatic drug metabolism and aging. Clinical Pharmacokinetics 1990; 19: 359
5. Vestal RE, Montamat SC, Nielson CP. Drugs in special patient groups: the elderly. In: Melmon, Morrelli, Hoffman, et al., editors. Clinical pharmacology - basic principles in therapeutics. 3rd ed. New York: McGraw-Hill, 1992: 851
6. Health Care Financing Administration, Office of the National Cost Estimates, National health expenditures, 1988. Health Care Financing Review 1990; 11: 1-41.
7. Ho PC, Triggs EJ. Drug therapy in the elderly. Australian and New Zealand Journal of Medicine 1984; 14: 179
8. Beard K. Adverse reactions as a cause of hospital admission for the aged. Drugs & Aging 1992; 2: 356
9. Grymonpre RE, Mitenko PA, Sitar DS, et al. Drug-associated hospital admissions in older medical patients. Journal of the American Geriatric Society 1988; 36: 1092

10. Hale WE, May FE, Marks RG, et al. Drug use in an ambulatory elderly population: a 5-year update. Drug Intelligence and Clinical Pharmacy 1987; 21: 530
11. Helling DK, Lemke JH, Semla TP, et al. Medication use characteristics in the elderly: the Iowa 65+ rural health study. Journal of the American Geriatric Society 1987; 35: 4
12. Williamson J, Chopin JM. Adverse reactions to prescribed drugs in the elderly: a multicentre investigation. Age and Ageing 1980; 9: 73
13. Nolan L, O'Malley K. Prescribing for the elderly. Part I: sensitivity of the elderly to adverse drug reactions. Journal of the American Geriatric Society 1988; 36: 142
14. Gurwitz GH, Avorn J. The ambiguous relation between aging and adverse drug reactions. Annals of Internal Medicine 1991; 114: 956
15. Carbonin P, Pahor M, Bernabei R, et al. Is age an independent risk factor of adverse drug reactions in hospitalized medical patients? Journal of the American Geriatric Society 1991; 39: 1093
16. Chrischilles EA, Segar ET, Wallace RB. Self-reported adverse drug reactions and related resource use: a study of community-dwelling persons 65 years and older. Annals of Internal Medicine 1992; 117: 634
17. Manton KG, Stallard E. Medical demography: interaction of disability dynamics and mortality. In: Martin & Preston, editors. Demography of aging. Washington: National Academy Press, 1994: 217.
18. Vestal RE, Dawson GW. Pharmacology and aging. In: Finch & Schneider, editors. Handbook of the biology of aging. 2nd ed. New York: Van Nostrand, 1985: 744.
19. Kekki M, Samloff IM, Ihamäki T, et al. Age- and sex-related behaviour of gastric acid secretion at the population level. Scandinavian Journal of Gastroenterology 1982; 17: 737
20. Bender AD. Pharmacologic aspects of aging: a survey of the effect of age on drug activity in adults. Journal of the American Geriatric Society 1964; 12: 114
21. Parsons RL. Drug absorption in gastrointestinal disease with particular reference to malabsorption syndromes. Clinical Pharmacokinetics 1977; 2: 45
22. Welling PG. Interactions affecting drug absorption. Clinical Pharmacokinetics 1984; 9: 404
23. Castleden CM, George CF. The effects of aging on the hepatic clearance of propranolol. British Journal of Clinical Pharmacology 1979; 7: 49
24. Vestal RE, McGuire EA, Tobin JD, et al. Aging and ethanol metabolism. Clinical Pharmacology & Therapeutics 1977; 21: 343
25. Klotz U, Avant GR, Hoyumpa A, et al. The effect of age and liver disease on the disposition and elimination of diazepam in adult man. Journal of Clinical Investigation 1975; 55: 347
26. Brandfonbrener M, Landowne M, Shock NW. Changes in cardiac output with age. Circulation 1955; 12: 557
27. Woodhouse KW, Wynne HA. Age-related changes in liver size and hepatic blood flow: the influence on drug metabolism in the elderly. Clinical Pharmacokinetics 1988; 15: 287
28. Lindeman RD. Changes in renal function with aging: implications for treatment. Drugs & Aging 1992; 2: 423
29. Bender AD. The effect of increasing age on the distribution of peripheral blood flow in man. Journal of the American Geriatric Society 1965; 13: 192
30. Sjöqvist F, Alván G. Aging and drug disposition - metabolism. Journal of Chronic Diseases 1983; 36: 31
31. Woodhouse KW, Mutch E, Williams FM, et al. The effect of age on pathways of drug metabolism in human liver. Age and Ageing 1984; 13: 328
32. Schmucker DL, Woodhouse KW, Wang RK, et al. Effects of age and gender on in vitro properties of human liver microsomal monooxygenases. Clinical Pharmacology & Therapeutics 1990; 48: 365
33. Vestal RE, Norris AH, Tobin JD, et al. Antipyrine metabolism in man: influence of age, alcohol, caffeine and smoking. Clinical Pharmacology & Therapeutics 1975; 18: 425
34. Greenblatt DJ, Allen MD, Harmatz JS, et al. Diazepam disposition determinants. Clinical Pharmacology & Therapeutics 1980; 27: 301
35. Kruse WHH. Problems and pitfalls in the use of benzodiazepines in the elderly. Drug Safety 1990; 5: 328
36. Farah F, Taylor W, Rawlins M, et al. Hepatic drug acetylation and oxidation: effects of aging in man. British Medical Journal 1977; 11: 155
37. Korrapati MR, Sorkin JG, Andres R, et al. Acetylator phenotype in relation to age and gender in the Baltimore Longitudinal Study of Aging. Clinical Pharmacology & Therapeutics 1995; 53: 192
38. Pearson MW, Roberts CJC. Drug induction of hepatic enzymes in the elderly. Age and Ageing 1984; 13: 313
39. Vestal RE, Wood AJ. Influence of age and smoking on drug kinetics in man: studies using model compounds. Clinical Pharmacokinetics 1980; 5: 309
40. Vestal RE, Cusack BJ, Crowley JJ, et al. Aging and the response to inhibition and induction of theophylline metabolism. Experimental Gerontology 1993; 28: 421
41. Vestal RE, Wood AJ, Shand DG. Reduced beta-adrenoceptor sensitivity in the elderly. Clinical Pharmacology & Therapeutics 1979; 26: 181
42. Scarpace PJ, Tumer N, Mader SL. β-Adrenergic function in aging: basic mechanisms and clinical implications. Drugs & Aging 1991; 1: 116
43. Feldman RD, Limbird LE, Nadeau J, et al. Alterations in leukocyte beta-receptor affinity with aging. New England Journal of Medicine 1984; 310: 815
44. Castleden CM, George CF, Marcer D, et al. Increased sensitivity to nitrazepam in old age. British Medical Journal 1977; 1: 10
45. Reidenberg MM, Levy M, Warner H, et al. The relationship between diazepam dose, plasma level, age and central nervous system depression in adults. Clinical Pharmacology & Therapeutics 1978; 23: 371
46. Cusack B, Vestal RE. Clinical pharmacology. In: Abrams WB, Beers MH, Berkow R, editors. The Merck Manual of Geriatrics. 2nd ed. Whitehouse Station, New Jersey: Merck Research Laboratories, 1995: 255
47. Greenblatt DJ, Haematz JS, Shapiro L, et al. Sensitivity to triazolam in the elderly. New England Journal of Medicine 1991; 324: 1691
48. Clark BA, Sharron RP, Rose RM, et al. Increased susceptibility to thiazide-induced hyponatremia in the elderly. Journal of the American Society of Nephrology 1994; 5: 1106
49. Epstein M, Hollenberg NK. Age as a determinant of renal sodium conservation in normal men. Journal of Laboratory and Clinical Medicine 1976; 87: 411
50. Crane JG, Harris JJ. Effect of aging on renin activity and aldosterone excretion. Journal of Laboratory and Clinical Medicine 1976; 87: 947
51. Gribben B, Pickering TG, Sleight P, et al. Effect of age and high blood pressure on baroreflex sensitivity in man. Circulation Research 1971; 24: 424

52. Young JB, Rowe JW, Pallotta JA, et al. Enhanced plasma norepinephrine reponse to upright posture and oral glucose administration in elderly human subjects. Metabolism 1980; 29: 532
53. Burr ML, King S, Davies HEF, et al. The effects of discontinuing long term diuretic therapy in the elderly. Age and Ageing 1977; 6: 38
54. Learoyd BM. Psychotropic drugs and the elderly patients. Medical Journal of Australia 1972; 1: 1311
55. Beers MH, Ouslander JG, Rollinger I, et al. Explicit criteria for determining inappropriate medication use in nursing home residents. Archives of Internal Medicine 1991; 151: 1825
56. Finlayson RE, Davis LJ. Prescription drug dependance in the elderly population: demographic and clinical features of 100 inpatients. Mayo Clinic Proceedings 1994; 69: 1137
57. Stewart RB. Noncompliance in the elderly: is there a cure? Drugs & Aging 1991; 1: 163
58. Nanada C, Fanale JE, Kronholm P. The role of medication noncompliance and adverse drug reactions in hospitalizations of the elderly. Archives of Internal Medicine 1990; 150: 841
59. Schwartz D, Wang M, Feitz L, et al. Medication errors made by elderly, chronically ill patients. American Journal of Public Health 1962; 52: 2018
60. Parkin DM, Henney CR, Quirk J, et al. Deviation from prescribed drug treatment after discharge from hospital. British Medical Journal 1976; 2: 686
61. Mazullo JM. The nonpharmacologic basis of therapeutics. Clinical Pharmacology & Therapeutics 1972; 13: 157
62. Plein JB, Plein EM. Ageing and drug therapy. Annual Review of Gerontology 1981; 2: 211
63. Ouslander JG. Drug therapy in the elderly. Annals of Internal Medicine 1981; 95: 711
64. Eisen SA, Miller DK, Woodward RS, et al. The effect of prescribed daily dose frequency on patient medication compliance. Archives of Internal Medicine 1990; 150: 1881
65. Ayd FJ. Once-a-day neuroleptic and tricyclic antidepressant therapy. International Drug and Therapeutics Newsletter 1972; 7: 33
66. Ayd FJ. Single daily dose of antidepressants. Journal of the American Medical Association 1974; 230: 263
67. Davison W. Drug hazards in the elderly. British Journal of Hospital Medicine 1971; 6: 83
68. Law R, Chambers C. Medicines and elderly people: a general practice survey. British Medical Journal 1976; 1: 565
69. Morrow D, Lierer V, Sheikh J. Adherence and medication instructions: review and recommendations. Journal of the American Geriatric Society 1988; 36: 1147
70. Murray MD, Birt JA, Manatunga AK, et al. Medication compliance in elderly outpatients using twice-daily dosing and unit-of-dose packaging. Annals of Pharmacotherapy 1993; 27: 616
71. Wong BS, Norman DC. Evaluation of a novel medication aid, the calender blister-pak, and its effect on drug compliance in a geriatric outpatient clinic. Journal of the American Geriatric Society 1987; 35: 21
72. Mackowiak ED, O'Connor Jr TW, Thomason M, et al. Compliance devices preferred by elderly patients. American Pharmacist 1994; 34: 47
73. Wandless I, Davie JW. Can drug compliance in the elderly be improved? British Medical Journal 1977; 1: 359
74. Burns E, Austin CA, Box NDS. Elderly patients' understanding of their drug therapy: the effect of cognitive function. Age and Ageing 1990; 19: 236
75. Gerstinblith G, Weisfeldt ML, Lakatta EG. Disorders of the heart. In: Andres et al., editors. Principles of geriatric medicine. New York: McGraw-Hill, 1985: 515
76. Malenka DJ, Baron JA. Cholesterol and coronary heart disease: the importance of patient-specific attributable risk. Archives of Internal Medicine 1988; 148: 2247
77. Denke MA, Grundy SM. Hypercholesterolaemia in elderly persons: resolving the treatment dilemma. Annals of Internal Medicine 1990; 112: 780
78. Manolio TA, Furberg CD, Wahl PW, et al. Eligibility for cholesterol referral in community-dwelling older adults. The Cardiovascular Health Study. Annals of Internal Medicine 1992; 116: 641
79. Santinga JT, Rosman HS, Rubenfire M, et al. Efficacy and safety of pravastatin in the long-term treatment of elderly patients with hypercholesterolemia. American Journal of Medicine 1994; 96: 509
80. Boccuzzi SJ, Bocaenegra TS, Walker JF, et al. Long-term safety and efficacy profile of simvastatin. American Journal of Cardiology 1991; 68: 1127
81. Applegate WB. Hypertension in elderly patients. Annals of Internal Medicine 1989; 110: 901
82. Amery A, Birkenhäger W, Brixko P, et al. Mortality and morbidity results from the European Working Party on High Blood Pressure in the Elderly trial. Lancet 1985; 1: 1349
83. Coope J, Warrender TS. Randomized trial of treatment for hypertension in elderly patients in primary care. British Medical Journal 1986; 293: 1145
84. Dahlof B, Lindholm LH, Hansson L, et al. Morbidity and mortality in the Swedish trial in old patients with hypertension. Lancet 1991; 338: 1281
85. SHEP Cooperative Research Group. Presentation of stroke by antihypertensive drug treatment in older persons with isolated systolic hypertension. Journal of the American Medical Association 1991; 265: 3255
86. Ying CY, Tifft CP, Gavras H. Renal revascularization in the azotemic hypertensive patient resistant to therapy. New England Journal of Medicine 1984; 311: 1070
87. Bühler FR, Burkart F, Lutold BE, et al. Antihypertensive beta-blocking action as related to renin and age: a pharmacologic tool to identify pathogenic mechanisms in essential hypertension. American Journal of Cardiology 1975; 36: 653
88. Dall JLC, Gardiner HS. Dietary intake of potassium by geriatric patients. Gerontologia Clinica 1971; 13: 119
89. Jellett LB. Potassium therapy: when is it indicated? Drugs 1978; 16: 88
90. Helderman JH, Vestal RE, Rowe JW, et al. The response of arginine vasopressin to intravenous ethanol and hypertonic saline in man: the impact of aging. Journal of Gerontology 1978; 33: 39
91. Booker JA. Severe symptomatic hyponatremia in elderly outpatients: the role of thiazide therapy and stress. Journal of the American Geriatric Society 1984; 32: 108
92. Caird FI, Andrews GR, Kennedy RD. Effect of posture on blood pressure in the elderly. British Heart Journal 1973; 35: 527
93. Myers MG, Kearns PM, Kennedy DS, et al. Postural hypotension and diuretic therapy in the elderly. Canadian Medical Association Journal 1978; 119: 581
94. Beard K, Bulpitt CJ, Mascie-Taylor H, et al. Management of elderly patients with sustained hypertension. British Medical Journal 1992; 304: 412

95. Greenblatt DJ, Koch-Weser J. Adverse reactions to propranolol in hospitalized medical patients: a report from the Boston Collaborative Drug Surveillance Program. American Heart Journal 1973; 86: 478
96. Schneck DW, Luderer JR, Pritchard JF, et al. A comparison of the intrinsic clearance of propranolol in young and elderly subjects. Clinical Pharmacology & Therapeutics 1980; 27: 284
97. Quarterman CP, Kendall MJ, Jack DB. The effect of age on the pharmacokinetics of metoprolol and its metabolites. British Journal of Clinical Pharmacology 1981; 11: 287
98. Rubin PC, Scott PJ, McLean K, et al. Atenolol disposition in young and elderly subjects. British Journal of Clinical Pharmacology 1982; 13: 235
99. Kelly JG, McGarry K, O'Malley K, et al. Bioavailability of labetalol increases with age. British Journal of Clinical Pharmacology 1982; 14: 304
100. Topol EJ, Traill TA, Fortuin NJ. Hypertensive hypertrophic cardiomyopathy of the elderly. New England Journal of Medicine 1985; 312: 277
101. Simon AC, Safar MA, Levenson JA, et al. Systolic hypertension: hemodynamic mechanism and choice of antihypertensive treatment. American Journal of Cardiology 1979; 44: 505
102. Koch-Weser J. Hydralazine. New England Journal of Medicine 1976; 295: 320
103. Rubin PC, Scott PJ, Reid JL. Prazosin disposition in young and elderly subjects. British Journal of Clinical Pharmacology 1981; 12: 401
104. Kelly JG, O'Malley K. Calcium antagonists in the elderly. Drugs & Aging 1993; 3: 400
105. Bühler FR. Calcium antagonists as first line antihypertensive monotherapy. Proceedings of the Second World Conference on Clinical Pharmacology and Therapeutics. American Society for Pharmacology and Experimental Therapeutics, Bethesda, 1984.
106. Psaty BM, Heckbert SR, Koepsell TD, et al. The risk of myocardial infarction associated with antihypertensive drug therapies. Journal of the American Medical Association 1995; 274: 620
107. Applegate WB, Phillips HL, Schnaper H, et al. A randomized controlled trial of the effects of three antihypertensive agents on blood pressure control and quality of life in older women. Archives of Internal Medicine 1991; 151: 1817
108. Cushman WC, Khatri I, Materson BJ, et al. Treatment of hypertension in the elderly. III. Response of isolated systolic hypertension to various doses of hydrochlorothiazide: results of a Department of Veterans Affairs cooperative study. Archives of Internal Medicine 1991; 151: 1954-60
109. Materson BJ, Comenii JR, Cushman WC. Single drug therapy for hypertension in men: a comparison of six antihypertensive agents with placebo. New England Journal of Medicine 1993; 328: 914
110. Mader SL, Josephson KR, Rubenstein LZ. Low prevalence of postural hypotension among community-dwelling elderly. Journal of the American Medical Association 1987; 258: 1511
111. Lipsitz LA. Orthostatic hypotension in the elderly. New England Journal of Medicine 1989; 321: 952
112. Robertson D, Davis TL. Recent advances in the treatment of orthostatic hypotension. Neurology 1995; 45: 526
113. Holtdke RD, Streeten DH. Treatment of orthostatic hypotension with erythropoietin. New England Journal of Medicine 1993; 329: 611
114. Freedman SB, Richman DR, Ashley JJ. Verapamil kinetics in normal subjects and patients with coronary artery spasm. Clinical Pharmacology & Therapeutics 1981; 30: 644
115. Ridker PM, Manson JE, Gaziano JM, et al. Low-dose aspirin therapy for chronic stable angina. Annals of Internal Medicine 1991; 114: 835
116. Nwasakwa ON, Koss JH, Friedman JH, et al. Bypass surgery for chronic stable angina: predictors of survival benefit and strategy for patient selection. Annals of Internal Medicine 1991; 114: 1035
117. Willard JE, Lange RA, Hillis LD. The use of aspirin in ischemic heart disease. New England Journal of Medicine 1992; 327: 175
118. Théroux P, Ouimet H, McCans J, et al. Aspirin, heparin, or both to treat acute unstable angina. New England Journal of Medicine 1988; 319: 1105
119. Volpi A, DeVita C, Grazia Franzosi M, et al. Determinants of 6-month mortality in survivors of myocardial infarction after thrombolysis. Circulation 1993; 88: 416
120. Battershill PE, Benfield P, Goa KL. Streptokinase: a review of its pharmacology and therapeutic efficacy in acute myocardial infarction in older patients. Drugs & Aging 1994; 4: 63
121. ISIS-2 (Second International Study of Infarct Survival) Collaborative Group. Randomized trial of intravenous streptokinase, oral aspirin, both or neither among 17,187 cases of suspected acute myocardial infarction: ISIS-2. Lancet 1988; 2: 349
122. Krumholz HM, Pasternack RC, Weinstein MC, et al. Cost effectiveness of streptokinase in elderly patients with suspected acute myocardial infarction. New England Journal of Medicine 1992; 327: 7
123. GUSTO Investigators. An international randomized trial comparing four thrombolytic strategies for acute myocardial infarction. New England Journal of Medicine 1993; 329: 673
124. Fibrinolytic Therapy Trialists (FTT) Collaborative Group. Indications for fibrinolytic therapy in suspected acute myocardial infarction: collaborative overview of early mortality and major morbidity results from all randomised trials of more than 100 patients. Lancet 1994; 343: 311
125. Williamson BD, Muller DWM, Topol EJ. Should older patients with acute myocardial infarction receive thrombolytic therapy? Drugs & Aging 1992; 2: 461
126. Gurwitz JH, Gore JM, Goldberg RJ, et al. Recent age-related trends in the use of thrombolytic therapy in patients who have had acute myocardial infarction. Annals of Internal Medicine 1996; 124: 283
127. Gruppo Italiano per lo Studio della Sopravvivenza nell'infarto Miocardico. GISSI-3: effects of lisinopril and transdermal glyceryl trinitrate singly and together on 6-week mortality and ventricular function after acute myocardial infarction. Lancet 1994; 343: 1115-22
128. ISIS-4 (Fourth International Study of Infarct Survival) Collaborative Group. ISIS-4: a randomised factorial trial assessing early oral captopril, oral mononitrate and intravenous magnesium sulfate in 58,050 patients with suspected acute myocardial infarction. Lancet 1995; 345: 669-85
129. Krumholz HM, Radford MJ, Ellerbeck EF, et al. Aspirin for secondary prevention after myocardial infarction in the elderly: prescribed use and outcomes. Annals of Internal Medicine 1996; 124: 292
130. Bourassa MG, Guene O, Bangdiwala SI, et al. Natural history and patterns of current practice in heart fail-

ure. Journal of the American College of Cardiology 1993; 22 Suppl. A: 14A

131. Rodeheffer RJ, Gerstenblith G, Becker LC, et al. Exercise cardiac output is maintained with advancing age in healthy human subjects: cardiac dilation and increased stroke volume compensate for a diminished heart rate. Circulation 1984; 69: 203
132. Cody RJ, Torre S, Clark M, et al. Age-related hemodynamic, renal and hormonal differences among patients with congestive heart failure. Archives of Internal Medicine 1989; 149: 1023-8
133. Altus P. Timolol induced congestive heart failure. Southern Medical Journal 1981; 74: 88
134. Munroe WP, Rindone JP, Kershner RM. Systemic side effects associated with ophthalmic administration of timolol. Drug Intelligence and Clinical Pharmacy 1985; 19: 85
135. Cusack B, Kelly J, O'Malley K, et al. Digoxin in the elderly: pharmacokinetic consequences of old age. Clinical Pharmacology & Therapeutics 1979; 25: 772-6
136. Nelson RD, Ezri MD, Denes P. Arrhythmia and conduction disturbances in the elderly. In: Messerli, editor. Cardiovascular disease in the elderly. Boston: Martinus Nijhoff, 1984: 83
137. Trivalle C, Doucet J, Chessagne P, et al. Differences in the signs and symptoms of hyperthyroidism in older and younger patients. Journal of the American Geriatric Society 1996; 44: 50
138. Camm AJ, Evans KE, Ward DE. The rhythm of the heart in active elderly subjects. American Heart Journal 1980; 99: 598
139. Echt DS, Liebson PR, Mitchell LB, et al. Mortality and morbidity in patients receiving encainide, flecainide, or placebo. New England Journal of Medicine 1991; 327: 1818
140. Mason JW, for the Electrophysiological Study versus Electrocardiographic Monitoring Investigators. A comparison of seven antiarrhythmic drugs in patients with ventricular tachyarrhythmias. New England Journal of Medicine 1993; 329: 452.
141. Donovan MD, Castleden CM, Pohl JEF. The effect of age on digitoxin pharmacokinetics. British Journal of Clinical Pharmacology 1981; 11: 401
142. Passmore AP, Johnston GD. Digoxin toxicity in the aged: characterizing and avoiding the problem. Drugs & Aging 1991; 1: 364
143. Kernan WN, Castellsague J, Perlman GD, et al. Incidence of hospitalization for digitalis toxicity among elderly Americans. American Journal of Medicine 1994; 96: 426
144. Klein HO, Kaplinsky E. Digitalis and verapamil in atrial fibrillation and flutter: an update. Drugs 1986; 31: 185
145. Ochs HR, Greenblatt DJ, Woo E, et al. Reduced quinidine clearance in elderly persons. American Journal of Cardiology 1978; 42: 481
146. Drayer DE, Hughes M, Lorenzo B, et al. Prevalence of high 3-hydroxyquinidine/quinidine ratios in serum and decreased clearance of quinidine in cardiac patients with age. Clinical Pharmacology & Therapeutics 1980; 27: 72
147. Coplen SE, Antman EM, Berlin JA, et al. Efficacy and safety of quinidine therapy for maintenance of sinus rhythm after cardioversion: a meta-analysis of randomized controlled clinical trials. Circulation 1990; 82: 1106
148. Reidenberg MM, Camacho MC, Kluger J, et al. Aging and renal clearance of procainamide and acetylprocainamide. Clinical Pharmacology & Therapeutics 1980; 28: 732
149. Bonde J, Petersen LE, Bodtker S, et al. The influence of age and smoking on the elimination of disopyramide. British Journal of Clinical Pharmacology 1985; 20: 453
150. Cusack B, O'Malley K, Lavan J, et al. Protein binding and disposition of lignocaine in the elderly. European Journal of Clinical Pharmacology 1985; 29: 233
151. Nation RL, Triggs EJ, Selig M. Lignocaine kinetics in cardiac patients and aged subjects. British Journal of Clinical Pharmacology 1977; 10: 439
152. Lie KI, Wellens HJ, Van Capelle FJ, et al. Lidocaine in the prevention of primary ventricular fibrillation. New England Journal of Medicine 1974; 291: 1324
153. Pfeifer HJ, Greenblatt DJ. Clinical use and toxicity of intravenous lidocaine. American Heart Journal 1976; 92: 168
154. Grech-Belanger O, Barbeau G, Kishka P, et al. Pharmacokinetics of mexiletine in the elderly. Journal of Clinical Pharmacology 1989; 29: 311
155. Roden DM. Risks and benefits of antiarrhythmic therapy. New England Journal of Medicine 1994; 331: 785
156. Ishizaki T, Hirayama H, Tawara K, et al. Pharmacokinetics and pharmacodynamics in young normal and elderly hypertensive subjects: a study using sotolol as a model drug. Journal of Pharmacology and Experimental Therapeutics 1980; 212: 173
157. Hyatt RH, Sinha B, Vallon A, et al. Non-cardiac side-effects of long-term oral amiodarone in the elderly. Age and Ageing 1988; 17: 116
158. Shetty HGM, Woodhouse KW. Use of amiodarone for elderly patients. Age and Ageing 1992; 21: 233
159. Antiplatelet Trialists' Collaboration. Secondary prevention of vascular disease by prolonged antiplatelet treatment. British Medical Journal 1988; 296: 320
160. Matchar DB, McCrory DC, Barnett HJM, et al. Medical treatment for stroke prevention. Annals of Internal Medicine 1994; 121: 41
161. Sivenius J, Riekkinen PJ, Laakso M, et al. European Stroke Prevention Study (ESPS): antithrombotic therapy is also effective in the elderly. Acta Neurologica Scandinavica 1993; 87: 111-4
162. The Dutch TIA Trial Study Group. A comparison of two doses of aspirin (30 vs. 283 mg a day) in patients after a transient ischemic attack or minor ischemic stroke. New England Journal of Medicine 1991; 325: 1261
163. Noble S, Goa KL. Ticlopidine: a review of its pharmacology, clinical efficacy and tolerability in the prevention of cerebral ischaemia and stroke. Drugs & Aging 1996; 8: 214-32
164. Albers GW. Stroke prevention in nonvalvular atrial fibrillation. Annals of Internal Medicine 1991; 115: 727
165. Stroke Prevention in Atrial Fibrillation Investigators. Warfarin versus aspirin for prevention of thromboembolism in atrial fibrillation: Stroke Prevention in Atrial Fibrillation II Study. Lancet 1994; 343: 687
166. European Atrial Fibrillation Trial Study Group. Secondary prevention in non-rheumatic atrial fibrillation after transient ischaemic attack or minor stroke. Lancet 1993; 342: 1255
167. Lipsey JR, Robinson RG, Pearlson GD, et al. Nortriptyline treatment of post-stroke depression: a double-blind study. Lancet 1984; 1: 297
168. Porter JM, Cutler BS, Lee BY, et al. Pentoxifylline efficacy in the treatment of intermittent claudication:

multicenter controlled double-blind trial with objective assessment of chronic occlusive arterial disease patients. American Heart Journal 1982; 104: 66
169. Frampton JE, Brogden RN. Pentoxifylline (oxpentifylline): a review of its therapeutic efficacy in the management of peripheral vascular and cerebrovascular disorders. Drugs & Aging 1995; 7: 480-503
170. Hirsh J, Genton E, Hull R, editors. Venous thromboembolism. New York: Grune and Stratton, 1981
171. Carson JL, Kelley MA, Duff A, et al. The clinical course of pulmonary embolism. New England Journal of Medicine 1992; 326: 1240-5
172. Clagett GP, Anderson FA, Heit J, et al. Prevention of venous thromboembolism. Chest 1995; 108: 312S
173. Gruber UF, Saldeen T, Brokop T, et al. Incidence of fatal postoperative pulmonary embolism after prophylaxis with dextran 70 and low dose heparin: an international multicentre study. British Medical Journal 1980; 280: 69
174. Leyvraz PF, Richard J, Bachmann F, et al. Adjusted versus fixed-dose subcutaneous heparin in the prevention of deep vein thrombosis after total hip replacement. New England Journal of Medicine 1983; 309: 954
175. Levine MN, Hirsh J, Gent M, et al. Prevention of deep vein thrombosis after elective hip surgery. A randomized trial comparing low molecular weight heparin with standard unfractionated heparin. Annals of Internal Medicine 1991; 114: 545
176. Salzman EW, Ploetz J, Bettman M, et al. Intraoperative external pneumatic calf compression to afford long-term prophylaxis against deep vein thrombosis in urological patients. Surgery 1980; 87: 239
177. Hull R, Delmore TJ, Hirsh J. Effectiveness of intermittent pulsatile elastic stockings for the prevention of calf and thigh vein thrombosis in patients undergoing elective knee surgery. Thrombosis Research 1979; 16: 37
178. Mohr DN, Silverstein MD, Ilstrup DM, et al. Venous thromboembolism associated with hip and knee arthroplasty: current prophylactic practices and outcomes. Mayo Clinic Proceedings 1992; 67: 861
179. Coon WW, Willis III PW. Hemorrhagic complications of anticoagulant therapy. Archives of Internal Medicine 1974; 133: 386
180. Jick H. Efficacy and toxicity of heparin in relation to age and sex. New England Journal of Medicine 1968; 179: 284
181. Landefeld CS, Beyth RJ. Risk for anticoagulant-related bleeding: a meta-analysis. American Journal of Medicine 1993; 95: 315
182. Jones BR, Baran A, Reidenberg MM. Evaluating patients' warfarin requirements. Journal of the American Geriatric Society 1980; 28: 10
183. Shepherd AMM, Hewick DS, Moreland TA, et al. Age as a determinant of sensitivity to warfarin. British Journal of Clinical Pharmacology 1977; 4: 315
184. Shepherd AMM, Wilson N, Stevenson IH. Warfarin sensitivity in the elderly. In: Crooks & Stevenson, editors. Drugs in the elderly. Baltimore: University Park Press 1979; 44: 505.
185. O'Malley K, Stevenson IH, Ward C. Factors influencing anticoagulant control - an epidemiologic study in drug interactions. In: Morselli et al., editors. Drug interactions. New York: Raven Press, 1974: 309
186. Cipolle RJ, Seifert RD, Neilan BA, et al. Heparin kinetics: variables related to disposition and dosage. Clinical Pharmacology & Therapeutics 1982; 29: 387
187. Cruickshank MK, Levine MN, Hirsh J, et al. A standard heparin nomogram for the management of heparin therapy. Archives of Internal Medicine 1991; 151: 333
188. O'Connor GT, Sparrow D, Segal MR. Smoking, atopy and methacholine airway responsiveness among middle-aged and elderly men: the normative aging study. American Review of Respiratory Diseases 1989; 140: 1520
189. Robin ED. Death rate from bronchial asthma. Chest 1988; 93: 614
190. Connolly MJ, Selly C, Walters EH, et al. An assessment of methacholine inhalation tests in elderly asthmatics. Age and Ageing 1988; 17: 123
191. Connolly MJ, Crowley JJ, Charan NB, et al. Impaired bronchodilator response to albuterol in healthy elderly men and women. Chest 1995; 108: 401-6
192. Ullah MI, Newman GB, Saunders KB. Influence of age on response to ipratropium bromide and salbutamol in asthma. Thorax 1981; 36: 523
193. Diggory P, Bailey R, Vallon A. Effectiveness of inhaled bronchodilator delivery system for elderly patients. Age and Ageing 1991; 20: 379
194. Cusack B, Kelly JG, Lavan J, et al. Theophylline kinetics in relation to age: the importance of smoking. British Journal of Clinical Pharmacology 1980; 10: 109
195. Vestal RE, Cusack BJ, Crowley JJ, et al. Aging and the response to inhibition and induction of theophylline metabolism. Experimental Gerontology 1993; 28: 421
196. Crowley JJ, Cusack BJ, Jue SG, et al. Aging and drug interactions, II: effect of phenytoin and smoking on the oxidation of theophylline and cortisol in healthy men. Journal of Pharmacology and Experimental Therapeutics 1988; 245: 513
197. Shannon M. Predictors of major toxicity after theophylline overdose. Annals of Internal Medicine 1993; 119: 1161
198. Sessler CN. Theophylline toxicity: clinical features of 116 consecutive cases. American Journal of Medicine 1990; 88: 567-76
199. Shannon M, Lovejoy FH. The influence of age vs peak serum concentration on life threatening events after chronic theophylline intoxication. Archives of Internal Medicine 1990; 150: 2045
200. Juniper EF, Kline PA, Vanzieleghem MA, et al. Long term inhaled steroids for asthmatics. American Review of Respiratory Disease 1990; 142: 832
201. Sambrook P, Birmingham J, Kelly P, et al. Prevention of corticosteroid osteoporosis: a comparison of calcium, calcitriol, and calcitonin. New England Journal of Medicine 1993; 328: 1747
202. Liberman UA, Weiss SR, Bröll J, et al. Effect of oral alendronate on bone mineral density and the incidence of fractures in postmenopausal women. New England Journal of Medicine 1995; 333: 1437
203. Gross NJ. Ipratropium bromide. New England Journal of Medicine 1988; 319: 486-94
204. Dompeling E, Van Schayck CP, van Grunsven PM, et al. Slowing the deterioration of asthma and COPD observed during bronchodilator therapy by adding inhaled corticosteroids: a 4-year prospective study. Annals of Internal Medicine 1993; 118: 770
205. Nichol KL, Margolis KL, Wuorenma J, et al. The efficacy and cost effectiveness of vaccination against influenza among elderly persons living in the community. New England Journal of Medicine 1994; 331: 778
206. Mokshagundam S, Barzel US. Thyroid disease in the elderly. Journal of the American Geriatric Society 1993; 41: 1361

207. Berglund J, Christensen SB, Hallengren B. Total and age specific incidence of Graves' thyrotoxicosis, toxic nodular goiter, and solitary toxic adenoma in Malmo, 1970-74. Journal of Internal Medicine 1990; 227: 137
208. Tibaldi JM, Barzel US, Albin J, et al. Thyrotoxicosis in the very old. American Journal of Medicine 1986; 81: 619
209. Gregerman RI, Katz MS. Thyroid diseases. In: Hazzard et al., editors. Principles of geriatric medicine and gerontology. New York: McGraw Hill, 1994: 807
210. Davis PJ, Davis FB. Hyperthyroidism in patients over the age of 60 years. Medicine 1974; 6: 83
211. Rosenbaum RL, Barzel US. Levothyroxine replacement dose for primary hypothyroidism decreases with age. Annals of Internal Medicine 1982; 96: 53
212. Petri MP, Gatling W, Petri LM, et al. Diabetes in the elderly, an epidemiological perspective. Practical Diabetes 1986; 3: 152
213. Harris MI. Epidemiology of diabetes mellitus among the elderly in the United States. Clinics in Geriatric Medicine 1990; 6: 703
214. Ilarde A, Tuck M. Treatment of non-insulin dependent diabetes mellitus and its complications: a state of the art review. Drugs & Aging 1994; 4: 470
215. Morley JE. Diabetes mellitus: new approaches to management. Clinical Geriatrics 1996; 4: 75
216. Robertson DA, Home PD. Problems and pitfalls of sulphonylurea therapy in older patients. Drugs & Aging 1993; 3: 510
217. Melander A, Sartor G, Whalin E, et al. Serum tolbutamide and chlorpropamide concentrations in patients with diabetes mellitus. British Medical Journal 1978; 1: 142
218. Goldberg AP, Coon PJ. Diabetes mellitus and glucose metabolism in the elderly. In: Hazzard et al., editors. Principles of geriatric medicine and gerontology. New York: McGraw Hill, 1994: 825
219. Berger W. 88 schwere hypoglykamiezwishenfalle unter der behandlung mit sulfonylharnstoffen. Schweizerische Medizinishe Wochenschrift 1971; 71: 1013
220. Brodows RG. Benefits and risks with glyburide and glipizide in elderly NIDDM patients. Diabetes Care 1991; 15: 75
221. Turkington RW. Encephalopathy induced by oral hypoglycemic drugs. Archives of Internal Medicine 1977; 137: 1082
222. Slade IH, Iosefa RN. Fatal hypoglycemic coma from the use of tolbutamide in elderly patients: report of two cases. Journal of the American Geriatric Society 1967; 15: 948
223. De Fronzo RA, Goodman AM, and The Metoformin Multicenter Study Group. Efficacy of metformin in patients with non-insulin dependent diabetes mellitus. New England Journal of Medicine 1995; 333: 541.
224. Orskov H, Christiansen NJ. Plasma disappearance rate of injected human insulin in juvenile diabetic, maturity-onset diabetic and nondiabetic subjects. Diabetes 1969; 18: 653
225. Minaker KL, Rowe JW, Tonino R, et al. Influence of age on clearance of insulin in man. Diabetes 1982; 31: 851
226. Coscelli C, Calabrese G, Fedele D, et al. Use of premixed insulin among the elderly: reduction of errors in patient preparation of mixtures. Diabetes Care 1992; 15: 1628
227. Albanese AA, Edelson AH, Lorenze EJ, et al. Problems of bone health in elderly: ten year study. New York State Journal of Medicine 1975; 75: 326
228. Riggs AL, Melton LJ. Involutional osteoporosis. New England Journal of Medicine 1986; 314: 1676
229. Frumar AM, Melorum OR, Geola F, et al. Relationship of fasting urinary calcium to circulating estrogen and body weight in postmenopausal women. Journal of Clinical Endocrinology and Metabolism 1980; 50: 70
230. Conference Report. Consensus development conference: diagnosis, prophylaxis and treatment of osteoporosis. American Journal of Medicine 1993; 94: 646
231. Kiel DP, Felson DP, Anderson JJ, et al. Hip fracture and the use of estrogens in postmenopausal women: the Framingham Study. New England Journal of Medicine 1987; 317: 1169
232. Cauley JA, Seeley DG, Ensrud K, et al. Estrogen replacement therapy and fractures in older people. Annals of Internal Medicine 1995; 122: 9
233. Chapuy MC, Arlot ME, Duboeuf F, et al. Vitamin $D_3$ and calcium to prevent hip fractures in elderly women. New England Journal of Medicine 1992; 327: 1637
234. Reckler RR. Calcium absorption and achlorhydria. New England Journal of Medicine 1985; 313: 70
235. Slovik DM, Adams JS, Neer RM, et al. Deficient production of 1,25-dihydroxy vitamin D in elderly osteoporotic females. New England Journal of Medicine 1981; 305: 372
236. Shoemaker ES, Forney JP, MacDonald PC. Estrogen treatment of postmenopausal women: benefits and risks. Journal of the American Medical Association 1977; 238: 1524
237. Weiss NS. Decreased risk of fractures of the hip and lower forearm with post-menopausal use of estrogen. New England Journal of Medicine 1980; 303: 1195
238. Gordon GS, Picchi J, Roof BS. Antifracture efficacy of long-term oestrogens for osteoporosis. Transactions of the Association of American Physicians 1973; 86: 326
239. Boston Collaborative Drug Surveillance Program. Surgically confirmed gallbladder disease, venous thromboembolism, and breast tumours in relation to postmenopausal estrogen therapy. New England Journal of Medicine 1974; 290: 15
240. Ziel HK, Finkle WD. Increased risk of endometrial cancer among users of conjugated estrogens. New England Journal of Medicine 1975; 293: 1167
241. Paterson MEL, Wade-Evans T, Sturdee DW, et al. Endometrial disease after treatment with estrogen and progestins in the climacteric. British Medical Journal 1980; 1: 822
242. Reginster J-Y. Calcitonin for prevention and treatment of osteoporosis. American Journal of Medicine 1993; 95 Suppl. 5A: 5A
243. Storm T, Thamsborg G, Stenicke T, et al. Effect of intermittent cyclical etidronate therapy on bone mass and fracture rate in women with postmenopausal osteoporosis. New England Journal of Medicine 1990; 322: 1265
244. Jackson RD, Harris ST, Garant HK, et al. Cyclical etidronate treatment of post-menopausal osteoporosis: 4 year experience. Bone and Mineral 1992; 17 Suppl. 1: 154
245. Cuny G, Royer RJ, Mur JM, et al. Pharmacokinetics of salicylates in the elderly. Gerontology 1979; 25: 49

246. Montgomery PR, Sitar DS. Increased serum salicylate metabolites with age in patients recieving chronic acetylsalicylic acid therapy. Gerontology 1981; 27: 329
247. Traeger A, Kunze M, Stein G, et al. Zur Pharmacokinetik von indomethacin bei alten menschen. Zeitschrift für Alternsforschung 1973; 27: 151
248. Poe WD, Holloway DA. Arthritis and its treatment. In: Poe WD, Holloway DA, editors. Drugs and the aged. New York: McGraw Hill, 1980: 115-27
249. Davies DM, editor. Textbook of adverse drug reactions. Oxford: Oxford University Press, 1977. (137)
250. Clive DM, Stoff JS. Renal syndromes associated with nonsteroidal antiinflammatory drugs. New England Journal of Medicine 1984; 310: 563
251. Blackshear JL, Davidman M, Stillman T. Identification of risk for renal insufficiency from nonsteroidal anti-inflammatory drugs. Archives of Internal Medicine 1983; 143: 1130
252. Nesher G, Moore TL. Rheumatoid arthritis in the aged: incidence and optimal management. Drugs & Aging 1993; 3: 487
253. Kean WF, Bellamy N, Brooks PM. Gold therapy in the elderly rheumatoid arthritis patient. Arthritis & Rheumatism 1983; 26: 705
254. Kean WF, Anastassiades TP, Dwosh IL, et al. Efficacy and toxicity of D-penicillamine for rheumatoid arthritis in the elderly. Journal of the American Geriatric Society 1982; 30: 94
255. Porro GB, Lazzaroni M. Prescribing policy for antiulcer treatment in the elderly. Drugs & Aging 1993; 3: 308
256. Hawkey CJ. Non-steroidal, anti-inflammatory drugs and peptic ulcers: facts and figures multiply, but do they add up? British Medical Journal 1990; 300: 278
257. Griffin MR, Ray WA, Schaffer W. Nonsteroidal anti-inflammatory drug use and death from peptic ulcer disease. Annals of Internal Medicine 1988; 109: 359
258. Lind T, Cederberg C, Olavsson M, et al. Omeprazole in duodenal ulcer patients: relationship between reduction in gastric acid secretion and plasma fasting gastrin. European Journal of Clinical Pharmacology 1991; 40: 557
259. Small RE, Atwell DR, Garnett WR. Utilization of cimetidine in extended care facilities. Abstracts, St Louis: American Pharmaceutical Association Annual Meeting, 1981.
260. Sirgo MA, Mills R, Enles A, et al. The safety of ranitidine in elderly versus nonelderly patients. Journal of Clinical Pharmacology 1993; 33: 78
261. Jensen DM, Cheng S, Kovacs TOG, et al. A controlled study of ranitidine for prevention of recurrent hemorrhage from duodenal ulcer. New England Journal of Medicine 1994; 330: 382
262. Graham DY, Lew GM, Klein PD, et al. Effect of treatment of *Helicobacter pylori* infection on the long term recurrence of gastric ulcer or duodenal ulcer: a randomized, controlled trial. Annals of Internal Medicine 1992; 116: 705
263. Whitehead WE, Drinkwater D, Cheskin J, et al. Constipation in the elderly living at home: definition, prevalence and relationship to lifestyle and health status. Journal of the American Geriatric Society 1989; 37: 423
264. Harari D, Gurwitz JH, Minaker KL. Constipation in the elderly. Journal of the American Geriatric Society 1993; 41: 1130
265. Newman HF, Freeman J. Physiologic factors affecting defacatory sensation. Journal of the American Geriatric Society 1974; 22: 553
266. Read NW, Abouzekry L, Read MG, et al. Anorectal function in elderly patients with fecal impaction. Gastroenterology 1985; 89: 959-66
267. Cerulli MA, Nikoomanesh P, Schuster MM. Progress in biofeedback conditioning for fecal incontinence. Gastroenterology 1979; 76: 742
268. Orne MT. The efficacy of biofeedback therapy. Annual Review of Medicine 1979; 30: 499
269. Chutka DS, Fleming KC, Evans MP, et al. Urinary incontinence in the elderly population. Mayo Clinic Proceedings 1996; 71: 93
270. Ouslander JG. Geriatric urinary incontinence. Disease-a-Month 1979; 38: 67
271. Williams ME, Fitzhugh CP. Urinary incontinence in the elderly. Annals of Internal Medicine 1982; 97: 895
272. Sourander LB. Treatment of urinary incontinence: the place of drugs. Gerontology 1990; 36 Suppl. 2: 19
273. Malone-Lee JG, Wagg A, Mundy A, et al. Science of urinary incontinence. Lancet 1994; 344: 311
274. Yarker YE, Goa KL, Fitton A. Oxybutynin: a review of its pharmacodynamic and pharmacokinetic properties and its therapeutic use in detrusor instability. Drugs & Aging 1995; 6: 243-62
275. Wein AJ. Pharmacological treatment of incontinence. Journal of the American Geriatric Society 1990; 38: 317
276. Castleden CM, George CF, Renwick AG, et al. Imipramine: a possible alternative to current therapy for urinary incontinence in the elderly. Journal of Urology 1980; 125: 318
277. Palmer JH, Worth PHL, Exton-Smith AN. Flunarizine: a once-daily therapy for urinary incontinence. Lancet 1981; 2: 279
278. Langtry HD, McTavish D. Terodiline: a review of its pharmacological properties and therapeutic use in the treatment of urinary incontinence. Drugs 1990; 40: 748-61
279. Walter S, Wolf H, Barlebo H, et al. Urinary incontinence in post-menopausal women treated with estrogens. Urology International 1978; 33: 135
280. Stewart BH, Banowsky LHW, Montague DK. Stress incontinence: conservative therapy with sympathomimetic drugs. Journal of Urology 1976; 115: 558
281. Larsson B, Andersson K-E, Batra S, et al. Effects of estradiol on norepinephrine-induced contraction, alpha-adrenoceptor number, and norepinephrine content in the female rabbit urethra. Journal of Pharmacology and Experimental Therapeutics 1984; 229: 557
282. Morley JE, Kaiser FE. Impotence in elderly men. Drugs & Aging 1992; 2: 330
283. Morales A, Condra M, Owen JA, et al. Is yohimbine effective in the treatment of organic impotence? Results of a controlled trial. Journal of Urology 1987; 137: 1168
284. De Palma RG. New developments in the diagnosis and treatment of impotence. Western Journal of Medicine 1996; 164: 54
285. Korenman SG, Viosca SP, Kaiser FE, et al. Use of a vacuum tumescence device in the management of impotence. Journal of the American Geriatric Society 1990; 28: 217
286. Stanisic TH, Francisco GE. Impotence. In: Bressler & Katz, editors. Geriatric gerontology. New York: McGraw-Hill, 1993: 263.
287. Helms PM. Efficacy of antipsychotics in the treatment of the behavioral complications of dementia: a review

of the literature. Journal of the American Geriatric Society 1985; 33: 206

288. Salzman C. Treatment of the elderly agitated patient. Journal of Clinical Psychiatry 1987; 48 Suppl.: 19
289. Smith JM, Baldessarini RJ. Changes in prevalence, severity and recovery in tardive kinesia with age. Archives of General Psychiatry 1980; 37: 1368
290. Salzmann C, Shader RI, Van der Kolk BA. Clinical psychopharmacology and the elderly patient. New York State Journal of Medicine 1976; 76: 71
291. Gleason RP, Schneider LS. Carbamazepine treatment of agitation in Alzheimer's outpatients refractory to neuroleptics. Journal of Clinical Psychiatry 1990; 51: 115
292. Thapa PB, Meador KG, Gideon P, et al. Effects of antipsychotic withdrawal in elderly nursing home patients. Journal of the American Geriatric Society 1994; 42: 280
293. Wagstaff AJ, McTavish D. Tacrine: a review of its pharmacodynamic and pharmacokinetic properties and therapeutic efficacy in Alzheimer's disease. Drugs & Aging 1994; 4: 510
294. Davis KL, Powchik P. Tacrine. Lancet 1995; 345: 625
295. Blazer D. Depression in the elderly. New England Journal of Medicine 1989; 320: 164
296. von Moltke LL, Greenblatt DJ, Shader RI. Clinical pharmacokinetics of antidepressants in the elderly: therapeutic implications. Clinical Pharmacokinetics 1993; 24: 141
297. Abernethy DR, Greenblatt DJ, Shader DJ. Imipramine and desipramine disposition in the elderly. Journal of Pharmacology and Experimental Therapeutics 1985; 232: 183
298. Reynolds III CF. Treatment of depression in late life. American Journal of Medicine 1994; 97: 39S-46S
299. Preskhorn SH. Recent pharmacological advances in antidepressant therapy in the elderly. American Journal of Medicine 1993; 94 Suppl. 5A: 2S
300. Heydorn WE. Nefazadone: a summary of the available data on a new antidepressant agent. Expert Opinion on Investigational Drugs 1995; 4: 131
301. Holliday SM, Benfield P. Venlafaxine: a review of its pharmacology and therapeutic potential in depression. Drugs 1995; 49: 280
302. Woods SW, Tesar GE, Murray GB, et al. Psychostimulant treatment of depressive disorders secondary to medical illness. Journal of Clinical Psychiatry 1986; 47: 12
303. Hewick DS, Newbury P, Hopwood S, et al. Age as a factor affecting lithium therapy. British Journal of Clinical Pharmacology 1977; 4: 201
304. Cole MG. The prognosis of depression in the elderly. Canadian Medical Association Journal 1990; 143: 633
305. Man Son-Hing M, Wells G. Meta-analysis of efficacy of quinine for treatment of nocturnal leg cramps in elderly people. British Medical Journal 1995; 310: 13
306. Mullan E, Katona C, Bellew M. Patterns of sleep disorders and sedative hypnotic use in seniors. Drugs & Aging 1994; 5: 49
307. Ritschel WA. Age dependent disposition of amobarbital: analog computer evaluation. Journal of the American Geriatric Society 1978; 26: 540
308. World Health Organization. Health care in the elderly. Drugs 1981; 22: 279
309. Cook PJ, Huggett A, Graham-Pole R, et al. Hypnotic accumulation and hangover in elderly inpatients: a controlled double-blind study of temazepam and nitrazepam. British Medical Journal 1983; 286: 100
310. Greenblatt DJ, Allen MD, Shader RI. Toxicity of high-dose flurazepam in the elderly. Clinical Pharmacology & Therapeutics 1977; 21: 355
311. MacDonald JB, MacDonald ET. Nocturnal femoral fractures and continued widespread use of barbiturate hypnotics. British Medical Journal 1977; 2: 483
312. Ray WA. Psychotropic drugs and injuries in the elderly: a review. Journal of Clinical Pharmacology 1992; 12: 386-96
313. Wadworth AN, McTavish D. Zoplicone: a review of its pharmacological properties and therapeutic efficacy as an hypnotic. Drugs & Aging 1993; 3: 441
314. Langtry HD, Benfield P. Zolpidem: a review of its pharmacodynamic and pharmacokinetic properties and therapeutic potential. Drugs 1990; 40: 291-313
315. Monane M, Glynn RJ, Avorn J. The impact of sedative hypnotic use on sleep symptoms in elderly nursing home residents. Clinical Pharmacology & Therapeutics 1996; 59: 83
316. Von Hoff DD, Layard MW, Basa P, et al. Risk factors for doxorubicin-induced congestive heart failure. Annals of Internal Medicine 1979; 91: 710
317. Hutchins LF, Lipschitz DA. Cancer, clinical pharmacology, and aging. Clinics in Geriatric Medicine 1987; 3: 483
318. Begg CB, Carbone PP. Clinical trials and drug toxicity in the elderly: the experience of the Eastern Cooperative Oncology Group. Cancer 1983; 52: 1986
319. Kinzell T, Feleppa V. Minimising the side effects of cancer chemotherapy in senior patients. Drugs & Aging 1992; 2: 137
320. Crocker I, Prosnitz L. Radiation therapy of the elderly. Clinics in Geriatric Medicine 1987; 3: 473
321. Palmberg S, Hirsjarvi E. Mortality in geriatric surgery. Gerontology 1979; 25: 103
322. Ferrell BA. Pain management in elderly people. Journal of the American Geriatric Society 1991; 39: 64
323. Durnas C, Cusack BJ. Salicylate intoxication in the elderly: recognition and recommendations on how to prevent it. Drugs & Aging 1992; 2: 20
324. Miller DR. Treatment of nonsteroidal anti-inflammatory drug-induced gastropathy. Clinical Pharmacy 1992; 11: 690
325. Langman MJS, Weil J, Wainwright P, et al. Risk of bleeding peptic ulcer associated with individual non-steroidal anti-inflammatory drugs. Lancet 1994; 343: 1075
326. Rodriquez LAG, Jick H. Risk of upper gastrointestinal bleeding and perforation associated with individual non-steroidal anti-inflammatory drugs. Lancet 1994; 343: 769
327. Graham DY, White RH, Moreland LW, et al. Duodenal and gastric ulcer prevention with misoprostol in arthritis patients taking NSAIDs. Annals of Internal Medicine 1993; 119: 257
328. Sandler DP, Burr R, Weinberg CR. Nonsteroidal anti-inflammatory drugs and the risk for chronic renal disease. Annals of Internal Medicine 1991; 115: 165
329. Gurwitz GH, Avorn J, Ross-Degnan D, et al. Nonsteroidal anti-inflammatory drugs - associated azotemia in the very old. Journal of the American Medical Association 1990; 264: 471
330. Flanagan RJ, Johnston A, White AST, et al. Pharmacokinetics of dextropropoxyphene and nordextropropoxyphene in young and elderly volunteers after single and multiple dextropropoxyphene dosage. British Journal of Clinical Pharmacology 1989; 28: 463

331. Kaiko RF, Wallenstein SL, Rogers AG, et al. Narcotics in the elderly. Medical Clinics of North America 1982; 66: 1079
332. Kaiko RF. Age and morphine analgesia in cancer patients with postoperative pain. Clinical Pharmacology & Therapeutics 1980; 28: 823
333. Chan K, Kendall MJ, Mitchard M, et al. The effect of aging on plasma pethidine concentration. British Journal of Clinical Pharmacology 1975; 2: 297
334. Holdsworth M, Forman WB. Pain control. In: Bressler R, Katz MD, editors. Geriatric pharmacology. New York: McGraw-Hill, 1993: 207
335. Roy RC. Anesthesia for the elderly patient. In: Hazzard WR, Bierman EL, Blan JP, et al., editors. Principles of geriatric medicine and gerontology. 3rd ed. New York: McGraw-Hill, 1994: 287
336. Muravchick S. Physiologic processes of aging in the central nervous system. In: Wilson-Kretchel, editor. Anesthesia and the geriatric patient. Orlando: Grune and Stratton, 1984: 1-9
337. Stanski DR, Maitre PO. Population pharmacokinetics and pharmacodynamics of thiopental: the effect of age revisited. Anesthesiology 1990; 72: 412-22
338. Gregory GA, Eger EI, Munson ES. The relationship between age and halothane requirement in man. Anesthesiology 1969; 30: 488
339. Stevens WD, Dolan WM, Gibbons RT. Minimum alveolar concentrations (MAC) of isoflurane with and without nitrous oxide in patients of various ages. Anesthesiology 1975; 42: 197
340. Katoh T, Suguro Y, Ikeda T, et al. Influence of age on awakening concentrations of sevoflunane and isoflurane. Anesthesia and Analgesia 1993; 76: 348
341. Marsh RHK, Chmielewski AT, Goat VA. Recovery from pancuronium: a comparison between young and old patients. Anesthesia and Analgesia 1980; 35: 1193
342. Koscielmiak-Nielson ZJ, Bevan JC, Popovic V, et al. Onset of maximum neuromuscular block following succinylcholine or vecuronium in four age groups. Anesthesiology 1993; 79: 229
343. Matteo RS, Ornstein E, Schwartz AE, et al. Pharmacokinetics and pharmacodynamics of rocuronium in elderly surgical patients. Anesthesia and Analgesia 1993; 77: 1193
344. Lien CA, Matteo RS, Ornstein E, et al. Distribution elimination and action of vecuronium in the elderly. Anesthesia and Analgesia 1991; 73: 39
345. Park WY, Massengale M, Kim SI, et al. Age and the spread of local anesthetic agent in the epidural space. Anesthesia and Analgesia 1980; 59: 768
346. Ellison N, Mull TD. Unique anesthetic problems in the elderly patient coming to surgery for fracture of the hip. Orthopedic Clinics of North America 1974; 5: 493

Chapter 5

# Therapeutic Drug Monitoring: The Strategy of Target Concentration Intervention

*N.H.G. Holford* and *S. Tett*

## Synopsis of Important Principles

1) Knowledge of drug concentrations can provide important assistance to a clinician in making quantitative therapeutic decisions. Clinical effects are more closely related to drug concentration than to drug dose. Drug concentrations can be used as surrogates for both therapeutic and adverse effects. For many drugs, the outcome of therapy is improved if concentrations are used as targets for dose adjustment intervention.

2) Interpretation of drug concentrations requires an understanding of both the pharmacokinetics and pharmacodynamics of the drug.

3) Comparison of the expected concentration of a drug with the measured value provides the greatest understanding of the absorption, distribution and elimination of the drug in that individual.

4) The interpretation of drug concentrations is made easier if simple dosage regimens are adhered to in conjunction with optimum timing of blood sampling. If the prior dosage history is vague, a concentration measurement should be used as a substitute for an accurate history by providing a starting point for the interpretation of subsequent measurements.

5) A drug concentration measured shortly after the first dose will be most useful for estimating the individual's volume of distribution. A further sample between 1 and 2 expected half-lives after commencing maintenance dosages may be used to assess clearance. If the clearance is substantially different from the initial prediction, the dosage can be changed to avoid inappropriately low or high concentrations. After 4 half-lives have elapsed, clearance can be estimated from a sample taken when the concentration is expected to be at the average value within the dosage interval – most commonly at the mid-point of the interval.

6) The magnitude of the difference between the measured and predicted concentration can be used to indicate if the individual's pharmacokinetic parameters are similar to those expected (in which case no revision of the parameters is necessary), or are different because of individual variation from the population mean (calling for a change in the individual's expected parameters). If the difference between measured and predicted values is unreasonably large, then the assumptions that have been made about dosage, concentration measurements, and the patient's disease state must be critically reviewed.

7) Altered plasma protein binding is an important cause of artefactual changes in drug concentration. Recognition of the direction and magnitude of the change and suitable adjustment of the measured value is an essential step in the interpretation of concentrations for drugs that are highly protein bound. This is particularly important for phenytoin and lidocaine (lignocaine).

8) Drug concentrations must always be interpreted in conjunction with clinical assessment of the patient. The quoted therapeutic range of a drug is not a range of 'normal values'. The therapeutic range is an expression of the probability of beneficial effects with an acceptable risk of toxicity in a population of patients. It may bear little relationship to the effects at a particular concentration in a particular individual.

The use of therapeutic drug monitoring has become widespread but its potential benefit may not have been achieved because of the passive approach implicit in the term 'monitoring'. Taking a blood sample, measuring the concentration and doing nothing because the measurement is within the laboratory 'therapeutic range' denies the patient the benefit of a more critical interpretation and active intervention. We believe that a more appropriate description for the optimum use of drug concentrations in clinical practice is *'target concentration intervention'*.

The rational series of steps involved in achieving the desired therapeutic outcome in an individual is known as the *target concentration strategy*. These steps are:

1) Select a target concentration (see section 4; table I).

2) Predict clearance and volume of distribution values for the patient based on population pharmacokinetic parameters (e.g. those in appendix A) and observable individual characteristics (e.g. weight, renal function).

3) Calculate a loading dose and maintenance dose rate to achieve the target concentration (for relevant equations, see section 1.2).

4) Administer the doses and measure drug concentrations.

5) Use the measured concentrations to predict individualised values of clearance and volume of distribution for the patient.

6) If appropriate, revise the target concentration for the individual based on clinical assessment.

7) Revert to step 3.

The target concentration should be considered as a *surrogate effect,* i.e. a convenient substitute for the desired therapeutic outcome. In this sense, it is similar to a target blood pressure in a hypertensive patient who is at increased risk of cardiovascular disease. In many situations, the therapeutic benefit of a drug is difficult to assess in the short term, in which case, step 6 (above) may not be feasible. The target concentration can provide some assurance that treatment is adequate even if the therapeutic benefit cannot (yet) be observed.

By intervening with a dose adjustment to achieve a specific target concentration, a major source of the variability in the dose-response relationship can be reduced, i.e. the variability in concentration when the same dose is given to different people due to interindividual differences in pharmacokinetics.

Given an accurate dosage history and one or more drug concentrations, it is possible to describe the pharmacokinetic processes of distribution and elimination quite precisely in an individual and make accurate predictions of concentrations at future points in time, whatever dosage regimen is used. The ability to interpret drug concentrations and extract the information so that future concentrations can be predicted, and a rational dosage scheme instituted, requires a different kind of intellectual effort from that needed to interpret, say, a plasma glucose concentration. This is most immediately interpreted by reference to a so-called 'normal range' – usually the 95% confidence interval based upon measurements from a sample of a 'normal' population. Under most circumstances, if the plasma glucose concentration is within the 'normal range', little further attention is paid to it. If it is outside the 'normal range' diagnostic efforts are made to appreciate what pathophysiological process is disturbed. The precise value, however, will be used only in a semiquantitative fashion, e.g. 'high', 'very high', or 'extremely high', or in reference to some previously defined diagnostic threshold value; for example, diabetes mellitus may be diagnosed if a random plasma glucose concentration is greater than 11 mmol/L.

On the other hand, a very different approach is necessary for the optimum use of drug concentrations. There is no equivalent 'normal range' based on 95% confidence intervals from a 'normal' population for drug concentrations. Quantitative interpretations are essential to maximise opportunities for beneficial therapeutic outcomes while minimising the risks of drug toxicity.

The quantitative approach to therapeutic decision making is relatively new to the art of medicine. Most clinicians will not have learned pharmacokinetics at medical school and may have only a very hazy idea of the quantitative decisions that form the basis of rational therapeutics. The young clinician may be misled into thinking that the pharmacokinetics he or she was taught in medical school and material in textbooks such as this are irrelevant to modern medicine, because senior colleagues pay no attention to pharmacokinetic detail and make therapeutic decisions in a seemingly capricious fashion. Such a conclusion would be quite incorrect because therapeutic decisions made by an experienced clinician are founded upon a wide base of knowledge gained from treating many similar patients. This prior knowledge of the characteristics of the population being treated provides an empirical, but nevertheless frequently satisfactory, guide to making an appropriate quantitative and qualitative therapeutic decision.

Recognition of the value of such prior information when faced with an individual patient about whom little is known, is the basis of techniques of rational, quantitative, pharmacokinetic and pharmacodynamic forecasting. For the person who must make a therapeutic choice on behalf of an individual patient, the application of quantitative pharmacokinetic principles can enhance the advice of a more experienced colleague. For all clinicians, young and old, these same principles can be applied to new therapeutic entities and reduce the suffering of patients who would otherwise be exposed to the vagaries of a trial and error approach.

Target concentration intervention is based upon the collaboration between a care giver (clinician, pharmacist, nurse) responsible for making quantitative and qualitative decisions about drug treatment, and the clinical laboratory providing analytical services for the measurement of drug concentrations. The collaborative team approach encourages optimum use of the therapeutic skills of all health professionals involved.

## 1. Concept of Target Concentration Intervention

The idea that drug concentrations could be measured and used to guide therapeutic decisions was first applied to quinidine when it was used to convert the cardiac rhythm of patients with atrial fibrillation to sinus rhythm.[1] Although quinidine is rarely used for this purpose today because of the advent of DC cardioversion, this study is still almost unique because it defined a *target concentration* based upon both the probability of therapeutic success and toxicity. A concentration of 8 mg/L was shown to have an 80% chance of converting to sinus rhythm and a 20% chance of some serious toxicity. No attention was paid to pharmacokinetics – the target concentration was chosen on the basis of pharmacodynamics, i.e. the effects, both good and bad, seen at particular concentrations.

*Rational therapeutics* can be defined as giving the appropriate dose to achieve the desired effect (fig. 1). Pharmacokinetics is the science

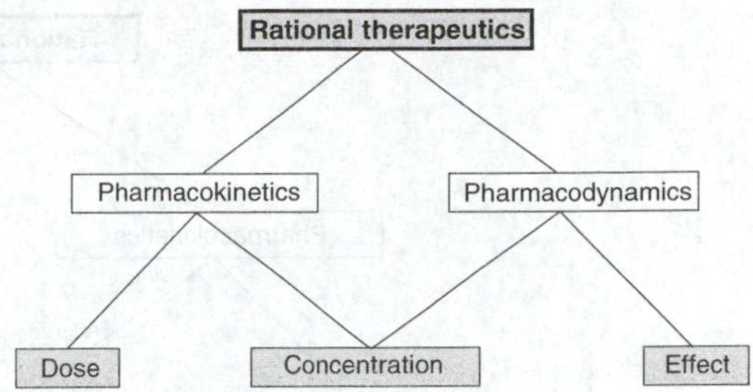


**Fig. 1.** *Rational therapeutics:* the aim of rational therapeutics is to achieve the correct effect with the correct dose. The foundation of decision making is based on pharmacokinetics and pharmacodynamics which provide the rational principles to link dose and effect through drug concentration.

that links dose and concentration by defining the processes of drug distribution (volume of distribution) and elimination (clearance). Pharmacodynamics, on the other hand, is the science linking concentration to effect by defining the maximum effect of the drug ($E_{max}$) and the sensitivity of the target organ ($EC_{50}$).

*Target concentration intervention* can now be placed at the centre of this therapeutic triangle (fig. 2). This strategy takes information about doses, concentrations and effects in an individual and integrates them to estimate more precisely the pharmacokinetic (volume of distribution, clearance) and pharmacodynamic ($E_{max}$, $EC_{50}$) parameters in that individual. These new values can then be used to predict the consequences of future dosage decisions and lead to the selection of an appropriate dose to achieve the desired effect, i.e. rational therapeutics.

### 1.1 Pharmacodynamics: The Concentration-Effect Relationship

The selection of a target concentration for a drug is based upon what is known of the relationship between concentration and effects, both desired (therapeutic effects) and undesired (adverse effects). There is, unfortunately, a paucity of information about the clinical pharmacodynamics of most drugs on which to base such a decision. Further complications are introduced by the judgements that must be made in weighing up the relative merits of increased therapeutic effects against the increased risk of adverse effects.

As an example, consider how the target concentration for theophylline might be defined. Theophylline is a bronchodilator often used in the acute management of severe bronchospasm

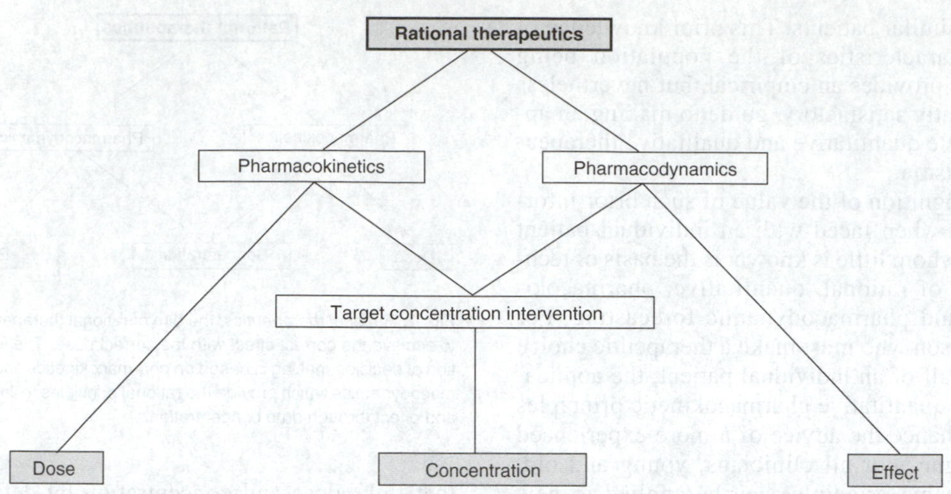


**Fig. 2.** *Target concentration intervention:* the individualisation of drug dose to achieve the desired therapeutic effect is aided by the measurement of drug concentration. Target concentration intervention integrates dose, concentration, and effect in order to understand more precisely the pharmacokinetics and pharmacodynamics of the drug in an individual.

due to asthma. Studies performed in a small number of asthmatics recovering from an acute attack of asthma have examined the increase in forced expiratory volume in 1 second ($FEV_1$), which is inversely related to the degree of airways obstruction. The relationship between the theophylline concentration and change in $FEV_1$ is not a straight line (fig. 3). As concentrations rise, the increase in $FEV_1$ is proportionately less and approaches a maximum response ($E_{max}$). Half of the maximum improvement is achieved at a concentration of 10 mg/L – the $EC_{50}$. Notice that doubling the concentration to 20 mg/L produces less than 20% further improvement over that at 10 mg/L, and it can be predicted that concentrations of 40 mg/L are required to obtain 80% of the maximum response (equation 1):

$$\text{Effect} = \frac{E_{max} \cdot \text{Concentration}}{EC_{50} + \text{Concentration}} \quad \text{(Eq. 1)}$$

For example, if $E_{max}$ = 100% and $EC_{50}$ = 10 mg/L, the effect at 40 mg/L will be:

$$\text{Effect} = \frac{100\% \cdot 40\ \text{mg/L}}{10\ \text{mg/L} + 40\ \text{mg/L}}$$

$$= 80\%$$

The above calculations do not, however, consider adverse effects. In a study in patients with acute asthma treated with intravenous theophylline and randomly assigned to a target concentration of either 10 or 20 mg/L, the greatest difference in peak expiratory flow rate was small but 5 times as many patients assigned to 20 mg/L experienced vomiting (12% of those assigned to this target concentration).[4] The question is therefore whether a small improvement in relief of bronchospasm justifies a 5-fold increase in the risk of vomiting. Such a decision must be made by each clinician caring for a patient based upon the particular circumstances. The general principle to be learned from this example is the diminishing therapeutic gains from increased concentrations which must be

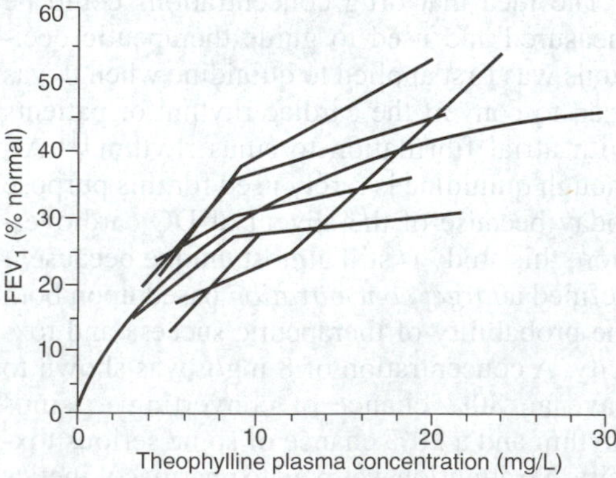


**Fig. 3.** *Theophylline pharmacodynamics:* the effects of increasing concentrations of theophylline on the change in forced expiratory volume in 1 second ($FEV_1$ – expressed as a percentage of the predicted normal $FEV_1$ for each individual) are shown.[2,3] A maximum response is approached at higher concentrations ($E_{max}$). Half of the maximum response is achieved at a theophylline concentration of 10 mg/L ($EC_{50}$). Note that the maximum response ($E_{max}$) is less than the predicted $FEV_1$.

weighed against the enhanced risks of adverse effects.

Guidance in establishing the target concentration can be obtained from a knowledge of the $E_{max}$ and $EC_{50}$ because these define the extent of the therapeutic response that can be expected and the steepest part of the concentration-response curve where the most gain can be expected for the smallest increase in concentration.[5] The target concentration can only be defined on the basis of pharmacodynamics; it is quite independent of the determinants of concentration – i.e. dose and pharmacokinetics.

### 1.2 Pharmacokinetics: The Dose-Concentration Relationship

The selection of the dose needed to achieve the target concentration rests upon pharmacokinetics. In particular, the choice of a *loading dose* can be determined from the volume of distribution:

$$\text{Loading dose} = \text{Volume of distribution} \cdot \text{Concentration} \qquad \text{(Eq. 2)}$$

For example, the volume of distribution of theophylline is about 35L in a 70kg person. If the target concentration is 10 mg/L, then the loading dose is:

$$\text{Loading dose} = 35\text{L} \cdot 10\ \text{mg/L} = 350\text{mg}$$

The *maintenance dose rate,* on the other hand, can be predicted from the clearance:

$$\text{Maintenance dose rate} = \text{Clearance} \cdot \text{Concentration} \qquad \text{(Eq. 3)}$$

The clearance of theophylline is about 3 L/h in a 70kg person. For a target concentration of 10 mg/L, the maintenance dose is:

$$\begin{aligned}\text{Maintenance dose rate} &= 3\ \text{L/h} \cdot 10\ \text{mg/L}\\ &= 30\ \text{mg/h}\\ &= 720\ \text{mg/day}\end{aligned}$$

In practice, this might be administered as 350mg every 12 hours, using a slow release preparation (see chapter 23; sect. 3.1.1 and 3.2).

These elementary principles of pharmacokinetics relating dose to concentration emphasise that a major goal of target concentration intervention is to estimate the volume of distribution and clearance in an individual. Once this has been done, other useful derived parameters such as the half-life can be obtained to assist in determining appropriate dosage intervals or the time needed to reach steady-state (see also chapter 1; sect. 2.3):

$$\text{Half–life} = \frac{0.7 \cdot \text{Volume of distribution}}{\text{Clearance}} \qquad \text{(Eq. 4)}$$

In the above example for theophylline, the half-life is:

$$\begin{aligned}\text{Half–life} &= \frac{0.7 \cdot 35\text{L}}{3\ \text{L/h}}\\ &\approx 8\ \text{hours}\end{aligned}$$

Thus, the expected time to achieve 90% of the steady-state theophylline concentration (around 4 half-lives) is 32 hours.

### 1.3 Why Measure Plasma Concentrations?

It is sometimes argued that the value of measuring drug concentrations in plasma is limited because the site of drug action is not in plasma and concentrations at the active site are quite different. It is probably true that the concentration in plasma and the concentration at a receptor are different but for most practical purposes this is irrelevant. What is important is to understand that the concentrations in plasma and at the receptor will usually be directly proportional to each other at steady-state. If the plasma concentration increases 2-fold, the receptor concentration will also increase 2-fold. If concentrations are not changing rapidly, an individual's pharmacodynamics can be understood quite easily from plasma concentration measurements.

More complex situations can also be described and understood in terms of the equivalent steady-state concentration by defining the kinetics of an effect compartment which accounts for the delay in equilibration between plasma and effect site, or by considering the kinetics of a physiological intermediate.[2]

### 1.4 Therapeutic Range or Target Concentration?

Most people involved with therapeutic drug monitoring know what is meant by the term 'therapeutic range', but few would agree on a common definition that would apply reliably to all drugs. The origins of the therapeutic range can be attributed to the close liaison between clinical pharmacologists who have developed and used drug assays for research studies of pharmacokinetics, and clinical laboratories that have offered a therapeutic drug monitoring service and added drug assays to their repertoire of techniques. All clinical laboratories provide some kind of reference values or normal range for the substances they measure. With the exception of drugs and poisons, these substances are present normally in the body and a normal range can be defined using simple statistical methods applied to measurements made in a representative sample of the normal population. However, no such normal range exists for drugs, although a range of concentrations can be defined which reflects the typical values seen in most patients who appear to be adequately treated and not suffering from excessive adverse effects.

Unfortunately, there is no simple, reliable and consistent statistical procedure applicable to the task of defining the therapeutic range for drugs that is like that used for defining the normal range of natural substances. The therapeutic range is therefore rather loosely and even arbitrarily defined. Ranges tend to be copied by authors from one reference to another, which gives a false sense of consistency and correctness if several different texts are scanned. Most commonly, the origins of a therapeutic range are in the earliest publications describing the measurement of concentrations in a small number of patients at doses which appeared to be effective or toxic. The upper limit of the therapeutic range is defined by levels at which no patient exhibited unacceptable toxicity, and the lower limit by the lowest concentration at which patients appeared to be effectively treated. Limits defined in this way are quite sensible but are subject to considerable error because of the sampling errors arising from such small numbers of patients. They reflect the variation in sensitivity of individuals to the therapeutic and toxic effects of a drug but provide no insight into the steepness of the concentration-response curve within a typical patient.

In the case of theophylline, the pharmacodynamics of which were discussed above, the desired therapeutic effect is graded and continuous. A therapeutic range of 10 to 20 mg/L is almost universally cited. This can be justified in terms of population pharmacodynamics by noting that half of the maximum possible response is achieved at about 10 mg/L[5] and toxicity at this concentration is usually mild. Doubling the concentration to 20 mg/L produces a small enhancement of the therapeutic effect, while the toxicity, although more severe, is not usually life-threatening. The therapeutic range for theophylline can be interpreted to mean that there is little difference in the desired therapeutic effect within the range and no advantage can be expected by exceeding the upper limit because toxicity will outweigh any benefit. Nevertheless, it should be recognised that one-third of the maximal benefit is expected at a concentration of 5 mg/L and almost no adverse effects are likely at this level. A reasonable case could therefore be made for a 4-fold therapeutic range (5 to 20 mg/L) instead of the traditional 2-fold range (10 to 20 mg/L).

On the other hand, an antiarrhythmic drug, such as amiodarone, has pharmacodynamics which are effectively quantal, i.e. all or none. The patient either has an arrhythmia or does not. The target concentration for such a drug is easy to define in principle. It is the concentration which just exceeds the threshold concentration at which the arrhythmia is suppressed. Any higher and the risk of toxicity increases with no offsetting benefit; any lower and the drug is ineffective yet still potentially toxic. For an individual patient, there is no such thing as a therapeutic range for an antiarrhythmic drug, only a target concentration. When a sample of patients is studied, a population target can be defined at which the benefit is reasonably high and toxicity relatively low (fig. 4). From these data, a target concentration of 1.5 mg/L for amiodarone would seem to be reasonable. But what about a therapeutic range? No doubt there are those who will wish to use information such as that in figure 4 to create a therapeutic range, but there is no real justification for it. Others have questioned whether there is any merit in measuring amiodarone concentrations.[6] Overall, for a given patient, the antiarrhythmic benefit is present only when the concentration is above a critical value and is absent below it. There is no graded response for the individual as there is for theophylline.

We believe that attention to a range in a fashion similar to the normal range in clinical chemistry is unwise and in many cases unhelpful in the process of dose optimisation. The specificity and sensitivity of the usual upper limits of therapeutic ranges in the detection of clinical toxicity has been evaluated.[8,9] For theophylline, the misclassification rate using 20 mg/L as the upper limit of 'normal' was estimated to be

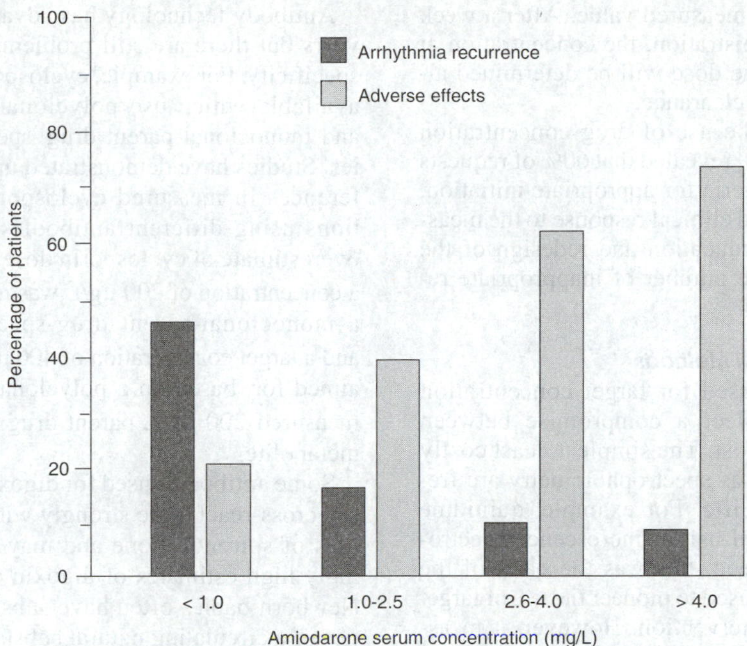


**Fig. 4.** *Amiodarone target concentration:* the chance of arrhythmia decreases with concentration but the chance of toxicity increases. Between 1 and 2 mg/L, the benefits appear to be quite high (80%) and the toxicity acceptably small (40%). A target concentration of 1.5 mg/L is therefore reasonable (after Rotmensch et al.[7]).

16%, i.e. 1 in 6 patients was deemed to have toxicity, based on the concentration measurement, when in fact they had no signs or symptoms of theophylline toxicity.

Dosage calculations for an individual are based on a target concentration, not a range (see equations 2 and 3). The concentration is determined by clinical assessment of the patient and knowledge about the probabilities of benefit and toxicity of the drug in relation to concentration. Therefore target concentrations, and interventions based on these, should be the focus for health professionals involved in individualising dosages.

## 1.5 Cost Effectiveness of Target Concentration Intervention

It is difficult to evaluate the effectiveness of concentration measurements in terms of cost and benefit.[10] A cost-benefit analysis of target concentration intervention for gentamicin has claimed a benefit of nearly $9 for each $1 spent on a pharmacokinetic service.[11] Others have also claimed substantial cost savings.[12]

In general, a concentration measurement provides a substantial piece of information that reflects the use of a particular drug in a particular patient. The detection of noncompliance with recommended treatment, for example, is one common application. Although it is difficult to cost the benefit of this particular piece of information, it certainly enhances the ability of a clinician to understand the response (or lack of it) in a particular setting.

## 1.6 Potential Problems in the Use of Drug Concentrations

### *1.6.1 Missing Information*

In order to interpret a measured drug concentration, certain information is essential. Drug concentrations may vary widely over a dosage interval. For example, gentamicin has a half-life of about 2 hours if renal function is normal. The dosage interval is rarely less than 8 hours, so that at least a 16-fold variation in concentration is expected after each dose. If a gentamicin measurement is made without an accurate record of the time of the sample collection in relation to the last dose, almost all useful information from the measurement is lost.

The second key piece of information is the recent dosage history. As a rule of thumb, all doses within 4 expected half-lives must be known. The interpretation of a digoxin concentration taken 12 hours after the first dose will focus on the role of volume of distribution in determining the measured value. After a week of regular administration, the concentration at 12 hours after the dose will be determined almost entirely by clearance.

An audit of the use of drug concentration measurements[13] revealed that 60% of requests did not fulfil criteria for appropriate initiation, interpretation and clinical response to the measurement. After education and redesign of the request form, the number of inappropriate requests fell to 26%.

#### *1.6.2 Analytical Methods*

Most assays used for target concentration intervention reflect a compromise between specificity and cost. The simplest, least costly techniques such as spectrophotometry are frequently nonspecific. For example, quinidine may be measured using fluorescence spectrophotometry. Indeed, this was the basis of the original method used to pioneer the use of target concentration intervention. However, it measures all fluorescent substances in the plasma and may give seriously misleading overestimates of quinidine concentrations in patients taking other drugs which fluoresce or have fluorescent metabolites (such as aspirin or furosemide). This problem may be particularly important in patients with impaired renal function, who may accumulate drugs and metabolites.

##### Immunoassay Techniques

Radioimmunoassay is often used because it is capable of measuring very low concentrations. In comparison with some other automated techniques it can, however, be relatively expensive because of intensive labour costs. Perhaps the most widely used techniques involve combinations of immunoassay with spectrophotometry, linking the sensitivity of immunoassay with the convenience of spectrophotometry. Such techniques include fluorescence polarisation immunoassays and enzyme multiplied immunoassays. These are simple to perform, require little or no preparation of the samples, and use small plasma volumes (e.g. 50μl). The machines are fully automated and many samples can be assayed at one time. Sample turnaround time is rapid, so that urgent results can be available within 30 minutes of sample receipt by the laboratory. However, these newer techniques are still susceptible to problems of specificity. Fluorescence polarisation immunoassay methods for quinidine are currently no more specific than the older fluorescence spectrometry technique.

Antibody technology has advanced in recent years but there are still problems with lack of specificity. For example, cyclosporin assays are available which use polyclonal, monoclonal and monoclonal-parent drug–specific antibodies. Studies have demonstrated up to 400% differences in measured cyclosporin concentrations using different antibodies.[14] A 2-fold overestimate of cyclosporin dose could occur if a concentration of 200 μg/L was measured using a monoclonal-parent drug-specific antibody and a target concentration of 400 μg/L was being aimed for, based on a polyclonal assay which measured 200 μg/L parent drug and 200 μg/L metabolite.

Some antibodies used for digoxin immunoassay cross-react quite strongly with the metabolites of spironolactone and may give misleadingly high estimates of digoxin concentration. Newborn babies often have substantial quantities of a circulating natural substance that is indistinguishable from digoxin using many radioimmunoassays. They may appear to have low therapeutic concentrations of digoxin, even when they are not receiving the drug.[15] Similar problems have been reported for some of the immunoassays used to quantify phenytoin concentrations in uraemic patients.[16]

There are also kits available, based on immunoassay methods, which enable drug concentrations to be assayed visually, rather than with a machine. These provide results very quickly, taking less than half an hour to complete, and have the potential to be very useful in sites such as accident and emergency units.[17]

##### GC and HPLC Methods

The most specific methods used in target concentration intervention are gas chromatography (GC) or high-pressure liquid chromatography (HPLC). These are generally more time consuming and costly but have the advantage of greater specificity and can be used to measure both drugs and their metabolites.

##### Interferences with Drug Assays

There are numerous examples of interferences with drug assays by other substances.[18] Clinical laboratories measuring drug concentrations have a good knowledge of likely interferences with their assays. By inclusion of laboratory staff as members of a therapeutics team, such problems can be readily identified and strategies developed to overcome them.

#### 1.6.3 Altered Plasma Protein Binding

Nothing is more difficult to explain and likely to confuse those new to target concentration intervention than the effects of altered plasma protein binding on the interpretation of drug concentrations. For reasons of convenience and expense, routine measurements of drug concentrations are based on the total concentration of drug in plasma or serum. The total concentration is the sum of the drug bound to plasma proteins and the unbound drug, but drug effects are determined solely by the concentration of unbound drug. Bound drug is pharmacologically inactive but, unfortunately, for several important agents it contributes the largest fraction of the total drug concentration.

The main relevance of plasma protein binding is in the *interpretation* of measured concentrations. For example, the unbound drug concentration in a patient with a normal plasma protein concentration given 300mg phenytoin per day is about 1 mg/L. The unbound concentration is therefore expected to be the same, i.e. 1 mg/L, even if plasma protein concentrations are reduced, e.g. in a patient with chronic renal failure.

With normal plasma protein concentrations and affinity, the bound concentration of phenytoin is typically 9 mg/L at an unbound concentration of 1 mg/L. In renal failure, because of the lower albumin concentration and decreased affinity, only 4 mg/L is bound at the same unbound concentration. Thus in the patient with normal protein binding, the total drug concentration (bound + unbound) will be 9 mg/L + 1 mg/L, i.e. 10 mg/L. On the other hand, the patient with renal failure with reduced protein binding will have a total drug concentration of 4 mg/L + 1 mg/L, i.e. 5 mg/L.

Patients with and without renal failure taking the same dose of phenytoin can therefore be expected to have the same unbound drug concentration (1 mg/L) but a 2-fold difference in the total concentration (10 mg/L *vs* 5 mg/L). Because only the unbound drug is pharmacologically active, both patients can be expected to have similar antiepileptic effects. The patient with normal renal function with a total concentration of 10 mg/L will generally be considered 'within the therapeutic range', and no change in dose would be considered (unless he or she was still having convulsions). However, the patient with renal failure with a total concentration of 5 mg/L is at risk because it may be thought that the concentration is 'below the therapeutic range' and the dose accordingly increased. This could be quite inappropriate because the unbound concentration is just as likely to be 'within the therapeutic range' as in the patient with normal renal function, and an increase in dose may simply produce toxicity with no increased effectiveness.

*Drug interactions* can also contribute to this problem of interpreting unbound drug concentrations. Valproic acid competes with phenytoin for plasma protein binding sites. If the two drugs are combined in a patient with epilepsy, the same principles used to understand the consequences of renal failure on phenytoin protein binding apply. Valproic acid does not change the clearance of phenytoin; therefore if the dose of phenytoin is unchanged, the unbound drug concentration at steady-state will remain the same. Because phenytoin binding is reduced by valproic acid, the bound drug concentration will be lower and so will the total drug concentration that is measured. Typically, the total drug concentration will fall from 10 to 6.6 mg/L and the bound concentration from 9 to 5.6 mg/L, while the unbound concentration will remain the same at 1 mg/L. However, this is the case only when steady-state has been re-established. Immediately after valproic acid is started, some phenytoin will be displaced from plasma proteins and the unbound concentration will rise. If the body was a closed system, the total concentration would be expected to stay the same, even though more drug is now in the unbound form. However, the body is continually eliminating drug and the sudden increase in unbound drug concentration without a change in maintenance dose will mean that the elimination rate will be increased and exceed the maintenance dose rate until the unbound concentration has fallen to its previous level (i.e. 1 mg/L) and steady-state is re-established. As the unbound drug concentration falls, so must the bound drug and the total drug concentration so that eventually, the total drug concentration is substantially lower than before valproic acid was started but the pharmacological effect of the phenytoin will be unchanged.

In some circumstances, the binding of drugs may be enhanced; for example, in association with acute inflammatory responses, there is a rise in the acute phase reactant, $\alpha_1$-acid glycoprotein. This protein has a high affinity for many basic drugs, e.g. lidocaine, quinidine. Total drug concentrations measured when $\alpha_1$-acid glycoprotein concentrations are increased will therefore be higher but if clearance is unchanged, the unbound drug concentration and drug effect will remain the same.

The situation is somewhat more complex for lidocaine. It has a high hepatic extraction ratio (see chapter 1; sect. 3.3.2 and 5.4.3) and clearance of unbound lidocaine is expected to be determined not only by *intrinsic clearance* (unchanged by plasma protein binding) but also by the rate of *drug delivery* to the liver. After myocardial infarction, the plasma protein binding of lidocaine is increased.[19] This means that drug delivery to the liver is increased, even though blood flow may not change, and clearance of unbound drug should increase. If this happened, then total lidocaine concentrations in blood should not change very much because, although the bound fraction is increased, the unbound concentration decreases. In fact, total lidocaine concentrations do increase and there is even a small increase in the unbound lidocaine concentration, which means the unbound clearance is lower.[20] There is no simple explanation for this. The pitfall for the unwary, who may measure lidocaine concentrations after a myocardial infarction when $\alpha_1$-acid glycoprotein concentrations may be increased, is to misinterpret the elevated total drug concentration as being 'above the therapeutic range' and reduce the lidocaine dose, which may allow an arrhythmia to break through.

These examples of altered protein binding and the potential for inappropriate dosage adjustments highlight the need to assess the patient's response to treatment and not to focus too much attention on the drug concentration. If the patient with chronic renal failure receiving phenytoin is not having seizures, there is no need to increase the dose because the measured plasma concentration seems low. Conversely, if the patient receiving an infusion of lidocaine because of an arrhythmia after a myocardial infarction has a drug concentration that seems high but has no signs or symptoms of toxicity, the dose should not be reduced on these grounds alone.

Special care must be taken in the interpretation of concentrations of highly protein bound drugs in patients who have low albumin concentrations (e.g. severe liver disease, malabsorption, renal failure), high $\alpha_1$-acid glycoprotein concentrations (e.g. acute inflammatory conditions such as after surgery or myocardial infarction), or those receiving other drugs which may cause displacement from plasma proteins.[21,22]

#### *1.6.4 Presence of Active Metabolites*

Several drugs involved in target concentration intervention produce significant quantities of metabolites which may be detectable and resolved from the parent compound using a specific assay. Procainamide, for example, has an acetylated metabolite, acecainide (*N*-acetylprocainamide; NAPA), the formation of which depends on the acetylator capacity of the individual; this property is bimodally distributed in the population (so-called fast and slow acetylators) [see also chapter 1; sect. 5.3]. Acecainide is itself an active antiarrhythmic compound. Estimates of its potency vary but when used alone, concentrations required to suppress arrhythmias are 5 to 6 times greater than comparably effective concentrations of procainamide. Acecainide is eliminated almost entirely by the kidney, whereas procainamide is eliminated only about 50% by this route. Patients with renal impairment may therefore accumulate significant quantities of acecainide, particularly if they are fast acetylators, which should be taken into account when assessing the response to a given procainamide concentration.

Quinidine also produces a variety of metabolites, some of which appear to be pharmacologically active. Nonspecific assays measure these metabolites as if they were quinidine. In some ways this is desirable because the apparent 'quinidine' concentration will more closely reflect the total contribution of pharmacologically active substances in the plasma than a specific assay that measures quinidine alone. Furthermore, the therapeutic range for quinidine has largely been established on measurements using nonspecific analytical methods so that attempts to define a therapeutic range for specifically measured quinidine are fraught with difficulty. However, attempts to understand an individual's pharmacokinetics will be simpler and more reliable if a specific assay is used and this method is to be preferred for dose forecasting.

For further discussion of the clinical implications of active drug metabolites, see review by Garattini.[23]

#### *1.6.5 Stereoisomerism*

Some drugs are administered as a racemic mixture of stereoisomers or enantiomers. Because the body can discriminate between different 3-dimensional structures, frequently one isomeric form or enantiomer is more potent than the other.[24] Furthermore, the pharmacokinetics of the two enantiomers may be quite different.[25]

Administering a racemate is like giving a mixture of two different drugs. Measurements of drug concentration will usually quantify the concentration of the racemate. For example, verapamil is usually supplied as a racemic mixture. When it is administered orally, the relative metabolism of the isomers is different from that when given intravenously. This leads to a relative enhancement of the plasma concentration of the less active isomer after oral administration. The target concentration for verapamil after intravenous administration, based on measurements of racemic verapamil, is therefore much lower than that after oral verapamil.[26,27]

#### 1.6.6 Quality Control

The reproducibility and accuracy of drug concentration measurements are central to therapeutic decision making based on these measurements. Quality control schemes not only provide the means for individual laboratories to maintain a high standard and comparability with other sites, but can also help in identifying potential sources of bias and unreliable analytical methods.

Most clinical laboratories participate in external quality assurance programmes. Those designed for target concentration intervention vary widely in the range of drugs that are offered and the numbers of subscribers. If there are relatively few laboratories participating with a particular drug, it becomes impossible to attach any statistical significance to the performance of an individual laboratory, which makes it difficult to know who is wrong if there is systematic disagreement among laboratories assaying the same reference materials.

#### 1.6.7 Units for Drug Concentrations, Volume of Distribution and Clearance

##### Drug Concentrations

There continues to be debate about the most suitable units for reporting drug concentrations.[28-30] Many clinical laboratories have adopted molar units for all their test results. Various arguments are put forward for this but they usually focus on matters of aesthetics rather than practical benefits. The ease of stoichiometric conversions is sometimes cited but as there are few real examples of stoichiometric applications in clinical practice for naturally occurring substances, this argument carries little weight.

There is, however, one area in which the stoichiometry between the quantity of substance administered and the concentration that is measured is paramount – i.e. in target concentration intervention. All drugs in common use today are formulated, packaged and prescribed in gravimetric units, and nearly always in terms of the milligram. The natural, practical unit for amount of drug in target concentration intervention is therefore the milligram, and concentrations are readily expressed in milligrams per litre (mg/L). When drugs are dispensed in molar units, it will be natural and practical to report concentrations using moles for the amount. Meanwhile, laboratories that currently report concentrations in molar units force upon those attempting to interpret them the need to convert from moles to milligrams.

##### Volume of Distribution

A practical unit for volume of distribution is the litre. Most volumes of distribution are then easily manipulated whole numbers between 10 and several thousand and most commonly in the low hundreds of litres.

##### Clearance

Practical units for clearance are litres per hour. This fits readily with volumes in litres and concentrations in milligrams per litre. The choice of the hour as the unit of time is also more practical than the minute or the day for most dose rate calculations. Typical values for clearance range from 1 to 50 L/h.

For ease of calculation, is it suggested that all data be converted to milligram-litre-hour units before attempting to estimate pharmacokinetic parameters and calculate a rational dosage regimen. This will result in convenient units of milligrams for loading doses, milligrams per hour for maintenance dose rates, and hours for half-lives.

##### Body Size

Values for volume of distribution and clearance are sometimes reported per kilogram of bodyweight. This implies that these parameters are linearly proportional to weight but while this may be reasonable for volume of distribution, it is not for clearance. The clearance of drugs and many functional attributes of the body, e.g. metabolic rate, are best described by a power function of weight. For this reason, it is not usually appropriate to apply a clearance per kilogram value obtained from an adult to predict the clearance in a child. To avoid this error and to demonstrate more clearly actual values of volume of distribution and clearance, it is preferable to cite values that are typical of a standard 70kg individual.[31]

#### *1.6.8 Blood Collection Procedures*

The way that blood is collected from a patient may lead to errors in measurement of drug concentrations. If a drug is administered by infusion, it is important not to collect blood for concentration measurement from the same cannula even if several hours have elapsed since the last time a dose was given. Local concentrations of drug are frequently higher because of stagnation of blood adjacent to the cannula and adsorption to the cannula and vessel wall.

Diurnal variation in concentrations has been reported for some drugs (e.g. cyclosporin).[32] A consistent sampling time may be helpful if repeated measurements are to be comparable. There have also been reports of drug concentrations being affected by exercise or posture (e.g. digoxin).[33] It might therefore be advisable to recommend a standard procedure where possible: for example, 10 minutes rest before blood collection from a seated or semirecumbent position.

The use of serum separator tubes offers advantages to the clinical chemistry laboratory in processing time for serum specimens. However, some drugs, e.g. tricyclic antidepressants, may bind to the gels used in these tubes.[34] If possible, the use of serum separator tubes should be avoided.

#### *1.6.9 Blood, Plasma, Serum or Unbound Concentrations?*

For most purposes, the terms plasma concentration and serum concentration may be considered equivalent. Usually the unqualified term drug concentration refers without distinction to either plasma or serum samples. However, there are some exceptions. Serum concentrations of chloroquine have been reported to be twice as high as plasma concentrations because of drug which has accumulated in platelets being released during the clotting process.[35] Similar phenomena may occur for other drugs; for example, amiodarone concentrations have been reported to be 15% higher in serum.[36]

As a matter of convenience, most clinical laboratories use serum, whereas most research laboratories use plasma because it is more rapidly separable from blood cells (but requires the addition of an anticoagulant). However, this is not recommended for all drugs. For example, cyclosporin accumulates in red blood cells. This is a temperature-sensitive process and cyclosporin is released into serum (or plasma) after blood has been collected. This contributes importantly to variability in measured concentrations and it is generally accepted that whole blood should be used for cyclosporin measurement.

The introduction of methods for measuring the unbound drug concentration provides the potential for enhanced interpretation of concentration measurements (see section 2.3). Many laboratories can measure phenytoin unbound concentrations when requested. This is clinically the most important drug where unbound concentrations are helpful. The target concentration for unbound phenytoin is 1 mg/L. Specialised laboratories can also provide a similar service for unbound concentrations of other antiepileptic drugs.

The magnitude of volume of distribution and clearance will depend upon the precise fluid referred to for measuring concentration. The default fluid is plasma or serum. Occasionally, it is valuable to refer to pharmacokinetics with reference to blood, e.g. when comparing clearance with organ blood flow. Volumes of distribution expressed in terms of unbound drug (free water concentrations) are helpful for appreciating the extent of tissue binding and uptake of a drug.

In some situations, there may be quite large discrepancies between arterial and venous drug concentrations.[37] However, these are generally only relevant to drug samples taken during the distribution phase. Most drug concentration measurements for clinical purposes are taken after distribution is essentially complete.

## 2. Target Concentration Intervention in Clinical Practice

### 2.1 Which Drugs Should Be Monitored?

The primary reasons for target concentration intervention are that the desired therapeutic effect is itself difficult to monitor and the drug has a relatively narrow therapeutic index. For instance, when using an antiepileptic drug, it is not sufficient to know that the patient is not actually having a seizure at the time of review. Epileptic fits may be quite infrequent yet devastating when they occur. The absence of seizures is not an adequate measure of efficacy until a sufficiently long interval has elapsed, e.g. a year without a seizure. In the meantime, the patient and clinician would like some reassurance of a reasonable chance that therapeutic effectiveness is likely to be achieved. If antiepileptic drugs had a wide therapeutic index, like most antibiotics, it would be sufficient to give large doses to all patients in the knowledge that the concentrations would always be sufficient to suppress seizure activity irrespective of the interpatient variability in pharmacokinetics. However, this is not the case. Target concentrations for most antiepileptic drugs are frequently close to those producing significant adverse effects.

For similar reasons, the absence of an arrhythmia when using an antiarrhythmic drug, the absence of mania or depression when using lithium, or the absence of signs of transplant rejection when using cyclosporin, coupled with the significant risk of toxicity when using these drugs in effective doses makes them prime candidates for target concentration intervention.

The indications for other drugs rely on softer criteria. The bronchodilator response to theophylline is readily measurable but the flat concentration-response curve above 10 mg/L (fig. 3) and the real risk of serious toxicity at concentrations only twice this value make the measurement of concentrations valuable in assessing whether a further increase in dose, and by how much, is likely to bring therapeutic reward. The effectiveness of digoxin in controlling atrial fibrillation is simply assessed by taking the pulse and cardiac auscultation. Like theophylline, however, if the response is inadequate, a decision to increase the dose, and to what extent, is made easier if the current concentration is known.

The response to adequate treatment with an aminoglycoside antibiotic may be clear cut, e.g. by rapid resolution of fever and a fall in leucocyte count, but the occurrence of nephrotoxicity or ototoxicity may be delayed for some days after a therapeutic response is apparent. The early measurement of drug concentrations can forestall excessive treatment and possibly prevent subsequent toxicity.

In general, most drugs whose concentrations are widely measured have been in clinical use for many years.[38] Newer drugs generally have a wider therapeutic index (although there are exceptions such as some of the newer immunosuppressants now being developed). Drugs which may have needed concentration measurements for their effective use may therefore have been sidelined during development, which may explain why there are few examples of drugs introduced in recent years that are thought to require concentration measurements.

## 2.2 When Should Samples Be Taken for Drug Concentration Measurement?

The best time to obtain samples for concentrations depends upon what information is desired. The type of information that may be determined may be classified as follows.

### 2.2.1 Pharmacodynamic Applications

If a patient reports a symptom or exhibits a sign that may be due to a drug effect, whether therapeutic or toxic, then obtaining a sample for measurement of the drug concentration at that time can be quite useful. By considering the concentration along with the patient's clinical picture, it is possible to make a more reasonable judgement as to whether the drug is contributing to the signs and symptoms. For example, if a patient is taking theophylline and complains of not feeling well and has a headache, it is possible that the drug is the cause of the problems, or alternatively, some intercurrent illness or dietary indiscretion may be responsible. If the theophylline concentration is less than 5 mg/L, one can be reasonably confident that the drug is not causing the problems. On the other hand, if the concentration is over 15 mg/L, there is a very good chance that theophylline is the culprit. In between these concentrations, the situation is not well resolved but one would tend to put more weight on a drug cause at a higher drug concentration. Making a decision based on the drug concentration and the prior probability of the signs and symptoms occurring at that concentration is a commonsense approach that can be formalised (see Holford & Sheiner[39] for a fuller discussion). The use of formal decision analysis has been advocated.[8]

Alternatively, if the drug is an antiarrhythmic agent and the patient is to have 24-hour electrocardiographic monitoring of the cardiac rhythm, it would be useful to measure the concentration on the day of the study just before each dose. If subsequent analysis revealed that significant arrhythmias were absent throughout the recording period, the trough concentrations could be used as an upper limit of the target concentration for that drug. But if the arrhythmia recurred at times when the concentration was low during the dosage interval, these concentrations would be less than the target concentration for this individual. The application of simple pharmacokinetic principles can predict the likely range of peak to trough concentrations, and a reasonable guess can be made of the patient's target concentration. Many antiarrhythmic drugs (e.g. quinidine, procainamide, disopyramide) are administered as slow release formulations every 8 to 12 hours. If these preparations are used, the peak to trough fluctuation is likely to be less than 50%. If better antiarrhythmic control is needed, the dose should not need to be more than doubled if it seems that control is achieved for some of the time on the current regimen.

A final pharmacodynamic application for measuring a drug concentration is to improve one's knowledge of the patient's pharmacodynamic parameters ($E_{max}$, $EC_{50}$) when the drug effect is readily quantified. This may be done in conjunction with a pharmacokinetic analysis and may provide the means to forecast the most appropriate dose to obtain the desired effect. However, there is no widespread application of such techniques at present.

#### 2.2.2 Pharmacokinetic Applications

The most widespread use of drug concentration measurements is to find out its relationship to the therapeutic range. Some clinicians interpret drug concentration in 1 of 3 ways:

1) If the concentration is within the therapeutic range, they do nothing further.

2) If it is above the range, they reduce the dose in proportion to the degree that the measured concentration exceeds that desired.

3) If it is below the range, they increase the dose along similar lines.

If the previous dosage has been constant long enough to achieve steady-state and the drug is given by intravenous infusion (e.g. theophylline) or as a slow release preparation (e.g. quinidine), or if it has a long half-life in relation to the dosage interval (e.g. digoxin), this course of action is likely to be effective (as long as it is consistent with clinical assessment of the patient) and the procedure is simple to follow and apply. It may, however, lead to important delays in effective treatment if all that is done is to change the maintenance dose rate. For instance, if a digoxin concentration of 0.5 μg/L (ng/ml) is measured in a patient who continues to have uncontrolled atrial fibrillation and the dose is doubled, it will take at least a week before the new steady-state level is reached and if this is not enough, the dose will need to be increased again and perhaps another week will pass before the treatment is effective. This particular situation calls for use of a loading dose whose size can be calculated using simple pharmacokinetic principles (see section 1.2 and also appendix G).

On the other hand, if there is marked fluctuation of concentrations or a sample is taken shortly after initiation of treatment or a change of dose, then knowledge of the timing of the sample is crucial.

The simplest underlying pharmacokinetic goal of measuring drug concentrations is to estimate values of *volume of distribution* and *clearance* in an individual (see section 1.2). These can then be used to predict further loading doses or the maintenance dose rate needed to reach and sustain the target concentration. Samples drawn early in a dosage interval or shortly after starting treatment will mainly reflect the volume of distribution. As steady-state is approached, the contribution of clearance becomes overwhelming as a determinant of the concentration.

For practical reasons, only one or two blood samples are usually collected from a patient. There have been suggestions that multiple concentrations are measured to allow a more precise estimate of drug exposure, e.g. using the area under the concentration-time curve (AUC).[40-42] The merits of these approaches are still being evaluated but the successes achieved by Rodman and Evans[42] in the treatment of paediatric cancer are very impressive.

The need to obtain concentrations at steady-state and/or concentrations at special times after the dose has largely been made redundant by the availability of computer programs for concentration interpretation. Using simple pharmacokinetic models, it is possible to use the information from any blood sample as long as its timing and an accurate dosage history are available. Nevertheless, attention to sampling at optimal times can enhance the quality of the information gained; for example, two aminoglycoside concentrations sampled at an interval of 1 hour (with no intervening dose) are less useful than samples taken with an interval of 3 half-lives.

The ideal times for sampling in order to estimate volume of distribution and clearance will depend upon the usual pattern of dose administration and the expected half-life of the drug. The principles may be illustrated by the following examples:

##### Theophylline

If a patient with an acute attack of asthma, who has already been taking an oral theophylline preparation, is given an intravenous loading dose of theophylline, it is often useful to obtain blood samples immediately before the intravenous dose and 20 minutes or so after the dose is given (usually 1 hour after the preload sample because theophylline loading doses are given over at least 20 to 30 minutes). If the concentrations are measured promptly, further dose adjustment can be made based on an estimate of the patient's volume of distribution (see further section 4.1). It is important to understand that these concentrations do not reflect theophylline clearance. The typical half-life of theophylline is about 8 hours, so, in 1 hour, less than 5% of the drug will have been eliminated and the concentration provides almost no information about theophylline clearance. This illustrates why these early levels should not be used to adjust the maintenance dose rate, which depends upon an accurate estimate of clearance.

A blood sample drawn about 4 hours after starting a constant infusion of theophylline may be used with the postload measurement, to make an early adjustment of the maintenance dose rate. At 4 hours (half of the expected half-life), about 30% of the dose administered will have been eliminated and reflect the patient's clearance to this extent. Subsequently, samples should be obtained within 24 hours and then every day until it is clear that the desired target concentration has been achieved.

If theophylline therapy is started less urgently using the oral route, it is often reasonable to omit the loading dose and simply start out with the maintenance dose using a slow release preparation, e.g. 200 to 400mg twice a day. Because the fluctuation after each dose is likely to be less than 15% of the mean, the exact sampling time is not critical but at least 32 hours should pass (4 half-lives) so that the measured concentration is at steady-state and will reflect the clearance. The measured level at this time will essentially provide no information about the volume of distribution because the average steady-state concentration is determined only by the dose rate and clearance (see Equation 3, section 1.2). Under these circumstances, however, a knowledge of the volume of distribution is unimportant because the principal goal is to adjust the maintenance dose to achieve the target concentration, and the use of a loading dose is not required.

Sampling immediately before the next dose is often recommended (the trough concentration) because this is a well-defined point in the dosage interval, and from a pharmacodynamic perspective it can function as a measure of the lowest effective concentration. When slow release preparations are used, the timing within the dosage interval is less critical but the actual moment of sampling in relation to the last dose is frequently valuable to assess if the measured value is likely to be above or below the mean concentration (which reflects the clearance).

#### Digoxin

Digoxin takes some hours to distribute into the tissues. The concentration immediately after rapid intravenous administration of a loading dose may easily reach 20 μg/L (ng/ml), but within 6 to 8 hours will have reached a concentration of 2 μg/L. Even after oral administration, it takes an appreciable time for digoxin to be absorbed and distributed in the body. Samples for digoxin concentration measurement should always be drawn at least 6 hours after the last dose. To make this easier, it is helpful if digoxin is administered in the evening so that samples may be drawn in the morning for despatch to the laboratory.

The elimination half-life of digoxin is typically nearly 2 days. Therefore it takes at least a week to reach steady-state. Care with interpretation is needed if samples are drawn earlier than 1 week after a change in dose or initiation of treatment. It is commonly believed that the administration of a loading dose prior to the use of a maintenance dose leads more quickly to the establishment of steady-state. However, this is quite incorrect. If, by good fortune, exactly the right loading dose and maintenance dose rate are chosen and drug concentrations are essentially constant all the time after the loading dose has been given, it is still the case that the concentration prior to the elapse of 1 half-life is predominantly determined by the volume of distribution; concentrations measured early on are unreliable guides to clearance and thus the maintenance dose.

If, as is more common, the maintenance dose is not appropriately matched to the loading dose, serious errors can arise in predicting the eventual steady-state concentration. Suppose the maintenance dose is too large, such that the eventual concentration will exceed the target, yet the loading dose was a good guess. If a concentration is only 30% higher than the target at less than one half-life after the loading dose, e.g. at 24 hours in the case of digoxin, then one might accept that all will be well with the current maintenance dose. But in fact, the eventual steady-state concentration could be more than twice as high as the target value. This is a par-

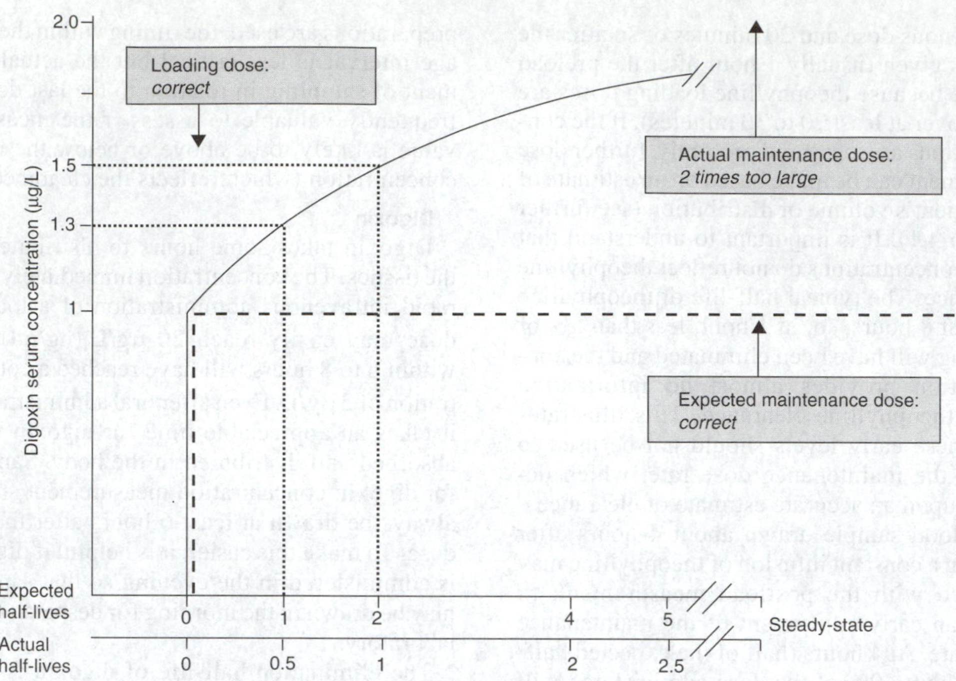


**Fig. 5.** A loading dose does not affect the time to steady-state: samples drawn at 1 expected half-life after initiation of treatment with a loading dose and a maintenance dose may seriously mislead. In this example, typical of digoxin, the concentrations after an idealised loading dose and maintenance dose rate that were exactly correct to achieve and sustain the target concentration of 1 μg/L are shown (broken line). If a sample is obtained within 2 days of starting treatment (equal to or less than 1 expected half-life), the concentration will be exactly on target. On the other hand, if the clearance is really half the expected value, the actual half-life will be twice as long and the eventual steady-state concentration will be twice the target (continuous line). In this case, a sample obtained at the same time will be about 30% greater than the target. Coupled with the expected measurement error of 15 to 20%, it is easy to understand how this early concentration may be misinterpreted and it would not be recognised that the maintenance dose should be halved.

ticular problem when the clearance has been underestimated, because the half-life will be longer than expected and a sampling time that might be expected to be adequate if the half-life had been normal, will in fact be too early and underestimate the eventual steady-state level (fig. 5).

#### Aminoglycoside Antibiotics

Traditionally, the aminoglycoside antibiotics (e.g. gentamicin) are administered by short intravenous infusion over 20 to 30 minutes at intervals of 8 hours. The typical half-life of gentamicin in a patient with good renal function is about 2 hours. In the 8-hour interval between doses (for the moment ignoring the 20 to 30 minutes taken for the infusion), a period of 4 half-lives will elapse and a peak concentration which may have been 8 mg/L will be only 0.5 mg/L just before the next dose. If there is a 16-fold variation in concentration in the dosage interval, the question of the ideal sampling time becomes important.

If the goal of sampling were simply to estimate clearance, a case could be made for taking a single sample about 1.5 times the expected half-life after the dose is given, e.g. at 3 hours in the case of gentamicin. It can be shown mathematically that the concentration in a sample drawn at this time after the first dose (with the further assumption that there is negligible loss of drug during the loading infusion) is determined almost entirely by the size of the loading dose and the clearance. This principle has been used to justify the use of single concentrations, drawn after the first dose, for prediction of the maintenance dose.[43] While this may be successful in some cases, it is dependent upon having a good estimate of the expected half-life. But, of course, if the half-life is known well, the clearance will also be known well, and this makes the concentration measurement effectively redundant. This kind of single concentration method fails when it is needed most, i.e. in the patient whose pharmacokinetics are markedly different from those expected.

Most commonly, two samples will be taken for the measurement of aminoglycoside concentrations. The first, often referred to as 'the peak', is taken 20 to 30 minutes after the short infusion has finished. This delay after the true peak concentration (which necessarily occurs at the moment the infusion ceases) allows time for the drug to distribute into the extracellular space, which is the effective volume of distribution. This postdistributional concentration (post-dose) can be used with a second concentration sampled just before the second dose is started (pre-dose) to estimate the patient's volume of distribution and clearance.

Whenever possible, the post-dose and pre-dose samples should be taken after the first dose is given. This will mean the results of the analysis are available at the earliest possible time and have the greatest influence on the subsequent doses the patient will receive. A second advantage of taking the samples after the first dose is the simpler pharmacokinetic calculations that are required because the contribution of earlier doses does not have to be considered.

If a patient is thought to have good renal function and the half-life is expected to be short, it is not necessary to wait until just before the next dose. A sample drawn 4 hours after the post-dose sample will provide useful information about the patient's pharmacokinetics. In such a patient with a short half-life, the concentration just before the next dose may be less than 0.5 mg/L and below the sensitivity of most assays. It may take up to 24 hours for the laboratory to report an 'undetectable' concentration and valuable time will have been lost before a rational dosage decision can be made.

Aminoglycosides are frequently combined with a penicillin. When this is done, care must be taken to administer the penicillin immediately after the post-dose sample has been obtained. This is because many penicillins combine chemically with aminoglycosides. Samples which are left for 12 to 24 hours awaiting analysis, even if refrigerated, will slowly lose aminoglycoside activity. The measured concentration may therefore be substantially lower than that which actually existed in the patient, and pharmacokinetic calculations based on such concentrations will be invalid. By giving the penicillin immediately after the post-dose sample, the penicillin concentration, and therefore the extent of *in vitro* inactivation, will be at its lowest when the post-dose and pre-dose samples are obtained. In patients with severely impaired renal function, there may be some *in vivo* inactivation because both classes of drugs are renally eliminated and will have long half-lives, which means the concentrations of both drugs will tend to be high throughout the dosage interval. If samples are analysed promptly, the *in vitro* inactivation can be ignored and the measured values will not only reflect clearance due to the usual routes of elimination, but also that due to penicillin inactivation, which may necessitate a somewhat larger dose than would otherwise be needed.

Recent studies have shown that equally good therapeutic benefits and perhaps diminished toxicity can be achieved with *once daily administration* of aminoglycosides (see further section 4.8.1).[44-47] This offers important practical advantages. The target concentration concept needs to be revised for once daily administration. In its simplest form, it would be reasonable to aim for an initial peak concentration 3 times higher than that used for 8-hourly administration but aim for the same average steady-state concentration of 3 mg/L. The timing of blood sampling also needs attention. It will usually be a waste of time to take a pre-dose concentration 24 hours after the last dose because the concentration is likely to be too low to be measured (unless the patient has impaired clearance). However, a sample taken about 3 half-lives after the dose, in conjunction with the previously described post-dose sample, will provide useful information for estimating clearance and volume of distribution.

**Phenytoin**

The sampling time problem is particularly acute for phenytoin. Because of its concentration-dependent elimination (Michaelis-Menten kinetics), the concept of half-life becomes vague and ill-defined. One can define a sort of half-life at a particular concentration but it does not possess the useful predictive property it has for drugs with simple first-order elimination. For instance, the 'half-life' at typical therapeutic concentrations (10 to 20 mg/L) is said to be about 15 to 24 hours, which might imply that it would take no longer than 4 days to approach steady-state. But this is not the case; it can be shown to take nearly 2 weeks to reach 90% of steady-state with typical values for $V_{max}$ (maximum elimination rate), Km (concentration at which the rate of elimination is one-half of maximum), and volume of distribution.[48] Furthermore, a reasonable basis for estimation of the $V_{max}$ and Km in an individual requires two measurements of steady-state concentrations at different maintenance dose rates (other less demanding sampling times may be used but the methods required for interpretation are more complex). Therefore, it may take about a month before one can have any confidence in predicting the dose required to reach a target concentration. The use of a computer program incorporating Bayesian forecasting methods (see section 3.3.3) may be helpful in shortening the time to estimate an individual patient's parameters.[49,50]

In a typical situation when a patient is started on phenytoin, a loading dose will have been given to achieve rapid protection against further seizures. Whether this is given by slow intravenous infusion or, if the patient is sufficiently alert, as the rapidly absorbed oral elixir, it is very useful to obtain a sample an hour or so after the dose has been given. This has two purposes: firstly, it can document that a sufficiently large dose has been given for a reasonable probability of seizure control and if the concentration is low, a further loading dose can be given. Secondly, it serves to define a reference point for the eventual steady-state concentration. If a maintenance dose regimen is continued after the loading dose and samples are taken at the same time each day, it is possible within a few days to determine if concentrations are falling or rising. If they are falling from the postload level, one can be sure that the eventual steady-state level will be lower and one may wish to increase the maintenance dose right away to achieve the target concentration. On the other hand, if the concentrations are rising, it is difficult to predict just how high they will go (or even if a steady-state will ever be reached). For this reason, it is a good idea to give a sufficiently large loading dose so that the postload concentration is somewhat higher than the desired target concentration. If concentrations are not falling while on the maintenance dose, one can be sure, at an early stage, that the maintenance dose rate is too high.

### 2.3 Use of Unbound Drug Concentrations

For historical and practical reasons, almost all target concentration interventions are based on the measurement of total drug concentrations. When plasma protein binding is changed by disease or drug interactions, the relationships of dose and effect to the total drug concentration are changed (see section 1.6.3). Such complications could be abolished very simply if only unbound concentrations were measured. Phenytoin is the most common drug, with an assay readily available, for which such problems can affect clinical management. The phenomenon of drug binding to plasma protein should be regarded as an artefact obscuring the truth from those attempting to understand pharmacokinetics and pharmacodynamics.[22,51,52]

### 2.4 Interpretation of Drug Concentrations in Special Populations

A multitude of factors may modify the interpretation of drug concentrations in disease. The more obvious ones are related to altered clearance secondary to renal, hepatic or cardiac impairment and changes in plasma protein binding. These and other factors have been reviewed by Perucca et al.[53] and Ladero et al.[54] Other factors include ethnicity[55] and age.[56,57] For example, neonates do not appear to form morphine 6-glucuronide, an active metabolite of morphine. This has been suggested as a reason why neonates require higher morphine concentrations for sedation than older children.[56] Particular problems associated with drug concentration measurement in children have been reviewed by Gilman.[58]

### 2.5 Drug Monitoring in Renal Replacement Therapy

When renal failure develops, either acute or chronic, a major drug eliminating organ is lost. Estimating the clearance of a drug in an individual with renal failure can usually be predicted from the serum creatinine concentration (see appendix G), but can occasionally be extremely difficult. Changes in volume of distribution can occur, with changes in both concentration and affinity of drug binding proteins; for example, digoxin's volume of distribution is reduced in renal failure. Accumulation of fluid may also be important for drugs such as the aminoglycoside antibiotics which are distributed largely in extracellular fluids. As these changes can occur quickly or slowly, repeated, frequent measurement of drug plasma concentrations with recalculation of pharmacokinetic parameters may be necessary to maintain optimum therapy. Changes in renal function are an indication to consider another measurement of drug concentration. It is useful to bear in mind that because aminoglycosides have a volume of distribution about half that of creatinine but have about the same clearance value, they have a shorter half-life and will reflect changes in renal function more quickly than the serum creatinine.

Patients with chronic renal failure are treated with intermittent haemodialysis or continuous ambulatory peritoneal dialysis, whereas those with acute renal failure are mainly treated using continuous haemofiltration or dialysis. These forms of dialysis eliminate drugs from the body, as well as endogenous wastes. The amount of drug eliminated during dialysis can be estimated by measuring the drug concentration in the filtrate or dialysate effluent and multiplying this by the volume of fluid. If desired, this amount of drug can then be directly replaced. However, this is not commonly done because reasonable estimates can be made from the changes in plasma concentration and an estimate of the volume of distribution. Certain predictions about the elimination of drugs during dialysis are possible by consideration of the type of renal replacement used (and the kind of membrane used because of possible drug-membrane interactions), and the physicochemical properties of the particular drug.

#### 2.5.1 Intermittent Haemodialysis

A loading dose for a patient with renal failure can be calculated by estimation of the volume of distribution (Equation 2; section 1.2). Maintenance dose calculation will depend upon the patient's clearance of the drug. Clearance will be determined by two very different sets of conditions; the periods of dialysis and the times between dialysis. Drugs that are usually mainly renally eliminated (e.g. digoxin, the aminoglycoside antibiotics and cimetidine), can remain in the body at quite high concentrations during the periods between haemodialysis with very little elimination. Drug clearance during dialysis can be estimated by obtaining blood samples for drug concentration measurement before and after the dialysis period.

Guidelines have been devised to assist in dosage adjustment in patients receiving intermittent haemodialysis (for reviews, see Mac-Kay et al.[59] and Reetze-Bonorden et al.[60]).

#### 2.5.2 Continuous Ambulatory Peritoneal Dialysis

Drug-membrane interactions are not a consideration in this type of dialysis, as the membrane used is the endogenous peritoneal membrane. Estimates of volume of distribution, especially for drugs with low volumes of distribution (indicating distribution mainly into body water), and hence of the loading dose may need to be increased to allow for the extra volume of fluid present. Dialysis is continuous; therefore elimination is also continuous and drug clearance can be estimated in the usual manner from single, steady-state concentrations once a maintenance dose has commenced.

The initial choice of a maintenance dose may be different from that chosen for a patient with normal renal function, as active processes such as tubular secretion and reabsorption are lost in a patient with no kidney function. Drugs are eliminated by diffusion and filtration. However, guidelines are available to assist with initial dosage choice (for a review, see Keller et al.[61]).

#### 2.5.3 Continuous Haemodialysis or Haemoperfusion

To date, few studies have investigated the pharmacokinetics of drugs used in patients receiving continuous arteriovenous or venovenous haemofiltration or dialysis. However, the principles have recently been reviewed and guidelines for drug dosage in patients receiving continuous renal replacement therapy suggested.[60] As these methods are most commonly used for acute renal failure, regular measurement of drug concentrations is essential to ensure adequate therapy is maintained during a possibly rapidly fluctuating clinical course.

### 2.6 Monitoring of Drug Concentrations in Saliva

The discomfort of venepuncture and difficulties in obtaining blood samples, particularly in children, have led to the consideration of saliva as an alternative fluid for target concentration intervention. Saliva has the additional potential advantage of reflecting the unbound concentration of a drug rather than the total concentration, because diffusion into salivary glands is limited to the non-protein bound form. However, the concentration of a drug in saliva is also determined by the saliva flow rate, the source of saliva (e.g. parotid, sublingual, or mixed) and saliva pH (ion trapping). The variability in the saliva : plasma concentration ratio caused by these additional factors is so large that use of saliva for monitoring cannot be recommended, except for semiquantitative purposes.

For a review of drug monitoring in saliva, see Drobitch and Svensson.[62]

## 3. Use of Drug Concentrations for Dose Prediction

The use of target concentration intervention to predict the future dose requirements of an individual is known as forecasting. For reviews of available methods, see Vozeh and Steimer,[63] Buffington et al.[64] and Jelliffe et al.[65]

The basis of forecasting is a pharmacokinetic model for drug concentration. The parameters of this model (usually volume of distribution and clearance) must be estimated for an individual; then a prediction of future concentrations can be made. By trying different potential dosage schemes, it is possible to predict the concentrations and assess which dosage scheme is most likely to achieve the desired pattern of concentrations.

For the purposes of dose forecasting, the disposition of most drugs can be adequately described by a 1-compartment model (see chapter 1; sect. 2.2.4). This holds even for drugs like digoxin which clearly have a prolonged distribution phase even after oral administration. Provided drug concentrations are obtained when distribution is essentially complete, the 1-compartment model can be used.

### 3.1 Population Pharmacokinetics

Frequent reference has been made to the 'typical' population pharmacokinetic parameters of a drug. An obvious source for such parameters is appendix A in this textbook. The values listed here are based on a variety of sources and rely heavily upon the bias and expertise of the compiler.

For target concentration intervention, the important parameters are *clearance* and *volume of distribution*, and it is useful to know in quantitative terms how body size and disease states should be used to modify the 'standard' values. It is often valuable to know something of the variability of each parameter in the population in order to decide what are reasonable deviations from the population average. This variability can be expressed as a coefficient of variation, i.e. the measured standard deviation of the parameter in the population divided by the mean parameter value, expressed as a percentage. For example, if based on measured concentrations, the estimated clearance in an individual was 40% lower than the mean and the coefficient of variation of the clearance of the drug was 50%, then it would be reasonable to adjust the dose based on this new estimated clearance. However, if the coefficient of variation was only 10%, other reasons for the lower estimated clearance in the individual (such as poor compliance, checking the time of the last dose and blood sampling) would need to be sought before adjustment of the dosage regimen was undertaken. These estimates of variability are essential for the Bayesian feedback methods of dosage adjustment described below (section 3.3.3).

Estimates of variability can be obtained in a number of ways. Currently, the most common way is to conduct full pharmacokinetic studies in a number of individuals, calculate the pharmacokinetic parameters in each individual, and report the mean and standard deviation of these parameters. However, such studies are very labour intensive, requiring long study days for study participants, and often return visits for blood sampling, with multiple blood samples and drug concentration assays needed for each person. Of necessity, such studies can only be performed in a few individuals and are unlikely to be done in people receiving the drug therapeutically.

Methods that are becoming more popular and widespread now are the population pharmacokinetic methods,[66-68] which use sophisticated mathematical techniques to derive pharmacokinetic parameters for a drug using single (or just a few) drug concentration-time points from a number of individuals. These methods, including the NONMEM program, the P-Pharm program, and others, can utilise the sparse data collected, for example, in clinical trials or from a routine therapeutic drug monitoring service. Data can be obtained easily from people actually receiving the drug therapeutically. These methods give estimates of the pharmacokinetic parameters, such as clearance and volume of distribution, in the particular population from which the data derive, but more importantly, they also give estimates of the variability of those parameters both within and between individuals in the group. This is most useful for dosage prediction, as an estimate of how much, for example, clearance is likely to vary in the individual from time to time, as well as how much that individual might reasonably deviate from the population average value, can then be obtained.

### 3.2 Initial Predictions of Pharmacokinetic Parameters

The first step in forecasting drug concentration in an individual is to estimate the essential parameters of the model – the clearance and volume of distribution.

#### The *A Priori* Population Prediction

If the individual has never taken the drug before, the usual procedure is to use clearance and volume of distribution parameters typical of a population of patients similar to the individual in question. 'Typical' in this context usually involves knowing the average value of, say, clearance in a 'standard' patient, e.g. 70kg, normal renal, hepatic and cardiac function, nonsmoker, no other drug therapy. Adjustments to the 'standard' patient's clearance can then be made using information about the individual for whom a prediction is to be made.

For example, if the patient weighs 90kg, the 'standard' clearance would be increased by a factor of 90/70; if heart failure usually decreases clearance by a factor of 50%, then the 'standard' clearance would be halved if the patient has heart failure. The value of clearance obtained by applying these various factors to the 'standard' clearance will be 'typical' of a patient coming from a population with weight, cardiac function, etc. similar to the patient in question. The 'typical' parameter values can then be used to make an *initial* prediction of the concentrations which would be achieved if a given set of doses were administered to the patient. Because these initial estimates are representative of an average patient sharing the characteristics of the patient who is about to be given the drug, the predictions will be the most probable values, but in practice will be either too high or too low to the extent that the actual patient differs from the 'typical' patient. Estimates of clearance and volume of distribution obtained in this way are known as *a priori* population predictions.

The steps involved in predicting 'typical' total clearance values in individual patients are summarised in algorithm form in appendix G.

### 3.3 Revised Predictions of Pharmacokinetic Parameters

Once the drug has been given to the patient, and drug concentrations after a known dosage history are available, it is possible to use the concentrations to modify the expected pharmacokinetic parameters.

A wide variety of methods have been proposed to utilise measured concentrations to provide feedback in order to forecast future doses. They can be broadly classified into the one-point, least squares, and Bayesian methods.

#### *3.3.1 One-Point Feedback Method*

These methods are used to interpret a single drug concentration. The problem is how to use a single measurement to predict two unknowns, e.g. clearance and volume of distribution. The solution most commonly applied for nomogram feedback methods is to assume that the value for one of these parameters, say volume of distribution, is the same as the population prediction. Then it is possible to solve the pharmacokinetic model equations to determine a unique value for clearance that 'explains' the measured concentration.

The one-point methods are the most widely used and easiest to understand. They are used implicitly by most clinicians when they make a change in maintenance dose in proportion to the difference between the measured and target concentrations. If the concentration represents the average steady-state value, then the volume of distribution can be ignored and clearance calculated from the known dosage rate and the measured value (Equation 3; section 1.2). The steps involved in predicting 'typical' clearance and volume of distribution values in individual patients are summarised in appendix G.

The biggest drawbacks of this method are its reliance on a single measurement as if it were known without error and the assumption that other parameters are the same as the population predictions. When two concentrations are available, it may be possible to solve exactly for both volume of distribution and clearance but these predictions are still based on the assumption that the prediction error is negligible. The prediction error will be determined not only by the assay measurement error, which is often quite small (usually less than 10%), but also by errors in the dosage history and errors arising from a pharmacokinetic model which may be too simple (model mis-specification error). This latter error may easily be larger than the measurement error and be impossible to assess in the individual case.

#### *3.3.2 Least Squares Feedback Method*

If there are more concentrations available than the number of parameters that need to be estimated, it is possible to solve for all of the parameters, but some method must be used to resolve the different predictions that are obtained if different sets of concentrations are applied. This is nearly always done using the least squares method. It is based on statistical regression theory. The idea is to minimise the sum of the squared differences between the measured concentrations and those predicted by the pharmacokinetic model.

It is usually too difficult to use this method without the assistance of a computer program. The use of a computer has the disadvantage of making the prediction process more remote from the patient. Most commonly, the computer will be situated in the laboratory rather than on the ward or in the clinic, and the delays involved in transmitting the dosage history to the laboratory and communicating the results to the physician may remove any benefits that could accrue from this greater sophistication.

Like the one-point method, the least squares method may be seriously misled by over-emphasis on the precision of concentration measurements and ignoring the possibility of model mis-specification error (e.g. using a 1-compartment model for a sample drawn before drug distribution had equilibrated with the tissues). When there are many concentration measurements, it may be possible to choose among alternative models and so reduce the error arising from the use of an inappropriate model, but this situation is really a research investigation in clinical pharmacokinetics rather than a typical application of target concentration intervention.

### 3.3.3 Bayesian Feedback Method

A solution to the problem of obtaining reasonable individual predictions from a limited number of measured concentrations is provided by the Bayesian feedback method.[69-71] This is like the least squares method in searching for those parameter values that minimise the sum of squared differences between the measured and predicted concentrations. In addition, it attempts to minimise the sum of squared differences between the 'typical' population parameter values and those predicted for the patient.

The differences between the measured and predicted drug concentrations and the population and individually predicted pharmacokinetic parameters are scaled in proportion to the expected error in the prediction. For the concentration differences, this arises from model misspecification and measurement error and typically has a value of 20 to 30%. The error in the prediction of volume of distribution also has a typical value of 20 to 30%. The typical error for clearance, however, is often twice this size, maybe 50 to 60%.

This means that if there is a single concentration measurement and one wishes to estimate both clearance and volume of distribution, then the percentage difference between the population and individual prediction of clearance should be about twice the difference in the predictions for the volume of distribution.

For example, suppose a patient is expected to have *a priori* 'typical' population parameters for theophylline clearance (2.8 L/h) and volume of distribution (35L), and the theophylline concentration is measured to be 8 mg/L some hours after an intravenous loading dose. If the predicted concentration is 10 mg/L (25% greater than measured) with a volume of distribution of 44L (25% greater than predicted) and a clearance of 4.2 L/h (50% greater than predicted), this would satisfy the Bayesian method for trading off the relative contributions of deviations from the measured concentrations and the population pharmacokinetic parameters. This example is based on the further assumption that the volume of distribution and clearance contribute equally to the model prediction of concentration. If the level was measured at steady-state, then there could be no possible contribution from the volume of distribution, which would keep its population value. A compromise value of clearance would be needed to balance the likelihood of a deviation of the measured concentration from the predicted value and the likelihood that the individual's clearance differs from the population value.

The Bayesian method has some very useful properties in the setting of target concentration intervention. If no concentrations are available, it will predict the population pharmacokinetic parameters just like the *a priori* population prediction method. On the other hand, if there are many concentrations, it will effectively 'ignore' the *a priori* population predictions and come up with the same answers as the least squares method. When there are only 1 or 2 measured concentrations, it makes a more reasonable prediction than the one-point method because it will underemphasise measurements that require relatively large deviations from the population values. If, for example, because of a sample handling error, a concentration result is reported from the wrong patient and it is 10 times lower than expected using the population parameters, the Bayesian method will modify the parameters only a little but the one-point method could predict a clearance 10 times larger than the population value. If this was interpreted literally, the patient could be given a dose that was 10 times too large. The Bayesian method provides an automated way of making 'reasonable' predictions which may be difficult to do in any other way if the dosage history is complex and there are 2 or 3 concentrations to be interpreted.

A number of Bayesian forecasting programs are available for dose forecasting (e.g. Abbotbase PKS, Simkin, MWPharm; reviewed by Buffington et al.).[64] An ideal package would allow new drugs (e.g. those undergoing clinical development) to be included easily, allow flexible report writing, and save the dose and concentration observations in a way that would allow subsequent population-based analysis to improve knowledge of the drug and the variability of its parameters.

### 3.4 Individual Dose Prediction

The prediction of a suitable dose for an individual can be made from estimates of the patient's pharmacokinetic parameters. An additional piece of information is required – the target concentration. If the drug is to be given by continuous intravenous infusion, then the loading dose and the maintenance dose infusion rate can be calculated using the equations described above (section 1.2) [see also appendix G]. If the drug is given intermittently, it is helpful to look at a graph of time *versus* concentration for potential dosage schemes suggested by the clinician. The trade-off between excessive swings from peak to trough and the unacceptability of frequent administration is best made by taking into account the patient's previous response to the drug and attitude towards medication.

The provision of an excellent therapeutic drug monitoring service, also sometimes called a clinical pharmacokinetics service, based on continual assessment of the patient and revision of the optimum dosage advice can offer much to enhance individualised patient care.[72-74]

## 4. Monitoring of Individual Drugs

The general principles that determine the role of target concentration intervention and when to obtain samples have been discussed above. Individual agents or classes of drugs have special features that must be considered when measurement of their concentration is contemplated (see table I).

### 4.1 Theophylline

Several of the principles of target concentration intervention have already been illustrated with reference to theophylline (see section 2.2.2). It certainly satisfies one of the criteria for the use of drug concentration measurements: a narrow therapeutic index plus wide unpredictable variability in clearance which mandates individual dose adjustment. However, the other principal criterion, a therapeutic effect that is difficult to assess, is not so obviously supported.

The major aim of theophylline therapy is to relieve the symptoms of airways obstruction, and this is usually thought to depend upon bronchodilatation. It is simple for patients to monitor their own airway function using a peak flow meter, which can provide a regular, day-by-day, relatively objective measurement of the therapeutic effect. However, the action of theophylline is not so simple. There is a growing suspicion that some of the long term benefits of theophylline use depend upon reductions in airway reactivity rather than an acute bronchodilator effect. This more subtle action may take several weeks to develop. Furthermore, patients with chronic irreversible airway obstruction may obtain significant symptomatic relief of dyspnoea and improved exercise tolerance without any change in peak flow. Finally, even the bronchodilator effects of theophylline in an acute attack of airway obstruction may take many hours to develop.[75] The desired clinical effect may not be related immediately to the serum theophylline concentration, and therefore the effects cannot be relied upon, alone, to ensure that therapeutic benefit is likely.

The choice of a target concentration and the implementation of a target concentration strategy are important to achieve optimum results. Consider the situation described earlier (section 2.2.2) when a patient with an acute attack of asthma who is already taking an oral theophylline preparation is given an intravenous loading dose of theophylline[1] and the pre- and post-dose

1 For intravenous administration, theophylline is given as aminophylline, the dose of which is calculated by adding 25% to the theophylline dose (e.g. 350mg theophylline is equivalent to approximately 450mg aminophylline).

**Table I.** Commonly monitored drugs

| Drug | Sampling time(s) | Time to reach steady-state[a] | Usual minimum effective–maximum safe concentration range (mg/L[b]) | | Suggested target concentration (mg/L[b]) |
|---|---|---|---|---|---|
| | | | *Trough:* | *Peak:* | |
| **Aminoglycosides**[c] | | | | | |
| Amikacin | Peak concentration[d] and 8h later | 8 hours | 3-5 | 20-30 | 25 (peak)<br>9 (average) |
| Gentamicin | | 8 hours | 1-2 | 5-10 | 8 (initial)<br>3 (average) |
| Netilmicin | | 8 hours | 1-2 | 5-10 | 8 (initial)<br>3 (average) |
| Tobramycin | | 8 hours | 1-2 | 5-10 | 8 (initial)<br>3 (average) |
| **Antiarrhythmics** | | | | | |
| Amiodarone | Middle of dose interval | 1 month[e] | 1.0-2.5 | | 1.5 |
| Disopyramide | | 24 hours | 2-5 | | 3 |
| Flecainide | | 3 days | 0.25-0.9 | | 0.5 |
| Lidocaine | | 12 hours | 1.5-5 | | 3.5 |
| Mexiletine | | 2 days | 0.5-1.9 | | 1.5 |
| Procainamide | | 16 hours | 3.6-10 | | 6 |
| Quinidine | | 24 hours | 1-5[f] | | 1.5[f] |
| Sotalol | | 48 hours | 1.0-2.5 | | 1.5 |
| **Antiepileptics** | | | | | |
| Carbamazepine | Middle of dose interval | 2 weeks | 5-12 | | 8 |
| Clonazepam[g] | | 5 days | 0.025-0.075 | | 0.05 |
| Ethosuximide | | 8 days | 50-100 | | 75 |
| Phenobarbital | | 2 weeks | 15-40 | | 25 |
| Phenytoin | | >2 weeks | 10-20 | | 10 |
| Valproic acid[g] | | 40 hours | 50-100 | | 75 |
| **Antidepressants** | | | | | |
| Amitriptyline[h] | Middle of dose interval | 3 days | 0.1-0.25 | | 0.2 |
| Imipramine | | 2 days | 0.12-0.3 | | 0.2 |
| Nortriptyline | | 5 days | 0.05-0.15 | | 0.1 |
| **Antipsychotics** | | | | | |
| Haloperidol | Middle of dose interval | 3 days | 5.2-15 | | 10 |
| Lithium | 12h after last dose | 3 days | 5.5-7<br>(0.8-1 mmol/L) | | 6<br>(0.9 mmol/L) |
| **Others** | | | | | |
| Digoxin | At least 6-8h after last dose | 7 days | 1-2 μg/L | | 1 μg/L (heart failure)<br>2 μg/L (atrial fibrillation) |
| Salicylate | Middle of dose interval | 2-5 days | 150-300 | | 200 |
| Theophylline | Middle of dose interval | 36 hours | 10-20 | | 10 |
| Cyclosporin | Middle of dose interval | 3 days | 0.08-0.25[i] | | 0.15[i] |
| Vancomycin | Peak level (after infusion) and before next dose (trough) | | | | 20 (average) |

a Time to reach steady-state during normal therapeutic use of drug (starting or changing the dose).

b Unless specified otherwise.

c Concentrations shown apply for 8-hourly dosage regimens.

d 20-30 minutes after completion of first 30-minute infusion (or 15 minutes after completion of 1 hr infusion or < 60 min after IV bolus injection). If once-daily dosage regimens of aminoglycosides are employed, a sample taken 3 half-lives after the dose will provide useful information for estimating clearance and volume of distribution; an average steady-state concentration of 3 mg/L (for gentamicin, netilmicin and tobramycin) should be aimed for.

e Although the half-life of amiodarone is up to 10 weeks in some patients, the measured plasma concentration appears to reach a relatively constant value by 1 month.

f Concentrations measured using a specific assay for quinidine (see section 1.6.4).

g Concentration ranges for clonazepam and valproic acid are very approximate.

h Amitriptyline is the sum of amitriptyline plus nortriptyline.

i Whole blood should be used for cyclosporin (values refer to specific assay). Target concentrations depend on indication.

concentrations are measured. If one assumes a target concentration of 10 mg/L and the pre- and post-dose concentrations after a 350mg intravenous loading dose are 6 and 16 mg/L, respectively, the difference in concentration is 10 mg/L so the volume of distribution is 35L (350 mg ÷ 10 mg/L) which is typical for a 70kg person. The pre-dose concentration is compatible with an oral dose of 300mg of slow release theophylline twice daily if the patient smokes cigarettes (clearance 4.5 L/h) or a similar dose in a nonsmoking patient (clearance 2.8 L/h) who is not fully compliant with the prescribed dose. The post-dose concentration (16 mg/L) is higher than the target of 10 mg/L, so it would be prudent to stop the maintenance infusion of theophylline for about half a half-life to allow the concentration to fall by 30% to around 10 mg/L. If the patient is a nonsmoker, this would be 4 to 5 hours but only 3 hours for a smoker.

Suppose the concentration is checked after stopping the infusion for 4 hours (the patient is a nonsmoker), a maintenance infusion of 30 mg/h is started and the concentration is measured again 5 hours later. If the values at the start of the infusion and after 5 hours are 11 mg/L and 9 mg/L, respectively, one can be fairly confident that the patient has a clearance close to the typical value of 3 L/h (30 mg/h ÷ 10 mg/L) and can safely leave the infusion running until the concentration is checked again in 18 to 24 hours. However, if the levels are 12 mg/L and 14 mg/L, one should anticipate that the clearance is lower than expected (around 2.1 L/h) and be prepared to reduce the infusion rate accordingly (e.g. to about 20 mg/h) and measure the concentration again within a few hours.

If a higher target concentration is chosen, e.g. 20 mg/L, or if concentrations are to be interpreted in patients who have achieved concentrations similar to this, the clearance of theophylline may deviate from simple first-order predictions. There is a growing body of evidence to suggest that theophylline is at the border of first-order and concentration-dependent elimination, particularly in children. For adults, the Km has been estimated to be about 24 mg/L and $V_{max}$ about 2000 mg/day.[76]

### 4.2 Digitalis Glycosides

The use of concentration measurements for digoxin is widespread. Although digoxin is far more commonly used than digitoxin, there are still arguments made for the use of digitoxin based on its pharmacokinetic properties (very long half-life, nonrenal-dependent clearance). However, if the pharmacokinetics of digoxin are understood, these putative advantages fade away.

Concentrations of digoxin are commonly measured and are among the most easy to interpret in order to achieve a target concentration.[77] This is because digoxin's relatively long half-life (about 2 days) in relation to the usual dosage interval (1 day) makes the fluctuation in concentrations small. A sample taken at more or less any time during the dosage interval, but at least 6 hours after the last dose and a week after starting treatment, will reflect the average steady-state concentration. Any deviation from the target concentration can then be simply translated into a proportional change in the maintenance dose. The toxicity of digoxin is influenced by potassium and magnesium concentrations and the target concentration of digoxin needs to be lowered to achieve the desired beneficial outcome in an individual with a low serum potassium level. This viewpoint is not uniformly held and it has been asserted that the way digoxin concentrations are used in common practice is of doubtful value.[78]

The target concentration for digoxin required to control atrial fibrillation is higher (2 μg/L) than that for the treatment of heart failure. The value of maintaining digoxin concentrations at about 1 μg/L in patients with heart failure has been demonstrated.[79,80] Another useful application of digoxin plasma concentration measurements is in deciding whether further digoxin should be given to a patient who presents with worsening heart failure and an arrhythmia. If the digoxin concentrations are high, the probability of a digoxin-induced arrhythmia is increased and further digoxin should be given only with caution.[39]

### 4.3 Antiepileptic Drugs

The benefits of drug concentration measurements in the management of patients with epilepsy may still be disputed by some experienced neurologists, but for those without this clinical wisdom, the use of concentrations can provide reassurance that effective steps have been taken to control an intermittent, but often serious problem.[81]

#### *4.3.1 Phenytoin*

The problems associated with concentration-dependent elimination and alterations in protein binding of phenytoin have been discussed above (sections 1.6.3 and 2.2.2). Dosage prediction is further complicated by the great variability between individuals in the parameters describing elimination. It is not possible to make reliable predictions of the elimination capacity (i.e. the maximum elimination rate, $V_{max}$) or the concentration at which the rate of elimination is half of $V_{max}$ (Km) from patient characteristics such as weight. Dosage adjustment is often empirical, with the patient being exposed to either low concentrations and continued risk of a seizure, or high concentrations and often disabling toxicity. Small increments in phenytoin dose, e.g. 10 to 20%, can change concentrations from subtherapeutic to toxic and *vice versa* for small decrements.

Computer-assisted dosage prediction methods are now available and can greatly assist in rapidly determining the optimum dose of phenytoin.[50,82-84] A steady-state concentration is not necessary; adequate predictions of the required dose can be made from 2 or 3 properly timed concentrations prior to steady-state.

The usual therapeutic range quoted for phenytoin is 10 to 20 mg/L (40 to 80 μmol/L). An initial target concentration might be 15 mg/L with adjustment of the target based upon the patient's response.[85] Once daily administration in most adults will not cause excessive fluctuations once concentrations are above 10 mg/L, because the half-life of the drug is greater at concentrations above this level and fluctuations are therefore smaller.

#### 4.3.2 Valproic Acid (Sodium Valproate)

The use of concentrations to guide valproic acid therapy is complicated to some extent by saturable plasma protein binding, which means the rise in total drug concentration will be less than expected from an increase in dose. This phenomenon is not of much practical significance because its magnitude is similar to the intraindividual fluctuations in concentrations. It is doubtful if one could detect the effect of decreased fractional binding in an individual patient from a single sample at each dose level.

It has been suggested that the antiepileptic action of valproic acid is only partly explained by the plasma concentration and there is a more slowly developing action that may persist for some time after stopping the drug.[86] It is sometimes argued that there is little value in the use of valproic acid concentrations because of the rather weak relationship between concentration and antiepileptic activity. Nevertheless, even if the immediate association between concentration and effect is not discernible, the long term effects are most reasonably related to the average concentration. Valproic acid has been used successfully by basing dose adjustments simply on the response to treatment without the use of concentrations.[87] While this may be effective eventually, it has not been shown that the use of valproic acid concentrations would not help in achieving seizure control earlier. If for no other reason than documenting compliance, the use of target concentration intervention must contribute to the information available to the clinician in making a therapeutic decision.

#### 4.3.3 Carbamazepine

Carbamazepine, like phenytoin, is a potent inducer of hepatic enzymes. Not only does this lead to problems with the use of other drugs whose metabolism may be increased, but it also enhances its own metabolism by a factor of 4 (see appendix A). Attempts to predict the eventual dose requirement based upon concentrations measured only a few days after starting treatment will most likely be underestimates. At least 2 weeks should elapse after a dose adjustment before any confidence can be placed in the steady-state concentration estimate.

There have been models proposed which account for this autoinduction of carbamazepine metabolism,[88] but to date these are not programmed in any of the computer-assisted dosage prediction packages. The usual therapeutic range quoted for carbamazepine is 5 to 12 mg/L (20 to 50 μmol/L). These are the suggested steady-state concentrations and a reasonable initial target concentration to achieve after 2 to 3 weeks would be 8 mg/L. Administration might be instituted in a twice daily regimen, but after autoinduction, 3 times daily administration is often required to avoid excessive concentration fluctuations within a dosage interval.

#### 4.3.4 Phenobarbital/Primidone

The principal feature of phenobarbital concentration monitoring is related to its very low clearance. It has a long half-life (nearly 5 days) and takes 3 weeks to reach steady-state concentrations. Primidone is largely a prodrug which is metabolised to phenobarbital – the principal active form. The measurement of both primidone and phenobarbital concentrations does, however, give some additional information about compliance. At steady-state, the typical ratio of phenobarbital to primidone is about 3.

If a patient has generally been noncompliant but remembers to take the medication for a few days prior to seeing the doctor, the primidone concentration will reflect steady-state, but because of phenobarbital's long half-life, the latter will be disproportionately low. Conversely, if a patient has recently stopped taking primidone, the phenobarbital concentration will continue to be detectable and effective for several days after the primidone is no longer measurable.

#### 4.3.5 Other Antiepileptic Drugs

There are a number of new antiepileptic drugs either recently released or about to be released onto the market. Target concentration intervention has been considered for some of these. The pharmacokinetics of lamotrigine are variable between individuals, and interactions with other antiepileptic drugs occur, leading to either lower than predicted (with phenytoin and carbamazepine) or higher than predicted (with valproic acid) plasma concentrations of lamotrigine. A range of 1 to 4 mg/L has been suggested,[89] which implies a target of 2.5 mg/L.

Vigabatrin is administered as a racemate, with activity residing in one of the enantiomers (section 1.6.5). However, the mechanism of action of the drug is through covalent (irreversible) binding to a target enzyme; therefore the clinical activity is unlikely to be related to plasma concentrations.[90] For further discussion of the pharmacokinetics of these and other newer agents, see review by Bialer.[91]

### 4.4 Antiarrhythmic Drugs

Antiarrhythmic drugs, like antiepileptic drugs, are prime candidates for target concentration intervention (for reviews, see Follath et al.[92] Gillis & Kates,[93] and Latini et al.[94]). Because of their steep concentration-effect curves, an attempt should be made to define a target concentration for each individual rather than rely on a therapeutic range (see section 1.4). This may be done in conjunction with ambulatory electrocardiographic monitoring, although there are limitations to this method of assessment which arise from the inherent day-to-day variability in arrhythmia activity.

#### 4.4.1 Quinidine

An initial target concentration of 1.5 mg/L (using a specific assay for quinidine; see section 1.6.4) or 3 mg/L (using a nonspecific assay) should be aimed for with slow release oral formulations. Increases in $\alpha_1$-acid glycoprotein will increase quinidine plasma protein binding. Measured concentrations following an acute inflammatory event, such as myocardial infarction, should therefore be adjusted downwards by about 30% to reflect the unbound concentration.[95]

Although quinidine is usually given orally, it should be recognised that if the intravenous route is used, the target concentration of quinidine using a specific assay may be 50% higher because active metabolites formed during oral absorption contribute to the effects that have been used to define the target concentration after oral administration.[96] Even though the target concentration is based on a specific assay after oral administration, the antiarrhythmic effects are in part due to metabolites which are not present in such quantities after intravenous administration.

#### 4.4.2 Procainamide

The recommended target concentration for procainamide has increased in recent years with the realisation that toxicity was not commonly encountered at the lower concentrations advocated previously. An initial target of 6 mg/L is suggested. In patients with impaired renal function, the additional antiarrhythmic contribution of acecainide (*N*-acetylprocainamide; NAPA) should be recognised and may be converted to 'procainamide' equivalents by dividing its concentration by 5.

#### 4.4.3 Disopyramide

Using total drug concentrations, an initial target of 3 mg/L of disopyramide is recommended. Because of concentration-dependent plasma protein binding at typical therapeutic concentrations, the increase in total drug concentration will be less than predicted from a dose increase, but the unbound drug concentration will rise in proportion and so will the pharmacological effect.[97]

#### 4.4.4 Amiodarone

The pharmacokinetics of amiodarone are unusual because of its extensive tissue binding and, consequently, a large volume of distribution and very long half-life (for reviews, see Latini et al.[98] and Pourbaix et al.[99]). The terminal half-life has been estimated to be from 3 to 6 weeks, which implies that it may take up to 6 months to reach steady-state. However, because of the slow distribution of drug from plasma to tissues, the measured serum concentration may appear to reach a relatively constant value by 1 month.

The antiarrhythmic effect appears to have an early and a late component and it is not clear if these reflect the same pharmacological action. The late effect is related to the amiodarone concentration, and a target concentration of 1.5 mg/L is suggested.[7]

A metabolite of amiodarone, desethylamiodarone (DEA), is measured by some HPLC assays. Soon after initiation of treatment with amiodarone, the ratio of amiodarone to DEA is usually greater than 1 but as steady-state is approached, the ratio is about 1. This may be used as an indirect guide to compliance. If the ratio is greater than 1.5 after several weeks, it suggests that the patient may not be compliant with the prescribed dose. DEA may have some activity as an antiarrhythmic substance; however, it accounts for only a very small part of the extensive metabolism of amiodarone and is unlikely to contribute to the antiarrhythmic effects of amiodarone *in vivo*. Other, as yet unidentified, metabolites of amiodarone may also be active and may contribute to the discrepancy between the early and late antiarrhythmic response.

#### 4.4.5 Lidocaine

There is still considerable debate about the role of lidocaine in the treatment of arrhythmias. Some of the discrepancies between the various studies may be accounted for by the wide variation in concentrations in different patients. The short term pharmacokinetics of lidocaine are best described by a 2-compartment model because of the relatively long distribution phase in relation to elimination. This makes the interpretation of concentrations quite difficult and several groups have developed computer programs to assist with interpretation.[100] The use of a Bayesian forecasting method to achieve target concentrations of lidocaine more quickly and reliably may prove to be the key element in effective use of the drug.

An initial lidocaine target concentration of 3.5 mg/L has been suggested.[101]

#### 4.4.6 Other Antiarrhythmic Drugs

The pharmacokinetics and target concentration intervention aspects of a number of newer and less widely used antiarrhythmic drugs have been reviewed by Gillis and Kates,[93] including encainide, flecainide,[102] lorcainide, mexiletine, pirmenol, propafenone and tocainide.

### 4.5 Antidepressants

The use of target concentration intervention to guide the use of antidepressant drug dosage is controversial. Interpretation of the relationship between concentration and effect is difficult because depression is an episodic phenomenon with spontaneous improvement, and commonly used drugs such as amitriptyline and imipramine have active metabolites. It is claimed that the concentration-effect relationship for antidepressant effect does not approach and maintain a maximum value as the concentration increases but instead, the effect decreases when an optimum level is exceeded. This probably reflects the integration of several psychological phenomena, some positive and some negative. As the concentration increases beyond the optimum value, the negative influences on mood predominate.

An evaluation of the merits of tricyclic antidepressant concentration measurement by Perry et al.[103] concluded that the evidence is strongest for the use of nortriptyline. The evidence was weaker for imipramine and desipramine and weakest for amitriptyline. Similarly, there appears to be a poor relationship between plasma concentrations of dothiepin and metabolites and clinical effects.[104]

Nevertheless, the fact that most antidepressants are metabolised by the cytochrome P450 isoenzyme CYP2D6 and are therefore subject to polymorphic oxidation (see further chapter 1; sect. 5.2.2) has been advanced as a reason favouring the measurement of plasma concentrations of these drugs. The poor metaboliser phenotype (5 to 10% of caucasians) is at risk of drug accumulation at conventional doses while the ultrarapid metaboliser may develop subtherapeutic concentrations. In this respect, optimum ranges for some antidepressant drugs have been suggested: amitriptyline plus nortriptyline (an active metabolite) 100 to 250 μg/L; nortriptyline 50 to 150 μg/L; imipramine plus desipramine (an active metabolite) 120 to 300 μg/L. Initial target concentrations around the middle of these suggested ranges could be used, with subsequent target concentration revision and dosage adjustment based on the clinical response. Three to four weeks should be allowed for steady-state concentrations to be achieved.

Discrimination of nonresponders and responders to clomipramine therapy has been suggested based on measurement of parent drug plus demethylated and hydroxylated metabolites 2 weeks after initiation of therapy.[105]

### 4.6 Lithium

Lithium is always administered orally and usually at 12-hour intervals. The lithium ion takes several hours to distribute in body fluids and so the concentration in samples drawn in the first half of the dosage interval tends to be higher than would be expected if distribution were rapid. In order to remove the variability that arises from differences in the rates of distribution, it is recommended that samples be taken shortly before the next dose.[106] Dosage prediction for lithium, based on population values for clearance using the demographic variables age, weight and serum creatinine, has been found to be reasonably accurate.[107]

### 4.7 Antipsychotics

Wide interpatient variability in plasma concentrations of antipsychotic drugs (such as haloperidol and phenothiazines) and difficulties in evaluating the response to these drugs suggest that target concentration intervention would be valuable in achieving results more rapidly. However, the long term, fluctuating nature of severe psychotic illness has meant that empirical dose adjustment continues to be the most widely used method of dosage individualisation. Controlled studies of individual agents attempting to define a target concentration have generally been unsuccessful.[108]

Some support for measuring concentrations of specific agents has been provided by Balant-Georgia and Balant,[109] and its use in avoiding supratherapeutic concentrations of these drugs (e.g. in the poor metaboliser phenotype), and hence their Parkinsonian adverse effects, has also been advocated (see further chapter 1; sect. 5.2.2 and 6.2.1).

### 4.8 Antimicrobial Agents

The aminoglycoside antibiotics are widely prescribed and target concentration intervention is almost universally used to individualise their dosages. Most other antimicrobial agents have such a wide therapeutic index that little attention is paid to dose individualisation.

#### *4.8.1 Aminoglycosides*

Gentamicin, tobramycin, netilmicin and amikacin have essentially the same pharmacokinetic properties. Amikacin, however, differs in requiring target concentrations about 4 times greater than the others. The issue of a target concentration is vexed. Traditional dosage regimens have been intermittent (3 times daily) giving rise to wide fluctuations in concentration during a dosage interval (see section 2.2.2). More recently, once or twice daily regimens have been used. The rationale for these regimens is based on the 'post-antibiotic effect', i.e. inhibition of bacterial growth continues below the minimum inhibitory concentration (MIC) of the organism for that drug, and the concentration-dependent killing rate of aminoglycoside antibiotics (for reviews, see Gilbert;[44] Hustinx & Hoepelman[45]). It has also been suggested that adaptive resistance of organisms may occur, providing a further reason for once or twice daily administration.[44] Such data suggest that therapy may be improved if a high concentration is targeted initially, then a sufficient time allowed for most of the aminoglycoside to be eliminated from the body before another dose is given.

Many studies performed with 3 times daily administration have suggested that aminoglycoside efficacy and toxicity are related to peak and/or trough concentrations. The usual target concentrations recommended by such studies are peaks of 5 to 10 mg/L and troughs of 1 to 2 mg/L (or 20 to 30 mg/L and 3 to 5 mg/L, respectively, for amikacin), although there are difficulties in interpreting the results from different studies.[110] The duration of therapy is also important for development of toxicity and it is suggested that, for most patients, courses of aminoglycoside therapy should last no longer than 5 to 7 days.

A suggested strategy in 8-hourly dosage regimens is to aim for an initial concentration of 8 mg/L after the first dose and an average concentration of 3 mg/L with the maintenance dose regimen. In the case of amikacin, the corresponding target concentrations would be 25 mg/L (peak) and an average of about 9 mg/L. For once daily regimens, peak concentrations three times these values should be targeted, and individualised pharmacokinetic parameters calculated after the first dose (as described in section 2.2.2) for prediction of optimum subsequent doses.

It has been suggested that for once daily administration, a target area under the concentration-time curve (AUC) be used instead of a target concentration.[47] However, the target AUC is simply the target concentration multiplied by the dosage interval and offers no additional information. It should also be noted that the AUC approach has been shown to be invalid for predicting aminoglycoside toxicity (since toxicity is greater with shorter dosage intervals despite the same overall AUC), and currently has no experimental or theoretical basis for superior performance compared with a target based on an average concentration. Empirical support for improved therapy with aminoglycosides is based on manipulation of the dosage interval to achieve different concentration-time profiles. Neither the target AUC nor the target concentration approach offer any help in choosing the optimum profile. We prefer the target concentration approach because the same concept is applicable to other drugs and it is independent of the dosage interval. The same average steady-state target concentration of 3 mg/L (9 mg/L for amikacin) can be used for 8-hour or 24-hour dosage regimens.

### 4.8.2 Vancomycin

The use of concentration targeting for vancomycin is ill-defined. A survey of monitoring practices in Australasia reflected the confusion.[111] Current literature recommendations indicate a peak concentration target of 20 to 40 mg/L. The actual time of peak sampling after a dose, in the Australasian laboratories studied, ranged from 0 to 120 minutes after the end of an infusion. A concentration of 30 mg/L 2 hours after administration will arise from a completely different dosage regimen from that targeting 30 mg/L at the end of the infusion.

There is some evidence that nephrotoxicity is associated with trough concentrations above 10 mg/L, especially if vancomycin is used in conjunction with other nephrotoxic drugs and/or for a prolonged period of time (more than 21 days).[112,113]

By analogy with the recommendations made for aminoglycosides, it seems reasonable to propose a target concentration based on the average steady-state value. A patient with a clearance of 4 L/h given 1g every 12 hours would have an average concentration of about 20 mg/L. A target concentration of 20 mg/L is compatible with other recommendations,[111] and offers a unified approach along with the aminoglycosides.

### 4.8.3 Chloramphenicol

This drug is not widely used nowadays, except for the treatment of certain specific infections in which its benefits outweigh the risk of serious toxicity, especially blood dyscrasias. At least in part, bone marrow suppression is concentration-dependent and target concentrations around 10 mg/L have been suggested to try to reduce the risk of this complication. The 'grey baby' syndrome, which may occur at any age, is said to be associated with concentrations over 40 mg/L and provides another reason for using concentration measurements to guide therapy (for a review, see Ambrose[114]).

### 4.8.4 Antifungal Agents

#### Flucytosine

It is recommended that plasma concentrations of flucytosine do not exceed 70 mg/L. Bone marrow toxicity, including some reports of death, has been documented in patients with flucytosine concentrations exceeding 100 mg/L.[115] As concentrations of around 25 mg/L are necessary for antifungal efficacy, a suitable initial concentration target would be 50 mg/L. Particular attention to concentration measurement is needed in any patient with renal impairment, as this is the major route of elimination.

#### Azole Antifungal Drugs

Plasma concentration measurements of the azole antifungal drugs are not performed routinely at the moment, but there is some evidence that low concentrations may be associated with therapy failures. There are specific groups of patients for whom concentration targeting may be particularly useful to ensure efficacy, e.g. those with human immunodeficiency virus infection (low bioavailability of ketoconazole and itraconazole) and patients receiving multiple drugs (induction of itraconazole metabolism by some antiepileptic agents). For a review of the pharmacokinetics of antifungal drugs, see Schafer-Korting.[115]

### 4.8.5 Antiviral Agents

#### Zidovudine

There is preliminary evidence that the efficacy and toxicity of zidovudine may be related to intracellular concentrations of phosphorylated drug.[116] Zidovudine 5'-triphosphate is the active form of the drug, but the complexity of currently available assays to specifically measure intracellular concentrations of this active species precludes use as a routine test.[117] In the future, concentration targeting of this triphosphate and that of other antiretrovirals (e.g. didanosine and zalcitabine) may be possible to ensure maintenance of virustatic concentrations with minimal risk of adverse effects.

**Ganciclovir**

Ganciclovir inhibits human cytomegalovirus. There is some evidence that efficacy and toxicity are related to the plasma concentration,[118,119] although again, the active form of the drug is the triphosphate. In the future, optimal dosage design for ganciclovir could also be based on achieving specified target concentrations of the active form.

### 4.9 Antineoplastic Drugs

The complexity of multiple drug regimens, the protean manifestations of toxicity, and the usually slow onset of therapeutic response have made it very difficult to evaluate the relationship between plasma concentrations and effects for this class of drugs (for reviews, see Balis et al.[120] and Moore & Ehrlichman[121]).

Many of the drugs used in cancer chemotherapy, such as methotrexate, carboplatin, teniposide and others, could be considered suitable candidates for dosage adjustment based on target concentration interventions. Several of these agents have been demonstrated to show wide interindividual variability in pharmacokinetic parameters.[122,123] The difference between effective and toxic concentrations is also small for many of these drugs. The main problem to date, as for so many other drugs, has been the lack of rigorous studies demonstrating their concentration-effect relationships and thus providing target concentrations. Incorporation of these types of studies in phase I-III clinical trials of newer drugs has been strongly recommended to provide such data in the future.[122,124]

**Methotrexate**

Concentration monitoring of methotrexate, a folate antagonist, has become common to guide the use of folinic acid (leucovorin) 'rescue' therapy after high doses.[121] Patients with low methotrexate clearances are thus identified and 'rescue' therapy can continue until methotrexate concentrations fall below 0.1 mmol/L. Mortality has fallen dramatically since the introduction of methotrexate concentration determination for this indication.

There is also some evidence to support the use of a target concentration of methotrexate in the treatment of acute lymphocytic leukaemia. Therapeutic failure has been shown to be more likely if the concentration at the end of a 24-hour infusion of methotrexate is less than 16 μmol/L.[125]

### 4.10 Immunosuppressants

#### *4.10.1 Cyclosporin*

A major advance in the prevention of transplanted organ rejection has come from the introduction of cyclosporin therapy (see also chapter 28; sect. 2.1.3). Cyclosporin is also used as therapy for a number of other immunological disorders, such as rheumatoid arthritis, psoriasis and Behçet's syndrome. The narrow therapeutic index, marked interpatient variability in clearance (mainly by metabolism), low and variable bioavailability, and the large number of drug interactions that potentially affect cyclosporin concentrations make this drug an obvious candidate for dosage adjustment using concentration targeting techniques.

However, target concentrations are not well defined for cyclosporin, and reported optimum ranges vary from institution to institution. Different indications require different target concentrations, with cardiac transplant recipients generally maintaining higher concentrations than those with renal grafts, for example. It is also generally accepted that lower concentration targets are needed after a period of time than those targeted in the immediate post-transplant period. As an example, using a monoclonal (nonspecific) immunoassay, target cyclosporin concentrations for cardiac transplant recipients immediately after transplantation might be as high as 500 μg/L, whereas for long term care of a renal transplant recipient, a concentration of 150 μg/L would be appropriate.

A number of consensus documents are now available to guide the optimum use of cyclosporin concentration monitoring.[126-129] These guidelines indicate that concentrations should be determined in whole blood (because of the temperature-dependent cellular uptake of cyclosporin) and that parent drug concentrations should be measured as specifically as possible. Many of the older assays measured cyclosporin metabolites concurrently with parent drug, which made the determination of target concentrations difficult as metabolite ratios change with time after transplantation and are variable between individuals (for a review of assay methods, see Kivisto[130]).

There are also suggestions that measurement of more than one concentration in a dosage interval may be a better method of optimising dosage than the usual practice of monitoring trough concentrations.[41,131,132] However, it is yet to be demonstrated that the added inconvenience and cost are matched by significant improvements in clinical outcomes.

#### *4.10.2 Other Immunosuppressants*

A number of newer immunosuppressant drugs are due for release (or have recently been released) onto the market. These include tacrolimus (FK 506), gusperimus, rapamycin, mycophenolate mofetil and others (see chapter 28; sect. 2.1.1, 2.1.3). Already data are emerging about the distribution of these other agents between blood cells and plasma, and differences between analytical techniques.[133,134] It has been suggested that it may be better to measure total immunosuppression by measurement of binding proteins and receptors, rather than relying on determination of actual drug concentrations.[135] The lessons learned from the cyclosporin experience about optimum assay procedures, which biological samples to collect and, importantly, high quality studies to identify correlations of clinical outcomes with concentration need to be applied to these drugs to ensure that optimum dosage strategies are used.

### 4.11 Antirheumatic Drugs

#### *4.11.1 Disease-Modifying Antirheumatic Drugs (DMARDs)*

There is wide interindividual variability in the pharmacokinetic parameters of many of the disease-modifying antirheumatic drugs, including gold, hydroxychloroquine and sulfasalazine.[136,137] A relationship between blood concentrations and effect has been demonstrated for hydroxychloroquine[138] and it has been postulated that the characteristic variable response to all these agents may be due, at least in part, to variability in the steady-state concentrations arising from the standard dosage regimens used.[137]

#### *4.11.2 Salicylate*

The use of salicylate concentrations for target concentration intervention is unusual. When used for its antipyretic and analgesic actions, it is sufficient to observe the clinical response and adjust the dose on that basis. The use of salicylate in the treatment of rheumatic fever is traditional, and doses greater than those usually necessary may be used in an attempt to achieve a target concentration of 200 mg/L.[139]

The interpretation of salicylate concentration is complicated by two pharmacokinetic factors. Firstly, the metabolism of salicylate is complex with 2 of the 4 principal metabolites being formed by concentration-dependent (Michaelis-Menten) processes. Secondly, the plasma protein binding of salicylate is concentration-dependent. The former makes unbound drug concentrations rise more rapidly than increases in dose, while the latter makes total concentrations rise less rapidly than increases in unbound concentration. The net result may give rise to an approximately linear relationship between salicylate dose and total drug concentration.[140]

## References


1. Sokolow M, Ball RE. Factors influencing conversion of chronic atrial fibrillation with special reference to serum quinidine concentration. Circulation 1956; 14: 568-83
2. Holford NHG, Sheiner LB. Understanding the dose-effect relationship: clinical application of pharmacokinetic-pharmacodynamic models. Clinical Pharmacokinetics 1981; 6: 429-53
3. Mitenko PA, Ogilvie RI. Rational intravenous doses of theophylline. New England Journal of Medicine 1973; 289: 600-3
4. Holford NHG, Black P, Briant R, et al. Theophylline target concentration - comparison of 10 vs 20 mg/L in patients with airways obstruction requiring IV theophylline. Clinical Pharmacokinetics 1993; 25: 495-505
5. Holford NHG, Hashimoto Y, Sheiner LB. Time and concentration determine the response to theophylline. Clinical Pharmacokinetics 1993; 25: 506-15
6. Maling T. Amiodarone therapeutic plasma concentration monitoring: is it practical? Clinical Pharmacokinetics 1988; 14: 321-4
7. Rotmensch HH, Belhassen B, Swanson BN, et al. Steady state serum amiodarone concentrations: relationships with antiarrhythmic efficacy and toxicity. Annals of Internal Medicine 1984; 101: 462-9
8. Schumacher GE, Barr JT. Making serum drug levels more meaningful. Therapeutic Drug Monitoring 1989; 11: 580-4
9. Schumacher GE, Barr JT. Using population-based serum drug concentration cutoff values to predict toxicity: test performance and limitations compared with Bayesian interpretation. Clinical Pharmacy 1990; 9: 788-96
10. Vozeh S. Cost-effectiveness of therapeutic drug monitoring. Clinical Pharmacokinetics 1987; 13: 131-40
11. Bootman JL, Wertheimer AI, Zaske D, et al. Individualizing gentamicin dosage regimens in burn patients with Gram-negative septicemia: a cost-benefit analysis. Journal of Pharmaceutical Sciences 1979; 68: 267-72
12. Bertino JS, Rodvold KA, Destache CJ. Cost considerations in therapeutic drug monitoring of aminoglycosides. Clinical Pharmacokinetics 1994; 26: 71-81
13. Pearce GA, Day RO. Compliance with criteria necessary for effective drug concentration monitoring. Therapeutic Drug Monitoring 1990; 12: 250-7
14. Morris RG, Saccoia N, Ryall RG, et al. Specific enzyme-multiplied immunoassay and fluorescence polarization immunoassay for cyclosporin compared with cyclotrac ($^{125}$I) radioimmunoassay. Therapeutic Drug Monitoring 1992; 14: 226-33
15. Ray JE, Crisan D, Howrie DL. Digoxin-like immunoreactivity in serum from neonates and infants reduced by centrifugal ultrafiltration and fluorescence polarization immunoassay. Clinical Chemistry 1991; 37: 94-8
16. Roberts WL, Rainey PM. Interference in immunoassay measurements of total and free phenytoin in uremic patients: a reappraisal. Clinical Chemistry 1993; 39: 1872-7
17. Kino R, Day RO, Pearce G, et al. Bedside measurement of plasma theophylline concentration within the emergency

department. Australian Journal of Hospital Pharmacy 1991; 21: 292-4

18. Yosselson-Superstine A. Drug interferences with plasma assays in therapeutic drug monitoring. Clinical Pharmacokinetics 1984; 9: 67-87
19. Routledge PA, Shand DG, Barchowsky A, et al. Relationship between alpha-1-acid glycoprotein and lidocaine disposition in myocardial infarction. Clinical Pharmacology and Therapeutics 1981; 30: 154-7
20. Routledge PA, Stargel WW, Barchowsky A, et al. Factors affecting free (unbound) lignocaine concentration in suspected acute myocardial infarction. British Journal of Clinical Pharmacology 1989; 28: 593-7
21. Baird-Lambert J, Manglick MP, Wall M, et al. Identifying patients who might benefit from free phenytoin monitoring. Therapeutic Drug Monitoring 1987; 9: 134-8
22. du Souich P, Verges J, Erill S. Plasma protein binding and pharmacological response. Clinical Pharmacokinetics 1993; 24: 435-40
23. Garattini S. Active metabolites: an overview of their relevance in clinical pharmacokinetics. Clinical Pharmacokinetics 1985; 10: 216-27
24. Williams KM, Lee EJD. Importance of drug enantiomers in clinical pharmacology. Drugs 1985; 30: 333-54
25. Ariens EJ. Implications of the neglect of stereochemistry in pharmacokinetics and clinical pharmacology. Drug Intelligence and Clinical Pharmacy 1987; 21: 827-9
26. Vogelsang B, Echizen H, Schmidt E, et al. Stereoselective first-pass metabolism of highly cleared drugs: studies of the bioavailability of L- and D-verapamil examined with a stable isotope technique. British Journal of Clinical Pharmacology 1984; 18: 733-40
27. Holford NHG. Target effect or therapeutic range - what is the goal of antiarrhythmic therapy? In: Smith W, editor. Forum on the management of arrhythmias: the role of flecainide. Auckland: Adis Press, 1985: 15-32
28. Begg EJ. Units for drug concentrations in biological fluids. Lancet 1986; 1: 505
29. McInnes GT. The value of therapeutic drug monitoring to the practising physician - an hypothesis in need of testing. British Journal of Clinical Pharmacology 1989; 27: 281-4
30. Flanagan RJ. SI units - common sense not dogma is needed. British Journal of Clinical Pharmacology 1995; 39: 589-94
31. Holford NHG. A size standard for pharmacokinetics. Clinical Pharmacokinetics 1996; 30: 329-32
32. Ohlman S, Lindholm A, Hagglund H, et al. On the intraindividual variability and chronobiology of cyclosporine pharmacokinetics in renal transplantation. European Journal of Clinical Pharmacology 1993; 44: 265-9
33. Jogestrand T, Nordlander R. Serum digoxin determination in out-patients; need for standardisation. British Journal of Clinical Pharmacology 1983; 15: 55-8
34. Cai WM, Leader WG, Poert WH, et al. Influence of serum separator tubes on total and free phenytoin concentrations and dosages. Therapeutic Drug Monitoring 1993; 15: 427-30
35. Bergqvist Y, Domeij-Nyberg B. Distribution of chloroquine and its metabolite desethylchloroquine in human blood cells and its implication for the quantitative determination of these components in serum and plasma. Journal of Chromatography 1983; 272: 137-48
36. Siebers RWL, Chen CT, Ferguson RI, et al. Effect of blood sample tubes on amiodarone and desethylamiodarone concentrations. Therapeutic Drug Monitoring 1988; 10: 349-51
37. Chiou WL. The phenomenon and rationale of marked dependence of drug concentration on blood sampling site. Parts I and II. Clinical Pharmacokinetics 1989; 17: 175-99 and 275-90
38. Brown GR, Miyata M, McCormack JP. Drug concentration monitoring: an approach to rational use. Clinical Pharmacokinetics 1993; 24: 187-94
39. Holford NHG, Sheiner LB. The digoxin concentration: before and after the fact. American Heart Journal 1976; 94: 529-30
40. Johnston A, Sketris I, Marsden JT, et al. A limited sampling strategy for the measurement of cyclosporine AUC. Transplantation Proceedings 1990; 22: 1345-7
41. Grevel J, Napoli KL, Gibbone S, et al. Area-under-the-curve monitoring of cyclosporine therapy: performance of different assay methods and their target concentrations. Therapeutic Drug Monitoring 1990; 12: 8-15
42. Rodman JH, Evans WE. Targeted systemic exposure for paediatric cancer therapy. In: D'Argenio D, editor. Advanced methods of pharmacokinetic and pharmacodynamic systems analysis. New York: Plenum Press, 1991: 177-83
43. Slattery JT, Gibaldi M, Koup JR. Prediction of maintenance dose required to attain a desired drug concentration at steady-state from a single determination of concentration after an initial dose. Clinical Pharmacokinetics 1980; 5: 377-85
44. Gilbert DN. Once-daily aminoglycoside therapy. Antimicrobial Agents and Chemotherapy 1991; 35: 399-405
45. Hustinx WNM, Hoepelman IM. Aminoglycoside dosage regimens - is once a day enough? Clinical Pharmacokinetics 1993; 25: 427-32
46. Janknegt R. Aminoglycoside monitoring in the once- or twice-daily era. Pharmacy World and Science 1993; 15: 151-5
47. Begg EJ, Barclay ML, Duffull SB. A suggested approach to once-daily aminoglycoside dosing. British Journal of Clinical Pharmacology 1995; 39: 605-9
48. Vozeh S, Follath F. Nomographic estimation of time to reach steady-state serum concentration during phenytoin therapy. European Journal of Clinical Pharmacology 1980; 17: 33-5
49. Levine M, Chang T. Therapeutic drug monitoring of phenytoin: rationale and current status. Clinical Pharmacokinetics 1990; 19: 341-58
50. Pulver LK, Tett SE, Montgomery WS. Clinical evaluation of a predictive model (PHENDA) for phenytoin plasma concentrations. Australian Journal of Hospital Pharmacy 1991; 21: 303-7
51. Levy R, Shand D. Clinical implications of drug-protein binding. Clinical Pharmacokinetics 1984; 9 Suppl. 1: 1-104
52. Rolan PE. Plasma protein binding displacement interactions - why are they still regarded as clinically important? British Journal of Clinical Pharmacology 1994; 37: 125-8
53. Perucca E, Grimaldi R, Crema A. Interpretation of drug levels in acute and chronic disease states. Clinical Pharmacokinetics 1985; 10: 498-513
54. Ladero JM, Andres MP, Banares A, et al. Acetylator polymorphism in rheumatoid arthritis. European Journal of Clinical Pharmacology 1993; 45: 279-81
55. Darmansjah I, Muchtar A. Dose-response variation among different populations. Clinical Pharmacology and Therapeutics 1992; 52: 449-52
56. Chay PCW, Duffy BJ, Walker JS. Pharmacokinetic-pharmacodynamic relationships of morphine in neonates. Clinical Pharmacology and Therapeutics 1992; 51: 334-42
57. Oberbauer R, Krivanek P, Turnheim K. Pharmacokinetics of indomethacin in the elderly. Clinical Pharmacokinetics 1993; 24: 428-34
58. Gilman JT. Therapeutic drug monitoring in the neonate and paediatric age group. Clinical Pharmacokinetics 1990; 19: 1-10
59. Mac-Kay MV, Burson JS, Martinez-Lanao J, et al. Drug dosage in end-stage renal disease (ESRD) patients under-

going haemodialysis. Clinical Pharmacokinetics 1993; 25: 243-57

60. Reetze-Bonorden P, Bohler J, Keller E. Drug dosage in patients during continuous renal replacement therapy. Clinical Pharmacokinetics 1993; 24: 362-79
61. Keller E, Reetze P, Schollmeyer P. Drug therapy in patients undergoing ambulatory peritoneal dialysis: clinical pharmacokinetic considerations. Clinical Pharmacokinetics 1990; 18: 104-17
62. Drobitch RK, Svensson CK. Therapeutic drug monitoring in saliva, an update. Clinical Pharmacokinetics 1992; 23: 365-79
63. Vozeh S, Steimer JL. Feedback control methods for drug dosage optimisation: concepts, classification, and clinical application. Clinical Pharmacokinetics 1985; 10: 457-76
64. Buffington DE, Lampasona V, Chandler MHH. Computers in pharmacokinetics - choosing software for clinical decision making. Clinical Pharmacokinetics 1993; 25: 205-16
65. Jelliffe RW, Schumitzky A, Van Guilder M, et al. Individualizing drug dosage regimens: roles of population pharmacokinetic and dynamic models, Bayesian fitting and adaptive control. Therapeutic Drug Monitoring 1993; 15: 380-93
66. Aarons L. Population pharmacokinetics: theory and practice. British Journal of Clinical Pharmacology 1991; 32: 669-70
67. Balant LP, Rowland M, Aarons L, et al. New strategies in drug development and clinical evaluation: the population approach. European Journal of Clinical Pharmacology 1993; 45: 93-4
68. Sheiner LB, Ludden TM. Population pharmacokinetics/dynamics. Annual Reviews in Pharmacology and Toxicology 1992; 32: 185-209
69. Peck CC, D'Argenio DZ, Rodman JH. Analysis of pharmacokinetic data for individualizing drug dosage regimens. In: Evans et al., editors. Applied pharmacokinetics. 3rd ed. Vancouver: Applied Therapeutics, 1992: 91-103
70. Thomson AH, Whiting B. Bayesian parameter estimation and population pharmacokinetics. Clinical Pharmacokinetics 1992; 22: 447-67
71. El Desoky E, Meinshausen J, Buhl K, et al. Generation of pharmacokinetic data during routine therapeutic drug monitoring: Bayesian approach vs pharmacokinetic studies. Therapeutic Drug Monitoring 1993; 15: 281-7
72. Wilkinson DS. Establishing a therapeutic drug monitoring consultation service. Clinics in Laboratory Medicine 1987; 7: 473
73. Goode MA, Gums JG. Therapeutic drug monitoring in ambulatory care. Annals of Pharmacotherapy 1993; 27: 502-5
74. Tett SE, Day RO, Lauchlan R. Clinical pharmacy and clinical pharmacology. Australian Journal of Hospital Pharmacy 1993; 23: 207-10
75. Vozeh S, Kewitz G, Perruchoud A, et al. Theophylline serum concentration and therapeutic effect in severe acute bronchial obstruction: the optimal use of intravenously administered aminophylline. American Review of Respiratory Diseases 1982; 125: 181-4
76. Wagner JG. Theophylline. Pooled Michaelis-Menten parameters (Vmax and Km) and implications. Clinical Pharmacokinetics 1985; 10: 432-42
77. Mooradian AD. Digitalis: an update of clinical pharmacokinetics, therapeutic monitoring techniques and treatment recommendations. Clinical Pharmacokinetics 1988; 15: 165-79
78. Dobbs RJ, O'Neill CJA, Deshmukh AA, et al. Serum concentration monitoring of cardiac glycosides: how helpful is it for adjusting dosage regimens? Clinical Pharmacokinetics 1991; 20: 175-93
79. Lee DC-S, Johnson RA, Bingham JB, et al. Heart failure in outpatients - a randomized trial of digoxin versus placebo. New England Journal of Medicine 1982; 306: 699-705
80. Packer M, Gheorghiade M, Young JB, et al. Withdrawal of digoxin from patients with chronic heart failure treated with angiotensin-converting-enzyme inhibitors. New England Journal of Medicine 1993; 329: 1-7
81. Choonara IA, Rane A. Therapeutic drug monitoring of anticonvulsants. State of the art. Clinical Pharmacokinetics 1990; 18: 318-28
82. Ludden TM, Beal SL, Peck CC, et al. Evaluation of a Bayesian regression-analysis computer program for predicting phenytoin concentration. Clinical Pharmacy 1986; 5: 580-5
83. Godley PJ, Ludden TM, Clement WA, et al. Evaluation of a Bayesian regression-analysis computer program using non-steady state phenytoin concentrations. Clinical Pharmacy 1987; 6: 634-9
84. Garcia MJ, Gavira R, Buelga DS, et al. Predictive performance of two phenytoin pharmacokinetic dosing programs from non-steady state data. Therapeutic Drug Monitoring 1994; 16: 380-7
85. Schumacher GE, Barr JT, Browne TR, et al. Test performance characteristics of the serum phenytoin concentration (SPC): the relationship between SPC and patient response. Therapeutic Drug Monitoring 1991; 13: 318-24
86. Chadwick DW. Concentration-effect relationships of valproic acid. Clinical Pharmacokinetics 1985; 10: 155-63
87. Turnbull DM, Howel D, Rawlins MD, et al. Which drug for the adult epileptic patient: phenytoin or valproate? British Medical Journal 1985; 290: 815-9
88. Fletcher SC, Tett SE, Montgomery WS, et al. Clinical application of a predictive model for carbamazepine plasma concentrations. Australian Journal of Hospital Pharmacy 1991; 21: 10-5
89. Rambeck B, Wolf P. Lamotrigine clinical pharmacokinetics. Clinical Pharmacokinetics 1993; 25: 433-43
90. Rey E, Pons G, Olive G. Vigabatrin clinical pharmacokinetics. Clinical Pharmacokinetics 1992; 23: 267-78
91. Bialer M. Comparative pharmacokinetics of the newer antiepileptic drugs. Clinical Pharmacokinetics 1993; 24: 441-52
92. Follath F, Ganzinger U, Schuetz E, et al. Reliability of antiarrhythmic drug plasma concentration monitoring. Clinical Pharmacokinetics 1983; 8: 62-82
93. Gillis AM, Kates RE. Clinical pharmacokinetics of the newer antiarrhythmic agents. Clinical Pharmacokinetics 1984; 9: 375-403
94. Latini R, Maggioni AP, Cavalli A. Therapeutic drug monitoring of antiarrhythmic drugs: rationale and current status. Clinical Pharmacokinetics 1990; 18: 91-103
95. Verme CN, Ludden TM, Clementi WA, et al. Pharmacokinetics of quinidine in male patients. Clinical Pharmacokinetics 1992; 22: 468-80
96. Holford NHG, Coates PE, Guentert TW, et al. The effect of quinidine and its metabolites on the electrocardiogram and systolic time intervals: concentration-effect relationships. British Journal of Clinical Pharmacology 1981; 11: 187-95
97. Thibonnier M, Upton RA, Williams RL, et al. Pharmacokinetic-pharmacodynamic analysis of unbound disopyramide directly measured in serial plasma samples in man. Journal of Pharmacokinetics and Biopharmaceutics 1984; 12: 559-73
98. Latini R, Tognoni G, Kates RE. Clinical pharmacokinetics of amiodarone. Clinical Pharmacokinetics 1984; 9: 136-56
99. Pourbaix S, Berger Y, Desager JP, et al. Absolute bioavailability of amiodarone in normal subjects. Clinical Pharmacology and Therapeutics 1985; 37: 118-23
100. Vozeh S, Berger M, Wenk M, et al. Rapid prediction of individual dosage requirements for lignocaine. Clinical Pharmacokinetics 1984; 9: 354-63
101. Vozeh S, Uematsu T, Ritz R, et al. Drug level assisted lidocaine dosage: comparison between computerized fore-

casting technique and physician. Clinical Pharmacology and Therapeutics 1986; 39: 233
102. Holmes B, Heel RC. Flecainide: a preliminary review of its pharmacodynamic properties and therapeutic efficacy. Drugs 1985; 29: 1-33
103. Perry PJ, Pfohl BM, Holstad SG. The relationship between antidepressant response and tricyclic antidepressant plasma concentrations: a retrospective analysis of the literature using logistic regression analysis. Clinical Pharmacokinetics 1987; 13: 381-92
104. Ilett KF, Blythe TH, Hackett P, et al. Plasma concentrations of dothiepin and its metabolites are not correlated with clinical efficacy in major depressive illness. Therapeutic Drug Monitoring 1993; 15: 351-7
105. Noguchi T, Shimoda K, Takahashi S. Clinical significance of plasma levels of clomipramine, its hydroxylated and desmethylated metabolites: prediction of clinical outcome in mood disorders using discriminant analysis of therapeutic drug monitoring data. Journal of Affective Disorders 1993; 29: 267-79
106. Schou M. Serum lithium monitoring of prophylactic treatment: critical review and updated recommendations. Clinical Pharmacokinetics 1988; 15: 283-6
107. Yukawa E, Nimiyama N, Higuchi S, et al. Lithium population pharmacokinetics from routine clinical data: role of patient characteristics for estimating dosing regimens. Therapeutic Drug Monitoring 1993; 15: 75-82
108. Dahl SG. Plasma level monitoring of antipsychotic drugs: clinical utility. Clinical Pharmacokinetics 1986; 11: 36-61
109. Balant-Georgia AE, Balant L. Antipsychotic drugs: clinical pharmacokinetics of potential candidates for plasma concentration monitoring. Clinical Pharmacokinetics 1987; 13: 65-90
110. McCormack JP, Jewesson PJ. A critical reevaluation of the 'therapeutic range' of aminoglycosides. Clinical Infectious Diseases 1992; 14: 320-9
111. Duffull SB, Chambers ST, Begg EJ. How vancomycin is used in Australasia - a survey. Australian and New Zealand Journal of Medicine 1993; 23: 662-6
112. Rybak MJ, Albrecht LS, Boike SC, et al. Nephrotoxicity of vancomycin, alone and with an aminoglycoside. Journal of Antimicrobial Chemotherapy 1990; 16: 235-41
113. Matzke G. Vancomycin. In: Evans WE, Schentag JJ, Jusko WJ, editors. Applied pharmacokinetics, the principles of therapeutic drug monitoring. Vancouver: Applied Therapeutics Inc., 1992: 15.1-15.31
114. Ambrose PJ. Clinical pharmacokinetics of chloramphenicol and chloramphenicol succinate. Clinical Pharmacokinetics 1984; 9: 222-38
115. Schafer-Korting M. Pharmacokinetic optimisation of oral antifungal therapy. Clinical Pharmacokinetics 1993; 25: 329-41
116. Stretcher BN, Pesce AJ, Frame PT, et al. Correlates of zidovudine phosphorylation with markers of HIV disease progression and drug toxicity. AIDS 1994; 8: 763-9
117. Robbins BL, Rodman J, McDonald C, et al. Enzymatic assay for measurement of zidovudine triphosphate in peripheral blood mononuclear cells. Antimicrobial Agents and Chemotherapy 1994; 38: 115-21
118. Fletcher C, Sawchuk R, Chinnock B, et al. Human pharmacokinetics of the antiviral drug DHPG. Clinical Pharmacology and Therapeutics 1986; 40: 281-6
119. Laskin OL, Stahl-Bayliss CM, Kalman CM, et al. Use of ganciclovir to treat serious cytomegalovirus infections in patients with AIDS. Journal of Infectious Diseases 1987; 155: 323-7
120. Balis FM, Holcenberg JS, Bleyer WA. Clinical pharmacokinetics of commonly used anticancer drugs. Clinical Pharmacokinetics 1983; 8: 202-32
121. Moore MJ, Ehrlichman C. Therapeutic drug monitoring in oncology: problems and potential in antineoplastic therapy. Clinical Pharmacokinetics 1987; 13: 205-27
122. Galpin AJ, Evans WE. Therapeutic drug monitoring in cancer management. Clinical Chemistry 1993; 39: 2419-30
123. Madden T, Sunderland M, Santana VM, et al. The pharmacokinetics of high-dose carboplatin in pediatric patients with cancer. Clinical Pharmacology and Therapeutics 1992; 51: 701-7
124. Peck CC, Barr WH, Benet LZ, et al. Opportunities for integration of pharmacokinetics, pharmacodynamics and toxicokinetics in rational drug development. Clinical Pharmacology and Therapeutics 1992; 51: 465-73
125. Evans WE, Crom WR, Abramowitch M, et al. Clinical pharmacodynamics of high-dose methotrexate in acute lymphocytic leukaemia. New England Journal of Medicine 1986; 314: 471-7
126. Shaw LM, Bowers L, Demer L, et al. Critical issues in cyclosporine monitoring: report of the task force on cyclosporine monitoring. Clinical Chemistry 1987; 33: 1269-88
127. Shaw LM, Yatscoff RW, Bowers LD, et al. Canadian Consensus Meeting on cyclosporine monitoring: report of the consensus panel. Clinical Chemistry 1990; 36: 1841-6
128. Holt DW, Johnston A, Roberts NB, et al. Methodological and clinical aspects of cyclosporin monitoring: report of the Association of Clinical Biochemists' task force. Annals of Clinical Biochemistry 1994; 31: 420-46
129. Morris RG, Tett SE, Ray JE. Cyclosporin-A monitoring in Australia: consensus recommendations. Therapeutic Drug Monitoring 1994; 16: 570-6
130. Kivisto KT. A review of assay methods for cyclosporin: clinical implications. Clinical Pharmacokinetics 1992; 23: 173-90
131. Awni WM, Heim-Duthoy K, Kasiske BL. Monitoring of cyclosporine by serial post-transplant pharmacokinetic studies in renal transplant patients. Transplantation Proceedings 1990; 22: 1343-4
132. Regazzi MB, Rondanelli R, Gastaldi L, et al. Optimisation of sampling time for cyclosporine monitoring in transplant patients. Journal of Clinical Pharmacology 1992; 32: 978-81
133. Takada K, Katayama N, Kiriyama A, et al. Distribution characteristics of immunosuppressants FK506 and cyclosporin A in the blood compartment. Biopharmaceutics and Drug Disposition 1993; 14: 659-72
134. Warty V, Zuckerman S, Venkataramanan R, et al. FK506 measurement: comparison of different analytical methods. Therapeutic Drug Monitoring 1993; 15: 204-8
135. Paul K, Harding MW, Marks WH, et al. Cyclophilin binding: a more accurate measure of cyclosporine immunosuppressive activity after renal transplantation. Transplantation Proceedings 1991; 23: 974-5
136. Blocka KLN, Paulus HE, Furst DE. Clinical pharmacokinetics of oral and injectable gold compounds. Clinical Pharmacokinetics 1986; 11: 133-43
137. Tett SE. Clinical pharmacokinetics of slow-acting antirheumatic drugs. Clinical Pharmacokinetics 1993; 25: 392-407
138. Tett SE, Day RO, Cutler DJ. Concentration-effect relationship of hydroxychloroquine in rheumatoid arthritis - a cross-sectional study. Journal of Rheumatology 1993; 20: 1874-9
139. Dromgoole SH, Furst DE. Salicylates. In: Evans WE, Schentag JJ, Jusko WJ, editors. Applied pharmacokinetics, the principles of therapeutic drug monitoring. Vancouver: Applied Therapeutics Inc., 1992: 32.1-32.34
140. Furst DE, Tozer TN, Melmon KL. Salicylate clearance, the resultant of protein binding and metabolism. Clinical Pharmacology and Therapeutics 1979; 26: 380-9

Chapter 6

# Pharmacological Basis of Adverse Drug Reactions

*I.R. Edwards*

## Synopsis of Important Principles

1) The risks, extent of likely benefits and costs of drugs should be known and carefully considered before a prescribing decision is made.

2) Prescribers are the patient's partner in therapy: since the patient stands to gain the benefits, but also runs the risks, the prescriber's specialised knowledge of both must be shared as completely as possible.

3) The risk of adverse drug reactions is an inevitable consequence of drug use. Few reactions are life-threatening, but almost all effective drugs may cause serious adverse effects in some patients. A necessary skill of therapeutics is to anticipate the risk, and then use drugs in a way that minimises it.

4) The potential of a particular drug to cause adverse reactions, and the profile and seriousness of those reactions dictate both the choice of drugs and the risks that are acceptable. Sometimes however, a drug that is more toxic or less effective than the ideal may be the only one available because of selection restrictions (imposed for whatever reason).

5) All drug effects are the result of complex interaction between the drug, the patient, the illness, and extrinsic factors that can modify drug response.

6) Some adverse drug reactions may be avoided by knowledge of the pharmacological properties of a particular drug, the mechanisms of adverse effects, and an awareness of the predisposing factors, particularly those determining special susceptibility of an individual patient.

7) Adverse drug reactions can result from idiosyncratic patient responses (allergy, genetic factors and physiological variables), acquired diseases (the treated condition and other associated or intercurrent illness), anomalies of drug presentation and administration, or drug interactions. The developing fetus is at special risk. Pregnancy and labour are also times of altered drug responsiveness.

8) Important general predisposing factors include excessive drug dosages due to non-individualised dosage and extremes of age. Abnormalities of the organs involved in drug metabolism and excretion, primarily the liver and kidneys, may also predispose patients to adverse drug reactions.

9) The incidence of adverse reactions increases with the number of drugs prescribed. Only a few adverse effects of drugs can be attributed to drug interactions, but some important reactions are predictable and can be avoided rather than treated with other drugs.

10) The clinician has a responsibility to recognise the presence of a possible adverse drug reaction and to report clinically important adverse drug effects to a committee or registry responsible for deciding on drug formularies (local or national) and for advice on therapeutics.

Drugs are capable of modifying fundamental biological processes profoundly, and their use is associated with the risk of adverse drug reactions. National and international agencies and a number of hospital-based programmes have been established for monitoring the occurrence of reactions, collating the data, and then providing information and warnings to health care professionals. The aim has been to promote awareness of possible adverse reactions in all therapeutic fields and to assist in their early recognition. Complementary to the documentation and interpretation of adverse reaction data (an aspect of pharmacoepidemiology) is an adequate understanding of the processes underlying the occurrence of adverse drug reactions (clinical toxicology).

## 1. General Considerations

Most drugs are non-toxic, but serious and even life-threatening reactions can occur.[1,2] A few drugs have a small margin between the effective and toxic dose. The indications for use of such 'low therapeutic ratio' drugs must be very sound. All drugs may cause severe or occasionally fatal reactions, even when administered appropriately and (on the basis of present knowledge) for sound indications, the reactions being neither predictable nor avoidable. However, adverse drug reactions due to inappropriate or inadequately supervised therapy also occur, and these can be avoided.

Table I lists examples of adverse reactions included in lists of the 10 most important reactions by 10 clinical specialists and 10 drug regulatory physicians. Most of these are rare and not likely to be identified in premarketing clinical experience of new drugs. The message should therefore be clear: *take particular care in prescribing newly marketed drugs and be vigilant for unexpected unwanted effects.*

### 1.1 Basic Definitions of Adverse Drug Reactions and their Causality Assessment

Practicing clinicians must always consider adverse drug reactions as part of their clinical diagnosis. The causal relationship of a drug to a clinical event may be far from easy to distinguish from other candidates in the differential diagnosis. There is an extensive international literature on aids to the diagnosis of drug reactions which includes basic definitions, guidelines and causality algorithms.[4] Since there is controversy over the use of some of these aids, only the more widely accepted definitions will be mentioned here in detail. The definitions below are those adopted by national centres participating in the WHO International Drug Monitoring Programme, September 1991.[5]

#### Side Effect

Any unintended effect of a pharmaceutical product, occurring at doses normally used in humans, and related to the pharmacological properties of the drug.

#### Adverse Event/Adverse Experience

Any untoward medical occurrence that may present during treatment with a pharmaceutical

**Table I.** Frequency of identification of adverse reactions included in lists of the 10 most important reactions reported since thalidomide (after Venning).[3] *NB.* This table is based on opinion and may not reflect the overall public health impact of a reaction type

| Adverse reaction | Drug | No. of times included: | | |
|---|---|---|---|---|
| | | by 10 physicians in UK | by 10 physicians in regulatory agencies[a] | total (out of 20 lists) |
| Oculomucocutaneous syndrome | Practolol | 9 | 10 | 19 |
| Thromboembolism | Oral contraceptives | 10 | 7 | 17 |
| Nephropathy | Analgesics (especially phenacetin) | 7 | 5 | 12 |
| Lactic acidosis | Phenformin | 3 | 8 | 11 |
| Deaths from asthma | Sympathomimetic aerosols | 6 | 4 | 10 |
| Subacute myelo-optic neuropathy | Clioquinol | 5 | 5 | 10 |
| Vaginal cancer (in daughters) | Stilbestrol (diethylstilboestrol) [maternal] | 4 | 5 | 9 |
| Aplastic anaemia | Chloramphenicol | 1 | 5 | 6 |
| Jaundice | Halothane | 2 | 4 | 6 |
| Retroperitoneal fibrosis | Methysergide | 3 | 3 | 6 |
| Pseudomembranous colitis | Lincomycin, clindamycin | 2 | 4 | 6 |
| Aplastic anaemia | Phenylbutazone | 2 | 3 | 5 |
| Dyskinesia (especially tardive) | Phenothiazines | 2 | 3 | 5 |

a Australia, Canada, Germany, Holland, Italy, New Zealand, Sweden, UK (2), US (1 composite list from 6 physicians).

product but which does not necessarily have a causal relationship with this treatment.

#### Adverse Reaction

A noxious or unintended response to a drug, which occurs at doses normally used in humans for the prophylaxis, diagnosis, or treatment of disease, or for the modification of physiological function.

#### Unexpected Adverse Reaction

An adverse reaction, the nature or severity of which is not consistent with domestic labelling or market authorisation, or expected from the characteristics of the drug.

#### Signal

Reported information on a possible causal relationship between an adverse event and a drug, the relationship being unknown or incompletely documented previously. Usually more than one report is required to generate a signal, depending on the seriousness of the event and the quality of the information.

#### Causality Assessment of Suspected Adverse Reactions

***Certain:*** a clinical event, including laboratory test abnormality, occurring in a plausible time relationship to drug administration, and which cannot be explained by concurrent disease or other drugs or chemicals. The response to withdrawal of the drug (dechallenge) should be clinically plausible. The event must be definitive pharmacologically or phenomenologically, using a satisfactory rechallenge procedure if necessary.

***Probable/likely:*** a clinical event, including laboratory test abnormality, with a reasonable time sequence to administration of the drug, unlikely to be attributed to concurrent disease or other drugs or chemicals, and which follows a clinically reasonable response on withdrawal (dechallenge). Rechallenge information is not required to fulfil this definition.

***Possible:*** a clinical event, including laboratory test abnormality, with a reasonable time sequence to administration of the drug, but which could also be explained by concurrent disease or other drugs or chemicals. Information on drug withdrawal may be lacking or unclear.

***Unlikely:*** a clinical event, including laboratory test abnormality, with a temporal relationship to drug administration which makes a causal relationship improbable, and in which other drugs, chemicals or underlying disease provide plausible explanations.

***Conditional/unclassified:*** a clinical event, including laboratory test abnormality, reported as an adverse reaction, about which more data are essential for a proper assessment or the additional data are under examination.

***Unassessable/unclassifiable:*** a report suggesting an adverse reaction which cannot be judged because information is insufficient or contradictory, and which cannot be supplemented or verified.

Despite every care taken in therapy, adverse reactions may occur that may be difficult to diagnose. As mentioned above, the use of causality algorithms is advocated by some, and more recently computer-assisted methods using Bayesian logic and complex systems have been devised.[6] None of these have found general support and most are too time-consuming for clinical practice. What the development and testing of algorithms has shown is that many diagnostic failures – both erroneously blaming a drug for a reaction and failing to recognise a drug as a cause of a reaction – occur because clinical data required for a diagnosis are missing. Most importantly, this includes inadequate patient follow-up and lack of familiarity with the drug in question. With multiple therapy, the decision as to which, if any, drug is to blame is compounded by the possibility of drug interactions producing or aggravating the clinical condition.

#### Seriousness/Severity of Adverse Reactions

In addition to the above definitions, there is also widespread agreement on the definition of *seriousness and severity* of a reaction.

A ***serious reaction*** is any untoward medical occurrence that at any dose:

- Results in death
- Requires inpatient hospitalisation or prolongation of existing hospitalisation
- Results in persistent or significant disability/incapacity or is life-threatening.

Cancers and congenital anomalies or birth defects should also be regarded as serious, as should medical events that would be regarded as serious if they had not responded to acute treatment.

The term ***'severe'*** is often used to describe the intensity (severity) of a medical event, as in the grading 'mild', 'moderate' and 'severe'. Thus, a 'severe' skin reaction is not usually 'serious'.

#### 'Types' of Reactions

Adverse reactions may be of an expected and appropriate character, in keeping with the pharmacology of the drug, though perhaps of inordinate severity. Many are allergic or idiopathic in origin, may be bizarre in character and essentially unpredictable.[7] Some are the results of true cytotoxic effects of the drug or an active metabolite. Others do not fit easily into the two main categories above but may result in genetic effects causing birth defects, neoplasia, or even second generation effects not apparent at birth. Other reactions may be to the pharmaceutical form of the product such as oesophageal damage caused by a hard tablet, or a reaction to an excipient.

Drug abuse (except insofar as dependence may result from therapeutic use), accidental or suicidal self-administration, and homicidal use of drugs do not come under the heading of 'adverse drug reactions', but adverse effects of prescribed drugs that are inappropriate for a particular patient do. In fact, these effects constitute a very important, and avoidable, proportion of drug safety problems with some drugs.

As seen from the definitions above, it should not be thought that every adverse event associated with a drug is an adverse reaction in every situation. Sometimes effects that are not the main effect of the drug are welcomed by the patient. For example, the euphoria which accompanies the use of opioids for pain relief in patients with terminal illnesses is likely to add to their value to these patients, even though the same effect is a reason for their dependency potential in other situations.

### 1.2 Evaluating the Risk of Adverse Reactions Against the Benefits of Drug Use

The risks of serious reactions are generally acceptable if the disease being treated is itself very serious. Sometimes, however, the illness is trivial and the use of a drug that can cause a serious reaction, even if only rarely, becomes completely unacceptable. Some of the worst drug reactions have occurred during the use of potentially toxic drugs for trivial or inappropriate indications. Before prescribing chloramphenicol, the clinician should ask: 'Does this patient stand a greater than 1 in 24,500 to 40,800 chance of dying from this condition?' If the answer is 'no' then chloramphenicol should not be prescribed.[8] This is a simplified example, since there are usually many possible adverse reactions to consider and balance during treatment, and the incidence of a reaction is usually not so well defined as for aplastic anaemia with chloramphenicol.

The potential of a particular drug to cause adverse reactions, their profile and their seriousness dictate the risks which are acceptable and, therefore, the choice of drug. Sometimes a more toxic or less effective drug than the ideal may be the only one available because of selection restrictions imposed for budgetary or other reasons.

The information available on marketed drugs contains a wealth of detail on pharmacological actions, toxicology and clinical experience for each indication and this can provide a reasonable idea of how a patient's health may be improved by treatment. In addition, the chance of harm occurring in up to 1 in 1000 patients exposed to the drug may be known from premarketing studies with good controls. However, about 3000 patient exposures are needed to be fairly certain of finding an adverse reaction with a random incidence of 1 in 1000, if the background risk is zero.

The information missing on newly marketed drugs is, firstly, that which might identify people particularly at risk, i.e. clinical trials in certain subgroups of patients who are more likely to be using the drug or are at risk of adverse effects. However, this situation is changing. Recently, we have seen more clinical studies conducted in the elderly and in patients with disease states such as liver and renal disease (where these are clinically relevant) prior to marketing, but often there are no studies conducted at this time in children or women. This is sometimes said to be for ethical reasons, but may mean having to use a drug without scientific evaluation. Refraining from conducting research on children is claimed to deprive paediatric populations of the advantages of research while subjecting those who receive untested drugs to greater hazards than they would meet in a clinical trial.[9] We could at least require special monitoring and reporting when drugs are used in children, even if we do not want children used in clinical trials. However, methods for ensuring that drug studies are performed ethically and as safely as possible in children are available.[9,10] Less attention has been paid to ensuring that drug studies may be safely and ethically conducted in pregnant women, which may explain the lack of these studies.

The second major area of missing information after premarketing studies is the full nature and extent (i.e. expression) of the known harmful aspects of a drug. When a drug is marketed, experience with adverse effects occurring in less than 1 in 100 patients is often too limited to be certain of the full expression of a reaction. Attribution of causality might even be debatable for some events that have a high background incidence in the population. If events have an incidence of less than 1 in 1000 they may not even be seen in premarketing studies. Most experts agree that more extensive premarketing trials, before the drug is tried in normal clinical practice, would provide little or no greater security and would be at an unacceptable cost, both in financial terms and perhaps in terms of delaying the availability of a useful treatment option. Whether greater safety information should be required for new drugs developed for clinical indications where there are already adequate alternatives has to be debated.

The term *risk-benefit ratio* is often used as a general term linked to the use of a drug. To balance risk and benefit is, however, a very complex exercise. Usually, the risks of the drug are of a totally different nature and frequency compared with the benefits. For an individual patient, there is usually only a single benefit sought (and for most drugs the benefits are limited to a few indications) but the potential risks are multiple.

Perceptions of risk *versus* benefits are notoriously susceptible to the context in which they occur. Sometimes the risks of administered drugs are given greater emphasis by prescribers relative to the risks of disease because of a feeling of being causally responsible for the latter. Patients often have the misconception that drugs should be completely safe, which may lead them to dwell excessively on any risks to which their attention is drawn, unless their clinical situation is dire in which case they may accept hazardous and upsetting treatments with little question.

Perception of risk may therefore be different to actual risk (see also section 1.5 below). Ultimately, the acceptable risk-to-benefit balance is an individual judgement by a patient after consultation, or by the prescriber on behalf of a patient, in any given situation, but overall decisions are made by regulators as to which drugs have an acceptable risk-to-benefit balance and can therefore be made generally available. Prescribers make similar general decisions as to which drugs they are going to use in their regular drug armamentarium.

The above are just some of the aspects of risk-benefit judgements and against such a background, the term *risk-benefit ratio* gives an unwarranted impression of mathematical precision. Moreover, the weight of information for and against the use of a drugs is often not summarised by users of the term, so that only a loose impression of the pros and cons of the use of a particular drug is gained. The terms *risk-benefit balance* or *risk-benefit assessment* seem better, but even these terms have been criticised as judgemental (i.e. why not use *benefit-risk* to be more positive about drug therapy!). Perhaps a neutral term such as *merit assessment* would be more acceptable.

Disparate information is difficult to compare without introducing serious errors. (Apples and oranges can be compared by weight, but this misses other very important parameters for comparison such as taste and texture). Conversely, comparing and contrasting large amounts of information can lead to a complexity that stifles decision-making. Given certain contextual limits, however, it is possible to nominate the main concepts that need to be accounted for in any comparison. This will lead to an ability recognise and discuss the merits of a drug in any given context.

A merit assessment for drugs should be based on concepts that are clinically useful and can be used on both sides of the balance. Clinically, there are three main concepts related to any effect on the body: how great the effect is; its duration; and the incidence. Thus, there are three main aspects of risk:

- The seriousness and severity of the adverse reaction
- The duration of the adverse reaction
- The frequency of occurrence.

Similarly, there are three main aspects of benefit:

- The seriousness of the disease being treated, considered against the likely extent of improvement
- The chronicity of the disease, against the probable reduction in duration produced by treatment
- The frequency of the disease (in an individual 100%), against the frequency of improvement.

The above concepts can be used in a general sense, e.g. to compare drugs used in the same indication, and applied to individual patients. Considerable judgement is still required in the application of the concepts, but we can now generalise from the example cited above for chloramphenicol[8] to, for example: 'I have a patient with a serious infection with about 80% mortality and which may last for weeks if the patient does not die. Chloramphenicol is curative in 90% of cases and patients usually improve within days. Aplastic anaemia is the main adverse reaction to chloramphenicol with an incidence of about 1 in 18,000 and a mortality of, say, 30% and a protracted morbidity of months'. The simple clinical decision here would be to use chloramphenicol.

On the other hand, penicillin may be effective in the same condition in about 88% of cases, but because of penicillin resistance, there is a slightly slower improvement in those who recover. The most frequent adverse reaction to penicillin is skin rash in about 10% of patients, and the most serious is anaphylaxis in about 1 in 5000 patients, with death from anaphylaxis in about 10%. However, most patients recover from anaphylaxis very quickly. There is now a need to consider, given a consistent response with similar disease severity, that an additional 16 in 1000 patients may die using penicillin rather than chloramphenicol because of its lower effectiveness. The mortality from adverse reactions is 1 in 54,000 for chloramphenicol and 1 in 50,000 for penicillin. New questions now need to be asked when treating an individual patient: what is the chance of penicillin resistance? How can the better overall effectiveness of chloramphenicol be rated against the higher morbidity that is likely from chloramphenicol adverse reactions (the mortality from adverse reactions being about equal for the two drugs)? Is the patient penicillin-sensitive, which would considerably increase the chance of mortality from penicillin? A decision about the general availability of the two drugs for this indication is somewhat easier: the benefits and risks are quantitatively rather similar but qualitatively very different, and therefore both should be available for this indication.

Regulatory and professional decisions are continually being made on the availability and use of drugs. Examples of drug safety issues leading to regulatory action include:

1) *Felbamate:* this antiepileptic drug has been claimed to have special effectiveness in severe childhood epilepsy (Lennox-Gastaut syndrome). No cases of aplastic anaemia were seen prior to marketing but, when licenced, a 50-fold incidence over the expected rate led to a restriction in its use and a requirement for special monitoring of blood counts. Clearly, there is a balance to be considered between difficult-to-treat epilepsy with its morbidity and mortality and aplastic anaemia.

2) *Terodiline:* this agent was used to treat incontinence but was also prodysrhythmic, producing rare but fatal ventricular arrhythmias. The drug was not totally effective in arresting incontinence in the elderly but did lead to significant clinical improvements. In this case, a regulatory decision was made that the risk of fatal adverse reactions could not be allowed to be set against an incomplete and only symptomatic benefit (see further section 1.5 for an alternative view).

3) *Tiaprofenic acid:* suggestions have been made to remove this NSAID from the market because of reports of fibrosing cystitis. This adverse reaction is unique to tiaprofenic acid, which is about equally effective with most other drugs in the same group. On the other hand, tiaprofenic acid is about average among the NSAIDs in terms of causing gastrointestinal haemorrhage. Yet again, if the report rates of cystitis are added to the report rates of serious adverse reactions for a group of 7 representative NSAIDs, tiaprofenic acid is in the top three for causing adverse reactions with serious potential.

Lessons to be learned from the above examples are:

- The safety profile is incomplete when a drug is marketed, to the extent of missing importance incidences of serious adverse reactions
- Balancing slight or moderate benefit against a rare but serious risk is very difficult
- The total benefit and risk profiles of a drug for each of its indications must be used to determine its overall merit
- On the whole, merit assessments of one drug should be compared with other therapies to be useful
- Broad regulatory decisions may not adequately cover the needs of individual patients.

### 1.3 Awareness and Recognition of Adverse Reactions

The prescriber cannot be expected to memorise all the likely possibilities, but each time a drug is used, its risks should be ascertained and assessed. In follow-up with the patient, the clinician should be alert to the possibility of a drug as the cause of or a causative factor in the occurrence of disorders. Some adverse reactions to drugs are easily overlooked because they closely resemble naturally occurring conditions (e.g. digitalis-induced diarrhoea), or because the disorder is so unusual that it does not seem possible that it should be associated with the use of a drug (e.g. sclerosing peritonitis associated with practolol). In other instances, it may be particularly difficult to incriminate a drug as a cause of a particular reaction, e.g. skin eruptions (see chapter 17; sect. 22) and liver disease.

It is just as important for the clinician to consider an adverse drug reaction in the resolution of a diagnostic problem as it is to recognise malignant disease, septicaemia, or a metabolic abnormality. Prompt withdrawal of the drug may be essential to recovery from the drug-induced illness. With some types of reaction (e.g. hypersensitivity, genetic enzyme defects), avoidance of a drug may be necessary to prevent repeat illness in the future. Recognition of a potential adverse reaction may save the patient unnecessary and even hazardous investigation, looking for other causes.

### 1.4 Reporting of Reactions and Pharmacoepidemiology

The clinician has a duty to report to the appropriate committee or registry any adverse event with a new drug, however trivial, for it may be the first of its kind. Similarly, unexpected or serious reactions to established drugs should also be reported, for even if they are known, it is still important to accumulate sufficient information to assess their clinical significance. It is worth asking the following questions when reporting adverse reactions:

- Is a clear impression of the event conveyed in the report?
- Is the relationship of all drug therapy to the clinical event(s) clear?
- Did the event disappear when the drug was stopped (dechallenge)?
- Can part or all of the event be explained by underlying diseases or other drugs that are being used?
- If the event has occurred on previous exposure to the drug, i.e. this occasion is a re-exposure, can it be confirmed absolutely that the previous event and the brand of drug and dosage were the same? If so, this is a *rechallenge*, and is regarded by many to implicate the drug as almost certainly causal in the reaction.
- Is this a re-exposure in which either the nature of the first or second event has not been medically confirmed and/or the exact drug product and dose have not been identified as identical on the two occasions? If so, this cannot be regarded as a confirmed rechallenge.
- Can information required to answer these questions be readily acquired?

For further discussion of adverse reaction reporting, see reviews by McEwen[11] and Edwards.[12]

Quantitative assessment of the frequency of adverse reactions requires at least a knowledge of the extent of use of a drug to provide an incidence denominator of patients at risk. Even then, spontaneous adverse reaction reporting does not give a reliable numerator for incidence because of under-reporting. A realistic assessment of incidence is only possible with the use of comparative cohort studies (which are practical if the clinical event is common) or by case control studies. The latter are generally more useful in determining drug safety, because unknown adverse reactions to marketed drugs are comparatively rare. Targeted postmarketing studies of new drugs, which try to assemble very large cohorts of patients and collect information about all new clinical events, whether they are thought to be drug-related or not, provide event profiles that may give pointers to possible adverse drug reactions. However, since they are often uncontrolled, the information must be interpreted carefully, particularly with consideration of the background disease prevalence.

Information from epidemiological studies must be interpreted carefully because of the potential for bias and confounding and other methodological difficulties. More recently, pharmacoepidemiology has come to the fore in drug safety because cohort and case control studies, both prospective and retrospective, allow for quantitative risk estimation from controlled comparisons (see further chapter 9; sect. 4.2.5). The case control methodology has been seen as particularly attractive because data from existing disease databases, either multipurpose or specialised, can be used to obtain relatively quick and inexpensive results. Cohort studies are, on the whole, more expensive and take longer to produce information, but there are instances where the latter are scientifically more appropriate.

Given that pharmacoepidemiology has an important place in determining drug safety, a pivotal question is how quickly can an early signal of a problem with a drug be investigated using appropriate techniques. The only practical approach is to use data that are continuously and reliably collected and that will identify all relevant patient information, including all drug use and disease information. Hospital discharge registers, such as those first developed in the Nordic countries, have proved valuable for studies in pharmacovigilance. The multipurpose disease-based registers now being used increasingly for these sorts of studies in a more general patient population are available mainly in North America, but are also being developed in Europe. The use of patient cohorts derived from prescription monitoring, as used in New Zealand and Britain, has proved effective in compiling safety profiles for new drugs, and has the advantage of being able to assess benefits at the same time as risks, as well as determining secular trends for both. The experience of 25 years of monitoring for problems with drugs in the UK has been reviewed by Bem et al.[13] and this provides an overview of the general scope of drug monitoring. [For further information on pharmacoepidemiology and databases that can be used for drug safety investigations, see Strom].[14]

### 1.5 Communicating with the Patient

The clinician has a responsibility to warn the patient about possible important reactions (common and/or severe or serious), particularly those that may cause the patient to discontinue or modify medication, and to ask him or her to report any usual symptoms or premonitory signs of major adverse effects (e.g. fever, sore mouth, rash as a warning of marrow dysplasia with gold or carbimazole). The clinician must also make quite clear to the patient how the therapy should be used to obtain maximum benefit and minimum risk. The same information should be reinforced by other members of the medical team, particularly pharmacists and nurses.

It is well established that patients may not understand or remember information given to them, and reinforcement is therefore important. Adverse drug reaction information is particularly sensitive since patients may react badly to it and either suppress the idea that a drug may actually harm them or be frightened to use the drug. It is commonly proposed that disclosing information on adverse effects will make the patient more likely to experience or report them. However, apart from some anecdotal information, this is difficult to confirm because it is not simply the passing on of information that is involved, but also the context and mode of information. There is a world of difference between giving a patient a drug package insert containing closely typed medical terms amongst which is *gastrointestinal irritation* and a statement that 'stomach bleeding may occur and can be fatal' and telling the patient that 'these tablets have been known to upset the stomach, so if you have pain or vomiting you should stop the tablets and make an appointment – particularly if you vomit blood, which happens in a few patients, you should stop the tablets and contact me straight away since this can be serious'. On the whole, information on adverse effects is well received if:

a) It is provided in terms that a particular patient can understand.

b) The clinician is prepared to explain further anything that is unclear (e.g. a patient may ask what is 'a few' in the example above).

c) Clear advice is given about what to do in any particular situation.

Health professionals must, therefore, avoid any confusion caused by giving conflicting information and should attempt to put comments into the perspective of both the risks of the disease being treated and other well known risks. The patient has an absolute right to know and to be a full partner in his/her disease management, but this has to take into account the patient's background and understanding. Health professionals must be ready with open and honest answers to any questions about therapy at any time during treatment, even if the answer is: 'I don't know, but I'll try to find out'. This approach will give the patient more confidence in the treatment goals and may save the clinician from litigation.

It is important to bear in mind that what a clinician thinks is 'common','rare', 'serious' or 'trivial' may not be so for the patient. This difference in risk perception was well illustrated after a drug that improved urinary incontinence (terodiline) was removed from the market because of a rare incidence of fatal cardiac arrhythmia. A 90-year-old woman telephoned a 50-year-old drug regulator and asked why the drug that had helped her had been discontinued. When told of the risk of fatality she said: 'Young man, at my age, it is better to be dry than alive!'

**Table II.** Important determinants of adverse drug reactions

| |
|---|
| **The administered drug:** |
| • Physicochemical and pharmacokinetic characteristics |
| • Formulation characteristics |
| • Dose |
| • Rate and route of administration |
| **The patient and his/her condition:** |
| • Physiological variables |
| Age |
| Sex |
| Pregnancy |
| Malnutrition |
| • Pathological variables |
| Associated disease |
| Intercurrent illness |
| • Allergic state |
| • Genetic predisposition |
| **Additional extrinsic factors:** |
| • Other drugs given |
| • Alcohol consumption |
| • Environmental pollutants (heavy occupational exposure to insecticides) |
| • Cigarette smoking |

## 2. Determinants of Adverse Reactions

All drug effects are the result of complex interactions between the drug, the patient, the illness, and a number of known and/or unknown extrinsic factors that can modify the drug response (table II). In practical therapeutics, the emphasis must be on the individual patient and his or her disease. Thus, with a knowledge of the pharmacological characteristics of a particular drug (i.e. its actions, physicochemical and pharmacokinetic properties), and an appreciation of the possibility of special susceptibility of an individual patient under specific circumstances, many drug reactions may be avoided or at least mitigated.

### 2.1 Onset of Reactions

Abnormal responses to drugs can occur at any time during a course of treatment or after its completion. Many reactions occur early in the course of treatment (e.g. anaphylaxis or reactions due to genetic enzyme defects), even with the first dose. Alternatively, important reactions can develop insidiously over a prolonged period of treatment (e.g. corticosteroid-induced posterior or subcapsular cataracts, retroperitoneal fibrosis from methysergide). Other reactions (e.g. cancer related to immunosuppressants) may only become apparent long after the drug is discontinued. There is even one example of an adverse reaction (vaginal cancer in the female offspring of mothers using estrogens during pregnancy) occurring in the second generation and without any abnormality being present at birth.[15]

The level of risk may vary according to the type of reaction and length of time exposed to the drug: the risk of anaphylaxis is infinitesimal after the first doses, and blood dyscrasias are not likely to occur after the first 3 months of therapy. Consideration of the elimination half-life of a drug may be important: the half-life of acitretin used for psoriasis is about 50 hours and its teratogenic potential is persistent long after the drug is stopped. In fact, two years of adequate contraception is advised after completion of acitretin therapy to avoid this risk.[15]

Similar time scales apply to adverse drug interactions. Some, such as those involving nonselective monoamine oxidase inhibitors (MAOIs) [see chapter 7; sect. 3], occur with the first dose of an interactant, e.g. phenylpropanolamine. The effects of some drugs such as MAOIs or anticholinesterases such as ecothiopate eye drops, persist when they are discontinued and an interaction may still occur with a drug started several days or weeks (MAOIs) or months (ecothiopate) later (see also chapter 7, sect. 3).[15]

### 2.2 Amount of Drug Administered

Some drug effects are dose-related, but because of individual differences in pharmacokinetic handling of the drug (see chapter 1; sect. 5.3), a dosage tolerated by one patient may cause adverse effects in another. Particular care should be taken in prescribing for the very young, the elderly and those with diseases of the excretory organs (liver and kidney).

Medication errors may also lead to an excessive amount of a drug being given, as may differences in bioavailability due to substitution of products of the same drug substance (see section 6). In this respect, care should be taken when changing from standard to depot or sustained release preparations or *vice versa*.

It is quite possible to overdose a patient with a newly marketed drug, since dose-response data are usually obtained in a small, selected population: the first recommended dose of a new antihypertensive may be too high and cause hypotension and dangerous falls in a frail octogenarian (if indeed it is deemed necessary to treat the hypertension at all in patients of this age).

**Table III.** Examples of adverse drug reactions due to the influence of associated disease or intercurrent illness[a]

| Condition | Drug(s) | Possible effect or risk[b] | Mechanism |
|---|---|---|---|
| **Renal disease** (see also appendix D) | | | |
| Renal failure | Aminoglycoside antibiotics | Ototoxicity | PKe |
| | Colistin | Neuropsychiatric reactions in chronic renal failure (better tolerated in acute renal failure) | PKe<br>PDt |
| | Tetracyclines | Rise in blood urea, aggravation of renal insufficiency | PDd |
| | Digoxin | Digitalis toxicity | PKe |
| | Furosemide (frusemide)<br>Ethacrynic acid | Risk of ototoxicity (more likely with large doses) | |
| | Aspirin (acetylsalicylic acid) | Enhances bleeding tendency of uraemia and may itself cause blood loss due to gastric mucosal irritation | PDd |
| Nephrotic syndrome | Clofibrate | Myopathy | PKd |
| | Prednisolone | Increased incidence of adverse effects | PKd |
| | Diuretics | Incautious use can precipitate acute renal failure | PDd |
| **Liver disease** (see also appendix F) | | | |
| Hepatic precoma | Morphine | May precipitate encephalopathy | PDd |
| Cirrhotic oedema and ascites | Diuretics | Incautious use can precipitate encephalopathy | PDd |
| Obstructive jaundice<br>Hepatitis<br>Cirrhosis | Oral anticoagulants | Enhanced response | PDt |
| Cirrhosis | Lidocaine (lignocaine) | Severe CNS toxicity | PKm |
| Hepatitis | Ergot drugs | Ergot poisoning | PKm |
| **Gastroduodenal disease** | | | |
| Peptic ulcer | Corticosteroids<br>Nonsteroidal anti-inflammatory drugs (NSAIDs) [e.g. aspirin, indomethacin, phenylbutazone] | Risk of bleeding or perforation of a peptic ulcer | PDd |
| Acute gastroenteritis | Oral contraceptives | Pregnancy may result | PKa |
| **Cardiovascular disease** | | | |
| Heart failure | β-Adrenoceptor antagonists<br>Nonsteroidal anti-inflammatory drugs (NSAIDs)<br>Tricyclic antidepressants | Aggravate or precipitate heart failure | PDd |
| | Lidocaine | CNS toxicity if dose not reduced in advanced heart failure | PKm |
| Pulmonary heart disease | Digoxin | Digitalis toxicity | PDt |
| Myocardial ischaemia | Tricyclic antidepressants | Disturbances of cardiac rate, rhythm and conduction | PDd |
| | Digoxin | Arrhythmias | PDt |
| | Procainamide | Reduced cardiac output | PDd |
| Bradycardia<br>Conduction abnormality | Quinidine<br>Procainamide<br>Lidocaine<br>Propranolol | Cardiac standstill | PDd |
| Hypertension | Carbenoxolone<br>Oral contraceptives<br>Vasoconstrictors | Rise in blood pressure | PDd |
| | Phenothiazines<br>Nitroglycerin (glyceryl trinitrate) | Fall in blood pressure | PDd |
| | Tricyclic antidepressants<br>Amphetamines<br>Vasoconstrictors | Antagonise guanethidine-type antihypertensive agents with rise in blood pressure | PDd |
| **Haematological diseases** | | | |
| Bleeding disorders | Aspirin | Increased risk of haemorrhage | PDd |

**Table III.** *[Continued]*

| Condition | Drug(s) | Possible effect or risk[b] | Mechanism |
|---|---|---|---|
| Thromboembolic disorders | Oral anticoagulants | Many drugs can modify response of oral anticoagulants (see chapter 26) | PD<br>PK |
| Inherited abnormalities of erythrocytes | Many drugs | Haemolytic anaemia in those with G6PD deficiency | PDd |
| Megaloblastic anaemia | Cotrimoxazole (trimethoprim/sulfamethoxazole) | Haemopoietic depression | PDd |
| **Psychological disorders** | | | |
| Schizophrenia | Corticosteroids | May aggravate schizophrenia | PDd |
| **Neurological disorders** | | | |
| Myasthenia gravis | Aminoglycoside antibiotics<br>Polymixins<br>Penicillamine | Aggravate muscle weakness | PDd |
| Epilepsy | Nalidixic acid<br>Phenothiazines<br>Tricyclic antidepressants | May aggravate seizures | PDd |
| Cerebrovascular disease | Ergotamine | Ischaemic episodes | PDd |
| **Rheumatic disease** | | | |
| Systemic lupus erythematosus | Many drugs | Increased incidence of drug reactions in general | PDd |
| Hyperuricaemia | Thiazides | Attack of gout | PDd |
| **Respiratory disease** | | | |
| Asthma | β-Adrenoceptor antagonists<br>Dinoprost (prostaglandin $F_{2\alpha}$) | Acute bronchospasm | PDd |
| Pulmonary heart disease | Digoxin | Digitalis toxicity | PDt |
| **Endocrine disorders** | | | |
| Diabetes mellitus | Thiazides<br>Furosemide (frusemide)<br>Ethacrynic acid<br>Corticosteroids<br>Oral contraceptives | May aggravate diabetes or make control more difficult | PDd |
| Hypothyroidism | Digoxin<br>Oral anticoagulants | Enhanced response<br>Decreased response | PK/PD<br>PDt |
| Hyperthyroidism | Digoxin<br>Oral anticoagulants | Decreased response<br>Enhanced response | PK/PD<br>PDt |
| Hypopituitarism | Morphine and analogues | Precipitate coma | PDt |
| **Ocular disease** | | | |
| Glaucoma (narrow angle) | Anticholinergics | Risk of precipitating angle closure glaucoma | PDd |
| Glaucoma (open angle) | Corticosteroids (systemic) | Sudden rise in intraocular pressure | PDd |
| Infections | Corticosteroids (topical) | Exacerbate infection | PDd |

a Examples relating to drugs used in anaesthetic practice are given in chapter 12. For drug interactions, see also chapter 7 and appendix B.

b Some adverse reactions are predictable, others may not necessarily occur or occur in all patients. Many can be avoided by appropriate adjustment of dosage.

*Abbreviations:* PK = due to altered pharmacokinetic handling; PKa = inhibition of absorption; PKd = altered distribution; PKm = inhibition of hepatic metabolism; PKe = inhibition of renal excretion; PD = due to pharmacodynamic action of the drug; PDd = direct effect of drug; PDt = altered tissue sensitivity; CNS = central nervous system; G6PD = glucose-6-phosphate dehydrogenase.

## 2.3 Age

Adverse reactions are more likely to occur in the very young and the old. Physiological functions show certain deficiencies compared with those of young adults and older children, and elimination of some drugs is markedly delayed in elderly and newborn patients. Changes in distribution may also contribute to altered responsiveness. Tissue sensitivity and altered homeostasis are other contributory factors. In both of these age groups, a lower dosage than dictated by body size alone is generally indicated (see further chapters 3 and 4).

### 2.4 Disease and Pathophysiological Variables

The presence of associated disease or intercurrent illness may alter pharmacokinetic handling or tissue sensitivity and can markedly influence drug response and the occurrence of adverse drug reactions. Such variables are the most important determinants of drug reactions (table III).

Diseases of drug-eliminating organs, particularly the liver and kidney, increase the risk of adverse reactions of a predictable type, as well as occasionally contributing to unexpected abnormal responses such as neuropsychiatric reactions (see section 5). A special skill in therapeutics is to use a single drug to treat two or more conditions, sometimes taking advantage of the adverse effects of the drug. For example, if depression occurs in a patient with irritable bowel disease, then the usually unwanted anticholinergic effects of tricyclic antidepressants may improve the bowel symptoms.

Pregnancy and labour also change the response to drugs (see further chapter 18; sect. 1).

### 2.5 Gender

More adverse reactions are reported in women than in men. Some of the reactions in women are related to therapy for obstetric or gynaecological conditions. For example, oral contraceptives cause both morbidity and mortality due to thromboembolism, among other effects. Women show a greater tendency to seek medical attention and hence to receive drugs. They are also more likely than men to receive pain-relieving drugs in hospital wards; however, the reasons for this observation display considerable variability.

It is possible that a sex hormone-determined predisposition to drug reactions occurs in humans, comparable to the regularly observable differences in dose responses seen in experimental animals. Kellerman et al.[16] showed that the half-life of phenazone (antipyrine) varied significantly with the phase of the menstrual cycle. Giudicelli & Tillement[17] and Wilson[18] have reviewed a number of situations in which drug kinetics appeared to be significantly modified by gender.

Gender-linked genetic factors are other causes of differences, e.g. oxidant drug-induced haemolysis in glucose-6-phosphate dehydrogenase (G6PD) deficiency which affects males preponderantly (see section 4.2.2). Some reactions that occur more frequently in women, such as cough with ACE inhibitors, have so far not been entirely explained.[19]

**Table IV.** Incidence of adverse drug reactions in hospitalised patients in relation to previous history of reactions or drug allergy (after Smith et al.[21]; Hurwitz[22])

| Parameter | US study[21] (% of pts) | UK study[22] (% of pts) |
|---|---|---|
| History of prior reaction | 14.1 | 27.9 |
| No history of prior reaction | 9.0 | 8.6 |
| History of allergic disease | 12.5 | 28.4 |
| No history of allergic disease | 10.5 | 9.0 |

### 2.6 Previous History of Allergy or Reaction to Drugs

Adverse reactions are much more likely to occur in patients with a history of previous reaction to drugs. In a New Zealand hospital study, 28% of patients having an adverse reaction had experienced one before.[20] A history of allergic disease, including anaphylaxis, is also associated with an increased risk of adverse drug reactions (table IV), due primarily to a genetically determined liability to form inordinately large amounts of IgE.

### 2.7 Multiple Drug Therapy

The incidence of adverse reactions increases with the number of drugs given (table V). Studies conducted in the 1970s showed that the average inpatient in an American hospital received 9 drugs during hospitalisation compared with 6 for the average Israeli inpatient,[23] and about 5 for the average British one.[24] Patients in hospital in the US who experienced adverse drug reactions received on average 14 or 15 drugs.[25] Outpatients are also prescribed a number of drugs at the same time.[26] In some cases, reactions resulting from use of a larger number of drugs are partly due to severe or multiple disease processes for which multiple therapy is unavoidable. However, the necessity of prescriptions of 20 or more drugs at the same time, as has happened in an intensive care patient who even received two different brands of cotrimoxazole at the same time, must be questioned.

There is a considerable temptation to add drugs to existing treatments, particularly if the patient's current drugs were prescribed by someone else. In this situation, a clinician may fall into the trap of thinking that an earlier prescriber knew more about the situation. Even

**Table V.** Incidence of adverse drug reactions in hospitalised patients in relation to number of drugs given (after Smith et al.[21]; Hurwitz[22])

| US study[21] | | UK study[22] | |
|---|---|---|---|
| drugs given | adverse reaction rate (%) | drugs given | adverse reaction rate (%) |
| 0-5 | 4.2 | 1-5 | 3.3 |
| 6-10 | 7.4 | 6+ | 19.8 |
| 11-15 | 24.2 | | |
| 16-20 | 40.0 | | |
| 21+ | 45.0 | | |

though that may be so, it is important to review all of the patient's medications, including self-medications, herbal preparations and the like, before adding to them. Confusion over which drugs to take and when is also a problem. Safe storage is an issue with elderly patients who may leave drugs around the house where visiting grandchildren can find and take them as sweets. It is the elderly and the seriously or chronically ill who are most likely to experience these problems.

### 2.8 Genetic and Ethnic Factors

Inherited characteristics can lead to abnormal drug response or increased risk of adverse reactions, either by altering the pharmacokinetic handling of the drug, or by altering tissue responsiveness (see section 4.2). There are genetically determined differences in the rate of metabolism of many drugs. Differences in hepatic oxidation and acetylation of drugs occur between individuals, and the proportion of poor/slow metabolisers may vary among ethnic groups (see chapter 1; sect. 5.2, 5.3). Therapeutic monitoring by blood concentration measurement can therefore be very important with drugs that are metabolised via these pathways, particularly those with a small therapeutic window.

It therefore seems reasonable to determine the genotype or metabolic phenotype of individuals who have dose-related reactions to drugs whose metabolism is subject to genetic polymorphism. This may allow avoidance of unwanted responses to these and other drugs metabolised by the same pathway via individual tailoring of dosage regimens. However, whether this is a useful approach in routine clinical practice has still to be determined (see also chapter 1; sect. 5.2.4).[27]

Other genetic factors can lead to unique and unexpected responses, some of which may be fatal (e.g. malignant hyperpyrexia with general anaesthesia). A careful patient history including previous drug problems, family history, and racial background may allow the prevention of genetically determined reactions. For example, patients with genetic enzyme defects such as G6PD deficiency and porphyria should avoid certain drugs (see further section 4.2.2; and chapter 26; sect. 5.2.2).

Ethnicity, however, includes more than racial (or genetic) attributes. Cultural differences, and different medical practices and disease distributions may all influence the occurrence and reporting of adverse drug reactions. In fact, geneticists have shown that differences between the main racial groups are about 10% of total genetic variability; 6% of the total variability is between nations and 84% is between individuals. This does not mean that the 10% racial variability is unimportant, only that it is wrong to think that ethnic differences are largely genetic.[28,29]

## 3. Aetiological Basis of Adverse Drug Reactions

On an aetiological basis, adverse drug reactions can be classified as occurring due to:

1. *Inherent anomalies in patient response:* reactions resulting from allergy or idiosyncrasy, including those due to genetic factors, or physiological variables such as age, gender, pregnancy.

2. *Acquired patient abnormalities:* reactions due to the presence of associated disease states or intercurrent illnesses which may modify the response to the drug.

3. *Anomalies of drug presentation and administration:* reactions occurring as a consequence of excessive dosage, changed bioavailability characteristics such as a new dosage form or substitution of a drug product, altered drug excipients (the so-called inactive ingredients), inappropriate route or method of administration, medication errors.

4. *Interaction of drugs:* reactions resulting from the combined effects of more than one drug prescribed or taken at the same time.

5. *Indirect reactions:* those not affecting the person taking the drug directly but causing an effect on a second organism, e.g. where the reaction involves the fetus, a breast-feeding baby, or a saprophyte such as the bacterial flora of the gut (see further section 11).[30]

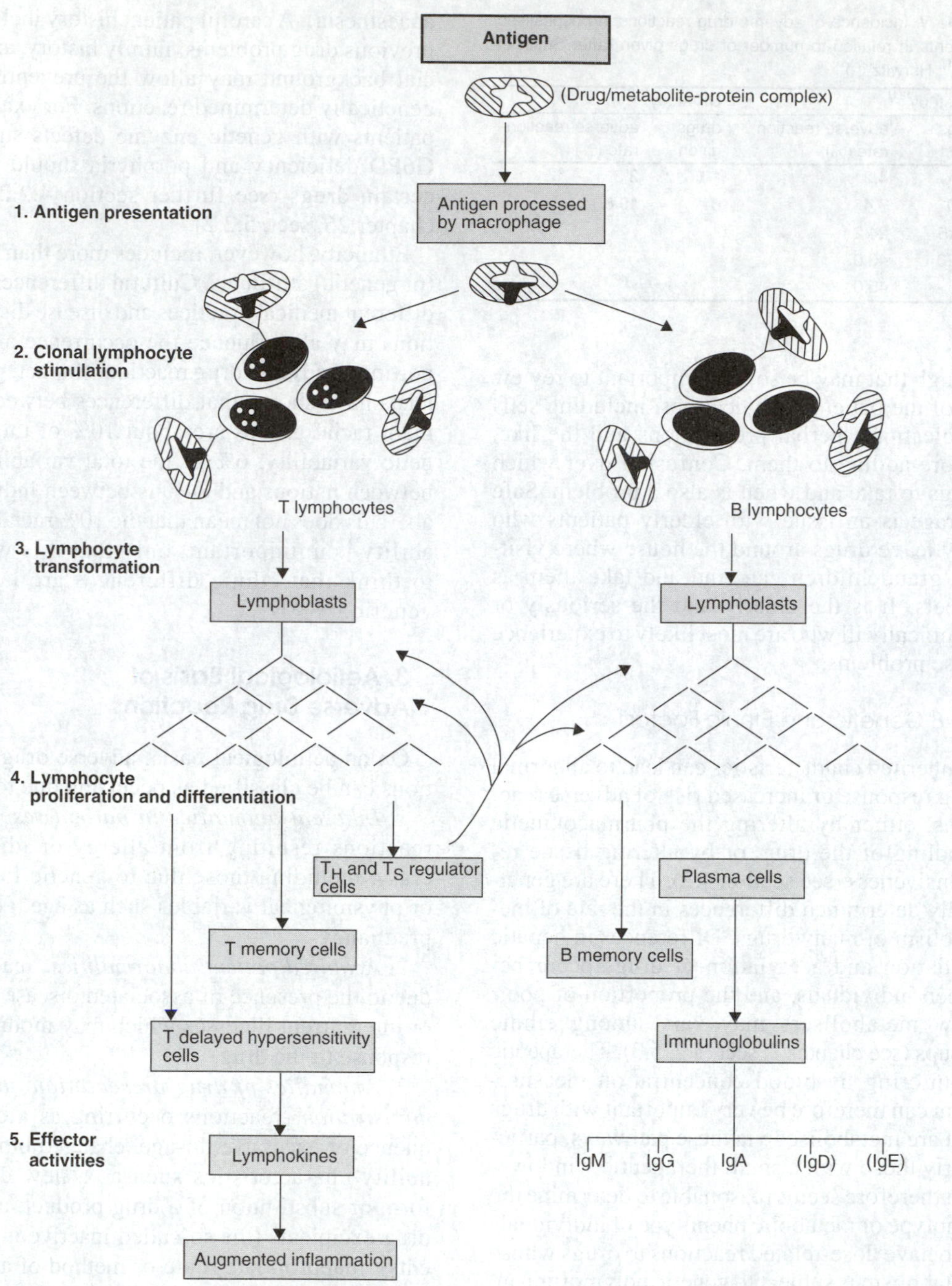


**Fig. 1.** Schematic representation of immune responses of B and T lymphocytes following the entry of an antigen (e.g. a drug or breakdown product) that is recognised as foreign. B lymphocytes are responsible for antibody-mediated immunity; sensitised B cells produce immunoglobulins (antibodies) that bind to the antigenic determinant. T lymphocytes are responsible for cell-mediated immunity; sensitised T cells cause release of inflammatory substances that act on the antigen. B and T memory cells provide a mechanism whereby a more rapid and heightened response occurs on re-exposure to the antigen (after McQueen[30]). *Abbreviations:* $T_H$ = T-helper cell; $T_S$ = T-suppressor cell.

## 4. Reactions Due to Inherent Anomalies in Patient Response

### 4.1 Drug Allergy

In categorising reactions under this heading, it is important to establish clearly what is intended by the term 'allergy'. Originally introduced by von Pirquet in 1906 to describe a state of 'changed reactivity' resulting from exposure to a foreign substance acting as an 'allergen', the allergic state is one of specifically altered potential reactivity to a particular chemically definable substance, in this case a drug or breakdown product of a drug.

Recognition of a drug reaction as allergic classically follows its conformity to the pattern characteristically associated with allergy:[31,32]

- There is a delay in the establishment of the allergic state following the initial exposure.
- Once an allergic state has been established, the allergic reaction can be precipitated by minute amounts of the drug.
- There is recurrence of the reaction on repeated exposure.
- The reaction does not resemble the pharmacological activity of the drug.
- The symptoms are suggestive of some form of allergic response, e.g. urticaria, serum sickness, anaphylaxis, etc., and may be accompanied by other stigmata such as eosinophilia or, more chronically, fibrosis.

None of these criteria is specific and differentiation from genetically determined anomalies of drug response may be difficult. Reactions believed to be due to an immune mechanism may prove to be due to enzymatic or other abnormalities in the patient. Anaphylactoid responses to aspirin and other nonsteroidal anti-inflammatory drugs (NSAIDs) may be a case in point (see section 4.1.4).

#### *4.1.1 Mechanisms of Drug Allergy*

All allergic mechanisms depend on interaction between a foreign antigen and host antibodies or sensitised lymphocytes.[32-36] The general mechanisms of immune responses are given in figure 1.

Drugs may induce immunotoxic reactions in 4 main ways:

1) The drug may be a protein and potentially immunogenic.

2) The drug or a metabolite may form a hapten by combination with endogenous proteins.

3) The drug or a metabolite may be involved in causing or potentiating a reaction between a modified self antigen and an antibody.

4) The drug or metabolite may cause the synthesis of autoantibodies, but its continued presence is not required for binding between the antibody and antigen to occur.

In Coombs-Gell ***type I*** (immediate) hypersensitivity, after an initial immunogenic exposure, the drug-protein or protein conjugate binds to specific IgE on the surfaces of basophils and mast cells (fig. 2a). This leads to degranulation of mast cells and basophils, massive mediator release and, clinically, urticaria, bronchospasm and, at the most severe end of the spectrum, anaphylactic shock related to increased vascular permeability.

***Type II*** (cytotoxic) hypersensitivity (fig. 2b) results when IgG or IgM antibody reacts to a drug-protein conjugate on cells such as blood cells or other specific tissues. Resultant complement release may lead to, for instance, thrombocytopenia, neutropenia or haemolysis, or type III hypersensitivity.

In ***type III*** (immune complex) hypersensitivity (fig. 2c), the protein complexes form insoluble matrices with IgG or IgM which trigger complement and cause localised vascular damage leading to serum sickness with fever, joint and muscle pain and lymphadenopathy. Examples are reactions to sulfhydryl-containing compounds, hydralazine, and penicillins.

***Type IV*** (delayed) hypersensitivity (fig. 2d) may occur if the drug-protein complex on a target cell is recognised by a T lymphocyte and causes direct cytotoxicity and/or activation of macrophages. Clinically, this results in reactions such as fixed drug eruptions or allergy to topical agents.

***Autoimmune reactions*** (fig. 2e), such as drug-induced lupus erythematosus, may be due to direct drug binding with nuclear proteins, particularly histone, which activates major histocompatibility complex (MHC) sites. Alternatively, they may be due to inflammation-activated monocytes metabolising the drug to a reactive metabolite, which in turn activates its own MHC sites, or to the drug inhibiting T suppressor function. In all 3 possible situations, the resulting enhanced helper cell activity leads to T cytotoxic cell proliferation and the formation of immunoglobulins.

The problems of drug allergy are complex and the type of response may depend on the route of administration, underlying immune

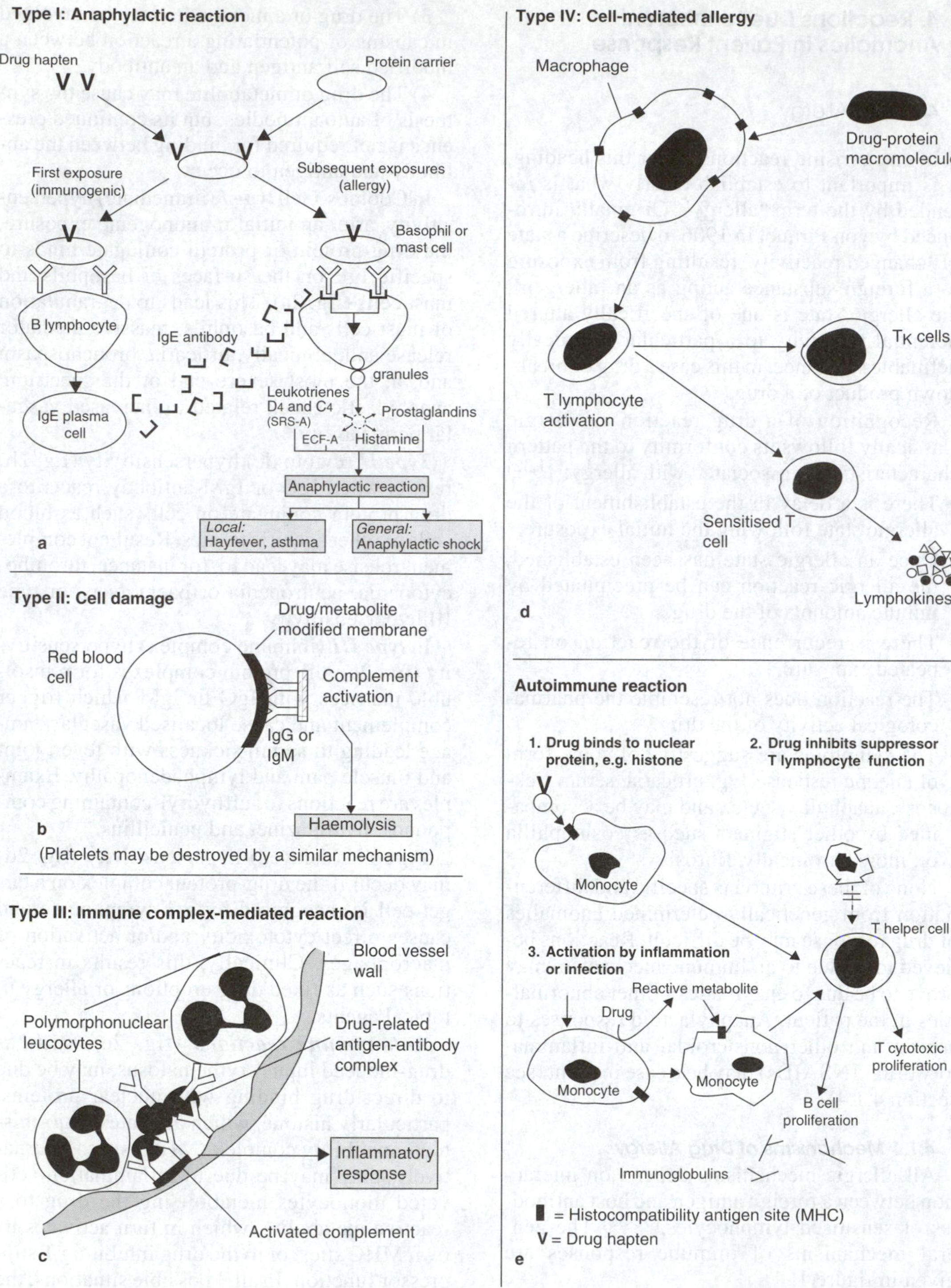


**Fig. 2.** Mechanisms of cell damage by allergic responses, representing: (a) type I, anaphylactic reaction; (b) type II, cell damage such as haemolysis; (c) type III, immune complex-mediated reaction such as serum sickness; (d) type IV, cell-mediated allergy such as skin reactions; (e) autoimmune reaction. *Abbreviation:* $T_K$ = T-killer cells.

disease such as atopy, the coadministration of immune modulators such as corticosteroids, or even physical stress.[37] In addition, leucocytes can metabolise a variety of drugs to reactive metabolites that may cause idiosyncratic reactions.[38] Moreover, the mechanisms described are not mutually exclusive. Common drug-induced cytotoxic, immune complex, delayed hypersensitivity and autoimmune responses have been reviewed by Gleichmann et al.[33] This review also draws attention to the fact that HLA phenotypes have been linked to certain adverse drug reaction situations, e.g. DR3 and DR4 phenotypes are associated with penicillamine glomerulonephritis, and DR1 and Bw35 phenotypes with penicillamine myasthenia.

It is worth considering further the common and rapidly life-threatening immediate (type I) hypersensitivity. In the case of penicillin, the unmodified molecule circulates bound to serum albumin, but in a loose readily dissociable combination not capable of acting as an antigen. A number of its breakdown products, however, readily couple with larger peptide or protein molecules by amide, carbonyl, or disulfide linkages to form a series of potent antigenic determinants.[39] Thus, antibodies that can be detected in the serum of patients receiving penicillin are not directed towards penicillin itself, but to its breakdown products, especially the penicilloyl group, which are capable of existing in covalent linkages to protein.[40]

A structural component of a drug shared with others may act as an antigenic determinant, such as the tertiary or quaternary ammonium groups possessed by a number of skeletal muscle relaxants, e.g. suxamethonium (succinylcholine), and also by choline.[41] The immunogenicity of the carrier itself seems to be important, since haptens combined with foreign proteins are more effective in promoting immune responses than haptens on native proteins. However, induction of allergic responsiveness is not determined by any specific chemical characteristic of the hapten, other than that it should have a degree of chemical reactivity. Precipitation of a reaction in the already sensitised patient, however, need not necessarily involve the complete macromolecular antigen necessary for creation of the allergic state. Thus, penicillin may precipitate anaphylactic shock by virtue of the polymeric complexes of the drug itself, which are already formed in the preparation prior to administration.[42]

As stated above, antibodies formed against drug-protein complexes may also be of the IgG or IgM types, which are circulating antibodies, whereas the IgE type coat cells and sequester in tissues. IgG and IgM may act as 'blocking antibodies', combining with antigen before it can reach fixed IgE antibodies, thereby preventing anaphylaxis. These antibodies only rarely cause a clinical syndrome themselves. They are very widespread, being found in non-allergic patients as often as in those with allergies. 'Blocking antibodies' may explain the discrepancies between the negative results of skin testing in patients who have documented acute anaphylaxis to the tested substance. Additionally, free drug or a non-conjugated metabolite may preempt binding sites on antibodies, denying access to complete antigens.

#### 4.1.2 Clinical Manifestations of Drug Allergy

Table VI lists examples of drug reactions known or suspected to be due to allergic mechanisms. Some of these reactions to particular drugs are discussed in the following sections to illustrate the clinical presentations of allergy.

##### Anaphylactic Reactions

As stated above, reactions of the immediate type are largely IgE-mediated (fig. 2a). They may be generalised, resulting in acute systemic anaphylactic shock, or localised.

*Localised reactions* are determined by the main site of interaction of the allergen with IgE, a target 'shock-organ' being involved. This may be the skin (with acute urticaria or angio-oedema), the respiratory tract (bronchial asthma), or the gastrointestinal tract (vomiting, abdominal pain and diarrhoea). The same pattern often repeats itself with repeated exposure in any given patient.

*Generalised systemic anaphylaxis* is acute and life-threatening, with hypotension, bronchospasm, urticaria, laryngeal oedema, etc., in various combinations or sometimes as isolated features. Anaphylaxis is most common with drugs given intramuscularly or intravenously, although it can occur after oral or percutaneous administration or even exposure through eye drops. The reaction typically develops rapidly (reaching a maximum within 5 to 30 minutes) and usually occurs at the start of treatment with a drug to which the patient has been exposed previously. Allergic symptoms may not necessarily have occurred during previous courses of treatment. Indeed, anaphylactic shock to penicillin has been known to occur with the 17th

**Table VI.** Examples of adverse immunological effects of drugs in humans (after Gleichmann et al.[33]). Compounds are listed alphabetically and not according to the frequency of adverse immunological effects they induce

| Reaction | Inducing drug(s) |
|---|---|
| **1. Immediate hypersensitivity (type I)** | |
| Anaphylaxis | Penicillins, dextrans, foreign antisera, iodinated radiocontrast media, intravenous anaesthetics and relaxants |
| **2. Drug-induced autoantibodies** | |
| Autoimmune chronic active hepatitis, virus-negative | Halothane |
| Autoimmune haemolytic anaemia (certain types) | Methyldopa, levodopa, captopril, cefalexin, mefenamic acid, penicillins |
| Goodpasture's syndrome | Penicillamine |
| Granulocytopenia (certain types) | Aminophenazone (aminopyrine), captopril, cefalexin, chloral hydrate, chlordiazepoxide, chlorpromazine, chlorpropamide, gold salts, mercurial diuretics, indomethacin, *p*-aminosalicylic acid, penicillins, sulfapyridine/sulfathiazole, thiouracils, tolazoline |
| Myasthenia gravis | Penicillamine, possibly gold salts |
| Pemphigus vulgaris | Penicillamine |
| Bullous pemphigoid | Penicillamine |
| Systemic lupus erythematosus | Gold salts, griseofulvin, hydralazine, phenytoin, penicillamine, procainamide, thiouracils |
| Immune complex type glomerulonephritis | Gold salts, penicillamine and other drugs with a sulfhydryl group |
| **3. Drug-induced immunological diseases of unknown pathogenesis** | |
| Aplastic anaemia (certain types) | Penicillamine, phenytoin, mepacine (quinacrine), oxyphenbutazone, phenylbutazone |
| Intrahepatic cholestasis/cholangitis | Chlorpromazine, chlorpropamide, erythromycin estolate, imipramine, nalidixic acid, nitrofurantoin |
| Hepatitis, nonviral | *p*-Aminosalicylic acid, amiodarone, captopril, isoniazid, phenytoin and other hydantoins |
| Hypogammaglobulinaemia | Gold salts, phenytoin |
| Infectious mononucleosis-like syndrome | *p*-Aminosalicylic acid, dapsone, phenytoin |
| Interstitial nephritis | Azathioprine, cefalosporins, furosemide, penicillins (esp. methicillin), phenindione, phenytoin, rifampicin, sulfinpyrazone, sulfonamides |
| Lymphadenopathy/(pseudo) lymphoma, non-Hodgkin | Phenytoin and other hydantoins, possibly gold salts |
| Peripheral neuritis | Colchicine, gold salts, nitrofurantoin, sulfonamides |
| Serum sickness | Penicillins, cefalosporins, streptomycin, sulfonamides |
| Skin (immunological drug reactions can mimic virtually *all* clinical and histological patterns of disease) | Antibiotics, barbiturates, diuretics, gold salts, hydantoins, tranquillosedatives |
| Thrombocytopenia (certain types) | Acetazolamide, aspirin, carbamazepine, cefalothin, chloramphenicol, digitoxin, gold salts, imipramine, levodopa, meprobamate, methyldopa, *p*-aminosalicylic acid, phenylbutazone, phenytoin, quinidine, quinine, rifampicin, spironolactone, stibophen, sulfonamides, sulphonylureas, thiazides |
| Vasculitis (different types) | Allopurinol, busulfan, indomethacin, isoniazid, iodides, penicillin, phenothiazines, phenylbutazone, tetracyclines, thiazides, thiouracils |
| **4. Examples of allergic reactions to chemicals** (only reactions against non-self antigens are involved) | |
| Allergic asthma and related conditions | Different types of allergen inhaled at the work place, such as the dust of manufactured antibiotics, ethylenediamine, formaldehyde, insecticides, isocyanates, salts of the heavy metals chromium, cobalt, mercury, nickel, platinum |
| Contact dermatitis | Many topically applied drugs, such as antibiotics, antihistamines, local anaesthetics; and a variety of other chemicals, including many different organic compounds and the salts of heavy metals, such as chromium, cobalt, mercury, and nickel |
| Food allergy | Many different types of food additive, chemical contaminations of food |

course of treatment, the previous 16 courses having been given without incident.[39] On the other hand, there may be no history of prior therapeutic exposure.

Some drugs that can cause anaphylaxis by allergic mechanisms are listed in table VI. Acute anaphylaxis may be related to any of the intravenous anaesthetics or relaxants (see chapter 12, sects 2.2.1, 5.6).[43]

#### Immunologically Mediated Reactions Against Specific Tissues

Many drugs cause autoimmune haemolysis (table VI), the mechanism in most cases being a combination of hapten with a surface cell membrane protein constituent to produce an antigen. Circulating antibodies interact with the cell surface antigen producing cell damage (fig. 2b) and activation of complement produces haemolysis.[44] Similarly, drug-platelet surface antigens combine with circulating antibodies to produce aggregation and sequestration of platelets. Although a number of drugs are responsible for either haemolysis or thrombocytopenia, there is consistency of the same reaction in a given patient. Specific involvement of the platelet as a component of the antigen was originally postulated by Ackroyd.[45] Rifampicin, however, can apparently produce either thrombocytopenia or haemolysis or both.[46]

Very high doses of some penicillins may result in Coombs' positive haemolysis (see section 4.1.4). Antineutrophil antibody activity may be demonstrable in patients with neutropenia associated with various drugs.[47]

Some drugs can induce an autoimmune state. Antibodies develop that are directed towards native antigens on the red cell surface and often have Rh specificity. The process is manifest by a positive Coombs' test, but only a minority of such patients develop overt haemolysis (see chapter 26; sect. 5.2.2). In a few patients, there may also be antinuclear antibodies.

Immunologically-mediated disturbances of hepatic function may also occur. These may be accompanied by fever, nausea, vomiting, diarrhoea and abnormalities of liver function tests, particularly alanine and aspartate aminotransferases (ALT and AST). Occasionally, the hepatic damage may be so severe as to resemble viral hepatitis.[48] High titres of antinuclear autoantibody can be demonstrated in drug-induced chronic active hepatitis.[49] Drugs that have been implicated include methyldopa, isoniazid, sulfonamides and nitrofurantoin.[50,51] An autoimmune myasthenic state may be induced by penicillamine, which in some patients promotes the development of antibodies to acetylcholine receptors at the neuromuscular junction and basement membrane proteins. The clinical state precisely resembles the spontaneous condition but remits with cessation of the drug.[32]

Other drug reactions, involving either entrapment of circulating immune complexes or the interaction of circulating antibodies with tissue-bound drug, may result in damage to the lungs, liver, locomotor system, heart, kidneys and peripheral nerves. Specific involvement of the liver might entail damage by the products of biotransformation of the drug in question. Involvement of the kidney could be associated with the trapping of circulating immune complexes.

Often, the drug antibodies have a high degree of specificity, e.g. most patients with quinine-sensitive thrombocytopenia do not react to the optical isomer quinidine, although some 20% may do so.[52] An oxidative derivative of both drugs (quininone) may then be responsible, but cross-allergy may be evident with structurally related drugs such as sulfonamides,[53] involving drug fever, dermatitis and conjunctivitis. Similarly, nitrofurantoin-induced eosinophilic pneumonitis may occur as a cross-reaction to furazolidone. Allergic reactions to cefalosporins in persons with penicillin allergy are as likely to be due to independent cefalosporin sensitivity as to cross-reactivity (see section 4.1.4).

#### Serum Sickness (Type III Hypersensitivity)

In the presence of a relative excess of antigen, immune complexes are small and not readily removed; they lodge in small blood vessels, leading to inflammation (fig. 2c). Such reactions may take the form of fever only, or may involve generalised lymphadenopathy and joint swellings and be accompanied by anaphylactic (IgE-mediated) features as well, such as bronchospasm, urticaria, and angio-oedema.[54] Neutropenia is likely to be evident early on; eosinophilia is not a feature of this condition, but thrombocytopenia may occur. Skin rashes are particularly common and may occur locally at a previous injection site. Glomerulonephritis, pericarditis, myocarditis, meningitis, meningoencephalitis, peripheral neuritis or myelitis may also occur.

Serum sickness may be the result of the classical foreign serum injection (e.g. ATS), or it may result from the injection of contaminant foreign proteins, e.g. egg protein in influenza vaccine. Penicillins are again a frequent cause, particularly the long-acting penicillins. Streptomycin, sulfonamides and a few other drugs (table VI) have also been implicated quite often.

In the initial exposure to a drug, symptoms of the serum sickness syndrome generally develop after a latent period of 6 days or more, reflecting the time taken to synthesise appreciable amounts of antibody. However, symptoms may first appear as long as 3 weeks after the last dose. Generally, symptoms last a few days to a week, but may persist for as long as 6 weeks.

#### Skin Reactions

Skin reactions include Coombs-Gell type I reactions, immune complex (type III) reactions, and cell-mediated (type IV) allergy (fig. 2a, c, d). Drug-induced cutaneous eruptions can occur as isolated manifestations or accompany reactions involving the viscera, e.g. the oculomucocutaneous practolol syndrome with extension to produce sclerosing serositis.[55] Urticaria and angio-oedema exemplify type I reactions.

An unpleasant, but fortunately very uncommon, type III reaction involving blood vessels in the skin and subcutaneous tissues may occur with oral anticoagulants, particularly with the coumarin derivatives but also with phenindione.[56] This reaction may lead to necrosis of large areas of skin and subcutaneous tissues, and it may be accompanied by acute renal failure due to renal cortical necrosis.

The delayed hypersensitivity-type reaction is a result of interaction between the drug and specifically sensitised cells and does not depend on the presence of circulating antibody. Localisation of these cell-mediated (type IV) allergic reactions such as fixed drug eruptions is often impossible to interpret.

#### Fever

Drug-induced pyrexia is allergic in origin in most instances.[57] It is usually mediated by circulating antibodies, particularly IgG, but may be a manifestation of cellular immunity. It is thought to be due to the release of endogenous pyrogens from granulocytes or mononuclear cells. Marked and sustained fever may be associated with inflammatory lesions of small vessels, and, if the drug is continued, serious visceral or cutaneous manifestations can result.

Drugs most commonly involved in causing fever include sulfonamides, penicillins, cefalosporins and their analogues, quinidine, methyldopa, phenytoin, captopril, and amphotericin B. Fever is also caused by some anticancer drugs, e.g. bleomycin. In the case of the latter, it possibly results from liberation of pyrogens released by damaged neoplastic cells. Similarly, pyrogenic endotoxins released from dying organisms may be responsible for Jarisch-Herxheimer reactions that follow antibiotic treatment for spirochaetal diseases. The special case of malignant hyperpyrexia is discussed in section 4.2.2.

### *4.1.3 Factors Influencing the Occurrence of Allergic Drug Reactions*

The factors that determine the likelihood of an allergic reaction to a drug can be classified as follows.[39]

#### Duration and Number of Courses of Treatment

In general, the likelihood of a reaction increases with the number of courses of treatment. For example, a patient may have been given penicillin on a number of occasions without incident, but then experiences anaphylactic shock with the first injection of the next course. With drugs given in a single course over a prolonged period, the likelihood of a reaction is much greater in the first days or within 2 weeks, although reactions may occur later, even after years of treatment. In any one course, anaphylaxis should not be a problem once treatment is under way, provided that different batches of the drug are of comparable purity.

#### Route of Administration

Any route of administration can result in allergic manifestations; with topical application, the site of entry is usually the main target area for the reaction. Anaphylaxis is, however, much less common with oral than with parenteral administration.[58] Occasionally, absorption from a topical application, such as eye drops, may result in anaphylaxis.

#### Atopy

Anaphylaxis to injected drugs seems to occur with about the same frequency in the general population as in atopic individuals. However, anaphylaxis following administration by other routes (oral, inhalation) occurs considerably more often in atopic than in non-atopic individuals.

#### Previous History of Allergic Reactions

The likelihood of another reaction is greater in those who have suffered a previous allergic reaction, but the allergy may not persist indefinitely. Cross-allergy can occur between chemically related drugs (see table VI).

#### Age

Allergic reactions to drugs seem less common in children. The reason for this may be that they have a lower degree of exposure to drug antigens than adults. However, fatal anaphylaxis may occur even in neonates, possibly as a result of passive sensitisation from maternal blood or milk.

#### Coexisting Disease States

Patients with infectious mononucleosis, lymphoid leukaemia, or hyperuricaemia (whether or not receiving allopurinol therapy) have a very much greater likelihood of maculopapular rash with ampicillin. This may result from a reaction involving polymeric adducts of penicillin, which have the capacity to induce lymphocyte proliferation in abnormal lymphocytes.[59] It appears that the incidence of the rash can be reduced by use of polymer-free ampicillin.

Despite the reduction in immune responsiveness in AIDS patients, they seem to be particularly prone to allergic drug reactions, e.g. with cotrimoxazole. Assessing any abnormal drug response in AIDS patients is difficult because of their susceptibility to a wide range of secondary problems and the use of multiple drug therapies to treat them.[60]

Impaired renal function increases the risk of haemolytic anaemia occurring with high-dose penicillin therapy (see section 4.1.2). However, in patients with systemic lupus erythematosus, there does not seem to be an increased prevalence of drug allergy.[61]

#### Other Drugs

It has been suggested that an increased risk (and severity) of anaphylaxis may be present in patients taking β-adrenoceptor blocking agents. This could be due to the limitation of sympathetic responsiveness by these drugs. It may also be present with other antihypertensive drugs such as calcium antagonists, presumably because of a general exacerbation of hypotension. For a review, see Anderson.[36]

### *4.1.4 Clinically Significant Allergies to Commonly Used Drugs*

#### Penicillin Allergy

Penicillins can cause many types of allergic reactions (table VI; for reviews, see Girard & Cueras[62] and Sogn[63]). Its peculiarly high capacity to generate allergens is possibly because a proteinaceous fermentation residue may be present in commercial penicillins, certified as pure by ordinary standards, with which penicilloyl groups and minor determinants conjugate readily. This may explain why life-threatening anaphylactic responses are characteristically observed with natural benzylpenicillin. The deacylation and replacement of side chains which are involved in manufacture of the semisynthetic penicillins presumably remove the proteinaceous residue.

Acute anaphylaxis is less common when drugs are given orally, because alimentary digestion may also remove proteinaceous allergens. However, acute anaphylaxis may occur with ampicillin, even when given orally. Precipitation of an allergic reaction in a sensitised patient does not necessarily require complete antigen and may be elicited by polymeric complexes forming spontaneously in solutions of penicillins (see section 4.1.1).

Penicillins are a frequent cause of acute immunologically mediated reactions, though they cause anaphylaxis infrequently. The risk of anaphylactic reactions to penicillin is 2 to 3 times greater in atopic patients than in the general population, but individuals who experience anaphylactic reactions to drugs need not have a personal or family history of allergy. The incidence of allergic reactions to cefalosporins in patients not hypersensitive to penicillin is about 1.7%, while the incidence in patients who are hypersensitive to penicillin is about 8.2%.[64] This does not necessarily mean that there is cross-allergenicity, but it does mean that allergic reactions to cefalosporins are about 5 times more common in patients with a history of penicillin allergy. This is not far from the 6-fold increase in reactions noted among patients with bacterial endocarditis who were treated with penicillin itself, despite a history of allergy to penicillin.[65] Thus, the incidence of cefalosporin reactions in penicillin-sensitive patients probably reflects that expected in an atopic population.

At excessively high blood concentrations of penicillin (e.g. with doses of 15 MU/day in patients with tubular blockade and/or renal disease), circulating red cells become modified by hapten and bind antihapten antibody (IgG or IgM), resulting in a positive Coombs' test. Under these circumstance, they are primed to undergo phagocytosis and lysis.[39] Penicillin-induced haemolytic anaemia has also been described as occurring at low dosages,[66,67] and cefalothin-induced haemolysis with a positive Coombs' test occurs at regular dosages in the absence of renal disease.[68,69]

#### Sensitivity to Aspirin and Other NSAIDs

In sensitised individuals, bronchospasm accompanied by rhinorrhoea, conjunctival congestion, and flushing of the head and neck may occur within minutes or hours of the ingestion of aspirin. The condition may be so severe as to be comparable to anaphylactic shock and is occasionally fatal. Females, and people aged 40 years or more seem to be affected more frequently and may have a history of vasomotor rhinitis with polyposis and the subsequent development of asthma. Other NSAIDs are likely to precipitate attacks in such individuals.

Precipitation of attacks by drugs which have structures differing markedly from one another seems incompatible with true drug allergy. It has been suggested[70] that the action these drugs share – i.e. the inhibition of the cyclo-oxygenase step in the pathway of prostaglandin synthesis – may divert arachidonic acid metabolism towards production of the bronchiolar constricting leukotrienes $LTC_4$ and $LTD_4$. Alternative pathogenetic factors are also possible,[71] including discharge of granules from mast cells through a direct chemical rather than an immunological mechanism, and activation of complement with formation of C3a anaphylatoxin.

#### Anaesthetic Agents and Drugs Used in Intensive Care

Most reactions occurring during anaesthesia can be shown to be of immunological origin. The cardinal feature of major incidents is cardiovascular collapse, with or without bronchospasm, the latter particularly involving asthmatic patients. Cutaneous and mucosal oedema are usual accompaniments, and angio-oedema is particularly dangerous if it affects the glottis. Such reactions are more common in young adults than in other age groups, and in females more than males. Interaction with IgE of the antigenic determinant concerned and consequent histamine release seems to be the major pathogenetic factor. In addition, there may be activation of the complement cascade and generation of the C5a and C3a anaphylatoxins. It has been suggested[41] that the IgE antibodies concerned may be directed against quaternary ammonium ion determinants, thus explaining the frequent cross-sensitivity between skeletal muscle relaxants.[72]

'Anaphylactoid' reactions may present with features resembling those of genuine allergic reactions (bronchospasm, urticaria, etc.) following administration of certain drugs which act directly as histamine releasers (i.e. by a pharmacological mechanism). Intravenous opioids (e.g. heroin, codeine, morphine) may produce this effect, as may intravenous dextran, which, however, is a potent allergen as well. This type of reaction is also common during anaesthetic procedures and may cause confusion as to its true nature. Careful assessment of possible anaesthetic agent reactions is necessary before attributing causality, since an erroneous assessment may result in useful drugs being wrongly withheld.

Anaesthetic use and intensive care units provide the best places to see pharmacology in action, because of the use of powerful, rapidly acting drugs under circumstances where physiological responses are often well monitored. They are also, however, areas where therapeutic disasters are likely to occur if due care is not taken. For an authoritative guide to the background, investigation and management of immediate anaesthetic reactions, see review by Watkins & Levy.[73]

#### Radiographic Contrast Media

These agents are increasingly used by injection, with adverse effects that relate partly to the agents but also to the techniques of administration. Many of the adverse effects are due to allergy (5 to 20%) and include anaphylaxis. However, some of these and certain other reactions may be pseudoallergic, resulting from the drugs crossing the blood-brain barrier, damaging the vascular endothelium, and causing vasodilatation. The incidence of adverse effects is about 33% for ionic contrast media and 5% for non-ionic agents.

Many of the effects are vascular, particularly with ionic contrast media, and include vascular spasm, feelings of heat and hypotension. The serious true allergic reactions seem to be similar for both kinds of agents; apparently it is the milder vascular disturbances that are related to the physicochemical properties of the ionic agents. Fatal reactions occur at a frequency of between 1 in 10,000 to 1 in 100,000 examinations.[74]

#### Pharmaceutical Excipients

These occur in all drug products and include aerosol propellants, antimicrobial preservatives, colouring agents, emulsifying, solubilising and wetting agents, perfumes, ointment bases, solvents, sweeteners, tablet and capsule binders and disintegrants, and antioxidants. These categories include many chemicals, which are commonly believed to be inert, but this is far from true. Many, but by no means all, of the reactions due to these agents have an allergic basis.

Some excipients, such as sulfites used as preservatives and the yellow colouring agent tartrazine, have been replaced wherever possible with less troublesome agents because of the frequency with which they have caused allergy and, in particular, severe asthma attacks. On the other hand, the 'safer' preparations may still cause problems. For instance, Sunset Yellow, which has commonly been used to replace tartrazine, may provoke asthma and some individuals exhibit cross-sensitivity to the two agents. Both are azo dyes, and cross-sensitivity in patients reacting to tartrazine with other azo dyes has been recorded at a level as high as 60%.[75]

There are increasing calls from the public for complete disclosure of information on all constituents so that known hypersensitivity can be avoided. For the moment, it is important for health professionals to consider excipients (not only in drugs, but also in prepared foods) whenever an allergic response is investigated.

**Cytotoxic Drugs**

While these drugs are well known for a variety of toxic reactions related to their effects on rapidly dividing cells (mainly haematological and gastrointestinal toxicity), most have also been implicated in a variety of allergic responses. Causality is often difficult to determine because patients with cancer are usually taking many drugs. Asparaginase has been implicated as causing hypersensitivity symptoms in between 6 and 43% of patients studied; however, other drugs appear less prone to cause problems.[35,76]

#### *4.1.5 Diagnosis and Management of Drug Hypersensitivity*

It must be emphasised that a good clinical history is essential before prescribing any drug. Careful questioning about previous diseases treated is often more revealing than direct questions about drugs taken; a patient will probably remember that they had appendicitis, but may not recall what drugs they were given at that time and certainly may not relate one of those drugs to a skin rash. The factors outlined in section 4.1.3 should be borne in mind.

In general, clinical rechallenge with a suspect drug should be avoided because of the possibility of a much more severe, even life-threatening, reaction. This is particularly true of immediate allergy, and if the use of a suspect drug is essential, then great care must be taken, using a test dose(s) and with full pharmacological and physical resuscitative procedures available.[77]

*In vivo* skin tests must be approached with similar precautions to clinical rechallenge; even the minute amounts injected may be dangerous, and a preceding scratch test should be used when the risk seems great. Nevertheless, skin tests may be useful in diagnosing IgE-mediated reactions. Type IV photosensitivity and contact dermatitis may be diagnosed by patch tests.

*In vitro* tests have been developed and have the clear advantage of avoiding dangerous patient exposure. The radioallergosorbent test (RAST) and enzyme-linked immunosorbent assay (ELISA) can provide measures of IgE. Good positive and negative controls are required; false positives due to nonspecific binding and false negatives due to blocking antibodies have made some researchers doubt the usefulness of these tests. Measurement of specific IgG and IgM antibodies and complement is possible, but the tests have not yet found a real role in clinical practice: complement measurements are not specific for drug hypersensitivity.

For guidance on the diagnosis of anaesthetic reactions, see review by Watkins and Levy.[73] It should be noted that no single test gives all the answers. For overviews of diagnostic methods and the management of hypersensitivity to common drugs, see reviews by Weiss[35] and Blaiss & deShazo,[78] respectively.

### 4.2 Genetically Determined Adverse Drug Reactions

Individual patients vary widely in their response and reaction to drugs. Even if allowance has been made for the patient's age, gender, bodyweight, disease state and concurrent drug regimens, there is still variation between individuals. The patient's unique genetic constitution is one contribution to this variability. Depending on the drug, some patients do not obtain the desired therapeutic effect, while others experience severe adverse reactions when given what is considered to be the average and safe dose. The discipline of pharmacogenetics deals with those variations in drug response that are under hereditary control (see chapter 1; sect. 5.2). These can be divided into 2 types: those due to altered pharmacokinetic handling of the drug in the body and those due to altered tissue responsiveness (which, hence, are pharmacodynamic in origin).

Variability in the response to a drug in the general population may take the form of a unimodal distribution curve or a polymodal curve. Multiple genetic influences presumably determine the unimodal type of variability. The polymodal type gives bimodal or even trimodal distributions and suggests a simpler genetic system, but it can also indicate extraneous influences or even artefacts.

Other genetic terms relevant to a basic understanding of pharmacogenetics include the phenotype and genetic polymorphism. The phenotype is the manifestation of the genetic constitution, or genotype, of an individual which, in the case of a 'gene of large effect' can produce manifest characteristics, or characteristics which can be discovered by examination (e.g. acetylation phenotype of isoniazid or dapsone).

Polymorphism is a type of variation in which individuals with sharply distinct qualities (i.e. polymodal variability) coexist as members of a population (fig. 3). Genetic polymorphism is a property of the population which has in it different genotypes. A genetic polymorphism is maintained from one generation to the next by inheritance of the appropriate allelic genes. Allelic genes are alternative genes which can occupy the same locus on a chromosome. Anomalous drug responses due to genetic variability derive from the extremes of normal distribution curves or from sharply polymodal variation in genetically determined frequency distributions. It is in the latter area that the most dramatic manifestations, which may still merit the term 'idiosyncrasy', occur.

#### *4.2.1 Genetically Determined Pharmacokinetic Reactions*

As discussed in chapter 1 (section 5) differences between individuals in drug absorption, distribution, metabolism and excretion can have profound effects on the response to drugs. Genetic factors have not been shown to be important in influencing drug absorption and distribution. Similarly, genetic factors do not seem to be directly related to altered rates of renal excretion, although genetic disorders associated with abnormal renal function (e.g. renal tubular acidosis) may influence drug excretion indirectly.

Drug metabolism, however, is markedly influenced by genetic factors. Wide interindividual differences exist in the rate of drug elimination, and there are also individual differences in the pattern of drug metabolites. For a variety of drugs, wide differences in steady-state plasma concentrations exist between individuals given the same dose of the drug. Such differences may explain why some patients have a poor therapeutic response and others have severe adverse effects on a standard dosage of the drug. Moreover, drug metabolites may have pharmacological or toxic potential themselves. Genetically determined differences in metabolism have been shown to be of particular importance for a number of drugs initially metabolised by hydrolysis, acetylation or oxidation pathways.

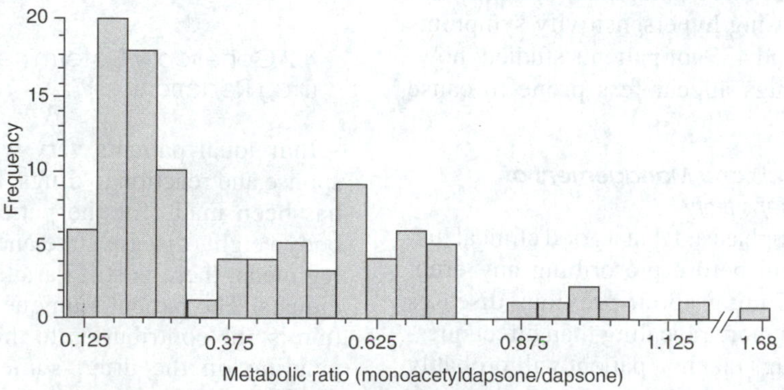


**Fig. 3.** Frequency distribution histogram showing trimodal distribution of dapsone acetylation metabolic ratios in a randomly selected sample of 102 individuals in the Newcastle upon Tyne, UK, area (after Clark[79]). The dapsone acetylation metabolic ratio is determined by measuring the ratio of monoacetyldapsone to dapsone in plasma 3 hours after oral administration of dapsone 100mg. Possible antimodes are at 0.35 and 0.85. The antimode at 0.35 separates homozygous slow acetylators of dapsone from heterozygous fast acetylators.

**Table VII.** Adverse reactions according to acetylation (metabolism) phenotype (after Lunde et al.[81]; Drayer & Reidenberg[82]; Clark[79])

| Drug | Phenotype | Adverse effects[a] |
|---|---|---|
| Isoniazid | Slow | Increased incidence of peripheral neuropathy (overcome by pyridoxine)<br>Systemic lupus syndrome more likely<br>Increased risk of interaction with phenytoin<br>Increased risk of hepatitis when combined with rifampicin |
| Hydralazine | Slow | Systemic lupus syndrome more likely, particularly with high doses<br>Other unwanted effects more common than in rapid acetylators |
| Procainamide | Slow | Systemic lupus syndrome more likely and of earlier development |
| Phenelzine | Slow | ?Severe reactions more likely |
| Sulfasalazine[b] | Slow | Adverse effects due to sulfapyridine component more likely when large doses used |
| Dapsone | Slow | ?Haematological effects more likely |

a See also text (section 4.2.1).

b Sulfasalazine is metabolised by colonic bacteria to 5-aminosalicylic acid and sulfapyridine, which are both metabolised in the liver by the enzyme *N*-acetyltransferase. Sulfapyridine also undergoes metabolism by hydroxylation followed by glucuronide conjugation.[83, 84]

#### Drugs Metabolised by Hydrolysis

An example of altered drug response as a result of individual differences in metabolism by hydrolysis is suxamethonium (succinylcholine) apnoea. Suxamethonium usually exerts its neuromuscular blocking effect for only a few minutes. It is rapidly inactivated by hydrolysis catalysed by plasma butyrylcholinesterase, which exists in several genetically determined forms. There are 4 allelic genes at the principal genetic locus, 1 common and 3 uncommon. Of the latter, one determines the presence of a butyrylcholinesterase of low suxamethonium affinity. In persons who are homozygous for this allele (about 1 in 2500 of a UK population), suxamethonium apnoea may last 30 minutes or even 2 to 3 hours. Apnoea may be somewhat prolonged in heterozygotes for this gene. Individuals who are homozygous for one of the other genes have no detectable butyrylcholinesterase at all, again giving rise to serious problems of apnoea.

The occurrence of the atypical genes shows marked racial variation. The frequency of the low-affinity enzyme genes is low in Africans and Japanese, high in Jews in some areas, and intermediate in Caucasians. Apart from these genetic differences, liver disease, malnutrition, other drugs and occupational exposure to organophosphorus insecticides can also influence the activity of plasma cholinesterase (see chapter 12; sect. 2.2.1).

Atypical resistance to suxamethonium has also been described as occurring due to the presence of a form of cholinesterase with an activity 3 times that of the usual enzyme.

#### Drugs Metabolised by Acetylation

A number of drugs are metabolised by acetylation. The rate at which these drugs are acetylated (e.g. isoniazid and dapsone) varies widely between individuals and shows a bimodal or trimodal distribution in the population, so that individuals are termed either 'slow' or 'rapid' acetylators (fig. 3).[79] The variability is mainly due to differences in activity of the liver enzyme *N*-acetyltransferase. Slow acetylators are homozygous for an autosomal recessive gene. Fast acetylators are either heterozygous or homozygous for a dominant gene.

Other drugs metabolised polymorphically by *N*-acetyltransferase include hydralazine, procainamide, phenelzine, sulfadimidine (sulfamethazine) and sulfapyridine; other sulfonamides are *N*-acetylated by a different enzyme. The amine metabolite of nitrazepam is also subject to polymorphic acetylation.

The plasma half-life of isoniazid in rapid acetylators ranges from 45 to 80 minutes, but in slow acetylators from 140 to 200 minutes (see chapter 1; sect. 5.2.1). In rapid acetylators, only 3% of a dose is excreted unchanged whereas slow acetylators may excrete 30% as the unchanged drug.[80] The clinical consequences of these differences in rate and pattern of metabolism are that the neuropathic effects of isoniazid are more common in slow acetylators than in rapid acetylators (table VII). This can, however, be overcome by administration of pyridoxine.

Slow acetylators of isoniazid are also more susceptible to certain drug interactions involving drug metabolism. Thus, phenytoin toxicity with concurrent isoniazid treatment is confined to slow acetylators,[85] while the risk of liver

**Table VIII.** Distribution of rapid acetylation phenotype according to ethnic origin (after Ellard & Gammon [87]; Lunde et al.[81]; Motulsky[92]; Vivien et al.[93])

| Ethnic group | Rapid acetylators (%) |
|---|---|
| **Asiatic origin** | |
| Canadian Eskimo | 95-100 |
| New Zealand Polynesian | 93 |
| Korean | 89 |
| Japanese | 88-90 |
| Ainu | 87 |
| Ryukyuan | 85 |
| Saame Lapp | 80 |
| Alaskan Eskimo | 79 |
| American Indian | 79 |
| Chinese | 78-85 |
| Thai | 72 |
| Filipino | 72 |
| Canadian Indian | 63 |
| Burmese | 62 |
| Skolt Lapp | 50 |
| Hindu Indian | 40 |
| **African origin** | |
| South African Negro | 59 |
| American Negro | 49-58 |
| African | 43-51 |
| Sudanese Negro | 35 |
| Ethiopian Negro | 20-50 |
| **European origin** | |
| Latin American | 67 |
| Italian | 51 |
| Norwegian | 44 |
| US White | 43-48 |
| German | 43 |
| French | 41 |
| US Greek | 40 |
| Czechoslovakian | 40 |
| Swiss | 39 |
| British | 38-40 |
| Finn | 36-39 |
| US Italian | 36 |
| US Scandinavian | 33 |
| Swede | 32-49 |
| Canadian | 30-41 |
| **Mediterranean origin** | |
| US Askenazi | 45 |
| Israeli Askenazi | 33 |
| Israeli non-Askenazi | 31 |
| Israeli Baghdad Jew | 25 |
| Egyptian | 18 |

toxicity with antituberculosis regimens containing isoniazid and rifampicin appears to be increased in those who are slow acetylators of isoniazid (table VII). There is some doubt as to whether susceptibility to hepatitis is greater among fast[86] than among slow acetylators when isoniazid is used alone. Formation of the highly reactive acetylated metabolite acetylhydrazine, which is thought to be responsible for hepatotoxicity, is likely to be more rapid in fast acetylators. However, acetylhydrazine is itself polymorphically acetylated to diacetylhydrazine and this process occurs more rapidly in fast acetylators who excrete much more acetylhydrazine as diacetylhydrazine than do slow acetylators.[87,88]

There is a more frequent association and earlier development of procainamide-induced systemic lupus erythematosus with slow acetylation than with fast. Similarly, slow acetylators receiving hydralazine are much more likely to develop lupus erythematosus than fast acetylators.[89,90]

With hydralazine, two other genetically determined traits are important in the pathogenesis of systemic lupus erythematosus. Hydralazine-induced lupus erythematosus affects females 4 times as frequently as males and the HLA-DR4 phenotype is evident significantly more often in patients with lupus than in controls.[91] Procainamide- or hydralazine-induced systemic lupus erythematosus is likely to be mild, but this is usually due to prevention of its full development by prompt withdrawal of the drug. However, where withdrawal is impractical, the full pathological picture including the typical renal changes may be seen.

Adverse reactions to the sulfapyridine component of sulfasalazine are more common in slow than in fast acetylators (see chapter 22; sect. 9.1).

The proportion of rapid and slow acetylators in a given population varies according to the ethnic group. Rapid acetylation is most common among Eskimos, Polynesians and Asians and lowest among some Mediterranean Jews and Egyptians (table VIII). Acetylation status can be determined by giving the patient a single dose of sulfadimidine and measuring the proportions of free and acetylated drug that appear in the plasma and urine.[94,95] The possibility that other factors such as pathophysiological states may also affect the acetylator phenotype must be considered, since patients with renal failure often appear to be slow acetylators.[81]

#### Drugs Metabolised by Oxidation

Oxidation is the major initial step in the metabolism of a large number of drugs. The rate of oxidation of a particular drug can vary considerably between individuals, but for most drugs

**Table IX.** Examples of genetically determined adverse reactions of pharmacodynamic origin (after La Du[99]; World Health Organization[5])

| Condition | Drug | Effects |
|---|---|---|
| **1. Quantitatively abnormal reactions** | | |
| Angle closure glaucoma | Atropine | Intraocular pressure increased |
| Down's syndrome | Atropine | Response increased |
| Muscular subaortic stenosis | Digitalis | Decreased cardiac output |
| **2. Qualitatively abnormal reactions** | | |
| Erythrocyte enzymatic deficiencies: | | |
| • Glucose-6-phosphate dehydrogenase | Oxidant drugs[a] | Haemolytic anaemia |
| • Methaemoglobin reductase | Oxidant drugs[a]<br>Nitrites | Methaemoglobinaemia |
| Haemoglobin variants: | | |
| • Haemoglobin H | Oxidant drugs[a] | Haemolytic anaemia |
| • Haemoglobin Zurich | Sulfonamides | Haemolytic anaemia |
| Malignant hyperpyrexia | General anaesthetics (halothane)<br>Muscle relaxants (suxamethonium) | Hyperthermia with prolonged muscle rigidity, acidosis |
| Genetic predisposition to open angle glaucoma, diabetes, pre-diabetes, certain myopes | Topical corticosteroids | Increased intraocular pressure. This may also make underlying open angle glaucoma more difficult to treat |
| Porphyria (hepatic) | Barbiturates[b]<br>Griseofulvin | Precipitate attack of porphyria |

a See text (section 4.2.2).
b See text (section 4.2.5) and table XI for other drugs.

the distribution curve is unimodal and the control of oxidative enzyme activity polygenetic. However, as with acetylation, population studies of the rates of oxidation of certain drugs have demonstrated a bimodal distribution, indicating oxidative polymorphism (see further chapter 1; sect. 4.2.2).

The best characterised example of polymorphic oxidation occurs with the antihypertensive drug debrisoquine. Mahgoub et al.[96] demonstrated two distinct phenotypes, 'extensive metabolisers' and 'poor metabolisers' of debrisoquine. Similar findings were reported for the antihypertensive (and oxytocic) agent sparteine,[97] and it was found that these two characteristics were related and controlled by the same genetic locus or two closely linked loci.[98] The incidence of the poor oxidiser phenotype is between 5 and 10% in Caucasians, but there are significantly different proportions in other populations.

There is evidence to suggest that a number of other clinically important drugs are affected by this polymorphism, including several β-adrenoceptor blocking drugs (e.g. metoprolol), tricyclic antidepressants (e.g. nortriptyline and desipramine), propafenone and possibly perhexiline and encainide. In addition, genetic polymorphism in other oxidative pathways not associated with the debrisoquine/sparteine polymorphism has been reported for an increasing number of drugs (see further chapter; 1 sect. 4.2.3).

The ability to genotype and phenotype patients for their ability to oxidise a variety of drugs is an area of active research, but the importance to safe and effective drug use of establishing the phenotype of a given patient where drugs with polymorphic oxidation are to be used is still a matter for debate. However, information obtained by the sparteine method that a patient is a poor metaboliser of perhexiline might allow some of the potentially serious adverse effects of that drug (e.g. peripheral neuropathy) to be avoided.[27,79]

#### *4.2.2 Genetically Determined Pharmacodynamic Reactions*

Genetically determined adverse reactions may be either normal responses that occur to an exaggerated extent (i.e. quantitatively abnormal) or novel pharmacodynamic effects (i.e. qualitatively abnormal) [table IX]. The latter are well illustrated by acute haemolytic anaemia precipitated by oxidant drugs.

Drug-induced haemolytic anaemia depends on several genetically determined aspects of red cell metabolism. The best known of these is an autonomous sex-linked deficiency of G6PD activity (table X). G6PD in sufficient amounts is required for the stability of red blood cells, particularly to protect them against the oxidative

**Table X.** Populations with more than 1% frequency of glucose-6-phosphate dehydrogenase (G6PD) deficiency in males (after World Health Organization[5])

| |
|---|
| African |
| All populations with African ancestry (i.e. American Negro, Puerto Rican) |
| Arabs (Egyptian, Kuwaiti, Lebanese) |
| Filipino |
| Greek |
| Indians (from Indian subcontinent) |
| Indonesian |
| Jew (primarily Oriental and Sephardic) |
| Kurd |
| Malaysian |
| Papua-New Guinean |
| Pakistani |
| Persian |
| Romanian |
| Sardinian |
| Sicilian |
| Southern Chinese |
| Thai |

stresses of substances which include the 8-aminoquinoline antimalarial, primaquine, many sulfonamides, nitrofurans (e.g. nitrofurantoin), sulfones (e.g. dapsone), quinine, and a variety of other drugs and chemicals, including naphthalene (see also chapter 26; sect. 5.2.2). Affected males carry the defect on their one X chromosome. Heterozygous females show intermediate sensitivity as both the defective gene on one of the X chromosomes and the normal allele on the other give expression, the latter reducing the effects of the former.

There is a great degree of genetic heterogeneity of G6PD, more than 80 different variants being recognised. Thus, the severity and duration of the haemolytic anaemia varies.[100] The African (A– type) variant, and the Mediterranean (B– type) variant have been studied in most detail.

The Mediterranean type, which is found in Greeks, Sardinians, Sephardic Jews, and Asian and northwest Indian peoples, is the more severe deficiency. It is affected by the widest range of drugs, and haemolytic episodes are not necessarily self-limiting. The variants of G6PD that are common in East and Southeast Asia (i.e. Canton and Union variants) differ from the Mediterranean and A– types, but it is likely that at least some of these may be as severe as the Mediterranean types. In patients with the A– type variant, haemolytic episodes may stop at intermediate levels of haemoglobin, even with continuation of a precipitating drug, and affect the older red cells which are destroyed in the initial haemolysis and replaced with younger ones. In the Mediterranean type, red cells of all ages are destroyed. The offending drug should be discontinued in both types.

Individuals with haemolytic anaemia due to the Mediterranean type deficiency may require transfusion. Acute infection, diabetic acidosis, liver failure and uraemia may also promote haemolysis. In some variants, the G6PD defect is associated with spontaneous haemolysis.

A deficiency of G6PD can lead to marked neonatal jaundice. In some cases, this may appear spontaneously, but other factors, particularly drugs, are usually involved. Any patient with haemolytic episodes (e.g. shivers, fever, often with back pain and dark urine due to free haemoglobin), particularly after administration of an oxidant drug, should be suspected of having G6PD deficiency. Family studies should be undertaken in proven cases and affected individuals given appropriate advice about medication to avoid, and also genetic counselling.[5] A number of tests are available for detecting G6PD deficiency; of these, the fluorescent spot test on blood collected on filter paper is the most specific and simple to perform.[101,102]

Other genetically determined red cell abnormalities, including unstable haemoglobin mutants (e.g. haemoglobin variants 'H' and 'Zurich'), may result in the production of haemolysis by drugs (see chapter 26; sect. 5.7.3); e.g. haemolysis induced by oxidant drugs in patients with haemoglobin H and by sulfonamides and primaquine in patients with haemoglobin Zurich. Several inherited biochemical lesions of the red blood cell are associated with the development of methaemoglobinaemia following administration of oxidant drugs. A deficiency of the enzyme methaemoglobin reductase may result in the development of methaemoglobinaemia and cyanosis when a patient is given drugs such as primaquine, chloroquine and dapsone, but anyone may develop methaemoglobinaemia and a degree of haemolysis when challenged with a sufficient dose of a strongly oxidant drug.

Malignant hyperpyrexia is a rare complication of general anaesthesia which presents as an emergency demanding immediate and expert management (see chapter 12; sects 2.2.1, 5.6). The basic defect is probably related to an abnormality of calcium regulation within voluntary muscle cells. The condition is inherited in all or at least a substantial number of cases. Affected members of a family usually have high resting serum creatine phosphokinase activity. The possibility cannot be excluded that some cases might occur without genetic predisposition. For a review of the whole area of drug-induced rhabdomyolysis, which is one of the severe complications of malignant hyperthermia, see Köppel.[103]

Continuous use of topical corticosteroid eye drops may produce a marked rise in intraocular pressure in some individuals (see chapter 15; sect. 3.10). The extent of increase in intraocular pressure is greater in those over 40 years, and also varies with genotype. Caucasian population studies have shown a trimodal distribution, 66% with low, 29% with intermediate and 5% with high pressure changes.[104]

#### *4.2.3 Genetic Factors and Drug Idiosyncrasy*

Metabolites of drugs may be responsible for hypersensitivity reactions, and therefore phenotypic differences in metabolism may result in variation in differential risk from hypersensitivity. The arene oxide metabolites of antiepileptic drugs such as phenytoin, phenobarbital and carbamazepine are probably responsible for the reaction of fever, skin rash, and lymphadenopathy which may proceed to hepatitis, nephritis and haematological abnormalities. There are genetic differences in epoxide hydroxylase activity, which may make some individuals unable to detoxify such metabolites. A predictive assay, based on patients' lymphocytes showing toxic drug metabolites generated in a mouse hepatic microsomal system, has been developed. Patients whose lymphocytes lack epoxide hydroxylase (and therefore show toxic damage in the test) correlate well with those who had exhibited the hypersensitivity syndrome. Patients with glutathione transferase deficiency may also be identified using a similar technique.[105]

The liver damage from halothane is of 2 types: a mild form occurring in about 25 to 30% of cases with disturbances of transaminases and glutathione-*S*-transferase only, and a second form which seems to be immune-mediated and results in severe liver necrosis. The incidence of this severe type is about 1 in 3500 to 1 in 35,000. It seems that there may be genetic differences in reductive metabolism to account for some of these cases. The metabolism of sulfonamides has been mentioned previously (see section 4.2.1), but in addition to problems of slow acetylation, defective hydroxylamine detoxification may be linked to hypersensitivity to these drugs.[106]

#### *4.2.4 Possible Genetically Determined Reactions of Undetermined Origin*

Jaundice with oral contraceptives is rare, except in Sweden[107] and Chile.[108] A genetically determined increased risk of developing hormonal steroid-induced cholestasis is possible.

Erythropoiesis may be impaired, often after the second week, in patients receiving chloramphenicol but usually recovers quickly when the drug is stopped. This is associated with an impairment of incorporation of iron into haem. There is another mechanism operating in patients who develop aplastic anaemia, which is either irreversible or which recovers only after a prolonged period.[109] This may be related to a chloramphenicol metabolite, nitrosochloramphenicol, which inhibits DNA synthesis. Although reducing compounds produced by the effect of gut flora on chloramphenicol may contribute to this toxicity, genetic variation in metabolism or some other genetic defect is suggested by its occurrence in identical twins exposed to chloramphenicol.[110]

Phenothiazine-induced agranulocytosis tends to occur early in treatment.[111] If the patient has not developed this adverse effect within 3 months, it is not likely to develop. Low-dose phenothiazines, such as prochlorperazine, produce agranulocytosis less often than those with which higher dosage is required, such as chlorpromazine. Chlorpromazine-sensitive patients may have a cellular defect, involving the final step of DNA synthesis, which limits incorporation of thymidine triphosphate into DNA. This type of reaction may occur in patients with limited proliferative potential of bone marrow cells, thus reducing the compensatory bone marrow response during treatment with a drug which ordinarily has little bone marrow toxicity.

The introduction of the antipsychotic drug clozapine into Finland was shortly followed by a disconcerting incidence of agranulocytosis, despite extensive prior safe use elsewhere in Europe.[112,113] This drug can, however, be used safely by monitoring the white blood count weekly for 18 weeks and then monthly, taking action as appropriate to the cell count. The tetracyclic antidepressant mianserin has also been reported as producing a higher incidence of agranulocytosis in Finland and New Zealand than in many other countries.[114]

**Table XI.** Drugs reported as hazardous in porphyria[a]

| |
|---|
| **Antimicrobial agents:** |
| Dapsone |
| Griseofulvin |
| Pyrazinamide |
| Sulfonamides |
| **Anaesthetic agents:** |
| Barbiturates[b] |
| **Antiepileptics:**[c] |
| Barbiturates[c] |
| Hydantoins (phenytoin, mephenytoin) |
| Carbamazepine |
| Succinimides |
| **Antianxiety drugs/hypnosedatives:**[c] |
| Glutethimide |
| Methyprylon |
| Meprobamate |
| **Antidiabetic agents:** |
| Sulphonylureas |
| **Antihypertensives:** |
| Methyldopa |
| **Opioid analgesics:** |
| Pentazocine |
| **Nonsteroidal anti-inflammatory drugs/analgesics:** |
| Propyphenazone (isopropylphenazone) |
| Aminophenazone (amidopyrine) |
| Phenazone (antipyrine) |
| Phenylbutazone |
| **Miscellaneous:** |
| Ethanol |
| Oral contraceptives[d] |

a This table is not comprehensive, and because of the criteria applied for inclusion of drugs, it is conservative (see text).

b Attacks are generally more severe when multiple barbiturate therapy is given to porphyric patients than when single drugs are used. Exposure to thiopental and phenobarbital does not always lead to an acute attack. A past history of uneventful usage of a drug does not guarantee freedom from danger on subsequent exposure.

c 'At risk' individuals should be advised that over-the-counter medicines may contain potentially dangerous tranquillosedative agents.

d Oral contraceptives are among the most common identifiable precipitating factors in the acute porphyric attack.

Extreme inherent susceptibility may also be encountered from time to time, e.g. to anticoagulants.[115] Although such reactions are of the same character as the intended therapeutic effect, the potentially highly dangerous and even fatal effects that may result from extreme susceptibility must lead them to be regarded as adverse reactions.

#### *4.2.5 Genetic Diseases Associated with Abnormal Responses to Drugs*

An important example of genetic disorders with altered drug sensitivity is precipitation of porphyria by drugs.[116,117] The hepatic porphyrias constitute several genetically distinct disorders which involve the metabolic pathway of porphyrins and haem biosynthesis in the liver. One feature of the disorders is overproduction of the rate-limiting enzyme δ-aminolevulinic acid (ALA) synthetase in the liver. Variation in an operator gene which is poorly responsive to the normal repressor (haem) may underlie the disorder. A number of drugs which induce hepatic ALA synthetase may precipitate clinical attacks when given in usual therapeutic doses to patients in remission or with latent disease. A list of the major drugs that may precipitate attacks of porphyria is given in table XI.[118]

Three types of porphyria, acute intermittent, variegate and porphyria cutanea tarda may be drug-induced. The clinical features include combinations of abdominal colic, vomiting and severe constipation, peripheral neuritis, severe psychological disturbances, and cutaneous photodermatoses. An attack may be precipitated by a single dose of one of the drugs listed in table XI but may not necessarily occur each time it is taken or, in another patient, may require a number of relatively large doses. Porphyrinogenic drugs may lead to profound quadriplegia and bulbar involvement, resulting, without adequate support, in respiratory failure and death.

### 4.3 Other Reactions Due to Inherent Patient Susceptibility

#### *4.3.1 Age*

Elderly patients are at risk from drug toxicity when the very substantial reductions in clearance that occur with increasing age are not appreciated and adjustments are not made to dosage (see further chapter 4; sect. 2.1.3). This is particularly likely to occur when the normal plasma half-life of the drug is long. An example is piroxicam, which has a normal half-life of 48 hours that extends to 72 hours in patients over 70 years of age. With daily administration of piroxicam for 2 weeks, the body content would be about 4 times that after the first dose. Serious side effects could be avoided only by a substantial reduction of the dose after the first week or a substantial increase of the dosage interval.

Young infants, particularly neonates, are also susceptible to drug toxicity by virtue of their incompletely developed hepatic and renal mechanisms for drug elimination (see further chapter 3; sect. 2.4). Young people may also be peculiarly susceptible to some drug-induced effects. The severity that dystonic side effects from phenothiazines may assume in healthy young people is quite astonishing, not to say frightening for the patient (and the clinician) and includes oculogyric crises and opisthotonus. Females appear to be more susceptible than males, and children under 15 years of age show the most severe and most bizarre neuromuscular symptoms.[119]

#### 4.3.2 Asthma

If the existence of an asthmatic tendency is overlooked and a β-blocker is prescribed, the results may be disastrous. Even relatively $\beta_1$-selective agents can have significant $\beta_2$-adrenoceptor blocking properties. Between attacks, this may not seem to alter the patient's well-being, but during an acute attack, the severity of bronchospasm may be much greater. It has also been suggested that anaphylaxis in the presence of a β-blocker may be worsened and more difficult to treat. In this instance, it is both the bronchospasm and the hypotension that may be worsened.

#### 4.3.3 Pregnancy

There are physiological changes in pregnancy that may affect drug disposition (see further chapter 2, sect. 4.1 and chapter 18; sect. 1). In general, the changes are more likely to alter drug handling in such a way as to reduce effectiveness, and perhaps therefore some dose-related adverse effects. For example, the plasma volume increases by a mean maximum of about 40%, and the interstitial fluid volume is proportionately less in the first 2 trimesters. There is an accelerated expansion of the latter in the third trimester, and then a slow reduction to normal in the first 2 postpartum months. These effects generally mean that the doses of water soluble drugs may need to be increased during pregnancy. In this regard, the NSAIDs will enhance fluid retention and should be used with caution.

Cardiac output and renal blood flow are increased during pregnancy (up to 25% in the first 2 trimesters and then falling in the third) with an increase in glomerular filtration of about 50%; consequently, the renal clearance of some drugs is enhanced. Although slower gastic emptying and reduced intestinal motility are a feature of pregnancy, there seems to be no clinically significant alteration in drug absorption.

Changes in liver function, particularly in the third trimester, may influence the occurrence of adverse effects. Sulfation and oxidation are decreased, even though other enzyme activity is increased. There is also a special drug-induced 'acute fatty liver of pregnancy' associated with the tetracyclines and valproic acid. Much more needs to be learned about these effects, but it is clear that care should be taken with drugs that are metabolised in the liver, particularly late in pregnancy.

Care should also be taken late in pregnancy with drugs that might impair blood clotting. Clearly, fibrinolytics and anticoagulants need very special consideration and are generally to be avoided. Heparin is a safer anticoagulant to use with its short half-life and reversibility. Aspirin and probably other NSAIDs will increase blood loss during parturition.

The physiological changes of pregnancy may result in particular medical problems such as vomiting, heartburn, constipation, urinary tract infection, hypertension, convulsions, and diabetes. Drug treatments may therefore be necessary, but should *always* be considered with great care (see further chapter 2).

## 5. Reactions Due to Acquired Patient Anomalies

By altering the pharmacokinetic handling of or tissue response to a drug, the pathophysiological condition of the patient can increase the susceptibility to adverse reactions. Thus, an associated disease (i.e. a disease for which treatment is not primarily intended) or intercurrent illness must always be considered to have the potential to modify the effects of existing treatment. In particular, hepatic and renal disease may alter the pharmacokinetic handling of many drugs and may result in abnormal drug responses. However, it should be noted that hypoalbuminaemia and changes in protein binding do not usually result in altered drug responses since in the absence of concomitant changes in intrinsic clearance (i.e. hepatic metabolism or renal excretion), such changes do not lead to altered unbound drug concentrations (see further chapter 1; sect. 3.2.3 and chapter 5; sect. 1.6.3).

### 5.1 Liver Disease

An increased susceptibility to drug reactions in liver disease can occur as a result of altered pharmacokinetic handling not only because of decreased hepatic clearance, but also possibly as a result of altered sensitivity due in part to the general metabolic disturbance. The processing of drugs by the liver to permit their elimination from the body gives the liver a central role. Consequently, liver disease is of particular importance as a potential source of untoward reactions resulting from excessively high plasma concentrations of drugs mainly eliminated by this route.

It is not easy to predict which patients with hepatic disease will have impaired drug metabolism, and indeed many such patients may react normally to drugs.[120] Although some mechanisms such as bilirubin secretion may be impaired, liver enzymes may continue to metabolise drugs normally. It appears that the efficiency with which a drug is metabolised by the liver, the extent of binding to blood constituents, and the aetiology and stage of hepatic disorder are all important in determining whether significant alterations in drug disposition will occur. If liver disease is severe (as in hepatic cirrhosis), the rate of metabolism of drugs such as lidocaine can be markedly impaired and there are other occasional examples of excessive clinical susceptibility to adverse reactions (see table III).[121]

Abnormal responses to drugs in liver disease may also occur as a result of susceptibility to the action of the drug. It is a common clinical experience that morphine may precipitate coma and that hypnotics may cause profound sleep in patients with severe hepatic disease.[122,123] Patients with cirrhosis are also extremely sensitive to chlorpromazine and to MAOIs.[124] Incautious diuretic therapy can precipitate hepatic coma in susceptible patients with cirrhotic oedema and ascites.[121,125]

It is not surprising that it is difficult to recommend useful tests for predicting an extent of liver injury that will result in problems of drug handling. Hepatic enzymes may be very elevated without real impairment of liver function; tests of liver metabolic capacity such as the prothrombin time and bilirubin level are better indicators, but still may not relate to altered drug elimination. The difficulty is probably related to the multiplicity of metabolic operations the liver performs and the fact that some may be preserved depending on the kind of liver damage existing. A reasonable rule is to be cautious if prothrombin metabolism is impaired (this is a simple test available almost anywhere), and to be very careful when the clinical picture indicates global liver damage, such as in cirrhosis or when the bilirubin level is rising and albumin levels are falling.

The pharmacological basis for adverse drug effects in liver disease is discussed in more detail in chapter 22 (sect. 12.4). That chapter also gives a number of examples of untoward effects and provides guidelines for safe prescribing in liver disease. Appendix F provides guidelines for modification of drug dosage in liver disease.

### 5.2 Renal Disease

Diseases of the kidney may profoundly alter drug kinetics and occasionally alter sensitivity to drugs. In addition, some drugs may themselves exacerbate renal disease. Thus, renal disease frequently leads to adverse reactions, especially when renal excretion contributes importantly to elimination of the particular drug or its pharmacologically active metabolite (see further chapter 24; sect. 1).

Digoxin clearance is approximately equivalent to creatinine clearance and when the latter is reduced, a dosage appropriate for patients with normal renal function will inevitably lead to high plasma concentrations with serious risk of digitalis toxicity. Aminoglycoside antibiotic ototoxicity is likely in patients with renal insufficiency, unless appropriate dosage adjustment is made. Some adverse drug reactions are virtually confined to patients with impaired renal function. Peripheral neuritis due to nitrofurantoin occurs almost (although not quite) exclusively in patients with impaired renal function.[126] Cyanide toxicity resulting from the use of sodium nitroprusside (a vasodilator used in hypertensive emergencies) is much more likely in patients with severe renal disease.[127]

Patients with chronic renal failure are especially prone to neuropsychiatric reactions.[128] This is thought to be due partly to an accumulation of drugs normally excreted by the kidney, and partly to susceptibility of the central nervous system in uraemic patients (e.g. synergism between uraemic somnolence and the CNS depressant effects of opioid drugs). Synergism between pathological substrates in uraemia, the presence of electrolyte and acid-base disturbance, and drugs which increase myocardial irritability may promote arrhythmias. It is possible that in uraemic patients, the body membranes may be generally altered so that drugs may enter anatomical areas from which they are normally excluded.[128,129]

Polar drug derivatives ordinarily eliminated promptly by the kidney may accumulate in the presence of renal disease, e.g. the glucuronide conjugates of clofibrate.[130,131] Additional examples of enhanced susceptibility to drug toxicity in renal disease are discussed in chapter 24 (sect. 9). Guidelines for modification of usual drug dosages and the principles of safe prescribing of drugs in renal disease are also given in chapter 24 (sect. 11), and in appendices D and E.

### 5.3 Acquired Drug Receptor Anomalies

Occasionally, acquired drug receptor anomalies may result in altered sensitivity. The basis of this may be some metabolic alteration of the target organ. Examples include enhanced susceptibility to the toxic effects of digoxin in the presence of potassium depletion, and the excessive depressant effects which may result from hypnotics in patients with respiratory depression or hypopituitarism. Other examples are given in table III.

## 6. Reactions Due to Anomalies of Drug Presentation

Substitution of drug products with different bioavailabilities is an important potential cause of toxicity with certain drugs. This is illustrated by the epidemic of phenytoin intoxication that occurred some years ago in Australia[132] and New Zealand[133] due to increased absorption following removal of calcium sulfate from the capsule excipient. A more obvious problem is the substitution of sustained release for standard preparations without careful consideration of dosage (and clear instructions to the patient). Different sustained release products of the same active drug may behave differently.

Outdated and poorly stored products may also cause toxicity.[134] Poorly formulated liquid preparations permitting unduly rapid sedimentation of the active ingredient may lead to dangerous inequality of dosage.

Counterfeiting of drugs is now a problem in many countries. Containers and labels are often well reproduced, but the active ingredients may be altered or even missing and tablets may often crumble in their falsified packages or be so hard as to totally survive passage through the gastrointestinal tract.

Very serious results may follow the accidental introduction of therapeutic substances intra-arterially. Most often this has involved accidental introduction of intravenous anaesthetic agents into the brachial artery,[135] but it has occurred following injection of penicillin into the buttock,[136] with local gangrene and severe damage to the lower limb. The problem is also common among drug addicts who inject themselves in many body sites. One such person in my experience who, after failing to keep patent veins in his arms, legs and penis, accidentally injected his temporal artery, experienced scalp necrosis.

Unduly rapid infusion is a potential cause of reactions, some of which may be of an unexpected character, e.g. hypocalcaemic tetany from rapid intravenous infusion of tetracyclines[137] and cardiac arrhythmias from rapid intravenous infusion of lincomycin.[138]

With some drugs, frequency of dosage may be more important in determining adverse reactions than total dosage. For example, in patients receiving methotrexate for treatment of recalcitrant psoriasis, the prevalence of cirrhosis and fibrosis is significantly greater in those treated with frequent small doses than in those treated with intermittent large doses, even though the dose level (in mg/month) and the therapeutic effect is similar in both groups.[139] With low-dose methotrexate, greater cumulative dosage is associated with hepatic toxicity over a long period of time. However, use of low initial doses and good monitoring allow this toxic drug to be used in severe psoriasis.[140]

## 7. Drug Withdrawal Reactions

Sudden cessation of treatment may have serious results, sometimes due to alterations in receptor responsiveness that occurs during therapy. Most notorious are those resulting from the withdrawal of opioids (see chapter 30; sect. 12.3). However, sudden withdrawal of antiepileptics or even benzodiazepine hypnosedatives may also precipitate withdrawal syndromes that may include worsened symptoms of underlying diseases, as well as severe convulsions even in those whose primary disease was not epilepsy.

Abrupt discontinuation of tricyclic antidepressants and lithium may also lead to a recurrence of underlying disease. Sudden withdrawal of clonidine for hypertension can cause a rapid rise in blood pressure to pretreatment levels, although serious rebound with significant risk of a cerebrovascular accident seems likely only when fairly large doses have been used. Sudden cessation of methyldopa has also been followed

**Table XII.** Stereoselective drug interactions with warfarin: effects on individual enantiomer clearance (after Scott[143])

| Interacting drug | *R*-warfarin clearance | *S*-warfarin clearance |
|---|---|---|
| Amiodarone | ↓ | ↓ |
| Cimetidine | ↓ | |
| Cotrimoxazole (trimethoprim/sulfa-methoxazole) | ↑ | ↓ |
| Enoxacin | ↓ (6-hydroxylation) | |
| Metronidazole | | ↓ |
| Phenylbutazone | Complex effects | ↓ |
| Rifampicin | ↑ | ↑ |
| Sulfinpyrazone | ↑ | ↓ |

*Symbols:* ↓ = reduced; ↑ = increased.

occasionally by severe rebound hypertension, while abrupt withdrawal of β-blockers in ischaemic heart disease may be followed by tachycardia, relative ischaemia and myocardial damage. There have also been a few reports of a similar rebound effect to that seen with the β-blockers when calcium antagonists such as diltiazem and verapamil are suddenly withdrawn.

The sudden withdrawal of corticosteroids may result in an adrenal crisis if greater than 'replacement' doses are used, i.e. 5 to 7.5mg of prednisolone daily or equivalent for more than a few days. In addition, intercurrent illness may necessitate an increase in dosage. Apart from the above, recrudescence of treated disease may occur, psychological dependence on corticosteroids has been reported, and children have developed a syndrome with benign raised intracranial pressure on drug withdrawal. Patients on long term corticosteroids should carry a card warning that they are on those drugs and of the need to continue or even increase therapy in an emergency.

Discontinuation of antipsychotic drugs may result in extrapyramidal syndromes and psychiatric disturbances, and sudden withdrawal of anti-Parkinsonian drugs, particularly amantadine, may be followed by severe, even life-threatening exacerbation of the underlying condition.[141]

## 8. Reactions Due to Interaction of Drugs

There are many potential interactions possible, based on theoretical considerations, animal experiments or documented cases, but few have real clinical significance (see further chapter 7 and appendix B). However, the reality of the risk of interaction must always be borne in mind when more than one drug is being prescribed, particularly if they share the same metabolic pathways for their degradation or have effects on the same target, e.g. the use together of β-adrenoceptor agonists and antagonists – a fairly nonproductive therapeutic exercise.

As shown in table V, the incidence of adverse reactions increases with the number of drugs in use. Drug interactions, however, appear to make up only a small proportion of all adverse reactions. In reports to the New Zealand Committee on Adverse Drug Reactions, interactions accounted for only some 2%. In a published report of interaction frequency,[142] of 3600 reactions involving 83,200 drugs administered, 6.9% were considered to be due to drug interactions.

The mechanisms and determinants of adverse drug interactions are discussed in chapter 7.

## 9. Stereoisomerism (Chirality) and Adverse Reactions

Several drugs exist as enantiomeric mixtures (racemates). Sometimes one enantiomer has the beneficial effect while the other is toxic or has toxic potential. A couple of examples will suffice to show the nature of the problem. Table XII lists some of the drugs that interact with *R*- and *S*-warfarin. *S*-Warfarin is more rapidly cleared than *R*-warfarin but is about 3 times more potent as an anticoagulant. From the table it is clear that an interaction involving metronidazole will have a much greater effect than one with enoxacin.

A more obvious problem occurs with verapamil. *l*-Verapamil is extensively metabolised in the first pass through the liver and is the enantiomer which is most potently negatively inotropic and chronotropic. It follows that if the drug is given intravenously rather than orally, for the same vasodilating effect there will be greater cardiac depression, since first-pass hepatic metabolism is bypassed (see fig. 4). Thus, intravenous verapamil is likely to be associated with hypotension, bradycardia, heart block and asystole if not used cautiously. For a review of this topic, see Scott.[143]

## 10. Secondary Drug Problems (in a Treated Individual)

In clinical practice, the primary adverse reaction may be hidden or have been missed. A secondary clinical problem might then consid-

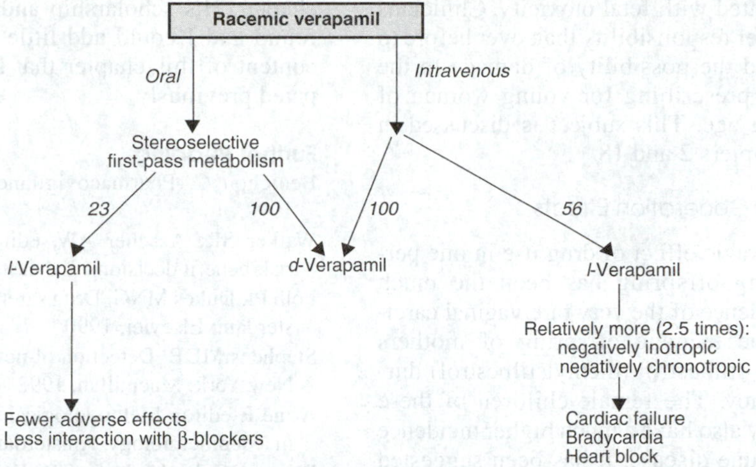


**Fig. 4.** Stereoselective pharmacokinetics and pharmacodynamics of verapamil. The numbers represent the relative amounts of the *d*- and *l*-enantiomers found in the systemic circulation following oral and intravenous administration (after Scott[143]).

erably confuse the issue and lead to missed diagnoses. Some examples will illustrate the problem. If an elderly person falls and fractures a hip, the fact that he or she is taking a benzodiazepine hypnotic or amiodarone may go unremarked in a busy surgical ward. However, daytime somnolence after a benzodiazepine or ataxia from amiodarone may have been the basic cause of the accident.

As a second, more complex, example, an 83-year-old man was given furosemide for mild cardiac failure. This resulted in the rare complication of vasculitis. Since he was disabled following a previous stroke, the vasculitis affecting his feet was at first mistaken for bed sores. The pain from the lesions was intense enough to need morphine sedation, which in turn led to respiratory depression, bronchopneumonia and death. Here, early recognition of the real problem and discontinuation of the furosemide might have avoided the use of morphine.

***Effects of drugs on endogenous microflora:*** diarrhoea, or even pseudomembranous colitis, are hazards of the use of broad-spectrum antibacterial agents (see further chapter 22; sect. 10.2.1). So, too, are oral and genital candidiasis. Again, clinicians must anticipate the possibility of complications of this type when prescribing antibacterial drugs.

Use of inhaled corticosteroids may result in overgrowth of *Candida* sp. in the mouth and nasopharynx, while use of systemic and topical corticosteroids may result in candidal overgrowth in skin folds and the genitalia.

## 11. Indirect Reactions (on a Third Party, not the Treated Patient)

### 11.1 Fetal Malformations

The thalidomide disaster focused attention on the whole problem of adverse drug reactions, and avoidance of fetal malformations assumed paramount importance in regulatory decisions on the release of medicines for marketing. Until relatively recently, evidence of teratogenicity in animal studies precluded further progression of a drug's development.

However, a relaxation of this prohibition has allowed two drugs with known potential as animal teratogens to be marketed: the retinoic acid derivatives etretinate and isotretinoin have been shown to be extremely effective in conglobate acne and psoriasis resistant to other treatments. Despite instances of malformation in infants of women who had taken each of these medicines during the vulnerable early weeks of pregnancy (even though they had signed informed consent that they had been warned to use adequate contraception during and after the use of these drugs), they join other drugs, which by reason of inescapable need such as warfarin and antiepileptics, have continued in use despite the potential risk.

Other currently used drugs that also have an acknowledged capacity to cause damage to the developing fetus include the tetracyclines and aminoglycosides. The tetracyclines can cause staining of developing teeth, while aminoglycosides such as kanamycin and streptomycin have been associated with fetal otoxicity. Clinicians have a greater responsibility than ever before to bear in mind the possibility of damage to the fetus when prescribing for young women of childbearing age. This subject is discussed in detail in chapters 2 and 18.

### 11.2 Third Generation Effects

Another tragic effect of drug use in one person affecting offspring has been the much greater incidence of the very rare vaginal carcinoma in the teenage offspring of mothers treated with stilbestrol (diethylstilbestrol) during pregnancy. The female children of these mothers may also have a much higher incidence of autoimmune disease. It has been suggested that these effects may also be seen in the third generation offspring.[144]

### 11.3 Effects of Drug Treatment on Other Third Parties

There are several reports of aggressive behaviour and even homicide related to such apparently innocuous drugs as antihistamines, benzodiazepines and cimetidine. These cases are relatively rare and as such, form the subject of contentious legal wrangles and scientific debate over causality.[145]

It is also clear that drugs may affect a patient's control of machinery or their driving ability, and this may result in injury to third parties. Allergies are also possible in third parties following contact with topical preparations, e.g. vaginal creams and pessaries.

## 12. Responsibilities of the Prescriber

It is important to conclude this chapter with the revelation that in one study of 30,195 hospital inpatients, 3.7% had disabling injuries due to their therapy.[146] Of these injuries, 19% were due to drugs and thus formed the most common adverse event group. In 58% of the total adverse events, there appeared to be errors in management, nearly half of which were adjudged 'negligent'. Not only should we try to minimise all errors in judgement in the choice and use of treatment, but we should also remember again that a positive approach to the patient, adequately explaining the why, how and when of treatment as well as its benefits and risks, will achieve the best results in the end.

**Acknowledgement**

I wish to express my admiration for Professor Garth McQueen, the previous author of this chapter. His scholarship and wisdom are profound and I could add little to the layout and content of this chapter that he had not anticipated previously.

### Further Reading

Benichou C. Pharmacovigilance. Editions Pradel, 1992.

Walker SR, Asscher AW, editors. Medicines and risk/benefit decisions. Lancaster: MTP Press, 1987

Folb PI, Dukes MNG. Drug safety in pregnancy. Amsterdam: Elsevier, 1990

Stephens MDB. Detection of new adverse reactions. New York: Macmillan, 1992

Arme P, editor. Methodological approaches in pharmacoepidemiology. Amsterdam: Elsevier, 1993

Briggs GG, Bodendorfer TW, Freeman RK, et al., editors. Drugs in pregnancy and lactation. Baltimore: Williams & Wilkins, 1993

Folb PI, editor. Drug safety in clinical practice. Berlin: Springer-Verlag, 1984

Vestal RE, editor. Drug treatment in the elderly. Sydney: ADIS Health Science Press, 1984

Strom BL, editor. Pharmacoepidemiology. 2nd edition. New York: John Wiley & Sons, 1994

### Reference Texts

Dollery C, Davies DM, editors. Textbook of adverse drug reactions, Vol. 2, Oxford: Oxford University Press, 1991

Dukes MNG, editor. Meyler's side effects of drugs, Vol. 12 and Annual supplements. Amsterdam: Excerpta Medica, 1992

Watkins J, Levy CJ. Guide to immediate anaesthetic reactions. Butterworths, 1988

### References

1. Jick H. Adverse drug reactions. The magnitude of the problem. Journal of Allergy and Clinical Immunology 1984; 74: 555
2. Koch-Weser J. Fatal reactions to drug therapy. New England Journal of Medicine 1974; 291: 302
3. Venning GR. Rare and serious adverse reactions. Medical Toxicology and Adverse Drug Experience 1987; 2: 235
4. Stephens MDB. Detection of new adverse drug reactions. 3rd ed. New York: Macmillan, 1992
5. World Health Organization. Technical Report Series No. 524. Pharmacogenetics. Geneva: WHO, 1973
6. Naranjo CA, Lanctôt KL. Recent developments in computer-assisted diagnosis of putative adverse drug reactions. Drug Safety 1991; 6: 315
7. Rawlins MD, Thompson JW. Mechanism of adverse drug reactions. In: Davies DM, editor. Textbook of adverse drug reactions. 4th ed. Oxford: Oxford Medical Publications, 1991: 18-45
8. Flegg P, Cheong I, Welsby PD. Chloramphenicol - are concerns about aplastic anaemia justified? Drug Safety 1992; 7: 167
9. Kauffman RE, Kearns GL. Pharmacokinetic studies in paediatric patients: clinical and ethical considerations. Clinical Pharmacokinetics 1992; 23: 10-29

10. Gilman JT, Gal P. Pharmacokinetic and pharmacodynamic data collection in children and neonates: a quiet frontier. Clinical Pharmacokinetics 1992; 23: 1-9
11. McEwen J. Improving adverse drug reaction monitoring. Medical Toxicology and Adverse Drug Experience 1987; 2: 398
12. Edwards IR. Adverse drug reaction monitoring - the practicalities. Medical Toxicology and Adverse Drug Experience 1987; 2: 405
13. Bem JL, Wood SM, West L, et al. 25 years of the Committee on Safety of Medicines - an international perspective of the benefits. Drug Safety 1990; 5: 161
14. Strom BL, editor. Pharmacoepidemiology. 2nd ed. New York: John Wiley & Sons, 1994
15. Dukes MNG, editor. Meyler's side effects of drugs. Vol. 12 and Annual Supplements. Amsterdam: Excerpta Medica, 1992
16. Kellerman G, Luyten-Kellermann M, Homing MG, et al. Elimination of antipyrine and benzo(a)pyrene metabolism in cultured human lymphocytes. Clinical Pharmacology and Therapeutics 1976; 20: 72
17. Giudicelli JF, Tillement JP. Influence of sex on drug kinetics in man. Clinical Pharmacokinetics 1977; 2: 157
18. Wilson K. Sex-related differences in drug disposition in man. Clinical Pharmacokinetics 1984; 9: 189
19. Coulter DM, Edwards IR. Cough associated with captopril and enalapril. British Medical Journal 1987; 294: 1521-3
20. Smidt NA, McQueen EG. Adverse reactions to drugs: a comprehensive hospital inpatient survey. New Zealand Medical Journal 1972; 76: 397
21. Smith JW, Seidl LG, Cluff LE. Studies on the epidemiology and adverse drug reactions. Annals of Internal Medicine 1966; 65: 629
22. Hurwitz N. Predisposing factors in adverse reactions to drugs. British Medical Journal 1969; 1: 536
23. Levy M, Nir I, Birnbaum D, et al. Adverse reactions to drugs in hospitalised medical patients. Israel Journal of Medical Sciences 1973; 9: 617
24. Lawson DH, Jick H. Drug prescribing in hospitals: an international comparison. American Journal of Public Health 1976; 66: 644
25. May FE, Stewart RB, Cluff LE. Drug interactions and multiple drug administration. Clinical Pharmacology and Therapeutics 1977; 22: 322
26. Kellaway GS, McCrae E. Intensive monitoring for adverse drug effects in patients discharged from acute medical wards. New Zealand Medical Journal 1973; 78: 525
27. Clark DWJ, Edwards IR. Adverse drug reaction reporting and retrospective phenotyping for oxidation polymorphism. Medical Toxicology and Adverse Drug Experience 1988; 3: 241
28. McKenzie KJ, Crowcroft NS. Race, ethnicity, culture and science. British Medical Journal 1994; 309: 286-7
29. Senior PA, Bhopal R. Ethnicity as a variable in epidemiological research. British Medical Journal 1994; 309: 327-30
30. McQueen EG. Pharmacological basis of adverse drug reactions. In: Speight TM, editor. Drug treatment. 3rd ed. Auckland: Adis Press, 1987: 223-54
31. Barkow R, editor. The Merck Manual, 16th ed. Rahway: Merck Research Laboratories, 1992: 342
32. Mitchell JA, Gillam EMJ, Stanley LA, et al. Immunotoxic side-effects of drug therapy. Drug Safety 1990; 5: 168
33. Gleichmann E, Kimber I, Purchase IFH. Immunotoxicology: suppressive and stimulatory effects of drugs and environmental chemicals on the immune system. Archives of Toxicology 1989; 63: 257
34. Coleman JW. Allergic reactions to drugs: current concepts and problems. Clinical and Experimental Allergy 1990; 20: 79
35. Weiss ME. Drug allergy. Medical Clinics of North America 1992; 76: 857
36. Anderson JA. Allergic reactions to drugs and biological agents. Journal of the American Medical Association 1992; 268: 2845
37. Thomassen D. Effect of stress on drug hypersensitivity. Drug Safety 1991; 6: 235
38. Uetrecht JP. The role of leukocyte-generated reactive metabolites in the pathogenesis of idiosyncratic drug reactions. Drug Metabolism Reviews 1992; 24: 299
39. Parker CW. Drug allergy. New England Journal of Medicine 1975; 292: 511, 732, 957
40. Batchelor FR, Dewdney J, Feinberg JG, et al. A penicilloylated protein impurity as a source of allergy to benzylpenicillin and 6-aminopenicillanic acid. Lancet 1967; 1: 1175
41. Harle DG, Baldo BA, Fisher MM. Detection of IgE antibodies to suxamethonium after anaphylactoid reactions during anaesthesia. Lancet 1984; 1: 930
42. Stewart GT. Allergenic residues in penicillins. Lancet 1967; 1: 1177
43. Bird AG. 'Allergic' drug reactions during anaesthesia. Adverse Drug Reactions Bulletin Feb, 1985; No. 110: 408
44. Beutler E. Drug-induced haemolytic anaemia. Pharmacological Reviews 1969; 21: 73
45. Ackroyd JF. The role of Sedormid in the immunological reaction that results in platelet lysis in Sedormid purpura. Clinical Science 1954; 13: 409
46. Pujet J-C, Homberg J-C, Decroix G. Sensitivity to rifampicin: incidence, mechanism and prevention. British Medical Journal 1974; 2: 415
47. Weitzman SA, Stossel TP. Drug-induced immunological neutropenia. Lancet 1978; 1: 1068
48. Husseri FE, Messerli FH. Adverse effects of antihypertensive drugs. Drugs 1981; 22: 188
49. Lindberg J, Lindholdm A, Lundin P, et al. Trigger factors and HL-A antigens in chronic active hepatitis. British Medical Journal 1975; 4: 77
50. Maddrey WC, Boitnott JK. Drug-induced chronic liver disease. Gastroenterology 1977; 72: 1348
51. Zimmerman HJ. Drug-induced liver disease. Drugs 1978; 16: 25
52. Horowitz HI, Nachman RL. Drug purpura. Seminars in Haematology 1965; 2: 287
53. Goldstein A, Aronow L, Kalman SM, editors. Principles of drug action. 2nd ed. New York: Wiley, 1974
54. Coombs RRA, Gell PGH. Classification of allergic reactions responsible for clinical hypersensitivity and disease. In: Gell & Coombs, editors. Clinical aspects of immunology. 2nd ed. Oxford: Blackwell, 1968: 575
55. Brown P, Baddeley H, Read AE, et al. Sclerosing peritonitis, an usual reaction to a β-adrenergic-blocking drug (practolol). Lancet 1974; 2: 1477
56. Koch-Weser J. Coumarin necrosis. Annals of Internal Medicine 1968; 68: 1365
57. Lipsky BA, Hirschmann JV. Drug fever. Journal of the American Medical Association 1981; 245: 851
58. Simmonds J, Hodges S, Nicol F, et al. Anaphylaxis after oral penicillin. British Medical Journal 1978; 2: 1404
59. Parker AC, Richmond J. Reduction in incidence of rash using polymer-free ampicillin. British Medical Journal 1976; 1: 998
60. Bayard PJ, Berger TG, Jacobson MA. Drug hypersensitivity reactions and human immunodeficiency virus disease. Journal of Acquired Immune Deficiency Syndromes 1992; 5: 1237
61. Becker LC. Allergy in systemic lupus erythematosus. Johns Hopkins Medical Journal 1973; 133: 38
62. Girard JP, Cueras M. Clinical and immunologic analysis of 1047 allergic reactions to penicillin. Schweizerische Medizinische Wochenschrift 1975; 105: 953
63. Sogn DD. Penicillin allergy. Journal of Allergy and Clinical Immunology 1984; 74: 589

64. Petz LD. Immunologic reactions of humans to cephalosporins. Postgraduate Medical Journal 1971 Feb; 47 Suppl. 64
65. Green GR, Peters GA, Geraci JE. Treatment of bacterial endocarditis in patients with penicillin hypersensitivity. Annals of Internal Medicine 1966; 64: 1170
66. Dove AF, Thomas DJB, Aronstam A, et al. Haemolytic anaemia due to penicillin. British Medical Journal 1975; 3: 684
67. McPherson AJ, Parkin JD, Hope R. Penicillin-induced haemolytic anaemia associated with microangiopathy. Australian and New Zealand Journal of Medicine 1976; 6: 152
68. Gralnick HR, McGuiness M, Elton W, et al. Haemolytic anaemia associated with cephalothin. Journal of the American Medical Association 1971; 217: 1102
69. Rubin RN, Burka ER. Anti-cephalothin antibody and Coombs-positive hemolytic anemia. Annals of Internal Medicine 1977; 86: 64
70. Szczeklik A, Gryglewski RJ. Asthma and anti-inflammatory drugs: mechanisms and clinical patterns. Drugs 1983; 25: 533
71. Stevenson DD. Diagnosis, prevention and treatment of adverse reactions to aspirin and non-steroidal anti-inflammatory drugs. Journal of Allergy and Clinical Immunology 1984; 74: 617
72. Youngman PR, Taylor KM, Wilson JD. Anaphylactoid reactions to neuromuscular blocking agents: a commonly undiagnosed condition. Lancet 1983; 2: 597
73. Watkins J, Levy CJ. Guide to immediate anaesthetic reactions. London: Butterworths, 1988
74. Westhoff-Bleck M, Bleck JS, Jost S. The adverse effects of angiographic radiocontrast media. Drug Safety 1991; 6: 28
75. Michaëlsson G, Juhlin L. Urticaria induced by preservative and dye additives in food and drugs. British Journal of Dermatology 1973; 88: 525-32
76. O'Brian MER, Souberbielle BE. Allergic reactions to cytotoxic drugs - an update. Annals of Oncology 1992; 3: 605
77. Bochner BS, Lichtenstein LM. Anaphylaxis. New England Journal of Medicine 1991; 324: 1785
78. Blaiss MS, deShazo RD. Drug allergy. Pediatric Clinics of North America 1988; 35: 1131
79. Clark DWJ. Genetically determined variability in acetylation and oxidation. Drugs 1985; 29: 342
80. Evans DAP, Manley KA, McKusick VA. Genetic control of isoniazid metabolism in man. British Medical Journal 1960; 2: 485
81. Lunde PKM, Frislid K, Hansteen V. Disease and acetylation polymorphism. Clinical Pharmacokinetics 1977; 2: 182
82. Drayer DE, Reidenberg MM. Clinical consequences of polymorphic acetylation of basic drugs. Clinical Pharmacology and Therapeutics 1977; 22: 251
83. Cowan GO, Das KM, Eastwood MA. Further studies of sulphasalazine metabolism in the treatment of ulcerative colitis. British Medical Journal 1977; 2: 1057
84. Das KM, Dubin R. Clinical pharmacokinetics of sulphasalazine. Clinical Pharmacokinetics 1976; 1: 406
85. Kutt H, Brennan R, Dehejia H, et al. Diphenylhydantoin intoxication: a comparison of isoniazid therapy. American Review of Respiratory Disease 1970; 101: 377
86. Mitchell JR, Thorgeirsson UP, Black M, et al. Increased incidence of isoniazid hepatitis in rapid acetylators: possible relation to hydrazine metabolites. Clinical Pharmacology and Therapeutics 1975; 18: 70
87. Ellard GA, Gammon PT. Pharmacokinetics of isoniazid metabolism in man. Journal of Pharmacokinetics and Biopharmaceutics 1976; 4: 83
88. Ellard GA, Gammon PT. Acetylator phenotyping of tuberculosis patients using matrix isoniazid on sulphadimidine and its prognostic significance for treatment with several intermittent isoniazid-containing regimens. British Journal of Clinical Pharmacology 1977; 4: 5
89. Cameron HA, Ramsay LE. The lupus syndrome induced by hydralazine: a common complication with low dose treatment. British Medical Journal 1984; 289: 410
90. Uetrecht JP, Woosley RL. Acetylator phenotype and lupus erythematosus. Clinical Pharmacokinetics 1981; 6: 118
91. Batchelor JR. Genetic role in autoimmunity. Triangle 1984; 23: 77
92. Motulsky AG. Pharmacogenetics. Progress in Medical Genetics 1964; 3: 49
93. Vivien JN, Thiebier R, Lepeuple A. La pharmacocinetique de l'isoniazide dans la race blanche. Revue Française des Maladies Respiratoires 1973; 1: 753
94. Evans DAP. An improved and simplified method of detecting the acetylator phenotype. Journal of Medical Genetics 1969; 6: 405
95. Eze LC, Evans DAP. The use of the autoanalyser to determine the acetylator phenotype. Journal of Medical Genetics 1972; 9: 57
96. Mahgoub A, Idle JR, Dring LC, et al. Polymorphic hydroxylation of debrisoquine in man. Lancet 1977; 2: 584
97. Eichelbaum M, Spannbrucker N, Steincke B, et al. Defective N-oxidation of sparteine in man: a new pharmacogenetic effect. European Journal of Clinical Pharmacology 1979; 16: 183
98. Eichelbaum M, Bertilsson L, Sawe J, et al. Polymorphic oxidation of sparteine and debrisoquine: related pharmacogenetic entities. Clinical Pharmacology and Therapeutics 1982; 31: 184
99. La Du BN. Pharmacogenetics: defective enzymes in relation to reactions to drugs. Annual Review of Medicine 1972; 23: 453
100. Panick V. Glucose-6-phosphate dehydrogenase deficiency. Part 2. Topical Asia. Clinical Haematology 1981; 10: 800
101. Beutler E. Screening for glucose-6-phosphate dehydrogenase deficiency. Israel Journal of Medical Sciences 1973; 9: 1350
102. Dow PA, Mozellar B, Petteway BA, et al. Simplified method for G6PD screening using blood collected on filter paper. American Journal of Clinical Pathology 1974; 61: 333
103. Köppel C. Clinical features, pathogenesis and management of drug-induced rhabdomyolysis. Medical Toxicology and Adverse Drug Experience 1989; 4: 108
104. Armaly MF. Genetic factors related to glaucoma. Annals of the New York Academy of Sciences 1968; 151: 861
105. Shear NH, Spielberg SP. Anticonvulsant hypersensitivity syndrome. Journal of Clinical Investigation 1988; 82: 1826
106. Lennard MS. Genetically determined adverse drug reactions involving metabolism. Drug Safety 1993; 9: 60-77
107. Sotaniemi E, Krens KE, Schinin TM. Oral contraception and liver damage. British Medical Journal 1964; 2: 1264
108. Popper H. Cholestasis. Annual Review of Medicine 1968; 19: 39
109. Yunis AA. Chloramphenicol-induced bone marrow suppression. Seminars in Haematology 1973; 10: 225
110. Nagao T, Mauer AM. Concordance for drug-induced aplastic anaemia in identical twins. New England Journal of Medicine 1969; 281: 7
111. Pisciotta V. Drug-induced agranulocytosis. Drugs 1978; 15: 132
112. Idänpään-Heikkilä J, Alhava E, Olkinuora M, et al. Agranulocytosis during treatment with clozapine. European Journal of Clinical Pharmacology 1977; 11: 193
113. Anderman B, Griffith RW. Clozapine-induced agranulocytosis: a situation reported up to August 1976. European Journal of Clinical Pharmacology 1977; 11: 199
114. Coulter DM, Edwards IR. Mianserin and agranulocytosis in New Zealand. Lancet 1990; 336: 785-7
115. Bochner F, Hooper WD, Eadie MJ, et al. Decreased capacity to metabolize diphenylhydantoin in a patient with hy-

persensitivity to warfarin. Australian and New Zealand Journal of Medicine 1975; 5: 462

116. de Matteis F. Disturbances of liver porphyrin metabolism caused by drugs. Pharmacological Reviews 1967; 19: 523
117. Moore MR, Disler PB. Drug induction of the acute porphyrias. Adverse Drug Reactions and Acute Poisoning Reviews 1983; 2: 149
118. Folb PI, editor. Drug safety in clinical practice. Berlin: Springer-Verlag, 1984
119. Ayd FJ. Toxic somatic and psychopathologic reactions to antidepressant drugs. Journal of Neuropsychiatry and Clinical Neurosciences 1961; 2 Suppl. 1: 119
120. Blaschke TF. Protein binding and kinetics of drugs in liver disease. Clinical Pharmacokinetics 1977; 2: 32
121. Naranjo CA, Busto U, Mardones R. Adverse drug reactions in liver cirrhosis. European Journal of Clinical Pharmacology 1978; 13: 429
122. Laidlaw J, Read AE, Sherlock S. Morphine tolerance in hepatic cirrhosis. Gastroenterology 1961; 40: 389
123. Sherlock S. Drugs and the liver. British Medical Journal 1968; 1: 227
124. Read AE, Laidlaw J, McCarthy CF. Effects of chlorpromazine in patients with hepatic disease. British Medical Journal 1969; 3: 497
125. Sherlock S, Senewirante B, Scott A, et al. Complications of diuretic therapy in hepatic cirrhosis. Lancet 1966; 1: 1049
126. Toole JF, Parrish ML. Nitrofurantoin polyneuropathy. Neurology 1973; 23: 554
127. Rauscher A, Hurst JM, Collins GM. Nitroprusside toxicity in a renal transplant patient. Anesthesiology 1978; 49: 428
128. Richet G, Lopex de Novales E, Verroust P. Drug intoxication and neurological episodes in chronic renal failure. British Medical Journal 1970; 2: 394
129. Schreiner G, Maher JF. Drugs and the kidney. Annals of the New York Academy of Sciences 1965; 123: 326
130. Faed EM, McQueen EG. Measurement of clofibric acid (CPIB) metabolites in plasma of patients on clofibrate therapy. Clinical and Experimental Pharmacology and Physiology 1979; 6: 267
131. Gugler R. Clinical pharmacokinetics of hypolipidaemic drugs. Clinical Pharmacokinetics 1978; 3: 425
132. Tyrer JH, Eadie MJ, Sutherland JM, et al. Outbreak of anticonvulsant intoxication in an Australian city. British Medical Journal 1970; 4: 271
133. McQueen EG. Phenytoin intoxication. New Zealand Medical Journal 1968; 68: 332
134. Fulop M, Drapkin A. Potassium-depletion syndrome secondary to nephropathy caused by 'outdated tetracycline'. New England Journal of Medicine 1965; 272: 986
135. Cohen SM. Accidental intra-arterial injection of drugs. Lancet 1948; 2: 361, 409
136. Knowles JA. Accidental intra-arterial injection of penicillin. American Journal of Diseases of Children 1966; 3: 552
137. Azarnoff DL, Hurwitz A. Drug interactions. Pharmacology for Physicians 1970; 4 (2): 1
138. Paturaud J-P, Gut J-P. Cardiac arrest following the rapid intravenous injection of lincomycin. Nouvelle Presse Medicale 1975; 4: 1593
139. Bahl MGC, Gregory MM, Scheuer PJ. Methotrexate hepatotoxicity in psoriasis - comparison of different dose regimens. British Medical Journal 1972; 1: 654
140. Conaghan PG, Brooks PM, Quinn DI, et al. Hazards of low-dose methotrexate. Australian and New Zealand Journal of Medicine 1995; 25: 670-3
141. George CF, Robertson D. Clinical consequences of abrupt drug withdrawal. Medical Toxicology and Adverse Drug Experience 1987; 2: 367
142. Boston Collaborative Drug Surveillance Program. Adverse drug reactions. Journal of the American Medical Association 1972; 220: 1238
143. Scott AK. Stereoisomers and drug toxicity. Drug Safety 1993; 8: 149
144. Lynch HT, Quinn T, Severin MJ. Diethylstilboestrol, teratogenesis and carcinogenesis: medical/legal implications of its long-term sequelae, including third-generation effects. International Journal of Risk and Safety Medicine 1990; 1: 171
145. Berry M. Criminal behaviour following drug treatment for psychiatric disorders: medicolegal and ethical issues. CNS Drugs 1994; 2: 301-12
146. Leape LL, Brennan TA, Laird N, et al. The nature of adverse events in hospitalized patients. New England Journal of Medicine 1991; 324: 377

Chapter 7

# Clinically Important Drug Interactions

*D.I. Quinn* and *R.O. Day*

### Synopsis of Important Principles

**1)** The effects of one drug can be increased or decreased or a quite new effect produced by the previous, concurrent or subsequent administration of another.

**2)** Many drug interactions can be predicted if the pharmacodynamic effects, pharmacokinetic properties and mechanisms of action of the interacting agents are known. Most can be avoided by the application of this knowledge.

**3)** Drug interactions with a pharmacodynamic basis involve actions on the same receptors or physiological systems. Alternatively, they may involve modification of drug response as a result of changes brought about by compensatory homeostatic responses to changes produced by drugs. Pharmacokinetic interactions are caused by the effect of one drug on the absorption, distribution, metabolism or excretion of another.

**4)** Pharmacokinetic and pharmacodynamic interactions observed *in vitro* or in animals will not necessarily occur in humans.

**5)** Interactions will not necessarily occur in all patients receiving a given combination of drugs known to have potential for interaction in humans.

**6)** Many clinically important interactions, especially pharmacokinetic interactions, depend on a variety of factors in addition to the drugs given.

**7)** Pharmacokinetic drug interactions demonstrated with one drug combination should not be extrapolated to other combinations involving closely related drugs. However, care should be taken in using these latter combinations until experience determines whether interactions are likely.

**8)** The increasing number of drugs available and the increasing use of multidrug therapeutic regimens enhance the potential for drug interactions. However, in clinical practice, most interactions are either not significant or rarely of significance.

**9)** The most common interactions are those involving mutual pharmacodynamic potentiation of central nervous system (CNS) depression by benzodiazepines, barbiturates, antidepressants, alcohol (ethanol), opioid analgesics, sedating antihistamines, antiepileptics and other centrally-acting drugs.

**10)** The most obvious interactions are those producing altered pharmacokinetics of oral anticoagulants, antidiabetic drugs, cardiac glycosides, nonsedating antihistamines, benzodiazepines and immunosuppressant and cytotoxic drugs. These drugs have a low therapeutic ratio and an altered response may be potentially lethal. Interactions involving certain antihypertensive and antiepileptic drugs also can be important.

Modern therapeutic agents are more powerful and specific in action than their predecessors, but often have complex mechanisms of action and multiple effects. Given this inherent complexity and multiplicity of actions, it is not surprising that these agents have enormous potential to quantitatively or qualitatively change the effects of drugs which are administered concurrently. In some situations, changes in effects may result from the prior or subsequent administration of an agent with interacting potential. The net effect of the combination may be:

- Synergism of effect of one or more of the drugs.
- Antagonism of effect of one or more of the drugs.
- Alteration of effect of one or more drugs or production of idiosyncratic effects such that a clinical event occurs which is not normally associated with the usage of those agents.

A drug interaction may be defined as occurring when the 'pharmacological or clinical response to the administration of a drug combination is different from that anticipated from the known effects of the two agents given alone'.[1]

**Table I.** Examples of drugs commonly used together with synergistic intent

| Condition | Examples of drugs with potential for use in combination |
|---|---|
| Post-transplantation immunosuppression | Corticosteroids<br>Azathioprine<br>Cyclosporin<br>Tacrolimus (FK 506)<br>Monoclonal antibodies (e.g.muromonab CD3) |
| Malignancy | Alkylating agents (e.g. cyclophosphamide)<br>Anthracyclines (e.g. doxorubicin, daunorubicin)<br>Antimetabolites (e.g. methotrexate, cytarabine, fluorouracil)<br>Biological response modifiers (e.g. interferon-α) |
| Infection | β-Lactam antibiotics (e.g. penicillins, cefalosporins)<br>Aminoglycosides (e.g. gentamicin, tobramycin) |
| Systemic hypertension | α-Adrenoceptor blocking agents (e.g. prazosin, terazosin)<br>β-Adrenoceptor blocking agents (e.g. metoprolol, atenolol)<br>ACE inhibitors (e.g. captopril, enalapril, lisinopril)<br>Calcium antagonists (e.g. nifedipine, felodipine, amlodipine, verapamil, diltiazem)<br>Diuretics [e.g. thiazides, furosemide (frusemide)] |
| Asthma | Corticosteroids (inhaled or systemic)<br>$\beta_2$-Adrenoceptor agonists<br>Ipratropium bromide<br>Sodium cromoglycate (cromolyn sodium) |

*Abbreviation:* ACE = angiotensin converting enzyme.

**Table II.** Incidence of adverse drug reactions in medical hospital patients in relation to the number of drugs prescribed concurrently (after May et al.[3])

| Parameter | Number of drugs prescribed | | | |
|---|---|---|---|---|
| | 0-5 | 6-10 | 11-15 | 16-20 |
| Number of patients | 4009 | 3861 | 1713 | 641 |
| Number of reactions | 142 | 397 | 478 | 347 |
| Adverse reaction rate | 4% | 10% | 28% | 54% |

More simply, they occur 'when the effects of one drug are changed by the presence of another drug, food, drink or by some environmental chemical agent'.[2]

Potentiating or synergistic effects of various combinations are commonly used with the intent of obtaining a therapeutic goal while reducing toxicity. They also were used where the therapeutic effect of a single agent has peaked but the therapeutic goal has not been reached. Good examples of these include multiple agents used in post-transplantation immunosuppression, combination chemotherapy for malignancy, antimicrobial treatment of certain infections, and treatment of systemic hypertension and asthma (table I).

Antagonistic effects can be useful. Opioid antagonists, such as naloxone, are useful in treating opioid overdose, while anticholinergic agents such as trihexyphenidyl (benzhexol) and benztropine are useful in the treatment of extrapyramidal syndromes associated with the use of antiemetics and antipsychotics.

Only the unintentional or undesirable consequences of drug interactions will be considered in detail in this chapter.

Drug interactions represent a major problem in day-to-day practice. The incidence of adverse reactions increases almost exponentially as the number of drugs coprescribed rises, and this is in part due to interactions (table II).[3] Critically ill, chronically ill and elderly patients are particularly at risk of clinically manifest drug interactions. This is not only because these patients are likely to be taking more medications, but also because of impaired homeostatic mechanisms that might otherwise counteract some of the unwanted effects of drugs and drug interactions.[4-6]

## 1. General Considerations

Drug interactions are an important cause of therapy-related toxicity. Unfortunately, awareness and recognition of adverse drug interactions by doctors is low.[7] Over-the-counter nonprescription medications, herbal or home remedies, and combination prescription products add to the potential for drug interactions to occur in settings over which clinicians have little control.[8] Unfortunately, even with a good knowledge of pharmacodynamics and pharmacokinetics and an awareness of potential interactions, factors can conspire against the most erudite clinician. Patients are commonly unaware of some or all of their medications, often because they do not consider nonprescription drugs as part of drug therapy, they omit to mention drugs given by non-oral routes, such as transdermal or inhaled drugs, or they cannot remember what they have taken. Furthermore, they may have multiple clinicians involved in their care, each primarily responsible for the treatment of one system or ailment. The role of clear communication with the patient and with the primary care clinician in such instances can never be understated.[9] Asking patients to bring all medications with them to a consultation can help reduce confusion and improve compliance.

### 1.1 Incidence of Important Drug Interactions

The incidence of clinically significant drug interactions is difficult to assess. Studies in this area are impaired by the lack of an agreed definition for drug-drug interactions and the lack of an agreed standard list of drug-drug interactions against which hospital admissions can be correlated. A number of pharmacy-based databases have been designed in an attempt to define the incidence of clinically important interactions more accurately.[10]

The incidence of prescription of drugs with potential for interaction is probably around 4 to 5% among hospital inpatients.[11,12] However, most of these potential interactions either do not occur or go unrecognised. A major surveillance programme revealed an incidence of reported adverse drug reactions of 3600 in 83,000 drug exposures (4.3%). Of those, 234 (6.9%) were attributed to drug interactions.[13] More recent data suggest that drug-drug interactions probably cause between zero and 1.0% of hospital admissions.[14] However, these figures underestimate drug-drug interactions as a problem because:

- Most therapeutic interventions or adjustments occur in ambulatory or outpatient settings.[15]
- The incidence of hospitalisation secondary to adverse drug reactions is low (about 3%).[16]
- The annual rate of illnesses serious enough to warrant admission is less than 1 per 1000 persons exposed to any given drug per year.[17]

A study of drug interactions related to prescriptions presented to community pharmacists in the US revealed an overall incidence of 4.1%.[18] In defined groups taking particular medications with routinely measurable serum concentrations, the incidence of biochemical and clinical toxicity is more easily evaluated. One study in epileptic patients suggested that 6% of cases of drug toxicity involved drug interactions as a contributory factor.[19] The elderly have a higher incidence of clinically evident drug interactions for a variety of reasons, including use of more drugs per person than younger individuals and deficient homeostatic compensatory mechanisms when adverse effects occur. Some studies have found an incidence of drug interactions of up to 88% in certain nonambulatory geriatric populations, although the real incidence in most groups of patients is considerably less than this number.[6]

### 1.2 Consequences of Drug Interactions

Drug interactions are only important for the patient and clinician when they interfere with the efficacy or diminish the safety of treatment.[20] The Harvard Medical Practice Study examined adverse events in inpatients of non-psychiatric acute care hospitals. 20% of adverse events were drug related; of those, 8% were considered due to a drug-drug interaction, suggesting that such interactions are responsible for less than 2% of adverse events in this patient group.[21] The obvious gravity of potentially lethal interactions involving anticoagulants, antidiabetic agents and antineoplastic drugs makes them highly important. However, drug interactions affecting therapeutic control are far more likely to be confronted in daily practice than in hospitals.

Drug interactions are more likely to have serious consequences when they affect elderly or severely ill patients. Certain drugs require careful attention, especially those with narrow therapeutic indices, self-inducible or saturable metabolic pathways, or steep dose-response curves (see chapter 1, sect. 1, 3, 6; chapter 5, sect. 2.1, 4).

The small but not insignificant number of clinically important drug-drug interactions (see appendix B) must be distinguished from the larger number which are for the most part only of academic interest. The necessary coadministration of many interacting drugs is possible and safe provided that the effects are monitored closely and dosage is modified appropriately.

### 1.3 Drug Usage

Interactions between commonly used drugs, or drugs often given together in the treatment of specific conditions, are clearly more important than those occurring with rarely used drugs. This is a particular problem with some drugs available without prescription. For instance, alcohol, tobacco, antacids and nonsteroidal anti-inflammatory drugs have the potential to interact with many drugs, yet are widely consumed and may not be thought of as drugs by those consuming them.[8,22-24]

### 1.4 Documentation and Reliability of Clinical Data

The clinical significance of many interactions described in the literature is grossly overstated. Some authors have described interactions with far reaching clinical implications which have not been confirmed by others in subsequent studies, and many 'interactions' included in exhaustive lists have never been shown to occur in humans or only do so rarely. In this regard, too much credence has been placed on reports of:

- Interactions in one or a few patients with a multitude of variable factors, including coexistent disease states and other medications[25]
- Interactions in animals
- Trials of drug combinations in healthy volunteers.

Information from each of these sources is extremely important in highlighting drugs with potential for clinically important interactions. However, the significance of a drug interaction is only finally evaluable when the combination is used in the population for which the drugs were intended, i.e. in the 'population at risk'. Studies in the group likely to use a drug may be technically and ethically difficult. To balance this, most countries have set up reporting systems to allow systematic review of adverse drug reactions and interactions. Even when an interaction is seen to occur in that population, it may only occur in selected patients and may be avoided by scheduling times of administration based on knowledge of the pharmacokinetics and pharmacodynamics (see further appendix B).

### 1.5 Individual Variation

Interactions may occur in some individuals but not in others.[26] Although diltiazem almost invariably results in an increase in plasma cyclosporin concentrations, the dosage of diltiazem and the degree of change in cyclosporin concentrations for a given diltiazem dosage varies greatly between individuals.[27,28] Indeed, some interactions involving both selective and nonselective monoamine oxidase inhibitors (MAOIs) seem only to occur in a very small proportion of patients at risk.[29] The effects of interactions involving drug metabolism may vary greatly in different patients because of individual differences in the initial rates of drug metabolism and in susceptibility to microsomal enzyme induction (see chapter 1; sect. 3.3).

The ability of individuals to metabolise certain subsets of drugs varies on a genetic basis.[30,31] Humans are classifiable as either poor or extensive or slow or fast metabolisers with respect to the activity of their individual P450 microsomal and acetylator enzyme subsets (see also chapter 1, sect. 5.2 and chapter 6, sect. 2.8).[32] An elevated concentration of a drug in a slow acetylator may have effects on the metabolism of other drugs, such as when an elevated isoniazid concentration is seen to inhibit the metabolism of phenytoin, with the potential for phenytoin toxicity, whereas this is rarely seen in rapid acetylators of isoniazid. Significant interactions between antibiotics and digoxin occur in only about 10% of patients taking these drugs at the same time.[33,34]

Given significant interindividual variability in pharmacokinetics and effects of drugs, the evaluation of new drugs to define population pharmacokinetics and the degree of variance is important.[35] Having achieved this, the subsequent delineation of drug interactions and prediction of their clinical importance becomes much easier.

### 1.6 Effects of Disease

Some interactions are likely to be modified by disease states, but there is very little reliable information on this point. Muscle weakness caused by the combination of aminoglycoside antibiotics (e.g. kanamycin, gentamicin, tobramycin) and non-depolarising muscle relaxants (e.g. tubocurarine, pancuronium, vecuronium) is increased by coexistent myopathy, hypokalaemia or renal impairment.[36-38] Acute febrile illnesses, influenza vaccination, hepatitis, hepatic ischaemia or hepatic congestion due to right heart failure may diminish the ability of hepatic P450 microsomal enzymes to metabolise drugs such as theophylline, cyclosporin and warfarin.[39-42] In this situation, inhibitors of drug metabolism may have a synergistic effect in elevating serum concentrations of the metabolised drug. The inhibitory effect of cimetidine on hepatic microsomal enzymes is greater in patients with chronic liver disease.[43] The hepatotoxic effect of paracetamol (acetaminophen) is magnified by the coexistence of chronic liver disease and by the coadministration of enzyme inducers such as long term alcohol (ethanol) as well as by concurrent isoniazid therapy.[8,44]

**Table III.** Mechanisms of drug interactions

1. Pharmaceutical incompatibility
2. *In vivo* binding of drug with loss of effect
3. Mutual antagonism or potentiation of drugs acting at the same site or influencing the same physiological system
4. Competition at receptor sites
5. Changes in electrolyte or fluid balance
6. Intracellular transport (interference with amine uptake by sympathetic neurons)
7. Interference with absorption:
   a) Change in pH of GI fluids
   b) Effects on gastric emptying and GI motility
   c) Binding and chelation of drugs
   d) Competition for active absorption sites
   e) Toxic effects on GI tract
8. Drug distribution (tissue binding displacement; see section 2.3.2)
9. Modification of drug metabolism:
   a) Induction
   b) Inhibition
   c) Changes in hepatic blood flow
10. Interference with biliary excretion and enterohepatic circulation
11. Modification of renal excretion:
    a) Interference with renal excretion due to drug-induced renal impairment
    b) Competition for active renal tubular secretion
    c) Changes in urine pH
12. Miscellaneous:
    a) Monoamine oxidase inhibition
    b) Antagonism of antibacterial and antiviral drugs
13. Interactions with no proven mechanism

*Abbreviation:* GI = gastrointestinal.

## 2. Mechanisms of Drug Interaction

Drugs may interact on a pharmaceutical (physical), pharmacodynamic or pharmacokinetic basis. Pharmaceutical interactions may occur when drugs are mixed inappropriately in syringes and infusion fluids prior to administration, while pharmacodynamic interactions arise with drugs acting on the same receptors, sites of action or physiological systems. With pharmacokinetic interactions, one drug interferes with the absorption, transport, distribution or elimination of another. Some mechanisms of interaction are listed in table III, while some examples likely to be of potential clinical significance are given in table IV.

Since the first edition of this book in 1976, there have been hundreds of further drug interaction reports. Although many are isolated anecdotal accounts of doubtful significance, others are clearly of great importance. It is becoming increasingly difficult to provide a balanced comprehensive summary of such reports. Those unlikely to influence the result of drug therapy have generally been omitted from this discussion, even if adequately documented in humans, and none have been included solely on the basis of animal or *in vitro* studies. The interactions listed in table IV are intended only to illustrate important principles. For a more comprehensive list of potentially clinically important drug interactions, see appendix B.

A number of drugs may interact simultaneously at different sites so that it may be difficult to attribute an interaction to a single mechanism. For instance, aspirin (acetylsalicylic acid) could interfere with the absorption and active renal tubular secretion of other acidic drugs. It also might increase the toxicity of oral anticoagulants through effects on the bleeding time, capillary fragility, platelet adhesiveness, intrinsic inhibition of clotting factor synthesis, and production of gastrointestinal erosions and ulcers which may bleed. Alcohol can also alter both the pharmacodynamics and pharmacokinetics of other drugs.[45,46] Amiodarone increases the serum concentration of digoxin principally through inhibition of renal excretion, but also by inhibition of hepatobiliary excretion, and possibly by displacement from tissue binding sites and increasing its absorption.[47-49]

Many lists of interactions extrapolate reactions demonstrated with one compound to other combinations involving closely related drugs.

**Table IV.** Mechanisms and examples of potential drug interactions. It is important to realise that a particular interaction may not occur in all patients (see text and appendix B)

| Mechanism | Effect | Examples[a] |
|---|---|---|
| Pharmaceutical incompatibility | Inactivation of the drug *in vitro* | Inactivation of carbenicillin by gentamicin; reaction between hydrocortisone or penicillin and heparin, and between penicillins and phenytoin when drugs are mixed in syringes and infusion bottles |
| | | Many other examples are known, including incompatibilities with solutions containing amino acids or proteins, fat emulsions, complex sugars, mannitol and sodium bicarbonate |
| *In vivo* binding of drug with loss of effect | Binding and formation of an inert complex | Inactivation of heparin by protamine and of lead by edetic acid (EDTA) |
| Mutual potentiation or antagonism by drugs acting at the same site or influencing the same physiological system | Exaggerated or reduced effects | Potentiation of central nervous system (CNS) depression caused by alcohol (ethanol), hypnotics, sedatives, tranquillisers, antidepressants, opioid analgesics, antiepileptics, antihistamines, methyldopa, clonidine, marijuana and miscellaneous drugs |
| | | Non-depolarising muscle relaxants potentiated by aminoglycoside antibiotics, cyclosporin, magnesium infusions, local anaesthetics and quinidine |
| | | Risk of severe hypotension if diazoxide is given with other potent antihypertensive agents, especially vasodilators such as hydralazine, minoxidil, ACE inhibitors and calcium antagonists |
| | | Potentiation of antihypertensive agents by CNS depressants, anaesthetic drugs and diuretics |
| | | Potentiation of the peripheral vasoconstrictive effects of ergotamine with ischaemia when used in combination with β-adrenoceptor blockers, dopamine and/or adrenaline (epinephrine), and erythromycin |
| | | Antagonism of some antihypertensive agents by sympathomimetics, tricyclic antidepressants and NSAIDs |
| | | Potentiation of antidiabetic agents by salicylates, anabolic steroids and nonselective MAOIs |
| | | Antagonism of antidiabetic agents by thiazide diuretics, diazoxide, corticosteroids and oral contraceptives |
| | | ACE inhibitors potentiate insulin and oral antidiabetic drugs by increasing cellular uptake and utilisation of glucose |
| | | Increased risk of aminoglycoside antibiotic ototoxicity with furosemide (frusemide) and ethacrynic acid |
| | | Clofibrate and thyroxine potentiate effects of coumarin anticoagulants |
| | | Potentiation of anticoagulants (increased risk of bleeding) by aspirin (acetylsalicylic acid) and other NSAIDs |
| | | Antagonism of warfarin effect by nafcillin and sucralfate |
| | | Bradycardia and atrioventricular block with combinations including β-adrenoceptor blockers, verapamil, diltiazem, digoxin, disopyramide, flecainide, tacrine and adenosine |
| | | Antagonism of levodopa or bromocriptine effect by haloperidol, phenothiazines and tiapride |
| | | Tremor, confusion and extrapyramidal reactions when lithium is combined with haloperidol or methyldopa |
| | | Long term use of oral or topical nitrates (e.g. isosorbide dinitrate) without a daily 'nitrate free period' results in tolerance and reduced therapeutic response to sublingual nitroglycerin (glyceryl trinitrate) |
| | | Antagonism of the effects of methotrexate by folic acid or folinic acid |
| Competition at receptor sites | Usually antagonism | Naloxone is a specific opioid antagonist |
| | | Flumazenil is a specific benzodiazepine antagonist |
| | | Neostigmine and pyridostigmine antagonise non-depolarising muscle relaxants (e.g. tubocurarine) and potentiate polarisation block caused by suxamethonium (succinylcholine) |
| | | Mutual antagonism of β-adrenoceptor agonists (e.g. salbutamol) and β-adrenoceptor blockers (e.g. propranolol) |
| | | Vitamin K antagonises coumarin anticoagulants |
| | | Anabolic steroids thought to potentiate oral anticoagulants by altering receptor affinity for vitamin K (other mechanisms suggested include increased rate of decay or impaired synthesis of clotting factors). Thyroxine may act similarly |

**Table IV.** *[Continued]*

| Mechanism | Effect | Examples[a] |
|---|---|---|
| Changes in electrolyte or fluid balance | Antagonism or potentiation | Potentiation of effects of digoxin and non-depolarising muscle relaxants by hypokalaemia induced by diuretics and amphotericin B<br>Prolonged paralysis after suxamethonium in patients given lithium<br>Precipitation of lithium toxicity by thiazide diuretics and NSAIDs<br>Therapeutic failure of lithium if renal excretion enhanced by high sodium intake (e.g. sodium bicarbonate)<br>Ventricular arrhythmias in patients receiving digoxin caused by release of $K^+$ following injection of suxamethonium, especially in patients with trauma, burns or muscle disorders<br>Antagonism of antiarrhythmic and potentiation of proarrhythmic actions of lidocaine (lignocaine), quinidine, procainamide, disopyramide, amiodarone and sotalol by drugs which cause hypokalaemia<br>Hyperkalaemia if ACE inhibitors given with potassium supplements or NSAIDs<br>Antagonism of effects of antihypertensive agents and diuretics by NSAIDs |
| Interference with amine uptake by sympathetic neurons | Potentiation of neurotransmitter effect | Potentiation and prolongation of the pressor effects of adrenaline (epinephrine) and noradrenaline (norepinephrine) by tricyclic antidepressants<br>Serotonergic syndrome in some patients given combinations of proserotonergic drugs such as lithium, fluoxetine, MAOIs, carbamazepine and tricyclic antidepressants |
| Interference with drug absorption | Increased or decreased rate of absorption or amount of drug absorbed | |
| a) Change in pH of gastrointestinal fluids | | Sodium bicarbonate reduces absorption of tetracycline, increases absorption of levodopa and increases the rate of absorption of aspirin<br>Antacids, cimetidine, ranitidine and didanosine reduce bioavailability of ketoconazole and itraconazole<br>Omeprazole may inhibit cyanocobalamin (vitamin $B_{12}$) absorption<br>Some antacids increase levodopa absorption<br>Magnesium hydroxide, $H_2$-receptor antagonists and omeprazole increase the absorption of ibuprofen, glibenclamide (glyburide), tolbutamide and glipizide |
| b) Effects on gastric emptying and gastrointestinal motility | | Anticholinergics such as propantheline and other antispasmodic drugs such as mebeverine slow absorption of alcohol, paracetamol (acetaminophen), diazepam, propranolol, phenylbutazone and lithium (slow release tablets), and decrease absorption of levodopa<br>Opioid analgesics such as diamorphine (heroin), morphine, pethidine (meperidine) and pentazocine strongly inhibit gastric emptying and greatly reduce the rate of absorption of paracetamol (and probably many other drugs). Morphine and diamorphine slow down and reduce the absorption of mexiletine in patients with myocardial infarction. Similar effects are likely with other oral antiarrhythmic drugs<br>Aluminium hydroxide gel decreases isoniazid absorption<br>Prokinetic drugs such as metoclopramide and cisapride accelerate absorption of paracetamol, alcohol, diazepam, propranolol, cyclosporin, mefloquine and lithium (slow release tablets), and increase overall absorption of cyclosporin |
| c) Binding or chelation of drugs | | Kaolin-pectin reduces digoxin and quinidine absorption. Some antacids reduce digoxin absorption<br>Cholestyramine interferes with absorption of warfarin, propranolol, thyroxine, cyclosporin, digoxin and digitoxin; colestipol reduces absorption of digitoxin and propranolol<br>$Fe^{++}$ diminishes the absorption of levodopa, levodopa/carbidopa combinations, and methyldopa<br>Tetracycline and fluoroquinolone absorption reduced by $Ca^{++}$, $Mg^{++}$, $Al^{+++}$, $Fe^{++}$, colloidal bismuth subcitrate (tripotassium dicitrato bismuthate), sucralfate and didanosine<br>Magnesium hydroxide increases the absorption of dicoumarol and some oral antidiabetic agents |
| d) Competition for active absorption sites | | Amiloride decreases absorption of dipeptide β-lactam antibiotics such as amoxicillin and cefalexin |

*[Continued over]*

**Table IV.** *[Continued]*

| Mechanism | Effect | Examples[a] |
|---|---|---|
| e) Toxic effect on gastrointestinal tract | | Mefenamic acid, aminosalicylic acid, neomycin, and colchicine may cause malabsorption syndromes |
| | | Neomycin interferes with penicillin, cyanocobalamin and digoxin absorption |
| | | Cytotoxic chemotherapy, particularly with regimens which include cisplatin or anthracyclines, results in decreased absorption of many drugs, including phenytoin for 5 to 7 days after its administration |
| f) Effects on gut bacterial flora | Increased or decreased drug effects | Erythromycin, tetracycline and other broad-spectrum antibiotics increase digoxin bioavailability and plasma concentrations by inhibiting its intestinal bacterial metabolism |
| | | Antibiotics may reduce the efficacy of oral contraceptives by inhibiting bacterial hydrolysis of estrogen conjugates secreted into the bile and thereby reducing their enterohepatic circulation |
| g) Unknown | | Aluminium hydroxide reduces absorption of propranolol, isoniazid and indomethacin; phenytoin, cimetidine, ranitidine and chlorpromazine absorption reduced by antacids |
| | | Phenytoin absorption reduced by furosemide; digoxin by sulfasalazine; phenobarbital interferes with griseofulvin absorption; clarithromycin decreases the absorption of zidovudine; octreotide decreases the absorption of cyclosporin |
| Plasma protein binding displacement | Very rarely clinically significant | Few clinically important examples. Most interactions reputed to involve protein binding displacement are caused largely by other mechanisms (e.g. inhibition of drug metabolism) [see text; section 2.3.2] |
| Tissue binding displacement | Potentiation of effects of displaced drug | Quinidine increases steady-state plasma concentrations of digoxin |
| Induction of drug metabolism | Increased rate of drug metabolism. Drug effects are usually reduced, but are enhanced if metabolites are more active than the parent drug; similarly, increased or decreased toxicity | Accelerated metabolism and reduced effects of oral anticoagulants, antiepileptics, barbiturates, opioid analgesics, antidepressants, digitoxin, some β-adrenoceptor blockers, corticosteroids, cyclosporin and many other drugs possible with administration of enzyme-inducing agents such as barbiturates (especially phenobarbital), phenytoin, primidone, carbamazepine, rifampicin (rifampin) and griseofulvin |
| | | *NB.* If drug dose is increased to regain initial response, overdosage will occur 1 to 3 weeks after the inducing drug is discontinued. This effect is particularly hazardous with oral anticoagulants |
| | | Transplant rejection in patients receiving cyclosporin may occur if enzyme-inducing agents taken as well |
| | | Toxicity caused by metabolic activation may be increased in patients taking inducing drugs. Induction of carbamazepine metabolism by lamotrigine or valproic acid can produce high plasma concentrations of the toxic metabolite, carbamazepine-10,11-epoxide with clinical toxicity in the presence of normal or low plasma carbamazepine concentrations |
| Inhibition of drug metabolism | Reduced rate of drug metabolism; usually prolonged action, accumulation and toxicity | Reduced metabolic clearance of many drugs, including tolbutamide, phenytoin, warfarin, theophylline, terfenadine, astemizole and midazolam by inhibitors of oxidative drug metabolism such as cimetidine, phenylbutazone, sulfinpyrazone, some sulfonamides and macrolide antibiotics, chloramphenicol, azole antifungal agents, verapamil, diltiazem, fluoxetine, fluvoxamine, isoniazid, dextropropoxyphene, disulfiram and alcohol (short term consumption) |
| | | Reduction in hepatic blood flow by β-adrenoceptor blockers increases the oral bioavailability of high clearance drugs such as lidocaine, chlormethiazole and morphine |
| | | Serious potentiation of azathioprine and mercaptopurine by allopurinol |
| | | Suxamethonium paralysis prolonged by ecothiopate, demecarium, phenelzine, pyridostigmine and tacrine |
| | | Disulfiram-like syndrome following alcohol in some patients receiving chlorpropamide, metronidazole, ketoconazole, procarbazine, and some cefalosporins [e.g. latamoxef (moxalactam), cefamandole, cefoperazone, cefotetan] |
| Interference with biliary excretion | Prolonged drug action | Inhibition of hepatic uptake and delayed plasma clearance of rifampicin by probenecid in some individuals |
| | | Probenecid reduces non-renal clearance of indomethacin, possibly by reducing biliary clearance |
| | | Verapamil, amiodarone and quinidine decrease the biliary clearance of digoxin |

**Table IV.** *[Continued]*

| Mechanism | Effect | Examples[a] |
|---|---|---|
| Interference with renal excretion due to drug-induced renal impairment | Reduced renal clearance, prolonged effects, cumulation and toxicity | Increased serum digoxin and flucytosine concentrations in renal impairment induced by aminoglycosides, amphotericin B, captopril or cyclosporin |
| Competition for active renal tubular secretion | Reduced renal clearance, prolonged effects, cumulation and toxicity | Phenylbutazone and dicoumarol cause accumulation of chlorpropamide with hypoglycaemia<br>Salicylate, high-dose penicillin, NSAIDs, probenecid and sulfonamides inhibit excretion of methotrexate<br>Probenecid reduces the renal clearance of penicillins, cefalosporins, zidovudine, dapsone, furosemide and sulfinpyrazone<br>Salicylate (low doses) inhibits the actions of uricosuric drugs<br>Quinidine, amiodarone and verapamil reduces the renal clearance of digoxin; cimetidine and ranitidine reduce the renal clearance of procainamide |
| Changes in urine pH | Renal clearance of basic drugs (pKa 7.5 to 10) increased in acid urine; clearance of acidic drugs (pKa 3 to 7.5) enhanced in alkaline urine, decreased in acid urine | Renal excretion of amphetamine and ephedrine, increased in acid urine, decreased in alkaline urine (e.g. following administration of sodium bicarbonate or acetazolamide)<br>Renal clearance of quinidine is decreased in an alkaline urine<br>Renal clearance of salicylate and barbiturates enhanced in alkaline urine (e.g. following antacid therapy) |
| Monoamine oxidase inhibition | Hypertensive reactions, coma and hyperpyrexia; potentiation of antidiabetic agents and antihypertensive drugs; interactions more common with older nonselective MAOIs than newer selective MAOIs | Acute hypertensive crisis or exaggerated and prolonged rise in blood pressure following foods containing tyramine or dopamine (matured cheese, chianti-type wine, yeast extracts, pickled herrings, broad beans), pressor agents (amphetamine, mephentermine), nasal decongestants (ephedrine), proprietary cold 'cures' (phenylpropanolamine, pseudoephedrine) and levodopa<br>Central excitation with methyldopa<br>Hypotension, agitation, tremor, convulsions, hyperpyrexia and coma in minority of patients given pethidine, tricyclic antidepressants and anaesthetics<br>Serotonergic syndrome in some patients receiving concurrent fluoxetine, clomipramine or tryptophan<br>Potentiation of some antidiabetic and antihypertensive agents |
| Antagonism of antibacterial and antiviral agents | Reduced antibacterial or antiviral activity | Mutual antagonism between bactericidal and bacteriostatic drugs when both drugs used at minimum effective levels, e.g. penicillins and tetracycline<br>Ribavirin antagonises the antiviral effect of zidovudine |
| Mechanisms unknown | Antagonism or potentiation | Antagonism of effects of levodopa by pyridoxine<br>Antagonism of effect of warfarin by sucralfate<br>Paradoxical rise in blood pressure in some patients when clonidine combined with sotalol<br>Increased nephrotoxicity of methoxyflurane in patients receiving tetracycline<br>Potentiation of aminoglycoside-related ototoxicity by furosemide and ethacrynic acid |

a Examples given which refer only to the mechanism involved (e.g. reduced rate of absorption, inhibition of metabolism) may not necessarily be of clinical significance.

*Abbreviations:* ACE = angiotensin converting enzyme; MAOIs = monoamine oxidase inhibitors; NSAIDs = nonsteroidal anti-inflammatory drugs.

Such extrapolations might be relevant when an interaction involves a pharmacodynamic mechanism, but should not normally be made with pharmacokinetic interactions.[50] Indeed, pharmacodynamic interactions involving one drug should generally be anticipated with other related drugs, even though confirmation in humans is lacking. For example, cardiovascular effects attributed to propranolol may well be observed with other β-blockers. However, the situation is often different with interactions involving pharmacokinetic mechanisms.

Drugs have characteristic physicochemical and pharmacokinetic properties. For example, pharmacokinetic interactions that can occur with cimetidine rarely occur with other $H_2$-receptor antagonists. Similarly, the interaction between terfenadine or astemizole and ketoconazole or itraconazole cannot be extrapolated to apply to all nonsedating antihistamines and azole antifungal agents.[51-54]

Considerable efforts are made in the preclinical evaluation of new drugs to predict potential for interaction in clinical use, but these only provide a guide for subsequent clinical studies.[55,56] It must be emphasised that interactions will not necessarily occur in all patients receiving a given combination of potentially interacting drugs. This is not only because of individual variation (see section 1.5), but also because the occurrence of a clinically important interaction often depends on a variety of factors additional to the combination of drugs given, including genetics, age, pre-existent disease and use of nonprescribed agents.[20,57-59]

Many pharmacodynamic interactions are potentially predictable and could be avoided with knowledge of the actions of drugs and the use of common sense. It should come as no surprise to find that the combined use of full doses of potent vasodilators such as diazoxide and hydralazine can cause catastrophic hypotension, that combinations of hypnosedatives, antidepressants and opioid analgesics may cause depression, gait disturbance and confusion in the elderly, and that dopamine and ergotamine combined may cause peripheral vasoconstriction resulting in gangrene of the extremities. Strategies to avoid such adverse reactions include avoidance of the combination or institution of therapy by a process of careful serial dosage increments after the effects of the previous dose are observed (see further appendix B).

## 2.1 Pharmaceutical Incompatibility

Drugs may be inactivated or precipitated from solution if mixed in syringes or added to blood or infusion fluids prior to administration. Phenytoin has a pKa of around 8.0 to 8.3 and may precipitate in many types of crystalloid solution, which have a lower pH, but is more likely to do so in 5% dextrose than 0.9% saline solution.[60] This means that when intravenous phenytoin is required, it should be administered in 0.9% saline and with vigilance for precipitation. Thiopental has a high pKa and may produce a precipitate if mixed with a number of commonly administered anaesthetic drugs that produce a lower pH when made soluble. These include suxamethonium (succinylcholine), pancuronium, atracurium and ketamine. Amphotericin B when administered intravenously in the non-liposomal form is prone to precipitate in electrolyte-containing solutions and so should be given in 5% dextrose.[61] Hydrocortisone may inactivate penicillins, heparin or kanamycin given concurrently. Some drugs are inactivated by exposure to light (sodium nitroprusside) or by binding the plastic of their containers or giving sets [nitroglycerin (glyceryl trinitrate)].

The interaction of gentamicin and carbenicillin is a specific incompatability that is quite commonly encountered, and is important in terms of interpretation of gentamicin concentrations (see further chapter 5; sect. 2.2.2).

Interactions of this type are not limited to drugs administered by the intravenous route. If soluble (rapid acting) insulin is coadministered subcutaneously with slower acting insulins containing either zinc or protamine, then the onset of effect of the rapid acting insulin may be markedly delayed, probably due to the formation of slowly soluble complexes with the protamine or zinc.[62] The use of soda lime (a mix of hydroxides of sodium or potassium with calcium hydroxide) with a number of inhalational anaesthetic agents can result in degradation, absorption and altered solubility of the anaesthetic gas. This has a variety of potential outcomes. When soda lime is used with older anaesthetic agents such as chloroform and trichloroethylene, it can result in the production of toxic products such as phosgene and dichloroacetylene. This has not been a problem with more modern inhalational anaesthetics, but their use with soda lime can result in diminished anaesthetic delivery and delayed onset of anaesthesia, particularly where halothane and sevoflurane are used.[63,64] This effect can be minimised by ensuring adequate water content of the soda lime used.[65]

Numerous physical incompatibilities have been demonstrated and drugs should never be mixed unless the absence of reaction has been clearly established.[66-69]

## 2.2 Pharmacodynamic Interactions

Pharmacodynamic interactions involving additive, synergistic or antagonistic effects of drugs acting on the same receptors or physiological systems probably account for most clinically important drug interactions, although they have not received the attention they deserve. The greatest problems appear to be caused by multiple prescription of drugs acting on the central nervous system (CNS).[13] This is a particular problem in elderly patients.

Many psychotherapeutic drugs and their active metabolites have very long elimination half-lives, and since the full effects may not become apparent for several weeks, neither the patient nor the clinician may associate slow deterioration with drug therapy. The inappropriate prescription of CNS depressants with antidepressants, convulsants [e.g. high-dose penicillins, imipenem, lidocaine (lignocaine)] with antiepileptics, and even β-adrenoceptor blockers with β-adrenoceptor agonists is not uncommon. Interaction between psychotherapeutic drugs, alcohol and a variety of illicit drugs is a major problem and contributes significantly to death and injury in road traffic accidents.[70-73]

An enormous number of interactions could be included in table IV, but only representative examples of the most important types are listed.

### *2.2.1 Interactions at Receptors*

One drug may have a greater affinity than another for a receptor. If it has little or no intrinsic activity, the actions of the second drug are antagonised (see chapter 1; sect. 1.2). This is a common mechanism of drug action, and drugs such as atropine and tubocurarine act by combining reversibly with receptors and thus prevent access to the normal physiological transmitter (acetylcholine). Since the drug-receptor combination is reversible, it is possible to overcome the antagonism by increasing the amount of agonist at the receptor. Thus, muscle paralysis induced by non-depolarising relaxants such as tubocurarine, atracurium, pancuronium or vecuronium can be reversed by neostigmine or edrophonium which inhibit cholinesterase and increase the concentration of acetylcholine at receptors.[66,74]

Many other interactions occur at receptors and familiar examples include the antagonism of opioid analgesics by naloxone, and the competition for β-adrenoceptors between catecholamines such as adrenaline (epinephrine) and β-blockers such as propranolol. In the latter case, use of adrenaline as an inotropic drug in patients receiving β-adrenoceptor blocking agents can result in severe hypertension as well as peripheral ischaemia due to vasoconstriction from peripheral $\alpha_1$-adrenoceptor effects that would usually be opposed by peripheral β-adrenoceptor action.[75-77] Individuals on β-blockers may also be relatively resistant to the effects of adrenaline in the treatment of anaphylaxis.[78-80]

Serious interactions characterised by extrapyramidal syndromes and irreversible dementia have been reported with lithium combined with methyldopa or haloperidol, and with methyldopa combined with haloperidol.[81-83] The mechanisms are unknown, but all 3 drugs act on central dopaminergic receptors. However, in the case of the former, the possibility of lithium intoxication should always be excluded.[84] Similarly, many antidepressant drugs have effects on the central serotonergic system and their use in combination can result in a potentially fatal serotonin syndrome in a small number of individuals (see section 3).[85,86] Other examples include bradycardia and atrioventricular conduction defects with calcium antagonists (e.g. verapamil, diltiazem) given in combination with β-adrenoceptor blockers such as propranolol or with digoxin,[87-89] and potentiation of some neuromuscular blocking agents by aminoglycoside antibiotics and some calcium antagonists.[37,90,91]

Some drugs may alter the pharmacodynamic effects of another drug either by altering receptor sensitivity or by an action on another receptor that results in synergistic or antagonistic effects within the cell concerned or at another 'downstream' site. One example of this is in the induction of anaesthesia where opioids potentiate the sedative response to benzodiazepines.[92-94] The opioid antagonist naloxone has been shown to diminish the sedative effects of diazepam.[95] Benzodiazepines exert their sedative effects by interacting with the γ-aminobutyric acid subtype A ($GABA_A$) receptor/chloride ionophore complex on the cell membrane of CNS neurones, whereas opioids interact with their own receptors that may be present on the same or adjacent neurons to induce sedation and analgesia. It has been suggested that opioids and benzodiazepines may produce synergistic effects on the CNS either by a combined effect on intracellular ('downstream') cyclic adenosine monophosphate (cyclic-AMP) concentrations or by opioids altering $GABA_A$ receptor subunit phosphorylation through a cyclic-AMP dependent process.[96] While this effect is useful in anaesthesia, the combined sedative effect of benzodiazepines and opioids on the CNS in the non-anaesthetic setting may be potentially fatal. Acute alcohol ingestion also potentiates $GABA_A$ receptor effects in a selection of CNS neurons which have the long chain variant of this receptor, and this accounts for some of its sedative effects and explains the additive sedative effect seen when it is combined with benzodiazepines and/or opioids.[97,98]

Many other drugs are known to produce additive sedative effects when used in combination including antihistamines, some antidepressants and antiepileptics. Some of these, such as phenytoin are well known to interact at the level of the $GABA_A$ receptor while others appear to produce sedation by actions at other sites within the CNS.

#### *2.2.2 Drugs Acting at the Same Site or on the Same Physiological System*

Combinations of drugs acting at the same site or influencing the same physiological system may cause reduced or exaggerated responses. Diuretics, drugs with β-blocking effects, MAOIs, anaesthetics and CNS depressants may potentiate the blood pressure-lowering effects of antihypertensive agents.[99] There is great potential for interactions involving the cardiovascular and the central and peripheral nervous systems in anaesthetic practice.[38,100-102] This type of pharmacodynamic interaction is exemplified by the hypotension seen in some patients on angiotensin converting enzyme (ACE) inhibitors at the induction of general anaesthesia.[103,104]

Such interactions are not limited to prescribed drugs: the deleterious effects of cocaine and cigarette smoking in reducing myocardial oxygen supply (coronary artery vasoconstriction) and increasing demand (as measured by the cardiac rate pressure product) are synergistic when these agents are taken together, as is commonly the case.[105]

#### *2.2.3 Changes in Fluid and Electrolyte Balance*

Changes in electrolyte balance may alter the effects of drugs, particularly those acting on the myocardium, neuromuscular transmission and on the kidney. An important interaction is the potentiation of the action of cardiac glycosides by diuretic-induced hypokalaemia.[106] The proarrhythmic potential of some antiarrhythmic drugs, particularly sotalol, amiodarone, quinidine and disopyramide, is potentiated by hypokalaemia due to concurrently administered diuretics.[107-109] The sudden release of potassium from muscle following the injection of suxamethonium (succinylcholine) may cause ventricular arrhythmias in patients receiving digitalis.[110,111] Non-depolarising muscle relaxants may produce prolonged paralysis in the presence of hypokalaemia in patients taking potassium-depleting diuretics; hypokalaemia causes hyperpolarisation of the motor end-plate and thereby antagonises the action of acetylcholine.

Potassium chloride is obviously contraindicated in patients also taking potassium-sparing diuretics. This combination can cause fatal hyperkalaemia in patients with impaired renal function.[112] Nevertheless, in one study, no less than 42% of 245 patients on spironolactone were also prescribed potassium chloride and of these, 52% developed hyperkalaemia.[11] Angiotensin converting enzyme (ACE) inhibitors may increase plasma potassium concentrations and there is a risk of hyperkalaemia if these drugs are used with potassium supplements, particularly in patients with impaired renal function and/or diabetes mellitus.[113,114] NSAIDs may produce fluid retention, hyperkalaemia, renal impairment and loss of blood pressure control if coadministered with ACE inhibitors. This occurs through the ability of NSAIDs to inhibit prostaglandins G and H synthetase, which reduces the renal synthesis of these vasodilator prostaglandins.[115-117] Aspirin has relatively weak inhibitory effects on renal prostaglandins when given in low doses[118] but may elevate blood pressure slightly. When aspirin is given in moderate to high dosages, it can abolish the beneficial effects of enalapril on the cardiovascular system (reduction in systemic vascular resistance, left ventricular filling pressure and total pulmonary resistance) in patients with severe heart failure.[119,120]

There is a direct relationship between lithium excretion and sodium balance. Lithium intoxication can be precipitated by the use of diuretics, particularly thiazides and thiazide-like agents, including metolazone.[121,122] Lithium intoxication may also be produced by the concurrent administration of some NSAIDs.[123-125] This is due principally to the inhibition by NSAIDs of prostaglandin-dependent renal excretion mechanisms for lithium. NSAIDs also impair renal function and cause sodium and wa-

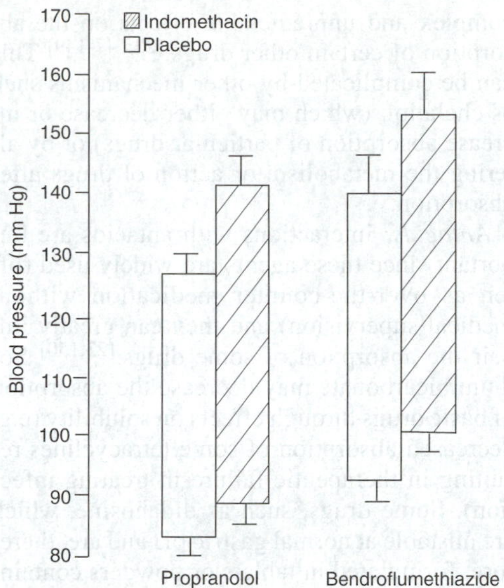


**Fig. 1.** Changes in fluid and electrolyte balance after adding either indomethacin 100mg daily for 3 weeks or placebo to regimens of either bendroflumethiazide (bendrofluazide) [n = 5] or propranolol (n = 8) in patients with hypertension. The upper and lower margins of each bar represent mean supine systolic and diastolic pressures, respectively (after Watkins et al.[127]).

ter retention, and may give rise to other interactions both as a result of this effect and impaired renal synthesis of vasodilator prostaglandins.[126] Thus, NSAIDs antagonise the effects of most diuretics and antihypertensive drugs and there have been numerous reports of such interactions occurring in oedematous and hypertensive patients (see fig. 1).[14,128,129] The combination of indomethacin and triamterene appears particularly hazardous as it may result in acute renal failure.[130]

NSAIDs may also interfere with the beneficial effects of diuretics and ACE inhibitors in patients with cardiac failure.[116,129,131] However, some evidence suggests that sulindac has less potential than other NSAIDs for renal-based interaction with other drugs. It may, therefore, be the NSAID of choice in patients being treated for cardiac failure or hypertension or with lithium.[132,133]

#### 2.2.4 Interference with Intracellular Transport Mechanisms

One drug may interfere with the uptake and transport of another to intracellular sites of action. Many aromatic amines are taken up into sympathetic nerve endings by an active transport mechanism which can be blocked competitively by sympathomimetic amines and other compounds. For example, therapeutic doses of ephedrine, amphetamines, phenylpropanolamine, pseudoephedrine, phenylephrine, chlorpromazine, amitriptyline, imipramine and desipramine can inhibit the blood pressure-lowering action of adrenergic neuron blocking drugs such as guanethidine and bethanidine.[99]

Tricyclic antidepressants such as imipramine may potentiate the pressor effects of adrenaline and nonadrenaline (see also chapter 12, sect. 6.1.2). ACE inhibitors and perhexiline (a drug useful in some patients with refractory angina) may induce hypoglycaemia in diabetic patients receiving antidiabetic medication.[134-138] The mechanism of this effect (and its relative clinical importance) has been greatly debated but it probably occurs secondary to enhanced glucose uptake and utilisation, which in the case of ACE inhibitors has been postulated to relate to increased kinin levels enhancing glucose transport.[139-141]

### 2.3 Pharmacokinetic Interactions

#### 2.3.1 Drug Absorption Interactions

Drug absorption depends on a number of factors including formulation, pKa and lipid solubility which should be considered contiguously with splanchnic blood flow and intestinal pH, motility, bacterial flora and the metabolic capacity of the gastrointestinal tract. A drug may alter the rate of absorption or the degree of absorption of other drugs in the gastrointestinal tract. The mechanisms involved in these interactions vary with the individual drugs, their methods and rates of absorption, and with variations in formulation. These variables make prediction of drug absorption interactions very difficult.[142-144]

It is important to differentiate between interactions which alter the *rate* of drug absorption and those which increase or decrease the total *amount* of drug absorbed (i.e. alter bioavailability), since the consequences may be quite different.

A change in the rate of absorption of a drug with a plasma half-life which is long in relation to its dosage interval, such as warfarin (plasma half-life approximately 36 hours; dosage interval 24 hours), would have little or no effect if the total amount of the drug administered were eventually absorbed. A change in the total amount absorbed, however, may lead to significant complications for the patient. Conversely, if the rate of absorption of a drug with a short plasma half-life relative to its dosage interval such as procainamide (plasma half-life approximately 3 hours; dosage interval 4 to 8 hours) is reduced, then therapeutic plasma concentrations may never be reached. Delayed absorption is also important when a rapid effect is required as a function of a rapid, high peak concentration, e.g. with analgesics, hypnotics and some antibiotics. Lack of effect may result where the plasma half-life of the drug is short relative to the duration of absorption due to lack of attainment of a peak concentration or, alternatively, where the plasma half-life of the drug is long relative to the duration of absorption, when the peak in plasma concentration may be delayed with consequent delayed onset of the clinical effects of the drug.

Some adverse effects are dependent on the speed of absorption, such as the tachycardia seen with nifedipine in its standard capsule dosage form. This tachycardia is only rarely seen with the more recently introduced sustained-release preparation, despite the overall extent of absorption being similar.[145]

In the setting of drug interactions, this is exemplified when metoclopramide is given concurrently with slow-release theophylline. The result is a more rapid rate but similar overall extent of theophylline absorption. Adverse effects such as headache and nausea are 3 times more common in individuals receiving concurrent metoclopramide and theophylline. The sensitivity of these adverse effects to the absorption rate is perhaps a reflection of the narrow therapeutic index of theophylline.[146]

#### Change in pH of Gastrointestinal Fluids

The rate of absorption of many drugs is limited by the rate at which the drug passes into solution from its ingested form. Many slow- or extended-release compounds make use of this. Basic drugs are more soluble in acid gastrointestinal contents and acidic drugs are more soluble in alkaline fluids. On the other hand, basic drugs will tend to be ionised and less lipid soluble in acid solution and hence are absorbed less rapidly, but these theoretical concepts do not always hold in practice. For example, weak acids such as aspirin are absorbed more rapidly from buffered alkaline solutions (e.g. in the small intestine) than from unbuffered solutions at pH 2.8 (e.g. in the stomach). Drugs that alter pH, such as antacids, $H_2$-receptor antagonists and proton pump inhibitors may therefore have complex and unpredictable effects on the absorption of certain other drugs.[23,147-149] This can be complicated by other mechanisms such as chelation (which may either decrease or increase absorption of particular drugs) or by altering the metabolism or action of drugs after absorption.

*Antacids:* interactions with antacids are important since these agents are widely used (often as over-the-counter medication without medical supervision) and they can greatly impair the absorption of some drugs.[23,150] Sodium bicarbonate may decrease the absorption of basic drugs through effects on solubility (e.g. decreased absorption of some tetracyclines resulting in therapeutic failure in treating infection). Some drugs, such as didanosine, which are unstable at normal gastric pH and are, therefore, formulated in tablets or powders containing antacid buffers that can increase gastric pH, may alter the absorption of other drugs administered in the subsequent 2 to 3 hours.[151,152]

Magnesium hydroxide has a particular propensity for increasing the rate and sometimes extent of absorption of weak acids such as ibuprofen, glibenclamide (glyburide), tolbutamide and glipizide.[153] With the latter three drugs, there is a potential for hypoglycaemia if the patient mistimes a meal relative to a dose of their oral antidiabetic agent.

Magnesium-containing antacids may decrease the absorption of ciprofloxacin by formation of a less soluble chelation product, whereas their chelation with dicoumarol increases its absorption. The bioavailability of cefpodoxime proxetil and cefuroxime axetil are decreased when drugs which increase the gastric pH are coadministered, probably because these antibiotics are prodrugs that require an acid environment for de-esterification before absorption.[154,155] This is not seen with other commonly used cefalosporins such as cefalexin or cefaclor.

*$H_2$-Receptor antagonists and acid (proton) pump inhibitors:* $H_2$-receptor antagonists inhibit gastric acid secretion and cause the same pH-dependent absorption interactions as antacids, but without chelation or binding effects. Thus, $H_2$-antagonists and antacids greatly reduce the absorption of the antifungal agents ketoconazole and itraconazole, both of which are weak bases and require an acid environment for optimal solubility and absorption.[156,157] The effect of omeprazole and other acid (proton) pump inhibitors on ketoconazole or itra-

conazole absorption has not been widely studied but absorption would be expected to be reduced to a similar extent to that seen with other antiulcer drugs.[158] However, the absorption of fluconazole is not significantly altered by changes in gastric pH.[157,159]

Like magnesium-containing antacids, $H_2$-receptor antagonists and omeprazole may also increase the extent of absorption of glibenclamide (glyburide), glipizide and tolbutamide, with the potential for hypoglycaemia in some circumstances.[160-162] Reductions in serum cyanocobalamin (vitamin $B_{12}$) levels have been reported with omeprazole therapy of greater than 3 years' duration, while a dose-related decrease in the absorption of cyanocobalamin has been demonstrated over a 2-week period of omeprazole therapy.[163,164]

*Sucralfate:* this antiulcer agent has minimal effects on pH but rather acts by coating the upper gastrointestinal mucosa. It produces a small decrease in the absorption of ketoconazole and a significant decrease in levothyroxine absorption through intraluminal binding via the sucralfate polyanion.[165-167] Even though it is poorly absorbed, sucralfate may also antagonise the effects of warfarin without altering warfarin absorption or metabolism (a probable pharmacodynamic effect).[168-172]

#### Effects on Gastric Emptying and Gastrointestinal Motility

Drugs that alter gastrointestinal motility or the rate of gastric emptying often have significant effects on the rate of absorption, but less commonly alter the extent of absorption of other drugs.[143,173] Drugs are absorbed much more rapidly from the small intestine than from the stomach. It follows therefore that agents that alter the rate of gastric emptying may influence the rate of absorption of other drugs given at the same time.[148,174,175] Drugs such as levodopa are metabolised by the gastric mucosa, and if gastric emptying is delayed, less unchanged drug is available for absorption.[176] Other drugs such as digoxin and some penicillins may be degraded by prolonged exposure to gastric acid.[174] On the other hand, very rapid gastrointestinal transit may decrease the absorption of poorly soluble drugs (e.g. nitrofurantoin and digoxin) or drugs that are actively absorbed from a limited area of the intestine (e.g. riboflavin).[177-179]

Pharmaceutical excipients such as mannitol and sodium acid pyrophosphate (SAPP), which decrease small intestinal transit time, may decrease the absorption of drugs that are formulated in them.[180] This has been demonstrated with an effervescent oral form of ranitidine containing SAPP[181] and may be a feature of drugs formulated in chewable or dissolvable effervescent forms where a variety of excipients are used to disguise the taste of the drug. Similar reductions in absorption might be predicted to occur if rapid gastrointestinal transit occurs with medications formulated for slow release, including calcium antagonists and theophylline preparations. However, these medications are well absorbed from most parts of the gastrointestinal tract. Therefore, studies to delineate reductions in absorption with drugs that increase intestinal transit have not shown changes likely to be of clinical significance.

Paracetamol (acetaminophen) is used as a model for drug absorption studies because it is a weak acid (pKa 9.5) that is largely non-ionised in both gastric and intestinal fluids and its rate of absorption in humans is directly related to the gastric emptying rate. *Anticholinergic drugs* such as propantheline and other antispasmodic agents such as *mebeverine* decrease gastrointestinal motility and slow the rate of absorption of paracetamol (fig. 2), but do not affect the total amount of drug absorbed.[183,184] Anticholinergic drugs are commonly used in combination therapy for Parkinson's disease and to treat extrapyramidal effects of antipsychotic medication, but they delay gastric emptying, reducing the bioavailability of levodopa by as much as 50% and reduce plasma chlorpromazine concentrations significantly.[185,186]

On the other hand, the bioavailability of poorly absorbed drugs such as dicoumarol may be increased by concomitant *tricyclic antide-*

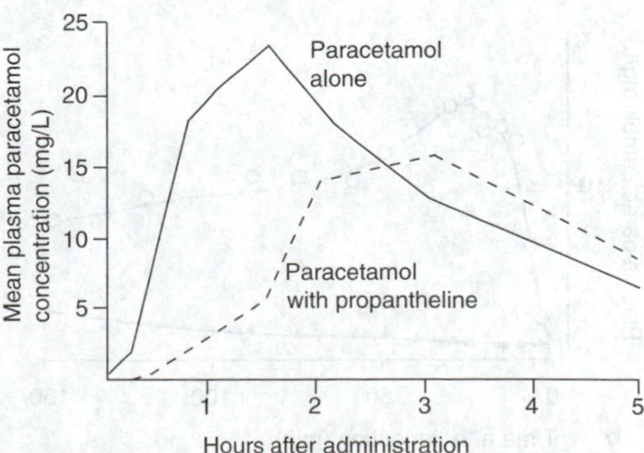


**Fig. 2.** Reduction in the rate of absorption of oral paracetamol (acetaminophen) 1.5g caused by intravenous propantheline 30mg (after Nimmo et al.[183]).

*pressants* in some individuals.[50] Tricyclic antidepressants have marked anticholinergic effects which probably slow gastrointestinal motility. This may increase the time available for dissolution and absorption of dicoumarol. A similar effect has been suggested with slowly dissolving preparations of digoxin after administration of propantheline.[177,178] Other drugs with anticholinergic activity which might influence gastrointestinal motility include antipsychotic drugs (e.g. phenothiazines), and certain sedating antihistamines (e.g. diphenhydramine, promethazine).

*Antacids* such as aluminium hydroxide gel delay gastric emptying and can decrease the rate of absorption of highly soluble and rapidly absorbed drugs such as pentobarbital and isoniazid.[147] β-*Adrenoceptor agonists* and *antagonists* decrease and increase, respectively, the rate of paracetamol absorption, presumably through effects on gastric emptying.[187]

*Opioid analgesics* such as pethidine (meperidine), morphine, diamorphine (heroin), buprenorphine and pentazocine can produce a marked delay in gastric emptying and slow the rate of

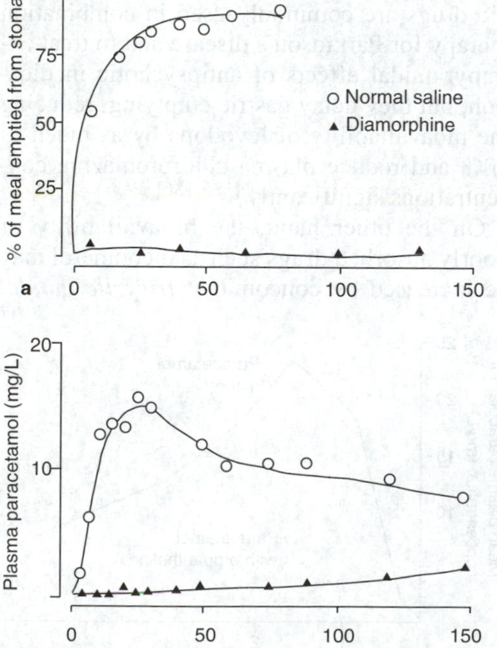


**Fig. 3.** Changes in rates of (a) gastric emptying and (b) drug (paracetamol) absorption are exemplified by the effect of diamorphine (heroin) [10mg intramuscularly] compared with that of saline injection in a healthy individual (after Nimmo et al.[182]).

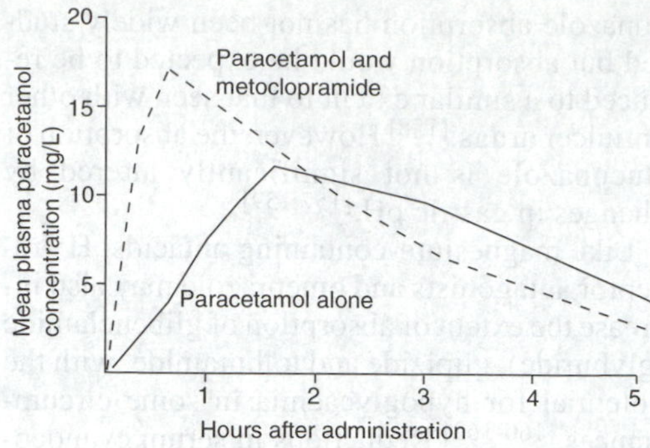


**Fig. 4.** Changes in the rate of absorption of oral paracetamol (1.5g) caused by intravenous metoclopramide 10mg (after Nimmo et al.[183]).

absorption of paracetamol (fig. 3).[188-190] Codeine, which is frequently administered in combination with paracetamol, however, has no significant pharmacokinetic effects on the latter drug.[191] The inhibitory effect of strong analgesics on gastric emptying contributes to slow absorption of oral antiarrhythmic agents and therapeutic failure in patients with acute myocardial infarction.[192] The slowing effects on gastric emptying produced by opioid analgesics are reversed by intravenous metoclopramide and cisapride and intramuscular cisapride, but not intramuscular metoclopramide or oral dosages of either agent.[182,188,193,194]

*Metoclopramide* and *cisapride* accelerate gastric emptying. Metoclopramide has been shown to increase the rate of absorption and peak plasma concentrations of a number of drugs including paracetamol (fig. 4), diazepam, propranolol, alcohol, lithium from slow-release tablets, slow-release theophylline, mefloquine, cyclosporin and others.[146,174,195,196] Cisapride can markedly increase the rate of absorption of a number of drugs, including $H_2$-receptor antagonists, alcohol, disopyramide, flecainide, cyclosporin, sustained-release morphine and possibly oral anticoagulants.[197] However, the overall extent of absorption of these drugs when coadministered with prokinetic agents is usually not significantly increased. An exception to this is cyclosporin, which normally has slow and erratic absorption. Prokinetic drugs may greatly increase its overall absorption, with the potential for resultant toxicity.[195,198] Conversely, plasma concentrations of digoxin from slowly dissolving tablets are decreased with metoclopramide coadministration, possibly as a result of the decreased time available for disso-

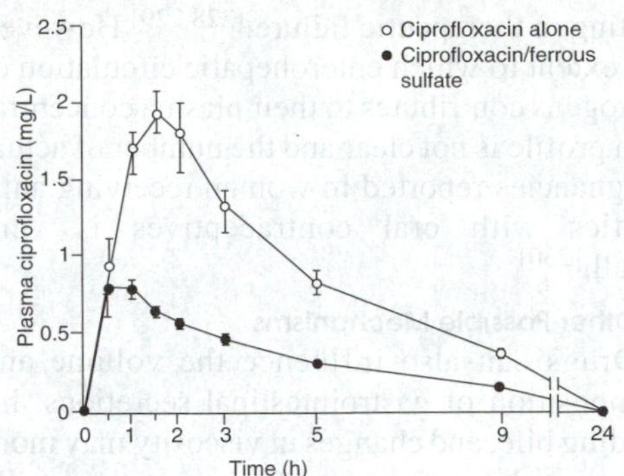


**Fig. 5.** Interference with drug absorption, where reduced absorption of ciprofloxacin is caused by simultaneous ingestion of ferrous sulfate (after Lehto et al.;[201] by permission of author and editor).

lution and absorption of digoxin, a poorly soluble drug.[177,178,199] Similar findings have been reported with chlorothiazide.[200]

The results of interactions involving changes in gastrointestinal motility may depend critically on dissolution characteristics. Depending on whether the drug is readily or poorly soluble, and whether release of the drug from its formulation is rapid or slow, there may be significant variation in its rate and extent of absorption.

#### Binding or Chelation of Drugs

Drugs may react directly within the gastrointestinal tract to form insoluble chelates which cannot be absorbed, e.g. iron and quinolone antibiotics such as ciprofloxacin[201] (fig. 5) or aluminium-, calcium- or magnesium-containing antacids and tetracycline or ciprofloxacin.[149,169,202,203] In some cases, more rapidly absorbed soluble complexes are formed (e.g. caffeine and ergotamine). The absorption of dicoumarol is increased by the formation of a more soluble complex with magnesium hydroxide,[204] while the absorption of penicillamine is decreased by the formation of less soluble chelates when it is coadministered with aluminium- and magnesium-containing antacids, food and iron preparations.[205] The absorption of levodopa, levodopa/carbidopa combinations and methyldopa is diminished by the concurrent use of iron supplements, with resultant loss of efficacy.[206,207]

Absorption of drugs may also be reduced if they are given with adsorbents such as kaolin or charcoal, or anionic exchange resins such as cholestyramine and colestipol. Digoxin absorption is seriously impaired by some antacids and by kaolin-pectin combinations.[208] Propranolol, digoxin, warfarin, tricyclic antidepressants, cyclosporin and thyroxine absorption is reduced by colestipol and cholestyramine.[209-212] Sucralfate interferes with absorption of ciprofloxacin, thyroxine, phenytoin and a number of other drugs.[149,166,213,214] Orally administered adsorbents may also interrupt the enterohepatic circulation of some drugs (see further section 2.3.6).

Bisphosphonates such as etidronate are often coprescribed with calcium supplements in the treatment of osteoporosis. If these preparations are ingested at the same time, the bioavailability of both is significantly reduced – a potential unrecognised cause of therapeutic failure.[215] This may be avoided either by giving etidronate in the morning and calcium supplements at night, or by alternating treatment with etidronate for 2 weeks and calcium supplements for 10 weeks in a given 12-week period.[216] Many potential chelation and adsorption interactions can in fact be avoided by separating doses of the respective drugs by 2 hours or more.

#### Competition for Active Absorption Mechanisms

Drugs that are analogues of naturally occurring purines, pyrimidines, sugars and amino acids (e.g. mercaptopurine, levodopa, methyldopa) may be absorbed by specialised active transport systems that exist primarily in the small intestine, and absorption of these agents can be inhibited on a competitive basis. Amino β-lactam antibiotics such as amoxicillin and cefalexin are, in effect, analogues of the dipeptide D-alanyl-D-alanine and are actively transported by the small intestinal dipeptide carrier. Inhibition of the absorption of these drugs by others using the transporter has been demonstrated, as has potentiation of their absorption by coadministration of nifedipine.[217] The efficiency of the dipeptide carrier depends on the pH gradient generated by sodium/hydrogen ion exchange across the brush border of the small intestine. Amiloride is an inhibitor of sodium/hydrogen exchange and has been shown to diminish the bioavailability of oral amoxicillin (fig. 6).[218]

#### Toxic Effects on the Gastrointestinal Tract

Patients receiving therapy with neomycin, mefenamic acid and colchicine may develop a malabsorption syndrome. In such circumstances, the absorption of other drugs might be impaired. Thus, colchicine may cause megaloblastic anaemia by interfering with ileal

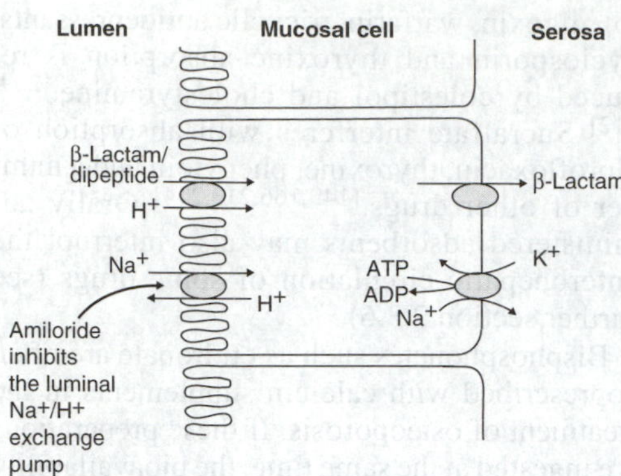


**Fig. 6.** Competition for active absorption mechanisms is exemplified by the dependence of transmucosal absorption of amino β-lactam antibiotics such as amoxicillin and cefalexin on the activity of the sodium/hydrogen ($Na^+/H^+$) ion exchange pump. Amiloride inhibits the sodium/hydrogen ion exchange pump, resulting in reduced bioavailability of coadministered amoxicillin or cefalexin (after Catnach et al.;[217] by permission of author and publisher).

cyanocobalamin (vitamin $B_{12}$) absorption, while neomycin diminishes the absorption of phenoxymethylpenicillin (penicillin V), cyanocobalamin and digoxin.[219-221]

Antineoplastic agents may change the mucosal absorptive surface, alter motility of the upper gastrointestinal tract, and decrease the bioavailability of a number of drugs including phenytoin, digoxin and verapamil.[222-224] Mucosal absorptive abnormalities return to normal approximately one week after combination chemotherapy.[223]

### Changes in Gut Bacterial Flora

Some drugs are metabolised extensively (sulfasalazine) or in part (levodopa) by the gut bacterial flora.[34,225] This process may be altered by concurrent administration of antibacterial drugs. Suppression of the gut bacterial flora by antibiotics may limit the metabolic conversion of sulfasalazine to its active component.[226,227] In about 10% of individuals, digoxin is extensively metabolised by gut bacteria. Inhibition of these organisms by antibiotics such as erythromycin, tetracycline and other broad-spectrum antibiotics can double the plasma concentration of digoxin, the effect being greatest with poorly absorbed oral formulations of digoxin.[33,34]

Antibiotics may also prevent the intestinal bacterial hydrolysis of drug conjugates secreted into bile and, thus, reduce reabsorption of the active parent drug. In this way, antibiotics may reduce the enterohepatic circulation of ethinylestradiol in oral contraceptives, potentially resulting in therapeutic failure.[228,229] However, the extent to which enterohepatic circulation of estrogens contributes to their plasma concentration profile is not clear and the number of actual pregnancies reported in women receiving antibiotics with oral contraceptives is very small.[230]

### Other Possible Mechanisms

Drugs can also influence the volume and composition of gastrointestinal secretions, including bile, and changes in viscosity may modify drug absorption. Interference with micelle formation may limit the solubility of lipids, e.g. inhibition of absorption of cholesterol, bile acids and retinol (vitamin A) by long term neomycin therapy. Other possible mechanisms include changes in portal blood flow and permeability of the gastrointestinal epithelium. The mechanisms of many other drug absorption interactions are unknown.

Many new drugs with powerful effects on gastrointestinal function have the potential to alter the absorption of other drugs. The somatostatin analogue *octreotide* has multiple effects on the gastrointestinal tract including acceleration of gastric emptying, reduction in splanchnic blood flow, diminished pancreatic and gastric acid secretion, and increased intestinal transit time.[231] Studies examining the interactive potential of octreotide have yet to be performed, but case reports suggest it has the potential to reduce the oral bioavailability of cyclosporin.[232]

*Acarbose* competitively inhibits intestinal α-glucosidases and delays release of glucose from complex carbohydrates and disaccharides, and thereby improves postprandial blood sugar control in patients with diabetes mellitus.[233-235] It has been found to slow the absorption of concurrently administered metformin, although overall bioavailability may not be altered.[236] This does not appear to adversely affect blood sugar control. The mechanism of reduced metformin absorption is unclear, but may relate either to decreased gastrointestinal transit time secondary to malabsorbed sugar in the gut lumen, or interference with enzymes involved in active metformin uptake.[236,237] Studies have shown that the pharmacokinetics of digoxin, propranolol and glibenclamide (glyburide) are not altered by concurrent acarbose therapy.[238,239] However, the effects of acarbose on the absorption of other drugs with more labile bioavailability such as cyclosporin are not easily predicted and, therefore, studies of its effects on other coadministered drugs of this type are needed.

#### 2.3.2 Drug Distribution Interactions

One drug may change the distribution of another, but the effect of changes (such as displacement of drugs from plasma protein binding sites) on concentrations of unbound drug is negligible because changes in distribution do not alter drug clearance. The net effect of clearance of unbound drug is to return the unbound drug concentration to predisplacement levels. In the *tissues*, displacement of one drug from tissue binding sites by another may alter pharmacokinetics by reducing the volume of distribution of the displaced drug (see chapter 1, sect. 3.2.3); however, the capacity of tissue binding sites is huge, so that such displacement may have only a transient effect on the unbound drug concentration. Longer term changes in steady-state concentrations depend on other interactive mechanisms such as inhibition of metabolism or excretion.

The importance of plasma protein binding interactions as a cause of clinically relevant drug interactions has been overestimated in the past. There are very few, if any, plasma protein binding interactions that produce clinically important changes in drug action.[240]

##### Plasma Protein Binding Displacement

Many drugs and drug metabolites are highly bound to plasma proteins. Generally, acidic drugs bind predominantly to albumin, though not necessarily to the same site (see chapter 1; sect. 3.2.1), while basic drugs such as tricyclic antidepressants, lidocaine, disopyramide and propranolol bind to the acute phase reactant protein $\alpha_1$-acid glycoprotein (AAG) as well as albumin. The addition of another drug to a primary drug regimen may, under certain circumstances, result in displacement of the primary drug from its plasma binding site, leading to altered kinetics and potentially, in some instances (see below), to altered drug effects in the patient.

However, while protein binding displacement has been implicated as the causative mechanism in many drug interactions, its importance has generally been overstated, being based largely on *in vitro* data. Since displacement makes more unbound (free) drug available for metabolism or glomerular filtration and the displaced drug can normally distribute out of the plasma compartment, increased unbound drug concentrations are usually only transient and, therefore, do not commonly give rise to altered pharmacological effects in the patient. It is the *intrinsic clearance* of a drug that determines steady-state unbound drug concentrations for a given dosage rate, and protein binding displacement interactions do not normally alter intrinsic clearance. Therefore, steady-state unbound drug concentrations remain essentially unaltered. Those interactions formerly considered to occur via displacement from plasma binding sites usually have another interaction mechanism involved, e.g. decreased liver metabolism or renal elimination.[240-244]

For further discussion of plasma protein binding displacement interactions and their clinical significance, see chapter 1, section 3.2.3 and chapter 5, section 1.6.3.

##### Tissue Binding Displacement

Interactions can occur if one drug displaces another from binding sites (other than receptors) in the tissues. However, because of the huge capacity of tissue binding sites, transient increases in unbound drug concentration rather than longer lasting alterations are the more common result of drug-induced tissue binding displacement.

Quinidine, verapamil, nifedipine and amiodarone cause a variable but often very significant increase in steady-state plasma concentrations of digoxin. Not only does quinidine decrease the total clearance of digoxin, but it also appears to decrease its volume of distribution, perhaps by displacing it from tissue binding sites (see also section 2.3.8).[245,246]

The contribution of the various mechanisms of interaction to the overall increase in serum digoxin concentrations is debated. The mechanism by which an apparent increase in volume of distribution for digoxin occurs after the addition of these other drugs is unknown. The slow increase in serum digoxin concentrations that results from these interactions does not suggest that displacement from tissue binding sites is the dominant mechanism, because there is no abrupt increase. The volume of distribution certainly appears to decrease but this could be a misleading phenomenon due to the assumption implicit in all methods of computing volume of distribution from plasma concentrations that all elimination is from the central compartment. If elimination changes in a peripheral compartment then there will appear to be a change in the volume of distribution. The decrease in renal and non-renal components of clearance may indeed reflect a change in elimination from a non-central compartment. In any case, it appears that alterations in volume of distribution are less important than effects on digoxin excretion once a new steady-state concentration is approached. The contribution of tissue binding displacement to the interaction may be transient and important only in the first few days after the introduction of the interacting agent. The quinidine-digoxin interaction may be anticipated and many clinicians work on the assumption that the dose of digoxin should be halved when quinidine is added.

### 2.3.3 Induction of Drug Metabolism

Many lipid soluble drugs and foreign compounds stimulate drug metabolism through induction of metabolising enzymes present in the liver and gastrointestinal mucosa. Thus, long term exposure to enzyme-inducing agents such as barbiturates, phenytoin, carbamazepine, aminoglutethimide, alcohol, rifampicin (rifampin), griseofulvin and insecticides such as dicophane (DDT) and lindane causes stimulation of not only their own metabolism, but also the metabolism of many other unrelated drugs and endogenous hormones that are substrates for these enzymes.[247-249] Cigarette smoking also causes induction of the metabolism of drugs including theophylline, propranolol, tricyclic antidepressants and heparin and should, as a consequence, be considered a contributory factor in drug interactions.[250-254] The induction effect of tobacco smoking is probably mediated through polycyclic hydrocarbons which are systemically absorbed.[255]

Depending on drug dosage and half-life, induction usually develops over a period of several days or weeks, and persists for a similar period following withdrawal of the enzyme-inducing agent. The time course of enzyme induction will depend in part on the pharmacokinetic characteristics of the inducer but may be determined more by the kinetics of the enzyme that is induced, e.g. if the half-life of the enzyme is 3 days it will take approximately 12 days for the enzyme to reach a new steady-state level as a consequence of its increased rate of synthesis. Enzyme-inducing drugs with shorter half-lives (e.g. rifampicin) will induce metabolism more quickly than drugs with longer half-lives (e.g. phenytoin or phenobarbital) because they reach steady-state concentrations more rapidly. The diminishment of induction effects of drugs with shorter half-lives is also more rapid than those with longer ones. The effects of chlorinated hydrocarbon insecticides such as dicophane and lindane are more persistent since they are stored in body fat and have very long elimination half-lives.

Induction of drug metabolism is a complex, dose-related phenomenon. It requires the inducer to reach a critical concentration at an intranuclear receptor or regulation point from which upregulation of messenger RNA occurs with consequent increases in enzyme protein production.[248] At the start of administration of the drug, there may be transient inhibition. Mixed-function oxidase (cytochrome P450; CYP) is not one enzyme, but rather a group of closely related isoenzymes with different, but often overlapping, specificities which are localised predominantly in the liver and mucosa of the upper gastrointestinal tract.[256,257] Thus, an enzyme-inducing agent may stimulate the metabolism of some drugs but not others, even though they share the same metabolic route.[247,258] In the case of drugs affecting warfarin metabolism, their effect may be on the metabolism of either enantiomer or both. Phenobarbital and rifampicin increase the clearance of both the *R* and *S* isomers (metabolised by cytochrome P450 subtypes CYP1A2 and CYP2C9/10, respectively),[259,260] whereas the inhibitory effects of a number of drugs on warfarin metabolism may be relatively stereoselective (see section 2.3.4). Complex reciprocal interactions may occur between antiepileptic drugs, in which stimulation or inhibition of metabolism may occur.[261-263]

The effects of drugs whose metabolites have little or no pharmacological activity are reduced by enzyme-inducing drugs. This may partly explain the development of tolerance to some agents. On the other hand, drug effects may be enhanced if metabolites are more active than the parent compound. Sometimes toxicity is caused by drug metabolites and toxicity may be enhanced by previous exposure to enzyme-inducing agents. Experimental paracetamol hepatotoxicity is increased by some enzyme-inducing agents and many reports attest to the increased toxicity of paracetamol (metabolised by CYP2E1) in patients who have a significant long term alcohol intake.[8,59,264] Acute hepatic necrosis has been reported in patients previously taking enzyme-inducing drugs following anaesthesia with halothane.[265-267]

The induction in carbamazepine metabolism (metabolised predominantly by CYP3A4) produced by lamotrigine and valproic acid may result in clinical toxicity secondary to elevated concentrations of its epoxide metabolite in the presence of normal serum carbamazepine concentrations.[268-270] It has been suggested that hepatitis in patients on isoniazid is caused by the metabolite, acetylhydrazine and that the induction of metabolising enzymes by phenytoin in slow acetylators of isoniazid results in increased production of this metabolite with an increased incidence of hepatitis.[271]

Stimulation of the metabolism of warfarin (metabolised by CYP2C9/10) and other oral anticoagulants by barbiturates, phenytoin, carbamazepine and rifampicin is one of the most important enzyme-induction interactions.[172,272] If barbiturates are administered to a patient on long term warfarin therapy, the anticoagulant effect is reduced over 1 to 4 weeks and the dose of warfarin may have to be increased between 2- and 10-fold to regain the original effect on prothrombin time. Satisfactory control can usually be maintained with the higher dosage. However, the patient's life is endangered if the enzyme-inducing drug is suddenly withdrawn. Drug metabolising enzyme activity returns to normal in 1 to 4 weeks, and unless the dose of warfarin is correspondingly reduced, the patient is at risk of haemorrhage.

Induction interactions can be particularly difficult to recognise since the enhanced effect of one drug occurs gradually days or weeks after stopping another unrelated drug. When barbiturates are discontinued, warfarin dosages must be progressively reduced over several months to a small fraction of the previous maximum dose. The propensity of barbiturates to interact with other drugs and the development of hypnosedatives and antiepileptic drugs with less interactive potential and better therapeutic : toxic concentration ratios has resulted in diminished use of barbiturates in recent years. While this has reduced the incidence of the warfarin/barbiturate interaction, it still occurs with significant frequency.

***Oral contraceptives and enzyme-inducing drugs:*** interactions involving possible failure of oral contraceptive therapy through enzyme induction (ethinylestradiol is metabolised by CYP3A4 as well as CYP2C and CYP2E1 to varying degrees in different individuals) are of great concern, particularly in family planning clinics and primary care practices. There are reports of unplanned pregnancies and intermenstrual bleeding with the concurrent use of primidone, phenobarbital, phenytoin, carbamazepine, griseofulvin and rifampicin with combination contraceptives, probably due to induction of estrogen metabolism.[228-230,273,274] While these reports suggest that unplanned conception is an uncommon occurrence when these drugs are given in combination, the clinician and patient should be aware that concurrent therapy may diminish the efficacy of the contraceptive pill. Intermenstrual bleeding or irregularity in the onset of menstrual bleeding may be a warning of an inadequate estrogen effect for contraception to be effective. The strategy used in patients taking oral combination contraceptive agents who require therapy with an inducing agent might include:

- The selection of drugs which have not been demonstrated to induce estrogen metabolism, e.g. valproic acid (sodium valproate) or lamotrigine rather than other antiepileptics.[275,276] Finding alternatives for griseofulvin may be difficult as ketoconazole and fluconazole have been reported to be associated with unplanned pregnancies and irregular bleeding, although the mechanism of such an interaction is unclear. Suitable alternatives to rifampicin may also be difficult to identify as many antibiotics have been reported in association with unplanned pregnancies and irregular bleeding in patients on the combination contraceptive pill (through mechanisms that are not fully understood).[230]
- Using an alternative method of contraception (such as a barrier method) for the duration of the enzyme-inducing drug and several weeks after its cessation.
- Using supplemental ethinylestradiol so that the daily dose is increased from 50μg to 100μg either at the commencement of the enzyme-including drug or in response to irregular bleeding.[274,277]

Each of these strategies carries with it particular challenges for the patient and clinician by way of compliance and risk of pregnancy.

Most studies of potential interactions with oral contraceptives have concentrated on the estrogen component and generally progestagen components are less likely to be involved in clinically significant interactions. However, the progestagen-only pill or 'minipill' has not been well studied in the setting of enzyme-in-

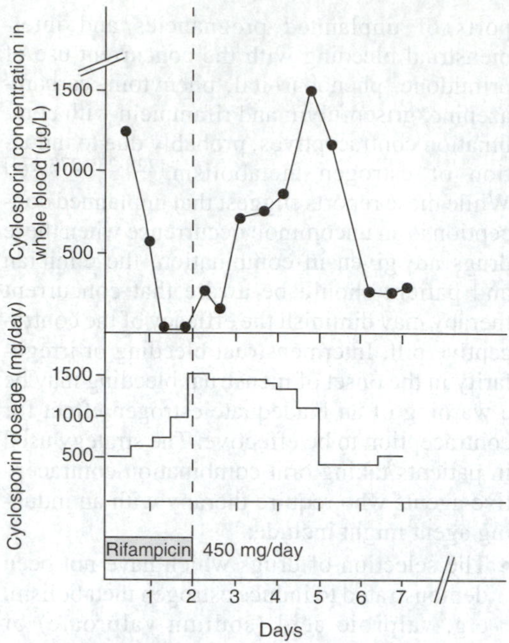


**Fig. 7.** Induction of drug metabolism resulting in therapeutic concentrations of cyclosporin not being attained in a renal transplant patient who also received rifampicin (rifampin). Following cessation of rifampicin (dotted vertical line), cyclosporin concentrations rise to levels required to suppress transplant rejection (after Langhoff & Madsen;[278] by permission of author and publisher).

ducing drugs and therefore does not provide a suitable alternative to combination pills. Some newer contraceptive agents may be less prone to interaction and therefore may provide further alternatives in these patients, although this will require pharmacokinetic evaluation and postmarketing surveillance for each new compound.

Other important induction interactions that may occur with enzyme-inducing drugs include organ transplant rejection in patients receiving cyclosporin for immunosuppression (fig. 7),[278-280] methadone withdrawal reactions in patients on maintenance programmes,[281] and therapeutic failure with digoxin and digitoxin.[246,282,283]

Stimulation of drug metabolism can also have significant effects on the amount of unchanged drug reaching the systemic circulation after an oral dose. This effect is particularly marked with drugs that are extensively metabolised in the first pass through the gastrointestinal tract and liver following absorption (see chapter 1; sect. 3.3). Thus, administration of phenobarbital 100 mg/day for 10 to 14 days had no significant effect on the clearance of alprenolol, but the amount of an oral dose reaching the circulation unchanged was reduced almost 5-fold.[284] Similar changes occur in the pharmacokinetics of oral cyclosporin when the cytochrome P450 enzyme-inducer rifampicin is coadministered.[285,286] This is because a significant proportion of the P450 enzyme subtype responsible for cyclosporin metabolism is present in the mucosa of the upper gastrointestinal tract, where it metabolises orally ingested cyclosporin and is subject to the effects of enzyme-inducing (as well as inhibiting) agents.[34,225,287] Most of the remainder of this enzyme subtype is present in the liver, where it both contributes to first-pass metabolism and increases the clearance of cyclosporin independently of its route of administration. This probably explains the greater effect of inducers of cyclosporin metabolism when cyclosporin is given orally rather than intravenously.[279,280]

#### 2.3.4 Inhibition of Drug Metabolism

Inhibition of drug metabolism may result in exaggerated and prolonged responses, with an increased risk of toxicity. Many interactions of this type involve liver and upper gastrointestinal mucosa drug metabolising enzymes of the cytochrome P450 (CYP) group, and mechanisms[286,288-291] include:

- Reversible competition for enzyme binding sites (e.g. by quinidine)
- An enzyme/substrate product which binds the enzyme tightly but not irreversibly to form an inactive complex (e.g. by macrolide antibiotics)
- Enzyme destruction (e.g. by vinyl chloride)
- Inhibition of enzyme synthesis (by some metallic ions)
- Interference with drug transport (e.g. for digoxin).

Of these mechanisms of enzyme inhibition, reversible competition is probably the most common.

The onset of inhibition through reversible competition occurs once sufficient concentrations of inhibitor accumulate at the site(s) of enzyme action (usually the liver). The inhibitory effect is maximal within the first 24 hours of administration and dissipates rapidly after cessation.[292] Inhibition of drug metabolism may be stereospecific. For example, metronidazole, phenylbutazone, sulfinpyrazone and cotrimoxazole inhibit the metabolism of the *S*(–) enantiomer of warfarin (metabolised by

CYP2C9/10) but have little or no effect on the *R*(+) form (metabolised by CYP1A2).[172,272]

*Cimetidine* is an important inhibitor of oxidative drug metabolism and prolongs the half-life of many drugs including phenazone (metabolised by CYP1A2), phenytoin (CYP2C9/10), diazepam (CYP2C19), nitrazepam (CYP2C19), warfarin (CYP2C9/10), and theophylline (CYP1A2).[293-297] The onset and offset of inhibition of oxidative metabolism by cimetidine are rapid; the effect is dose-related and greater in patients with impaired liver function.[43,293] Cimetidine has a differential effect on different pathways of theophylline metabolism, and inhibition is more marked in smokers than nonsmokers.[295] It seems to have no important effects on conjugation reactions.

Inhibition of drug metabolism by cimetidine does not depend on its $H_2$-receptor blocking action. Other $H_2$-receptor antagonists such as ranitidine and famotidine do not inhibit oxidative metabolism significantly (see also appendix B).[158] Cimetidine contains an imidazole ring within its structure.[298] This ring is also present in other enzyme inhibitors such as metronidazole and azole antifungals.[299-301] It probably represents a critical structural element in the interaction of these drugs with metabolising enzymes and the subsequent inhibition of enzyme metabolising capacity.[301] Critical structural elements in other drugs with enzyme-inhibiting capacity have not been defined.

Some interactions arise through inhibition of other enzymes. For example, hexafluorenium prolongs muscle paralysis produced by suxamethonium (succinylcholine) by competing with it for plasma cholinesterase. This enzyme is also irreversibly inhibited by cholinesterase inhibitors such as ecothiopate and demecarium.[66,302] It might be expected that others drugs with anticholinesterase activity, such as pyridostigmine (used in myasthenia gravis) and tacrine (used in Alzheimer's disease), might be able to prolong the effect of suxamethonium used to induce muscle paralysis.[303,304]

Mercaptopurine is metabolised by xanthine oxidase, and its toxicity is enhanced if xanthine oxidase is inhibited by *allopurinol*. Azathioprine is converted in the body to mercaptopurine, and like the latter drug, must be given in reduced dosage (to about 33%) in patients receiving allopurinol.[305,306]

The clinical significance of interactions due to inhibition of drug metabolism depends on the therapeutic ratio of the drug involved and on the initial plasma concentration before the inhibiting drug is given. If, for example, the steady-state plasma concentration of phenytoin in a patient on long term therapy is 5 mg/L and this increases to 15 mg/L when an enzyme inhibiting drug such as chloramphenicol, amiodarone or cimetidine is added, the increase in plasma concentration would probably result in better control of seizures rather than toxicity. However, if the initial concentration of phenytoin had been 15 mg/L, an increase beyond the desirable therapeutic range (upper limit 20 mg/L) to 60 mg/L would have caused severe toxicity (see chapter 5, sect. 2.2.2 and 4.3.1; chapter 29, sect. 4.3.1). Inhibition of the metabolism of phenytoin and other drugs with saturable metabolism is likely to cause a disproportionate increase in plasma concentrations and pharmacological effects (see also chapter 1; sect. 2.2.8).[307-309]

Inhibition of the metabolism of low extraction ratio drugs such as warfarin results in prolongation of the plasma half-life, but with high extraction ratio drugs (e.g. propranolol), oral bioavailability may be increased (due to reduced first-pass metabolism in the gut mucosa), with little effect on plasma half-life. Some subgroups of metabolising enzymes are present in significant quantities in the upper gastrointestinal mucosa.[34,225,310] These enzymes may be subject to inhibition by other drugs in much the same way as are similar enzymes in the liver. Such interactions produce important changes in first-pass metabolism in drugs taken orally, while having less effect on drugs given intravenously. An example of this is where oral cyclosporin is coadministered with erythromycin, with resultant marked increases in cyclosporin concentrations compared with a much smaller increase if cyclosporin is given intravenously.[311] The enzyme responsible for cyclosporin metabolism (CYP3A4) is present in significant quantities in the small bowel mucosa[310] and is subject to inhibition and induction of its activity by drugs at that site.[285,287]

Particular care is needed with known inhibitors of drug metabolism[260,299,312-325] such as:

- Cimetidine
- Some calcium antagonists (diltiazem, verapamil)
- Amiodarone
- Phenylbutazone
- Sulfinpyrazone
- Some sulfonamides

- Some macrolide antibiotics (erythromycin, troleandomycin, clarithromycin)
- Chloramphenicol
- Azole antifungals (ketoconazole, itraconazole, miconazole)
- Isoniazid
- Dextropropoxyphene
- Fluoxetine
- Fluvoxamine
- Disulfiram
- Alcohol (short term consumption)
- Metronidazole
- Allopurinol
- Grapefruit juice.

Enzyme inhibition interactions that involve commonly used drugs and which may have important consequences include:

1) Inhibition of terfenadine and astemizole metabolism (CYP3A4) by ketoconazole, itraconazole, erythromycin and clarithromycin. The result is an increase in terfenadine or astemizole serum concentrations to levels where they may induce torsades de pointes, a potentially fatal cardiac arrhythmia.[51,52,54,326,327]

2) Inhibition of the metabolism of the short-acting benzodiazepine, midazolam (CYP3A4) by diltiazem, verapamil, ketoconazole and itraconazole (fig. 8). The result is an extended duration and increased depth of sedation in patients undergoing procedures that require either brief sedation or anaesthesia that reverses rapidly allowing early discharge home.[328,329]

3) Inhibition of cyclosporin metabolism (CYP3A4) by diltiazem, verapamil, azole antifungal agents, erythromycin and clarithromycin with resultant potential for renal, hepatic and CNS toxicity.[279,280,330-333]

It should be noted that inhibitors of cyclosporin metabolism may be administered with cyclosporin in organ transplant recipients with the aim of producing a similar degree of immunosuppression with a lower dose of cyclosporin and hence significant cost savings as well as other benefits.[334]

#### *2.3.5 Changes in Hepatic Blood Flow*

Hepatic blood flow is an important determinant of the elimination of drugs that are extensively and rapidly removed from the plasma by the liver [e.g. propranolol and lidocaine (lignocaine)], such that their disposition can be affected by drug-induced changes in blood flow to the liver.[335,336] As a consequence of the reduced cardiac output that they cause, propranolol and other β-blockers not only decrease hepatic blood flow and affect their own clearance, but also decrease the plasma clearance of other concomitantly administered drugs with high hepatic extraction ratios (e.g. lidocaine).[101,337,338]

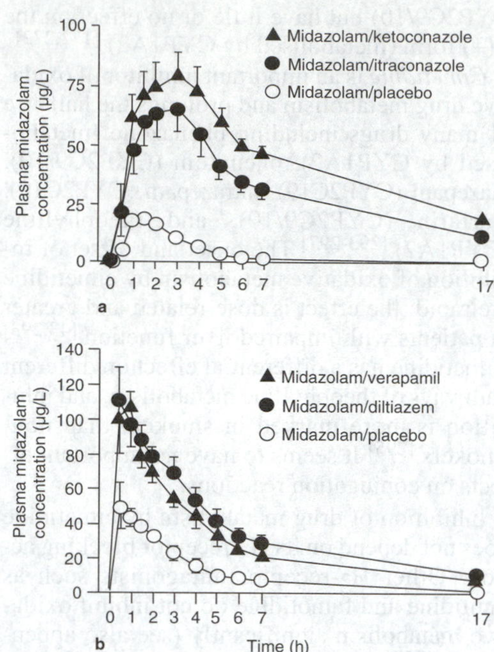


**Fig. 8.** Inhibition of drug metabolism resulting in (a) ketoconazole and itraconazole inducing an increase in plasma midazolam concentrations after a single oral midazolam dose (after Olkkola et al.;[329] by permission of author and editor), and (b) diltiazem and verapamil inducing increases in plasma midazolam concentrations after a single oral midazolam dose (after Backman et al.;[328] by permission of author and editor).

Some vasoactive drugs such as glucagon and isoprenaline (isoproterenol) increase hepatic blood flow and can increase the rate of elimination of propranolol and lidocaine. Phenobarbital also increases hepatic blood flow. When drugs are administered intravenously, a change in blood flow may have a greater role than enzyme induction in enhancing drug clearance. Hydralazine also influences liver blood flow and increases the oral bioavailability of drugs such as propranolol and metoprolol; this effect can be avoided by reducing the substrate delivery rate with a sustained-release formulation.[339] Verapamil and nifedipine increase hepatic blood flow and may alter the pharmacokinetic profile of high extraction drugs such as propranolol.[88,340,341]

The potential interactive effects of drugs that decrease splanchnic and hepatic blood flow such as octreotide have not yet been evaluated.[342] Thus, some interactions can be understood and predicted only by taking into account possible effects on hepatic blood flow as well as enzyme activity. In this regard, haemodynamic effects of drug interactions may be potentiated in acutely ill patients who receive drugs intravenously, where the liver blood flow may be diminished by a variety of factors including neuromuscular blocking drugs.[335,343,344] Liver blood flow may also be diminished during general anaesthesia.[101,344] Halothane and possibly other volatile anaesthetics decrease liver blood flow as well as inhibiting P450 microsomal enzymes.[345]

Some agents may alter the distribution of blood flow within the liver and hence alter therapeutic response. Verapamil may potentiate the cellular effects of anthracycline anticancer chemotherapy.[346] However, verapamil may also cause a diminution of blood flow to hepatic metastases, resulting in reduced delivery of the anthracycline drug to cancer cells and increased delivery to surrounding normal hepatic tissue.[347]

#### *2.3.6 Interference with Biliary Excretion and Enterohepatic Circulation*

Many polar compounds with molecular weights above about 400D are actively secreted into bile either unchanged or conjugated (e.g. with glucuronide or glutathione). Drugs and their metabolites may compete for biliary excretion or for the essential preliminary conjugation step. Thus, probenecid may reduce the biliary excretion of rifampicin and indomethacin,[348-350] while quinidine, amiodarone and verapamil reduce the biliary clearance of digoxin.[47,351-353]

Some drug conjugates are hydrolysed (sometimes by bacteria) in the intestine and the parent drug is then reabsorbed and undergoes enterohepatic circulation which may greatly prolong its half-life. Such enterohepatic circulation can be interrupted by suppression of intestinal bacteria with broad-spectrum antibiotics[34,354] and by preventing reabsorption of the original drug by administration of a binding agent such as cholestyramine. The latter drug may significantly increase total clearance and therefore reduce the half-lives of warfarin, digoxin, digitoxin and amiodarone by this mechanism.[209,355,356]

#### *2.3.7 Interference with Renal Excretion Due to Drug-Induced Renal Impairment*

A number of drugs may induce renal impairment by decreasing the glomerular filtration rate with a resultant decrease in creatinine clearance and increase in serum creatinine and a corresponding diminished excretion of a variety of drugs or their metabolites (see chapter 6; sect. 5.2). Aminoglycoside antibiotics may induce renal impairment, particularly if trough concentrations are elevated (see also chapter 5, sect. 2.2.2; chapter 24, sect. 11.1).[357] This may result in accumulation of the aminoglycoside antibiotic itself as well as a number of other drugs which depend on renal excretion, including digoxin. Similarly, cyclosporin and captopril reduce the renal clearance of digoxin in proportion to their effect in reducing creatinine clearance[358,359] and renal impairment secondary to amphotericin B results in elevated concentrations of coadministered flucytosine with resultant potential for bone marrow suppression.[360] It has been also suggested that lithium may sensitise the kidney to the effects of ACE inhibitors, with a resultant increase in the incidence of renal impairment in patients coprescribed these drugs.[361]

There may also be synergism in the production of drug-induced renal impairment when one drug with the potential to cause renal impairment is added to another. This may occur when aminoglycoside antibiotics are used in patients receiving NSAIDs or amphotericin B.[131,362] Concurrent use of amphotericin B and pentamidine may result in a rapid onset of acute renal failure and should be avoided.[363]

Drugs that alter the distribution of blood flow within the kidneys, such as NSAIDs, ACE inhibitors, cyclosporin and tacrolimus (FK 506), may have the potential to alter the excretion of other drugs disproportionately to their effect on creatinine clearance. However, clinical studies to support this supposition are lacking.

#### *2.3.8 Competition for Active Renal Tubular Secretion*

Many acidic drugs and drug metabolites share the same proximal tubular active transport system and can compete with each other for secretion.[364,365] One drug may, therefore, interfere with the renal excretion of another and cause accumulation and toxicity (fig. 9). The onset and offset of this inhibitory effect is often rapid and concentration-dependent, due to its competitive nature.

Drugs that may interact by this mechanism include sulfonamides, acetazolamide, thiazide diuretics, diazoxide, chlorpropamide, indomethacin, salicylate, sulfinpyrazone, probenecid, penicillins, cefalosporins, dicoumarol and methotrexate. Such competition between drugs can be used to therapeutic advantage when, for example, probenecid is given to increase the serum concentration of penicillins and cefalosporins by delaying their renal excretion.[367,368] The clearance of penicillins is also significantly decreased by phenylbutazone, sulfinpyrazone, aspirin, indomethacin and sulfaphenazole.[369]

Salicylates antagonise the actions of uricosuric drugs and complex interactions may occur between these therapeutic agents.[370,371] Severe toxicity has been observed in patients given high-dose methotrexate together with nonsteroidal anti-inflammatory drugs.[372-374] Although competition for the renal tubular secretion of methotrexate is the probable mechanism, a contributing factor may be the adverse effects of nonsteroidal anti-inflammatory drugs on renal function and renal blood flow (see also section 2.3.7).[131]

There is a separate active renal tubular transport system for organic bases and similar competitive interactions may occur at this site. Thus, cimetidine and, to a lesser extent, ranitidine (but not famotidine) inhibit the renal clearance of procainamide by this mechanism.[227,375,376] Similarly, the tubular secretion of digoxin is inhibited by quinidine and amiodarone and possibly transiently by verapamil.[47,353,377,378]

Lithium is subject to some of the same renal handling mechanisms as sodium. Drugs that produce a compensatory increase in proximal tubular resorption of sodium, such as thiazide diuretics, also tend to cause retention of lithium with potential for lithium toxicity (see also sections 2.2.3 and 2.3.7).[125,379]

### *2.3.9 Change in Urine pH*

The renal clearance of weak organic bases with pKa values of 7.5 to 10 is increased if the urine is made acid and decreased in alkaline urine. Conversely, the clearance of weak organic acids (pKa 3.0 to 7.5) is higher in alkaline than acid urine.[380] Strong acids and bases are virtually completely ionised over the physiological range of urine pH and their clearance is unaffected by changes in pH. With a few exceptions, interference with pH-dependent renal excretion is of no clinical significance because most weak organic acids and bases are inactivated by hepatic metabolism rather than renal excretion. Even if the amount of drug excreted

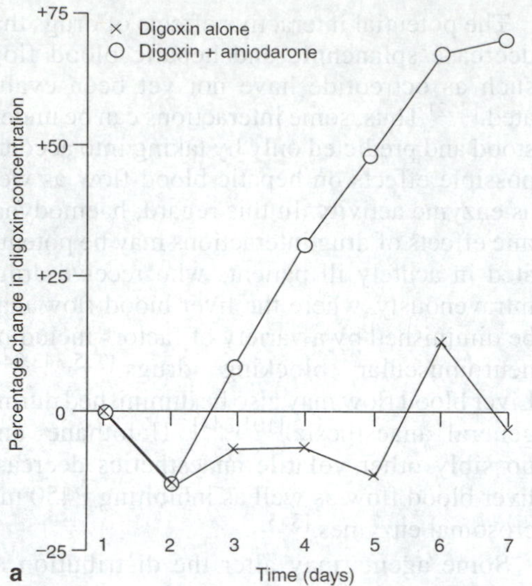


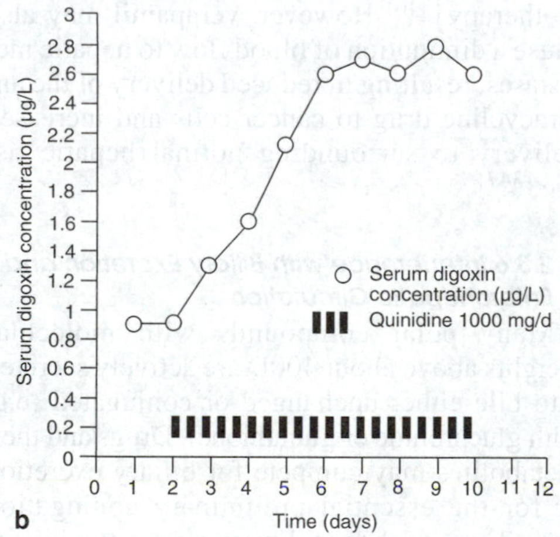


**Fig. 9.** Serum digoxin concentrations may be increased by other drugs via multiple mechanisms: (a) Mean percentage change in digoxin concentration in 7 patients receiving digoxin and amiodarone and 6 patients on digoxin alone (after Moysey et al.;[366] by permission of the publisher); (b) Serum digoxin concentrations in a typical patient on a stable digoxin regimen who is then given quinidine 1000 mg/day with no change in the digoxin dosage. Initial serum digoxin concentrations in the patient are stable at around 0.9 μg/L, but rise to a new equilibrium at around 2.7 μg/L after 5 days of quinidine therapy. In practice, clinicians adding quinidine to a stable digoxin regimen usually decrease the dosage of digoxin by 50% in anticipation of this interaction.

in the urine is increased from 2 to 20%, the effect on clearance would be of no practical importance. Furthermore, it is rarely necessary to prescribe drugs that produce large changes in urine pH.

A few basic drugs (e.g. amphetamine) are normally excreted unchanged in the urine to a significant extent (more than 30%), and their effects may be prolonged if the urine is made strongly alkaline. Alkaline diuresis is commonly used in patients with severe salicylate or phenobarbital intoxication. In the case of salicylate, changes in urine pH have a much greater effect on removal of the drug than changes in urine flow rate (see also chapter 8, sect. 6.4.1).[381] Therapeutic doses of antacids such as aluminium and magnesium hydroxide, and sodium bicarbonate also markedly decrease serum concentrations of salicylate, as a consequence of increased renal clearance caused by the rise in urinary pH.[382,383]

Acetazolamide and other carbonic anhydrase inhibitors render the urine alkaline by interfering with bicarbonate reabsorption. The urinary excretion of calcium is thereby increased and this may lead to renal calculi and aggravation of osteomalacia induced by long term antiepileptic drug therapy.[384]

## 3. Interactions Involving Monoamine Oxidase Inhibitors (MAOIs)

Nonselective irreversible inhibitors of monoamine oxidase may be involved in serious drug interactions with a range of drugs and foods through a number of different mechanisms.[385,386] While the extent of their interaction potential has probably been overestimated, interactions resulting in death or serious morbidity are by no means uncommon. Inhibition of monoamine oxidase results in the accumulation of large amounts of noradrenaline in sympathetic nerve endings, and a decrease in the rate of intracellular metabolism of biogenic amines such as catecholamines, dopamine and serotonin (5-hydroxytryptamine).

If a patient receiving a monoamine oxidase inhibitor is given indirect-acting sympathomimetic agents such as amphetamine, phenylpropanolamine, pseudoephedrine or tyramine, large amounts of noradrenaline may be released, causing an alarming reaction, with severe headache, marked hypertension, and in some cases acute left ventricular failure or fatal intracerebral haemorrhage. This is the basis of the notorious 'cheese reaction'.[387] Foods such as matured cheese, Chianti and Alicante type wines, yeast extracts and pickled herrings can contain large amounts of tyramine.[385,388] Dietary tyramine is normally metabolised by monoamine oxidase in the intestinal mucosa and the liver before it can reach the systemic circulation, but in patients receiving MAOIs it is absorbed intact and releases large amounts of stored noradrenaline, causing a hypertensive crisis (see also chapter 12, sect. 6.1.2). Similar hypertensive reactions have occurred following ingestion of fava beans or pods of broad beans, which contain dopamine rather than tyramine.[388] Such reactions should be treated by intravenous injection of an α-adrenoceptor blocking agent such as phentolamine.[389]

Other serious interactions characterised by agitation, hypotension, tachycardia, hyperpyrexia, convulsions, and coma have occasionally been observed in patients taking MAOIs after administration of tricyclic antidepressants, anaesthetics and pethidine (meperidine). This central excitatory syndrome may be mediated in part by the central effects of excess serotonin and is potentially related to the serotonin syndrome seen with combinations of selective serotonin reuptake inhibitors, clomipramine and other drugs (see also section 2.2.1 and appendix B).[85,386] In addition, MAOIs may potentiate antihypertensive drugs, insulin and sulphonylurea antidiabetic agents (see also appendix B).[390]

Interactions involving MAOIs are unpredictable and some, such as those with tricyclic antidepressants,[385,391,392] occur only in a very small proportion of patients at risk. They are important because of their severity, and since the enzyme is irreversibly inhibited, can occur up to 3 weeks after the drugs are discontinued (see also chapter 12, sect. 6.1.1). Notwithstanding these comments, serious interactions with nonselective MAOIs are rare and the risks with sensible prescribing have probably been overestimated.[385,393,394]

The advent of selective inhibitors of MAO A and B enzyme subtypes brought predictions of therapeutic response without the need for dietary restriction and with less potential for serious drug interactions. While this is largely true, it is evident that selective inhibitors of MAO A used in depression (e.g. moclobemide) and inhibitors of MAO B used in extrapyramidal disorders (e.g. selegiline) carry with them the potential for serious interactions in a small number of patients (see appendix B).[29,395,396] It is, therefore, wise to exercise caution when drugs with β-adrenoceptor or serotonergic actions are coadministered with inhibitors of MAO, whether those inhibitors have a selective, reversible effect on MAO or not.

Reactions related to the ingestion of tyramine-rich food are probably less common in individuals receiving selective MAOIs than in those on nonselective MAOIs. Nevertheless, tyramine reactions have been described in patients on selective MAOIs and it may be prudent to advise patients of the potential for this reaction when commencing the medication, despite the fact that a strict tyramine exclusion diet seems unnecessary.[29,397]

## 4. Miscellaneous Interactions

Many drug interactions cannot be classified because the mechanisms involved are not entirely clear. Examples include antagonism of the action of levodopa by pyridoxine (vitamin $B_6$)[398] and the increased risk of renal failure in patients receiving tetracycline when methoxyflurane is used for anaesthesia.[399]

## 5. Conclusions

It is difficult to assess the true incidence and ultimate clinical significance of drug interactions. Published clinical reports represent only the tip of an enormous iceberg, and it is particularly difficult to know how often drug interactions are responsible for therapeutic failure. Not all drug interactions are predictable, and the results of studies in experimental animals cannot be extrapolated directly to humans because of species differences. The dangers of multiple drug therapy may have been exaggerated and clinicians are confused rather than helped by exhaustive tabulations of largely theoretical and unconfirmed interactions.

It is unrealistic to expect clinicians to be familiar with all known interactions. However, particular care is needed with patients receiving anticoagulants, cardiac glycosides, and antidiabetic, antihypertensive, antiepileptic, psychotherapeutic, immunosuppressant and cytotoxic drugs. Such patients can be at special risk if other drugs are added or discontinued without consideration of the potential for interaction. This occurs most commonly when an anti-infective agent such as a macrolide antibiotic or azole antifungal agent is prescribed for a set course and then ceased in individuals previously on stable therapeutic regimens.

Most importantly, the incidence of drug interactions could be greatly reduced by a therapeutic approach which uses the smallest number of drugs in individual patients.

### Further Reading

Gibson GG, Skett P. Introduction to drug metabolism. London: Chapman & Hall, 1994

McInnes GT, Brodie MJ. Drug interactions that matter: a critical appraisal. Drugs 1988; 36: 83-110

Pond SM. Pharmacokinetic drug interactions. In: Benet et al. editors. Pharmacokinetic basis of drug treatment. New York: Raven Press, 1984: 195

Stockley IH. Drug interactions. 3rd ed. Oxford: Blackwell Scientific, 1994

### References

1. Tatro DS, Olin BR. Drug interaction facts. Facts and Comparisons. 3rd ed, St Louis: Lippincott, 1992
2. Stockley IH, editor. Drug interactions. 3rd ed. Oxford: Blackwell Scientific Publications, 1994
3. May FE, Stewart RB, Cluff LE. Drug interactions and multiple drug administration. Clinical Pharmacology and Therapeutics 1977; 22: 322
4. Cardieux RJ. Drug interactions in the elderly. Postgraduate Medicine 1989; 86: 179-86
5. Hansten PD, Horn JR, editors. Drug interactions and updates. 8th ed. Vancouver: Applied Therapeutics, 1993
6. Lipton JL, Bero LA, McPhee SJ. The impact of clinical pharmacist consultations on physicians' geriatric drug prescribing. Medical Care 1992; 30: 646-58
7. Petrie JC, Howie JGR, Dumo D. Awareness and experience of general practitioners of selected drug interactions. British Medical Journal 1974; 2: 262
8. Strom BL. Adverse reactions to over the counter analgesics taken for therapeutic purposes. Journal of the American Medical Association 1994; 272: 1866-67
9. McInnes GT, Helenglass G. The performance of clinics for outpatient control of anticoagulation. Journal of the Royal College of Physicians of London 1987; 21: 42-5
10. Jankel CA, Speedie SM. Detecting drug interactions: a review of the literature. DICP - Annals of Pharmacotherapy 1990; 24: 982-9
11. Simborg DW. Medication prescribing on a university medical service: the incidence of drug combinations with potential adverse interactions. Johns Hopkins Medical Journal 1976; 139: 23
12. Tinawi M, Alguire P. The prevalence of drug interactions in hospitalized patients. Clinical Research 1992; 40: 773A
13. Boston Collaborative Drug Surveillance Program. Adverse drug interactions. Journal of the American Medical Association 1972; 220: 1238-9
14. Jankel CA, Fitterman LK. Epidemiology of drug-drug interactions as a cause of hospital admission. Drug Safety 1993; 9: 51-9
15. Koch KM. Drug utilization in office practice by age and sex of the patient: national ambulatory medical care survey 1980. Advance Data 1982; 81: 1-2

16. Karch FE, Lasagna L. Adverse drug reactions: a critical review. Journal of the American Medical Association 1975; 231: 1236-41
17. Jick H. Adverse drug reactions: the magnitude of the problem. Journal of Allergy and Clinical Immunology 1984; 74: 555-7
18. Rupp MT, De Young M, Schondelmeyer SW. Prescribing problems and pharmacist interventions in community practice. Medical Care 1992; 30: 926-40
19. Manson-Espaillat R, Burnstine TH, Remler B, et al. Antiepileptic drug intoxication: factors and their significance. Epilepsia 1991; 32: 96-100
20. Koch-Weser J, Greenblatt DJ. Drug interactions in clinical perspective. European Journal of Clinical Pharmacology 1977; 11: 405
21. Leape LL, Brenan TA, Laird N, et al. The nature of adverse events in hospitalised patients: results of the Harvard Medical Practice Study II. New England Journal of Medicine 1991; 324: 377-84
22. Seixas FA. Alcohol and its drug interactions. Annals of Internal Medicine 1975; 83: 86
23. Gugler R, Allgayer H. Effects of antacids on the clinical pharmacokinetics of drugs. Clinical Pharmacokinetics 1990; 18: 210-9
24. Henry D, Dobson A, Turner C. Variability in the risk of major gastrointestinal complications from nonaspirin nonsteroidal anti-inflammatory drugs. Gastroenterology 1993; 105: 1078-88
25. Sjöqvist F, Alexanderson B. Drug interactions: a critical look at their documentation and clinical importance. In: Baker & Neuhaus, editors. Proceedings of the European Society for the Study of Drug Toxicity, Vol. 13. Toxicology problems of drug combinations. Amsterdam: Excerpta Medica, 1972: 167
26. Vessell ES, Passananti GT, Glenwright P. Anomalous results of studies of drug interaction in man. Pharmacology 1975; 13: 481
27. Maddux MS, Veremis SA, Bauma WD, et al. Significant drug interactions with cyclosporin. Hospital Therapy 1987; 12: 56-70
28. Roy LF, East DS, Brownings FM, et al. Short term effects of calcium antagonists on hemodynamics and cyclosporine pharmacokinetics in heart transplant patients. Clinical Pharmacology and Therapeutics 1989; 46: 657-67
29. Livingstone MG. Interactions with selective MAOIs. Lancet 1995; 345: 533-34
30. Alvan G. Genetic polymorphisms in drug metabolism. Journal of Internal Medicine 1992; 231: 571-3
31. Kalow W, editor. Pharmacogenetics of drug metabolism. Oxford: Pergamon Press, 1992
32. Gonzalez FJ, Idle JR. Pharmacogenetic phenotyping and genotyping: present status and future potential. Clinical Pharmacokinetics 1994; 26: 59-70
33. Lindenbaum J, Rund DG, Butler VP, et al. Inactivation of digoxin by the gut flora: reversal by antibiotic therapy. New England Journal of Medicine 1981; 305: 789
34. Ilett KF, Tee LBG, Reeves PT, et al. Metabolism of drugs and other xenobiotics in the gut lumen and wall. Pharmacology and Therapeutics 1990; 46: 67-93
35. Sheiner LB, Benet LZ. Premarketing observational studies of population pharmacokinetics of new drugs. Clinical Pharmacology and Therapeutics 1985; 38: 481-7
36. Regan AG, Perumbetti PPV. Pancuronium and gentamicin interaction in patients with renal failure. Anesthesia and Analgesia 1980; 59: 393
37. Dupuis JY, Martin R, Tetrault JP. Atracurium and vecuronium interaction with gentamicin and tobramycin. Canadian Journal of Anaesthesia 1989; 36: 407-11
38. Abel M, Book WJ, Eisenkraft JB. Adverse effects of nondepolarising neuromuscular blocking agents: incidence, prevention and management. Drug Safety 1994; 10: 420-38
39. Kramer P, Tsuru M, Cook CE, et al. Effect of influenza vaccine on warfarin anticoagulation. Clinical Pharmacology and Therapeutics 1984; 35: 416-8
40. Farrell GC. Drug metabolism in extrahepatic diseases. Pharmacology and Therapeutics 1987; 35: 375-404
41. Hirsh J. Oral anticoagulant drugs. New England Journal of Medicine 1991; 324: 1865-75
42. Chen YL, Vraux VL, Leneveu A, et al. Acute-phase response, interleukin-6, and alteration of cyclosporine pharmacokinetics. Clinical Pharmacology and Therapeutics 1994; 55: 649-60
43. Nelson DC, Avant GR, Speeg Jr KV. The effect of cimetidine on hepatic drug elimination in cirrhosis. Hepatology 1985; 5: 305-9
44. Crippin JS. Acetaminophen hepatotoxicity: potentiation by isoniazid. American Journal of Gastroenterology 1993; 88: 590-2
45. Sellers EM, Holloway MR. Drug kinetics and alcohol ingestion. Clinical Pharmacokinetics 1978; 3: 440
46. Lane EA, Guthrie S, Linnoila M. Effects of ethanol on drug and metabolite pharmacokinetics. Clinical Pharmacokinetics 1985; 10: 228-47
47. Fenster PE, White NW, Hanson CD. Pharmacokinetic evaluation of the digoxin-amiodarone interaction. Journal of the American College of Cardiology 1985; 5: 108-12
48. Santostasi G, Fantin M, Marango I, et al. Effects of amiodarone on oral and intravenous digoxin kinetics in healthy subjects. Journal of Cardiovascular Pharmacology 1987; 9: 385-90
49. Robinson K, Johnston A, Walker S, et al. The digoxin-amiodarone interaction. Cardiovascular Drugs and Therapy 1989; 3: 25-8
50. Pond SM, Graham GG, Birkett DJ, et al. Effect of tricyclic antidepressants on drug metabolism. Clinical Pharmacology and Therapeutics 1975; 18: 191
51. Honig PK, Wortham DC, Zamani K, et al. Effect of erythromycin, clarithromycin and azithromycin on the pharmacokinetics of terfenadine. Clinical Pharmacology and Therapeutics 1993; 53: 161
52. Honig PK, Wortham DC, Zamani K, et al. Terfenadine-ketoconazole interaction: pharmacokinetic and electrocardiographic consequences. Journal of the American Medical Association 1993; 269: 1513-8
53. Kivisto KT, Neuvonen PJ, Klotz U. Inhibition of terfenadine metabolism: pharmacokinetic and pharmacodynamic consequences. Clinical Pharmacokinetics 1994; 27: 1-5
54. Simons FE, Simons KJ. The pharmacology and use of $H_1$-receptor-antagonist drugs. New England Journal of Medicine 1994; 330: 1663-70
55. Tucker GT. The rational selection of drug interaction studies: implications of recent advances in drug metabolism. International Journal of Clinical Pharmacology and Therapeutics 1992; 30: 550-3
56. Houston JB. Utility of in vitro drug metabolism data in predicting in vivo metabolic clearance. Biochemical Pharmacology 1994; 47: 1469-79
57. Vestal RE, Norris AH, Tobin JD, et al. Antipyrine metabolism in man: influence of age, alcohol, caffeine

and smoking. Clinical Pharmacology and Therapeutics 1975; 18: 425-32
58. Perucca E, Hedges A, Makki KA, et al. A comparative study of the relative enzyme-inducing properties of anticonvulsant drugs in epileptic patients. British Journal of Clinical Pharmacology 1984; 18: 401-10
59. Whitcomb DC, Block GD. Association of acetaminophen hepatotoxicity with fasting and ethanol use. Journal of the American Medical Association 1994; 272: 1845-50
60. Carmichael RR, Mahoney CD, Jeffrey LP. Solubility and stability of phenytoin sodium when mixed with intravenous solutions. American Journal of Hospital Pharmacy 1980; 37: 95-8
61. Khoo SH, Bond J, Denning DW. Administering amphotericin B - a practical approach. Journal of Antimicrobial Chemotherapy 1994; 33: 203-13
62. Colagiuri S, Villalobos S. Assessment of the effect of mixing insulins in subjects with diabetes mellitus using the glucose clamp technique. Diabetes Care 1986; 9: 579-86
63. Grodin WK, Epstein MAP, Epstein RA. Mechanisms of halothane absorption by dry soda-lime. British Journal of Anaesthesia 1982; 54: 561-5
64. Strum DP, Johnson BJ, Eger II EI. Stability of sevoflurane in soda lime. Anesthesiology 1987; 67: 779-81
65. Strum DP, Eger II EI. The degeneration, absorption, and solubility of volatile anaesthetics in soda lime depend on water content. Anaesthesia and Analgesia 1994; 78: 340-8
66. Davie IT. Specific drug interactions in anaesthesia. Anaesthesia 1977; 32: 1000
67. Kramer W, Inglott A, Cluxton R. Additive review: some physical and chemical incompatibilities of drugs for IV administration. Drug Intelligence and Clinical Pharmacy 1971; 5: 211
68. Joint Formulary Committee. Appendix 6: Intravenous additives. In: British National Formulary. London: British Medical Association and The Pharmaceutical Press, 1995: 584-94
69. Trissel LA. Handbook on injectable drugs. 8th ed. Bethesda: American Society of Hospital Pharmacists, 1994
70. Seppala T, Linnoila M, Mattila MJ. Drugs, alcohol and driving. Drugs 1979; 17: 389
71. Gjerde H, Kinn G. Impairment in drivers due to cannabis in combination with other drugs. Forensic Science International 1991; 50: 57-60
72. Brookoff D, Cook CS, Williams C, et al. Testing reckless drivers for cocaine and marijuana. New England Journal of Medicine 1994; 331: 518-22
73. Angell M, Kassirer JP. Alcohol and other drugs: toward a more rational and consistent policy. New England Journal of Medicine 1994; 331: 537-9
74. Donati F, Smith CE, Bevan DR. Dose-response relationships for edrophonium and neostigmine as antagonists of moderate and profound atracurium blockade. Anesthesia and Analgesia 1989; 68: 13-9
75. Hansbrough JF, Near A. Propranolol-epinephrine antagonism with hypertension and stroke. Annals of Internal Medicine 1980; 92: 717
76. Houben H, Thien T, van't Laar A. Effect of low-dose epinephrine infusion on hemodynamics after selective and nonselective beta-blockade in hypertension. Clinical Pharmacology and Therapeutics 1982; 31: 685-94
77. Gandy W. Severe epinephrine-propranolol interaction. Annals of Emergency Medicine 1988; 18: 98-9
78. Newman BR, Schultz LK. Epinephrine resistant anaphylaxis in a patient taking propranolol hydrochloride. Annals of Allergy 1981; 47: 35-7
79. Toogood JH. Beta blocker therapy and the risk of anaphylaxis. Canadian Medical Association Journal 1987; 136: 929
80. Lang DM. Anaphylactoid and anaphylactic reactions: hazards of β-blockers. Drug Safety 1995; 12: 299
81. Cohen WJ, Cohen NH. Lithium carbonate, haloperidol and irreversible dementia. Journal of the American Medical Association 1974; 230: 1283
82. Thornton WE. Dementia induced by methyldopa with haloperidol. New England Journal of Medicine 1976; 294: 1222
83. Addonizio G. Rapid induction of extrapyramidal side effects with combined use of lithium and neuroleptics. Journal of Clinical Psychopharmacology 1985; 5: 296-98
84. Amdisen A. Lithium and drug interactions. Drugs 1982; 24: 133
85. Sternbach H. The serotonin syndrome. American Journal of Psychiatry 1991; 148: 705-13
86. Lejoyeux M, Ades J, Rouillon F. Serotonin syndrome: incidence, symptoms and treatment. CNS Drugs 1994; 2: 132-43
87. Hutchinson SJ, Lorimer AR, Lakhdar A, et al. β-Blockers and verapamil: a cautionary tale. British Medical Journal 1984; 289: 659
88. McCourty JC, Silas JH, Tucker GT, et al. The effect of combined therapy on the pharmacokinetics and pharmacodynamics of verapamil and propranolol in patients with angina pectoris. British Journal of Clinical Pharmacology 1988; 25: 349-57
89. LeWinter MM, Crawford MH, O'Rourke RA, et al. The effects of oral propranolol, digoxin and combination therapy on the resting and exercise electrocardiogram. American Heart Journal 1977; 93: 202-9
90. Durant NN, Nguyen N, Katz RL. Potentiation of neuromuscular blockade by verapamil. Anesthesiology 1984; 60: 298
91. Wali FA. Interactions of nifedipine and diltiazem with muscle relaxants and reversal of neuromuscular blockade with edrophonium and neostigmine. Journal of Pharmacology and Experimental Therapeutics 1986; 17: 244-53
92. Vinik HR, Bradley Jr EL, Kissin I. Midazolam-alfentanil synergism for anesthetic induction in patients. Anesthesia and Analgesia 1989; 69: 213-7
93. Goodchild CS. GABA receptors and benzodiazepines. British Journal of Anaesthesia 1993; 71: 127-33
94. Michalowski P, Rosow CE. Perioperative drug interactions. Journal of Clinical Anesthesia 1993; 5 Suppl. 1: 29S-33S
95. Stella L, Crescenti A, Torri G. Effect of naloxone on the loss of consciousness induced by IV anaesthetic agents in man. British Journal of Anaesthesia 1984; 56: 369-73
96. Moss SJ, Smart TG, Blackstone CD, et al. Functional modulation of $GABA_A$ receptors by cAMP-dependent protein phosphorylation. Science 1992; 257: 661-5
97. Ticku MK. Alcohol and GABA-benzodiazepine receptor function. Annals of Medicine 1990; 22: 241-6
98. Nutt DJ, Peters TJ. Alcohol: the drug. British Medical Bulletin 1994; 50: 5-17
99. Crook JE, Nies AS. Drug interactions with antihypertensive drugs. Drugs 1978; 15: 72
100. Grogono AW, Seltzer JL. A guide to drug interactions in anaesthetic practice. Drugs 1980; 19: 279

101. Wood M. Pharmacokinetic drug interactions in anaesthetic practice. Clinical Pharmacokinetics 1991; 21: 285-307
102. Berthoud MC, Reilly CS. Adverse effects of general anaesthetics. Drug Safety 1992; 7: 434-59
103. McConachie I, Healy TEJ. ACE inhibitors and anaesthesia. Postgraduate Medical Journal 1989; 65: 273-4
104. Littler C, McConachie I, Healy TEJ. Interaction between enalapril and propofol. Anaesthesia and Intensive Care 1989; 17: 514-5
105. Moliterno DJ, Willard JE, Lange RA, et al. Coronary-artery vasoconstriction induced by cocaine, cigarette smoking, or both. New England Journal of Medicine 1994; 330: 454-9
106. Steiness E, Olesen KH. Cardiac arrhythmias induced by hypokalaemia and potassium loss during maintenance digoxin therapy. British Heart Journal 1976; 38: 167
107. McKibben JK, Pocock WA, Barlow JB, et al. Sotalol, hypokalaemia, syncope, and torsade de pointes. British Heart Journal 1984; 51: 157-62
108. Levine JH, Morganroth J, Kadish AH. Mechanisms and risk factors for proarrhythmia with type 1a compared with 1c antiarrhythmic drug therapy. Circulation 1989; 80: 1063-9
109. Leatham EW, Holt DW, McKenna WJ. Class III antiarrthymics in overdose: presenting features and management principles. Drug Safety 1993; 9: 450-62
110. Dreifus LS, de Azevedo IM, Watanabe Y. Electrolyte and antiarrhythmic drug interaction. American Heart Journal 1974; 88: 95
111. Evers W, Racz GB, Dobkin AB. A study of plasma potassium and electrocardiographic changes after single dose and succinylcholine. Canadian Anaesthetists Society Journal 1969; 16: 273
112. Greenblatt DJ, Koch-Weser J. Adverse reactions to spironolactone: a report from the Boston Collaborative Drug Surveillance Program. Journal of the American Medical Association 1973; 225: 40
113. Hansten PD, Horn JR. Captopril drug interactions. Drug Interactions Newsletter 1985; 5: 15
114. Todd PA, Heel RC. Enalapril: a review of its pharmacodynamic and pharmacokinetic properties, and therapeutic use in hypertension and congestive heart failure. Drugs 1986; 31: 198
115. Johnson AG, Nguyen TV, Day RO. Do nonsteroidal anti-inflammatory drugs affect blood pressure? A meta-analysis. Annals of Internal Medicine 1994; 112: 289-300
116. Oates JA, Fitzgerald GA, Branch RA, et al. Clinical implications of prostaglandin and thromboxane A2 formation. New England Journal of Medicine 1988; 319: 761-7
117. Motwani JG, Struthers AD. Interactive effects of indomethacin, angiotensin II and frusemide on renal haemodynamics and natriuresis in man. British Journal of Clinical Pharmacology 1994; 37: 355-61
118. Muniz P, Barrow SE, Cockroft JF, et al. Effects of nonsteroidal anti-inflammatory drugs on prostacyclin and thromboxane biosynthesis in patients with mild essential hypertension. British Journal of Pharmacology 1990; 30: 519-26
119. Hall D, Zeitler H, Rudolph W. Counteraction of the vasodilator effects of enalapril by aspirin in severe heart failure. Journal of the American College of Cardiology 1992; 20: 1549-55
120. Patrono C. Aspirin as an antiplatelet drug. New England Journal of Medicine 1994; 330: 1287-94
121. Kerry RK, Ludlow JM, Owen G. Diuretics are dangerous with lithium. British Medical Journal 1980; 281: 371
122. Dorevitch A, Baruch E. Lithium toxicity induced by combined amiloride hydrochloride-hydrochlorothiazide administration. American Journal of Psychiatry 1986; 143: 257-8
123. Reimann IW, Diener U, Frolich JC. Indomethacin but not aspirin increases plasma lithium ion levels. Archives of General Psychiatry 1983; 40: 283
124. Ragheb M. The clinical significance of lithium-nonsteroidal anti-inflammatory drug interactions. Journal of Clinical Psychopharmacology 1990; 10: 350-4
125. Harvey NS, Merriman S. Review of clinically important drug interactions with lithium. Drug Safety 1994; 10: 455-63
126. Herschuelz A, Derenne F, Deger F, et al. Interaction between non-steroidal anti-inflammatory drugs and loop diuretics: modulation by sodium balance. Journal of Pharmacology and Experimental Therapeutics 1989; 248: 1175-81
127. Watkins J, Abbott CE, Hensby CN, et al. Attenuation of hypotensive effect of propranolol and thiazide diuretics by indomethacin. British Medical Journal 1980; 281: 702
128. Favre L, Glasson P, Riondel A, et al. Interactions of diuretics and non-steroidal anti-inflammatory drugs in man. Clinical Science 1983; 64: 407
129. Webster J. Interactions of non-steroidal anti-inflammatory and antihypertensive drugs. Drugs 1985; 30: 32
130. Favre L, Glasson P, Vallotton MB. Reversible acute renal failure from combined triamterene and indomethacin. Annals of Internal Medicine 1982; 96: 317
131. Tonkin AL, Wing LMH. Interactions of non-steroidal anti-inflammatory drugs. Ballieres Clinical Rheumatology 1988; 2: 455-83
132. Brooks PB, Day RO. Nonsteroidal antiinflammatory drugs - differences and similarities. New England Journal of Medicine 1991; 324: 1716-25
133. Stockley IH. Interactions between lithium and NSAIDs. Canadian Medical Association Journal 1995; 152: 152-3
134. Ferriere M, Lachkar H, Richard JL, et al. Captopril and insulin sensitivity. Annals of Internal Medicine 1985; 102: 134-5
135. Arauz-Pacheco C, Ramirez LC, Rios JM, et al. Hypoglycaemia induced by angiotensin-converting enzyme inhibitors in patients with non-insulin-dependent diabetes receiving sulfonylurea therapy. American Journal of Medicine 1990; 89: 811-3
136. Button IK, Davies HR, Zeitz CJ, et al. Adverse reactions to perhexiline during short and long-term therapy. Australian and New Zealand Journal of Medicine 1993; 23: 599
137. Horowitz JD, Button IK, Wing L. Is perhexiline essential for optimal management of angina pectoris? Australian and New Zealand Journal of Medicine 1995; 25: 111-3
138. Herings RMC, de Boer A, Stricker BHC, et al. Hypoglycaemia associated with use of inhibitors of angiotensin converting enzyme. Lancet 1995; 345: 1195-8
139. Vaughan Williams EM. Anti-arrhythmic action and the puzzle of perhexiline. London: Academic Press, 1980
140. Jauch KW, Hartl W, Guenther B, et al. Captopril enhances insulin responsiveness of forearm muscle tissue in non-insulin dependent diabetes mellitus. European Journal of Clinical Investigation 1987; 17: 448-54

141. Donnelly R, Morris AD. Drugs and insulin resistance: clinical methods of evaluation and new pharmacological approaches to metabolism. British Journal of Clinical Pharmacology 1994; 37: 311-20
142. Prescott LF, Nimmo WS, Heading RC. Drug absorption interactions. In: Grahame-Smith, editor. Drug interactions. London: Macmillan, 1977: 45
143. Greiff JMC, Rowbotham D. Pharmacokinetic drug interactions with gastrointestinal motility modifying agents. Clinical Pharmacokinetics 1994; 27: 447-61
144. Sadowski DC. Drug interactions with antacids: mechanisms and clinical significance. Drug Safety 1994; 11: 395-407
145. Kleinbloesem CH, Van Brummelen P, Danhof M, et al. Rate of increase in the plasma concentration of nifedipine as a major determinant of its hemodynamic effects in humans. Clinical Pharmacology and Therapeutics 1987; 41: 26-30
146. Steeves RA, Robinson D, McKenzie MW, et al. Effects of metoclopramide on the pharmacokinetics of a slow-release theophylline product. Clinical Pharmacy 1982; 1: 356-60
147. Hurwitz A. Antacid therapy and drug kinetics. Clinical Pharmacokinetics 1977; 2: 269
148. Welling PG. Interactions affecting drug absorption. Clinical Pharmacokinetics 1984; 9: 404
149. Nix DE, Watson WA, Lener M, et al. Effects of aluminium and magnesium hydroxide and ranitidine on the absorption of ciprofloxacin. Clinical Pharmacology and Therapeutics 1989; 46: 700-5
150. Naggar VF, Khalil SA. Effect of magnesium trisilicate on nitrofurantoin absorption. Clinical Pharmacology and Therapeutics 1979; 25: 857
151. Hartman NR, Yarchoan R, Pluda JM, et al. Pharmacokinetics of 2'-3'-dideoxyinosine in patients with severe human immunodeficiency virus infection II: the effects of different oral formulations and the presence of other medications. Clinical Pharmacology and Therapeutics 1991; 50: 278-85
152. Morris DJ. Adverse effects and drug interactions of clinical importance with antiviral drugs. Drug Safety 1994; 10: 281-91
153. Neuvonen PJ, Kivisto KT. Enhancement of drug absorption by antacids: an unrecognised drug interaction. Clinical Pharmacokinetics 1994; 27: 120-8
154. Sommers DK, Van Wyk KM, Moncrieff J, et al. Influence of food and reduced gastric emptying on the bioavailability of cefuroxime axetil. British Journal of Clinical Pharmacology 1984; 18: 535-9
155. Hughes GS, Heald DL, Barker KB, et al. The effects of gastric pH and food on the pharmacokinetics of a new oral cephalosporin, cefpodoxime proxetil. Clinical Pharmacology and Therapeutics 1989; 46: 674-85
156. Van Peer A, Woestenborghs R, Heykants J, et al. The effects of food and dose on the oral systemic availability of itraconazole in healthy subjects. European Journal of Clinical Pharmacology 1989; 36: 423-6
157. Blum RA, D'Andrea DT, Florentin BM, et al. Increased gastric pH and the bioavailability of ketoconazole and fluconazole. Annals of Internal Medicine 1991; 114: 755-7
158. Hansten PD. Drug interactions with antisecretory drugs. Alimentary Pharmacology and Therapeutics 1991; 5 Suppl. 1: 121-8
159. Baciewicz AM, Baciewicz FA. Ketoconazole and fluconazole drug interactions. Archives of Internal Medicine 1993; 153: 1970-6
160. Archambeaud-Mouveroux F, Nouille Y, Nadalon S, et al. Interaction between gliclazide and cimetidine. European Journal of Clinical Pharmacology 1987; 31: 631
161. Leek K, Mize R, Lowenstein SR. Glyburide-induced hypoglycaemia and ranitidine. Annals of Internal Medicine 1987; 107: 261
162. Feely J, Collins WCJ, Cullen M, et al. Potentiation of the hypoglycaemic response to glipizide in diabetic patients by histamine $H_2$-receptor antagonists. British Journal of Clinical Pharmacology 1993; 35: 321
163. Koop H. Review article: metabolic consequences of long-term inhibition of acid secretion by omeprazole. Alimentary Pharmacology and Therapeutics 1992; 6: 399-406
164. Marcuard SP, Albernaz L, Khazanie PG. Omeprazole therapy causes malabsorption of cyanocobalamine (vitamin B12). Annals of Internal Medicine 1994; 120: 211-5
165. Goss TF, Piscitelli SC, Schentag JJ. Evaluation of ketoconazole bioavailability interactions with sucralfate and ranitidine using gastric pH monitoring. Clinical Pharmacology and Therapeutics 1991; 49: 128
166. Sherman SI, Tielens ET, Ladenson PW. Sucralfate causes malabsorption of L-thyroxine. American Journal of Medicine 1994; 96: 531-5
167. Hoeschele JD, Roy AK, Pecoraro VL, et al. In vitro analysis of the interaction between sucralfate and ketoconazole. Antimicrobial Agents and Chemotherapy 1994; 38: 319-25
168. O'Reilly RA. Comparative interaction of cimetidine and ranitidine and racemic warfarin in man. Archives of Internal Medicine 1984; 144: 989-91
169. Nix DE, Watson WA, Handy L, et al. The effect of sucralfate pretreatment on the pharmacokinetics of ciprofloxacin. Pharmacotherapy 1989; 9: 377-80
170. Neuvonen PJ. The effect of magnesium hydroxide on the oral absorption of ibuprofen, ketoprofen and diclofenac. British Journal of Clinical Pharmacology 1991; 31: 263-6
171. Neuvonen PJ, Kivisto KT. The effects of magnesium hydroxide on the absorption and efficacy of two glibenclamide preparations. British Journal of Clinical Pharmacology 1991; 32: 215-20
172. Hirsh J, Fuster V. Guide to anticoagulant therapy: Part 2: oral anticoagulants. Circulation 1994; 89: 1469-80
173. Riley SA, Sutcliffe F, Kim M, et al. The influence of gastrointestinal transit on drug absorption in healthy volunteers. British Journal of Clinical Pharmacology 1992; 34: 32-9
174. Nimmo WS. Drugs, diseases and altered gastric emptying. Clinical Pharmacokinetics 1976; 1: 189-203
175. Prescott LF. Gastric emptying and drug absorption. British Journal of Clinical Pharmacology 1974; 1: 189
176. Rivera-Calimlim L, Dujorne CA, Morgan JP, et al. L-DOPA treatment failure: explanation and correction. British Medical Journal 1970; 4: 93-4
177. Manninen V, Apajalahti A, Simonen H, et al. Effect of propantheline and metoclopramide on absorption of digoxin. Lancet 1973; 1: 1118
178. Manninen V, Melin J, Apajalahti A, et al. Altered absorption of digoxin in patients given propantheline and metoclopramide. Lancet 1973; 1: 398
179. Jaffe JM. Effects of propantheline on nitrofurantoin absorption. Journal of Pharmaceutical Sciences 1975; 64: 1729
180. Adkin DA, Davis SS, Sparrow RA, et al. The effects of pharmaceutical excipients on small intestinal transit.

British Journal of Clinical Pharmacology 1995; 39: 381-7
181. Koch KM, Parr AF, Tomlinson JJ, et al. Effect of sodium acid pyrophosphate on ranitidine bioavailability and gastrointestinal transit time. Pharmaceutical Research 1993; 10: 1027-30
182. Nimmo WS, Heading RC, Wilson J, et al. Inhibition of gastric emptying and drug absorption by narcotic analgesics. British Journal of Clinical Pharmacology 1975; 2: 509
183. Nimmo WS, Heading RC, Tothill P, et al. Pharmacological modification of gastric emptying effects of propantheline and metoclopramide on paracetamol absorption. British Medical Journal 1973; 1: 587
184. Clark JM, Seager SJ. Gastric emptying following premedication with glycopyrrolate or atropine. British Journal of Anaesthesia 1983; 55: 1195-9
185. Rivera-Calimlim L, Nasrallah H, Strauss J, et al. Clinical response and plasma levels: effect of dose, dosage schedules and drug interaction on plasma chlorpromazine levels. American Journal of Psychiatry 1976; 133: 646
186. Algeri S, Cerletti C, Cucio M, et al. Effect of anticholinergic drugs on gastrointestinal absorption of L-dopa in rats and man. European Journal of Pharmacology 1976; 35: 293-9
187. Clark RA, Holdsworth CD, Rees MR, et al. The effect on paracetamol absorption of stimulation and blockade of beta-adrenoceptors. British Journal of Clinical Pharmacology 1980; 10: 555
188. Nimmo WS, Wilson J, Prescott LF. Narcotic analgesics and delayed gastric emptying during labour. Lancet 1975; 1: 890-3
189. Park GR, Weir D. A comparison of the effect of oral controlled release morphine and intramuscular morphine on gastric emptying. Anaesthesia 1984; 39: 645-8
190. Trotter TN, Rowbotham DJ, Windram I, et al. Effect of sublingual buprenorphine on gastric emptying of a liquid meal. British Journal of Anaesthesia 1991; 67: 748-50
191. Dougall JR, Cunningham B, Nimmo WS. Paracetamol absorption from Paramax, Panadol and Solpedeine. British Journal of Clinical Pharmacology 1983; 15: 487-9
192. Pottage A, Campbell RWF, Achuff SC, et al. The absorption of oral mexiletine in coronary care patients. European Journal of Clinical Pharmacology 1978; 13: 393
193. Rowbotham DJ, Bamber PA, Nimmo WS. Comparison of the effect of cisapride and metoclopramide on morphine-induced delay in gastric emptying. British Journal of Clinical Pharmacology 1988; 26: 741-6
194. McNeill MJ, Ho EJ, Kenny GN. Effect of iv metoclopramide on gastric emptying after opioid premedication. British Journal of Anaesthesia 1990; 640: 450-2
195. Wadhwa NK, Schroeder TJ, O'Flaherty E, et al. The effect of oral metoclopramide on the absorption of cyclosporine. Transplantation 1987; 43: 211-3
196. Na Bangchang KNA, Karbwang J, Bunnag D, et al. The effect of metoclopramide on mefloquine pharmacokinetics. British Journal of Clinical Pharmacology 1991; 32: 640-1
197. Wiseman LR, Faulds D. Cisapride: an updated review of its pharmacology and therapeutic efficacy as a prokinetic agent in gastrointestinal motility disorders. Drugs 1994; 47: 116-52
198. Finet L, Westeel PF, Hary L, et al. Effects of cisapride on intestinal absorption of cyclosporine in renal transplant patients. Gastroenterology 1991; 100 (5 Pt 2): A209
199. Johnson BF, Bustrack JA, Urbach DR, et al. Effect of metoclopramide on digoxin absorption from tablets and capsules. Clinical Pharmacology and Therapeutics 1984; 36: 724-30
200. Osman MA, Welling PG. Influence of propantheline and metoclopramide on the bioavailability of chlorothiazide. Current Therapeutic Research 1983; 34: 404
201. Lehto P, Kivisto KT, Neuvonen PJ. The effect of ferrous sulphate on the absorption of norfloxacin, ciprofloxacin and ofloxacin. British Journal of Clinical Pharmacology 1994; 37: 82-5
202. Neuvonen PJ. Interactions with the absorption of tetracyclines. Drugs 1976; 11: 45
203. Frost RW, Lasster KC, Noe AJ, et al. Effects of aluminium hydroxide and calcium carbonate on the bioavailability of ciprofloxacin. Antimicrobial Agents and Chemotherapy 1992; 36: 830-2
204. Ambre JJ, Fischer LJ. Effect of coadministration of aluminium and magnesium hydroxides on absorption of anticoagulants in man. Clinical Pharmacology and Therapeutics 1973; 14: 231-7
205. Osman MA, Patel RB, Schuna A, et al. Reduction in oral penicillamine absorption by food, antacid and ferrous sulphate. Clinical Pharmacology and Therapeutics 1983; 33: 465
206. Campbell NRC, Paddock V, Sundaram R. Alteration of methyldopa absorption, metabolism and blood pressure control caused by ferrous sulfate and ferrous gluconate. Clinical Pharmacology and Therapeutics 1988; 43: 381-6
207. Campbell NRC, Ranfine D, Goodridge AE, et al. Sinemet-ferrous sulphate interactions in patients with Parkinson's disease. British Journal of Clinical Pharmacology 1990; 30: 599-605
208. Brown DD, Juhl RP. Decreased bioavailability of digoxin due to antacids and kaolin-pectin. New England Journal of Medicine 1976; 295: 1034
209. Janhchen E, Meinertz T, Gilfrich HJ, et al. Enhanced elimination of warfarin during treatment with cholestyramine. British Journal of Clinical Pharmacology 1978; 5: 437-40
210. Hibbard DM, Peters JR, Hunninghake DB. Effects of cholestyramine and colestipol on the plasma concentrations of propranolol. British Journal of Clinical Pharmacology 1984; 18: 337
211. Keogh A, Day R, Critchley L, et al. The effect of food and cholestyramine on the absorption of cyclosporine in cardiac transplant patients. Transplantation Proceedings 1988; 20: 27-30
212. Farmer JA, Gotto Jr AM. Antihyperlipidaemic agents: drug interactions of clinical significance. Drug Safety 1994; 11: 301-9
213. Mandel SJ, Brent GA, Larsen PR. Levothyroxine therapy in patients with thyroid disease. Annals of Internal Medicine 1993; 119: 492-502
214. Smart HL, Somerville KW, William J, et al. The effect of sucralfate upon phenytoin absorption in man. British Journal of Clinical Pharmacology 1985; 20: 238-40
215. Fogelman I, Smith L, Mazess R, et al. Absorption of oral diphosphonates in normal subjects. Clinical Endocrinology 1986; 24: 57-62
216. Compston JE. The therapeutic use of bisphosphonates. British Medical Journal 1994; 309: 711-5
217. Catnach SM, Fairclough PD, Hammond SM. Intestinal absorption of peptide drugs: advances in our understanding and clinical implications. Gut 1994; 35: 441-4

218. Westphal JF, Jehl F, Brogard JM, et al. Amoxicillin intestinal absorption reduction by amiloride: possible role of the $Na^+$-$H^+$ exchanger. Clinical Pharmacology and Therapeutics 1995; 57: 257-64
219. Cheng SH, White A. Effect of orally administered neomycin on absorption of penicillin V. New England Journal of Medicine 1962; 267: 1296-7
220. Faloon WW, Chodos RB. Vitamin $B_{12}$ absorption studies using colchicine, neomycin and continuous $^{37}Co$ $B_{12}$ administration. Gastroenterology 1969; 56: 1251
221. Lindenbaum J, Maulitz RM, Butler Jr VP. Inhibition of digoxin absorption by neomycin. Gastroenterology 1976; 71: 399-404
222. Sylvester RK, Lewis FB, Caldwell KC, et al. Impaired phenytoin bioavailability secondary to cisplatinum, vinblastine and bleomycin. Therapeutic Drug Monitoring 1984; 6: 302-5
223. Kuhlmann J, Zilly W, Wilke J. Effects of cytostatic drugs on plasma level and renal excretion of beta-acetyldigoxin. Clinical Pharmacology and Therapeutics 1981; 30: 518-27
224. Kuhlmann J, Woodcock B, Wilke J, et al. Verapamil plasma concentrations during treatment with cytostatic drugs. Journal of Cardiovascular Pharmacology 1985; 7: 1003-6
225. Back DJ, Rogers SM. Review: first pass metabolism by the gastrointestinal mucosa. Alimentary Pharmacology and Therapeutics 1987; 11: 275-8
226. Houston JB, Day J, Walker J. Azo reduction of sulphasalazine in healthy volunteers. British Journal of Clinical Pharmacology 1982; 14: 395-8
227. Klotz U. Clinical pharmacokinetics of sulphasalazine, its metabolites and other prodrugs of 5-aminosalicyclic acid. Clinical Pharmacokinetics 1985; 10: 285-302
228. Back DJ, Breckenridge AM, Crawford FE, et al. Interindividual variation and drug interactions with hormonal steroid contraceptives. Drugs 1981; 21: 46
229. Shenfield GM. Oral contraceptives: are drug interactions of clinical significance? Drug Safety 1993; 9: 21-37
230. Back DJ, Grimmer SFM, Orme ML'E, et al. Evaluation of Committee on Safety of Medicines yellow cards on oral contraceptive drug interactions with anticonvulsants and antibiotics. British Journal of Clinical Pharmacology 1988; 25: 527-32
231. Harris AG. Somatostatin and somatostatin analogues: pharmacokinetic and pharmacodynamic effects. Gut 1994; 35 Suppl. 3: S1-S4
232. Landgraf R, Landgraf-Leurs MMC, Nusser J, et al. Effect of somatostatin analogue (SMS 201-995) on cyclosporin levels. Transplantation 1987; 44: 724-5
233. Lebowitz H. Oral antidiabetic drugs: the emergence of the alpha-glucosidase inhibitors. Drugs 1992; 44 Suppl. 3: 21-8
234. Conniff RF, Shapiro JA, Seaton TB. Long term efficacy and safety of acarbose in the treatment of obese subjects with non insulin dependent diabetes mellitus. Archives of Internal Medicine 1994; 154: 2442-8
235. Krentz AJ, Ferner RE, Bailey CJ. Comparative tolerability profiles of oral antidiabetic agents. Drug Safety 1994; 11: 223-41
236. Scheen AJ, Fereira Alves de Magalhaes AC, Salvatore T, et al. Reduction of the acute bioavailability of metformin by the alpha-glucosidase inhibitor acarbose in man. European Journal of Clinical Investigation 1994; 24 Suppl. 3: 50-4
237. Ladas SD, Frydas A, Papadopoulos A, et al. Effects of alpha-glucosidase inhibitors on mouth to caecum transit time in humans. Gut 1992; 33: 1246-8
238. Gerard J, Lefebvre PJ, Luyckx AS. Glibenclamide pharmacokinetics in acarbose treated type 2 diabetics. European Journal of Clinical Pharmacology 1984; 27: 233-6
239. Hillebrand I, Graefe KH, Bischoff H, et al. Serum digoxin and propanolol levels during acarbose treatment. Diabetologia 1981; 21: 282
240. Rolan PE. Plasma protein binding interactions - why are they still regarded as clinically important? British Journal of Clinical Pharmacology 1994; 37: 125-8
241. McElnay JC, D'Arcy PF. Protein binding displacement interactions and their clinical importance. Drugs 1983; 25: 495
242. MacKichan JJ. Pharmacokinetic consequences of drug displacement from blood and tissue proteins. Clinical Pharmacokinetics 1984; 9 Suppl. 1: 32
243. MacKichan JJ. Protein binding drug displacement interactions: fact or fiction? Clinical Pharmacokinetics 1989; 16: 65-73
244. Sansom IN, Evans AM. What is the true clinical significance of plasma protein binding displacement interactions. Drug Safety 1995; 12: 227
245. Fichtl B, Doering W. The quinidine-digoxin interaction in perspective. Clinical Pharmacokinetics 1983; 8: 137
246. Rodin SM, Johnson BF. Pharmacokinetic interactions with digoxin. Clinical Pharmacokinetics 1988; 15: 227-44
247. Park BK, Breckenridge AM. Clinical implications of enzyme induction and enzyme inhibition. Clinical Pharmacokinetics 1981; 6: 1
248. Okey AB. Enzyme induction in the cytochrome P-450 system. Pharmacology and Therapeutics 1990; 45: 241-98
249. George J, Farrell GC. Role of human hepatic cytochromes P450 in drug metabolism and toxicity. Australian and New Zealand Journal of Medicine 1991; 21: 356-62
250. Ogilvie RI. Smoking and theophylline dose schedules. Annals of Internal Medicine 1978; 88: 263-4
251. Fox K, Jonathan A, Williams H, et al. Interaction between cigarettes and propranolol in the treatment of angina pectoris. British Medical Journal 1980; 281: 191-3
252. Linnoila M, George L, Guthrie S, et al. Effect of alcohol consumption and cigarette smoking on antidepressant levels of depressed patients. American Journal of Psychiatry 1981; 138: 841-2
253. Cipolle RJ, Seifert RD, Neilen BA, et al. Heparin kinetics: variables related to disposition and dosage. Clinical Pharmacology and Therapeutics 1981; 29: 387-93
254. Schein JR. Cigarette smoking and clinically significant drug interactions. Annals of Pharmacotherapy 1995; 29: 1139
255. Jusko WJ. Influence of cigarette smoking on drug metabolism in man. Drug Metabolism Reviews 1979; 9: 221-36
256. Guengerich FP. Cytochrome P-450 enzymes and drug metabolism. In: Bridges JW, Chasseaud LF, Gibson GG, editors. Progress in drug metabolism. London: Taylor and Francis, 1987: 1-54
257. Perucca E, Richens A. Drug interactions with phenytoin. Drugs 1981; 21: 120
258. Murray M. P450 enzymes: inhibition mechanisms, genetic regulation and effects of liver disease. Clinical Pharmacokinetics 1992; 23: 132-46

259. Heimark LD, Gibaldi M, Trager WF, et al. The mechanism of warfarin-rifampin drug interactions in humans. Clinical Pharmacology and Therapeutics 1987; 42: 388-94
260. Orme M, Breckenridge AM, Cook P. Warfarin and Distalgesic interaction. British Medical Journal 1976; 1: 200
261. Levy RH, Koch M. Drug interactions with valproic acid. Drugs 1982; 24: 543
262. Perucca E. Pharmacokinetic interactions and antiepileptic drugs. Clinical Pharmacokinetics 1982; 7: 57
263. Harden CL. New antiepileptic drugs. Neurology 1994; 44: 787-95
264. Seeff LB, Cuccherine BA, Zimmerman HJ, et al. Acetaminophen hepatotoxicity in alcoholics: a therapeutic misadventure. Annals of Internal Medicine 1986; 104: 399-404
265. Hoft RH, Bunker JP, Goodman HI, et al. Halothane hepatitis in three pairs of closely related women. New England Journal of Medicine 1981; 304: 1023-4
266. Nomura F, Hatano H, Ohnishi K, et al. Effects of anticonvulsant agents on halothane-induced liver injury in human subjects and experimental animals. Hepatology 1986; 6: 952-6
267. Ray DC, Drummond GB. Halothane hepatitis. British Journal of Anaesthesia 1991; 67: 84-99
268. Rambeck B, Salke-Treumann A, May TH, et al. Valproic acid induced carbamazepine-10,11-epoxide toxicity in children and adolescents. European Neurology 1990; 45: 474-7
269. Brodie MJ. Lamotrigine. Lancet 1992; 339: 1397-1400
270. Wagner ML, Remmel RP, Graves NM, et al. Effect of felbamate on carbamazepine and its major metabolites. Clinical Pharmacology and Therapeutics 1993; 53: 536-43
271. Evans DAP. N-acetyltransferase. Pharmacology and Therapeutics 1989; 42: 157
272. Freedman MD, Otalidoye AG. Clinically significant drug interactions with the oral anticoagulants. Drug Safety 1994; 10: 381-94
273. Back DJ, Orme ML'E. Pharmacokinetic drug interactions with oral contraceptives. Clinical Pharmacokinetics 1990; 18: 472-84
274. Crawford P, Chadwick DJ, Martin C, et al. The interaction of phenytoin and carbamazepine with combined oral contraceptive steroids. British Journal of Clinical Pharmacology 1990; 30: 892
275. Crawford P, Chadwick DJ, Martin C, et al. The lack of effect of sodium valproate on the pharmacokinetics of oral contraceptive steroids. Contraception 1986; 3: 23
276. Holdich T, Whiteman P, Orme M, et al. Effect of lamotrigine on the pharmacology of the combined oral contraceptive pill. Epilepsia 1991; 32 (Suppl. 1): 96
277. Editorial. Drug interactions with oral contraceptive steroids. British Medical Journal 1980; 3: 93
278. Langhoff E, Madsen S. Rapid metabolism of cyclosporin and prednisone in kidney transplant patient receiving tuberculostatic treatment. Lancet 1983; 2: 1031
279. Yee GC, McGuire TR. Pharmacokinetic drug interactions with cyclosporin (Pt 1). Clinical Pharmacokinetics 1990; 19: 319-22
280. Yee GC, McGuire TR. Pharmacokinetic drug interactions with cyclosporin (Pt 2). Clinical Pharmacokinetics 1990; 19: 400-15
281. Maurer PM, Bartkowski RR. Drug interactions of clinical significance with opioid analgesics. Drug Safety 1993; 8: 30-48
282. Boman G, Eliasson K, Odar-Cederlöf I. Acute cardiac failure during treatment with digitoxin: an interaction with rifampicin. British Journal of Clinical Pharmacology 1980; 10: 89
283. Gault H, Longerich L, Dawe M, et al. Digoxin-rifampicin interaction. Clinical Pharmacology and Therapeutics 1984; 35: 750
284. Alvan G, Piafsky K, Lind M, et al. Effect of pentobarbitone on the disposition of alprenolol. Clinical Pharmacology and Therapeutics 1977; 22: 316
285. Hebert MF, Roberts JP, Prueksaritanont T, et al. Bioavailability of cyclosporine with concomitant rifampin administration is markedly less than predicted by hepatic enzyme induction. Clinical Pharmacology and Therapeutics 1992; 52: 453-7
286. Slaughter RL, Edwards DJ. Recent advances: the cytochrome P450 enzymes. Annals of Pharmacotherapy 1995; 29: 619
287. Kolars JC, Schmiedlin-Ren P, Schuetz JD, et al. Identification of rifampin-inducible P450 3A4 (CYP3A4) in human small bowel enterocytes. Journal of Clinical Investigation 1992; 90: 1871-8
288. Testa B, Jenner P. Inhibitors of cytochrome P450s and their mechanism of action. Drug Metabolism Reviews 1981; 12: 1-117
289. Okudaira K, Sawada Y, Sugiyama Y, et al. Effects of basic drugs on the hepatic transport of cardiac glycosides in rats. Biochemical Pharmacology 1988; 37: 2949-55
290. Park BK, Kitteringham NR. Relevance and means of assessing induction and inhibition of drug metabolism in man. In: Gibson CC, editor. Progress in drug metabolism. London: Taylor and Francis, 1988: 1-60
291. Babany G, Larrey B, Pessayre D. Macrolide antibiotics as inducers and inhibitors of cytochrome P-450 in experimental animals and man. In: Gibson GG, editor. Progress in drug metabolism. London: Taylor & Francis, 1988: 61-97
292. Dossing M, Pilsgaard H, Rasmussen B, et al. Time course of phenobarbital and cimetidine mediated changes in hepatic drug metabolism. European Journal of Clinical Pharmacology 1983; 25: 215-22
293. Bartle WR, Walker SE, Shapero T. Dose dependent effect of cimetidine on phenytoin kinetics. Clinical Pharmacology and Therapeutics 1983; 33: 649-55
294. Gough PA, Curry SH, Araujo OE, et al. Influence of cimetidine on oral diazepam elimination with measurement of subsequent cognitive change. British Journal of Clinical Pharmacology 1982; 14: 739
295. Grygiel JJ, Miners JO, Drew R, et al. Differential effects of cimetidine on theophylline metabolic pathways. European Journal of Clinical Pharmacology 1984; 26: 335
296. Ochs HR, Greenblatt DJ, Gugler R, et al. Cimetidine impairs nitrazepam clearance. Clinical Pharmacology and Therapeutics 1983; 34: 227
297. Shinn AF. Clinical relevance of cimetidine drug interactions. Drug Safety 1992; 7: 245-67
298. Rendic S, Kajfez F, Ruf HH. Characterisation of cimetidine, ranitidine and related structures' interaction with cytochrome P450. Drug Metabolism and Disposition: The Biological Fate of Chemicals 1983; 11: 137-42
299. Lau AH, Lam NP, Pisctelli SC, et al. Clinical pharmacokinetics of metronidazole and other nitroimidazole anti-infectives. Clinical Pharmacokinetics 1992; 23: 328-64

300. Brown MW, Maldonado AL, Meredith CG, et al. Effect of ketoconazole on hepatic oxidative drug metabolism. Clinical Pharmacology and Therapeutics 1985; 37: 290-7
301. Ritter JK, Franklin MR. Induction and inhibition of rate hepatic drug metabolism by N-substituted imidazole drugs. Drug Metabolism and Disposition: The Biological Fate of Chemicals 1987; 15: 335-43
302. Donati F, Bevan DR. Controlled succinylcholine infusion in a patient receiving echothiopate eye drops. Canadian Anaesthetists Society Journal 1981; 28: 488-90
303. Hunter AR. An appraisal of tacrine extended suxamethonium. British Journal of Anaesthesia 1970; 42: 155-62
304. Mirakhur RK, Lavery TD, Briggs LP, et al. Effects of neostigmine and pyridostigmine on serum cholinesterase activity. Canadian Journal of Anaesthesia 1982; 29: 55-8
305. Rundles RW, et al. Effects of a xanthine oxidase inhibitor on thiopurine metabolism, hyperuricaemia and gout. Transactions of the Association of American Physicians 1963; 76: 126
306. Zimm S, Collins JM, O'Neill D, et al. Inhibition of first-pass metabolism in cancer chemotherapy: interaction of 6-mercaptopurine and allopurinol. Clinical Pharmacology and Therapeutics 1983; 34: 810-7
307. Nation RL, Evans AM, Milne RW. Pharmacokinetic drug interactions with phenytoin (Pt 1). Clinical Pharmacokinetics 1990; 18: 37-60
308. Nation RL, Evans AM, Milne RW. Pharmacokinetic drug interactions with phenytoin (Pt 2). Clinical Pharmacokinetics 1990; 18: 131-50
309. Graves NM. Neuropharmacology and drug interactions in clinical practice. Epilepsia 1995; 36 Suppl. 2: S27-S33
310. Watkins PB, Wrighton SA, Scheutz EG, et al. Identification of glucocorticoid-inducible cytochromes P-450 in the intestinal mucosa of rats and man. Journal of Clinical Investigation 1987; 80: 1029-36
311. Gupta SK, Bakran A, Johnson RWG, et al. Cyclosporin-erthromycin interaction in renal transplant patients. British Journal of Clinical Pharmacology 1989; 27: 475-81
312. Hansen JM, Christensen LK. Drug interactions with oral sulphonylurea hypoglycaemic drugs. Drugs 1977; 13: 24
313. Koup JR, Gibaldi M, McNamara P, et al. Interaction of chloramphenicol with phenytoin and phenobarbital. Clinical Pharmacology and Therapeutics 1978; 24: 571
314. Linnoila M, Matilla MJ, Kitchell BS. Drug interactions with alcohol. Drugs 1979; 19: 299
315. Pedersen AK, Jakobsen P, Kampmann JP, et al. Clinical pharmacokinetics and potentially important drug interactions of sulphinpyrazone. Clinical Pharmacokinetics 1982; 7: 42
316. Pond SM, Birkett DJ, Wade DN. Effect of tricyclic antidepressants on drug metabolism: phenylbutazone, oxyphenbutazone, sulphaphenazole. Clinical Pharmacology and Therapeutics 1977; 22: 573
317. Rolan PE, Somogyi AA, Drew MJR, et al. Phenytoin intoxication during treatment with parenteral miconazole. British Medical Journal 1983; 287: 1760
318. Wright JM, Stokes EF, Sweeney VP. Isoniazid-induced carbamazepine toxicity and vice versa. New England Journal of Medicine 1982; 307: 1325
319. Bailey DG, Spence JD, Munoz C, et al. Interaction of citrus juices with felodipine and nifedipine. Lancet 1991; 337: 357-62
320. Periti P, Mazzei T, Mini E, et al. Pharmacokinetic interactions of macrolides. Clinical Pharmacokinetics 1992; 23: 106-31
321. Como JA, Dismukes WE. Oral azole drugs as systemic antifungal therapy. New England Journal of Medicine 1994; 330: 263-72
322. Altamura AC, Moro AR, Percudani M. Clinical pharmacokinetics of fluoxetine. Clinical Pharmacokinetics 1994; 26: 201-14
323. Bertschy G, Baumann P, Eap CB, et al. Probable metabolic interaction between methadone and fluvoxamine in addict patients. Therapeutic Drug Monitoring 1994; 16: 42-5
324. Van Harten J. Clinical pharmacokinetics of selective serotonin reuptake inhibitors. Clinical Pharmacokinetics 1993; 24: 203-20
325. Yee GC, Stanley DL, Pessa LJ, et al. Effect of grapefruit juice on blood cyclosporin concentrations. Lancet 1995; 345: 955-6
326. Monahan BP, Ferguson CL, Killeavy ES, et al. Torsades de pointes occurring in association with terfenadine use. Journal of the American Medical Association 1990; 264: 2788-90
327. Honig PK, Woolsley RL, Zamani K, et al. Changes in the pharmacokinetics and electrocardiographic pharmacodynamics of terfenadine with concomitant administration of erythromycin. Clinical Pharmacology and Therapeutics 1992; 52: 231-8
328. Backman JT, Olkola KT, Aranko K, et al. Dose of midazolam should be reduced during diltiazem and verapamil treatment. British Journal of Clinical Pharmacology 1994; 37: 221-5
329. Olkkola KT, Backman JT, Neuvonen PJ. Midazolam should be avoided in patients receiving the systemic antimycotics ketoconazole or itraconazole. Clinical Pharmacology and Therapeutics 1994; 55: 481-5
330. Wagner K, Phillip T, Heinemeyer HH, et al. Interaction of cyclosporin and calcium antagonists. Transplantation Proceedings 1989; 21: 1453-6
331. Schlanz KD, Myre SA, Bottorff MB. Pharmacokinetic interactions with calcium channel antagonists (Pt 1). Clinical Pharmacokinetics 1991; 21: 344-56
332. Schlanz KD, Myre SA, Bottorff MB. Pharmacokinetic interactions with calcium channel antagonists (Pt 2). Clinical Pharmacokinetics 1991; 21: 448-60
333. Spicer ST, Liddle C, O'Connell P. Mechanism of interaction of clarithromycin and cyclosporine A [abstract]. Annual Scientific Meeting of the Australasian Society of Nephrology, Canberra, March, 1995
334. Keogh A, Spratt P, McCosker C, et al. Ketoconazole to reduce the need for cyclosporin after cardiac transplantation. New England Journal of Medicine 1995; 333: 628
335. Nies AS, Shand DG, Wilkinson GR. Altered hepatic blood flow and drug disposition. Clinical Pharmacokinetics 1976; 1: 135
336. Wilkinson GR, Shand DG. A physiological approach to hepatic drug clearance. Clinical Pharmacology and Therapeutics 1975; 18: 377-90
337. Conrad KA, Byers JM, Finley PR, et al. Lidocaine elimination: effects of propranolol and of metoprolol. Clinical Pharmacology and Therapeutics 1983; 33: 133
338. Wood AJJ, Feely J. Pharmacokinetic drug interactions with propranolol. Clinical Pharmacokinetics 1983; 8: 253

339. Byrne AJ, McNeil JJ, Harrison PM, et al. Stable oral availability of sustained release propranolol when co-administered with hydralazine or food: evidence implicating substrate delivery rate as a determinant of presystemic drug interaction. British Journal of Clinical Pharmacology 1984; 17: 45S

340. Lauer LA, Murray K, Horn JR, et al. Influence of nifedipine therapy on indocyanine green and oral propranolol pharmacokinetics. European Journal of Clinical Pharmacology 1989; 37: 257-60

341. Avignina P, Sansoe G, Martini M, et al. Effects of nifedipine on functional liver plasma flow in normal subjects and in patients with cirrhosis. Clinical Pharmacology and Therapeutics 1993; 53: 368-73

342. Lin HC, Tsai YT, Lee FY, et al. Hemodynamic evaluation of octreotide in patients with hepatitis B related cirrhosis. Gastroenterology 1992; 103: 229-34

343. Koch-Weser J. Drug interactions in cardiovascular therapy. American Heart Journal 1975; 90: 93

344. Cowan RE, Jackson BT, Grainger SL, et al. Effects of anesthetic agents and abdominal surgery on liver blood flow. Hepatology 1991; 14: 1161-6

345. Reilly CS, Wood AJJ, Koshakji RP, et al. The effect of halothane on drug disposition contribution of intrinsic drug metabolising capacity and hepatic blood flow. Anesthesiology 1985; 63: 70-6

346. Kessel D, Wilberding C. Anthracycline resistance in P388 murine leukemia and its circumvention by calcium antagonists. Cancer Research 1985; 45: 1687-91

347. Ramirez LH, Munck J-N, Zhao Z, et al. Verapamil-reversing concentrations induce blood flow changes that could counteract in vivo the MDR-1-modulating effects. Cancer 1994; 74: 810-6

348. Kenwright S, Levi AJ. Impairment of hepatic uptake of rifamycin antibiotics by probenecid and its therapeutic implications. Lancet 1973; 2: 1401

349. Baber N, Halliday L, Sibeon R, et al. The interaction between indomethacin and probenecid: a clinical and pharmacokinetic study. Clinical Pharmacology and Therapeutics 1978; 24: 298

350. Sinclair H, Gibson T. Interaction between probenecid and indomethacin. British Journal of Rheumatology 1986; 25: 316-7

351. Hager WD, Fenster P, Mayersohn M, et al. Digoxin-quinidine interaction: pharmacokinetic evaluation. New England Journal of Medicine 1979; 300: 1238-41

352. Angelin B, Arvidsson A, Dahlqvist R, et al. Quinidine reduces biliary clearance of digoxin in man. European Journal of Clinical Investigation 1987; 17: 262-5

353. Hedman A, Angelin B, Arvidsson A, et al. Digoxin-verapamil interaction: reduction of biliary but not renal digoxin clearance in humans. Clinical Pharmacology and Therapeutics 1991; 49: 256-62

354. Hamalainen E, Korpela JT, Aldercreutz H. Effect of oxytetracycline administration in intestinal metabolism of oestrogens and on plasma sex hormones in healthy men. Gut 1987; 28: 439-45

355. Brown DD, Schmid J, Long RA, et al. A steady-state evaluation of the effects of propantheline bromide and cholestyramine on the bioavailability of digoxin when administered as tablets or capsules. Journal of Clinical Pharmacology 1985; 25: 360-4

356. Nitsch J, Luderitz B. Beschleunigte elimination von amiodaron durch colestyramine (enhanced elimination of amiodarone by cholestyramine). Deutsche Medizinische Wochenschrift 1986; 111: 1241-4

357. Humes HD. Aminoglycoside toxicity. Kidney International 1988; 33: 900-11

358. Dorian P, Strauss M, Cardella C, et al. Digoxin-cyclosporine interaction: severe digitalis toxicity after cyclosporine treatment. Clinical and Investigative Medicine 1988; 11: 108-12

359. Cleland JGF, Dargie HJ, Pettigrew A, et al. The effects of captopril of serum digoxin and urinary area and digoxin clearances in patients with congestive heart failure. American Heart Journal 1986; 112: 130-5

360. Stamm AM, Diasio RB, Dismukes WE, et al. Toxicity of amphotericin B plus flucytosine in 194 patients with cryptococcal meningitis. American Journal of Medicine 1987; 83: 236-42

361. Lehmann K, Ritz E. Angiotensin-converting enzyme inhibitors may cause renal dysfunction in patients on long-term lithium. American Journal of Kidney Diseases 1995; 25: 82-7

362. Churchill DN, Seely J. Nephrotoxicity associated with combined gentamicin-amphotericin B. Nephron 1977; 19: 176-81

363. Antoniskis D, Larsen RA. Acute, rapidly progressive renal failure with simultaneous use of amphotericin B and pentamidine. Antimicrobial Agents and Chemotherapy 1990; 34: 470-2

364. Rennick BR. Renal tubular transport of organic cations. American Journal of Physiology 1981; 240: F83-9

365. Kosoglou T, Vlasses PH. Drug interactions involving renal transport mechanisms: an overview. Drug Intelligence and Clinical Pharmacy: Annals of Pharmacotherapy 1989; 23: 116-22

366. Moysey JO, Jaggarao NSV, Grundy EN, et al. Amiodarone increases plasma digoxin concentrations. British Medical Journal 1981; 282: 272

367. Griffiths RS, Black HR, Brier GL, et al. Effect of probenecid on blood levels and urinary excretion of cefamandole. Antimicrobial Agents and Chemotherapy 1977; 11: 809-12

368. Allen MB, Gitzpatrick RW, Barratt A, et al. The use of probenecid to increase the serum amoxycillin levels in patients with bronchiectasis. Respiratory Medicine 1990; 84: 143-6

369. Kampmann J, Molholm Hansen J, Sierboek-Nielsen K, et al. Effect of some drugs on penicillin half life in blood. Clinical Pharmacology and Therapeutics 1972; 13: 516

370. Regal RE. Aspirin and uricosurics: interaction revisited. Drug Intelligence and Clinical Pharmacy 1987; 21: 219-20

371. Miners JO. Drug interactions involving aspirin (acetylsalicylic acid) and salicylic acid. Clinical Pharmacokinetics 1989; 17: 327-44

372. Ellison NM, Servi RJ. Acute renal failure and death following sequential intermediate dose methotrexate and 5FU; a possible adverse effect due to concomitant indomethacin administration. Cancer Treatment Reports 1985; 69: 342-3

373. Daly H, Boyle J, Roberts C, et al. Interaction between methotrexate and non-steroidal anti-inflammatory drugs. Lancet 1986; 1: 557

374. Johnson AG, Seideman P, Day RO. Adverse drug reactions with nonsteroidal anti-inflammatory drugs (NSAIDs): recognition, management and avoidance. Drug Safety 1993; 8: 99-127

375. Somogyi A, Bochner F. Dose and concentration dependent effects of ranitidine on procainamide disposition and renal clearance in man. British Journal of Clinical Pharmacology 1984; 18: 175

376. Rodvold KA, Paloucek FP, Jung D, et al. Interaction of steady state procainamide with $H_2$-receptor antagonists cimetidine and ranitidine. Therapeutic Drug Monitoring 1987; 9: 378-83
377. Leahey EB, Reiffel JA, Giardina EG, et al. The effect of quinidine and other oral antiarrhythmics drugs on serum digoxin: a prospective study. Annals of Internal Medicine 1980; 92: 605-8
378. Pedersen KE, Dorph-Pedersen A, Hvidt S, et al. The long term effect of verapamil on plasma digoxin concentration and renal digoxin clearance in healthy subjects. European Journal of Clinical Pharmacology 1982; 22: 123-7
379. Price LH, Heninger GR. Lithium in the treatment of mood disorders. New England Journal of Medicine 1994; 331: 591-8
380. Milne MD, Scribner BH, Crawford MA. Non-ionic diffusion and the excretion of weak acids and bases. American Journal of Medicine 1958; 24: 709
381. Prescott LF, Balali-Mood M, Critchley JAJH, et al. Diuresis or urinary alkalinisation for salicylate poisoning? British Medical Journal 1982; 285: 1383
382. Gibaldi M, Grunhofer B, Levy G. Effects of antacids on pH of urine. Clinical Pharmacology and Therapeutics 1974; 16: 520
383. Levy G, Lampman T, Kamath BL, et al. Decreased serum salicylate concentrations in children with rheumatic fever treated with antacid. New England Journal of Medicine 1975; 293: 323
384. Mallette LE. Acetazolamide-accelerated anticonvulsant osteomalacia. Archives of Internal Medicine 1977; 137: 1013
385. Lippman SB, Nash K. Monoamine oxidase inhibitor update: potential food and drug interactions. Drug Safety 1990; 5: 195-204
386. Blackwell B. Monoamine oxidase inhibitor interactions with other drugs. Journal of Clinical Psychopharmacology 1991; 11: 55-9
387. Blackwell B, Marley E, Price J, et al. Hypertensive interactions between monoamine oxidase inhibitors and foodstuffs. British Journal of Psychiatry 1967; 113: 349
388. McCabe BJ. Dietary and other pressor amines in MAOI regimens: a review. Journal of the American Dietetic Association 1986; 76: 1059-64
389. Stack CG, Rogers P, Linter SPK. Monoamine oxidase inhibitors and anaesthesia: a review. British Journal of Anaesthesia 1988; 60: 222-7
390. Sjöqvist F. Interaction between monoamine oxidase (MAO) inhibitors and other drugs. Proceedings of the Royal Society of Medicine 1965; 58: 967
391. Goldberg RS, Thornton WE. Combined tricyclic MAOI therapy for refractory depression: a review with guidelines for appropriate usage. Journal of Clinical Pharmacology 1978; 18: 143
392. Spiker DG, Pugh DD. Combining tricyclic and monoamine oxidase inhibitor antidepressants. Archives of General Psychiatry 1976; 33: 828
393. McGilchrist JM. Interactions with monoamine oxidase inhibitors. British Medical Journal 1975; 3: 591
394. Sargent W. Interactions with monoamine oxidase inhibitors. British Medical Journal 1975; 4: 101
395. Neuvonen PJ, Pohjola-Sintonen S, Tacke U, et al. Five fatal cases of serotonin syndrome after moclobemide-citalopram or moclobemide-clomipramine overdoses. Lancet 1993; 342: 1419
396. Lefebvre H, Noblet C. Moore N, et al. Pseudo-phaeochromocytoma after multiple drug interactions involving the selective monoamine oxidase inhibitor selegiline. Clinical Endocrinology 1995; 42: 95-9
397. McGrath PJ, Stewart JW, Quitkin FM. A possible deprenyl induced hypertensive reaction. Journal of Clinical Psychopharmacology 1989; 9: 310-1
398. Yahr MD, Duvoisin RC. Pyridoxine and levodopa in the treatment of parkinsonism. Journal of the American Medical Association 1972; 220: 861
399. Kuzucu EY. Methoxyflurane, tetracycline, and renal failure. Journal of the American Medical Association 1970; 211: 1162

Chapter 8

# Drug Overdosage and Poisoning

*J.A. Vale* and *A. Proudfoot*

## Synopsis of Important Principles

1) The majority of poisoned patients recover with measures to ensure adequate gas exchange in the lungs, an adequate cardiac output and, when necessary, control of complications such as seizures and arrhythmias.

2) Specific antidotal therapy is available for relatively few poisons. Mechanisms include pharmacological antagonism, inhibition of metabolism to toxic metabolites, inactivation of highly reactive alkylating intermediates, chelation, and binding with drug-specific antibodies.

3) With some important exceptions, the management of poisoning is not altered by knowledge of plasma drug concentrations. However, serial estimations of plasma concentrations may be helpful in the assessment of prognosis and the efficacy of treatment.

4) The routine use of any gut decontamination procedure (induced emesis, gastric lavage, activated charcoal, whole bowel irrigation) is inappropriate as there is no evidence that their use improves outcome and they may cause significant morbidity.

5) Gastric lavage should be considered only if a patient has ingested a life-threatening amount of a toxic substance within one hour of presentation. Even then, clinical benefit has not been confirmed in controlled studies.

6) Multiple-dose activated charcoal effectively increases the total body clearance of a number of drugs, and this technique should be considered if a patient has ingested a life-threatening amount of phenobarbital, carbamazepine, theophylline, quinine, dapsone or salicylate. With all of these drugs, there are clinical data to confirm enhanced elimination, though a reduction in morbidity and mortality has not been demonstrated in controlled studies.

7) Forced diuresis can increase the renal clearance of reabsorbed compounds and may be employed in the absence of renal impairment. However, there are no controlled studies demonstrating clinical benefit and its role is limited, probably to cases of mild lithium poisoning.

8) The renal clearance of some toxins may be dramatically increased by appropriate manipulation of urine pH. However, the renal excretion of most drugs is insignificant in relation to metabolic clearance. In clinical practice, alkaline diuresis is largely restricted to poisoning with salicylates and phenoxyacetate herbicides.

9) Peritoneal dialysis increases the elimination of poisons such as ethylene glycol, methanol and salicylates but is much less efficient than haemodialysis.

10) Haemodialysis significantly enhances the elimination of salicylates, lithium, methanol, isopropanol, ethylene glycol and ethanol, and should be considered in all cases of severe poisoning with these substances.

11) Haemoperfusion significantly increases the elimination of barbiturates, carbamazepine, disopyramide, ethchlorvynol, glutethimide, meprobamate, methaqualone, theophylline and trichloroethanol derivatives but, in many cases, multiple-dose activated charcoal is of similar value.

Accidental and deliberate self-poisoning with drugs and toxic substances remains a common reason for hospital admissions and deaths in many countries.[1,2] Successful management depends on an understanding of the pharmacodynamics, toxicology and pharmacokinetic principles involved. However, there are many practical difficulties. The number of toxic substances likely to be taken is enormous and includes not only drugs, but also the whole range of household, agricultural and industrial chemicals, and animal and plant toxins. No single clinician could possibly have the necessary knowledge and experience to deal with even a tiny fraction of these, and poisons information centres have been established in many countries to provide emergency information.

With many of the less common poisons, clinical and toxicological data are very limited. Household products are most often taken by young children but, contrary to popular belief, rarely cause serious trouble.[3,4] Drugs that could be lethal when taken in small amounts by small children include tricyclic antidepressants, quinine and other antimalarials, methyl salicylate, theophylline and phenothiazines.[5] It must also be remembered that the pattern of drugs used for self-poisoning changes with time and the prescribing habits of doctors.

## 1. General Principles

Therapeutic measures for acute poisoning should be assessed by the same strict scientific criteria as other medical treatment. Unfortunately, this is rarely practical because of ethical constraints on the use of controls and difficulty in obtaining adequate numbers of patients for clinical trials in any one centre. Moreover, clinical desperation may drive clinicians to resort to measures which are unproven, ineffective or illogical but survival is not proof of the efficacy of treatment since the great majority of poisoned patients recover with supportive therapy alone.[6,7]

The basis of drug toxicity in poisoning often differs from that encountered with adverse reactions from the therapeutic use of drugs. So-called 'hypersensitivity' and immunological reactions are rarely seen, and most forms of acute toxicity represent exaggerated therapeutic responses, expected dose-related adverse effects, secondary pharmacological actions, drug-specific organ toxicity, and interference with vital enzyme systems. Some examples of the different types of toxicity in drug overdosage and poisoning are shown in table I.

In practice, the issue is more complex since about 40% of patients take 2 or more drugs in overdosage. For example, dextropropoxyphene (propoxyphene) when combined with paracetamol (acetaminophen) in the same formulation may cause rapid death from respiratory depression; those who survive then run the risk of severe liver damage, sometimes fatal, from the paracetamol component. In addition, alcohol is taken beforehand by some 70% of men and 40% of women (in the UK) and has great potential for toxic interactions, particularly with drugs such as tricyclic antidepressants, opioid analgesics and benzodiazepines which depress the central nervous system. There is obviously considerable individual variation in susceptibility to toxicity depending on such factors as rate of absorption (which is influenced by food and alcohol), age, genetic factors, underlying disease, drug metabolising enzyme activity, tolerance, and previous drug therapy, not to mention other drugs and alcohol taken at the same time.

Many drugs and poisons produce reversible effects. Some are nonspecific while others are

**Table I.** Examples of different types of toxicity in drug overdosage and poisoning

| Mechanism | Drug or poison | Action/use | Manifestations of poisoning |
|---|---|---|---|
| Exaggerated therapeutic effect | Amobarbital (amylobarbitone) | Sedative/hypnotic | Deep coma, respiratory depression, hypothermia |
| | Propranolol | β-Adrenoceptor blocker | Bradycardia, hypotension |
| Secondary pharmacological actions | Morphine<br>Dextropropoxyphene | Analgesic | Coma, severe respiratory depression |
| | Amitriptyline | Antidepressant | Anticholinergic syndrome |
| Drug-specific organ toxicity | Paracetamol (acetaminophen) | Antipyretic/analgesic | Acute hepatic necrosis |
| | Paraquat | Herbicide | Progressive pulmonary fibrosis |
| Enzyme inhibition | Cyanide | Industrial | Inactivation of cytochrome oxidase |
| | Organophosphorus compounds | Insecticide | Inhibition of acetylcholinesterase |

**Table II.** Some compounds for which measurements of plasma concentrations may be helpful in the management of poisoning

| Indication | Drug or poison |
| --- | --- |
| Specific antidotal therapy | Paracetamol (acetaminophen)<br>Iron salts |
| Specific antidotal therapy and active removal | Methanol<br>Ethylene glycol |
| Assessment of prognosis and risk of complications | Paraquat<br>Quinine |
| Severe poisoning where active removal is being considered | Salicylates<br>Phenobarbital<br>Lithium<br>Medium-duration of action barbiturates (e.g. amobarbital, butobarbital)<br>Glutethimide<br>Meprobamate<br>Ethchlorvynol<br>Chloral hydrate and trichloroethanol derivatives<br>Theophylline |

caused by stimulation or blockade of receptors. In the latter cases, the severity of intoxication is, within limits, related to the concentration at the sites of action, and the duration of intoxication depends on the rate of elimination of the toxin from the body. Other compounds, however, behave as 'hit and run' poisons and features of toxicity may not become apparent until most of the poison has disappeared (e.g. carbon tetrachloride).

Specific antidotal therapy is available for relatively few drugs and poisons. For that reason, the basic approach to the management of poisoning is *intensive supportive therapy*, by which is meant the appropriate use of drugs and mechanical techniques to maintain vital body functions. Its primary objective is to ensure an adequate cardiac output and gas exchange in the lungs, so that oxygen delivery to the tissues is such that cellular processes may proceed as normally as possible while the toxin is eliminated. Additional measures include removal of unabsorbed drug from the gastrointestinal tract (gut decontamination) and enhancement of elimination of poisons from the body by diuresis, haemodialysis and haemoperfusion.

## 2. Drug/Toxin Identification and Measurement

Identification of a poison (normally a drug) and measurement of its plasma concentration is often thought to be of value in the management of poisoning. However, there are relatively few situations (table II) where treatment is actually influenced by this knowledge[8] since concentrations usually correlate poorly with clinical toxicity.

### 2.1 Identification of the Poison

The nature of the poison is usually suspected from a combination of the patient's history (if he/she is an older child or adult) and circumstantial evidence and, in some cases, will be supported by the finding of compatible symptoms and signs. However, poor correlation between what patients state they have taken and what can be detected analytically in the plasma or urine[9,10] provides objective support for the widespread belief amongst clinicians that poisoned patients are notoriously unreliable historians in respect of both what, and how much, has been taken. An alternative, less palatable, explanation for such discrepancies is that clinicians are not as assiduous in their history taking as they think! Whatever the truth, emergency and supportive treatment must never be delayed pending laboratory confirmation of poisoning. In most cases, the toxicology laboratory provides reassurance for the clinician rather than benefit for the patient.

Drug identification and measurement of plasma concentrations is necessary for the proper treatment of intoxication with the compounds listed in table II. It is also necessary or, at least, highly desirable, before attempting to induce an alkaline diuresis or undertaking such measures as peritoneal dialysis, haemodialysis and haemoperfusion. Serial estimations are helpful in the assessment of prognosis and the efficacy of treatment.

Comprehensive screening for the identification of drugs and their metabolites in urine is generally not possible[11] but may occasionally be useful to determine what has been taken, and is frequently essential for the diagnosis of non-accidental poisoning of children (sometimes referred to as Munchausen syndrome by proxy).[12] Otherwise, it is of little or no clinical value. In a survey of 287 paediatric patients referred for toxicological investigation, a diagnosis of poisoning was confirmed as a result of the analysis in only 17%.[13] Toxicological results are often accepted by clinicians without question, but there may be major discrepancies between the findings of different laboratories.[14]

### 2.2 Interpretation of Plasma Concentrations

The concept of 'toxic' and 'lethal' plasma or blood concentrations of drugs and poisons is inappropriate and misleading. Because of individual variation in susceptibility, frequent ingestion of more than one drug, and common use of nonspecific analytical methods, such data are often meaningless in practical clinical terms. There are many pitfalls in the interpretation of plasma drug concentrations in poisoned patients, and the relationship between concentrations and toxicity is complex. Previous consumption of some drugs may result in marked tolerance, and there is often cross tolerance between central nervous system depressants including ethanol. Several drugs may be contributing to toxicity and it is pointless to measure one but not the others. There may also be doubt concerning continuing absorption. Moreover, the use of nonspecific analytical methods that measure metabolites in addition to the parent compound may give highly misleading results. Many metabolites of commonly used drugs have little or no pharmacological activity but sometimes their concentrations in plasma may be high.

Occasionally, however, active metabolites may contribute to toxicity. For example, delayed prolonged, deep coma in mesuximide (methsuximide) overdosage has been attributed to increasing concentrations of the metabolite methylphenylsuccinimide rather than the parent drug.[15]

With poisons that produce delayed toxicity and are rapidly eliminated (e.g. paracetamol) or are rapidly taken up into tissues (e.g. paraquat), plasma concentrations can only be interpreted in relation to the time of ingestion, and serial estimations are desirable. They form the basis of widely used treatment and prognostic concentration/time curves.[16,17] Prediction of the duration of coma on the basis of a single estimation of the concentration of a central nervous system depressant is unreliable as there is great individual variation in the rate of drug elimination, and acute tolerance may occur. In overdosage, barbiturates cause induction of hepatic microsomal enzymes with a progressive shortening of their plasma half-lives.[18] The metabolism of drugs such as salicylate and phenytoin is dose-dependent because of saturation of drug metabolising enzymes, and the rate of elimination is initially slow but increases rapidly with the transition from mixed-order to first-order kinetics. The kinetics of many other drugs may also be dose-dependent following overdosage.

In severely poisoned patients, reduced cardiac output and tissue perfusion, and multiple organ failure may make drug disposition grossly different from that encountered with normal therapeutic doses.[19]

## 3. General Management of Drug Overdosage and Poisoning

Most deaths from poisoning occur outside hospital and, when due to central nervous system depressants, are usually the result of respiratory obstruction and/or depression. In the hospital setting with expert nursing care and minimal medical interference, the overall mortality from poisoning is very low and deaths in hospitalised patients are more likely to be secondary to cardiac arrhythmias, gross myocardial depression, liver failure or irreversible hypoxic brain damage sustained before admission. Inevitably, multiple organ failure is present in some cases. It is clear therefore that with the important exception of appropriate and early administration of naloxone, and possibly flumazenil, the resuscitation and management of poisoned patients differ very little from that of any other ill patient.

### 3.1 Emergency Respiratory Management

Cardiorespiratory arrest may be present on arrival at hospital and is dealt with conventionally. In less serious cases, respiratory obstruction initially requires only simple measures, including the removal of dentures and secretions from the oropharynx and the use of the chin-lift and jaw-thrust manoeuvre to clear an airway blocked by the tongue falling back. Endotracheal intubation may be required when coma is deep. It has 3 benefits: (1) it helps maintain a clear airway; (2) it facilitates removal of secretions when atelectasis, infection or pulmonary oedema is present; and (3) it reduces the respiratory dead space and increases alveolar ventilation, thus improving oxygenation and removal of carbon dioxide. Oxygenation is further enhanced by increasing the inspired oxygen concentration and ventilation must be assisted if it is obviously inadequate.

Naloxone (1.2mg for an adult) should then be given intravenously (or down the endotracheal tube if venous access is difficult) if there is the slightest suspicion of opioid intoxication. When naloxone is ineffective or the adequacy of spontaneous ventilation is not an immediate concern, the results of arterial blood gas analysis should be awaited before making a decision to ventilate.

### 3.2 Management of Hypotension

Hypotension is likely to be the single most important cardiac problem encountered when poisoned patients arrive at hospital. The aetiology of hypotension in acute poisoning is complex and often multifactorial, and the likely factors in individual cases must be identified if management is to be optimal. In poisoning with CNS depressants, cardiac output falls, normal cardiovascular reflexes are impaired, and the venous return to the heart is reduced because loss of venous tone results in a disproportion between vascular capacity and blood volume. The resultant hypotension often causes alarm but is rarely, if ever, of consequence in the presence of warm extremities. It usually responds promptly to elevating the foot of the bed and, failing that, infusion of plasma or a plasma substitute. Only when poisoning with CNS depressants is severe, does cardiac output fall to such an extent that it is inadequate. In these cases, in addition to the measures already mentioned, infusion of dopamine and/or dobutamine may be required to achieve an acceptable blood pressure and perfusion of vital organs.

Other toxins may cause hypotension by different means. Drugs such as β-adrenoceptor blocking agents depress the myocardium, while envenomation or ingestion of corrosives, colchicine and paraquat produce hypovolaemia due to considerable blood or fluid loss into the tissues or gut. Less commonly, hypotension is the consequence of extreme brady- or tachyarrhythmias. In all cases, significant hypotension leads to impaired tissue perfusion and oxygen delivery and, in turn, to metabolic acidosis which further compromises cardiac function.

### 3.3 Management of Cardiac Arrhythmias

Cardiac arrhythmias complicating acute poisoning are commonly caused by tricyclic antidepressant and theophylline overdosage and, less commonly, by chloral hydrate and recreational drugs which stimulate the central nervous system – mainly cocaine, amphetamines, 'ecstasy' (methylenedioxymethamphetamine) and phencyclidine. Sinus tachycardia may occasionally be extreme (e.g. with theophylline and amphetamines) and, if associated with hypotension, may require treatment with a β-adrenoceptor blocker provided the patient is not asthmatic. Chloral hydrate-induced supraventricular tachycardia can be expected to respond rapidly to similar treatment.

Arrhythmias complicating *tricyclic antidepressant* poisoning pose the greatest problems. These drugs have sympathomimetic, anticholinergic and quinidine-like actions, and increasing toxic doses produce a sinus tachycardia, and progressively prolong the P-R (causing eventual disappearance of 'P' waves) and QRS intervals, the resultant appearances being easily mistaken for ventricular tachycardia.[20,21] In the first instance, hypoxia, metabolic acidosis and electrolyte balance must be corrected and may be all the treatment that is required. Intravenous sodium bicarbonate (1 mmol/kg bodyweight) may also have a beneficial action, even in the absence of metabolic acidosis.[22] The dilemma is to know when to use antiarrhythmic agents since their unnecessary administration may merely depress cardiac activity further. Ventricular fibrillation must clearly be treated on its merits but, otherwise, the use of antiarrhythmic drugs is usually only indicated when the arrhythmia is seriously reducing cardiac output. Ventricular tachycardia is rare after tricyclic antidepressant overdosage and is best treated by administering as little lidocaine (lignocaine) intravenously as is necessary to produce the desired response. Lidocaine is the treatment of choice since it has a short half-life and its adverse actions, if any, will be transient.

Infusion of magnesium sulfate may be beneficial for the torsade de pointes variety of ventricular tachycardia.[23,24] Cardiac pacing may be required in some cases but may not be effective because of a high pacing threshold and/or severely impaired myocardial contractility. Prolonged external cardiac massage and mechanical devices (e.g. intra-aortic balloon counterpulsation) have been used successfully in rare cases.[25]

### 3.4 Control of Convulsions

Convulsions occur in a variety of intoxications[26] and their presence may pose a major threat to the patient's airway, cardiac rhythm and oxygenation, in addition to exacerbating any metabolic acidosis. The associated hypoxia may, in turn, precipitate cardiac arrhythmias, especially when a cardiotoxin has been ingested, and make maintenance of a clear airway difficult, particularly if vomiting is also present.

Fortunately, most seizures are isolated, short-lived events and routine administration of an anticonvulsant is unnecessary and potentially dangerous since it may further depress respiration. However, repeated or prolonged convulsions must be controlled and intravenous diazepam is currently the drug of choice. Status epilepticus or a combination of seizures and vomiting may be better managed by neuromuscular blockade and assisted ventilation than by large doses of diazepam. This approach ensures that the airway, ventilation and oxygenation are secure but, if adopted, cerebral function should then be monitored at the bedside and electrical seizure activity suppressed with diazepam, thiopental or some other anticonvulsant.

### 3.5 Continuing Care

Once the poisoned patient has been resuscitated and a stable clinical state achieved, vital functions must be maintained while the spontaneous elimination of the poison proceeds and recovery follows.[7] In the majority of cases, this requires the application of intensive care principles. Seriously ill patients are nursed in an intensive care area where the airway, and cardiac and respiratory function can be closely monitored and any necessary intervention implemented immediately and its efficacy rapidly assessed. Control of electrolyte and fluid balance is an integral part of the process and expert nursing is essential. The latter includes frequent turning of unconscious patients, attention to skin pressure areas, prompt removal of bronchial secretions, passive limb movements, physiotherapy, and care of the mouth and eyes. Routine bladder catheterisation is unnecessary since the bladder can usually be emptied satisfactorily by fundal pressure and only a small proportion of poisoned patients are unconscious for longer than 12 hours.

A close watch should be kept for signs of infection but there is no case for the prophylactic use of antibiotics, except perhaps in aspiration pneumonia. Administration of unnecessary drugs in an already seriously ill patient can turn a critical situation into a disaster and medical interference must be kept to an absolute minimum.

### 3.6 Management of Complications

Acid-base and electrolyte disturbances and abnormalities of glucose homeostasis are common in acute poisoning and are caused by many toxins. Respiratory and metabolic acidosis, hypoglycaemia, hypokalaemia, hyperkalaemia and hypocalcaemia are the most dangerous and may require appropriate treatment.

#### *3.6.1 Acid-Base Disturbances*

The management of respiratory failure and acidosis is reviewed above (sections 3.1 and 3.3). Metabolic acidosis is most often secondary to impaired tissue perfusion which, itself, is secondary to a reduction of cardiac output and hypotension. Management of the latter (see section 3.2) should correct acidosis from this cause, and administration of alkali is generally inappropriate. Seizures commonly exacerbate a metabolic acidosis by causing additional hypoxia.

Less commonly, metabolic acidosis is due to ingestion of an acidic compound, although some acids are so weak that they contribute little to the acidosis associated with poisoning (e.g. with salicylic acid derived from hydrolysis of aspirin). In other cases, metabolic acidosis results from metabolism of the substance ingested to toxic intermediates, e.g. methanol to formate and ethylene glycol to glycolate and possibly oxalate.[27] In these cases, correction of acidosis with intravenous sodium bicarbonate is essential and very large amounts may be necessary.

#### *3.6.2 Hypoglycaemia*

Hypoglycaemia is usually due to overdosage with insulin or an oral antidiabetic drug[28] and may develop in the course of massive, toxin-induced, hepatic necrosis. Anticipation of its development is essential for correct management, and bedside monitoring should be carried out. Hypoglycaemia is an uncommon complication of poisoning with salicylates (particularly in children) and ethanol.[29]

#### *3.6.3 Electrolyte Disturbances*

Potassium disturbances occur in acute poisoning either because of a direct effect of the poison on extrarenal potassium control mechanisms, or indirectly as a result of complications arising.[30] The stimulation of $Na^+/K^+$ ATPase activity by $\beta_2$-agonists or its inhibition by digoxin are examples of direct effects. Complications of poisoning such as severe diarrhoea and vomiting will increase gastrointestinal potassium loss, whereas rhabdomyolysis, which involves the disruption of muscle cell membranes with release of the high intracellular potassium content into the extracellular space, produces hyperkalaemia.

Acid-base disturbances precipitate cellular potassium shifts as part of the acute defence mechanism to maintain a neutral metabolic environment without disrupting the membrane electrical potential. Hence a systemic acidosis involves the outward movement of potassium from cells to compensate for the cellular uptake of hydrogen ions. The reverse occurs in a systemic alkalosis and hypokalaemia results. These acute changes in potassium distribution are reversed once renal compensating mechanisms have resumed acid-base neutrality.

Unless renal function is impaired or rhabdomyolysis is severe, hyperkalaemia is a relatively uncommon metabolic complication of poisoning. In contrast, significant hypokalaemia is a more common problem and may have serious sequelae.

#### *3.6.4 Hypothermia*

Hypothermia is a common complication of poisoning with central nervous system depressants, particularly if alcohol has also been taken. It almost always responds to a warm environment and simple commonsense measures to minimise further heat loss. Active rewarming is rarely, if ever, necessary.

#### *3.6.5 Hyperthermia*

Body temperature frequently overshoots normal during recovery from prolonged, deep coma with hypothermia but, in this context, is not a matter for concern or administration of antibiotics unless there is associated infection.

More importantly, in present day clinical practice, some widely used 'recreational' drugs can cause severe hyperthermia when taken in excess.[31-33] Other drugs and non-drug substances can also raise body temperature including theophylline and its derivatives, monoamine oxidase inhibitors, salicylates and pesticides such as pentachlorophenol and dinitrophenol which uncouple oxidative phosphorylation. Frequently, convulsions, greatly increased muscle tone, and rhabdomyolysis and its complications are associated with hyperthermia. Pharmacological measures to control convulsions (see section 3.4), induce cooling (chlorpromazine), and reduce exaggerated muscle activity (dantrolene) may therefore be required in addition to cold sponging.

#### *3.6.6 Other Complications*

Other complications such as cerebral and pulmonary oedema, and renal and hepatic failure are treated conventionally (see chapters 29, 23, 24 and 22, respectively). Skin blisters should be treated as thermal burns. Rhabdomyolysis may require alkalinisation of the urine (to minimise the risk of acute renal tubular necrosis), and fasciotomy if a muscle compartment syndrome develops.

## 4. Antidotal Therapy

Unfortunately, specific antidotes or antagonists are available for very few commonly taken drugs and poisons. Furthermore, their usefulness is sometimes limited because they must be given very soon after ingestion to be effective. Toxicity may be reversed by several different mechanisms and some examples are shown in table III.

### 4.1 Reversal of Toxicity Due to Drug-Receptor Interactions

The effects of compounds that produce toxicity by stimulation or blockade of specific receptors can sometimes be reversed by the appropriate pharmacological antagonists or agonists, respectively. The result of the combined action of an agonist and an antagonist depends on their relative concentrations, affinities for the receptor, and intrinsic activities. The correct dose to reverse toxicity thus depends on the actual drugs involved and the severity of intoxication.

#### *4.1.1 Opioid Analgesics and Benzodiazepines*

Coma and respiratory depression induced by opioid analgesics and benzodiazepines can be reversed with *naloxone* and *flumazenil*, respectively. However, the dose of naloxone recommended for reversal of the effects of a therapeutic dose of morphine (0.4mg) cannot be expected to reverse severe opioid analgesic intoxication. In the example shown in figure 1, severe central nervous system and respiratory depression caused by dipipanone was not reversed by 'therapeutic' doses of naloxone and a larger dose was eventually required. Adults require a minimum dose of 1.2mg and frequently more. An increased dose will also be necessary if an agonist-antagonist opioid drug such as pentazocine has been taken[34] but the effects of buprenorphine cannot be reversed by even high doses of naloxone.

**Table III.** Specific antidotal therapy for poisoning

| Drug or poison | Specific therapy | Mechanism |
|---|---|---|
| Opioid analgesics, including pentazocine and dextropropoxyphene | Naloxone | Pharmacological antagonist |
| Paracetamol (acetaminophen) | Acetylcysteine, L-methionine | Sulfhydryl donors; inactivation of toxic metabolite |
| Iron salts | Deferoxamine (desferrioxamine) | Chelation |
| Metoclopramide, phenothiazines, butyrophenones (extrapyramidal reactions) | Anticholinergics (e.g. benztropine, procyclidine, orphenadrine) | Restoration of balance between dopaminergic and cholinergic activity in CNS |
| β-Adrenoceptor blockers | Atropine | Inhibition of vagal activity |
| | Isoprenaline (isoproterenol) | Pharmacological antagonist |
| | Glucagon | |
| | Prenalterol | |
| Sympathomimetics | β-Adrenoceptor blockers | Pharmacological antagonist |
| Methanol | Ethanol | Inhibition of conversion to toxic metabolites |
| Ethylene glycol | | |
| *Heavy metals:* | | |
| Arsenic | Dimercaprol (BAL) | Chelation |
| | Dimercaptosuccinic acid (DMSA; succimer) | Chelation |
| Copper | Penicillamine | Chelation |
| Lead | Sodium calcium edetate | Chelation |
| | Dimercaptosuccinic acid (DMSA; succimer) | Chelation |
| Mercury | Dimercaptopropane sulfonate (DMPS; unithiol) | Chelation |
| | Dimercaptosuccinic acid (DMSA; succimer) | Chelation |
| Thallium | Prussian blue | Chelation |
| Cholinesterase inhibitors | Atropine | Pharmacological antagonism |
| | Pralidoxime | Regeneration of acetylcholinesterase |
| | Obidoxime | |
| Cyanide | Dicobalt edetate | Chelation |
| | Sodium nitrite | Methaemoglobinaemia |
| | Sodium thiosulfate | Provision of sulfur for metabolism to thiocyanate |
| Oxidising agents causing methaemoglobinaemia | Methylene blue | Reduction of $Fe^{+++}$ to $Fe^{++}$; conversion of haemoglobin |
| Coumarin anticoagulants | Clotting factors | Replacement of clotting factors |
| | Vitamin $K_1$ (phytomenadione) | Pharmacological antagonist |
| Methotrexate | Folinic acid | Bypass of inhibited enzyme reaction |

Similarly, the dose of flumazenil used to reverse benzodiazepine sedation given for minor investigative procedures (0.2mg) is unlikely to improve an adult who is unconscious and in respiratory failure after massive overdosage. However, most will respond satisfactorily to doses of 2 to 3mg.[35]

Two points are important in the use of both naloxone and flumazenil in acutely poisoned patients:

1) Their durations of action are considerably shorter than those of the drugs for which they are given and recurrence of toxicity shortly after the last administration of the antidote should be expected.[35-37] Repeated doses or an intravenous infusion may therefore be necessary,[37] possibly for as long as 48 to 72 hours in poisoning with long-acting opioid analgesics such as dipipanone and methadone.

2) Their administration may produce an acute withdrawal reaction, including convulsions, in some patients dependent on opioids or benzodiazepines.[35] Fortunately, the incidence of such effects is very low with modest doses of naloxone (up to 0.8mg) and not of sufficient concern to prohibit prehospital use by paramedics.[38] Prehospital use of flumazenil has not yet been assessed formally.

#### *4.1.2 β-Adrenoceptor Blockers*

Bradycardia and myocardial depression in mild poisoning with β-adrenoceptor blockers can often be reversed with *atropine* and *isoprenaline (isoproterenol)*, but these agents have lit-

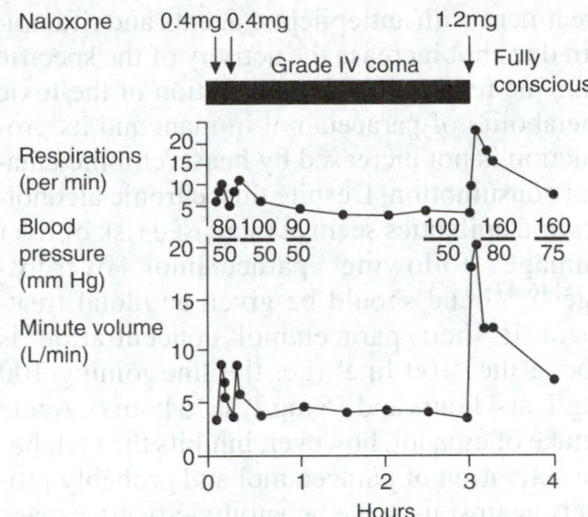


**Fig. 1.** The effect of naloxone on coma, respiratory depression and blood pressure in a patient with severe dipipanone intoxication. Note the slight transient response to inadequate doses of 0.4mg and subsequent complete reversal of toxicity with 1.2mg.

tle or no effect in gross overdosage. In such circumstances, myocardial function can be considerably improved with *glucagon* which is the treatment of choice for severe poisoning.[39] It probably activates adenyl cyclase by a mechanism different from that of isoprenaline.

*Prenalterol* is thought to have a wider safety margin than isoprenaline in large doses, and has also been used in severe poisoning with β-adrenoceptor blockers,[40] though it is only available in a few countries.

#### 4.1.3 Theophylline and Central Nervous System Stimulants

*β-Adrenoceptor blockers* can be used as antidotes in intoxication with central nervous system stimulants, including recreational substances such as amphetamines and cocaine, and commonly used bronchodilators such as theophylline[41] and $\beta_2$-agonists.[42] β-Blockers slow the heart rate and may reverse the flux of potassium into cells, thus obviating the need for intravenous potassium supplements.[41,42]

#### 4.1.4 Tricyclic Antidepressants

*Physostigmine* acts to antagonise many of the effects of anticholinergic agents such as tricyclic antidepressants. Being a cholinesterase inhibitor, it increases acetylcholine concentrations at synapses and therefore has a greater opportunity of occupying receptors. Unfortunately, physostigmine does not seem to reverse the effects of tricyclic antidepressants on atrioventricular conduction or their serious quinidine-like action on the heart. This therapeutic limitation, together with its ability to cause convulsions and asystole, has led to it being abandoned.

### 4.2 Reversal of Toxicity Due to Enzyme Inhibition

Toxicity may be caused by inhibition of vital enzymes, e.g. cyanide inactivates cytochrome oxidases; organophosphorus and carbamate insecticides inhibit acetylcholinesterase; and salicylate uncouples oxidative phosphorylation and thereby interferes with the function of enzymes dependent on adenosine triphosphate. If a single enzyme is inhibited, it may be possible to restore function by increasing the concentration of the substrate or administration of the product of the inhibited reaction. Thus, the toxicity of the antifolate drug methotrexate can be reduced by *folinic acid*.

The toxicity of organophosphorus compounds is related to inhibition of acetylcholinesterase (AChE) activity in the blood, brain and other tissues, thereby allowing acetylcholine to accumulate at autonomic and some central synapses and at the autonomic postganglionic and skeletal efferent nerve endings. The rate of spontaneous reaction of alkyl-phosphorylated AChE depends on the chemical structure of the organophosphorus compound.[43] Most of the commonly used organophosphorus insecticides carry either 2 methyl (e.g. demeton-*S*-methyl, dichlorvos, dimethoate, malathion) or 2 ethyl (e.g. chlorpyrifos, diazinon, parathion) ester groups attached to the phosphorus atom, so that dimethyl phosphorylated AChE or diethyl phosphorylated AChE, respectively, will be generated. Spontaneous reactivation of dimethyl phosphorylated AChE proceeds quite rapidly so that the patient's condition should improve even without oxime therapy. Unless oximes (see below) are employed, there is no such expectation of rapid recovery for patients intoxicated with diethyl phosphoryl insecticides.

Oximes such as *pralidoxime* and *obidoxime* are able to reverse enzyme inhibition as long as the inhibited AChE remains in the 'unaged' form. It is commonly, but erroneously, believed that within one day of intoxication virtually all of the inhibited AChE will be in the 'aged' form so that oxime therapy, if employed, would be useless. However, there are good biochemical reasons for suggesting that as soon as an effective concentration of an oxime is achieved *in vivo*, the balance of 'aging' and reactivation reaction rate for inhibited AChE is altered in favour of the latter.[43] Thus, progress towards complete inhibition may be slowed markedly. It is probable that benefit will ensue even if oxime therapy is commenced or continued several days after intoxication has occurred.[44]

*Atropine* antagonises the effect of accumulated acetylcholine at muscarinic receptors. Atropine sulfate 2mg intravenously should be given as soon as possible in moderately or severely poisoned patients. Repeated injections of atropine may have to be given over the first few hours of therapy; the dose should be titrated to control peripheral muscarinic signs, principally bronchospasm and bronchorrhoea. In severe cases, particularly when oximes are not administered, 100mg or more may be required to control symptoms.

### 4.3 Reversal of Toxicity Caused by Toxic Metabolites

Many compounds are converted to toxic metabolites. It therefore follows that it may be possible to reduce toxicity by inhibiting the biotransformation of the parent compound or by giving agents that inactivate the toxic metabolite. Paracetamol (acetaminophen) is the most important example in present day clinical practice; other compounds with important metabolites whose toxicity may be reduced by such measures include methanol and ethylene glycol.

#### 4.3.1 Paracetamol

Paracetamol in overdosage can be fatal; it causes acute hepatic and, less commonly, renal tubular necrosis. When taken in therapeutic doses, about 5 to 10% of paracetamol is converted by cytochrome P450-dependent mixed-function oxidases to a toxic alkylating intermediate metabolite, *N*-acetyl-*p*-benzoquinonimine (NABQI) which is then inactivated by preferential conjugation with hepatic reduced glutathione.[45] When hepatotoxic doses are taken, however, glutathione is rapidly depleted and the excess metabolite binds covalently to liver macromolecules causing cell damage and necrosis. There is evidence that individuals with heavy consumption of ethanol or drugs such as barbiturates, antiepileptic agents and rifampicin are at increased risk of paracetamol hepatotoxicity. It was assumed that microsomal enzyme induction allows the rate of production of NABQI to outstrip that of glutathione synthesis. However, treatment with antiepileptic agents and rifampicin does not increase the activity of the specific enzyme responsible for generation of the toxic metabolite of paracetamol in man, and its production is not increased by heavy chronic ethanol consumption. Despite this, chronic alcoholics and epileptics seem at increased risk of liver damage following paracetamol overdosage[46,47] and should be given antidotal treatment if their paracetamol concentration is above the '100 line' (i.e. the line joining 100 mg/L at 4 hours and 15 mg/L at 15 hours). Acute intake of ethanol, however, inhibits the metabolic activation of paracetamol and probably protects against its acute hepatotoxicity after overdosage.[48]

Paracetamol hepatotoxicity can be prevented by the oral or intravenous administration of *acetylcysteine* (*N*-acetylcysteine)[49-51] and the oral administration of *L-methionine*,[52] which act primarily by facilitating glutathione synthesis. Currently 4 different treatment protocols are in use internationally and each offers virtually complete protection, provided it is started within 8 to 10 hours of ingestion of the overdose.[53] However, some degree of liver damage becomes increasingly likely if the start of treatment extends beyond 10 hours; according to different series, 26 to 63% of patients in this category will develop severe hepatotoxicity as defined by a serum alanine or aspartate aminotransferase activity of 1000 IU/L or greater. The activity of these enzymes increases significantly the longer the delay in antidote administration.[49-52] However, acetylcysteine still appears to confer some benefit even after 1 to 2 days, although the mechanism by which it does so is probably quite different from that when it is given early.[54]

Fortunately, only a minority of patients are at risk of severe liver damage but they cannot be identified from the features of toxicity at the time at which antidotes would be expected to provide maximum protection. Unnecessary treatment of patients not at risk is to be avoided in principle and because the antidotes, particularly acetylcysteine given intravenously, are not without adverse effects. It has therefore become clinical practice to identify at-risk patients by assessing their plasma paracetamol concentration in relation to the time from ingestion of the overdose. Various 'treatment' or 'danger' lines have been devised (fig. 2). The one most commonly used joins plots of plasma paracetamol concentrations of 200 mg/L at 4 hours and 30

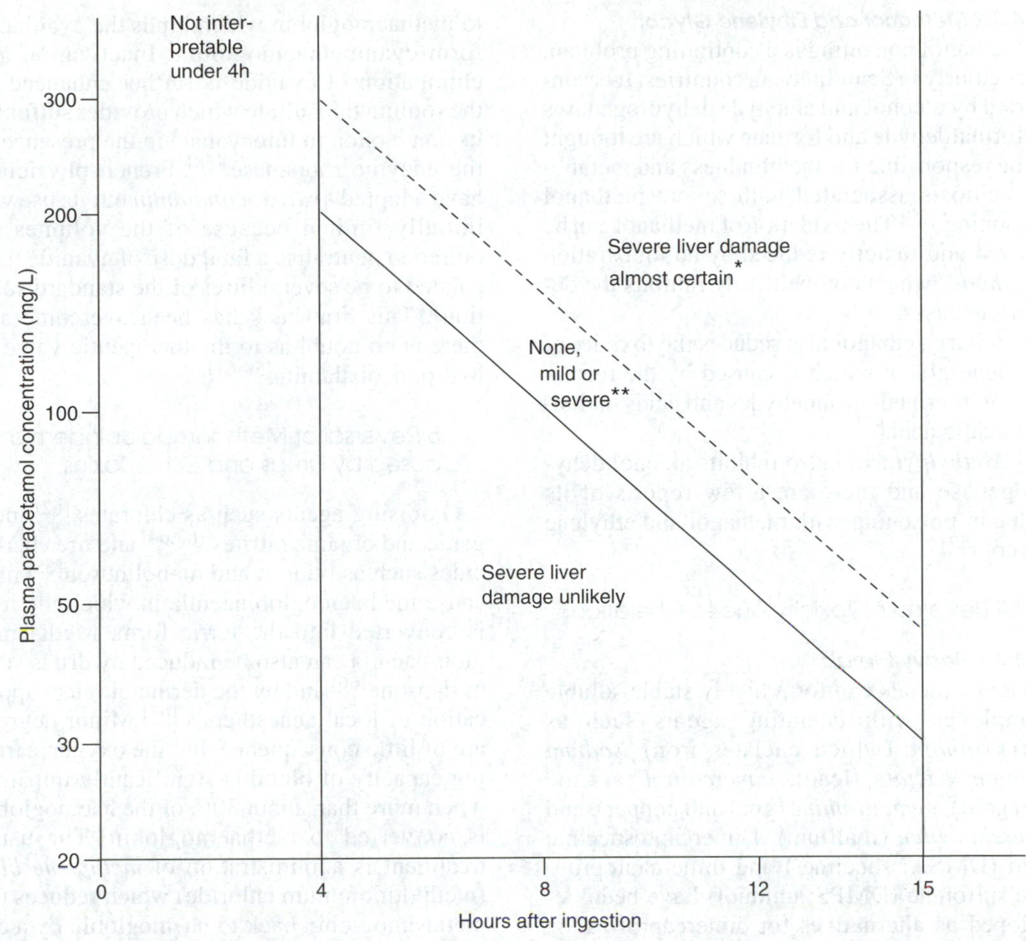


**Fig. 2.** Relationship between plasma paracetamol concentrations, time after ingestion, and risk of liver damage following overdosage. Treatment with antidote (e.g. acetylcysteine) is indicated in patients with values above the lower solid line. * 90% of untreated patients will develop ALT/AST >1000 IU/L. ** 60% of untreated patients will develop ALT/AST >1000 IU/L. *Abbreviations:* AST = aspartate amino transferase; ALT = alanine amino transferase.

mg/L at 15 hours after ingestion, on a semilogarithmic graph.[49] Paracetamol concentrations measured within 4 hours of ingestion are potentially misleading because absorption and distribution of the drug is still continuing. Another line which lies parallel and starts at 150 mg/L is widely used in the US.[50,51] This method of identifying at-risk patients has the clinical advantages of ready availability and speed so that treatment is not unduly delayed. However, it is not without flaws;[7] accurate estimation of the ingestion/presentation interval is especially critical, but the age of the patient, interindividual variations in handling paracetamol, the possibility of enzyme induction, and co-ingestion of other toxins are all potential confounding factors. Clinicians should therefore not be surprised if prognostic lines occasionally predict wrongly.

Reduced glutathione plays a vital protective role against attack by reactive electrophilic metabolites and radicals. As well as preventing acute paracetamol-induced liver damage by facilitating glutathione synthesis, acetylcysteine, L-methionine and other sulfhydryl compounds also protect against ionising radiation and the toxicity of heavy metals, cytotoxic alkylating agents, and halogenated hydrocarbons such as chloroform and bromobenzene.[55] However, the hepatotoxicity of carbon tetrachloride is not glutathione-dependent and acetylcysteine does not prevent liver damage following exposure to this agent in man.[56]

#### *4.3.2 Methanol and Ethylene Glycol*

Methanol poisoning is a continuing problem, particularly in Scandinavian countries. It is converted by alcohol and aldehyde dehydrogenases to formaldehyde and formate which are thought to be responsible for the blindness and metabolic acidosis associated with severe methanol poisoning.[27] The oxidation of methanol can be slowed and toxicity reduced by administration of *ethanol* which competitively inhibits the dehydrogenases.

Similarly, ethanol also reduces the toxicity of ethylene glycol which is caused by the formation of intermediate aldehydes and acids including oxalic acid.[27]

*4-Methylpyrazole* also inhibits alcohol dehydrogenase and there are a few reports of its value in poisoning with methanol and ethylene glycol.[57]

### 4.4 Reversal of Toxicity Due to Chelation

#### *4.4.1 Heavy Metals*

Heavy metals can form highly stable soluble complexes with chelating agents such as *deferoxamine* (which chelates iron), *sodium calcium edetate* (lead), *dimercaprol* (arsenic and gold), *penicillamine* (gold and copper), and *Prussian blue* (thallium). Dimercaptosuccinic acid (DMSA; succimer) and dimercaptopropane sulfonate (DMPS; unithiol) have been developed as alternatives for dimercaprol in the treatment of mercury and arsenic poisoning and for sodium calcium edetate in lead poisoning.

The toxicity of these metals can be reduced by early administration of chelating agents but their efficacy is reduced once the metals have become firmly bound in the tissues. Iron poisoning is relatively common, especially in young children and, irrespective of age, intravenous deferoxamine is indicated if the plasma iron concentration exceeds the predicted total iron binding capacity.

#### *4.4.2 Cyanide*

Cyanide is a very rapidly acting poison that inhibits cell respiration by combining with cytochrome oxidase. It is avidly bound by many compounds containing cobalt, but the current treatment of choice for cyanide poisoning varies from one country to another. In the UK and France, *dicobalt edetate* is preferred, while in the US, intravenous *sodium nitrite* and *sodium thiosulfate* are employed (as dicobalt edetate is not available). The rationale for use of sodium nitrite is that the nitrite converts haemoglobin to methaemoglobin which binds the cyanide to form cyanmethaemoglobin. Inactivation and elimination of cyanide is further enhanced by the sodium thiosulfate which provides sulfur for its conversion to thiocyanate in the presence of the enzyme rhodanase.[58] French physicians have adopted *hydroxocobalamin* but its use was initially limited because of the volumes required to neutralise a fatal dose of cyanide (calculated to be several litres of the standard solution). This drawback has been overcome and there is no doubt as to the therapeutic value of hydroxocobalamin.[59-61]

### 4.5 Reversal of Methaemoglobinaemia Caused by Drugs and Other Toxins

Oxidising agents such as chlorates,[62] inorganic and organic nitrites,[63,64] and urea herbicides such as linuron and monolinuron[65] may cause methaemoglobinaemia in which the iron is converted into the ferric form. Methaemoglobinaemia can also be induced by drugs such as dapsone[66] and by the dermatological application of local anaesthetics.[67] Minor degrees are of little consequence, but the oxygen carrying capacity of blood is significantly impaired when more than about 30% of the haemoglobin is converted to methaemoglobin. The usual treatment is administration of *methylene blue* (methylthioninium chloride) which reduces the methaemoglobin back to haemoglobin by a cyclic reaction involving conversion of the dye to its colourless form, leucomethylene blue.

### 4.6 Reversal of Toxicity by Immunotherapy

Immunotherapy is a recent and important advance in clinical toxicology. It involves the use of *anti-drug antibodies* to bind and inactivate drugs. To date, its main application has been in severe digoxin intoxication where it has been highly successful.[68] Not surprisingly, it has also been used in poisoning with digitoxin and in serious toxicity resulting from ingestion of plants such as yew[69] and oleander species[70] which have toxins chemically similar to cardiac glycosides. The antibodies are digoxin-specific and raised in sheep but only their Fab fragments are used in clinical practice. Limited experience suggests that repeated administration is possible and safe.[71]

Similar antibodies are being developed for poisoning with colchicine,[72] paraquat[73,74] and tricyclic antidepressants but, as yet, there is very little clinical experience with them. However, clinical trials of Fab antibody fragments against envenomation by the European adder *(Vipera berus)* have shown promising results.[75]

Antibody therapy for digoxin toxicity is usually dramatically effective and produces an immediate fall in plasma digoxin concentrations and rapid reversal of life-threatening complications such as hyperkalaemia and cardiac arrhythmias. The dose of antibody is calculated according to the estimated amount of digoxin to be found on an equimolar basis. Unfortunately, this dose is usually large and the antibody is expensive.

## 5. Methods to Reduce Drug Absorption

It is logical to assume that removal of unabsorbed drug from the gastrointestinal tract ('gut decontamination') is beneficial, yet the efficacy of current methods remains unproven and efforts to remove small amounts of 'safe' drugs are clearly not worthwhile.

### 5.1 Gastric Lavage

Gastric lavage has been employed widely for some 180 years. However, evidence of substantial clinical benefit accruing to the majority of poisoned patients undergoing lavage is lacking. Few adequate clinical studies have been performed and therefore, the value of gastric lavage remains controversial. Yet 'to advocate abandoning it is to attack one of the very pillars of the management of poisoning by ingestion and cannot be supported lightly. However, endorsement by common usage should not blind physicians to its limitations or protect it from critical appraisal'.[76]

#### *5.1.1 Clinical Effectiveness*

Gastric emptying studies in experimental animals have shown no impressive drug recovery[77-80] even when undertaken within one hour of administration, circumstances which are not likely to prevail in most poisoned patients who arrive at a treatment facility at a later time after overdose. Volunteer studies also provide no support for the use of gastric lavage,[81-83] while an endoscopic study performed in poisoned patients showed that after lavage, most patients (88%) still had residual intragastric solid.[84] Gastric lavage may also cause gastric contents to be discharged into the small bowel, thereby increasing the amount of drug available for absorption.[85] Continued absorption of drug after lavage is known to occur[86,87] and drug concretions may be found in the stomach[88,89] or at post-mortem examination[90] even after gastric lavage.

Clinical studies in patients poisoned with a number of agents have not demonstrated any major benefit from the use of gastric lavage to limit drug absorption. Lavage has been shown to remove only small quantities of ingested drug or significant amounts in only a minority of patients in studies with paracetamol,[91] salicylate,[92] tricyclic antidepressants,[93] and barbiturates.[92,94,95] In barbiturate poisoning, more than 200mg of drug was recovered in around 40 to 50% of patients in whom lavage was carried out within 4 hours of ingestion, but in very few of those lavaged after this time.[92,95] Overall, the best results were obtained in deeply unconscious patients, presumably reflecting the fact that unconscious patients are more severely poisoned and have therefore ingested more drug.

In unselected cases of poisoning, poor recovery of drug has been reported if lavage is performed more than 2 hours after overdosage.[87] A comparison with activated charcoal treatment in patients with paracetamol poisoning showed gastric lavage to be inferior to activated charcoal in limiting drug absorption.[91] However, the use of gastric lavage in conjunction with activated charcoal produced a better outcome than activated charcoal alone in unselected cases of poisoning if the latter was administered within one hour of overdosage.[96]

#### *5.1.2 Complications*

The potential complications of gastric lavage are well documented though, in practice, serious sequelae occur only rarely. Laryngospasm has been observed[94] particularly when a semiconscious patient is resisting the procedure, either intentionally or as a consequence of the agent ingested. Mechanical injury to the gut is very uncommon, though oesophageal perforation has been observed rarely.[92,96-99] In our clinical experience, perforation has only occurred once in some 15,000 lavages. Gastric haemorrhage has also been reported very rarely.

Other complications reported include a fall in partial pressure of oxygen; this fall was significantly greater in conscious than unconscious patients, in smokers than in non-smokers, and was most marked in male smokers aged 45 years or older.[100] Aspiration pneumonia is particularly likely to ensue if petroleum distillates have been ingested or lavage is carried out in a semicomatose patient without an endotracheal tube *in situ*, though aspiration has been reported even when hydrocarbons are not involved.[92,101,102] Tension pneumothorax and charcoal empyema have also been described after lavage and the administration of charcoal via the tube.[98]

A significant rise in pulse rate has been observed during lavage,[100] the rise being greater in conscious than unconscious patients. Small conjunctival haemorrhages are observed commonly and are particularly likely to occur in those who are not fully cooperative with the procedure for whatever reason. Hypernatraemia due to lavage with large quantities of saline has been described and water intoxication has been reported as a result of over-zealous lavage,[103] particularly in children.

The possible adverse psychological impact of lavage should also be recognised.[104] However, the impact of gastric lavage does not reduce the likelihood of repeat overdose.[105]

#### *5.1.3 Place of Lavage in the Management of Poisoning*

Gastric lavage should not be employed *routinely* in the management of poisoned patients, as there is no certain evidence that its use improves outcome and it may cause significant morbidity. Since the efficacy with which gastric lavage removes gastric contents decreases with time, lavage should only be considered if a patient has ingested life-threatening amounts of a toxic agent up to one hour previously. Even then, it is possible that drug absorption may be enhanced by its use. Although reports indicate that impressive recoveries of drug are occasionally achieved, there is no strong clinical evidence to support the view that, overall, lavage later than one hour after a toxic ingestion will benefit patients, including those who have ingested a tricyclic antidepressant or aspirin.

### 5.2 Activated Charcoal: Single Dose

Charcoal is prepared from vegetable matter and petroleum and 'activation' creates a highly developed internal pore structure, thereby increasing the surface area from 2 to 4 $m^2/g$ to more than 1000 $m^2/g$. Activated charcoal is able to adsorb a wide variety of drugs and toxic agents; the exceptions are listed in table IV.

Although a few reports of the use of activated charcoal in volunteers suggest no benefit in reducing drug absorption,[83,106,107] others have shown that, when given 30 to 60 minutes after

**Table IV.** Toxins which are poorly adsorbed by activated charcoal

| |
|---|
| Acids and alkalis |
| Ethanol (alcohol) |
| Ethylene glycol |
| Iron |
| Lithium |
| Methanol |

ingestion, a single dose of activated charcoal reduces the absorption of aminophylline,[108] ampicillin,[82] aspirin,[109,110] carbamazepine,[111] digoxin,[109] doxepin,[112] mefenamic acid,[113] paracetamol,[114] phenobarbital,[111] phenytoin,[109] tetracycline,[108] theophylline,[115] and tolfenamic acid.[106] However, all these studies were performed in fasting volunteers given non-toxic doses and a comparatively large dose of charcoal (usually 50g). The results are therefore of doubtful relevance to poisoned patients in whom an uncertain – but usually larger – amount of drug has been taken after food and often in association with alcohol and other drugs. Comparative studies in volunteers have indicated that activated charcoal is better than either syrup of ipecac[108,110,116,117] or gastric lavage[82] in reducing drug absorption.

A significant reduction in drug absorption has been observed in only one clinical study and this involved patients poisoned with paracetamol.[91] Activated charcoal was superior to gastric lavage and syrup of ipecac in reducing absorption, though its use has not yet been shown to reduce the need for an antidote in paracetamol poisoning.

### 5.3 Syrup of Ipecac and Other Emetics

A number of measures for induction of emesis in poisoned patients have been studied. Stimulation of the pharynx with the fingers is safe, though its efficacy is low. Saline emetics should not be used as fatal hypernatraemia may ensue. Apomorphine commonly produces CNS and respiratory depression and therefore cannot be recommended.

***Syrup of ipecac*** is derived from the dried root of *Cephaelis ipecacuanha* and *C. acuminata*, and contains the active alkaloids emetine and cephaeline. Emetine has a direct irritant action on the gastric mucosa which causes vomiting within 30 minutes of ipecac administration; subsequent vomiting results from the central action of both alkaloids. Provided the dose is appropriate, almost all patients given syrup of ipecac will vomit within 25 to 30 minutes. However, there is little evidence that its use prevents significant absorption of toxic material. In volunteer studies, syrup of ipecac administered half to one hour after drug administration did not have any significant effect on the absorption of paracetamol and theophylline[108] or of salicylate;[110] in both cases, activated charcoal was superior. No clinical studies have demonstrated its efficacy.

There are a number of objections to the routine use of syrup of ipecac, particularly in children. Firstly, only a small percentage of children presenting to hospital develop toxic symptoms and therefore, in most of these patients, treatment of any kind including the routine administration of an emetic is inappropriate. Secondly, the use of ipecac in patients who are asymptomatic on presentation may result in persistent vomiting, diarrhoea, lethargy and drowsiness. This is not only unpleasant for the child but may also make diagnosis more difficult, and is likely to be without therapeutic benefit. Thus, in our opinion, syrup of ipecac should be abandoned as an emetic as there is no good clinical evidence that it significantly reduces drug absorption and its adverse effects may complicate diagnosis.

### 5.4 Whole Gut Lavage

Theoretically, the more rapidly a poison passes through the gut, the less it will be absorbed. Whole bowel irrigation using physiological saline was originally introduced to prepare patients for bowel surgery. In recent years, polyethylene glycol electrolyte solutions have been used for this purpose; these solutions do not result in absorption of fluid and electrolytes, even though large volumes are administered rapidly via a nasogastric tube.

Although 3 volunteer studies[118-120] have shown a significant reduction in drug absorption after whole bowel irrigation, no adequate studies have been performed to assess the value of whole gut lavage in poisoned patients. It has been recommended for patients who have ingested substantial amounts of iron, lithium and modified-release drugs, but there is no evidence that its use improves outcome.

### 5.5 Cathartics

Cathartics have been used alone and in conjunction with activated charcoal. Although the use of a cathartic is traditional, this measure alone has not been shown to reduce drug absorption in poisoned patients. However, there is evidence from volunteer studies[121,122] that the combination of sorbitol and activated charcoal does reduce drug absorption. Currently, cathartics cannot be recommended as there is no clinical evidence of efficacy and, moreover, clinically significant adverse effects have occasionally been reported with their use.

### 5.6 Other Binding Agents

Other agents have been used in attempts to bind unabsorbed drug or chemical in the gastrointestinal tract. Fullers' earth and bentonite have been employed traditionally in paraquat poisoning but activated charcoal is superior in this situation.[123]

Cholestyramine binds acidic drugs and can reduce the absorption of paracetamol (acetaminophen) taken at the same time, but there are no adequate clinical data to support its use..

## 6. Methods to Enhance Drug Elimination

### 6.1 General Principles

Haemodialysis, peritoneal dialysis, haemoperfusion, exchange transfusion, alkaline diuresis and multiple-dose activated charcoal have all been used in attempts to increase the rate of removal of poisons from the body. However, the amount of active drug removed is often disappointingly small, and the indications for the use of such measures are very limited. None of these methods has been shown in a controlled clinical trial to reduce morbidity or mortality. This is not to say that such measures are never necessary, or indeed sometimes life-saving, but rather that a more critical appraisal of their role is required.

The efficacy of these techniques for drug removal in poisoned patients can be predicted from well established toxicological and pharmacokinetic principles.[124-128] They obviously have no place following overdosage with 'safe' drugs such as benzodiazepines or drugs such as paracetamol or opioid analgesics for which specific antidotal therapy is available (see sections 4.1.1 and 4.3.1). Also, they are unlikely to be helpful for rapidly acting metabolic poisons (e.g. cyanide) and poisons that inhibit enzyme activity (e.g. organophosphorus insecticides). Whatever the mechanisms and time-course of toxicity, the ultimate pharmacokinetic criteria for the effectiveness of assisted removal is that drug clearance by the technique used should be similar to, or greater than, endogenous total body clearance. From a clinical point of view, the use of such measures can only be justified by the results of controlled clinical trials or analytical evidence of removal of toxicologically significant amounts of active drug.

### 6.2 Multiple-Dose Activated Charcoal

Multiple-dose activated charcoal is thought to produce its beneficial effects by:

1) Adsorbing any unabsorbed material still present in the gut. This may be particularly relevant in the case of slow-release preparations (e.g. theophylline) or drugs that are slowly absorbed because of decreased gastric motility (e.g. tricyclic antidepressants).

2) Adsorbing drugs that are secreted in bile, thereby preventing intestinal reabsorption.

3) Binding any drug that diffuses from the circulation into the gut lumen. After absorption, a drug will re-enter the gut by passive diffusion provided the concentration there is lower than in the blood. The rate of passive diffusion depends on the concentration gradient and the intestinal surface area, permeability and blood flow. Exceptionally, drugs such as digoxin may, in addition, be actively secreted by the intestinal mucosa, though this process is unlikely to contribute more than passive diffusion to the effect of activated charcoal on drug clearance. Under these 'sink' conditions, a concentration gradient is maintained and drug passes continuously into the gut lumen where it is adsorbed to charcoal.

Drugs with a small volume of distribution (<1 L/kg bodyweight), a clearance of less than 0.1 L/h/kg, low pKa (which maximises transport across membranes), and a prolonged elimination half-life following overdose, are particularly likely to have their elimination enhanced by multiple-dose activated charcoal. In addition, multiple-dose activated charcoal will also make a considerable contribution to total body clearance of the drug ingested in overdose when endogenous processes are compromised by liver and/or renal failure.

#### *6.2.1 Clinical Effectiveness*

In animal studies, multiple-dose activated charcoal has been shown to reduce the elimination half-life and increase the total body clearance of phenobarbital,[129] phenytoin[130] and theophylline.[129,131,132] However, the elimination of salicylate[133] was not enhanced.

Studies in volunteers have demonstrated that multiple-dose activated charcoal increases the elimination of phenobarbital,[111,134,135] carbamazepine,[111] phenytoin,[136,137] theophylline,[115,121,138-143] dapsone,[144] quinine,[145] dextropropoxyphene (proproxyphene),[146] phenylbutazone,[111] piroxicam,[147] digitoxin,[148,149] nadolol,[150] sotalol,[151] and disopyramide.[152] The elimination of salicylate was found to be increased by multiple-dose activated charcoal in 2 studies,[153,154] but not in 2 others,[155,156] probably for methodological reasons. In other studies, multiple-dose activated charcoal therapy did not increase the elimination of mefenamic acid,[157] valproic acid (sodium valproate),[158] tobramycin,[159,160] vancomycin,[161] or chlorpropamide.[162]

The elimination half-life of amitriptyline,[163] but not that of imipramine[164] or doxepin,[112] was also reduced in volunteer studies. However, there are good pharmacokinetic reasons to suggest that in the case of tricyclic antidepressants, a clinically significant increase in total body clearance is unlikely to result from the use of this treatment, even though the half-life may be shortened.

Although the elimination of digoxin was enhanced in volunteer studies[148,149,165] and in 2 case reports[166,167] by the use of multiple-dose activated charcoal, it is unlikely that the increase in total body clearance of digoxin will be of clinical significance. Moreover, severe digoxin poisoning can be treated effectively with digoxin-specific antibody fragments (see section 4.6).

Studies in poisoned patients have confirmed those in volunteers demonstrating that the elimination of phenobarbital, carbamazepine, theophylline, quinine and dapsone is enhanced by multiple-dose activated charcoal. There is also evidence to suggest that, contrary to the findings in one animal and 2 volunteer studies, multiple-dose activated charcoal also increases the elimination of salicylate.

**Phenobarbital Poisoning**

There is good evidence from studies in poisoned patients that the elimination of phenobarbital is significantly enhanced by multiple-dose activated charcoal therapy.[168-171] Increases in the total body clearance of the drug or reductions in its elimination half-life have been reported in these studies. The theoretical value of

**Table V.** Elimination techniques in phenobarbital poisoning

| Management | Phenobarbital clearance (L/h) | Reference |
|---|---|---|
| Untreated | 0.25 | Goodman & Gilman[172] |
| Alkaline diuresis | 0.4 | Jacobsen et al.[173] |
| Haemodialysis | 3.6 | Berman et al.[174] |
| Haemoperfusion | 4.6 | Vale;[175] Jacobsen et al.[173] |
| Multiple-dose activated charcoal | 5.0 | Boldy et al.[169] |

multiple-dose activated charcoal in phenobarbital poisoning may be judged by comparing the efficacy of various elimination therapies on its clearance (table V); charcoal therapy is the most impressive and the simplest to initiate. Although there is some clinical evidence that the time to recovery from phenobarbital poisoning might be reduced by this therapeutic approach,[169] this needs to be confirmed in further studies.

#### Carbamazepine Poisoning

In patients poisoned with carbamazepine, multiple-dose activated charcoal therapy has been shown to reduce the mean elimination half-life of the drug to 8.6 hours;[176] in comparison, in patients treated only with supportive measures, the mean elimination half-life was approximately 19 hours. In terms of increasing the drug's total body clearance, multiple-dose activated charcoal has proved as effective as charcoal haemoperfusion[177-179] and superior to dialysis.[180,181] However, a significant reduction in morbidity and mortality has not yet been demonstrated.

#### Theophylline Poisoning

The elimination of theophylline has been found to be increased by multiple-dose activated charcoal treatment in patients with theophylline poisoning. A number of studies and case reports have indicated that the elimination half-life of theophylline is reduced from 17 to 35 hours to around 5 to 8 hours or less.[139,142,182-185] However, further studies are required to confirm that morbidity and mortality are reduced by charcoal therapy.

#### Salicylate Poisoning

Although 2 volunteer studies did not demonstrate increased salicylate clearance with multiple-dose activated charcoal therapy (see above), there is suggestive evidence from clinical studies that it increases salicylate elimination in poisoned patients. Substantial reductions in the elimination half-life of the drug have been reported with multiple-dose activated charcoal given alone or in conjunction with sodium bicarbonate to maintain an alkaline urine.[170,186,187] In one study, the mean 'maximum' elimination half-life of salicylate in patients who had received multiple-dose activated charcoal was estimated as 3.2 hours; in comparison, the mean elimination half-life in a control group of patients who were treated with oral fluids alone was 27 hours.[187]

#### Dapsone and Quinine Poisoning

Reductions in the elimination half-lives of dapsone (from 77 to 12 hours[188]) and quinine (from 26 hours in patients treated supportively to 8.1 hours[189,190]) have been reported in poisoned patients treated with multiple-dose activated charcoal. However, with quinine, further studies are required to confirm that the serious sequelae encountered in poisoning due to this drug are abolished or even reduced by charcoal therapy.

### *6.2.2 Complications*

Treatment with multiple-dose activated charcoal is relatively free from serious adverse effects, although transient constipation is common. Occasionally, bowel obstruction has been reported, necessitating manual evacuation or surgical intervention.[191-193] Regurgitation of charcoal into the lungs in a semiconscious patient, particularly when extubated or given an emetic, or direct instillation of charcoal into the lungs as a result of a misplaced nasogastric tube, has led rarely to severe pulmonary complications and death.[194-201]

### *6.2.3 Place of Multiple-Dose Activated Charcoal in Management of Poisoning*

The use of multiple-dose activated charcoal should be considered if the patient has ingested a life-threatening amount of phenobarbital, carbamazepine, theophylline, quinine, aspirin or dapsone. Clearance values achieved by multiple-dose activated charcoal in the case of phenobarbital, carbamazepine, theophylline and dapsone poisoning are similar, or superior, to those achieved by haemodialysis or haemoperfusion.

It may be difficult in clinical practice to administer substantial doses of activated charcoal because of drug-induced vomiting such as occurs with theophylline in overdose. In these circumstances, it is usually necessary to give either intravenous ondansetron or high doses of metoclopramide to ensure satisfactory administration of charcoal, even by a nasogastric tube. In addition, in patients who are semiconscious or confused, it may be necessary to administer a benzodiazepine such as diazepam intravenously, both to allow insertion of the nasogastric tube and to reduce the risk of the patient removing it.

### 6.3 Forced Diuresis

The filtrate produced by the glomeruli has a composition similar to that of plasma water but excludes molecules with a molecular weight of more than 66,000D (which includes drug-protein complexes). Thus, only that fraction of the drug which is free (non-protein-bound) is filtered. Some drugs are secreted actively into the proximal renal tubules against the concentration gradient. These include acidic drugs such as the penicillins, sulfonamides, phenobarbital, salicylates, phenylbutazone and probenecid, and organic bases such as quinine, quinidine, amphetamine and procainamide.

Drugs may also be eliminated by passive diffusion across the epithelium of the tubule into the lumen. As water is progressively reabsorbed from the tubular fluid as it passes distally, a favourable concentration gradient is created for the reabsorption of these dissolved substances back into the blood stream.

Tubular reabsorption is influenced by urinary flow rate. Diuresis therefore increases renal clearance of drugs that are passively reabsorbed since the concentration gradient is reduced. Potentially, therefore, drugs excreted largely unchanged by the kidney may be removed in significant quantities by increasing urinary flow. If reabsorption is complete, the concentration of drug in the plasma and final urine are the same and the renal clearance then equals the urine flow rate.[202]

#### 6.3.1 Clinical Effectiveness

Forced diuresis has been shown to increase the clearance of phenobarbital,[203,204] an increase in mean clearance from 0.1 to 0.8 L/h (1.8 to 14 ml/min) and a maximum excretion rate of 121.2 mg/h being achieved in one study in which the clearance of phenobarbital was found to be directly related to urine flow.[204] However, the increase in clearance achieved by this procedure is less than that obtained by multiple-dose activated charcoal therapy, haemodialysis and haemoperfusion. There is also evidence that the clearance of phenytoin is increased by forced diuresis (from 0.3 to 1.2 L/h[205]), although this is less impressive than that achieved by body clearance alone (1 L/h).

In patients with lithium poisoning, sodium chloride diuresis has been proposed as a useful means of increasing lithium excretion.[206] Although the renal clearance of lithium was shown to be enhanced by this procedure in one study,[207] in 2 other studies, no significant increases in lithium elimination were demonstrated.[208,209] The use of low-dose dopamine has also been advocated in lithium intoxication on the basis that dopamine increases sodium excretion by a specific action on the proximal tubule;[210] however, this observation remains to be confirmed.

### 6.4 Forced Diuresis With pH Manipulation

Most drugs are weak electrolytes which, at physiological pH, exist partly as undissociated molecules. The extent of ionisation is a function of the ionisation constant (Ka) of the drug and the pH of the medium in which it is dissolved. Ionisation constants are expressed in the form of their negative logarithms, pKa (see appendix A for a compilation of pKa values). Hence, the stronger an acid, the lower its pKa, and, the stronger a base, the higher the pKa. The relationship between pKa and the proportion of total drug in ionised form is represented by the Henderson-Hasselbach equation:

*For weak acids:*

$$\mathrm{pH} - \mathrm{pKa} = \log \frac{\text{Ionised drug}}{\text{Non–ionised drug}}$$

*For weak bases:*

$$\mathrm{pH} - \mathrm{pKa} = \log \frac{\text{Non–ionised drug}}{\text{Ionised drug}}$$

Thus, when pKa = pH, the concentrations of ionised and non-ionised drug are equal.

Cell membranes are more permeable to substances that are lipid soluble and in the non-ionised, rather than the ionised form. Thus, the rate of diffusion from the renal tubular lumen back into the circulation is decreased when a drug is maximally ionised. Because ionisation of weak acids is increased in an alkaline environment, as is that of basic drugs in an acid solution, manipulation of the urinary pH can enhance renal excretion. For acidic drugs, there is a greater degree of ionisation at pH 8 than 7.4 and, for basic drugs, a greater degree of ionisation at pH 6 than 7.4. Thus, elimination of weak acids by the kidneys is increased in alkaline urine if the pKa of the drug concerned lies in the range 3.0 to 7.4; for weak bases, elimination is increased in acid urine if the pKa of the drug lies in the range 7.5 to 10.5.

Since pKa is a logarithmic function then, theoretically, a small change in urine pH could have a disproportionate effect on clearance, especially for those drugs that have pKa values close to blood pH. Thus, for each change in urine pH of one unit, there is theoretically a 10-fold change in renal clearance, whereas at best, the renal clearance of a reabsorbed drug varies directly with the urine flow rate. The effectiveness of alkaline diuresis depends on the relative contribution of renal clearance to the total body clearance of active drug. If only 1% of an ingested dose is normally excreted unchanged in the urine, even a 20-fold increase in renal clearance will have no clinically significant effect on the overall rate of removal. The elimination of salicylate (pKa 3.5) is increased in alkaline urine, while urinary acidification will increase the elimination of amphetamine (pKa 9.8). If urine pH is decreased to 5.5, the elimination of amphetamine is increased some 7 times as compared with its elimination in individuals with uncontrolled urinary pH (see below).

It is now recognised that the urine pH is of far greater importance than the urine volume in enhancing elimination.[211,212] To achieve maximum excretion of salicylate, a urine pH above 7.5 (ideally between 8.0 and 8.5) is necessary. Rather than using a standard 'cocktail' as recommended by Lawson et al.[86] the regimen should be adjusted for the individual patient. Only then will the optimum elimination of poison be achieved.

### *6.4.1 Clinical Effectiveness of Alkaline Diuresis*

#### Phenobarbital Poisoning

Studies in animals have shown that alkalinisation of the urine increases the renal clearance of phenobarbital, which rises sharply as the urine pH exceeds 7.5.[213,214] However, in studies in poisoned patients, changes in urinary pH had little effect on tubular reabsorption, as indicated by the ratio of the urine to plasma concentrations.[204] Moreover, the maximum renal clearance of phenobarbital achieved by alkaline diuresis is of the order of only 0.4 to 0.9 L/h,[173,215] which compares poorly with that found after multiple-dose activated charcoal therapy and is similar to endogenous clearance.[173]

#### Salicylate Poisoning

Salicylate elimination is highly dose-dependent because of early saturation of the mechanisms for conjugation with glycine to form salicyluric acid.[216] In adults, a single therapeutic dose is eliminated with a half-life of about 3 hours, irrespective of urine flow and pH, since about 80 to 90% is metabolised to salicyluric acid which is actively secreted by the renal tubules. Following high therapeutic and toxic doses, salicylurate conjugation is saturated, plasma concentrations of this metabolite are no higher than with therapeutic doses, and the salicylate half-life is 20 to 30 hours. However, with increasing blood concentrations, the elimination of salicylate by the kidney assumes increasing importance. A 4-fold increase in renal clearance of salicylate for each rise of one unit in urine pH has been demonstrated.[217] Renal salicylate clearance increased from 1 to 3.8 L/h (16 to 64 ml/min) as urine pH increased from 6.5 to 7.5. The renal clearance of salicylate also increased with increasing urine flow, an effect that diminished as urine pH rose.

Other investigations have shown that initial salicylate concentrations can be reduced from 800 to 900 mg/L to 300 to 400 mg/L with 8 hours of alkaline diuresis.[218] In a comparison of the value of alkaline diuresis, forced diuresis and oral fluids alone, the respective mean renal clearances of salicylic acid were 1.4, 0.26 and 0.08 L/h and the respective half-lives were 5.0, 8.0 and 19.4 hours.[212] Despite these encouraging results, alkaline diuresis has not been shown to reduce the morbidity or mortality from salicylate poisoning.

#### Poisoning with Phenoxyacetate Herbicides

Alkaline diuresis greatly increases the renal clearance of 2,4-D (2,4-dichlorophenoxyacetic acid), with a concomitant rapid fall in plasma concentration (half-life 3.7 hours compared with 143 hours) and corresponding clinical improvement.[219] The effect on mecoprop elimination was similar but less dramatic.[219] With alkaline diuresis, the renal clearance of 2,4-D rose from 0.008 to 3.8 L/h (0.14 to 63 ml/min) and for each increase of 1 pH unit, the renal clearance of 2,4-D rose almost 5-fold (fig. 3). In the case of mecoprop, the renal clearance in-

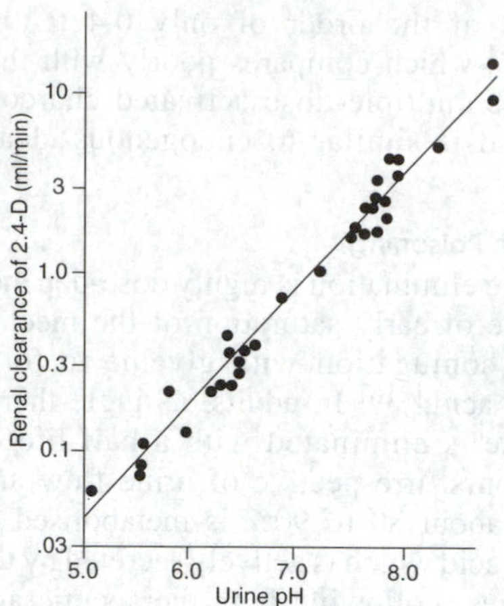


**Fig. 3.** The renal clearance of 2,4-dichlorophenoxyacetic acid (2,4-D) in relation to urine pH in a poisoned patient. The renal clearance was corrected to a urine flow of 1 ml/min.

creased 2-fold for each 1 unit pH rise. More recent evidence[220-223] confirms the value of alkaline diuresis, not only in the case of poisoning with 2,4-D and mecoprop, but also in the case of dichlorprop.

**Chlorpropamide Poisoning**

The elimination of chlorpropamide is greatly increased by making the urine alkaline with sodium bicarbonate;[162] however, these data have not been confirmed in poisoned patients.

### *6.4.2 Clinical Effectiveness of Acid Diuresis*

**Amphetamine Poisoning**

Studies in volunteers have indicated that 57 to 66% of an administered dose of amphetamine is recovered unchanged over a period of 6 hours in urines with pH values ranging from 4.8 to 5.15;[224] less than 5% of the drug was recovered when the urine was alkalinised to a pH of 7.6 to 8.3. Similarly, the plasma half-life of amphetamine has been found to be shorter with acid (pH 5.5 to 6.0) urine than with alkaline (pH 7.5 to 8.0) urine (8 to 10 hours *vs* 16 to 31 hours).[225] In patients with amphetamine psychoses, the plasma half-life of the drug in those in whom the urine was acidified was 7 to 14 hours and symptoms cleared rapidly; by contrast, the plasma half-life in those in whom the urine was alkalinised was 19 to 34 hours and the psychosis was prolonged.[226] Other studies have also shown that acid diuresis increases amphetamine elimination in patients with amphetamine poisoning.[227] Rarely, however, rhabdomyolysis complicates amphetamine intoxication and acid diuresis may increase the risk of the associated renal failure.

As forced acid diuresis is a difficult technique to undertake and, as it may increase morbidity in patients with amphetamine poisoning, it should only be considered in those few patients who do not respond to sedation, either with diazepam, chlorpromazine or droperidol. Its value remains unproven.

**Fenfluramine Poisoning**

Urinary acidification increases the renal elimination of fenfluramine,[228] but has never been employed widely and there are no published clinical data on its efficacy. Some findings suggest that the amount of drug recovered in the urine is small. Furthermore, sedation with diazepam or chlorpromazine is invariably sufficient once the risk of early cardiac arrest has passed.

**Phencyclidine Poisoning**

Acid diuresis has been shown to increase the urinary clearance of phencyclidine from 2.2 to 16.3 L/h,[229] but, surprisingly, there was little effect on either plasma concentrations of the drug or the time to clinical recovery. Moreover, acid diuresis may potentiate the toxicity of phencyclidine by increasing the risk of renal failure secondary to rhabdomyolysis.

**Quinine Poisoning**

Contrary to earlier reports, it has now been demonstrated that quinine elimination is not enhanced by the use of acid diuresis.[190]

### *6.4.3 Complications of Alkaline and Acid Diuresis*

Forced diuresis with or without pH manipulation is potentially hazardous, particularly in poisoning in the elderly and in patients with impaired cardiac and renal function. Complications include fluid overload, pulmonary oedema, cerebral oedema, disturbances of acid-base and electrolyte balance (hypokalaemia, hypocalcaemia). Deaths from cerebral oedema have also been recorded following forced diuresis.[230] On the other hand, diuresis may protect against renal damage, and administration of alkali and acidifying agents may have a beneficial effect on redistribution of drug from the tissues to the blood.[213]

## 6.5 Dialysis

The rate of transfer of drugs across a dialysis membrane depends on many factors including molecular size and weight, concentration gradient, permeability and surface area of the dialysis membrane, blood and dialysate flow rates, and pH differences between blood and dialysate. Within limits, which depends on molecular size, the clearance by haemodialysis increases with the flow rate. Drugs with molecular weights exceeding about 350D cross most membranes poorly and the clearance is not increased with flow rates above 12 to 18 L/h (200 to 300 ml/min).[231] The properties required of a drug for rapid removal from the body by haemodialysis are summarised in table VI.

If a drug has a small volume of distribution (e.g. salicylate, about 0.15 L/kg), the fraction of the drug in the circulation is high and there is a high concentration gradient between blood and dialysate. Plasma protein binding may limit the clearance by dialysis, although binding is usually less at higher plasma concentrations.[125]

The amount of drug actually removed by haemodialysis is the product of the haemodialysis clearance, plasma concentration and duration of dialysis. An impressive value for clearance therefore means little if the fraction of the drug in the circulation is very low (in relation to the total amount of drug in the body). Thus, the clinical effectiveness of haemodialysis depends on the apparent volume of drug distribution (see chapter 1). It is virtually useless for compounds such as digoxin, tricyclic antidepressants and paraquat which are extensively taken up by tissues, since at steady-state only a small fraction of the dose is in the circulation. Removal by haemodialysis is further impeded by slow redistribution from peripheral tissues to blood. The clearance of drugs by haemodialysis rarely exceeds 6 L/h (100 ml/min) and there is considerable variation, depending on the actual drug and the haemodialysis system used. A further disadvantage is that haemodialysis is, of necessity, an intermittent procedure.

Claims for clinical effectiveness are sometimes based on a shortening of the plasma half-life during haemodialysis. As can be seen from figure 4, unless concentrations are followed

**Table VI.** Properties required for rapid removal of a drug or poison from the body by haemodialysis or haemoperfusion

| |
|---|
| Low molecular size and weight |
| Rapid diffusion across dialysis membrane or rapid absorption to charcoal in haemoperfusion column |
| Rapid transfer from tissues to blood |
| Small volume of distribution |
| Haemodialysis or haemoperfusion clearance greater than endogenous total body clearance |
| Toxicity directly related to concentration of drug in body |

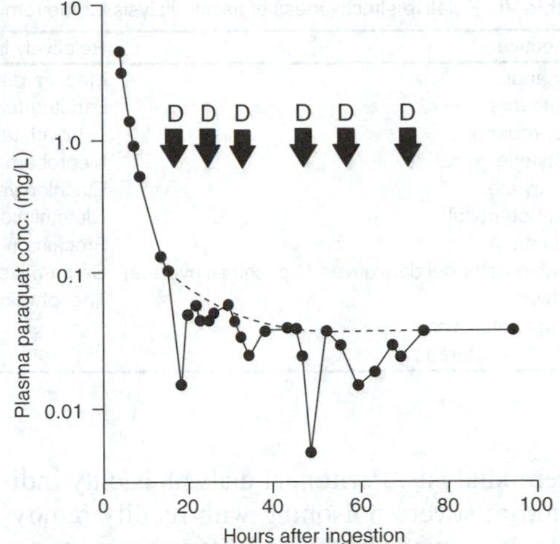


**Fig. 4**. Lack of effect of repeated haemodialysis (D) on the overall plasma concentration-time curve in a patient with paraquat poisoning. Note the logarithmic scale and the very low steady-state paraquat concentration.

during the period after dialysis is discontinued, the rebound rise will be missed, giving a false impression of efficacy. A similar phenomenon has been observed with other compounds[232] and there may be clinical improvement during dialysis followed by relapse after it is stopped.

### 6.5.1 Indications for Haemodialysis

Clearcut indications for haemodialysis are difficult to define. The decision must rest primarily on the clinical state of patient, the anticipated prognosis and the effectiveness of dialysis in the removal of the particular drug or poison. Failure of spontaneous improvement with adequate intensive supportive therapy within a reasonable time, old age, serious complications such as severe pneumonia, and impairment of normal mechanisms of elimination caused by underlying cardiac, hepatic and renal disease, are also factors that must be taken into account. The drug should be identified if possible and its plasma concentration measured before, during and after dialysis. A decision to undertake haemodialysis should not be based solely on the plasma concentration (see table VII).

### 6.5.2 Indications for Peritoneal Dialysis

The clearance of drugs by peritoneal dialysis is much less than by haemodialysis and rarely exceeds 1.2 L/h (20 ml/min). However, unlike haemodialysis, it is a continuous process which can be kept going for days. The same general principles regarding drug removal apply as for

**Table VII.** Relative effectiveness of haemodialysis for the removal of some drugs and poisons from the body

| Effective | Relatively ineffective | Ineffective |
|---|---|---|
| Ethanol | Medium duration of action | Digoxin |
| Methanol | barbiturates (e.g. amobarbital, | Amphetamines |
| Isopropanol | butobarbital) | Antidepressants |
| Ethylene glycol | Meprobamate | Phenothiazines |
| Salicylates | Ethchlorvynol | Butyrophenones |
| Phenobarbital | Glutethimide | Chloroquine |
| Barbital | Procainamide | Colchicine |
| Trichloroethanol derivatives (e.g. chloral hydrate) | Carbamazepine | Dextropropoxyphene (propoxyphene) |
| Lithium | Theophylline | Paraquat |
| Many antibiotics | | Phenytoin |
| ? Sulphonylureas | | Atropine |

haemodialysis. Peritoneal dialysis is only indicated in severe poisoning with readily removable drugs when haemodialysis or haemoperfusion is not available.

#### *6.5.3 Clinical Effectiveness of Dialysis*

**Barbiturate Poisoning**

The clearance of barbiturates with peritoneal dialysis rarely exceeds 0.6 L/h (10 ml/min)[233,234] which, in the case of phenobarbital, is unimpressive compared with values achieved by multiple-dose activated charcoal therapy (see table V, section 6.2). Although phenobarbital clearance during haemodialysis is greater than with peritoneal dialysis,[126,174] multiple-dose activated charcoal is again superior.

Short- and medium-acting barbiturates are not amenable to haemodialysis because of their high lipid solubility.

**Ethchlorvynol Poisoning**

In patients with acute ethchlorvynol intoxication, mean clearance values of 1.1 and 3.8 L/h (18.5 and 64 ml/min) were found in one study during peritoneal and haemodialysis, respectively.[235] However, haemoperfusion is a more efficient method of removal (see section 6.6.1).

**Glutethimide Poisoning**

Peritoneal dialysis and haemodialysis are unimpressive in poisoning due to this agent and produce clearance values of only 1 L/h (17 ml/min)[236] and 2 to 3.8 L/h (34 to 63 ml/min),[237] respectively, though higher values have been reported occasionally.[236] Again, haemoperfusion is preferred (see section 6.6.1).

**Poisoning Due to Trichloroethanol Derivatives**

Chloral hydrate is metabolised to trichloroethanol and trichloroacetic acid. While there are no data on the efficacy of peritoneal dialysis, clearances of 7.2 to 9.7 L/h (120 to 162 ml/min) have been achieved during haemodialysis.[238,239]

**Meprobamate Poisoning**

In patients with poisoning due to this drug, peritoneal dialysis produces a clearance of only 1.6 L/h (27 ml/min). Haemodialysis is more impressive and clearances as high as 3.7 L/h (62 ml/min) have been reported.[240]

**Carbamazepine Poisoning**

Since carbamazepine is extensively metabolised and highly protein bound, peritoneal and haemodialysis are of little value in enhancing its elimination.[180,181] Multiple-dose activated charcoal treatment is as effective as or superior to dialysis.[176]

**Salicylate Poisoning**

Peritoneal dialysis has been shown to lower plasma salicylate concentrations. Although less efficient than alkaline diuresis (see section 6.4.1), it can be employed in the presence of renal impairment. Haemodialysis is 4 times more effective.[231]

**Ethanol Poisoning**

A calculated dialysate clearance of 0.6 to 1.2 L/h was achieved during peritoneal dialysis in a patient who presented with a blood ethanol concentration of 15,000 mg/L and survived.[241] Haemodialysis is the preferred elimination technique in that it is more efficient than both peritoneal dialysis and charcoal haemoperfusion, and it should be considered if the blood ethanol concentration is 5000 mg/L and/or if severe metabolic acidosis is present.

**Methanol Poisoning**

In studies of methanol intoxication in dogs, the spontaneous methanol half-life of over 70 hours was reduced by a factor of 10 with peritoneal dialysis.[242] Peritoneal dialysis removes 3 times as much methanol as renal excretion.[242] In patients with admission blood methanol concentrations ranging from 960 to 1980 mg/L, a 13% reduction in methanol concentrations was achieved by peritoneal dialysis after 8 hours compared with a 66% reduction by haemodialysis in other patients.[243] One death and one case of permanent blindness occurred in those treated by peritoneal dialysis whereas all patients treated by haemodialysis survived.

Methanol is easily removed by haemodialysis.[244] Clearance values lie between 9 and 12 L/h, depending on the blood flow and surface area of the dialyser. In addition, haemodialysis may also remove formate;[245,246] clearance values for formate range from 8.4 to 9 L/h (140 to 150 ml/min).

#### Ethylene Glycol Poisoning

Peritoneal dialysis removes ethylene glycol, albeit at a slower rate than haemodialysis.[247] Since ethylene glycol has a low molecular weight (62D) and a volume of distribution of 0.7 to 0.8 L/kg, this glycol should be dialysable, though it is less so than methanol.[248-250] Dialysis of glycolate (8.4 L/h), a metabolite of ethylene glycol, has also been demonstrated in one patient.[251]

#### Isopropanol Poisoning

Isopropanol has a low molecular weight and a low volume of distribution, and dialysis is therefore likely to be of clinical benefit. Haemodialysis is considerably more effective than peritoneal dialysis, both in removing isopropanol and in shortening the duration of coma in intoxicated patients.[252-256]

#### Lithium Poisoning

Lithium can be removed by peritoneal dialysis,[208,257] although this technique is less efficient than haemodialysis. Clearances of 0.8 to 0.9 L/h (13 to 15 ml/min) have been achieved with peritoneal dialysis[19] compared with haemodialysis clearance values of 3.6 to 7.9 L/h (60 to 132 ml/min).[208,209,258-260] However, after haemodialysis, there is often a rebound increase in serum lithium concentrations due to slow diffusion of the drug across cell membranes.

Haemodialysis is the treatment of choice in severe lithium intoxication, though there has been debate recently on when it should be employed and for what period.[261,262] Following an acute overdose of lithium, haemodialysis may prevent lithium diffusion into the brain and the onset of severe toxicity. In contrast, those patients who develop intoxication during long term therapy may require long periods of dialysis to produce clinical improvement.

#### Theophylline Poisoning

Peritoneal dialysis produces a theophylline clearance of the same order as the endogenous clearance: in children aged 18 months and 34 months, it was 0.08 L/h and 0.31 L/h, respectively.[263,264] In a study in adults, theophylline clearance during dialysis was less than 0.7 L/h (12 ml/min), and only 4mg was removed over a 48-hour period.[265] Similar clearance values (0.6 L/h) were reported in another study.[266]

Thus, peritoneal dialysis is much less effective than haemodialysis which can achieve clearances of 6.7 L/h (112 ml/min) in adults if blood flow is maintained.[267] When it is not, clearances between 2 and 5.3 L/h (33 and 88 ml/min) are obtained.[268,269] Haemodialysis can therefore be expected to double the total body clearance of theophylline but is less effective than haemoperfusion (see section 6.6.1).

### *6.5.4 Complications of Dialysis*

Complications of peritoneal dialysis include perforation, peritonitis, adhesions, and disturbances of acid-base, electrolyte and fluid balance. Although haemodialysis is a relatively safe elective procedure, there are well recognised though uncommon hazards, including air embolism, haemolysis, haemorrhage and disturbances of electrolyte and fluid balance. These risks may be increased with emergency dialysis, particularly if a seriously ill patient is suicidal.

### *6.5.5 Place of Dialysis in Management of Poisoning*

Haemodialysis is an efficient technique for the removal of salicylate, ethanol, methanol, ethylene glycol, isopropanol and lithium. Peritoneal dialysis is much less efficient in these circumstances than haemodialysis, and should only be considered if haemodialysis is unavailable. Dialysis has not been shown in controlled clinical trials to reduce morbidity or mortality, though this is likely to be the case in patients severely poisoned with the above agents.

## 6.6 Haemoperfusion

Drugs can also be removed by passing heparinised blood through a column packed with adsorbents such as activated charcoal or exchange resins. Charcoal is coated (e.g. with acrylic hydrogel) to reduce the risk of embolism, damage to blood cells and pyrexial reactions.[270]

**Table VIII.** Examples of drugs and poisons which can and cannot be effectively removed by haemoperfusion

| Removed effectively | Not removed |
|---|---|
| Barbiturates | Camphor |
| Carbamazepine | Chloroquine |
| Dapsone | Digitoxin |
| Glutethimide | Inorganic mercury |
| Meprobamate | Paraquat |
| Salicylate | Podophyllin |
| Theophylline | Quinine |
| | Tricyclic antidepressants |

Apart from the question of efficient adsorption by the charcoal or exchange resin, the pharmacokinetic basis for drug removal by haemoperfusion is similar to that for haemodialysis (table VI). Haemoperfusion is most effective for drugs that have a low clearance and small volume of distribution.

The clearance of many drugs by haemoperfusion, including barbiturates, glutethimide and salicylate is considerably greater than can be achieved by haemodialysis, and barbiturate clearances of 6 to 7.5 L/h (100 to 125 ml/min) have been obtained with flow rates of about 12 L/h (200 ml/min).[231,270,271] Even more efficient removal of drugs has been reported with haemoperfusion through ion exchange resins such as Amberlite XAD-2 and XAD-4.[272] Unlike charcoal haemoperfusion, saturation of the column is not usually encountered and the clearances of barbiturates and glutethimide may approach the blood flow rate.[231,273]

Some drugs and poisons that can be removed effectively by haemoperfusion are shown in table VIII.

### *6.6.1 Clinical Effectiveness*

#### Barbiturate Poisoning

In phenobarbital poisoning, there is good evidence that charcoal haemoperfusion produces more impressive drug clearances than endogenous elimination alone, alkaline diuresis, or dialysis (table IX), but multiple-dose activated charcoal is as efficient as charcoal haemoperfusion.[169]

#### Glutethimide Poisoning

Haemoperfusion results in a more impressive clearance of glutethimide than haemodialysis (table IX). A significant rebound in plasma concentration occurs in some patients and repeated haemoperfusion may be necessary.

#### Ethchlorvynol Poisoning

Resin haemoperfusion effectively removes ethchlorvynol and is superior to haemodialysis (table IX).[275]

#### Meprobamate Poisoning

Meprobamate clearance values of 4.8 to 18 L/h (80 to 300 ml/min) have been achieved using charcoal and resin haemoperfusion with very high blood flow rates.[276] These values are superior to those achieved by peritoneal and haemodialysis (table IX).

#### Poisoning Due to Trichloroethanol Derivatives

Mean trichloroethanol clearances of 11.9 L/h (198 ml/ min) have been achieved with haemoperfusion.[276] Haemoperfusion is therefore more effective than haemodialysis in removing trichloroethanol and its derivatives.

#### Carbamazepine Poisoning

Charcoal haemoperfusion has been shown to produce carbamazepine clearance values of 4.8 to 7.7 L/h (80 to 129 ml/min)[177-179] and elimination half-lives during perfusion of 8.6 to 10.7 hours,[178] although these values are similar to those achieved by multiple-dose activated charcoal therapy.[176]

#### Theophylline Poisoning

Of the various invasive techniques available, charcoal haemoperfusion has proved the most effective in theophylline poisoning, increasing its clearance 4-fold.[277] Haemoperfusion should be considered if plasma theophylline

**Table IX.** Mean clearances (L/h) of various drugs achieved by forced diuresis, peritoneal dialysis, haemodialysis and haemoperfusion

| Drug | Forced diuresis[a] | Peritoneal dialysis[a] | Haemodialysis[a] | Haemoperfusion[b] |
|---|---|---|---|---|
| Amobarbital | 0.3 | 0.6 | 1.8 | 4.5 |
| Butobarbital | 0.3 | 0.6 | 1.8 | 4.5 |
| Phenobarbital | 1.2 | 0.6 | 3.6 | 4.6 |
| Meprobamate | | 1.6 | 3.7 | 7.5 |
| Glutethimide | | 1.0 | 3.0 | 7.5 |
| Ethchlorvynol | 1.2 | 1.1 | 3.8 | 11.0 |
| Trichloroethanol | | | 7.2-9.7 | 11.2-13.3 |

a Data obtained from literature.
b Data from Vale et al.[270,274] and unpublished data.

concentrations are greater than 100 mg/L following an acute overdose, or greater than 60 mg/L in a patient receiving theophylline long term. However, the use of supportive measures (including the correction of electrolyte and metabolic abnormalities) and multiple-dose oral activated charcoal (see section 6.2.1) usually obviates the need for haemoperfusion.

#### Disopyramide Poisoning

There is evidence that Amberlite XAD-4 resin (but not charcoal) haemoperfusion together with inotropic support may increase the elimination of disopyramide sufficiently to prevent a fatal outcome in cases of severe poisoning,[278] although inotropic support alone may be sufficient, even in very severely poisoned patients.

#### Phenylbutazone Poisoning

XAD-4 resin haemoperfusion proved unimpressive in removing phenylbutazone in an *in vivo* study.[271] However, it has been employed clinically[279,280] and success for its use has been claimed. Clinical experience is too limited to know whether haemoperfusion is more effective than multiple-dose activated charcoal.

### 6.7 Exchange Transfusion and Plasmapheresis

These methods are of very limited value for enhancing drug elimination. Exchange transfusion can only remove drug present in the blood and is of little benefit even with drugs that have a small volume of distribution.[281,282] It is of no value for the removal of extensively distributed drugs such as digoxin.[283]

Plasmapheresis only removes drug in plasma and bound to plasma proteins. Phenytoin is extensively bound but in one study, only 10% of the total in the body was removed by a 2 plasma volume exchange.[284]

## Acknowledgement

The authors gratefully acknowledge the contribution of Professor L.F. Prescott in the preparation of this chapter.

## References

1. Charlton J, Dunnell K, Evans B, et al. Suicide deaths in England and Wales: trends in factors associated with suicide deaths. Population Trends 1993; 71: 34
2. Meredith TJ. Epidemiology of poisoning. Pharmacology and Therapeutics 1993; 59: 251
3. Sibert JR, Routledge PA. Accidental poisoning in children: can we admit fewer children with safety? Archives of Disease in Childhood 1991; 66: 263
4. Litovitz TL, Holm KC, Clancy C, et al. Annual Report of the American Association of Poison Control Centers Toxic Exposure Surveillance System. American Journal of Emergency Medicine 1993; 11: 494
5. Koren G. Medications which can kill a toddler with one tablet or teaspoonful. Clinical Toxicology 1993; 31: 407
6. Agarwal SK, Tiwari SC, Dash SC. Spectrum of poisoning requiring haemodialysis in a tertiary care hospital in India. International Journal of Artificial Organs 1993; 16: 20
7. Proudfoot AT. Acute poisoning. Diagnosis and management. 2nd ed. Oxford: Butterworth-Heinemann, 1993
8. Mahoney JD, Gross PL, Stern TA, et al. Quantitative serum toxic screening in the management of suspected drug overdose. American Journal of Emergency Medicine 1990; 8: 16
9. Kellerman AL, Fihn SD, LoGerfo JP, et al. Impact of drug screening in suspected overdose. Annals of Emergency Medicine 1987; 16: 1206
10. Ray JE, Reilly DK, Day RO. Drugs involved in self-poisoning: verification by toxicological analysis. Medical Journal of Australia 1986; 144: 455
11. Wiley JF. Difficult diagnoses in toxicology: poisons not detected by the comprehensive drug screen. Pediatric Clinics of North America 1991; 38: 725
12. Lacey SR, Cooper C, Runyan DK, et al. Munchausen syndrome by proxy: patterns of presentation to pediatric surgeons. Journal of Pediatric Surgery 1993; 28: 827
13. Flanagan RJ, Huggett A, Saynor DA, et al. Value of toxicological investigation in the diagnosis of acute drug poisoning in children. Lancet 1981; 2: 682
14. Ingelfinger JA, Isakson G, Shine D, et al. Reliability of the toxic screen in drug overdose. Clinical Pharmacology and Therapeutics 1981; 29: 570
15. Karch SB. Methsuximide overdose: delayed onset of profound coma. Journal of the American Medical Association 1973; 223: 1463
16. Prescott LF, Newton RW, Swainson CP, et al. Successful treatment of severe paracetamol overdosage with cysteamine. Lancet 1974; 1: 588
17. Proudfoot AT, Stewart MS, Levitt T, et al. Paraquat poisoning: significance of plasma-paraquat concentrations. Lancet 1979; 18: 330
18. Forrest AH, Roscoe P, Stevenson IH, et al. Abnormal drug metabolism following barbiturate and paracetamol overdosage. Scottish Medical Journal 1974; 19: 157
19. Rosenberg J, Benowitz NL, Pond S. Pharmacokinetics of drug overdose. Clinical Pharmacokinetics 1981; 6: 161
20. Pellinen TJ, Farkkila M, Heikkila J, et al. Electrocardiographic and clinical features of tricyclic antidepressant intoxication: a survey of 88 cases and outlines of therapy. Annals of Clinical Research 1987; 19: 12
21. Caravati EM, Bossart PJ. Demographic and electrocardiographic factors associated with severe tricyclic antidepressant toxicity. Clinical Toxicology 1991; 29: 31
22. Hoffman JR, Votey WR, Bayer M, et al. Effect of hypertonic sodium bicarbonate in the treatment of moderate-to-severe cyclic antidepressant overdose. American Journal of Emergency Medicine 1993; 11: 336
23. Leor J, Harman M, Rabinowitz B, et al. Giant U waves and associated ventricular tachycardia complicating astemizole overdose: successful treatment with intra-

venous magnesium. American Journal of Medicine 1991; 91: 94

24. Hasan RA, Zureikat GY, Nolan BM. Torsade de pointes associated with astemizole overdose treated with magnesium sulfate. Pediatric Emergency Care 1993; 9: 23
25. McVey FK, Corke CF. Extracorporeal circulation in the management of massive propranolol overdose. Anaesthesia 1991; 46: 744
26. Olson KR, Kearney TE, Dyer JE, et al. Seizures associated with poisoning and drug overdose. American Journal of Emergency Medicine 1993; 11: 565
27. Jacobsen D, McMartin KE. Methanol and ethylene glycol poisonings: mechanisms of toxicity, clinical course, diagnosis and treatment. Medical Toxicology and Adverse Drug Experience 1986; 1: 309
28. Seltzer HS. Drug-induced hypoglycemia. Endocrinology and Metabolism Clinics of North America 1989; 18: 163
29. Sporer KA, Ernst AA, Conte R, et al. The incidence of ethanol-induced hypoglycemia. American Journal of Emergency Medicine 1992; 10: 403
30. Bradberry SM, Vale JA. Disturbances of potassium homeostasis in poisoning. Clinical Toxicology 1995; 33: 295
31. Merigian KS, Roberts JR. Cocaine intoxication: hyperpyrexia, rhabdomyolysis and acute renal failure. Clinical Toxicology 1987; 25: 135
32. Menashe PI, Gottlieb JE. Hyperthermia, rhabdomyolysis, and myoglobinuric renal failure after recreational use of cocaine. Southern Medical Journal 1988; 81: 379
33. Tehan B, Hardern R, Bodenham A. Hyperthermia associated with 3,4-methylenedioxyethamphetamine ('Eve'). Anaesthesia 1993; 48: 507
34. Challoner KR, McCarron MM, Newton EJ. Pentazocine (Talwin) intoxication: report of 57 cases. Journal of Emergency Medicine 1990; 8: 67
35. Spivey WH, Roberts RJ, Derlet RW. A clinical trial of escalating doses of flumazenil for reversal of suspected benzodiazepine overdose in the emergency department. Annals of Emergency Medicine 1993; 22: 1813
36. Chern T-L, Hu S-C, Lee C-H, et al. Diagnostic and therapeutic utility of flumazenil in comatose patients with drug overdose. American Journal of Emergency Medicine 1993; 11: 122
37. Winkler E, Almog S, Kriger D, et al. Use of flumazenil in the diagnosis and treatment of patients with coma of unknown etiology. Critical Care Medicine 1993; 21: 538
38. Yealy DM, Paris PM, Kaplan RM, et al. The safety of prehospital naloxone administration by paramedics. Annals of Emergency Medicine 1990; 19: 202
39. Taboulet P, Cariou A, Berdeaux A, et al. Pathophysiology and management of self-poisoning with beta-blockers. Clinical Toxicology 1993; 31: 531
40. Freestone S, Thomas HM, Bhamra RK, et al. Severe atenolol poisoning: treatment with prenalterol. Human Toxicology 1986; 5: 343
41. Amin DN, Henry JA. Propranolol administration in theophylline overdose. Lancet 1985; 1: 520
42. Connell JMC, Cook GM, McInnes GT. Metabolic consequences of salbutamol poisoning reversed by propranolol. British Medical Journal 1982; 285: 779
43. Johnson MK, Vale JA. Clinical management of acute organophosphate poisoning: an overview. In: Ballantyne B, Marrs TC, editors. Clinical and experimental toxicology of organophosphates and carbamates. Oxford: Butterworth-Heinemann, 1992: 528
44. Casey PB, Blakey L, Bradberry SM, et al. Late reactivation of erythrocyte cholinesterase activity by pralidoxime in a case of chlorpyrifos poisoning. Przeglad Lek 1995; 52: 206
45. Albano E, Rundgren M, Harvison PJ, et al. Mechanisms of *N*-acetyl-*p*-benzoquinone imine cytotoxicity. Molecular Pharmacology 1985; 28: 306
46. Bray GP, Mowat C, Muir DF, et al. The effect of chronic alcohol intake on prognosis and outcome in paracetamol overdose. Human and Experimental Toxicology 1991; 10: 435
47. Bray GP, Harrison PM, O'Grady JG, et al. Long-term anticonvulsant therapy worsens outcome in paracetamol-induced fulminant hepatic failure. Human and Experimental Toxicology 1992; 11: 265
48. Prescott LF, Critchley JA. Drug interactions affecting analgesic toxicity. American Journal of Medicine 1983; 75: 113
49. Prescott LF, Illingworth RN, Critchley JAJH, et al. Intravenous N-acetylcysteine: the treatment of choice for paracetamol poisoning. British Medical Journal 1979; 2: 1079
50. Smilkstein MJ, Knapp GL, Kulig KW, et al. Efficacy of oral N-acetylcysteine in the treatment of acetaminophen overdose. New England Journal of Medicine 1988; 319: 1557
51. Smilkstein MJ, Bronstein AC, Linden C, et al. Acetaminophen overdose: a 48-hour intravenous N-acetylcysteine treatment protocol. Annals of Emergency Medicine 1991; 20: 1058
52. Vale JA, Meredith TJ, Goulding R. Treatment of acetaminophen poisoning: the use of oral methionine. Archives of Internal Medicine 1981; 141: 394
53. Vale JA, Proudfoot AT. Paracetamol (acetaminophen) poisoning. Lancet 1995; 346: 547
54. Harrison PM, Keays R, Bray GP, et al. Improved outcome of paracetamol-induced fulminant hepatic failure by late administration of acetylcysteine. Lancet 1990; 335: 1572
55. Flanagan RJ, Meredith TJ. Use of N-acetylcysteine in clinical toxicology. American Journal of Medicine 1991; 91 Suppl. 3C: 131S
56. Ruprah M, Mant TGK, Flanagan RJ. Acute carbon tetrachloride poisoning in 19 patients: implications for diagnosis and treatment. Lancet 1985; 1: 1027
57. Harry P, Turcant A, Bouachour G, et al. Efficacy of 4-methylpyrazole in ethylene glycol poisoning: clinical and toxicokinetic aspects. Human and Experimental Toxicology 1994; 13: 61
58. Chen KK, Rose CL. Nitrite and thiosulfate therapy in cyanide poisoning. Journal of the American Medical Association 1952; 149: 113
59. Baud FJ, Barriot P, Toffis V, et al. Elevated blood cyanide concentrations in victims of smoke inhalation. New England Journal of Medicine 1991; 325: 1761
60. Forsyth JC, Mueller PD, Becker CE, et al. Hydroxycobalamin as a cyanide antidote: safety, efficacy and pharmacokinetics in heavily smoking normal volunteers. Clinical Toxicology 1993; 31: 277
61. Meredith TJ, Jacobsen D, Haines JA, et al. Antidotes for poisoning by cyanide. IPCS/CEC Evaluation of Antidotes Series, Vol 2. Cambridge University Press, 1994
62. Steffen C, Wetzel E. Chlorate poisoning: mechanism of toxicity. Toxicology 1993; 84: 217

63. Bradberry SM, Gazzard B, Vale JA. Methemoglobinemia caused by the accidental contamination of drinking water with sodium nitrate. Clinical Toxicology 1994; 32: 173
64. Bradberry SM, Whittington RM, Parry DA, et al. Fatal methemoglobinemia due to inhalation of isobutyl nitrite. Clinical Toxicology 1994; 32: 179
65. Casey PB, Buckley BM, Vale JA. Methemoglobinemia following ingestion of a monolinuron/paraquat herbicide (Gramonol). Clinical Toxicology 1994; 32: 185
66. Hansen DG, Challoner KR, Smith DE. Dapsone intoxication: two case reports. Journal of Emergency Medicine 1994; 12: 347
67. Eldadah M, Jaffe JP. Methemoglobinemia due to skin application of benzocaine. Clinical Pediatrics 1993; 32: 687
68. Banner W, Bayer MJ, Smith TW. Digitalis intoxication: update on clinical recognition and management. American Journal of Emergency Medicine 1991; 9 Suppl. 1
69. Cummins RO, Haulman J, Quan L, et al. Near-fatal yew berry intoxication treated with external cardiac pacing and digoxin-specific FAB antibody fragments. Annals of Emergency Medicine 1990; 19: 38
70. Shumaik GM, Wu AW, Ping AC. Oleander poisoning: treatment with digoxin-specific Fab antibody fragments. Annals of Emergency Medicine 1988; 17: 732
71. Bosse GM, Pope TM. Recurrent digoxin overdose and treatment with digoxin-specific Fab antibody fragments. Journal of Emergency Medicine 1994; 12: 179
72. Terrien N, Urtizberea M, Scherrmann JM. Influence of goat colchicine specific antibodies on murine colchicine disposition. Toxicology 1989; 59: 11
73. Nagao M, Takatori T, Wu B, et al. Immunotherapy for the treatment of acute paraquat poisoning. Human Toxicology 1989; 8: 121
74. Chen KW, Wu MH, Huang JJ, et al. Bilateral spontaneous pneumothoraces, pneumopericardium, pneumomediastinum, and subcutaneous emphysema: a rare presentation of paraquat intoxication. Annals of Emergency Medicine 1994; 23: 1132
75. Karlson-Stiber C, Persson H. Antivenom treatment in Vipera berus envenoming: report of 30 cases. Journal of Internal Medicine 1994; 235: 57
76. Proudfoot AT. Abandon gastric lavage in the accidental and emergency department? Archives of Emergency Medicine 1984; 2: 65
77. Arnold FJ, Hodges JB, Barta RA. Evaluation of the efficacy of lavage and induced emesis in treatment of salicylate poisoning. Pediatrics 1959; 23: 286
78. Abdallah AH, Tye A. A comparison of the efficacy of emetic drugs and stomach lavage. American Journal of Diseases of Children 1967; 113: 571
79. Corby DG, Lisciandro RC, Lehman RH, et al. The efficiency of methods used to evacuate the stomach after acute ingestions. Pediatrics 1967; 40: 871
80. Burton BT, Bayer MJ, Barron L, et al. Comparison of activated charcoal and gastric lavage in the prevention of aspirin absorption. Journal of Emergency Medicine 1984; 1: 411
81. Tandberg D, Diven BG, McLeod JW. Ipecac-induced emesis versus gastric lavage: a controlled study in normal adults. American Journal of Emergency Medicine 1986; 4: 205
82. Tenenbein M, Cohen S, Sitar DS. Efficacy of ipecac-induced emesis, orogastric lavage, and activated charcoal for acute drug overdose. Annals of Emergency Medicine 1987; 16: 838
83. Danel V, Henry JA, Glucksman E. Activated charcoal, emesis, and gastric lavage in aspirin overdose. British Medical Journal 1988; 296: 1507
84. Saetta JP, Quinton DN. Residual gastric content after gastric lavage and ipecacuanha-induced emesis in self-poisoned patients: an endoscopic study. Journal of the Royal Society of Medicine 1991; 84: 35
85. Saetta JP, Marsh S, Gaunt ME, et al. Gastric emptying procedures in the self-poisoned patients: are we forcing gastric content beyond the pylorus? Journal of the Royal Society of Medicine 1991; 84: 274
86. Lawson AAH, Proudfoot AT, Brown SS, et al. Forced diuresis in the treatment of acute salicylate poisoning in adults. Quarterly Journal of Medicine 1969; 38: 31
87. Comstock EG, Faulkner TP, Boisaubin EV, et al. Studies on the efficacy of gastric lavage as practiced in a large metropolitan hospital. Clinical Toxicology 1981; 18: 581
88. Sharman JR, Cretney MJ, Scott RD, et al. Drug overdoses: is one stomach washing enough? New Zealand Medical Journal 1975; 81: 195
89. Schwartz HS. Acute meprobamate poisoning with gastrotomy and removal of a drug-containing mass. New England Journal of Medicine 1976; 295: 1177
90. Victor LB, Gordon EI, Greendyke RM. Therapeutic implications of autopsy findings in acute barbiturate intoxication. New York State Journal of Medicine 1968; 68: 2090
91. Underhill TJ, Greene MK, Dove AF. A comparison of the efficacy of gastric lavage, ipecacuanha and activated charcoal in the emergency management of paracetamol overdose. Archives of Emergency Medicine 1990; 7: 148
92. Matthew H, Mackintosh TF, Tompsett SL, et al. Gastric aspiration and lavage in acute poisoning. British Medical Journal 1966; 1: 1333
93. Watson WA, Leighton J, Guy J, et al. Recovery of cyclic antidepressants with gastric lavage. Journal of Emergency Medicine 1989; 7: 373
94. Allan BC. The role of gastric lavage in the treatment of patients suffering from barbiturate overdose. Medical Journal of Australia 1961; 2: 513
95. Wright JT. The value of barbiturate estimations in the diagnosis and treatment of barbiturate intoxication. Quarterly Journal of Medicine 1955; 24: 95
96. Kulig K, Bar-Or D, Cantrill SV, et al. Management of acutely poisoned patients without gastric emptying. Annals of Emergency Medicine 1985; 14: 562
97. Askenasi R, Abramowicz M, Jeanmart J, et al. Esophageal perforation: an unusual complication of gastric lavage. Annals of Emergency Medicine 1984; 13: 146
98. Justiniani FR, Hippalgaonkar R, Martinez LO. Charcoal-containing empyema complicating treatment for overdose. Chest 1985; 87: 404
99. Wald P, Stern J, Weiner B, et al. Esophageal tear following forceful removal of an impacted oral-gastric lavage tube. Annals of Emergency Medicine 1986; 15: 80
100. Thompson AM, Robins JB, Prescott LF. Changes in cardiorespiratory function during gastric lavage for drug overdose. Human Toxicology 1987; 6: 215
101. Harstad E, Moller KO, Simesen MH. Über den wert der magenspülung bei der behandlung von akuten vergiftungen. Acta Medica Scandinavica 1942; 112: 478
102. Spray SB, Zuidema GD, Cameron JL. Aspiration pneumonia: incidence of aspiration with endotracheal tubes. American Journal of Surgery 1976; 131: 701

103. Leclerc F, Martin V, Gaudier B. Intoxication par l'eau secondaire au lavage d'estomac. Nouvelle Presse Médicale 1981; 10: 1149
104. Oswald I. Poisoning treatment centres. British Medical Journal 1972; 4: 430
105. Kennedy P. Poisoning treatment centres. British Medical Journal 1972; 4: 670
106. Olkkola KT, Neuvonen PJ. Do gastric contents modify antidotal efficacy of oral activated charcoal? British Journal of Clinical Pharmacology 1984; 18: 663
107. Scolding N, Ward MJ, Hutchings A, et al. Charcoal and isoniazid pharmacokinetics. Human Toxicology 1986; 5: 285
108. Neuvonen PJ, Vartiainen M, Tokola O. Comparison of activated charcoal and ipecac syrup in prevention of drug absorption. European Journal of Clinical Pharmacology 1983; 24: 557
109. Neuvonen PJ, Elfving SM, Elonen E. Reduction of absorption of digoxin, phenytoin and aspirin by activated charcoal in man. European Journal of Pharmacology 1978; 13: 213
110. Curtis RA, Barone J, Giacona N. Efficacy of ipecac and activated charcoal/cathartic: prevention of salicylate absorption in a simulated overdose. Archives of Internal Medicine 1984; 144: 48
111. Neuvonen PJ, Elonen E. Effect of activated charcoal on absorption and elimination of phenobarbital, carbamazepine and phenylbutazone in man. European Journal of Clinical Pharmacology 1980; 17: 51
112. Scheinin M, Virtanen R, Iisalo E. Effect of single and repeated doses of activated charcoal on the pharmacokinetics of doxepin. International Journal of Clinical Pharmacology Therapy and Toxicology 1985; 23: 38
113. El-Bahie N, Allen EM, Williams J, et al. The effect of activated charcoal and hyoscine butylbromide alone and in combination on the absorption of mefenamic acid. British Journal of Clinical Pharmacology 1985; 19: 836
114. McNamara RM, Aaron CK, Gemborys M, et al. Sorbitol catharsis does not enhance efficacy of charcoal in a simulated acetaminophen overdose. Annals of Emergency Medicine 1988; 17: 243
115. Lim DT, Singh P, Nourtsis S, et al. Absorption inhibition and enhancement of elimination of sustained-release theophylline tablets by oral activated charcoal. Annals of Emergency Medicine 1986; 15: 1303
116. Neuvonen PJ, Olkkola KT. Activated charcoal and syrup of ipecac in prevention of cimetidine and pindolol absorption in man after administration of metoclopramide as an antiemetic agent. Clinical Toxicology 1984; 22: 103
117. Cordonnier J, Van Den Heede M, Heyndrickx A. Activated charcoal and ipecac syrup in prevention of tilidine absorption in man. Veterinary and Human Toxicology 1987; 29 Suppl. 2: 105
118. Tenenbein M, Cohen S, Sitar DS. Whole bowel irrigation as a decontamination procedure after acute drug overdose. Archives of Internal Medicine 1987; 147: 905-7
119. Kirshenbaum LA, Mathews SC, Sitar DS, et al. Whole bowel irrigation versus activated charcoal in sorbitol for the ingestion of modified-release pharmaceuticals. Clinical Pharmacology and Therapeutics 1989; 46: 264-71
120. Smith SW, Ling LJ, Halstenson CE. Whole bowel irrigation as a treatment for acute lithium overdose. Annals of Emergency Medicine 1991; 20: 536-9
121. Goldberg MJ, Spector R, Park GD, et al. The effect of sorbitol and activated charcoal on serum theophylline concentrations after slow-release theophylline. Clinical Pharmacology and Therapeutics 1987; 41: 108-11
122. Keller RE, Schwab RA, Krenzelok EP. Contribution of sorbitol combined with activated charcoal in prevention of salicylate absorption. Annals of Emergency Medicine 1990; 19: 654-6
123. Meredith TJ, Vale JA. Treatment of paraquat poisoning in man: methods to prevent absorption. Human Toxicology 1987; 6: 49
124. Gibson TP, Atkinson AJ. Effect of changes in intercompartment rate constants on drug removal during hemoperfusion. Journal of Pharmaceutical Sciences 1978; 67: 1178
125. Gwilt PR, Perrier D. Plasma protein binding and distribution characteristics of drugs as indices of their hemodialyzability. Clinical Pharmacology and Therapeutics 1978; 24: 154
126. Takki S, Gambertoglio JG, Honda DH, et al. Pharmacokinetic evaluation of hemodialysis in acute drug overdose. Journal of Pharmacokinetics and Biopharmaceutics 1978; 6: 427
127. Pond S, Rosenberg J, Benowitz NL, et al. Pharmacokinetics of haemoperfusion for drug overdose. Clinical Pharmacokinetics 1979; 4: 329
128. Tilstone WJ, Winchester JF, Reavey PC. The use of pharmacokinetic principles in determining the effectiveness of removal of toxins from blood. Clinical Pharmacology and Therapeutics 1979; 4: 23
129. Arimori K, Nakano M. Accelerated clearance of intravenously administered theophylline and phenobarbital by oral doses of activated charcoal in rats: a possibility of the intestinal dialysis. Journal of Pharmacobio-Dynamics 1986; 9: 437
130. Arimori K, Nakano M. The intestinal dialysis of intravenously administered phenytoin by oral activated charcoal in rats. Journal of Pharmacobio-Dynamics 1987; 10: 157
131. Kulig KW, Bar-Or D, Rumack BH. Intravenous theophylline poisoning and multiple-dose charcoal in an animal model. Annals of Emergency Medicine 1987; 16: 842
132. Chyka PA, Mandrell TD, Holley JE, et al. Evaluation of a porcine model to study repeat-dose activated charcoal therapy. Veterinary and Human Toxicology 1993; 35: 367
133. Johnson D, Eppler J, Giesbrecht E, et al. Effect of multiple-dose activated charcoal on the clearance of high-dose intravenous aspirin in a porcine model. Annals of Emergency Medicine 1995; 26: 569
134. Berg MJ, Berlinger WG, Goldberg MJ, et al. Acceleration of the body clearance of phenobarbital by oral activated charcoal. New England Journal of Medicine 1982; 307: 642
135. Berg MJ, Rose JQ, Wurster DE, et al. Effect of charcoal and sorbitol-charcoal suspension on the elimination of intravenous phenobarbital. Therapeutic Drug Monitoring 1987; 9: 41
136. Mauro LS, Mauro VF, Brown DL, et al. Enhancement of phenytoin elimination by multiple-dose activated charcoal. Annals of Emergency Medicine 1987; 16: 1132
137. Rowden AM, Spoor JE, Bertino JS. The effect of activated charcoal on phenytoin pharmacokinetics. Annals of Emergency Medicine 1990; 19: 1144
138. Berlinger WG, Spector R, Goldberg MJ, et al. Enhancement of theophylline clearance by oral activated char-

coal. Clinical Pharmacology and Therapeutics 1983; 33: 351
139. Mahutte CK, True RJ, Michiels TM, et al. Increased serum theophylline clearance with orally administered activated charcoal. American Review of Respiratory Disease 1983; 128: 820
140. Park GD, Radomski L, Goldberg MJ, et al. Effects of size and frequency of oral doses of charcoal on theophylline clearance. Clinical Pharmacy and Therapeutics 1983; 34: 663
141. Park GD, Spector R, Goldberg MJ, et al. Effect of the surface area of activated charcoal on theophylline clearance. Journal of Clinical Pharmacology 1984; 24: 289
142. Radomski L, Park GD, Goldberg MJ, et al. Model for theophylline overdose treatment with oral activated charcoal. Clinical Pharmacology and Therapeutics 1984; 35: 402
143. Ilkhanipour K, Yealy DM, Krenzelok EP. The comparative efficacy of various multiple-dose activated charcoal regimens. American Journal of Emergency Medicine 1992; 10: 298
144. Neuvonen PJ, Elonen E, Mattila MJ. Oral activated charcoal and dapsone elimination. Clinical Pharmacology and Therapeutics 1980; 27: 823
145. Lockey D, Bateman DN. Effect of oral activated charcoal on quinine elimination. British Journal of Clinical Pharmacology 1989; 27: 92
146. Karkkainen S, Neuvonen PJ. Effect of oral charcoal and urine pH on dextropropoxyphene pharmacokinetics. International Journal of Clinical Pharmacology Therapy and Toxicology 1985; 23: 219
147. Laufen H, Leitold M. The effect of activated charcoal on the bioavailability of piroxicam in man. International Journal of Clinical Pharmacology Therapy and Toxicology 1986; 24: 48
148. Reissell P, Manninen V. Effect of administration of activated charcoal and fibre on absorption, excretion and steady state blood levels of digoxin and digitoxin: evidence for intestinal secretion of the glycosides. Acta Medica Scandinavica 1982; 668 Suppl.: 88
149. Park GD, Goldberg MJ, Spector R, et al. The effects of activated charcoal on digoxin and digitoxin clearance. Drug Intelligence and Clinical Pharmacy 1985; 19: 937
150. Du Souich P, Caillé G, Larochelle P. Enhancement of nadolol elimination by activated charcoal and antibiotics. Clinical Pharmacology and Therapeutics 1983; 33: 585
151. Karkkainen S, Neuvonen PJ. Effect of oral charcoal and urine pH on sotalol pharmacokinetics. International Journal of Clinical Pharmacology Therapy and Toxicology 1984; 22: 441
152. Arimori K, Kawano H, Nakano M. Gastrointestinal dialysis of disopyramide in healthy subjects. International Journal of Clinical Pharmacology Therapy and Toxicology 1989; 27: 280
153. Barone JA, Raia JJ, Huang YC. Evaluation of the effects of multiple-dose activated charcoal on the absorption of orally administered salicylate in a simulated toxic ingestion model. Annals of Emergency Medicine 1988; 17: 34
154. Kirshenbaum LA, Mathews SC, Sitar DS, et al. Does multiple-dose charcoal therapy enhance salicylate excretion? Archives of Internal Medicine 1990; 150: 1281
155. Ho JL, Tierney MG, Dickinson GE. An evaluation of the effect of repeated doses of oral activated charcoal on salicylate elimination. Journal of Clinical Pharmacology 1989; 29: 366
156. Mayer AL, Sitar DS, Tenenbein M. Multiple-dose charcoal and whole-bowel irrigation do not increase clearance of absorbed salicylate. Archives of Internal Medicine 1992; 152: 393
157. Allen EM, Buss DC, Williams J, et al. The effect of charcoal on mefenamic acid elimination. British Journal of Clinical Pharmacology 1987; 24: 830
158. Al-Shareef A, Buss DC, Shetty HGM, et al. The effect of repeated-dose activated charcoal on the pharmacokinetics of sodium valproate in healthy volunteers. British Journal of Clinical Pharmacology 1990; 30: 331P
159. Watson WA, Jenkins TC, Velasquez N, et al. Repeated oral doses of activated charcoal and the clearance of tobramycin, a non-absorbable drug. Clinical Toxicology 1987; 25: 171
160. Davis RL, Koup JR, Roon RA, et al. Effect of oral activated charcoal on tobramycin clearance. Antimicrobial Agents and Chemotherapy 1988; 32: 274
161. Davis RL, Roon RA, Koup JR, et al. Effects of orally administered activated charcoal on vancomycin clearance. Antimicrobial Agents and Chemotherapy 1987; 31: 720
162. Neuvonen PJ, Karkkainen S. Effects of charcoal, sodium bicarbonate, and ammonium chloride on chlorpropamide kinetics. Clinical Pharmacology and Therapeutics 1983; 33: 386
163. Karkkainen S, Neuvonen PJ. Pharmacokinetics of amitriptyline influenced by oral charcoal and urine pH. International Journal of Clinical Pharmacology Therapy and Toxicology 1986; 24: 326
164. Goldberg MJ, Park GD, Spector R, et al. Lack of effect of oral activated charcoal on imipramine clearance. Clinical Pharmacology and Therapeutics 1985; 38: 350
165. Lalonde RL, Deshpande R, Hamilton PP, et al. Acceleration of digoxin clearance by activated charcoal. Clinical Pharmacology and Therapeutics 1985; 37: 367
166. Lake KD, Brown DC, Peterson CD. Digoxin toxicity: enhanced systemic elimination during oral activated charcoal therapy. Pharmacotherapy 1984; 4: 161
167. Boldy DAR, Smart V, Vale JA. Multiple doses of charcoal in digoxin poisoning. Lancet 1985; 2: 1076
168. Pond SM, Olson KR, Osterloh JD, et al. Randomized study of the treatment of phenobarbital overdose with repeated doses of activated charcoal. Journal of the American Medical Association 1984; 251: 3104
169. Boldy DAR, Vale JA, Prescott LF. Treatment of phenobarbitone poisoning with repeated oral administration of activated charcoal. Quarterly Journal of Medicine 1986; 61: 997
170. Mofenson HC, Caraccio TR, Greensher J, et al. Gastrointestinal dialysis with activated charcoal and cathartic in the treatment of adolescent intoxications. Clinical Pediatrics 1985; 24: 678
171. Inotsume N, Kimoto A, Katsuya H, et al. Accelerated elimination of phenobarbital by oral activated charcoal suspensions with alkaline diuresis in an overdose patient. Japanese Journal of Clinical Pharmacology and Therapeutics 1988; 19: 779
172. Goodman LS, Gilman A. In: Gilman AG, Rall TW, Neis AS, et al. (editors). Goodman and Gilman's the pharmacological basis of therapeutics. 8th ed. New York: Pergamon Press, 1990: 1698
173. Jacobsen D, Wilk-Larsen E, Dahl T, et al. Pharmacokinetic evaluation of haemoperfusion in phenobarbital

poisoning. European Journal of Clinical Pharmacology 1984; 26: 109

174. Berman LB, Jeghers HJ, Schreiner GE, et al. Hemodialysis, an effective therapy for acute barbiturate poisoning. Journal of the American Medical Association 1956; 161: 820
175. Vale JA. The medical management of acute poisoning: an evaluation of charcoal haemoperfusion. MD Thesis: University of London, 1980
176. Boldy DAR, Heath A, Ruddock S, et al. Activated charcoal for carbamazepine poisoning. Lancet 1987; 1: 1027
177. Leslie PJ, Heyworth R, Prescott LF. Cardiac complications of carbamazepine: treatment by haemoperfusion. British Medical Journal 1983; 286: 1018
178. De Groot G, van Heijst ANP, Maes RA. Charcoal hemoperfusion in the treatment of two cases of acute carbamazepine poisoning. Clinical Toxicology 1984; 22: 349
179. Nilsson C, Sterner G, Idvall J. Charcoal hemoperfusion for treatment of serious carbamazepine poisoning. Acta Medica Scandinavica 1984; 216: 137
180. Gruska H, Peyer K-H, Kubicki S, et al. Klinik toxicologie und Therapie einer Schweren Carbamazepinvergiftung. Archives of Toxicology 1971; 27: 193
181. Lee C-SC, Wang LH, Marbury TC, et al. Hemodialysis clearance and total body elimination of carbamazepine during chronic hemodialysis. Clinical Toxicology 1980; 17: 429
182. True RJ, Berman JM, Mahutte CK. Treatment of theophylline toxicity with oral activated charcoal. Critical Care Medicine 1984; 12: 113
183. Gal P, Miller A, McCue JD. Oral activated charcoal to enhance theophylline elimination in an acute overdose. Journal of the American Medical Association 1984; 251: 3130
184. Sessler CN, Glauser FL, Cooper KR. Treatment of theophylline toxicity with oral activated charcoal. Chest 1985; 87: 325
185. Ohning BL, Reed MD, Blumer JL. Continuous nasogastric administration of activated charcoal for the treatment of theophylline intoxication. Pediatric Pharmacology 1986; 5: 241
186. Vale JA. Methods to increase poison elimination. In: Catto GRD, editor. New clinical applications: nephrology, drugs and the kidney. Lancaster: Kluwer Academic Publishers, 1990: 65-111
187. Hillman RJ, Prescott LF. Treatment of salicylate poisoning with repeated oral charcoal. British Medical Journal 1985; 291: 1472
188. Neuvonen PJ, Elonen E, Haapanen EJ. Acute dapsone intoxication: clinical findings and effect of oral charcoal and haemodialysis on dapsone elimination. Acta Medica Scandinavica 1983; 214: 215
189. Prescott LF, Hamilton AR, Heyworth R. Treatment of quinine overdosage with repeated oral charcoal. British Journal of Clinical Pharmacology 1989; 27: 95
190. Bateman DN, Blain PG, Woodhouse KW, et al. Pharmacokinetics and clinical toxicity of quinine overdosage: lack of efficacy of techniques intended to enhance elimination. Quarterly Journal of Medicine 1985; 54: 125
191. Watson WA, Cremer KF, Chapman JA. Gastrointestinal obstruction associated with multiple-dose activated charcoal. Journal of Emergency Medicine 1986; 4: 401
192. Ray MR, Padin DR, Condie JD, et al. Charcoal bezoar: small-bowel obstruction secondary to amitriptyline overdose therapy. Digestive Diseases and Sciences 1988; 33: 106
193. Atkinson SW, Young Y, Trotter GA. Treatment with activated charcoal complicated by gastrointestinal obstruction requiring surgery. British Medical Journal 1992; 305: 563
194. Pollack MM, Dunbar BS, Holbrook PR, et al. Aspiration of activated charcoal and gastric contents. Annals of Emergency Medicine 1981; 10: 528
195. Harsch HH. Aspiration of activated charcoal. New England Journal of Medicine 1986; 314: 318
196. Menzies DG, Busuttil A, Prescott LF. Fatal pulmonary aspiration of oral activated charcoal. British Medical Journal 1988; 297: 459
197. Rau NR, Nagaraj MV, Prakash PS, et al. Fatal pulmonary aspiration of oral activated charcoal. British Medical Journal 1988; 297: 918
198. Benson B, VanAntwerp M, Hergott T. A fatality resulting from multiple dose activated charcoal therapy. Veterinary and Human Toxicology 1989; 31: 335
199. Elliot GG, Colby TV, Kelly TM, et al. Charcoal lung: bronchiolitis obliterans after aspiration of activated charcoal. Chest 1989; 96: 672
200. Givens T, Holloway M, Wason S. Pulmonary aspiration of activated charcoal after tricyclic antidepressant overdose. Veterinary and Human Toxicology 1990; 32: 375
201. Harris CR, Filandrinos D. Accidental administration of activated charcoal into the lung: aspiration by proxy. Annals of Emergency Medicine 1993; 22: 1470
202. Prescott LF. Mechanisms of renal excretion of drugs (with special reference to drugs used by anaesthetists). British Journal of Anaesthesia 1972; 44: 246
203. Mawer GE, Lee HA. Value of forced diuresis in acute barbiturate poisoning. British Medical Journal 1968; 2: 790
204. Prescott LF. Limitations of haemodialysis and forced diuresis. The poisoned patient: the role of the laboratory. Ciba Foundation Symposium No. 26. Amsterdam: Excerpta Medica, 1974: 269-82
205. Bochner F, Hooper WD, Sutherland JM, et al. The renal handling of diphenylhydantoin and 5-(p-hydroxphenol)-5-phenylhydantoin. Clinical Pharmacology and Therapeutics 1973; 14: 791
206. Thomsen K. The effect of sodium chloride on kidney function in rats with lithium intoxication. Acta Pharmacologica et Toxicologica 1973; 33: 92
207. Dyson EH, Simpson D, Prescott LF, et al. Self-poisoning and therapeutic intoxication with lithium. Human Toxicology 1987; 6: 325
208. Hansen HE, Amdisen A. Lithium intoxication. Quarterly Journal of Medicine 1978; 47: 123-44
209. Jacobsen D, Aasen G, Frederichsen P, et al. Lithium intoxication: pharmacokinetics during and after terminated haemodialysis in acute intoxications. Clinical Toxicology 1987; 25: 81
210. Macdonald TM, Cotton M, Prescott LF. Low dose dopamine in lithium poisoning. British Journal of Clinical Pharmacology 1988; 26: 195
211. Meredith TJ, Vale JA. Salicylate poisoning. In: Vale JA, Meredith TJ, editors. Poisoning: diagnosis and treatment. London: Update Books, 1981: 97-103
212. Prescott LF, Balali-Mood M, Critchley JAJH, et al. Diuresis or urinary alkalinisation for salicylate poisoning? British Medical Journal 1982; 285: 1383
213. Waddell WJ, Butler TC. The distribution and excretion of phenobarbital. Journal of Clinical Investigation 1957; 36: 1217

214. Bloomer HA. A critical evaluation of diuresis in the treatment of barbiturate intoxication. Journal of Laboratory and Clinical Medicine 1966; 67: 898
215. Hadden J, Johnson K, Smith S, et al. Acute barbiturate intoxication: concepts of management. Journal of the American Medical Association 1969; 209: 893
216. Levy G, Tsuchiya T. Salicylate accumulation kinetics in man. New England Journal of Medicine 1972; 287: 430
217. Morgan AG, Polak A. The excretion of salicylate in salicylate poisoning. Clinical Science 1971; 41: 475
218. Dukes DC, Blainey JD, Cumming G, et al. The treatment of severe aspirin poisoning. Lancet 1963; 1: 329
219. Prescott LF, Park J, Darrien I. Treatment of severe, 2,4-D and mecoprop intoxication with alkaline diuresis. British Journal of Clinical Pharmacology 1979; 7: 111
220. Onyon LJ, Liddle A, Flanagan RJ. Acute toxicology of chlorinated phenoxy herbicides in man. Human Toxicology 1986; 5: 127
221. Wells WDE, Wright N, Yeoman WB. Clinical features and management of poisoning with 2,4-D and mecoprop. Clinical Toxicology 1981; 18: 273
222. Friesen EG, Jones GR, Vaughan D. Clinical presentation and management of acute 2,4-D oral ingestion. Drug Safety 1990; 5: 155
223. Flanagan RJ, Meredith TJ, Ruprah M, et al. Alkaline diuresis for acute poisoning with chlorophenoxy herbicides and ioxynil. Lancet 1990; 335: 454
224. Beckett AH, Rowland M, Turner P. Influence of urinary pH on excretion of amphetamine. Lancet 1965; 1: 303
225. Davis JM, Kopin IJ, Lemberger L, et al. Effects of urinary pH on amphetamine excretion. Annals of the New York Academy of Sciences 1971; 179: 493
226. Anggard E, Johnson L-E, Hogmark A-L, et al. Amphetamine metabolism in amphetamine psychosis. Clinical Pharmacology and Therapeutics 1973; 14: 870
227. Gary NE, Saidi P. Methamphetamine intoxication: a speedy new treatment. American Journal of Medicine 1978; 64: 537
228. Beckett AH, Brookes LG. The absorption and urinary excretion in man of fenfluramine and its main metabolite. Journal of Pharmacy and Pharmacology 1967; Suppl. 19: 41S
229. Done AK. Ion trapping in the pathogenesis and treatment of poisoning. Veterinary and Human Toxicology 1980; 22 Suppl. 2: 2
230. Muhlendahl KE, Krienke EG, Bunjes R. Fatal overtreatment of accidental childhood intoxication. Journal of Paediatrics and Child Health 1978; 93: 1003
231. Winchester JF, Forbes CD, Courtney JM, et al. Effect of sulphinpyrazone and aspirin on platelet adhesion to activated charcoal and dialysis membranes in vitro. Thrombosis Research 1977; 11: 443
232. Welch LT, Bower JD, Ott CE, et al. Oil dialysis for ethchlorvynol intoxication. Clinical Pharmacology and Therapeutics 1972; 13: 745
233. Berman LB, Vogelsang P. Removal rates for barbiturates using two types of peritoneal dialysis. New England Journal of Medicine 1964; 270: 77
234. Kennedy AC, Briggs JD, Young N, et al. Successful treatment of three cases of very severe barbiturate poisoning. Lancet 1969; 1: 995
235. Teehan BP, Maher JF, Carey JJH, et al. Acute ethchlorvynol (Placidyl) intoxication. Annals of Internal Medicine 1970; 72: 875
236. De Myttenaere M, Schoenfeld L, Maher JF. Treatment of glutethimide poisoning: a comparison of forced diuresis and dialysis. Journal of the American Medical Association 1968; 203: 885
237. Stein G, Kangas L, Traeger A, et al. In-vitro- und in-vivo-Dialysance-Untersuchungen von Psychopharmaka, Hypnotika und Lithium. Deutsche Gesundh-Wesen 1977; 32: 1952
238. Vaziri ND, Kumar KP, Mirahmadi K, et al. Hemodialysis in treatment of acute chloral hydrate poisoning. Southern Medical Journal 1977; 70: 377
239. Stalker NE, Gambertoglio JG, Fukumitsu CJ, et al. Acute massive chloral hydrate intoxication treated with hemodialysis: a clinical pharmacokinetic analysis. Journal of Clinical Pharmacology 1978; 18: 136
240. Lobo PI, Spyker D, Surratt P, et al. Use of hemodialysis in meprobamate overdosage. Clinical Nephrology 1977; 7: 73
241. O'Neil LS, Tipton KF, Prichard JS, et al. Survival after high blood alcohol levels: associated with first order elimination kinetics. Archives of Internal Medicine 1984; 144: 641
242. Schreiner GE. Dialysis of poisons and drugs: annual review. Transactions of the American Society for Artificial Internal Organs 1970; 16: 544
243. Keyvan-Larijarni H, Tannenberg AM. Methanol intoxication: comparison of peritoneal dialysis and hemodialysis treatment. Archives of Internal Medicine 1974; 134: 293
244. Jacobsen D, Jansen H, Wilk-Larsen E, et al. Studies on methanol poisoning. Acta Medica Scandinavica 1982; 212: 5
245. McMartin KE, Ambre JJ, Tephly TR. Methanol poisoning in human subjects. American Journal of Medicine 1980; 68: 414
246. Jacobsen D, Ovrebo S, Sejersted OM. Toxicokinetics of formate during haemodialysis. Acta Medica Scandinavica 1983; 214: 409
247. Vale JA, Prior JG, O'Hare JP, et al. Treatment of ethylene glycol poisoning with peritoneal dialysis. British Medical Journal 1982; 284: 557
248. Peterson CD, Collins AJ, Himes JM, et al. Ethylene glycol poisoning. New England Journal of Medicine 1981; 304: 21
249. Jacobsen D, Ostby N, Bredesen JE. Studies on ethylene glycol poisoning. Acta Medica Scandinavica 1982; 212: 11
250. Rothman A, Normann SA, Manoguerra AS, et al. Short-term hemodialysis in childhood ethylene glycol poisoning. Journal of Pediatrics 1986; 108: 153
251. Jacobsen D, Ovrebo S, Ostborg J, et al. Glycolate causes the acidosis in ethylene glycol poisoning and is effectively removed by hemodialysis. Acta Medica Scandinavica 1984; 216: 409
252. Freireich AW, Cinque TJ, Xanthaky G, et al. Hemodialysis for isopropanol poisoning. New England Journal of Medicine 1967; 277: 699
253. King HL, Kent PB, Shires DL. Hemodialysis for isopropyl alcohol poisoning. Journal of the American Medical Association 1970; 211: 1855
254. Dua SL. Peritoneal dialysis for isopropyl alcohol poisoning. Journal of the American Medical Association 1974; 230: 235
255. Mecikalski MB, Depner TA. Peritoneal dialysis for isopropanol poisoning. Western Journal of Medicine 1982; 137: 322
256. Rosansky SJ. Isopropyl alcohol poisoning treated with hemodialysis: kinetics of isopropyl alcohol and acetone removal. Clinical Toxicology 1982; 19: 265

257. Wilson JHP, Donker AJM, Van Der Hem GK, et al. Peritoneal dialysis for lithium poisoning. British Medical Journal 1971; 2: 749
258. Von Hartitzsch B, Hoenich NA, Leigh RJ, et al. Permanent neurological sequelae despite haemodialysis for lithium intoxication. British Medical Journal 1972; 4: 757
259. Clendeninn NJ, Pond SM, Kaysen G, et al. Potential pitfalls in the evaluation of the usefulness of hemodialysis for the removal of lithium. Clinical Toxicology 1982; 19: 341
260. Jaeger A, Sauder PH, Kopferschmitt J, et al. Toxokinetics of lithium intoxication treated by hemodialysis. Clinical Toxicology 1985-86; 23: 501
261. Bismuth C, Baud FJ, Buneaux F, et al. Spontaneous toxokinetics of lithium during a therapeutic overdose with renal failure. Clinical Toxicology 1986; 24: 261
262. Jaeger A, Sauder PH, Kopferschmitt J, et al. When should dialysis be performed in lithium poisoning? A kinetic study in 14 cases of lithium poisoning. Clinical Toxicology 1993; 31: 429
263. Miceli JN, Bidani A, Aronow R. Peritoneal dialysis of theophylline. Clinical Toxicology 1979; 14: 539
264. Miceli JN, Clay B, Fleischmann LE, et al. Pharmacokinetics of severe theophylline intoxication managed by peritoneal dialysis. Developmental Pharmacology and Therapeutics 1980; 1: 16
265. Brown GS, Lohr TO, Mayor GH, et al. Peritoneal clearance of theophylline. American Journal of Kidney Diseases 1981; 1: 24
266. Lee C-SC, Peterson JC, Marbury TC. Comparative pharmacokinetics of theophylline in peritoneal dialysis and hemodialysis. Journal of Clinical Pharmacology 1983; 23: 274
267. Woo OF, Pond SM, Benowitz NL, et al. Benefit of hemoperfusion in acute theophylline intoxication. Clinical Toxicology 1984; 22: 411
268. Levy G, Gibson TP, Whitman W, et al. Hemodialysis clearance of theophylline. Journal of the American Medical Association 1977; 237: 1466
269. Lee CS, Marbury TC, Perrin JH, et al. Hemodialysis of theophylline in uremic patients. Journal of Clinical Pharmacology 1979; 19: 219
270. Vale JA, Rees AJ, Widdop B, et al. Use of charcoal haemoperfusion in the management of severely poisoned patients. British Medical Journal 1975; 1: 5
271. Okonek S. Intoxication with pyrazolones. British Journal of Clinical Pharmacology 1980; 10: 385S
272. Rosenbaum JL, Kramer MS, Raja R. Resin hemoperfusion for acute drug intoxication. Archives of Internal Medicine 1976; 136: 263
273. Gibson TP, Matusik E, Nelson LD, et al. Artificial kidneys and clearance calculation. Clinical Pharmacology and Therapeutics 1976; 20: 720
274. Vale JA, Thomas T, Widdop B, et al. Use of charcoal haemoperfusion in poisoned patients: a review of 20 cases. Proceedings of the European Society of Artificial Organs 1975; 2: 239
275. Benowitz N, Abolin C, Tozer T, et al. Resin haemoperfusion in ethchlorvynol overdose. Clinical Pharmacology and Therapeutics 1980; 27: 236
276. De Groot G. Haemoperfusion in clinical toxicology. A pharmacokinetic evaluation. Published thesis: University of Utrecht, 1982
277. Heath A, Knudsen K. Role of extracorporeal drug removal in acute theophylline poisoning: a review. Medical Toxicology and Adverse Drug Experience 1987; 2: 294
278. Gosselin B, Mathieu D, Chopin C, et al. Acute intoxication with disopyramide: clinical and experimental study by hemoperfusion on Amberlite XAD-4 resin. Clinical Toxicology 1980; 17: 439
279. Strong JE, Wilson J, Douglas JF, et al. Phenylbutazone self-poisoning treated by charcoal haemoperfusion. Anaesthesia 1979; 34: 1038
280. Berlinger WG, Spector R, Flanigan MJ, et al. Hemoperfusion for phenylbutazone poisoning. Annals of Internal Medicine 1982; 96: 334
281. Yakatan GJ, Smith RB, Leff RD, et al. Pharmacokinetic considerations in exchange transfusion in neonates. Clinical Pharmacology and Therapeutics 1978; 24: 90
282. Lindahl S, Westerling D. Detoxification with peritoneal dialysis and blood exchange after diphenylhydantoin intoxication. Acta Paediatrica Scandinavica 1982; 71: 665
283. Keller F, Kreutz G, Vohringer HF, et al. Effect of plasma exchange on the steady-state kinetics of digoxin and digitoxin. Clinical Pharmacokinetics 1985; 10: 514
284. Lui E, Rubenstein M. Phenytoin removal by plasmapheresis in thrombotic thrombocytopenic purpura. Clinical Therapeutics 1982; 31: 762

Chapter 9

# Principles and Practice of Pharmacoepidemiology

*T.R. Einarson, U. Bergman* and *B.-E. Wiholm*

## Synopsis of Important Principles

1) Pharmacoepidemiology is used to answer clinical pharmacological questions by applying epidemiological methods that are mainly nonexperimental, i.e. do not involve an intervention, such as a random assignment of treatment, but are observations of what occurs in populations given different treatments.

2) Pharmacoepidemiology describes the distribution of usage of medicines in the population and the effects of such use with regard to morbidity, mortality, and health economics, most often with special emphasis on negative effects.

3) Observational data may be used to detect new adverse drug reactions, to estimate and delineate risk groups, as well as to compare risks with different medications.

4) Research designs include single groups (e.g. case reports, case series, cross-sectional studies) or comparative studies (e.g. case control, cohort studies).

5) Concentration-effect and time-risk relationships are important considerations in pharmacoepidemiology and are rarely linear.

6) Under special circumstances, effectiveness rates may be measured by prospective cohorts. The advantage of this method is that it is the only observational study design whereby incidence rates can be directly measured and compared.

Pharmacoepidemiology is a relatively new field of study, with concepts, methods and applications that have made increasing contributions to healthcare as the field has evolved over the past few decades. This chapter describes the potential of this field, in terms of what it can achieve, the strengths, weaknesses and limitations of pharmacoepidemiological models, and projections for future developments of this area of science.

## 1. Pharmacoepidemiology: Definitions and Scope

Pharmacoepidemiology is the study of the use of and the effects of medicines in large numbers of people.[1] It falls within the area of clinical pharmacology as well as epidemiology, and may be seen as the application of the principles of epidemiology to drug effects and drug use. Studies range in focus from very specific to very broad. They may examine a single individual (e.g. a case report of a rare drug reaction), or huge groups of people followed for many years. Information is gathered and analysed to identify possible causation and related factors that can be applied in clinical practice to groups of people and also to individuals undergoing treatment. Table I identifies the focus of pharmacoepidemiology and the related fields of drug utilisation and clinical pharmacology. In general, clinical pharmacology is concerned with drug effects in individual patients, drug utilisation focuses on drug usage patterns and appropriateness of drug use in groups, and pharmacoepidemiology examines the relationship between drug exposure and health outcomes in defined populations.

### 1.1 Origins and Evolution of Pharmacoepidemiology

Modern pharmacotherapy has developed largely during the 20th century. However, as modern effective drugs became increasingly available and used in large populations, appreciation of their potential for producing adverse drug reactions (ADRs) emerged, as well as other therapeutic problems including drug resistance, abuse and unexplained variations in rates of clinical effectiveness.

The awareness of the potential for drugs to cause adverse effects became abruptly evident in 1961 when case reports in the literature associated maternal use of thalidomide with malformations (i.e. limb reductions) in the offspring.[2] Although not the first drug to produce serious ADRs, the nature of the effect was so dramatic that much attention became focused on the detection, prevention, and management of ADRs. It also began the era of pharmacoepidemiology.

To identify ADR problems, spontaneous reporting and other surveillance systems have been created in many countries. Classic examples detected through such systems include the association of grey baby syndrome with chloramphenicol and of vaginal cancer in adolescent offspring of women who took diethylstilbestrol (stilbestrol) in pregnancy.[1,3-5] More recent events of concern include associations of birth defects with isotretinoin,[6] central nervous system (CNS) disturbances with triazolam,[7] suicidal ideation with fluoxetine,[8] deaths with fenoterol,[9] and venous thromboembolism with oral contraceptives.[10-12] Not all of these have been substantiated. Table II lists examples of some of the events associated with drug use that resulted in withdrawal of the drug from the market in at least 1 country.

In some instances, drugs have been re-introduced for use (e.g. dipyrone) or reserved for special situations (e.g. thalidomide and clozapine). Clozapine is an interesting example, because at the time of withdrawal, it was estimated to cause agranulocytosis in 1 in every 5000 patients. It was later found to cause severe neu-

**Table I.** Focus of pharmacoepidemiology and related areas of study

| Discipline | Focus | Indicator of drug exposure | Result studied |
|---|---|---|---|
| Clinical pharmacology | Individual patient | Clinical effect | Drug effectiveness |
| | | Adverse reaction | Drug toxicity |
| Drug utilisation | Groups | Utilisation patterns | Excessive or inadequate use |
| | | Appropriateness of use | Quality of care |
| | | Correlation with outcome | Drug safety, possible relationships |
| Pharmacoepidemiology | Populations (defined) | Exposure-outcome relationship | Causality |
| | | Comparative effectiveness | Quantification of benefit |
| | | Comparative toxicity | Quantification of risk |

**Table II.** Drugs associated with adverse events that led to withdrawal from the market in at least one country

| Drug | Adverse reaction | Frequency of occurrence |
|---|---|---|
| Thalidomide | Phocomelia | 1/4 |
| Clozapine | Agranulocytosis | 1/200 |
| Terodiline | Torsades de pointes | 1/1000 |
| Phenformin | Lactic acidosis | 1/1500 |
| Nomifensine | Haemolysis | 1/3000 |
| Temafloxacin | Haemolysis | 1/5000 |
| Zimelidine | Guillain-Barré syndrome | 1/6000 |
| Phenylbutazone | Stevens-Johnson syndrome, blood dyscrasias | 1/100,000 |
| Dipyrone | Agranulocytosis | 1/1,000,000 |
| Zomepirac | Anaphylactic shock | 1/1,000,000 |
| Benoxaprofen | Liver toxicity, phototoxicity | ? |
| Practolol | Fibrosis, ocular toxicity | ? |
| Clioquinol | SMON (subacute myelo-optic neuropathy) | ? |

tropenia at a much higher incidence of ≈1 in 200, but this was a manageable risk and clozapine was found to have unique benefits. In other cases, the size of the risk when later evaluated was so low that the relevance of withdrawal may be questioned. On the other hand, some more toxic drugs have not been removed from the market. Examples include isotretinoin, which has a higher rate of teratogenicity than thalidomide, and many cancer drugs that suppress bone marrow virtually 100% of the time; however, these agents have unique benefits and the risks can be managed. There are also examples where old drugs suspected of having a negative benefit-risk balance are left on the market because there are insufficient data to warrant their removal.

At the same time, a need has been recognised to develop further methods to study the effects of drugs, both negative and positive, in populations. To discuss, develop and disseminate information about pharmacoepidemiological methods, an international society (i.e. The International Society for Pharmacoepidemiology; ISPE) was formed, and at least 2 textbooks on pharmacoepidemiology have now been published.[1,13]

The related field of drug utilisation developed in parallel with the study of ADRs. It began in the early 1960s both in North America and Europe.[14] Previously, drug utilisation studies had been conducted mostly for marketing purposes and data were not available for use by academic researchers or health authorities. The increased interest was in recognition of the virtual explosion in the marketing of new drugs, the wide variations in the patterns and extent of drug prescribing, the growing concern about ADRs and the cost of drugs. The development of pharmacoepidemiological methods, however, has emerged along 2 different lines in Europe and in North America, as discussed below, nowadays approaching each other, and strongly influenced by the different availability of data sources.

The World Health Organization (WHO) defines *drug utilisation* as the 'marketing, distribution, prescription, and use of drugs in a society, with special emphasis on the resulting medical, social, and economic consequences'.[15] In Europe, drug utilisation research developed at the national and international level with a common methodology for comparative drug utilisation studies, exploiting relatively inexpensive and readily available sources of drug statistics.[14,16-19]

In North America, drug utilisation research has developed on a smaller scale, primarily at institutional or local health programme levels, and greater emphasis has been placed on the qualitative aspects of prescribing, particularly with respect to antibiotics. Drug utilisation review (DUR) has been defined[20] as 'an authorized, structured and continuing program that reviews, analyses and interprets patterns of drug use against predetermined standards'. Such drug utilisation studies focus on the drug; they aim to evaluate the appropriateness of therapy using approved criteria and to develop programmes to intervene and correct deficiencies in the drug use process.

Simultaneously, the *medical audit* concept[21] was implemented in Europe. Audit was defined in drug use or therapeutic audits as 'a searching examination of the way in which drugs are used in clinical practice carried out at intervals frequent enough to maintain a generally accepted standard of prescribing'.[21,22] The audit focuses on medical practitioners, with the aim of improving the rational use of medicines as therapeutic agents. The medical audit and drug utilisation review concepts are essentially the same. Both depend on the use of criteria for the evaluation of drug use and tend to be situation-specific, with feedback for improvement.

## 1.2 Why Pharmacoepidemiology?

Several reasons exist for the evolution of interest in the observational methods used in pharmacoepidemiology. Firstly, in the investigation of some drug events, other models are not possible. A pertinent example is pregnancy. If the sole purpose of the study were to ascertain the possible teratogenic effects of a new medicine, it would be unethical to enrol pregnant (or soon to be pregnant) women in a trial, administer a drug to one group and placebo to another, and then compare the outcome as in a randomised controlled trial (RCT). However, information on drugs in pregnancy is vital. Pharmacoepidemiology provides an alternative approach that addresses the question in a meaningful way.

Secondly, RCTs are often inadequate to answer questions about drug safety, because they lack adequate statistical power. In premarketing studies of drug effectiveness, the RCT represents the usual model for evaluation (see chapter 11, sect. 2). Generally, from 500 to 6000 patients are exposed to a drug during phase III trials. Although adequate for establishing effectiveness, these sample sizes are inadequate to detect less common ADRs.

Moreover, premarketing studies are normally conducted on highly selected patients with no other disease conditions and who are taking no other drugs. Study groups seldom include elderly, paediatric or pregnant patients, and usually, a single indication is investigated. Therefore, the approach taken today fails to provide adequate information to answer questions concerning both the safety of medicines and their effectiveness under non-trial conditions and in other indications.

Pharmacoepidemiological models offer alternative approaches to the evaluation of drug effects. They are observational (i.e. nonexperimental) and can be retrospective, taking advantage of many sources of data.

## 1.3 Aims and Applications of Pharmacoepidemiology

### *1.3.1 Aims*

The three aims of pharmacoepidemiology are signal generation, quantification of risk or benefit, and hypothesis testing.

#### Signal Generation

Through signal generation, new (sometimes serious) ADRs can be identified. Signal generation is most often associated with ADRs, but can be used to detect new applications for medicines. For example, minoxidil was first indicated for hypertension, but case reports (i.e. signals generated) soon identified that it produced hirsutism in a number of patients. That side effect was investigated and, subsequently, minoxidil was marketed for that purpose, namely, stimulation of hair growth.

#### Risk Quantification

Risk quantification of ADR rates often requires large sample sizes. The 'rule of three' indicates if an event occurs in 1 of every 5000 exposed persons, $3 \times 5000$ (i.e. 15,000) people would be needed in a sample to be 95% certain that the sample would include one case. This one case might not be detected unless a clinically significant sign appeared, such as the patient turning blue. This has not yet happened, but the patient might have turned yellow, indicating the development of jaundice. To be detected, the practical number of 3 cases is probably a minimum. Since there are common diseases such as cholelithiasis that cause jaundice, statistically significant differences in incidence rates are also needed. This multiplies the sample size required by one order of magnitude. Pharmacoepidemiological models can be applied for that purpose (see further section 4 below). Similarly, beneficial effects such as cure rates may be quantified.

#### Hypothesis Testing

Hypothesis testing requires the use of comparison groups to determine whether there are differences in variables of interest (risk factors, traits, characteristics, drug exposure or clinical conditions). Statistical methods are used to assess whether the observed differences could have occurred by chance alone. Conclusions about the relationship between exposure to a drug and a clinical event are thus based on the ability to reject the null hypothesis, postulating that the 2 groups are no different with regard to either the drug exposure or the clinical event.

Statistical methods cannot, by themselves, however, show the nature of associations found to be statistically significant. The designs used, namely, cohort and case control studies, are discussed in section 4.2.5.

### *1.3.2 Applications*

Broadly speaking, pharmacoepidemiology provides both qualitative and quantitative information about medicines. The information falls into 2 categories, which are descriptive and analytical, both of which aim to improve therapeutic choices.

*Descriptive data* are generated from drug utilisation studies, drug utilisation reviews or evaluations, and prescription audits. The aim is to identify and, if possible, correct irrational drug use. The focus of drug utilisation review may be on the prescribers, the users, or a combination of both. Prescription audits may incorporate criteria for appropriateness or may simply involve a survey to identify high volume prescribers and users of drugs. Reasons for apparently excessive use may then be investigated and problems rectified. This type of approach has been used in North America[23-25] and in Europe.[26-28]

A more macro approach has used the same concept and applied it to drug use at the national level.[29,30] It has in common with drug utilisation review the application of criteria to drug use, thereby creating qualitative data. In 2 studies,[29,30] the most widely sold products in 5 countries were evaluated using criteria to determine their effectiveness as proven in controlled clinical trials, representing evidence-based medicine. These studies identified a considerable wastage of money in some countries on the basis of use of questionable drugs.

*Quantitative studies* includes hypothesis testing, risk quantification and intervention trials. These models are used to strengthen and verify signals generated from case reports and other suggestions of possible associations.

#### Estimation of the Risks of Drug Use

The most common use of epidemiological data is in the estimation of risk. Included are case control and cohort studies (see also section 4.2.5) as well as randomised controlled trials. It is in the interest of all parties, including manufacturers, prescribers, consumers, healthcare personnel, financial officers and policy makers alike, that risks involved in drug use be quantified. Thus, the benefits and risks of use of a given drug may be weighed.

Risk estimation may also be used to identify risk situations. When triazolam was introduced, case reports of psychiatric disturbances soon appeared. The drug was withdrawn in some countries, but not in others. Since reactions seemed to be dose-related, a lowering of recommended dosages was required and the problem seems to have abated.[31]

#### Use in Patient Counselling

Another application of pharmacoepidemiological data is in counselling patients. For example, a pregnant patient may wish to terminate a pregnancy if there is a substantial risk for producing a seriously malformed child (see chapter 2, sect. 5) but would also wish to proceed with the pregnancy if that risk is low. Collecting and analysing observational data from other such exposures provides a means for addressing that issue.[32,33] Other studies have attempted to determine the exact incidence of adverse events in populations using quantitative methods outlined below (see section 4.2). In Sweden, a system for classification of teratogenic risk for drugs has been developed for the Swedish physicians manual comparable to that seen in the US Physicians Desk Reference (PDR).[34]

#### Formulation of Public Health Policy Decisions

From the point of view of public health, pharmacoepidemiology can provide information to address many issues. Both qualitative and quantitative information may be used to guide policy decisions. For example, if prescribers have high rates of inappropriate prescribing, regulatory agencies could require educational intervention or impose restrictions on specific drugs or on practitioners. Those engaged in policy making could use such data to assess whether a drug should be withdrawn from the market or allowed to remain. Without the facts (i.e. evidence-based medicine), such judgements could not be made rationally. To be effective and efficient, healthcare policy options must be based on sound scientific evidence.[35]

#### Formulation of Therapeutic Guidelines and Discovery of New Indications

Drug experience from large samples of the population can be used to examine the effectiveness of drugs in groups of people not included in phase III trials. In particular, elderly and paediatric patients, and those with concomitant diseases and/or using other medications can be examined, and lessons can be learned from these experiences, with the results used to guide therapeutics in such people. New indications for drugs may also be discovered which can be tested in RCTs.

**Facilitation of Pharmacoeconomic Evaluations**

Data from pharmacoepidemiological studies can be used to measure the effects of drugs on overall healthcare costs and resource consumption. For example, drugs may cause serious adverse effects that lead to hospitalisation,[36,37] which is costly in monetary terms and in terms of resource consumption, especially since such effects are avoidable to a large extent. These data are also fundamental for all kinds of pharmacoeconomic evaluations (see further chapter 10) as they can provide real life estimates of effectiveness, compliance and ADR rates.

**Other Applications**

Observational studies also point to areas that may be fruitful for bench scientists to investigate. Pharmacoepidemiology can identify where and when phenomena occur, but is seldom able to determine why or how.

## 2. Measurement of Outcomes in Pharmacoepidemiology

The measurement and reporting of patient outcomes is becoming an important area of study. Included are studies on functional status (i.e. level of functioning, supervision required, ability to work), symptom status (e.g. days free of pain), patient satisfaction with various aspects of care (e.g. delivery of care, effects on daily activities or life satisfaction), and quality of life studies.

Therapeutic outcomes may be classified as cure, improvement, no change, or deterioration. Alternatively, they could be categorised as successes or failures, with a variety of possible definitions that must be stated explicitly, especially if comparisons are to be made. In any event, clinical judgement is required in establishing outcomes.

Perhaps the most commonly used measures of outcome are morbidity and mortality as well as avoidance of those outcomes. Morbidity is measured as the number of cases of disease or events that occur per unit of population (e.g. per 1000 or per million inhabitants), unit of time (e.g. events per year) or both (e.g. events per 1000 inhabitants per year). Other measures of morbidity are the number of hospitalisations resulting from drug use or prevented by drug use, or days of hospitalisation (or days avoided), and deaths due to or prevented by the use of drugs.[38]

### 2.1 Outcome Measures

The occurrence of pharmacoepidemiological outcomes is commonly expressed by such measurements as prevalence, cumulative incidence, and incidence rate. Incidence measures focus on events while prevalence is concerned with disease states.

*Prevalence* is the proportion of people affected with a disease or exposed to a particular drug in a population at a given time. It is a cross-sectional measure that is usually determined by surveying the population of interest. Prevalence varies between 0 and 1, but can also be expressed as a percentage. For example, it might be said that the prevalence of schizophrenia is 1% in Europe. That means that, at a given time, 1 out of every 100 persons is affected by the disorder.

The *cumulative incidence* is a longitudinal measure. It is the number of new cases of a disease or outcome that occur in a population during a specified amount of time (usually 1 year) divided by the initial number of people in that population. It is the average risk of the individual developing the outcome in a specified time interval,[39] and is expressed either as a percentage or in cases per 1000 or multiples thereof, depending on the rarity of the occurrence.

The *incidence rate* is defined as the ratio of new cases to the person-time at risk. The denominator is the sum of all exposures multiplied by the length of those exposures and may be expressed in person-days or person-years. The incidence rate may be expressed as the number of cases per person-year of exposure (or any other time unit).

Incidence and prevalence measures can be used to compare disease occurrence between areas, over time, or between drug exposures within a given area. They can also be used to monitor the effectiveness of a drug or programme (e.g. immunisation).

### 2.2 Drug Use Measures

For any of the above measures, a baseline of the use in the population is needed. A number of different sources on drug use are available and can be applied in different situations.[14,17]

#### *2.2.1 Monetary Units*

Drug use has been measured in monetary units to quantify the amounts being consumed by populations. It can indicate the burden on a society from drug use. Monetary units (e.g. dollars, pounds, etc.) are convenient and can be converted to a common unit such as the ECU (Euro-) or US dollar, which then allows for international comparisons. This approach was taken in a comparison of drug expenditures among European countries expressed in ECU/person.[40] However, there are several disadvantages, in that quantities of drugs actually consumed are not known and prices may vary widely, especially for different strengths and package sizes of drugs.

#### 2.2.2 Numbers of Prescriptions

Numbers of prescriptions have been used in research due to the availability and ease of use of this method. The problem is that quantities dispensed vary greatly, as does the duration of treatment. Without a diagnosis and these other data, the use of prescription numbers is at best a rough estimate of use. For short term treatments like antibiotics, the number of prescriptions may, however, provide a fairly good estimate of the number of people exposed and of the number of treatment episodes.

#### 2.2.3 Units of Drug Dispensed

Like the prescription, units of drug dispensed (e.g. packs, tablets) is easy to obtain and can be used to compare usage trends within countries. However, as with all sources on drug use, no information is available on the quantity actually taken by the patient (e.g. 1 or 4 tablets may be taken daily). Thus, it is difficult to determine the actual number of patients exposed to the drug. Patterns can, however, be compared and hypotheses generated about excessive use or underuse in some areas.

#### 2.2.4 Defined Daily Doses

The concept of defined daily doses (DDDs) was developed to produce a standard measure of drug utilisation that avoids the problems of the methods mentioned in sections 2.2.1, 2.2.2 and 2.2.3. The DDD is the estimated average maintenance dose per day of a drug when used in its major indication.[14,17] Utilisation is normally expressed as DDDs/1000 inhabitants/day, which allows for comparisons between countries or regions.[41] A variation adapted for use in hospitals is the DDD/100 bed-days, adjusted for occupancy.[42]

This method has been useful in describing and comparing patterns of drug utilisation, and provides denominator data for estimation of adverse reaction rates, performing epidemiological screening for problems in drug utilisation, and monitoring the effects of informational and regulatory activities. The advantage of the method is its usefulness for working with readily available drug statistics at various levels of the health chain. As a standardised unit of measurement, it allows comparisons between drugs in the same therapeutic class, between different healthcare settings or geographic areas, and evaluations of trends over time. It is also relatively easy and inexpensive to use. For chronic diseases such as diabetes and Parkinson's disease, the concept of DDD/1000 inhabitants/day also provides a rough estimate of the prevalence of the drug-treated population.[17]

The DDD methodology also has some significant limitations. The DDD is not a recommended dose, but rather a technical unit of comparison. Many drugs have not yet been assigned DDDs, but guidelines have been published by the WHO Collaborating Centre For Drug Statistics Methodology in Oslo[43] for defining DDDs under these circumstances. Paediatric uses are usually not considered in any calculations. Problems can also arise when doses vary widely, such as with antibiotics or when there is more than 1 major indication for a drug. One example is aspirin (acetylsalicylic acid), which may be used in low doses to avoid cardiac events, moderate doses for pain, and high doses for inflammatory conditions. On the other hand, the usefulness of the methodology was demonstrated in a comparison of antibiotic utilisation in a surgery department, a hospital and a catchment area, relating the findings to the development of resistance.[44] In this retrospective survey, antimicrobial agents primarily used for outpatients in the catchment area seemed to have had more influence on the susceptibility of micro-organisms isolated from postoperative infections than did agents primarily used in the hospital.

#### 2.2.5 Prescribed Daily Doses

The prescribed daily dosage (PDD) is the average daily dose of a drug that has actually been prescribed.[14,17] It is calculated from a representative sample of prescriptions. Although useful for validating the DDD, there may be problems in that the drug may be used for different indications (see section 2.2.4). It also does not indicate how many people are exposed. However, it may provide a refined estimate of the number of person-days (or years) of

**Table III.** Schematic presentation of data from cohort and case control studies

| Factor status | Outcome | | Total |
|---|---|---|---|
| | AE | No AE | |
| Exposed | A | B | $e_1$ |
| Not exposed | C | D | $e_0$ |
| Total | $c_1$ | $c_0$ | N |

*Abbreviations:* AE = adverse event; $e_1$ = total number of people exposed to the drug; $e_0$ = total number of people not exposed to the drug; $c_1$ = total number of cases of the outcome (such as an AE); $c_0$ = total number of people who did not have the outcome; N = total number of people in the study.

exposure, such as in risk calculations with antidepressants.[38] Such analyses have shown that newer less toxic antidepressants were found more often than older compounds in cases of suicide.

### 2.3 Diagnosis and Therapy Surveys

Another source of information useful in pharmacoepidemiology is survey data that describe prescribing patterns of individual clinicians and rates of diseases encountered in practice. The international company IMS has published a National Disease and Therapeutic Index annually in the US and other countries.[14] Similarly, annual data from the Swedish Diagnosis and Therapy Survey have been published by the National Corporation of Pharmacies for many years.[45] Such data, combined with the national sales and prescription surveys, have provided a comprehensive assessment of the use of drugs in Sweden.[14,46]

## 3. The Concept of Risk

An adverse event is any negative medical occurrence that is associated in time with drug therapy. An adverse drug reaction (ADR) is an adverse event attributed to a drug.[1] A distinction should also be made between *risk* and *harm.* Risk refers to the probability of developing an outcome, regardless of severity. Harm is a more descriptive term, and includes not only frequency of occurrence, but also severity and duration. Thus, agranulocytosis and aplastic anaemia are 2 rare disorders that can be elicited by drugs. They also have roughly the same risk, but cause very different harm. Agranulocytosis has a mortality rate of about 9% and 50% of patients recover within 8 days.[47] Aplastic anaemia has a fatality rate of 30 to 50% during the first 2 years of this usually chronic disorder.

The International Committee on Harmonisation has further distinguished *serious* from *severe* reactions. The former relates to outcomes of ADRs while the latter is a grading of the degree of any ADR.[48] As an example, severe pruritus is not a serious ADR,[48] since 'serious' usually denotes that a reaction is life-threatening.

The Council for International Organizations of Medical Sciences (CIOMS) has suggested a scale of risk level terms. In their terminology, *very common* is an event that occurs in ≥1 in 10 exposures; those that occur <1 in 10 but ≥1 in 100 exposures are *common*, <1 in 100 but ≥1 in 1000 exposures are *uncommon*, <1 in 1000 but ≥1 in 10,000 exposures are *rare*, and <1 in 10,000 exposures are *very rare*.[49]

The WHO has developed categories of likelihood for causal associations of exposure-event relationships.[48] Included are *certain, probable/likely*, *possible*, *unlikely*, *conditional* and *unclassifiable*, depending on the strength of the available evidence.

Many research groups have suggested different algorithms for evaluating causality.[50,51] These algorithms vary from simple[50] to very complex.[51] Some have been demonstrated to increase conformity between evaluators (i.e. reliability), but none has been proven to identify the truth (i.e. validity).

### 3.1 Measurement of Risk

The risk of an adverse reaction from a drug is expressed in a number of ways. When a single group is studied, the rate is described as a percentage (cases/total exposures). However, that rate fails to account for the baseline risk, which can be substantial. Consequently, risks are usually expressed in comparison with an unexposed control group.

Table III illustrates the presentation of data from a comparative pharmacoepidemiological study. In the table, 'A' represents the number of persons exposed to a drug who experience the outcome of interest (e.g. an ADR), and 'B' is the number of exposed persons who did not develop the ADR. 'C' and 'D' are the parallel numbers among the nonexposed persons. More complex models have been developed and may be found in standard epidemiology texts such as that by Rothman.[39]

#### *3.1.1 Attributable Risk*

A useful approach to expressing the magnitude of problems is the attributable risk (AR), also referred to as the risk difference or excess risk. It is the difference between the risk in the exposed group and the baseline risk in an unexposed population. Thus, it is the risk in excess of the baseline risk that may be attributed to exposure to the drug. Figuratively, it may be expressed as:

AR = [A/(A + B)] – [C/(C + D)]

For example, if 26 people among 1000 exposed (2.6%) and 36 out of 2000 not exposed (1.8%) developed a rash, the AR would be 2.6% – 1.8%, or 0.8%.

An interesting variant is the *number needed to treat (NNT)*.[52] This is the reciprocal of the risk difference (1/AR) and determines the number of people who would have to be treated to produce 1 more case of the outcome. In this case, NNT = 1/0.008 = 125, i.e. 125 people would need to be treated to produce 1 additional case of rash.

### *3.1.2 Relative Risk*

The relative risk (RR), also referred to as the risk ratio, is the ratio of the risk rate in the exposed group to the risk rate in the nonexposed group. In other words, it is the probability of experiencing an outcome in a group of exposed persons relative to the baseline risk that would occur in the population of unexposed individuals. It is calculated in cohort studies that measure incidences of ADRs or other patient outcomes in exposed and nonexposed patients. Using the terminology in table III, the RR would be expressed as follows:

RR = [A/(A + B)] / [C/(C + D)]

Figure 1 demonstrates the presentation of results expressed as the RR (and the odds ratio, discussed in section 4.2.5). Results are expressed on a logarithmic scale. The horizontal line having a relative risk of 1 (i.e. unity) means that the risks are identical between groups. An RR of 2 means that the exposed group has twice the risk (i.e. 100% increase over baseline) of experiencing the ADR and is the usual minimum to generate concern (i.e. clinical importance) in observational studies. In the example presented above, where the incidence rates were 2.6% and 1.8% respectively, the RR was 1.44, meaning that there was a 44% increase in risk in persons exposed to the drug.

It should be noted that pharmacoepidemiological studies measure the association between exposure and outcome. Causality can be established only by the RCT. However, a high relative risk (RR) is suggestive of causation. Without a mechanistic explanation with biological plausibility, a causal relationship remains a hypothesis. For example, there is currently a debate as to whether third-generation oral contraceptives (i.e. containing desogestrel or gestodene) cause venous thromboembolism more often than second-generation oral contraceptives; the odds ratio (see section 4.2.5 for calculation of this value) was approximately 2 when compared with second-generation (containing levonorgestrel) oral contraceptives.[10-12] The relative risk or odds ratio is the minimum required to generate concern. It means that women exposed to third-generation drugs have twice the risk of developing venous thromboembolism than women exposed to second-generation drugs. However, when the low baseline risk is considered, little impact in terms of public health would be expected. The debate is further complicated by the findings of a nonsignificant odds ratio, which is an estimate of the RR (see section 4.2.5), of 0.4 for third- *versus* second-generation oral contraceptives against myocardial infarction.[53]

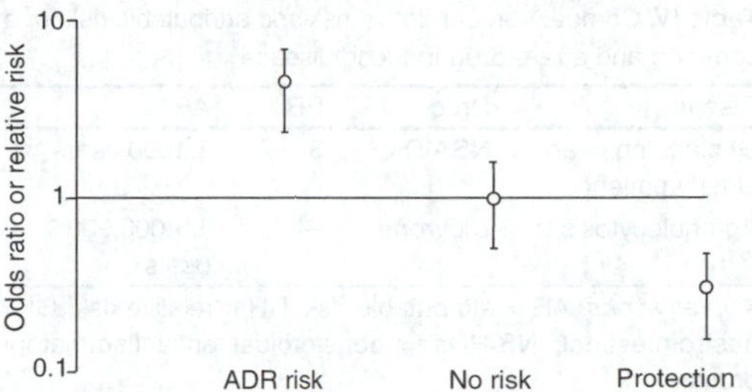


**Fig. 1.** Data presentation for pharmacoepidemiological studies. *Abbreviation:* ADR = adverse drug reaction.

Relative risk values of less than unity indicate that the drug is protective against the outcome of interest. For example, an RR of 0.5 means that exposed persons experience a 50% reduction in risk and an RR of 0.2 indicates an 80% reduction.

With all statistics, a measure of dispersion is always included to evaluate results. In the case of the RR, as well as related statistics such as the odds ratio (see section 4.2.5), the 95% confidence interval (CI) is presented. This means that the true value of the relative risk lies between the 2 limits 95% of the time. Intervals that cross unity (i.e. 1 lies within the interval) indicate that, statistically, there is less than a 5% probability of a real difference between the groups. The example in the centre of figure 1

**Table IV.** Comparison of relative risk and attributable risk for a common and a rare drug-induced disease

| Disease | Drug | RR | AR |
|---|---|---|---|
| GI bleeding in an elderly patient | NSAIDs | 3 | 1/1000 users |
| Agranulocytosis | Dipyrone | 24 | 1/1,000,000 users |

*Abbreviations:* AR = attributable risk; RR = relative risk; GI = gastrointestinal; NSAIDs = nonsteroidal anti-inflammatory drugs.

illustrates a nonsignificant result. Intervals that lie completely above the line (such as the example on the left in figure 1) indicate a significant adverse effect and those completely below the line (figure 1, example on the right) indicate a protective effect. Note that, due to the log scale, confidence intervals are asymmetrical.

In the example above, the RR is 1.44 with a 95% CI from 0.88 to 2.38. Since 1 is in the interval, the RR does not differ significantly from 1 (i.e. there is no difference between groups), so we can conclude that the drug is not associated with the outcome.

To evaluate the relevance or importance of the findings, both the frequency of occurrence and the seriousness of the outcome must be considered. A relatively small increase in risk of a disorder that occurs frequently may have a greater effect in terms of morbidity than a large relative risk for a disorder that occurs rarely. Table IV illustrates the problem. Nonsteroidal anti-inflammatory drugs (NSAIDs) are widely consumed and are associated with frequently occurring gastric irritation and bleeding. It has been calculated[3] that the modest increase in relative risk of 3 for an elderly person taking an NSAID to develop a gastrointestinal bleed translates to an attributable risk of about 1 per 1000 users.[3] Dipyrone, on the other hand, carries a high relative risk (RR = 24) for inducing agranulocytosis, but the attributable risk is only 1 per million users in a week since the background rate of agranulocytosis ($3\text{-}5 \times 10^{-6}$ per year) is so low. The clinician may be most interested in the RR associated with a particular exposure when treating a patient, whereas for health authorities, the attributable risk should be the basis for appropriate policy decisions.[3,35]

### 3.2 Time-Risk Relationships

The classic measure *incidence rate* implies that the risk is independent of time, i.e. the risk is the same for the first week, second week, etc., but this is rarely true in pharmacoepidemiology. In fact, the risk varies with time in a number of different ways that are dependent on the drug and/or the type of ADR that it produces. In figure 2, some different time-risk relationships are depicted. These phenomena demonstrate that exposure time must always be considered and the risk should ideally be expressed as a function of time. In practice, this may be difficult, since the type of function may not be known. To explore what model should be used, the exposure duration in a large number of cases can be investigated. The risk must at least be estimated for different time segments.

There are several mechanisms for the different shapes of the time-risk curves. Early adaptation of homeostatic mechanisms may explain first-dose or early symptoms. For immunological mechanisms, it takes a certain amount of time for the immune system to become activated and to synthesise antibodies. If there are susceptible subgroups in the population, depletion of these individuals will be seen as a decrease in population risk with increased exposure duration. Lastly, for fibrotic lesions as well as cancers there is usually an induction time of months to years.

For example, the use of oral contraceptives has been measured in person-years.[54] The relative risk (see section 3.1.2) for developing breast cancer was found to increase with the duration of exposure from 1.1 to 1.7 after 9 years ($p = 0.002$). The authors concluded that for women taking estrogens, the risk of developing breast cancer was increased only slightly (by 10% overall) and was time related, increasing to an excess (i.e. attributable) risk of 70% after more than 10 years of exposure.

## 4. Pharmacoepidemiological Methods

The methods used in pharmacoepidemiology involve both descriptive (i.e. qualitative) and analytical (i.e. quantitative) approaches. The former are generally aimed at evaluating how drugs are being prescribed and used, and may be used as part of a quality assurance programme. These programmes attempt to improve prescribing through medical audit and drug utilisation review (DUR). Qualitative methods attempt to provide explanations for drug-related events (i.e. ADRs). Tables V and VI list the applications of pharmacoepidemiology and the

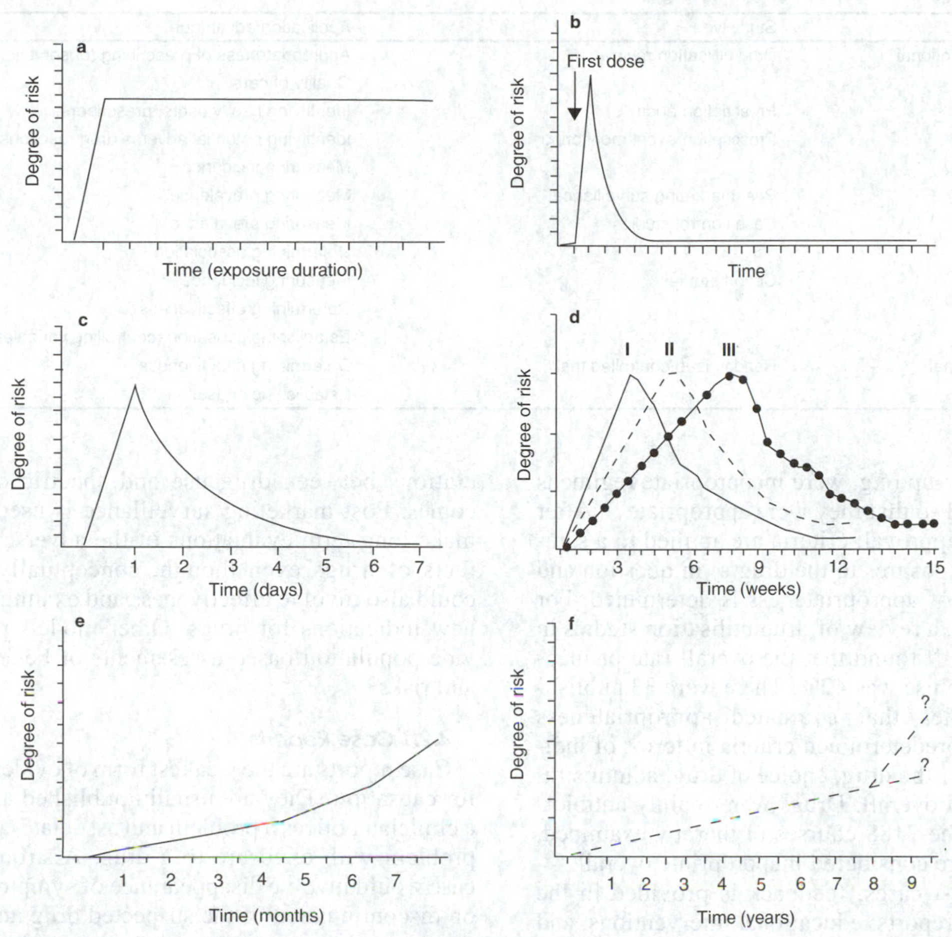


**Fig. 2.** Some examples of time-risk relationships. a) Risk constantly elevated. There are few good examples of this, except perhaps for the occurrence of seizures with tricyclic antidepressants. b) First-dose phenomena, e.g. hypotension with clonidine. c) Early adaptive phenomena, e.g. gastric mucosal microbleeds with aspirin (acetylsalicylic acid). d) I = type I allergic reactions; II = many other immunological reactions, e.g. Guillain-Barré syndrome with zimelidine, agranulocytosis with sulfasalazine; III = toxic metabolites. e) Fibrotic reactions, e.g. liver fibrosis with methotrexate. f) Cancers, e.g. breast cancer with oral contraceptives.

strengths and weaknesses of the different models used.

## 4.1 Qualitative Models: Drug Utilisation Review (DUR)

As mentioned before, the concept of drug utilisation review (DUR) was developed in hospitals to assess how well drugs were being used.[20] The usual approach is to identify a drug or class of drugs that warrants such examination. Drugs that have been the focus of the most attention have been those with high costs such as third-generation cefalosporins,[55] parenteral ranitidine[56] or biotechnology agents.[57,58] Reviews have also been performed on medicines that have widespread use (e.g. cardiac drugs or diuretics),[59] a narrow margin of safety (e.g. aminoglycosides),[60] or are prone to misuse or overuse (e.g. antibiotics).[61] Serum concentrations of drugs or indicators of toxicity (e.g. serum creatinine) have also been the focus of these reviews.[62]

Criteria of appropriateness are developed after analysis of the literature and from the input of clinical experts.[63] They are developed for different aspects of drug use including appropriateness of indication (i.e. is the drug right for this patient?), regimen (i.e. dose, interval, duration, route), monitoring (e.g. blood concentrations of drug, serum enzymes, kidney function),

**Table V.** Applications of pharmacoepidemiology

| Category | Study type | Application/advantage |
|---|---|---|
| Noninterventional | Drug utilisation review | Appropriateness of prescribing (observational) |
| | | Quality of care |
| | Prescription audit | Identifying heavy users, prescribers |
| | Prescription event monitoring | Identifying potential adverse drug reactions |
| | | Measuring incidence |
| | Post-marketing surveillance | Measuring prevalence |
| | Case control studies | Measuring prevalence |
| | | Determining association |
| | Cohort studies | Measuring incidence |
| | | Determining effectiveness |
| | | Establishing causation (controlling variables) |
| Interventional | Randomised controlled trial | Determining effectiveness |
| | | Establishing causation |

or follow-up (e.g. were inappropriate regimens modified so that they were appropriate?). After official approval, criteria are applied to a sample of exposures to the drug(s) in question and the rate of appropriateness is determined. For example, a review of drug utilisation studies in Canada[64] found that the overall rate of inappropriate use was 42%. There were 33 published studies that evaluated appropriateness against predetermined criteria in terms of indication for the drug, choice of drug, administration, and overall. Drugs were mainly antibiotics. Of the 2188 courses of therapy examined, 42% were considered inappropriate overall.

In most cases, feedback is provided in the form of reports, educational interventions, and (in problem cases) restrictions on use, with varying degrees of success.[65] Often, this approach is part of quality assurance programmes in hospitals.

## 4.2 Quantitative Models

Two types of drug effects are of interest in pharmacoepidemiology, i.e. safety and effectiveness. The ideal model for evaluation of effectiveness is the double-blind randomised controlled trial. However, for methodological, practical and economic reasons, this method is rarely applied in post-marketing drug surveillance. A number of nonexperimental methods have therefore been applied to marketed drugs. Quantitative models have been borrowed from the field of epidemiology and applied to drug use. All models are useful in some way, but each has its unique application, advantages, and disadvantages.

The aim is to assess drug use so that patterns may be examined to identify and quantify associations between drug use and specific outcomes. Post-marketing surveillance is used to make long term evaluations of the adverse effects of drugs even though, conceptually, it could also involve effectiveness and examining new indications for drugs. Other models provide population based assessments of benefits and risks.

### *4.2.1 Case Reports*

Case reports are the weakest form of evidence for causation. They are usually published after a clinician notices a problem and associates that problem with exposure to a drug. A stronger case would involve disappearance of symptoms on discontinuation of the suspected drug and a recurrence of symptoms on rechallenge. A case report can also be strengthened by relating ADRs to drug concentrations in the body.

Problems remain with this simplistic model in that other explanations for the findings must be ruled out before causation can be established. Often, that cannot be done, and interpretation of the importance of the report must be performed cautiously. The case remains a single episode among an unknown number of exposures.

This does not mean, however, that the case report is without value. In fact, pharmacoepidemiology began with the publishing of case reports.[2] These reports serve as an alerting mechanism for clinicians, investigators and others that a drug or group of drugs could produce a given effect. It prompts clinicians to be aware of the potential problem and to report other such occurrences. By identifying issues that warrant closer scrutiny, case reports stimulate research into such problems so that accurate risk estimates can be made. They may directly lead to hypothesis generation that can guide research.

In fact, most new serious ADRs have been detected by a collection of single case reports.

#### *4.2.2 Case Series*

The case series is a group or cluster of case reports that may be generated by a single clinician, group of clinicians, a hospital, pharmaceutical company, or (most importantly and, perhaps, most commonly) a regulatory agency. When series are reported, cases can be compared to note similarities between them so that a syndrome, if present, may be identified. This was the case with thalidomide-induced phocomelia and the fetal alcohol syndrome, where the same type of malformations occurred consistently among exposed (susceptible) individuals. Another example was the development of Guillain-Barré syndrome with the antidepressant drug zimelidine.[66]

Such reports allow a closer examination of the problem, but provide little insight into the rates of occurrence or extent of the problem. Causation may still be difficult to establish, but the likelihood of a causal relationship is enhanced if a consistent syndrome exists. Occasionally, case series may produce a false alarm when the relationship is strictly spurious. Such was the case with the antiemetic doxylamine/pyridoxine ('Bendectin'), where original case series suggested it was a teratogen, but this was not confirmed by analysis of all available data.[67]

#### *4.2.3 Surveys of Drug Use*

Historically, due to limitations in the availability of data, studies take a very simplistic approach and provide only crude utilisation data for large areas. Sales data are often used, as are numbers of prescriptions dispensed or total number of pills consumed. These have been referred to as 'drug use surveys',[68] also called 'single group cohort studies'. Examples are the lists of top 100 drugs used in a country that are produced by IMS and seen in publications such as *Scrip*. Such studies are interesting, but of limited use from a pharmacoepidemiological point of view, and find application largely in marketing.

Such sales and prescription data have been refined for pharmacoepidemiological purposes through the application of DDD and PDD methodologies (see sections 2.2.4 and 2.2.5), and combined with diagnostic information when relevant. Wide variations seen in the use of drugs such as antidiabetic, psychotropic and antihypertensive agents have been identified between as well as within countries, and are not fully explained by differences in disease prevalence.[14,18,19,69,70] Consumption of antihypertensive drugs among Nordic countries showed dramatically different patterns of use.[41] More recent studies indicate significant international differences in approaches to drug treatment of schizophrenia,[71] therapy for gastric ulcers (where low use of $H_2$-receptor antagonists was associated with a high incidence of gastric surgery) [Kiivet et al., personal communication],

**Table VI.** Strengths and weaknesses of different pharmacoepidemiological models

| Model | Strength | Weakness |
|---|---|---|
| Case report | Signal generation | No causation |
| Case series | Confirm relationship | No causation |
| Cross-sectional study | Identify correlating factors | Confounding variables |
| | Estimate of prevalence | |
| Longitudinal study | Trends over time detected | Confounding variables |
| | Can measure effect of events (before-after comparison) | |
| Nonexperimental comparison | Suggests causation | Confounding variables |
| Case control study | Measures strength of relationship | Causation not certain |
| | Least costly model | Controls a single variable |
| | Study multiple exposures | Recall bias |
| Cohort study | Measures incidence | Costly |
| | Measures strength of relationship | Time-consuming |
| | Controls multiple factors | |
| | Study multiple outcomes | |
| Randomised controlled trial | Establishes causation | Generalisability |
| | Controls all factors | Costly |
| | The only experimental model | Focus on a single factor |

and also in approaches to treatment of diabetes[72] and related to the degree of metabolic control.[73]

Utilisation data can also be monitored over time, noting changes in patterns. For example, a study comparing longitudinal usage data of psychotropic drugs in the UK[74] noted an upward overall trend over time. Of special interest was the effect of changes in legislation or reimbursement on drug use patterns. This type of model has been used to examine the effect of delisting antacids from the Ontario Drug Benefit Formulary in Canada.[75] The study found that the utilisation of prescription antiulcer drugs did not increase following the termination of reimbursement for prescribed antacids. Therefore, savings from delisting the latter were not offset by increases in alternative more costly drugs.

A further option is to compare drug utilisation data with outcome data for the same area over the same time period to identify possible associations. For example, the media attention to doxylamine/pyridoxine ('Bendectin') and its possible teratogenicity was examined in a follow-up ecological study.[76] Utilisation patterns of antinauseants (i.e. doxylamine/pyridoxine) were compared over time with patterns of hospitalisation for hyperemesis gravidarum and also to rates of birth defects in Canada. No relationships were found.

#### *4.2.4 Cross-Sectional Studies*

Cross-sectional studies involve determining the proportion of use of drugs in a defined population. Pioneering studies were conducted in Czechoslovakia and Sweden in the late 1960s,[77,78] and two databases of 17,000 (Jämtland) and 22,000 (Tierp) persons in Sweden have been developed for this purpose. One such study compared the heavy use of drugs in elderly patients in Canada and Sweden and found a high degree of concordance among the 20 most frequently prescribed drugs.[79] However, these databases are limited in size and cannot provide populations large enough for analytical pharmacoepidemiology. They may, however, be used to compare drug use between countries or different areas.[79] Studies such as this can identify differences in patterns and suggest closer scrutiny of the reasons for these differences.

#### *4.2.5 Cohort and Case Control Studies*

For analytical purposes, such as for strengthening or testing a hypothesis, cohort and case control study designs are the most powerful of pharmacoepidemiological tools. The choice between them depends on the question(s) to be answered, the frequency of the disease and the exposure(s) under study. In both designs, cases of the outcome under study are identified and exposure status is determined. In *cohort studies*, the procedure is to identify all, or a specified proportion, of patients who are, or have been, exposed to a certain medicine and compare the occurrence of the outcome under study among these individuals with the occurrence among patients who were not exposed but who are otherwise similar. In *case control studies*, the same cases are identified and their exposure status is determined but compared with the exposure status of a random sample of disease-free individuals from the source population. Thus, the main difference is that in case control studies, for reasons of efficiency, only a sample of the study base (source population) is recruited.

In cohort studies, incidence rates can be directly calculated and therefore both relative and attributable risk may be determined, but in case control studies only the relative risk can be directly estimated (through the odds ratio) and attributable risk must be derived indirectly. Another practical difference is that a cohort study directly gives information on a number of different outcomes for one or a group of drugs, while a case control study is more suitable if the risk of one or few outcomes is to be compared for many drugs. Both designs can be prospective (cases are identified as they develop) or retrospective (cases have already occurred).

As an example, the relationship between oral contraceptive use and the development of breast cancer was examined in a cohort of 23,244 women.[54] There was a relative risk of 1.1 (95% CI 1.0 to 1.3) when compared with non-exposed women from the same area. The mean follow-up time in this study was 5.7 years. In this cohort study, the authors measured the cumulative incidence and incidence rate of cancer. They found that there were 253 cases in 23,244 women, which equals a cumulative incidence of 1.09%. Since there were 133,375 woman-years of exposure to estrogens, the incidence rate was 253/133,375 or 1.90 per 1000 woman-years of exposure. This latter value was compared with the rate of 1.67 per 1000 woman-years in a group of unexposed women who were otherwise similar. Thus, the authors were able to directly measure incidence and excess (i.e. attributable) risk.

One disadvantage is that cohort studies require large (often huge) numbers of patients. It is difficult to recruit and monitor large numbers of patients, and many are expected to drop out over time. Large cohort studies are costly and take a long time to generate results. Often, variables change over time so that results from a longitudinal study may not be relevant because of these changes (e.g. the study drugs are no longer used in general practice).

The advantage of a case control design is that rare events can be studied at a lower cost. For example, a case control study design[80] was used to evaluate the relationship between Guillain-Barré syndrome and exposure to a wide range of drugs in 146 cases and 291 controls. A positive relationship was found with bacterial vaccines, with an odds ratio of 8.2.

#### Calculation of Odds Ratio

The odds ratio (OR) is an estimate of the RR. Figuratively, it may be expressed as:

OR = AD/BC

where the symbols are as defined in table III and section 3.1. The OR and RR are interpreted in the same way and are identical if there is a large number of observations, but they can diverge considerably if the numbers of observations are smaller. For example, 1 study[81] had values of A = 12, B = 9, C = 184, and D = 398. It produced an odds ratio of 2.88 (95% CI 1.19 to 6.97), but the relative risk found with the same data was 1.81 (95% CI 1.23 to 2.67). In this case, the results are reasonably similar (i.e. both are statistically significant), but the discrepancy warrants caution in interpretation of the results. In the example given in section 3.1.1, the relative risk was 1.44 (95% CI 0.88 to 2.38). Since the number of observations was reasonably large, the odds ratio was a very good approximation at 1.46, with only a slightly wider confidence interval of 0.87 to 2.43.

The case control approach has, however, a number of problems associated with the data collection. Missing data are always a problem. For example, hospital charts often do not record outcomes. If patients are interviewed, there may be recall bias. This is especially true in researching birth defects.[82] It has been found that women who give birth to malformed children spend a great deal of time thinking about possible causes for the defect, and hence have better recall than mothers of normal offspring (see chapter 2, section 1.3.2). Some researchers have found a partial solution to the recall bias problem. Assuming that a drug would cause a specific defect or syndrome, they matched neonates born with specific defects with those having other defects known to be caused by factors other than drugs. In this way, the influence of recall bias was minimised.[83]

#### *4.2.6 Case-Cohort Studies*

A pharmacoepidemiological design that has recently been employed is a hybrid of cohort and case control studies. A series of cases is identified and exposure status is determined, as in a case control study. As a comparison group, a cohort of exposed individuals is used, and their outcomes are determined.[84] For example, the risk of breast cancer from estrogens in 2 groups of women was examined in one study.[54] The first series included women who had developed cancer and were sent a questionnaire to determine exposure status. The second group consisted of a cohort of exposed women selected from a computerised database with linkages to a cancer registry. The data from the cases were compared with the data from the cohort and a statistically significant relationship was found.

The advantage of the case-cohort approach is that very rare phenomena may be examined (as in a case control study), but there is more statistical power due to the large cohort used in the comparison group. Disadvantages are similar to other models, with an added problem that the statistics are somewhat more complex to calculate.

### 4.3 Meta-Analysis Models

Meta-analysis is the combination of results from a group of studies to arrive at a summary (overall) estimate of effect (i.e. effectiveness of a drug or risk of an adverse reaction). It involves a variety of methods for aggregating results and may be applied to randomised controlled trials, case control or cohort studies. A variety of effect sizes may be used to produce summary results. The odds ratio is commonly used with epidemiological studies, as is the risk (or rate) difference,[67,85] which is identical to the attributable risk (see sect. 3.1.1). Methods have also been presented[13] for calculating the summary relative risk from a series of cohort studies.

These techniques may be used to resolve controversies when there are conflicting results in the literature, by comparing the magnitude of differences between treatments with respect to effectiveness or adverse reaction risk. The Prospective Studies Collaboration[86] has used meta-analysis to examine the relationship between cholesterol concentrations and the occurrence of stroke in 450,000 patients. Another application is to provide summary estimates of risk or effectiveness that may be used as inputs into pharmacoeconomic analyses or to verify therapeutic guidelines.[87]

When using meta-analysis techniques on observational data, extreme caution must be applied in both performing the analysis and interpreting the results, since the studies are often much more heterogeneous than data from randomised controlled trials.

## 5. Systems for Studying Drug Effects in Populations

### 5.1 Spontaneous Reporting

Most countries in the developed world (and some developing countries) have instituted spontaneous reporting systems to record suspected adverse drug reactions (ADRs). Clinicians are encouraged (or, in some countries, mandated) to report any and all reactions that they believe may be associated with drug use. Usually, attention is focused on new drugs and serious ADRs, the reporting of which is mandatory in some countries.[1,88-90]

In 1968, the WHO established a system for collecting reports of ADRs. It now has centres in 45 countries that have documented 1.4 million cases of possible drug-related events. This database has been of benefit in signalling possible new ADRs.[48] Recent examples include tachycardia from cisapride[91] and drug-induced pancreatitis.[92]

These systems alert clinicians and regulators to possible drug-related problems. They provide an early warning signal that indicates where attention should be given. For example, they can identify series of similar ADRs that can be further investigated. The systems are generally inexpensive and simple to operate and do not interfere with clinical practice to any great extent.

On the other hand, it is difficult to establish causation using these systems. The information obtained is often incomplete, unverified, and inadequate. Spontaneous reports have proven to be excellent sources for identifying new ADRs, but the voluntary nature means that many are never reported. Because under-reporting is common, the true extent of the problem can never be ascertained. Moreover, under-reporting gives room for selective reporting, which can lead to bias when ADR rates for different drugs are compared.

### 5.2 Prescription Event Monitoring

Prescription event monitoring (PEM) was developed in the UK[93-95] at the Drug Safety Research Unit to study large cohorts of drug users. Unlike voluntary reporting systems or programmes in hospitals, PEM is a method for generating and testing hypotheses about ADRs in defined populations of users. PEM has the advantage of providing estimates of the incidence of events over a defined follow-up period. The Prescription Pricing Authority identified patients who have been prescribed monitored drugs, which includes virtually all new chemical entities. Criteria include:

- A new chemical entity
- A new pharmacological principle
- Predicted widespread use
- Suspected problems
- Identified but unquantified risks.

Information on the first 5000 to 18,000 prescriptions for that drug are then obtained from the National Health Service. Prescribers are contacted with a questionnaire to determine subsequent events or clinical outcomes. Experiences with the drugs can then be examined and the incidence of various events can be estimated. Comparisons have been made between periods before and after drug use.[96] One example examined in this way is the occurrence of jaundice with erythromycin estolate.[97]

In 1965, New Zealand established a surveillance system that had an academic, rather than governmental or regulatory, focus.[98] The Medicines Adverse Reactions Committee (MARC) is responsible for monitoring ADRs through a spontaneous reporting system. Pharmacists participate in monitoring large cohorts for 3 to 4 years. The MARC sends follow-up questionnaires to physicians to determine outcomes. For selected drugs, they have introduced an intensified spontaneous reporting system. Physicians are requested to report all 'adverse events' occurring in patients receiving listed drugs. Events include death from any cause, deterioration of a pre-existing condition, referral to a specialist, hospital admission, changes in laboratory values, possible drug interactions, and fetal malformations. In a cohort of 3926 patients taking perhexiline and 2837 taking labetalol, 25% of all patients discontinued taking their drug.

ADRs were the reason for stopping in 20 and 43% for each drug, respectively.

### 5.3 Post-Marketing Surveillance

Post-marketing surveillance studies were originally designed to detect and quantify adverse reactions of drugs after entry into the market. Most often, they are conducted by the pharmaceutical manufacturer and are performed as a single group follow-up (cohort) study where, by tradition, a cohort of 5000 to 10,000 patients are followed during some months to years. One of the first such studies was a large follow-up of patients who were prescribed cimetidine when it was a new medicine.[99] At first, there appeared to be an association with gastric cancer before it was determined that the drug had been prescribed to treat what were later found to be the early symptoms of cancer. This example demonstrates one of the many problems of interpretation of the results of a cohort study without a comparison group.

It is essential that legitimate post-marketing studies that seek scientific information be distinguished from those intended for marketing or promotional efforts.[100] The American Society for Clinical Pharmacology[101] has issued a position statement that clearly delineates the features of a legitimate study. All companies are mandated to maintain records of ADRs reported in association with the use of their products and make the information available to drug regulatory agencies, clinicians and researchers.

### 5.4 Record Linkage Systems

In 1946, H.L. Dunn wrote, 'Each person in the world creates a book of life. This book starts with birth and ends with death. Its pages are made of the records of the principal events in life. Record linkage is the name given to the process of assembling the pages of this book into a volume'.[102] With the advent of computer technology, record linkage systems have been heralded as the ideal approach for researching and monitoring the effects of drug use. Providing useful information requires a diagnosis, patient information, and outcomes. Table VII lists some of the databases available for pharmacoepidemiological research. These databases can provide readily accessible information on thousands of patients, thereby reducing the time required for examining relationships between drug exposures and outcomes. All 3 types of studies (i.e. cohort, case control, and case-cohort) can be performed using record linkage databases.

**Table VII.** Examples of computerised databases used for pharmacoepidemiological research

| Database | Location |
|---|---|
| General Practice Research Database (formerly VAMP) | UK |
| Group Health Cooperative of Puget Sound | Seattle, US |
| Kaiser Permanente | California, US |
| Medicaid | US (several states) |
| Odense | Denmark |
| Ontario Drug Benefit | Ontario, Canada |
| Saskatchewan | Saskatchewan, Canada |

A study in which data from a linked database were compared with a large clinical trial demonstrated the equivalence of the two approaches in reporting adverse events.[103] This evidence supports the use of such linked systems as a cost-effective alternative to clinical megatrials. For example, in the UK, the *General Practice Research Database* (formerly the VAMP System) provides data on 4.4 million patients and 680 practices, including 2333 general practitioners.[104] Complete information is available for each patient available, including the medical and drug history. Researchers have investigated arrhythmias from terodiline, suicides after antidepressant use, and liver disease occurring with NSAIDs.

Database research is not however, without its drawbacks and limitations. In several cases, research produced results that were often inaccurate or led to incorrect conclusions.[105] Problems existed in establishing actual exposure to drugs or the duration of use. Some databases have inadequate numbers of patients to allow for examination of rare events and some were designed for the sole purpose of claims reimbursement and thus have minimal patient information available.[106]

Often, with a patient identifier, patient records may be linked with other databases so that a relationship may be determined between drug exposure and patient outcomes. Examples are records of hospitalisation, medical records (e.g. surgery performed, infections developed, etc.), pharmacy prescriptions, death records, or birth defect registries. In using record linkage databases, it is vital to have a validation process built in to each study to verify the accuracy of the data.

*Medicaid* was developed in the US to pay for healthcare, including drugs, required by the poor.[106,107] It operates throughout the country, paying for prescribed drugs for millions of recipients. Its advantage is that it contains a great deal of drug-related information on millions of people so that even very rare phenomena may be examined. Data are readily accessible, while patient confidentiality is maintained. On the other hand, generalisability to non-Medicaid patients may be a problem. As well, people may leave the system, resulting in incomplete records. A further problem with databases in general is in the validity of the data due to the potential for entry errors.[106] One example of research from Medicaid was a validation study reported by Carson et al.[107] They examined Medicaid claims of 414 patients who had an ICD-9 (International Classification of Disease) code consistent with acute hepatitis. When they retrieved patient charts and compared the data, they found that 89.4% of the cases were confirmed.

The Canadian province of *Saskatchewan* has produced a fairly complete computerised database for almost all of its residents (population about 1 million).[23] The database is able to access data on prescription drugs received, hospital services rendered, physician services and laboratory testing, and contains a cancer registry. Many cross-sectional and longitudinal studies have been conducted using this database. For example, Suissa et al.[108] examined the relationship between β-agonist inhaler use and death in a large cohort of these patients.

A unique programme that applies the methods of pharmacoepidemiology is the *Motherisk* programme at the Hospital For Sick Children in Toronto (see also chapter 2).[32,33] It is both a counselling service providing information on drug (as well as other) exposures in pregnancy and a research programme. Women who contact the service about drug exposures in pregnancy are monitored in 2 ways. Those who are perceived to be at risk due to the nature of the exposure are invited to attend a special clinic where a detailed history is taken. Periodic follow-up is then routine so that outcomes, some of which are long term, can be documented. Others are contacted by telephone after delivery of the neonate to ascertain the outcome. Results are then compared with matched controls.[32] The group has published more than 100 reports on drugs and other exposures (e.g. solvents, radiation, electric shock) in pregnancy (see also chapter 2).

In Sweden, a register has been established that contains information on drug exposures in all women participating in the official programme of pregnancy follow-up. These data from about 110,000 pregnancies per year can be linked to outcome data in the same region, to the birth register for immediate outcomes, or to the malformation register.

## 6. Advantages and Disadvantages of Pharmacoepidemiological Models

### 6.1 Advantages

Pharmacoepidemiological methods can be used in many cases where other models cannot. They allow examination of such groups as elderly, pregnant or paediatric patients, and those having concomitant diseases or using other drugs. They can be used to study people over time and the effects that drugs have on these people.

These approaches can generate effectiveness data, i.e. they can examine drug use under everyday conditions, rather than the artificial environment of a randomised controlled trial. The effects of concomitant diseases or drug use can be examined as can the effects of varying rates of adherence to prescribed treatment regimens.

These types of studies can be used to alert clinicians, manufacturers, and regulators of potential problems. They act as signal generators to direct further research and indicate new areas to explore.

Models allow for comparison of drug use patterns between areas, allowing for the identification of drug-related problems. Excessive prescribing or abuse can be identified, sometimes with minimal information. Programmes can be used for monitoring drug use by healthcare providers, health authorities, or in the regulation of clinical practice.

Pharmacoepidemiological models have a great deal of flexibility in that they can use data from a variety of sources. This includes patient records and charts, patient interviews and computerised databases.

### 6.2 Disadvantages

Data derived from pharmacoepidemiological studies are mostly nonexperimental and tend to be correlational; hence, causation is difficult to establish. A number of biases and confounding variables can threaten the validity of pharmacoepidemiological data, and have been categorised[109] as selection bias, information bias and confounding. *Selection bias* is related to recruitment of study participants or loss to follow-up. *Information bias* relates to the accuracy of data collected. *Confounding* refers to correlative factors that make causation by the drug being investigated unclear. Techniques are available to deal with issues of bias, and must be incorporated into the research design.[109]

Often, there may be confounding by indication, whereby patients are selected because of the severity of their disease and are then observed to have a higher rate of a specific outcome than comparison groups. Thus, these studies may make it impossible to know whether the difference was due to the treatment or the disease. Solutions include the stratification of disease severity, restriction of patient types, or (best) when possible, an RCT. The recent studies and debate on the possible difference in thrombophilic tendency related to oral contraceptives with different progestagens provides a wide variety of possible problems with biases in observational studies.

Some models (e.g. cohort studies) still require huge sample sizes to provide meaningful information, are expensive, and may take many years to complete. Researchers have documented recall bias in retrospective studies (i.e. when patients are interviewed), and in retrolective studies (when charts are read or databases used). Incomplete records and missing data are also common problems. In rare diseases, the sample sizes are often very small, with anecdotal information, making confirmation of results difficult.

## 7. The Future of Pharmacoepidemiology

One problem with the evaluation of ADRs is that a variety of definitions and approaches exist. Many researchers and clinicians have suggested the standardisation of terminology.[48] To this end, the Council for International Organizations of Medical Sciences (CIOMS) has established a working group.[110] In the first project, a routine form for the expedited reporting of single cases was developed. The second project set standards for international reporting of periodical drug safety update summaries. The third project developed guidelines for preparing core clinical-safety information on drugs.[49] This group is continuing to work as a think tank for the International Committee on Harmonisation (ICH) on procedures for the standardisation and harmonisation of issues in the field of drug safety. Presently, guidelines for benefit-risk evaluations are being developed.

Verification of new ADRs is essential, and methods must address that issue. It has been suggested[93,94] that data be collected on at least the first 10,000 patients exposed to a new chemical entity and that follow-up be conducted on as many of these patients as possible. This number would permit the identification of all events that occurred in 1 in 1000 exposed individuals (or more frequently), while allowing for dropouts and losses to follow-up. A system of continuous case control surveillance of rare drug-induced diseases that most often lead to drug withdrawal (e.g. blood dyscrasias, liver damage, etc.) has been suggested.[90] This system is now being tested in Sweden and parts of other European countries with the help of a grant from the European Economic Commission.

Special attention should be paid to developing countries and their special problems (see chapter 34), including parasitic diseases, infections, and drug resistance.[111] A relatively unexplored area is that of herbal medicines and traditional remedies. The WHO has just begun a project to examine the safety of these products, which are widely used but little understood.[112]

It appears that pharmacoepidemiology is destined to expand. It is anticipated that there will be a great deal of development of new techniques for research design and statistical analysis. This field offers the best approach to monitoring the use of new drugs released on the market and will probably find application in that area. The most promising application for pharmacoepidemiology is in providing the basis for pharmacoeconomic analyses, especially in modelling and forecasting cost effectiveness in different countries.

As is evident from the above examples, there are many methods that can be used in pharmacoepidemiological studies. No single method will cover all needs; each method has its advantages and disadvantages. Evaluating the effects of drug use (both beneficial and adverse) requires a comprehensive approach that combines the various available methods. Such an approach will need to include descriptive surveys of patterns of drug utilisation, means of identifying possible new and rare ADRs (spontaneous reporting, case control and cohort surveillance), and instruments for testing hypotheses.[14]

## Further Reading

Strom BL. Pharmacoepidemiology, 2nd ed. New York: John Wiley & Sons, 1994

Hartzema AG, Porta MS, Tilson HH. Pharmacoepidemiology: an introduction, 2nd ed. Cincinnati: Harvey Whitney Books, 1991

## References


1. Strom BL. Pharmacoepidemiology. 2nd ed. New York: John Wiley & Sons, 1994
2. McBride WG. Thalidomide and congenital abnormalities. Lancet 1961; 2: 1358
3. Lee D, Bergman U. The quantification of drug risks in practice. In: Dukes MNG, editor. Drug utilization studies: methods and uses. Copenhagen: World Health Organization, 1993: 79-95
4. Inman W, Pearce G. Prescriber profile and post-marketing surveillance. Lancet 1993; 342: 658-61
5. Herbst AL, Ulfelder H, Poskanzer DC. Adenocarcinoma of the vagina: association of maternal stilbestrol therapy with tumor appearance in young women. New England Journal of Medicine 1971; 284: 878-81
6. Stern RS. When a uniquely effective drug is teratogenic: the case of isotretinoin. New England Journal of Medicine 1989; 320: 1007-9
7. Editorial. Triazolam's status in the European community. Lancet 1991; 338: 1586-7
8. Teicher MH, Gold C, Cole J. Emergence of intense suicidal preoccupation during fluoxetine treatment. American Journal of Psychiatry 1990; 147: 207-10
9. Crane J, Flatt A, Jackson R, et al. Prescribed fenoterol and death from asthma in New Zealand 1981-83. Lancet 1989; 1: 917-22
10. World Health Organization Collaborative Study of Cardiovascular Disease and Steroid Hormone Contraception. Venous thromboembolic disease and combined oral contraception: results of international multicentre case-control study. Lancet 1995; 346: 1575-82
11. World Health Organization Collaborative Study of Cardiovascular Disease and Steroid Hormone Contraception. Effect of different progestagens in low oestrogen oral contraceptives with differing progestagen components. Lancet 1995; 346: 1582-8
12. Spitzer WO, Lewis MA, Heinemann LAJ, et al. Third generation oral contraceptives and risk of venous thromboembolic disorders: an international case-control study. British Medical Journal 1996; 312: 83-8
13. Hartzema AG, Porta MS, Tilson HH. Pharmacoepidemiology: an introduction. 2nd ed. Cincinnati: Harvey Whitney Books, 1991
14. Lee D, Bergman U. Studies of drug utilization. In: Strom BL, editor. Pharmacoepidemiology. 2nd ed. New York: John Wiley & Sons, 1994: 379-93
15. World Health Organization Expert Committee. The selection of essential drugs. Geneva: World Health Organization, 1977
16. Bergman U, Elmes P, Halse M, et al. The measurement of drug consumption: drugs for diabetes in Northern Ireland, Norway and Sweden. European Journal of Clinical Pharmacology 1975; 8: 83-89
17. Bergman U, Sjöqvist F. Measurement of drug utilization in Sweden: methodological and clinical implications. Acta Medica Scandinavica 1984; Suppl. 683: 15-22
18. Bergman U, Grisson A, Wahba AHW, et al., editors. Studies in drug utilization: methods and applications. WHO Regional Publications, European Series No. 8. Copenhagen: World Health Organization, 1979
19. Dukes MNG, editor. Drug utilization studies: methods and uses. WHO Regional Publications, European Series No. 45. Copenhagen: World Health Organization, 1993
20. Brodie DC. Drug utilization review: planning. Hospitals 1972; 46: 103-12
21. Crooks J. Methods of 'audit' in drug use. In: Duchene-Marullaz P, editor. Advances in pharmacology and therapeutics. Proceedings of the 7th international congress of pharmacology, Paris 1978. Oxford: Pergamon Press, 1979: 189-95
22. Anonymous. Auditing drug therapy: approaches towards rationality at reasonable costs. Stockholm: Swedish Pharmaceutical Press, 1992
23. Strand LM. Drug epidemiology resources: the Saskatchewan data base. Drug Information Journal 1985; 19: 253-5
24. Strom BL, Morse ML. Use of computerized databases to survey drug utilization in relation to diagnoses. Acta Medica Scandinavica 1988; Suppl. 721: 13-20
25. Soumerai SB, Lipton HL. Evaluating and improving physician prescribing. In: Strom BL, editor. Pharmacoepidemiology. 2nd ed. New York: John Wiley & Sons, 1994: 396-412
26. Sjöqvist F. Auditing drug therapy, why and how? Proceedings from an International Symposium: auditing drug therapy - approaches towards rationality at reasonable costs. Stockholm: Swedish Pharmaceutical Press, 1992; 28-34
27. McGavock H. Peer-review audit of GP prescribing in N Ireland: techniques and results. In: Auditing drug therapy: approaches towards rationality at reasonable costs. Stockholm: Swedish Pharmaceutical Press, 1992: 93-103
28. de Vries T. Auditing drug therapy through peer review; the Dutch experience. In: Auditing drug therapy: approaches towards rationality at reasonable cost. Stockholm: Swedish Pharmaceutical Press, 1992: 104-9
29. Garattini S, Garattini L. Pharmaceutical prescriptions in four European countries. Lancet 1993; 342: 1191-2
30. Laporte JR, Porta M, Capella D. Drug utilization studies: a tool for determining the effectiveness of drug use. British Journal of Clinical Pharmacology 1983; 16: 301-4
31. Inman W. 30 years in post-marketing surveillance. In: Inman W, editor. Drug Safety Research Unit PEM News. Southampton: Hamble Valley Press, 1993: 19-60
32. Koren G, Feldman Y, Shear N. Motherisk: a new approach to drug/chemical teratogenicity. Veterinary and Human Toxicology 1986; 28: 563-5
33. Koren G, MacLeod SM. Monitoring and avoiding drug and chemical teratogenicity. Canadian Medical Association Journal 1986; 135: 1079-81
34. Sannerstedt R, Lundborg P, Danielsson BR, et al. Drugs during pregnancy: an issue of risk classification and information to prescribers. Drug Safety 1996; 14: 69-77
35. Anderson GM, Spitzer WO, Weinstein MC, et al. Benefits, risks, and costs of prescription drugs: a scientific basis for evaluating policy options. Clinical Pharmacology and Therapeutics 1990; 48: 111-9

36. Bergman U, Wiholm BE. Drug-related problems causing admission to a medical clinic. European Journal of Clinical Pharmacology 1981; 20: 193-200
37. Einarson TR. Drug related hospital admissions. Annals of Pharmacotherapy 1993; 27: 832-40
38. Isacsson G, Holmgren P, Wasserman D, et al. Use of antidepressants among people committing suicide in Sweden. British Medical Journal 1994; 308: 506-9
39. Rothman KJ. Modern epidemiology. Boston: Little, Brown and Company, 1986
40. Haaijer-Ruskamp FM, Dukes MNG. The economic aspects of drug use. In: Dukes MNG, editor. Drug utilization studies: methods and uses. Copenhagen: World Health Organization Regional Publications, 1993: 125-45
41. Baksaas I. Patterns of drug utilization - national and international aspects: antihypertensive drugs. Acta Medica Scandinavica 1984; Suppl. 683: 59-66
42. Bergman U, Christenson I, Janson B, et al. Auditing hospital drug utilization by means of defined daily doses per bed-days. European Journal of Clinical Pharmacology 1980; 17: 183-7
43. Anonymous. Guidelines for DDD. Oslo: World Health Organization Collaborating Centre for Drug Statistics Methodology (PO Box 100, Veitvet N-0518, Oslo 5, Norway; Fax: +4722-169818), 1991
44. Sjöstedt S, Levin P, Kager L, et al. Hospital and catchment area antibiotic utilization and bacterial sensitivity in primary infections following gastric surgery in Huddinge, Sweden. European Journal of Clinical Pharmacology 1990; 39: 211-6
45. Nordenstam I, Wennberg M, Kristoferson K. Svensk Läkemedels-Statistik. Stockholm: Apoteksbolaget, 1995
46. Isacsson G, Redfors I, Wasserman D, et al. Choice of antidepressants: questionnaire survey of psychiatrists and general practitioners in two areas of Sweden. British Medical Journal 1994; 309: 1546-9
47. Kaufman DW, Kelly JP, Levy M, et al. The drug etiology of agranulocytosis and aplastic anemia. Monographs in Epidemiology and Biostatistics, Volume 18. Oxford: Oxford University Press, 1991
48. Edwards IR, Biriell C. Harmonisation in pharmacovigilance. Drug Safety 1994; 10: 93-102
49. Report of the CIOMS Working Group III. Guidelines for preparing core clinical-safety information on drugs. Geneva: CIOMS, 1995
50. Naranjo C, Busto U, Sellers E. A method for estimating the probability of adverse drug reactions. Clinical Pharmacology and Therapeutics 1981; 30: 239-45
51. Karch FE, Lasagna L. Adverse drug reactions. A critical review. Journal of the American Medical Association 1975; 234: 1236-41
52. Laupacis A, Sackett DL, Roberts RS. An assessment of clinically useful measures of the consequences of treatment. New England Journal of Medicine 1988; 318: 1728-33
53. Lewis MA, Spitzer WO, Heinemann LAJ, et al. Third generation oral contraceptives and risk of myocardial infarction: an international case-control study. British Medical Journal 1996; 312: 88-90
54. Bergkvist L, Adami HO, Persson I, et al. The risk of breast cancer after estrogen and estrogen-progestin replacement. New England Journal of Medicine 1989; 321: 293-7
55. Strong DK, Dupuis LL, Domaratzki JL. Pharmacist intervention in prescribing of cefuroxime for pediatric patients. American Journal of Hospital Pharmacy 1990; 47: 1350-3
56. Santora J, Kitrenos JG, Green ER. Pharmacist intervention program focused on IV ranitidine therapy. American Journal of Hospital Pharmacy 1990; 47: 1346-9
57. Krichbaum DW, Grabavoy G, Finley RC, et al. Use of alteplase for myocardial infarction in two community hospitals. American Journal of Hospital Pharmacy 1990; 47: 1535-40
58. Nishimura LY, Shane RR, Saltiel E. Prospective physician review of orders for colony stimulating factor. American Journal of Hospital Pharmacy 1992; 49: 2722-7
59. Bjornson DC, Rector TS, Daniels CE, et al. Impact of a drug use review program intervention on prescribing after publication of a randomized clinical trial. American Journal of Hospital Pharmacy 1990; 47: 1541-6
60. Nightingale C, Chaffee BW, Colvin CL, et al. Retrospective evaluation of vancomycin use in a university hospital. American Journal of Hospital Pharmacy 1987; 44: 1807-9
61. Menczel E, Hershkovitz A, Levy D, et al. Inpatient antimicrobial use in two hospitals near Tel Aviv. American Journal of Hospital Pharmacy 1992; 49: 659-63
62. Jackevicius C, Einarson TR. Utilization review of serum digoxin levels at Toronto General Hospital. Canadian Journal of Hospital Pharmacy 1990; 43: 273-80
63. Knapp DA. Development of criteria for drug utilization review. Clinical Pharmacology and Therapeutics 1991; 50: 600-2
64. Einarson TR, Segal HJ, Mann JL. Drug utilization in Canada: a literature analysis. Journal of Social and Administrative Pharmacy 1989; 6: 69-82
65. Soumerai SB, McLaughlin TJ, Avorn J. Improving drug prescribing in primary care. Millbank Quarterly 1989; 67: 268-317
66. Fagius J, Osterman PO, Siden Å, et al. Guillain-Barré syndrome following zimelidine treatment. Journal of Neurology, Neurosurgery and Psychiatry 1985; 48: 65-9
67. Einarson TR, Leeder JS, Koren G. A method for meta-analysis of epidemiologic studies. Drug Intelligence and Clinical Pharmacy 1988; 22: 813-24
68. Rosman AW, Sawyer WT. Population-based drug use evaluation. Topics in Hospital Pharmacy Management 1988; 8(2): 76-92
69. Sjöqvist F, Agenäs I, editors. Drug utilization studies: implications for medical care. Acta Medica Scandinavica 1984; Suppl. 683: 7-9
70. Kiivet RA, Bergman U, Sjöqvist F. The use of drugs in Estonia compared to the Nordic countries. European Journal of Clinical Pharmacology 1992; 42: 511-5
71. Kiivet RA, Llerena A, Dahl ML, et al. Patterns of drug treatment of schizophrenic patients in Estonia, Spain, and Sweden. British Journal of Clinical Pharmacology 1995; 40: 467-76
72. Groop PH, Klaukka T, Reunanen A, et al. Antidiabetic drugs in the Nordic countries. Reasons for variation in their use. (English summary). Helsinki: Folkpensionsanstaltens Publikationer ML105, 1991
73. Stålhammar J, Bergman U, Boman K, et al. Metabolic control in diabetic subjects in three Swedish areas with high, medium, and low sales of antidiabetic drugs. Diabetes Care 1991; 14: 12-19
74. King DJ, Griffiths K. Patterns in drug utilization - national and international aspects: psychoactive drugs

1966-80. Acta Medica Scandinavica 1984; Suppl. 683: 71-7

75. Bradley CA, Einarson TR. Impact of delisting of antacids from the Ontario Drug Benefit Formulary on prescription anti-ulcer drug usage. Poster presented at the 11th International Conference on Pharmacoepidemiology, Stockholm, Sweden, AU 27-30, 1995
76. Neutel CI, Johansen HL. Measuring drug effectiveness by default: the case of Bendectin. Canadian Journal of Public Health 1995; 86: 66-70
77. Bergman U. Pharmacoepidemiologic perspectives. Journal of Clinical Epidemiology 1992; 45: 313-7
78. Boethius G. Approaches to assessing the rationality of drug usage in a developed country. Acta Medica Scandinavica 1988; Suppl. 721: 21-6
79. Sitar DS, Boethius G, Bergman U, et al. Prescribing patterns for elderly community-dwelling heavy medicinal drug users in Manitoba, Canada and Jämtland, Sweden. Journal of Clinical Epidemiology 1995; 48: 825-31
80. Stricker BHC, van der Klauw MM, Ottervanger JP, et al. A case-control study of drugs and other determinants as potential causes of Guillain-Barré syndrome. Journal of Clinical Epidemiology 1994; 47: 1203-10
81. Golding J, Vivian S, Baldwin JA. Maternal anti-nauseants and clefts of lip and palate. Human Toxicology 1983; 2: 63-73
82. Feldman Y, Koren G, Mattice D, et al. Determinants of recall and recall bias in studying drug and chemical exposure in pregnancy. Teratology 1989; 40: 37-45
83. Mitchell AA, Schwingl PJ, Rosenberg L, et al. Birth defects related to Bendectin use in pregnancy I: oral clefts and cardiac defects. Journal of the American Medical Association 1981; 245: 2311-14
84. Feldmann U. Design and analysis of drug safety studies, with special reference to sporadic use and acute adverse reactions. Journal of Clinical Epidemiology 1993; 46: 237-44
85. DerSimonian R, Laird N. Meta-analysis in clinical trials. Controlled Clinical Trials 1986; 7: 177-88
86. Prospective Studies Collaboration. Cholesterol, diastolic blood pressure, and stroke: 13000 strokes in 450000 people in 45 prospective cohorts. Lancet 1995; 346: 1647-53
87. Rovers JP, Ilersich AL, Einarson TR. Meta-analysis of parenteral clindamycin dosing regimens. Annals of Pharmacotherapy 1995; 29: 852-8
88. Faich GA. Adverse drug reaction monitoring. New England Journal of Medicine 1986; 314: 1589-92
89. Wiholm BE, Olsson S, Moore N, et al. Spontaneous reporting systems outside the United States. In: Strom BL, editor. Pharmacoepidemiology. 2nd ed. New York: John Wiley & Sons, 1994: 139-55
90. Wiholm BE. Postmarketing surveillance of ADRs by spontaneous reporting and register data: the Swedish approach. In: Strom BL, Velo G, editors. Drug epidemiology and post marketing surveillance. New York: Plenum Press, 1992: 9-20
91. Olsson S, Edwards IR. Tachycardia during cisapride treatment. British Medical Journal 1992; 341: 748-9
92. Bergholm U, Langman M, Rawlins M, et al. Drug-induced pancreatitis. Pharmacoepidemiology and Drug Safety 1995; 4: 329-34
93. Inman WHW. Postmarketing surveillance of adverse drug reactions in general practice I: search for new methods. British Medical Journal 1981; 282: 1131-2
94. Inman WHW. Postmarketing surveillance of adverse drug reactions in general practice II: prescription event monitoring at the University of Southampton. British Medical Journal 1981; 282: 1216-7
95. Rawson NSB, Pearce GL, Inman WHW. Prescription-event monitoring: methodology and recent progress. Journal of Clinical Epidemiology 1990; 43: 509-22
96. Inman WHW. Prescription-event monitoring. Acta Medica Scandinavica 1984; Suppl. 683: 119-26
97. Inman WHW, Rawson NSB. Erythromycin estolate and jaundice. British Medical Journal 1983; 286: 1954-5
98. Coulter DM, Edwards IR, McQueen EG. New Zealand. In: Inman WHW, editor. Monitoring for drug safety, 2nd ed. pp. 119-33. Lancaster, UK: MTP Press, 1986
99. Colin-Jones DG, Langman MJS, Lawson DH, et al. Postmarketing surveillance of the safety of cimetidine: 12 month mortality report. British Medical Journal 1983; 286: 1713-6
100. Stephens MDB. Marketing aspects of company-sponsored postmarketing surveillance studies. Drug Safety 1993; 8: 1-8
101. American Society for Clinical Pharmacology and Therapeutics. Position paper on the use of purported postmarketing drug surveillance studies for promotional purposes. Clinical Pharmacology and Therapeutics 1990; 48: 598
102. Dunn HL. Record linkage. American Journal of Public Health 1946; 36: 1412
103. West of Scotland Coronary Prevention Study Group. Computerised record linkage: compared with traditional patient follow-up methods in clinical trials illustrated in a prospective epidemiological study. Journal of Clinical Epidemiology 1995; 48: 1441-52
104. Mann RD. The VAMP System and the detection of risk, some examples. Pharmacoepidemiology and Drug Safety 1994; 3: 313-9
105. Shapiro S. The role of automated record linkage in the postmarketing surveillance of drug safety: a critique. Clinical Pharmacology and Therapeutics 1989; 46: 371-86
106. Ray WA, Griffin MR. Use of Medicaid data for pharmacoepidemiology. American Journal of Epidemiology 1989; 129: 837-49
107. Carson JL, Strom BL, Duff A, et al. The feasibility of studying acute hepatitis using Medicaid data. Clinical Pharmacology and Therapeutics 1992; 52: 214-9
108. Suissa S, Ernst P, Boivin JF, et al. A cohort analysis of excess morbidity in asthma and the use of inhaled beta-agonists. American Journal of Respiratory and Critical Care Medicine 1994; 149: 604-10
109. Collet JP, Boivin JF, Spitzer WO. Bias and confounding in pharmacoepidemiology. In: Strom BL, editor. Pharmacoepidemiology. 2nd ed. New York: John Wiley & Sons, 1994: 609-27
110. Castle WM, Chen D. The three CIOMS working groups on drug safety. In: Bankowski Z, Dunne JF, editors. Drug surveillance: international cooperation past, present, and future. Geneva: CIOMS, 1994: 99-108
111. Nunn P, Felten M. Needs in developing countries: surveillance of resistance to anti-tuberculosis drugs. In: Bankowski Z, Dunne JF, editors. Drug surveillance: international cooperation past, present, and future. Geneva: CIOMS, 1994: 141-7
112. Edwards IR. Monitoring the safety of herbal remedies: WHO project is underway. British Medical Journal 1995; 311: 1569

Chapter 10

# Pharmacoeconomics and Drug Prescribing

*P.G. Davey, M. Malek, T. Dodd* and *T. MacDonald*

## Synopsis of Important Principles

1) Pharmacoeconomics was originally established as a subdiscipline of health economics. Its ultimate objective is to assist in making informed clinical decisions by providing information about costs and consequences of alternative methods of treatment.

2) The pharmaceutical industry has been quick to recognise the relevance of pharmacoeconomic analysis to strategic planning, both in early drug development and in determining the likely prices of future drugs. Likewise, healthcare providers and government agencies have recognised the potential of systematic research in this area to examine the link between the costs and quality or value of individual healthcare measures.

3) The basic principle underlying pharmacoeconomic evaluation of treatment programmes is the simultaneous measurement of costs and outcomes, such that decisions can be made regarding allocation of resources between different programmes.

4) In comparing the costs and outcomes of 2 or more healthcare measures, 4 different types of pharmacoeconomic analysis may be undertaken: (1) cost-minimisation analysis (CMA), where alternatives that achieve a major outcome equally are compared in terms of cost; (2) cost-effectiveness analysis (CEA), where cost : outcome ratios are compared in terms of physical units of effectiveness; (3) cost-benefit analysis (CBA), where cost : outcome ratios of alternatives with fundamentally different outcomes are compared in monetary terms; and (4) cost-utility analysis (CUA), where cost : outcome ratios are compared in terms of utilities such as improved quality of life (QOL).

5) In any pharmacoeconomic evaluation, it is important that the perspective of the analysis is made clear from the outset, i.e. from whose perspective the costs and outcomes are being evaluated – that of society, community health services or patients.

6) The relationship between pharmacoepidemiology and pharmacoeconomics is important, because pharmacoeconomics relies heavily on good clinical and epidemiological data. Despite the limitations of current pharmacoepidemiology databases in providing data on drug utilisation and outcomes, such databases are an invaluable component in pharmacoeconomic analysis.

7) The process of costing in pharmacoeconomic analyses involves the identification, measurement and valuation of all relevant costs, and this separation should be maintained throughout the analysis. Variations in costs (and in medical practices) both within and between individual countries exist, and it is important to be aware of this when interpreting economic analyses performed in other settings.

8) Decision analysis is used for identifying the points of decision or uncertainty about a treatment programme and for modelling the consequences of the decisions. This technique is particularly relevant to decisions about inclusion of drugs in formularies.

9) Health-related quality of life (HRQOL) is an appropriate outcome measure in pharmacoeconomic analyses as it examines 'health status' and allows comparison of treatments of different conditions.

10) There is growing recognition of the need for a long term perspective in healthcare that is based equally on the costs and efficiency of individual treatment measures. Only by doing so can they be fully appreciated for the value they contribute rather than the costs they generate.

Just a few years ago, very few people would have been familiar with the discipline of pharmacoeconomics or would have acknowledged the relevance of the topic to every day clinical practice. However, there has been a silent revolution in the thinking, if not yet practising, of medicine with the invasion of health economists into territories previously occupied exclusively by clinicians. Economic evaluation studies are growing exponentially.[1] That the intrusion has not been entirely welcomed by clinicians is quite understandable given the philosophical and methodological differences between the 2 disciplines, not to mention the loss of monopoly power of clinicians facing a discipline like economics, with its notorious imperialistic reputation. However, the inroad of economics into medicine has not been without benefit. The 2 disciplines have gained from the experience, have mutually enriched their research methodologies, and are gradually coming to some form of understanding. The result of this exchange include, for example, economists using the methodology of matching countries to study the effects of adopting similar economic strategies, a method of investigation used by clinicians in matching patients with similar conditions to study the effectiveness of medical interventions.[2] The traffic, therefore, has not been just in the direction of economics into medicine, and the scientific community has benefited from the exchange of ideas, methods and debate on issues of mutual concern.

This chapter provides an overview of the issues and theory that lie at the heart of pharmacoeconomics, and indicates how these can be applied in practice to decisions about drug therapy. The ultimate objective of pharmacoeconomics is to assist informed clinical decisions, and some practical examples explaining the link between the presentation of pharmacoeconomics results and decision making are provided. In addition, the importance of outcome measures with regard to some popular indices currently applied in assessing the impact of medical interventions on the quality of life of patients are discussed.

## 1. Evolution of Pharmacoeconomics

Pharmacoeconomics is a subdivision of health economics and is a result of that discipline coming of age through consolidation to diversification. Health economics as a branch of economics is itself relatively young. Few systematic references to it can be found before the mid-1960s and the first book on this subject was published in 1973.[3]

The premises on which both health economics and pharmacoeconomics are based are virtually identical to those of mainstream economics. The central problem in economics is to find a socially acceptable solution to people's unlimited demands and society's limited ability to respond to these demands with the production of goods and services, i.e. 'economics is the study of how society decides *what* gets produced, *how*, and for *whom*'.[4]

It is important to note that this definition emphasises the role of society and societal views on *what, how,* and for *whom* goods and services are produced. An extended definition of economics by Samuelson contains all of the above elements and more, i.e. 'economics is the study of how men and society end up choosing, with or without the use of money, to employ scarce productive resources that could have alternative uses, produce various commodities and distribute them for consumption, now or in future, among various people and groups in society. It analyses the costs and benefits of improving patterns of resource allocation'.[5]

Some of the important issues raised in the above definition are recurring sources of confusion and misunderstanding as to what economics is about. These are:

1) Resources everywhere, no matter how rich a society is, are limited.

2) There are unlimited competing demands on these limited, scarce, productive resources.

3) Individuals and society have choices about how resources are used for production, distribution or other purposes.

4) With each choice comes a cost associated with that choice. The cost is that resources, once used, cannot be used again or to be more precise, there is an 'opportunity cost' associated with economic decisions. 'Opportunity cost' is the amount lost by not using economic resources (labour, capital, building, management, etc.) in its best alternative use.

5) The aim of economics is to define the most efficient use of our limited resources, recognising the costs associated with the choices made. Health economics is the discipline of economics as applied to the topic of health, and as such is more than a bag of tools – it is a way of thinking about the problems and dealing with them.[6] Health economics treats healthcare as an economic commodity, while acknowledging the fact that there are significant differences be-

tween healthcare and other conventional economic commodities.[7]

As indicated above, pharmacoeconomics was originally established as a subdiscipline of health economics and there are still health economists who regard the growth of pharmacoeconomics as an unnecessary overspecialisation. As a discipline still in the process of evolving, any definition would become outdated by the time this book is published. The earliest definitions of pharmacoeconomics focus very narrowly on the 'analysis of the costs of drug therapy to healthcare systems and society'.[8] This perception of pharmacoeconomic research is solely concerned with costs and does not consider the outcome from the use of pharmaceutical products. Others have taken a much broader view of what pharmacoeconomic research is about, i.e. as assessing the implications of *projected* outcomes and costs of pharmaceutical products for the decision whether to continue or stop development of a drug and for global pricing strategy.[9] This expanded definition has the advantage of incorporating pharmacoeconomic research into the process of drug development from inception (pre-phase I) to phase IV when postmarketing surveillance is undertaken.

Of course, the role of pharmacoeconomics does not remain the same during the different phases of drug development. For example, during the early phases it helps to identify commercially viable options and find the market niche that could be commercially exploited, while in the later stages it permits informed decision making with regard to the appropriate use of drugs that have been developed. Thus, pharmacoeconomics is a tool of management that may be applied to strategic and operational decisions about pharmaceutical development, production or consumption. The focus of emphasis in the earliest phase is on making informed decisions about product development (essentially 'go/no-go' decisions), while the emphasis at later stages shifts to rational prescribing and utilisation. The aim throughout is to ensure the most efficient use of limited resources.

## 2. Relevance of Pharmacoeconomics to the Pharmaceutical Industry

The pharmaceutical industry has an important role to play in society that some argue is out of proportion to its size.[10,11] Its importance stems from its joint responsibility with the health professions for the maintenance of health, which in itself is a valuable asset, as well as being an important determinant of the productivity of human resources in the economy.[12]

Specifically, the industry is expected to discover and develop new drugs, which it then converts into useful therapeutic products as rapidly and safely as possible, experiencing very high research and development (R&D) costs in the process (see also chapter 11). It is then expected to undertake the manufacture and distribution of these products. Within this function, there are opportunities for individual companies to exploit the market due to information imperfections and certain unique characteristics of the market.

### 2.1 Factors Influencing the Demand for Pharmaceutical Products

One of the most striking features of the pharmaceutical market is that in many countries, access to drugs is controlled by the health service. It follows that the demand function for prescription pharmaceuticals involves an unusual separation of the consumer from the decision maker. Imperfect information for the patient (the consumer) means his/her knowledge of the therapeutic and other properties of drug products is inadequate for determining what treatment is required, what drugs are available, and in what form and dosage. The patient therefore approaches the clinician who acts as an agent, an expert with the desired knowledge. It is the clinician who advises which product is appropriate for each case.

The demand for pharmaceutical products is a *derived* demand as they are wanted for the benefits they are perceived to provide (not for their own value, in the sense that the demand for cars is derived from the demand for transportation), and also a *directed* demand, as the patient has no choice but to take the prescribed drug or none at all. As drugs are often a necessity, the patient's demand for products is almost perfectly price inelastic up to levels of prohibitively high prices. In simpler terms, a price increase will not chase many customers out of the market, while a price decrease may not attract customers to the market.

Very few pharmaceutical products are appropriate for the treatment of more than a limited range of medical conditions, i.e. they are disease-specific with limited possibilities for substitution. The pharmaceutical market therefore consists of a large number of separate submarkets that are often constricted in size. The potential demand for a drug or group of related drugs consists of the total need for medication for the particular illnesses they can treat. Total effective demand at given drug prices may, however, be lower than the total physical need if patients do not have access to welfare or sufficient resources to obtain drugs. Alternatively, total effective demand may exceed total physical need if individuals are prescribed such products when they are not appropriate or necessary. The actual relevant market comprises the total effective demand for medication from patients who have consulted a clinician and who have a disorder for which the clinician may be persuaded to prescribe the particular drug.[11]

Such price inelasticity is reinforced by the isolation of clinicians in this market. When making a decision, the clinician is concerned with efficacy, safety and quality. As the decision-maker and not the purchaser, the clinician is not primarily concerned with prices. In a market where a number of identical drug products may be present and offered at very different prices, the clinician will choose that which is regarded as the best, often regardless of the price. To keep abreast of all the latest developments in products, indications, formulations and dosages, clinicians rely on various sources of information, one of which is promotional literature produced by the pharmaceutical industry. As the clinician puts efficacy, safety and quality first, the availability of promotional material may shift the clinician's 'demand curve' from one product to another, without any reference to price. The clinician has little motivation for prescribing the lowest priced product available on the market nor is he or she formally required to even be aware of the prices charged.

## 2.2 Factors Influencing the Supply of Pharmaceutical Products

Although demand in the pharmaceutical industry is price inelastic, it does not necessarily follow that a monopoly will result. With some exceptions, drugs are not expensive to manufacture and, compared with other industries, there are not major economies of scale to be made with respect to drug manufacture.[11,13] The steady growth in the number of companies involved in the manufacture of medicines after the expiry of patents suggests that full competition occurs at this point. In comparison with manufacture of generic drugs, new drug development represents a higher risk project that may prevent smaller companies from entering the market; nonetheless, innovative companies continue to arise. In general therefore, it appears that economies of scale are no more a barrier to entry into the pharmaceutical market than in any other industry. Therefore, full competition seems a plausible and desirable possibility despite the inelastic price demand.

### 2.2.1 Requirement to Achieve an Adequate Return on R&D Investment

If prices were kept close to manufacturing costs, the return on the R&D investment by innovative companies would be negligible. While one company might invest millions on research and development, another may enter the market, copy existing products at a marginal cost, and sell them at much lower prices. If this occurred, there would be no incentive for innovative companies to undertake the expensive and time-consuming research that stimulates the industry. Society would suffer as new drug treatments would not be forthcoming, with the exception of discoveries made by academia or government research bodies. However, these facilities tend to be severely limited by a lack of financial resources; hence the number of discoveries would probably fall dramatically while development times would increase significantly.

### 2.2.2 Patent Protection

The patent system is therefore used by the innovative pharmaceutical industry to ensure competitive returns and to encourage continued R&D. A patent confers on the owner the specific right to exclude others from using the protected know-how for commercial purposes for a defined period after filing of the patent. It gives the company with a new innovation a temporary monopoly over the supply of a product or process. This is a temporary privilege as otherwise serious inefficiencies from continuous monopoly pricing could occur. There is a delicate dividing line concerning the length of patent protection. If the privilege is permitted for too long, inefficiencies from monopoly pricing would result; however, if the protection period is too short, there will be inefficiencies from inadequate innovation.

The patent privilege introduces a barrier to entry and so restricts competition on the supply side for the drug market. Research and develop-

**Table I.** Phases of drug development, their mean duration and approximate cost (after Anon[16] and DiMasi et al.[17]). The duration of each phase is based on a study of both successful and unsuccessful compounds, as well as some overlap between the phases

| Phase of drug development | Time from phase to start of approval (mos) | Capitalised expected costs (1987 $US millions) | Approximate number of compounds completing the process |
|---|---|---|---|
| Screening of compounds and preclinical testing leading to approval for clinical trials | Not quantified | 155.6 | 10,000 screened:<br>20 undergo preclinical testing<br>10 approved for clinical trial |
| Phase I clinical trials | 98.9 | 17.8 | 10 compounds enter clinical trials |
| Phase II clinical trials | 82.7 | 21.4 | |
| Long term and reproductive animal toxicology | 78.7 | 8.9 | |
| Phase III clinical trials | 60.2 | 27.1 | 1 compound completes clinical trials and is submitted for licensing |

ment is a major determinant of competitive behaviour as it establishes the potential market power of a company, but also sets in motion the forces that may result in competitive price behaviour in the future.[14]

### *2.2.3 Competitive Research Pressures*

In reality, successful new drugs may only hold a commanding position for approximately 5 years, after which they may be replaced by a presumably better rival.[15] This may be a drug with a similar mechanism of action but that has potential advantages in terms of safety (e.g. the introduction of ranitidine after cimetidine), or it may be a drug with a new mechanism of action which has similar therapeutic effects (e.g. the introduction of omeprazole after ranitidine). When one company finds a new compound that becomes a new major product, others will intensify their research in the same areas, perhaps improving on the original product until it is 'competed out' of the market. This competitive research can have benefits to society by increasing the chances of significant discoveries; however, there are possible drawbacks from duplicative R&D efforts.

### *2.2.4 Joint Ventures and Licensing Agreements*

Due to the high costs of research, development and marketing, large financial resources are required for success in the pharmaceutical industry. Although smaller companies may make innovative discoveries, the current competitive climate is such that small companies often do not have the funds to develop and market their discoveries rapidly. A considerable number of joint ventures and licensing agreements with larger firms have therefore resulted. These larger firms then dominate the market, becoming multinational in the process. As the demand for pharmaceuticals is global and the costs involved considerable, it is in the interests of the companies to take advantage of this huge market potential and develop an international character.

### *2.2.5 Likelihood of Success in Developing New Compounds*

It has been estimated that of approximately 10,000 preparations that may be synthesised and tested for therapeutic potential, only 20 will enter the preclinical stage. Of these 20 agents, only 10 will successfully complete this stage and pass the regulatory (e.g. FDA) review to enter clinical trials. From phase I trials, 5 compounds will pass through to phase II trials, of which only 2 will enter phase III trials. After all this, only one product may be put forward by the company for approval as a new drug and will hopefully reach the market (table 1).[16] The proportion of new chemical entities (NCEs) tested in each stage diminishes as the various characteristics of the tested compounds are discovered and products abandoned due to adverse effects or other undesirable features.

Not only is the probability of getting a new compound onto the market small for the companies, but the probability of that product becoming a success and recovering R&D costs is slim. It has been estimated that there is a 1 in 4000 chance of a compound investigated for biological activity ever becoming a marketed drug, a 1 in 21,000 chance of the product entering the market and becoming a moderate success, while only a 1 in 60,000 chance of that product becoming highly successful.[18]

2.3 Applications of Pharmacoeconomics

Duplication of R&D and production of 'me too' pharmaceuticals has implications for loss of welfare, given the huge costs involved in the process of R&D. The welfare loss is due to the opportunity cost of production of 'me toos' using scarce productive resources, which could have usefully been allocated to production of genuinely beneficial products. As such, strategic use of pharmacoeconomics at early stages of drug development provides a new mechanism for preventing wastage of resources and redirecting these resources to more socially desirable and commercially viable areas. This will ensure that what is optimum from a commercial point of view will also turn out to be optimum from the consumer's point of view. Consequently, it is a vital component of the management of risks in the development, production and marketing of pharmaceutical products.

## 3. Definition of Terms and Basic Methodology of Economic Evaluation

Economists are very fond of using *models* in describing and analysing the problems of the real world. An economic model is a simplified picture of reality and provides a useful framework for understanding the nature of the important parameters involved in achieving a certain outcome. A simple economic model used in describing the process of production is the production function, in which various inputs are combined together to produce some outputs (fig. 1). The same analogy can be applied to any healthcare programme whether at local, national or international level, or indeed at an individual level.

In the context of healthcare, inputs into the production process include labour (clinical staff, auxiliary staff, professions allied to health, managerial staff, etc.), equipment, buildings, and consumables such as drugs. Inside the shaded box in figure 1, these factors are combined and organised to provide certain levels of care that will lead to an improvement in the health status of the population for whom the programme has been designed – which could be a single patient, or a segment of the population or the total national population. The basic principle underlying the economic evaluation of health programmes is relatively simple as it seeks to identify, measure and value their costs and outcomes *simultaneously.* The simultaneous measurement of costs and outcomes is the key to understanding the purpose and indeed the *raison d'etre* of economic evaluation. The ultimate objective of economic evaluation is to provide a menu of choice for decision making regarding allocation of resources between different programmes. To do this, the analysis has to include health costs and outcomes of at least 2 alternatives, or else the evaluation will be only partial and incomplete (fig. 2).

As there are potential conflicts of interest between different segments of the population and/or the majority of the population and that of a minority, it is important to make the *perspective* of the analysis clear before opting for a certain type of analysis. The simple question to ask is, from whose perspective are the costs and outcomes being evaluated? Is this from a general practitioner's point of view or that of a hospital manager? Different answers to the same question could be obtained from different interest groups, as the categories of costs to be included differ from one group to the other. From a patient's perspective, it may not matter if the relative cost of a drug therapy is quite high compared with alternative therapy, but a hospital manager may have a quite different view. Ideally, the analysis should always include the

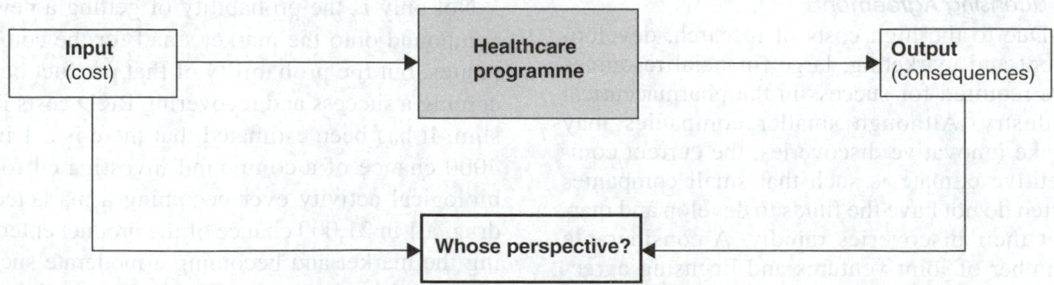


**Fig. 1.** A simple model of economic analysis of healthcare.

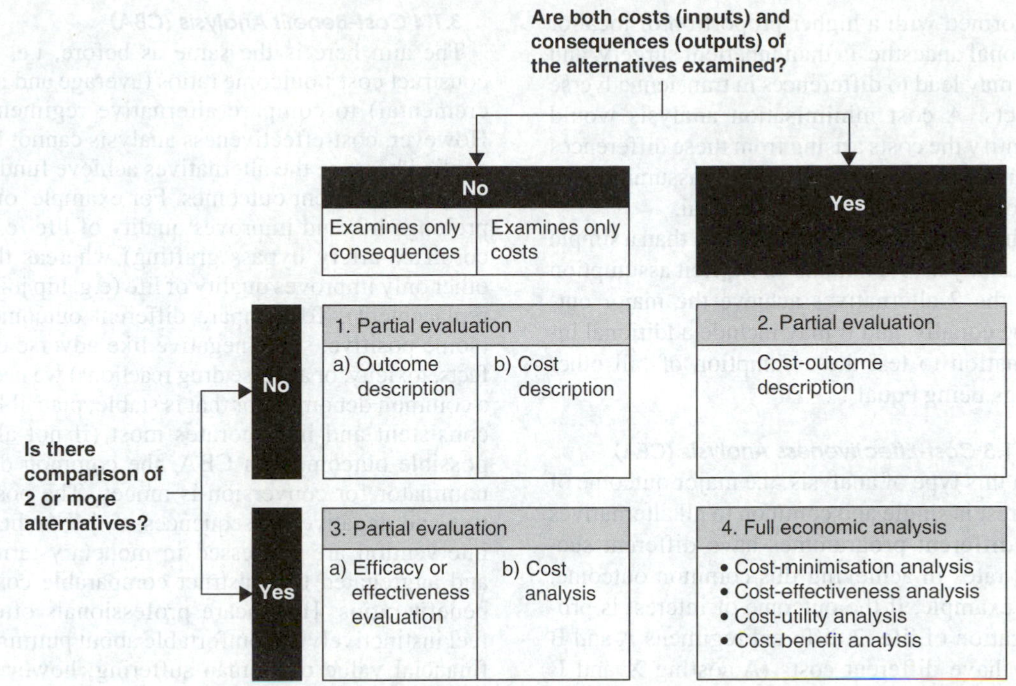


**Fig. 2.** Distinction between partial and complete economic analysis based on the answer to 2 questions: (1) Does the analysis compare 2 or more alternatives? (2) Does the analysis include both costs and outcomes?

perspective of society, thus comparing the social cost with the social consequences of alternative programmes.

## 3.1 Types of Economic Evaluation

There are 4 types of economic evaluation, all of which can be applied to pharmaceutical products. In order of sophistication and level of complexity, these are:

- Cost-minimisation analysis (CMA)
- Cost-effectiveness analysis (CEA)
- Cost-benefit analysis (CBA)
- Cost-utility analysis (CUA).

The ultimate objective of all 4 methods is to compare the cost and outcome of alternative regimens, ideally by generating a single index or cost : outcome ratio. Issues related to cost and cost models are discussed in section 6 below. The nature of outcome measurement is the all important factor determining both the level of complexity and sophistication, as well as the reliability and validity of a comparison of alternative regimens.

### *3.1.1 The Common Components of All Economic Analyses*

A full economic analysis will always address the following 2 questions:

1) Are 2 or more alternatives being considered?
2) Are both the costs and consequences of each alternative being considered?

If the answer to either question is no, the study is not a full economic analysis (fig. 2). Two or more alternatives must be considered, otherwise the analysis is merely a description of costs and/or outcome.

### *3.1.2 Cost-Minimisation Analysis (CMA)*

In this type of analysis, the major outcome of interest is the same and is achieved equally by the alternative regimens, thus allowing the evaluators of the programme to concentrate on the cost side of the equation and choose the alternative that has the lowest costs. An example is minor surgery for adults that can be done either as an inpatient or outpatient procedure without any significant difference in the clinical outcome. All other things being equal, economic efficiency requires choosing the option that allows the maximum number of operations for a given budget. The key to successful cost minimisation is that the comparators must be shown to have equal clinical efficacy before the analysis is carried out. Furthermore, although the 2 options must achieve the major outcome of interest equally, they may still have other outcomes that differ. For example, day-case surgery may be performed with a higher proportion of local or regional anaesthesia than inpatient surgery, and this may lead to differences in transient adverse effects. A cost minimisation analysis would quantify the costs arising from these differences in anaesthetic technique, while assuming that the outcome of surgery is identical.

Thus, cost minimisation is more than a simple cost analysis. It contains an explicit assumption that the 2 alternatives achieve the major outcome equally, and it may include additional information to test the assumption of 'all other things being equal'.

#### *3.1.3 Cost-Effectiveness Analysis (CEA)*

In this type of analysis, the major outcome of interest is single and common to all alternatives but different programmes have different success rates in achieving this common outcome. For example, if the outcome of interest is prolongation of life, 2 different regimens A and B may have different costs (A costing X and B costing Y) and prolong life to a different degree (A producing a gain of M life years, B producing a gain of N life years).

It would be possible to construct the cost : outcome ratios of X ÷ M and Y ÷ N and thus compare the 2 regimens A and B in terms of costs per life years gained. Alternatively, M ÷ X could be used as life years gained per unit of currency (pound, dollar, etc.) spent on each regimen. This process will provide *average* ratios to assist decision making in allocating resources.

If possible, it is preferable to use *marginal* (or *incremental*) cost-effectiveness ratios for making a comparison. In all likelihood, the marginal ratios would be different from the averages. Constructing marginal ratios would involve considering what the cost and outcome would be if an additional unit of output is produced. If it is known that regimen B is both more expensive and more effective than regimen A, the question for the decision maker is whether or not to shift resources from A to B. In this case, the cost per additional life year saved by regimen B would be calculated as:

$$\text{Cost/additional life year saved} = \frac{(Y - X)}{(N - M)}$$

The difference between the *average* and *marginal* cost is considered in more detail in section 7.1.

#### *3.1.4 Cost-Benefit Analysis (CBA)*

The aim here is the same as before, i.e. to construct cost : outcome ratios (average and incremental) to compare alternative regimens. However, cost-effectiveness analysis cannot be applied because the alternatives achieve fundamentally different outcomes. For example, one prolongs life and improves quality of life (e.g. coronary artery bypass grafting) whereas the other only improves quality of life (e.g. hip joint replacement). To compare different outcomes (some positive, some negative like adverse effects, toxicity, or adverse drug reactions) we need a common denominator that is stable, plausible, consistent and incorporates most (if not all) possible outcomes. In CBA, the common denominator for conversion is money. The positive and negative consequences of the medical intervention are expressed in monetary terms and aggregated to construct comparable cost-benefit ratios. Healthcare professionals often feel instinctively uncomfortable about putting a financial value on human suffering; however, the function of money is quite simply to allow society to compare the value of totally different commodities.

The most controversial aspect of CBA is putting a value on items that are perceived to be inherently unsuitable for valuation by healthcare professionals, e.g. the loss of vision, impairment of hearing, renal failure or even loss of human life. However, this practice is well established in the insurance industry, and indeed, is neither new nor exclusive to this industry.

CBA is not very common in pharmacoeconomics and where performed, the investigators usually calculate the costs and benefits that can be easily (and noncontroversially) expressed in monetary terms. Alternatively, there are techniques for quantifying the strengths of individual preferences for alternatives. These include *willingness to pay* and the *standard gamble* technique, in which hypothetical examples are used to ask individuals how much they would be willing to pay to secure improvements in treatment.[19]

#### *3.1.5 Cost-Utility Analysis (CUA)*

In CUA, a different measure of value derived directly from economics is used to measure an outcome called utility. The basic principle underlying CUA is that one purpose of medical intervention is to improve the quality of life of patients, and that changes in quality of life can be measured alongside measures of increase in

**Table II.** Impact of discounting on economic analysis: the importance of distribution of costs and outcomes. Drug costs tend to be distributed evenly over time, whereas for programmes such as surgery or screening almost all costs are incurred at the start of the programme. Treatment of established disease tends to result in immediate benefits, whereas the benefits of primary or secondary prevention occur in the future

| Source of uneven distribution of costs and outcomes of alternatives in the analysis | Example | Effect of applying a discount rate to both costs and outcomes | Effect of applying a discount rate to costs only |
|---|---|---|---|
| Costs occur at different times | Surgery *vs* drug treatment for peptic ulcer | Makes drug treatment more attractive | Makes drug treatment more attractive |
| Benefits occur at different times | Drug treatment of hypertension *vs* drug treatment of established hypertensive heart failure | Makes treatment of established heart failure more attractive | No effect on treatment costs. Will discount long term savings on healthcare costs (e.g. prevention of future strokes by drug treatment of hypertension) |
| Costs and benefits occur at different times | Screening and treatment of hyperlipidaemia *vs* coronary artery bypass grafting for established coronary artery disease | Could go either way: discounting future costs favours drug treatment of hyperlipidaemia; discounting future benefits favours surgery because the benefits occur immediately | Makes screening for hyperlipidaemia more attractive by discounting future drug costs |

life expectancy. Therefore, the comparative efficacy of the alternative treatments is captured and measured through their contribution to the quality of life of the individuals undergoing such treatments. This is an important concept that deserves a more detailed explanation and is discussed further in section 8. However, despite the obvious theoretical advantages of CUA, there are major practical difficulties in establishing the exact utility attached to different health states.

### 3.2 Discounting of Future Costs and Benefits

A consideration relevant to all 4 methods of economic evaluation is the problem of discounting, based on the 'time preference principle' derived directly from mainstream economics. This principle, put in simple terms, states that even if there were no bank charges or inflation, people would still prefer to receive what is due to them as early as possible, and defer their debt payment to a later time, indeed the later the better. Since not all costs and consequences of the alternative regimens necessarily occur at the same time, discounting becomes relevant to both costs and consequences, at least on *theoretical grounds*.

The process of discounting involves determining the present value of the costs and outcomes of alternative methods of intervention by choosing an appropriate discount rate. Although there is no general agreement on what constitutes an appropriate discount rate, in principle there is agreement that costs should be discounted.[20,21] However, there has been much discussion on the question of whether health benefits should be discounted as well.[20,22,23]

In practice, discounting is only an issue if the costs or outcomes of alternative regimens occur at different times (table II). Fortunately, this is usually not the case in pharmacoeconomic studies. We believe that the best solution is to include discounting in a sensitivity analysis, a practice endorsed in some national guidelines on pharmacoeconomic analysis (see section 4.1). A range of discount rates should be applied to both costs and outcomes. Results should be presented in 3 formats: firstly, results with a zero rate of discount applied to both costs and outcomes; secondly, with a range of discount rates applied to costs alone; thirdly, with a range of discount rates applied to both costs and outcomes. The final analysis should then make it clear that the conclusion is or is not sensitive to the application of discount rates from x% to y%, applied either to costs alone or to both costs and outcomes.

Table II gives examples of analyses in which future outcomes would need to be discounted, and the effect that discounting would have on the result of the analysis. The second example compares drug treatment of hypertension with drug treatment of established heart failure. Suppose that one of the outcome measures is quality of life. Drug treatment of hypertension is unlikely to have any immediate beneficial effect on quality of life; indeed, it may have a negative effect on current quality of life. However, drug treatment of hypertension may prevent events like cerebrovascular accidents, which would have a devastating negative effect on future quality of life. Conversely, drug treatment of established heart failure is likely to achieve immediate improvements in current quality of life. Inclusion of a discount rate applied to future outcomes will magnify these differences, because the improvement in future quality of life by treatment of hypertension will be discounted (i.e. diminished) relative to the immediate improvement in quality of life achieved by treatment of heart failure. Essentially, application of discounting to future outcomes will reduce the apparent value of any healthcare programme that has a strong preventative component.

## 4. Guidelines for Pharmacoeconomic Evaluations

The relative youth of health economics and pharmacoeconomics and the sudden rush to produce economic evaluations by the pharmaceutical industry, healthcare providers and government agencies around the world has caused an explosion in the number of papers generated and submitted to journals. Unfortunately, lack of proper expertise in reviewing these papers has meant that some of the earlier studies failed to stand up to the normal scrutiny of a peer reviewed journal. Add to this some general misconceptions about the reliability of economic end-points and it is not surprising that there is a degree of suspicion about the validity of pharmacoeconomic research.[24,25] There has also been concern over the sponsorship of research in this area by the pharmaceutical industry and the use of such studies for marketing purposes. The analogy between the use of standard clinical trials *vs* economic evaluations for pharmaceutical marketing has been explored.[26,27]

In 1990, the UK Department of Health also issued advice to the industry, encouraging it to provide economic data for its new products. Four years later, this was followed by guidelines from the Department of Health for conducting economic evaluations of pharmaceuticals. Despite the claims that these guidelines are pioneering, there is considerable overlap between them and the original 10-question checklist proposed 7 years earlier.[19] The most significant aspect of the UK guidelines was that they were drawn up by a joint working group from the Department of Health and the Association of the British Pharmaceutical Industry. These guidelines are relatively brief and provide a good summary of currently accepted practice for economic evaluation of drugs. They are reproduced here as an example, rather than the last word on good practice.

### 4.1 Guidelines on Good Practice in the Conduct of Economic Evaluations of Medicines (Issued by the UK Department of Health)

1) The question being addressed by the study, including the demographic characteristics of the target population group, should be identified and set out at the start of the report of the study.

2) The conceptual and practical reasons for choosing the comparator should be set out and justified in the report of the study.

3) The treatment paths of the options being compared should be identified, fully described, placed in the context of overall treatment, and reported. Decision analytic techniques can be helpful in this regard.

4) The perspective of the study should ideally be societal, identifying the impact on all parts of society, including patients, the National Health Service (NHS), other providers of care, and the wider economy. However, costs and outcomes should be reported in a disaggregated way so that the recipients of costs and outcomes can be identified. Attention should be drawn to any significant distributional implications. Indirect costs should normally be included in a societal perspective, although care should be taken to avoid any double-counting and results should be reported including and excluding these costs.

5) The study should use a recognised technique. These include cost-minimisation analysis (CMA), cost-effectiveness analysis (CEA), cost-utility analysis (CUA), and cost-benefit analysis (CBA). Any one of these could be appropriate according to the purpose of the study. The report of the study should include justification of the technique chosen.

6) In choosing the method of data capture and analysis, the use of one of, or a combination of, prospective or retrospective randomised clinical trials, meta-analysis, observational data and modelling should be considered. The reason for choice of method and, where relevant, for the choice of trials should be reported.

7) Assessment of the question should include determining and reporting what additional ben-

efit is being provided at what extra cost using incremental analysis of costs and outcomes.

8) Outcome measures should be identified and the basis for their selection reported. Where CUA is used, proven generic measures of quality of life are preferred.

9) All relevant costs should be identified, collected and reported. Physical units of resource use should be collected and reported separately from information about the costs of the resources. Costs should reflect full opportunity cost, including the cost of capital and administrative and support costs where relevant. Average cost data are often acceptable as a proxy for long run marginal cost.

10) Discounting should be undertaken on 2 different bases:

a) all costs and outcomes discounted at the prevailing rate recommended by the Treasury, currently 6% per annum; and

b) all costs and monetary outcomes discounted at the Treasury rate, currently 6%, but nonmonetary outcomes not discounted.

Both sets of results should be reported. The physical units and values of costs and outcomes prior to discounting should also be reported.

11) Sensitivity analysis should be conducted and reported. The sensitivity of results to all uncertainty in the study should be explored. This should involve the use of confidence intervals and/or ranges for key parameters, as appropriate. The ranges and choice of parameters to vary should be justified.

12) Comparisons with results from other studies should be handled with care. Particular attention should be paid to differences in methodology (such as the treatment of indirect costs) or differences in circumstances (such as different population groups).

## 5. Relationship Between Pharmacoeconomics and Pharmacoepidemiology

Pharmacoepidemiology provides data about drug utilisation and outcomes in everyday clinical practice (see further chapter 9). The behaviour of clinicians and patients in clinical trials is inevitably influenced by the protocol. Computerised databases provide the opportunity to study drug utilisation in large numbers of patients and some provide data that may be used to assess the outcome of treatment. However, it is easy to be impressed by the sheer size of these databases and forget their obvious limitations, particularly for studying the effectiveness of drug treatment.[32]

In 1989, the US Agency for Health Care Policy and Research created 15 patient outcomes research teams (PORTs) to combine findings from the literature with information from computerised databases in order to identify effective treatments for a range of conditions. The problem with routine databases is that it is impossible to exclude confounding effects of disease severity, accompanying disease, concomitant treatment, etc. and the only way to satisfactorily exclude confounding variables is through a prospective, randomised clinical trial.[32] Nonetheless, provided that these limitations are acknowledged explicitly, we believe that pharmacoepidemiology databases provide an invaluable component in pharmacoeconomic analysis. For example, in assessing the cost effectiveness of antibiotic treatment in the community, the possibility that failure of antibiotic treatment results in hospital admission is clearly important, as are unscheduled repeat visits to community health services.[33] To design clinical trials that incorporate these events as endpoints, their frequency must be measured and, if possible, high risk groups identified who may be most likely to benefit from a new intervention.[34,35] Observational data may be used in critical analysis of priorities for clinical trials. For example, if a new intervention is unlikely to be more cost effective than current treatment under even highly optimistic assumptions derived from observational data, then it is unlikely to prove more cost effective in a clinical trial.[33]

Pharmacoepidemiology databases can also provide information about patient behaviour in the real world[36] and help to identify patients for clinical study, including identifying groups for clinical trials.[37] Consequently, pharmacoepidemiology provides a vital link between randomised clinical trials and clinical practice, provided that the limitations of computerised databases are well understood.

## 6. Cost Models and Cost-Effectiveness Analysis

### 6.1 Cost Models

#### 6.1.1 Top-Down Versus Bottom-Up Models

***Top-down cost models*** estimate the overall economic burden of diseases and are often referred to as *cost of illness* studies.[38] The most commonly used method is based on an estimate of the prevalence of a particular disease (the number of people who have the disease in any given year) and an estimate of the costs accrued during that year. Alternatively, the cost of illness may be estimated from information about the incidence of disease (the number of new cases that occur in 1 year) and the estimated lifetime costs accrued by these patients. Clearly, the second approach is more difficult to execute because it requires information about the rate of progression of disease and the incremental costs incurred as the disease progresses. However, a longitudinal model of disease progression facilitates discussion about the relative merits of strategies such as primary or secondary prevention *vs* treatment of established disease.[39]

The majority of top-down disease models are based on data about prevalence of illness.[38] The principal application of these studies is in highlighting the importance of a particular disease in order to influence policy makers about allocation of healthcare resources or research funding. What additional information do such studies provide in comparison with traditional epidemiological estimates of morbidity and mortality? Cost-of-illness studies may give additional information about morbidity, particularly if this is not physically disabling (e.g. days lost from work because of migraine). However, major concerns have been expressed about the quality of information cost of illness studies provide,[38] the 2 principal objections being that:

1) Most studies use loss of productivity as an estimate of costs to society and this focuses attention on diseases that affect people of working age.

2) Measurement of cost of illness is not a good guide to allocation of healthcare resources because it cannot provide information about the comparative effectiveness of interventions to prevent the disease.[38] Economic analysis should be based on definition of need in terms of capacity to benefit from treatment, as opposed to severity of illness alone.[40,41]

***Bottom-up cost models*** are based on prospective collection of data about individual patients. A bottom-up cost model has 2 principal aims. The first is to quantify costs and the second is to allocate them to the appropriate person(s) or budget(s). In practice, it is essential to separate 3 phases:

- Identification of the items to be included
- Measurement of each item in natural units such as days of hospitalisation
- Financial valuation of each item.

Identification of costs should include a range of perspectives (e.g. hospital health services, community health services, social services, the patient). All guidelines about pharmacoeconomic analysis recommend that costs should be presented in a disaggregated manner, which can only be fully achieved by a bottom-up cost model that clearly identifies and allocates the components of overall costs.

#### Classification of Costs

In health economics, it is usual to separate 3 broad categories of costs:

1) Healthcare costs, i.e. financial costs that fall on the health services (e.g. drug acquisition costs, days in hospital). Healthcare costs are usually subdivided as follows:

a) variable costs, i.e. costs that vary immediately according to the number of patients treated (e.g. drug acquisition costs, costs of other consumables such as needles and syringes); and

b) fixed costs, i.e. costs that do not vary with the number of patients treated, at least in the short term, usually 1 year (e.g. capital costs of building or equipment and staff salaries).

2) Other financial costs, i.e. costs that fall outside the health services (e.g. prescription charges or other treatment expenses incurred by the patient; the cost of the patients' or carers' travel to and from hospital, costs of providing social services, loss of productivity).

3) Intangible costs, i.e. costs that are difficult to value financially (e.g. pain, anxiety and loss of energy; time given up by voluntary carers).

#### Direct Costs, Indirect Costs and Overheads

The terms *direct* and *indirect* costs appear frequently in the pharmacoeconomic literature but, unfortunately, they are used somewhat differently by accountants and economists. Accountants use the term indirect costs to describe costs that do not arise directly from a single treatment, investigation or service. These are essentially overhead costs (e.g. the cost of providing the heating or lighting for a building, the cost of training staff, or the cost of renewing or servicing equipment). Various methods for allocating these costs have been devised but it must be understood that the principal aim of all methods is to ensure that the organisation recovers all of its operating costs.[42]

Accurate allocation of costs to individual patients or treatments is not necessarily a priority and all of the methods used inevitably involve some cross-subsidisation.[42] For example, the pharmacy delivers drugs, which are bought from a wholesaler and passed on to the patient. This process includes a number of additional costs (e.g. safe storage, reconstitution or preparation, dispensing in a form that will be administered safely, patient education and therapeutic drug monitoring). Some of these additional costs are relatively easy to allocate to particular drugs (e.g. preparation costs for intravenous injections, therapeutic drug monitoring of aminoglycosides) but there will always be a residue of general overhead costs that do not arise directly from any one particular drug. These overhead costs are usually recovered by calculating a surcharge, or dispensing fee for each drug. This is a fixed fee and it is inevitable that it involves some averaging across patients. For example, the time taken to show an asthmatic patient how to use an inhaler properly is unlikely to be charged directly to the patient, so that patients who are prescribed drugs that do not require special instructions are effectively subsidising other patients. The important point to understand is that a nonprofit organisation must recover all of its operating costs, which inevitably involves addition of an overhead cost to the actual cost of a particular treatment. It is this overhead cost that an accountant would call the *indirect cost* of a treatment or service.

In contrast, economists tend to use the term *indirect costs* to describe social costs such as loss of productivity that are only indirectly related to healthcare.[19] However, indirect costs are not synonymous with nonmedical financial costs because economists also use a category of 'direct nonmedical costs'.[19] This includes out-of-pocket expenses for the patient or carers that arise directly from healthcare (e.g. travel expenses, copayment for drugs or other treatments).

We believe that the terms 'direct' and 'indirect' costs are potentially confusing and imprecise, because it is not clear whether they are being used to distinguish costs arising directly or indirectly from a particular treatment *vs* costs that are directly or indirectly related to healthcare. If these terms are used in an economic analysis, then it is crucial that they are defined precisely. Alternatively, the information can be conveyed precisely by distinguishing between healthcare costs *vs* other financial costs, and further distinguishing between variable *vs* fixed costs.

#### 6.1.2 Planning a Cost Model

Before a cost model can be constructed, the crucial question that must be answered is, *from whose perspective will the analysis be conducted?* An analysis conducted from the perspective of a hospital budget holder might be restricted to the costs incurred by the hospital and is likely to yield different results compared with an analysis conducted from the perspective of community health services or the patient. For example, consider home administration of intravenous drugs. Even if the hospital continues to pay for the drugs, there are obvious resource savings to be made from early discharge of the patient because the bed becomes available to treat another patient, nursing time is made available for other patients, and so on. It is also easy to identify several advantages for the patient, such as reduced risk of hospital-acquired infection or other hospital-related complications and improved quality of life.[43,44] Nonetheless, the patient is likely to have some concerns, particularly if complications occur in the home.[45] There are also likely to be financial costs for the patient, particularly if the healthcare system reimburses a lower proportion of costs incurred outside the hospital.[46]

Despite these negative aspects, many patients prefer to receive treatment outside the hospital.[46] A successful home intravenous service should be based on a thorough analysis of the home environment and the likely consequences for the patient of earlier discharge from hospital.[47] This will facilitate preparation of the patient for all of the implications of earlier discharge.

#### 6.1.3 The Three Stages of Costing: Identify, Measure, Value

The process of costing should be divided into 3 clear stages (table III) and this separation should be maintained throughout the analysis up to and including reporting of the results. This will allow readers to understand fully the separate elements in the model and, if necessary, to adjust the model to suit their own perspective.

Classification of the costs of drug administration is relatively straightforward, but the same classification is equally applicable to the costs of adverse drug effects or failure of treatment (see examples in table III). Provided the stages of identification, measurement and valuation are separated, the requirements for data collection should become clear.

**Table III.** Examples of the identification, measurement and valuation of costs. These are intended to be illustrative rather than exhaustive

| Costing stage | Hospital intravenous drug administration | Gentamicin ototoxicity |
|---|---|---|
| **Identify** | *Healthcare:* drug acquisition; consumables; staff time; laboratory tests<br>*Non-healthcare financial:* travel costs of patient's visitors<br>*Intangible:* discomfort from intravenous canula | *Healthcare:* tests; treatment; extra days in hospital; staff time; litigation costs<br>*Non-healthcare financial:* travel costs; reduction in income, loss of productivity<br>*Intangible:* deafness or impaired balance |
| **Measure** | Number of consumables<br>Hours of staff time<br>Number of tests<br>Number of hospital visits by family<br>Visual analogue scale for pain measurement | Number of tests<br>Hours of staff time<br>Extra days in hospital<br>Working days affected<br>Degree of hearing loss<br>Change in mobility |
| **Value** | Obtain financial values for all direct and indirect costs<br>Depending on the reimbursement system, calculate implied value of reducing any or all of the following:<br>• fixed direct costs<br>• indirect costs<br>• intangible costs<br>Consider other methods for valuation of intangible costs:<br>• willingness to pay to avoid intangible costs<br>• standard gamble or other measures of risk averseness<br>• quality of life or other utility measures | |

The most difficult step is valuation of intangible costs. A crude, but relatively simple method is implied valuation. For example, in comparing a non-ototoxic antibiotic with gentamicin, a thorough analysis of healthcare costs, including therapeutic drug monitoring of gentamicin, may show that the non-ototoxic drug costs \$50 more per patient treated. If the incidence of symptomatic deafness caused by gentamicin is 1%, then a decision to use the nonototoxic drug implies that the decision maker believes that it is worth investing at least \$5000 to prevent 1 case of deafness, because 1 case will be avoided per 100 patients treated, at a total additional cost of \$5000 (\$50 × 100). Sometimes the implied value generated can be compared with resources that are already committed by society to prevention of similar disability in another setting. In the above hypothetical example, it would be relevant to obtain data about the costs of preventing noise-induced hearing loss in industry or about compensation awards for industrial or other causes of established hearing loss.[48] Unfortunately, in most cases, there are no such readily available comparative data. Nonetheless, implied valuation still serves as a crude first step to making decisions based on intangible costs.

Financial valuation of short term intangible costs is also achieved by measuring patients' willingness to pay to avoid them.[19] The same technique may be applied to long term problems. However, long term disability can also be quantified by measurements of utility or quality of life. These are dealt with in more detail in section 8.

### 6.2 Sources of Variation in Healthcare Costs

There are genuine variations in the costs of treatments both within and between individual countries. It is important to be aware of this when interpreting economic analyses that have been performed in other settings and also in planning the sensitivity analysis for new economic analyses. Sources of variation in costs associated with drug treatment include accounting and reimbursement systems, economies of scale, the sample size and method of statistical analysis, and medical practice variation.

#### *6.2.1 Accounting Systems*

Fixed costs (staff salaries and buildings or other capital equipment costs) account for the majority of any healthcare budget. Accounting practices for allocation of these fixed costs vary considerably. In the UK, quoted hospital drug costs equate with the drug *acquisition cost*. This is usually derived from sources such as the British National Formulary, and is likely to be higher than most hospitals currently pay because they are able to negotiate discounts. However, no allowance is made for pharmacy services provided by the hospital for dispensing, preparation or clinical monitoring. In contrast, in the US, there is a tendency to allocate some fixed costs to drug utilisation, although practices vary considerably between hospitals. In a survey of 71 hospitals, it was found that 93% charged a preparation fee, 63% charged a dispensing fee, and 68% charged an additional variable markup, particularly for drugs like gentamicin that require intensive monitoring by clinical pharmacy services. This markup often exceeded the acquisition cost of the drug, the maximum being a 961% markup on the acquisition cost of gentamicin. The scale of other charges also varied considerably, for example from \$0.80 to \$31.50 for preparation fees.[49] Similar variation in accounting practices has been reported for other consumables, such as intravenous lines and minibags.[50,51]

Drug wastage is another potential source of accounting variation. Wastage occurs because drugs cannot be used due to incorrect preparation or breach of sterility or lapsed expiry date, or if a drug is prepared for a patient who does not receive it because of a change in treatment, or the dosage or presentation size is greater than the required dose.[52,53] Wastage rates genuinely vary between hospitals and are likely to be lowest in those hospitals that use a centralised intravenous additive service.[54] In addition to genuine variation, there is variation in the ability to track and record wastage rates accurately.[55] Clearly therefore, the accounting method used to recover the costs of drug wastage is another source of variation in drug costs between hospitals.

#### *6.2.2 Reimbursement Systems*

Reimbursement systems that pay per patient treated make it relatively easy to allocate fixed costs to individual patients or treatments administered. For example, in the US, decreasing length of hospital stay allows the hospital to treat more patients, which will increase revenue because the hospital can charge for each individual patient that is treated. In other healthcare systems, however, hospitals receive a total annual budget or a fixed block contract for treating a specified number of patients. Under these systems, it is more difficult to achieve savings through earlier discharge of patients. In fact, reducing hospital stay is likely to increase the average cost per day in the hospital (fig. 3). This paradox occurs because treatment costs are not distributed evenly throughout a patient's admission. They are likely to be higher early in the admission, when investigation and treatment

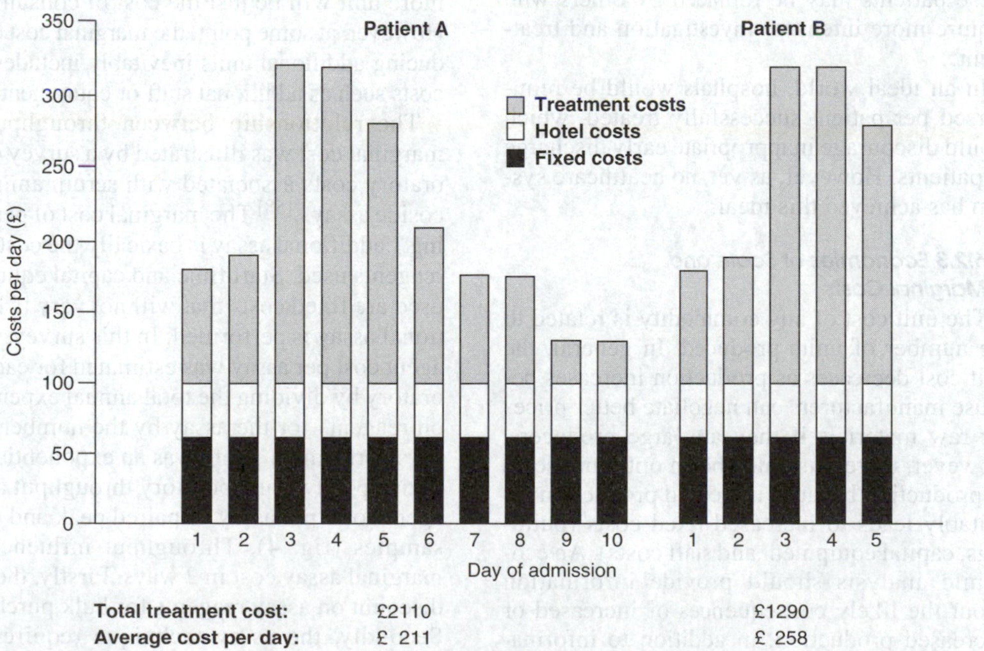


**Fig. 3.** Components of the costs of hospitalisation, their distribution during an individual patient's admission, and the likely impact of shortening the length of hospital stay. Fixed costs include capital equipment and professional salaries; hotel costs include catering, laundry and ancillary staff salaries; treatment costs include costs of drugs, investigations, surgery etc. (after Lowson[56]).

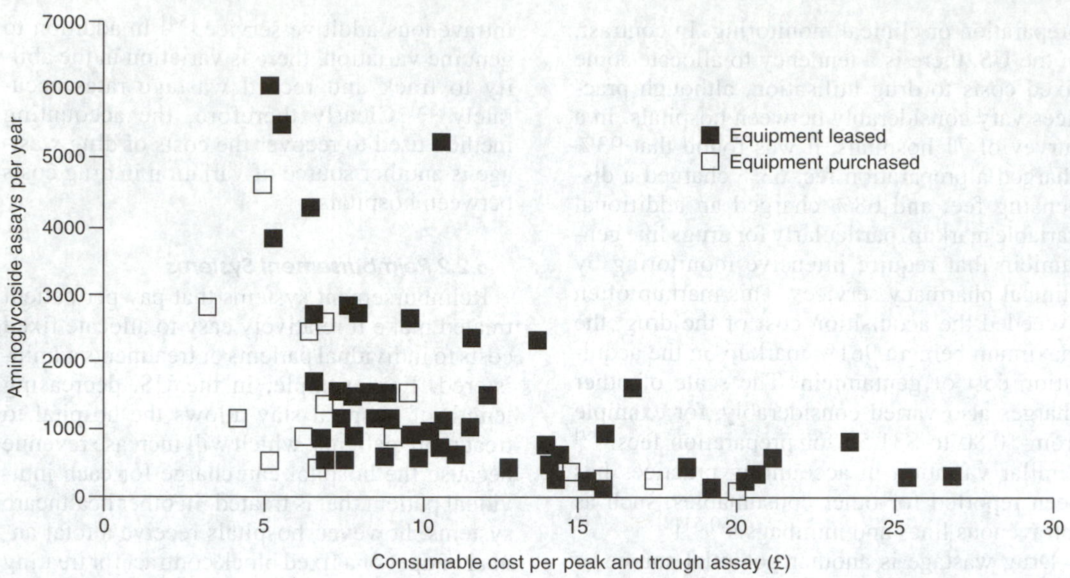


**Fig. 4.** Cost of serum aminoglycoside assay by laboratory throughput and method of payment for capital equipment. The cost includes only the cost of reagents used to perform the assay (after Vacani et al.[58]).

are usually more intense.[56,57] Consequently, programmes such as home intravenous drug administration result in earlier discharge of patients whose diagnosis has been established and these patients may be replaced by others who require more intensive investigation and treatment.

In an ideal world, hospitals would be reimbursed per patient successfully treated, which would discourage inappropriate early discharge of patients. However, as yet, no healthcare system has achieved this ideal.

### *6.2.3 Economies of Scale and Marginal Costs*

The unit cost of any commodity is related to the number of units produced. In general, the unit cost decreases as production increases because manufacturers can negotiate better prices for raw materials if they are large producers. However, there must also be an optimum scale of production because increased production inevitably leads to increased fixed costs (buildings, capital equipment and staff costs). An economic analysis should provide information about the likely consequences of increased or decreased production, in addition to information about cost effectiveness at current levels of production. The term *marginal cost* is used to describe the cost of producing additional units of output. Most production processes have a mixture of fixed costs (buildings, equipment, staff salaries) and variable costs (consumables). In general, the marginal cost of producing 1 more unit will be just the cost of consumables. However, at some point, the marginal cost of producing additional units inevitably includes fixed costs such as additional staff or equipment.

The relationship between throughput and marginal cost was illustrated by a survey of laboratory costs associated with serum aminoglycoside assays.[58] The marginal cost of performing 1 additional assay is basically the cost of the reagents used. Staff time and capital equipment used are fixed costs that will not vary if 1 additional assay is performed. In this survey, the reagent cost per assay was estimated for each laboratory by dividing the total annual expenditure on reagents for the assay by the number of assays performed. There was an exponential relationship between laboratory throughput and reagent costs per assay of paired peak and trough samples (fig. 4). Throughput influences the marginal assay cost in 2 ways. Firstly, there is a discount on assay reagents for bulk purchasers. Secondly, the assay technique requires consumption of a fixed amount of reagent in order to calibrate the equipment. Clearly, the more assays that can be performed at one time, the lower the amount of reagent used per sample assayed. Another source of cost variation identified in this study was the method of payment for capital equipment. Laboratories that had purchased their equipment were able to negotiate lower reagent costs than laboratories that leased their equipment from the reagent manufacturers (fig. 4).

Economies of scale also affect the cost of consumables used for drug preparation and administration[50] and the costs of the drugs themselves. Awareness amongst purchasers of healthcare of economies of scale may make it difficult for small departments to survive. However, the importance of a local, personal service should not be forgotten and it is likely that this will result in small hospitals continuing to maintain their own laboratories or pharmacies. This is the healthcare equivalent of the survival of small, local greengrocers, bakers and butchers in competition with large supermarket chains. For the foreseeable future therefore, there will continue to be genuine variation in healthcare costs produced by economies of scale.

#### 6.2.4 Sample Size and Method of Statistical Analysis

Distribution of healthcare costs is often skewed and this has important implications for data analysis and interpretation.[59] Furthermore, the amount of information available to the decision maker may be quite small and the reliability of an estimate of the mean or median should be quantified by calculation of the 95% confidence intervals (CI) [fig. 5].

These statistics have important practical implications. The 95% CIs indicate that the mean or median of a second sample from the same population is 95% likely to lie between these extremes. Therefore, the mean and median are at best very approximate descriptions of the population. The median is the cost incurred by at least 50% of the sample, and therefore is a reasonable estimate of the cost likely to be incurred by an individual patient. The mean is influenced by outlying patients with unusually high costs, and therefore is a better guide to total cost over a period of time. Which statistic should be used? As stated above, it depends on the perspective from which the analysis is being performed. If the analysis is being performed from the perspective of a budget holder, we believe that the *mean* is appropriate, because budget holders need to take outliers into account in their calculations. For this reason, it may also be appropriate to provide the range of values obtained. The issue of measurement of central tendency should be addressed early in the design of any cost analysis, and it is also important that readers of economic analyses understand the implications of different measures.[59]

Finally, in addition to information about the additional cost per patient, budget holders need information about the number of patients who

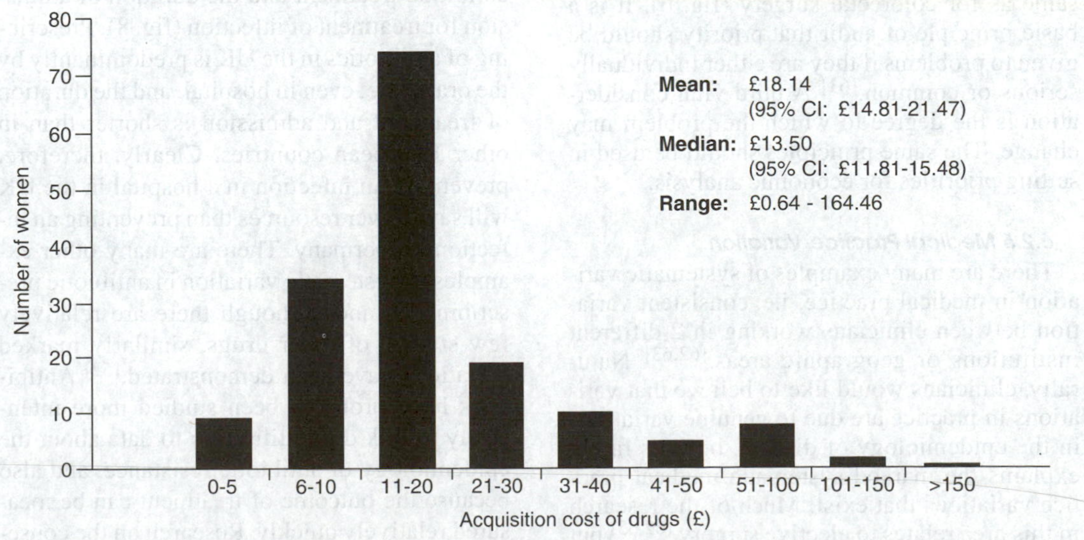


**Fig. 5.** Costs of antibiotics administered to 162 women for infection after caesarean sections: an example of a skewed distribution of healthcare costs and the impact on the mean and median of the distribution. *Abbreviation:* CI = confidence interval.

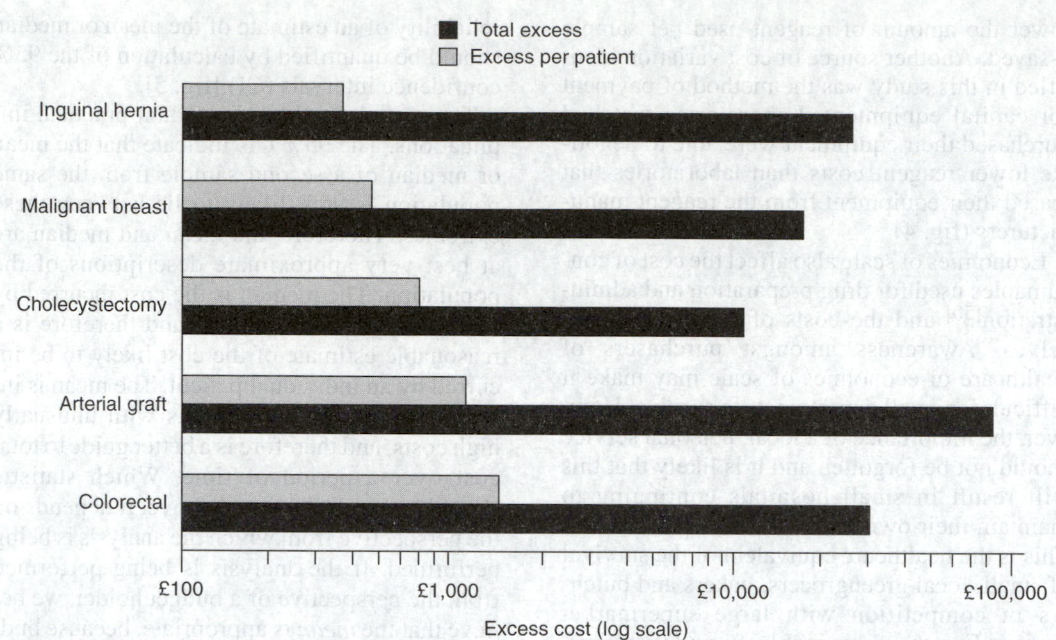


**Fig. 6.** Data on excess costs of treating wound infections presented either as excess cost per infected case or as total excess cost per year (after Lynch et al.[60]).

are likely to incur costs, because these may give different insights into priorities for intervention. In the comparison of excess costs associated with wound infection after different operations shown in figure 6, inguinal hernia appears relatively unimportant if the excess cost per patient is considered but, because it is a common procedure, the contribution of inguinal hernia to total excess costs is almost the same as for colorectal surgery (fig. 6). It is a basic principle of audit that priority should be given to problems if they are either individually serious or common.[61] A third vital consideration is the degree to which the problem may change. The same principles should be used in setting priorities for economic analysis.

### *6.2.5 Medical Practice Variation*

There are many examples of systematic variation in medical practice, i.e. consistent variation between clinicians working in 2 different institutions or geographic areas.[62,63] Naturally, clinicians would like to believe that variations in practice are due to genuine variations in the epidemiology of disease, but this rarely explains the marked systematic medical practice variations that exist. Much of the research in this area relates to elective surgery,[62,63] but a few examples related to antibiotic therapy in hospitals will serve to illustrate the potential impact of medical practice variation on pharmacoeconomic analysis (table IV).

Intravenous formulations of drugs are almost always more expensive than oral formulations, often by a factor of 10.[52] The proportion of antibiotic doses that are administered by the intravenous route varies markedly between countries in Europe (fig. 7), as does the duration of antibiotic treatment and the duration of admission for treatment of infection (fig. 8). Prescribing of antibiotics in the UK is predominantly by the oral route, even in hospital, and the duration of treatment and admission is shorter than in other European countries. Clearly, therefore, preventing an infection in a hospital in the UK will save fewer resources than preventing an infection in Germany. There are many other examples of systematic variation in antibiotic prescribing[65] and, although there are relatively few studies of other drugs, similarly marked variations have been demonstrated.[52] Antibiotics have probably been studied more intensively to link drug utilisation to data about the epidemiology of antibiotic resistance, and also because the outcome of treatment can be measured relatively quickly. Research on the consequences of medical practice variation for other drugs should be given a higher priority.

**Table IV.** Reasons for medical practice variation (after Anderson & Mooney;[62] McPherson[63])

| |
|---|
| Genuine differences in epidemiology of disease |
| The clinician's judgement of beneficial and adverse outcomes |
| The clinician's judgement of the probability of these outcomes |
| The utilities attached to these outcomes by clinician and patient |
| The attitude to risk of the clinician and patient |
| The degree of paternalism or autonomy in the clinician-patient relationship |
| The availability and cost of facilities |
| The nature of the clinician's reward system |
| The nature of systems for defining and penalising medical malpractice |

The impact of medical practice variation on pharmacoeconomic studies can be illustrated by comparing the costs of antibiotics administered to treat infections occurring after hysterectomy or caesarean section in UK hospitals in comparison with reported costs from the US (table V). The published figures for the US are sometimes 100-fold higher than those in the UK. To some extent, this discrepancy is related to different accounting systems, because the costs of drugs reported in the US are likely to include costs of pharmacy services, whereas costs quoted in the UK are the acquisition costs of the drugs alone. However, the major source of the discrepancy is that practitioners in the US routinely prescribe 7 days of intravenous drug treatment, whereas in the UK the majority of infections are managed with oral drugs, which are in general 10-fold cheaper than equivalent intravenous formulations.[52]

## 7. Application of Pharmacoeconomics in Decision Making

### 7.1 Cost Effectiveness, Incremental Analysis and Programme Budgeting

#### *7.1.1 Use of Implied Values in Cost-Effectiveness Analysis*

Cost-effectiveness analysis (CEA) is the simplest method for beginning to assess the value of differences in outcome between treatments. Having completed the cost model, it is possible to express the results in terms of cost per life year saved, cost per case of cancer detected, etc. (see section 3).

Another method for presenting results and debating the consequences of decisions is to calculate an implied value. For example, suppose that drug A is more effective in preventing complications in hospitalised patients than drug B, and that a cost-effectiveness analysis has measured the net costs of both regimens and shown that patients who receive drug A are discharged 4 days earlier than patients who receive drug B. If drug A costs £200 per patient treated more than drug B, a decision to use drug A implies that the decision maker believes that it is worth investing £50 in variable costs to gain 1 hospital bed day by earlier discharge. Conversely, continuing to use drug B implies that the decision maker does not believe that the resources gained by using drug A justify the investment.

As discussed above, in most healthcare systems, it is in fact quite difficult to increase hospital revenue through early discharge of patients (see section 6.2.2). Calculation of implied value clarifies the implications of a decision and facilitates development of a long term plan for healthcare. In this case, the decision maker may decide to use drug A, recognising that in the short term, this decision will increase variable healthcare costs, having also set out a long term plan for reallocation of the resources saved. This could include changing the structure of the ward unit (e.g. increasing the number of day beds or closing some beds) or redeployment of inpatient staff to provide new outpatient or

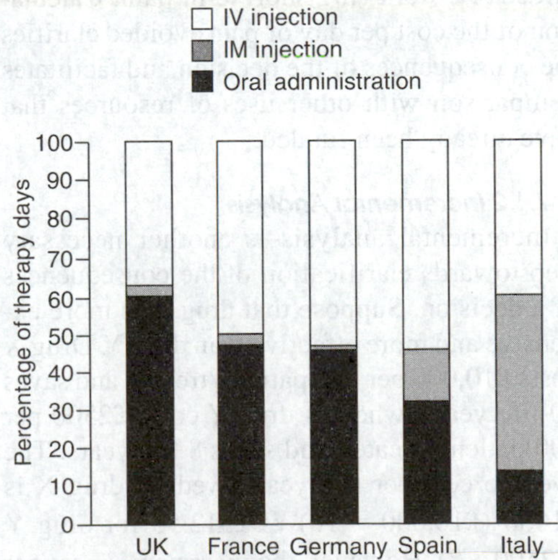


**Fig. 7.** Route of administration of antibiotics in hospital in selected European countries (after Halls[64]). *Abbreviations:* IV = intravenous; IM = intramuscular.

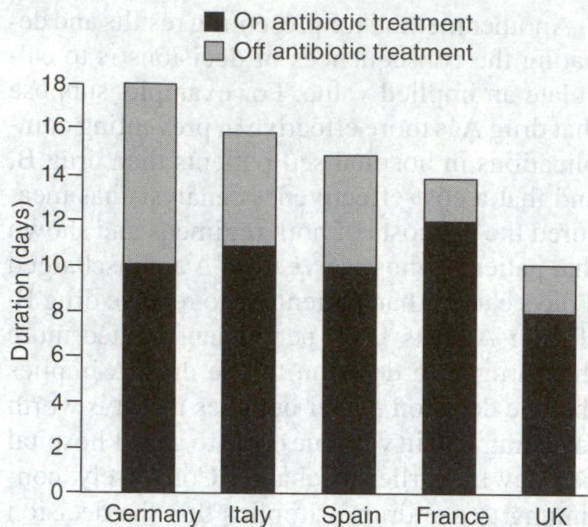


**Fig. 8.** Duration of hospital admission (days) and duration of antibiotic treatment in selected European countries (after Halls[64]).

homecare facilities. Whatever use is made of the resources saved through early discharge, provided the value of the resources gained by earlier discharge of patients exceeds the investment of £50 per hospital day saved, the decision to use drug A will have been justified.

Calculation of implied values can also be applied to intangible costs (see section 6.1.3 and table III). In this case, the decision maker is presented with the fact that drug C is more expensive than drug D after consideration of all healthcare costs, fixed and variable, but is more effective at relieving short term pain. Calculation of the cost per day of pain avoided clarifies the consequences of the decision and facilitates comparison with other uses of resources that have already been funded.

#### *7.1.2 Incremental Analysis*

Incremental analysis is another necessary step towards clarification of the consequences of a decision. Suppose that drug X is more expensive and more effective than drug Y. Drug X costs £10,000 per 100 patients treated and saves 10 life years, whereas drug Y costs £2500 per 100 patients treated and saves 8 life years. The average cost per life year saved by drug X is £1000 (£10,000 ÷ 10) *vs* £312.50 for drug Y (£2500 ÷ 8). However, the *incremental cost per additional life year saved* by drug X is £3750, which is calculated by dividing the difference in costs by the difference in outcome as follows:

$$[£10,000 - £2500] \div [10 - 8] = £7500 \div 2 = £3750$$

The average cost per life year saved therefore gives a misleadingly optimistic impression of the cost effectiveness of a new treatment that is both more expensive and more effective than the comparator. All guidelines on pharmacoeconomic analysis recommend presentation of incremental costs and outcomes rather than averages.

#### *7.1.3 Programme Budgeting*

Programme budgeting recognises that the decision maker rarely has the opportunity to increase the available budget for healthcare; in fact, it is more likely that there is pressure to reduce the budget. Programme budgeting involves identification of a short list of effective treatments that are currently not funded, but that would have the highest priority if additional funds could be provided. A second list is then made of treatments that are currently funded, but that are considered to be the least valuable treatments in the programme and that would be the first to be given up if the budget was reduced. Comparison of the 2 lists then gives the decision maker the option of ceasing to provide some treatments from the negative list in order to free resources that can be used to provide some of the treatments in the positive list.

### 7.2 Decision Analysis

So far, we have dealt with reasonably simple problems, where there is only one major difference between 2 drugs. In reality, this is rarely the case. Moreover, the consequences of a decision are likely to be influenced by uncertainty about the probability of an event happening and about the consequences of the event. For example, if maintenance treatment for peptic ulcer fails, what is the probability that the patient will have recurrent symptoms and what is the probability that the clinician will refer the patient for an endoscopy? Decision analysis is a technique for identifying the points of decision or uncertainty and modelling the consequences of decisions.[68-70]

For reviews of the application of decision analysis to pharmacoeconomics with particular reference to making decisions about drug formularies, see Nash et al.,[71] Lipsy,[72] and Schechter.[73]

**Table V.** Contrasting costs of management of suspected infection in women following caesarean section from studies conducted in the US[66] and UK.[67] Not surprisingly, the authors of the two studies reached opposite conclusions about the cost-effectiveness of giving preoperative prophylaxis to prevent infection

| Source of cost | US study | UK study |
|---|---|---|
| Isolation of mother | $447 × 5 days = $2235 | Not practised |
| Isolation of baby | $614 × 5 days = $3070 | Not practised |
| Investigations | $570 | £6 to £10 |
| Drug acquisition costs | $1251 | £14 |
| Additional costs of preparation, administration and monitoring of intravenous drugs | $316 | Almost all doses prescribed orally |
| Total cost per woman with suspected infection | $7442 | £20 to £34 |

## 8. Outcome Measures and Quality of Life

Using outcome measures to evaluate the benefits of medical intervention is not all that new to clinicians. Furthermore, since the primary objective of medical practice is to improve the quality of life of patients, the choice of quality of life as an outcome measure seems to be appropriate. Before describing methods that have been developed for quantification of quality of life, it is worth reflecting on why it is necessary to try to quantify such a nebulous concept.

### 8.1 Clinical Judgement *vs* Quantification of Response to Treatment

Clinicians are liable to say that assessment of a patient's response to treatment is complex, depends on multiple factors and should be left to clinical judgement. While respecting the importance of considering the individuality of patients, we believe that progress can only be made if clinicians assess the need for and response to treatment based on a standardised data set with an agreed method for weighting the information. Systematic study of clinical decision making can be made by presentation of the same data to a group of clinicians. In one example, 48 rheumatologists judged the change in disease activity in 50 sets of patient data drawn from real life and presented as examples.[74] Each set comprised 2 values, recorded a year apart, for 10 commonly measured clinical variables. The rheumatologists recorded the magnitude of the improvement or deterioration on a visual analogue scale (VAS) and whether the change was clinically important or not. Clinical judgement policies were modelled using linear regression of the clinical variables on the VAS score. It was found that only 14 of the 48 specialists agreed about the response to treatment of individual variables. However, even these 14 specialists showed little agreement over which patients had improved and which had not; indeed in a few cases, one or more specialists said that the same patient had deteriorated whereas others said that they had improved (fig. 9).

Possible reasons could be discovered by inspecting their judgement policies. The weights attributed to the clinical variables differed considerably between specialists. Furthermore, the weights they believed they attached to the variables frequently differed from the weights in the regression models generated by the decisions that they made. In particular, the specialists believed that they ranked the patients' own assessment as the second most important variable, whereas their decisions implied that they ranked it 9th out of 10.[74]

Clearly, there is a need for consensus about aggregation of several outcome variables into a single outcome measure. Most clinicians are now familiar with disease-specific scoring systems, which have arisen from a general recognition of the desirability of systematic assessment of treatment outcome. Measurement of quality of life simply takes the process a step further and seeks to develop measures that will allow comparison of treatments of different conditions.

### 8.2 Health-Related Quality of Life

The relationship between illness and quality of life (QOL) is both complex and asymmetrical. To start with, it is obvious that illness (lack of health) affects a patient's QOL. However, QOL is a broad term that includes health status and other attributes such as environment, income, living standard, etc. On the whole, QOL is a vague term without conceptual clarity[75] that lacks focus and precision.[76] The aim of measuring QOL is to provide information about the well-being of the population at large. The United Nations Human Development Index

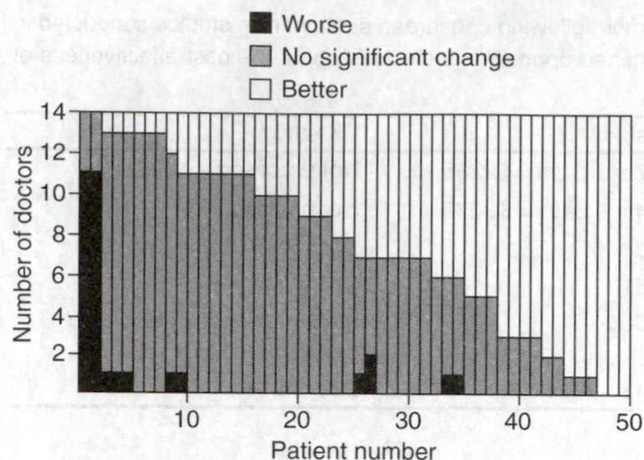


**Fig. 9.** Assessment by 14 rheumatologists of the response to treatment of 50 individual patients (after Chaput de Saintonge et al.[74]).

(HDI) is a typical example.[76] The World Health Organization (WHO) is also developing an instrument to measure quality of life (WHOQOL). According to the WHO, quality of life is defined as 'an individual's perception of their position in life in the context of the culture and value systems in which they live and in relation to their goals, expectations, standards and concerns'.[77]

Since QOL is such a broad term, most pharmacoeconomic analyses focus on health-related quality of life (HRQOL), which is a narrower term used to examine 'health status' alone. Among these methods, the approach of *quality adjusted life years* (QALYs) occupies a prominent position. The QALY approach assumes that a valid, reliable and acceptable cardinal scale for valuing all possible health states and death can be created, for example with full health at 1.0 and death at 0.0. In this approach, the basic unit is the life year. Two procedures may extend life, but if these extra years are filled with pain, on the one hand, and pain-free, on the other, the second procedure is held to be worth more than the first. Applying a fraction to the number of years increase in survival, which values these years relative to full healthy years (1.0), makes a 'quality adjustment', and produces a figure for the procedure's impact expressed in 'quality-adjusted life years' or QALYs.

Broadly speaking, HRQOL measures are divided into 2 distinct categories: generic and disease-specific measures.

### *8.2.1 Generic Instruments for Measuring Health-Related Quality of Life*

Generic instruments are designed to apply broadly across types of disease, across patient groups (e.g. children or the elderly), across different medical interventions (e.g. drug therapy or surgery), and cover a range of functions, moods, and distress. Some commonly used generic tests include the Sickness Impact Profile (SIP), Nottingham Health Profile (NHP), Psychological Adjustment to Illness Scale (PAIS), Activities of Daily Living (ADL) and Medical Outcomes Study Short Form (SF-36).

#### Sickness Impact Profile (SIP)

This is one of the best known instruments based on a psychometric approach.[78] It examines health status by a descriptive profile of changes in a person's behaviour due to sickness. The SIP consists of 136 items divided into 12 different categories of functional behaviour. Examples of the application of the SIP include assessment of cardiac rehabilitation,[79] total hip joint replacement,[80] and treatment of back pain.[81]

The SIP provides global subscale scores that have been well researched and validated. The major disadvantage of the SIP is that it is long and some patients will have difficulties answering such a lengthy questionnaire. It may also be insensitive to mild dysfunction.

#### Nottingham Health Profile (NHP)

The NHP consists of 38 statements divided into 6 problem areas: energy, pain, emotional reactions, sleep, social isolation and physical mobility.[82] This measure has been extensively used in the measurement of quality of life across different countries and diseases. Its main advantage is that it is relatively quick to complete, is easy to understand, and it has been extensively researched and validated. Its major disadvantage is that because it requires 'yes/no' responses, the zero scores cannot be improved, and hence it emphasises negative aspects of health.[83,84]

#### SF-36

The Medical Outcomes Study Short Form (SF-36) was developed and validated originally in the US. The 36 items included in the 8 subscales were derived from 108 items that were originally included in another measure of outcome. The 8 dimensions are physical functioning (10 items), social functioning (2 items), impairment to role activities due to emotional problems (3 items), impairment to role activities due to physical problems (4 items), pain (2 items), mental health (5 items), energy (4 items) and general health perception (5 items). There is also one item about changes in health over the preceding year. There are an expanding number of authorised translations of SF-36 that are being validated in different countries.[85,86]

The main advantages of SF-36 are that it is the briefest of the generic measures described here and can be completed without supervision or interview, yet it remains comprehensive. On the other hand, relatively little work has been done to test its sensitivity to clinical changes. There is little doubt that we shall see more of it in years to come.

#### 8.2.2 Specific Instruments for Measuring Health-Related Quality of Life

These instruments have been designed to cover specific functions (e.g. the Hospital Anxiety and Depression Scale [HADS]), specific diseases (e.g. the Arthritis Impact Measurement Scale [AIMS]), or specific populations (e.g. the Pediatric Functional Independence Measure [wee FIM]). There are in excess of 300 specific instruments available for assessment of health-related quality of life, each emphasising the particular parameters that are of significance to the population group or the disease under study. For example, AIMS contains 66 questions grouped in a Cuttman-type format where responses form a continuum of increasing levels of intensity or severity. There are 3 domains (physical, psychological and pain) in which items such as mobility, physical activity, dexterity, ability to perform household tasks, social life, pain and stress are included. It has been properly validated and is a well researched, reliable instrument that is disease (arthritis) specific.

#### 8.2.3 Desirable Properties of Any Measurement of Health-Related Quality of Life

There are 3 properties that all instruments for assessment of quality of life, whether generic or specific, must possess. These are:

1) ***Reliability:*** the instrument must be reliable in that it measures something in a consistent and reproducible fashion.

2) ***Validity:*** this can be established in different ways and must address several independent aspects of the scale for measuring quality of life. In general, the aim is to clarify what the scale measures and how well it does so. A critical appraisal of the content and validity of 4 questionnaires used to assess quality of life in patients with respiratory disease has been published.[87] This appraisal distinguishes 3 major categories of validity: criterion, content and construct. *Criterion validity* means that the new test is assessed against an external criterion that is an objective measurement, e.g. a psychological assessment of job suitability might be measured against the objective criterion of work output. There is no objective measure that represents health; therefore criterion validity cannot be applied to tests of health-related quality of life. *Content validity* is an assessment of the degree to which the questionnaire covers the range of topics that it purports to measure (e.g. symptoms, physical activity and emotions). *Construct validity* assumes the existence of a construct or theoretical entity that the questionnaire is measuring. The construct validity of the new test can be assessed in a number of ways. One is measurement of the impact of experimental interventions (i.e. response to treatment) and a second is examination of the internal consistency of the questionnaire.

These abstract terms are difficult to grasp without reference to the performance of specific tests of quality of life.[87] The important point to emphasise is that measurement of health-related quality of life poses formidable problems and therefore design and assessment of the instruments should be done in close collaboration with psychologists.

3) ***Responsiveness or sensitivity:*** this refers to whether the instrument is capable of detecting a clinically important change, even when these changes are marginal and small.

### 8.3 Use and Abuse of Cost-Utility Data

The aim of any economic analysis is to provide information about the costs and consequences of alternative uses for scarce resources. Whether they like it or not, decision makers have to allocate resources between fundamentally different healthcare programmes, and

**Table VI.** Major methodological concerns about using cost per quality-adjusted life year (QALY) league tables as a method for allocation of healthcare resources

| |
|---|
| 1. Is this a theoretically sound method for deciding priorities? |
| 2. Are the instruments for measuring quality of life robust? |
| 3. From what data were the QALYs derived? |
| 4. From what data were the costs derived? |
| 5. What is the precision and statistical distribution of the cost and QALY data? |
| 6. Are the results sensitive to discounting? |

there is an understandable hunger for any form of apparently objective information that would ease the pain of making these difficult decisions. The possibility of providing decision makers with a league table of priorities for funding is a very laudable idea. However, serious doubts have been expressed about the validity of league tables derived from cost-utility studies.[22,88-98] These objections focus on 6 major issues (table VI):

***1) Is this a theoretically sound method for deciding priorities?*** The concept requires acceptance of maximisation of utility as the primary priority for allocation of scarce resources.[96] Aggregation of individual utility values is not a theoretically sound method for deriving a community health outcome measure.[97] The available techniques for measurement of utility do not take account of patient preferences.[97] A true community health outcome measure should be based on surveys that allow members of the community to compare and value several different states of health.

***2) Are the instruments for measuring quality of life robust?*** The instruments may be biased against certain groups, particularly the elderly.[95] There has been insufficient discussion about the weighting of individual items used to derive an overall estimate of health-related quality of life and the potential bias that is the inevitable result of such weighting.[88,99]

***3) From what data were the quality-adjusted life years (QALYs) derived?*** In descending order of merit, there are 3 major options for data collection:[92]

a) prospective measurement of QALYs before and after an intervention;

b) single interview after an intervention with retrospective estimate of the pre-intervention quality of life; and

c) derivation of QALY estimates by the researcher based on previously collected clinical data that did not directly measure health-related quality of life.

Unfortunately, the majority of published cost per QALY estimates use the third method.[92] If data are to be aggregated from several studies, a formal method must be used based on accepted standards for meta-analysis.[98] Also, wherever possible, outcomes should be stratified for risk.[35,100]

***4) From what data were the costs derived?*** If it is accepted that cost-utility analysis is a method for allocating a healthcare budget, then it follows that costs should be restricted to healthcare costs.[96] Comparisons should be based on recently collected cost data derived from the same healthcare system.[91] Medical practice variation and other factors produce massive variations in costs between different healthcare systems (see section 6.2.5).

***5) What is the precision and statistical distribution of the cost and QALY data?*** Very few published studies provide any statistical analysis of costs or QALYs.[93] The estimates should be analysed and confidence intervals for the estimates reported.[101]

***6) Are the results sensitive to discounting?*** There continues to be debate about whether or not it is appropriate to apply discounting to future QALY gains.[22] Estimates of cost per QALY are often highly sensitive to discounting of either future cost or future QALYs, yet few past estimates explicitly analyse the impact of discounting.[93]

**Table VII.** An example of the presentation of cost per quality-adjusted life year (QALY) data in a clinical trial which overcomes many of the concerns set out in table VI (after Oldridge et al.[101]). A range for the estimate of cost per QALY is presented, derived from the estimates of both cost and outcome. The comparison is with recent studies of related (cardiovascular) healthcare programmes which were conducted in a similar setting (US or Canada)

| Parameter | Cost per QALY gained (1991 $US) |
|---|---|
| **Subject of the clinical trial reported:** | |
| Cardiac rehabilitation after myocardial infarction: | |
| • mean | 6800 |
| • range | 3200 to 18,000 |
| **Previously published contemporary estimates from related programmes in a similar environment:** | |
| Coronary artery bypass grafting for left main vessel disease | 7900 |
| Treatment of severe diastolic hypertension (>104mm Hg) in a 40-year-old man | 17,700 |
| Treatment of mild diastolic hypertension (95-104mm Hg) in a 40-year-old man | 35,900 |
| Coronary artery bypass grafting for 1-vessel disease in patients with mild angina | 68,200 |

**Table VIII.** Factors which lead to international variation in drug pricing (after Wertheimer & Grumer;[102] Andersson[104])

| Global factors | National factors |
|---|---|
| Development costs | ***Factors influencing the unit price of the drug:*** |
| Costs of making the drug (raw materials and manufacturing) | Government regulations |
| Distribution costs (e.g. 'cold chain' storage for vaccines) | Requirements for inclusion of the drug in formularies or other limited lists |
| Promotion and advertising costs | Application of value added tax or other retail taxes |
| Advantages of the drug over competitive products | Availability of parallel imports or pirate versions of the same drug |
| Availability of other (nondrug) therapies to treat the same condition | Exchange rate and cost of living |
| Patent life of the drug | ***Factors influencing the perceived price per patient treated:*** |
| Estimated current and future market size | Regulations about retail and hospital discounting of drug prices |
| | Regulations about pack size |
| | Local medical practice variations about unit dose or duration of therapy |

Provided the limitations of cost-utility analysis are understood, we believe that these techniques can and should be used in debates about priorities. Before starting an economic analysis, the quality of clinical information should be discussed to distinguish 2 broad groups of treatments: those of proven effectiveness *vs* those of potential value. The first is essentially a list that must be ranked in order of priority for implementation, whereas the second must be used to discuss priorities for evaluation and research.[98] Even if the clinical data are sound within the context of specific trials, the patients studied may not be the same as the patients who are being considered for implementation of the intervention.

Some form of incremental analysis is required to adjust cost-utility ratios for risk.[100] Cost per QALY gained has been used to estimate the incremental cost-utility of changing to non-ionic radiographic contrast media. The overall estimate was US$65,000 per QALY gained; however, the range was from US$23,000 per QALY gained for high-risk patients to US$220,000 per QALY gained for low-risk patients.[100] The ideal is that the data used to construct cost-utility ratios should be collected prospectively, the statistical uncertainty of both costs and utilities should be analysed, and the cost-utility ratios should be compared with recent data derived from the same healthcare system. A recent study has shown that this is an achievable ideal,[101] but even so, the authors of this excellent study were careful to confine their comparisons to interventions for cardiovascular disease (table VII). Given all of these strictures about the methods of data collection, we believe that cost-utility ratios and league tables may assist the decision maker in allocating resources between broadly similar healthcare programmes. In economic terminology, the appropriate use of the information is to maximise utility gains within a healthcare budget.[96]

Everyone concerned with decision making based on cost-utility data must realise that any measurement of HRQOL is sensitive to assumptions and value judgements. It would be a tragedy if such useful measures become discredited because they are used to camouflage difficult ethical decisions behind an apparently objective numerical score.

## 9. The Future of Pharmacoeconomics

### 9.1 Changes in Drug Pricing and Reimbursement

Pharmaceutical companies have been quick to recognise the relevance of pharmacoeconomic analysis to strategic planning, both in early drug development and in determining the likely prices of future drugs.[9] Governments have been well aware of the 'drug pricing Tower of Babel',[102] but have so far made little progress, even through cooperative trade groups like the European Economic Community (EEC).[102] The academic community has been slow to recognise either the complexity of factors determining drug pricing (table VIII) or the potential for systematic research in this area. Most governments have developed some form of price regulation, with Australia probably having the strictest price control of all,[102] whereas the US has virtually no government control, allowing the market to determine price.[102,103] In this regard, the mechanism of price control is worthy of note. Although the UK has a comprehensive pharmaceutical pricing system, this is

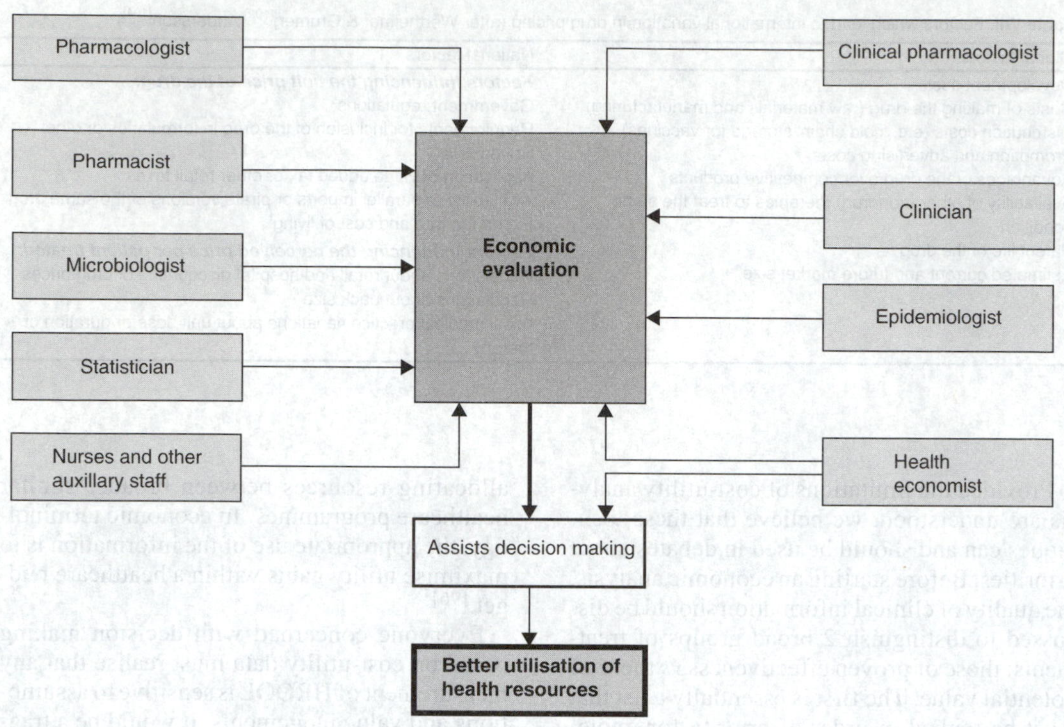


**Fig. 10.** Multidisciplinary nature of economic evaluation.

based on target points for voluntary price restraint that are in turn based on the contribution of the company to the UK economy, i.e. the system explicitly recognises the cost and value of research and development. Consequently pharmaceutical companies continue to invest in UK research, whereas there is very little investment in Australia.[102]

The challenge for future research is to examine the links between pricing and prescribing or more importantly, between pricing and efficiency.[104] The evolution of managed care systems may offer the opportunity to conduct such research. Currently, most systems try to contain costs over at most an 18-month perspective.[103] As managed care matures, there is growing recognition of the need for a longer term perspective that is based equally on consideration of cost and quality or value. Only by doing so will pharmaceuticals be fully appreciated for the value they contribute, rather than the costs they generate.[103]

### 9.2 Copayment For Drugs and Availability of Over-the-Counter Medications

Copayment is another method for attempting to reduce a government's contribution to drug costs, and simply means that the patient pays part or all of the cost of the medication received. Making drugs available over-the-counter (OTC) means that the patient pays the full cost of the medication. In addition, the patient no longer requires access to a clinician to obtain a prescription, leading to further potential reductions in healthcare costs. Clinicians have been quick to point out the potential disadvantages of reduced control of drug prescribing, and perhaps the clearest example is OTC availability of antibacterial drugs, which has been linked to high rates of drug resistance amongst bacteria in developing countries.[105-110] There is also some evidence that the availability of OTC medications for asthma leads to undertreatment and poorer patient outcomes.[111] Nonetheless, it must be recognised that clinicians have a strong vested interest in maintaining control of prescribing, and that community pharmacists have an equally strong vested interest in encouraging OTC availability.[112] From the patients' perspective, OTC availability increases convenience and allows individuals to take control of their treatment, which may in turn increase the number of patients who are treated.[113] An analysis conducted from the economic theory of consumer surplus concluded that, from the perspectives of the individual patient or society as a whole, the benefits of shifting drugs from prescription-only to OTC status may outweigh the costs.[113]

Clarification of the long term costs and benefits of changes in copayment and in availability of OTC medication is a further challenge for pharmacoeconomic research. As with pricing, the key issue is the impact of the intervention on the overall efficiency of the healthcare system.

## 9.3 A Research Agenda for the Future

The development of pharmacoeconomics from health economics provides a sound theoretical structure that is in turn based on knowledge derived from the evolution of economics. The time is now right to test this theoretical base in controlled clinical trials. Drugs are the major variable cost in healthcare but still consume only a small part of the total healthcare budget, the major part being consumed by fixed costs (buildings, staff and equipment). There is increasing evidence to show that drugs can be used to reduce fixed costs and that these resources can be redeployed to provide new services. The challenge for the future is to show that pharmacoeconomic analysis increases the efficiency of allocation of healthcare resources. This will only be achieved by integration of health economics into the multidisciplinary structure of health services research (fig. 10).

The disciplines discussed in this chapter are meant to be illustrative rather than exhaustive. The key points are, firstly, that many disciplines should shape an economic analysis and, secondly, that the aim of the analysis is to help someone to make a decision about the allocation of healthcare resources. The analysis cannot make the decision but it should make clear to the decision maker the likely costs and consequences of the available alternatives.

## References


1. Backhouse ME, Backhouse RJ, Edey SA. Economic evaluation biliography. Health Economics 1992; Suppl. 1
2. Harrigan J, Mosley P. Evaluating the impact of world bank structural adjustment lending: 1980-87. In: Malek M, editor. Contemporary issues in European development aid. London: Gower, 1991
3. Cooper MH, Culyer AJ. Health economics. London: Penguin, 1973
4. Fischer S, Dornbusch R. Economics. New York: McGraw Hill, 1983
5. Samuelson PA. Economics. New York: McGraw Hill, 1976
6. Mooney G, editor. Economics, medicine and health care. London: Harvester Wheatsheaf, 1992
7. McGuire A, Henderson J, Mooney G, editors. The economics of health care. London: Routledge & Kegan Paul, 1988
8. Townsend RJ. Post-marketing research and development. Drug Intelligence and Clinical Pharmacy 1987; 21: 134-6
9. Clemens K, Garrison Jr LP, Jones A, et al. Strategic use of pharmacoeconomic research in early drug development and global pricing. PharmacoEconomics 1993; 4: 315-22
10. Steele H. Monopoly and competition in the ethical drugs market. Journal of Law and Economics 1962; 5: 131-63
11. Smith M. Pharmaceutical marketing strategy and cases. London: Pharmaceutical Products Press, The Haworth Press Inc., 1991
12. Wiggins S. The pharmaceutical industry. Texas: A&M University, 1985
13. Reekie D, Wells N. Pharmaceuticals. In: Johnson P, editor. The structure of British industry. London: Unwin Hymen, 1988
14. Cocks D. Product innovation and the dynamic elements of competition in the ethical pharmaceutical industry. In: Helms RB, editor. Drug development and marketing. Washington: American Enterprise Institute, 1975
15. Tesler L. The supply response to shifting demand in the ethical pharmaceutical industry. In: Helms RB, editor. Drug development and marketing. Washington: American Enterprise Institute, 1975
16. Anonymous. The story of a new medicine. Basel: Ciba Geigy Pharmaceuticals, 1991
17. DiMasi JA, Hansen RW, Grabowski HG, et al. Cost of innovation in the pharmaceutical industry. Journal of Health Economics 1991; 10: 107-42
18. Mossinghoff G. Pharmaceutical research is expensive but well worth the cost. Journal of Endocrinology 1991; 128: 3-5
19. Drummond MF, Stoddart GL, Torrance GW. Methods for the economic evaluation of health care programmes. Oxford: Oxford University Press, 1987
20. Drummond M, Brandt A, Luce B, et al. Standardizing methodologies for economic evaluation in health care. International Journal of Technology Assessment in Health Care 1993; 9: 26-36
21. Spackman M. Discount rates and rates of return in the public sectors. Economic Issues, Working Paper 113. London: Government Economic Service, 1991
22. Parsonage M, Neuberger H. Discounting and health benefits. Health Economics 1992; 1: 71-9
23. Cairns J. Discounting and health benefits: another perspective. Health Economics 1992; 1: 71-9
24. Davey P, Malek M, Dodd T. Pharmacoeconomics: the truth. Lancet 1993; 341: 1097-8
25. Malek M. Pharmacoeconomics: science or fad? Scottish Medicine 1993; 13: 12-13
26. Drummond M. Australian guidelines for cost-effectiveness studies of pharmaceuticals. The thin end of the boomerang? York: Centre for Health Economics, Discussion Paper 88, 1991
27. Drummond MF. Economic evaluation of pharmaceuticals: science or marketing? PharmacoEconomics 1992; 1: 8-13

28. Hillman AJW, Eisenberg JM, Pauly MV, et al. Avoiding bias in the conduct and reporting of cost-effectiveness research sponsored by pharmaceutical companies. New England Journal of Medicine 1991; 324: 1362-5
29. Mitchell A, Henry D. Potential for bias in economic analyses. New England Journal of Medicine 1991; 325
30. Commonwealth of Australia. Draft guidelines for the pharmaceutical industry on preparation of submissions to the pharmaceutical benefits committee, including submissions involving economic analyses. Canberra: Department of Health, Housing and Committee Services, 1990
31. Detsky AS. Guidelines for economic analysis of pharmaceutical products: a draft document for Ontario and Canada. PharmacoEconomics 1993; 3: 354-61
32. Sheldon TA. Please bypass the PORT. Observational studies of effectiveness run a poor second to randomised controlled trials. British Medical Journal 1994; 309: 142-3
33. Davey P, Rutherford D, Graham B, et al. Repeat consultations after antibiotic prescribing for respiratory infection in one general practice. British Journal of General Practice 1994; 44: 509-13
34. Tallis R, Hall G, Craig I, et al. How common are epileptic seizures in old age? Age and Ageing 1991; 20: 442-8
35. Davey Smith G, Egger M. Who benefits from medical interventions? British Medical Journal 1994; 308: 72-4
36. Beardon PHG, McGilchrist MM, Mckendrick AD, et al. Primary noncompliance with prescribed medication in primary care. British Medical Journal 1993; 307: 846-8
37. Wheeldon NM, MacDonald TM, Flucker CJ, et al. Echocardiography in chronic heart failure in the community. Quarterly Journal of Medicine 1993; 86: 17-23
38. Drummond M. Cost-of-illness studies: a major headache? PharmacoEconomics 1992; 2: 1-4
39. Weiss KB, Sullivan SD. The economic costs of asthma. PharmacoEconomics 1993; 4: 14-30
40. Donaldson C, Mooney G. Needs assessment, priority setting and contracts for health care: an economic view. British Medical Journal 1991; 303: 1529-30
41. Normand C. Economics, health and the economics of health. British Medical Journal 1991; 303: 1572-7
42. Finkler SA. The distinction between cost and charges. Annals of Internal Medicine 1982; 96: 102-9
43. Williams DN, Bosch D, Boots J, et al. Safety, efficacy and cost savings in an outpatient intravenous antibiotic program. Clinical Therapeutics 1993; 15: 169-79
44. Rubinstein E. Cost implications of home care on serious infections. Hospital Formulary 1993; 28 Suppl. 1: 46-50
45. Graham DR. Nosohusial infections: complication of home intravenous therapy. Infectious Diseases in Clinical Practice 1993; 2: 158-61
46. Poretz DM, Woolard D, Eron LJ, et al. Outpatient use of ceftriaxone: a cost-benefit analysis. American Journal of Medicine 1984; 77 Suppl. 4C: 77-83
47. Sharp JW. Social work in a home intravenous antibiotic therapy program. Social Work in Health Care 1986; 12: 93-101
48. Davey P, Hernanz C, Lynch W, et al. Human and non-financial costs of hospital-acquired infection. Journal of Hospital Infection 1991; 18 Suppl. A: 79-84
49. McCue JD, Hansen C, Gal P. Hospital charges for antibiotics. Reviews of Infectious Diseases 1985; 7: 643-5
50. Tanner DJ, Nazarian MQ. Cost containment associated with decreased parenteral antibiotic administration frequencies. American Journal of Medicine 1984; 77 Suppl. 4C: 104-10
51. Knodel LC, Goldspiel BR, Gibbs RS. Prospective cost analysis of moxalactam versus clindamycin plus gentamicin for endomyometritis after cesarean section. Antimicrobial Agents and Chemotherapy 1988; 32: 853-7
52. Parker SE, Davey PG. Pharmacoeconomics of intravenous drug administration. PharmacoEconomics 1992; 1: 103-15
53. Birdwell SW. Direct costs of intravenous delivery systems. PharmacoEconomics 1993; 4: 8-13
54. Newhouse JG, Paul VM, Waugh NA, et al. Reducing IV waste to under 2.25%. Hospital Pharmacy 1988; 23: 241-7
55. Birdwell SW, Meyer GE, Scheckelhoff DJ, et al. Survey of wastage from intravenous admixture in US hospitals. PharmacoEconomics 1993; 4: 271-7
56. Lowson K. Health economics for clinician managers. Clinician in Management 1993; 2: 9-12
57. Shulkin DJ, Kinosian B, Glick H, et al. The economic impact of infections: an analysis of hospital costs and charges in surgical patients with cancer. Archives of Surgery 1993; 128: 449-52
58. Vacani PF, Malek MMH, Davey PG. Cost of gentamicin assays carried out by microbiology laboratories. Journal of Clinical Pathology 1993; 46: 890-5
59. Polgar S, Thomas SA. Measures of central tendency and dispersion. In: Polgar S, Thomas SA, editors. Introduction to research in the health sciences. Melbourne: Churchill Livingstone, 1991
60. Lynch W, Malek M, Davey PG, et al. Costing wound infection in a Scottish hospital. PharmacoEconomics 1992; 2: 163-70
61. Crombie IK, Davies HTO, Abraham SCS, et al., editors. The audit handbook - improving health care through clinical audit. Chichester: John Wiley & Sons, 1993
62. Andersen TF, Mooney G. Medical practice variations: where are we? In: Anderson TF, Mooney G, editors. The challenges of medical practice variations. Basingstoke: Macmillan Press, 1990
63. McPherson K. Why do variations occur? In: Andersen TF, Mooney G, editors. The challenges of medical practice variations. Basingstoke: Macmillan Press, 1990
64. Halls GA. The management of infections and antibiotic therapy: a European survey. Journal of Antimicrobial Chemotherapy 1993; 31: 985-1000
65. Davey PG, Parker SE, Malek MM. Pharmacoeconomics of antibacterial treatment. PharmacoEconomics 1992; 1: 409-37
66. Ford LC, Hammil HA, Lebherz TB. Cost-effective use of antibiotic prophylaxis for cesarean section. American Journal of Obstetrics and Gynecology 1987; 157: 506-10
67. Keane D, James D. Prophylactic antibiotics at caesarean section do not reduce costs. Health Trends 1993; 25: 84-7
68. Thornton JG, Lilford RJ, Johnson N. Decision analysis in medicine. British Medical Journal 1992; 304: 1099-103

69. Schumacher GE. Multiattribute evaluation in formulary decision making as applied to calcium-channel blockers. American Journal of Hospital Pharmacy 1991; 48: 301-8
70. De Vries TPGM. Presenting clinical pharmacology and therapeutics: a problem based approach for choosing and prescribing drugs. British Journal of Clinical Pharmacology 1993; 35: 581-6
71. Nash DB, Catalano ML, Wordell CJ. The formulary decision-making process in a US academic medical centre. PharmacoEconomics 1993; 3: 22-35
72. Lipsy RJ. Institutional formularies: the relevance of pharmacoeconomic analysis to formulary decisions. PharmacoEconomics 1992; 1: 265-81
73. Schechter CB. Decision analysis in formulary decision making. PharmacoEconomics 1993; 3: 454-61
74. Chaput de Saintonge DM, Kirwan JR, Evans SJ, et al. How can we design trials to detect clinically important changes in disease severity? British Journal of Clinical Pharmacology 1988; 26: 355-62
75. Kongpatanakul S, Strom BL. Quality of life, health status and clinical drug research. PharmacoEconomics 1992; 1: 8-14
76. United Nations. The human development report. Oxford: Oxford University Press, 1994
77. WHOQOL Group. Study protocol for the World Health Organization Project to develop a quality of life assessment instrument (WHOQOL). Quality of Life Research 1993; 2: 153-9
78. Bergner M, Bobbitt RA, Carter WB. The sickness impact profile: development and final revision of a health status measure. Medical Care 1981; 19
79. Ott CR, Sivarajan ES, Newton KM. A controlled randomised study of early cardiac rehabilitation: the sickness impact profile as an assessment tool. Heart and Lung 1983; 12
80. Liang MH, Larson MC, Cullen KE. Comparative measurement efficacy and sensitivity of five health status instruments for arthritis research. Arthritis and Rheumatism 1985; 28: 542-7
81. Dayo RA, Diehl AK, Rosenthal M. How many days of bed rest for acute low back pain? A randomised clinical trial. New England Journal of Medicine 1986; 315
82. Hunt SM, McKenna SP, McEwen J. A quantitive approach to perceived health status: a validation study. Journal of Epidemiology and Community Health 1980; 34: 281-6
83. Jenkinson C, Fitzpatrick R, Argyle M. The Nottingham Health Profile: an analysis of its sensitivity in differentiating illness groups. Social Science and Medicine 1988; 27: 1411-4
84. Jenkinson C, Fitzpatrick R. Measurement of health status in patients with chronic illness: comparison of the Nottingham Health Profile and General Health Questionnaire. Family Practice 1990; 7: 121-4
85. Brazier JE, Harper R, Jones NMB. Validating the SF 36 health survey questionnaire: new outcome measure for primary care. British Medical Journal 1992; 305
86. Jenkinson C, Coulter A, Wright L. Short form 36 (SF36) health survey questionnaire: normative data for adults of working age. British Medical Journal 1993; 306: 1437-40
87. Hyland ME. Quality-of-life assessment in respiratory disease: an examination of the content and validity of four questionnaires. PharmacoEconomics 1992; 2: 43-53
88. Hyland ME. Selection of items and avoidance of bias in quality of life scales. PharmacoEconomics 1992; 1: 182-90
89. Spilker B. Standardisation of quality of life trials: an industry perspective. PharmacoEconomics 1992; 1: 73-5
90. Jaeschke R, Guyatt GH, Cook D. Quality of life instruments in the evaluation of new drugs. PharmacoEconomics 1992; 1: 84-93
91. Mason J, Drummond M, Torrance G. Some guidelines on the use of cost effectiveness league tables. British Medical Journal 1993; 306: 570-2
92. Coast J. Developing the QALY concept: exploring the problems of data acquisition. PharmacoEconomics 1993; 4: 240-6
93. Petrou S, Malek M, Davey PG. The reliability of cost-utility estimates in cost-per-QALY league tables. PharmacoEconomics 1993; 3 Suppl. 5: 345-53
94. Hopkins A, editor. Measures of the quality of life and the uses to which such measures may be put. London: Royal College of Physicians of London, 1992
95. Grimley-Evans J. Quality of life assessments and elderly people. In: Hopkins A, editor. Measures of the quality of life and the uses to which such measures may be put. London: Royal College of Physicians of London, 1992
96. Gerard K, Mooney G. QALY league tables: handle with care. PharmacoEconomics 1993; 2: 59-64
97. Mehrez A, Gafni A. Preference based outcome measures for economic evaluation of drug interventions: quality adjusted life years (QALYs) versus health years equivalents (HYEs). PharmacoEconomics 1992; 1: 338-45
98. Simes RJ, Glasziou PP. Meta-analysis and quality of evidence in the economic evaluation of drug trials. PharmacoEconomics 1992; 1: 282-92
99. Nord E. Towards quality assurance in QALY calculations. International Journal of Technology Assessment in Health Care 1993; 9: 37-45
100. Goel V, Deber RB, Detsky AS. Nonionic contrast media: economic analysis and health policy development. Canadian Medical Association Journal 1989; 140: 389-95
101. Oldridge N, Furlong W, Feeny D, et al. Economic evaluation of cardiac rehabilitation soon after acute myocardial infarction. American Journal of Cardiology 1993; 72: 154-61
102. Wertheimer AI, Grumer SK. Overview of international pharmacy pricing. PharmacoEconomics 1992; 2: 449-55
103. Navarro RP. Regulation of pharmaceutical prices: a managed care perspective. PharmacoEconomics 1993; 3: 179-82
104. Andersson F. Methodological aspects of international drug price comparisons. PharmacoEconomics 1993; 4: 247-56
105. Obaseiki-Ebor EE, Akerele JO, Ebea PO. A survey of antibiotic outpatient prescribing and antibiotic self-medication. Journal of Antimicrobial Chemotherapy 1987: 759-63
106. Thamlakitkul V. Antibiotic dispensing by drug store personnel in Bangkok, Thailand. Journal of Antimicrobial Chemotherapy 1988; 21: 125-31
107. Montefiore D, Rotimi VO, Adeyemi-Doro FAB. The problem of bacterial resistance to antibiotics among strains isolated from hospital patients in

Lagosand Ibadan, Nigeria. Journal of Antimicrobial Chemotherapy 1989; 23: 641-51

108. Lepage PB. Multiresistant *Salmonella typhimurium* systemic infection in Rwanda: clinical features and treatment with cefotaxime. Journal of Antimicrobial Chemotherapy 1990; 26 Suppl. A: 53-7
109. Lamikanra A, Ndep RB. Trimethoprim resistance in urinary tract pathogens in two Nigerian hospitals. Journal of Antimicrobial Chemotherapy 1989; 23: 151-4
110. Clendennen TE, Hames CS, Kees ES, et al. In vitro antibiotic susceptibilities of *Neisseria gonorrhoeae* isolates in the Philippines. Antimicrobial Agents and Chemotherapy 1992; 36: 277-82
111. Gibson P, Henry D, Francis L, et al. Association between availability of non-prescription $\beta_2$-agonist inhalers and undertreatment of asthma. British Medical Journal 1993; 306: 1514-8
112. Ryan M, Bond C. Dispensing physicians and prescribing pharmacists: economic considerations for the UK. PharmacoEconomics 1994; 5: 8-17
113. Andersson F, Hatziandreu E. The costs and benefits of switching a drug from prescription-only to over-the-counter status: a review of methodological issues and current evidence. PharmacoEconomics 1992; 2: 388-96

Chapter 11

# Drug Development and Approval Processes

*B. Spilker*

## Synopsis of Important Principles

1) In the development of a new drug, adherence to high standards in the conduct, analysis and interpretation of all preclinical and clinical studies is vital to ensure its smooth passage through the development and regulatory approval phases to eventual marketing. Carefully developed strategies as well as experienced and dedicated staff are also required.

2) To guide the development process, it is important to establish minimally acceptable criteria for an agent's performance.

3) In creating the overall development plan, it is important to distinguish between those studies that are *desirable* to conduct, and those that are *necessary* to conduct, and to include only the latter. However, the distinction between these two broad types of studies may change during a drug's development.

4) The design of a clinical trial depends on the specific primary objectives that have been set. Trial objectives that are to be addressed must be clearly established and described.

5) A strategy for monitoring and auditing a clinical trial should be planned at the time of its initiation. This should include what will be monitored, how it will be monitored, and who will monitor it, and when and where it will be monitored. The role of auditing is to ensure that both the investigators and monitors are carrying out their functions appropriately, and that Good Clinical Practices (GCP) guidelines are being followed.

6) Interpretation of the data obtained from a clinical trial involves not only an evaluation of its statistical significance, but also its clinical significance and the trial's relevance for medical practice. Evaluation of the clinical significance of data requires experienced clinical judgement and involves comparisons with standard treatments or placebo.

7) Important requirements of regulatory submissions include conciseness, clarity, correctness (in terms of the data provided), completeness and consistency of organisation. Problems must not be buried in applications but discussed openly. Computer-assisted new drug applications (CANDAs) are currently viewed as a controversial method of improving the speed of regulatory reviews.

Drug development is principally undertaken by research-based pharmaceutical companies, but development-oriented pharmaceutical companies, research institutes, academic centres and contract research organisations also act as sponsors of drug development. The term development is defined differently in different situations. It may refer specifically to the technical aspects of chemical scale-up, analytical procedures, and pharmaceutical development of a dosage form or a specific formulation. Alternatively, or in addition, the term development may

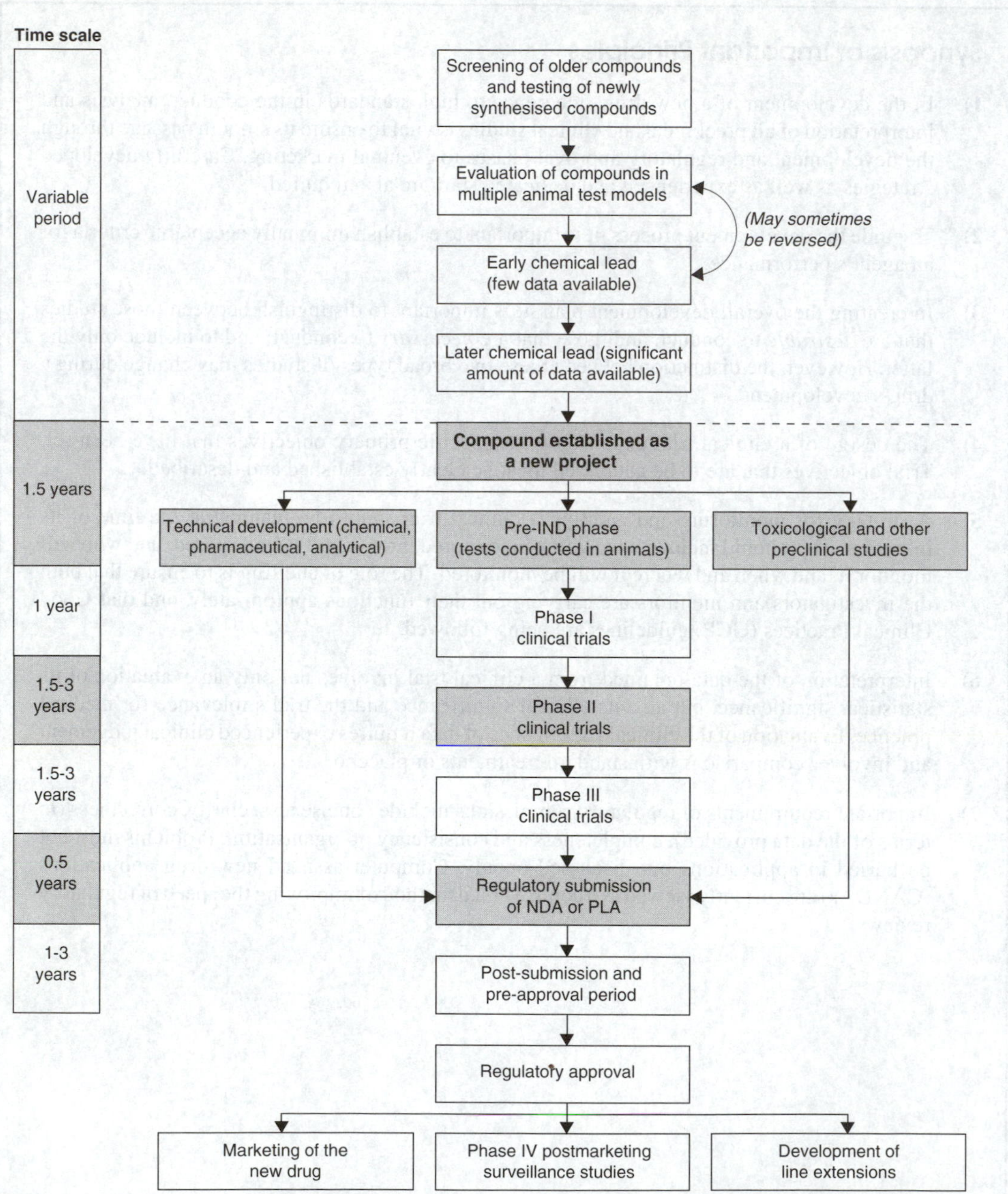


**Fig. 1.** Stages of drug discovery (above the dotted line) and development (below the dotted line). Note that various feedback loops exist, especially during the initial stages of drug discovery (IND = Investigational New Drug; NDA = New Drug Application; PLA = Product License Application) [after Spilker;[1] with permission]. The lowest time scale (1 to 3 years) refers to regulatory review, and the time above it the time to assemble the regulatory dossier.

refer to the entire process of taking a newly discovered compound through regulatory approval to the point of marketing (fig. 1). This broad definition will be used in this chapter.

Adherence to high standards in the conduct, analysis and interpretation of all preclinical and clinical trials with a new agent is vital. Poorly planned or conceived studies will often raise questions that may be difficult to explain. This in turn will create the need for additional trials that might not have been necessary to conduct. Obtaining and analysing the additional data such studies generate will generally delay regulatory submissions.

## 1. Important Steps in the Development Process

### 1.1 Deciding Which Compounds to Develop as New Drugs

To enable this decision to be made, criteria should be established for all research efforts directed at discovering a new agent. When a chemical compound is found that meets these criteria, then it is (usually) developed as a medicine. The compound continues to be developed until events demonstrate that some of the criteria (primarily safety and efficacy) cannot be met and that a medically and commercially viable medicine is no longer likely or possible to achieve.

Because research programmes in one therapeutic area may lead to discovery of a compound that has activity in another area, carefully developed criteria are not always present when a new direction in a drug's development is debated. Considerations as to whether to develop the compound for a new use include determining how the compound fits into the company's strategies and portfolio for current and future drug development. This includes evaluation of old product line extensions, entrance into new product lines, perceived medical need, perceived commercial gains, plus the patent situation on the new compound.

In addition to the company's basic strategies, other important issues to consider include the resources necessary to test and develop a new drug. Will it be relatively straightforward to evaluate its efficacy, as with a diuretic or neuromuscular blocking agent, or will it be much more complex and expensive, as with an antipsychotic? Is the path to regulatory approval different from that for an 'average' medicine? For example, chemical classes of drugs with

**Table I.** Research and development criteria to evaluate a new compound for potential development as a medicine[a] (after Spilker,[2] with permission)

1. Likelihood of technical success
2. Estimated time to develop the drug to NDA[b] status
3. Time to reach a go/no-go decision[c]
4. Anticipated technical development problems (e.g. stability of the product)
5. Availability in desired dosage forms
6. Presence of skills to develop the drug
7. Degree of medical need for the type of drug
8. Medical advantages of the drug compared with alternative therapies
9. Actual or potential restrictions on the drug's use
10. Cost of development in comparison to predicted third-year sales or profits (may be calculated in terms of time to pay back the investment)
11. Number of potential indications
12. Any known limitations or problems not covered above

a A number of additional criteria are described in the text.
b NDA = New Drug Application.
c This point usually occurs during phase II.

toxicity known to be greater than that of others in the same therapeutic class are not looked on favourably by some regulatory authorities. In addition, each regulatory authority may require different types and degrees of proof of efficacy. This may make a drug's development far more complex and costly for one country than for another.

Depending on the answers to these (and other) questions (table I), the company may decide to go all out, to go ahead with a limited programme, to develop the agent for certain countries only, to license it to another company, or to take a totally different course of action.

### 1.2 Determining the Appropriate Scope of a Drug Development Plan

A preclinical and clinical programme of appropriate and well designed studies should be planned to address all pertinent issues. A company may attempt to do this by developing a plan that emphasises any desired approach varying from a *'lean'* one that eliminates all studies that are not absolutely essential, to a *'fat'* approach that includes all possible considerations and studies. If the approach chosen is too lean and incomplete, it may not achieve regulatory approval in some or all of the target countries. Conversely, a plan that is far in excess of what is necessary to meet regulatory requirements would not only take extra years to complete, but would generate excessive data that would require additional time for processing, analysis, interpretation, and report writing.

In arriving at an appropriate balance between these extremes, the following decisions need to be made:

1) Determine if it would be reasonable to conduct any of the clinical trials after the drug is marketed.

2) Determine what would be lost if each study on the list were deleted. Which studies are mandatory to conduct?

3) Review the size of each study with a statistician. Could any be abbreviated?

4) Review the clinical plan in detail with the appropriate regulatory authorities.

Additional steps might be:

a) to evaluate the number and nature of studies conducted on recently approved drugs of the same type;

b) to discuss the issue with knowledgeable consultants; and

c) to develop alternative stepwise plans.

The master plan must distinguish between studies that are ***desirable*** to conduct and those that are ***necessary*** to conduct – whether they are clinical, toxicological, metabolic, pharmacokinetic or fit other categories of studies. The distinction between these two broad types of studies often changes during the development of a new drug. Although the master plan represents the blueprint for a drug's development, the plans must periodically be reassessed and necessary changes made.

### 1.3 Establishing Criteria for a Drug's Performance During its Development

Compounds that have achieved the criteria established during the drug discovery period are advanced into the development phase. Even if clear criteria have not been established during the discovery period, it is important to set criteria during development. This is primarily to know when the drug's development should be terminated.

Criteria established at an early stage of development to judge each drug's future performance should include medical, technical and commercial considerations. If the drug falls below or otherwise fails to meet these standards, then its termination should be considered. This does not mean that a company would not develop it as an 'orphan' drug (i.e. a drug useful in a limited patient population) in which case the company's management might agree to accept lower minimal medical and/or commercial criteria (e.g. smaller profits and a lower return on its investment). However, appropriate standards should still be set for 'orphan' drugs, just as for other medicines. If appropriate medical and commercial criteria are established (see Spilker[1] for an extensive discussion of the types of criteria that may be established), a project's termination would be expedited if the drug's characteristics are such that the minimally acceptable criteria could not be met.

The criteria used to determine whether a drug passes the go/no-go decision point in phase II of its development may be set to a particularly high or low standard. Either approach may be desirable from a marketing viewpoint. For example, the company's marketing group may believe they do not want to sell a new drug unless it is 'sensational' medically, or conversely, they may believe that it is desirable to have the drug available for sale, even if it is not as effective (or safe) as the medical staff and managers hoped it might have been. Nonetheless, there are major differences among the types of criteria that may be created (e.g. ideal, desirable, realistic and minimally acceptable) for any drug and I believe that minimally acceptable criteria should almost always be used.[1]

An important new drug with great medical value may be of limited commercial benefit to a company if actual sales are small or modest, but this type of agent often provides numerous other benefits to a company (e.g. by enhancing its reputation, educating sales forces in a new area, and obtaining clinical experience in a new area). The company's overall reaction to possibly developing this type of drug depends to a large degree on their original expectations. These expectations are reflected in the criteria established for the drug's development.

### 1.4 Transfer of a Project from Preclinical to Clinical Development and from Clinical Development to Marketing and Production

As a drug progresses along the development pipeline and is marketed, various individuals and functions control the progress and decision-making about the drug. A transfer of responsibility occurs at discrete times as the drug moves forward. An important principle is that a minimum number of major transfers (e.g. preclinical to clinical) should be made within the company as a drug proceeds along the development pipeline. Each time a drug project is transferred from one department to another, it creates the opportunity for a person (or the department) to hold on to it too long and thereby delay its development. The opposite problem, in which the compound (or drug) is transferred too soon, is also a serious problem that could complicate its development. The person (or team) taking over at the next stage may or may not be ready to act expeditiously and appropriately to develop the agent, as it requires a period of time for a person or group to become sufficiently familiar with its details to ensure that full development speed is established and maintained. Thus, the more transfers that occur during development, the longer will be the nonproductive time. This process will be expedited if the new leader is a member of the team that had been developing the drug.

It is theoretically possible to have transfers occur when the project is formed and when the drug enters each new clinical phase (i.e. phases I to IV). This process would create a total of five development leaders, plus those in production and marketing. This is clearly an excessive number of transfers and would be highly inefficient. I believe that a more efficient system is for a single project manager to lead the project from its initiation to market launch, when it is turned over to someone in the marketing group.

### 1.5 Should a Drug Also Be Tested for Other Indications?

If a drug is available in appropriate dosage form(s) to treat patients with a particular disease and its formulation is appropriate in terms of stability, bioavailability and other technical considerations, important questions concerning its possible evaluation for other indications include:

1) What clinical evidence already exists that the drug is also effective in patients with the other diseases being considered and how convincing is this evidence?

2) What animal data already exist to indicate that the drug will be effective in these other diseases?

3) What is the medical need for a new drug to treat patients with these diseases?

4) What is the potential commercial value for a new agent in these indications?

5) What is the status of the research on the drug to treat the disease for which it was originally developed?

6) Does treating one or more additional diseases represent a tangent or part of the agreed-on development plan?

7) How will studies on other diseases affect resources allocated to the original project goals and the dates for achieving the original milestones?

**Table II.** Activities performed on marketed drugs in research departments (after Spilker;[2] with permission)

**1. Any research department**
a) Additional evaluation of the drug's mechanism of action
b) Training of sales representatives
c) Support marketing, medical, legal, production and other departments with information
d) Participate in writing and reviewing promotional materials
e) Participate in writing and reviewing technical materials for compendia
f) Answer requests for relevant information

**2. Organic chemistry**
Synthesis of additional compounds for patent protection of marketed drugs. Important structural relatives of marketed drugs must be made to protect them from the inevitable intense research conducted in the same chemical areas by competitors as well as to seek successor drugs

**3. Medicinal biochemistry**
a) Measure drug concentrations in samples obtained in clinical studies that are evaluating new indications
b) Conduct biochemical or metabolic studies to evaluate the basis for adverse reactions
c) Monitor drug concentrations in life-threatening situations
d) Refine and report on assay methodologies that may be used by outside laboratories
e) Participate in interlaboratory validation of methods
f) Expand the database in specific patient populations (e.g. neonates)
g) Conduct studies to help develop new formulations

**4. Pharmacology**
a) Investigation of drug-drug interactions that are reported in the literature or to the company
b) Investigation of a newly found therapeutic indication

**5. Toxicology**
a) Carcinogenicity or other toxicological studies dictated by clinical effects observed before or after marketing
b) Limited toxicology studies on new formulations

**6. Medical**
a) Conduct postmarketing trials
b) Develop new indications
c) Conduct other trials

**7. Other departments**
a) Assay of clinical samples of patients participating in clinical studies, especially in pursuit of added indications
b) Assay of samples from nonstudy patients treated with the drug
c) Assistance to outside laboratories in setting up assays
d) Pharmacokinetic studies in special patient groups (e.g. dialysis patients)
e) Computer assistance for analysis of assay data collected by other laboratories
f) Resistance studies

**Table III.** Activities performed on marketed drugs in technical development and regulatory affairs departments (after Spilker;[2] with permission)

**1. Library and information services[a]**
a) Monitor published literature for relevant papers
b) Perform *ad hoc* searches on the published literature
c) Prepare bibliographies for submission to regulatory authorities (e.g. the FDA[b] in the US).

**2. Pharmaceutical research and development laboratories**
a) Provide technical support for production
b) Improve various processes
c) Develop improved formulations or additional dosage forms
d) Conduct stability studies
e) Evaluate new packaging components and prepare submissions
f) Prepare drug materials for clinical trials
g) Validate equipment and processes
h) Prepare documents on formulation/manufacturing procedures and stability data for annual reports to regulatory authorities
i) Evaluate new equipment/materials
j) Participate in establishing release guidelines and revised specifications for marketed products

**3. Chemical development laboratories**
a) Provide technical support for chemical production (e.g. troubleshoot problem batches or process steps, optimisation/fine-tuning of processes, and reuse or recover waste)
b) Search for and develop improved synthetic route
c) Provide regulatory affairs with documents supporting manufacturing changes
d) Develop alternative sources of key raw materials or intermediates

**4. Analytical development laboratories**
a) Maintain and update development standards and analytical standards for reports to regulatory authorities
b) Convert development standards to analytical standards where applicable
c) Validate and file modifications to assays and other tests procedures with the regulatory authority
d) Validate and file modifications to analytical procedures found necessary as the result of improved formulations
e) Validate and file modifications to the testing methods for raw materials, intermediates, and bulk drug
f) Prepare pharmacopoeia-style monographs for the drug and dosage forms
g) Troubleshoot products to minimise problems and back orders

**5. Regulatory affairs department**
a) Submit annual reports to the regulatory authority on each product, describing serious adverse reactions and ongoing clinical trials
b) Compile, submit and track all submissions on marketed drugs to the regulatory authority for new indications, formulations, new routes of synthesis, labelling changes, and manufacturing control supplements
c) Provide support for state/regional formulary activities
d) Submit adverse reactions reports to the regulatory authority as required by law
e) Assist the legal department in relevant activities including recalls and liability actions
f) Maintain official records on all marketed drugs

a This group is usually situated organisationally in research and development.
b FDA = Food and Drug Administration.

8) What is the marketing perspective on pursuing these other indications?

9) How easy or difficult will it be to obtain regulatory approval for the proposed new indications?

10) How expensive will it be in terms of money, time and resources to complete a regulatory submission for each disease?

### 1.6 Activities Performed on Marketed Drugs by Research and Development Departments

Once a new agent has reached the point of marketing, the major activities performed by research departments and by technical and regulatory affairs departments are shown in tables II and III. The total quantity of work often increases after a drug is marketed for various reasons (e.g. new indications, new dosage forms, and technical questions that arise).

## 2. Design and Conduct of Clinical Trials

### 2.1 Classification and Description of Phases I to IV Studies

A classification of phase I, II, III and IV studies and the various activities that are undertaken at each stage is shown in table IV. The various types of clinical trials that may be conducted are shown in table V.

#### *2.1.1 Prospective versus Retrospective Trials*

There are three possible types of clinical trials, in terms of the period of time evaluated: prospective, retrospective, or a combination of both approaches within the same clinical trial (fig. 2). Numerous references show how retrospective trials often lead to false conclusions since effects may be blamed on the wrong causes, the correct probabilities may be poorly understood, and many biases and confounding factors may enter the trial, which can be neither purged nor fully understood. Thus, unless there are strong reasons to the contrary, clinical trials should use a prospective design whenever possible.

#### *2.1.2 Single Patient Group Designs*

In some open-label or single-blind clinical trials, all patients are treated with the same drug throughout the study. Criteria may be established to allow for dosage reductions (e.g. for adverse effects) or dosage increases (e.g. for lack of optimal improvement). Thus, a single

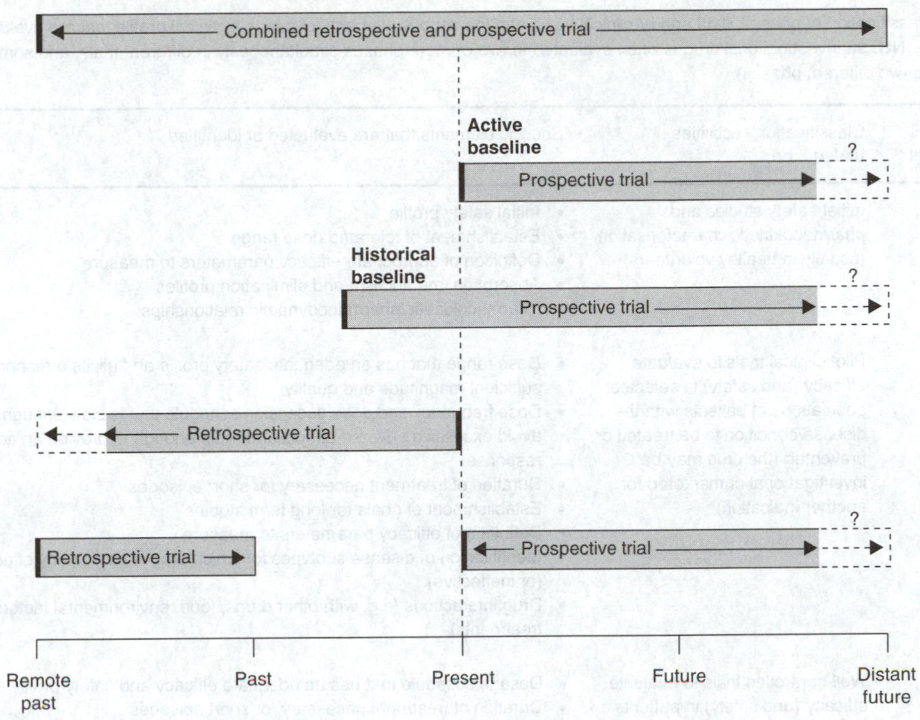


**Fig. 2.** Clinical trial timeline, illustrating the various types of retrospective and prospective trials (after Spilker;[2] with permission).

homogeneous group of patients at the start of a clinical trial may complete the trial as a heterogeneous group because each was treated with a different dose regimen.

Study designs using historical controls for comparative purposes can be considered as either single patient group or two patient group trials. However, in this discussion, studies using historical controls will be considered as designs with two groups of patients.

#### 2.1.3 Cross-Sectional versus Longitudinal Trials

##### Definitions

Cross-sectional trials are usually short term trials in which a cross section of the patient population of interest is evaluated for a period of up to 10 weeks. Longer cross-sectional trials are possible, but are less common. Patients are usually placed into one of two or more treatment groups and the data obtained from each group are then compared.

Longitudinal trials are usually long term clinical trials conducted for several months or longer. Placebos and/or active drug controls are seldom used, although a 'usual care' or 'no treatment' group may be included as a control group. The patients' data are generally compared with their own baseline values to identify changes. If a control group is included in the clinical trial, then a between-group comparison is conducted as well.

Although most longitudinal trials are long term, they may also be conducted over short periods. This may be the case, for example, in a longitudinal trial of a bronchodilator used by patients 4 times over the course of a day in which serial forced expiratory volume in 1 second ($FEV_1$) values are measured.

##### Uses of Cross-Sectional and Longitudinal Trials

Most efficacy and safety assessments of investigational drugs are conducted in short term cross-sectional trials, but a few long term longitudinal trials are often conducted as well, primarily during late phase II and phase III of development. Many epidemiological population studies conducted during phase IV are longitudinal studies. These include the well-known Framingham epidemiological study and many other large cohort studies of patients followed for more than a year.

**Table IV.** Classification of phase I, II, III and IV clinical trials, and the various elements of a drug's clinical profile that are evaluated at each phase (**NB.** an investigational drug is often evaluated in two or more phases simultaneously in different trials, and some trials may overlap two different phases)

| Phase of development | Classification / activities undertaken | Specific elements that are evaluated or identified |
|---|---|---|
| **I** | Initial safety studies and pharmacokinetic characterisation (usually in healthy volunteers) | • Initial safety profile<br>• Establishment of tolerated dose range<br>• Definition of appropriate efficacy parameters to measure<br>• Absorption, metabolism and elimination profiles<br>• Pharmacokinetic/pharmacodynamic relationships |
| **IIa** | Pilot clinical trials to evaluate efficacy (and safety) in selected populations of patients with the disease/condition to be treated or prevented (the drug may be investigational or marketed for another indication) | • Dose range that has an adequate safety profile and elicits a response of sufficient magnitude and quality<br>• Dose frequency and dose ascension schedule that is slow enough to avoid excessive adverse effects and rapid enough to provide an adequate response<br>• Duration of treatment necessary for short episodes<br>• Establishment of goals for long term studies<br>• Definition of efficacy parameters to measure<br>• Identification of disease subtypes for which drug is particularly effective (or ineffective)<br>• Drug interactions (e.g. with other drugs, food, environmental factors, other treatments) |
| **IIb** | Well-controlled trials to evaluate efficacy (and safety) in patients with the disease/condition to be treated or prevented (usually small scale studies) | • Dosage schedule that has an adequate efficacy and safety profile<br>• Duration of treatment necessary for short episodes<br>• Establishment of goals for long term studies<br>• Identification of disease subtypes for which drug is particularly effective (or ineffective)<br>• Comparisons with placebo and other (standard) drugs<br>• Drug interactions (e.g. with other drugs, food, environmental factors, other treatments) |
| **IIIa** | Controlled and uncontrolled trials in relatively large numbers of patients, or in special groups (e.g. those with renal failure) [conducted after demonstration of efficacy but prior to regulatory submission] | • Dosage schedule that has an adequate efficacy and safety profile (initial risk: benefit assessment)<br>• Identification of disease subtypes for which drug is particularly effective (or ineffective)<br>• Evaluation in special populations (e.g. elderly, renally impaired)<br>• Comparisons with other (standard) drugs<br>• Pharmacokinetic comparisons of 2 or more formulations/dosage forms |
| **IIIb** | Clinical trials that supplement or complete earlier trials, or new types of trials (conducted after regulatory submission but prior to approval and launch) | • Further evaluation of efficacy and safety profile<br>• Identification of disease subtypes for which drug is particularly effective (or ineffective)<br>• Comparisons with other (standard) drugs<br>• Quality of life studies (may be conducted in other phases)<br>• Pharmacoeconomic studies (may be conducted in other phases) |
| **IV** | Studies or trials to provide additional efficacy and safety data (conducted after marketing) | • Confirmation of efficacy and safety profile in larger numbers of patients and in everyday clinical practice<br>• Postmarketing surveillance studies to establish incidence of adverse reactions, detect previously unkown or inadequately quantified adverse reactions, and define risk factors<br>• Further comparisons with other drugs<br>• Additional evaluation of overdosage characteristics and treatments<br>• Drug interactions (e.g. with other drugs, food, environmental factors, other treatments)<br>• Identification of new indications (which are then evaluated in phase II or III trials)<br>• Evaluations of different formulations, dosages, durations of treatment<br>• Evaluations in different age groups and other types of patients<br>• Drug utilisation patterns |

Ideally, more clinical trials should be longitudinal, but this approach is often impractical and most trials are cross-sectional instead. One of the dangers of cross-sectional trials is that if they are conducted in one area only, the data obtained may only be relevant to the population living in that particular area. The ability to extrapolate data to other patients with the same or other characteristics should always be considered when deciding on how homogeneous the study group should be.

#### *2.1.4 Two Patient Group Designs*

The two most common designs using two groups of patients are parallel groups (non-crossover) and crossover designs.

**Parallel Group Trials**

The parallel group design is applicable to most experimental situations. It is 'robust' (i.e. tolerant) enough for many kinds of problems that often occur in clinical trials (e.g. missed visits, missing data). In such trials, patients are randomised to one of two treatment groups and usually receive the assigned treatment during the entire trial. This may be either the trial drug or placebo, one of two different trial drugs, or one of two doses of the same trial drug. Two placebo medications could also be evaluated.

One (of many) variations of the parallel group design is for each group of patients to receive alternating (and escalating) doses of the same drug.

**Crossover Trials**

In the crossover design, each patient receives both treatments being compared in the clinical trial. If one of the treatments is placebo, then the effect of the trial drug may be expressed as the difference between responses to the two treatments. The variability of data obtained with this design is less than that associated with the parallel group design. Whereas within-patient differences are used to assess treatment differences in a crossover trial, between-patient differences are used to assess treatment differences in a parallel group trial.

The crossover design requires fewer patients than the parallel group design to detect the same effect, as it is more sensitive in detecting differences between the two treatments. However, the analysis of data obtained with a crossover design is adversely affected by patient dropouts and missing data, since it is not as 'robust' as the parallel group design. Analysis should also evaluate carryover effects from one treatment period on the next, and also period effects where

**Table V.** Types (designs) of clinical trials conducted in phases I to III (after Spilker;[2] with permission)

**1. Prospective or retrospective**

**2. Single group of patients**

**3. Two groups of patients**
a) Parallel cross-sectional
b) Parallel longitudinal
c) Crossover
d) Matched pairs
e) Historical controls
f) Sequential

**4. Multiple groups of patients**

**5. Trial designs for evaluating prophylactic activity**

**6. Design variations**
a) Withdrawal of treatment trials
b) Single-patient clinical trials
c) Chart review trials
d) Factorial designs
e) Novel trial designs based on variations in informed consent or randomisation
– pre-randomisation method
– double-consent pre-randomisation method
– deferred consent process
– two-tiered consent process

**7. Run-in period designs**
a) Placebo run-in
b) Compliance run-in
c) No-treatment run-in
d) Combination type of run-in
e) Dose ascension

**8. Other trial designs that attempt to avoid ethical problems[a]**
a) Fail-safe designs
b) Dose-response designs
c) Concentration-response designs
d) Designs with escape clauses or rescue treatments
e) Alternative designs
f) Comparison with nondrug therapy

**9. Designs in specific therapeutic areas or situations**
a) Oncology
b) Surgery
c) Antibiotics
d) Medical devices
e) Pharmacokinetics
f) Compassionate plea

a This category specifically refers to situations when it is not ethically acceptable to maintain patients on placebo medications.

patients may do better in the first (or second) period regardless of the treatment.

#### *2.1.5 Clinical Studies Conducted During Phases I to III*

The types of clinical studies conducted during a drug's investigational period (i.e. phases I to III) are listed in table IV. Although some trials (e.g. pharmacoeconomics, quality of life) could be conducted in phases IIa, IIb, IIIa, IIIb or IV, they are most appropriately conducted in phase IIIa if the data are required as part of regulatory approval and during phase IIIb if the data are needed instead to have the drug placed on a formulary after it is approved for marketing.

A drug does not necessarily have to pass through all phases to receive regulatory approval for marketing. The definition of each phase is primarily functional and not necessarily chronological (e.g. a phase I pharmacokinetic trial may be conducted at any point in a drug's development or marketing history).

The appropriate definitions of each phase of clinical development are often distorted by various groups. For example, both stock analysts and companies often describe phase IIb trials as phase III trials in order to give investors the idea of progress on a drug.

#### *2.1.6 Clinical Studies Conducted During Phase IV*

Phase IV studies include much more than just postmarketing surveillance and other types of pharmacoepidemiology studies. Marketing-oriented 'seeding' trials, comparative trials *versus* other drugs, and clinically oriented trials to learn more about the agent are also part of phase IV (see table IV). In fact, almost any type of clinical study or trial may be conducted during phase IV.

##### Purposes of Clinical Studies Conducted During Phase IV

The purposes of clinical trials and studies conducted during phase IV are to:

1) Address questions that arose during phases I to III, but which have not yet been completely answered or adequately addressed. These clinical trials include comparisons with other drugs, cost-effectiveness studies, quality of life trials, mechanism of action studies, and trials that explore specific hypotheses.

2) Continue clinical trials initiated but not completed during phase III.

3) Investigate interactions with other drugs, food, environmental factors, and non-drug treatments.

4) Expose more patients to the new drug to confirm its efficacy.

5) Expose more patients to the new drug to confirm and better understand its safety (e.g. delayed effects, prolonged use effects) and quantify rates of known adverse reactions. In addition, the drug should generally be evaluated in special patient populations (e.g. children, pregnant women, nursing mothers, elderly, immunosuppressed) who have not previously been exposed to it or not exposed in sufficient numbers.

6) Determine if the results obtained at tertiary care and special hospitals during phases I to III can be confirmed in other hospitals, as well as when the drug is used in everyday clinical practice by a large number of new clinicians.

7) Evaluate whether any rare but serious adverse reactions occur.

8) Discover new indications that may then be explored and developed in phase II and phase III trials. These discoveries may occur through serendipity or via informal tests by private clinicians.

9) Evaluate the pattern of a drug's utilisation in a specific or general population.

10) Study the clinical characteristics of overdosage and the means of counteracting this problem.

11) Assess the costs of adverse reactions to various sectors of society and possibly develop an approach to meet these costs.

The primary goals of pharmacoepidemiology studies in phase IV are to discover previously unknown adverse reactions caused by the drug, identify specific risk factors for the occurrence of adverse effects, and estimate their overall frequency. This information is then used to assess the benefit-to-risk relationship for the drug, to decrease the risks to patients, and ultimately to improve the quality of medical treatment. The field of pharmacoepidemiology addresses broad therapeutic questions that cannot easily be addressed in phase I to III clinical studies, or in other phase IV studies (see further chapter 9).

##### Categories of Phase IV Studies

Phase IV studies can be divided into five categories as follows:

- ***Descriptive studies:*** these provide information on the pattern of disease occurrence in populations according to demographic and prognostic characteristics. The data used are from routinely collected epidemiological intelligence which is analysed to identify the occurrence of rare adverse reactions or to generate an hypothesis. Passive monitoring of events and reports is an important method for collecting data included in descriptive studies.

- ***Cross-sectional studies:*** these are also called *surveys or prevalence studies*, and usually involve a statistically-based random sampling of a target population. Data are classified according to reported exposure to the drug and the observed outcomes. Results pertain to a single time-point, and this type of study is therefore like a snapshot in time. If such studies were conducted retrospectively, it may be unclear whether exposure truly preceded the outcome.
- ***Case control studies:*** these are always retrospective. Cases have the disease and controls do not. Data are collected by looking backward in time to determine differences between the two groups in the past. Each case is matched for specific confounding factors (e.g. age, sex) with one or more controls. Multiple controls are sometimes used to increase the efficiency of matching for each case included, as it is difficult, if not impossible, to identify a single control that has all factors. Cases could also have some, but not all factors of interest. In some situations, it is difficult to find appropriate controls (e.g. for psychotic patients), and the information obtained is often incomplete and subject to recall bias.
- ***Cohort studies:*** a cohort is a group that is exposed, and followed forward to a point in time when its members are evaluated retrospectively to look for differences in the frequency of one or more outcomes from a control unexposed group. If the case and controls both come from the same study population, the results of the study are more easily validated. It is important to determine that both cases and controls have the same disease status at the start of the observation period.
- ***Controlled clinical studies and trials:*** the term 'controlled' in this context refers to the trial's adherence to a tightly designed protocol, the purpose of which is to reduce the variability of the many factors and biases that might influence the result. Control features include the double-blind procedure, where neither the patient nor the investigator is aware of which treatment the patient is receiving, but are not confined to this; others include the adequacy of the group(s) used as controls. The greater the number of factors of the study or trial design that are specified and the more tightly delineated they are, the greater the degree of control that is built into the study.

## 2.2 Objectives of Clinical Trials

After one of the above broad types of clinical trials has been identified as appropriate to meet the specific goals that have been set, the trial objectives that are to be addressed within the framework of the trial type must be clearly established.

Clinical trial objectives are concise statements of the major and minor questions that the trial is designed to answer. The trial protocol author should reflect on the objectives and confirm that they represent valid and proper questions, or series of questions, to answer. If an underlying question is the basis of the proposed objective, then it may be desirable to modify the objective to reflect the underlying consideration. The overall trial goals (purposes) are differentiated from the objectives in that the former represent the type of trial to be conducted whereas the objectives are the concise statements that will enable the appropriate design to be chosen to achieve the goals.

### 2.2.1 Why is it Critical to Express Clinical Trial Objectives Precisely?

The objectives of a clinical trial are the questions the trial asks and tries to answer. In all areas of research, asking the right question is perhaps the most important part of the research. How the research problem is stated determines the trial design used, the data that are collected, the analyses conducted, and the conclusions (i.e. interpretation) that can be drawn. It is therefore essential that the objective(s) be clearly, completely and concisely expressed. If they are not, then the rest of the enterprise may be irrelevant and represent a significant waste of research effort.

### 2.2.2 How Should Trial Objectives be Stated?

In all types of clinical trials, the objective should be stated as specifically and succinctly as possible in the protocol. It is not appropriate to state that the objective is 'to determine the mechanism of action of drug X,' or 'to evaluate the efficacy of drug X,' since these objectives are too general, vague, and merely restate the overall goal of the trial. Rather, it is preferable to state that the trial objective is to evaluate the effects of daily dose T of drug X in population W on parameters Y and Z by continuous or daily recording of results obtained in tests A and B during time period C, as compared with drug D at dose E, under the same experimental conditions.

If too many questions (i.e. objectives) are posed in the protocol, a number of methodological and statistical problems may result. Posing many questions often creates an excessive number of subgroups of data, some of which may be insufficient in quantity to answer the particular question(s). In addition, posing many questions often makes the clinical trial difficult to conduct and decreases the probability of the trial being successfully completed. Nonetheless, one must be sensitive to the large number of potential questions from which the most important ones are chosen, and be aware of the many potentially informative analyses that may provide valuable insights that could be evaluated in future trials.

#### 2.2.3 Primary and Secondary Objectives

A clinical trial often has both primary and secondary objectives, and these should be identified as such in the protocol. Ideally, no more than one or two of each should be included in a clinical trial. The more objectives posed, the less the chance that a single clinical trial design will adequately address each objective. Also, a large number of objectives will complicate the protocol and conduct of the clinical trial and make it less likely to be completed successfully, and moreover, the analysis and interpretation of data will be compromised. Thus, the inclusion of numerous objectives should be avoided whenever possible. Certain groups of people (e.g. PhD scientists who design clinical protocols and marketers) are prone to seek an excessive number of objectives. One reason why scientists are prone to make this mistake is that they are able to control more parameters and conditions in animal or biological experiments than may be reasonably controlled in a clinical trial.

### 2.3 Choosing Efficacy and Safety Parameters

#### 2.3.1 Criteria for Evaluating Efficacy

Various types of criteria may be used to measure efficacy (or safety) parameters. They include:

1) ***Presence or absence criteria,*** i.e. a symptom, sign, lesion or other manifestation of a disease that is either present or not. Operational definitions may be established to define the existence of the effect.

**Table VI.** Types of end-points used to measure efficacy of a drug in clinical trials (after Spilker;[2] with permission)

1. Time for an important parameter to improve by a fixed percentage (e.g. 75%, 100%)
2. Time to recurrence of symptoms after treatment is stopped (e.g. return to 50% or 75% of baseline)
3. Time to a new episode of disease while treatment continues
4. Degree of recurrence of symptoms after treatment is stopped
5. Duration of improvement while on maintenance therapy
6. Magnitude of improvement noted at a fixed time (e.g. 1 week or month) after therapy is initiated
7. Any calculated parameter related to efficacy that is calculated from parameters measured[a] (e.g. ejection fraction, integrated area under the curve, dp/dt of left ventricular end-diastolic pressure)
8. Any subjective parameter of improvement
9. Any quality of life domain or component
10. Any objective parameter (e.g. number of deaths)

a Any of the end-points listed could be used for the calculated parameter.

2) ***Graded or scaled criteria:*** these include both Likert scales (i.e. where descriptive categories such as much better, somewhat better, unchanged, or worse, are used) and visual analogue scales. Graded scales can be applied to both subjective and objective clinical symptoms and signs. A number of scales have become well established in clinical medicine (e.g. cardiac murmurs are graded from 0 to 6, and neurological reflexes are graded from 0 to 4).

3) ***Relative change criteria:*** these refer to measurements in specific tests that are expressed as degree of change (e.g. percent, number of units of measure) and provide direct or indirect indications of efficacy.

4) ***Global criteria:*** these enable the overall evaluation of a patient's disease status or changes in the disease itself (e.g. its severity or global improvement) to be assessed. The individual factors that this aggregate evaluation is based on may or may not be specified. Specific (or general) criteria, or a scoring system, may also be developed to rate each of the factors.

The pros and cons of each efficacy parameter incorporated into the study should be reviewed. The potential value of data obtained from each efficacy test must be evaluated against the increase it will create in time requirements, personal efforts, financial costs, and overall complexity of the trial. At some point in virtually all clinical trials, adding tests becomes counterproductive, and the trial becomes inefficient. Types of end-points used to measure efficacy are listed in table VI.

### 2.3.2 Assessing Efficacy in Preventive Therapy

Most clinical trials assess one or more therapies for treating a disease, syndrome or condition; fewer trials assess the efficacy of preventive therapy. The three types of preventive therapy and the criteria that will need to be assessed in evaluating efficacy are:

**Type 1 (Prevention of Disease Occurrence)**

In this type, therapy is aimed at preventing patients from contracting the disease, which is, for example, the purpose of many vaccines (e.g. tetanus, diphtheria and pertussis vaccines). Vaccines are often given to normal children prior to any direct threat of disease, as well as being given after a presumptive threat has been experienced (e.g. a puncture wound that may lead to tetanus), or to patients at high risk of contracting a disease (e.g. pneumonia).

**Type 2 (Prevention of Disease Episodes)**

In this case, therapy is given to patients so that the number, duration or severity of disease episodes are decreased. This type of preventive therapy is illustrated by many drugs that are given to patients with chronic diseases (e.g. asthma, epilepsy).

**Type 3 (Prevention of Progression of Underlying Disease)**

In this type, therapy is given to delay or prevent disease progression. This is the aim of treatment with drugs used to prevent more serious sequelae of the disease in patients who are either asymptomatic (e.g. lowering blood pressure in hypertensive patients, decreasing lipids in patients with hyperlipidaemias) or symptomatic [e.g. decreasing blood sugar in diabetic patients, treating mildly and moderately symptomatic patients who are human immunodeficiency virus (HIV)-positive with antiviral drugs to slow the progression of acquired immune deficiency syndrome (AIDS)].

### 2.3.3 Risk Factors as Clinical End-Points

Risk factors for a disease are often used as clinical end-points in clinical trials. They may be used to define subpopulations of patients with a disease, including those who may benefit from a particular treatment. Risk factors may be measured to identify an individual's risk of having a particular disease, and are often used as a prognostic factor to stratify patients entering a clinical trial.

### 2.3.4 Assessment of Safety

A selected list of examinations and tests commonly used to assess the safety of drugs is given in table VII. Although many of these tests are not performed in most clinical trials, the list provides a checklist of possible tests to consider for inclusion.

Choosing the appropriate safety parameter(s) for a clinical trial depends on a number of factors. An assessment of the quantity and quality of data previously obtained with the drug is es-

**Table VII.** Selected list of examinations and tests used to evaluate safety (after Spilker;[2] with permission)

**1. Clinical examinations**
- a) Physical
- b) Vital signs (usually considered as part of the physical examination)
- c) Height and weight
- d) Neurological or other specialised clinical examinations

**2. Clinical laboratory examinations**
- a) Haematology
- b) Clinical chemistry
- c) Urinalysis
- d) Virology (viral cultures or viral serology)
- e) Immunology or immunochemistry (e.g. immunoglobins, complement)
- f) Serology (e.g. VDRL)
- g) Microbiology (including bacteriology and mycology)
- h) Parasitology (e.g. stool for ova and protozoa)
- i) Pulmonary function tests (e.g. arterial blood gas)
- j) Other biological tests (e.g. endocrine, toxicology screen)
- k) Stool for occult blood (Hemoccult® or guaiac method)
- l) Skin tests for immunological competence[a]
- m) Drug screen (usually in urine) for detection of illegal or non-protocol-approved agents
- n) Bone marrow examination
- o) Gonadal function (e.g. sperm count, sperm motility)
- p) Genetics studies (e.g. evaluate chromosomal integrity)
- q) Stool analysis using *in vivo* dialysis

**3. Probes for adverse reactions**

**4. Psychological and psychiatric tests and examinations**
- a) Psychometric and performance examinations
- b) Behavioural rating scales
- c) Dependence liability

**5. Examinations requiring specialised equipment (selected examples)**
- a) Audiometry
- b) Electrocardiogram (ECG)
- c) Electroencephalogram (EEG)
- d) Electromyography (EMG)
- e) Stress test
- f) Endoscopy
- g) Computed tomography (CT) scans
- h) Ophthalmological examination
- i) Ultrasound
- j) x-Rays

a Examples are *Candida albicans*, Tricophyton and dinitrochlorobenzene.

sential. The choice of which safety parameters to measure requires consideration of areas where there are potential (or actual) safety problems, as well as areas of special interest such as the collection of tolerance data on the new drug. Until a sufficient body of safety data has accumulated, more laboratory parameters of safety are generally included than will be needed at a later date. The nature of the efficacy tests used may dictate that certain safety parameters should or should not be included. For example, in testing a new anticancer agent, it may be necessary to perform a bone marrow biopsy and smear to confirm the lack of toxicity, and in assessing an agent used in anaesthetised patients, the appropriate tests to ensure the patients' safety while under anaesthesia should be performed.

If, on the basis of preclinical pharmacological or toxicological data, any toxicity is either anticipated or considered possible, then an attempt should be made to evaluate patients for those possible problems. The anticipated use(s) of a drug will also influence which safety parameters are chosen for evaluation (e.g. ophthalmological tests would be included for agents intended for ocular use).

#### *2.3.5 Measuring Safety Parameters*

After specific safety parameters have been chosen, it is necessary to determine how thorough the evaluation of each parameter should be. It is possible that different types of a single test or examination would be suitable at different points of a clinical trial. For example, a physical examination may include only some measurements at some patient visits, as a complete examination may not be necessary at each visit.

Vital signs may be measured with the patient in a supine, seated, and/or erect position. Both supine and erect positions are usually used if orthostatic changes are being evaluated. The need for such data will depend on the situation, but the position of the patient for this examination, as well as the period of time desired for stabilisation, should be specified in the protocol.

#### *2.3.6 Parameters that Measure Either Safety or Efficacy*

Certain parameters may be viewed as being either safety or efficacy parameters. The electroencephalogram (EEG) is one example (although there is some controversy as to its true adequacy as an efficacy parameter) and blood pressure is another. Therefore, it is important to establish clearly in the protocol whether each parameter is being incorporated in the protocol for safety or efficacy evaluations (or possibly both).

### 2.4 Sample Size Considerations

The number of patients required for a clinical trial (i.e. the sample size) refers to the number of patients who finish a trial rather than the number who enter. Thus, in planning a trial, the definition of a 'completed' patient is important to establish, as is the expected rate of patient dropouts and discontinuations. An important result may not be detected if too few patients complete a trial.

Another problem that may occur if too few patients complete a clinical trial is a false-positive result. The chances of this happening are higher when fewer patients are enrolled than intended. Numerous biases and errors in a clinical trial may be minimised by increasing the number of patients entered until adequate power is obtained.

#### *2.4.1 Fixed or Sequential Sample Size?*

There are two main types of sample sizes to consider: fixed and sequential. When a fixed sample size is used in a clinical trial, the number of patients in each group may be fixed:

a) At a defined number
b) Within a narrow or broad range
c) By a minimum number; or
d) By a maximum number.

In a sequential trial design, the final number of patients enrolled will depend on analyses performed throughout the trial. In this design, a significant result can be obtained more rapidly and probably with fewer patients than with a fixed sample size, provided that there is a real difference to be detected.

#### *2.4.2 Multiple Sample Sizes Within a Single Clinical Trial*

If multiple objectives (e.g. both safety and efficacy) are included in a clinical trial protocol, then each will probably require a different sample size. The larger the expected difference in magnitude of the effect between a drug and placebo or between two drugs, the smaller the sample size required to detect this difference. Thus, a clinical trial generally requires larger sample sizes to demonstrate the small differences expected in safety parameters between a drug and placebo, and smaller sample sizes to demonstrate the large differences expected in efficacy parameters. On the other hand, low variability in the data obtained (e.g. with some vital signs) may mitigate against the requirement for larger sample sizes to show small differences.

When multiple sample sizes are computed, the most reasonable one should be utilised. This often requires compromises and identifying the most important objectives to be addressed.

### *2.4.3 Determining the Sample Size*

In the past, clinically experienced investigators often estimated the number of patients to include in a clinical trial on the basis of their judgement and clinical expertise. However, these 'guesstimates' of sample size are invalid and scientifically unacceptable for controlled clinical trials, no matter how experienced the guessers. For all trials, the required sample size is usually determined by statisticians on the basis of:

1) The magnitude of the effect expected (or desired).

2) The variability (often estimated) of the specific parameters being analysed.

3) The desired probability (power) of observing that effect with a defined significance level.

A power of 80% (0.8) is usually chosen as adequate for most controlled trials, although some groups prefer to use a higher power.

#### Equal versus Unequal Sample Sizes

In determining sample size, a suitable ratio of patients between the two treatment groups needs to be established. There are basically two choices: using either equal-sized samples in all treatment groups or unequal but proportional-sized groups (e.g. a 2 : 1 ratio that assigns 12 patients to receive the active drug and 6 to receive placebo). The general rule to follow is that groups of equal size are preferable from a statistical perspective for clinical trials, although not all statisticians would require equal-sized groups in all situations. An advantage of using equal-sized treatment groups is that the clinical trial gains in power. However, with unequal-sized groups, the resultant loss of power is not great and may be acceptable if the ratios are no more than 2 or 3 to 1. A disadvantage of using equal-sized groups is that less information may be gained on patient responses to a new drug in comparison with unequal-sized groups, since less patients receive the trial drug.

Some statisticians advocate that all patients should have an equal chance of receiving a clinical trial drug and thus would assign patients in a trial of a high- and low-dose group and a placebo group in the ratio of 1 : 1 : 2 (i.e. twice the number in the placebo group as in either of the other groups). However, from a practical and often ethical point of view, patients are usually more willing to enrol in a drug trial when the chance of their receiving the active agent is greatest. Thus, this particular apportionment of patients would make the clinical trial more difficult to initiate than an equal distribution of patients among the groups, or an apportionment in favour of the drug group. The relative importance of the patients' attitudes in determining the ratio of group size in a trial depends to a large degree on the particular disease studied and the severity of its symptoms. A patient with severe or moderate pain will be less willing to enter a trial in which the chances of receiving placebo are 50% than one in which the chances of this are about 10%.

#### Influence of Placebo Responsiveness on Sample Size

The magnitude of the placebo effect that will be observed in a clinical trial is useful to know when planning the trial, as this impacts greatly on the sample size and often represents the difference between a clinical trial that demonstrates a clinical effect and one that does not. Placebo responsiveness is estimated to be about 35% in most clinical trials, regardless of therapeutic area. However, the actual magnitude of the placebo responses reported in the literature varies over an enormous range (even for double-blind clinical trials), and is almost totally independent of therapeutic area. Many factors are responsible for this variation, which is observed even when objective end-points and measures are used. Use of subjective end-points and measures does not necessarily mean that a large placebo response will be obtained, but it does appear to facilitate this finding.

## 2.5 Ethical Requirements and Guidelines

Many national, international and professional guidelines and regulations describe and protect the patient's right to an informed consent before he or she may be given an experimental therapy. Before 1900, the only ethical guidelines for performing experimentation related to the clinician's need to adhere to acceptable medical standards in designing and conducting a clinical trial. The issue of a patient's agreement was never addressed. It may be argued, however, that there has always been an ethical responsibility on the part of the clinician to adequately inform a patient who has been enrolled in a clinical trial and received an experimental treatment and to obtain that patient's consent.

Major milestones for informed consent include:

1) The Nuremberg code (1949), which was an outcome of World War II.

2) The Helsinki Doctrine of the World Medical Association (1964).

3) Legislation in the US regarding Institutional Review Boards (Volume 46 *Federal Register* 8975, January 27, 1981, 21 Code of Federal Regulations 56) and informed consent (45 FR 36390, May 30, 1980 21 CFR 50).

### 2.5.1 Obtaining Informed Consent

The regulations governing informed consent do not cover many of the nuances relating to the individual who actually obtains it. For example, if a nurse, research coordinator or other individual obtains the informed consent but is not able or qualified to discuss the details of the protocol or alternative treatments, then the signed consent form may not be legally valid if it is ever challenged.

Variations on the traditional methods of providing information to patients and obtaining informed consent that have been suggested[3] include:

1. Holding a group meeting of patients
2. Testing patient comprehension
3. Including relatives in the discussions.

These are among the techniques that can improve patient comprehension of the benefits and risks inherent in a trial. It should be noted that in the US, informed consent is not required if:

a) The patient is confronted by a life-threatening situation necessitating use of an investigational medicine.

b) The patient is unable to communicate and family members are not present or available.

c) There is insufficient time to obtain informed consent.

d) There is no alternative method of acceptable treatment available and therapy must be initiated rapidly.

### 2.5.2 Elements of Informed Consent

Investigators should be familiar with their national guidelines on informed consent and the procedures under which this obligation is carried out. Those that apply in the US are summarised in table VIII. The trial protocol should state that the purpose of the clinical trial will be explained to the patient in the presence of a witness (plus the parent or legal guardian for trials in children) and an informed consent obtained.

**Table VIII.** Elements of informed consent: summary of the US Food and Drug Administration (FDA) regulations (after Spilker;[2] with permission)

An informed consent must be written by the investigator, approved by the Institutional Review Board (IRB) [or Ethics Committee], signed by the subject (patient or volunteer) or authorised representative, and witnessed

**1. Points that must be included in all informed consents:**

a) A statement that the study involves research, an explanation of the purpose of the research and the expected duration, a description of the procedures, and identification of any procedures that are experimental

b) A description of any reasonably foreseeable risks or discomforts to the patient

c) A description of the benefits to the patient or to others that may be expected from the research

d) A disclosure of appropriate alternative procedures or courses of treatment, if any, that might be advantageous to the patient

e) A statement describing the extent, if any, to which confidentiality of the records identifying the patient will be maintained and that the regulatory authority may inspect the records

f) For research involving more than minimal risk, an explanation as to whether any compensation will be paid and whether any medical treatments are available if injury occurs, and what those treatments are; information should also be provided on how further information about this study may be obtained

g) An explanation of whom to contact for answers to questions and whom to contact in the event of a research-related injury

h) A statement that participation is voluntary, that refusal to participate will involve no penalty or loss of benefits to which the patient is otherwise entitled, and that the patient may discontinue participation at any time without penalty

**2. Additional elements of informed consent that must be present when appropriate:**

a) A statement that the particular treatment or procedure may involve risks to the patient or to the fetus (if the patient is pregnant) that are currently unforeseeable

b) Anticipated circumstances under which the patient's participation may be terminated by the investigator

c) Any additional costs to the patient resulting from participation in the research

d) The consequences and procedures for withdrawing from the research

e) A statement that significant new findings (such as new hazards) developed during the research will be provided to the patient

f) The approximate number of patients who will be enrolled in the clinical trial

Although a witness is only required (in the US) if the informed consent is obtained orally or in a summary written form, including a witness in the informed consent procedure is generally prudent.

#### *2.5.3 Ethics Committee/Institutional Review Board Review of the Trial Protocol and Informed Consent Procedure*

In the US, an Institutional Review Board (IRB) must review and approve an investigator's protocol and informed consent form before the study may be initiated. Other countries that have a comparable review group (i.e. an Ethics Committee) have similar regulations. In the US, the IRB must comprise at least five members including at least one physician and at least one person who must be unaffiliated with the institution. The IRB may not be composed entirely of men or women of one profession, and at least one member must be a nonscientist. Nonvoting consultants may also be included. The experiences of Ethics Committees in the UK have been reviewed by Wells and Griffin.[4]

IRBs may be institutional or independent and they may be formed on either a nonprofit or profit basis. Their primary role is to consider the ethical acceptability of clinical trial protocols and informed consent forms, along with various other responsibilities. In reviewing the investigator's written informed consent form, the IRB must confirm that it includes all information required by law (see table VIII). The IRB may also consider the informed consent form in the light of the following questions:

- Does the informed consent form contain all of the information that most doctors in the community would provide to their patients under similar circumstances?
- Does the informed consent form contain all of the information that the patient who is considering enrolment in this clinical trial would want to know?

Depending on the nature of the clinical trial, the Ethics Committee/IRB may request the investigator to provide them with periodic updates that focus primarily on informed consent issues, in addition to periodic updates relating to the conduct of the trial.

### 2.6 Legal Considerations

This section does not purport to provide legal advice relating to clinical trials but raises points that may be discussed further with legal advisors or other individuals who are familiar with the specific details in particular situations and the local laws governing them. Important issues include:

1) The informed consent form cannot contain any exculpatory language that would waive or appear to waive any of the patient's legal rights or releases, or appear to release the investigator, the sponsor, the institution or its agents from liability for negligence.

2) Personal injury may result during treatment in the clinical trial; however, the occurrence of injury does not indicate that any liability attaches.

3) The investigator's legal obligations towards the patient include obtaining a voluntary informed consent from the patient or the patient's guardian, adhering to a proper and adequate clinical trial design and protocol that is approved by an Ethics Committee/IRB, and exercising due care in conducting the trial.

4) Indemnification agreements may be entered into between sponsors and institutions, and between institutions and investigators.

5) Guidelines for compensation for medicine-induced injuries have been proposed in the UK by the Association of the British Pharmaceutical Industry.[5,6]

### 2.7 Monitoring and Auditing of Clinical Trials

Monitoring in this context refers to the overseeing of the planning, initiation, conduct, and data processing of clinical studies. Individuals who are appointed as monitors check and confirm that the execution of each step of the study follows the agreed-on plans.

#### *2.7.1 Specific Functions of Monitors*

Clinical trial monitors have a wide variety of backgrounds both in their disciplines of training and in their experience with clinical medicine. Although many monitors perform similar functions, they do so at highly different levels of expertise. The broad functions of monitors include participation in most or all of the following activities:

- Planning clinical trials
- Writing protocols
- Initiating trials
- Assessing the conduct of trials
- Assisting in their termination
- Assisting in data editing and analysis
- Assisting in data interpretation and extrapolation.

More specific functions of medical monitors during the conduct of a clinical trial may include:

- Observing what is being done

- Assessing or evaluating the quality of the trial's conduct
- Comparing the quality to preset standards
- Discussing results with the groups being monitored, as well as with other monitors and supervisors
- Proposing improvements to be made to the trial or proposing solutions to problems.

One of the rarely perceived functions of monitoring is to help maintain and improve the morale and enthusiasm of the staff. The means of achieving this vary among clinical trials and individual monitors, but some attention should be devoted to this aspect by all monitors. It should be noted that investigators of unsponsored trials are also concerned with internal monitoring. Thus, the comments below are applicable to both sponsors and clinical investigators (of sponsored and unsponsored trials), even though various aspects will require modification.

#### 2.7.2 Developing a Monitoring Strategy

A basic monitoring strategy should be planned at the time of initiation of a clinical trial. This strategy will contain a number of different elements. Although a monitoring function may suggest that the trial is a sponsored one, in fact all unsponsored trials involve monitoring through periodic review and internal checks of performance and results.

In developing an overall monitoring strategy for a trial, it is essential to determine the answers to several questions, including:

a) What will be monitored?
b) How will it be monitored?
c) Who will monitor it?
d) Where will it be monitored? and
e) When will it be monitored?

The answer to the question of *what* to monitor depends on the functions of the particular monitor(s). In general, there are four basic areas that must be periodically assessed. These involve confirmation that:

1. The facilities remain adequate
2. The trial is proceeding according to the protocol
3. The investigator and other trial personnel are fulfilling their various obligations
4. The data in the data collection forms are accurate and complete.

The question of *how* to monitor is answered differently for each trial and for each monitor, while the question of *who* will monitor is generally an obvious one. Monitors may be associated with the investigator, sponsor or contract organisation setting up the trial for a sponsor, or they may function independently and not be directly associated with either the sponsor or investigator. This last method is sometimes used in large multicentre trials, for which an independent monitoring group may be established. The numbers and functions of each monitor and blinding of the relevant monitors must also be considered. Monitors include individuals with various backgrounds and experience, ranging from college graduates to PhDs, MDs, and medical specialists who monitor one aspect of a trial (e.g. pathologists, radiologists).

The question of *where* to monitor depends on the number of trial sites; monitoring must be performed at each site where the trial is being conducted, in addition to the monitor's own institution. While it may be more comfortable and convenient for monitors to rely on telephones, remote data entry, letters, electronic mail and facsimiles rather than direct visits, this temptation must be avoided as otherwise, monitors may be greatly misled about a trial's true status.

The question of *when* to monitor refers to the timing of the visits to each site. Each clinical trial has its own appropriate times for visits (e.g. after the first two patients are entered, every 6 weeks, at 50% completion, or during the entire clinical trial).

#### 2.7.3 Principles of Medical Auditing

A major principle of any audit is that the auditor is independent of the auditee. Otherwise, a conflict of interest will almost certainly develop if problems are found by the auditor. This principle does not imply that one cannot audit one's own work, the work of one's superior, or the work of someone who at some point in the administrative hierarchy reports to one's superior. However, it does mean that if the audit is to be credible to an outside group (e.g. the public or a regulatory agency), then a strong degree of independence of the two groups is required. Thus, quality assurance (QA) auditors of a company's manufacturing processes do not report to production personnel, and Good Laboratory Practices (GLP) auditors who audit toxicology data do not report to toxicology personnel. Good Clinical Practices (GCP) auditors should also not report to personnel responsible for sponsoring, conducting or monitoring the clinical trial.

##### Purposes of Auditing

The precise role of clinical auditors should be established prior to initiating this function

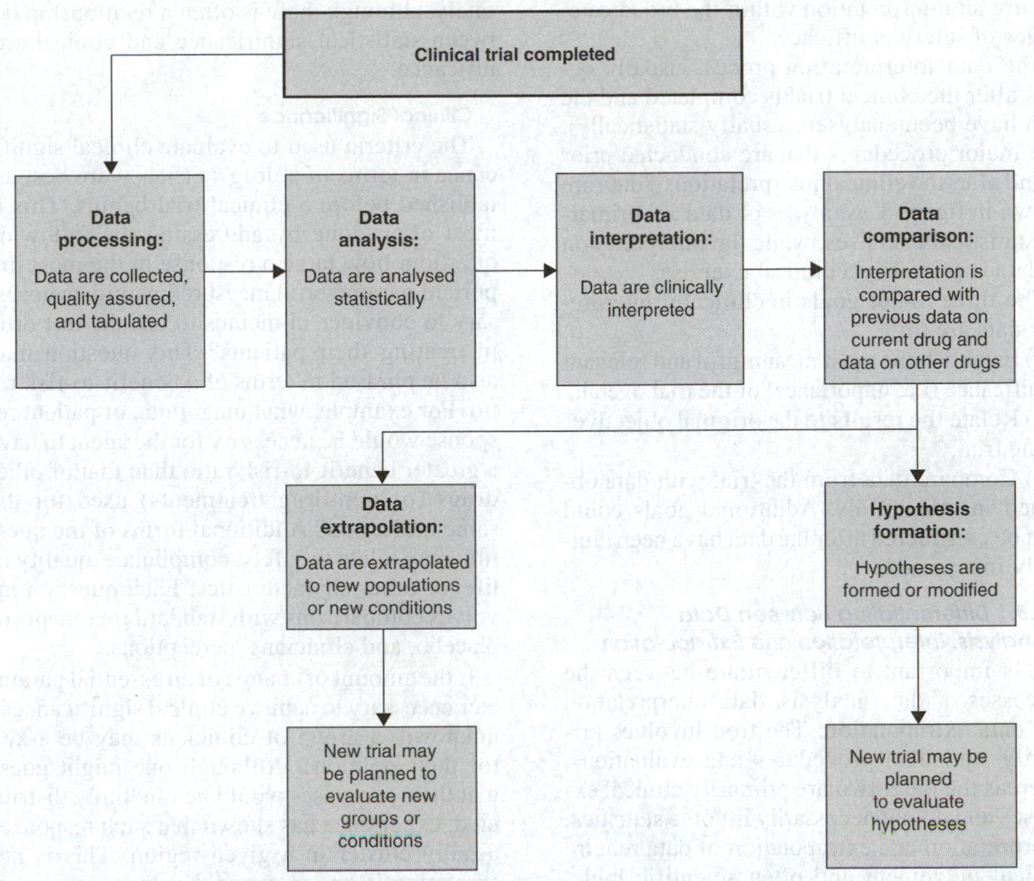


**Fig. 3.** Procedures to conduct after completion of a clinical trial (after Spilker;[2] with permission). The initiation of data processing often occurs while the trial is still in progress.

within an organisation. Specific purposes of auditing a clinical trial include ensuring that:

1) The investigators (and their staff) and clinical monitors are carrying out their functions appropriately.

2) Regulatory authority inspections will be smooth and uneventful.

3) The data obtained will be suitable for regulatory submission.

4) The clinical development process is conducted as efficiently as possible.

### Adherence to Good Clinical Practices (GCP) Guidelines

Good clinical practices (GCP) guidelines form the basis for determining what processes and activities should be audited. GCP guidelines are being developed by several groups worldwide, and most appear to be generally similar in content and approach. They include the following aspects of clinical research:

1) Requirements for regulatory authority submissions necessary to initiate clinical trials (e.g. Investigational New Drug [IND] Applications).

2) Requirements of Institutional Review Boards (IRBs)/Ethics Committees.

3) Requirements for obtaining informed consent.

4) Obligations of sponsors and monitors regarding clinical trials.

5) Obligations of investigators regarding clinical trials.

## 2.8 Interpreting Clinical Trial Data

Interpretation denotes the process of discerning the clinical meaning or significance of, or providing an explanation for the data being evaluated. The term *data* usually refers to data collected from patients entered in a clinical trial. Numerous aspects of clinical data usually require an interpretation within the broad categories of safety or efficacy.

The data interpretation process usually occurs after the clinical trial is completed and the data have been analysed (usually statistically). The major procedures that are conducted prior to and after the clinical interpretation of data are shown in figure 3. Analyses of data are primarily statistical exercises, while the interpretation of data is primarily a clinical exercise.

The three major goals in clinically interpreting data are to:

1) Establish the most meaningful and relevant significance (i.e. importance) of the trial overall.

2) Relate the results to the original objectives of the trial.

3) Compare data from the trial with data obtained in other trials. Additional goals could then be considered after the data have been clinically interpreted.

#### *2.8.1 Differentiating Between Data Analysis, Interpretation and Extrapolation*

It is important to differentiate between the processes of data analysis, data interpretation and data extrapolation. The first involves primarily statistical procedures and evaluations, whereas the latter two are primarily clinical exercises and do not necessarily involve statistics. Interpretation and extrapolation of data require clinical judgement and often scientific logic. Although different individuals usually carry out these processes, they may be performed by the same individual. The three processes for any one trial are usually conducted in the order of analysis, interpretation, and then extrapolation, although feedback loops often occur.

#### *2.8.2 Major Perspectives in Data Interpretation*

The three major perspectives in establishing an appropriate interpretation of a trial's data are:

1. Statistical significance
2. Clinical significance
3. Relevance for medical practice.

Interpretation usually begins when a clinical trial is completed; the data have been collected, edited and entered into a computer; appropriate statistical tests have been used to analyse the data; and the statistical report has been prepared.

##### Statistical Significance

Statistical significance on its own does not provide information on whether a data set is important for patients, and if so, how important. Clinical significance must be evaluated separately, although there is often a relationship between statistical significance and clinical significance.

##### Clinical Significance

The criteria used to evaluate clinical significance in terms of a drug's efficacy are best established before a clinical trial begins. This is most often done by addressing the following question: how large a response in the most important parameter(s) measured would be necessary to convince clinicians to use the test drug in treating their pátients? This question may also be phrased in terms of a benefit-to-risk ratio. For example, what magnitude of patient response would be necessary for the agent to have a greater benefit-to-risk ratio than that of other drugs (or non-drug treatments) used for the same indication? Additional forms of the question may relate to safety, compliance, quality of life, or other characteristics. Each question involves comparisons with standard treatments or placebo, and clinicians' perceptions.

If the amount of change of an essential parameter necessary to achieve clinical significance is unknown, a group of clinicians may be asked for their opinions. Although one might guess that their responses would be randomly distributed, experience has shown that such responses usually cluster in a given region. This is not surprising if one assumes that there is a value for a parameter's change that is clinically significant. If this exercise is conducted prior to a clinical trial, it generally yields a response related to the specific disease being treated, and not to the specific drug being tested.

Thus, the amount of change of a critical parameter caused by any new drug must equal or surpass the change caused by existing therapy. Exceptions might be for agents with an important advantage not possessed by existing therapy, such as an improved quality of life or improved safety profile.

##### Relevance for Medical Practice

The relevance of data for medical practice means its implications for treating other patients, i.e. its extrapolation to new situations, new patients, and new conditions. Posing the question of how important or relevant the data are for other clinical situations may lead to a different interpretation from that based on the group of patients treated. For example, a new antihypertensive may lower blood pressure by a statistically significant amount versus placebo. This change may also be highly clinically sig-

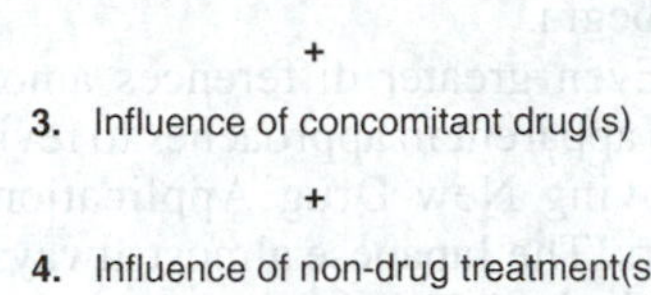


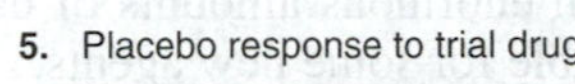


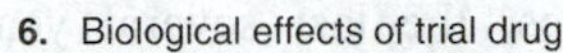


**Fig. 4.** Major components of the overall clinical response. The overall magnitude of the clinical response varies during the trial. There may be changes in the magnitude of any individual component during the trial, and there may be interactions between these components that will influence the observed clinical effect. The '?' symbol indicates that clinical deterioration does not usually result from that cause. The source of the deterioration (e.g. concomitant drug or non-drug treatment) is usually removed after being identified. The observed clinical effect at any one time equals the overall sum of the components shown (after Spilker;[2] with permission).

nificant, but the relevance for medical practice may be nil because of all the other drugs available.

#### 2.8.3 Differentiating Between the Components of the Overall Clinical Response

Although the clinical response of a specific patient is usually measured by single or multiple end-points and/or parameters, an overall clinical response will be observed by the investigator. A patient's overall clinical response is usually composed of two or more factors, such as those illustrated in figure 4. Each of these factors may lead to either improvement or deterioration, although some, such as the placebo response, usually lead to an improvement. Not only is the patient's overall clinical response a summation of a number of these factors, but there may be a complex interaction between any two (or more) that makes it difficult, if not impossible, to separate out and accurately measure each individual factor.

Using separate treatment groups or specifically chosen trial designs is the most common method of obtaining information on the importance and relevant role of each specific factor.

#### 2.8.4 Ten-Step Approach for Data Interpretation

A general 10-step approach to the interpretation of clinical data, which is proposed for use after all data have been edited, processed and analysed statistically, is as follows:

1) Compare the treatment groups in terms of demographic characteristics and prognostic factors. Statistically significant differences in demographics between the groups do not mean that the differences are clinically significant, but any differences mean that the major trial parameter(s) should be carefully assessed using subgroup analyses based on the differences in demographics. Differences in a critical prognostic factor may mean that the entire set of clinical trial data are worthless, or nearly so. Any demographic characteristic or prognostic disease factor that is considered critical to the outcome of the clinical trial should be used as a basis for randomisation (e.g. mild and severe cases, or men and women, or low risk factor and high risk factor patients may be randomised separately). Alternatively, a different randomisation system (e.g. minimisation) may be used. Other alternatives may be used (e.g. patient exclusion) to avoid having an important factor represented unequally in the treatment groups, which could invalidate the entire clinical trial.

2) Consider whether the data affirm or refute the primary objective(s) of the clinical trial. This is the real heart of the interpretation. It is important, therefore, that the objective(s) be clearly specified in the protocol before the trial is initiated.

3) Evaluate whether the data affirm or refute the secondary objective(s) of the trial.

4) Consider all the specific factors that may have influenced or biased the data and the conclusion(s) reached.

5) Discuss the interpretation(s) with a statistician and other colleagues to determine whether any additional analyses or subgroup analyses should be conducted.

6) Adopt the 'devil's advocate' perspective and strongly criticise one's own interpretation. Then evaluate each criticism and determine how it may be refuted or addressed. These evaluations or counter-arguments will be helpful in the discussion section of the publication or report that is generated to present the trial results.

7) Compare the interpretations and data with those obtained using standard drugs or treatments. These may be obtained from data in the same clinical trial or from results in the published literature.

8) Discuss the interpretation with others and seek their input and reaction. These may be same or other people than consulted within step number 5 above.

9) Extrapolate the interpretations to as many different patient populations, types of physicians, settings, levels of organisation as may be justified and appropriate (see Spilker[1] for a detailed discussion).

10) Develop hypotheses or plans to evaluate further any relevant new questions, issues or models in future clinical trials.

## 3. Regulatory Authority Approval Processes

The discovery and development of a new drug does not inevitably lead to its marketing and use for treating patients. A major step in the development of any agent is its approval by regulatory authorities. These are usually governmental agencies. Traditionally, regulatory authorities have been primarily charged with assuring the safety of drugs already on the market and are less concerned with approval of new medicines. However, there is evidence that this orientation is changing.

Although a regulatory authority's most important role in terms of new drugs is the decision to approve an agent for marketing, most authorities also approve initial tests in humans. Authorities in some countries, such as France, play little part in this, while others, including the FDA in the US want to be involved in the development process and make themselves available for important discussions. Most regulatory authorities discourage meetings with industry representatives before submission of an application for marketing. The regulatory authority in Canada used to insist on approving each clinical protocol before allowing any trial to begin.

Even greater differences among authorities are apparent in approaches to reviewing and approving New Drug Application (NDA) dossiers. The Japanese almost always insist on new clinical trials being conducted in Japan, even though enormous amounts of data are already available for some new agents.

Despite the differences among regulatory authorities, the last several years have been marked by a trend toward more similar approaches and cooperation among various regulatory groups. This has been referred to as 'harmonisation'; formal meetings are being held to advance this process and true progress is being made. Such cooperation promises to benefit patients, healthcare professionals and those who evaluate data and decide which research to pay for and how much to pay for it.

### 3.1 Developing Regulatory Strategies

A simplified approach to creating regulatory strategies is to answer the following questions. The answers to each may be thought of as points on a spectrum or as discrete choices for each question.

1) ***Should the regulatory submission contain data for a 'lean' or a 'fat' development plan?*** The terms 'lean' and 'fat' refer to the number of studies conducted in each area of development (e.g. toxicology, medical, preclinical), the number of patients or animals in each study, and the amount of data collected on each subject. The answer to this question is ideally based on a risk-benefit assessment for the drug, the special status or need for it (e.g. an important 'orphan' drug *versus* a 'me-too' drug), as well as on special regulations that may apply (e.g. Treatment – IND). Because all data available from anywhere in the world must be filed on a new drug with most regulatory authorities, the choice of a 'fat' versus 'lean' plan must be considered at the outset of a new drug's development (see further section 1.2). Nonetheless, a submission may be 'lean' in some areas and 'fat' in others. Failure to plan a drug's development internationally may generate undesirable data and

force a company to adopt a regulatory strategy different from the preferred one.

2) ***Should separate regulatory submissions for marketing authorisation be made for different indications or should they be combined?*** The answer to this question is often a matter of senior research and development managers trying to second-guess the reviewing policy of a specific regulatory authority, as well as marketing managers trying to second-guess the reception of the drug for each indication in the marketplace. Second-guessing the actions of a regulatory authority is seldom possible, despite sophisticated reviews by regulatory affairs personnel. A limiting factor is that many companies are unable to codevelop multiple indications simultaneously and submit applications at the same (or nearly the same) time.

3) ***Should the initial regulatory submission for marketing authorisation be made in the country in which: (a) the fastest approval is expected; (b) the least amount of data are required; (c) the largest market exists; or (d) the best opportunity exists to obtain postmarketing data; or should the submission be delayed until it can be submitted to many countries simultaneously?*** It is desirable to follow the last approach whenever possible, but regulatory applications in Japan usually follow a few years later for practical reasons.

By submitting a similar dossier containing the same data to many countries simultaneously, one avoids the problem of having to rewrite expert reports for new dossiers when additional data become available. This could create major problems if different interpretations are reached in multiple versions of an expert's report, or in reports written by different experts at different times. In Europe, this is becoming less of an issue because new regulations allow a dossier to be submitted to all members states of the European Economic Community at one time. In addition, more countries are seeking membership in that organisation, which will further simplify the regulatory submission process. For many other countries, the question of resolving differences between submissions still exists, but this issue is less relevant in almost all countries that receive submissions several years after the initial ones are submitted.

4) ***Assuming that a core package of data is assembled, how large should it be? Should it be as small as possible or quite large with many modules that may be used in multiple submissions?*** A large core package without modules should be avoided. The question of core size should be addressed at the outset of a new drug's development. (For a review of the issues surrounding this question, see Spilker[2]).

5) ***Should an electronic submission be made, and if so what part(s) of the application should be submitted electronically?*** There is a wide range of possible options for electronic submission, from submitting an optical disk of the reports, which is essentially a hard copy that cannot be manipulated, to a submission enabling word-processing functions to be carried out, to supplying raw data (plus reports) that enable the regulatory authority to freely explore new analyses. If a Computer-Assisted New Drug Application (CANDA) is to be used (see further section 3.4), then planning (and, preferably, interaction with the regulatory authority) should begin early in the development process. The decision-making role of the regulatory affairs groups in the area of electronic submission varies considerably among companies, but recommendations should always be sought from this group.

6) ***Should a company proactively interact with a regulatory authority at all stages of the development process, or should it adopt a totally reactive position – only responding to questions from the authority?*** It is particularly important to prepare the regulatory authority to view an application on a novel agent or a request for information in the way intended. In the US, there are specified times during a drug's development when it is appropriate to present and discuss data and plans with the FDA. These occur usually at the end of phases I and II and at the pre-NDA stage, although meetings at other times (e.g. pre-IND) are often possible. My strong bias in this regard is to be as proactive as possible with regulatory authorities to obtain feedback on proposed strategies and development plans.

7) ***How should a company respond to questions from regulatory authorities about a regulatory submission?*** The company may decide how to respond to each request for information, or it may have established specific (or general) standard operating procedures for responding to regulatory questions. Letters requesting data and information can be assigned to a task force or to an individual who can prepare a written response or coordinate the work needed to provide an answer. An organised systematic approach is a more efficient process than adopting

an *ad hoc* response to each request for information.

8) ***How and when should a company prepare draft labelling for new medicines?*** At some stage of drug development, it is necessary to prepare a proposed package label for new investigational medicines. The copy submitted to the FDA in the US must be fully annotated, i.e. each statement in the draft label must be referenced to a specific item, volume and page in the NDA or other appropriate place (e.g. Federal Register) that supports the statement.

The contents of the label may be driven by requirements for class labelling or by a particular style that the regulatory authority desires. A committee may be formed about a year prior to the expected submission date to develop the label. One person may prepare an early draft and after committee review, the draft could be circulated to the company's experts within medical, marketing, legal, regulatory affairs and other relevant divisions for further comment and revision. Spilker[1] discusses many reasons why it is counter-productive to develop a draft label early in a drug's development.

9) ***Should regulatory strategies be designed to achieve regulatory success or to achieve commercial success?*** The former type of strategy focuses on obtaining approvals as rapidly as possible. The latter type involves planning symposia, developing an approach to publications, and conducting appropriate clinical trials on quality of life and pharmacoeconomic endpoints. Ideally, the regulatory strategies chosen will attain both goals, but companies should be certain that they do not focus on regulatory success and not pay adequate attention to commercial success.

### 3.2 Preparing/Publishing Documents for Regulatory Submissions

The format and content of all documents submitted must be evaluated to ensure that they comply with all appropriate regulations. Although regulations differ around the world, major steps toward 'harmonisation' are occurring. Preparing and submitting regulatory documents to a regulatory authority may be viewed as a publication activity. This activity involves collecting manuscripts and reports, and then copy editing them, indexing the contents, adding cross-references, copying and binding them, and distributing the copies. This is an extremely complex and difficult process to carry out rapidly and efficiently. Documents must be well organised and written in a style that is easy to read and understand. The submission should also be easy for reviewers to follow in terms of scientific logic and internal consistency (e.g. always proceed in order of small to large animals in presenting results for toxicology, metabolism and pharmacokinetic studies). The style of expert reports should adhere to the preferences of the regulators.

### 3.3 Interacting With Regulatory Authorities

The scope of interactions between regulatory affairs professionals in pharmaceutical companies and regulatory authorities depends on the country involved, the company and the type of interaction. Regulatory affairs professionals often act as a liaison between personnel in the company and regulatory authorities. This coordinating role is crucial because it circumvents individuals in the company independently or semi-independently interacting with regulatory authorities.

All interactions with regulatory authorities should be documented by the regulatory affairs department. Regulatory affairs personnel should also document all interactions.

### 3.4 Computer-Assisted New Drug Applications

The goals of a computer-assisted NDA (CANDA) are to:

1) Increase the accuracy of information transmission to and within regulatory authorities.

2) Increase the efficiency of the regulatory review.

3) Shorten the time for a regulatory decision.

4) Reduce the amount of paper used; and

5) Improve the quality of the regulatory application.

To achieve these goals, a CANDA should contain:

- An indexing, filing and cataloguing system of the NDA's contents
- A word processing system of the text file to help the regulatory authority prepare its reports (e.g. Summary Basis of Approval)
- A database to query. This is intended to provide the regulatory authority with a high degree of comfort with the quality and accuracy of the data presented.

#### What Form Should CANDAs Take?

There is no single type of CANDA submission, and a wide range currently exists. One extreme is to provide the regulatory authority with a laser disk that merely substitutes for (or supplements) hard copy. At the other extreme, an interactive computer program is given to a regulatory authority so that they may theoretically bypass the company and obtain raw data directly from the investigator(s).

Each NDA must be carefully considered as to whether it is a candidate for a CANDA. If so, then the company should determine where it best fits along the electronic spectrum. In addition, the sponsor should interact with the regulatory authority (if possible) to ensure that they agree with the company's plans.

#### Pros and Cons of CANDAs

In an analysis of the time for CANDAs to be approved by the FDA as compared with non-CANDAs, the mean approval time for 10 CANDAs submitted during the period 1987 to 1990 was found to be 3.1 years, which was 10% longer than the mean time for 64 non-CANDAs.[7] CANDAs permit FDA reviewers to check raw data more easily in the sponsor's database. To date, the fear of some people that 'data dredging' and unwarranted analyses of data by regulatory agencies might occur has not been realised. Although such analyses are theoretically possible with the hard copy data the agencies currently receive, they are not commonly performed by most regulatory authorities. Rather, the agency usually requests the company to conduct additional analyses, although if the company believes a request for additional analyses is unreasonable or inappropriate, they may challenge such a request.

Another as yet unresolved issue regarding electronic submissions is that a regulatory authority may only have one type of computer system while pharmaceutical companies often have several different types. Thus, a company's electronic data may have to be converted to a different format so that it is compatible with the system at the regulatory authority. This often takes a great deal of time and effort. Moreover, if electronic data are to be sent to multiple regulatory authorities, it is likely that multiple conversions of the data would have to be made.

### 3.5 Major Reasons for Delays in Drug Approval

Some of the reasons for delays in drug approval rest primarily with the regulatory authority and others (to a greater or lesser degree) with the submitting company. A few of the reasons for delays in approval that can be influenced or controlled by the pharmaceutical company are given below. Appropriate attention to each point enhances the probability that the application will be reviewed rapidly.

1) ***The submission is a poorly organised document that is not clear to the reviewers:*** if the scientific and medical rationales for the clinical or other studies are not clear to reviewers or if the material is not presented in a logical order, some reviewers will cease reviewing the submission (and thereby delay the application), rather than immediately asking the sponsor for clarification. Sponsors should therefore keep in touch with the regulators to follow the status of their applications and to develop an appropriate rapport with the reviewers assigned.

2) ***The clinical trials conducted were poorly designed:*** not only should individual clinical trials be well designed, but the overall clinical programme should also create a clear picture of what was done and why each trial was conducted.

3) ***One or more important clinical trials were not conducted:*** if a drug is primarily eliminated from the body by the kidneys, it is important to evaluate how patients with poor kidney function will handle it. Similarly, if a drug is to be used in conjunction with another agent in clinical practice, it is important to determine the extent and nature of any interactions between them.

4) ***Clinical trials were poorly conducted, and the data were poorly or inappropriately analysed:*** these points are self-explanatory.

5) ***The submission appears to bury or inadequately discuss problems:*** reviewers who detect major deficiencies or problems that they believe are purposely buried in an application usually react strongly and may become frustrated and delay progress of the application. Actual or potential problems should be dealt with openly and honestly by the sponsor and the company's perspective presented. Any major problems with the drug should be discussed in pre-NDA meetings so that the regulatory authority's perspective is obtained. This information should help the company present the problem in the most appropriate manner.

When drug-related issues are raised by preclinical, clinical or technical development scientists, it is important that all three (or more) groups should comment on the implications, if any. This also provides the regulatory authority with some assurance that the NDA or Product

License Application (PLA) document is a whole and not three (or more) separate documents written by people who do not communicate with one another.

6) ***Developing a 'me-too' product with little clinical benefit in comparison with presently available therapy:*** it often takes a long time (i.e. many years) to review an application for a drug considered to be of little therapeutic importance.

7) ***Submitting additional data to a regulatory authority after an NDA or PLA application is submitted:*** some companies submit additional (unsolicited) data several times to the regulatory authority. This is naturally annoying to the agency, which is attempting to review the specific set of data originally submitted.

8) ***Submitting a large amount of 'dirty or noisy' data in an application:*** the more these kinds of data are included in the application, the slower the review will be. If the pivotal trials (i.e. generally the most well-controlled clinical trials) are not 'clean', then the delays are almost certain to be long ones. One exception would be if only case studies were submitted for certain 'orphan' drugs or drugs indicated for previously untreatable conditions. There is no guarantee, however, that case studies are acceptable on their own, without a controlled trial, to have such a drug approved.

9) ***Submitting an NDA and PLA prematurely so that the drug can join the queue for review at the agency:*** regulatory authorities strongly dislike obviously inadequate submissions that are prematurely submitted. A company that uses this technique usually does so in the hope of obtaining a shopping list of inadequacies to address. When they receive the list, they will presumably have completed the studies in the meantime and can therefore obtain a rapid approval of their drug. However, this practice only holds up the review of more complete applications. To deal with this issue expeditiously, agencies can 'refuse to file' an NDA. This practice is becoming more widely used by the FDA and is truly in the industry's interests.

10) ***Requesting approval for too many indications:*** in most instances, this approach will delay the entire submission because the data supporting each indication are judged on their own.

11) ***Using inexperienced regulatory personnel:*** company staff who do not follow written and unwritten procedures for dealing with regulatory authority personnel may easily delay the company's applications. For example, labelling conferences vary from 'give and take' negotiations to situations where fixed class labels are required, to situations where the regulatory authority adopts inflexible positions. The procedure for a particular situation depends on the type of drug (e.g. are there 10 other similar medicines available, how strong are the data and how safe is it?), and on the personalities of the negotiators.

12) ***Delaying responses to regulatory questions:*** there is no question that some delays in approving drugs relate to the time taken by a company to respond to a request from a regulatory authority. Some companies who are convinced of the strength of their data overlook the fact that the data must be able to convince others who review it with a critical perspective. In such cases, there is a potential danger that the company may not present the data as well or as convincingly as possible.

### 3.6 Five Basic Rules of Regulatory Applications

The following list of rules (also known as 'the five Cs') is only one of several mnemonics to help guide the approach to preparing regulatory applications:

- ***Concise submission*** – make the applications easy to read and follow.
- ***Clearly written*** – do not dilute the text or add excessive materials that do not enhance the value of the submission.
- ***Correct information*** – ensure the application is carefully reviewed for errors.
- ***Complete documents*** – review the application to make certain there are no major omissions.
- ***Consistent organisation*** – ensure that the application is logically and consistently organised.

### 3.7 Techniques for Speeding Approval of Regulatory Submissions

One technique to help speed regulatory approval is to have experts from outside the company review a summary of the regulatory application and write an opinion letter. Such as letter should be a critical analysis of the data and not a summary. This might be especially useful for regulatory applications that are basically weak. For example, if the application primarily uses historical data as controls or uses data from compassionate plea trials, experts may express the degree to which the application contains substantial data and evidence that will convince clinicians working in the same therapeutic area. The experts should only comment on the part of the application that they are most familiar with (e.g. clinical interpretation and importance, technical issues, social need).

A wise practice is to provide a desk copy of the relevant part(s) of the application for the reviewer's personal use. This will allow the reviewer to mark it up freely. Some reviewers within the regulatory authority like to have personal interactions with company representatives to discuss the NDA, but others discourage such interactions. In situations where interactions are either acceptable or desired by the regulatory agency, it is critical to determine who the most appropriate contact person or group at the company should be. It is often desirable for one person to be appointed to fill this role. The person chosen should have a good rapport with the reviewer and be at the appropriate decision-making level within the company.

As pointed out above, ensuring the adequacy the data submitted is vital. For example, efficacy data on a new drug given at different doses is extremely important. If dose-response data are not submitted in an NDA, there should be a good reason for this. There should also be an adequate number of patients who have received full therapeutics doses of a new drug before the regulatory dossier is submitted.

A few other recommendations that may help to speed approval of a regulatory submission are:

1) Engage a consultant with excellent knowledge of the approval process.

2) Adopt an open, non-confrontational attitude.

3) Discuss the company's regulatory approach with the authority at the earliest practical opportunity.

4) Discuss the issues with all relevant areas of the regulatory authority (e.g. if the agent is a biological product, then discuss issues with both the offices of medicine research and biologics research).

5) Do not change the formulation used in a major way during later stages of clinical trials (if possible).

6) Use only one name (generic) for the drug throughout the application.

7) Prepare reviewer-friendly types of documents that lead the reviewer step by step through the logic and the data in the application.

8) When responding to questions from regulatory authorities, ensure that the information the reviewer is actually looking for is provided.

A principle observed by some companies is that taking an extra 6 to 12 months to assemble a first-class NDA will save regulatory review time and yield a more rapid approval overall. Attention to detail, good medical practice and good ethics is an appropriate formula to achieve commercial success.

### *Acknowledgement*

Portions of the text in this chapter have previously been published in 'Multinational Pharmaceutical Companies: Principles and Practices (2nd Edition, 1994)' and 'Guide to Clinical Trials (1991)', both published by Raven Press (New York, NY). I am grateful to the publisher for permission to republish them here.

### Further Reading

Spilker B. Guide to clinical trials. New York: Raven Press, 1991

Spilker B. Multinational pharmaceutical companies: principles and practices. 2nd ed. New York: Raven Press, 1994

### References

1. Spilker B. Multinational pharmaceutical companies: principles and practices. 2nd edition. New York: Raven Press, 1994
2. Spilker B. Guide to clinical trials. New York: Raven Press, 1991
3. Hassar M, Weintraub M. 'Uninformed' consent and the healthy volunteer: an analysis of patient volunteers in a clinical trial of a new anti-inflammatory drug. Clinical Pharmacology and Therapeutics 1976; 20: 379-86
4. Wells FO, Griffin JP. Ethics committees for clinical research experience in the United Kingdom. Drugs 1989; 37: 229-32
5. Association of the British Industry. Compensation and drug trials. Guidelines: Clinical trials - compensation for medicine induced injury. British Medical Journal 1983; 287: 675
6. Diamond AL, Laurence DR. Commentary. British Medical Journal 1983; 287: 676-7
7. Kaitin KI, Walsh HL. Are initiatives to speed the new drug approval process working? Drug Information Journal 1992; 26: 341-9

Chapter 12

# Drugs in Anaesthetic Practice and Analgesia

*W. McCaughey* and *R.K. Mirakhur*

### Synopsis of Important Principles

1) The main aims of anaesthesia are the prevention of pain during surgery and at other times, together with maintenance of the patient's physiological functions at these times.

2) Anaesthesia involves a balanced approach, in which the individual patient's psyche and pathophysiology are taken into account and drugs are used to modify and control any aspect as required.

3) Any associated disease or pathophysiological abnormality should be treated or corrected before operation, and potentially dangerous physiological disturbances avoided during and after anaesthesia.

4) Drugs used in anaesthesia are often characterised by a rapid onset of action and rapid elimination. Knowledge of their pharmacokinetics is essential in making best use of these properties.

5) Rapid action may be accompanied by rapid development of adverse effects. Especially in elderly and critically ill patients, slow titration of drug to desired effect is important to minimise this danger.

6) Anaesthetic drugs are relatively nontoxic, but there are some important idiosyncratic effects. Halothane has lost favour because of rare development of hepatitis. Malignant hyperpyrexia, a rare but potentially fatal disorder of muscle, can be triggered by several drugs used in anaesthesia in genetically susceptible individuals.

7) Management of chronic pain and management of the critically ill in the intensive care unit (ICU) are largely subspecialties of anaesthesia in many countries.

8) In the ICU, although mechanical support of ventilation is often a mainstay of treatment, drugs of many classes are used for support of failing body systems.

9) Pain perception is an individual sensation. Symptomatic treatment of acute pain should not therefore be based on a concept of the painfulness of certain conditions, although some analgesics may be more appropriate for the pain of certain conditions.

10) Chronic pain may have multiple causes, requiring psychotherapy, nerve blocking or nerve stimulation techniques, and psychotropic drugs as well as analgesic drugs given by various routes. Invasive treatments should be used last.

Anaesthesia, i.e. 'artificially induced insensibility to pain', was partially achieved by pharmacological means even in prehistoric times, by use of plant products such as the hallucinogenic mandrake and datura. However, reliable anaesthesia awaited the introduction of ether by Morton in 1846. Since that time, anaesthesia has developed and been refined considerably, and several important milestones are worthy of recall. These include the discovery of the local anaesthetic actions of cocaine by Koller in 1884 and its use for spinal anaesthesia by Bier in 1898, the perfection of endotracheal anaesthesia by Magill and Rowbotham around 1920, the introduction of the first barbiturate for induction of anaesthesia in 1932, and the introduction of curare in 1942.

## 1. General Considerations

Over the past quarter century, the specialty of anaesthesia has been broadened, although its scope is still well described in a definition provided for the US Department of Labor 30 years ago,[1] i.e.:

'Anesthesiology is a practice of medicine dealing with:

1) The management of procedures for rendering a patient insensible to pain during surgical procedures.

2) The support of life functions under the stress of anesthetic and surgical manipulations.

3) The clinical management of the patient unconscious from whatever cause.

4) The management of problems in pain relief.

5) The management of problems in cardiac and respiratory resuscitation.

6) The application of specific methods of inhalational therapy.

7) The clinical management of various fluid, electrolyte and metabolic disturbances.'

The skills described here are those that have led to the key position now occupied by anaesthetists in the intensive care unit (ICU) and pain clinic, as well as in the operating theatre.

Modern anaesthesia uses a balanced approach, in which the whole of the patient's psyche and pathophysiology are taken into account, and drugs are used to modify and control any aspect as required. Thus, as well as local and general anaesthetic agents, drugs of many classes – tranquillisers, analgesics, muscle relaxants, drugs affecting the autonomic nervous system, etc. – all fall within the sphere of interest of the anaesthetist.

## 2. Clinical Pharmacology of Drugs Used in Anaesthesia

The general principles of rational drug therapy, based on pharmacokinetic principles and knowledge or experience of the actions of drugs, apply to anaesthetic practice as to other disciplines. Many drugs used in anaesthesia are potent and may have a relatively low therapeutic index. In common with other situations where this occurs, e.g. cytotoxic drug therapy, it is important to tailor dosages closely to the needs of the individual patient. Thus, most drugs used in anaesthetic practice will be given on a mg per kg basis rather than by the broader dose recommendations used in other situations. Inhalational drugs are an exception, due to the pharmacokinetics of their uptake and distribution.

### 2.1 General Anaesthetic Agents

The mechanism by which anaesthetic drugs produce unconsciousness is still unknown. However the unifying central concept is that action occurs at membrane level.[2] The Meyer and Overton rule describes the close correlation that is observed between the anaesthetic potency and hydrophobic solubility of chemically related series of anaesthetic drugs, thus suggesting a lipid site of action. This relationship applies to inhaled anaesthetics with potency over a 100,000-fold range and across species as varied as goldfish and humans, and has been described as one of the most powerful correlations in biology. On the other hand, evidence from different sources also supports action at various synapses, at neurotransmitter receptors, or in or at ion channels. No anaesthesia receptor has been described and it is unclear whether one or a number of mechanisms are involved. For reviews, see Tinker[3] or Halsey.[2]

#### *2.1.1 Inhalational Agents*

Anaesthetic practice is unique in that a high proportion of the drugs are administered by the inhalational route. Such drugs must either be gaseous, or the vapours of volatile liquids. Their general properties are shown in table I.

Of the original 3 inhalational agents – nitrous oxide, ether and chloroform – the first 2 are still in use today. Research has been driven by the disadvantages of existing drugs. Flammability was a major problem with many of the earlier gases and volatile liquids, and the introduction of halothane in 1956 was an important advance. The main trend in newer volatile agents has

**Table I.** A summary of the major clinical pharmacological properties of inhalational anaesthetics

| Agent | Physical characteristics | MAC (%v/v) | Blood/gas partition coefficient | Cardiovascular effect | Respiratory effect | Elimination | Degree of metabolism (%) | Notes (see also table IV) |
|---|---|---|---|---|---|---|---|---|
| Nitrous oxide | Non-flammable gas | 104 (see text) | 0.47 | Stable (see text) | Mild respiratory depression | Lungs | Minimal | Weak anaesthetic unless supplemented; good analgesic |
| Ether | Volatile, flammable liquid | 1.92 | 12 | BP stable CO ↑ | Tracheobronchial irritation | Lungs; hepatic metabolism and renal excretion (minor) | | Analgesic in subanaesthetic concentrations |
| Halothane | Volatile, non-flammable liquid | 0.8 | 2.4 | BP ↓, bradycardia CO ↓ (minor) Sensitises myocardium to adrenaline (epinephrine) | Respiratory depression | Lungs; hepatic metabolism and renal excretion | 20% | Increases intracranial pressure; inhibits uterine contractility. Hepatitis (rare) |
| Enflurane | Volatile, non-flammable liquid | 1.68 | 1.9 | BP ↓ CO ↓ (minor) Sensitises myocardium to adrenaline (epinephrine) | Respiratory depression | Lungs; hepatic metabolism and renal excretion | 2% | Convulsions a risk in epileptic patients; inhibits uterine contractility |
| Isoflurane | Volatile, non-flammable liquid | 1.15 | 1.4 | BP ↓ | Marked respiratory depression | Lungs; minimal biotransformation | 0.2% | |
| Desflurane | Volatile, non-flammable gas/liquid | 7.5 | 0.42 | BP ↓ | Tracheobronchial irritation | Lungs; minimal biotransformation | 0.02% | Boiling point below room temperature |
| Sevoflurane | Volatile, non-flammable liquid | 2 | 0.69 | BP ↓ | | Lungs; hepatic metabolism | 3% | |

*Abbreviations and symbols:* MAC = minimum alveolar concentration; BP = blood pressure; CO = cardiac output; ↓ = reduced; ↑ = increased.

been in the development of drugs requiring less metabolism in the body, with the expectation of a reduction in the hepatic and renal toxicity which has been linked to metabolic products of inhaled anaesthetics.

### Pharmacokinetics of Uptake and Distribution

The same principles underlie the pharmacokinetics of inhaled anaesthetic drugs as of those administered by other routes. However, the situation is complicated by several factors that make it difficult to apply some of the same mathematical concepts. In particular, the lung changes from being the route for delivery of the drug to being the principal organ of excretion depending of the relationship between inspired, alveolar and blood concentration. Likewise, the drug is not given as a specific dose nor as an infusion at a predetermined rate, but at a rate depending on factors outlined briefly below.

Depth of anaesthesia is determined by the effective gas tension (partial pressure) of the drug in the brain. When a constant concentration of the anaesthetic is inhaled, the concentration in the alveoli rises gradually toward the inhaled level. How quickly it rises will depend on:

1) The concentration of inhaled cases.

2) The ventilation of the alveoli (which may be reduced if the drug is irritant or depresses respiration).

3) The rate at which the drug is taken up into the blood from the alveoli.

Movement of anaesthetic drug from alveolus to blood reduces alveolar concentrations and thus maintains the concentration gradient from inspired to alveolar gas. If the solubility (blood/gas solubility coefficient) of the drug is high, then it will take longer for equilibrium to be attained, because: (a) more of the drug needs to be dissolved in the blood for a given tension to be reached; and (b) the more rapid removal of the drug from the alveoli reduces the concentration there and, therefore, reduces the gradient driving it from alveolus to capillary.

The rate of removal of drug into the circulation will also depend on cardiac output, which may be influenced by the drug itself. Finally, the rate at which blood tension reaches that in alveoli will also depend on the rate at which it is distributed to other tissues, not only the target organ (brain), but also muscle, fat depots, etc. Differences in this respect between neonates and adults help to explain the more rapid uptake of inhalational anaesthetics in the neonate.[4,5]

The *anaesthetic potency* of the drug is obviously an important factor in production of anaesthesia. This is commonly expressed as the MAC, i.e. the minimal alveolar concentration of the drug which under equilibrium conditions will produce anaesthesia (prevention of movement in response to a painful stimulus, such as skin incision) in 50% of patients. This term is used to compare the potency of different inhalational drugs. Concentrations of anaesthetic gases and vapours of volatile agents are commonly expressed as percentages by volume (v/v). The relationship between this and the mass of agent can be calculated using Avogadro's hypothesis – that 1 mole of saturated (i.e. 100%) vapour occupies 22.4L at standard temperature and pressure.

The attributes that will lead to rapid induction of and emergence from anaesthesia are: high potency, low blood solubility, low fat solubility (all of which reduce the mass of the drug that needs to be transferred from alveoli to blood), lack of irritant and respiratory depressant effect (so that ventilation is maintained without interruption), lack of cardiac depressant effects, and in the case of a volatile liquid, a relatively low boiling point so that adequate vapour pressure can be attained. To achieve equilibrium rapidly, anaesthesia is induced using a relatively high concentration of inhaled drug (overpressure technique), to create a relatively high concentration gradient from alveoli to tissues. This concentration is gradually reduced, usually over 5 to 10 minutes, to a maintenance level around or above 1.5 MAC depending on the surgical stimulus and the use of other anaesthetic or analgesic agents. This is in essence the same principle as the use of a loading and maintenance dose or infusion with other drugs. The blood concentration of drug will increase as a first-order process, giving an exponential 'wash in' curve (provided that coughing, breath holding, etc. do not interfere with the process). Required maintenance concentrations also depend on how long and how fast drug continues to pass from the blood to more peripheral compartments, i.e. its volume of distribution (Vd), and rate constants for transfer between compartments.

Inhalational drugs can leave the body by the same route they enter, but a proportion – varying from a minimal amount in the case of nitrous oxide to over 20% for halothane (table I) – is metabolised. There is an association between the biotransformation of inhalational anaesthetics and the development of toxicity.[6] For a more complete review of the pharmacokinetics of anaesthetic agents, see Dale and Brown.[7]

#### Nitrous Oxide

Nitrous oxide is a weak anaesthetic and in the absence of hypoxia will not by itself produce anaesthesia in all patients. Its MAC is 104%,[8] i.e. it can only produce anaesthesia in 50% of patients if the partial pressure of nitrous oxide is greater than atmospheric pressure, and this can only be achieved under hyperbaric conditions (in 19th century Paris, a horse-drawn hyperbaric chamber was used for this purpose). It is commonly used in a 50 to 70% concentration with oxygen as a carrier gas for more potent volatile agents. In subanaesthetic concentrations, it is analgesic and is used in obstetrics in a 50% mixture with oxygen, and as a sedative in dentistry at 25% – this is known as 'relative analgesia'. As it is largely insoluble in blood and tissues, its action is rapid and recovery time short; the rapidity of action is helped by it being non-irritant and almost without odour.

Nitrous oxide is relatively nontoxic, but it does have a direct myocardial depressant effect that may be masked by a sympathomimetic action. Bone marrow depression occurs after a few hours of exposure, and is due largely to inactivation of cyanocobalamin (vitamin $B_{12}$), which is the bound cofactor of methionine synthase.[9,10]

#### Ether

Ether (diethyl ether) is still used for anaesthesia, especially in developing countries; its low cost and relative safety justify this continuing use. Ether is a volatile liquid, flammable in air and explosive in oxygen. It is a potent anaesthetic (MAC 1.92%), but is irritant to the tracheobronchial tree and is relatively unpleasant to inhale. Since it is highly soluble in blood and in tissues, the concentration in blood builds up only slowly, and induction of anaesthesia is slow, as is recovery. Ether is a comparatively safe drug to use, being less depressant to the heart and cardiovascular system than halothane, and because respiratory depression in overdosage will become apparent before there is dangerous depression of the circulation. However, this cardiovascular stability depends on it stimulating the release of catecholamines from the adrenal medulla, which counteract myocardial depression caused by ether, and thus its use in the presence of β-blockade may lead to cardiovascular depression. Clinically, ether is used in concentrations of 10 to 20 volumes percent. Despite its good features, its flammability and slowness of action have led to its virtual abandonment in the developed world.

**Halothane**

Halothane, introduced in 1956, was the first of the new generation of halogenated anaesthetic compounds in which fluorine was incorporated in the molecule. It is a volatile liquid with a fairly low boiling point of 50.2°C, potent (MAC around 0.8%), has a sweet and not unpleasant odour, and allows rapid induction and recovery. It is highly soluble in blood, with a solubility coefficient of 0.8, which compares with 0.47 for nitrous oxide and 0.62 for isoflurane. It is also nonflammable, and rapidly became the most popular general anaesthetic in use. It was, for many years, and in some respects still is the standard by which other anaesthetics are judged.

The adverse effects of halothane are few but important. It is a potent vasodilator, and its use is accompanied by a reduction in blood pressure and some myocardial depression. This varies with the conditions of use, but some studies have shown reductions in mean blood pressure of 11 to 15%, while myocardial contractility was reduced by 30 to 50%.[11,12] There is also a negative chronotropic and dromotropic effect, partly due to increased vagal tone. Halothane also sensitises the heart to the arrhythmogenic effects of catecholamines, whether administered exogenously or generated endogenously by a raised carbon dioxide level, but in the absence of either of these the problem rarely arises. The question of halothane-associated hepatitis remained controversial for many years but it is now apparent that 2 types of liver damage may occur:[6]

- *Type I:* abnormal liver function tests may occur in up to 20% of patients, the incidence increasing with each subsequent halothane exposure.[13] This type of damage may be exacerbated by hypoxic conditions or by enzyme induction, but is generally mild and not important. It is also dose-related and reproducible, in contrast to the second type, and does not appear to progress to this.[14]
- *Type II:* massive hepatic necrosis, with a mortality of up to 50%, is an extremely rare phenomenon following halothane anaesthesia, occurring in about 1 in 35,000 exposures.[15] There have been a number of theories as to its cause. Damage has occurred even more rarely following enflurane or isoflurane anaesthesia, and the incidence of clinical reports correlates with the extent of metabolism of the different drugs. Thus, it seems likely that products of metabolism play in integral part in hepatotoxicity.

An immune mechanism has also been proposed to explain the occasional nature of the type II syndrome. Currently, attention is focused on a combination of these mechanisms. Halothane, and to a correspondingly lesser extent other halogenated volatile anaesthetics, is metabolised to trifluoroacetyl (TFA) halide, which binds covalently to and, thus, modifies microsomal proteins of hepatocytes. Antibodies to such modified proteins have been found in the sera of patients with a histologically proven clinical diagnosis of halothane hepatitis.[16] However, although all halothane-exposed individuals metabolise halothane to TFA and produce TFA-labelled proteins, only in rare 'susceptible' individuals is there an immune response.[16] This may suggest a genetically-determined susceptibility, and raises the possibility in the future of a test to identify those who are potentially at risk.

Until such a test is available, prevention of halothane hepatitis may be difficult, and the only clear way of reducing the incidence is to avoid re-exposure to halothane in those patients who have had a previous adverse reaction to the drug, demonstrated either by unexplained pyrexia or by jaundice. Halothane should also be avoided in those patients who have a family history of sensitisation to the drug. In such cases, halothane-free equipment should be used, and exposure to other volatile anaesthetics should also be avoided.[17]

It is now difficult to justify the routine use of halothane unless a case can be made that it offers greater safety than available alternatives in the individual patient. This may, indeed, often be the case in paediatric anaesthesia, where halothane-associated hepatitis appears to be very rare, and perhaps also with ischaemic heart disease[18] and in some other circumstances in adults.

#### Enflurane and Isoflurane

Enflurane and isoflurane are isomers; both are halogenated ethers, as was methoxyflurane, which has virtually dropped out of use.

***Enflurane*** entered clinical practice around 1978, helped by concerns over possible hepatotoxicity of halothane and nephrotoxicity of methoxyflurane. It is potent, although less so than halothane (MAC 1.68%;[19] blood gas partition coefficient 1.9), and fairly pleasant to inhale. It causes a similar degree of myocardial depression to other volatile anaesthetics, but, like ether, it relies to some extent for cardiovascular stability on circulating catecholamines to counter its cardiovascular depressant effects, and should used only with extreme caution in patients receiving β-adrenoceptor blocking drugs.

Although enflurane does sensitise the heart to catecholamines, it is much less likely to provoke arrhythmias than is halothane. Unlike halothane, it has an excitatory or even convulsant effect on the central nervous system (CNS), and is inappropriate for use in epileptic patients. It is metabolised much less than halothane (comparative rates are halothane 20%; enflurane 2%; isoflurane 0.2%) and although prolonged anaesthesia can lead to raised serum inorganic fluoride concentrations, these are not likely to cause renal dysfunction unless there is pre-existing renal disease.[20]

***Isoflurane:*** despite its greater cost than halothane or enflurane, isoflurane is used widely because of its low rate of metabolism. Hepatic and renal toxicity are unlikely, although isolated reports have occurred.[21] Its potency is similar to enflurane (MAC 1.15%[22]), but despite low blood gas solubility, pungency makes inhalational induction of anaesthesia less pleasant than with halothane, especially in children, and may lead to breath-holding and hypoxic episodes.

Cardiovascular stability is a feature of isoflurane. Although blood pressure is reduced, cardiac output is well maintained. There has been controversy as to whether isoflurane has a greater propensity to cause 'steal' from cardiac ischaemic regions. Evidence is still contradictory on this point.[23] It is reasonable to avoid isoflurane in patients with multivessel disease.[24] In neurosurgery, isoflurane has 2 advantages. Firstly, it reduces both electrical activity and oxygen consumption of the brain, which may have a protective effect. Secondly, effects on cerebral blood flow and intracerebral pressure are absent up to 1.1 MAC, and are less than those of halothane or enflurane at higher levels.

Isoflurane has been used in low concentrations for long term sedation in the ICU.[25]

#### Desflurane

Desflurane is closely related chemically to isoflurane and continues the logical progress to lower rates of metabolism, being less metabolised again than isoflurane by a factor of 10.[26] Its effects on the cardiovascular, respiratory and nervous systems closely resemble those of isoflurane. Its potential advantages lie in low tissue solubility which leads to rapid recovery, and low potential for hepatic and renal toxicity. However, there are disadvantages: special vapourisers are required because a boiling point of 23.5°C, i.e. around room temperature, means that without these it could be above or below boiling point depending on small variations in ambient temperature. Its potency is low, MAC is about 7.5% in $O_2$, 4.0% in 60% $N_2O$,[27] and pungency makes inhalational induction of anaesthesia difficult.

#### Sevoflurane

Sevoflurane has recently been introduced into worldwide clinical practice. In contrast to desflurane, it is potent (MAC 2%), pleasant to inhale, and has a boiling point of 58.5°C – similar to enflurane – but it is metabolised to a greater extent than enflurane, and thus there are concerns over possible toxicity which only time will resolve.[28] A low blood-gas partition coefficient (0.69) together with lack of irritant properties allows rapid induction of anaesthesia, and indeed the most obvious place for its use may be for inhalational induction of anaesthesia in children.

### 2.1.2 Intravenous Anaesthetic Agents

The intravenous route is simple and pleasant for the patient. As the drugs enter the circulation directly, the effects are rapid in onset and can be readily controlled. Unlike inhalational agents, anaesthetic drugs given by this route depend mainly on hepatic and renal mechanisms for their metabolism and/or elimination. The dosage may, therefore, need to be modified according to the age, organ function and general condition of the patient, being reduced in the elderly, and in patients in shock or with poor risk profiles.

**Table II.** A summary of the main clinical pharmacological properties of intravenous anaesthetics

| Agent | Onset of action | Duration (single dose) | Recovery[a] | Cardiovascular effects[b] | Respiratory or other effects |
|---|---|---|---|---|---|
| Thiopental | Rapid | Short | Moderately rapid | BP ↓<br>CO ↓ | Marked respiratory depression, laryngospasm, bronchospasm |
| Methohexital | Rapid | Short | Moderately rapid | BP ↓<br>CO ↓<br>Tachycardia | Respiratory depression, abnormal muscle movements, cough, hiccough |
| Etomidate | Rapid | Short | Moderately rapid | Minimal | Marked muscle movements, pain on injection |
| Propofol | Rapid | Short | Moderately rapid | BP ↓<br>CO ↓ | Respiratory depression, pain on injection |
| Diazepam | Slow | Long | Very slow | Minimal | Mild respiratory depression, marked amnesia |
| Midazolam | Slow | Long | Slow | Minimal | Mild respiratory depression, marked amnesia |
| Ketamine[c] | Slow | Moderately long | Slow | BP ↑<br>CO ↑<br>Tachycardia | Transient respiratory depression; increases intracranial pressure; hallucinations, dreams on recovery |
| Eltanolone | Moderately rapid | Short | Moderately rapid | BP ↓ | Movement or hypertonus |

a Not an indication of elimination half-life.

b See also table IV.

c Can also be given intramuscularly to induce anaesthesia.

*Abbreviations and symbols:* BP = blood pressure; CO = cardiac output; ↓ = reduced; ↑ = increased; rapid onset = 30-60 sec; slow onset = 2-5 min; short duration = 4-8 min; long duration = ≈30 min or more.

Intravenous anaesthetic agents are widely used for the induction of anaesthesia and as sole agents for short procedures, but for operations longer than a few minutes, maintenance of anaesthesia is commonly continued by inhalational agents. For this reason, intravenous anaesthetic drugs are mainly described as intravenous induction agents. However, total intravenous anaesthesia has now become more popular due to the availability of suitable agents. With careful regard for the pharmacokinetics of the individual drug, a loading dose or loading infusion is followed by a maintenance infusion of the drug.

The barbiturates were introduced as intravenous anaesthetic agents in 1932, and remained virtually unchallenged until the late 1960s. Thiopental (thiopentone) remains one of the most commonly used intravenous induction agents, but the use of methohexital has decreased. Several newer non-barbiturate drugs are now available (table II).[29,30]

#### Formulation Considerations

While barbiturates used as induction agents possess both water solubility required for injection into the bloodstream and high lipid solubility required for rapid access to the brain, several non-barbiturate agents, notably propanidid, alfaxalone/alfadolone acetate ('Althesin') and propofol, are not water soluble. These agents were therefore formulated with a solubilising agent, 'Cremophor EL'; however, it seems likely that 'Cremophor EL' was responsible for most of the hypersensitivity reactions that occurred with these agents, and led to their withdrawal or, in the case of propofol, reformulation. Other preparations (e.g. etomidate which is formulated with propylene glycol) do not have this problem, but are associated with a high incidence of venous damage. An alternative is to use an emulsion (similar to 'Intralipid') as the vehicle. Diazepam in this form has been available for some time, while propofol is now available in an emulsion containing 10% soy bean oil.

#### Pharmacokinetic Characteristics

Intravenous anaesthetics comprise a variety of drugs that differ in chemical structure, but share a suitable combination of physical properties that confer ready penetration of the blood-brain barrier. Lipid solubility is particularly important in this respect. Rapid entry into the brain is associated with rapid distribution and redistribution in the body for most of these drugs, and this terminates their clinical effect. They all readily cross the placenta to the fetus. The rate of elimination varies between the rapidly biotransformed drugs like etomidate and the slowly metabolised agents like thiopental, diazepam and its major active metabolite nordazepam (*N*-desmethyldiazepam). The liver is the main site of biotransformation for intravenous anaes-

**Table III.** Pharmacokinetic parameters of some intravenous anaesthetics (after Burch & Stanski;[35] Ghoneim et al.;[31] Arden et al.;[36] Cockshott et al.;[37] Carl et al.[38])

| Drug | Dose (mg/kg) | Half-life[a] | | | $Vd_{ss}$ (L) [per 70kg] | CL (L/h) |
|---|---|---|---|---|---|---|
| | | $\pi$ (min) | $\alpha$ (min) | $\beta$ (min) | | |
| Thiopental | 6.0 | 6.8 | 59.0 | 719 | 164 | 14.3 |
| Methohexital | 2.0 | | 1.8 | 231 | 128 | 36.5 |
| Etomidate | 0.35 | 0.93 | 12.1 | 324 | 329 | 76.9 |
| Propofol | 2.5 | 2.9 | 27.5 | 225[b] | 287 | 121.8 |
| Diazepam | 5-10mg | | | 92.4 | 147 | 1.42 |
| Midazolam | 0.75 | | 0.3 | 2.3h | 49 | 19.02 |
| Ketamine | 2.2 | 0.5 | 7.8 | 135 | 125 | 58.8 |
| Eltanolone | 0.6 | 0.3-2.0 | 12-29 | 72-212 | 126-378 | 112.1-160.9 |

a $\pi$ = initial distribution half-life; $\alpha$ = redistribution half-life; $\beta$ = terminal elimination half-life.

b Terminal half-life may be 5 to 7 times longer after the use of longer term infusions.

*Abbreviations:* CL = clearance; $Vd_{ss}$ = steady-state volume of distribution.

thetics, with the exception of etomidate, which is hydrolysed by esterases in the plasma and liver.

Biotransformation leads to the formation of active metabolites in the case of ketamine and diazepam. Recovery of mental and psychomotor functions depends on redistribution and hepatic metabolism, and takes longer than with the inhalational anaesthetics. Use of intravenous anaesthetics, therefore, needs to take into account the individual pharmacokinetic properties of the various agents (see table III and appendix A).[31-34]

#### Tolerability

Adverse reactions include induction complications, such as tissue irritation and damage (by the drug or the solvents used for insoluble drugs); pain on injection and venous complications; recovery complications; and hypersensitivity or idiosyncratic reactions, which can be caused by most of the drugs administered intravenously during anaesthesia.

Hypersensitivity reactions are being increasingly reported (see further section 5.6). The precise mechanism of the hypersensitivity response with the individual agents remains to be clarified, but may be due to direct pharmacological effects causing histamine release (thiopental and methohexital cause an increase in the plasma histamine concentration, but etomidate does not appear to stimulate histamine release); or chemical activation of complement C3 leading to histamine release. Other amines and peptides may also be involved in many of these reactions.

Several of these drugs, including thiopental, methohexital and etomidate (but not ketamine) may induce δ-aminolaevulinic acid synthetase activity and precipitate an attack of acute intermittent porphyria in susceptible individuals (tables II and IV).[39-43]

#### Thiopental and Methohexital

These rapid-acting barbiturates cross the blood-brain barrier very rapidly, and induce sleep in a single arm-to-brain circulation time. This time will vary between 8 to 10 seconds in patients with a hyperdynamic circulation, but can be up to 2 minutes in patients with cardiac disease or in shock. Acidosis favours penetration of the drug through the blood-brain barrier while alkalosis has the opposite effect. This is due to changes in ionisation, acidosis resulting in reduced ionisation and alkalosis in increased ionisation.[44]

With average doses (4 to 6 mg/kg for thiopental or 1.6 to 2.0 mg/kg for methohexital) sleep will last for a few minutes, and the patient will reawaken as the drug concentration decreases due to redistribution to other parts of the body, particularly muscle (and later to fat depots in the case of thiopental). The dose requirements are higher in children and lower in the elderly. In hypovolaemia, the blood flow to the muscles and other tissues to which thiopental is redistributed is diminished, leading to high concentrations in the circulation and possibly leading to marked cerebral and cardiac depression. Hepatic metabolism is not important in the immediate recovery from thiopental, but contributes significantly to the more rapid initial recovery from methohexital.[45] If anaesthesia is maintained by giving incremental small doses of the drug, these will become progressively smaller as the sites of redistribution (the tissues) become saturated (a reflection of accumulation). Since this method leads to slow recovery, barbiturates are not commonly used to maintain anaesthesia.

**Table IV.** Drug reactions and interactions and some special risk situations with anaesthetic drugs

| Drug | Secondary drug or clinical situation | Site/mechanism and potential result | Notes |
|---|---|---|---|
| **Inhalational anaesthetics** | | | |
| Halothane/other halogenated volatile anaesthetics<br>Cyclopropane | Adrenaline (epinephrine) and other sympathomimetics | (S) Anaesthetic sensitises myocardium to adrenaline; risk of severe ventricular arrhythmias | Adrenaline solutions should be dilute and not given IV<br>Avoid hypercarbia |
| Methoxyflurane<br>Enflurane<br>?Sevoflurane | Renal disease | (M) Renal toxicity from inorganic fluoride | Avoid prolonged exposure in patients with pre-existing renal disease |
| | Tetracycline | (S) Increased risk of renal toxicity | |
| Ether<br>Enflurane | β-Adrenoceptor blockers | Blockade of normal compensation for cardiodepressant effects; risk of myocardial depression and hypotension | |
| Ether<br>Enflurane | Epilepsy | (S) Risk of seizures | |
| Halothane, enflurane, etc. | Nondepolarising relaxants | (S) Potentiation of neuromuscular blockade | Reduction in dosage requirement |
| All volatile anaesthetics | Patients with malignant hyperpyrexia | (S) May trigger malignant hyperthermia | |
| **Intravenous anaesthetics** | | | |
| Thiopental | Renal failure<br>Cirrhosis | (B) Enhanced activity of thiopental | Reduce rate of administration |
| | Metabolic acidosis | (B) Enhanced activity | |
| Thiopental<br>Methohexital | Acute intermittent porphyria | (M) Induction of δ-aminolaevulinic acid synthetase by barbiturates; precipitation of attacks | |
| Methohexital | Epilepsy | (S) Risk of seizures | |
| Thiopental<br>Methohexital | Allergy<br>Asthma | (S) Hypersensitivity; increased risk of anaphylactic response and bronchospasm | |
| Etomidate | Prolonged use | Blockade of corticosteroid synthesis | Impaired stress response, especially in ICU patients |
| **Local anaesthetics** | | | |
| All local anaesthetics | Metabolic acidosis | (B) Increased risk of toxicity | |
| Tetracaine (amethocaine), procaine | Low serum cholinesterase activity | (M) Prolonged activity | |
| Prilocaine | Large or repeated doses<br>Neonates and infants | (M) Methaemoglobinaemia | Care with dosage |
| **Neuromuscular blocking agents** | | | |
| Suxamethonium | Severe liver disease<br>Anticholinesterases | (M) Reduced serum cholinesterase levels leading to prolonged block | |
| | Procaine | (M) Competition for plasma cholinesterase leading to prolonged block | |
| Nondepolarising agents | Diuretics<br>Hypokalaemia | (S) Potentiation of neuromuscular block; danger of prolonged paralysis | |
| | *Antibiotics:*<br>Aminoglycosides<br>Polymixins<br>Tetracyclines<br>Lincomycin<br>Clindamycin | (?S) Depending on group, either or both pre- and postganglionic block and potentiation of nondepolarising muscle relaxants (prolonged block) | Rare muscle weakness caused by antibiotic alone |
| | Calcium antagonists | (S) Preganglionic block; possible potentiation of block | |

*[Continued over]*

**Table IV.** [continued]

| Drug | Secondary drug or clinical situation | Site/mechanism and potential result | Notes |
|---|---|---|---|
| **Analgesic drugs** | | | |
| a) *Opioids:* | | | |
| Morphine, etc. | Diazepam and other CNS depressants | (S) Additive effect | Titrate doses carefully |
| | Opioid antagonists and agonist-antagonists | (S) Competitive antagonism; precipitation of abstinence syndrome in addicts | |
| Pethidine (meperidine) | MAOIs (nonselective) | (?) Possibly due to increased serotonin level in brain (a certain critical level may have to be reached); severe, potentially fatal reaction in some patients | See text (section 6.1.1) |
| | Phenobarbital and other enzyme inducers | (M) Increased production of norpethidine; increased sedation, danger of seizures | |
| Alfentanil | Erythromycin | (M) Reduced clearance of alfentanil (prolongation of its effect) | |
| b) *Others:* | | | |
| NSAIDs | Surgery | (S) Inhibition of prostaglandins: (i) in platelets – risk of bleeding (ii) in kidney – risk of acute renal failure | |

*Abbreviations and symbols:* CNS = central nervous system; ICU = intensive care unit; IV = intravenous; MAOIs = monoamine oxidase inhibitors; NSAIDs = nonsteroidal anti-inflammatory drugs; (S) = at or near site of action; (M) = occurs via alteration of metabolism; (B) = binding.

The barbiturates produce depression of the heart, cardiovascular reflexes and respiration. They are administered directly into the bloodstream, so their effects will often be more marked than with inhalational agents, particularly if the intravenous injection is rapid or if the circulatory state is already precarious.

Thiopental should not be given extravenously, since it may cause local tissue necrosis. Also, should it be given intra-arterially, thrombosis of the artery with distal gangrene often occurs. This is less likely with weaker solutions (2.5%). If this occurs, immediate treatment in the form of vasodilatation and anticoagulation is necessary. Some tissue damage is almost inevitable after intra-arterial injection of thiopental.

#### Etomidate

Etomidate is chemically unrelated to other anaesthetic drugs. It is a mixture of optical isomers – interestingly of different potency, perhaps evidence for a stereospecific anaesthesia receptor, the hypnotic activity being principally due to the dextro isomer.[46] Although soluble in water, the preparation is unstable. The drug is, therefore, formulated with propylene glycol. This causes a significant incidence of pain on injection and postoperative venous sequelae. Following injection, etomidate is rapidly inactivated, being mainly hydrolysed by esterases in both the liver and plasma.[47] While an elimination half-life of 70 minutes has been reported,[47] much longer values of over 200 minutes have been noted in other studies following administration of almost similar doses.[36,48,49] 98% of the drug is excreted as metabolites and only 2% as the unchanged form in the urine.

Etomidate produces a rapid induction of anaesthesia, although this is somewhat marred by frequent involuntary muscle movements. However, smoothness may be improved by giving etomidate after an opioid, e.g. fentanyl, alfentanil or sufentanil. It has a high therapeutic ratio due to a relative lack of cardiovascular or respiratory depression[50,51] and, particularly when combined with fentanyl or alfentanil, is suitable for use in 'poor risk' patients, such as in those with cardiovascular or respiratory disease. Like thiopental, it also reduces intracranial pressure and is suitable for neurosurgical anaesthesia.

Etomidate, being rapidly metabolised, would be suitable for use as an infusion in continuous intravenous anaesthesia. However, it inhibits corticosteroid formation by the adrenal cortex.

In the past, when etomidate infusions were used for sedation in ICU patients, this suppression of the stress response led to increased mortality in these patients.[52] Thus, etomidate is no longer advocated for use in maintenance of anaesthesia.

Etomidate administration is not associated with significant histamine release. It is virtually devoid of hypersensitivity and other adverse reactions and is, overall, one of the safest induction agents.[53] Although the successful use of etomidate has been described in a patient with acute intermittent porphyria,[54] it should be regarded as a potential porphyrogenic agent on the basis of experimental studies in rats.[39] The average induction dose of 0.3 mg/kg in adults is increased in children and lower in the elderly.

#### Fentanyl, Alfentanil and Sufentanil

These short-acting opioids have been used to induce anaesthesia alone or as adjuncts to other drugs. They can be given before thiopental to provide analgesia in the balanced anaesthesia technique, and to reduce the induction dose. They also reduce the excitatory adverse effects of methohexital and etomidate. As a group, the short-acting opioids have a minimal depressant effect on the cardiovascular system and larger doses are given in anaesthesia for cardiac operations. However, they are not as reliable as thiopental in inducing loss of consciousness and are usually given with a benzodiazepine or a primary induction agent. Large doses cause rigidity of the chest wall, and difficulty in breathing and inflating the lungs. They invariably cause respiratory depression, so it is rational to administer a neuromuscular blocking drug and control the ventilation.

#### Remifentanil

Remifentanil is the newest of the short-acting opioids and is characterised by a rapid onset of effect and a very short duration of action (a few minutes only). Its elimination half-life is about 10 minutes due to its rapid metabolism by esterases in the plasma.

#### Propofol

Propofol, a substituted phenol, has a therapeutic index similar to that of thiopental, but is more rapidly metabolised. It is about twice as potent as thiopental (induction dose 1.5 to 2.5 mg/kg). The commercially available preparation is formulated in an emulsion containing 10% soy bean oil.[55]

Propofol is rapidly and extensively distributed, with a large apparent volume of distribution. It is predominantly metabolised in the liver and is excreted in the urine as the glucuronide and as conjugates of the corresponding quinal metabolite. Less than 0.3% is excreted as the unchanged drug. The terminal elimination half-life is relatively long (200 to 300 minutes), due probably to the slow return of drug from a poorly perfused deep compartment;[56] this may be even longer after continuous infusions.

Arterial hypotension occurs frequently and is due to a combination of peripheral vasodilatation and myocardial depression.[57] Respiratory depression with apnoea, and pain at the injection site are also common with propofol use, but are not a major problem. In general, the drug is well tolerated.

Relatively rapid and clear-headed recovery has made propofol the drug of choice for use by continuous infusions for maintenance of anaesthesia. The incidence of postoperative nausea and vomiting is low with its use. It is currently a popular drug for use in short stay surgery (for reviews, see Langley & Heel;[58] Various authors[59]).

#### Eltanolone

Eltanolone (pregnanolone) is a naturally occurring metabolite of progesterone. Like propofol, it is not soluble in water, but has been formulated as a stable oil-in-water emulsion in the same way as propofol. The dosage for induction of anaesthesia appears to be 0.8 to 1.0 mg/kg compared with 2.1 mg/kg for propofol.[60] Whereas there is a 20% incidence of pain on injection with propofol, pain on administration of eltanolone is rarely observed. However, excitation on induction of anaesthesia shown as twitching of extremities or slight hypertonus occur more frequently with eltanolone than with propofol.

The recovery from eltanolone anaesthesia is also slower than after propofol. Induction of anaesthesia is achieved in 1 to 2 minutes and the duration of action in healthy individuals after a 0.6 mg/kg dose is between 6 and 13 minutes.[38] The terminal half-life is between 72 and 212 minutes, and there is rapid total body clearance. Some reduction in arterial pressure occurs if the drug is administered rapidly or if a higher dose is used.

#### Ketamine

Ketamine is a cyclohexylamine derivative with actions that are different from those of other general anaesthetic agents, tranquillisers or droperidol.[29] Its produces depression of the neocortex and thalamus, but may also stimulate parts of the limbic system. This produces a state of dissociative anaesthesia. Ketamine administration is associated with profound analgesia, but the patient's eyes may remain open during anaesthesia with it. In addition, some degree of nystagmus, hypertonus of the skeletal musculature, and muscle movement are often present. Lacrimation and salivation also occur frequently.

Ketamine is highly lipid soluble (much more so than thiopental) and it crosses the blood-brain barrier and placenta rapidly. The drug undergoes *N*-demethylation, hydroxylation and glucuronidation to form water soluble metabolites. Although norketamine has been shown to have some anaesthetic potency in animals, little is known about the effects of metabolites of ketamine in humans.[34] Clearance of ketamine and biotransformation to its active *N*-dealkyl metabolite is inhibited by diazepam, resulting in prolongation of its half-life and increasing the duration of anaesthesia. Sedative effects of diazepam may also contribute to prolonged anaesthesia. Halothane also slows the redistribution (responsible for termination of its action) and hepatic metabolism of ketamine.

Since ketamine readily crosses the placenta, this may account for the CNS depression of the neonate after relatively large doses of the drug given to the mother. Also, there is little metabolism of ketamine in the neonate.[61]

Unlike other anaesthetic agents, ketamine has a cardiovascular stimulating effect (tables II and III), although it acts as a myocardial depressant in isolated heart preparations *in vitro*. In humans, there is often an increase in heart rate, cardiac output and arterial pressure when ketamine is administered. This is due to a central effect and the release of noradrenaline (norepinephrine). This cardiovascular stimulation has popularised the use of ketamine in patients with compromised cardiovascular function. Ketamine relaxes bronchial smooth muscle, probably due to a sympathetic stimulating effect. The cerebral blood flow and intracranial pressure are increased by the drug.

Ketamine is absorbed rapidly following intramuscular injection, and has a bioavailability of 86 to 99%.[34] It is, therefore, unique in being able to produce anaesthesia within 5 to 7 minutes when given by the intramuscular route. The dose must, however, be about 5 times the usual intravenous dose (about 10 mg/kg compared with 2 mg/kg intravenously). The high intramuscular dose is required to produce anaesthesia within a reasonable period of time with a duration of about 20 minutes. Although the bioavailability of ketamine after intramuscular administration is high, peak concentrations similar to those after intravenous administration are attained only with larger doses.[62]

Recovery from ketamine is often complicated by delirium or excitement, which can be minimised by intravenous diazepam shortly before the conclusion of anaesthesia. Alternatively, a benzodiazepine, given preoperatively, will reduce the incidence of such sequelae.[63] More troublesome are perceptual disturbances during recovery. Patients may have hallucinations and dreams, which may be pleasant or unpleasant, sometimes terrifying. These, however, appear much less often in children and in elderly patients. Reflex activities, including maintenance of a good airway, are generally only slightly depressed by ketamine in comparison with other general anaesthetic drugs, but this cannot be relied on, and both airway obstruction and aspiration of vomit can occur.

The adverse effects of ketamine are too marked for it to be used widely in routine anaesthesia, but it is valuable in certain limited fields. It is very useful for surgical procedures requiring multiple frequent anaesthetics, such as dressing of burns, especially in children. It would also appear to be very suitable for mass numbers of casualties, and it is a good choice in some procedures such as cardiac catheterisation, where it is an advantage for the patient to breathe air. Ketamine has been used in obstetric practice, but the uncertainty of the competence of the laryngeal reflex is a danger in this context. It may, however, be a first-line agent for patients with asthma.

Ketamine infusions have been investigated, but while they are very effective when given with neuromuscular blocking drugs, the possibility of hepatotoxicity with large doses of ketamine must be considered.[64]

#### Benzodiazepines

Benzodiazepines act at specific receptors that are linked to the γ-aminobutyric acid (GABA) receptor and chloride channels. The duration of action of all benzodiazepines as tranquillisers, hypnotics, antiepileptics or for induction of anaesthesia depends on their pharmaceutical preparation and on their pharmacokinetics.

With the exception of midazolam, the benzodiazepines are not water soluble, and special preparations are required for injection. In the case of diazepam, these include solubilising agents such as propylene glycol, a 'micelles' preparation, and an emulsion preparation with soy bean oil ('Diazemuls'). The water solubility of midazolam is pH dependent; an imidazole ring is open at the pH of the pharmaceutical preparation (<4), resulting in water solubility, and closed at the pH of plasma so as to enhance lipid solubility.

The effects of benzodiazepines vary from anxiolysis with smaller doses to sedative, antiepileptic, amnesic and hypnotic effects as the dose is increased. On injection, anaesthesia induction is slow and may take 30 to 60 seconds or longer. There is wide variation in the response of patients: a dose of diazepam ranging from 0.2 to 2.0 mg/kg was required in one study;[65] an average dose might be 0.5 mg/kg. Midazolam is about 1.5 to 2 times more potent than diazepam, an induction dose of 0.3 mg/kg midazolam being adequate for most patients. Elderly patients are more sensitive and require a lower dose; however, plasma concentrations of midazolam after a given dose are similar in the young and the elderly.[66–68] The effect may also last longer in the elderly due to reduced clearance and an increased elimination half-life.[69] Clinically, benzodiazepines are rarely used as sole agents for induction of anaesthesia, but are often used in combination with other drugs like opioids and the more traditional intravenous anaesthetics.

The benzodiazepines have a marked amnesic effect, which to some extent compensates for the unreliability of induction. This effect also greatly enhances the usefulness of intravenous benzodiazepines as part of a sedative-hypnotic technique for uncomfortable procedures such as cardioversion, endoscopy or dental treatment. In these cases, the patient does not lose consciousness, but will be largely amnesic for events occurring 20 minutes or longer after injection. Airway protective reflexes are relatively intact, but this cannot be relied on, especially if other drugs have been given, and so verbal contact with the patient should not be lost. The initial midazolam dose in this application should not exceed 0.2 mg/kg, and smaller doses are preferable. Recovery after the use of benzodiazepines is also slow and with diazepam, dizziness may persist for up to 24 hours, although patients may be essentially normal 3 hours after moderate doses of midazolam.

The pharmacokinetic properties of the benzodiazepines have been well studied and have important implications for their use in clinical practice (see reviews by Nilsson;[70] Davis & Cook;[33] Ghoneim & Korttila;[71] and Mandelli et al.[72]). Midazolam is cleared relatively rapidly from plasma, with a half-life of 1.5 to 5 hours, whereas that of diazepam ranges from 20 to 70 hours,[70] and can be up to 90 hours in the elderly.[73] The duration of action of diazepam is further increased in the elderly because its major metabolite, nordazepam, accumulates in the plasma after repeated doses (due to its long half-life of 51 to 120 hours), and can reach concentrations up to 2 to 3 times those of the parent drug.[74] In contrast, the major metabolite of midazolam, hydroxymidazolam, although active, has a shorter half-life than the parent drug and does not prolong its activity.

There is a consistent rise in the plasma concentration of diazepam (but not midazolam) 6 to 8 hours after administration, and this is accompanied by the subjective recurrence of drowsiness.[75] The mechanism of this second peak effect is not clear. It may be a result of enterohepatic recirculation of diazepam. The clearance of diazepam may be delayed in hepatic disease, while, contrary to expectation, that of midazolam seems to be unaffected.[76] Neither drug is significantly affected by renal disease.[77] Placental transfer of diazepam occurs and the fetal to maternal concentration ratio has been reported as 1.3 to 1.[78] This may suggest the possibility of accumulation in the fetus, particularly with administration of larger doses. Elimination of diazepam is slower in premature neonates and mature neonates at term than in older infants, children and adults, and the nature of the diazepam metabolites formed varies according to age.

Several other benzodiazepines have been administered intravenously, including lorazepam and flunitrazepam,[79,80] but have no real advantage over midazolam or the newer preparations of diazepam.

#### *2.1.3 Antagonists to Benzodiazepines*

Although physostigmine and aminophylline have been used clinically on occasion in the past as benzodiazepine antagonists, neither is a specific antagonist of their central nervous system (CNS) actions. However, *flumazenil*, a specific benzodiazepine receptor antagonist,[81] reverses the CNS effects of benzodiazepines without producing agonistic effects, although these have been reported in experimental settings to a small extent. After intravenous administration, flumazenil has a rapid onset of effect.

Its elimination half-life (about 1 hour) is shorter than that of commonly used benzodiazepines.

Flumazenil is used clinically to treat benzodiazepine overdose and in anaesthesia to enhance recovery from benzodiazepines. It is recommended that small incremental doses of 0.1 to 0.2mg are used. A total dose of 1 to 2mg flumazenil is usually enough to counteract the effects of diazepam or midazolam.[70] Its administration may need to be repeated if very large doses of benzodiazepines are being countered.[82] Additional doses should be given with care in patients with circulatory impairment.

## 2.2 Skeletal Muscle Relaxants and their Antagonists

### *2.2.1 Neuromuscular Blocking Agents*

#### Mechanism/Site of Action

Muscle relaxation or paralysis results from an interruption in the pathways for nervous impulses between the nervous system and the muscle (fig. 1). Muscle relaxants in use in anaesthetic practice act at the neuromuscular junction, mainly postjunctionally at the acetylcholine receptor, which is an ion channel in the postjunctional membrane. Most drugs may also exert a variable degree of prejunctional effect. The channel opens when both the receptor sites on the α-subunits of the membrane-spanning protein are occupied simultaneously by an agonist, usually acetylcholine (fig. 2).

Classically, the neuromuscular blocking drugs are described as belonging to 1 of 2 groups, nondepolarising (competitive blocking) or depolarising (table V). Nondepolarising drugs, e.g. tubocurarine, occupy one or both of the receptor sites and thus prevent depolarisation by denying acetylcholine access to the receptors. These drugs can be antagonised by anticholinesterase agents such as neostigmine, which prevent breakdown of acetylcholine so that more of it is present to compete with the relaxant drug.

Among the depolarising drugs, suxamethonium (succinylcholine) is the only one currently used. It acts by causing a prolonged depolarisation of the muscle end-plate, making it unresponsive to acetylcholine. Such a block is not antagonised by neostigmine (except in the circumstances of a 'dual' block, where the type of myoneural block changes to a competitive type). Anticholinesterase drugs, in fact, prolong a suxamethonium block. For a more extensive review of the clinical types and pharmacology of neuromuscular blockade and factors that may alter neuromuscular function or responses to muscle relaxant drugs, see Bowman.[83]

#### Pharmacokinetic Characteristics

All neuromuscular blocking agents have 1 or 2 quaternary ammonium groups (except gallamine which has 3) and are ionised and positively charged irrespective of the pH and, thus, are poorly lipid soluble. Because of this they do not readily cross the blood-brain barrier, cell membranes or placenta. The pharmacokinetics

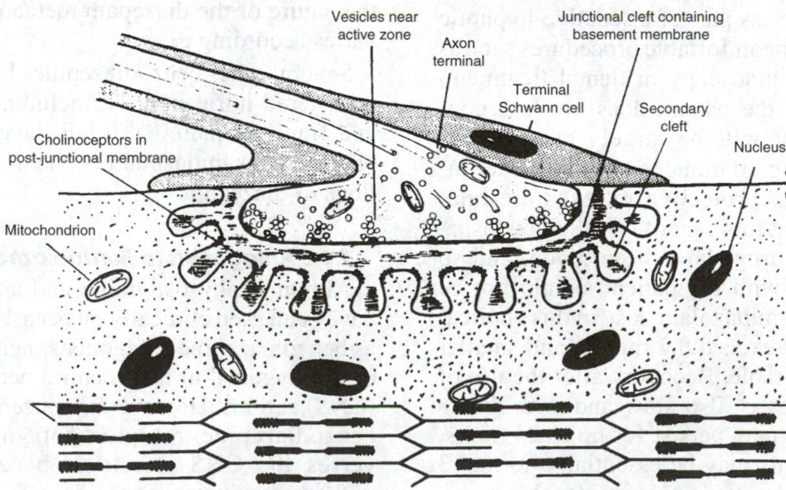


**Fig. 1.** Schematic representation of the neuromuscular junction. The actual receptors are located on the shoulders of the clefts (reproduced with permission from Bowman[83]).

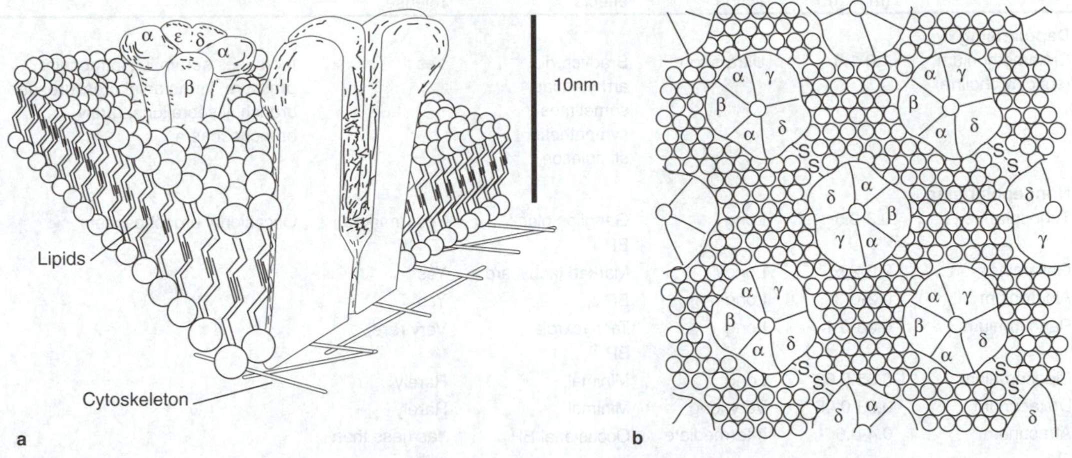


**Fig. 2.** Structure of the receptor showing the individual subunits and the ion channel (reproduced with permission from Bowman[83]).

of relaxants are described by 2- or 3-compartment models. The volume of distribution of these drugs is relatively small due to their poor lipid solubility.

Changes in cardiac output and muscle blood flow affect the time to onset of block due to the effect on the rate of delivery of the relaxants to their sites of action. Neuromuscular blockade with nondepolarising agents wears off because of biotransformation and/or excretion. Only when the inactive sites of uptake have been saturated (e.g. after an excessive single dose or repeated fractional doses) will elimination processes become the rate-determining factors for clearance of the drug and termination of the neuromuscular block.[84] This has important implications when repeated doses of these agents are used in patients with poor renal or hepatic function when accumulation may occur.

Neuromuscular block with suxamethonium is terminated by rediffusion into plasma, where the drug is relatively rapidly hydrolysed by plasma cholinesterase. The main pharmacokinetic variables of the individual agents are summarised in table VI.[85,86]

#### Tolerability

As with intravenous anaesthetics (see section 2.1.2), hypersensitivity reactions to neuromuscular blocking agents are being increasingly reported; these reactions may be due to direct pharmacological effects causing histamine release (which are minimal in the case of vecuronium), or immune-mediated type I anaphylactic reactions.[88-90] Suxamethonium has been implicated most frequently in adverse reactions to muscle relaxants.[91] Other important reactions are summarised in table V. A variety of drugs may modify, usually enhance, the neuromuscular blocking effects of the muscle relaxants (see section 6.3).

#### Clinical Application

Neuromuscular blocking drugs are used mainly as part of balanced anaesthesia to produce profound muscular paralysis and facilitate surgical procedures. Their use to block the reflex arc at the neuromuscular level will mean that less general anaesthesia is required, although ventilation of the lungs and endotracheal intubation will be necessary. The depolarising drug, suxamethonium, is used to provide rapid paralysis of short duration for intubation of the trachea, or for electroconvulsive therapy. Although suxamethonium can be given intermittently or by infusion for longer procedures, it is usual to employ nondepolarising relaxants when prolonged neuromuscular blockade is required. Neuromuscular blockers are also used, although less frequently now, in ICUs to facilitate controlled ventilation when oxygenation is difficult to maintain otherwise, or in rare patients with tetanus. Their principal clinical pharmacological properties are summarised in table V.

Tubocurarine, gallamine, and alcuronium are not commonly used in clinical practice nowa-

**Table V.** Principal clinical pharmacological properties of neuromuscular blocking agents

| Agent | Dose (mg/kg)[a] | Duration of action | Cardiovascular effects | Histamine release | Other effects[b] |
|---|---|---|---|---|---|
| **Depolarising** | | | | | |
| Suxamethonium (succinylcholine) | 1.0-1.5 | Ultra-short | Bradycardia, arrhythmias, sometimes sympathetic stimulation | Yes | Increases serum $K^+$, intraocular pressure, intracranial pressure, and bronchial secretions; rarely bronchospasm |
| **Nondepolarising** | | | | | |
| Tubocurarine | 0.3-0.5 | Long | Ganglion block BP ↓ | Yes (marked) | Occasional bronchospasm |
| Gallamine | 2.0-2.5 | Long | Marked tachycardia | Yes | |
| Alcuronium | 0.2-0.3 | Long | BP ↓ | Yes | |
| Pancuronium | 0.08-0.1 | Long | Tachycardia BP ↑ | Very rare | |
| Pipecuronium | 0.05-0.08 | Long | Minimal | Rarely | |
| Doxacurium | 0.03-0.06 | Very long | Minimal | Rarely | |
| Atracurium | 0.4-0.6 | Intermediate | Occasional BP ↓ | Yes (less than with tubocurarine) | |
| Cisatracurium | 0.1-0.15 | Intermediate | Minimal | | |
| Vecuronium | 0.08-0.1 | Intermediate | Minimal | Rarely | |
| Rocuronium | 0.5-0.6 | Intermediate | Slight tachycardia | Minimal | |
| Mivacurium | 0.15-0.2 | Short | Slight BP ↓ | Yes | |
| ORG 9487 | 1.0-1.5 | Short | ?Slight tachycardia | Not known (likely to be minimal) | |

a Dosage should be reduced when using potent volatile anaesthetics.

b See also table IV.

*Abbreviations and symbols:* BP = blood pressure; ↑ = increased; ↓ = decreased; ultra-short duration = <10 min; short duration = about 20 min; intermediate duration = about 30 min; long duration = about 60 min; very long duration = 1-2 hours.

days, but are included in this discussion for the sake of completeness.

### Tubocurarine

Tubocurarine, introduced in 1942, is the active principle of 'tube' curare, while toxiferine is isolated from 'calabash' or 'gourd' curare. Following an intravenous dose of 0.3 to 0.6 mg/kg, tubocurarine provides good relaxation for 40 to 60 minutes, although complete spontaneous recovery takes much longer. It causes a reduction in blood pressure, mainly due to histamine release and ganglion blockade.

Tubocurarine is eliminated mostly unchanged in the bile and urine. In patients with impaired renal function, the duration of neuromuscular blockade is only modestly increased after standard doses of tubocurarine, but can be markedly prolonged after large or repeated doses when the decreased rate of clearance becomes important. Dosages should be reduced in anephric patients.[92] A newly transplanted kidney can eliminate tubocurarine effectively, but the rate of excretion is slow, although this can be augmented by furosemide (frusemide).[93,94]

Although it does cross the placenta in small amounts, tubocurarine can be used in obstetric practice. The clinical dose is 0.4 to 0.5 mg/kg (1 × $ED_{95}$, i.e. dose effective in 95% of patients). Neonates are more sensitive than children and adults to tubocurarine (see further section 3.1). A dose of 0.25 mg/kg can be used in neonates at birth, increasing to 0.5 mg/kg at age 28 days, with reduction of dosage in the event of prematurity, acidosis or hypothermia.[95]

### Gallamine

Gallamine, a synthetic drug, has the advantage of a shorter duration of action than tubocurarine, but because of vagolytic properties it causes tachycardia. It is almost entirely excreted unchanged by the kidney. There is, therefore, a significant prolongation of blockade following its use in patients with renal failure. The elimination half-life is increased markedly in such patients and gallamine is therefore contraindicated in renal disease of any severity.

### Alcuronium

Alcuronium (diallylnortoxiferine) was initially claimed to have a shorter duration of action than tubocurarine, to be more readily reversed by neostigmine, and to cause a smaller reduction in blood pressure. However, more extensive use has shown that any differences between alcuronium and tubocurarine are very small.

### Pancuronium

Pancuronium[96] is an aminosteroid (free from hormonal activity) muscle relaxant that has no significant histamine-liberating properties.[97] Its duration of action is similar to that of tubocurarine, although its onset is slightly more rapid when used in a dose of 0.08 to 0.1 mg/kg (1.2 to 1.7 × $ED_{95}$). Unlike tubocurarine, its use is not associated with a decrease in arterial pressure. In fact, it usually causes a slight increase, due to sympathetic stimulation. This is an advantage in many situations, such as in cardiac surgery or in patients who are in shock or hypovolaemic. However, it consistently causes some tachycardia due to a vagolytic effect.

As with tubocurarine, pancuronium is mainly eliminated via the kidneys and to a smaller extent via the liver (10%). It is metabolised in the liver and its 3-hydroxy metabolite possesses some muscle relaxant activity. Prolongation of pancuronium blockade and delayed elimination has been reported in patients with renal failure following usual dosages.[98,99] Patients with liver disease require a high initial dose for adequate muscle relaxation due to an increased volume of distribution (due to their tendency to retain large amounts of water), but repeated doses should be smaller because of delayed elimination and the risk of prolongation of pancuronium blockade.[100]

Pancuronium does not appear to cross the placenta in appreciable amounts.[101,102] Prolonged corticosteroid therapy and therapy with antiepileptic drugs may cause resistance to its action.[103,104]

**Table VI.** Pharmacokinetic parameters of some neuromuscular blocking agents (after Booij;[86] Cook et al.[87])

| Drug | $Vd_{ss}$ (L) [per 70kg] | CL (L/h) | $t_{1/2}$ (min) |
|---|---|---|---|
| **Long-acting drugs** | | | |
| Alcuronium | 24.5 | 5.6 | 143 |
| Doxacurium | 15.4 | 11.6 | 99 |
| Gallamine | 14.0 | 5.0 | 134 |
| Pancuronium | 18.2 | 7.6 | 132 |
| Pipecuronium | 21.7 | 9.7 | 137 |
| Tubocurarine | 17.5 | 10.1 | 84 |
| **Intermediate-acting drugs** | | | |
| Atracurium | 14.7 | 27.7 | 21 |
| Rocuronium | 14.7 | 15.5 | 97 |
| Vecuronium | 18.9 | 21.8 | 71 |
| **Short-acting drugs** | | | |
| Mivacurium | 7.7 | 294 | 18[a] |
| Suxamethonium (succinylcholine) | | | 6 |

a The elimination half-lives of the *cis-trans* and *trans-trans* isomers (94% of the injected drug) are 2 to 3 minutes.

*Abbreviations:* CL = clearance; $t_{1/2}$ = elimination half-life; $Vd_{ss}$ = steady-state volume of distribution.

### Doxacurium

Doxacurium[105] is a benzylisoquinolinium compound from the same series as atracurium and mivacurium. It is the most potent nondepolarising neuromuscular blocking agent currently available, with an $ED_{95}$ of approximately 30 µg/kg. Doxacurium has a very slow onset and a long and variable duration of action. The onset of action of a dose of 30 to 60 µg/kg (1 to 2 × $ED_{95}$) may vary from 4 to 10 minutes, with a duration of clinical relaxation of over 2 hours.[106,107] The duration of clinical relaxation is longer in elderly patients. Antagonism of its neuromuscular block is also slow.

Doxacurium is mainly eliminated via the kidneys and the duration of action is, therefore, prolonged in patients with renal disease. This is associated with a significant reduction in clearance and an increase in the elimination half-life.[108]

The major advantage of doxacurium is its lack of cardiovascular effects. This has been observed with dosages of up to 80 µg/kg.[109,110] These advantages have been confirmed in more recent studies.[111]

### Pipecuronium

Pipecuronium is a bisquaternary steroid like pancuronium, but slightly more potent. It resembles pancuronium in many of its neuromuscular blocking effects, but lacks its sympathetic stimulating and vagolytic effects.[112] Pipecuronium has a long duration of action and some variability in response. Elimination occurs mainly via the kidneys, although an additional nonrenal pathway may also exist.[113] The onset of action after a dose of about 50 µg/kg is 4 to 5 minutes, making it a relatively slow-acting drug; the duration of action is similar to that of pancuronium. Adequate antagonism of block is attained provided that sufficient spontaneous recovery has taken place. The elimination half-life and clearance of this drug are similar to those of doxacurium (table VI).

Both pipecuronium and doxacurium have few advantages in terms of neuromuscular blocking effects. Their use may, however, be advantageous in patients undergoing cardiac surgery or surgery of long duration, particularly in the presence of cardiovascular problems.

#### Vecuronium

Vecuronium is a monoquaternary analogue of pancuronium. It is consequently more lipophilic and has a more rapid onset of action, although like atracurium, this is still slower than for suxamethonium. Vecuronium is virtually devoid of cardiovascular effects and histamine release is minimal. Elimination, which is mainly in the bile and to a smaller extent via the kidneys, is much more rapid than with pancuronium. The duration of clinical neuromuscular blockade is thus short, about 20 to 40 minutes. This is similar to that of atracurium at equipotent doses, even though the terminal elimination half-life of vecuronium is much longer. Vecuronium is, thus, a suitable drug for use in short surgical procedures. Its duration of action is increased in severe hepatic disease, but not in renal disease unless large doses are used.

#### Atracurium

Atracurium is a unique drug in that its molecule was designed specifically to have the property of spontaneous degradation. It is broken down by 2 purely chemical mechanisms, the Hofmann elimination pathway (a nonenzymatic base-catalysed reaction) and ester hydrolysis, although some organ uptake has also been demonstrated. The molecule is relatively stable as formulated at a pH of 3.5, but at body temperature and pH it is rapidly degraded.[114] Its action is predictable, with an elimination half-life of 21 minutes. Thus, it is suitable for short surgical procedures. Like vecuronium, but unlike other nondepolarising relaxants, when repeated doses are given to prolong its action, no sign of accumulation is seen, perhaps due to a short elimination half-life and the unique mode of metabolism, which is not dependent on organ function. It may, thus, be administered by repeated bolus doses or by continuous infusion[115] without recovery from the final dose being any longer than from a single dose.

Cardiovascular effects with atracurium are minimal, but it can on occasions cause histamine release. As its breakdown is independent of renal or hepatic mechanisms, the drug can be given without dosage adjustment in patients with renal or hepatic insufficiency.

#### Rocuronium

Rocuronium, a newer compound in the aminosteroid series of muscle relaxants, is structurally related to vecuronium. Its main features are its low potency, and its rapid onset of effect.[116] The onset of action of rocuronium is at least twice as rapid as that of vecuronium, but with a duration of muscle relaxation that is similar to that of atracurium and vecuronium. The rapid onset of effect is mainly responsible for the provision of better intubating conditions at an earlier time with this drug than with any other currently available nondepolarising relaxant.[117] The dose commonly used clinically is 0.6 mg/kg. This provides a clinical duration of approximately 30 minutes, with total spontaneous recovery in about 1 hour. Little accumulation has been reported. The lack of significant cardiovascular effects with rocuronium is not as marked as with vecuronium, and usual clinical doses may produce a 10 to 15% increase in heart rate.[118] Higher doses (unlikely in clinical practice) are likely to produce a significant increase in heart rate. As with other aminosteroids, rocuronium does not liberate histamine, even in doses of up to 1.2 mg/kg.[119] The reversibility of rocuronium is easy, provided that some spontaneous recovery has taken place.

Like all aminosteroids, elimination of rocuronium from the body is principally via hepatic metabolism. Although initial studies in cats suggested that renal elimination of the drug was unimportant, studies in humans suggest that approximately one-third of a rocuronium dose may be eliminated via the kidney.[120,121] Patients with renal failure tend to show greater interindividual variability in response to the effects of rocuronium, along with a decreased rate of clearance.[122] The duration of action is prolonged in patients with liver disease and in the elderly, mainly due to a decrease in clearance of the drug.[82,123]

Unlike vecuronium, rocuronium is stable in solution and, so far, metabolites have not been detected in plasma. The drug appears to be promising as a relaxant for rapid sequence intubation in situations where the use of suxamethonium may be contraindicated.[124]

#### Cisatracurium

Cisatracurium is an isomer of atracurium that has been isolated and evaluated as a muscle relaxant in itself. It is about 4 times more potent than atracurium ($ED_{95}$ 0.05 mg/kg) and a common clinical dose is 0.1 mg/kg.[125] The onset of action is slightly slower than with atracurium and the duration of effect is slightly longer. In general, however, cisatracurium resembles atracurium. Like atracurium, the main mechanism of elimination of cisatracurium is via the Hofmann pathway.

The main advantage of cisatracurium is lack of significant histamine liberation compared with atracurium.[125] Because of the similar unique mode of breakdown, the pharmacokinetics of cisatracurium are not significantly different from those of atracurium, with an elimination half-life of just over 20 minutes.[126]

#### Mivacurium

Mivacurium is a bisquaternary benzylisoquinolinium compound, structurally similar to atracurium. Unlike other nondepolarising relaxants, mivacurium is hydrolysed by plasma cholinesterase at a slightly lower rate than suxamethonium. However, the effects of the drug can also be antagonised by the administration of anticholinesterase drugs.[127,128]

The main feature of mivacurium is its relatively short duration of action compared with other nondepolarising relaxants. Following a dose of 0.15 to 0.2 mg/kg, the maximum block occurs within 2 to 3 minutes, with a clinical duration of approximately 15 minutes and total spontaneous recovery time of 25 to 30 minutes. The brevity of action, however, does not approach that of suxamethonium. Since mivacurium is relatively slow-acting, like vecuronium and atracurium, the time to attain good intubating conditions with mivacurium is similar to that with the latter two drugs.

Because mivacurium is metabolised by plasma cholinesterase and is short acting, it has been found that antagonism of residual block does not achieve much saving in time compared with spontaneous recovery.[127,129] It is more convenient to administer mivacurium by continuous infusion, the dose requirement being 5 to 6 μg/kg/min.

One of the disadvantages of administering mivacurium is its potential for histamine liberation. Because of this, the drug needs to be administered slowly and perhaps in doses of 0.2 mg/kg or less. Rapidly administered doses of 0.2 mg/kg may lead to a significant decrease in arterial pressure, mainly due to histamine liberation.[130]

The pharmacokinetics of mivacurium are complicated by the fact that the drug is a mixture of 3 isomers. Two of these, the *cis-trans* and the *trans-trans* isomers have elimination half-lives of approximately 2 minutes, while the *cis-cis* isomer has an elimination half-life of about 1 hour. The *cis-cis* isomer, however, contributes to only about 6% of the activity of mivacurium. The clearance of the *cis-trans* and *trans-trans* isomers is very high compared with the *cis-cis* isomer. Since the drug is metabolised by plasma cholinesterase, there are several case reports of prolonged duration of action in patients with abnormal plasma cholinesterase enzymes. The effects of the drug are also prolonged in patients with hepatic and renal disease, although the extent of prolongation is not the same as with other muscle relaxants.[131] Its effects are also prolonged in elderly patients, due to a reduced plasma cholinesterase activity in this age group.[132] For reviews, see Mirakhur[106] and Frampton & McTavish.[133]

#### ORG 9487

ORG 9487 is a new aminosteroid compound in the same series as vecuronium and rocuronium. It is undergoing evaluation as a possible replacement for suxamethonium. Preliminary studies with ORG 9487 have shown that a dose of 1.5 mg/kg produces complete block in about 1.5 minutes, with a clinical duration of 9 minutes and complete spontaneous recovery in about 25 minutes.[134] Intubating conditions with this agent are similar to those of suxamethonium within 1 minute and the neuromuscular effects of the drug can be antagonised within 2 minutes. Wider clinical experience with ORG 9487 is awaited, but it holds the prospect of being a nondepolarising relaxant with an onset and duration of action similar to that of suxamethonium.

#### Suxamethonium

Suxamethonium (succinylcholine) is the most commonly used depolarising relaxant, producing paralysis lasting 8 to 10 minutes after a dose of 1 to 1.5 mg/kg. As well as acting at the neuromuscular junction, it also has significant cardiovascular effects. Suxamethonium can exert a parasympathomimetic effect, producing slowing of the heart rate, which is particularly seen with a second dose and is commonly seen in children; this is abolished by anticholinergic drugs. It may also increase the heart rate by producing an increase in circulating catecholamines.

Suxamethonium is normally hydrolysed relatively rapidly by the enzyme plasma (pseudo) cholinesterase, and its action may be prolonged if the concentration of this enzyme is very low. This occasionally occurs in patients with malnutrition, uraemia or liver disease, after occupational exposure to anticholinesterase drugs such as the organophosphorus insecticides, procaine, or if the patient's cholinesterase is an abnormal genetic variant, which occurs as an hereditary condition (see further chapter 6; sect. 4.2.1).[135] In such cases, the dose of suxamethonium should be reduced by as much as a factor of 10 or more[136] or preferably avoided altogether.

On a mg per kg basis, less suxamethonium is required to obtain a desired degree of neuromuscular blockade as the age of the patient increases; infants require more than children or adults. This may be due to changes in the relative volumes of extracellular fluid in the different age groups (see also section 3.1; and chapter 3; sect. 2.3.1). Although plasma cholinesterase concentrations in the neonate are about one-half those in the older child, recovery rates are comparable in infants and older children. This suggests that redistribution of suxamethonium from the neuromuscular junction in a limited muscle mass into a large extracellular fluid volume compensates well for the low plasma cholinesterase concentrations.[137] Few data are available on the placental transfer of suxamethonium in humans, but a dose of 1 mg/kg during obstetric anaesthesia should not endanger the fetus, provided that repeated doses are not needed or atypical plasma cholinesterase is not encountered. This is, however, based on an experimental study only.[138]

When suxamethonium is administered to a patient, transient muscle contraction, seen as fasciculations, occurs before paralysis. Some patients have muscular aches postoperatively, which may be related to this phenomenon. It is thought to be due to direct damage to the muscle during the period of fasciculation and it can be reduced by pretreatment with small doses of nondepolarising drugs, which also minimise fasciculations.[139] An increase in serum potassium concentrations may occur when suxamethonium is given,[140] but this is only important in burned and traumatised patients, those with muscular disorders and in some with central nervous system lesions, where the rise in serum potassium can be quite large and lead to cardiac arrest.[141,142] Suxamethonium also leads to an increase in intraocular and intracranial pressures.

The incidence of anaphylactic reactions among the relaxants is highest with suxamethonium. Occasionally, jaw relaxation may appear inadequate with the use of suxamethonium due to the occurrence of masseter muscle spasm. Suxamethonium is also a known trigger of malignant hyperpyrexia, and a significant proportion of patients who have masseter spasm may prove to be susceptible to malignant hyperpyrexia (see also section 5.5).

Because of its rapid and short duration of action, suxamethonium is often used for short procedures such as intubation of the trachea, particularly during a rapid sequence induction. Intermittent doses or administration by continuous infusion have also been used for procedures of longer duration. In these situations, the block produced by suxamethonium may begin to change to a competitive type.

Due to its significant adverse effects and the availability of rapid-acting intermediate-duration agents, the use of suxamethonium has decreased markedly. However, it remains the only really rapid and short-acting relaxant.

### 2.2.2 Antagonists to Muscle Relaxants

#### Neostigmine

Neostigmine is the most commonly used antagonist of muscle relaxants. It acts predominantly through its anticholinesterase activity, although there is an element of direct stimulation of the postjunctional nicotinic receptors, as well as a prejunctional effect involving mobilisation and liberation of acetylcholine.[143] The elimination half-life of neostigmine in commonly used doses of 2.5 to 5mg is between 24 and 80 minutes, and is not dose-related. Neostigmine combines with both the anionic and the ester sites on acetylcholinesterase. If administered in the absence of a non-depolarising agent, muscle fibrillations and a depolarising block may develop. In clinical practice, the speed with which neostigmine antagonises neuromuscular block depends on the depth of the block when antagonism is attempted and on the muscle relaxant that has been used.

Neostigmine and all other anticholinesterase agents used to reverse neuromuscular block also exert muscarinic effects, which can be prevented by the use of anticholinergic agents, such as atropine or glycopyrronium bromide (glycopyrrolate).[144] The principal muscarinic adverse effects to be antagonised include bradycardia and occurrence of secretions. Neostigmine and glycopyrronium bromide form an ideal combination from the point of view of cardiovascular stability, although atropine has also been used. This is because the peak actions of neostigmine and glycopyrronium on one hand and those of atropine and edrophonium on the other hand occur at similar times, thus minimising fluctuations in the heart rate. Atropine is therefore a more logical choice for use with edrophonium.[145]

Neostigmine and the allied drug, pyridostigmine, are also used outside of anaesthesia, in the management of myasthenia gravis (see further chapter 29; sect. 8.2).

#### Pyridostigmine

Pyridostigmine is approximately one-fifth as potent as and is slower in onset than neostigmine.[146] The duration of action of pyridostigmine is slightly longer than that of neostigmine. This may make it a useful agent to reverse the neuromuscular block of long-acting agents such as tubocurarine and pancuronium and the new agents, doxacurium and pipecuronium. Its mode of action is similar to that of neostigmine.

Because of its slower onset of action and the more frequent use of intermediate-acting relaxants, pyridostigmine is not commonly used as a decurarising agent. However, it retains its place in the treatment of myasthenia gravis (see chapter 29; sect. 8.2). Its pharmacokinetics are similar to those of neostigmine when used in doses of 0.25 mg/kg.

#### Edrophonium

Edrophonium has been classically thought to be too short-acting for use as a decurarising agent. However, edrophonium can be useful as an antagonist to neuromuscular blocking agents provided that doses of 0.5 to 1.0 mg/kg are used and that the block is not too profound.[145,147,148] On average, edrophonium is 20 to 30 times less potent than neostigmine. The pharmacokinetics of edrophonium are not significantly different from those of neostigmine in doses that antagonise neuromuscular block effectively. The advantages of using edrophonium are its rapid onset of effect and occurrence of less severe muscarinic adverse effects. Edrophonium has, however, been found ineffective in antagonising deep blocks adequately.

Edrophonium may be more suitable for antagonism of neuromuscular block induced by intermediate and short-acting agents when the block is not very deep. It differs from neostigmine in producing much less suppression of acetylcholinesterase and plasma cholinesterase activities.[149,150] Neostigmine administration resulted in greater than 80% suppression of the activities of plasma cholinesterase and acetylcholinesterase at its peak effect, compared with <10 to 15% with edrophonium. This has led to the belief that edrophonium exerts its decurarising effects only partly by inhibiting cholinesterase and partly by a presynaptic action.

#### Physostigmine

Physostigmine was the first anticholinesterase agent isolated, but it has been found to be an unreliable antagonist of muscle relaxants.[151] Being a tertiary compound, it crosses the blood-brain barrier, and has been used to improve the level of consciousness, treat overdosage of atropine, and tachyarrhythmias occurring after tricyclic antidepressant drug overdose. It has also been claimed to be useful in arousing patients from drowsiness following tranquillisers and antihistamines, but not anaesthetic drugs.[152]

### 2.3 Drugs Used in Preoperative Preparation

Premedication was introduced in the 1860s to make the induction of anaesthesia easier by the methods then in use. With changing surgical and anaesthetic practice, premedication needs have changed. Fear of anaesthesia and surgery remain, and allaying anxiety is still a major aim. Traditionally, a combination of an opioid with an atropine-like drug was used, but currently benzodiazepines have largely replaced these. It should not be forgotten that the preoperative visit can be as effective an anxiolytic as pharmacological premedication.[153]

Vagal blockade using atropine or another anticholinergic drug was important when ether was the main anaesthetic agent, but use of these agents in adults has declined over the past 20 years, and they would now normally be given intravenously only where specifically indicated, usually to prevent bradyarrhythmias. In the UK, a recent survey found that anticholinergic premedication was used by only 36% of anaesthetists in adults and 56% in children.[154]

*Antacid therapy* may be indicated in patients at risk of aspiration of gastric contents – in particular, obstetric patients (see section 3.4), obese patients, and those with peptic ulcer or hiatus hernia. The most common treatment is with histamine $H_2$-receptor blocking drugs, such as ranitidine.

### 2.3.1 Drugs Used for Preoperative Sedation

#### Barbiturates

The barbiturates are now largely of historical interest. Rectal thiopental is still used in children, but preoperative hypoxaemia is a danger and premedicated patients require experienced supervision.[155]

#### Benzodiazepines

This group are by far the most popular of the sedative-hypnotic drugs used in premedication. They differ mainly in their pharmacokinetic characteristics. Pharmacodynamically, they are similar, acting at the GABA-benzodiazepine receptor, but there is great variation in the individual patient response. Adverse effects are few, although heavy sedation with benzodiazepines in elderly patients can contribute to hypoxaemia, e.g. during regional anaesthetic procedures.[156]

*Diazepam* is less used now because of its prolonged elimination and active metabolites. It is rapidly absorbed orally, and 10 to 20mg is the usual adult dose. Intravenously, the emulsion preparation ('Diazemuls') is preferred because of its low incidence of venous sequelae.

*Temazepam* is available as capsules and elixir, but not for parenteral administration. Absorption is rapid, its half-life is short (5.1 to 15.3 hours), and it has no active metabolites. This makes it particularly suitable for day surgery. Adult doses of 10 to 30mg are used, while for children, use of the elixir in a dose of 1 mg/kg gives effective anxiolysis.[157]

*Lorazepam* has a slower onset of action and longer duration (elimination half-life 14 hours) than temazepam. It is usually given on the preoperative night as well as before surgery. Lorazepam has a more pronounced amnesic effect than other benzodiazepines, and is favoured by some clinicians for particularly nervous individuals.

*Midazolam* is used as an oral premedicant in some countries, although its main use is by the intravenous route. A 10mg dose is equivalent to 20mg temazepam.

#### Opioid Drugs

Morphine and pethidine (meperidine), usually combined with atropine or scopolamine (hyoscine), were the mainstay of premedication for the first half of this century. Nowadays, opioids are still used in some circumstances, for example, as part of a combination regimen given before cardiac surgery, and they are still probably the most reliable premedicant for children.[158] Newer methods of administering opioids include oral transmucosal fentanyl citrate ('fentanyl lollipop'), which has been assessed for premedication in children and found to provide good sedation, although there can be a significant incidence of nausea or vomiting, and some respiratory depression.[159]

#### Other Sedative Drugs

Other drugs such as hydroxyzine and zopiclone have also been used. The phenothiazines have proved generally unsatisfactory; however, alimemazine (trimeprazine) in a dose of 3 to 4 mg/kg is fairly widely used in children, and normally gives good sedation and some antiemetic action, but occasional idiosyncratic reactions have occurred.[160,161]

### 2.3.2 Anticholinergic (Antiparasympathetic) Drugs

The use of these drugs in premedication is no longer routine, and they are only given if specifically needed. Indications for their use include premedication for ketamine administration.

*Atropine* blocks the action of acetylcholine at parasympathetic nerve endings. Its main effects are drying of secretions and tachycardia, and it is also a mild cerebral stimulant. The adult dose is 0.5 or 0.6mg for most purposes, such as treatment of bradycardia, but at least 2mg is required for nearly complete vagal blockade; a dose of 1 to 1.2mg is given when used with neostigmine or edrophonium (see section 2.2.2).

*Scopolamine (hyoscine)* differs from atropine chiefly in having a cerebral depressant effect, and it may cause confusion in elderly patients. It is more antiemetic than atropine and, unlike the latter, has little effect on the heart.

*Glycopyrronium bromide (glycopyrrolate),* a synthetic quaternary ammonium compound, is about twice as potent as atropine, and has the advantage of being active when given orally. When used with neostigmine, it is given in a dose of 10 μg/kg, i.e. 0.6mg in an adult. In this situation, it provides greater cardiovascular stability than atropine.[162]

### 2.3.3 Other Drugs Used in Premedication

$\alpha_2$-Adrenoceptor agonists such as *clonidine* have characteristics which are desirable in a premedicant: anxiolysis, analgesia and sedation.[163] They appear to reduce the incidence of hypertensive episodes during anaesthesia, such as the response to laryngoscopy and intubation.[164,165] However, it is recognised that this may be at the expense of an increased incidence of hypotension and bradycardia at other times perioperatively[166] and, thus, their routine use is inadvisable.

## 2.4 Local Anaesthetic Drugs

The major properties of the local anaesthetics are shown in table VII.

### *2.4.1 Mechanism/Site of Action*

Sensory information, including pain, travels to the brain along nerves, the action potential being propagated by a local flow of sodium ions into and potassium ions out of the axon. Local anaesthetic drugs can cause a localised and reversible block to conduction by interfering with the opening of the sodium channel.[169,170] It seems most likely that the drugs act at a site at the inner end of the sodium channel after diffusing inward through the plasma membrane.

### *2.4.2 Pharmacokinetic Characteristics*

When administered by infiltration, local anaesthetics do not depend on the circulation to carry them to their sites of action on the nerve membrane or in the neural fluids. Instead, penetration from their site of injection into the nerve is an important determinant of the characteristics of their action. However, uptake into the systemic circulation is the major factor both in terminating their action and in leading to toxic and other systemic effects.

#### Pharmacokinetics of Onset of Action

Chemically, local anaesthetics are classified as amides or esters. This is an important distinction, affecting several aspects of their behaviour, but most drugs now in use are amides. Local anaesthetics are weak bases, with pKa values between 7.8 (lidocaine) and 9.0 (procaine). The rate at which they diffuse to their site of action will depend on the non-ionised fraction, the lipid solubility of this fraction, and the unbound concentration.[171] The product of these factors has been described as the 'lipid diffusion index'.[172] This correlates well with the relative rates of onset of action of different local anaesthetic drugs. Since the solutions are usually acidic, and pKa high, alkalinisation should in theory speed onset, although, the available studies are inconsistent.

All nerve fibres are not equally sensitive to local anaesthetics. The approximate order of sensitivity is: sympathetic > pain/temperature > proprioception > coarse touch > motor. This may be due in part to the differing sizes of the fibres, the smaller fibres offering less of an obstacle to diffusion. One explanation[173] relates it to the length of nerve exposed to local anaesthetic without the protection of myelination.

The pharmacokinetics of spinal and epidural anaesthesia are complicated by the anatomy of this region,[174] with uptake into fat and blood vessels being a significant factor. Permeation into the dura is more dependent on molecular weight of the agent than other factors,[175] but the molecular weights of local anaesthetics range from only 220 to 288D, so in practice this has little influence.

#### Pharmacokinetics of Systemic Disposal

Local anaesthetic action is terminated by the decrease in concentration at the nerve as the drug both diffuses away and is taken up by the vasculature. Diffusion will be slower for the more potent drugs of the series, which are generally more lipid soluble and also more highly bound to tissues, which reduces the concentration gradient for unbound drug. Otherwise, the rate of uptake is related mainly to the vascularity of the site and the regional blood flow and, thus, any vascular effects of the local anaesthetic or adjuvant drug are important. Adrenaline (epinephrine) is frequently used to prolong the action of local anaesthetics by its vasoconstrictor action; however, it should not be used for anaesthetising any extremity as this could lead to ischaemia. Local anaesthetic drugs may themselves also be vasoactive – for example, the lower toxicity of ropivacaine compared with bupivacaine may be partly due to their respective vasoconstrictor and vasodilator actions.

Following most regional anaesthetic procedures, maximum arterial blood concentrations of local anaesthetics occur within about 10 to 25 minutes, as typified by epidural administration.[176] Thus, the most intensive surveillance of the patient should be during the first half hour after local anaesthetic injection.

The ester drugs are broken down in the blood by plasma (pseudo) cholinesterase and red cell esterases, as well as in the liver, and they have short half-lives ranging from 10 to 20 seconds for chloroprocaine to a few minutes for tetracaine (amethocaine). This contributes to safety after inadvertent overdose, although high plasma concentrations may saturate metabolising enzymes and prolong the half-lives.[177]

Amides depend principally on hepatic metabolism for their elimination, and have terminal half-lives of 1.5 to 3 hours. Their clearance may be reduced both by reduced hepatic blood flow and by inhibition of metabolising enzymes. Slower elimination is found in neonates, and in patients with hepatic cirrhosis and cardiovascu-

**Table VII.** Major clinical pharmacological properties of local anaesthetics (after Mather & Cousins;[418] Concepcion & Covino;[167] Akerman et al.[168])

| Agent | Lipid solubility | pKa | Plasma protein binding (%) | Equianaesthetic concentration (lidocaine = 1) | Onset of action | Duration (single dose) | Principal uses[a] | Primary site of metabolism |
|---|---|---|---|---|---|---|---|---|
| **Amide type** | | | | | | | | |
| Bupivacaine | High | 8.1 | 95 | 0.25 | Slow | Long | Infiltration, minor and major nerve blocks, epidural block, spinal block | Liver |
| Dibucaine (cinchocaine) | High | ? | ? | 0.25 | Rapid | Long | Spinal | Liver |
| Etidocaine | High | 7.7 | 94 | 0.5 | Rapid | Long | Infiltration, minor and major nerve blocks, epidural block, spinal block | Liver |
| Lidocaine (lignocaine) | Medium | 7.9 | 64 | 1 | Rapid | Medium | Infiltration, minor and major nerve blocks, epidural block, spinal block | Liver |
| Mepivacaine | Medium | 7.6 | 78 | 1 | Slower | Medium | Infiltration, minor and major nerve blocks, epidural block | Liver |
| Prilocaine | Medium | 7.9 | 55 | 1 | Slower | Medium | Infiltration, minor and major nerve blocks, epidural block; intravenous block | Liver |
| Ropivacaine | Moderate | 8.1 | 95 | 0.25 | Slow | Long | Infiltration, minor and major nerve blocks, epidural block; intravenous block | Liver |
| **Ester type** | | | | | | | | |
| Tetracaine (amethocaine) | High | 8.5 | ? | 0.25 | Slow | Long | Spinal, topical (use limited by high systemic toxicity) | Plasma |
| Cocaine | Medium | ? | ? | 1 | Slow | Medium | Topical (high systemic toxicity) | Liver |
| Procaine | Low | 8.9 | ? | 2 | Slow | Short | Infiltration, spinal (first-line drug in porphyria) | Plasma |

a Surgical indication for regional anaesthetic techniques:
*Infiltration anaesthesia:* (a) extravascular: superficial surgical procedures; (b) intravascular (tourniquet occluded limb): short surgical procedures of hand and foot.
*Peripheral nerve blockade:* (a) minor nerve blocks: hand or foot surgery; (b) major nerve blocks or plexus blocks: surgery of the upper or lower extremities.
*Epidural:* (a) thoracic: segmental anaesthesia involving middle and lower thoracic dermatomes, for upper abdominal surgery, and for postoperative analgesia following thoracic or upper abdominal procedures; (b) lumbar: lower abdominal surgery (alone or in combination with light general anaesthesia), surgery of the pelvis, perineum, lower extremities, and obstetric procedures, postoperative analgesia; (c) caudal: pelvic and perineal surgery and vaginal delivery.
*Spinal (subarachnoid):* as for lumbar epidural or caudal anaesthesia, but not commonly used for postoperative analgesia.

lar disease, but not in pregnancy, old age or renal disease.[171]

### *2.4.3 Tolerability*

Hypersensitivity reactions are rare, and account for only 1% of adverse reactions to local anaesthetics.[178] Allergic responses are much more common with ester than with amide type local anaesthetics, as the former, which are little used today, are hydrolysed by esterases to metabolites that are capable of acting as haptens. Allergy may also be caused by preservatives such as methylhydroxybenzoate.[179]

The most important risks associated with local anaesthetics are dose- or plasma concentration–related CNS and cardiovascular toxicity. Signs and symptoms of CNS toxicity include seizures, followed by coma and respiratory depression. Seizures are due to disinhibition of nervous conduction, probably by an action at the GABA receptor complex,[180] while depressant effects, which predominate at higher doses, are due to blockade of sodium channels. CNS toxicity is potentiated by hypoxia and hypercarbia, so acute management must minimise these.

Cardiovascular toxicity also involves sodium channel blockade, reducing contractility and interfering with conduction.[181] Bupivacaine differs from lidocaine in the sudden occurrence of dangerous ventricular arrhythmias, including fibrillation, at subconvulsant doses.

### *2.4.4 Properties of Individual Drugs*

#### Esters

Esters are little used in the UK, but *tetracaine (amethocaine)* is a standard drug for spinal anaesthesia in the US, and is most commonly used as a hyperbaric solution. It is metabolised slowly by plasma cholinesterase, which contributes to its relatively long duration of action of 2 to 3 hours (4 to 6 hours if given with adrenaline). It is rarely administered by other routes because of toxicity when used in higher doses.

#### Amides

Of the amides, *lidocaine* was the first to be introduced, and remains the most commonly used drug. Qualities include rapid onset, moderate toxicity and topical anaesthetic activity. Solutions of 0.5 to 2% are used for infiltration or nerve blocks, and 4 to 5% for topical application and for subarachnoid injection.

*Bupivacaine* has achieved popularity because of its potency, long duration of action and an ability to give a degree of differential block, sparing some motor function while blocking pain. A low fetal to maternal ratio of bupivacaine relative to lidocaine may contribute to safety[182] and together with the above features make it particularly suitable for epidural injection, either for surgery or for analgesia for labour. Solutions of 0.25 to 0.5% are used; stronger solutions are available, but have raised concerns about possible cardiotoxicity.[183,184]

*Ropivacaine*[168] is a newer amide local anaesthetic with cardiotoxicity intermediate between lidocaine and bupivacaine, but potency similar to bupivacaine. Lower toxicity is associated with the fact that it is a pure *S*-enantiomer, while bupivacaine is a mixture of 2 stereoisomers. There are no major differences between the pharmacokinetics of bupivacaine and ropivacaine.[167,185]

*Prilocaine* is the least toxic of the amide local anaesthetics. Its properties are generally similar to lidocaine, but as it causes less vasodilatation, its duration of effect is longer. Methaemoglobinaemia may occur after large doses (800mg in adults). Lower cardiotoxicity makes it a first-line drug for use with a tourniquet for intravenous local analgesia (Bier's block).

*'EMLA' cream* is an aqueous preparation containing prilocaine 25 mg/g with lidocaine 25 mg/g and is used for topical analgesia of intact skin.[186] The eutectic mixture of the two drugs in this form allows absorption through intact skin. The cream should be applied at least 60 to 90 minutes before skin anaesthesia is required. 'EMLA' has proved useful in preventing pain with venepuncture and cannulation, especially in children, and can also be used for minor dermatological surgery. It should not be used in infants under 6 months of age because of a small risk of methaemoglobinaemia.

A preparation of *tetracaine (amethocaine)* for topical application has recently become available.

## 2.5 Drugs Used to Control Cardiovascular Function in Anaesthesia

In anaesthetic practice, and in the ICU, it is frequently necessary to modify cardiovascular parameters such as blood pressure or cardiac output by pharmacological means.

The autonomic nervous system (sympathetic and parasympathetic) controls the automatic functions of the body, including the cardiovascular system. From controlling centres in the midbrain, autonomic fibres leave the central nervous system, and synapse once before reaching their ultimate destination. The parasympathetic outflow is in cranial nerves and sacral nerve roots; the sympathetic outflow is in the thoracolumbar region and synapses mainly in the ganglia of the sympathetic chain. The neurotransmitter in the intermediate synapses, at parasympathetic endings and at a few sympathetic endings is acetylcholine, while at most sympathetic endings it is noradrenaline (norepinephrine).

The important cardiovascular effect of the parasympathetic system is vagal activity on the heart, causing slowing that may be antagonised by atropine.

### 2.5.1 Sympathomimetic Agents

The sympathetic nervous system is the body's main mechanism for controlling cardiac output, blood pressure and distribution of blood flow. Drugs may act at adrenergic receptors in the sympathetic ganglia or at nerve endings. The adrenergic receptors may be subdivided into 6 or perhaps 8 subtypes ($\beta_1$, $\beta_2$, $\alpha_{1A}$, $\alpha_{1B}$, $\alpha_{2A}$, $\alpha_{2B}$) and dopamine into 2 subtypes ($D_1$ and $D_2$). Receptor activity of different adrenergic agonists is shown in table VIII.

#### Inotropic Drugs

The use of positive inotropic drugs in the intensive care setting is described in chapter 13 (section 3.1.3). Anaesthesia in the critically ill patient is a continuum with their ICU management and the same therapies may be used in the operating theatre. Dopamine, in a low dose of around 3 μg/kg/min may also be used for its renal protective effect during the stress of major surgery.

**Table VIII.** Receptor activity of different adrenoceptor agonists

| Agent | $\alpha_1$ | $\alpha_2$ | $\beta_1$ | $\beta_2$ | $D_1$ | $D_2$ |
|---|---|---|---|---|---|---|
| Phenylephrine | ++++ | ? | +/– | 0 | 0 | |
| Noradrenaline (norepinephrine) | ++++ | ++++ | +++ | 0 | 0 | |
| Adrenaline (epinephrine) | ++++ | +++ | ++++ | ++ | 0 | |
| Isoprenaline (isoproterenol) | 0 | 0 | ++++ | ++++ | 0 | |
| Dopamine | + to ++++ | ? | ++++ | ++ | ++++ | +++ |
| Dobutamine | 0 to + | ? | ++++ | ++ | 0 | |
| Dopexamine | 0 | 0 | + | ++++ | ++ | ++ |
| Ephedrine | ++ | ? | +++ | ++ | 0 | 0 |

*Abbreviations:* 0 = no activity; + to ++++ = minor to major activity.

### Vasopressor Agents

During epidural and spinal anaesthesia, it may be necessary to use a vasopressor in addition to fluid therapy to maintain blood pressure and cardiac output in the face of the vasodilatation caused by extensive sympathetic nerve blockade.

***Ephedrine:*** a mixed α- and β-adrenoceptor agonist, this drug is the most commonly used vasopressor in this situation, especially in obstetrics, mainly because it is believed to have little effect on uterine blood flow. Studies of the effect of ephedrine on human placental blood flow[187] have confirmed earlier animal work[188] showing that whereas a pure α-agonist (methoxamine) transiently reduces flow, ephedrine does not. However, in humans, the choice of vasopressor is relatively unimportant compared with the avoidance of hypotension.[187]

Either bolus doses of 3 to 10mg ephedrine, or an infusion of 1 to 2 mg/min[189] can be used, taking care to avoid hypertension.

### 2.5.2 Drugs Inducing Controlled Hypotension

Deliberate lowering of blood pressure is used as an aid to surgery, e.g. during middle ear surgery. The approach is multifactorial: sedation reduces afferent input to the vasomotor centre; deep anaesthesia does this as well and also causes reduced cardiac output and vasodilatation, but the principal mechanism employed is reduction of vascular tone. Sympathetic blockade has long been used: $\alpha_1$-adrenoceptor blockade by drugs such as phenoxybenzamine was an early method. β-Adrenoceptor blocking drugs are also often used as a part of the hypotensive technique, particularly to slow heart rate as well. These drugs are often given orally before operation.

***Labetalol:*** this drug has a combined α- and β-adrenoceptor blocking action and is useful in both hypotensive anaesthesia and management of hypertensive crises. Doses of 25mg intravenously can augment the hypotensive action of isoflurane. Sympathetic ganglion blockade using trimetaphan or pentolinium is less popular now.

***Nitroglycerin (glyceryl trinitrate) and sodium nitroprusside:*** these drugs both act directly on the smooth muscle of blood vessels via the second messenger pathway of nitric oxide (endothelium-derived relaxing factor, EDRF), and relax both resistance and capacitance vessels. Whereas sodium nitroprusside has a relatively balanced action on arteriolar and venous dilatation, nitroglycerin has a more marked action on the venous side of the circulation. The latter has been used to induce hypotension in anaesthesia[190] and in the ICU. Since its preferential action on preload leads to greater maintenance of diastolic pressure, nitroglycerin is probably preferable to sodium nitroprusside in patients with impaired coronary or cerebral perfusion. It produces a rapid and controllable effect, as it is metabolised rapidly, with a half-life of about 4 minutes.[191]

Sodium nitroprusside has an even more evanescent action, so that direct monitoring of arterial pressure is mandatory. It is given as an infusion, usually starting at 0.5 to 5 μg/kg/min, and the rate is titrated to effect. Metabolism to cyanide occurs in red blood cells and plasma, and cyanide is mostly further metabolised by rhodanase in the liver to thiocyanate. To avoid toxicity, which is manifest by tachyphylaxis, metabolic acidosis and reduced tissue oxygen extraction, a maximum dose of 1.5 mg/kg[192] or 10 μg/kg/min[193] should be observed. Sodium thiosulfate or hydroxocobalamin may be used in prophylaxis and treatment of cyanide toxicity.[194] Sodium nitroprusside is usually used against a background of a hypotensive anaesthetic technique, including drugs such as isoflurane or tubocurarine.

## 2.6 Antiemetic Drugs

Nausea and vomiting are a particular problem in two areas of medical practice: in the postoperative period, and in patients receiving chemotherapy or radiotherapy. The physiological background to emesis is complex.[195,196] Afferent impulses from a number of different regions are integrated in the brainstem, in what is conveniently referred to as the vomiting or emetic centre. This comprises areas such as the nucleus tractus solitarius and the parvicellular reticular formation. The main sources of emetic stimuli in postoperative nausea and vomiting are the gastrointestinal tract, with afferents in the vagus nerve, and the area postrema or chemoreceptor trigger zone. This is a small structure in the caudal part of the fourth ventricle, and lies outside the blood-brain barrier, so that it is ideally located to respond to circulating messenger molecules. The vestibular apparatus is the origin of input leading to motion sickness, and may contribute to postoperative emesis. Input from higher centres and psychological factors are also important.

A number of different receptor types are found in these areas – dopamine, opioid and serotonin (5-hydroxytryptamine, 5-HT) in the area postrema and enkephalin, histamine and muscarinic-cholinergic in the nucleus tractus solitarius.[196] This distribution should predict the drugs that will be effective in treating nausea and vomiting.[197,198] This remains a problem area, as controlled studies of many of the drugs described in this section have shown only small differences between active drug and placebo, while comparisons between active drugs often give contradictory results in different trials.[199,200]

### 2.6.1 Metoclopramide

Metoclopramide is a prokinetic drug which increases motility and hastens gastrointestinal emptying. It has a central and peripheral antidopaminergic action, and its most important adverse effects are related to this: dysphoria and agitation are not uncommon and extrapyramidal effects can also occur. It is widely used, but is of limited efficacy, although it does seem to be reasonably effective in treating opioid-induced nausea and vomiting.[201]

### 2.6.2 Phenothiazines

Phenothiazines have a number of actions, again including an antidopaminergic effect. *Prochlorperazine* and *perphenazine* are the most commonly used agents for postoperative nausea and vomiting, and have been studied widely. Their adverse effects include sedation and occasional extrapyramidal reactions.

### 2.6.3 Butyrophenones

*Droperidol* is the only butyrophenone used in anaesthesia. It is a moderately effective antiemetic, and is used in single doses ranging from 0.25 to 1.25mg. Some studies[202] have suggested that the lower dose is at least as effective as the higher. Adverse effects include sedation or prolongation of recovery from anaesthesia; dysphoria may also occur, with restlessness and apprehension, but extrapyramidal effects are rare. A slight α-adrenoceptor blocking effect may cause hypotension in some patients.

### 2.6.4 Anticholinergic Drugs

Anticholinergic drugs with antiemetic effects include both atropine and scopolamine (hyoscine). Atropine is not used specifically for this purpose, but its inclusion in an anaesthetic regimen lowers the incidence of postoperative emesis.

***Scopolamine*** is the antiemetic usually given as premedication (0.4mg). Its main adverse effects are drowsiness and dryness of the mouth, although confusion may also occur in the elderly. A transdermal scopolamine preparation is now available.[203] Absorption from the transdermal patch is slow, and steady-state plasma concentrations are not achieved until after 5 hours, so that the patch needs to be applied early. Studies have again shown only moderate efficacy in postoperative nausea and vomiting, but adverse effects are slight.

### 2.6.5 Antihistamines

Of these agents, only *cyclizine* is widely used. This drug acts on the muscarinic cholinergic receptors, and in a dose of 50mg is a reasonably effective antiemetic. Since its adverse effects are also slight, it is a drug of choice for postoperative nausea and vomiting.

### 2.6.6 Serotonin$_3$ (5-HT$_3$) Antagonists

Drugs of this group include ondansetron, granisetron and tropisetron.

*Ondansetron* has proved extremely effective in the management of vomiting associated with chemotherapy and radiotherapy.[204] 5-HT$_3$ receptors occur centrally in the area postrema and nucleus tractus solitarius, and peripherally on mucosal vagal afferent fibres.[205] Ondansetron is well absorbed orally, with a bioavailability of 80%, and is eliminated mainly by hydroxylation and conjugation, with an elimination half-life of 3 hours; this increases to around 5.4 hours in

**Table IX.** Alteration in drug response in paediatric anaesthetic practice

| Class | Drug | Response compared with adult |
|---|---|---|
| Inhalational anaesthetics | Halothane | MAC lower in neonates but higher in infants and children (not for use in cardiovascular and respiratory depression) |
| | Isoflurane, etc. | Uptake and distribution rapid; high alveolar ventilation<br>Respiration more easily depressed than in adult |
| Intravenous anaesthetics | Thiopental (thiopentone) | Increased brain uptake in neonates leads to increased sensitivity, delayed recovery; therefore, avoid this agent<br>Metabolised rapidly in older children, but induction dose only marginally greater |
| | Propofol | Increased volume of distribution leads to increased induction dose<br>Cardiovascular stability good<br>Pain on injection may be a problem |
| | Ketamine | Larger dose in mg/kg in infants. Atropine premedication advised to prevent salivation problem |
| Neuromuscular blocking agents | Suxamethonium (succinylcholine) | Dose in neonates is larger if based on mg/kg but unchanged if based on surface area comparison (distribution effect produces increased volume of distribution from increased extracellular fluid; also immature neuromuscular system) |
| | Nondepolarising | Dose based on mg/kg unchanged, on surface area decreased.<br>Same effect on neuromuscular transmission, but both decreased when response measured is depression of respiratory function |
| Opioid drugs | Morphine<br>Alfentanil, etc. | Greater sensitivity of neonates and younger children (morphine crosses immature blood-brain barrier more easily). Reduce doses. Immature metabolic pathways produce slower clearance, prolonged half-life |

*Abbreviation:* MAC = minimum alveolar concentration.

patients over 75 years of age. As well as orally, it may also be administered intravenously, by slow injection or infusion. A dose of 8mg has been found effective in prophylaxis and treatment of postoperative nausea and vomiting.[206]

Ondansetron and the other 5-$HT_3$ antagonists are still finding their place in the management of postoperative nausea and vomiting. Although there is no doubt as to their effectiveness in comparison with placebo for treatment of postoperative nausea and vomiting, there are as yet few comparative studies of their effectiveness *versus* other antiemetic drugs.

## 3. Anaesthesia in Various Settings

### 3.1 Paediatric Anaesthesia

Neonates, infants under the age of 1 year, and young children all differ from each other and from adults in their physiology and in the pharmacodynamics and pharmacokinetics of drugs used (see further chapter 3). The main physiological differences lie in the immaturity of various systems, and many of these have important pharmacological consequences. Major alterations in drug responses in paediatric anaesthetic practice are listed in table IX.

#### 3.1.1 Physiological Differences

*Central nervous system:* inability to communicate with the neonate has led to a belief that analgesia is relatively unnecessary. Evidence for this is lacking, although higher concentrations of circulating endorphins in the neonate might support the hypothesis. However, studies have suggested that neonates do suffer pain[207] and that analgesics reduce the stress responses to surgery.[208]

Reluctance to use opioid drugs is encouraged by the greater sensitivity of neonates and younger children to them. Brain concentrations of morphine are 2 to 4 times higher in infants than in older children or adults, probably because of the immaturity of the blood-brain barrier and immaturity of glucuronide metabolism. However, the same relative sensitivity is not seen with more lipid soluble opioids, such as fentanyl, which enter the brain easily in either age group. In addition, plasma concentrations for the same bodyweight-related dose of drug may be higher in the infants due to lower clearance (see also section 7.1.1).[209]

*Respiratory system:* CNS immaturity also leads to potential respiratory problems. Periodic respiration and a tendency to apnoea are common in premature infants and the danger is compounded by sensitivity to opioids. The anatomical differences in young infants also leads to a reduction in respiratory reserve, and these are factors in the frequent decision to use controlled ventilation in the neonate and infant.

*Cardiovascular system:* the changes from fetal to adult circulation at birth are important, but following this, there remains a reduced reserve capacity in the neonate, particularly to increase stroke volume. Thus, cardiac output is relatively rate-dependent, and the infant will not cope well with bradycardia. This is relevant to use of the newer muscle relaxant drugs such as vecuronium and atracurium, which do not antagonise vagal overactivity.

*Hepatic and renal function:* hepatic metabolic pathways are immature, particularly in the first 3 months, although this affects phase II more than phase I metabolic processes (see further chapter 1; sect. 3.3.4). Renal function is also not fully developed, glomerular filtration being inefficient. All these factors contribute to reduced clearance of drugs.

#### 3.1.2 Pharmacokinetic Differences

A relative increase in extracellular fluid contributes to increased volumes of distribution of drugs in very young patients. Smaller fat stores and increased permeability of the blood-brain barrier (especially to lipophilic drugs) can also lead to increased CNS concentrations and effects after a given dose of drug. Some differences between age groups can be large. For example, a group of premature infants receiving intensive care demonstrated a bodyweight-adjusted apparent volume of distribution of alfentanil almost twice that seen in older children, a clearance less than half, and an elimination half-life prolonged from a mean of 60 to 525 minutes.[210]

#### 3.1.3 Use of Inhalational Anaesthetics

Inhalational induction is commonly used, especially in the younger infant. Higher concentrations will be needed than in older individuals, because of rapid alveolar uptake and rapid distribution. As a consequence, induction is also rapid. MACs are higher in infants and children than in adults,[211,212] although the heart and respiration do not share this relative resistance, so that cardiovascular and respiratory depression may easily occur in small children, and thus higher concentrations of volatile agents must be used with care. In contrast, MACs are lower in neonates. Halothane is still an accepted drug for use in children, partly because of the pungency of isoflurane (see section 2.1.1), but sevoflurane is likely to supplant both of them.

#### 3.1.4 Use of Intravenous Anaesthetics

In older children, dose requirements are slightly higher than in adults (e.g. thiopental 4 to 6 mg/kg), but in neonates and young children doses are lower (2 to 3 mg/kg), probably due to more rapid uptake into the brain, and recovery may be prolonged. Propofol is used in older children, but pain on injection is a disadvantage. Ketamine is particularly useful for repeated anaesthesia, e.g. when dressing burns.

#### 3.1.5 Use of Muscle Relaxants

There is reputed to be a relative resistance in neonates and infants to the effects of suxamethonium but sensitivity to nondepolarising relaxants, although interpretation of the available data depends on whether the comparison with adults is made on the basis of bodyweight or body surface area. The dose of suxamethonium on a surface area basis is the same in adults and infants,[213] while the dose of tubocurarine is the same on a bodyweight basis.[214]

#### 3.1.6 Use of Local Anaesthetics

Concern over the depressant effects of opioids has led to increased use of regional anaesthetic techniques, often combined with general anaesthesia.[215,216] As in adults, bupivacaine is the most commonly used drug for most techniques. Peak plasma concentrations occur more rapidly than in adults, and in the first 6 months of life, blood concentrations are higher than in adults mainly because of reduced metabolism.[217] Venepuncture in children has become much more acceptable with the use of surface analgesia by application of a preparation such as 'EMLA' (prilocaine/lidocaine) cream applied topically some 2 hours previously.

### 3.2 Anaesthesia in the Elderly

Although there are consistent changes in physiology with increasing age, the main problems encountered by the anaesthetist are those of associated disease. Patients are also likely to be receiving drugs for other diseases, and adverse effects may be associated with them. The major changes in drug responses in anaesthetic practice in the elderly are listed in table X.

#### 3.2.1 Physiological Differences

In the healthy elderly patient, there is slowing of some mental skills, but many intellectual functions, in particular language skills, are well preserved. Following anaesthesia, any postoperative mental deterioration is brief and no greater in elderly than in young patients.[218] Changes in the cardiovascular system in health are probably slight, but the incidence of cardiovascular disease is high. Autonomic impairment with age leads to less stable control of the car-

**Table X.** Alteration in drug response in anaesthetic practice in the elderly

| Class | Drug | Response compared with younger patient |
|---|---|---|
| General anaesthetics | Inhalational agents | MAC decreases with age. More rapid induction, slower recovery, so reduced dose requirement |
| | | Greater risk of hypotension |
| | Intravenous agents | Reduced dose of thiopental (changed distribution due to slower intercompartmental distribution) |
| | | Slower rate of injection of thiopental, propofol (slower circulation time) recommended |
| Benzodiazepines | | Increased sensitivity to CNS depressant effects |
| Neuromuscular blocking agents | Suxamethonium | Slower onset of maximum block for intubation (slower circulation) |
| | Pancuronium Tubocurarine | Slower clearance, prolonged effect |
| | Atracurium | No significant age-related changes in clearance |
| | All agents | Reduced dose due to degenerative changes in neuromuscular function |
| Local anaesthetics | Lidocaine (lignocaine) | Decreased clearance |
| | Bupivacaine | Increased risk of toxicity |
| Opioid analgesics | Morphine and analogues | Reduced dose requirement due to increased CNS sensitivity and reduced clearance |

*Abbreviations:* CNS = central nervous system; MAC = minimum alveolar concentration.

diovascular system, and lability of blood pressure. Respiratory changes include reduction in the power of respiratory musculature, increased chest wall stiffness and increased ventilation-perfusion mismatch. The ability to detoxify and excrete drugs is reduced both because of a reduction in liver blood flow (with decreased clearance of high extraction ratio drugs), and a decrease in renal function. This includes reduced renal plasma flow, glomerular filtration rate, and other functions.

Drug-induced confusion is common in the elderly; drugs known to cause this (e.g. scopolamine) should be avoided, and other psychotherapeutic drugs (e.g. benzodiazepines in premedication) should be used cautiously. The elderly are particularly sensitive to the depressant effects of midazolam; the dose required is half or less than that in younger adults, and must be administered very slowly. Heavy premedication can contribute to hypoxaemia during regional anaesthesia,[156] and at other times during the perioperative period.

#### 3.2.2 Pharmacokinetic Differences

Drug handling is not consistently different in the elderly, but reduced body water and reduced plasma albumin concentrations will alter distribution, while reduction in renal function is important with some drugs that are eliminated by the kidneys (see further chapter 4; sect. 2.1). The main changes are summarised in table XI.

#### 3.2.3 Choice of Anaesthetic Technique

There is no overall difference in safety between general and regional anaesthesia when used appropriately.[221] Doses of most systemic drugs will be reduced for the reasons outlined above, and slower administration is also necessary in many cases because of slower circulation and often increased pharmacodynamic sensitivity. MAC of inhalational anaesthetic agents decreases with age, in parallel with reduction in oxygen consumption and neuronal density.[22,222]

Local anaesthetics such as lidocaine (lignocaine) and bupivacaine show reduced elimination in the elderly,[223,224] with an increased risk of toxicity. On the other hand, the dose requirement for epidural anaesthesia is reduced by about 40% in the elderly, probably because less escapes through intervertebral foraminae.[225,226]

In general, therefore, there are few specific recommendations, but the choice of a drug dosage is more critical, and often should be considerably reduced in the elderly patient.

**Table XI.** Main pharmacokinetic changes in the elderly (after Dundee;[219] Ramsay & Tucker[220]) [see also chapter 4; sect. 2.1]

| Change | Effect |
|---|---|
| Reduced bodyweight | Standard dose gives greater mg/kg |
| Reduced body water | Water soluble drugs have initial higher blood concentrations because of a smaller volume of distribution |
| Increased body fat | Lipid soluble drugs have initial lower blood concentrations because of a greater volume of distribution |
| Metabolism | Oxidative processes reduced; some reduction in first-pass metabolism |
| Excretion | Glomerular filtration and tubular secretion decline with age |

## 3.3 Day Surgery

An increasing proportion and range of surgical procedures are being carried out on a day-stay basis. This makes specific demands on anaesthetic and pain relief techniques. Safe discharge of patients requires rapid recovery of cognitive and psychomotor skills, and adequate control both of pain and of nausea or vomiting. The choice of technique is important, although the time to return to normal depends more on the duration of anaesthesia than the anaesthetic drug used.[227] Reaction times can be prolonged for up to 48 hours after anaesthesia, even if the patient feels perfectly normal the next day.[228]

### 3.3.1 Premedication

Premedication is not given routinely in most centres in the belief that it may delay recovery,[229] although with short-acting drugs such as temazepam, studies have generally found little evidence of this.[230]

### 3.3.2 Choice of Anaesthetic Technique

Anaesthesia is usually induced intravenously, and propofol is a first-line agent in this setting. Recovery is more rapid than with barbiturates,[231] and it also has a slight antiemetic action. Maintenance of anaesthesia is usually with nitrous oxide/oxygen and a volatile agent. Despite the physical and pharmacokinetic differences, there is little detectable difference in recovery times between halothane, enflurane and isoflurane following brief procedures, such as minor gynaecological operations lasting under 10 minutes,[232] although isoflurane shows an advantage in longer operations.[233] Desflurane also gives good recovery, but no major advantage over older drugs. Total intravenous anaesthesia with propofol has good recovery characteristics and is a useful alternative.

Regional anaesthesia is often used, and is highly appropriate for many operations. Although spinal or epidural techniques are also practised, these can impair mobility and discharge may not be any faster than after general anaesthesia.

### 3.3.3 Use of Opioid Drugs

Opioids should be used with caution in day surgery. Intraoperative analgesia with a short-acting opioid such as alfentanil, fentanyl or sufentanil can shorten recovery time by reducing the anaesthetic requirement, and help with pain on awakening, but care must be taken that this is not offset by increased emesis. A single dose of alfentanil does not increase morbidity, but conversely has questionable benefit on the quality of anaesthesia.[234]

### 3.3.4 Use of Antiemetic Drugs

These agents are used prophylactically by many anaesthetists for procedures and patients with a high likelihood of postoperative emesis. The preferred drug regimens are those with few sedative effects, such as low-dose droperidol (0.25 to 1.25mg) or one of the 5-$HT_3$ antagonists (see section 2.6.6).

### 3.3.5 Postoperative Pain Control

Postoperative pain control is important, and usually a combined approach is used. Strong opioid drugs are usually not indicated, although they may be useful in the earliest postsurgical stage. A nonsteroidal anti-inflammatory drug (NSAID) such as diclofenac may be given perioperatively, or alone or in combination with codeine postoperatively.

Local anaesthetics are also useful as part of a combined approach. Local application or nerve blocks or infiltration may be used, and should have few drawbacks.

## 3.4 Obstetric Anaesthesia

In obstetric anaesthesia, the requirements of both the mother and fetus must be considered, as well as the altered disposition of drugs during pregnancy and labour (see further chapter 2; sect. 4, 7.1.3). Most drugs, including intravenous and inhalational anaesthetics, opioids and local anaesthetics cross the placenta and their use must be controlled to prevent depression of the neonate. However, muscle relaxant drugs do not cross the placenta in significant amounts.

Analgesia for labour has traditionally been provided by a combination of the use of an intramuscular opioid (pethidine) in the first stage and inhalation of nitrous oxide/oxygen as delivery approaches. While this remains the most common method of systemic analgesia, epidural analgesia now sets the standard for pain relief. It requires skilled and experienced personnel for safe institution and management, with the aim of blocking T11 and T12 during the first stage of labour, and in addition S2 to S4 in the second stage. Epidural analgesia is particularly indicated in patients with pre-eclampsia.[235] Analgesia for labour is discussed further in section 7.2.3.

For operative procedures, including caesarian section, regional anaesthetic techniques (epidural or spinal), are being used increasingly, with a corresponding reduction in the number of general anaesthetics employed.

The main problem presented by general anaesthesia during labour is the risk of pulmonary aspiration of stomach contents during induction of anaesthesia. This danger is enhanced by delayed emptying of the stomach, a low pH of stomach contents, and incompetence of the lower oesophageal sphincter. Antacid therapy is a mainstay of prevention of aspiration pneumonitis (Mendelson's syndrome). Particulate antacids such as magnesium trisilicate are themselves capable of causing pulmonary tissue damage if aspirated[236] and have been succeeded by nonparticulate preparations. Probably the best protection is afforded by a combination of $H_2$-receptor blockade (e.g. ranitidine) and a single oral dose of sodium citrate or bicarbonate.[237,238] Omeprazole has also been investigated, but offers no advantage over $H_2$-blockade, being less effective in reducing volume and acidity of stomach contents when given in a single preoperative dose.[239]

Rapid intravenous induction of anaesthesia with intubation of the trachea under the action of a rapidly acting muscle relaxant, usually suxamethonium, and the use of cricoid pressure affords the other means of protection of the lungs at induction of anaesthesia. Anaesthesia is continued with nitrous oxide/oxygen (50 to 66% $O_2$), which is supplemented by low concentrations of a volatile anaesthetic agent. The MAC values of these agents are reduced in pregnancy,[240] and 0.6% enflurane or 0.75% isoflurane have been shown to prevent awareness without causing uterine relaxation or neonatal depression,[241,242] although higher concentrations may have these effects. An opioid drug may be given following delivery.

Regional anaesthesia has advantages in avoiding the dangers of induction of general anaesthesia and in generally producing less neonatal depression, although if there is fetal acidosis then ion trapping can lead to higher concentrations of bupivacaine in the fetal circulation. *Bupivacaine* is the most commonly used drug. Typical doses used for management for labour are 8ml of 0.375% solution followed by an infusion of 0.1% solution given epidurally. For caesarian section, typical doses are about 20ml of 0.375 to 0.5% solutions, although recommendations are changing with its increasing use in combination with opioids. *Lidocaine* (2%) is unsuitable for use in labour because of its short duration of action and the development of tachyphylaxis,[243] but its more rapid onset of action can make it useful alone or in combination with bupivacaine for anaesthesia for caesarian section. The main danger of epidural anaesthesia is the occurrence of hypotension as a result of sympathetic blockade.

Spinal anaesthesia remains the most frequent choice for caesarian section in the US, and is gaining popularity in the UK.[244] The dose requirement is less than in the nonpregnant patient, and 2.5ml of bupivacaine 0.5% can be expected to give a block to T2. However, the onset is rapid and hypotension is common if measures are not taken to prevent this (e.g. prophylactic volume loading and use of a vasopressor such as ephedrine, see section 2.5.1). Use of small doses of opioid drugs in combination with local anaesthetics is becoming standard practice,[245] e.g. fentanyl 12.5 to 25μg in spinal block, or 100μg epidurally.

Drugs given for anaesthesia during labour and delivery, with the possible exception of long-acting benzodiazepines and high doses of pethidine, do not, in general, cause any problems to the mother or neonate in the puerperium.[67]

## 4. Anaesthesia in the Presence of Associated Disease

Whenever possible, concurrent disease should be treated and an attempt made to correct any pathophysiological abnormality before operation. Patients with disease who are receiving drug treatment may often respond differently to operation and anaesthesia, and require modification in their management, with avoidance of some drugs or drug combinations, and changes in the dosages of others.

### 4.1 Cardiovascular Disease

Significant cardiovascular disease is present in perhaps one-fifth of patients undergoing anaesthesia for major surgery. Several schemes have been devised to assess cardiac risk, but the only factors that are constant predictors of increased morbidity are recent myocardial infarction, the presence of congestive heart failure, and major vascular surgery on the aorta. The presence or absence of angina is a less reliable risk index because silent ischaemia is relatively common[246] and may be more dangerous than actual angina. Most cardiac complications occur in the first 24 to 48 hours postoperatively,[247] and prevention requires more attention to be paid to this period.[248]

#### *4.1.1 Use of Preoperative Medication*

In patients with cardiovascular disease undergoing noncardiac operations, an increased demand is placed on the heart without the operation improving cardiac performance. The main factor likely to lead to complications such as reinfarction or congestive failure is an imbalance in oxygen supply and demand in the heart. Preoperatively, appropriate premedication can help to reduce tachycardia, but excessively high doses of opioids or sedatives can lead to hypoxaemia.

In general, cardiovascular drug therapy should be optimised before an operation and treatment continued through surgery. Antihypertensive drugs should be continued, with some cautions. Calcium antagonists have a negative inotropic and vasodilator action that may be additive to that of the volatile anaesthetic agents.[249,250] β-Adrenoceptor blockade improves cardiovascular stability, but may mask ischaemia during preoperative exercise testing.[251] Angiotensin-converting enzyme (ACE) inhibitors may be associated with hypotension at induction or in the postoperative period, but there is no consensus as to whether to stop them before operation.[252,253]

#### *4.1.2 Use of Anaesthetic Agents*

At induction of anaesthesia, the stress of intubation of the trachea is frequently accompanied by transient hypertension and ischaemic electrocardiographic changes. These can be attenuated or prevented by fentanyl or alfentanil.[254] Other drugs including lidocaine and clonidine, and β-blockers such as esmolol, have also been used for this purpose, but have other unwanted effects.

Intravenous induction agents should be titrated cautiously in patients with cardiovascular disease to avoid hypotensive episodes, since they all tend to a differing extent to cause myocardial depression, and most cause some vasodilatation. There has been continuing controversy in the literature over the effects of different volatile agents on the heart and coronary circulation. In particular, the evidence for coronary steal with isoflurane in comparison with other inhalational agents still stimulates discussion.[255] However, although there is evidence in several studies of maldistribution of myocardial blood flow during isoflurane anaesthesia, it now appears that the choice of anaesthetic agent is not important in determining the outcome of the operation.[256]

High epidural anaesthesia appears to improve the dynamics of coronary blood flow[257] and should in theory protect a compromised heart from the stress of operation, provided that coronary filling pressure is maintained. Despite this, present evidence suggests that the choice of general or epidural anaesthesia does not seem to affect the outcome of surgery in either way. However, epidural analgesia has a major contribution in protecting the patient from pain, tachycardia and hypoxaemia in the dangerous postoperative period, which may be the most important factors in the patient's long term outcome.[258]

### 4.2 Respiratory Disease

Chronic obstructive airways disease is the most common respiratory problem encountered in surgical patients. Measurement of forced expiratory volume in 1 second ($FEV_1$) has been suggested as a screening test, and arterial blood gases may be measured in any patient in whom the $FEV_1$ is below 50% of predicted values.[259] As well as airway obstruction, hypercarbia or hypoxaemia may be found in these investigations. The implications of these tests for the pharmacological treatment of the patient are obvious. Drugs that depress ventilation will exacerbate blood gas abnormalities, and this applies not only to opioid drugs, but also tranquillo-sedatives and volatile inhalational agents. However, the bronchodilator effect of halothane or isoflurane can be of benefit in counteracting bronchospasm, especially in asthmatic patients, and these agents have been used in the ICU setting in treatment of resistant status asthmaticus.[260,261] Opioids should be used cautiously, and the use of pethidine should be considered in view of its atropine-like bronchodilator action.

The anaesthetic technique will depend on the individual circumstances. Preoperative treatment, both physiotherapy and drug therapy using $\beta_2$-agonists, methylxanthines, etc. as indicated, may improve the patient's respiratory condition. Epidural analgesia can have a major role in postoperative care, allowing free respiration and coughing.

### 4.3 Endocrine Disease

#### *4.3.1 Diabetes Mellitus*

In patients with diabetes mellitus, the aim is to maintain control of diabetes in the operative and postoperative period, avoiding hyper- or hypoglycaemic episodes. Modern anaesthetic drugs have little effect on blood sugar.

Patients who are satisfactorily controlled on diet have no special anaesthetic requirements. Patients receiving oral antidiabetic drugs undergoing minor surgery should stop taking the drug on the day of surgery, or if it is a long-acting agent, stop taking it on the day before surgery. Blood glucose should be monitored. Patients on oral medication undergoing major surgery should change to an insulin regimen before surgery and during recovery.

Patients controlled on insulin undergoing minor operations can be managed satisfactorily by delaying both the morning dose of insulin and breakfast until after surgery, which is carried out early in the day. A more formal routine is needed for major procedures or in patients with brittle diabetes. Most popular is the use of an infusion containing insulin 2U, KCl 2 mmol and glucose 10g in 100ml each hour (i.e. glucose 10% 500ml with added insulin 10U and KCl 10 mmol at 100 ml/h).[262,263] The more traditional methods using subcutaneous insulin injections are, however, comparable in effectiveness,[264] provided of course that they are carefully managed.

#### 4.3.2 Conditions Requiring Corticosteroid Therapy

All patients who have had or are still receiving systemic corticosteroids should be assessed and observed carefully. However, routine prophylactic cover is only necessary for those who have ceased corticosteroids recently.

#### 4.3.3 Thyroid Disease

In the past, thyroidectomy carried the risk of 'thyroid crisis' induced by increased circulating thyroxine ($T_4$) due to surgical manipulation. This is exceedingly rare now as patients are prepared medically before operation. Anaesthesia does have a small but probably unimportant effect on thyroid-stimulating hormone (TSH) and $T_4$ levels. If preoperative preparation has included β-adrenoceptor blockade, this should be continued and a dose given with any premedication. The premedication should be strongly sedative; atropine should be avoided as it may produce unwanted tachycardia.

Patients who are hypothyroid do not respond well to the stress of surgery, and if possible, the operation should be postponed until the patient has been rendered euthyroid.

### 4.4 Renal Disease

In established renal failure, many of the problems encountered are related to water and electrolyte balance and acid-base disturbance, or to anaemia which accompanies the disease. There are also major changes in the pharmacokinetics of many of the drugs used in anaesthesia, due to reduced renal excretion and some changes in hepatic metabolism. The plasma half-lives of drugs eliminated by the kidney are usually only slightly affected by deteriorating renal function until the glomerular filtration rate has fallen to 0.6 to 1.2 L/h (10 to 20 ml/min),[265] and then half-lives increase rapidly.

Patients who are maintained on haemodialysis will be more sensitive to hypotension immediately after dialysis, when their circulating volume is lower. For minor procedures, such as establishment of arteriovenous shunts, local nerve block techniques are often suitable.

#### 4.4.1 Use of Muscle Relaxants

The action of suxamethonium (succinylcholine) may be slightly prolonged, but the main problem with this drug is the rise in serum potassium that it causes. Although this is no greater in renal failure than in normal patients, it may be dangerous where there are already raised potassium concentrations, and suxamethonium should then be avoided.

Nondepolarising drugs are excreted to a variable extent by the kidneys. The elimination of gallamine is markedly prolonged in renal failure, and it should be avoided. Pancuronium, tubocurarine, alcuronium, doxacurium, pipecuronium and vecuronium show a small but significant decrease in excretion, so that prolongation of block is likely. Although they may be used with careful monitoring of neuromuscular function, they are best avoided if possible (see also section 2.2). However, atracurium,[266] which is mainly metabolised by Hofmann degradation and ester hydrolysis, and mivacurium which is metabolised by plasma esterases, can be used safely during renal failure. Although there is accumulation of laudanosine from atracurium metabolism,[267] this has not been shown to be clinically important.

#### 4.4.2 Use of Opioid Drugs

Morphine does not accumulate in renal failure, but its active metabolite morphine-6-glucuronide does,[268] and this leads to a prolonged morphine action in renal failure. Norpethidine, the convulsant metabolite of pethidine, also accumulates, and normorphine may have a similar effect.[269] Any changes in the action of fentanyl, alfentanil and sufentanil appear to be small.

#### 4.4.3 Use of Anaesthetic Agents

The duration of action of thiopental is prolonged in patients with uraemia.[270] Slow administration of the drug minimises this effect, allowing the end-point of sleep to be identified before a relative overdose is given.

Several of the halogenated volatile anaesthetics are metabolised to inorganic fluorides, raised concentrations of which may result in renal failure. In the case of methoxyflurane, high output renal failure was not uncommon with prolonged anaesthesia.[271] Enflurane, sevoflurane and isoflurane are less extensively metabolised; however, inorganic fluoride concentrations might be significant in patients with pre-existing renal disease receiving enflurane and sevoflurane.[28,272]

#### 4.4.4 Nonsteroidal Anti-Inflammatory Drugs

These drugs are a common cause of drug-induced acute renal failure. This is because their action in inhibiting prostaglandin synthesis stops the action of vasodilator prostaglandins that maintain renal perfusion in patients with raised concentrations of vasoconstrictor hormones (see section 7.1.2). They should therefore be avoided in patients with any degree of renal failure.

### 4.5 Hepatic Disease

Full assessment and careful management are as important for patients with liver disease as for those with cardiac or renal impairment.[273] Cirrhosis is the most common cause of severe liver disease in Western countries and, when surgery is required, mortality can range from 30 to 80%. However, management of ascites and nutritional status can improve the chances of survival.

**Table XII.** Pharmacokinetic changes in severe liver disease (see also appendix F)

| Pathophysiological change | Pharmacokinetic effect |
|---|---|
| Reduction in portal blood flow | Decreased drug absorption from gut |
| Reduction in plasma albumin | Increased free drug fraction in circulation but no change in unbound concentration (unless intrinsic hepatic eliminating capacity is reduced) |
| Sodium retention, increased extracellular fluid | Increased volume of distribution of some drugs (e.g. tubocurarine) with decreased effect |
| Enzyme induction (early alcoholism) | Increased phase I metabolism |
| Enzyme inhibition (late cirrhosis) | Decreased phase I metabolism |

The pharmacokinetics of drugs are altered, often drastically, by liver disease (table XII). In addition, pharmacodynamic sensitivity varies. In early alcoholic cirrhosis, there is CNS tolerance to anaesthetic and sedative drugs (although not cardiovascular tolerance). Later, possibly due to an increase in blood-brain barrier permeability or to changes in brain amine concentrations, the action of such drugs may be prolonged and much more profound.

Anaesthetic management principally requires careful monitoring, with avoidance as far as possible of opioids and sedatives. Light inhalational anaesthesia with an agent such as isoflurane is preferred. Although the action of suxamethonium can be prolonged if plasma cholinesterase is reduced, this need not be a problem. Resistance to nondepolarising relaxants can be allowed for by increasing the initial dose, but further doses should be reduced because elimination is likely to be delayed.

### 4.6 Neurological and Neuromuscular Disease

#### 4.6.1 Epilepsy

Epileptic patients usually tolerate anaesthesia without incident, but occasionally they present problems. There is not only a risk of convulsions in susceptible patients given certain anaesthetics (methohexital, ether, enflurane, ketamine), but also a possibility of antiepileptic drug neurotoxicity, particularly with phenytoin (diphenylhydantoin),[274] as a result of the depressant effect of general anaesthesia on hepatic drug elimination processes. It is therefore wise to monitor phenytoin concentrations prior to elective surgery and to adjust the dosage to attain the minimum effective concentration (see also section 6.1.3).

#### 4.6.2 Myasthenia Gravis

In this autoimmune disease, there is a loss of 70 to 90% of functional acetylcholine receptors at the neuromuscular junction. If anaesthesia is required, the patient's treatment should be optimised preoperatively, and anticholinesterase therapy continued. Regional anaesthesia will avoid some of the problems that occur with general anaesthesia, but it may not always be appropriate. Since muscle power is reduced, it may be possible to use an inhalational agent such as isoflurane as the sole anaesthetic for anaesthesia maintenance, thus avoiding the use of neuromuscular blocking agents.

Myasthenic patients are resistant to suxamethonium, so that increased doses will be required, but the picture is complicated because a nondepolarising block can occur after suxamethonium use.[275] There is sensitivity to nondepolarising relaxants, so that the dose required will be reduced, and a more prolonged block may also result. Short-acting drugs should be used; the dose of vecuronium is reduced by 50%,[276] and that of atracurium to 20% of the usual,[277] with considerable variation between individual patients.

## 5. Toxicity of Anaesthetic Drugs

Virtually all drugs produce undesired effects as well as those for which they are prescribed, and anaesthetic drugs are no exception.

### 5.1 Effects of Anaesthetics on Cell Division, and Occupational Exposure

Bone marrow depression can occur after prolonged administration of nitrous oxide and in animals, similar effects have been seen with other anaesthetic agents. Teratogenicity has not been shown with any anaesthetic agent in humans (although an effect on cell division in human cell cultures has been demonstrated), but many substances including nitrous oxide, ether, cyclopropane, and methoxyflurane have produced congenital abnormalities in chick embryos. Nitrous oxide and halothane are also capable of producing abnormalities in the rat.[278] The only inference that can be drawn at present is that anaesthetic drugs, like all other drugs, are relatively contraindicated during the first trimester of pregnancy.

Long term exposure to trace amounts of anaesthetic agents is a different situation.[279] Several surveys have suggested that operating theatre personnel have a higher incidence of disease than control groups. However, the validity of the results of many of these studies can be seriously questioned.[280] The chemical structures of halogenated anaesthetics, in particular, show a similarity to known carcinogens,[281] but in several studies of mortality in anaesthetists there was no outstanding difference in death rate from cancers between anaesthetists and other doctors,[282] and rates were low in comparison with men of similar social standing.[283] A recent study[284] found abnormal metabolism of folic acid in patients exposed to 70% nitrous oxide for 90 minutes or more, but no evidence of this in a group of 10 anaesthetists. There may be an increase in spontaneous abortion rates among female operating room staff.[285,286] However, while it has not been shown unequivocally that waste anaesthetics are responsible for an increase in disease among exposed personnel, it seems highly desirable to scavenge all exhaust gases from anaesthetic circuits and the theatre atmosphere and vent them to the outside air. Maximum allowable concentrations of these gases have now been laid down in several countries.

Studies of the effect of trace quantities of anaesthetics on mental performance have been inconsistent, but some have suggested a measurable decrease in performance of psychological tests by volunteers exposed to as little as 50 ppm (parts per million) of nitrous oxide or 1 ppm halothane. Halothane is metabolised to various substances including bromide, and after exposure to a typical anaesthetic dose, bromide concentrations rise to the psychoactive range by the second day and are still high after 9 days.[287]

### 5.2 Oxygen Toxicity

Oxygen in high concentrations is commonly used in anaesthesia, as well as in the ICU. Oxygen, although vital to life, is also highly toxic and in humans affects mainly 3 systems: the CNS, the lung, and the lens of the neonatal eye.[288,289] Breathing 80 to 100% oxygen produces signs of pulmonary oxygen toxicity within 24 hours, with substernal pain and reductions in both vital capacity and lung compliance. With hyperbaric therapy, these changes will occur more rapidly, and at over 2.5 atmospheres (1600mm Hg), central nervous system toxicity with convulsions occurs. In the neonate, retrolental fibroplasia can occur if arterial oxygen tension is not carefully monitored.

Toxicity is believed to be due to production of partially reduced metabolites of oxygen – oxidant free radicals.[290-292] While metabolically active organs of the body, e.g. the liver and kidney, have enzymatic and other mechanisms to protect against damage from free radicals produced by metabolism, the lung is poorly provided with defences. Toxicity can be potentiated by agents that increase the metabolic rate (thyroxine, adrenaline) or pyrexia, by exogenous factors (paraquat, ionising radiation), or by deficiency of substances such as selenium, copper, ascorbic acid (vitamin C), tocopherol (vitamin E) or sulfur-containing amino acid, all of which are involved in defence.[288]

Despite this, high oxygen concentrations are believed to have greater benefit than risk during routine anaesthesia. With more prolonged exposure, as in the ICU, careful monitoring is necessary, and the inspired oxygen concentration should exceed 40% only when this is strictly necessary to maintain acceptable oxygenation of arterial blood.

### 5.3 Renal Toxicity

Few drugs used in anaesthesia have any directly damaging effect on the function of the kidneys, and by far the most common cause of damage during operation and anaesthesia is inadequate renal blood flow.[293] The body reacts to hypovolaemia by constricting the splanchnic (including renal) blood vessels, and this may lead to acute tubular necrosis. The response to haemorrhage is different in conscious and anaesthetised animals, and renal vasoconstriction may be relatively more marked during anaesthesia.[294]

Vasoconstrictor drugs may exacerbate the problem, although low-dose (2 to 5 μg/kg/min) dopamine is a selective renal vasodilator and is used for renal protection. NSAIDs remove the protective effect of renal vasodilator prostaglandins (see further section 7.1.2). In susceptible patients, e.g. those with obstructive jaundice, mannitol may be given during surgery to maintain renal blood flow by producing an osmotic diuresis.

Damage to the kidneys from metabolites of volatile anaesthetic agents is discussed in section 2.1.1.

### 5.4 Hepatic Toxicity

Although anaesthetic drugs are relatively nontoxic to the liver as compared with many other groups of drugs, liver damage during anaesthesia may occur by several mechanisms,[6,295,296] including the following.

1) Indirectly due to drugs, anaesthetic technique or surgery, via effects such as hypoxia, hypercarbia, or underperfusion due to splanchnic vasoconstriction in states of shock, or to hypotension after sympathetic block in hypotensive techniques or spinal anaesthesia, or prolonged hypotension from any cause.

2) A direct toxic effect of a drug or a metabolite. Chloroform is generally acknowledged to be toxic to the liver, and severe damage has often occurred, so it is now little used. Clinical doses of intravenous agents are not toxic, but liver dysfunction can occur after large doses of thiopental.[297] These effects occur with the first exposure, are dose-related, and predictable.[6]

3) Unpredictably, e.g. fulminant hepatic failure following exposure to halothane or less commonly other halogenated volatile anaesthetics. A previous exposure is usually identifiable, and the severity is not dose-related. There are 2 main theories to explain this: toxicity due to a metabolite or an immune reaction. The hypothesis that a genetic susceptibility exists to trifluoroacetyl (TFA) halide-labelled liver cell proteins incorporates both of the latter mechanisms. This is discussed in more detail in section 2.1.1.

### 5.5 Malignant Hyperpyrexia

Some susceptible patients who suffer from an inherited abnormality in muscle membranes, develop fulminating and often fatal hyperpyrexia when given certain anaesthetic drugs and depolarising muscle relaxants.[298,299] Most patients develop muscle contracture, acidosis and hyperkalaemia. Unexplained tachypnoea, tachycardia, sweating, cyanosis, or increases in expired $CO_2$ may be nonspecific early warning signs. A working clinical definition of malignant hyperpyrexia is an unexplained fever during anaesthesia in which the body temperature rises at a rate of at least 2°C an hour. However, sometimes the rise in body temperature can be a late sign.

Malignant hyperpyrexia is due to an abnormality in the calcium channel of the muscle sarcolemma or sarcoplasmic reticulum. This is inherited, probably in an autosomal dominant manner, and an abnormality has been traced to a gene on the long arm of chromosome 19.[300] However, the abnormality in some families investigated appears to lie at a different chromosome location, which not only indicates a more complicated pattern of inheritance, but delays the development of a routine simple test for susceptibility.[301] At present, firm diagnosis requires muscle biopsy.

The incidence of the condition as diagnosed lies between 1 in 6000 and 1 in 200,000 patients. This range indicates different criteria for diagnosis in the absence of a readily available diagnostic test. Mortality in the UK was around 24%,[302] but is improving as increased $O_2$ and $CO_2$ monitoring allows earlier diagnosis. Triggering agents include:

- Volatile anaesthetic agents
- Cyclopropane
- Suxamethonium.

In addition, there is doubt about ketamine, phenothiazines, tricyclic and other antidepressants, and monoamine oxidase inhibitors, although this may be because of confusion between malignant hyperthermia and neuroleptic malignant syndrome, which is now known to be a separate entity.[303] Drugs that are not associated with hyperpyrexia include all local anaesthetics, opioids, nitrous oxide, all nondepolarising muscle relaxants, atropine and neostigmine.

Management of the condition consists first in discontinuation of the triggering agent, and symptomatic management including cooling and treatment of the hyperkalaemia which can be the fatal event. *Dantrolene sodium* is the specific treatment. It is a direct-acting muscle relaxant that acts by dissociating excitation-contraction coupling in the muscle through inhibition of calcium ion release from the sarcoplasmic reticulum. The site of action may be on the transverse tubular-sarcoplasmic reticulum coupling, on the sarcoplasmic reticulum directly, or both.[304,305] A dose of 2.4 mg/kg intravenously appears to be adequate for prophylaxis or initial treatment.[278,306] The dose may be infused until a therapeutic effect is achieved or a total dose of 10 mg/kg is reached. A further prophylactic dose of 2.4 mg/kg after 10 to 12 hours may be considered.[307]

### 5.6 Hypersensitivity Reactions

Hypersensitivity reactions are not uncommon in anaesthetics, although severe reactions are unusual, with an incidence of between 1 in 5000 and 1 in 20,000 exposures to general anaesthetics as a whole.[308] The most common groups of agents associated with hypersensitivity are muscle relaxants, intravenous induction agents and plasma volume expanders.

There are several possible mechanisms for these reactions. They may be anaphylactic (immune-mediated phenomena involving previous sensitisation of the patient), but the more general term 'anaphylactoid' is more appropriate when the history and mechanism are not certain. The clinical features often resemble the effects of histamine release, and they also need to be distinguished from cases where histamine is released simply as part of the normal spectrum of action of a drug, as with morphine, tubocurarine or thiopental, which are also capable of causing anaphylactic reactions.

Hypersensitivity reactions to drugs may be classified as type I to IV depending on their mechanism (see further chapter 6; sect. 4.1). Type I, involving IgE or IgG antibodies, is the main mechanism involved in most hypersensitivity to anaesthetic drugs, but type IV cellular responses mediated by sensitised lymphocytes may account for up to 80% of *local anaesthetic* allergic reactions.[309] Type I reactions require a previous exposure, but this is not necessary for 'anaphylactoid' reactions involving complement activation by alternative pathways or in other 'histaminoid' reactions where there is direct pharmacological release of histamine.

Hypersensitivity reactions are more likely to occur in patients with a personal or family history of asthma or eczema, and in those known to be sensitive to other drugs.[310] Particularly low or high IgE concentrations may predispose patients to reactions by different mechanisms.[311] Severe reactions mainly involve acute hypotension and bronchospasm. The latter can be very severe and difficult to treat. In cardiovascular collapse, plasma loss of up to 35% of circulating blood volume may occur within 10 minutes due to capillary permeability, and rapid replacement, preferably using colloid, is indicated. Adrenaline (epinephrine), infused intravenously with electrocardiographic monitoring, is the drug treatment of choice. When adrenaline and adequate volume replacement do not produce improvement, noradrenaline (norepinephrine) may be lifesaving. Antihistamines and corticosteroids have little effect in the acute stages, although they are worth trying as second-line drugs.[312]

Identification of the causative agent is not likely to be simple, and some guidelines for the procedure to be followed have been suggested.[313]

## 6. Clinically Important Drug Interactions in Anaesthesia

The general principles underlying drug interactions are described in chapter 7. Anaesthesia requires polypharmacy, and therefore many interactions may occur, most occurring predictably and as part of the planned treatment of the patient. However, some are not planned, and table IV lists the principal adverse effects and interactions of anaesthetic drugs that are likely to be of importance to the anaesthetist. Some of these, and a few others are discussed in this section.

## 6.1 Interactions with Psychoactive Drugs

### 6.1.1 Monoamine Oxidase Inhibitors (MAOIs)

Monoamine oxidase (MAO) inactivates monoamine substances, many of which are, or are related to, neurotransmitters. The central nervous system mainly contains MAO-A, the substrates of which are adrenaline, noradrenaline, metanephrine and serotonin (5-hydroxytryptamine, 5-HT), whereas extraneuronal tissues such as the liver, lung and kidney contain mainly MAO-B, which metabolises β-phenylethylamine, phenylethanolamine *o*-tyramine and benzylamine.[314] Apart from behavioural changes, the main effect of MAO inhibition is a generalised reduction in sympathetic tone, with lower resting blood pressure and a reduced ability to respond to stresses such as postural change.

There are no serious interactions with the commonly used anaesthetic agents, but problems have occurred with pethidine (meperidine). When a patient receiving an older nonselective MAOI (e.g. phenelzine, isocarboxazid, tranylcypromine) is inadvertently given pethidine, either at induction of anaesthesia or postoperatively, there follows a reaction characterised by hypertension, hyperthermia, decreased level of consciousness or coma, and even convulsions. This is unlikely to occur with other opioids unrelated to pethidine, although data are scarce. It is less well recognised that, in addition to this excitatory response, a 'depressive' type of reaction can occur due to reduced metabolism, resulting occasionally in an increased and prolonged response to drugs such as morphine.[315]

Newer monoamine oxidase inhibitor drugs such as moclobemide are selective for the MAO-A subtype of the enzyme, and are less likely to interact with foods or other drugs than the older MAOIs.

Withdrawal of monoamine oxidase inhibitors can result in severe anxiety, agitation, pressured speech, sleeplessness or drowsiness, hallucinations, delirium and paranoid psychosis,[316] and thus should not be undertaken lightly. The older nonselective MAOIs cause irreversible inhibition of MAO, and it is advisable to stop treatment at least 1 week before operation. The newer MAO-A selective inhibitors may be reversible in 24 to 48 hours, although with careful selection of anaesthetic management, it should usually be possible to avoid drugs likely to interact with them.

### 6.1.2 Tricyclic Antidepressants and Phenothiazines

The cardiovascular effects of noradrenaline and adrenaline (particularly adrenaline-induced heart rate and rhythm changes) are likely to be hazardously potentiated in patients taking tricyclic antidepressants or phenothiazines. This is because these drugs inhibit the noradrenaline uptake mechanism into nerve endings. In local anaesthetic solutions, felypressin would seem to be a safer alternative vasoconstrictor in such patients.

### 6.1.3 Antiepileptic Drugs

Antiepileptic drugs such as the barbiturates and phenytoin are well known inducers of hepatic enzymes and may increase the dosage requirements of many drugs, including fentanyl.[317] They may also cause resistance to nondepolarising muscle relaxants (except atracurium), but the mechanism of this interaction is unclear; it may be pharmacodynamic, perhaps due to a change in the sensitivity of acetylcholine receptors.[318]

## 6.2 Interactions with Cardiovascular Drugs

### 6.2.1 Calcium Antagonists

These drugs are generally without hazard during anaesthesia, but the volatile anaesthetics can interact adversely with calcium antagonists. Experimentally, halothane and enflurane have direct cardiac inhibitory effects similar to verapamil and diltiazem, whereas the properties of isoflurane seem closer to those of the dihydropyridines (e.g. nifedipine and nicardipine), the dominant action of which is vasodilatation. Interactions may cause an additive effect on conduction with isoflurane[249] or halothane.[250]

Combined therapy using calcium antagonists with β-blockers is increasingly common and is probably safest if undertaken with dihydropyridines. Synergy occurs, which can lead to marked interference with conduction, leading further to bradycardia or even sinus arrest.[319] Caution is needed during operations in patients receiving such a combination, as conduction disturbances can occur,[320] although very careful monitoring of the electrocardiograph will usually minimise any problems.[321]

#### 6.2.2 β-Adrenoceptor Blocking Drugs

Bradycardia, hypotension and bronchospasm are the main hazards in β-blocker recipients undergoing anaesthesia. However, continuation of β-blockade up to and including the day of operation results in improved perioperative haemodynamic stability and avoids the rebound effect that can result from their abrupt withdrawal.[322] There may be a risk of bradycardia following neostigmine administration in patients receiving β-blockers,[323] and it is advisable to give an anticholinergic drug first rather than mixed with the anticholinesterase.

#### 6.2.3 Other Antihypertensive Drugs

It is usually recommended that *ACE inhibitors* be continued perioperatively in common with other antihypertensive agents. It has been suggested that they improve haemodynamic stability during operation,[324] but there is also evidence that ACE inhibitors may predispose to hypotension during anaesthesia[252,253] and that they reduce cerebral blood flow during any period of systemic hypotension.[325] Their use should therefore be regarded with caution.

*Clonidine* appears to reduce the incidence of hypertensive episodes during anaesthesia, such as the response to laryngoscopy and intubation.[165] However, this may be at the expense of an increased incidence of hypotension and bradycardia at other times perioperatively,[166] with bradycardia being somewhat resistant to atropine.

### 6.3 Interactions with Neuromuscular Blockers

A number of antibiotics possess neuromuscular blocking activity and may potentiate the effect of nondepolarising muscle relaxants. The aminoglycoside, polymixin, lincosamide and tetracycline groups are those most commonly involved, while the penicillins, cefalosporins and erythromycin have not caused clinical problems. The aminoglycosides act mainly at prejunctional sites, while the polymixins, tetracyclines and lincosamides act mainly at postjunctional sites. There are also considerable differences between individual drugs of each group. Because of these complexities, antagonism of this type of block is uncertain and although, in the experimental setting, calcium can achieve a 75% reversal of the effect of aminoglycosides, clinically it is usually safer to continue ventilation until adequate muscle power has returned. Less difficulty might be expected with the newer nondepolarising drugs such as atracurium and vecuronium, but clinical concentrations of aminoglycosides (e.g. gentamicin, tobramycin) can prolong the duration of blockade with these drugs.[326]

The calcium antagonists verapamil and nifedipine have been shown to potentiate the effect of the commonly used nondepolarising muscle relaxants, including vecuronium and atracurium.[327] Magnesium sulfate, used in the management of pre-eclampsia, has a similar effect, and magnesium sulfate and nifedipine in combination may themselves cause neuromuscular block.[328]

Suxamethonium breakdown may be delayed by drugs that reduce plasma cholinesterase concentrations or compete as substrates. Many of the drugs that do this, such as procaine or propanidid, are mainly of historical interest, but metoclopramide, which is often given before obstetric anaesthesia, prolongs the duration of action of suxamethonium by as much as 50%.[329]

## 7. Pain Relief

Pain is a defence mechanism. However, excess pain interferes with normal body function. Therefore, the body also has an endogenous ability to modulate the appreciation of pain. Activation of analgesic mechanisms results from an interaction between specific neurotransmitters, such as enkephalin, serotonin or noradrenaline, and specific receptors located on the neurons that transmit pain. Opioid drugs, such as morphine, interact with opioid receptors and produce analgesia by the same mechanisms as enkephalin, i.e. hyperpolarisation of interneurons and depressing the release of transmitters associated with transmission of pain. Adrenergic drugs can also interact with specific receptors to produce analgesia, and there is interaction between the systems. Pain may be considered as physiological (somatic or visceral) or pathological.

Pain resulting from, for example, a surgical incision originates at peripheral nociceptors where a number of chemical mediators (e.g. bradykinins) are involved in initiating the nociceptive signal. The resulting nerve impulse, carried by small unmyelinated C fibres and by the delta group of A fibres in afferent neurons, passes via the dorsal horn of the spinal cord, the opposite lateral spinothalamic tract and the thalamus, to the cerebral cortex, where it is consciously felt. However, this description is false in its simplicity. The pathway synapses a number of times and an immense number of interconnections between neurons allows processing of the signal at several levels. This involves a number of local receptor systems, including opioid, $\alpha_2$-adrenergic and, to a lesser extent, serotonin, $GABA_B$, neuropeptide Y, cholinergic, adenosine, and the *N*-methyl-D-aspartate (NMDA)-glutamate site.[330] A malfunction of signal processing is the basis for the development of pathological pain states in which a slight stimulus is perceived as severe pain, or where a sensation of pain arises or is maintained entirely within the nervous system itself.

The main thrust of pain management in anaesthetic practice is directed toward acute physiological pain occurring intra- and postoperatively. Management of pathological, often chronic pain syndromes requires a multidisciplinary approach in which anaesthetists play a leading role.

The pain pathway may be modified at several points (fig. 3). Local anaesthetic drugs can be used to block transmission at any point up to spinal cord level, and some other drugs act at spinal level. Drugs given systemically might be considered in 3 groups:

1) Drugs that are not analgesic, but reduce pain by treating its cause, e.g. nitroglycerin (glyceryl trinitrate) in angina.

2) Analgesic drugs that act mainly peripherally, e.g. aspirin (acetylsalicylic acid) and paracetamol (acetaminophen).

3) Analgesic drugs that act mainly centrally in the brain and spinal cord. Enkephalinergic, noradrenergic, serotonergic and cholinergic pathways all contribute to modulation of pain perception, and interact with each other. However, the opioids are the most important strong analgesic drugs, acting on receptors in the brain and spinal cord to modify both the transmission of pain and its perception by the brain.

With the complex interactions referred to in section 6, it is not surprising that analgesia may sometimes be enhanced by drugs that are not considered primarily as analgesics. This is referred to here in the context of the treatment of chronic pain (see section 7.2.2).

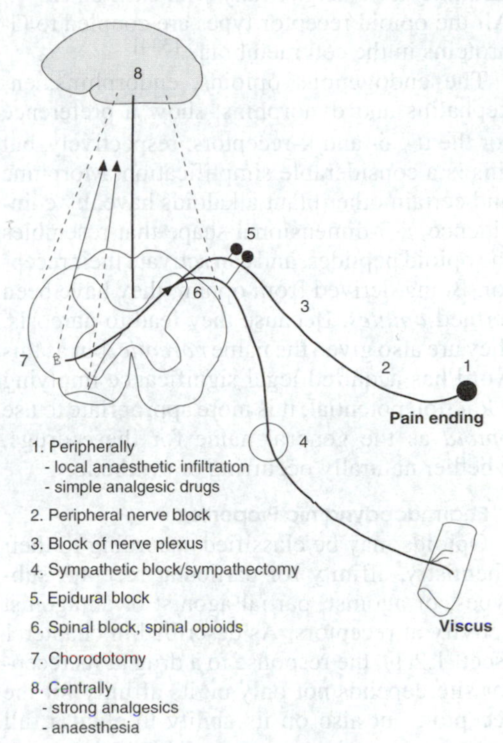


**Fig. 3.** Simplified concept of the pain pathway, showing points where it may be interrupted.

## 7.1 Clinical Pharmacology of Analgesic Drugs

### *7.1.1 Opioid Analgesics*

Receptor sites exist in the brain, spinal cord and elsewhere, at which opioids such as morphine act to produce analgesia and their other actions. The endogenous ligands for these are peptides, often loosely described as endorphins, but classified as endorphins, enkephalins and dynorphins. The receptor sites are heterogeneous and their classification is difficult. Behavioural criteria were used by Martin et al.[331] in the earliest attempt at classification, while binding studies and more recently cloning have been used.

Three major classes of opioid receptors defined are mu ($\mu$), kappa ($\kappa$), and delta ($\delta$) [table XIII]. Current knowledge suggests that $\mu$-receptors can be further subclassified into 2 distinct subtypes ($\mu_1$ and $\mu_2$), as can $\delta$-receptors ($\delta_1$ and $\delta_2$). The $\kappa$-receptors have been subdivided into $\kappa_1$, $\kappa_2$ and $\kappa_3$ subtypes. All of these subtypes modulate pain perception, with the exception of the $\kappa_2$-receptor, which has not been adequately examined. Supraspinal systems have been described for $\mu_1$-, $\kappa_3$- and $\delta_2$-receptors while $\mu_2$-, $\kappa_1$- and $\delta_1$-receptors modulate pain at the spinal level. In addition to their ability to act independently, the various systems also interact synergistically with each other.[333] All the opioid receptor types are coupled to G-proteins in the cell membrane.[334]

The endogenous opioids, endorphins, enkephalins and dynorphins, show a preference for the μ-, δ- and κ-receptors, respectively, but this is a considerable simplification. Morphine and certain other plant alkaloids have, by coincidence, a 3-dimensional shape that resembles the opioid peptides, and can activate their receptor. Being derived from opium, they have been termed *opiates*. Because they lead to narcosis, they are also given the name *narcotic*, but as this word has acquired legal significance implying addiction potential, it is more appropriate to use *opioid* as the general name for these drugs, whether naturally occurring or synthetic.

#### Pharmacodynamic Properties

Opioids may be classified according to their chemistry, affinity for particular receptor subtypes, or agonist, partial agonist or antagonist activity at receptors. As described in chapter 1 (sect. 1.2.1), the response to a drug at its receptor site depends not only on its affinity for the receptor, but also on its ability to elicit a full response from the receptor and, thus, there may be a full spectrum of activity of different drugs. A pure agonist such as morphine can (in adequate concentrations) elicit a maximum response from the receptor. However, a partial agonist such as buprenorphine, even in high concentrations, can only cause a partial response. The general properties and principal uses of the opioid analgesics are listed in table XIV.

Most opioids in clinical use (morphine, pethidine, methadone, fentanyl and its derivatives, and most older opioids) are pure agonists at the μ-receptor. A number of drugs including pentazocine, nalbuphine and others are partial agonists at the κ-receptor, but they are able to antagonise the action of morphine at the μ-receptor; they are thus usually classified as agonist-antagonists. Buprenorphine and propiram are regarded as partial μ-agonists.[335,336]

Although there is evidence that different receptor subtypes may be responsible for different aspects of opioid action,[333] the expectation that this finding would lead to development of opioid analgesic drugs without adverse effects has yet to bear clinical fruit. Thus, for all the drugs described here, however much they may differ in potency, maximum efficacy and dose-response characteristics, their analgesic and toxic effects (e.g. respiratory depression) occur in proportion to each other and cannot be separated.

#### Pharmacokinetic Characteristics

The main differences between the many μ-agonists are pharmacokinetic. Morphine and alfentanil lie toward the opposite ends of a spectrum – morphine is relatively lipophobic and thus penetrates the brain slowly, whereas alfentanil has higher lipid solubility, a pKa favouring the unionised state at body pH, and a small volume of distribution, all of which favour rapid equilibration from plasma to site of effect. The differences between fentanyl, alfentanil, sufentanil and remifentanil are discussed further below. With some exceptions, e.g. the newer agents propiram and tramadol,[336,337] oral absorption of the opioid analgesics is poor and bioavailability is low and variable, as they undergo extensive first-pass metabolism, mainly in the liver. There is also wide interindividual variation in plasma concentrations and rates of elimination after parenteral administration. Since there is also a wide variation in patients' perception of pain and in the plasma concentration of opioid needed to provide analgesia, it is essential to use individualised schedules for opioid analgesics.

Although most opioids undergo significant first-pass hepatic metabolism following single doses, their bioavailabilities may increase with long term administration at higher doses as me-

**Table XIII.** Opioid receptors and subtypes (after Pasternak[332])

| Receptor | Agonist | Second messenger | Subtypes | Analgesia |
|---|---|---|---|---|
| μ | Morphine | Cyclic-AMP ↓ | $m_1$ | Supraspinal |
| | Endorphins | $K^+$ channels ↑ | $m_2$ | Spinal |
| κ | Pentazocine | Cyclic-AMP ↓ | $k_1$ | Spinal |
| | Dynorphins | $K^+$ channels ↑ | $\kappa_2$ | |
| | | | $\kappa_3$ | Supraspinal |
| δ | Enkephalins | $Ca^{++}$ channels ↓ | $d_1$ | Spinal |
| | | | $\delta_2$ | Supraspinal |

*Symbols:* ↑ = increased; ↓ = decreased.

**Table XIV.** Properties and principal uses of the strong opioid analgesics

| Drug | Usual IM dosage[a] (mg) | Duration of single IM dose (h) | Oral efficacy for severe pain | Usual oral dosage (mg) | Principal indications[b] | Main adverse effects[c] and interactions |
|---|---|---|---|---|---|---|
| **Natural opioids** | | | | | | |
| Morphine[d] | 8-16 | 4-6 | Good | 5-30 | Acute pain, myocardial infarction, chronic pain, terminal malignancy | Respiratory depression<br>Nausea and vomiting<br>Dependence; ?interaction with MAOIs (see text; section 6.2.1) |
| Papaveretum[d] | 20 | 3-4 | Poor | | | |
| **Semisynthetic** | | | | | | |
| Diamorphine[d] (heroin) | 4-8 | 2 | Good | 5-10 | Myocardial infarction, chronic pain, terminal malignancy | Respiratory depression<br>Nausea and vomiting<br>Dependence; ?interaction with MAOIs (see text section 6.2.1) |
| Oxymorphone[d] | 1-3 | 4-6 | | | | |
| Oxycodone[d] | 10 | 4-6 | Good | 5-20 | | |
| **Synthetic** | | | | | | |
| Buprenorphine[e] | 0.3-0.6 | 6-8 | Good (sublingual) | 0.4-0.8 | | Low dependence liability |
| Butorphanol[f] | 1-4 | 3-4 | Poor[g] | | | Low dependence liability |
| Dextromoramide[d] | 5-8 | 2-3 | Good | 5-10 | | |
| Dezocine[f] | 5-15 | 2-4 | | | | Nausea, vomiting, sommolence, ? low dependence liability |
| Levorphanol[d] | 2-4 | 4-6 | Good | 1.5-4.5 | Postoperative pain | As for morphine |
| Meptazinol[d] | 75-100 | 3-4 | Fair | 200 | Postoperative pain, labour | Nausea, vomiting, low dependence liability |
| Methadone[d] | 5-15 | 6-8 | Good | 5-10 | Postoperative pain, chronic pain | Risk of accumulation with repeated doses |
| Pentazocine[f] | 20-40 | 2-4 | Fair | 75-100 | Labour, moderate postoperative or chronic pain | Low dependence liability, but inappropriate use has led to abuse<br>Hallucinations |
| Nalbuphine[f] | 20 | 2-4 | | | Moderately severe postoperative or chronic pain | Low dependence liability |
| Pethidine[d] (meperidine) | 75-125 | 3-4 | Poor | 50-100 | Labour, renal and biliary colic | Respiratory depression, nausea and vomiting<br>Interaction with MAOIs |
| Phenazocine[f] | 2-4 | 4-6 | Good (sublingual) | 10-20 | Labour | |
| Propiram[e] | | | Good | 50-100 | | Nausea, vomiting, dizziness, drowsiness;? low dependence liability |
| Tramadol[d] | 100 | 5-6 | Good | 50-100 | | Nausea, dizziness, sedation, dry mouth;? low dependence liability |

a Dosages of opioids should be reduced if any other respiratory depressant drug has been given, in patients with reduced respiratory reserve, elderly patients, neonates and infants under 1 year (older infants and children tolerate opioids well), and in patients with impaired renal or liver function. Some patients with uraemia are extremely sensitive to depressant effects of strong analgesics (see appendix D). Note that in the presence of hypovolaemia (e.g. trauma, burns), IM medications may be poorly absorbed and dosages should be titrated intravenously.

b Indications given are those where drugs are generally first choices. Other agents may be used as alternatives for specified indications (see also section 7.2).

c Adverse effects of morphine apply to all other opioid analgesics; see also section 7.1.1.

d Pure agonist.

e Partial agonist.

f Agonist-antagonist.

g A transnasal formulation of butorphanol has proved effective (usual dose via this route, 1-2mg).

*Abbreviations and symbols:* IM = intramuscular; MAOIs = monoamine oxidase inhibitors.

tabolic pathways become saturated. Hepatic metabolism of morphine gives rise to 2 glucuronides, morphine-6-glucuronide (M6G), which has analgesic activity, and morphine-3-glucuronide (M3G), which is inactive. A significant proportion of the analgesic action of morphine is in fact due to M6G. Opioid studies have revealed individual differences in the metabolism of morphine to its 3- and 6-glucuronides; patients with pain that responds poorly to morphine or diamorphine probably have a high ratio of M3G to M6G concentrations. Methadone may be useful in such patients, because it is not metabolised to glucuronides.[338]

Patients with cirrhosis may be unduly sensitive to the depressant action of opioids and, with pethidine, cumulative toxicity may occur due to slow elimination of the more toxic metabolite, norpethidine.[339] Norpethidine has occasionally been associated with convulsions. It, and methadone (a variable proportion of which, up to 20% or more, is excreted in the urine) may also accumulate during renal failure. Accumulation of morphine due to reduced hepatic metabolism may also occur in critically ill patients,[340] while in renal insufficiency, increased concentrations of the active morphine metabolite M6G may develop.

Dosages of opioid analgesics should be reduced in the elderly, not only because of increased sensitivity to the drug effects, but also because increased plasma concentrations occur, as seen with morphine and pethidine.[341,342]

Neonates are also more sensitive to the actions of opioid analgesics. Morphine clearance is much lower in the neonate, reaching adult values by age 6 months to 2.5 years.[209] Paradoxically, neonates may require higher plasma concentrations of morphine for sedation, perhaps because of the low concentration of circulating M6G.[343]

#### Opioid Agonists (Morphine and Related Drugs)

***Morphine*** has long been the standard with which other opioid analgesics are compared. It acts, as described above, on opioid receptors, both by reducing transmission along the pain pathways and modifying the central perception of pain. The central action also contributes to drowsiness and euphoria (though occasional dysphoria can occur). It depresses respiration (a $\mu_2$-receptor action), mainly by reducing the response to carbon dioxide, and overdose is characterised by extremely low respiratory rates. Stimulation of the vomiting centre leads to prolonged nausea and vomiting in a proportion of patients.

Morphine and related drugs strongly inhibit gastric emptying and decrease intestinal motility. Gastric, pancreatic and biliary secretions are reduced. The effects on intestinal motility can result in marked constipation or may impair the absorption of orally administered drugs. Constipation is a particular problem in the management of terminal care patients receiving high oral doses of opioids. The tone in the anal and ileocolic sphincters and in the sphincter of Oddi is increased, and marked increases in biliary pressure may occur, even to the extent of causing biliary colic. Ureteric tone and contractions are increased, as is the tone of the detrusor muscle, which in association with increased tone of the vesicular sphincter occasionally causes difficulty in micturition. This is more marked when the drug is given intraspinally. Bronchoconstriction may follow large doses of morphine, but is rarely seen after therapeutic doses. All these effects on smooth muscle are less pronounced with pethidine. Further information can be gleaned from reviews of this field.[344-347]

Morphine and diamorphine (heroin) have little effect on cardiovascular haemodynamics, either in healthy individuals or following myocardial infarction. However, some postural hypotension may occur as a result of peripheral vasodilatation, and with morphine, transient hypotension may result from histamine release. On the other hand, pethidine in large doses can cause significant myocardial depression.

As is well known, morphine and its analogues are drugs of dependence, and although this is not a problem in short term treatment, such as in relief of postoperative pain, dependence and associated tolerance (which leads to a need for increasing doses), it becomes a serious problem in managing chronic pain. This should not, however, lead clinicians to be reluctant to prescribe adequate analgesia in terminal or cancer pain simply because of a misplaced fear of addiction.

***Diamorphine (heroin)*** is very rapidly hydrolysed to morphine in the plasma, so that it is essentially a prodrug. However, its high lipid solubility leads to more rapid absorption and onset of action. It is more potent than morphine (by 1.5-fold), but has a shorter duration of action and greater dependence potential.

***Pethidine (meperidine)*** [75 to 100mg ≡ morphine 10mg] is chemically a piperidine derivative, which produces smooth muscle relaxant activity to offset the smooth muscle stimulation of its opioid action. Thus, it has a specific place in management of pain associated with spasm (e.g. renal or biliary colic, acute pancreatitis) and in treating acute pain in patients with obstructive airways disease. It is also widely used for analgesia in labour, and is the most popular alternative to tranquillisers as a sedative premedicant. Pethidine has a shorter duration of action than morphine and is somewhat more toxic, causing more nausea, vomiting and hypotension.

***Methadone*** [10mg ≡ morphine 10 to 15mg] is a synthetic opioid chemically unrelated to morphine or pethidine. Metabolism is by *N*-demethylation in the liver, and since it is not conjugated, it may be useful in some patients with morphine-resistant pain. It has a long duration of action (up to 35 hours[348]), which can produce prolonged postoperative analgesia, but there is a danger of accumulation when repeated doses are given. Methadone is used to treat postoperative and chronic pain, and is also used in the management of opioid withdrawal (especially diamorphine) in addicts.

***Tramadol:*** this newer opioid agonist is a synthetic agent of the aminocyclohexanol class. It is reasonably well absorbed when given orally and its bioavailability after single doses is approximately 68% but this increases to 90 to 100% after multiple doses, possibly due to saturable first-pass hepatic metabolism. Tramadol is administered parenterally, orally or rectally. Following intravenous or intramuscular administration in patients with moderate to severe postoperative pain, tramadol has proved to be equivalent in analgesic potency to pethidine. Intravenous tramadol 50 to 150mg was also equivalent in analgesic effectiveness to morphine 5 to 15mg in patients with moderate pain following surgery. It appears to have a good tolerability profile in short term use, and evidence to date suggests that there is only a low incidence of respiratory depression.[337] It is probably best not used as part of a balanced anaesthetic technique, since some (though not all) studies have suggested an increased risk of awareness.[349,350]

#### Fentanyl and Related Drugs

***Fentanyl*** and its derivatives are phenylpiperidines structurally similar to pethidine. At the μ-receptor, fentanyl is 2 to 5 times as potent as morphine, yet clinically it is 60 to 80 times as potent on a milligram basis. This is due to its high lipid solubility, which allows rapid access across the blood-brain barrier. Fentanyl has a rapid onset of action, and when administered in small doses, has a short duration of action of around 20 to 30 minutes, due to rapid redistribution. However, at larger doses, it becomes a long-acting drug as its elimination is relatively slow with a terminal elimination phase half-life of about 4 hours. Cardiovascular stability is excellent, especially as histamine release is minimal, and this group of drugs is used widely in cardiac anaesthesia.

Their adverse effects are similar to those of morphine. Muscle rigidity may follow rapid administration. This is a central effect of opioids and is presumably seen with fentanyl derivatives because of the rapidity of their penetration of the CNS.

Fentanyl has been shown to diffuse across the oral mucosa and an oral transmucosal formulation (a 'fentanyl lollipop') has been assessed for premedication in children. It provides good sedation, although there can be a significant incidence of nausea or vomiting, and some respiratory depression.[159] Delivery of fentanyl by the transdermal route is also under investigation,[351] but is unlikely to be useful as a sole analgesic method (see also section 7.2.1).[352]

***Alfentanil*** is some 40 to 75 times less potent than fentanyl,[353] but its main distinction lies in its very short duration of action. A pKa of 6.8 means that it is 89% non-ionised (as compared with 9% for fentanyl), and this combined with a moderate lipid solubility and small volume of distribution leads to very rapid receptor occupancy. As well as having a rapid onset of action, alfentanil has a short duration of action, due to both rapid redistribution and elimination (plasma half-life 1.5 hours). A single bolus dose of alfentanil will provide intense but short-lived analgesia, which may be appropriate for extremely short procedures (e.g. day surgery). For longer operations, doses must be repeated at frequent intervals, and infusion is the logical means of administration. It is used in this way in cardiac surgery, and alfentanil infusion is particularly appropriate for short term sedation in the ICU.[354]

***Sufentanil*** is the most potent member of this group currently available. It is 8 to 10 times more potent than fentanyl, and has extremely high affinity for the μ-receptor. Both its pharmacokinetics and clinical effects are intermediate between fentanyl and alfentanil.[355]

**Table XV.** Time for plasma concentrations of fentanyl and related opioids to decrease by 50% after infusions of different durations. Values are derived from computer simulations using the program PK-SIM (Specialized Data Systems, Jenkintown, USA) [modified from Bovill, personal communication]

| Infusion duration (min) | Half-time (min) | | | |
|---|---|---|---|---|
| | fentanyl | sufentanil | alfentanil | remifentanil |
| 60 | 20 | 20 | 33 | 5.4 |
| 120 | 39 | 28 | 50 | 5.4 |
| 360 | 230 | 43 | 60 | 5.4 |

Haemodynamic stability during major surgery is excellent, and sufentanil has achieved popularity, especially in cardiac and neurosurgery.

***Remifentanil*** is a new μ-agonist opioid with similar potency to fentanyl. It is structurally unique among the opioids in having an ester linkage, so that it is rapidly metabolised by non-specific plasma and tissue esterases in the same way as the β-blocker esmolol. It has an elimination half-life of around 10 minutes, and unlike other opioids, this does not increase even after constant infusion of up to 3 [356]hours.

It is useful to compare the pharmacokinetic behaviour of fentanyl, sufentanil, alfentanil and remifentanil as they change between bolus administration and infusions of increasing duration. Alfentanil has a very rapid onset of action, the half-life for equilibration between plasma and site of effect being 1.5 minutes, compared to 5 to 6 minutes for fentanyl or sufentanil.[357] This is accompanied by rapid recovery as it is redistributed to the central compartment. However, after an infusion as short as 10 minutes, this difference is lost and there is no real difference in recovery from the 3 drugs over the next 90 minutes. After longer infusions, recovery from sufentanil becomes more rapid than from either fentanyl or alfentanil – this is the 'context-sensitive half-time' (table XV).[358] These differences cannot be predicted by simply considering figures for plasma half-lives, but become apparent using computer simulations that take into account all the intercompartmental movements involved.

### Opioid Partial Agonist Drugs

***Buprenorphine*** is a partial agonist at the μ-receptor.[335] It also binds to δ- and κ-receptors, and has some antagonist activity.[359] A very high affinity for the μ-receptor and slow dissociation from this, rather than pharmacokinetic factors, probably accounts for its prolonged duration of action compared with morphine. Antagonism of its respiratory depressant effect by naloxone is incomplete, although a noncompetitive respiratory stimulant such as doxapram can be used for this purpose. An infusion of doxapram is preferable to a single dose, in view of the prolonged action of buprenorphine. High binding affinity can also mean that doxapram will deny receptor access to a full agonist drug, thus reducing its analgesic effect.

Buprenorphine 0.3 to 0.6mg given parenterally is equivalent to morphine 10 to 15mg, but being a partial agonist, its action reaches a plateau at around 0.6 to 1.2mg in adults. It is, thus, about 30 times more potent than morphine at these doses, but like other partial agonists, efficacy in treating more severe pain in inadequate. The bioavailability of buprenorphine following oral administration is low, due to significant hepatic first-pass metabolism. However, it has been made available in a preparation for *sublingual administration*, and when given in this way it is reasonably well absorbed, with bioavailability averaging around 55%.[360]

***Propiram:*** this newer partial agonist drug shows relatively specific activity for the μ-receptor and is inactive at δ-receptors. Unlike buprenorphine, absorption of propiram following oral administration is virtually complete, and its bioavailability after oral doses of 25 to 100mg is >97%. The onset of action of propiram appears rapid, and it has proved an effective analgesic in moderate to severe postoperative pain when administered orally, its effect in doses of 50 to 100mg being comparable to that of standard doses of other orally administered opioids, e.g. pentazocine and pethidine.[336]

### Opioid Agonist-Antagonist Drugs

The opioid agonist-antagonists are a heterogeneous group of drugs, in that they act at different receptors.

***Pentazocine*** and ***nalbuphine*** are partial agonists at the κ-receptor and antagonists at the μ-receptor. For moderate pain, pentazocine 30 to 60mg or nalbuphine 10 to 15mg are equipotent to morphine 10mg, but there is a relatively low ceiling to both their analgesic and respiratory depressant effects. They also act at the σ-receptor (not an opioid receptor) to produce dysphoric and occasionally hallucinogenic effects. Dysphoria and emetic adverse effects may be fewer with nalbuphine.

Nalbuphine has a place in management of myocardial infarction, but pentazocine is contraindicated as it can cause an increase in pulmonary artery pressure and an increase in left ventricular workload. Nalbuphine has also been used to antagonise respiratory depression caused by pure opioid antagonists such as fentanyl, and may avoid the problems sometimes encountered with complete reversal of opioid action by naloxone.[361]

***Butorphanol:*** like pentazocine and nalbuphine, this agent also has agonist activity at the κ-receptor and antagonist activity at the μ-receptor. Its analgesic potency following intramuscular or intravenous administration is 4 to 8 times that of morphine, 30 to 40 times that of pethidine and 16 to 24 times that of pentazocine, and it has proved useful in relieving moderate to severe postoperative pain, primarily after abdominal or orthopaedic surgery. Initially, butorphanol was formulated only for parenteral administration as significant first-pass metabolism occurs after oral administration. Recently, however, absorption via the nasal mucosa has been demonstrated, and a *transnasal formulation* has been found to provide analgesia comparable to that of intramuscular pethidine in postsurgical pain, and comparable to or greater than that of intramuscular methadone in migraine headache.[362] The tolerability of transnasal butorphanol appears to parallel that of the injectable form.

***Dezocine:*** this newer agonist-antagonist agent has broad structural similarities to pentazocine, and has an analgesic potency equivalent to that of morphine. Following parenteral administration, it has proved at least as effective an analgesic as morphine, pethidine and butorphanol in moderate to severe postoperative pain.[363]

#### Opioid Antagonists

The *N*-allyl opioid derivatives *nalorphine* and *levallorphan*, which have an agonist-antagonist profile, have been used for many years to antagonise overdosage of opioids.

***Naloxone***, the *N*-allyl derivative of oxymorphone, is more potent than either nalorphine or levallorphan and longer lasting than the latter. Unlike these drugs, it is a pure antagonist, with no intrinsic agonist activity. As well as respiratory depression, it will also antagonise other opioid effects, including analgesia. Thus, it is best titrated in small doses to avoid the danger of sudden arousal of the patient into a painful awareness, and to obtain a suitable balance between reversal of ventilatory depression and maintenance of analgesia. On rare occasions, there have been problems associated with sudden reversal, including pulmonary oedema or cardiac arrest.[364,365] This may be due to the release of sudden intense sympathetic activity. Alternatives to naloxone include the nonspecific respiratory stimulant doxapram, which will not antagonise analgesia, and mixed agonist-antagonists such as nalbuphine.[366]

***Naltrexone***, a newer opioid antagonist, has a longer duration of action than naloxone. It is more potent in blocking μ- than κ-receptor activity.[367] Naltrexone is rapidly absorbed after oral administration but undergoes substantial first-pass metabolism, so that its oral bioavailability is around 20%. Plasma concentrations decrease slowly (initial half-life 10.3 hours, terminal elimination half-life 96 hours), and its major metabolite, naltrexol, may also contribute to its long duration of action. This metabolite is a weaker antagonist than its parent, but is present in the plasma in higher concentrations.[360] Naltrexone is used in long term treatment of addiction to diamorphine (heroin) and other opioids, and appears to be a useful adjunct in patients who are well motivated and have strong psychological support systems available. Like naloxone, it is also used as an investigational drug in opioid receptor research, and has shown promise in both investigating and treating conditions that may involve abnormalities of opioid pathways, such as Gilles de la Tourette's syndrome[368] or self-injurious behaviour.

#### 'Spinal' Opioids

The substantia gelatinosa in the dorsal horn of the spinal cord contains opioid receptors that modulate pain pathways, so that administration of opioid drugs either epidurally or intrathecally should have a selective effect. In practice, excellent analgesia can be achieved with relatively small doses of opioids given in this way. For example, equivalent analgesic doses of morphine are: systemic 10 to 15mg, epidural 2 to 4mg, and intrathecal 0.06 to 0.12mg.[369]

The relevant pharmacokinetics of these intraspinal routes differ from those of systemic administration. Opioids are absorbed from the epidural space into the circulation as rapidly as from intramuscular injection, and this contributes a central component to analgesia. About 1 to 2% of an epidural dose enters the cerebrospinal fluid.[370] Analgesia following morphine, which has relatively low lipid solubility, lasts for 12 to 18 hours after a single dose (depending on dose and intensity of pain), but is much shorter for more lipid soluble drugs such as fentanyl, which have a faster onset of action and are removed more rapidly from the site of action and from cerebrospinal fluid. A consequence of this is that delayed respiratory depression, due to circulation of drug through cerebrospinal fluid to reach the brain, is more common with morphine. The risk of late respiratory depression, which can occur 3 to 12 hours after administration, is the main limiting factor in clinical use of the intraspinal route for opioids.

Other adverse effects not unique to intraspinal use but which are more severe than with systemic use are pruritus, urinary retention, and nausea. The incidence of clinically important respiratory depression is approximately 1 in 1100 patients after epidural administration and 1 in 275 patients after intraspinal morphine,[371] but is much lower with more lipophilic drugs such as diamorphine, fentanyl, sufentanil or alfentanil. Thus, patients must be nursed in a ward where this complication will be detected.

Morphine and fentanyl are the most commonly used drugs, but many others are effective, differences being related mainly to their lipid solubility. While a lack of sympathetic blockade is seen as an advantage over local anaesthetics, the latter are now often given in combination with opioids, reducing the dosage of both in the hope of reducing the adverse effects of each.[372] The risk of adverse effects may also be lower when an infusion rather than a bolus dose is used. There is evidence that fentanyl gives equally good analgesia with a lower total dose if patient-controlled administration is used.[373]

#### Mild Opioid Analgesics

Some of the less potent compounds related to morphine (codeine, dihydrocodeine, etc.) may be used in the treatment of less severe pain. However, most drugs used for this purpose (e.g. aspirin, paracetamol) are unrelated to the opioids (table XVI).

***Codeine***, a naturally occurring constituent of opium, shares the characteristic pharmacological properties of morphine. It has a low affinity for opioid receptors which leads to low potency (about one-sixth that of morphine). It is relatively more effective when administered orally than when given parenterally. This is partly because methylation at the C3 position protects it from rapid conjugation, but also because about 10% of an oral dose is demethylated to norcodeine and to morphine, which may contribute to its analgesic effect. Codeine has a plasma elimination half-life of 2.5 to 3 hours.[374]

The combination of codeine with aspirin or paracetamol has a synergistic analgesic effect. Codeine is particularly valuable for pain associated with coughing, as it has an antitussive effect. Its main adverse effects are nausea and sometimes vomiting, dizziness, drowsiness, and constipation (it can be used to treat diarrhoea).

***Dihydrocodeine*** is a semisynthetic derivative of codeine, which is more potent (30mg ≡ morphine 10mg), and may be of use in management of moderately severe chronic pain, although stubborn constipation is often a problem. Other adverse effects are similar to but relatively greater than those seen with codeine.

***Dextropropoxyphene*** is chemically related to methadone. It is still a widely prescribed mild analgesic, often given in combination with paracetamol. It is a drug of primary abuse,[375] and a common cause of death in cases of drug overdosage.[376] Overdosage of combinations of dextropropoxyphene and paracetamol are particularly dangerous; respiratory failure and convulsions may occur early from the dextropropoxyphene component followed later by hepatic failure from paracetamol.[377]

### *7.1.2 Aspirin and Other Nonsteroidal Anti-Inflammatory Drugs (NSAIDs)*

The prototype of the NSAID drugs is *aspirin*. The analgesic, antipyretic and anti-inflammatory actions of the NSAIDs have all been attributed to inhibition of prostaglandin synthesis.[378] However, this mechanism may not underlie all their actions. There is now good evidence that inhibition of white cell adhesion by blocking G-protein mediated signal transduction is the action underlying the anti-inflammatory effect of NSAIDs, and there are probably several other mechanisms by which signal transduction at the cell membrane is altered.[379]

The NSAIDs belong to several distinct chemical classes (see further chapter 25; sect. 3.1.2) with no obvious structural similarity between them and, thus, they cannot all be expected to

**Table XVI.** Properties and principal uses of the mild analgesics

| Drug | Usual oral dosage (mg)[a] | Principal indications[b] | Main adverse effects and interactions[c] | Dependence liability |
|---|---|---|---|---|
| **Peripherally acting** | | | | |
| Aspirin (acetylsalicylic acid)[d] | 300-600 | Continuous aching pain<br>Acute pain of bone, joint trauma, tissue inflammation | Gastric irritation, haemorrhage; ?nephropathy (long term abuse)<br>Inhibits platelet aggregation (see chapter 26, sect. 3.1.1) | Nil |
| Paracetamol[d] (acetaminophen) | 500-1000 | Pain, fever in children; alternative to aspirin | Hepatic necrosis in overdosage | Nil |
| **Centrally acting** | | | | |
| Codeine | 30-60 | Visceral pain, cough with pain; synergistic with aspirin, paracetamol | Constipation, dizziness, nausea, vomiting | Low (morphine-like) |
| Dihydrocodeine | 30-60 | Moderately severe chronic pain | As for codeine (? better tolerated) | Low (morphine-like) |
| Dextropropoxyphene | 65-100 | Visceral pain | Dizziness, nausea, vomiting, skin rash; in overdosage coma, convulsions, respiratory depression | Low (morphine-like) |
| Flupirtine[d,e] | 100-200 | Moderately severe acute pain; chronic pain of musculoskeletal origin (short term use) | Drowsiness, dizziness, dry mouth, GI upset | ? Nil |
| Nefopam[d] | 30-60 | Moderately severe acute and chronic pain | Nausea, dizziness, dry mouth, sedation | ? Nil |

a See chapter 3 (table VII) for dosages in infants and children.
b Indications given are those where drugs are generally first choices (see also section 7.2).
c Refer also to sections 7.1.1, 7.1.2, 7.1.3 and chapter 7, section 2 and appendix B.
d Non-opioid agent.
e Flupirtine also produces muscle relaxant activity (possibly mediated via GABA-ergic mechanisms).

have the same range or ratio of effects. They are sometimes termed mild analgesics, but this does not imply that they have no role in more severe pain. Indeed, some acute conditions, particularly those involving tissue inflammation or bone and joint trauma, may produce extremely severe pain that responds well to these drugs. In the management of postoperative pain, the NSAIDs have recently enjoyed a resurgence of popularity, either used alone or in combination with opioid analgesics and local anaesthetics, although they have adverse effects that suggest caution if used in surgical patients.

The main benefits of NSAIDs derive from their opioid-sparing effect (e.g. reduction in perioperative nausea and vomiting and improvement in ventilation), although there may be an enhanced quality of analgesia from the combination compared with either NSAID or opioid alone.[380] The majority of their adverse effects are related to prostaglandin inhibition and include gastrointestinal irritation, which may occasionally result in profuse bleeding. However, cumulative data from controlled studies of perioperative treatment with NSAIDs do not suggest an increased risk of gastroduodenal complications such as bleeding or perforation in the first 7 days.[381]

Inhibition of platelet adhesiveness may exacerbate haemorrhagic problems, but this property has a major therapeutic potential in prevention of cardiovascular disease. Aspirin with its acetyl group causes irreversible platelet inactivation because it acetylates prostaglandin synthetase, while others inhibit prostaglandins reversibly. However, in patients with normal haemostatic function prior to NSAID administration, almost all indices of coagulation remain within the normal range after NSAID treatment, and most studies of perioperative blood loss have reported no significant effect of NSAIDs.[382]

Renal function may be compromised acutely by NSAIDs. Patients who are 'stressed' by hypovolaemia, cardiac or hepatic failure, or surgery, have an active renin-angiotensin system and increased vasoconstrictor hormone activity. This effect on renal circulation is opposed by locally produced vasodilator prostaglandins which maintain renal perfusion, but may be inhibited by NSAIDs. Although renal blood flow is temporarily reduced in normovolaemic patients during surgery, renal insufficiency is likely to occur only in patients who are hypovolaemic, septic or have coexisting disease.

#### Aspirin

In usual therapeutic doses, aspirin has no significant effect on the circulation or respiration. Overdosage, however, is characterised by hyperventilation and respiratory alkalosis, and later by metabolic acidosis, which is seen particularly in children with fever and dehydration. A few patients are allergic to aspirin, and aspirin-induced asthma is a potentially lethal complication. Prostaglandin $F_{2\alpha}$ may be implicated in development of bronchospasm in aspirin sensitive asthmatics.[383] Aspirin is contraindicated in small children because of a causal link with Reye's syndrome.

#### Other NSAIDs

Of the very large number of NSAIDs available, only those that have been widely used for management of perioperative pain are described here. Of these, currently the two most popular are diclofenac and ketorolac. Both of these drugs are members of the acetic acid group of NSAIDs.

***Diclofenac*** has been used widely for postoperative pain,[384] either as the main analgesic after minor surgery, or to supplement opioids in more major procedures. Diclofenac may be given rectally (100mg), intramuscularly (75mg) or intravenously (75mg), though it is not licensed for intravenous use in all countries, and intramuscular use can cause sterile abscesses. Absorption of diclofenac after intramuscular or rectal use is rapid, with peak plasma concentrations reached in about 90 minutes, and it is eliminated with a half-life of $< 2$ hours.

Although study results differ, diclofenac 75mg will generally reduce morphine requirements by about 10mg in the first 24 hours after operation.[385] After tonsillectomy, rectal diclofenac has been found to be equally effective as pethidine.[386] It is commonly used for day-surgery procedures, as it causes fewer adverse effects such as sedation and emesis than the opioids.

The adverse effects of diclofenac are similar to those of NSAIDs in general. Although it has an antiplatelet effect and may produce increased skin bleeding times,[387] this has not been found to cause significant problems. Diclofenac causes temporary deterioration in renal function during major surgery[388] accompanied by a reduction in renal blood flow, and as with other NSAIDs, it is best avoided in patients with renal failure.

***Ketorolac*** (as the tromethamine salt) is available for use orally, intramuscularly or intravenously. When given orally, ketorolac is absorbed rapidly (peak plasma concentrations reached in about 45 minutes) and virtually completely (bioavailability 80 to 100%). It is mainly eliminated by metabolic conjugation and renal excretion, with a terminal elimination half-life of 4 to 6 hours.[389,390]

The analgesic efficacy of ketorolac in treating postoperative pain has been at least as good as with diclofenac. However, most studies have used a dose of 30mg, and this has been associated with serious adverse effects including gastrointestinal bleeding and renal impairment. In some countries, this has resulted in a warning by regulatory authorities and a reduction in the recommended parenteral starting dose to 10mg. Contraindications to its use[391] include a history of conditions that may involve bleeding, such as peptic ulceration, gastrointestinal bleeding, haemorrhagic diathesis, cerebrovascular bleeding (confirmed or suspected), operations involving a high risk of haemorrhage, or the use of anticoagulants or other NSAIDs. In addition, pregnant women, patients with asthma, moderate or severe renal impairment, hypovolaemia, dehydration or hypersensitivity to NSAIDs should not be given ketorolac.

While these contraindications have been specified for ketorolac, the principles involved apply to use of any NSAID. Since both the analgesic efficacy of an NSAID and its adverse effect profile are related to effects on prostaglandin synthesis, more efficacious drugs are unfortunately also likely to have a worse safety profile,[392] although the relationship does not always hold.

### 7.1.3 Other Analgesics

#### Paracetamol (Acetaminophen)

Paracetamol also appears to cause analgesia by prostaglandin inhibition, but in contrast to aspirin, paracetamol-induced analgesia is centrally mediated.[393] It is also an effective antipyretic, but has little anti-inflammatory effect. Paracetamol has replaced aspirin for the treatment of mild pain in children. Gastrointestinal tolerability is better than for aspirin and, since paracetamol does not interfere with haemostasis, it is preferable to aspirin in patients with any bleeding tendency. Overdosage of paracetamol often leads to severe hepatic damage due to formation of a toxic metabolite (see further chapter 8; sect. 4.3.1).

#### Nefopam

Nefopam is a non-opioid benzoxazocine compound structurally related to the anti-Parkinsonian drug orphenadrine and the antihistamine diphenhydramine. It is effective by the oral and parenteral routes; oral administration of nefopam 30 to 60mg produces analgesia comparable to aspirin (60mg ≡ aspirin 600mg), dextropropoxyphene and pentazocine, while intramuscular (15 to 30mg) or intravenous (10 to 15mg) nefopam produces analgesia comparable to moderate doses of morphine, pethidine or pentazocine. However, at higher dose levels, morphine and pethidine are usually more effective. Nefopam does not have respiratory depressant effects and does not cause gastrointestinal blood loss. The most frequent adverse effects are nausea, dizziness and sedation.[394]

#### Flupirtine

Flupirtine is a non-opioid, centrally-acting analgesic with muscle relaxant properties (possibly mediated via GABA-ergic mechanisms). It is given orally and rectally, and has proved at least as effective as codeine, dihydrocodeine and pentazocine and the NSAIDs diclofenac, suprofen and ketoprofen in relieving pain due to surgery, traumatic injury, dental procedures, headache/migraine and abdominal spasm. Flupirtine has also proved as effective as pentazocine in short term studies in patients with muscular or neuralgiform pain, soft tissue rheumatism or cancer pain. In comparison with opioid drugs, flupirtine appears to produce fewer CNS effects, and no respiratory or cardiovascular depression. The most common adverse effects are drowsiness, dizziness, dry mouth and various gastrointestinal disturbances.[395]

## 7.2 Optimum Treatment of Pain

### *7.2.1 Acute Pain*

Where pain persists after treatment of the precipitating cause, symptomatic management is required, and analgesic drugs are commonly used. Each patient must be considered individually, rather than on the basis of a concept of the painfulness of the condition. Timing of analgesia may be important. Early treatment may have a pre-emptive effect, so that less pain is experienced and less analgesia required.[396]

In general, mild analgesics (see table XVI) will suffice for lesser degrees of pain, whereas for more severe pain, strong analgesics (see table XIV) will be required, or a combination of approaches may be employed.

#### Routes and Regimens of Administration

The oral route is commonly used for mild analgesics, but oral opioid analgesics are not often employed for acute pain relief, although sustained-release morphine tablets have had a limited use for this purpose (but are probably more effective as a 'second day' analgesic, i.e. used when the degree of pain has become less acute and the patient is able to take oral preparations). Use of sublingual or transnasal formulations avoids the first-pass effect and sublingual buprenorphine or transnasal butorphanol could be considered.

Opioid drugs are traditionally given according to a fixed dosage schedule and by intramuscular injection. Although this can be adjusted according to the patient's age, bodyweight, etc., and to allow for the known pharmacokinetic parameters of the drug used, there is still at least a 4-fold interindividual variation in analgesic requirements between patients, which cannot be anticipated. More individual treatment may be achieved by using the intravenous route.

A constant-rate intravenous infusion can produce relatively steady plasma concentrations of analgesic drugs, but interindividual differences in needs are still a problem. A loading dose can be titrated to achieve a suitable balance of analgesia and adverse effects, either to treat an acute pain episode such as renal colic, or to achieve adequate postoperative pain relief. Following this, a low-dose constant infusion may be suitable in some patients, especially children,[397] provided that adequate supervision is available. Incremental intravenous boluses will be needed in most, to individualise the analgesic regimen. This may be undertaken by a nurse in an ICU, but is more commonly administered by use of a patient-controlled analgesia system.

***Patient-controlled analgesia*** (PCA) systems are available either as programmable electronic or disposable units. They allow the patient, at the press of a button, to administer intravenous increments of drug (within the limits set by the clinician). Programmable units also allow bolus doses to be given together with a background steady-rate infusion if desired, although there now seems to be little advantage to this background dosage.[398,399] PCA systems provide more adequate analgesia than intermittent intramuscular injections postoperatively. However, good analgesia administered by either method may be at the expense of more frequent episodes of low oxygen saturation,[400] especially during sleep, and continued oxygen administration is desirable.

***Transdermal fentanyl*** administration is an alternative way of providing a 'background' level of analgesia, and has received limited approval by the FDA for use in cancer pain, but is as yet unsuitable for acute pain.[401] The patches which have been tested have all shown great interindividual variation in fentanyl absorption rates and plasma concentrations.[402] This results in a significant risk of respiratory depression, and there have been patient deaths. Therefore, the FDA has not approved the use of transdermal fentanyl in the treatment of acute and postoperative pain.

***Local anaesthetic techniques*** are being increasingly used as part of a combined approach to pain relief. Extradural block using local anaesthetics is often the most effective means of providing postoperative pain relief, but the danger of adverse effects, in particular hypotension from an extensive block, limits its use to patients who can be nursed in a high-dependency environment. It is especially useful following thoracic and upper abdominal surgery, in patients with respiratory diseases and in the management of chest injuries. Extradural or intrathecal use of morphine, fentanyl or other opioids (table XVII) can give excellent and long lasting analgesia.[403,404] However, use of these routes is limited by the danger of delayed onset of respiratory depression.[405] This is less with more lipid soluble drugs such as fentanyl. Longer-lasting pain relief can be provided in some cases, e.g. in thoracotomy, by cryotherapy to intercostal nerves, but there is a 10% incidence of analgesia dolorosa occurring some 6 months later, which is difficult to manage.

***Inhalational analgesia:*** this route is used widely in obstetrics, and is also suitable for procedures such as burns dressings. While volatile agents have been used, the most commonly used drug is nitrous oxide. In obstetric practice, this is in a 50% mixture with oxygen and self-administered, while in dental practice, a maximum of 25% is used for 'relative analgesia'.

### *7.2.2 Chronic Pain*

Chronic pain management is often complex, and requires attention to both physical and psychological factors, so that a multidisciplinary team approach is often appropriate.

Pain may be chronic because the cause persists, but also changes may occur in the nervous system both peripherally and centrally, leading to hyperalgesia at the site of injury as well as pain referred to or hyperalgesia in other sites. There are many patterns and causes of such pathological pain, and many pharmacological and other approaches to management. Cancer pain is one of the most common problems, and this section deals mainly with the pharmacological aspects of *terminal cancer pain*.[406]

#### General Measures

These include attention to comfort, explanation, good nursing, and drug treatment of distressing accompaniments such as vomiting, constipation, etc.

#### Analgesic Drugs

Analgesic drugs should preferably be given orally and in adequate dosage. A common failure is the clinician's unwillingness to use adequate doses of opioid drugs, which are the mainstay of management of severe pain and, in particular, pain of malignant origin. The concept of an analgesic ladder, starting with mild analgesics and moving progressively to the more potent drugs, is important. While the mild analgesics are unlikely to be adequate for any length of time, NSAIDs often have a place in combination with opioids, especially when secondary bony metastases occur. Drug therapy should be administered on a regular basis and the next dose given before the last has worn off.

***Morphine*** may be administered by several routes, and is the opioid of choice in most cases. Oral sustained-release morphine (with appropriate concomitant laxative treatment) is used to give a background level of pain relief, with increasing doses if tolerance develops. The bioavailability of sustained-release morphine tablets is adequate, since the proportion lost to first-pass metabolism does not increase with increasing dosages.[407] Use of other opioids such as methadone, dipipanone, etc. has probably decreased, but these drugs are possible alternatives to morphine. Breakthrough pain can be managed with more rapidly acting preparations, such as morphine solution, diamorphine (heroin) elixir, or transmucosal fentanyl.[408] In more severe pain, and in late terminal care, other systemic routes are used, including subcutaneous and intravenous infusion.

**Table XVII.** Suggested intraspinal dose ranges for some opioids

| Drug | Extradural bolus | Extradural infusion | Intrathecal dose |
|---|---|---|---|
| Morphine | 2-5mg | 0.5-2 mg/kg/h | 0.2-0.5mg |
| Diamorphine (heroin) | 1-5mg | 0.4-0.8 mg/kg/h | 0.5-1mg |
| Pethidine | 25-50mg | | 0.1 mg/kg |
| Fentanyl | 1-2 μg/kg | 0.3-0.5 μg/kg/h | |
| Sufentanil | 0.1-0.2 μg/kg | 0.15-0.5 μg/kg/h | 0.1-0.2 μg/kg |
| Alfentanil | 15-30 μg/kg | 15-30 μg/kg/h | |

Intraspinal (epidural or intrathecal) opioids (table XVII) are used increasingly in specialised centres, and can give excellent analgesia with little central effect, but are invasive. Implantable devices may be used for administration.

Adverse effects of opioids include constipation, and nausea and vomiting. Antiemetic drugs are likely to be needed only in the early stages, perhaps because of the antiemetic effect of opioids on the vomiting centre.[409] Fixed-dose combinations with drugs such as phenothiazines (e.g. Brompton Hospital Cocktail) should be avoided and drug dosages adjusted independently.

Opioid drugs are addictive, but this is not a problem in terminal care. The use of long term opioid treatment in nonmalignant chronic pain is more debatable.

#### Nerve Blocks

An effective nerve block can often remove pain completely, whereas systemic drug therapy can only diminish it. However, it is not always possible to block the appropriate pain pathway, nor is it possible to block only pain without involving other modes of sensation. In some cases, the loss of sensation can be as distressing as the original pain.

*Local anaesthetic drugs* (see section 2.4) act only for a short time, but the patient often experiences pain relief even after the drugs have worn off, making them worth trying. More permanent blocks are achieved using substances that destroy nerves, such as *phenol* and *alcohol (ethanol)*. These are most successful when used intrathecally to block carefully chosen dorsal nerve roots. Any such procedure must only be undertaken after careful consideration of the anatomy of the pain, and the probable adverse effects of the block. Many pain clinicians now use invasive techniques less often than in the past. Lumbar sympathetic blockade for ischaemic limb pain, using a neurolytic solution, is less controversial and will help many patients for whom surgery is not an option.

#### Other Drugs

A number of drugs acting by other mechanisms have a place in the treatment of pathological pain states. Most do not have a clearly defined role, nor are the mechanisms of their analgesic action always clearly understood.

***Capsaicin***, derived from capsicum or peppers, is an irritant. However, repeated application desensitises the C-fibre nociceptors and blocks conduction in their axons. This may be of use in postherpetic neuralgia.

***Tricyclic antidepressants*** such as amitriptyline have an effect on centrally-mediated pain which is independent of their antidepressant effect.[410,411] This may be due to a selective noradrenergic mechanism. The tricyclic antidepressants also appear useful in the treatment of postherpetic neuralgia.[412]

***GABA agonists***, e.g. benzodiazepines: the anxiolytic effect of these drugs may be of use in certain patients. They also have a modulating action on central pain transmission, and a central muscle relaxant action. Other drugs with this ability include *baclofen* which is used mainly to treat spasticity in different conditions (see further chapter 29; sect. 8.1). Baclofen may be given orally, or in severe spasticity, by intraspinal injection or infusion. It also has some efficacy in the treatment of trigeminal neuralgia.

***Membrane stabilising drugs***, such as *mexiletine* or *lidocaine* which block sodium channels, are of use in some cases of neuropathic pain,[413] as are antiepileptics such as *carbamazepine* or *valproic acid*.

***Corticosteroids*** are useful for their anti-inflammatory effect in a number of chronically painful syndromes.

### 7.2.3 Obstetric Analgesia

Pain associated with childbirth differs from other types in that it is intermittent in type and increases in severity as labour progresses. The patient's background, emotional status and her pain threshold are important factors in the response it evokes, and this varies markedly. Consequently, some patients may give birth without requiring analgesia while others may find labour a very distressing experience.[414]

#### Opioid Analgesics

Labour is often managed using parenteral analgesics in the early stages, changing to inhalational analgesia as the time of delivery approaches. Opioids are usually given intramuscularly; intravenous administration may cause transient high plasma concentrations of the drug with resultant placental transmission of larger amounts to the fetus, while patient-controlled analgesia is not suited to the intermittent nature of the pain.

***Pethidine (meperidine)*** is the most widely used parenteral agent, and the average dose of 100mg may be repeated at 2-hourly intervals. However, if given late in labour, or in excessive amounts, depression of the neonate may occur (see chapter 2; sect. 7.1.1). Nausea and dizziness are the two most frequent adverse effects. Almost all the other potent opioid analgesic drugs have been used for obstetric analgesia, but none has been shown to possess clear advantages over pethidine. Pethidine concentrations in the neonate peak 2 to 3 hours after administration to the mother.[415]

If respiratory depression is induced by opioids in the neonate, naloxone may be administered.

#### Inhalational Analgesia

Premixed cylinders containing 50% nitrous oxide in oxygen are available in some countries. Nitrous oxide is available in a 50% mixture with oxygen ('Entonox') to provide analgesia during labour. Because it is relatively insoluble, uptake and excretion are rapid and it is therefore suitable for intermittent use, providing satisfactory pain relief in about 50% of mothers. It is used in management of both first and second stages of labour.

#### Extradural Analgesia

This is now used in approximately 22% of all deliveries in the UK.[416] It is indicated most in primiparous patients if a difficult labour is anticipated, in others who have such a history, or in pre-eclampsia and some other medical conditions. A successful epidural analgesic will completely remove the pain and effort of the second stage of labour. Extradural techniques require the services of a skilled anaesthetist and a 24-hour service can be both demanding and expensive.

***Bupivacaine*** has superseded the use of other local anaesthetics, mainly because of its longer duration of action and lack of tachyphylaxis. Use in a concentration of 0.5% is giving way gradually to lower strengths (0.375%), often combined with a small dose of fentanyl 50 to 70μg. After establishing analgesia, an infusion of a lower concentration of bupivacaine or a bupivacaine-fentanyl mixture will prolong analgesia. One regimen is 0.1 or 0.125% bupivacaine with or without fentanyl 1 μg/ml. Use of mixtures leads to lower bupivacaine requirements and a lower incidence of hypotension, with some hospitals now allowing patients to walk about during labour (with assistance). Although bupivacaine has relatively little effect on the fetus, it should be given in the lowest effective dose and concentration. Fetal acidosis favours increased drug ionisation and leads to ion trapping and increased concentrations of the drug in the fetal circulation, with an increased risk of CNS and cardiac toxicity.[417]

While the obstetrician can do much to relieve labour discomfort by the use of drugs, it should be remembered that antenatal training, sympathetic understanding and constant reassurance can do much to help the patient. The effect of labour and delivery on the disposition of drugs is discussed in chapter 18 (section 1.1.6).

### Further Reading


Nunn JF, Utting JE, Brown Jr BR, editors. General anaesthesia. 5th ed. London: Butterworth, 1989

Miller RD, editor. Anesthesia. 4th ed. New York: Churchill Livingstone, 1995

Nimmo WS, Rowbotham DJ, Smith G, editors. Anaesthesia. 2nd ed. London: Blackwell Scientific Publications, 1994


### References


1. Dripps RD. Objective analysis of a medical specialty: the anaesthesia survey. In: White, editor. Medical education and anaesthesia. Oxford: Blackwell, 1966: 1
2. Halsey MJ. Molecular interactions of anaesthetics with biological membranes. General Pharmacology 1992; 23: 1013-6
3. Tinker JH. Voices from the past - from ice crystals to fruit flies in the quest for a molecular mechanism of anaesthetic action [editorial]. Anesthesia and Analgesia 1993; 77: 1-3
4. Cook DR. Paediatric anaesthesia: pharmacological considerations. Drugs 1976; 12: 212
5. Eger EI, Bahlman SH, Munson ES. The effect of age on the rate of increase of alveolar anesthetic concentration. Anesthesiology 1971; 35: 365
6. Elliott RH, Strunin L. Hepatotoxicity of volatile anaesthetics. British Journal of Anaesthesia 1993; 70: 339-48
7. Dale O, Brown Jr BR. Clinical pharmacokinetics of the inhalational anaesthetics. Clinical Pharmacokinetics 1987; 12: 145-67
8. Hornbein TF, Eger II EI, Winter PM, et al. The minimal alveolar concentration of nitrous oxide in man. Anesthesia and Analgesia 1982; 61: 553-6

9. Deacon R, Lumb M, Perry J, et al. Inactivation of methionine synthase by nitrous oxide. European Journal of Biochemistry 1980; 104: 419-23
10. Royston BD, Nunn JF, Weinbren HF, et al. Rate of inactivation of human and rodent methionine synthase by nitrous oxide. Anesthesiology 1988; 48: 213-6
11. Morrow DH, Morrow AG. The effects of halothane on myocardial contractile force and vascular resistance. Anesthesiology 1961; 22: 537-41
12. Kaplan JA, Miller ED, Bailey DR. A comparative study of enflurane and halothane using systolic time intervals. Anesthesia and Analgesia 1976; 55: 263-8
13. Fee JPH, Black GW, Dundee JW, et al. A prospective study of liver enzyme and other changes following repeat administration of halothane and enflurane. British Journal of Anaesthesia 1979; 51: 1133
14. Neuberger JM, Williams R. Halothane anaesthesia and liver damage. British Medical Journal 1984; 289: 1136-9
15. Ray DC, Drummond GB. Halothane hepatitis. British Journal of Anaesthesia 1991; 67: 84-99
16. Kenna JG, Jones RM. A national database on hepatitis after exposure to inhaled anaesthetics. British Journal of Anaesthesia 1992; 69: 228-9
17. Neuberger JM. Halothane and hepatitis: incidence, predisposing factors and exposure guidelines. Drug Safety 1990; 5: 28-38
18. Merin RG. Physiology, pathophysiology and pharmacology of the coronary circulation with particular emphasis on anesthetics. Anaesthesiologie und Reanimation 1992; 17: 5-26
19. Gion H, Saidman LJ. The minimum alveolar concentration of enflurane in man. Anesthesiology 1971; 35: 361-4
20. Cohen EN. Toxicity of inhalational anaesthetics. British Journal of Anaesthesia 1978; 50: 665
21. Scheider DM, Klygis LM, Tsang TK, et al. Hepatic dysfunction after repeated isoflurane administration. Journal of Clinical Gastroenterology 1993; 17: 168-70
22. Stevens WC, Dolan WM, Gibbons RT, et al. Minimum alveolar concentration (MAC) of isoflurane with and without nitrous oxide in patients of various ages. Anesthesiology 1975; 42: 197-200
23. Priebe HJ. Coronary circulation and factors affecting coronary 'steal'. European Journal of Anaesthesiology 1991; 8: 177-95
24. Becker LC. Is isoflurane dangerous for the patient with coronary artery disease? (Editorial). Anesthesiology 1987; 66: 259-61
25. Spencer EM, Willats SM. Isoflurane for prolonged sedation in the intensive care unit; efficacy and safety. Intensive Care Medicine 1992; 18: 415-21
26. Sutton TS, Koblin DD, Gruenke LD, et al. Fluoride metabolites after prolonged exposure of volunteers and patients to desflurane. Anesthesia and Analgesia 1991; 73: 180-5
27. Rampil IJ, Lockhart SH, Zwass MS, et al. Clinical characteristics of desflurane in surgical patients: minimum alveolar concentration. Anesthesiology 1991; 74: 429-33
28. Mazze RI. The safety of sevoflurane in humans (editorial). Anesthesiology 1992; 77: 1062-3
29. Dundee JW, Wyant GM. Intravenous anaesthesia. 2nd ed. Edinburgh: Churchill Livingstone, 1986
30. Dundee JW, Zacharias M. Etomidate. In: Dundee JW, editor. Current topics in anaesthesia: intravenous anaesthetic agents. London: Arnold, 1979
31. Ghoneim MM, Chiang CK, Schoenwald RD, et al. The pharmacokinetics of methohexital in young and elderly subjects. Acta Anaesthesiologica Scandinavica 1985; 29: 480-2
32. Duvaldestin P. Pharmacokinetics in intravenous anaesthetic practice. Clinical Pharmacokinetics 1981; 6: 61
33. Davis PJ, Cook DR. Clinical pharmacokinetics of the newer intravenous anaesthetics. Clinical Pharmacokinetics 1986; 11: 18
34. Gepts E, Camu F. Pharmacokinetics of intravenous induction agents. Baillieres Clinical Anaesthesiology 1991; 5: 513-42
35. Burch PG, Stanski DR. The role of metabolism and protein binding in thiopental anesthesia. Anesthesiology 1983; 58: 146-52
36. Arden JR, Holley FO, Stanski DR. Increased sensitivity to etomidate in the elderly: initial distribution versus altered brain response. Anesthesiology 1986; 65: 19-27
37. Cockshott ID, Briggs LP, Douglas EJ, et al. Pharmacokinetics of propofol in female patients: studies using single bolus injection. British Journal of Anaesthesia 1987; 59: 1103-0
38. Carl P, Hogskilde S, Lang-Jensen T, et al. Pharmacokinetics and pharmacodynamics of eltanolone (pregnanolone) a new steroid intravenous anaesthetic in humans. Acta Anaesthesiologica Scandinavica 1994; 38: 734-41
39. Harrison GG, Moore MR, Meissner TM. Porphyrogenicity of etomidate and ketamine as continuous infusions: screening in the DDC-primed rat model. British Journal of Anaesthesia 1985; 57: 420
40. Parikh RK, Moore MR. Effect of certain anaesthetic agents on the activity of δ-aminolaevulinate synthase. British Journal of Anaesthesia 1978; 50: 1099
41. Clarke RSJ. Adverse effects of intravenously administered drugs used in anaesthetic practice. Drugs 1981; 22: 26
42. Whitwam JG. Adverse reactions to IV induction agents. British Journal of Anaesthesia 1978; 50: 677
43. Watkins J, Ward AM, editors. Adverse responses to intravenous drugs. London: Academic Press; New York: Grune and Stratton, 1978.
44. Ghoneim M, Spector R. Pharmacokinetics of drugs administered intravenously. In: Scurr C, Feldman S, editors. Scientific foundations of anaesthesia. 3rd ed. London: Heinemann Medical, 1982: 415-24
45. Breimer DD. Pharmacokinetics of methohexitone following intravenous infusion in humans. British Journal of Anaesthesia 1976; 48: 643
46. Dundee JW, Wyant GM. Etomidate. In: Dundee JW, editor. Intravenous anaesthesia. 2nd ed. London: Churchill Livingstone, 1988: 160-71
47. Heykants JJP, Meuldermans WES, Michiels LJM, et al. Distribution, metabolism and excretion of etomidate, a short-acting hypnotic drug in the rat. Archives Internationales Pharmacodynamie et de Therapie 1975; 216: 113
48. van Hamme MJ, Ghoneim MM, Ambre JJ. Pharmacokinetics of etomidate, a new intravenous anesthetic. Anesthesiology 1978; 49: 274-7
49. de Ruiter G, Popescu DT, De Boer AG. Pharmacokinetics of etomidate in surgical patients. Archives Internationales de Pharmacodynamie et de Therapie 1981; 249: 180-8
50. Choi SD, Spaulding BC, Gross JH, et al. Comparison of the ventilatory effects of etomidate and methohexitone. Anesthesiology 1985; 62: 442

51. Gooding JM, Corssen G. Effect of etomidate on the cardiovascular system. Anesthesia and Analgesia 1977; 56: 717
52. Ledingham IMcA, Watt I. Influence of sedation on mortality in critically ill multiple trauma patients. Lancet 1983; 1: 1270
53. Watkins J. Etomidate: an 'immunologically safe' anaesthetic agent. Anaesthesia 1983; 38 Suppl.: 34
54. Famewo CE. Induction of anaesthesia with etomidate in a patient with acute intermittent porphyria. Canadian Anaesthetists Society Journal 1985; 32: 171-3
55. Cummings DC, Dixon J, Kay NH, et al. Dose requirements of ICI 35,868 (propofol, 'Diprivan') in a new formulation for induction of anaesthesia. Anaesthesia 1984; 39: 1168
56. Cockshott ID. Propofol ('Diprivan') pharmacokinetics and metabolism - an overview. Postgraduate Medical Journal 1985; 61 Suppl. 3: 45
57. Phillips AS, McMurray TJ, Mirakhur RK, et al. Propofol-fentanyl anaesthesia in cardiac surgery: a comparison in patients with good and impaired ventricular function. Anaesthesia 1993; 48: 661-3
58. Langley MS, Heel RC. Propofol: a review of its pharmacodynamic and pharmacokinetic properties and use as an intravenous anaesthetic. Drugs 1988; 35: 334-72
59. Various authors. Anaesthesia 1988; Suppl. 43: 1-121.
60. Kallela H, Haasio J, Korttila K. Comparison of eltanolone and propofol in anesthesia for termination of pregnancy. Anesthesia and Analgesia 1994; 79: 512-6
61. Chang T, Glazko T. Biotransformation and distribution of ketamine. International Anesthesiology Clinics 1974; 12: 157
62. Grant IS, Nimmo SW, McNicol LR. Ketamine disposition in children and adults. British Journal of Anaesthesia 1983; 55: 1107
63. Lilburn JK, Dundee JW, Nair SG, et al. Ketamine sequelae: evaluation of the ability of various premedicants to attenuate its psychic actions. Anaesthesia 1978; 33: 307
64. Lilburn JK, Dundee JW, Moore J. Ketamine infusions: observations on technique, dosage and cardiovascular effects. Anaesthesia 1978; 33: 315
65. Brown SS, Dundee JW. Clinical studies of induction agents. XXXV: diazepam. British Journal of Anaesthesia 1968; 40: 108
66. Sjovall S, Kanto J, Himberg J-J, et al. CSF penetration and pharmacokinetics of midazolam. European Journal of Clinical Pharmacology 1983; 25: 247-51
67. Kanto J, Aaltonen L, Himberg J-J. Midazolam as an intravenous induction agent in the elderly: a clinical and pharmacokinetic study. Anesthesia and Analgesia 1986; 65: 15-20
68. Halliday NJ, Dundee JW, Loughran PG, et al. Age and plasma proteins influence the action of midazolam. Anesthesiology 1984; 61: A357
69. Harper KW, Lowry KG, Elliott P, et al. Age and nature of operation influence the pharmacokinetics of midazolam. British Journal of Anaesthesia 1985; 57: 866-71
70. Nilsson A. Pharmacokinetics of benzodiazepines and their antagonists. Baillieres Clinical Anaesthesiology 1991; 5: 615-34
71. Ghoneim MM, Korttila K. Pharmacokinetics of intravenous anaesthetics: implications for clinical use. Clinical Pharmacokinetics 1977; 2: 344
72. Mandelli M, Tognoni G, Garattini S. Clinical pharmacokinetics of diazepam. Clinical Pharmacokinetics 1978; 3: 72
73. Klotz U, Avant GR, Hoyumpa A, et al. The effects of age and liver disease on the disposition and elimination of diazepam in adult man. Journal of Clinical Investigation 1975; 55: 347
74. Gamble JAS, Dundee JW, Gray RC. Plasma diazepam concentrations following prolonged administration. British Journal of Anaesthesia 1976; 48: 1087
75. Gamble JAS, Dundee JW, Assaf RAE. Plasma diazepam levels after single dose oral and intramuscular administration. Anaesthesia 1975; 30: 164
76. Dundee JW, Halliday NJ, Harper KW, et al. Midazolam: a review of its pharmacological properties and therapeutic use. Drugs 1984; 28: 519
77. Vinik HR, Reves JG, Greenblatt DJ, et al. The pharmacokinetics of midazolam in chronic renal failure patients. Anesthesiology 1983; 59: 390
78. Gamble JAS, Moore J, Lamki H, et al. A study of plasma diazepam levels in mother and infant. British Journal of Obstetrics and Gynaecology 1977; 84: 588
79. Ameer B, Greenblatt DJ. Lorazepam: a review of its clinical pharmacological properties and therapeutic use. Drugs 1981; 21: 161
80. Mattila MAK, Larni HM. Flunitrazepam: a review of its pharmacological properties and therapeutic use. Drugs 1980; 20: 353
81. Brogden RN, Goa KL. Flumazenil: a preliminary review of its benzodiazepine antagonist properties, intrinsic activity and therapeutic use. Drugs 1988; 35: 448-67
82. Matteo RS, Ornstein E, Schwartz A, et al. Pharmacokinetics and pharmacodynamics of rocuronium (ORG 9426) in elderly surgical patients. Anesthesia and Analgesia 1993; 77: 1193-7
83. Bowman WC. Pharmacology of neuromuscular function. London: Wright-Butterworth, 1990
84. Foldes FF. The rational use of neuromuscular blocking agents: the role of pancuronium. Drugs 1972; 4: 153
85. Shanks CA. Pharmacokinetics of muscle relaxants and cholinesterase inhibitors. Baillieres Clinical Anaesthesiology 1991; 5: 567-91
86. Booij LHDJ. Pharmacokinetics of muscle relaxants. Baillieres Clinical Anaesthesiology 1994; 8: 349-67
87. Cook DR, Wingard LB, Taylor FH. Pharmacokinetics of succinylcholine in infants, children and adults. Clinical Pharmacology & Therapeutics 1976; 20: 493-8
88. Clarke RSJ, Fee JPH, Dundee JW. Factors predisposing to hypersensitivity reactions to intravenous anaesthetics. Proceedings of the Royal Society of Medicine 1977; 70: 782
89. Fisher MMcD. Anaphylactic reactions to gallamine triethiodide. Anaesthesia in Intensive Care 1978; 6: 62
90. Fisher MMcD, Hallowes R-C, Wilson RM. Anaphylaxis to alcuronium. Anaesthesia in Intensive Care 1978; 6: 125
91. Clarke RSJ, Mirakhur RK. Adverse effects of muscle relaxants. Advances in Drug Reactions and Toxicology Reviews 1994; 13: 23-41
92. Ali HH, Savarese JJ. Monitoring of neuromuscular function. Anesthesiology 1976; 45: 216
93. Miller RD, Sohn YJ, Matteo RS. Enhancement of d-tubocurarine neuromuscular blockade by diuretics in man. Anesthesiology 1976; 45: 442
94. Miller RD, Matteo RS, Benet LZ, et al. The pharmacokinetics of d-tubocurarine in man with and without

renal failure. Journal of Pharmacology and Experimental Therapeutics 1977; 202: 1

95. Bennett EJ, Ignancio A, Patel K, et al. Tubocurarine and the neonate. British Journal of Anaesthesia 1976; 48: 687
96. Speight TM, Avery GS. Pancuronium bromide: a review of its pharmacological properties and clinical application. Drugs 1972; 4: 163
97. Bodman RI. Pancuronium and histamine release. Canadian Anaesthetists Society Journal 1978; 25: 40
98. Miller RD, Stevens WC, Way WL. The effect of renal failure and hyperkalaemia on the duration of pancuronium neuromuscular blockade in man. Anesthesia and Analgesia 1972; 52: 661
99. Somogyi AH, Shanks CA, Triffs EI. The effect of renal failure on the disposition and neuromuscular blocking action of pancuronium bromide. European Journal of Clinical Pharmacology 1977; 12: 23
100. Duvaldestin P, Agoston S, Henzel D, et al. Pancuronium pharmacokinetics in patients with liver cirrhosis. British Journal of Anaesthesia 1978; 50: 1131
101. Booth PN, Watson MJ, McLeod K. Pancuronium and the placental barrier. Anaesthesia 1977; 32: 320
102. Duvaldestin P, Demetriou M, Henzen D, et al. The placental transfer of pancuronium and its pharmacokinetics during caesarean section. Acta Anaesthesiologica Scandinavica 1978; 22: 327
103. Laflin MJ. Interaction of pancuronium and corticosteroids. Anesthesiology 1977; 47: 471
104. Erkola O. Complications of neuromuscular blockers: interactions with concomitant medications and other neuromuscular blocks. Anesthesia Clinics of North America 1993; 11: 427-4
105. Faulds D, Clissold SP. Doxacurium: a review of its pharmacology and clinical potential in anaesthesia. Drugs 1991; 42: 673-89
106. Mirakhur RK. Newer neuromuscular blocking drugs: an overview of their clinical pharmacology and therapeutic use. Drugs 1992; 44: 182-99
107. Maddineni VR, Cooper AR, Stanley JC, et al. Clinical evaluation of doxacurium chloride. Anaesthesia 1992; 47: 554-7
108. Cook DR, Freeman JA, Lai AA, et al. Pharmacokinetics and pharmacodynamics of doxacurium in normal patients and in those with hepatic or renal failure. Anesthesia and Analgesia 1991; 72: 145-50
109. Stoops CM, Curtis CA, Kovach DA, et al. Haemodynamic effects of doxacurium chloride in patients receiving oxygen-sufentanil anaesthesia for coronary artery bypass grafting or valve replacement. Anesthesiology 1988; 69: 365-70
110. Emmott RS, Bracey BJ, Goldhill DR, et al. Cardiovascular effects of doxacurium, pancuronium and vecuronium in anaesthetised patients presenting for coronary artery bypass surgery. British Journal of Anaesthesia 1990; 65: 480-6
111. Searle NR, Sahab B, Blain R, et al. Haemodyamic and pharmacodynamic comparison of doxacurium and high dose vecuronium during coronary artery bypass surgery: a cost-benefit study. Journal of Cardiothoracic and Vascular Anesthesia 1994; 8: 490
112. Stanley JC, Carson IW, Gibson FM, et al. Comparison of the haemodynamic effects of pipecuronium and pancuronium during fentanyl anaesthesia. Acta Anaesthesiologica Scandinavica 1991; 35: 262-6
113. Ornstein E, Matteo RS, Schwartz AE, et al. Pharmacokinetics and pharmacodynamics of pipecuronium bromide (Arduan) in elderly surgical patients. Anaesthesia 1992; 74: 841-4
114. Stenlake JB, Waigh RD, Urwin J, et al. Atracurium: conception and inception. British Journal of Anaesthesia 1983; 55: 3S
115. Eager BM, Flynn PJ, Hughes R. Infusion of atracurium for long surgical procedures. British Journal of Anaesthesia 1984; 56: 447
116. Bowman WC, Rodger IW, Houston J, et al. Structure-action relationship among some desacetoxy analogs of pancuronium and vecuronium in the anesthetised cat. Anesthesiology 1988; 69: 57-62
117. Cooper AR, Mirakhur RK, Clarke RSJ, et al. Comparison of intubating conditions after administration of ORG 9426 (rocuronium) and suxamethonium. British Journal of Anaesthesia 1992; 69: 269-73
118. McCoy EP, Maddineni VR, Elliott P, et al. Haemodynamic effects of rocuronium during fentanyl anaesthesia: comparison with vecuronium. Canadian Journal of Anaesthesia 1993; 40: 703-8
119. Levy JH, Davis GK, Duggan J, et al. Determination of the haemodynamics and histamine release of rocuronium (ORG 9426) when administered in increased doses under N2O/O2-sufentanil anesthesia. Anesthesia and Analgesia 1994; 78: 318-21
120. Khuenl-Brady K, Castagnoli KP, Canfell PC, et al. The neuromuscular blocking effects and pharmacokinetics of ORG 9426 and ORG 9616 in the cat. Anesthesiology 1990; 72: 669-74
121. Wierda JMKH, Kleef UW, Lambalk LM, et al. The pharmacodynamics and pharmacokinetics of ORG 9426, a new nondepolarising neuromuscular blocking agents in patients anaesthetised with nitrous oxide/halothane. Canadian Journal of Anaesthesia 1991; 38: 430
122. Cooper AR, Maddineni VR, Mirakhur RK, et al. Time course of neuromuscular effects and pharmacokinetics of rocuronium bromide (ORG 9426) during isoflurane anaesthesia in patients with and without renal failure. British Journal of Anaesthesia 1993; 71: 222-6
123. Magorian T, Wood P, Caldwell J, et al. The pharmacokinetics and neuromuscular effects of rocuronium bromide in patients with liver disease. Anesthesia and Analgesia 1995; 80: 754-9
124. Various authors. Rocuronium bromide investigators' workshop. European Journal of Anaesthesiology 1994; 11 Suppl. 9: 1-140.
125. Lepage JY, Malinovsky JM, Malinge M, et al. Pharmacodynamics and histamine releasing potency of high dose of 51W89. Anesthesiology 1994; 81: A1077
126. Tullock W, Scott V, Smith DA, et al. Kinetics/dynamics of 51W89 in liver transplant patients and in healthy patients. Anesthesiology 1994; 81: A1076
127. Savarese JJ, Ali HH, Basta SJ, et al. The clinical neuromuscular pharmacology of mivacurium chloride (BW B1090U), a short acting nondepolarising ester neuromuscular blocking drug. Anesthesiology 1988; 68: 723-32
128. Maddineni VR, Mirakhur RK, McCoy EP. Recovery of mivacurium block with or without anticholinesterases following administration by continuous infusion. Anaesthesia 1994; 49: 946-8
129. Connolly FM, Mirakhur RK, Loan PB, et al. Antagonism of mivacurium block with edrophonium from various degrees of spontaneous recovery. British Journal of Anaesthesia 1995; 74: 229-30

130. Loan PB, Elliott P, Mirakhur RK, et al. Comparison of the haemodynamic effects of mivacurium and atracurium during fentanyl anaesthesia. British Journal of Anaesthesia 1995; 74: 330
131. Head-Rapson AG, Devlin JC, Parker CJ, et al. Pharmacokinetics of the three isomers of mivacurium and pharmacodynamics of the chiral mixture in hepatic cirrhosis. British Journal of Anaesthesia 1994; 73: 613-8
132. Maddineni VR, Mirakhur RK, McCoy EP, et al. Neuromuscular and haemodynamic effects of mivacurium in elderly and young adult patients. British Journal of Anaesthesia 1994; 73: 608-12
133. Frampton JE, McTavish D. Mivacurium: a review of its pharmacology and therapeutic potential in general anaesthesia. Drugs 1993; 45: 1066-89
134. Wierda JMKH, van den Broek L, Proost JH, et al. Time course of action and endotracheal intubating conditions of ORG 9487, a new short-acting steroidal muscle relaxant: a comparison with succinylcholine. Anesthesia and Analgesia 1993; 77: 579-84
135. Kalow WM, Gunn DR. Some statistical data on atypical cholinesterase of human serum. Annals of Human Genetics 1959; 23: 239
136. Lee-Son S, Pilon RN, Nahor A, et al. Use of succinylcholine in the presence of atypical cholinesterase. Anesthesiology 1975; 43: 239
137. Cook DR, Fischer CG. Neuromuscular blocking effects of succinylcholine in infants and children. Anesthesiology 1975; 42: 662
138. Drabkova J, Crul JF, Van der Kleigne. Placental transfer of 14C-labelled succinylcholine in near-term macaca malatta monkeys. British Journal of Anaesthesia 1973; 45: 1086-8
139. Bali IM, Dundee WJ, Doggart JR. The source of increased plasma potassium following succinylcholine. Anesthesia and Analgesia 1975; 54: 680
140. Gronert GA, Theye RA. Pathophysiology of hyperkalaemia induced by succinylcholine. Anesthesiology 1975; 43: 89
141. Cooperman LH. Succinylcholine-induced hyperkalaemia in neuromuscular disease. Journal of the American Medical Association 1970; 213: 1867
142. Mazze RI, Escue HM, Houston JB. Hyperkalaemia and cardiovascular collapse following administration of succinylcholine to the traumatised patient. Anesthesiology 1969; 32: 540
143. Mirakhur RK, McCarthy GJ. Basic pharmacology of reversal agents. Anesthesia Clinics of North America 1993; 11: 237-50
144. Mirakhur RK, Dundee JW, Jones CJ, et al. Reversal of neuromuscular blockade: dose determination studies with atropine and glycopyrrolate given before or in a mixture with neostigmine. Anesthesia and Analgesia 1981; 60: 557-62
145. Mirakhur RK. Antagonism of neuromuscular blockade. Baillieres Clinical Anaesthesiology 1994; 8: 461-81
146. Miller RD, Van Nyhuis LS, Eger II EI, et al. Comparative times to peak effect and durations of action of neostigmine and pyridostigmine. Anesthesiology 1974; 41: 27-33
147. Bevan DR. Reversal of pancuronium with edrophonium. Anaesthesia 1979; 34: 614-9
148. Kopman AF. Recovery times following edrophonium and neostigmine reversal of pancuronium, atracurium and vecuronium steady state infusions. Anesthesiology 1986; 65: 572-8
149. Sakuma N, Hasimoto Y, Iwatsuki M. The effects of neostigmine and edrophonium on human erythrocyte acetyl cholinesterase activity. British Journal of Anaesthesia 1992; 68: 316-7
150. McCoy EP, Mirakhur RK. Comparison of the effects of neostigmine and edrophonium on the duration of action of suxamethonium. Acta Anaesthesiologica Scandinavica 1995; 39: 744
151. Baraka A. Antagonism of neuromuscular block by physostigmine in man. British Journal of Anaesthesia 1978; 50: 1075-7
152. Brebner J, Hadley L. Experiences with physostigmine in the reversal of adverse post-anaesthetic effects. Canadian Anaesthetists Society Journal 1976; 23: 574
153. Egbert LD, Battit GE, Turndorff H, et al. The value of the preoperative visit by an anaesthetist. Journal of the American Medical Association 1963; 185: 553
154. Mirakhur RK. Preanaesthetic medication: a survey of current usage. Journal of the Royal Society of Medicine 1991; 84: 481-3
155. Raftery S, Warde D. Oxygen saturation during inhalation induction with halothane and isoflurane in children: effect of premedication with rectal thiopentone. British Journal of Anaesthesia 1990; 64: 167-9
156. Munoz HR, Dagnino JA, Rufs JA, et al. Benzodiazepine premedication causes hypoxemia during spinal anesthesia in geriatric patients. Regional Anesthesia 1992; 17: 139-42
157. Furness G, Boyle MM, Fee JPH. Temazepam elixir for premedication in paediatric ENT operations. British Journal of Anaesthesia 1986; 58: 811P
158. Morgan-Hughes JO, Bangham JA. Pre-induction behaviour of children: a review of placebo-controlled trials of sedatives. Anaesthesia 1990; 45: 427-35
159. Nelson PS, Streisand JB, Mulder SM, et al. Comparison of oral transmucosal fentanyl citrate and an oral solution of meperidine, diazepam, and atropine for premedication in children. Anesthesiology 1989; 70: 616-21
160. Loan W, Cuthbert D. Adverse cardiovascular response to trimeprazine in children. British Medical Journal 1985; 290: 1548-9
161. Chambers FA, O'Leary E, Gormley PK, et al. Delayed profound respiratory depression after premedication with trimeprazine. Anaesthesia 1992; 47: 585-6
162. Cozanitis DA, Dundee JW, Merrett JD, et al. Evaluation of glycopyrrolate and atropine as adjuncts to reversal of non-depolarising neuromuscular blocking agents in a 'true-to-life' situation. British Journal of Anaesthesia 1980; 52: 85
163. Maze M, Tranquillo W. Alpha-2 adrenoceptor agonists: defining their role in clinical anesthesia. Anesthesiology 1991; 74: 581-605
164. Ghignone M, Noe C, Calvillo O, et al. Anesthesia for ophthalmic surgery in the elderly: the effects of clonidine on intraocular pressure, operative hemodynamics and anesthetic requirement. Anesthesiology 1988; 68: 707-16
165. Flacke JW, Bloor BC, Flacke WE, et al. Reduced narcotic requirement by clonidine with improved hemodynamic and adrenergic stability in patients undergoing coronary bypass surgery. Anesthesiology 1987; 67: 11-9
166. Wright PMC, Carabine UA, McClune S, et al. Preanaesthetic medication with clonidine. British Journal of Anaesthesia 1990; 65: 628-32

167. Concepcion M, Arthur GR, Steele SM, et al. A new local anesthetic, ropivacaine: its epidural effects in humans. Anesthesia and Analgesia 1990; 70: 80-5
168. Akerman B, Hellberg IB, Trossvik C. Primary evaluation of the local anaesthetic properties of the amino amide agent ropivacaine (LEA 103). Acta Anaesthesiologica Scandinavica 1988; 32: 571-8
169. Covino BG. Pharmacology of local anaesthetics. British Journal of Anaesthesia 1986; 58: 701-16
170. Butterworth JF, Strichartz GR. Molecular mechanisms of local anesthesia: a review. Anesthesiology 1990; 72: 711-34
171. Tucker GT. Local anaesthetic drugs: mode of action and pharmacokinetics. In: Nimmo WS, Rowbotham DJ, Smith G, editors. Anaesthesia. 2nd ed. London: Blackwell, 1994
172. Hull CJ. The pharmacokinetics of opioid analgesics, with special reference to patient-controlled administration. In: Hamer M, Rosen M, Vickers MD, editors. Patient-controlled analgesia. Oxford: Blackwell Scientific Publications, 1985
173. Fink BR. Mechanisms of differential axial blockade in epidural and subarachnoid anesthesia. Anesthesiology 1989; 70: 851
174. Burm AGL. Clinical pharmacokinetics of epidural and spinal anaesthesia. Clinical Pharmacokinetics 1989; 16: 283-311
175. Moore RA, Bullingham RES, McQuay HJ, et al. Dural permeability to narcotics: in vitro determination and application to extradural administration. British Journal of Anaesthesia 1982; 54: 1117-28
176. Tucker GT, Mather LE. Pharmacokinetics of local anaesthetics. British Journal of Anaesthesia 1975; 47: 213-4
177. Seifen AB, Ferrari AA, Seifen AA, et al. Pharmacokinetics of intravenous procaine infusion in humans. Anesthesia and Analgesia 1979; 58: 382-86
178. Assem ES, Punnia-Moorthy A. Allergy to local anaesthetics: an approach to definitive diagnosis: a review with an illustrative study. British Dental Journal 1988; 164: 44-7
179. McCaughey W. Adverse effects of local anaesthetics. Drug Safety 1992; 7: 178-89
180. Stone WE, Javid MJ. Anticonvulsive and convulsive effects of lidocaine: comparison with those of phenytoin, and implications for mechanism of action concepts. Neurological Research 1988; 10: 161-8
181. Moller R, Covino D. Cardiac electrophysiological effects of lidocaine and bupivacaine. Anesthesia and Analgesia 1988; 67: 107-14
182. Reynolds F. Adverse effects of local anaesthetics. British Journal of Anaesthesia 1987; 59: 78-95
183. Albright GA. Cardiac arrest following regional anesthesia with etidocaine or bupivacaine. Anesthesiology 1979; 51: 285
184. Writer WDR, Davies JM, Strunin L. Trial by media: the bupivacaine story. Canadian Anaesthetists Society Journal 1984; 31: 1
185. Katz JA, Bridenbaugh PO, Knarr DC, et al. Pharmacodynamics and pharmacokinetics of epidural ropivacaine in humans. Anesthesia and Analgesia 1990; 70: 16-21
186. Buckley MM, Benfield P. Eutectic lidocaine/prilocaine cream: a review of the topical anaesthetic/analgesic efficacy of a eutectic mixture of local anaesthetics (EMLA). Drugs 1993; 46: 126-51
187. Wright PM, Iftikhar M, Fitzpatrick KT, et al. Vasopressor therapy for hypotension during epidural anesthesia for cesarean section: effects on maternal and fetal flow velocity ratios. Anesthesia and Analgesia 1992; 75: 56-63
188. Ralston DH, Shnider SM, de Lorimer AA. Effects of equipotent ephedrine, metaraminol, mephentermine and methoxamine on uterine bloodflow in the pregnant ewe. Anesthesiology 1974; 40: 354-70
189. Gajraj NM, Victory RA, Pace NA, et al. Comparison of an ephedrine infusion with crystalloid administration for prevention of hypotension during spinal anesthesia. Anesthesia and Analgesia 1993; 76: 1023-6
190. Fahmy NR. Nitroglycerin as a hypotensive drug during general anaesthesia. Anaesthesia 1978; 49: 17
191. Hill NS, Antman EM, Groen LH, et al. Intravenous nitroglycerin: a review of pharmacology, indications, therapeutic effects and complications. Chest 1981; 79: 69
192. Vesey CJ, Cole PV, Simpson PJ. Sodium nitroprusside in anaesthesia. British Medical Journal 1975; 3: 229
193. Tinker JH, Michenfelder JD. Sodium nitroprusside. Anesthesiology 1976; 45: 340
194. Krapez JR, Vesey CJ, Adams L, et al. Effects of cyanide antidotes used with sodium nitroprusside infusion: sodium thiosulphate and hydroxycobalamin given prophylactically to dogs. British Journal of Anaesthesia 1981; 53: 793-804
195. Andrews PRL. Physiology of nausea and vomiting. British Journal of Anaesthesia 1992; 69: 2-19
196. Watcha MF, White PF. Postoperative nausea and vomiting: its etiology, treatment and prevention. Anesthesiology 1992; 77: 162-84
197. Peroutka SJ, Snyder SH. Antiemetics: neuroreceptor binding predicts therapeutic action. Lancet 1982; 1: 658-9
198. Harris AL. Cytotoxic-therapy-induced vomiting is mediated via enkephalin pathways. Lancet 1982; 1: 714-6
199. Rowbotham DJ. Current management of postoperative nausea and vomiting. British Journal of Anaesthesia 1992; 69: 46-59
200. Rowbotham DJ. Gastric emptying, postoperative nausea and vomiting, and antiemetics. In: Nimmo WS, Rowbotham DJ, Smith G, editors. Anaesthesia. 2nd ed. Oxford: Blackwell Scientific Publications, 1994: 350-70
201. Gralla RJ. Metoclopramide: a review of antiemetic trials. Drugs 1983; 25 Suppl. 1: 63-73
202. O'Donovan N, Shaw J. Nausea and vomiting in daycare dental anaesthesia: the use of low-dose droperidol. Anaesthesia 1984; 39: 1172-6
203. Clissold SP, Heel RC. Transdermal hyoscine (scopolamine): a preliminary review of its pharmacodynamic properties and therapeutic use. Drugs 1985; 29: 189-207
204. Markham A, Sorkin EM. Ondansetron: an update of its therapeutic use in chemotherapy-induced and postoperative nausea and vomiting. Drugs 1993; 45: 931-52
205. Bunce KT, Tyers MB. The role of 5-HT in postoperative nausea and vomiting. British Journal of Anaesthesia 1992; 69 Suppl. 1: 60-2
206. Kenny GN, Oates JD, Leeser J. Efficacy of orally administered ondansetron in the prevention of postoperative nausea and vomiting: a dose ranging study. British Journal of Anaesthesia 1992; 68: 466-70
207. Owens ME, Todt EH. Pain in infancy: neonatal reaction to a heel lance. Pain 1984; 20: 77-86
208. Anand KJS, Sippell WG, Aynsley-Green A. Randomised trial of fentanyl anaesthesia in preterm neonates undergoing surgery: effects on the stress response. Lancet 1987; 1: 62

209. McRorie TI, Lynn AM, Nespeca MK, et al. The maturation of morphine clearance and metabolism. American Journal of Diseases of Children 1992; 146: 972-6
210. Davis PJ, Killian A, Stiller RL, et al. Pharmacokinetics of alfentanil in newborn premature infants and older children. Developmental Pharmacology and Therapeutics 1989; 13: 21-7
211. Gregory GA, Eger II EL, Munson ES. The relationship between age and halothane requirement in man. Anesthesiology 1969; 30: 488
212. Katoh T, Ikeda K. Minimum alveolar concentration of sevoflurane in children. British Journal of Anaesthesia 1992; 68: 139
213. Walts LF, Dillon JB. The response of newborns to succinylcholine and d-tubocurarine. Anesthesiology 1969; 31: 35
214. Fisher DM, O'Keefe C, Stanski DR, et al. Pharmacokinetics and pharmacodynamics of D-tubocurarine in infants, children and adults. Anesthesiology 1982; 57: 203-8
215. Arthur DS, McNicol LR. Local anaesthetic techniques in paediatric surgery. British Journal of Anaesthesia 1986; 58: 760-8
216. Yaster M, Maxwell LG. Pediatric regional anesthesia. Anesthesiology 1989; 70: 324-8
217. Hatch DJ. Paediatric anaesthesia. In: Nimmo WS, Rowbotham DJ, Smith G, editors. Anaesthesia. 2nd ed. Oxford: Blackwell Scientific Publications, 1994: 912-43
218. Chung F, Seyone C, Dyck B, et al. Age-related cognitive recovery after general anesthesia. Anesthesia and Analgesia 1990; 71: 217-4
219. Dundee JW, McMillan CM. Positive evidence for P6 acupuncture antiemesis. Postgraduate Medical Journal 1991; 67: 417-22
220. Ramsay LE, Tucker GT. Drugs and the elderly. British Medical Journal 1981; 282: 125-7
221. Jones MJ, Piggott SE, Vaughan RS, et al. Cognitive and functional competence after anaesthesia in patients aged over 60: controlled trial of general and regional anaesthesia for elective hip or knee replacement. British Medical Journal 1990; 300: 1683-7
222. Krechel SW. Anaesthesia and the elderly patient. In: Nimmo WS, Rowbotham DJ, Smith G, editors. Anaesthesia. London: Blackwell Scientific Publications, 1994: 1301-20
223. Abernethy DR, Greenblatt DJ. Impairment of lidocaine clearance in elderly male subjects. Journal of Cardiovascular Pharmacology 1983; 5: 1093-6
224. Veering BTH, Burm AGL, Spierdijk J. Spinal anesthesia with hyperbaric bupivacaine: effects of age on neural blockade and pharmacokinetics. British Journal of Anaesthesia 1988; 60: 187-94
225. Bromage PR. Aging and epidural dose requirements. British Journal of Anaesthesia 1969; 41: 10-6
226. Hirabayashi Y, Shimizu R. Effect of age on extradural dose requirement in thoracic extradural anaesthesia. British Journal of Anaesthesia 1993; 71: 445-6
227. Editorial. Following up day case anaesthesia in general practice. Drugs and Therapeutics Bulletin 1990; 28: 81-2
228. Herbert M, Healy TE, Bourke JB, et al. Profile of recovery after general anaesthesia. British Medical Journal 1983; 286: 1539-42
229. Ogg TW. Use of anaesthesia: implications of day-case surgery and anaesthesia. British Medical Journal 1980; 281: 212-4
230. Beechey APG, Eltringham RJ, Studd CJ. Temazepam as premedication in day surgery. Anaesthesia 1981; 36: 10-5
231. O'Toole DP, Milligan KR, Howe JP, et al. A comparison of propofol and methohexitone as induction agents for day case isoflurane anaesthesia. Anaesthesia 1987; 42: 373-6
232. Carter JA, Dye AM, Cooper GM. Recovery from day-case anaesthesia. Anaesthesia 1985; 40: 545-8
233. Valanne J, Korttila K. Recovery following general anaesthesia with isoflurane or enflurane for outpatient dentistry and oral surgery. Anaesthesia Progress 1988; 35: 48-52
234. Bagshaw ON, Singh P, Aitkenhead AR. Alfentanil in daycase anaesthesia: assessment of a single dose on the quality of anaesthesia and recovery. Anaesthesia 1993; 48: 476-81
235. Ramanathan J. Anesthetic considerations of preeclampsia. Clinical Perinatology 1991; 18: 875-9
236. Gibbs CP, Schwartz DJ, Wynne JW, et al. Antacid pulmonary aspiration in the dog. Anesthesiology 1979; 51: 380
237. McAuley DM, Moore J, Dundee JW, et al. Oral ranitidine in labour. Anaesthesia 1984; 39: 433
238. Thompson EM, Loughran PG, McAuley DM, et al. Combined treatment with ranitidine and saline antacids prior to obstetric anaesthesia. Anaesthesia 1984; 39: 1086
239. Orr DA, Bill KM, Gillon KR, et al. Effects of omeprazole, with and without metoclopramide, in elective caesarian section. Anaesthesia 1993; 48: 114-9
240. Gin T, Chan MTV. Decreased minimum alveolar concentration of isoflurane in pregnant humans. Anesthesiology 1994; 81: 829-32
241. Coleman AJ, Downing JW. Enflurane anaesthesia for caesarian section. Anesthesiology 1975; 43: 354-7
242. Warren TM, Datta S, Ostheimer GW, et al. Comparison of maternal and neonatal effects of halothane, enflurane and isoflurane. Anesthesia and Analgesia 1983; 62: 516-20
243. Greiff J, Cousins MJ. Subarachnoid and extradural anaesthesia. In: Nimmo WS, Rowbotham DJ, Smith G, editors. Anaesthesia. London: Blackwell Scientific Publications, 1994: 1436-7
244. Kestin IG. Spinal anaesthesia in obstetrics. British Journal of Anaesthesia 1991; 66: 596-607
245. Naulty JS. Continuous infusions of local anesthetics and narcotics for epidural analgesia in the management of labor. International Anesthesiology Clinics 1990; 28: 17-24
246. Muir AD, Reeder MK, Foëx P, et al. Preoperative silent myocardial ischaemia: incidence and predictors in a general surgical population. British Journal of Anaesthesia 1991; 67: 373-7
247. Seegobin RD, Goodland FC, Wilmshurst TH, et al. Postoperative myocardial damage in patients with coronary artery disease undergoing major non cardiac surgery. Canadian Journal of Anaesthesia 1991; 38: 1005-1
248. Mangano DT, Browner W, Hollenberg M, et al. Association of perioperative myocardial ischemia with cardiac morbidity and mortality in men undergoing noncardiac surgery. New England Journal of Medicine 1990; 323: 1781-8
249. Leon A, Graftieaux JP. Interaction between nimodipine and isoflurane and peroperative sinus node deficiency. Annales Francaises d'Anesthesie et de Reanimation 1991; 10: 93

250. Yokota S. Comparative effects of inhalational anesthetics on atrioventricular conduction with and without calcium entry blockers. Hokkaido Igaku Zasshi - Journal of Medical Science 1989; 64: 43-54
251. Cunningham AJ. Anaesthesia for abdominal aortic surgery: a review. Canadian Journal of Anaesthesia 1989; 36: 426-3, 568-77
252. Selby DG, Richards JD, Marshman JM. ACE inhibitors. Anaesthesia in Intensive Care 1989; 17: 110
253. Colson P, Saussine M, Séguin JR, et al. Hemodynamic effects of anesthesia in patients chronically treated with angiotensin-converting enzyme inhibitors. Anesthesia and Analgesia 1992; 74: 805
254. Chraemmer-Jhrgensen B, Hoilund-Carlsen PF, Bjerre-Jepson K, et al. Does alfentanil preserve left ventricular pump function during rapid sequence induction of anaesthesia? Acta Anaesthesiologica Scandinavica 1992; 36: 362-8
255. Priebe HJ. Isoflurane and coronary hemodynamics. Anesthesiology 1989; 71: 960-76
256. Tuman KJ, McCarthy RJ, Spiess BD, et al. Does choice of anesthetic agent significantly affect outcome after coronary artery surgery? Anesthesiology 1989; 70: 189-98
257. Blomberg S, Emanuelsson H, Kvist H, et al. Effects of thoracic anesthesia on coronary arteries and arterioles in patients with coronary artery disease. Anesthesiology 1988; 73: 840-7
258. Mangano DT, Siliciano D, Hollenberg M, et al. Postoperative myocardial ischaemia: therapeutic trials using intensive analgesia following surgery. Anesthesiology 1992; 76: 342-53
259. Milledge JS, Nunn JF. Criteria of fitness for anaesthesia in patients with chronic obstructive lung disease. British Medical Journal 1975; 3: 670
260. Saulnier FF, Durocher AV, Deturck RA, et al. Respiratory and haemodynamic effects of halothane in status asthmaticus. Intensive Care Medicine 1990; 16: 104-7
261. Johnston RG, Noseworthy JW, Friesen EG, et al. Isoflurane therapy for status asthmaticus in children and adults. Chest 1990; 97: 698-701
262. Thomas DJB, Platt HS, Alberti GMM. Insulin-dependent diabetes during the perioperative period: an assessment of continuous glucose-insulin-potassium infusion, and traditional treatment. Anaesthesia 1984; 39: 629-37
263. Alberti KMM, Hockaday TDR. Diabetes mellitus. In: Weatherall DJ, Ledingham JGG, Warrell DA, editors. Oxford textbook of medicine. Oxford: Oxford University Press, 1987: 9.51-9.101
264. Hall GM, Desborough JP. Diabetes and anaesthesia - slow progress. Anaesthesia 1988; 43: 531-2
265. Kunin CM. A guide to use of antibiotics in patients with renal disease. Annals of Internal Medicine 1967; 67: 151-8
266. Hunter JM, Jones RS, Utting JE. Comparison of vecuronium, atracurium and tubocurarine in normal patients and in patients with no renal function. British Journal of Anaesthesia 1984; 56: 941-51
267. Ward S, Boheimer N, Weatherley BC, et al. Pharmacokinetics of atracurium and its metabolites in patients with normal renal function, and in patients in renal failure. British Journal of Anaesthesia 1987; 59: 697-706
268. Sear J, Hand CW, Moore RA, et al. Studies on morphine disposition: influence of renal failure on the kinetics of morphine and its metabolites. British Journal of Anaesthesia 1989; 62: 28-32
269. Glare PA, Walsh TD. Normorphine, a toxic metabolite? Lancet 1990; 335: 725-6
270. Dundee JW, Annis D. Barbiturate narcosis in uraemia. British Journal of Anaesthesia 1955; 27: 114-23
271. Mazze RI, Hitt BA. Methoxyflurane metabolism. Anesthesiology 1976; 44: 369
272. Wickstrom I. Enflurane in living donor renal transplantation. Acta Anaesthesiologica Scandinavica 1981; 25: 263-9
273. Farman J. Anaesthesia and perioperative care for patients with liver disease. British Journal of Hospital Medicine 1986; 36: 448-52
274. Karlin JM, Kutt H. Acute diphenylhydantoin intoxication following halothane anesthesia. Pediatrics 1970; 76: 941
275. Wainwright AP, Brodrick PM. Suxamethonium in myasthenia gravis. Anesthesiology 1987; 42: 950-7
276. Eisenkraft JB, Book WJ, Papatestas AE. Sensitivity to vecuronium in myasthenia gravis: a dose-response study. Canadian Journal of Anaesthesia 1990; 37: 301-6
277. Bell CF, Florence AM, Hunter JM, et al. Atracurium in the myasthenic patient. Anaesthesia 1984; 39: 961-8
278. Tuchmann-Duplessis H. Drug effects on the fetus. Sydney: Adis Press, 1975: 162.
279. Spence AA. Environmental pollution by inhalational anaesthetics. British Journal of Anaesthesia 1987; 59: 96-103
280. Tannenbaum TN, Goldberg RJ. Exposure to anaesthetic gases and reproductive outcome: a review of epidemiologic literature. Journal of Occupational Medicine 1985; 27: 659-8
281. Corbett TH. Anaesthetics: are they carcinogens? American Society of Anesthesiologists. Abstracts. Refresher Course 1976, San Francisco, Paper 211. Philadelphia: JB Lipincott, 1976.
282. Doll R, Peto R. Mortality among doctors in different occupations. British Medical Journal 1977; 1: 1433-6
283. Neil HAW, Fairer JG, Coleman MP, et al. Mortality among male anaesthetists in the United Kingdom 1957-83. British Medical Journal 1987; 295: 360-2
284. Armstrong P, Rae PW, Gray WM, et al. Nitrous oxide and formiminoglutamic acid: excretion in surgical patients and anaesthetists. British Journal of Anaesthesia 1991; 66: 163-9
285. Vessey MP. Epidemiological studies of the occupational hazards of anaesthesia: a review. Anaesthesia 1978; 33: 430-8
286. Spence AA, Wall RA, Nunn JF. Environmental safety of the anaesthetist. In: Nunn JF, Utting JE, Brown BRJ, editors. General anaesthesia. 5th ed. London: Butterworth, 1989
287. Tinker JH, Gandolfi J, Van Dyke RA. Elevation of plasma bromide levels in patients following halothane anesthesia. Anesthesiology 1976; 44: 194
288. Clark JM, Lambertson CJ. Pulmonary oxygen toxicity: a review. Pharmacology Reviews 1971; 23: 37-134
289. Editorial. The pulmonary toxicity of oxygen. British Journal of Anaesthesia 1974; 46: 325
290. Stogner SW, Payne DK. Oxygen toxicity. Annals of Pharmacotherapy 1992; 26: 1554-62
291. Risberg B, Smith L, Ortenwall P. Oxygen radicals and lung injury. [Review]. Acta Anaesthesiologica Scandinavica 1991; Suppl. 95: 106-6
292. Frank L. Developmental aspects of experimental pulmonary oxygen toxicity. [Review]. Free Radical Biology and Medicine 1991; 11: 463-94

293. Rosen SM. Effects of anaesthesia and surgery on renal haemodynamics. British Journal of Anaesthesia 1972; 44: 252
294. Vatner SF, Braunwald E. Cardiovascular control mechanisms in the conscious state. New England Journal of Medicine 1975; 293: 970
295. Clarke RSJ, Doggart JR, Lavery T. Changes in liver function after different types of surgery. British Journal of Anaesthesia 1976; 48: 119
296. Strunin L. The liver and anaesthesia. London: Saunders, 1977
297. Dundee JW, editor. Thiopentone and other thiobarbiturates. Edinburgh: Churchill Livingstone, 1956
298. Denborough MA, Lovell RRH. Anaesthetic deaths in a family. Lancet 1960; 2: 45
299. Ellis FR, Halsall PJ. Malignant hyperpyrexia. British Journal of Hospital Medicine 1980; 24: 318
300. McCarthy TV, Healy TM, Heffron JJ, et al. Localisation of the malignant hyperthermia susceptibility locus to human chromosome 19q 12-13.2. Nature 1990; 343: 562-4
301. Hopkins PM, Halsall PJ, Ellis FR. Diagnosing malignant hyperthermia susceptibility. (Editorial). Anaesthesia 1994; 49: 373-4
302. Simpson KH, Ellis FR. Inherited metabolic diseases and anaesthesia. In: Nimmo WS, Rowbotham DJ, Smith G, editors. Anaesthesia. 2nd ed. London: Blackwell Scientific Publications, 1994: 1113-29
303. Krivosic-Horber R, Adnet P, Guevart D, et al. Neuroleptic malignant syndrome and malignant hyperthermia. British Journal of Anaesthesia 1987; 59: 1554-6
304. Morgan KG, Bryant SH. The mechanism of action of dantrolene sodium. Journal of Pharmacology and Experimental Therapeutics 1977; 201: 138
305. Harrison GC. Dantrolene sodium: pharmacodynamics and pharmacokinetics. British Journal of Anaesthesia 1988; 60: 279-86
306. Kolb ME, Horne ML, Martz R. Dantrolene in human malignant hyperthermia. Anesthesiology 1982; 56: 254-62
307. Harrison GC. Malignant hyperthermia. In: Nunn JF, Utting JE, Brown BRJ, editors. General anaesthesia. 5th ed. London: Butterworth, 1989
308. Fisher MM, Moore DG. The epidemiology and clinical features of anaphylactoid reactions in anaesthesia. Anaesthesia in Intensive Care 1981; 9: 226-34
309. Adriani J, Zepernick R. Allergic reactions to local anesthetics. Southern Medical Journal 1981; 74: 694-9
310. Dundee JW, Fee JPH, McDonald JR, et al. Frequency of allergy and atopy in an anaesthetic patient population. British Journal of Anaesthesia 1978; 50: 793-8
311. Watkins J, Wild G, Clarke RSJ. Allergy, plasma IgE level and anaphylactoid response: a hypothesis. Anaesthesia 1985; 40: 362
312. Fisher MMcD. Clinical observations on the pathophysiology and treatment of anaphylactic cardiovascular collapse. Anaesthesia in Intensive Care 1986; 14: 17-21
313. Laxenaire M-C, Moneret-Vautrin DA, Watkins J. Diagnosis of the causes of anaphylactoid anaesthetic reactions. Anaesthesia 1983; 38: 147
314. Glover V, Sandler M. Clinical chemistry of monoamine oxidase. Cell Biochemical Functions 1986; 4: 89-97
315. Stack CG, Rogers P, Linter SP. Monoamine oxidase inhibitors and anaesthesia: a review. British Journal of Anaesthesia 1988; 60: 222-7
316. Dilsaver SC. Monoamine oxidase inhibitor withdrawal phenomena: symptoms and pathophysiology. Acta Psychiatrica Scandinavica 1988; 78: 1-7
317. Tempelhoff R, Modica PA, Spitznagel Jr EL. Anticonvulsant therapy increases fentanyl requirements during anaesthesia for craniotomy. Canadian Journal of Anaesthesia 1990; 37: 327
318. Ornstein E, Matteo RS, Schwartz AE, et al. The effect of phenytoin on the magnitude and duration of neuromuscular block following atracurium or vecuronium. Anesthesiology 1987; 67: 191-6
319. Misra M, Thakur R, Bhandari K. Sinus arrest caused by atenolol-verapamil combination. Clinical Cardiology 1987; 10: 365-7
320. Hartwell BL, Mark JB. Combinations of β-blocker and calcium channel blockers: a case of malignant perioperative conduction disturbance. Anesthesia and Analgesia 1986; 65: 905-7
321. Henling CE, Slogoff S, Kodali SV, et al. Heart block after coronary artery bypass - effect of chronic administration of calcium-entry blockers and β-blockers. Anesthesia and Analgesia 1984; 63: 515-20
322. Lehot JJ, Foëx P, Durand PG. Beta blockers and anesthesia. Annales Francaise d'Anesthesie et de Reanimation 1990; 9: 137-52
323. Eldor J, Hoffman B, Davidson JT. Prolonged bradycardia and hypotension after neostigmine administration in a patient receiving atenolol. Anaesthesia 1987; 42: 1294-7
324. Yates AP, Hunter DN. Anaesthesia and angiotensin-converting enzyme inhibitors: the effect of enalapril on peri-operative cardiovascular stability. Anaesthesia 1988; 43: 935-8
325. Jensen K, Bunemann L, Riisager S, et al. Cerebral blood flow during anaesthesia: influence of pretreatment with metoprolol or captopril. British Journal of Anaesthesia 1989; 62: 321
326. Dupuis JY, Martin R, Tétrault JP. Atracurium and vecuronium interaction with gentamicin and tobramycin. Canadian Journal of Anaesthesia 1989; 36: 407-11
327. Bikhazi GB, Leung I, Flores C, et al. Potentiation of neuromuscular blocking agents by calcium channel blockers in rats. Anesthesia and Analgesia 1988; 67: 1-8
328. Snyder SW, Cardwell MS. Neuromuscular blockade with magnesium sulfate and nifedipine. American Journal of Obstetrics and Gynecology 1989; 161: 35-6
329. Kao YJ, Tellez J, Turner DR. Dose-dependent effect of metoclopramide on cholinesterases and suxamethonium metabolism. British Journal of Anaesthesia 1990; 65: 220-4
330. Sosnowski M, Yaksh TL. Spinal administration of receptor-selective drugs as analgesics: new horizons. Journal of Pain Symptom Management 1990; 5: 204-13
331. Martin WR, Eades CG, Thompson JA, et al. The effects of morphine and nalorphine-like drugs in the nondependent and morphine-dependent spinal dog. Journal of Pharmacology and Experimental Therapeutics 1976; 197: 517
332. Pasternak GW. Pharmacological mechanisms of opioid analgesics. Clinical Neuropharmacology 1993; 16: 1-18
333. Pasternak GW. Multiple morphine and enkephalin receptors, and the relief of pain. Journal of the American Medical Association 1988; 259: 1362-7
334. Childers SR. Opioid receptor-coupled second messenger system. Life Sciences 1991; 48: 1991-2003
335. Martin WR. The pharmacology of opioids. Pharmacology Reviews 1984; 35: 283

336. Goa KL, Brogden RN. Propiram: a review of its pharmacodynamic and pharmacokinetic properties, and clinical use as an analgesic. Drugs 1993; 46: 428-5
337. Lee RC, McTavish DM, Sorkin EM. Tramadol: a preliminary review of its pharmacodynamic and pharmacokinetic properties, and therapeutic potential in acute and chronic pain states. Drugs 1993; 46: 313-40
338. Bowsher D. Pain syndromes and their treatment. Current Opinion in Neurology and Neurosurgery 1993; 6: 257-63
339. Pond SM, Tong T, Benowitz NL, et al. Presystemic metabolism of meperidine to normeperidine in normal and cirrhotic subjects. Clinical Pharmacology & Therapeutics 1981; 30: 183
340. Burns AM, Shelly MP, Park GR. The use of sedative agents in critically ill patients. Drugs 1992; 43: 507-15
341. Berkowitz BA. The relationship of pharmacokinetics to pharmacological activity: morphine methadone and naloxone. Clinical Pharmacokinetics 1976; 1: 219
342. Mather LE, Meffin PJ. Clinical pharmacokinetics of pethidine. Clinical Pharmacokinetics 1978; 3: 352
343. Chay PC. Pharmacokinetic-pharmacodynamic relationships of morphine in neonates. Clinical Pharmacology & Therapeutics 1992; 51: 334-42
344. Bovil JG. Pharmacokinetics and pharmacodynamics of opioid agonists. Anaesthetic Pharmacology Reviews 1993; 1: 122
345. Pleuvry B. Opioid receptors and their relevance to anaesthesia. British Journal of Anaesthesia 1993; 71: 119
346. Rawal N. Spinal and epidural opioids. Anaesthetic Pharmacology Reviews 1993; 2: 168
347. Shafer SL, Varvel JR. Pharmacokinetics, pharmacodynamics and rational opioid selection. Anesthesiology 1992; 74: 53-63
348. Gourlay GK, Wilson PR, Glynn CJ, et al. Pharmacodynamics and pharmacokinetics of methadone during the postoperative period. Anesthesiology 1982; 57: 458-67
349. Eggers KA, Power I. Tramadol. British Journal of Anaesthesia 1995; 74: 247-9
350. Coetzee JF, Maritz JS, Du Toit JC. Effect of tramadol on depth of anaesthesia. British Journal of Anaesthesia 1996; 76: 415-8
351. Rowbotham DJ, Wyld R, Peacock JE, et al. Transdermal fentanyl for the relief of pain after upper abdominal surgery. British Journal of Anaesthesia 1989; 63: 56-9
352. Nimmo WS. The promise of transdermal drug delivery. British Journal of Anaesthesia 1990; 64: 7-10
353. Bovill JG. Which potent opioid? Drugs 1987; 33: 520-30
354. Bodenham A, Park GR. Alfentanil infusions in patients requiring intensive care. Clinical Pharmacokinetics 1988; 15: 216-6
355. Monk JP, Beresford R, Ward A. Sufentanil: a review of its pharmacological properties and therapeutic use. Drugs 1988; 36: 286-313
356. Kapila A, Glass PS, Jacobs JR, et al. Measured context-sensitive half-times of remifentanil and alfentanil. Anesthesiology 1995 'Nov; 83: 968-75
357. Shafer SL, Varvel JR. Pharmacokinetics, pharmacodynamics and rational opioid selection. Anesthesiology 1991; 74: 53
358. Hughes MA, Glass PS, Jacobs JR. Context-sensitive half-time in multicompartment pharmacokinetic models for intravenous anesthetic drugs. Anesthesiology 1992; 76: 334-41
359. Heel RC, Brogden RN, Speight TM, et al. Buprenorphine: a review of its pharmacological properties and clinical efficacy. Drugs 1979; 17: 81
360. Bullingham RES, McQuay HJ, Moore RA. Clinical pharmacokinetics of narcotic agonist-antagonist drugs. Clinical Pharmacokinetics 1983; 8: 332
361. Magruder MR, Delaney RD, DiFazio CA. Reversal of narcotic-induced respiratory depression with nalbuphine hydrochloride. Anesthesiology Review 1982; 9: 34
362. Gillis JC, Benfield P, Goa KL. Transnasal butorphanol: a review of its pharmacodynamic and pharmacokinetic properties, and therapeutic potential in acute pain management. Drugs 1995; 50: 157-75
363. O'Brien JJ, Benfield P. Dezocine: a preliminary review of its pharmacodynamic and pharmacokinetic properties, and therapeutic efficacy. Drugs 1989; 38: 226-48
364. Andree RA. Sudden death following naloxone administration. Anesthesia and Analgesia 1980; 59: 782
365. Brimacombe J, Archdeacon J, Newell S, et al. Two cases of naloxone-induced pulmonary oedema - the possible use of phentolamine in management. Anaesthesia in Intensive Care 1991; 19: 578-80
366. Cohen SE, Ratner EF, Kreitzman TR, et al. Nalbuphine is better than naloxone for treatment of side effects after epidural morphine. Anesthesia and Analgesia 1992; 75: 747-52
367. Preston KL, Bigelow GE. Differential naltrexone antagonism of hydromorphone and pentazocine effects in human volunteers. Journal of Pharmacology and Experimental Therapeutics 1993; 264: 813-23
368. Kurlan R, Majumdar L, Deeley C, et al. A controlled trial of propoxyphene and naltrexone in patients with Tourette's syndrome. Annals of Neurology 1991; 30: 19-23
369. Yamaguchi H, Watanabe S, Harukuni I, et al. Effective doses of epidural morphine for relief of postcholecystectomy pain. Anesthesia and Analgesia 1991; 72: 80-3
370. Nordberg G. Epidural versus intrathecal route of opioid administration. International Anesthesiology Clinics 1986; 24: 93-111
371. Rawal N, Arner S, Gustafsson LI, et al. Present state of extradural and intrathecal opioid analgesia in Sweden. British Journal of Anaesthesia 1987; 59: 791-9
372. George KA, Chisakuta AM, Gamble JA, et al. Thoracic epidural infusion for postoperative pain relief following abdominal aortic surgery: bupivacaine, fentanyl or a mixture of both? Anaesthesia 1992; 47: 388-94
373. Ferrante FM, Lu L, Jamieson SB, et al. Patient-controlled epidural analgesia: demand dosing. Anesthesia and Analgesia 1991; 73: 547-2
374. Findlay JWA, Jones EC, Butz RF, et al. Plasma codeine and morphine concentrations after therapeutic oral doses of codeine-containing analgesics. Clinical Pharmacology & Therapeutics 1978; 24: 60
375. Ng B, Alvear M. Dextropropoxyphene addiction - a drug of primary abuse. American Journal of Drug and Alcohol Abuse 1993; 19: 153-8
376. Kaa E, Dalgaard JB. Fatal dextropropoxyphene poisonings in Jutland, Denmark. Zeitschrift fur Rechtsmedizin - Journal of Legal Medicine 1989; 102: 107-5
377. Whittington RM. Dextropropoxyphene (Distalgesic) overdosage in the West Midlands. British Medical Journal 1977; 2: 172
378. Ferreira SH, Vane JR. New aspects of the mode of action of nonsteroid anti-inflammatory drugs. Annual Review of Pharmacology and Toxicology 1974; 14: 57
379. Weissmann G. Aspirin. Scientific American 1991; 264: 58-64

380. Mather LE. Do the pharmacodynamics of the nonsteroidal anti-inflammatory drugs suggest a role in the management of postoperative pain? Drugs 1992; 44 Suppl. 5: 1-12
381. Kehlet H, Dahl JB. Are perioperative nonsteroidal anti-inflammatory drugs ulcerogenic in the short term? Drugs 1992; 44 Suppl. 5: 38-41
382. Kenny GN. Potential renal, haematological and allergic adverse effects associated with nonsteroidal anti-inflammatory drugs. Drugs 1992; 44 Suppl. 5: 31-6
383. Williams WR, Pawlowicz A, Davies BH. Aspirin-sensitive asthma: significance of the cyclooxygenase-inhibiting and protein-binding properties of analgesic drugs. International Archives of Allergy and Applied Immunology 1991; 95: 303-8
384. Todd PA, Sorkin EM. Diclofenac sodium: a reappraisal of its pharmacodynamic properties, and therapeutic efficacy. Drugs 1988; 35: 244-85
385. Moffat AC, Kenny GN, Prentice JW. Postoperative nefopam and diclofenac: evaluation of their morphine-sparing effect after abdominal surgery. Anaesthesia 1990; 45: 302-5
386. Watters CH, Patterson CC, Mathews HMI, et al. Diclofenac sodium for post-tonsillectomy pain in children. Anaesthesia 1988; 43: 641-3
387. Power I, Chambers WA, Greer IA, et al. Platelet function after intramuscular diclofenac. Anaesthesia 1990; 45: 916
388. Power I, Cumming AD, Pugh GC. Effect of diclofenac on renal function and prostacyclin generation after surgery. British Journal of Anaesthesia 1992; 69: 451-6
389. Brocks DR, Jamali F. Clinical pharmacokinetics of ketorolac. Clinical Pharmacokinetics 1992; 23: 415-27
390. Buckley MM-T, Brogden RN. Ketorolac: a review of its pharmacodynamic and pharmacokinetic properties and therapeutic potential. Drugs 1990; 39: 86-109
391. Committee on Safety of Medicines. Ketorolac: new restrictions on dose and duration of treatment. Current Problems in Pharmacovigilance 1993; 19: 5-6
392. Fowler PD. Aspirin, paracetamol and non-steroidal anti-inflammatory drugs: a comparative review of side effects. Medical Toxicology and Adverse Drug Experience 1987; 2: 338-66
393. Piletta P, Porchet HC, Dayer P. Central analgesic effect of acetaminophen but not of aspirin. Clinical Pharmacology & Therapeutics 1991; 49: 350-4
394. Heel RC, Brogden RN, Pakes GE, et al. Nefopam: a review of its pharmacological properties and therapeutic efficacy. Drugs 1980; 19: 249
395. Friedel HA, Fitton A. Flupirtine: a review of its pharmacological properties, and therapeutic efficacy in pain states. Drugs 1993; 45: 548-69
396. Dahl JB, Kehlet H. The value of pre-emptive analgesia in the treatment of postoperative pain. British Journal of Anaesthesia 1993; 70: 434-9
397. Pounder DR, Steward DJ. Postoperative analgesia: opioid infusions in infants and children. Canadian Journal of Anaesthesia 1992; 39: 969-74
398. Owen H, Plummer JP, Szekely S, et al. Varying the variables of patient controlled analgesia. II: concurrent infusion. Anaesthesia 1989; 44: 11-3
399. Hill HF, Mather LE. Patient-controlled analgesia: pharmacokinetic and therapeutic considerations. Clinical Pharmacokinetics 1993; 24: 124-40
400. Wheatley RG, Shepherd D, Jackson IJ, et al. Hypoxaemia and pain relief after upper abdominal surgery: comparison of IM and patient-controlled analgesia. British Journal of Anaesthesia 1992; 69: 558-61
401. Sevarino FB, Naulty JS, Sinatra R, et al. Transdermal fentanyl for postoperative pain management in patients recovering from abdominal gynecologic surgery. Anesthesiology 1992; 77: 463-6
402. Fiset P, Cohane C, Browne S, et al. Biopharmaceutics of a new transdermal fentanyl device. Anesthesiology 1995; 83: 459-69
403. Behar M, Magora F, Olshwang D, et al. Epidural morphine in treatment of pain. Lancet 1979; 1: 527
404. Bromage PR, Camporesi E, Chestnut D. Epidural narcotics for postoperative analgesia. Anesthesia and Analgesia 1980; 59: 473
405. McCaughey W, Graham JL. The respiratory depression of epidural morphine: time course and effect of posture. Anaesthesia 1982; 37: 990
406. Schug SA, Dunlop R, Zech D. Pharmacological management of cancer pain. Drugs 1992; 43: 44-53
407. Säwe J. High-dose morphine and methadone in cancer patients: clinical pharmacokinetic considerations of oral treatment. Clinical Pharmacokinetics 1986; 11: 97
408. Fine PG, Marcus M, De Boer AJ, et al. An open label study of oral transmucosal fentanyl citrate (OTFC) for the treatment of breakthrough cancer pain. Pain 1991; 45: 149-53
409. Costello DJ, Borison HL. Naloxone antagonises narcotic self blockade of emesis in the cat. Journal of Pharmacology and Experimental Therapeutics 1977; 203: 222-30
410. Watson CP, Evans RJ, Reed K, et al. Amitriptyline versus placebo in postherpetic neuralgia. Neurology 1982; 32: 671-3
411. Watson CP, Chipman M, Reed K, et al. Amitriptyline versus maprotiline in postherpetic neuralgia: a randomized, double-blind, crossover trial. Pain 1992; 48: 29-36
412. Magni G. The use of antidepressants in the treatment of chronic pain: a review of the current evidence. Drugs 1991; 42: 730-48
413. Brose WG, Cousins MJ. Subcutaneous lidocaine for treatment of neuropathic cancer pain. Pain 1991; 45: 145-8
414. Moir DD, Thorburn J, editors. Analgesia and anaesthesia. 3rd ed. London: Baillière-Tindall, 1986
415. Kuhnert BR, Linn PL, Kennard MJ, et al. Effects of low doses of meperidine on neonatal behaviour. Anesthesia and Analgesia 1985; 64: 335-42
416. Davies MW, Harrison JC, Ryan TD. Current practice of epidural analgesia during normal labour: a survey of maternity units in the United Kingdom. Anaesthesia 1993; 48: 63-5
417. Dodson WE. Local drug intoxication: local anesthetics. Pediatric Clinics of North America 1974; 23: 307
418. Mather LE, Cousins MJ. Local anaesthetics and their current clinical use. Drugs 1979; 18: 185-205

Chapter 13

# Drug Use in the Critically Ill

*N.L. Benowitz, P. Pentel* and *J. Leatherman*

## Synopsis of Important Principles

1) Critical illnesses are often associated with circulatory, respiratory, hepatic and/or renal dysfunction which may alter the pharmacokinetics and/or pharmacodynamics of drugs.

2) Decisions about routes of administration and doses of drugs used during medical emergencies must consider the physiological status of the patient, the pharmacokinetic and pharmacodynamic characteristics of the particular drug, and how the two interact.

3) Adverse drug reactions and interactions are more likely in critically ill patients due to the effect of the disease on drug kinetics, the decreased toxic-therapeutic ratio due to severe underlying illness, and the large number of medications that such patients receive. Adverse reactions to drugs should be considered when unexplained deterioration or failure to respond to therapy are encountered.

4) Preservation of function of vital organs is a fundamental concept of critical care therapeutics. In addition, measures to reduce complications such as infections, gastric stress erosions and ulcers, acute respiratory distress syndrome, pulmonary emboli, and haemostatic disorders are also an important part of management.

5) Shock can be produced by many different processes including myocardial infarction, hypovolaemia, sepsis, drug overdose, burns, hypothermia, spinal cord transection and anaphylaxis. Optimum treatment of shock depends on knowledge of the pathophysiology of the shock state and the pharmacology of the drugs used.

6) Features of acute drug intoxication include coma, agitated delirium, seizures, hypo- and hyperthermia, shock, arrhythmias, aspiration and pulmonary oedema. Successful therapy of acute drug intoxication depends on the integration and application of knowledge of the pharmacology of both the intoxicating drug and the drugs used in therapy, as well as the principles of supportive critical care.

Drug therapy of emergencies differs in several respects from that of stable medical conditions. Because of the urgency of the patient's condition, therapeutic drug concentrations must be achieved rapidly, often within minutes. To accomplish this, a route of administration that allows prompt drug absorption and delivery to target organs must be chosen. Most critical illnesses are associated with some degree of circulatory, respiratory, hepatic and/or renal dysfunction that may in turn alter the pharmacokinetics and/or pharmacodynamics of therapeutic agents. Drug dosage regimens must be tailored to accommodate these changes. The clinical status of the acutely compromised patient often changes rapidly, requiring adjustment of drug dosages. The acutely ill patient can also be expected to tolerate toxic drug effects poorly, so that avoidance of excessive dosages is important.

During medical emergencies, time often does not permit the measurement of drug concentrations in blood for use as a guide to dosage. Decisions about drug doses must frequently be made on the basis of knowledge of the pharmacokinetic characteristics of a particular drug, the physiological status of the patient, and an appreciation of how the two interact.

## 1. Clinical Pharmacological Considerations in Critically Ill Patients

### 1.1 Cardiovascular Emergencies/Circulatory Failure

#### *1.1.1 Pathophysiology of Circulatory Failure*

Circulatory failure, or the inability of the heart to provide sufficient cardiac output to satisfy tissue metabolic requirements, is the most important and most common cause of altered pharmacokinetics during cardiac emergencies. Circulatory failure may result from decreased myocardial contractility, arrhythmias that allow insufficient time for diastolic filling or impair atrioventricular synchrony, circulatory stresses such as increased afterload or hypovolaemia, valvular dysfunction, tamponade, or a variety of less common insults.

Regardless of the aetiology, circulatory failure elicits characteristic compensatory haemodynamic adjustments, mediated in large part by activation of the sympathetic nervous system (fig. 1).[1,2] Enhanced sympathetic tone increases cardiac contractility and peripheral vascular resistance, both of which serve to maintain arterial blood pressure. The increase in peripheral vascular resistance, however, is not uniform among different vascular beds. Organs with high metabolic requirements such as the heart and brain exhibit autoregulation; despite sympathetic stimulation, the vessels in these organs remain relatively vasodilated as a result of the local effects of hypoxia, lactic acid or other products of anaerobic metabolism that accumulate when organ perfusion is reduced. Blood flow to the heart and brain tends to be preserved, while vasoconstriction decreases blood flow in other organs such as the liver, gut, skin and muscle. Thus, a disproportionate fraction of the available cardiac output is delivered to the heart and brain.

**Pathophysiology of Cardiopulmonary Resuscitation (CPR)**

Cardiac output during cardiopulmonary resuscitation (CPR) is severely compromised; in humans, the mean arterial pressure is less than 50% of normal,[3,4] and cardiac output in dogs is less than 30% of normal.[5] Haemodynamic measurements are difficult to obtain in patients during CPR, but animal data suggest that changes in blood flow distribution are qualitatively similar to those observed with circulatory failure and spontaneous circulation. Blood flow during CPR in anaesthetised, electrically fibrillated dogs is reduced to all organs, but is least reduced to the brain and next least to the heart.[5]

For the purpose of pharmacokinetic considerations, CPR and circulatory failure with spontaneous circulation can be considered to be similar, in that total cardiac output is reduced and the pattern of blood redistribution during promptly initiated CPR resembles that seen in circulatory failure.

#### *1.1.2 Circulatory Failure and Drug Absorption*

Circulatory failure may alter pharmacokinetics in several ways (fig. 2). For example, the absorption of oral mexiletine and disopyramide are slowed in acute myocardial infarction, and the absolute bioavailability of disopyramide is reduced.[6,7] Absorption of drugs from sites with impaired blood flow is slow, sometimes incomplete, and subject to changes in circulatory status. Thus, the oral, subcutaneous and intramuscular routes of administration may not be reliable in acute cardiac emergencies, and an intravascular route is preferred. When intravascular access cannot be established rapidly, however, intratracheal or intramuscular drug administration may be useful. The pulmonary tree

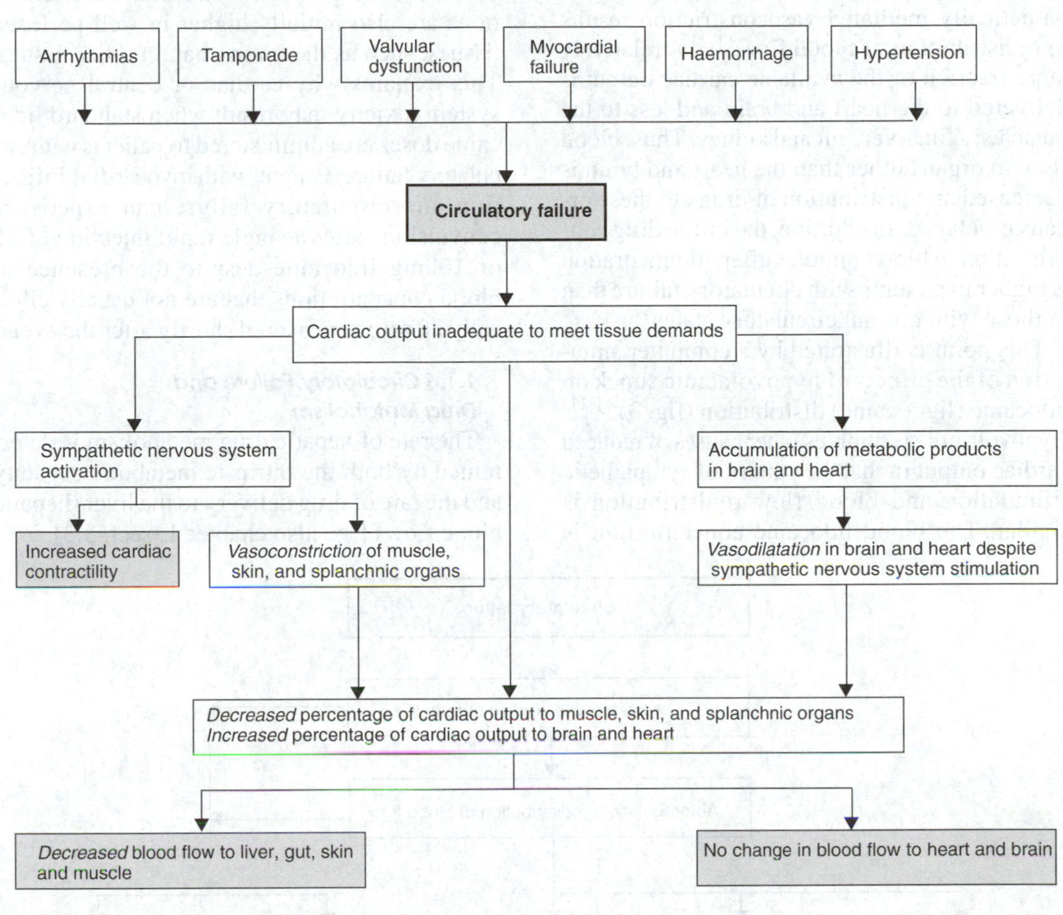


**Fig. 1.** Effects of circulatory failure on blood flow distribution (after Pentel & Benowitz[1]).

provides an extensive surface for drug absorption and pulmonary venous blood empties directly into the heart. Consequently, some drugs [e.g. adrenaline (epinephrine), lidocaine][8] appear to be absorbed from this site, even when cardiac output is markedly decreased. However, the absorption of adrenaline from endotracheal tubes is variable, and higher than usually recommended doses may be necessary.[9,10]

### *1.1.3 Circulatory Failure and Drug Distribution*

The magnitude of the therapeutic or toxic effects of most drugs is determined by their concentration at the target organ. At steady-state (see chapter 1; sect. 2.3), when the concentration of drug in blood is in equilibrium with the concentration of drug in tissues, the tissue concentration is proportional to the blood concentration. For most cardioactive drugs, the blood concentration of drug at steady-state correlates with the magnitude of its effect and can be used as a predictor of therapeutic efficacy or toxicity. However, because all drugs take time to distribute from blood to tissues, the blood concentration of a drug may not correlate with the tissue concentration immediately after its administration. Thus, it is important to consider the disequilibrium between drug concentrations in blood and tissue immediately after administration in designing and monitoring drug dosages in acute situations.

In response to impaired cardiac output, sympathetically mediated vasoconstriction results in redistribution of blood flow.[1,2] A relatively large fraction of the available cardiac output is delivered to the heart and brain and less to the muscles, skin, liver, gut and kidney. Thus, blood flow to organs other than the heart and brain is decreased and distribution of drugs to these organs is delayed. In addition, the initial drug concentration in blood minutes after administration is higher in patients with circulatory failure than in those with normal circulatory states.

This point is illustrated by a computer simulation of the effects of hypovolaemic shock on lidocaine (lignocaine) distribution (fig. 3).[1,11] Hypovolaemia resembles other causes of reduced cardiac output in that the pattern of sympathetic stimulation and blood flow redistribution is similar. The blood lidocaine concentration is higher than normal minutes after drug administration during haemorrhage due primarily to reduced muscle perfusion. Lidocaine concentrations are also initially higher in well perfused tissues, such as the brain, than in other tissues. This explains why cardiac or central nervous system toxicity may result when standard lidocaine doses are administered to patients with circulatory failure. Patients with myocardial infarction and circulatory failure can experience convulsions after a single rapid injection of 75 or 100mg lidocaine despite the presence of blood concentrations that are not usually clinically effective measured shortly after the event.

#### *1.1.4 Circulatory Failure and Drug Metabolism*

The rate of hepatic drug metabolism is determined by both the intrinsic metabolic capacity and the rate of drug delivery to the liver (hepatic blood flow) [see also chapter 1; sect. 3.3].

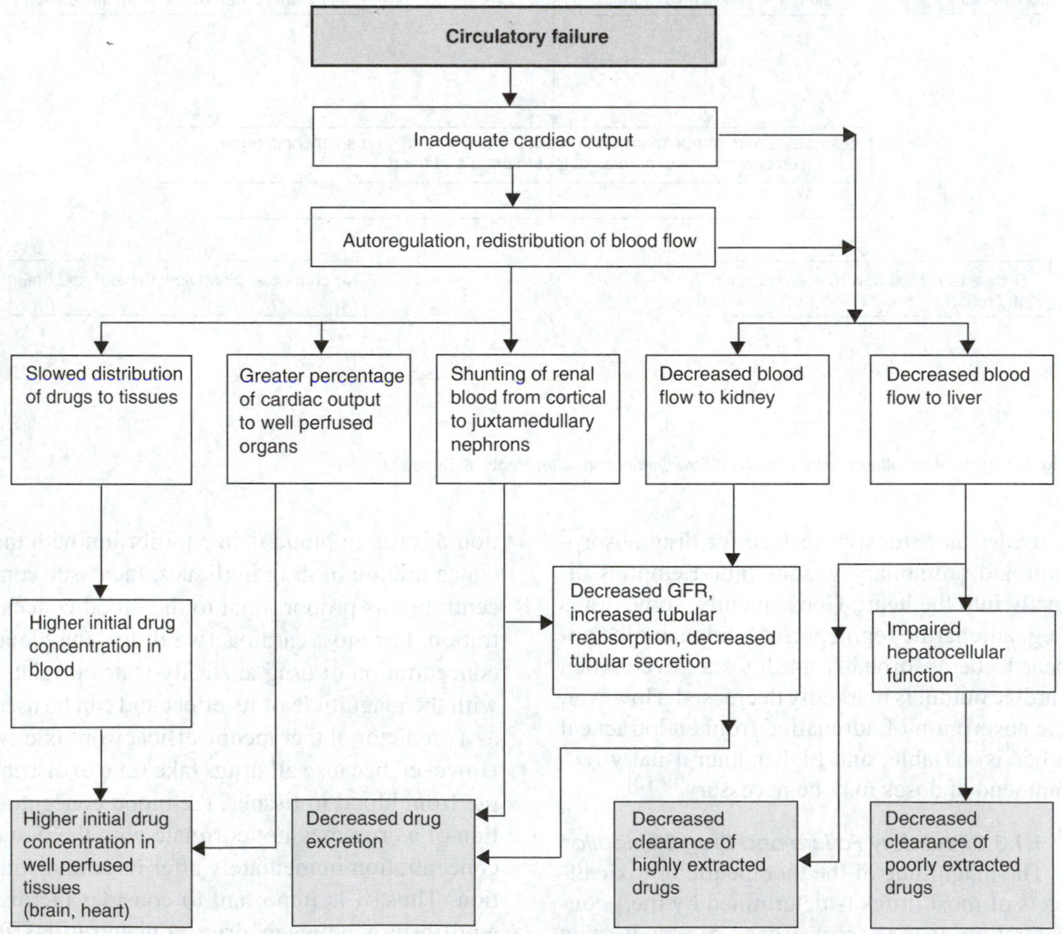


**Fig. 2.** Pharmacokinetic consequences of circulatory failure (GRF = glomerular filtration rate) [after Pentel & Benowitz[1]].

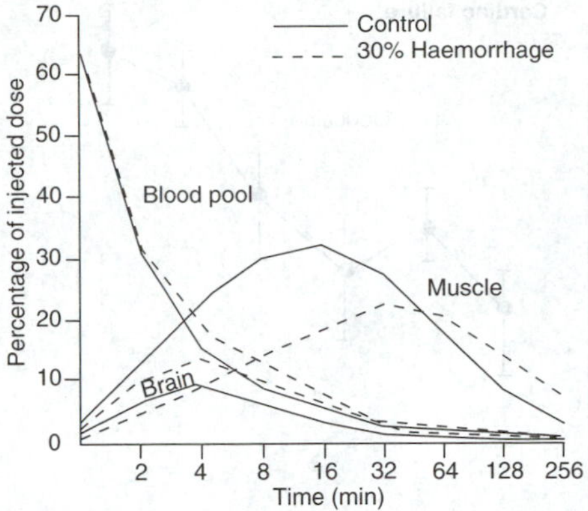


**Fig. 3.** Computer simulation based on a perfusion model of the distribution of lidocaine to various tissues after a 1-minute intravenous infusion of 100mg in a 70kg person (after Benowitz et al.[11]).

Drugs for which the intrinsic hepatic metabolising capacity is high are rapidly and extensively cleared from hepatic blood, and their rate of metabolism is dependent primarily on hepatic blood flow. Lidocaine is such a drug; in circulatory failure, decreased cardiac output is associated with a roughly proportional decrease in hepatic blood flow and the metabolic clearance of lidocaine is therefore diminished. This may have substantial therapeutic implications. The elimination half-life of lidocaine is prolonged up to 3-fold in patients with myocardial infarction without overt cardiac failure and up to 6-fold in those with overt cardiac failure (fig. 4).[12] In one series of patients with excessive plasma lidocaine concentrations during infusion, congestive heart failure or shock was responsible for elevated concentrations in 51 of 72 cases.[13] Likewise, the metabolic clearance of midazolam and morphine is reduced in states of reduced liver blood flow.[14,15]

Drugs such as digoxin and quinidine, for which the intrinsic hepatic metabolising capacity is low, are, by contrast, slowly and incompletely cleared from hepatic blood. Their rates of metabolism are relatively independent of hepatic blood flow and are determined primarily by the intrinsic metabolic capacity of the liver. Injury to hepatocytes due to reduced perfusion, arterial hypoxaemia, or passive congestion can decrease hepatic enzyme function and hence impair the intrinsic metabolic capacity and slow the metabolic clearance of such drugs.[16]

#### *1.1.5 Circulatory Failure and Drug Excretion*

Circulatory failure, with a resulting decrease in renal blood flow, may have important effects on the renal excretion of drugs. The kidney does have a modest capacity for autoregulation, and when renal blood flow is moderately reduced (10 to 20%), the glomerular filtration rate does not fall. However, further reductions in renal blood flow lower the glomerular filtration rate and reduce tubular secretion, and consequently slow the excretion of drugs cleared by the kidney, such as procainamide and digoxin.[17]

#### *1.1.6 Circulatory Failure and Protein Binding*

Changes in the plasma protein binding of drugs used in critically ill patients may be caused by changes in the concentration of the plasma proteins to which they are bound.

One factor which can alter the protein binding of drugs during acute myocardial infarction is a change in the serum concentration of $\alpha_1$-acid glycoprotein. This serum protein is an acute phase reactant to myocardial necrosis, and a major binding protein for basic drugs such as lidocaine and propranolol.[18] Increases in the concentration of $\alpha_1$-acid glycoprotein in serum, which occur over 24 to 48 hours, change the fraction of lidocaine unbound in the plasma. The result is a higher total plasma concentration for any given unbound (active) drug concentration. This change has implications for plasma concentration monitoring (see chapter 5).

### 1.2 Altered Fluid Balance

Hypovolaemia may influence drug kinetics by inducing circulatory insufficiency as discussed above (section 1.1). Fluid retention is also seen in patients with chronic cardiac, liver or kidney disease, as well as in patients with hypoproteinaemia due to malnutrition or burns, and in trauma and postoperative patients. Fluid retention may increase the volume of distribution of water soluble drugs.

Hypoproteinaemia may result in decreased plasma protein binding and thereby increase the volume of distribution of highly protein bound drugs, or increase the hepatic clearance of poorly extracted ones. In general, however, changes in protein binding do not require changes in drug dosages, but they do have implications for interpretation of plasma concentrations in the context of therapeutic drug monitoring (e.g. phenytoin) [see further chapter 5].

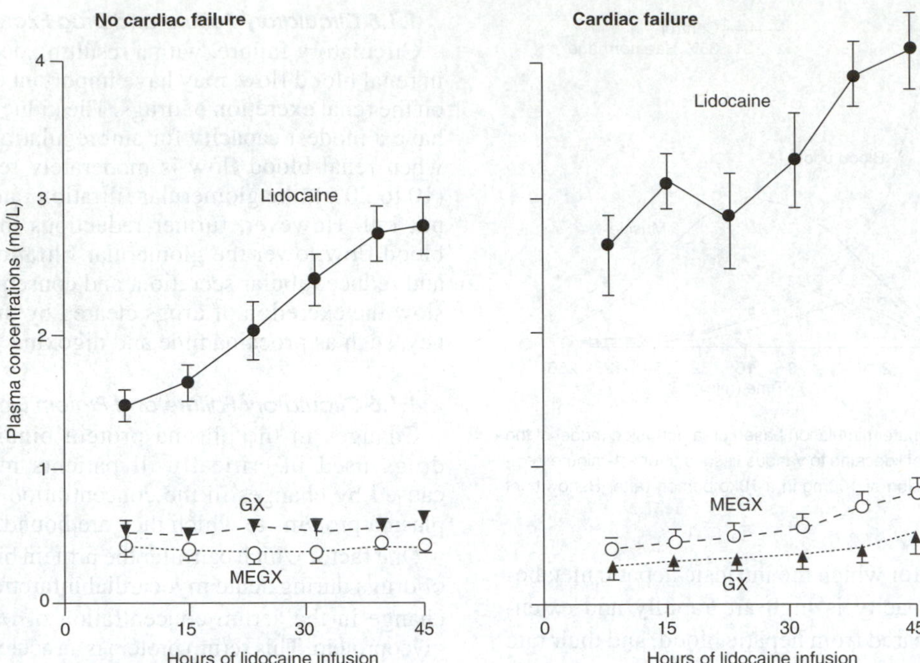


**Fig. 4.** Mean (± SE) plasma concentrations of lidocaine, monoethyl glycine xylidide (MEGX) and glycine xylidide (GX) in patients in a coronary care unit with (n = 7) and without (n = 6) cardiac failure during a constant infusion of lidocaine 1.4 mg/min (after Prescott et al.;[12] with permission).

## 1.3 Hepatic Failure

Pathophysiological consequences of hepatic failure which may influence drug disposition include:

- Depressed synthetic function with decreased serum albumin concentrations
- Accumulation of endogenous compounds which may displace drugs from protein binding sites
- Formation of ascites and peripheral oedema
- Development of portal-systemic shunts
- Decreased liver blood flow
- Depressed drug metabolising activity.

In addition to causing pharmacokinetic disturbances (see also chapter 22; sect. 1.4), hepatic failure may also enhance the patient's sensitivity (i.e. organ responsiveness to a given concentration) to some drugs, such as hypnosedatives and opioids.[19] Central nervous system depression is particularly prominent in patients with a prior history of encephalopathy.

### *1.3.1 Hepatic Failure and Oral Bioavailability*

Liver disease may substantially increase the oral bioavailability of drugs that are subject to extensive first-pass metabolism. For drugs that are completely absorbed from the gastrointestinal tract, bioavailability (F) is determined by liver extraction (E):

$$F = 1 - E$$

Extraction may be decreased as a result of decreased drug metabolising activity and/or portal-systemic shunting. In patients with cirrhosis and portal hypertension, more than 50% of portal blood flow may be shunted.

The bioavailability of some drugs increases by up to 250% in the presence of cirrhosis.[20] Drugs for which increased oral bioavailability in cirrhotic patients has been demonstrated include labetalol, metoprolol, propranolol, pethidine (meperidine), pentazocine, diltiazem and verapamil. To avoid toxicity, oral doses of drugs with known first-pass metabolism need to be reduced in patients with severe liver disease.

### *1.3.2 Hepatic Failure and Drug Distribution*

The presence of fluid accumulation in ascites or peripheral oedema may increase the volume of distribution of water soluble drugs such as amikacin.[21] The decreased protein binding of drugs may also influence distribution. For highly bound drugs, decreased binding means a greater fraction of the drug in plasma is available to enter the tissues and the apparent volume of distribution increases. In the context of plasma concentration monitoring, the implications are that for any given total drug concentration, the pharmacological effect will be greater.

An increased volume of distribution may also increase the half-life of certain drugs such as tolbutamide.[22] Whether or not changes in protein binding influence the half-life depends on how binding influences clearance (see section 1.3.3 below).

#### 1.3.3 Hepatic Failure and Drug Elimination

Severe liver disease, by decreasing enzyme activity and/or decreasing liver blood flow, reduces the clearance of many drugs which are extensively metabolised. For such drugs, doses must be reduced during long term therapy (see appendix F) or alternative drugs, which are eliminated primarily by the kidney, should be selected. Exceptions are drugs such as oxazepam and lorazepam, which are metabolised by conjugation with glucuronic acid.[23] The clearance of these drugs is not affected by even severe liver disease.

It is not possible to predict the extent of impairment of metabolism from liver function tests. However, abnormal liver function, particularly decreased albumin and increased prothrombin time, or clinical evidence of severe liver disease such as ascites, jaundice, or hepatic encephalopathy indicate that some dosage adjustments may be required for susceptible drugs. A reasonable approach in such circumstances is to lower the dose and monitor drug concentrations where possible, closely observing the patient for evidence of drug toxicity.

### 1.4 Renal Failure

Acute renal failure may follow severe traumatic injury or prolonged hypotension. Chronic renal failure is a risk factor for a variety of life-threatening medical illnesses and is common in critically ill patients in general.

Renal failure is primarily of concern in slowing the clearance of drugs eliminated by the kidney, but renal failure can also result in abnormal distribution, metabolism and pharmacodynamics of drugs.

#### 1.4.1 Renal Failure and Drug Distribution

Chronic renal failure is associated with reduced serum albumin concentrations, resulting in reduced binding of drugs normally bound to albumin (see also chapter 1; sect. 5.4.2; and chapter 24; sect. 1.2). Accumulation of endogenous substances may compete with plasma proteins for the binding of drugs such as phenytoin.[24] As a consequence, the fraction of unbound phenytoin increases. Binding may decrease from 90 to 80%, which means the unbound percentage increases from 10 to 20%. Since the concentration of unbound phenytoin during long term therapy at stable dosage remains the same (see chapter 5, sect. 1.6.3), the total plasma concentration will be 50% lower than expected for the particular dose. The therapeutic implications are that the total concentration of phenytoin in the blood will be lower for the same free drug concentration, but the daily dose requirement is unchanged.

The tissue distribution of digoxin appears to be decreased in renal failure, resulting in higher than expected blood concentrations after a single dose.[25]

#### 1.4.2 Renal Failure and Drug Metabolism

Chronic renal failure accelerates the metabolism of some drugs like phenazone (antipyrine), but impairs the acetylation of several agents and slows the hydrolysis of procaine (see also chapter 24; sect. 1.3).[26]

The magnitude of the effect of renal failure on the metabolism of most drugs is however, relatively small, and dosage adjustments for drugs which are primarily metabolised are not generally required. The exception is when drugs are metabolised to active metabolites, which are renally excreted. Some examples are morphine, pethidine and procainamide, the active metabolites of which are morphine 6-glucuronide, norpethidine and acecainide, respectively.

#### 1.4.3 Renal Failure and Drug Excretion

Renal failure is associated with a reduced glomerular filtration rate (GFR) and a reduced clearance of drugs whose excretion is primarily by the kidney. For some drugs, such as the aminoglycosides, changes in clearance are proportional to changes in GFR. The maintenance dose of such drugs is decreased in proportion to the reduction in GFR.

Many drugs are secreted or reabsorbed by the renal tubules. These processes are also affected by renal failure, although they are often proportionally less affected than the decrement in GFR. The modification in maintenance dose for drugs primarily excreted by tubular secretion may be less than the fall in GFR.

Renal failure may also lead to accumulation of toxic drug metabolites. For example, accumulation of the pethidine metabolite norpethidine in patients with renal insufficiency may cause sedation, myoclonus or seizures.[27] Likewise, morphine 6-glucuronide can accumulate and produce respiratory depression when morphine is administered in patients with chronic renal failure.[28]

For most drugs, renal failure does not require a change in loading dose, but maintenance doses for renally excreted drugs need to be reduced. This may be achieved by giving smaller doses at the usual dosage intervals or, as is commonly done for the aminoglycosides, by giving the same maintenance dose at longer intervals. For example, 50% of the loading dose is given every half-life, and the change in half-life is computed according to the change in GFR. Dosage guidelines based on serum creatinine or creatinine clearance have been developed for many drugs (see appendices D and E).

## 1.5 Acute Pulmonary Insufficiency

Pulmonary insufficiency influences drug kinetics primarily by causing hypoxia, or by haemodynamic consequences of treatment such as with positive-pressure mechanical ventilation.

### 1.5.1 Pulmonary Insufficiency and Drug Absorption and Distribution

Drugs such as bronchodilators and corticosteroids are often administered by inhalation to patients with acute pulmonary insufficiency. Aerosolised drugs are absorbed via the tracheal and bronchial mucosa. Although it is theoretically possible that severe bronchial disease might impair the absorption of such drugs, there is no evidence to date that this is a clinical problem.

Severe hypoxia and/or hypotension, which is sometimes present in patients requiring positive-pressure ventilation, results in the activation of sympathetic reflexes and redistribution of blood flow as described above (section 1.1.1). Positive pressure ventilation itself may decrease venous return to the heart and lower cardiac output.[29] In such patients, absorption from intramuscular or subcutaneous sites is expected to be slow. As in cardiac failure, a consequence of reduced blood flow to the muscle and skin may be central nervous system or cardiac toxicity after rapid intravenous administration of drugs.

### 1.5.2 Pulmonary Insufficiency and Drug Elimination

Pulmonary failure can affect drug elimination in several ways. Acute severe hypoxia ($PO_2$ <40mm Hg) can directly impair the function of drug metabolising enzymes and decrease the metabolic rate.[30,31] Cardiovascular consequences of positive-pressure ventilation include decreased liver blood flow and a reduced glomerular filtration rate,[32] both of which can slow drug elimination. Reduced clearance of lidocaine during mechanical ventilation has been reported.[33]

While it is difficult to determine which abnormality is responsible, acute respiratory failure is known to be associated with a 2- to 3-fold decrease in theophylline clearance.[34] In such patients, it is prudent to begin theophylline maintenance therapy with 50% of the dose predicted on the basis of body weight and smoking history, and to adjust the dose according to subsequently measured blood concentrations.

## 1.6 Infections/Fever

Hepatic drug metabolism may be depressed by the presence of infection. Febrile respiratory viral illnesses have been reported to depress the metabolism of theophylline.[35,36] Malaria and pneumococcal pneumonia are associated with depressed hepatic clearance of quinine and phenazone (antipyrine), respectively.[37,38] Fever, induction of interferon, and bacterial endotoxins have each been shown to impair hepatic drug metabolism and may contribute to reduced

**Table I.** Physiological changes resulting from burns that could affect drug kinetics[a]

| Phase | Physiological alteration | Effect on drug kinetics |
|---|---|---|
| **Early** (<24h post-burn) | Hypovolaemic shock with:<br>• Decreased renal blood flow<br>• Decreased hepatic blood flow<br>• Peripheral vasoconstriction | Decreased renal drug excretion<br>Decreased hepatic clearance of highly extracted drugs<br>Decreased volume of distribution |
| | Increased serum $\alpha_1$-acid glycoprotein concentration | Increased protein binding of basic drugs |
| **Late** (>1 week post-burn) | Increased glomerular filtration rate | Increased renal drug excretion |
| | Decreased serum albumin concentration | Decreased protein binding of acidic drugs |
| | Increased hepatic blood flow | Increased hepatic clearance of highly extracted drugs |

a The clinical importance of some of these mechanisms has not been established (see table II).

**Table II.** Changes in drug kinetics and dynamics in humans and animals as a result of extensive burns

| |
|---|
| **Humans** |
| Enhanced elimination due to increased glomerular filtration rate: |
| • Cimetidine |
| • Ranitidine |
| • Aminoglycoside antibiotics: |
| Tobramycin |
| Gentamicin |
| Amikacin |
| Vancomycin |
| Decreased drug effect on target organ: |
| • Neuromuscular blocking drugs (tubocurarine) |
| Decreased clearance due to decreased hepatic metabolism: |
| • Pethidine (meperidine) |
| • Quinidine |
| • Lidocaine (lignocaine) |
| **Animals** |
| Increased protein binding (lower free drug fraction) of drugs that bind to $\alpha_1$-acid glycoprotein: |
| • Quinidine |
| • Lidocaine (lignocaine) |
| Decreased volume of distribution – mechanism uncertain: |
| • Quinidine |
| • Lidocaine (lignocaine) |
| • Pethidine (meperidine) |

metabolic clearance in patients with infections.[39]

## 1.7 Burns/Multiple Organ Failure

Burns can affect a drug's action by altering its pharmacokinetics or by effects on target organs (tables I and II). These changes are most prominent with extensive burns involving 15 to 25% of the body surface area. Relatively few drugs have been well studied in burn patients. However, knowledge of the physiological alterations observed in burn patients does allow anticipation of the types of drugs and magnitude of dosage changes that may be required.[40]

### 1.7.1 Early Physiological Changes (<24 Hours After Burn)

Shock may develop rapidly after extensive burns as a result of sequestration of fluid in the burned tissues (burn oedema) at the expense of intravascular volume. Fluid sequestration results from at least 3 distinct mechanisms:

1) Cellular swelling resulting from changes in cell membrane permeability.

2) Release of osmotically active substances from injured tissues.

3) Increased vascular permeability of burned tissue.

Increased permeability may be mediated in part by vasoactive substances such as histamine and prostaglandins.

The physiological consequences of shock due to burns are similar to those of other types of hypovolaemic shock. Systemic vascular resistance increases, tissue perfusion is impaired, and lactic acidosis may occur. Renal blood flow and glomerular filtration rate may be decreased markedly. Since shock due to burns is usually readily corrected by fluid administration, the duration of shock and its physiological consequences are generally brief. However, if shock is complicated by acute tubular necrosis and renal failure, renal function may be impaired for much longer periods of time.

The early post-burn period is also accompanied by an increase in the serum concentration $\alpha_1$-acid glycoprotein (AAG), necessitating extra attention to interpreting measured total concentrations of basic drugs for which therapeutic drug monitoring is undertaken.

### 1.7.2 Late Physiological Changes (>7 Days After Burn)

By one week post-burn, blood pressure is usually normal or high. Fluid requirements are increased because of evaporative losses from burned tissues but, with adequate fluid administration, circulatory function is not impaired. Cardiac output is often increased, perhaps because of the hypermetabolic state and increased body temperature associated with extensive burns. The glomerular filtration rate increases markedly. A mean creatinine clearance of 172 ml/min (10.32 L/h; normal is 125 ml/min or 7.5 L/h) was measured in one group of patients between the fourth and thirty-fifth day post-burn.[41]

Impaired liver function following burns is common.[42] Impaired metabolism of pethidine (in humans), quinidine and lidocaine (in rats) has been described. In contrast to these cytochrome P450-mediated metabolic pathways, the clearance of lorazepam and morphine via conjugation appears to be unaffected by burns.[43,44]

Plasma protein concentrations fall in the late post-burn period, with albumin concentrations often as low as 2 to 3 g/100ml.

### 1.7.3 Effects of Burns on Drug Kinetics

The effects of burns on drug disposition vary greatly from patient to patient and over time. When changes in drug kinetics are anticipated, the most practical approach is to individualise dosage by monitoring the drug effect or drug concentrations in plasma.

The effects of hypotension or shock resulting from burns on drug disposition would be expected to be similar to those of other types of hypovolaemic shock. However, few drugs have been studied specifically in the early post-burn period. Initial doses of some drugs may need to be reduced because of impaired tissue perfusion and the resulting decreased volume of distribution. Decreased renal drug excretion and decreased hepatic metabolism of highly extracted drugs may be anticipated but their importance will be minimised if the duration of hypotension is brief. In rats, the unbound fraction of the basic drugs quinidine and lidocaine in plasma decreases 24 hours post-burn, because of an increase in the plasma $\alpha_1$-acid glycoprotein concentration.[45] While this could lead to altered drug metabolism or magnitude of drug effect, the clinical importance of this mechanism in patients is unclear.

In the late post-burn period, the increased glomerular filtration rate clearly influences drug elimination. Shortened half-lives have been demonstrated for tobramycin, gentamicin, amikacin, vancomycin, cimetidine and ranitidine.[41,46-49] For each of these drugs, the change in half-life is sufficient to require increased drug doses to maintain therapeutic plasma drug concentrations. For the aminoglycosides, dosage can be individualised by measurement of serum/plasma concentrations. In the case of cimetidine or other $H_2$-blockers, monitoring of gastric pH and attempting to maintain it at >4 as a measure of efficacy, or using antacids or sucralfate are alternatives to drug concentration monitoring.[46]

The unbound fraction of phenytoin, a drug that binds to albumin, is increased 2- to 3-fold in burned patients with hypoalbuminaemia.[50] Since phenytoin is poorly extracted by the liver and only unbound drug is metabolised, the increase in unbound fraction enhances the total plasma clearance of the drug and decreases the total plasma concentration (although the unbound clearance does not change). The decreased phenytoin binding in plasma also increases its volume of distribution. As a result of these changes, the concentration of free, pharmacologically active drug in plasma is difficult to predict.

#### 1.7.4 Effects of Burns on Pharmacodynamics

Aside from their effects on pharmacokinetics, extensive burns may change target organ sensitivity to drugs. The non-depolarising neuromuscular blocking drug tubocurarine is less potent in burn patients, and plasma concentrations 2- to 5-fold greater than normal are required to produce muscular relaxation. This effect cannot be accounted for by changes in drug protein binding, and is probably due to burn-related changes at the neuromuscular junction.[51]

### 1.8 Acid-Base Disturbances

Acidaemia is a common feature of circulatory and respiratory states, sepsis, seizures and renal failure. Alkalaemia is occasionally seen during assisted ventilation in patients with underlying metabolic alkalosis and sometimes during cardiopulmonary resuscitation when excessive doses of sodium bicarbonate are administered.

Acid-base disturbances may influence both drug distribution and elimination. The primary effects of acid-base disturbances on drug kinetics depend on the effect on ionisation of a particular drug. Unionised drugs are able to penetrate lipid membranes more easily than ionised drugs. The extent of ionisation depends on the pH of the blood or tissue and the pKa of the drug (see chapter 1; sect. 1.1). Weak acids are more extensively ionised at a high pH, and weak bases are more extensively ionised at a low pH. Specific examples in critical care where acid-base disorders influence pharmacokinetics are described below.

#### 1.8.1 Acid-Base Disturbances and Drug Distribution

The tissue distribution of many weakly basic and acidic drugs is influenced by systemic acid-base disturbances. For example, the development of systemic acidaemia is associated with aggravation of the CNS toxicity associated with salicylate intoxication. Salicylate is less ionised in acid conditions and crosses membranes into tissues, including the brain. Conversely, treatment with an alkali to correct acidaemia is a critical component of successful management of salicylate poisoning.

Differences in pH between blood and body tissues may influence the penetration of drugs into those tissues. One example is the effect of seizures on the uptake of antiepileptic drugs into the brain. During seizures, both the brain and blood become more acidic than normal, the fall in pH being more pronounced for blood than for the brain. As a consequence, the penetration into the brain of phenobarbital, a weak acid, is greater during seizures than in non-seizure conditions.[52] By contrast, the penetration of the weak base lidocaine is reduced during seizures.[53]

#### 1.8.2 Acid-Base Disturbances and Drug Excretion

For a number of drugs, renal excretion is influenced by urinary pH. Weak acids, such as phenobarbital and salicylate, are excreted to a greater extent in alkaline urine. Weak bases, such as amphetamines and quinidine, are excreted to a greater extent in acid urine (see also chapter 1, sect. 3.4; chapter 24, sect. 1.4.2).

### 1.9 Drug Interactions in Critically Ill Patients

Certain drug interactions are particularly common in critically ill patients because of the large number of medications they typically receive. For example, cimetidine and antacids are used widely in the management or prophylaxis of gastrointestinal stress ulceration. Cimetidine inhibits the oxidative metabolism of many drugs, including lidocaine, theophylline and warfarin (see also chapter 22; sect. 4.2.2 and appendix B).[54] When cimetidine is used, doses of other interacting drugs need to be reduced appropriately; however, this is not a problem with other $H_2$-blockers. Antacids may interfere with the gastrointestinal absorption of a number of drugs (see chapter 22; sect. 4.2.1 and appendix B) and may, in large doses, produce an alkaline urine which can affect the renal excretion of drugs, as described above (section 1.8.2).

Antibiotic use is quite common in critically ill patients. Erythromycin may inhibit the metabolism of theophylline,[55] and in some patients reduces the clearance of digoxin.[56] Many broad-spectrum antibiotics are capable, particularly in malnourished patients, of eliminating vitamin K synthesising bacteria in the gastrointestinal tract, making patients more sensitive to the hypoprothrombinaemic action of warfarin.

Vasoactive drugs used to manage shock or other circulatory problems may influence the distribution and elimination of other drugs. For example, infusion of noradrenaline (norepinephrine) will reduce blood flow to the muscles, skin, liver and kidney, slowing the distribution and elimination of other drugs.[11] Conversely, infusion of isoprenaline (isoproterenol), by increasing liver blood flow, might accelerate the hepatic metabolism of drugs such as lidocaine.

Other drugs used in critically ill patients that are subject to significant drug interactions include digoxin, calcium antagonists, β-adrenoceptor blockers, antiarrhythmic drugs, anticoagulants and cyclosporin (see appendix B for further information).

## 2. General Principles of Critical Care Management

### 2.1 Preservation of Cardiovascular, Respiratory and Metabolic Function

#### 2.1.1 Physiological Monitoring

Physiological measurements in combination with clinical assessment provide the basis for therapeutic intervention. Routine monitoring of critical care patients includes frequent vital signs and central nervous and electrocardiographic monitoring. Where blood pressure is unstable, intra-arterial catheters provide continuous assessment of blood pressure. Frequent measurements of arterial blood gases and pH, $PO_2$ by transcutaneous oximetry, and serum electrolytes are useful in monitoring respiratory and metabolic function. In the presence of cardiac or respiratory disease with circulatory dysfunction, central venous or pulmonary arterial catheters are useful to guide optimum fluid resuscitation and vasoactive drug therapy. Intracranial pressure monitoring is used to guide therapy in patients with head trauma, mass lesions or some infectious processes of the brain. Electroencephalographic recording is useful in managing status epilepticus, particularly when patients are paralysed.

#### 2.1.2 Preservation of Cardiovascular Function

Preservation of cardiovascular function requires prompt attention to fluid and electrolyte status, and prompt recognition and correction of arrhythmias and shock (see section 3.1). Preservation of the myocardium in acute myocardial infarction is most effectively achieved by early use of thrombolytic agents such as streptokinase or alteplase (tissue-type plasminogen activator; t-PA), or by emergency coronary angioplasty when thrombolytics are contraindicated (see also chapter 20). In addition, blood pressure control and use of β-adrenoceptor blockers will reduce myocardial oxygen demand and may help limit the extent of permanent myocardial damage. The use of angiotensin-converting enzyme (ACE) inhibitors after acute myocardial infarction reduces long term morbidity and mortality by preventing progressive deterioration of ventricular function (ventricular remodelling), and appears to reduce short term mortality, at least in patients not receiving thrombolysis as well.[57,58]

#### *2.1.3 Preservation of Respiratory Function*

Major respiratory complications in critically ill patients include pulmonary oedema, due to fluid overload and/or increased pulmonary capillary permeability (acute respiratory distress syndrome; ARDS), and pneumonia, both bacterial and due to aspiration. Prolonged exposure to high levels of oxygen can also induce pulmonary injury. Preservation of respiratory function requires the cautious use of fluids and the use of oxygen concentrations only as necessary to maintain reasonable oxygenation, i.e. arterial $PO_2 \geq 60$mm Hg. A major cause of ARDS is sepsis.[59] Prompt recognition and management of infection may reduce the risk of this pulmonary complication. Meticulous nursing care, protection of the airway, and gastric suction will reduce the risks of pneumonia.

#### *2.1.4 Attention to Metabolic Factors*

Optimisation of circulatory and respiratory function provides the best chance of maintaining adequate hepatic and renal function. In the presence of liver failure, restriction of protein intake, use of lactulose and avoidance of hypnosedative drugs may prevent or reduce the severity of hepatic encephalopathy (see also chapter 22; sect. 8.3.3, 12.4). With acute renal failure, haemodialysis may be necessary to treat fluid overload, electrolyte disturbances or manifestations of uraemia (see chapter 24; sect. 6.1). Hyperglycaemia and hypoglycaemia due to diabetes and/or stress and liver disease and/or malnutrition are relatively common. These conditions are managed with insulin and glucose as described in chapter 19 (sect. 3).

Critically ill patients are often catabolic and unable to take adequate nutrition. Malnutrition impedes healing and makes patients more susceptible to infection. Critically ill patients should therefore receive adequate nutrition within 2 to 3 days of admission. Adequate nutrition may be achieved by the enteral or parenteral route. The enteral route is preferred, because of lower cost, fewer complications, and better preservation of intestinal mucosal integrity. If enteric nutrition is impossible, the use of parenteral nutrition is recommended.[60,61] The goal of parenteral nutrition is to establish a positive nitrogen balance.

### 2.2 Fluid Therapy

The goal of fluid therapy in critically ill patients is to replete intravascular volume. Common causes of intravascular volume depletion include haemorrhage, vomiting, diarrhoea, excessive diuresis (due to drugs or diabetes), inadequate fluid intake, and redistribution of fluid out of the vascular space (e.g. in anaphylaxis, sepsis, burns). A relative deficiency of intravascular volume may also occur due to vasodilatation, without fluid loss. The consequences of intravascular volume depletion are hypotension and inadequate organ perfusion. A systolic blood pressure of 90mm Hg is usually adequate, but assessment of end organ function is a better measure of tissue perfusion. Adequate perfusion of the brain (in the absence of complicating factors) is indicated by a normal level of consciousness and mentation. Administration of fluid is usually continued until clinical signs of inadequate perfusion are no longer evident, or until the central venous pressure is at least 12 to 15cm $H_2O$.

In the presence of cardiac disease, central venous pressure may not accurately reflect filling pressures in the left ventricle, and a pulmonary artery catheter is helpful. Fluid replacement should continue until adequate blood pressure and organ perfusion are achieved, or until the pulmonary capillary wedge pressure is 15 to 18mm Hg. In patients with the acute respiratory distress syndrome (see section 3.4), it may be necessary to limit the pulmonary capillary wedge pressure to avoid aggravating pulmonary oedema.

Fluid replacement may be accomplished using crystalloid (isotonic solutions such as normal saline or Ringer lactate), colloid (albumin, dextran, hetastarch) or blood components. Crystalloid is used most commonly because it is readily available and inexpensive. The principal disadvantage of crystalloid is that it readily distributes out of the vascular space. Colloid solutions remain in the intravascular space longer than crystalloid, but do enter tissues to some extent along with water. In most clinical settings, an advantage of colloid over crystalloid has not been established. To achieve the same degree of expansion of intravascular volume, one must infuse a much larger (3- to 4-fold) amount of crystalloid than colloid. However, there is no convincing evidence that either crystalloid or colloid is superior when resuscitation is targeted to a constant end-point, e.g. a specific central venous or pulmonary capillary wedge pressure. There is no advantage to the use of colloids in the setting of non-cardiogenic pulmonary oedema, because the leaky pulmonary capillaries allow the infused colloids to enter the lung interstitium. The principal use of colloid solutions is in the treatment of haemorrhagic shock when crystalloid is not effective and blood is not readily available.

Blood is the most effective fluid for expanding intravascular volume, and is the only fluid that can provide oxygen carrying capacity. It is indicated for haemorrhagic shock, but is generally not used in situations where crystalloid or colloid are effective because of the risk of transfusion reactions, transmission of infection, and cost.

### 2.3 Cerebral Protection

Brain injury or death is a common cause of morbidity or mortality in critically ill patients. Protection of cerebral function requires the maintenance of cerebral blood flow with adequate oxygenation and glucose, sufficient to meet the metabolic demands of the brain. Cerebral blood flow depends on mean systemic blood pressure and intracranial pressure. Effective cerebral perfusion pressure is the difference between the two. Circulatory support, maintaining adequate oxygenation and blood glucose, and control of intracranial hypertension are necessary to preserve cerebral blood flow. Specific management of brain injury is discussed in section 3.5.

Reducing the metabolic demands of the brain may be critical to preserving brain function. Prompt control of seizures and hyperthermia, both of which increase the metabolic activity of the brain, is essential.

### 2.4 Anti-Infective Therapy

Critically ill patients have a high risk of infection because of impaired host defences and multiple invasive procedures. Diseases predisposing to infection include severe trauma, renal failure, diabetes and leukaemia. Therapy with drugs which suppress the immune system or bone marrow, such as those used in patients with organ transplants, cancer or vasculitis, or the presence of acquired immune deficiency due to malnutrition or viral infections (e.g. human immunodeficiency virus, HIV) also present a high risk. Iatrogenic sources of infection include endotracheal tubes, indwelling bladder or intravenous catheters, and contaminated nebulisers for inhalational drug therapy.

Prophylaxis against acquired infections requires vigorous handwashing and adherence to principles of sterility in the placement and maintenance of intravenous and bladder catheters, and the regular sterilisation of and use of sterile solutions in nebulisers. Prophylactic antibiotic therapy in critically ill patients has not been shown to be effective.

The evaluation of infection is often difficult in critically ill patients. Fever may be due to tissue injury, central nervous system dysfunction or drug allergy rather than infection. Conversely, patients with sepsis are often afebrile or hypothermic. Similarly, leucocytosis is nonspecific; it can result from severe tissue injury. Some infected patients are neutropenic. Sudden changes in mental status, unexplained tachypnoea, hypotension or hypothermia are important, although nonspecific, clues to the development of sepsis.

The management of specific infections is discussed in other chapters in this book. The selection of antibiotics depends on the presumed site of infection and the particular experience of individual hospitals with respect to types and antibiotic sensitivities of bacteria. However, when patients are critically ill and sepsis is suspected, it is often prudent to begin antibiotic therapy on an empirical basis. Combination antibiotic therapy to cover both Gram-negative and Gram-positive bacteria is commonly employed in critically ill patients or compromised hosts. Antibiotics should be appropriately adjusted when bacterial cultures and sensitivities become available.

### 2.5 Prophylaxis against Gastric Stress Erosions and Ulcers

Gastric erosions, resembling erosive gastritis, are common in patients with critical illnesses. Although only a small percentage of patients develop frank gastrointestinal haemorrhage, when they do haemorrhage it is associated with substantial mortality. The risk of significant gastric bleeding is greatest in patients who require mechanical ventilation or have a coagulopathy.[62] The prophylactic use of either $H_2$-blockers (e.g. cimetidine) or sucralfate for such patients is common practice. Of note, however, is a recent study showing no benefit of cimetidine or sucralfate compared with placebo in preventing gastric haemorrhage in medical intensive care patients.[63] The prophylactic use of $H_2$-blockers appears to be associated with an increased risk of nosocomial pneumonia, which is believed to be caused by microaspiration of gastric contents that have been colonised with bacteria that normally would not survive at a more acid pH. An increase of nosocomial pneumonia in patients receiving $H_2$-blockers has been reported in some studies but not in others.[63-65]

### 2.6 Pulmonary Embolism

In addition to the problems discussed above, critically ill patients are prone to develop complications such as pulmonary embolism because of prolonged immobility, tissue injury and/or activation of coagulation. Deep vein thrombosis was present in 58% of patients with major trauma in one large series.[66] When prolonged bed rest is required and there is no contraindication (such as recent surgery, head trauma or gastrointestinal haemorrhage), prophylactic treatment with subcutaneous heparin (5000 units 2 or 3 times daily) is often instituted.[67] However, when the thrombotic risk is very high, as with total hip or knee replacement, subcutaneous heparin may be ineffective in preventing venous thromboembolism. In this situation, effective prophylaxis may be achieved with use of low molecular weight heparin (e.g. enoxaparin in a dose of 30mg subcutaneously twice daily).[68] The management of acute pulmonary embolism is discussed further in chapter 23 (sect. 11).

When more rapid resolution of emboli is necessary, as in the case of hypotension or clinical evidence of low cardiac output, a thrombolytic agent is indicated. Alteplase (tissue-type plasminogen activator; t-PA) in a dose of 100mg over 2 hours is superior to standard doses or urokinase.[69] Emergency embolectomy is seldom indicated, but should be considered for shock due to massive embolism when thrombolysis is contraindicated or is ineffective.

### 2.7 Avoiding Drug-Induced Complications

Adverse drug reactions are common enough in patients in general, but critically ill patients are particularly susceptible because of the multiple number of drugs used, the presence of multiple organ dysfunction, and the difficulty in predicting the pharmacokinetics and altered sensitivity of organs to drug effects. The presence of severe disease makes it difficult to diagnose drug-induced organ dysfunction, and critically ill patients are often less able to tolerate drug toxicity. A common example is the problem of aminoglycoside-induced nephrotoxicity in patients with sepsis and pre-existing renal failure.

To minimise the occurrence of adverse drug reactions, the following are recommended:

1) Consider the effects of the presence of organ dysfunction on pharmacokinetics and adjust initial drug doses accordingly.

2) Set specific end-points for therapy where possible.

3) Monitor drug concentrations if possible.

4) Monitor patients carefully for early evidence of toxicity.

5) Review medication records in total on a regular basis to detect possible adverse drug interactions.

## 3. Management of Specific Critical Care Conditions

Selected disorders which are particularly relevant to the care of critically ill patients are discussed below. For a more complete discussion of critical care management, see review by Chernow.[70]

### 3.1 Non-Cardiogenic Shock

Shock is a state of reduced blood flow that is inadequate to meet the metabolic requirements of vital organs. Shock may be caused by intravascular volume depletion, impaired myocardial performance, or dilatation of arteries or veins due to released vasoactive substances during bacterial sepsis or to the actions of drugs. When impaired cardiac pump function is the principal cause of shock, it is termed cardiogenic (see further chapter 20). Other types of shock are collectively termed non-cardiogenic (table III). Regardless of cause, shock is typically manifested by profound arterial hypotension, impaired mentation, decreased urine output, and lactic acidosis. Therapy is directed at:

1) Alleviating the precipitating cause of shock.

2) Treating the haemodynamic and metabolic consequences.

3) Managing secondary medical complications such as renal failure and pulmonary oedema.

#### *3.1.1 Features Common to all Types of Shock*

Shock is often reversible if the underlying cause is corrected and the haemodynamic disturbances are managed appropriately. If shock persists, it may be complicated by injury to vital organs and may eventually become irreversible.

**Table III.** Common causes of shock

| |
|---|
| **Cardiogenic:** |
| Mechanical |
| • Regurgitant lesions |
| • Obstruction of blood flow |
| Arrhythmias |
| Myopathic |
| • Infarction |
| • Cardiomyopathy |
| **Non-cardiogenic:** |
| Intravascular volume depletion |
| • Haemorrhage |
| • Dehydration |
| • Burns |
| • Anaphylaxis |
| Vasodilatation |
| • Sepsis |
| • Spinal shock |
| **Obstructive lesions:** |
| Pericardial tamponade |
| Pulmonary embolus |
| **Drugs:** |
| Many mechanisms (see table IV) |

An important and common consequence of persistent shock is impaired cardiac performance. Factors contributing to impaired cardiac performance include ischaemia due to hypotension and decreased coronary artery blood flow, increased cardiac workload due to increased systemic vascular resistance (primarily a problem in cardiogenic shock), and arrhythmias that impair cardiac filling. Acidosis and circulating substances such as myocardial depressant factor may also contribute to cardiac dysfunction. In patients with severe and persistent shock, impaired cardiac contractility may contribute to the shock state becoming irreversible.

Lactic acidosis caused by impaired tissue perfusion and the resulting anaerobic metabolism is common in patients with shock. Acidosis may be detrimental because it may decrease cardiac contractility or cause or aggravate ventricular arrhythmias and/or attenuate the pressor actions of catecholamines and sympathomimetic amines used to treat shock. However, the use of bicarbonate in lactic acidosis is controversial. Animal studies have demonstrated worsening of myocardial contractility when bicarbonate was given in the setting of hypoxic lactic acidosis, perhaps because of a reduction in intracellular pH.[71] Hypertonic bicarbonate or other solutions also dilate arteries resulting in reduced coronary blood flow, which can also impair myocardial performance.[72] A prospective, randomised study found neither benefit nor harm from administration of bicarbonate to humans with shock and lactic acidosis.[73]

Shock may be accompanied by non-cardiogenic pulmonary oedema (see section 3.4). If hypoxaemia results, it may further compromise cardiac performance or contribute to the development of arrhythmias.

### 3.1.2 Common Types of Non-Cardiogenic Shock

#### Hypovolaemic Shock

Hypovolaemic shock is caused by depletion of intravascular volume. This may be due to loss of blood (haemorrhage), loss of body water (dehydration), or redistribution of body water out of the vascular space (anaphylaxis, burns). Loss of intravascular volume impairs cardiac output by decreasing cardiac filling and stroke volume. Systemic vascular resistance is increased due to increased sympathetic nervous system tone. Increasing the systemic vascular resistance increases the cardiac workload and may further compromise cardiac output. Cardiac contractility may become impaired in the late stages of hypovolaemic shock.

Septic shock is usually due to overwhelming infection with Gram-negative or Gram-positive bacteria, fungi, rickettsiae or viruses.[74,75] Endotoxins derived from cell walls of Gram-negative bacteria appear to be a cause of septic shock. The condition is characterised by both low systemic vascular resistance and impaired cardiac contractility. Cardiac output is often increased, despite impaired cardiac contractility, because of the low vascular resistance.

#### Drug Overdose

Drug overdosage may cause shock by producing arrhythmias, decreased cardiac output, or vasodilatation.[76] Drug-induced shock may therefore have features of both cardiogenic and non-cardiogenic shock. Individual drugs may act by more than one mechanism, or toxicity may be due to more than one drug. When the responsible drug is known, the mechanism of shock can often be anticipated and appropriate therapy initiated (table IV).

#### Burns

Burns are associated with oedema of the injured tissues and sequestration of fluids in these areas at the expense of intravascular volume. Factors contributing to burn oedema include cellular swelling due to increased cell membrane permeability, local release of osmotically active substances, and increased vascular permeability of burned tissue (see section 1.7).

### Spinal Shock

Spinal shock is a condition seen in patients with acute spinal cord injury, usually involving the cervical spine. Intravascular volume is normal in such patients, but because of a functional sympathectomy they have reduced vascular tone such that blood pools in the venous system. Bradycardia may potentiate the shock state, and hypothermia is common.

### Hypothermia

Hypothermia may cause hypotension when the core body temperature is lower than 30°C (86°F); a core temperature of ≥33°C (91°F) rarely causes haemodynamic compromise.[77] Hypothermia decreases the heart rate and, at very low temperatures, impairs cardiac contractility. Hypotension is further aggravated by loss of fluid from the vascular space into tissues. It is important to note that hypothermia decreases the metabolic requirements of tissues and thereby enhances their ability to withstand periods of poor perfusion. Patients with severe hypothermia may survive prolonged periods of profound hypotension (sometimes with no measurable blood pressure) and recover fully.

## *3.1.3 Clinical Pharmacology of Drugs Used in Treatment of Non-Cardiogenic Shock*

### Catecholamines and Sympathomimetic Amines

These drugs act on adrenergic receptors, producing a variety of cardiac and vascular effects that may be useful in the treatment of shock (table V). Their actions differ considerably, so that no single drug is appropriate for all forms of shock. The initial choice of a drug is based on the clinical setting and the expected

**Table IV.** Mechanisms and management of drug-induced shock

| Drug | Mechanism of shock | Specific antidote(s) | Supportive measures |
|---|---|---|---|
| Opioid drugs | Vasodilatation<br>Bradycardia | Naloxone | Fluids |
| Tricyclic antidepressants and other membrane-depressant drugs (e.g. quinidine, procainamide) | Decreased cardiac contractility<br>Vasodilatation<br>Arrhythmias | Sodium bicarbonate (hypertonic) | Fluids<br>Inotropic agents<br>Vasopressors |
| Hypnosedatives (barbiturates, ethanol) | Vasodilatation<br>Decreased cardiac contractility | | Fluids<br>Inotropic agents<br>Vasopressors<br>Enhancement of elimination of some hypnosedatives by haemodialysis or haemoperfusion |
| β-Adrenoceptor antagonists (β-Blockers) | Decreased cardiac contractility<br>Bradycardia | β-Agonists<br>Glucagon | Fluids |
| Calcium antagonists | Decreased cardiac contractility<br>Bradycardia<br>Vasodilatation | Calcium chloride or calcium gluconate | Fluids<br>Inotropic agents<br>Vasopressors |
| Antipsychotics (chlorpromazine, thioridazine) | Vasodilatation | | Fluids<br>Vasopressors |
| Theophylline | Vasodilatation<br>Tachyarrhythmias | | Fluids<br>β-Blockers<br>Vasopressors<br>Enhancement of drug elimination by haemoperfusion |
| Sympatholytic antihypertensive drugs (clonidine, methyldopa, reserpine) | Vasodilatation<br>Bradycardia | | Fluids<br>Vasopressors |
| Cholinergic agents (organophosphates, carbamate insecticides, physostigmine) | Bradyarrhythmias<br>Vasodilatation | Atropine<br>Pralidoxime | Fluids<br>Cardiac pacemaker |
| Digitalis glycosides | Arrhythmias<br>Atrioventricular block<br>Hyperkalaemia | Drug-specific Fab antibody fragments | Atropine<br>Cardiac pacemaker<br>Phenytoin, lidocaine |
| Carbon monoxide | Myocardial ischaemia with arrhythmias or decreased cardiac contractility | Oxygen, 100% or hyperbaric | Fluids<br>Inotropic agents<br>Antiarrhythmic drugs |

**Table V.** Receptor-mediated drug actions of importance in the treatment of shock

| Receptor | Cardiac effects | Vascular effects | Principal clinical effects |
|---|---|---|---|
| $\beta_1$-Adrenergic | Increased heart rate<br>Increased cardiac contractility<br>Enhanced atrioventricular conduction<br>Increased automaticity | | Increased cardiac output |
| $\beta_2$-Adrenergic | Increased heart rate | Vasodilatation (arterial) | Decreased systemic vascular resistance |
| $\alpha_1$-Adrenergic | | Vasoconstriction (arterial and venous) | Increased systemic vascular resistance<br>Increased venous return to the heart |
| $\alpha_2$-Adrenergic (postsynaptic) | | Vasoconstriction (arterial and venous) | Increased systemic vascular resistance<br>Increased venous return to the heart |
| $D_1$-Dopaminergic | | Vasodilatation (renal, mesenteric) | Increased renal and mesenteric blood flow |

haemodynamic lesion. If shock persists, placement of a pulmonary artery catheter is useful. Such a catheter allows measurement of cardiac output, pulmonary artery wedge pressure and systemic vascular resistance, which can help determine whether fluids, inotropic drugs, vasopressors, or a combination of these is needed (table VI). For example, if left ventricular filling pressure, reflected by pulmonary capillary wedge pressure, is low then fluids are indicated. If cardiac output is low, inotropic agents and/or vasodilators are indicated; if systemic vascular resistance is low, vasoconstrictors are indicated.

Sympathomimetic drugs may act directly by stimulating adrenergic receptors or indirectly by stimulating the release of stored catecholamines from adrenergic neurons. Drugs that act directly are preferred because neuronal stores of catecholamines may be reduced in patients with shock. The dose of catecholamines or sympathomimetic amines required by patients with shock differs markedly from patient to patient, and may change over time in a single patient. The most satisfactory method of dosage is to choose drugs for which blood concentrations and magnitude of effect can be adjusted rapidly. Dosage is then determined by titration and is adjusted according to the patient's response. The catecholamines and sympathomimetic amines discussed below all have very short half-lives of 2 to 4 minutes, so that blood concentrations produced by intravenous infusion can be adjusted rapidly. Correction of acidaemia may be necessary when using catecholamines and sympathomimetic amines to treat shock, since these drugs may be less effective in acidaemic patients. The primary treatment for acidosis is correction of hypotension and restoration of normal tissue perfusion. As described below, the routine use of sodium bicarbonate in treating lactic acidosis is controversial.

***Adrenaline (epinephrine)*** is the primary therapy for anaphylactic shock because it combines both α- and β-adrenergic effects (see table VII). For all other types of shock, more selective adrenoceptor agonists are preferred (see section 3.1.4).

***Noradrenaline (norepinephrine)*** stimulates vascular $\alpha_1$ and $\alpha_2$ adrenoceptors and is used primarily as a vasopressor (vasoconstrictor). Arterial constriction increases systemic vascular resistance, while venous constriction increases venous return to the heart. Noradrenaline is also a weak $\beta_1$-adrenoceptor agonist and may produce a modest increase in heart rate and cardiac contractility in patients with shock. The primary indication for noradrenaline in patients with shock is low systemic vascular resistance. Noradrenaline is particularly useful in the early stages of septic shock when arterial vasodilatation predominates and cardiac function is not markedly depressed. Noradrenaline has also been used as a supplemental measure for patients with hypovolaemic shock until sufficient fluid replacement can be accomplished.

The lowest infusion rate of noradrenaline that produces haemodynamic effects in healthy volunteers is 4 to 8 μg/min.[78] When time permits, therapy should be initiated at this dose and the rate increased every 5 to 10 minutes as needed.

***Isoprenaline (isoproterenol)*** is a non-selective β-adrenoceptor agonist. Its $\beta_1$ action increases heart rate and contractility and enhances atrioventricular conduction, while its $\beta_2$ action produces vasodilatation and decreases systemic vascular resistance. The usefulness of isoprenaline in patients with shock is limited because decreasing systemic vascular resistance can worsen hypotension, and the cardiac effects result in greatly increased myocardial oxygen consumption. Isoprenaline is indicated for hypotension due to bradycardia, atrioventricular block, or certain arrhythmias such as polymorphic ventricular tachycardia associated with long Q-T interval (torsades de pointes). The usual starting dose is 0.5 μg/min, increased at 5- to 10-minute intervals as needed.

***Dopamine*** is the most widely used drug for all types of shock. Its actions are complex and dose-dependent. At low infusion rates (1 to 5 mg/kg/min), dopamine increases cardiac contractility through its $\beta_1$-adrenoceptor agonist activity and increases renal and mesenteric blood flow through its dopaminergic ($D_1$) agonist activity. At higher infusion rates (5 to 10 μg/kg/min), its α-adrenoceptor agonist activity results in increased systemic vascular resistance.

Compared with noradrenaline, dopamine has more $\beta_1$-adrenoceptor agonist activity and is preferred when both vasopressor and inotropic actions are needed. However, dopamine is less useful than noradrenaline when the predominant haemodynamic disturbance is a profound reduction in systemic vascular resistance.[79] Dopamine maintains renal blood flow better than noradrenaline, but may have adverse effects on splanchnic oxygen delivery. Dopamine may increase gut mucosal oxygen requirements while redistributing blood flow within the gut, resulting in reduced mucosal blood flow and worsening ischaemia.[80] In contrast, noradrenaline improves splanchnic oxygen utilisation in patients with hyperdynamic sepsis.

Selection of an initial dopamine infusion rate depends on the cause of hypotension. If dopamine is used primarily as an inotropic agent, an initial rate of 1 μg/kg/min is often sufficient. If it is used primarily as a vasopressor, an initial rate of 5 μg/kg/min is necessary.

***Dobutamine,*** a synthetic catecholamine with relatively selective inotropic activity, is used primarily in patients with cardiogenic shock (see further chapter 20). Because patients with non-cardiogenic shock usually require some vaso-

**Table VI.** Inotropic and vasopressor drugs used to treat shock

| Drug | Usual starting dose[a] | Receptor activity | Primary actions | Indications | Toxicity |
|---|---|---|---|---|---|
| Noradrenaline (norepinephrine) | 4-8 μg/min IV, increased as needed | $\alpha_1$, $\alpha_2$ weak $\beta_1$ | Vasoconstriction | Low systemic vascular resistance<br>Venodilatation | Decreased tissue perfusion<br>Increased cardiac workload |
| Adrenaline (epinephrine) | (see table VII) | | | | |
| Dopamine | 1 μg/kg/min for inotropic effect; 5 μg/kg/min for vasopressor effect, then increase as needed. Max. rate usually 10-15 μg/kg/min but up to 40 μg/kg/min has been used | Dose-related; dopamine $D_1$, $\beta_1$, $\beta_2$, α | Increased cardiac contractility<br>Increased systemic vascular resistance<br>Renal blood flow preserved (at lower infusion rate) | Low cardiac contractility<br>Low systemic vascular resistance | Tachyarrhythmias<br>Increased cardiac workload with high-dose infusions similar to noradrenaline |
| Dobutamine | 2.5 μg/kg/min, increased as needed. Max. rate usually 15 μg/kg/min but up to 50 μg/kg/min has been used | $\beta_1$, $\beta_2$, α | Increased cardiac contractility | Low cardiac contractility<br>Useful when increased heart rate and systemic vascular resistance not desired | Increased myocardial oxygen demand<br>Tachyarrhythmias |
| Isoprenaline (isoproterenol) | 0.5 μg/min, increased as needed | $\beta_1$, $\beta_2$ | Increased heart rate, cardiac contractility<br>Decreased systemic vascular resistance<br>Enhanced atrioventricular conduction | Bradycardia<br>Atrioventricular block<br>Torsades de pointes | Ventricular irritability<br>Tachyarrhythmias<br>Worsening of hypotension |

a Loading doses not needed because of short half-lives of these drugs; allow 5 to 10 minutes to approximate steady-state before changing the infusion rate.

*Abbreviation:* IV = intravenous.

**Table VII.** Drugs used in the treatment of anaphylaxis

| Drug | Dose | Mechanism | Clinical indications | Comments |
|---|---|---|---|---|
| Adrenaline (epinephrine) | *Mild reactions:* 0.3-0.5mg SC *Severe reactions:* 5-10 μg/min IV infusion; double rate every 5 min *or* 1.0ml of 1 : 10,000 solution (100μg) IV over 5-10 min *or* 100μg in 10ml normal saline per endotracheal tube | • Inhibits mediator release by mast cells and basophils • Bronchodilator • Vasopressor in large doses | Hypotension Angioedema, particularly oedema of upper airway Bronchospasm | • Primary drug therapy for anaphylaxis. Rapid onset of action. May be ineffective for hypotension unless adequate fluids administered • For insect stings in an extremity, injection of part of the dose SC locally may slow absorption of allergen |
| Inhaled $\beta_2$-agonist [e.g. salbutamol (albuterol)] | 2.5-5mg every 1-2h as needed (salbutamol) | Bronchodilator | Bronchospasm | |
| Antihistamines | Diphenhydramine 25-50mg IV over 1 min | Antagonises $H_1$ actions of histamine | Same as adrenaline (above) | Adjunctive therapy; rarely effective alone for severe anaphylaxis Role of $H_2$ blockers not established |
| Corticosteroids | Equivalent of hydrocortisone 200-300mg IV | Unclear | Bronchospasm ? Hypotension, oedema | Onset of action delayed 12-24h |

*Abbreviations:* IV = intravenous; SC = subcutaneous.

constriction, dobutamine is rarely used initially in this setting. It is useful primarily for patients already receiving a sympathomimetic drug who require additional inotropic support. The usual starting dose of dobutamine is 2.5 μg/kg/min. At infusion rates of up to 15 μg/kg/min, dobutamine produces little change in heart rate or systemic vascular resistance. Higher doses are occasionally used but may result in sinus tachycardia or other arrhythmias.

***Other sympathomimetic drugs:*** *phenylephrine* is a selective α-adrenoceptor agonist with little, β-adrenoceptor activity. It is theoretically preferable to noradrenaline in patients who require only vasoconstriction and is sometimes used for this purpose. An example would be therapy of spinal shock. Noradrenaline, however, is a satisfactory vasopressor for most situations because its weak $\beta_1$-adrenoceptor action is desirable in preventing a reflex decrease in cardiac output. *Methoxamine* is also more selective than noradrenaline, but it acts in part indirectly and may be less effective in patients with reduced neuronal stores of catecholamines.

### Other Drugs

***Glucagon*** increases cardiac contractility and rate through non-adrenergic mechanisms. It is useful in treating hypotension in patients with β-blocker overdose, who may not respond to β-agonists, and possibly in verapamil overdose. In other situations, glucagon offers no advantage over sympathomimetic agents, is more difficult to titrate because of its longer half-life, and often produces nausea and vomiting.

***Naloxone*** is a specific opioid antagonist that has been shown to be beneficial in several experimental models of shock. Large doses of naloxone (1 to 10 mg/kg) increased blood pressure in animals with septic, hypovolaemic or spinal shock.[81,82] Reversal of shock in animals is associated with an increase in cardiac contractility and cardiac output, with little or no change in vascular resistance. A controlled trial of naloxone in septic shock in humans showed only a small effect in increasing blood pressure and no effect on survival.[83]

***Corticosteroids*** have been studied as an adjunct to the use of inotropic and vasopressor drugs for septic shock. Their efficacy, as well as their proposed mechanisms of action, are controversial; inhibition of complement-mediated aggregation and resultant endothelial injury, and inhibition of the release of β-endorphin are current theories of their mechanism of action. However, controlled studies have not indicated a beneficial effect of high-dose corticosteroid therapy in treating septic shock.[84,85] Hence, there is no established role for corticosteroids in the treatment of shock, except shock caused by adrenal insufficiency.

#### 3.1.4 Optimum Treatment of Common Types of Non-Cardiogenic Shock

##### Hypovolaemic Shock

The primary therapy for hypovolaemic shock is volume replacement (see section 2.2). Drug therapy alone is ineffective; the roles for drug therapy are:

1) As an adjunct when maximum volume replacement alone is not rapidly effective; or

2) When hypovolaemic shock is prolonged and cardiac contractility is secondarily impaired.

The drugs most commonly used to supplement fluids in treating hypovolaemic shock are vasopressors such as noradrenaline and dopamine. These drugs increase systemic blood pressure by adding to the patient's already elevated systemic vascular resistance, and venoconstriction may increase venous return to the heart. However, perfusion of the kidneys, viscera and muscle may be further impaired by vasopressors, worsening organ injury and acidosis. Dopamine may be preferable to noradrenaline because, at least in low doses, it spares renal blood flow. Dopamine is also a more potent inotropic agent than noradrenaline and may be more useful when cardiac contractility is impaired. Overall, however, the contribution of vasopressors and inotropic agents to the treatment of hypovolaemic shock is limited.

Mechanical support of the circulation, in the form of pneumatic trousers, has been used as an adjunct to fluid administration for patients with haemorrhagic shock. It is most useful in the prehospital setting, before adequate fluid administration is possible. This device inflates over the patient's legs and increases vascular resistance in the compressed extremities. Blood pressure increases as a result of the increased total systemic vascular resistance. Inflation of the abdominal portion of the device may be useful in tamponading abdominal injuries and minimising bleeding. The use of pneumatic trousers for other types of shock is less well studied.

##### Septic Shock

Primary therapy for septic shock is treatment of the underlying infection. Support of blood pressure in the interim can be accomplished with fluids and drugs. Fluid administration may increase the blood pressure in patients with decreased systemic vascular resistance, and may increase cardiac output in patients with impaired cardiac contractility by increasing the left ventricular filling pressure. Vasopressors such as noradrenaline or dopamine may be used to increase systemic vascular resistance if fluid administration alone does not restore blood pressure. The combined use of dobutamine and noradrenaline provides both inotropic and vasopressor support.[86] A recent randomised study found that reversal of septic hypotension due to a profound reduction in systemic vascular resistance was achieved much more frequently by noradrenaline than by dopamine, and that patients who failed to respond to dopamine subsequently responded to noradrenaline.[79] A pulmonary artery catheter is often helpful to assess the relative need for fluids, vasopressors and inotropic agents. Unfortunately, the mortality from septic shock remains high.

In recent years, there has been great interest in the potential role of antibodies to endotoxins in the treatment of patients with presumed Gram-negative sepsis. However, controlled trials of antiendotoxin monoclonal antibodies have shown no benefit.[87] Similarly, preliminary results of trials using an antibody to tumour necrosis factor (TNF) or an antagonist to the interleukin-1 receptor have also demonstrated no clear benefit.[88] The disappointing results in these clinical trials of antiendotoxin and anticytokine therapies highlight the complexity of the sepsis syndrome. It is doubtful that a single 'magic bullet' will be found to effectively treat patients with overwhelming sepsis.

##### Drug-Induced Shock

Management of shock due to drug ingestion includes minimising drug absorption by gastric decontamination and administration of activated charcoal (see chapter 8; sect. 6.2). Subsequent therapy depends upon the mechanism of action of the particular drug. When the identity of the ingested drug is not known, initial therapy must be empirical. If shock is due to an arrhythmia, therapy is directed at correction of the arrhythmia. If cardiac rhythm is not the cause of shock, initial therapy is a fluid challenge, e.g. 200ml increments of normal saline, until a total of 1 to 2 litres has been administered over 1 hour or the patient develops signs of fluid overload. If fluid administration does not improve blood pressure, pharmacological support should be added. Dopamine is often used initially because its combination of inotropic and vasopressor effects is appropriate for many common types of drug overdose.

When the identity of the ingested drug is known, more specific measures may be available to treat toxicity. Antidotes may rapidly and completely reverse the toxic effect of some drug, e.g. naloxone reversal of opioid toxicity. For other drugs, antidotes may be less than completely effective and the patient may still require blood pressure support with fluids and drugs (table IV). Enhancement of drug elimination by haemodialysis or haemoperfusion may be effective in decreasing the severity or duration of some types of drug toxicity (see further chapter 8).

Mechanical support of the circulation using aortic balloon counterpulsation or partial cardiopulmonary bypass as treatment for intractable drug-induced shock may have a role, although this has not been well studied. Shock due to drugs is potentially reversible if adequate perfusion of vital organs can be maintained. A case of massive lidocaine overdose has been treated successfully by supporting the blood pressure with cardiopulmonary bypass until a satisfactory cardiac rhythm was obtained.[89] When all other therapies have failed, mechanical support of the circulation should be considered to allow additional time to institute specific therapy.

#### Burns

Burn shock is due to sequestration of fluid in injured tissues resulting in intravascular volume depletion. Therapy is fluid replacement, large amounts often being required in the acute phase. Haemodynamic monitoring may be useful in this situation. Colloid solutions may be superior to isotonic saline because they increase plasma oncotic pressure more effectively and reduce the loss of water into burn tissues. Thus, smaller volumes of fluid are needed to correct hypotension, and burn oedema is less likely to be aggravated.

Since burn shock is usually readily corrected by fluid administration, sympathomimetic drugs are generally not needed. Although burn oedema may be due in part to the actions of histamine and prostaglandins, pharmacological antagonism of these mediators has not been shown to be of benefit.

#### Hypothermia

Hypotension due to hypothermia differs from shock in that treatment of the circulatory disturbance *per se* is not always necessary. Decreased metabolic requirements of tissues allow hypothermic patients to survive prolonged periods of reduced or absent blood pressure. Mild hypotension in hypothermic patients is usually not treated, and blood pressure improves as the patient is warmed. Core rewarming (warmed saline gastric or peritoneal lavage, haemodialysis or partial cardiopulmonary bypass) is preferable to surface warming (warm water immersion), because surface warming may cause cutaneous vasodilatation and thereby worsen hypotension.[77] Severe hypotension is best treated by partial cardiopulmonary bypass, the most rapid method of rewarming. This procedure also supports the blood pressure until the patient's haemodynamic status improves.

Sympathomimetic drugs are generally ineffective in increasing blood pressure in hypothermic patients. Bretylium may be particularly useful as an antiarrhythmic agent in hypothermic patients.[77]

#### Spinal Shock

Spinal shock usually responds to the administration of fluids along with α-adrenoceptor agonists such as phenylephrine or noradrenaline. Bradycardia may be treated with atropine.

## 3.2 Anaphylaxis

Anaphylaxis is a potentially life-threatening reaction of abrupt onset caused by exposure of sensitised individuals to specific allergens.[90] Signs and symptoms may include bronchospasm and laryngeal oedema that together may lead to respiratory failure, increased vascular permeability and third-spacing of fluid leading to shock, cardiac arrhythmias, urticaria, rhinorrhoea, abdominal pain, nausea, vomiting and diarrhoea. Signs and symptoms are due primarily to the release of chemical mediators from mast cells and basophils. Non-antigenic stimuli may also trigger the release of mediators from these cells, resulting in a clinically identical syndrome (anaphylactoid reaction). Prompt recognition and treatment of anaphylaxis and anaphylactoid reactions may be life-saving.

### *3.2.1 Pathophysiology of Anaphylaxis*

The leading causes of anaphylaxis include drugs (most notably penicillin and other antibiotics; see chapter 6; sect. 4.1), foods (nuts, fish, shellfish), insect stings, and extracts of allergens used for desensitisation. Susceptible individuals produce IgE antibody directed against these antigens, and this antigen-specific IgE binds to the surface of mast cells and basophils.[90] Upon subsequent exposure, antigen binds to and crosslinks with the tissue-bound IgE, triggering the release of various compounds stored in secretory granules.

The best studied of these mediators, histamine, interacts with both $H_1$- and $H_2$-receptors:

the binding to pulmonary histamine receptors causes bronchospasm; the binding to vascular histamine receptors causes a rapid and marked increase in vascular permeability. Actions on $H_2$-receptors cause dilatation of some vascular beds which may also contribute to hypotension.

In addition to the release of preformed mediators, the binding of antigen to cell surface IgE stimulates the synthesis of mediators. Leukotrienes, prostaglandins and other mediators have actions similar to histamine and may contribute to increased vascular permeability and bronchospasm. Allergens can also activate complement (C3a and C5a, also known as anaphylotoxins), directly increase vascular permeability, and further stimulate mast cells to produce the mediators of anaphylaxis.

The release of mediators from mast cells can also be triggered by non-antigenic stimuli (without the participation of IgE). The resulting anaphylactoid reaction is clinically identical to anaphylaxis and responds to the same therapies. The most common causes of anaphylactoid reactions are intravenous radiographic contrast media, opioids, aspirin and nonsteroidal anti-inflammatory drugs (see also chapter 6; sect. 4.1).

#### *3.2.2 Clinical Presentation*

Increased vascular permeability and loss of plasma from the vascular space have two important consequences: depletion of intravascular volume and tissue oedema. Loss of intravascular volume may occur within minutes of exposure to antigens, resulting in hypovolaemic shock. Haemoconcentration is common, resulting in haematocrits of 60% or greater. Intravascular volume depletion is confirmed by low central venous and pulmonary artery pressures. Reduced cardiac output is due to inadequate venous return to the heart and/or haemodynamic consequences of acute pulmonary hypertension. Peripheral vascular resistance is usually normal or increased, indicating that arteriolar dilatation is not a major contributor to hypotension.

Leakage of fluid into tissues causes oedema. In the skin, this is manifested by urticaria. Swelling of deeper tissues is referred to as angioedema. When oedema involves the pharynx or vocal cords it can cause acute upper airway obstruction. Leakage of fluid into the lungs may occur, but respiratory compromise is usually due to either upper airway obstruction or severe bronchospasm.

#### *3.2.3 Optimum Treatment of Anaphylaxis*

Treatment of anaphylaxis is directed at:

1) Antagonising the effects of chemical mediators.

2) Preventing further release of mediators.

3) Minimising exposure to the inciting agent.

**Non-Pharmacological Therapy**

Upper airway obstruction requires immediate, definitive therapy by placement of an endotracheal tube. Less severe oedema of the upper airway (e.g. hoarseness without stridor or respiratory insufficiency) may be treated with adrenaline (see below). Tracheal intubation is necessary for management of respiratory failure due to bronchospasm.

Hypotension is mainly due to rapid, massive loss of intravascular volume. Placing the patient in the Trendelenberg (feet up) position may be helpful. The primary therapy for hypotension is fluid administration. Fluid requirements may be massive, up to 4 to 6 litres in the first few hours.

**Drug Therapy**

***Adrenaline (epinephrine)*** is the primary drug therapy for treatment of anaphylaxis. It acts by several mechanisms (table VII):

1) Through its $\beta_2$-adrenoceptor agonist action, adrenaline inhibits the release of chemical mediators from stimulated mast cells and basophils, presumably by increasing the concentration of intracellular cyclic-AMP. By blocking this critical event, adrenaline can rapidly limit the severity of anaphylaxis.

2) Stimulation of $\beta_2$-adrenoceptors on bronchial smooth muscle producing bronchodilatation.

3) At high concentrations, adrenaline also has a vasoconstrictor effect due to its $\alpha$-adrenoceptor agonist action. Vasoconstriction may increase blood pressure in patients with anaphylactic shock.

Administration of adrenaline should be initiated as soon as possible, concurrently with any other therapies that are indicated. In mild cases (e.g. urticaria, angioedema without airway obstruction, or bronchospasm without respiratory failure), adrenaline can be administered subcutaneously in a dose of 0.3 to 0.5mg. The onset of effect is usually within 3 to 5 minutes and the dose can be repeated once or twice at 5- to 10-minute intervals if needed. In severe anaphylaxis, the onset of action of subcutaneous adrenaline is too slow. Absorption may be delayed due to poor perfusion of muscle and subcutaneous tissue (see section 1.1.2). Intravenous adrenaline is therefore preferred in this situation. The drug can be administered as 50 to

100μg intravenous boluses, dosed over several minutes, followed by an infusion starting at a rate of 10 to 20 μg/min and the rate doubled every 5 minutes if necessary.

In the prehospital setting where controlled intravenous infusion is difficult, 1ml of 1 : 10,000 solution (100μg) can be administered intravenously over several minutes as needed.[91] More rapid administration or the use of larger doses can precipitate ventricular tachycardia and fibrillation. For patients in whom intravenous access cannot be obtained, intratracheal adrenaline can be administered. Therapy by this route has been studied primarily in patients during cardiac arrest, but should also be effective for patients with anaphylaxis. A suitable dose can be delivered by diluting 1ml of 1 : 10,000 solution (100μg) to 10ml with normal saline and administering it through an endotracheal tube.

It must be emphasised that adrenaline cannot reverse depletion of intravascular volume or tissue oedema that has already occurred. As a result, the drug may be ineffective in treating hypotension unless fluids are administered, and adrenaline cannot replace endotracheal intubation in managing upper airway obstruction.

***$\beta_2$-Adrenoceptor agonists*** [e.g. salbutamol (albuterol) and orciprenaline (metaproterenol)] given by inhalation may be useful when anaphylaxis is associated with bronchospasm. Either nebulisation or use of a metered-dose inhaler can be used to deliver the $\beta_2$-agonist. There is no convincing evidence that addition of theophylline to optimal inhaled bronchodilator therapy is of any benefit.

***Antihistamines:*** $H_1$-receptor blocking drugs antagonise the increased vascular permeability and bronchospasm caused by histamine. These drugs are rarely effective alone for severe anaphylaxis, but may be useful as an adjunct to therapy with fluids and adrenaline. Diphenhydramine is the most commonly used antihistamine (table VII). $H_2$-Receptor blockers have been used in combination with $H_1$-receptor blockers for the prophylaxis of allergic reactions, but a role for $H_2$-receptor blockers in the treatment of anaphylaxis is not established.

***Corticosteroids*** are commonly administered to patients with anaphylaxis, although their efficacy in treating anaphylaxis is unproven. As the onset of their therapeutic effect is delayed for 12 to 24 hours, they are of no value in the initial management of anaphylaxis. Nevertheless, some patients continue to have bronchospasm for several days after the onset of anaphylaxis and might benefit from the early administration of corticosteroids.[92]

***Vasopressors*** (noradrenaline, methoxamine) have been used to treat hypotension in patients with anaphylaxis. The rationale for using these drugs is to provide venoconstriction and increased venous return of blood to the heart, or to increase peripheral vascular resistance if it is low.

#### Minimising Absorption of Allergen

A venous tourniquet is often recommended for anaphylaxis resulting from insect stings on an extremity. Subcutaneous injection of part of the adrenaline dose at the site of the sting to cause local vasoconstriction and slow absorption of the allergen has also been recommended.[93] While these manoeuvres seem reasonable, their efficacy is unproven and appropriate systemic therapy should also be administered.

When anaphylaxis is caused by recently ingested drugs or foods, persistence of signs or symptoms could be due to continuing exposure to allergens in the gastrointestinal tract. In this situation, it may be useful to empty the stomach by gastric lavage using a large bore tube. Activated charcoal slurry (50g) can then be administered via the gastric tube to bind the allergen remaining in the stomach or intestine. However, as with the use of venous tourniquets, the clinical efficacy of gastric emptying and activated charcoal is unproven.

### 3.3 Acute Respiratory Failure

Acute respiratory failure may be a complication of chronic obstructive lung disease, the acute respiratory distress syndrome (see section 3.4), severe pulmonary infection, diaphragmatic muscular weakness or paralysis, massive obesity, or central nervous system dysfunction due either to brain injury or to drug overdose. The clinical manifestations may include confusion, somnolence, disorientation or coma, depressed respiration, and cyanosis. Because many of the symptoms are nonspecific, the diagnosis is made by arterial blood gas analysis revealing hypoxaemia, carbon dioxide retention, or both abnormalities.

Therapy for acute respiratory failure is based on the severity of arterial blood gas abnormalities and their responses to treatment. Treatment may include the following:

1) Low flow oxygen by nasal cannula or mask is appropriate in patients with mild hypoxae-

mia. If progressive carbon dioxide retention develops with oxygen therapy or if respiration is severely depressed, mechanical ventilation is required. Recently, use of noninvasive ventilatory support via a face mask has been shown to obviate the need for endotracheal intubation in selected patients.[94]

2) Higher concentrations of oxygen delivered via an endotracheal tube with mechanical ventilation care are required for patients with more severe hypoxaemia and hypercapnia that are unresponsive to less invasive therapy.

3) Specific precipitating events such as acute bronchitis, pneumonia or pneumothorax should be treated with antibiotics or a chest tube, respectively.

4) Bronchodilators, particularly inhaled $\beta_2$-agonists, are administered to patients with chronic obstructive lung disease or with other evidence of bronchospastic disease.

5) Corticosteroids may be of benefit in treating acute respiratory failure due to asthma or chronic obstructive pulmonary disease.

The management of acute respiratory failure is discussed further in chapter 23 (sect. 5).

### 3.4 Acute Respiratory Distress Syndrome (Non-Cardiogenic Pulmonary Oedema)

#### 3.4.1 Pathophysiology and Clinical Presentation

Most cases of pulmonary oedema are cardiogenic in nature, i.e. they are a result of elevated hydrostatic pressure due to elevated pulmonary venous pressures. Because the pulmonary capillary endothelium is intact, the oedema fluid in cardiogenic pulmonary oedema is transudative and has a low protein content.

The acute respiratory distress syndrome (ARDS) is a form of pulmonary oedema which results from injury to the pulmonary capillary endothelial cells and to the epithelial cells that line the alveolus and provide the tightest barrier to fluid and protein movement. As a result of this injury, fluid leaks into the alveoli. The protein concentration may be as high as in plasma.

Causes of ARDS include sepsis, trauma, shock, burns, aspiration pneumonia, drug overdosage, inhalation of toxic chemicals, oxygen toxicity and fat embolism.[59] Clinically, ARDS is similar to cardiogenic pulmonary oedema except for the lack of findings of venous hypertension (such as distension of neck veins and dependent oedema). Early ARDS is manifested by decreased lung compliance and evidence of progressive hypoxaemia due to perfusion/ventilation mismatch and intrapulmonary shunting. Arterial blood gases typically show hypoxia, hypocarbia and respiratory alkalosis. Chest x-ray shows diffuse infiltration. Physical examination reveals rales and rhonchi, although these findings may occur late.

The development of ARDS is associated with substantial mortality. An important concept is prevention of iatrogenic worsening of oxygenation by restricting fluid therapy to only what is absolutely necessary to maintain cardiovascular and renal function.

#### 3.4.2 Optimum Treatment of ARDS

The treatment of ARDS is primarily nonpharmacological:

1) Oxygen administered by mask or by mechanical ventilation as necessary to maintain adequate oxygenation (arterial $PO_2$ 70 to 80mm Hg).

2) Positive end-expiratory pressure (PEEP) or continuous positive airway pressure (CPAP) administered by face mask or mechanical ventilation with a cuffed endotracheal tube. The mechanism of benefit is believed to be inflation of the collapsed alveoli and redistribution of extravascular lung water with a resultant reduction in ventilation-perfusion mismatch and shunt and improved oxygenation.

3) Haemodynamic monitoring may be necessary to guide fluid therapy. A normal or low pulmonary capillary wedge pressure, reflecting the left ventricular filling pressure, is desirable. With concurrent shock, therapy is difficult as the clinician must try to balance the adverse consequences of inadequate intravascular volume against worsening of the pulmonary oedema.

4) There is no clear role for drug therapy in ARDS. With evidence of fluid overload, diuretics are indicated to reduce pulmonary arterial pressures. The use of vasodilators for preload and afterload reduction is being evaluated but cannot be recommended routinely. Sometimes pressor drugs, such as dopamine, are used in place of fluids for treatment of concurrent shock.

5) Predisposing and complicating illnesses such as sepsis or pneumonia should be treated. However, there is no role for prophylactic antibiotics for ARDS in the absence of evidence of infection. Corticosteroids have not been shown to be of benefit.[95]

### 3.5 Brain Injury

#### *3.5.1 Pathophysiology of Brain Injury*

Brain injury due to trauma, cerebrovascular disease, infection, anoxia such as carbon monoxide poisoning, or global ischaemia such as postcardiac arrest or severe shock, may present a clinical situation where some neurons are at risk but still viable. Thus, there is the potential to salvage brain function through appropriate medical care.

An important consideration in the treatment of cerebral injury is the concept of supply and demand. It is imperative that the demand of the brain for nutrients is adequately supplied. An imbalance may occur because of inadequate cerebral perfusion or excessive metabolic demand. Cerebral autoregulation, the ability to maintain constant cerebral blood flow despite changes in systemic blood pressure, is lost in brain injury. Since the cerebral perfusion pressure is equal to the mean systemic arterial pressure minus intracranial pressure, inadequate cerebral perfusion may be due to systemic arterial hypotension or intracranial hypertension, as discussed below. Excessive metabolic demand may be a consequence of seizures or hyperthermia. Support of oxygenation and circulatory function and prompt control of seizures and hyperthermia are critical aspects of cerebral protection. Treatment of seizures and hyperthermia are discussed further in sections 4.3 and 4.4.

Acute intracranial hypertension (intracranial pressure greater than 15mm Hg) can be the consequence of space-occupying lesions such as a tumour, abscess or haematoma, or generalised brain oedema. Cerebral oedema may directly impede microcirculatory perfusion in ischaemic areas of the brain. It can also cause injury directly by inducing transtentorial herniation with brain stem compression.

#### *3.5.2 Clinical Pharmacology of Drugs Used in Treatment of Cerebral Oedema*

##### Osmotic Agents

*Mannitol* and *glycerol* are neutral polar molecules which do not or only slowly cross membranes and therefore act as osmotic agents (see also chapter 29; sect. 6.1.1). They result in osmotic diuresis as well as dehydrating the brain. These actions are dependent upon elevation of serum osmotic pressure, commonly to the 310 to 320 mOsm/L range. Prolonged use of osmotically active agents, particularly where there is a breakdown of the blood-brain barrier, may result in the entry of osmotically active agents into the brain. This results in a diminished dehydrating action and possibly rebound intracranial hypertension after their use is discontinued.

Mannitol (20% solution) is the most frequently prescribed osmotic agent. Single doses of 0.25 to 1.0 g/kg, or continuous infusions of 0.05 to 0.1 g/kg/h, are commonly used. Doses are titrated to a serum osmolality of 310 to 320 mOsm/L. Mannitol is excreted entirely by filtration in the kidney. *Furosemide* (40 to 80mg) decreases cerebrospinal fluid formation, and in combination with mannitol may yield a more sustained reduction in intracranial pressure than mannitol alone.[96]

The principal adverse effect of mannitol is excessive diuresis. In addition, intravascular volume expansion can result in pulmonary oedema in patients with cardiac disease or renal failure.

##### Corticosteroids

The pharmacology and adverse effects of corticosteroids are discussed in chapter 19 (sect. 7.1.1). The beneficial action of glucocorticoids in treating brain oedema appears to be their effects of suppressing inflammation and decreasing capillary permeability. Dexamethasone is the agent most commonly used because it has negligible mineralocorticoid activity. Large doses, typically 4 to 8mg every 6 hours, are used, although there are few dose-response data to establish optimum dose levels.

##### Barbiturates

The beneficial action of barbiturates in treating brain injury is believed to be a reduction in cerebral metabolic activity, which improves the ratio of oxygen supply to demand and also increases cerebral blood flow. Although animal studies have shown promising results, there is currently little evidence of benefit in patients who have suffered stroke or traumatic brain injury. A controlled study of thiopental therapy in survivors of cardiac arrest showed no beneficial effect on neurological outcome.[97]

Barbiturates are commonly used to treat cerebral oedema in Reyes' syndrome. The major problem with barbiturate therapy in treating brain injury is the worsening of hypotension resulting from increased venous pooling. Hypotension can itself aggravate brain injury and may outweigh any benefits.

#### 3.5.3 Optimum Treatment of Intracranial Hypertension

The management of intracranial hypertension includes:

1) Careful monitoring of neurological status, intracranial pressure and intra-arterial pressure. Cerebral perfusion pressure can be estimated as the difference between the mean arterial pressure and the intracranial pressure. A cerebral perfusion pressure of less than 50mm Hg may lead to brain injury or death. Intracranial pressure greater than 40mm Hg is associated with a poor prognosis.

2) Normalising metabolic functions, i.e. maintaining adequate oxygenation and blood glucose concentrations.

3) Ensuring adequate venous drainage (so that intracranial blood volume does not increase) with the patient at a 30° head-up tilt.

4) Surgical decompression of amenable mass lesions.

5) Hyperventilation for the short term management of intracranial hypertension. Hyperventilation induces hypocarbia which causes cerebral vasoconstriction and reduces cerebral blood flow. The $PaCO_2$ should not be reduced below 20mm Hg, and a target value of 25mm Hg is most appropriate.

6) Antioedema therapy, including the infusion of 20% mannitol or 10% glycerol and the use of diuretics such as furosemide (frusemide) [see also section 3.5.2 and chapter 29; sect. 6.1].

7) Corticosteroids in high doses are useful primarily for brain oedema due to brain tumour or abscesses, and possibly inflammatory processes such as meningitis (see also chapter 29; sect. 12.). However, they have not been shown to be of benefit for global ischaemia or head trauma.[98]

### 3.6 Disorders of Haemostasis

#### 3.6.1 Pathophysiology of Bleeding Disorders in Critically Ill Patients

Critically ill patients may acquire defective haemostasis as a result of deficiencies in coagulation factors, deficiencies in platelet numbers or function, and/or excessive fibrinolysis. Clotting factor deficiencies are seen in patients with acute or chronic liver disease or vitamin K deficiency, the latter being due to poor dietary intake, plus the use of broad-spectrum antibiotics.

Thrombocytopenia is seen with a variety of diseases where there is defective platelet production or excessive destruction and/or sequestration (such as in the spleen), and may also be induced by reactions to drugs. Assuming normal platelet function, severe bleeding is usually a problem only with platelet counts below 30,000/µl. At counts below 10,000/µl, spontaneous intracerebral haemorrhage is of concern. Abnormal platelet function may result in bleeding at higher platelet counts. The most important cause of platelet dysfunction is drugs, primarily the nonsteroidal anti-inflammatory drugs (including aspirin), but also some of the cefalosporins such as cefamandole, cefoperazone and latamoxef (moxalactam).

Disseminated intravascular coagulation (DIC) is a syndrome seen in critically ill patients, particularly as a consequence of Gram-negative sepsis, massive tissue trauma, prolonged shock and obstetric complications. The process is one of accelerated intravascular clotting. This results in thrombotic occlusions of small vessels in various organs and consumption of coagulation factors and platelets, resulting in a bleeding state.

The diagnosis of DIC is based on the finding of an unexplained decrease in platelet counts associated with a prolongation of the prothrombin, activated partial thromboplastin, and thrombin times, and findings of a decreased plasma concentration of fibrinogen and the presence of fibrin-split products. The finding of fragmented red blood cells on a peripheral blood smear is evidence of injury of red cells passing through partially occluded capillaries.

#### 3.6.2 Optimum Treatment of Haemostatic Disorders

The treatment of haemostatic disorders in critically ill patients is as follows:

1) The underlying disorder must be diagnosed and treated. For example, sources of infection need to be identified and sepsis treated. Shock must be controlled. After placental abruption, the uterus must be evacuated.

2) For bleeding due to deficient vitamin K-dependent clotting factors, e.g. in liver or biliary disease or malnutrition, treatment with phytomenadione (vitamin $K_1$; 10 to 20 mg/day) and, if necessary, fresh frozen plasma is indicated.

3) For patients with thrombocytopenia due to decreased production, platelet transfusions are indicated for platelet counts below 20,000/µl or with higher counts when associated with bleeding. For patients with accelerated destruction of platelets, such as with idiopathic thrombocytopenic purpura, corticosteroids are often

administered (see also chapter 26; sect. 4.2.3). Drugs which inhibit platelet function should be avoided.

4) For disseminated intravascular coagulation (DIC), heparin may slow the intravascular coagulation process, but aggravate bleeding. Heparin is best used to treat thrombotic complications, rather than bleeding *per se*. Low doses, such as a 2000 unit loading dose with a maintenance dose of 200 to 500 units per hour, should be used to reduce the risk of excessive bleeding. With uncontrolled bleeding, replacement of coagulation factors and platelets may also be necessary. Antithrombin III concentrate has been used as therapy for severe DIC.[99] However, this therapy is very expensive and a beneficial effect on patient outcome has not been established. The pharmacology of heparin and the management of bleeding disorders are discussed further in chapter 26.

## 4. Complications of Drug Intoxications

Drug intoxication is often accompanied by acute, life-threatening complications. In general, the initial care of patients with life-threatening drug toxicity resembles that of other acutely ill patients. However, if the identity of the drug responsible for the toxicity is known, specific antidotes may be available. If the identity of the drug(s) responsible for the toxicity is not known, pharmacological therapy is particularly challenging because of the risk of unanticipated drug interactions.

Management of drug intoxication is an example of a therapeutic circumstance in which a successful outcome depends on the integration of knowledge of the pharmacology of the intoxicating drug and drugs used in treatment with principles of supportive critical care. The general management of drug overdosage is discussed in chapter 8. This section focuses on the initial management of medical emergencies associated with drug toxicity.

### 4.1 Drug-Induced Coma

#### *4.1.1 Causes*

A depressed level of consciousness is commonly observed after overdosage with hypnosedatives, opioids and various anticholinergic drugs, but may also be due to a wide variety of other agents. Central nervous system depression may be due to a direct effect of the drug, or to hypoxia, hypotension or a postictal state.

#### *4.1.2 Complications of Coma*

The most important complications of central nervous system depression are pulmonary. Respiratory drive is blunted, resulting in hypoventilation or respiratory arrest. Inability to protect the airway may lead to aspiration and subsequent pneumonitis. Prolonged pressure on muscles because of lying immobile may cause rhabdomyolysis and myoglobinuric renal failure. Hypothermia may also result, particularly after overdoses of barbiturates, phenothiazines or ethanol.

#### 4.1.3 Optimum Treatment of Drug-Induced Coma

The initial management of central nervous system depression includes protecting the airway by endotracheal intubation, and supporting respiration.

Drug therapy of coma is available for a limited number of poisonings. Coma due to opioid drugs is rapidly reversed by the specific opioid antagonist *naloxone*. Naloxone is administered in doses of 0.4 to 2mg intravenously, which may be repeated at 2- to 3-minute intervals until the opioid effects are reversed. If no response is achieved after a total of 10 to 15mg, the diagnosis of opioid intoxication should be questioned. Naloxone should be titrated carefully in opioid-dependent patients, in whom opioid withdrawal symptoms may be precipitated. Patients intoxicated with long-acting opioids, such as methadone, may experience recurrent intoxication as the effect of naloxone wears off (over 1 to 2 hours), requiring repeated naloxone administration.

Coma due to benzodiazepines can be rapidly reversed by the specific benzodiazepine antagonist *flumazenil*. Flumazenil is administered in a dose of 0.2mg intravenously; subsequent doses of 0.3mg, then 0.5mg repeated every 30 to 60 seconds may be given up to a total of 3 mg. Flumazenil should be given with extreme caution, if at all, in benzodiazepine-dependent patients who may develop severe withdrawal symptoms. Flumazenil may also precipitate seizures in patients with combined benzodiazepine and tricyclic antidepressant (or other proconvulsant drug) intoxications. Patients with intoxications due to long-acting benzodiazepines may experience recurrent sedation after the effects of flumazenil dissipate (1 to 5 hours).

Coma may also be due to hypoglycaemia in patients exposed to ethanol, insulin, oral antidiabetic agents or salicylates. *Glucose* (50g intravenously) should therefore be administered to all patients with coma of unknown aetiology. The resulting increase in blood glucose concentrations will not harm patients, even if the initial blood glucose was high. *Thiamine* (aneurine; vitamin $B_1$) should also be administered to patients with coma of unknown aetiology. In alcoholic patients who are poorly nourished, intravenous glucose may precipitate Wernicke's syndrome if thiamine is omitted. In addition, Wernicke's syndrome itself may present as coma.

*Physostigmine* is a cholinesterase inhibitor that crosses the blood-brain barrier. It can increase the central nervous system concentration of acetylcholine and thereby reverse coma due to anticholinergic drugs. However, unlike the drugs discussed above, physostigmine may have potentially serious adverse effects, the most common of which is seizures. In patients who have ingested membrane depressant drugs such as tricyclic antidepressants, physostigmine may cause severe bradycardia or asystole.[100] For these reasons, physostigmine should not be used routinely to awaken patients with known anticholinergic drug overdosage or to determine whether an anticholinergic drug has been ingested. Coma due to an anticholinergic drug can be treated with general supportive measures without incurring the risks associated with the use of physostigmine.

In addition to its specific effect of reversing anticholinergic coma, physostigmine may partially reverse coma from unrelated drugs such as benzodiazepines. The magnitude of arousal is small and the risk of administering physostigmine in this setting seem to outweigh any potential benefit.

Other stimulant drugs, termed analeptic agents (e.g. doxapram), have been used to reverse drug-induced coma. These drugs have no demonstrated benefit, and have no role in the management of poisonings.

### 4.2 Drug-Induced Agitated Delirium

#### 4.2.1 Causes

Delirium with agitated, uncooperative, combative or psychotic behaviour may be caused by stimulant drugs (amphetamines, cocaine, caffeine, phencyclidine), drugs with anticholinergic properties (antipsychotic drugs, tricyclic depressants, antihistamines), hallucinogens (lysergic acid diethylamide, mescaline), salicylates, lithium, and alcohol or hypnosedative drug withdrawal.

#### 4.2.2 Complications of Delirium

The consequence of agitated behaviour include inadvertent injury to the patient and difficulty in delivering medical care. Excessive muscular activity may contribute to hyperthermia, acidosis or rhabdomyolysis.

#### 4.2.3 Optimum Treatment of Drug-Induced Delirium

Physical restraints may be helpful and, initially, necessary but often make the patient even more agitated. Reassuring the patient and providing a secure, non-threatening environment (talking the patient down) is helpful for patients with agitation due to hallucinogens, but is less useful for other types of intoxications. Few specific therapies for toxic delirium are available. *Physostigmine* may be rapidly and dramatically effective for anticholinergic delirium, but has a short duration of action and potentially lethal adverse effects (see section 4.1.3). Its use should be restricted to patients for whom the diagnosis of anticholinergic delirium is well established and toxicity is otherwise unmanageable.

Delirium due to alcohol or hypnosedative drug withdrawal occurs when patients who are dependent on these drugs discontinue their use abruptly, and may be indistinguishable from delirium due to drug intoxication. The substitution of another hypnosedative drug such as diazepam or clomethiazole (chlormethiazole) will control agitation, although confusion or hallucinations may persist.

When specific therapy is not available, sedation is often accomplished using *benzodiazepine* or *antipsychotic drugs*. The use of either of these classes of drugs should be undertaken cautiously because of the potential for adverse interactions with the drugs responsible for the delirium. Benzodiazepines generally have few adverse cardiovascular effects and are useful for patients in whom cardiac toxicity is a consideration. The major risk associated with the use of intravenous benzodiazepines is respiratory depression, and facilities for endotracheal intubation and mechanical ventilation must be available if these drugs are given. Antipsychotic drugs are often effective in controlling agitated behaviour, and are less likely than the benzodiazepines to produce respiratory depression. However, their $\alpha$-adrenoceptor blocking effects may cause vasodilatation and hypotension, and their anticholinergic properties may increase the heart rate or contribute to hyperthermia. Antipsychotic drugs with weak anticholinergic and α-adrenoceptor blocking activity such as haloperidol minimise but do not eliminate these risks.

Patients who are intubated and who require sedation can be managed with benzodiazepines or opioids. The choice of agent may be dictated by its adverse effects, e.g. patients with ileus should not receive opioid drugs. Benzodiazepines with longer half-lives such as diazepam (half-life 60 to 80h) are appropriate for long term sedation (weeks), while those with shorter half-lives such as lorazepam (half-life 15h) are more appropriate for shorter periods. Midazolam (half-life 3 to 6h) or propofol are useful for short term sedation. Constant intravenous infusions of midazolam or propofol have been used for longer term sedation,[101] but are very expensive and offer no distinct advantage over longer acting drugs. The choice of drug for agitated patients who cannot be otherwise managed therefore depends on the clinical presentation and the type of drug causing the toxicity.

## 4.3 Drug-Induced Seizures

### 4.3.1 Causes

Drugs that most commonly cause seizures include theophylline, caffeine, sympathomimetic amines, cocaine, phencyclidine, tricyclic antidepressants, antipsychotics, salicylates, isoniazid, and cholinesterase inhibitors.[102] Seizures can also result from the secondary effects of poisonings such as hyperthermia or hypoxia.

### 4.3.2 Complications of Seizures

Seizures due to drug toxicity may compromise respiration, particularly if they are generalised and prolonged. Emesis may occur and lead to aspiration if the airway is not protected. The intense muscular activity accompanying seizures generates lactic acid, and marked acidaemia is common. Prolonged seizures can also cause rhabdomyolysis with myoglobinuria and acute renal failure. Status epilepticus lasting more than 2 hours may lead to irreversible brain injury.

While the metabolic consequences of seizures may contribute, brain injury can occur even when hypoxia, acidosis and other metabolic derangements are controlled.

### 4.3.3 Optimum Treatment of Drug-Induced Seizures

In treating seizures, both the secondary consequences and the cortical seizure activity must be considered. Endotracheal intubation is useful to prevent aspiration, and mechanical ventilation may be needed. Hyperthermia may be treated with appropriate cooling measures such as sponging with tepid water and fanning, iced gastric or colonic lavage, or ice water immersion.[103] If seizures cannot be controlled rapidly, treatment of hyperthermia may require paralysis with neuromuscular blocking drugs. Paralysis also prevents further rhabdomyolysis and acidosis. It does not, however, stop the cerebral seizure activity, and brain injury may ensue unless specific anticonvulsant therapy is administered. Monitoring with electroencephalography may be needed to determine whether seizures persist in the paralysed patient.

Specific therapy is available for only a few types of drug-induced seizures. *Pyridoxine* (vitamin $B_6$) may prevent seizures due to isoniazid toxicity. Seizures caused by cholinesterase inhibiting (organophosphate) pesticides may be treated by reactivating cholinesterase using *pralidoxime*. Alcohol or hypnosedative drug withdrawal seizures usually respond to administration of another hypnosedative such as *diazepam*.

For other types of seizures, specific therapies are not available and standard anticonvulsants are used. Commonly, *lorazepam* 4 to 8mg or *diazepam* 10mg intravenously over 2 to 5 minutes is administered. Benzodiazepines may arrest status epilepticus, but their effects are brief. Therefore *phenytoin* or *phenobarbital* should be administered immediately following the diazepam trial. The loading dose of phenytoin is 18 mg/kg given by slow intravenous infusion at a rate of not greater than 100 mg/min. The dose of phenobarbital is 20 mg/kg given intravenously at a rate of 100 mg/min. Both phenytoin and phenobarbital may aggravate or cause hypotension.

If the above drugs are ineffective, third-line drugs, including *paraldehyde* and *lidocaine* or general anaesthesia with *pentobarbital*, *thiopental* or *amobarbital* are indicated. Prompt sequential therapy optimises the probability of seizure control and minimises the risk of brain injury. However, some drug-induced seizures are notably resistant to anticonvulsant therapy. Seizures due to theophylline or salicylate toxicity are among these, and the control of these seizures often requires enhancement of drug elimination using haemoperfusion or haemodialysis.

## 4.4 Drug-Induced Hyperthermia

### 4.4.1 Causes

Hyperthermia is a potentially fatal complication of drug overdose; patients with a rectal temperature greater than 105°F as a result of drug intoxication usually either do not survive or develop severe neurological sequelae.[104] Hyperthermia may be caused by increased heat generation and/or decreased heat dissipation. Stimulant drugs such as amphetamines, cocaine, theophylline and caffeine may increase heat production by producing agitated behaviour or seizures. Salicylates uncouple oxidative phosphorylation and lead to excessive metabolic heat generation. Drugs such as tricyclic antidepressants, antipsychotics, or antihistamines with anticholinergic properties inhibit sweating and dissipation of heat. Sympathomimetics may also inhibit heat dissipation by vasoconstricting cutaneous vessels.

The greatest risk of hyperthermia comes from drugs that increase the body temperature by more than one mechanism, such as tricyclic antidepressants which have anticholinergic properties and also cause seizures.

#### 4.4.2 Complications of Hyperthermia

Severe hyperthermia may be fatal if left untreated.[103] Common sequelae include disseminated intravascular coagulation, lactic acidosis, hypotension, cardiac arrhythmias, acute renal failure, coma and seizures. It is important to recognise that due to cutaneous vasoconstriction, hyperthermic patients may feel cool to the clinician. Thus, hyperthermia may go undetected unless core temperature is monitored.

#### 4.4.3 Optimum Treatment of Drug-Induced Hyperthermia

The primary therapy of hyperthermia is treatment of its cause. Seizures should be controlled promptly, using paralysis if necessary; agitated patients should be sedated. Active cooling is indicated for all patients with elevated temperatures because the core temperature can rise as rapidly as 3°C per hour. For mild hyperthermia, external cooling using cooling blankets or ice water may be effective. For temperatures greater than 39°C or where there is a rapidly rising temperature, these methods can be supplemented with evaporative cooling (wetting the patient and enhancing evaporation with a fan), or with ice water gastric lavage using a large bore gastric tube. The rectal temperature should be monitored at least every 15 minutes to assess the adequacy of cooling.

*Dantrolene* and *bromocriptine* are useful in treating malignant hyperthermia and possibly for the neuroleptic malignant syndrome, which are distinct entities caused by therapeutic rather than toxic drug doses (see chapter 12, sect. 5.5; chapter 30, sect. 3.1.5).

### 4.5 Drug-Induced Hypertension

#### 4.5.1 Causes and Consequences of Drug-Induced Hypertension

Drug-induced hypertension may be due to sympathomimetic drugs with a-adrenoceptor agonist properties (amphetamines, phenylpropanolamine, ephedrine), cocaine, phencyclidine, occasionally anticholinergic drugs, or hypnosedative drug withdrawal. Previously normotensive patients with acute hypertension may develop encephalopathy or intracranial haemorrhage at lower blood pressures than patients with chronic hypertension because autoregulation of cerebral blood flow has not had time to adjust to the high pressures. A blood pressure of greater than 170mm Hg systolic or 110mm Hg diastolic caused by drugs should therefore be treated as a medical emergency.

#### 4.5.2 Optimum Treatment of Drug-Induced Hypertension

Hypertension due to α-adrenoceptor agonists may be treated with an intravenous infusion of the α-adrenoceptor blocking drug *phentolamine*. If the identity of the ingested drug is not known, intravenous infusion of *sodium nitroprusside* is effective, regardless of the aetiology of the hypertension. Intravenous agents with short half-lives are preferred to intramuscular or oral agents because the dosage rate can be rapidly titrated to the patient's needs.

### 4.6 Drug-Induced Aspiration Pneumonia

#### 4.6.1 Causes

Any drug overdose that impairs the level of consciousness may limit the patient's ability to protect his or her airway. Aspiration of oral secretions or gastric contents may result. Drug-induced seizures are often accompanied by vomiting, and aspiration is common. Furthermore, the administration of syrup of ipecac to induce emesis in patients who are stuporous increases the risk of aspiration. Because ipecac generally takes 20 to 30 minutes to produce emesis, its administration to patients whose level of consciousness is deteriorating or who are at risk for seizures may also contribute to aspiration.

#### 4.6.2 Complications of Aspiration

Aspiration of acidic gastric contents produces a chemical pneumonitis. Secondary bacterial infection may subsequently develop in the area of pneumonitis. Aspiration of gastric contents is also a common contributing factor in the development of the acute respiratory distress syndrome [see section 3.4]. The aspiration of activated charcoal does not appear to be more hazardous than aspiration of gastric contents alone.

#### 4.6.3 Optimum Treatment of Drug-Induced Aspiration

Aspiration may be prevented by the proper positioning of the comatose patient (lying prone or on the side with head down), or by protecting the airway by tracheal intubation. If a known caustic substance has been ingested, gastric emptying by lavage or administration of syrup of ipecac is generally contraindicated because aspiration of such material produces unusually severe pulmonary injury. Suction through the endotracheal tube may remove some aspirated material. If aspiration is extensive or obstruction of the large airways is suspected because of diminished breath sounds or volume loss on the chest x-ray, bronchoscopy is useful to help clear aspirated material.

Although *corticosteroids* are sometimes recommended for patients with aspiration of gastric contents, there are no convincing data to support their use after aspiration has occurred. Infection is not an invariable consequence of aspiration of gastric contents, and it is not clear that *antibiotics* confer benefit to patients who do not have fever, leucocytosis, and purulent sputum. Nonetheless, it is often unclear whether the pulmonary process represents only chemical pneumonitis or chemical pneumonitis plus infection. For this reason, empiric antibiotics are often given to patients who have a significant aspiration injury. Bacterial infection following aspiration is usually due to Gram-positive aerobic and anaerobic organisms from the pharynx. Satisfactory treatment can be accomplished using a variety of antibiotics such as penicillin or clindamycin. Elderly patients and those in hospitals or nursing homes may also harbour Gram-negative organisms, and additional antibiotic coverage for these organisms is indicated.

### 4.7 Drug-Induced Pulmonary Oedema

Overdose patients are particularly prone to developing the acute respiratory distress syndrome (ARDS) because of the frequent occurrence of aspiration and hypotension. The pulmonary alveolar-capillary membrane may also be directly injured by inhalation of irritant fumes or aspiration after ingestion of caustic materials. Some drugs, most notably salicylates, have a specific toxic effect on the alveolar-capillary membrane that may result in pulmonary oedema.

The management of drug-induced ARDS is similar to that for ARDS of other aetiologies (see section 3.4.2).

### 4.8 Drug-Induced Arrhythmias

#### 4.8.1 Causes

Drugs may cause arrhythmias by their direct cardiac effects or indirectly by altering autonomic tone. Anticholinergic drugs commonly cause sinus tachycardia. Sympathomimetic amines such as amphetamines and cocaine produce tachyarrhythmias by directly stimulating cardiac $\beta_1$-adrenoceptors, or releasing noradrenaline from and/or blocking its reuptake by adrenergic neurons.

β-Adrenoceptor blocking drugs and calcium antagonists (verapamil and diltiazem) may cause bradyarrhythmias or atrioventricular heart block. Membrane depressant drugs (tricyclic antidepressants, type I antiarrhythmic agents such as quinidine and procainamide) may prolong the electrocardiographic QRS duration, slow atrioventricular conduction, and cause brady- or tachyarrhythmias. Sinus tachycardia with aberrant conduction (prolonged QRS duration), due to a combination of anticholinergic and membrane depressant actions, is common with tricyclic antidepressant toxicity and may be difficult to distinguish from ventricular tachycardia. Recording the electrocardiogram via an oesophageal electrode to accentuate P waves is sometimes helpful in distinguishing supraventricular from ventricular arrhythmias. Differentiating these rhythms is important because sinus tachycardia with aberration is usually benign, while ventricular tachycardia requires immediate intervention.

Some membrane depressant drugs cause abnormal repolarisation and prolongation of the Q-T interval. These drugs are occasionally associated with torsades de pointes, a ventricular tachycardia with changing QRS axis. Cholinergic agents may cause bradyarrhythmias or atrioventricular block.[76]

#### 4.8.2 Complications of Arrhythmias

Severe bradyarrhythmias may compromise cardiac output leading to hypotension and shock. Rapid rate tachyarrhythmias may do the same by limiting the time available in diastole for ventricular filling. Some arrhythmias are in themselves not compromising, but indicate a high risk of developing more detrimental arrhythmias or other complications of drug overdose. QRS prolongation after tricyclic antidepressant overdose, for example, identifies patients at greatest risk of developing ventricular tachycardia, hypotension or seizures.[105]

#### 4.8.3 Optimum Treatment of Drug-Induced Arrhythmias

Sinus tachycardia is usually well tolerated and does not require therapy. Rarely, the heart rate is rapid enough to cause hypotension. Sinus tachycardia due to drugs such as theophylline or caffeine may be slowed using a *β-adrenoceptor blocking drug*. Sinus tachycardia due to anticholinergic drugs may be transiently slowed using the cholinesterase inhibitor *physostigmine*, but physostigmine may cause bradyarrhythmias or asystole if membrane depressant drugs have been ingested (see section 4.1.3).

Paroxysmal atrial tachycardia may respond to carotid sinus pressure, *adenosine* or *verapamil*. For atrial fibrillation or flutter with a rapid ventricular response, *digoxin, verapamil* or *diltiazem* may be useful for slowing the ventricular rate. For persistent paroxysmal atrial tachycardia, atrial fibrillation or atrial flutter, electrical cardioversion may be needed. When patients have ingested many drugs or the identity of the drug ingested is not known, cardioversion is often safer than pharmacotherapy.

Ventricular tachycardia due to drug toxicity is often accompanied by hypotension and requires prompt therapy. Ventricular tachycardia due to sympathomimetic drugs may respond to a *β-blocker*. Drug-induced torsades de pointes often responds to magnesium, electrical pacing, or to infusion of *isoprenaline*.

Ventricular tachyarrhythmias due to tricyclic antidepressants may respond to *hypertonic sodium bicarbonate* or *sodium lactate*. This therapy is also useful for ventricular tachyarrhythmias due to membrane depressant drugs such as quinidine. Tricyclic antidepressant-induced arrhythmias should not be treated with other membrane depressant drugs (e.g. procainamide) because this may aggravate toxicity. Antiarrhythmic drugs that do not slow conduction, such as *lidocaine*, may be used if hypertonic sodium bicarbonate is not effective.

Ventricular arrhythmias due to digoxin sometimes respond to lidocaine. Arrhythmias may be aggravated by hypo- or hyperkalaemia, and these conditions should be corrected. Digoxin specific Fab antibody fragments are the treatment of choice for life-threatening ventricular arrhythmias.[106]

Drug-induced bradyarrhythmias or heart block are best treated with a pacemaker. *Atropine* may be sufficient for bradyarrhythmias due to digoxin or cholinergic agents. Bradyarrhythmias due to β-blockers may respond to a $\beta_1$-agonist such as *isoprenaline* or to *glucagon*; the latter increases the heart rate by a non-adrenergic mechanism. Bradyarrhythmias due to verapamil or diltiazem may respond to calcium.[107]

### Further Reading

Carlson RW, Gehab MA, editors. Principles and practice of medical intensive care. Philadelphia: Saunders, 1993

Chernow B, editor. The pharmacologic approach to the critically-ill patients, 3rd edition. Baltimore: Williams & Wilkins, 1994

Hall JB, Schmidt GA, Wood LDH, editors. Principles of critical care. New York: McGraw-Hill, 1991

Shoemaker WC, Ayres S, Gronvik A, et al. The society of critical care medicine: textbook of critical care. 2nd ed. Philadelphia: Saunders, 1989

### References

1. Pentel P, Benowitz N. Pharmacokinetic and pharmacodynamic considerations in drug therapy of cardiac emergencies. Clinical Pharmacokinetics 1984; 9: 273
2. Benowitz NL, Meister W. Clinical pharmacokinetics of lidocaine. Clinical Pharmacokinetics 1978; 3: 177
3. Chandra N, Snyder LD, Weisfeldt JL. Abdominal binding during cardiopulmonary resuscitation in man. Journal of the American Medical Association 1981; 246: 351
4. McDonald JL. Systolic and mean arterial pressures during manual and mechanical CPR in humans. Critical Care Medicine 1981; 9: 382
5. Voorhees WD, Babbs CF, Tacker WA. Regional blood flow during cardiopulmonary resuscitation in dogs. Critical Care Medicine 1980; 8: 134
6. Pentikainen PJ, Huikuri H, Jounela AJ, et al. Disopyramide pharmacokinetics in patients with acute myocardial infarction. European Journal of Clinical Pharmacology 1985; 28: 45-51
7. Pentikainen PJ, Halinen MO, Helin MJ. Pharmacokinetics of oral mexiletine in patients with acute myocardial infarction. European Journal of Clinical Pharmacology 1983; 25: 773-7
8. Roberts JR, Greenberg MI, Knaub MA, et al. Blood levels following intravenous and endotracheal epinephrine administration. Journal of the American College of Emergency Physicians 1979; 8: 53
9. Quinton DN, O'Byrne G, Aitkenhead AR. Comparison of endotracheal and peripheral intravenous adrenaline in cardiac arrest. Is the endotracheal route reliable? Lancet 1987; 1: 828-9
10. Crespo SG, Schoffstall JM, Fuhs LR, et al. Comparison of two doses of endotracheal epinephrine in a cardiac

arrest model. Annals of Emergency Medicine 1991; 20: 230-4

11. Benowitz NL, Forsyth RP, Melmon KL, et al. Lidocaine disposition kinetics in monkey and man. II. Effects of hemorrhage and sympathomimetic drug administration. Clinical Pharmacology and Therapeutics 1974; 16: 99
12. Prescott LF, Adjepon-Yamoah KK, Talbot RG. Impaired lignocaine metabolism in patients with myocardial infarction and cardiac failure. British Medical Journal 1976; 1: 939
13. Davison R, Parker M, Atkinson Jr AJ. Excessive serum lidocaine levels during maintenance infusions: mechanisms and prevention. American Heart Journal 1982; 104: 203
14. Shelly MP, Mendel L, Park GR. Failure of critically ill patients to metabolise midazolam. Anaesthesia 1987; 42: 619
15. MacNab MSP, Macrae OJ, Guy E, et al. Profound reduction in morphine clearance and liver blood flow in shock. Intensive Care Medicine 1986; 12: 366
16. Lambert C, Halpert JR, Rouleau J, et al. Effect of congestive heart failure on the intrinsic metabolic capacity of the liver in the dog. Drug Metabolism and Disposition 1991; 19: 985
17. Duchin KL, Schrier RW. Interrelationship between renal haemodynamics, drug kinetics and drug action. Clinical Pharmacokinetics 1978; 3: 58
18. Routledge PA, Stargel WW, Wanger GS, et al. Increased alpha-1-acid glycoprotein and lidocaine disposition in myocardial infarction. Annals of Internal Medicine 1980; 93: 701
19. Branch RA, Morgan MH, James J, et al. Intravenous administration of diazepam in patients with chronic liver disease. Gut 1976; 17: 975
20. Pond SM, Tozer TT. First pass elimination: basic concepts and clinical consequences. Clinical Pharmacokinetics 1984; 9: 1
21. Lanao JM, Dominguez-Gil A, Macias JG, et al. The influence of ascites on the pharmacokinetics of amikacin. International Journal of Pharmacology, Therapy and Toxicology 1980; 18: 57
22. Williams RL, Blaschke TF, Meffin PJ, et al. Influence of acute viral hepatitis on disposition and plasma binding or tolbutamide. Clinical Pharmacology and Therapeutics 1977; 23: 301
23. Shull HJ, Wilkinson GR, Johnson R, et al. Normal disposition of oxazepam in acute viral hepatitis and cirrhosis. Annals of Internal Medicine 1976; 84: 420
24. Reidenberg MM, Drayer DE. Alteration of drug protein binding in renal disease. Clinical Pharmacokinetics 1984; 9: 18
25. Aronson JK. Clinical pharmacokinetics of digoxin. Clinical Pharmacokinetics 1980; 5: 137
26. Reidenberg MM. The biotransformation of drugs in renal failure. American Journal of Medicine 1977; 62: 482
27. Szeto HH, Inturrisi CE, Houde R, et al. Accumulation of normeperidine, an active metabolite of meperidine, in patients with renal failure or cancer. Annals of Internal Medicine 1977; 86: 738
28. Osborne RJ, Joel SP, Slevin ML. Morphine intoxication in renal failure: the role of morphine-6-glucuronide. British Medical Journal 1986; 292: 1548
29. Luce JM. The cardiovascular effects of mechanical ventilation and positive end-expiratory pressure. Journal of the American Medical Association 1984; 252: 807
30. du Souich P, McLean AJ, Lalka D, et al. Pulmonary disease and drug kinetics. Clinical Pharmacokinetics 1978; 3: 257
31. Kishimoto I, Tanigawara Y, Okumura K, et al. Blood oxygen tension-related change of theophylline clearance in experimental hypoxemia. Journal of Pharmacology and Experimental Therapeutics 1989; 248: 1237
32. Bonnet F, Richard C, Glaser P, et al. Changes in hepatic flow induced by continuous positive pressure ventilation in critically ill patients. Critical Care Medicine 1982; 10: 703
33. Richard C, Berdeaux A, Delion F, et al. Effect of mechanical ventilation on hepatic drug pharmacokinetics. Chest 1986; 90: 837
34. Vozeh S, Powell RJ, Riegelman S, et al. Changes in theophylline clearance during acute illness. Journal of the American Medical Association 1978; 240: 1882
35. Kraemer MJ, Furukawa CT, Koup JR, et al. Altered theophylline clearance during an influenza B outbreak. Pediatrics 1982; 69: 476
36. Koren G, Greenwald M. Decrease in theophylline clearance causing toxicity during viral epidemics. Journal of Asthma 1985; 22: 75
37. Trenholme GM, Williams RL, Rieckman KH, et al. Quinine disposition during malaria and during induced fever. Clinical Pharmacology and Therapeutics 1976; 19: 459
38. Sonne J, Dossing M, Loft S, et al. Antipyrine clearance in pneumonia. Clinical Pharmacology and Therapeutics 1985; 37: 701
39. Williams SJ, Baird-Lambert JA, Farrell GC. Inhibition of theophylline metabolism by interferon. Lancet 1987; 2: 939
40. Bonate PL. Pathophysiology and pharmacokinetics following burn injury. Clinical Pharmacokinetics 1990; 18: 118
41. Loirat P, Rohan J, Baillet A, et al. Increased glomerular filtration rate in patients with major burns and its effect on the pharmacokinetics of tobramycin. New England Journal of Medicine 1978; 299: 915
42. Czaja AJ, Rizzo TA, Smith WR, et al. Acute liver disease after cutaneous thermal injury. Journal of Trauma 1975; 15: 887
43. Martyn JAJ, Greenblatt DJ. Lorazepam conjugation is unimpaired in burn trauma. Clinical Pharmacology and Therapeutics 1988; 43: 250
44. Perry S, Inturrisi CE. Analgesia and morphine disposition in burn patients. Journal of Burn Care and Rehabilitation 1983; 4: 276
45. Fruncillo RJ, Digregorio GJ. Pharmacokinetics of pentobarbital, quinidine, lidocaine and theophylline in the thermally injured rat. Journal of Pharmaceutical Sciences 1984; 73: 1117
46. Martyn JAJ, Greenblatt DJ, Abernethy DR. Increased cimetidine clearance in burn patients. Journal of the American Medical Association 1985; 253: 1288
47. Martyn JAJ, Bishop AL, Oliveri MF. Pharmacokinetics and pharmacodynamics of ranitidine after burn injury. Clinical Pharmacology and Therapeutics 1992; 51: 408
48. Zaske DE, Sawchuck RJ, Gerding DN, et al. Increased dosage requirements of gentamicin in burn patients. Journal of Trauma 1976; 16: 824
49. Garrelts JC, Peterie JD. Altered vancomycin dose vs. serum concentration relationship in burn patients. Clinical Pharmacology and Therapeutics 1988; 44: 9
50. Bowdle TA, Heal GD, Levy RH, et al. Phenytoin pharmacokinetics in burned rats and plasma protein binding of

phenytoin in burned patients. Journal of Pharmacology and Experimental Therapeutics 1980; 213: 97
51. Martyn JAJ, Szyfelbein SK, Ali HH, et al. Increased d-tubocurarine requirement following major thermal injury. Anesthesiology 1980; 52: 352
52. Simon RP, Benowitz NL, Hedlund R, et al. Influence of the brain-blood pH gradient on brain phenobarbital uptake during status epilepticus. Journal of Pharmacology and Experimental Therapeutics 1985; 234: 830
53. Simon RP, Benowitz NL, Culala S. Motor paralysis increases brain uptake of lidocaine during status epilepticus. Neurology 1984; 34: 384
54. Shinn AF. Clinical relevance of cimetidine drug interactions. Drug Safety 1992; 7: 245
55. LaForce DF, Miller MF, Chai H. Effect of erythromycin on theophylline clearance in asthmatic children. Journal of Pediatrics 1981; 99: 153
56. Lindenbaum J, Rund DG, Butler VP, et al. Inactivation of digoxin by the gut flora: reversal by antibiotic therapy. New England Journal of Medicine 1981; 305: 789
57. Pfeffer MA, Braunwald E, Moyé LA, et al. Effect of captopril on mortality and morbidity in patients with left ventricular dysfunction after myocardial infarction: results of the Survival and Ventricular Enlargement Trial. New England Journal of Medicine 1992; 327: 669
58. Ambrosioni E, Borghi C, Magnani B. The effect of angiotensin-converting-enzyme inhibitor zofenopril on mortality and morbidity after anterior myocardial infarction. New England Journal of Medicine 1995; 332: 80
59. Kollef MH, Schuster DP. The acute respiratory distress syndrome. New England Journal of Medicine 1995; 332: 27
60. Driscoll DF, Blackburn GL. Total parenteral nutrition 1990: a review of its current status in hospitalised patients, and the need for patient-specific feeding. Drugs 1990; 40: 364
61. McMahon MM, Farnell MB, Murray MJ. Nutritional support of critically ill patients. Mayo Clinic Proceedings 1993; 68: 911
62. Cook DJ, Fuller HD, Guyatt GH, et al. Risk factors for gastrointestinal bleeding in critically ill patients. New England Journal of Medicine 1994; 330: 377
63. Ben-Menachem T, Fogel R, Patel RV, et al. Prophylaxis for stress-related gastric hemorrhage in the medical intensive care unit: a randomized, controlled single-blind study. Annals of Internal Medicine 1994; 121: 568
64. Cook DJ, Laine LA, Guyatt GH, et al. Nosocomial pneumonia and the role of gastric pH: a meta-analysis. Chest 1991; 100: 7
65. Prod'hom G, Leuenberger P, Koerfer J, et al. Nosocomial pneumonia in mechanically ventilated patients receiving antacid, ranitidine, or sucralfate and prophylaxis for stress ulcer: a randomized controlled trial. Annals of Internal Medicine 1994; 120: 653
66. Geerts WH, Code KI, Jay RM, et al. A prospective study of venous thromboembolism after major trauma. New England Journal of Medicine 1994; 331: 1601
67. Weinmann EE, Salzman EW. Deep-vein thrombosis. New England Journal of Medicine 1994; 331: 1630
68. Spiro TE, Johnson GJ, Christie MJ, et al. Efficacy and safety of enoxaparin to prevent deep venous thrombosis after hip replacement surgery. Annals of Internal Medicine 1994; 121: 81
69. Goldhaber SZ, Heit J, Sharma GVRK, et al. Randomised controlled trial of recombinant tissue plasminogen activator versus urokinase in the treatment of acute pulmonary embolism. Lancet 1988; 6: 293
70. Chernow B, editor. The pharmacologic approach to the critically-ill patient. 3rd ed. Baltimore: Williams & Wilkins, 1994
71. Graf H, Leach W, Arieff AI. Evidence for detrimental effect of bicarbonate therapy in hypoxic hepatic lactic acidosis. Science 1985; 27: 754
72. Kette F, Weil MH, Gazmuri RJ, et al. Buffer solutions may compromise cardiac resuscitation by reducing coronary perfusion pressure. Journal of the American Medical Association 1991; 266: 2121
73. Cooper DJ, Walley KR, Wiggs BR, et al. Bicarbonate does not improve hemodynamics in critically ill patients who have lactic acidosis. Annals of Internal Medicine 1990; 112: 492
74. Bone RC. The pathogenesis of sepsis. Annals of Internal Medicine 1991; 115: 457
75. Parrillo JE. Pathogenetic mechanisms of septic shock. New England Journal of Medicine 1993; 328: 1471
76. Benowitz NL, Golschlager N. Cardiac disturbances. In: Haddad & Winchester, editors. Clinical management of poisoning and drug overdose. 2nd ed. Philadelphia: Saunders, 1990: 63
77. Danzl DF, Pozos RS. Accidental hypothermia. New England Journal of Medicine 1994; 331: 1756
78. Silverberg AB, Shah SD, Haymond MW, et al. Norepinephrine: hormone and neurotransmitter in man. American Journal of Physiology 1978; 234: 252
79. Martin C, Papazian L, Perrin G, et al. Norepinephrine or dopamine for the treatment of hyperdynamic septic shock. Chest 1993; 103: 1826
80. Marik PE, Mohedin M. The contrasting effects of dopamine and norepinephrine on systemic and splanchnic oxygen utilization in hyperdynamic sepsis. Journal of the American Medical Association 1994; 272: 1354
81. Faden AI, Jacobs TP, Holaday JW. Opiate antagonist improves neurologic recovery after spinal injury. Science 1981; 211: 493
82. Grull NJ, Reynolds DG, Vargish T, et al. Naltrexone improves survival rate and cardiovascular function in canine hemorrhagic shock. Journal of Pharmacology and Experimental Therapeutics 1982; 220: 625
83. Safani M, Blair J, Ross D, et al. Prospective, controlled randomized trial of naloxone infusion in early hyperdynamic septic shock. Critical Care Medicine 1989; 17: 1004
84. Bone RC, Fisher CJ, Clemmer TP, et al. (Methylprednisolone Severe Sepsis Study Group). A controlled clinical trial of high-dose methylprednisolone in the treatment of severe sepsis and septic shock. New England Journal of Medicine 1987; 317: 653
85. Hinshaw L, et al. The Veterans Administration Systemic Sepsis Cooperative Study Group. Effect of high-dose glucocorticoid therapy on mortality in patients with clinical signs of systemic sepsis. New England Journal of Medicine 1987; 317: 659
86. Martin C, Saux P, Eon B, et al. Septic shock: a goal-directed therapy using volume loading, dobutamine and/or norepinephrine. Acta Anaesthesiologica Scandinavica 1990; 34: 413
87. McCloskey RV, Straube RC, Sanders C, et al. Treatment of septic shock with human monoclonal antibody HA-1A. Annals of Internal Medicine 1994; 121: 1
88. Natanson C, Hoffman WD, Suffredini AF, et al. Selected treatment strategies for septic shock based on

proposed mechanisms of pathogenesis. Annals of Internal Medicine 1994; 120: 771
89. Noble DJ, Kennedy DJ, Lattimer RD, et al. Massive lignocaine overdose during cardiopulmonary bypass. British Journal of Anaesthesia 1984; 56: 1439
90. Bochner BS, Lichtenstein LM. Anaphylaxis. New England Journal of Medicine 1991; 324: 1785
91. Barach EM, Norvak RM, Tennyson GL, et al. Epinephrine for treatment of anaphylactic shock. Journal of the American Medical Association 1984; 251: 2118
92. Stark BJ, Sullivan TJ. Biphasic and protracted anaphylaxis. Journal of Allergy and Clinical Immunology 1986; 78: 76
93. Patterson R, Valentine M. Anaphylaxis and related allergic emergencies including reactions due to insect stings. Journal of the American Medical Association 1982; 248: 2632
94. Bott F, Carroll MP, Conway FJ, et al. Randomized controlled trial of nasal ventilation in acute ventilatory failure due to chronic obstructive airway disease. Lancet 1993; 19: 341
95. Bernard GR, Luce LM, Sprung CL, et al. High dose corticosteroids in patients with adult respiratory distress syndrome. New England Journal of Medicine 1987; 317: 1565-70
96. Schettini A, Stahurski B, Young H. Osmotic and osmotic-loop diuresis in brain surgery. Journal of Neurosurgery 1982; 56: 679
97. Brain Resuscitation Clinical Trial I Study Group. Randomized clinical study of thiopental loading in comatose survivors of cardiac arrest. New England Journal of Medicine 1986; 314: 397
98. Jastremski M, Sutton-Tyrrell K, Vaagenes P, et al. Glucocorticoid treatment does not improve neurological recovery following cardiac arrest. Journal of the American Medical Association 1989; 262: 3427
99. Fourrier F, Lestavel P, Chopin C, et al. Meningococcemia and purpura fulminans in adults: acute deficiencies of proteins C and S and early treatment with antithrombin III concentrates. Intensive Care Medicine 1990; 16: 121
100. Pentel P, Peterson CD. Asystole complicating physostigmine treatment of tricyclic antidepressant overdose. Annals of Emergency Medicine 1980; 9: 588
101. Burns AM, Shelly MP, Park GR. The use of sedative agents in critically ill patients. Drugs 1992; 43: 507
102. Olson KR, Kearney TE, Dyer J, et al. Seizures associated with poisoning and drug overdose. American Journal of Emergency Medicine 1993; 11: 565
103. Olson K, Benowitz NL. Environmental and drug-induced hyperthermia pathophysiology, recognition and management. Emergency Medicine Clinics of North America 1984; 2: 459
104. Rosenberg J, Pentel P, Pond SM, et al. Hyperthermia associated with drug intoxication. Critical Care Medicine 1986; 14: 964-9
105. Boehnert MT, Lovejoy FH. Value of the QRS duration versus the serum drug level in predicting seizure and ventricular arrhythmias after an acute overdose of tricyclic antidepressants. New England Journal of Medicine 1985; 313: 474
106. Smith RW. Review of clinical experience with digoxin immune fab (ovine). American Journal of Emergency Medicine 1991; 9: 1
107. Pearigen PD, Benowitz NL. Poisoning due to calcium antagonists: experience with verapamil, diltiazem and nifedipine. Drug Safety 1991; 6: 408

Chapter 14

# Ear, Nose and Throat Diseases

*R.T. Jackson, N.W. Todd* and *J.S. Turner Jr*

## Synopsis of Important Principles

1) Drug therapy in ear, nose and throat disease is a balance between the practical and scientific bases for drug selection and use.

2) In bacterial infections of the ear, nose or throat, good evidence as to which is the most likely causative organism is available in various situations. With this knowledge, the appropriate agent for initial therapy can be selected with confidence.

3) Systemic therapy with phenoxymethylpenicillin (penicillin V), erythromycin or, when *Haemophilus influenzae* is likely to be involved, amoxicillin/clavulanic acid, cotrimoxazole (trimethoprim/sulfamethoxazole) or cefaclor, and topical use of gentamicin, cover the common causative organisms.

4) Measures directed at attaining a clear ear canal or nasal airway, and enhancing eustachian tube function, are also important in a number of disorders involving the ear or nose.

5) Allergy can be implicated in some nasal disorders and is often associated with secretory otitis media.

6) Treatment of vertigo is guided on the basis of a careful history and investigation such that the most likely cause can be identified and an appropriate antivertigo drug (or other treatment) selected.

7) Some drugs can cause ototoxicity, most cases being associated with aminoglycoside antibacterial drugs and loop diuretics used in patients with impaired renal function.

This chapter addresses both practical and scientific aspects of pharmacological therapies of otorhinolaryngological conditions. Problems in this field involve microbial, allergic and immunological processes, inflammation, and altered vascular perfusion. Drug treatments include antimicrobial agents (against bacteria, viruses and fungi), antihistamines ($H_1$-receptor antagonists), sympathomimetics, corticosteroids, vasodilators and suppressors of the statokinetic system.

## 1. Clinical Pharmacological Considerations and General Principles of Treatment

The drugs most often prescribed for ear, nose and throat diseases fall into the following classes: antimicrobial agents, antihistamines, antivertigo drugs, sympathomimetics, corticosteroids and vasodilators.

### 1.1 Antimicrobial Agents

Knowledgeable clinicians can intelligently predict the likely organism or class of organism to be treated in many given situations in otolaryngology, and need not await cultures to initiate therapy (see section 2.1 and table I). However, as a rule, cultures should be taken when treating severe infections, chronic infections not responsive to treatment, infections in immunocompromised patients (e.g. with immunodeficiency, diabetes mellitus, cystic fibrosis), or infections that produce life-threatening complications (e.g. suppurative labyrinthitis). The selection of a suitable agent, its dosage and route of administration are functions of the these considerations, which, along with the pharmacological properties and activity of antibacterial drugs, are discussed further in chapter 31.

Use of antibacterial and antiviral agents for routine uncomplicated cases of colds and upper respiratory symptoms of other viral diseases is to be condemned (see further section 2.1). Once started, an antimicrobial agent should be used in an adequate dosage for sufficient time to completely control infection, and the patient (or parent of a young child) should be educated in the need to comply with medication instructions and to complete the prescribed course.

### 1.2 Antihistamines ($H_1$-Receptor Antagonists)

For many years, antihistamines have been used to treat immediate hypersensitivity reactions such as allergic rhinitis. The introduction of the second-generation of antihistamines has already had a significant effect on the treatment of some inflammatory and allergic diseases.

The *first-generation* antihistamines can cause 3 types of adverse central nervous system (CNS) effects (stimulatory, neuropsychiatric and suppressive) in addition to peripheral ad-

**Table I.** Systemic antibacterial drugs for initial treatment of common ear, nose and throat infections

| Indication | Causative organisms[a] | First-line drugs[b] | Usual dosage and duration[c] |
|---|---|---|---|
| Acute rhinosinusitis | *Streptococcus pneumoniae* (pneumococcus)<br>*Streptococcus pyogenes* | Phenoxymethylpenicillin (penicillin V) | 250mg (6.25 mg/kg) qid for ≥10 days (parenteral benzylpenicillin if severe) |
| Pharyngitis | β-Haemolytic streptococci | Phenoxymethylpenicillin | 250mg (6.25 mg/kg) qid ≥10 days |
| Acute furunculosis | Staphylococci<br>*Staphylococcus pyogenes* | Dicloxacillin<br>Cloxacillin<br>Flucloxacillin | 125mg (3.125 mg/kg) qid ≥10 days<br>500mg (12.5 mg/kg) qid ≥10 days<br>250mg (6.25 mg/kg) qid ≥10 days (parenteral cloxacillin if severe) |
| Acute otitis media | *Staphylococcus pneumoniae*<br>*S. pyogenes*<br>*Haemophilus influenzae* | Amoxicillin | 250mg (6.25 mg/kg) tid ≥10 days |
| | *H. influenzae* (β-lactamase–producing)[d]<br>*Moraxella catarrhalis* | Amoxicillin + clavulanic acid | 250mg + 125mg (6.25 mg/kg amoxicillin) tid ≥10 days |

a Those most likely to predominate. See text for situations when culture is necessary.

b In cases of penicillin allergy, erythromycin (250mg or 10 mg/kg qid), clarithromycin (250mg or 7.5 mg/kg bid) or, when *H. influenzae* is involved, cotrimoxazole [trimethoprim/sulfamethoxazole 160/800mg (i.e. 2 tablets) twice daily] can be used.

c Oral unless stated otherwise. Childrens' dosages are given in parentheses (see also chapter 3, table VII). Give penicillin and cloxacillin 1 hour before meals.

d The incidence of amoxicillin/ampicillin resistance by β-lactamase-producing strains of *H. influenzae* is ≥20% in some areas. In such areas, use of amoxicillin + clavulanic acid is preferred to amoxicillin alone. In cases of penicillin allergy, cotrimoxazole [160/800mg (i.e. 2 tablets) twice daily] can be used.

*Abbreviations:* bid = twice daily; tid = 3 times daily; qid = 4 times daily.

**Table II.** Pharmacokinetic properties of some commonly used $H_1$-antihistamines (after Desager & Horsmans;[8] Kontou-Fili;[9] Simons & Simons[10])

| Drug | Chemical class | Pharmacokinetic parameters | | | | Principal route of elimination | Active metabolites |
|---|---|---|---|---|---|---|---|
| | | F (%) | CL (L/h) | Vd (L/70kg) | $t_{1/2}$ (h) | | |
| **First-generation agents (sedating)** | | | | | | | |
| Chlorpheniramine (chlorphenamine) | Alkylamine | | 7.2 | 238 | 20-30 | Hepatic | Yes |
| Diphenhydramine | Ethanolamine | 42 | 47 | 280 | 5-9 | Hepatic | Yes (possibly active) |
| Diphenylpyraline | Ethanolamine | | | | 32 | Hepatic | Yes (possibly active) |
| Hydroxyzine | Piperazine | | 41 | | 20 | Hepatic | Yes [cetirizine] |
| **Second-generation agents (nonsedating)** | | | | | | | |
| Acrivastine | Pyridine | 18 | 18.2 | 52.5 | 1.4-2.1 | Renal/ hepatic | Yes |
| Astemizole | Piperidine-imidazole | | 90 | ≈17,500 | 20 [456[a]] | Hepatic | Yes [demethyl-astemizole] |
| Azelastine[c] | Phthalazinone | 82 | 35.7 | | 22 | Hepatic | Yes |
| Cetirizine | Piperidine | | 3 | 35 | 6.5-10 | Renal[b] | No |
| Levocabastine[c] | Piperidine | 60-80[d] 30-60[e] | | | 35-40 | Renal | No |
| Loratadine | Piperidine | | 722 | | 7.8-11 [17.3-24[a]] | Hepatic | Yes [decarbo-ethoxy-loratadine] |
| Terfenadine | Piperidine | | 36-42[a] | | 16-23 [17[a]] | Hepatic | Yes [terfenadine carboxylate] |

a Data for active metabolite.
b Some faecal elimination also (mainly as unchanged drug).
c Azelastine and levocabastine are administered topically (as a nasal spray and/or eye drops).
d After nasal administration.
e After ocular administration.
*Abbreviations:* F = bioavailability; CL = total plasma clearance; Vd = volume of distribution; $t_{1/2}$ = elimination half-life.

verse effects. In some studies, sedation or drowsiness occurred in 10 to 25% of antihistamine users.[1] These effects are usually dose-related. A plot of the adverse and beneficial effects of these antihistamines *vs* dosage follows a normal (bell-shaped) distribution and varies with the drug and the patient. For example, some antihistamines such as diphenhydramine are used in over-the-counter sleeping pills and would be expected to cause sedation in more people than some other agents.

There are several techniques used to objectively and subjectively assess the safety of antihistamines. Sleep latency, self-awareness, the P300 response (an electroencephalographic measure of sustained attention and processing speed), visual function, visual-motor coordination, reaction time and various driving functions can be measured. Concerns have been expressed about the safety of antihistamine-alcohol and antihistamine-tranquilliser combinations, and these studies are now performed on newer antihistamines before they reach the market.

The *second-generation* antihistamines such as terfenadine,[2] astemizole,[3] loratadine,[4] cetirizine,[5] ebastine,[6] and acrivastine (table II)[7] cause little fatigue, lassitude, drowsiness or sedation. They also do not act synergistically with alcohol, diazepam or other CNS suppressive substances.[11] These drugs should be considered 'antiallergic agents' because they inhibit the release of inflammatory mediators such as histamine and block inflammatory cell migration, in addition to blocking histamine receptors.[12] As well as the above second-generation oral antihistamines, there are also two second-generation agents that are used topically: levocabastine[13,14] and azelastine.[15] The possibility of using a locally acting antihistamine may significantly increase treatment options in rhinitis (see section 2.4).

There is conjecture as to why the older antihistamines induce drowsiness. An attractive notion stems from the fact that the sedative properties of these drugs are consistent with the blockade of central histaminergic neurons that control sleep and wakefulness. These neurons set the overall excitability level of the telencephalon. Blockade of their function with antihistamines would, therefore, cause sedation.[16,17] Studies performed with the second-generation, nonsedating agents indicate that they do not readily cross the blood-brain barrier (for reviews, see Desager & Horsmans;[8] Kontou-Fili;[9] and Simons & Simons[18]).

The new second-generation compounds are considerably more expensive than the older agents and it is reasonable to question whether they are worth the additional cost.[11] Clinical experience has indicated that most patients are not sedated by the older drugs; others are sedated for only a few days. Some use the sedative effect to help them get to sleep at night. Conversely, there are patients who experience marked sedation with first-generation antihistamines and become noncompliant with treatment. For machinists, drivers and others with occupations involving working with machinery, even a small a degree of sedation or CNS impairment may be dangerous. The clinician must discuss these problems with the patient so as to choose the best agent.

Both $H_1$- and $H_2$-receptors have been found in the nasal mucosal blood vessels.[19] There is some clinical evidence that the *combined use of $H_1$- and $H_2$-antagonists* blocks the actions of histamine more effectively than either agent alone. Topical chlorpheniramine (chlorphenamine) and ranitidine were studied alone and in combination to determine their effect on topically applied histamine in human nasal mucosa.[20] The 2 agents together were more effective than either agent alone. Oral chlorpheniramine and cimetidine were similarly tested and found to have an additive effect.[21] Studies with levocabastine and ranitidine[22] showed that the $H_2$-antagonist alone produced a significant effect on rhinorrhoea caused by nasal allergen challenge but not on the sneeze effect. An adverse effect appeared to occur with cimetidine in one study.[23] Mucosal swelling and nasal blockade are usually not helped by either type of antihistamine. Combined $H_1$- and $H_2$-blockade suppresses skin test reactions better than $H_1$-blockade alone.

It was hypothesised early that $H_2$-receptors may mediate vasodilatation and thus vascular engorgement might be prevented by $H_2$-antagonists. Evidence suggests that intravenous doses of cimetidine induce great improvement in the symptoms of allergy and a clear decrease in the serum IgE concentrations in 70% of patients.[24] However, the authors of that report did not think their evidence suggested strong vascular effects of cimetidine. More recently, cetirizine 10mg was compared with a combination of cetirizine and cimetidine 800mg.[25] The combination produced a more significant reduction in nasal airway resistance and an increase in nasal air flow. It is unfortunate that the evidence for both efficacy and mechanism is not clear in this potentially useful drug combination.

The second-generation antihistamines appear to be generally quite well tolerated when administered in standard doses. However, with terfenadine and astemizole, a few cases of adverse cardiovascular effects such as torsades de pointes and other ventricular arrhythmias have been reported. Terfenadine and astemizole are contraindicated in patients taking ketoconazole, itraconazole or erythromycin (because of CYP3A4 inhibition), those with severe hepatic dysfunction, or those already receiving drugs known to cause QT interval prolongation (e.g. antiarrhythmics such as quinidine or procainamide) who may be especially prone to the adverse cardiovascular effects of these drugs.

Histamine is not the only mediator of inflammation released in infected or allergic tissue.[12] Other mediators such as kinins, prostaglandins, leukotrienes, lysosomal enzymes, cytokines and toxins elaborated by micro-organisms are partially responsible for symptoms of the inflammatory response. Also involved are T cells, eosinophils, basophils, neutrophils, platelets, mast cells and agents produced by these cells. It is unrealistic to expect that antihistamines could suppress the action of all these mediators of inflammation and the actions of all these cell types.

Besides being inhibitors of histamine, antihistamines can also have a number of other actions, including a weak anticholinergic effect (minimal or absent with the second-generation agents), local anaesthetic effects, vasoconstrictor effects, and the ability to prevent or control motion sickness and disequilibrium or vertigo; they can also be used as sedatives. The second-generation agents also inhibit the release of histamine from mast cells and basophils (for reviews, see Kontou-Fili;[9] and Simons & Simons[10]).

### 1.3 Antivertigo Drugs

Vertigo is a symptom produced by a complex system for the maintenance of balance and posture, and the awareness of the body's position in space. Vertigo can be caused by malfunction in the peripheral labyrinth, the eighth cranial nerve, or the nerve's connections in the brain stem, cerebrum and cerebellum. Visual tracts are involved, as are spinal tracts related to posture, especially those from the cervical stretch receptors. Unbalanced neuronal activity in any of these components can lead to dizziness or vertigo. In addition, extrinsic disorders (haemodynamic, metabolic or psychological) can affect this system. Logically, drugs used to treat vertigo would:

1) Interact with neuronal transmitters in this system (of which there are many).

2) Increase blood flow to ischaemic tissue.

3) Treat a biochemical pathology (e.g. Ménière's disease).

4) Treat an extrinsic disorder.

Thus, drugs used to treat vertigo are of many different types and actions, and their selection depends on the suspected diagnosis (see further section 4). However, it should be remembered that not all causes of vertigo or dizziness are treatable by drugs or surgery. For a review of the pharmacology of antivertigo drugs, see Rascol et al.[26]

### 1.4 Sympathomimetic Drugs

Sympathomimetic drugs are used in otorhinolaryngology mainly for their effects on inflamed nasal, sinus and eustachian tube mucosa. Normal nasal patency depends on a constant flow of sympathetic nerve impulses [and noradrenaline (norepinephrine)] to nasal blood vessels. This sympathetic vasoconstrictor 'tone' usually alternates between nostrils in a variable rhythm (the nasal cycle). Interruption of this flow by drugs that inhibit sympathetic transmission will produce vasodilatation. Thus, certain drugs such as reserpine (which depletes noradrenaline stores) and guanethidine (which inhibits noradrenaline release) produce a restricted nasal airway or stuffy nose. Augmentation of noradrenaline release (e.g. by cocaine) or use of topical or systemic decongestants opens the nasal airway. The sympathetic tone has not been described in the vasculature of the sinus and eustachian tube mucosa.

Most common decongestants are classified as ***α-adrenoceptor agonists.*** Two types of α-receptor, $\alpha_1$ and $\alpha_2$, have been described.[19] $\alpha_1$-Receptors are postsynaptic, i.e. located on the surface of the vascular smooth muscle, while $\alpha_2$-receptors are both postsynaptic and presynaptic. In general, the presynaptic receptors regulate the release of neurotransmitters. Stimulation of postsynaptic receptors, either $\alpha_1$ or $\alpha_2$, produces a smooth muscle contraction and an open nasal airway. Thus, α-adrenoceptor agonists acting at either $\alpha_1$- or $\alpha_2$-receptors may be useful as decongestants. There are several agents that are commonly used for this purpose because of long term familiarity and their relative lack of cardiovascular and CNS stimulation. They include *pseudoephedrine* and *phenylpropanolamine* for oral use, and *phenylephrine, oxymetazoline* and *xylometazoline* for topical use. Some of these agonists act *directly* on the α-receptors on the vascular smooth muscle surface (e.g. oxymetazoline), while others act *indirectly* by exerting an effect on the release of noradrenaline from the nerve terminal (e.g. pseudoephedrine). Topical decongestants are effective and seldom cause difficulty if their use is restricted to less than 5 days. Beyond that time, their potential for causing rebound congestion becomes important.

In rebound congestion, the patient notes that after weeks of using topical nasal sprays, the drug is no longer effective. The clinician may see that nasal tissue appears worse than it did before treatment. In former times, this tachyphylaxis was thought to be due to the use of indirect-acting agonists such as pseudoephedrine. Long term use of the drug depletes 'releasable' stores of noradrenaline. Others believed that rebound was reactive hyperaemia. A tissue depleted of oxygen and substrates by intense and long term constriction produces substances that cause vasodilatation. Part of the problem might be the relatively high concentration of the drug itself and the effects of preservatives and stabilising agents, which could act as chemical irritants. Newer work has shown that high concentrations of adrenergic agents can lead to decreased numbers of receptors or 'downregulation' and a decreased response to the drug and to the vasomotor tone. Stern warnings against excessive use coupled with the use of paediatric dosages of drugs in adults might be partially effective in postponing rebound.

The oral agents are more likely to cause systemic effects because they stimulate α-adrenoceptors in other parts of the body.

β-***Adrenoceptor agonists*** are seldom used in otorhinolaryngology and have little effect on nasal function.[27] However, they tend to dilate peripheral blood vessels and are occasionally used in attempts to increase blood flow in the labyrinth.

### 1.5 Vasoactive Peptides

The discovery and elucidation of a host of vasoactive neuropeptides in nasal mucosa has drastically changed the physiological framework.[28] Trigeminal sensory neurons can signal pain and produce wheal and flare responses to heat, acid, bradykinin or histamine. Neurotransmitters such as calcitonin gene-related peptide (CGRP), substance P and neurokinin A are found in these neurons.[29] Parasympathetic neurons contain vasoactive peptide; sympathetic neurons contain neuropeptide Y. Extremely potent vasoconstrictors such as *endothelin*[30] have been isolated from blood vessels and shown to be active in human nasal mucosa. The ways that we explain some normal behaviour of the nasal mucosa, drug effects and nasal pathologies are undergoing serious revision. We can no longer think of noradrenaline and acetylcholine as the only two neurotransmitters controlling upper respiratory mucosa. At present, however, there are few drugs that have been developed to control or interact with these neuropeptides. Perhaps the first will antagonise bradykinin and substance P.

### 1.6 Vasodilator Drugs

These drugs are used to treat sudden hearing loss (see section 6) and certain types of vertigo (see section 4). They dilate blood vessels and thereby increase blood flow. However, the use of these drugs raises two questions. Firstly, do they actually increase blood flow to the inner ear? Secondly, if the blood flow does increase, can a therapeutic effect be reasonably expected?

There is a great deal of controversy about the effectiveness of these drugs, especially on intracranial vessels.[31] Many pharmacologists believe that only a few vascular beds (e.g. skin) are readily affected by vasodilators, since autoregulatory mechanisms (local changes in pH, $pO_2$ and $pCO_2$) have already adjusted blood flow as much as possible in ischaemic areas. Besides local regulation, it is difficult to promote significant changes in blood flow to intracranial vessels because of baroreceptor reflexes originating in the carotids and elsewhere. However, animal studies have shown that several agents (e.g. carbon dioxide, histamine, papaverine) induce increased otic blood flow if given in adequate dosages.[32,33] These data form the experimental basis for treating ischaemic inner ear disease with such drugs. If this medication is effective in the patient, and clinical experience suggests that at times it is, it may be that blood flow is restricted by functional (nervous or humoral) rather than structural (sclerotic) changes. The pharmacologist's cynicism is usually engendered by claims of relieving ischaemia during long term treatment of degenerative vascular diseases.

### 1.7 Corticosteroids

Corticosteroids are commonly used in otorhinolaryngology to treat allergic rhinitis, nasal polyposis, rhinitis in pregnancy, postoperative nasal oedema, rhinitis medicamentosa, vocal process ulcers, forms of laryngeal and tracheal injuries, and ulcers. They are also used for ear barotrauma, certain kinds of eustachian tube congestion, autoimmune ear disease, and sudden hearing loss.

Corticosteroids modulate the humoral and cellular mechanisms of the inflammatory response. They inhibit the activation and infiltration of eosinophils, basophils and mast cells into the inflammatory site and reduce the production and release of many mediators of inflammation. They also inhibit the production of prostaglandins and leukotrienes by inhibiting the production or arachidonic acid, and are potent vasoconstrictors. Corticosteroids work best if given before the start of the allergic reaction but usually improve rhinitis symptoms within 3 days if given after the inflammation begins.

Although the potential for adrenal suppression occurs whenever corticosteroids are used, topical agents such as beclomethasone dipropionate,[34] flunisolide,[35] budesonide,[36,37] and fluticasone propionate[38] are poorly absorbed systemically if the dosage regimen is followed. Intranasal injection of depot corticosteroid preparations such as triamcinolone acetonide or methylprednisolone acetate may be used when a rapid onset and prolonged duration of action with a relative lack of systemic effects are desired. However, a rare complication of intranasal injection of corticosteroids is visual loss.[39]

## 2. Upper Respiratory Tract Conditions

### 2.1 General Principles of Treatment

Upper respiratory tract dysfunction often reflects an alteration in local ventilation and in the ciliated secretory epithelium that lines the tract from the nose to the lungs. This mucociliary epithelium is phylogenetically old and generally robust, withstanding and rebuffing infection, allergy, anatomical factors, trauma, tumours, drug-related processes or any combinations thereof. Despite the continuity of the upper respiratory epithelium, studies have demonstrated, within respiratory regions, a wide range of responses to infectious organisms. There is also a variation in the response to drugs.

Drug treatment of upper respiratory conditions is generally 2-fold in nature. The initial goal is to resolve the inflammatory symptoms. This is accomplished by shrinking the swollen mucous membranes and reducing the profuse secretions associated with the process. Concomitantly, treatment may be directed at eliminating the offending causative agent with appropriate systemic therapy.

An organism responsible for the infection should be identified, at least presumptively, before choosing an antimicrobial drug. Identification may be by intelligent guesswork based on clinical evidence (table I), or by definitive culture isolation. The specimen obtained for bacteriological study must be representative of those in the infected site. The meticulous collection of pus is often facilitated by direct visualisation and use of a small (e.g. Alden-Senturia) suction trap.

The normal bacterial flora of the pharynx may include such usual pathogens as *Haemophilus influenzae* and *Streptococcus pneumoniae*. The nose may have the same organisms but the paranasal sinuses, middle ear and mastoid areas are thought to be normally sterile. A very large number of viruses have been isolated from the upper respiratory tract and shown to have pathogenic potential. The routine use of viral cultures or acute and convalescent antibody titres is, however, not generally performed and at present is of limited value in daily practice. Specific antiviral treatment is generally wanting. However, effective prevention and treatment of some viral infections is possible (see further chapter 32; sect. 3).

Most acute infections causing morbidity are in the upper respiratory tract, and most of these are viral in origin (e.g. the common cold) and do not benefit from *routine* use of antibacterial drugs.[40,41] The common cold may result from any of a large number of potential viral pathogens, most commonly from rhinoviruses. It is generally a self-limiting illness requiring only symptomatic treatment. However, some patients present with a progression of symptoms that is suggestive of secondary bacterial involvement. Consequently, the use of antibacterial agents in these *more complicated* cases has gained favour among many clinicians.

It should be emphasised that functional anatomy is of paramount importance in all disorders of the middle ear, nose and paranasal sinuses. Complete resolution of infectious disorders in these areas is generally precluded unless adequate ventilation and drainage pathways are established. This may involve only pharmacological shrinkage of oedematous tissues with re-establishment of physiological drainage, or may require surgical creation of drainage or ventilation pathways.

### 2.2 Acute Rhinosinusitis

Most nasal inflammatory disorders also involve, to a greater or lesser degree, the paranasal sinuses. The sinuses are formed as embryological and developmental outgrowths of nasal structures and, thus, have the same general histological and pharmacological properties as the nasal mucosa.[42,43]

Acute rhinosinusitis presents as a mucoid or purulent discharge. The nature of the discharge forms the basis for an initial differential diagnosis. A thin mucoid discharge is typical of vasomotor, allergic or viral infectious states. Purulent discharge is typical of bacterial infection.

#### *2.2.1 Optimum Treatment*

**Initial Symptomatic Treatment**

Acute allergic, vasomotor or viral disorders are generally treated initially with topical decongestant nasal sprays or oral decongestants (see section 1.4). Supplemental moisture is helpful and is conveniently supplied by spinning disc atomisers, ultrasonic or pneumatic nebulisers or steam vaporisers. Night-time augmentation of water-laden air is especially important. Warm air must have a much greater water content (absolute humidity) to have the same relative humidity as cool air. The nose must raise the temperature of the air to near 37°C, and then raise its relative humidity to near 100%.

**Table III.** Guide to the differential diagnosis of the stuffy nose (after May & West[45])

| Nasal passage | Local causes | Systemic causes |
|---|---|---|
| Obstructed | *Infection:* viral, bacterial, diphtheria, leprosy<br>Allergic rhinitis<br>Environmental dryness or heat<br>*Congenital:* atresia, asymmetry<br>*Acquired:* trauma, crooked nose, foreign body<br>*Neoplasm:* polyps, adenoids, malignancies<br>*Mucociliary anomalies:* immotile cilia syndrome, cystic fibrosis | *Drugs:* reserpine, guanethidine, methyldopa, antithyroid drugs, oral contraceptives<br>Diabetes mellitus<br>Hypothyroidism<br>Pregnancy, menses<br>*Systemic disorders:* sarcoidosis, Wegener's granulomatosis |
| Open | Localised atrophic rhinitis<br>*Iatrogenic:* surgery, cautery scarring<br>Trauma<br>Irritants (e.g. chromium, smoke) | Generalised atrophic rhinitis<br>Age >65 years<br>Sjögren's syndrome |

Topical sprays of decongestants such as *oxymetazoline* or *xylometazoline* are recommended for a period of not more than 5 to 7 days. The commonly available oral decongestants may contain only vasoconstrictors (e.g. sympathomimetic amines such as phenylpropanolamine, pseudoephedrine, phenylephrine) or may be combined with antihistamines. Well designed clinical studies have demonstrated the efficacy and synergism of oral sympathomimetic amines combined with antihistamines in the treatment of nasal mucosal congestion due to infection or allergy.[44] The sense of nasal obstruction relates to the velocity of air flow through the nose being either too fast or too slow. Stuffiness can occur with actual obstruction or with widely patent nasal passages that have a slow flow of air across the nasal mucosa (table III).

Topical decongestants have the advantage of selective site of action and more rapid action than oral agents. However, all topical vasoconstrictor and mucolytic agents damage the mucociliary flow apparatus. The most serious objection to their use is the rebound or reactive hyperaemic state known as rhinitis medicamentosa that develops with repeated use.[39,46] Particular attention should be directed to the medically unsupervised use of nose drops in infants and children. Systemic effects such as tachycardia, somnolence and shock-like states have been reported in infants and children after administration of a large number of drops.[47,48]

#### Treatment of Secondary Bacterial Infection

Persistence of congestion for over 7 to 10 days and the appearance of purulent discharge are indicative of progression of disease to secondary bacterial involvement. Once bacterial infection has supervened, systemic antibacterial drugs should be administered for 10 to 14 days. Persisting or worsening symptoms and signs after 2 to 5 days of antibacterial therapy are an indication for paranasal sinus radiography and consideration for establishing mechanical drainage.

Penicillin remains the drug of choice for the initial treatment of acute upper respiratory bacterial conditions (table I).

#### Treatment of Recurrent Bouts of Acute Rhinosinusitis

Incompletely resolved bacterial infections or recurrent bouts of acute rhinosinusitis may give rise to mucosal ulcerations, inflammatory metaplasia and progressive fibrosis with resultant obstruction of the drainage orifices of the sinuses. Unless adequate drainage and ventilation are re-established, the mucosa ultimately becomes irreversibly damaged and surgical intervention is required. Early drug treatment during this progression can sometimes halt the process. Saline lavage of the maxillary antrum is helpful, both in mechanically removing inspissated secretions and for identification of the predominant bacterial species.

Presumptive drug treatment for this condition should include antibacterial cover for *H. influenzae* which (table I), along with anaerobic streptococci, are the predominant organisms in chronic rhinosinusitis. Second-line antibiotic therapy, as for otitis media, is commonly amoxicillin/clavulanic acid, cotrimoxazole (trimethoprim/sulfamethoxazole) and cefaclor. Antihistamines are also indicated in allergic patients.

Development of tolerance to a particular class of antihistamine or undesirable adverse effects such as somnolence can be a problem in drug treatment of chronic rhinosinusitis. Periodic changes among chemical classes of antihistamines (see table II) may achieve the desired physiological effect while minimising undue adverse effects. The use of nonsedating antihistamines (e.g. astemizole, terfenadine, loratadine or cetirizine) may obviate the problem of drowsiness.

Patients with recurrent sinusitis should be carefully checked for causative factors. These may include dental infection, tumours, nasal foreign body, deviated nasal septum or cystic fibrosis.[49]

### 2.2.2 Complications

Intracranial and orbital extension are the most serious and life-threatening complications of suppurative diseases of the nose and paranasal sinuses.[50] Meningitis, extradural, subdural and multifocal brain abscesses may complicate paranasal infections (for treatment of these infections, see chapters 29 and 31). Mild headache, malaise and low grade fever may be the only symptoms of cryptogenic intracranial infection.

## 2.3 Vasomotor Rhinitis

Vasomotor rhinitis is a poorly understood disease that is characterised by chronic nasal congestion, usually with an accompanying thin viscid rhinorrhoea associated with a hypertrophic red to red-blue mucosa. Some call it nasal hyper-reactivity[51] or non-allergic perennial rhinitis. The most common cause is thought to be an imbalance between the secretory-vasodilatory effect of the parasympathetic nerve supply and the drying-vasoconstrictive effect of the sympathetic nerve supply. Some clinicians believe that the term 'vasomotor rhinitis' is confusing, only vaguely descriptive and falsely attributes cause. The diagnosis of vasomotor rhinitis is perhaps equivalent to idiopathic rhinitis. Since the diagnosis of vasomotor rhinitis is usually one of exclusion, a diligent search to explain the rhinitis is indicated (see table III; section 2.2).

#### Optimum Treatment

Drug treatment is usually started with oral decongestants (see section 1.4). Many patients with this disorder abuse topical decongestant sprays and rhinitis medicamentosa typically results. Complete cessation of topical decongestants and frequent nasal spraying with normal saline containing glycerin 0.125% may be helpful in restoring the nasal mucosa to a more physiological state. Perhaps more effective is the use of an *intranasal aerosol corticosteroid* such as beclomethasone dipropionate, 1 puff to each nostril 4 times daily.[34,52] Dexamethasone phosphate, flunisolide, budesonide or fluticasone propionate aerosols can be used as alternatives. The anti-inflammatory action of these corticosteroids is useful in restoring physiological function to the atrophic, denuded nasal mucosa which occurs as an end-stage of vasomotor and allergic rhinitis.

In patients exposed to cold dry air[53] and those with chronic watery rhinorrhoea as the dominating symptom, intranasal *ipratropium bromide* has proved useful in reducing the hypersecretion.[54,55] Topical atropine in a low dose (≈0.08mg to each nostril) can have the same effect.[56]

## 2.4 Allergic Rhinitis

Allergic rhinitis may begin at any age and is generally categorised as either seasonal or perennial. The common symptoms are bilateral nasal stuffiness, watery discharge, sneezing, and itching of the eyes and nose; epistaxis may also occur. Signs include a purple, boggy nasal mucosa, bridging strands of mucus and 'allergic shiners' (especially in children). Smears of nasal mucus in typical cases show more than 20% of the leucocytes as eosinophils. Offending inhalant allergens in genetically predisposed patients have the capacity to alter the immune system. The resulting antigen-antibody reaction triggers the release of chemical mediators of inflammation, most notably histamine. The severity of the symptoms depends on the amount of allergen exposure and the sensitivity of the nasal mucous membrane. Aspirin (acetylsalicylic acid) may cause rhinitis, asthma and polyposis in certain allergic individuals.

### 2.4.1 Optimum Treatment

Therapy of allergic rhinitis may be considered to be in tiers dictated by the severity of the process and the responsiveness to therapy. The principles of management include allergen avoidance, pharmacotherapy and immunotherapy. Avoidance can include air-conditioning with filters, use of fibre masks when performing outdoor work during pollen seasons, careful house cleaning, plastic casings over pillows and mattresses, elimination of thick rugs and other dust collectors, and outdoor segregation of pets. Sometimes, many or all of these may be impractical or ineffective.

#### Immunotherapy

Immunotherapy is usually reserved for severe cases of rhinitis and those refractory to pharmacotherapy. Immunotherapy attempts to decrease the allergic response by injecting increasing doses of specific allergen extracts. The injec-

**Table IV.** Some commonly used drugs in the treatment of rhinitis (Simons & Simons[10,57])

| Drug | Usual dosage |
|---|---|
| **Oral antihistamines** | |
| Chlorpheniramine (chlorphenamine) | *Children:* 0.35 mg/kg/day<br>*Adults:* 8-12mg bid |
| Astemizole | *Children:* 0.2 mg/kg/day<br>*Adults:* 10mg once daily |
| Cetirizine | *Adults:* 5-10mg once daily |
| Loratadine | *Children 2-12 years:* 5 mg/day; *>12 years:* 10 mg/day<br>*Adults:* 10mg once daily |
| Terfenadine | *Children 3-6 years:* 15mg bid; *7-12 years:* 30mg bid<br>*Adults:* 60mg bid or 120mg once daily |
| **Intranasal antihistamines** | |
| Levocabastine (0.5 mg/ml solution) | 2 sprays (50μg each) bid |
| Azelastine (0.1% solution) | 2 sprays (137 μg each) once or twice daily |
| **Intranasal sympathomimetics[a]** | |
| Oxymetazoline (0.025% paediatric and 0.05% solutions) | 2-3 sprays or drops/nostril once to 3 times daily |
| Xylometazoline (0.05% paediatric and 0.1% solutions) | 1-2 sprays q8-12h |
| Phenylephrine (0.5% solution) | 1-2 sprays q4h |
| Tetryzoline (tetrahydrozoline) [0.1% solution] | 1-2 sprays q4h |
| **Oral sympathomimetics** | |
| Pseudoephedrine | *Children:* 15-30mg tid<br>*Adults:* 60mg tid or 120mg bid |
| Phenylpropanolamine | *Adults:* 25mg q4h or 75mg sustained release q12h |
| Phenylephrine | *Adults:* 10mg q4h |
| **Mast cell stabilisers** | |
| Sodium cromoglycate (cromolyn sodium) | *Adults and children >6 years:* 1 spray (5.2mg)/nostril 3-6 times daily |
| **Corticosteroids - intranasal** | |
| Beclomethasone dipropionate | *Adults and children >6 years:* 2 sprays (50μg each)/nostril bid |
| Flunisolide | *Children 6-14 years:* 1 spray (25μg)/nostril tid<br>*Adults:* 2 sprays (25μg each)/nostril bid or tid, then 1-2 sprays bid |
| Budesonide | *Adults and children >6 years:* 2 sprays (50μg each)/nostril bid |
| Fluticasone propionate | *Adults and children >12 years:* 2 sprays (50μg each)/nostril once daily |
| **Anticholinergics – intranasal** | |
| Atropine sulfate (1 mg/ml solution) | *Adults:* 1 spray/nostril tid |
| Atropine methonitrate (0.13% solution) | *Adults:* 1 spray/nostril tid |
| Ipratropium bromide | *Children:* 1-2 sprays (20μg each)/nostril bid-tid<br>*Adults:* 2 sprays (20μg each)/nostril tid-qid |

a Restrict to 10-day maximum use.

*Abbreviations:* bid = twice daily; tid = three times daily; qid = 4 times daily.

tions induce IgG-blocking antibodies to the allergens, which results in less mediator release and reduced inflammatory response.

### Drug Treatment

Table IV lists the several classes of agents commonly used to treat allergic rhinitis. In general, if the rhinitis is sporadic and not severe, antihistamines, antihistamines combined with oral or topical decongestants,[58] or anticholinergic agents[59,60] are suitable. If the rhinitis is not severe, but occurs daily or seasonally, nonsedating antihistamines and/or mast cell stabilisers[61,62] can be used. If the rhinitis is chronic and more severe, topical corticosteroids are usually used.[63] For a review, see Horak.[12]

***Antihistamines and decongestants:*** antihistamines are effective in the management of seasonal and perennial allergic rhinitis symptoms such as rhinorrhoea, oedema, nasal itching and sneezing. They are not as useful against nasal blockage caused by vasodilation, which appears to be either under greater control of $H_2$-receptors or caused by mediators other than histamine. Control is accomplished in practice by the use of decongestants. Decongestants stimulate α-adrenergic receptors on nasal blood vessels and induce vasoconstriction. Oral decongestants commonly used include *pseudoephedrine, phenylephrine* and *phenylpropanolamine*. Systemic adverse reactions with these drugs include tachycardia, palpitations, nervousness, tremor, insomnia and hypertension in predisposed individuals.[64]

Topical nasal decongestants have a place in both seasonal and perennial allergies, but when overused can induce rhinitis medicamentosa. Therefore, long term relief of nasal congestion should be obtained by other approaches, with nasal sprays being used only for brief periods (5 to 10 days) during acute exacerbations.

The combined use of an antihistamine and an oral decongestant is helpful and combats the drowsiness of daytime doses of first-generation antihistamines.

Dosages of some commonly used antihistamines are given in table IV. *Terfenadine* and *loratadine* appear to have a somewhat faster onset of action and are probably better suited to use on an 'as-needed' basis. *Astemizole* may be more appropriately used for conditions that require a daily dose for a long period. The half-life of terfenadine is about 17 hours, while that of the active metabolite of astemizole (demethylastemizole) is about 19 days during long term therapy. Although such a long half-life would interfere with skin allergy testing, it implies that once a patient has taken astemizole for a few weeks, missing the drug for a day or two would have little effect because the blood concentration would still be high.

***Mast cell stabilisers:*** *sodium cromoglycate (cromolyn sodium)* used as drops, spray or powder is a safe topical intranasal drug that protects against the effects of antigen challenge. It stabilises mast cells, thus inhibiting release of chemical mediators. However, since it is effective only when used prophylactically before allergen challenge and because administration is required about every 6 hours, intranasal corticosteroids are often preferred.

***Intranasal corticosteroids:*** the intranasal corticosteroids (i.e. beclomethasone dipropionate, budesonide, flunisolide, fluticasone propionate, dexamethasone phosphate and triamcinolone acetonide) are effective in both seasonal and perennial allergic rhinitis. As would be expected, these preparations have little effect on eye symptoms. For maximum effectiveness, the intranasal formulation must reach all or most of the nasal mucosa. For this reason, polyps may need to be removed surgically prior to such therapy. Since the nasal mucosal shrinkage begins anteriorly and progresses posteriorly, several days of treatment are often necessary before the onset of symptomatic relief. Some clinicians recommend the use of oral decongestants for the first 3 days of treatment to overcome this delay. Long term high-dose intranasal corticosteroid use produces increased capillary fragility and mucosal atrophy. However, there have been no important local or systemic adverse effects with clinical use at usually recommended dosages.

Depot corticosteroids injected into nasal turbinates and polyps can be effective, but since blindness has arisen from this treatment, it is recommended that this treatment be used only by those skilled in the technique.[65]

***Intranasal anticholinergic drugs:*** intranasal application of anticholinergic drugs such as *atropine*[60] or *ipratropium bromide* aerosol may prove useful in reducing hypersecretion seen in allergy, rhinovirus infections, vasomotor rhinitis and the inhalation of cold, dry air.[66] In using atropine, the dose must be kept below 0.5mg or adverse effects will occur.

#### Surgical Management

Surgical management may be required in cases with anatomical nasal obstruction (e.g. polyps, deviated nasal septum) or hyperplastic sinusitis. However, when irreversibly damaged tissues have been removed and adequate drainage and ventilation re-established, medical management is usually successful.

### 2.5 Fungal Infections of the Nasal Cavity

Mucormycosis of the nasal and paranasal tissues is almost always found in immunocompromised patients [e.g. those with poorly controlled diabetes mellitus, renal failure, acquired immune deficiency syndrome (AIDS), or those receiving cancer chemotherapy]. The organisms are commensal or saprophytic fungi. For a timely diagnosis, there must be a high index of clinical suspicion, a thorough intranasal examination, and a microscopic examination of drainage and biopsy tissue. Clinically, such mycotic infections are more aggressive than the more common bacterial infections.

Treatment includes control of underlying systemic disease states, local surgical removal of infected tissues and a systemic antifungal agent, such as amphotericin B at as high a dosage as the patient's renal function will allow (see chapter 31; sect. 6.1.1).

### 2.6 Nasal Furuncles

Furuncles are often found in the nasal vestibular area and may recur chronically. Effective treatment consists of warm soaks and local incision and drainage after maturation has occurred. Topical antibacterial agents such as *povidone iodine* or *bacitracin* are helpful prophylactic measures. Neomycin preparations should be used with caution because sensitisation may occur. Treatment usually lasts 10 or more days. Persistent or progressive furunculosis demands the use of systemic antibacterials. Since penicillinase-producing *Staphylococcus aureus* and streptococci are the usual organisms, a penicillinase-resistant penicillin (table I) is indicated.

### 2.7 Pharyngitis

Acute sore throat is a common illness; it has numerous causes including not only many infectious agents but also nonspecific irritants and chemical pollutants. After diphtheria has been ruled out (by a history of adequate immunisation and physical examination not revealing a pharyngeal adherent grey-white membrane, the removal of which causes bleeding), the clinician must usually decide between viral and streptococcal infection. In addition to streptococci, pharyngitis may also be due to *Mycoplasma pneumoniae, Chlamydia pneumoniae, Neisseria gonorrhoeae* or *Candida* spp. Except in epidemics or in cases of scarlet fever, experienced clinicians can distinguish between streptococcal and non-streptococcal pharyngitis with only about 75% accuracy. For this reason, a bacteriological test of the tonsillar surface should be considered.[67]

#### Optimum Treatment

Individual clinicians differ in their approach to treatment (and in their enthusiasm for throat culture). Some administer antibacterial drugs empirically to all patients complaining of sore throat, but this is not the generally recommended authoritative practice. Many sore throats are of viral or irritant aetiology and respond to supportive therapy and avoidance of the offending irritant. Symptomatic treatment consists of warm saline throat irrigations, throat lozenges and analgesics such as aspirin (acetylsalicylic acid) or paracetamol (acetaminophen).

***Antibacterial drugs*** are effective not only in preventing the rheumatic sequelae of streptococcal pharyngitis, but also in early symptomatic relief of bacterial pharyngitis.[68] In some geographical areas, bacteria are seasonally the predominant cause of sore throat. Group A haemolytic streptococci are the more prevalent cause of bacterial sore throat. The usual therapy is phenoxymethylpenicillin (penicillin V) for 10 days. The result of culture of the tonsil surface may not be representative of the flora within the tissue of the tonsil. Sometimes streptococci persist in the tonsil even after treatment with penicillin, an occurrence probably explained by a penicillin-prompted shift in the pharyngeal flora. This can cause the emergence of β-lactamase-producing strains of *H. influenzae, S. aureus* and *Bacteroides* spp.[69] Therefore, patients with persistent sore throats may benefit from empirical treatment with a β-lactamase-resistant antibiotic. A search for sources of recurring streptococcal exposure (e.g. close personal contacts, pets) may be rewarding.

Any viral infectious diseases, infectious mononucleosis in particular, may present as a pharyngitis. The treatment is symptomatic. Attention should be directed to hepatosplenomegaly and the other protean manifestations of this disease. If tonsillar enlargement compromises the airways, high doses of corticosteroids (e.g. prednisone 40 to 80 mg/day for an adult patient) are indicated for 2 to 4 days and then rapidly tapered. If acute tonsillar enlargement obstructs the airways and endotracheal intubation or tracheotomy are required, consideration should be given to acute tonsillectomy.

***Tonsillectomy:*** the role of tonsillectomy in the treatment of recurrent tonsillitis continues to be controversial.[70] The indication for tonsillectomy is often a social one, i.e. when the risk and expense of school or work absence exceed the risk and expense of tonsillectomy, surgery is recommended. In general, 6 or more clinical episodes of tonsillitis in 1 year in a child, and 4 or more in 1 year in an adult, should prompt consideration of tonsillectomy. Of course, obstructing tonsils causing sleep apnoea or cor pulmonale, and consideration of tonsillar malignancy are indications for tonsillectomy.

Peritonsillar abscesses are the most common parapharyngeal suppurative infections of the neck. They are rarely seen in children, but typically occur in teenagers and young adults. The usual history is several days of sore throat, progressive difficulty with swallowing and talking, and development of trismus and fever. Most of these infections are unilateral and involve streptococci and anaerobic bacteria. Treatment consists of an antibiotic (a penicillin) plus aspiration, surgical drainage or immediate tonsillectomy.[71] Although the risk of subsequent recurrent peritonsillar abscess is low, many clinicians recommend tonsillectomy 6 to 8 weeks after an abscess.

Treatment of pertussis is discussed in chapter 3 (section 4.2.5).

## 3. Ear Infections

### 3.1 Otitis Externa

Drugs that control disease in the external auditory canal are basically medications for various forms of dermatitis.[72,73] The skin of the ear canal should have an acidic surface pH, and variations in pH may lead to disease states. Therapy involves a thorough cleaning of the skin and is directed towards the restoration of pH, reduction of swelling, elimination of infection and removal or control of predisposing causes, especially prevention of scratching or rubbing in and around the ear.

Five classifications of external ear disease requiring drug therapy are:

1) Acute oedematous otitis externa (swimmer's ear).

2) Eczematoid dermatitis with secondary infection.

3) True otomycosis.

4) Acute furunculosis.

5) Malignant otitis externa.

#### *3.1.1 Acute Oedematous Otitis Externa (Swimmer's Ear)*

Swimmer's ear is a common affliction in humans. Inflammation and oedema of the ear canal and adjacent structures usually develop when the patient has been exposed to frequent water contamination as may occur during swimming or in climates with high constant humidity. Diabetic patients and those with recurrent skin disorders such as eczema seem more susceptible to this disease. Infection is usually with saprophytic agents such as *Pseudomonas* or *Proteus* spp. Secondary inflammation from *Candida* may also occur.

**Optimum Treatment**

Gentle and meticulous cleansing with a suction apparatus or with extremely small wire (e.g. dental broaches) cotton-tipped applicators is needed. The usual wooden applicator stick is far too large and should not be used. A hydrocellulose sponge or, alternatively, cotton wick is gently inserted into the ear canal. It should be saturated with an acetic acid-corticosteroid or antibacterial-corticosteroid solution, and the patient instructed to apply the same solution as topical ear drops 4 times a day. The sponge or wick is usually removed after 4 days, and the drops often continue for a few more days. Since the infection is often due to Gram-negative bacilli, antibacterial-corticosteroid preparations containing neomycin, framycetin, polymixin B, gentamicin or ciprofloxacin may be used. Occasional allergic responses to these agents have been reported.

Severe swelling may require the use of systemic corticosteroids for a few days to reduce the oedema and pain. A systemic antipruritic agent (e.g. cyproheptadine) is often beneficial.

Otitis externa, for example in competitive swimmers or professional scuba divers, may be prevented by avoiding the precipitating factor by evaporating residual ear canal water with a blow (hair) dryer and by use of 2 to 5% acetic acid in 50 to 90% alcohol (ethanol) after immersion (the higher percentage alcohol can be painful). This is done to dry the skin, kill bacteria and fungi, and maintain the normal acidity of the canal skin.

#### *3.1.2 Infected Eczematoid Dermatitis*

This condition involves secondary infection of an existing neurodermatitis and is commonly induced by scratching skin with infected nails.

**Optimum Treatment**

Following careful ear cleaning by suction and wiping of the ear canal with 70 to 95% alcohol, a cotton or hydrocellulose gauze wick is gently inserted into the external ear canal with a small wire applicator and is saturated with aluminium acetate (Burow's) solution. The patient should be treated with these drops 3 times daily for 48 to 72 hours. The aluminium acetate solution should then be stopped, the wick removed and antibacterial-corticosteroid ear drops used for 1 week, together with an oral antipruritic agent at night (see section 3.1.1).

Recurrent crusting or itching of the meatus after the drops have been stopped may necessitate application of a topical corticosteroid or a corticosteroid plus antibacterial/antifungal ointment for a prolonged period of time as a prophylactic measure.

#### 3.1.3 Otomycosis

True fungus infection of the ear canal is not seen often (although it may be frequently mentioned by the patient as the primary complaint). Actual growth of fungus from the canal is rarely accomplished.

##### Optimum Treatment

If inspection indicates probable mycelia, or a blackish accumulation, then the ear canal should be cleansed carefully with applicators and suction (see section 3.1.1), and should be wiped several times with an antifungal solution such as tolnaftate 1% or 'Cresylate' solution, which contains merthiolate, *m*-cresyl acetate, propylene glycol, boric acid and alcohol. The ear canal may then be painted with a solution of gentian violet (10%); or an antifungal powder such as nystatin or clioquinol (iodochlorhydroxyquinoline) may be insufflated into the canal. Usually, the application of this powder once weekly will keep the fungal infection under control. An occasional resistant case may require tolnaftate to be applied daily (1 drop twice daily). The patient should be repeatedly instructed to keep the ears exquisitely dry and to avoid any picking, scratching or rubbing in and around the ear.

Clotrimazole 1% can also be used topically for Aspergillus and Candida infections. Oral ketoconazole or fluconazole may help resistant cases.

#### 3.1.4 Acute Furunculosis

Acute infection around hair follicles in the ear canal may develop with subsequent boil formation and sudden onset of severe burning pain in one ear, with this pain increasing rapidly in severity.

##### Optimum Treatment

Unlike acute mastoiditis (see section 3.3), acute furunculosis is not related to a history of upper respiratory infection and acute otitis media. Opioid analgesics such as morphine and pethidine (meperidine) may be needed in the beginning, but after the first 24 hours, aspirin with codeine is often adequate. Careful cleansing of the ear canal should be carried out with suction and 70% alcohol. A hydrocellulose or cotton wick saturated with aluminium acetate (Burow's) solution or gentamicin 0.1 to 0.3% topical ointment or 0.3% ophthalmic solution is inserted otically.

Since most of these infections are due to staphylococcal or sometimes streptococcal organisms, the patient should be started on oral antibiotics such as cloxacillin, flucloxacillin or erythromycin (table I). In severe cases with signs of systemic spread (e.g. lymphadenitis, fever), parenteral administration of cloxacillin or flucloxacillin is necessary. Surgical incision and drainage of obvious abscess is necessary. Patients should be treated for 7 to 10 days.

#### 3.1.5 Malignant Otitis Externa

The proper management of this rapidly progressive disorder[74] involves the rigid control of diabetes mellitus, with which it is usually associated. The disease can also occur in children with malnutrition and anaemia.[75]

##### Optimum Treatment

In most cases, parenteral gentamicin in maximum dosages short of toxicity is required. This usually involves a dosage of 3 mg/kg/day, but some clinicians use 5 mg/kg/day, reducing to 3 mg/kg/day when a healing response occurs, or 80mg 3 times daily given with carbenicillin 4g 6 times daily. Maximum dosages of gentamicin are determined by using these dosages until tinnitus, oscillopsia or vertigo occurs.[76-78] This therapy should be given for a minimum of 2 weeks and then lower, preventative dosages should be maintained for longer periods (e.g. 3 to 4 weeks).[78] The condition may be due to *Pseudomonas* strains resistant to gentamicin, and alternative therapy with intravenous ticarcillin or piperacillin may be indicated by sensitivity studies. Ciprofloxacin has also been used successfully, and metronidazole has been used in cases involving anaerobes.

Local cleansing is mandatory. Extensive resection of infected cartilage and devitalised skin and soft tissue is held in reserve until the effects of 14 days' intravenous antibiotic therapy are assessed.

Repeated daily treatment with local gentamicin 0.3% solution is also helpful. After the immediate severe local infection is controlled, the patient should be placed on long term prophylaxis with topical application of gentamicin drops and/or oral ciprofloxacin. This infection usually involves *Pseudomonas* spp. or *Proteus* spp. and careful attention to recurrent infection must be maintained. After all infection has subsided, 70 to 90% alcohol drops in the ear canal once daily should be continued indefinitely.

### 3.2 Otitis Media

Inflammation of the middle ear is a common problem in infants, usually manifesting as acute suppurative otitis media (i.e. pus in the middle ear cleft) or middle ear effusion (generally sterile fluid in the middle ear). Although most children outgrow the problem by the age of 2 or 3 years, in some it persists, usually manifesting as middle ear effusion (also known as serous or secretory otitis, or middle ear catarrh). Those who continue having problems as teenagers or adults usually have atelectatic otitis, perforation of the tympanic membrane (so-called 'chronic suppurative otitis media'), or cholesteatoma. The problem is bilateral, although not necessarily symmetrical in its manifestations. A comparatively small mastoid air cell system is generally found in otitis media patients.

There is no generally accepted explanation as to why some children have the problem and most do not; nor why most outgrow the problem and some do not. Anatomical and allergic involvement of the eustachian tube are commonly invoked.

#### Optimum Treatment

Diagnostic and management guidelines for otitis media are shown in table V. Some discussion of the 'masterful inactivity' approach to treating acute otitis media is appropriate. This approach, which is not universally accepted, involves use of an analgesic, and limited or no use of an antibiotic unless the illness progresses or persists beyond 3 or 4 days. The reports supporting this approach[79,80] must be interpreted carefully: infants were excluded from the studies and otological consultation was readily available. This approach to treatment is discussed more fully in a recent review.[81]

Adequate tympanoscopy is necessary, preferably including visualisation during pneumatic movement of the tympanic membrane. Acute otitis media typically follows closely after a viral respiratory infection.[82] Worldwide, bacteria can be found in about 75 to 80% of acute otitis ears. The more common bacteria are *Streptococcus pneumoniae, Haemophilus influenzae, Streptococcus pyogenes* and *Staphylococcus aureus*.[83] The same bacteria can be found in the middle ear fluid of some children (perhaps 45%) with middle ear effusion.[84] Other organisms that have been implicated include *Moraxella (Branhamella) catarrhalis,* which has been isolated with increasing frequency in recent years; most strains of this organism appear to produce β-lactamase.

*Prophylactic antibiotics* (see table V) seem useful in decreasing recurrences of otitis media. However, the magnitude of the effect is limited, requiring treatment of 9 children to show an improved outcome in 1 child.[85] The benefit to the individual patient *versus* society's burden caused by increasing antibiotic resistance prompts careful selective use of prolonged, repeated courses of antibiotics.[86]

Although decongestants and antihistamines, either alone or in combination, have long been used in the treatment of otitis media, evidence for their clinical efficacy is lacking.[87] However, decongestants are usually effective in the eustachian tube if there is a minor problem with changes in barometric pressure such as occurs during aircraft descents. In controlled studies with relatively long treatment periods, the effects of decongestants appear to be no different from those of placebo.

Some clinicians have advocated a short course of *systemic corticosteroids* in the treatment of persistent middle ear effusion. While some have found that their usefulness is minimal and probably synergistic with systemic antibiotic therapy,[88] others consider that reports of the efficacy of corticosteroids are encouraging and support the hypothesis that drugs that counteract inflammatory mediators promote effective clearance in otitis media with effusions.[89]

*Adenoidectomy* (carried out in the hope of improving eustachian tube function) has been shown, on average, to lessen otitis media. Although *pneumococcal vaccines* have not been found to prompt an adequate antibody response in children under 2 years of age, a single injection administered to a child with persistent otitis media should be considered. The avoidance of known contributors to the occurrence or persistence of otitis media is also reasonable, e.g.:

- Supine bottle feeding[90]
- Barotrauma (during the barotrauma challenge of the descent portion of aircraft or mountain travel, sleeping and reclining persons are particularly likely to get otitis media)[91]
- Inhaled irritants and allergens.[92]

*Tympanotomy tube insertion* has become the most commonly performed minor surgical procedure in the US. It may be better to restrict tympanotomy tube insertion to two general indications:

**Table V.** Management approach in otitis media

| Diagnosis | Criteria | Management |
|---|---|---|
| Acute suppurative otitis media | Erythematous eardrum: early = red pars flaccida; late = bulging red eardrum without landmarks; decreased mobility; pain in the ear; fever | **Look for causative factors**<br>**Look for complications of acute otitis:**<br>• Facial paralysis<br>• Labyrinthitis: nystagmus, nausea, vomiting<br>• CNS inflammation; altered mental status, stiff neck<br>• Acute mastoiditis<br>• Draining pus through acute perforation:<br>a) Clean the debris<br>b) Instil antibiotic-corticosteroid drops<br>**Administer antibacterial drugs** - either:<br>• Amoxicillin 250mg tid × 10 days (children 50 mg/kg/day in 3 divided doses). In regions with a high incidence of β-lactamase-producing strains of *Haemophilus influenzae,* or *Moraxella catarrhalis*: amoxicillin 250mg + clavulanic acid 125mg tid (children 20-40 mg/kg/day amoxicillin + clavulanic acid in 3 divided doses)<br>• Erythromycin 250mg qid *plus* sulfafurazole (sulfisoxazole) 0.5g qid × 10 days (children 40/120 mg/kg/day in 4 divided doses)<br>• Cefaclor 250mg tid × 10 days (children 20-40 mg/kg/day in 3 divided doses)<br>• Cotrimoxazole (trimethoprim-sulfamethoxazole) 160/800mg (2 tablets) bid × 10 days (children 8/40 mg/kg/day in 2 divided doses)<br>**Decongestant:** at discretion of the clinician<br>**Re-examine in 2 weeks:**<br>• Normal<br>• Abnormal:<br>a) Fluid in middle ear, erythematous eardrum, patient remains symptomatic with ear complaints – myringotomy for Gram stain, culture and sensitivity then treat as bacteriology dictates<br>b) Fluid in middle ear and erythematous eardrum but patient is asymptomatic – 10-day course of another antibiotic<br>c) Fluid in middle ear, but no erythema of drum – recheck in 2 weeks: If abnormal – antibacterial prophylaxis with cotrimoxazole for 2 weeks |
| Recurrent acute suppurative otitis media | 2 bouts in first 12 months of life | **Look for causative factors**<br>**Antibacterial prophylaxis:** amoxicillin 20 mg/kg/day or sulfafurazole (sulfisoxazole) 250mg twice daily for 3 months<br>**If acute bout while on prophylaxis:**<br>• Myringotomy, Gram stain, culture and sensitivity<br>• If myringotomy, Gram stain, culture and sensitivity not feasible, treat as acute suppurative otitis media |
| Serous/secretory otitis media | Nonsuppurative fluid in middle ear; dull, retracted eardrum with decreased mobility; conductive hearing loss | **Look for causative factors**<br>**Use decongestant** (at discretion of clinician)<br>**Ventilating manoeuvre:** modified Valsalva, Politzer, Frenzel<br>**Recheck in 1 month:**<br>• Normal<br>• Abnormal: empirical course of amoxicillin or erythromycin *plus* sulfafurazole (sulfisoxazole) |
| Chronic suppurative otitis media | Tympanic membrane perforation present for more than 3 weeks with active drainage | **Look for complications of acute suppurative otitis media**<br>**If febrile, treat as acute suppurative otitis media** (see above)<br>**Institute water precautions**<br>**Clean debris and drainage** (microscopic suction is preferred)<br>**Topical therapy:**<br>• Marked mucosal inflammation: antibiotic-corticosteroid drops qid × 4 days<br>• Moderate mucosal inflammation: sulfacetamide/prednisolone/phenylephrine drops qid × 4 days<br>• Minimal inflammation: drops of 1 : 40 aluminium acetate (Burow's) solution or 0.25% acetic acid solution qid × 4 days |
| | No active drainage | **Keep water and all other substances out of ear** |

*Abbreviations:* bid = twice daily; tid = 3 times daily; qid = 4 times daily.

1) Patients with persistent (more than 2 months) middle ear effusion with delayed language acquisition and/or demonstrable hearing loss.

2) Atelectatic otitis when there is a risk of developing cholesteatoma.

Diagnosis is essential before medical treatment of a chronically draining ears begins. This may require microscopic suction removal of cerumen, pus and other debris. The usual bacteria are Gram-negative coliforms. Some clinicians use topical aminoglycoside antibiotics, although others consider that these drugs, being ototoxic, may cause hearing loss even after topical use.[93]

Allergy in the nose or respiratory tract is sometimes associated with serous/secretory otitis media. Suitable antiallergy treatment (e.g. a milk-free diet, avoidance of dust and animals, hyposensitisation to airborne allergens), including antihistamines or intranasal beclomethasone dipropionate or sodium cromoglycate, and treatment of obvious cases of allergic rhinitis (see section 2.4), may be required as indicated by appropriate testing measures.[94,95]

#### Clinical Outcome and Economic Considerations

Insufficient data are available to determine economic cost effectiveness for individual patients' with otitis media.[81,96,97] Cost effectiveness of treatment of otitis media may be measured by examining:

1) Quality-adjusted life years.
2) Costs per unit of hearing improvement.
3) Costs saved with a given treatment.

For data to be sufficient to form a rational conclusion, investigators must also consider the natural history of the disease (which is usually outgrown in childhood), the life-long consequences of inadequately treated otitis media (e.g. in terms of the patient's abilities to communicate), and of course, the end-stage aspects of atelectasis-adhesive otitis and cholesteatoma.

The complexity of determining cost effectiveness is exemplified by the hypothetical case of a 13-month-old boy with 6 weeks of persistent 'asymptomatic' bilateral middle ear effusion.[97] It was concluded that an additional course of antibiotic plus corticosteroid, followed by a third course of antibiotic, is cost effective. If the effusions persist despite a fourth antibiotic course, then tympanostomy tube placement was the most cost-effective treatment.

### 3.3 Mastoiditis

In acute mastoiditis, unlike acute furunculosis (see section 3.1.4), there is definite progression from upper respiratory infection to acute otitis media to acute mastoiditis, and the deafness that occurs with the stage of otitis media is frequently severe.

#### Optimum Treatment

Once a diagnosis of acute mastoiditis has been made, initial intravenous antibiotics followed by several weeks of maintenance oral antibiotic therapy should be given. If no culture information is available, ampicillin 8g daily or amoxicillin 4g daily should be started in adults; children's dosages would be intravenous ampicillin 100 mg/kg/day or oral amoxicillin 50 mg/kg/day. Appropriate surgical procedures should also be performed. Certain cases of acute mastoiditis may respond without surgery if adequate middle ear drainage is established. Chronic mastoiditis in association with any persistent purulent ear exudate requires surgical management.

### 3.4 Perichondritis

Inflammation and infection of the cartilage of the ear occurs from trauma, postoperative ear surgery effects or progressive infection of the skin of the ear canal. Insidious swelling and subtle tenderness may develop over several weeks. The poor vascularisation of cartilage makes ordinary antibiotic treatment ineffectual. The inflammation is more common in diabetic and immunocompromised patients and is seldom seen postoperatively now. A high index of suspicion is needed to diagnose perichrondritis early before extensive involvement of the canal and pinna cartilage occurs.

#### Optimum Treatment

Immediate incision and drainage of the infected pinna is necessary to separate the infected skin and cartilage and permit infusion of antibacterial agents into the relatively avascular cartilage. Perforated plastic or rubber drains should be inserted between the skin and cartilage and irrigation of a topical antibiotic solution should be made through these drains at least twice a day.

Most infections associated with perichondritis are due to *Pseudomonas* spp. or *Proteus* spp. Systemic antibacterials are generally not effective. Occasionally, a topical solution of acetic acid 0.25% will be effective in eliminating the infection. More rapid resolution can usually be obtained by irrigating with a gentamicin, colistin, polymixin B, ticarcillin or chloramphenicol solution. Supplemental parenteral dosages of these drugs, in maximum amounts below the level of toxicity (maximum dosage recommended by the manufacturer), for a period of 2 to 4 weeks may also be useful. More recently, ciprofloxacin has been used orally at a dosage of 750mg twice daily.

Debriding agents such as topical trypsin may also be helpful. Resection of infected cartilage

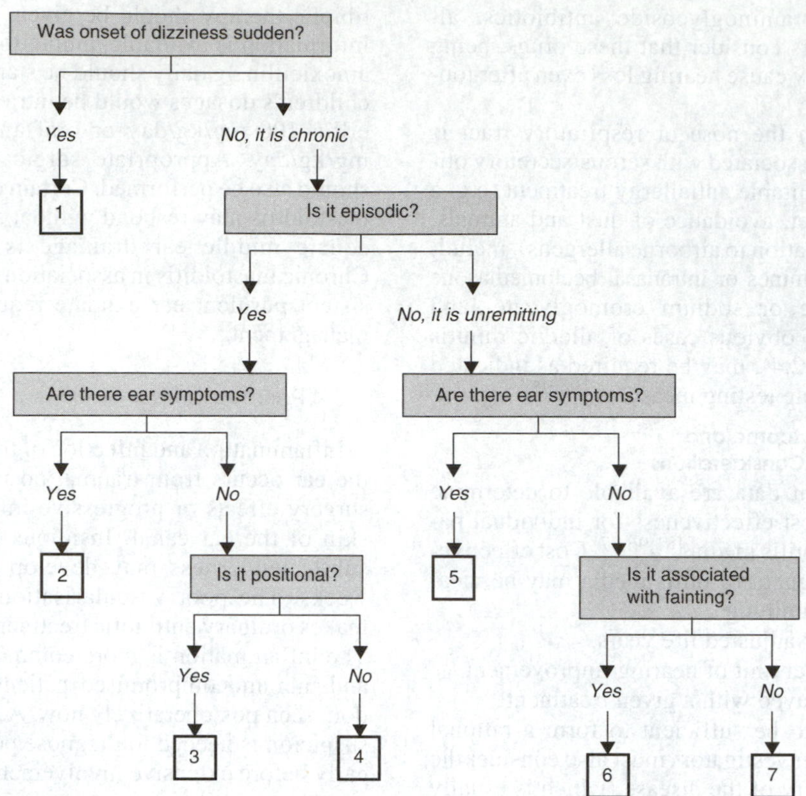


**Fig. 1.** Diagnostic approach to patient with vertigo and key to possible diagnoses that influence treatment (after Turner;[101] with permission). (1) Exertional vertigo, vestibular neuronitis, labyrinthitis, vascular disorder of inner ear. (2) Chronic suppurative otitis media or mastoiditis, Ménière's disease, acoustic neurinoma. (3) Benign positional vertigo (e.g. head injury), cervical spine lesions. (4) Drugs, hyperventilation, trauma to cervical spine, menopause, migraine. (5) Acoustic neurinoma or other cerebello-pontine angle tumour. (6) Vertebrobasilar artery insufficiency, or orthostatic hypotension, paroxysmal cardiac arrhythmias, carotid arteriosclerosis, carotid sinus sensitivity. (7) Psychoneurosis, diabetes mellitus, thyroid disease, anaemia, hypertension, leukaemia.

may become necessary if the measures described above do not yield results after a 2-week period.

## 4. Vertigo

Vertigo is a symptom, not a disease, and essentially denotes an hallucinatory sensation of movement.[98-100] A more common term is dizziness. Patients with 'vertigo' do not always have neat descriptive symptoms such as 'the world is spinning'. They may feel as if they are falling or swinging; or they may have oscillopsia or feel that the ground is moving. They may also have a vague lightheadedness or feel that they are walking on pillows. These patients must be differentiated from those who have syncope.

As mentioned in section 1.3, there are a large number of conditions that can cause 'vertigo'. Vertigo or dizziness can be classified in more than one way, but a scheme based on a symptomatic investigation which progresses to the most likely cause (fig. 1) is practical for treatment purposes.[101] Vertigo is usually not life-threatening, but it sometimes heralds serious disease such as multiple sclerosis, intracranial tumours or focal epilepsy. The clinician should attempt to rule out the dangerous causes, deal with treatable causes (e.g. diabetes, mastoiditis), and use drugs or vestibular exercises to reduce the symptoms of the remainder.

A variety of drugs have been used for vertigo (for a review, see Rascol et al.[26]). Those that are considered most useful are listed in table VI. Selection should be based on the cause of the condition, whenever possible. However, since the causes of vertigo often cannot be determined, a consideration of possible pathological mechanisms should lead to intelligent trial and error treatment.

### 4.1 Vertigo of Sudden Onset

A sudden, severe, primary attack of vertigo in a patient less than 50 years of age is usually due to a labyrinthitis or vestibular neuronitis as a sequel to bacterial or viral infection or metabolic disturbance (e.g. hypoglycaemia). Most viral labyrinthine infections occur after upper respiratory infections. Bacterial labyrinthitis is serious, destroys the end organ, and can lead to meningitis, but fortunately is rare. Most labyrinthine infections are viral.

**Optimum Treatment**

Viral end-organ or neuronal disease is self-limiting and treatment consists of bed rest and oral labyrinthine suppressants such as prochlorperazine or dimenhydrinate (table VI) for a few weeks. Corticosteroids (table VI) given at the onset of symptoms may reduce the damage caused by the virus. The patient may be left with a sensitive labyrinth and require mild sedatives such as diazepam 2mg when travelling. If a patient with sudden vertigo has an associated severe and persistent headache, meningitis should be ruled out.

In a patient more than 50 years of age, sudden vertigo is more likely to be due to a vascular disorder involving the labyrinthine blood supply. This includes a plexus of small arteries branching from the vertebral-basilar system. A previous history of peripheral arteriosclerotic or hypertensive vascular disease suggests such a mechanism. Treatment includes hospitalisation and vasodilatation by an intravenous infusion of histamine 1 μg/kg/min or papaverine 0.5 mg/kg/min. Inhalation of 5% carbon dioxide and 95% oxygen, from a tight fitting anaesthesia mask with a large reservoir and 1-way valve, is also effective. However, there is no evidence that nicotinic acid increases brain or otic blood flow.

A sudden, unprecedented attack of vertigo with hearing loss may follow physical activity (extreme exertion, intercourse), middle ear pressure changes (flying, scuba diving) or emotional stress. Otological examination for round window rupture and complete bed rest are required. Oral diazepam 10mg every 6 hours is helpful in relieving symptoms.

### 4.2 Chronic, Episodic Vertigo with Ear Symptoms

#### 4.2.1 Recurrent Vertigo due to Otological Causes

If the patient admits to associated ear symptoms (e.g. fullness in one ear, tinnitus or hearing loss), the cause of vertigo is probably otological. Obvious chronic suppurative otitis media, with or without mastoiditis, is treated with local secretion aspiration, mechanical cleaning, antibacterial drugs and often surgery. Bacterial flora vary, so it is wise to take cultures in these chronic disorders.

#### 4.2.2 Ménière's Disease (Endolymphatic Hydrops)

Only a few patients with recurrent vertigo have Ménière's disease. The classical symptoms are a unilateral, fluctuating hearing loss, episodic vertigo (often with nausea), fullness of the ear, and tinnitus. The latter is usually a roaring or low frequency tinnitus. These can be accompanied by diplacusis (perception of a single auditory stimulus as two separate sounds) and loudness intolerance. It is possible to have labyrinthine hydrops without hearing loss, and *vice versa*. Skilled audiometry is necessary to confirm the diagnosis when hearing loss is present and it will also help differentiate unilateral hearing loss from that due to acoustic neuroma.[105] Further reviews of the pathophysiology of this condition are available.[106-110]

**Optimum Treatment**

Medical treatment reduces the morbidity of Ménière's disease but treatment at an early stage may not prevent advance of the condition. Surgical treatment is reserved for cases refractory to medical treatment. Ménière's disease has more than one causative or precipitating factor, although the pathological finding (distension of the endolymphatic space) is the same in all patients. Cigarettes, coffee and other CNS stimulants should be prohibited. Abnormalities of glucose metabolism (e.g. hyper- or hypoglycaemia) are corrected with the appropriate dietary modification (see chapter 19; sect. 3). Lipid metabolism variations, as reflected in high triglyceride concentrations, are similarly corrected by appropriate dietary modification (see further chapter 20; sect. 4). A suspected allergic diathesis should be confirmed by appropriate testing and corrected as far as possible by hyposensitisation and allergen withdrawal.

The pathophysiological events leading to hydrops are not precisely known. Drug therapy is empirical.[111] It currently centres on *diuretics* (see table VI) or a salt restriction-diuretic regimen to remove water from the body, with the aim of decreasing the supposed elevated intralabyrinthine fluid pressure. Symptomatic antivertiginous antihistamines such as *mecloz-*

**Table VI.** Drugs used in treatment of vertigo (see also Haid;[102] Elbaz;[103] Uijtdehaage et al.[104])

| Action | Drug | Initial dosage[a] | Notes |
|---|---|---|---|
| **Labyrinthine suppressants** | | | |
| *Antihistamines (most also have an anticholinergic and sedative effect)*[b] | | | |
| Suppress vestibular end-organ receptors and inhibit activation of histaminergic and cholinergic pathways | Cinnarizine | 15mg q4-6h | |
| | Cyclizine | 50mg q4-6h | |
| | Dimenhydrinate | 50mg q4-6h | |
| | Diphenidol (NB. not an antihistamine) | 50mg q4-6h | Hallucinations may occur; use initially only in hospital |
| | Meclozine | 25-50mg q24h | |
| | Promethazine | 25mg q12h | |
| | Astemizole | 10mg od | Useful for chronic vertigo |
| *Antiemetic phenothiazines* | | | |
| Suppress central vestibular pathways | Prochlorperazine | 10mg q4h | Useful when nausea or vomiting prominent |
| | Thiethylperazine | 10mg q8-24h | |
| *Anticholinergics* | | | |
| Inhibit activation of central cholinergic pathways? | Atropine sulfate | 0.4mg IM | Useful in preventing motion sickness |
| | Scopolamine (hyoscine) hydrobromide | 0.6mg q3h | |
| **Vasodilators** | | | |
| Improve blood flow to labyrinth and brain stem; useful when vascular ischaemia suspected (e.g. sudden hearing loss and vertigo), but probably not when atherosclerosis limits blood flow | Histamine (diphosphate) | 2.5mg/250ml saline IV | Given after a meal at 16-60 drops/min to produce flushing. Blood pressure must not fall > 10-15mm Hg |
| | 5% $CO_2$ + 95% $O_2$ | Breathe over 20 min bid-qid | Use tight fitting mask (see section 4.1) |
| | Betahistine | 32-48 mg/day in 3-4 doses | |
| | Cyclandelate | 200mg q6-8h; up to 1200 mg/day if needed | |
| | Flunarizine | 10-60 mg/day | |
| | Papaverine | 0.5 mg/kg/min IV or 150mg q12h (long-acting capsule) | |
| **Diuretics** | | | |
| ?Decrease intralabyrinthine fluid pressure | Chlorothiazide | 250 mg/day | Useful in women with premenstrual fluid retention (salt restriction alone may suffice) |
| | Hydrochlorothiazide (or equivalent) | 25 mg/day | Potassium supplements may be necessary if given long term |
| **Psychotherapeutic drugs** | | | |
| Central sedation or brainstem-cerebellar inhibition | | | Useful in some cases of Ménière's disease, vasomotor labyrinthitis, psychogenic dizziness |
| *Antianxiety agents* | | | |
| Central sedation or brainstem-cerebellar inhibition | Chlordiazepoxide | 30 mg/day | When anxiety is the predominant response to vertigo |
| | Diazepam | 6-15 mg/day | |
| **Corticosteroids** | | | |
| Suppress labyrinthine oedema and swelling due to virus infection | Methylprednisolone | 40-80 mg/day × 4-5 days, then 20 mg/day × next 4 days | May lessen damage of acute viral labyrinthitis if given within 1 or 2 days |
| **Antibacterial drugs** | | | |
| Combat direct bacterial infection of labyrinth | Penicillin (or per culture results) | High doses (10-20MU penicillin daily) by IV infusion | Used in suppurative labyrinthitis (life-threatening illness) and in vertigo associated with chronic suppurative otitis media and mastoiditis |

a The usual adult oral (unless specified) dosage for initial treatment. Some dosages (e.g. labyrinthine suppressants, vasodilators) may need to be reduced for maintenance treatment (i.e. decreased dose or less frequent dosage interval).

b Not astemizole.

*Abbreviations:* IV = intravenous; IM = intramuscular; od = daily; bid = twice daily; qid = 4 times daily.

*ine* or *astemizole*, and *psychotherapeutic drugs* are used to offset attacks (table VI). Correction of metabolic aberrations, where relevant, rounds out these choices. While several drugs are often used simultaneously, it is not known whether combinations are more efficacious than each agent by itself. Potassium supplementation may be required if diuretics are used long term. If attacks occur, maintenance dosages of vestibulosuppressive but not diuretic drugs should be increased. After 2 weeks' freedom from vertigo, the usual maintenance dosage of vestibulosuppressive drugs should be resumed.

Drug therapy of Ménière's disease has been of little or no benefit in conservation or improvement of hearing, but treatment can affect the disabling vertigo. Several investigators have reported the use of ototoxic antibiotics such as streptomycin or gentamicin in the treatment of progressive Ménière's disease that is unresponsive to other medical therapy. The rationale for this therapy is that careful treatment with low doses destroys cells that produce endolymph and vestibular hair cells before it destroys cochlear hair cells.

For unilateral Ménière's, some clinicians[112,113] have applied gentamicin locally to the round window by means of a tube into the middle ear. Others[114] give streptomycin intramuscularly for bilateral disease. Some otologists surgically expose a semicircular canal and introduce small doses of streptomycin into the perilymph.[115,116] These techniques appear to greatly reduce the disabling vertigo and can stabilise hearing. However, they also can cause ataxia and oscillopsia if not performed cautiously.

### 4.3 Chronic, Episodic Vertigo without Ear Symptoms but Related to Position

Vertigo that occurs within seconds of assuming certain head positions and is reproducible, can usually be confirmed as benign positional vertigo by positional testing. Detailed neurological and medical examination may, however, be necessary to rule out vertigo due to cervical spine lesions, multiple sensory deficit, or malignant posterior fossa lesions.

#### Optimum Treatment

Benign positional vertigo, which includes post-traumatic vertigo following head injury, may improve spontaneously, usually within weeks. An antianxiety agent and reassurance that adaptation to the head position will occur in time is generally sufficient, but in some cases labyrinthine suppressants (table VI) may be more effective. If benign positional vertigo persists, exercises to habituate the vertiginous mechanism,[117] or single neurectomy add to the available options.

### 4.4 Chronic, Episodic Vertigo without Ear Symptoms and Not Related to Position

Overdosage of antiepileptic drugs (e.g. phenytoin) can cause severe imbalance and nystagmus indistinguishable from a posterior fossa syndrome, which may be prevented by phenytoin concentration monitoring. Overdosage of streptomycin or gentamicin may lead to severe imbalance and vertigo occurring after sudden movements (see section 8.1.1, table VII). A careful history may show drugs such as antihypertensives, diuretics or other agents to be the cause of the dizziness.[118] Relief in these cases can be achieved by discontinuing the drug or reducing the dosage. Oral contraceptives may also cause dizziness in some women, and in such cases a change to a low-dose preparation may help.

Other causes include trauma to the cervical spine or periodic dizziness associated with menopause. The dizziness associated with migraine headaches often responds to ergotamine.

### 4.5 Chronic, Unremitting Vertigo without Ear Symptoms or Fainting

Psychoneurotic patients may complain of lightheadedness or vertigo, sometimes over a period of years, and may be shown on clinical examination to be anxious or depressed. More serious disorders must, however, be ruled out before a diagnosis of psychogenic dizziness is made. Such conditions include CNS disease, uncontrolled or poorly controlled diabetes mellitus, and untreated thyroid disease, anaemia or hypertension, and we find in our university practice that these affect 5 to 10% of patients with vertigo.

Treatment of psychogenic dizziness consists of an explanation of the relationship of patients' dizziness to their environmental stress. In some cases, benzodiazepines such as diazepam are recommended for anxiety or tricyclic antidepressants such as amitriptyline for depression. However, it is not recommended that these agents be used without careful consideration, since they carry a high risk of dependence and adverse effects [see further chapter 30].[119]

### 4.6 Chronic Idiopathic Vertigo

Patients who have experienced dizziness for more than 6 weeks and show spontaneous or positional nystagmus are often treated with *meclozine* and/or *diazepam* on a long term basis. Most of this treatment is empirical and has not been confirmed as being specific or efficacious. Two newer agents, *flunarizine* and *astemizole*, are promising alternatives. Flunarizine, an antihistamine and calcium antagonist, has been used successfully in dosages ranging from 10 to 60 mg/day for vertigo of central and peripheral origin.[120] Astemizole, a nonsedating antihistamine, reduced nystagmus and symptoms of dizziness in 60% of patients in a pilot study,[121] and showed a slightly higher rate of control in a double-blind, 3-dose-level comparison with placebo.[122] In this latter study, 20 mg/day proved to be more effective than the 10mg dose used in the previous study. The drug appeared to be effective only in cases of dizziness with peripheral causes. It is important to tell the patient that astemizole often needs to be taken for 15 to 20 days before it is effective. If it is not effective after 5 weeks, its use should be discontinued.

## 5. Motion Sickness

The subjective sensation in motion sickness is one of malaise rather than of vertigo.

#### Optimum Treatment

Evaluation of motion sickness drugs has greatly benefited by the sustained, practical interest of the armed services of many countries. Efficacy has been tested both subjectively and objectively, and the effectiveness of any one drug was shown to have no relationship to its efficacy in other types of nausea and vomiting.[123,124] The most effective single drug has proved to be *scopolamine (hyoscine) hydrobromide* 0.6mg, which is about one-third more effective than dimenhydrinate 50mg in inhibiting experimentally-induced motion sickness. Surprisingly, amphetamine 10 to 20mg is equivalent to scopolamine or better than antihistamines such as dimenhydrinate or promethazine. The most effective and best tolerated regimen is a combination of promethazine 25mg with dexamphetamine 10mg, or scopolamine 0.6mg with dexamphetamine 10mg. Thus, drugs with central anticholinergic actions (e.g. scopolamine, promethazine) and drugs with central sympathomimetic activity (e.g. dexamphetamine) are effective against motion sickness and a combination of these actions produces a synergistic effect.

A skin patch formulation containing *scopolamine* 1.5mg, designed to be released over a 3-day period, is used extensively and is effective in reducing nausea and vomiting due to motion sickness.[125] Although the incidence of adverse effects is less than with oral scopolamine hydrobromide, it causes dry mouth and/or blurred vision in more than 50% of patients. Cutting the patch in half or into quarters reduces these adverse effects, especially with long term use. Removal of the patch does not cause rapid resolution of adverse effects, because a drug depot builds up in the skin and takes time to dissipate. However, this preparation is not effective in patients who use it for chronic dizziness.

Scopolamine is also effective when given after symptoms of motion sickness have begun. An intramuscular injection of scopolamine hydrobromide 0.2mg is effective within 15 to 30 minutes and its effects last for about 4 hours.

*Cinnarizine*, a calcium antagonist and vasodilating agent, has also been used with some success in the prevention of motion sickness. A dosage of 15mg 3 times a day for adults and half this dose for children aged 5 to 12 years has been suggested.[126] The drug is started 1 day before sailing or other activities that induce motion sickness.

## 6. Sudden, Sensorineural Hearing Loss

Sudden sensorineural hearing loss is an abrupt loss of hearing that usually occurs over less than a few hours or is noticed on awakening. The loss is significant, often by as much as 50dB and occasionally by as much as 90dB. Speculation favours viral infection as a cause in patients under 50 years of age, and ischaemia and intracochlear membrane rupture in those over 50 years. Acoustic neuroma, demyelinating disease, trauma and syphilis are also speculated as causes. Most cases (85%) are idiopathic.

#### Optimum Treatment

The rationale for drug treatment of this condition is beset with problems.[127] It is known that viruses can damage the cochlea and that viral infection often parallels sensorineural hearing loss, but it is very difficult to demonstrate that a particular patient has this infection. A review by Wilson & Gulya[128] presents some of the newer evidence linking viral infection with sudden hearing loss. Occasionally, patients will report that their hearing loss was preceded by symptoms of a viral upper respiratory tract infection. However, the absence of an obvious viral infection does not rule out this cause for the loss. Temporal bone studies[129,130] have shown histopathological findings compatible with virus infections. There do not appear to have been any controlled trials of antiviral agents such as aciclovir or ribavirin in sudden hearing loss, but the study by Dickens et al.[131] suggests that aciclovir may be an effective treatment. Corticosteroids have proved to be effective in some cases.[132,133] The usual dosage of prednisone is 80mg daily for 3 to 4 days, thereafter reducing the dose in a stepwise manner over 10 days to 10 mg/day.

Partial or complete interruption of the blood supply to the cochlea results in partial or complete loss of cochlear function. In patients with sensorineural hearing loss, the interruption could conceivably be caused by vascular spasm, thrombosis or capillary sludging, perhaps induced by hypercoagulopathy or hyperlipidaemia. Attempts to increase cochlear blood flow have provided mixed results. Some consider that complete or good recovery occurs in 65% of cases of sensorineural hearing loss, independent of any type of medication.[134] However, disagreements abound. What constitutes a vasodilator or antispasmodic agent to one investigator is considered a placebo by another. Some investigators do not specify their vasodilator or its dose. Others give agents that are known to have no influence on intracranial blood flow, e.g. nicotinic acid. However, a mixture of either 5 or 10% carbon dioxide in oxygen has been shown by many investigators to significantly increase otic and brain blood flow in animals.[33] These gas mixtures have been reported to yield significantly better results than other treatments in patients with sensorineural hearing loss.[135] High viscosity syndromes have been treated by plasmapheresis and haemodilution with rheological agents such as dextrans.[136] Others have had success with pentoxifylline.[137]

In general, improvement is more likely to occur after low frequency losses, absent or slight vertigo, and associated tinnitus.[138]

## 7. Immune Inner Ear Disease

Immune inner ear disease is a relatively new and distinct clinical entity that produces unexplained rapidly progressive bilateral sensorineural hearing loss. There are at least 4 possible mechanisms for autoimmune disease of the inner ear:[139]

- Specific or cross-reacting autoantibodies may react with specific autoantigens in the inner ear.
- Circulating immune complexes from bacterial or viral antibodies may deposit in the ear.
- There may be cell-mediated immune responses involving cytotoxic T cells for specific ear targets.
- Autoantibodies directed against type-II collagen may be important.

Some of the problems inherent in these studies are discussed by Veldman et al.[140] Not all patients have cross-reacting antibodies or cochlea specific antigens.

The diagnosis is based on clinical manifestations, positive immune laboratory testing, and beneficial responses to corticosteroids. Cyclophosphamide has also been used alone and in combination with other agents for this disorder. Immunological test results should always be considered whenever this line of therapy is to be used and treatment should be based on collagen, vascular or other immune disorders, abnormal nonspecific serum screening test results, and positive testing for cellular and humoral immunity (if this is available).

Initial corticosteroid therapy should be prednisone 80 mg/day, with tapering of the dosage over a 10-day period. When cyclophosphamide is used, 100 mg/day for several weeks should be tried. A white blood cell count should be performed every 2 weeks. Prolongation of therapy depends on the response to treatment. The lowest possible effective dosage of corticosteroid should be used (e.g. prednisone 5 to 10 mg/day). A lack of response after several weeks should dictate the end of treatment.[141]

## 8. Drug-Induced Ear, Nose and Throat Disorders

### 8.1 Ototoxicity

A number of drugs have been associated with impaired auditory or vestibular function, sometimes permanently (see section 4.4).[142-145]

The risk of ototoxicity is greatly increased in patients with impaired renal function, and in general is more likely in elderly patients, following a high dose or a large total dose of an ototoxic drug over a prolonged period of time, and if there has been a previous course or concurrent administration of another ototoxic drug.

High noise levels and hyperthermia also potentiate damage if they occur concurrently with the ototoxic drug. Some of the most important ototoxic drugs are also potentially nephrotoxic; thus, it is highly desirable to adjust the dose of an ototoxic drug on the basis of renal function. Because the patient may sometimes not become aware of hearing loss until after the drug treatment is completed, it is prudent to regularly test auditory function when using certain ototoxic drugs (e.g. kanamycin, loop diuretics in renal failure). The initial effects of aminoglycosides will be on the high frequencies. Ideally, hearing should be tested between 8 and 20 kHz for signs of damage. However, these values are beyond the limits of usual audiometry.

#### *8.1.1 Antibacterial Agents*

Antibacterial agents are the most important ototoxic drugs, particularly the aminoglycosides. However, even agents normally considered to be well tolerated may be associated with ototoxicity; for example, temporary hearing loss has been reported on rare occasions following large doses of erythromycin, usually in patients with impaired renal function,[146] although this does not affect dosages,[147] and minocycline sometimes causes troublesome dizziness or vertigo, particularly in women.[148] Other antibacterial drugs which have been more often associated with important ototoxicity include vancomycin (affects auditory function only) and capreomycin and the polymixins (mainly affect vestibular function). Others such as viomycin, ristocetin or dihydrostreptomycin are either little used nowadays or have been discontinued.[149]

All aminoglycosides share the capacity to damage the auditory and vestibular hair cells, sometimes irreversibly.[147,150] Streptomycin, gentamicin and sisomicin mainly affect vestibular function, while kanamycin, amikacin, neomycin, framycetin and paromomycin mainly affect auditory function. However, decreased auditory capacity can occur with gentamicin and hearing loss in young children has been attributed to use of streptomycin in infancy. Tobramycin and netilmicin, like gentamicin, can affect both auditory and vestibular function (table VII). Netilmicin appears to be associated with fewer audiovestibular adverse effects than other currently available aminoglycosides.[151]

The early clinical features of ototoxicity differ with the individual aminoglycosides (table VII). In the case of streptomycin, there is often a high pitched tinnitus and vertigo. In time, there is usually some compensation for the vestibular disturbance, which is replaced by a chronic condition of uncertainty of balance in which only sudden movements cause vertigo. Loss of hearing (mainly high frequencies) with the aminoglycosides, particularly kanamycin, tends to appear after a latent period and usually becomes worse if treatment is continued. In some cases, the onset of hearing loss may not occur until some time after treatment is discontinued, or may continue to progress even when treatment is stopped. There are clinical reports documenting unilateral ototoxicity in patients receiving aminoglycosides.[152]

The risk of ototoxicity is greatly increased in the presence of impaired renal function. It is also more likely in the elderly, after excessive dosages or a large total dose, or following a previous course or concurrent administration of another ototoxic drug.[153,154] The aminoglycosides are excreted unchanged in the urine and their ototoxicity is related to a prolonged high concentration in the inner ear. Their renal clearance is the same as that of creatinine and hence any impairment of creatinine clearance will be reflected in impaired excretion of the aminoglycoside. Thus, the rate of excretion by the kidney and the fact that the aminoglycosides are slowly reabsorbed from the endolymph once they have been secreted into it[155] are the most important

**Table VII.** Differential ototoxicity of aminoglycoside antibacterial drugs (relative effects)

| Drug | Vestibular toxicity | Auditory toxicity | Early symptoms | |
|---|---|---|---|---|
| | | | tinnitus | vertigo |
| Streptomycin | +++ | + | + | + |
| Gentamicin | ++ | + | + | + |
| Tobramycin | + | + | ?+ | ?+ |
| Amikacin | + | ++ | ?+ | ? |
| Kanamycin | + | +++ | ++ | ? |
| Neomycin | ++ | ++++ | ? | 0 |
| Netilmicin | + | + | ?+ | ?+ |
| Sisomicin | ++ | + | + | + |

factors in determining ototoxicity. High dosages and the use of ordinary doses in patients with renal failure will predictably cause ototoxic effects. In such cases, pretreatment and regular in-treatment tests with otoacoustic emissions should be conducted and the dosage reduced as indicated by hearing changes. Data on confounding factors (e.g. acidosis, hypoxaemia, electrolyte imbalance, genetic predisposition) are not available to allow specific guidelines on aminoglycoside dosage reduction. If a life-threatening infection demands therapy with a drug that can cause deafness, this adverse event may be tolerable. Deafness of cochleotoxic origin is treatable by cochlear implantation.

Ototoxicity is not necessarily limited only to parenteral administration. Hearing loss has occurred with neomycin following irrigation of surgical wounds, superficial dressing of severe burns, aerosol inhalation, rectal and colonic irrigation, or even after oral administration.[153,156] Systemic absorption of neomycin is high following its use as an irrigating solution and probably only low-strength solutions should be used.[157,158] Absorption of neomycin from the gastrointestinal tract is minimal. However, when there are gastric mucosal abnormalities (e.g. ulcerative colitis, gastroenteritis) or when large doses are used for prolonged periods (e.g. prophylaxis in chronic portal systemic encephalopathy), particularly if the patient also has impaired renal function, the amount absorbed and retained in the endolymph is sufficient to cause ototoxic effects.

Use of ototoxic antibiotics topically in the ear appears to be relatively safe if they are administered properly and for correct indications.[159,160] Severe ototoxicity has been associated with *direct* application (transtympanic) of streptomycin to the inner ear,[161] as can also be readily demonstrated with direct application of aminoglycosides, polymixins, chloramphenicol and erythromycin to the inner ears of experimental animals.[155,162] If an otic suspension of polymixin B, neomycin, hydrocortisone and propylene glycol is introduced directly or through tympanostomy tubes into the middle ear of experimental animals, local inflammatory responses and ototoxicity can occur.[163] Recent studies have shown, however, that 94% of US otolaryngologists use topical preparations in the presence of tubes or drum perforations[93] and a 3% incidence of sensory hearing loss has been reported. Merifield et al.[164] tested gentamicin, neomycin, colistin and polymixin as commercial preparations and found no statistically significant change in bone conduction thresholds in 70 ears.

Ototoxic antibiotics should not be used locally during, or as preoperative prophylaxis before, inner ear surgery.

#### *8.1.2 Diuretics*

Transient and occasionally permanent hearing loss has been observed in some patients receiving the loop diuretics ethacrynic acid and furosemide (frusemide). Deafness from ethacrynic acid may follow an intravenous dose or large oral doses in patients with impaired renal function, especially if given along with an aminoglycoside antibacterial drug.[165,166] Hearing loss from furosemide has also occurred only in patients with impaired renal function, generally after rapid intravenous administration of a high dose,[167] but gradually progressive and permanent deafness has developed up to 6 months after treatment with relatively small repeated doses of furosemide,[168] and transient deafness has followed use of large oral doses in the nephrotic syndrome.[169]

Since uraemic patients are at special risk, it would seem prudent to monitor hearing during treatment with loop diuretics in these patients. This is especially true if patients are also receiving or have recently received ototoxic antibacterial drugs (see section 8.1.1).

#### *8.1.3 Salicylates*

Symptoms of hearing loss, tinnitus and vertigo are observed with high doses of salicylates and much less frequently with other nonsteroidal anti-inflammatory drugs, particularly in patients with rheumatoid arthritis. Deafness and tinnitus are almost always reversible within a few days after cessation of the drug.[170]

#### *8.1.4 Chloroquine, Quinine and Quinidine*

Chloroquine can cause tinnitus and perceptive deafness. Hearing loss may become apparent after the drug has been discontinued; it tends to occur after long term high dosage and is usually irreversible.[171] Vertigo, tinnitus and hearing loss can also occur with large doses or prolonged treatment with quinine. The ototoxic symptoms are, however, usually reversible. Congenital deafness has been noted in infants born of mothers who attempted to induce abortion with high doses of quinine.[172] Vertigo, tinnitus, and, rarely, reversible mild hearing loss can occur with usual doses of quinidine.[173]

### 8.1.5 Miscellaneous Agents

Vertigo has been attributed to use of oral contraceptives and other commonly used drugs (see section 4.4). Regional perfusion of chlormethine (mustine) may cause vestibular symptoms and sometimes hearing loss.[153] Bleomycin may cause ototoxicity when used in high dosage,[174] as may cisplatin.

General poisons such as arsenic, lead, mercury, cadmium disulfide, phosphorus and carbon monoxide can cause deafness, tinnitus and vertigo. Quaternary ammonium compounds such as benzalkonium and chlorhexidine are unsuitable as skin antiseptics before surgery on or in the region around the ear, especially for repair of a perforated eardrum, as total and permanent deafness has been reported.[175] Tinnitus and dizziness have also occurred. Other antiseptics such as povidone iodine can have an ototoxic effect if applied to the round window.

Gradual development of reversible deafness has been observed with the now withdrawn β-adrenoceptor blocking drug practolol, in association with, but months to years after the appearance of, the oculomucocutaneous syndrome seen with this drug.[176]

## 8.2 Nasal Congestion

It is well recognised that drugs can cause nasal congestion.[177] Nasal blood vessels are kept in a state of partial constriction by a tonic sympathetic discharge. Any drug that interferes with sympathetic transmission will induce a degree of nasal congestion, e.g. reserpine and drugs such as guanethidine and methyldopa. β-Adrenoceptor agonist drugs such as isoprenaline (isoproterenol) are often used in the treatment of asthma. Although these drugs dilate the lower airway, they are capable of inducing both vasodilatation and congestion of the nasal passage and the eustachian tube.

High circulating concentrations of female sex hormones, as occur with some oral contraceptives, can produce nasal congestion. The mechanism is unknown but is thought to be associated with fluid retention and increased blood volume. Conversely, oral contraceptives can produce a patulous eustachian tube.[178] Allergic rhinitis has also been reported, usually in women with a history of perennial rhinitis or pollinosis.[179]

As discussed in section 2.2.1, vasoconstrictors used in topical nasal sprays or drops will inevitably induce a rebound nasal congestion if used for prolonged periods. Some investigators feel that the rebound is due to reactive hyperaemia. Part of the rebound congestion may be due to the toxic effect of some drugs on the nasal mucosa. Several common topical nasal decongestants (but not 0.1% and 0.25% phenylephrine) have been shown to be ciliotoxic when tested in tracheal organ culture.[180]

## Further Reading

De Weese DD, Saunders WH. Textbook of otolaryngology, 7th edition. St Louis: Mosby, 1993

Fairbanks DWF. Pocket guide to antimicrobial therapy in otolaryngology head neck surgery, 7th edition. Alexandria, VA: American Academy OHNS, 1993

Turner JS. Diseases of the ear, nose and throat. In: Hurst JW, editor. Medicine for the practising physician. Section 22, 3rd edition. Boston: Butterworths, 1992

## References

1. Meltzer EO. Comparative safety of $H_1$ antihistamines. Annals of Allergy 1991; 67: 625-33
2. McTavish D, Goa KL, Ferrill M. Terfenadine: an updated review of its pharmacological properties and therapeutic efficacy. Drugs 1990; 39: 552-74
3. Richards DM, Brodgen RN, Heel RC, et al. Astemizole: a review of its pharmacodynamic properties and therapeutic efficacy. Drugs 1984; 28: 38-61
4. Haria M, Fitton A, Peters DH. Loratadine: a reappraisal of its pharmacological properties and therapeutic use in allergic disorders. Drugs 1994; 48: 617-37
5. Spencer CM, Faulds D, Peters DH. Cetirizine: a reappraisal of its pharmacological properties and therapeutic use in selected allergic disorders. Drugs 1993; 46: 1055-80
6. Wiseman LR, Faulds D. Ebastine: a review of its pharmacological properties and clinical efficacy in the treatment of allergic disorders. Drugs 1996; 51: 260-77
7. Brogden RN, McTavish D. Acrivastine: a review of its pharmacological properties and therapeutic efficacy in allergic rhinitis, urticaria and related disorders. Drugs 1991; 41: 927-40
8. Desager JP, Horsmans Y. Pharmacokinetic-pharmacodynamic relationships of $H_1$-antihistamines. Clinical Pharmacokinetics 1995; 28: 419-32
9. Kontou-Fili K. $H_1$-receptor antagonists in the management of allergic rhinitis: a comparative review. Clinical Immunotherapeutics 1994; 2: 352-75
10. Simons FER, Simons KJ. The pharmacology and use of $H_1$-receptor-antagonist drugs. New England Journal of Medicine 1994; 330: 1663-70
11. Simons FER. New $H_1$ receptor antagonists: worth the price? Annals of Allergy 1992; 69: 163-5
12. Horak F. Seasonal allergic rhinitis. Drugs 1993; 45: 518-27
13. Dechant KL, Goa KL. Levocabastine: a review of its pharmacological properties and therapeutic potential as a topical antihistamine in allergic rhinitis and conjunctivitis. Drugs 1991; 41: 202-4
14. Noble S, McTavish D. Levocabastine: an update of its pharmacology, clinical efficacy and tolerability in the

topical treatment of allergic rhinitis and conjunctivitis. Drugs 1995; 50: 1032-49

15. McTavish D, Sorkin EM. Azelastine: a review of its pharmacodynamic and pharmacokinetic properties and therapeutic potential. Drugs 1989; 38: 778-800
16. Schwartz J-C, Barbin G, Duchemin A-M, et al. Histamine receptors in the brain and their possible functions. In: Ganelin & Parsons, editors. Pharmacology of histamine receptors. Bristol: Wright-PSG, 1982: 351
17. Wada H, Inagaki N, Yamatodani A, et al. Is the histaminergic neuron system a regulatory center for whole-brain activity? Trends in Neurosciences 1994; 14: 415-8
18. Simons FER, Simons KJ. Pharmacokinetic optimisation of histamine $H_1$-receptor antagonist therapy. Clinical Pharmacokinetics 1991; 21: 372-93
19. Ichimura K, Jackson RT. H-1 and H-2 histamine receptors in the in vitro nasal mucosa. Acta Oto-Laryngologica 1985; 99: 610
20. Secher C, Kirkegaard J, Borum P, et al. Significance of $H_1$ and $H_2$ receptors in the human nose: rationale for topical use of combined antihistamine preparations. Journal of Allergy and Clinical Immunology 1982; 70: 211-8
21. Carpenter GB, Bunker-Soler AL, Nelson HS. Evaluation of combined $H_1$- and $H_2$-receptor blocking agents in the treatment of seasonal allergic rhinitis. Journal of Allergy and Clinical Immunology 1983; 71: 412-7
22. Holmberg K, Pipkorn U, Bake B, et al. Effects of topical treatment with $H_1$ and $H_2$ antagonists on clinical symptoms and nasal vascular reactions in patients with allergic rhinitis. Allergy 1989; 44: 281-7
23. Brooks CD, Butler D, Metzler C. Effect of $H_2$ blockade in the challenged allergic nose. Journal of Allergy and Clinical Immunology 1982; 70: 373-6
24. Testa B, Mesolella C, Filippini P, et al. The role of $H_2$ antagonists in perennial allergic rhinitis. Laryngoscope 1993; 103: 1013-9
25. Wang D, Clement P, Smitz J. Effect of $H_1$ and $H_2$ antagonists on nasal symptoms and mediator release in atopic patients after nasal allergen challenge during the pollen season. Acta Oto-Laryngologica 1996; 116: 91-6
26. Rascol O, Hain TC, Brefel C, et al. Antivertigo medications and drug-induced vertigo: a pharmacological review. Drugs 1995; 50: 777-91
27. Stewart EJ, Cinnamond MJ, Nicholls P, et al. The influence of beta receptors on nasal mucosal function. Rhinology 1993; 31: 121-4
28. Lundberg JM, Lundblad L, Martling CR, et al. Coexistence of multiple peptides and classic transmitters in airway neurons: functional and pathophysiologic aspects. American Review of Respiratory Disease 1987; Suppl. 136: S1-83
29. Raphael GD, Baraniuk JN, Kaliner MA. How and why the nose runs. Journal of Allergy and Clinical Immunology 1991; 87: 457-67
30. Ichimura K, Okita W, Tanaka T. Vasoactivity of endothelin in nasal blood vessels. Rhinology 1991; 29: 125-35
31. Kuvayama A, Zervas NT, Shintani A, et al. Papaverine hydrochloride and experimental hemorrhagic cerebral arterial spasm. Stroke 1972; 3: 27
32. Ohlsen A, Hultorantz E, Engstrom B. The effect of topical application of vasodilating agents on cochlear electrophysiology. Acta Oto-Laryngologica 1993; 113: 55-61
33. Pollock RA, Jackson RT, Clairmont AA, et al. Carbon dioxide as an otic vasodilator. Archives of Otolaryngology - Head and Neck Surgery 1974; 100: 309
34. Brogden RN, Heel RC, Speight TM, et al. Beclomethasone dipropionate: a reappraisal of its pharmacodynamic properties and therapeutic efficacy after a decade of use in asthma and rhinitis. Drugs 1984; 28: 99
35. Pakes GE, Brogden RN, Heel RC, et al. Flunisolide: a review of its pharmacological properties and therapeutic efficacy in rhinitis. Drugs 1980; 19: 397
36. Clissold SP, Heel RC. Budesonide: a preliminary review of its pharmacodynamic properties and therapeutic efficacy in asthma and rhinitis. Drugs 1984; 28: 485
37. Brogden RN, McTavish D. Budesonide: an updated review of its pharmacological properties, and therapeutic efficacy in asthma and rhinitis. Drugs 1992; 44: 375-407
38. Bryson HM, Faulds D. Intranasal fluticasone propionate: a review of its pharmacodynamic and pharmacokinetic properties, and therapeutic potential in allergic rhinitis. Drugs 1992; 43: 760-5
39. Mabry RL. Rhinitis medicamentosa: the forgotten factor in nasal obstruction. Southern Medical Journal 1982; 75: 817-9
40. Soyka LF, Robinson DS, Lachant N, et al. The misuse of antibiotics for treatment of upper respiratory tract infections in children. Pediatrics 1975; 55: 552
41. Taylor B, Abbott GD, Kerr MMcK, et al. Amoxycillin and co-trimoxazole in presumed viral respiratory infections of childhood: placebo-controlled trial. British Medical Journal 1977; 2: 552
42. Chapnick JS, Bach MC. Bacterial and fungal infections of the maxillary sinus. Otolaryngologic Clinics of North America 1976; 9: 43
43. Kutnick SL, Keith JD. Acute sinusitis and otitis: their complications and surgical treatment. Otolaryngologic Clinics of North America 1976; 9: 689
44. Aschan G. Decongestion of nasal mucous membranes by oral medication in acute rhinitis: a rhinomanometric study to demonstrate synergism between antihistamines and adrenergic substance. Acta Oto-Laryngologica 1974; 77: 433
45. May M, West JW. The 'stuffy' nose. Otolaryngologic Clinics of North America 1973; 6: 655-74
46. Walker JS. Rhinitis medicamentosa. Journal of Allergy and Clinical Immunology 1952; 23: 183
47. Geimer M, Geimer R. Zur Wirksamkeit, Vertraglichkeit und therapeutischen Anwendung moderner Nasentropfen unter besonderer Berucksichtigung von Adrianol. Nasen-tropfen für Sauglinge und Kleinkinder. Monatsschrift fur Kinderheikunde 1966; 114: 553
48. Wick H. Ueber Tyzine-Vergiftung. Praxis 1966; 55: 791
49. Dayal VS, Jones J, Noyek AM. Management of odontogenic maxillary sinus disease. Otolaryngologic Clinics of North America 1976; 9: 213
50. Chandler JR, Lagenbrunner DJ, Stevens ER. The pathogenesis of orbital complications in acute sinusitis. Laryngoscope 1970; 80: 1414
51. Hallen H, Juto J-E. An objective method to record changes in nasal reactivity during treatment of nonallergic nasal hyperreactivity. ORL - Journal of Oto-Rhino-Laryngology and its Related Specialities 1994; 56: 92-5
52. Lofkvist T, Svensson G. Treatment of vasomotor rhinitis with intranasal beclomethasone dipropionate (Becotide). Results from a double-blind crossover study. Acta Allergologica 1976; 31: 227
53. Jankowski R, Philip G, Togias A, et al. Demonstration of bilateral cholinergic secretory response after uni-

lateral nasal cold, dry air challenge. Rhinology 1993; 31: 97-100

54. Borum P, Mygind N, Schultz Larsen F. Ipratropium treatment for rhinorrhoea in patients with perennial rhinitis: an open follow-up study of efficacy and safety. Clinical Otolaryngology 1983; 8: 267
55. Sjögren I, Juhaz J. Ipratropium in the treatment of patients with perennial rhinitis. Allergy 1984; 39: 457
56. Jackson RT, Teichgraeber J. Low-dose topical atropine for rhinorrhea. Archives of Otolaryngology - Head and Neck Surgery 1981; 107: 288
57. Simons FER, Simons KJ. Optimum pharmacological management of chronic rhinitis. Drugs 1989; 38: 313-
58. Empey DW, Medder KT. Nasal decongestants. Drugs 1981; 21: 438-43
59. Dockhorn R, Grossman J, Posner M, et al. A double-blind, placebo-controlled study of the safety and efficacy of ipratropium bromide nasal spray versus placebo in patients with the common cold. Journal of Allergy and Clinical Immunology 1992; 90: 1076-82
60. Gaffey MJ, Gwaltney JM, Dressler WE, et al. Intranasally administered atropine methonitrate treatment of experimental rhinovirus colds. American Review of Respiratory Disease 1987; 135: 241-4
61. Corrado OJ, Gomez E, Baldwin DL, et al. The effect of nedocromil sodium on nasal provocation with allergen. Journal of Allergy and Clinical Immunology 1987; 80: 218-2
62. King HC. Mast cell stabilizers. Otolaryngology - Head and Neck Surgery 1992; 107: 841-4
63. Lindqvist N, Andersson M, Bende M, et al. The clinical efficacy of budesonide in hay fever treatment is dependent on topical nasal application. Clinical and Experimental Allergy 1989; 19: 71-6
64. Dushay ME, Johnson CE. Management of allergic rhinitis: focus on intranasal agents. Pharmacotherapy 1989; 9: 338-50
65. Mabry RL. Intranasal steroids in rhinology: the changing role of intraturbinal injection. ENT Journal 1994; 73: 242-6
66. Spector SL, et al. Intranasal anticholinergic treatment of nasal disorders. Journal of Allergy and Clinical Immunology 1992; Suppl. 90: 1041-86
67. Lang SDR, Singh K. The sore throat: when to investigate and when to prescribe. Drugs 1990; 40: 854-62
68. Krober MS, Bass JW, Michels GN. Streptococcal pharyngitis: placebo-controlled double-blind evaluation of clinical response to penicillin therapy. Journal of the American Medical Association 1985; 253: 1271
69. Brook I, Yocum P, Friedman EM. Aerobic and anaerobic bacteria in tonsils of children with recurrent tonsillitis. Annals of Otology Rhinology and Laryngology 1981; 90: 261
70. Paradise JL, Bluestone CD, Bachman RZ, et al. Efficacy of tonsillectomy for recurrent throat infection in severely affected children. New England Journal of Medicine 1984; 310: 674
71. Weinberg E, Brodsky L, Stanievich J, et al. Needle aspiration of peritonsillar abscess in children. Archives of Otolaryngology - Head and Neck Surgery 1993; 119: 169-72
72. Ruddy J, Bickerton RC. Optimum management of the discharging ear. Drugs 1992; 43: 219-35
73. Cassisi N, Cohn A, Davidson T, et al. Diffuse otitis externa. Annals of Otology Rhinology and Laryngology 1977; 86 Suppl. 39: 1
74. Rubin J, Yu V. Malignant otitis externa: insights into pathogenesis, clinical manifestations, diagnosis and therapy. American Journal of Medicine 1988; 85: 391-8
75. Joachims HZ. Malignant external otitis in children. Archives of Otolaryngology - Head and Neck Surgery 1976; 102: 236
76. Selesnick SN. Otitis externa: management of the recalcitrant case. American Journal of Otology 1994; 15: 408-12
77. Amorosa L, Mudugno GC, Pirodda A. Malignant external otitis: review and personal experience. Acta Oto-Laryngologica 1996; Suppl. 521: 3-16
78. Uri N, Kitzes R, Meyer W, et al. Necrotizing external otitis, the importance of prolonged drug therapy. Journal of Laryngology and Otology 1984; 98: 1083-5
79. Meistrup-Larsen K-I, Sorensen H, Johnsen H-J, et al. Two versus 7 days penicillin treatment for acute otitis media: a placebo-controlled trial in children. Acta Oto-Laryngologica 1983; 96: 99
80. van Buchem FL, Peeters MF, van't Hof MA. Acute otitis media: a new treatment strategy. British Medical Journal 1985; 290: 1033
81. Sagraves R, Maish W. Therapy of acute otitis media: clinical and economic aspects. PharmacoEconomics 1994; 6: 202-14
82. Henderson FW, Collier AM, Sanyal MA, et al. A longitudinal study of respiratory viruses and bacteria in the etiology of acute otitis media with effusion. New England Journal of Medicine 1982; 306: 1377
83. Fujita K, Iseki K, Yoshioka H, et al. Bacteriology of acute otitis media in Japanese children. American Journal of Diseases of Children 1983; 137: 152
84. Riding KH, Bluestone CD, Michaels RH, et al. Microbiology of recurrent and chronic otitis media with effusion. Journal of Pediatrics 1978; 93: 739
85. Williams RL, Chalmers TC, Strange KC, et al. Use of antibiotics in preventing recurrent acute otitis media and in treating otitis media with effusion: a meta-analytic attempt to resolve the brouhaha. Journal of the American Medical Association 1993; 270: 1344-51
86. Murray BE. Can antibiotic resistance be controlled? New England Journal of Medicine 1994; 330: 1229-30
87. Cantekin EI, Mandel EM, Fria TJ, et al. Lack of efficacy of a decongestant-antihistamine combination for otitis media with effusion ('secretory' otitis media) in children. New England Journal of Medicine 1983; 308: 297
88. Macknin ML, Jones PK. Oral dexamethasone for treatment of persistent middle ear effusion. Pediatrics 1985; 75: 329
89. Brown DT, Potsic WP, Marsh RR, et al. Drugs affecting clearance of middle ear secretions: a perspective for the management of otitis media with effusion. Annals of Otology Rhinology and Laryngology 1985; 117 Suppl: 94
90. Saarinen UM. Prolonged breast feeding as prophylaxis for recurrent otitis media. Acta Paediatrica Scandinavica 1982; 71: 567
91. Randel HW. Aerospace medicine, 2nd edition. Baltimore: Williams and Wilkins, 1971: 89
92. Kraemer MJ, Richardson MA, Weiss NS, et al. Risk factors for persistent middle ear effusions. Journal of the American Medical Association 1983; 249: 1022
93. Lundy LB, Graham MD. Ototoxicity and ototopical medications: a survey of otolaryngologists. American Journal of Otology 1993; 14: 141-6
94. Dees SC, Lefkowitz D. Secretory otitis media in allergic children. American Journal of Diseases of Children 1972; 124: 364

95. Phillips MJ, Knight NJ, Manning H, et al. IgE and secretory otitis media. Lancet 1974; 2: 1176
96. Gates GA. Cost-effectiveness considerations in otitis media treatment. Otolaryngology - Head and Neck Surgery 1996; 114: 525-30
97. Berman S, Roark R, Luckey D. Theoretical cost effectiveness of management options for children with persisting middle ear effusions. Pediatrics 1994; 43: 353-63
98. Dix MR. Vertigo. Practitioner 1973; 211: 295
99. Oosterveld WJ. Vertigo: current concepts in management. Drugs 1985; 30: 278
100. Roydhouse N. Vertigo and its treatment. Drugs 1973; 7: 297
101. Turner JS. A practical guide to the patient with vertigo: an outline of diagnosis and management for the nonspecialist. Southern Medical Journal 1975; 68: 241
102. Haid T. Evaluation of flunarizine in patients with Ménière's disease. Acta Oto-Laryngologica 1988; Suppl. 460: 149-53
103. Elbaz P. Flunarizine and betahistine. Acta Oto-Laryngologica 1988; Suppl. 460: 143-8
104. Uijtdehaage SHJ, Stern RM, Koch KL. Effects of scopolamine on autonomic profiles underlying motion sickness susceptibility. Aviation Space and Environmental Medicine 1993; 64: 1-8
105. Turner JS. Diseases of the ear, nose and throat. In: Hurst JW, editor. Medicine for the practising physician. Section 22, 3rd ed. Boston: Butterworths, 1992: 777-91
106. Nadol JB, editor. Meniere's disease, pathogenesis, pathophysiology, diagnosis and treatment. Berkeley, CA: Kugler & Ghedini, 1989
107. Green JD, Blum DJ, Harner SG. Longitudinal follow-up of patients with Meniere's disease. Otolaryngology - Head and Neck Surgery 1991; 104: 783-8
108. Turner JS. Diseases of the ear, nose and throat. In: Hurst JW, editor. Medicine for the practising physician. 4th ed. Norwalk CT: Appleton & Lange, 1996
109. Dereberg MJ, Srinavasa Rao V, et al. Meniere's disease: an immune complex-mediated illness? Laryngoscope 1991; 101: 225-9
110. Merchant SW, Rauch SD, Nadol JB. Meniere's disease. European Archives of Oto-Rhino-Laryngology 1995; 252: 63-75
111. Santos PM, Hall RA, Snyder JM, et al. Diuretic and diet effect on Ménière's disease evaluated by the 1985 Committee on Hearing and Equilibrium Guidelines. Otolaryngology - Head and Neck Surgery 1993; 109: 680-9
112. Lange G. Gentamicin and other ototoxic antibiotics for the transtympanic treatment of Ménière's disease. Archives of Otorhinolaryngology 1989; 246: 269-70
113. Yamazaki T, Hayaski M, Komatsuzaki A. Intratympanic gentamicin therapy for Ménière's disease placed by a tubal catheter with systemic isosorbide. Acta Oto-Laryngologica 1991; 481: 613
114. Langman AW, Kemink JL, Graham MD. Titration streptomycin therapy for bilateral Ménière's disease: follow-up report. Annals of Otology Rhinology and Laryngology 1990; 99: 923-6
115. Monsell EM, Shelton C. Labyrinthotomy with streptomycin infusion: early results of a multicentre study. American Journal of Otology 1992; 13: 416-22
116. Norris CH, Aubert A, Amedee RG. Acute and chronic effects of streptomycin applied to the lateral semicircular canal. American Journal of Otology 1993; 14: 373-9
117. Parnes LS, Price-Jones RG. Particle repositioning maneuver for benign paroxysmal positional vertigo. Annals of Otology Rhinology and Laryngology 1993; 102: 325-1
118. Wennmo K, Wennmo C. Drug related dizziness. Acta Oto-Laryngologica 1988; 455: 11-3
119. Marriott S, Tyrer P. Benzodiazepine dependence. Drug Safety 1993; 9: 93-103
120. Holmes B, Brogden RN, Heel RC, et al. Flunarizine: a review of its pharmacological and pharmacokinetic properties and therapeutic use. Drugs 1984; 27: 6
121. Turner JS, Jackson RT. Astemizole: its use in patients with chronic vertigo and ENG signs: a pilot study of a new drug. Laryngoscope 1983; 93: 898
122. Jackson RT, Turner Jr JS. Astemizole: its use in management of patients with chronic vertigo. Archives of Otolaryngology - Head and Neck Surgery 1987; 113: 536-42
123. Wood CD, Graybiel A. A theory of motion sickness based on pharmacologic reactions. Clinical Pharmacology and Therapeutics 1970; 11: 621
124. Wood CD, Graybiel A. Theory of antimotion sickness drug mechanisms. Aerospace Medicine 1972; 43: 249
125. Clissold SP, Heel RC. Transdermal hyoscine (scopolamine): a preliminary review of its pharmacodynamic properties and therapeutic efficacy. Drugs 1985; 29: 189
126. Tristram SJ. The role of cinnarizine in the prophylaxis of sea sickness. In: Cinnarizine and the vertiginous syndrome: Royal Society of Medicine International Congress and Symposium Series No. 33. London: Academic Press, 1980: 39
127. Norris CH. Drugs affecting the inner ear. Drugs 1988; 36: 754-2
128. Wilson WR, Gulya AJ. Sudden sensorineural hearing loss. In: Cummings CW, editor. Otolaryngology, head and neck surgery, 2nd ed., vol 4. St Louis: Mosby Year Book, 1993: 3103-12
129. Schuknecht HF, Donovan ED. The pathology of idiopathic sudden sensorineural hearing loss. Archives of Otorhinolaryngology 1986; 243: 1-15
130. Yoon TH, Paparella MM, Schachern PA. Systemic vasculitis: temporal bone histopathologic study. Laryngoscope 1990; 99: 600-9
131. Dickens JRE, Smith JT, Graham SS. Herpes zoster oticus, treatment with intravenous acyclovir. Laryngoscope 1988; 98: 776-9
132. Wilson WR, Byl FM, Laird N. Efficacy of steroids in the treatment of idiopathic sudden hearing loss: a double-blind clinical study. Archives of Otolaryngology – Head and Neck Surgery 1980; 106: 772-6
133. Moskowitz D, Lee KJ, Smith HW. Steroid use in idiopathic sudden sensorineural hearing loss. Laryngoscope 1984; 94: 664
134. Mattox DE, Simmons FB. Natural history of sudden sensorineural hearing loss. Annals of Otology Rhinology and Laryngology 1977; 86: 463
135. Fisch U. Management of sudden deafness. Otolaryngology – Head and Neck Surgery 1983; 91: 3
136. Wilhelm HJ, Jung F, Kiesewetter H, et al. Hemidilution therapy for patients with sudden loss of hearing: clinical and rheological results. Klinische Wochenschrift 1986; 64: 1058-61
137. Laskawi R, Shrader B, Schroder M, et al. Zur therapie des horsturzes - naftidrofuryl (Dusodril) and pentoxifylline (Trental) im vergleich. Laryngologie Rhinologie Otologie 1987; 66: 242-5
138. Byl Jr FM. Sudden hearing loss: eight years experience and suggested prognostic table. Laryngoscope 1984; 94: 647

139. Bernstein JM. The immunobiology of autoimmune disease of the inner ear. In: Bernstein J, Ogra P, editors. Immunology of the ear. 2nd ed. New York: Raven Press, 1987
140. Veldman JE, Hanada T, Neeuwsen F. Diagnostic and therapeutic dilemmas in rapidly progressive sensoriheural hearing loss and sudden deafness. Acta Oto-Laryngologica 1993; 113: 303-6
141. Hughes GB, Moscicki R, Barna BP, et al. Laboratory diagnosis of immune inner ear disease. American Journal of Otology 1994; 15: 198-202
142. Tran Ba Huy P, Deffrennes D. Aminoglycoside ototoxicity: influence of dosage regimen on drug uptake and correlation between membrane binding and some clinical features. Acta Oto-Laryngologica 1988; 105: 511-5
143. Brummett RE, Jackson RT. Age related changes influencing the effects of drugs and other xenobiotics on sensorineural hearing. Pharmacology and Therapeutics 1994; 26: 209-19
144. Gendeh BS, Said H, Gibb AG, et al. Gentamicin ototoxicity in continuous peritoneal dialysis. Journal of Laryngology and Otology 1993; 107: 681-5
145. Brummett RE. Drug-induced ototoxicity. Drugs 1980; 19: 412
146. van Marion WF, van der Meer JWM, Kalff MW, et al. Ototoxicity of erythromycin. Lancet 1978; 2: 214
147. Chiodo AA, Alberti PW. Experimental, clinical and preventive aspects of ototoxicity. Archives of Otorhinolaryngology 1994; 251: 375-92
148. Gump DW, Ashikaga T, Fink TJ, et al. Side effects of minocycline: different dosage regimens. Antimicrobial Agents and Chemotherapy 1977; 12: 642
149. Wersall J, Lundquist P-G. Ototoxic drugs. In: Herxheimer A, editor. Drugs and sensory functions. London: Churchill, 1968: 142
150. Gorlin RJ, Wester DC, Carey JC. Genetic hearing loss associated with renal disorders. In: Gorlin RJ, Toriello HV, Cohen MM, editors. Hereditary hearing loss and its syndromes. New York: Oxford University Press, 1995: 234-7
151. Kahlmeter G, Dahlager JI. Aminoglycoside toxicity - a review of clinical studies published between 1975 and 1982. Journal of Antimicrobial Chemotherapy 1984; 13 Suppl. A: 9
152. Brummett RE, Harris RF, Lindgren JA. Detection of ototoxicity from drugs applied topically to the middle ear space. Laryngoscope 1976; 86: 1177
153. Ballantyne J. Ototoxic drugs. In: Hinchcliffe & Harrison, editors. Scientific foundations of otolaryngology. Chicago: Year Book Medical Publishers, 1976
154. Jackson GG, Arcieri G. Ototoxicity of gentamicin in man. A survey and controlled analysis of clinical experience in the United States. Journal of Infectious Diseases 1971; 124: S130
155. Stupp H, Kupper K, Lagler F, et al. Inner ear concentrations and ototoxicity of different antibiotics in local and systemic application. Audiology 1973; 12: 350
156. Kalbian VV. Deafness following oral use of neomycin. Southern Medical Journal 1972; 65: 499
157. Anderson MG. Neomycin ototoxicity associated with wound irrigation in the local treatment of osteomyelitis. Journal of the Florida Medical Association 1978; 65: 20
158. Weinstein AJ, McHenry MC, Gavan TL. Systemic absorption of neomycin irrigating solution. Journal of the American Medical Association 1977; 238: 152
159. McKelvie P, Johnstone I, Jamieson I, et al. The effect of gentamicin ear drops on the cochlea. British Journal of Audiology 1975; 9: 45
160. Turner JS, Staats E, Store H, et al. Preparation of the chronically infected ear for tympanoplastic surgery. Southern Medical Journal 1966; 59: 94
161. Schuknecht HF. Ablation therapy in the management of Ménière's disease. Acta Oto-Laryngologica 1957; Suppl. 132: 1
162. Mittleman H. Ototoxicity of 'ototopical' antibiotics: past, present, and future. Transactions of the American Academy of Ophthalmology and Otolaryngology 1972; 76: 1432
163. Wright CG, Meyerhoff WL. Ototoxicity of otic drops applied to the middle ear in the chinchilla. American Journal of Otolaryngology 1984; 5: 166
164. Merifield DO, Parker NJ, Nicholson NC. Therapeutic management of chronic suppurative otitis media with otic drops. Otolaryngology - Head and Neck Surgery 1993; 109: 77-82
165. Matz GL. The ototoxic effects of ethacrynic acid in man and animals. Laryngoscope 1976; 86: 1065
166. Mathog RH. Vestibulotoxicity of ethacrynic acid. Laryngoscope 1977; 87: 1791
167. Rupp W. Pharmacokinetics and pharmacodynamics of Lasix. Scottish Medical Journal 1974; 19: 5
168. Quick C, Hoppe W. Permanent deafness associated with furosemide. Annals of Otology Rhinology and Laryngology 1975; 84: 94
169. Rifkin SI, de Quesada AM, Pickering MJ, et al. Deafness associated with oral furosemide. Southern Medical Journal 1978; 71: 86
170. Brien J. Ototoxicity associated with salicylates. Drug Safety 1993; 9: 143-8
171. Toone EC, Hayden GD, Ellman HM. Ototoxicity of chloroquine. Arthritis and Rheumatism 1965; 8: 475
172. McKinna AJ. Quinine induced hypoplasia and the optic nerve. Canadian Journal of Ophthalmology 1966; 1: 261
173. Rosketh R, Storstein O. Quinidine therapy of chronic auricular fibrillation. Archives of Internal Medicine 1963; 111: 184
174. Dal I, Edsmyr R, Stahle J. Bleomycin therapy and ototoxicity. Acta Oto-Laryngologica 1973; 75: 323
175. Bicknell PG. Sensorineural deafness following myringoplasty operations. Journal of Laryngology and Otology 1971; 85: 957
176. McNab Jones RF, Hammond VT, Wright D, et al. Practolol and deafness. Journal of Laryngology and Otology 1977; 91: 963
177. Capel LH. Rhinotoxic drugs. In: Hinchcliffe & Harrison, editors. Scientific foundations of otolaryngology. Chicago: Year Book Medical Publishers, 1976: 862
178. Schiff M. The 'pill' in otolaryngology. Transactions of the American Academy of Ophthalmology and Otolaryngology 1968; 72: 76
179. Pelikan Z. Possible immediate hypersensitivity reaction of the nasal mucosa to oral contraceptives. Annals of Allergy 1978; 40: 211
180. Dudley JP, Cherry JD. Effects of topical nasal decongestants on the cilia of a chicken embryo tracheal organ culture system. Laryngoscope 1978; 88: 110

Chapter 15

# Ocular Diseases

*R.S. Abel Jr* and *A.D. Abel*

## Synopsis of Important Principles

1) Vision is an important factor in patient well-being and livelihood.

2) Optimum management of ocular disease involves screening (for diabetic retinopathy, open angle glaucoma), rapid diagnosis and treatment (corneal ulcer, injury, narrow angle glaucoma), and forming a partnership with the patient (cataract, dry eye) to determine the most appropriate options.

3) Systemic conditions giving rise to ocular disease should be treated and recommendations for nutritional supplementation (e.g. vitamins, zinc, where appropriate) made for degenerative diseases of the eye.

4) For drugs administered topically to the eye, both the physicochemical properties of the drug (and its vehicle) and the physiological state of the eye affect penetration into ocular structures.

5) Therapeutic drug concentrations in the cornea and aqueous humour can be maintained or increased by prolonging drug contact with the eye by means of ointments, gels, controlled-release inserts, contact lenses or collagen shields.

6) Intraocular drug concentrations adequate for the treatment of anterior segment disease can usually be achieved by topical administration. Higher concentrations in the eye can be achieved with subconjunctival or subtenon injections, soaked collagen shields or contact lenses, or (rarely) intravenous treatment.

7) The therapy of posterior ocular disorders requires retrobulbar or systemic drug therapy. Occasionally, vitrectomy and intraocular drugs are necessary.

8) Drug-induced ocular disease may be produced by a wide variety of drugs used systemically and locally to treat diseases in all systems of the body, as well as in the eye. Locally and systemically administered corticosteroids and systemic phenothiazines are important examples; however, there are numerous photosensitising drugs that may accelerate cataract formation.

9) The benefits and risks of long term intraocular medication must be weighed against those of surgical interventions. Topical eye medications, particularly those used in glaucoma therapy, can be responsible for systemic adverse effects.

10) Laser and surgical interventions provide alternatives in the therapy of cataract, glaucoma and certain retinal disorders. The choice is determined by urgency, cost and individual variation.

The eye is an organ that is readily available for examination by virtue of its transparency, and many parameters of ophthalmic function can be quantified. A therapeutic effect in the eye can be achieved by drugs given topically, by local injection, or systemically. In administering drugs topically, it should be remembered that they can have remote effects in organs other than the eye and should therefore be considered as systemic medications.

An epidemiological study in Nottingham, UK found that 1 in 14 patients visiting a clinician did so because of an eye problem. Among these individuals, one-third presented to a hospital casualty department while the remainder were seen by primary care and specialist clinicians.[1]

## 1. Clinical Pharmacological Considerations

### 1.1 Ability of Drugs to Penetrate the Eye

Many factors determine the ability of a drug to penetrate into the eye (table I). These include the type of agent, its physicochemical properties such as differential solubility in water and lipids (partition coefficient) and dissociation constant, its concentration and the pH of the vehicle, and the nature of the ocular structure.[2]

When administered topically, drugs can be absorbed through the cornea or through the conjunctiva and sclera. Subconjunctival or subtenon deposits of medication tend to penetrate through the cornea. Retrobulbar injections pass through the sclera, and systemically administered drugs must pass through the blood-eye barrier, which in many ways is similar to the blood-brain barrier.

The corneal epithelium and endothelium are readily penetrated by lipid-soluble substances and the stroma by water-soluble agents. Therefore, substances combining polar (water-soluble) and nonpolar groups penetrate the cornea more freely than totally polar or nonpolar compounds. Weak acids and bases have different lipid and water solubilities in their two different ionic states, depending on the pH of the vehicle.

The physicochemical properties of the drug, its concentration, and the osmolarity and pH of the vehicle will, therefore, influence ocular absorption. Hypotonic solutions tend be more permeable. Wetting agents such as benzalkonium chloride, a commonly used preservative in ophthalmic medications, lower surface tension and can improve corneal permeability.

**Table I.** Factors which influence penetration of drugs into ocular structures

**Nature of the drug:**
- Chemical structure
- Molecular weight (occasionally)
- Physicochemical properties (lipid: water solubility ratio or partition coefficient; polarity; ionisation)

**Nature of the pharmaceutical preparation:**
- Drug concentration
- Vehicle characteristics (pH; osmolarity; inclusion of agents to lower surface tension; viscosity)

**Method of administration:**
- Systemic
- Topical – increased duration of contact with eye (vehicle viscosity – ointment *vs* drops; continuous irrigation; diminution of tear production; prolonged drug release system; cotton pledgets soaked in solution of drug; soft contact lenses and collagen shields)
- Subconjunctival, subtenon or retrobulbar injection
- Carotid perfusion (only experimentally in the case of certain ocular tumours)

**Nature of the ocular structure:**
- Integrity of corneal epithelium (particularly polar compounds) – abrasion; ulceration
- Inflammation (dilated vasculature). Increases the permeability of ciliary and iris vessels and increases drug concentration in the eye
- Status of lacrimal outflow passages and conjunctival vasculature (which carry drug away from the eye)
- Status of the gonioangle (ability to be deepened or closed)
- Presence of the lens (influences drug penetration into the vitreous body)

For a review of pharmacokinetic considerations in ocular drug delivery, see Schoenwald.[3]

### 1.2 Vehicle and Drug Delivery System

The topical route is effective for administering all alkaloids, corticosteroids, local anaesthetics and various antibiotics and antiviral agents to the eye. Therapeutic drug concentrations in contact with the cornea, aqueous humour and cul-de-sac can be maintained or increased by prolonging contact with the eye via ointments.

Petrolatum and lanolin are viscous vehicles commonly used as bases in ophthalmic ointments. However, these bases are toxic to the corneal endothelium and generally are not used before intraocular surgery. Also, there is conflicting evidence as to whether ointments affect the healing of corneal abrasions. Nonetheless, ointments protect the eye from exposure, soften discharges and are less diluted by tears than are suspensions, powders and solutions.

Newer bases have been used to enhance penetration of medication [e.g. timolol (in a gel-forming base) and dorzolamide (in 0.5% hydroxyethylcellulose)] into the eye. Drugs may also be administered on cotton pledgets soaked with ophthalmic solutions and inserted for a short time into the inferior cul-de-sac to facilitate mydriasis on a short term basis.

Liposomes, soluble drug inserts, hydrophilic contact lenses and drug-soaked porcine collagen shields[4] can serve as drug reservoirs and maintain better intraocular drug concentrations.

Sterility of all commercially available ophthalmic products is essential, since barriers to infection are frequently compromised when these products are used. Most ophthalmic products include preservatives.

### 1.3 Physiological State of the Eye

The intraocular concentration of drugs is also determined by the rate of removal by the conjunctival and episcleral circulations and by the physiological egress of aqueous humour through the trabecular meshwork. The dilated vasculature in the inflamed eye facilitates penetration[5] but also hastens the removal of medication. Thus, drugs indicated for treatment of ocular inflammation require more frequent topical application.

Since 80% of eye drops diffuse into the general circulation, drugs administered by this route may exert systemic effects, even at very low concentrations.[6] The lacrimal pump facilitates this diffusion of eye drops into systemic circulation. This is also the route by which topical medication administered into one eye can affect the contralateral eye.

Gentle lid closure to eliminate rapid blinking and digital occlusion of the lower punctum will negate rapid tear dilution and minimise systemic uptake. The corneal nervous supply determines the degree of discomfort of topically applied medications.

### 1.4 Animal Models for Eye Disease

The rabbit eye has historically been chosen as an investigative model of ocular therapeutics and toxicity[3] because of its size, sensitivity and the cost of maintaining laboratory facilities. However, anatomical, physiological and immunological differences have led to discrepancies in predictability. This has also been the case with the use of guinea-pig, rat, cat and even monkey models.[7,8]

## 2. General Principles of Treatment

Drug treatment in ophthalmology is largely directed to one of the following approaches:

1) Reduction of inflammation by prompt and intensive treatment of microbial infection, or by identification and removal of the predisposing factor.

2) Reduction of raised intraocular pressure.

3) Removal of an opacified corneal epithelium.

4) Physiological replacement of tears.

5) Use of dye solutions, and mydriatic and cycloplegic drugs for diagnosis and investigative procedures.

6) Intraocular fluid replacement.

7) Enhancement of extraocular and intraocular surgical or laser procedures.

### 2.1 Inflammation and Infection

The sequelae of an infective process can have a marked effect on vision. Even minimal scarring in the central pupillary zone of the cornea can markedly decrease visual acuity. Therefore, the treatment of acute ophthalmological inflammatory disorders such as blepharitis, conjunctivitis, corneal ulcer and endophthalmitis consists of prompt and intensive antimicrobial therapy. In bacterial infections of the conjunctiva (which are less common than seborrhoeic or viral infections), this means frequent topical application, i.e. at least hourly during the daytime and frequently at night for the first 2 to 3 days. Topical (ointment or solution) and sometimes systemic therapy should be used for corneal infections, depending on the extent of the infection (table II).[9] Both ointments and solutions can be highly effective in treatment,[10,11] and the choice may depend on market availability of the dosage form or patient convenience. Subconjunctival injection should be considered if a higher antibacterial concentration is required. It is often necessary to start broad-spectrum antibacterial coverage on initial suspicion of bacterial infection and subsequently alter therapy on clinical grounds. Ideally, the pathogen should be identified by cultures and its sensitivity determined, but this is not always practical.

Combined topical corticosteroid and antibacterial preparations should be used cautiously in superficial infections of the eye, because suppression of inflammation by the corticosteroid may falsely suggest that the infection is being controlled. In blepharitis, a corticosteroid-antibacterial drug combination often results in a

**Table II.** Usual route(s) of corticosteroid administration in ocular inflammation

| Condition | Route |
|---|---|
| Blepharitis | Topical |
| Conjunctivitis | Topical |
| Episcleritis | Topical |
| Scleritis | Topical and/or systemic |
| Keratitis | Topical |
| Anterior uveitis | Topical and/or periocular |
| Posterior uveitis | Systemic and/or periocular |
| Endophthalmitis | Systemic/periocular, intravitreal |
| Optic neuritis | Systemic or periocular |
| Cranial arteritis | Systemic |
| Sympathetic ophthalmia | Systemic and topical |

dramatic response when an antibacterial agent alone does not.

The treatment of chronic conjunctivitis is aimed at eliminating predisposing factors (keratoconjunctivitis sicca, seborrhoea, trichiasis, abnormalities of the lid margins, heavy alcohol intake, and exophthalmic eyes) wherever possible, as well as treating any microbial pathogen. The treatment of seborrhoea is discussed in section 3.6. Staphylococcal hypersensitivity, caused by the organism's exotoxin, is treated by appropriate antibacterial therapy in conjunction with topical corticosteroids.[12]

The treatment of uveitis and optic neuritis is based on careful diagnostic evaluation, and specific therapy is used whenever possible. However, nonspecific therapy [corticosteroids, nonsteroidal anti-inflammatory drugs (NSAIDs), mydriatics] is usually given, even when the cause is known (see further section 6). Corticosteroid therapy is initiated and ocular and systemic health are monitored for improvement, deterioration or adverse effects so that treatment can be altered as necessary.

### 2.2 Raised Intraocular Pressure

A number of pharmacological approaches are used to control intraocular pressure (IOP) in chronic glaucoma. Topical β-adrenoceptor blocking drugs such as timolol, betaxolol, carteolol, levobunolol and metipranolol, which act by decreasing aqueous humour production, have replaced miotics as initial therapy (see further section 5.1). However, since miosis changes the configuration of the angle structures, thereby allowing a greater outflow of aqueous humour into the canal of Schlemm, miotic therapy remains useful for both angle closure and open angle types of glaucoma. Other agents used in glaucoma are discussed in section 5.1.

Anticholinergic drugs, sympathomimetics and even topical vasoconstrictors have been known to precipitate an acute attack of glaucoma. This usually occurs in people over 60 years of age who are far-sighted (hyperopic) and have early cataracts. Therefore, clinicians should ask patients who wear bifocal spectacles if they have a history of narrow angle glaucoma. Patients who are receiving therapy for glaucoma will rarely be disturbed by these drugs.

### 2.3 Corneal Oedema

Corneal oedema resulting from intractable glaucoma, corneal degenerations and corneal dystrophies can be reduced with hypertonic agents. However, it should always be ascertained first that active infection is not present. Glycerol can be used in acute conditions to evaluate the chamber angle and intraocular function. For long term use, sodium chloride 2 to 8% solutions or ointments are well tolerated. A soft contact lens may facilitate the use of these agents and serve as a therapeutic ocular bandage.[13]

### 2.4 Removal of Opacified Corneal Epithelium

Epitheliolytic iodine, trichloroacetic acid and ether solutions can be used to remove the corneal epithelium in the treatment of refractory herpes simplex keratitis and before decalcification treatment for band keratopathy, although manual removal is easier.

Chelating agents, primarily edetic acid (ethylenediamine tetra-acetic acid; EDTA) are used to decalcify Bowman's membrane in band keratopathy. After the epithelium is pharmacologically or manually removed, a swab immersed in the edetic acid solution is applied to the cornea for several minutes, then the solution is washed off. Calcium ions become bonded to the inner ring of the molecule. Hypercalcaemia should be ruled out as a cause of band keratopathy.

### 2.5 Dry Eyes

Tear replacement for keratoconjunctivitis sicca or neuroparalytic keratitis (which often necessitates a tarsorrhaphy) consists of physiological replacement using a moist solution containing various electrolytes. Drops (e.g. of polyvinyl alcohol, hypromellose, carmellose) or ointments (e.g. paraffin/mineral oil) are generally applied every hour or less frequently, but in warmer climates drops may have to be applied more often. It is often necessary to try several agents until the patient's discomfort has been alleviated.[14] New tear substitutes (e.g. hydroxypropylcellulose ocular inserts) and punctal occlusion are improving the comfort of patients with dry eye syndromes. Lubricants and wetting agents are also often necessary for people who wear contact lenses and prostheses.

Mucolytic agents such as acetylcysteine can be used to break up ropy mucoid secretions which are often a feature of this condition. Acetylcysteine (10% solution) and edetic acid (0.1 to 1.0 mol/L) may also have a role in binding the destructive collagenase enzymes produced by species of *Pseudomonas*, *Streptococcus* and *Clostridium*, and after severe chemical burns when the cornea fails to re-epithelialise.

## 2.6 Diagnostic and Investigative Procedures

### *2.6.1 Use of Mydriatic and Cycloplegic Drugs*

#### Fundus Examination

The mydriatic drugs phenylephrine (2.5 to 10%) and tropicamide (0.5%) are routinely used to examine the fundus oculi. Cycloplegic agents such as cyclopentolate (1%), homatropine (5%) and atropine (1%) may be used during refraction, especially in young children.

Pupillary size may return to normal in as little as 2 hours (tropicamide) or as long as several days (cyclopentolate). Patients should be informed about the possibility of large pupils for several days, since many people become concerned about them.

Phenylephrine and cyclopentolate may cause the shedding of iris pigment cells, leading to an erroneous diagnosis of iritis. Caution should be used when administering these agents to children because of their rapid absorption and relatively large dosages. Cyclopentolate, particularly with repeated instillation, can cause fever, convulsions and disorientation. Phenylephrine 10% has been associated with subarachnoid bleeding in infants, and cardiac arrest and myocardial infarction in adults,[15] while atropine 1% can cause fever, rash, disorientation and dehydration, particularly when several drops are applied. It is important to tell all patients to be mindful of unusual symptoms.

#### Cycloplegia

The sympathomimetic drugs (e.g. phenylephrine) are weaker mydriatics and dilate the pupil without affecting accommodation, whereas the anticholinergic agents (e.g. cyclopentolate, homatropine, atropine, tropicamide) are longer acting and produce cycloplegia as well as mydriasis. These actions are essential for performing retinoscopy in paediatric ophthalmology, are helpful in determining the refractive error in young people, and may allow a better ophthalmoscopic examination.

Cyclopentolate exerts its maximum effect in less than 1 hour and usually exerts an effect for 4 to 24 hours. However, strict attention to dosage is necessary to avoid potentially serious adverse effects. Children under 2 years of age should have only one drop of a 1% solution instilled in each eye, while one drop of a 2% solution is used in older children. Tropicamide is a weaker cycloplegic agent, acting within 15 to 20 minutes and lasting for 2 to 4 hours.

### *2.6.2 Use of Diagnostic Dyes*

Fluorescein solutions are dyes that reveal corneal epithelial defects. Rose bengal solution stains devitalised cornea and conjunctiva; it is used as part of the evaluation of keratoconjunctivitis sicca. The Schirmer filter paper test is a valuable adjunct in evaluating tear film disorders.

## 2.7 Intraocular Fluid Replacement

Ophthalmic irrigating solutions available for use during surgical procedures include sterile physiological solutions of sodium chloride, potassium chloride, calcium chloride, magnesium chloride and sodium citrate dihydrate, such as 'Balanced Salt Solution'. This solution is isotonic to the tissues of the eye and contains essential ions for normal cell metabolism.

A preparation of a highly purified non-inflammatory fraction of hyaluronic acid may be used as a substitute for aqueous or vitreous humour in anterior segment and vitreous surgical procedures. This agent forms a viscoelastic solution in water at physiological pH and ionic strength. It has a high molecular weight and is nonantigenic, highly viscous and transparent. Other viscoelastic substances contain chondroitin sulfate or methylcellulose. Their viscous nature provides mechanical protection for cell layers such as the corneal endothelium and other intraocular structures exposed to mechanical damage during intraocular surgery.

In retinal detachment surgery, intravitreal gases (e.g. air) can also be used to maintain the volume of the globe when a large amount of subretinal fluid must be drained.

**Table III.** Some currently available topical antibiotics and their principal uses

| Drug | Dosage form(s) | Indications for use | |
|---|---|---|---|
| | | blepharitis and conjunctivitis | corneal ulcer |
| Chloramphenicol | Solution 0.5%; ointment 0.5% or 1% | | + |
| Ciprofloxacin | Solution 0.3% | | + |
| Erythromycin | Ointment 0.5% | + | |
| Gentamicin | Solution, ointment 0.3% | | + |
| Norfloxacin[a] | Solution 0.3% | + | |
| Ofloxacin | Solution 0.3% | | + |
| Sulfacetamide | Solution, ointment 10% or 15% | + | |
| Sulfafurazole (sulfisoxazole) | Solution 4% | + | |
| Tetracycline | Ointment 1% | + | |
| Tobramycin | Solution, ointment 0.3% | | + |
| **Combination preparations:** | | | |
| Bacitracin/polymixin B | Ointment 500U/10,000U per g | + | |
| Bacitracin/polymixin B/neomycin | Ointment 400U/10,000U/3.5mg per g | + | |
| Gramicidin/polymixin B/neomycin | Solution 0.025mg/10,000U/1.75mg per ml | | + |
| Polymixin B/trimethoprim | Solution 10,000U/1mg per ml | + | |

a The difference between indications for this agent and other quinolones is due to their differential effects on *Streptococcus* spp.

## 3. Ocular Inflammation and Ocular Infections

### 3.1 Acute Conjunctivitis

This condition may be bacterial, viral or chlamydial in origin. It must be treated early and adequately because of occasional epidemics it can cause.

In many cases, especially of viral conjunctivitis, there are concomitant systemic symptoms. This applies particularly to infections due to *Staphylococcus aureus*, which can chronically colonise the lid margins and involve the peripheral cornea. Samples of exudate should be obtained for bacteriological examination and empirical therapy started before the results are available. Rarely, serological and fluorescent immunological studies are important in making the diagnosis of a viral disease.

#### Optimum Treatment

*Staphylococcus* species, *Streptococcus pneumoniae*, *Streptococcus pyogenes*, and occasionally *Haemophilus aegyptius* (Koch-Weeks bacillus) are among the more common bacterial causes of conjunctivitis. Topical sulfonamides [e.g. sulfacetamide or sulfafurazole (sulfisoxazole)], neomycin-polymixin B or bacitracin or gramicidin-neomycin-polymixin B combinations, or tetracycline preparations are usually adequate treatment. Tobramycin 0.3% and gentamicin 0.3% solutions and the quinolones (e.g. ciprofloxacin 0.3% or ofloxacin 0.3%) are reserved for more refractory cases (table III).

Drops should be instilled frequently during the day (at least hourly for the first 2 to 3 days) and an ointment applied at night for about a week.

Chloramphenicol is no longer mainstream therapy for this condition (at least in the US), due to the rare association with aplastic anaemia and availability of safer agents. However, because of its effectiveness and low cost, chloramphenicol is still used sparingly in other countries.

### 3.2 Dacryocystitis

Dacryocystitis can be caused by any of the common external ocular pathogens, the most frequently implicated organism being *S. pneumoniae*. For treatment, oral and occasionally parenteral antibiotics are required to attain therapeutic drug concentrations, while decongestant nose drops and lacrimal sac massage are useful adjuncts.

### 3.3 Bacterial Corneal Ulcers

Bacterial organisms responsible for corneal ulceration include Gram-positive and Gram-negative cocci, and less frequently Gram-negative bacilli. There is an increased incidence of microbial keratitis in people who wear hydrophilic contact lenses. Any infiltrate in the cornea of a patient wearing contact lenses must be suspected as being infectious, the use of the lens should be discontinued, and topical antibiotics should be intensively administered (see table III).

In addition to bacteria, viruses (herpes simplex, vaccinia) and fungi (*Aspergillus, Fusarium, Cephalosporium* and *Candida* spp.) may also be implicated in a corneal ulceration, and should be considered especially when there are differences in symptoms (watery discharge with viruses) and onset (delayed with fungal keratitis).

#### Optimum Treatment

For corneal ulcers, appropriate antibacterial agents must be started immediately after examining the corneal scrapings and while specimens are being cultured. For some cases of bacterial keratitis, an initial subconjunctival injection and full dosage parenteral therapy may be necessary to avoid such complications as diffuse scarring, perforation and endophthalmitis. Topical antibacterial solutions should also be instilled every 10 to 60 minutes. Occasionally, a conjunctival flap, superficial keratectomy or penetrating keratoplasty are performed to ameliorate a refractory ulceration.

Table III indicates the topical antibiotics that are recommended for acute bacterial corneal ulceration. Occasionally, 'fortified' antibiotics (i.e. concentrated solutions made from intravenous preparations) are necessary to achieve better concentrations; however, a non-epithelialised ulcer will readily absorb a topical antibiotic. Rarely, a soft contact lens or cyanoacrylate glue may be necessary if there is marked corneal thinning or perforation, and topical edetic acid (EDTA) or acetylcysteine are useful in chelating calcium to minimise collagenolysis.

### 3.4 Fungal Keratitis

Mycotic infections are seen as vegetable and plant contaminants. *Candida* and *Aspergillus* spp. predominate in the northern US, whereas *Penicillium, Fusarium* and *Cephalosporium* spp., among others, are seen in less temperate climates. The symptoms of fungal corneal ulcers are marked injection (redness), severe pain, hypopyon and polypoid ulceration with frequent satellite lesions. Delayed onset, especially after the use of topical antibiotics and corticosteroids, is an important differentiating feature between fungal and bacterial corneal ulcers.

#### Optimum Treatment

In the treatment of keratitis due to *Candida* spp. and other yeast-like fungi, topical amphotericin B 0.15% (1.5 mg/ml) drops every hour or topical nystatin (100,000 U/ml) solutions every 2 hours can be used. Clotrimazole 1% (10 mg/ ml) drops are active against both dermatophytes and yeast-like fungi and has also been used successfully in ocular infections, especially *Aspergillus* infections.[16] Conjunctival flaps and lamellar keratoplasty may be of some value in refractory conditions.

Oral ketoconazole (200 to 400mg daily) or intravenous miconazole are indicated for intraocular fungal infections. Occasionally, vitrectomy may be necessary when pharmacological therapy is delayed or ineffective; intravitreous miconazole can be administered at that time.

### 3.5 Ophthalmia Neonatorum

Ophthalmia neonatorium refers to acute conjunctivitis in the first 4 weeks in the life of a child and manifests as purulent ocular discharge. This worldwide problem may be caused by Chlamydia (inclusion blenorrhoea), bacteria (*Neisseria gonorrhoeae, S. aureus, S. pneumoniae, S. pyogenes* and *Haemophilus influenzae*), or herpes simplex virus.

Infection due to *N. gonorrhoeae* is the most serious form because of the potential of this organism to rapidly invade the eye, leading to blindness. *Chlamydia trachomatis*, while not as destructive, can cause severe inflammation and in some cases infection can persist for many years.

#### Optimum Treatment

Neonates born to mothers with active gonococcal infection should receive a single aqueous benzylpenicillin (penicillin G) intramuscular injection (20,000U for those less than 2kg or 50,000U for those over 2kg). Bacterial conjunctivitis requires only topical therapy. Exposure keratopathy should be identified, especially if *Pseudomonas* is present, and patching should supplement hourly antibiotic ointment administration. Oral erythromycin (10 mg/kg 3 times daily) combined with topical tetracycline or sulfonamide drops or erythromycin ointment 4 times daily is recommended for *Chlamydia* for 2 to 3 weeks. For herpetic involvement, intravenous aciclovir 10 mg/kg every 8 hours for 10 days and topical trifluridine 5 times daily are advised.[17]

Current prophylaxis consists of applying tetracycline 1% ointment or erythromycin ointment 0.5% in the eyes of all at-risk neonates. Credé prophylaxis (1% silver nitrate solution) is no longer used in most locations.

### 3.6 Blepharitis and Other Lid Lesions

Blepharitis is usually caused by *Staphylococcus* spp. and less commonly by parasites such as lice and *Demodex folliculorum*. It may also present as an angular form. Rare causes such as anthrax, glanders, chancroid or tetanus may be seen in endemic areas.

#### Optimum Treatment

Since eye drops do not penetrate the upper lid, ointments are the major form of therapy for blepharitis, but even then penetration is still relatively poor.

***Staphylococcal blepharitis*** is generally treated with a topical sulfonamide (e.g. sulfacetamide 10% solution) or erythromycin 0.5% eye ointment, and by removal of crusts and manual expression of the meibomian glands. Recurrences are treated by the addition of topical corticosteroids (see table IV), long term topical and sometimes oral antibiotics, and shampooing of the eyelids.

***Allergic blepharitis*** usually responds to topical antihistamines (e.g. levocabastine, antazoline, pheniramine) and dilute corticosteroid preparations (e.g. prednisolone 0.12%), and may also respond to the use of mast cell stabilisers (e.g. sodium cromoglycate, lodoxamide) and topical nonsteroidal anti-inflammatory drugs (e.g. diclofenac 0.1%, ketorolac tromethamine 0.5%). Corticosteroids must be used with care, because of the risk of steroid-induced glaucoma, particularly with the more potent topical preparations.

***Angular blepharitis***, which is often due to the Morax-Axenfeld Gram-negative bacillus, responds to sulfacetamide, zinc sulfate, or gentamicin, topically applied several times daily.

***Chronic blepharitis*** is frequently a mixture of seborrhoeic, staphylococcal and sicca forms (appropriately termed 'triple S' syndrome). Some clinicians consider that the fungus *Pityrosporum ovale* may be a causative factor and should be carefully searched for in the smear, but this organism is very difficult to culture. Treatment is by removal of crusts and scales, shampooing the hair (e.g. with selenium sulfide suspension) and even the eyelids (e.g. using baby shampoo or, in more severe cases, 0.5% selenium sulfide and hydrocortisone). The blepharitis responds to a combination of sulfacetamide 10% and prednisolone 0.2 or 0.5%. Expression of the meibomian glands can be attempted by capable patients.

A ***hordeolum (stye)*** is a staphylococcal infection of the sebaceous glands of the eyelids. It is usually self-limiting. Hot moist compresses, sometimes removal of lashes to expedite drainage, and antibacterial eye ointments (if needed) are the basis of therapy.

***Granulomatous lid lesions*** are usually seen as a chalazion (a sterile inflammation of the meibomian glands due to obstruction of the duct) or meibomianitis in the acute diffuse form. Warm moist compresses are usually adequate therapy, but systemic tetracycline therapy does reduce the inflammation in the meibomian glands.

**Table IV.** Some currently available topical corticosteroid preparations

| |
|---|
| **Corticosteroids alone** |
| Betamethasone sodium phosphate |
| Dexamethasone and dexamethasone sodium phosphate |
| Fluorometholone and fluorometholone acetate[a] |
| Hydrocortisone and hydrocortisone acetate |
| Medrysone[a] |
| Prednisolone acetate |
| Prednisolone sodium phosphate |
| **Corticosteroid-antibacterial drug combinations** |
| Betamethasone sodium phosphate + neomycin |
| Dexamethasone + neomycin and polymixin B |
| Dexamethasone + gramicidin and framycetin |
| Dexamethasone + tobramycin |
| Dexamethasone sodium phosphate + neomycin |
| Fluorometholone + sulfacetamide |
| Hydrocortisone + bacitracin, neomycin and polymixin |
| Hydrocortisone + neomycin and polymixin B |
| Hydrocortisone acetate + chloramphenicol |
| Hydrocortisone acetate + chloramphenicol and polymixin B |
| Prednisolone + chloramphenicol |
| Prednisolone acetate + gentamicin |
| Prednisolone acetate + neomycin and polymixin B |
| Prednisolone acetate + sulfacetamide |

a Fluorometholone and medrysone have a lower propensity to raise intraocular pressure than other topical corticosteroids.

### 3.7 Viral Infections

Viral lesions of the lids, conjunctiva and cornea can be caused by a number of different viruses such as varicella-zoster, vaccinia, molluscum contagiosum and herpes simplex.

Primary ocular infection with herpes simplex virus occurs early in life and usually causes blepharoconjunctivitis. Recurrent disease usually takes the form of dendritic or geographical corneal ulceration, but may also manifest as stromal inflammation or uveitis. More often, stromal disease follows corneal ulceration and may precede corneal destruction or scarring.

**Table V.** Currently available antiviral agents for use in ocular viral infections

| Drug | Dosage form(s) | Indications for use | Usual dosage (adults) |
|---|---|---|---|
| **Topical agents** | | | |
| Aciclovir | Ophthalmic ointment 3% | Herpes simplex keratitis | Apply 1cm 5 times daily |
| Idoxuridine | Ophthalmic solution and ointment 0.1% | Herpes simplex keratitis | *Solution:* 1 drop every hour during the day and, if severe, every 2 hours during night<br>*Ointment:* apply 5 times daily |
| Trifluridine | Ophthalmic solution 1% | Herpes simplex keratitis | 1 drop every 2 hours (maximum, 9 doses/day) |
| Vidarabine | Ophthalmic ointment 3% | Herpes simplex keratitis | Apply 1.5cm 5 times daily |
| **Systemic agents** | | | |
| Aciclovir[a] | Oral capsules/tablets<br>IV injection | Herpes simplex keratitis<br>Herpes zoster ophthalmicus | 200mg PO 5 times daily for 7-10 days[b]<br>600-800mg PO 5 times daily for 10 days[b]<br>Consider IV administration if patient is immunocompromised (10 mg/kg by infusion over 1h every 8h)[b] |
| Foscarnet[a] | IV injection | CMV retinitis in AIDS patients | By IV infusion only, either via central or peripheral vein: *Induction,* 60 mg/kg over 1h every 8h for 14-21 days[b]<br>*Maintenance,* 90-120 mg/kg over 2h once daily[b] |
| Ganciclovir[a] | IV or intravitreous injection | CMV retinitis in immunocompromised patients (including AIDS) | *Intravenous:* Induction, 5 mg/kg over 1h every 12h for 14-21 days. Maintenance, 5 mg/kg over 1h once daily on 7 days/week ***or*** 6 mg/kg once daily on 5 days/week[b]<br>*Intravitreous:* 200μg |

a See chapter 32 (section 2) for further discussion on the properties and clinical usage of antiviral drugs.

b Reduce dosage in presence of renal impairment.

*Abbreviations:* AIDS = acquired immune deficiency syndrome; CMV = cytomegalovirus; IV = intravenous; PO = oral.

#### Optimum Treatment

***Herpes zoster ophthalmicus*** is treated with oral aciclovir (for dosage, see table V) and a topical antibiotic/corticosteroid ointment.

***Molluscum contagiosum*** responds best to excision or cauterisation of lid lesions. ***Herpes simplex lid infections*** can be treated with topical antiviral agents (table V), as can vaccinia lid and corneal lesions.

***Acute herpes simplex keratitis*** requires special consideration and patients presenting with this condition should be promptly referred to an ophthalmologist. Topical antiviral agents (table V) are effective for surface disease and are usually applied 5 times daily for the initial week or until re-epithelialisation, and for 3 to 7 days after healing is complete. Aciclovir appears to be the best tolerated of the topical medications currently available. Cross-resistance, cross-toxicity and cross-hypersensitivity between antiviral agents are rare.

***Herpetic stromal keratitis*** is treated with a topical antiviral agent (table V), with or without a topical corticosteroids. Corticosteroids should never be used alone in the treatment of this disease because they can exacerbate the epithelial component of the disease. Topical corticosteroids are used for disciform stromal swelling and for iritis. Oral aciclovir has been recommended for severe or refractive forms of corneal ulceration.

***Epidemic keratoconjunctivitis*** (usually caused by adenovirus type 8) can be suppressed but not cured by topical corticosteroids and thus there may be rebound after corticosteroids are withdrawn, prolonging the course of the disease. Therefore, it is recommended that only artificial tears (see section 2.5) or topical sulfacetamide solution be used in the acute phase of the disease. In the rare case of iritis or with post-infectious corneal opacities in the visual axis, suppressive corticosteroid therapy may be helpful. A long established treatment using 1% silver nitrate is extremely effective for neutralisation of the acute conjunctival reaction.

***Other viral infections:*** intravenous foscarnet and ganciclovir have been used for necrotising retinitis and severe uveitis and in the treatment of cytomegalovirus retinopathy (see further section 7.6).

### 3.8 Trachoma and Inclusion Conjunctivitis

Trachoma and inclusion conjunctivitis are caused by chlamydiae, obligate intracellular organisms that can invade the conjunctiva and cornea.

#### Optimum Treatment

Trachoma responds to treatment with systemic or topical tetracyclines given for 3 to 6 weeks. Topical tetracycline ointment 1% applied 3 to 4 times daily is useful for mass prophylaxis programmes in endemic areas.

Systemically administered tetracyclines provide more constant tissue drug concentrations, but are more costly and have a greater incidence of adverse effects. Systemic administration should, however, be used for recurrences and progressive disease.

Intramuscular benzathine benzylpenicillin and erythromycin given once a week for 3 weeks has also provided good results. In many areas, communicable ophthalmia is caused by a combination of chronic trachoma and bacterial superinfection. Treatment must be directed against both infectious entities, and fly control, since an increased density of fly populations is associated with an increased incidence of trachoma.[18]

## 3.9 Parasitic Infestations

### 3.9.1 Pediculosis and Scabies Infestations of the Eyelids

Infestations by *Phthirus palpebrum* (crab louse) or *P. pubis* (pubic louse) and *Scarcoptes scabiei* (scabies mite) are effectively treated by shampooing the cilia with lindane (gamma benzene hexachloride) or selenium sulfide and repeating the application in 5 to 7 days. Lindane 1% cream may be used as an alternative, applied to the lid margins and repeated in 5 to 7 days. Lid infection is associated with infection of abdominal skin and pubic areas, which should also be treated with lindane shampoo. Newer preparations include permethrin 1% cream and pyrethrins/piperonyl butoxide shampoo. Sex partners should also be treated.

Physostigmine and dyflos (isoflurophate) solutions have also been used in treatment, but produce uncomfortable adverse effects due to ciliary spasm and miosis.

### 3.9.2 Demodex folliculorum Infestation

*D. folliculorum*, a tenacious mite that resides in eyelid hair shafts, may contribute to chronic blepharitis, but responds to the same treatment as for louse infection (section 3.9.1). If this fails, the cholinesterase inhibitor ecothiopate iodide eye drops can be used.

### 3.9.3 Toxoplasmosis

*Toxoplasma gondii* can cause acute or chronic chorioretinal infection and requires early diagnosis and rapid therapy. Traditional therapy is with pyrimethamine plus a sulfonamide (e.g. sulfadiazine or sulfadoxine) or clindamycin, which affect the parasite at a ribosomal level. If a pyrimethamine-sulfonamide combination is used, oral calcium folinate (calcium leucovorin) 5mg should also be given twice weekly to reduce the risk of haematological toxicity. For a review of the management of toxoplasmosis, see St Georgiev.[19]

### 3.9.4 Acanthamoebic Keratitis

Acanthamoebic keratitis has been seen in temperate and subtropical areas around the world in conjunction with contamination of soft contact lenses. The chronic pain and delayed onset of infection make diagnosis difficult. Results of therapy with propamidine 0.1%, framycetin 0.5%, and imidazole drugs have been inconsistent. Oral paromomycin, oral ketoconazole and topical polyhexamethylene biguanide 0.02% have been used with limited success.[20] Penetrating keratoplasty is often the only effective treatment for eradicating this amoebic organism.

## 3.10 Allergic External Ocular Diseases

Ocular allergic disease is the most frequent ocular condition seen in general medical practice. Seasonal allergic conjunctivitis, perennial allergic conjunctivitis and giant papillary conjunctivitis are confined to the conjunctiva and eyelids and carry a good prognosis.

Seasonal allergic conjunctivitis is seen concomitantly with seasonal allergic rhinitis, with symptoms of pruritus, watery discharge and scleral injection in addition to lid oedema, injected bulbar conjunctiva with conjunctival thickening, and occasional chemosis.

Perennial allergic conjunctivitis is very similar to seasonal conjunctivitis, but occurs year-round, produces milder symptoms, and house-dust mites are usually the cause.

Giant papillary conjunctivitis is caused by a foreign body in the ocular surface, i.e. contact lens, ocular prosthesis or exposed suture, and generates itching, mucopurulent discharge and contact lens intolerance. The upper tarsal conjunctiva is the most common site of involvement and it becomes hyperaemic and thickened with a marked giant papillary reaction.[21]

Vernal keratoconjunctivitis, a rare chronic allergic condition in children, and atopic keratoconjunctivitis in adults involve the cornea and can cause blindness. They both demonstrate pruritus, photophobia, blepharospasm, diplopia and a stringy discharge. The upper tarsal conjunctiva demonstrates thickening, hyperaemia and a giant papillary reaction in the vernal form.

**Optimum Treatment**

Allergic external ocular diseases are ubiquitous and can be treated using the same general concepts. Possible contact allergens, including contact lens wetting solutions, should be eliminated wherever possible. Desensitisation may be beneficial where there is history of atopic allergy, but is rarely used because of cost, patient noncompliance, and a limited number of allergies against which it is effective.

*Topical antihistamines* (e.g. levocabastine,[22] antazoline or pheniramine), often in combination with a vasoconstrictor, may be useful for minimal and infrequent symptoms. *Mast cell stabilisers*, such as sodium cromoglycate (cromolyn sodium) 2 or 4% and lodoxamide 0.1% have proved useful if given before the development of conjunctival redness and swelling.

*Topical corticosteroids* (table IV) may be used in severe, sight-threatening disease but caution is urged because of their potential toxicity (cataract, glaucoma) in susceptible individuals and the chronic nature of the allergic condition. For long term use, ophthalmological consultation is advised. Fluorometholone, medrysone and the newer agent rimexolone have the lowest propensity to raise intraocular pressure, but are the weakest agents and prednisolone or dexamethasone may be needed for acute severe inflammation.

Recently, topical *nonsteroidal anti-inflammatory drugs* have proved effective for relief of seasonal allergic conjunctivitis. Available preparations include diclofenac 0.1%,[23] ketorolac tromethamine 0.5%, and suprofen 1%.

For a review of therapeutic options in ocular allergic disease, see Hingorani and Lightman.[21]

### 3.1 Keratoconjunctivitis Sicca

Keratoconjunctivitis sicca can be caused by deficiency of tear production (with or without Sjögren's syndrome) and may be seen in many people over the age of 50 years. It may also be due to mucin deficiency caused by the scarring of the conjunctiva that may occur with cicatricial trachoma, Stevens-Johnson syndrome, ocular pemphigoid, irradiation, drug therapy (e.g. dyflos) and chemical burns.

**Optimum Treatment**

Treatment consists of artificial tear solutions (see section 2.5) or sometimes bland ointments. The second line of defence is occlusion of the inferior and perhaps superior punctum to maintain the current level of tear function. Often artificial tear solutions containing no preservatives are helpful in these patients.

Rarely, tarsorrhaphy is necessary to shorten the palpebral fissure. Soft contact lenses may be beneficial in conjunction with tear substitutes in selected cases.

## 4. Cataracts

A cataract is defined as any opacity in the crystalline lens of the eye. A It is responsible for half the cases of blindness in the world. In the US, the prevalence of cataracts in 50- to 85-year-olds has been estimated at 12%,[24] while 13.6% (9.7% of men and 16.8% of women) of persons over 40 years of age have cataracts.[25]

### 4.1 Prevention

Cataract formation is multifactorial in nature. Since cataract-related blindness is significant in developing nations, efforts to reduce the incidence should include improving nutrition, reducing diarrhoea and malabsorption, and wearing sunglasses. Ultraviolet light (UV) contributes to the formation of cataracts, and the role of acute light damage, such as sunburn of the eyelids, photokeratitis and solar retinopathy, is acknowledged. However, only recently has long term sunlight exposure been implicated in epidemiological studies as being associated with cataracts, pterygium and age-related macular degeneration.[26,27]

There is a growing list of photosensitising drugs that contribute to UV light-induced ocular damage. Even young children should be recommended to wear sunglasses with sufficient ultraviolet block for both acute and chronic sunlight exposure.

### 4.2 Optimum Treatment

#### *4.2.1 Medical Treatment*

Topical solutions for treatment of cataract (e.g. retinol, ascorbic acid, pantothenic acid and herbal agents) have attracted attention around the world, but none has demonstrated reproducible results in studies.

*Bendazac lysine* (an oxyacetic acid with anti-inflammatory properties) has been shown to inhibit the denaturation of proteins. Although preliminary studies using bendazac lysine 0.1% eye drops or oral therapy with 500mg 3 times daily have suggested that the drug may be useful in delaying the progression of cataract, there is little evidence that it is capable of reversing existing opacity.[28]

#### 4.2.2 Cataract Surgery

The only currently recognised therapy for cataracts is surgical removal. The surgical procedure has undergone considerable evolution, with decreases in the incision size and number of sutures enabled by changes in intraocular lens design and wound management technique. The incidence of complications continues to decrease, especially with the use of topical anaesthesia.

After much research into the legitimacy of cataract surgery, it has been realised that the most important consideration is the needs of the individual patients. Some patients with posterior subcapsular cataracts require surgery very early while others require early intervention because of their work. It is recognised that elderly people who have hip fractures frequently experience ocular problems. Thus, appropriate intervention should be determined on an individual basis.

##### Drugs Used in Cataract Surgery

***Nonsteroidal anti-inflammatory drugs*** (e.g. diclofenac[23]): these agents are often applied preoperatively to prevent constriction of the pupil. They inhibit prostaglandin synthesis and limit surgically-induced miosis. NSAIDs also reduce ocular inflammation without changing intraocular pressure, and may reduce the occurrence and severity of postoperative cystoid macular oedema.

***Topical antibiotics:*** patients with chronic eyelid disease should receive a short course of topical antibiotic therapy to reduce the possibility of postoperative intraocular infection.

***Intraoperative antibiotics:*** intraoperative antibiotics (e.g. gentamicin) have generally been used subconjunctivally at the end of an operation; this remains the surgeon's choice. A common practice is to soak a collagen shield or a hydrophilic contact lens in tobramycin and dexamethasone solution and place it on the eye at the end of the procedure; the antibiotic and the corticosteroid are thus the only prophylaxis administered. Long term studies are necessary to confirm the feasibility of topical *versus* subconjunctival prophylactic therapy.

***Postoperative anti-inflammatory agents:*** postoperatively, patients are given topical corticosteroids (with or without antibiotics) or nonsteroidal anti-inflammatory drugs for 1 to 4 weeks. With the advent of topical cataract anaesthesia without the need for stitches or patches, the patient's convalescence has been further shortened.

***Local anaesthetics:*** bupivacaine 0.25 to 0.75%, lidocaine (lignocaine) 1 to 4%, mepivacaine 1 to 2%, or etidocaine 1% are the standards for regional ocular anaesthesia. Mepivacaine has an inherent vasoconstrictor effect, whereas bupivacaine 0.25 to 0.75% probably has the longest duration of action [480 to 720 minutes without the need for adrenaline (epinephrine)].

### 4.3 Newer Treatment Possibilities

There will always be controversies and new frontiers in the cataract field. The age of oral and topical pharmaceutical agents to block cataract formation is just beginning.[26] Glutathione, sorbitol-lowering agents and herbal products are currently being studied. It is hoped that such therapies will have the potential to reduce the need for cataract surgery and minimise the high cost borne by individuals and health systems.

## 5. Glaucoma

Glaucoma is a group of diseases that share a characteristic, progressive form of optic nerve excavation. The optic nerve damage is usually associated with elevated intraocular pressure (IOP) and any patient with an IOP greater than 21mm Hg should be suspected of having glaucoma. However, the mere presence of elevated IOP is not synonymous with glaucoma, since many patients with elevated pressure do not demonstrate any loss of vision.

Glaucoma may be conveniently discussed in terms of angle closure (or narrow angle), primary open angle, and other types. The diagnosis of acute *angle closure glaucoma* can be made almost immediately when a patient presents with blurred vision, coloured haloes, a painful eye, mid-dilated pupil, intense ciliary injection, and variably elevated IOP.

In contrast, the diagnosis of *open angle glaucoma* may be difficult. The diurnal variation in IOP, visual fields, the gonioangle, and optic cupping must be carefully assessed and followed for diagnostic and treatment purposes. Ophthalmologists use a number of criteria for initiating treatment, such as an enlarging optic cup, progressive visual field changes, or the existence of other risk factors (myopia, pigment on the corneal endothelium or positive family history).

Estimates of the prevalence of glaucoma vary. In the US, up to 2 million patients have the disease, and an additional 5 to 10 million have an elevated IOP. It has been estimated that 50% of patients with glaucoma may be unaware that they have the disease.[29] In the UK, the prevalence of glaucoma in the general population has been estimated at 0.24%, with around 200,000 individuals having the disease.[30]

Since glaucoma is progressive, elderly patients have an increased risk of developing the condition. It has been estimated[31] that 3% of the US population aged 65 years or older has glaucoma. It is particularly common in people over 75 years of age.[32]

### 5.1 Clinical Pharmacology of Drugs Used in Treatment

The various classes of drugs used in the treatment of glaucoma, their mechanisms of action, intraocular pressure (IOP) lowering efficacy, frequency of use, and adverse effects are summarised in table VI.

#### *5.1.1 β-Adrenoceptor Antagonists (β-Blockers)*

Topically applied β-blockers are the most frequently prescribed drugs for the treatment of open angle glaucoma; they reduce IOP by decreasing the rate of aqueous humour production. The currently available agents (table VI) have all proven effective in the treatment of glaucoma when administered twice or in some cases once daily. Timolol is the best studied agent and has been shown to impart significant additional reduction of IOP when added to miotics, but its combination with adrenaline (epinephrine) appears to offer only small additional benefit. Long term studies have shown that timolol retains its effectiveness when used for periods of 5 years or more. A gel-forming preparation of timolol which remains in the precorneal tears film much longer than the drops has recently become available. With this formulation, once-daily administration is possible.

Although the topical β-blockers are generally well tolerated by the eye, several potentially serious systemic adverse effects have been reported in patients using these drugs and are the main reason for discontinuation of therapy. They include bronchospasm, bradycardia or heart failure in predisposed individuals.[33] All ocular β-blockers can potentially cause these systemic effects, although betaxolol, being a relatively $\beta_1$-selective agent, appears to be largely free of adverse respiratory effects.[34,35] However, this may be dose-related and caution should still be exercised in patients with a history of respiratory illness. Stinging on instillation may occur with ocular β-blockers, as may local allergy on rare occasions.

For further information on the clinical pharmacology of ocular β-blockers, see reviews by Brooks & Gillies,[35] Buckley et al.[34] and Chrisp & Sorkin.[36]

#### *5.1.2 $\alpha_2$-Adrenoceptor Agonists (Apraclonidine)*

Apraclonidine, a topically active derivative of the antihypertensive drug clonidine, has been shown to lower IOP by decreasing aqueous humour production. It has proved useful in treating IOP elevations following various anterior segment laser surgical procedures and cataract surgery, and also appears useful in the treatment of glaucoma when used as an adjunct to other medications. In patients with open angle glaucoma receiving timolol 0.5%, twice-daily administration of apraclonidine 0.5% provided significant additional reduction of IOP in a long term study and was as effective in this regard as a higher strength (1%) apraclonidine solution.[37]

Intolerable local adverse effects may, however, limit the long term usefulness of apraclonidine. Allergic conjunctival reactions, which appear to be related to the drug itself and not to preservatives,[38] have been reported in a significant percentage of patients (10 to 30%) during continued usage.

#### *5.1.3 Sympathomimetics*

The sympathomimetics (adrenaline and its prodrug dipivefrine) are less commonly used nowadays because of the emergence of more effective/better tolerated agents.

*Adrenaline (epinephrine)* lowers IOP by increasing trabecular as well as uveoscleral aqueous outflows. It is administered in concentrations ranging from 0.25 to 2%, and may be employed in addition to pilocarpine in patients not responding sufficiently to the latter. Because of its ability to dilate the pupil, adrenaline is contraindicated in patients with angle closure glaucoma.

*Dipivefrine (dipivalyl adrenaline)* is an ester prodrug of adrenaline that is converted to the active form by corneal esterases. Esterification of adrenaline with two pivalic acid groups increases its lipid solubility and corneal absorption 10- to 17-fold. A 0.1% solution of dipivefr-

**Table VI.** Properties of drugs currently used in the medical management of glaucoma

| Drug | Mechanism of action | Dosage form(s) | IOP lowering efficacy | Frequency of use | Adverse effects/notes |
|---|---|---|---|---|---|
| **Miotics – topical** | | | | | |
| Pilocarpine | *Parasympathomimetic:* increased trabecular aqueous outflow | Ophthalmic solution 0.5%, 1%, 2%, 3%, 4%, 5%, 6%, 8%, 10% | ++± | 3-4 × daily | Local irritation, blurred vision, ciliary spasm, headache. Tolerance develops after a while (increase strength, switch miotics or add a topical sympathomimetic or β-blocker) |
| | | Ophthalmic gel[a] 4% | +± | Once daily | Similar adverse effects as above. Less frequent administration may improve patient compliance |
| | | Ocular insert ('Ocusert')[b] 20 μg/h, 40 μg/h | ++± | Once weekly | Reduced incidence of pilocarpine adverse effects and improved effectiveness due to greater convenience for patient, though some unable to keep insert in the eye or do not tolerate foreign body sensation |
| Carbachol | *Parasympathomimetic:* increased trabecular aqueous outflow | Ophthalmic solution 0.75%, 1.5%, 2.25%, 3%. | ++ | 3 × daily | Local irritation, blurred vision, ciliary spasm, headache. Stronger than pilocarpine because of some anticholinesterase effect, but does not penetrate well. Irregular effectiveness and more rapid development of resistance |
| Ecothiopate iodide | *Cholinesterase inhibitor:* increased trabecular aqueous outflow | Ophthalmic solution 0.03%, 0.06%, 0.125%, 0.25% | ++± | 2 × daily | Local irritation, ciliary and conjunctival injection, browache, blurred vision. More potent and prolonged effect than direct-acting parasympathomimetics and tolerance takes longer to develop, but adverse effects limit usefulness. Systemic absorption may lead to toxic effects (abdominal cramps, sweating, bradycardia, bronchospasm in asthmatic patients). *NB.* Discontinue use 4 to 6 weeks prior to elective surgery |
| **β-Adrenoceptor antagonists – topical** | | | | | |
| Betaxolol | *All agents:* decreased aqueous humour production | Ophthalmic solution 0.25%, 0.5% | ++ | 2 × daily | *All agents:* transient stinging, tearing. Systemic absorption can occur and may lead to adverse effects such as bronchospasm (risk appears less with betaxolol), bradycardia and heart failure in predisposed individuals |
| Carteolol | | Ophthalmic solution 1%, 2% | ++ | 2 × daily | |
| Levobunolol | | Ophthalmic solution 0.25%, 0.5% | ++± | 1-2 × daily | |
| Metipranolol | | Ophthalmic solution 0.3% | ++± | 2 × daily | |
| Timolol | | Ophthalmic solution 0.25%, 0.5% | ++± | 2 × daily | |
| | | Gel-forming solution 0.25%, 0.5% | ++± | Once daily | |
| **$\alpha_2$-Adrenoceptor agonists – topical** | | | | | |
| Apraclonidine | Decreased aqueous humour production | Ophthalmic solution 0.5% | ++ | 2-3 × daily | Allergic reactions in 10-30% of patients (e.g. pruritus, hyperaemia, tearing, oedema of lids/conjunctiva). Useful adjunctive therapy in patients receiving maximally tolerated doses of other antiglaucoma agents |

**Table VI.** *[Continued]*

| Drug | Mechanism of action | Dosage form(s) | IOP lowering efficacy | Frequency of use | Adverse effects/notes |
|---|---|---|---|---|---|
| **Sympathomimetics – topical** | | | | | |
| Adrenaline (epinephrine) | Increased trabecular and uveoscleral aqueous outflow | Ophthalmic solution 0.25%, 0.5%, 1%, 2% | + | 1-3 × daily | Local irritation, hyperaemia, blurred vision; conjunctival or corneal pigmentation (prolonged use). Reasonably effective when combined with miotics |
| Dipivefrine (dipivalyl adrenaline) | As for adrenaline | Ophthalmic solution 0.1% | +± | 2 × daily | As for adrenaline. Addition of 2 pivalyl side chains makes dipivefrine a prodrug of adrenaline (more lipophilic than adrenaline, and better absorbed and tolerated) |
| **Carbonic anhydrase inhibitors (CAIs) – topical** | | | | | |
| Dorzolamide | Decreased aqueous humour production | Ophthalmic solution 2% | ++ | 3 × daily | Mild stinging, burning, bitter taste; local allergic reactions (caution in sulfonamide-sensitive patients). Few systemic adverse effects reported |
| **Carbonic anhydrase inhibitors (CAIs) – systemic** | | | | | |
| Acetazolamide | *All agents:* decreased aqueous humour production | Tablet 125mg, 250mg SR capsule 500mg | ++ | 2-4 × daily (*Usual dose*: 125-250mg 1 to 4 × daily)[c] | Paraesthesias, anorexia, GI distress, drowsiness, metabolic acidosis, hyperuricaemia, renal calculi, skin rash, blood dyscrasias (rarely); caution in sulfonamide-sensitive patients. Long term usefulness limited by adverse effects |
| Diclofenamide (dichlorphenamide) | | Tablet 50mg | ++ | 2-4 × daily (*Usual dose*: 100mg twice daily initially, then 25 to 50mg 1-3 × daily) | As for acetazolamide but less metabolic acidosis. More renal potassium loss, but not likely to be clinically significant |
| Methazolamide | | Tablet 25mg, 50mg | ++ | 2-3 × daily (*Usual dose*: 50mg 2-3 × daily) | As for acetazolamide but GI disturbances and renal calculi appear less frequent. Penetrates the CSF and aqueous humour 3 to 5 times more rapidly than acetazolamide |

a High viscosity acrylic acid polymer vehicle (provides different results from other formulations).

b Elliptically shaped controlled-release system designed to release pilocarpine continuously following placement into the upper or lower conjunctival sac.

c Sustained-release (SR) formulation of acetazolamide is administered 12-hourly.

*Abbreviations and symbols:* CSF = cerebrospinal fluid; GI = gastrointestinal; CAI = carbonic anhydrase inhibitor; SR = sustained release; IOP = intraocular pressure; + = mild IOP lowering effect; ++ moderate IOP lowering effect; +++ = marked IOP lowering effect.

ine has an approximately equivalent IOP lowering effect as a 2% solution of adrenaline, and is associated with fewer ocular and systemic adverse effects. Dipivefrine is occasionally used as the primary agent in open angle glaucoma, and it has an additive effect when given with other agents. Its twice-daily administration schedule is an advantage, but the relatively high incidence of delayed local allergy must be considered.

#### *5.1.4 Miotics*

This group includes the direct-acting parasymathomimetics pilocarpine and carbachol, and the indirect-acting anticholinesterase drug ecothiopate iodide.

The parasympathomimetic agents have historically been the primary topical therapy for glaucoma. By mimicking the action of acetylcholine on parasympathetic postganglionic nerve endings, they lower IOP by increasing trabecular aqueous outflow. *Pilocarpine* and *carbachol* eye drops have similar durations of activity and are normally administered 3 or 4 times daily. Adverse effects associated with their use include local irritation, frontal headache and blurring of vision due to their effects on accommodation.

The use of pilocarpine ocular inserts ('Ocuserts'), which are inserted on a weekly basis, will usually lower IOP as effectively as daily instillation of pilocarpine drops. However, some patients are not able to keep the insert in the eye and others may not tolerate the foreign body sensation. The 'Ocusert' system would seem to be most useful for some patients who have marked adverse effects with pilocarpine eye drops and for unreliable users of eye drops.

Another pilocarpine formulation available is a 4% aqueous gel in which the vehicle is a high viscosity polymer of acrylic acid. This allows slow release of the active drug and a prolonged duration of effect on IOP, thus permitting once-daily administration.

*Ecothiopate iodide* is the most commonly used ocular anticholinesterase drug. It has a more potent and prolonged effect than the parasympathomimetics and tolerance takes a longer time to develop, but it frequently causes adverse effects (see table V) which may necessitate cessation of therapy. Nevertheless, ecothiopate iodide is still very valuable in selected cases that require maximal medical therapy.

#### *5.1.5 Carbonic Anhydrase Inhibitors*

##### Systemic Agents

The systemic carbonic anhydrase inhibitors (acetazolamide, methazolamide and diclofenamide) act by decreasing the formation of aqueous humour; the precise mechanism of this effect is known, but may involve decreasing sodium efflux into the aqueous humour, secondary to decreasing formation of bicarbonate.[31] The carbonic anhydrase inhibitors are used orally in primary and secondary open angle glaucoma when IOP cannot be controlled with topical agents, but up to 50% of patients are unable to tolerate them because of their adverse effects (see table V). Acetazolamide is the most commonly used agent and is usually given in a dosage of 125 to 250 mg 1 to 3 times daily; a sustained release capsule formulation of acetazolamide is also available and is usually given in a dosage of 500mg twice daily. Methazolamide appears to cause less anorexia and gastrointestinal disturbances, but still has the potential to cause long term adverse effects (e.g. hypokalaemia, renal calculi, paraesthesias, blood dyscrasias, abdominal discomfort, backache, etc.). Diclofenamide (dichlorphenamide) is not chemically related to the other two agents, but all are non-bacteriostatic sulfonamide derivatives and may cause allergic reactions in patients with sulfonamide hypersensitivity.

##### Topical Agents

*Dorzolamide* is a newer carbonic anhydrase inhibitor that is effective in lowering IOP when administered topically. It is specific for carbonic anhydrase II, the isoenzyme involved in the ciliary process. A 2% solution of dorzolamide administered 3 times daily appears to provide good control of IOP in glaucoma patients,[39] and has been shown to have an additive effect when given with timolol and probably other agents.[29] Dorzolamide is associated with some local stinging and burning upon instillation, and some patients experience a bitter taste; however, none of the systemic adverse effects associated with oral carbonic anhydrase inhibitors has been reported.

#### *5.1.6 Other Drugs*

##### Prostaglandins

*Latanoprost* (PhXA41) is one of several topical prostaglandin analogues that is capable of reducing IOP, even in normotensive eyes. Solutions of 0.0035%, 0.006% and 0.0115% administered twice daily have been found to reduce elevated IOP by up to 38% in short term clinical studies.[29] The prostaglandins appear to act via a different mechanism from that of other antiglaucoma agents, and it has been postulated that they increase the amount of fluid leaving the eye by uveoscleral pathways. This suggests that their effects may be additive to those of other agents, and this possibility is currently under investigation. The adverse effects of latanoprost appear to be only topical, consisting of conjunctival redness and occasional headache.

##### Antimetabolite Drugs

*Fluorouracil* injected subconjunctivally, and *mitomycin* applied topically via an applicator, reduce scleral healing and render trabeculectomy more reliable. By identifying a deficiency in glaucoma surgery, clinical researchers have adopted a pharmacological solution.

##### Moxisylyte (Thymoxamine)

This agent is an α-adrenoceptor antagonist. A 0.5% solution of moxisylyte has been used in the acute treatment of angle closure glaucoma.

### 5.2 Optimum Treatment

#### *5.2.1 Angle Closure Glaucoma*

In eyes with anatomically narrow angles, dilatation (spontaneous or drug-induced) may allow the peripheral iris to close off the drainage system from the anterior chamber and cause an acute rise in IOP. In an acute angle closure attack, therapy is aimed at pulling the iris away from the chamber angle. Medical treatment is given until the pressure is normalised and the patient can be carefully evaluated; thereafter, treatment with laser iridectomy is standard. Pilocarpine 2 to 4% is administered every few minutes until the pressure is controlled, then less frequently. Concomitantly, other topical agents (e.g. a β-blocker and apraclonidine) and a carbonic anhydrase inhibitor (e.g. acetazolamide 500mg per day orally) are given until normal or subnormal IOP is attained. For a summary of management, see figure 1.

The advent of argon and Nd : YAG laser technology has made surgical intervention the most frequently employed option for well equipped facilities. Besides being 97% effective, the treatment is rapid and the course of illness is abbreviated.

In certain cases, vigorous mydriasis will help halt the attack. However, the pupils of elderly patients do not dilate well. Topical corticosteroids may be required to reduce inflammation (*NB.* monitor IOP closely; see section 10.1). Occasionally, argon or YAG laser therapy may be used for the immediate treatment of an attack of angle closure glaucoma.

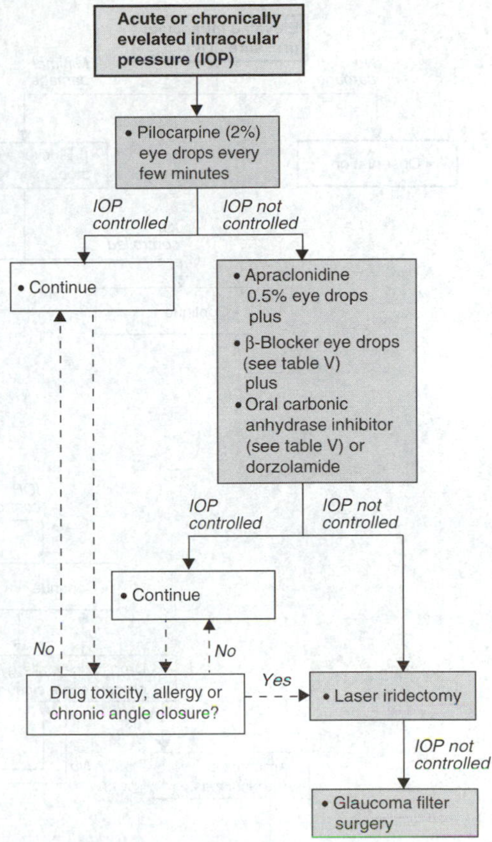


**Fig. 1.** Management of angle closure glaucoma.

### 5.2.2 Primary Open Angle Glaucoma

Most individuals with chronic open angle glaucoma have primary disease. However, other entities with an open chamber angle may be encountered, such as pigmentary glaucoma, pseudoexfolliation glaucoma and conditions where the angle is clogged with inflammatory cells, blood or lens products or active vascularisation (neovascular glaucoma). Therapy for these other types of glaucoma is discussed in section 5.2.3.

Figure 2 summarises the stepwise management of open angle glaucoma. With multiple treatment options available, patients can now have therapy customised to their needs. β-Blockers have become the most popular therapy although their cardiorespiratory adverse effects must be considered, particularly in elderly patients and those with respiratory disease. Pilocarpine remains the least expensive treatment but may affect accommodation, night vision and may increase the risk of cataracts. However, its use may be considered in older individuals, patients who have had intraocular lens replacement, and more refractory cases.

Argon laser trabeculoplasty is moderately effective in lowering IOP for several years. This laser technique for chronic open angle glaucoma is equivalent to one of the stronger topical medicines. For a significant long term decrease in IOP, trabeculoplasty with or without mitomycin (0.4 mg/ml) is advised, especially for progressive cases with limited time to try multiple drop interventions.

### 5.2.3 Other Types of Open Angle Glaucoma

Trauma, inflammation, rubeosis (neovascularisation of the iris and trabeculum), extraocular venous congestion, pseudoexfolliation, Fuchs' heterochromic cyclitis, essential iris atrophy (iridocorneal endothelial syndrome), and phakomatoses may cause unilateral open angle glaucoma. Early chronic simple glaucoma must also be ruled out.

***Secondary glaucoma*** is managed by controlling the primary ocular condition and by following the general treatment rules for open angle glaucoma (see section 5.2.2). Pupillary dilata-

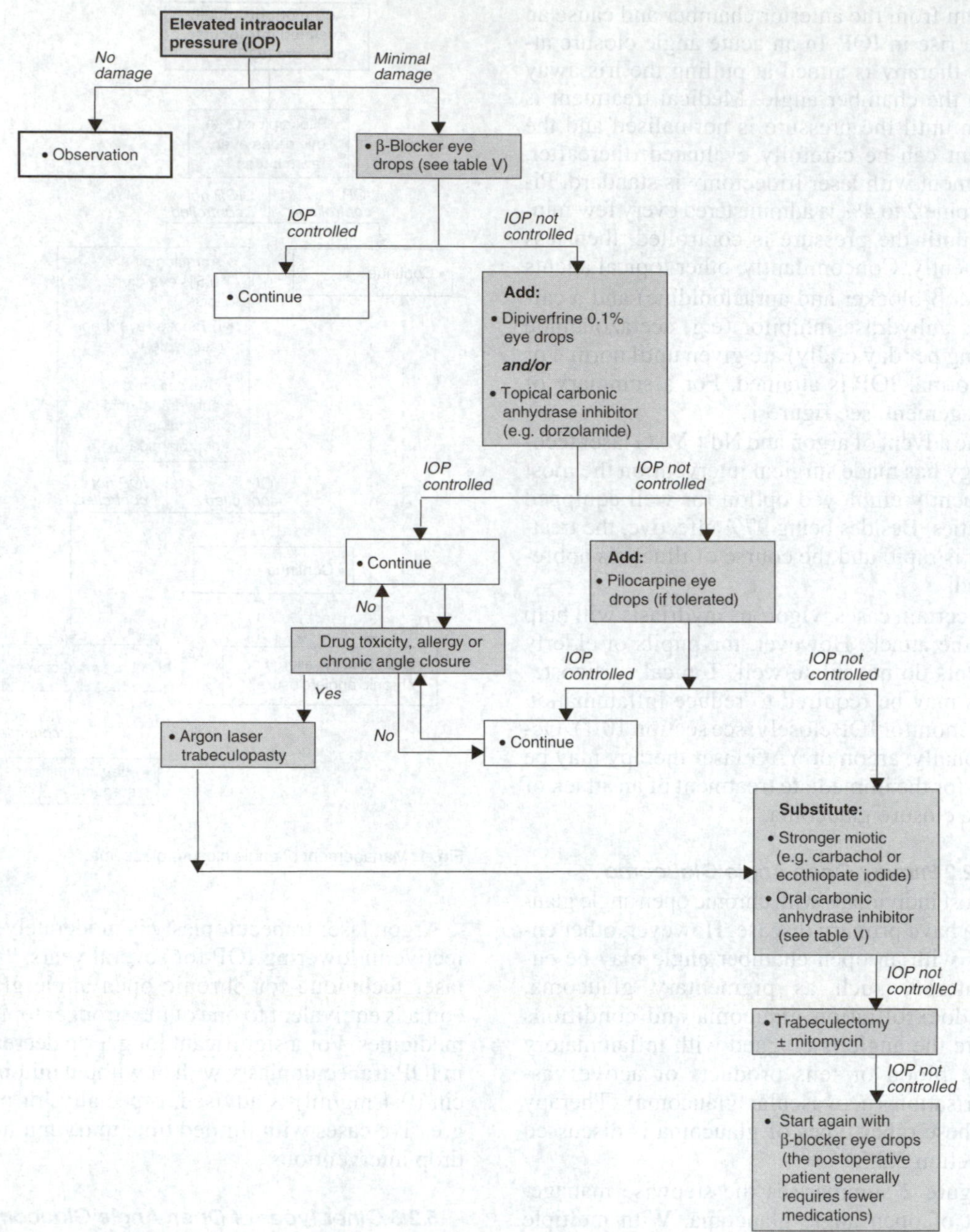


**Fig. 2.** Management of open angle glaucoma.

tion is preferable in cases where intraocular inflammation is present.

***Low tension glaucoma*** (when normal intraocular pressure is associated with progressive disc and visual field changes because of vascular insufficiency) must be considered in certain cases of open angle glaucoma. Intraocular pressure should be lowered, but the prognosis for continuing visual field loss is not good.

***Children*** with glaucoma may present with eye rubbing, photophobia, excess tearing, corneal enlargement and opacification, and abnormal anatomy of the trabeculum, iris or cornea. After infancy, headache and coloured haloes around lights are prominent symptoms; optic cupping and visual field changes may be observed. Trabeculectomy is usually preferable to medical management in this age group.

***Malignant glaucoma*** following intraocular surgery is treated by vigorous dilatation (with care not to create significant mydriasis in a susceptible fellow eye) with acetazolamide. A flat (postoperative) anterior chamber must be reformed. Occasionally, rupture of the hyaloid face must be used to break pupillary block. Transient pressure elevations may follow intraocular surgery.

### 5.3 Clinical Outcome and Economic Considerations

Since glaucoma is usually a long term disease, economic considerations are important, particularly as the elderly population (in whom glaucoma is most prevalent) is increasing in size and improvements in diagnostic techniques may increase the total number of patients with identified disease. In the US, it has been estimated that the cost of glaucoma care will quadruple over the period from 1988 to 2000 if there are no cost constraints.[40] In the UK, the total economic burden of glaucoma in 1990 was estimated as follows: direct medical costs £61 million; direct non-medical costs (residential care) £26 million; and indirect costs in lost production £132.5 million.[30] It may be possible to decrease the total costs attributable to glaucoma care by changing the way that care is provided, and by better definition of the costs and benefits associated with the currently available treatment options to assist in decisions regarding the timing of surgical and drug therapy.

In this respect, improved screening programmes to detect glaucoma are an important consideration. While an opportunistic screening programme would lead to additional healthcare costs, from both the screening procedure itself and the follow-up and treatment of patients who would not otherwise have been identified as having glaucoma, this must be balanced against potential reductions in the need for surgery and in improved visual health of the population (with consequent reductions in direct and indirect costs). Detection may allow patients to receive drug therapy early enough to reduce the requirement for hospitalisation and surgical intervention.[30] Therefore, regular eye examinations after the age of 35 years are to be encouraged, particularly in individuals with predisposing conditions (family history, diabetes, cardiovascular disease, hypertension, thyroid disease, chronic obstructive pulmonary disease, hyperlipidaemia, etc.), and in populations that currently receive little health care.

## 6. Uveitis

The term 'uveitis' signifies any inflammation of the uveal (vascular) coat of the eye and includes a variety of conditions such as iritis, cyclitis, iridocyclitis, peripheral retinitis, choroiditis, and chorioretinitis. However, while these various classifications of uveitis are useful for descriptive and diagnostic purposes, they do not always indicate specific therapeutic regimens.

An anatomical classification dividing uveitis into anterior, posterior and mixed correlates with the knowledge that topical and subconjunctival administration of corticosteroids produces high drug concentrations in the anterior segment of the eye and that retrobulbar and systemic routes provide adequate drug concentrations in the posterior segment.

A histopathological classification[41] divides uveitis into exogenous and endogenous, suppurative and non-suppurative, and the latter into granulomatous and non-granulomatous lesions. Exogenous uveitis is due to the introduction of foreign material or pathogens into the eye and is generally suppurative. Endogenous uveitis may be related to idiopathic ocular disease or systemic disorders, and is generally non-suppurative.

The most frequent causes of uveitis are trauma, idiopathic, and systemic disease, in that order. Idiopathic iritis (uveitis) may recur and become refractory.

### 6.1 Optimum Treatment

The diagnosis and treatment of uveitis conditions is frequently perplexing and frustrating. Table VII lists the more common specific causes of uveitis and specific treatment (where this is possible). It cannot be overemphasised that a thorough and continuing evaluation of a given patient's medical history and general health, combined with a discerning approach to therapy, is basic to successful management.

#### Nonspecific Treatment

Topical *cycloplegics* (see section 2.6.1) and *corticosteroids* (table IV) are the mainstay of nonspecific therapy and are frequently sufficient to stop the anterior segment uveal reaction. Solutions of 0.2 to 0.5% scopolamine (hyoscine), 1% atropine or 5% homatropine are used to achieve pupillary dilatation and relaxation of the ciliary body; atropine also decreases

**Table VII.** Causes and treatment of uveitis

| Cause | Notes and guide to treatment |
|---|---|
| Infection (gonococcal, toxoplasmosis, herpes, etc.) | Appropriate systemic antimicrobial agent in full dosage |
| Associated systemic disease (rheumatoid arthritis, ankylosing spondylitis, systemic lupus erythematosus, sarcoidosis, etc.) | Treat underlying condition, or use topical corticosteroids, cycloplegia and occasionally systemic corticosteroid/antimetabolite therapy |
| Trauma | Uveitis usually acute, anterior and responsive to topical corticosteroids and cycloplegia |
| Allergy (drug, foreign protein or bacterial hypersensitivity) | Treat as nonspecific uveitis (see section 6.1); antihistamines usually not very effective |
| Toxicity (external, intraocular foreign body) | Remove any foreign substances (especially iron and copper) whenever possible |
| Sympathetic ophthalmia | Prophylaxis (surgery) may be only means of cure.<br>For active sympathetic uveitis: cycloplegia, analgesics, intensive systemic or topical corticosteroids, cytotoxic agents |
| Primary intraocular disease | Often refractory to treatment, but spontaneous remissions and exacerbations occur (pars planitis or peripheral uveitis, cyclitis), or is generally benign (heterochromic iridocyclitis). Some conditions may require maximum therapy as for sympathetic ophthalmia. Most cases are idiopathic in origin |

vascular permeability. Dexamethasone 0.1% or prednisolone 1.0% drops should be instilled frequently during the day and their ointment forms applied at night.

Topical NSAIDs (e.g. diclofenac 0.1%) may be effective in both the prevention and treatment of postoperative iritis and cystoid macular oedema. Oral NSAIDs or antimalarial drugs (e.g. hydroxychloroquine) may be effective for accompanying arthritis in selected cases (see further chapter 25; sect. 3.1.3).

The use of subconjunctival, subtenon, and retrobulbar corticosteroid injections may provide higher intraocular concentrations for several days to several weeks. These routes are used for acute exacerbations, for focal chorioretinal lesions, to decrease the frequency of application of topical agents, and to avoid the requirement for systemic corticosteroids. The latter are necessary for chronic refractory uveitis. The corticosteroid dose should be kept to a minimum and gradually reduced whenever possible. Guidelines for the duration or cessation of therapy are not rigidly established. Relapses and rebound phenomena are common. Failure to respond to one corticosteroid preparation may rarely be overcome by changing to another.

Immunosuppressive agents have been used in selected cases of refractory ocular inflammatory conditions, including uveitis. *Methotrexate* and *cyclophosphamide* have been successfully employed in the treatment of sympathetic ophthalmia, cystoid macular oedema due to chronic pars planitis, scleromalacia perforans, Wegener's granulomatosis and Behçet's disease.[42] However, corticosteroids have remained the mainstay of therapy for chronic inflammatory conditions.

*Cyclosporin* therapy[43-47] may be useful in chronic iritis or graft rejection, and in cases that have proven refractory to systemic corticosteroids and cytotoxic agents.

## 7. Diseases of the Retina

### 7.1 Age-Related Macular Degeneration

Macular degeneration in elderly patients is an increasing occurrence in our society. Exposure to ultraviolet light, nutritional factors (decreased gastrointestinal absorption), age, smoking and systemic diseases (e.g. hyperlipidaemia, diabetes, hypertension and atherosclerosis) contribute to the growing numbers of people with degeneration in the centre of the retina.[48,49] 15.3% of Caucasian Americans 40 years of age and older have been diagnosed as having some degree of age-related macular degeneration.[25]

#### Optimum Treatment

A small percentage of patients with macular degeneration (approximately 10%) have the exudative or leakage type of the disease. In these individuals, photocoagulation may be effective in stabilising the disease if the centre of the macula has not been disrupted. There is also an entity known as subretinal neovascularisation, which can occur rapidly and destroy vision. Early recognition allows appropriate intervention with argon or krypton laser photocoagulation.

Efforts at containing and possibly treating age-related macular degeneration have largely been nutritional. The use of oral zinc in combination with other vitamins and minerals has been recommended. Laboratory and early clinical studies have shown some dramatic improvement with the use of intravenous retinol, ascorbic acid and tocopherol (vitamins A, C and E), selenium and zinc. A review of the literature has shown the value of mineral supplementation.[48,49] Nevertheless, we must await the results of controlled clinical studies to confirm the effectiveness of this approach. In the meantime, it is recommended that elderly people be encouraged not to smoke, and to control their medical diseases, exercise, stabilise their nutrition, and consider taking vitamin and mineral supplementation.

### 7.2 Diabetic Retinopathy

Patients with either insulin-dependent (IDDM) and non-insulin-dependent diabetes mellitus (NIDDM) may eventually develop leakage in the macula and surrounding retina (nonproliferative retinopathy) or neovascularisation (proliferative retinopathy). In 1990, 13.4% of Americans 40 years of age and older were diabetic, and 5.1% of this population were found to have diabetic retinopathy.[25]

#### Optimum Treatment

Good glycaemic control is often associated with a better long term prognosis for patients with diabetes (see further chapter 19; sect. 3.3). Nonetheless, any diabetic patient can slowly or rapidly develop macular oedema or neovascularisation, making this disease the leading cause of blindness among working-age Americans.[50] An annual eye examination with dilated ophthalmoscopy is important, but may miss a percentage of diabetic retinopathy. Therefore, annual stereoscopic fundus photography has become the standard for detection and staging of diabetes and the fundus.

Retinal photocoagulation for proliferative retinopathy and macular oedema reduces visual loss by 50% in these two conditions.[51] Furthermore, early detection and treatment of eye disease in both IDDM and NIDDM patients has been shown to be cost saving.[50] Early intervention can reverse neovascularisation and avoid associated haemorrhage, scarring and tractional retinal detachment. The Early Treatment of Diabetic Retinopathy Study[52] showed that focal macular photocoagulation was effective for clinically significant macular oedema.

### 7.3 Retinal Vascular Disease

Patients with retinal vascular disease should be carefully evaluated for underlying conditions before therapy is initiated.

#### Optimum Treatment

Retinal vasculitis can be treated with corticosteroids, or anticoagulants when vascular occlusion is imminent, and by discontinuing drugs such as oral contraceptives.

Retinal vein occlusion is occasionally treated with inhibitors of platelet aggregation (see chapter 26; sect. 3.1.1) and monitored for the delayed appearance of haemorrhagic glaucoma. Laser photocoagulation has proven effective for branch vein occlusions, macular oedema or neovascular complications. Argon and krypton laser photocoagulation may be effective in the exudative type of senile macular degeneration. If patients are taking oral contraceptives, these should be discontinued. Alteplase (rt-PA) is being studied for use in removal of large subretinal clots.

Retinal arterial occlusions, when diagnosed immediately, are treated with anterior chamber paracentesis or carbon dioxide rebreathing. However, the visual loss is generally irreversible because therapy is ineffective after 15 minutes of occlusion.[53]

### 7.4 Macular Oedema

Swelling in the centre of the retina is called cystoid macular oedema. The usual cause is inflammation and may be the result of cataract surgery, intraocular inflammation, long standing uveitis, light toxicity or perhaps even certain medications.

#### Optimum Treatment

The treatment of cystoid macular oedema consists of topical NSAIDs (e.g. diclofenac 0.1%), corticosteroids or oral carbonic anhydrase inhibitors. However, a small percentage of lesions will remain refractory and may respond either to nothing or to vitrectomy.

Trauma can lead to a number of retinal and vascular disorders. Berliner's macular oedema seems to be reversible, whereas chorioscleral rupture leads to permanent visual impairment. Vitreous haemorrhage, secondary to ocular trauma, usually resolves but may be associated with a traumatic peripheral retinal tear which, if not diagnosed in time, can lead to retinal detachment.

### 7.5 Retinopathy of Prematurity

Prematurity itself is the leading cause of blindness among premature infants. Cryotherapy reduces the likelihood of blindness, as demonstrated by one study in which sight was saved in 321 out of 1000 cases by this form of treatment.[54] Therefore, monthly screening of all premature infants is recommended to identify the early changes in the retina and to start therapy.[54]

### 7.6 Acquired Immune Deficiency Syndrome (AIDS) and the Eye

The anterior segment manifestations of human immunodeficiency virus (HIV) infection are numerous. The most frequent of these is dry eye syndrome, but various infections also occur, including herpes simplex keratitis, herpes zoster, ulcerative keratitis, molluscum contagiosum and microsporidiosis, while Kaposi's sarcoma can also cause eye problems.[55]

Before the AIDS epidemic, cytomegalovirus (CMV) retinitis was rarely seen in other than immunosuppressed individuals. Initial complaints in patients with CMV retinitis include light flashes, multiple floaters, foggy vision and loss of peripheral and central vision. Haemorrhage and necrosis in the retina can progress to total retina destruction and blindness if untreated. *Ganciclovir* and *foscarnet* (see table V) have proved useful in this condition but long term maintenance therapy is usually required (see further chapter 32; sect. 3.2).

At least a dozen other infectious agents have caused retinal (or choroidal) disease in AIDS patients. These include varicella-zoster virus, herpes simplex virus, *Toxoplasma gondii*, *Pneumocystis carinii*, *Cryptococcus neoformans*, *Mycobacterium avium* and *Mycobacterium tuberculosis*.[55] Concern for systemic disease with each of these entities as well as the potential for spread is valid; therefore, rapid identification and therapy is important.

### 7.7 Retinal Degenerations and Dystrophies

Retinitis pigmentosa appears to be a degenerative disease related to abnormal recycling of outer photoreceptor segment and is associated with increased vision loss with time.

#### Optimum Treatment

Up to 30,000IU of retinol (vitamin A) daily may slow the disease in patients who are affected by the different forms of retinitis pigmentosa. In these individuals, 400IU of tocopherol (vitamin E) daily appears to be as good as oral retinol.[56]

Retinal dystrophies remain a therapeutic enigma. It is hoped that a specific enzyme deficiency can be isolated for the amaurotic familial idiocies, macular dystrophies, the mucolipidoses and the mucopolysaccharidoses.

## 8. Diseases of the Optic Nerve

### 8.1 Papilloedema

Papilloedema may be caused by increased intracranial pressure (see further chapter 29; sect. 6) and less frequently by increased intraorbital pressure or sudden decreased intraocular pressure. Thorough radiological (computed tomography scans and nuclear magnetic resonance imaging) and laboratory evaluation is imperative. Pharmacological causes of benign intracranial hypertension (e.g. tetracycline, triamcinolone, retinol excess) should be eliminated. Infectious causes should be immediately identified and treated, wherever possible.

#### Optimum Treatment

Intracranial pressure can be rapidly lowered with intravenous mannitol (or other hyperosmotic agents; see further chapter 29; sect. 6.2), and fluorescein angiography may demonstrate the reversal of some of the optic nerve inflammatory response.

The sudden appearance of papilloedema and papillitis due to leptomeningeal infiltration (e.g. leukaemias and lymphomas) has been dramatically reversed with localised radiotherapy, systemic corticosteroids, and specific intrathecal chemotherapy. Radiation therapy and chemotherapy may be useful in the treatment of solid CNS metastases.[57]

### 8.2 Optic Neuritis

Optic neuritis should be carefully studied and treated before nerve fibre oedema is replaced by gliosis, leading to optic atrophy. Cranial arteritis may respond to corticosteroid therapy (see further chapter 25; sect. 6.1), while vascular insufficiency in suitable cases may be improved by carotid endarterectomy. Drug-induced optic neuritis is another presentation.

The diagnosis of multiple sclerosis as the cause of optic neuritis can be made by magnetic resonance scanning of the brainstem, where more than one area of opacification may be diagnostic. Corticosteroids are no longer recommended as the first-line of treatment and have been replaced by supportive therapies, including a low-fat diet.

Non-arteritic optic neuritis doesn't respond well to treatment. Arteritic optic neuropathy can be caused by circulatory disorders. Vasculitis, such as cranial arteritis, must be ruled out, but may be amenable to treatment.

## 9. Miscellaneous Ophthalmological Disorders

### 9.1 Thyrotoxic Exophthalmos

The pathogenesis of thyrotoxic or thyrotrophic exophthalmopathy remains unexplained and may be more frequently encountered after medical rather than surgical management of Graves' disease. When the exophthalmos becomes 'malignant', causing optic nerve compromise, multiple extraocular muscle pareses or exposure keratitis, several procedures have been used. These include high-dose systemic corticosteroids,[58] low-dose radiation,[59] orbital decompression, and short term cyclophosphamide.

### 9.2 Orbital Pseudotumour

Orbital pseudotumour, a cause of proptosis diagnosed by exclusion and biopsy, is also treated with corticosteroids and orbital decompression. Computed tomography scans are helpful in the diagnosis of proptosis and exophthalmos.

### 9.3 Intraocular Tumours

Drug therapy is usually the last choice in treatment of intraocular tumours. For retinoblastoma, the affected eye or worse eye (when the disease is binocular) is often enucleated and supravoltage radiation is given for involvement of the second eye and for metastases. Genetic investigation and counselling are essential. If diagnosis of a choroidal melanoma is convincing, enucleation or local excision are often the treatments of choice, depending on the size of the tumour.[60]

Ocular wall resection of localised choroidal melanomas and localised cobalt plaque is being performed at several centres. Vincristine, carmustine and dacarbazine are combined for treating a melanoma in an only eye or for metastatic disease (see further chapter 27). Photocoagulation to the adjacent retina has been used to contain an overlying retinal detachment.

Ocular complications may be associated with autoimmune disorders, leukaemia and lymphomas. The haematogenous neoplasms can infiltrate the conjunctiva, retina (leukaemia), orbit, and rarely the cornea (leukaemia) and choroid (lymphoma). Treatment is usually directed at the systemic disease (see chapter 27). Orbital involvement usually responds to radiation.

## 10. Use of Drugs in the Presence of Associated Ocular Disease

### 10.1 Glaucoma

The systemic administration of agents such as corticosteroids and anticholinergics (e.g. anti-Parkinsonian drugs, tricyclic antidepressants, and the antiarrhythmic drug disopyramide) and the topical use of corticosteroids and sympathomimetics (e.g. adrenaline and phenylephrine) may sometimes have adverse effects in patients with associated ocular diseases which are often unsuspected. The susceptibility to angle closure and open angle glaucoma should always be anticipated when these agents are being used. Glaucoma is most likely to occur in the elderly patient who has hyperopia (farsightedness) and is developing early cataractous changes (see further section 2.2).

Adrenaline (epinephrine) and phenylephrine dilate the pupil when applied topically, and may also induce angle closure glaucoma in predisposed patients. The effect of systemically administered sympathomimetic drugs (e.g. anorexiants, common cold remedies) is unclear, but is probably only significant in those with very shallow anterior chambers and probably only rarely so.

The use of systemic anticholinergic drugs is much less of a problem in patients with chronic open angle glaucoma, since their anterior chambers are much deeper, allowing pupillary dilatation without the danger of precipitating angle closure glaucoma. In only a minority of patients with chronic open angle glaucoma have systemic anticholinergic drugs caused a significant rise in intraocular pressure, and this has usually been readily controlled by adjustment of the glaucoma treatment. Thus, systemic anticholinergic drugs may be safely given to most patients with open angle glaucoma if the management is shared between the clinician and ophthalmologist. If the patient is already receiving miotic drug therapy for glaucoma, the risk of pupillary dilatation with these drugs is infinitesimally small.

Systemic corticosteroids may sometimes make glaucoma more difficult to control in patients with chronic open angle disease. Topical corticosteroids certainly carry a risk of inducing a sudden rise in intraocular pressure in patients with open angle glaucoma and their use must be closely supervised. Alternatively, agents such as medrysone, fluorometholone or rimexolone which have lesser potential to raise intraocular pressure could be used for treatment of external inflammatory and allergic conditions.

### 10.2 Infections

In patients with bacterial infections, herpes simplex or vaccinia keratitis, topical corticosteroids may exacerbate the condition and are therefore contraindicated until antimicrobial control has been achieved. Some ophthalmologists do, nevertheless, use topical corticosteroids in herpes simplex keratitis, especially with stromal involvement and iritis, but only in conjunction with an antiviral agent (see section 3.7). Topical corticosteroids will, however, temporarily fade the subepithelial opacities of epidemic keratoconjunctivitis, quell the iritis of herpes zoster ophthalmicus, and ameliorate the symptoms of Thygeson's punctate keratopathy.[61]

If a hypersensitivity-induced blepharitis, conjunctivitis, or keratitis is suspected, it is prudent not to treat the condition with any of the more sensitising topical antimicrobial preparations (e.g. neomycin, bacitracin, sulfonamides) or to use agents such as dipivefrine or apraclonidine.

## References

1. Sheldrick JH, Vernon SA, Wilson A, et al. Prospective study of diagnostic accord between general practitioners and an ophthalmologist in 1103 patients over a twelve month period. British Medical Journal 1992; 304: 1096-8
2. Benson H. Permeability of the cornea to topically applied drugs. Archives of Ophthalmology 1974; 91: 313
3. Schoenwald RD. Ocular drug delivery: pharmacokinetic considerations. Clinical Pharmacokinetics 1990; 18: 255-69
4. Johnston WH, Wellish KL, Beltran F, et al. Collagen shields. International Ophthalmology Clinics 1993; 33: 93-107
5. Cox WV, Kupferman A, Leibowitz HM. Topically applied steroids in corneal disease: I. The role of inflammation in stromal absorption of dexamethasone. Archives of Ophthalmology 1972; 88: 308
6. Hugues F-C, LeJeunne C. Systemic and local tolerability of ophthalmic drug formulations. Drug Safety 1993; 8: 365-80
7. Rank RG, Whittum-Hudson JA. Animal models for ocular infections. Methods of Enzymology 1994; 235: 69-83
8. Engerman RL, Kern TS. Retinopathy in animal models of diabetes. Diabetes Metabolism Reviews 1995; 11: 109-20
9. Jones DB. Early diagnosis and therapy of bacterial corneal ulcers: external ocular diseases, diagnosis and current therapy. International Ophthalmology Clinics 1973; 13: 1
10. Hobden JA, O'Callaghan RJ, Insler MS, et al. Ciprofloxacin ointment versus ciprofloxacin drops for therapy of experimental Pseudomonas keratitis. Cornea 1993; 12: 138-41
11. McCloskey RV. Topical antimicrobial agents and antibiotics for the eye. Medical Clinics of North America 1988; 72: 717-22
12. Leibowtiz HM, Pratt MJ, Flagstad LJ, et al. Human conjunctivitis. II. Treatment. Archives of Ophthalmology 1976; 94: 1752
13. Abel Jr R. Therapeutic indications for soft contact lenses. Delaware Medical Journal 1975; 47: 515
14. Holly FJ, Lemp MA. Tear physiology and dry eyes. Survey of Ophthalmology 1977; 22: 69
15. Fraunfelder FT, Scafidi AF. Possible adverse effects from topical ocular 10% phenylephrine. American Journal of Ophthalmology 1978; 85: 447
16. Friedberg MA, Rapuano CJ. Wills Eye Hospital office and emergency room diagnosis and treatment of eye disease. Philadelphia: JB Lippincott, 1990
17. O'Hara MA. Ophthalmia neonatorum. Pediatric Clinics of North America 1993; 40: 715-25
18. Jones BR, Darougar S, Mohsenine H, et al. Communicable ophthalmia: the blinding scourge of the Middle East. British Journal of Ophthalmology 1976; 60: 492
19. St Georgiev V. Management of toxoplasmosis. Drugs 1994; 48: 179-88
20. Asbell PA, Torres MA. Therapeutic dilemmas in external ocular disease. Drugs 1991; 42: 606-15
21. Hingorani M, Lightman S. Therapeutic options in ocular allergic diseases. Drugs 1995; 50: 208-21
22. Noble S, McTavish D. Levocabastine: an update of its pharmacology, clinical efficacy and tolerability in the topical treatment of allergic rhinitis and conjunctivitis. Drugs 1995; 50: 1032-49
23. Goa KL, Chrisp P. Ocular diclofenac: a review of its pharmacology and clinical use in cataract surgery, and potential in other inflammatory ocular conditions. Drugs & Aging 1992; 2: 473-86
24. Kahn HA, Milton RC. Revised Framingham eye study prevalence of glaucoma and diabetic retinopathy. American Journal of Epidemiology 1980; 111: 769-76
25. Prevent Blindness America. Vision Problems in the US: a report on blindness and vision impairment in adults age 40 and older. Washington: Prevent Blindness America, 1994
26. Roh S, Weiter JJ. Light damage to the eye. Journal of the Florida Medical Association 1994; 81: 248-51
27. Harding JJ. Pharmacological treatment strategies in age-related cataracts. Drugs & Aging 1992; 2: 287-300
28. Balfour JA, Clissold SP. Bendazac lysine: a review of its pharmacological properties and therapeutic potential in the management of cataracts. Drugs 1990; 39: 575-96
29. Serle JB. Pharmacological advances in the treatment of glaucoma. Drugs & Aging 1994; 5: 156-70
30. Coyle D, Drummond M. The economic burden of glaucoma in the UK: the need for a far-sighted policy. PharmacoEconomics 1995; 7: 484-9

31. Hurvitz LM, Kaufman PL, Robin AL, et al. New developments in the drug treatment of glaucoma. Drugs 1991; 41: 514-32
32. Klein BEK, Klein R, Sponsel WE, et al. Prevalence of glaucoma: the Beaver Dam eye study. Ophthalmology 1992; 99: 1499-504
33. Fraunfelder FT, Meyer SM. Systemic reactions to ophthalmic drug preparations. Medical Toxicology and Adverse Drug Experience 1987; 2: 287-93
34. Buckley MMT, Goa KL, Clissold SP. Ocular betaxolol: a review of its pharmacological properties, and therapeutic efficacy in glaucoma and ocular hypertension. Drugs 1990; 40: 75-90
35. Brooks AMV, Gillies WE. Ocular β-blockers in glaucoma management: clinical pharmacological aspects. Drugs & Aging 1992; 2: 208-21
36. Chrisp P, Sorkin EM. Ocular carteolol: a review of its pharmacological properties, and therapeutic use in glaucoma and ocular hypertension. Drugs & Aging 1992; 2: 58-77
37. Stewart WC, Ritch R, Shin DH, et al. The efficacy of apraclonidine as an adjunct to timolol therapy. Archives of Ophthalmology 1995; 113: 287-92
38. Butler P, Mannschreck M, Lin S, et al. Clinical experience with the long-term use of 1% apraclonidine. Archives of Ophthalmology 1995; 113: 293
39. Weinreb RN, Kass MA, Lippa EA, et al. MS-507 vs MK-417: comparative efficacy of two topically active carbonic anhydrase inhibitors. Ophthalmology 1990; 97 Suppl. 1: 124
40. Lee P. Economic concerns in glaucoma management in the 21st century. Journal of Glaucoma 1993; 2: 148-51
41. Hogan MJ, Zimmerman LE. Ophthalmic pathology, 2nd ed. Philadelphia: WB Saunders Co. 1962: 373
42. Yazici H, Barnes CG. Practical treatment recommendations for pharmacotherapy of Behcet's syndrome. Drugs 1991; 42: 796-804
43. Whitcup SM, Salvo Jr EC, Nussenblatt RB. Combined cyclosporine and corticosteroid therapy for sight-threatening uveitis in Behcet's disease. American Journal of Ophthalmology 1994; 118: 39-45
44. Naussenblatt RB, de Smet MD, Rubin B, et al. A masked, randomized, dose-response study between cyclosporine A and G in the treatment of sight-threatening uveitis of noninfectious origin. American Journal of Ophthalmology 1993; 115: 583-91
45. Atmaca LS, Batioglu F. The efficacy of cyclosporin-a in the treatment of behcet's disease. Ophthalmic Surgery 1994; 25: 321-7
46. Martin DF, DeBarge LR, Nussenblatt RB, et al. Synergistic effect of rapamycin and cyclosporin A in the treatment of experimental autoimmune uveoretinitis. Journal of Immunology 1995; 142: 992-7
47. Faulds D, Goa KL, Benfield P. Cyclosporin: a review of its pharmacodynamic and pharmacokinetic properties, and therapeutic use in immunoregulatory disorders. Drugs 1993; 45: 953-1040
48. Richer S. Multicenter ophthalmic and nutritional age-related macular degeneration study - part 2: antioxidant intervention and conclusions. Journal of the American Optometric Association 1996; 67: 30-49
49. Richer S. Multicenter ophthalmic and nutritional age-related macular degeneration study - part 1: design, subjects and procedures. Journal of the American Optometric Association 1996; 67: 12-29
50. Javitt JC, Aiello LP, Chiang Y, et al. Preventive eye care in people with diabetes is cost saving to the Federal Government. Diabetes Care 1994; 17: 909-17
51. Singer DE, Nathan DM, Fogel HA, et al. Screening for diabetic retinopathy. Annals of Internal Medicine 1992; 116: 660-71
52. Early Treatment of Diabetic Retinopathy Study Research Group. Photocoagulation for diabetic macular edema. Early Treatment of Diabetic Retinopathy Study Report Number 1. Archives of Ophthalmology 1985; 103: 1796-806
53. Ffytche TJ. A rationalization of treatment of central retinal artery occlusion. Transactions of the Ophthalmological Societies of the United Kingdom 1974; 94: 468
54. Javitt JC, Cas RD, Chiang V. Cost-effectiveness of screening and cryotherapy for threshold retinopathy of prematurity. Pediatrics 1993; 91: 859-66
55. Stenson SM, Friedberg DN, editors. AIDS and the eye. New Orleans: Contact Lens Association of Ophthalmology, 1995
56. Berson E. Visual function testing: clinical correlations. Journal of Clinical Neurophysiology 1994; 11: 472-81
57. Wright DC, Delaney TF, Buckner JC. Treatment of metastatic cancer. In: de Vita Jr V, Hellman S, Rosenberg SA, editors. Cancer: principles and practice of oncology. 4th ed. Philadelphia: JB Lippincott, 1993
58. Hiromatsu Y, Tanaka K, Sato M, et al. Intravenous methylprednisolone pulse therapy for Graves' ophthalmopathy. Endocrine Journal 1993; 40: 63-72
59. Prummel MF, Mourits MP, Blank L, et al. Randomized double-blind trial of prednisone versus radiotherapy in Graves' ophthalmopathy. Lancet 1993; 342: 949-54
60. Shields JA. Advances in management of intraocular tumors. Highlights of Ophthalmology 1994; 22: 73-82
61. Hyndiuk RA, Chin GN. Corticosteroid therapy in corneal disease: I. International Ophthalmology Clinics 1973; 13: 112

Chapter 16

# Diseases of the Oral Mucosa

*D.J. Zegarelli*

## Synopsis of Important Principles

1) As in other areas of medicine, accurate diagnosis of oral disease is an important prerequisite to effective therapy.

2) Due to the interaction of the oral cavity with diseases elsewhere in the body and the effect on the oral mucosa of medications used to treat other illnesses, consultation between medical and oral medicine/dental practitioners is often necessary.

3) Many oral mucosal illnesses are benign, inflammatory and self-limiting, though incurable. The clinician must recognise this and advise the patient accordingly, and be satisfied for the moment with controlling the lesions rather than permanently curing them.

4) During the past decade, the incidence of oral candidiasis has increased dramatically. The clinician should be continually alert to the clinical signs and symptoms of oral candidal infection and the numerous factors that predispose to it, particularly medications given to treat other illnesses.

5) The impact of human immunodeficiency virus (HIV) infection and acquired immune deficiency syndrome (AIDS) continues to increase. Oral lesions found in AIDS patients include candidiasis, hairy leukoplakia, aphthae, HIV-related gingivitis/periodontitis, herpetic infection and Kaposi's sarcoma. Treatment of these conditions is basically the same as in the absence of HIV infection, but relapses are common and vigilant follow-up is necessary.

As many as 500 diseases may occur in the mouth. These diseases can be divided anatomically into those that are primarily mucosal, submucosal, odontogenic, intraosseous and paraoral. Specific oral diseases most likely to be encountered by clinicians are those that occur on mucosal surfaces. This is true whether the patient is symptomatic and self-referred, is a referral to an otorrhinolaryngological or dermatological specialist, or is simply an asymptomatic patient presenting for routine examination.

## 1. Clinical Pharmacological Considerations

Oral mucosal involvement may be seen in diseases that are local, systemic, inflammatory, infectious, autoimmune, neoplastic, painful, painless, incurable, etc. Therefore, knowledge of a wide variety of medications is needed to effectively treat these conditions. Medications may be given topically, by sublesional injection, or systemically. In the case of topical administration, the particular characteristics of the oral mucosa may give rise to a number of problems. These characteristics and the difficulties they create include:

1) The wet nature of the oral mucosa which makes direct application difficult and the adherence of medication short-lived.

2) Its movable nature, which may dislodge topically applied agents.

3) The presence of saliva, which tends to digest drugs applied to the mucosa.

As a result of these factors, the search for an ideal topical vehicle has been an arduous and ongoing one. An alternative method for placement and retention of topical medications is the use of dental prostheses as stents, e.g. the application of topical medication to the undersurface of a denture in order to treat an underlying lesion.

In the case of sublesional injection, there are several problems associated with delivering a drug by this route, the major one being the discomfort of the procedure. This is further compounded when the injection is preceded by a local anaesthetic injection. If the lesion is widespread or multifocal, several injections may in fact be necessary to adequately anaesthetise and treat the condition. A second problem is the delivery of injectable medications into thin, taut, dense, bound-down tissues, e.g. the gingiva and hard palate. It is difficult to deposit therapeutic amounts of medication sublesionally into these masticatory mucosal sites. In addition, although some patients can be adequately trained to self-deliver injectable medications into non-oral sites, patients cannot be expected to inject themselves intraorally.

Systemic therapy for oral disease is usually the easiest to administer and generally the most effective. On an outpatient basis, systemic medications for oral mucosal disease are almost always given in tablet or liquid form. Problems with such treatment usually involve systemic adverse effects. Some medications (e.g. corticosteroids, antibiotics, xerostomic agents) can alter the oral cavity environment, making it prone to oral candidal infection, while others can give rise to oral lichenoid lesions. Also, some systemic medications have well-documented oral adverse effects (e.g. gingival hypertrophy with cyclosporin).

## 2. General Principles of Treatment

The oral cavity surface is highly innervated, packed with exceedingly sharp and powerful movable structures, and wet. Unfortunately, it is also dark and emphasis must be placed on adequate lighting to properly visualise all intraoral structures before, during and after instituting treatment regimens. By definition, oral mucosal lesions are surface phenomena and thus the clinician needs to use direct vision to detect a lesion. It is unnecessary to employ sophisticated internal imaging devices to discover and follow-up an oral surface lesion.

Laboratory diagnostic corroboration of an oral mucosal lesion can usually be performed quickly and easily. Most surface phenomena can be diagnosed by a cytological smear, a culture, or small biopsy. The first two procedures can be performed painlessly in less than 2 minutes. Following the delivery of a local anaesthetic, most incisional or excisional intraoral biopsies can be performed in less than 10 minutes.

The following sections of this chapter review the more common intraoral diseases. These conditions in fact represent around 95% of all patients presenting with oral mucosal disease. While some are very common (e.g. oral lichen planus, aphthae, oral candidiasis), others are relatively rare (e.g. pemphigus vulgaris) but have been included because of their unique clinical presentation and therapy, together with their potential morbidity and mortality. Patients presenting with surface skin lesions vastly outnumber those with surface oral lesions. This is one factor that has led to greater pharmacological research in dermatology than in oral medicine. Hence, it is not unusual for oral medicine specialists to borrow medications developed for dermatology and other specialities, and to utilise them orally (e.g. beclomethasone dipropionate aerosol spray).

As in other areas of medicine, there are still many benign inflammatory diseases involving the oral mucosa that are not curable and can only be controlled. Corticosteroids are often prescribed to decrease the intensity of an oral lesion, or perhaps to eradicate it for a brief period of time. Clinicians should therefore become thoroughly familiar with the use of corticosteroids, whether delivered in topical, injectable or systemic dosage forms (for a discussion of the clinical pharmacology of corticosteroids, see chapter 19; sect 7.1.1). Often, intraoral candidal infection presents secondary to a corticosteroid-treated dermatosis. Clinicians treating such combined lesions should therefore be familiar not only with corticosteroids, but also with antifungal agents, and combination corticosteroid/antifungal preparations.

Some patients with chronic oral mucosal disease may simply be diagnosed initially and reexamined periodically without receiving active treatment, particularly those with lesions that are benign, self-limiting or incurable. For lesions that do not compromise the patient's appearance or oral functioning (e.g. oral lichen planus), treatment is not needed unless the patient is also symptomatic.

## 3. Oral Ulcerative Lesions

An oral ulcer is an area of surface epithelial denudation. The ulcerated zone presents with an inflamed surface mesenchyme instead of stratified squamous epithelium.

There are numerous diseases and lesions that can be classified as being ulcerative, or that present at some stage with surface ulceration. However, in this section, the discussion is limited to traumatic ulcers and recurrent aphthous stomatitis. Other ulcerating diseases such as lichen planus, mucosal pemphigoid and pemphigus vulgaris are described in section 4.

### 3.1 Traumatic Ulcers

Traumatic ulcers result from a severe insult to the surface oral mucosa. The insult may be physical (mechanical), chemical, thermal, or a combination of all three. If the insult is severe enough to denude the surface epithelium, there is resultant, usually intense, inflammation. Traumatic ulcers can occur at any age, in either gender, and at any intraoral site. The lesion is painful and can exist singly or in groups. Microscopic examination demonstrates nonspecific ulceration and inflammation. Since the pathological diagnosis is nonspecific, diagnostic accuracy depends on clinical appearance and a thorough clinical history.

#### *3.1.1 Physical (Mechanical) Traumatic Ulcers*

Physically (mechanically)-induced traumatic ulcers can be caused by dentition (cheek, lip, tongue biting), sharp edges on dental fillings, rough denture surfaces, etc. Usually the ulcers are flat, with a grey necrotic centre surrounded by a rim of erythema. If chronic, mechanical ulcers may be crateriform in appearance. When a mechanically-induced ulcer is caused by a chronic nervous habit such as lip biting, the lesion is said to be factitial.

**Optimum Treatment**

The primary treatment of a traumatic ulcer is to eliminate the offending agent. In a dental surgery, this may include smoothing a sharpened tooth cusp or filing or grinding away a roughened denture surface. Once the offending agent is removed, the ulcer should heal in 3 to 10 days. Although the use of drug therapy to eradicate a mechanical ulcer is generally of secondary importance, there are times when a topical corticosteroid may be useful. Beclomethasone dipropionate aerosol (50 μg/puff)[1] sprayed 4 to 12 times a day, and fluocinonide 0.05% cream applied 4 times daily have both proved helpful. For relief of pain, lidocaine (lignocaine) 2% viscous solution or 5% ointment may be used.

Some chronic mechanical ulcers have depressed centres and can appear clinically very similar to a squamous cell carcinoma, particularly when caused by a biting episode involving the posterior lateral tongue. In such cases, surgical excision may be the preferred treatment.

#### *3.1.2 Chemical Traumatic Ulcers*

Some patients may present with chemically-induced traumatic ulcers. Two commonly offending agents are aspirin (acetylsalicylic acid) and, in the US, a phenol/benzocaine/alcohol gel preparation ('Anbesol') which is used topically

1 In the US, beclomethasone dipropionate inhaler is stated to deliver 42 μg/metered dose, since 8μg of the standard 50μg dose delivered by the valve is lodged on the inside of the inhaler device with each actuation.

for toothache pain, aphthous ulcer pain, or even a traumatic ulcer from a denture or sharp filling, etc. Following long term application of these agents to the oral mucosa, the mucosa may eventually slough leaving an ulcerated painful surface. If the phenol/benzocaine/alcohol gel preparation is applied just prior to a surgery visit, the clinician may detect a characteristic pungent medicinal odour. Patients using this preparation often apply it repetitively, since the topical anaesthetic benzocaine provides temporary symptomatic relief as the phenol component causes mucosal ulceration.

#### Optimum Treatment

The treatment of chemically-induced traumatic ulcers is directed primarily at eliminating the cause. Healing should then occur in 3 to 10 days. Other treatment measures should be considered of secondary importance. Lidocaine 2% viscous solution or 5% ointment can be used for relief of pain.

### *3.1.3 Thermal Traumatic Ulcers*

Excessive heat application to the oral mucosa can cause tissue necrosis with subsequent ulceration and pain. Examples include hot liquids such as coffee and tea, as well as hot solid foods such as the classic palatal ulcer caused by hot pizza.

#### Optimum Treatment

Again, treatment should be directed at eliminating the cause. Palliative medications (e.g. lidocaine 2% viscous solution or 5% ointment) should also be considered.

## 3.2 Recurrent Aphthous (Ulcerative) Stomatitis

Recurrent aphthae are very common in the general population. Aphthae have been classified into 4 subtypes:[1] (1) minor; (2) herpetiform; (3) major; and (4) aphthae associated with Behçet's syndrome. Their precise aetiology still remains unknown, but factors that have been proposed as being involved in their aetiology/genesis include heredity, viral disease, L-forms of streptococci, food allergies, emotional stress, menstruation, minor mucosal trauma, and deficiencies of cyanocobalamin (vitamin $B_{12}$), folic acid and iron.[2]

Aphthous lesions of the minor and herpetiform subtypes are characterised by a small mucosal ulcer, usually between 1 and 5mm in diameter. The centre has a grey-white superficial necrotic slough and there is surrounding, usually intense, erythema. If a biopsy is performed, examination will reveal nonspecific ulceration and inflammation, sometimes accompanied by a slight increase in eosinophils. Pain varies from patient to patient, and in some cases can be quite extreme. Lesions come and go and generally persist for 4 to 14 days. Some patients have 2 bouts a year and others have continuous lesions occurring in waves, with previous ulcers waning as a fresh new group arises. Some adults note that lesions are absent for years but then recur.

Minor forms of aphthae usually consist of 2 to 6 small lesions scattered about the oral mucosa. Persons of all ages and either gender can be affected, but young females constitute the highest prevalence group. Although some clinicians consider that true aphthae rarely occur on oral bound-down tissues such as the gingiva and hard palate, in my experience, aphthae may be seen in many patients widespread throughout the oral cavity.

Herpetiform aphthae consist of clusters of numerous tiny lesions that sometimes coalesce into one or more large ulcers. The major form, which is also referred to as recurrent ulcerative scarifying stomatitis, Sutton's disease, or periadenitis mucosa necrotica recurrens, consists of one or more deep crateriform lesions that persist for long periods and, because of extensive deep tissue destruction, heal by secondary intention with scarification. The lesions of Behçet's syndrome have extraoral involvement as well, involving particularly the eyes, genitalia and skin.

#### Optimum Treatment

Since little is known about the aetiology of aphthae, with numerous diverse and sometimes compounded theories being proposed, and since they affect millions of people, it is not surprising that a wide variety of treatment regimens have been used. Some consider that patients with oral aphthae may have lesions generated by food substances. In one investigation,[3] patients were placed on strict elimination diets supplemented with a number of permitted foods and vitamins. On such a regimen, if lesions disappear after starting the diet, it is presumed that a particular food substance served as an allergen and caused the aphthae. Gradually, the patient is then brought back to normal diet status by introducing one food item at a time over 4-day periods. When reintroduction of a specific item causes new lesions, that substance is considered causal. Problems with this approach include the reluctance of patients to participate in such a restrictive diet, despite the intensely painful oral lesions. Moreover, certain crisp, hot or spicy foods may further exacerbate lesions already present, and the patient may mistakenly think they are causal.

A treatment regimen consisting of an antibacterial agent such as tetracycline is preferred by some, the theory being that the antibiotic will eliminate the overlying bacteria, whether they are causal or secondarily infect the aphthae. A tetracycline suspension containing 250mg/5ml has been used:[4] patients are instructed to rinse (for 2 minutes) and then swallow 5ml 4 times daily for 5 to 7 days, discontinuing treatment when lesions are absent. However, children should not take tetracycline because of its potential to cause tooth discolouration. Some investigators[5,6] have used lower tetracycline concentrations of 125mg/5ml, while others have advocated using chlorhexidine gluconate mouthwash - which has been shown to inhibit bacterial plaque formation on teeth and bacterial counts in saliva. A significant reduction in the incidence, duration and discomfort of aphthae treated with chlorhexidine mouthwash has been reported;[7] usually it is prescribed as a 0.12% chlorhexidine gluconate solution, with patients rinsing 15ml for 30 seconds (and then expectorating) twice daily.

Another approach, and the one that I favour, is to commence treatment of aphthae with topical corticosteroid therapy. Beclomethasone dipropionate spray (50 μg/puff)[8] is preferred when there are a few scattered minor aphthae. The patient uses 2 puffs 4 times daily after meals and at bedtime, directing the spray onto the oral lesion(s) with instructions not to inhale as an asthmatic patient would. If the lesions are more numerous and widespread, oral dexamethasone elixir (0.5mg/5ml) may be given with the patient rinsing 5ml for 2 minutes (and then expectorating) 4 times daily after meals and before bedtime. Occasionally, a patient may present with 1 or 2 deep crateriform major aphthae which may have begun as minor aphthae that became chronic and deep secondary to an added physical insult such as trauma from a repetitive lip-biting habit, rubbing against a sharp filling, etc. In such instances, rapid and complete resolution is usually obtained by giving a single sublesional injection of a depot corticosteroid such as methylprednisolone acetate suspension (40 or 80 mg/ml); a dose of 0.3 to 0.8ml of the 40 mg/ml or 80 mg/ml suspension is deposited immediately beneath the lesion. In patients with extremely painful aphthae that compromise important social and/or professional obligations, systemic corticosteroid therapy may be given, e.g. prednisone 30mg daily for the first week, 15mg daily for the second week, and 5mg daily for the third and final week.

Other corticosteroid regimens that have been used for control of aphthae include topical triamcinolone acetonide 0.1% in 'Orabase',[9] and 5ml triamcinolone acetonide 0.1% or 0.2% aqueous suspension rinsed 4 times daily alone or together with oral prednisone 40 mg/day in the morning for 5 days, followed by 20 mg/day every alternate day for an additional week.[2] This systemic regimen is very effective in the control of aphthae and is reported to cause minimal suppression of the HPA (hypothalamic-pituitary-adrenal) axis. The successful use of a combination of azathioprine (50mg twice daily) and dexamethasone 0.5mg/5ml elixir (5ml as a 1-minute rinse 4 times daily) has also been reported in a 32-year-old woman with an extremely severe bout of lingual major aphthous ulceration.[10] The lesion completely resolved over a 3-month period.

***Other therapy:*** *levamisole*, an immunostimulating agent (see chapter 28; sect. 2.2.5) has been found to be effective in controlling aphthae in some studies (see review by Miller[11]). The dosage of levamisole used in these studies was 150mg daily in 3 divided doses given at lesion onset for 3 days, followed by an 11-day period of no drug therapy. The adverse effects of this agent include dysgeusia, hyperosmia and nausea.

There has been recent interest in the use of *colchicine* for treatment of recurrent aphthae.[12] The initial dosage of this drug is 0.6mg 3 times daily which is then increased if necessary, although adverse effects including severe and persistent diarrhoea may eventually emerge. When colchicine is taken long term (e.g. for several years), discontinuation of therapy is often followed by abrupt recurrence. Ulcerations associated with Behçet's syndrome have also been reported to improve with colchicine therapy[13] and it has been suggested that an anti-polymorphonuclear leucocyte effect is responsible for its therapeutic benefit.

Another drug that has been used in the treatment of aphthae is *thalidomide*. In a study of its use in 40 patients,[14] 75% experienced at least marked improvement. Mild cases were treated with thalidomide 100 mg/day initially, this dosage being reduced to 50 mg/day and eventually withdrawn after control was obtained. Severe cases were treated with 300 mg/day with eventual reduction to maintenance dosages of around 100 mg/day. When the aphthae disappeared, the medication was stopped. It must be remembered that thalidomide has well-known teratogenic effects and should be avoided in women of child-bearing potential.

Some attempts at therapeutic control of aphthae have been entirely empirical, and there are a wide range of other topical and systemic preparations available. One that I have used with some success is 7% tannic acid in alcohol ('Zilactin') as a topical adherent protective film. However, it can only be easily applied to anterior oral cavity lesions and it is readily dislodged during the next meal.

Finally, the numerous theories concerning the aetiology of minor aphthae, together with the documented reports of their successful treatment using a wide variety of therapeutic agents, point to the possibility that minor aphthae may not reflect one disease entity, but instead several, each presenting with similar clinical features.

## 4. Oral Dermatoses (Diseases Involving Both the Oral Mucosa and Skin)

Since the oral mucosa is covered by stratified squamous epithelium, it is not surprising that a large number of patients with dermatological diseases are diagnosed and treated in an oral medicine clinic. In fact, a more appropriate term for this practice may be 'oral dermatology'. Dermatological diseases with oral manifestations covered in this section include lichen planus, mucosal pemphigoid, pemphigus vulgaris, and erythema multiforme.

### 4.1 Lichen Planus

Lichen planus is one of the most commonly encountered oral mucosal diseases. Because of its high prevalence and somewhat predictable response to corticosteroid medication, ulcerative lesions of oral lichen planus serve as a general model for corticosteroid therapy of oral ulcerative disease.

The aetiology of oral lichen planus is unknown. Factors such as stress, micro-organisms, heredity, immunological factors, similarities to graft-versus-host disease, and drug reactions have all been implicated at one time or another. It appears to be more common in women than men, with an average age of onset in the 50s, although the disease has been found in patients between the ages of 15 and 80 years. Although it can be found at any oral site, the buccal mucosa and gingivae are most commonly involved. Oral lichen planus can be *multiforme* in clinical appearance and it may present simultaneously in 1 or more of the following 6 forms:

1) *Papular:* the basic lesion in this form is a small, flat, white adherent keratotic dot, approximately 1mm in greatest dimension.

2) *Lacey:* the classic clinical appearance of this form is of linear, flat, adherent and often intersecting lacey white lines. Intersecting foci are called striae of Wickham. A single lace represents a continuum of lichen planus papules forming a line and having the width of a single papule.

3) *Plaquey:* this refers to the presentation of lichen planus in adherent, flat, white patches which have an area, being measured in length and width. It forms when numerous tightly clustered laces fuse into a single white patch.

4) *Ulcerative:* in this form, the surface squamous epithelium of lichen planus is lost, being sloughed away as a result of an intense chronic inflammatory infiltrate immediately beneath the surface epithelium. Clinically, pain is possible and usually the lesion presents with a flat, grey-white adherent surface slough with a peripheral erythematous rim.

5) *Erosive:* typically, erosive lesions are flat and intensely red. The erythema reflects an overlying thinned epithelium with underlying intense chronic inflammation. This form may be painful.

6) *Vesicular:* this is the least common form, and appears as a small blister. However, because of the heat, humidity and almost constant movement of the oral cavity, the thin epithelial covering of a vesicle is ruptured, transforming it into a painful ulcer.

The papular, lacey and plaquey forms have intact surface squamous epithelial coverings. Thus, while there is an intense chronic inflammatory cell infiltrate immediately beneath the surface epithelium in each case, these forms of oral lichen planus are almost always asymptomatic (painless). However, ulcerative, erosive and vesicular forms are usually symptomatic (uncomfortable or frankly painful). Since multiple forms of oral lichen planus can exist simultaneously at any oral site, the painful form merges and often mixes with painless forms. Pain is emphasised in any discussion of the condition because symptoms usually dictate when lichen planus should be treated and which medications should be prescribed.

Biopsy corroboration of oral lichen planus is strongly encouraged. As in most oral cavity lesions, histopathology is the best and most appropriate confirmatory procedure. This is particularly appropriate in oral lichen planus because most oral pathologists accept the premise that the condition is associated with oral squamous cell carcinoma in approximately 1 to 2% of patients. Thus, although oral lichen planus is properly not considered a premalignant lesion for a variety of sound medical reasons, the affected patient should be forewarned of a small but real potential for developing oral cancer. The 3 microscopic features of oral lichen planus are: (1) overlying keratotic material; (2) an underlying band-like layer of chronic inflammatory cells that hugs the overlying epithelium; and (3) liquefaction degeneration of the epithelial basal cell zone.

#### Optimum Treatment

Treatment of oral lichen planus involves 3 basic principles. Firstly, patients should return at least annually for re-examination, to ascertain whether dysplastic change has occurred. This principle should be maintained whether the patient is being actively treated or not. Secondly, the possibility that lichen planus may have been caused by another drug should be considered and that a dosage reduction or cessation of this treatment may improve the condition. However, drug cessation or decreased dosages are not always possible, since the prescribed agent(s) may be controlling diseases that are potentially more harmful than oral lichen planus. Furthermore, cessation of the offending drug does not guarantee elimination of oral lichen planus or that it will be reduced in a particular time period.

The third principle is that drug therapy is not always required, e.g. in patients who are asymptomatic - mostly those with papular, lacey and plaquey forms. Why prescribe medications to patients when they are pain-free, when there are no cosmetic compromises (lesions are intraoral), when there are no functional compromises involving eating, drinking, talking, etc., and when the disease itself is incurable?

Patients presenting with erosive and ulcerative forms may have pain and thus treatment should be offered. Corticosteroids are used for their anti-inflammatory effects and can control but not cure the lesions; however, recurrence is possible following cessation of corticosteroid therapy. Beclomethasone dipropionate spray (50 μg/puff) is helpful in controlling one or more small and medium-sized lesions,[8] the usual dosage being 2 to 4 puffs 4 times daily after meals and at bedtime. Since application is easy, patient compliance is usually better than with corticosteroid creams and ointments. If beclomethasone dipropionate spray is not helpful or if the lesions are numerous and large, a multimodality corticosteroid regimen may be used.[8,15] This comprises:

- 2 to 4 puffs of beclomethasone dipropionate spray 4 times daily after meals and at bedtime, for 3 weeks (*NB.* the patient should be instructed to direct the spray onto the lesions but not to inhale).
- Sublesional injection of 0.5 to 1.5ml methylprednisolone acetate suspension (40 or 80 mg/ml) once weekly for 3 weeks.
- Oral prednisone 30 mg/day for the first of 3 weeks, 15 mg/day for the second week, and 5 mg/day for the third and final week.

Corticosteroid injections are contraindicated in gingival and hard palate sites because it is very difficult to deliver therapeutic amounts to these bound-down, thin mucosal structures.

Beclomethasone dipropionate spray alone or the multimodality corticosteroid regimen will achieve considerable improvement in more than 90% of symptomatic oral lichen planus patients. This is a rather predictable benefit that can be obtained in less than 3 weeks. Some patients with oral lichen planus have secondary oral candidiasis or will develop candidiasis as a result of the corticosteroid regimen. Consequently, it is often necessary to prescribe antifungal agents in conjunction with the corticosteroid therapy (see further section 5.1).

***Other therapy:*** if corticosteroids are unsuccessful in controlling oral lichen planus, some clinicians prescribe *griseofulvin* therapy, which may benefit surface squamous epithelium and keratin, although its exact mechanism of action remains unknown. Considerable improvement in oral lichen planus has been noted in studies with griseofulvin administered in dosages of 500 mg/day for 4 to 8 weeks[16,17] or 500mg twice daily for 8 to 10 weeks.[18] However, in other studies with griseofulvin, only limited improvement[19] or worsening of the condition[20] has been reported.

Another approach has been to use retinoid analogues. *Tretinoin* 0.1% cream has been found to produce dramatic reductions in lesion size in patients with asymptomatic white lesions of oral lichen planus (papular, lacey and plaquey forms), though this was followed by almost immediate recurrence after withdrawal of the medication.[21] Tretinoin cream is administered as a thin film application once daily at bedtime; however, excessive amounts can cause mucosal irritation and its use is probably best reserved for white, keratotic, mildly dysplastic oral lesions (see further section 7). In other studies with retinoids, significant improvement in oral lichen planus has also been reported with topical *isotretinoin* 0.1% gel applied twice daily, but relapses were again noted following withdrawal of treatment.[22] Similarly, systemic retinoid therapy with *etretinate* 25mg 3 times daily produced a marked beneficial effect in one study,[23] although adverse effects required discontinuation of therapy in about 20% of patients. Results with oral *isotretinoin* (10 to 60 mg/day for 8 weeks) were not nearly as impressive, producing only slight improvement and troublesome adverse effects in one study.[24]

There has been recent interest in treating oral lichen planus with the immunosuppressant drug *cyclosporin*. In two studies in which patients rinsed for 5 minutes (and then expectorated) 5ml of cyclosporin oral solution (100 mg/ml) 3 times daily for 8 weeks, marked improvement was noted in all cases.[25,26] However, it should be noted that this form of therapy is expensive.

Since oral lichen planus often presents with widespread clinical involvement, surgical excision is rarely considered. However, a small percentage of patients will present with 1 or 2 small lacey foci and surgical excision of these lesions is possible.

### 4.2 Mucosal Pemphigoid

The pemphigoid group of skin and mucosal diseases is generally divided into 2 forms, bullous and benign mucous membrane; the latter is also referred to as cicatricial pemphigoid or mucosal pemphigoid. There is still debate over whether the 2 diseases are closely related processes or separate entities. Since overlapping cases have been noted, most now consider them to be similar diseases along a single spectrum. Mucosal pemphigoid can involve the eye, oral cavity, upper aerodigestive tract structures, genitalia and skin. Patients in whom the oral cavity is affected are generally between 40 and 70 years of age and more often female. Intraorally, gingival sites are predominant but other sites may be involved such as the buccal mucosa, palate, etc.

Mucosal pemphigoid is considered to be autoimmune in aetiology with antigen/antibody activity at the epithelial basement membrane. Oral pemphigoid is benign, inflammatory and incurable. Thus, treatment is again aimed at controlling rather than curing the condition. In the US, the incidence of mucosal pemphigoid is lower than that of oral lichen planus but higher than that of oral pemphigus.[27]

The most common clinical presentation of oral mucosal pemphigoid is one of gingival involvement, the affected gingival tissues being flat or slightly swollen and bright red. The lesions are usually generalised and involve large areas of gingivae - maxillary and mandibular as well as buccal and lingual. No other intraoral lesion desquamates with the ease of mucosal pemphigoid, at times only the slightest touch provoking sheets of surface epithelial detachment and desquamation. During a biopsy procedure, sometimes the slightest drag of the scalpel blade passing cleanly through affected gingival tissues will cause the adjacent mucosa to peel. The clinically reddened lesion is covered by a thinned and usually intact squamous epithelium and although patients may complain of pain, this symptom occurs less frequently than might be expected. Patients complain instead of discomfort and bleeding tendencies when brushing their teeth. Frank ulcerations may be present and painful, presenting as grey-white sloughs with peripheral erythema. Blisters and vesicles can also be present, but they are almost always short-lived. Usually there is a positive Nikolsky's sign (i.e. rubbing causes a lesion, e.g. desquamation or a blister).

Diagnostic corroboration involves biopsy and immunofluorescence. Biopsy of a lesion reveals a thinned layer of surface squamous epithelium often devoid of rete pegs, with an underlying nonspecific chronic inflammatory cell infiltrate. Areas of subepithelial separation from the underlying inflamed mesenchyme are also noted. Direct immunofluorescence reveals activity at the basement membrane.

#### Optimum Treatment

Treatment is usually commenced with corticosteroids, using topical, injectable, systemic or multiple forms. For mild non-painful gingival lesions, beclomethasone dipropionate spray (50 μg/puff), 2 to 3 puffs directed onto the lesions 4 times daily after meals and at bedtime, can be used. For only 1 or 2 small lesions, gentle application of fluocinonide 0.05% cream 3 or 4 times daily may help. In using topical creams or gels, a form-fitting plastic or rubber gingival tray, made to the exact outline of the maxillary and/or mandibular alveolar ridges, should be considered. The soft, thin custom-made tray is used to carry the topical agent as a thin film 4 to 6 times a day, being held by the dentition directly against the affected gingivae.[28] Similar methods can be used to hold topical medication to the tongue surface.[29]

If topical therapy is ineffective, systemic corticosteroids may be considered. A combined regimen comprising topical corticosteroids in conjunction with oral prednisone burst therapy (40mg once daily in the morning for 5 consecutive days followed by 20mg every alternate day for 2 to 3 weeks) has been used.[30] After clinical control is achieved, maintenance therapy can be provided by the topical corticosteroid alone. If necessary, sublesional injections of a depot corticosteroid can be utilised, as for oral lichen planus (see section 4.1). Again, candidiasis can be problematic and consideration should be given to simultaneous antifungal therapy.

Another approach that has been successfully used in managing mucosal pemphigoid is the use of *dapsone*.[31,32] An initial dose of 25 to 50 mg/day, with a slow increase to 125 to 150 mg/day has been used. Beneficial effects may not be evident for 6 weeks, and ultimately some form of maintenance therapy is likely to be necessary. The slow dose increase may allow the patient's bone marrow to adapt to the adverse haemolytic effects of dapsone. Dapsone is contraindicated in patients with glucose-6-phosphate dehydrogenase (G6PD) deficiency because of the risk of haemolysis and methaemoglobinaemia.

Mucosal pemphigoid is less responsive to corticosteroid treatment than oral lichen planus. Fortunately, patients with oral mucosal pemphigoid appear overall to be less symptomatic than those with oral lichen planus.

### 4.3 Pemphigus Vulgaris

Pemphigus vulgaris is an autoimmune vesiculobullous disease that involves both the skin and oral mucosa. It usually occurs in adults, the average age of onset being in the early 50s. There is an almost equal male/female distribution, although some reports suggest a slightly greater prevalence in females, and others in males. Intraoral lesions can occur anywhere and in some patients many intraoral sites are simultaneously involved. In one study,[33] the buccal mucosa, palate, and gingivae were the most commonly involved intraoral sites. Pemphigus vulgaris tends to be more common in certain ethnic groups (e.g. people of Jewish or Mediterranean origin). There are 4 basic types of pemphigus: vulgaris, vegetans, foliaceous and erythematosus. Many consider vulgaris and vegetans as variants of one another, and so too the foliaceous and erythematosus types. Regardless of classification, almost all patients with oral pemphigus have the vulgaris type.

Intraoral lesions generally consist of multiple, sometimes widespread, flat, irregularly sized and shaped painful ulcers covered by a white slough and often having little surrounding erythema. If secondarily irritated or infected, the lesions may exhibit intense redness. Pemphigus vulgaris lesions are persistent, and while some may heal spontaneously, others replace them beforehand, so the patient usually has a continual pool of painful lesions. The lesions can begin in the throat as well as the oral cavity, causing complaints of persistent sore throat, tonsillitis, etc. It is not unusual for lesions to be so numerous, large and persistent that patients have difficulty eating and suffer weight loss. When the lesions involve only the oral cavity and not (yet) the skin, clinical diagnosis can be difficult. This may cause months of delay with an ever worsening condition being inappropriately treated or not treated at all.

Diagnostic corroboration is provided by biopsy and immunofluorescence. A biopsy demonstrates intraepithelial, usually suprabasilar clefting and acantholysis. Immunofluorescence, whether direct or indirect, yields antigen-antibody activity between epithelial cells within the surface squamous epithelium. In fact, with the indirect method, antibody titres often correlate with clinical activity.

Although there has been a vast improvement in the survival of patients with pemphigus vulgaris over the past 50 years, the disease remains a potentially lethal one, or at least one associated with considerable morbidity due to the medications needed for control.

#### Optimum Treatment

Unlike some diseases and lesions covered elsewhere in this chapter, the treatment of oral pemphigus vulgaris, and pemphigus vulgaris in general, is not well standardised. The reasons for this include:

1) The fact that pemphigus vulgaris is rare. Few investigators have been able to accumulate a sufficiently large number of patients to conduct meaningful therapeutic trials.

2) The disease is potentially lethal. Consequently, initiating double-blind studies with a placebo arm is usually inappropriate.

3) The severity of the disease may vary between patients. Some patients may have inherently mild forms, while others have much more severe forms, and in some the disease may have the potential to undergo self-remission.[34]

4) Pemphigus vulgaris is still widely considered to be incurable; hence treatment is directed at long term control with its potential for flare-ups, medication adverse effects, etc.

5) Treatment often involves several medications being delivered simultaneously. Consequently, the efficacy of any one drug may be impossible to determine. Agents and procedures that have been used in the last 20 years include corticosteroids, cyclophosphamide, azathioprine, methotrexate, gold, dapsone, cyclosporin, photophoresis and plasmapheresis. Many of these have been used simultaneously and reported in small series and single case reports.

***Systemic corticosteroids:*** most investigators advocate the use of systemic corticosteroids as primary therapy, either alone or combined with immunosuppressant drugs such as *azathioprine, cyclophosphamide,* or *cyclosporin.* Corticosteroid therapy is usually initiated in high doses (e.g. prednisolone 20 to 120 mg/day) and increased if necessary, depending on clinical progression.[35] Once most lesions have healed, the dose can then be gradually reduced to a maintenance level of around 10mg prednisolone per day or every alternate day. In patients in whom corticosteroid therapy alone is unsuccessful, azathioprine 100 mg/day or cyclophosphamide 50 mg/day have been added to the regimens and then reduced gradually (along with the corticosteroid dosage) once control is achieved.[34]

The concomitant use of corticosteroids and immunosuppressants from the outset has been reported by some investigators, e.g. initial doses of methylprednisolone 80 to 200 mg/day plus azathioprine 2 to 3 mg/kg[36] and prednisone 200 mg/day plus cyclophosphamide 100 to 200 mg/day,[37] these doses being reduced gradually to maintenance levels once clinical improvement is achieved. Others have advocated the simultaneous use of cyclosporin and corticosteroids.[38] In using these immunosuppressants, their adverse effects need to be borne in mind; with azathioprine adverse effects include leucopenia, alopecia and hepatitis, while with cyclophosphamide they include haemorrhagic cystitis, alopecia, leucopenia and possible carcinogenesis (long term use), and with cyclosporin, gingival hypertrophy, hypertrichosis and renal function impairment. However, offsetting this, immunosuppressant drugs have valuable steroid-sparing properties and permit lower doses of corticosteroids to be used, thereby lessening the risk of long term corticosteroid adverse effects such as hypertension, osteoporosis, diabetes mellitus, duodenal ulcer, Cushingoid facies, etc.

In patients not responding to combined use of corticosteroids and azathioprine, the use of *dapsone* together with a corticosteroid and cyclophosphamide has been advocated.[39]

***Other therapy:*** following initial treatment with corticosteroids, the use of *gold therapy* has been advocated.[40] The recommended initial dosage is sodium aurothiomalate 50mg per week intramuscularly until: (a) clinical improvement occurs; (b) toxicity forces cessation of therapy; or (c) a total dose of 1g has been delivered and the systemic corticosteroid dose cannot be reduced. Maintenance doses vary considerably, generally ranging from 50mg every 2 weeks to 50mg monthly. Gold therapy is also potentially toxic and the dosage should be reduced whenever possible. Its mechanism of action is unknown but is thought to be via decreasing circulating antibody titres. The simultaneous use of plasma exchange and corticosteroids has been reported.[41] Each plasma exchange in this study reduced intercellular antibody levels by a mean of 2 dilutions.

As with the management of oral lichen planus and mucosal pemphigoid (see sections 4.1 and 4.2), oral candidiasis may emerge at some time during therapy and hence concomitant antifungal medication may be appropriate. Early diagnosis, particularly when only oral lesions are present, often leads to the use of quantitatively less medication for pemphigus vulgaris. Hence, early accurate diagnosis influences treatment and prognosis.

Topical corticosteroids and injectable sublesional depot corticosteroids may also be used for oral pemphigus vulgaris lesions, e.g. beclomethasone dipropionate spray, fluocinonide 0.05% cream, and dexamethasone 0.5mg/5ml elixir (for dosages, see sections 3.2, 4.1, 4.2).

Corticosteroid creams can be applied topically to oral pemphigus vulgaris lesions via the use of custom-made trays.[28,29] The use of sublesional corticosteroid therapy is described in sections 3.2 and 4.1.

### 4.4 Erythema Multiforme

Erythema multiforme, like lichen planus, mucosal pemphigoid and pemphigus vulgaris, may involve the oral cavity solely or the oral cavity, skin and other surface tissues. Erythema multiforme is widely considered to be an acute hypersensitivity reaction. Causes of the reaction include: (1) micro-organisms such as herpes simplex virus (HSV) and *Mycoplasma pneumoniae;* (2) drugs, including the sulfonamides, penicillin, phenytoin, barbiturates, etc; and (3) other systemic diseases and neoplasms. In many patients with erythema multiforme, the exact aetiological agent is never identified. A drug hypersensitivity reaction is suggested by the observation of a patient developing characteristic erythema multiforme lesions 1 to 3 weeks after initial exposure to a particular medication, and when a subsequent eruption begins just hours or 1 to 2 days after a second exposure to the same drug.

The clinical severity of oral and generalised erythema multiforme may vary widely. Some consider that mild oral erythema multiforme is similar to severe forms of oral aphthae (see section 3.2); indeed, oral aphthae and severe erythema multiforme (Stevens-Johnson syndrome) may be at opposite ends of the same long clinical spectrum. Typical oral erythema multiforme lesions consist of multiple, flat, irregularly sized and shaped painful ulcers, some having grey-white surface sloughs with peripheral intense erythema and others being simply erythematous. The condition is frequently diagnosed when characteristic black encrusted lip lesions are present. Its onset (unlike that of lichen planus, mucosal pemphigoid and pemphigus vulgaris) is generally sudden, with an affected patient being in distress in a matter of hours or 1 to 2 days. In one study,[42] the recurrent lesions returned in some patients at 3-week intervals and in others annually, and each cycle lasted 10 to 42 days. Pain was so severe that patients lost weight as a result of being unable to eat. Characteristic skin lesions are described as 'iris or target lesions'. Variants of erythema multiforme are sometimes described according to their clinical activity and severity. Less severe forms are referred to as erythema multiforme minor, and very severe forms, sometimes leading to considerable morbidity or eventually death, as erythema multiforme major; the latter include Stevens-Johnson syndrome and toxic epidermal necrolysis.

Unlike lichen planus, mucosal pemphigoid and pemphigus vulgaris, the diagnosis of oral erythema multiforme lesions cannot always be corroborated histologically. Although occasional oral biopsies reveal microscopic findings suggestive of erythema multiforme, most are diagnosed simply as nonspecific ulceration and inflammation. Immunofluorescent findings in erythema multiforme specimens may also be nonspecific or demonstrate blood vessel insult. Nevertheless, when immunofluorescent findings in erythema multiforme are nonspecific, they do not display the characteristic features of pemphigoid or pemphigus, two oral lesions that may be confused clinically with erythema multiforme. Thus, routine histopathology and immunofluorescence may help to confirm the diagnosis of erythema multiforme by eliminating lichen planus, mucosal pemphigoid and pemphigus vulgaris.

#### Optimum Treatment

Before prescribing drug therapy, the clinician should attempt to identify the causative agent and eliminate it, if possible. This may mean the cessation of a particular drug regimen, or treating an infection (e.g. *Mycoplasma pneumoniae* infection with a macrolide antibiotic or HSV infection with aciclovir). Although there is still some controversy regarding the efficacy of systemic corticosteroids in treating erythema multiforme, most clinicians favour their use. Some advise systemic corticosteroid therapy early in the course of the disease, considering that corticosteroids are less effective later and may give rise to secondary infections.[43] Dosage regimens that have been used include prednisone or methylprednisolone 1 to 2 mg/kg/ day[43] or prednisone 40 to 60 mg/day[42] initially, tapering downward over 2 to 3 weeks. Topical corticosteroids such as dexamethasone elixir 0.5mg/ 5ml, fluocinonide 0.05% cream, and beclomethasone dipropionate spray may also be used (see sections 3.2, 4.1 and 4.2 for appropriate regimens). Recently, the successful use of cyclosporin (10 mg/kg/day) in conjunction with prednisone has been reported in 1 patient.[44] After control was achieved, dosages of both medications were tapered.

**Table I.** Relative daily costs of commonly used agents in the treatment of oral dermatoses and oral ulcerative lesions

| Drug | Relative treatment cost (per day) |
|---|---|
| **Corticosteroids:** | |
| Beclomethasone dipropionate aerosol spray (8 puffs × 50μg) | ++ |
| Fluocinonide 0.05% cream (from 15g tube[a]) | + |
| Triamcinolone acetonide 0.1% in 'Orabase' (from 5g tube[a]) | ++ |
| Dexamethasone elixir 0.5 mg/5ml (20ml) | + |
| Methylprednisolone sublesional injection, 80 mg/ml (1ml) | +++ |
| Prednisone tablet (5mg) | + |
| Prednisolone tablet (5mg) | + |
| **Others:** | |
| Dapsone tablet (100mg) | + |
| Griseofulvin tablet (500mg) | ++ |
| Tetracycline suspension 125 mg/5ml (20ml) | + |

a Estimated cost.

*Symbols:* + = low; ++ = low-medium; +++ = medium; ++++ = high.

Treatment regimens for erythema multiforme must be integrated with the overall care of the patient. Those with minor forms and oral lesions only may be treated on an outpatient basis. However, patients with severe forms such as Stevens-Johnson syndrome should be hospitalised and treated with appropriate systemic corticosteroid regimens and supportive care.

The relative daily costs of drugs commonly used in oral dermatoses and oral ulcerative lesions are shown in table I.

## 5. Diseases of Microbial Origin

Inflammatory oral disease confined to the periodontium (caries leading to pulpitis, periapical infection, periodontal inflammatory disease) and caused by bacteria is still very common in dental practice. However, bacterial infection involving the oral mucosa is uncommon. Indeed the non-periodontal oral mucosa appear to be more resistant to bacteria than to fungi and viruses. Consequently, this section focuses primarily on oral fungal infection, particularly candidiasis and oral herpetic infection, both primary and secondary forms. However, acute necrotising ulcerative gingivitis is also discussed as this bacterial infection can cause a mild fever and regional lymphadenitis, and it is sometimes associated with a debilitated medical status.

### 5.1 Candidiasis

Candidiasis (moniliasis) is basically synonymous with oral fungal infection; only rarely are fungi other than Candida involved. However, within the Candida family there are many strains besides *Candida albicans* that can cause candidiasis, including *C. torulopsis glabrata, C. tropicalis, C. parapsilosis, C. guilliermondii, C. lipolytica* and *C. krusei*.[45,46] Candidal organisms are ubiquitous and thus it is not surprising that a high proportion of healthy adults have Candida in their normal mouth flora. Consequently, a positive oral candidal culture does not necessarily imply a diagnosis of candidiasis; characteristic lesions of oral fungal infection must be visible. Inherently, candidal organisms are considered to be insufficiently virulent to cause infection; they infect only when the appropriate opportunity arises, e.g. in a compromised host. Hence most of the population is never threatened with candidal infection. Factors leading to candidiasis can be local or systemic. Local factors include use of topical corticosteroids and antibiotics, the wearing of dentures, decreased salivation, and smoking; systemic causes include diabetes mellitus, pernicious anaemia,[47] systemic corticosteroid and antibiotic treatment, acquired immune deficiency syndrome (AIDS), and various debilitating illnesses.

Oral fungal infections generally occur at the extremes of age, in the very young and the very old, with healthy middle-aged people often being spared. Oral candidiasis is more common in females than in males, but this may simply reflect a gender predilection based on the observation that some compromising oral diseases that lead to oral candidiasis (e.g. lichen planus) are also more common in females than in males. Oral candidiasis can occur anywhere, and it is often widespread (involving an extensive oral surface area) and multifocal. Two oral sites that appear to be predisposed to the development of oral candidiasis are the hard palate and the dorsal tongue. The hard palate, particularly when covered by an upper complete denture, is frequently infected with Candida. The dorsal tongue, with its extensive network of filiform papillae, provides ideal conditions for the entrapment and proliferation of the organism.

Oral candidiasis is usually divided into 4 subtypes,[48] i.e. the pseudomembranous, erythematous, denture erythematous and hyperplastic forms. Although the subtypes were previously modified with the terms acute or chronic, these modifiers are best avoided as it is often impossible to determine how long particular lesions have been present and, since they are intraoral and difficult to detect by the patient, are often asymptomatic as well.

*Pseudomembranous* lesions are flat, often large, and may be uni- or multifocal. They have a red base and multiple, movable, superficial white dots, commonly referred to as 'milk curds', which consist of fungal hyphae, desquamated cells, debris, etc. When symptomatic, the patient usually complains of 'burning' symptoms. *Erythematous* lesions are similar to pseudomembranous lesions, the main difference being an absence of white, movable milk curds. Characteristically, the dorsal tongue appears bald, erythematous and atrophic, reflecting a temporary loss of filiform papillae. The papillae usually return promptly after successful anticandidal therapy. Sometimes pseudomembranous lesions convert to erythematous lesions as the candidiasis is being successfully treated. Erythematous lesions can also burn.

*Denture erythematous* lesions, often referred to as denture stomatitis, usually occur beneath an upper complete or partial denture. The affected mucosa is vividly red and the flat lesion follows the denture outline. Patients are often asymptomatic and unaware of the lesion. The *hyperplastic* variant is unilateral or bilateral, usually occurring at the internal angles of the mouth. It is an adherent white lesion fulfilling a definition of leukoplakia (clinical adherent white patch). It is usually asymptomatic and chronic.

Two other lesions are also included under a widened definition of oral candidiasis: *median rhomboid glossitis* and *angular cheilitis*. Previously, these entities were classified as other than 'candidiasis',[49] but median rhomboid glossitis is now basically accepted as being a form of chronic oral candidiasis, and angular cheilitis is very often related to candidal organisms. Median rhomboid glossitis is found in the midline of the dorsal tongue surface, anterior to the circumvallate papillae. It is usually flat, red, oval shaped and may have a white keratotic component. Originally, median rhomboid glossitis was considered a developmental defect, but more recent studies have confirmed a fungal presence. Angular cheilitis is found uni- or bilaterally at the mouth angles. It is a red and sometimes crusted lesion that can be painful, particularly when the mouth is stretched widely. Very often it is candidal in origin, but cases have been reported implicating vitamin deficiency and bite overclosure.

It should be borne in mind that 2 or more clinical forms of oral candidiasis can exist simultaneously.

Diagnostic corroboration of oral candidiasis can be performed in several ways. Since a high proportion of healthy people harbour oral candidal organisms, a positive culture does not always indicate candidiasis. However, a positive culture taken from 1 of the 6 clinical lesion types would confirm oral candidiasis. Further substantiation can be obtained by simultaneous treatment using an antifungal agent. If the characteristic lesions improve with antifungal treatment, then the diagnosis is confirmed. In fact, many clinicians never take a culture, their diagnosis being corroborated by the patient's favourable response to the antifungal regimen. A potential disadvantage of fungal culture methodology is the often lengthy (2-week) period for completion and analysis.

In addition to diagnostic confirmation by treatment alone, and by treatment combined with culture, a third method of confirmation involves a fungal smear. The smear, prepared as a KOH preparation or spray-fixed and stained with periodic acid-Schiff (PAS), has the advantages of speed and of identifying the organism in its more virulent hyphal form. A slight disadvantage is its lack of precision for strain identification. Of course, this method can also be coupled with simultaneous treatment. A fourth method is biopsy confirmation, whereby the diagnosis may be accidental, the surgeon not expecting a histopathological diagnosis of candidiasis. Nevertheless, the presence on biopsy of fungal hyphae penetrating the surface squamous epithelium is the most confirmatory method.

#### Optimum Treatment

Treatment of oral candidiasis should include a search for and elimination of the background local or systemic factors that originally facilitated the onset of candidiasis. This may mean adequate control of diabetes or anaemia or prescribing sialologues in a xerostomic patient. Sometimes it is impossible to eliminate the underlying cause, e.g. in a patient with a maxillary full denture. Often a patient with oral candidiasis caused by wearing a complete upper denture will not, for aesthetic and functional reasons, stop using the denture.

In the past, the most commonly used antifungal agent for patients with pseudomembranous, erythematous and denture erythematous forms was *nystatin* (in various different dosage forms). However, with the advent of the azole derivatives, regimens such as *clotrimazole* lozenges and systemically administered agents such as *ketoconazole, fluconazole* and *itraconazole* are now preferred. Regardless of the antifungal regimen used, treatment should be given for at least 2-weeks.[50] If candidal lesions return soon after the cessation of successful antifungal therapy, it can be concluded that the underlying causative factor has not been rectified. Some patients with severe host compromise (e.g. AIDS patients) have only partial resolution of candidal lesions during antifungal therapy, and fungal hyphae can still be cultured while treatment is ongoing.

If nystatin is used, it may be given as an oral suspension or as lozenges (pastilles). The suspension is prepared at a concentration of 100,000 U/ml, and the patient should be instructed to rinse for 2 minutes (and then expectorate) 5ml 4 times daily after meals and at bedtime. Alternatively, nystatin lozenges (200,000U), 1 dissolved in the mouth 5 times per day, may be used. Nystatin's mode of action is thought to involve a change in fungal cell membrane permeability, leading to leakage of intracellular components. The disadvantages of nystatin include: (1) some formulations cause oral burning sensations, a symptom already noted in oral candidiasis; and (2) it is not as effective as the azole antifungal agents. Nevertheless, nystatin can be used to combat pseudomembranous, erythematous and denture erythematous lesions; in the case of the latter, the patient should be directed to remove his/her denture while treating the condition.

Clotrimazole lozenges (oral troches) are prescribed in 2-week regimens, one being dissolved in the mouth 5 times per day. Clotrimazole's mode of action involves inhibition of fungal growth by altering cell membrane permeability. It has the advantage of being more effective than nystatin and having better patient compliance than nystatin suspension, but the disadvantage of causing occasional liver enzyme changes such that periodic liver function tests should be undertaken if long term use is contemplated. Clotrimazole is effective in treating pseudomembranous, erythematous and denture erythematous forms. Again, when lesions exist beneath a denture, the denture must be removed before applying topical medication.

Ketoconazole and fluconazole are the most commonly used agents for systemic therapy. Ketoconazole is given in a dosage of 200 mg/day for 2 weeks. It has the advantage of being a very effective antifungal agent with excellent patient compliance, but as with clotrimazole, it has the potential to cause liver enzyme changes and periodic liver function tests should be performed if therapy is prolonged. As a systemic agent, it can be used against all 6 forms of oral candidiasis.

Fluconazole has also been successfully used in oral candidiasis. Following successive treatment failures using nystatin, clotrimazole, ketoconazole and amphotericin B in an AIDS patient, fluconazole therapy has been found to be effective.[51] It is prescribed as 100mg tablets, 2 being taken on the first day then 1 daily thereafter for 2 weeks. Like clotrimazole and ketoconazole, it has the potential to cause hepatic enzymes changes. Fluconazole can be used to eradicate all 6 clinical forms of oral candidiasis. However, resistance to this agent has been reported as a problem in treatment.[52]

Denture erythematous and angular cheilitis lesions can be treated with topical antifungal preparations. Nystatin cream 100,000 U/g or clotrimazole cream 1% may be used, applied as a thin film beneath an upper denture or at the mouth angles 4 times daily. If there is an additional need for a topical corticosteroid, e.g. in an oral lichen planus patient with secondary candidiasis, triamcinolone acetonide/nystatin cream or betamethasone/clotrimazole cream can be used. Denture disinfection with 0.2 to 2% chlorhexidine solution has also been advocated.[53]

In patients with lichen planus, mucosal pemphigoid and pemphigus vulgaris (see sections 4.1, 4.2 and 4.3), it should be noted that oral candidiasis may occur simultaneously. Since these oral dermatoses are generally treated with corticosteroids, the absence of an adjunctive antifungal agent may worsen the condition. As the dermatosis is being controlled with corticosteroids, the oral candidiasis progresses with formation of pseudomembranous and erythematous lesions accompanied by burning symptoms. Consequently, antifungal agents should be prescribed prophylactically if it is suspected that oral candidiasis may develop during corticosteroid treatment.

**Table II.** Relative daily costs of commonly used antifungal regimens

| Drug | Relative treatment cost (per day) |
|---|---|
| Nystatin oral suspension 100,000 U/ml (20ml) | ++ |
| Nystatin lozenges 200,000U | +++ |
| Clotrimazole lozenges 10mg | +++ |
| Ketoconazole tablet 200mg | ++ |
| Fluconazole tablet 100mg | ++++ |

*Symbols:* + = low; ++ = low-medium; +++ = medium; ++++ = high.

Some forms of oral candidiasis may be resistant to drug therapy, particularly those that are chronic. These include hyperplastic candidiasis and median rhomboid glossitis for which consideration should be given to surgical excision of a small lesion (if practical) after systemic antifungal therapy. Also, some otherwise healthy patients may present with therapy-resistant chronic oral candidal lesions which may persist for long periods.

The relative daily costs of the commonly used antifungal medications are shown in table II.

## 5.2 Oral Herpes Infections

### *5.2.1 Primary Herpetic Gingivostomatitis*

Primary herpetic gingivostomatitis is caused by herpes simplex virus type 1 (HSV-1), although HSV-2 has also been implicated, albeit less frequently. The primary infection generally occurs in children but adults can be infected as well. Many primary infections are subclinical and go unnoticed, or have such mild features as to be almost ignored by the patient. A full blown primary oral infection is characterised by sudden onset of lesions, unlike the onset of painful ulcerative lesions of lichen planus, mucosal pemphigoid and pemphigus vulgaris. Usually, herpetic lesions commence as tiny vesicles that rapidly break down to painful ulcers. The ulcers are aphthae-like having white necrotic centres surrounded by intense peripheral erythema. Usually they vary between 1 and 3mm in diameter but many may coalesce to create a single lesion covering several square centimetres. The lesions are painful and the patient might wince and recoil his/her head backward when touched during the clinical examination. Characteristically, the gingivae are swollen and reddened. The painful lesions cause a tender submandibular lymphadenopathy and there may be a concomitant sore throat. The entire process is accompanied by fever and malaise. The primary infection generally lasts from 7 to 14 days.

Diagnostic corroboration is provided in several ways. Firstly, a fresh lesion can be gently scraped (sometimes with the aid of a local anaesthetic) and smeared on a glass slide which is then spray-fixed and subsequently stained in H & E (haematoxylin and eosin); characteristic viral balloon cells are identified. Secondly, if lesions are not clinically diagnostic, a biopsy is performed and again viral balloon cells are noted. Thirdly, along with a viral smear, a fresh lesion(s) can be cultured and a culture report can be received in 24 to 72 hours. In addition, sequential antibody testing can be performed which will detect a change from negative to positive, or a several-fold increase in titre when comparing the onset titre with the convalescent titre.

#### Optimum Treatment

Primary treatment should be supportive and palliative.[54,55] Antipyretic/analgesics such as aspirin and paracetamol (acetaminophen) and topical anaesthetics can be helpful. Bed rest and fluid intake should be encouraged. Antibacterial and/or antifungal agents should be prescribed if secondary infection is suspected.

Treatment with the antiviral drug *aciclovir* may also be considered, provided it is commenced early in the course of the infection; the mode of action of this drug involves its *in vivo* conversion to the triphosphate form which inhibits viral DNA synthesis.[56] If, during the first visit, the patient reveals that his/her infection has been present for 5 to 7 days and there has been some improvement in the last 24 hours, palliative and supportive care only should be provided and there is no need for systemic antiviral therapy. However, if the infection is still at an early stage and worsening, oral aciclovir 200 to 400mg 5 times per day for 7 to 10 days may be given. In one study in which patients were treated with aciclovir 2000 mg/day for 10 days,[54] lesion results were not significantly different from those achieved previously with palliative care only. However, viral shedding time was decreased from an average of 23 days to 7 days.

### *5.2.2 Recurrent Herpetic Infection (Intraoral and Labial)*

In the oral region, recurrent herpetic infection can exist strictly intraorally or on the outer skin surface of the lips. Recurrent intraoral lesions begin as vesicles that rapidly convert to ulcerative lesions. Some reports suggest they are more prevalent on the bound-down intraoral tissues of the hard palate and gingiva. In my experience, intraoral secondary herpetic lesions are much less common than recurrent aphthae. Extraoral lesions of herpes labialis begin as papules that evolve to vesicles and then ulcers and finally to scab-covered inflammatory lesions. Both intraoral and extraoral lesions are painful. Herpes labialis is sometimes preceded by prodromal signs of pain, burning, itching and tingling. A variety of factors are considered causal, including trauma (e.g. a dental visit with lip manipulation), sunlight (fever blisters), and cold (cold sores).

Usually, a clinical diagnosis is sufficient although some clinicians seek laboratory confirmation via a viral culture or smear.

**Optimum Treatment**

If the lesions are mild and tolerable, treatment may simply be to allow them to run their natural course. Alternatively, a variety of topical medications may be used. Since herpes labialis is often solar generated, the prophylactic use of a sunscreen may be helpful, e.g. a lipstick preparation, a white opaque physical sunscreen such as zinc oxide, or a chemical sunscreen (e.g. a preparation containing *p*-aminobenzoic acid).[57]

Systemic and topical *aciclovir* therapy have also been used in the treatment of herpes labialis. As in primary herpetic infections, aciclovir therapy should be commenced early after recurrence if clinical benefit is to be expected. However, secondary herpetic development may be well under way on a cellular and microscopic level before the patient is clinically aware of this.[58] Orally administered aciclovir 200mg 5 times daily for 5 days has been shown to produce significant improvement in patients with herpes labialis;[59] however, most reports of the use of aciclovir 5% ointment or cream indicate that topical therapy is not as effective as systemic therapy. Poor penetration of the drug to the site of viral replication may be the reason.

For recurrent intraoral herpetic infection, similar treatment regimens as for recurrent herpes labialis may be given. Treatment should commence early after recurrence with either oral aciclovir 200mg 5 times daily (for severe cases) or topical aciclovir 5% ointment or cream applied 4 times daily (for mild cases). However, prior to commencing treatment for any recurrent oral ulcerative lesion, it should be remembered that diagnostic confusion exists between recurrent herpes and recurrent aphthae and that the latter are much more common in the general population.

Topical idoxuridine 0.5% ointment has also been used in herpes labialis but, as with topical aciclovir, it appears to have only slight clinical benefit.

### 5.3 Acute Necrotising Ulcerative Gingivitis (Vincent's Disease, Trench Mouth)

Acute necrotising ulcerative gingivitis is a periodontal bacterial infection that is multifactorial in aetiology. Micro-organisms associated with this illness include *Treponema* spp., *Selenomonas* spp., *Fusobacterium* spp. and *B. intermedius*.[60] Host susceptibility is necessary for infection. Predisposing factors include emotional stress, smoking and poor oral hygiene.[61] It has been suggested that stress-induced increases in steroid concentrations in acute necrotising ulcerative gingivitis patients may lead to decreased neutrophil and lymphocyte responses in these individuals. Systemic illnesses such as blood dyscrasias, terminal cancer, malnutrition and AIDS have also been known to be causal.[62]

Clinically, the infection is typically encountered in young adults, characteristically between 18 and 30 years of age. Affected individuals of university and military age develop the lesions during particularly intense periods of stress such as when entering military service or going on leave. Its association with soldiers engaged in trench warfare during World War I is well known and its incidence then was so high that many erroneously thought it to be contagious.

The characteristic finding in acute necrotising ulcerative gingivitis is necrosis of marginal gingivae, particularly of one or more interdental papillae. Naturally, the necrosis leads to an ulcerated surface. The ulcerated surface is covered by a grey-white slough which is commonly referred to as a pseudomembrane. This is often accompanied by a marked tendency of the affected gingival tissues to bleed, particularly after the slightest mechanical provocation. The lesions are usually painful, and moderate to severe cases may even have an accompanying fever and regional lymphandenitis. Patients may also complain of a metallic taste and a malodour.

Some diagnostic confusion exists between acute necrotising ulcerative gingivitis and acute herpetic gingivostomatitis and, certainly, there is clinical overlap between the two diseases. However, a typical herpes infected patient will have nongingival affected sites as well as gingival sites. These extragingival sites found only in herpes infected patients include the buccal mucosa, floor of the mouth, soft palate, tongue, etc. Typically, herpetic gingivostomatitis patients will have oral vesicles leading to flat ulcers, while necrotising gingivitis patients do not present with vesicles.

Microscopically, a biopsy of affected tissue shows nonspecific mostly acute and chronic inflammation. Bacterial colonies are often identified, and more peripherally affected tissues may demonstrate a concentration of chronic inflammatory cells and granulation tissue.

#### Optimum Treatment

Treatment of acute necrotising ulcerative gingivitis is 3-fold:

1) Mechanical debridement via periodontal instruments at affected gingival sites.

2) Elimination of the infection. Appropriate systemic therapy includes phenoxymethylpenicillin (penicillin V) 250mg 4 times daily for 7 days[61] and metronidazole 250mg 3 times daily for 7 days.[60] In patients who are hypersensitive to penicillins, erythromycin 250mg 4 times daily can be substituted. Some clinicians also advocate the use of rinses such as hydrogen peroxide (3% mixed with an equal amount of warm water[63]) and chlorhexidine (0.12% solution).

3) Counselling during and following treatment, and instructions regarding oral hygiene and preventive measures.

## 6. Common Benign Lesions of the Tongue

There are 3 common, benign, self-limiting lesions of the tongue which may be of concern to an affected patient. These entities are benign migratory glossitis (geographic tongue), fissured tongue and hairy tongue. More than one can occur simultaneously in a patient and 1 of the 3 (benign migratory glossitis) is sometimes associated with painful burning symptoms.

### 6.1 Benign Migratory Glossitis (Geographic Tongue)

This tongue lesion is very common. Its aetiology is unknown, but in some cases may be related to psoriasis, candidiasis, stress, atopy and genetic factors.[64,65] It is found more frequently in women than in men. Characteristically, lesions form as one or more variable sized and shaped flat, denuded red patches with thin, linear white rims; the red patches reflect loss of or a reduced size of filiform papillae. Over time, the lesions come and go and wax and wane. Although most lesions are asymptomatic, some patients complain of burning symptoms. Sensitivity to hot and/or spicy foods is also possible.[66] Geographic lesions are usually present on the dorsal and/or lateral tongue surfaces but can also be detected less frequently on the ventral tongue and ectopically, involving the cheeks, palate and lip mucosa. Symptomatic geographic lesions often occur in patients experiencing considerable stress.

Since most patients present with classic clinical lesions, there is no need for biopsy confirmation. When a biopsy is performed, the microscopic pattern is described as being psoriasiform. Neutrophilic microabscesses similar to Munro microabscesses of psoriasis are noted in the superficial regions of the surface squamous epithelium. Periodic acid-Schiff stains are negative for *Candida*.

#### Optimum Treatment

Asymptomatic patients need not be treated at all. Instead, the patient should be given a thorough description of this benign, inflammatory, self-limiting, harmless, incurable nuisance phenomenon. If the patient is symptomatic, the same reassuring descriptions should again be provided, but pressures may be brought to prescribe some form of medication. In such cases, palliative agents such as topical anaesthetics, analgesics, or even topical corticosteroid preparations may be given. Systemic corticosteroids, with their attendant adverse effects, should be avoided. If treatment appears to provide improvement, this may in fact be coincidental, as geographic tongue lesions wax and wane spontaneously.

If patients with geographic lesions appear overly stressed, referral for counselling may be appropriate along with use of antianxiety agents.

### 6.2 Fissured Tongue (Cerebriform Tongue, Scrotal Tongue)

Clinically, a fissured tongue is a mild tongue malformation with a variable number of grooves arranged on the dorsal tongue surface. Sometimes the grooves arise from a midline dorsal groove that extends anteriorly-posteriorly from the tongue tip region. There are several theories concerning the aetiology of fissured tongue, more recent ones citing genetic factors.[64,65]

An association of fissured tongue with geographic tongue has been noted, with both conditions present simultaneously in the same patient. Prevalences of fissured tongue without geographic tongue of 2.1% in Saudi Arabia[65] and 5% in the US[67] have been cited. The fissures vary so widely from patient to patient that they defy classification.

Since a fissured tongue is of no pathological concern, there is no need for treatment. Rarely, entrapped food or debris may cause mild discomfort necessitating water lavages or gauze sponge cleansing.

### 6.3 Hairy Tongue

This entity occurs on the tongue dorsum. It consists of an elongation/hypertrophy of filiform papillae without epithelial desquamation. The hypertrophy may be so extensive as to simulate a clinical hairy appearance of the dorsal surface. Furthermore, the elongated hair-like papillae may be stained yellow, white, brown or black. Its exact aetiology is unknown and many causative factors have been suggested, including broad-spectrum antibiotics, systemic corticosteroids, oxygenating agents (e.g. hydrogen peroxide), intensive smoking, and head and neck radiation therapy. One or more of these factors may be related to an alteration of oral flora favouring an overgrowth of chromagenic bacteria and fungi.[67]

Clinically, a brown, black, yellow and/or white stained hypertrophy of the dorsal tongue filiform papillae is seen, creating the characteristic hairy appearance. This may be a solitary patch measuring 1 $cm^2$, or it may cover almost the entire dorsum. Staining can vary from site to site. The lesion is entirely asymptomatic, at most causing a mild gagging or tickling sensation in a small percentage of patients.

#### Optimum Treatment

Treatment consists of a thorough description of this benign entity along with reassurance of its harmless clinical course. Attempts at reversal include a search for and elimination of the likely causative factors. Additionally, patients might attempt reversal by tooth-brushing the affected dorsum with a water-moistened brush. Some clinicians have advocated 25 or 50% trichloroacetic acid and 1% podophyllin applications. My initial approach is to try to avoid therapy, reassuring the patient of its benign harmless nature. However, if patients insist on treatment, excision of the elongated filiform papillae can be undertaken with surgical scissors. If the papillae are properly and superficially excised, this effective and painless procedure requires no anaesthetic.

## 7. Oral Leukoplakic Lesions

Leukoplakia is an enigmatic term that causes confusion among clinicians and patients alike. This confusion is caused by the multiple definitions used to describe intraoral leukoplakic lesions:

1) Leukoplakia may be defined as any white adherent intraoral lesion (the word, which is of Greek origin, literally means white patch).

2) A second common definition is intraoral white lesion demonstrating microscopic premalignancy (unfortunately, some oral premalignant lesions are red clinically, and some are red and white).

3) A third common definition describes leukoplakia as any white adherent lesion which histologically demonstrates hyperkeratosis, hyperplasia, and/or dysplasia and which cannot be classified clinically or histologically as any other specific disease.

In any discussion of leukoplakia, it should be made clear which definition is being applied.

### 7.1 Premalignant Lesions and Hyperkeratosis

Oral surface premalignant lesions (sometimes referred to as epithelial dysplasia) are thought to be caused by a variety of agents, including tobacco, excessive alcohol consumption, and viruses such as human papilloma virus and herpes simplex virus. However, tobacco in any of its several forms is of primary importance. Men are more often affected than women, and usually the affected patient is over 50 years of age. Although premalignant lesions and hyperkeratosis can be found anywhere intraorally, dysplastic lesions and subsequent oral squamous cell carcinomas are most often found on lateral tongue surfaces and the floor of the mouth. Clinically, the dysplastic lesion can be red, white, or red and white. It is usually flat or slightly raised and generally has greater firmness than the adjacent normal mucosa. When palpated, premalignant lesions can be painful.

Diagnostic corroboration of a dysplastic lesion is obtained microscopically. An incisional or excisional biopsy is performed, and if significant epithelial atypism is detected, the lesion can be defined as epithelial dysplasia. Epithelial dysplasia can be defined further as being mild, moderate or severe, respectively, if atypism is restricted to the basal 25%, the basal 50%, or the basal 75%. If epithelial dysplasia is maximal and presents through full thickness epithelium, the lesion is carcinoma *in situ*. If it is also invasive, it is a squamous cell carcinoma. Finally, if a clinically white lesion demonstrates overlying keratin and no epithelial atypism, it is diagnosed as hyperkeratosis.

### Optimum Treatment

Treatment of premalignant leukoplakic lesions varies considerably. A biopsy should almost always be performed to corroborate a specific diagnosis. If atypism is absent or only very mildly present, treatment may consist of removal of possible causative agents (e.g. tobacco) and waiting a short time to see if lesion reversal occurs. Alternatively, a leukoplakic lesion may be surgically excised, particularly if it is small and accessible. Another treatment method which is being increasingly used is chemoprevention with retinoids. In some cases, it may be appropriate to use more than one method in tandem or simultaneously. If premalignancy is documented, patient safety requires periodic reexaminations.

***Retinoids:*** there has been considerable interest recently in the treatment of oral leukoplakia with retinol (vitamin A) and its numerous derivatives. The commonly used analogues include *isotretinoin, β-carotene* and *tretinoin.* Currently, isotretinoin is the best studied derivative and it has an established benefit in this condition. In a 12-month study comparing isotretinoin with β-carotene in terms of their ability to prevent progression of leukoplakic lesions to squamous cell carcinoma, patients receiving isotretinoin (maintenance dose 0.5 mg/kg/day) fared better than those receiving β-carotene (30 mg/day).[68] In a similar study in patients with a prior history of oral carcinoma,[69] isotretinoin proved significantly more effective than placebo in preventing the development of second primary tumours. However, in using retinoids, it should be noted that cessation of such therapy may often result in lesion recurrence.[21]

The mechanism of action of retinoids is similar to that of steroid hormones.[70,71] Retinol and retinoic acid are bound to intracellular retinoid-binding proteins and transported to the nucleus where 4 genetic nuclear receptors are present; these genes play a critical role in normal cell growth and function. The adverse effects of the retinoids are significant, although most are dose-related and reversible (except for their teratogenic effects). Adverse effects include cheilitis, dry skin, xerostomia, conjunctivitis, hyperostosis, hepatotoxicity and increased serum triglycerides. Naturally occurring retinol analogues such as β-carotene tend to have fewer adverse effects.

The relative costs of retinoid preparations are shown in table III.

**Table III.** Relative daily costs of retinoid preparations used in the treatment of oral mucosal conditions

| Drug | Relative treatment cost (per day) |
|---|---|
| Tretinoin cream 0.1% (from 20g tube[a]) | + |
| β-Carotene tablet (30mg) | ++ |
| Etretinate capsule (75mg) | ++++ |
| Isotretinoin capsule (60mg) | ++++ |

a Estimated cost.

*Symbols:* + = low; ++ = low-medium; +++ = medium; ++++ = high.

## 8. Symptomatic Disorders that are Sometimes Psychogenic

In oral medicine, patients are sometimes referred with symptoms unassociated with any space-occupying morphological disease. If attempts to relate symptoms to organic disease fail, the symptoms are often regarded as being perceptual or psychogenic. Such symptoms include a burning mouth (stomapyrosis), altered taste perception (dysgeusia), and a dry mouth (xerostomia). These symptoms can be caused by organic disease as well, but in many instances they are not.

### 8.1 Burning Mouth Syndrome (Stomapyrosis)

A patient with a burning mouth complaint is presenting with a symptom and not necessarily a lesion. Known causes of burning mouth include pernicious anaemia, diabetes mellitus, hypothyroidism, oral fungal infection, geographic tongue, submucous fibrosis, lingual arteritis, simple trauma, medications such as levodopa/carbidopa, and psychological disorders. Every attempt should be made to detect organic space-occupying disease before accepting a psychogenic cause.[72] In fact, a psychogenic origin is accepted in part via exclusion of the other entities already noted and any others detected or suspected during the medical work-up. Further corroboration such as the patient being under psychiatric care, or having a behavioural disorder is meaningful and helpful.

Patients with psychogenic-induced oral burning symptoms are mostly female, postmenopausal, and over 50 years of age. The oral mucosa appears completely normal and there is no medical evidence to substantiate organic disease in symptom generation. By the time patients visit an oral medicine clinic, most have had blood tests, refuting diagnoses of pernicious anaemia, diabetes mellitus, etc. Typically, the patient complains of a burning mouth or a hot or scorched oral sensation. When questioned, many patients describe periods of stress, depression, loss, etc., prior to symptom onset. The symptoms can occur anywhere intraorally but commonly involve the anterior tongue, anterior palate and lips.

#### Optimum Treatment

Treatment begins with a thorough explanation of the clinical findings. The absence of a space-occupying morphological disease should be mentioned, but it should be pointed out that psychogenic factors (stress, tension, anxiety, depression, loss) may be related to the burning symptoms. At this juncture, some patients feel helped and need no further treatment; some want simply to be reassured that they do not have oral cancer. Others remain symptomatically uncomfortable and require therapy. Patients in this category may need to be referred for counselling.

Some clinicians[73] prescribe mood-altering drugs, e.g. chlordiazepoxide 5 to 10mg 3 times daily or diazepam 6 to 15 mg/day. The tricyclic antidepressant amitriptyline can also be used, beginning with 25mg at bedtime and increasing gradually to 75mg over 2 to 3 weeks. However, these drugs may cause drowsiness. Significant improvement in some patients with specific vitamin B deficiencies given daily supplements of thiamine (vitamin $B_1$) 300mg, riboflavin (vitamin $B_2$) 20mg and pyridoxine (vitamin $B_6$) 150mg has also been reported.[74]

### 8.2 Taste Aberration (Dysgeusia)

Some patients present with a chief complaint of taste aberration (dysgeusia), which may be described as metallic, salty, bitter, sweet, sour, etc. Others claim a total lack of taste (ageusia), a diminished taste (hypogeusia), or a 'lousy' taste (cacogeusia). There are numerous causes of taste aberration,[75,76] including aging, radiation, dental restorations and lack of oral hygiene, craniofacial abnormalities, psychiatric disorders, cerebral tumours, cerebral trauma, diabetes mellitus, Sjögren's syndrome, chronic renal failure, liver cirrhosis, vitamin B deficiency, zinc deficiency, and numerous drugs (for a review of drug-induced taste disturbances, see Henkin[77]). This can be complicated further when recalling that senses of taste and smell are often intimately related.

#### Optimum Treatment

A thorough oral examination must be performed in attempting to identify a relationship of dysgeusia with a correctable oral problem. Also, a detailed history should be taken to identify local or systemic disease, medications, or psychiatric disorders that may possibly be causal. Treatment should begin with rectifying, if possible, any detectable cause(s). In my experience, more than 50% of patients with dysgeusia also have oral burning symptoms and most have no known physical causative factors related to these symptoms. Furthermore, two-thirds of the patients with burning mouth and dysgeusia are middle-aged women, the group most represented in purely psychogenic burning mouth patients. Thus, it has been suggested that psychogenic factors may be involved in a significant percentage of cases of dysgeusia.[73,78]

If a correctable oral problem is identified, treatment may involve adjusting a dental prosthesis or treating a mucositis. Referral to an internist or neurologist may be advisable to confirm or rule out systemic illness, including CNS disorders. Zinc therapy (e.g. zinc-supplemented vitamin capsules or tablets) has been advocated in the treatment of dysgeusia and may be worth a trial.

### 8.3 Dry Mouth (Xerostomia)

In patients presenting with a complaint of dry mouth, the most common causes are likely to be drug therapy, irradiation of the head and neck region, and systemic disease.[79] A frequently overlooked local cause is mouth breathing. Some patients do not have a truly dry mouth, but instead have dry mouth symptoms and may be better placed in a burning mouth syndrome category.[78] The burning mouth syndrome has a triad of oral symptoms that include burning mouth, dry mouth and altered taste.

A work-up for xerostomia should first emphasise a medication history with subsequent referral to appropriate texts, if necessary, to verify any xerostomic qualities of suspect drugs. Whether a drug-related cause is detected or not, questions regarding symptoms and illnesses related to Sjögren's syndrome should be asked. Appropriate laboratory testing for Sjögren's syndrome, including lip biopsy, should be performed when appropriate, and the patient should be questioned about prior therapeutic head and neck radiation.

An oral examination might reveal a truly dry or normally wet mouth. If doubt exists, the clinician can insert a Lashley cup to collect and evaluate (quantitatively and qualitatively) stimulated and unstimulated saliva. This procedure verifies whether there is a normal or truly dry mouth. Xerostomic mouths feel dry, may be slightly reddened due to secondary candidiasis, and may be associated with significant dental decay.

#### Optimum Treatment

Treatment of a true xerostomia must be directed initially at the cause, which should be sought and eliminated if possible. Attempts at stimulating salivation locally by frequent use of sugar-free candy and gum may be made, and the patient should be advised to sip water frequently and to use artificial saliva preparations, e.g. 'Salivart' and 'Xerolube'. The patient can also be referred to a dentist for construction of fluoride gel trays. A variety of stannous fluoride gel preparations are available to help prevent dental decay.

If xerostomia persists despite intensive local therapy, consideration should be given to systemic salivary stimulation, the most frequently prescribed drug for this purpose being *pilocarpine*. This parasympathomimetic agent stimulates human exocrine glands, resulting in sweating, salivation, lacrimation, and gastric and pancreatic secretion. In one study involving xerostomic patients,[80] 44% improved while on pilocarpine 5mg 3 times daily as compared with 25% on placebo. Pilocarpine can be given as a solution containing 1 mg/ml, 5ml being administered 4 times daily. A newer agent that has been successfully used in treating xerostomia is *anethole trithione*.[79]

## 9. Oral Mucosal Diseases in Patients with Acquired Immune Deficiency Syndrome (AIDS)

Human immunodeficiency virus (HIV) infection and AIDS have had a major impact on healthcare in the past 15 years. This section discusses HIV- and AIDS-related oral lesions and their appropriate treatment. For further discussion of the management of AIDS patients, see chapter 28 (sect. 3.2) and chapter 32 (sect. 3.1). For a recent review of this subject, see Foltyn and Marriott.[81]

Oral lesions found in AIDS patients include candidiasis, hairy leukoplakia, aphthae, HIV-related gingivitis/periodontitis, herpetic infection and Kaposi's sarcoma.[82,83]

### 9.1 Candidiasis

The most common oral lesion in AIDS patients is candidiasis, particularly the pseudomembranous form. The clinical and diagnostic features of this condition and its treatment are outlined in section 5.1. Treatment consists of nystatin suspension or lozenges, clotrimazole lozenges, or oral ketoconazole or fluconazole therapy. Candidal relapse is frequent on discontinuation of treatment and severe cases unresponsive to therapy have been reported.

### 9.2 Hairy Leukoplakia

Hairy leukoplakia is a unilateral or bilateral adherent white keratotic lesion(s) of the lateral tongue. It has a corrugated surface contour often imparting the appearance of hair-like projections. This Epstein-Barr virus–related lesion has a characteristic almost pathognomonic microscopic appearance.

Antiviral chemotherapy with aciclovir has been used with some success. In one study,[84] 5 of 6 patients treated with aciclovir 3.2 g/day for 20 days achieved clinical regression of lesions, but recurrences were seen following cessation of therapy. Lesion reduction has also been associated with zidovudine therapy.

### 9.3 Aphthae

Some patients with HIV infection and some with AIDS develop lesions identical to oral aphthae. These lesions may be minor, major or herpetiform.[85] Treatment for AIDS-related aphthae is basically the same as for patients with aphthae in the absence of HIV infection (see section 3.2). Topical and systemic corticosteroids have been successfully used, as has tetracycline suspension.[86] Some investigators[87] have used a liquid corticosteroid preparation plus sucralfate 1g for treating major aphthae involving the oesophagus; the success of this regimen may have been due in part to the coating action of sucralfate.

### 9.4 Gingivitis

HIV-positive patients may have an associated gingivitis, which can progress to a painful HIV-related periodontitis. Treatment of HIV-related periodontal inflammatory disease has 4 components,[88] i.e. debridement, local antimicrobial therapy, immediate follow-up care, and regular long term maintenance.

Povidone iodine solution is helpful in debriding gingivitis lesions during the immediate treatment phase. Local antimicrobial therapy may consist of twice daily chlorhexidine (0.12% solution) rinses. When indicated, systemic antimicrobial therapy usually consists of metronidazole 250mg 4 times daily for 4 to 5 days.

### 9.5 Primary and Secondary Herpetic Infections

Primary and secondary herpetic infections are also associated with HIV infection (see sections 5.2.1 and 5.2.2 for clinical, laboratory and therapeutic considerations). Typically, the patient is treated with aciclovir. The duration of infection in immunocompromised patients may be prolonged and relapses may occur following treatment withdrawal.

### 9.6 Kaposi's Sarcoma

Recognition of Kaposi's sarcoma is important in confirming a diagnosis of AIDS. Typical Kaposi's sarcoma lesions occur intraorally, particularly on the gingiva and maxillary half of the oral mucosa. In one study of patients with oral Kaposi's sarcoma, some received benefit from low-dose radiation or chemotherapy;[89] radiation treatment consisted of 800 cGy or equivalent fractionated therapy, while chemotherapy was intralesional vinblastine (0.2 mg/ml solution), given as multiple injections of 0.1ml per 0.5cm lesion. More than 50% regression of oral Kaposi's sarcoma was noted in 80% of the patients treated with radiation or with intralesional vinblastine.

## Acknowledgements

I wish to express my gratitude to the Miles Hodsdon Vernon Foundation, Marta J. Brooks (PharmD), and Laurie A. Towle (PhD).

## References

1. Shafer WG, Hine MK, Levy BM. A textbook of oral pathology. 4th ed. chapter 6. Philadelphia: WB Saunders, 1983
2. Vincent SD, Lilly GE. Clinical, historic, and therapeutic features of aphthous stomatitis. Oral Surgery Oral Medicine and Oral Pathology 1992; 74: 79
3. Hay KD, Reade PC. The use of an elimination diet in the treatment of recurrent aphthous ulceration of the oral cavity. Oral Surgery Oral Medicine and Oral Pathology 1984; 57: 504
4. Graykowski EA, Barile MF, Lee WB, et al. Recurrent aphthous stomatitis. Journal of the American Medical Association 1966; 196: 129
5. Zegarelli DJ. Mouthwashes in the treatment of oral disease. Drugs 1991; 42: 171
6. Burgess JA, Johnson BD, Sommers E. Pharmacological management of recurrent oral mucosal ulceration. Drugs 1990; 39: 54
7. Addy M, Tapper-Jones L, Seal M. Trial of astringent and antibacterial mouthwashes in the management of recurrent aphthous ulceration. British Dental Journal 1974; 136: 452
8. Zegarelli DJ. The treatment of oral lichen planus. Annals of Dentistry 1993; 52: 3
9. Graykowski EA, Holroyd SV. Therapeutic management of primary herpes, recurrent labial herpes, aphthous stomatitis, and Vincent's infection. Dental Clinics of North America 1970; 14: 721
10. Brown RS, Bottomley WK. Combination immunosuppressant and topical steroid therapy for treatment of recurrent major aphthae. Oral Surgery Oral Medicine and Oral Pathology 1990; 69: 42
11. Miller MF. Use of levamisole in recurrent aphthous stomatitis. Drugs 1980; 19: 131
12. Ruah CB, Stram JR, Chasin WD. Treatment of severe recurrent aphthous stomatitis with colchicine. Archives of Otolaryngologic Head and Neck Surgery 1988; 114: 671
13. Muzulu SI, Walton S, Keczkes K. Colchicine therapy in Behcet's syndrome - a report of five cases. Clinical and Experimental Dermatology 1989; 14: 298
14. Grinspan D. Significant response of oral aphthosis to thalidomide treatment. Journal of the American Academy of Dermatology 1985; 12: 85
15. Zegarelli DJ. Multimodality steroid therapy of erosive and ulcerative oral lichen planus. Journal of Oral Medicine 1983; 38: 127
16. Sehgal VN, Abraham GJ, Malik GB. Griseofulvin therapy in lichen planus. British Journal of Dermatology 1972; 87: 383
17. Sehgal VN, Bikhchandani R, Koranne RV, et al. Histopathological evaluation of griseofulvin therapy in lichen planus. Dermatologica 1980; 161: 22
18. Aufdemorte TB, DeVillez RL, Gieseker DR. Griseofulvin in the treatment of three cases of oral erosive lichen planus. Oral Surgery Oral Medicine and Oral Pathology 1983; 55: 459
19. Massa MC, Rogers RS. Griseofulvin therapy of lichen planus. Acta Dermato-Venereologica 1981; 61: 547
20. Bagan JV, Silvestre FJ, Mestre S, et al. Treatment of lichen planus with griseofulvin. Oral Surgery Oral Medicine and Oral Pathology 1985; 60: 608
21. Zegarelli DJ. Treatment of oral lichen planus with topical vitamin A acid. Journal of Oral Medicine 1984; 39: 186
22. Giustina TA, Stewart JC, Ellis CN, et al. Topical application of isotretinoin gel improves oral lichen planus. Archives of Dermatology 1986; 122: 534
23. Hersle K, Mobacken H, Sloberg K, et al. Severe oral lichen planus: treatment with an aromatic retinoid

(etretinate). British Journal of Dermatology 1982; 106: 77
24. Camisa C, Allen CM. Treatment of oral erosive lichen planus with systemic isotretinoin. Oral Surgery Oral Medicine and Oral Pathology 1986; 62: 393
25. Eisen D, Ellis CN, Duell EA, et al. Effect of topical cyclosporine rinse on oral lichen planus. New England Journal of Medicine 1990; 323: 290
26. Eisen D, Griffiths CE, Ellis CN, et al. Cyclosporin wash for oral lichen planus. Lancet 1990; 335: 535
27. Zegarelli DJ, Sabbagh E. Relative incidence of intraoral pemphigus vulgaris, mucus membrane pemphigoid and lichen planus. Annals of Dentistry 1989; 47: 5
28. Aufdemorte TB, DeVillez RL, Parel SM. Modified topical steroid therapy for the treatment of oral mucous membrane pemphigoid. Oral Surgery Oral Medicine and Oral Pathology 1985; 59: 256
29. Zegarelli DJ. Ulcerative and erosive lichen planus. New York State Dental Journal 1987; 53: 23
30. Vincent SD, Lilly GE, Baker KA. Clinical, historic, and therapeutic features of cicatricial pemphigoid. Oral Surgery Oral Medicine and Oral Pathology 1993; 76: 453
31. Hanson RD, Olsen KD, Rogers RS. Upper aerodigestive tract manifestations of cicatricial pemphigoid. Annals of Otology Rhinology and Laryngology 1988; 97: 493
32. Rogers RS, Seehafer JR, Perry HO. Treatment of cicatricial (benign mucous membrane) pemphigoid with dapsone. Journal of the American Academy of Dermatology 1982; 6: 215
33. Zegarelli DJ, Zegarelli EV. Intraoral pemphigus vulgaris. Oral Surgery Oral Medicine and Oral Pathology 1977; 44: 384
34. Bystryn JC. Adjuvant therapy of pemphigus. Archives of Dermatology 1984; 120: 941
35. Lamey PJ, Rees TD, Binnie WH, et al. Oral presentation of pemphigus vulgaris and its response to systemic steroid therapy. Oral Surgery Oral Medicine and Oral Pathology 1992; 74: 54
36. Aberer W, Wolff-Schreiner EC, Stingl G, et al. Azathioprine in the treatment of pemphigus vulgaris. Journal of the American Academy of Dermatology 1987; 16: 527
37. Fellner MJ, Katz JM, McCabe JB. Successful use of cyclophosphamide and prednisone for initial treatment of pemphigus vulgaris. Archives of Dermatology 1978; 114: 889
38. Barthelemy H, Frappaz A, Cambazard F, et al. Treatment of nine cases of pemphigus vulgaris with cyclosporine. Journal of the American Academy of Dermatology 1988; 18: 1262
39. Ahmed AR, Hombal S. Use of cyclophosphamide in azathioprine failures in pemphigus. Journal of the American Academy of Dermatology 1987; 17: 437
40. Penneys NS, Eaglstein WH, Frost P. Management of pemphigus with gold compounds. Archives of Dermatology 1976; 112: 185
41. Roujeau JC, Andre C, Fabre MJ, et al. Plasma exchange in pemphigus. Archives of Dermatology 1983; 119: 215
42. Bean SF, Quezada RK. Recurrent oral erythema multiforme. Journal of the American Medical Association 1983; 249: 2810
43. Renfro L, Grant-Kels JM, Feder HM, et al. Controversy: are systemic steroids indicated in the treatment of erythema multiforme? Pediatric Dermatology 1989; 6: 43
44. Wilkel CS, McDonald CJ. Cyclosporine therapy for bullous erythema multiforme. Archives of Dermatology 1990; 126: 397
45. Zegarelli DJ, Zegarelli-Schmidt EC. Oral fungal infection. Journal of Oral Medicine 1987; 42: 76
46. Budtz-Jorgensen E. Histopathology, immunology and serology of oral yeast infections. Acta Odontologica Scandinavica 1990; 48: 37
47. Zegarelli DJ. Burning mouth: an alternative explanation for some patients with diabetes mellitus and pernicious anemia. Annals of Dentistry 1987; 46: 23
48. Zegarelli DJ. Fungal infections of the oral cavity. Otolaryngologic Clinics of North America 1993; 26: 1069
49. Zegarelli EV. Diseases of the oral cavity. In: Speight TM, editor. Avery's drug treatment. 3rd ed. Auckland: Adis Press, 1987: 418
50. Epstein JB. Antifungal therapy in oropharyngeal mycotic infections. Oral Surgery Oral Medicine and Oral Pathology 1990; 69: 32
51. Lucatorto FM, Franker C, Hardy WD, et al. Treatment of refractory oral candidiasis with fluconazole. Oral Surgery Oral Medicine and Oral Pathology 1991; 71: 42
52. Hoepelman IM; Dupont B. Oral candidiasis: the clinical challenge of resistance and management. International Journal of Antimicrobial Agents 1996; 6: 155-159
53. Fotos PG, Vincent SD, Hellstein JW. Oral candidosis: clinical, historical and therapeutic features of 100 cases. Oral Surgery Oral Medicine and Oral Pathology 1992; 74: 41
54. Poland JM. The spectrum of HSV-1 infections in nonimmunosuppressed patients. Compendium 1988; Suppl. 9: 310
55. Straus SE, Rooney JF, Sever JL, et al. Herpes simplex virus infection: biology, treatment and prevention. Annals of Internal Medicine 1985; 103: 404
56. Whitley RJ, Gnann JW. Acyclovir: a decade later. New England Journal of Medicine 1992; 327: 782
57. Lundeen RC, Langlais RP, Terezhalmy GT. Sunscreen protection for lip mucosa: a review and update. Journal of the American Dental Association 1985; 111: 617
58. Rowe NH. Diagnosis and treatment of herpes simplex virus disease. Compendium 1988; Suppl. 9: 292
59. Raborn GW, McGaw WT, Grace M, et al. Oral acyclovir and herpes labialis: a randomized double-blind, placebo-controlled study. Journal of the American Dental Association 1987; 115: 38
60. Lindhe J. Textbook of clinical periodontology (chapter 7). 2nd ed. Copenhagen: Munksgaard, 1989
61. Johnson BD, Engel D. Acute necrotizing ulcerative gingivitis: a review of diagnosis, etiology, and treatment. Journal of Periodontology 1986; 57: 141
62. Genco RJ, Goldman HM, Cohen DW. Contemporary periodontics (chapter 38). Philadelphia: CV Mosby, 1990
63. Schluger S, Yuodelis R, Page RC, et al. Periodontal diseases: basic phenomena, clinical management, and occlusal and restorative interrelationships (chapter 9). 2nd ed. Philadelphia: Lea & Febiger, 1990
64. van der Wal N, van der Kwast WA, van Dijk E, et al. Geographic stomatitis and psoriasis. International Journal of Oral and Maxillofacial Surgery 1988; 17: 106
65. Mani NJ. Occurrence of fissured tongue, geographic tongue and filiform atrophy among dental patients in Saudi Arabia. Annals of Dentistry 1985; 44: 14
66. Brooks JK, Balciunas BA. Geographic stomatitis: review of the literature and report of five cases. Journal of the American Dental Association 1987; 115: 421

67. Regezi JA, Sciubba J. Oral pathology clinical-pathological correlations. 2nd ed, chapters 3 and 4. Philadelphia: WB Saunders, 1993
68. Lippman SM, Batsakis JG, Toth BB, et al. Comparison of low-dose isotretinoin with beta-carotene to prevent oral carcinogenesis. New England Journal of Medicine 1993; 328: 15
69. Hong WK, Lippman SM, Itri L, et al. Prevention of second primary tumors with isotretinoin in squamous-cell carcinoma of the head and neck. New England Journal of Medicine 1990; 323: 795
70. Lippman SM, Hong WK. Retinoid chemoprevention of upper aerodigestive tract carcinogenesis. In: Important advances in oncology. Philadelphia: JB Lippincott, 1992
71. Bollag W. Vitamin A and retinoids: from nutrition to pharmacotherapy in dermatology and oncology. Lancet 1983; 1: 860
72. Zegarelli DJ. Burning mouth: an analysis of 57 patients. Oral Surgery Oral Medicine and Oral Pathology 1984; 58: 34
73. Gorsky M, Silverman S, Chinn H. Clinical characteristics and management outcome in the burning mouth syndrome. Oral Surgery Oral Medicine and Oral Pathology 1991; 72: 192
74. Lamey PJ, Hammond A, Allam BF, et al. Vitamin status of patients with burning mouth syndrome and the response to replacement therapy. British Dental Journal 1986; 160: 81
75. Ship JA. Gustatory and olfactory considerations: examination and treatment in general practice. Journal of the American Dental Association 1993; 124: 55
76. Schiffman SS. Taste and smell in disease. New England Journal of Medicine 1983; 308: 1275
77. Henkin RI. Drug-induced taste and smell disorders: incidence, mechanisms and management related primarily to treatment of sensory receptor dysfunction. Drug Safety 1994; 11: 318-77
78. Grushka M. Clinical features of burning mouth syndrome. Oral Surgery Oral Medicine and Oral Pathology 1987; 63: 30
79. Fox PC. Systemic therapy of salivary gland hypofunction. Journal of Dental Research 1987; 66: 689
80. Johnson JT, Ferretti GA, Nethery WJ, et al. Oral pilocarpine for post-irradiation xerostomia in patients with head and neck cancer. New England Journal of Medicine 1993; 329: 390
81. Foltyn P, Marriott D. HIV and oral disease. Medical Journal of Australia 1996; 164: 357-359
82. Phelan JA. Oral health complications. In: Criteria for the medical care of adults with HIV infection. New York State Department of Health, 1993
83. Phelan JA, Saltzman BR, Friedland GH, et al. Oral findings in patients with acquired immunodeficiency syndrome. Oral Surgery Oral Medicine and Oral Pathology 1987; 64: 50
84. Resnick L, Herbst JS, Ablashi DV, et al. Regression of oral hairy leucoplakia after orally administered acyclovir therapy. Journal of the American Medical Association 1988; 259: 384
85. MacPhail LA, Greenspan D, Greenspan JS. Recurrent aphthous ulcers in association with HIV infection. Oral Surgery Oral Medicine and Oral Pathology 1992; 73: 283
86. Phelan JA, Eisig S, Freedman PD, et al. Major aphthous-like ulcers in patients with AIDS. Oral Surgery Oral Medicine and Oral Pathology 1991; 71: 68
87. Sokol-Anderson ML, Prelutsky DJ, Westblom TU. Giant esophageal aphthous ulcers in AIDS patients: treatment with low-dose corticosteroids. AIDS 1991; 5: 1537
88. Winkler JR, Robertson PB. Periodontal disease associated with HIV infection. Oral Surgery Oral Medicine and Oral Pathology 1992; 73: 145
89. Epstein JB, Scully C. HIV infection: clinical features and treatment of thirty-three homosexual men with Kaposi's sarcoma. Oral Surgery Oral Medicine and Oral Pathology 1991; 71: 38

Chapter 17

# Skin Diseases

*S. Weltfriend* and *H.I. Maibach*

## Synopsis of Important Principles

1) There is no great mystery about treatment of skin diseases, as the same rules apply to the management of inflammation, infection, allergy and neoplasia as elsewhere in the body.

2) In other disease processes that are specific to the skin, there are some equally logical treatments; for example, in psoriasis, effective control can be achieved by drugs directed, at least partially, towards reducing the abnormally high epidermal cell turnover.

3) In planning rational treatment, it is important to know whether the disease is confined to the skin, and when other organs are involved, to know whether the primary fault is internal or in the skin.

4) Especially when the disease is confined to the skin, topical as well as systemic treatment can often be used.

5) There is usually some good reason if topical treatment is unsatisfactory, e.g. the drug is irritant or sensitising, or does not adequately penetrate the skin.

6) The base in which a drug is applied to the skin is important. In general, lotions and pastes are best for weeping lesions and greasy ointments for dry lesions, while creams are suitable for either.

7) In some skin diseases, considerable reliance is placed on symptomatic treatment.

8) The placebo effect is large in a number of skin diseases but if a placebo is to be used, it should be harmless.

9) Drug-induced skin disease is common; there are few drugs that have never caused a skin eruption. Drug rashes are of many different types. Only a few are produced by a known immunological mechanism.

10) Proof that a given drug is responsible for a rash is often difficult to obtain. Nevertheless, in general, it is important to stop the drug or drugs thought most likely to be responsible, especially when the drug is known to have severe effects on the skin or adverse systemic effects.

Dermatological therapeutics has seen great recent advances with the development of treatments specifically for skin disease, including photochemotherapy and the retinoid group of drugs. Previously, there had been only empirical remedies such as tar and calamine lotion and drugs originally intended for non-dermatological disease, such as the corticosteroids, antihistamines, antimitotics and antibacterials.

Placebos remain an essential part of dermatological treatment, and it is reasonable to use them provided they are recognised for what they are and are used only when there is nothing better to offer. Placebos should preferably be harmless and inexpensive.

Many dermatological treatments, however, remain symptomatic. Corticosteroids are widely used to control symptoms in inflammatory dermatoses, and antipruritic agents (such as sedative antihistamines) are valuable in the management of itch. Similarly the application of simple emollients to dry scaly eruptions, or of calamine lotion to acute lesions such as sunburn, produces symptomatic relief.

## 1. Clinical Pharmacological Considerations and General Principles of Treatment

The rational therapy of skin disorders is based on similar fundamental principles to those applied in the treatment of diseases of other systems.

### 1.1 Underlying Disease Mechanisms

As with disorders of other organs, the ideal treatment of skin disease corrects, permanently, the underlying abnormality. Thus, infective dermatoses can often be effectively eradicated with appropriate antimicrobials. Alternatively, in conditions with 'trigger' factors that precipitate specific eruptions, removal of the precipitant may prevent relapses. For example, withdrawal of sensitising agents in patients with allergic contact dermatitis, or prevention of recurrent streptococcal infections in individuals prone to guttate psoriasis,[1] will usually ameliorate these disorders. Even in these instances, however, it is clear that patients susceptible to such conditions often have some underlying constitutional abnormality that remains unresolved. In some dermatological disorders, although inactivation of the underlying abnormality may be impossible, sufficient knowledge is available about the disease process to indicate the manner in which effective pharmacological control might be achieved. Thus, many forms of urticaria can be treated with antihistamines, even though the nature of the underlying abnormality remains poorly understood. Similarly, drugs that reduce epidermal cell turnover can be used in the treatment of psoriasis, despite lack of knowledge about the mechanism of how epidermal cell turnover is increased in this condition.

### 1.2 Relationship of Skin Disease and Systemic Disease

In a patient with a rash, the skin may be the only organ involved, but often the rash is associated with a systemic disease. When other organs are involved, it is essential to know the relationship between the skin disease and the disease of the other organs, for only in this way can treatment be planned intelligently. Skin disease and systemic disease can be related in 4 different ways:[2]

1) *Where the skin disease is due to an internal disease;* for example, when dermatomyositis arises as a consequence of an internal carcinoma, when dry skin results from malabsorption or other wasting diseases, or when a purpuric rash is caused by thrombocytopenia. Here it is essential to treat the primary cause and, if this can be done effectively, the rash will disappear. Topical treatment of the skin is only symptomatic.

2) *Where the skin disease causes disease of other organs;* for example, when shunting of blood through the vessels of inflamed skin results in high output 'heart failure'. In this situation, prompt treatment of the rash is essential; treatment of the heart failure will not be fully effective until the skin is dealt with. The systemic effects of skin disease are many and varied and, while not all are serious, some are of practical importance in management. For example, the hypoferraemia caused by eczema and psoriasis, like the hypoferraemia of infection, is not due to deficiency of iron but to inability to release it from the body stores where it is present in abundance. The hypoferraemia should be recognised for what it is, since it is not necessary or desirable to treat it by administration of iron, and indeed oral iron is not effective in increasing the serum iron concentration.

3) *Where the skin disease and internal disease have a common cause or a common pathology;* for example, in the so-called 'collagen vascular' diseases, the skin is often affected along

with internal organs. If an effective treatment is available to deal with the basic cause, the skin and internal organs will both respond. Often, however, e.g. in most cases of systemic sclerosis, all that can be done is to treat the symptoms.

4) *Where the skin disease and the internal disease are related indirectly;* i.e. when they occur together more commonly than would be expected by chance, and yet relationships 1, 2 and 3 above do not apply. For example, the epilepsy which arises from glial proliferation in 80% of cases of tuberous sclerosis (epiloia) needs treatment in its own right, independently of anything that is done to the hyperplastic vascular lesions of the skin.

## 1.3 Appropriate Route of Administration

The skin is ideally suited for topical therapy and, at least when it is primarily implicated, this would seem the logical route of administration. The effectiveness of topically applied drugs, however, is dependent on several factors, and this route of administration also produces its own problems.

### *1.3.1 Ability of the Applied Drug to Penetrate the Skin Adequately*

Numerous factors pertaining to the pharmaceutical preparation and also to the patient and his/her environment determine whether a medicament applied topically will penetrate to the required level in the skin and will act when it reaches there. Many (see table I) are poorly understood or their practical clinical importance ill defined (for reviews, see Bronaugh & Maibach;[3] Bronaugh & Maibach[4]). Penetration through the intact stratum corneum is a key rate-limiting step in percutaneous absorption of a drug, as once this barrier is passed, the drug usually disperses freely through the rest of the epidermis and the dermis and thence into its blood vessels. There is a 'reservoir' in the stratum corneum[5] where some drugs are held for a variable time to be absorbed later when conditions of keratin hydration or temperature change. Drugs can also pass into the body through pilosebaceous follicles and sweat glands, and although this movement can be rapid, it is usually minimal compared with absorption through the intact stratum corneum.[6-8]

**Table I.** Factors that influence the penetration of a drug into and through the skin

| |
|---|
| **Physicochemical properties of the drug:** |
| • Polarity |
| • Solubility in pharmaceutical base |
| • Solubility in lipid |
| • Stability |
| **Nature of the pharmaceutical preparation:** |
| • Drug concentration |
| • Composition and physicochemical properties of the base |
| • Incompatible mixtures |
| **Method of application (occlusion)** |
| **Nature of the skin:** |
| • Integrity of horny cell layer of epidermis |
| • Flexural surfaces |
| • Age (penetration greater in infants, elderly) |
| **External factors:** |
| • Temperature |
| • Ambient water vapour pressure |

As a rule, nonpolar (lipid soluble) compounds are more easily absorbed than highly polar (water soluble) ones, though this depends to some extent on the base in which the compound is applied and the partition coefficient between the base and the epidermis. Esterification, which renders polar compounds more lipid soluble, may result in enhanced penetration, though the extent to which this increases its pharmacological effect depends on the rate of local hydrolysis, and the activity of the esterified molecule itself. Increasing the concentration of drug in its base also increases the amount absorbed, although the proportionate quantity tends to fall, i.e. the percent absorption decreases but the mass absorbed increases.[9]

In clinical practice, there are other ways of increasing percutaneous absorption:

1) Applying the drug under polythene occlusion for prolonged periods as, for example, in the case of corticosteroids.

2) Applying the drug with enhancers such as dimethylsulfoxide (DMSO), which enhances absorption without damaging the skin, as for example in the case of idoxuridine in cutaneous herpes simplex infection (see section 2.2.2).[10] This approach has been extensively documented.[11]

3) Mixing the drug with substances which damage the stratum corneum and remove its barrier action, e.g. salicylic acid, sodium lauryl sulfate.

Quite apart from adding 'active' substances to enhance absorption from a base, the composition of the base itself can alter absorption; for example, propylene glycol in bases as a solvent for corticosteroids increases their release and therapeutic effectiveness, but a base with an optimum amount of propylene glycol for one corticosteroid is not necessarily suitable for another.[12] The type of base may also affect absorption; for example, betamethasone benzoate is more active in a gel than in a cream or lotion,[13] fluocinolone acetonide is more active in an ointment than in a gel or cream,[14] while betamethasone valerate ointment is more active than the cream.[13,15] Usually it is not possible to forecast the best vehicle for penetration, and each new corticosteroid preparation has to be assayed in several vehicles.[16]

Just as there are 'incompatible' mixtures in internal medicine (see chapter 7), so there are substances which should not be mixed in topical preparations; for instance, salicylic acid combines with zinc to form zinc salicylate, which no longer has the effect on the skin of salicylic acid. When dithranol (anthralin) is used in zinc paste, the zinc oxide of the paste combines with the dithranol to form an inert compound, though in this case, the presence of salicylic acid is helpful in preventing the unwanted interaction between dithranol and zinc.[17] Another undesirable effect of mixing is seen with dimethylsulfoxide, for although it enhances absorption of many substances, including corticosteroids, it may reduce the therapeutic effectiveness of certain corticosteroids when it is mixed with them; presumably there is a chemical alteration in the steroids.

There are also regional differences in percutaneous absorption and some are related to differences in regional anatomy. The palms and soles are relatively resistant to topical applications; topical corticosteroids, for example, which are effective without occlusion on other parts of the body, may have to be applied with occlusion to be equally effective on these parts. This is true regardless of the numerous eccrine glands opening onto the palms and soles, which suggests that this latter anatomical peculiarity is relatively unimportant. Regional differences in the construction of the stratum corneum probably explains the increased permeability of facial skin compared with that of forearm skin.[18] The flexures are well known sites for enhanced absorption, partly because flexural skin is relatively thin and partly because of the occlusive effect of the apposing surfaces. Non-cornifying mucous membranes are other sites of increased absorption. For further information, see reviews by Wester & Maibach,[8] and Guy & Maibach.[19]

The age of the skin affects percutaneous absorption too, and in general, the skin of premature infants is more permeable[20] while the skin of individuals older than 70 years may be less permeable.[21]

Damaged skin, whether as a result of experimental cellulose tape stripping, burns, disease, or the application of substances that break down the stratum corneum, may be more permeable than normal skin. This can be clinically important, as in the case of boric acid, which, in quantities that do not have toxic effects when applied to intact skin, produces systemic toxicity when added to excoriated skin of the diaper area. Burnt skin also readily leads to enhanced percutaneous absorption, as in a case of fatal encephalopathy following use of hexachlorophane emulsion for an uncomplicated burn.[22] For a review of this topic, see Moon & Maibach.[23]

Since the ability of drugs to penetrate skin is probably reduced by the presence of scale and crust, it seems logical to remove 'heaped-up' scale before starting more specific treatment; for example, in scalp psoriasis, a preparation such as salicylic acid ointment or mineral oil can be used. In impetigo, however, there is no evidence from controlled studies that removing the crust increases the effectiveness of topical antibiotics.

#### *1.3.2 Undesirable Local Effects of Drugs When Used Topically*

The topical route of administration is liable to induce immunologically mediated hypersensitivity phenomena to drugs that only rarely give rise to such reactions after systemic use. This is possibly due in part to the unique 'antigen-processing' properties of cutaneous Langerhans cells, and frequently results in contact dermatitis after topical application of antihistamines, local anaesthetics, and certain antibiotics (e.g. penicillin, streptomycin). The use of such drugs in dermatology is generally limited to oral or parenteral administration.

Some drugs have an adverse effect on the skin whether given systemically or topically. The deleterious effect of corticosteroids on the skin is a good example, whether they are produced as part of a Cushing's syndrome following systemic administration, or purely as the result of a local effect when applied to the skin directly.[24-26]

In certain diseases (e.g. severe eczema) in which the choice may lie between treatment with a topical or a systemic corticosteroid, it may be that the adverse effects on the skin will prove to be greater with the topical preparation than with the systemic preparation given in the dose required to produce the same therapeutic effect. Thus, in certain special situations where adverse effects on the skin are particularly undesirable, the systemic route of administration might then be the one of choice.

#### 1.3.3 Lack of Effect of Some Drugs Used Topically

In some cases, local treatment is relatively unsatisfactory for reasons which are not understood. In severe eczema and certain bullous dermatoses of the pemphigus group, a systemic corticosteroid is often effective in cases where a topical corticosteroid is not, even though it can be calculated that the amount of corticosteroid reaching the skin is much less in the case of the systemically administered drug. It is not known why this should be so but there are several possible explanations. One possibility is that a systemic as well as a local action of the corticosteroid is necessary for maximum effect. The effectiveness of methotrexate in psoriasis (see section 6.1.2) also depends on its being given systemically, although *in vitro* it has a direct effect on epidermal cells, reducing their rate of turnover. The fact that it has been found to be ineffective when used topically is partly due to lack of penetration of the epidermis,[27] but the additional possibility that its action in psoriasis is due in part to the production of folic acid deficiency in the body as a whole has not been entirely ruled out.

### 1.4 Which Drug?

As with therapeutic choices in other systems, drug selection in dermatology is determined by the nature and severity of the clinical condition. Treatments are also conditioned by the site of the lesion, and secondary pharmacological actions may also play an important role. The antipruritic and hypnotic properties of the so-called 'sedative' antihistamines (histamine $H_1$-receptor antagonists) [e.g. trimeprazine, chlorphenamine] may be useful, especially at night, in patients with eczematous eruptions. By contrast, in patients with urticaria, nonsedating antihistamines (e.g. terfenadine, astemizole, loratadine, cetirizine, acrivastine) are better tolerated by patients.

The choice of a topical corticosteroid can be even more difficult. Numerous preparations exist (see table II) and the active drug is sometimes available in several dilutions and in different bases, as well as in combination with various antimicrobial agents. The task of the clinician

**Table II.** Relative activities of topical corticosteroid preparations[a] (after Niedner & Schopf[28])

| Drug | Concentration(s) |
|---|---|
| **Very strong** | |
| Betamethasone dipropionate (propylene glycol base) | 0.05% |
| Clobetasol propionate | 0.05% |
| Diflucortolone valerate | 0.3% |
| Halobetasol (ulobetasol) propionate | 0.05% |
| **Strong** | |
| Amcinonide | 0.1% |
| Betamethasone dipropionate | 0.05% |
| Betamethasone valerate | 0.1% |
| Desoximethasone | 0.25% |
| Diflorasone diacetate | 0.05% |
| Diflucortolone valerate | 0.1% |
| Fluocinolone acetonide | 0.025% |
| Fluocinonide | 0.05% |
| Fluocortolone/fluocortolone hexanoate | 0.5%[b] |
| Fluticasone propionate (cream base) | 0.05% |
| Fluticasone propionate (ointment base) | 0.005% |
| Halcinonide | 0.1% |
| Mometasone furoate | 0.1% |
| Triamcinolone acetonide | 0.5% |
| **Moderately strong** | |
| Alclomethasone dipropionate | 0.05% |
| Betamethasone benzoate | 0.025% |
| Betamethasone valerate | 0.05% |
| Clobetasone butyrate | 0.05% |
| Clocortolone pivalate/hexanoate | 0.2%[b] |
| Desonide | 0.05%, 0.1% |
| Desoximethasone | 0.05% |
| Dexamethasone | 0.05%, 0.08%, 0.1% |
| Flumethasone pivalate | 0.02% |
| Fluocinolone acetonide | 0.01% |
| Fluocortolone | 0.2%[b] |
| Fluprednidene acetate | 0.05%, 0.1% |
| Flurandrenolone (flurandrenolide) | 0.025%, 0.05% |
| Halcinonide | 0.025% |
| Hydrocortisone aceponate | 0.1% |
| Hydrocortisone butyrate | 0.1% |
| Prednicarbate | 0.25% |
| Triamcinolone acetonide | 0.025%, 0.1% |
| **Mild** | |
| Clocortolone pivalate/hexanoate | 0.06%[b] |
| Dexamethasone | 0.012%, 0.03%, 0.035% |
| Fluocortin butylester | 0.75% |
| Hydrocortisone | 0.25-2% |
| Hydrocortisone acetate | 0.25-1% |
| Prednisone | 0.4% |
| Triamcinolone acetonide | 0.0018% |

a Approximate guide only, based on activity in vasoconstrictor assays. Note that the distinction between the various groups is not well defined, and varies with the concentration of the conticosteroid and the vehicle in which it is formulated.

b Total concentration (as mixed esters or ester plus base).

**Table III.** Properties and uses of common dermatological bases (after Hunter[30,31])

| Surface, disease | Base | Effect | Examples/notes |
|---|---|---|---|
| Dry and scaly (e.g. psoriasis, dry eczema, ichthyosis) | Ointment | Occlusive emollient | Soft white or soft yellow paraffin<br>Emulsifying ointment<br>Synthetic bases<br>Lanolin (*NB.* may sensitise) |
| Moist or dry (e.g. eczema in various stages) | Cream | Cooling emollient and moisturising | Oily cream<br>Aqueous cream<br>Cetomacrogol cream<br>Synthetic bases (*NB.* preservatives may sensitise) |
| Acutely inflamed; wet and oozing (e.g. weeping eczema and other bullous diseases) | Lotions | Drying, soothing and cooling | Saline solution<br>Calamine lotion<br>Aluminium acetate solution<br>Potassium permanganate solution |
| Lichenified (e.g. eczema); oozing (e.g. eczema) | Pastes | Protective, prevent spreading of active ingredient<br>Drying effect on wet areas | Zinc compound paste<br>Lassar's paste<br>Coal tar paste-impregnated bandages protect eczema from scratching<br>Pastes used as vehicle for dithranol in psoriasis |
| Flexures, especially if sore and moist (e.g. intertrigo, flexural eczema and psoriasis, candidiasis) | Dusting powders | Lessen friction and are drying | Talc dusting powder; zinc starch and talc can be used as a vehicle for antifungal drugs |
| Flexures (e.g. intertrigo, candidiasis, ulcers) | Paints | Drying | Castellani's magenta paint<br>Better than powders for very moist areas |

in choosing the appropriate preparation is not straight forward and data quoting results of clinical trials require expert knowledge for correct interpretation. Therapeutic trials of topical preparations need planning to take into account several factors, of which choosing the right endpoint, the right base, the right disease and inclusion of an adequate number of patients are particularly important.[29] The vasoconstrictor assay, often used in screening and comparing topical corticosteroids, is not necessarily a measure of their therapeutic effectiveness in a given disease; for example, while fluocinonide cream causes more vasoconstriction than either betamethasone valerate cream or ointment, it is inferior therapeutically to the ointment of betamethasone although superior to betamethasone cream.[15] The choice of a suitable corticosteroid is discussed below (see sections 6.1.1, 7.1.1 and table II).

## 1.5 Which Base?

Many factors should be considered and some have already been mentioned (see section 1.3.1 and table III). In general, it is best to prescribe a lotion or a paste for application to a weeping skin surface and a greasy ointment for application to a dry, cracked surface. Creams are convenient, since to some extent they can be used for either dry or wet surfaces, and have the advantage over ointments of being cosmetically elegant. Many ointments contain lanolin or wool alcohols, and patients not uncommonly develop contact sensitivity to these substances when they are applied to leg ulcers. Creams less often contain lanolin, but usually contain a preservative or stabiliser; the ones in general use (e.g. parabens or ethylenediamine hydrochloride) are known to be occasional sensitisers.[32,33] Thus, choice of a base will be limited if the patient develops a contact dermatitis to one of its constituents. Manufacturers change the constituents of their bases from time to time, so it is always wise to check the current formulation before advising those with known contact sensitivity.

The boundary line between creams and ointments has to some extent become blurred by the introduction of certain synthetic bases, e.g. fatty alcohol propylene glycol (FAPG), which is said to have 'the properties of a cream and an ointment'. Early impressions that they are not routinely satisfactory when a truly greasy preparation is required have not altered with time.

Lotions are preferable to greasy applications for flexural sites, e.g. the groin and toe clefts. Sprays are expensive and on the whole not to be recommended.

The choice of a base will, to some extent, be influenced by the drug in question, for as already mentioned, corticosteroids (for example) perform better in one base than in another.

## 2. Skin Infections

### 2.1 Bacterial Infections

#### *2.1.1 Impetigo*

This is a superficial infection of the skin caused by staphylococci, a mixture of staphylococci and streptococci or, less often, streptococci alone.[34]

**Optimum Treatment**

Because the lesion is so superficial, it would be reasonable to expect it to respond to topical antibiotics – and indeed it usually does so – but systemic antibiotics are preferable in many cases, particularly in young children (see below). Ideally, the choice of antibiotic should be based on knowledge of the sensitivity of the organism but in practice this information is not always available and the choice of the topical antibiotic is then often a personal one. Antibiotics which are used topically carry the risk of producing allergic contact dermatitis, but in impetigo, where the period of time over which application is required is short, this is not often a problem. Antibiotics which may later be needed for treatment of a systemic illness should be avoided (when practical) for topical use, in order to minimise development of resistant organisms – particularly as the skin is a site likely to predispose to development of such resistance (see also chapter 31, sect. 2.3).[35] Thus, fusidic acid and gentamicin are best not used topically but reserved for systemic use in serious infections.

*Mupirocin* is an antibacterial agent that is active against many Gram-positive and some Gram-negative organisms. Because of its rapid systemic metabolism, mupirocin can only be used topically and this, together with the fact that it is chemically unrelated to other antibiotics and only rarely appears to sensitise the skin, makes it a theoretically valuable agent for skin infections. When used as a 2% ointment, good success rates above those of the vehicle have been reported in patients (usually children) with impetigo.[36] Although its precise clinical role remains unclear, it may prove to be an ideal treatment for impetigo.[37] Other topical preparations such as *0.5% neomycin, 1.5% framycetin, 0.025% gramicidin, or 3% chlortetracycline* have also been found to be effective and are cosmetically acceptable. These agents should not be routinely used in combination with corticosteroids; it is neither necessary nor desirable to use a corticosteroid in impetigo.

Patients with impetigo who present to hospital clinics often do so because they have failed to respond to topical antibiotics for one reason or another. It should first be determined that there is no underlying skin condition such as scabies, pediculosis, human immunodeficiency virus (HIV) infection or herpes simplex. If there is not, information about the identity and sensitivity of the bacterial organism is especially desirable, but again it cannot always be obtained. In any case, the choice of antibacterial agent must be influenced by the fact that cases of nephritis following streptococcal infections of the skin have been described.[38,39] Consequently, the antibacterial agent should be effective against streptococci as well as against staphylococci. The incidence of nephritis seems to be particularly great in certain geographic areas and in children aged 1 to 11 years, particularly if the rash is extensive.[38]

When there is a case for treating impetigo with systemic antibiotics, one of the penicillinase-resistant penicillins such as *cloxacillin* or *flucloxacillin* is the first-line of treatment, with *erythromycin* or *cotrimoxazole* (trimethoprim/sulfamethoxazole) as alternatives for patients with known penicillin allergy. The full oral dosage, correspondingly reduced for small children, should be given and treatment continued for approximately 10 days. The potential problem of resistant strains of bacteria readily emerging does not arise with penicillins or cotrimoxazole, and bacteriologists do not seem concerned about it arising with erythromycin, provided it is used only occasionally.

As a general rule, topical antibiotics (see above) should be used, except in the following groups of patients who should have systemic treatment:

- Children up to 11 years of age, except those with a very small area of skin involved
- Anyone who has not responded to topical treatment
- Those with coexisting eczema
- Those immunosuppressed by drugs or disease and those receiving systemic or topical corticosteroids
- Those who develop systemic symptoms (e.g. pyrexia) and/or adenopathy
- Those with existing renal and heart disease and those who have previously had guttate psoriasis
- Those who develop proteinuria, haematuria, oedema, hypertension or have a low third

component of complement (C3) level in the serum
• In 'epidemics' of dermatogenic nephritis.

Clinicians are often confused by the results of antimicrobial sensitivity assays in impetigo. Most patients are clinically improved when the laboratory report becomes available. Presumably the natural history of spontaneous remission combined with the high concentrations of drug (especially with topical preparations) that may pool in the lesion favours clinical resolution, despite *in vitro* resistance.

#### *2.1.2 Erysipelas*

This is an infection of the skin and the superficial parts of the subcutaneous tissues by *Streptococcus pyogenes*. It differs from streptococcal cellulitis, since in this condition the deeper tissues are also involved. The infecting bacteria usually enter through a small crack in the skin surface. Systemic symptoms are frequent.

##### Optimum Treatment

Treatment should be with a systemic antibiotic. Oral *phenoxymethylpenicillin (penicillin V)* is the drug of choice and should be given in full dosage for 7 days, with *erythromycin* or a *sulfonamide* substituted for individuals with penicillin allergy. Recurrent attacks of erysipelas may occur in patients who, for one reason or another, have inadequate lymphatic drainage of the part concerned. Whether this is due to congenital hypoplasia of the lymphatics or to damage to the lymphatics from the infection itself is usually impossible to determine, but in any case the situation will be made worse by recurrent attacks of infection, and in such patients long term maintenance therapy with low doses of penicillin (or erythromycin) should be given. Often, administration for approximately 5 to 7 days per month is adequate although placebo-controlled studies are not available.

#### *2.1.3 Recurrent Boils (Furunculosis)*

A furuncle or boil is an acute infection of a hair follicle in which staphylococci are usually involved. While diabetes mellitus, an underlying immunological abnormality or uraemia are well known causes, boils most often occur in otherwise healthy individuals. Staphylococci of the same phage type may be isolated from the boil as from other parts of the skin and from the nose, throat and perineum. The role of these 'carrier' sites in the production of skin infection can be overstressed and in some cases there is evidence that the appearance of a given bacterium in the skin predates its appearance in the nose and throat. Nevertheless, if infection (clinical or subclinical) persists at any site after clearing of skin lesions, it is reasonable to deal with it. In this regard, *mupirocin* ointment and other topical antibacterial agents have been reported to clear the nose of staphylococci.[40,41]

##### Optimum Treatment

In the acute stage, boils may be treated with full dosage of an appropriate antibacterial agent, as indicated by sensitivity studies, e.g. cloxacillin, flucloxacillin, erythromycin (and other macrolides), and the fluoroquinolones. Guidelines for the use of systemic antibiotics in acute furunculosis remain imprecise. The overwhelming majority of boils resolve spontaneously. Incision and drainage of a pointing lesion decreases pain. Patients with significant underlying disease, signs of systemic response (pyrexia) or adenopathy, and those with lesions that might lead to cavernous sinus thrombosis, are candidates for systemic therapy. Patients who develop boils at frequent intervals may need long term treatment. Topical antibacterial preparations can also be used if it is decided to treat the 'carrier' state.[42]

The role of antiseptics such as chlorhexidine applied to the skin as a cream or added to a bath is not proven, but they may help to reduce skin carriage of bacteria, and the spread of infection.[43]

Bacterial interference therapy with *Staphylococcus aureus* strain 502 A may induce remissions when other techniques fail.[44,45]

#### *2.1.4 Tuberculosis of the Skin*

Lupus vulgaris is the only tuberculous infection now seen with any frequency in dermatological clinics, and even this is uncommon. It is a low grade infection in an individual who has previously acquired some immunity and some hypersensitivity to the organism. In affected patients, tuberculosis may be present at sites other than the skin but this is by no means usual. The course of the skin lesion is often chronic and slowly progressive with a tendency to self-healing, and when some cases are referred for treatment, the disease has already been present for many years and has run an entirely benign course over this period. The few cases in which the infection is more aggressive leave little doubt, however, that all patients should be treated. The risks of leaving the disease untreated are mainly those of local extension. Spread to other organs is rare and, although cases of carcinoma arising at the site of previous lupus vulgaris in the absence of treatment with irradiation or ultraviolet light are documented, there is no proof that carcinoma can be caused by lupus vulgaris itself.

#### Optimum Treatment

Treatment requires an accurate diagnosis, with confirmation by mycobacterial growth on solid media (i.e. Lowenstein-Jensen, Middlebrook 7H11). The BACTEC system (radiometric detection of carbon dioxide produced by growing organisms) advocated by many laboratories, provides a more rapid detection of *Mycobacterium tuberculosis*.[46] All isolates of *M. tuberculosis* warrant testing for antimicrobial drug sensitivity.

Extrapulmonary/cutaneous tuberculosis requires the same therapy as pulmonary tuberculosis.[47,48] The regimens in current use consist of 2 phases. An initial phase, using at least 3 drugs for 8 to 12 weeks, is designed to reduce the population of viable organisms as quickly as possible. A continuation phase, with fewer drugs, continues for several months thereafter. Drugs in present use include the following:

- *Isoniazid* (usually 300mg daily) for the full 6 months. Pyridoxine 50mg daily is given in addition, to prevent isoniazid-induced peripheral neuropathy
- *Rifampicin* (450mg daily for those weighing less than 50kg and 600mg daily for those above this weight) for the full 6 months
- *Pyrazinamide* for the first 2 months (1.5g daily for those weighing less than 50kg, 2.0g daily for those weighing between 50 and 74kg, and 2.5g daily for those over 75kg); and
- *Ethambutol* for the first 2 months (15 mg/kg bodyweight daily).

The use of streptomycin is probably rarely justifiable in tuberculosis confined to the skin, and when *p*-aminosalicylic acid is prescribed, a high proportion of patients with lupus vulgaris refuse to take it (see chapter 23; sect. 9.1.1).

Some cases of lupus vulgaris respond dramatically to treatment but others, including some in whom the bacterial sensitivities are known and the appropriate antituberculosis drugs have been given in full doses, continue unabated. In some of these, intralesional injection of a corticosteroid such as triamcinolone acetonide is helpful, antituberculosis drugs being given at the same time.

## 2.2 Viral Infections

### *2.2.1 Warts*

Fortunately, the majority of warts do not need treatment, as they undergo spontaneous regression in time. In one hospital, for example, in 50% of patients with warts placed on a waiting list for 6 months, treatment was no longer necessary at the end of this time because of spontaneous regression.[49] Warts are infectious, especially in children, who presumably have little or no immunity to the virus which is almost ubiquitous. Public health measures such as banning from swimming baths those with plantar warts are not very effective in stopping spread and are possibly best abandoned. The main indications for treatment are pain, uncertainty of diagnosis, and serious cosmetic disability. Genital and perianal warts also usually need treatment.

#### Optimum Treatment

Once a decision to treat a wart has been made, therapy can be by destroying it by heat, cold, acid, alkali, etc., or by surgical removal. The chosen procedure will depend to some extent on the number of warts to be dealt with and on the local facilities available for treatment. Warts should never be excised but should be removed by curettage. If this is done properly, scarring will be minimal if at all. Any treatment that requires general anaesthesia is rarely justifiable and, similarly, radiotherapy is not an acceptable treatment for this benign condition.

Common methods of destroying a wart include *liquid nitrogen, trichloroacetic acid,* or *phenol;* more than one application may be required. All can produce scarring if used injudiciously. *Salicylic acid* is the active constituent of most general purpose wart paints that patients buy themselves, a typical formula being salicylic acid 1 part, lactic acid 1 part, flexible collodion 4 parts. *Formaldehyde* and *podophyllin* are helpful in the management of plantar warts, although 5% formaldehyde soaks can lead to overdrying of the skin or to contact dermatitis, and podophyllin paint can lead to painful blistering and sloughing. *Gluteraldehyde* 10% is a possible alternative.[50]

***Genital and perianal warts:*** 0.5% *podophyllotoxin (podofilox)* solution or a 25% solution of *podophyllin* in spirit or compound benzoin tincture is the treatment of choice in anogenital warts. If weekly painting with these formulations fails, curettage under anaesthesia is usually required. Podophyllotoxin has been shown to be more effective than its vehicles in genital warts.[51] General purpose wart paints should not be used on the face or anogenital regions, and podophyllin or podophyllotoxin should only be used on a limited area of skin, and not at all in pregnancy because of their toxicity and possible teratogenic effects.[52]

Exceptionally, for example in extensive warts in immunosuppressed patients, painting with *dinitrochlorobenzene* solution (after first sensitising the patient), systemic *interferon-α* therapy,[53,54] and intralesional *bleomycin* have been used with some success, but all have potentially serious adverse effects.

For anogenital warts in children, as well as treating with topical measures, it is necessary to be aware of the fact that such warts are associated with a likelihood of previous sexual molestation.

### 2.2.2 Herpes Simplex

The human herpes simplex virus consists of two closely related viruses – herpes simplex virus type 1 (HSV-1) and herpes simplex virus type 2 (HSV-2). Both viruses cause a wide variety of mucocutaneous infections and produce both primary and recurrent infections. The primary infection is defined as the first infection with herpes simplex virus in a seronegative patient. It occurs primarily by direct exposure through mucocutaneous contact with another infected individual. The primary infection is usually more severe and has a different natural history. Recurrent infection is usually milder and of shorter duration than primary infection. Certain triggering events, such as exposure to sunlight, severe stress, and neurosurgical manipulation of the ganglia will cause the latent virus to reactivate.

#### Optimum Treatment

Topical aciclovir (cream or ointment)[55,56] and *idoxuridine* (solution)[10] have both proved of marginal value in the treatment of herpes simplex infections of the skin. Idoxuridine, a derivative of deoxyuridine, appears to be introduced into viral DNA and results in the formation of an unstable nucleotide which produces aberrant protein synthesis (see chapter 32; sect. 2.17). To enhance its penetration into the skin, idoxuridine is formulated as a solution in dimethylsulfoxide.

Aciclovir is a guanine analogue and requires phosphorylation by a viral thymidine kinase to an active metabolite which inhibits virus DNA polymerase (see chapter 32; sect. 2.8). In patients with recurrent herpes labialis infections, early application of 5% aciclovir in a cream formulation has proved marginally effective in decreasing the healing time and duration of symptoms in some studies,[57,58] though not in others.[59] Results with the 5% ointment formulation, however, have been less conclusive.[56]

Systemic *aciclovir* therapy rather than topical treatment is indicated in extensive mucocutaneous infection, particularly in immunocompromised individuals. The oral dose is 200mg 5 times a day for 5 days initially.[60-62] Short term prophylactic therapy with aciclovir may benefit some patients with recurrent herpes labialis. However, there are no data regarding the use of long term treatment for the prevention of herpes labialis.[63] In practice, oral therapy is the standard, with topical therapy being considered of marginal value.

Treatment directed at 'drying up' the lesion may help the patient symptomatically, and surgical spirit or calamine lotion are suitable applications for this purpose. The role of topical corticosteroids remains to be determined. Treatment of herpes simplex of the eye should be undertaken by ophthalmologists (see chapter 15; sect. 3.7).

### 2.2.3 Varicella and Herpes Zoster

Varicella and herpes zoster are distinct clinical entities caused by varicella-zoster virus (VZV). The differences between these two diseases are in the host and circumstances of infection. Varicella is an acute, contagious exanthem which follows primary exogenous VZV infection and occurs most often in childhood. It is characterised by a short prodromal period and a generalised pruritic vesicular eruption. Systemic symptoms and serious complications occur in adults and in immunocompromised individuals.

Herpes zoster occurs most often in elderly people following an earlier attack of varicella. Herpes zoster is the result of reactivation of an endogenous infection that had persisted in latent form within sensory ganglia. The disease is characterised by unilateral radicular pain and grouped vesicles on an erythematous and oedematous base, limited to the distribution of nerves from one or more posterior ganglia. In immunocompromised individuals, bacterial superinfection, scarring and cutaneous dissemination are frequent.

**Optimum Treatment**

Infections due to varicella-zoster virus seem less responsive to topical *aciclovir* and *idoxuridine* than herpes simplex infections; both drugs used topically have proved only marginally beneficial. An appropriate formulation and dose regimen of idoxuridine can be effective in shortening healing time and reducing the duration of symptoms in cutaneous herpes zoster.[64,65] Similarly, topical aciclovir applied as a 5% ointment has been reported to be effective in shortening healing time in localised herpes zoster in a trial in immunocompromised patients.[66]

*Systemic aciclovir* therapy has been used to treat acute localised or disseminated herpes zoster in both immunocompromised and immunocompetent individuals (for reviews, see Richards et al.;[55] O'Brien & Campoli-Richards;[56] Whitley & Gnann[63]). In the latter, both intravenous aciclovir (5 mg/kg or 250 mg/m$^2$ 8-hourly for 5 days)[67,68] and oral aciclovir (800mg 5 times daily for 7 days)[69-72] have been found to shorten the healing time and decrease the pain of herpes zoster if started within 48 to 72 hours of the onset of rash. In addition, early treatment of acute herpes zoster with oral aciclovir appears to reduce both the incidence and duration of subsequent postherpetic neuralgia.[73] In a trial in immunocompromised patients, intravenous aciclovir (500 mg/m$^2$ 8-hourly for 7 days) decreased both cutaneous dissemination and the development of visceral complications.[74]

Other antiviral drugs that have been used in the treatment of herpes zoster include *famciclovir*, the oral prodrug of penciclovir, and *valaciclovir*, the L-valyl ester of aciclovir which is rapidly converted to the parent compound (aciclovir) following oral administration (see further chapter 32; sections 2.9 and 2.10). A comparative study of famciclovir (250, 500 and 750mg 3 times daily) and aciclovir (800mg 5 times daily) given for 7 days in uncomplicated herpes zoster in immunocompetent patients has shown the two drugs to be equieffective in accelerating healing of cutaneous lesions and reducing the duration of pain.[75] Although the less frequent dosage regimen of famciclovir may be an advantage, no clinical benefit of this drug over and above that seen with aciclovir has been demonstrated.

Valaciclovir has also proved comparable in effectiveness to aciclovir, dosages of 1g 3 times daily being as effective as aciclovir 800mg 5 times daily in reducing the appearance of new lesions, time to crusting, and time to 50% healing in a trial in immunocompetent patients with localised herpes zoster.[76] Valaciclovir was somewhat more effective than aciclovir in decreasing the duration of pain in this study, and it also significantly reduced the duration of postherpetic neuralgia and the proportion of patients with pain persisting for 6 months.

In practice, when antiviral chemotherapy is used in acute herpes zoster, it should be oral or, in immunocompromised patients, intravenous, and given early after the onset of symptoms. Topical therapy is considered of marginal benefit only, and not cost-effective.

Whether systemic corticosteroids should be given to patients with herpes zoster remains controversial. Short courses of high-dose corticosteroids have been reported to reduce the incidence and duration of postherpetic neuralgia,[77,78] and at present, there is no evidence that this treatment given to patients who are otherwise fit leads to an increased liability of the infection to disseminate. A recent study suggested that the addition of prednisolone may confer additional benefit in reducing the incidence and severity of pain during the first few weeks of illness but has no appreciable influence on postherpetic neuralgia; however, since the addition of a short course of this corticosteroid is not without adverse effects, even in patients with no contraindications, the indiscriminate use of corticosteroids is not advocated.[79]

#### *2.2.4 Kaposi's Varicelliform Eruption*

This term was formerly used to describe a widely disseminated infection of the skin with the herpes simplex or the vaccinia virus, but the latter is now only of historical interest. Such infections were most common in patients with atopic eczema, and it was on this evidence that the advice not to vaccinate atopic individuals without good reason was based.

The treatment of disseminated herpes simplex infection in an atopic individual should be with systemic aciclovir as described in section 2.2.2.

### 2.3 Fungal Infections

#### *2.3.1 Candidiasis*

Mucocutaneous candidiasis is almost invariably caused by *Candida albicans*, although other *Candida* species may also be involved. *Candida albicans* rarely, if ever, invades intact skin of normal individuals, but patients with intertrigo and chronic paronychia as well as patients who have recently been treated with immunosuppressive drugs and certain antibiotics, or who are suffering from infectious diseases are notoriously prone to Candida infection. Oral candidiasis is most commonly seen in children, but increasingly so in HIV-positive patients. The napkin area in infants, finger web spaces, and the submammary region in obese women are the more commonly involved sites. In some patients who have an underlying systemic disease, the infection is particularly chronic and extensive, and rarely Candida granulomata may develop.

#### Optimum Treatment

Management should include attention to the underlying condition, when possible. *Nystatin* or *amphotericin B* can be used topically as a cream, ointment, lotion, powder, oral suspension or lozenges. Oral administration, except in massive dosage, is only of use in clearing the intestinal tract of the yeast, as both drugs are poorly absorbed. Nystatin 1,500,000 units daily for 3 weeks is usually sufficient; vaginal treatment (pessary or cream) should be given for the same length of time as oral treatment.

Mucocutaneous candidiasis can also be effectively treated by topical application with one of the broad-spectrum *imidazole* antifungal agents [e.g. clotrimazole, econazole, ketoconazole (cream), miconazole, isoconazole, tioconazole, bifonazole or sulconazole] or the substituted pyridone antimycotic *ciclopirox olamine*.[80] Oral *ketoconazole*, 200 to 400 mg/day, has been used to treat chronic mucocutaneous candidiasis (for a review, see Gupta et al.[81,82]). Oral lesions usually respond within days and cutaneous lesions within weeks. However, ketoconazole may cause hepatotoxicity in some individuals and its administration should be accompanied by regular clinical and biochemical monitoring for evidence of liver damage. Ketoconazole also impairs the metabolism of cyclosporin,[83] and plasma concentrations of the latter should be closely monitored when the two drugs are given together. Similarly, coadministration of ketoconazole and terfenadine may lead to arrhythmias and QT interval prolongation on the ECG (see further chapter 7 and appendix B).

Newer azole antifungal drugs such as *fluconazole* and *itraconazole* are likely to prove more efficacious and require therapy for a shorter period. Itraconazole 100 to 200 mg/day for 15 days or a single dose of fluconazole 150mg are recommended for oral candidiasis, and itraconazole 200 mg/day for 3 days or a single dose of fluconazole 150mg for vaginal involvement. Mucocutaneous candidiasis has been effectively treated with itraconazole 100 mg/day for 3 to 12 weeks or fluconazole 50 mg/day.[81,82] Adverse effects are similar to those seen with ketoconazole but are probably less common (for reviews of fluconazole and itraconazole, see Grant & Clissold[84,85]).

*Terbinafine* is the newest antifungal agent and belongs to a class of drugs known as allylamines. It has broad-spectrum antifungal activity, but its *in vitro* activity against Candida is more variable and species dependent. Terbinafine is fungicidal against *Candida parapsilosis* but fungistatic against *Candida albicans*.[81,82] Terbinafine 250mg daily proved superior to placebo when given for 4 but not 2 weeks in cutaneous candidiasis.[86]

### *2.3.2 Ringworm*

The mycoses caused by dermatophytes are called ringworm, tinea or dermatophytosis. The infection is usually superficial and limited to a depth of 1 or 2mm. The skin appendages, namely, the hair and nails, are also involved in these infections. Nystatin and amphotericin B are not effective in infections by these filamentous fungi (i.e. dermatophytes). In 1958, *griseofulvin became the first significant oral antifungal agent available for the treatment of dermatophytosis.*

***Griseofulvin:*** the mechanism of action of this drug is not fully understood,[81,82] but it is active only where new keratin is being formed. Consequently, it deals with the fungal hyphae present at this site only and treatment has to be continued until all affected keratin has been shed. Absorption of griseofulvin from the gastrointestinal tract is markedly affected by the particle size of the drug, smaller particle sizes producing higher plasma concentrations (table IV).[87] Absorption is also increased if the drug is taken with a fatty meal. The concentration of griseofulvin in the stratum corneum exceeds by several-fold the concentration in plasma sampled at the same time.[88] Most of the drug is eliminated in the urine as metabolites, but about 18 to 36% of a dose is excreted in the faeces.

The standard dose of microsize griseofulvin is 500mg once daily or as 2 divided doses, taken with a fatty meal for maximum absorption.[89] With ultramicrosize griseofulvin preparations, the usual dose is 330 to 375mg once daily or as 2 divided doses. It is, on the whole, a safe drug but some patients may complain of headache or

**Table IV.** Absorption and systemic availabilities of some currently available microsize and ultramicrosize griseofulvin formulations (after Faergemann & Maibach[89]). Note the higher dose-adjusted $C_{max}$ and AUC values for the ultramicrosize formulations

| Formulation | $t_{max}$ (h) | $C_{max}$ (mg/L) | AUC (mg/L•h) | Usual dosage (adults) |
|---|---|---|---|---|
| **Microsize formulations** | | | | |
| Tablets, 500mg[a] | 4.6-6.9 | 0.7-0.9 | 16.8-26.0 | 500mg daily (as 1 or 2 divided doses); maximum 1g daily |
| Suspension, 500mg/20ml[b] | 4.4 | 0.9 | 24.0 | |
| **Ultramicrosize formulations** | | | | |
| Tablet, 125mg[c] | 3.8 | 0.86 | 17.5 | 330-375mg daily (as 1 or 2 divided doses); maximum 750mg daily |
| Tablet, 330mg[d] | 5.1 | 0.75 | 15.0 | |
| Tablet 250mg[d] | 3.3 | 0.79 | 17.1 | |

a Data for 'Grisovin', 'Fulvicin U/F', 'Grifulvin V' and 'Grisactin' brands (range of values).

b Data for 'Grifulvin V' suspension.

c Data for 'Gris-PEG'.

d Data for 'Fulvicin P/G'.

*Abbreviations:* $C_{max}$ = peak plasma concentrations; $t_{max}$ = time to peak concentration; AUC = area under the plasma concentration-time curve.

gastrointestinal disturbances. Rarely, griseofulvin may cause photosensitivity reactions and, by reducing absorption, it may decrease the effect of coumarin anticoagulants such as warfarin in some patients.[90,91]

***Newer systemic antifungal agents:*** during the last few years, newer systemic antifungal agents have become available. The major classes are the azoles, which include the imidazoles *(ketoconazole)* and triazoles *(fluconazole, itraconazole)*, as well as the recently introduced allylamines *(terbinafine)* [table V]. These agents act primarily by interfering with the formation of the fungal cell membrane.[92]

***Topical antifungal agents*** effective against dermatophytes include the broad-spectrum *imidazoles* (see table V), *naftifine*,[93] *terbinafine*,[94] *haloprogin*,[95] *tolciclate, tolnaftate, ciclopirox olamine*,[80] *undecenoic (undecylenic) acid*, and *amorolfine*.[81,82] Older effective topical fungicides include Castellani's magenta paint, which is particularly useful for flexural sites like toe webs and the groin, and Whitfield's ointment (ung. benzoic acid co.), which is a convenient preparation for other sites. Comparative costs for some of the available topical agents are shown in table VI.

#### Optimum Treatment

***Head/scalp (tinea capitis):*** topical therapy in tinea capitis is often unsuccessful. *Griseofulvin* has been considered a first-line therapy. The optimum dosage of griseofulvin (microsize) is 500mg once daily and of griseofulvin (ultramicrosize) 250 to 375mg once daily. In children, 7.27 mg/kg/day (3.3 mg/lb/day) of ultramicrosize griseofulvin is given. Treatment should continue for 4 to 6 weeks. Oral ketoconazole 200 to 400mg daily for 2 to 8 weeks or 5 mg/kg/day is an alternative to griseofulvin. *Itraconazole* and *terbinafine* may also be useful in the treatment of tinea capitis. *Selenium sulfide shampoo*, *prednisone* and *oral antibiotics* are frequently used as adjunctive therapy.

In a *kerion*, or inflammatory ringworm (which is usually transmitted from cattle or horses), fungal elements are relatively sparse and, although it is usual to treat with griseofulvin, it is not always effective. Similarly, topical fungicides are not very effective. Fortunately, the natural history is such that spontaneous healing occurs, but often there is considerable scarring in the process. The usefulness of systemic or intralesional corticosteroids in treatment of a kerion is not established, but there are theoretical reasons why they might be expected to be efficacious.

***Tinea corporis:*** when only one or two patches occur, topical treatment is sufficient; *Castellani's magenta paint* is particularly useful for flexural sites like the groin. Systemic therapy is primarily indicated for widespread disease and in immunocompromised patients. *Griseofulvin* (microsize) 500mg or griseofulvin (ultramicrosize) 250 to 375mg once daily is the treatment of choice. Oral *ketoconazole* 200 to 400mg daily is as effective as griseofulvin. *Itraconazole* 100mg daily for 30 days or 200mg daily for 7 days, *fluconazole* 150mg per week (1 to 4 treatments) and *terbinafine* 250mg daily for 2 to 4 weeks are also convenient and effective treatment options for tinea corporis.

**Table V.** Antifungal agents available for the treatment of superficial fungal infections

| Drug/class | Route of administration | Indications |
|---|---|---|
| **Imidazoles** | | |
| Clotrimazole | Topical | Cutaneous dermatophyte and candidal infections |
| Econazole | Topical | |
| Ketoconazole | Oral[a]/topical | |
| Miconazole | Topical | |
| Oxiconazole | Topical | |
| Sulconazole | Topical | |
| Tioconazole | Topical | |
| **Triazoles** | | |
| Fluconazole | Oral | Widespread and/or recurrent cutaneous mycoses |
| Itraconazole | Oral | |
| **Allylamines** | | |
| Naftifine | Topical | Cutaneous dermatophyte infections |
| Terbinafine | Oral/topical | Dermatophyte infections of the skin and nails |
| **Polyenes** | | |
| Nystatin | Topical | Cutaneous candidosis |
| **Others** | | |
| Amorolfine | Topical | Dermatophyte infections of the skin and nails[b] |
| Ciclopirox olamine | Topical | Dermatophyte and candidal infections of the skin and nails[b] |
| Griseofulvin | Oral | Dermatophyte infections of the scalp and nails |
| Tolciclate | Topical | Cutaneous dermatophyte infections |
| Tolnaftate | Topical | Cutaneous dermatophyte infections |

a Oral ketoconazole treatment is indicated in widespread and/or recurrent cutaneous mycoses.
b As nail lacquers.

***Tinea pedis:*** tinea pedis is the most widespread form of mycosis in humans, and is most often seen in adult men. The primary lesions consist of maceration between the fourth and fifth toes, slight scaling and occasional vesiculation. Management should include attention to the presence of inflamed skin or secondary pyogenic infection. Conventional topical fungicidal agents have proved to be effective, but treatment has to be continued as a prophylactic measure for months. Oral therapy should be considered in topical treatment failure and in immunocompromised patients. *Griseofulvin* (microsize) 500mg or griseofulvin (ultramicrosize) 250 to 375mg twice daily for 4 to 8 weeks is effective. Oral *terbinafine* 250mg daily for 2 to 6 weeks, *itraconazole* 100mg daily for 30 days or *fluconazole* 150mg per week (up to 4 doses) can also be considered.

***Tinea unguium:*** dermatophytes, yeasts and moulds are the causative organisms of fungal nail infections. Traditional topical agents used as monotherapy for onychomycosis are only able to inhibit the growth of fungal nail infections. Surgical avulsion may be used in conjunction with either topical or systemic antifungal therapy. An alternative, efficacious topical treatment involves applying antifungal agents concurrently or sequentially with the chemical removal or debridement of the infected nail structures.

The application of antifungal lacquers to fingernail and toenail fungal infections may be effective for the treatment of less severe forms of onychomycosis without nail matrix involvement. *Ciclopirox olamine* 8% in a lacquer base applied once daily for 6 months has proved effective for mild distal subungual onychomycoses and superficial white onychomycoses. This hydroxypyridone agent has several modes of action, primarily interfering with the uptake and accumulation of products required for cell membrane synthesis. It also has anti-inflammatory activity, inhibits synthesis of prostaglandins and leukotrienes, and possesses both fungistatic and fungicidal activity *in vitro*.

*Amorolfine* 5% nail lacquer applied once or twice a week for 6 months in fingernail infections and 12 months for toenail onychomycosis is also effective in onychomycosis without matrix involvement. Amorolfine is fungicidal; it inhibits sterol synthesis which leads to ergosterol deprivation, with accumulation of squalene, ignosterol and ergosta-8,14,24(28)-trien-3b-o1. Adverse effects with topical antifungal lacquers include local events such as burning, erythema, pruritus and scaling.

The systemic treatment of fungal infections has changed considerably over the past decade. Oral griseofulvin has been the first-line drug in the therapy of dermatophyte onychomycosis for many years. However, even when used long term, it has a cure rate that seldom exceeds 40%. The standard dose of griseofulvin (microsize) is 500mg once daily or as 2 divided doses, taken with a fatty meal for maximum absorption (table IV).[89] Ketoconazole 200mg daily is as effective as griseofulvin in dermatophyte nail infections. Oral ketoconazole, like griseofulvin, requires long term therapy. This may be for as long as one year or more in the case of the toenails.

Recently, newer systemic antifungal agents which include the *triazoles* and *allylamines* have become available. These agents act primarily by interfering with the formation of the fungal cell membrane (table V).[92] They diffuse more rapidly into the stratum corneum and nail and are more effective with short term treatment. *Terbinafine* 250mg daily is particularly effective in the treatment of dermatophyte onychomycosis. Short term cure rates of well over 80% have been noted in fingernail and toenail infections with treatment periods of 6 and 12 weeks, respectively. Terbinafine may cause gastrointestinal disturbances as well as headache, skin reactions, hypogeusia/dysgeusia and erectile dysfunction. There have also been rare instances of reversible hepatic damage. Most adverse effects have been noted during the first weeks of therapy. In addition, at therapeutic concentrations of terbinafine, the potential for drug interaction is much less likely than with the azole antifungals.[81,82]

**Table VI.** Comparative costs of commonly used topical drugs to treat tinea of the skin[a] (after Chren[96])

| Drug | Relative cost (per course) |
|---|---|
| **Usually recommended regimens** (4-week courses) | |
| Miconazole | + |
| Tolnaftate | + |
| Oxiconazole | ++ |
| Ketoconazole | ++ |
| Naftifine | ++ |
| Clotrimazole | ++ |
| Econazole | ++ |
| Ciclopirox olamine | +++ |
| Sulconazole | +++ |
| Terbinafine | ++++ |
| **Alternative regimens** (shorter courses) | |
| Clotrimazole (2 weeks) | + |
| Econazole (2 weeks) | + |
| Ketoconazole (2 weeks) | + |
| Terbinafine (1 week) | ++ |
| Terbinafine (2 weeks) | ++++ |

a Assuming application of 15 g/week for drugs used once a day and 30 g/week for drugs used twice a day.

*Key:* + = up to US$20; ++ = US$21-40; +++ = US$41-60; ++++ = > US$60.

*Itraconazole* 200mg daily has been noted to be similarly effective in the same treatment period.[81,82] Pulse therapy consisting of monthly 1-week cycles of 400mg itraconazole daily for 3 to 4 months may offer a new option for treatment.[97] Recently, *fluconazole* as a single daily dose of 100mg for a period of 6 months was shown also to be effective.[98]

#### 2.3.3 Tinea (pityriasis) Versicolor

Tinea (pityriasis) versicolor results from the proliferation of the lipophilic skin commensal *Malassezia furfiur (Pityrosporon orbiculare)*. It is particularly common in patients with Cushing's syndrome, but occurs in healthy individuals as well. Lesions are seen most commonly on the trunk and consist of scaling hypo- or hyperpigmented patches.

**Optimum Treatment**

The usual topical fungicide preparations (see section 2.3.2 above) are used in its treatment and are reasonably effective. *10% sodium thiosulphate solution* applied to the whole upper trunk and upper arms every day for 3 weeks is also useful. Alternatively, a *2.5% selenium sulphide lotion* may be used.

Systemic therapy is primarily indicated for extensive lesions, resistance to topical treatment, and for frequent relapse. *Ketoconazole* 400mg orally as a single dose, *itraconazole* 200mg daily for 7 days, or a single oral dose of *fluconazole* 400mg have provided good results. The risk of adverse effects is minimised with short term treatment.[99]

## 3. Skin Infestations

### 3.1 Scabies

*Sarcoptes scabiei* var. *hominis* is a mite, the female of which lays her eggs in burrows in the skin. These are especially common in the finger webs and on the wrist flexures but are also found on the palms, soles, breasts and penis. Lesions on other parts of the body are mostly due to 'sensitivity' reactions to the mite, or to secondary infection. Human scabies is spread from person to person by close contact only. An exception is the extremely infectious crusted scabies, where all skin lesions are teeming with mites, and minimal contact with the patient or his/her clothing, bedding or furniture can lead to infestation, for example, of medical and nursing personnel.[100]

#### Optimum Treatment

*Benzyl benzoate* remains an effective treatment as long as attention is paid to details of application. For this reason, precise instructions should always be given to the patient. A 25% emulsion of benzyl benzoate should be painted on all areas of the skin except that of the face, head and neck, where the mites are very rarely found. The application should be painted on the dried skin after a hot bath and left on for 24 hours, after which time another application should be made but without a further bath. At the end of the total of 48 hours, all the emulsion should be washed off. All sarcoptes will have been killed. As benzyl benzoate is a highly irritant substance, it is imperative that its application should not be continued. Thus, it is important to explain to the patient that the itch may persist sometimes for as long as 3 weeks, but even so, benzyl benzoate should not be reapplied. It is important too that all members of the affected family or bedmates should be considered for treatment at the same time, or reinfestation will occur ('ping pong scabies'). For a review on the issue of whether or not to treat asymptomatic contacts, see Orkin & Maibach.[101]

It is customary to tell patients to change their clothes and sheets after treatment, but, as the scabies mite cannot survive for long outside the human skin, this is probably not very important except in crusted scabies (see above). It may be necessary to treat secondary infection, e.g. impetigo, as well (see section 2.1.1), but this will not usually respond until the antiscabetic treatment has been given.

Several other antiscabetic preparations have been advocated in an attempt to avoid the inconvenience and irritant effect of benzyl benzoate. *Crotamiton* is a weak antiscabetic and not to be recommended for use on its own; *monosulfiram* is effective but absorption can lead to severe symptoms in those who have taken alcohol. The most widely used agents are lindane (gamma benzene hexachloride), permethrin 5% cream, and sulfur.

*Lindane* (gamma benzene hexachloride) is used as a 1% preparation and has to be applied as meticulously as benzyl benzoate, though it is slightly less messy and less irritant. Because of enhanced percutaneous absorption[102] and consequent risk of toxicity (CNS disturbances, convulsions, respiratory failure) in infants, some clinicians do not use lindane in infants or young children. It should be avoided in pregnant women and used with caution in patients with massively excoriated skin. Lindane is used after a bath or shower, but to avoid excessive percutaneous absorption, it should be applied after the skin has been allowed to dry and cool. A cool bath or shower 24 hours later to remove the insecticide is also recommended in an attempt (not proven) to decrease percutaneous penetration.[103]

*Permethrin* 5% cream is an effective agent with low toxicity. It should be applied and left on the skin for 10 hours before being washed off. Some clinicians repeat the treatment in 1 week, although there are no controlled studies showing that two applications are more effective than one.[101]

*Sulfur*, which is usually prescribed as precipitated sulfur (5 to 9%) in petrolatum, is applied nightly for 3 nights (washing off previous applications before reapplying new applications), and is then washed off thoroughly 24 hours after the last application.[101]

### 3.2 Pediculosis

Three varieties of pediculi commonly attack man, although others infest lower animals and may become temporarily deposited on human hosts. The three variants are *Pediculus humanus var. capitis* (head louse), *P. humanus var. corporis* (body louse), and *P. phthirus pubis* (pubic or crab louse). Each of the varieties of pediculi has a predilection for certain parts of the skin. In piercing the skin, the parasites exude a poisonous salivary secretion. This, together with the mechanical puncture, produces a pruritic dermatitis.

#### Optimum Treatment

Preparations containing 5% *dicophane (DDT)* and 1% *lindane* (gamma benzene hexachloride) have been the insecticides traditionally used to kill head, body and pubic lice. The hair or body is washed and the preparation applied daily for

4 or 5 days. Any secondary infection or exudative lesions should be treated before using insecticides. Lice putatively resistant to lindane have emerged.

*Malathion:* in contrast, resistance has not been reported with this agent. It is less irritant to the skin and also kills ova, so repeated applications are not required.[104] Malathion has been used mainly for infestations with head lice as a 1% shampoo, but a 0.5% lotion can be used to treat body and pubic lice as well. Thorough personal hygiene is essential and clothing and bedding must be disinfested, by steam autoclaving or liberal application of malathion or other insecticide powders, especially to garment seams. The chlorinated hydrocarbon insecticides have powerful metabolic effects, and they should never be taken by mouth.

*Permethrin* is a synthetic pyrethroid that is photostable, highly effective against a wide variety of insects and mites, and demonstrates extremely low toxicity. It is recommended that permethrin 1% cream rinse be applied undiluted to affected areas of pediculosis for 10 minutes and then rinsed off with warm water. Adverse reactions to permethrin include transient burning, stinging, and pruritus.[105]

Other effective agents in the treatment of head and body lice include *pyrethrins/piperonyl butoxide* shampoo. The treatment of pubic lice is discussed further in chapter 33 (section 5.3.1).

## 4. Acne

Acne is a common skin disorder and indeed most teenagers have it in some degree. As a rule, it regresses with time but while it lasts it can, in its severe forms, be extremely disfiguring and can result in scarring. Thus, patients often ask for treatment of their acne and although to some extent this is still symptomatic and empirical, it is, with increasing knowledge, becoming more and more directed to specific aspects of the pathogenesis. The following are believed to be factors in production of acne:

- *Grease:* an important abnormality is that the skin contains more oil (sebum) than normal. In addition, the composition of the sebum differs from normal although the significance of this remains uncertain.[106]
- *Bacteria:* the anaerobic bacterium *Propionibacterium acnes* (*Corynebacterium acnes*) and other bacteria, which are usually not regarded as pathogens, are found on the surface of the skin and in the lesions of acne.
- *Lipolysis: P. acnes* and other bacteria are able to split fats in sebum to form irritant fatty acids which probably contribute to pus formation.
- *Blocking of ducts of sebaceous glands:* this is manifest clinically by the blackhead or comedone and may be important in the production of other lesions such as pustules and cysts.
- *Increased sensitivity of the skin end organs to androgens.*

Of these, the increased sebum production is especially important and the most effective treatment, isotretinoin, causes shrinkage of the sebaceous glands and a decrease in sebum excretion. This drug is, however, neither necessary nor desirable in any but the most severe cases of acne.

### 4.1 Optimum Treatment

#### 4.1.1 First-line Measures

Most patients who ask for treatment do need it and many patients seen by dermatologists need systemic treatment, usually with a tetracycline. Cleansers and peeling agents (see below) may well have been used alone before specialist referral.

***Cleansers:*** removal of sebum by proprietary products or frequent gentle washing with soapy water may be helpful, but these methods have not been convincingly demonstrated to be useful in controlled trials.

***Peeling agents:*** these presumably help by unblocking follicles. *Sulfur, benzoyl peroxide* and sunlight produce peeling and probably work this way; benzoyl peroxide may also act by an antibacterial action, thereby suppressing *P. acnes*.[107] *Tretinoin* (all-*trans*-retinoic acid; vitamin A acid), which is available as a cream, gel and lotion, produces irritation to a greater extent than the other agents, as well as peeling, and patients must be warned to reduce the frequency of application, e.g. to twice a week, if this occurs, since a marked peeling effect is not needed for therapeutic benefit.[108,109] Used correctly, tretinoin is an effective topical agent for acne. It can be applied in conjunction with systemic tetracycline.

***Azelaic acid:*** this agent is a naturally-occurring saturated dicarboxylic acid, which on application as a 20% cream, has been reported to have an effect on the process of keratinisation and to cause a significant decrease in the follicular bacterial population.[110] Applied twice daily, it has proved effective in comedonal and inflammatory acne, and has comparable anti-acne effectiveness to topical tretinoin, benzoyl peroxide and erythromycin, and oral tetracycline. Azelaic acid is well tolerated, with adverse effects generally limited to mild and transient local irritation.[111]

***Topical antibiotics***, e.g. 1% clindamycin and 2% erythromycin solutions: these agents act by suppressing *P. acnes* and are effective in milder cases of acne. They are often used prior to systemic antibiotics.[112]

***Systemic tetracycline therapy***: this is the most useful single measure in moderately severe acne. The mechanism of action of tetracycline is not known, but it probably involves reduction of bacterial lipolysis; it does not reduce sebum secretion. Tetracycline is given orally in a dosage of 500mg daily half an hour before breakfast for maximal absorption; in this low dosage, toxic effects are almost unknown[113] but vaginal candidiasis may occur in a small number of cases.[114] Alternatively, minocycline in a dosage of 50mg twice daily or doxycycline 100mg daily can be given. The treatment should be continued for at least 3 months and longer if new lesions are still appearing or if they do so on stopping the drug. Tetracycline has been known to cause phototoxic reactions.[115] It should not be given in pregnancy or in young children because of staining of the teeth (see chapter 3; sect. 4.1.2), and it should not be used in those with impaired renal function.

#### 4.1.2 Further Measures

The above 3 methods of treatment are satisfactory in the majority of cases; only rarely is it necessary to resort to other measures.

***Other systemic antibacterial agents:*** if tetracyclines are contraindicated or ineffective, other antibacterial drugs active against *P. acnes* can be given systemically in an equivalent dose, e.g. *erythromycin* 250mg daily and *cotrimoxazole* 960mg (2 tablets) daily. Cotrimoxazole should be used as a second choice, and only in patients with severe acne who do not respond to other antibiotics, due to the possibility of severe eruptions. All patients given long term cotrimoxazole therapy must also be monitored for potential haematological suppression. Alternatively, in resistant cases, tetracycline can be given in full dosage, up to 2000mg daily,[116] although often this is no more effective than the smaller dose and patients cannot always tolerate it for long. Such a regimen may, however, serve as a useful temporary measure. Intracranial hypertension has been reported in adolescents on higher dose tetracycline regimens.[117,118]

***Antiandrogens*** (e.g. cyproterone): these drugs have been used in severe acne and are effective. They should never be given in pregnancy because they may cause feminisation of the male fetus. In men, their general antiandrogenic effects make them unacceptable in all but those with the most severe acne.

***Isotretinoin*** (13-*cis*-retinoic acid): this drug is a derivative of vitamin A which has been used for treating acne since 1979 (for reviews, see Ward et al.;[119] Cunliffe[120]). The pharmacological profile of isotretinoin suggests that it acts primarily by reducing sebaceous gland size and sebum production, and as a result alters skin surface lipid composition; bacterial skin microflora populations are also reduced. It is an effective drug but its adverse effects preclude its use as a first-line treatment, and it should be reserved for severe pustular and nodulocystic acne when other measures have failed. Isotretinoin is used in a dosage of 0.5 to 2.0 mg/kg/day according to severity, response and patient tolerability, and improvement should be obvious within 2 months. Treatment should be continued for approximately 20 weeks in the first instance and after withdrawal of the drug, the skin will remain clear in most patients.

Isotretinoin is well absorbed following oral administration. Its elimination half-life is relatively short (10 to 20 hours) in comparison with the long elimination half-life of the related retinoid analogue etretinate (see section 6.1.2). About 20 to 30% of an isotretinoin dose isomerises *in vivo* to tretinoin. The other major metabolites in humans are 4-oxo-isotretinoin and 4-oxo-tretinoin. The parent drug, its stereoisomer and oxidised metabolites undergo conjugation with glucuronic acid, biliary excretion and enterohepatic recirculation.[121,122]

The adverse effects of isotretinoin are generally little more than annoying to the patient. They are usually dose-related and reversible on stopping the drug or reducing the dose and include:

- Ubiquitous dryness and cracking of mucosae sometimes with bleeding
- Routine dryness and peeling of the skin
- Initial flare-up of acne with inflammation and granuloma formation
- Diffuse hair loss.

More important adverse effects of isotretinoin are:

1) *Teratogenicity:* isotretinoin is highly teratogenic (see chapter 2; sect. 6) and must never be given to women capable of bearing children without assurance that effective contraceptive measures are being taken. It is recommended that pregnancy should not occur for 2 months after cessation of treatment.

2) *Hyperlipidaemia:* isotretinoin produces a rise in serum triglycerides and, in particular, in very-low-density lipoprotein (VLDL) cholesterol. The changes are reversible on stopping treatment and it is unlikely with the short courses of isotretinoin used in acne that this finding is of serious clinical import.

3) *Skeletal abnormalities:* premature closure of epiphyses and changes resembling diffuse idiopathic skeletal hyperostosis (DISH) syndrome have been reported in patients taking isotretinoin, but are more likely to be clinically significant with longer courses of the drug than those used for acne.

4) *Abnormalities of liver enzymes:* these have also been reported with isotretinoin but their clinical relevance is uncertain.

***Other treatment:*** sparingly soluble corticosteroids such as triamcinolone acetonide can be used for local injection into acne cysts but otherwise, should rarely be used in acne. Plastic surgery in the form of dermabrasion for severe scarring may be satisfactory in some cases of 'burnt out' acne.

#### 4.1.3 General Measures

There is no evidence that diet influences acne significantly, but if patients are convinced that a particular food (e.g. chocolate) makes their acne worse, they should be advised not to eat it. Local conditions (e.g. industrial oil, greasy make-up, hot damp conditions), which often make acne worse, should obviously be avoided. Some drugs can also aggravate acne (table X; section 22).

## 5. Rosacea

Rosacea is a disease which affects an older age group than acne. It is characterised by a marked tendency of the skin to flush and by the formation of papules and pustules. Some cases are iatrogenic and have resulted from long term application of strong topical corticosteroids to the face.[123] The mechanism of the production of the disorder is not known. The histological appearances of a papule resemble those seen in a tuberculoid granuloma, although there is no evidence that the disease is a manifestation of tuberculosis. *P. acnes* is often found in the skin and may be important there. The presence of *Demodex folliculorum* is not thought to be important in pathogenesis. The skin is not always greasy.

#### Optimum Treatment

The most effective treatment for rosacea is *tetracycline* 500mg daily orally (given before food), and as with acne, therapy may have to be continued for months or years.[124] If corticosteroids are being used, they should be stopped immediately, and the patient should be warned that temporary worsening may follow.[123] It is not logical to use topical corticosteroids in rosacea; any temporary improvement will often be followed by worsening.

Apart from systemic tetracycline, treatment can include the use of emulsifying ointment instead of soap for washing. Extremes of temperature and excess of sunlight as well as peeling agents (see section 4.1.1) often aggravate the condition and should be avoided. Topical sunscreens may help.

Topical *metronidazole gel* has been demonstrated to be effective in rosacea. The mechanism of action of this agent is unknown, but it may relate to the inhibitory effects of metronidazole on *Demodex brevis*. Its use during pregnancy, by nursing mothers and by children is not recommended. Adverse local effects include dryness, burning and stinging.[105,125]

Other measures which can be used, especially in cases where tetracycline is contraindicated or ineffective, include systemic *metronidazole*, *cotrimoxazole* (only as a last choice because of potential adverse effects[126] [see section 4.1.2] and, in extreme cases, *isotretinoin*.[127] There is no need to put patients on a diet, although if foods and drinks which produce extreme flushing make the condition worse, they are best omitted. Eye complications such as keratitis and corneal ulcers will need specialist advice, and rhinophyma can be dealt with by plastic surgery.

## 6. Psoriasis

Psoriasis is one of the most common dermatoses for which patients request specialist treatment, but in most cases, *albeit* usually the milder ones, they put up with their affliction without seeking any advice. The large hereditary element in type I psoriasis and the idea of 'trigger' factors producing overt disease in those with a predisposed hereditary background have been mentioned in section 1.1.[128,129] The only 'triggers' known at present to have any relevance to prevention and treatment are streptococcal infections and trauma. Streptococcal infections, especially in children, can produce attacks of guttate psoriasis, and if such infections can be prevented, then further attacks of psoriasis may be prevented too.[1] Localised trauma to the skin, e.g. sunburn, vaccination, or an operation incision will often produce psoriasis at its site, but the practical application of this 'Koebner phenomenon' to prevention and treatment of psoriasis is obviously limited.

Extensive information is available about the many abnormalities that can be found in the skin and elsewhere in psoriasis.[2,130,131] The majority, however, are the result and not the cause of the disease. A near fundamental feature is that epidermal cell 'turnover' is increased to about 10 times the rate found in normal skin. Drugs such as the cytotoxic agent methotrexate, which reduce epidermal turnover, certainly help psoriasis,[132] and psoralens in combination with long-wave length ultraviolet light (UVA) act by inhibiting DNA synthesis.[133,134] Most currently available effective treatments are capable of inhibiting epidermal mitosis, although in many cases (e.g. corticosteroids) there is no evidence that this is their mechanism of action.

It should be noted that all measures available to treat psoriasis will suppress the disease while they are being used, but when they are stopped, there is a good chance that the lesions will recur, although the time taken for this recurrence varies. There is no evidence that permanent 'cure' is effected by any form of treatment, so that when the lesions remain absent after treatment, it is possibly because of a coincidental natural remission or because the treatment has altered homeostatic mechanisms. Fortunately, this occurs.

There are two separate problems in the treatment of psoriasis. The first is to clear the lesion, which can usually be achieved. The second is to prevent recurrence of the rash, which, with few exceptions, is an impossible task. For further information, see Roenigk & Maibach.[135]

## 6.1 Optimum Treatment

### *6.1.1 Topical Therapy*

Dithranol (anthralin), tar, calcipotriol, and the stronger topical corticosteroids (table II) are the four forms of treatment available. For the most part it is not known why they work. The anti-inflammatory action of the corticosteroids may not be the only mechanism or indeed the main mechanism by which they exert their effect in psoriasis. Dithranol appears to act by the formation of free radicals which interfere with DNA synthesis, but little is known about the mechanism of the action of tar in psoriasis.

The choice of dithranol, tar, calcipotriol or topical corticosteroids in a given case of psoriasis will depend on many factors. For example, dithranol, which stains the skin brown, is not normally acceptable for treatment of the face. If topical corticosteroids are to be used over long periods, the undesirable adverse effect of skin atrophy must be weighed against the beneficial effect upon the lesions. If treatment is to be carried out by the patient at home, he/she may find messy applications like dithranol and tar so impracticable as to be useless. Different treatment centres tend to concentrate on either the dithranol or the tar regimens as the mainstay of treatment for chronic psoriasis; thus, since both forms of treatment depend for their success upon attention to detail, it is usually better to prescribe a treatment which is familiar to the local clinicians and nurses who are administering it.

#### Clinical Use of Dithranol

***Ingram regimen***: dithranol is an irritant substance but it is less irritant to psoriatic lesions than to clinically unaffected skin. The Ingram regimen[136] aims at confining the application to psoriatic plaques by using dithranol in stiff Lassar's paste of which starch, zinc oxide, salicylic acid and hard paraffin are all essential ingredients; powdering the paste after it is applied also helps to stop it spreading.[137] The concentration of dithranol that can be tolerated varies from individual to individual. It tends to be greater as treatment continues, and varies from site to site, but strengths from 0.05 to 0.4% are usually satisfactory.

The dithranol paste is applied accurately to psoriatic plaques after the patient has had a bath to which 120ml coal tar solution (liquor picis carbonis) and 30ml of liquid detergent (or proprietary tar-detergent preparation) have been added. After the bath and before the application of the dithranol, the patient is exposed to intermediate wavelength ultraviolet light (UVB), either as sunlight or in a light box. The patient wears dressings until the next day when the whole procedure is repeated.

***Short contact regimens:*** efforts have been made to replace the Ingram regimen by a simpler dithranol regimen. Following work showing that dithranol penetrates damaged skin quickly and therefore need only be left on for short periods to reach therapeutic concentrations,[138] new interest arose and has continued. Many short contact or 'minutes' methods are in use involving the application of different concentrations of dithranol in different bases and applied for different durations. Contact times of 30 minutes or less are adequate and concentrations about 10 times as high as for the Ingram regimen are used; the base is easy to apply and to remove and does not have to be confined accurately to psoriatic lesions. One regimen[139] uses 2 to 16% dithranol in emulsifying ointment with 0.5% salicylic acid added; it is left on for 15 minutes and washed off in a shower or bath containing a liquid detergent.

This regimen and the Ingram regimen have proved equally effective when clearance times are compared. It can be used by patients at home, and in hospital it shortens nursing times in outpatient departments and wards. Burning of uninvolved skin, initially a problem, becomes less so with experience. The great disadvantage is staining of clothes, floors, etc. if the dithranol is not completely removed from the skin in the shower or bath.

***Scalp applications:*** the scalp can be treated with dithranol too, though in fair haired people it may produce discoloration of the hair; stiff pastes are unsuitable for the scalp and a 'pomade' containing emulsifying ointment and a wetting agent such as polysorbate 20 ('Tween 20') is a better vehicle for the dithranol, which is used at a 0.2 or 0.4% concentration. The choice of shampoo is probably not important; many liquid detergents are effective in removing scale and old pomade.

#### Clinical Use of Tar

Coal tar, usually as a 2 to 5% paste, is used in conjunction with UVB radiation.[140-142] The variation between different treatment centres in the preparations of tar used, as well as the methods of applying them and the number of times the preparation and the ultraviolet light are applied during the day, all mean that there is no standard regimen. There is no evidence that, in good hands, tar is inferior to dithranol; however, few centres use the two regimens with equal enthusiasm, so that no real comparisons are available.

The so-called Goeckerman regimen has proved a reliable and safe regimen in patients with severe psoriasis who have not responded to simpler forms of treatment. This consists of daily applications of crude coal tar and exposure to UV light (after the tar has been removed from the psoriatic plaques). Widespread psoriasis can be cleared in 2 to 3 or more weeks with this regimen (for a review, see Farber & Nall[143]). The theoretical risk of carcinogenesis with tar has not been reflected in clinical practice despite decades of use and careful follow-up, other than for a few isolated case reports.[144] Tar is available as various coal tar solutions, bath oils, shampoos, lotions and ointment preparations.

#### Clinical Use of Topical Corticosteroids

The stronger topical corticosteroids (e.g. betamethasone valerate 0.1%, fluocinolone acetonide 0.025%, clobetasol propionate 0.05%) are usually effective in psoriasis and are even more so if they are applied under polythene occlusion.[5,145] This can be effected in localised areas such as the hands and feet, by polythene gloves or polythene bags, and in the case of large areas, by a polythene suit. However, occlusion encourages infection of the underlying skin, and whole body occlusion is perhaps the form of dressing most likely to lead to dangerous overheating of the patient in cases of widespread skin disease in which temperature control is already abnormal. The great disadvantage of occlusion is that it enhances the local and systemic toxicity of corticosteroids, to an extent depending on duration and extent of use. Systemic absorption, although it undoubtedly occurs, is not often of serious consequence unless large amounts of topical corticosteroids are applied over a large body surface area.[146] The risk of clinically important absorption is greatest in infants[147,148] (see also chapter 3; sect. 2.1.3). For a review of the dermatopharmacokinetics of topical corticosteroids, see Korting & Maibach.[26]

The principal indications for using topical corticosteroids in psoriasis are as follows:

1) In cases where the skin is particularly 'sore' or likely to be irritated by other applications. In some instances, a topical corticosteroid can be used together with dithranol or tar to decrease their irritant effect and to enable higher concentrations of these agents to be used than

would otherwise be possible.[149] However, more controlled studies are needed in this area to confirm this observation.

2) As a possible adjunct to systemic corticosteroid treatment in cases of erythrodermic psoriasis. Here, diminution of the inflammation of the skin is an urgent matter because if allowed to continue, it can be expected to have adverse systemic consequences such as hypothermia and heart failure.

3) For a limited period of use in particular areas of the body or in particular patients where other applications are cosmetically unacceptable. Note, however, that application, of strong corticosteroids to the face – usually over long periods – produces a clinical picture indistinguishable from that of rosacea.[123]

There is no doubt that a strong topical corticosteroid can be effective and can produce a rapid and dramatic improvement in appearance in some cases of psoriasis. There is, however, an impression, although this has not been proved, that this rapid clearing is followed, when treatment is stopped, by a more rapid return of the lesions than after the standard treatment with dithranol or tar.[150]

#### Calcipotriol

Calcipotriol is a synthetic vitamin $D_3$ analogue that can regulate cell differentiation and proliferation and suppress lymphocyte activities (for a review, see Murdoch & Clissold[151]). Compared with the natural hormone 1$\alpha$,25-dihydroxyvitamin $D_3$, calcipotriol is about 100 to 200 times less potent in its effects on calcium metabolism. At present, calcipotriol in an ointment base represents an alternative to treatment with topical corticosteroids and dithranol.[152,153]

### *6.1.2 Systemic Treatment*

Treatment with systemic drugs is necessary in certain severe or recalcitrant cases of psoriasis, but is not advised outside hospital or without specialist dermatological supervision. Treatment with psoralen and long-wave ultraviolet light (PUVA) has to some extent reduced the need for systemic corticosteroids and cytotoxic drugs in psoriasis.

#### Corticosteroids

These should rarely be given in chronic psoriasis, but have some part to play in erythrodermic, generalised pustular and severe arthropathic psoriasis. There is no good evidence regarding the relative effectiveness, dose for dose, of the different corticosteroids in psoriasis – despite claims, based mainly on clinical impressions, that triamcinolone is the preferred drug. In the absence of such evidence, there is no reason to use corticosteroids other than prednisone or prednisolone. Doses of the order of 80 to 100mg daily of these agents may be required initially, but every effort should be made to reduce the dose gradually and to stop the drug as soon as possible. The risks and benefits of such treatment have been reviewed by Lahti and Maibach.[154]

Rapid dose reduction of corticosteroids is liable to result in a flare-up of the psoriasis. Patients should be told about the potential hazards of systemic corticosteroids and should carry a 'corticosteroid card' (see further chapter 19; sect. 7.1.1).

#### Cytotoxic Drugs

Cytotoxic drugs have a place in the treatment of the following types of psoriasis:

- Erythrodermic psoriasis
- Generalised pustular psoriasis
- Extensive chronic or recurrent plaque psoriasis which cannot be controlled by other means.

The decision to use these drug should never be taken without full consideration of their undesirable effects. Although many cytotoxic agents have been shown to be effective in psoriasis, those used regularly in clinical practice are *methotrexate, hydroxycarbamide (hydroxyurea)* and *azathioprine*. Methotrexate, which is the agent most commonly used, competitively inhibits dihydrofolate reductase. By inhibiting the conversion of folate to tetrahydrofolate, it impairs the biosynthesis of thymidylate and purines. Hydroxycarbamide inhibits ribonucleotide reductase, resulting in the impairment of DNA synthesis, while azathioprine inhibits purine synthesis. All 3 compounds are myelotoxic, and both methotrexate and azathioprine may produce liver damage. Cytotoxic therapy should not be given when pregnancy is a possibility. Many cytotoxic drugs are genotoxic carcinogens; methotrexate, however, appears (from both animal and human evidence) to lack this potential, and it is for this reason, in particular, that it is considered the cytotoxic agent of first choice in the management of psoriasis not responding to other measures.

Methotrexate can be given orally or by intramuscular injection and a dose of 2.5 to 5mg weekly is a reasonable one to start with in patients with good renal, hepatic and bone marrow function. If this dose produces no clinical improvement and there are no adverse effects, the dose can be increased to a maximum of approximately 30mg weekly, but it should be reduced as soon as possible. Intermittent therapy is less toxic to the liver than continuous therapy.[155] Provided only severe psoriasis is treated with methotrexate, the risk of liver toxicity is acceptable, although it may be greater in those with a high alcohol intake. Biopsy to assess liver architecture before treatment is wise, as is regular follow-up in patients receiving the drug for more than a few months. Acute toxicity, e.g. bone marrow suppression and mucosal ulceration, is usually reversible and folinic acid should be given if this occurs. Guidelines for clinical use of methotrexate have been reviewed by Tung & Maibach.[156]

*Thioguanine*, a purine analogue structurally related to mercaptopurine and azathioprine, inhibits purine synthesis and interconversions by thioguanine ribonucleotide. Its elimination is primarily by hepatic metabolism. Thioguanine is a valuable agent in the management of refractory psoriasis, and it has been particularly useful for patients who fail to respond to methotrexate. However, because of the hazard of severe bone marrow depression, it is not recommended as a first-line treatment.[157]

#### Oral Psoralens and Long-Wave Ultraviolet Light (PUVA)

Photochemotherapy[158,159] is used in most major dermatological centres. Its therapeutic effect depends upon the binding with DNA in the skin of the photosensitising drugs methoxsalen (8-methoxypsoralen; 8-MOP), 5-methoxypsoralen (5-MOP), or trioxsalen (trimethylpsoralen) in the presence of long-wave ultraviolet light (UVA) at 320 to 400nm. This suppresses skin cell division, which is its putative mechanism of action.

*Methoxsalen* is generally given orally in a dosage of about 0.6 mg/kg 2 hours before irradiation, although general rules about timing are not entirely satisfactory in view of interindividual[160,161] and interproduct[162] variation in absorption and peak concentrations in blood and skin. The presence of food has also been shown to impair the absorption of methoxsalen. The drug has a short half-life (0.5 to 2 hours) and undergoes extensive biotransformation in the liver. There is a large interpatient variability in the clearance of methoxsalen which is at least partly due to differences in first-pass metabolism. Individuals with a high methoxsalen clearance and low peak plasma concentration usually show less biological sensitivity to PUVA (in terms of the minimal phototoxic dose of UVA) and frequently, a less favourable clinical response (for a review, see de Wolff & Thomas[163]).

In contrast to methoxsalen, *trioxsalen* is usually applied topically, mainly in the form of baths. When given orally, trioxsalen appears to be less well absorbed than methoxsalen and produces a lesser photosensitivity response.

Special lamps are necessary to deliver the UVA and are relatively expensive. The dose of UVA is adjusted to the patient's history of burning and/or tanning on exposure to natural sunlight[164] and a number of different regimens are in use. Generally, patients are treated 2, 3 or 4 times a week until clearance occurs and in most this takes longer than with a dithranol regimen.[165,166] Patients relapse without maintenance treatment but with maintenance therapy once a week, or even once every 3 weeks, relapse is postponed.[167]

Patients intolerant of or resistant to dithranol and patients who have previously needed cytotoxic drugs are among those who do well on PUVA therapy.[166] However, with the usual regimens, psoriasis of the scalp, nails and flexures does not as a rule respond well, and joint symptoms (psoriatic arthritis) do not respond at all. Great care has to be taken with erythrodermic and generalised pustular psoriasis,[168] although some patients eventually improve in skilled hands.

Undesirable effects of PUVA therapy with methoxsalen on the liver, kidneys and blood have not been significant,[164] and although pruritus and nausea occur, they have not often interfered with treatment. Accidental burns are serious but should not occur with skilled operators. Hyperpigmentation, although attractive and unavoidable, is undesirable as it interferes with the subsequent response to treatment. Cataracts, a feature of high-dose psoralens and UVA in animals, have not been seen in large-scale clinical trials in humans. Accelerated aging of the skin due to collagen damage occurs, and it is likely that there will be an increase in skin cancer in treated individuals (see below), but internal cancer and significant effect on germ cells seem unlikely.

Patients likely to become pregnant should not receive PUVA therapy and those with significant disease of the liver (where psoralens are metabolised) should be treated with caution. Great care should be taken to protect the eyes and prevent burning of the skin. The patient should wear goggles which protect from UVA, e.g. 'Hazemaster' (American Optical), 'Cool-Ray' (Polaroid)[169] during treatment and for at least 8 hours afterwards (the duration of significant psoralen levels in the blood and skin); the skin should also be protected by clothes for 8 hours after treatment from extraneous UVA in natural sunlight. Long term follow-up of eyes for cataract and skin for cancer is essential.

***PUVA and skin cancer:*** from animal studies and other laboratory experiments, it is to be expected that treatment with PUVA will increase the risk of skin cancer. Most experience in the US (e.g. Stern & Lange)[170] demonstrates a strong association between cumulative exposure to PUVA and an increased risk of squamous cell carcinoma of the skin. Comparable increases in relative risk were noted in patients of all skin types, irrespective of prior ionising radiation exposure. A modest dose-dependent increase in the risk for the development of basal cell carcinoma was observed in patients who received more than 200 treatments compared with those who had received fewer than 160 treatments within the same time period. Tumours detected exhibit biological behaviour similar to non-melanoma skin cancers associated with sun exposure.

***Selection of patients for PUVA:*** this technique will rarely be first-line treatment in psoriasis, although there is no reason why it should not be so in the elderly. In all those whose disease is not satisfactorily controlled by dithranol and tar, it should be considered. The younger the patient, the less enthusiastic one will be about using PUVA, but the young are the very ones in whom extensive disease and messy applications cause the greatest distress, and each case should be considered on its merits. PUVA with whole-body radiation should not normally be given to those with less than 20% of the body surface involved.

***Topical psoralens with UVA:*** topical psoralen lotions, creams or ointments have been shown to be useful in the treatment of localised forms of the disease, and the phototherapeutic effects induced by UVA are achieved with short treatment times. However, this may result in patchy hyperpigmentation and increased risk of unwanted phototoxic erythema and blistering. Alternative means of delivering psoralens have been used, where both methoxsalen and trioxsalen have been delivered in bathwater. A dilute psoralen solution is made in the bathwater; the patient soaks in the psoralen bath and then undergoes UVA phototherapy.[134]

**Etretinate and Acitretin**

*Etretinate* is less effective than isotretinoin in acne but more effective in several diseases where there is abnormal keratinisation, including psoriasis (for reviews, see Ward et al.;[171] Cunningham & Geiger[172]). The pharmacological profile of etretinate suggests that it acts by normalising pathological changes in dermal and epidermal skin, particularly by inhibiting hyperkeratinisation and cell differentiation, although its specific mode of action in psoriasis remains to be established. Following oral administration, the bioavailability of etretinate is about 40%. The drug undergoes substantial first-pass hydrolysis to a biologically active carboxylic acid metabolite which, along with its corresponding phenol, undergoes glucuronidation and excretion in the bile; other (inactive) metabolites are also formed by oxidation and demethylation and these are eliminated in the urine.[121] Pharmacokinetically, the main difference between etretinate and isotretinoin is the much longer elimination half-life of etretinate (120 days *versus* 10 to 20 hours for isotretinoin), and it has been suggested that this represents storage of etretinate in a 'deep tissue compartment' from which it slowly returns to the central compartment. This characteristic has major implications in terms of its clinical and adverse effect profiles. The dermatopharmacokinetics of etretinate have been reviewed by Orfanos et al.,[122] Gollnick et al.,[173] and Geiger & Saurat.[174]

Etretinate can be used in psoriasis on its own or in combination with other treatments, especially PUVA. Used alone, it is still not clear which types of psoriasis respond best, although severe erythrodermic and pustular psoriasis are said to, and pustular psoriasis of the palms and soles certainly does,[175] only to relapse quickly when the drug is stopped. In combination with PUVA, etretinate reduces the time to clearance of lesions to an extent that is certainly worthwhile in palmoplantar psoriasis.[176] As with isotretinoin, the dose of etretinate ranges from 0.5 to 1 mg/kg/day. Adverse effects are similar to those occurring with isotretinoin (see section 4.1.2), but as treatment is likely to be required for longer than with acne, effects on serum lipids, liver enzymes and bones have to be considered more seriously, though it is still not known how clinically important they are. The chief limitation in the use of etretinate lies in its teratogenic effect (see chapter 2; sect. 6), and because of its long half-life, pregnancy should not be allowed to occur for 2 years after stopping the drug.

*Acitretin* is the main metabolite of etretinate. It is less lipophilic and more rapidly eliminated (half-life 50 to 60 hours *versus* 120 days for etretinate),[177,178] but in terms of therapeutic activity, acitretin resembles etretinate. The dose ranges from 10 to 50mg per day in a single dose. Adverse effects are similar to those occurring with isotretinoin (see section 4.1.2). For a review of the pharmacology and therapeutic use of acitretin, see Pilkington & Brogden.[178]

#### Cyclosporin

This drug, now fully established for its action on T cells and its prevention of organ rejection after transplantation (see further chapter 28; sect. 2.1.3), was found by chance to be effective in clearing psoriasis.[179,180] In the first double-blind trial, cyclosporin given in a dosage of 14 mg/kg/day for 4 weeks produced significantly better improvement than placebo in a small group of patients with severe plaque psoriasis.[181] In subsequent psoriasis studies, the dose of cyclosporin was reduced, and lower doses were shown to be effective.[182] Cyclosporin doses ranging from 2 to 5 mg/kg/day are appropriate for the treatment of psoriasis. The therapeutic response is dose-dependent: higher doses clear psoriasis more quickly and more effectively than lower doses. Tachyphylaxis does not occur.

The use of cyclosporin requires careful patient selection and close clinical monitoring.[180,183,184] For further discussion of the use of cyclosporin in psoriasis, see Faulds et al.[185]

## 7. Dermatitis (Eczema)

Dermatitis or eczema is an inflammation of the skin which has special clinical and histological features. It may be caused by an external irritant or allergen, or it may be of unknown aetiology, in which case it is sometimes called 'constitutional' or 'endogenous'. Atopic dermatitis is a form of 'constitutional' dermatitis: it is associated with circulating IgE antibodies to one or more of a wide variety of antigens, although these antigens usually bear no obvious relationship to production of clinical disease. Recent work in certain aspects of the atopic state, including the role of early antigen exposure, has suggested possible new ways of managing atopic eczema. The effect of avoidance of antigen, especially cow's milk protein, on its development has not yet been fully assessed:[186,187] the great practical inconvenience involved makes it unjustifiable to recommend this method of management until more is known. Sodium cromoglycate, which is effective in the treatment of allergic asthma (see chapter 23; sect. 3.1.2), has not proved useful in atopic eczema, according to most clinical dermatologists,[188] although one report suggests that it can be effective in some children.[189] Thus, at the present time, the treatment of this common form of eczema is still mainly symptomatic.

### 7.1 Optimum Treatment

Different types of dermatitis need treatments that differ in some respects (table VII), but the basic drug therapy is common to all types. Nearly always, an anti-inflammatory agent is required. At present, corticosteroids are the most appropriate agents; topical nonsteroidal anti-inflammatory agents such as bufexamac have not proved satisfactory[190] in double-blind controlled trials, although their clinical popularity in Europe indicates that further study is warranted.

#### *7.1.1 Topical Therapy*

#### Topical Corticosteroids

In all but exceptional cases, if corticosteroids are to be used, they are used topically. The particular proprietary preparation chosen is largely a matter of personal preference. Nevertheless, some preparations 'suit' one patient better than another, and this depends on numerous factors, including the character of the base (see section 1.5) as well as the potency and strength of the corticosteroid.[24,28] Many cases of dermatitis respond readily to 1% hydrocortisone or milder fluorinated corticosteroid preparations (see table II) and it is obviously desirable to use these if they work. Nevertheless, it is useless to continue with mild preparations that are having no effect and, especially in hospital practice, stronger corticosteroids may be required temporarily to bring severe dermatitis under control.

The adverse effects of topical corticosteroids on the skin (see table VIII) make it imperative that once the dermatitis is under control, attempts should be made to stop the corticosteroid, or to reduce its concentration to the weakest which is effective, especially when used on the face.[24,192] In severe chronic dermatitis, one may have to choose between progressive skin atrophy and continuing eczema. This

**Table VII.** Therapeutic measures to be used in addition to general ones (see text) in different types of dermatitis

**Atopic:**
- Deal with dryness of skin, with itch and with secondary infection when it occurs. Paste bandages helpful in children

**Seborrhoeic:**
- Antibacterial and less often anticandidal drugs may be necessary

**Discoid:**
- Antibacterial measures may be necessary

**Varicose:**
- Bandages which reduce oedema and support varicose veins may be needed. Paste bandages sometimes aid healing of dermatitis.
- Contact dermatitis to applied medicaments should be watched for

**Contact:**
- Patch testing for delayed hypersensitivity in cases of allergic contact dermatitis is extremely helpful in diagnosis and thus in management. Offending allergens should be removed.
- Patch testing is not helpful in diagnosis of non-allergic irritant dermatitis, but removal of irritants is equally important in management of these types of dermatitis

choice may not be easy, although most patients, if they are asked, seem to prefer the atrophy.

#### Other Topical Agents

Because of the adverse effects of continued use of corticosteroids, a critical reappraisal is warranted of some of the treatments for dermatitis that were used in precorticosteroid days. Of these, *tar* preparations may prove the most rewarding. They are effective in some hands, but it is not known which of their many constituents are the active ones, or how tar is best used. The colour and smell of tar make it unacceptable to many patients but it may be that in the future, both can be removed from the crude coal tar preparations without reducing effectiveness.

Other topical preparations that are effective in dermatitis include tap water compresses (which are useful for 'drying' acute weeping lesions), certain occlusive bandages (which are useful as a mechanical barrier to scratching), and certain preparations which counteract the dryness of the skin that accompanies some types of dermatitis. In the latter group of preparations, simple lipoidal mixtures like emulsifying ointment are commonly used.

### *7.1.2 Systemic Therapy*

#### Corticosteroids

Systemic corticosteroids have no place in the routine treatment of dermatitis, but are certainly effective in acute disease. Situations in which they can reasonably be used are:

1) *Acute contact dermatitis*, where, if the offending substances can be identified and removed, the condition will not recur. Systemic corticosteroids will rapidly reduce the discomfort of the acute stage and the question of continuing the corticosteroid for more than a few days will not arise. A dose of 30mg prednisone daily is a reasonable one to start with and it is usually possible to stop the drug within 10 to 14 days.

2) *Widespread or erythrodermic dermatitis*, in which, regardless of the cause of the dermatitis, the patient is at risk from the systemic consequences of the inflammation, e.g. hypothermia and heart failure. Here, an initial large dose of up to 100mg prednisone may be required in an emergency. The dose must be reduced gradually and only when the dermatitis is under control, or the condition will recur. A small 'maintenance' dose of 10 to 15mg daily usually has to be given for several months or even longer.

3) *Certain cases of severe atopic dermatitis*, in which additional factors, e.g. the presence of severe asthma, influence the decision to give systemic corticosteroids.

#### Other Agents

The part played by other systemic treatments in dermatitis is unproven. Obviously, if sleep is a problem, some form of sedation should be given. *Antihistamines* with a strong sedative action are usually satisfactory for this purpose, and in addition they reduce itch, possibly by virtue of their local anaesthetic action. However, antihistaminic activity is not important in dermatitis, as in this disease the inflammation is usually not mediated by histamine. Topical antihistamines should be used with caution to minimise the risk of sensitisation; because of the frequency with which they produce contact dermatitis, the systemic route is preferred. Children tolerate antihistamines well. A small baby with atopic dermatitis may, for instance, need and tolerate 30 to 50mg trimeprazine at night, while an adult will need only 10 to 20mg.

*Systemic antibacterials*, e.g. cloxacillin/flucloxacillin, are useful alternatives to topical antibiotics in infected dermatitis, especially when it is severe or extensive or when there is evidence of contact sensitivity to topical preparations.

### *7.1.3 Treatment of Napkin (Diaper) Dermatitis*

Psoriasiform napkin (diaper) dermatitis of babies is infrequently true psoriasis, but is usu-

**Table VIII.** Principal adverse effects of topical corticosteroids applied to the skin (after Burry;[191] Sneddon[24])

| Adverse effect | Influencing factors/notes |
|---|---|
| Epidermal and dermal atrophy, manifest by clinical thinning of the skin, telangiectasia, corticosteroid purpura and striae | Prolonged use of strong corticosteroids<br>More likely when occlusive dressings used, or waterproof plastic pants in babies treated for napkin eruptions and in deeper skin folds<br>Combined dermal and epidermal atrophy is the most common form |
| Rosacea-like 'corticosteroid face' and 'perioral dermatitis' | Here the signs of atrophy with telangiectasia and corticosteroid purpura are accompanied by pustulation<br>Corticosteroids, especially the stronger ones, applied to the face can produce this picture whatever the primary facial condition |
| Impeded healing | Particularly ulcers |
| Local hypertrichosis | Usually only after prolonged use<br>Most noticeable on the face |
| Masking of spread of infection | When used in presence of fungal, viral or bacterial infection |
| Systemic absorption | Application in large quantities to large areas, particularly under occlusion. Risk of adrenal suppression greatest in infants |
| Glaucoma | Can occur in susceptible individuals, especially when strong corticosteroids are applied around the eyes |

ally a severe form of seborrhoeic dermatitis with secondary candidal infection. As such, it responds to a mild corticosteroid cream, topical anticandidal agents (see table V), and measures directed towards eliminating *Candida albicans* from the gut (e.g. nystatin oral suspension).

#### 7.1.4 Treatment of Seborrhoeic Dermatitis

Seborrhoeic dermatitis, an inflammatory dermatosis that principally affects the scalp and sebaceous rich areas of the face and trunk, may be related to the presence of the yeast *Pityrosporum ovale*. It commonly affects adults and infants within the first months of life. Topical therapy with corticosteroids, although generally effective, may be associated with several unwanted effects. Nonfluorinated topical corticosteroid preparations or corticosteroid/antifungal drug combinations may not always be needed, except in resistant or florid cases.

The development of alternative non-corticosteroid-based therapies may enable patients to avoid the use of topical corticosteroids. Imidazole agents are known to be more than just antifungal; they can also block leukotriene synthesis both *in vitro* and *in vivo* and, therefore, exert some anti-inflammatory effects.[193] Usually, 2% preparations in the form of creams and shampoos are used. *Ketoconazole* 2% emulsion or cream has been found to be superior to placebo in the treatment of seborrhoeic dermatitis of the face, scalp and trunk,[194,195] and the 2% cream has proved comparable in effectiveness to hydrocortisone 1% cream.[196] *Topical metronidazole* up to 2% in a cream base has also been recommended.[197]

Shampoos containing *selenium sulfide, imidazoles* and *zinc pyrithione* are all effective for scalp involvement. Topical corticosteroid scalp lotions should be used only for a limited period.

#### 7.1.5 Treatment of Secondary Infections

Some forms of dermatitis are particularly prone to secondary infection;[198-200] topical or systemic antibacterial or anticandidal agents (see sections 2.1 and 2.3) are then prescribed as required. Some topical corticosteroid preparations include an antibacterial and/or anticandidal agent. These agents should be used with discretion as they add little, if anything, to the efficacy of routine treatment, and some increase the risk of contact dermatitis, especially in cases of stasis dermatitis and ulcers.[201] The contact sensitivity to the antibacterial agent is to some extent masked by the corticosteroid, and often the only evidence of sensitisation will be the persistence of the dermatitis. Patch testing to the antibacterial agent alone, i.e. without the corticosteroid, is necessary for diagnosis, and cross-sensitivity (e.g. between neomycin and framycetin) is common.

## 8. Pruritus Vulvae and Pruritus Ani

The irritation in these regions that concerns the dermatologist is that due to skin disease which happens to be in these areas. In some instances, other areas of skin will also be involved and examination of the skin as a whole may well lead to the finding of typical lesions elsewhere which help in diagnosis.

### 8.1 Local and Systemic Conditions

Local conditions, such as tumours, warts and herpes simplex virus infections, occasionally cause itch, and examination including proctoscopy and colposcopy should always be performed. In children especially, threadworms may be present. Care should be taken to exclude systemic disease such as diabetes mellitus (especially in the case of pruritus vulvae) and altered gut flora from broad-spectrum antibiotics (especially in the case of pruritus ani).

Pediculosis of pubic hair is unlikely to give rise to true vulval or perianal itch.

### 8.2 Skin Conditions

***Dermatitis:*** this is not an uncommon site for atopic dermatitis, and lichenification often occurs from persistent itch and scratching. Contact dermatitis, e.g. to proprietary creams (especially those containing local anaesthetics), suppositories and contraceptives, is another common cause of dermatitis here. Management is as for dermatitis elsewhere (see section 7.1). Topical corticosteroids are best used as lotions or creams and clioquinol is a useful mild anticandidal agent in these conditions.

***Psoriasis:*** treatment is as for flexural psoriasis elsewhere. Usually, dithranol is not well tolerated and topical corticosteroids have to be used (see section 6.1.1).

***Candidiasis:*** this may produce pruritus from genital tract or alimentary candidiasis, and these conditions should be treated when appropriate, in addition to treatment of the skin. Topical preparations such as nystatin or a topical imidazole preparation are suitable (see table V).

***Lichen sclerosus:*** this is a relatively rare but important disease of the vulva which can extend to involve perianal skin and very occasionally can be complicated by carcinoma. Topical corticosteroids are usually effective in relieving the itch, and carefully used topical testosterone has been shown to be effective in controlled trials.[202] The oral retinoids etretinate and acitretin have been reported to have beneficial effects in severe disease.[203]

## 9. Ichthyosis

Ichthyosis occurs in inherited and acquired forms. The common form is inherited as an autosomal dominant characteristic and is common in atopic individuals. The rarer sex-linked recessive form is confined to males. Acquired ichthyosis can be secondary to changes in climatic conditions but should also give rise to suspicion about underlying wasting diseases such as a malabsorption or malignant disease.

### Optimum Treatment

Some cases of acquired ichthyosis, e.g. those after small bowel resection, respond to topical linoleic acid (as sunflower seed oil), of which there is presumed to be a deficiency.[204] Otherwise, the treatment of ichthyosis is usually symptomatic with the application of grease (e.g. emulsifying ointment or soft paraffin), or hygroscopic agents (e.g. glycerin, urea or alpha-hydroxyacids, e.g. glycolic acid).

***Retinoids:*** isotretinoin, etretinate and acitretin are effective in some patients with various types of inherited ichthyosis.[119,171] The results of different clinical trials with isotretinoin have been contradictory.[122] However, good therapeutic results have been achieved with *etretinate* in the treatment of both the autosomal dominant and the sex-linked recessive form of ichthyosis vulgaris. Therapy is usually started with moderate initial doses (0.5 to 0.6 mg/kg/day) and continued at the lowest possible maintenance level over months or years.[122] Obviously, the condition must be severe for it to merit such treatment (for discussion of adverse effects, see section 6.1.2), especially as many of the patients are children. Possible effects of the retinoid drugs on, for example, serum lipids, liver function and bone, which may not be important when they are used short term, may be serious in the long term, and have to be weighed very carefully against the beneficial effects in each individual case.

## 10. Urticaria

Urticaria is a common condition which may be acute or chronic. Certain different clinical patterns of rash are seen (e.g. papular urticaria, giant urticaria), but there is always some degree of whealing and some erythematous flare, so that the basic lesion mimics that produced by experimental intradermal injection of histamine.

The causes of urticaria include pressure on the skin (dermographism), heat, cold, ingestion of food allergens and systemic administration of drugs and antisera (see section 22.3.1). The mechanisms whereby they produce histamine release in the skin are many and varied, only a few urticarias being the end result of a 'type I' hypersensitivity reaction. Urticaria can be a manifestation of the atopic state, i.e. it can occur in families with dermatitis, hay fever and asthma. In such patients, circulating antibodies of the IgE class (reagins) are found, although the relationship of a specific reagin – or of the antigen that produces it – to the urticaria is not a simple one of cause and effect.

### 10.1 Acute Urticaria

Usually, the cause is obvious to patients who know, for instance, that they have eaten shellfish or had a penicillin injection to which they are allergic. Future trouble is prevented by avoiding the offending substance. Intradermal testing is unnecessary and unlikely to elicit any more useful information than a good history; in addition, of course, it can be dangerous. Drug challenge may be helpful if the agent has not been identified. For a review of oral provocation, see Kauppinen & Alanko.[205]

#### Optimum Treatment

Treatment of attacks is with an oral *non-sedating antihistamine* such as astemizole,[206-208] terfenadine,[209] loratadine,[210] cetirizine,[211] and acrivastine.[212] Occasionally it may be necessary to give an antihistamine intramuscularly; as parenteral preparations of non-sedating antihistamines are not currently available, other (sedating) antihistamines such as chlorpheniramine (10 to 20mg intramuscularly) or diphenhydramine (25 to 50mg intramuscularly) may be administered.

**Angioedema,** which may accompany acute urticaria or occur without the rash, requires urgent treatment. When this involves or threatens to involve the mouth or upper respiratory passages, it is a life-threatening condition and if the patient is already showing signs of respiratory distress, a tracheotomy should be done. In any case, attempts should be made to reduce the swelling and to deal with accompanying effects of histamine release such as hypotension. The following treatments should be given in this order:

1) Adrenaline (epinephrine) by intramuscular injection at a dosage of 0.5ml of 1 : 1000 solution.

2) Hydrocortisone sodium succinate 100mg intravenously, preferably in a saline 'drip' so that fluid and more hydrocortisone can be given if necessary; and

3) An antihistamine, e.g. chlorpheniramine 10mg or diphenhydramine 25mg intramuscularly.

### 10.2 Chronic Urticaria

In chronic urticaria, it is usually much more difficult to find a cause and indeed it is rare for the cause to be proven. Intradermal testing with suspected allergens is, in general, not productive; some positive reactions are to be expected in atopic individuals and give no clue to the cause of the urticaria.

Infections such as candidiasis and food additives such as azo dyes are sometimes blamed, but the response of the patient to elimination of the infection or withdrawal of the food is difficult to evaluate in this disease, whose natural history is one of eventual spontaneous remission.

#### Optimum Treatment

Treatment is with adequate doses of a *non-sedating antihistamine* ($H_1$-receptor antagonist) such as astemizole, terfenadine, loratadine, cetirizine or acrivastine. Astemizole is usually given in a dose of 10mg once daily, but higher doses may be required to control symptoms.[213] Both $H_1$ and $H_2$ histamine receptors are present in cutaneous blood vessels and $H_2$-receptor antagonists such as cimetidine or ranitidine may therefore be useful as adjunctive therapy in patients who remain symptomatic after adequate doses of $H_1$-receptor antagonists.[214,215]

Systemic corticosteroids are rarely effective in chronic urticaria and are not a recommended form of treatment. Topical applications such as calamine lotion serve only to 'cool' the skin. Nonspecific worsening of urticaria (of whatever cause) by aspirin is a common phenomenon, and patients with urticaria should be advised not to take aspirin (see also section 22.3.1).

### 10.3 Cholinergic Urticaria

This is a clinically recognisable variant of chronic urticaria which is seen particularly in fit young men after exercising or bathing, often in association with sweating. Although the lesions resemble those produced by injection of cholinergic drugs, the mechanism of their production is not known.

#### Optimum Treatment

The attacks can sometimes be minimised by regular or periodic oral antihistamines. Anticholinergic drugs such as propantheline bromide can be used in addition, although when given alone they usually produce too many adverse effects if used at clinically effective doses.

### 10.4 Familial Angioedema

This is a rare condition inherited as an autosomal dominant trait. It is not related to allergic or other urticarias or angioedemas, and a useful diagnostic point is that the submucosal and subcutaneous swellings that occur are not usually accompanied by urticaria. There is a deficiency of the inhibitor of the enzyme Cl esterase, one of the components of complement. One of the consequences of the defect is that kinins are released and oedema results, though why this occurs in attacks is not fully understood. Local trauma is often a provoking factor and this is of course particularly dangerous if the mouth, neck or throat are traumatised. Death from respiratory obstruction often occurs in early adult life so that life expectancy is considerably reduced in affected individuals.

#### Optimum Treatment

Treatment is by prompt relief of respiratory obstruction and by correcting the enzyme deficiency with a transfusion of fresh frozen or freeze-dried plasma.[216] Adrenaline (epinephrine) and other measures used for allergic angioedema are not effective and should not be administered. Few clinicians have enough experience of treating these patients to enable any alternatives to plasma infusions to be assessed properly, but ε-*aminocaproic acid or tranexamic acid*, both inhibitors of Cl esterase (see chapter 26; sect. 4.1.1), are reported to control spontaneous attacks and can be used as (expensive) long term maintenance treatment when this is required.[217]

*Danazol*, a synthetic antigonadotrophic agent with anabolic and weak androgenic activity, is currently considered the treatment of choice for preventing attacks, though in an acute attack it is not effective and should not be relied upon. Danazol can be given long term in doses of 200 to 600mg daily, but should be avoided in pregnant women, and in growing children in whom it may cause premature closing of epiphyses. Danazol appears to act by increasing the synthesis of the inhibitor of the first component of complement.[218-220]

### 10.5 Contact Urticaria Syndrome

Contact urticaria syndrome consists of an immediate-type response (minutes to an hour or so). The primary lesion consists of wheal and flare, although subvisible lesions may demonstrate only itch. At least two mechanistic forms, non-immunological (NICU) and immunological (ICU), exist. The former produces localised lesions only, whereas ICU may, in severe forms, involve generalised urticaria, angioedema, anaphylaxis and death. Treatment is best directed to diagnosis and avoidance. For reviews, see Maibach & Johnson;[221] Lahti et al.;[222] and Lahti & Maibach.[223]

## 11. Lichen Planus

Lichen planus is a disease of unknown aetiology, except that rashes similar to it have been seen after bone marrow transplantation as part of a graft-*versus*-host reaction. Rashes indistinguishable from lichen planus can be caused by drugs such as the antimalarial agents and gold. Contact with chemicals used in colour photography processing occasionally produces a similar rash. There is no evidence that infection or emotional upsets produce the disease. Mouth lesions are common (see chapter 16; sect. 4.1), and among other mucosal surfaces known to be involved, the glans penis is the most common. An attack of lichen planus usually lasts several months or more, and some patients have recurrent attacks.

#### Optimum Treatment

The necessity to treat the condition depends on the extent of the rash and the amount of irritation present. Often only reassurance or symptomatic treatment is required. Both systemic sedative antihistamines and topical corticosteroids, with or without occlusion, will help to relieve the itch, and a strong topical corticosteroid, if necessary applied under polythene occlusion, will improve the appearance of the rash.

Occasionally, a systemic corticosteroid is required if the rash is extensive: oral prednisone in a dose of about 40mg daily initially should suppress the rash but does not appear to alter the natural history of the disease.

## 12. Bullous Diseases

### 12.1 Pemphigus and Pemphigoid

In these diseases, the extensive blistering of the skin means that patients may lose heat, water, electrolytes and protein through the skin and consequently are in danger of death from their disease, especially if they are elderly. Diagnosis is based on morphology, dermatopathology and the demonstration of antibodies by immunofluorescence in a skin biopsy. In pemphigus, these are directed towards the intercellular cement substance between the epidermal cells, and in pemphigoid, to a component of the basement membrane at the dermoepidermal junction. It is not known for certain that these antibodies are the cause rather than a result of the disease.

#### Optimum Treatment

Corticosteroids in large doses, usually about 100mg prednisone daily, are generally needed to control the blistering, and the maintenance dose required, though lower, may well be of an order likely to produce serious adverse effects.

Immunosuppressive drugs, especially azathioprine and methotrexate, are also useful in treatment when used in a dosage of about 150mg daily (2.5 mg/kg bodyweight) assuming renal function is normal.[224] Azathioprine is relatively safe, although leucopenia and deterioration in liver function are occasional complications. At this dosage a 'corticosteroid-sparing' effect is possible,[225] and in some cases it is even possible to take the patient off corticosteroids and maintain him/her on azathioprine alone. Methotrexate use is discussed in section 6.1.2. Exceptionally, especially in severe pemphigus, plasmapheresis,[226] gold therapy,[227] and cyclosporin[228,229] have been used. Intramuscular gold may be effective for both pemphigus vulgaris and pemphigus foliaceus patients. Most patients treated with gold are also treated with corticosteroids. However, gold may have potentially life-threatening adverse effects.

General measures directed towards replacing lost fluid, electrolytes and protein and maintaining a normal temperature are obviously required in severe cases. An extensively blistered skin is extremely uncomfortable and the application of 'spread dressings' of a corticosteroid such as betamethasone valerate is soothing. Potassium permanganate baths to dry up the blisters and oozing surfaces also help.

### 12.2 Benign Mucous Membrane Pemphigoid

Blisters occur in the mouth in the majority of patients with pemphigus and in some patients with pemphigoid; occasionally, mouth lesions predate skin lesions by months or even longer (see chapter 16; sect. 4.2). Benign mucous membrane pemphigoid has clinical and immunological differences from the other bullous diseases, although it is most closely related to pemphigoid. In some cases, the skin is not involved at all and in most patients the skin lesions are the least important feature of the disease. Mouth, genital and other mucosal lesions can be extremely troublesome but it is in the eye that the disease is most serious for it can result in blindness.

#### Optimum Treatment

A topical corticosteroid may be all that is required to control the rash; otherwise systemic corticosteroids and immunosuppressive agents can be used as in pemphigoid and pemphigus (see section 12.1). However, controlled clinical trials are not available. Treatment of the eye and mouth lesions is best left to the specialist in those fields.

### 12.3 Dermatitis Herpetiformis

This is a blistering disease with some resemblance to pemphigoid but usually without the extensive large blisters. It does not as a rule respond to corticosteroids or to immunosuppressive drugs. Autoantibodies to particular components of skin have not been demonstrated, although characteristic deposits of IgA are found in the dermis.

#### Optimum Treatment

The rash of dermatitis herpetiformis is completely and promptly suppressed by sulfonamides and sulfones. *Dapsone* is the drug most commonly used, the minimal effective dose ranging from 50mg weekly to 500mg daily in different individuals and also varying considerably from time to time in a given individual. Dapsone should always be used in the smallest dose required to produce a clinical effect. Laboratory evidence of haemolysis can be found in most people who take the drug, but in the absence of clinically important anaemia, this is not an indication that it must be stopped.

Dapsone is well absorbed and peak plasma concentrations occur within a few hours of an oral dose, but the drug is still detectable in the blood 4 days later, partly because of its excretion in the bile and enterohepatic recirculation. It is distributed into all body tissues and secretions (including breast milk) and is concentrated in red cells, one of its main targets for toxicity, but not apparently in skin apart from the granulomatous lesions of leprosy. Dapsone is strongly protein bound (70 to 90%) and extensively metabolised, both by acetylation and hydroxylation. Acetylation results in monoacetyldapsone (MADDS) and the acetylation ratio (MADDS : dapsone) shows a genetically determined bimodal distribution which allows the definition of 'slow' and 'rapid' acetylators (see chapter 1; sect. 5.2.1); however, no clear relationship between acetylation capacity and either the clinical response or the incidence of adverse effects has been demonstrated. Following oral administration, the parent drug, some MADDS and their hydroxylated metabolites are found in the urine, partly conjugated – mainly as glucuronides and to a lesser extent *N*-sulfates. The elimination half-life of both dapsone and MADDS is around 30 hours.[230] Rifampicin increases the metabolic clearance of dapsone while probenecid decreases its renal clearance.

Dapsone has been shown to have many effects but its mechanism of action in dermatitis herpetiformis is not known. It is an enzyme inhibitor and inhibition of the myeloperoxide $H_2O_2$ iodide system is a suggested mode of action in this disease. Dapsone also has a number of immunological effects including inhibition of complement activation by the 'alternative' pathway.

Although depression, rashes, leucopenia and neuropathy occur, the main undesirable effects of dapsone are on red cells. These are detectable in nearly all patients taking the drug and are clinically important in a few cases.[231,232] Oxidation of haemoglobin results in the formation of methaemoglobin, and this is the main cause of the blue colour and in more extreme cases, shortness of breath. Oxidation of globin results in the formation of Heinz bodies which are frequently found in patients' blood films. Oxidation of the red cell membrane results in haemolysis. This is dose-related but, in addition, is worse in those with glucose-6-phosphate dehydrogenase deficiency (see chapter 26; sect. 5.2.2). Severe haemolytic anaemia and severe methaemoglobinaemia will mean that dapsone must be stopped, but care should be taken to see that anaemia in patients with dermatitis herpetiformis that is dapsone-induced is not confused with that due to coeliac disease (see below). Dapsone therapy should be closely supervised because of potential for clinical toxicity.

#### Dermatitis Herpetiformis and Coeliac Disease

The discovery that at least two-thirds of patients with dermatitis herpetiformis have structural changes in the small intestinal mucosa indistinguishable from those of coeliac disease[233,234] raised hopes that the rash, like the bowel, might respond to a gluten-free diet. This has not universally been the case, even in those whose bowel has returned to normal on the diet. Although most patients are able to reduce the dose of dapsone or do without it altogether, some have been reported to develop dermatitis herpetiformis for the first time while on a gluten-free diet for coeliac disease. Putting patients on a 'gluten-free diet' has effects other than simple withdrawal of gluten and there may be other factors involved in the production of the rash.

Patients with dermatitis herpetiformis who also have coeliac disease should of course be put on a gluten-free diet. Those without gut symptoms should be similarly treated if the structural changes in the bowel are severe or there is biochemical evidence of malabsorption. It is not known whether putting those with minor changes on a gluten-free diet will decrease the risk of small bowel lymphoma, which is a complication of coeliac disease. Even in those with a normal bowel, a gluten-free diet is certainly worth trying for its effect on the rash, especially in patients in whom dapsone is ineffective or is producing adverse effects, but many patients prefer taking dapsone to life on a strict gluten-free diet.[235]

### 12.4 Erythema Multiforme

This disease and its severe variant, the Stevens-Johnson syndrome, is presumably an immunological reaction to one of a number of insults. Some of the more common ones are infections such as herpes simplex virus;[236] drugs such as antibiotics (see section 22.3.8); and malignant disease, especially after treatment which results in tissue destruction.

In the Stevens-Johnson syndrome there is fever, soreness or ulceration of the mouth, eyes and genitalia, as well as a rash: the classical rash consists of 'target' or 'iris' lesions especially of the hands and feet, but erythematous, urticated, purpuric and bullous rashes also occur. Associated nephritis can result in death.

#### Optimum Treatment

Treatment of the severe form, whatever its cause, is with oral *prednisone* 40mg daily. If an infection is thought to be the cause, the appropriate antibacterial or antiviral agent must also be given and any drug thought to be responsible must, of course, be stopped. Symptomatic treatment, including mouthwashes, soothing baths for the genital lesions, and bathing the eyes, is also important in the severe forms.

## 13. Collagen Vascular Diseases

The skin is one of the organs most commonly involved in these diseases and consequently the dermatologist may be called upon to supervise treatment, especially in the less acute forms. All have in common the ability to produce skin abnormalities as a result of blockage of blood vessels of various sizes with resulting livedo reticularis, Raynaud's phenomenon, vasculitic purpura and gangrene. Some are amenable to treatment by vasodilators, anticoagulants and lowering of blood viscosity. Other skin manifestations which are not particularly associated with vascular disease need different treatment, depending upon the particular collagen vascular disease involved.

### 13.1 Systemic Lupus Erythematosus

A variety of nonspecific rashes occur in this disease, often in light-exposed areas (e.g. the butterfly area of the face).

#### Optimum Treatment

Some patients are helped by the application, especially in summer, of sunscreen preparations (see further section 21). The rash is usually helped by *hydroxychloroquine* in a dose of 200 to 400mg daily and this may also improve other aspects of the systemic disease. This drug and chloroquine itself have toxic effects, of which those on the retina, which can lead to blindness, are the most important. They should never be given without good reason, or for too long, or without frequent expert ophthalmological supervision. For this reason, *mepacrine* (quinacrine) may be preferred in spite of the fact that it stains the skin yellow.

The skin lesions of systemic lupus erythematosus rarely warrant other systemic treatment such as corticosteroids and immunosuppressive drugs, although they will respond if these drugs are used for other reasons. When skin lesions of discoid lupus erythematosus occur in the course of systemic lupus erythematosus, they should be treated like all other lesions of discoid lupus (see section 13.4).

### 13.2 Systemic Sclerosis

Scleroderma in this condition is usually most obvious on the fingers and the face. It is not treated in the absence of other abnormalities.

#### Optimum Treatment

Measures directed towards treating the vascular and internal aspects of systemic sclerosis rarely help the scleroderma. Antimalarial drugs are not effective and systemic corticosteroids are less useful than in other collagen vascular diseases, and should be restricted to patients with inflammatory myopathy or symptomatic serositis.[237] Immunosuppressive drugs have been used, with some success claimed in severe cases, though placebo-controlled studies are not available. Penicillamine has been shown to improve skin sclerosis and prolong survival of patients with early, rapidly progressive disease,[238] and isotretinoin has been found to improve systemic sclerosis lung disease.[239]

Immunomodulating therapies such as plasmapheresis, extracorporeal photochemotherapy, and interferon have also been used. The results of the available studies are encouraging and indicate that further clinical trials are warranted.[237]

### 13.3 Dermatomyositis

In adults, this collagen vascular disease is more often than not a skin manifestation of underlying malignancy.

#### Optimum Treatment

Removal of the tumour, if this is practicable, will result in improvement of the rash and the myopathy. In other cases, it may not be necessary to treat the rash but the myopathy will need treatment when there is clinically important weakness of the proximal limb and trunk muscles, or dysphagia from weakness of the muscles for swallowing. In such cases, the rash will improve with topical corticosteroids, systemic corticosteroids or immunosuppressive therapy, while for the myopathy, large doses of corticosteroids (e.g. prednisone 100mg daily) may be required initially. As maintenance therapy, a smaller dose with or without an immunosuppressive drug such as azathioprine or methotrexate is usually effective.[240,241] Plasmapheresis has been used effectively in both children and adults in combination with a corticosteroid and a cytotoxic agent. Improvement is often not apparent until 2 to 3 weeks after plasmapheresis is started.[242] However, some controlled studies have reported no benefit from plasmapheresis in polymyositis or dermatomyositis.[243]

A high dose of intravenous immune globulin has been shown to be effective as a corticosteroid-sparing agent in patients with refractory disease.[244]

### 13.4 Discoid Lupus Erythematosus and Morphoea

These are conditions related to the collagen vascular diseases. Usually they are confined to the skin and so only rarely are they of more than cosmetic importance.

#### *13.4.1 Discoid Lupus Erythematosus*

This can occur as one of the skin manifestations of systemic lupus, and a minority of cases of discoid lupus do go on to develop systemic lupus. Nevertheless, discoid lupus erythematosus usually occurs in patients who are otherwise fit. The rash, like that of systemic lupus, is often on light-exposed areas, especially the face. Unlike the nonspecific and often transient rashes of systemic lupus, it progresses to scarring, and when this occurs on the scalp, it results in permanent baldness.

**Optimum Treatment**

In severe and widespread discoid lupus, antimalarial drugs or systemic corticosteroids may be necessary, as for systemic lupus, but usually topical treatment with corticosteroids is sufficient. Hydrocortisone does not work, and stronger preparations like betamethasone valerate or clobetasol propionate or their equivalents (see table II) have to be used. Occlusion, when needed, enhances their efficacy. Their use, even on the face, is completely justifiable in this potentially scarring condition. An alternative route of administration of corticosteroids is by intradermal injection, and triamcinolone is a convenient preparation for this. Sunscreen creams may also help.

#### *13.4.2 Morphoea (Localised Scleroderma)*

This form of scleroderma usually occurs in otherwise fit people, although it is occasionally seen in systemic sclerosis. Its only effects on internal structures are mechanical, e.g. if the chest wall is involved with large plaques, they will interfere with respiration.

**Optimum Treatment**

Lathyrogenic agents like penicillamine have been used to 'dissolve' the collagen,[245] but are only to be recommended in severe cases, as they are likely to cause collagen breakdown in vital organs as well as in the skin. Autoimmune disorders, haematological and gastrointestinal disturbances, renal disorders, and cutaneous and systemic allergies have been reported. Application of a strong topical corticosteroid or intralesional triamcinolone injection may help, but the effects are difficult to assess in this disease whose natural history is one of slow regression.

Intralesional injection of triamcinolone acetonide can be done through a needle or with a 'Dermojet' painless injector. The quantity injected will vary according to the size and nature of the lesion, but it is reasonable to start with 0.5ml of a 10 mg/ml suspension and to repeat it in 2 or 3 weeks if necessary. Atrophy of subcutaneous tissue can occur and if there are any signs of this, the injections should be stopped.

## 14. Leg Ulcers

Leg ulcers have many causes, but most result from arterial or arteriolar disease or venous 'stasis'. Often arterial and venous disease occur in the same patient.

### 14.1 Optimum Treatment

**Surgery and Systemic Therapy**

Only rarely is it possible to improve the mechanical state of the blood vessels to any degree, and operations (e.g. stripping of varicose veins) should be undertaken only by experts after due consideration of the 'pros' and 'cons'. The relief most patients with leg ulcers obtain from vascular surgery is negligible. In the case of venous ulcers, venous drainage can be improved by raising the legs at night and when sitting down, by wearing elastic stockings or tights, and by various external 'pumps'. Normal walking should usually be encouraged. Occasionally, in arterial and arteriolar disease, the patients are helped by vasodilators, sympathectomy and lowering of blood viscosity. Obviously, coexisting diabetes mellitus and other contributory disease should be treated, and drugs such as corticosteroids, which impede healing, should not be given (except in some cases of arteritis, when they may be necessary).

Zinc is essential for wound healing, but this does not mean that it will heal leg ulcers, and trials designed to test its efficacy have produced differing results.[246] Zinc deficiency is difficult to assess,[247] but on the present evidence it is reasonable to give oral zinc sulfate 220mg twice daily with or after meals for a few weeks, in those with a low serum zinc concentration.[248]

Systemic antibiotics should not be administered routinely for colonisation of leg ulcers with such organisms as *Pseudomonas aeruginosa*, but when clinical erysipelas or cellulitis occur around the ulcer, systemic antistreptococcal drugs such as penicillin should be given. Pain should be treated with analgesics.

**Topical Therapy**

Possibilities for topical treatment are extremely numerous and only a few are discussed here.

***Cleaning the ulcer:*** this can be done with normal saline solution, hydrogen peroxide or a solution of potassium permanganate. The use of hydrogen peroxide requires caution because of its cytotoxic effects observed in cell culture media.[249] Occasionally, slough has to be removed surgically or by proteolytic enzymes (e.g. *trypsin, collagenase*[250]), *urea* cream, or substances that act by adsorbing exudate, etc. on a large surface (e.g. *dextranomer*).[251-253]

***Topical antibacterials:*** silver nitrate solution, vital dyes (e.g. gentian violet) and clioquinol (iodochlorhydroxyquinoline) are among the preparations used, but antibiotics are probably preferable as long as the general rules for use of topical antibiotics are observed (see section 2.1). *Mupirocin* may also have a role here.[36] In chronic leg ulcers, contact sensitivity to antibiotics and ointment bases is a considerable risk and may delay ulcer healing; it should always be watched for.[201,254]

***Dressings:*** constant changing of dressings is detrimental to healing and unless discharge and/or pain dictate otherwise, the ulcer can be occluded for days or weeks at a time, either with traditional non-stick polyester film dressings or hydrocortisone and silicone cream-impregnated bandages. Firm crepe or elastic bandages should be applied on top to help reduce oedema, to support varicose veins, and to protect the legs from further trauma.

Covering the ulcer with various preparations of porcine skin, which acts as a framework for epithelisation, does not seem as satisfactory as skin grafting and this is successful in some cases.[255,256]

***Oxygen therapy:*** a variety of techniques have been used to provide supplemental oxygen to cutaneous ulcers on the basis that oxygen stimulates phagocytosis, granulation tissue growth and bacteriostasis. Success has been claimed in leg ulcers with hyperbaric oxygen,[257] and with application of dressings saturated in a 20% benzoyl peroxide emulsion.[258]

## 15. Pressure Sores

Many of the principles of treatment of leg ulcers (see section 14) apply to management of pressure sores. They are best prevented by frequent turning and, where possible, ambulation of incontinent, paralysed and immobile patients. If, in spite of this, sores do develop, maximum activity is more than ever necessary. Special 'hammocks' and water beds are available for easier nursing.

## 16. Burns

Burns are the concern of the dermatologist only if they are superficial or of limited extent. Topical corticosteroids such as fluocinolone acetonide cream applied early on may be helpful, especially in sunburn (see section 21.1.1). Exceptionally, a course of systemic corticosteroids may be required, and these should be given as soon as possible after the appearance of the burn. Non-stick polyester film dressings should then be applied. Light pressure dressings seem to prevent subsequent keloid formation. Systemic analgesics can be used as required in more severe cases.

Infection should be treated as it arises and lost fluid, electrolytes and protein should be replaced. Many of the principles of treating leg ulcers (see section 14) apply to management. Surgical intervention may be necessary for grafting, prevention of contractures and dealing with established keloid formation.

## 17. Acrodermatitis Enteropathica

Acrodermatitis enteropathica is a rare disease, but an interesting and an important one to recognise and treat. Affected children 'fail to thrive' and have diarrhoea, alopecia and recurrent blistering with secondary *Candida albicans* infections of the nail folds, mouth and perineum ('acrodermatitis').

#### Optimum Treatment

Previously, treatment with di-iodohydroxyquinoline produced dramatic improvement, although the mechanism of action of this agent was not known and the children were at risk of developing optic atrophy from absorbed drug. It is now known that patients with acrodermatitis enteropathica have a low serum zinc concentration and the condition is completely controlled by *zinc sulfate* 3 mg/kg/ day.[259,260]

## 18. Vitiligo

This abnormality of pigmentation is probably of autoimmune aetiology. It is most unusual for spontaneous recovery to occur and treatment is unsatisfactory.

### 18.1 Optimum Treatment

#### Symptomatic Treatment

Symptomatic treatment of vitiligo consists of:

1) Sunscreen preparations (see section 21.1.2) which prevent burning of the depigmented skin.

2) Cosmetic disguise with covering creams and commercially available paints (e.g. artificial tanning preparations) or with dihydroxyacetone in 50 : 50 water and acetone.

The concentration of dihydroxyacetone used determines the resultant skin colour and so it should be adjusted to suit the patient. Starting concentrations should be 1 to 2%.[261]

#### Attempts to Produce Repigmentation

These are usually not satisfactory, which is not surprising considering the fact that melanocytes are destroyed, but photochemotherapy has been used. *Trioxsalen* (trimethylpsoralen) is the synthetic psoralen most used for photosensitising the skin in vitiligo. In sunny parts of the world, it can be used with natural sunlight, but in Western Europe and in many parts of the US, this is unsatisfactory. The oral dose of psoralen must be followed in 2 hours by exposure to long-wave ultraviolet light (UVA) from an artificial source. Management of the patient and precautions to be taken are similar to those of patients with psoriasis treated with PUVA therapy (see section 6.1.2). Trioxsalen is used in a dosage of 40mg orally and the treatment is given 2 or 3 times a week for about a year.[158,262] A minority of patients show significant repigmentation in this time. Alternatively, trioxsalen can be used as a paint, the application being followed 2 hours later by exposure to UVA.

#### Attempts to Counteract Autoimmune Reaction

This is a possible mechanism for the action of topical corticosteroids, especially 0.05% clobetasol propionate which has been used in vitiligo and has been claimed to produce partial repigmentation, but only when used in amounts that also produced dermal atrophy.[263]

#### Attempts to Produce Depigmentation of Remaining Normal Skin

Permanent depigmentation can be produced by monobenzone (monobenzylether of hydroquinone).[264] This is only to be recommended in extensive vitiligo, or that which because of its site is particularly cosmetically disabling. A 20% paint is used twice daily and depigmentation usually takes from 3 to 12 months. Allergic contact dermatitis is a possible complication.

## 19. Alopecia

There are many causes of hair loss, which may be diffuse or patchy, scarring and non-scarring. The treatment of drug-induced alopecia, scalp ringworm, and the scarring alopecia of discoid lupus erythematosus are discussed elsewhere (sections 22.2.3, 13.4.1). Other aspects are discussed below.

### 19.1 Alopecia Areata

This condition is related to the autoimmune group of diseases and as might be expected, corticosteroids influence regrowth of hair. Except in large doses, however, systemic corticosteroid therapy does not alter the natural history of the disease and so the hair falls out again when the corticosteroid is stopped, and this continues until spontaneous remission occurs.[265] Thus, systemic corticosteroids can only rarely be justified in this disease.

#### Optimum Treatment

Intralesional triamcinolone injection can be used (see section 13.4.2) and corticosteroid creams can be tried. The immunopotentiating agent dinitrochlorobenzene, as a topical solution or ointment, and diphenylcyclopropenone have been used with success claimed in persistent refractory cases.[266-268]

*Minoxidil* is a vasodilator which produces hypertrichosis as a side effect, and for this reason it has been tried topically for treating alopecia. However, in most cases, the hair growth is not cosmetically useful.[269] There is some evidence that the response is dose-related, but caution needs to be exercised because of possible toxic effects from absorption (for reviews, see Clissold & Heel;[270] and Tsai et al.[271]).

### 19.2 Male Pattern Alopecia

This requires the presence of circulating androgens as well as genetic factors for its production. The distribution of the hair loss with frontal recession and balding on the vertex is well known and these areas of scalp are most androgen-sensitive.

#### Optimum Treatment

The success of hair transplants in this condition depends upon the fact that hair transplanted from the back (androgen-insensitive) area to the bald area retains its properties at its new site and thus survives.

*Minoxidil* has produced slightly more impressive results in this condition, approximately one-third of patients achieving a cosmetically acceptable result within 1 year with topical treatment applied twice daily (Clissold & Heel;[270] De Villez;[272] Olsen et al.[273]). Unfortunately, the best responses appear to have been in the milder cases who are least in need of treatment.

### 19.3 Chronic Diffuse Alopecia

This type of alopecia is most troublesome in women and often has a hereditary basis so that results of treatment are extremely poor. It is important not to miss the relatively rare treatable causes of the condition, namely hypothyroidism and hypoferraemia. These should be treated by appropriate replacements. Topical minoxidil has proved significantly more effective than placebo in the treatment of female androgenetic alopecia.[274]

### 19.4 Telogen Effluvium

The synchronous precipitation of hair into the resting (telogen) phase and its subsequent shedding is a not uncommon occurrence following serious illness or parturition. The prognosis is excellent and no treatment is required.[275]

## 20. Skin Tumours and Naevi

Tumours both benign and malignant can arise from all anatomical components of skin including blood vessels, nerves, connective tissue, pigment cells and epidermis. Often, histological examination is necessary for diagnosis. Thus, excision biopsy is the treatment of choice for the majority of solitary small tumours. Multiple benign tumours like skin tags and seborrhoeic warts (basal cell papillomata) can be removed by curettage or destroyed by heat, cold, acid or alkali.

### 20.1 Malignant and Premalignant Tumours

Exposure to actinic radiation over the years is a common predisposing cause as in 'sailor's skin' and 'farmer's skin'. Those occupationally exposed to the sun should be encouraged to wear protective clothing or to use an effective sunscreen. Exposure to x-rays, contact with mineral oils, inorganic arsenic ingestion and hereditary factors are important in other cases. It is not uncommon for malignant epidermal tumours to be multiple and for premalignant tumours such as solar or senile keratoses to coexist.

#### Optimum Treatment

Excision, radiotherapy and local destruction, e.g. by deep curettage and cautery, all have a role in treatment of malignant and premalignant tumours, but where they are multiple, chemotherapy is especially useful. *Fluorouracil* cream (5%) is a commonly used preparation and is worth a trial in solar and senile keratoses, intraepidermal carcinomas and superficial basal cell carcinomas.[276,277] It should not be used for squamous cell carcinomas as these metastasise rapidly and require urgent treatment of a more radical nature. Most basal cell carcinomas will not respond to chemotherapy either. Fluorouracil cream is irritant and patients should be told that inflammation may follow its use, although this is rarely severe enough to warrant stopping treatment.

Most important in management of malignant melanoma and in improving prognosis are early diagnosis and adequate excision. Current recommendations for surgical excision are resection margins ranging from about 1 to 3cm. Excisions should extend into subcutaneous fat with primary closure considered most desirable.[278] Other measures such as radiotherapy, chemotherapy and immunotherapy are for advanced disease and are to some degree experimental. In ideal practice, they should never be needed.

### 20.2 Vascular Naevi

These constitute a considerable cosmetic problem whether they are of the 'strawberry' cavernous type or the 'port wine' capillary type.

#### Optimum Treatment

The 'strawberry' naevus, although unsightly in infants, is likely to disappear within the first decade of life. The end result is best when the lesion is left to regress spontaneously, but in certain situations (e.g. near the eye) active treatment with systemic corticosteroids, x-rays or plastic surgery may be necessary.

The 'port wine' naevus does not as a rule regress, and may increase in size with time. Usually, surgical removal is not practical, and radiotherapy is ineffective. Treatment with lasers is time consuming and can produce scarring if used injudiciously, but it remains the treatment of choice. In recent years, 13 major lasers (at 15 different wavelengths) have been used. Argon (continuous), KTP (pseudocontinuous), krypton (continuous), and argon-pumped tunable dye (continuous) are in use for thick 'port wine' stains in adults. Flashlamp-pumped dye (long-pulsed) is used for flat 'port wine' stains and those in children.[279] Fortunately, the lesion is, as a rule, flat, and special opaque cosmetics give satisfactory disguise, although they take time to apply properly: professional instructions in their use enhance acceptability. Over-tattooing with flesh-coloured pigments is a possible alternative.

### 20.3 Cutaneous T-Cell Lymphoma (CTCL)

Cutaneous T-cell lymphoma (CTCL) is a neoplasm of helper T cells. The disease is initially confined to the skin, but may progress to involve lymph nodes, peripheral blood and visceral organs.

#### Optimum Treatment

Treatments for CTCL include topical corticosteroids for limited patch-stage disease, chlormethine (mechlorethamine; nitrogen mustard) and carmustine (BCNU) for patch-stage and superficial- to intermediate-depth plaque-stage disease. UVB radiation can provide good responses in patients with patch-stage disease, and PUVA (see section 6.1.2) is useful in patch- and early plaque-stage disease. Total skin electron beam is particularly valuable for patients with extensive, deeply infiltrated plaques and tumours, whereas conventional orthovoltage x-ray or other ionising radiation is effective in eradicating individual tumour lesions.

Erythrodermic CTCL is treated with low-dose methotrexate, interferon, extracorporeal photopheresis, and single or combined chemotherapeutic agents. Treatments for systemic disease include interferon, chemotherapy, and combined modalities. Several adenosine analogues and retinoids have shown activity but their optimal use remains uncertain. Promising preliminary results have also been seen with interleukin-2 fusion toxins and several antibody conjugates.[280,281]

## 21. Dermatological Conditions Arising from Adverse Effects of Sunlight

Sunlight has both acute and chronic effects on the skin. The acute ones are burning, the development of new rashes and the exacerbation of existing rashes; the chronic ones are hyperpigmentation, collagen degeneration and neoplasia. The precise wavelength involved is not always known but, except in industrial processes involving UVC (200 to 290nm), UVB (290 to 320nm) and/or UVA (320 to 400nm) and, exceptionally, even visible light are to blame. The wavelength responsible for some diseases is specific and can have important diagnostic and therapeutic consequences, e.g. radiation of wavelength 400nm produces the rash of porphyria and is transmitted through window glass, while light of shorter wavelength responsible for some other rashes is filtered off by window glass.

### 21.1 Acute Conditions

#### *21.1.1 Sunburn*

When sunburn results from natural sunlight it is due to UVB, but high intensity UVA light as part of PUVA treatment (see section 6.1.2) can produce a clinically similar (but pharmacologically different) response. Those with a relative or complete lack of protective melanin are particularly liable to sunburn and this includes fair skinned races, albinos and those with vitiligo. Those taking photosensitising drugs (table X) are also susceptible to sunburn.

#### Optimum Treatment

Sunburn is most unpleasant. Prevention is far preferable to treatment and susceptible individuals should be particularly careful. It is most unwise to expose the skin to bright sunlight for long periods of time until a protective tan has developed, and some people never do tan. A number of sunscreen preparations (see section 21.1.2) are available which do give some protection and aid tanning, but they do not prevent burning completely in the susceptible. It is not safe for normal people to take antimalarials such as chloroquine, or psoralens (to produce a tan) merely to prevent sunburn.

The principles of treatment of sunburn are discussed in section 16.

#### *21.1.2 Photodermatoses*

Rashes precipitated or made worse by the sun (photodermatoses) are summarised in table IX.[282,283]

#### Optimum Treatment

Management involves protection of the skin from radiation, identification and treatment of specific photodermatoses and, in some conditions, use of systemic agents.

1) *Treat the specific disease,* e.g. porphyria cutanea tarda with venesection; photosensitive drug eruptions by stopping the drug.

2) *Protect skin from radiation* with clothing and sunscreen preparations.[284,285] Sunscreens can be divided into those that protect by physical and those that protect by chemical means. Physical sunscreens like zinc oxide, titanium dioxide and red veterinary petrolatum are effective but are often cosmetically unacceptable.

Chemical agents are divided into UVA and UVB absorbers. *p*-Aminobenzoic acid (PABA) and its derivatives, cinnamates, and salicylates are effective only in the ultraviolet light wavelength range 280 to 320nm. The major types of UVA-absorbing sunscreens are the benzophenones, anthranilates, and dibenzoylmethanes. Padimate-O, a PABA ester, and oxybenzone are the most widely used UVB and UVA-absorbing agents, respectively. Parsol 1789 (avobenzone), a dibenzoylmethane, is the most recent agent to become available and has been found to be effective throughout the UVA spectrum.[286] The effectiveness of a sunscreen preparation is indicated by its sun protective factor, usually 4 to 30. For example, a sun protective factor of 8 means that burning will take about 8 times as long to occur as when the skin is left unprotected.

3) *Use of systemic drugs:* β-carotene has been used in a number of photodermatoses but it is probably effective only in erythropoietic protoporphyria.[287] To be effective, it has to be used in doses that produce yellow discolouration of the skin. In an adult, a reasonable starting dose would be 100mg daily.

*Antimalarial drugs* are occasionally used as in lupus erythematosus (see section 13.1), but are contraindicated in porphyria.

*Indomethacin* is an inhibitor of prostaglandin synthetase and in certain experimental situations is effective against UVB in preventing erythema. However, its clinical usefulness has not been proven. *Antihistamines* are effective in some cases of solar urticaria.[288] Photochemotherapy with PUVA, starting with a small dose and building up, will produce 'tolerance' and prevent subsequent photosensitivity in some patients.

#### Use of Tretinoin in Photodamaged Skin

In several well controlled clinical trials, 0.01% or 0.05% tretinoin cream has been shown to be effective in reversing epidermal atrophy and clinically diminishing fine wrinkling, mottled hyperpigmentation and skin roughness. Tretinoin cream may not offer a solution to gross solar damage, but it may be useful as combination therapy with fluorouracil in the treatment and eradication of premalignant skin growths such as actinic keratoses.[289]

### 21.2 Chronic Conditions

Chronic effects of sunlight include hyperpigmentation, especially chloasma and poikiloderma of Civatte, collagen degeneration (e.g. 'solar elastosis') and, importantly, malignant and premalignant changes. Solar keratoses, squamous cell carcinomas, basal cell carcinomas and possibly malignant melanomas are most common in light-exposed skin. Patients with xeroderma pigmentosum, who have a genetic defect of DNA repair after ultraviolet light damage, are particularly liable to develop these skin cancers.

It is not known precisely what wavelengths are responsible for all the skin effects of chronic ultraviolet light exposure in man, but susceptible individuals should be advised to use sunscreens which absorb over a wide range of the spectrum.

**Table IX.** Rashes precipitated or aggravated by exposure to sunlight

| |
|---|
| **Rashes precipitated by sunlight:** |
| Lupus erythematosus (see section 13.1) |
| Porphyria cutanea tarda (PCT) and erythropoietic protoporphyria (EPP) |
| Solar urticaria |
| Photosensitive drug eruptions (see section 22.3.11) |
| Pellagra |
| Polymorphic light eruption |
| Some herpes simplex virus infections |
| **Rashes aggravated by sunlight:** |
| Eczema – especially atopic and seborrhoeic; 'actinic reticuloid' |
| Rosacea |
| Dermatomyositis |
| Psoriasis (occasionally) |

## 22. Drug-Induced Skin Disease

The adverse effects of drugs on the skin are legion (see Felix et al.),[290] and the changes they produce are not always explicable on the basis of known pathological mechanisms: certainly, only a minority are strictly immunological reactions. Proof that a given drug is responsible is often extremely difficult to obtain, although in the majority of cases with careful history and examination and – where indicated – rechallenge, it is possible to make a clinical diagnosis with some degree of confidence.

Some of the more common dermatological reactions to drugs and those agents that have most often been implicated are summarised in table X.

## 22.1 Diagnosis

Some of the difficulties that arise in the diagnosis of drug-induced rashes, and particularly in allocating the blame to a given drug, are as follows:

1) The rashes are rarely specific, so that a given drug is capable of producing different skin effects in different patients, and even in the same patient in different situations. The reverse is also true, since drugs of different chemical structures and pharmacological actions are capable of producing the same rash.

2) Direct proof that a given drug is responsible for a given rash is often difficult to obtain. Few patients are given one drug at a time (see chapter 6). Thus, even when it is fairly certain on morphological grounds that the rash is drug-induced, it may be impossible to identify the culprit. Sometimes, the relationship in time of the appearance of the rash to the administration of the drug helps, but often it does not. Some rashes, e.g. those due to penicillin, have even been known to develop after the drug has been stopped. Diagnosis by stopping all drugs and then reintroducing them one by one may be possible, but it is not entirely without its problems and dangers.

Some drugs, such as ampicillin, may produce a rash in a given individual on one occasion but not necessarily on another, e.g. patients with infectious mononucleosis are prone to ampicillin rashes at that time.[291,292] In the case of serious drug reactions, systemic rechallenge may well be dangerous and this also applies to *in vivo* skin testing. *In vivo* skin testing in other situations may be unreliable, and unfortunately, of the many *in vitro* tests that have been tried, none has proved infallible as a simple method of identifying the drug which produced the rash. Nevertheless, in centres where the drug challenge principles defined by Kauppinen and colleagues are followed, such challenge has proved of great value in defining causation.[205] Certainly, even after taking all the known facts into consideration, it may still be impossible to say that the rash was not due to a given drug.

3) Many of the diseases for which drugs are given can themselves produce rashes. For instance, erythema multiforme and erythema nodosum, which are relatively common types of drug reactions, can be produced both by infections and by antibiotics and other drugs used to combat them.

## 22.2 General Effects of Drugs on the Skin

### 22.2.1 Change in Skin Colour

When drugs do affect the skin, they may do so by producing a diffuse or patchy change in skin colour. This may be due to deposition of the drug or its metabolites in the skin, as for instance in the case of amiodarone, silver and mepacrine, or to production of excessive melanin pigmentation as in the 'raindrop' pigmentation of arsenical poisoning. Often, the colour change is due to both accumulation of the drug and increased melanin pigmentation, and this is known to be the case with iron and chlorpromazine.

Other colour changes in the skin are not due to alteration in the skin itself but reflect an alteration in the colour of the blood flowing through it. Such is the case in the various drug-induced jaundices as well as in methaemoglobinaemia and sulfhaemoglobinaemia caused by drugs such as the sulfonamides and sulfones (e.g. dapsone).

### 22.2.2 Skin Cancer and Infections

Drugs like arsenic and tar may predispose to skin cancer and produce precancerous lesions. Other drugs make the skin less resistant to infection with viruses, bacteria or fungi, such as can follow the use of both immunosuppressive and corticosteroid drugs (see further section 2).

### 22.2.3 Effects on the Hair

Heparin, the coumarins, cytotoxic drugs, carbimazole, trimethadione (troxidone), oral contraceptives, retinoids, lithium, thallium and overdosage with vitamin A can all produce diffuse alopecia. With vitamin A intoxication, alopecia is accompanied by excessive dryness of the scalp and hair. In the case of the coumarin anticoagulants, there is shedding of large numbers of club, resting or telogen hairs, while with cytotoxic drugs the hair is arrested in the growing or anagen phase, and then breaks off.[293] Thallium is no longer used in therapeutics but cases of poisoning occasionally occur, and the resulting alopecia seems to be the result of hairs being shed in both anagen and telogen phases.

Two types of alopecia have been described with oral contraceptives – a 'male pattern' alopecia with preparations containing the more androgenic progestagens, and an excessive shedding of telogen hairs after stopping the more estrogenic preparations.[294,295] However, considering the numbers of contraceptive pills consumed at the present time, these adverse effects

**Table X.** Some dermatological reactions to drugs used systemically and topically

| Skin reaction | Examples of implicated drugs (*NB.* see also text. Not a comprehensive list) |
|---|---|
| Urticaria (possibly with accompanying angioneurotic oedema) | Penicillin; aspirin; sulfonamides; barbiturates; morphine; captopril; enalapril |
| Erythematous rash | Barbiturates; aspirin; antibacterial agents |
| Acne or aggravation of existing acne | Corticosteroids; androgenic and anabolic steroids; phenobarbital; phenytoin; oral contraceptives (some); bromides; iodides; cytotoxic drugs; isoniazid; PUVA therapy; lithium; danazol |
| Eczema from systemic drug (exfoliative dermatitis) | Gold; organic arsenic |
| Eczema from contact with drug (contact urticaria) | Topical antimicrobials (penicillin, streptomycin, chloramphenicol, neomycin, sulfonamides); topical local anaesthetics (except amide types); topical antihistamines; cream and lotion preservatives; lanolin |
| Purpura (non-thrombocytopenic or thrombocytopenic) | Corticosteroids; anticoagulants; aspirin; carbromal; meprobamate; barbiturates; thiazides; sulfonamides; sulfonylureas; cytotoxic drugs and other drugs which cause bone marrow suppression or thrombocytopenia |
| Bullous reactions | Barbiturates (coma); phenylbutazone (toxic epidermal necrolysis); penicillamine (pemphigus); nalidixic acid (photosensitivity); furosemide (photosensitivity; high doses in chronic renal failure); rifampicin; captopril; NSAIDs; PUVA |
| Erythema multiforme (Stevens-Johnson syndrome; *NB.* may be bullous) | Penicillin; sulfonamides; barbiturates; NSAIDs; thiazides; phenytoin; allopurinol |
| Lichenoid eruptions | Gold; antimalarials; amiphenazole; *p*-aminosalicylic acid; quinine; labetalol; thiazides |
| Fixed drug eruptions | Phenolphthalein; barbiturates; phenylbutazone; aspirin; sulfonamides; quinine; tetracyclines |
| Photosensitivity from systemic and/or topical administration | Tetracyclines (e.g. demeclocycline); phenothiazines (including some antihistamines); griseofulvin; nalidixic acid; sulfonamides; thiazides; sulphonylureas; furosemide (high doses in chronic renal failure); psoralens; oral contraceptives (rarely); NSAIDs; topically applied sulfonamides; halogenated salicylanilide antiseptics (e.g. soaps) |
| Systemic lupus erythematosus-like reaction | Hydralazine; procainamide; phenytoin; isoniazid |
| Discolouration[a] (except due to drug-induced jaundice, methaemoglobinaemia) | *Brown:* ACTH; oral contraceptives (chloasma); hydroxycarbamide (hydroxyurea); iron; silver; arsenic<br>*Purple:* chlorpromazine<br>*Blue:* chloroquine; hydroxychloroquine; amodiaquine; amantadine (elderly Parkinsonian patients)<br>*Yellow:* β-carotene; mepacrine (quinacrine) [greenish-bluish-grey discolouration of ears, nose, nail beds on prolonged use]<br>*Grey:* amiodarone |
| Alopecia | Anticoagulants; cytotoxic drugs; carbimazole; trimethadione; ethionamide; oral contraceptives; vitamin A (overdosage); retinoids, lithium, thallium (not now used in therapeutics) |

a May be due to increased melanin deposition or to presence of drug or its metabolites in the skin. Sometimes drug and melanin are deposited together (e.g. haemosiderosis).

*Abbreviations:* ACTH = adrenocorticotrophic hormone; NSAID = nonsteroidal anti-inflammatory drug; PUVA = psoralen and long-wave ultraviolet light.

are seen in only a very small proportion of the population at risk.

The prognosis in drug-induced alopecias is excellent if the drug can be stopped, and patients should be persuaded not to patronise expensive 'hair clinics' which have little to offer that time will not also provide. A wig may be necessary during the acute episode. For a review, see Reeves & Maibach.[275]

Drugs that can cause hypertrichosis include minoxidil,[296] oral diazoxide,[297] cyclosporin, phenytoin, streptomycin, penicillamine, danazol, systemic corticosteroids, and occasionally topical corticosteroids, usually after prolonged use.

#### *22.2.4 Rashes*

The greatest diagnostic difficulties arise with actual rashes induced by drugs. Here, an opinion from a dermatologist is worthwhile. As discussed in section 22.1, the dermatologist's task may well be impossible and he/she can perhaps do no more than make an intelligent guess at the offending drug. This 'informed guess' may be no better than that of non-dermatological colleagues. A dermatologist can, however, describe the reaction in precise dermatological terms and allocate it to one of the clinical types (see section 22.3), which may be useful for future reference. The dermatologist is also usually the best person to advise on the management of the reaction which, in severe cases, may be so serious that the correct treatment for the skin can make all the difference between life and death.

Drug challenge may be used as a method for detecting the causative agent (e.g. with severe erythroderma, toxic epidermal necrolysis). It should be performed in controlled circumstances and preferably in hospitalised patients.[205]

## 22.3 Clinical Types of Skin Reactions

Individual lesions may be urticarial, erythematous, acneform, eczematous, purpuric, bullous and lichenoid. Clinically recognisable patterns include erythema multiforme, erythema nodosum, the 'fixed' eruption, and rashes which involve predominantly the light-exposed areas of the skin. Rarely, drugs may 'induce' lupus erythematosus or porphyria and then the rashes characteristic of these diseases may appear. In psoriatic individuals, any rash, including one produced by a drug, may take on psoriatic features.

### 22.3.1 Urticaria

Many drugs can produce urticaria and this is one of the most common skin reactions produced by drugs. Such reactions are potentially dangerous since there may be accompanying swelling of the mouth and larynx from angioedema, as well as bronchospasm and hypotension. Some urticarias are produced by an allergic mechanism. Apart from the various antisera which may be responsible, penicillin and aspirin are two of the most common drug causes. In such patients, death may follow injection of as little as a few molecules in the course of skin testing, so these tests should never be carried out unless full resuscitative measures, including intravenous hydrocortisone succinate, are available. Urticaria can also be produced by drugs which act as histamine liberators, for example, aspirin and morphine. Thus aspirin is one of the drugs that can cause urticaria by allergic or non-allergic mechanisms. Furthermore, patients with non-allergic aspirin-induced urticaria may also develop similar eruptions with other nonsteroidal anti-inflammatory drugs.[298]

### 22.3.2 Erythema

Erythematous rashes of various patterns are another common form of drug rash. Barbiturates, aspirin and antibiotics are common culprits. In general, the rashes, although uncomfortable, are not dangerous and some disappear even with continued use of the drug responsible.

### 22.3.3 Acne

Corticosteroids, cytotoxic drugs and androgens produce acne, as do isoniazid, iodides and bromides when given over relatively long periods of time. Phenobarbital and phenytoin appear to aggravate existing acne. Some progestagens (e.g. certain oral contraceptive formulations) may also make acne worse.

### 22.3.4 Dermatitis (Eczema)

Eczematous reactions to drugs are most often produced by contact with the drug by topical application, or by handling of the drug. Medications most likely to produce contact sensitivity are topical antibiotics, especially penicillin, streptomycin, chloramphenicol and neomycin; sulfonamides; local anaesthetics (except amide types such as lidocaine); and antihistamines. Preservatives in creams and lotions (e.g. parabens, chlorocresol;[299] diazolidinyl urea;[300] isothiazolinones;[301,302]) or their stabilisers (e.g. ethylenediamine hydrochloride)[33] may occasionally cause contact sensitivity. Among drugs handled by nurses, streptomycin and chlorpromazine have produced much trouble from contact sensitivity in the past, but now that the problem is recognised and efforts are made to prevent contact with the nurse's skin, such undesirable effects of these drugs should be almost completely preventable.

Contact dermatitis is one of the few adverse reactions of the skin to drugs in which it is relatively easy to make a firm diagnosis as a result of challenge with the suspected drug – in this case by patch testing with a small amount of the suspected substance. (The exact amount and concentration suitable for patch testing, and the form and base in which it should be applied, is known for most substances as a result of previous trial and error, and this information is available in standard textbooks dealing with the subject.) An eczematous reaction present at 48 to 96 hours after applying the substance under an occlusive dressing indicates a 'delayed' type of hypersensitivity reaction to that substance.[303] Eczematous reactions to drugs are not all due to 'delayed' hypersensitivity, however, and some are due to nonspecific irritation by the substance. Formalin, for example, can produce a nonspecific irritant dermatitis as well as allergic contact sensitivity. Patch testing is not designed to diagnose these nonspecific reactions. Furthermore, numerous agents have been reported to cause immediate contact reactions, e.g. topical antimicrobials, local anaesthetics, and topical antihistamines.[223]

Allergic contact dermatitis is less often produced by drugs given systemically. Occasionally, there is 'lighting up' of a patch of contact dermatitis when the allergen or a related substance is given systemically. This may occur, for instance, in a dermatitis due to contact with nickel when at a later date, a blood transfusion is given through a needle which contains nickel. Other eczematous reactions to systemic medication also occur, and an extreme example of this is the exfoliative dermatitis which sometimes follows injections of gold. These reactions can be extremely serious and can result in death.

#### 22.3.5 Vasculitis and Purpura

Drug-induced purpura can arise from a number of different mechanisms, e.g. by depression of platelet formation in the bone marrow as with the cytotoxic drugs or chloramphenicol, or by destruction of formed platelets by an allergic mechanism. In either case, there will be thrombocytopenia. In cases where the platelet count is normal, the drug may interfere with other aspects of the clotting mechanism, or there may be damage to the blood vessel walls or their supporting ground substance. Aspirin is an example of a drug which causes purpura partly by interfering with prothrombin formation.

Numerous drugs can produce vasculitis, and purpura resembling that of Henoch-Schönlein disease will result if small blood vessels are affected. The capillaries of the skin are often affected in drug reactions and the purpuras which then result are associated with a decreased capillary resistance, as shown by a positive Hess' test. One of the most easily recognisable drug eruptions was that produced by carbromal. The rash consisted of fine purpura ('cayenne pepper') and scaling and was usually most marked on the lower legs. Histologically, eczema and capillaritis were present. Meprobamate and barbiturates occasionally produce an identical rash. Corticosteroids, by virtue of a deleterious action on the collagen of the ground substance which supports the capillaries, can produce purpura, which clinically resembles senile purpura.[304] Corticosteroids have this effect whether they are used topically or systemically.

#### 22.3.6 Bullous Reactions

Blisters are not uncommonly seen in unconscious patients. The impression that such blisters are particularly common when the unconsciousness is due to a barbiturate is probably false, as blisters are seen in patients unconscious from other causes. The 'scalded skin' syndrome or toxic epidermal necrolysis (Lyell's disease) is characterised by extensive superficial blistering of the skin.[305,306] The disease is extremely serious, as a number of affected patients, especially adults, die. In adults, most of the cases are due to drugs, and phenylbutazone is one of those most commonly responsible. A similar clinical picture can occur in children, in whom it is more likely to be due to a staphylococcal infection that is eminently treatable by large doses of an appropriate antibiotic such as flucloxacillin. Blisters also occur in the course of eczematous and urticarial drug reactions and of erythema multiforme, in 'fixed' drug reactions and in rashes induced by sunlight. Some drugs, e.g. griseofulvin, can produce blisters by precipitating porphyria in those with latent disease.[307]

Pemphigus has been associated with a variety of drugs.[308] Penicillamine is the most common drug implicated in causing pemphigus,[309] which can present with both oral and cutaneous lesions.[310] Rifampicin and captopril may also produce pemphigus-like eruptions.[311,312] Large doses of furosemide (frusemide) in patients with chronic renal failure can produce blisters in areas exposed to sunlight.[313,314]

#### 22.3.7 Lichenoid Eruptions

Rashes indistinguishable from lichen planus may be induced by drugs, e.g. gold, antimalarials, labetalol, and amiphenazole.

#### 22.3.8 Erythema Multiforme

The characteristic lesions consist of concentric circles of erythema and are 'target'- or 'iris'-like. They are usually most numerous on the hands and feet. Occasionally, blisters and purpura are seen. In the severe variant, the Stevens-Johnson syndrome, there is in addition pyrexia and lesions of the eyes, mouth and genitalia. The disease may be precipitated by an infection or by drugs, and it may be difficult to decide whether to blame the infection or the drug given for the infection. The disease may be extremely serious and patients may die from renal involvement. Treatment is discussed in sections 12.4 and 22.4.2.

#### 22.3.9 Erythema Nodosum

This may be drug-induced, but streptococcal infection, sarcoidosis and tuberculosis, as well as less common causes like ulcerative colitis, should be excluded.

#### 22.3.10 'Fixed' Drug Eruption

This is a localised skin lesion in which there are plaques, usually of a dusky colour, which reappear in exactly the same site each time a drug is given systemically, i.e. the site is fixed. The plaques occasionally blister and afterwards leave areas of hyperpigmentation. The drug most often involved is probably phenolphthalein which the patient has taken as a constituent of one of a number of proprietary purgatives. Many other drugs have been implicated (e.g. barbiturates, phenylbutazone, salicylates, sulfonamides and derivatives).[315]

#### 22.3.11 Rashes on Light-Exposed Areas

Photosensitivity may be induced by a drug applied to the skin or by a drug given systemically.[316,317] The drug-induced photosensitivities are usually eczematous. In some, there is evidence of an immunological reaction but in others there is not. Many of the drug-induced photosensitivities are caused by ultraviolet light of longer wave length, i.e. about 350nm. In some cases, the wave length which does the damage corresponds to the maximum absorption spectrum of the drug. Drugs which induce lupus erythematosus (e.g. hydralazine, procainamide) or porphyria (e.g. griseofulvin) will also lead to photosensitivity in those so predisposed.

Topically applied drugs which produce UV light sensitivity reactions include antihistamines, sulfonamides and the halogenated salicylanilide antiseptics. Systemically administered drugs which produce photosensitivity include the tetracyclines, especially demeclocycline (demethylchlortetracycline) and doxycycline, the phenothiazines, some antihistamines and psoralens, nalidixic acid, furosemide (high doses in chronic renal failure), sulfonamides and their derivatives (e.g. oral sulphonylureas, thiazides), and some nonsteroidal anti-inflammatory drugs. Oral contraceptives may occasionally cause photosensitivity.[318]

#### 22.3.12 Adverse Local Effects of Topical Corticosteroids

The adverse effects on the skin of topically applied corticosteroids are summarised in table VIII (for a review, see Lauerma & Maibach).[319]

### 22.4 Management of Rashes Induced by Drugs

#### 22.4.1 Diagnosis by Challenge

The difficulty of precise diagnosis in a large number of cases has been discussed above. In general, it is not only the bedside diagnosis that is difficult, for laboratory tests as well as intradermal and patch tests (except in cases of contact dermatitis) on the patient at a later date rarely help. The decision whether or not to challenge the patient with a drug that is suspected of causing the reaction is sometimes difficult, and must ultimately depend upon the individual case.

If the initial drug reaction has been serious, e.g. a severe exfoliative dermatitis or a toxic epidermal necrolysis, it would be extremely unwise to give even a small dose of the suspected drug again. The usual advice is not to give the patient the implicated drug on any future occasion. Occasionally, however, it might be vital to know which of several possible drugs has caused a reaction so that it becomes necessary to challenge the patient, e.g. in a patient who had reacted to a combination of drugs he or she was taking for tuberculosis.

With less serious reactions, challenge would almost certainly be a completely safe procedure. In all cases in which challenge is made, its limitations must of course be borne in mind. If a patient does not respond to the challenge, it does not rule out the possibility that the initial reaction was caused by the drug.[205]

#### 22.4.2 Optimum Treatment

The most important part of treatment is usually to stop the drug suspected of causing the rash. In the case of severe reactions, however, other measures may be required. Urgent treatment will of course be needed in severe urticarial reactions accompanied by collapse or difficulty in breathing. Intravenous hydrocortisone succinate should be given together with adrenaline (epinephrine), and measures should be taken to ensure that an airway is maintained, if necessary by tracheotomy (see section 10.1). Simple urticarial drug reactions, whether they are allergic or not, will nearly always be suppressed by adequate doses of a systemic antihistamine.

Cases of toxic epidermal necrolysis as well as severe cases of exfoliative dermatitis, Stevens-Johnson syndrome and 'allergic vasculitis' due to drugs may require systemic corticosteroids; unfortunately, prospective placebo-controlled studies are not available. Other treatment is symptomatic. If the rash is inflammatory and itches, a corticosteroid cream can be applied and an antihistamine given by mouth. When it is essential for a drug to be continued, even though it is known to be responsible for a rash, it may be possible to suppress the reaction by giving systemic corticosteroids at the same time. Remember that the skin is not necessarily the only organ which is reacting adversely and it is important not to assume that because the rash has disappeared, more important organs such as the kidneys, eyes, liver or bone marrow are necessarily free from the adverse effects. If these are left unheeded, the patient may die from toxic effects of the drug. On the other hand, in some cases, the appearance of a rash in a patient taking a drug may be important in drawing attention to impaired renal function and the need to modify the dosage of the drug.

## Further Reading

Rook A, Wilkinson DS, Ebling FJG, et al. Textbook of dermatology. 5th edition. Oxford: Blackwell Scientific, 1993

## References

1. Whyte HJ, Baughman RD. Acute guttate psoriasis and streptococcal infection. Archives of Dermatology 1964; 89: 350
2. Shuster S, Marks J, editors. Systemic effects of skin disease. London: Heinemann, 1970
3. Bronaugh RL, Maibach HI, editors. Percutaneous absorption: mechanisms-methodology-drug delivery. 2nd ed. New York: Marcel Dekker Inc., 1989
4. Bronaugh RL, Maibach HI, editors. In vitro percutaneous absorption: principles fundamentals and application. Boston: CRC Press, 1991
5. Vickers CFH. Existence of reservoirs in the stratum corneum. Archives of Dermatology 1963; 59: 10
6. Scheuplein RJ. Percutaneous absorption after twenty-five years: or 'old wine in new wineskins'. Journal of Investigational Dermatology 1976; 69: 31
7. Scott R. In vitro absorption through damaged skin. In: Bronaugh RL, Maibach HI, editors. In vitro percutaneous absorption: principles, fundamentals and application. Boston: CRC Press, 1991
8. Wester RC, Maibach HI. Individual and regional variation with in vitro percutaneous absorption. In vitro percutaneous absorption: principles, fundamentals and applications (chapter 4). Boston: CRC Press, 1991: 25.
9. Wester RC, Maibach HI. Relationship of topical dose and percutaneous absorption in Rhesus monkey and man. Journal of Investigational Dermatology 1976; 67: 518
10. MacCallum FO, Juel-Jensen BE. Herpes simplex virus skin infections in man treated with idoxuridine in dimethyl sulphoxide. British Medical Journal 1966; 2: 805
11. Smith E, Maibach HI, editors. Percutaneous penetration enhancers. Boca Ratan: CRC Press, 1995
12. Poulson BJ, Young E, Coquilla V, et al. Effect of topical vehicle composition on the *in vitro* release of fluocinolone acetonide and its acetate ester. Journal of Pharmaceutical Science 1968; 57: 928
13. Stoughton RB. Bioassay system for formulations of topically applied glucocorticosteroids. Archives of Dermatology 1972; 106: 825
14. Coldman MF, Lockerbie L, Laws EA. The evaluation of several topical corticosteroid preparations in the blanching test. British Journal of Dermatology 1971; 85: 381
15. Munro DD, Robinson TWE, duVivier AWP, et al. Betamethasone valerate ointment compared with fluocinonide FAPG: use in the treatment of psoriasis and eczema. Archives of Dermatology 1977; 113: 599
16. Stoughton RB. Corticosteroids in psoriasis. In: Farber & Cox, editors. Psoriasis: Proceedings of the International Symposium. Stanford: Stanford University Press, 1971
17. Comaish JS, Smith J, Seville RH. Factors affecting the clearance of psoriasis with dithranol (anthralin). British Journal of Dermatology 1971; 84: 282
18. Craig FN, Cummings EG, Sim VM. Environmental temperature and the absorption of a cholinesterase inhibitor, XV. Journal of Investigational Dermatology 1977; 68: 357
19. Guy RH, Maibach HI. Calculations of body exposure from percutaneous absorption data. In: Bronaugh RL, Maibach HI, editors. Percutaneous absorption: mechanisms-methodology-drug delivery. 2nd ed. New York: Marcel Dekker, 1989: 391
20. Maibach HI, Bouits E, editors. Neonatal skin: structure and function. New York: Marcel Dekker, 1982: 279
21. Roskos KV, Guy RH, Maibach HI. Percutaneous absorption in the aged. Dermatology Clinics 1986; 4: 455
22. Chilcote R, Curley A, Loughlin HH, et al. Hexachlorophene storage in a burn patient associated with encephalopathy. Pediatrics 1977; 59: 457
23. Moon KC, Maibach HI. Percutaneous absorption in diseased skin: relationship to the exogenous dermatoses. In: Menne T, Maibach HI, editors. Exogenous dermatoses: environmental dermatitis. Boston: CRC Press, 1990: 217
24. Sneddon IB. Clinical use of topical corticosteroids. Drugs 1976; 11: 193
25. Maibach HI, Surber C, editors. Topical corticosteroids. Basel: Karger, 1992
26. Korting HC, Maibach HI, editors. Topical glucocorticoids with increased benefit/risk ratio: current problems in dermatology. 2nd ed. vol. 21. New York: Karger, 1993
27. McCullough JL, Snyder DS, Weinstein GD, et al. Factors affecting human percutaneous penetration of methotrexate and its analogues in *vitro*. Journal of Investigational Dermatology 1976; 66: 103
28. Niedner R, Schopf E. Clinical efficacy of topical glucocorticoid preparations and other types of dermatics in inflammatory diseases, particularly in atopic der-

matitis. In: Burg G, editor. Topical glucocorticoids with increased benefit/risk ratio: current problems in dermatology. New York: Karger, 1993: 157
29. Wilson L. The clinical assessment of topical corticosteroid activity. British Journal of Dermatology 1976; 91 Suppl. 12: 33
30. Hunter JAA. The basis of skin therapy. British Medical Journal 1973; 4: 411
31. Hunter JAA. The structure and function of skin in relation to therapy. British Medical Journal 1973; 4: 340
32. Bandman NH, Calnan CD, Cronin E, et al. Dermatitis from applied medicaments. Archives of Dermatology 1972; 106: 335
33. White MI, Douglas WS, Main RA. Contact dermatitis attributed to ethylenediamine. British Medical Journal 1978; 1: 415
34. Esterly NB, Markowitz M. The treatment of pyoderma in children. Journal of the American Medical Association 1970; 212: 1667
35. Noble WC, Naidoo J. Evolution of antibiotic resistance in *Staphylococcus aureus.* The role of the skin. British Journal of Dermatology 1978; 98: 481
36. Ward A, Campoli-Richards DM. Mupirocin: a review of its antibacterial activity, pharmacokinetic properties and therapeutic use. Drugs 1986; 32: 425
37. Leyden JJ. Review of mupirocin ointment in the treatment of impetigo. Clinical Pediatrics 1992: 549
38. Anthony BF, Perlman LV, Wannamaker LW. Skin infection and acute glomerulonephritis in American Indian children. Pediatrics 1967; 39: 263
39. Bassett DCJ. Streptococcal pyoderma and acute nephritis in Trinidad. British Journal of Dermatology 1971; 86 Suppl. 8: 55
40. Dacre JE, Emmerson AM, Jenner EA. Nasal carriage of gentamicin and methicillin resistant *Staphylococcus aureus* treated with topical pseudomonic acid. Lancet 1983; 2: 1036
41. Leyden JJ. Mupirocin: a new topical antibiotic. Seminars in Dermatology 1987; 6: 48
42. Aly R. The pathogenic staphylococci. Seminars in Dermatology 1990; 9: 292
43. Aly R, Maibach HI. Effect of antimicrobial soap containing chlorhexidene on the microbial flora of skin. Applied Environmental Microbiology 1976; 31: 931
44. Maibach HI, Strauss WG, Shinefield H. Bacterial interference relating to chronic furunculosis in man. British Journal of Dermatology 1969 Suppl. 1: 69
45. Aly R, Shinefield H, editors. Bacterial interference. Boca Ratan: CRC Press, 1982
46. Gart GS, Forstall GJ, Tomecki KJ. Mycobacterial skin disease: approaches to therapy. Seminars in Dermatology 1993; 12: 352
47. Kakakhel KU, Fritsch P. Cutaneous tuberculosis. International Journal of Dermatology 1989; 28: 355
48. Van Scoy RE, Wilkowske CJ. Antituberculous agents. Mayo Clinic Proceedings 1992; 67: 179
49. Marks J, Rawlins MD. Skin diseases. In: Speight TM, editor. Drug treatment. 3rd ed. Auckland: Adis Press, 1987: 446
50. Allenby CF. The treatment of viral warts with glutaraldehyde. British Journal of Clinical Practice 1977; 31: 12
51. Beutner KR, von Krogh G. Current status of podophyllotoxin for the treatment of genital warts. Seminars in Dermatology 1990; 9: 148
52. Chamberlain MJ, Reynolds AL, Yeoman WB. Toxic effect of podophyllin application in pregnancy. British Medical Journal 1972; 3: 391
53. Bunney MH, editor. Viral warts: their biology and treatment. Oxford: Oxford University Press, 1982
54. Stadler R, Ruszczak Z. Interferons: new additions and indications for use. Dermatology Clinics 1993; 11: 187
55. Richards DM, Carmine AA, Brogden RN, et al. Acyclovir: a review of its pharmacodynamic properties and therapeutic efficacy. Drugs 1983; 26: 378
56. O'Brien JJ, Campoli-Richards DM. Acyclovir: an updated review of its antiviral activity, pharmacokinetic properties and therapeutic efficacy. Drugs 1989; 37: 233-309
57. Fiddian AP, Yeo JM, Stubbings R, et al. Successful treatment of herpes labialis with topical acyclovir. British Medical Journal 1983; 286: 1699
58. Van Vloten WA, Swan RNJ, Pot F. Topical acyclovir therapy in patients with recurrent orofacial herpes simplex infections. Journal of Antimicrobial Chemotherapy 1983; 12 Suppl. B: 89
59. Shaw M, King M, Best JM, et al. Failure of acyclovir cream in treatment of recurrent herpes labialis. British Medical Journal 1985; 291: 7
60. Thomas RHM, Dodd HJ, Yeo JM, et al. Oral acyclovir in the suppression of recurrent non-genital herpes simplex virus infection. British Journal of Dermatology 1985; 113: 731
61. Beutner KR. Rational use of acyclovir in the treatment of mucocutaneous herpes simplex virus and varicella zoster virus infections. Seminars in Dermatology 1992; 11: 256
62. Sasadeusz JJ, Sacks SL. Systemic antivirals in herpesvirus infections. Dermatology Clinics 1993; 11: 171
63. Whitley RJ, Gnann JW. Acyclovir: a decade later. New England Journal of Medicine 1992; 327: 782
64. Juel-Jensen BE, MacCallum FO, Mackenzie AMR, et al. Treatment of zoster with idoxuridine in dimethyl sulphoxide. British Medical Journal 1970; 4: 776
65. Llorca MA. Treatment of herpes zoster with topical 5-iodo-2-deoxyuridine: a double-blind controlled study. Current Therapeutic Research 1985; 37: 472
66. Levin MJ, Zaia JA, Hershey BJ, et al. Topical acyclovir treatment of herpes zoster in immunocompromised patients. Journal of the American Academy of Dermatology 1985; 13: 590
67. Bean B, Braun C, Balfour Jr HH. Acyclovir therapy for acute herpes zoster. Lancet 1982; 2: 118
68. Peterslund NA, Seyer-Hansen K, Ipsen J, et al. Acyclovir in herpes zoster. Lancet 1981; 2: 287
69. Huff JC, Bean B, Balfour Jr HH, et al. Therapy of herpes zoster with oral acyclovir. American Journal of Medicine 1988; 85 Suppl. 2A: 84-9
70. McKendrick MW, McGill JI, White JE, et al. Oral acyclovir in acute herpes zoster. British Medical Journal 1986; 293: 1529-32
71. Morton P, Thomson AN. Oral acyclovir in the treatment of herpes zoster in general practice. New Zealand Medical Journal 1989; 102: 93-5
72. Wood MJ, Ogan PH, McKendrick MW, et al. Efficacy or oral acyclovir treatment of acute herpes zoster. American Journal of Medicine 1988; 85 Suppl. 2A: 79-83
73. Crooks RJ, Jones DA, Fiddian AP. Zoster-associated chronic pain: an overview of clinical trials with acyclovir. Scandinavian Journal of Infectious Disease 1991; 78 (Suppl.): 62-8
74. Balfour Jr HH, Bean B, Laskin OL, et al. Acyclovir halts progression of herpes zoster in immunocompromised patients. New England Journal of Medicine 1983; 308: 1448

75. Degreef H, et al. (Famciclovir Herpes Zoster Clinical Study Group). Famciclovir, a new oral antiherpes drug: results of the first controlled clinical study demonstrating its efficacy and safety in the treatment of uncomplicated herpes zoster in immunocompetent patients. International Journal of Antimicrobial Agents 1994; 4: 241-6.
76. Beutner KR, Friedman DJ, Forszpaniak C, et al. Valacyclovir compared with acyclovir for improved therapy for herpes zoster in immunocompetent adults. Antimicrobial Agents and Chemotherapy 1995; 39: 1546-53
77. Eaglstein WH, Katz R, Brown JA. Use of steroids in herpes zoster. Journal of the American Medical Association 1970; 21: 1
78. Keczkes K, Basheer AM. Do corticosteroids prevent post-herpetic neuralgia? British Journal of Dermatology 1980; 102: 551
79. Wood MJ, Johnson RW, McKendrick MW, et al. A randomized trial of acyclovir for 7 days or 21 days with and without prednisolone for treatment of acute herpes zoster. New England Journal of Medicine 1994; 330: 896
80. Jue SG, Dawson GW, Brogden RN. Ciclopirox olamine 1% cream: a preliminary review of its antimicrobial activity and therapeutic use. Drugs 1985; 29: 330
81. Gupta AK, Sauder DN, Shear NH. Antifungal agents: an overview. Part I. Journal of the American Academy of Dermatology 1994; 30: 677
82. Gupta AK, Sauder DN, Shear NH. Antifungal agents: an overview. Part II. Journal of the American Academy of Dermatology 1994; 30: 911
83. Ferguson RM, Sutherland DER, Simmons RL, et al. Ketoconazole, cyclosporin metabolism and renal transplantation. Lancet 1982; 2: 882
84. Grant SM, Clissold SP. Itraconazole: a review of its pharmacodynamic and pharmacokinetic properties, and therapeutic use in superficial and systemic mycoses. Drugs 1989; 37: 310-44
85. Grant SM, Clissold SP. Fluconazole: a review of its pharmacodynamic and pharmacokinetic properties, and therapeutic potential in superficial and systemic mycoses. Drugs 1990; 39: 877-916
86. Vilars V, Jones TC. Present status of the efficacy and tolerability of terbinafine (Lamisil) used systemically in the treatment of dermatomycoses of skin and nails. Journal of Dermatology Treatment 1990; 1: 33-8
87. Lin C, Symchowicz S. Absorption, distribution, metabolism and excretion of griseofulvin in man and animals. Drug Metabolism Reviews 1975; 4: 75
88. Epstein WL, Shah WP, Riegelman S. Griseofulvin levels in stratum corneum: study after oral administration in man. Archives of Dermatology 1972; 106: 344
89. Faergemann J, Maibach HI. Griseofulvin and ketoconazole: a review with special emphasis on dermatology. Seminars in Dermatology 1987; 6: 31
90. Cullen SI, Catalano PM. Griseofulvin-warfarin antagonism. Journal of the American Medical Association 1967; 199: 582
91. Koch-Weser J, Sellers EM. Drug interactions with coumarin anticoagulants. New England Journal of Medicine 1971; 285: 487-547
92. Leyden JJ, Aly R. Tinea pedis. Seminars in Dermatology 1993; 12: 280
93. Monk JP, Brodgen RN. Naftifine: a review of its antimicrobial activity and therapeutic use in superficial dermatomycoses. Drugs 1991; 42: 659-72
94. Balfour JA, Faulds D. Terbinafine: a review of its pharmacodynamic and pharmacokinetic properties, and therapeutic potential in superficial mycoses. Drugs 1992; 43: 259-84
95. Gupta AK, Sauder DN, Shear NH. Antifungal agents: an overview. Part I. Journal of the American Academy of Dermatology 1994; 30: 667-98
96. Chren MM. Costs of therapy for dermatophyte infections. Journal of the American Academy of Dermatology 1994; 31: 103
97. De Doncker P, Decroix J, Pierard GE, et al. Antifungal pulse therapy for onychomycosis. A pharmacokinetic and pharmacodynamic investigation of monthly cycles of 1-week pulse therapy with itraconazole. Archives of Dermatology 1996; 132: 34-41
98. Smith SW, Sealy DP, Schneider E, et al. An evaluation of the safety and efficacy of fluconazole in the treatment of onychomycosis. Southern Medical Journal 1995; 88: 1217-20
99. Faergemann J. Pityriasis versicolor. Seminars in Dermatology 1993; 12: 276
100. Carslaw RW, Dobson RM, Hood AJK, et al. Mites in the environment of cases of Norwegian scabies. British Journal of Dermatology 1975; 92: 333
101. Orkin M, Maibach HI. Scabies therapy - 1993. Seminars in Dermatology 1993; 12: 22
102. Ginsburg CM, Lowry W, Reisch JS. Absorption of lindane (gamma benzene hexachloride) in infants and children. Journal of Pediatrics 1977; 91: 998
103. Solomon LM, Fahmer L, West DP. Gamma benzene hexachloride toxicity. Archives of Dermatology 1977; 113: 353
104. Meinking TL, Taplin D, Kalter DC, et al. Comparative efficacy of treatments for pediculosis capitis infestations. Archives of Dermatology 1986; 122: 267-71
105. Robertson DB, Maibach HI. Dermatologic pharmacology. In: Basic and clinical pharmacology, 5th ed. Katzung BG, 1992.
106. Downing DT, Stewart ME, Wertz PW, et al. Essential fatty acids and acne. Journal of the American Academy of Dermatology 1986; 14: 221
107. Anderson AS, Gaidys GI, Green RC, et al. Improved reduction of cutaneous bacteria and free fatty acids with new benzoyl peroxide gel. Cutis 1975; 16: 307
108. Heel RC, Brogden RN, Speight TM, et al. Vitamin A acid: a review of its pharmacological properties and therapeutic use in the topical treatment of acne vulgaris. Drugs 1977; 14: 401
109. Verschoore M, Bouclier M, Czernielewski, et al. Topical retinoids: their uses in dermatology. Dermatology Clinics 1993; 11: 107
110. Gollnick H. A new therapeutic agent: azaleic acid in acne treatment. Journal of Dermatology Treatment 1990; 1 Suppl. 3: 523
111. Fitton A, Goa KL. Azelaic acid: a review of its pharmacological properties and therapeutic efficacy in acne and hyperpigmentary skin disorders. Drugs 1991; 41: 780-98
112. Cunliffe WJ. Topical erythromycin: clinical and laboratory studies. In: Marks R, editor. Topical antibiotics in acne. London: Martin Dunitz, 1989
113. Gould DJ, Cunliffe WJ. The long-term treatment of acne vulgaris. Clinical and Experimental Dermatology 1978; 3: 249
114. Hall JH, Lupton ES. Tetracycline therapy for acne: incidence of vaginitis. Cutis 1977; 20: 97
115. Bjellerups M, Ljunggren B. Double-blind cross-over studies on photoxicity to three tetracycline deriva-

tives in human volunteers. Photodermatology 1987; 4: 281
116. Baer RL, Leshaw SM, Shalita AR. High dose tetracycline therapy in severe acne. Archives of Dermatology 1976; 112: 479
117. Monaco F, Agnelti V, Mutani R. Benign intercranial hypertension after minocycline therapy. European Neurology 1978; 17: 48
118. Stuan BH, Litt IF. Tetracycline-associated intercranial hypertension in an adolescent: a complication of systemic acne therapy. Journal of Pediatrics 1978; 92: 679
119. Ward A, Brogden RN, Heel RC, et al. Isotretinoin: a review of its pharmacological properties and therapeutic efficacy in acne and other skin disorders. Drugs 1984; 28: 6
120. Cunliffe WJ. Evolution of a strategy for the treatment of acne. Journal of the American Academy of Dermatology 1987; 16: 591
121. Lucek RW, Colburn WA. Clinical pharmacokinetics of the retinoids. Clinical Pharmacokinetics 1985; 10: 38
122. Orfanos CE, Ehlert R, Gollnick H. The retinoids: a review of their clinical pharmacology and therapeutic use. Drugs 1987; 34: 459
123. Sneddon IB. Adverse effect of topical fluorinated corticosteroids in rosacea. British Medical Journal 1969; 1: 671
124. Knight AG, Vickers CFH. A follow-up of tetracycline-treated rosacea with special reference to rosacea keratitis. British Journal of Dermatology 1975; 93: 577
125. Gamborg Nielsen P. Treatment of rosacea with 1% metronidazole cream: a double-blind study. British Journal of Dermatology 1983; 108: 327
126. Pye RJ, Bunon JL. Treatment of rosacea by metronidazole. Lancet 1976; 1: 121
127. Plewig G. Action of isotretinoin in acne, rosacea, and Gram negative folliculitis. Journal of the American Academy of Dermatology 1982; 6: 766
128. Watson W, Cann HM, Farber EM, et al. The genetics of psoriasis. Archives of Dermatology 1972; 105: 197
129. Farber EM, Nall L, editors. Epidemiology: natural history and genetics: Psoriasis. 2nd ed. New York: Marcel Dekker, 1991: 209
130. Tickner A. The biochemistry of psoriasis. British Journal of Dermatology 1961; 73: 87
131. Pittelkow MR, editor. Keratinocyte abnormalities: Psoriasis. 2nd ed. New York: Marcel Dekker, 1991: 305
132. Roenigk Jr HH, Maibach HI. Methotrexate. In: Psoriasis, 2nd ed. New York: Marcel Dekker, 1991: 563.
133. Walter JF, Voorhees JJ, Kelsey WH, et al. Psoralen plus black light inhibits DNA synthesis. Archives of Dermatology 1973; 107: 861
134. Lowe NJ. Psoralen ultraviolet A (PUVA) therapy: systemic psoralens. In: Practical psoriasis therapy. 2nd ed. New York: Mosby - Year Book, 1993: 121
135. Roenigk Jr HH, Maibach HI. In: Psoriasis. 2nd ed. New York: Marcel Dekker, 1991.
136. Ingram IT. Approach to psoriasis. British Medical Journal 1953; 2: 591
137. Seville RH. Dithranol paste for psoriasis. British Journal of Dermatology 1966; 78: 269
138. Schaefer H, Farber E, Goldberg L, et al. Limited application period for dithranol in psoriasis. British Journal of Dermatology 1980; 102: 571
139. Marsden J, Coburn P, Marks J, et al. Response to short term application of dithranol in psoriasis. British Journal of Dermatology 1983; 108: 243
140. Perry HO, Soderstrom CW, Schulze RW. The Goeckerman treatment of psoriasis. Archives of Dermatology 1968; 98: 178
141. Grupper C. The chemistry, pharmacology and use of tar in the treatment of psoriasis. In: Farber & Cox, editors. Psoriasis: proceedings of the International Symposium. Stanford: Stanford University Press, 1971.
142. Hjort N, Norgaard M, editors. Tars. Psoriasis. 2nd ed. New York: Marcel Dekker, 1991: 473
143. Farber EM, Nall L. Psoriasis: a review of recent advances in treatment. Drugs 1984; 28: 324
144. Zachheim HS. Should therapeutic coal-tar preparations be available over-the-counter? Archives of Dermatology 1978; 114: 125
145. Vickers CFH. Dam, reservoir or filter. Transactions of the St Johns Hospital Dermatological Society 1973; 59: 10
146. Scoggins RB, Kliman B. Percutaneous absorption of corticosteroids: systemic effects. New England Journal of Medicine 1965; 273: 831
147. Feiwel M. Percutaneous absorption of topical steroids in children. British Journal of Dermatology 1969; 81 Suppl. 4: 113
148. Keipen JA. Therapeutic implications of percutaneous absorption of topical corticosteroids in infancy and childhood. Medical Journal of Australia 1971; 2: 315
149. Ashton RE, Lowe NJ, editors. Anthralin therapy of psoriasis: practical psoriasis therapy. 2nd ed. St. Louis: Mosby - Year Book, 1993
150. Knudsen EA. Fluocinolone-plastic treatment in severe psoriasis: a comparative study. Acta Dermatologica Venereologica 1965; 45: 50
151. Murdoch D, Clissold SP. Calcipotriol: a review of its pharmacological properties and therapeutic use in psoriasis vulgaris. Drugs 1992; 43: 415-29
152. Menne T, Larsen K. Psoriasis treatment with vitamin D derivatives. Seminars in Dermatology 1992; 11: 278
153. Kragballe K, Iversen L. Calcipotriol: a new topical antipsoriatic. Dermatology Clinics 1993; 11: 137
154. Lahti A, Maibach HI, editors. Systemic corticosteroids: Psoriasis. 2nd ed. New York: Marcel Dekker, 1991
155. Dahl MGC, Gregory MM, Scheuer PJ. Methotrexate hepatotoxicity in psoriasis - comparison of different dose regimens. British Medical Journal 1972; 1: 654
156. Tung JP, Maibach HI. The practical use of methotrexate in psoriasis. Drugs 1990; 40: 697
157. Zachheim HS, Glogau RG, Fisher DA, et al. 6-Thioguanine treatment of psoriasis: experience in 81 patients. Journal of the American Academy of Dermatology 1994; 30: 452
158. Parrish JA, Fitzpatrick TB, Tanenbaum L, et al. Photochemotherapy of psoriasis with oral methoxsalen and long wave ultraviolet light. New England Journal of Medicine 1974; 291: 1207
159. Wolff K, Fitzpatrick RB, Parrish JA. Photochemotherapy for psoriasis with orally administered methoxsalen. Archives of Dermatology 1976; 112: 943
160. Steiner I, Prey T, Gschnait F, et al. Serum levels of 8-methoxypsoralen 2 hours after oral administration. Acta Dermermatologica et Venereologica 1978; 58: 185
161. Thune P. Plasma levels of 8-methoxypsoralen and phototoxicity studies during PUVA treatment of psoriasis with meladinin tablets. Acta Dermatologica et Venereologica 1978; 58: 149
162. Polano MK, Schothorst AA. Difference in the efficiency of two delivery forms of 8-methoxypsoralen. Dermatologica 1977; 154: 216

163. de Wolff FA, Thomas TV. Clinical pharmacokinetics of methoxsalen and other psoralens. Clinical Pharmacokinetics 1986; 11: 62
164. Wolff K, Gschnait F, Honigsmann H, et al. Phototesting and dosimetry for photochemotherapy. British Journal of Dermatology 1977; 96: 1
165. Morrison WI, Parrish JA, Fitzpatrick TB. Controlled study of PUVA and adjunctive therapy in management of psoriasis. British Journal of Dermatology 1978; 98: 125
166. Rogers S, Marks J, Briffa DV, et al. Comparison of photochemotherapy and dithranol in the treatment of chronic plaque psoriasis. Lancet 1979; 1: 455
167. Vella Briffa D, Greaves MW, Wann AP, et al. Relapse rate and long-term management of plaque psoriasis after treatment with photochemotherapy and dithranol. British Medical Journal 1981; 282: 937
168. Honigsmann H, Gschnait F, Konrad K, et al. Photochemotherapy for psoriasis (Von Zumbusch). British Journal of Dermatology 1977; 97: 119
169. Wennersten G. Photoprotection of the eye in PUVA therapy. British Journal of Dermatology 1978; 98: 137
170. Stern RS, Lange R. Non-melanoma skin cancer occurring in patients treated with PUVA five to ten years after first treatment. Journal of Investigational Dermatology 1988; 91: 120
171. Ward A, Brogden RN, Heel RC, et al. Etretinate: a review of its pharmacological and therapeutic efficacy in psoriasis and other skin disorders. Drugs 1983; 26: 9
172. Cunningham WJ, Geiger JM. Practical use of retinoids in psoriasis. Seminars in Dermatology 1992; 11: 291
173. Gollnick H, Bauer R, Brindley C. Acitretin versus etretinate in psoriasis: clinical and pharmacokinetic results of a German multicenter study. Journal of the American Academy of Dermatology 1988; 19: 458
174. Geiger JM, Saurat JH. Acitretin and etretinate: how and when they should be used. Dermatology Clinics 1993; 11: 17
175. White SI, Marks JM, Shuster S. Etretinate in pustular psoriasis of palms and soles. British Journal of Dermatology 1985; 113: 581
176. Lawrence C, Marks J, Parker S. A comparison of PUVA-etretinate and PUVA-placebo for palmo-plantar pustular psoriasis. British Journal of Dermatology 1984; 110: 221
177. Brindley C. An overview of recent clinical pharmacokinetic studies with acitretin (RO 10-1670, etretin). Dermatologica 1989; 178: 79
178. Pilkington T, Brogden RN. Acitretin: a review of its pharmacological and therapeutic use. Drugs 1992; 43: 597-627
179. Harper JI, Keat ACS, Staughton RCD. Cyclosporin for psoriasis. Lancet 1984; 2: 981
180. Silverman AK, Emmett M, Menter A. Can maintenance cyclosporine be used in psoriasis without decreasing renal function? Seminars in Dermatology 1992; 11: 302
181. Ellis CN, Gorsulowsky DC, Hamilton TA, et al. Cyclosporine improves psoriasis in a double-blind study. Journal of the American Medical Association 1986; 256: 3110
182. Timonen P, Friend D, Abeywickrama K, et al. Efficacy of low-dose cyclosporine A in psoriasis: results of dose finding studies. British Journal of Dermatology 1990; 122 Suppl. 36: 33-9
183. Meinardi MMHM, Bos JD. Cyclosporine maintenance therapy in psoriasis. Transplantation Proceedings 1988; 20 Suppl. 4: 42-9
184. Griffiths CEM, Powels AV, McFadden J, et al. Long term cyclosporine for psoriasis. British Journal of Dermatology 1989; 120: 253-60
185. Faulds D, Goa KL, Benfield P. Cyclosporin: a review of its pharmacodynamic and pharmacokinetic properties, and therapeutic use in immunoregulatory disorders. Drugs 1993; 45: 953-1040
186. Matthew DJ, Norman AP, Taylor B, et al. Prevention of eczema. Lancet 1977; 1: 321
187. Vandenplas Y. Pathogenesis of food allergy in infants. Current Opinion in Pediatrics 1993; 5: 567
188. Thirumoorthv T, Greaves MW. Disodium cromoglycate ointment in atopic eczema. British Medical Journal 1978; 2: 500
189. Haider SA. Treatment of atopic eczema in children: clinical trial of 10% sodium cromoglycate ointment. British Medical Journal 1977; 1: 1570
190. Christiansen JV, Gadborg E, Kieiter I, et al. Efficacy of bufexamac (NFN) cream in skin diseases: a double-blind multicentre trial. Dermatologica 1977; 154: 177
191. Burry JN. Adverse effects of fluorinated corticosteroid creams and ointments. Medical Journal of Australia 1973; 1: 393
192. Sneddon IB. Perioral dermatitis. British Journal of Dermatology 1972; 87: 430
193. Beetens JR, Loots W, Somers Y, et al. Ketoconazole inhibits the biosynthesis of leukotriene *in vitro* and *in vivo*. Biochemical Pharmacology 1986; 35: 883-91
194. Green CA, Farr PM, Shuster S. Treatment of seborrhoeic dermatitis with ketoconazole. British Journal of Dermatology 1987; 116: 217-21
195. Pierard GE, Pierard-Franchimont C, Van Cutsem J, et al. Ketoconazole 2% emulsion in the treatment of seborrheic dermatitis. International Journal of Dermatology 1991; 30: 806-9
196. Stratigos JD, Antoniou C, Katsambas A, et al. Ketoconazole 2% cream versus hydrocortisone 1% cream in the treatment of seborrheic dermatitis. A double-blind comparative study. Journal of the American Academy of Dermatology 1988; 19: 850-3
197. Fitzpatrick TB, Eisen AZ, Wolff K, et al., editors. Dermatology in general medicine. 4th edition. New York: McGraw-Hill, 1993: 1573
198. Leyden JJ, Kligman AH. The case of steroid-antibiotic combinations. British Journal of Dermatology 1977; 96: 179
199. Aly R. Bacteriology of atopic dermatitis. Acta Dermatologica et Venereologica 1980; Suppl. 92: 16
200. Svejgaard E. The role of microorganisms in atopic dermatitis. Seminars in Dermatology 1990; 9: 255
201. Wereide K. Neomycin sensitivity in atopic dermatitis and other eczematous conditions. Acta Dermatologica et Venereologica 1970; 50: 114
202. Ayhan A, Urman B, Yuce K, et al. Topical testosterone for lichen sclerosus. International Journal of Gynaecology and Obstetrics 1989; 30: 253
203. Bousema MT, Romppanen U, Geiger JM, et al. Acitretin in the treatment of severe lichen sclerosus et atrophicus of the vulva: a double-blind, placebo-controlled study. Journal of the American Academy of Dermatology 1994; 30: 225
204. Prottey C, Hartop PJ, Pross M. Correction of the cutaneous manifestations of fatty acid deficiency in man by application of the sunflower-seed oil. Journal of Investigational Dermatology 1975; 64: 223
205. Kauppinen K, Alanko K. Oral provocation: uses. Seminars in Dermatology 1989; 8: 187

206. Sorkin EM, Heel RC. Terfenadine: a review of its pharmacodynamic properties and therapeutic efficacy. Drugs 1985; 29: 34
207. Richards DM, Brogden RN, Heel RC, et al. Astemizole: a review of its pharmacodynamic properties and therapeutic efficacy. Drugs 1984; 28: 38
208. Soter NA. Treatment of urticaria and angioedema: low sedating H1-type antihistamines. Journal of the American Academy of Dermatology 1991; 24: 1084
209. McTavish D, Goa KL, Ferrill M. Terfenadine: an updated review of its pharmacological properties and therapeutic efficacy. Drugs 1990; 39: 552-74
210. Haria M, Fitton A, Peters DH. Loratadine: a reappraisal of its pharmacological properties and therapeutic use in allergic disorders. Drugs 1994; 48: 617-37
211. Spencer CM, Faulds D, Peters DH. Cetirizine: a reappraisal of its pharmacological properties and therapeutic use in selected allergic disorders. Drugs 1993; 46: 1055-80
212. Brogden RN, McTavish D. Acrivastine: a review of its pharmacological properties and therapeutic efficacy in allergic rhinitis, urticaria and related disorders. Drugs 1991; 41: 927-40
213. Monroe EW. Nonsedating H1 antihistamines in chronic urticaria. Annals of Allergy 1993; 71: 585
214. Greaves M, Marks R, Robinson I. Receptors for histamine in human skin blood vessels: a review. British Journal of Dermatology 1977; 97: 225
215. Choy M, Middleton RK. Cimetidine in idiopathic urticaria. Drug Intelligence and Clinical Pharmacy 1991; 25: 609
216. Frank MM, Gelfand JA, Atkinson JP. Hereditary angioedema: the clinical syndrome and its management. Ann Intern Med 1976; 84: 580
217. Sheffer AL, Austen KF, Rosen FS. Tranexamic acid therapy in hereditary angioneurotic edema. New England Journal of Medicine 1972; 287: 452
218. Agostoni A, Marasoni B, Licardi M, et al. Intermittent therapy with danazol in hereditary angiodema. Lancet 1978; 1: 453
219. Gelfand JA, Shenns RJ, Alling DW, et al. Treatment of hereditary angioedema with danazol: reversal of clinical and biochemical abnormalities. New England Journal of Medicine 1976; 295: 1444
220. Cicardi M, Bergamaschini L, Cugno M, et al. Long-term treatment of hereditary angioedema with attenuated androgens: a survey of a 13-year experience. Journal of Allergy and Clinical Immunology 1991; 87: 768
221. Maibach HI, Johnson HL. Contact urticaria syndrome: contact urticaria to diethyltoluamide (immediate type hypersensitivity). Archives of Dermatology 1975; 111: 726
222. Lahti A, von Krogh G, Maibach HI. Contact urticaria syndrome: an expanding phenomenon. In: Stone J, editor. Dermatologic immunology and allergy. St Louis: Mosby, 1985: 379
223. Lahti A, Maibach HI. Contact reactions: contact urticaria syndrome. Seminars in Dermatology 1987; 6: 313
224. Greaves MW, Bunon JL, Marks J, et al. Azathioprine in treatment of bullous pemphigoid. British Medical Journal 1971; 1: 144
225. Burton JL, Harman RRM, Peachey RDG, et al. Azathioprine plus prednisone in treatment of pemphigoid. British Medical Journal 1978; 2: 1190
226. Bystryn JC. Plasmapheresis therapy of pemphigus. Archives of Dermatology 1988; 124: 1702
227. Poulin Y, Perry HO, Muller SA. Pemphigus vulgaris: results of treatment with gold as a steroid-sparing agent in a series of thirteen patients. Journal of the American Academy of Dermatology 1984; 11: 851
228. Barthelemy H, Frappaz A, Cambazard F, et al. Treatment of nine cases of pemphigus vulgaris with cyclosporine. Journal of the American Academy of Dermatology 1988; 18: 1262
229. Lapidoth M, David M, Ben-Amitai D, et al. The efficacy of combined treatment with prednisone and cyclosporine in patients with pemphigus: preliminary study. Journal of the American Academy of Dermatology 1994; 30: 752
230. Zuidema J, Hilbers-Modderman ESM, Merkus FWHM. Clinical pharmacokinetics of dapsone. Clinical Pharmacokinetics 1986; 11: 299
231. Cream JJ, Scott GL. Anemia in dermatitis herpetiformis: the role of dapsone induced haemolysis and malabsorption. British Journal of Dermatology 1970; 82: 333
232. Cockburn EM, Wood SM, Waller PC, et al. Dapsone-induced agranulocytosis spontaneous reporting data. British Journal of Dermatology 1993: 702
233. Marks J, Shuster S, Watson AJ. Small bowel changes in dermatitis herpetiformis. Lancet 1966; 2: 1280
234. Fry L, Seah P, Harper P, et al. The small intestine in dermatitis herpetiformis. Journal of Clinical Pathology 1974; 27: 817
235. Kadunce DP, McMurry MP, Avots-Avotinos A, et al. The effect of an elemental diet with and without gluten on disease activity in dermatitis herpetiformis. Journal of Investigational Dermatology 1991; 97: 175
236. Krezemien D, Weston WL, Brice SL, et al. Detection of a herpes simplex virus DNA in cutaneous lesions of erythema multiforme. Journal of Investigational Dermatology 1989; 93: 183
237. Perez MI, Kohn SR. Systemic sclerosis. Journal of the American Academy of Dermatology 1993; 28: 525
238. Jimenez SA, Sigal SH. A 15-year prospective study of treatment of rapidly progressive systemic sclerosis with D-penicillamine. Journal of Rheumatology 1991; 18: 1496
239. Bunker CB, Mauric PDL, Little S, et al. Isotretinoin and lung function in systemic sclerosis. Clinical and Experimental Dermatology 1991; 16: 11
240. Malaviya AN, Many A, Schwanz RS. Treatment of dermatomyositis with methotrexate. Lancet 1968; 2: 485
241. Bunch TW. Long-term follow-up of azathioprine for polymyositis. Arthritis & Rheumatism 1980; 23: 658
242. Dau PC. Plasmapheresis in idiopathic inflammatory myopathy: experience with 35 patients. Archives of Neurology 1981; 38: 544
243. Campion EW. Desperate diseases and plasmapheresis. New England Journal of Medicine 1992; 326: 1425
244. Dalakas MC, Illa I, Dambrosia JM, et al. A controlled trial of high-dose intravenous immune globulin infusions as treated for dermatomyositis. New England Journal of Medicine 1993; 329: 1993
245. Nimni ME. Mechanism of inhibition of collagen cross-linking by penicillamine. Proceedings of the Royal Society of Medicine 1977; 70 Suppl. 3: 65
246. Agren MS. Studies on zinc in wound healing. Acta Dermatologica et Venereologica 1990; Suppl. 154: 1
247. Hawkins T, Marks JM, Plummer VM, et al. Whole body monitoring of zinc 65 retention in patients with leg ulceration and minimal dermatoses. Clinical and Experimental Dermatology 1976; 1: 243

248. Phillips A, Davidson M, Greaves MW. Venous leg ulceration: evaluation of zinc treatment, serum zinc and rate of healing. Clinical and Experimental Dermatology 1977; 2: 395
249. Polansky JR, Fauss DJ, Hydorn T, et al. Cellular injury from sustained *vs* acute hydrogen peroxide exposure in cultured human corneal endothelium and human lens epithelium. CLAO Journal 1990; 16 Suppl. 1: S23-8
250. Nierman MM. Treatment of dermal and decubitus ulcers. Drugs 1978; 15: 226
251. Floden CH, Wikstrom K. Controlled clinical trial with dextranomer (Debrisan) on venous leg ulcers. Current Therapeutic Research 1978; 24: 753
252. Heel RC, Morton P, Brogden RN, et al. Dextranomer: a review of its general properties and therapeutic efficacy. Drugs 1979; 18: 89
253. Wilson I, Cameron J, Powell SM, et al. High incidence of contact dermatitis in leg-ulcer patients - implications for management. Clinical and Experimental Dermatology 1991; 16: 250
254. Perera P. An investigation of varicose ulcers. Transactions of the St Johns Hospital Dermatological Society 1970; 56: 175
255. Millard LG, Robens MM, Gatecliffe M. Chronic leg ulcers treated by the pinch graph method. British Journal of Dermatology 1977; 97: 289
256. Kanj LF, Phillips TJ. Management of leg ulcers. Fitzpatrick's Journal of Clinical Dermatology 1994 Sep/Oct
257. Olejniczak S, Zielinsh A. Topical oxygen promotes healing of leg ulcers. Resident and Staff Physician 1977; 23: 165
258. Pace WE. Treatment of cutaneous ulcers with benzoyl peroxide. Canadian Medical Association Journal 1976; 115: 1101
259. Moynahan EJ. Acrodermatitis enteropathica: a lethal inherited human zinc deficiency disorder. Lancet 1974; 2: 399
260. Prendiville JS, Manfredi LN. Skin signs of nutritional disorders. Seminars in Dermatology 1992; 11: 88
261. Maibach HI, Kligman AM. Dihydroxyacetone: a suntan-stimulating agent. Archives of Dermatology 1960; 82: 505
262. Nordlund JJ, Halder RM, Grimes P. Management of vitiligo. Dermatology Clinics 1993; 11: 27
263. Clayton R. Treatment of vitiligo with clobetasol propionate. British Journal of Dermatology 1977; 96: 71
264. Mosher DB, Pamsh JA, Fitzpatrick TB. Monobenzylether of hydroquinone: a retrospective study of 18 vitiligo patients and a review of the literature. British Journal of Dermatology 1977; 97: 669
265. Winter RJ, Kem F, Blizzard RM. Prednisone therapy for alopecia areata: a follow-up report. Archives of Dermatology 1976; 112: 1549
266. Happle R, Echternacht K. Induction of hair growth in alopecia areata with DNCB. Lancet 1977; 2: 1002
267. Daman LA, Rosenberg EW, Drake L. Treatment of alopecia areata with dinitrochlorobenzene. Archives of Dermatology 1978; 114: 1036
268. Shapiro J. Alopecia areata: update on therapy. Dermatology Clinics 1993; 11: 35
269. Weiss VC, West DP, Fu TS, et al. Alopecia areata treated with topical minoxidil. Archives of Dermatology 1984; 120: 457
270. Clissold SP, Heel RC. Topical minoxidil: a preliminary review of its pharmacodynamic properties and therapeutic efficacy in alopecia areata and alopecia androgenetica. Drugs 1987; 33: 107
271. Tsai JC, Flynn GL, Weiner N, et al. Influence of application time and formulation reapplication on the delivery of minoxidil through hairless mouse skin as measured in Franz diffusion cells. Skin Pharmacology 1994; 7: 270
272. De Villez RL. Topical minoxidil therapy in hereditary androgenetic alopecia. Archives of Dermatology 1985; 121: 197
273. Olsen EA, Weiner MS, Amara IA, et al. Five-year follow-up of men with androgenetic alopecia treated with topical minoxidil. Journal of the American Academy of Dermatology 1990; 22: 643
274. De Villez RL, Jacobs JP, Szpunar CA, et al. Androgenetic alopecia in the female: treatment with 2% topical minoxidil solution. Archives of Dermatology 1994; 130: 303
275. Reeves JRT, Maibach HI. Drug and chemical-induced hair loss. In: Marzulli FN, Maibach HI, editors. Dermatotoxicology, 3rd ed. Washington: Hemisphere, 1987: 553
276. Belisano JC. Topical cytotoxic therapy of solar keratoses with 5-fluorouracil. Medical Journal of Australia 1969; 2: 1136
277. Klein E. Tumours of the skin. IX. Local cytotoxic therapy of cutaneous and mucosal premalignant and malignant lesions. New York State Journal of Medicine 1968; 68: 886
278. Ho VC, Sober AJ. Therapy for cutaneous melanoma: an update. Journal of the American Academy of Dermatology 1990; 22: 159
279. Anderson RR, Hruza G. A brief guide to surgical lasers. Fitzpatrick's Journal of Clinical Dermatology 1993 Nov/Dec: 52
280. Zachheim HS. Treatment of cutaneous T-cell lymphoma. Seminars in Dermatology 1994; 13: 207
281. Bunn PA, Hoffman SJ, Norris D, et al. Systemic therapy of cutaneous T-cell lymphomas (mycosis fungoides and the Sezary syndrome). Annals of Internal Medicine 1994; 121: 592
282. Ramsay CA. Photosensitivity and the skin. British Journal of Hospital Medicine 1975; 13: 536
283. Kerker BJ, Morison WL. The photoaggravated dermatoses. Seminars in Dermatology 1990; 9: 70
284. Lane-Brown M. New concepts in prevention and treatment of sunburn. Drugs 1977; 13: 366
285. Poh-Fitzpatrick MB. The biologic actions of solar radiation on skin with a note on sunscreens. Journal of Dermatological Surgery and Oncology 1977; 3: 199
286. Stiller MJ, Davis IC, Shupack JL. A concise guide to topical sunscreens: state of the art. International Journal of Dermatology 1992; 31: 540
287. Pollitt N. β-Carotene and the photodermatoses. British Journal of Dermatology 1975; 93: 721
288. Soter NA. Physical urticaria/angiodema. Seminars in Dermatology 1987; 6: 302
289. Noble S, Wagstaff AJ. Tretinoin: a review of its pharmacological properties and clinical efficacy in the topical treatment of photodamaged skin. Drugs & Aging 1995; 6: 479-96
290. Felix RH, Smith AG, Stevenson CJ. Skin disorders. In: Davies, editor. Textbook of adverse drug reactions. 3rd ed. Oxford: Oxford University Press, 1985: 445
291. Almeyda I, Levantine A. Adverse cutaneous reactions to the penicillins - ampicillin rashes. British Journal of Dermatology 1972; 87: 294

292. McKenzie H, Parratt D, White RG. IgM and IgG antibody levels to ampicillin in patients with infectious mononucleosis. Clinical and Experimental Immunology 1976; 26: 214
293. Van Scott EJ, Reinenson RP, Steinmuller R. The growing hair roots of the human scalp and morphologic changes therein following amethopterin therapy. Journal of Investigational Dermatology 1957; 29: 197
294. Cormia FE. Alopecia from oral contraceptives. Journal of the American Medical Association 1967; 201: 635
295. Editorial: Hair loss and contraceptives. British Medical Journal 1973; 2: 499.
296. Earhan RN, Ball J, Nuss DD, et al. Minoxidil-induced hypertrichosis: treatment with calcium thioglycolate depilatory. Southern Medical Journal 1977; 70: 442
297. Burton JL, Schutt WH, Caldwell I. Hypertrichosis due to diazoxide. British Journal of Dermatology 1976; 93: 707
298. Bigby M. Nonsteroidal anti-inflammatory drug reactions. Seminars in Dermatology 1989; 8: 182
299. Shorr WF. Paraben allergy. Journal of the American Medical Association 1968; 204: 859
300. Hectorne KJ, Fransway AF. Diazolidinyl urea: incidence of sensitivity, patterns of cross-reactivity and clinical relevance. Contact Dermatitis 1994; 30: 16
301. Rietschel RL, Nethercott JR, Emmett EA, et al. Methylchloroisothiazolinone-methylisothiazolinone reactions in patients screened for vehicle and preservative hypersensitivity. Journal of the American Academy of Dermatology 1990; 22: 734
302. Menne T, Frosch PJ, Veien NK, et al. Contact sensitization to 5-chloro-2-methyl-4-isothiazolin-3-one and 2-methyl-4-isothiazolin-3-one (MCI/MI): a European multicenter study. Contact Dermatitis 1991; 24: 334
303. Bruynzeel DP, van Ketel WG. Patch testing in drug eruptions. Seminars in Dermatology 1989; 8: 196
304. Shuster S, Scarborough H. Corticosteroid purpura. Quarterly Journal of Medicine 1961; 30: 33
305. Lyell A. A review of toxic epidermal necrolysis in Britain. British Journal of Dermatology 1967; 79: 662
306. Roujeau JC, Chosidow O, Saiag P. Toxic epidermal necrolysis (Lyell syndrome). Journal of the American Academy of Dermatology 1990; 23: 1039
307. Felsher BF, Redeker AG. Acute intermittent porphyria: effect of diet and griseofulvin. Medicine (Baltimore) 1967; 46: 217
308. Anhalt GJ. Drug-induced pemphigus. Seminars in Dermatology 1989; 8: 166
309. Marsden RA, Ryan TJ, Vanhegan RI, et al. Pemphigus foliaceus induced by penicillamine. British Medical Journal 1976; 2: 1423
310. Hay KD, Muller HK, Reade PC. D-penicillamine-induced mucocutaneous lesions with features of pemphigus. Oral Surgery Oral Medicine and Oral Pathology 1978; 45: 385
311. Gauge RW, Rhodes EL, Edwards CP, et al. Pemphigus induced by rifampicin. British Journal of Dermatology 1976; 95: 445
312. Parfrey PS, Clement M, Vandenburg MJ, et al. Captopril-induced pemphigus. British Medical Journal 1980; 281: 194
313. Burry JN, Lawrence JR. Phototoxic blisters from high frusemide dosage. British Journal of Dermatology 1976; 94: 495
314. Heydenreich G, Pinddborg T, Schmidt H. Bullous dermatitis among patients with chronic renal failure on high dose frusemide. Acta Medica Scandinavica 1977; 202: 61
315. Sehgal VN, Rege VL, Kharangate VN. Fixed drug eruptions caused by medications: a report from India. International Journal of Dermatology 1978; 17: 78
316. Pathak M, Fitzpatrick TB. Photosensitivity caused by drugs. Rational Drug Therapy 1972 (Jun); 6: 1
317. Epstein JH, Wintroub BU. Photosensitivity due to drugs. Drugs 1985; 30: 42
318. Erickson LR, Peterka ES. Sunlight sensitivity from oral contraceptives. Journal of the American Medical Association 1968; 203: 980
319. Lauerma AI, Maibach HI. Contact allergy to natural human compounds: steroids. Cosmetics and Toiletries 1993; 108: 47

Chapter 18

# Obstetric and Gynaecological Disorders

*M.H. Hall* and *J. Webster*

## Synopsis of Important Principles

1) Drug use in pregnancy requires a careful assessment of the risks of not giving the drug against any potential harm from its use. There should be a clear indication of benefit to mother or fetus.

2) The desired (or adverse) effects of some drugs occur in the periconceptual period. As conception cannot always be planned, preconceptual use of (or abstinence from) drugs is necessary. This may be also important for fathers.

3) In the first trimester, only essential drugs should be given because of the risk of teratogenesis.

4) As pregnancy advances, maternal absorption, distribution and elimination of drugs may be altered.

5) Labour is a time of special therapeutic problems. When delivery approaches, administration of drugs should be cautious, not only because of altered maternal disposition of drugs, but also because of the immature metabolic or excretory capacity of the fetus and neonate.

6) Drugs may be used to modify the risk of maternal-fetal transmission of infection.

7) In the puerperium, drugs administered to the mother may occasionally be excreted in breast milk in sufficient amounts to cause harmful effects in the breast fed infant.

8) Fertility control by drugs has brought simple and effective contraception within the reach of millions of women. Many adverse effects have been described, but all are uncommon and most are minor.

9) Drugs are extensively used in infertility practice, especially in assisted reproduction.

10) Hormone therapy should not be prescribed for gynaecological disorders without careful assessment to exclude other pathology. Even where a hormonal abnormality is definitely present, hormones may not be the treatment of choice.

11) There are important pharmacoeconomic considerations in long term use of hormone replacement therapy, and a paucity of prospective randomised trials on which to judge safety and effectiveness.

The safe and rational use of drugs in pregnancy requires knowledge of the potential harm to the fetus and neonate. Relatively few drugs given during pregnancy are of direct benefit to the fetus and the benefits to the mother need to be clearly established. Pregnancy, labour and the puerperium may each alter the pharmacokinetics and pharmacodynamics of therapeutic drugs. Oral contraceptives remain the most effective and most widely used form of reversible fertility control. Adverse effects are important but are heavily outweighed by the advantages. Assisted reproduction is important for a relatively small number of women but advances in drug therapy have made an important contribution. Medical termination of pregnancy is now an alternative to surgical methods in a substantial number of cases, but the potential for abuse must be recognised.

Hormone replacement therapy is emerging as one of the most effective preventative health strategies for women, but it deserves thorough evaluation in prospective randomised trials so that recommendations for its use can be based on unequivocal evidence.

## 1. Clinical Pharmacological Considerations

Much research on the effectiveness and safety of drugs has been done only in men, sometimes because the relevant condition is commoner in men. However, conclusions from such research will not necessarily apply to women. Women are smaller than men, with a greater fat to muscle ratio. Women have a longer life expectancy than men in developed countries, but mature gonadal function is in place for a shorter duration than in men (usually for about 35 years, from age 15 to 50 years).

During menstrual life, cyclical hormonal changes may affect drug administration, and may cause symptoms. Menstruation itself is associated with considerable dysfunction in respect of blood loss and pain in some women. Estrogen production during reproductive life seems to protect women from many conditions to which men are subject, such as arteriosclerotic heart disease, but their longer life expectancy means they may require more drug therapy for conditions associated with old age. There are also psychological differences between men and women which may affect the appropriate threshold for initiating drug therapy, and compliance with a treatment regimen.

Infertility in women is more likely to be amenable to drug therapy than infertility in men.

### 1.1 Pregnancy and the Puerperium

The use of drugs in pregnancy and the puerperium requires special consideration for a number of reasons:

- Teratogenesis and other adverse effects on the developing embryo may occur
- Transplacental passage of drugs may lead to adverse effects on the fetus later in pregnancy
- Pregnancy alters both the pharmacokinetics of drugs and the maternal response to drugs
- Labour is a time of special therapeutic problems
- Drugs administered to the mother may be excreted in breast milk.

#### *1.1.1 Teratogenesis and Other Embryopathic Effects*

Very early in pregnancy, particularly in the preimplantation period, drugs may kill the embryo or cause abortion. There is evidence that occupational exposure of mothers to cytotoxic drugs may increase the rate of spontaneous abortion,[1] and possibly also of ectopic pregnancy.[2] During the period of organogenesis, drugs may produce major structural abnormalities (teratogenesis) [see chapter 2; sect. 2]. Later in pregnancy, drug-induced teratogenic effects are less obvious, but more subtle effects can be equally serious, such as growth retardation, virilisation and abnormalities of brain development.

Some harmful effects of drugs used during pregnancy may not become apparent until some time after delivery. In the case of substances of addiction such as heroin, barbiturates and alcohol, a withdrawal syndrome may occur in the neonate hours or days after delivery. Some adverse effects may take much longer to become manifest. Tetracycline given in the latter half of pregnancy can lead to the discolouration of the deciduous teeth of the child. Vaginal tumours have occurred in girls whose mothers had been given stilbestrol (diethylstilbestrol) as treatment for threatened spontaneous abortion 10 to 15 years before.[3] Long term follow-up confirms that this form of treatment has no beneficial effects on the outcome of pregnancy, but induces a wide variety of unfavourable outcomes in the sons, daughters and also in the mothers themselves.[4]

Predicting the teratogenic potential of a drug is very difficult, because of the multifactorial nature of this problem. Such factors include:

1. Mechanism(s) of action of the drug
2. Dosage and duration of therapy
3. Timing of administration in relation to gestational age
4. Genetic susceptibility
5. Maternal nutritional status
6. Underlying disease and concomitant medication.

Species differences mean that animal data cannot be directly extrapolated to humans. Lack of specificity of effect also leads to difficulty in interpretation. One drug may produce a multiplicity of malformations, e.g. isotretinoin. Conversely, one malformation may result from the effect of a variety of different drugs, e.g. craniofacial abnormalities with antiepileptic drugs. Where such a malformation occurs spontaneously without drug exposure, occurs with only a slight increase in frequency in the offspring of patients exposed to the drug, and occurs with a variety of agents used to treat the underlying disease, it may be very difficult to prove a cause and effect relationship. In addition, other factors may confound the association between drug and malformation:

- The illness for which the drug is used may itself be teratogenic (this is almost certainly the case in respect of epilepsy and diabetes mellitus)
- The drug may inhibit the abortion of a malformed fetus
- Combinations of drugs may confuse the picture, either by way of a drug interaction or the wrong drug being implicated.

On the other hand, some teratogenic effects in humans can be predicted with reasonable confidence from known effects in animals, as in the case of isotretinoin. The tragedy is that even though this drug was clearly shown to have powerful teratogenic effects in animals and was predicted to have the potential to exhibit similar effects in humans (and was licensed with very explicit warnings against its use in young women unless they were sterilised or taking strict contraceptive precautions), many cases of multiple malformations due to isotretinoin and its analogues have occurred.[5] This drug now rivals thalidomide in potency as a human teratogen.

Thalidomide itself did not appear harmful in early animal tests, but in humans caused a very unusual constellation of abnormalities, including phocomelia, in a high proportion of cases in which it was given at the critical stage of gestation.[6] As a result, the association was detected at a relatively early stage (4 years after marketing), but even then not until thousands of affected offspring had been born. This drug is still widely available in Brazil for the treatment of lepra reaction, and deformities continue to occur.[7]

**Table I.** Some drugs to be avoided or given with caution in pregnancy (see also chapter 2)

| Early pregnancy (fetotoxicity/teratogenesis) | Later pregnancy (fetal and neonatal effects) | Throughout |
|---|---|---|
| **High risk:** | **Avoid:** | **Avoid:** |
| Etretinate/acitretin | ACE inhibitors | Sex hormones |
| Isotretinoin | Chloramphenicol | Tetracyclines |
| Methotrexate | Indomethacin | Mifepristone |
| Sex hormones | Iodides | Misoprostol |
| Thalidomide | Sulfonamides | |
| Warfarin | Sulphonylureas | |
| | Warfarin | |
| **Increased risk:** | | |
| Carbamazepine | **Use with care:** | |
| Phenytoin | Antithyroid drugs | |
| Valproic acid | Aspirin (acetylsalicylic acid) | |
| Retinol (vitamin A) | Barbiturates | |
| | Benzodiazepines | |
| **Possibly increased risk:** | Corticosteroids | |
| Inhalational anaesthetics | Heparin | |
| Salicylates | Lithium | |
| | Opioids | |
| | Phenothiazines | |

The experience with thalidomide can be said to have laid the foundation for the discipline of clinical pharmacology and for much of our current practices in relation to preclinical toxicology testing of new drugs. Some drugs with known or suspected adverse effects on the embryo, fetus and neonate are shown in table I.

In women with a previous history of *neural tube malformation* in her offspring, a major reduction in the recurrence of such malformations can be achieved by the administration of folic acid 4mg daily preconceptually and in the early weeks of pregnancy, as shown in a large randomised trial.[8] The question of whether a smaller dose would be effective remains unanswered. Another contentious issue is whether first occurrences of neural tube defect can be prevented by administration of folic acid to women who might be planning a pregnancy. A Hungarian trial[9] reported a significantly lower incidence of neural tube defects in 2394 women receiving preconceptual multivitamins including folic acid 0.8 mg/day than in 2310 women receiving trace elements only. However, other trials and observational studies suggest that a dose of 0.4 mg/day will suffice, and the lower dose would reduce the risk of precipitation of subacute combined degeneration of the cord if supplementation was long term in a woman with undiagnosed pernicious anaemia. The pharmacological evidence of effectiveness is not conclusive[8] and the target group difficult to identify, but prophylactic periconceptual folic acid 0.4 mg/day is recommended in the UK and in the US.[10]

Therapy may also be used to correct vitamin deficiency, either in all women or in selected groups with metabolic abnormalities such as hyperhomocysteinaemia.[11] It is not known if folic acid will prevent the development of neural tube defects associated with some antiepileptic drugs (see section 3.12), but it does seem sensible to offer such supplements to all epileptic patients on antiepileptic therapy who may be embarking on a pregnancy.

Vitamin supplementation is not entirely innocuous, however, and should only be considered where benefit has been firmly established, as in the case of folic acid. By contrast, there is now evidence that excessive dietary retinol (vitamin A) may be associated with congenital abnormalities.[12,13] Pregnant women should avoid use of over-the-counter (OTC) supplements containing retinol, and also ingestion of liver.

Effects on the fetus of paternal exposure to therapeutic drugs (as opposed to environmental chemicals) seem to be confined to cyclophosphamide and possibly other cytotoxic drugs.[14]

#### *1.1.2 Transplacental Passage of Drugs*

The placenta is not a barrier to the transfer of drugs from the maternal to the fetal organism and most drugs cross the placenta by simple diffusion to a greater or lesser extent from as early as the 5th week of embryonic life (see also chapter 2; sect. 4.2.1). Some drugs, such as thiopental, cross the placenta so readily that the fetus has circulating concentrations almost as high as those in the mother. Other drugs, particularly those of high molecular weight, do not cross the placenta to any appreciable extent, e.g. heparin. Insulin does not cross the placenta but glucose does and may stimulate islet cell hyperplasia in the fetal pancreas. The resultant fetal hyperinsulinaemia may result in macrosomia, visceromegaly and neonatal hypoglycaemia. Oral antidiabetic drugs cross the placenta and may also cause neonatal hypoglycaemia. Neither thyroxine[15,16] nor triiodothyronine[17] cross the placenta very efficiently, but iodine and antithyroid drugs do. One notable exception to the general rule that larger molecular weight compounds do not cross the placenta is thyroid-stimulating immunoglobulin, which is readily transported and may cause transient neonatal hyperthyroidism and goitre.[18]

#### *1.1.3 Fetal Metabolism and Excretion*

During most of pregnancy, even if a drug does cross the placenta, maternal metabolism and excretion mechanisms ensure that clearance of the drug from both the mother and fetus is maintained. After delivery, the neonate may be unable to metabolise adequately and excrete some drugs that were administered to the mother. The less mature the fetus, the less competent its capacity for drug elimination, so that a neonate born prematurely while its mother is receiving drugs that it cannot adequately eliminate, such as benzodiazepines, may be in serious difficulty.

Drugs administered to the mother at parturition may also affect the metabolic capacity of the neonate. Antenatal use of corticosteroids has been shown to enhance the ability of the fetal lung to produce surfactant and to reduce the risk of respiratory distress syndrome (see also section 5.2). On the other hand, therapeutic doses of corticosteroids administered for maternal indications may cause temporary adrenal suppression in the neonate.

#### 1.1.4 Maternal Drug Disposition

Pregnancy is a time of continual physiological adjustment which may influence the pharmacokinetics of drugs as pregnancy advances. The effects of the various physiological changes on the principal determinants of maternal pharmacokinetics (absorption, distribution, metabolism and excretion) are discussed in chapter 2 (section 4.1).

#### 1.1.5 Maternal Responses to Drugs

Most women gain 10 to 15kg during pregnancy, so that some drugs not normally prescribed on a bodyweight basis may be prescribed in subtherapeutic doses. In addition plasma volume expands, and the attainment of adequate plasma concentrations of drugs with relatively low volumes of distribution may require larger doses for this reason.

During pregnancy, sensitivity to the toxic effects of some drugs may increase. For example, acute fatty liver of pregnancy has been precipitated by the administration of tetracycline or valproic acid (sodium valproate).[19] When β-agonists are given in pregnancy as tocolytic agents for premature labour, tachycardia, myocardial ischaemia and pulmonary oedema may occur. Susceptibility may be enhanced by the concomitant administration of saline and possibly by corticosteroids. This remains an important and avoidable cause of maternal morbidity and mortality.[20]

The therapeutic efficacy of a drug can be altered by the effect of pregnancy on the disease for which it is administered. For example, the insulin requirement of a diabetic patient will alter as pregnancy advances. In the second and third trimesters, increased production of endogenous (cortisol, prolactin) and placental (progesterone, human placental lactogen) hormones leads to relative insulin resistance, while in the last 4 weeks, carbohydrate tolerance may improve as a result of fetal 'siphoning' of glucose.[21]

#### 1.1.6 Problems in Labour

During labour, there is a delay in gastric emptying and vomiting may occur, which may be exacerbated by the use of opioid analgesics.[22] The absorption of most drugs by the oral route may be affected, and parenteral administration is more reliable. In addition, it is necessary in some situations, e.g. hypertensive crises, to use drugs with a rapid onset of action.

Elimination of drugs such as pethidine (meperidine) may be prolonged at the time of delivery and pathways of metabolism may be altered in labour, although the clinical implications of these alterations are uncertain.

Where the drug is potentially harmful to the fetus, e.g. opioid analgesics or sedatives, the dosage must be kept to a minimum and if possible other methods of analgesia such as epidural block should be considered. Drugs that are not cleared by hepatic metabolism, those without active metabolites, and intrinsically short-acting drugs may be preferred if there is a risk of neonatal toxicity from drug accumulation. However, if a drug is considered essential to save the life of the fetus, such as an antibiotic in the case of intrauterine infection, then of course every effort should be made to use a drug that will readily cross the placenta and appear in adequate concentrations in liquor and fetal blood. In such circumstances, dosages should take account of the increased renal clearance that occurs in pregnancy and the drug should be administered by a route that ensures effectiveness.

#### 1.1.7 Excretion of Drugs in Breast Milk

Most drugs are not selectively excreted in breast milk and for this and other reasons relating to the physicochemical and pharmacokinetic characteristics of the particular drug, the neonate will receive a much smaller dose of the drug than the mother (see further appendix C). Nevertheless, even when drugs pass into breast milk in only small amounts, the neonate may be more sensitive to the drug than the mother, as in the case of laxatives, and may also be less able to metabolise and excrete some other drugs, such as those metabolised by glucuronidation (e.g. nalidixic acid). The age and maturity of the neonate also needs to be taken into account. In the case of allergenic antibiotics, such as penicillins, the infant may be sensitised to the risk of subsequent hypersensitivity. Furthermore, even small doses of antimicrobials may be sufficient to alter the bowel flora of the feeding infant and predispose to superinfection. Despite these concerns, few commonly prescribed drugs have been shown to be harmful to the breast fed infant. A list of drugs that are not recommended or need to be used with extra care in the breast feeding mother is shown in table II.

**Table II.** Drugs not recommended in breast feeding mothers or which need to be used with caution because of possible adverse effects in the infant

| Precaution | Drug/group | Notes |
|---|---|---|
| Avoid | Radioiodine | Concentrated in milk |
| | | Thyroid cancer risk |
| Use with care | Amiodarone | Thyroidal uptake |
| | Carbimazole | Hypothyroidism |
| | Chloramphenicol | Aplastic anaemia |
| | Cytotoxic drugs | Immunosuppression |

Radioiodine is the only drug that is absolutely contraindicated in lactating mothers, as it is concentrated in milk with a milk : plasma ratio of 70 : 1 and is further concentrated in the fetal thyroid gland, with a subsequent increase in the risk of permanent hypothyroidism and possibly thyroid cancer.

## 2. General Principles of Drug Prescribing in Women

Indications for the prescription of drugs for women should be determined by research conducted in women. The possible effect of any drug on sexual function, on current or future fertility, or on an unsuspected pregnancy should be considered, as should possible interactions with any over-the-counter medicine used for menstrual dysfunction.

Another problem relates to the inadvertent or self administration of drugs in the early weeks of pregnancy, perhaps before the woman or her doctor realises that she is pregnant. The risks involved can only be avoided by a sensible prescribing policy and by the recognition that any woman of childbearing age may become pregnant. It is the responsibility of the prescriber to make the appropriate enquiries in all such cases.

### 2.1 Pregnant Women

Administration of drugs in pregnancy requires a careful assessment of the risks of not giving the drug against any potential harm from its use. Despite this admonition, drugs continue to be widely used during pregnancy. In a study in the US in the 1970s, the average number of drugs taken was 6.4, 3.2 of them being self-prescribed.[23] A later study in Glasgow showed much lower levels of consumption of drugs in pregnancy[24] and it is possible that there is now a greater awareness of the desirability of restricting such use to a minimum. Even so, under-reporting and self-medication remain common and the use of so-called 'recreational' drugs and drugs of addiction in certain sections of the community adds a new and much more sinister dimension to this problem.[25]

There is little doubt that some drugs if taken by the mother can, under certain circumstances, affect the fetus or neonate profoundly, but most drugs probably do not affect it at all. For most drugs prescribed or self-administered during pregnancy, the incidence of congenital abnormalities in the infants of mothers taking them appears to be only marginally greater than the incidence of abnormalities in infants of mothers not taking these drugs. The overall incidence of major congenital abnormalities is around 2%; thus, most infants born to mothers taking 'low risk' drugs during the first trimester of pregnancy are likely to be normal. Nevertheless, the use of drugs in pregnant women should be avoided unless there are clearcut clinical indications and the drug is of proven benefit.

The following guidelines for drug prescribing are recommended:

- Consider the possibility of pregnancy when prescribing for women of childbearing age
- Consider the possibility of drug ingestion when caring for pregnant women or women of childbearing age
- During the first trimester of pregnancy, avoid the use of any drug that is not absolutely necessary and of proven benefit
- After the first trimester, bear in mind that drugs have a potential to affect the fetus or neonate, even its later physiological and behavioural development
- Bear in mind that the maternal response to drugs can be modified by pregnancy or the puerperium.

Further discussion of prescribing during pregnancy is presented in chapter 2.

## 3. Medical Conditions Requiring Treatment in Pregnancy

### 3.1 Anaemias

The diagnosis of anaemia in pregnancy is complicated by the disproportionate expansion in the plasma volume that occurs early in pregnancy. This expansion probably persists until near term, so that a haemoglobin concentration that would be pathologically low in the non-pregnant state may be normal in pregnancy, and in fact can be associated with a more than adequate oxygen carrying capacity. In the diagnosis of pregnancy anaemia, it is wise, therefore, to give due attention to the packed cell volume, the mean cell haemoglobin concentration and the morphology of the cells, as well as to the actual haemoglobin concentration, which should be measured at the time of first consultation, and then again at 30 and 36 weeks' gestation as a minimum. A low serum ferritin concentration may indicate depleted iron stores even in the absence of anaemia. The red cell folate concentration is the best index of folate deficiency, but red cell morphology (macrocytosis, or rarely megaloblastosis) may indicate the need to measure the red cell folate.

### *3.1.1 Optimum Treatment*

#### Iron Deficiency Anaemia

Iron deficiency is common in pregnancy even in developed countries. Initial treatment is with 130mg of elemental iron daily which is usually acceptable and effective, and should be continued for 3 months. Intramuscular iron is indicated only if there is a suspicion of poor compliance or of malabsorption. Intramuscular injection of iron sorbitol (iron sorbitol citric acid complex) 100mg daily for 7 to 10 days may occasionally cause a pyrexial response and an apparent relapse in patients with chronic pyelonephritis.

The necessity for *routine prophylaxis* with oral iron during pregnancy in developed countries is questionable.[26] Most women are not iron deficient and although it is true that the haemoglobin level will rise in normal women if iron supplements are taken (as a result of its erythropoietic effect), there is no evidence of an improved outcome for the mother or fetus.

Routine oral iron supplements should, however, be prescribed in areas where iron deficiency is common (e.g. due to dietary deficiency, or gastrointestinal blood loss from hookworm infestation), and possibly in the second and third trimester for women in low socioeconomic groups, or who have a history of iron deficiency. In developing countries, the addition of retinol (vitamin A) 2.4 mg/day to iron therapy improves its efficacy, probably by its antimicrobial properties.[27]

#### Folate Deficiency Anaemia

In developed nations, megaloblastic anaemia (which is due in pregnancy to folic acid deficiency) is uncommon. Treatment is by oral folic acid 5mg 3 times a day. Routine folate supplements during pregnancy are not indicated to prevent anaemia[28] and there is no good evidence that they reduce pregnancy complications that were at one time thought to be due to folate deficiency. Routine supplements of at least 0.4 mg/day of folic acid are, however, necessary where dietary deficiency of folate is common or where folate requirements are increased by malarial haemolysis and/or haemoglobinopathies. In these circumstances, this inexpensive drug may provide huge benefits in terms of reduction in blood transfusion and maternal mortality.

The use of folic acid supplements to prevent neural tube defects (see section 1.1.1 and also chapter 2; sect. 1.3.5) is a separate issue not related to the treatment or prophylaxis of anaemia.

#### Refractory Anaemia

Refractory anaemia in pregnancy may occasionally be due to consumption of toxic substances due to pica, where the main aim of treatment is to prevent consumption of the toxin. It may also occur due to chronic infection, often in the urinary tract, which inhibits the erythropoietic response to haematinics, when treatment of the infection is important. Iron is not indicated as iron stores may already be increased, but unavailable for haemoglobin synthesis. In developed countries, such anaemias are seldom severe enough to require transfusion.

#### Haemoglobinopathies

In patients of African, Southeast Asian or Mediterranean descent, the possibility of haemoglobinopathy due to genetic enzyme defects should always be considered (see further chapter 26; sect. 5.2.2).

## 3.2 Urinary Tract Infection in Pregnancy

Urinary infection is particularly likely to occur during pregnancy and the puerperium because of the ureteric dilatation and consequent stasis that appears early in pregnancy and persists for several weeks after delivery.

#### Optimum Treatment

The usual organism is *Escherichia coli* and initial therapy with two 3g doses of amoxicillin (12 hours apart) is recommended – if oral therapy can be tolerated. Other drugs (see chapter 2; sect. 7.5.1) should be reserved for treatment failure or known penicillin hypersensitivity. Where vomiting precludes oral therapy, intravenous therapy may be given.

Therapy of urinary infection should always be preceded by urine culture and the response checked by culture 7 to 10 days after treatment and then monthly, or again at 6 months if continuous therapy is given for refractory infections. Where the culture shows that the infecting organism is insensitive or resistant to amoxicillin, then the appropriate antibacterial drug should be chosen of the basis of sensitivity results, remembering that certain agents are relatively or completely contraindicated in pregnancy:

1) Even a few doses of a tetracycline in the second half of pregnancy can cause discolouration of unerupted teeth and possibly enamel hypoplasia. These drugs may also impair fetal bone growth, and so should never be administered in pregnancy (see chapter 2; sect. 7.5.3).

2) Sulfonamides should be avoided in late pregnancy because of the increased risk of kernicterus in the neonate (see also chapter 2; sect. 7.5.2). Sulfonamides (and nitrofurantoin) may also cause haemolytic anaemia in infants who are glucose-6-phosphate dehydrogenase (G6PD) deficient. The combination of a sulfonamide with trimethoprim (i.e. cotrimoxazole, trimethoprim/sulfamethoxazole) is no longer widely used as a first-line antimicrobial in the UK, although it is still commonly prescribed worldwide. Although it has not been linked with fetal growth inhibition or teratogenesis, there are theoretical reasons why this combination should be avoided if possible in pregnancy because of its effect on folate metabolism.

3) Aminoglycosides should be used with caution because of the possibility of 8th cranial nerve damage. Congenital ototoxicity (both cochlear and vestibular) has been linked to *in utero* exposure to streptomycin and kanamycin,[29] though not to the newer agents amikacin, gentamicin, netilmicin or tobramycin. Pregnancy *per se* would not contraindicate their use in severe infection.

If the urinary tract infection is not eradicated or recurs after initial therapy, a further 5- to 7-day course of therapy should be given. The possibility of continuing with a nightly dose of nitrofurantoin until the puerperium should also be considered.

***Asymptomatic bacteriuria*** occurs in 2 to 10% of pregnant women. Because these women are at increased risk of clinical urinary infection in pregnancy, antibacterial therapy has been suggested where the incidence is high.[30] This will reduce the incidence of clinical infection. A single-dose treatment may suffice.[31] If such a programme is being costed, elements to be included would be the cost of urine screening, prophylactic and therapeutic antibiotics, and possible savings on the cost of admissions avoided.

A more contentious issue is whether bacteriuria is the cause of other complications such as preterm delivery and low birthweight. There is no evidence that treatment with antibiotics will reduce these problems.[32]

### 3.3 Hypertension in Pregnancy

Hypertension is one of the most frequent complications of pregnancy, and remains one of the commonest causes of maternal death, even in advanced countries such as the UK[33] and the US.[34] *Essential* or *secondary hypertension* may be known about in advance and should be suspected if the blood pressure at first visit exceeds 140/90mm Hg. *Gestational hypertension* is present when the blood pressure exceeds 140/90mm Hg after 20 weeks of gestation. *Pre-eclampsia* is present when hypertension is complicated by the development of proteinuria >0.5 g/day. Pre-eclampsia may supervene in both pre-existing or gestational hypertension.

Irrespective of the cause of hypertension, both the mother and the fetus are at risk of complications, although the risks are greatest when pre-eclampsia occurs. Maternal complications include: eclampsia, stroke, renal failure, thrombocytopenia, microangiopathic haemolytic anaemia, abnormal liver function, placental abruption and antepartum haemorrhage. Fetal complications include growth retardation, intrauterine death, and increased perinatal morbidity and mortality as a result of immaturity.

#### *3.3.1 Optimum Treatment*

Antihypertensive therapy should be prescribed with a realistic expectation of what can be achieved. Most antihypertensive drugs will prevent increases in blood pressure, though the evidence that they greatly influence other outcomes is lacking. Severe hypertension *per se*, whatever the cause or mechanism, merits treatment as this will protect the mother from the risk of cerebral haemorrhage. The level of blood pressure that merits intervention remains a matter of debate, but as a general rule the higher the pressure, the greater the likely net benefit. Few would hesitate to initiate therapy in a patient with pressures sustained at levels in excess of 160mm Hg (systolic) and/or 110mm Hg (diastolic). At lower levels of blood pressure, the benefits of treatment are less certain, largely because most studies in this blood pressure range have lacked the statistical power to provide con-

**Table III.** Advantages and disadvantages of antihypertensive agents used during pregnancy

| Drugs | Advantages | Disadvantages/adverse effects |
|---|---|---|
| **Central $\alpha_2$-adrenoceptor agonists** | | |
| Methyldopa | Safe for fetus | *Central adverse effects:* drowsiness, lethargy, fatigue, depression, psychotic reactions (rare), nasal stuffiness, positive Coomb's test (haemolysis rare), jaundice |
| **β-Adrenoceptor antagonists** (β-blockers) | | |
| Acebutolol<br>Atenolol<br>Labetalol<br>Metoprolol<br>Oxprenolol<br>Propranolol | Good safety/efficacy if used in third trimester | Fetal growth retardation if used for prolonged periods from early pregnancy, airways obstruction, cold extremities, tremulousness (labetalol) |
| **Vasodilators** | | |
| Hydralazine | Good safety record (oral/intramuscular/intravenous) | Flushing, headache, tachycardia |
| Nifedipine | Good efficacy data | Flushing, headache, tachycardia, chest pain, leg oedema; wide interindividual variation in dosage requirements |
| Prazosin | Safety record good | Limited experience |
| Nitroglycerin (glyceryl trinitrate) | Intravenous in emergency only for speed/efficacy/rapid titration | Tolerance |
| **Thiazide diuretics** | | |
| Bendroflumethiazide<br>Chlorothiazide<br>Hydrochlorothiazide | Good safety record | Hyperuricaemia (dose-related) |

vincing results. In addition, several antihypertensive agents are known to have adverse effects and these must be balanced against the expected benefits.

In all forms of hypertension in pregnancy, there is little evidence that antihypertensive treatment consistently improves the fetal outcome in terms of growth retardation, intrauterine death or perinatal morbidity/mortality.[35] There are limited data to show that antihypertensive therapy with thiazides prevents the emergence of pre-eclampsia.[36] Once proteinuria has developed, antihypertensive therapy has little if any effect on fetal outcome, though some protection against maternal complications may still be achieved. In this situation, the role of antihypertensive therapy is principally to provide temporary maternal protection until delivery can be expedited.

Delivery of the placenta often results in rapid resolution of the hypertension, although in a significant number of patients the blood pressure may take days or weeks to resolve, and may never do so entirely if there had been antecedent hypertension. In eclampsia, it is important to include specific anthypertensive therapy as part of the treatment regimen (note that anticonvulsant medications do little themselves to reduce the blood pressure). Advances in obstetric anaesthesia and the judicious use of caesarean section or expedited delivery under epidural analgesia have had a major effect on maternal and fetal morbidity and mortality from this disease, though worldwide it remains a major management problem.

The clinical pharmacology of antihypertensive drugs is discussed in greater detail in chapter 21 (section 3). The principal advantages and disadvantages of the major drug groups used in pregnancy are summarised in table III, and several broad clinical scenarios are outlined below. For a discussion of the safety of antihypertensive drugs in pregnancy, see chapter 2 (section 7.2.1).

**Hypertension During Early Pregnancy**

*Methyldopa* remains first-line therapy for treatment of hypertension during early pregnancy. This centrally-acting drug is reasonably effective, though multiple daily doses and stepwise dosage titration is necessary. Initial data suggested that it might protect against midtrimester fetal death,[37] but this has not been confirmed.[38] Symptomatic maternal adverse effects can be troublesome but most women are prepared to tolerate the central effects of drowsiness, lassitude and nasal stuffiness for the duration of pregnancy. It is the only antihypertensive agent that has been shown to be safe for the fetus, and studies following offspring up to school age are reassuring that no adverse developmental effects occur.[39] However, the numbers of patients and studies showing this are relatively small.

β-*Adrenoceptor blocking drugs* should be avoided at this stage in pregnancy as there is some evidence that prolonged use may lead to fetal growth retardation.[40] *Thiazide diuretics* are not widely used at present, but may be more useful than is generally thought[36] and have a good record of safety and tolerability, particularly if used in low dosages.

*Angiotensin-converting enzyme (ACE) inhibitors* have proved fetotoxic in animal studies, may be associated with teratogenesis, and have adverse homeostatic effects on the fetus in late pregnancy, particularly on renal function (see further chapter 2; sect. 7.2.1). They are therefore contraindicated in pregnancy.

Some *dihydropyridine calcium antagonists* (e.g. nifedipine and nisoldipine) have shown a fetotoxic and teratogenic potential in animals,[41,42] and it would be prudent to bear this in mind when treating hypertension in young women. However, it is probable that high dosages of these drugs are necessary to produce these effects and their relevance to use in humans is unknown. Nevertheless, until further human data are available, the dihydropyridines are probably best avoided in early pregnancy.

#### Gestational Hypertension

Treatment should be started on the basis of perceived maternal risk. Any additional effects that may accrue, such as less time in hospital, less chance of developing proteinuria, should be regarded as a bonus rather than a major reason to start therapy. *Methyldopa* may be used, as at earlier stages, but β-blockers such as *atenolol, oxprenolol* and *labetalol* have all been shown to be as effective and probably as safe when prescribed in the third trimester. Nifedipine appears promising, but may be poorly tolerated and remains a second-line agent until further trials are reported and more experience obtained.

*Thiazide diuretics* are no longer widely used but many of their perceived disadvantages are theoretical rather than real. At least in essential hypertension, their long term blood pressure-lowering effect is attributable to a reduction in total peripheral resistance rather than to a sustained effect on plasma volume, and can be achieved by low dosages of thiazides that do not cause adverse biochemical or metabolic effects.[43,44] In pregnancy, it is possible that thiazides may restrict the normal increase in plasma volume but there is no evidence that this is harmful. Low-dose diuretic therapy has not been adequately evaluated in pregnancy-related hypertension. A recent meta-analysis of available trial data[36] concluded that there is overwhelming evidence to suggest that they prevent the rise in blood pressure, but these drugs are currently not favoured as first-line therapy. There is no clear evidence of benefit in respect of proteinuria, perinatal deaths, or stillbirth.

#### Pre-Eclampsia

Antihypertensive therapy may be used as in gestational hypertension, but it is essential to be alert to deterioration in the patient's condition and that of her fetus as conservative measures may need to be abandoned in favour of early delivery. In severe pre-eclampsia, parenteral antihypertensive therapy is often required. Intramuscular or intravenous *hydralazine* is commonly used despite its decline in popularity in non-obstetric practice. Disadvantages include lack of precision in controlling the response, uncertain duration of action, and reflex tachycardia with headache. Advantages are its long established use and absence of known serious fetal toxicity.

Oral or sublingual *nifedipine* has shown considerable promise in this situation.[45] Its effectiveness is, however, counterbalanced by dihydropyridine-related vasodilator adverse effects, such as flushing, headache, chest pain and peripheral oedema, some of which mimic the symptoms of pre-eclampsia itself. The magnitude and duration of response is also unpredictable and this is undesirable, particularly in patients requiring epidural anaesthesia which can itself lower the blood pressure.

Intravenous *nitroglycerin* has much to commend it – rapid onset, high efficacy, ready minute to minute dosage titration and lack of serious toxicity. Tachyphylaxis may occur after continuous infusion for several days, but this is not usually a problem in the context of pre-eclampsia. A relative dearth of clinical trial data[46] and unfamiliarity in obstetric circles currently limits its applicability.

*Labetalol* is a useful adjunct in this situation as it can be administered orally or by intravenous bolus or infusion and can have a useful complementary effect when combined with any of the vasodilators mentioned above.[38]

***Antiplatelet therapy in pre-eclampsia:*** severe pre-eclampsia may be complicated by a syndrome of haemolysis, intravascular platelet consumption, and abnormal liver function (HELLP syndrome). A falling platelet count in pre-eclampsia is usually regarded as an ominous prognostic feature. Attempts have been made to interrupt or reverse this process by using antiplatelet agents, including *aspirin* (acetylsalicylic acid) and *epoprostenol* (prostacyclin; prostaglandin $I_2$), but while early anecdotal experience was promising, this approach has not become established as a useful therapeutic option. When this syndrome develops, there is a strong case for early delivery rather than continued conservative management.[47]

Interest has also been generated in the hypothesis that less florid degrees of platelet consumption, possibly triggered by a fundamental disturbance in endothelial cell function, may predispose patients to the development of pre-eclampsia.[48] Several early uncontrolled studies[49,50] suggested that low-dose aspirin, administered to mothers perceived to be at high risk of developing pre-eclampsia, might prevent the onset of the syndrome and of the associated intrauterine growth retardation (IUGR). These initial hopes were subsequently dampened by a randomised study in 2985 normotensive primigravidae showing that although the use of aspirin decreased the incidence of pre-eclampsia (relative risk 0.7), it may have led to a slight increase in the risk of abruptio placentae.[51] A recent large multicentre trial has cast further doubts on the value of this form of therapy.[52] This study recruited women either with clinical features of pre-eclampsia or IUGR, or who were considered by their clinician to be at risk of developing such problems. The use of aspirin 60 mg/day was associated with a nonsignificant (12%) reduction in the risk of pre-eclampsia, with no useful effect on IUGR or on stillbirths and neonatal deaths. There was, however, a significant reduction in preterm delivery (14%). No adverse bleeding consequences were observed and aspirin was generally safe for the fetus and neonate.

The use of aspirin for this purpose can no longer be justified on a wide scale, although it is possible that in selected patients, low-dose aspirin may be of benefit in early onset pre-eclampsia. In their discussion of the results of this trial,[52] the investigators made the important observation that strikingly beneficial results from early small trials may have given a misleading impression of the true overall benefit from this form of therapy as a result of publication bias – those early studies with strongly positive results finding their way into the literature, while studies with negative or equivocal results did not.

### Eclampsia

In eclampsia, drugs are usually required for control of blood pressure, control of seizures, analgesia and sometimes anaesthesia. Rapid control of blood pressure is essential and the drugs suggested above for the management of severe pre-eclampsia are all appropriate. Epidural or spinal analgesia for urgent vaginal or operative delivery is often indicated, though its use is sometimes constrained by the presence of thrombocytopenia. This technique in itself will lower the blood pressure, sometimes to an unpredictable degree, and it is prudent to chose an antihypertensive regimen that can be readily titrated against the patient's response. General anaesthesia suffers the major disadvantage in this context of being accompanied by substantial increases in blood pressure, particularly during induction and endotracheal intubation.

Convulsions must also be controlled. Until recently, there was divergence of opinion and practice as how this should be achieved. In the US, there is a widespread preference for the use of parenteral *magnesium sulfate*. Although there is uncertainty about its mechanism of action, an empirical regimen based largely on the extensive experience with this drug at the Parkland Memorial Hospital in Dallas has become established practice.[53] A standard dosage is 4g intravenously plus 10g intramuscularly, followed by 5g intramuscularly every 4 hours. Impressive mortality data have been reported from specialist centres using this regimen, though these data may owe at least as much to the detailed protocols and intensive monitoring and other supportive care that such units provide. Excessive dosage of magnesium sulfate is characterised by disappearance of deep tendon reflexes and lethal respiratory depression can occur.

Other anticonvulsants that have been used include intravenous *diazepam* (10mg over 10 min followed by infusion of 3 mg/kg over 24 hours) and also *phenytoin*. A large randomised multicentre controlled trial of magnesium sulfate *versus* diazepam or phenytoin in women with eclampsia demonstrated the superiority of magnesium sulfate over these agents.[54] Not only did magnesium sulfate lower the risk of recurrent convulsions to a significantly greater extent than either diazepam or phenytoin, but it was also associated with a trend towards lower maternal mortality, and in comparison with phenytoin, lower fetal morbidity. Treatment can be intravenous or intramuscular, and routine monitoring of blood concentrations is not necessary. Because of the rarity of eclampsia, there are benefits in having available treatment packs with drugs and giving sets ready for use.

Prophylactic use of magnesium sulfate in the patient with features of impending eclampsia (clouding of consciousness, hyper-reflexia, liver tenderness, uncontrolled blood pressure) has not yet been properly evaluated and a multicentre trial is required. In hypertensive women who had not had a seizure, prophylactic magnesium sulfate was compared with phenytoin in a randomised trial.[55] Ten of 1089 women randomly assigned to phenytoin had eclamptic convulsions, as compared with none of 1049 women assigned to magnesium sulfate. Maternal and infant outcomes were similar in the 2 groups. A notable feature of this study was that eligible patients included those with a systolic blood pressure of at least 140mm Hg and diastolic blood pressure of at least 90mm Hg. Thus a large number of pregnant women – as many as 5% of all deliveries – might need to be treated to prevent approximately 1 seizure in 100 women at risk. This prophylactic regimen remains firmly established in the US, but there may be some resistance to its implementation elsewhere because of the logistical implications. If the patients at greatest risk could be identified, that would greatly increase the acceptance of this regimen.

#### *3.3.2 Clinical Outcome and Economic Considerations*

In the long term treatment of hypertension in the nonpregnant patient, the costs of therapy are of considerable importance because of the need for lifelong therapy (see further chapter 21). For the duration of a pregnancy, however, these costs are of much lesser significance compared with the costs of prolonged hospitalisation,[56] frequent clinic visits and the dire maternal consequences (albeit uncommon) of uncontrolled hypertension. A drug that protects the mother and improves the prognosis for the fetus would have additional economic advantages, whereas a drug that protects the mother but leads to even a slight increase in the risk of IUGR, premature delivery and perinatal morbidity might well have major adverse cost implications, particularly if the surviving offspring required prolonged intensive care support and/or lifelong special care. At present, there is little evidence that antihypertensive medication in pregnancy has much effect on fetal outcome.

The hope that aspirin might represent an inexpensive and widely applicable prophylaxis against the development of pre-eclampsia and IUGR has not been realised. However, the data from the CLASP study[52] suggest that this might still be useful in a selected cohort of women at risk of early onset of the syndrome. This form of therapy will almost certainly be cost effective, although identification of the women at risk seems likely to be an imperfect, difficult and relatively expensive process for the foreseeable future.

### 3.4 Oedema in Pregnancy

Oedema is physiologically normal in pregnancy and although in severe cases, it may be temporarily uncomfortable and disfiguring for the mother, it is not harmful to the fetus. Although oedema often occurs in association with pre-eclampsia, it is not pathognomonic of this syndrome.

In a recent meta-analysis of the prophylactic use of *diuretics* in normotensive women or in women without oedema or excessive weight gain,[36] overwhelming evidence was found for prevention of 'any form of pre-eclampsia', although there was no effect on the development of proteinuria or on the risk of perinatal death. It is suggested that this probably reflects the ability of diuretics to reduce blood pressure rather than any other mechanism.

There is little evidence to show that the use of diuretics in pregnancy to treat oedema *per se* is of any benefit. The use of loop diuretics may lead to an unnecessary and theoretically disadvantageous reductions in plasma volume and to troublesome secondary aldosteronism with hypokalaemia and rebound oedema. The use of low-dose thiazides to treat hypertension in pregnancy may be more useful and less harmful than previously thought (see section 3.3.1), but formal prospective studies are required to confirm this.

## 3.5 Thromboembolic Disease in Pregnancy

### *3.5.1 Venous Thromboembolism*

Thromboembolic disease remains an important cause of maternal morbidity and mortality in pregnancy and the puerperium. Pulmonary embolism is the commonest cause of maternal death during pregnancy in the UK.[33] Risk factors include increasing age, obesity, severe varicose veins, multiparity, immobility, thrombophilia, and a previous history of thromboembolism. The greatest risk occurs in the postpartum period, and in women requiring caesarean section the risk increases up to 5-fold.[57]

Objective confirmation of the diagnosis is essential. In the case of suspected deep vein thrombosis, this will usually require duplex ultrasound scanning, which is accurate for ileofemoral thrombi, supplemented by ascending venography if uncertainty remains. In the case of suspected pulmonary embolism, ventilation perfusion scanning is mandatory. Indeterminate lung scans may need to be supplemented by duplex ultrasound scanning of leg veins and pulmonary angiography if there is residual uncertainty.

#### Optimum Treatment

Treatment should be started with intravenous *heparin* in full dosage for 7 days to achieve a 2-fold prolongation of the activated partial thromboplastin time (APTT). Continuation of therapy depends on the stage of pregnancy. If the thromboembolism occurs antepartum, heparin should be continued for the duration of pregnancy by switching to subcutaneous injections. In patients who cannot tolerate this approach, warfarin may be substituted. Two weeks prior to term, the patient should be hospitalised and changed back to continuous intravenous heparin, which can be discontinued 4 hours before delivery to minimise the risks of bleeding, restarted within 4 hours after delivery, and either continued for 6 weeks postpartum or until a therapeutic dosage of warfarin has been reintroduced. If the thromboembolism occurs postpartum, the initial therapy with heparin should be followed by warfarin therapy for a minimum of 3 months. Warfarin therapy is not a contraindication to breast feeding.

***Prophylaxis*** should be considered in all women with a previous history of venous thromboembolism, and in those with known thrombophilia or additional risk factors. Timing and duration will depend on individual circumstances. In most cases, prophylaxis should be continued postpartum for a minimum of 6 weeks, usually with warfarin. If antepartum prophylaxis is required, subcutaneous heparin should be used (7500 to 10,000IU every 12 hours). Early ambulation, intermittent pneumatic calf compression or graduated elastic stockings may also be helpful.

Authoritative guidelines on these issues have recently been published (see THRIFT Consensus Group[58]; Scottish Intercollegiate Guidelines Network[59]; Royal College of Gynaecologists & Obstetricians[60]).

### *3.5.2 Prosthetic Heart Valves*

Bioprosthetic valves do not normally require anticoagulation unless the patient is in atrial fibrillation. This had been considered a potential advantage of this type of valve in young women, but it is now recognised that these valves deteriorate alarmingly during pregnancy and should no longer be used in this age group. A recent audit showed that in patients with mechanical heart valves, warfarin treatment was safe and effective and was not associated with embryopathy.[61] In the same survey, heparin was associated with more thromboembolic complications and episodes of bleeding, including maternal fatalities. Warfarin dosage should be tailored to the type of prosthesis used, with lower intensity of anticoagulation required for second generation valves, aiming for tight control within an international normalised ratio (INR; see chapter 26; sect. 3.1.5) range of 2 to 3.

### *3.5.3 Avoiding Problems with Anticoagulants in Pregnancy*

Reported spontaneous abortion rates vary widely between series, but it is likely that both warfarin and heparin may increase the risk by predisposing patients to placental haemorrhage. Assiduous control of dosages should minimise the risk. High dosages of warfarin may have an added direct fetotoxic effect. In later pregnancy, heparin probably carries little risk to the fetus.

Thrombocytopenia occurs in about 0.3% of patients given porcine heparin. If heparin is given for more than 5 days, platelet counts must be monitored regularly and if the problem persists, heparin must be stopped. Low molecular weight (LMW) heparins are mixtures of oligosaccharides with molecular weights in the range 2500 to 8000D, compared with a range of 5000 to 30,000D for standard heparins (see further chapter 26; sect. 3.1.4).[62] Compared with standard heparins, LMW preparations have improved bioavailability from subcutaneous sites and a longer, more predictable, elimination half-life and duration of action. They also have less effect on platelets. It is unlikely that even LMW heparins would cross the placenta, but experience with these drugs in pregnancy is limited. The most uncertain problem with long term heparin use in pregnancy is osteoporosis, which is difficult to predict and to detect.

Warfarin readily crosses the placenta and has been associated with embryopathy.[63] Exposure between 6 and 12 weeks' gestation has been linked with a number of abnormalities, including nasal hypoplasia and chondrodysplasia punctata.[64] Exposure during later pregnancy is linked with a variety of central nervous system (CNS) abnormalities, but these are probably rare. In both situations, it is possible that a common mechanism relates to haemorrhage into the respective tissues. Debate continues on the exact risk of these abnormalities. It is possible that published reports reflect a bias in favour of reporting abnormal findings; several recent audits have failed to detect warfarin embryopathy. It is still prudent, however, to aim for the tightest possible quality of control.

Warfarin increases the risks of maternal haemorrhage from the uterus, episiotomy and abdominal incisions at the time of delivery and postpartum, and fetal intracranial haemorrhage, especially if delivery is traumatic or premature. For this reason, it is preferable to switch temporarily to intravenous heparin to cover the anticipated time of delivery, since its anticoagulant effect is easier to control and reverse.

#### *3.5.4 Clinical Outcome and Economic Considerations*

In terms of direct pharmacy costs, neither unfractionated heparin nor warfarin are expensive drugs. LMW heparins are more expensive, but there are few indications for their use in pregnancy. The main costs attributable to either warfarin or heparin use relate to the need for monitoring the anticoagulant response. For low-dose prophylactic heparin, no monitoring is usually necessary (except perhaps antepartum). During pregnancy, it is recommended that monitoring of full-dose heparin and warfarin be even more intense than usual and that tight control is maintained. Evidence that this strategy is cost-effective is lacking, but it makes good sense if only as an arbitrary measure to ensure a satisfactory fetal outcome.

A recent report indicated that, excluding spontaneous abortions, delivery of a healthy neonate should be possible in over 80% of pregnancies in patients with mechanical heart valves.[61] However, women with mechanical heart valves given heparin instead of warfarin during pregnancy run a substantial risk of valve thrombosis, systemic embolism and death. Even without a formal economic analysis, there seems little doubt that the preferred management of these patients includes warfarin, especially if there is little risk of embryopathy with good control.

There is wide consensus that prophylaxis with anticoagulants against venous thromboembolism is both life-saving and cost-effective in reducing the risks of nonfatal symptomatic thromboembolism.

### 3.6 Nausea and Vomiting of Pregnancy

Nausea and vomiting in the first trimester of pregnancy are common, but are due to physiological changes in most cases and usually do not require drug therapy.

#### Optimum Treatment

When symptoms are troublesome, an antiemetic may be necessary. Dicyclomine/doxylamine/pyridoxine was a popular choice, but it was withdrawn for medicolegal reasons, although there is no evidence that it was teratogenic. A doxylamine/pyridoxine combination is still available in Canada for use in nausea and vomiting of pregnancy (see chapter 2; sect. 7.3).

Alternatives include *pyridoxine,* antihistamines such as *cyclizine,* or phenothiazines such as *prochlorperazine*.[65] With the latter, dystonic reactions may occur in a small number of cases, especially if treatment is prolonged.

Prompt outpatient treatment may be cost effective if it reduces the need for admission and intravenous fluid replacement.

### 3.7 Heartburn of Pregnancy

This occurs in the second and third trimester of pregnancy, probably as a result of relaxation of the lower oesophageal sphincter by progesterone.

#### Optimum Treatment

Attention to diet, correction of obesity and avoidance of bending or a supine posture usually help, but a number of women will also need antacid therapy. In refractory cases, a histamine $H_2$-receptor antagonist such as *cimetidine* or *ranitidine* may be used. These drugs are also of value in reducing the volume and acidity of gastric secretions in women about to undergo operative delivery, when they may reduce the risk of aspiration pneumonitis.[66]

Metoclopramide is not recommended because of its propensity to induce dystonic reactions in young women.[67] The safety of omeprazole has not been established in pregnancy, and misoprostol is absolutely contraindicated because it causes abortion and fetal malformations.

## 3.8 Asthma

This is a common condition and its associated morbidity and mortality remains a cause for serious concern. Asthma worsens during pregnancy in a significant proportion of patients[68] and about 10% of pregnant women with asthma will experience exacerbations during labour. Maternal asthma is associated with increased perinatal mortality and intrauterine growth retardation.[69] There is a small but important risk of maternal death, particularly with severe disease. An adverse outcome is more likely if asthma is poorly controlled. It is, thus, important to be aware of the diagnosis, to assess its severity accurately and objectively and to ensure rapid and aggressive treatment of exacerbations and complications.

### Optimum Treatment

In general, asthma management should follow the guidelines recommended for the nonpregnant patient (see chapter 23; sect. 3.2). There is no clear evidence that $\beta_2$-agonists or corticosteroids are teratogenic or fetotoxic and these drugs should form the mainstay of therapy – given by inhalation, orally or intravenously as appropriate in usual dosages.

***Avoiding problems in treatment:*** when an asthmatic mother is receiving long term oral corticosteroid therapy, she may suffer adrenocortical insufficiency when subjected to the stress of delivery or its complications and may require supplemental doses. Both hydrocortisone and prednisolone are metabolised by placental enzyme activity to inactive metabolites and as a result, the risks of fetal pituitary suppression are slight, although careful monitoring of the neonate should be undertaken to ensure that hypoadrenalism does not go undetected. Certain other elementary precautions should be observed in the asthmatic patient, e.g. avoidance of drugs that may precipitate airway obstruction, such as β-blockers, aspirin and dinoprost (prostaglandin $F_{2\alpha}$).

## 3.9 Other Conditions Requiring Corticosteroid Therapy

Conditions other than asthma that may require corticosteroid therapy during pregnancy include inflammatory bowel disease, systemic lupus erythematosus, lymphoreticular malignancies, uveitis, renal transplantation and a variety of chronic inflammatory diseases. As a general rule, if the diagnosis is secure and the indication for corticosteroid therapy firmly established, then these drugs should be prescribed as in the nonpregnant patient, observing the precautions mentioned in section 3.8.

The use of corticosteroids in preterm labour is discussed in section 5.2.

## 3.10 Diabetes Mellitus

In a normal pregnancy, carbohydrate tolerance improves in the first trimester. In the second and third trimester, insulin resistance develops as a result of increasing concentrations of progesterone, human placental lactogen, cortisol and prolactin. In the last few weeks, the rapidly growing fetus may consume so much glucose that maternal carbohydrate tolerance improves again. These changes are reflected in the changing insulin requirements of diabetic patients during pregnancy.[21] Most diabetic patients who become pregnant are insulin-dependent, although a small number of older women will have non-insulin-dependent diabetes. Gestational diabetes mellitus develops in up to 10% of pregnancies, depending on the definitions used. Apart from the usual maternal complications of diabetes, the fetus is also at risk.

There is evidence that hyperglycaemia at the time of conception results in an increased incidence of congenital malformations. In later pregnancy, fetal hyperinsulinaemia may cause increased growth, organomegaly and neonatal hypoglycaemia.[70]

### Optimum Treatment

In all diabetic patients, strict dietary measures and insulin are the mainstays of management. Various management strategies have been proposed, but the preferred regimen incorporates human insulin administered as intensified conventional therapy (see further chapter 19; sect. 3.3.2).[21]

***Avoiding problems in treatment:*** management of the pregnant diabetic patient should always be undertaken in consultation with a specialist in that disease. Ideally, prepregnancy counselling and planning should be undertaken to ensure maximum understanding of the disease and compliance with therapy. Strict euglycaemic control reduces the risks of malformation and perinatal morbidity.[71] This may be at the expense of maternal hypoglycaemia and some reversible deterioration in background retinopathy in early pregnancy. Drugs that may impair glucose tolerance, such as $\beta_2$-agonists, are contraindicated and oral antidiabetic drugs are no longer used during pregnancy.

### 3.11 Hyperthyroidism

Graves' disease is by far the most common cause of this problem in pregnant women.

#### Optimum Treatment

Hyperthyroidism is treated in the same way as in nonpregnant patients, except that radioiodine cannot be used (see chapter 19; sect. 5.2.2). Carbimazole crosses the placenta and although this may be useful in controlling presumed coincidental fetal hyperthyroidism, it may cause hypothyroidism and goitre in the fetus. Dosages should be kept to a minimum and if possible stopped 4 weeks before delivery, to avoid fetal hypothyroidism at the time of maximum brain growth and development. Subtotal thyroidectomy can be undertaken with reasonable safety in the second trimester, but definitive thyroid ablative therapy is best postponed until after delivery.

Carbimazole may appear in significant concentrations in breast milk, although there is little evidence that this is harmful to the infant. The excretion of propylthiouracil into breast milk is negligible.

### 3.12 Epilepsy

Seizures may become more frequent in pregnancy, particularly during labour and in the puerperium. Offspring are at increased risk of stillbirth, mental retardation and congenital malformations, as well as epilepsy in later life. The risk of teratogenesis increases with the number of seizures and with the number of antiepileptic drugs used.

#### Optimum Treatment

Every attempt should be made to control seizures using monotherapy (see further chapter 29; sect. 4.2). *Phenytoin* is highly effective, but causes hirsutism and gum hyperplasia that may be undesirable in young women. It has also been implicated in the development of cleft lip and palate and, rarely, in a fetal hydantoin syndrome. *Phenobarbital* may share some of these teratogenic effects and in addition causes a neonatal withdrawal syndrome and may predispose to haemorrhagic disease of the neonate.

*Valproic acid* has been linked with neural tube defects, and has been associated with the development of menstrual disturbances, polycystic ovaries and hyperandrogenism in a high proportion of women with epilepsy.[72] These problems raise serious concerns about the use of this otherwise effective drug in the treatment of women in their reproductive years.

*Carbamazepine* does not share the adverse cosmetic effects of phenytoin or the endocrine effects of valproic acid, but it does cause sedation, unsteadiness and mild cognitive impairment at higher dosages. Until recently, it was thought not to be implicated in teratogenesis when used as monotherapy but this may not be correct. Carbamazepine has been reported to be associated with a syndrome of minor craniofacial abnormalities, fingernail hypoplasia and developmental delay in a substantial proportion of offspring.[73] Perhaps more disturbingly, this drug has also been implicated in an increased risk of spina bifida.[74] In this report, the 'background' risk of spina bifida was quoted as 1 in 1500, whereas for a pooled estimate of the risk in offspring of mothers on carbamazepine it was 1 in 109, and on valproic acid 1 in 68.

It is possible that no antiepileptic drug is entirely free from teratogenic potential. Prepregnancy counselling and optimisation of therapy is recommended. All women receiving antiepileptic drugs and planning to become pregnant should be offered prophylactic folic acid (see section 1.1.1). Screening by ultrasound and measurement of $\alpha$-fetoprotein concentrations should be made available to pregnant women at risk.

### 3.13 Human Immunodeficiency Virus (HIV) Infection in Pregnancy

Because pregnant women and neonates are routinely offered blood tests, anonymous non-attributable HIV screening has been done in the UK to estimate the population prevalence of positivity. In areas of high prevalence, attributable screening may be offered, to allow counselling of the mother about: (a) the theoretical possibility of exacerbation of the disease because of immunological changes in pregnancy; (b) about the 15% risk that the fetus may be infected;[75] and (c) the possibility that the neonate may be infected by breast feeding.[76]

Some mothers may chose to terminate the pregnancy. For those who continue, the risk of vertical transmission may be reduced by two-thirds by *zidovudine* 100mg 5 times daily.[77] However, the long term outcomes of this therapy are not yet known. The cost implications of screening and treating at risk patients are substantial.[78]

## 4. Threatened Miscarriage

Because the cause of most miscarriages is not known even after investigations are complete, any therapy is speculative. Treatment with progesterone was widely practised for many years, but seems on meta-analysis of controlled trials, not to be effective.[79] Inadequate data are available on the value of human chorionic gonadotrophin (hCG). Immunotherapy became fashionable in the 1980s, but has now been shown to be ineffective.[80] Much more research in this area is needed.

## 5. Preterm Labour

### 5.1 Tocolytic Therapy

Uterine contractions associated with inappropriate preterm labour may be inhibited by $\beta_2$-adrenoceptor agonists such as *salbutamol, fenoterol, terbutaline, ritodrine* or *isoxsuprine* given by intravenous infusion in dosages that inhibit contractions. Unfortunately, the dosages required are relatively high and induce maternal adverse effects including tachycardia, hypotension, vomiting, hyperglycaemia, hypokalaemia and, more seriously, myocardial ischaemia, arrhythmias and pulmonary oedema.[20] Numerous fatalities have been reported.

Meta-analysis of randomised controlled trials[81] shows that these drugs do prolong pregnancy, but with no consequent benefit in terms of perinatal outcome. Because of the maternal hazards, they should, therefore, be used only short term (e.g. for transfer to a delivery setting with neonatal intensive care facilities or to allow time for corticosteroid administration to facilitate lung maturation in the soon-to-be-delivered premature infant), and only under the most careful maternal monitoring. The concomitant administration of large volumes of intravenous fluids, particularly saline, probably contributes to the risk of pulmonary oedema and death.

Indomethacin prolongs gestation,[82] but may cause premature closure of the ductus arteriosus, in addition to necrotising enterocolitis and intracranial haemorrhage.[83] Similarly, nifedipine has been used for this purpose, but its safety and effectiveness have not yet been clearly established. This effect of nifedipine could be an advantage in a hypertensive patient at risk of preterm labour, but may diminish uterine tone sufficiently to be a disadvantage in a patient in whom a prompt delivery is desirable. A recent report suggests that nitroglycerin (glyceryl trinitrate) transdermal patches may delay the onset of labour for up to a month, with minimal adverse effects.[84] If this observation is confirmed by prospective randomised trial, it may prove to be a major advance in the treatment of this condition.

### 5.2 Corticosteroids and Thyrotrophin-Releasing Hormone

Where preterm delivery (either spontaneous or planned) is anticipated and cannot be averted, antenatal administration of *betamethasone* 24mg over 48 hours will significantly reduce the incidence and severity of neonatal respiratory distress syndrome (RDS),[85] with consequent reduction in perinatal mortality. It is not, as was thought earlier, contraindicated in women with hypertension. There is conflicting evidence on whether the use of thyrotrophin-releasing hormone (TRH; protirelin) in addition to corticosteroids may further reduce the incidence of neonatal RDS, and more trials are needed.[86]

Because the care of very-low birthweight neonates is enormously expensive, it is likely that the use of corticosteroids may be cost-effective. However, a detailed analysis would have to include the cost of care for handicaps in a proportion of survivors.

## 6. Induction and Augmentation of Labour

Induction of labour may be required for maternal reasons, e.g. to prevent further deterioration in fulminating pre-eclampsia, or because of fetal compromise. It is also recommended in post-term pregnancy,[87] where a modest reduction in perinatal mortality has been reported, with no increase in the caesarian section rate.

Augmentation of labour has been advocated in nulliparae to reduce the caesarian section rate. However, a recent randomised trial has shown no such effect, although labour was shorter.[88]

In women with prelabour rupture of the membranes at term, a large prospective randomised trial compared induction of labour using either intravenous oxytocin or vaginal dinoprostone (prostaglandin $E_2$) with expectant management. No significant differences were observed in the rates of neonatal infection or caesarian section. Induction of labour with oxytocin resulted in a lower risk of clinical chorioamnionitis and a reduced need for antibiotic therapy. Women given oxytocin also experienced shorter labour.[89]

### 6.1 Oxytocin Administration

If the cervix is ripe, induction of labour is usually performed by forewater rupture, followed after 2 to 3 hours by intravenous oxytocin if labour does not become established. The intravenous route is chosen to allow titration of the dosage according to the uterine response, so that regular contractions of good tone and duration are achieved without hypertonus, which may cause fetal anoxia or even uterine rupture. Infusion pumps are used to control the dosage (with fluid restriction to avoid water intoxication from the antidiuretic effect), and uterine contractions must be monitored by external or internal tocography. Continuous monitoring of the fetal heart is essential.

### 6.2 Prostaglandins

If the cervix is unripe, the vaginal administration of *dinoprostone* (prostaglandin $E_2$) in tablet or gel form will improve the cervical score and in some cases will actually start labour.[82] However, there is a risk of gastrointestinal adverse effects (diarrhoea) and of uterine hypertonus. Fetal heart rate monitoring is essential.

When vaginal prostaglandins are compared with intravenous oxytocin,[90] the caesarean section rate is lower, but there are more gastrointestinal adverse effects. Mothers may prefer a vaginal preparation to an intravenous infusion (as more 'natural' and allowing more mobility), but fetal monitoring is essential.

### 6.3 Antiprogestagens

*Mifepristone* (RU486) has been successfully used before induction of labour in cases of intrauterine death. In a dosage of 200mg twice daily it shortens the interval to delivery,[91] which is a great benefit for distressed women who would otherwise tend to have long labour. This drug has also been tried for induction of labour in normal women,[92] but more information is required on neonatal outcome before it can be recommended for routine use. For a review of mifepristone, see Brogden et al.[93]

### 6.4 Clinical Outcome and Economic Considerations

Provided that adverse effects can be averted or minimised, shortening of labour would have important economic benefits in terms of saving staff costs, though the need for monitoring and hospital confinement need to be taken into consideration.

## 7. Third Stage of Labour

The mechanism of haemostasis in the third stage of labour is uterine contraction. While this does happen naturally, blood loss at delivery can be reduced by the use of oxytocic drugs. These drugs have been used since the 1950s, but routine use was only subjected to formal evaluation relatively recently. Meta-analysis of all identifiable trials[94] shows conclusively that routine oxytocic use reduces the rate of postpartum haemorrhage, but increases maternal blood pressure.

The available drugs are *ergometrine*, an ergot alkaloid that can be given by intramuscular or intravenous routes (alone or in combination with oxytocin), and *oxytocin*, which can also be given alone by either route. The intramyometrial route may also be used in severe postpartum haemorrhage. A comparison of oxytocin alone *versus* oxytocin and ergometrine in a randomised controlled trial showed that for routine prophylactic use, oxytocin alone is preferable, because there are fewer adverse effects (nausea, vomiting, hypertension) and no difference in the haemorrhage rate.[95] In the event of significant postpartum haemorrhage, evidence from clinical trials is more difficult to obtain, but intravenous ergometrine should be used despite its adverse effects.

## 8. Lactation Enhancement and Suppression

### 8.1 Enhancement

Lactation can be enhanced by the use of *sulpiride,* a dopamine antagonist,[96] but this is not widely used, and natural methods of increasing milk supply (by increasing suckling frequency) are to be preferred.

### 8.2 Suppression

Some women wish to suppress lactation despite the advantages of breast feeding. Lactation can be suppressed naturally by not suckling the infant, with supportive measures such as binders and mild analgesics. However, drug treatment, although expensive, may be indicated if lactation is contraindicated, e.g. by prior breast sepsis or surgery, or if there has been a late miscarriage or perinatal death. Dopamine receptor agonists such as *bromocriptine* or *cabergoline* have replaced all other methods of drug inhibition of lactation. They appear to be specific at the pituitary level in preventing the release of prolactin. The dosage of bromocriptine is 2.5mg twice daily for 2 weeks. Cabergoline has a longer duration of action and can be given as a single oral dose of 1mg after delivery. Nausea, headaches and dizziness may be a problem, but are less likely with cabergoline. Prompt attention to contraception is necessary, as ovulation is expedited.

## 9. Induced Abortion

Although surgery is still widely used, developments in pharmacology have resulted in a wider choice of methods for the procedure of abortion, including the option of medical methods alone at certain durations of gestation.

The major innovation has been the introduction of *mifepristone,* a synthetic norsteroid which has a high affinity for progesterone receptors in the uterus.[97] It therefore removes the inhibitory effect of progesterone on uterine activity, causes uterine contractions and increases the sensitivity of the uterus to prostaglandin administration. Neither drug alone is as effective as the 2 combined, and mifepristone is most effective when given 24 to 48 hours before the prostaglandin. There are no significant adverse effects except antiglucocorticoid activity, and nausea and vomiting in a few cases.

*Misoprostol,* a prostaglandin $E_1$ analogue, is marketed primarily as a treatment for peptic ulcer disease (see chapter 22; sect. 4.2.3). When used in combination with mifepristone, it results in abortion in a high proportion of pregnancies.[98] Because of its widespread availability in non-obstetric practice, there is a serious potential for its abuse as an abortifacient under unsupervised conditions, particularly in underdeveloped countries.[99-101] Used on its own, misoprostol causes expulsion of the fetus in less than half of cases, the survivors then being exposed to the substantial teratogenic effects of the drug.[102]

### 9.1 Therapeutic Abortion

Early in gestation (up to 9 weeks), many women prefer surgical termination by vacuum extraction, but medical termination should be available for women who prefer it or who are unsuitable for general or local anaesthesia. A single dose of oral *mifepristone* 600mg is given, followed 48 hours later by *gemeprost* (a prostaglandin $E_1$ analogue) 1mg vaginally or *misoprostol* orally or vaginally (note that misoprostol has a lower acquisition cost than gemeprost). The prostaglandin will then result in a complete evacuation of the uterus within 4 to 6 hours in 98% of women.[103] Abdominal cramps often develop and some form of analgesia is usually required. If an opioid analgesic is used, the patient should be monitored for signs of hypotension. Medical abortion is less expensive than surgical, according to Henshaw et al.[104]

From 9 to 13 weeks' gestation, the preferred method of termination is vacuum aspiration under local or general anaesthesia. If the woman is 17 years of age or less, or has a pregnancy of more than 10 weeks' gestation, the cervix should be primed, or rendered easier to dilate surgically, by using *gemeprost* 1mg vaginally 4 hours preoperatively, or *mifepristone* 200mg orally 36 hours preoperatively or 600mg vaginally 4 hours preoperatively. This reduces the force required to dilate the cervix and reduces the operative blood loss.[103,105]

Second trimester termination can be performed surgically, but medical methods are increasingly preferred, especially since *mifepristone* has become available. It is given in a dose of 600mg 24 to 48 hours before commencing a 4-hourly course of *gemeprost, meteneprost* or *misoprostol* pessaries, and significantly reduces the rate of abdominal pain, diarrhoea and vomiting and the prostaglandin to abortion interval.[106]

### 9.2 Nonviable Pregnancy

Where ultrasonic scanning has shown a nonviable pregnancy, evacuation may be accomplished within 3 days by the use of oral mifepristone 600mg. This method may in time become preferable to surgical evacuation.

## 10. Fertility Control

Although a number of other contraceptive techniques are available, and indeed commonly used, hormonal steroid contraception is overwhelmingly the most widely used reversible method in developed countries. This is mainly because it is the most effective method in terms of pregnancy rates, but also because it is simple and convenient, does not interrupt the sexual act, and is taken by women who are naturally better motivated to adopt effective contraceptive techniques.

### 10.1 Hormonal Steroid Preparations

#### *10.1.1 Continuous Low-Dose Oral Progestagens*

Several progestagens (progestins; progestogens) are available in continuous low-dose formulations, including *norethisterone* (norethindrone), *ethynodiol diacetate* and *levonorgestrel*. The mode of action of progestagens is complex and may include effects on cervical mucus, endometrial function and tubal transport mechanisms. Pregnancy rates are slightly higher than with combined estrogen/progestagen preparations and it is essential that women take these formulations within a narrow dosage window of a few hours on a daily basis.

The main symptomatic adverse effect of low-dose progestagens is irregular menstrual bleeding, and in some women the worry that they may have missed a period and could be pregnant is a considerable strain. This form of contraception is particularly suited to lactating mothers and to women in whom estrogens are contraindicated, such as hypertensive or diabetic patients, women with a history of venous thromboembolism, and smokers over the age of 35 years.

#### *10.1.2 Depot Progestagens (Injectable and Subdermal)*

##### Injectable Preparations

Intramuscular *medroxyprogesterone acetate* is administered in a dosage of 150mg every 3 months. Intramuscular *norethisterone* is given in a dosage of 200mg every 2 months for the first 4 injections and then every 3 months.

Menstrual irregularities are inevitable and amenorrhoea is common with these agents, but they are otherwise highly effective, safe and convenient.[107] The main factor that has limited their more widespread use is the observation that high doses of depot medroxyprogesterone acetate may cause breast tumours in beagles, but this is no longer considered to be relevant to use in humans. This reassurance was reflected by the granting of official FDA approval for the use of medroxyprogesterone acetate for this indication in 1992.

Depot progestagens act primarily by inhibiting ovulation. Consistent, clinically significant disturbances in carbohydrate or lipid metabolism or in blood coagulation have not been observed. Depot medroxyprogesterone acetate does not increase the risk of breast, ovarian or cervical cancer, and may even reduce the risk of endometrial cancer.[108] This method of contraception is suitable for women susceptible to anaemia, particularly if haemoglobinopathy is present.[109] There may also be advantages from this method in women with epilepsy requiring antiepileptic medication.[110]

##### Subdermal Implants

Recently, *levonorgestrel* has become available for subdermal implantation ('Norplant'). This formulation releases the progestagen to provide a contraceptive effect over 5 years. A trocar is used to place the capsules under the skin of the upper arm under local anaesthetic. These must be removed in the case of pregnancy or intercurrent thromboembolic disease. Initial experience suggests that many women request that the capsules be removed within the 5-year lifespan of the implant, and to some extent this negates the main advantage of the technique – i.e. its long duration of action.

The main problem with this form of contraception, not seen with other forms, is infection at the site of implantation. In some patients, such as those with diabetes, this can cause major problems, and excision of the implanted area may be needed if an abscess forms. This is a relatively expensive form of contraception, especially taking into account the trained staff required to supervise the insertion and removal of the implants, and it has limited applicability at the present time.

#### *10.1.3 Vaginal Long-Acting Progestagens*

Vaginal silicone rings can be impregnated with a progestagen or a combination of an estrogen and a progestagen. This gives slow release, constant blood steroid concentrations, good compliance and maximum local effects with minimal systemic effects.[111] These agents probably act by a local effect on the uterus. Vaginal rings need to be changed every 3 to 6 months, but this is often an acceptable alterna-

**Table IV.** Adverse effects of hormonal contraceptives

| Effect | Comment[a] |
|---|---|
| Liver function abnormalities | Minor abnormalities, probably not harmful; avoid estrogens in overt jaundice or cholestasis |
| Porphyria | Estrogens may exacerbate hepatic, variegate or acute intermittent porphyrias |
| Psychological | Progestagens may cause depression and/or loss of libido |
| Hypertension | Estrogens often cause increased blood pressure, occasionally to hypertensive levels, rarely to accelerated phase. Reversal of blood pressure rise may take months. In hypertensive women, avoid estrogens and monitor regularly while using alternatives |
| Venous thromboembolism | Risk directly related to estrogen dose, but occasionally reported even with 25 μg/day preparations. Third-generation preparations containing desogestrel or gestodene appear to carry an increased relative risk (see section 10.2.1). Previous deep venous thrombosis, obesity, venous insufficiency, thrombophilia and major surgery increase the risk |
| Myocardial infarction[b] | Oral contraceptives join other risk factors including smoking, hyperlipidaemia, hypertension, family history, diabetes, age over 35 years |
| Stroke[b] | Increased risk of thrombotic stroke, even with low-dose estrogen preparations. Very slight increase in risk of subarachnoid haemorrhage. |
| Neoplasia | *Breast cancer:*[c] impressive evidence of no increase in risk, except possibly with long term oral contraceptive use in patients <35 years |
| | *Cervical cancer:* increase in risk of *in situ* and invasive disease; mechanism may relate to sexual habits; cytological screening recommended |
| | *Hepatic tumours:* substantially increased risk of adenomas; large interethnic variation in prevalence of hepatocellular carcinoma makes risk of oral contraceptive use difficult to ascertain; increased relative risk from long term use in developed countries (where absolute risk is low) |

a Most risk relationships ascertained by cohort or case control studies in women on combined sequential pills with relatively high estrogen content. Data about low-dose preparations, including biphasic and triphasic formulations, are sparse. Changing patterns of oral contraceptive-attributable disease may be due as much to changes in awareness, screening procedures and selection of patients as to changes in formulation. The relative risk of venous thromboembolism associated with low-dose estrogen products containing desogestrel or gestodene, compared with products containing norethisterone or levonorgestrel, is 2-fold. The absolute risk remains low at ≈30 events per 100,000 woman-years. The influence of third-generation oral contraceptives on the risks of myocardial infarction and stroke has yet to be ascertained.

b Risk of myocardial infarction and thrombotic stroke is largely confined to current users only. Risk of myocardial infarction and thrombotic stroke is additive or synergistic with cigarette smoking, particularly in women over 35 years of age.

c Breast cancer remains a major source of anxiety. Although no definite cause-and-effect relationship has been established, concerns persist about effects in women who start oral contraceptives at a young age and use them for long periods of time. The interval between such use and emergence of clinical signs may be such that we are only now about to see the effects of extensive long term use in the cohort of women approaching late middle age.

tive to regular tablet taking or intermittent injections.

### *10.1.4 Copper and Progestagen-Containing Intrauterine Contraceptive Devices (IUCDs)*

In general, modern copper-containing IUCDs are simple to use, with good long term effectiveness and few adverse effects, and are particularly useful for multiparous women. Many devices contain copper, which has a local action without systemic effects. The main disadvantages of such devices are a slight increase in the risk of ectopic pregnancy, a definite increase in the risk of pelvic inflammatory disease, and an increase in blood loss at menstruation.

Progestagen-containing IUCDs (e.g. *levonorgestrel*) do not suffer from the disadvantage of increasing menstrual blood loss and may even decrease it.[112] This appears to be a highly effective method but is still undergoing clinical evaluation in the UK. Because of the relatively large size of the device, it is recommended that first insertions be done during menstruation or immediately after pregnancy termination, when the cervix is dilated. Expulsion rates are no higher than with conventional IUCDs.

### *10.1.5 Combined Estrogen/Progestagen Oral Contraceptives*

This is by far the most widely used type of oral contraceptive in the UK. The progestagen component (19-nortestosterone derivatives such as *norethisterone, norgestrel, levonorgestrel, norgestimate, ethynodiol diacetate, desogestrel* and *gestodene*) is present in daily doses of 0.075 to 2mg, and the estrogen component (*ethinylestradiol* or *mestranol*) in daily doses of 0.02 to 0.05mg. These preparations act primarily by inhibiting secretion of follicle-stimulating hormone (FSH) and luteinising hormone (LH), thereby suppressing ovulation. Additional actions on the endometrium, tubal motility and cervical mucus enhance the contraceptive effect. Effectiveness is maintained and estrogenic adverse effects minimised by using daily doses of less than 0.05mg estrogen. Fixed ratio combinations may be given either as 21 to 22 days of active medication or as continuous medication with prepackaged placebo for 7 days to optimise compliance. Lower total doses may be achieved by the use of biphasic or triphasic preparations, in which the dosages of both estrogen and progestagen are altered throughout the cycle.

The adverse effects of oral contraceptive steroids are discussed further in section 10.2 and are summarised in table IV.

#### 10.1.6 Post-Coital Regimens

Most sexually active women require long term contraception, but there is a place for post-coital administration of hormones where the woman has been exposed to unprotected coitus, failed barrier contraception or rape. A well tried treatment is *ethinylestradiol* 100μg combined with *norgestrel* 1mg given within 72 hours of coitus and repeated 12 hours later. This has a low failure rate of around 1%. However, an even better method is now available – *mifepristone* 600mg within 72 hours of coitus.[113] Several series have reported no pregnancies with this regimen.[114] The onset of the next period is delayed.

Great care should be taken not to use either of these treatments when women are already pregnant, and to make sure that advice and therapy is given about long term contraception.

### 10.2 User Acceptability and Adverse Effects of Hormonal Contraceptives

The effectiveness of any contraceptive method depends on its acceptability to the user, and on the care with which it is used. While some adverse effects of hormonal contraceptives are of major importance (table IV), many are no more than a nuisance (table V). All are extremely uncommon, particularly since the advent of low-dose preparations. For most young women seeking a reliable contraceptive, they offer a reasonable solution. Combined estrogen/progestagen oral contraceptives are the most acceptable and effective method of temporary contraception and most women are probably at lower risk of adverse events using these than other less reliable methods.

Ascertainment of adverse (or beneficial) effects of oral contraceptives cannot be made by randomised placebo-controlled trials. Randomised parallel-group comparative trials of sufficient power require such large numbers as to be unmanageable. Retrospective case control studies or prospective cohort studies give information that is always susceptible to confounding and difficulties in interpretation. Recent events have illustrated some of these difficulties.

#### 10.2.1 Venous Thromboembolism and Third-Generation Oral Contraceptives

In October 1995, the UK Committee on Safety of Medicines (CSM) announced that it had become aware that 3 epidemiological studies had indicated that oral contraceptives (OCs) containing desogestrel and gestodene (i.e. third-generation OCs) were associated with an approximate 2-fold increase in the risk of venous thromboembolism. The excess risk of thrombosis compared with users of OCs containing levonorgestrel, norethisterone or ethynodiol was 15 cases per 100,000 women per year. The Committee advised that combined OCs containing gestodene or desogestrel should not be used by women with risk factors for venous thromboembolism, including obesity, varicose veins

**Table V.** Some minor adverse effects of hormonal steroid contraceptives and their management by manipulation of the dose and/or ratio of estrogen/progestagen

| Adverse effect | Cause | Management |
|---|---|---|
| Breakthrough bleeding in late cycle | Estrogen excess | Increase progestagen |
| Menorrhagia/dysmenorrhoea | Estrogen excess | Increase progestagen |
| Amenorrhoea | Progestagen excess | Increase estrogen or decrease progestagen |
| Nausea and vomiting | Estrogen excess | Decrease estrogen |
| Fluid retention | Estrogen excess | Decrease estrogen |
| Acne/oily skin and hair | Progestagen excess | Decrease progestagen/increase estrogen |
| Weight gain | Progestagen excess | Decrease progestagen |
| Breast tenderness/enlargement | Estrogen and/or progestagen excess | Decrease estrogen and progestagen |
| Irritability/depression | Progestagen excess | Decrease progestagen |
| Decreased libido | Progestagen excess | Decrease progestagen |

or previous history of thrombosis. These OCs should only be used in women who are intolerant of other OCs and who are prepared to accept an increased risk of thrombosis. The UK product licences for these preparations were not withdrawn, however, and licensing authorities in several other countries have so far declined to take action on this issue.

Subsequent publication of the data on which the CSM announcement was based has allowed a more detached consideration of the issues involved. The published evidence confirms the concerns of the CSM, with a pooled estimate of relative risk of venous thromboembolism of about 2 [95% confidence interval (CI) 1.4, 2.7].

The World Health Organization (WHO) Collaborative Study of Cardiovascular Disease and Steroid Hormone Contraceptives[115] investigated 1143 patients and 2998 age-matched controls in 21 hospital centres in Africa, Asia, Europe and Latin America. Patients were aged 20 to 44 years, with a hospital discharge diagnosis of deep vein thrombosis (DVT) or pulmonary embolism (PE); 42% of suspected DVTs and 25% of PEs were confirmed 'definite' by objective tests. Current use of OCs was associated with a significant increase in risk of first episode of venous thromboembolism, with an overall odds ratio of 4.0, at the lower end of the range previously reported for OC use. The risk appeared to be fully developed within 4 months of starting OCs and resolved within 3 months of stopping the drugs, but did not differ according to whether the estrogen dosage was greater or less than 50 μg/day. A surprising and novel observation was that the risk was much higher in users of third-generation progestagens.

This unexpected relationship between venous thromboembolism events and third-generation progestagens was further explored in a separate analysis of a subset of the original study population by the WHO Collaborative Group[116] in 769 cases and 1979 age-matched controls. In this analysis, the risk of venous thromboembolism associated with low-dose estrogen OCs containing levonorgestrel (137 cases, 203 patients) was compared with the risk in users of desogestrel (35 cases and 28 controls) and gestodene (36 cases and 28 controls). The ratio of risk, compared with levonorgestrel, was 2.6 for the third-generation agents (range 1.1 to 4.8). The excess risk of venous thromboembolism for users of desogestrel or gestodene over levonorgestrel-containing OCs was 11 per 100,000 woman-years (CI 1.2, 22.7).

The concern generated by these data prompted separate analyses of the UK General Practice Database in a cohort of 303,470 otherwise-healthy women.[116] The second analysis examined the risk of venous thromboembolism. A cohort analysis was undertaken, together with a nested case control study in which 80 cases requiring hospital admission for suspected nonfatal venous thromboembolism were compared with 300 controls (64% of cases had the diagnosis confirmed by objective tests). The adjusted relative risk estimates for venous thromboembolism, compared with levonorgestrel users, were 1.9 (desogestrel) and 1.8 (gestodene) in the cohort analysis, and 2.2 (desogestrel) and 2.1 (gestodene) in the nested case control analysis. Excess risks for venous thromboembolism associated with the third-generation OCs were similar between agents, at 16 per 100,000 women years.

A further analysis was performed by the Transnational Research Group in Germany and the UK in 471 cases and 1772 controls.[117] All cases were identified in hospital and were said to have been 'confirmed by imaging procedures', although the details are not presented. The odds ratio for risk of venous thromboembolism, compared with users of second-generation OCs, were 1.5 (1.0 to 2.2) for desogestrel and 1.5 (1.1 to 2.1) for gestodene. The probability of death due to venous thromboembolism was 5/million/year for non-OC users, 14/million/year for women using second-generation OCs and 20/million/year for women using third-generation OCs.

The risks of cardiovascular disease have been assessed in 2 of these projects. In the first,[118] the risk of idiopathic cardiovascular death was low in groups taking levonorgestrel, desogestrel and gestodene and there were no large differences between them. The death rate among current users of levonorgestrel was 4.3 per 100,000 and the adjusted combined relative risk for third-generation OCs was 0.9 (0.3 to 2.4). In the second,[119] the relative risk of myocardial infarction was 0.36 (0.1 to 1.2) for third-generation OC use. In other words, gestodene and desogestrel had either a neutral or cardioprotective influence. This particular issue remains unresolved, but is highly relevant to public health policy, because of the much higher case fatality from myocardial infarction and stroke than from venous thromboembolism.

If, as is still possible, the third-generation OCs reduce the risk of arterial disease, this

**Table VI.** Risks of nonfatal venous thromboembolism associated with oral contraceptives (OCs)

| | Pregnancy | OCs containing: | | Non-users of OCs |
|---|---|---|---|---|
| | | gestodene or desogestrel | norethisterone or levonorgestrel | |
| Absolute risk (per 100,000 woman-years)[a] | 60 | 30 | 15 | 5 |
| Relative risk | 12 | 6 | 3 | 1 |
| Women free from thrombosis (%) | 99.94 | 99.97 | 99.985 | 99.995 |

a Data from Mills et al.[123]

could transform the balance of risk in favour of these preparations. One of the greatest dangers of the current controversy is that it may have compromised completion of the studies that had hoped to elucidate this issue.

Several conclusions can now be drawn from the published data. The original warning by the CSM can now be seen to have been based on highly consistent results from 4 independent sources showing an increased risk of venous thromboembolism associated with the use of third-generation OCs. The relative risk is approximately 2-fold. However, the absolute risk and the case-fatality rates are small and much less than the risks of venous thromboembolism associated with pregnancy.

In a separate, but highly informative publication, the risk of DVT was assessed in respect of OC use and carriership of factor V Leiden mutation (activated protein C resistance) as a marker of thrombophilia.[120] As in the other case control studies, OC use increased the risk of DVT approximately 4-fold. Factor V Leiden mutation increased the risk of DVT 8-fold. The risk of DVT for the combination was increased 30- to 50-fold. In a follow-up report,[121] the apparent multiplication of risk was most obvious for OCs containing desogestrel (2.5-fold higher than for all other OC types examined. Among 10,000 women followed for a year, the attributable risk of DVT would be 3 cases for OC use, 7 for factor V Leiden carrier status, and 19 for OC-using carriers.

Following the publication of these papers and the public debate on this issue, attempts have been made to reassure prescribers and patients on the remarkable safety record of all modern combined oral contraceptives, and guidelines have been offered for prescribing.[122,123] The safety of oral contraceptives in respect of venous thromboembolism is illustrated in table VI, which draws on published data,[123] but also includes the all-important concept of absolute *versus* relative risk.

In prescribing oral contraceptives, the issues have been summarised succinctly by McPherson:[124] 'a careful personal and family history for increased risk of venous thromboembolism is essential, followed where appropriate by screening for thrombophilia. Women with risk factors for venous thromboembolism should probably not start taking third-generation pills; but once informed of the small excess risk, women already taking them satisfactorily may choose to continue using them.'

#### 10.2.2 Other Considerations

Depot injections of progestagen are finding an increasing role, now that they have been shown to have a low rate of adverse effects, good effectiveness and reversibility, and are particularly useful when motivation or compliance with regular tablet ingestion may be a problem. None of these methods offer protection against transmission of HIV infection and alternative or additional barrier methods should be recommended for women at risk.

It has usually been regarded as essential that hormonal contraceptives be available only on prescription, and that all women using them be subjected to repeated intensive observation during their use. However, it has been suggested that such procedures inhibit many of the women most in need from using them, that screening should be reduced to a minimum except for selected cases, or indeed that medical intervention should occur only if the woman has a complaint. Paramedical personnel such as nurses, health visitors, midwives and pharmacists have been trained to provide oral contraception in many countries, but their use is still controversial in developed countries. This debate has recently been reopened, with a suggestion that oral contraceptives should be more widely available as OTC medication.[125] The clinical, economic, legal and ethical issues are complex, but on safety grounds alone, there is a strong case for this approach.

The most important single issue that remains unresolved is the risk of breast cancer. This is not only of considerable clinical and public health importance, but also carries with it major emotive overtones for many women and their families. The risks of this problem will need to be more accurately assessed and quantified before oral contraceptives are made more widely available on a nonprescription basis.

### 10.3 Additional Benefits

Beneficial side effects of combined oral contraceptives include a reduction in menstrual flow (of considerable importance in areas where women often suffer from iron deficiency anaemia), regularity of menstruation and almost invariable absence of dysmenorrhoea. Functional ovarian cysts may also be less frequent.

Autoimmune thyroid disease may be less frequent, as may rheumatoid arthritis, although this needs confirmation. Oral contraceptive use provides some protection against pelvic inflammatory disease, possibly by a local action in the uterus, and convincingly reduces the risk of both endometrial and ovarian cancer.

### 10.4 Avoiding Problems with Therapy

The most common problem associated with the use of oral contraceptives remains forgetfulness and/or poor compliance on the part of the woman, with resultant breakthrough bleeding and risk of pregnancy. Patient instruction remains paramount, and illiteracy, education and motivation must be taken into account in recommending a method of contraception. If a combined pill is more than 12 hours late, the next pill should be taken immediately and administration resumed as normal when the next dose is due and continued without a break, using a new packet if necessary and omitting inactive pills. If a progestagen-only pill is more than 3 hours late, the missed pill should be taken immediately and administration resumed as normal when the next dose is due. In both instances, additional contraceptive precautions should be taken for 7 days. Similar precautions are advisable if vomiting or diarrhoea have occurred.

Minor adverse effects are not uncommon, but are often amenable to manipulation of the dosage and ratio of estrogen to progestagen (table V).

Major adverse effects are uncommon, given the massive scale on which these drugs are prescribed, but the implications for the individual patient can be substantial, and still constitute important reasons for discontinuing or avoiding the use of these forms of contraception.

### 10.5 Drug Interactions with Hormonal Contraceptives

These are of particular importance with oral contraceptives.

#### *10.5.1 Effect of Contraceptives on Other Drugs*

Oral contraceptive steroids are weak inhibitors of hepatic microsomal drug metabolising enzymes and may inhibit the metabolism of other drugs, though the magnitude of this effect is of doubtful clinical importance, particularly as low doses of estrogen are now favoured. Possibly the only major drug group for which this might be relevant are benzodiazepines that undergo hydroxylation, such as alprazolam, chlordiazepoxide, diazepam, nitrazepam and triazolam.[126] Even a slight impairment in reaction time or coordination may be important in certain occupations or while driving. Lorazepam, oxazepam and temazepam do not share this interaction and may be preferred.

Long term oral contraceptive usage results in a significantly reduced clearance of prednisolone.[127] The reported pharmacokinetic changes were substantial, but it is not known if they are of clinical importance. Another interaction of this type is between norethisterone and cyclosporin;[128] the latter drug may accumulate if its metabolism is inhibited.

#### *10.5.2 Effect of Other Drugs on Oral Contraceptives*

Most of these interactions relate to the effect of other drugs on the pharmacokinetics and pharmacodynamics of ethinylestradiol, leading to diminished efficacy of the estrogen. This may result in breakthrough bleeding (common) or pregnancy (rare). The commonest predisposing factors to inadvertent pregnancy occurring in women on oral contraceptives are missed tablets, gastrointestinal disturbances and drug interactions. The most important groups of drugs interacting in this way are antibiotics and antiepileptics.[126]

##### Antibiotics

The most important mechanism of interaction is antibiotic-stimulated enzyme induction, resulting in increased clearance and lower plasma estrogen concentrations. There is little doubt that rifampicin is capable of doing this and this interaction has been implicated in numerous unplanned pregnancies.[129] Thus, oral contraceptives should not be relied on if rifampicin is coadministered. Griseofulvin may also share this effect.[130]

With other antibiotics, there does seem to be something of a discrepancy between experimental evidence that has failed to show objective signs of either pharmacokinetic or pharmacodynamic interaction, and numerous anecdotal case reports indicating that this is an occasional problem. Methodological problems beset many of the formal studies, however, and it does seem likely that some women may be at particular risk, especially those characterised by high first-pass metabolism of estrogens,[131] and possibly those taking triphasic pills.

From a pragmatic point of view, women should be counselled about the potential risks and advised to take extra contraceptive precautions if taking concurrent antibiotics for the first time or if they have experienced breakthrough bleeding on such drugs in the past. This precaution should certainly be offered in the case of broad-spectrum penicillins and tetracyclines, which may interfere with intestinal absorption of estrogens by altering the bowel flora and also by their tendency to cause diarrhoea. Erythromycin is a metabolising enzyme inhibitor and would be a good alternative choice, with little risk of attenuating the estrogen effect.

**Antiepileptic Drugs**

Carbamazepine, phenobarbital and phenytoin are all powerful enzyme inducers and reduce plasma concentrations of oral contraceptives. If a combined oral contraceptive is used in an epileptic patient receiving any of these antiepileptics, a dosage of at least 50μg and preferably 100μg of estrogen daily may be required.[132] Valproic acid does not share this effect, but has the disadvantage of causing neural tube defects in offspring and menstrual irregularities in a high proportion of women.

Alternative forms of contraception such as depot progestagens should be considered in patients receiving antiepileptics, particularly as there is evidence that control of epilepsy may be improved by such measures.[110]

### 10.6 Medical Sterilisation

A method has been developed whereby mepacrine (quinacrine) pellets can be inserted into the uterine cavity using a modified IUCD inserter.[133] When given as 2 doses 1 month apart during the proliferative phase of the menstrual cycle, this causes fibrotic occlusion of the fallopian tubes. Recently, experience from Vietnam in a series of over 30,000 women showed that this procedure was inexpensive, well tolerated, and as safe as surgical sterilisation, with a failure rate of about 2% at 1 year.[134] This is identical with the rate for surgical sterilisation in Vietnam,[135] though higher than that for surgical sterilisation in the developed world (usually <1%). Success with this technique is highly operator dependent, but it may be a feasible and cost-effective method of family planning in developing countries. However, toxicology testing is incomplete[136] and there have been alarming reports of genetic damage in *in vitro* systems.[137]

## 11. Gynaecological Disorders

The sequence of events in the normal menstrual cycle can be summarised as follows. Basal secretion of follicle stimulating hormone (FSH) and luteinising hormone (LH) stimulate the theca interna cells of the developing graafian follicle to produce increasing concentrations of estradiol. When an estrogen peak is reached in mid-cycle, this causes, by a positive feedback mechanism, a brief surge in gonadotrophin output (especially LH) mediated by hypothalamic releasing factors. Ovulation occurs and is followed by granulosa cell hypertrophy in the developing corpus luteum, which is then invaded by theca interna cells and secretes increasing concentrations of progesterone that characterise the 14-day luteal phase of the cycle. At the end of this phase, the hypertrophied endometrium is receptive to implantation of the fertilised egg, but if this does not occur, menstruation ensues and the cycle restarts. The secretion of gonadotrophins is in turn controlled by preceding pulsatile secretion of gonadotrophin-releasing hormone (GnRH) from the hypothalamus. Figure 1 depicts the hormone changes in the human menstrual cycle.

Hormonal profiles of abnormal menstrual cycles are less complete. The elucidation of these abnormal changes has nevertheless facilitated the diagnosis of disorders of menstrual function such as unopposed estrogen secretion in the anovulatory cycles of women with menorrhagia due to cystic glandular hyperplasia, or failure of ovulation as a cause of infertility. Many therapeutic developments have followed, such as the use of contraceptive steroids to inhibit ovulation (see section 10), the treatment of infertility

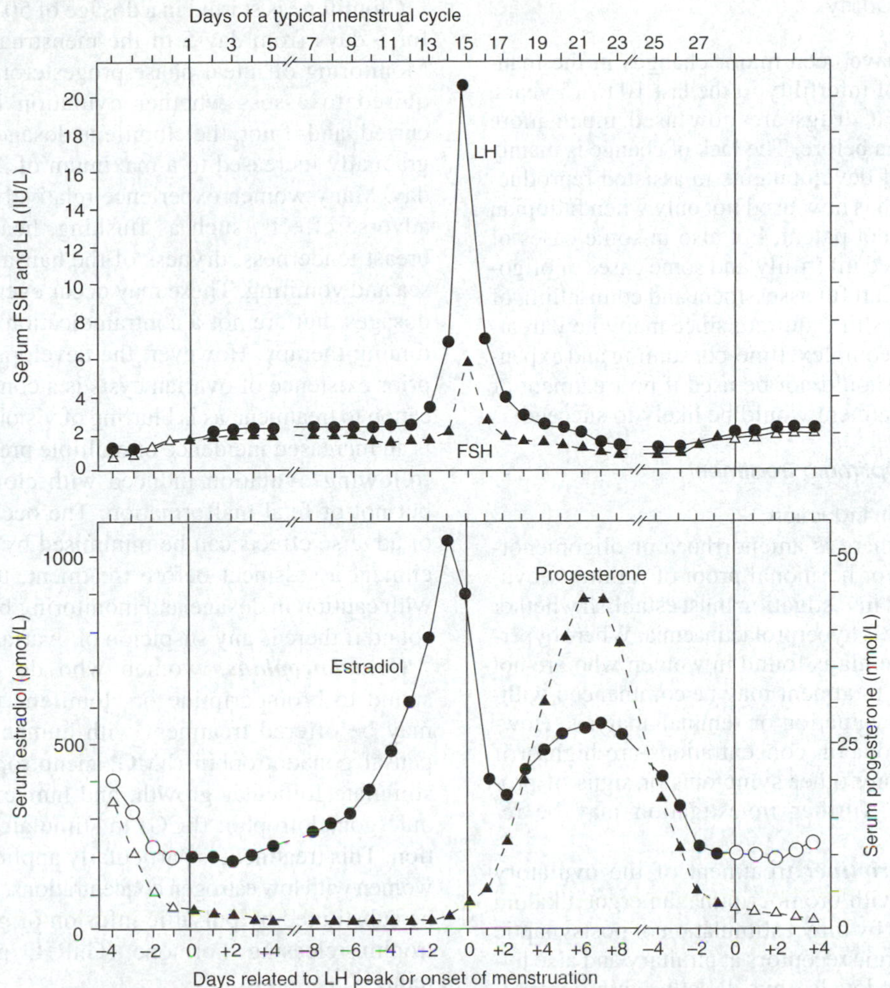


**Fig. 1.** Hormone patterns in the human menstrual cycle (after Hull[138]).

(bromocriptine, clomifene), and more recently, the introduction of GnRH agonists (e.g. buserelin, goserelin, leuprorelin, nafarelin, triptorelin) for the treatment of infertility and menstrual disorders, as well as a means of 'medical castration' for men with prostatic carcinoma.

## 11.1 General Principles of Hormone Therapy

Hormonal therapy should never be prescribed without careful assessment of the patient. This should include a history, general and pelvic examination, investigation, often including endometrial biopsy, hysteroscopy, transvaginal ultrasonic scan, or hormone assays. The assessment is important because carcinoma of the cervix or uterus, or even incomplete miscarriage, may masquerade as menstrual dysfunction, or a pituitary adenoma as hypothalamic amenorrhoea.

Even where a hormonal abnormality is undoubtedly present, hormones may not be the treatment of choice. In women who have completed childbearing who are 35 years of age or over or in whom other pathology such as cervical intraepithelial neoplasia or pelvic inflammatory disease has been diagnosed, endoscopic surgery or hysterectomy may be preferred to hormones as a treatment for menorrhagia. Definite contraindications to hormonal steroid therapy exist, e.g. a previous history of venous thromboembolism will usually preclude the use of estrogens, except in very low dosages.

Most hormone preparations have adverse effects, so that careful supervision of patients on hormone therapy is essential.

## 11.2 Infertility

There have been major changes in the management of infertility in the last 10 to 15 years, except that drugs are now used much more widely than before. The lack of change is mainly because of developments in assisted reproduction, which is now used not only when fallopian tubes are not patent, but also in some cases of unexplained infertility and some cases of oligospermia. Careful assessment and counselling of couples is still required, since many new treatments are complex, time-consuming and expensive, and should not be used if no treatment or simple treatment would be likely to succeed.

### 11.2.1 Optimum Treatment

#### Ovulation Induction

Where there is amenorrhoea or oligomenorrhoea and/or hormonal proof of failure to ovulate, initial investigation must establish whether or not there is hyperprolactinaemia. Where hyperprolactinaemia is found in women who are not ovulating, treatment may be commenced without tubal evaluation or seminal analysis. However, if prolactin concentrations are high or if there are any other symptoms or signs of prolactinoma, further investigation may be required.

***Bromocriptine:*** treatment of the ovulatory failure is with bromocriptine, an ergot alkaloid which acts by direct stimulation of postsynaptic dopaminergic receptors at pituitary and also hypothalamic levels, thus directly inhibiting prolactin release (see also chapter 19, sect. 9.1.3). Common adverse effects of bromocriptine are nausea and vomiting, dizziness, constipation and cold extremities. These maybe minimised by increasing the dosage gradually to the usual level of 5 mg/day. Regular menstruation is usually rapidly restored, and there is no increased likelihood of multiple pregnancy. When pregnancy is confirmed, bromocriptine therapy can be stopped.

***Clomifene:*** if a woman with ovulatory failure has normal prolactin concentrations and has no other endocrine abnormality, treatment is with clomifene. This synthetic nonsteroidal compound is a 1: 1 mixture of *cis-* and *trans*-clomifene and binds to the estrogen receptor.[139] It acts mainly by displacing estrogen from hypothalamic estrogen receptors and causing increased GnRH secretion, but may also act at the pituitary level, and on the ovary by decreasing ovarian aromatase activity.[140]

Clomifene is started in a dosage of 50 mg/day for 5 days from day 5 of the menstrual cycle. Monitoring of luteal phase progesterone is required to assess whether ovulation has occurred, and if not, the clomifene dosage can be gradually increased to a maximum of 200 mg/day. Many women experience relatively minor adverse effects, such as flushing, headaches, breast tenderness, dryness of the hair and nausea and vomiting. These may occur even at low dosages, but are not a contraindication to continuing therapy. However, the development or prior existence of ovarian cysts is a contraindication to treatment, as is blurring of vision. There is an increased incidence of multiple pregnancy following ovulation induced with clomifene, but not of fetal malformation. The occurrence of adverse effects can be minimised by careful clinical assessment before treatment, together with caution in dosage and monitoring by ultrasound if there is any suspicion of ovarian cysts.

***Gonadotrophins:*** women who do not respond to bromocriptine or clomifene therapy may be offered treatment with human menopausal gonadotrophin (hMG; menotropins) to stimulate follicular growth, and human chorionic gonadotrophin (hCG) to stimulate ovulation. This treatment is particularly applicable to women with low estrogen concentrations, and can be substituted by pulsatile infusion of gonadotrophin-releasing hormone (GnRH; gonadorelin).[141]

Because of the major risk of twin and higher multiple pregnancy, which results in much higher rates of cerebral palsy,[142] and the risk of ovarian hyperstimulation, these treatments should be offered only in centres with daily access to urgent hormone assays and/or ultrasound scanning. The syndrome of ovarian hyperstimulation is characterised by massive ovarian cysts, ascites, pleural effusion, thrombosis and hypoproteinaemia, and can be fatal.

*hMG* is given intramuscularly in dosages of 75 to 150IU of FSH daily or on alternate days until an adequate but not excessive ovarian response is observed (assessed by measurement of estrogen concentrations or growth of a single follicle). Ovulation can then be induced by a single intramuscular injection of *hCG* 5000 to 10,000IU. Conception can then be attempted 24 to 48 hours later. In the event of an excessive ovarian response, hCG should be withheld.

**Tubal Infertility**

This can be treated surgically or by assisted reproduction (see below).

**Assisted Reproduction**

The many different techniques now in use are beyond the scope of this chapter, but although *in vitro* fertilisation can be performed in physiological cycles where the indication for treatment is tubal impatency, the more usual technique is superovulation, especially where the indication for treatment is unexplained infertility or male infertility.

Superovulation is almost always preceded by downregulation using *GnRH (gonadorelin)*, to allow advanced scheduling of retrieval procedures, which is more convenient and cost effective for patients and staff. GnRH agonists such as *buserelin, goserelin* or *nafarelin* are administered either by subcutaneous injection or nasal spray to suppress spontaneous ovarian activity before the start of a fixed schedule of ovulation induction with hMG. The purpose of superovulation is to maximise the gain from the (expensive) oocyte retrieval process. As many follicles as possible are stimulated with a view to cryopreservation of gametes, not for immediate replacement. Hence a larger dosage of hMG is normally used than in ovulation induction (see above). Even with careful monitoring, there is a risk of hyperstimulation. The multiple pregnancy rate is determined by the number of oocytes or embryos replaced rather than by the characteristics of the drug therapy. There have been isolated reports of ovarian granulosa-cell tumours after superovulation,[143] but further studies are needed to determine the degree to which this is a problem.

**Male Infertility**

The treatment of male infertility is discussed in chapter 19 (section 8.3.5). In some cases of oligospermia, *in vitro* fertilisation (IVF) or other treatments may be of value.

#### *11.2.2 Clinical Outcome and Economic Considerations*

Since infertility is not an illness, economic appraisal involves philosophical assumptions about the benefits of treatment. An assumption that the issue of treatment (the offspring) is the beneficiary can permit comparisons with other medical treatments.[144,145] However, studies do not always fully consider the costs of care for children with cerebral palsy resulting from multiple pregnancies.

When comparing one method of infertility treatment with another, drug costs (though substantial for drugs such as GnRH and hMG) may pale into insignificance compared with the costs of necessary monitoring. There may, of course, be savings in expensive surgery such as tubal microsurgery.

## 11.3 Disorders of Menstrual Function

Disorders of menstrual function are common, but it is often not possible to reach a precise diagnosis, and there is no consensus as to how to quantify the severity of problems not associated with demonstrable pathology.

#### *11.3.1 Menorrhagia*

Heavy menstrual flow is often associated with menstrual irregularity (usually menstrual periods that last unusually long or occur more frequently, or both) and/or with dysmenorrhoea. Appropriate investigation and management will depend on the combination of presenting features, the obstetric and contraceptive history, and the findings on clinical examination. Endometrial biopsy is necessary in women over 40 years of age, and laparoscopy is needed if dysmenorrhoea is severe. Transvaginal scanning and hysteroscopy can be helpful in identifying abnormalities in the uterine cavity.

Common underlying causes are uterine fibroids, adenomyosis, endometrial polyps and an intrauterine contraceptive device. Uncommon causes are endometrial, cervical or ovarian malignancy, concomitant anticoagulant therapy, or occasionally retained products of conception or pelvic sepsis. However, most cases have no specific pathology and there is controversy as to whether the problem should be treated only when there is evidence of heavy menstrual loss as shown by anaemia or objective evidence of blood loss, or whether to be guided by the woman's own perception of her health status.

**Optimum Treatment**

The dosages and adverse effects of the various drugs used for menorrhagia are summarised in table VII. If not contraindicated, a combined (estrogen/progestagen) oral contraceptive should be the first-line treatment, as it is inexpensive and gives good cycle control and relief of dysmenorrhoea. Oral progestagens are comparatively ineffective, but may be useful where estrogens are contraindicated, e.g. by a history of venous thromboembolism. Adverse effects often limit their use to the short term. The pro-

**Table VII.** Reduction in menstruation achieved, dosages and adverse effects of used drugs for menorrhagia

| Drug | Reduction in menstruation[a] (%) | Dosage | Main adverse effects |
|---|---|---|---|
| Combined oral contraceptives | 50 | Ethinylestradiol 50μg + norethisterone 1-3mg in a 21-day cycle | Headaches, weight gain, migraine, breast tenderness, nausea, cholestatic jaundice, thromboembolism (see also table IV) |
| Oral progestagens (e.g. norethisterone) | 12 | 30 mg/day decreasing to 5-10 mg/day for 21 days per cycle | Weight gain, nausea, bloating, oedema, headaches, acne, depression, exacerbation of epilepsy and migraine |
| Levonorgestrel intrauterine contraceptive device | 90 | | Amenorrhoea, spotting |
| Danazol | 60 | 200 mg/day | Headaches, weight gain, acne, rashes, virilisation, mood changes, flushes, reduced levels of high-density lipoprotein (HDL) cholesterol |
| Tranexamic acid | 50 | 500g bid-tid during menses | Nausea, vomiting, diarrhoea, dizziness, ?cerebral thrombosis |
| Nonsteroidal anti-inflammatory drugs (e.g. ibuprofen) | 30 | 200mg (ibuprofen) bid during menses | Nausea, vomiting, dyspepsia, peptic ulceration, gastrointestinal bleeding, diarrhoea, headache, dizziness, rashes, bronchospasm, fluid retention, renal impairment, hypertension |
| GnRH agonists (e.g. goserelin) | 100 | Injection every 28 days | Flushes, hypoestrogenic effects, osteoporosis |

a Estimated by objective measurement of menstrual blood loss, usually by extracting haemoglobin from menstrual protection materials.

*Abbreviations:* bid = twice daily; tid = 3 times daily.

gestagen-containing IUCD[112] seems to be much more effective, though it does have some of the same adverse effects.

*Danazol*[146] and the related gonadotrophin release inhibitor *gestrinone* are effective, but at the cost of adverse effects that are unacceptable to many women, and they are also expensive drugs. *Tranexamic acid* (see chapter 26, sect. 4.1.1), a fibrinolytic inhibitor, is effective for women in whom hormone therapy is unacceptable or contraindicated, but does not help dysmenorrhoea or irregularity.

*Nonsteroidal anti-inflammatory drugs* (NSAIDs), given only during menstruation, are also helpful in the relief of dysmenorrhoea.[147] It has become apparent that, although their effectiveness is generally similar, there are substantial differences in the gastrointestinal adverse effect profile of these drugs and this aspect should influence selection.[148] *Ibuprofen* is inexpensive, widely available as an OTC medication, and a low dosage of this drug should normally be the first-line therapy because of its tolerability and safety record.

The most drastic drug therapy is to abolish ovarian function altogether by giving *goserelin* (see chapter 19, sect. 8.2.3), a semisynthetic GnRH agonist. In repeated large dosages, this drug causes desensitisation of the pituitary with secondary ovarian atrophy. This is not acceptable as a long term therapy but may be useful in the short term, or to reduce the size of a fibroid when surgery is proposed.[149]

Hysterectomy (abdominal or vaginal) is a well tried treatment for refractory or severe menorrhagia. It may still be required in a proportion of cases, but is to some extent being replaced by conservative surgery in the form of endometrial resection, ablation or coagulation. These procedures are often preceded by hormone therapy to thin the endometrium. The drugs in use are goserelin, combined oral contraceptives and danazol, but no good evidence is available to show which is more effective or least expensive. The prothrombotic effect of estrogens should be taken into account, particularly in women at risk of venous thromboembolism.

#### *11.3.2 Endometriosis*

Ectopic endometrium will normally bleed cyclically into the peritoneal cavity and, if extensive, may cause the formation of cysts ('chocolate cysts'), adhesions, bowel or urinary tract haemorrhage, and scarring. Common symptoms are secondary dysmenorrhoea, dyspareunia and infertility. The diagnosis must be confirmed at laparoscopy since the symptoms and signs are not exclusive to endometriosis. Asymptomatic disease need not be treated.

#### Optimum Treatment

The definitive treatment of endometriosis is surgical, including bilateral oophorectomy, but as the condition often occurs in young women who wish to preserve fertility, drug treatment is often used to suppress menstruation, although there is no evidence that this actually improves fertility. Drugs may be used to render surgery easier by shrinking endometrial deposits. The drugs available are danazol, progestagens, GnRH and its agonists, and combined estrogen/progestagen preparations.

*Danazol* is an androgen agonist that inhibits ovarian estrogen production and causes atrophy of endometrial deposits if given continuously in a dosage sufficient to abolish menstruation (usually 200 to 800 mg/day). Pregnancy must be avoided, as the drug might cause pseudohermaphroditism in a female fetus. Serious adverse effects are common, including virilisation and bodyweight gain,[150] but if not troublesome, treatment may be continued for 6 months or more. *Gestrinone* has a similar net effect.

*Progestagens* such as norethisterone, medroxyprogesterone, dydrogesterone and megestrol can cause decidual change in endometriotic deposits and thus relieve symptoms in some women. However, they are not effective if breakthrough bleeding persists, and often have adverse effects, including depression and bloating. If well tolerated, they should also be continued for at least 6 months.

*GnRH (gonadorelin)* and *GnRH agonists* are successful in abolishing menstruation when given continuously by intramuscular injection or nasal spray, but because it is accompanied by the inevitable consequences of hypoestrogenism (hot flushes, accelerated bone loss, etc.), treatment must be of limited duration. These agents are most useful as pretreatment for surgery.

*Combined estrogen/progestagen preparations* can suppress menstruation if given continuously, but may be less effective than the drugs mentioned above because the estrogen component may stimulate the endometrium. Nevertheless, this treatment has fewer adverse effects than others and gives better contraceptive protection than danazol and progestagens, and will therefore be appropriate for some women.

### *11.3.3 Dysmenorrhoea*

Dysmenorrhoea (pain with periods) may be of uterine or extrauterine origin. When of uterine origin, it may be due to muscular spasm, intramyometrial bleeding (in adenomyosis) or to uterine colic during expulsion of clots, or rarely to pedunculated submucous fibroids. Pain of extrauterine origin may be due to inflammation of the fallopian tubes, or to haemorrhage into pelvic deposits of endometriosis.

#### Optimum Treatment

Primary dysmenorrhoea seems to occur only in ovulatory cycles, and the most rational treatment, if the condition is severe enough to require treatment, is suppression of ovulation by cyclical *combined estrogen/progestagen preparations* (such as oral contraceptives). However, if the patient wishes to retain her fertility during treatment, then cyclical treatment with the progestagen *dydrogesterone* 10mg twice daily may be tried, although it is less likely to be effective. Should cyclical hormone therapy fail to help the symptoms, menstruation may be abolished altogether by continuous therapy. It may be wise to stop treatment every few months to establish whether remission has occurred.

*Nonsteroidal anti-inflammatory drugs* (NSAIDs): the strong uterine contractions recorded may be due to increased prostaglandin production which may be inhibited by prostaglandin synthetase inhibitors (e.g. NSAIDs). It is likely that most of these drugs are equally effective and selection will be governed principally by their record of safety and tolerability.[148] NSAIDs have proved effective in relieving symptoms when given at the onset of pain and continued for about 3 days.

Secondary dysmenorrhoea is more likely to have a specific cause, such as endometriosis, and an attempt should be made to estimate the extent of this prior to therapy. Surgery may be required, but cyclical hormone therapy is often effective. In dysmenorrhoea secondary to the presence of an intrauterine device, NSAIDs are effective and also diminish excessive blood loss.

## 11.4 Menopausal Disturbances

Both the menopause itself (the time of cessation of menstruation) and the postmenopausal era of life bring inevitable changes, which may constitute medical problems. The median age at menopause is around 51 years, but some women undergo a menopause praecox much earlier, and others have gonadal dysgenesis, or are castrated, often at the time of hysterectomy. There are certainly cultural and possibly biological variations in the prevalence of symptoms such as flushes, which, for example, are rarely reported in Japanese women.[151] However, the main problem in ascertaining this is that surveys often involve clinic attenders rather a general population.[152] It is important to distinguish between therapy and prophylaxis, and in the context of prophylaxis, between universal treatment and selective treatment of high risk groups.

The physiology of the menopause and postmenopause are different. The menopause is a time of transition, whereas the postmenopause is a more or less steady state of relative estrogen deficiency. The menopause is characterised by vasomotor disturbances thought to be due to downward setting of the central thermostat of the hypothalamic thermoregulatory centres. These flushes are most common around the menopause, but can occur premenopausally, and gradually decline in frequency in the following years.[153] The diagnosis of the menopause may be confirmed by assay of FSH and LH, which will be elevated, or by an interval of 1 year since the last period. The postmenopause is characterised by gradual atrophy of tissues that are targets for estrogen (vagina, vulva, uterus, bladder trigone, breasts, skin); by trabecular bone loss, and by increasing arteriosclerosis, possibly due to an increase in low-density lipoprotein cholesterol and possibly also due to a direct effect on vascular endothelium.[154] Diabetes may also become more frequent after the menopause.

#### 11.4.1 Clinical Pharmacology of Drugs Used in Treatment

##### Estrogens

When 'replacement' therapy is prescribed to treat or prevent perimenopausal or postmenopausal problems, a constant component of therapy is estrogen, which may be given systemically or locally as *ethinylestradiol, estradiol valerate, 17β-estradiol, estrone, estropipate* or *conjugated estrogens*. Estrogens have numerous pharmacological effects, including increasing plasma estradiol, lowering of FSH and LH concentrations, inhibiting osteoclastic bone resorption, reducing plasma lipids, preserving endothelial function and a protective effect on the uterus. Systemic estrogen therapy is given orally or by transdermal patches, percutaneous gel or subcutaneous implants (all estradiol). In administering estrogens, treatment needs to be individualised, the dosage being reduced if estrogenic adverse effects occur (e.g. nausea, breast tenderness) or increased if menopausal symptoms are not controlled. Administration is continuous, but the need for ongoing treatment should be regularly assessed.

In women with cholelithiasis or previous deep vein thrombosis, it may be preferable to give estrogen by subcutaneous implant or transdermal patches. By circumventing the portal system in this way, some of the potentially adverse metabolic effects of the estrogen may be minimised. Such patches should not be administered at a site close to the breasts, to avoid undue local influences of estrogen and because of uncertainty about the risks of breast cancer (NB. progestagens may also be given transdermally).[155] Concerns have been expressed that even the low dosages of estrogen used in hormone replacement therapy may have adverse effects on blood pressure, lipid profile and haemorrheology in hypertensive patients. However, there is no convincing evidence that this is the case and such patients should not be denied the benefits of replacement estrogen, although it is prudent to ensure regular monitoring of the blood pressure.

Because of the risk of endometrial cancer resulting from unopposed estrogen, a cyclical progestagen must be given for at least 12 days/month, usually by the oral route, to all women with an intact uterus. A recent study has shown that neither medroxyprogesterone acetate nor norgestrel when used in combination with conjugated estrogens, significantly impairs the beneficial effects of estrogen on lipid profiles and fibrinogen.[156] Contrary to previous reports, combined preparations are actually tolerated better by women. Withdrawal bleeds will occur with cyclical combinations, and may be seen by women as a serious disadvantage. This problem can be circumvented by the use of *continuous* combined oral regimens or by intrauterine levonorgestrel,[157] although experience is more limited with these techniques.

It is common practice to judge the estrogen dosage (or the frequency of implants) by the frequency of flushes, but there have been reports of 'tachyphylaxis' where supraphysiological serum concentrations of estradiol can be found after estradiol implants, and yet women still experience flushes. Endometrial stimulation can last for many months after treatment has been stopped.[158] This suggests that the dosage should not be monitored by the frequency of flushing, but by measurement of estradiol concentrations.

Absolute contraindications to estrogen treatment are active liver disease and current venous thrombosis. It has been suggested that a previous history of venous thromboembolism is not a contraindication to therapy,[159] but some concerns remain about this. A history of breast cancer is a relative contraindication (see further section 11.4.2).

#### Tibolone

Tibolone is a synthetic steroid structurally related to the progestagens norethisterone and norethynodrel.[160] It has weak progestagenic, estrogenic and androgenic activity, and is useful in controlling hot flushes, sweating and headache. At a daily dose of 2.5mg, tibolone probably does not stimulate the endometrium. This makes it an attractive alternative to estrogen in women with an intact uterus, although it is recommended that the patient be amenorrhoeic for a year before starting this drug. However, long term experience with tibolone is limited, and although it looks promising, further data, particularly on safety and in respect of its effect on cardiovascular disease, bone density and breast cancer, are required before it can be recommended for widespread use.

### 11.4.2 Optimum Treatment

#### Symptomatic Treatment

Some women present around the menopause with a variety of symptoms, such as tiredness and depression, which are not specific to the menopause. Flushing can be treated with estrogens with or without progestagens for as long as desired, but will tend to recur when treatment is withdrawn. *Clonidine* (50μg twice daily) is less effective than estrogens but may be useful if hormone therapy is contraindicated or poorly tolerated.

Vaginal dryness may cause dyspareunia and may also predispose patients to infection. It can be treated with oral estrogens, with or without progestagens, but may more conveniently be managed with repeated short courses of *local vaginal estrogens*. However, systemic absorption does occur with large doses, and might theoretically cause endometrial hyperplasia. The low-dose estradiol vaginal ring seems to be as effective as, and more acceptable than vaginal cream.[161]

Trigonitis and frequent urinary infection are common in postmenopausal women and can be prevented to some extent by local vaginal estrogens.[162]

#### Prophylactic Therapy

Prophylactic hormone replacement therapy (HRT) is often advocated because of its assumed beneficial effects on osteoporosis (and resulting fractures) and atherosclerosis (and risk of myocardial infarction and stroke). Unfortunately, however, there are few randomised placebo-controlled trials on those topics, nor on the potentially most serious adverse effect, an increase in breast cancer. Selection bias in prescribing may have caused case control studies to underestimate the risk of breast cancer and to overestimate the potential for preventing fractures.[163] In addition, a review of recent meta-analyses suggests that inadvertent selection of relatively healthy individuals may have resulted in low rates of cardiovascular disease with resultant exaggeration of the potential benefits of hormone replacement.[164] Selective reporting in the medical literature might also tend to bias opinion in favour of 'positive' results.

#### Benefits of Prophylactic Hormone Replacement Therapy

*Prevention of osteoporosis:* there is good evidence that estrogens commenced at the time of the menopause prevent both osteoporosis and fractures. However, this effect is maximal only during estrogen use and declines rapidly thereafter at a rate similar to that after the normal menopause.[165] The problem is that the peak incidence of fractures is much later (median for hip fracture 80 years) and prolonged therapy would be required to have a significant effect.[166] Even treatment for 10 years soon after the menopause has been shown to have little influence on bone density after the age of 75 years, and is unlikely to prevent fractures in the age group at greatest risk.[167] Routine prophylactic therapy is unlikely to represent cost-effective expenditure in respect of preservation of bone mass.[168] Screening by available bone density measurements to identify women at high risk is currently neither effective nor economical,[169] although the use of such technology is advancing both our knowledge of the disease and the identification of risk groups.

In women with *established osteoporosis*, estrogens increase bone density and this strategy can certainly be recommended.[170] Other categories of patients known to be at increased risk include those on corticosteroid therapy, undergoing immobilisation or with strong family histories of osteoporosis (see further table VIII). Low bone mass measurements *per se*, particularly in such high risk groups, may also be con-

**Table VIII.** Risk factors for osteoporosis (after Dempster & Lindsay;[171] Notelovitz[172])

| |
|---|
| **Genetic:** |
| White or Asian ethnicity |
| Petite/small body frame (<58kg) |
| Family history of osteoporosis |
| **Lifestyle:** |
| Cigarette smoking |
| Alcohol abuse |
| Physical inactivity/immobilisation |
| Excessive exercise (producing amenorrhoea) |
| **Nutritional:** |
| Life-long inadequate dietary calcium intake |
| High animal protein intake |
| Eating disorders/anorexia nervosa |
| Malabsorption syndromes |
| **Gynaecological:** |
| Nulliparity |
| Early natural menopause |
| Late menarche |
| Oligohypomenorrhoea |
| Previous hysterectomy |
| Hyperprolactinaemia |
| **Medical conditions:** |
| Chronic renal failure |
| Hyperparathyroidism |
| Thyrotoxicosis |
| Cushing's syndrome |
| Diabetes mellitus, insulin-dependent |
| Gastrectomy and intestinal bypass |
| Rheumatoid arthritis |
| Ankylosing spondylitis |
| Prolactinoma |
| Mastocytosis |
| Haemolytic anaemia, haemochromatosis, thalassaemia |
| **Drug therapy:** |
| Corticosteroids (long term) |
| Antiepileptic drugs (long term) |
| Thyroid replacement therapy |
| Antacids (aluminium-containing) |
| Anticoagulants (heparin) |
| Lithium (long term) |

sidered an indication for prophylactic treatment. Attention to other measures, such as exercise, diet, smoking cessation and calcium supplements should be implemented in these patients. Progestagens, if required, may slightly augment the beneficial effects of estrogens on bone density.[173]

*Prevention of atherosclerosis:* it was thought until recently that hypertension, hyperlipidaemia or otherwise increased risk of myocardial infarction were contraindications to hormone replacement therapy. However, there is now a great deal of evidence from case control studies to indicate that unopposed estrogens are of benefit, particularly in respect of coronary heart disease.[174,175] Epidemiological data indicate that unopposed estrogen replacement therapy may reduce the risk of fatal and nonfatal myocardial infarction by 50% over 10 years.[176] The benefits may be even greater in women with established coronary disease.[177] It is not clear, however, what the optimum dosage, formulation or duration of therapy should be, whether the simultaneous use of progestagens will influence these beneficial effects (recent evidence suggests a favourable effect of the combination),[178] nor indeed whether the perceived benefits are magnified by selection or reporting bias.[179]

Coronary heart disease is the most common cause of death in postmenopausal women and any treatment that influences this in a major way is bound to have profound implications. However, for a problem of this magnitude it is essential to have accurate, unbiased information on the potential ratio of risks to benefits, and widespread prophylaxis should await the results of prospective controlled clinical trials, such as that currently being coordinated by the National Institutes of Health in the US.[180] Unfortunately, the results of this project will not be known by the end of this century. As an interim measure, guidelines have been published.[181,182] At the very least, women will need to be fully informed of the risks as well as the potential benefits of prolonged hormone replacement therapy before embarking on this form of prophylaxis.

#### Risks of Hormone Replacement Therapy

***Breast cancer:*** there appears to be a modest increase in the risk of breast cancer with long term replacement therapy both with unopposed and opposed estrogens.[183-185] The relative risk is of the order of 1.3 to 1.6, and is greater in older women. The most recent data from the US Nurses' Health Study showed a relative risk of 1.71 (95% CI 1.34, 2.18) in women aged 60 to 64 years who had been using hormone replacement therapy for over 5 years compared with non-users.[185] The relative risk of death from breast cancer was 1.45 in this subgroup.

The risk of breast cancer may be outweighed in absolute terms in respect of morbidity and mortality by the benefit from protection against coronary heart disease, stroke and osteoporosis, although there is some concern that the risk of breast cancer may have been underestimated as a result of selective prescribing in the past.[186] Breast cancer carries with it major fears and anxieties not shared with these other diagnoses and is probably a common reason for women's reluctance to comply with therapy. They should certainly be informed of this potential risk before being put on long term therapy. Many prescribers will regard the residual uncertainty over this issue as the main reason to use this form of treatment sparingly until formal trial results are available.

In women who have already been treated for breast cancer, replacement therapy has usually been considered contraindicated. This embargo may be waived in selected cases if there are strong indications.[187,188] If, in a patient who is free of metastatic disease and the local disease is under control, menopausal flushing is intolerable despite simple remedies or progestagen therapy, combined replacement therapy with low-dose continuous estrogen and progestagen for up to 12 months may be considered. Women who have had small tumours detected by mammography (who would normally have a good prognosis) and who have established coronary heart disease may be considered for longer-term prophylactic hormone replacement therapy, as long as they are aware of the absence of sound data on this subject.

***Endometrial and ovarian cancer:*** the available evidence indicates that the risk of endometrial cancer with estrogens can be reduced by simultaneous progestagen therapy.[189] Preliminary results from the US Postmenopausal Estrogen/Progestin Interventions (PEPI) trial, which was coordinated by the US National Institutes of Health Woman's Health Initiative,[190] showed that endometrial hyperplasia developed in 62% of women given conjugated estrogens 0.625 mg/day for up to 3 years, but the addition of a progestagen effectively abolished this effect. The investigators suggested that unopposed estrogen therapy would result in complex or atypical hyperplasia after about 5 years in the majority of women. On the basis of these observations, the investigators discontinued the use of unopposed estrogen therapy to women in this trial who have an intact uterus.

There are conflicting reports, and no consensus, on whether the risk of ovarian cancer is increased or decreased.[169]

#### *11.4.3 Clinical Outcome and Economic Considerations*

Estimates of the cost of screening programmes, the cost of short or long term therapy and the likely savings or costs associated with fractures, myocardial infarction or strokes avoided or breast cancer induced, are difficult to make in view of the long time scale involved. It is to be hoped that current trials will include full economic assessment, and long term follow-up.

It is also to be hoped that guidelines on the frequency of physical examination and mammography and other investigations in patients receiving hormone replacement therapy will be developed. If treatment is prescribed, it is clear, however, that oral therapy is less expensive and more appropriate for most women than transdermal or subcutaneous therapy.

For a review of pharmacoeconomic considerations in using hormone replacement therapy, see Whittington and Faulds,[191,192] who report cost effectiveness in women with major risk factors or severe symptoms.

#### *11.4.4 Risks versus Benefits of Routine Prophylaxis*

While awaiting evidence from randomised controlled trials, weighing up of risk and benefit can be done only using the results of observational studies, preferably prospective cohort studies but also case control studies. Apart from the issue of possible noncomparability of cases and controls, the principal uncertainty in calculating net years of life gained springs from doubt about the duration of risk (or benefit) after cessation of therapy. It has been pointed out[193] that if the cardiovascular benefit considerably outlasts cessation of hormone replacement therapy, and the breast cancer risk returns immediately to baseline after cessation, then that would result in a net gain in years of life. However, the converse is equally possible. Also, long term policy on therapy would need to take account of current trends in baseline risk, which show a reduction for coronary heart disease and an increase for breast cancer. Further imprecision arises from the paucity of studies on the long term effects of added progestagens, and on the effects of non-oral estrogen therapy.[194]

There is a compelling need for prospective randomised trials of postmenopausal hormone replacement therapy.[169,186] Until such results are available, we recommend that routine or widespread prescription should be avoided.

There is, however, a strong case for therapy in high-risk women such as those with surgical castration, premature menopause or gonadal dysgenesis, at least until the age of 50 years. Women with established coronary heart disease should also be considered for hormonal prophylaxis.

### 11.5 Premenstrual Syndrome

The premenstrual syndrome is a term used to describe a group of adverse symptoms associated with the premenstrual 14 days of the cycle. However, because there is no clear evidence as to the underlying pathology, and because there is a marked placebo effect with therapies that have been tried, a conservative approach is appropriate, with drug treatment (if any) being tailored to the predominant symptoms.

#### Optimum Treatment

*Diuretics* are sometimes used for bloating and bodyweight gain, but secondary aldosteronism often develops and leads to 'rebound' oedema on attempted withdrawal of these drugs. Their adverse biochemical and metabolic effects are considerable, especially at higher dosages, and this form of therapy should be avoided if at all possible.

If breast discomfort is a problem, either *bromocriptine, danazol* or *tamoxifen* may be helpful, but there are doubts as to whether long term therapy with these agents is safe. Low dosages of *pyridoxine* (50mg daily) may help some women with depressive symptoms, but high dosages may cause peripheral neuropathy. *Nonsteroidal anti-inflammatory drugs* (NSAIDs) may be helpful if pain is the main complaint.

A variety of hormone treatments, including progesterone, progestagens, and combined estrogen-progestagen oral contraceptives have been used, with conflicting reports of their effectiveness. The woman's aspirations to fertility, and the usual contraindications, must be taken into account.

### 11.6 Hirsutism

Full investigation of women presenting with hirsutes is required, particularly if they also have oligomenorrhoea or amenorrhoea, to identify the cause. Most such women are found to have constitutional or idiopathic hirsutes, and while the response to treatment is often disappointing, some improvements can be achieved.

#### Optimum Treatment

The most effective treatment seems to be a combined estrogen-progestagen preparation such as *ethinylestradiol* 30μg plus *ethynodiol diacetate* 2mg, given cyclically. The estrogen acts primarily by reducing ovarian steroidogenesis. The ethynodiol component has little androgenic activity and may in addition act locally in the skin to inhibit the conversion of testosterone to dihydrotestosterone.

*Cyproterone,* a synthetic antiandrogenic steroid, has also been used in hirsutism, generally in combination with an estrogen, either in a regular cyclical fashion with a low dosage of cyproterone (2mg daily), or in a reverse sequential regimen with a much larger dosage (100mg daily) given from days 5 to 14 of the cycle, while the estrogen (ethinylestradiol) is given from days 5 to 25. The latter method of administration gives measurable benefit in terms of reduction in hirsutes,[195,196] but increases plasma triglycerides and lowers high density lipoproteins. Long term administration may therefore be unwise, particularly if there are other cardiovascular risk factors.

*Spironolactone* impairs both the synthesis and peripheral action of testosterone (see also chapter 19; sect. 7.1.3 and 10.2.3). It has been used in hirsute women with beneficial effects,[197] but is not approved for this use in either the UK or the US.

## 12. Sexually Transmissible Diseases

The treatment of sexually transmissible diseases is discussed in detail in chapter 33 and only the principles of management of female patients are outlined in the following sections.

### 12.1 Gonorrhoea and *Chlamydia trachomatis* Infections

In the treatment of gonorrhoea, the choice of regimens for uncomplicated infections depends largely on the pattern of resistance. Ideally all treatment should be administered under supervision, but patients are prone to default from follow-up. The resultant problem of failed compliance with therapy can be avoided by the use of a single-dose treatment given by intramuscular injection (e.g. *ceftriaxone* 125mg). A regimen active against *Chlamydia trachomatis* is also recommended (see below), since this organism is often present concurrently.

To treat *C. trachomatis* infection, multiple-dose regimens of a tetracycline (e.g. *doxycy-*

*cline* 100mg twice daily), *erythromycin* (500mg 4 times daily) given for 7 days, or single-dose *azithromycin* 1g are first-line therapy. In pregnant patients, of course, tetracyclines should be avoided.

### 12.2 Pelvic Inflammatory Disease

Pelvic inflammatory disease in women is a common cause of acute and chronic pelvic pain but, perhaps more significantly, also an important cause of sterility by damaging the fallopian tubes. Prompt appropriate treatment is therefore essential. Apart from tuberculosis, infection of the upper genital tract is usually sexually transmitted. Some asymptomatic infected women will be detected as contacts of infected men, and conversely, the partners of presenting women should be offered treatment. Women with intrauterine contraceptive devices are at increased risk.

Careful clinical examination is essential, sometimes including laparoscopy, and treatment should ideally be based on microscopy and culture results. Most cases of pelvic inflammatory disease are probably caused by more than one organism, including *Neisseria gonorrhoeae*, *C. trachomatis*, *Mycoplasma hominis*, and Gram-negative anaerobes and aerobes. It may be necessary to start treatment before full bacteriological results are available and, in such cases, a treatment regimen that is active against the broadest range of pathogens associated with the condition should be given. Appropriate regimens are given in chapter 33 (section 4.3). If the infection is severe, treatment should be initiated with intravenous therapy.

All patients with pelvic inflammatory disease should be carefully followed clinically and microbiologically after treatment.

### 12.3 Genital Herpes

Both primary lesions and recurrences of genital infection with herpes simplex virus may be treated with oral *aciclovir* (200mg 5 times daily for 7 to 10 days) to reduce the duration of viral shedding and of symptoms. In severe cases, intravenous therapy may be used.

The cost-effectiveness of prophylactic therapy with aciclovir (400mg twice daily) has not been fully evaluated, and this should certainly be reserved for cases with frequent recurrences (see also chapter 33; sect. 5.2.1).

## 13. Vaginitis

Vaginitis is a common condition, but not every woman who presents with vaginal discharge has vaginitis. Other causes that need to be considered include 'physiological' discharge, atrophic vaginitis and reaction to topical deodorants.

### 13.1 Vaginal Candidiasis

The treatment of vaginal candidiasis requires an accurate diagnosis and a highly specific agent. *Imidazole derivatives* (e.g. miconazole, clotrimazole, econazole, ticonazole, terconazole, butaconazole and isoconazole) are now standard treatment in short courses (see further chapter 33; sect. 5.1.2). Investigation of the partner and the possibility of underlying diabetes or concurrent bowel infection should be considered in recurrent cases.

### 13.2 Trichomoniasis and Bacterial Vaginosis

In the case of trichomoniasis and *Gardnerella vaginalis* infection, care should be taken to exclude other concurrent sexually transmissible diseases, and to investigate the partner(s), since these infections are usually sexually acquired. Treatment of both conditions is with *metronidazole* 400 to 500mg twice daily for 7 days. Alternatively, in the treatment of trichomoniasis, single-dose regimens of *metronidazole* 2g, *tinidazole* 2g or *ornidazole* 1.5g may be used (see also chapter 33; sect. 5.1.1 and 5.1.3).

## References


1. Selevan SG, Lindbohm M-L, Hornung RW, et al. A study of occupational exposure to antineoplastic drugs and fetal loss in nurses. New England Journal of Medicine 1985; 313: 1173
2. Saurel-Cubizolles MJ, Job-Spira N, Estryn-Behar M. Ectopic pregnancy and occupational exposure to antineoplastic drugs. Lancet 1993; 341: 1169-71
3. Herbst AL, Cole P, Colton T, et al. Age-incidence and risk of DES-related clear cell adenocarcinoma of the vagina and cervix. American Journal of Obstetrics and Gynecology 1977; 128: 43
4. Chalmers I. Diethylstilboestrol in pregnancy, No 2891. In: Enkin MW, Keirse MJNC, Renfrew MJ, et al. editors. Cochrane database of systematic reviews: pregnancy and childbirth module. Cochrane Update on Disc, 2nd ed. Oxford: Oxford Update Software, 1993
5. Lammer EJ, Chen DT, Hoar RM, et al. Retinoic acid embryopathy. New England Journal of Medicine 1985; 313: 837
6. Yaffe SJ, Stern L. Clinical implications of perinatal pharmacology. In: Mirkin B, ed. Perinatal pharmacology and therapeutics. New York: Academic Press, 1976: 355

7. Cutler J. Thalidomide revisited. Lancet 1994; 343: 795-6
8. Expert Advisory Group. Folic acid and the prevention of neural tube defects. Edinburgh: Department of Health, Scottish Office; Home and Health Department, Welsh Office; Department of Health and Social Services, Northern Ireland, 1992
9. Czeizel AE, Dudas I. Prevention of the first recurrence of neural tube defects by periconceptual vitamin supplementation. New England Journal of Medicine 1992; 327: 1832-5
10. Morbidity and Mortality Weekly Report. Atlanta, Georgia: Centers for Disease Control, 1992: RR-14
11. Steegers-Theunissen RPM, Boes GHJ, Trijbeis FJM, et al. Maternal hyperhomocysteinaemia: a risk factor for neural tube defects. Metabolism 1994; 43: 1457-80
12. Rosa FW, Wilk AL, Kelsey FO. Teratogen update: vitamin A congeners. Teratology 1986; 33: 355-64
13. Hathcock JH, Hattan DG, Jenkins MY, et al. Evaluation of vitamin A toxicity. American Journal of Clinical Nutrition 1990; 52: 183-202
14. Robaire B, Hales BF. Paternal exposure to chemicals before conception. British Medical Journal 1993; 307: 341-2
15. Ramsay I, Kaur S, Krassas G. Thyrotoxicosis in pregnancy: results of treatment by antithyroid drugs combined with T4. Clinical Endocrinology 1983; 18: 73
16. Vulsma T, Gans MH, de Viljder JJ. Maternal-fetal transfer of thyroxine in hypothyroidism due to total organification defect or thyroid agenesis. New England Journal of Medicine 1989; 321: 13
17. Ibbertson AK, Seddon RJ, Croxson MS. Fetal hypothyroidism complicating medical treatment of thyrotoxicosis in pregnancy. Clinical Endocrinology 1975; 4: 521
18. La Franchi S, Mandel SH. Graves' disease in the neonatal period and childhood. In: Braverman LE, Utiger RD, editors. Werner and Ingbar's The thyroid: a fundamental and clinical text, 6th ed. Philadelphia: JB Lippincott Company, 1991: 1237-46
19. Editorial. Acute fatty liver of pregnancy. Lancet 1983; 1: 339
20. Hankins GDV. Complications of beta-sympathomimetic tocolytic agents. In: Clark SL, Cotton DB, Hankins GDV, et al. editors. Critical care obstetrics, 2nd ed. Boston: Blackwell Scientific Publications, 1991: 223-50
21. Crombach G, Siebolds M, Mies R. Insulin use in pregnancy: clinical pharmacokinetic considerations. Clinical Pharmacokinetics 1993; 24: 89-100
22. Nimmo WS, Wilson J, Prescott LF. Narcotic analgesics and delayed gastric emptying in labour. Lancet 1975; 1: 890
23. Hill RM, Craig JP, Chanet MD, et al. Utilization of over the counter drugs during pregnancy. Clinical Obstetrics and Gynecology 1977; 20: 381
24. Rubin PC, Craig GF, Gavin K, et al. Prospective survey of use of therapeutic drugs, alcohol and cigarettes during pregnancy. British Medical Journal 1986; 292: 81
25. Vega WA, Kolody B, Hwang J, et al. Prevalence and magnitude of perinatal substance exposures in California. New England Journal of Medicine 1993; 329: 850-4
26. Mahomed K. Routine iron supplementation in pregnancy, No 3157. In: Enkin MW, Keirse MJNC, Renfrew MJ, et al. editors. Cochrane database of systematic reviews: pregnancy and childbirth module. Cochrane Updates on Disc, 2nd ed. Oxford: Oxford Update Software, 1993
27. Suharno D, West CE, Muhilal, et al. Supplementation with vitamin A and iron for nutritional anaemia in pregnant women in West Java, Indonesia. Lancet 1993; 342: 1325-8
28. Mahomed K. Routine folate supplementation in pregnancy, No 3158. In: Enkin MW, Keirse MJNC, Renfrew MJ, et al. editors. Cochrane database of systematic reviews: pregnancy and childbirth module. Cochrane Updates on Disc, 2nd ed. Oxford: Oxford Update Software, 1993
29. Briggs GG, Bodendorfer TW, Freeman RK, et al. Drugs in pregnancy and lactation: a reference guide to fetal and neonatal risk. Baltimore: Williams & Wilkins, 1994
30. Smaill F. Antibiotic versus no treatment for asymptomatic bacteriuria, No 3170. In: Enkin MW, Keirse MJNC, Renfrew MJ, et al. editors. Cochrane database of systematic reviews: pregnancy and childbirth module. Cochrane Updates on Disc, Oxford: Oxford Update Software, 1993
31. Masterton RG, Evans DC, Strike PW. Single dose amoxycillin in the treatment of bacteruria in pregnancy and the puerperium: a controlled trial. British Journal of Obstetrics and Gynaecology 1985; 92: 498
32. Editorial. Urinary tract infection during pregnancy. Lancet 1985; 2: 190
33. Report on confidential enquiries into maternal deaths in the United Kingdom 1988-1990. London: HMSO, 1994
34. Kaunitz AM, Hughes JM, Grimes DA, et al. Causes of maternal mortality in the United States. Obstetrics and Gynecology 1985; 65: 605-12
35. Redman CWG. Controlled trials of antihypertensive drugs in pregnancy. American Journal of Kidney Disease 1991; 17: 149-53
36. Collins R, Duley L. Diuretics for prevention of pre-eclampsia. No 4393. In: Enkin MW, Keirse MJNC, Renfrew MJ, et al. editors. Cochrane database of systematic reviews, 2nd ed. Oxford: Oxford Update Software, 1993
37. Redman CWG, Beilin LJ, Bonnar J, et al. Fetal outcome of antihypertensive treatment in pregnancy. Lancet 1976; 2: 753-6
38. Sibai BM, Mabie WC, Shamsa F, et al. A comparison of no medication versus methyldopa or labetalol in chronic hypertension during pregnancy. American Journal of Obstetrics and Gynecology 1990; 162: 960-7
39. Cockburn J, Moar VA, Ounsted M, et al. Final report of study on hypertension during pregnancy: the effects of specific treatment on the growth and development of the children. Lancet 1982; 1: 647-9
40. Butters L, Kennedy S, Rubin PC. Atenolol in essential hypertension during pregnancy. British Medical Journal 1990; 301: 587-9
41. Dollery CT, editor. Nifedipine. In: Therapeutic drugs. Vol. 2. Edinburgh: Churchill Livingstone, 1991: N80-N87
42. Detzer K. Toxicological investigations with nisoldipine. In: Lichtler PR, Hugenholz PG, editors. Nisoldipine. Stuttgart: Schattauer, 1988: 3-10
43. Carlsen JE, Kober L, Torp-Pedersen C. Relation between dose of bendrofluazide, antihypertensive effect, and adverse biochemical effects. British Medical Journal 1990; 300: 975-8
44. Burris JF, Weir MR, Oparil S. An assessment of diltiazem and hydrochlorothiazide in hypertension. Journal of the American Medical Association 1990; 263: 1507-12

45. Walters BNJ, Redman CWG. Treatment of severe pregnancy-associated hypertension with the calcium antagonist nifedipine. British Journal of Obstetrics and Gynaecology 1984; 91: 330-6
46. Cotton DB, Longmire S, Jones MM, et al. Cardiovascular alterations in severe pregnancy-induced hypertension: effects of intravenous nitroglycerin coupled with blood volume expansion. American Journal of Obstetrics and Gynecology 1986; 154: 1053-9
47. Dildy GA, Phelan JP, Cotton DB. Complications of pregnancy-induced hypertension. In: Clark SL, Cotton DB, Hankins GDV, et al. editors. Critical care obstetrics, 2nd ed. Boston: Blackwell Scientific Publications, 1991: 251-88
48. Wallenburg HCS. Changes in the coagulation system and platelets in pregnancy-induced hypertension and pre-eclampsia. In: Sharp & Symonds, editors. Hypertension in pregnancy: proceedings of the sixteenth study group of the Royal College of Obstetricians and Gynaecologists, New York: Perinatology Press, 1987: 227-48
49. Goodlin RC, Haesslein HO, Fleming J. Aspirin for the treatment of recurrent toxaemia. Lancet 1978; 2: 51
50. Wallenburg HCS, Dekker GA, Makovitz JW, et al. Low-dose aspirin prevents pregnancy-induced hypertension and pre-eclampsia in angiotensin-sensitive primigravidae. Lancet 1986; 1: 1-3
51. Sibai BM, Caritis SN, Thom E, et al. Prevention of pre-eclampsia with low-dose aspirin in healthy, nulliparous pregnant women. New England Journal of Medicine 1993; 329: 1213-8
52. CLASP Collaborative Group. CLASP: a randomised trial of low-dose aspirin for the prevention and treatment of pre-eclampsia among 9364 pregnant women. Lancet 1994; 343: 619-29
53. Pritchard JA, Pritchard SA. Standardized treatment of 154 consecutive cases of eclampsia. American Journal of Obstetrics and Gynecology 1975; 123: 543-52
54. Eclampsia Trial Collaborative Group. Which anticonvulsant for women with eclampsia?: evidence from the Collaborative Eclampsia Trial. Lancet 1995; 345: 1455-63
55. Lucas MJ, Levene KJ, Cunningham FG. A comparison of magnesium sulphate with phenytoin for the prevention of eclampsia. New England Journal of Medicine 1995; 333: 201-5
56. Twaddle S, Harper V. Economic evaluation of daycare in the management of hypertension in pregnancy. British Journal of Obstetrics and Gynaecology 1992; 94: 459-563
57. Rutherford SE, Phelan JP. Deep venous thrombosis and pulmonary embolism. In: Clark SL, Cotton DB, Hankins GDV, et al. editors. Critical care obstetrics, 2nd ed. Boston: Blackwell Scientific, 1987: 150-79
58. Thromboembolic Risk Factors (THRIFT) Consensus Group. Risk of and prophylaxis for venous thromboembolism in hospital patients. British Medical Journal 1992; 305: 567-74
59. Scottish Intercollegiate Guidelines Network. Prophylaxis of venous thromboembolism. Edinburgh: Royal College of Physicians, 1995
60. Royal College of Obstetricians and Gynaecologists. Report of Royal College of Obstetricians and Gynaecologists Working Party on prophylaxis against thromboembolism in obstetrics and gynaecology. London: Royal College of Obstetricians and Gynaecologists, 1995
61. Sbarouni E, Oakley CM. Outcome of pregnancy in women with valve prostheses. British Heart Journal 1994; 71: 196-201
62. Holmer E. Low molecular weight heparin. In: Lane DA, Lindahl U, editors. Heparin: chemical and biological properties, clinical applications, London: Edward Arnold, 1989: 573-95
63. Ginsberg JS, Hirsh J. Optimum use of anticoagulants in pregnancy. Drugs 1988; 36: 505-12
64. Iturbe-Alessio I, del Carmen Fonseca M, Mutchinik O, et al. Risks of anticoagulant therapy in pregnant women with artificial heart valves. New England Journal of Medicine 1986; 315: 1390-3
65. Jewell MD. Benzylamide and Dramamine for nausea in pregnancy, No 3350. Phenothiazines for nausea in pregnancy, No 3388. Piperazine for nausea in pregnancy, No 4428. Pyridoxine for nausea in pregnancy, No 7703. In: Enkin MW, Keirse MJNC, Renfrew MJ, et al. editors. Cochrane database of systematic reviews: pregnancy and childbirth module. Cochrane Updates on Disc, 2nd ed. Oxford: Oxford Update Software, 1993
66. Andrews AD, Brock-Utne JG, Downing JW. Protection against pulmonary acid aspiration with ranitidine. Anaesthesia 1982; 37: 22
67. Bateman DN, Rawlins MD, Simpson JM. Extrapyramidal reactions with metoclopramide. British Medical Journal 1985; 291: 930
68. Turner ES, Greenberger PA, Patterson R. Management of the pregnant asthmatic. Annals of Internal Medicine 1980; 6: 905-18
69. Gordon M, Niswander KR, Berendes H, et al. Fetal morbidity following potentially anoxigenic obstetric conditions: bronchial asthma. American Journal of Obstetrics and Gynecology 1970; 106: 421-9
70. Weiss PAM. Gestational diabetes: a survey and the Graz approach to diagnosis and therapy. In: Weiss & Coustan, editors. Gestational diabetes. Vienna-New York: Springer, 1994: 1-55
71. Skyler JS. Diabetes and pregnancy: consensus and controversy. In: Sutherland HW, editor. Carbohydrate metabolism in pregnancy and the newborn, 4th ed. Berlin-Heidelberg: Springer, 1989: 363-72
72. Isojvari JIT, Laatikainen TJ, Pakirinen AJ, et al. Polycystic ovaries and hyperandrogenism in women taking valproate for epilepsy. New England Journal of Medicine 1993; 329: 1383-8
73. Jones KL, Lacro R, Johnson KA, et al. Pattern of malformations in the children of women treated with carbamazepine during pregnancy. New England Journal of Medicine 1989; 320: 1661-6
74. Rosa FW. Spina bifida in infants of women treated with carbamazepine during pregnancy. New England Journal of Medicine 1991; 324: 674-7
75. Ades AE, Davison CF, Holland FJ, et al. Vertically transmitted HIV infection in the British Isles. British Medical Journal 1993; 306: 1296-9
76. Dunn DT, Newell ML, Adas ED, et al. Risk of human immunodeficiency virus type 1 transmission through breast-feeding. Lancet 1992; 340: 585-8
77. AIDS Clinical Trials Information Service. Washington DC: National Institutes of Health, 1994
78. Banatvala JE, Chrystie IL. HIV screening in pregnancy; UK lags. Lancet 1994; 343: 1113-4
79. Goldstein PA, Sacks MS, Chalmers TC. Hormone administration for the maintenance of pregnancy. In: Chalmers I, Enkin MW, Keirse MJNC, editors. Effec-

tive care in pregnancy and childbirth. Oxford: Oxford University Press, 1989

80. Fraser EJ, Grimes DA, Schulz KF. Immunization as therapy for recurrent spontaneous abortion: a review and meta-analysis. Obstetrics and Gynecology 1993; 82: 854-9
81. King JF, Grant AM, Keirse MJNC, et al. Beta-mimetics in preterm labour: an overview of the randomised controlled trials. British Journal of Obstetrics and Gynaecology 1988; 95: 211-22
82. Keirse MJNC, Van Oppen ACC. Preparing the cervix for induction of labour. In: Chalmers I, Enkin MW, Keirse MJNC, editors. Effective care in pregnancy and childbirth. Oxford: Oxford University Press, 1989
83. Norton ME, Merrill J, Cooper BAB, et al. Neonatal complications after administration of indomethacin for preterm labor. New England Journal of Medicine 1993; 329: 1602-7
84. Lees C, Campbell S, Jauniaux E, et al. Arrest of preterm labour and prolongation of gestation with glyceryl trinitrate, a nitric oxide donor. Lancet 1994; 343: 1325-6
85. Crowley P, Chalmers I, Keirse MJNC. The effects of corticosteroid administration before preterm delivery: a review of the evidence from controlled trials. British Journal of Obstetrics and Gynaecology 1990; 97: 11-25
86. Chiswick M. Antenatal TRH. Lancet 1995; 345: 872
87. Hannah ME, Hannah WJ, Hellman J, et al. Induction of labour as compared with serial antenatal monitoring in post-term pregnancy: a randomised controlled trial. New England Journal of Medicine 1992; 326: 1587-92
88. Frigoletto FD, Lieberman E, Lang JM, et al. A clinical trial of active management of labor. New England Journal of Medicine 1995; 333: 745-50
89. Hannah ME, Ohlsson A, Farine D, et al. Induction of labor compared with expectant management for prelabor rupture of the membranes at term. New England Journal of Medicine 1996; 334: 1005-10
90. Keirse MJNC, Van Oppen ACC. Comparison of prostaglandins and oxytocin for inducing labour. In: Chalmers I, Enkin MW, Keirse MJNC, editors. Effective care in pregnancy and childbirth. Oxford: Oxford University Press, 1989
91. Cabrol D, Dubois C, Cranje H, et al. Induction of labour with mifepristone (RU 486) in intrauterine death. American Journal of Obstetrics and Gynecology 1990; 163: 540-2
92. Frydman R, Baton C, Lelandier C, et al. Mifepristone for induction of labour. Lancet 1991; 337: 488-9
93. Brogden RN, Goa KL, Faulds D. Mifepristone: a review of its pharmacodynamic and pharmacokinetic properties and therapeutic potential. Drugs 1993; 45: 384-409
94. Prendeville WJ. Progestogens in pregnancy, No 3284. In: Enkin MW, Keirse MJNC, Renfrew MJ, et al. editors. Cochrane database of systematic reviews: pregnancy and childbirth module. Cochrane Updates on Disk, 2nd ed. Oxford: Oxford Update Software, 1993
95. McDonald SJ, Prendiville WJ, Blair E. Randomised controlled trial of oxytocin alone versus oxytocin and ergometrine in active management of third stage of labour. British Medical Journal 1993; 307: 1167-77
96. Aono T, Shioji T, Hirota K, et al. Augmentation of puerperal lactation by oral administration of sulpiride. Journal of Clinical Endocrinology and Metabolism 1979; 48: 478
97. Spitz IM, Bardin CW. Drug therapy: mifepristone (RU 486) - a modulator of progestin and glucocorticoid action. New England Journal of Medicine 1993; 329: 404-12
98. Norman JE, Thong KJ, Baird DT. Uterine contractility and induction of abortion in early pregnancy by misoprostol and mifepristone. Lancet 1991; 338: 1233-6
99. Schonhofer PS. Brazil: misuse of misoprostol as an abortifacient may induce malformations. Lancet 1991; 337: 1534-5
100. Costa SH, Vessey MP. Misoprostol and illegal abortion in Rio de Janeiro, Brazil. Lancet 1993; 341: 1258-61
101. Coelho HLL, Teixeira AC, Santos AP, et al. Misoprostol and illegal abortion in Fortaleza, Brazil. Lancet 1993; 341: 1261-3
102. Fonseca W, Alencar AJC, Mota FSB, et al. Misoprostol and congenital malformations. Lancet 1991; 338: 56
103. El-Refaey H, Calder L, Wheatley DN, et al. Cervical priming with prostaglandin E1 analogues, misoprostol and gemeprost. Lancet 1994; 343: 1207-9
104. Henshaw RC, Templeton AA, Naji SA, et al. Medical abortion. British Medical Journal 1992; 304: 914
105. Henshaw RC, Templeton AA. Pre-operative cervical preparation before first trimester vacuum aspiration: a randomised controlled comparison between gemeprost and mifepristone (RU 486). British Journal of Obstetrics and Gynaecology 1991; 98: 1025-30
106. Thong KJ, Baird DT. A study of gemeprost alone, dilapan or mifepristone in combination with gemeprost for the termination of second trimester pregnancy. Contraception 1992; 46: 11-7
107. Kaunitz AM, Rosenfield A. Injectable contraception with depot medroxyprogesterone acetate. Drugs 1993; 45: 857-65
108. World Health Organization. WHO collaborative study of neoplasia and steroid contraceptives: endometrial cancer. International Journal of Cancer 1991; 49: 186-90
109. Cuelar KD, Gruber C, Hayes R, et al. Medroxyprogesterone acetate and homozygous sickle-cell disease. Lancet 1982; 2: 229-31
110. Mattson RH, Cramer JA, Caldwell BV, et al. Treatment of seizures with medroxyprogesterone acetate: preliminary report. Neurology 1984; 34: 1255-8
111. Weisberg E, Fraser IS, Mishell Jr DR, et al. The acceptability of a combined oestrogen-progestagen contraceptive ring in different populations. Contraception 1995; 51: 39-44
112. Thiery M, Vander Pas H, Delborge W, et al. The levonorgestrel intrauterine device. Geburoshilfe und Frauenheilkund 1989; 49: 186-8
113. Glasier A, Thong KJ, Dewar M, et al. Mifepristone (RU 486) compared with high-dose estrogen and progestogen for emergency postcoital contraception. New England Journal of Medicine 1992; 327: 1041-4
114. Webb AMC, Russell J, Elstein M. Comparison of Yuspe regimen, danazol and mifepristone (RU 486). British Medical Journal 1992; 305: 927-31
115. World Health Organization Collaborative Study of Cardiovascular Disease and Steroid Hormone Contraception. Venous thromboembolic disease and combined oral contraceptives: results of international multicentre case-control study. Lancet 1995; 346: 1575-82
116. World Health Organization Collaborative Study of Cardiovascular Disease and Steroid Hormone Contraception. Effect of different progestagens in low oestrogen oral contraceptives on venous thromboembolic disease. Lancet 1995; 346: 1582-8
117. Spitzer WO, Lewis MA, Heinemann LAJ, et al. on behalf of Transnational Research Group on Oral Con-

traceptives and the Health of Young Women. Third generation oral contraceptives and risk of venous thromboembolic disorders: an international case-control study. British Medical Journal 1996; 312: 83-8
118. Jick H, Jick SS, Gurewich V, et al. Risk of idiopathic cardiovascular death and nonfatal venous thromboembolism in women using oral contraceptives with differing progestagen components. Lancet 1995; 346: 1589-93
119. Lewis MA, Spitzer WO, Heinemann LAJ, et al. Third generation oral contraceptives and risk of myocardial infarction: an international case-control study. British Medical Journal 1996; 312: 88-90
120. Vandenbroucke JP, Koster T, Briet E, et al. Increased risk of venous thrombosis in oral contraceptive users who are carriers of factor V Leiden mutation. Lancet 1994; 344: 1453-7
121. Bloemenkamp KWM, Rosendaal FR, Helmerhorst FM, et al. Enhancement by factor V Leiden mutation of risk of deep-vein thrombosis associated with oral contraceptives containing a third-generation progestagen. Lancet 1995; 346: 1593-6
122. Guillebaud J. Advising women which pill to take. British Medical Journal 1995; 311: 1111-2
123. Mills AM, Wilkinson CI, Bromham DR, et al. Guidelines for prescribing combined oral contraceptives. British Medical Journal 1996; 312: 121-2
124. McPherson K. Third generation oral contraceptives and venous thromboembolism. British Medical Journal 1996; 312: 68-9
125. Editorial. OCs O-T-C? Lancet 1993; 342: 565-6
126. Shenfield GM. Oral contraceptives: are drug interactions of clinical significance? Drug Safety 1993; 9: 21-37
127. Legler UF, Benet LZ. Marked alterations in dose-dependent prednisolone kinetics in women taking oral contraceptives. Clinical Pharmacology and Therapeutics 1986; 39: 425-9
128. Ross WB, Roberts D, Griffen PJA, et al. Cyclosporin interaction with danazol and norethisterone. Lancet 1986; 1: 330
129. Back DJ, Breckenridge AM, Orme ML'E. Drug interactions involving oral contraceptive steroid therapy. In: Petrie JC, Cluff L, editors. Clinically important drug interactions, Amsterdam: Elsevier, 1984: 305-7
130. Cote J. Interaction of griseofulvin and oral contraceptives. Journal of the American Academy of Dermatology 1990; 22: 124-5
131. Back DJ, Grimmer SFM, Orme ML'E, et al. Evaluation of Committee on Safety of Medicines yellow card reports on oral contraceptive-drug interactions with anticonvulsants and antibiotics. British Journal of Clinical Pharmacology 1988; 25: 527-32
132. Orme ML'E, Back DJ. Oral contraceptive steroids: pharmacological issues of interest to the prescribing physician. Advances in Contraception 1991; 7: 325-31
133. Zipper J, Cole LP, Goldsmith A, et al. Quinacrine hydrochloride pellets: preliminary data on a nonsurgical method of female sterilization. International Journal of Gynaecology and Obstetrics 1980; 18: 275-9
134. Hieu DT, Tan TT, Tan DN, et al. 31781 cases of nonsurgical female sterilization with quinacrine pellets in Vietnam. Lancet 1993; 342: 213-7
135. Hieu WB, Tan TT, Tan DN, et al. Non-surgical female sterilization. Lancet 1993; 342: 870-1
136. World Health Organization. Progress in human reproductive research. Geneva: World Health Organization, 1995
137. Family Health International. FH1 quinacrine studies. Network 1995; 16 (1): 27
138. Hull MGR. Monitoring the ovarian cycle for in vivo and in vitro fertility in insemination. In: Thompson et al., editors. In vitro fertilisation and donor insemination. London: Royal College of Obstetrics and Gynaecology, 1984
139. Dollery CT, editor. Clomiphene. In: Therapeutic drugs. Edinburgh: Churchill Livingstone, 1991: C290-C293
140. Adashi EY. Clomiphene citrate: mechanisms and sites of action - hypothesis revisited. Fertility and Sterility 1984; 62: 331-44
141. Fraser HM. GnRH and its analogues. Drugs 1984; 27: 187
142. Petterson B, Nelson KB, Watson L, et al. Twins, triplets and cerebral palsy in births in Western Australia. British Medical Journal 1993; 307: 1239-43
143. Willemsen W, Kruitwagen R, Bastiaans B, et al. Ovarian stimulation and granulosa-cell tumour. Lancet 1993; 341: 986-8
144. Page H. Economic appraisal of in-vitro fertilisation: discussion paper. Journal of the Royal Society of Medicine 1989; 82: 99-102
145. Page H, Brazier J. Benefits of in-vitro fertilisation. Lancet 1989; 334: 1327-8
146. Low RA, Roberts AD, Lees DA. A comparative study of various dosages of danazol in the treatment of endometriosis. British Journal of Obstetrics and Gynaecology 1984; 91: 167-71
147. Dockeray CJ, Sheppard BL, Bonnar J. Comparison between mefenamic acid and danazol in the treatment of established menorrhagia. British Journal of Obstetrics and Gynaecology 1989; 96: 840-4
148. Langman MJS, Weil J, Wainwright P, et al. Risks of bleeding peptic ulcer associated with individual non-steroidal anti-inflammatory drugs. Lancet 1994; 343: 1075-8
149. Healy DL. The use of LHRH analogues in the treatment of uterine fibroids. Gynecology & Endocrinology 1989; 3 Suppl. 2: 33-49
150. Barbieri RL, Evans S, Kistner RW. Danazol in the treatment of endometriosis: analysis of 100 cases with a 4 year follow-up. Fertility and Sterility 1982; 37: 737-46
151. Lock M. Contested meanings of the menopause. Lancet 1991; 337: 1270-2
152. McKinley SM, Brambilla DJ, Avis NE, et al. Women's experience of the menopause. Current Obstetrics and Gynaecology 1991; 1: 3-7
153. Oldenhave A, Jaszmann LJB, Haspels AA, et al. Impact of climacteric on well-being: a survey based on 5213 women 39-60 years old. American Journal of Obstetrics and Gynecology 1993; 168: 772-80
154. Oldenhave A, Netelenbos C. Pathogenesis of climacteric complaints: ready for the change? Lancet 1994; 343: 649-53
155. Whitehead MI, Fraser D, Schenkel L, et al. Transdermal administration of oestrogen/progestagen hormone replacement therapy. Lancet 1990; 335: 310-2
156. Medical Research Council's General Practice Research Framework. Randomized comparison of oestrogen versus oestrogen plus progestagen hormone replacement therapy in women with hysterectomy. British Medical Journal 1996; 312: 473-8
157. Rees M. On menstrual bleeding with hormone replacement therapy. Lancet 1994; 343: 250-1
158. Gangar KF, Fraser D, Whitehead MI, et al. Prolonged endometrial stimulation associated with oestradiol implants. British Medical Journal 1990; 300: 436-8

159. Forbes CD, Greer IH. Hormone replacement therapy is not a risk for venous thrombosis. Scottish Medical Journal 1994; 39: 165-6
160. Dollery CT, editor. Tibolone. In: Therapeutic drugs. Vol. 2. Edinburgh: Churchill Livingstone, 1994: 257-61
161. Ayton RA, Darling GM, Murkies AL, et al. A comparative study of safety and efficacy of continuous low dose oestradiol released from a vaginal ring compared with conjugated equine oestrogen cream in the treatment of postmenopausal urogenital atrophy. British Journal of Obstetrics and Gynaecology 1996; 103: 351-8
162. Raz R, Stamm WE. A controlled trial of intravaginal estriol in postmenopausal women with recurrent urinary tract infection. New England Journal of Medicine 1993; 329: 753-6
163. Hemminki E, Sihvo S. A review of postmenopausal hormone therapy recommendations: potential for selection bias. Obstetrics and Gynecology 1993; 82: 1021-8
164. Posthuma WFM, Westendorp RGJ, Vandenbrouke JP. Cardioprotective effect of hormone replacement therapy in postmenopausal women: is the evidence biased? British Medical Journal 1994; 308: 1268-9
165. Lindsay R. Why do oestrogens prevent bone loss? Bailliere's Clinical Obstetrics and Gynaecology 1991; 5: 837-52
166. Ettinger B, Grady D. The waning effect of postmenopausal estrogen therapy on osteoporosis. New England Journal of Medicine 1993; 329: 1192-3
167. Felson DT, Zhang Y, Hannan MT, et al. The effect of postmenopausal estrogen therapy on bone density in elderly women. New England Journal of Medicine 1993; 329: 1141-6
168. Law MR, Wald NJ, Meade TW. Strategies for prevention of osteoporosis and hip fracture. British Medical Journal 1991; 303: 453-9
169. Jacobs HS, Loeffler FE. Postmenopausal hormone replacement therapy. British Medical Journal 1992; 305: 1403-8
170. Lufkin EG, Wahner HW, O'Fallon WM, et al. Treatment of postmenopausal osteoporosis with transdermal estrogen. Annals of Internal Medicine 1992; 117: 1-9
171. Dempster DW, Lindsay R. Pathogenesis of osteoporosis. Lancet 1993; 341: 797-801
172. Notelovitz M. Osteoporosis: screening, prevention and management. Fertility and Sterility 1993; 59: 707-25
173. Gallagher JC, Kable WT, Goldgar D. Effect of progestin therapy on cortical and trabecular bone: comparison with estrogens. American Journal of Medicine 1991; 90: 171-8
174. Stampfer MJ, Colditz GA, Willett WC, et al. Postmenopausal estrogen therapy and cardiovascular disease. New England Journal of Medicine 1991; 325: 756-62
175. Stampfer MJ, Colditz GA. Estrogen replacement therapy and coronary heart disease; a quantitative assessment of the epidemiological evidence. Preventative Medicine 1991; 20: 47-63
176. Grady D, Rubin SM, Petitti DB, et al. Hormone therapy to prevent disease and prolong life in postmenopausal women. Annals of Internal Medicine 1992; 117: 1016-37
177. Sullivan JM, Zwaag RV, Hugus JP, et al. Estrogen replacement and coronary artery disease. Effect on survival in postmenopausal women. Archives of Internal Medicine 1990; 150: 2557-62
178. Nabulsi AA, Folsom AR, White A, et al. Association of hormone-replacement therapy with various cardiovascular risk factors in postmenopausal women. New England Journal of Medicine 1993; 328: 1069-75
179. Martin KA, Freeman MF. Postmenopausal hormone-replacement therapy. New England Journal of Medicine 1993; 328: 1115-7
180. Healy B. The Yentl syndrome. New England Journal of Medicine 1991; 325: 274-6
181. American College of Physicians. Guidelines for counselling postmenopausal women about preventative hormones. Annals of Internal Medicine 1992; 117: 1038-41
182. Belchetz PE. Hormone treatment of postmenopausal women. New England Journal of Medicine 1994; 330: 1062-71
183. Steinberg KK, Thacker SB, Smith SJ, et al. A meta-analysis of the effect of estrogen replacement therapy on the risk of breast cancer. Journal of the American Medical Association 1991; 265: 1985-90
184. Persson I, Yuen J, Bergkvist L, et al. Combined oestrogen-progestogen replacement therapy and breast cancer risk. Lancet 1992; 340: 1044
185. Colditz GA, Hankinson SE, Hunter DJ, et al. The use of estrogen and progestins and the risk of breast cancer in postmenopausal women. New England Journal of Medicine 1995; 332: 1589-93
186. te Velde ER, van Leusden HAIM. Hormonal treatment for the climacteric: alleviation of symptoms and prevention of postmenopausal disease. Lancet 1994; 343: 654-8
187. Disaia P, Odicino F, Grosen EA, et al. Hormone replacement therapy in breast cancer. Lancet 1993; 342: 1232
188. Eden JA. Estrogen replacement therapy in survivors of breast cancer: a risk-benefit assessment. Drugs & Aging 1996; 8: 127-33
189. Persson I, Adami H, Bergkvist L, et al. Risk of endometrial cancer after treatment with oestrogen alone or in conjunction with progestogens: results of a prospective study. British Medical Journal 1989; 298: 147-51
190. Writing Group for the PEPI trial. Effects of hormone replacement therapy on endometrial histology in postmenopausal women: the Postmenopausal Estrogen/Progestin Intervention (PEPI) trial. Journal of the American Medical Association 1996; 275: 370-5
191. Whittington R, Faulds D. Hormone replacement therapy. I: a pharmacoeconomic appraisal of its therapeutic use in menopausal symptoms and urogenital estrogen deficiency. PharmacoEconomics 1994; 5: 419-45
192. Whittington R, Faulds D. Hormone replacement therapy. II: a pharmacoeconomic appraisal of its role in the prevention of postmenopausal osteoporosis and ischaemic heart disease. PharmacoEconomics 1994; 5: 513-54
193. McPherson K. Breast cancer and hormone supplements in post-menopausal women. British Medical Journal 1996; 311: 669-70
194. LaRosa JC. Has HRT come of age? Lancet 1995; 345: 76-7
195. Chapman MG. Management of hirsutism. Hospital Medicine 1981; 270
196. Fraser IS, Shearman RP, Allen JK, et al. Cyproterone acetate and the treatment of hirsutism. Australian and New Zealand Journal of Obstetrics and Gynaecology 1983; 23: 93
197. Barth JH, Cherry CA, Wojnarow SKAF, et al. Spironolactone is an effective and well-tolerated systemic antiandrogen therapy for hirsute women. Journal of Clinical Endocrinology & Metabolism 1989; 68: 966-70

# Chapter 19

# Endocrine Diseases

*I.D. Caterson, S.C. Boyages, B. Brooks, F. Capstick, R. Donnelly, J. Feely, D.J. Handelsman, M. Lewitt, X. Qu, K.S. Steinbeck, S. Swaraj, J.R. Turtle* and *D.K. Yue*

## Synopsis of Important Principles

1) Precise diagnosis of endocrine disorders is possible and necessary to institute appropriate therapy.

2) The physiological control mechanisms of the endocrine system help with diagnosis of the site of endocrine disease.

3) The aim of endocrine therapy is normalisation of hormonal and physiological function, and this can be achieved in most situations.

4) The therapy of endocrine disease is long term and generally provided to ambulatory patients (i.e. hospitalisation is rarely required).

5) The pharmacokinetics of some drugs are altered by uncontrolled or poorly controlled diabetes and thyroid disease.

6) Conversely, some drugs may alter endocrine function. This is particularly true in diabetes, where glucocorticoids, diuretics and growth hormone therapy may precipitate the disorder or make its control more difficult.

7) The metabolic and nutritional basis underlying normal growth and development must be remembered when treating patients with diabetes or obesity, and appropriate nutritional management and exercise plans implemented.

8) Drugs can alter the normal endocrine physiological control mechanisms (e.g. after prolonged courses with pharmacological doses of glucocorticoids) or induce endocrine disease (e.g. lithium- or amiodarone-induced thyroid disease).

9) Some drugs alter endocrine testing and hormonal levels.

10) Better and more appropriate therapy of disorders of the male endocrine system is possible and necessary. It should be remembered that 'anabolic' steroids are androgens.

Endocrinology has developed extensively as a discipline over the past few years. With the advent of specific immunoassays for hormones, and the general availability of computed tomography (CT) and magnetic resonance imaging (MRI), precise diagnosis of endocrine conditions is possible. As immunoassays become automated, diagnosis is ever more rapid. Endocrinology also has a strong physiological and biochemical background and research in these areas continues, so there is better understanding of endocrine disorders as each year passes. New hormones, growth factors and binding proteins are being found continually. These, coupled with genetic studies, will allow even better understanding of the causes and mechanisms of endocrine disease. There is also a wide range of hormone replacements, specific drugs and modes of therapy that allow appropriate long term treatment of all endocrine disorders.

In the treatment of endocrine disease, two aspects require special emphasis. Firstly, the aim of therapy is to produce a normal life and lifespan, and this is possible in most disorders. Secondly, endocrine diseases are chronic, and there are additional skills required for their long term therapy.

## 1. Clinical Pharmacological Considerations

The endocrine system exerts a major influence on the individual, the body and its processes. It is a major control system that acts at the cellular level to affect metabolic and biosynthetic processes of the cells. In most instances, hormones bind to cellular receptors either on the cell surface (membrane) or within the cell cytoplasm. Steroid hormones tend to bind to the latter type of receptors, which belong to a 'superfamily' of nuclear binding receptors to which thyroid hormones, vitamin D and retinoic acid may also bind (see sections 7.1.1 and 8.2). Once the hormone is bound to a receptor, a series of biochemical events may be initiated from the cell membrane, or the receptor may translocate to the cell nucleus, bind to DNA and initiate or block DNA transcription. Such hormone binding can then alter the metabolic processes of cells. The hormone effect may be tissue specific or have effects throughout the body.

The action of the endocrine system is regulated by the principle of negative feedback. Secretion of hormones from the pituitary gland is controlled by releasing and inhibitory hormones from the hypothalamus. There is a short feedback loop of anterior pituitary hormones to the hypothalamus. The anterior pituitary trophic hormones, in turn, induce peripheral target glands to produce hormones. These hormones feed back, in a long feedback loop, to the hypothalamus and, to a lesser extent, to the pituitary gland itself, and modulate trophic hormone secretion (fig. 1). Using the negative feedback principle and with current abilities to measure many hormones, it is possible to determine where disordered hormone secretion is occurring. Endocrine disease may be caused by over-, under- or inappropriate secretion of trophic or peripheral hormones. Changes in hormone secretion may be due to disease of the endocrine gland itself, replacement of the gland with abnormal tissue, or to alterations in hormone secretion or metabolism caused by disease in other organs.

A broad outline of the regulation of carbohydrate and lipid metabolism and control of thyroid and adrenal gland secretion is presented to allow a better understanding of the rationale for endocrine drug therapy.

### 1.1 Regulation of Carbohydrate and Lipid Metabolism and Insulin Secretion

The major macronutrients in the diet are protein (11 to 15% in Western diets), carbohydrates (45 to 55%) and fats (≈40%). The cells use these macronutrients for energy and to maintain their structure and integrity. In energy metabolism, there is a reciprocal relationship between the use of fat and carbohydrate, known as the 'glucose fatty acid cycle', which was first described in 1963.[1]

#### *1.1.1 Lipid Metabolism*

Fats are absorbed from the gut, resynthesised and formed into chylomicrons that enter the circulation via the thoracic duct. These large lipid particles interact with lipoprotein lipase, liberating free fatty acids that can enter cells that use them for energy, store them as triglyceride or, in the case of the liver, export them in a smaller set of triglyceride rich lipid particles (very-low-density lipoprotein or VLDL). In most physiological situations, except for refeeding after prolonged fasting, it is unusual for humans to synthesise fats as they rely on dietary intake for this nutrient. Animals synthesise fats more readily. While it is believed that most fats diffuse into cells, a number of fatty acid binding proteins have been recently described and may play a significant role in transport and metabolism. Within the cell, fatty acids may be stored as triglyceride (with the 3-carbon backbone coming from carbohydrates), oxidised for energy or incorporated into membranes. There are at least 2 oxidation paths, the major one being β-oxidation within the mitochondrion, but there also are perioxsomal pathways.

### *1.1.2 Carbohydrate Metabolism*

Carbohydrates may be ingested as monosaccharides, disaccharides or more complex carbohydrates and starches. Before being absorbed, they are broken down to monosaccharides in the gut. These carbohydrates are then transported into cells where they are metabolised for energy and a small amount will be stored as glycogen. Glucose is the most important carbohydrate. It is actively transported into cells by several specific transporters. The transporters vary from cell type to cell type, but in most cells, the insulin-sensitive transporter is GLUT 4. Within the cell, there is a small amount of free glucose, but most is rapidly phosphorylated to glucose-6-phosphate (G6P) by hexokinase or glucokinase and this molecule cannot escape from the cells. There are a number of subsequent metabolic paths.

Glycogen (storage carbohydrate) may be synthesised or G6P may be further metabolised in the glycolytic or pentose phosphate pathways. Stored glycogen contains far less energy than the major fat stores, but is important in providing energy for rapid movement (muscle) and maintaining blood glucose levels during fasting (liver glycogen), since the brain does not use fat as a metabolic fuel routinely. Anaerobic glycolysis provides energy and 3-carbon units that may then be metabolised in the oxidative citric acid cycle. In periods of fasting or of energy excess, gluconeogenesis may take place from amino acids and smaller 2-, 3- and 4-carbon carbohydrates, with energy provided from oxidation of lipids. Gluconeogenesis takes place mainly in the liver and serves to replace liver glycogen and maintain blood sugar concentrations.

A number of hormones have major effects on these processes. Insulin stimulates glucose transport into cells by enhancing transporter ac-

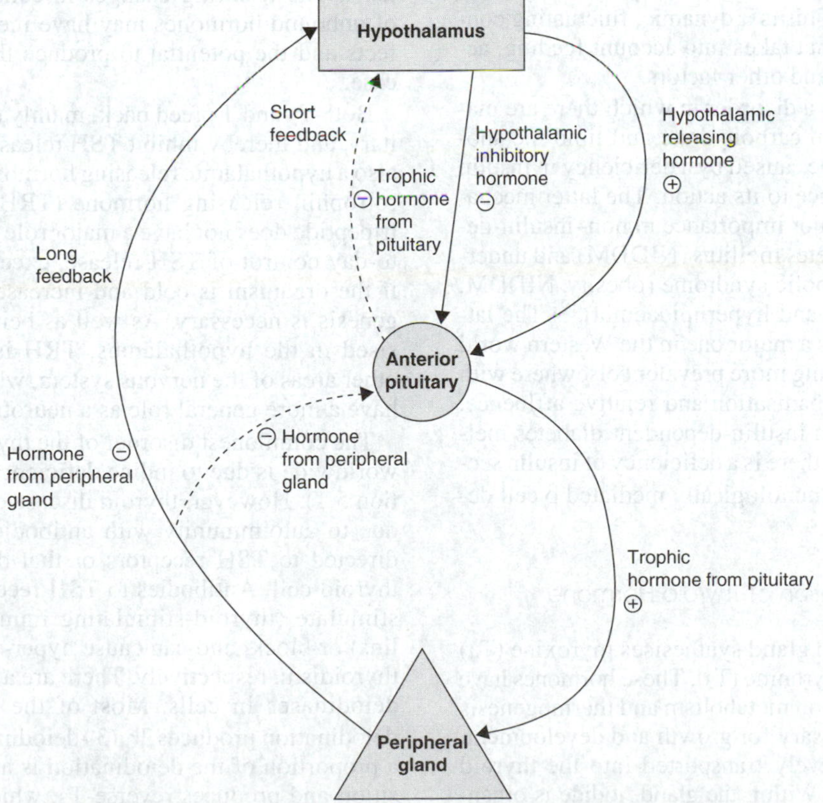


**Fig. 1.** Schematic representation of control of endocrine secretion. Hormones may be either stimulatory (+) or inhibitory (–). Other hormones or factors not shown in this diagram may also modulate hypothalamic or pituitary secretion.

tivity and recruiting transporters from the interior of the cell. It also stimulates metabolic processes, glycolysis, glucose oxidation, glycogen synthesis and lipogenesis, among other processes, and stimulates synthetic processes within the cells. Insulin binds to a specific receptor on the cell surface; these receptors aggregate and are internalised. The metabolic signal starts with phosphorylation of the receptor by an intrinsic kinase. The signal is passed through many associated proteins and enzymes in an ever-expanding net to stimulate metabolic processes.

#### *1.1.3 Insulin Secretion*

Insulin secretion from the β cells of the islets of Langerhans is stimulated by glucose, amino acids and medium chain triglycerides in humans as well as by glucagon, other gastrointestinal hormones and vagal stimulation. Hormones such as glucagon, catecholamines, insulin-like growth factor-I (IGF-I; somatomedin-C), growth hormone and glucocorticoids also affect either the same metabolic processes as insulin or cause glycogen breakdown and lipolysis (fat breakdown). The control of metabolism is exerted by these messengers and by the sympathetic nervous system. This is a dynamic, fluctuating control system that takes into account feeding, activity, stress and other factors.

Diabetes is a disorder in which there are major changes in carbohydrate and lipid metabolism. It may be caused by a deficiency in insulin or by resistance to its action. The latter mechanism is of major importance in non–insulin-dependent diabetes mellitus (NIDDM) and underlies the metabolic syndrome (obesity, NIDDM, hypertension and hyperlipidaemia).[2] The latter problem is a major one in the Western world and is becoming more prevalent elsewhere with increasing urbanisation and relative affluence. In contrast, in insulin-dependent diabetes mellitus (IDDM) there is a deficiency of insulin secondary to immunologically mediated β cell destruction.

### 1.2 Regulation of Thyroid Hormone

The thyroid gland synthesises thyroxine ($T_4$) and tri-iodothyronine ($T_3$). These hormones have major effects on metabolism and thermogenesis and are necessary for growth and development. Iodide is actively transported into the thyroid from plasma. Within the gland, iodide is organified, attached to tyrosine, and two molecules of iodinated tyrosine then couple to form $T_4$ or $T_3$. These hormones are then stored in the thyroid follicle bound to thyroglobulin.

The control of thyroxine synthesis is mediated by thyroid-stimulating hormone (TSH or thyrotrophin), which is released from the pituitary. This glycoprotein has specific receptors on the membrane of thyroid cells that activate adenyl cyclase and $T_4$ synthesis. As well, $T_4$ and $T_3$ are released from stores to the plasma. Here, most is bound to proteins [thyroxine binding globulin (TBG), albumin and thyroid binding prealbumin] with only a small fraction (<1%) unbound. It is the unbound (free) hormone that interacts with cells to produce the effects of the thyroid hormones, and there are a number of specific nuclear receptors (see section 5.1.1). Unbound $T_3$ is the active hormone. Within cells, there are deiodinases that remove an iodide from $T_4$ to form the active hormone.

The mechanism of action of thyroid hormone remains unclear, but is related to synthesis of specific messenger RNAs and proteins. Many drugs alter either the concentration of thyroid binding proteins in the blood (e.g. estrogens increase TBG) or the binding of $T_4$ to these proteins. The resulting changes in concentrations of unbound hormones may have metabolic effects and the potential to produce thyroid disease.

Both $T_3$ and $T_4$ feed back, mainly to the pituitary, and thereby inhibit TSH release. There is also a hypothalamic releasing hormone, i.e. thyrotrophin releasing hormone (TRH), but this tripeptide does not have a major role in the day-to-day control of TSH release, except perhaps if the organism is cold and increased thermogenesis is necessary. As well as being synthesised in the hypothalamus, TRH is found in other areas of the nervous system, where it may have a more general role as a neurotransmitter.

The commonest disorder of the thyroid gland worldwide is due to iodine deficiency (see section 5.1). However, thyroid disease can also be due to autoimmunity with antibodies that are directed to TSH receptors or that destroy the thyroid cell. Antibodies to TSH receptors may stimulate (thyroid-stimulating immunoglobulins) or block, and can cause hyper- and hypothyroidism, respectively. There are a number of deiodinases in cells. Most of the peripheral deiodination produces $T_3$ (3′-deiodination), but a proportion of the deiodination is at the 3-position and produces reverse-$T_3$, which is inactive in adults. In severe illness, starvation, anaesthesia and certain other conditions, the relative activity of deiodinases can be altered with production of less $T_3$ and more reverse-$T_3$. As the illness becomes more severe or prolonged, there may be suppression of TSH. This has been called the 'euthyroid-sick' syndrome, since patients are clinically euthyroid. With recovery from severe illness, there may be a transient increase in TSH.

### 1.3 The Hypothalamic-Pituitary-Adrenal Axis

The actions of glucocorticoids are discussed further in section 7.1.1. The discussion here concentrates on control of this system as an example of negative feedback.

There is diurnal secretion of corticotrophin-releasing hormone (CRH) from the hypothalamus. In addition to diurnal rhythms, factors such as stress lead to the production of CRH in the hypothalamus and its secretion into the portal system to the anterior pituitary. Vasopressin is produced and secreted in parallel with CRH. CRH stimulates the basophil cells of the pituitary to synthesise pro-opiomelanocortin (POMC), of which corticotrophin (adrenocorticotrophic hormone, ACTH) is a small part, as are the endorphins and melanocyte-stimulating hormone (MSH). Corticotrophin is secreted and stimulates the adrenal cortex to synthesise and secrete glucocorticoids. Corticotrophin secretion also inhibits CRH production (via a short feedback loop). The glucocorticoids exert their action throughout the body and feed back to the hypothalamus to reduce CRH and subsequent corticotrophin secretion. There are at least 2 forms of glucocorticoid receptor in the hypothalamus and they are part of the nuclear binding receptor superfamily (see section 7.1.1).

Disorders of the hypothalamic-pituitary-adrenal (HPA) axis can occur in the hypothalamus, pituitary or adrenal cortex, with either over- or underproduction of the hormones at any site depending on the pathological process. For example, with an adenoma of the adrenal cortex overproducing cortisol, concentrations of CRH and corticotrophin will be suppressed due to the negative feedback of the high cortisol levels. Conversely, when the adrenal cortex is destroyed by tuberculosis (which occurs commonly in many parts of the world), there will be low cortisol but high corticotrophin and CRH levels. Note that peripheral concentrations of CRH are not usually measured in clinical situations due to its short half-life and the lack of a routine assay.

### 1.4 Pharmacokinetics in Endocrine Disorders

Little definitive information is available on drug disposition in endocrine and metabolic disorders, but the kinetics of some drugs may be altered. In some cases, altered disposition can be related to changes in the status of the endocrine disorder. The clinical implications of many of these changes has not been studied.

#### *1.4.1 Influence of Diabetes Mellitus on Pharmacokinetics*

Untreated diabetes and exogenous insulin seem capable of altering the metabolism of drugs. For most drugs, oral absorption is unaffected, but poorly controlled IDDM (though not well controlled NIDDM) and autonomic neuropathy reduce the absorption of ampicillin and tolazamide, respectively.[3]

Hepatic biotransformation appears occasionally to be impaired in patients with uncontrolled diabetes. For example, the acetylation of caffeine, but not the oxidation of debrisoquine, has been found to be altered in IDDM.[4] The former led to the erroneous suggestion that acetylator phenotype was a risk factor for diabetes; genotyping has subsequently refuted this possibility.[5] In a small study, the rate of conversion of phenacetin (acetophenetidin) to paracetamol (acetaminophen) and its subsequent conjugation was impaired in untreated diabetic patients. Metabolism reverted toward normal when the diabetes was well controlled by insulin, but became impaired again if insulin was withdrawn.[6] Conversely, clearance of paracetamol, which is primarily conjugated, was no different in NIDDM, but sulfation of the drug appeared to be reduced.[7] While clearance of theophylline was normal in IDDM, it was positively correlated with glycated haemoglobin ($HbA_{1c}$).[8]

In patients with poorly-controlled IDDM, decreased albumin concentrations, elevated free fatty acids and glycosylation of plasma proteins may explain the observed reduction in protein binding of a variety of drugs bound to either albumin (sites I and II) or $\alpha_1$-acid glycoprotein, including diazepam, sulfafurazole (sulfisoxazole),[9] warfarin, lidocaine (lignocaine), phenytoin and valproic acid.[10,11] It would be anticipated that such changes would be of clinical importance only for highly bound drugs such as warfarin and diazepam, where the studies show a 20% and 40% increase, respectively.

Elimination of renally excreted drugs can also be altered in insulin-treated diabetic children. Glomerular filtration rate and clearance of intravenous penicillin and carbenicillin are increased, along with a marked decrease in serum concentrations.[12,13] Decreased serum concentrations have also been noted with kanamycin and amikacin in insulin-treated diabetic children.[14] These patients require larger than normal doses of antibiotics that are excreted by the kidneys. Absorption of intramuscular benzylpenicillin (penicillin G) is impaired in some adults with diabetes mellitus and has been associated with therapeutic failure.[15,16] Aminoglycoside absorption may also be slower in diabetic patients.[3] Early in IDDM, the glomerular filtration rate may be elevated, but as the disease progresses, renal function declines. Therapeutic drug monitoring, particularly of the aminoglycosides, is therefore recommended in the diabetic patient (see further chapter 5).

### 1.4.2 Influence of Thyroid Disease on Pharmacokinetics

Thyroid dysfunction can alter the disposition of certain drugs but whether changes occur or are important depends on the pharmacokinetic properties of the particular drug and the patient's thyroid status (for a review, see Shenfield[17]). There is a need to alter dosage of some drugs as thyroid disease is treated and requirements change.

Thyroid disease is associated with disturbances of gastrointestinal motility and function that may influence absorption of orally administered drugs, but very few data are available. Some patients with hyperthyroidism have steatorrhoea or increased intestinal motility, and the bioavailability of poorly soluble drugs such as digoxin has been shown to be decreased in some hyperthyroid patients.[18] The rate of absorption of paracetamol and propranolol is more rapid in hyperthyroid than hypothyroid patients[19,20] and absorption of atenolol may be reduced.[21]

Hepatic metabolism of drugs may be altered in untreated thyroid disease, as shown by increased phenazone (antipyrine) clearance in hyperthyroidism and decreased clearance in hypothyroidism (by approximately one-third and two-thirds, respectively), and this changes to normal with effective treatment of either dysfunction.[22,23] Glucaric acid excretion, a measure of hepatic microsomal glucuronidation capacity, is increased in some hyperthyroid patients.[24] The clearance of paracetamol[20] and oxazepam,[25] which are primarily eliminated by glucuronidation, increases in hyperthyroid patients (by approximately 25%) and decreases in hypothyroidism.[26] In contrast, the pharmacokinetics of diazepam[27] are not altered. Thus, drugs with pharmacokinetic properties different from phenazone or metabolised by different primary pathways may behave differently in thyroid disease.

While the rate of elimination of tolbutamide and theophylline is increased in hyperthyroidism (by about 20%), the clearance of phenytoin is unaffected by either hyperthyroidism or hypothyroidism.[23,28] Studies with thiamazole (methimazole) and propylthiouracil (for a review, see Cooper et al.[29]) suggest that their elimination is not enhanced in hyperthyroidism; earlier studies with these drugs were flawed because of nonspecific analytical techniques.

#### β-Adrenoceptor Blockers

β-Adrenoceptor blocking drugs (β-blockers) are commonly used in thyroid disorders and show concentration-related effects, so the influence of thyroid disease on their disposition is important (for reviews, see Feely and Peden;[30] O'Connor and Feely[31]).

In *hyperthyroidism,* the clearance of intravenous propranolol is increased by approximately 50%, an effect that may be attributed to the marked increase in hepatic blood flow.[32] Following single oral doses, the clearance of propranolol has been reported to be either unchanged or increased, but there is increased clearance during long term oral therapy, presumably due to increased hepatic drug metabolising enzyme activity.[33] However, the elimination half-life of the drug is unaltered during both single dose and long term therapy, in part because of an increased apparent volume of distribution. The clearance of metoprolol, which like propranolol undergoes extensive hepatic metabolism, is also increased in hyperthyroidism (by 50%).[34]

The wide interindividual variation in propranolol plasma concentrations,[35] which is largely attributed to age and smoking habits, may explain the reported cases of thyroid crisis, particularly after surgery in patients receiving fixed dosage regimens. In the latter situation, thyroid surgery may markedly alter the disposition of propranolol. Plasma propranolol concentrations rise 2- to 3-fold after thyroidectomy,[30] presumably as a result of increased drug binding and impaired hepatic metabolism for some days following surgery.[36]

The effect of *hypothyroidism* on the disposition of β-blockers has not been definitively studied. In hypothyroidism, the elimination half-life of propranolol after a single oral dose may be prolonged, although clearance appears to be unaffected. However, possibly because bioavailability increases, steady-state plasma propranolol concentrations are elevated (by about two-thirds) during long term therapy. The degree of plasma protein binding of propranolol is increased in hypothyroidism but decreased in hyperthyroidism. In comparison, that of warfarin is also decreased in hyperthyroidism (which may in part explain the exaggerated response to anticoagulation in this condition), but is unchanged in hypothyroidism.[37] These changes may be due to parallel changes in $\alpha_1$-acid glycoprotein (which binds to basic drugs like propranolol) and a decrease in albumin (which binds to acidic drugs like warfarin) in hyperthyroidism.[25,37]

Glomerular filtration is decreased in hypothyroidism, and there is evidence that renal plasma flow is increased in hyperthyroidism and decreased in hypothyroidism.[38] However, apart from β-blockers and digoxin (see below), there is no information on disposition in thyroid disease of drugs that are mainly eliminated unchanged in the urine (e.g. aminoglycoside antibiotics). The oral clearance of renally excreted β-blockers such as sotalol and atenolol is not altered in hyperthyroidism,[39] nor is that of atenolol in hypothyroidism.[21]

#### Digitalis

The response to digitalis glycosides is influenced by the patient's thyroid status and has been attributed to both altered tissue responsiveness and altered digitalis kinetics.[40,41] The response to a given dose is increased in hypothyroidism and decreased in hyperthyroidism. Serum concentrations of both digitoxin and digoxin are lower in hyperthyroidism and higher in hypothyroidism than in healthy individuals or euthyroid patients.[42,43] The reasons for this are not clear but may include changes in distribution,[43,44] renal digoxin clearance,[45] metabolism and biliary excretion, particularly of digitoxin, or malabsorption.[18] Altered skeletal and cardiac muscle binding of digoxin and the number of $Na^+/K^+$-ATPase pumps have been suggested as other possible explanations.[17]

Whatever the mechanisms, plasma concentrations may change as thyroid dysfunction is effectively treated. It is, therefore, important to monitor serum concentrations of digoxin during therapy, at least until biochemical control of thyroid disease has been attained.

#### Other Drugs

The elimination half-lives of thyroxine, triiodothyronine and cortisol are reduced in hyperthyroidism and prolonged in hypothyroidism,[17] presumably reflecting changes in the activity of hepatic enzyme systems that metabolise drugs.

In hyperthyroid patients, the metabolic clearance of prednisolone is enhanced, resulting in reduced systemic availability of prednisolone after administration of oral prednisone. This is accompanied by reduced inhibition of allogenically stimulated lymphocytes, so higher prednisone and prednisolone dosages are recommended for patients with hyperthyroidism.[46]

### *1.4.3 Influence of Obesity on Pharmacokinetics*

Obesity might be expected to alter the distribution and plasma concentration of drugs as a consequence of increased distribution into body fat or, since fat contains less extracellular fluid than other tissues, decreased distribution into extracellular fluid (for reviews, see Abernethy and Greenblatt;[47] Cheymol[48]). In general, highly lipid soluble drugs (benzodiazepines, verapamil, thiopental, halothane, enflurane) distribute extensively into excess bodyweight whereas drugs with intermediate lipid solubility (e.g. aminoglycosides, atracurium, vecuronium, phenazone, paracetamol, theophylline) distribute to a lesser extent into excess bodyweight than into ideal bodyweight, producing a reduced weight-related volume of distribution. Being hydrophilic, digoxin does not distribute into excess bodyweight. However, it should be noted that the degree of lipophilicity may only partially explain increased distribution of some drugs in obesity. Other complex factors may also be involved.

Changes in drug distribution in obesity may alter the elimination half-life. The metabolic clearance of drugs that are primarily oxidised (e.g. diazepam, alprazolam, theophylline, phenazone and caffeine) and that of high clearance drugs (verapamil, lidocaine, midazolam) is generally not significantly affected. However, clearance of paracetamol, lorazepam and oxazepam is increased, suggesting enhanced hepatic glucuronidation.[49,50] Renal clearance of some drugs (aminoglycosides, unmetabolised procainamide) is increased while that of other drugs (e.g. digoxin) is unchanged. Plasma protein binding of phenytoin and benzodiazepines is unaltered in obese patients, although there may be a slight decrease in diazepam binding in morbidly obese (>190% of ideal bodyweight) patients. In contrast, the binding of propranolol is increased, in part because of elevated $\alpha_1$-acid glycoprotein concentrations.[51]

There is little information available on whether dosages of drugs with low therapeutic ratios should be based on ideal bodyweight or actual (total) bodyweight. For more lipid soluble drugs and those distributed equally between lean and fat tissues (e.g. theophylline), loading doses are best based on actual bodyweight. However, due to the increased volume of distribution and prolonged half-life of theophylline in obesity, the maintenance dosage should be based on ideal bodyweight.[52] For less soluble drugs (e.g. atracurium, $H_2$-receptor antagonists) and some drugs (e.g. cyclosporin) restricted to lean tissues, loading doses should be based on ideal bodyweight.[48]

The rate of uptake of halothane and recovery time are increased in obesity, being most marked in younger patients.[53] Biotransformation of methoxyflurane, and to a lesser extent of halothane, to ionic fluoride seems to be increased in obesity[54] (see also chapter 12, sect. 2.1.1). Obese patients need the same dose of digoxin, a hydrophilic drug, to achieve similar plasma concentrations before and after bodyweight reduction. The dosage of digoxin in obesity should, therefore, be based on ideal bodyweight and not on actual bodyweight.[55]

Plasma concentrations of gentamicin and tobramycin, drugs that are distributed mainly to extracellular fluid, are increased in obesity when dosage is based on actual bodyweight. The dosages of these drugs should, therefore, be based on ideal bodyweight but serum concentrations should be monitored to ensure that therapeutic concentrations are attained.[56,57] The total systemic and renal clearance of cimetidine is increased in obese patients without a change in the volume of distribution, suggesting that dosage of this drug should be based on actual bodyweight.[58] Presumably, this reflects increased glomerular filtration.[48] For lithium,[59] clearance is increased, suggesting the need for larger maintenance doses.

The plasma half-lives of tolbutamide, sulfafurazole (sulfisoxazole) and isoniazid are not altered in obesity or during fasting, but the rate of renal excretion of sulfafurazole is decreased with fasting.[60] Endogenous corticosteroid production is increased in obesity, but clearance of unbound prednisolone is enhanced, suggesting that dosage adjustments should reflect actual bodyweight.[61] However, clearance of methylprednisolone and dexamethasone[62] is reduced, suggesting dosage based on ideal bodyweight.

Following intestinal bypass operations for gross obesity, plasma concentrations of norethisterone and to a lesser extent norgestrel in oral contraceptives are reduced, apparently as a result of decreased hepatic synthesis of sex hormone binding globulin.[63] Steady-state plasma concentrations of digoxin are unaltered, but the area under the plasma concentration-time curve is reduced in most patients after intestinal bypass operations,[64] suggesting that bioavailability may be decreased if intestinal transit is unduly rapid.

#### *1.4.4 Influence of Other Endocrine Disorders on Pharmacokinetics*

Perturbations of other hormones (e.g. sex hormones, evinced from changes brought about by pregnancy and oral contraceptives) would be expected to alter drug disposition. However, for most endocrine disorders, limited information is available and usually no consistent trend is discernible. Treatment of children with human growth hormone is associated with changes to the elimination half-life of amobarbital (prolonged) and theophylline (reduced), but there is no change in phenazone clearance.[65]

In some patients, hydrocortisone infusions increase the oxidation of phenylbutazone and phenazone,[66] although the latter finding has not been confirmed.[67]

## 2. General Principles of Treatment

### 2.1 Diagnosis

It is now possible to diagnose endocrine disorders precisely and quickly. Immunoassays for hormones are very specific, widely available and many have been automated so that results can be obtained within hours. Many disorders can be diagnosed from a basal blood sample, but the limitations of this approach must be recognised. The diurnal rhythms of many hormones, the stage of growth and development of the individual being tested, and the stage of the menstrual cycle may affect the results. There are also specific stimulatory and inhibitory tests for hormones that can be applied to aid diagnosis. To interpret hormone assays, it is necessary to remember that the endocrine system, in general, operates on a principle of negative feedback and that it is appropriate to consider a stimulatory test if the hormone of interest is at a low concentration, and an inhibitory test if the hormone is present at excessive concentrations. Also, newer methods of imaging (CT and MRI scanning, nuclear scanning, ultrasound) can aid visualisation and precise location of endocrine glands and abnormalities within them. The pancreas remains the least accessible gland.

### 2.2 Aims of Therapy

Where possible, normal physiological function should be restored. If that is not possible, for example in IDDM, the aim should be a lifestyle as normal as possible within the constraints of therapy and the prevention of complications. The goals of treatment in specific endocrine diseases are discussed further below.

### 2.3 Ambulatory Care

With developments in diagnosis and treatment, patients with endocrine diseases rarely need to be admitted to hospital. This, and the fact that most endocrine disorders are chronic or require regular review, has lead to the development of ambulatory care centres (particularly for diabetes) where appropriate diagnosis, management and on-going care can be undertaken under one roof. Such centres have reduced the need for hospital admission.

## 3. Diabetes Mellitus

### 3.1 General Principles and Specific Aims of Treatment

Diabetes is a major medical and economic problem. The World Health Organization estimated that there were 6 million people with IDDM worldwide in 1992.[68] It also estimated that the worldwide population of individuals with NIDDM is increasing and may reach 100 million by 2000 AD.

Diabetes is associated with increased mortality and a high risk of vascular, renal, retinal and neuropathic complications. To prevent these complications, available evidence strongly supports maintaining normal blood glucose, lipid and blood pressure levels as desirable goals of treatment of both types of diabetes. Although dietary changes and exercise are important, individually they are often insufficient to enable patients to attain these goals. Therefore, pharmacological agents still play a major role in the treatment of diabetes and its complications.

### 3.2 Clinical Pharmacology of Drugs Used in Treatment

#### *3.2.1 Oral Antidiabetic Drugs*

There are 2 major classes of oral antidiabetic drugs commonly used in the treatment of diabetes mellitus: the sulphonylureas and biguanides (table I). Some newer agents are also mentioned in section 3.3.1 on treatment of NIDDM.

The sulphonylureas act predominantly by stimulating insulin secretion. However, the antihyperglycaemic effect of the biguanide drug metformin is independent of any change in insulin concentrations: it works primarily by inhibiting hepatic glucose production and improving peripheral insulin sensitivity.

**Sulphonylureas**

***Mechanism/site of action:*** despite being the first class of oral antidiabetic agents in common clinical usage, the precise mechanisms of action of sulphonylureas have continued to be a matter for debate. Undoubtedly, in short term usage they stimulate insulin secretion, both directly and by sensitising the β cells to nutrients. These actions are initiated by the drug binding to a cell surface receptor. This causes closure of $K^+$ channels that then triggers opening of $Ca^{++}$ channels. The resultant increase in intracellular $Ca^{++}$ concentration increases secretion of insulin. During long term usage of sulphonylureas, circulating insulin concentrations decrease, leading to the suggestion that stimulation of insulin secretion is not an important mechanism in their mode of action. However, this conclusion fails to account for the lower glucose concentrations while the patient is taking a sulphonylurea.

Extrapancreatic actions of sulphonylureas have also been invoked to account for some of their hypoglycaemic effects, but since sulphonylureas are not effective in the absence of β cells, it seems clear that their main action is in normalisation of insulin secretion.

***Pharmacokinetic characteristics and clinical use:*** there are a number of sulphonylureas available commercially. They vary in their pharmacokinetic characteristics and dosages (table I),

**Table I.** Pharmacokinetic characteristics, dosages and duration of clinical effect of some currently available oral antidiabetic drugs

| Drug | Pharmacokinetic parameters | | | Elimination | Dosage (mg/day) | | Duration of clinical effect | Risk of hypoglycaemia[d] |
|---|---|---|---|---|---|---|---|---|
| | CL (L/h) | $t_{1/2}$ (h) | Vd (L) [per 70kg] | | initial (usual) | maximum | | |
| **Sulphonylureas** | | | | | | | | |
| Chlorpropamide | 0.13 | 40 | ≈10.5 | Variable hepatic metabolism[a] and renal excretion of unchanged drug (6 to 60%) | 250 | 500 | Long | Moderate |
| Glibenclamide (glyburide) | 5.5 | 6-10 | 10.5 | Hepatic metabolism[b] and biliary excretion | 5 | 20 | Medium/long | Moderate |
| Gliclazide | 0.8 | 6-12 | 21 | Hepatic metabolism and some renal excretion of unchanged drug (<20%) | 80 | 320 | Medium | Mild |
| Glimepiride | | ?9-10 | | Hepatic metabolism and renal excretion of metabolites | 1-2 | 8 | Medium/long | ?Mild |
| Glipizide | 2.5 | 5 | 14 | Hepatic metabolism[c] | 5 | 20 | Short | Uncommon |
| Tolazamide | | 7 | | Hepatic metabolism[b] | 250 | 1000 | Medium | Moderate |
| Tolbutamide | ≈1 | 7 | 10.5 | Hepatic metabolism[a] | 500 | 3000 | Short | Uncommon |
| **Biguanides** | | | | | | | | |
| Metformin | 26-42 | 1.5-4.5 | 70-280 | Renal excretion of unchanged drug | 500-850 | 3000 | Medium | Very uncommon |

a Contribution of metabolites to activity probably minimal.
b Metabolites may have some pharmacological activity (less than parent drug).
c Metabolites probably inactive (and are excreted rapidly in urine).
d Risk of hypoglycaemia indicates relative risk of drug producing hypoglycaemia, particularly in the elderly.

but with some minor exceptions (see below) do not differ greatly in clinical usage. Most drugs are formulated conveniently so that a dosage of half to 3 tablets per day can be used to treat most NIDDM patients. Second-generation agents such as gliclazide and glipizide have significant advantages over the earlier compounds (e.g. chlorpropamide) in having shorter half-lives and a duration of effect that mimics physiological patterns of insulin release more closely. There is some suggestion that exceeding the maximum recommended dosages of sulphonylureas rarely adds to their effectiveness and in some case may impair insulin secretion.[69]

*Tolerability:* hypoglycaemia is a well recognised adverse effect of sulphonylurea therapy, particularly with the longer acting drugs. To minimise the risk of hypoglycaemia, irrespective of whether the drug is eliminated primarily by the liver or by both the liver and kidney, sulphonylureas should be used more cautiously in elderly patients and in those with impaired renal or hepatic function. This is particularly so for glibenclamide (glyburide), whereas glipizide is less hazardous in these situations because of its shorter duration of action.

Serious adverse reactions with sulphonylureas have proved to be very uncommon. Although the University Group Diabetes Program (UGDP) study conducted in the US some years ago caused great concern in showing that the use of tolbutamide may be associated with more cardiovascular disease than a placebo,[70,71] it is now widely accepted that the study used controls that are inadequate by modern standards.

*Drug interactions potential:* numerous other drugs may potentiate the effects of the sulphonylureas. For a summary of potentially clinically significant interactions involving these drugs, see appendix B.

#### Biguanides

Metformin is the only commonly used drug in this class. Its predecessor, phenformin, was phased out in most countries because of its association with lactic acidosis. In contrast, despite initial caution, oral metformin is exceedingly well tolerated if its use is avoided in patients with significantly raised creatinine or severely abnormal liver function.

*Mechanism/site of action:* metformin acts principally by increasing insulin sensitivity. How it does this is uncertain, but the result is increased peripheral glucose utilisation and decreased hepatic glucose production. Because it does not increase insulin secretion, metformin virtually never causes hypoglycaemia when used alone, and has little or no glucose-lowering effect in non-diabetic patients.

***Pharmacokinetic characteristics:*** unlike the sulphonylureas, metformin is principally eliminated unchanged by renal excretion. Its renal clearance is strongly correlated with creatinine clearance, but the values are well in excess of those for creatinine clearance suggesting that some active tubular secretion takes place.[72] Pharmacokinetic parameters for metformin are shown in table I.

***Tolerability:*** the most common adverse effects of metformin are nausea and diarrhoea; these may be minimised by starting therapy slowly and taking the drug after food. The main risk with metformin is lactic acidosis, which occurs most often (but not exclusively) in patients with renal impairment and higher circulating metformin concentrations.

***Drug interactions potential:*** there are relatively few drug interactions of clinical significance with metformin. Alcohol (ethanol) may increase the risk of hyperlacticacidaemia.

#### 3.2.2 Insulin Preparations

The various types of insulin available and their action profiles are shown in table II. However, the latter should only be regarded as guidelines; in reality, the actions of the various insulins are much less predictable. The different action profiles of insulin preparations are due to their different rates of absorption rather than the innate action of insulin. Severe renal impairment, however, can prolong insulin action by delaying clearance.

For practical purposes, most patients can be satisfactorily treated with any combination of short- and intermediate-acting insulins. However, mixing a short-acting insulin with lente or ultralente insulins can result in a time-dependent loss of short-acting insulin activity. Thus, if this combination is used, it should be injected immediately after mixing. For this reason, current trends are to use isophane insulin, an intermediate-acting insulin that is not prone to this time-dependent problem. It is also shorter in duration of action than lente and, therefore, is more suited to a twice-daily regimen. It should be noted that bovine ultralente insulin is much longer acting than its human equivalent. Therefore, it should be specified if indeed the intention is to use a very long acting insulin to provide a basal insulin level.

Premixed insulins are convenient to inject, especially for people with difficulty mastering the techniques of mixing insulins, e.g. elderly patients. However, these insulins are not suitable for patients who require tight metabolic control throughout the day, because the proportion of short- and long-acting insulins cannot be altered easily.

**Table II.** Types and action profiles of insulin preparations

| Insulin type | Peak effect | Duration of action |
|---|---|---|
| **Short-acting** | | |
| Soluble insulin | 2-5h | 6-8h |
| **Intermediate-acting** | | |
| Isophane insulin (NPH) | 4-12h | 16-24h |
| Lente insulin | 7-15h | 22-24h |
| Soluble and isophane[a] (premixed) | 2-12h | 16-24h |
| **Long-acting** | | |
| Human ultralente | 6-24h | 24-28h |
| Bovine ultralente | 10-30h | 36-38h |

a Short and intermediate-acting.

#### Human Insulins

Human insulins have been available for the past 10 years and are now the predominant type of insulin used in developed countries. This preparation of insulin is absorbed more rapidly, but overall its only significant benefit over animal insulins is the very low incidence of allergy associated with its use. The main impetus for the worldwide use of human insulins is that they are produced by recombinant DNA techniques using either *Escherichia coli* or yeast, which is economically more efficient for manufacturers.

Since the use of human insulin became widespread, there has been controversy whether it reduces patients' awareness of hypoglycaemia or increases the frequency of hypoglycaemic episodes. Recently, a comprehensive survey has been conducted of 39 clinical studies and 12 epidemiological reports comparing porcine and human insulin.[73] Symptoms and physiological response to acute hypoglycaemia and the incidence of hypoglycaemia were the same with the 2 types of insulin.

A small number of patients do, however, report alterations in symptoms following a change to human insulin, so it is good clinical practice to warn patients of this.[74] In rare cases, clinicians and patients prefer to continue using animal insulins, but the availability of these insulins on commercial markets is diminishing.

#### Insulin Analogues

In healthy individuals, ingestion of food results in rapid secretion of insulin to control the postprandial rise in blood glucose. Currently, the available insulins are incapable of reproducing this response. After a subcutaneous injection of conventional short-acting insulin, plasma concentrations do not reach a peak until 90 to 120 minutes after injection and can be sustained for several hours. The result is an exaggerated rise in postprandial blood glucose excursion. Attempts to minimise postprandial hyperglycaemia by increasing short-acting insulin dosages can produce hypoglycaemia a few hours after meals. To counteract these problems associated with delayed absorption, insulin is traditionally injected 30 minutes before a meal. However, patients often do not recognise the importance of this and may ignore the instruction, finding it too disruptive to their lifestyles.

Recombinant DNA techniques have allowed modification of the amino acid sequence of insulin to produce analogues that can overcome this problem. Native insulin self-associates in a hexameric form that must dissociate before absorption. Insulin analogues that remain in monomeric form may be absorbed more rapidly into the bloodstream. One product in clinical trials is Lys-Pro insulin, where the lysine and proline residues on amino acid positions B28 and B29 are reversed. This affects the site of association on the insulin molecule and maintains it in the monomeric state. In pharmacokinetic studies and clinical trials, Lys-Pro insulin was absorbed rapidly after injection and reduced the postprandial rise in blood glucose.[75] It can be given immediately before food, a convenience factor that is likely to ensure wide acceptance by patients.

## 3.3 Optimum Treatment

### *3.3.1 Non-Insulin-Dependent Diabetes Mellitus (NIDDM)*

#### Aims of Treatment

While this section deals mainly with control of hyperglycaemia, clinicians should keep in mind that in the overall management of NIDDM, it is also necessary to maintain a normal blood pressure and lipid profile (see further sections 3.4.3 and 3.4.4 below).

Maintenance of normoglycaemia in patients with NIDDM has the dual aims of symptomatic relief and prevention of diabetic complications. Although oral antidiabetic agents and insulin have been available for years, there is little information on optimum strategies for use of these agents to derive long term benefits. This deficiency is being addressed in the UK Prospective Diabetes Study (UKPDS)[76] in which more than 5000 patients have been randomised to either diet, metformin, a sulphonylurea or insulin treatment. By 1998, after about 12 years of follow-up, it is hoped that there will be concrete information about the best way for NIDDM patients to achieve good metabolic control and prevent diabetic complications. In addition, the ongoing Veterans' Affairs Cooperative Study (CSDM)[77] is examining the effects of intensive insulin treatment for NIDDM patients. Until the results of these trials are available, most guidelines for treatment of NIDDM are based on clinical experience and the good evidence from cross-sectional studies that maintenance of normoglycaemia can reduce diabetic complications in these patients. Clinicians should consider that macrovascular diseases are the major complications in NIDDM and that it is uncertain that they can be modified by better glycaemic control.

#### When to Introduce Oral Antidiabetic Agents

Exercise and dietary modification are accepted first-line treatments for patients with NIDDM. However, diet and exercise are rarely sufficient to induce or maintain normoglycaemia. Indeed, in the UKPDS study, preliminary results have indicated that only 17% of patients attain normoglycaemia without drug treatment and these responsive patients usually had only modest hyperglycaemia initially. Therefore, treatment with oral agents should not be delayed beyond 3 months of dietary therapy if sufficient metabolic control is not achieved.

In individuals with symptoms or severe hyperglycaemia, oral agents should be introduced earlier. However, in elderly and frail patients, some degree of hyperglycaemia is acceptable if symptoms are not severe.

#### Selecting an Oral Antidiabetic Agent

Sulphonylureas and metformin have proved about equal in effectiveness when compared in various studies. It is common clinical practice to use sulphonylureas in normal or underweight patients, and metformin in overweight patients, but there is little concrete evidence that this is the correct approach. Due to the ability of metformin to reduce insulin resistance and hyperinsulinaemia (and therefore minimise possible vascular risk factors), there may be a theoretical advantage in using it first. There is also some evidence that even at early phases, combined sulphonylurea and metformin treatment may be more effective, although this remains to be confirmed. The use of shorter-acting sulphonylureas in patients with renal or hepatic disease is established.

Failure to respond to oral agents initially (primary failure) is often due to severe underlying insulin deficiency. In this situation, insulin therapy is required. However, many patients may not respond to oral agents because of severe initial hyperglycaemia. At blood glucose concentrations >15 mmol/L (270 mg/dl), glucose toxicity impairs both the response of β cells to stimuli and the absorption of sulphonylureas. During this early phase, a much higher dosage of oral antidiabetic agents may be needed but it can be reduced subsequently. If hyperglycaemia is successfully lowered by any means, e.g. insulin therapy, responsiveness to oral agents may be regained. Recognition of this phenomenon can spare patients years of unnecessary insulin treatment because, to the best of current knowledge, as long as optimal control can be attained, oral agents are not inferior to insulin in the treatment of NIDDM.

#### Dosage Adjustments

The UKPDS study[76] has shown that in the natural history of NIDDM, progressively higher blood glucose concentrations develop over the first few years of diabetes, and presumably are a manifestation of worsening insulin deficiency. If maintenance of normoglycaemia is accepted as a desirable goal, dosages of oral antidiabetic agents must be increased accordingly, or a second agent added. This is a common and logical clinical practice, but persistent use of sulphonylureas may desensitise the β cell, with consequent reduction in insulin secretion. If this sequence of events is the underlying mechanism, it is theoretically best dealt with by changing temporarily to insulin therapy to allow the β cells to recover. Currently, there is no scientific evidence to indicate which is the correct approach.

#### Treatment of Secondary Failure of Oral Antidiabetic Drugs

In most NIDDM patients, after 5 to 10 years of diabetes, normoglycaemia can no longer be maintained by oral antidiabetic agents alone, a phenomenon known as 'secondary failure'. In this situation, to maintain normoglycaemia, insulin is usually instituted unless the general prognosis of the patient is poor. However, there is little information about how this treatment should be implemented. Some favour stopping the oral antidiabetic agents abruptly and replacing them with insulin; others maintain oral agents at half the original dose and add insulin to the regimen either in the morning or before bed.[78] If insulin is used alone, a higher dosage and twice-daily regimen is often required. This presumably reflects the fact that oral agents have not failed completely. Generally, the advantage of combining oral agents and insulin is greatest in overweight patients with a relatively short duration of diabetes.

A major problem of insulin treatment in NIDDM is that it often makes patients put on weight without gaining improvements in metabolic control. The precise mechanism underlying this combination of events is unclear, but it is a constant reminder that insulin therapy is not a panacea in this type of patient. This clinical scenario can sometimes be improved by using insulin in combination with metformin.

#### Additional Therapeutic Agents

The current treatment of NIDDM is far from perfect, so efforts to find new and useful agents are continuing.

*Acarbose* is an α-glucosidase inhibitor that reduces the rate of disaccharide breakdown and subsequent absorption.[79,80] Acarbose decreases disaccharide absorption, which in turn decreases postprandial glycaemia by approximately 3 mmol/L. When used as monotherapy, it decreases mean $HbA_{1c}$ levels by 0.6 to 1.0%. When used as an additional agent in NIDDM patients with inadequate control on sulphonylureas or insulin therapy, there is an additional decrease in $HbA_{1c}$ of 0.4 to 0.6%.[81] Most of its adverse effects are gastrointestinal in nature, including diarrhoea, bloating, flatulence and nausea, but may decrease with continued treatment and by reducing the amount of sucrose in the diet. Its role in the treatment of NIDDM is not firmly established. Although acarbose has been advocated as a first-line treatment,[82] its gastrointestinal adverse effects and relatively low effectiveness suggest it is more likely to find a place as an adjunct to conventional therapy.

*Dexfenfluramine* (see further section 4.2.2) is also useful in this context. It improves glycaemic control in obese NIDDM patients in whom conventional treatment with oral antidiabetic agents and insulin is inadequate.[83,84]

*Troglitazone* is a thiazolidinedione derivative that acts by increasing insulin sensitivity, and has been shown to have antihyperglycaemic effects in patients with NIDDM.[85] Its clinical role has yet to be established.

Well formulated, very low energy (low kilocalorie or kilojoule) diets have also been found to be useful and safe in treating obese NIDDM patients.

### 3.3.2 Insulin-Dependent Diabetes Mellitus (IDDM)

Insulin treatment in IDDM has 2 separate aims:

1) To keep the patient alive, since IDDM patients will die from ketoacidosis unless treated with insulin.

2) To maintain good glycaemic control, since the experience of the Diabetes Control and Complications Trial[86,87] has shown that this reduces diabetic complications.

#### Treatment and Prevention of Ketoacidosis

In patients with ketoacidosis, short-acting insulin is best given by intravenous infusion at a dosage of 2 to 5 U/h. Although insulin plays a central role in treatment, it must be supported by other measures such as rehydration, electrolyte replacement and control of infection. When facilities for intravenous infusion are not available, ketoacidosis may be treated with hourly intramuscular injections of short-acting insulin.

In newly-diagnosed IDDM patients, there may be hyperglycaemia and ketonuria, but no overt dehydration and acidosis. In this situation, insulin still needs to be commenced immediately, but hospitalisation is not required if facilities to support ambulatory stabilisation are available. Initially, the patient and relatives should be instructed in basic survival skills such as how to give an insulin injection, monitor blood glucose and test for urinary ketones. Insulin dosages and selection of insulin types must be individualised. However, it is usual to give 10 to 20U of a premixed insulin twice daily, supplemented with short-acting insulin every 4 to 6 hours, depending on results of blood glucose monitoring and ketonuria. For most patients, it is not necessary to teach them how to mix insulin on the first day. It is also not necessary to aim for normoglycaemia immediately, the emphasis being more on clearing ketones from the urine. As the metabolic disturbance settles, usually over a period of 1 to 2 days, patients are stabilised on twice-daily insulin injections. After a few visits, most of the stabilisation process can be conducted over the phone. Ambulatory stabilisation is cost-effective and adjustment is made while the individual is carrying out normal routine activity.

In patients with established IDDM, ketoacidosis may develop during intercurrent illness. This is often precipitated by patients mistakenly omitting insulin (for fear of inducing hypoglycaemia) when they have reduced their food intake. It is vital for patients to be taught routinely that during illness they must continue to take insulin and monitor urine for significant ketonuria. When this is present, they should administer additional short-acting insulin every 1 to 2 hours until ketonuria abates.

#### Conventional Maintenance Therapy

In conventional maintenance therapy of IDDM, insulin is usually administered twice daily. The total dosage required varies between individuals. Patients must be told that dosage does not reflect the severity or seriousness of their disease. Generally, a good basic regimen is:

- Two-thirds of the total daily dose given in the morning with the remainder administered before the evening meal
- Each injection consists of both intermediate- and short-acting insulins, approximately in the ratio of 2 to 1.

Naturally, treatment must be individualised for each patient. Adjustments to the insulin regimen can be made according to the following principles:

1) *Total insulin dosage:* this is best determined by accounting for both the glycated haemoglobin ($HbA_{1c}$) result and the prevailing frequency of hypoglycaemia. A high $HbA_{1c}$ concentration suggests that an increase in insulin dosage is necessary if the patient does not already have an unacceptable frequency of hypoglycaemic episodes. However, near normal $HbA_{1c}$ in the presence of hypoglycaemic episodes indicates that the insulin dosage is too high. The magnitude of change in insulin dosage that can be made at each adjustment depends on many factors, but generally should not exceed 4 to 6U every few days.

2) *Distribution in timing and type of insulin:* this is best determined by examining the profile of blood glucose concentrations performed by the patient. Another useful practice is to ask the patient what time of the day they are most likely to find high or low blood glucose readings. Adjustment of the proportion of morning *versus* afternoon and intermediate *versus* short-acting insulins can then be made accordingly.

Inherent in the philosophy of conventional therapy is that fixed doses of insulin are administered each day at predetermined times. The patient then attempts to have a regular diet and exercise pattern each day to balance the insulin action and attain good glycaemic control. Adjustments to insulin dosage are only made when there are major changes in clinical response and usually occur at medical consultations. Many patients with regular lifestyles find this an acceptable method of managing their diabetes. Glycaemic control attained by this method can be very good, but is often suboptimal, because the inflexibility of the regimen does not cater for achievement of near normoglycaemia.

#### Use of Multiple Insulin Injections

An alternative to conventional treatment (see above) is the multiple insulin injection regimen. This means injection of a short-acting insulin before each of the 3 main meals, with additional intermediate or long-acting insulin administered before bedtime. This combination attempts to mimic postprandial and night-time basal release of insulin in normal individuals. Delaying injection of intermediate- or long-acting insulin until just before bedtime reduces the chance of nocturnal hypoglycaemia because its peak action occurs at about 5 to 6am, when blood glucose concentration normally rises as a result of the dawn phenomenon.

This regimen is popular amongst young IDDM patients because it allows a more flexible lifestyle, especially in relation to timing of the meals. This type of treatment provides better flexibility and more even distribution of insulin but, unless combined with intensive treatment methods, does not achieve near normal glycaemic control. It should, therefore, not be considered identical to the intensive therapy used in the Diabetes Control and Complications Trial.[86,87] This type of treatment has been described in a separate section (see below) to emphasise the differences.

#### Intensive Insulin Therapy

In intensive therapy, patients are required to have at least 4 injections of insulin daily or use an insulin infusion pump. The expense associated with an insulin pump and its imperfect technology have meant that most patients use the multiple injection technique. In this treatment, patients must monitor their blood glucose frequently, usually at least 4 to 7 times daily. They need to learn from theoretical knowledge and practical experience how their blood glucose concentrations might fluctuate in response to changes in physical activity and food consumption. Then, the patient makes frequent adjustments to the insulin dosage; if necessary, changing each injection. The aim is to keep blood glucose concentrations as near normal as possible. This management method requires a great deal of patient education and is most easily conducted where there is close involvement between patients and a multidisciplinary healthcare team.

In the Diabetes Control and Complications Trial (DCCT) experience,[86,87] intensive treatment reduced $HbA_{1c}$ by about 2% and reduced both the development and progression of diabetic complications by 35 to 76%. However, it was also associated with a 3-fold higher incidence of severe hypoglycaemic episodes. Hence, it should be used with caution in patients prone to hypoglycaemia. Many patients also find the demand of managing diabetes on an hour-to-hour basis too much of a psychological burden. Thus, counselling and selection of patients for intensive treatment must be conducted carefully by experienced healthcare professionals.

#### Treatment of Hypoglycaemia with Glucagon

In most cases, hypoglycaemic episodes can be treated effectively by ingesting any form of simple sugar. However, if the patient cannot respond to commands and medical help is not immediately available, intramuscular glucagon could be administered by a friend or family member. Glucagon stimulates the breakdown of hepatic glycogen stores. The dose of glucagon is 1mg (1IU) and it can be administered intramuscularly or subcutaneously. There is no preferred site for injection of glucagon and relatives should not be given excessive details that might confuse them and delay administration. If there is no response within 10 to 15 minutes, medical assistance should be sought. All patients with IDDM should be encouraged to have a friend or family member learn how to inject glucagon and should be advised to keep a supply at home.

### 3.4 Long Term Complications of Diabetes Mellitus and their Pharmacological Management

The DCCT trial[86,87] proved conclusively that good glycaemic control reduces microvascular and neuropathic complications in IDDM.

Studies are ongoing [e.g. the UKPDS[76] and the CSDM[77] trials] to determine if this conclusion is also applicable to NIDDM. Unfortunately, optimal glycaemic control is difficult to achieve in many IDDM and NIDDM diabetic patients. Therefore, early detection and treatment of complications remain important aspects of patient care.

#### *3.4.1 Diabetic Neuropathy*

Diabetic peripheral neuropathy is one of the most common complications of diabetes and it is predominantly sensory in type. There are 2 related but separate clinical problems:

- Progressive nerve fibre damage causing sensory loss and ulcer formation, usually at sites of increased pressure at the sole of the feet
- Distressing symptoms of pain, numbness and paraesthesia.

The aims of drug therapy for diabetic peripheral neuropathy therefore reflect attempts to counter these problems.

##### Drugs to Prevent and Allay Nerve Fibre Damage

***Aldose reductase inhibitors*** *(e.g. tolrestat, epalrestat, zopolrestat):* aldose reductase is the enzyme that converts glucose to sorbitol and subsequently to fructose. Excessive flux of this pathway in hyperglycaemia has been implicated in the pathogenesis of peripheral neuropathy, so a class of agents known as aldose reductase inhibitors has been developed to interrupt this sequence, with the hope of preventing nerve damage.[88] However, extensive study of aldose reductase inhibitors in the treatment of diabetic peripheral neuropathy has not shown substantial benefits. This is partly because end-points used in clinical trials (symptoms and nerve conduction velocity) are neither sufficiently objective nor sensitive. It may also be because clinical trials have been performed on patients with moderately severe neuropathy, at a stage when it has become irreversible. However, it does seem fair to conclude from available evidence that the magnitude of improvement in these indices, if any, is small.

Early studies using aldose reductase inhibitors involved *sorbinil* which had a number of toxic effects and was eventually withdrawn from clinical trials. More recent research has mainly involved *tolrestat*. In a meta-analysis of its effectiveness in clinical trials,[89] tolrestat was found to produce improvement in peripheral nerve function similar in magnitude to that obtained by intensive insulin therapy. A non-comparative trial examining nerve biopsy findings in patients treated with tolrestat for several years concluded that tolrestat may improve nerve regeneration.[90] Overall, the benefits of tolrestat have not been considered sufficiently definitive for it to be accepted for routine clinical care. To gain more precise information about the response to aldose reductase inhibitors, a prospective clinical trial is underway, which will use the more quantitative (and invasive) technique of measuring morphometric changes in sural nerve biopsies as an end-point.

Until more definitive guidelines become available, the decision to use tolrestat must be individualised and made after discussing with patients the available evidence of its effectiveness so that they can make an informed choice. In general, it seems most suitable for patients with definite evidence of early clinical neuropathy, e.g. those with absent ankle jerks and mild sensory loss, but before the stage of developing chronic neuropathic ulceration. Patients should also be informed that although tolrestat has been shown to relieve paraesthesia better than a placebo in controlled clinical trials,[91] its use is unlikely to produce great symptomatic improvement. Fortunately, tolrestat is not a particularly hazardous drug. Apart from elevation of liver enzymes in about 3% of patients, it has no obvious clinical toxicity.

***γ-Linolenic acid:*** peripheral neuropathy can develop and progress in patients with apparently good diabetic control, so factors other than hyperglycaemia have been suggested as playing a role in pathogenesis of this condition. Disturbances of n-6 essential fatty acids in diabetes are believed to cause a variety of microvascular and other abnormalities that lead to reduced bloodflow and neural hypoxia. It has been suggested that treatment with γ-linolenic acid can restore these defects in essential fatty acid biochemistry. In a multicentre study,[92] in which patients were randomly allocated to take γ-linolenic acid or placebo for 12 months, γ-linolenic acid significantly improved both neurophysiological and neurological parameters compared with placebo. The investigators concluded that patients with lower $HbA_{1c}$ concentrations are likely to have better responses to γ-linolenic acid treatment. However, these observations were made in patients with relatively mild neuropathy.

### Drug Therapy to Relieve Symptoms of Diabetic Neuropathy

Clinicians and patients have been frustrated by the lack of a completely satisfactory treatment to allay the distressing symptoms of neuropathy. Pharmacological agents described in this section have been used to alleviate discomfort but have no known effect on slowing the progression of disease. They should, therefore, be used in combination with measures to improve metabolic control and possibly with drugs described in the previous section.

***Tricyclic antidepressants*** are among the most common therapies used to reduce neuropathic symptoms. They are thought to relieve neuropathic pain by blocking the reuptake of the neurotransmitters noradrenaline (norepinephrine) or serotonin, which are released by pain-modulating systems descending from the brain stem to the spinal cord. In a well controlled study[93] in patients with painful neuropathy in which amitriptyline was compared with desipramine (a more selective blocker of noradrenaline uptake), the selective serotonin reuptake inhibitor fluoxetine, and placebo, amitriptyline and desipramine were found to be more effective than either fluoxetine or placebo in relieving pain. However, symptoms improved in patients randomised to placebo, which highlights the difficulties of performing clinical effectiveness studies in chronically painful conditions. A moderate relief of pain was obtained in 74% of patients receiving amitriptyline compared with 61% of patients receiving desipramine. The difference was not statistically significant, suggesting that desipramine is an alternative for patients who cannot tolerate amitriptyline. High doses (50 to 100 mg/day) of tricyclic antidepressants are often needed to alleviate discomfort. Unfortunately, effective treatment may be limited by adverse effects, such as orthostatic hypotension, urinary retention and cardiac arrhythmias. For maximum benefit, patients should be monitored closely so the dosage can be adjusted to achieve symptom relief without untoward effects.

***Mexiletine:*** neuropathic pain is thought to depend on the flow of sodium ions into the nerve. Mexiletine is primarily used as an antiarrhythmic agent, and its sodium channel blocking effect is thought to be the mechanism by which it reduces discomfort. Earlier studies showed that the analgesic effects of intravenous lidocaine (lignocaine) lasted 3 to 21 days. However, lidocaine treatment required hospital admission, so subsequent studies used mexiletine, an oral analogue of lidocaine. A multicentre study showed no difference between mexiletine and placebo in pain relief,[94] but mexiletine was superior to placebo in a subset of patients whose symptoms were characterised by stabbing or burning pain and heat sensations. No electrocardiographic abnormalities were detected, but there was a high incidence of gastrointestinal and CNS adverse effects (33%) when the maximum dosage (675 mg/day) was used. Since adverse events were increased at the higher dose, the recommended dosage is 450 mg/day.

***Topical capsaicin:*** this agent is an alkaloid found in capsicum peppers. Its local application to peripheral nerves is believed to reduce conduction in type C fibres, rendering them less sensitive to stimuli. The initial response to capsaicin can result in local warmth, redness, burning and increased pain. However, with continued application, the patient gradually becomes desensitised to these stimuli and experiences subsequent relief of discomfort. Most studies of capsaicin included patients unresponsive or intolerant to conventional pain relief therapy. Results indicate that application of topical capsaicin 0.075% can significantly reduce pain.[95] However, while the results are encouraging, there are inherent difficulties in performing double-blind, placebo-controlled trials of capsaicin because it induces a mild burning sensation when first applied.

### Therapy for Diabetic Autonomic Neuropathy

Autonomic neuropathy is a disabling and potentially serious complication of diabetes. By the time clinical features appear, this complication of diabetes is already very advanced. Treatment is only for symptomatic relief and often is not completely successful. Postural hypotension can be reduced by expanding vascular volume with fludrocortisone (see also chapter 4; sect. 4.1.3). Cisapride, metoclopramide and erythromycin can increase gastric emptying and, therefore, reduce the feeling of fullness and nausea, and make food absorption more regular.

Cholinergic agents are useful in increasing contractility of an atonic bladder. Penile injection of alprostadil (prostaglandin $E_1$) gives a good response in patients troubled by impotence (see further section 8.2.5).

### 3.4.2 Diabetic Foot Problems: Use of Antibiotics in Management

Amputation of the lower limb remains a leading cause of morbidity and healthcare cost in diabetes. A common sequence of events is that a minor trauma in the presence of peripheral neuropathy and/or vascular disease causes formation of an ulcer that becomes infected. Failure to eradicate the infection leads to tissue destruction, bone infection and abscess formation, culminating in amputation. Thus, early control of infection is crucial, although improvement of circulation, reduction of pressure at the ulcer site and meticulous wound care are also essential.

#### Common Pathogens and Antibiotic Selection

*Staphylococcus aureus* is the most common pathogen causing infection in the feet of diabetic patients. *Streptococcus* spp., *Enterococcus* spp. and other species of *Staphylococcus* may also be responsible. The more serious infections are often due to a combination of aerobic and anaerobic organisms. With recurrent infections and repeated use of antibiotic therapy, the microbial flora become more complex.

Ideally, antibiotic therapy should be targeted to the specific pathogen. However, in diabetic foot infections it is difficult to identify the major offender by wound swabbing. Clinical judgement is often the best guide. For simple, localised infection, *flucloxacillin* or *cefalexin* are often effective. If anaerobic infection is suspected because of the presence of odour, necrosis or profuse discharge, these two agents can be used in combination with *metronidazole*. Alternatively, standard combinations of *amoxicillin* and *clavulanic acid* can be tried. Clavulanic acid broadens the spectrum of activity of amoxicillin to include penicillinase-producing *Staphylococcus* spp. When infections fail to respond or if patients have penicillin allergy, *clindamycin* and *ciprofloxacin* can be used alone or in combination. For patients with infection due to staphylococci resistant to multiple antibiotics, fusidic acid and/or rifampicin may be used.

In patients with spreading cellulitis or more deep-seated infection, parenteral antibiotic therapy becomes necessary. Due to reduction in numbers of hospital beds in many countries, many of these infections are now treated without hospital admission, either by a nurse administering the antibiotics at home or the patient visiting an ambulatory care facility each day. The third-generation cefalosporin *ceftriaxone* has the advantage in this situation because it can be administered once daily.

A controversy in diabetic foot infection treatment is the question of how often they are accompanied by coexisting osteomyelitis. A US study[96] found that when bone biopsy and white cell scan are used as diagnostic tools, osteomyelitis is associated with 60 to 70% of foot ulcers, even when conventional x-rays are normal. Subclinical osteomyelitis can be eradicated by several months of oral antibiotic treatment. If confirmed, the US study suggests a need for routine white cell bone scan to determine the length of antibiotic therapy required.

### 3.4.3 Diabetic Nephropathy and Hypertension

Hypertension is about twice as common in patients with diabetes and its early treatment is essential to prevent vascular disease. Hypertension accelerates progression of established nephropathy (characterised by proteinuria >0.5 g/day) and progression of the earlier phase of diabetic kidney disease, microalbuminuria (albumin excretion 30 to 300 mg/day). Treatments of hypertension and diabetic kidney disease are so interrelated that they will be considered together here. To add to the complexity of this area, there is now evidence that the *angiotensin-converting enzyme (ACE) inhibitors*, a commonly used class of antihypertensive agents (see also chapter 21; sect. 3.4), may have renoprotective effects in diabetes above and beyond those explained by their antihypertensive actions.

Hypertension occurs at a different phases of the natural history of IDDM and NIDDM. Patients with IDDM are usually normotensive until they develop renal disease. In contrast, NIDDM patients are often hypertensive at diagnosis. The association of NIDDM, hypertension, central obesity and hyperlipidaemia has been referred to as 'syndrome X' or the 'metabolic syndrome', and insulin resistance is thought to be the common thread underlying these abnormalities[97] (see also section 4 below).

There has been a general trend to diagnose and treat hypertension in diabetes at a lower threshold. For example, the JNC-V criteria[98] adopted by the American Diabetes Association regard hypertension as present if systolic blood pressure is >140mm Hg and/or diastolic blood pressure is >90mm Hg. This is more sensitive than the older WHO criterion that has a threshold of systolic blood pressure at 160mm Hg and of diastolic blood pressure at 95mm Hg. While medically sound, it causes a significant increase in the prevalence of hypertension (IDDM 26 to 51%, NIDDM 61 to 80%), and in particular, isolated systolic hypertension in NIDDM.[99] This has major healthcare cost implications.

#### Patients With Established Diabetic Nephropathy

Patients with established diabetic nephropathy are usually hypertensive. Effective antihypertensive therapy is the most important factor in preserving renal function in patients with established diabetic nephropathy. Diuretics, β-adrenoceptor blockers, vasodilators and ACE inhibitors have all been used successfully in this regard. In a study[100] spanning 4 years, the ACE inhibitor *captopril* was compared with other antihypertensive agents in patients with diabetic nephropathy. When matched for blood pressure control achieved, captopril was shown to be 50% more effective in retarding increases in serum creatinine and more effective in reducing proteinuria. These advantages of captopril were observed even when the initial blood pressure was lower than 140/90mm Hg. The investigators concluded that captopril has renoprotective effects independent of its antihypertensive action. This conclusion was supported by a meta-regression analysis of 100 studies on antihypertensive treatment in diabetes.[101]

Thus, ACE inhibitors seem to be the logical choice of antihypertensive agents in diabetic patients with established nephropathy. It also suggests that ACE inhibitors should be prescribed in these patients even in the absence of hypertension. Captopril is the best studied drug in this regard. It is not clear whether this holds for all ACE inhibitors.

#### Patients with Microalbuminuria

Diabetic patients with microalbuminuria have, as a group, slightly higher blood pressure than patients without microalbuminuria. Although the elevation is modest, antihypertensive treatment can lower albumin excretion rate in this group of patients. There are limited data that suggest that this can reduce the development of overt proteinuria. While it is logical to assume that antihypertensive treatment will, therefore, lead to less decline in renal function, this remains to be proven. The meta-regression analysis discussed above[101] found that *ACE inhibitors* reduced albumin excretion in patients with microalbuminuria to an extent not explained by their antihypertensive action alone.

In another study,[102] enalapril was compared with placebo in normotensive NIDDM patients with microalbuminuria; if needed, blood pressure increases in both groups were treated with long-acting nifedipine. After 5 years of follow-up, the enalapril group had significantly less proteinuria and a smaller increase in serum creatinine. However, the difference from placebo was small, which is not surprising considering the mild degree of existing renal abnormalities. Even for patients with overt nephropathy,[100] the advantage of captopril over placebo was only obvious in patients with more severe renal impairment. A similar study in patients with microalbuminuria who usually have perfectly normal renal function will require at least 10 to 20 years of follow-up to reach similar end-points.

#### Patients with Hypertension and Normal Albumin Excretion

In diabetic patients with hypertension but no microalbuminuria or overt proteinuria, there is no clear evidence that any antihypertensive agent is superior in improving long term prognosis. The meta-regression analysis performed by Kasiske et al.[101] found all classes of antihypertensive agents to be similar in their ability to reduce blood pressure. Therefore, factors other than blood pressure reduction become important in the choice of antihypertensive agents. *ACE inhibitors* and *calcium antagonists* are recommended as first-line agents by some authorities because they do not have detrimental effects on lipids and insulin sensitivity. This enthusiasm for ACE inhibitors should be tempered with the recent report[103] that suggests that ACE inhibitors may significantly increase the risk of severe hypoglycaemia. However, neither this problem nor alteration in diabetes control have been reported in other trials.[104] Clearly, prospective trials are needed to clarify this point.

β-Blockers can cause hyperlipidaemia (although changes are minimal with some agents), aggravate peripheral vascular disease, impair glucose counter-regulation and affect sexual potency. In theory, use of relatively $\beta_1$-selective agents may minimise some of these problems, but in practice their advantage is uncertain. Therefore, in patients with diabetes, β-blockers are considered by some to be indicated only where there is cardiac disease such as angina pectoris and arrhythmias. Diuretics may cause hypokalaemia that can affect insulin secretion, an adverse effect that is minimised if the dosage is kept low, or if indapamide (1.25 to 2.5mg daily) is prescribed.[105,106] However, full dosages of diuretics are needed in diabetic patients with fluid accumulation as well as hypertension.

In many patients, hypertension cannot be controlled by monotherapy. A general approach is to use an *ACE inhibitor* as first-line therapy and add a *calcium antagonist* and *low-dose diuretic* sequentially as indicated by the blood pressure response. In the enthusiasm to use new antihypertensive agents, it should be borne in mind that there is no evidence that ACE inhibitors are renoprotective in patients with normal albumin excretion. In fact, β-blockers and diuretics have been proven in large clinical trials to reduce vascular disease. Furthermore, ACE inhibitors can themselves aggravate proteinuria, hyperkalaemia and renal perfusion in patients with renal artery stenosis.

### 3.4.4 Hyperlipidaemia (Dyslipidaemia) in Diabetes

The most common pattern of lipid abnormalities in NIDDM patients is elevated plasma triglycerides occurring together with reduced high-density lipoprotein (HDL) cholesterol concentrations. Some patients with this pattern also have elevated low-density lipoprotein (LDL) cholesterol (mixed dyslipidaemia). In others, only LDL-cholesterol is elevated, although this is no more common than in the general population. These lipid abnormalities are often observed even when diabetes appears mild or well controlled. The most common lipid abnormality in IDDM patients is elevated plasma triglyceride concentrations, which is usually associated with poor glycaemic control.

Diabetic patients have a higher incidence of vascular disease. Thus, the importance of lipid abnormalities is highlighted by the observation that multiple risk factors cause a striking cumulative increase in cardiovascular mortality.[107] Despite this, there is no concrete evidence of benefits of normalising lipid concentrations in diabetic patients because these patients are systematically excluded from many large lipid intervention studies. Therefore, strategies to treat hyperlipidaemia in diabetes are based on the logical but unproven assumption that lipid abnormalities in diabetic patients should be treated aggressively because diabetes itself is a profound risk factor of vascular disease.

As in the general population, lifestyle modifications are important in the management of hyperlipidaemia in diabetes. If lifestyle changes together with improvement of glycaemic control fail to achieve optimal lipid concentrations, drug intervention is indicated (see further chapter 20). What is uncertain is the extent to which the threshold for treatment should be lowered for diabetic patients. However, there is good agreement that lipid-lowering treatment should be implemented aggressively in patients with existing clinical vascular disease (secondary prevention).

#### Hypertriglyceridaemia with Low HDL-Cholesterol

The fibric acid derivative *gemfibrozil* is generally considered first-line treatment to normalise both of these abnormalities. In the Helsinki Heart Study,[108] gemfibrozil was shown to reduce the incidence of cardiac events in the subset of patients with this lipid profile. The older preparation, clofibrate, is less effective and now largely superseded. When gemfibrozil by itself is insufficient to lower triglyceride to the optimal concentration, fish oil containing omega-3 fatty acids could be added.[109]

*Nicotinic acid* is one of the few agents with a significant ability to raise HDL-cholesterol, but unfortunately it can aggravate glucose intolerance. *Acipimox*, an analogue of nicotinic acid, has a more sustained action on free fatty acids and is less diabetogenic than nicotinic acid.[110]

Although it is traditional to try dietary therapy for several months before embarking on drug treatment, gemfibrozil should be prescribed early in patients with grossly elevated triglycerides (e.g. >10 mmol/L), which is associated with increased risk of acute pancreatitis.

#### Hypercholesterolaemia

This abnormality is best treated by inhibitors of 3-hydroxy-3-methylglutaryl-coenzyme A (HMG-CoA) reductase (e.g. *simvastatin, pravastatin, lovastatin*), the rate-limiting enzyme of cellular cholesterol synthesis. In comparison with older drugs, these agents are highly effective therapy for patients with elevated cholesterol concentrations and have less unpleasant adverse effects.[111] They have been shown to be effective in reducing macrovascular events in nondiabetic patients. When insufficient by themselves to lower cholesterol to a satisfactory concentration, the HMG-CoA reductase inhibitors can be used in conjunction with a bile acid-binding resin (e.g. cholestyramine or colestipol) [see also chapter 20].

#### Mixed Dyslipidaemia

This condition often poses a special problem in management. There is no consensus whether *gemfibrozil* or *HMG-CoA reductase inhibitors* should be the chosen first-line therapy. Neither are ideal in normalising the lipid abnormalities of this syndrome because the ability of gemfibrozil to lower LDL-cholesterol is relatively modest, while HMG-CoA reductase inhibitors are less effective in lowering triglycerides and raising HDL-cholesterol. The combined use of gemfibrozil and an HMG-CoA reductase inhibitor increases their individual adverse effects on skeletal muscle (e.g. myopathy) and should not be prescribed without careful consideration. Clinicians must make an arbitrary decision about which lipid abnormalities is to be treated first.

*Fenofibrate* is similar to gemfibrozil, but may be more effective in decreasing LDL-cholesterol.

### 3.5 Clinical Outcome and Economic Considerations

There is little doubt that diabetes is a major health care burden in both developed and developing countries. In the US alone, it has been estimated that the annual combined direct and indirect costs of diabetes are in excess of US$20 billion. There is also no argument that diabetes is a major cause of increased morbidity and mortality. What is less certain is the most cost-effective way of achieving good health outcomes. In the foreseeable future, primary prevention aiming to reduce the incidence of NIDDM and secondary or tertiary measures to reduce the effects of diabetic complications are needed in parallel.

Since diabetes is a chronic condition with morbidity and mortality occurring late in the natural history of disease, it has been extremely difficult to evaluate outcomes of any treatment strategy. Despite a mean follow-up of 6.5 years at a cost of several hundred million dollars, the DCCT trial[86,87] has only managed to follow the study cohort up to the stage of developing relatively mild complications. Many of the conclusions regarding development of severe complications were based on extrapolations from epidemiological studies. The UKPDS study follow-up has already been extended, but is not due to be reported until 1998. Thus, there is a paucity of data to allow scientific calculation of the cost-effectiveness of various treatment strategies. Even when data are available, the conclusions of clinical trials based on highly selected groups of patients cannot be extended directly to the population at large, because patient preferences, genetic and environmental factors, and skills of the healthcare team may all modify outcomes. Therefore, collection of data on treatment outcomes in settings outside of clinical trials are also important.

Until more facts are available, many healthcare decisions in diabetes management will have to be made on the basis of best guess estimates from available data. From a drug intervention perspective, maintenance of good diabetic control through the optimal use of oral antidiabetic agents and insulin is a good investment. From the findings of the DCCT trial[86,87] and a meta-analysis of the literature,[121] the association between hyperglycaemia and diabetic complications is undoubted. With modern technology, both classes of therapeutic agents can be produced inexpensively.

The early use of antihypertensive agents is also likely to be cost-effective (see section 3.4.3 above). Hypertension is associated with poor prognosis in diabetic patients and its treatment is a proven strategy to lower the incidence of vascular disease. Evidence is also accumulating that lipid-lowering agents are effective in preventing vascular disease after a relatively short period of treatment of at-risk individuals.

## 4. Obesity

Obesity and overweight are common disorders. They are increasingly prevalent in societies as they become urbanised, more affluent and adopt more Western diets. In many Western countries, the prevalence of obesity ranges from 9 to 15% of the adult population, with a far greater proportion of the population being overweight.[113] However, in some societies or groups, particularly in the South Pacific, far greater proportions of the population are obese. Despite their prevalence, and the acknowledgment that they are a significant public health problem, obesity and overweight remain difficult to treat.

Obesity and overweight are associated with increased mortality and morbidity.[114-116] They are independent cardiovascular risk factors, and are associated with increased hypertension. There is a mild myocardial dysfunction, seen on echocardiography, caused by obesity that is reversed by weight loss. There are also a number of associated metabolic problems, including non–insulin-dependent diabetes mellitus

(NIDDM), hyperlipidaemias, fatty liver and gall bladder disease. Obese individuals may have high serum cortisol concentrations, but these are suppressed with low-dose dexamethasone. The combination of NIDDM, abdominal obesity, hypertension and hypertriglyceridaemia is now called the 'metabolic syndrome or 'syndrome X', and hyperinsulinaemia (insulin resistance) is thought to be a common linking or causative factor.

There are several mechanical problems associated with obesity. These include sleep apnoea (associated with hypertension, arrhythmias and sudden death, and leading to pulmonary hypertension and right heart failure),[117] osteoarthritis and other musculoskeletal problems. Infertility is a problem in obese patients, and obesity is a surgical risk. Furthermore, obesity is a factor in psychosocial problems, including low self-esteem, difficulty in getting employment and psychological illness.

It is not weight *per se* that is associated with these problems, but adiposity and, in particular, abdominal adiposity.[118,119] Adiposity cannot be measured directly and the techniques used (underwater weighing, dual x-ray absorptiometry, bioelectrical impedance) may not be easily available. Instead, an indirect measure of adiposity is commonly used, i.e. the *body mass index* (BMI). This is the mathematical expression of bodyweight (in kilograms) divided by the square of the height (in meters). It gives a reasonable measure of adiposity except at extremes of age and in very fit and muscular individuals. The problems of obesity occur with BMI >27,[120] though lower cutoff points have been suggested. While the BMI gives a good practical measure of adiposity and its risks, it has been developed for Europeans and may not be valid for other populations and ethnic groups. In addition, abdominal adiposity can be assessed simply by measuring waist and hip circumferences and calculating the waist to hip (W/H) ratio, which should be <0.8 in women and <1.0 in men. A waist measurement of 100cm in men and 95cm in women denotes increased risk.

### 4.1 Aetiology of Obesity

It has become obvious that there is a substantial genetic basis to obesity,[121,122] which may account for 25 to 40% of the problem. Abdominal obesity seems to be more strongly inherited. There is no single gene responsible, but 23 have been described associated with obesity. One of the more recent is the obese gene,[123] which was originally described in the ob/ob mouse, but has been found in the human genome. The mechanisms through which the genes act are not known, but it has been suggested that there may be changes in resting metabolic rate, diet-induced thermogenesis, satiety and/or control of metabolism through the hypothalamic-pituitary adrenal axis, to give but a few mechanisms. A number of specific genetic syndromes may cause obesity. Prader Willi syndrome (involving a deletion in the short arm of chromosome 15) is perhaps the best known and most common.

It is obvious, however, that genetic change is not sufficient for obesity to occur. Environmental factors also play a role, e.g. affluence, urbanisation and Westernisation of diet. While additional energy intake is important, this may not be just due to overeating, but may be due to 'stress eating', wherein the diet may be appropriate most of the time. The quality of the diet is also important, with increased proportions of fat in the diet predisposing individuals to weight gain. In addition, as society becomes more affluent and with industrialisation and mechanisation, less exercise is performed. These 3 factors are major contributors to the development of overweight and obesity.

Other causes are medical treatment, either in the reduction of activity by prescription (as for arthritis), or caused by drugs (e.g. β-blockers, which reduce exercise capacity). Other drugs may cause patients to increase food intake, including glucocorticoids, phenothiazines, many antidepressants (either directly or as a result of the depression), cyproheptadine and pizotifen. In some individuals, estrogens also increase food intake.

Endocrine conditions are often blamed for obesity, but in reality they rarely cause obesity and in general only produce a 5 to 8kg weight gain. Endocrine disorders associated with increased weight are Cushing's syndrome, hypothyroidism and acromegaly. Hyperprolactinaemia produces an increase in adiposity, while hyperinsulinaemia is part of the 'metabolic syndrome'. Hypothalamic damage (following trauma, tumour, infection or surgery) may also alter eating patterns and produce obesity. Another common cause of increased weight is smoking cessation, wherein women tend to gain more weight than men. Conversely, smokers as a group are lighter than nonsmokers, which is due in part to stimulation of the metabolic rate while asleep. The risks of smoking are greater than the risks of any weight gained on ceasing smoking.

## 4.2 Optimum Treatment

### 4.2.1 Basic Therapy

Treatment of obesity is both possible and effective when behaviour modification and follow-up are included.[124] There are many recent reviews of therapy (e.g. Bray & Gray,[125] Caterson[126] and Dyer[127]). The initial step in treatment should be the setting (and recording) of goals specific for the patient. These obviously include weight loss and a reduction in risk factors, but may include control of diabetes, increased mobility, the ability to have an operation and other individual goals. The attainment of goals should be noted. Diet, exercise and behaviour modification are the starting points of therapy.

#### Behaviour Modification

Behaviour modification is very important in maintaining weight loss. It involves changing habits, improving self-esteem, reducing guilt inherent in eating, and early recognition of behaviour and stresses that predispose patients to obesity. Among the techniques used are diary-keeping, stimulus control and cognitive restructuring. Patients may be asked to record what is eaten and what exercise is performed, and to recognise stresses and stimuli that predispose them to eating, then to alter these stimuli or the environment. In patients who have tried to lose weight and failed, these techniques remove guilt often associated with both eating and food.

#### Dietary Measures

A healthy eating plan rather than a specific diet is a necessary part of weight loss therapy. Diets end, but individuals keep on eating. The plan can be developed from the food logs kept by the patient. Rather than counting kilojoules or kilocalories, it is sufficient to prescribe a low-fat eating programme. Steps to be taken include removal of visible fat from meats, grilling rather than frying, use of less oil in cooking and on salads, low-fat dairy products, and so on. This type of eating should be encouraged for the whole family.

Some clinicians may prescribe a specific diet. It is generally not necessary to prescribe diets that contain less than 1200 kcal/day in women or 1500 kcal/day in men to achieve adequate weight loss. Young men may need special attention and nutritional education. Alcohol consumption may be sufficient to impede weight loss. Rather than forbidding it entirely, appropriate alternatives such as low alcohol beer may be recommended. Many obese individuals do not overeat all the time, but binge or eat while under stress. Attention should be paid to the stresses that cause overeating and to finding alternative ways of dealing with them.

#### Role of Exercise

Exercise is also important. It is not necessary to be as fit as a trained athlete to alter weight and metabolic parameters.[119,128] Continuous, lower intensity exercise appears to achieve the same effect. Individual programmes should be prescribed. For patients with arthritis starting exercise programmes, adequate pain treatment and hydrotherapy (exercising in a pool) can be a great help. Exercise does not produce major weight loss (changes in dietary intake are needed for that), but it does produce some weight loss, improves well-being and increases mobility.

### 4.2.2 Adjunctive Therapies

Adjunctive therapies should be used in conjunction with a basic therapy programme, because while these therapies may be successful in the short term in their own right, there is no evidence that they provide long term weight loss (with the possible exception of gastric surgery).[129,130]

#### Drug Therapy

A number of anorectic agents have been used to treat obesity and overweight. In general, they are either amphetamine-related compounds or agents that require patients to have an intact serotonergic system.

***Amphetamine-related drugs:*** in this class are *amfepramone* (diethylpropion), *phentermine* and *mazindol* (for a review of their use, see Greenaway & Caterson[131]). Older amphetamine-like agents (e.g. dexamphetamine, methamphetamine) have been abandoned as therapy for obesity due to their adverse effects and abuse potential. In general, these agents act on central mechanisms that control appetite. As a class, they are effective in producing weight loss in the short term (over 3 months),[114] but may have stimulatory adverse effects on both the CNS and cardiovascular systems. Because of these stimulatory effects, psychological dependence, rather than true physical dependence, may occur, although it is infrequent amongst those who are taking them as part of a weight loss programme. Tolerance to these drugs has been shown to occur after variable periods.

Amfepramone (diethylpropion) has a low adverse effect profile and has been studied extensively. Phentermine is usually given intermittently, which minimises its adverse effects. It has been suggested that mazindol acts by inhibiting axonal noradrenaline uptake and by stimulating peripheral catecholamine receptors, but there is no evidence that it is more effective than the other drugs in this group.

***Agents that require patients to have an intact serotonergic system:*** these include *fenfluramine* and its racemic derivative *dexfenfluramine*. Both are effective in producing weight loss in the short to medium term (3 to 15 months),[132,133] but after cessation of therapy (as with all anorectic drugs) weight tends to be regained. Although usually taken as an indication of failure to change habits, weight gain may also occur because the drugs have a continuing effect, the mechanism of which is not known.

Fenfluramine and dexfenfluramine should be used as part of a weight loss programme, and in this setting they produce some 30% extra weight loss.[132] Adverse effects (tiredness, fatigue and sleepiness, dry mouth, diarrhoea and depression) tend to be transient and mild. In young women, a risk of pulmonary hypertension has been suggested, particularly in those who use anorectics (of any class) intermittently, but more data are needed to confirm this. Dexfenfluramine is also useful in patients with NIDDM who need to lose weight as it has mild antihyperglycaemic activity, improves diabetic control,[83] and also exerts mild antihypertensive activity.[134] It has been suggested that combination therapy with fenfluramine and phentermine in low doses may be more effective and may cause less adverse effects than either drug used alone.[135]

Other drugs that act via a serotonin-related mechanism include *fluoxetine*, an antidepressant (see also chapter 30; sect. 5.1) which produces weight loss in depressed patients,[130] and appears to be of particular use in this situation

***Other drugs:*** a number of newer agents are being studied as anorectics. They include $\beta_3$-adrenoceptor agonists with thermogenic activity and pancreatic lipase inhibitors, such as *orlistat* (tetrahydrolipstatin). Other drugs shown to have some effect on obesity include benzocaine lozenges and methylcellulose as a bulking agent, but neither are in routine use because of their adverse effects or the small weight losses achieved. Other agents, such as thyroxine, human chorionic gonadotrophin (hCG), dinitrophenol and amylase inhibitors have proven to be ineffective (or dangerous) and should not be used in obesity treatment.

#### Very Low Energy Diets

Very low energy (i.e. low calorie or low kilojoule) diets contain between 400 and 800 kcal/day. The food intake is mostly of protein with essential fatty acids, vitamins and minerals and very little carbohydrate. These diets are extremely effective at producing rapid and early weight loss in very obese patients (BMI >40). The quality of protein used in these diets has improved and early problems reported with this therapy are no longer seen. They should be used under close supervision, as part of a broader weight loss programme.

Patients on these diets continue their normal activities, including work, but must have regular follow-up and should be prescribed a regular exercise programme. Some problems include lightheadedness, precipitation of gout and constipation. In addition, care should be taken to prevent gastric irritation if patients are receiving nonsteroidal anti-inflammatory drugs (NSAIDs). A further problem may be hunger, which can be treated by adding vegetables or dexfenfluramine to the regimen.

After a planned time on a very low energy diet, normal eating should reintroduced. Tissue glycogen is depleted during the time on these diets, so when normal eating begins, replenishment of glycogen stores may produce a slight weight gain because glycogen is osmotically active. Part of this weight loss can be prevented by increasing carbohydrate intake gradually over time.

#### Surgery

Surgery to treat obesity is not performed as often as it was in the past. Gastric banding is still effective in carefully selected patients, but is no longer a common procedure.[130] Plastic surgery, in the form of breast reduction, local liposuction or lipectomy, is useful in selected patients.

### 4.3 Preventive Therapy

Because of the genetic predisposition to obesity of much of the population, a preventive approach is needed.[127] Many therapies have been tried, but as yet none has been shown to be effective. If effective programmes can be found, in the future these approaches should be targeted to specific population subgroups. There will probably be a greater emphasis on physical activity than nutrition education in many of these approaches.

## 5. Thyroid Disease

Disorders of the thyroid gland can be broadly divided into those that present with a predominant abnormality of function, either hypothyroidism or hyperthyroidism, or those with a predominant abnormality of morphology, i.e. an enlargement of part or the whole of the thyroid. The latter group of disorders may be either diffuse or nodular and may occur in the absence of functional abnormalities. The advent of sensitive thyroid function testing, in particular the reliability of testing for unbound thyroid hormone concentrations and the introduction of second- and third-generation tests for serum TSH (thyrotrophin), has made diagnosis and management of hypothyroidism and hyperthyroidism relatively simple. It is essential to exclude thyroid malignancy in any patient with a dominant thyroid nodule. The most sensitive and specific test is fine needle biopsy.[136]

### 5.1 Hypothyroidism

The principles of therapy in any patient with hypothyroidism are to establish the severity of hypothyroidism, identify its cause, and institute appropriate thyroid hormone replacement without causing significant adverse effects. The introduction of increasingly sensitive assays for TSH, which have the ability to discriminate between normal and suppressed TSH concentration, allows the tailoring of therapy to achieve physiological replacement of thyroid hormone or suppression of TSH production. The introduction of these new assays has also led to concern regarding the safety of suppressive TSH therapy, with fears about over-replacement and possible osteoporosis.

Causes of hypothyroidism are listed in table III. The most common cause in developed countries is autoimmune thyroid disease, either primary atrophic hypothyroidism or Hashimoto's thyroiditis. Iodine deficiency is the commonest cause of hypothyroidism on a global basis, and prevention should be the first goal of its management.[137]

#### 5.1.1 Clinical Pharmacology of Drugs Used in Treatment

There are 4 different preparations available for oral thyroid hormone replacement therapy – thyroxine, liothyronine, thyroglobulin and dry or desiccated thyroid. Of these, thyroxine (levothyroxine) is the most commonly prescribed and recommended treatment for hypothyroidism.[138] Liothyronine (L-tri-iodothyronine) may be used in special circumstances (e.g. as short term replacement therapy or in the rare situation of myxoedema coma) but there is no longer a recognised role for thyroglobulin or desiccated thyroid.

**Table III.** Causes of primary hypothyroidism

| |
|---|
| **Congenital:** |
| • Agenesis |
| • Ectopic |
| • Dyshormonogenesis |
| **Iodine deficiency disorders:** |
| • Dietary goitrogens (cassava, sorghum, maize and millet) |
| **Autoimmune thyroid disease:** |
| • Primary atrophic hypothyroidism |
| • Hashimoto's thyroiditis |
| **Subacute thyroiditis-recovery phase** |
| **Post-radioactive iodine** |
| **Drugs:** |
| • Goitrogens (phenylbutazone, sulfonamides, sulphonylureas, resorcinol and thiocyanate) |
| • Iodine-induced hypothyroidism (e.g. kelp; potassium iodide; amiodarone; topical iodine antiseptics) |
| **Post-surgery** |

***Pharmacokinetic characteristics:*** thyroid hormones are rapidly absorbed from the gastrointestinal tract. Liothyronine is readily absorbed, whereas absorption of thyroxine can be variable, with a bioavailability ranging from 50 to 80%, but this is considered adequate for replacement therapy by the oral route.[139] Both thyroid hormones are tightly protein bound, principally to thyroxine binding globulin, transthyretin (tri-iodothyronine only) and albumin. Only the unbound hormone component is active, and thyroxine (99.95%) is more tightly bound than tri-iodothyronine (99.5%). The half-life of thyroxine is 1 week, compared with 1 day for liothyronine. Thus, it takes about 1 month to reach steady-state concentrations after initiating or altering thyroxine therapy.

Following absorption, thyroxine is metabolised to its active form tri-iodothyronine and to inactive reverse tri-iodothyronine, which then undergo further deiodination principally to inactive metabolites.[140] Tri-iodothyronine binds to at least 3 different types of intranuclear receptors. Further metabolites result from the deamination and decarboxylation of thyroxine and tri-iodothyronine to tetrac and tiratricol (triac), respectively. Thyroxine undergoes enterohepatic recycling and excretion in the faeces.

Until recently, it was thought that thyroid hormones did not readily cross the placenta. More recent data suggest that in some circumstances, particularly in the first trimester before fetal thyroid gland function is established or if fetal thyroid function is compromised or delayed, maternal thyroid hormone may play an important developmental and protective role in the fetus.[141] Nevertheless, the amounts transferred appear to be small and cannot compensate fully for a lack of fetal thyroid hormone.[142] The minimal amounts of thyroid hormone excreted in breast milk are insufficient to meet the needs of a suckling infant with a nonfunctioning thyroid gland.

### 5.1.2 Optimum Treatment

#### Overt Hypothyroidism

Several factors must be considered during treatment of patients with clinically overt hypothyroidism:

1) The age and health status of the patient is important in determining the starting dose of thyroxine.

2) Patients may have other coexisting endocrine disorders that can affect or be affected by thyroid hormone therapy.

3) Patients may be taking other drugs that can interact with thyroid hormone.

4) The level of endogenous thyroid hormone activity should be considered, since it may change the starting dose of thyroxine, e.g. in patients who are hypothyroid after treatment of Graves' disease.

Treatment of a young, healthy adult with classic features of hypothyroidism is relatively straightforward. *Thyroxine* can be started at close to a total replacement dose, at a mean of 100 to 150 μg/day or 2 μg/kg/day, without the need for an incremental rise in dosage. The dosage can be adjusted after 6 to 8 weeks to maintain serum TSH concentrations in the normal range, i.e. between 0.5 to 3.5 mIU/L. The drug should be taken once daily. Once concentrations have stabilised, routine measurement of thyroid hormones should be undertaken once or twice a year.

Treatment of all other patients should begin with a smaller initial dose, no higher than 50 μg/day. This is particularly the case in elderly patients and those with potential cardiac disease. In patients with established coronary artery disease, therapy should start with 12.5 μg/day or even 12.5μg on alternate days. Intensive therapy of the underlying coronary artery disease should also be undertaken. The dosage of thyroxine should be adjusted incrementally by 25μg every 4 to 6 weeks. If adrenal insufficiency is suspected, the hypothalamic-pituitary-adrenal axis should be tested and glucocorticoids added to the regimen if needed.

Patients receiving warfarin or other anticoagulants should be treated with additional caution, since restoration to the euthyroid state will further prolong the prothrombin time, increasing the risk of haemorrhage. Glucose intolerance may worsen when thyroid hormone concentrations improve, and concomitant diabetic therapy may need adjustment. Also, some drugs alter the absorption of thyroxine, e.g cholestyramine, soy-based milk products, and aluminium hydroxide–containing antacids and administration of these drugs should be separated from thyroxine administration by 4 to 5 hours if possible.

#### Subclinical Hypothyroidism

Controversy exists as to whether patients with subclinical hypothyroidism, i.e. normal unbound thyroid hormone concentrations but elevated serum TSH, benefit from thyroid hormone replacement. Many of these patients are detected incidentally after investigation of nonspecific symptoms or in follow-up after therapy for chronic autoimmune thyroid disease. Results of studies suggest that these patients may exhibit subtle biochemical and physiological indicators of tissue thyroid hormone deficiency.[29,143] If abnormal thyroid function tests are confirmed on more than one occasion, thyroxine therapy may be given, particularly in patients with a prior history or current biochemical evidence of autoimmune thyroid disease. Up to 50% of patients report clinical improvement after the start of therapy.[29] However, it is important to lessen the expectations of patients who may seek to attribute their symptoms to subtle thyroid hormone changes.

#### Transient Hypothyroidism

Most patients with hypothyroidism require lifelong therapy. However, hypothyroidism may be transient, particularly in the recovery phases of subacute thyroiditis and painless postpartum thyroiditis. Rarely, chronic lymphocytic thyroiditis may remit spontaneously.

Transient hypothyroidism is common in neonates, due either to iodine excess[144] or deficiency,[137] or to transplacental TSH receptor blocking antibodies.[145]

#### Hypothyroidism in Pregnancy

All women of childbearing age receiving long term thyroxine therapy should be advised to seek medical advice before becoming pregnant, to ensure that thyroid hormone concentrations are in the normal range before conception. The effect of maternal hypothyroidism on fetal development (in the absence of concomitant fetal hypothyroidism) is debated, but may be detrimental to neurological development. In addition, if there is a history of autoimmune thyroiditis or Graves' hyperthyroidism, then TSH receptor and/or blocking antibodies should also be measured to ensure there is no risk of fetal hyperthyroidism or hypothyroidism.[146]

When pregnancy is confirmed, the patient should seek medical attention early in the pregnancy so that thyroid hormone dosages can be adjusted. Patients should be reviewed at each trimester and then 6 to 8 weeks after delivery. Increased thyroid hormone requirements are seen in approximately 75% of women. The average thyroxine dosage increase in one series was 52 μg/day.[147] Serum TSH concentrations should be maintained in the normal range, except in patients with a history of thyroid cancer, in whom the goal of therapy should be to suppress serum TSH concentrations.

#### Conditions Requiring Suppression of TSH

There are clinical circumstances in which the aim of therapy is not to maintain serum TSH in the normal range, but to suppress TSH concentrations to below normal, i.e. below the detection limit of a second-generation TSH assay, usually <1 mIU/L. Unbound thyroid hormone concentrations are usually at the upper limits of normal or just above the normal range in this situation. The strongest indication for suppressive TSH thyroxine therapy is in the management of patients with differentiated thyroid cancer. Although this form of therapy has also been employed to achieve regression of nodular thyroid disease, it is generally unsuccessful either for solitary or multiple thyroid nodules.[148,149] It should not be routinely advocated except in circumstances of goitrous autoimmune Hashimoto's thyroid disease. Apart from its lack of effectiveness, there is also increasing concern regarding the adverse effects of excessive thyroxine therapy.

#### Fetal and Neonatal Hypothyroidism

Thyroid hormone exerts multiple effects on cellular metabolism, but its most important effects may be those on the development and differentiation of the brain during fetal and neonatal life, as well as its interaction with other trophic hormones to promote growth and concordant pubertal development during childhood. Thyroid hormone deficiency at critical phases of development will cause severe mental disability, shortness of stature, delayed epiphyseal closure (with secondary bone deformity) and discordant pubertal development, as well as other typical clinical signs of hypothyroidism. Depending on the timing of the insult, some or all of these clinical features may be present.

Until recently, the fetus was thought to be insensitive to the prenatal action of thyroid hormone. Although this is probably still correct for the growth of the fetus, the fetal brain appears to depend on thyroid hormone for normal development. Direct experimental evidence from animal studies and indirect evidence from clinical studies indicate that thyroid hormone plays a vital role in processes involved in the maturation of the brain at different stages. There appear to be 2 periods when the brain is vulnerable, corresponding to its main growth spurts. The first phase comprises the neuronal multiplication that occurs between 12 and 18 weeks of gestation and is completed by about mid-gestation, a period critical for the formation of the cerebral cortex, basal ganglia and of the cochlea of the inner ear. The second period constitutes the main growth spurt and includes glial cell multiplication and migration, myelination, development of dendritic arborisations and synaptic connections. This second phase begins in mid-pregnancy, is maximal around birth and 6 months after birth.

Placental transfer of maternal thyroid hormone may be important in the first phase of brain growth (before the fetal thyroid gland begins to function) and assumes greater importance for later brain development if fetal thyroid gland function is compromised.[141] In the postnatal period, the brain depends on normal concentrations of thyroid hormone for at least the first 6 months and probably for the first 2 to 3 years of life. Somatic development, including puberty, depends on normal thyroid gland function until growth is completed.

The causes of paediatric primary hypothyroidism are, therefore, best considered in 3 categories: (1) those resulting in maternal and fetal

**Table IV.** Causes of hypothyroidism at different stages of paediatric development

| Maternal and fetal hypothyroidism | Fetal/neonatal hypothyroidism | Late postnatal hypothyroidism |
|---|---|---|
| Severe iodine deficiency (endemic cretinism)<br>Maternal thyroid-stimulating hormone (TSH) receptor blocking autoantibodies | Thyroid agenesis or dysgenesis (sporadic congenital hypothyroidism)<br>Thyroid dyshormonogenesis<br>Antithyroid drug therapy<br>Accidental $^{131}$I thyroid ablation<br>Thyroid hormone resistance<br>Maternal TSH receptor blocking autoantibodies<br>Iodine deficiency | Autoimmune thyroid disease<br>Iodine deficiency |

hypothyroidism; (2) fetal/neonatal hypothyroidism alone; and (3) those resulting in late postnatal hypothyroidism.[150] Major causes according to this classification are listed in table IV. Clinical situations where both maternal and fetal thyroid gland function are disturbed (e.g. severe iodine deficiency) or where the target tissues do not respond to thyroid hormone (e.g. thyroid hormone resistance syndrome) will lead to irreversible neurological damage.

Prevention strategies should be the mainstay of therapy in these situations. Fetal or neonatal hypothyroidism, if adequately treated, will generally lead to normal neurological and somatic development. Hypothyroidism in later childhood and adolescence does not impair neurological functioning and presents mainly as disturbances of growth and or puberty. A schedule of thyroxine replacement dosages for different ages is shown in table V.

#### *5.1.3 Management of Excessive Thyroxine Therapy*

Patients given excessive thyroxine dosages generally develop symptoms of hyperthyroidism, in particular tremor and palpitations. The diagnosis is made by the finding of a suppressed serum TSH concentration and concurrently elevated peripheral thyroid hormone concentrations. If the patient is symptomatic, thyroxine therapy should be stopped until symptoms abate and then restarted at a lower dose. If the patient is asymptomatic, the daily dose should be reduced by 25μg to restore TSH concentrations to normal. Recent evidence has shown that patients with suppressed serum TSH but with normal thyroid hormone concentrations may be at risk of complications of therapy. Longstanding overt or subclinical hyperthyroidism may result in a higher prevalence of atrial arrhythmias and pose an additional risk factor for osteoporosis. The latter has been a source of controversy, but may be a particular problem for postmenopausal female patients.

**Table V.** Thyroxine dosage schedule for hypothyroidism of infancy and childhood[a]

| Age | Dosage (μg/kg/day) | Usual range (μg/day) |
|---|---|---|
| Birth to 6 months | 10 | 25 to 50 |
| 6 to 12 months | 6 to 10 | 50 to 75 |
| 1 to 5 years | 5 to 6 | 75 to 100 |
| 6 to 12 years | 3 to 5 | 75 to 125 |
| >12 years | 2 to 3 | 100 to 150 |

a Dosage is adjusted to keep serum TSH normal. Many clinicians commence at the lower end of the range stated.

Suppressive TSH thyroxine therapy (see section 5.1.2) should only be used to treat patients with differentiated thyroid cancer or goitrous Hashimoto's thyroiditis.

### 5.2 Thyrotoxicosis and Hyperthyroidism

Effective therapy of hyperthyroidism or thyrotoxicosis requires an accurate diagnosis of the underlying cause. Thyrotoxicosis is not a disease in itself, but represents the clinical findings that arise when peripheral tissues receive and respond to an excess of thyroid hormone. Hyperthyroidism occurs in a subset of patients with thyrotoxicosis due to primary or secondary hyperfunction of the thyroid. The pathogenesis in each of these conditions is different (table VI). The most common causes in Western society are Graves' disease, autonomous single nodule (toxic hot nodule) or multiple functioning nodules (toxic multinodular goitre), and subacute thyroiditis. Initial therapy is similar and centres around the use of antithyroid drugs to block the peripheral effects of thyroid hormone excess at the tissue level and/or reducing thyroid hormone overproduction where present. Subsequent definitive therapy (see section 5.2.2), i.e. surgery or radioactive iodine therapy, is dictated by the pathophysiology of the disorder and the likelihood of spontaneous disease remission.

### 5.2.1 Clinical Pharmacology of Drugs Used in Treatment

#### Antithyroid Drugs

The most commonly prescribed antithyroid drugs belong to the thioureylene family of compounds and include thiourea, thiouracil, methylthiouracil, propylthiouracil (PTU), thiamazole (methimazole) and carbimazole. The drugs most commonly used in clinical practice are the *thionamides* propylthiouracil, thiamazole and carbimazole. Carbimazole is rapidly metabolised to the active agent thiamazole and hence behaves in a similar fashion to this agent.[29] The clinical pharmacological properties of these drugs are listed in table VII.

***Mechanism/site of action and pharmacodynamic properties:*** the antithyroid drugs block the production of thyroid hormones by virtue of a shared thiocarbamide group (S=C-N) which acts to inhibit thyroid peroxidase. This leads to inhibition of oxidation of iodide and of iodination of tyrosyl groups of thyroglobulin. There is also inhibition of coupling of iodotyrosines to form the iodothyronines. The thionamides have no effect on the release or secretion of thyroid hormone; hence, clinical effects of these drugs are only apparent when the preformed hormones are depleted and circulating thyroid hormone concentrations are lowered. It has been suggested that these agents may also possess direct immune modulatory effects and recent data suggest that they may also have antiproliferative properties.[151] An added advantage of propylthiouracil is its inhibition of the peripheral deiodination of thyroxine to form the more active hormonal agent, tri-iodothyronine.[29]

***Pharmacokinetic characteristics:*** the thionamide compounds are rapidly absorbed from the gut, with peak plasma concentrations occurring 1 to 2 hours after an oral dose. The absorption and fate of carbimazole and thiamazole (methimazole) can be considered together since carbimazole is rapidly metabolised to the latter compound.[152] All the antithyroid drugs concentrate in the thyroid. Propylthiouracil is strongly protein bound whereas thiamazole is not protein bound. The plasma elimination half-life of thiamazole is 3 to 6 hours, as compared with 1 to 2 hours for propylthiouracil, but the duration of action of these agents is longer than would be predicted from plasma half-lives, being closely related to the intrathyroid concentrations. Prolonged antithyroid activity makes single daily doses possible, particularly with thiamazole.

Both thiamazole and propylthiouracil are extensively metabolised, probably by the liver, and excreted in the urine as the parent drug and metabolites. The elimination half-life may be prolonged in hepatic and renal impairment. Both drugs both cross the placenta and are excreted in breast milk. Because propylthiouracil is more ionised at pH 7.4, it crosses the placenta and enters breast milk less readily than thiamazole.[152]

***Clinical use/effectiveness:*** no fundamental differences exist between the antithyroid drugs in terms of rate of response to therapy, of remission in patients with Graves' hyperthyroidism, or adverse effects. Thus, the choice of therapy may be based on personal preference, predicted patient compliance, and special circumstances such as pregnancy and lactation.[153] Treatment is generally started with 10 to 30 mg/day of thiamazole or carbimazole or with 150 to 300 mg/day of propylthiouracil. In pregnancy and lactation, propylthiouracil is preferred, starting at dosages of 50 to 100 mg/day.

Under normal circumstances, antithyroid agents are given in 3 to 4 divided doses daily at the start of therapy. The dose and frequency should be reduced after 4 to 6 weeks of therapy, depending on clinical and biochemical improvement, and then adjusted at 2- to 3-month intervals to maintain normal thyroid hormone secretion. The usual maintenance dose of thiamazole or carbimazole is 5 to 10 mg/day and of

**Table VI.** Common disorders associated with thyrotoxicosis

| Disorder | Pathogenic mechanism | Natural history |
|---|---|---|
| Graves' disease | Stimulating antibody to thyroid-stimulating hormone receptor | Disease remission in 15 to 75% |
| Toxic multinodular goitre | Multiple foci of functional autonomy | Progressive |
| Toxic hot nodule | Single focus of functional autonomy | Progressive |
| Iodine-induced hyperthyroidism | Loss of iodine autoregulation, usually in the setting of a multinodular gland | May be self-limiting |
| Subacute thyroiditis | Leakage of stored thyroid hormone | Self-limiting |
| Thyrotoxicosis factitia | Hormone ingestion | Self-limiting |

**Table VII.** Clinical pharmacological properties of the antithyroid drugs

| Feature | Propylthiouracil | Thiamazole (methimazole) | Carbimazole |
|---|---|---|---|
| Mechanism of action | Inhibition of thyroid peroxidase | Inhibition of thyroid peroxidase | Inhibition of thyroid peroxidase |
| Other pharmacodynamic effects | Inhibition of peripheral conversion of $T_4$ to $T_3$ | | |
| Time course of drug effect (hours) | 1-2 | 3-6 | 3-6 |
| Clearance (L/h) | 7 | 10 | ...[a] |
| Elimination half-life (hours) | 1.5 | 4 | ...[a] |
| Volume of distribution (L) | ≈28 | ≈42 | ...[a] |
| Protein binding (%) | 70-80 | 0 | ...[a] |
| Principle route of elimination | Hepatic/renal | Hepatic/renal | Hepatic/renal |
| Active metabolites | No | No | Yes (thiamazole) |
| Dosage adjustment in renal failure | Yes[b] | Yes[b] | Yes |
| Dosage adjustment in hepatic failure | Yes | Yes | Yes |
| Route of administration | Oral | Oral | Oral |
| Frequency of administration | 2-3 ×/day | 1-3 ×/day | 1-3 ×/day |
| Therapeutic effectiveness | Excellent/rapid relief of symptoms | Excellent/rapid relief of symptoms | Excellent/rapid relief of symptoms |
| Adverse effects | Rash; hepatotoxicity; vasculitis; lupus-like syndrome; agranulocytosis | Rash; hepatotoxicity; vasculitis; lupus-like syndrome; agranulocytosis | Rash; hepatotoxicity; vasculitis; lupus-like syndrome; agranulocytosis |

a As for thiamazole.

b See appendix D for dosage adjustments in varying degrees of renal failure.

propylthiouracil 50 to 100 mg/day, given in 2 divided doses. If compliance is poor, single daily doses of thiamazole may be used.[154]

***Tolerability:*** serious adverse effects may occur in 1 to 3 of every 1000 patients, irrespective of the antithyroid compound used. Dose-related neutropenia may occur, necessitating a switch to another antithyroid agent. Agranulocytosis is the most serious adverse effect;[29] it is idiosyncratic and occurs most commonly in patients >40 years of age. It usually presents in the first few weeks of therapy, but may occur with a second course of treatment. Patients receiving antithyroid therapy should be alerted to the possibility of this effect and instructed to discontinue the drug and seek medical attention if they develop symptoms such as fever, sore throat and mouth ulceration. Since the adverse effect is idiosyncratic, routine measurement of white cell count is not helpful or predictive. The mild neutropenia that may occur in patients with Graves' hyperthyroidism should not be confused with agranulocytosis. Further courses of antithyroid therapy are contraindicated in patients who have developed agranulocytosis.

Other adverse effects include hepatotoxicity, vasculitis and lupus-like syndrome. Development of a maculopapular or urticarial skin rash is common. Skin rash may develop in up to 5% of patients and is thought to be a hypersensitivity reaction. Spontaneous resolution of the rash may occur despite continuation of therapy. Switching to an alternative thionamide compound may be also useful in these patients, although cross-sensitivity does occur.

#### Adjunctive Therapy

***β-Adrenoceptor blockers (β-blockers):*** these drugs block the peripheral effects of thyroid hormone excess and the peripheral conversion of thyroxine to tri-iodothyronine. Most experience has been with propranolol (40mg every 8 hours), although other β-blockers such as metoprolol, atenolol and nadolol have also been used. Atenolol (50 to 100mg daily) may be useful in patients with poor compliance because of its once-daily administration schedule. Other β-blockers such as sotalol or esmolol may be useful because of their selectivity and shorter half-lives in patients with arrhythmias and these drugs can be used intravenously to control such problems, e.g. as an adjunct to radioiodine therapy in patients not adequately controlled prior to thyroidectomy, and in thyroid crisis. β-Blockers may be given in conjunction with the thionamide drugs as first-line therapy, or on their own in patients with subacute thyroiditis. However, they are contraindicated in patients with asthma or chronic obstructive lung disease, while cardiac failure arising secondary to thyrotoxicosis is a relative contraindication. The dose of β-blockers is usually adjusted according to the clinical response (degree of symptoms, particularly tachycardia). The benefit of adding a β-blocker to a thionamide agent is that it alleviates many of the signs and symptoms of hyperthyroidism but has little effect on the fundamental disease process. This is a useful interim measure while awaiting a response to the effects of the thionamide.

***Iodine:*** this can be given just before surgery to reduce the vascularity of the thyroid, or rarely as adjunctive therapy for a thyroid crisis. The usual dose of Lugol's iodine solution (which contains 50mg iodine/ml) is 0.1 to 0.3ml and that of a saturated solution of potassium iodide is 60mg in a glass of milk or water twice daily. Iodide is of short term benefit only and precludes the use of radioactive iodine therapy in the short term.

***Iodinated radiocontrast agents*** (e.g. sodium ipodate) are useful second-line agents in the management of thyrotoxicosis. They are usually used in patients who are allergic to the thionamide agents. They have the advantage over iodide of inhibiting the conversion of thyroxine to tri-iodothyronine.

***Lithium carbonate:*** in a dose of 600 to 1200 mg/day, lithium carbonate inhibits thyroid hormone release. It is a second-line drug for use in patients allergic to the usual drugs and has the advantage of not blocking radioactive iodine uptake.

#### *5.2.2 Optimum Treatment*

There are 3 forms of primary therapy for hyperthyroidism in common use:

1) Blockade of hormone synthesis and action by antithyroid drugs and β-blockers to reduce symptoms.

2) Ablation of the thyroid by radioactive iodine.

3) Partial or total surgical ablation of the thyroid gland (after control of the disease process with antithyroid drugs).

Selection of the optimum therapy depends upon a multiplicity of considerations; in particular, the underlying pathophysiology needs to be considered. Diffuse hyperplasia due to Graves' disease has the potential for long term remission following treatment with antithyroid therapy, whereas nodular thyroid disease, either multinodular or solitary, has no long term prospects for disease remission with medical therapy alone. Other considerations in terms of moving from medical therapy to definitive therapy are the availability of a competent surgeon, emotional concern/anxiety about the hazards of radioactive iodine therapy, and the patient's compliance with a strict medical regimen. Therapy with antithyroid drugs is used as the initial treatment in all patients with hyperthyroidism prior to a decision being made to undertake definitive therapy with either surgery or radioactive iodine. A treatment plan is presented in figure 2.

#### Antithyroid Therapy

The duration of treatment with antithyroid drugs is dictated by the pathophysiology of the disorder (table VII). Graves' disease is an autoimmune disorder characterised by spontaneous remission and relapse. There are no strong and reliable predictors of long term disease remission and reported rates vary from 10 to 75%. Patients with milder disease, absence of thyroid-stimulating immunoglobulins at the end of therapy, and smaller thyroid glands are more likely to remain in disease remission. The duration of therapy also appears to predict durable remission, with remission improving from 31% in patients treated for 6 months to 82% in those treated for 2 years.[156]

A 'block and replace' (i.e. high-dose thionamides plus thyroxine replacement) technique may be used to counter the problems of fluctuating thyroid hormone concentrations. This technique is also thought to result in a higher rate of sustained remission.[157] In most cases, therapy usually continues for 12 to 24 months, depending on patient compliance, patient preference and adverse effects. All patients require medical antithyroid therapy to render them euthyroid before definitive therapy (see below) with surgery or radioactive iodine may be undertaken. Follow-up in 2 months, 6 months, and 1 year is advised. Most relapses occur within the first 6 months. Long term antithyroid therapy is an option in patients not wishing to proceed to definitive therapy.

In patients with toxic adenoma or toxic multinodular goitre, antithyroid drugs are usually administered until the patient is rendered euthyroid. This usually takes 6 to 8 weeks. Because spontaneous remission is unlikely, the treatment of choice is definitive therapy (see below), preferably with radioiodine. Subacute thyroiditis is usually treated with β-blockers if hyperthyroidism is present. Short term salicy-

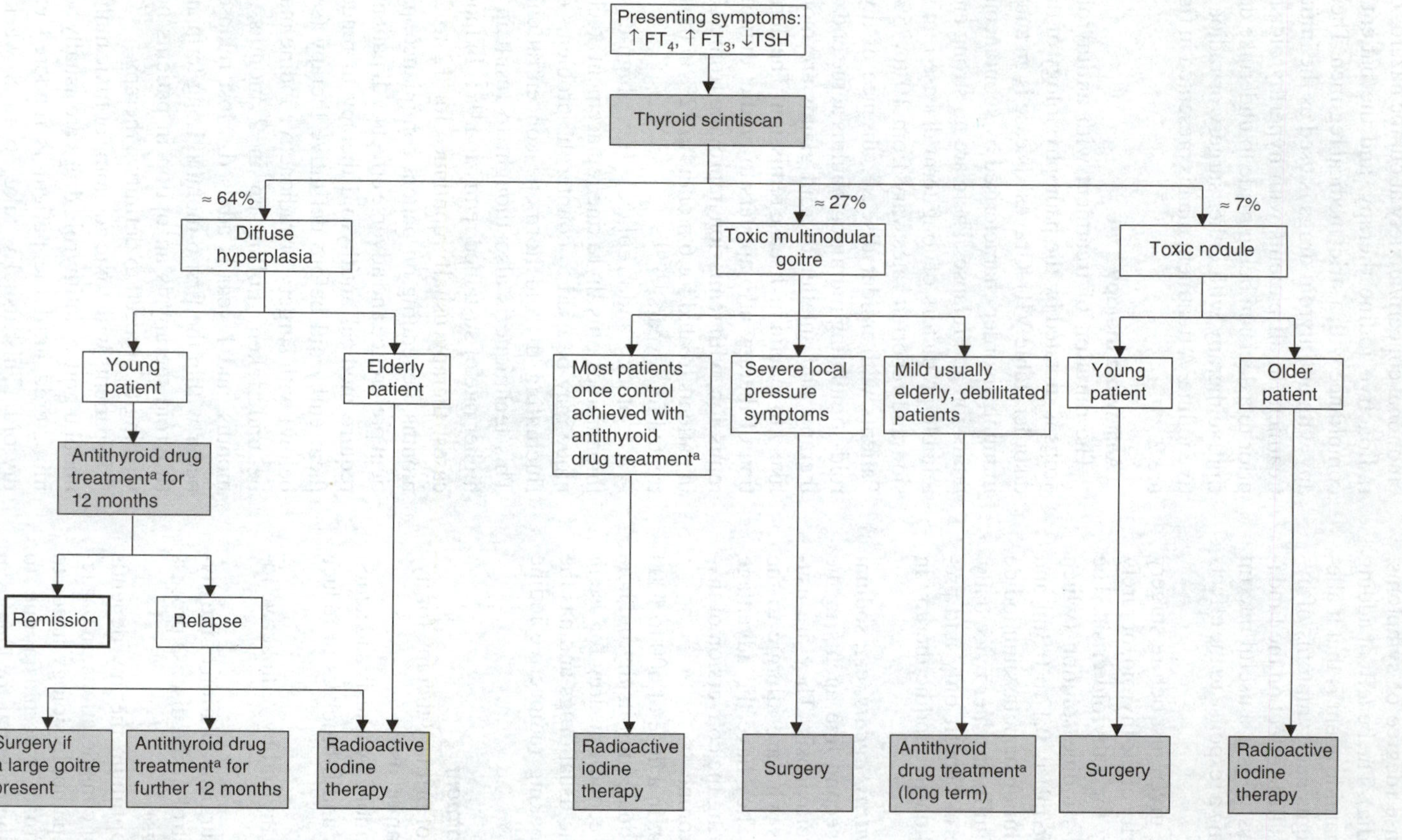


**Fig. 2.** Treatment of thyrotoxicosis (after Brownlie[155]). The patient's general health will influence management and reluctance to undergo radioactive iodine therapy or surgery may change the therapeutic plan. *Abbreviations:* $FT_4$ = free thyroxine; $FT_3$ = free tri-iodothyronine; TSH = thyroid-stimulating hormone.

late or glucocorticoid therapy may be necessary to relieve thyroid pain.

#### Definitive Therapy

The two choices for definitive therapy are surgery (usually subtotal thyroidectomy) or radioactive iodine therapy. There are no hard or fast rules to dictate the choice of therapy and, more often than not, this is governed by the preferences of the patient and the clinician.

***Radioactive iodine:*** this agent provides an effective cure after a single dose of therapy in 70 to 90% of patients. Many centres give a moderate dose of iodine (15 mCi) to ensure adequate ablation of the thyroid gland. At this dose, the patient does not require hospital admission. The patient must understand that they may be rendered permanently hypothyroid and will then require lifelong thyroid hormone replacement. The patient is instructed to cease antithyroid therapy 4 days before the dose of radioactive iodine and restart it 2 days after therapy. Some patients experience transient pain over the thyroid and salivary glands and some experience a dry mouth. A pregnancy test should be performed in women of childbearing age before administering radioactive iodine. Most patients (85%) are rendered hypothyroid 4 to 6 weeks after therapy, although a response may not be seen for 4 to 6 months. Thus, patients are continued on maintenance doses of antithyroid therapy that is slowly withdrawn. Thyroxine is started once hypothyroidism is established.

### *5.2.3 Treatment in Special Circumstances*

#### Iodine-Induced Hyperthyroidism

This is commonly an iatrogenic disorder and follows exposure of patients with multinodular glands to large iodine loads. For unexplained reasons, the normal autoregulatory systems of the thyroid fail and the patient is rendered hyperthyroid. The commonest sources of iodine are radiocontrast agents and amiodarone. Amiodarone may also cause thyrotoxicosis by causing a specific form of focal thyroiditis.[158] Patients with this disorder present with similar features to those with a toxic multinodular gland, except that they are extremely resistant to standard doses of antithyroid therapy. Doses of thiamazole or carbimazole of 20mg 4 times daily or propylthiouracil 200mg 4 times daily may be needed.

Perchlorate 200mg 3 times daily to block iodine uptake has been suggested as being useful. Glucocorticoid therapy (prednisone 20 to 60 mg/day) may be useful in patients with amiodarone-induced thyrotoxicosis.

#### Thyroid Crisis or Storm

Thyrotoxic crises occur very rarely during appropriate management of hyperthyroidism. Patients require medical antithyroid therapy to render them euthyroid before definitive therapy with surgery or radioactive iodine is undertaken. A thyroid crisis is usually seen in patients who have not been appropriately treated, or those with another underlying illness (e.g. myocardial infarction, respiratory illness). Inappropriate treatment refers to situations where a patient has undergone surgery or radioactive iodine therapy without prior medical therapy. Thyroid crisis is a life-threatening condition in which the typical signs and symptoms of Graves' disease are exaggerated. Many patients have vomiting, diarrhoea, dehydration, fever and confusion. They usually have severe tachycardia and heart failure, and coma may also occur.

There is almost always a precipitating factor and treatment is aimed at correcting both the severe thyrotoxicosis and the precipitating, illness and providing general supportive care. Large doses of propylthiouracil (1200mg daily) or either thiamazole or carbimazole (120mg daily) are given by mouth or by nasogastric tube in divided doses. Propylthiouracil is preferred because it can inhibit peripheral conversion of thyroxine to tri-iodothyronine. A β-blocker is usually given in a high dosage either intravenously (e.g. propranolol 2 to 5mg every 4 hours) or orally (propranolol 80mg 4 times daily). Glucocorticoids and iodide (e.g. Lugol's solution or sodium ipodate) are also given. In addition, because of the hypermetabolic state, the patient will require nutritional supplementation and vitamins.

#### Hyperthyroidism in Pregnancy

While hyperthyroidism often results in infertility, the start of antithyroid therapy may result in unplanned pregnancy. Women of childbearing age should be warned of this potential risk. The management of hyperthyroidism in pregnancy is difficult.[159] Fortunately, as in most other autoimmune disorders, the severity of the illness tends to wane as pregnancy progresses. A postpartum flare is, however, likely. Propylthiouracil is the antithyroid agent of choice in pregnancy, as this agent crosses the placenta less readily than either thiamazole or carbimazole. The smallest effective dose of propylthiouracil is used, usually 50 to 100mg daily, and thyroid function should be kept at the upper limit of normal. TSH receptor antibodies, thyroid-stimulating immunoglobulins and other thyroid antibodies are monitored to determine the risk of neonatal thyrotoxicosis, which occurs in about 1 of every 100 pregnancies involving Graves' hyperthyroidism. Fetal heart rate and thyroid size can be monitored in the second and third trimesters of pregnancy. Surgery, if needed, may be undertaken in the second trimester of pregnancy. However, radioactive iodine is absolutely contraindicated.

Propylthiouracil is the drug of choice in lactating mothers as it appears in breast milk in only small amounts and does not appear to affect thyroid function in infants of mothers who are breast feeding.

## 6. Parathyroid Disease

### 6.1 Hyperparathyroidism

Primary hyperparathyroidism may present either on a sporadic basis or be part of an inherited group of disorders, multiple endocrine neoplasia (MEN) types 1, 2A and 2B. It may present asymptomatically on routine biochemical testing or occur with symptoms attributable to hypercalcaemia and hypercalciuria, such as polyuria, polydipsia, confusion and renal colic.[160-163] Hypercalcaemia of hyperparathyroidism must be differentiated from other causes of hypercalcaemia, in particular from humoral hypercalcaemia of malignancy (mediated by parathyroid hormone-like peptide PTHrP), vitamin D toxicity and familial hypocalciuric hypercalcaemia.[164]

The most common cause of primary hyperparathyroidism is a solitary adenoma of the parathyroid glands, with hyperplasia being less common and parathyroid carcinoma most rare of all. Secondary hyperparathyroidism most commonly refers to hyperplasia of the parathyroid glands found in patients with longstanding chronic renal failure and hypocalcaemia. Tertiary hyperparathyroidism denotes the development of hypercalcaemia following secondary hyperparathyroidism and indicates development of an autonomous parathyroid adenoma.

The diagnosis of primary hyperparathyroidism is readily made by the finding of an inappropriate (i.e. normal or elevated) parathyroid hormone (PTH) concentration through the use of an assay directed against the whole PTH molecule, in the presence of elevated serum calcium. The 24-hour urinary calcium concentration is usually elevated in primary hyperparathyroidism. Low urinary calcium usually indicates familial hypocalciuric hypercalcaemia; treatment of this condition is rarely necessary. Many localisation techniques have been used to detect a parathyroid adenoma, but no single technique is adequately sensitive or specific. Operative localisation is more reliable than preoperative imaging.

#### Optimum Treatment

There is currently no medical therapy for primary hyperparathyroidism. Surgery offers the only opportunity for long term cure. However, many patients with mild or moderate hyperparathyroidism who are asymptomatic and lack evidence of end-organ damage (nephrolithiasis, osteopenia) may be observed for prolonged pe-

**Table VIII.** Medical therapy of hypercalcaemia due to primary hyperparathyroidism

| Feature | Phosphates | Calcitonin | Bisphosphonates (e.g. pamidronate) | Plicamycin (mithramycin) |
|---|---|---|---|---|
| Mode of action | Inhibition of 1α,25-dihydroxy-cholecalciferol production, decreasing GI calcium absorption | Inhibits osteoclastic bone resorption activity and suppresses renal tubular reabsorption | Inhibits osteoclastic activity | Inhibits osteoclastic activity by impairing the production of new osteoclasts |
| Administration | PO | SC | IV infusion | IV infusion |
| Dosage | *Sodium acid phosphate:* 2 g/day | *Salmon calcitonin:* 50-200U q12h<br>*Human calcitonin:* 0.5mg q12h | *Pamidronate:* 15-60mg as a single infusion over at least 4h | 15 to 25 µg/kg/day for 3 or 4 days |
| Adverse effects | Diarrhoea, renal calculi, muscle cramps, soft tissue calcification | Flushing, nausea, vomiting | Nausea, rarely hypocalcaemia | Liver damage, renal failure, rarely thrombocytopenia |
| Duration of action | Short | Short | Prolonged | Moderate |
| Acquisition cost | Low | Medium | High | High |

*Abbreviations:* GI = gastrointestinal; IV = intravenous; SC = subcutaneous; PO = oral.

**Table IX.** Dosages and duration of activity of vitamin D preparations

| Preparation | Time until peak activity (weeks) | Duration of action (weeks) | Usual daily dose |
|---|---|---|---|
| Cholecalciferol (vitamin $D_3$) | 4-8 | 4-16 | 400-1000IU |
| Ergocalciferol (vitamin $D_2$) | 4-8 | 4-16 | 50,000IU |
| Calcifediol (25-hydroxycholecalciferol) | 2-4 | 4-12 | 5-200μg |
| Calcitriol (1α,25-dihydroxycholecalciferol) | 0.1 - 0.4 (1-3 days)[a] | 0.1 - 0.4 (1-3 days)[a] | 0.5-1μg |
| Dihydrotachysterol | 1-2 | 1-3 | 0.2-1mg |

a Individual variability exists between peak activity and duration of action.

riods without significant morbidity.[160,161] Some postmenopausal women with mild to moderate disease respond well to estrogen replacement therapy.

Drug therapy is required for patients with *severe hypercalcaemia* before surgery or in those for whom surgery is contraindicated. There are 4 broad classes of agents that may be used: phosphates, calcitonin, bisphosphonates and plicamycin (mithramycin). The mechanisms of action, dosages and adverse effects of these therapies are shown in table VIII. Rehydration and the use of loop diuretics are sometimes required to lower serum calcium rapidly.

### 6.2 Hypoparathyroidism

This disorder most commonly occurs following thyroid surgery and may be either transient or permanent. Other causes include congenital absence of the glands, irradiation, infiltration, hypomagnesaemia and autoimmunity. The most common manifestation is hypocalcaemia which presents clinically as cramping, muscle fasciculation, seizures and cardiac arrhythmias.

#### Optimum Treatment

The principles of therapy include an assessment of the severity and expected reversibility of the disorder, with the aim of normalising the serum ionised calcium concentrations.

When symptoms are severe and acute, intravenous calcium therapy should be used. *Calcium gluconate* 10% (10 to 20ml) is administered over 5 to 10 minutes, and may be repeated until symptoms have abated. If symptoms fail to respond to calcium infusion, then magnesium deficiency should be excluded. When magnesium deficiency is severe, magnesium should be administered by infusion (as magnesium sulfate 5g in 500ml isotonic saline infused over 5 hours). Regular intermittent or continuous calcium infusions may be used after the acute symptoms have been controlled.

Oral administration of calcium is used in chronic hypoparathyroidism or after correction of the acute disorder. Calcium may be administered as the carbonate, glubionate, gluconate, citrate or lactate salts. Carbonate salts are the least expensive, while citrate and gluconate are the most expensive. The most common adverse effects of calcium preparations are gastrointestinal disturbance, bloating, flatulence and constipation; calcium citrate is probably the best tolerated agent. A dose of 1.5 to 4g elemental calcium per day is given in 3 divided doses. However, in most patients with hypoparathyroidism, calcium therapy alone is not sufficient to restore calcium concentrations to normal and a *vitamin D* preparation is also required. Several vitamin D preparations are available (table IX) but the most reliable and least toxic (because of its short half-life) is *calcitriol* (1α,25-dihydroxycholecalciferol).[165]

## 7. Adrenal Disease

The adrenal cortex secretes 3 principal hormone types: aldosterone, cortisol and the adrenal androgens. Aldosterone is a mineralocorticoid, its primary role being sodium and potassium homeostasis via a direct effect on the renal tubule. Sodium is retained and potassium excreted. Cortisol, a glucocorticoid, promotes body fuel availability via its catabolic effects on glucose, fat and protein intermediary metabolism; cortisol is a stress hormone. Adrenal androgens are less potent than testicular androgens, but are a major source of androgens in females.

Endocrine diseases of the adrenal gland are due to either over- or underproduction of one or more hormones, particularly aldosterone and cortisol. All 3 principal hormones are controlled by classical negative feedback loops, with the controlling factors varying in type and degree: hypothalamic-pituitary corticotrophin-releasing hormone/corticotrophin for cortisol and androgens; the renin-angiotensin system for aldosterone; corticotrophin, possibly not alone, for adrenal androgens. Adrenocortical disease can thus be primary, with the hormonal disorder being a direct result of adrenal pathophysiology, or secondary, with the hormonal disorder occurring at the level of external control. Adrenocortical disease may affect single or multiple hormones, e.g. 3 hormone abnormalities in autoimmune hypoadrenalism or congenital adrenal hyperplasia, but a single hormone abnormality in hyporeninaemic hypoaldosteronism or glucocorticoid-producing adrenal adenoma. The potential for cure or control is greater if the defect is primary, e.g. mineralocorticoid excess secondary to tumour or hyperplasia.

The adrenal medulla produces a proportion of body catecholamines; it is under the control of the autonomic nervous system and is physiologically totally separate from the adrenal cortex.

## 7.1 Clinical Pharmacology of Drugs Used in Treatment

### *7.1.1 Glucocorticoids (Glucocorticosteroids)*

Glucocorticoids have widespread application in clinical practice, primarily in conditions not involving a deficiency of glucocorticoid. The dosages of glucocorticoids used for non-physiological replacement therapy regimens are far in excess of physiological production rates. Therefore, a thorough understanding of the multiple actions of these agents is needed if optimal effectiveness is to be obtained with minimal adverse effects.

#### Mechanism/Site of Action

Some glucocorticoid compounds function as a pure glucocorticoid, while others have some mineralocorticoid activity. This is because these activities are mediated by separate but closely related receptors: a high affinity, low capacity type I mineralocorticoid receptor and a low affinity, greater capacity type II glucocorticoid receptor. Drugs may bind to either receptor with varying affinity. The glucocorticoid receptor is present in the cell cytoplasm and translocates to the nucleus after glucocorticoid binding. Translocation without glucocorticoid binding appears to be inhibited by a cytoplasmic complex with a heat shock protein (HSP). In the nucleus, the glucocorticoid receptor binds to DNA at specific hormone receptor elements to start gene transcription.[166] Because of the catabolic actions of glucocorticoids, many of their effects in extrahepatic tissues are to reduce protein (enzyme) synthesis, while in the liver there is stimulation of enzyme synthesis, with hepatocytes displaying significant increases in mRNA, e.g. in gluconeogenesis.

***Effects on carbohydrate metabolism:*** glucocorticoids are associated with insulin resistance, resulting in reduced peripheral glucose uptake that is at least partly a result of impaired glucose transport.[167] There are increases in plasma glucose and insulin concentrations and hepatic gluconeogenesis. The hyperglycaemia resulting from glucocorticoid therapy is, therefore, a result of both underutilisation and overproduction of glucose. Any glucocorticoid effect on glucose metabolism is enhanced by other insulin resistant states, including NIDDM and obesity.

***Effects on lipid metabolism:*** VLDL, HDL, LDL and triglycerides can all be increased with glucocorticoid usage. Lipid abnormalities are due to both increased hepatic synthesis and reduced clearance, the latter primarily as a result of lipoprotein lipase deficiency and LDL receptor defects. Non–insulin-dependent diabetes mellitus (NIDDM), obesity and hypothyroidism amplify this glucocorticoid effect.[168]

***Effects on protein metabolism:*** glucocorticoids induce loss of lean body mass, even if adequate protein intake is provided. There is an increase in plasma amino acids, including gluconeogenic precursors. The mobilisation of protein is indiscriminate and affects skin, tendons, muscle and bone.[169] Glucocorticoids have multiple effects on bone mineral metabolism, including inhibition of intestinal calcium absorption, reduction of renal calcium absorption (resultant secondary hyperparathyroidism) and suppression of osteoblastic function by inhibiting cell replication, as well as the synthesis of collagen and growth factors. The effect is more pronounced for trabecular bone.

***Effects on lean body mass and fat mass:*** the overall effect of glucocorticoids is to alter the proportions of lean and fat masses and the distribution of fat to central and deeper visceral stores. The mechanism for this latter finding is unclear. Both effects are reversible with reduced exposure to glucocorticoid. Abdominal adiposity is associated with hyperinsulinaemia, thought to be secondary to the large metabolically active adipocytes producing increased free fatty acid turnover in the portal circulation.

***Effects on energy expenditure and bodyweight:*** the resting metabolic rate does not appear to alter with glucocorticoid use, if corrected for changes in lean body mass.[170] Glucocorticoids appear to stimulate increased energy intake and there is weight gain with consequent increased daily energy expenditure.

***Gastrointestinal tract effects:*** it is controversial whether glucocorticoids increase the prevalence of peptic ulceration. The proposed mechanisms are reduction in mucosal defence mechanisms and a possible effect on gastric acidity.[171]

***Renal effects:*** glucocorticoids have a significant physiological action on the distribution and excretion of body water. There is a maintenance of intravascular water. Renal water excretion is affected by suppression of antidiuretic hormone, an increased rate of glomerular filtration and direct effects on the renal tubule, the net result being an increase in free water clearance. Glucocorticoids have varying but weak mineralocorticoid function and, when given in sufficiently high doses, act at the renal tubule to promote sodium retention and potassium loss.

***Effects on the hypothalamus and pituitary:*** there is a central suppressive effect on gonadotrophin-releasing hormone (GnRH) and gonadotrophins that produce anovulation and irregular menstrual periods in women and, at high doses, reduce spermatogenesis in men. Inhibition of growth hormone secretion and an even more profound effect on growth factors, including IGF-I production, may have growth retardation effects.

***Effects on cerebral function:*** psychosocial well-being and psychological functioning are enhanced by normal cortisol action. Increased and decreased glucocorticoid concentrations impair cognition and promote mood disturbance, presumably by effects on neurotransmitters.

***Effects on the immune system:*** an increase in endogenous glucocorticoid production is a normal response to physical and nonphysical stress and provides the appropriate metabolic milieu for the body to combat stress. The anti-inflammatory effects of glucocorticoids may play a role in containing the physical response to stress. These effects of glucocorticoids are also the major reason for their pharmacological usage, in which glucocorticoid concentrations that are greatly in excess of levels found in the endogenous response to stress are provided. The anti-inflammatory effects are multifactorial and directed at both microvasculature and cellular components, the latter by both alteration of location and function. The greater the glucocorticoid dose, the greater the effect.

Suppression of the immune response has the unwanted effect of increasing opportunistic or nosocomial infection. Glucocorticoids enhance vascular responsiveness to circulating vasoconstrictor factors and reduce the capillary permeability that characterises acute infection. Glucocorticoids reduce neutrophil migration into tissues, with resultant blood neutrophilia, by altering the production and action of migration inhibiting factor (MIF). Thymus-derived or T lymphocytes, responsible for delayed or cell-mediated immunity, are also reduced, secondary to a hastening of immature lymphocyte death and the inhibition of T cell proliferation/activation by suppression of interleukin-2 production and interleukin-2 dependent signal transduction.

Glucocorticoids alter the macrophage production of cytokines including tumour necrosis factor-$\alpha$ (TNF-$\alpha$) and interleukins-3, -4, -6 and interferon-$\gamma$. There is thus a shift from inflammatory $T_H1$ to helper $T_H2$ responses. Glucocorticoids inhibit IgE-mediated histamine release from basophils and there is a reduction in the number of circulating eosinophils, the cells responsible for acute allergic response mediation. At pharmacological dosages they also suppress antibody production and stabilisation of lysosomal (storage) membranes occurs, limiting proteolytic release of stored antibody. Increased catabolism of immunoglobulins may also modify the immune response by glucocorticoids.[172]

For further discussion on the effects of glucocorticoids on the immune system, see chapter 28, section 2.1.2.

#### Pharmacodynamic Properties

Glucocorticoids are vital to the normal function of the human body. Once given in pharmacological rather than physiological dosage, there is a dose-related increase in effects that may be both desirable (e.g. immune suppression) and undesirable (e.g. bone demineralisation and effects on glucose metabolism). Synthetic glucocorticoids have been designed to have higher glucocorticoid potency, reduced mineralocorticoid effects and longer durations of action.

***Onset of action:*** peak concentrations of oral glucocorticoids are achieved in the blood within 1 to 2 hours of administration. The therapeutic response is apparent within the first 24 to 48 hours, although it may take up to 7 days for a maximal response to be achieved. Several groups have elucidated the concentration-effect relationship of glucocorticoids in recent years. Models of indirect pharmacodynamic responses have been created and are quite different from conventional pharmacodynamic models. In particular, the outcome as a drug effect or indicator is described as a balance between such variables as drug concentration, volume of distribution, and drug dosage.[173] The onset and dissipation of action is also governed at a molecular level by such characteristics as receptor occupancy, binding and recycling, and mRNA/protein synthesis.[174]

***Dose-response relationships:*** glucocorticoids are prescribed in pharmacological doses for a wide variety of medical conditions including autoimmune disease (rheumatoid arthritis, systemic lupus erythematosus, dermatomyositis), allergic conditions, severe asthma, lymphomatous neoplastic conditions, inflammatory eye disease (including optic neuritis), blood dyscrasias, inflammatory bowel disease and the nephrotic syndrome. The glucocorticoids with longer durations of action are preferred because of the need for fewer daily doses. The dose-response relationship is somewhat individual, but in general, the higher the dose, the more likely a therapeutic response is to be achieved. As doses are increased, there should be some objective clinical measure or response that is used as a marker or sign of a positive therapeutic effect (see further below). Assays for glucocorticoids other than the specific radioimmunoassay for cortisol are not routine and do not provide therapeutic guidance.

***Maximal dosages:*** the maximum glucocorticoid dosage to achieve pharmacological rather than replacement concentrations is dictated by a balance between the therapeutic effect and adverse effects to a degree that is not usually seen with other drugs, except perhaps cytotoxic agents. Because of this, prednisone is unlikely to be given at greater than 120 mg/day and the dose is rapidly tapered to the lowest possible clinically effective dose over the shortest possible time (ideally 7 to 10 days). Dexamethasone is unlikely to be used at greater than 20 mg/day. It is safer to use higher doses if the disease process is acute and self-limiting.

***Hypothalamic-pituitary-adrenal axis (HPA) suppression:*** it is possible to use high-dose glucocorticoids for up to 3 weeks without adrenal suppression occurring, but longer usage usually produces adrenal suppression. It is reasonable, particularly in patients treated for months to years, to reduce the dose to replacement concentrations and then test for adrenal responsiveness before ceasing glucocorticoid therapy. HPA suppression is influenced by the potency of the glucocorticoid, its dose, duration of therapy, the time of day the dose is given (suppression is greater if the dose is given in the evening closer to the physiological surge of corticotrophin), if the regimen is daily rather than given on alternate days, and the route of administration (oral doses produce greater HPA suppression than topical, inhaled or intra-articular doses[175]).

***Physiologically normal production:*** 10 to 12mg of cortisol per $m^2$ body surface area is produced by the adrenal cortex in a normal adult each day. Cortisol is secreted in a pulsatile or episodic fashion and its plasma concentrations vary predictably over a 24-hour period, the highest concentrations occurring in the early morning and the lowest at midnight (diurnal circadian rhythm). The normal plasma concentration at 8am is 100 to 250 μg/L (270 to 600 nmol/L) and it reaches a nadir at midnight.[176]

#### Pharmacokinetic Characteristics

***Absorption and bioavailability:*** mean cortisol concentrations are lower after oral cortisone acetate administration than after hydrocortisone; the mean bioavailability of cortisone is about 80% of that of hydrocortisone. There is wide individual variability in bioavailability for these 2 compounds, ranging from 25 to 90%,[177] but there appears to be less difference in bioavailability between prednisolone and prednisone, individual bioavailabilities for which range between 50 and 90%.[178] The bioavailabilities of prednisone and prednisolone are closely correlated intraindividually (due to hepatic interconversion of one compound to the other), which suggests that substituting one for the other may have no clinical advantage. Cortisone and prednisone are converted in the liver to their active metabolites, cortisol and prednisolone, respectively. There have been no consistent effects of antacids, foodstuffs or bile salt binding resins on the absorption of these agents.

***Protein binding:*** under normal conditions, approximately 90% of cortisol is reversibly bound to plasma proteins [10% to albumin and 80% to a high affinity, low capacity $\alpha_2$-globulin, transcortin or corticosteroid-binding globulin (CBG)]; 10% circulates free or unbound. The unbound fraction determines the biological activity of the hormone. At low or normal plasma concentrations, cortisol is largely bound to CBG. With increasing concentrations, the globulin-bound cortisol changes little, but the fraction of unbound and albumin-bound cortisol increases. In addition, glucocorticoids in high dosages decrease CBG concentrations,[42] Synthetic analogues of cortisol bind less avidly to transcortin (approximately 70%) and diffuse more completely into the tissues.[179] In patients with hypoalbuminaemia, e.g. those with liver or renal disease, there is a consequent diminution in storage capacity for glucocorticoids resulting in a higher unbound fraction, although the unbound drug concentration will be unchanged.

***Elimination:*** hydrocortisone disappears rapidly from the circulation through hepatic metabolism and excretion in the urine, mainly as inactive glucuronide metabolites. Synthetic analogues of cortisol are metabolised in the liver more slowly than cortisol, the result being a prolongation of plasma half-life. Prednisolone is metabolised mainly by glucuronidation, although other pathways including hydroxylation also exist. The latter pathway is more likely to be impaired in chronic hepatic disease. Elimination of the metabolites is both renal and hepatic.

11β-Hydroxysteroid dehydrogenase is responsible for the inactivation of prednisolone to prednisone. Tissues with a high enzyme content, such as the kidney, will therefore have lower prednisolone : prednisone concentration ratios which may be a determinant of the local intrarenal immunosuppressive effect of prednisolone at pharmacological doses.[180]

***Half-life and clearance:*** the plasma half-lives of cortisol and cortisone are similar, at approximately 90 minutes. This means that on a twice-daily cortisone dosage schedule, cortisol concentrations decrease to pretreatment values before the next dose. The half-life of prednisone and prednisolone is close to 3.5 hours. Prednisolone clearance increases with increasing concentrations of the drug, due largely to saturable protein binding. In addition, the hepatic interconversion of prednisolone to prednisone is saturable at high doses of prednisolone, and incomplete conversion of methylprednisolone sodium succinate to methylprednisolone is likewise seen with high doses. Prednisolone clearance (both total and unbound) is about 20% higher in female than in male individuals.[181]

The clearance of glucocorticoids may be enhanced in patients with severe acute asthma receiving these drugs. The half-lives of the glucocorticoids are much longer as a result of post-glucocorticoid receptor events.

Typical pharmacokinetic parameters for the commonly used glucocorticoids are given in appendix A.

#### Clinical Use/Effectiveness

For replacement therapy, the shorter acting glucocorticoids, cortisone and hydrocortisone, are preferred, being more physiological in their action and having a reduced risk of excessive dosage. Intravenous hydrocortisone is first-line therapy when high-dose stress treatment is required in hospitalised patients, patients with vomiting (where the oral dose is not retained), or in any other short term situation where oral administration is inconvenient or undesirable.

Suppressive therapy to modify immune responses requires more potent, longer-acting glucocorticoids to produce pharmacological, as opposed to physiological, effects. Generally, this effect can be obtained with prednisone but careful consideration should be given to the use of longer-acting derivatives because of the increased risk and severity of adverse effects. For similar reasons, oral glucocorticoids are preferred to intramuscular corticotrophin to stimulate endogenous glucocorticoid production, because of the difficulty in moderating the dose of the latter, the high frequency of severe Cushingoid features, the intramuscular injection route, and the occurrence of HPA suppression with the injection regimen.

To modify the immune response in chronic, severe disease, consideration should be given to other (nonsteroidal) immune modifiers, such as methotrexate, cyclophosphamide or interferons. Cyclosporin has significant steroid-sparing effects, particularly in transplantation.

Nonsystemic disease should not be treated with systemic glucocorticoids without an adequate trial of an inhaled or topical glucocorticoid where such treatment is possible. If glucocorticoids are successful in pharmacological doses, limitations may be the effects produced by the iatrogenic Cushingoid state: hypertension, diabetes, psychosis, osteoporosis, opportunistic infection, myopathy, skin fragility and superficial ulceration, hirsutism, acne, and peptic ulceration.

Pharmacological glucocorticoid doses are contraindicated in patients with systemic fungal infections, active tuberculosis (except in fulminant, disseminated disease where glucocorticoids form part of the therapeutic regimen), and other uncontrolled infections until adequately treated. Relative contraindications and conditions requiring caution in their usage include ocular herpes simplex (due to the risk of corneal perforation), ulcerative colitis (to avoid perforation and abscess formation), severe osteoporosis, poorly controlled diabetes, major psychosis, disseminated carcinoma (unless used to treat hypercalcaemia), recent major abdominal surgery and peptic ulceration (unless treated with omeprazole or an $H_2$-antagonist). Glucocorticoids inhibit long bone growth and the benefits must be carefully weighed before being used long term in growing children because of the permanent loss of height potential.

Before high-dose glucocorticoid therapy is commenced, outcome indicators should be clearly delineated. Specific indicators such as a decrease in erythrocyte sedimentation rate (ESR), antinuclear antibody (ANA), urinary protein or active phase proteins should be used rather than nonspecific indicators such as increased well-being or reduction in fever. For example, serum creatinine, ESR and C3 and C4 complement components have been used as significant biological markers for the activity of lupus nephritis treated with methylprednisone,[182] and the ESR and serum amyloid A apolipoprotein can be used as indicators of the activity of the inflammatory process in giant cell arteritis and polymyalgia rheumatica.[183] Very high-dose therapy should be rapidly tapered to the lowest possible effective dose once these outcomes have been achieved. The natural history of the disease should be considered, as the most commonly treated diseases are often those of exacerbation and remission and it is important to re-evaluate dose reduction to low maintenance or dose cessation at regular intervals. If there has been no clear improvement in the disease process within 7 to 10 days, consideration should be given as to whether the initial diagnosis was correct, the dose of glucocorticoid was inadequate, the patient is not taking or not absorbing the drugs, or there has been exacerbation of infection or other disease process.

***Alternate-day therapy:*** while this should not be considered for primary adrenal failure, it can be effective in a number of conditions requiring glucocorticoid therapy and should be considered in patients who will need long term high-dose therapy. Alternate-day therapy is effective in allowing relatively normal height growth in children.[184] Other advantages of alternate-day therapy are that the total dose of glucocorticoid over a period of time is lower and suppression of the HPA axis is reduced because of the 48-hour recovery period. Alternate-day therapy is generally used in less severe or less acute disease. Intermediate-acting corticosteroids (e.g. prednisone, prednisolone) are the usual first choice agents. The dose should be given in the morning, after the peak of corticotrophin secretion. Alternate-day therapy should not be started until the disease process has been controlled by daily therapy. The change to alternate-day therapy should be made as soon as possible and, if initial therapy was twice daily, a single daily dosage should be used first. The use of steroid-sparing agents (e.g. NSAIDs or inhaled glucocorticoids such as those inhaled in asthma), should also be considered, particularly on the 'off' day. The severity and prevalence of adverse effects are reduced with such regimens.[185]

***Termination of therapy:*** the longer and higher the dose, the longer the tapering of therapy should be. A number of clinical tests can be performed to provide a more objective assessment of recovery of the HPA. The simplest but least reliable is an early morning plasma cortisol and corticotrophin determination immediately before the next dose. A normal tetracosactide stimulation test will indicate adequate adrenal steroidogenesis, but the HPA axis might still be unable to respond adequately. Corticotrophin therapy will not hasten HPA recovery.

Insulin-induced hypoglycaemia to test the whole HPA is the best test, but even this can provide false positive results. Once glucocorticoid therapy has been withdrawn, the patient must be considered relatively glucocorticoid deficient for the next 6 months and given supplementary glucocorticoids when under stress.

***Dosage modification in associated disease states and old age:*** excessive effects or an inadequate response to glucocorticoid therapy may result from individual differences in the metabolism of these drugs. While this is extremely unlikely in the absence of significant organ disease, some situations may necessitate changes to prescribed doses.[186]

In *liver disease* there is reduced metabolism of glucocorticoids, and a reduction in CBG and albumin, all of which increase systemically available glucocorticoid. Reduced nonrenal clearance may also influence dosage requirements. In practice, however, hepatic failure must be severe before dosage reduction is required. Liver function tests are not able to accurately predict dosage reduction requirements.

In *renal disease* the situation is also complex because of the different factors involved. Renal excretion of prednisolone is not well understood, with the total metabolites measured in urine (and faeces) being significantly lower than the administered dose. In the nephrotic syndrome with lowered albumin, unbound prednisolone is not elevated, unless there is associated hepatic disease. However, renal transplantation may reduce the clearance of prednisolone. Haemodialysis removes negligible amounts of prednisolone.

In *hyperthyroidism,* the nonrenal clearance of glucocorticoids may be enhanced. Conversely, although the evidence is limited, severe *hypothyroid states* are likely to reduce glucocorticoid clearance.

In *elderly patients,* dosage modifications may be needed if their bodyweight is low, due to a lower metabolic clearance and the possibility of increased adverse effects with comorbidity and, drug interactions (see below). The normal loss of bone mineral density with age may be exacerbated and the fracture risk increased.

**Tolerability and Drug Interactions Potential**

The frequency of adverse effects, varying from relatively mild effects such as weight gain, skin fragility and striae, and altered physical appearance, to major ones such as diabetes, psychosis and osteoporosis, is close to 100% in nonphysiological glucocorticoid use. Their severity increases with higher doses, and these adverse effects often limit tolerability of therapy, despite effectiveness in treating the condition, and a dosage compromise may need to be reached. Most adverse effects are reversible, but growth retardation and osteoporosis are not. Interestingly, the newer prednisolone derivative *deflazacort* appears to be associated with a lower risk of osteoporosis than prednisolone or prednisone, and may also have less negative impact on growth rate in children requiring glucocorticoid therapy.[187] However, further long term trials are required to confirm this.

The main drug interactions with glucocorticoids are with hepatic enzyme inducers, including phenobarbital, primidone, phenytoin, carbamazepine and rifampicin. With these drugs, the clearance of the glucocorticoid is increased and dosage requirements may be greater. Estrogen preparations can decrease glucocorticoid clearance via an increase in CBG. The potential for aspirin-induced haemorrhage is increased by glucocorticoids if the patient is hypoprothrombinaemic. Conversely, glucocorticoids may enhance aspirin metabolism.

Due to their effects on glucose metabolism, glucocorticoids may reduce the effectiveness of oral antidiabetic agents and insulin. During disease exacerbation, patients with NIDDM may need to be changed to insulin therapy. Glucocorticoids also antagonise the action of pancuronium and anticholinesterase drugs used in myasthenia gravis.

Prednisone is the drug of choice for necessary pharmacotherapy in pregnancy. A very few cases of transient fetal adrenal suppression have occurred in such circumstances. Some prednisone is excreted in the breast milk but is generally considered insignificant in terms of neonatal HPA suppression.[188]

### *7.1.2 Mineralocorticoids*

The only synthetic mineralocorticoid available for therapeutic use, i.e. *fludrocortisone*, is available only as an oral preparation. This is not a therapeutic limitation, since (if nasogastric administration is contraindicated) adequate salt retention can be achieved by intravenous saline administration in severely ill patients. Mineralocorticoid secretion is predominantly controlled by the renin-angiotensin system which in turn is sensitive to sodium/potassium flux and plasma volume. Corticotrophin plays a lesser role. Mineralocorticoid therapy has fewer applications than glucocorticoid therapy, being confined to replacement therapy and to syndromes of severe postural hypotension.

**Mechanism/Site of Action**

Fludrocortisone is a 9α-fluorinated derivative of hydrocortisone. Its mineralocorticoid effect is 30 times that of its glucocorticoid activity. The hormone receptor mechanisms are similar to those described for glucocorticoids (see section 7.1.1). There are, therefore, 2 potential receptors (type I and type II) in the kidney. The primary site of action is the distal tubule, where sodium and water retention are increased and potassium excretion promoted. A fludrocortisone dose elicits a similar magnitude of antinatriuretic and kaliuretic responses, but hypertension and bodyweight increase require higher dosages.[189]

Renin activity and aldosterone secretion are suppressed by fludrocortisone, whereas at usual therapeutic dose levels, there is no corticotrophin suppression. Fludrocortisone also suppresses sympathetic nervous activity and reactivity.[190] In larger dosages, inhibition of endogenous adrenal glucocorticoids, suppressed immune responses, deposition of hepatic glycogen, and negative nitrogen balance (particularly if protein intake is inadequate) may occur.

**Pharmacodynamic Properties**

The onset of action of fludrocortisone occurs within hours of ingestion. Mineralocorticoids are unusual pharmacotherapeutic agents, in that the dosage is not at all dependent on the size or age (if a child) of the patient. The dose-response relationship is consistent, provided that there is an adequate sodium intake. There is no mineralocorticoid effect in patients who are sodium depleted.[191] The general dosage range is 50 to 200 μg/day for replacement therapy. Lower doses, including alternate-day therapy, have been used when sodium retention is a clinical problem. Higher doses may be used for autonomic dysfunction and postural hypotension.

Limitations to therapy with fludrocortisone include hypokalaemia, hypertension and clinical oedema. Intrinsic patient variability, presumably at the receptor level, may mean that replacement glucocorticoid therapy has a more potent mineralocorticoid effect than expected and the dose of the mineralocorticoid can be reduced.

Assessment of the effectiveness of mineralocorticoid therapy is generally based on clinical signs, blood pressure and any postural change, and the presence of oedema. Plasma renin activity is a guide to dose adequacy, but should not be used as the sole determinant. Serum electrolytes are not a therapeutic guide, but serum potassium should be measured after starting therapy and monitored if there is a tendency towards hypokalaemia. In hot climates and with intense physical activity, the dosage may need to be increased, combined with an adequate salt intake to counteract sweat losses.

Dosage modifications will likely be needed in disease states where sodium and water retention is a feature, including congestive cardiac failure, hypertension, hypokalaemia and particularly with diuretic usage. In elderly patients, dosage modification is more likely, because of the increased prevalence of these conditions and of subclinical renal impairment.

**Pharmacokinetic Characteristics**

The principal route of elimination of fludrocortisone is hepatic, although there is a renal component as well.[192] Its plasma half-life is approximately 200 minutes.

**Tolerability and Drug Interactions Potential**

Patient tolerability of mineralocorticoid therapy is high. The use of diuretics, either potassium-losing or potassium-sparing, should be carefully considered in patients on fludrocortisone because of an increased risk of electrolyte imbalance. Consideration should be given to modifying the fludrocortisone dose instead. Spironolactone must not be used with fludrocortisone as it is a direct antagonist.

Lithium may inhibit the action of fludrocortisone in the distal renal tubule.

### *7.1.3 Other Drugs Used in Adrenal Disease*

These agents are discussed in other sections and are considered here in their specific adrenal context. Their principal adrenal uses are in Cushing's syndrome, either to improve the physical status of the patient before definitive therapy or if other therapies are contraindicated, and in adrenal carcinoma.

**Mitotane**

Mitotane is an isomer of *p,p′*DDD, an insecticide. Cortisol synthesis is blocked by inhibition of 11β-hydroxylation, and cholesterol side-chain cleavage by interference with cytochrome P450. Mitotane is highly lipid soluble, accumulates in fat and continues to act several weeks after discontinuation of therapy. It is the only adrenolytic antiadrenal agent.

The dosage and duration of therapy with mitotane depend on the condition treated, but adverse effects generally become intolerable above 10 g/day.[193] Patients develop primary hypoadrenalism on this drug and full glucocorticoid replacement therapy should be started when mitotane treatment is begun, with an appropriate increase for any stresses. Ataxia, decreased attention span, lethargy, skin rashes, fevers, nausea and diarrhoea are common adverse effects. There is often an increase in serum cholesterol due to the reduced production of oxysterols (downregulators of HMG CoA reductase) by the hepatic cytochrome P450.[194]

**Aminoglutethimide**

Aminoglutethimide inhibits the conversion of cholesterol to pregnenolone, as well as inhibiting several other steps of steroid synthesis including the C11, C21 and C18 hydroxylases and hydroxylations in the aromatisation of androgens to estrogens.[138] Cortisol, aldosterone and estrogen synthesis are reduced by inhibition of cytochrome P450 complexes and this inhibition is reversible within a few days. Aminoglutethimide is rapidly and almost completely absorbed after an oral dose and at least 50% is excreted unchanged in the urine. Its half-life is approximately 12 hours, but this decreases with duration of therapy, suggesting that aminoglutethimide accelerates its own clearance. Approximately 20% is bound to plasma proteins.

Hypoadrenalism may occur with aminoglutethimide and replacement therapy with a glucocorticoid (not dexamethasone, the metabolism of which is accelerated by aminoglutethimide) and fludrocortisone is required. Patients with impaired renal function require a reduction in the aminoglutethimide dose. The drug is contraindicated in patients with inducible porphyria.

As well as its effect in enhancing dexamethasone metabolism, aminoglutethimide reduces the effectiveness of oral antidiabetic agents and coumarin anticoagulants. Lethargy, dizziness, skin rashes, nausea and vomiting are common adverse effects and bone marrow suppression has been reported. Abnormal liver function tests may also occur and compensated primary hypothyroidism may result from inhibition of thyroxine synthesis in the early stages of treatment.[195]

#### Ketoconazole

Ketoconazole is a synthetic imidazole derivative, primarily used as an antifungal agent. It also inhibits adrenal and gonadal cytochrome P450 pathways, particularly androgen synthesis. Peak plasma concentrations are achieved 1.5 hours after oral administration and there is a biphasic disposition pattern. There is extensive postabsorption metabolism of ketoconazole and the major route of excretion is via the faeces. In plasma, at least 85% is protein bound.

Ketoconazole may be used as a means of temporary management in Cushing's syndrome. Primary adrenal failure may occur if doses larger than those used for antifungal therapy are used. Common adverse effects are gastrointestinal disturbances and skin rash. Necrotic hepatocellular dysfunction has been reported and is mostly seen in prolonged use, older women and associated liver disease. Dosages of cyclosporin, coumarin anticoagulants, methylprednisolone and busulfan need to be reduced if administered with ketoconazole due to its inhibitory effect on the cytochrome P450 isonenzyme CYP3A4[196] (see also chapter 6 and appendix B).

#### Metyrapone

This antiadrenal agent was formerly used as a diagnostic agent. It acts on the cytochrome P450 enzyme responsible for 11β-hydroxylation, the final step in cortisol production. Its onset of action is within hours and multiple daily doses are required. Metyrapone is likely to be effective in Cushingoid states where there is no overproduction of pituitary corticotrophin. Overproduction of adrenal androgens limits its usefulness in long term treatment in women.[197]

#### Spironolactone

Spironolactone is a specific antagonist of aldosterone.[198] It acts via competitive binding at the mineralocorticoid (aldosterone) receptors in the distal tubule of the nephron. Spironolactone has a weaker heat shock protein-receptor interaction and rapidly disassociates from the receptor. While its major use is as a diuretic, spironolactone has a potential role in the therapy of primary hyperaldosteronism. Its other endocrine effect is inhibition of ovarian androgen synthesis and inhibition of androgen activity at the receptor level.

The bioavailability of spironolactone exceeds 70% after an oral dose and plasma concentrations peak at 3 hours. Both spironolactone and its major metabolite canrenone are 90% plasma protein bound. Metabolites of spironolactone are excreted primarily in urine, but also in bile.

Spironolactone is contraindicated in impaired renal function and hyperkalaemic states. It decreases the elimination of digoxin by reducing its renal clearance.[199] Gynaecomastia, diarrhoea, headache, menstrual irregularity and skin rashes are potential adverse effects. The maintenance dosage of spironolactone for primary hyperaldosteronism is between 100 and 400 mg/day in divided doses. The therapeutic response can be judged by the blood pressure response and resolution of hypokalaemia.

## 7.2 Optimum Treatment

### *7.2.1 Adrenal Insufficiency*

Primary adrenal insufficiency is due to destruction of the adrenal glands as a result of autoimmune disease, tuberculosis or fungal infections, haemorrhage or iatrogenic causes. Secondary insufficiency is due to inadequate corticotrophin stimulation as a result of a pituitary and/or hypothalamic lesions. The conditions are generally chronic with lifelong dependency on corticosteroid replacement.

#### Glucocorticoid Therapy

The general therapeutic principle in using glucocorticoids is to imitate normal diurnal cortisol rhythm, with the highest concentrations in the early morning and the lowest in the evening (within the limits of oral medication). To do this, short-acting glucocorticoids such as cortisone or hydrocortisone are preferred so that there is a peak and nadir of steroid activity over 24 hours. Prednisone is sometimes used but has the disadvantages of potential over-replacement because of its longer half-life and minimal mineralocorticoid activity.

The usual adult daily replacement dose is 20 to 30mg hydrocortisone or 25 to 37.5mg cortisone acetate. For children, 9.5 to 15.5 mg/m$^2$ hydrocortisone (cortisol) has been used, the mean dose being 12.5 mg/m$^2$/day; however, recent studies suggest that this may be an overestimate.[200] The dose is generally divided as two-thirds in the morning and one-third late afternoon or early evening. A third dose, equivalent to one-quarter of the total, may be required if the person is under stress or very physically active. Individual variation in clearance also plays a role in the dosage required. Assessment of the adequacy of replacement is generally made on clinical, rather than biochemical grounds. The patient should lose all symptoms related to adrenal insufficiency.

There are several other important management principles in using glucocorticoids:

1) The patient should wear a bracelet to identify steroid dependency and the contact number for emergency care.

2) In periods of physical (strenuous exercise, trauma, surgery, infection) or psychological stress, there is an absolute requirement for an increase in the glucocorticoid dosage to mimic the normal increased cortisol response to stress (the normal capacity is >5-fold output). Febrile illnesses, infective symptoms for longer than 1 day, boils or significant skin infections and any medical condition more serious than a simple upper respiratory tract infection will require a temporary increase in the glucocorticoid dosage (sick day schedule). A basic guide is 3 times the usual dosage in 3 divided doses to be continued until symptoms start to resolve. The dosage can then be tapered rapidly over 3 days to the usual maintenance level. All patients should have a parenteral dose of glucocorticoid and syringe at home to administer if they have a vomiting illness. Persistent vomiting will require hospitalisation for parenteral therapy.

3) Glucocorticoids are generally taken with food. Their exact relation to peptic ulceration, especially at physiological dosages, is unclear. If there is persistent upper abdominal discomfort, a trial of $H_2$-antagonist therapy is indicated, after appropriate investigation.

4) Exacerbation of glucose intolerance by physiological glucocorticoid doses is unlikely, but in patients with a family history of NIDDM, an increased glucocorticoid dosage for any reason may induce elevated blood glucose concentrations.

5) Vigilance should be maintained for overmedication as a cause of the appearance of Cushingoid features.

An exception to standard glucocorticoid replacement is post-craniopharyngioma removal in children. Much less glucocorticoid is required, no more than hydrocortisone 10 mg/m$^2$, otherwise growth will be severely inhibited.

### Mineralocorticoid Therapy

Mineralocorticoid replacement therapy varies from fludrocortisone 0.05 to 0.2 mg/day. Very young children may be relatively mineralocorticoid-resistant and require higher doses than older children or adolescents.[201] If the total dose exceeds 0.1mg this should be divided and given twice daily. In general, twice-daily dosage is advantageous in hotter climates and with strenuous bouts of exercise. Twice-daily dosage also reduces problems with nausea and fluid retention. With febrile illness and excessive sweating, mineralocorticoid doses may need to be increased, although generally the obligatory increase in glucocorticoid confers adequate increase in mineralocorticoid activity. The adequacy of replacement is based on postural blood pressure changes, weight fluctuation and assessment of hydration. Serum sodium and potassium, and plasma renin activity may clarify situations of over- or under-replacement.

In secondary adrenal insufficiency, because aldosterone is predominantly under the control of the renin-aldosterone system, mineralocorticoid replacement is rarely required. However, the same guidelines as for increasing glucocorticoid dosages with stress apply, and replacement doses are similar to those in primary adrenal failure. Because of persisting mineralocorticoid secretion, life-threatening crises with steroid withdrawal are unlikely.

### Chronic *vs* Acute Adrenal Insufficiency

Acute adrenal insufficiency, a life-threatening situation, may be due to:

- First presentation of primary adrenal failure, usually with intercurrent infection

- Cessation of therapy, particularly in primary adrenal failure
- Failure to increase glucocorticoid with stress
- Acute destruction of the adrenal glands with haemorrhage associated with septicaemia or anticoagulant therapy.

The treatment principles are as follows:

1) Do not wait for confirmatory laboratory evidence; treatment will have no lasting ill effects if there was an incorrect diagnosis, but withholding treatment may be fatal.

2) Commence an intravenous solution of 0.9% (normal) saline. As the patient will be absolutely salt- and water-depleted, 4 to 6L in 24 hours will be required. Do not stop intravenous saline until oral intake is adequate. Dextrose may be required in addition if hypoglycaemia is present initially.

3) Give 100mg hydrocortisone intravenously immediately and every 6 hours thereafter for the first 24 hours, reducing the dose as the patient improves. Avoid intramuscular injection as absorption may be variable.

4) Do not stop parenteral glucocorticoid therapy until the patient is eating and drinking normally.

5) Taper the glucocorticoid dose to high replacement levels over about 10 days.

6) Add oral mineralocorticoid therapy (fludrocortisone) when the glucocorticoid (hydrocortisone) dose is between 75 and 50 mg/day.

7) Treat intercurrent infections aggressively.

8) Ensure that there is a conclusive diagnosis of adrenal insufficiency and that these details are given to the patient. This procedure allows future clinicians to be reminded of the diagnosis, so that steroid replacement is not ceased.

For patients with adrenal insufficiency who are to undergo major surgery, special precautions are required (for short day-stay procedures, adopt the sick day schedule). Parenteral hydrocortisone 400mg in divided doses should be given in the first 24 hours, intravenously while an access line is inserted. The sicker the patient is, the longer the high dose should be maintained.

### *7.2.2 Congenital Adrenal Hyperplasia*

While there are 6 possible inherited enzyme deficiencies producing congenital adrenal hyperplasia, this condition is classified under hypoadrenalism because there is failure of both cortisol and aldosterone production in the most common type, 21-hydroxylase deficiency. The low plasma cortisol stimulates pituitary corticotrophin production which is ineffective in increasing cortisol production because of the enzymatic block. However, the high corticotrophin level stimulates excess adrenal androgen production as this biosynthetic pathway is unaffected. The clinical presentation is variable, from female genital virilisation at birth or life-threatening neonatal hyponatraemia, through to precocious pubertal changes in the male and precocious adrenarche in the female. If inadequately treated, the excess androgen causes premature epiphyseal closure and short stature.

Glucocorticoids are given to suppress corticotrophin. This is generally as a twice-daily dosage, but sometimes thrice-daily cortisone is needed to provide adequate control in growing children. Prednisone, with its longer duration of action, may be used if suppression is inadequate with cortisone and is particularly effective as a night-time dose to suppress the early morning corticotrophin surge. Dexamethasone can be used nocturnally and sometimes as a once-daily dosage, but the risk of Cushingoid adverse effects is high and it is not recommended as first-line therapy. Mineralocorticoid therapy is added in patients with aldosterone deficiency and has the additional effect of improving adrenal suppression without the need to increase glucocorticoid dosage. Glucocorticoid dosages vary from 10 to 40mg of hydrocortisone depending on size, and on the severity of enzyme deficiency. Mineralocorticoid replacement varies between fludrocortisone 0.05 to 0.2 mg/day. Glucocorticoids must be increased with physical stress.

Appropriate replacement is indicated by normal growth rate and bone maturation (in children), together with suppressed 17-hydroxyprogesterone and testosterone concentrations (in children and adult females) and plasma renin activity.[202]

### *7.2.3 Isolated Adrenal Mineralocorticoid Underproduction*

Most cases are secondary to renin underproduction (hyporeninaemic hypoaldosteronism). The patient is generally an adult with diabetes complicated by renal impairment. The usual presentation is with dizziness, postural hypotension and hyperkalaemia and this must be differentiated from autonomic neuropathy. Renin and aldosterone concentrations fail to rise in the face of salt restriction, and hyperkalaemia may be exacerbated.

Fludrocortisone may be used to restore electrolyte balance and diminish symptoms, but patients may be relatively resistant to treatment and need up to 0.4 mg/day. This dose may produce hypertension and a risk of renal damage, for which a potassium-losing diuretic such as furosemide (frusemide) and a reduction in fludrocortisone dosage may be considered. ACE inhibitors should not be used in this situation because of their ability to exacerbate hyperkalaemia[203] (see also section 10.2.4).

#### 7.2.4 Adrenal Hyperfunction

Primary adrenal hyperfunction is the result of autonomous adrenal steroid overproduction and may be due to adenoma, carcinoma or bilateral hyperplasia in the absence of corticotrophin excess. Secondary adrenal hyperfunction results from excess corticotrophin production. The latter may be pituitary in origin (Cushing's disease) or produced by certain malignancies, including small cell carcinoma of the lung. Such ectopic corticotrophin syndromes are the most common form of adrenal hyperfunction and are ideally treated by complete tumour removal. If this fails, glucocorticoid blockers may be used (e.g. ketoconazole, metyrapone or aminoglutethimide). The most common cause of Cushing's syndrome is iatrogenic, accompanying pharmacological-dose glucocorticoid therapy, but this is not true adrenal hyperfunction.

##### Glucocorticoid (and Androgen) Overproduction

***Adrenal adenoma:*** the usual method of treatment is surgical removal. The HPA axis will be profoundly suppressed and replacement glucocorticoid therapy may be required for over 12 months until central adrenal control resumes. Adrenal enzyme blockade (see above) may rarely be used to improve the physical status of a severely Cushingoid patient before surgery.

***Adrenal carcinoma:*** these tumours have multiple hormone excesses and the tumour tissue often has steroidogenic enzyme blocks. The tumours are aggressive and progress rapidly. This means that the patient often does not have time to develop the classic features of Cushing's syndrome, and virilisation in the female, hypertension, local mass and pain are the predominant symptoms. Surgical removal or at the very least, debulking, is initial therapy. The tumours are insensitive to radiotherapy and standard solid tumour chemotherapy. Mitotane 8 to 10 g/day in divided doses is palliative rather than curative in most cases and may also be effective against metastases.

##### Bilateral Adrenal Hyperplasia

***Pituitary dependent – Cushing's disease:*** therapy in this condition is directed at the pituitary with trans-sphenoidal removal of a microadenoma. A second operation may be necessary. Radiotherapy is second-line treatment and has the disadvantage of taking months to have an effect. Adrenal blocking agents may be used as a temporary measure in this situation while waiting for radiotherapy to be effective and to improve physical symptoms before surgery. Aminoglutethimide 1 to 4 g/day is given in divided doses. Ketoconazole 200 to 1200 mg/day has also been used.[204]

***Ectopic corticotrophin syndrome:*** if therapy directed at the primary tumour is ineffective, adrenal blocking agents may be used. Aminoglutethimide, ketoconazole and metyrapone have all been used. However, the onset of mitotane is considered too delayed for use under these conditions. *Octreotide,* a somatostatin analogue, has been stated to be effective in reducing ectopic corticotrophin production.

***Autonomous bilateral adrenal hyperplasia:*** the treatment of choice for this non–corticotrophin–dependent condition is bilateral adrenalectomy and lifelong replacement therapy, as for Addison's disease.

### 7.3 Clinical Outcome and Economic Considerations

#### 7.3.1 Adrenal Insufficiency

The medications used to treat this condition are relatively inexpensive. Quality of life is excellent in primary adrenal insufficiency provided that adequate replacement is used and the patient is familiar with self-management of sick-day regimens. The association of additional autoimmune diseases such as IDDM, primary hypothyroidism, pernicious anaemia and premature ovarian failure may make therapy schedules complex and arduous. Secondary adrenal insufficiency is more likely to be associated with multiple pituitary deficiency and the underlying cause often dictates the quality of life achieved.

#### 7.3.2 Adrenal Hyperfunction

Hypercortisolism, if not successfully managed, has major morbidity and mortality from hypertensive disease, infection and suicide. Cushing's disease, while uncommon, is the condition most likely to require multiple and repeated therapy, but not generally prolonged and expensive pharmacotherapy. Adrenal blockers (see section 7.1.3) are costly, cause significant adverse effects and should only be employed as a temporary measure before definitive therapy is undertaken or when there are no other treatment options.

## 8. Testicular Disease

Sexual function and fertility are among the most deeply valued human needs. Disorders of male reproduction have particularly great impact on the well-being of otherwise healthy men during the peak productive epoch of their lives. In addition, consideration of the impact of disease and treatment on male sexual function and fertility is a paramount consideration in the general medical care of men. Knowledgeable and skilful medical management can achieve a satisfactory outcome for virtually all disorders of male reproduction, although, as many treatments remain empirical and suboptimally effective, improvements are still needed.

### 8.1 Testicular Physiology

The testis is the endocrine organ most accessible to clinical examination. It has 2 interdependent but distinct functions: steroidogenesis by interstitial Leydig cells culminating in secretion of testosterone, the body's major anabolic hormone; and spermatogenesis occurring in the seminiferous tubules producing viable male gametes, the spermatozoa. Disturbances can result in androgen deficiency (including sexual dysfunction) and/or male infertility. The term 'hypogonadism' is ambiguous and more specific functional terms are preferable.

#### *8.1.1 Testosterone Production and Action*

The principal goal of androgen replacement therapy (ART) is to replace the physiological effects of endogenous testosterone through replication of its circulating concentrations with exogenous testosterone. Consequently, understanding of the normal physiology of testosterone, the principal androgen in men, is an essential basis for androgen pharmacology.

After puberty, testosterone is secreted almost exclusively from the testis at a production rate of 3 to 10 mg/day. It has active metabolites, with 4% converted to dihydrotestosterone and 0.2% aromatised to estradiol, but most is rapidly inactivated by hepatic oxidation and conjugation before urinary and biliary excretion. Dihydrotestosterone is a more potent androgen formed by enzymatic 5$\alpha$-reduction of testosterone within the prostate and, to a lesser extent, in other tissues (e.g. liver, skin). Although dihydrotestosterone circulates at about 10% of testosterone concentrations, its major effects are through local formation. Aromatisation occurs in liver, muscle, brain and fat to permit androgen action via the estrogen receptor. The extent to which testosterone metabolites are critical to androgen action in various tissues remains unclear. The avid hepatic inactivation of unmodified testosterone leads to both low oral bioavailability and a short duration of action when injected parenterally. These features dictate the need to develop parenteral depot testosterone formulations or oral synthetic androgens to achieve practical, sustained androgenic effects.

In the blood, testosterone circulates at concentrations above its aqueous solubility by binding to circulating plasma proteins. Most (60 to 70%) is avidly bound to sex hormone binding globulin (SHBG) while the remainder is bound to lower-affinity, high-capacity binding sites (albumin, $\alpha_1$-acid glycoprotein, transcortin) and 2% remains unbound. SHBG is an hepatic protein, the concentrations of which are increased by estrogens, thyroxine, chronic liver disease (cirrhosis, hepatitis) and androgen deficiency, and decreased by obesity, supraphysiological (especially oral) doses of glucocorticoids or androgens, protein-losing states and genetic SHBG deficiency.[205] The readily diffusible unbound fraction of testosterone is the most biologically active, with the loosely protein-bound fraction constituting a large and accessible buffer for the unbound fraction.

The metabolic clearance of testosterone is governed mainly by circulating SHBG concentrations as well as hepatic function and blood flow.[206,207] Theoretically, drugs influencing hepatic mixed-function oxidase activity or SHBG binding could alter metabolism of testosterone, but such interactions have not been described. Blood testosterone concentrations have circhoral (hourly) and diurnal rhythms of small magnitude without clear physiological importance. After middle age, circulating testosterone concentrations decline gradually as gonadotrophin and SHBG concentrations increase.[208] These trends are accelerated by any coexisting chronic illness.[209]

Androgen deficiency of sufficiently severe degree will lead to subnormal blood testosterone concentrations. If the primary lesion is in the testis, blood luteinising hormone (LH) concentrations will increase reflexly in rough proportion to the degree of androgen deficit, reaching castrate levels eventually. Less severe, but clinically significant androgen deficiency can be accompanied by a state of compensated Leydig cell failure characterised by low-normal testosterone concentrations with persistently elevated LH concentrations. If the primary lesion is in the hypothalamus and/or pituitary, there may be little or no increase in LH.

#### 8.1.2 Spermatogenesis and Fertility

Sperm are produced within the seminiferous tubules of the testis that constitute >90% of testicular volume. Spermatogenesis is tightly governed by Sertoli cells that form the scaffolding and the distinctive interior fluid milieu of the seminiferous tubules. They also regulate proliferation and differentiation of the germinal epithelium that is sequestered within the diffusion-tight blood testis barrier. Hormonal control, including initiation and maintenance, of spermatogenesis is exerted via Sertoli cells which express key hormone receptors [for follicle-stimulating hormone (FSH) and androgen] whereas the germinal cells do not. During early puberty, the progressive increase in pituitary FSH and LH and testicular testosterone secretion leads to the initiation of spermatogenesis. Spermarche, the time sperm first appear, occurs at about the age of 14 as judged by the first appearance of sperm in morning urine samples.

The full cycle of spermatogenesis takes 75 days and consequently any hormonal treatments aiming to influence sperm output must be evaluated over sufficiently long periods, usually at least 3 months, to allow evaluation of effects on the early stages of spermatogenesis. After puberty, spermatogenesis persists into late life, but is sensitive to many noxious environmental influences. Sperm output fluctuates markedly within and between healthy individuals. Severe direct damage to spermatogenesis by any means leads to a reciprocal rise in circulating FSH concentrations in azoospermic men with small testes. Although the physiological mechanism of this reciprocal relationship remains controversial, blood FSH concentrations represent a useful clinical guide to spermatogenesis.

Practical management of disorders of spermatogenesis is best achieved by distinguishing the more readily treatable pretesticular (gonadotrophin deficiency) and post-testicular (vas, epididymal or ejaculatory ductal obstruction) lesions from the more frequent but rarely treatable testicular level lesions.

### 8.2 Clinical Pharmacology of Drugs Used in Treatment

#### 8.2.1 Androgens

Androgens and antiandrogens are defined pharmacologically by their binding to and activation or blockade, respectively, of the androgen receptor. The androgen receptor is a nuclear protein of 919 amino acids specified by a single X chromosome gene, a member of the steroid receptor gene superfamily.[210] Androgen binding to the C-terminal hormone-binding domain of the receptor causes receptor activation, leading to DNA binding. Androgen action is exerted by the androgen receptor acting as a ligand-activated DNA transcriptional factor.

Testosterone is the model androgen. A number of testosterone derivatives have been developed to enhance its intrinsic androgenic potency, prolong the duration of action and/or improve oral bioavailability.

##### Injectable Testosterone Esters

The most widely used testosterone formulation is *mixed testosterone esters* (resulting from esterification of testosterone with fatty acids of various chain lengths and composition) which are injected intramuscularly in a vegetable oil (sesame, castor or arachis) vehicle. This depot formulation relies on retarded release of the testosterone esters from the oil vehicle injection depot by hydrophobic partitioning. Following release, the esters undergo rapid hydrolysis by ubiquitous esterases to liberate free testosterone into the circulation. The pharmacokinetics of testosterone esters are, therefore, primarily determined by ester side-chain length and hydrophobicity. These dictate the rate-limiting ester release via physicochemical partitioning of the testosterone ester between the hydrophobic oil vehicle and the aqueous extracellular fluid.

*Testosterone propionate*, a short aliphatic side-chain ester, has a short duration of action requiring injections of 25 to 50mg at 1- to 2-day intervals for androgen replacement. In contrast, *testosterone enanthate* has a medium duration of action so that it is routinely administered at doses of 200 to 250mg every 10 to 14 days for androgen replacement therapy.[211,212] Other testosterone esters (cypionate, cyclohexanecarboxylate) alone or in mixtures have virtually identical pharmacokinetics to the enanthate[213] and are used at comparable doses and frequency, but none approaches desirable zero-order release kinetics.

Intramuscular injections often cause local pain or bruising. Accidental injection of vegetable oil vehicle into the dermis is highly irritating, causing pain, inflammation or even dermal necrosis, whereas vascular oil microembolisation can cause transient coughing or fainting.[214] Allergy to the oil vehicle is exceptionally rare and even patients allergic to peanuts may tolerate arachis oil without incident.

An important recent advance is the development of *testosterone buciclate*, a novel insoluble testosterone ester in an aqueous suspension, the first truly long-acting testosterone ester formulation. Release of testosterone from the buciclate ester is rate-limited by steric hindrance to ester side-chain hydrolysis, providing steady testosterone release for up to 4 months after an intramuscular injection of 1000mg in hypogonadal men.[215]

### Other Testosterone Formulations

Unmodified testosterone is used in a variety of formulations. Fused cylindrical pellets of crystalline testosterone provide stable, physiological testosterone concentrations for 4 to 6 months after a single implantation of 3 to 6 pellets of 200mg each.[216] However, despite near ideal depot properties, this testosterone dosage form is not widely used. The minor surgery of the implantation procedure and its infrequent but operator-dependent complications (extrusion 5%, bleeding <1%) are limitations.[217]

Testosterone-impregnated adhesive transdermal patches can maintain physiological testosterone concentrations when worn continuously (>22 hours/day) and applied daily to a clean, dry, shaved and adequately sized scrotum. The highly vascular, thin scrotal skin still requires relatively large transdermal patches (40 and 60 $cm^2$ containing 10 and 15mg testosterone) to allow sufficient testosterone delivery (4 or 6 mg/day), and blood dihydrotestosterone concentrations are disproportionately increased by 5α-reduction of testosterone during trans-scrotal passage.[218] Apart from minor skin irritation, scrotal patches are well tolerated and effective except in men with scrotal malformation or those who use them irregularly.

Alternative nonscrotal patches applied to less steroid-permeable truncal skin require potentially irritating absorption enhancers.[219] Compared with the scrotal patches, the nonscrotal patches deliver similar testosterone profiles without increasing blood dihydrotestosterone concentrations. In Europe, dermal 2.5% hydroalcoholic gels containing either testosterone[220] or dihydrotestosterone[221] are applied on the trunk at a once-daily dose of 5g gel (125mg of the steroid) without occlusive dressing and this rapidly evaporates without residue. Equivalent dermal preparations can be simply made by mixing steroid powder into a standard cream base. Transdermal gels provide effective androgen replacement, but are absorbed variably making administration inaccurate. They may also unintentionally transfer androgen to the female partner by skin contact.[222]

The implants and transdermal preparations have in common the stability of testosterone concentrations, and are preferred by many patients who dislike the wide swings in symptoms caused by testosterone ester injections.

### Oral Agents

Oral *testosterone undecanoate,* an oleic acid suspension of the ester, is administered in dosages of 160 to 240mg per day in 3 to 4 divided doses. The hydrophobic, long aliphatic chain ester in an oil vehicle favours preferential absorption into chylomicrons entering the gastrointestinal lymphatics and partially bypassing hepatic first-pass metabolism during portal absorption. Testosterone undecanoate has low and erratic oral bioavailability, a short duration of action and causes gastrointestinal intolerance, making it a second choice testosterone formulation[212] unless parenteral therapy is undesirable or intolerable (e.g. bleeding disorders or anticoagulation, adolescents with delayed puberty).

The recent reintroduction of *sublingual testosterone* in a novel cyclodextrin formulation increases blood testosterone for such short times (<2 hours) that multiple daily doses are needed to maintain physiological testosterone concentrations, making it unlikely to be useful for long term androgen replacement.[223] *Micronised testosterone* has low oral bioavailability requiring high daily doses (200 to 400mg) to maintain physiological concentrations. Such heavy androgen loading causes prominent hepatic enzyme induction and is, therefore, little used.

Most other oral androgens are 17α-alkylated derivatives [e.g. *methyltestosterone, fluoxymesterone, oxymetholone, oxandrolone, ethylestrenol, stanozolol, metandienone* (methandrostenolone), *norethandrolone, danazol*] and have class-specific hepatotoxicity that renders them unsuitable for routine androgen replacement therapy (ART) in men with full life expectancy. The 1-methyl androgen, *mesterolone,* functionally an oral dihydrotestosterone analogue, is free of hepatotoxicity, but is rarely used for ART due to uncertain effectiveness and the need for multiple daily doses.

#### 8.2.2 Anabolic Steroids

The term 'anabolic steroid' is a vestigial misnomer from the failed search in the 1950s for an androgen derivative with myotrophic but not virilising properties. The recent identification of a single gene and protein for the androgen receptor explains the inability to separate these 2 intrinsic aspects of androgen action. This also explains the physiological observation that all androgens, at equivalent doses, have essentially identical biological effects apart from variability in time-course between tissues.[224] Consequently, the term 'anabolic steroid' is functionally synonymous with the term 'androgen'. The false distinction of the 2 names merely perpetuates semantic confusion in pharmacology and, as scientifically obsolete terminology, should be abandoned.

#### 8.2.3 Androgen Antagonists

##### Antiandrogens

Antiandrogens consist of steroidal and nonsteroidal drugs that are androgen antagonists acting by competitive binding to and blockade of the androgen receptor. *Cimetidine* and *spironolactone* are weak antiandrogens, useful only in women with low blood testosterone concentrations not maintained by specific closed-loop reflex mechanisms as in men.

*Cyproterone,* a progestagen and androgen receptor antagonist, has greater antiandrogenic potency in eugonadal men due its dual action of progestagen-related inhibition of gonadotrophin secretion in conjunction with its competitive blockade of the androgen receptor.[225] Used at doses of 100 mg/day, it has few consistent serious adverse effects apart from hepatotoxicity related to its 17$\alpha$-substitution. Other mostly outmoded antiandrogenic steroids such as medroxyprogesterone and megestrol are predominantly progestagens with glucocorticoid adverse effects. They inhibit androgen action mainly by gonadotrophin suppression rather than via androgen receptor antagonism.

The nonsteroidal pure antiandrogens, including *flutamide*[226] *nilutamide*[227] and *bicalutamide*, are androgen receptor antagonists without agonist activity. However, they cause reflex gonadotrophin increases due to their inhibition of negative hypothalamic feedback of endogenous testosterone. Flutamide (active metabolite hydroxyflutamide) is used at a dose of 250mg 3 times daily. Nilutamide (150 to 300 mg/day) and bicalutamide (50 to 150 mg/day) are given once daily due to their long plasma half-lives. Their major adverse effects include gastrointestinal intolerance, hepatotoxicity, tender gynaecomastia, flushing, and decreased libido and potency. In addition, nilutamide causes delayed light-dark visual adaption, alcohol intolerance and interstitial pneumonitis. When used alone in men with an intact HPG axis, pure antiandrogens are only partially effective in blocking androgens, due to reflex increases in gonadotrophins and testosterone secretion.[225] Their use is more logical pharmacologically and effective clinically when the closed negative feedback loop is abrogated (e.g. postorchidectomy or with GnRH analogues).

##### 5$\alpha$-Reductase Inhibitors

Avid local formation of dihydrotestosterone from testosterone by the enzyme 5$\alpha$-reductase, which is largely restricted to the prostate, has allowed the development of azasteroid 5$\alpha$-reductase inhibitors. These prevent amplification of testosterone action on urogenital sinus derivatives like the prostate without inhibiting systemic androgenic effects.[228] The novel class of 4-azasteroid 5$\alpha$-reductase inhibitors, exemplified by *finasteride,* bind competitively and inhibit type II (prostate) 5$\alpha$-reductase without significant binding to the androgen receptor or SHBG.

Finasteride is maximally effective and well tolerated at the standard oral dose of 5mg once daily. It is well absorbed orally and is extensively metabolised, with a half-life of 6 to 8 hours. It causes few significant adverse effects in long term treatment of benign prostatic hyperplasia, at present its only widely registered indication. For a review of the pharmacological properties of finasteride, see Peters and Sorkin.[229]

Finasteride has little deleterious effect on sexual function. No more than 5% of men taking finasteride (*vs* 2% of those on placebo) report decreased libido and sexual function.[228] It is moderately effective in reducing prostate size and symptoms, but is not recommended either in patients with very large prostates or to relieve prostatic urinary retention (see also chapter 24; sect. 8).

Wider application of finasteride and its congeners may include treatment and/or prevention of prostate cancer and treatment of benign androgen-dependent disorders such as acne, hirsutism and male-pattern alopecia. Topical dermal application may also be possible, but therapeutic applications in women of reproductive age are overshadowed by the risk of interference with fetal masculinisation.

#### Gonadotrophin-Releasing Hormone (GnRH) Agonists

GnRH agonists are administered to produce medical castration by paradoxical inhibition of pituitary gonadotrophin and, thereby, of testicular testosterone secretion. They act initially to overstimulate and then to desensitise pituitary GnRH receptors and gonadotrophin secretion. During the first 1 to 2 weeks of treatment, testosterone concentrations may actually increase before testosterone is inhibited to castration levels. This transient overstimulation creates the rare but serious 'flare' phenomenon, whereby bony metastases may grow to worsen bone pain or spinal cord compression. The risk of flare is reduced by concurrent use of nonsteroidal antiandrogens such as flutamide, nilutamide or bicalutamide and would be eliminated by the new generation of pure GnRH antagonists, such as cetrorelix (currently in development).

This reversible, medical castration is increasingly used to treat androgen-dependent disorders including precocious puberty, prostate diseases and possibly in the future, androgen-dependent alopecia and acne. The highly specific site of action of short peptide analogues confers freedom from serious adverse effects apart from androgen deficiency (flushing, mood and behavioural changes), which are expected effects.

The available GnRH agonists include *buserelin*,[230] *goserelin*,[231] *histrelin*,[232] *leuprorelin*,[233] *nafarelin*,[234] and *triptorelin*. They differ only in the artificial amino acid substituted into the GnRH decapeptide molecule that protects against proteolytic degradation, increasing the plasma half-life and/or enhancing GnRH receptor affinity. All are available as daily injections, or monthly depot injections or implants (table X). Buserelin and nafarelin are also available as nasal sprays used 2 or 3 times daily. Although they differ in intrinsic molar potency, at equally effective doses as marketed, they have essentially indistinguishable pharmacological features, including effectiveness and safety. The clinical pharmacology of the GnRH agonists is discussed further in section 9.1.2.

### 8.2.4 Gonadotrophins and GnRH (Gonadorelin)

In men, the only established medical indication for gonadotrophin therapy is treatment of gonadotrophin-deficient (hypogonadotrophic) patients to induce spermatogenesis and fertility. A less clear indication is the induction of testicular maturation and spermatogenesis in gonadotrophin-deficient adolescents not seeking immediate fertility. In some gonadotrophin-deficient men who have not undergone puberty, inducing testicular growth is psychologically reassuring and their sperm can be cryopreserved for future use. Subsequent induction of spermatogenesis is also generally faster and treatment, therefore, is more cost-effective. When fertility is required in gonadotrophin-deficient men, spermatogenesis can usually be initiated by treatment with gonadotrophins,[235] or if the pituitary gonadotropes are intact, with pulsatile GnRH (gonadorelin).[206]

#### Gonadotrophins

Gonadotrophin therapy is usually started with *human chorionic gonadotrophin* (hCG) treatment alone for up to 6 months. Chorionic gonadotrophin purified from the urine of pregnant women is used as a natural long-acting analogue of luteinising hormone (LH), having an identical α-subunit and a highly homologous β subunit. However, the chorionic gonadotrophin β-subunit has a C-terminal 32–amino acid extension that confers greatly prolonged circulating residence time on the chorionic gonadotrophin molecule. Consequently, the circulating half-life of chorionic gonadotrophin greatly exceeds that of LH, allowing a 2- to 3-day dosage interval for chorionic gonadotrophin. Recombinant hCG is likely to supplant urine-derived hCG in the near future.

***Clinical use:*** the chorionic gonadotrophin dose is 1500IU 2 or 3 times weekly by self-administered subcutaneous or intramuscular injections, with the former route being more convenient. Monitoring of therapy is by measuring trough testosterone concentrations, which should be in the eugonadal range immediately before the next injection, in conjunction with clinical evaluation of androgen replacement on sexual and other function. If both are not adequate then the dosage interval can be adjusted to alternate daily and subsequently the dose may be increased to a maximum of 3000IU per injection.

**Table X.** Currently available GnRH (gonadorelin) agonists and their properties and principal indications/uses

| Drug | Amino acid substitutions in GnRH molecule | | Pharmacokinetic parameters[a] | | | Principal indications/uses | Formulations | Frequency of administration |
|---|---|---|---|---|---|---|---|---|
| | position 6 | position 10 | CL (L/h) | Vd (L) | $t_{1/2}$ (h) | | | |
| Buserelin | D-*t*-Butyl-serine | Ethylamide | | | 1.3 | Prostate cancer<br>Endometriosis[b]<br>Controlled ovarian hyperstimulation[c] | Nasal spray, 0.15 mg/dose<br>Injection (SC), 1 mg/ml | 3 x daily<br>1-3 × daily |
| Goserelin | D-*t*-Butyl-serine | Azaglycine | 8 | 13.7 | 4-5 | Prostate cancer<br>Advanced breast cancer<br>Endometriosis[b]<br>Uterine fibroids | Depot implant (for SC injection), 3.6mg | q4wk |
| Histrelin | D-bzl-Histidine | Ethylamide | | | | Central precocious puberty | Injection (SC) | od |
| Leuprorelin (leuprolide) | D-Leucine | Ethylamide | 9.1 | 27.4-37.1 | 3.6 | Prostate cancer<br>Central precocious puberty<br>Endometriosis[b]<br>Uterine fibroids | Injection (SC), 5 mg/ml<br>Depot injection (lyophilised microspheres for IM or SC injection), 3.75mg and 7.5mg | od<br>q4wk |
| Nafarelin | D-Naphthylala-nine | | | | 2-3 | Central precocious puberty<br>Endometriosis[b]<br>Ovulation induction[c] | Nasal spray, 0.2 mg/dose | 2 × daily |
| Triptorelin | D-Tryptophan | | | | | Prostate cancer<br>Endometriosis[b]<br>Uterine fibroids | Depot injection (biodegradable polymer for IM injection), 3.75mg | q4wk |

a No data available for some agents.
b See further chapter 18 (sect. 11.3.2) for use in endometriosis.
c In combination with gonadotrophins in *in vitro* fertilisation techniques.

*Abbreviations:* od = once daily; q4wk = every 4 weeks; IM = intramuscular; SC = subcutaneous; CL = clearance; Vd = volume of distribution; $t_{1/2}$ = half-life.

Resistance to chorionic gonadotrophin at these doses for periods of months is usually only observed in men with additional severe testicular defects, notably cryptorchidism and small pretreatment testis size (<4ml), who have a poor prognosis for induction of spermatogenesis and fertility. Very rarely, neutralising antibodies to chorionic gonadotrophin may cause secondary failure to maintain testosterone secretion during treatment. Chorionic gonadotrophin therapy is generally well tolerated, produces relatively stable testosterone concentrations and usually produces fewer androgenic adverse effects (acne, weight gain, gynaecomastia) than testosterone ester treatment, but it is more expensive.

Adequate spermatogenesis is induced by chorionic gonadotrophin treatment alone only in men with partial and/or postpubertal onset of gonadotrophin deficiency. Most gonadotrophin-deficient infertile men require the addition of *follicle-stimulating hormone* (FSH). FSH treatment is usually started after an adequate trial, usually 6 months, of chorionic gonadotrophin treatment alone. Where the prognosis for induction of spermatogenesis is poor (small testes, cryptorchidism, poor testosterone response to chorionic gonadotrophin), treatment with FSH may be commenced earlier. FSH is either purified from urine of postmenopausal women (uFSH, menotrophins) or recombinant (rhFSH). Pituitary FSH (pFSH) is no longer used due to the rare but catastrophic risk of Creutzfeldt-Jakob disease.

The traditional pharmacopoeial requirements to standardise the LH content of menotrophins (urinary gonadotrophins with FSH activity) means that commercial grade of clinical menotrophins containing 75IU of uFSH also contains 75IU of uLH, the latter being clinically negligible. The FSH dosage generally starts with 75IU 3 times weekly and doses can be combined in the same syringe with chorionic gonadotrophin doses that, for practical reasons, are harmonised in frequency. Monitoring is by monthly semen analysis and blood testosterone measurement. If sperm are not present after 3 months, the FSH dose can be increased at 3-month intervals to 150IU 3 times weekly and then to daily dosage. Female fertility should be evaluated and any readily treatable defects (anovulation, tubal obstruction) either ruled out or corrected before starting gonadotrophin treatment.

The outcome for induction of spermatogenesis and fertility by gonadotrophin treatment is usually excellent but slow, with the average treatment course exceeding 12 months. Despite prolonged treatment, normal testis size and sperm output are rarely achieved and fertilisation often occurs at low sperm output after sufficient cycles. Major prognostic factors include negative features (cryptorchidism, small pretreatment testis size [<4ml]) indicative of severe gonadotrophin deficiency or testicular dysgenesis, and positive features such as postpubertal onset of gonadotrophin deficiency and prior successful gonadotrophin treatment. The time to fertilisation is usually less with subsequent treatments than with the first treatment. In case gonadotrophin therapy fails, the couple's attitude to donor insemination and adoption should be evaluated empathetically and appropriate advice provided regarding likely outcomes and waiting times for such alternatives to infertility treatment.

**GnRH (Gonadorelin)**

Pulsatile GnRH therapy is appropriate in gonadotrophin-deficient men who have normal pituitary function, such as men with idiopathic hypogonadotrophic hypogonadism with (Kallman's syndrome) or without anosmia. It is unsuitable for most men with pituitary tumours or haemochromatosis. In the rare situation where pituitary responsiveness is unclear, a limited GnRH priming study involving a 1-week trial of the pump with determination of LH, FSH and testosterone responses can verify or exclude the possibility of nonresponsive pituitary gonadotrophs.

***Clinical use:*** pulsatile GnRH therapy is administered by a small portable pump worn on the hip under clothing. It gives regular boluses of GnRH solution through a cannula placed subcutaneously under the abdominal skin. Although intravenous delivery of GnRH produces more physiological LH responses and is more effective at ovulation induction in women with hypothalamic amenorrhoea, the much longer duration of treatment required for gonadotrophin deficient men and the consequent higher risks of bacteraemia with use of the intravenous route means that such treatment is usually not practical. The dosage of GnRH required varies from 2.5 to 20 mg/pulse administered subcutaneously at a frequency of 1 pulse every 60 to 120 minutes.

The response to pulsatile GnRH therapy is monitored as for gonadotrophin therapy by measuring blood testosterone concentrations and regular, usually monthly, semen analysis to determine the need for dose increases. Mechanical problems of pump malfunction and cannula problems need regular surveillance, but otherwise the adverse effects, prognostic factors and outcomes (sperm output, fertility) of pulsatile GnRH are similar to those for gonadotrophin therapy. Neutralising antibodies to GnRH that interfere with its effectiveness are rare. Although pulsatile GnRH therapy is more physiological, with possibly faster and greater testis growth, it is much more complex and, outside investigational centres, this demanding protocol is suitable only for highly motivated men or after failure of conventional gonadotrophin therapy.

For reviews on the clinical use of gonadotrophins and GnRH, see Kleisch et al.,[236] Burris et al.,[237] Delemarre-van der Waal[238] and Finkel et al.[239]

#### *8.2.5 Vasodilators Used in Erectile Failure*

The development in the last decade of treatment for erectile dysfunction by self-administered intracavernosal injections of vasodilators has been a significant therapeutic advance in the management of sexual dysfunction. The vasodilators used in these regimens include *papaverine, phentolamine* and *alprostadil* (prostaglandin $E_1$, $PGE_1$), either alone or in various combinations. The earliest regimens used papaverine alone and later with phentolamine (which reduces the papaverine dose requirement), but recently alprostadil has become first-line therapy. It is equally or more effective and is associated with a lower risk of priapism or long term fibrosis. Priapism with these drugs is dose-related, but vasodilator sensitivity is highly variable between men, although relatively consistent within any patient. Consequently, all men starting treatment require individual dose-titration under supervision of an experienced urologist to determine the optimal dosage to produce an adequate erection lasting less than 60 minutes.[240,241]

The optimal alprostadil dosage ranges from 5 to 40μg among men with idiopathic (mostly vascular) impotence, but is significantly lower among men with neurogenic and psychogenic erectile failure. In the former group, alprostadil doses start at 5 to 10μg, escalating in 5μg increments. In the latter group, doses start at 1 to 2μg, escalating at 1 to 2μg increments until an adequate erection is achieved. With papaverine, doses range from 20 to 80mg as monotherapy and 5 to 30mg when combined with phentolamine 0.5 to 1mg.

The complications of intracavernosal therapy are mostly local pain, bruising or haematoma, priapism or cavernosal fibrosis. Systemic complications such as hypotension are rare unless large doses (>40mg papaverine) are used. The most serious problem is prolonged erections, occurring in 5 to 10% of men during supervised dose titration, but much less frequently (<1%) during self-administration. Priapism is treated urgently by blood aspiration and/or intracavernosal injection of an α-adrenoceptor agonist (e.g. phenylephrine) if the erection lasts 6 hours to avoid permanent damage to corpora cavernosae. Intracavernosal injection of an α-adrenoceptor agonist requires continuous blood pressure monitoring as it may cause severe systemic hypertension.

Pain due to a variety of factors including needle trauma, acidic solutions and unknown factors is more common following injection of alprostadil than papaverine/phentolamine. Bruising, needle site haematoma or, rarely, uretheral bleeding can occur following cavernosal injection and systemic anticoagulation or a bleeding disorder is a relative contraindication to this therapy. Long term use of papaverine/phentolamine may cause cavernosal fibrosis, producing nodules, plaques or shaft deviation, but fibrosis is uncommon with alprostadil. Continuation rates on intracavernosal self-injection programmes, however, drop to 50% within 6 to 24 months of starting the treatment for various reasons unrelated to technical success at inducing erections.

## 8.3 Optimum Treatment

### 8.3.1 Androgen Replacement Therapy (ART)

ART is required to rectify androgen deficiency of any cause that has been sufficient to produce clinical consequences in psychosexual function or anabolic effects on bone, muscle, blood-forming marrow and other androgen-responsive tissues.[242] The clinical features of androgen deficiency depend on the severity, chronicity and epoch of life at presentation. They include ambiguous genitalia, microphallus, delayed puberty, sexual dysfunction, infertility, osteoporosis, anaemia, flushing, excessive fatigueability or incidental biochemical diagnosis.[243]

Since the underlying disorders are mostly irreversible, life-long ART after the age of puberty is required. ART can rectify all clinical features of androgen deficiency apart from inducing spermatogenesis, which requires gonadotrophin replacement in gonadotrophin-deficient men. Once fertility is no longer required, ART usually reverts to the simpler and less expensive use of testosterone, while preserving the subsequent ability to reinitiate spermatogenesis by gonadotrophin replacement. Preliminary studies suggest that androgen supplementation in aging men with partial androgen deficiency may ameliorate age-related deterioration in bone and muscle function.[244] However, larger and longer studies and better definition of target populations are required to clarify the effectiveness and safety of long term androgen supplementation in aging before it can be generally recommended.[245]

*Testosterone* and its esters should be used in preference to synthetic androgens by virtue of safety and effectiveness, ease of dose titration and assay monitoring. The hepatotoxicity of synthetic 17α-alkylated androgens[246] makes them unsafe for long term androgen administration. The practical goal of ART is to maintain stable, physiological testosterone concentrations for prolonged periods. Treatment usually commences with testosterone ester injections and may be switched to alternative formulations (see section 8.2.1) depending on clinician experience and patient preference. Factors to consider include cost, convenience, availability and familiarity with alternatives, and tolerability of frequent injections. Crossover studies have indicated that the stable testosterone concentrations and smoother clinical effects provided by implants[212] or transdermal formulations[218] are preferred to the wide fluctuations in testosterone concentrations and androgen effects seen with intramuscular testosterone ester injections.[211-213,247] Long-acting depot testosterone preparations with zero-order release patterns are likely to supplant injectable testosterone esters as the mainstays of ART if convenient and affordable products become available.

### Monitoring of Therapy

Monitoring of ART involves serial clinical observation of changes in presenting features of androgen deficiency, together with hormonal assays taken at suitable times in relation to doses. Androgen deficient patients may report subjective improvements in energy, mood, well-being, psychosocial drive, initiative and assertiveness as well as in sexual activity (especially libido and ejaculation frequency), increased sexual hair and muscular strength and endurance. Tissue thresholds for androgen action vary, with that for restoration of sexual function being the lowest, making adequate sexual function a necessary but not sufficient condition for clinically adequate androgen replacement.

Hormonal monitoring has a limited role in routine monitoring of ART, particularly during initiation of treatment and in evaluating adequacy of replacement. Trough circulating LH, FSH and testosterone concentrations immediately before the next dose can be a valuable guide to adequacy of androgen replacement. In men with hypergonadotrophic hypogonadism, suppression of blood LH concentrations into the eugonadal range indicates adequate ART, whereas persistent nonsuppression of LH and FSH after 3 to 6 months of treatment indicates inadequate testosterone dosage. However, in hypogonadotrophic hypogonadism, impaired hypothalamo-pituitary function renders blood gonadotrophin concentrations uninterpretable in regard to androgen effects.

In men with systemic disorders, drug intake, or other conditions that alter circulating SHBG concentrations, total testosterone concentrations can be altered, leading occasionally to diagnostic confusion. In this setting, measuring free testosterone concentrations can help clarify androgen status. Where direct measurement of free testosterone is not available, a free testosterone index calculated as the ratio of total testosterone to SHBG concentrations provides an approximation of free testosterone levels, but unfortunately this index is less reliable clinically when SHBG changes are extreme and when it is most needed.

Although testosterone is indeed the active ingredient in the undecanoate ester, the day-to-day inconsistency of its oral bioavailability, the dependence of plasma testosterone concentrations after the last dose on the sampling time, and the erratic pharmacokinetics make plasma testosterone concentrations useless in the monitoring of androgen replacement therapy with testosterone undecanoate. Other indices of androgen action (e.g. haemoglobin, SHBG, HDL-cholesterol concentrations)[242] are too insensitive and mostly reflect only excessive androgen effects, and so have no use in practical monitoring of ART.

### Adverse Effects

The long term effects of ART on cardiovascular and prostate diseases have been inadequately described. Low blood testosterone concentrations are part of the constellation of interrelated epidemiological risk factors for atherosclerotic cardiovascular disease.[248,249] However, the cardiovascular risks of frank androgen deficiency and ART have not been defined and do not seem consistent with classical epidemiological interpretation of hyperlipidaemia in androgen deficiency.[250] Hence, the cardiovascular effects of pharmacological androgen therapy remain unclear.

Although chronic androgen deficiency is protective against prostatic disease, hypogonadal men receiving androgen replacement require surveillance for prostatic disease (as do eugonadal men of comparable age). Evaluation of symptoms, digital rectal examination of the prostate (or preferably transrectal prostatic ultrasonography) and prostate-specific antigen (PSA) measurements should be performed regularly in men >50 years of age and annually among those >60 years. Monitoring lipids and blood pressure should be comparable with eugonadal men of similar age. Serial evaluation of bone density (especially vertebral trabecular bone) by quantitative computed tomography or photon absorptiometry at biannual intervals may verify the adequacy of androgen effects.

Serious adverse effects from testosterone treatment are uncommon, apart from its use in inappropriate settings (e.g. women, children) or the hepatotoxicity of the 17α-alkylated androgens. Previously untreated older hypogonadal men and/or their wives may find unfamiliar libidinal effects of androgens disturbing; more gradual introduction with half the usual testosterone dose may be useful. Seborrhoea and acne in a predominantly truncal distribution (in contrast to facial acne of adolescents) is common during testosterone ester injections, but is readily managed with topical measures and, rarely, intermittent broad-spectrum antibiotics (see further chapter 17; sect. 4.1). Weight gain reflecting anabolic effects on muscle and/or fluid retention is also common. Increased truncal hair and temporal hair loss or balding may also occur. Gynaecomastia may be seen during use of aromatisable androgens such as testosterone. Androgenic adverse effects are rapidly reversible on cessation of treatment, apart from vocal and terminal body hair changes that are irreversible.

***Hepatotoxicity,*** involving biochemical liver damage or hepatic tumour formation, is a well recognised adverse effect of the 17α-alkylated androgens (see further section 8.2.1), but not of other synthetic androgens or testosterone.[246] In fact, it precludes the continued clinical use of 17α-alkylated derivatives in men with a normal life expectancy as safer and equally effective alternatives are available. Biochemical hepatotoxicity with either a cholestatic or hepatitic pattern usually abates with cessation of the steroids. Androgen-related hepatic tumours include peliosis hepatis (blood-filled cysts), adenoma or carcinoma. Unlike safer androgens, regular biochemical monitoring of liver function is necessary if 17α-alkylated androgens are used. Structural lesions should be identified by radionuclide scanning, ultrasound or abdominal computed tomography scan before hepatic biopsy because severe, even fatal, bleeding can occur during hepatic biopsy of peliosis hepatis.

#### Contraindications and Precautions

Prostate or breast cancer are absolute contraindications to androgen therapy because the tumours may be androgen-responsive. Precautions and/or careful monitoring of androgen use is required in:

1) Older men starting androgen treatment who may not tolerate unfamiliar increases in libido or precipitation of urinary obstruction.

2) Competitive athletes who may be subject to disqualification.

3) Patients with bleeding disorders or receiving anticoagulant therapy when parenteral administration may cause severe bruising or bleeding.

4) Sex steroid-sensitive epilepsy or migraine.

5) Patients with cardiac or renal failure or severe hypertension susceptible to fluid overload from sodium and fluid retention.

6) Men with obstructive sleep apnoea that may be exacerbated by exogenous androgens.[145]

Excessive androgen doses before completion of puberty may risk premature epiphyseal closure leading to foreshortened final adult stature and/or precocious sexual development, and are thus to be avoided.

### 8.3.2 Delayed Puberty

Delayed puberty may be due to either constitutional delay (wherein spontaneous puberty will eventually occur and androgen therapy is needed only temporarily) or permanent hypogonadotrophic hypogonadism (where life-long androgen therapy is needed to induce puberty and maintain androgenisation). The distinction between these 2 situations remains difficult and the indication to commence androgen therapy is based on delay in virilisation, its psychological impact and chronological age.

Adolescent boys without evidence of testicular growth as an indication of entering puberty by the chronological age of 14 years, or earlier if developmental immaturity is causing psychological distress, warrant androgen administration. This is given in 6- to 12-month periods with intervening 3-month breaks to determine the progress of underlying endogenous pubertal mechanisms. *Testosterone enanthate* 50 to 100 mg/month intramuscularly or oral *testosterone undecanoate* 40 to 80 mg/day is usually started and gradually increased to full adult doses at a rate dependent on desired speed of maturation with monitoring of physical and psychic androgen effects.

The use of hepatotoxic oral 17α-alkylated androgens (e.g. oxandrolone) in healthy children is difficult to justify given the availability of safer oral or parenteral testosterone preparations.

### 8.3.3 Pharmacological Androgen Therapy

Pharmacological androgen therapy can be used in anaemia due to marrow or renal failure, osteoporosis, estrogen-receptor positive breast cancer, hereditary angio-oedema (C1 esterase inhibitor deficiency), excessively tall stature in boys, and muscular diseases. However, these applications represent second-line empirical therapy that will be rendered obsolete eventually by more specific treatments for the underlying conditions; for example, epoetin (recombinant erythropoietin) has supplanted androgen therapy for anaemias where testosterone acts primarily by stimulating endogenous erythropoietin secretion.[251]

Pharmacological androgen therapies have often used orally active 17α-alkylated androgens. However, due to their inherent hepatotoxicity (see section 8.2.1), therapy with these agents is now justified only in patients with limited life expectancy or who are unable to take safer testosterone formulations. Despite transient increases in nitrogen balance and bodyweight in eugonadal men, androgens have no proven role in sustaining improved nitrogen balance during catabolic states or in preventing muscular atrophy after injury or during limb immobilisation.

#### 8.3.4 Medical Castration

*GnRH agonists* (table X) are used to reduce endogenous testosterone to concentrations equivalent to orchidectomy where medical castration is intended such as in prostate cancer, precocious puberty, transsexuals or sexual criminality. The most widely used role for GnRH agonists is as an accepted alternative to orchidectomy for hormonal palliation of prostate cancer. They are administered as daily injections or by monthly biodegradable depot injections or implants, the latter improving therapeutic compliance. All have comparable effectiveness, safety and cost. Both medical and surgical castration lead equally to acute (hot flushing, impotence) and chronic (osteoporosis, mental disturbances) features of androgen deficiency. The major advantage of using GnRH agonists is avoidance of the surgical and psychological consequences of orchidectomy, although they are more expensive.

Due to the risk of a 'flare' reaction during initiation of treatment with GnRH agonists (see section 8.2.3), the addition of a nonsteroidal antiandrogen (e.g. flutamide or nilutamide) during the first few weeks of treatment may prevent temporary worsening of bone pain or cord compression from growth of bony metastases precipitated by the transient rise in testosterone concentrations. The use of antiandrogens alone in prostate cancer is generally limited as they are only partially effective in the closed-loop feedback situation with an intact HPA axis. More controversially, antiandrogens are increasingly used as an adjunct after medical or surgical castration intended to eradicate the biological effects of residual (5%) extratesticular androgens arising from peripheral interconversion of androgen precursors.[252]

*Precocious puberty* due to premature central activation of pituitary gonadotrophin secretion and testicular function is best treated with GnRH agonists as they are more effective and have fewer adverse effects than steroidal antiandrogens (e.g. cyproterone or medroxyprogesterone). Treatment is monitored clinically and by testosterone concentrations, aiming to maintain suppression to infantile levels until an appropriate chronological age. Gonadotrophin-independent precocious puberty, where GnRH agonists are ineffective, such as androgen-secreting tumours of the adrenals or testis, are best treated surgically, whereas the rare familial gonadotrophin-independent precocious puberty due to activating mutations of the LH receptor or G-proteins is treated with antiandrogens.

In *male-to-female transsexuals*, androgen blockade, mainly with cyproterone, is used prior to orchidectomy to facilitate the change of morphological gender while their adjustment to transgender life is evaluated. The use of medical castration with either GnRH agonists or steroidal antiandrogens as part of criminal punishment for sexual crimes remains controversial due to the inherent coercion of consent for a nontherapeutic medical treatment that may indeed be deleterious, even fatal.

#### 8.3.5 Male Infertility

Optimal management of male infertility depends on skilled recognition of underlying conditions for which specific treatments are available (10 to 15%). For the remainder of patients in whom untreatable testicular failure is present, management requires appropriate advice on timing, expectations and selection of empirical treatment, including the increasingly complex array of expensive assisted reproductive techniques. Male-factor *in vitro* fertilisation (IVF) and related techniques have diminished the role of empirical medical treatments, none of which were effective in placebo-controlled trials with appropriate end-points.[253] These unproven or failed treatments include gonadotrophins, androgens (mesterolone, testosterone undecanoate, fluoxymesterone, testosterone rebound), antiestrogens (clomifene, tamoxifen), miscellaneous nonhormonal drugs, and physical treatments (testicular cooling, varicocele surgery). None can presently be recommended as effective and some may be deleterious.

Medical treatments for male subfertility include gonadotrophin or pulsatile GnRH therapy for gonadotrophin deficiency (see section 8.2.4), immunosuppressive doses of prednisone for sperm autoimmunity and, possibly, antibiotics for accessory gland infection. Cytoprotective treatments to minimise bystander germ cell killing by cytotoxic regimens are being developed to augment or supersede sperm cryopreservation that is the only form of fertility insurance currently available.

The advent of male-factor IVF procedures that allow assisted fertilisation with very few, even single or immature, sperm has revolutionised management of male infertility. Although expensive, relatively inefficient and stressful, procedures such as microepididymal sperm aspiration and/or intracytoplasmic sperm injection can achieve fertilisation even in azoospermic men for whom paternity was previously considered impossible. The assisted reproductive techniques create a new opportunity for pharmacological treatment of sperm *in vitro*, thereby avoiding adverse corporeal effects of drugs. However, the potential teratogenic and embryotoxic effects of such treatments requires careful evaluation. The ability to fertilise most oocytes by intracytoplasmic injection of sperm largely circumvents the need to fertilise by natural means. Adoption or donor insemination are last resort alternatives for men with untreatable azoospermia, complete lack of gametes (e.g. orchidectomy), or failure of sperm to fertilise oocytes. Consideration of donor insemination requires careful advice, personal reflection and professional counselling, and is acceptable to only a minority of eligible couples. In future, germ cell transplantation[254] may become an alternative to donor insemination, allowing otherwise irreversibly infertile men to conceive without gamete manipulation.

#### *8.3.6 Sexual Dysfunction*

##### Erectile Failure

The community prevalence of erectile failure increases more than 10-fold between the ages of 40 and 65 years, reaching 25%. Among men with long-standing diabetes the prevalence exceeds 50%. Although the cause is poorly understood, irreversible degenerative vascular disease is believed to be a major factor. A substantial minority of patients have correctable underlying causes including psychogenic erectile failure (10 to 30%) and endocrine disorders (<5%). Men with primarily psychogenic erectile failure usually have performance anxiety that can be effectively treated with sensate-focus behavioural therapy by a skilled psychotherapist. Correctable endocrine causes include androgen deficiency, which is usually effectively treated with ART, and hyperprolactinaemia, which may respond to bromocriptine alone, but usually requires pituitary surgery and/or irradiation, and ART. In some men with compensated Leydig cell dysfunction, the diagnosis of partial androgen deficiency can be difficult. As a last resort, a carefully explained but strictly limited (3-month) trial of androgen therapy is occasionally justified to determine whether sustained benefits from androgen therapy can be obtained. Such individual therapeutic trials, however, can be overshadowed by placebo reactions which manifest as transient therapeutic benefits.

In most psychologically well adjusted eugonadal men with idiopathic erectile failure, empirical treatments can be rewarding. However, long term continuation rates drop sharply despite technically effective treatment, indicating limitations of this therapy. Self-injection therapy (see section 8.2.5) must be considered against physical alternatives such as external mechanical devices, which are inexpensive and simple, but not very effective, and penile prosthetic implants, which are expensive, involve surgical implantation of foreign materials and are thus a last resort. Currently, intracavernosal therapy (see section 8.2.5) is favoured as more effective and less traumatic than either mechanical treatments. Autoinjection programmes must be supervised by clinicians experienced in determining the optimal dose, after which most patients can accomplish regular self-injection.

##### Ejaculatory Failure

Ejaculatory failure, including anejaculation and retrograde ejaculation, is usually due to interruption of neural pathways facilitating ejaculation, as in autonomic neuropathy (especially long term diabetes), post-transurethral prostatectomy, retroperitoneal lymph node dissection, or bowel surgery. Sympathomimetic drugs or tricyclic antidepressant agents may be used for symptoms or to assist in obtaining sperm for assisted fertilisation procedures.

### 8.4 Clinical Outcome and Economic Considerations

Disorders of male reproductive function occur during the peak productive epoch of life and have great effects on the psychosocial health and well-being of not only the individual but also his immediate and extended family and his working life. Nevertheless, estimating the cost-effectiveness of treating testicular disorders is exceptionally difficult because most disorders, with the exception of prostate and testicular cancers, are not directly fatal. Although crude estimates of direct (medical, nursing, drug) costs are feasible, realistic quantification of attendant disabilities and their repair by treatment is not possible due to lack of data, making meaningful costings of the benefits impracticable. Even disregarding any calculation of emotional costs, only for male infertility, where there exists a standard and reasonably costed empirical treatment (male-factor IVF), can plausible estimates be attempted.

#### 8.4.1 Male Infertility

Male infertility is common, constituting a major factor in 30 to 50% of the 24% of all married couples who experience subfertility.[255] Medical treatment of male infertility has a limited role but can be measured against the cost of a successful pregnancy from a conventional IVF programme (AU$40,000). Costs for male-factor IVF (see section 8.3.5) would be significantly higher. The direct costs of a successful pregnancy for gonadotrophin treatment for hypogonadotrophic hypogonadism [assuming effectiveness in 80% of men and a 13-month mean duration of treatment[256]] is AU$10,000 per pregnancy, of which drugs constitute nearly 90%. Costs for pulsatile GnRH are higher, mainly due to more labour-intensive supervision being required. Other medical treatments are usually less expensive, but when absent or unproven effectiveness is considered, their costs per successful pregnancy become exorbitant.

#### 8.4.2 Androgen Deficiency

Classical androgen deficiency, with a community prevalence of 0.5%, is the most frequent hormone deficiency state among men, even before including the partial androgen deficiency of male aging. The subtle clinical features and usually insidious onset of postpubertal androgen deficiency contribute to the underdiagnosis of this condition. In addition, androgen deficiency with onset from puberty may never have provided men with any opportunity to notice changes. Such underdiagnosis denies men simple and effective medical treatment. Untreated androgen deficiency is compatible with a long but poor quality of life. Economic effects of treating androgen deficiency can only be measured against the quality of life during productive young and middle years of working life rather than in terms of prolonging life in retirement. The direct costs of ART are AU$1.00 to $1.50/day for medium duration testosterone ester injections and testosterone implants, AU$2.00 to $3.00/day for transdermal patches, and AU$4.00/day for oral testosterone undecanoate. The costs of no or inadequate treatment and the extent to which treatment rectifies sequelae have not been quantified.

#### 8.4.3 Medical Castration

Medical castration is most widely used in palliative hormonal treatment of disseminated prostate cancer where it can be compared with the standard surgical treatment of orchidectomy. Over the average life expectancy of men with disseminated prostate cancer, direct costs of continuous medical androgen blockade are progressively higher than surgical costs, but the psychological impact of surgical castration is difficult if not impossible to cost. There are insufficient long term data to determine whether the late physical and mental sequelae of prolonged androgen deficiency are similar for these 2 treatment modalities.

#### 8.4.4 Sexual Dysfunction

Male sexual dysfunction is another nonfatal disorder with often devastating psychological effects. While direct treatment costs can be calculated, the deleterious effects of no treatment are exceptionally difficult to quantify or cost meaningfully.

## 9. Pituitary and Growth Disorders

Pituitary disease is characterised by signs and symptoms of hormone excess or deficiency, or may present with manifestations of a pituitary mass. There is a diverse clinical spectrum, including short stature, precocious puberty and infertility, disorders that have significant medical, social and economic implications. The anterior pituitary secretes at least 6 trophic hormones; somatotrophin or growth hormone (GH) and the gonadotrophins luteinising hormone (LH), follicle-stimulating hormone (FSH), thyrotrophin (TSH), corticotrophin (ACTH), and prolactin. These pituitary hormones are regulated by hypothalamic releasing hormones, growth hormone-releasing hormone (GHRH), gonadotrophin-releasing hormone (GnRH), thyrotrophin-releasing hormone (TRH), and corticotrophin-releasing hormone (CRH). The releasing hormones are synthesised in the median eminence of the hypothalamus and transported to the pituitary via the hypothalamic-hypophyseal portal venous system. Deficiency of these releasing hormones will lead to pituitary hormone deficiency. The main control of prolactin secretion is by the tonic inhibitory effect of dopamine. Multiple factors are responsible for neural regulation of hypothalamic releasing hormones and include sleep rhythms, stress and monoaminergic neurotransmitters. Feedback to the hypothalamus and pituitary from target gland hormones is an important aspect of regulation.

The hypothalamic and pituitary hormones are polypeptides and most are secreted in a pulsatile fashion. Therefore, direct replacement in deficiency states requires complex regimens of parenteral administration. Replacement of the hormone secreted by the target organ, such as adrenal steroid or thyroid hormone, is a more simple and convenient approach. Gonadal steroid replacement with estrogen or testosterone is also more practical, but more elaborate regimens employing GnRH are appropriate when fertility is required (see section 8.2.4). Management of pituitary hormone excess is more complex than that of deficiency and is mainly based on the development of agonists and antagonists of hypothalamic releasing factors. Availability of pure hypothalamic releasing hormones has improved diagnostic assessment of hypothalamic-pituitary-target organ function.

## 9.1 Clinical Pharmacology of Drugs Used in Treatment

### *9.1.1 Growth Hormone (GH; Somatropin)*

Human GH is a 191–amino acid protein, secreted in a pulsatile fashion from the anterior pituitary under dual hypothalamic control; it is stimulated by GHRH and inhibited by somatostatin. GH has multiple actions directly though GH receptors and indirectly via secretion of insulin-like growth factors (IGFs) that are in turn regulated in a complex fashion by the IGF-binding proteins, one of which is under GH control.[257] A dual-effector hypothesis for GH action has been proposed, such that GH stimulates differentiation of precursor cells and the IGFs then act as mitogens to stimulate clonal growth of the differentiated cells.[258]

Purified GH was first available for therapeutic use in the 1950s and 1960s.[259] Its use was limited by the supply of cadaveric pituitaries, and the exclusive indication was treatment of children with GH-deficiency. Development of recombinant preparations accelerated after the discovery that pituitary GH was a source of the agent causing Creutzfeldt-Jakob disease.[260] The first recombinant preparations had an additional methionyl group at the carboxyl terminus of the molecule (somatrem) but were therapeutically equivalent to the natural sequence now available.[261] The half-life of exogenously administered GH is short, approximately 10 minutes.[262]

#### Clinical Effectiveness

Growth hormone therapy clearly increases final adult height in children with GH deficiency and Turner's syndrome. A knowledge of its effectiveness in other conditions associated with short stature awaits the results of current clinical trials. It has been proposed that GH be used for disorders other than short stature since it improves metabolic status, being anabolic for protein homeostasis and anti-insulin like in its actions on fat and carbohydrate metabolism. Recent studies suggest that GH replacement of adults with GH deficiency is appropriate.[263] It preserves body nitrogen stores in a range of catabolic states including burns, long term critical illness and AIDS.[264]

Of interest is the possible use of GH in conjunction with IGF-I (insulin-like growth factor-I; somatomedin-C), which would minimise the complications of carbohydrate intolerance.[265] Further studies of the effectiveness of GH treatment for ovulation induction and lactation failure are also required.[264]

#### Tolerability

Use of recombinant GH has reduced the risk of transmission of Creutzfeldt-Jakob disease. However, the incubation period for this infection is 10 to 20 years, so there are still many patients worldwide at risk of the disease. Antigenicity is not a problem with the use of recombinant GH. Even with GH purified from human pituitaries, antibody formation was rarely of clinical significance.[261] If the growth response is poor in a clearly GH-deficient child, it is more likely that hypothyroidism is also present.

Growth hormone is generally well tolerated.[266] Reported risks of GH treatment include slipped capital femoral epiphysis, which may not be an adverse effect of GH treatment *per se*, as it is also common in healthy rapidly growing children. An early report of an excess incidence of leukaemia in GH-treated patients has not been confirmed. There will always be concern over theoretical risks, based on the knowledge of the role of GH and IGFs in malignancy and immune function. The problems of insulin resistance, sodium and water retention, and acromegalic features are dose-related and should not present problems in GH replacement. However, there is a tendency toward GH-induced carbohydrate intolerance and fluid imbalance in older individuals already prone to these problems.

### 9.1.2 GnRH and its Analogues

Gonadotrophin-releasing hormone (GnRH) is a decapeptide released in a pulsatile fashion from the hypothalamus. It acts on specific receptors on pituitary gonadotrophs and stimulates the synthesis and secretion of LH and FSH. It has a circulating half-life of 2 to 4 minutes.[267] Synthetic analogues of GnRH have been developed with increased receptor affinity and improved resistance to enzymatic degradation (see also sections 8.2.3 and 8.2.4). They are, therefore, long acting, have greater potency (15 to 200 times that of GnRH) and lead to GnRH receptor downregulation and a hypogonadal state.[268] In some patients there is also an initial period of stimulation (see section 8.2.3). Several GnRH agonists are available, including *leuprorelin*,[233] *goserelin*,[231] *buserelin*,[230] *nafarelin*,[234] *histrelin*,[232] and *triptorelin* (table X). They require parenteral administration and are effective when given as daily subcutaneous injections or monthly depot injections. Other routes of administration have been developed and include nasal sprays (e.g. buserelin and nafarelin), subcutaneous implants, and transvaginal preparations.

#### Clinical Effectiveness

There is a wide range of clinical applications of GnRH and its analogues.[269] The use of GnRH (gonadorelin) as a provocative test of LH and FSH secretion is well established. Pulsatile GnRH therapy is effective in inducting puberty and in the management of fertility in men and women with hypothalamic disorders and impaired GnRH secretion (e.g. isolated hypogonadotrophic hypogonadism and postirradiation damage to the CNS).

When administered continuously, *GnRH agonists* induce biochemical castration and are effective in managing GnRH-dependent precocious puberty and some hormone-dependent tumours, such as prostatic carcinoma. GnRH agonist therapy is also useful in the treatment of endometriosis (see further chapter 18; sect. 11.3.2), allowing administration of lower doses of progestational agents. They can also be used to treat uterine fibroids, either as primary therapy or in preparation for surgery. When used in long term treatment of polycystic ovarian disease, it is appropriate to supplement GnRH analogues with sex steroids to avoid the complications of hypoestrogenism. In assisted fertilisation, GnRH agonists allow exogenous gonadotrophins to induce ovulation without causing premature rupture of ovarian follicles.

Some GnRH analogues are antagonistic at the GnRH receptor and, therefore, block its action. They suppress gonadotrophin production and lack the unwanted initial stimulatory phase of GnRH agonists. Initial use of these agents was associated with significant histamine release. Newer generation antagonists are proving hopeful.[269]

#### Tolerability

GnRH and its derivatives have low toxicity. Very rarely, local and systemic allergic reactions occur. Gonadal suppression is fully reversed within weeks to months, even after several years of treatment, so that long term fertility is preserved.[270] Long term use will lead to prolonged hypogonadism and reduced bone mineral density. Undertreatment with a GnRH agonist will result in stimulation of the hypothalamic-pituitary-gonadal axis, rather than suppression. To avoid this, it is important to monitor the response closely to determine that gonadotrophins decrease to the prepubertal range and that no progression of sexual maturation occurs.[270]

### 9.1.3 Dopamine Agonists

Dopamine is the dominant physiological prolactin inhibitory factor. Released from dopaminergic neurones of the hypothalamus into the portal circulation, it stimulates dopamine receptors on lactotrophs and tonically inhibits prolactin secretion.[271] Long-acting dopamine agonists are established in the management of hyperprolactinaemia. *Bromocriptine* is a semisynthetic ergot alkaloid, first introduced in 1971 for the treatment of hyperprolactinaemia.[271] Other agonists which have longer half-lives are now available and include *lisuride, pergolide, metergoline* and *cabergoline*. A long-acting injectable preparation of bromocriptine, employing polyactic acid microspheres, has been used to suppress prolactin secretion for up to 6 weeks.

When given orally, bromocriptine is 40 to 90% is absorbed, but only 6% reaches the circulation after first-pass hepatic metabolism. Peak concentrations are reached in 2 to 3 hours and the drug is 90 to 95% bound to plasma proteins. Although its plasma half-life is 3 hours, the biological effect of a single 2.5mg dose may persist for up to 24 hours, suggesting prolonged binding to or activation of the dopamine receptor.[271]

#### Clinical Effectiveness

Bromocriptine is effective in patients with microprolactinomas and most macroprolactinomas. A reduction in tumour size occurs in many cases and may lead to improvement in visual field and cranial nerve abnormalities, and restoration of gonadal function and other anterior pituitary hormone deficits.[271] Dopamine agonists are also used in pathological hyperprolactinaemia of other origin and in postpartum galactorrhoea.

Although dopamine agonists stimulate GH release acutely in healthy humans, they inhibit GH in acromegaly by an unknown mechanism.[272] High-dose bromocriptine (10 to 30 mg/day) reduces GH secretion in approximately 50% of patients with acromegaly, although only rarely are GH concentrations normalised. There is also an effect on nonfunctioning pituitary tumours when high doses are used. In addition, the dopamine agonists have documented effectiveness in Parkinson's disease (see chapter 29; section 7.1). Bromocriptine has also been used in premenstrual syndrome, cyclical mastalgia, luteal phase insufficiency and portal-systemic encephalopathy, but these applications require further clinical trials.[271]

#### Tolerability

Activation of dopamine receptors may lead to a range of adverse effects, including nausea and orthostatic hypotension, which are transient and dose-related. These symptoms can be minimised by starting with a small dose (e.g. bromocriptine 1.25mg), increasing slowly over several days and taking the tablets with food. Gastrointestinal adverse effects are minimised by intravaginal[273] and long-acting injectable[271] preparations. Headache, fatigue and constipation may also occur. Hallucinations and psychosis have been reported, but tend to occur only at higher doses used in acromegaly and Parkinson's disease. There are occasional reports of vasospasm including coronary artery spasm.[274] The safety of these agents during pregnancy is not established. There is no clear evidence that they are teratogenic, but if possible they should be ceased during pregnancy.

### 9.1.4 Somatostatin Analogues

Somatostatin is a tetradecapeptide produced in the hypothalamus and acting via a specific receptor on pituitary somatotrophs to suppress GH secretion. It is also present in the pancreas and gastrointestinal tract, where it inhibits a range of gut-related hormones including insulin. The therapeutic use of somatostatin is limited by its short half-life of less than 3 minutes, the need for parenteral administration and a rebound effect after cessation of the drug. Long-acting somatostatin analogues have been developed that resist degradation and, therefore, have a longer duration of action than the native peptide.[275]

*Octreotide* has a half-life of about 90 minutes and *lanreotide* of 10 to 14 days. Octreotide is an octapeptide that suppresses GH for up to 8 hours in normal and acromegalic patients. Absorption after subcutaneous injection is rapid, with 100% bioavailability. Peak plasma concentrations occur 20 to 30 minutes after administration and it is 65% bound to lipoproteins in the circulation. Octreotide has a relatively selective effect on GH secretion, being at least 20 times more effective than somatostatin in suppressing GH release, but has little effect on insulin release.

#### Clinical Effectiveness

In addition to acromegaly, somatostatin analogues have shown some effectiveness in thyrotrophin-secreting adenomas and other hormone-secreting tumours such as glucagonomas and carcinoid tumours. Octreotide is effective in controlling GH secretion in most patients with acromegaly and reduces the size of the pituitary tumour in about one-third of patients. The dose required for a response varies from 300 to 1500 μg/day and is most effective when given as a continuous infusion. The effectiveness of intranasal octreotide is currently being investigated.

#### Tolerability

Adverse effects with octreotide occur in one-third of patients.[275] Nausea, cramps and steatorrhoea usually improve within the first week of use. Pain at the injection site occurs in 5%. Although the effect on insulin secretion is not as profound as that on GH, insulin concentrations are reduced for about 3 hours after injection and can lead to postprandial hyperglycaemia. Octreotide inhibits gallbladder contractility and, thus, facilitates the formation of biliary sludge and gallstones.[272] Long term studies report a 30 to 50% incidence of gallstones.[275] To minimise this, it is best to administer the dose 2 to 3 hours after meals. *Ursodeoxycholic acid* may be used concurrently.

#### 9.1.5 Serotonin Antagonists

Serotonergic mechanisms are involved in the stimulation of corticotrophin, GH and prolactin secretion. *Cyproheptadine* potently antagonises serotonin, and also histamine and acetylcholine, and has produced satisfactory outcomes in patients with Cushing's disease and Nelson's syndrome.[276] Adverse effects include increased appetite and weight gain.

#### 9.1.6 Other Hypothalamic and Pituitary Hormones

Synthetic preparations of the hypothalamic releasing hormones have a well established place in the testing of pituitary responsiveness. They have short plasma half-lives of minutes. Peak trophic responses occur 1 to 2 hours after an intravenous or intramuscular bolus. *Thyrotrophin-releasing hormone* (TRH) 500μg (7 μg/kg in children) is used as a test of pituitary TSH responsiveness. It is also effective in releasing prolactin in healthy individuals and growth hormone in patients with active acromegaly. Some patients experience a transient urge to urinate, a metallic taste, nausea or lightheadedness. Transient hypertension occasionally occurs. *GnRH (gonadorelin)* 100μg is used to determine gonadotrophin responsiveness and is of particular use in distinguishing between constitutional delayed puberty and hypogonadotrophic hypogonadism. Adverse effects occur rarely and include headache, abdominal discomfort and flushing.

*Corticotrophin-releasing hormone* (CRH) 1 μg/kg may be used to distinguish Cushing's disease from ectopic corticotrophin production. Adverse effects include transient facial flushing and dyspnoea. *Growth hormone-releasing hormone* (GHRH; somatorelin) 1 to 2 μg/kg has been used as a test of GH responsiveness. Rarely, patients notice facial flushing or stinging at the injection site. GHRH and its analogues may promote growth in some individuals.

Synthetic pituitary hormone preparations are also useful. A synthetic corticotrophin preparation, *tetracosactide*, is well established in the testing of adrenal function. Cortisol and aldosterone concentrations are usually measured after a 0.25mg bolus. 17-Hydroxyprogesterone concentrations increase in response to corticotrophin in 21-hydroxylase deficiency. Corticotrophin can also be used as a replacement of pituitary deficiency when the adrenal is intact, but in general the use of the adrenal steroids is as effective and more convenient.

*Thyroid-stimulating hormone* (TSH) has been used as a diagnostic tool to stimulate radioiodine uptake and distinguishing between primary and secondary hypothyroidism and the euthyroid state. It is sometimes used to enhance radioiodine uptake for the ablation of metastatic thyroid carcinoma. Apart from the symptoms of hyperthyroidism, thyroid tenderness, soreness at the injection site, allergy or nausea may occasionally occur.

Preparations containing *follicle-stimulating hormone* (FSH) are used in the induction of ovulation in women and spermatogenesis in men (see section 8.2.4 and also chapter 18).

#### 9.1.7 Other Agents

##### Ketoconazole

Ketoconazole, an orally active substituted imidazole derivative, suppresses gonadal and adrenal steroidogenesis at several steps, importantly at the cytochrome P450 isoenzyme CYPC17, blocking conversion of 17-hydroxyprogesterone to androstenedione. Doses of 400 to 600 mg/day lead to a clinical response within days. There is a mild decrease in cortisol secretion which may lead to adrenal insufficiency in some individuals. Long term use of ketoconazole can cause hepatic injury which is, usually mild and reversible, but in 0.1% of patients is severe (see also section 7.1.3).

##### Testolactone

Testolactone is a derivative of testosterone that competitively inhibits the cytochrome P450 isoenzyme aromatase, leading to a reduction in the conversion of androstenedione to estrone and testosterone to estradiol. It has been used effectively in McCune-Albright syndrome in a dosage of 20 to 40 mg/kg daily,[277] and has also been used in combination with spironolactone 2 to 4 mg/kg daily in familial testotoxicosis.[278]

## 9.2 Optimum Treatment

### 9.2.1 Growth Disorders

Classical GH deficiency in children is a clear indication for GH therapy, whether it occurs as an isolated hormonal deficiency, as part of hypopituitarism or as a consequence of central nervous system tumours or cranial irradiation. GH is usually effective at a total dose of 0.6 IU/kg/week, administered as a daily subcutaneous injection.[264,279] The height gained in early years of therapy represents the major catch-up to be attained with treatment. Growth responsiveness appears to wane over time. Puberty has a crucial impact on the overall response. The later puberty begins, the greater the final height. GH may itself affect the tempo of puberty, shortening it, and thus limiting the height gain.[280] It is important to monitor thyroid function in this group of patients since initiation of GH therapy may unmask hypothyroidism.

With recombinant DNA technology and a plentiful supply, the role of GH therapy in disorders other than childhood deficiency can be considered.[263] A response to GH therapy has clearly been demonstrated in Turner's syndrome, where abnormalities of GH secretion or action have been postulated but never documented.[264,279] In this disorder, the cause of short stature appears to be multifactorial, with intrauterine growth retardation, skeletal abnormalities and lack of sex steroids at puberty contributing to final adult height. There are other groups of apparently non-GH deficient patients who also respond to GH therapy, many of whom have subtle GH secretory dysfunction.

Most clinical trials of GH (somatropin) in normal variant short stature or idiopathic short stature demonstrate an acceleration of growth rate over the short term, decreasing with each additional year. Overall, however, there does not seem to be any significant benefit in terms of final adult height.[263] Chronic renal failure is characterised by abnormalities of the GH/IGF axis and a favourable response to GH has been documented.[281] In other, non-GH deficient syndromes such as Silver-Russell, Noonan, Downs and Prader-Willi, no firm conclusion on GH therapy has yet been reached and further long term studies are required. The largest group of children with short stature have maturational delay; GH therapy is not indicated in this group. In most cases, it is appropriate to give no drug treatment, although occasionally, low-dose androgens may be used in boys.

Laron dwarfism is a hereditary disorder characterised by molecular defects of the GH receptor, and there are high circulating GH concentrations, low IGF-I concentrations and short stature. These individuals do not respond to GH, but grow in response to IGF-I therapy.[265]

### 9.2.2 Precocious Puberty

The treatment of precocious puberty depends on the cause. If it is a variation of normal (premature thelarche or adrenarche), clearly no drug intervention will be required. If congenital adrenal hyperplasia is the cause, glucocorticoids are indicated (see further section 7.2.2). Tumours producing chorionic gonadotrophin should be removed and intracranial lesions may require surgery.

Central or true precocious puberty is GnRH-dependent and is characterised by an exaggerated gonadotrophin response to GnRH. Drug therapy is, thus, directed toward the HPA axis and *GnRH agonists* (table X) are the treatment of choice. Antiandrogens may be used in the first weeks of therapy to prevent the effects of the transient increase in LH and FSH produced by GnRH agonists (see sections 8.2.3 and 8.3.4). Gonadotrophin concentrations decrease and reach the prepubertal range within 2 to 4 weeks in girls and 6 weeks in boys. Height velocity can be expected to decrease by 60% in the first year of therapy and then should become appropriate for bone age. Skeletal maturation slows during the first 3 years and an improvement in height potential has been reported.[270] Recent indications are that the improvement in final adult height may not be as great as originally thought.[282] The best growth response is seen in children treated before the bone age is far advanced.

It is of particular importance not to undertreat with GnRH agonists as this may aggravate sexual precocity. *Medroxyprogesterone* and *cyproterone* are effective in halting the progression of secondary sexual characteristics in true precocious puberty, but have virtually no effect on final height. Medroxyprogesterone is a progestagen that in oral doses of 5 to 10mg twice daily (or intramuscular doses of 100 to 200 mg/m$^2$ every 2 weeks) inhibits GnRH pulses and gonadotrophin production. It also has glucocorticoid actions and may, therefore, lead to Cushingoid features and adrenal suppression with long term use.[270] Oral cyproterone 5 to 50 mg/m$^2$ twice daily (or intramuscular doses of 100 to 200 mg/m$^2$ every 2 weeks) has antiandrogenic, antigonadotrophic and progestational actions. It may also lead to secondary adrenal insufficiency.

In peripheral, or GnRH-independent, sexual precocity, gonadal oversecretion is independent of hypothalamic-pituitary control. Girls with autonomous ovarian follicular cysts, boys with familial testotoxicosis, and the McCune-Albright syndrome are examples. Management of these disorders involves the inhibition of sex steroid production or metabolism with agents such as *medroxyprogesterone, ketoconazole* (see section 9.1.7), *testolactone* (see section 9.1.7), and androgen antagonists such as *cyproterone* (see section 8.2.3) and *spironolactone* (see section 8.2.3). However, these approaches to peripheral precocious puberty have no significant impact on final adult height. Possibly due to the priming effects of prior androgen exposure, some individuals exhibit true precocious puberty after control on these agents that may be managed with GnRH agonists.[270]

#### 9.2.3 Galactorrhoea

Prolactin is of primary importance in establishing and maintaining lactation. Where suppression of lactation is required, *bromocriptine* (see section 9.1.3) is the drug of choice and should be given continuously for 3 weeks (2.5mg twice daily for 2 weeks, then 2.5 mg/day for 1 week) to avoid a rebound. Galactorrhoea occurs in men and women with hyperprolactinaemia, and is often due to a prolactinoma, although other causes should be excluded, such as primary hypothyroidism and medications such as dopamine-depleting drugs (methyldopa, reserpine) and dopamine receptor blocking agents (phenothiazines, haloperidol, metoclopramide). In the remaining cases, whether or not a tumour can be identified, treatment with a dopamine agonist is usually successful.

Bromocriptine is effective in doses of less than 7.5 mg/day (in 3 divided doses). Prolactin concentrations return to normal and menses resume in 70 to 100% patients. Fertility is restored in most. It is advisable to confirm that the prolactin concentrations are normal after 1 to 2 months. Most studies recommend periodic cessation of bromocriptine to assess for remission of hyperprolactinaemia.[271] If pregnancy occurs, bromocriptine should be ceased, although no study has demonstrated effects on pregnancy or the fetus, and the drug can be reintroduced in patients with pituitary tumour enlargement during pregnancy.[271] Apart from troublesome galactorrhoea and infertility, it is appropriate to normalise the high prolactin concentrations to prevent the loss of bone mineral density due to the hypoestrogenaemic state.[283] In patients not desiring pregnancy and without galactorrhoea, estrogen in a combined oral contraceptive will achieve the same result.

#### 9.2.4 Acromegaly

The morbidity and mortality of acromegaly are considerable and reversible with treatment. The goals of management are the return of GH secretion to normal, as reflected by serum IGF-I concentrations, resolution of clinical signs and symptoms, and reduction in mass effects of the tumour. Although surgery and radiotherapy are first-line measures, many patients are not adequately controlled with these approaches and require subsequent drug treatment.

There are 2 options for drug therapy. *Octreotide* (see section 9.1.4) suppresses GH concentrations to below 5 μg/L and normalises IGF-I concentrations in 50% of patients, and shrinks 60% of tumours.[272] High-dose *bromocriptine* (see section 9.1.3) suppresses GH concentrations to below 5 μg/L and normalises IGF-I concentrations in 10 to 20%, and shrinks 10 to 20% of tumours.[272] Up to 50% of patients using *bromocriptine* experience some symptom improvement.[271]

### 9.3 Clinical Outcome and Economic Considerations

#### 9.3.1 Growth Disorders

Growth hormone treatment is prolonged and expensive. In the US, it costs in excess of US$20,000 to treat a child for a year. In idiopathic GH deficiency, the clinical benefit is indisputable. There is more of an ethical dilemma in cases of short stature without classical GH deficiency. Here, the actual benefit of a small increase in final adult height is difficult to quantify and the cost of treatment and concerns about adverse effects are significant in the equation. For some individuals, social pressures are so disabling that a short term height gain may be worth the cost and risks. Appropriate counselling is crucial and may be more important than drug therapy. Attention to psychosocial issues is also a cornerstone of therapy of precocious puberty.

#### 9.3.2 Acromegaly

Although bromocriptine produces a lower tumour shrinkage rate than octreotide (see section

9.2.4), it is cheaper (20 mg/day costs US$3800/year) and can be administered orally, and it could be argued that it should be prescribed first. Then, if the response is inadequate, octreotide (600 μg/day which costs US$17,500/year) should be commenced. One study has suggested that a combination of these 2 agents is effective because of increased bromocriptine bioavailability.[284]

## 10. Endocrine Hypertension

### 10.1 Clinical and Pathological Features

Endocrine disease accounts for 1 to 3% of all hypertension, and a variety of hormonal disorders are associated with an increase in blood pressure (table XI). The diagnosis can be easily overlooked, but the presence of 1 or more of the following clues should raise suspicion of an underlying endocrine disorder in a hypertensive patient:

1) Hypertension in a young patient without a family history.

2) Accelerated hypertension or hypertension refractory to standard triple therapy.

3) Presence of hypokalaemia.

4) Presence of unusual symptoms and/or evidence of other endocrine disease (e.g. multiple endocrine neoplasia).

#### *10.1.1 Primary Aldosteronism*

About 70% of cases of primary aldosteronism are caused by adrenal adenomas (Conn's syndrome). The remaining 30% are due to bilateral adrenal hyperplasia of the zona glomerulosa. The cause of multinodular hyperplasia is unknown, although a glycoprotein pituitary adrenal-stimulating factor has been implicated. In rare instances, the aldosterone hypersecretion is corticotrophin-dependent and dexamethasone suppressible. Primary aldosteronism can also be mimicked by ingestion of liquorice or carbenoxolone, which have metabolites with mineralocorticoid activity. Both types of primary aldosteronism present with hypertension and hypokalaemic alkalosis, although up to 20% of patients may have plasma potassium concentrations in the low normal range (i.e. 3.5 to 4.2 mmol/L) initially. There are usually few symptoms; severe manifestations such as tetany, muscle weakness and nocturia are uncommon. In general, the clinical and biochemical manifestations of aldosterone-secreting adenomata tend to be more pronounced than those of multinodular hyperplasia.

The classical biochemistry of primary aldosteronism shows hypokalaemic alkalosis, increased plasma aldosterone, suppressed plasma renin activity and inappropriately high urinary potassium excretion (>30 mmol/day) for a hypokalaemic state. All drugs should be stopped before measurements are taken of plasma aldosterone and renin activity. Distinguishing the 2 main causes of primary aldosteronism may be difficult. The accuracy of computed tomography scans depends on resolution; 10 to 40% of small adenomas may be missed. Adrenal scintillation scans with [$^{131}$I]iodocholesterol may distinguish unilateral uptake (Conn's) from more diffuse bilateral uptake (hyperplasia), but the radiation dose is high. A dexamethasone suppression test will identify the subgroup with dexamethasone suppressible aldosteronism.

#### *10.1.2 Congenital Adrenal Hyperplasia*

Congenital adrenal hyperplasia (see also section 7.2.2) is an inborn error of steroid metabolism and can produce a rare form of mineralocorticoid hypertension. Two enzyme defects may cause hypertension. An 11β-hydroxylation

**Table XI.** Causes of endocrine hypertension

| |
|---|
| **Estrogens** (e.g. in hormone replacement therapy) |
| **Glucocorticoids** (Cushing's syndrome): |
| • Pituitary dependent |
| • Ectopic corticotrophin |
| • Adenoma/carcinoma |
| • Iatrogenic |
| **Angiotensin II** (renal artery stenosis) |
| • Atheroma |
| • Fibromuscular hyperplasia |
| **Catecholamines** (phaeochromocytoma) |
| **Mineralocorticoids** |
| *Primary aldosteronism:* |
| • Adenoma |
| • Bilateral hyperplasia |
| • Glucocorticoid suppressible |
| • Carcinoma |
| *Pseudo-aldosteronism:* |
| • Liquorice |
| • Carbenoxolone |
| • Fludrocortisone excess |
| • Mineralocorticoid nasal sprays |
| **Diabetes** |
| *Insulin-dependent:* |
| • Nephropathy |
| • Coincident essential hypertension |
| *Non-insulin-dependent:* |
| • Obesity |
| • Coincident essential hypertension |
| **Growth hormone** (acromegaly) |
| **Others** |
| • Primary hyperparathyroidism |
| • Primary hypothyroidism |
| • Thyrotoxicosis |

defect causes decreased cortisol production, corticotrophin-dependent accumulation of the mineralocorticoid hormones, 11-deoxycorticosterone and 11-deoxycortisol, and gives rise to hypertension. The rarer defect in 17-hydroxylation is associated with high corticotrophin and hypersecretion of mineralocorticoid precursors.

#### 10.1.3 Cushing's Syndrome

40 to 75% of patients with Cushing's syndrome have hypertension, but the mechanism by which glucocorticoid hormones raise blood pressure is uncertain. Although glucocorticoids increase synthesis of renin substrate (angiotensinogen), hypertension in Cushing's syndrome is not usually associated with hyperactivity of the renin-angiotensin system. However, since Cushing's syndrome is associated with considerable cardiovascular morbidity, aggressive treatment of hypertension is indicated. Treatment is usually similar to that for essential hypertension.

#### 10.1.4 Phaeochromocytoma

Hypertension in phaeochromocytoma is the result of hypersecretion of catecholamines. Most phaeochromocytomas (80 to 90%) develop in the adrenal glands (10% are bilateral), but they can occur anywhere along the sympathetic chain: 3% occur outside the abdomen, about 10% are malignant and 25% are multiple. Most tumours synthesise noradrenaline predominantly, but some produce equal amounts of both adrenaline and noradrenaline. The important clinical characteristic of a phaeochromocytoma is paroxysmal hypertension, often accompanied by symptoms of catecholamine overactivity, e.g. palpitations, sweating, flushing and tremor. Catecholamine-induced diabetes or impaired glucose tolerance is also common. Although most patients (90%) are hypertensive most of the time, blood pressure profiles may be widely variable or truly paroxysmal, with blood pressure decreasing to normal or below-normal between attacks.

The diagnosis can usually be made by measuring elevated urinary catecholamine metabolites, e.g. vanillylmandelic acid or metanephrine. If three 24-hour collections are within the normal range (especially if symptoms and hypertension are present), a diagnosis of phaeochromocytoma is unlikely. Most tumours are fairly large and visible on computed tomography scanning. Additional scanning with [$^{131}$I]metaiodobenzylguanidine (MIBG) is helpful in confirming and locating the tumour(s), but false-negative scans occur in up to 10% of cases. Preoperative venous sampling and arteriography are performed less frequently than in the past.

#### 10.1.5 Thyroid Disease

There is still debate as to whether hypertension is associated with primary hypothyroidism. If an association does exist, the hypertension is only mild and blood pressure appears to settle with adequate thyroxine replacement. In thyrotoxicosis, systolic hypertension is particularly common, with a wide pulse pressure. Cardiac output is high but peripheral vascular resistance is low (presumably because of the increased metabolic demands of the tissues), and diastolic run-off is, therefore, high. The haemodynamic changes resolve quickly once hyperthyroidism has been controlled. Nonselective β-adrenoceptor blockers, e.g. nadolol or propranolol, are effective in controlling the cardiovascular features of thyrotoxicosis, while antithyroid drugs achieve biochemical euthyroidism (see further section 5.2).

#### 10.1.6 Primary Hyperparathyroidism

Hypercalcaemia, especially when due to hyperparathyroidism (see section 6.1), is reported to be associated with an increased prevalence of hypertension. Furthermore, blood pressure often fails to settle after parathyroidectomy and these patients require long term antihypertensive therapy.

#### 10.1.7 Acromegaly

Hypertension is seen in about one-third of patients with acromegaly (see section 9.2.4), and this is sometimes (but not always) reversed by surgery or bromocriptine therapy.

#### 10.1.8 Estrogen Therapy

Most women show an increase in blood pressure when starting an estrogen-containing regimen, although the increase does not usually produce hypertension by WHO criteria. The rise in blood pressure, which is probably dose-dependent, is about 7/4mm Hg after 1 year on ethinylestradiol 20 to 30mg daily. Evidence about whether patients with previous pregnancy-induced hypertension or positive family histories are more likely to become hypertensive on estrogen therapy is conflicting, and the mechanism of the rise in blood pressure is still unclear. Estrogens cause an increase in synthesis of renin substrate by the liver and this results in generation of increased quantities of angiotensin II. However, there is no correlation between increased renin-angiotensin system activity and hypertension associated with oral contraceptives; nor can the hypertension be explained by sodium or water retention.

## 10.2 Clinical Pharmacology of Drugs Used in Treatment

The clinical pharmacology of antihypertensive drugs in general is discussed in chapter 21, but consideration of drugs with specific reference to endocrine hypertension is given here.

### *10.2.1 α-Adrenoceptor Antagonists*

The main effect of α-adrenoceptor blocking drugs is to produce peripheral vasodilatation and a reduction in blood pressure, but in turn this triggers reflex tachycardia due to unopposed sympathetic drive to cardiac β-receptors. The increase in heart rate and cardiac output tends to counteract the decrease in blood pressure. Nonselective (i.e. $\alpha_1$ and $\alpha_2$) adrenoceptor antagonists, e.g. *phentolamine* and *phenoxybenzamine*, as well as inhibiting postjunctional responses, block prejunctional $\alpha_2$-receptor-mediated feedback inhibition of noradrenaline release at sympathetic terminals. Thus, release of noradrenaline (norepinephrine) from vasomotor nerve endings increases. Furthermore, transmitter release from cardiac sympathetic nerves is increased by blockade of the prejunctional α-adrenoceptors. This explains why vasoconstrictor responses to circulating noradrenaline are blocked more effectively than responses to noradrenaline released from sympathetic endings, and why reflex tachycardia is more pronounced with nonselective α-adrenoceptor blocking drugs than with selective $\alpha_1$-adrenoceptor blockers such as prazosin, doxazosin and terazosin (see chapter 21, sect. 3.3).

The unwanted effects of α-adrenoceptor blockers include postural hypotension, nasal congestion, red sclerae and failure of ejaculation.

#### Phentolamine

This is a short-acting drug that blocks both $\alpha_1$- and $\alpha_2$-adrenoceptors by competitive, reversible antagonism. It is only suitable for intravenous use, and tends to be reserved for intraoperative management of hypertensive crises during surgery to remove a phaeochromocytoma. Intravenous injections of 2 to 5mg can be repeated as necessary. With such a short duration of action, there is minimal risk of inducing prolonged hypotension after removal of the tumour. Typical adverse effects include gastrointestinal disturbance, as well as the cardiovascular risks of hypotension and occasionally arrhythmias.

#### Phenoxybenzamine

This is a competitive irreversible α-adrenoceptor antagonist with a prolonged duration of action. It is given orally to patients with phaeochromocytoma in the period leading up to surgery. The usual starting dose is 10mg once daily, with gradual titration to 1 to 2 mg/kg/day in 2 divided doses. The adverse effects of postural hypotension and nasal congestion are shared with other α-blockers, but additional adverse effects of phenoxybenzamine include dry mouth, drowsiness and sedation. The mechanism of these CNS effects is not clear since the drug does not appear to cross the blood-brain barrier.

### *10.2.2 β-Adrenoceptor Antagonists*

β-Adrenoceptor antagonists (β-blockers) still form the mainstay of antihypertensive therapy in patients with essential hypertension (see chapter 21; sect. 3.2). They reduce heart rate and cardiac output, and inhibition of renin release (a $\beta_2$ effect) may also contribute to the antihypertensive mechanism. There is no significant difference between the various drugs in the magnitude of blood pressure reduction.

There are 2 situations in the context of endocrine hypertension where β-blockers are particularly effective: phaeochromocytoma and thyrotoxicosis. In both conditions, a nonselective β-blocker is preferred, to attenuate both the central (cardiac) and peripheral cardiovascular manifestations and, at least theoretically, drugs with partial agonist activity (see chapter 21; table II) are likely to be less effective. Nonselective β-blockers include propranolol, oxprenolol, nadolol and timolol. Oxprenolol is the only one of these with partial agonist activity, while nadolol is the most water soluble agent and is eliminated unchanged in the urine. All β-blockers are contraindicated in patients with airflow limitation. Propranolol or nadolol are often preferred in patients with thyrotoxicosis (see section 5.2), while propranolol is often the drug of choice in phaeochromocytoma after adequate α-adrenoceptor blockade has been established with phenoxybenzamine.

### *10.2.3 Potassium-Sparing Diuretics*

Drugs in this class include spironolactone, amiloride and triamterene (see also chapter 21; sect. 3.1). Their use in conjunction with potassium-losing diuretics such as the thiazides in essential hypertension is seldom necessary as the low doses of these agents used nowadays cause little if any fall in plasma potassium concentrations. However, they are helpful in potassium-losing states associated with endocrine forms of secondary hypertension.

#### Spironolactone

The biological activity of spironolactone is due to competitive inhibition of aldosterone at the distal nephron, in particular the cortical and medullary collecting tubules. The net effect of the drug is to reduce $H^+$ and $K^+$ loss in the urine, as well as producing natriuresis and diuresis, and the patient develops a hyperkalaemic acidosis. Since spironolactone is a competitive inhibitor, the dose required to produce an adequate response depends on the circulating aldosterone concentration. The magnitude of the natriuresis and diuresis is greater if aldosterone concentrations are high. Provided that adequate doses are given, spironolactone has a significant antihypertensive effect (comparable to that of thiazide diuretics) in all hypertensive patients, but it is particularly useful in patients with primary aldosteronism.

***Pharmacokinetic characteristics:*** following oral administration, spironolactone is well absorbed and peak plasma concentrations occur after 2 hours. It is extensively metabolised to a large number of steroid derivatives of which 50% are excreted in urine and up to 30% are eliminated in faeces and bile. 80% is converted to canrenone, which is metabolised further, and many of the metabolites are biologically active. Canrenone is 98% protein bound in plasma and has a half-life of 10 to 35 hours in healthy volunteers. In single-dose studies, most biological activity appears to be due to the parent compound, or some intermediates in the conversion of spironolactone to canrenone, but during multiple-dose administration, canrenone accounts for 75% of the biological activity.

***Tolerability:*** spironolactone is well tolerated in short term studies, but troublesome adverse effects limit its suitability for long term use. These adverse effects are largely due to the steroid nature of the parent compound and, in particular, the progesterone-like activity of metabolites. Gynaecomastia affects 30% of males during long term use, and a large proportion of women will experience menstrual irregularities, hirsutism and deepening of the voice. 20% of patients complain of gastrointestinal irritation, nausea and vomiting, and the incidence of impotence is as high as 30% when spironolactone is used in high doses in males. These effects tend to be dose-related. Unlike the thiazide diuretics, spironolactone has no detrimental effect on glucose and insulin metabolism.

#### Amiloride

Amiloride acts directly on the luminal side of cortical and medullary collecting tubules. Inhibition of distal nephron transport of sodium causes $K^+$ and $H^+$ retention. The reduction in blood pressure is largely due to its effect on sodium balance, but doses required to achieve an antihypertensive effect are usually associated with hyperkalaemia and acidosis.

Amiloride is well absorbed orally and excreted unchanged in the urine. The effects of a single dose last for up to 12 hours. Because of the risks of hyperkalaemia and acidosis, amiloride is contraindicated in renal impairment and should be used with caution in elderly patients and those with congestive heart failure. Nevertheless, the adverse effects of amiloride make it more suitable than spironolactone for long term therapy, e.g. in patients with primary aldosteronism due to adrenal hyperplasia.

#### Triamterene

Triamterene is a pteridine derivative chemically related to folic acid. It is a relatively weak diuretic and antihypertensive that acts from the lumen of the distal tubule. Although its pharmacological profile has some similarities to amiloride, the only role for triamterene is in combination with a thiazide diuretic to maintain normal potassium balance in essential hypertension. It is unsuitable for monotherapy in patients with endocrine hypertension.

### *10.2.4 Angiotensin-Converting Enzyme (ACE) Inhibitors*

Angiotensin-converting enzyme (ACE) is a dipeptide carboxypeptidase that cleaves the terminal amino acids (His-Leu) from angiotensin I to form the potent vasoconstrictor peptide angiotensin II. It is now established that, in addition to the classic endocrine renin-angiotensin system (RAS) in the circulation, there is a local RAS in many tissues, e.g. brain, heart, blood vessels and kidney, that serves autocrine and paracrine functions. Thus, tissue as well as circulating ACE is the primary target of ACE inhibitors. Consistent with the pathophysiological data showing many unwanted effects of local RAS activation, e.g. in the heart, blood vessels and kidneys, there is good evidence from clinical trials showing that sustained ACE inhibition improves organ function and retards the progression of heart failure, diabetic nephropathy and vascular dysfunction associated with hypertension and atheroma. Accordingly, inhibition of the local autocrine effects of the tissue RAS is now thought to play a crucial role in the long term benefits of ACE inhibitor therapy.

With a few minor exceptions (e.g. in elimination characteristics), the clinical pharmacological properties of all ACE inhibitors are generally similar (see chapter 21; sect. 3.5) and on clinical grounds there are no major differences between the various drugs of this class. Apart from captopril and lisinopril, they are all prodrugs that require conversion in the liver to active diacid metabolites for ACE inhibitory activity. ACE inhibitors lower blood pressure via a reduction in peripheral vascular resistance, but (unlike other arteriolar vasodilators) their effects are not accompanied by a reflex rise in heart rate. An irritating dry cough is the most common adverse effect during chronic therapy and affects 10 to 15% of all patients.

ACE inhibitors are particularly suitable for hypertension associated with diabetes, mainly because of their neutral (or favourable) metabolic profile and renoprotective effects. They are also particularly effective in high renin states of hypertension, although a satisfactory antihypertensive effect is not dependent on the underlying renin status of the patient. For example, in primary aldosteronism, ACE inhibitors are effective in lowering blood pressure (even though renin concentrations are suppressed) and their potassium-conserving effects improve hypokalaemia.

## 10.3 Optimum Treatment

### *10.3.1 Primary Aldosteronism*

Adenomas should be removed if the patient is fit for surgery. *Spironolactone* 300 to 400 mg/day should always be used before surgery to restore total body potassium to normal. About 60% of patients will be rendered normotensive after surgery; 20% will be improved but may require some antihypertensive treatment, and 20% will show little change. However, the electrolyte abnormalities are always corrected. The response of blood pressure to removal of an aldosterone-secreting adenoma correlates well with the effects of spironolactone 400 mg/day for 3 to 4 weeks. If blood pressure does not respond to spironolactone, there is a strong case for adding other drugs rather than proceeding to surgery.

Unless there is doubt about the location of the tumour, a posterior surgical approach is preferred, being associated with less morbidity than laparotomy. Transient hyperkalaemia may occur as the contralateral zona glomerulosa is suppressed, so potassium supplements should be stopped before operation. In patients unfit for surgery, adrenal ablation can be performed by retrograde instillation of *ethanolamine* as a sclerosant into the adrenal vein. This procedure is successful in 50% of cases.

With bilateral adrenal hyperplasia, the primary goal is to reduce blood pressure using drug therapy. Initial treatment should be with *spironolactone* 50 to 400 mg/day. Spironolactone is often poorly tolerated (adverse effects include nausea, rashes, abdominal pain, gynaecomastia, impotence and menstrual disturbance), particularly at higher doses (>200 mg/day), in which case *amiloride* 10 to 40 mg/day may be preferable. Spironolactone has been associated with tumours in rats and although the relevance of this finding to its clinical use is uncertain, long term use of the drug is no longer generally advised. Combinations of drugs are necessary in many patients, and both inhibitors and calcium antagonists are often effective in controlling blood pressure and (to a lesser extent) reversing hypokalaemia.

### *10.3.2 Phaeochromocytoma*

The treatment of phaeochromocytoma is surgical excision of the tumour(s), the only exception being disseminated malignant disease. The role of drug therapy is to control blood pressure before surgery (during the period of investigation to localise the tumours) and intraoperatively. The aim is to block the effects of catecholamines at $\alpha_1$- and $\alpha_2$-adrenoceptor sites in the vasculature and at cardiac $\beta$-adrenoceptors. Thus, a combination of $\alpha$- and $\beta$-blockade is usually achieved with the nonselective $\alpha$-blocker, *phenoxybenzamine*, and a $\beta$-blocker such as *propranolol*. Phenoxybenzamine is preferable to selective $\alpha_1$-adrenoceptor antagonists, e.g. prazosin, in phaeochromocytoma because circulating catecholamines exert their vasoconstrictor effects via both $\alpha_1$- and $\alpha_2$-adrenoceptors. $\beta$-Blockers must not be given without adequate $\alpha$-blockade, because of the hazards of intense peripheral vasoconstriction.

In the preoperative control of hypertension, *phenoxybenzamine* should be started at a dose of 20 to 30 mg/day orally, increasing gradually to a maximum of 80 to 200 mg/day. Postural hypotension is the main dose-limiting adverse effect. A β-blocker should be added to the regimen once adequate α-blockade has been established. Intraoperative blood pressure control can be difficult due to dramatic swings in blood pressure, particularly when the tumour is handled. All patients should be well established on maximum tolerated doses of α- and β-blockers before surgery. An intravenous infusion of *phentolamine* and/or *sodium nitroprusside* should be titrated to blood pressure to control hypertensive peaks during the operation. Both agents have the advantage of fairly short half-lives. Precipitous decreases in pressure may occur after removal of the tumour or when venous drainage of the tumour is clamped. In anticipation of this, blood pressure may need to be maintained using pressor agents, e.g. *angiotensin II*. Arrhythmias occurring during the surgical procedure can be treated with intravenous *propranolol*.

In patients with disseminated malignant phaeochromocytoma, *metirosine* (α-methyl-*p*-tyrosine) may be used. This agent is an inhibitor of the rate-limiting enzyme in catecholamine biosynthesis, tyrosine hydroxylase. It causes a marked reduction in tumour synthesis of catecholamines and a reduction in blood pressure, but is reserved for patients in whom surgery is impractical.

## 11. Use of Drugs in the Presence of Associated Endocrine Diseases

Endocrine disease states may contribute to treatment failure or toxicity of drugs used to treat other diseases by influencing their pharmacokinetics or tissue action. Furthermore, certain drugs used in the presence of endocrine disease may aggravate the underlying condition or cause complications that might not otherwise have occurred.

### 11.1 Diabetes Mellitus

Both nonselective and relatively $\beta_1$-selective β-blockers inhibit sympathetic responses to hypoglycaemia, such as tachycardia and palpitations, and may decrease the warning signals and awareness of acute hypoglycaemia. Nonselective β-blockers drugs such as propranolol can also interfere with metabolic and cardiovascular responses to hypoglycaemia in patients with poorly controlled diabetes. Blockade of hepatic and skeletal muscle $\beta_2$-receptors impairs sympathetic stimulation of glycogenolysis and gluconeogenesis. This can lead to hypoglycaemia in patients with depleted liver glycogen stores, e.g. after prolonged fasts or in diffuse hepatocellular disease. Rarely, hypertensive crisis occurs during the hypertensive response to hypoglycaemia when $\beta_2$-receptor-mediated vasodilatation is blocked, leaving unopposed α-mediated vasoconstriction. Relatively $\beta_1$-selective β-blockers such as metoprolol and atenolol are less likely to cause hypoglycaemia and severe hypertensive responses.[285]

### 11.2 Thyroid Disease

Thyroid hormone status may alter absorption, metabolism and tissue sensitivity to drugs, often necessitating dose modification. Plasma digoxin concentrations are increased in the hypometabolic state of hypothyroidism and dose reductions may be needed to avoid toxicity. The reverse is true of hyperthyroidism, wherein plasma concentrations may be harder to maintain in the therapeutic range. Furthermore, digoxin may not be as effective as a β-blocker in controlling atrial fibrillation caused by thyrotoxicosis. Diabetic patients treated with insulin who become hypothyroid are at risk of hypoglycaemia due to decreased insulin metabolism and may require insulin dose reduction. Conversely, diabetic control may worsen in patients who becomes thyrotoxic and additional insulin may be required.

Hypothyroidism may render patients more sensitive to central nervous system depressants. The anticoagulant action of coumarin drugs is decreased in hypothyroidism due to decreased degradation of the vitamin K-dependent clotting factors. In hyperthyroid states, warfarin doses may need reduction and the prothrombin time must be closely monitored.

### 11.3 Other Endocrine Disease

The risk of digoxin toxicity is increased in patients with hypercalcaemia or hypokalaemia from any cause. Extra caution should be taken in monitoring for adverse effects and in monitoring plasma digoxin concentrations in these patients.

Digoxin toxicity is also more likely in patients with catecholamine-induced myocardial irritability due to phaeochromocytoma. The use of β-blockers in these patients without adequate, prior α-blockade can precipitate dangerous hypertensive crises due to blockade of compensatory, $\beta_2$-mediated vasodilatation in the limbs (table XII).

**Table XII.** Drugs that may precipitate hypertensive crises in patients with phaeochromocytoma

| |
|---|
| β-Adrenoceptor blockers |
| Opioids |
| Corticotrophin (ACTH) |
| Saralasin |
| Glucagon |
| Metoclopramide |
| Pancuronium |
| Radiocontrast media (intravascular) |
| Tricyclic antidepressants |

## 12. Drugs Causing or Exacerbating Endocrine Disorders

### 12.1 Hypoglycaemia

After insulin, sulphonylurea drugs (see section 3.2.1) are the most common cause of clinically significant hypoglycaemia. Especially at risk are elderly patients with NIDDM[286] or patients with renal disease. Agents such as chlorpropamide and glibenclamide (glyburide) have a long plasma half-lives and can cause hypoglycaemia for several days after cessation of the drug. Precipitating factors for hypoglycaemia in elderly patients include missed meals or reduced ability to eliminate the drugs due to renal or hepatic impairment. Agents with shorter half-lives such as tolbutamide or glipizide should be less likely to cause these problems in such patients.

The antimalarial drug quinine may cause hypoglycaemia when given intravenously to treat severe malaria. Similarly, the antibiotic pentamidine, used to treat *Pneumocystis carinii* infection in human immunodeficiency virus (HIV) infected patients, acts as a β cell toxin, stimulating insulin release initially and thereby causing hypoglycaemia. Diabetes may develop subsequently if sufficient β cells are damaged.[287]

### 12.2 Hyperglycaemia

Long term treatment of hypertensive patients with thiazide and loop diuretics can impair glucose tolerance in nondiabetic individuals and even precipitate diabetes in susceptible people. Islet cell dysfunction due to diuretic-induced hypokalaemia may be a causative mechanism. However, while caution is required, diabetes should not be regarded as a contraindication to the use of diuretics.

Glucocorticoids, by promoting hepatic glycogenolysis and impairing glucose utilisation by muscle, can precipitate diabetes in susceptible individuals or necessitate dose adjustments in the therapy of established diabetes. Some oral contraceptives can impair glucose tolerance in susceptible people.[288] This effect is mainly due to the progestagen component and is most often noted with nandrolone derivatives such as norgestrel and least with medroxyprogesterone.[289]

Increased insulin doses may be required in women with IDDM commenced on hormonal contraceptives. The low-dose hormone preparations currently used as oral contraceptives rarely cause glucose intolerance and in most cases glucose metabolism is normal after 6 months of use.[290]

Nonselective β-blocking drugs such as propranolol can exacerbate insulin resistance and impair glucose tolerance[291] and, in combination with drugs such as the thiazides, can lead to loss of glycaemic control in diabetic patients.

$\beta_2$-Agonist drugs such as salbutamol (albuterol) used intravenously to treat premature labour, can promote lipolysis and so increase the substrate for ketone body formation. When given in conjunction with corticosteroids to accelerate fetal lung maturity, they can precipitate ketoacidosis in pregnant diabetic women.

### 12.3 Thyroid Disease

Many nonthyroidal drugs can induce hypothyroidism, hyperthyroidism or abnormal thyroid function test results (see table XIII). Lithium, used to treat bipolar affective disorders, is a common cause of goitrous hypothyroidism. As a monovalent ion, it competes with iodide for thyroid gland uptake and inhibits release of thyroxine, resulting in low serum thyroxine and elevated TSH concentrations.

The antiarrhythmic agent amiodarone may cause complex changes to thyroid status due to its high iodine content (75mg iodine per 200mg tablet). Depending on the individual's state of iodine repleteness or deficiency, amiodarone may cause hypothyroidism or hyperthyroidism. In patients taking the drug, the large iodine load may be sufficient to block thyroxine release as well as its peripheral conversion to tri-iodothyronine. Being lipophilic, amiodarone is redistributed to adipose tissue where it can remain for several months. Hence, hyperthyroidism may manifest several months after cessation of the drug.

Long term therapy with phenytoin can decrease serum thyroxine levels through induction of hepatic enzymes. Serum TSH levels do not usually rise in response to the fall in thyroxine and this may be due to an effect of phenytoin at the pituitary level in blocking the TSH response to TRH. The presence of heparin in the serum can lead to a transient elevation in free thyroxine due to the stimulation of lipoprotein lipase, which leads to higher free fatty acid concentrations in the serum and competition with thyroxine ($T_4$) and tri-iodothyronine ($T_3$) for albumin binding sites,[292] with subsequent elevation of free thyroid hormone levels.

Intravenous furosemide in doses of 80mg or greater can cause a similar transient effect on free thyroid hormone concentrations but TSH is usually normal in this situation. Dopamine (above 1 μg/kg/min), dexamethasone (above 0.5 mg/day) and octreotide (above 100 μg/day) suppress TSH secretion and, in critically ill patients, can produce low free hormone concentrations with low TSH levels, which mimics pituitary insufficiency.[293] Corticosteroids also decrease TBG concentrations and inhibit peripheral deiodination of $T_4$ to $T_3$.[294]

**Table XIII.** Drugs causing abnormal thyroid function tests

| Drug | $FT_4$ | $FT_3$ | TSH | TBG |
|---|---|---|---|---|
| Lithium | ↓ | ↓ | ↑ | ↔ |
| Amiodarone | ↑ | ↑,↔ or ↓ | ↑ or ↓ | ↔ |
| Heparin | ↑ | ↔ | ↔ | ↔ |
| Phenytoin | ↓ | ↔ | ↔ | ↔ |
| Corticosteroids | ↔ | ↓ | ↓ | ↓ |

*Abbreviations and symbols:* $FT_4$ = free thyroxine; $FT_3$ = free tri-iodothyronine; TSH = thyroid-stimulating hormone; TBG = thyroxine-binding globulin; ↑ = increased; ↓ = decreased; ↔ = no change.

### 12.4 Pituitary and Adrenal Function

Synthetic glucocorticoids are used frequently in the treatment of inflammatory, immune and neoplastic disorders. Supraphysiological doses of these steroids can suppress hypothalamic corticotrophin-releasing hormone (CRH) production and pituitary corticotrophin secretion with resulting decreased cortisol secretion and atrophy of the adrenal cortex. The duration of therapy required to produce suppression depends on the dosage and varies with differing rates of steroid metabolism in individuals. Although it may be possible to demonstrate inadequate responses to exogenous corticotrophin for brief periods after stopping the glucocorticoid, clinical adrenal insufficiency is rare in patients treated for less than 3 weeks.[295]

Similarly, suppression is rare in individuals taking less than 10mg of prednisone or its equivalent for any length of time.[296] Patients who have been on pharmacological doses of glucocorticoids for 3 weeks or more can have suppression that may take several months to recover and are at risk of acute adrenal insufficiency if therapy is stopped abruptly.[175] Glucocorticoid doses must therefore be tapered steadily. In patients receiving these agents long term, the withdrawal process may require several weeks to months. During this period, patients require regular observation for signs of cortisol deficiency with provision of supplemental glucocorticoids for times of stress. Patients should be alerted to the possibility of acute adrenal insufficiency during intercurrent illness.

Glucocorticoid doses greater than the daily endogenous cortisol secretion rate can produce all the features of Cushing's syndrome including glucose intolerance, weight gain, muscle wasting and depressive illness. Long term use of systemic glucocorticoids, both oral and inhaled (e.g. in the treatment of asthma), can cause all the features of Cushing's disease as well as arrest of linear growth in children. With high-dose therapy, Cushingoid features may be seen within 4 weeks of starting treatment. Certain features are more common in iatrogenic Cushing's syndrome, including osteoporosis, aggravation of glaucoma, cataract formation and aseptic necrosis of the femoral head.[297] Alternate-day regimens are sometimes used in an attempt to prevent or alleviate Cushingoid adverse effects in patients stable enough to cope without any glucocorticoid for 24 hours. More than twice the usual daily glucocorticoid dose is given on alternate days, avoiding evening doses to prevent suppression of the next morning endogenous cortisol secretion.[296] With this regimen, the exposure time of the HPA axis to the glucocorticoid is reduced and suppression may be less likely.

As discussed in section 7.1.3, ketoconazole inhibits the 11β-hydroxylation step of steroid synthesis[298] and can be used to reduce excess cortisol production in patients with Cushing's disease. It can also lead to adrenal insufficiency in patients with limited reserve taking the drug long term. Patients taking glucocorticoid replacement for pituitary or adrenal insufficiency can become hypoadrenal when they start phenytoin or rifampicin which can induce hepatic metabolism of cortisol. In contrast, oral contraceptives can increase concentrations of corticosteroid-binding globulin, increasing bound hormone and decreasing the rate of steroid elimination from the plasma. A rare but potential cause of drug-induced adrenal failure is haemorrhage into the adrenal glands during anticoagulant therapy with heparin or warfarin.

Elevation of prolactin can be found in asymptomatic individuals taking dopamine antagonists such as phenothiazines. Galactorrhoea and amenorrhoea may occur and persist for several years after medication is stopped (table XIV).

**Table XIV.** Drugs causing hyperprolactinaemia

| |
|---|
| Metoclopramide |
| Chlorpromazine |
| Prochlorperazine |
| Thioridazine |
| Amitriptyline |
| Amphetamines |
| Estrogens |
| Androgens |

### 12.5 Drugs Affecting Dynamic Tests of Endocrine Function

Certain drugs may interfere with the sensitivity and specificity of stimulation and suppression tests of the HPA axis. Pharmacological doses of glucocorticoids, theophylline and chlorpromazine can decrease the growth hormone response to insulin-induced hypoglycaemia during pituitary stimulation testing. Concurrent estrogen therapy may cause an enhanced GH response.

The response of the HPA axis to metyrapone stimulation is reduced in the presence of estrogen and phenytoin. Chronic, excessive ethanol ingestion or phenytoin treatment can increase the metabolism of dexamethasone in dexamethasone suppression testing, providing false positive results. Amphetamines, benzodiazepines and NSAIDs can be associated with normal suppression (i.e. false negative tests) of cortisol concentrations in Cushing's disease (table XV).[298]

Phenytoin may cause a diminished TSH response to TRH[299] as well as reduced thyroxine concentrations due to increased hepatic metabolism. Hence, in patients taking phenytoin, TSH may be an unreliable correlate of a low $T_4$. Other drugs that may influence TSH response are levodopa, dopamine and aspirin.

### 12.6 Sexual and Reproductive Dysfunction

Disorders of sexual and reproductive function may be caused by drugs in the presence of normal hypothalamic and pituitary function. The imidazoles such as ketoconazole and metronidazole and the aldosterone antagonist spironolactone all inhibit testosterone production in the testis. Gynaecomastia may occur in males taking these drugs. Spironolactone also blocks the binding of androgen to its receptor and up to 50% of men receiving spironolactone 150 mg/day develop gynaecomastia.[300] The $H_2$-receptor blocker cimetidine also blocks androgen-receptor binding, producing gynaecomastia (see table XVI) and occasionally impotence. Digoxin can cause gynaecomastia in up to 10% of men after 1 year of treatment due to its weak agonist effect at the estrogen receptor.

Antihypertensive agents, in particular β-blockers and thiazide diuretics, may cause erectile dysfunction. Aside from lowering pressures in the pudendal artery, thiazides may have an effect on smooth muscle relaxation. Centrally-acting sympatholytic drugs such as methyldopa and clonidine may cause erectile difficulties in 30 to 40% of patients.[301] Cimetidine may cause impotence, and digoxin and clofibrate have also been associated with this problem.

Drug-induced infertility, without other endocrine dysfunction, is often due to alkylating agents, in particular, cyclophosphamide. Males treated with this agent in childhood for nephrotic syndrome or as adults for Hodgkins' disease may develop azoospermia as a result of damage to the testicular germinal epithelium. This is more common after cumulative doses of >6 to 10g and spermatogenesis returns within 3 years in about half of patients who develop azoospermia during treatment. Aside from antineoplastic agents, sulfonamide compounds are the only other prescribed drugs reported to cause oligospermia, in particular the anti-inflammatory drug sulfasalazine. Normal spermatogenesis frequently returns on cessation of these drugs. The continued use of androgenic steroids by young men hoping to enhance athletic performance can lead to azoospermia and even irreversible depletion of the germinal epithelium. The mechanism for this depletion is

**Table XV.** Drugs affecting the dexamethasone suppression test

| False positive test | False negative test |
|---|---|
| Phenytoin | Amphetamines |
| Barbiturates | Benzodiazepines |
| Carbamazepine | Nonsteroidal anti-inflammatory drugs |
| Opioids | |
| Alcohol (ethanol) | |
| High-dose estrogen-containing oral contraceptives | |

disruption of the negative feedback loop between the testis and the pituitary, depriving the testis of gonadotrophin stimulation and the high local testosterone concentrations needed for normal spermatogenesis.[302]

The stimulation of male-pattern hair growth in females or hirsutism is an adverse effect of therapeutic doses of phenytoin, glucocorticoids and androgens (used by female athletes).[303] Drugs such as cyclosporin and diazoxide tend to cause hypertrichosis or increased generalised body hair rather than the dark, thick terminal hair seen in androgen-sensitive areas. Minoxidil can also cause hair growth.

### 12.7 Weight Gain

Significant weight gain is a common adverse effect limiting the long term use of many psychoactive agents such as antidepressants, lithium and phenothiazines. It is not uncommon for weight to increase by several kilograms in the course of 1 to 2 years of treatment with antidepressants. The mechanism of weight gain is possibly via antagonism at the serotonin and histamine receptor. Serotonin is implicated as a central (hypothalamic) mediator of appetite and food choice; hence antiserotonergic drugs may stimulate hunger and craving for carbohydrates. This effect is seen in migraine patients on serotonin antagonists such as pizotifen and cyproheptadine. Most currently marketed tricyclic and tetracyclic antidepressants stimulate hunger and cravings for complex carbohydrates and sweets. In addition, their anticholinergic adverse effects of dry mouth and thirst lead to ingestion of large amounts of sweet beverages. The agent most implicated with food craving is amitriptyline, while desipramine and fluoxetine are the least associated with weight gain.[304]

Careful dietary advice before commencing therapy may diminish the extent of the problem and, once established, changing to a different antidepressant will frequently halt the increase in weight. Being essentially devoid of antihistaminic and anticholinergic activity, fluoxetine has been reported to facilitate weight loss through decreasing appetite and carbohydrate craving. However, the larger dosage required for this effect (40 to 60 mg/day) compared with the antidepressant dose (20 mg/day) may cause symptoms of anxiety and insomnia. Patients with bipolar affective disorders treated with lithium can experience increased hunger and weight gain, and this is compounded by fluid retention. Long term use of psychotropic drugs can produce weight gain by similar mechanisms to those of tricyclic antidepressants. The drugs causing most weight gain are the phenothiazines chlorpromazine and thioridazine, while the least implicated is the butyrophenone haloperidol.

Increased abdominal adiposity is a well recognised adverse effect of long term glucocorticoid treatment. The anabolic effect of testosterone replacement in hypogonadal males produces weight gain due to increased lean body mass.

### 12.8 Bone and Mineral Metabolism

Drugs in common usage such as glucocorticoids, thyroxine and heparin may cause or exacerbate osteoporosis when used long term, increasing the incidence of fractures and, hence, adding to the morbidity and cost of this common condition to the community. Osteoporosis-related fractures occur in 30 to 50% of patients who receive glucocorticoids. The most rapid loss of skeletal mass often occurs in the first 6 months of therapy. Several mechanisms are likely and include reduced intestinal calcium absorption, increased urinary calcium excretion, and inhibition of osteoblasts. Strategies to prevent glucocorticoid-induced osteoporosis include estrogen replacement therapy in postmenopausal women to help reduce and delay bone loss.[305] Calcium supplements should be recommended and cholecalciferol (vitamin $D_3$) supplementation may be used if serum 25-hydroxycholecalciferol concentrations are low. If hypercalciuria is present, a thiazide diuretic may correct the loss of calcium.

**Table XVI.** Drugs causing gynaecomastia

| | |
|---|---|
| Ketoconazole | Busulfan |
| Metronidazole | Methyldopa |
| Spironolactone | Isoniazid |
| Cimetidine | Tricyclic antidepressants |
| Digoxin | Penicillamine |
| Cyproterone | Captopril |
| Flutamide | Calcium antagonists |

**Table XVII.** Drugs influencing serum calcium concentrations

| Hypercalcaemia | Hypocalcaemia |
|---|---|
| Cholecalciferol (vitamin $D_3$) | Bisphosphonates |
| Thiazides | Corticosteroids |
| Lithium | Cisplatin |
| Tamoxifen | Antiepileptics |

Excessive thyroxine dosage can lead to osteoporosis through stimulation of bone remodelling units.[306,307] Long term heparin therapy is associated with loss of bone mass, possibly through potentiation of parathyroid hormone action. No similar reduction in bone density is seen with warfarin therapy.[308]

Hypercalcaemia with consequent nephrocalcinosis and renal failure can result from excessive doses of cholecalciferol used to treat hypoparathyroidism and renal osteodystrophy (table XVII). Due to its long half-life, cholecalciferol intoxication may persist for months. However, cessation of the drug and treatment with glucocorticoids will lower serum calcium in most patients. Thiazides may also cause hypercalcaemia since unlike other natriuretic agents, they increase renal tubular calcium resorption. In addition, thiazides may potentiate parathyroid hormone effects as well as having a direct effect on bone. If hypercalcaemia is noted during thiazide therapy, the drug should be discontinued before a more extensive search for the cause.

Calcium-lowering agents such as the bisphosphonates, calcitonin and plicamycin (mithramycin) are discussed in section 6.2. Rarely, hypocalcaemia is also seen in patients receiving high-dose glucocorticoids and prolonged antiepileptic drug therapy. The antineoplastic agent cisplatin causes renal tubular damage that can impair calcium resorption and lead to hypocalcaemia.

### 12.9 Extracellular Fluid Balance

Diabetes insipidus may occur as an adverse effect of lithium, demeclocycline and methoxyflurane general anaesthesia. Lithium, in serum concentrations within the therapeutic range for bipolar affective disorders (0.5 to 1.5 mmol/L), can cause antidiuretic hormone (ADH)-resistant diabetes insipidus in 12 to 30% of patients. Cessation of lithium will usually return the urine concentrating capacity to normal.[309]

Demeclocycline, which is occasionally used in treatment of the syndrome of inappropriate ADH (SIADH), causes a reversible nephrogenic diabetes insipidus by inhibiting the action of ADH at the distal renal tubule. The antidiabetic agent chlorpropamide exerts an ADH-like action at the distal tubule and, along with the thiazides, clofibrate, carbamazepine and oxcarbazepine, may contribute to a dilutional hyponatraemia.

## References


1. Randle PJ, Garland PB, Hales CN, et al. The glucose-fatty acid cycle: its role in insulin sensitivity and the metabolic disturbances of diabetes mellitus. Lancet 1963; 1: 785-9
2. Reaven GM. Role of insulin resistance in human disease (syndrome X): an expanded definition. Annual Review of Medicine 1993; 44: 121-31
3. Gwilt PR, Nahhas RR, Tracewell WG. The effects of diabetes mellitus on pharmacokinetics and pharmacodynamics in humans. Clinical Pharmacokinetics 1991; 20: 477-90
4. Bechtel YC, Joanne C, Grandmottet M, et al. The influence of insulin-dependent diabetes on the metabolism of caffeine and the expression of the debrisoquin oxidation phenotype. Clinical Pharmacology and Therapeutics 1988; 44: 408-17
5. Mrozikiewicz RM, Drakoulis N, Roots I. Polymorphic arylamine N-acetyltransferase (NAT2) genes in children with insulin-dependent diabetes mellitus. Clinical Pharmacology and Therapeutics 1994; 56: 626-34
6. Dajani RM, Kayyali S, Saheb SE, et al. A study of the physiological disposition of acetophenetidin by the diabetic man. Comparative General Pharmacology 1974; 5: 1
7. Kamali F, Thomas SHL, Ferner RE. Paracetamol elimination in patients with non-insulin dependent diabetes mellitus. British Journal of Clinical Pharmacology 1993; 35: 58-61
8. Korrapati MR, Vestal RE, Cho-Ming L. Theophylline metabolism in healthy nonsmokers and in patients with insulin-dependent diabetes mellitus. Clinical Pharmacology and Therapeutics 1995; 57: 413-8
9. Ruiz-Cabello F, Erill S. Abnormal serum protein binding of acidic drugs in diabetes mellitus. Clinical Pharmacology and Therapeutics 1984; 36: 691
10. Barry MG, Collins WJC, Feely J. Plasma protein binding of drugs in insulin-dependent diabetes mellitus. British Journal of Pharmacology 1986; 89: 719
11. O'Byrne S, Barry MG, Collins WCJ, et al. Plasma protein binding of lidocaine and warfarin in insulin-dependent and non-insulin-dependent diabetes mellitus. Clinical Pharmacokinetics 1993; 24: 183-6
12. Madacsy L, Bokor M, Matusovits L. Penicillin clearance in diabetic children. Acta Paediatrica Academiae Scient-Hungaricae 1975; 16: 139
13. Madacsy L, Bokor M, Kozocsa G. Carbenicillin half-life in children with early diabetes mellitus. International Journal of Clinical Pharmacology and Biopharmacy 1976; 14: 155
14. Garcia G, de Vidal EL, Trujilio H. Serum levels and urinary concentrations of kanamycin, bekanamycin and amikacin (BB-KS) in diabetic children and a control group. Journal of International Medical Research 1977; 5: 322
15. Lerner PI, Weinstein L. Abnormalities of absorption of benzylpenicillin G and sulfisoxazole in patients with

diabetes mellitus. American Journal of the Medical Sciences 1964; 248: 37

16. Weinstein L, Meade RH. Absorption and excretion of penicillin injected into the muscles of patients with diabetes mellitus. Nature 1961; 192: 987
17. Shenfield GM. Influence of thyroid dysfunction on drug pharmacokinetics. Clinical Pharmacokinetics 1981; 6: 275
18. Huffman DH, Klaassen CD, Harman CR. Digoxin in hyperthyroidism. Clinical Pharmacology and Therapeutics 1977; 22: 533
19. Bell JM, Russell C, Nelson JK, et al. Studies of the effect of thyroid dysfunction on the elimination of β-adrenoceptor blocking drugs. British Journal of Clinical Pharmacology 1977; 4: 79
20. Forfar JC, Pottage A, Toft AD, et al. Paracetamol pharmacokinetics in thyroid disease. European Journal of Clinical Pharmacology 1980; 18: 269
21. Levesque H, Richard MO, Fresel J, et al. Evolution of atenolol pharmacokinetics when hypothyroidism is corrected. European Journal of Clinical Pharmacology 1990; 38: 185-8
22. Crooks J, Hedley SJ, Macnee C, et al. Changes in drug metabolising ability in thyroid disease. British Journal of Pharmacology 1973; 49: 156P
23. Eichelbaum M. Drug metabolism in thyroid disease. Clinical Pharmacokinetics 1976; 1: 339
24. Varadi A, Foldes J. Serum digoxin in patients with thyroid disease. British Medical Journal 1976; 175
25. Scott AK, Khir ASM, Bewsher PD, et al. Oxazepam pharmacokinetics in thyroid disease. British Journal of Clinical Pharmacology 1984; 17: 49
26. Sonne J, Boesgaard S, Enghusen Poulsen H, et al. Pharmacokinetics and pharmacodynamics of oxazepam and metabolism of paracetamol in severe hypothyroidism. British Journal of Clinical Pharmacology 1990; 30: 737-42
27. Ochs H, Greenblatt DJ, Kaschell H, et al. Diazepam kinetics in patients with renal insufficiency or hyperthyroidism. British Journal of Clinical Pharmacology 1981; 12: 829
28. Hansen JM, Skovsted J, Lumholtz BI, et al. Unaltered metabolism of phenytoin in thyroid disorders. Acta Pharmacologica et Toxicologica 1978; 42: 343
29. Cooper DS, Halpern R, Wood LC, et al. L-thyroxine therapy in subclinical hypothyroidism: a double blind, placebo-controlled trial. Annals of Internal Medicine 1984; 101: 18
30. Feely J, Peden N. Use of β-adrenoceptor blocking drugs in hyperthyroidism. Drugs 1984; 27: 425
31. O'Connor P, Feely J. Clinical pharmacokinetics and endocrine disorders: therapeutic implications. Clinical Pharmacokinetics 1987; 13: 345-64
32. Wells PG, Feely J, Nadeau J, et al. Effect of thyrotoxicosis on liver blood flow and propranolol disposition after long term dosing. Clinical Pharmacology and Therapeutics 1983; 33: 603
33. Feely J. Clinical pharmacokinetics of β-adrenoceptor blocking drugs in thyroid disease. Clinical Pharmacokinetics 1983; 8: 1
34. Nilsson OR, Melander A, Tedler L. Effects and plasma levels or propranolol and metoprolol in hyperthyroid patients. European Journal of Clinical Pharmacology 1980; 18: 315
35. Feely J, Forrest AL, Gunn A, et al. Beta-blocking drugs and thyroid function. British Medical Journal 1977; 4: 1352
36. Elfstrom J. Drug pharmacokinetics in the postoperative period. Clinical Pharmacokinetics 1979; 4: 16
37. Feely J, Stevenson IH, Crooks J. Altered plasma protein binding of drugs in thyroid disease. Clinical Pharmacokinetics 1981; 6: 298
38. Bradley SE, Stephen F, Coelho JB, et al. The thyroid and the kidney. Kidney International 1974; 6: 346
39. Aro A, Antilla M, Korhonen T, et al. Pharmacokinetics of propranolol and sotalol in hyperthyroidism. European Journal of Clinical Pharmacology 1982; 21: 373
40. Doherty JE, Perkins WH. Digoxin metabolism in hypo- and hyperthyroidism: studies with tritiated digoxin in thyroid disease. Annals of Internal Medicine 1966; 46: 489
41. Morrow DH, Gaffney TE, Braunwald E. Studies on digitalis. VII. Influence of hyper- and hypothyroidism on the myocardial response to ouabain. Journal of Pharmacology and Experimental Therapeutics 1963; 140: 324
42. Englebienne P. The steroid transport proteins: biochemistry and clinical significance. Molecular Aspects of Medicine 1984; 7: 313-9
43. Shenfield GM, Thompson J, Horn DB. Plasma and urinary digoxin in thyroid dysfunction. European Journal of Clinical Pharmacology 1977; 12: 437
44. Bonelli J, Haydl H, Hruby K, et al. The pharmacokinetics of digoxin in patients with manifest hyperthyroidism and after normalisation of thyroid function. International Journal of Clinical Pharmacology and Therapeutics 1978; 16: 302
45. Croxson MS, Ibbertson HK. Serum digoxin in patients with thyroid disease. British Medical Journal 1975; 3: 566
46. Frey FJ, Horber FF, Frey BM. Altered metabolism and decreased efficacy of prednisolone and prednisone in patients with hyperthyroidism. Clinical Pharmacology and Therapeutics 1988; 44: 510-21
47. Abernethy DR, Greenblatt DJ. Pharmacokinetics of drugs in obesity. Clinical Pharmacokinetics 1982; 7: 108
48. Cheymol G. Clinical pharmacokinetics of drugs in obesity: an update. Clinical Pharmacokinetics 1993; 25: 103-14
49. Abernethy DR, Greenblatt DJ. Drug disposition in obese humans: an update. Clinical Pharmacokinetics 1986; 11: 199
50. Abernethy DR, Todd EL, Schwartz JB. Caffeine disposition in obesity. British Journal of Clinical Pharmacology 1985; 20: 61
51. Benedek IH, Fiske WD, Griffen WO, et al. Serum $\alpha_1$-acid glycoprotein and binding of drugs in obesity. British Journal of Clinical Pharmacology 1983; 16: 751
52. Gal P, Juski WJ, Yurchak AM, et al. Theophylline disposition in obesity. Clinical Pharmacology and Therapeutics 1978; 23: 438
53. Saraiva RA, Lunn JN, Mapleson WW, et al. Adiposity and the pharmacokinetics of halothane: the effect of adiposity of the maintenance of and recovery from halothane anaesthesia. Anaesthesia 1977; 32: 240
54. Young SR, Stoetling RK, Peterson C, et al. Anesthetic biotransformation and renal function in obese patients during and after methoxyflurane or halothane anesthesia. Anesthesiology 1975; 42: 451
55. Ewy GA, Groves BM, Ball MF, et al. Digoxin metabolism in obesity. Circulation 1971; 44: 810

56. Hull JH, Sarubbi FA. Gentamicin serum concentrations: pharmacokinetic predictions. Annals of Internal Medicine 1976; 85: 183
57. Schwartz SN, Pazin GJ, Lyon JA, et al. A controlled investigation of the pharmacokinetics of gentamicin and tobramycin in obese subjects. Journal of Infectious Diseases 1978; 138: 499
58. Bauer LA, Wareing-Tran C, Edwards WAD, et al. Cimetidine clearance in the obese. Clinical Pharmacology and Therapeutics 1985; 37: 425
59. Reiss RA, Haas CE, Karki SD, et al. Lithium pharmacokinetics in the obese. Clinical Pharmacology and Therapeutics 1994; 55: 392-8
60. Reidenberg MM. Obesity and fasting-effects on drug metabolism and drug action in man. Clinical Pharmacology and Therapeutics 1977; 22: 729
61. Milsap RL, Pliasance KI, Jusko WJ. Prednisolone disposition in obese man. Clinical Pharmacology and Therapeutics 1984; 36: 824
62. Dunne TE, Ludwig EA, Slaughter RL, et al. Pharmacokinetics and pharmacodynamics of methylprednisolone in obesity. Clinical Pharmacology and Therapeutics 1991; 49: 536-49
63. Johansson EDB, Kral JG. Oral contraceptives after intestinal bypass operations. Journal of the American Medical Association 1976; 236: 2847
64. Marcus FI, Horton H, Jacobs S, et al. The effect of jejunoileal bypass in patients with morbid obesity on the pharmacokinetics of digoxin in man. Cardiology 1976; 37: 154
65. Rifkind AB, Saenger P, Levine LS, et al. Effects of growth hormone on antipyrine kinetics in children. Clinical Pharmacology and Therapeutics 1981; 30: 127
66. Aarbakke J, Bending MR, Davies DS. Increased oxidation of phenylbutazone during hydrocortisone infusion in man. British Journal of Clinical Pharmacology 1977; 4: 621
67. Shively CA, Gagliardi CL, Hartshorn RD, et al. Failure of hydrocortisone to alter acutely antipyrine disposition. Clinical Pharmacology and Therapeutics 1977; 23: 408
68. Karvonen M, Tuomilehto J, Libman I, et al. A review of the recent epidemiological data on the worldwide incidence of type 1 (insulin-dependent) diabetes mellitus. World Health Organization DIAMOND Project Group. Diabetologia 1993; 36: 883-92
69. Stenman S, Melander A, Groop P-H, et al. What is the benefit of increasing the sulfonylurea dose? Annals of Internal Medicine 1993; 118: 169
70. University Group Diabetes Program. A study of the effects of hypoglycemic agents on vascular complications in patients with adult-onset diabetes. Diabetes 1970; 19 (Suppl. 2): 747
71. University Group Diabetes Program. A study of the effects of hypoglycemic agents on vascular complications in patients with adult onset diabetes. VI. Supplementary reports on nonfatal events in patients treated with tolbutamide. Diabetes 1976; 25: 1129
72. Tucker GT, Casey C, Phillips PJ, et al. Metformin kinetics in healthy subjects and in patients with diabetes mellitus. British Journal of Clinical Pharmacology 1981; 12: 235
73. Nelleman Jorgensen L, Dejgaard A, Pramming SK. Human insulin and hypoglycaemia: a literature survey. Diabetic Medicine 1994; 11: 925
74. Everett J, Kerr D. Changing from porcine to human insulin. Drugs 1994; 47: 286-96
75. Vignati L, Anderson J, Brunelle R. Efficacy of [Lys(B28), Pro(B29)] human insulin in a one year global randomized clinical trial [abstract]. Diabetes 1994; 43: 78a
76. UK Prospective Diabetes Study Group. UK Prospective Diabetes Study (UKPDS). VIII. Study design, progress and performance. Diabetologia 1991; 34: 877
77. Abraira C, Emanuele N, Colwell J, et al. Glycaemic control and complications in type II diabetes: design of a feasibility trial. Diabetes Care 1992; 15: 1560
78. Lebovitz HE. Sulphonylureas: basic aspects and clinical uses. In: Alberti K, De Fronzo R, Keen H, et al. editors. International textbook of diabetes mellitus. Chichester: John Wiley & Sons, 1992
79. Clissold SP, Edwards C. Acarbose: a preliminary review of its pharmacodynamic and pharmacokinetic properties and therapeutic potential. Drugs 1988; 35: 214
80. Balfour JA, McTavish D. Acarbose: an update of its pharmacology and therapeutic use in diabetes mellitus. Drugs 1993; 46: 1025-54
81. Coniff R. Results of US trials with acarbose in the treatment of NIDDM. FDA Application, 1991
82. Hanefeld M, Fischer S, Schulze J, et al. Therapeutic potentials of acarbose as first-line drug in NIDDM insufficiently treated with diet alone. Diabetes Care 1991; 14: 732
83. Willey KA, Molyneaux LM, et al. The effects of dexfenfluramine on blood glucose control in patients with type 2 diabetes. Diabetic Medicine 1992; 9: 341-3
84. Willey KA, Molyneaux LM, Yue DK. Obese patients type 2 diabetes poorly controlled by insulin and metformin: effects of adjunctive dexfenfluramine therapy on glycaemic control. Diabetic Medicine 1994; 11: 701
85. Donnelly R, Morris AD. Drugs and insulin resistance: clinical methods of evaluation and new pharmacological approaches to metabolism. British Journal of Clinical Pharmacology 1994; 37: 311
86. DCCT Research Group. Epidemiology of severe hypoglycaemia in the Diabetes Complications and Control Trial. American Journal of Medicine 1991; 90: 450
87. Diabetes Control and Complications Trial Research Group. The effect of intensive treatment of diabetes on the development and progression of long-term complications in insulin-dependent diabetes mellitus. New England Journal of Medicine 1993; 329: 977
88. Greene DA, Lattimer SA, Sima AAF. Sorbitol, phosphoinositides and the sodium-potassium ATPase in the pathogenesis of diabetic complications. New England Journal of Medicine 1987; 316: 599
89. Macleod A, Sonksen P. The effect of the aldose reductase inhibitor tolrestat on diabetic polyneuropathy: a meta-analysis. Diabetes 1991; 40 Suppl. 1: 555a
90. Sima AAF, Greene DA, Brown MB, et al. Effect of hyperglycaemia and the aldose reductase inhibitor tolrestat on sural nerve biochemistry and morphometry in advanced diabetic peripheral polyneuropathy. Journal of Diabetes and its Complications 1993; 7: 157
91. Boulton AJ, Levin S, Comstock J. A multicentre trial of the aldose-reductase inhibitor, tolrestat, in patients with symptomatic diabetic neuropathy. Diabetologia 1990; 33: 431
92. Keen H, Payan J, Allawi J, et al. Treatment of diabetic neuropathy with linolenic acid. Diabetes Care 1993; 16: 8

93. Max MB, Lynch SA, Muir J, et al. Effects of desipramine, amitriptyline, and fluoxetine on pain in diabetic neuropathy. New England Journal of Medicine 1992; 326: 1250
94. Stracke H, Meyer U, Schumacher HE, et al. Mexiletine in the treatment of diabetic neuropathy. Diabetes Care 1992; 15: 1550
95. Tandan R, Lewis GA, Krusinski PB, et al. Topical capsaicin in painful diabetic neuropathy. Diabetes Care 1988; 15: 8
96. Newman LG, Waller J, Palestro CJ, et al. Unsuspected osteomyelitis in diabetic foot ulcers: diagnosis and monitoring by leukocyte scanning with indium in 111 oxyquinoline. Journal of the American Medical Association 1991; 266: 1246
97. Reaven GM. Banting lecture: role of insulin resistance in human disease. Diabetes 1988; 37: 1595
98. Joint National Committee on Detection, Evaluation and Treatment of High Blood Pressure. The fifth report of the Joint National Committee on Detection, Evaluation and Treatment of High Blood Pressure (JNC V). Archives of Internal Medicine 1993; 153: 154
99. Tarnow L, Rossing P, Gall MA, et al. Prevalence of arterial hypertension in diabetic patients before and after the JNC V. Diabetes Care 1994; 17: 1247
100. Lewis EJ, Hunsicker LG, Bain RP, et al. The effect of angiotensin-converting-enzyme inhibition on diabetic nephropathy. New England Journal of Medicine 1993; 329: 1456
101. Kasiske BL, Kalil RS, Ma JZ, et al. Effect of antihypertensive therapy on the kidney in patients with diabetes: a meta-regression analysis. Annals of Internal Medicine 1993; 118: 129
102. Ravid M, Savin H, Jutrin I, et al. Long-term stabilizing effect of angiotensin-converting enzyme inhibition on plasma creatinine and on proteinuria in normotensive type II diabetic patients. Annals of Internal Medicine 1993; 118: 577
103. Herings RMC, de Boer A, Stricker BH, et al. Hypoglycaemia associated with use of inhibitors of angiotensin converting enzyme. Lancet 1995; 345: 1195
104. Feher MD, Amiel S. ACE inhibitors and hypoglycaemia. Lancet 1995; 346: 125
105. Beling S, Vukovich RA, Neiss ES, et al. Long term experience with indapamide. American Heart Journal 1983; 106: 258
106. Raggi U, Palumbo P, Mero B, et al. Indapamide in the treatment of hypertension in non-insulin dependent diabetes. Hypertension 1985; 7: 157
107. Stamler J, Vaccaro O, Neaton JD, et al. Diabetes, other risk factors and 12-yr cardiovascular mortality for men screened in the Multiple Risk Factor Intervention Trial. Diabetes Care 1993; 16: 434-44
108. Frick MH, Heinonen OP, Huttunen JK, et al. Efficacy of gemfibrozil in dyslipidaemic subjects with suspected heart disease: an ancillary study in the Helsinki Heart Study frame population. Annals of Medicine 1993; 25: 41
109. Phillipson BE, Rothrock DW, Connor WE, et al. Reduction of plasma lipids, lipoproteins and apoproteins by dietary fish oils in patients with hypertriglyceridemia. New England Journal of Medicine 1985; 312: 1210
110. Koev D, Zlateva S, Susuc M, et al. Improvement of lipoprotein lipid composition in type II diabetic patients with concomitant hyperlipoproteinaemia by acipimox treatment. Results of a multicentre trial. Diabetes Care 1993; 16: 1285
111. Grundy SM. HMG-CoA reductase inhibitors for treatment of hypercholesterolaemia. New England Journal of Medicine 1988; 319: 24
112. Wang P, Lau J, Chalmers T. Meta-analysis of intensive blood glucose control on late complications of type I diabetes. Lancet 1993; 341: 1306
113. Hodge AM, Zimmet PZ. The epidemiology of obesity. Clinical Endocrinology and Metabolism 1994; 8: 577-99
114. Black D, James WPT, et al. Obesity: a report of the Royal College of Physicians. Journal of the Royal College of Physicians of London 1983; 17: 5-65
115. NIH Consensus Panel. Health implications of obesity. Annals of Internal Medicine 1985; 103: 1073-7
116. Pi-Sunyer X. Medical hazards of obesity. Annals of Internal Medicine 1993; 119: 655-60
117. Grunstein RR, Wilcox I. Sleep-disordered breathing and obesity. Clinical Endocrinology and Metabolism 1994; 8: 601-28
118. Vague J. La differenciation sexuelle, facteur determinant des formes de l'obesite. Presse Medicale 1947; 30: 339-40
119. Despres JP. Dyslipidaemia and obesity. Clinical Endocrinology and Metabolism 1994; 8: 629-60
120. Report of the Task Force on the Treatment of Obesity. Health Services and Promotion Branch, Health and Welfare Canada, 1991
121. Stunkard AJ, Sorenson TI, Hanis C, et al. An adoption study of human obesity. New England Journal of Medicine 1986; 314: 193-8
122. Bouchard C, Despres J-P, et al. Genetic and non-genetic determinants of regional fat distribution. Endocrine Reviews 1993; 14: 72-93
123. Zhang Y, Proenca R. Positional cloning of the mouse obesity gene and its human homologue. Nature 1994; 372: 425-31
124. Bjorvell H, Rossner S. A ten-year follow-up of weight change in severely obese subjects treated in a combined behavioural modification programme. International Journal of Obesity 1992; 16: 623-5
125. Bray GA, Gray DS. Treatment of obesity: an overview. Diabetes Metabolism Reviews 1988; 4: 653-79
126. Caterson ID. Management strategies for weight control: eating, exercise and behaviour modification. Drugs 1990; 39 Suppl. 3: 20-32
127. Dyer RG. Traditional treatment of obesity: does it work? Clinical Endocrinology and Metabolism 1994; 8: 661-88
128. Despres JP, Lamarche B. Effects of diet and physical activity on adiposity and body fat distribution: implications for the prevention of cardiovascular disease. Nutrition Research 1993; 6: 137-59
129. Richman RM, Steinbeck KS, et al. Severe obesity: the use of very low energy diets or standard kilojoule restriction. Medical Journal of Australia 1992; 156: 768-70
130. Scheen AJ, Desaive C. Therapy for obesity - today and tomorrow. Clinical Endocrinology and Metabolism 1994; 8: 705-27
131. Greenaway TM, Caterson ID. Anorexiants - weighed carefully. Current Therapeutics 1989; 30: 55-69
132. Guy-Grand B, Crepaldi G, Lefebvre P, et al. International trial of long-term dexfenfluramine in obesity. Lancet 1989; 2: 1142-5
133. O'Connor HT, Richman RM, Steinbeck KS, et al. Dexfenfluramine treatment of obesity: a double blind trial with post trial follow up. International Journal of Obesity 1995; 19: 181-9

134. Kolanowski J, Younis LT, et al. Effect of dexfenfluramine treatment on body weight, blood pressure and noradrenergic activity in obese hypertensive patients. European Journal of Clinical Pharmacology 1992; 42: 599-606
135. Weintraub M, Hasday JD, et al. A double blind clinical trial in weight control: use of fenfluramine and phentermine alone and in combination. Archives of Internal Medicine 1984; 114: 1143
136. Boyages SC, Cheung NW. Goitre in Australia. Medical Journal of Australia 1996; 162: 488-9
137. Boyages SC. Iodine deficiency disorders. Journal of Clinical Endocrinology and Metabolism 1993; 77: 587
138. Toft AD. Thyroxine therapy. New England Journal of Medicine 1994; 331: 174-80
139. Wenzel KW, Kirschsieper HE. Aspects of the absorption or oral L-thyroxine in normal man. Metabolism: Clinical and Experimental 1977; 26: 1
140. Pittman CS, Chambers Jr JB, Read VH. The extrathyroidal conversion rate of thyroxine to triiodothyronine in normal man. Journal of Clinical Investigation 1971; 50: 1187
141. Vulsma T, Gons MH, de Vijlder JJM. Maternal-fetal transfer of thyroxine in congenital hypothyroidism due to a total organification defect or thyroid agenesis. New England Journal of Medicine 1989; 321: 13
142. Sack J, et al. Maternal-fetal transfer of thyroxine. New England Journal of Medicine 1989; 321: 1549
143. Nystrom E, Caidahl K, Fager G, et al. A double blind, cross-over 12 month study of L-thyroxine treatment of women with 'subclinical' hypothyroidism. Clinical Endocrinology 1988; 29: 63
144. Smerdely P, Lim A, Boyages SC, et al. Topical iodine antiseptics cause hypothyroidism in very low birthweight infants. Lancet 1989; 2: 661
145. Matsumoto A, Sandblom RE, Schoene RB, et al. Testosterone replacement in hypogonadal men: effects on obstructive sleep apnea, respiratory drives and sleep. Clinical Endocrinology 1985; 22: 713
146. Matsuura N, Yamada Y, Nohara Y, et al. Familial neonatal transient hypothyroidism due to maternal TSH-binding inhibitor immunoglobulins. New England Journal of Medicine 1980; 303: 738
147. Mandel SJ, Larsen PR, Seely EW, et al. Increased need for thyroxine during pregnancy in women with primary hypothyroidism. New England Journal of Medicine 1990; 323: 91
148. Gharib H, James EM, Charboneau JW, et al. Suppressive therapy with levothyroxine for solitary thyroid nodules: a double blind controlled clinical study. New England Journal of Medicine 1987; 317: 70
149. Mazzaferri E. Management of a solitary thyroid nodule. New England Journal of Medicine 1993; 328: 553
150. Boyages SC. Pediatric primary hypothyroidism and endemic cretinism. In: Bardin W, editor. Current therapy of endocrinology and metabolism. St Louis: Mosby - Year Book, 1994: 94-8
151. Smerdely P, Pitsiavis V, Boyages SC. Methimazole inhibits FRTL5 thyroid cell proliferation by inducing S-phase arrest of the cell cycle. Endocrinology 1993; 133: 2403
152. Kampmann JP, Hansen JEM. Clinical pharmacokinetics of antithyroid drugs. Clinical Pharmacokinetics 1981; 6: 401
153. Franklyn JA. The management of hyperthyroidism. New England Journal of Medicine 1994; 330: 1731
154. Mashio Y, Beniko M, Ikota A, et al. Treatment of hyperthyroidism with a small single daily dose of methimazole. Acta Endocrinologica 1988; 119: 139
155. Brownlie BEW. Thyrotoxicosis. In: Speight T, Sutherland J, editors. New Ethicals disease index, 4th ed. Auckland: Adis International 1995: 159-62
156. Tamai H, Nakagawa T, Fukino O, et al. Thionamide therapy in Graves' disease: relation of relapse rate to duration of therapy. Annals of Internal Medicine 1980; 92: 448
157. Hashizume K, Ichikawa K, Sakurai A, et al. Administration of thyroxine in treated Graves' disease: effects on the level of antibodies to thyroid stimulating hormone receptors and on the risk of recurrence of hyperthyroidism. New England Journal of Medicine 1991; 324: 947
158. Bartalena L, Brogioni S, Grasso L, et al. Interleukin-6: a marker of thyroid-destructive processes? Journal of Clinical Endocrinology and Metabolism 1994; 79: 1424
159. Momotani N, Noh J, Oyanagi H, et al. Antithyroid drug therapy for Graves' disease during pregnancy: optimal regimen for fetal thyroid status. New England Journal of Medicine 1986; 315: 24
160. NIH Conference. Diagnosis and management of asymptomatic primary hyperparathyroidism: consensus development conference statement. Annals of Internal Medicine 1991; 114: 593
161. Harrison BJ, Wheeler MH. Asymptomatic primary hyperparathyroidism. World Journal of Surgery 1990; 15: 724
162. Horowitz M, Wishart JM, Need AG, et al. Primary hyperparathyroidism. Clinical Geriatric Medicine 1994; 10: 757
163. Mollerup CL, Bollerslev J, Blichert-Toft M. Primary hyperparathyroidism: incidence and clinical and biochemical characteristics: a demographic study. European Journal of Surgery 1994; 160: 485
164. Bilezikian JP. Clinical review 51: management of hypercalcemia. Journal of Clinical Endocrinology and Metabolism 1993; 77: 1445
165. Halabe A, Arie R, Mimran D, et al. Hypoparathyroidism - a long-term follow-up experience with 1$\alpha$-vitamin D3 therapy. Clinical Endocrinology 1994; 40: 303
166. Smith DF, Toft DO. Steroid receptors and their associated proteins. Molecular Endocrinology 1993; 7: 4-11
167. Bowes SB, Benn JJ, Scobie, et al. Glucose metabolism in patients with Cushing's syndrome. Clinical Endocrinology 1991; 34: 311-6
168. Hromadova M. The role of hormones in the regulation of lipoprotein metabolism. Endocrinologia Experimentalis 1985; 19: 318-30
169. Gennari C. Glucocorticoid induced osteoporosis. Clinical Endocrinology 1994; 41: 273-4
170. Chong PKK, Jung RT, Scrimgeour CM, et al. The effect of pharmacological dosages of glucocorticoids on free living total energy expenditure. Clinical Endocrinology 1994; 40: 577-81
171. Piper JM, Ray WA, Daugherty JR, et al. Corticosteroid use and peptic ulcer disease. Annals of Internal Medicine 1991; 114: 735-40
172. Boumpas DT, Chrousos GP, Wilder RL, et al. Glucocorticoid therapy for immune-mediated diseases: basic and clinical correlates. Annals of Internal Medicine 1993; 119: 1198-208
173. Dayneka NL, Garg V, Jusko WJ, et al. Comparison of four basic models of indirect pharmacodynamic re-

sponses. Journal of Pharmacokinetics and Biopharmaceutics 1993; 21: 457-78

174. Jusko WJ. Receptor mediated pharmacodynamics of corticosteroids. Progress in Clinical and Biological Research 1994; 387: 261-70
175. Helfer E, Rose LJ. Corticosteroids and adrenal suppression: characterising and avoiding the problem. Drugs 1989; 38: 838
176. Esteban NV, Loughlin T, Yergey AL, et al. Daily cortisol production rate in man determined by stable isotope dilution/mass spectrometry. Journal of Clinical Endocrinology and Metabolism 1991; 71: 39-45
177. Heazelwood VJ, Galligan JP, Cannell GR, et al. Plasma cortisol delivery from oral cortisol and cortisone acetate: relative bioavailability. British Journal of Clinical Pharmacology 1984; 17: 55-9
178. Frey BM, Frey FJ. Clinical pharmacokinetics of prednisone and prednisolone. Clinical Pharmacokinetics 1990; 19: 126-46
179. Dhuly RG, Newmark SR, Lauler DP, et al. Pharmacology and chemistry of adrenal glucocorticoids. In: Azarnoff D, editor. Steroid Therapy. Philadelphia: W.B. Saunders, 1975: 1
180. Escher G, Frey FJ, Frey BM. 11β-Hydroxy steroid dehydrogenase accounts for low prednisolone/prednisone ratios in the kidney. Endocrinology 1994; 135: 101-6
181. Meffin PJ, Brooks PM, Sallusto BC. Alterations in prednisolone disposition as a result of administration, gender and dose. British Journal of Clinical Pharmacology 1984; 17: 395-404
182. Bertoni M, Brugnolo F, Bertone E, et al. Long term efficacy of high dose intravenous methyprednisolone pulses in active lupus nephritis. A 21 month prospective study. Scandinavian Journal of Rheumatology 1994; 23: 82-6
183. Hachulla E, Saile R, Parra HJ, et al. Serum amyloid A concentrations in giant-cell arteritis and polymyalgia rheumatica. Clinical and Experimental Rheumatology 1991; 9: 157-63
184. McEnery PT, Gonzalez LL, Martin LW. Growth and development of children with renal transplants. Use of alternate day steroid therapy. Journal of Paediatrics and Child Health 1973; 83: 806-14
185. Fitzsimons R, Grammer LC, Halwig JM, et al. Prevalence of adverse effects in corticosteroid dependent asthmatics. New England and Regional Allergy Proceedings 1988; 9: 157-62
186. Kawai S, Ichikawa Y, Homma M. Differences in metabolic properties among cortisol, prednisolone and dexamethasone in liver and renal diseases; accelerated metabolism of dexamethasone in renal failure. Journal of Clinical Endocrinology and Metabolism 1985; 60: 848-54
187. Markham A, Bryson HM. Deflazacort: a review of its pharmacological properties and therapeutic efficacy. Drugs 1995; 50: 317-33
188. Rayburn WF. Glucocorticoid therapy for rheumatic diseases: maternal, fetal and breast-feeding considerations. American Journal of Reproductive Immunology 1992; 28: 138-40
189. Whitworth JA, Saines D, Scoggins BA. Potentiation of ACTH hypertension in man with salt loading. Clinical and Experimental Pharmacology and Physiology 1985; 12: 239-43
190. Izzo JL, Horwitz D, Lawton WJ, et al. Fludrocortisone suppression of sympathetic nervous activity. Clinical Pharmacology and Therapeutics 1983; 33: 102-6
191. Whitworth JA, Saines D, Thatcher R. Differential blood pressure and metabolic effects of 9 alpha flurocortisol in man. Clinical and Experimental Pharmacology and Physiology 1983; 10: 351-4
192. Oelkers W, Buchen S, Diedrich S, et al. Impaired renal 11 beta hydroxylation of 9 alpha flurocortisol: an explanation of its mineralocorticoid potency. Journal of Clinical Endocrinology and Metabolism 1994; 78: 928-32
193. Luton JP, Cerdas S, Billaud L, et al. Clinical features of adrenocortical carcinoma, prognostic features and the effect of mitotane therapy. New England Journal of Medicine 1990; 322: 1195-201
194. Maher VMG, Trainer PJ, Scoppola A, et al. Possible mechanisms and treatment of o,p'DDD induced hypercholesterolaemia. Quarterly Journal of Medicine 1992; 84: 671-9
195. Lonning PE, Kvinnsland S. Mechanisms of action of aminoglutethimide as endocrine therapy of breast cancer. Drugs 1988; 35: 685-710
196. Sonino N, Boscaro M, Paoletta A, et al. Ketoconazole treatment in Cushing's syndrome - experience in 34 patients. Clinical Endocrinology 1991; 35: 347-52
197. Verhelst JA, Trainer PJ, Howlett TA, et al. Short and long term responses to metyrapone in the medical management of 91 patients with Cushing's syndrome. Clinical Endocrinology 1991; 35: 169-78
198. Skluth HA, Gums JG. Spironolactone - a re-examination. DICP - Annals of Pharmacotherapy 1990; 24: 52-9
199. Hedman A, Angelin B, Arvidsson A, et al. Digoxin interactions in man: spironolactone reduces renal but not biliary digoxin clearance. European Journal of Clinical Pharmacology 1992; 42: 481-5
200. Lindner B, Esteban NV, Yergey AL, et al. Cortisol production rates in children and adolescence. Journal of Pediatrics 1991; 117: 892-6
201. Miller WL. Congenital adrenal hyperplasias. Endocrinology and Metabolism Clinics of North America 1991; 20: 721-49
202. Miller WL. Clinical review 54: genetics, diagnosis and management of 21-hydroxylase deficiency. Journal of Clinical Endocrinology and Metabolism 1994; 78: 41-6
203. Williams ME. Endocrine crises: hyperkalemia. Critical Care Clinics 1991; 7: 155-74
204. Miller JW, Crapo L. The medical treatment of Cushing's syndrome. Endocrine Reviews 1993; 14: 443-58
205. von Schoultz B, Carlstrom K. On the regulation of sex-hormone-binding globulin: a challenge of an old dogma and outlines of an alternative mechanism. Journal of Steroid Biochemistry and Molecular Biology 1989; 32: 327
206. Southren AL, Gordon GG, Tochimoto S. Further studies of factors affecting metabolic clearance rate of testosterone in man. Journal of Clinical Endocrinology and Metabolism 1968; 28: 105
207. Petra P, Stanczyk FZ, Namkung PC, et al. Direct effect of sex-steroid binding protein (SBP) of plasma on the metabolic clearance rate of testosterone in the rhesus macaque. Journal of Steroid Biochemistry and Molecular Biology 1985; 22: 739
208. Vermeulen A. Androgens and male senescence. In: Nieschlag E, Behre HM, editors. Testosterone: action deficiency substitution. Berlin: Springer-Verlag, 1990
209. Nieschlag E, Lammers U, Freischem CW, et al. Reproductive function in young fathers and grandfathers.

Journal of Clinical Endocrinology and Metabolism 1982; 55: 676

210. Quigley CA, DeBellis A, Marschke KB, et al. Androgen receptor defects: historical, clinical and molecular perspectives. Endocrine Reviews 1994; 16: 271-321
211. Snyder PJ, Lawrence DA. Treatment of male hypogonadism with testosterone enanthate. Journal of Clinical Endocrinology and Metabolism 1980; 51: 1335
212. Conway AJ, Boylan LM, Howe C, et al. A randomised clinical trial of testosterone replacement therapy in hypogonadal men. International Journal of Andrology 1988; 11: 247
213. Behre HM, Oberpenning F, Nieschlag E. Comparative pharmacokinetics of androgen preparations: application of computer analysis and simulation. In: Nieschlag E, Behre HM, editors. Testosterone: action deficiency substitution. Berlin: Springer-Verlag, 1990
214. Mackey MA, Conway AJ, Handelsman DJ. Tolerability of intramuscular injections of testosterone ester in an oil vehicle. Human Reproduction 1995; 10: 862-5
215. Behre HM, Nieschlag E. Testosterone buciclate (20 Aet-1) in hypogonadal men: pharmacokinetics and pharmacodynamics of the new long-acting androgen ester. Journal of Clinical Endocrinology and Metabolism 1992; 75: 1204
216. Handelsman DJ, Conway AJ, Boylan LM. Pharmacokinetics and pharmacodynamics of testosterone pellets in man. Journal of Clinical Endocrinology and Metabolism 1990; 71: 216
217. Handelsman DJ. Pharmacology of testosterone pellet implants. In: Nieschlag H, Behre M, editors. Testosterone: action deficiency substitution. Berlin: Springer-Verlag, 1990
218. Place VA, Atkinson L, Prather DA, et al. Transdermal testosterone replacement through genital skin. In: Nieschlag E, Behre HM, editors. Testosterone: action deficiency substitution. Berlin: Springer-Verlag, 1990
219. Meikle AW, Mazer NA, Moellmer JF, et al. Enhanced transdermal delivery of testosterone across nonscrotal skin produces physiological concentrations of testosterone and its metabolites in hypogonadal men. Journal of Clinical Endocrinology and Metabolism 1992; 74: 623
220. Guerin JF, Rollet J. Inhibition of spermatogenesis in men using various combinations of oral progestagens and percutaneous or oral androgens. International Journal of Andrology 1988; 11: 187
221. Chemana D, Morville R, Fiet J, et al. Percutaneous absorption of 5α-dihydrotestosterone in man. II Percutaneous administration of 5α-dihydrotestosterone in hypogonadal men with idiopathic haemochromatosis; clinical, metabolic and hormonal effectiveness. International Journal of Andrology 1982; 5: 595
222. Delanoe D, Fougeyrollas B, Meyer L, et al. Androgenisation of female partners of men on medroxyprogesterone acetate/percutaneous testosterone contraception. Lancet 1984; 1: 276
223. Stuenkel CA, Dudley RE, Yen SSC. Sublingual administration of testosterone hydroxyypropyl-β-cyclodextrin inclusion complex simulates episodic androgen release in hypogonadal men. Journal of Clinical Endocrinology and Metabolism 1991; 72: 1054
224. Wilson JD. The use and misuse of androgens. Metabolism: Clinical and Experimental 1980; 29: 1278
225. Knuth UA, Hano R, Nieschlag E. Effect of flutamide or cyproterone actetate on pituitary and testicular hormones in normal men. Journal of Clinical Endocrinology and Metabolism 1984; 59: 963
226. Brogden RN, Chrisp P. Flutamide: a review of its pharmacodynamic and pharmacokinetic properties, and therapeutic use in advanced prostatic cancer. Drugs & Aging 1991; 1: 104-15
227. Harris MG, Coleman SG, Faulds D, et al. Nilutamide: a review of its pharmacodynamic and pharmacokinetic properties, and therapeutic efficacy in prostate cancer. Drugs & Aging 1993; 3: 9-25
228. Rittmaster RS. Finasteride. New England Journal of Medicine 1994; 330: 120-5
229. Peters DH, Sorkin EM. Finasteride: a review of its potential in the treatment of benign prostatic hyperplasia. Drugs 1993; 46: 177-208
230. Brogden RN, Buckley MMT, Ward A. Buserelin: a review of its pharmacodynamic and pharmacokinetic properties, and clinical profile. Drugs 1990; 39: 399-437
231. Chrisp P, Goa KL. Goserelin: a review of its pharmacodynamic and pharmacokinetic properties, and clinical use in sex hormone-related conditions. Drugs 1991; 41: 254-88
232. Barradell LB, McTavish D. Histrelin: a review of its pharmacological properties and therapeutic role in central precocious puberty. Drugs 1993; 45: 570-88
233. Plosker GL, Brogden RN. Leuprorelin: a review of its pharmacology and therapeutic use in prostatic cancer, endometriosis and other sex hormone-related disorders. Drugs 1994; 48: 930-67
234. Chrisp P, Goa KL. Nafarelin: a review of its pharmacodynamic and pharmacokinetic properties, and clinical potential in sex hormone-related conditions. Drugs 1990; 39: 523-51
235. Finkel DM, Phillips JL, Snyder PJ. Stimulation of spermatogenesis by gonadotropins in men with hypogonadotropic hypogonadism. New England Journal of Medicine 1985; 313: 651
236. Kleisch S, Behre HM, Nieschlag E. High efficacy of gonadotrophin or pulsatile gonadotrophin-releasing hormone treatment in hypogonadotrophic hypogonadism. European Journal of Endocrinology 1994; 131: 347-54
237. Burris AS, Rodbard HW, Winters SJ, et al. Gonadotropin therapy in men with isolated hypogonadotropic hypogonadism: the response to human chorionic gonadotropin is predicted by initial testicular size. Journal of Clinical Endocrinology and Metabolism 1988; 66: 1144-51
238. Delemarre-van der Waal HA. Induction of testicular growth and spermatogenesis by pulsatile intravenous administration of gonadotrophin-releasing hormone in patients with hypogonadotrophic hypogonadism. Clinical Endocrinology 1993; 38: 473-80
239. Finkel DM, Phillips JL, Snyder PJ. Stimulation of spermatogenesis by gonadotrophins in men with hypogonadotropic hypogonadism. New England Journal of Medicine 1985; 313: 651-5
240. Linet OI, Orginc FG. Efficacy and safety of intracavernosal alprostadil in men with erectile dysfunction. New England Journal of Medicine 1996; 334: 873-7
241. Porst H. The rationale for prostaglandin $E_1$ in erectile failure - a survey of worldwide experience. Journal of Urology 1996; 155: 802-15
242. Mooradian AD, Morley JE, Korenman SG. Biological actions of androgens. Endocrine Reviews 1987; 8: 1

243. Nieschlag E, Behre HM. Pharmacology and clinical use of testosterone. In: Nieschlag E, Behre HM, editors. Testosterone: action deficiency substitution. Berlin: Springer-Verlag, 1990
244. Tenover JS. Effects of testosterone supplementation in the aging male. Journal of Clinical Endocrinology and Metabolism 1992; 75: 1092
245. Tenover JS. Androgen administration to aging men. In: Bremner WJ, editor. Clinical andrology. Endocrinology and Metabolism Clinics of North America. Philadelphia: WB Saunders, 1994
246. Ishak KG, Zimmerman HJ. Hepatotoxic effects of the anabolic-androgenic steroids. Seminars in Liver Disease 1987; 7: 230
247. Lawrence JR, Sumner DJ, Kalk WJ, et al. Digoxin kinetics in patients with thyroid dysfunction. Clinical Pharmacology and Therapeutics 1977; 22: 7
248. Barrett-Connor E. Lower endogenous androgen levels and dyslipidemia in men with non-insulin-dependent diabetes mellitus. Annals of Internal Medicine 1992; 117: 807
249. Plymate SR, Swerdloff RS. Androgens, lipids and cardiovascular risk. Annals of Internal Medicine 1992; 117: 871
250. Oppenheim DS, George SL, Zervas NT, et al. Elevated serum lipids in hypogonadal men with and without hyperprolactinemia. Annals of Internal Medicine 1989; 111: 288
251. Gardner FH, Besa EC. Physiologic mechanisms and the hematopoietic effects of the androstanes and their derivatives. Current Topics in Hematology 1983; 4: 123
252. Crawford ED, De Antonio EP, Labrie F, et al. Endocrine therapy of prostate cancer: optimal form and appropriate timing. Journal of Clinical Endocrinology and Metabolism 1995; 80: 1062
253. O'Donovan P, Vandekerchkhove P, Lilford RJ, et al. Treatment of male infertility: is it effective? Review and meta-analysis of published randomised controlled trials. Human Reproduction 1993; 8: 1209-22
254. Brinster RL, Avarbock MR. Germline transmission of donor haplotype following spermatogonial transplantation. Proceedings of the National Academy of Sciences of the United States of America 1994; 91: 11303
255. Greenhall E, Vessey M. The prevalence of subfertility: a review of the current confusion and a report of two new studies. Fertility and Sterility 1990; 54: 978
256. Kliesch S, Behre HM, Nieschlag E. High efficacy of gonadotrophin or pusatile gonadotrophin-releasing hormone treatment in hypogonadotrophic hypogonadal men. European Journal of Endocrinology 1994; 131: 347
257. Baxter RC, Lewitt MS, Martin JL. Insulin-like growth factor binding proteins: regulators of IGF action. In: Mornex R, Jaffiol C, Leclère J, editors. Progress of endocrinology. Camforth: Parthenon, 1993: 248-51
258. Green H, Morikawa M, Nixon TA. A dual effector theory of growth-hormone action. Differentiation 1985; 29: 195-8
259. Raban MS. Clinical use of human growth hormone. New England Journal of Medicine 1962; 266: 82-6
260. Koch TK, Berg BO, De Armond SJ, et al. Creutzfeldt-Jakob disease in a young adult with idiopathic hypopituitarism: possible relationship to administration of cadaveric human growth hormone. New England Journal of Medicine 1985; 313: 731-3
261. Jorgensen JOL. Human growth hormone replacement therapy: pharmacological and clinical aspects. Endocrine Reviews 1991; 12: 189-207
262. Hindmarsh PC, Matthews DR, Brain CE, et al. The half-life of exogenous growth hormone after suppression of endogenous growth hormone secretion with somatostatin. Clinical Endocrinology 1989; 30: 443-50
263. Allen DB, Brook CG, Bridges NA, et al. Growth hormone (GH) treatment of non-GH deficient subjects. Journal of Clinical Endocrinology and Metabolism 1994; 79: 1239-48
264. Lippe BM, Nakamoto JM. Conventional and nonconventional uses of growth hormone. Recent Progress in Hormone Research 1993; 48: 179-235
265. Clemmons DR, Underwood LE. Uses of human insulin-like growth factor-I in clinical conditions. Journal of Clinical Endocrinology and Metabolism 1994; 79: 4-6
266. Ritzen EM, Czernichow P, Preece M, et al. Safety of growth hormone therapy. Hormone Research 1993; 39: 92-3
267. Handelsman DJ, Swerdloff RS. Pharmacokinetics of gonadotropin-releasing hormone and its analogs. Endocrine Reviews 1986; 7: 95-105
268. Karten MJ, Rivier JE. Gonadotropin-releasing hormone analog design: structure-function studies toward the development of agonists and antagonists: rationale and perspective. Endocrine Reviews 1986; 7: 44-66
269. Conn PM, Crowley WF. Gonadotropin-releasing hormone and its analogs. Annual Review of Medicine 1994; 45: 391-405
270. Wheeler MD, Styne DM. The treatment of precocious puberty. Endocrinology and Metabolism Clinics of North America 1991; 20: 183-90
271. Ho KY, Thorner MO. Therapeutic applications of bromocriptine in endocrine and neurologic diseases. Drugs 1988; 36: 67-82
272. Jaffe CA, Barkan AL. Acromegaly: recognition and treatment. Drugs 1994; 47: 425-45
273. Kletzky OQ, Vermesh M. Effectiveness of vaginal bromocriptine in treating women with hyperprolactinemia. Fertility and Sterility 1989; 51: 269-72
274. Larrazet F, Spaulding C, Lobreau HJ, et al. Possible bromocriptine-induced myocardial infarction. Annals of Internal Medicine 1993; 18: 199-200
275. Chanson P, Timsit J, Harris AG. Clinical pharmacokinetics of octreotide: therapeutic applications in patients with pituitary tumours. Clinical Pharmacokinetics 1993; 25: 375-91
276. Editorial. Cyproheptadine. Lancet 1978; 1: 367-8
277. Feuillan PP, Foster CM, Pescovitz OH, et al. Treatment of precocious puberty in the McCune-Albright syndrome with the aromatase inhibitor testolactone. New England Journal of Medicine 1986; 315: 1115-9
278. Laue L, Kenigsberg D, Pescovitz OH, et al. Treatment of familial male precocious puberty with spironolactone and testolactone. New England Journal of Medicine 1989; 320: 496-502
279. Neely EK, Rosenfeld RG. Use and abuse of human growth hormone. Annual Review of Medicine 1994; 45: 407-20
280. Darendeliler F, Hindmarsh PC, Preece MA, et al. Growth hormone increases rate of pubertal maturation. Acta Endocrinologica 1990; 122: 414-6
281. Mehls O, Tonshoff B, Haffner D, et al. The use of recombinant human growth hormone in short children with chronic renal failure. Journal of Pediatric Endocrinology 1994; 7: 107-13
282. Kletter GB, Kelch RP. Effects of gonadotropin-releasing hormone analog therapy on adult stature in preco-

cious puberty. Journal of Clinical Endocrinology and Metabolism 1994; 79: 331-4

283. Klibanski A, Greenspan SI. Increase in bone mass after treatment of hyperprolactinemic amenorrhea. New England Journal of Medicine 1986; 315: 542-6
284. Flogstad AK, Halse J, Grass P, et al. A comparison of octreotide, bromocriptine, or a combination of both drugs in acromegaly. Journal of Clinical Endocrinology and Metabolism 1994; 79: 461-5
285. Brass EP. Effect of antihypertensive drugs on endocrine function. Drugs 1984; 27: 447-52
286. Seltzer HS. Drug-induced hypoglycaemia: a review of 1418 cases. Endocrinology and Metabolism Clinics of North America 1989; 18: 163-83
287. Grinspoon S, Donovan D, Bilesekian J. Aetiology and pathogenesis of hormonal and metabolic disorders in HIV infection. Balliere's Clinical Endocrinology and Metabolism 1994; 8: 4-24
288. Skouby S, Jesperson J. Oral contraceptives in the nineties: metabolic aspects – facts and fiction. American Journal of Obstetrics and Gynecology 1990; Suppl. 163: 276-82
289. Belchetz PE. Hormonal treatment of post-menopausal women. New England Journal of Medicine 1994; 330: 1067-74
290. Baird D, Glasier A. Hormonal contraception. New England Journal of Medicine 1993; 328: 1543-7
291. Weidmann P, Boehlen LM, de Courten M, et al. Antihypertensive therapy in diabetic patients. Journal of Human Hypertension 1992; 6 (Suppl 2): 523-36
292. Chopra IJ, Teco GNC. Displacement of free thyroid hormones from binding proteins by FFA. Journal of Clinical Endocrinology and Metabolism 1985; 60: 980-4
293. Surks MI, Sievert R. Drugs and thyroid function. New ENgland Journal of Medicine 1995; 333: 1688-94
294. Evans PJ. Circulating TSH levels measured with an immunochemiluminetric assay in patients taking drugs interfering with biochemical thyroid status. Clinical Endocrinology 1987; 26: 717-21
295. Carella MJ. HPA axis function one week after a short burst of steroid therapy. Journal of Clinical Endocrinology and Metabolism 1993; 76: 1188
296. Orth DN, Kovacs WJ, Debold CR. The adrenal cortex. In: Wilson JD, Foster DW, editors. Williams' textbook of endocrinology. 8th ed. Philadelphia: WB Saunders, 1992
297. Baxter JD. Minimising the effects of glucocorticoid therapy. Advances in Internal Medicine 1990; 35: 173-93
298. Burch EA. Drug intake and the DST. Journal of Clinical Psychiatry 1986; 47: 144-6
299. Surks MI. Diphenylhydantoin inhibits the TSH response to TRH in man and rat. Journal of Clinical Endocrinology and Metabolism 1983; 56: 940-5
300. Jeunemaitre X. Efficacy and tolerance of spironolactone in essential hypertension. American Journal of Cardiology 1987; 60: 820-5
301. Carrier S. Erectile dysfunction in clinical andrology. Endocrine and Metabolic Clinics of North America 1994; 23
302. Jones TM. Infertility. In: DeGroot LJ, editor. Endocrinology. 2nd ed. Vol. 3. Philadelphia: WB Saunders, 1989: 2192-206
303. Malarkey WB. Endocrine effects in female weight lifters who self administer testosterone and anabolic steroids. American Journal of Obstetrics and Gynecology 1971; 165: 1385-90
304. Bernstein JG. Management of psychotropic drug-induced obesity. In: Bijorntorp & Brodoff, editors. Obesity. Philadelphia: Lippincott, 1992: 445-53
305. Sambrook P, et al. Prevention of corticosteroid induced osteoporosis. New England Journal of Medicine 1993; 329: 1747-52
306. Mosekilde L, Eriksen EF. Effects of thyroid hormones on bone and mineral metabolism. In: Tiegs RD, editor. Metabolic bone disease. Endocrinology and Metabolism Clinics of North America 1990; 19: 35
307. Greenspan SL, Greenspan FS, Resnick NM, et al. Skeletal integrity in premenopausal and post-menopausal women receiving long term L-thyroxine therapy. American Journal of Medicine 1991; 91: 5-14
308. Aurbach GD, Marx SJ, Spiegel AM. Parathyroid hormone, calcitonin and the calciferols. In: Wilson JD, Foster DW, editors. Williams' textbook of endocrinology. 8th ed. Philadelphia: WB Saunders, 1992: 1453-5
309. Reeves WB, Andreoli TE. The posterior pituitary and water metabolism. In: Wilson JD, Foster DW, editors. Williams' textbook of endocrinology. 8th ed. Philadelphia: WB Saunders, 1992

Chapter 20

# Cardiovascular Disorders

*J.J. McNeil* and *H. Krum*

## Synopsis of Important Principles

1) Hypertension, hyperlipidaemia and cigarette smoking are important risk factors for the future development of coronary heart disease because they are strongly predictive and potentially susceptible to medical and public health intervention. Prediction of coronary risk can be considerably strengthened by considering the additive effects of the major risk factors. Cost effective prevention of coronary heart disease requires both community-wide changes to diet and smoking habits, together with more intensive interventions directed towards those individuals at highest risk.

2) Lipid-lowering therapy with HMG CoA reductase inhibitors has been shown to reduce mortality over about 5 years in individuals both with and without pre-existing heart disease. Unlike other available lipid-lowering drugs, these agents are well tolerated and appear not to be associated with increases in nonvascular mortality, at least in the short to medium term. Lipid-lowering therapy should be considered in all patients with evidence of cardiovascular disease, even if their plasma cholesterol concentrations are within normal limits.

3) ACE inhibitors (usually given with diuretics) have been shown to improve survival in patients with mild, moderate and severe degrees of systolic dysfunction, and also to reduce recurrent myocardial infarction. The use of these drugs should be routine in all patients with symptomatic systolic dysfunction.

4) Digoxin is widely used in patients with atrial fibrillation and cardiac failure. Although it has no apparent influence on survival among cardiac failure patients in sinus rhythm, it produces an overall improvement in well-being.

5) Angina is frequently worsened by underlying cardiac or extracardiac disease. When drug treatment is required, long-acting nitrate formulations are usually chosen as initial therapy. Calcium antagonists or β-blockers may also be used alone or in combination with nitrates.

6) The early drug treatment of severe unstable angina usually involves combination therapy with heparin, aspirin, nitrates and β-blockers.

7) Early management of acute myocardial infarction is directed towards restoration of blood flow and the minimisation of myocardial damage. Thrombolytic drugs and aspirin administered early after the onset of pain have the potential to reduce early mortality by 30 to 40%. This represents a saving of up to 40 lives per 1000 patients treated.

8) Mortality in the years following a myocardial infarction can be substantially reduced by the routine use of β-blockers and aspirin. Verapamil may be an adequate substitute for those intolerant of β-blockers. ACE inhibitors should be administered to those with even transient evidence of left ventricular dysfunction, while HMG CoA reductase inhibitors should be used to lower plasma cholesterol concentrations (even when the cholesterol concentration is relatively normal).

9) In patients with cardiac arrhythmias, most antiarrhythmic drugs, apart from β-blockers and probably amiodarone, produce more harm than benefit when used long term.

Cardiovascular diseases are the most common cause of death and morbidity in Western countries. Despite the increasing application of surgery and a renewed emphasis on prevention, the cornerstone of management of most patients with established cardiac disease remains drug therapy. Over recent years, several new drug groups have been introduced including calcium antagonists, angiotensin-converting enzyme (ACE) inhibitors and a variety of new thrombolytic and lipid-lowering agents. Much remains to be learned about the optimum use of these agents, especially the definition of subgroups of patients particularly responsive to one or other agents or at increased risk of adverse effects.

## 1. Clinical Pharmacological Considerations

### 1.1 Drug Absorption in Cardiovascular Disease

In cardiac failure, and in other forms of cardiac disease, a number of alterations take place which may affect the rate of absorption and the bioavailability of an orally administered drug. The extent of these changes depends largely on the severity of the cardiovascular disease and may also be influenced by other drug therapy commonly administered in this clinical setting.

The principal factors likely to influence drug absorption are a reduced mesenteric blood flow and a reduction in intestinal motility. Both of these may result from the increased sympathetic tone found in patients with cardiac failure. The reduction in intestinal motility may be enhanced by the actions of opioid analgesics and drugs with anticholinergic properties (e.g. disopyramide). In severe cardiac failure, oedema of the intestinal mucosa may also be present together with impaired hepatic function. The latter may be sufficient to reduce the presystemic extraction and increase the bioavailability of drugs that are normally extensively metabolised.[1] The influence of changes in blood flow on drug elimination are discussed in section 1.3 (below).

The consequences of changes in drug absorption are most apparent for drugs such as analgesics, antiarrhythmics and diuretics when these are given for an immediate effect. In the presence of cardiac failure, or after myocardial infarction, a delay in absorption of up to 1 to 2 hours might be anticipated and parenteral administration may therefore be more appropriate, although it should be noted that reduced muscle blood flow may also impair absorption from intramuscular injection sites. Delays of this order have been documented with digoxin, procainamide, quinidine and mexiletine and may be anticipated with most other agents.

### 1.2 Drug Distribution in Cardiovascular Disease

The plasma concentration of a drug (and in most cases the intensity of its effect) is determined by the amount of drug present within the body and the extent to which it is concentrated in extravascular tissues, and by the rates of drug distribution and elimination. The extent to which it is concentrated in extravascular tissues is measured indirectly by the drug's apparent volume of distribution (see chapter 1; sect. 2.2.2). With some drugs, intracellular protein binding or tissue sequestration may leave only a small fraction of the drug in plasma, in which case the drug's volume of distribution is high.

The properties of a drug that favour accumulation in extravascular sites are not well understood, but appear to include high lipid solubility, minimal binding to plasma proteins, and a basic pKa. In theory therefore, alterations such as a decrease in plasma protein binding or a shift in plasma pH might affect the volume of distribution, leading to higher or lower plasma concentrations after a given total dose (see further chapter 1; sect. 3.2). Distribution into oedema fluid, if sufficiently marked, may also increase the volume of distribution of some drugs, particularly water soluble agents with a volume of distribution largely restricted to the extracellular fluid.

The effect of *cardiac failure* on the volume of distribution of a number of drugs widely used in cardiovascular disease has been studied; these include, lidocaine (lignocaine), disopyramide, procainamide, and quinidine. In general, the volumes of distribution of these agents have been found to be reduced by 25 to 40%. In the absence of other compensatory changes, a difference of this magnitude should mandate a lower loading dose at the commencement of therapy. The smaller volume of distribution will result in an increase in the concentration of the drug in the plasma and adequately perfused tissues. A decreased rate of elimination may also occur if hepatic (lidocaine) or renal (procainamide) blood flow is decreased. Thus, maintenance dose requirements of these drugs will also be decreased (see further section 8.2.2).

As well as giving lower doses in patients with cardiac failure or shock, it is necessary to administer them more slowly. In both of these conditions, there is a redistribution of blood flow from skin and muscle towards the brain, heart and other vital organs. The uptake of drug into the more slowly perfused tissues is likely to be reduced, thereby increasing plasma concentrations occurring shortly after administration. This effect has been shown experimentally with digoxin and in computer simulated models with lidocaine. This probably explains the increased incidence of lidocaine toxicity noted shortly after administration of standard doses in patients with circulatory failure[2] (see also chapter 13; sect. 1.1.3).

Finally, abnormalities of plasma protein binding have been noted in some patients with cardiac disease. Myocardial infarction produces an inflammatory response with increased circulating acute phase reactants such as $\alpha_1$-acid glycoprotein. The latter binds basic drugs such as lidocaine and may be responsible, at least in part, for the progressive increase in plasma lidocaine concentrations observed during the first 48 hours of continuous infusion in patients with a myocardial infarction (see also chapter 13; sect. 1.1.6).

### 1.3 Drug Elimination in Cardiovascular Disease

#### 1.3.1 Hepatic Metabolism

The rate of elimination of drugs metabolised by the liver is influenced both by the activity of drug metabolising enzymes and by the rate of delivery of drug to the liver by the blood (see also chapter 1; sect. 5.4.3; chapter 13; sect. 1.1.4). When a drug has a high extraction ratio (indicating avid removal), then changes in liver blood flow may alter its clearance. Liver blood flow is commonly reduced by 20 to 40% in patients with uncompensated cardiac failure, cardiogenic shock and in those receiving β-adrenoceptor blocking drugs. This pattern of events results in reduced clearance of lidocaine and probably contributes to the relatively high plasma concentrations of the drug observed during infusions in patients with circulatory failure. (As noted above, other factors, such as an increase in $\alpha_1$-acid glycoprotein binding may also contribute.) A similar pattern might be expected with other high clearance drugs, such as morphine, pethidine and propranolol.[3]

For various other drugs which are much less avidly removed, hepatic clearance is relatively insensitive to changes in blood flow, but is often affected by alterations in enzyme activity. This may be reduced by hepatic congestion, hypoperfusion or hypoxaemia (leading to impaired microsomal drug oxidation). In advanced cardiac failure, these influences would be expected to affect drugs such as theophylline, tolbutamide and warfarin. Reduced liver enzyme activity may also contribute to the reduced elimination of lidocaine in patients with cardiac failure.

#### 1.3.2 Renal Excretion

Cardiac failure may affect renal clearances of drugs by a number of mechanisms. Renal blood flow and glomerular filtration rate are decreased and there may be increased tubular reabsorption due to redistribution of intrarenal blood flow[4] and/or reduced urine flow. The decreased renal blood flow is correlated with the reduced cardiac output.

### 1.4 Altered Tissue Responsiveness in Cardiovascular Disease

The pathophysiological state of the heart in cardiovascular disease may also influence cardiac responsiveness to the pharmacological actions of the drug.[5] This is discussed further in section 10.1.

## 2. General Principles of Treatment

1) ***Prompt diagnosis and treatment:*** acute myocardial infarction must be diagnosed and treated as soon as it occurs. Prompt transfer to a coronary care unit probably offers the best chance of reducing mortality from infarction. Acute pulmonary oedema and acute pulmonary embolism are other examples of medical emergencies that must be diagnosed and treated promptly (see further section 7.2 and chapter 26; sect. 3.2.1 and 3.2.2).

2) ***Remove the cause:*** the first therapeutic approach in diseases such as angina pectoris, congestive heart failure and secondary hyperlipidaemia is to search for and correct the precipitating causes (see sections 4.3, 5.5, 6.2).

3) ***Individualised treatment:*** in the treatment of cardiac arrhythmias, the dosage of antiarrhythmic drugs and digoxin should be adjusted according to individual requirements and tolerance, particularly factors that can modify the response to the drug. Plasma concentration estimations are a valuable aid to therapy with certain antiarrhythmic drugs and in some circum-

stances with digoxin, but are not intended to replace careful monitoring and follow-up of the patient's clinical status. Rigid adherence to a laboratory determination of what constitutes a therapeutic concentration, without evaluation of the clinical status of the patient, is unwise. The aim of therapeutics is to treat the individual patient not a plasma concentration (see further sections 5.5 and 8.3).

4) ***Review of therapy:*** heart failure may become poorly controlled because of a lessening effect of diuretics in the face of electrolyte loss or development of secondary hyperaldosteronism, or because of inadequate ACE inhibitor or digoxin dosage, or digoxin toxicity (see further sections 5.4.1, 5.4.3).

5) ***Multiple drug therapy:*** while concurrent use of more than one drug is often needed and is of much benefit in cardiovascular therapy, adverse interactions between drugs can occasionally occur. Such adverse interactions can often be avoided or anticipated, but this requires familiarity with the pharmacokinetic properties and important therapeutic and toxic actions of each drug (see further section 10.2).

## 3. Prevention of Coronary Heart Disease

### 3.1 Primary Prevention

In most Western countries, coronary heart disease is responsible for approximately one-quarter of all deaths. Despite a persistent decline of about 2% per year, coronary heart disease still ranks fourth in the US and Australia in years of life lost prior to age 65, highlighting the impact of life lost in the early and middle years.[6] Approximately one man in 10 dies of the condition before 65 years of age.[7]

#### *3.1.1 Causes and Clinical Presentation of Coronary Heart Disease*

The cause of coronary heart disease is coronary atherosclerosis which begins relatively early in life as a streaky deposition of lipid beneath the intima of the major arteries. With advancing years, these deposits slowly enlarge, provoking a fibrotic and vascular reaction which culminates in the development of thickened scarred plaques. Arterial occlusion may occur, either by slow growth of the lesion, haemorrhage into it, or by thrombosis on its surface.[8]

The common clinical presentations of coronary heart disease are angina pectoris, myocardial infarction and sudden death. Less commonly, it presents as congestive cardiac failure or an arrhythmia. Since up to 50% of deaths from the disease occur within one hour of the onset of symptoms, and since there are often no premonitory warning symptoms, prevention must play a major part in its control.

#### *3.1.2 Risk Factors for Development*

The development of coronary atherosclerosis is determined largely by environmental influences. Evidence for this is seen with immigrant groups moving from low incidence to high incidence countries. These migrants quickly develop a level of risk similar to that of their hosts.[9] However, a high risk is not a necessary accompaniment of technological progress, as evidenced by the low incidence of the condition among the Japanese.[10]

A major achievement of epidemiological research has been the identification of a number of personal characteristics referred to as *risk factors* whose presence correlates with the future development of coronary heart disease. Among these, hypertension, hyperlipidaemia and cigarette smoking are important because they are strongly predictive and potentially susceptible to prevention and control measures. A variety of weaker links have been found with other factors such as physical inactivity, obesity, low socioeconomic status, abstinence from alcohol and oral contraceptive use. In many instances, these are interrelated, being components of the overall 'web of causation.'[11]

#### *3.1.3 Primary Prevention Strategies*

The primary prevention of coronary heart disease in Western communities requires two major strategies. The aim of the first is to produce a community-wide change in those aspects of lifestyle responsible for an increased disease risk. Since the bulk of coronary heart disease develops in the large proportion of people with small to moderately increased risk (rather than in the much smaller proportion with high risk), this strategy has the greatest chance of producing a major fall in disease incidence. It involves community-wide measures designed to reduce cigarette smoking, physical inactivity, obesity and animal fat consumption.[9]

The second strategy involves the identification of individuals at high risk of developing coronary heart disease and the provision of appropriate advice and/or drug treatment. The identification step involves a screening or case-finding programme which includes measurement of blood pressure and plasma lipids, and determination of smoking habit and other relevant personal characteristics. The risk prediction can be strengthened considerably by taking into account the results of these measurements simultaneously by considering their interactions.

#### 3.1.4 Treatment of Hypertension and Hyperlipidaemia

Aspects of the relationship between blood pressure and cardiovascular disease are discussed in chapter 21. Effective treatment of hypertension leads to a significant reduction in cardiovascular mortality and morbidity.

As pointed out above, hyperlipidaemia is an important risk factor for the development of coronary heart disease. The nature of this relationship and the optimum use of lipid-lowering therapy in decreasing the risk are discussed in section 4 below.

### 3.2 Secondary Prevention Following a Myocardial Infarction

About 10 to 15% of individuals who sustain a myocardial infarction experience a fatal or nonfatal recurrent infarction during the subsequent 2 years. Several risk factors that help identify those at greatest risk have been identified: these are dominated by measures of the severity of cardiac muscle damage. A variety of strategies designed to prevent further coronary occlusion and death in patients after myocardial infarction have been evaluated. These strategies are discussed in section 7.2.2 and include the use of low-dose aspirin (or other antiplatelet drugs), β-adrenoceptor blockers, ACE inhibitors, lipid-lowering drugs and antioxidants. The use of lipid-lowering drugs (particularly the HMG CoA reductase inhibitors) in secondary prevention is discussed in more detail in section 4.3.2 below.

## 4. Hyperlipidaemia/Atherosclerosis

Lipid abnormalities are important risk factors for coronary heart disease. Although the traditional medical focus has been on the plasma total cholesterol concentration, this has been largely because of its ease of measurement and its incorporation into early epidemiological studies. Modern knowledge of lipid physiology has led to an interest in other components of the lipid transport system as potential markers of increased coronary risk.

Because lipids are not soluble in blood, they are carried between the gut, liver and tissues in complex macromolecules known as lipoproteins. These spherical complexes have an outer coat consisting principally of proteins (apolipoproteins) and the amphophilic (charged) ends of phospholipid molecules. The inner core consists of varying proportions of cholesterol esters and triglycerides. Five major types of lipoprotein exist:

- Chylomicrons
- Very-low-density lipoproteins (VLDL)
- Intermediate-density lipoproteins (IDL)
- Low-density lipoproteins (LDL)
- High-density lipoproteins (HDL).

The lipoproteins transport fats between the sites of their absorption, utilisation and storage. Two pathways exist (fig. 1):

1) An *exogenous pathway* which involves the transport of fats from the intestine to the liver and peripheral tissues. After absorption, fats are reconstituted as chylomicrons which transport triglycerides to adipose tissue for storage and to muscles for use as an energy source. Chylomicron remnants, which contain cholesterol esters, are removed by catabolism in the liver.

2) An *endogenous pathway* which begins with the secretion of triglyceride-rich lipoprotein particles from the liver that are rapidly transformed into VLDL particles. Subsequently, the loss of triglycerides and some apoproteins leads to their transformation to LDL, which is composed largely of cholesterol esters and a surface apoprotein (apoprotein B). These particles circulate in the blood with a half-life of about 2 to 5 days before being removed from the circulation by binding to LDL receptors mainly in the liver.[13]

Cells of both the liver and peripheral tissues can synthesise cholesterol for use in membrane synthesis and in the production of steroid hormones. However, if adequate cholesterol becomes available by LDL receptor-mediated uptake, the rate of synthesis of LDL receptors is reduced and the critical enzyme (HMG CoA reductase) involved in cholesterol synthesis is inhibited.

### 4.1 Lipids and Coronary Heart Disease Risk

Most of the detailed information about the relationship between lipid levels and cardiovascular disease comes from large cohort studies conducted in the US and UK. Among 350,000 US males screened for the Multiple Risk Factor Intervention Trial (MRFIT), there was an approximately curvilinear relationship between

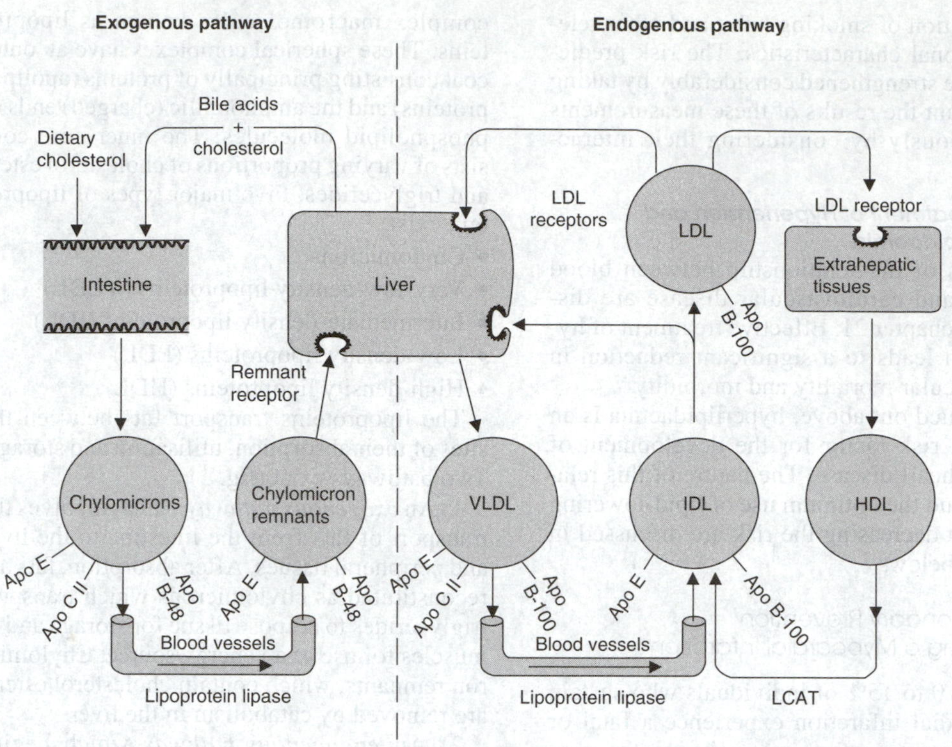


**Fig. 1.** Schematic representation of exogenous and endogenous pathways of cholesterol metabolism (after Comai et al.;[12] with permission). *Abbreviations:* HDL = high-density lipoprotein; IDL = intermediate-density lipoprotein; LCAT = lecithin/cholesterol acyltransferase; LDL = low-density lipoprotein; VLDL = very-low-density lipoprotein.

the plasma total cholesterol concentration and the subsequent risk of symptomatic or fatal coronary heart disease.[14] Those whose total cholesterol concentration exceeded 6.8 mmol/L (263 mg/dl) had four times the risk of coronary heart disease as those whose level was less than 4.7 mmol/L (182 mg/dl). However, the risk of cerebrovascular or peripheral vasular disease is less strongly correlated with high cholesterol concentrations.

This relationship between plasma cholesterol concentrations and coronary heart disease risk is also supported by:

1) The strong relationship observed between the average plasma cholesterol concentration within a country and the age-standardised incidence of coronary heart disease. Those countries at the upper and lower extremes of average plasma cholesterol concentrations (Finland and Japan, respectively) are also those with the extremes of coronary heart disease incidence.[15]

2) The contrasting coronary risk among US Seventh Day Adventists who are vegetarians, ovolactovegetarians and non-vegetarians.[16] While vegetarians avoid all animal products, ovolactovegetarians consume milk and milk products. After other risk factors are taken into account, coronary heart disease incidence is low in vegetarians, intermediate in ovolactovegetarians, and higher still in non-vegetarians in keeping with a similar gradient in plasma cholesterol concentrations.

3) Migration studies, particularly those comparing Japanese communities in Japan, Hawaii and the US.[17] Along with an increasing level of acculturation to a Western lifestyle, these communities demonstrate an increasing intake of dietary fat, an increasing average cholesterol concentration, and an increasing incidence of coronary heart disease.

Within any community, plasma cholesterol concentrations are normally distributed about mean levels that are dependent on community dietary preferences. High cholesterol concentrations may also arise as a result of genetic abnormalities or disease states (particularly hypothyroidism and nephrotic syndrome). The most common genetic abnormality results from impaired synthesis of receptors for the uptake of LDL into cells. In the homozygous condition (homozygous familial hypercholesterolaemia), concentrations above 20 mmol/L (773 mg/dl) are common and death from coronary heart disease usually occurs early in life. In the more common heterozygous condition, fewer than normal LDL receptors are produced and cholesterol concentrations are moderately raised.

The risk of coronary heart disease imparted by an elevated cholesterol level is strongly influenced by the presence or absence of other risk factors, particularly cigarette smoking, elevated blood pressure and diabetes.[18] For this reason, it is important to take account of the presence of other risk factors by intervening more aggressively to lower plasma cholesterol concentrations when other risk factors are present.

#### *4.1.1 Role of Cholesterol in Development of Atherosclerosis*

Elevated cholesterol concentrations are believed to contribute to the development of atheroma through the accumulation of oxidised LDL particles in the subintimal space. Unlike normal LDL, oxidised LDL is ingested by macrophages, and accumulates within them to form foam cells. The accumulation of foam cells leads to the formation of fatty streaks which represent the early stages of atheroma development.

Atheromatous lesions responsible for coronary artery disease are now thought to vary in their composition and their clinical sequelae. Some develop slowly, becoming calcified and fibrosed and produce gradual encroachment in the vessel lumen leading to progressive effort angina. At the other end of the spectrum are more rapidly developing lesions composed largely of a soft lipid core with a thin fibrous cover. The rupture or fissuring of such lesions is believed to be responsible for most cases of unstable angina and acute myocardial infarction.[19]

##### Rationale for Cholesterol-Lowering Therapy

Plasma cholesterol concentrations can be lowered by dietary modification or by various drugs. The dietary modifications principally involve a reduced intake of saturated animal fat. This is brought about by reducing the intake of meats, milk and other products derived from them. Although sustained dietary modification is effective, most hypercholesterolaemic patients find it difficult to maintain long term compliance with their prescribed diet, particularly when it is different to that of their family and friends.[20]

Several large clinical trials have now demonstrated that drug treatment is effective in producing a sustained reduction of plasma cholesterol concentrations, which leads to a reduced risk of coronary heart disease. However, studies using earlier drugs consistently demonstrated a small increase in nonvascular deaths. Although this may have been a chance finding, it has consistently led to some reluctance to use these agents except in high-risk patients. In recent studies with the newer agents (HMG CoA reductase inhibitors; see sections 4.2.1 and 4.3.2), no increase in nonvascular mortality has been observed.

Recent trials have also demonstrated the value of rapid cholesterol-lowering interventions in patients with established coronary heart disease (see section 4.3.2). The mortality reduction in these studies has appeared within 6 to 12 months of the commencement of treatment, suggesting that part of the benefit may result from a reduction in size of the soft lipid-rich lesions which underly acute coronary events. This finding provides a strong rationale to introduce effective lipid-lowering therapy as early as possible in patients at high risk, e.g. after a myocardial infarction.

Despite the demonstrated efficacy of the HMG CoA reductase inhibitors, their use is likely to be constrained by their cost and perhaps by some residual uncertainty about their long term safety. Nevertheless, it is likely that their use will increase rapidly among individuals at high risk of coronary heart disease, particularly those with pre-existing vascular disease. However, since the majority of new cases of coronary heart disease in Western countries arise from the bulk of the population with near normal lipid concentrations, their use is unlikely to substantially reduce the high incidence of coronary heart disease in Western communities. The future of community-based coronary heart disease prevention strategies will continue to rely heavily on a shift in the whole distribution of cholesterol concentrations (by sustained dietary change) rather than the use of drug therapy.

#### *4.1.2 Role of Triglycerides*

Triglycerides are present in the circulation in very-low-density lipoprotein (VLDL) and in chylomicron remnants. Their concentrations fluctuate considerably and proper interpretation requires a fasting blood sample. Triglyceride concentrations are elevated during acute illness (e.g. injury, burns) and in patients with diabetes, abdominal obesity, or a high alcohol intake. They are also elevated in certain familial lipoprotein disorders.

High fasting plasma triglyceride concentrations are associated with an increased risk of coronary heart disease.[21] However, this association may reflect the influence of the medical conditions with which they are associated.[22] It may also come about because of the frequent association between elevated triglyceride concentrations and low circulating HDL-cholesterol concentrations (see section 4.1.3 below) and high concentrations of the small dense LDL particles which are considered to be particularly atherogenic. In most epidemiological studies, triglyceride levels have not added substantially to the risk imparted by these other factors.

The approach to management of elevated triglyceride concentrations has been influenced by uncertainty about its status as an independent risk factor and by a lack of clinical trial evidence demonstrating that lowering triglyceride concentrations reduces morbidity and improves survival.[23] Interventions in patients with elevated triglyceride concentrations should therefore be directed towards weight control, improved management of concomitant diabetes, and reduction of excessive alcohol intake. Since elevated triglycerides are a marker of high coronary risk, any coexisting elevation in plasma cholesterol concentrations should be treated more aggressively. Unless triglyceride concentrations are exceptionally high (when a risk of pancreatitis may be a consideration), there is presently little rationale to use drug treatment in patients with isolated triglyceride elevations.

#### 4.1.3 Role of HDL-Cholesterol

High-density lipoprotein (HDL) is believed to assist in the transport of excess free cholesterol from peripheral tissues to the liver. High concentrations of HDL confer protection against coronary heart disease.[24] During their time in plasma, HDL particles of different sizes are formed, ranging from small and dense (HDL-4) to large and buoyant (HDL-1). In normal human plasma, HDL-3 makes up about two-thirds and HDL-2 one-third of the HDL present.

Measurement of HDL-cholesterol concentrations is technically difficult and frequently subject to error. Levels are influenced in part by familial factors but are decreased by obesity, inactivity and cigarette smoking. Several drugs increase HDL-cholesterol concentrations, particularly nicotinic acid (niacin), but no trials of therapy directed primarily towards increasing HDL-cholesterol concentrations have been reported.

In the presence of elevated LDL-cholesterol concentrations, a low HDL-cholesterol is a marker of increased risk and suggests the need for more intensive cholesterol-lowering therapy. The non-drug interventions available to raise HDL-cholesterol (e.g. physical exercise) should also be emphasised since these exert a generally beneficial effect on several aspects of cardiovascular risk. In the absence of supportive evidence from clinical trials, there would appear to be little indication to use drugs to increase HDL-cholesterol when this is an isolated finding.

#### 4.1.4 Role of Lp(a)

Lp(a) is a variant of low-density lipoprotein which consists of an LDL-like core bound to a large glycoprotein molecule that is structurally similar to plasminogen. It is believed that the molecule may exert a prothrombotic effect by competing with plasminogen for binding to endothelial cells. Although frequently cited as a risk factor for coronary heart disease, evidence for this is conflicting. Plasma Lp(a) concentrations appear to be influenced by some classes of lipid-lowering drugs, but the significance of this action is uncertain.

## 4.2 Clinical Pharmacology of Drugs Used in Treatment

#### 4.2.1 HMG CoA Reductase Inhibitors ('Statins')

Inhibitors of the enzyme HMG CoA (3-hydroxy-3-methylglutaryl coenzyme A) reductase are the newest of the lipid-lowering drugs and are considerably more active in reducing total and LDL-cholesterol concentrations than previously available drugs. Evidence is now available of their ability to improve survival in patients after a myocardial infarction and in those at high coronary risk but without established vascular disease (see section 4.3.2). Unlike most other lipid-lowering drugs, they have not been associated with an increase in nonvascular mortality in studies of up to 5 to 6 years' duration. These findings provide the background for the rapid increase in the use of these agents.

The HMG CoA reductase inhibitors currently in use include lovastatin,[25] simvastatin,[26] pravastatin[27] and fluvastatin.[28]

### Mechanism/Site of Action

The HMG CoA reductase inhibitors act by inhibiting the enzyme responsible for catalysing the conversion of 3-hydroxy-3-methylglutarate to mevalonate, which is an early rate-limiting step in the biosynthesis of cholesterol. As a consequence of the inhibition of intracellular cholesterol synthesis, hepatocytes increase the expression of LDL receptors which then promote the extraction of LDL-cholesterol from plasma. The drugs have no cholesterol-lowering activity in patients with homozygous familial hypercholesterolaemia who lack genes necessary for the synthesis of LDL receptors.[29]

### Pharmacokinetic Characteristics

The HMG CoA reductase inhibitors differ substantially in their pharmacokinetic behaviour (table I), although, as yet, few clinical consequences of these differences are obvious. Lovastatin and simvastatin are lipophilic compounds whereas pravastatin and fluvastatin are more hydrophilic and concentrate less in the central nervous system. Lovastatin and simvastatin are prodrugs and are hydrolysed in the liver to their active forms, while pravastatin has a metabolite with approximately 10% of the activity of the parent drug, and fluvastatin has no active metabolites.

Fluvastatin is the most extensively metabolised while pravastatin is the least (table I). Plasma elimination half-lives vary from 1 to 3 hours. The major cytochrome P450 isoenzyme responsible for their metabolism is CYP3A4, which is also responsible for the metabolism of erythromycin and cyclosporin (see also chapter 1; sect. 3.3.3 and 5).

The HMG CoA reductase inhibitors also vary substantially in their response to coadministration with food which reduces the bioavailability of pravastatin by about one-third, has little effect on simvastatin, and increases the bioavailability of lovastatin by about 50% (table I).

*Influence of disease states*: there are limited data on the effect of disease states on the pharmacokinetics of HMG CoA reductase inhibitors. Plasma concentrations are increased in liver disease, and in practice, the drugs are contraindicated in this situation. Lower initial doses are recommended in patients with moderate to severe renal failure.

### Clinical Effectiveness

The HMG CoA reductase inhibitors appear to be equally effective, maximal doses reducing LDL-cholesterol by 30 to 35% (table II), but the response is dose-dependent. They produce a lesser fall in plasma triglycerides (10 to 30%) by increasing the clearance of VLDL remnants by LDL receptors. The average HDL-cholesterol concentration is increased by 5 to 15%, but Lp(a) concentrations are not affected.[30] When compared on a weight-for-weight basis, simvastatin has about twice the potency of lovastatin and pravastatin.[31,32]

***Rationale for use in combination regimens:*** HMG CoA reductase inhibitors and bile acid sequestrants (see section 4.2.2) have complimentary modes of action and combinations of these drug classes exert an additive effect on LDL-cholesterol. This occurs despite the bile acid sequestrants causing a reduction in the oral bioavailability of the HMG CoA reductase inhibitors by up to 50%. In one study comparing fluvastatin and cholestyramine alone and in combination, cholestyramine alone (8 g/day) reduced LDL-cholesterol by 14%, fluvastatin alone by 19%, and the combination by 30%. However, the combination of HMG CoA reductase inhibitors with other lipid-lowering drugs

**Table I.** Pharmacokinetic parameters of HMG CoA reductase inhibitors (after Plosker & Wagstaff[28])

| Parameter | Fluvastatin | Lovastatin | Simvastatin | Pravastatin |
|---|---|---|---|---|
| Absorption (%) | 98 | 30 | 60-85 | 35 |
| Effect of food on absorption (% change in AUC) | ↓15-25 | ↑50 | 0 | ↓30 |
| Plasma protein binding (%) | ≥99 | ≥95[a] | 95-98[a] | 45 |
| Hepatic extraction (% of absorbed dose) | ≥70 | ≥70 | ≥80 | 45 |
| Crosses blood-brain barrier | No | Yes | Yes | No |
| Elimination half-life (h) | 1.2 | 3 | 1.9[b] | 3 |
| Renal excretion (%)[c] | 6 | 30 | 13 | 60 |

a For both parent drug and corresponding β-hydroxyacid metabolite.

b For main active metabolite.

c Renal excretion of radiolabelled parent drug plus metabolites is given as the percentage of an intravenous dose.

*Abbreviation and symbols:* AUC = area under the plasma concentration-time curve; ↓ = decreased; ↑ = increased.

is limited by a possible increased risk of myopathy (see further below).

#### Tolerability and Drug Interactions Potential

***Adverse effects:*** the HMG CoA reductase inhibitors are better tolerated than the earlier lipid-lowering drugs. The most common complaints at the commencement of therapy are nausea, epigastric fullness, distension, constipation or loose bowel actions, and headache. Mild elevations of liver enzymes (transaminases) are common and exceed the apparent safe level (3 times the upper limit of normal) in about 1.5% of patients. Liver function should therefore be monitored every 4 to 6 weeks during the first year of therapy and periodically thereafter.

*Myopathy:* a combination of muscle weakness with raised plasma creatine phosphokinase levels affects perhaps 1 or 2 per 1000 recipients of these drugs. On rare occasions, this has been reported to progress to rhabdomyolysis and myoglobinuria. It is believed that the risk of myopathy is greater when HMG CoA reductase inhibitors are administered concurrently with cyclosporin, erythromycin, gemfibrozil or nicotinic acid.[33,34]

*Other adverse effects:* a number of other rare or less well-defined adverse effects have also been reported. A few instances of hypotension have been noted, possibly resulting from interference with the synthesis of some steroidal hormones such as aldosterone.[35] A decrease in natural killer (NK) cells has also been described but the significance of this is unclear.

***Drug interactions:*** few clinically important drug interactions have been documented with the HMG CoA reductase inhibitors, other than those already noted. As mentioned above, bile acid sequestrants may decrease the bioavailability of HMG CoA reductase inhibitors, and if combined therapy is required, it is suggested that the HMG CoA reductase inhibitor be given at least 1 hour before or 4 hours after the bile acid sequestrant.

### *4.2.2 Bile Acid Sequestrants (Cholestyramine and Colestipol)*

Cholestyramine and colestipol are insoluble anion exchange resins. After oral administration they release chloride ions and bind bile acids in their place. The resulting bile acid complex is not absorbed and the bile acids are therefore largely excreted in the faeces.[36]

#### Mechanism/Site of Action

Under normal circumstances, 25 to 30g of bile acid passes through the liver daily as part of its enterohepatic circulation. When the cycle is interrupted by the administration of a bile acid sequestrant, the liver increases the synthesis of bile acids, using endogenous cholesterol as the substrate. The latter is derived partly from synthesis of cholesterol within liver cells and partly from the uptake of LDL-cholesterol from the plasma (by increasing surface LDL receptor numbers). If sufficient compensatory hepatic cell synthesis takes place, the efficacy of the bile acid sequestrant in lowering plasma cholesterol concentrations may be limited and this provides the rationale for the combination of cholestyramine with an HMG CoA reductase inhibitor[37] (see also section 4.2.1 above).

#### Clinical Effectiveness

In therapeutic doses, bile acid sequestrants decrease plasma total and LDL-cholesterol by 10 to 30%. HDL-cholesterol levels are usually not affected but very-low-density lipoproteins (mainly triglycerides) may increase.[38]

*Cholestyramine* is formulated as a powder which is usually taken with water or fruit juice. Sachets of the powder contain 4 or 8g of cholestyramine resin. The initial dose of 4 to 8g daily is increased to a usual maintenance level of 12 to 16g daily. *Colestipol* is formulated in 5g sachets and its usual maintenance dose is 15 to 30g daily. The timing of the dose in relation to meals is not important with either preparation.

#### Tolerability and Drug Interactions Potential

***Adverse effects:*** systemic adverse effects of cholestyramine are limited because the drug is not absorbed systematically. However, it produces unwanted symptoms in a high percentage of patients. These primarily affect the gastrointestinal tract and include constipation, heartburn, abdominal pain, belching, bloating and nausea.[39] The constipation may be countered by a high fibre diet, but occasionally a mild laxative may be required.

At doses above those normally recommended, there is at least a theoretical concern that the binding of bile salts may impair the absorption of fat soluble vitamins (A, D, E and K), and other substances such as iron and folate. Clinical evidence of such vitamin deficiencies is rare, although minor elevations in serum alkaline phosphatase are sometimes observed in young people and may represent an early sign of subclinical osteomalacia. Vitamin replacement has been advised for patients on long term high-dose therapy.[40]

***Drug interactions:*** the most significant drug interactions associated with bile acid sequestrants result from their ability to bind fat soluble drugs. This is clinically important when they are administered with drugs with a narrow therapeutic index such as anticoagulants, cardiac glycosides and thyroid hormones. The resins also bind other acidic drugs such as naproxen and thiazide diuretics but these are of less clinical importance since their dose can easily be adjusted to compensate for their reduced bioavailability. To minimise the risk of interactions, other drugs should be given at least one hour prior to the resin but in the case of thyroxine, an interval of 4 to 5 hours is recommended.[41]

#### 4.2.3 Probucol

Probucol is a lipid-lowering drug with strong antioxidant properties.[42] When administered in doses of 500mg twice daily, it reduces total cholesterol and LDL-cholesterol concentrations by about 10 to 20% without substantially affecting serum VLDL-cholesterol or triglyceride levels. The mechanism of its lipid-lowering action is uncertain but may be related to increased catabolism of LDL.[43]

In animal models of experimental atherosclerosis, probucol has been shown to reduce the number and extent of atheromatous lesions. In humans, LDL isolated from individuals treated with probucol has been found to be more resistant to oxidative modification than LDL from controls.[44] Despite these favourable findings, the drug failed to influence the progress of femoral atherosclerosis in patients with established atherosclerosis participating in the Swedish PQRST trial.[45] No other large-scale morbidity or mortality trials have been carried out with probucol and thus the balance of risks and benefits of long term therapy is uncertain. In the absence of such studies, and in view of the drug's adverse effect profile, there is probably little place for probucol in modern lipid-lowering therapy.

***Pharmacokinetic characteristics:*** probucol is a lipid soluble drug that concentrates in adipose tissue and is eliminated slowly with a half-life of between 20 and 50 days. During long term therapy, plasma drug concentrations rise slowly to a plateau level after 3 to 4 months and are very variable among different individuals.

***Adverse effects:*** probucol is generally well tolerated, with diarrhoea the most common adverse effect.[46] Other symptoms such as bloating, indigestion, heartburn, headache, arthralgia and erythema occur less often. Of most concern, however, is the drug's consistent effect in lowering plasma HDL-cholesterol concentrations (usually by 15 to 20%) and its effect in increasing the QT interval on the electrocardiogram.[47] In various animal species, probucol has been shown to predispose to arrhythmias and sudden death.

#### 4.2.4 Fibrates

The fibrates are a group of lipid-lowering drugs structurally and functionally related to clofibrate. *Clofibrate* and *gemfibrozil* have been the most commonly used members of the group, although others such as *fenofibrate, bezafibrate* and *ciprofibrate* are also available. The major property of this group of drugs is their ability to reduce plasma triglyceride concentrations by 20 to 30%. The reduction of total cholesterol concentrations is proportionally less (about 5 to 10%) while HDL-cholesterol concentrations generally increase by a similar proportion.[48]

##### Mechanism/Site of Action

The fibrates affect several aspects of lipoprotein metabolism but it is not yet clear which is the principal effect and which are secondary effects.[49,50] Lipoprotein lipase activity is increased, hepatic triglyceride production is decreased and there is a marked increase in the clearance of triglycerides from plasma. The increase in HDL-cholesterol is associated with an increase in the plasma concentration of HDL carrier apoproteins.

##### Pharmacokinetic Characteristics

The fibrates share many similarities in their pharmacokinetic characteristics. They are all well absorbed and highly protein bound in plasma. Clofibrate is a prodrug which is rapidly hydrolysed after oral administration to *p*-chlorophenoxyisobutyric acid (CPIB) which is the active substance. Similarly, fenofibrate is a prodrug which is rapidly hydrolysed to the active metabolite fenofibric acid. The elimination half-lives of the fibrates vary from 2 hours for bezafibrate, 2 to 7 hours for gemfibrozil, 15 hours for CPIB, and 19 to 26 hours for fenofibric acid. In most cases, their elimination is delayed in renal failure, and plasma concentrations are higher, leading to an increased risk of adverse reactions (particularly myopathy). The pharmacokinetic parameters of the fibrates are listed in appendix A, and their dosages schedules are shown in table II.

**Table II.** Mechanisms of action of lipid-lowering drugs, dosage schedules and changes in lipid concentrations produced

| Group/mechanism of action | Drugs | Daily dosage | Lipid changes (%) | | | |
|---|---|---|---|---|---|---|
| | | | LDL-C | VLDL | HDL-C | Lp(a) |
| **HMG CoA reductase inhibitors** | | | | | | |
| Inhibit intracellular cholesterol synthesis leading to an increase in hepatic LDL receptors. This results in increased clearance of cholesterol from plasma | Simvastatin | 10-40mg od | ↓30-35 | ↓10-30 | ↑5-15 | No effect |
| | Lovastatin | 20-80mg od | | | | |
| | Pravastatin | 10-40mg od | | | | |
| | Fluvastatin | 20-40mg od | | | | |
| **Bile acid sequestrants** | | | | | | |
| Bind bile acids in the gut which interrupts their enterohepatic recycling. This leads to increased synthesis of new bile acids by hepatic uptake of circulating cholesterol | Cholestyramine | 4g bid to 8g tid | ↓10-30 | ↓0-15 | No effect | No effect |
| | Colestipol | 5g bid to 10g tid | | | | |
| **Fibrates** | | | | | | |
| Major action uncertain. Increased lipoprotein lipax activity, reduced hepatic triglyceride synthesis and increased triglyceride clearance from plasma | Clofibrate | 500mg tid - qid | ↓5-10 | ↓20-30 | ↑5-10 | No effect |
| | Gemfibrozil | 600mg bid | | | | |
| | Bezafibrate | 200mg tid | | | | |
| | Fenofibrate | 100mg tid | | | | |
| **Nicotinic acid (niacin) derivatives** | | | | | | |
| Reduce hepatic VLDL production | Nicotinic acid | 0.5-1.5g tid | ↓15-25[a] | ↓15-40[a] | ↑15-25[a] | ↓5-10[a] |
| | Acipimox | 250mg bid-tid | | | | |

a Data for nicotinic acid.

*Abbreviations and symbols:* LDL-C = low-density lipoprotein cholesterol; HDL-C = high-density lipoprotein cholesterol; VLDL = very-low-density lipoprotein; od = once daily; bid = twice daily; tid = three times daily; qid = 4 times daily; ↓ = decreased; ↑ = increased.

#### Clinical Effectiveness

Unlike the HMG CoA reductase inhibitors, the role of the fibrates in lipid-lowering therapy is declining. This is partly because of uncertainty about the value of an intervention which primarily reduces plasma triglycerides and partly because of a small increase in nonvascular mortality seen in the large trials undertaken with both clofibrate and gemfibrozil. The more powerful cholesterol-lowering effect of the HMG CoA reductase inhibitors and their better results in large-scale mortality/morbidity trials is resulting in the displacement of fibrates from much of their previous clinical use, although they are still commonly used in patients with combined elevations of cholesterol and triglyceride.[51,52]

#### Tolerability and Drug Interactions Potential

***Adverse effects:*** the fibrates are generally well tolerated. Their most common immediate adverse effects are abdominal discomfort (5 to 10% of patients), epigastric fullness, nausea and mild diarrhoea. Occasional problems include weight increase, fluid retention, impotence, the provocation of cardiac arrhythmias, and gallstones resulting from an increase in the lithogenicity of bile.[53] Liver enzymes are sometimes slightly elevated and a syndrome of muscle tenderness with a raised serum creatine phosphokinase concentration has been observed, mainly in patients with the nephrotic syndrome.

***Drug interactions:*** the fibrates may potentiate the effect of sulphonylurea oral antidiabetic drugs and also that of warfarin (whose dose generally requires reduction by one-third to one-half)[54] [see further appendix B].

### 4.2.5 Nicotinic Acid (Niacin)

Nicotinic acid is a water soluble B group vitamin which at high doses favourably affects all plasma lipid subtypes.[55] It lowers plasma total and LDL-cholesterol concentrations, Lp(a) and triglycerides, and increases plasma HDL-cholesterol.[56] An analogue of nicotinic acid, *acipimox*, which has a more prolonged effect, is also available; however, nicotinic acid should not be confused with nicotinamide (niacinamide) which has no effect on lipids.

#### Clinical Effectiveness

Nicotinic acid reduces VLDL production in the liver and since VLDL is converted to LDL, the LDL-cholesterol concentration also falls.[57] However, a large dose is required to produce significant reductions. A dose of 1.5g generally produces a 10 to 15% average reduction in LDL-cholesterol and a 15 to 25% reduction is produced by a dose of 3g. This dose level also reduces plasma triglyceride concentrations by 5 to 30%.

The initiation of therapy with nicotinic acid must be undertaken with low dosages (e.g. 125mg twice daily with food) which is then slowly increased over 4 to 6 weeks to a usual maintenance level of 3 g/day in two or three divided doses (or a maximum of 4.5 g/day). Symptoms of flushing, tingling and headache (see below) are usually most troublesome during the initiation of treatment.[58] Aspirin (300 to 325mg) taken 30 minutes prior to a nicotinic acid dose lessens the intensity of these symptoms and considerably improves tolerance of the drug.[59] If therapy is interrupted, the drug should be reintroduced at lower doses.

#### Tolerability

Nicotinic acid is poorly tolerated by many patients. As mentioned above, its most frequent adverse effect is flushing but a variety of other symptoms including nausea, flatulence and diarrhoea are also common.[60] The drug may exacerbate peptic ulceration and gout and commonly produces a deterioration in glucose tolerance. For this reason, nicotinic acid is relatively contraindicated in gout and diabetes mellitus, despite its apparently favourable effect on the lipid abnormalities frequently encountered in diabetic patients.

The other important and serious adverse effect of nicotinic acid is hepatotoxicity.[61] Minor reversible abnormalities of liver function are common.[62] It is recommended that serum transaminases should be measured 3-monthly for the first year of nicotinic acid therapy and periodically thereafter. There have been several case reports of severe hepatic necrosis occurring, mainly affecting patients taking sustained-release forms of nicotinic acid, and concern over this problem has substantially limited the clinical acceptance of these preparations.

### *4.2.6 Antioxidant Vitamins*

The increasingly recognised role of oxidised LDL in the generation of atheromatous plaques (see section 4.1.1) has led to studies of the potential role of antioxidant vitamins (especially the fat soluble vitamin E and water soluble vitamin C) to slow the progression of atheroma. Early epidemiological studies suggested a benefit from vitamin E, especially when taken in high doses (up to 500 IU/day), but potential confounding of these results by other 'healthy lifestyle' practices raised questions about their reliability.[63,64] Two subsequent trials of vitamin E (one of low-dose supplementation [50 IU/day] in smokers and the other of high-dose supplementation [400 to 800 IU/day] in patients with established vascular disease) found a reduction in coronary vascular events without any beneficial effect on total mortality.[65,66] The role of antioxidant supplementation is therefore unclear, and will await the results of studies currently in progress.

## 4.3 Optimum Treatment

### *4.3.1 General Approach*

Patients with a lipid profile that indicates a high risk of coronary heart disease should be advised to reduce their intake of saturated fats, reduce bodyweight, and increase physical exercise. Contributory conditions such as diabetes, hypothyroidism, nephrotic syndrome and excessive alcohol intake should be looked for and treated appropriately. Unless the clinical situation is urgent (e.g. after a myocardial infarction), the introduction of drug therapy should be delayed until the effect of these interventions has been determined.

### *4.3.2 Drug Therapy*

The role of drugs in the management of increased cardiovascular risk is increasingly being determined by the results of large-scale clinical trials.

#### HMG CoA Reductase Inhibitors ('Statins')

The first of the major trials of the HMG CoA reductase inhibitors in reducing coronary heart disease risk was the Scandinavian Simvastatin Survival Study (4S study).[67] In this secondary prevention trial, 4444 patients with angina or a previous myocardial infarction (and a total cholesterol concentration of 5.5 to 8.0 mmol/L) were randomly allocated to *simvastatin* (20 to 40 mg/day) or placebo. After an average of 5.4 years of treatment, 12% of the placebo-treated patients had died compared with 8% of the simvastatin-treated group; there was no increase in nonvascular mortality. Subsequently, the CARE (Cholesterol and Recurrent Events) trial investigated whether the benefit achieved by lowering LDL-cholesterol concentrations extends to more typical coronary heart disease patients with average LDL-cholesterol levels. In this study, 4159 postmyocardial infarction patients with a mean LDL-cholesterol concentration of 3.5 mmol/L (139 mg/dl) and a mean total cholesterol concentration of 5.4 mmol/L (209 mg/dl) were randomly allocated to *pravastatin* (40 mg/day) or placebo.[68] After 5 years of treatment, 13.2% of the placebo group had suffered a fatal coronary event or a nonfatal myocardial infarction compared with 10.2% in the pravastatin group (i.e. a 24% reduction in risk with pravastatin). As with the 4S study, there was no significant difference in mortality from nonvascular causes.

Another major study with HMG CoA reductase inhibitors was the West of Scotland Coronary Protection Study (WESCOPS) which was conducted in patients mainly free of established coronary heart disease.[69] 6595 men aged 45 to 64 years with baseline LDL-cholesterol concentrations of 4.0 to 6.0 mmol/L were treated for an average of 4.9 years with *pravastatin* (40 mg/day) or placebo. Survival curves progressively diverged from 6 months after randomisation and at the end of follow-up, there were 22% less deaths among those treated with pravastatin. Again, there was no excess of nonvascular deaths.

Extrapolation of the results of the WESCOPS study to similar high-risk, middle-aged men free of pre-existing heart disease suggests that 5 years' therapy with HMG CoA reductase inhibitors has the potential to prevent around 20 nonfatal myocardial infarctions, 7 cardiovascular deaths and 18 revascularisation procedures per 1000 persons treated. These trials have dispelled most of the concerns about the risk : benefit ratio of HMG CoA reductase inhibitors when used in the medium term. However, issues such as tumourgenicity noted in studies in rodents and their immunological effects might still exert some influence on their use over long periods in relatively low risk patients. Overall, it is clear that the value of these drugs is well established in all settings where benefit from cholesterol-lowering can be expected over a 5- to 10-year time frame.

#### Bile Acid Sequestrants

The clinical value of the bile acid sequestrants has been examined in the Lipid Research Clinics Coronary Prevention (LRCCP) trial.[39,70] This study was conducted between 1973 and 1983 and involved 3806 middle-aged hypercholesterolaemic men aged 35 to 59 years and free of previous coronary heart disease. Half of the subjects were randomly allocated to treatment with cholestyramine (up to 24g daily) and the remainder received placebo. After 7 years of follow-up, there were 19% fewer cardiovascular events among those treated with cholestyramine. However, the smaller number of cardiovascular deaths was offset by a small excess of deaths from accidents, homicide and suicide so the overall mortality was similar in each group. With the small numbers involved, it is not possible to determine whether these excess 'nonvascular deaths' were related to the intervention or were a chance event. Despite the absence of any clearcut explanation, the finding has left some doubt about the risk : benefit ratio of long term cholestyramine therapy. No excess of malignancies were observed among the treated patients.

The greater effectiveness of the HMG CoA reductase inhibitors (and the absence of evidence of adverse effects with these drugs), and the poor tolerability of the bile acid sequestrants are relegating the latter to a second-line role in lipid-lowering therapy. However, they are commonly prescribed in addition to HMG CoA reductase inhibitors when maximum cholesterol-lowering activity is required, and they are also of value in the rare instances when HMG CoA reductase inhibitors are not tolerated.

#### Fibrates

The long term use of clofibrate and gemfibrozil has been examined in three large-scale morbidity/mortality studies. Clofibrate was evaluated in the World Health Organization Cooperative Trial[71] and in the Coronary Drug Project trial,[72] while gemfibrozil was studied in the Helsinki Heart Study.[52] In the WHO trial,[71] around 10,000 men aged 30 to 59 years were randomly allocated to double-blind treatment with either clofibrate 1.6 g/day or placebo and were followed for an average of 5.3 years. A reduction of total cholesterol concentrations in the clofibrate-treated group was accompanied by a 20% reduction in nonfatal myocardial infarction but this was more than offset by an increase in nonvascular mortality (which included an increase in malignancies). In both the Coronary Drug Project study[72] and the Helsinki Heart Study,[52] smaller increases in nonvascular mortality occurred. These increases were not statistically significant and the conditions responsible varied. However, the finding of an increase in malignancies (with clofibrate) is of potential significance because of the ability of the fibrates to induce tumours in rodents. These concerns, together with the failure of these drugs to reduce total mortality, has raised doubts about the wisdom of using them in other than high-risk patients.

#### Nicotinic Acid (Niacin)

It is doubtful that nicotinic acid would be used in the treatment of hyperlipidaemia without the results of the Coronary Drug Project trial.[73,74] A 15-year follow-up of patients in this study found the mortality to be lower in those who had originally been randomised to treatment with nicotinic acid compared with placebo. However, it is unclear how much of this apparent benefit results from nicotinic acid rather than concomitant therapy (e.g. aspirin). Nicotinic acid is rapidly being displaced by better tolerated and more effective drugs for the management of lipid abnormalities.

### 4.4 Clinical Outcome and Economic Considerations

Despite their effectiveness for the primary and secondary prevention of coronary heart disease (see section 4.3.2 above), the high cost of lipid-lowering drugs has raised concerns about their cost effectiveness. Direct costs associated with the use of these drugs include the cost of the drugs themselves together with the costs of medical supervision and laboratory monitoring. The benefits achieved include a prolongation of life and a reduction in medical costs associated with the investigation and treatment of coronary heart disease.

Information about the balance of costs and benefits was collected prospectively in the 4S study[67] as part of a cost analysis. Among the 2223 placebo-treated patients, there were 1905 episodes of hospitalisation for cardiovascular events lasting an average of 7.9 days. In the simvastatin-treated group, there were 1403 hospitalisations lasting an average of 7.1 days. The resulting reduction in hospitalisation costs over the 5.4 years of the trial amounted to US$3872 per patient or 88% of the cost of the medication. These results suggest that the reduction in hospital services (among patients with established vascular disease and hypercholesterolaemia) offsets most of the drug costs.[75]

Although the cost-effectiveness ratio among the high-risk patients included in the 4S study was relatively favourable, the benefit may be expected to be less pronounced in those at lower absolute risk. This was demonstrated in one recent study where the benefits of HMG CoA reductase inhibitor treatment were modelled over a 10-year period in men and women aged 45 to 64 years. Large differences in cost effectiveness were revealed, ranging from US$10,000 per year of life saved among men aged 55 to 64 years with a previous myocardial infarction and a plasma cholesterol concentration >7.2 mmol/L, to US$590,000 per year of life saved among women aged 45 to 54 years with angina and a plasma cholesterol concentration of 5.5 to 6.0 mmol/L.[76] In this study, it was concluded that currently available healthcare resources may be insufficient to provide these drugs to all who might benefit, and therefore careful risk stratification will be needed to ensure that they are targeted to those who will benefit most.

## 5. Cardiac Failure

Cardiac failure is a clinical syndrome of dyspnoea, fatigue and reduced effort tolerance that results from impaired cardiac ventricular function. This is accompanied by activation of neural and hormonal reflexes to maintain cardiac output and allow adequate tissue perfusion.

Cardiac failure accounts for about 5% of hospital admissions in Western countries and is primarily a disease of the elderly. In the Framingham epidemiological study, its incidence was found to increase sharply from 3 cases per 1000 in the 35- to 64-year age group to 10 cases per 1000 in those aged 65 to 94 years.[77] Despite a recent decline in age-specific incidence, the absolute number of cases presenting for treatment is increasing as a result of the aging of the population, greater survival after myocardial infarction and improved diagnostic techniques.

### 5.1 Causes and Categorisation of Cardiac Failure

The common causes of cardiac failure are shown in table III. Because of differences in pathophysiology, treatment and prognosis, ventricular dysfunction is now categorised on the basis of normal or abnormal systolic function, determined by a simple echocardiographic (or radionucleotide) assessment of the ejection fraction.[78] Systolic dysfunction refers to an ejection fraction of less than 40%, whereas in diastolic dysfunction, the ejection fraction is normal.

#### *5.1.1 Systolic Dysfunction*

Systolic or contractile dysfunction comprises the majority (over 70% of cases) of ventricular

**Table III.** Common causes of congestive cardiac failure

| |
|---|
| Coronary artery disease |
| Aortic stenosis |
| Systemic hypertension |
| Thyrotoxicosis |
| Anaemia |
| Post-viral infections |
| Toxins (e.g. alcohol) |
| Drugs (e.g. anthracyclines) |
| Unknown (idiopathic) |

dysfunction and has a worse prognosis than diastolic dysfunction.[79] The condition results from a reduction of ventricular contractile strength and a consequent inability of the ventricle to eject blood into the aorta. Haemodynamic changes within the kidneys coupled with a reduced glomerular filtration rate leads to sodium and water retention. This facilitates the utilisation of the Frank-Starling mechanism to maintain cardiac output. The increased left ventricular end-diastolic pressure results in increased pulmonary vascular pressure, leading to symptomatic pulmonary venous congestion.

The most common cause of systolic dysfunction is ischaemic heart disease. Following myocardial infarction, the degree of left ventricular dysfunction is directly proportional to the size of the infarct. A similar but more global depression of function may accompany other conditions such as viral cardiomyopathy and alcohol abuse.

The prognosis of established systolic dysfunction is one of inexorable deterioration. Among those with New York Heart Association (NYHA) class II or III symptoms (table IV), the annual mortality is about 15 to 20% while those in functional class IV have a 1-year mortality of approximately 50%.[80] About 40% of deaths are sudden and presumably result from arrhythmias. Another 40% result from deterioration in cardiac failure.

#### 5.1.2 Diastolic Dysfunction

Diastolic dysfunction refers to an impairment of ventricular filling resulting from hypertrophy, fibrosis or infiltration of the myocardium.[81] An increase in left atrial pressure is necessary to maintain adequate ventricular filling. As with systolic failure, this may be transmitted to the lungs resulting in pulmonary vascular congestion and signs similar to those of systolic dysfunction. The diagnosis is usually suggested by echocardiographic evidence of a normal or near normal ejection fraction in the presence of clinical evidence of pulmonary congestion. The annual mortality is approximately half that of systolic failure (i.e. about 8% per year) and is better still if coronary heart disease is absent.[82]

**Table IV.** New York Heart Association (NYHA) classification of cardiac failure

| | |
|---|---|
| Class I | No undue symptoms on ordinary activity<br>No limitation of physical activity |
| Class II | Slight limitation of physical activity<br>Patient comfortable at rest |
| Class III | Marked limitation of physical activity<br>Patient comfortable at rest |
| Class IV | Discomfort with any physical activity<br>Symptoms of cardiac insufficiency at rest |

### 5.2 Clinical Presentation

Systolic failure may develop rapidly in patients with previously normal hearts as a result of myocardial infarction, pulmonary embolism or viral myocarditis. In other settings, an acute event such as a respiratory infection or the development of atrial fibrillation may cause decompensation in a patient with previously stable but impaired systolic or diastolic function. Decompensation can also occur without apparent explanation in a patient whose heart has successfully coped with a volume or pressure overload over many years.

Signs and symptoms vary according to the predominant site of cardiac damage and its speed of development. Left ventricular failure is diagnosed when the predominant signs are those of pulmonary congestion resulting from left ventricular dysfunction, leading to a clinical picture dominated by dyspnoea, orthopnoea, paroxysmal nocturnal dyspnoea, and (in severe cases) pulmonary oedema. Right ventricular failure is manifested clinically by peripheral oedema, hepatomegaly and engorged neck veins. In the later stages, these symptoms may be accompanied by nausea, anorexia, abdominal distension, and right upper quadrant pain that may be mistaken for biliary or hepatic disease.

Although it is common for either right- or left-sided failure to predominate, early in the course of the disease combined right and left heart failure commonly develops as salt and water retention worsens.

### 5.3 Pathophysiology

Recent studies have emphasised the importance of neurohumoral activation in the pathophysiology of cardiac failure[83] (fig. 2). The sympathetic nervous system and the renin-angiotensin system become increasingly more active as the severity of the cardiac failure increases.[84] A wide variety of other hormonal systems also appear to be activated, as evidenced by high circulating levels of substances as diverse as arginine vasopressin, endothelin-1 and tumour necrosis factor-α (TNF-α).[85] The physiological compensation is disproportionate and results in peripheral vasoconstriction which further impairs cardiac output. This contributes

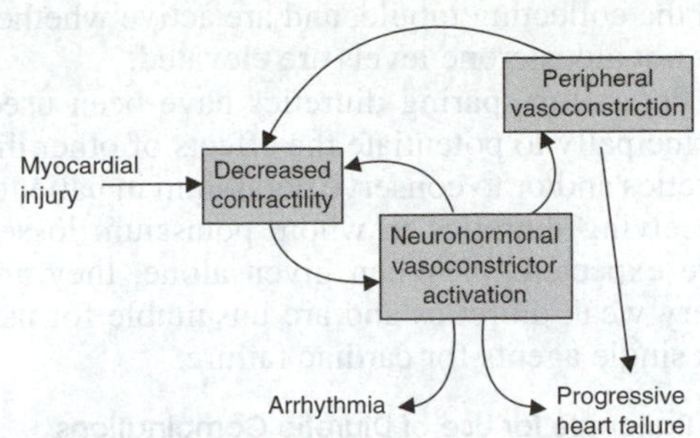


**Fig. 2.** Pathophysiology of congestive heart failure.

to the inexorable deterioration that is usual in this condition.

It is also increasingly evident that patients with cardiac failure are adversely affected by even small increases in afterload produced by vasoconstriction. While normal hearts can maintain a constant stroke volume in the presence of changing peripheral resistance, even small increases in peripheral resistance can markedly affect the stroke volume of the impaired heart.[86] Conversely, small reductions in peripheral resistance may lead to a disproportionately large improvement in cardiac function in patients with cardiac failure.

Recent interest has focused particularly on the possible role of TNF-α whose circulating levels have been found to be elevated in proportion to the severity of cardiac failure.[87] This substance is released from activated macrophages and may contribute to depressed myocardial function, and possibly helps explain the cachexia commonly observed in advanced cardiac failure.

## 5.4 Clinical Pharmacology of Drugs Used in Treatment

### *5.4.1 Diuretics*

Diuretics inhibit sodium and/or chloride reabsorption in the renal tubule, resulting in an increase in the urinary output of sodium chloride and water. They may be used alone or to potentiate the effect of other drugs. A large number of diuretics with different chemical structures are available. They are classified according to the site of the nephron at which they act[88] (see further chapter 24; sect. 5.1.1). Although diuretics share the general property of inhibiting sodium chloride reabsorption, there are differences in maximal effects, in the 'secondary' effects they produce, and in their adverse effects.

Understanding diuretic action requires a knowledge of the different mechanisms of sodium chloride reabsorption in the renal tubule.[89] In summary:

1) Approximately 70% of all sodium and 30% of bicarbonate filtered through the glomerulus is reabsorbed in the proximal tubule. This reabsorption is isotonic in that each molecule of sodium actively reabsorbed brings with it a molecule of chloride (to maintain electrical neutrality) and a molecule of water (to maintain isotonicity). Similarly, each molecule of bicarbonate reabsorbed brings with it a molecule of sodium and a molecule of water.

2) Approximately 25% of filtered sodium is reabsorbed in the ascending limb of the loop of Henle and the distal convoluted tubule. The process is different in this section of the tubule in that it is impermeable to water. The reabsorption mechanism involves the cotransport of $Na^+$, $K^+$ and $Cl^-$ while a positive electrical potential in the lumen provides an important driving force for the reabsorption of $Ca^{++}$ and $Mg^{++}$.

3) Approximately 5% of filtered sodium is absorbed in the collecting duct via an active transport mechanism which exchanges reabsorbed sodium ions for an ion of potassium or hydrogen ($H^+$). This exchange mechanism is stimulated by aldosterone and is subject to a degree of self-regulation in that an increase in sodium presented to the distal tubule will increase its activity.

#### Diuretic Classes Used in Cardiac Failure

***Loop diuretics:*** these agents inhibit the absorption of sodium chloride from the ascending limb of the loop of Henle. Since they have the potential to affect up to 25% of the filtered load of sodium, the maximal effect of the loop diuretics is much greater than that of thiazide diuretics.[90] The larger amount of sodium chloride and water reaching the collecting ducts (and the greater stimulation of aldosterone) leads to a greater degree of hypokalaemia and alkalosis than with the thiazides.

The loop diuretics in common use include furosemide (frusemide), bumetanide, piretanide, torasemide and ethacrynic acid.[91] Furosemide is by far the most widely used drug and is a relatively brief-acting agent. As well as having diuretic properties, furosemide alters blood flow through the kidney by redistributing flow to the renal cortex. Its structural analogues bumetanide and torasemide are longer acting, while ethacrynic acid has a very different chemical structure and is now rarely used except in subjects who develop allergies to other agents.

***Thiazide and thiazide-like diuretics:*** a large number of thiazide diuretics are in clinical use (e.g. chlorothiazide, hydrochlorothiazide, bendroflumethiazide, hydroflumethiazide, methyclothiazide, cyclopenthiazide and polythiazide).[92,93] In addition, a number of thiazide-like agents which are chemically dissimilar but act in a similar manner to the thiazides are also available (e.g. chlorthalidone, clorexolone, quinethazone, metolazone, mefruside, clopamide, indapamide and xipamide). The thiazide and thiazide-like agents inhibit sodium and chloride uptake in the upper part of the ascending limb of the loop of Henle and in the distal convoluted tubule. The increased presentation of sodium and chloride to the collecting duct leads to an increased $Na^+/H^+$ and $Na^+/K^+$ exchange, resulting in a concomitant loss of hydrogen and potassium in the urine. Consequently, thiazide and thiazide-like diuretics may produce a (mild) hypokalaemic alkalosis. As plasma volume falls, there is an increased aldosterone secretion, potentiating the loss of potassium and hydrogen.

Because they act on a limited segment of the distal tubule, the thiazide and thiazide-like agents are relatively weak diuretics and are therefore of limited value in cardiac failure. The various drugs have a similar maximal effect, and differ mainly in their potency (i.e. dose) and their duration of action.[91]

***Potassium-sparing diuretics:*** two types of potassium-sparing diuretics are used. The first of these is the competitive aldosterone antagonists of which *spironolactone* is the most commonly used agent. This is a synthetic steroid which competes with aldosterone for mineralocorticoid receptors that stimulate $Na^+$-$K^+/H^+$ exchange in the collecting ducts. The extent of its action depends on the amount of circulating aldosterone.[92] Spironolactone is most active in settings where renin-aldosterone activity is high, e.g. cardiac failure, ascites and nephrotic syndrome and in patients receiving drugs that activate the system. As part of its steroid-like activity, spironolactone reduces testosterone synthesis and inhibits dihydrotestosterone binding to androgen receptors, thereby producing a mild 'feminising' effect.[93]

The second type of potassium-sparing diuretics comprises *amiloride* and *triamterene*. These agents directly suppress $Na^+$-$K^+/H^+$ exchange in the collecting tubule, and are active whether or not aldosterone levels are elevated.

Potassium-sparing diuretics have been used principally to potentiate the effects of other diuretics and/or to conserve potassium in patients receiving diuretics in whom potassium losses are expected.[94] When given alone, they are very weak diuretics and are unsuitable for use as single agents for cardiac failure.

#### Rationale for Use of Diuretic Combinations

Thiazide and loop diuretics promote potassium loss as a result of the increased $Na^+$-$K^+/H^+$ exchange activity promoted as more sodium reaches the collecting duct from upstream in the renal tubule. The effect is enhanced by aldosterone secreted as a result of a diminution in plasma volume. The addition of a potassium-sparing agent (usually amiloride) counters this effect and also conserves potassium. In addition, the combination of furosemide and amiloride is commonly used to potentiate the effect of furosemide, especially in cases of refractory heart failure.[95] Without amiloride, some of the additional sodium that reaches the distal tubule is absorbed by the $Na^+$-$K^+/H^+$ pump, thereby reducing the efficacy of the loop diuretic. Amiloride stops this 'compensation' as well as providing its own diuretic effect, thereby potentiating the effect of furosemide.

In extreme cases of cardiac failure, a combination of a thiazide and a loop diuretic is used (usually with amiloride as well).[96] This combination can produce severe volume depletion and electrolyte loss and its volume-depleting effects may cause renal function to deteriorate.[97,98] For this reason, renal function must be monitored carefully.

#### Pharmacodynamic and Pharmacokinetic Characteristics

Thiazide and thiazide-like diuretics are organic acids that differ in their lipid solubilities and plasma half-lives[92,93] (see appendix A for pharmacokinetic parameters). Most are not metabolised but are excreted largely unchanged by the kidneys. Excretion is via the organic acid secretory system in the proximal tubule, thus raising uric acid levels by competing with uric acid for elimination. The most commonly used thiazide drug, *hydrochlorothiazide*, has a relatively long half-life, providing a 24-hour duration of action. In the presence of renal insufficiency, however, thiazide diuretics are ineffective and should not be used if serum creatinine concentrations are above 200 μmol/L (2.26 mg/dl).

*Furosemide* has a briefer and more intense action than the thiazides, but like the latter, this drug is largely excreted unchanged by the kidney.[94] When administered intravenously, it begins to act within 5 to 10 minutes and its action lasts about 2 hours. When given orally, furosemide has a wide range of effective dosages, ranging from 20mg up to 400mg (although the usual dosage is 20 to 40 mg/day). Its diuretic action usually begins within 1 hour and lasts up to 6 hours.

*Amiloride* is also eliminated unchanged and the effect of a single dose lasts about 24 hours. *Triamterene* is a shorter-acting agent, its effect lasting about 10 hours.

The principal pharmacodynamic and pharmacokinetic determinants of the response to diuretics, and factors that may give rise to *diuretic resistance* are discussed further in chapter 24 (section 5.1.2 and table VI).

#### Tolerability and Drug Interactions Potential

***Non-metabolic adverse effects:*** the non-metabolic adverse effects of diuretics include:

1) *Hypotension:* the severe sodium chloride and fluid loss that may accompany the use of furosemide can produce a sharp drop in blood pressure. Low doses must be used when introducing loop diuretics, especially in elderly patients where a 10 to 20mg starting dose of furosemide is appropriate.[99,100]

2) *Skin rash and other allergies:* thiazide and thiazide-like diuretics, furosemide, bumetanide, piretanide and torasemide are sulfur-containing agents which share some chemical similarities to other drug groups including antithyroid agents, sulphonylureas and sulfonamide antibacterials.[101] Like these other agents, they not infrequently cause skin rashes, which are often provoked by sunlight. Sometimes these rashes take the form of erythema multiforme (a specific rash characterised by small target lesions with a small blister found on sun-exposed surfaces).

3) *Cholecystitis, pancreatitis:* both of these are rare consequences of diuretic use, possibly resulting from increased viscosity of biliary or pancreatic secretions.[102]

4) *Impotence:* in a large clinical trial in which a thiazide was compared with placebo, the diuretic-treated group were found to experience an excess of impotence (about 2 cases per 1000 treatment-years).[103,104] This possibility should be considered, among many others, in patients complaining of impotence.

5) *Deafness:* this is sometimes seen with high doses of furosemide or other loop diuretics and may not be entirely reversible.[105] Subclinical effects such as high-tone deafness can also occur.

6) *Other adverse effects:* ethacrynic acid is more toxic to the gastrointestinal tract than other diuretics, producing nausea, vomiting and gastrointestinal haemorrhage in some patients.[106] Spironolactone has an antiandrogenic effect and may produce gynaecomastia, impotence and a loss of libido in men.[107] In women, it can cause breast soreness, voice deepening and menstrual irregularity.

***Metabolic adverse effects:*** the metabolic adverse effects of diuretics are generally dose-related and the present trend towards using much lower doses has reduced their significance.[70] Metabolic adverse effects include:

1) *Hypo- and hyperkalaemia:* both loop diuretics and the thiazide (and thiazide-like) diuretics induce a loss of potassium. In the case of the thiazides, the effect is usually mild but in certain patient groups, e.g. those with secondary hyperaldosteronism, or those on stimulant laxatives or corticosteroids, the effect can be more substantial. If significant hypokalaemia is present, these factors should be considered.[108] In patients receiving digoxin, even the relatively mild thiazide-induced hypokalaemia may potentiate serious digoxin toxicity and mild hypokalaemia may also exacerbate various cardiac arrhythmias. Because of their greater maximal effect, loop diuretics are likely to produce more significant degrees of hypokalaemia.

Hyperkalaemia may occur with potassium-sparing diuretics, particularly when these agents are used inadvertently in patients with renal dysfunction and especially if potassium supplements are also used. Combining amiloride and a potassium supplement in a patient with renal dysfunction is potentially dangerous.[109]

2) *Hyponatraemia:* although this is less of a problem since the move towards lower dose diuretic therapy, low sodium concentrations are still sometimes produced in elderly patients receiving more powerful diuretics (e.g. furosemide) or diuretic combinations (e.g. hydrochlorothiazide/amiloride).[110] At low sodium concentrations, evidence of mental confusion, poor peripheral circulation, postural hypotension and deterioration in renal function are seen.

3) *Hypercalcaemia/hypocalcaemia:* thiazide diuretics reduce calcium excretion and produce a mild increase in plasma calcium concentrations.[111] Surveys have shown that these drugs

cause about 25% of cases of hypercalcaemia observed in a general hospital. In contrast to the thiazides, loop diuretics cause a loss of calcium in the urine, and can lower plasma calcium concentrations. Both diuretic classes can also produce depletion of plasma magnesium, which may exacerbate the tendency to tachyarrhythmias in these patients.[112]

4) *Impaired glucose tolerance:* thiazide and loop diuretics worsen glucose tolerance and may lead to additional requirements for antidiabetic therapy. High-dose diuretic therapy produces a greater deterioration in glucose tolerance than low doses.[113]

5) *Hyperuricaemia:* thiazides and loop diuretics cause hyperuricaemia and may provoke gout.[114] They cause increased tubular reabsorption of uric acid and also compete with uric acid for tubular secretion. The effect is less pronounced when low doses are used.

6) *Hyperlipidaemia:* thiazide diuretics increase total cholesterol and triglyceride concentration in a dose-related fashion. The effect on triglycerides is proportionally much greater than the effect on cholesterol.[115] It is believed that these effects might counteract some of the beneficial preventive effects on cardiac disease resulting from the reduction in blood pressure. However, lipid changes produced by the low doses of these agents currently used are very small.

***Drug interactions:*** drugs that may cause clinically important drug interactions with diuretics include:

1) *Nonsteroidal anti-inflammatory drugs* (NSAIDs): these drugs block the production of vasodilating prostaglandins in the kidney. The consequent renal vasoconstriction may explain the ability of NSAIDs to partly antagonise the actions of diuretics.[116,117]

2) *Other potassium-losing drugs:* severe hypokalaemia may develop when thiazide or loop diuretics are combined with other drugs that promote potassium loss. Such agents include corticosteroids, stimulant laxatives, and excessive liquorice ingestion.[118]

3) *Lithium:* thiazide and loop diuretics impair lithium excretion (by inhibiting its tubular secretion) and may cause lithium intoxication.[119]

4) *ACE inhibitors:* thiazide and loop diuretics potentiate the blood pressure-lowering effect of ACE inhibitors. The initial dose of an ACE inhibitor should therefore be kept very low in patients receiving intensive diuretic therapy to avoid a severe drop in blood pressure.

5) *Digoxin:* toxicity from digoxin can take the form of virtually any arrhythmia and can occur even at normal digoxin concentrations in the presence of hypokalaemia. Low serum potassium concentrations cannot be tolerated in patients receiving digoxin.

### 5.4.2 Angiotensin-Converting Enzyme (ACE) Inhibitors

An ACE inhibitor administered concomitantly with a diuretic is now considered to be first-line therapy for systolic failure. The beneficial effects of these drugs have been demonstrated in mild, moderate and severe dysfunction. They have a particularly valuable role when cardiac failure develops during or after a myocardial infarction when they should be routinely used as part of the treatment regimen. The first agents of this class to become available were captopril and enalapril but a number of others have now been marketed including lisinopril, perindopril, fosinopril, ramipril, trandolapril, benazepril, cilazapril, delapril, moexipril, quinapril, spirapril and zofenopril (see also chapter 21; sect. 3.5).

#### Mechanism/Site of Action

ACE inhibitors inhibit the synthesis of angiotensin II and the breakdown of bradykinin[120] (fig. 3). This inhibition takes place in the circulation and in tissues such as the heart and vasculature where components of the renin-angiotensin system are located. Angiotensin II is a powerful vasoconstrictor, a stimulus to aldosterone release, and a promoter of cell growth in the heart and vasculature. Bradykinin, in contrast, is a vasodilator and cell growth inhibitor. The relative changes in concentration may represent an important stimulus to cardiac and vascular hypertrophy.

#### Pharmacodynamic Properties

Administration of an ACE inhibitor to a patient with systolic dysfunction produces an acute reduction in peripheral resistance and an increase in stroke volume and cardiac output, but relatively small changes in blood pressure, pulse rate and blood flow to the major organs.[121] These haemodynamic changes persist over the longer term and are relatively independent of circulating renin levels.

For further discussion on the pharmacodynamic properties of ACE inhibitors, see chapter 21; section 3.5.2.

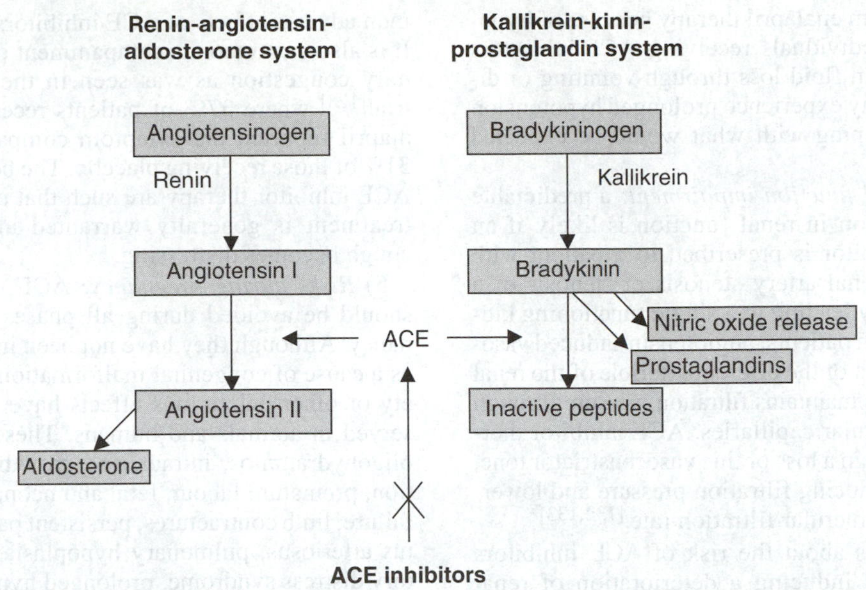


**Fig. 3.** Mechanism of action of ACE (angiotensin-converting enzyme) inhibitors.

#### Pharmacokinetic Characteristics

The pharmacokinetic characteristics of the ACE inhibitors are discussed in greater detail in chapter 21; section 3.5.3 (see table VI in this chapter for a compilation of their pharmacokinetic parameters). Few of the differences between them are of clinical significance apart from:

1) *Duration of action:* captopril has a shorter elimination half-life than most of the other agents, and this property may be useful when administering test doses at the commencement of therapy.

2) *Influence of food on absorption:* captopril, cilazapril and perindopril differ from the other ACE inhibitors in that food slows their absorption; in the case of captopril, bioavailability may be reduced by 30 to 40% if it is coadministered with food.[122]

3) *Route of elimination:* whereas most ACE inhibitors are eliminated principally by the kidneys, some agents such as fosinopril, spirapril and trandolapril are eliminated by both the kidneys and the liver, and hence are less likely to accumulate in renal insufficiency.[123-127]

#### Clinical Effectiveness

In the majority of studies in cardiac failure, ACE inhibitors have been used concomitantly with diuretic therapy. Because of the additive effect of this combination, it is appropriate to use diuretics in most instances where ACE inhibitors are administered. There is only limited information available about their effectiveness as monotherapy. The beneficial effects of ACE inhibitors in systolic dysfunction are seen in the presence or absence of most other drug therapy (e.g. β-blockers, vasodilators or calcium antagonists), although there is conflicting data about whether aspirin reduces their effect. This was suggested in the SOLVD trial[128] but not in the AIRE study[129] (see further section 5.5.2 below).

The beneficial effects of ACE inhibitors in systolic dysfunction are likely to be shared by all members of this class despite the fact that not all have been examined to the same extent in large-scale clinical trials.

#### Tolerability and Drug Interactions Potential

Exaggerated concerns about the incidence of adverse effects with ACE inhibitors have led to an underutilisation of these drugs in patients with cardiac failure. In practice, ACE inhibitors are very safe drugs provided appropriate attention is paid to monitoring their effects.[130] Adverse effects include:

1) *Hypotension:* a sharp drop in blood pressure may occur after the first dose of an ACE inhibitor – especially in the presence of volume depletion due to either disease states or prior diuretic therapy.[131] During long term therapy, blood pressure usually falls by a relatively small amount (5/4mm Hg systolic/diastolic in the SOLVD trial in mainly class II NYHA participants[128]). Among those with NYHA class IV symptoms (table IV), only 5% required with-

drawal from enalapril therapy because of hypotension. Individuals receiving ACE inhibitors who sustain fluid loss through vomiting or diarrhoea may experience prolonged hypotension out of keeping with what would be expected clinically.

2) *Renal function impairment:* a predictable deterioration in renal function is likely if an ACE inhibitor is prescribed to a patient with bilateral renal artery stenosis or stenosis of a renal artery leading to a single functioning kidney. In such patients, angiotensin-induced vasoconstriction of the efferent arteriole of the renal glomerulus maintains filtration pressure through the glomerular capillaries. ACE inhibitor therapy results in a loss of this vasoconstrictor tone, thereby reducing filtration pressure and lowering the glomerular filtration rate.[132,133]

Concerns about the risk of ACE inhibitors commonly inducing a deterioration of renal function have not been supported by data from large clinical trials. Among participants of the SOLVD trial,[128] the average serum creatinine concentration increased marginally [by 8.8 μmol/L (0.1 mg/dl)], while in the CONSENSUS trial,[134] renal insufficiency caused treatment to be withdrawn in only 1.5% more patients than in the placebo group. When renal function does deteriorate, consideration should be given to the possibility of prerenal failure resulting from inadequate renal perfusion which might respond to the correction of volume depletion. Because of the exclusion from large trials of patients with significant renal insufficiency, the efficacy of the drugs in such patients has not been clearly established.

3) *Hyperkalaemia:* serum potassium increases in patients receiving ACE inhibitors in association with inhibition of the renin-angiotensin-aldosterone system. The average increase in serum potassium is usually small. For example, in the SOLVD study,[128] the increase averaged only 0.2 mmol/L. More significant elevations may occur if these drugs are used in combination with potassium-sparing diuretics, particularly in the presence of renal failure and/or the administration of potassium supplements.[135] In general, ACE inhibitors should not be commenced in individuals whose serum potassium concentration exceeds 5.0 mmol/L, and potassium supplements should be avoided unless the serum potassium concentration falls below 3.5 to 4.0 mmol/L.

4) *Cough:* a dry persistent cough, sometimes accompanied by a wheeze, is one of the most common adverse effects of ACE inhibitors.[136-138] It is also a common accompaniment of pulmonary congestion as was seen in the SOLVD trial[128] where 37% of patients receiving enalapril reported the symptom compared with 31% of those receiving placebo. The benefits of ACE inhibitor therapy are such that continued treatment is generally warranted unless the cough becomes distressing.

5) *Risks during pregnancy:* ACE inhibitors should be avoided during all phases of pregnancy. Although they have not been implicated as a cause of congenital malformations, a variety of other deleterious effects have been observed in animals and humans. These include oligohydramnios, intrauterine growth retardation, premature labour, fetal and neonatal renal failure, limb contractures, persistent patent ductus arteriosus, pulmonary hypoplasia, respiratory distress syndrome, prolonged hypotension and neonatal death[139,140] (see also chapter 2; sect. 7.2.1)

*Other adverse effects:* rash, taste disturbance, neutropenia and proteinuria were commonly encountered when ACE inhibitors were used in much higher doses than is now usual, but are now rarely seen.[120] Angioedema refers to a well demarcated non-pitting area of oedema commonly involving the face, lips and tongue and occasionally the hands, feet, genitalia and mucous membranes. In some instances, it may cause respiratory distress due to laryngeal obstruction. Its occurrence requires withdrawal of ACE inhibitor therapy permanently.[140]

***Drug interactions:*** the most important drug interaction with ACE inhibitors in cardiac failure is with nonsteroidal anti-inflammatory drugs (NSAIDs). The combination of blockade of angiotensin II-mediated efferent renal arteriolar constriction (by ACE inhibition) and inhibition of renal vasodilator prostaglandins (by NSAIDs) may result in significant (sometimes irreversible) impairment in renal function in this setting.

#### 5.4.3 Digoxin

Digoxin has been a mainstay for the treatment of cardiac failure for many years and its role in patients with cardiac failure and atrial fibrillation is still widely accepted. However, in those with sinus rhythm, its value is the subject of continuing controversy. Its therapeutic ratio is particularly low in the elderly and in those with impaired renal function. Symptomatic patients with cardiac failure, whether taking ACE inhibitors or not, appear to derive symptomatic benefit from continuation of digoxin in comparison with those withdrawn from the drug. However, the overall effect of digoxin on mortality is neutral.[141] Therefore, its role in cardiac failure with sinus rhythm appears to be for symptom relief rather than prolongation of life.

#### Mechanism/Site of Action

Digoxin binds to and inhibits $Na^+/K^+$-ATPase (the sodium pump) which is the enzyme responsible for maintaining low sodium and high potassium concentrations within cells. Inhibition of this enzyme leads to an increase of the intracellular sodium concentration in myocardial cells, which in turns results in stimulation of a sodium-calcium exchange system in the cell membrane.[142,143] This increases calcium entry into the cell which becomes available for the contractile process.[144] The result is an increased force of cardiac contraction which subsequently results in a reduced end-systolic volume, reduced ventricular wall tension, reduced ventricular falling pressure and an increased stroke volume in patients with cardiac failure (little inotropic effect in normal individuals).

Another prominent effect of digoxin is its suppression of sympathetic nervous activity, manifested by a near halving of sympathetic nerve traffic to muscle, and a reduction of plasma noradrenaline (norepinephrine) concentrations.[145,146] Parasympathetic activity is enhanced, thus returning autonomic status in these patients towards normal.

Digoxin also exhibits a number of electrophysiological effects which include a slowing of the firing rate of the sinoatrial node and a slowing of conduction, and an increase in the refractory period of the atrioventricular node. These effects appear to result from vagal stimulation and a direct effect of the drug. Elsewhere in the specialised conducting system, conduction is also slowed (and the refractory period increased) but in the myocardium, the refractory period is shortened, as evidenced by a shortening of the QT interval on the electrocardiogram.[147]

#### Pharmacodynamic Factors Affecting the Response to Digoxin

Hypokalaemia resulting from concomitant diuretic or corticosteroid therapy enhances all of the cardiac effects of digoxin and increases the potential for toxicity. Other electrolyte abnormalities which may be associated with increased tissue sensitivity to digoxin include hypercalcaemia and hypomagnesaemia. Conversely, hypocalcaemia and hyperkalaemia may be associated with decreased sensitivity to the drug's effects.[148]

In addition to their influences on digoxin pharmacokinetics (see below), there is evidence that in hypothyroidism, sensitivity to digoxin is increased, while in hyperthyroidism, it is decreased. Chronic obstructive airways disease has also been reported to increase sensitivity to the drug's effects, but it is not clear whether extremes of age influence sensitivity.[148]

Sensitivity to the effects of digoxin also increases after cardioversion and this may lead to the development of serious arrhythmias. For this reason, digoxin should be stopped at least 3 days before cardioversion, and if this is not possible, low energy shocks should be used (10 to 20J initially).[149]

#### Pharmacokinetic Characteristics

Digoxin is administered either orally or intravenously. Following oral administration of digoxin tablets, peak plasma concentrations occur after 30 to 90 minutes, and the bioavailability of most currently available tablet formulations ranges from 60 to 75%. Coadministration with food may reduce peak concentrations and delay their attainment but does not generally affect bioavailability. In the past, outbreaks of toxicity have occurred following changes in tablet formulations and for this reason, guidelines relating to dissolution rates and '*in vitro*' bioavailability have been established.[150]

In the plasma, digoxin is 20 to 25% protein bound (principally to albumin). The drug is widely distributed and becomes concentrated in a number of extravascular sites, particularly skeletal muscle (65%), liver (13%) and the heart (4%). The apparent volume of distribution of digoxin is high (approximately 420L). It is eliminated largely by renal excretion with most of the drug recoverable in the urine as unchanged digoxin. A small amount is metabolised by gut bacteria to so-called 'digoxin reduction products' which are generally present in small quantities in the urine.[151] In individuals with normal renal function, the half-life of digoxin averages 40 hours.

#### Factors Influencing the Pharmacokinetics of Digoxin

*Physiological factors:* in the elderly, the creatinine clearance may be significantly reduced despite normal levels of serum creatinine. This subclinical renal impairment should be anticipated and smaller doses of digoxin used than in younger patients. Furthermore, elderly patients generally have a reduced volume of distribution and so loading doses should also be smaller.[150] In obesity, digoxin doses may be overestimated. Only low concentrations of the drug are present in adipose tissue and therefore dose calculations should be performed using ideal bodyweight.[152]

In pregnancy, digoxin crosses the placenta and at term, plasma concentrations in the fetus are similar to those in the mother. Breast milk concentrations are also similar to maternal plasma concentrations but as the total daily intake of a neonate is unlikely to exceed more than a few micrograms, breast feeding by women receiving the drug may be continued.

*Disease states:* in patients with impaired renal function, the half-life of digoxin increases in proportion to the degree of renal insufficiency, necessitating a reduction in the maintenance dose. The drug's volume of distribution is also reduced and it is recommended that the loading dose be reduced by 30 to 50% in patients with severe renal impairment. As haemodialysis produces only a small increase in total clearance of digoxin, this is not an efficient method of removing the drug from the body.[150]

The pharmacokinetics of digoxin are also altered in hypo- and hyperthyroidism. In hyperthyroidism, plasma drug concentrations are lower than in the euthyroid state and this may contribute to the 'digoxin resistance' seen in this condition. In hypothyroidism, plasma concentrations are on average higher than in the euthyroid state, with a lower volume of distribution and probably a reduced renal clearance.[148]

In patients with malabsorption due to disease of the small intestine, absorption of digoxin may be impaired. However, malabsorption due to pancreatic disease is not associated with reduced bioavailability.[147] Similarly, chronic liver disease appears to exert no major effect on the pharmacokinetics of digoxin.

#### Tolerability and Drug Interactions Potential

***Adverse effects/toxicity:*** few drugs in clinical medicine have a therapeutic index as narrow as that of digoxin. Surveys of hospitalised patients have revealed a prevalence of toxicity in 4 to 35% of recipients of the drug; however, the precise frequency is difficult to establish because the signs and symptoms of the condition cannot always be distinguished from those of the underlying disease.[148] The most common manifestations of digoxin toxicity are seen in the gastrointestinal tract and the central nervous system. However, the most serious and life-threatening effects are cardiac arrhythmias and disturbances of cardiac conduction. In a substantial proportion of cases, these may develop without prior warning.[153]

Anorexia is often an early manifestation of digoxin toxicity and is frequently accompanied by muscular weakness and lethargy. Vomiting, diarrhoea and abdominal pain are also common. These may be associated with a variety of central nervous system disturbances such as mental confusion, hallucinations, restlessness, insomnia, apathy, drowsiness, convulsions and, in occasional patients, a transient psychosis. Ophthalmic complaints are also common and include loss of visual acuity, hazy vision, and difficulty in red-green discrimination. Allergic skin reactions are observed only occasionally, while gynaecomastia is an uncommon adverse effect in men.[148]

Intramuscular administration of digoxin is painful, with tissue necrosis frequently produced by the propylene glycol solvent. The subsequent rise in plasma creatine phosphokinase concentrations may interfere with diagnosis of myocardial infarction.[150]

Arrhythmias caused by digoxin toxicity may take the form of virtually every known rhythm disturbance and it is likely that inhibition of $Na^+/K^+$-ATPase is the underlying cause. At high digoxin concentrations, this inhibition results in a progressive reduction of the resting membrane potential which leads to an increase in automaticity and a general slowing of conduction throughout the cardiac conducting system. Common arrhythmias observed with digoxin toxicity include supraventricular tachycardia with atrioventricular block, junctional escape rhythms, ventricular bigeminy or trigeminy, atrioventricular junctional tachycardia, unifocal or multifocal ventricular ectopic beats, and ventricular tachycardia. Sinus bradycardia is also common and is probably produced by a direct effect of the drug on the sinus node, as well as by stimulation of the vagal nerve. In occasional cases, sinoatrial arrest may occur.[154]

The atrioventricular node is also influenced, both by a direct effect of digoxin and by vagal stimulation. The principal effect is a slowing of the ventricular response in atrial flutter or atrial fibrillation. In patients with sinus rhythm, a first, second or third degree heart block may occur. In the presence of atrial fibrillation, clues to the presence of digoxin toxicity include bradycardia, atrioventricular escape beats, an atrioventricular junctional rhythm, or a type 1 exit block.[154]

***Treatment of overdosage:*** the treatment of ventricular tachyarrhythmias resulting from digoxin toxicity requires an antiarrhythmic agent capable of suppressing the automatic focus without worsening the impaired conduction through the cardiac conducting system. Quinidine and procainamide may further suppress the sinoatrial node and worsen the degree of atrioventricular block. *Propranolol* is often effective, but when administered intravenously, may cause asystole or depress myocardial contractility. *Lidocaine* (lignocaine) and *phenytoin* produce little suppression of atrioventricular conduction and may be effective.[147] Potassium replacement should also be given in those who are hypokalaemic.

Temporary pacing is often necessary in serious cases of atrioventricular block. In cases of severe digoxin intoxication, cardiac pacing and general supportive measures are the mainstay of treatment. Digoxin *antibodies* are now also available. These are raised in animals and the intact immunoglobulin is subsequently cleaved and digoxin-specific Fab fragments obtained. With their small mass, these distribute widely into tissues and are minimally immunogenic. Preliminary studies in patients with massive digoxin overdoses have suggested substantial efficacy with rapid reversal of signs and symptoms[155] (see also chapter 8; sect. 4.6).

***Drug interactions:*** digoxin is absorbed by passive diffusion and the extent of its absorption can be reduced by binding to certain other drugs within the gut. These include cholestyramine, colestipol, kaolin/pectin and activated charcoal. At least 2 hours should separate cholestyramine or colestipol and digoxin in patients receiving these drugs concomitantly.[156]

Administration of *quinidine* to patients receiving long term digoxin therapy may raise steady-state plasma concentrations of digoxin by 50% or more. This is brought about by a reduction in renal clearance and possibly displacement of digoxin from skeletal muscle. In addition, quinidine also reduces the nonrenal clearance of digoxin. Thus, if quinidine is added to the treatment regimen of a patient receiving digoxin, the digoxin dose should be halved and plasma digoxin concentrations monitored until a new steady-state concentration is achieved.[157]

Antiarrhythmic drugs with a similar action to quinidine such as procainamide, disopyramide and mexiletine do not appear to significantly affect digoxin plasma concentrations. However, the calcium antagonist *verapamil* has been shown to decrease both the total plasma clearance and volume of distribution of digoxin, leading to an increase of up to 50% in steady-state digoxin concentrations.[158] *Amiodarone* has also been reported to decrease the renal and nonrenal clearance of digoxin without changing its volume of distribution. As a consequence, a reduction in digoxin dosage is necessary.[159] Although early reports described alterations in steady-state digoxin concentrations after nifedipine was added to digoxin therapy, subsequent reports have indicated that no significant changes occur in the pharmacokinetics of digoxin.[160]

## 5.5 Optimum Treatment

### *5.5.1 General Approach*

The severity of cardiac failure may vary from a small reduction in exercise tolerance to an acute medical emergency with pulmonary oedema and/or shock. Regardless of the severity, the underlying principles of treatment involve:

1) Identification and removal of precipitating factors.

2) Improvement, where possible, of cardiac function.

3) Control of problems resulting from neurohumoral activation such as oedema and arrhythmias.[78,161]

*Precipitating factors* may be relatively subtle in conditions such as thyrotoxicosis, subacute bacterial endocarditis or a 'silent' myocardial infarction. Others which are relatively common include infections (especially respiratory infections), pulmonary embolism, arrhythmias and anaemia.

The contribution of drugs in precipitating or aggravating cardiac failure is often overlooked. Many drugs have a direct negative inotropic effect on cardiac muscle. Those most commonly implicated are the β-adrenoceptor blocking drugs, some calcium antagonists such as verapamil and diltiazem, and some antiarrhythmic agents (e.g. disopyramide). Other drugs, particularly antacids, contain substantial quantities of sodium and others such as nonsteroidal anti-inflammatory agents produce renal retention of sodium and water and may oppose the action of diuretics.[162]

Once external factors have been removed, other more specific measures require consideration. Bed rest has long been a fundamental component of any treatment regimen, although its contribution has never been studied systematically. However, considerable data now support the therapeutic benefit of increased exercise (e.g. low workload aerobic exercise) in these patients.[163]

A low-sodium diet is also a traditional part of therapy but in the absence of clinical trials to test its value, its role in the era of modern diuretic therapy is also unclear. Despite this uncertainty, it is common to advise sodium restriction to less than 3 g/day in symptomatic patients and to less than 2 g/day in resistant cardiac failure.[164] On the other hand, water restriction is appropriate in the presence of dilutional hyponatraemia (especially if the serum sodium concentration falls below 130 mmol/L) and oxygen therapy should be given to those with pulmonary oedema.

Despite the potential benefits of small daily quantities of alcohol, this should be avoided in heart failure patients (if possible) because of its direct myocardial toxic effect.

### 5.5.2 Drug Therapy

The choice of initial drug therapy for cardiac failure and the appropriate sequence for introducing additional medication is controversial. At present, the majority of clinicians choose a diuretic or an ACE inhibitor, the latter becoming increasingly popular because they are the only agents that have been shown to improve survival.[130] Digoxin is normally used if atrial fibrillation is present. However, in patients with sinus rhythm, it is not clear whether the modest improvements in cardiac function produced by digoxin outweigh the risk of toxicity. It is, therefore, a reasonable approach to give digoxin only if the patient remains symptomatic despite ACE inhibitors and diuretics.

#### Diuretics

In *acute pulmonary oedema*, furosemide is administered intravenously to reduce the extracellular volume and reduce pulmonary congestion. In patients likely to be sensitive to a diuretic (i.e. those not previously treated and those with normal renal function), a dose of 10 to 20mg furosemide should be used to avoid producing hypotension. Higher doses (20 to 40mg) are generally required in less sensitive patients.

In *chronic cardiac failure*, diuretics are still commonly used as first-line treatment, although ACE inhibitors may also be used and may be a more rational choice in the absence of evidence of salt and water retention. Thiazide diuretics may be used for mild cardiac failure and may be preferred to a loop diuretic because of their less abrupt onset of action. However, in most patients, loop diuretics are used because of their greater effectiveness and their activity in the presence of renal insufficiency.

Diuretic therapy in chronic cardiac failure must be undertaken carefully to avoid volume depletion and renal insufficiency, the patient's weight often providing a useful guide. Potassium replacement is usually required in patients on diuretics, particularly those not receiving ACE inhibitors and/or potassium-sparing diuretics concomitantly. Following initiation of diuretic therapy for this condition, serum potassium concentrations should be checked every 3 days or so until the patient is clinically stable, and periodically thereafter. In patients receiving potassium-sparing diuretics or ACE inhibitors (which oppose potassium loss) and in those with renal insufficiency, potassium supplements produce a risk of hyperkalaemia and must be used with caution.

In *refractory cardiac failure*, combinations of diuretics may be used to obtain a greater diuretic effect and to reduce potassium loss (see also section 5.4.1 above). Furosemide and amiloride are commonly combined for these reasons. In extreme cases, a thiazide diuretic may also be added. However, this combination may produce a substantial reduction in extracellular fluid volume, a fall in renal blood flow, and a progressive increase in serum creatinine.

#### ACE Inhibitors

Clinical trials have established that ACE inhibitors are effective in the treatment of mild, moderate and severe systolic dysfunction. They have been shown to improve symptoms, quality of life and exercise capacity, to reduce hospital admissions for cardiac failure treatment, and to reduce the incidence of myocardial infarction, sudden death, and death from progressive systolic failure among those treated. The available clinical studies suggest that while placebo administration produces symptomatic improvement in about 20% of individuals, ACE inhibitor treatment increases this percentage to approximately 80%. Other notable findings from these studies include:

1) In the CONSENSUS trial, which was conducted in patients with *severe* systolic dysfunction (NYHA class IV), ACE inhibitor therapy reduced the 12-month mortality rate from about 52% to around 36% (a 40% reduction).[134]

2) In the SOLVD trial in patients with *mild to moderately severe* cardiac dysfunction, a more modest benefit was seen, with the 4-year mortality reduced from 40% to 35%. However, over half the subjects in this trial were improved symptomatically by at least one NYHA class and the median survival increased by 6 months.[128]

3) In patients with *asymptomatic impairment* of left ventricular systolic function, treatment with ACE inhibitor therapy alone produced an 8% reduction in mortality (95% confidence interval −8 to +21%), but this was not statistically significant.[165]

4) The improvement in survival with ACE inhibitors results from reductions in both sudden death and progressive systolic failure.

5) In two of the major studies in patients with *mild to moderate* cardiac failure, those treated with ACE inhibitors experienced a 20% reduction in the incidence of acute myocardial infarction, suggesting that these drugs may impair atheroma progression. The explanation for this finding is unclear. It may result from a direct antiatherogenic property of ACE inhibitors, as has been demonstrated in some animal models.[166] New studies are now in progress to examine this further.

6) A slowing of the deterioration of renal function has been noted in diabetics which makes these drugs a desirable component of treatment in such patients[167] (see further chapter 19; sect. 3.4.3 and chapter 24; sect. 4.2).

***Patients with left ventricular dysfunction after myocardial infarction:*** in the postmyocardial infarction period, severe systolic dysfunction affects about 5% of individuals and mild to moderate dysfunction affects another 20%. The benefits of ACE inhibitor therapy in this setting have been studied extensively but with sometimes contradictory results. The present situation may be summarised as follows:

- Patients developing evidence of systolic dysfunction in the postmyocardial infarction period have benefited substantially from long term ACE inhibitor therapy, with a saving of 40 to 70 lives per 1000 patients treated over the subsequent 12 to 18 months.[129,168,169] Approximately half of this mortality reduction occurs in the first 24 hours of therapy.
- Routine administration to all patients in the early postmyocardial period is of lesser value, saving on average about 5 lives per 1000 patients during the period of hospital admission.[170,171] Most of this benefit probably originates from the high risk subgroup of patients with evidence of systolic dysfunction, and it may be detrimental to others (e.g. those with hypotension on presentation).[170]
- A pragmatic approach may be to administer ACE inhibitors early in the postmyocardial infarction period to those with clinical evidence of cardiac failure and a systolic blood pressure of 100mm Hg or more.[171]

***Clincal use of ACE inhibitors:*** when ACE inhibitor treatment is initiated, low doses are used to reduce the possibility of first-dose hypotension. Typically, captopril 6.25mg or enalapril 2.5mg is used and the blood pressure monitored for 2 to 3 hours. The likelihood of a marked blood pressure fall is greatest in the elderly receiving diuretics and those with clinical evidence of volume depletion (e.g. postural hypotension, a systolic blood pressure less than 100mm Hg or a serum sodium concentration below 135 mmol/L).[172] If the test dose is tolerated, an appropriate initial maintenance dosage is captopril 12.5mg three times daily or enalapril 2.5mg twice daily. Provided blood pressure levels remain satisfactory, these dosages may then be increased to target levels (i.e. captopril 50mg three times daily or enalapril 20 mg/day) over the next 2 to 4 weeks.

After one or two weeks of ACE inhibitor therapy, serum creatinine and potassium concentrations should be measured. The dosage may require a reduction if the serum creatinine has risen by more than 50 μmol/L (0.57 mg/dl) or the potassium concentration exceeds 5.0 mmol/L. Volume depletion induced by excessive diuretic therapy is a common cause of an increasing serum creatinine concentration.

#### Digoxin

Despite its long history of use, there is still controversy about the use of digoxin in cardiac failure. Most of the major clinical studies of the use of digoxin are withdrawal studies where individuals on long term therapies have been randomised to continue or to discontinue treatment. A recent example is the RADIANCE trial in which patients in sinus rhythm and NYHA class II and III symptoms (with an ejection fraction below 35%) were randomly allocated to continue or to discontinue digoxin therapy.[173] Diuretic and ACE inhibitor treatment was continued in both groups. The probability of clinical deterioration was greater among those withdrawn from digoxin therapy. This and other similar studies currently provide the most convincing evidence that digoxin adds to the therapeutic effects of combination ACE inhibitor/diuretic treatment.

Despite these results, there is, however, no information demonstrating that digoxin improves survival, and in this respect, the Digoxin Intervention Group mortality study was neutral.[141] There is also considerable uncertainty about the nature of the relationship between plasma digoxin concentrations and either its effectiveness or toxicity (see further below). In addition, it is unclear whether digoxin has any role in diastolic failure.[174]

In conditions where the underlying cause of cardiac dysfunction is a mechanical obstruction to blood flow, digoxin would not be expected to confer benefit. Such disorders include mitral stenosis with sinus rhythm, constrictive pericarditis, pericardial tamponade and cor pulmonale.[175] In idiopathic hypertrophic subaortic stenosis, digoxin may be deleterious because it may increase left ventricular outflow obstruction.

***Clinical use of digoxin:*** if a loading dose is not given, at least 7 days will elapse before steady-state plasma digoxin concentrations are reached. For this reason, it has been common to administer an initial oral loading dose of 0.75 to 1.5mg (depending on the size of the patient) divided into 2 or 3 doses over the first 24 hours of therapy.[149] If intravenous digitalisation is considered necessary, the loading dose should be reduced by 30% to allow for the increased systemic availability via this route. For long term therapy, oral maintenance doses of 0.125 to 0.25mg daily are sufficient to achieve therapeutic plasma concentrations in most patients of average weight and with normal renal function. In view of the frequency of toxicity induced by digoxin loading doses, there is now a tendency to digitalise patients more slowly except in emergency situations (such as with tachyarrhythmias).

***Interpretation of plasma digoxin concentrations:*** plasma concentrations can now be measured with a variety of commercially available assays. Blood specimens should be taken at least 6 hours after administration because of the slow equilibration of digoxin between the plasma and tissues. The usual therapeutic plasma concentration range is 0.8 to 2.0 μg/L, but because of individual differences in sensitivity to the drug, there is considerable overlap between therapeutic and toxic levels in different individuals.[176] Care is therefore necessary in the interpretation of a measured plasma concentration in any particular patient. For example, the time taken for the establishment of a new steady-state plasma concentration following a change in dose will depend on the half-life of the drug in that patient. In the average patient with normal renal function (half-life 40 hours), this might be expected to take about one week; however, it is likely to be considerably longer than this in the elderly and in those with renal insufficiency. Consequently, care should be taken not to make major dosage adjustments on the basis of levels measured before plasma concentrations have reached a new steady-state (see further chapter 5; sect. 4.2).

In a patient with a satisfactory response to a conventional dose regimen, routine plasma digoxin measurement is not necessary. However, if a digitalised patient develops toxic features, plasma concentrations together with other clinical data are often helpful in deciding on the appropriate dosage adjustment.

### 5.5.3 Other Drugs Used in Cardiac Failure

#### β-Adrenoceptor Blocking Drugs

β-Adrenoceptor blocking drugs (β-blockers) have traditionally been contraindicated in the presence of systolic cardiac failure because of their negative inotropic effects. Despite this, it has been noted in secondary prevention trials in postmyocardial infarction patients that the greatest benefit was evident in those with the largest infarcts and the greatest risk of ventricular dysfunction.[177]

Recently, several studies have been undertaken to examine the value of β-blockers in patients with systolic cardiac dysfunction.[178] Most of these show an increase in the average ejection fraction among those treated, but studies examining their effect on exercise tolerance have not shown consistent benefit, probably because of the heart rate reductions that accompany this therapy.

Three large-scale trials have examined the effect of β-blockers on morbidity and mortality. The first of these (with *bisoprolol*) showed a trend towards benefit (not statistically significant), but this study had low statistical power.[179] The second (with *metoprolol* in patients with idiopathic dilated cardiomyopathy) demonstrated a nonsignificant benefit in reducing the combined endpoint of death or requirement for transplantation.[180] A more recent trial (with the combined β-blocker/vasodilator *carvedilol*) showed a substantial benefit, raising the possibility that the outcome may depend on the particular properties of the agents involved.[181] Further clinical trials are presently underway to examine the effect of these drugs on survival.

#### Inotropic Agents

Results of studies using inotropic agents in cardiac failure have been almost uniformly negative.[182] These studies have generally involved the oral administration of inotropic drugs in an outpatient setting and may not reflect their value for short term use in intensive care settings where some agents have been shown to produce symptomatic benefit. The results have been interpreted as indicating that little therapeutic benefit is likely to be derived from stimulating an impaired myocardium. Some patients who remain symptomatic despite maximal therapy might be prepared to trade off some reduction in life expectancy for some symptomatic improvement.

A variety of inotropic agents have been studied in heart failure; these drugs belong to 4 principal classes:

- *β-Adrenoceptor agonists* – which increase intracellular calcium levels by stimulating cyclic-AMP (cyclic adenosine monophosphate)[183]
- *Phosphodiesterase inhibitors* – which increase intracellular calcium levels by preventing cyclic-AMP inactivation[184,185]
- *Ion channel agents* – which increase calcium delivery to the contractile elements
- *Calcium sensitisers* – which appear to increase the sensitivity of contractile proteins to calcium.

The specific agents that have been evaluated include:

1) ***Dobutamine*** – a β-adrenoceptor agonist that produces a positive inotropic and weak vasodilating effect. Dobutamine is most commonly used in the setting of cardiogenic shock occurring after myocardial infarction or cardiac surgery (see further chapter 13; sect. 3.1.3).

2) ***Xamoterol*** – a $\beta_1$-adrenoceptor agonist which has produced symptomatic benefit in short term studies but has increased mortality when administered over longer periods to patients with severe cardiac failure.[186]

3) ***Milrinone, amrinone*** and ***enoximone*** – these agents are phosphodiesterase inhibitors. They produce positive inotropic and vasodilating effects which, in turn, produce a large increase (10 to 50%) in cardiac index that persists with long term therapy. Unlike aminophylline, they exhibit selectivity for a subtype of phosphodiesterase localised mainly to the myocardium and vasculature and lead to increased levels of cyclic-AMP in these tissues. Although small differences exist in the pharmacological properties of these drugs, these differences have not been shown to be of clinical significance in the studies conducted to date.[187]

4) ***Vesnarinone***[188] – a complex drug with multiple actions including phosphodiesterase inhibition, action potential prolongation, calcium channel blockade, and inhibition of the potassium rectifier current. It also inhibits the action of tumour necrosis factor-α (TNF-α). A single mortality study with vesnarinone showed increased mortality at high doses, but improved mortality at low doses.[189] However, this was not confirmed in a subsequent mortality study.

5) ***Pimobendan*** – a calcium sensitiser with large and persisting haemodynamic effects which increases exercise tolerance.[190] This drug is presently under investigation.

#### Nitrates

Because of its short plasma half-life, ready reversibility and favourable haemodynamic effects, intravenous *nitroglycerin* (glyceryl trinitrate) is commonly included in regimens used to relieve cardiac failure in critical care settings, especially after myocardial infarction (see further sections 7.1.1 and 7.2.1). Its value is believed to arise from dilatation of capacitance vessels (which shifts blood from pulmonary to capacitance vessels) and reduction of afterload.

In longer term treatment, *isosorbide dinitrate* (160 mg/day) combined with *hydralazine* has been shown to reduce 2-year mortality in patients with NYHA class II and III cardiac failure by 34% compared with placebo. The contribution of nitrate therapy is unclear, although a second control group treated with the vasodilator drug prazosin (an $\alpha_1$-adrenoceptor blocker) showed no benefit. The combination of isosorbide dinitrate and hydralazine has not found widespread use because later studies have shown that ACE inhibitors provide more benefit. It has therefore been reserved for use in patients unable to tolerate ACE inhibitors.

#### Calcium Antagonists

*Verapamil* is contraindicated in cardiac failure because of its negative inotropic effect. Use of *diltiazem* has resulted in increased mortality in postmyocardial infarction patients with left ventricular dysfunction. The place of the *dihydropyridines* has been unclear with some expectation that their ability to reduce afterload might produce benefit. Addition of both *felodipine* and *amlodipine* to standard therapy in cardiac failure has resulted in improvements in exercise tolerance. However, a recent large-scale trial (V-HeFT-III) indicated no evidence of long term improvement in mortality with felodipine.[191] Similarly, the PRAISE mortality study with amlodipine was also neutral overall, although a mortality benefit was observed in a subgroup of patients with non-ischaemic cardiomyopathy.[192] This subgroup is being further evaluated in the PRAISE-2 study.

#### Antiarrhythmic Drugs

About 40% of deaths in patients with cardiac failure are sudden (and are therefore likely to be caused by cardiac arrhythmias). Following the adverse findings of the CAST trial,[193,194] class I antiarrhythmic agents (see section 8.2.2) now have little place in management.

Interest has therefore turned to the potential role of *amiodarone* which is a potent antiarrhythmic agent with low proarrhythmic potential and which is well tolerated haemodynamically. Two recent trials have come to different conclusions about the value of amiodarone in cardiac failure. In one, the GESICA trial[195] in patients with NYHA class II to IV cardiac failure, an improvement in survival was noted, whereas in another trial in patients with generally milder impairment, little benefit was noted except in a subgroup with tachycardia.[196] Until further evidence becomes available, there is little indication for amiodarone therapy, except perhaps in those at very high risk and when it is not feasible to use an implantable defibrillator.

Amiodarone is contraindicated in those with bradyarrhythmias or a history of torsades de pointes (in whom it produces a high risk of sudden death).

### 5.6 Clinical Outcome and Economic Considerations

Healthcare expenditure on cardiac failure accounts for between 1 and 2% of total healthcare costs in a number of industrialised nations. Between 67% and 75% of these costs are attributable to hospital care; therefore, treatments that substantially reduce hospitalisation may be expected to dramatically reduce attributable healthcare costs.

#### *5.6.1 ACE Inhibitors*

The most widely studied group of drugs in terms of their economic benefits in cardiac failure have been the ACE inhibitors. These drugs not only reduce mortality, but also significantly reduce morbidity and hospitalisation. Therefore, estimates of the cost effectiveness of this therapy can be made, based on cost per life-year gained (LYG).

A recent UK analysis of the SOLVD study[128] determined that if treatment with ACE inhibitors is initiated in hospital, the cost per life-year gained (LYG) was £747, whereas if it was initiated by a general practitioner (without hospitalisation) the cost saving was £11 per patient.[197] These findings are consistent with US, German and Dutch analyses. In addition, analysis of the V-HeFT trials has demonstrated an incremental cost-effectiveness for enalapril compared with hydralazine plus isosorbide dinitrate of US$9700 per life-year gained.[198]

The cost per life-year gained with ACE inhibitors in cardiac failure compares very favourably with other commonly used interventions in cardiovascular disease, including β-blockers and one-vessel coronary artery bypass grafting for myocardial infarction, and treatment of hypertension with β-blockers or ACE inhibitors.[199]

#### *5.6.2 Digoxin*

Based on data from the PROVED and RADIANCE studies with digoxin,[173,200] this drug has proved to be cost effective, principally by reducing hospitalisation. Cost-effectiveness data from the large DIG study[141] (where hospitalisations were reduced but there was a neutral effect on mortality) are awaited.

#### *5.6.3 β-Adrenoceptor Blocking Drugs*

A preliminary cost-effectiveness analysis of β-blockade with *carvedilol* in congestive cardiac failure has demonstrated a net cost saving with this drug due to reduced hospitalisations and morbidity/mortality outcomes.[201]

## 6. Stable Angina of Effort

Angina pectoris refers to a symptom complex, usually dominated by chest pain, which occurs when a portion of the myocardium receives less oxygen than is required for its level of activity. Myocardial oxygen requirements vary from moment to moment increasing, particularly when the heart rate accelerates during physical activity.[202] Oxygen requirements are also increased by a raised myocardial wall tension and by increased myocardial contractility. Conditions responsible for these changes may therefore exacerbate the severity of angina.

Since oxygen is highly extracted from blood in the coronary vessels during its passage through the myocardium, increased oxygen demand must be met largely from increased coronary blood flow. Under extreme circumstances, coronary vasodilatation allows cardiac perfusion to increase up to 4-fold.[202]

Coronary vascular resistance is modified by multiple neural, hormonal and metabolic factors. Nitric oxide derived from the endothelium is believed to provide an important vasodilating effect but its release may be impaired in vessels affected by atheroma or in the presence of hypercholesterolaemia.[203] Pharmacological restoration of coronary vasodilatation is therefore of potential importance in the management of angina.

## 6.1 Clinical Pharmacology of Drugs Used in Treatment

### 6.1.1 Nitrates

Nitrates are used principally for the treatment of angina pectoris.[204] Nitroglycerin (glyceryl trinitrate) has been the most widely used agent and is available in a variety of formulations for oral, transmucosal, transdermal and intravenous administration. Isosorbide dinitrate is available in sustained release oral formulations, as is isosorbide 5-mononitrate (5-ISMN), the major active metabolite of isosorbide dinitrate.[205]

The nitrates are very effective antianginal agents and are widely used to terminate effort angina and for its prophylaxis. They are also of value in the treatment of acute unstable angina (see section 7.1.1). Unlike β-blockers and calcium antagonists, they are not associated with a risk of worsening cardiac failure. In fact, their haemodynamic effects may be of benefit in patients with cardiac failure.

#### Mechanism/Site of Action

The nitrates are powerful dilators of veins, arteries and arterioles. The venodilating effect predominates at low doses and leads to pooling of blood outside the central circulation. The arterial dilating effect predominantly affects larger calibre vessels (including the coronary vessels). The vasodilating effects are produced by the intracellular conversion of nitrates to nitric oxide which stimulates guanylate cyclase. This, in turn, increases the intracellular concentration of cyclic guanosine monophosphate (cyclic-GMP) which subsequently reduces intracellular calcium levels and results in vasodilatation.[206] The nitrates also inhibit platelet aggregation,[207] which may be of benefit in preventing thrombus formation.

The conversion of organic nitrates to nitric oxide requires reduced sulfhydryl (SH) groups mainly derived from the amino acid cysteine. With continued administration, the supply of reduced sulfhydryl groups becomes depleted thus slowing the conversion to nitric oxide. This phenomenon may explain the development of clinical *nitrate tolerance*[208] (see further below).

Endothelial cells also provide a continued basal release of nitric oxide and several agents, including acetylcholine and serotonin, produce vasodilatation by stimulating the release of additional nitric oxide from the endothelium. In several clinical settings, including established atheroma and hypercholesterolaemia as well as in cigarette smokers, nitric oxide release is impaired and the same agents produce paradoxical vasoconstriction.[209,210] In the absence of a functional endothelium, organic nitrates may substitute for endothelial-derived nitric oxide to produce vasodilatation.

#### Pharmacokinetic Characteristics

***Oral and sublingual formulations:*** *nitroglycerin* (glyceryl trinitrate) sublingual tablets and spray are widely used for the immediate relief of angina symptoms. Nitroglycerin is highly lipid soluble and is rapidly absorbed through the mucosa of the mouth. The tablets may be sucked or chewed depending on the rapidity of the onset desired; they should not be swallowed because the drug is so extensively metabolised during first-pass metabolism that its bioavailability is negligible.

When administered sublingually, the onset of action of nitroglycerin occurs within 2 to 4 minutes (more rapidly with the spray), although the rate of absorption may be delayed in patients with reduced salivary flow. The plasma half-life of the parent drug is only a few minutes and its action wears off after 30 to 60 minutes. Nitroglycerin is volatile and is adsorbed onto packing materials; consequently, the tablets should be kept in a cool airtight container and only a small number should be carried by the patient. Tablets that have retained their potency will produce a burning or stinging sensation on the buccal mucosa.[204]

*Isosorbide dinitrate* (ISDN): this agent can be administered both sublingually (like nitroglycerin) and orally.[211] It is more slowly absorbed after sublingual administration than nitroglycerin and differs from the latter drug in having pharmacologically active metabolites.

After oral administration, about 60% of an isosorbide dinitrate dose is converted to isosorbide 2-mononitrate (half-life 2 hours) and isosorbide 5-mononitrate (half-life 5 hours). It is likely that for the first 1 to 2 hours after absorption, the antianginal effect of isosorbide dinitrate is largely attributable to the parent drug while its continued effect is attributable to the mononitrate metabolites.[211] The prolonged duration of action of isosorbide dinitrate allows this agent to be administered orally on a regular basis for angina prophylaxis.

*Isosorbide 5-mononitrate* is available as sustained-release tablets for long term oral administration.[212,213] Its properties include a higher bioavailability and a longer plasma half-life in comparison with isosorbide dinitrate (93% *vs* 30% and 4.4h *vs* 0.3h, respectively).

***Transdermal formulations:*** *nitroglycerin* is suited to topical administration because of its lipid solubility and its small molecular size. When absorbed through the skin, the drug does not undergo first-pass hepatic metabolism. Nitroglycerin is available for topical administration in the form of ointments and transdermal patches. The ointment formulation contains 2% nitroglycerin in a lanolin base,[214] while the transdermal patches consist of a nitroglycerin-impregnated silicone polymer disc bonded to a flexible adhesive bandage.[215] Various strengths are available, releasing 5mg, 7.5mg, 10mg or 15mg nitroglycerin over 24 hours.

***Parenteral formulations:*** intravenously administered nitroglycerin is used mainly in the management of acute coronary syndromes (see further sections 7.1.1 and 7.2.1). This route allows a rapid attainment of therapeutic blood concentrations and the drug's short half-life allows a rapid offset of effect. It is mainly used to relieve ischaemic cardiac pain and is also effective in the management of cardiac failure occurring in association with acute myocardial infarction and for perioperative hypertension. Intravenous nitroglycerin administration is typically commenced in a dosage of 5 μg/min and titrated upwards in increments of 5μg over 5 minutes (while monitoring blood pressure) until pain is relieved. The usual infusion rate is 30 to 80 μg/min.[216]

#### Tolerability

The major adverse effects of the nitrates are the unwanted effects of generalised vasodilatation such as headache and hypotension.[217] These are primarily concerns in the early days of treatment and generally become considerably less prominent with continued use. Apart from their tendency to produce these symptoms, the nitrates are relatively safe drugs and can be administered to all patients except those with clinically significant hypotension.

*Hypotension* is a common problem, especially in the elderly and in those taking drugs that interfere with normal haemodynamic compensatory mechanisms. The fall in blood pressure is usually most pronounced after the initial doses and results from vasodilatation. It is often associated with reflex tachycardia but on some occasions, bradycardia has been reported (presumably caused by vagal stimulation).

*Headaches:* these commonly occur in the early stages of therapy and are presumed to result from dilatation of cerebral vessels. They are most troublesome in individuals with a history of migraine. Patients are usually encouraged to control these headaches with simple analgesics with the knowledge that they will often resolve after 7 to 10 days. Despite this, 20 to 30% of patients are unable to tolerate nitrates because of headache.[217]

*Other adverse effects* include allergic contact dermatitis which may occur with the topical formulations and may represent an allergy to the drug, the ointment base or the adhesive used with the transdermal patches. Worsening hypoxaemia may accompany parenteral or oral therapy and presumably results from pulmonary vasodilatation increasing blood flow through under-ventilated areas of lung. Methaemoglobinaemia has been reported with oral overdosage but has not been reported as a clinical problem with intravenous administration, even with prolonged infusions.

***Nitrate tolerance:*** pharmacological tolerance to nitrates refers to an attenuation of their effect during long term administration, despite the presence of adequate blood concentrations. Tolerance to nitrates was demonstrated by the experience of munitions workers using organic nitrates in Europe during the early part of this century. These workers would typically develop severe headaches and fainting after commencing work on Mondays. However, these symptoms would abate with continued exposure. After leaving work at the weekend, rebound vasoconstriction sometimes led to chest pain (and occasionally infarction). The workers discovered that both the weekend symptoms and the Monday morning headaches could be eliminated by placing a small amount of nitrate in their headband, which maintained their exposure over the weekend.

The mechanism of nitrate tolerance is related to a loss of the relaxing effect on vascular smooth muscle. This occurs even in isolated smooth muscle exposed to nitrates *in vitro*. However, smooth muscle cells retain their response to cyclic-GMP, indicating that the step where tolerance occurs is proximal to this point. It is widely believed that tolerance develops because of exhaustion of the intracellular pool of reduced sulfhydryl groups required to produce nitric oxide from the organic nitrate.[218] It is recognised that tolerance develops very quickly (e.g. within 24 hours of commencing a nitrate infusion) and once it is established, little additional therapeutic effect can be gained by using higher doses. Development of tolerance to one nitrate preparation results in tolerance to them all and therefore will abolish the effect of sublingual nitroglycerin.

Because of the very valuable role of nitrates, various techniques have been used to maintain responsiveness to these drugs. In essence, these involve the provision of a 'nitrate-free' interval during which nitrate concentrations are very low and responsiveness can recover. This is usually provided by withdrawing therapy overnight when physical activity levels are low.[208]

#### 6.1.2 β-Adrenoceptor Antagonists (β-Blockers)

The β-blockers were introduced into clinical practice in the early 1960s after the unexpected observation that they reduced blood pressure.[219] They were subsequently found to be useful in the treatment of angina pectoris and in the early 1970s were shown to reduce mortality after myocardial infarction by about 20 to 30% (see further section 7.2.2). Initially, propranolol was the agent most commonly used but relatively $\beta_1$-selective drugs such as atenolol, metoprolol and celiprolol are now more widely used. A major drawback of this class of drugs is that they are unsuitable for use in the 20% or so of the population who have asthma or chronic bronchitis. Although still widely used, their place in hypertension is now being challenged by ACE inhibitors and calcium antagonists (see further chapter 21). Calcium antagonists and nitrates have also challenged their role in angina.

The clinical pharmacological properties and adverse effects of the β-blockers are discussed in greater detail in chapter 21 (section 3.2), and only the more commonly used drugs in angina are referred to here. For a listing of currently available β-blockers and their pharmacodynamic and pharmacokinetic characteristics, see chapter 21 (section 3.2 and table II).

***Atenolol** and **metoprolol:*** these are probably the most commonly used β-blocking drugs in angina. Both are relatively $\beta_1$-selective agents, i.e. they block $\beta_1$-adrenoceptors found predominantly in the heart and do not significantly block $\beta_2$-adrenoceptors located predominantly in the bronchi and peripheral blood vessels. Neither of these drugs has partial agonist (intrinsic sympathomimetic) activity and both may produce substantial slowing of the pulse rate.[220,221] Atenolol has a relatively long plasma half-life (6 to 9h *vs* 3.5h for metoprolol) which allows once daily administration and is also considerably less lipid soluble than metoprolol, leading to lower concentrations in brain tissue. However, it is not certain whether this confers any substantial clinical advantage.[220]

***Propranolol:*** this nonselective β-blocker is now used less often than relatively $\beta_1$-selective agents such as atenolol and metoprolol. Propranolol is unsuitable for use in individuals with any degree of asthma (because it blocks the action of $\beta_2$-agonist bronchodilators such as salbutamol or terbutaline) and for use in diabetics prone to hypoglycaemia as it delays recovery of the blood sugar level.

***Labetalol:*** this agent is also used in the treatment of hypertension (particularly in hypertensive emergencies where it can be administered as an infusion) and in hypertension of pregnancy[222] (see further chapter 21; sect. 4.4 and chapter 18; sect. 3.3). Labetalol exerts both nonselective β-adrenoceptor blocking properties and also weak α-adrenoceptor blocking properties. It must be commenced in low dosages and the dose escalated slowly. In high dosages, blockade of both α- and β-adrenoceptors is equivalent to a total sympathectomy resulting in severe postural hypotension.

***Pindolol:*** unlike most other commonly used β-blockers, pindolol possesses considerable partial agonist activity.[223,224] Although this property was once considered potentially useful (i.e. having less likelihood of precipitating cardiac failure or worsening symptoms of asthma or peripheral vascular disease), these expectations have not been borne out in therapeutic studies and it is doubtful whether this effect is relevant clinically.

***Celiprolol:*** this agent is a relatively $\beta_1$-selective β-blocker that also exerts vasodilator activity primarily through a $\beta_2$-adrenoceptor agonist effect and a weak $\alpha_2$-adrenoceptor antagonist effect. Clinical trials have suggested that celiprolol 200 to 600mg daily is at least equivalent in effectiveness to atenolol and propranolol in reducing the frequency of anginal attacks and improving exercise capacity in patients with ischaemic heart disease.[225]

***Carvedilol*** has some $\beta_1$-selectivity and, as with celiprolol, also possesses vasodilator activity which is due primarily to $\alpha_1$-adrenoceptor blockade. Like other β-blockers, carvedilol acts by reducing myocardial oxygen demand. In addition, its vasodilator properties lead to reductions, rather than increases, in peripheral resistance, further reducing myocardial oxygen demand. Carvedilol also possesses antiproliferative,[226] antioxidant[227] and antiplatelet[228] actions that may be of additional benefit in the treatment of patients with ischaemic heart disease. In clinical trials, carvedilol has been shown to be superior to placebo in the treatment of chronic stable angina. The drug increases total exercise time and time to 1mm ST segment depression.[229,230] Because it also possesses vasodilator properties, worsening of pre-existing heart failure (if present) is lessened; however, postural hypotension may be more of a problem.

***Other β-blockers:*** *timolol* is a nonselective β-blocking drug with properties similar to those of propranolol. It is also available in a formulation that can be applied topically (as a 0.25 or 0.5% solution) to reduce intraocular pressure in patients with glaucoma[231] (see further chapter 15; sect. 5.1). *Alprenolol* and *oxprenolol* are nonselective β-blockers that exert some partial agonist activity; however, in other features they are similar to propranolol. *Sotalol* (*dl*-sotalol) differs from other β-blocking drugs in that its *d*-isomer possesses the additional property of increasing the duration of the action potential in cardiac Purkinje fibres and in cardiac muscle fibres, thus resembling class III antiarrhythmic drugs[232] (see further section 8.3.3 below).

**Pharmacokinetic Characteristics**

The majority of β-blockers, including propranolol, metoprolol and labetalol, are lipid soluble drugs that are well absorbed from the gut and then subjected to extensive first-pass presystemic metabolism in the liver. Each of these drugs has an oral bioavailability of the order of 20 to 50%. Small variations in the extent of hepatic metabolism can lead to large variations in plasma concentrations and an unpredictable response to low dosages of these drugs.[233] This variability can be overcome by routinely prescribing doses sufficient to reach the upper plateau of the dose-response curve, even in those in whom the bioavailability is very low. For example, propranolol prescribed in a dosage of 20mg twice daily may produce an unpredictable effect whereas at 80mg twice daily, a suitable response can be expected in most patients.

Another consequence of the extensive first-pass metabolism of these drugs is that the intravenous dose is much smaller than the corresponding oral dose. For example, whereas 80mg twice daily of propranolol is a common oral dose, the intravenous dose is usually of the order of 5 to 10mg.

Because of their extensive hepatic metabolism, the plasma half-lives of metoprolol and labetalol are relatively short (approximately 4 hours). As a result, treatment of conditions such as angina which require a certain minimal plasma concentration of these drugs, necessitates dosing to be spaced on a twice or three times daily schedule. However, in hypertension, once-daily therapy appears to be satisfactory despite the short plasma half-life.[234]

Some β-blockers such as atenolol, celiprolol, nadolol and sotalol have relatively low lipid solubilities and differ from the drugs described above in that they undergo little or no first-pass hepatic metabolism and are mainly eliminated by renal excretion. In the case of atenolol, bioavailability is 50 to 60% (due to incomplete absorption rather than first-pass metabolism), and its half-life (approximately 6 to 9 hours) is long enough to allow once-daily dosing in most conditions.[220,221]

#### Tolerability

Many patients who are physically active find it difficult to undertake strenuous physical activity during β-blocker treatment; tiredness and diminished work capacity reduce the value of these drugs for the treatment of middle-aged physically active patients.

All β-blockers are contraindicated in asthmatics, including $\beta_1$-selective agents because this 'selectivity' is only relative. Unlike prazosin which has 10,000 times greater affinity for $\alpha_1$-adrenoceptors than $\alpha_2$-adrenoceptors, atenolol and metoprolol have only 10 to 20 times greater affinity for $\beta_1$-adrenoceptors than $\beta_2$-adrenoceptors.[235] For this reason, selectivity tends to be lost when higher doses of these drugs are used. The fact that over 10% of the β-adrenoceptors on bronchi are of the $\beta_1$ subtype (rather than $\beta_2$) also diminishes their selectivity.[236] Although a β-blocker administered to an asthmatic may occasionally produce a severe asthma attack, this is quite uncommon. More usually there will be a worsening of asthmatic symptoms which may be delayed until after an upper respiratory tract infection or a bout of physical exercise. In some instances, β-blockers may lead a previously undiagnosed asthmatic to develop cough and/or bronchospasm.

Relatively $\beta_1$-selective agents such as atenolol, metoprolol and celiprolol do, however, have an advantage over nonselective agents such as propranolol in that they do not block the action of $\beta_2$-agonist bronchodilators such as salbutamol (albuterol) or terbutaline. If asthma is precipitated in a patient receiving propranolol (or other nonselective agents) it can be difficult to treat, because the activity of $\beta_2$-agonists is blocked. It should be noted that timolol eye drops can precipitate asthma (see also chapter 15; sect. 5.1).

*Cardiac failure:* although it has been widely accepted that β-blockers decrease cardiac output because of their negative chronotropic and inotropic effects, recent studies suggest that certain agents (particularly those with additional vasodilating properties) may improve cardiac function and prolong survival.[237] However, worsening of heart failure or the development of heart failure in those with incipient heart failure who are dependent on a high sympathetic drive to maintain their cardiac output remains as a potential adverse effect, particularly when high initial dosages are used.

*Withdrawal symptoms:* during treatment with β-blockers such as atenolol and metoprolol, which are devoid of partial agonist activity, there is an up-regulation of β-receptor numbers which renders cells particularly sensitive to sympathetic stimulation if the β-blocker is withdrawn.[238,239] As a result, patients withdrawn suddenly from β-blocker therapy typically develop an exaggerated tachycardia on mild exertion. This may be associated with a sudden worsening of angina (and an increase in excess platelet aggregability[240]) that may result in myocardial infarction. For this reason, subjects should be withdrawn slowly from long term β-blocker therapy and should be advised to avoid physical exercise for several days after withdrawal.[241] It should also be noted that patients changed from β-blockers to alternative therapy frequently attribute these symptoms to their new treatment.

*Impaired peripheral circulation:* complaints of cold, white extremities are among the most common symptoms caused by β-blockers in cold climates.[242] They are caused by α-adrenoceptor-mediated vasoconstriction occurring in the absence of $\beta_2$-adrenoceptor-mediated vasodilatation. Such complaints are common in patients receiving either relatively $\beta_1$-selective or nonselective β-blockers and generally require symptomatic measures (e.g. gloves). In patients with peripheral vascular disease resulting from arterial occlusions, β-blockers may worsen symptoms because of reduced cardiac output. In general, these drugs should be avoided in such patients.

*Hypoglycaemia:* only relatively $\beta_1$-selective drugs should be used in diabetics prone to hypoglycaemia. This is because $\beta_1$-selective drugs produce less masking of the symptoms of hypoglycaemia, less delay in recovery towards normal blood sugar levels, and they are less likely to produce a rise in blood pressure accompanying the hypoglycaemia[243,244] (see further below).

*Hypertension:* in diabetic patients, hypoglycaemia is accompanied by substantial sympathetic hyperactivity and in those receiving nonselective β-blocking drugs (e.g. propranolol) the result may be intense vasoconstriction resulting from unopposed α-adrenoceptor stimulation, which leads to a rise in blood pressure.[245] A similar mechanism may produce hypertension in patients with a phaeochromocytoma or in those receiving treatment with certain sympathomimetic drugs; relatively $\beta_1$-selective drugs do not block the peripheral $\beta_2$-adrenoceptor-mediated vasodilatation and are therefore less likely to increase blood pressure in these circumstances. However, additional treatment with a vasodilator (e.g. phenoxybenzamine in phaeochromocytoma) is preferable.

*Lipid changes:* most (though not all) β-blocking drugs increase total triglyceride and reduce HDL-cholesterol concentrations. These changes may occur in patients receiving some relatively $\beta_1$-selective drugs, though to a lesser extent than with nonselective agents.[246] The significance of the lipid changes is unclear but it has been considered possible that they might contribute to the relatively poor cardiovascular results seen in large-scale trials of these drugs in the treatment of hypertension. β-Blockers that appear to have little or no adverse effects on plasma lipids include carvedilol and celiprolol.

*Bradycardia and heart block:* β-blockade with agents devoid of partial agonist activity may produce considerable degrees of bradycardia.[247] Pulse rates may be less than 50 beats/min. Although this frequently concerns the clinician, it is usually well tolerated. β-Blockers can also increase atrioventricular conduction time and are contraindicated in patients with second or third degree heart block. The use of sotalol has been linked to a rare form of ventricular tachycardia known as torsades de pointes (see further section 8.2.3).

*Sleep disturbances, depression and sexual dysfunction:* most β-blockers have been associated with a higher incidence of these symptoms, which are usually mild and resolve if the drug is stopped. Vivid dreams are a relatively common complaint, particularly with the more lipid soluble agents such as propranolol and oxprenolol, as are various sexual symptoms in males such as a loss of libido and impotence.[248-250] The latter symptoms appear to be as common in subjects receiving atenolol as they are among those receiving the more lipid soluble drugs.

### 6.1.3 Calcium Antagonists

The calcium antagonists (often referred to as calcium channel blockers) are a group of drugs used primarily for the treatment of hypertension, angina and certain cardiac arrhythmias. Their use in hypertension is discussed in chapter 21 (section 3.4).

#### Mechanism/Site of Action and Pharmacodynamic Properties

Despite widely differing chemical structures, the calcium antagonists share the ability to inhibit the inward passage of calcium ions through specific calcium channels in the membranes of cardiac muscles, conducting tissue and smooth muscle cells.[251,252] In cardiac conducting tissue, the origin of voltage changes, referred to as the cardiac action potential, differs in different regions of the heart. In most parts of the conducting system, the rapid upstrokes (phase 0) of the action potential is produced by rapid influx of sodium ions moving through 'fast' channels. In these fibres, movement of calcium also takes place through so-called 'slow' channels, but apart from its contribution to the plateau phase of the action potential, this is of minor significance.[253]

In the sinoatrial (SA) and atrioventricular (AV) nodes and in some areas of ischaemic damage, the depolarising current results from slow channel activation alone. Action potentials in these areas are characterised by a low resting membrane potential (–40mV compared with –80 to –90mV in fast fibres) and a slow rate of phase 0 depolarisation. The rate of impulse conduction in these areas is slow. Calcium antagonists retard this, thereby slowing the passage of the impulse through the AV node.[253] They may also slow the firing rate of the SA node, but this effect is often overridden by sympathetic nervous system activation.

Contraction of cardiac and vascular smooth muscle cells occurs when voltage-sensitive channels in the cell membrane are opened, allowing small amounts of extracellular calcium to enter the cell. The small increase in the level of free intracellular calcium initiates the release of larger amounts of calcium shared within the sarcoplasmic reticulum.[254] The subsequent high level of free intracellular calcium is necessary for contraction. The result is weaker contraction (of heart muscle) and vasodilatation (of blood vessels). Contraction of skeletal muscle relies almost entirely on intracellular calcium to initiate contraction and these drugs therefore have little effect on this type of muscle.

Various different groups of calcium antagonists are presently in use in angina, including:

- *Phenylalkylamines* (e.g. verapamil, gallopamil)
- *Benzothiazepines* (e.g. diltiazem)
- *Dihydropyridines* (e.g. nifedipine, felodipine, amlodipine, nicardipine, isradipine, nisoldipine and nilvadipine)

• *Diarylaminopropylamines* (e.g. bepridil).

The available drugs differ considerably in the site at which they exert their major activity.

***Verapamil*** affects all of the sites where membrane calcium influx occurs. It is a moderately powerful peripheral vasodilator, reduces the force of contraction of cardiac muscle and slows atrioventricular conduction. A decreased pulse rate may occur but this is usually overridden by a reflex increase in sympathetic activity.[255] Verapamil is commonly used in the treatment of hypertension, angina and cardiac arrhythmias.

***Dihydropyridines:*** drugs of this group (see above) are all powerful peripheral and coronary vasodilators that in normal doses have little effect on the myocardium or the cardiac conducting system. These pharmacological actions resemble those of other vasodilators (e.g. hydralazine) and when administered alone, they generally produce a substantial fall in blood pressure and a reflex increase in heart rate and cardiac output.[255] Some of these agents are 'more selective' for peripheral blood vessels than others and differences in pharmacokinetic behaviour exist among them (see further below). However, the clinical significance of these differences has not been established. The dihydropyridines are used for hypertension and as adjuncts in the treatment of angina, but are not useful for the treatment of cardiac arrhythmias.

***Diltiazem:*** the properties of this agent are intermediate between those of verapamil and nifedipine,[255] i.e. it is a powerful peripheral vasodilator and produces mild depression of atrioventricular conduction and a mild degree of negative inotropism at usual doses. It is mainly used as an antianginal and antihypertensive agent, but is also useful in some cardiac arrhythmias (see section 8.3).

***Bepridil:*** in contrast to other calcium antagonists, bepridil inhibits both receptor-operated and voltage-operated calcium channels in vascular smooth muscle; it also inhibits the potassium current and the intracellular calcium-calmodulin complex.[256] Bepridil produces only modest peripheral vasodilatation and causes little reflex tachycardia. Clinical experience with it has largely been confined to stable angina pectoris, and clinical trials have shown the drug to be of comparable effectiveness to nifedipine, verapamil, diltiazem, propranolol and nadolol in decreasing the frequency of anginal attacks and the consumption of nitroglycerin.[256]

***Mibefradil:*** this agent is a novel calcium antagonist that appears to act on T-type as well as L-type calcium channels.[1] It interacts competitively with verapamil binding sites but not with dihydropyridine binding sites. Mibefradil is associated with heart rate reductions (probably via a direct effect on the sinus node) as well as coronary vasodilatation; both of these properties may be of benefit in angina. In addition, the drug does not possess direct negative inotropic effects. Mibefradil has a long plasma half-life (10 to 17 hours) and high oral bioavailability (90%), and is suitable for once-daily administration. In clinical studies, beneficial effects have been demonstrated on exercise duration, time to onset of angina, time to 1mm ST segment depression and clinical symptoms. These benefits were observed in comparison with placebo when the drug was given as monotherapy as well as in addition to β-blockers or nitrates. The most common adverse effects of mibefradil are headache, dizziness, peripheral oedema, flushing and lightheadedness.

#### Pharmacokinetic Characteristics

Calcium antagonists are drugs whose pharmacological action corresponds relatively well with their plasma concentrations. Therefore, situations predisposing to higher than usual plasma concentrations generally require lower dosages and *vice versa*. Despite differences in their pharmacodynamic properties (see above), they have quite similar pharmacokinetic characteristics. For information on their pharmacokinetic parameters and the influence of old age and disease states on elimination of the various drugs, see chapter 21 (section 3.4 and table V).

***Verapamil*** is a lipid soluble drug with a large volume of distribution (indicating extensive tissue concentration),[257] and is eliminated by hepatic metabolism. With long term administration, its elimination half-life is about 6 hours, and twice-daily dosing is appropriate for most conditions. After oral administration, verapamil is extensively metabolised during its first-pass through the liver resulting in a bioavailability of 20 to 25%. This explains, in part, why the

1 Many calcium channel receptors have been identified, and they are classified as L, N and T channels. T channels activate upon weak depolarisation, whereas N and L channels require strong depolarising signals. L channels are blocked by verapamil, diltiazem and the dihydropyridines, while T channels may be blocked by mibefradil. N channels are insensitive to organic calcium antagonists.

dose given intravenously (e.g. to control arrhythmias) is only 5 to 10mg, whereas the corresponding oral dose is 40 to 80mg.

Commercially available verapamil is a mixture of its *d*- and *l*-isomers, and the *l*-isomer is 6 to 10 times more potent in slowing atrioventricular conduction than the *d*-isomer. The *l*-isomer is also eliminated twice as rapidly as the *d*-isomer,[258] and since greater metabolism of the *l*-isomer than of the *d*-isomer occurs during first-pass metabolism, intravenously administered verapamil exerts greater cardiac depression than the orally administered drug (see further chapter 6; sect. 9).

***Nifedipine and other dihydropyridines:*** these drugs are also largely eliminated from the body by hepatic metabolism.[257] The bioavailability of *nifedipine* is greater than that of verapamil (45% *vs* 20%) but its plasma half-life is relatively short (2 to 3.5 hours). Nifedipine is commercially available in various forms. The capsule form contains nifedipine in solution which is very rapidly absorbed with peak plasma concentrations often reached within 30 minutes after administration. This rapid absorption is sometimes utilised (e.g. for emergency lowering of blood pressure) but the sudden development of high plasma concentrations is often associated with reflex tachycardia, palpitations and hypotension. The duration of action of nifedipine capsules is relatively brief so that 3 or 4 times daily administration is required to provide an even effect. Nifedipine tablets are a different formulation which dissolve more slowly and provide peak plasma concentrations at 3 to 4 hours after administration. For most purposes, they are preferable to nifedipine capsules and when given twice daily, maintain adequate plasma drug concentrations.

Nifedipine is also available in a variety of sustained-release formulations, and the so-called *gastrointestinal therapeutic system* (GITS) is a recently developed formulation that slowly releases nifedipine (via an osmotically driven 'push-pull' mechanism) into the gastrointestinal lumen at a controlled rate over 24 hours.[259] With this formulation, once-daily administration of nifedipine is feasible in the treatment of both angina and hypertension.

*Felodipine* is also available as a conventional and extended-release formulation (referred to as felodipine ER).[260] Apart from a lower bioavailability (10 to 15%), and a somewhat longer plasma half-life (11.4 hours), felodipine is similar in its pharmacokinetic disposition to nifedipine.

*Amlodipine* has a relatively high oral bioavailability (60 to 65%) and does not appear to undergo extensive or variable presystemic elimination, although it is extensively metabolised by the liver.[261] In comparison with other calcium antagonists, amlodipine has a relatively long plasma half-life (≈35 hours) which permits once-daily administration.[261]

***Diltiazem:*** like other calcium antagonists, diltiazem is also eliminated by hepatic metabolism. Its bioavailability is 20 to 40%,[257] and its plasma half-life 4 to 6 hours. Diltiazem is usually administered in a three-times daily dosage regimen, although sustained-release formulations that can be administered once or twice daily are also available.

***Bepridil:*** this agent has a relatively high oral bioavailability (≈60%), an apparent volume of distribution of 560L, and a prolonged elimination half-life ranging from 1 to 2 days which permits once-daily administration. Again, like other calcium antagonists, bepridil undergoes extensive hepatic metabolism with <1% of the parent drug recovered unchanged in the urine and about 1% in the faeces. Several metabolites have been identified, but only one has been found to have pharmacological activity.[256]

***Influence of old age and disease states:*** because they are not dependent on the kidneys for their elimination, calcium antagonists are usually given in normal doses in patients with mild to moderate degrees of renal insufficiency. In the elderly, plasma concentrations tend to be higher due to a decrease in intrinsic clearance and hepatic blood flow and a decreased volume of distribution. The clearance of calcium antagonists is also decreased in patients with hepatic impairment, resulting in higher plasma concentrations.

#### Tolerability and Drug Interactions Potential

Adverse effects that may occur with calcium antagonists include:

1) *Constipation:* this is the single most common symptom associated with the use of verapamil, and it may also be caused by diltiazem.[262] This symptom presumably results from the relaxant effect of these drugs on smooth muscle. The prevalence of constipation is reduced by avoiding use of upper dosage levels.

2) *Cardiac failure:* verapamil and diltiazem suppress myocardial contractility and may precipitate or worsen cardiac failure.[263] This

event is more likely if high dosages are used or if they are used along with other cardiac depressant drugs, especially β-blockers.

3) *Disturbed cardiac conduction:* verapamil and diltiazem, but not nifedipine and the other dihydropyridines, suppress both the sinoatrial (SA) and atrioventricular (AV) nodes.[264] This can manifest as first or second degree AV block. The result can be sinus arrest, sinoatrial block, sinus bradycardia or third degree AV block. Verapamil and diltiazem can produce life-threatening arrhythmias in patients with accessory conducting pathways by diverting conduction through it.[265,266] This may precipitate ventricular fibrillation. In the case of bepridil, numerous cases of torsades de pointes have been documented,[256] and this drug is contraindicated in patients with proarrhythmic risk factors such as hypokalaemia, congenital QT interval prolongation or administration of other drugs that may prolong the QT interval (see section 8.3.7).

4) *Exacerbation of ischaemic chest pain:* initiation of treatment with nifedipine may be associated with a worsening of angina, possibly due to a reflex tachycardia and coronary steal phenomenon.[267]

5) *Peripheral odema:* patients receiving any of the calcium antagonists (but particularly the dihydropyridines) may develop peripheral oedema due to an effect of the drug on the microvessels, which does not readily respond to diuretic therapy.[262] The appropriate treatment is dosage reduction or cessation of treatment.

6) *Vascular headaches:* like any vasodilator, the calcium antagonists may cause headache in predisposed individuals.[268] This is mainly a problem at the commencement of therapy and is most common with nifedipine and other dihydropyridines. Flushing and postural hypotension may also occur.

***Drug interactions*** that may occur with the calcium antagonists include:

1) β-*Blockers:* although the combination of β-blockers and nifedipine is widely used in hypertension, it may produce excessive hypotension in a normotensive patient with angina.[269-271] The combination of a β-blocker and verapamil is less desirable, and this combination can be tolerated only if the patient has normal cardiac function. It may precipitate AV block as well as cardiac failure if myocardial function is borderline.[272] Intravenous verapamil should never be administered to a patient receiving β-blockers because of the danger of producing severe hypotension and cardiac failure.[273] Similar care should be taken with diltiazem.

2) *Digoxin:* verapamil raises plasma digoxin concentrations by 30 to 50% over a few weeks.[274] This may result in additive AV block. Other calcium antagonists may also increase digoxin concentrations but to a lesser degree. Plasma digoxin concentrations should be monitored in patients commencing on verapamil.

3) *Grapefruit juice:* concomitant intake of nifedipine with grapefruit juice (and possibly orange juice) increases the bioavailability of nifedipine and may result in hypotension.[275]

4) *Cytochrome P450 inhibitors:* calcium antagonists are metabolised by the cytochrome P450 isoenyzme CYP3A4 and may compete with other drugs metabolised via this pathway.[269] This may explain the increased plasma concentrations of drugs such as theophylline, cyclosporin and terfenadine. Plasma concentrations of the calcium antagonists may also be increased by these drugs.

5) *Lithium:* nifedipine increases lithium plasma concentrations.[276,277]

#### 6.1.4 Perhexiline

Perhexiline is believed to exert its antianginal effects via switching of myocardial metabolism from lipid to glucose substrate utilisation, thus improving myocardial energetics.[278] The drug may also possess calcium antagonist properties, but only at suprapharmacological doses.

##### Pharmacokinetic Characteristics

Following systemic absorption, perhexiline has a large volume of distribution and a prolonged plasma half-life, and steady-state concentrations of the drug are only achieved after 2 to 4 weeks of therapy. Perhexiline metabolism is readily saturable at usual dosages, and therefore small dosage adjustments may lead to large changes in plasma concentrations.

##### Tolerability

Because perhexiline distributes readily to tissues, a number of organs may be affected by its adverse effects in a dose-dependent manner. These adverse effects include peripheral neuropathy, elevations of liver enzymes (rarely, clinical hepatitis which is usually transient), unsteadiness, dizziness, and QT interval prolongation. These adverse effects can largely be prevented by maintenance of plasma concentrations within the therapeutic range for the drug (150 to 600 μg/L).[279] Monitoring of plasma concentrations is required following initiation of therapy as genetic variability in expression of the cytochrome P450 isoenzyme CYP2D6 leads to variable plasma concentrations among individual patients.[280]

#### *6.1.5 Nicorandil*

Nicorandil, like the antihypertensive drug pinacidil (see chapter 21; sect. 3.8), belongs to a class of compounds known as 'potassium channel activators'. It produces relaxation of vascular smooth muscle by 2 independently operating mechanisms: (1) increasing potassium flux through sarcolemmal potassium channels; and (2) a nitrate-like action, stimulating guanylate cyclase and increasing levels of cyclic-GMP. As a result, the drug exerts a vasodilatory action on both coronary and systemic vessels and also has antispasmolytic activity. Therapeutic doses of nicorandil appear to exert an antianginal action without significant cardiodepressant effects.[281] Clinical trials suggest that the drug has comparable effectiveness in stable angina to isosorbide dinitrate, propranolol, atenolol, nifedipine and diltiazem.[281]

##### Pharmacokinetic Characteristics

Nicorandil is well absorbed after oral administration and is not subject to extensive first-pass hepatic metabolism; its oral bioavailability is around 75%. The drug is rapidly eliminated with a half-life of around 50 minutes. The main route of elimination of nicorandil appears to be hepatic metabolism, with less than 1% of a dose eliminated unchanged in the urine. Its pharmacokinetics do not appear to be significantly altered in the elderly or in patients with renal impairment.[281]

##### Tolerability

As with the nitrates (see section 6.1.1), the most common adverse effect of nicorandil is headache which occurs most commonly in the early stages of therapy before diminishing with continued treatment. Other less common adverse effects include dizzinesss, palpitations and gastrointestinal disturbances. With high initial doses (≥40mg), postural hypotension leading to dizziness and syncope has been reported.[281]

### 6.2 Optimum Treatment

#### *6.2.1 General Approach*

In the management of angina, attention should be paid to coronary risk factors such as cigarette smoking, hypertension and hyperlipidaemia in the hope of slowing progression of the atherosclerotic disease process. Since angina is frequently worsened by underlying cardiac disease, patients presenting with this condition should be reviewed to assess and exclude such factors.

#### *6.2.2 Drug Therapy*

Drug therapy of angina depends on the severity of the condition and the presence or absence of cardiac dysfunction. At one extreme are patients who experience occasional attacks clearly related to exertion. If these activities cannot be avoided, sublingual *nitroglycerin* (glyceryl trinitrate) may hasten the relief of symptoms. In predictable situations, this drug may be administered as a prophylactic measure *before* exertion begins.

When the severity is such that sublingual nitroglycerin is used regularly, it is appropriate to consider long term prophylactic treatment. The choice usually involves long-acting nitrate formulations used alone or in combination with β-adrenoceptor blocking drugs or calcium antagonists.

There is also an increasing tendency to investigate patients with effort angina by angiography at an early stage with subsequent progression to angioplasty or coronary artery bypass grafting if lesions appropriate to these investigations are present.[282]

##### Nitrates

***Acute angina symptoms:*** the sublingual formulations of both *nitroglycerin* (usual dose 0.3 to 0.6mg) and *isosorbide dinitrate* (usual dose 5 to 10mg every 2 to 3 hours or as necessary) are valuable for the relief of angina that does not stop immediately upon cessation of exercise. They may also be used prophylactically in settings where angina occurs predictably (see below). Sensitivity to the nitrates varies considerably. When starting therapy, it is common to suggest that patients take one or two tablets at home when they are without chest pain in order to judge their sensitivity to the drug and its blood pressure-lowering and headache-inducing potential.

***Prophylaxis of angina:*** patients requiring sublingual nitrates regularly may be considered for oral nitrate therapy. A typical dosage of oral *isosorbide dinitrate* is 10mg 3 to 4 times daily, while *isosorbide 5-mononitrate* is given in a dosage of 1 sustained-release tablet (60mg) once daily, increased if necessary to 2 tablets once daily. Alternatively, transdermal formulations of *nitroglycerin* (ointment or patches) may be used. The dose of the ointment formulation is described in terms of the length of the extruded segment which is then spread over a skin area of approximately 15 × 15cm and covered with plastic. The patient should be advised to start with 1cm applied every 4 to 8 hours and the dose increased by 1cm at each application to a typical dose of 5cm. Doses up to 12.5cm have been used. The disadvantage of this formulation is its messiness. Transdermal patches are applied usually to hair-free areas on the chest or upper arm and left in place for 12 to 16 hours in each 24-hour period. Reduced doses of nitrates should be given in the presence of moderate to severe renal insufficiency.

Nitrates have been shown to be as effective as β-adrenoceptor blocking drugs or calcium antagonists and are not associated with a risk of worsening cardiac failure or asthma. They are also effective in reducing episodes of *silent ischaemia*.[283] To avoid adverse effects, especially headache, treatment with these agents should be initiated at low dosages. To avoid the development of tolerance, a 'nitrate-free' interval should be incorporated into the dosage regimen (see further section 6.1.1). If the patient continues to experience angina while receiving nitrate therapy, a calcium antagonist or β-adrenoceptor blocking drug should be added. Patients should also be told not to take more than 3 or 4 nitrate tablets for a single attack of pain. If pain is not relieved, a myocardial infarction should be suspected.[204]

#### β-Adrenoceptor Antagonists (β-Blockers)

β-Blockers are effective agents for the prophylaxis of angina. This results largely from their effectiveness in reducing heart rate and myocardial contractility, two of the major determinants of myocardial oxygen demand.[284] The effectiveness of these agents in secondary prevention of myocardial infarction (see section 7.2.2) has also contributed to their popularity as antianginal agents. In cases where single drug therapy is inadequate, a β-blocker may be combined with a nitrate or a calcium antagonist vasodilator (e.g. nifedipine, felodipine or amlodipine).

Patients receiving β-blockers on a long term basis are at risk of rebound angina (or even myocardial infarction) if treatment is stopped suddenly. For this reason, patients should be warned not to stop therapy except by a gradual reduction of dosage.

As in the treatment of hypertension, a substantial proportion of patients with angina are unsuited to treatment with β-blocker therapy. This includes patients who have asthma and those with cardiac failure. In the former group, a calcium antagonist such as verapamil is a useful alternative while in the latter group, nitrates are generally used. It should also be noted that β-blockers are not appropriate therapy for patients thought to be suffering from coronary spasm (in whom calcium antagonists or nitrates are preferred), while in cases of unstable angina, aspirin is a critical therapy (see further section 7.1.1).

#### Calcium Antagonists

*Verapamil* is at least as effective as the β-blockers in relieving effort angina and is also effective in relieving *variant angina* caused by coronary artery spasm.[285] The drug exerts its antianginal effect by decreasing afterload (via its vasodilator effect) and by blunting the heart rate response to exercise and stress, and possibly by reducing myocardial contractility. Verapamil has been shown in one study to have similar properties to β-blocking drugs in reducing the incidence of death and reinfarction during the 2 years following a myocardial infarction, although the result did not quite reach statistical significance.[286] This study has led to verapamil being considered a useful alternative preventive measure if atenolol is contraindicated (especially in asthmatics).

The *dihydropyridines* are also of value in patients with coronary artery spasm and for treating effort angina. When administered alone, nifedipine and other dihydropyridines may exacerbate angina initially because of reflex tachycardia; in some reports, 10% of subjects with stenotic coronary arteries have experienced aggravation of angina because of the reflex tachycardia and blood pressure fall. The combination of a dihydropyridine and a β-blocker avoids the reflex increase in heart rate but is only a suitable option in individuals with normal cardiac function (i.e. without heart failure). It should be noted that this combination can produce a substantial drop in blood pressure.[287]

Nifedipine has been studied in several secondary prevention trials and these have consistently shown a worse outcome in comparison with those receiving placebo.[288] Thus, the use of dihydropyridines as monotherapy (particularly high doses of short-acting formulations) should not be regarded as first-line therapy in patients with ischaemic heart disease; they should generally be used in combination with β-blockers.

*Diltiazem* is also an effective antianginal drug, and is useful in relieving both effort angina and variant angina due to coronary artery spasm.[289] Like verapamil, diltiazem possesses a negative inotropic effect and can worsen cardiac failure. In a single large trial in patients who had had a prior myocardial infarction, diltiazem showed no overall benefit.[290]

#### Other Drugs

***Perhexiline*** is a useful agent in the management of chronic angina refractory to standard drug therapy (nitrates, β-blockers, calcium antagonists), especially in patients unsuited to these agents or awaiting percutaneous transluminal coronary angioplasty (PTCA), coronary stenting or coronary artery bypass graft (CABG) surgery. Because it possesses modest vasodilator properties, perhexiline is a relatively safe drug in patients with ventricular dysfunction.

***Bepridil and nicorandil:*** the place of these agents in the management of stable angina is still being investigated. Both drugs are effective alternatives to the first-line agents described above, and may prove useful in patients who have failed to respond adequately to, or are intolerant of, other antianginal therapy.

## 7. Acute Coronary Syndromes

The acute coronary syndromes include unstable angina and acute myocardial infarction. Most cases have a common origin resulting from platelet aggregation and thrombosis occurring on a fissured or ruptured atherosclerotic plaque.[291] The plaques most likely to rupture in this manner are soft and contain abundant lipids. Prior to their rupture, they have often produced only minor or moderate luminal encroachment.

### 7.1 Unstable Angina

Unstable angina is a clinical syndrome intermediate between stable angina and acute myocardial infarction. It may develop in various clinical settings, including patients with or without previous stable angina and following a myocardial infarction or coronary artery bypass grafting or angioplasty.[292] The three common presentations of the condition are:

- Rest angina (usually of 20 minutes or more in duration)
- New onset angina (within the previous two months)
- Increasing severity of angina (more frequent, longer duration and lower threshold of onset).

The traditional definition of unstable angina has also been extended to include variant angina, non-Q-wave myocardial infarction, and postmyocardial infarction angina because of their similar underlying pathophysiology and the difficulty of distinguishing them in the early stages of their clinical presentation.

#### *7.1.1 Optimum Treatment*

The therapeutic approach to unstable angina is determined largely by the severity and the rate of progression of symptoms. At the more severe end of the spectrum, patients are at high risk of myocardial infarction and require urgent institution of treatment. The initial aim of therapy is to relieve pain, reverse ischaemia and prevent progression to infarction. Drug treatment is directed principally towards inhibition of platelet aggregation and blood coagulation at the site of plaque rupture.[293]

In the early stages of clinical presentation, it is often difficult to distinguish unstable angina from acute myocardial infarction. The distinction is important because thrombolytic therapy should be avoided in patients with unstable angina but no infarction. Treatment with thrombolytic drugs is indicated immediately in patients with acute ST segment elevation or left-bundle-branch block on their 12-lead electrocardiogram (ECG), but in those with ST depression or T-wave inversion, rapid CK-MB estimation or the use of new markers such as troponin-T appear to be useful in discriminating those at high risk who should receive thrombolytic therapy.[294]

The early drug treatment of unstable angina involves aspirin, heparin, nitrates and β-blockers.

#### Aspirin

All patients with unstable angina should receive aspirin (usual dose 300 to 600mg) as soon as possible after presentation, unless there is a definite contraindication to its use.[295] By inhibiting thromboxane $A_2$ formation, aspirin inhibits platelet aggregation on the surface of a disrupted plaque. Aspirin treatment has been shown to reduce mortality and myocardial infarction rates in unstable angina by about 50%.[295] Although there are no data comparing the efficacy of various doses of aspirin, when very low doses are used, the rate of onset of antiplatelet activity may be delayed. This was demonstrated in the RISC study when little benefit was found in the first two days of treatment with low-dose aspirin (75 mg/day).[296] Higher aspirin doses, however, are associated with a higher risk of gastrointestinal bleeding. For these reasons, maintenance doses of 100 to 325 mg/day are appropriate and should be continued long term.

#### Glycoprotein IIb/IIIa Antagonists

Newer antiplatelet drugs include the platelet glycoprotein (GP) IIb/IIIa receptor antagonists which block receptors responsible for the binding of platelets to fibrin (see also chapter 26; sect. 3.1.1). These receptors represent the 'final common pathway' through which the many known stimuli to platelet aggregation act. Three types of glycoprotein IIb/IIIa receptor blocking drugs are available including a receptor antibody (*abciximab*), synthetic peptides (e.g. *integrelin*), and several direct blocking agents (e.g. *lamifiban, tirofiban* and *xemlofiban*).[297] Abciximab differs from the other agents in having a prolonged duration of action which persists for several days after an infusion is ceased, and this may explain why it has appeared to be the most efficacious agent in clinical trials.[298,299]

The most promising results in patients with unstable angina have been reported with abciximab. After an early study (the EPIC trial[300]) reported a high incidence of bleeding, a second trial (EPILOG) was established using substantially lower doses of concomitant heparin.[301] When compared with patients receiving routine therapy with heparin and aspirin, those who received an additional 12-hour infusion of abciximab experienced an 88% reduction in death from myocardial infarction. Only 70% of the usual weight-adjusted dose of intravenous heparin was used and no excess serious bleeding was observed. Clinically significant, though less dramatic results have also been reported with abciximab when used to prevent death and reinfarction in patients undergoing coronary angioplasty.

#### Heparin

Intravenous heparin should be commenced as soon as a diagnosis of intermediate- or high-risk unstable angina is made. An initial intravenous bolus dose of 80 U/kg is recommended by the US National Institutes of Health (NIH), followed by a constant infusion of 18 U/kg/hour titrated to maintain the activated partial thromboplastin time (APTT) at 1.5 to 2.5 times control.[302]

Heparin is an anticoagulant drug which potentiates antithrombin III - an enzyme that inactivates thrombin and several other activated clotting factors (see also chapter 26; sect. 3.1.4). Clinical trial evidence has demonstrated that heparin is more effective than aspirin in preventing progression to acute myocardial infarction.[303] The addition of aspirin does not add to the effectiveness of heparin but without concomitant aspirin administration, rebound angina is more likely to occur when heparin infusion is stopped.[304] The combination of the two agents is therefore generally recommended.

Heparin should be given by intravenous infusion because this route of administration provides equivalent anticoagulant activity but with less risk of bleeding than with subcutaneous bolus administration. There is no evidence that newer direct-acting thrombin inhibitors such as hirudin or hirulog (bivalirudin) are more efficacious than heparin in this setting.

#### Nitrates

The US NIH guidelines recommend that patients whose symptoms are not fully relieved with three sublingual nitroglycerin (glyceryl trinitrate) tablets and the initiation of β-blocker therapy should receive intravenous nitroglycerin.[302] Nitroglycerin should be commenced in a dose of 5 to 10 μg/min every 5 to 10 minutes until symptoms are relieved or adverse effects [headache or hypotension (systolic BP <90mm Hg)] occur. Recommendations for the use of nitrates are based on their apparently favourable haemodynamic effects and accepted efficacy in relieving ischaemic pain. In large clinical trials that have examined the value of nitrates in acute myocardial infarction (e.g. GISSI-3 and ISIS-4[305,306]), a beneficial effect has been noted during the first 24 hours but not thereafter. The absence of sustained benefit is likely to result from 'nitrate tolerance' (see section 6.1.1) suggesting that the duration of nitrate use should be kept brief. Abrupt cessation of a prolonged nitrate infusion may be associated with rebound recurrence of ischaemia.[307]

These factors suggest that nitrates should be administered only for symptom relief, and intravenous nitroglycerin infusion should be converted to oral or topical therapy with appropriate 'nitrate-free intervals' after 2 to 3 days.

### β-Adrenoceptor Antagonists (β-Blockers)

The β-blockers (see section 6.1.2 and also chapter 21; sect. 3.2) reduce myocardial oxygen demand by reducing heart rate and cardiac contractility when administered in the acute phase of unstable angina. These drugs reduce the risk of progression to acute myocardial infarction by about 13%.[308]

The US NIH guidelines recommend that intravenous β-blocker therapy should be used in high-risk patients, while oral β-blockers should be used in intermediate- and low-risk patients.[302] Intravenous β-blocker therapy may take the form of:

- *Metoprolol* given in a dose of 5mg intravenously over 1 to 2 minutes, with the dose repeated every 5 minutes to a total initial dose of 15mg
- *Atenolol* given in a dose of 5mg intravenously over 1 to 2 minutes followed after 5 minutes by a second 5mg dose
- *Esmolol* given as an infusion commencing at 0.1 mg/kg/min and then increased by 0.05 mg/kg every 10 to 15 minutes provided the blood pressure remains stable.

Following the initial intravenous doses, therapy can be continued with an orally administered drug.

Patients should not receive intravenous β-blockers if they have cardiogenic shock, cardiac failure, significant atrioventricular (AV) block or asthma. In the presence of chronic obstructive airways disease or mild asthma, β-blockers may, however, be administered with caution. Low doses of relatively $\beta_1$-selective drugs (e.g. atenolol, metoprolol) or short-acting agents such as esmolol may be preferred in these situations.

### Other Drugs

***Morphine*** should be used to control pain when it is not adequately relieved by nitroglycerin. A dose of 2 to 5mg may be given intravenously and, if necessary, repeated periodically.[302] As well as relieving pain, morphine produces venodilatation and thereby reduces myocardial oxygen demand. Its principal adverse effects are nausea and hypotension.

***Ticlopidine:*** this antiplatelet drug (see also chapter 26; sect. 3.1.1) is a potential alternative to aspirin in patients who are hypersensitive to the latter or have experienced a recent bleeding peptic ulcer.[309] Ticlopidine exerts its antiplatelet effect by blocking the platelet fibrinogen receptor and inhibiting ADP-mediated platelet activation.[310] Unlike aspirin, it does not inhibit cyclo-oxygenase. In a large clinical trial in unstable angina, ticlopidine was found to significantly reduce vascular death and myocardial infarction.[309] However, it has not been compared directly with aspirin or heparin.

Despite its apparently similar efficacy, the pharmacokinetic profile and spectrum of adverse effects of ticlopidine have led to it being reserved for patients where aspirin is contraindicated or ineffective.[302] Unlike aspirin, ticlopidine has a prolonged elimination half-life of 4 to 5 days with continued administration, and with its usual dosage schedule, the onset of its antiplatelet effect is delayed for up to 3 days. It therefore has no role in the early acute management of unstable angina. When used to cover heparin withdrawal, it is necessary to commence ticlopidine treatment 2 to 3 days beforehand.

The principal adverse effects of ticlopidine are gastrointestinal upset and neutropenia. The gastrointestinal problems take the form of diarrhoea, abdominal pain, nausea and vomiting. Neutropenia affects about 2% of patients and may be severe. However, it usually resolves after discontinuation of the drug. Full blood examinations should be performed every 2 weeks during the first 3 months of therapy.[311]

***Dihydropyridine calcium antagonists:*** these drugs should *not* be used for the treatment of unstable angina in the absence of concurrent β-blocker therapy.[302] Their unopposed use in this setting is likely to increase cardiac work as a response to the powerful vasodilatation produced. In the HINT trial, which examined the value of nifedipine (administered alone) for unstable angina, mortality was 16% higher than in those receiving placebo.[312,313]

## 7.2 Acute Myocardial Infarction

Acute myocardial infarction is the leading cause of death in Western countries. It results from total occlusion of a coronary artery by a thrombus. The thrombosis usually forms on a ruptured or eroded atheromatous lesion. The lesions most often implicated have a soft lipid-laden core and a thin fibrous cap. Prior to their rupture, they often produce only mild levels of stenosis.[314]

The resulting myocardial necrosis progresses as a 'wave front' from the endocardium to the epicardium and may become complete and irreversible within 3 to 4 hours unless blood flow is restored.[315] Prognosis is largely dependent on the extent of the necrosis. When this is extensive and cardiogenic shock ensues, the in-hospital morbidity is close to 80%. More moderate necrosis may be accompanied by transient or permanent left ventricular dysfunction which signify a worse prognosis than when these are absent.

During the weeks and months after a myocardial infarction, the shape of the ventricle alters to compensate for the inactive necrosed segment. This process of 'remodelling' leads to a larger, more spherical ventricle which is less effective as a pump and is more prone to ventricular arrhythmias.[316]

### 7.2.1 Optimum Treatment

The *early management* of acute myocardial infarction is directed principally towards the restoration of blood flow through the infarct-related artery, and minimisation of the risk of reinfarction by reducing oxygen demand on the injured ventricle.[294] Myocardial infarction is unique for the large number of clinical trials that have evaluated various forms of drug therapy to achieve these goals.

*Primary angioplasty* has been advocated as an acute interventional approach to blood flow restoration during a myocardial infarction as an alternative to thrombolysis. This procedure is extremely costly and labour intensive and has thus far been reserved for high-risk patients, i.e. those with large anterior infarcts and/or cardiogenic shock.

#### Pain Relief

Cardiac pain of brief duration is best treated with sublingual *nitroglycerin* (0.6mg) provided the patient is not significantly hypotensive, i.e. the systolic blood pressure is not less than 100mm Hg.[317] Pain lasting longer than 20 minutes generally requires relief by an opioid analgesic. *Morphine* is generally regarded as the analgesic of choice and should be administered intravenously in doses of 2.5 to 5mg and repeated at intervals of 5 to 20 minutes up to a maximum dose of 20mg.

The major adverse effects of morphine administration are nausea and vomiting. These may be controlled by the concomitant administration of an antiemetic such as *metoclopramide* or *prochlorperazine*. Morphine also possesses parasympathomimetic activity and may induce bradycardia and atrioventricular block which can be treated with *atropine*. Respiratory depression may also occur, leading to hypoxia and worsening of serious ventricular rhythm disturbances. If this occurs, *naloxone* should be given to reverse the effect of morphine.

*Pethidine* (meperidine) is an alternative to morphine, although in standard doses it may provide less adequate analgesia. Its advantages over morphine include less nausea, and because of its relatively strong anticholinergic properties, there is less risk of bradycardia or atrioventricular block. *Pentazocine* is now rarely used because it tends to increase vascular resistance and therefore afterload.

It should be noted that all opioid analgesics tend to increase venous pooling and may therefore enhance the hypotensive effect of other vasodilator drugs.[318]

#### Aspirin

In patients presenting with symptoms suggestive of acute myocardial infarction, aspirin 300 to 600mg should be given at the earliest opportunity. This recommendation is based principally on the results of the ISIS-2 trial in which 162.5mg aspirin on admission (followed by 162.5mg daily for one month) reduced the 30-day mortality by 23% compared with placebo.[319] The combination of aspirin with streptokinase produced a 42% reduction in mortality which was markedly greater than with either agent alone, and this was achieved without an added risk of serious bleeding.

Low-dose aspirin therapy also reduces the rate of reocclusion after the completion of thrombolysis by about 50% and, in the longer term, reduces reinfarction by 20 to 30%. For these reasons, it is appropriate to continue aspirin administration (100 to 325mg daily) throughout the period of hospitalisation and beyond, unless very clear-cut contraindications exist.[320]

#### Thrombolytic Therapy

Thrombolytic drugs are used in acute myocardial infarction to lyse blood clots in an obstructed coronary artery. When blood flow is restored early on after the onset of acute myocardial infarction, myocardial necrosis is minimised, cardiac function is maintained and the chances of survival increases. Thrombolytic drugs can also be used to lyse clots in other settings such as acute pulmonary embolism and peripheral arterial embolism (see further chapter 26; sect. 3.2.2).

Prior to the advent of thrombolytic therapy, about 13% of patients admitted to hospital with acute myocardial infarction died within one month. When administered early after the onset of symptoms, thrombolytic agents have the potential to reduce mortality by up to 30 to 40% with benefits persisting for at least 5 years.[321] The proportional mortality reduction is similar among males and females with inferior, posterior and anterior infarcts, and in those with a first or subsequent infarct. However, thrombolytic therapy may worsen the prognosis of patients with unstable angina, and it should not be given to individuals with normal electrocardiograms or ST segment depression.

The most important determinant of the success of thrombolysis is the delay between onset of symptoms and receipt of the drug.[321] The overall mortality is reduced by about 62 lives per 1000 patients treated during the first hour after symptom onset, reducing to 35 to 40 lives between 1 and 2 hours, and 26 lives between 2 and 3 hours. At 6 to 12 hours, the benefit then reduces to 20 lives per 1000 patients treated and (perhaps) 10 lives per 1000 patients when administered between 12 and 18 hours. This strong time relationship has provided an impetus to investigate the feasibility of prehospital administration of these agents.

The available thrombolytic agents include *streptokinase, anistreplase* (anisoylated plasminogen-streptokinase activator complex, APSAC), *alteplase* (recombinant tissue-type plasminogen activator, rt-PA), *urokinase, saruplase* (recombinant single-chain urokinase-type plasminogen activator, pro-urokinase), and *reteplase* (recombinant plasminogen activator, r-PA) [for further discussion of the clinical pharmacological properties of these agents, see chapter 26; sect. 3.1.6]. Although little difference exists between the efficacy of the three most commonly used agents streptokinase, anistreplase and alteplase when administered by intravenous infusion, the recent GUSTO-1 trial has shown that *alteplase* (rt-PA) administered using the 'front loaded' regimen (see further below) leads to an additional reduction (over a conventional streptokinase regimen) of approximately 10 cardiac deaths per 1000 patients treated.[322] Although this regimen was associated with one additional fatal cerebral haemorrhage per 1000 patients treated, the net benefit of 9 lives per 1000 patients treated represents a small but distinct benefit. When used routinely, however, alteplase would typically incur an extra treatment cost of US$32,000 per year of life saved. Because of this high expense, clinicians in some countries have suggested reserving alteplase for those patients in whom the absolute benefit is likely to be greatest. These are primarily younger patients (under 75 years of age) with anterior infarcts in whom treatment is commenced within 6 hours after symptom onset. Alteplase should also be administered to individuals who have received streptokinase in the past 4 years because of the presence of antibodies.

*Elderly patients:* although the proportional mortality reduction appears to be less in this age group, the elderly should routinely receive thrombolytic therapy.[323] Their high baseline risk leads to an absolute mortality reduction that is similar to that occurring in younger patients. There is evidence that alteplase leads to a progressive increase in the risk of intracerebral haemorrhage, but no increase in risk with age is seen with streptokinase. For this reason, the advantages of alteplase may be lost in the older age groups.

• ***Clinical use of thrombolytic drugs***

*Streptokinase:* this agent is an enzyme derived from certain strains of β-haemolytic streptococci. It was the first thrombolytic drug to be used and is the most widely prescribed and least expensive of the agents in current use. It acts by binding to plasminogen and facilitates the conversion of plasminogen into plasmin. The resultant plasmin degrades fibrin and fibrinogen in the thrombus and throughout the circulation. Streptokinase has also been reported to reduce plasma viscosity and inhibit erythrocyte aggregation.[324]

In acute myocardial infarction, streptokinase is infused in a dose of 1.5MU over 30 to 60 minutes. This regimen produces a peak fibrinolytic effect within about 30 minutes which persists for about 36 hours. The drug is cleared by complexing with circulating antibodies and by uptake and metabolism of the streptokinase-plasminogen complex by the reticuloendothelial system. As a foreign protein, streptokinase is antigenic and is responsible for a variety of allergic reactions, including rash and hypotension. Low levels of pre-existing antibodies are common (presumably the result of previous bacterial infections), but these are usually insufficient to interfere with the drug's fibrinolytic effect. Following an initial decrease in titres during the first 24 hours of therapy, antibody levels increase within 3 to 4 days and remain elevated for at least 4 years.

*Alteplase* (rt-PA): this agent is chemically identical to tissue plasminogen activator which is produced in small quantities by the human endothelium.[325] The commercially available form is produced by recombinant DNA technology. Alteplase directly cleaves plasminogen to generate plasmin which subsequently degrades fibrin. The N terminal end of the molecule has a specific affinity for fibrin, leading to the expectation that it would act preferentially in the vicinity of thrombi, i.e. it would be clot specific. Despite producing briefer and less pronounced depression of plasma fibrinogen than streptokinase, hopes that this more localised action would reduce the incidence of serious haemorrhage have not been confirmed in clinical trials.

Alteplase is rapidly metabolised by the liver (elimination half-life 5 to 10 minutes) and therefore must be administered by infusion to ensure an adequate duration of effect. In earlier dosage regimens, the drug was infused in a dose of 100mg over 3 hours. Subsequent angiographic studies revealed improved arterial patency rates when alteplase was given in a 'front loaded' regimen. In this regimen, a bolus injection of 15mg is followed by an infusion of 0.75 mg/kg over 30 minutes, with the remainder of the 100mg total dose infused over 60 minutes. This regimen has resulted in a small but distinct improvement in survival beyond that achieved by streptokinase in the GUSTO-1 trial and has subsequently become the standard method of administration.[322] In contrast to streptokinase, the thrombolytic activity of alteplase resolves rapidly after the cessation of the infusion, allowing invasive procedures to be undertaken.

*Anistreplase* (APSAC): this agent is a complex of streptokinase and human *lys*-plasminogen which is gradually activated in the plasma following intravenous injection.[326] It was developed as a means of improving the fibrin specificity of streptokinase and of delivering sustained fibrinolytic activity after a single intravenous injection. In acute myocardial infarction, anistreplase is administered in a dose of 30U by intravenous injection over 3 minutes. The half-life of its fibrinolytic activity is 1 to 2 hours and its clearance from plasma is similar to that of streptokinase. In clinical trials, anistreplase has proven to be virtually identical to streptokinase in both its efficacy and adverse effect profile.

*Urokinase* is a plasminogen activator derived from human renal endothelial cells and obtained by extraction from urine or from cultures of human kidney cells.[327] Unlike streptokinase, urokinase acts directly on plasminogen to produce plasmin. It has the advantage over streptokinase of being less allergenic. Its main use has been in the management of acute pulmonary embolism and peripheral arterial embolism (see further chapter 26; sect. 3.2.2).

*Other thrombolytic drugs:* newer agents under investigation include *reteplase* (r-PA) which is derived from tissue plasminogen activator but has the advantage of a longer plasma half-life than alteplase; it provides the prospect of a thrombolytic agent that can be administered by bolus injection in a prehospital setting. *Saruplase* (prourokinase) and *staphylococcase* are other thrombolytic drugs being studied.[328] The ultimate aim is to produce compounds capable of more rapid and complete thrombolysis, more favourable pharmacokinetics allowing bolus administration in a prehospital setting, and less bleeding complications.

- ***Contraindications to thrombolytic therapy***

A large number of theoretical contraindications were incorporated into early studies of thrombolytic drugs but very few of these have entered clinical practice. In practice, there are relatively few situations where the risk outweighs the very substantial benefits to be gained, especially from early thrombolytic therapy. However, aortic dissection, acute pericarditis, acute severe bleeding, and a recent cerebral haemorrhage are *absolute* contraindications.[315] *Relative* contraindications which should be considered include pregnancy, liver disease, malignancy, history of a bleeding diathesis, and a potential focus of haemorrhage. In the latter situation, thrombolytic drugs are probably best avoided within 6 months of a previous stroke or gastrointestinal or urogenital haemorrhage or within 4 weeks of trauma, surgery or cardiopulmonary resuscitation. Proliferative diabetic retinopathy, a systolic blood pressure in excess of 200mm Hg, or a diastolic blood pressure over 120mm Hg are also relative contraindications.

- ***Adverse effects of thrombolytic drugs***

*Haemorrhage:* all thrombolytic drugs increase the risk of bleeding by lysing thrombi in blood vessels. Elevated plasma levels of plasmin also reduce circulating levels of fibrinogen and some coagulation factors (especially factors V and VIII), and the bleeding tendency is further enhanced by impaired platelet function and high levels of fibrin degradation products. Large trials have shown that these drugs cause about 7 major noncerebral bleeds per 1000 patients treated and the incidence is just as great with relatively fibrin-specific agents such as alteplase. Major haemorrhage frequently involves arterial puncture sites, the eyes (especially with diabetic retinopathy), the gastrointestinal tract and the retroperitoneal area. Spontaneous bruising, oozing from intravenous sites, epistaxis and haematuria are relatively common but are not usually serious. *Ranitidine* may be given for ulcer prophylaxis in patients with a past history of peptic ulcer.

*Cerebral haemorrhage:* this is the most serious complication of thrombolytic therapy, affecting 4 of every 1000 patients treated.[329] Two of these cases are fatal and are accounted for in the overall mortality comparison. Of the nonfatal cases, 1 is disabling while the other is minor. Overall therefore, the 1-month net survival benefit, which ranges between 10 and 40 lives per 1000 patients treated, is offset by 1 disabling case of cerebral haemorrhage.

Large-scale clinical trials have identified several factors that increase the risk of cerebral haemorrhage and may lead to a more finely balanced risk : benefit evaluation. These factors include female gender, those with a low bodyweight, elevated blood pressure at presentation or a previous history of hypertension, and those with a previous stroke.[329] The risk is also greater in the elderly when alteplase is used but apparently not when streptokinase is used.[330] Most of the increased risk occurs on the first day of therapy and is partly offset by a lower overall risk of ischaemic stroke in the subsequent month.

Results of the large GUSTO-1 trial[322] demonstrated that the risk of cerebral haemorrhage is slightly greater with the accelerated ('front loaded') alteplase regimen than with streptokinase, but it is unclear whether this can be attributed to alteplase itself or the intravenous heparin given with it. However, the increased risk of nonfatal but disabling cerebral haemorrhage of approximately 1 per 1000 patients treated must be set against an overall saving of 9 lives per 1000 patients treated with this regimen.[321]

*Allergy:* 3 to 5% of patients receiving streptokinase or anistreplase suffer minor allergic symptoms during the infusion or shortly afterwards.[319,331] These symptoms usually involve shivering, pyrexia and a skin rash, and have been attributed to a reaction between streptokinase and neutralising antibodies in the circulation. Alteplase, however, is relatively free of this complication since it is not a foreign protein.

Although anaphylactic reactions have been reported with thrombolytic drugs, they are rare; no cases were observed among 8000 patients treated in one large trial (ISIS-2).[319]

*Hypotension:* this occurs during streptokinase infusions in 10 to 12% of patients, but the incidence with the accelerated alteplase regimen is only 1 to 2%.[322] Hypotension is generally managed by slowing or temporarily interrupting the infusion. Since patients with haemodynamic disturbances resulting from their infarction have most to gain from thrombolysis, the presence of hypotension should not be considered a contraindication to therapy.

*Reperfusion arrhythmias:* these were noted frequently in animal models but have not been observed in most of the large trials in humans.[332]

- ***Concomitant aspirin therapy***

Early studies with thrombolytic drugs showed that they were associated with a higher incidence of reinfarction which was attributed to the potent activation of platelets by the partially lysed thrombus. When the effectiveness of aspirin (162.5mg daily) was studied in the large ISIS-2 trial, it was shown to reduce the 35-day mortality by almost as much as streptokinase and the combination of the two drugs almost doubled the effectiveness of either used alone.[319] As a result, it is now practice to routinely administer aspirin with all thrombolytic agents and to continue therapy on a daily basis indefinitely.

- ***Concomitant heparin therapy***

The value of heparin appears to vary depending on which thrombolytic drug is used. The effectiveness of streptokinase is not substantially increased by heparin but it may still be reasonable to add heparin when the risk of thromboembolism is high, e.g. in patients with anterior myocardial infarction, atrial fibrillation, cardiac failure or a history of thromboembolism. Subcutaneous administration of heparin is as effective as intravenous administration and appears to produce less risk of bleeding.[333,334]

Results of angiographic studies have shown that an aggressive heparin regimen increases the likelihood that coronary vessel patency will be achieved with alteplase therapy. Without heparin, the relatively short half-life of alteplase may lead to a greater risk of reocclusion and reinfarction than with streptokinase or anistreplase. This, and the favourable results of the GUSTO-1 trial,[322] have led to the routine use of intravenous heparin in a regimen that consists of:

- An intravenous bolus dose of 75 U/kg heparin at the start of the alteplase infusion
- An initial heparin maintenance dose of 1000 to 2000 U/hour
- Subsequent adjustment of the heparin dosage to maintain an activated partial thromboplastin time (APTT) of 1.5 to 2.0 times the baseline level
- Maintenance of this heparin regimen for 48 hours, but continued thereafter (usually subcutaneously) if there is a high risk of systemic or venous thromboembolism.

The most important practical disadvantage of heparin is its highly variable dose-response relationship (requiring careful dose titration and frequent monitoring of APTT levels).[335] Other, more theoretical disadvantages include its inability to inhibit thrombin bound to blood clots and the inhibition of its action by platelet factor 4. On the other hand, it possesses the ability to strongly inhibit several activated clotting factors in addition to its indirect antithrombin action.

*Hirudin* is a 65 amino acid peptide originally isolated from the leech, which binds to and directly inhibits thrombin activity.[336] A recombinant form (desulfatohirudin) is available for human administration, as is a smaller synthetic molecule with similar properties (*hirulog* [bivalirudin]). It was hoped that these agents would produce an anticoagulant effect without the disadvantages of heparin. Although early pilot studies with these drugs produced promising results, later large-scale studies revealed an excess of intracerebral haemorrhage without any suggestion of benefit beyond that achieved with heparin.[337,338] When these studies were continued using lower doses, the excess of intracerebral haemorrhage disappeared, but there remained no advantage over heparin.[339]

#### Nitrates

Oral, topical or parenteral nitrate therapy may be used during myocardial infarction to relieve chest pain, reduce blood pressure and assist in the relief of pulmonary venous congestion. By reducing left ventricular filling pressure (preload) and myocardial wall stress (afterload), these drugs might also be expected to limit ischaemic damage in the myocardium. This hope was supported by a meta-analysis published in 1990 which indicated a significant reduction in mortality associated with nitrate use.[340]

Subsequently, much larger studies (GISSI-3 and ISIS-4) have found that routine nitrate therapy produces little difference in mortality at 1 to 2 months after infarction.[305,306] The interpretation of data from these trials is complicated by the fact that 50 to 60% of patients received nitrates 'off-protocol.' At present, it does not appear that routine nitrate therapy has a place for mortality reduction but it will continue to be indicated for control of blood pressure, chest pain and pulmonary congestion.[315]

#### β-Adrenoceptor Antagonists (β-Blockers)

Intravenous β-blockers, e.g. atenolol and metoprolol, given early after the onset of symptoms to patients with acute myocardial infarction in the prethrombolytic era were shown to reduce the 7- to 14-day mortality by about 13% (equivalent to 6 to 7 lives saved for every 1000 treated).[341] In particular, the risk of sudden death resulting from cardiac rupture and from fatal cardiac arrhythmias is reduced.

The value of acute therapy with β-blockers in addition to thrombolytic agents was examined in the TIMI (Thrombolysis in Myocardial Infarction) II-B study, which found that they did not improve survival beyond that achieved with thrombolytic therapy alone.[342] However, the rate of intracranial bleeding was reduced by this intervention.

#### Angiotensin-Converting Enzyme (ACE) Inhibitors

ACE inhibitors should be administered early in the course of acute myocardial infarction to all patients with even transient signs of left ventricular dysfunction. This recommendation is based primarily on the results of the AIRE study in which 2006 patients with acute myocardial infarction complicated by left ventricular failure (even if transient) were randomly allocated to ramipril or placebo between days 3 and 10 after admission, in addition to full conventional treatment.[129] After 15 months of follow-up, the group receiving the ACE inhibitor experienced a 26% reduction in mortality, representing a saving of 45 premature deaths per 1000 patient years of treatment.

A smaller but identifiable reduction in mortality has also been seen when ACE inhibitors were given indiscriminately (i.e. regardless of evidence of left ventricular dysfunction) to normotensive patients within the first 24 hours after presentation. Benefits of 5 to 8 lives saved per 1000 patients treated were seen in these studies but on subgroup analysis, this benefit appeared largely derived from the high-risk patients (i.e. those with left ventricular dysfunction, anterior infarction or second or subsequent infarction).[294]

As a result of these studies, many clinicians now treat all patients with ACE inhibitors but stop therapy after about 6 weeks if ventricular function is normal. Others adopt a more selective approach, following the AIRE study[129] as a guideline. Data from the GISSI-3 study[305] suggest that ACE inhibitors commenced within 24 hours of presentation increase the incidence of hypotension from 4% to 9%, and thus should not be used in patients whose systolic blood pressure is less than 100mm Hg. However, the fact that half of the mortality benefit of these drugs occurs in the first 24 hours after symptom onset demonstrates the value of commencing treatment early in high-risk patients without contraindications.

#### Calcium Antagonists

Initiation of treatment with dihydropyridine calcium antagonists should be avoided during the early stages of a myocardial infarction.[343] Several trials have shown an increase in mortality when these drugs have been administered to patients with unstable angina or acute myocardial infarction. No studies have been conducted in this setting with verapamil or diltiazem; however, the negative inotropic and electrophysiological effects of these drugs contraindicates their use in patients with left ventricular dysfunction or high degrees of heart block.

#### Magnesium

The place of magnesium therapy in acute myocardial infarction has been the subject of debate. Following intravenous administration, it produces vasodilatation in the coronary and systemic vascular beds, inhibits platelet aggregation, exerts an antiarrhythmic effect and, in animal models, protects the myocardium from reperfusion injury.

The results of the LIMIT-2 study of magnesium sulfate administration in acute myocardial infarction supported the results of several smaller trials and showed a 24% reduction in 28-day mortality and a 25% reduction in the incidence of left ventricular failure.[344] In this study, magnesium sulfate was administered early (median 3 hours) after symptom onset in a dose of 2g over 5 minutes followed by 8g over 24 hours. Subsequently, the ISIS-4 study, which was conducted in 58,824 patients, demonstrated no survival advantage and a higher rate of cardiac failure among patients receiving treatment with magnesium, even in the subgroup receiving the drug within the first few hours after the onset of symptoms.[306] There seems little rationale to use magnesium except in the presence of low serum magnesium concentrations.

#### Antiarrhythmic Drugs

A meta-analysis of trials involving the routine use of intravenous lidocaine (lignocaine) in the presence of acute myocardial infarction showed no improvement in survival.[341] A reduction in ventricular fibrillation appears to be counterbalanced by an increase in fatal asystole. It is therefore appropriate to reserve parenteral lidocaine to those at very high risk of ventricular fibrillation and those with episodes of sustained ventricular tachycardia.

The only orally administered drugs with substantial antiarrhythmic efficacy (and without significant proarrhythmic potential) in this setting are the β-adrenoceptor blockers. Amiodarone may also prove beneficial but definitive studies are awaited. Other class I antiarrhythmic drugs such as procainamide, quinidine and flecainide should be avoided because of their potential proarrhythmic effects (see further section 8.2.2).

### *7.2.2 Secondary Prevention of Myocardial Infarction*

About 8 to 10% of patients who develop an acute myocardial infarction die within two years after discharge from hospital. The risk is greatest among those with more severe degrees of myocardial damage. A variety of interventions have been shown to reduce the risk of subsequent myocardial infarction and improve prospects for survival in these individuals (fig. 4). These interventions have been summarised by a consensus panel statement from the American Heart Association.[341]

#### β-Adrenoceptor Antagonists (β-Blockers)

Large morbidity/mortality trials using agents such as *propranolol, metoprolol* and *timolol* have shown that β-blockers reduce mortality during the first 1 to 2 years after a myocardial infarction by about 25%.[345-347] This is achieved by similar reductions in the incidence of sudden death and recurrent infarction. The reduction in sudden death appears to result from the antiarrhythmic effect of these drugs.

A consistent finding of the major trials with β-blockers has been that patients with severe or complicated myocardial infarction (including those with left ventricular dysfunction) derive the greatest benefit.[348]

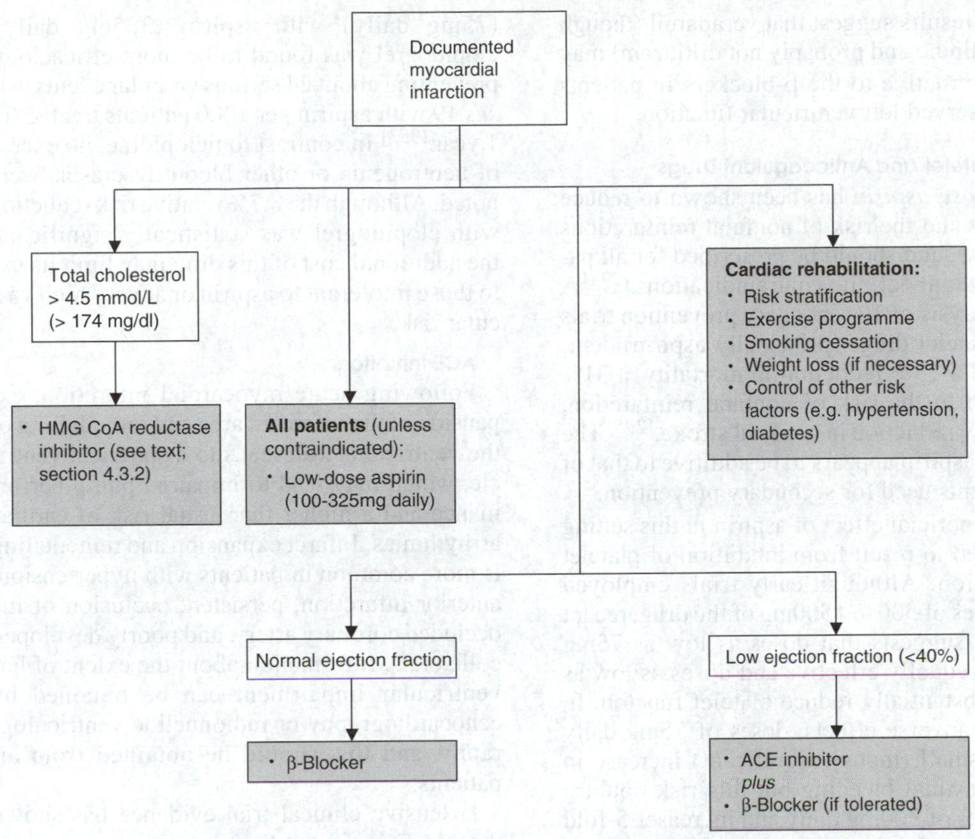


**Fig. 4.** Management of patients surviving a myocardial infarction.

It is likely that relatively β1-selective (e.g. *atenolol* and *metoprolol*) and nonselective (e.g. *propranolol*) β-blockers exert similar 'cardioprotective' effects, but it is less certain that this property is shared by drugs with partial agonist activity (e.g. pindolol).[349] Until the question of their effectiveness is resolved, the latter drugs should not be used for this indication.

It is also unclear how long treatment with β-blockers should be continued. In the trials with timolol and propranolol, the survival curves for the β-blocker and placebo groups diverged most rapidly in the early weeks to months after treatment commenced. Beyond that time, it is not clear whether the drugs exerted their effect or indeed are necessary for the continued survival of those who would not have survived without treatment. However, until more information is available, it would seem prudent to continue them indefinitely.

### Calcium Antagonists

Administration of *dihydropyridine calcium antagonists* to patients following a myocardial infarction has not been found to provide benefit. In fact, some trials have shown a small increase in mortality among those treated with these agents.[350]

*Diltiazem:* the effect of diltiazem in postmyocardial infarction patients was investigated in a multicentre trial where it was found to exert no overall effect on recurrent coronary events or on overall survival.[290] In a subgroup analysis, a beneficial effect among patients with good cardiac function appeared to be cancelled by a detrimental effect in those with impaired cardiac function.

*Verapamil:* a more encouraging result was noted in the DAVIT-II study in postmyocardial infarction patients in which verapamil was given orally (120mg three times daily) for 18 months commencing at least 7 days after the myocardial infarction.[286] A 20% reduction in mortality, which just failed to reach the 5% significance level, resulted. Again, a better result was found among those without impaired cardiac function.[286]

These results suggest that verapamil (though not nifedipine and probably not diltiazem) may be an alternative to the β-blockers in patients with preserved left ventricular function.

#### Antiplatelet and Anticoagulant Drugs

*Low-dose aspirin* has been shown to reduce mortality and the risk of nonfatal reinfarctions and stroke, and should be prescribed for all patients without definite contraindications.[295] A meta-analysis of 10 secondary prevention trials of antiplatelet drugs (principally aspirin) demonstrated a 13% reduction in mortality, a 31% reduction in the risk of nonfatal reinfarction, and a 42% reduction in nonfatal stroke.[295] The effect of aspirin appears to be additive to that of other agents used for secondary prevention.

The beneficial effect of aspirin in this setting is believed to result from inhibition of platelet aggregation. Although early trials employed daily doses of 500 to 1500mg of the drug, recent evidence suggests that doses as low as 75mg daily are equally effective and doses as low as 40mg substantially reduce platelet functon. In terms of adverse effects, doses of 75mg daily cause a small (though significant) increase in gastrointestinal bleeding but this risk doubles with doses of 300mg daily and increases 5-fold with doses of 1.8 to 2.4g daily. Thus, as low doses appear equally effective as high doses in preventing cardiovascular events, there is a strong rationale to employ doses within the low-dose range, i.e. 100 to 325mg daily or every alternate day.

Aspirin should be continued indefinitely in patients after myocardial infarction. Although most trials have progressed for 3 years or less, significant additional benefit has been discernible during the third year of treatment, suggesting that longer treatment might be more effective.[295]

High-risk patients unable to tolerate aspirin may be suited to treatment with alternative antiplatelet agents (e.g. *ticlopidine*) or with an oral anticoagulant (e.g. *warfarin*). However, the higher morbidity associated with these drugs limits their use to high-risk patients. There is no substantial evidence that *dipyridamole* adds to the effectiveness of aspirin given alone.[351]

*Clopidogrel* is a thienopyridine derivative which, like ticlopidine, blocks the activation of platelets by ADP[352] (see also chapter 26; sect. 3.1.1). In the CAPRIE study conducted among 19,185 patients at high risk of vascular disease, which compared the efficacy of clopidogrel (75mg daily) with aspirin (325mg daily), clopidogrel was found to be more efficacious, preventing about 24 serious vascular events *versus* 19 with aspirin per 1000 patients treated for 1 year.[353] In contrast to ticlopidine, no excess of neutropenia or other blood dyscrasias were noted. Although the 8.7% relative risk reduction with clopidogrel was statistically significant, the additional cost of this drug may limit its use to those intolerant to aspirin or at very high vascular risk.

#### ACE Inhibitors

Following acute myocardial infarction, expansion of the infarcted area and remodelling of the ventricular wall leads to a spherical ventricle, which may lead to impaired pump performance and a higher than usual risk of cardiac arrhythmias. Infarct expansion and remodelling is more common in patients with hypertension, anterior infarction, persistent occlusion of the occluded coronary artery, and poorly developed collaterals. Information about the extent of left ventricular impairment can be obtained by echocardiography or radionuclide ventriculography, and this should be obtained from all patients.

Extensive clinical trial evidence has shown that ACE inhibitor therapy given to patients with clinical evidence of heart failure (or an ejection fraction <40%) after a myocardial infarction leads to improved survival. It is unclear whether patients with normal ventricular function also benefit but, if so, the benefit is likely to be slight. Data from the SAVE trial with *captopril* indicate that the benefits derived from ACE inhibitors are additional to that achieved with aspirin and β-blockers.[354]

The benefits of ACE inhibitors have included an unexpected reduction in the rate of recurrent myocardial infarction.[355] This may be the consequence of a previously unrecognised effect of these drugs in delaying the progression of atheroma. Further information is needed before the implications of this finding are clarified.

A reduction in postmyocardial infarction mortality has been observed in studies using captopril, enalapril and ramipril, suggesting that this is a 'class' effect of these drugs. The doses used in these studies have been relatively high (i.e. captopril 50mg three times daily, enalapril 10 to 20mg twice daily and ramipril 5mg twice daily) but it is unclear whether doses of this magnitude are needed.[356] However, until further information is available, these should be regarded as target doses. Since no information is available about the optimum duration of therapy, it is appropriate that these drugs should be continued indefinitely.

#### Lipid-Lowering Drugs

Patients with even relatively 'normal' levels of LDL-cholesterol should receive a low-fat diet and be considered for immediate and intensive lipid-lowering therapy with an *HMG CoA reductase inhibitor*[357] (see section 4.2.1 above). Data from recent secondary prevention trials (see section 4.3.2) suggest that a survival advantage becomes apparent in treated patients within 6 months or so after the commencement of intensive therapy.[67] This early response may result from a reduction in the lipid content of soft lipid-laden plaques whose rupture is believed to be responsible for most cases of myocardial infarction, or perhaps from restoration of endothelial function.

There is ongoing debate about the level of LDL-cholesterol at which lipid-lowering therapy should be introduced. In general, patients with other risk factors (including low HDL-cholesterol levels) warrant treatment at lower LDL-cholesterol levels. Results of recent studies (e.g. the CARE study[68]) are likely to create pressure for the lowering of lipid levels previously considered normal in patients with established coronary disease, and a cost-effectiveness evaluation of this approach is required.

#### Antiarrhythmic Drugs

β-Adrenoceptor antagonists are the only antiarrhythmic agents with a proven beneficial effect after myocardial infarction. Class I antiarrhythmic drugs such as procainamide and flecainide should be avoided because of their proarrhythmic potential.[358] Amiodarone may have a role in selected patients but its place in this setting is still under investigation.

#### Other Interventions

The secondary prevention of myocardial infarction requires attention to the patient's overall risk factor profile. Attention should be given to reducing saturated fat in the diet, increasing physical fitness, maintaining weight and controlling blood pressure. Hormone replacement therapy (HRT) should be considered in postmenopausal women[359] (see further chapter 18; sect. 11.4).

## 8. Cardiac Arrhythmias

The place of antiarrhythmic drugs in the management of cardiac arrhythmias has altered substantially in recent years. The demonstration that these agents could induce serious or lethal arrhythmias through their proarrhythmic actions, while at the same time producing apparent improvement in electrocardiographic evidence of ventricular ectopy, has resulted in major changes in the recommended treatment of several common arrhythmias.[360] This finding has greatly reduced enthusiasm to prescribe drug treatment for asymptomatic or mildly symptomatic conditions such as palpitations and has increased the role of non-drug options such as electrical cardioversion, electrical ablation, pacemaker implantation and implantable defibrillators.[361]

### 8.1 Pathogenesis of Cardiac Arrhythmias

Cardiac arrhythmias result from a disturbance in the initiation or conduction of the cardiac impulse. They may be classified into those resulting from abnormal automaticity, those caused by disorders of impulse transmission and those caused by a mixture of both.[362] Abnormal automaticity may develop anywhere in the heart. If the rate of impulse generation is greater in one of these sites than in the sinoatrial node, then this site may take over pacemaker functions.

Disorders of impulse conduction range from simple obstruction to conduction (e.g. atrioventricular block) to 're-entry circuits' which probably represent the mechanism underlying most supraventricular and ventricular arrhythmias. Re-entry circuits are thought to involve the diversion of an impulse along two branches of the conducting system. In one limb, the impulse encounters a 'unidirectional' block and is halted. The impulse passing along the other limb recirculates to its point of origin, setting off repetitive impulse formation.[363]

#### The Action Potential

The normal cardiac impulse comprises a travelling wave of altered membrane conductance which briefly reverses membrane polarity.[364] Under normal circumstances, it originates in the sinoatrial (SA) node, spreads rapidly to the atrioventricular (AV) node (where it is delayed by approximately 0.2 sec), and then passes via the Purkinje system to the ventricles. The sequence of voltage changes accompanying the wave of depolarisation is referred to as the 'action potential'. The action potential of the specialised conducting tissue differs from that of myocardial cells by exhibiting automaticity, i.e. the resting membrane potential decays during the period between contractions until a critical threshold voltage is reached when spontaneous depolarisation occurs. Under normal circumstances, the rate of spontaneous depolarisation is greatest at the sinoatrial node and the cardiac impulse is therefore initiated at this site.

There are important differences in the nature of the depolarising current responsible for the rapid upstroke (phase 0) of the action potential in different regions of the heart. In most of the conducting system and in atrial and ventricular muscle, this current is produced principally by a rapid influx of sodium ions moving through 'fast channels'. In these fibres, movement of calcium also takes place through so-called 'slow channels' but this is of minor significance apart from its contribution to the plateau (phase 2) of the action potential.[365]

In the SA and AV nodes and in some areas of ischaemic damage, the polarising current results from slow channel activation alone. Action potentials in these areas are characterised by a low resting membrane potential (–40mV compared with –80 to –90mV in fast fibres) and a slow rate of phase 0 depolarisation. The rate of impulse conduction in these areas is slow.

Following depolarisation, myocardial cells are refractory to further stimuli until repolarisation is almost complete. The *absolute refractory period* refers to the delay that occurs until the earliest transient depolarisation can be produced, and the *relatively refractory period* refers to the time elapsing before a further propagated action potential can be elicited.

## 8.2 Clinical Pharmacology of Drugs Used in Treatment

### 8.2.1 Mechanisms/Sites of Action

Antiarrhythmic drugs are commonly classified according to their electrophysiological properties using the classification of Vaughan-Williams and Singh.[366] According to this classification, they can be divided into:

- ***Class I agents:*** these drugs slow the influx of sodium ions through cell membranes and therefore reduce the rate of spontaneous depolarisation, and slow the maximum rate of rise of phase 0 of the action potential. As a result, they reduce automaticity and generally slow the rate of impulse transmission. Class I drugs are further subdivided into a class IA agents which lengthen the action potential duration, class IB agents which shorten the action potential duration, and class IC agents which have little effect on the action potential duration.
- ***Class II agents:*** these drugs block the sympathetic nervous system by either β-adrenoceptor blockade or by reducing adrenergic neurotransmitter release. Since sympathetic nervous system stimulation increases the rate of spontaneous phase 4 depolarisation, a prominent effect of these agents is to reduce automaticity.
- ***Class III agents:*** these drugs, which include amiodarone and sotalol (the latter also possessing class II properties), increase the duration of the action potential and therefore also increase the action potential.
- ***Class IV agents:*** included in this class are drugs such as verapamil which inhibit the slow inward calcium current that carries the action potential in the SA and AV nodes and in some areas of marginally viable myocardium.

The following discussion focuses on antiarrhythmic drugs of classes I and III. For information on the clinical pharmacology of class II (β-adrenoceptor blockers) and class IV drugs (calcium antagonists), see sections 6.1.2 and 6.1.3 above and also chapter 21, sections 3.2 and 3.4.

### 8.2.2 Class I Antiarrhythmic Drugs

The clinical pharmacological properties of the currently available class I drugs are shown in table V. Some of the more commonly used members of this class are discussed individually below.

#### Quinidine

Quinidine is a dextroisomer of the antimalarial drug quinine, and was the first antiarrhythmic drug to be widely used.[367] In common with other drugs of this class, appreciation of its proarrhythmic potential has led to a greatly reduced role in therapeutics; however, prescribing surveys indicate that it is still widely used in medical practice. Much of this use has been directed towards the maintenance of sinus rhythm in patients with atrial flutter or fibrillation or for the prevention of ventricular tachycardia and ventricular fibrillation in patients at high risk of these arrhythmias. However, a meta-analysis of studies of the use of quinidine in supraventricular and ventricular arrhythmias suggests that the drug may reduce survival rather than improve it. Thus, there is little rationale for its continued use in long term therapy.[368,369]

***Pharmacodynamic properties:*** the antiarrhythmic activity of quinidine results from its action in depressing automaticity, slowing conduction and increasing the effective refractory period throughout the conducting system. These effects result from a slowing of sodium influx through sodium channels in the cell membrane. As with other class IA drugs, the time for recovery from block is intermediate between that of class IB drugs (short) and class IC drugs (prolonged). Slowing of repolarisation and a consequent prolongation of the QT interval also occurs. Quinidine also possesses moderate anticholinergic and α-adrenoceptor blocking activity.

The haemodynamic effects of quinidine are less pronounced than those of most other class I agents. A negative inotropic effect has been reported in *in vitro* studies, but has rarely been observed *in vivo*, possibly because it is countered by the drug's vasodilator activity.

***Pharmacokinetic characteristics:*** quinidine is used clinically as the sulfate, bisulfate, gluconate or polygalacturonate. Since the active form (quinidine base) makes up a different percentage by weight of these formulations, the doses required to provide equivalent amounts of quinidine base vary accordingly. The bioavailability of oral formulations averages 75%. Quinidine is mainly eliminated by hydroxylation in the liver, and its plasma half-life ranges from 5 to 12 hours.[370,371]

***Clinical use:*** the usual dose of quinidine sulfate is 200 to 300mg 4- to 6-hourly but a sustained-release preparation is available and is usually administered in a dose of 500mg 2 or 3 times daily. The therapeutic plasma concentration range is 2 to 5 mg/L (using a nonspecific assay; see chapter 5; sect. 4.4.1) but there is considerable overlap between therapeutic and toxic concentrations. Lower doses are required in settings where clearance is reduced, including the elderly and patients with renal or liver disease and cardiac failure. The drug is not administered intravenously because of the risk of hypotension.

***Tolerability:*** the most serious adverse effect of quinidine is its ability to produce various rhythm disturbances. About 2 to 8% of patients develop marked QT prolongation and torsades de pointes.[372] This proarrhythmic effect is probably responsible for the problem of 'quinidine syncope' which has long been recognised as occurring during the early stages of treatment and results from drug-induced ventricular tachycardia. The proarrhythmic risk is enhanced in patients with hypokalaemia and in those receiving concomitant therapy with drugs that prolong the QT interval.

Quinidine can also be hazardous if given to patients with atrial flutter or fibrillation.[373] The drug's anticholinergic effect can result in increased AV nodal transmission of impulses, leading to dangerous ventricular rates. This risk is reduced by prior administration of digoxin.

Other adverse effects of quinidine include diarrhoea, abdominal pain and anorexia which affect up to one-third of those given the drug.[374] Tinnitus, hearing loss, headache and blurred vision are also common and, when occurring together, are often referred to as 'cinchonism'. Less common adverse effects include drug fever (often with hepatic dysfunction), immune-mediated thrombocytopenia, lupus erythematosus, haemolytic anaemia, agranulocytosis and leucocytoclastic vasculitis.

***Drug interactions:*** quinidine is involved in clinically significant interactions with several other commonly used drugs.[375] Coadministration with digoxin generally leads to a near doubling of plasma digoxin concentrations as a result of both a reduced volume of distribution and a reduction in the renal and nonrenal clearance of digoxin. Cimetidine reduces the metabolism of quinidine and may increase quinidine plasma concentrations, while drugs that stimulate its metabolism (e.g. phenytoin and rifampicin) may decrease plasma concentrations (see further appendix B).

#### Procainamide

Procainamide is structurally similar to the local anaesthetic procaine but possesses an ester linkage that protects it from hydrolysis.[376] Its physiological actions are generally similar to those of quinidine but it lacks quinidine's anticholinergic and α-adrenoceptor blocking activity. Like quinidine, its use has substantially declined with the recognition of the proarrhythmic properties of class I antiarrhythmics. Although approved for use in the management of atrial and ventricular tachyarrhythmias and for prophylaxis against the recurrence of atrial fibrillation and flutter, the availability of more effec-

**Table V.** Principal actions, pharmacokinetic characteristics and adverse effects of commonly used antiarrhythmic drugs

| Class[a]/action | Drugs | Pharmacokinetic parameters | | | | | Route of elimination | Usual adult dosage[b] | Common adverse effects (other than proarrhythmic effects; see sections 8.2 and 9.3) |
|---|---|---|---|---|---|---|---|---|---|
| | | F (%) | CL (L/h) | $t_{1/2}$ (h) | Vd (L) [per 70kg] | protein binding (%) | | | |
| **Class IA:** prolong action potential duration; increase refractory period and QT interval | Cibenzoline[c] | 85 | 30-50 | 7.2 | 392 | 50-60 | Renal (mainly) and hepatic | 130mg twice daily | GI disturbances, blurred vision, dry mouth, urinary retention, hypotension, ↑ transaminases, ↓WBCs |
| | Disopyramide | 83 | 40[d] | 5.5[d] | 182[d] | 54-81[e] | Renal and hepatic | 250-300mg twice daily (as SR tablets) | Dry mouth, blurred vision, urinary retention, constipation, GI disturbances, dizziness, LV impairment |
| | Procainamide | 83 | 37[f] | 3[f] | 154 | 15 | Renal and hepatic[f] | 0.5-1g 3 times daily (as SR tablets) | GI disturbances, rash, pruritus, drug fever, muscle weakness, lupus erythematosus-like syndrome (risk greater in slow acetylators), haemolytic anaemia (rare) |
| | Quinidine | 78 | 18 | 6 | 175 | 90 | Hepatic (mainly); some renal | 500mg (as bisulfate SR tablets) twice daily | GI disturbances, tinnitus, hearing loss, headache, blurred vision, urticaria, rash, drug fever, thrombocytopenia, agranulocytosis, haemolytic anaemia, lupus erythematosus-like syndrome |
| **Class IB:** decrease action potential duration; shorten QT interval | Lidocaine (lignocaine) | 35 | 40 | 3.9 | 210 | 60 | Hepatic | 1 mg/kg IV bolus, then 1-3 mg/min by IV infusion (target plasma concentration 3.5 mg/L) | Nausea, paraesthesia, dizziness, blurred vision, disorientation, tremor, convulsions (more common with excessive plasma concentrations or over-rapid administration) |
| | Mexiletine | 85 | 27 | 10 | 350 | 70 | Hepatic (mainly); some renal | 200mg 3 times daily or 360mg SR tablet twice daily | GI disturbances, tremor, dizziness, blurred vision, ataxia, nystagmus, paraesthesia, drowsiness, confusion, hypotension, ↑ liver enzymes (rare) |
| | Tocainide | 100 | 10.9 | 15 | 224 | ≈50 | Renal and hepatic | 200-400mg 3 times daily | Nausea, tremor, dizziness, paraesthesia, confusion, rash, drug fever; abnormal liver function tests; agranulocytosis, thrombocytopenia, pancytopenia (occasionally) |
| **Class IC:** little effect on action potential duration; markedly prolong PR and QRS intervals | Flecainide | 95 | 42.8 | 12-27 | 588 | 52 | Hepatic (mainly); some renal | 50-150mg twice daily or 200mg SR capsule once daily | Dizziness, visual disturbances, nausea/vomiting, headache, ataxia, paraesthesia, ↑ liver enzymes (rare) |
| | Moracizine[g] (moricizine, ethmozine) | 34-38 | 78 | 2.8-4.3 | 185-210 | 81-90 | Hepatic | 200-300mg 3 times daily | GI disturbances, dizziness, blurred vision, headache, perioral paraesthesia, dyspnoea, hypoaesthesia, dry mouth |
| | Propafenone | 5-12[h] | 47-57[i] | 3.6-7.2[i] | 210 | 77->95 | Hepatic[i] | 150-300mg 3 times daily | Dizziness, GI and taste disturbances, blurred vision, headache, paraesthesia, skin rash, pruritus, cholestatic hepatitis (rare), azoospermia (rare), agranulocytosis (rare), exacerbation of asthma |

| | | | | | | | | | |
|---|---|---|---|---|---|---|---|---|---|
| **Class II:** block sympathetic nervous system, slowing conduction and increasing refractory period in AV node | β-Adrenoceptor antagonists (e.g. acebutolol, atenolol, metoprolol, pindolol, propranolol, timolol, etc.) | See section 6.1.2 and chapter 21; sect. 3.2 (table II) | | | | | | See text (sections 6.1.2, 8.3) | |
| **Class III:** prolong action potential duration and refractory period | Amiodarone | 40-50 | 8.6 | 14/ 1300[j] | 4970 | 96 | Hepatic (mainly); some intestinal metabolism | 200mg 3 times daily for 1 week, then 200mg twice daily for 1 week, then 200mg daily or less | Bradycardia, hypotension (IV administration), hypo- or hyperthyroidism, interstitial pneumonitis, GI and taste disturbances, skin rash, photosensitivity, grey/blue skin discolouration, peripheral neuropathy, tremor ataxia, ↑ liver enzymes, corneal microdeposits |
| | Bretylium | 23 | 47 | 7.8 | 574 | | Renal | 5 mg/kg IV bolus, then 10 mg/kg if needed | Transient hypertension followed by hypotension/postural hypotension; nausea/vomiting |
| | Sotalol | ≈100 | 10 | 10-17.7 | 105-126 | 20-40 | Renal (mainly); some hepatic | 80mg twice daily initially, increasing to 120-160mg twice daily | Dyspnoea, bradycardia, fatigue, asthenia, dizziness, headache, aggravation of cardiac failure |
| **Class IV:** block slow inward calcium current and slow conduction in AV node | Calcium antagonists (e.g. verapamil, diltiazem) | See section 6.1.3 and chapter 21; sect. 3.4 (table V) | | | | | | See text (sections 6.1.3, 8.3) | |
| **Other:** acts on purinergic receptors; transiently slows AV nodal conduction | Adenosine | | | 0.003 | | | Rapid metabolism in erythrocytes and blood vessel endothelial cells | 3mg by rapid IV bolus; if necessary a further 6mg IV after 1-2 mins, then 12mg IV after a further 1-2 mins if needed | Facial flushing, headache, hypotension, dry mouth, dyspnoea, chest pain, dizziness, paraesthesia, GI disturbances |

a Vaughan Williams-Singh electrophysiological classification.
b Oral dosage, unless otherwise specified.
c Cibenzoline also has limited class III and IV activity.
d Calculated from unbound plasma concentrations.
e Concentration-dependent.
f Acetylator phenotype-dependent. Approximately 50% of procainamide is metabolised to acecainide (*N*-acetylprocainamide) which exerts class III antiarrhythmic activity. The rate and extent of its *N*-acetylation to acecainide is bimodally distributed in the community (see further chapter 1; sect. 5.2.1).
g Although a class I antiarrhythmic drug, moracizine does not readily conform to any of the 3 subclasses (A, B or C).
h Dose-dependent.
i Hydroxylator phenotype-dependent (approximately 7% of Caucasians are poor metabolisers of propafenone).
j Half-life values shown are after single and multiple doses, respectively.
*Abbreviations and symbols:* CL = total plasma clearance; F = oral bioavailability; $t_{1/2}$ = elimination half-life; Vd = apparent volume of distribution; AV = atrioventricular; GI = gastrointestinal; IV = intravenous; LV = left ventricular; SR = sustained-release; WBCs = white blood cells; ↑ = increased; ↓ = decreased.

tive therapies has seen its clinical use largely superseded.

***Pharmacokinetic characteristics:*** procainamide can be administered either parenterally or orally. The oral formulation is rapidly absorbed and has a bioavailability of about 85%. Procainamide is eliminated by both renal excretion and hepatic metabolism with a plasma half-life of 2 to 5 hours. Conventional oral formulations of the drug must be given 3- to 4-hourly to avoid excessive fluctuation of plasma concentrations.[370]

Approximately 50% of procainamide is converted in the liver to the major metabolite, acecainide (*N*-acetylprocainamide; NAPA). This metabolite has significant class III antiarrhythmic activity,[377] and is eliminated mainly by renal excretion with a plasma half-life varying from 6 to 12 hours. The rate and extent of acetylation of procainamide to acecainide is genetically determined and is bimodally distributed in the community (along with acetylator phenotype). At any given dose of procainamide, rapid acetylators achieve higher concentrations of acecainide (and correspondingly lower concentrations of the parent drug) than slow acetylators. Acetylator status has no clear-cut effect on the drug's effectiveness, although lupus-like symptoms appear to be more common in slow acetylators.[378,379]

***Clinical use:*** conventional formulations of procainamide are typically administered in doses of 250 to 500mg 3- to 4-hourly, while sustained-release formulations are typically given in a dose of 500mg three times daily. The therapeutic plasma concentration range is 4 to 10 mg/L. The pharmacokinetic disposition of procainamide is altered in cardiac failure where renal elimination is slowed and the volume of distribution is decreased, necessitating lower doses. In patients with renal dysfunction, acecainide may accumulate and the dose of procainamide should therefore be reduced (see further appendix D).

Intravenous procainamide is typically administered in a dose of 50 mg/min to a total of 10 mg/kg bodyweight, followed by an infusion of 4 mg/min reducing to 2 mg/min over 2 hours and then continuing for 12 to 24 hours. When maintenance therapy is initiated without a loading dose, approximately 12 hours elapses before steady-state concentrations are achieved. Hypotension is likely to develop if the infusion rate is too rapid.

***Tolerability:*** procainamide produces a similar range of cardiac adverse effects as quinidine. High plasma concentrations may produce hypotension, AV block and a prolonged QT interval, and the drug is presumed to possess a similar likelihood of proarrhythmic activity as quinidine.[380] The major limitation to long term procainamide treatment, apart from its proarrhythmic potential, is the development of a systemic lupus erythematosus-like syndrome.[381] Antinuclear antibodies occur in 60 to 70% of patients receiving treatment for longer than 2 to 3 months, and symptomatic lupus syndrome involving arthralgia, arthritis, fever, rash, pericarditis and evidence of neutropenia or pancytopenia will develop in 20 to 30% of these patients if therapy is continued. The kidney and brain are rarely affected. Slow acetylators appear to be at a greater risk of developing the lupus syndrome. Antibodies develop more rapidly and at a lower total dose in this group than in rapid acetylators. It appears that the formation of antibodies and development of the lupus syndrome are related to the primary amino group of procainamide. This group is absent in the metabolite acecainide which does not cause the problem. The condition generally subsides spontaneously after withdrawal of procainamide.

Other adverse effects of procainamide include nausea, abdominal pain, diarrhoea, drug fever, Coombs' positive haemolytic anaemia, rash, hepatitis and confusional states. Granulomas in both the liver and the bone marrow have also been described and cerebellar ataxia and anticholinergic effects have been associated with the use of high doses of the drug for arrhythmia prophylaxis.

#### Disopyramide

Disopyramide is a class IA agent which has similar electrophysiological properties to quinidine and procainamide. Its principal distinguishing features are its strong anticholinergic and negative inotropic effects. In common with other class I agents, its use has declined in recent years;[382] however, the powerful anticholinergic effect of disopyramide has led to exploration of its use in the management of neurocardiogenic (vasovagal) syncope.

***Pharmacokinetic characteristics:*** orally administered disopyramide has a bioavailability of 80 to 90%. The drug is eliminated by both renal excretion and hepatic metabolism with a plasma half-life of 5 to 7 hours. About 70% of the drug is bound to plasma proteins, mainly to $\alpha_1$-acid glycoprotein, and the free fraction increases as the plasma concentration rises. The major metabolite of disopyramide is mono-*N*-desisopropyldisopyramide which has minor antiarrhythmic activity but pronounced anticholinergic properties.[370]

***Clinical use:*** the recommended oral dosage regimen of disopyramide comprises a loading dose of 300mg followed by 100 to 200mg 6- to 8-hourly with individual dose requirements varying from 300 to 800mg per day. The recommended intravenous dose is 2 mg/kg initially (maximum 150mg) administered over 10 to 15 minutes followed by a slow infusion of 0.4 mg/kg/hour up to a maximum of 800mg daily.

***Tolerability:*** the most significant adverse effect of disopyramide is impairment of left ventricular function. Its negative inotropic effect exceeds that of quinidine and procainamide, possibly because of disopyramide's tendency to increase peripheral resistance. During intravenous administration, hypotension may occur if the infusion rate is too rapid. Cardiac failure may develop weeks or months after commencement of long term oral treatment, and if there is a history of cardiac impairment, the incidence of this problem may approach 50%. Concomitant administration with other drugs with negative inotropic properties (such as β-blockers or verapamil) should be avoided wherever possible.

Other important adverse effects of disopyramide arise from its strong anticholinergic activity. These include urinary retention, blurred vision, dry mouth, constipation and urinary frequency. Less frequent adverse effects include reversible psychoses, cholestatic jaundice, hypoglycaemia, agranulocytosis and skin rashes.

Disopyramide is believed to have a similar proarrhythmic potential to other class I agents. Its other electrophysiological effects include atrioventricular block, widening of the QRS duration and prolongation of the QT interval.

#### Lidocaine (Lignocaine)

Lidocaine is a widely used local anaesthetic agent (see chapter 12; sect. 2.4) but also has antiarrhythmic activity; it is the prototype class IB antiarrhythmic agent.[383] Lidocaine has been used widely in coronary care units to suppress patterns of ventricular ectopy which were considered to be predictive of serious arrhythmias and cardiac arrest. However, more recent trials have established that suppression of ventricular ectopics with lidocaine (and other antiarrhythmic drugs) makes little difference to the subsequent development of serious arrhythmias. Routine use of lidocaine (e.g. in postmyocardial infarction patients) produces an increased incidence of hypotension and heart block with no overall benefit. Its use is now declining rapidly, although it is still widely used to terminate ventricular tachycardia or ventricular fibrillation.[384]

Like other class IB agents, lidocaine slows cardiac conduction and reduces automaticity. In contrast to the class IA drugs (which prolong the action potential duration), it shortens the action potential duration and the effective refractory period. However, its antiarrhythmic effect is reduced in the presence of hypokalaemia.

***Pharmacokinetic characteristics and clinical use:*** lidocaine is usually administered as a bolus intravenous injection of 75 to 100mg followed by an infusion of 4 mg/min for one hour and then continuing at a rate of 1 to 3 mg/min. The drug is eliminated very rapidly with 60 to 70% extracted during a single passage through the liver, producing a plasma half-life of 1.5 to 3 hours. Since lidocaine is a high clearance drug and its metabolism is blood flow-dependent, slower infusion rates are appropriate in patients whose cardiac output is depressed, e.g. in cardiac failure and shock.[385] Hepatocellular dysfunction also reduces lidocaine clearance, while the lower volume of distribution in patients with cardiac failure necessitates a smaller loading dose in this condition. In patients with cardiac failure or shock, a loading dose of 60mg followed by an infusion of 1 mg/min is appropriate.

The major metabolite of lidocaine is monoethylglycine xylidide (MEGX) which has similar antiarrhythmic activity and toxicity to lidocaine itself.[386] In most circumstances, plasma concentrations of MEGX are only about 20% of those of the parent drug. However, MEGX has a longer plasma half-life than lidocaine and has been reported to accumulate during prolonged infusions and in patients with shock, where it may contribute to both therapeutic effectiveness and toxicity.

Therapeutic plasma concentrations of lidocaine are considered to range from 2 to 6 mg/L at steady-state. Toxicity has been reported at concentrations between 5 mg/L and 9 mg/L and is common above 9 mg/L. When infusions are continued for 24 hours or longer, plasma concentrations of lidocaine may increase unless the infusion is slowed, possibly as a result of competition between lidocaine and MEGX for metabolising enzymes.[387]

Although lidocaine is well absorbed following intramuscular administration, the rate of absorption depends on the site of injection and its blood flow as well as on the concentration of the drug administered; therefore plasma concentrations with this route of administration cannot be predicted with confidence. An intramuscular dose of 200 to 300mg administered in the deltoid region has been reported to produce effective plasma concentrations after a delay of 5 to 15 minutes.

***Tolerability:*** the major adverse effects of lidocaine are neurological in origin and can generally be reduced by avoiding over-rapid administration and excessive doses. Nausea, paraesthesia, slurred speech, disorientation, hyperactivity and tremor are common and convulsions may occur, particularly if the plasma concentration exceeds 9 mg/L. At usual plasma concentrations, the drug produces few haemodynamic or electrophysiological changes and its potential for producing heart block is small. Despite this, over-rapid administration may produce heart block, bradycardia or tachycardia, hypotension and respiratory arrest. Sinus arrest has also been reported.

#### Mexiletine

Mexiletine is a class IB antiarrhythmic agent developed originally as an anticonvulsant. Its electrophysiological properties are similar to those of lidocaine, but unlike the latter, it is suitable for oral administration.[388] Mexiletine has been employed for the suppression of ventricular arrhythmias, but since publication of the CAST study,[193,194] its use has largely been curtailed.

***Pharmacokinetic characteristics and clinical use:*** following oral administration, peak plasma concentrations of mexiletine are usually achieved after 2 to 4 hours, although this may be delayed in the acutely ill. Its oral bioavailability is high (85 to 90%) and the apparent volume of distribution is large (>300L) indicating extensive tissue uptake. Mexiletine is approximately 70 to 75% bound to plasma proteins. The drug is primarily eliminated by hepatic metabolism, less than 20% of an oral dose being recovered unchanged in the urine. The remainder is recovered as metabolites (mainly parahydroxy- and hydroxymethyl-mexiletine and their corresponding alcohols). No pharmacologically active metabolites have been identified. The terminal elimination half-life of mexiletine is approximately 9 to 12 hours in healthy volunteers but is prolonged in the elderly and in individuals with cardiac failure, renal failure and chronic liver disease.

The therapeutic plasma concentration range for mexiletine has been reported to be 0.75 to 2.0 mg/L. Concentrations in this range will generally be achieved with oral dosages of 150 to 250mg 8-hourly. The higher dosage level is likely to be required in subjects receiving enzyme-inducing drugs such as phenytoin and rifampicin concomitantly. When administered by the intravenous route, an initial bolus dose of 250mg should be given over 10 minutes followed by an infusion of 0.5 to 1.0 mg/min. Assays for plasma concentrations are useful to confirm that an adequate dosage is being given and to help avoid toxicity, particularly in the elderly and the acutely ill.

***Tolerability:*** mexiletine has a narrow therapeutic ratio, with significant adverse effects occurring in up to 30 to 40% of patients.[389] Often, these occur while plasma drug concentrations are within the normal therapeutic range and are particularly common after intravenous administration. Gastrointestinal disturbances (usually nausea and vomiting) are the most commonly encountered problems. As with lidocaine, neurological symptoms are also prominent. A fine tremor is a frequent early sign commonly followed by nausea, dizziness, blurred vision, dysarthria, diplopia, ataxia, taste disturbances, nystagmus, drowsiness and a toxic confusional state.

Cardiovascular adverse effects are relatively uncommon with mexiletine, although after intravenous administration, hypotension, bradycardia and atrioventricular block have been reported, and the drug should be administered with caution to patients with an atrioventricular conduction delay or sinus node dysfunction. Widening of the QRS interval may also occur. However, at normal plasma concentrations, the drug has minimal negative inotropic effects. Mexiletine does not affect plasma digoxin concentrations.

#### Tocainide

Tocainide is an analogue of lidocaine with a pharmacokinetic profile that makes it suitable for oral administration.[390] It possesses electrophysiological properties virtually identical to lidocaine, and like lidocaine, it effectively suppresses ventricular ectopic activity.

***Pharmacokinetic characteristics and clinical use:*** the presently available formulation of tocainide is the racemate, the R(–) isomer being more potent in its electrophysiological effects but present in plasma in lower concentrations than the R(+) isomer. Following oral administration of tocainide, peak plasma concentrations are generally achieved after 0.5 to 4 hours. Absorption is delayed and a 40% reduction in peak concentrations has been reported when the drug is administered with food, but overall bioavailability is not affected. The bioavailability of tocainide is close to 100%.

Tocainide is approximately 50% protein bound in plasma and its apparent volume of distribution ranges from 112 to 224L. Elimination is both by excretion of unchanged drug via the kidney (approximately 50%) and by hepatic glucuronidation; the plasma half-life averages 15 hours in healthy subjects but in patients with cardiac failure, renal failure and hepatic cirrhosis, the half-life has been reported to be prolonged. In 9 patients whose creatinine clearance was less than 5 ml/min, the half-life was 22 hours (range 17 to 28 hours) and in 6 others with creatinine clearances of 10 to 55 ml/min, it ranged from 13 to 22 hours (mean 19 hours).[391] This suggests that the dose should be reduced by approximately 50% in severe renal disease, and in such patients plasma concentrations should be monitored.[391]

The recommended therapeutic plasma concentration range for tocainide is 3 to 10 mg/L. The initial oral dose should be 200 to 400mg 8-hourly; this may be increased every 3 to 4 days up to a maximum of 600mg 8- to 12-hourly.

***Tolerability:*** tocainide produces little deterioration of cardiac performance during long term oral therapy. Exacerbation of arrhythmias has been reported but there have been no reports of major QT interval prolongation or torsades de pointes. Noncardiac adverse effects require cessation of therapy in about 10% of patients and are more common if the plasma concentration exceeds 10 mg/L. Nausea and vomiting are common, but neurological symptoms, which progress from tremor and dizziness to paraesthesia, agitation, confusional states and convulsions, are also encountered. Confusional states, psychoses, hepatitis and fever have also been reported, but the development of antinuclear antibodies or lupus syndrome rarely occurs.[392,393] However, of most concern is the drug's reported association with agranulocytosis and other blood dyscrasias, some of which have proved fatal.[394] This has led to major restrictions on its use in some countries.

#### Flecainide

Flecainide, propafenone[395] and moracizine[396] are the most commonly used drugs of the IC class. Other members of this class such as encainide and lorcainide are now little used.

Flecainide is structurally similar to procainamide but differs from class IA agents in its spectrum of electrophysiological properties.[397] The distinguishing feature of flecainide's action (which leads to its classification as a type I agent) is its slow rate of dissociation from sodium channels between depolarising pulses. The drug exerts little effect on the action potential duration or the effective refractory period. The slowed impulse conduction is reflected in a prolongation of the PR interval and QRS duration on the electrocardiogram, although at normal doses, the QT interval is only minimally lengthened. Flecainide exerts a moderate negative inotropic effect, may suppress sinus node function, and produces a substantial increase in pacing threshold.

***Pharmacokinetic characteristics:*** flecainide is well absorbed with an oral bioavailability of over 90%.[398,399] The drug is a racemate but the individual enantiomers share similar electrophysiological and pharmacokinetic properties. About 70% of a dose is eliminated by hepatic metabolism and 30% is excreted unchanged in the urine. In the liver, the cytochrome P450 isoenzyme CYP2D6 converts the drug to largely inactive metabolites.

***Clinical use:*** flecainide may be administered either orally or intravenously. A typical intravenous dose is 2 mg/kg given over 3 minutes. The usual oral dose is 100 to 300 mg/day in two or three divided doses.

Flecainide reduces the frequency of ventricular arrhythmias ranging from ventricular premature complexes to nonsustained ventricular tachycardia. However, this effect is overshadowed by its ability to provoke other more lethal arrhythmias. As a result, long term administration is rarely indicated. The clinical use of flecainide is now largely confined to the management of supraventricular arrhythmias.[400] It is one of several agents usually effective at aborting supraventricular tachycardias, especially when caused by AV nodal re-entry or by an accessory pathway. Flecainide is effective in reverting recent onset atrial fibrillation to sinus rhythm in about 60% of cases but is substantially less effective than amiodarone in maintaining sinus rhythm in patients with paroxysmal atrial fibrillation.

***Tolerability:*** about 10% of patients discontinue flecainide early after commencement because of adverse effects. Dizziness and visual disturbances are the most common of these, affecting about one-third of patients. Headache, nausea, dyspnoea and chest pain are also common.[401]

The most serious adverse effects of flecainide are those resulting from its proarrhythmic properties.[402,403] The significance of these was demonstrated in the CAST (Cardiac Arrhythmia Suppression Trial) study[193] where flecainide and encainide were compared with a placebo in 1455 patients with asymptomatic ventricular arrhythmias after a myocardial infarction. The trial was stopped prematurely after 10 months when the rate of death or cardiac arrest was 7.6% among the drug-treated patients and 3.0% among those on placebo. Although most of the excess deaths among the drug-treated patients were sudden and presumably induced by arrhythmia, the number of deaths caused by other factors (particularly cardiac failure) was also higher in the drug-treated group. An excess of arrhythmic deaths occurred in most subgroups but particularly among those with recent non-Q-wave myocardial infarction – a subgroup at risk of continuing ischaemia. The mechanism by which flecainide exerts its proarrhythmic effects is unclear, although it is able to provoke an arrhythmia referred to as incessant ventricular tachycardia (because of the difficulty in treating it). A similar problem occurs with high plasma concentrations of quinidine and tricyclic antidepressant drugs.

Apart from its proarrhythmic and negative inotropic effects, the other major cardiovascular adverse effects of flecainide include sinus node dysfunction and worsening of cardiac failure.

#### Propafenone

Propafenone is a class IC antiarrhythmic drug that inhibits rapid sodium influx and slows cardiac conduction in a similar manner to flecainide.[404] However, propafenone also possesses other pharmacological properties including weak β-adrenoceptor blockade, potassium channel blockade and calcium channel blockade. It also produces an increase in the duration of the PR and QRS segments of the electrocardiogram but possesses only minor negative inotropic properties at low doses.

***Pharmacokinetic characteristics:*** following oral administration, propafenone is extensively metabolised in the liver through a saturable process involving the cytochrome P450 isoenzymes CYP2D6, CYP2A6/7 and CYP1A2.[405] The principal metabolite is 5-hydroxypropafenone which is at least as potent an antiarrhythmic agent as the parent drug. The 7% of Caucasians who possess the poor debrisoquine metaboliser phenotype metabolise propafenone slowly and have higher concentrations of the parent drug and lower concentrations of the metabolite.

Because of its extensive metabolism, propafenone undergoes extensive first-pass hepatic extraction after oral administration. It is extensively protein bound and its terminal elimination half-life averages approximately 6 hours. Insufficient data are available at present to adequately establish a concentration-effect relationship.

***Clinical use:*** propafenone has been shown to be effective in suppressing a wide spectrum of supraventricular and ventricular arrhythmias.[406] It appears to be particularly effective in suppressing arrhythmias associated with the Wolff-Parkinson-White syndrome. However, until proven otherwise, it must be assumed to share a similar proarrhythmic potential to other class I antiarrhythmic agents and its long term use restricted accordingly.

The usual intravenous dose of propafenone is 1 to 2.5 mg/kg by bolus injection followed by a maintenance infusion of 7 to 14 mg/kg/min. The standard oral dose is 150 to 300mg 8-hourly; lower doses should be used in elderly patients and in those with liver or renal disease.

***Tolerability:*** as with other class I antiarrhythmic agents, propafenone may produce a variety of adverse cardiovascular effects including proarrhythmic effects, worsening of cardiac failure, conduction disturbances and an increased ventricular rate when given to patients with atrial fibrillation.[404] Other common adverse effects include neurological symptoms (dizziness, taste disturbance, blurred vision, headache and paraesthesia) and gastrointestinal disturbances (nausea, anorexia, constipation). Occasional problems include cholestatic hepatitis, agranulocytosis, azoospermia and worsening of asthma (due to its β-adrenoceptor blocking action).

***Drug interactions:*** propafenone may inhibit the elimination of drugs metabolised by the same cytochrome P450 isoenzymes including cyclosporin, theophylline, cimetidine and desipramine.[405] Concomitant administration of these drugs may, at the same time, increase propafenone concentrations.

#### 8.2.3 Class III Agents

##### Sotalol

Sotalol is a racemate drug combining *d*- and *l*- isomers.[407] The *d*-isomer is a 'pure' class III antiarrhythmic agent. It is a potassium channel blocker which exerts its antiarrhythmic action by lengthening the duration of the action potential, leading to a prolongation of the effective refractory period. The *l*-isomer is a nonselective β-adrenoceptor antagonist.

The physiological effects of the racemate reflect its combined class III and β-blocking actions. It reduces resting and exercise heart rate, exerts a moderate negative inotropic effect, and lengthens the QT interval on the surface electrocardiogram (while having little effect on other electrocardiogram intervals).

***Pharmacokinetic characteristics:*** sotalol has low lipid solubility and an oral bioavailability close to 100%. It is eliminated almost entirely via the kidneys in unchanged form, its plasma half-life averaging 15 hours.

***Clinical use:*** a typical oral dose of sotalol is 80 or 160mg 12-hourly. When given intravenously, the usual dose is 1 to 2 mg/kg infused over 10 to 30 minutes; this dose may be repeated after a 10-minute interval and followed by an infusion of 80 to 160mg in 5% dextrose over 12 hours. In clinical trials, sotalol has been shown to abort and prevent a variety of supraventricular and ventricular arrhythmias and it is considerably more effective in this respect than conventional β-blocking drugs. Sotalol is effective in terminating most forms of supraventricular tachycardia (including Wolff-Parkinson-White syndrome) but is less effective in reverting atrial fibrillation and flutter.[408] During longer term therapy, the drug has appeared relatively effective for prophylaxis of recurrent supraventricular tachycardia or atrial fibrillation. However, it appears to be less effective as an antiarrhythmic agent in the setting of high sympathetic activity.

In ventricular arrhythmias, sotalol suppresses ventricular ectopy and higher grade arrhythmias up to ventricular fibrillation. However, the results of the SWORD (Survival With Oral *d*-Sotalol) study indicate that the net result may be an increase rather than a decrease in mortality, at least with *d*-isomer. This study investigated the value of *d*-sotalol in high-risk survivors of a myocardial infarction with impaired cardiac function.[409] The trial was stopped prematurely because of a significantly higher mortality in the *d*-sotalol treated group (4.6% *vs* 2.67%). The SWORD trial has demonstrated an unexpected hazard of 'pure' class III agents and suggests that long term therapy with these drugs should be avoided, at least in patients with left ventricular dysfunction.

***Tolerability:*** the most important adverse effect of sotalol is its proarrhythmic effect which was presumably responsible for the excess of sudden deaths observed in the SWORD study. Proarrhythmic effects associated with class III agents typically take the form of torsades de pointes which have been documented in about 2 to 3.5% of patients receiving sotalol.[410,411] This may convert spontaneously to ventricular fibrillation. The risk of developing torsades de pointes is greater among females (possibly because of their longer QT interval) than men, and among those with hypokalaemia or high plasma drug concentrations. Therefore, care must be taken to avoid high doses, particularly in patients with renal insufficiency.

Other adverse effects occurring with sotalol are principally those associated with its β-blocking activity and include exacerbation of asthma, dyspnoea, fatigue, bradycardia and aggravation of cardiac failure.[408,412]

##### Amiodarone

Amiodarone is the prototype class III antiarrhythmic drug.[413] It has a complex mixture of other properties including a powerful vasodilator effect. Amiodarone owes its antiarrhythmic activity to its ability to inhibit potassium ion fluxes during phases 2 and 3 of the normal action potential. This leads to a substantial prolongation of the action potential and effective refractory period which (in contrast to most class III drugs) persists at high heart rates.[414]

In addition to blockade of potassium channels, amiodarone also produces a weak blockade of sodium channels (thereby slowing impulse conduction) and calcium channels (thereby slowing the sinus rate and the rate of AV conduction). It also produces weak noncompetitive blockade of α- and β-adrenoceptors. The haemodynamic effects of amiodarone include peripheral and coronary vasodilatation and a slowed sinus rate. The drug possesses only mild negative inotropic properties which are normally offset by reflex sympathetic stimulation.

***Pharmacokinetic characteristics:*** amiodarone is a highly lipophilic drug with an oral bioavailability of around 40 to 50%.[415,416] It is eliminated principally by hepatic metabolism (involving the 3A family of cytochrome P450 enzymes) to an active metabolite (desethylamiodarone) whose pharmacological effects and plasma concentrations are similar to those of the parent drug. The plasma half-life of amiodarone during long term therapy is variable, ranging from 14 to 110 days, and it has a very high apparent volume of distribution (≈4970L). Because of its long half-life, it takes several weeks to achieve a steady-state level (and hence the full therapeutic effect) unless an oral loading dose is given. This also explains the slow disappearance of its effects after regular administration is ceased. Steady-state concentrations of amiodarone of the order of 1.0 to 2.5 mg/L have been associated with antiarrhythmic effects and acceptable toxicity.

***Clinical use:*** amiodarone may be administered either orally or intravenously. The *intravenous* formulation is usually administered as part of the acute management of sustained or nonsustained ventricular tachycardia. The usual dosage regimen involves an initial rapid infusion of 150mg over 10 minutes (15 mg/min) followed by 360mg over the next 6 hours (1 mg/min) and then 540mg (0.5 mg/min) over the next 18 hours. After the first 24 hours, a maintenance infusion of 0.5 mg/min may be continued for up to 3 weeks. Supplemental infusions of 150mg may be required for breakthrough arrhythmias; central lines should be used when the infused amiodarone concentration exceeds 2 mg/min.

It should be noted that amiodarone alters the surface properties of solutions resulting in, for example, a reduction in drop size. This may lead to an underdose of up to 30% if a drop counter is used to measure the infusion rate. The drug also binds to polyvinyl chloride (PVC) tubing and the dosage schedule should be designed to account for this adsorption.

*Oral* amiodarone is usually administered initially in a dose of 200 to 400mg 3 times daily for 2 weeks followed by a daily dose of 200 to 400mg as guided by plasma concentration estimations. When administered by the oral route, absorption is erratic; as the drug is lipid soluble, it concentrates in adipose tissue and in the highly perfused organs.

Because of its potential to cause serious toxicity, amiodarone should ideally be confined to indications where its value has been supported by large clinical trials. At present, it is widely recommended for use in the following clinical settings:[417]

- Attempted pharmacological cardioversion of recent onset atrial fibrillation. Amiodarone rarely produces reversion of established atrial fibrillation.
- Control of the heart rate in patients with atrial flutter or fibrillation, especially when urgent slowing is necessary and there is concern about the potential of alternative drugs to produce myocardial depression.
- Maintenance of sinus rhythm in patients with paroxysmal atrial fibrillation or after cardioversion. In small studies, success rates of about 80% have been reported compared with 50% for quinidine.
- Prophylaxis of recurrent supraventricular tachycardia, including that occurring by accessory pathways. However, because of the relatively young age of most affected patients and other dangers of long term amiodarone administration (see below), electrical ablation is generally the preferred therapy.
- Prophylaxis of sudden death in patients with ventricular arrhythmias after myocardial infarction or after resuscitation from ventricular tachycardia or fibrillation. β-Blockers are the preferred drugs in this setting but amiodarone may be of benefit in patients intolerant of β-blockers. Proper appraisal of its value is awaiting large studies.
- Systolic cardiac failure and ventricular arrhythmias. Two recently reported trials have provided conflicting results in this setting, with one unblinded study (conducted mainly in NYHA class III and IV patients) showing a 28% mortality reduction, while the other similar but blinded study in less seriously ill patients showed no benefit.[195,196] These results have led to the suggestion that amiodarone therapy is appropriate in patients with severely depressed left ventricular function, whereas alternative approaches (e.g. implantable defibrillation) may be more appropriate in patients with less impairment.

A reassuring finding from these studies has been the absence of an increased risk of death from proarrhythmic effects.

***Tolerability:*** adverse effects with amiodarone are common and sometimes serious, especially when higher doses are used.[417] They often develop after months or years of treatment, and because of the drug's long half-life, may take weeks to resolve on cessation of therapy. In 10 to 15% of those treated, it is necessary to stop treatment.

Several mechanisms contribute to the profile of adverse effects observed. They include accumulation of the parent drug, accumulation of iodine, intracellular accumulation of phospholipid as a result of phospholipase inhibition, free radical formation, and provocation of immunological reactions.[417] Adverse effects observed with amiodarone include the following:

1) *Cardiovascular effects:* the principal adverse cardiovascular effects produced by amiodarone are sinus bradycardia and atrioventricular block. Hypotension is seen in approximately 30% of patients when the drug is given intravenously, the risk of which is related to the rate of the infusion. Amiodarone also produces significant QT interval prolongation but proarrhythmic effects (torsades de pointes) are rare, unless other provoking features are present (e.g. hypokalaemia or coadministration of class I antiarrhythmic drugs).[418] Similarly, amiodarone produces a small negative inotropic effect but this is rarely of clinical significance.

2) *Pulmonary reaction:* these affect 6 to 8% of patients and represent the most serious noncardiac effect of amiodarone.[419] An acute syndrome, probably representing a hypersensitivity reaction, typically develops within weeks of the commencement of therapy with symptoms such as fever, dyspnoea, fatigue and cough. A delayed syndrome may develop after months or years of therapy, although this may also develop relatively suddenly. The chest x-ray generally reveals an interstitial infiltration or fibrosis. Treatment with corticosteroids has been recommended but without strong evidence of its value. Resolution of the process is usually very slow.

3) *Thyroid effects:* iodine makes up about 37% of the total weight of amiodarone and contributes to its effect of interfering with the conversion of thyroxine to tri-iodothyronine. A compensatory increase in plasma thyroid-stimulating hormone (TSH) levels is common.[420] Clinically significant hypo- or hyperthyroidism is seen in 5 to 10% of patients. When administered during pregnancy, amiodarone produces a small risk of congenital goitre and/or neonatal hypo- or hyperthyroidism.

4) *Gastrointestinal disturbances:* nausea, anorexia and other gastrointestinal symptoms are commonly seen when high loading doses are given.[417] Taste disturbances are occasionally encountered. Abnormal elevations of liver enzymes (especially serum aminotransferase and alkaline phosphatase) have occurred but clinically evident hepatitis is very rare.

5) *Skin reactions:* these are commonly caused by amiodarone and may take the form of an allergic rash, a photosensitivity reaction or a blue-grey skin discolouration.[421] Patients receiving amiodarone should restrict their exposure to sunlight.

6) *Neurological effects:* amiodarone may produce a peripheral neuropathy or other nonspecific symptoms including tremor, ataxia, fatigue and weakness.[422]

7) *Ocular effects:* corneal microdeposits result from the accumulation of amiodarone on the corneal surface.[423] They are seen in most patients and do not interfere with vision.

8) *Adverse effects on the fetus:* in addition to the risk of thyroid disturbances in neonates (see above), various other forms of developmental toxicity have been noted in animals.[424] Amiodarone should be administered during pregnancy only under compelling circumstances.

***Drug interactions:*** amiodarone interacts with several drugs that are often prescribed concurrently with it.[425] Of particular importance is its ability to slow the metabolism of *warfarin* and thereby potentiate its effects. Other potentially important drug interactions include:

- An increased risk of proarrhythmic effects when amiodarone is coadministered with drugs that increase the QT interval (particularly class I antiarrhythmics such as quinidine, procainamide, mexiletine and propafenone)
- Bradycardia and AV block with coadministration of amiodarone and a β-blocker, verapamil or diltiazem
- Hypotension and bradycardia when amiodarone is administered with anaesthetic agents
- Toxicity with digoxin as a result of amiodarone's capacity to decrease the clearance of digoxin and increase its plasma concentrations.

#### Bretylium

Bretylium is a quaternary amine with class III antiarrhythmic properties and an ability to interfere with the reuptake of noradrenaline (norepinephrine) into sympathetic nerve terminals.[426,427] It prolongs action potentials in normal cardiac tissue bringing these closer to those of ischaemic tissue. This reduces the heterogeneity of action potential durations which may underlie the development of re-entry circuits.

***Pharmacokinetic characteristics and clinical use:*** bretylium is used principally to treat ventricular fibrillation that has proved refractory to lidocaine. It is administered by rapid intravenous injection in a dose of 5 mg/kg. If fibrillation persists, the dose may be increased with a second bolus of 10 mg/kg. A response, if present, will usually be evident within 5 to 15 minutes.

Bretylium is eliminated unchanged via the kidneys and its plasma half-life is 7 to 12 hours.

***Tolerability:*** after intravenous administration, bretylium produces a transient release of noradrenaline that may cause an acute rise in blood pressure and heart rate.[426,427] Within 20 to 30 minutes, depletion of catecholamines leads to a reduction in vascular resistance and blood pressure which should be managed with fluid replacement.

#### 8.2.4 Adenosine

Adenosine is an endogenous nucleoside which, when administered as a rapid intravenous bolus, depresses atrioventricular (AV) nodal conduction resulting in a transient AV block of the anterograde AV nodal component of the re-entrance circuit.[428] A dose of 6 to 12mg adenosine is usually successful in aborting episodes of supraventricular tachycardia when these involve the AV node. Its effectiveness in converting these to sinus rhythm is at least as good as that of verapamil.[429]

***Pharmacokinetic characteristics and clinical use:*** adenosine has a very short plasma half-life in humans (less than 10 seconds).[429] This allows for rapid upward dose titration if initial doses are unsuccessful. Because of its specific action on the AV node, adenosine administration may be useful in determining the origin of broadened QRS complex tachycardia. The drug successfully terminates arrhythmias dependent on the AV node but has no effect on ventricular tachycardia.

Adenosine has also been used to induce vasodilatation in patients undergoing thallium-201 single photon emission computed tomography to evaluate suspected coronary artery disease. In this setting, adenosine is an alternative to physical exercise or dipyridamole in enhancing the display of ischaemic areas.

When used either for the diagnosis or treatment of supraventricular tachycardia, adenosine is generally administered rapidly (over 1 to 2 seconds) as an intravenous bolus of 6mg into a peripheral vein. If no effect is noted within 2 minutes, a further bolus of 12mg may be given after another 1 or 2 minutes, with subsequent upward dose titration every 1 to 2 minutes in 2.5 or 3mg increments. A maximum of 20mg has been used. Lower doses may be required if the drug is administered into a central vein.

***Tolerability:*** the principal adverse effects of adenosine are those resulting from its vasodilating properties and include flushing, dizziness, dyspnoea and chest pain.[429,430] Because of its short half-life, these usually last less than a minute.

### 8.3 Optimum Treatment of Specific Arrhythmias

#### 8.3.1 Atrial Flutter

This is a difficult arrhythmia to treat. It often originates from a re-entry circuit in the right ventricle and is frequently a complication of right-sided cardiac conditions such as right-sided congenital cardiac malformations. It is also common after cardiac surgery. The atrial rate is often about 300 beats/min (range 230 to 350 beats/min) which is conducted with a 2:1, 3:1 or 4:1 block producing ventricular rates of about 150, 100 or 75 beats/min, respectively.[431]

Atrial flutter rarely reverts spontaneously but rather transforms into atrial fibrillation if allowed to persist. Drug therapy rarely produces reversion to sinus rhythm. For this reason, when reversion is indicated, it is usually achieved by 'overdrive' pacing or (in an emergency) DC cardioversion.

There is little information about the comparative success of various drugs used to prevent recurrences of atrial flutter. If reversion is not attempted or is unsuccessful, then treatment should be directed towards rate control using the same strategies employed in atrial fibrillation (see section 8.3.2).

#### 8.3.2 Atrial Fibrillation

Atrial fibrillation (AF) results from a disorganised pattern of excitation whereby multiple wavelets circulate chaotically in the atria. The condition occurs in many clinical settings including acute illness, following cardiac surgery, or as an accompaniment to various forms of chronic heart disease. Chronic atrial fibrillation is more prevalent in the elderly, affecting about 10% of those over 70 years of age.[432]

The classical causes of atrial fibrillation are rheumatic heart valve disease (especially mitral stenosis) and thyrotoxicosis, but ischaemic heart disease is now the most common underlying condition. In about 15% of cases of sustained atrial fibrillation, no underlying heart disease or systemic disease can be found and the condition is then referred to as 'lone' atrial fibrillation.[433] Transient episodes of 'lone' atrial fibrillation occur more commonly in younger individuals, often during sleep or after meals when vagal activity may be higher than usual. These episodes rarely develop into established atrial fibrillation.

Atrial fibrillation requires intervention because:

1) The irregularity of the rhythm may produce uncomfortable palpitations.

2) A reduction in cardiac output may lead to dizziness, syncope, dyspnoea and angina, especially in patients with left ventricular dysfunction. Loss of atrial contraction leads to about a 20% reduction in ventricular filling and the uncoordinated ventricular contraction can depress it further. Patients with systolic cardiac failure who revert to sinus rhythm have been found to have an improvement in exercise tolerance.

3) The risk of thromboembolism may be increased (especially if underlying heart disease is present), resulting in an increased risk of stroke and peripheral emboli.

#### Rate Control

Control of the ventricular rate (usually aiming for an ideal rate at about 90 beats/min) will control palpitations and improve cardiac output.[431] *Digoxin* is the principal drug used for this purpose and to avoid a delay (often several days) in the onset of its effect, a loading dose is usually administered. Digoxin has positive inotropic properties and is therefore safe when cardiac output is low. To achieve optimal results, an adequate dose should be given (and plasma concentrations monitored), and potassium levels should be normalised.

Digoxin therapy alone may provide inadequate rate control, especially during periods of exercise, when inadequate ventricular filling may severely limit exercise tolerance. Provided their negative inotropic effects can be tolerated, low doses of *verapamil* (e.g. 40mg twice daily), *diltiazem* (e.g. 30mg three or four times daily), or *atenolol* (e.g. 25mg twice daily) may provide sufficient additional AV node blockade or may be used as alternatives to digoxin. *Amiodarone* (used alone or with digoxin) is another alternative which is also devoid of negative inotropic properties.

In some cases, the ventricular rate cannot be adequately controlled by drug therapy and additional measures are needed. Those currently popular include His bundle ablation and permanent adaptive rate ventricular pacing. Two surgical procedures to abolish the arrhythmia, i.e. the 'maze' procedure and the 'corridor' procedure, have also been described.

#### Cardioversion

Attempts to revert atrial fibrillation to sinus rhythm should be undertaken to improve cardiac function and to obviate the need for long term anticoagulant therapy.[434] Cardioversion is most likely to be successful in younger individuals with good ventricular function and a small left atrium. It is also more often successful when the duration of atrial fibrillation is short.

Pharmacological reversion is generally attempted after rate control has been achieved. Digoxin, β-blockers and calcium antagonists are effective in achieving rate control but have little antifibrillatory actions and should not be used for this purpose. On the other hand, several class I antiarrhythmic agents (including in particular intravenous *flecainide* and *propafenone*) and class III agents (including *sotalol* and *amiodarone*) are effective in 50 to 90% of cases. Because of their proarrhythmic effects, flecainide and propafenone should not be used in the presence of heart disease and amiodarone is the preferred drug in this setting.

In the presence of a haemodynamic compromise or following the failure of pharmacological reversion, electrical cardioversion using synchronised DC shocks may be attempted.[434] Prior to the intervention, the serum potassium concentration should be normalised and an anticoagulant administered for the preceding 2 weeks (unless a transoesophageal echocardiogram has excluded a left atrial thrombus). Recurrences after an initial successful cardioversion are common and in such cases, pretreatment with amiodarone may be of value.

#### Adjunctive Anticoagulant/ Antiplatelet Therapy

The most serious long term complications of atrial fibrillation are embolic stroke and peripheral embolism resulting from dislodgement of a thrombus in the left atrium.[435] The risk is particularly high in the case of rheumatic valvular heart disease, but is also substantial when any form of structural heart disease is present. On the other hand, the risk appears low in young patients without structural heart disease.

Several major trials have shown that anticoagulant treatment substantially reduces this risk, albeit at the cost of a small increase in cerebral haemorrhage and other bleeding complications. The most impressive result from the SPAF trial using low-dose *warfarin* [international normalised ratio (INR) targeted to 1.5 to 2.7] showed an 86% reduction in stroke incidence.[436] Several studies have investigated the value of *aspirin* which has also proved effective, though less so than warfarin (see further chapter 26; sect. 3.2). An appropriate policy is to use aspirin as stroke prophylaxis in settings where the risk of stroke is low or the risk of adverse effects from an anticoagulant is high.[437]

#### Treatment of Atrial Fibrillation in Various Clinical Settings

The treatment of atrial fibrillation depends on the clinical setting in which it occurs. In general, therapeutic options involve:

1) Control of the ventricular rate using drugs that slow conduction in the AV node, i.e. digoxin, a β-blocker or a calcium antagonist.

2) Attempted reversion to sinus rhythm using either drugs or electrical shock.

***Atrial fibrillation in acute illness:*** when atrial fibrillation occurs during an acute illness, it is likely to be self-limiting and to resolve with treatment of the underlying condition. Treatment is directed initially towards rate control with a loading dose of *digoxin* followed by maintenance therapy, but this regimen still takes some hours before its effect is noticeable. A *β-blocker* or *verapamil* is an alternative but their negative inotropic effects may contraindicate this approach. If the haemodynamic disturbance mandates more urgent therapy, then intravenous *amiodarone* or synchronised DC *cardioversion* may be required. When atrial fibrillation persists after an acute illness, cardioversion should be attempted.

***Paroxysmal episodes of atrial fibrillation:*** when patients experience paroxysmal episodes of atrial fibrillation, treatment is directed at reducing the frequency of these episodes. Digoxin has been shown to be ineffective while the increased mortality resulting from the proarrhythmic effects of quinidine, procainamide, disopyramide and flecainide probably make them an unacceptable risk. Low doses of *amiodarone* (200 mg/day) appear to be effective, but the long term risks are still unclear and this therapy should be used only when substantial clinical benefit ensues. When symptoms are incapacitating and control cannot be achieved with drugs, other interventions such as AV node ablation and pacing or surgical procedures may be considered.

When a paroxysm of atrial fibrillation becomes sustained or in cases where atrial fibrillation is of recent or unknown origin, pharmacological cardioversion should be attempted. *Amiodarone* is an appropriate drug for this purpose, especially in the presence of impaired cardiac function. Intravenous flecainide or propafenone are alternatives which may be used whenever cardiac function is normal. After reversion, amiodarone is generally effective in preventing reversions to atrial fibrillation.

***Chronic atrial fibrillation:*** in the usual situations of chronic atrial fibrillation, rate control is the appropriate treatment. *Digoxin* is most commonly used alone, although low doses of *verapamil, diltiazem* or *atenolol* may be added if rate control is inadequate. Antithrombotic therapy with either low-dose warfarin or aspirin (depending on the risk-benefit analysis; see above) should also be utilised.

### *8.3.3 Supraventricular Tachycardia*

Supraventricular tachycardia (SVT) refers to a tachyarrhythmia that relies on atrial or atrioventricular junctional tissue for initiation and maintenance.[438] These arrhythmias may arise from either a re-entry circuit, a focus of enhanced automaticity, or from ‘triggered activity’ which is another form of enhanced impulse initiation.

Over one-half of all cases of SVT arise from a re-entry circuit within the AV node (see further section 8.1 above). Accessory pathways are another relatively common cause of supraventricular tachycardia, e.g. the pathway associated with the Wolff-Parkinson-White (WPW) syndrome.[438] These pathways are abnormal bands of conducting tissue connecting the atria and ventricles that allow a re-entry circuit to be formed with the AV node. Supraventricular tachycardias associated with the WPW syndrome, e.g. atrial flutter or fibrillation, may be associated with dangerously high ventricular rates (because the atrial impulses can reach the ventricles without a delay in the AV node). Sudden death may result.

Supraventricular tachycardia may also result from re-entry circuits involving the SA node or from foci of enhanced automaticity in the AV node or within the atria. In the latter case, there is often underlying heart disease or acute illness. Digitalis intoxication is another occasional precipitant of atrial tachycardia and typically occurs with 2:1, 3:1 or variable atrioventricular conduction.

The clinical presentation of supraventricular tachycardia commonly involves palpitations, light-headedness, dyspnoea and sweating and these are often more common with underlying heart disease. More serious sequelae such as cardiac failure and myocardial infarction are rare. The diagnosis is confirmed by an electrocardiogram but it should be noted that in some cases, the impulses are conducted aberrantly in the ventricles, giving rise to a wide QRS tachycardia that may be mistaken for ventricular tachycardia.

#### Acute Management

Supraventricular tachycardias resulting from re-entry circuits that involve the AV node may be terminated by vagal stimulation (induced by carotid sinus massage or a Valsalva manoeuvre). Alternative therapy with adenosine or verapamil can be used to provide pharmacologically-induced AV blockade.

Intravenously administered *adenosine* is the therapy of choice.[438] This briefly active agent should be administered as a rapid bolus injection of 6mg followed 2 minutes later by 12mg and if necessary a subsequent dose of 18mg (see further section 4.2.4 above). The arrhythmia ceases in about 80% of cases but the drug commonly causes facial flushing, dyspnoea and chest pain. Adenosine is contraindicated in patients with atrial fibrillation and an anterograde conducting accessory pathway (because this may transmit impulses more rapidly when the AV node is blocked).

Intravenously administered *verapamil* causes reversion in a similar percentage of cases as adenosine.[438] Verapamil is administered in a dose of 1 mg/min intravenously up to a total dose of 15mg, with careful monitoring of blood pressure. There is a substantial risk of severe hypotension in patients receiving β-adrenoceptor blocking drugs and verapamil is contraindicated in this setting. Haemodynamic collapse may also occur if the drug is mistakenly administered to patients with ventricular tachycardia and, for this reason, it should not be used in patients with wide QRS complex tachycardia.

#### Treatment of Recurrent Episodes

When recurrent episodes of supraventricular tachycardia occur, the treatment of choice rests between radiofrequency ablation of the re-entrant circuit and the introduction of prophylactic drug therapy. *Verapamil* (typically 480mg daily) is the drug most commonly administered, although *digoxin* and β-*blockers* appear to be equally efficacious and sometimes these agents are best used in combination. If these drugs are poorly tolerated or are ineffective, class I antiarrhythmics (e.g. flecainide) may be introduced if the risk of proarrhythmic events is judged to be outweighed by the anticipated clinical benefit.

Ablation should be considered as a first step for WPW syndrome because of the disappointing response to drugs.[438] Unifocal atrial tachycardias also respond poorly to drug therapy, although a trial of verapamil or a β-blocker may be considered prior to the introduction of amiodarone or catheter ablation of the focus.

### *8.3.4 Ventricular Ectopic Beats*

Isolated ventricular ectopic beats (VEBs) represent one end of an arrhythmic continuum that progresses through unifocal and multifocal VEBs, to nonsustained ventricular tachycardia, sustained ventricular tachycardia and finally to ventricular fibrillation. Ambulatory monitoring has demonstrated that VEBs may occur in normal individuals where they convey little or no adverse prognostic implications.[439,440] However, they are more common in patients with heart disease.

VEBs occur commonly in patients after myocardial infarction and among those with cardiac failure. Their frequent presence during the days after a myocardial infarction has, in the past, led to attempts to suppress them with lidocaine. However, it was subsequently demonstrated that the routine use of lidocaine reduced the likelihood of ventricular fibrillation but this was unlikely to be related to its suppression of VEBs and was associated with a substantial risk of heart block and asystole.[384] For these reasons, the routine use of lidocaine has largely ceased.

In the later postinfarct period, the presence of a high frequency of VEBs (over 10/hour) is associated with a poor prognosis, principally due to an increased risk of sudden death. Class I drugs such as flecainide and encainide were effective at suppressing ectopics but the CAST study[193] demonstrated that they did not lead to an improved prognosis. Rather, this study was stopped prematurely because of an increased death rate in the treated group which presumably resulted from their proarrhythmic propensity. At the present time, only the β-*blockers* have been shown unequivocally to reduce the risk of sudden death in high-risk patients after myocardial infarction and are probably the treatment of choice in this setting.

In the presence of cardiac failure, VEBs also indicate a worse prognosis but again, little has been achieved by drugs which suppress them. Recent trials of β-blockers with additional vasodilating properties have indicated considerable benefit. Other studies with amiodarone have produced variable results but no evidence of an increased mortality. With either type of drug, it is not clear that VEB suppression provided benefit.

#### *8.3.5 Nonsustained Ventricular Tachycardia*

Nonsustained ventricular tachycardia refers to ventricular tachycardia lasting for at least four consecutive ventricular ectopic beats (VEBs) but persisting for less than 30 seconds. It may be asymptomatic or accompanied by dizziness, palpitations and syncope.[441] The condition occurs in up to 35% of patients during the acute phase of myocardial infarction (especially during reperfusion) and in 5 to 10% of those in the post-acute phase. It may also occur in patients with cardiac failure, but has also been recorded in persons with normal hearts.

When treatment is considered necessary, usually because of recurrent symptoms, a β-*blocker* is an appropriate first choice. Other treatments should be primarily directed towards the underlying heart disease.

#### *8.3.6 Sustained Ventricular Tachycardia*

Episodes of ventricular tachycardia (VT) lasting more than 30 seconds are most commonly encountered during the acute or post-acute phases of myocardial infarction and usually present with palpitations, dizziness and syncope.[442] Diagnosis may require differentiation from supraventricular tachycardia (SVT) with wide QRS complexes. An incorrect choice of drug therapy may be dangerous in this setting and, for this reason, it is safer, when in doubt, to treat as VT rather than SVT.

Sustained VT most commonly occurs after myocardial infarction when it originates at the border zone of the damaged myocardium. The clinical settings include dilated cardiomyopathy, mitral valve prolapse and hypertrophic cardiomyopathy. The condition may also occur in otherwise normal individuals.

The emergency treatment of ventricular tachycardia is generally cardioversion if the patient is haemodynamically compromised. In noncompromised patients, *lidocaine* or *amiodarone* administered intravenously will often suffice. β-Blockers and calcium antagonists should be avoided.

More prolonged treatment is controversial – *amiodarone* is currently popular with an implantable defibrillator as the alternative option.

#### *8.3.7 Torsades de Pointes*

Torsades de pointes are a form of ventricular tachycardia characterised by QRS complexes which in any electrocardiogram lead appear to revolve around the isoelectric line.[443,444] The tachycardia is usually brief but may be sustained long enough to produce syncope or degenerate into ventricular fibrillation and sudden death. Typically the rate is 180 to 250 beats/min.

Torsades de pointes develop in patients with a prolonged QT interval (usually greater than 500 msec) which can occur as a congenital anomaly or develop as a result of concomitant drug therapy and/or electrolyte disturbances.[445] Patients with the congenital form of QT interval prolongation usually present with syncope during childhood which often occurs after an exertion or a frightening experience. There is considerable variation between patients in the frequency of these episodes.

Acquired prolongation of the QT interval usually results from drugs that prolong repolarisation. Antiarrhythmic drugs including quinidine, procainamide, disopyramide, amiodarone and sotalol are frequently the cause and may precipitate the arrhythmia at plasma drug concentrations well within their therapeutic 'range'.[446] However, it is believed that some cases of torsades de pointes reported during procainamide therapy may have resulted from its active metabolite, acecainide (*N*-acetylprocainamide) which often accumulates in patients with renal insufficiency. Despite its class III actions, amiodarone rarely precipitates torsades de pointes.[445]

A variety of other drugs have also been associated with prolongation of the QT interval and torsades de pointes. They include phenothiazines, tricyclic and tetracyclic antidepressants, some $H_1$ antihistamines (e.g. terfenadine and astemizole), and some antibiotics, most notably erythromycin[445] (see also section 9.3 below). The likelihood of developing this arrhythmia is increased in the presence of hypokalaemia, hypomagnesaemia and starvation. It can also be precipitated by bradycardia, mitral valve prolapse, ventricular hypertrophy and the presence of acute neurological lesions such as intracerebral and subarachnoid haemorrhage.

Acute treatment of the condition involves intravenous *magnesium sulfate* 2g (i.e. 4ml of a 50% w/v solution) infused over 10 to 15 minutes followed if necessary by 0.5 to 0.75 g/hour (1 to 1.5ml) for 12 to 24 hours. *Atropine* (0.5 to 1.5mg) should be administered if any underlying bradycardia is present. Correction of electrolyte disturbances and withdrawal of possibly incriminated drugs should also be undertaken. Temporary atrial or ventricular pacing is an alternative choice of therapy but class IA, IC and III antiarrhythmic drugs should be avoided.[447,448]

If cessation of the precipitating drug and correction of metabolic disturbances does not abort subsequent episodes, longer term prophylaxis is usually undertaken with high doses of β-*blockers*. This is sometimes supplemented by left-sided cervicothoracic sympathetic ganglionectomy or permanent pacing. Implantation of an internal cardiovertor-defibrillator may be required in some patients who continue to be symptomatic despite these measures.

#### 8.3.8 Ventricular Fibrillation

Early defibrillation is the most important determinant of survival in this setting, and a standard sequence using energies of 200J, 200 to 300J, and 360J is widely accepted.[449] If this is unsuccessful, 1ml of 1:1000 *adrenaline* (epinephrine) solution should be given intravenously or into the endotracheal tube. This can be repeated every 5 minutes alternating with further defibrillations. If defibrillation after adrenaline is unsuccessful, *lidocaine* (75 to 100mg) should be given intravenously over 1 to 2 minutes with a second dose 3 minutes later. If successful, an infusion of lidocaine (4 mg/min) should be continued for one hour.

If adrenaline and lidocaine are unsuccessful, *bretylium* (5 mg/kg) should be given as a bolus intravenous injection and subsequent doses of 10 mg/kg should be given every 5 minutes. Sodium bicarbonate and calcium chloride are now considered potentially harmful in this setting.[449] Sodium bicarbonate should only be used after prolonged resuscitation or in the presence of confirmed acidosis. In this case, 1 mmol/kg (1ml of an 8.4% solution) should be administered over 5 to 15 minutes.

#### 8.3.9 Bradyarrhythmias

Sinus bradycardia is often caused by drugs such as β-blockers, digoxin, verapamil, diltiazem or amiodarone. Symptoms are rare at pulse rates in excess of 45 beats/min. When the condition results from sick sinus syndrome, pacing may be required.

Atrioventricular junctional rhythms usually represent an escape rhythm commonly resulting from suppression of sinus node function by increased vagal tone or from AV nodal block. If hypotension occurs, an adequate sinus rhythm can often be restored by vagal blockade using *atropine* (0.5 to 1.5mg given intravenously and repeated in 15 minutes if necessary). If atropine alone is insufficient, intravenously administered *isoprenaline* (isoproterenol) should be given as a slow injection of 20μg followed by an infusion at a rate of 1 to 4 μg/min.

#### 8.3.10 Atrioventricular (AV) Block

First degree atrioventricular (AV) block is manifested by a prolonged PR interval and does not require treatment. Similarly, second degree block rarely causes sufficient haemodynamic disturbance to warrant treatment (except fixed Mobitz type II block). Third degree block, however, commonly develops during acute myocardial infarction and management depends on the rate of the junctional escape rhythm and the site of the infarction. When third degree block develops acutely in a patient with an inferior myocardial infarction, a junctional escape rhythm with a rate of 50 to 60 beats/min commonly develops without a haemodynamic disturbance.

Temporary pacing is generally only required for slow escape rhythms associated with haemodynamic disturbance. After an anterior infarction, however, wide QRS escape rhythms are common and these usually require pacing because of the danger of ventricular standstill.

## 9. Drug-Induced Cardiovascular Disease

The heart may be adversely affected by many drugs, including some administered for the treatment of other forms of heart disease. This section discusses some of the more common drug-induced cardiovascular disorders.

### 9.1 Ischaemic Heart Disease

Drugs that increase the pulse rate may exacerbate angina in patients with stenotic lesions in major coronary vessels. *Nifedipine* capsules, whose active contents are rapidly released and absorbed, may cause profound hypotension and a reflex tachycardia which may, in turn, exacerbate angina in patients at risk.[350,450] Other drugs that may also provoke angina in this way include *diazoxide* and *hydralazine*.[451]

An exaggerated tachycardia may occur during mild exertion and is commonly experienced for 2 to 5 days after withdrawal of *β-blockers* devoid of partial agonist (intrinsic sympathomimetic) activity[452] (see also section 6.1.2 above). This results from an up-regulation of β-receptor numbers and leads to a reduced threshold for angina and, occasionally, myocardial infarction. An increase in platelet aggregation which occurs during β-blocker withdrawal may also contribute to these events.[240]

Worsened angina or myocardial infarction may also be induced by drugs with a direct coronary vasoconstrictor action such as *ergotamine, methysergide* and *bromocriptine*.[453] Consequently, these drugs are contraindicated in patients with pre-existing heart disease. Myocardial infarction is also a recognised complication of high-dose *estrogen* therapy in men. In contrast, in women, low-dose estrogen therapy appears to protect against the development of coronary atheroma (see further chapter 18; sect. 11.4.2).

Myocardial infarction is also a recognised complication of *cocaine* abuse.[454,455] Although the risk is greatest in patients with pre-existing coronary artery disease, it has also been reported in patients without pre-existing heart disease. The spectrum of cardiovascular effects of cocaine also includes fatal arrhythmias and cardiomyopathy (caused frequently by recurrent myocardial infarction).

Angina-like chest pain accompanies the administration of *sumatriptan* (an agonist at vascular serotonin$_1$-like receptors used in the treatment of migraine) in about 3 to 5% of recipients.[456] ECG monitoring has rarely provided evidence of myocardial ischaemia and the mechanism responsible for the symptoms is unclear. However, sumatriptan is contraindicated in patients with known ischaemic heart disease.

Constricting angina-like chest pain accompanied by nonspecific ST-T wave changes sometimes accompanies the intravenous infusion of *fluorouracil*.[457] The condition is unpredictable and usually resolves when the infusion is stopped. However, fatal ventricular fibrillation has been recorded, especially on rechallenge, and therefore it is not recommended that the drug be reintroduced in these patients. Fluorouracil administration may also cause acute or chronic ventricular systolic dysfunction.

### 9.2 Cardiomyopathy

*Doxorubicin* and *daunorubicin* are anthracycline derivatives used in the treatment of leukaemia and other malignancies (see further chapter 27). However, their use is limited by their ability to cause potentially fatal cardiomyopathy in 2 to 3% of recipients.[458] The risk appears to be partly dependent on the cumulative dose given and rises from approximately 1% among children who have received less than 500 mg/m$^2$ to up to 25% in those who have received much higher doses. Many patients develop transient ECG abnormalities during the administration of these drugs, but they usually resolve once treatment is stopped and do not bear a close relationship to the development of cardiotoxicity.[458] Once cardiomyopathy does develop, the prognosis is poor, with an 80% mortality reported in one study. Newer analogues of these drugs are now being developed with the hope of reducing the risk of cardiotoxicity.

Cardiotoxicity is also a well recognised but rare complication of therapy with cyclophosphamide and fluorouracil.

Drugs that may precipitate or aggravate cardiac failure are discussed in section 5.5.1 (above).

### 9.3 Arrhythmias

A wide variety of cardiac arrhythmias may be provoked by drug therapy. The most commonly implicated drugs are those with sympathomimetic properties including *theophylline, dopamine, dobutamine* and *levodopa*.[459] These drugs increase the sinus rate, increase the frequency of atrial and ventricular ectopic activity and, in particular settings, may induce more serious life-threatening arrhythmias. They have particular risks in patients with atrial fibrillation where an increase in ventricular rate may result in a sharp decline in cardiac output.

Theophylline toxicity is a common problem in emergency rooms which is partly a reflection of the drug's relatively low therapeutic index.[459] It is frequently administered to elderly patients with chronic obstructive airways disease who may also have additional features that decrease the rate of theophylline metabolism (e.g. cardiac failure, chronic liver disease). Under such circumstances, careful monitoring of theophylline plasma concentrations is mandatory to avoid theophylline toxicity, which commonly leads to serious arrhythmias, an uncontrolled ventricular rate (in atrial fibrillation), and sudden death. Hypokalaemia commonly contributes to the intractability of arrhythmias in this setting.

As discussed in section 8.3.7, certain other commonly prescribed drugs, including most antiarrhythmic drugs, may provoke torsades de pointes in which the mean QRS axis in any electrocardiographic lead appears to twist around the isoelectric line. Although commonly asymptomatic, this arrhythmia can occasionally transform into ventricular fibrillation and sudden death.[460] Among the antiarrhythmic drugs, *quinidine* and *sotalol* have been most commonly implicated in inducing this form of arrhythmia, although *procainamide, flecainide* and *disopyramide* are also recognised causes. Clinical experience suggests that the risk of this arrhythmia is less with amiodarone. Class I antiarrhythmic agents can also produce another form of ventricular tachycardia (often incessant) which is unrelated to QT prolongation.

Other drugs that have been associated with QT prolongation and torsades de pointes include the antihistamines ($H_1$-receptor antagonists) *terfenadine* and *astemizole*, the antibiotic *erythromycin*, the prokinetic agent *cisapride* and the antihypertensive drug *ketanserin*.[461,462] The risk with these drugs appears to be greater when plasma concentrations are high. For example, the risk appears higher during rapid intravenous infusion of erythromycin or when terfenadine or astemizole are coadministered with drugs that inhibit their metabolism (e.g. ketoconazole, itraconazole or erythromycin; see further chapter 7; sect. 2.3.4). The risk may also be enhanced by other factors associated with QT prolongation such as hypokalaemia or acute stroke (especially subarachnoid haemorrhage).[460]

A variety of other drugs may produce arrhythmias when taken in overdose. The alkaloid drug *emetine*, which is the principal ingredient of syrup of ipecac, is sometimes misused by bulimic individuals.[463] The result is a syndrome involving myopathy, lethargy and cardiotoxicity. The cardiovascular complications include myocardial cell necrosis and a ventricular tachycardia and fibrillation.

Overdosage of *tricyclic antidepressants* is also commonly complicated by ventricular arrhythmias. When doses in excess of 2g are ingested, the characteristic findings include hypotension, QT prolongation and ST-T segment abnormalities,[464] but the relationship between plasma concentrations and arrhythmia development is variable. Because of the anticholinergic effects of these drugs, gastric stasis may occur leading to a delay in absorption. This may explain why arrhythmias are sometimes delayed until 24 to 36 hours after their ingestion.

### 9.4 Myocarditis; Pericarditis

Drugs rarely implicated in causing myocarditis include *p*-aminosalicylic acid (PAS), sulfonamides, aspirin, phenylbutazone, benzathine benzylpenicillin, streptomycin and chlorpromazine.[465] In several cases, patients have exhibited simultaneous cutaneous lesions of urticaria, angioneurotic oedema, rash or purpura, and evidence of a generalised allergic drug reaction has been present in nearly all cases. A similar situation seems to exist with methyldopa.[466]

Drug-induced systemic lupus erythematosus may be associated with pericarditis, for example that occurring with *hydralazine*. Haemopericardium has been rarely associated with the use of *anticoagulants* in myocardial infarction. The antihypertensive drug *minoxidil* has been associated with pericardial effusions, particularly in patients with impaired renal function.[467]

### 9.5 Hypotension

Hypotension may be caused by a variety of drugs other than those used therapeutically to lower the blood pressure.[468] Drugs normally used to lower the blood pressure may, however, produce marked hypotension, particularly in patients with myocardial decompensation. Postural hypotension is a frequent adverse effect of the treatment of hypertension, e.g. with the $\alpha_1$-adrenoceptor antagonist *prazosin* (usually with an excessive first dose or rapid dose increment).[469]

*Morphine*, given intravenously, may produce hypotension in patients with acute myocardial infarction. *Quinidine* can also produce hypotension but this is related to both dosage and route of administration and is much more frequent when the intravenous route is used. Hypotension may be associated with intravenous injections of *phenytoin*, and appears to be related to the speed of injection. Only occasional minor reductions in blood pressure occur with slow infusion of phenytoin. β-*Blockers* given intravenously may cause hypotension in association with bradycardia. This may require correction with atropine in patients with acute myocardial infarction.[470] Hypovolaemia induced by potent diuretics may aggravate hypotension and low cardiac output in patients with myocardial infarction.

*Nitroglycerin* (glyceryl trinitrate) sometimes causes a fall in blood pressure and its combination with alcohol has led to cardiovascular collapse with marked hypotension.[471] Acute hypotension can occur after the use of *phenothiazine* antipsychotic drugs (notably chlorpromazine) in elderly or debilitated patients or after large parenteral doses. Postural hypotension is a potential hazard with the *tricyclic antidepressants* in the elderly and has resulted in physical injury due to falls, or possibly has precipitated myocardial infarction in those with cardiac disease.[472]

*Levodopa* commonly causes postural hypotension. This is likely to be more troublesome when the levodopa dosage is being increased.[473] This reaction is possibly reduced in incidence by combined use of levodopa and a decarboxylase inhibitor (see chapter 29; sect. 7.1.1).

## 10. Use of Drugs in the Presence of Associated Cardiac Disease

### 10.1 Altered Responsiveness to Drug Therapy

The presence of cardiac disease may alter both the pharmacokinetic disposition of, and the tissue sensitivity to various drugs. The extent of the alteration generally depends on the severity of the underlying disease and may fluctuate rapidly in conjunction with the clinical condition. The changes are of most relevance for drugs such as digoxin and some antiarrhythmic agents, where the margin between therapeutic effect and toxicity is generally small.

In the early stages of myocardial infarction, vagal tone is generally increased and this may be enhanced by the parasympathomimetic effect of morphine administered for pain relief. The resulting lack of salivary flow may interfere with the absorption of sublingual nitroglycerin and the associated slowing of gastric emptying may delay the absorption of orally administered drugs. These problems may be enhanced by drugs with anticholinergic properties such as the phenothiazines or disopyramide.

In both cardiac failure and shock states, blood flow to the organs of elimination is reduced. High clearance drugs (e.g. lidocaine), whose elimination is proportional to liver blood flow, are therefore eliminated more slowly in such patients and their plasma half-lives are increased. As a consequence, the maintenance dose should be reduced and a longer interval between dose modification and achievement of a new steady-state plasma concentration should be anticipated. Cardiac failure may also alter the volume of distribution of a drug. This has again been documented with lidocaine whose volume of distribution is reduced in this condition. For this reason, the loading dose of lidocaine should be reduced when treatment is commenced in a patient with cardiac failure (see also sections 1.2, 1.3 and 8.2.2; and chapter 13; sect. 1.1.4).

Cardiac diseases may also alter the sensitivity of organs to various drugs. Myocardial irritability for example, may be increased, particularly after myocardial infarction. Ventricular premature contractions and tachyarrhythmias may be precipitated by usual dosages of drugs such as aminophylline, levodopa, $\beta_2$-agonist bronchodilators and tricyclic antidepressants. If indicated, these agents should be administered cautiously and in low doses.

In patients with impaired myocardial contractility, drugs with negative inotropic properties must also be used with particular care since small doses may worsen cardiac function. A number of agents with this property are widely used in patients with cardiac disease. They include disopyramide, β-adrenoceptor blocking drugs and verapamil, all of which directly reduce the force of myocardial contraction. Other agents may precipitate overt failure in such patients by different mechanisms. For example, nonsteroidal anti-inflammatory drugs (NSAIDs) can induce sodium retention and various other drugs such as sodium-containing antacids and effervescent calcium preparations can substantially increase the sodium load.

Cardiac conduction disturbances frequently accompany myocardial damage and may be worsened by drugs whose effects are otherwise slight in patients free of cardiac disease. These agents include digoxin, β-adrenoceptor blocking drugs, certain calcium antagonists (verapamil and diltiazem), and antiarrhythmics such as quinidine, procainamide and disopyramide. Most of these drugs also depress automaticity and should be avoided in patients with sinus node dysfunction.

Tissue sensitivity to drug effects may also be influenced by fluid and electrolyte status. Digoxin toxicity, for example, is enhanced by hypokalaemia and hypercalcaemia. Similarly, hypokalaemia appears to reduce the effectiveness of many antiarrhythmic agents and should be corrected when arrhythmias are being treated.

Finally, important changes in drug sensitivity may be induced by withdrawal of therapy. An important example in cardiac disease is the hypersensitivity to adrenergic stimuli that may last for several days after the withdrawal of long term treatment with β-adrenoceptor blocking agents. Patients with pre-existing coronary artery disease should be withdrawn slowly from treatment with these drugs and warned to avoid exercise for some days after their cessation, since several reports have been published of 'rebound' angina, arrhythmias and myocardial infarction occurring during this period (see also sections 6.1.2 and 9.1).

### 10.2 Drug Interactions in Cardiovascular Therapy

Many patients with cardiovascular disease require treatment with multiple drugs. In some instances, combination therapy is used to increase the effectiveness or reduce the adverse effects of treatment. For example, the effectiveness of ACE inhibitors is increased substantially by diuretic-induced sodium depletion, and the antianginal effect of nifedipine (in effort angina) is enhanced by β-blockade. Similarly, the addition of amiloride to treatment with a thiazide or loop diuretic potentiates the natriuretic effect of the latter agents and reduces potassium loss. The addition of verapamil to digoxin to control the ventricular rate in atrial fibrillation is another example; here use is made of an additive effect of both agents in reducing atrioventricular conduction as well as a decrease in digoxin clearance by verapamil.

In some instances, the interactions produce deleterious effects. For example, a number of drugs which by themselves produce relatively minor depressions of ventricular function may precipitate severe failure when used in combination in patients with pre-existing heart disease. These agents include β-adrenoceptor blocking drugs, verapamil and disopyramide. This problem may be exacerbated by the administration of NSAIDs (whose actions include an interference with the natriuretic activity of diuretic therapy), or agents with a high sodium content.

Precipitation of conduction disturbances and arrhythmias is another problem sometimes provoked by multiple drug therapy. For example, digoxin, β-adrenoceptor blocking drugs, various antiarrhythmic agents (e.g. quinidine, disopyramide), and certain calcium antagonists (e.g. verapamil and diltiazem) independently reduce atrioventricular conduction. Careful monitoring of the PR interval of the electrocardiogram is therefore necessary when these drugs are used in combination (see also section 9.3 above).

Hypotension is another commonly recognised effect of certain drug combinations. It is frequently encountered in patients given β-adrenoceptor blocking drugs and vasodilators in combination, and may be pronounced if verapamil is administered parenterally to patients receiving β-adrenoceptor blocking drugs. It is also a common problem after the administration of ACE inhibitors to patients severely sodium-depleted by high doses of diuretics.

All clinicians should be aware of the important cardiovascular drugs whose simultaneous administration with other drugs requires special caution (see further appendix B).

## References


1. Pentel P, Benowitz N. Pharmacokinetic and pharmacodynamic consideration in drug therapy of cardiac emergencies. Clinical Pharmacokinetics 1984; 9: 273
2. Benowitz NL, Meister W. Pharmacokinetics in patients with cardiac failure. Clinical Pharmacokinetics 1976; 1: 389
3. Benowitz NL. Effects of cardiac disease on pharmacokinetics: pathophysiologic considerations. In: Benet LZ, et al. (editors) Pharmacokinetic basis for drug treatment. New York: Raven Press, 1984: 89
4. Barger AC. Renal hemodynamic factors in congestive heart failure. Annals of the New York Academy of Sciences 1966; 39: 276
5. Thomson PD. Alteration in pharmacologic response induced by cardiovascular disease. In: Melmon KL (editor) Cardiovascular drug therapy. Philadelphia: Davis, 1974

6. Centers for Disease Control. Years of life lost from coronary heart disease. Morbidity and Mortality Weekly Report 1986; 35: 653
7. Rose G. Ischaemic heart disease. Journal of Medical Genetics 1977; 14: 330
8. Ross R. The pathogenesis of atherosclerosis - an update. New England Journal of Medicine 1986; 344: 488
9. World Health Organization Expert Committee on Prevention of Coronary Heart Disease. Technical Report Series No. 678, 1982: 8
10. Rose G. International trends in cardiovascular disease - implications for prevention and treatment. Australian and New Zealand Journal of Medicine 1984; 14: 375
11. Criqui MH. Epidemiology of atherosclerosis - an updated overview. American Journal of Cardiology 1986; 57: 18C
12. Comai K, Feldman DL, Goldstein AL, et al. Atherosclerosis: an overview. Drug Development Research 1985; 6: 113-25
13. Brown MS, Goldstein JL. A receptor-mediated pathway for cholesterol homeostasis. Science 1986; 232: 34-47
14. Neaton JD, Blackburn H, Jacobs D, et al. Serum cholesterol level and mortality findings for men screened in the Multiple Risk Factor Intervention Trial. Archives of Internal Medicine 1992; 152: 1490-500
15. Keys A, Menotti A, Karvonan MJ, et al. The diet and 15-year death rate in the seven countries study. American Journal of Epidemiology 1986; 124: 903-15
16. Khan HA, Phillips RL, Snowdon DA, et al. Association between reported diet and all-cause mortality: twenty-one-year follow-up on 27,530 adult Seventh-Day Adventists. American Journal of Epidemiology 1984; 119: 775-87
17. Kagan A, Harris BR, Winkelstein Jr W, et al. Epidemiologic studies of coronary heart disease and stroke in Japanese men living in Japan, Hawaii and California: demographic, physical, dietary and biochemical characteristics. Journal of Chronic Diseases 1974; 27: 345-64
18. Kannel WB, Neaton JD, Wentworth D, et al. Overall and coronary heart disease mortality rates in relation to major risk factors in 325,348 men screened for the MRFIT. American Heart Journal 1986; 112: 825-36
19. Fuster V, Badimon L, Badimon JJ, et al. The pathogenesis of coronary artery disease and the acute coronary syndromes. New England Journal of Medicine 1992; 362: 242-50, 310-9
20. Grundy SM. Adherence to cholesterol-lowering diets. Archives of Internal Medicine 1992; 152: 1139
21. Brunzell JD, Austin MA. Plasma triglyceride levels and coronary disease [editorial]. New England Journal of Medicine 1989; 320: 1273-5
22. Avins AL, Haber RJ, Hulley SB. The status of hypertriglyceridemia as a risk factor for coronary heart disease. Clinics in Laboratory Medicine 1989; 9: 153-68
23. NIH Consensus Development Panel on Triglyceride, High-Density Lipoprotein and Coronary Heart Disease. Triglyceride, high-density lipoprotein, and coronary heart disease. Journal of the American Medical Association 1993; 269: 505-10
24. Wilson PW, Abbott RD, Castelli WP. High density lipoprotein cholesterol and mortality: the Framingham Heart Study. Arteriosclerosis 1988; 8: 737-41
25. Henwood JM, Heel RC. Lovastatin: a preliminary review of its pharmacodynamic properties and therapeutic use in hyperlipidaemia. Drugs 1988; 36: 429-54
26. Plosker GL, McTavish D. Simvastatin: a reappraisal of its pharmacology and therapeutic efficacy in hypercholesterolaemia. Drugs 1995; 50: 334-63
27. McTavish D, Sorkin EM. Pravastatin: a review of its pharmacological properties and therapeutic potential in hypercholesterolaemia. Drugs 1991; 42: 65-89
28. Plosker GL, Wagstaff AJ. Fluvastatin: a review of its pharmacology and use in the management of hypercholesterolaemia. Drugs 1996; 51: 433-59
29. Uauy R, Vega GL, Grundy SM, et al. Lovastatin therapy in receptor-negative homozygous familial hypercholesterolemia: lack of effect on low-density lipoprotein concentrations or turnover. Journal of Pediatrics 1988; 113: 387-92
30. Thiery J, Armstrong WW, Schleef J, et al. Serum lipoprotein Lp(a) concentrations are not influenced by an HMG-CoA reductase inhibitor. Klinische Wochenschrift 1988; 66: 462-3
31. Ditschuneit HH, Khun K, Ditschuneit H. Comparison of different HMG-CoA reductase inhibitors. European Journal of Clinical Pharmacology 1991; 40 (Suppl. 1): S27-32
32. Tobert JA. Efficacy and long-term effect pattern of lovastatin. American Journal of Cardiology 1988; 62: 28J-34J
33. Marais GE, Larson KK. Rhabdomyolysis and acute renal failure induced by combination lovastatin and gemfibrozil therapy. Annals of Internal Medicine 1990; 264: 71-5
34. Pierce LR, Wysowski DK, Gross TP. Myopathy and rhabdomyolysis associated with lovastatin-gemfibrozil combination therapy. Journal of the American Medical Association 1990; 264: 71-5
35. Jay RH, Sturley RH, Stirling C, et al. Effects of pravastatin and cholestyramine on gonadal and adrenal steroid production in familial hypercholesterolaemia. British Journal of Clinical Pharmacology 1991; 32: 417-22
36. Elnarsson K, Ericsson S, Ewerth S, et al. Bile acid sequestrants: mechanisms of action on bile acid and cholesterol metabolism. European Journal of Clinical Pharmacology 1991; 40 (Suppl. 1): S53-8
37. Fletcher GF, Fletcher BJ, Whitner JT, et al. Effect of variable doses and formulations of cholestyramine on elevated serum low-density lipoprotein cholesterol. American Journal of Cardiology 1995; 75: 738-9
38. Jones RJ, Dobrilovic L. Lipoprotein lipid alterations with cholestyramine administration. Journal of Laboratory and Clinical Medicine 1970; 75: 953-66
39. Lipid Research Clinics Program. The Lipid Research Clinics Coronary Primary Prevention Trials results. 1. Reduction in incidence of coronary heart disease. Journal of the American Medical Association 1984; 251: 351-64
40. Ginsberg HN, Arad Y, Goldberg IJ. Pathophysiology and therapy of hyperlipidemia. In: Antonaccio M, editor. Cardiovascular pharmacology. 3rd ed. New York: Raven Press, 1990: 485-513
41. Expert Panel on Detection, Evaluation, and Treatment of High Blood Cholesterol in Adults: Summary of the second report of the National Cholesterol Education Program (NCEP) Expert Panel on Detection, Evaluation, and Treatment of High Blood Cholesterol in Adults (Adult Treatment Panel II). Journal of the American Medical Association 1993; 269: 3015-23

42. Kuzuya M, Kuzuya F. Probucol as an antioxidant and antiatherogenic drug. Free Radical Biology and Medicine 1993; 14: 67-77
43. Buckley MM, Goa KL, Price AH, et al. Probucol: a reappraisal of its pharmacological properties and therapeutic use in hypercholesterolaemia. Drugs 1989; 37: 761-800
44. Reaven PD, Parthasarathy S, Belt WF, et al. Effect of probucol dosage on plasma lipid and lipoprotein levels and on protection of low density lipoprotein against in vitro oxidation in humans. Arteriosclerosis and Thrombosis 1992; 12: 318-24
45. Walldius G, Erikson U, Olsson AG, et al. The effect of probucol on femoral atherosclerosis: the Probucol Quantitative Regressive Swedish Trial (PQRST). American Journal of Cardiology 1994; 74: 875-83
46. Berg A, Baumstark MW, Frey I, et al. Clinical and therapeutic use of probucol. European Journal of Clinical Pharmacology 1991; 40 (Suppl. 1): S81-4
47. Klein L. QT-interval prolongation produced by probucol. Archives of Internal Medicine 1981; 141: 1102-3
48. Hunninghake DB, Peters JR. Effect of fibric acid derivatives on blood lipid and lipoprotein levels. American Journal of Medicine 1987; 83: 44-9
49. Saku K, Gartside PS, Hynd BA, et al. Mechanism of action of gemfibrozil on lipoprotein metabolism. Journal of Clinical Investigation 1985; 75: 1702-12
50. Grundy SM, Vega GL. Fibric acids: effects on lipids and lipoprotein metabolism. American Journal of Medicine 1987; 83: 9-20
51. Committee of Principal Investigators, World Health Organization. A co-operative trial in the primary prevention of ischaemic heart disease using clofibrate. British Heart Journal 1978; 40: 1069-118
52. Frick MH, Elo MO, Haapa K, et al. Helsinki Heart Study: primary-prevention trial with gemfibrozil in middle-aged men with dyslipidemia. Safety of treatment, changes in risk factors, and incidence of coronary heart disease. New England Journal of Medicine 1987; 317: 1237-45
53. Coronary Drug Project Research Group. Gallbladder disease as a side effect of drugs influencing lipid metabolism. New England Journal of Medicine 1977; 296: 1185-90
54. O'Reilly RA, Sahud MA, Robinson AJ. Studies on the interaction of warfarin and clofibrate in man. Thrombosis et Diathesis Haemorrhagica 1972; 27: 309-18
55. Henkin Y, Oberman A, Hurst DC, et al. Niacin revisited: clinical observations on an important but underutilized drug. American Journal of Medicine 1991; 91: 239-46
56. Grundy SM, Mok HY, Zach L. Influence of nicotinic acid on metabolism of cholesterol and triglycerides in man. Journal of Lipid Research 1981; 22: 24-36
57. Garg A, Grundy SM. Nicotinic acid as therapy for dyslipidemia in non-insulin-dependent diabetes mellitus. Journal of the American Medical Association 1990; 264: 723-6
58. Hunninghake DB, Probsfield JL. Drug treatment of hyperlipoproteinemia. In: Rifkind B, Levy R, editors. Hyperlipidemia: diagnosis and therapy. New York: Grune & Stratton, 1977: 327-62
59. Welan AM, Price SO, Fowler SF, et al. The effect of aspirin on niacin-induced cutaneous reactions. Journal of Family Practice 1992; 34: 165-8
60. Figge HL, Figg J, Souney PF, et al. Nicotinic acid: a review of its clinical use in the treatment of lipid disorders. Pharmacotherapy 1988; 8: 287-94
61. Mullin GE, Greenson JK, Mitchell MC. Fulminant hepatic failure after ingestion of sustained-release nicotinic acid. Annals of Internal Medicine 1989; 111: 253-5
62. Parsons WB. Studies of nicotinic acid use in hypercholesterolemia. Archives of Internal Medicine 1961; 107: 653-67
63. Rimm EB, Stampfer MJ, Ascherio A, et al. Vitamin E consumption and the risk of coronary heart disease in men. New England Journal of Medicine 1993; 328: 1450-6
64. Stampfer MJ, Hennekens CH, Mansion JE, et al. Vitamin E consumption and the risk of coronary heart disease in women. New England Journal of Medicine 1993; 328: 1444-9
65. The Alpha-Tocopherol Beta-Carotene Cancer Prevention Study Group. The effect of vitamin E and beta-carotene on the incidence of lung cancer and other cancers in male smokers. New England Journal of Medicine 1994; 33: 1029-35
66. Stephens NG, Parsons A, Schofiels PM, et al. Randomised controlled trial of vitamin E in patients with coronary disease: Cambridge Heart Antioxidant Study (CHAOS). Lancet 1996; 347: 781-6
67. The Scandinavian Simvastatin Survival Study Group. Randomised trial of cholesterol lowering in 4,444 patients with coronary heart disease: the Scandinavian Simvastatin Survival Study (4S). Lancet 1994; 344: 1383-9
68. Sacks FM, Pfeffer MA, Moye LA, et al. The effect of pravastatin on coronary events after myocardial infarction in patients with average cholesterol levels. New England Journal of Medicine 1996; 335: 1001-9
69. Shepherd J, Cobbe SM, Ford I, et al. Prevention of coronary heart disease with pravastatin in men with hypercholesterolaemia. New England Journal of Medicine 1995; 333: 1301-7
70. Lipid Research Clinics Program. The Lipid Research Clinics Coronary Primary Prevention Trial results. II. The relationship of reduction in incidence of coronary heart disease to cholesterol lowering. Journal of the American Medical Association 1984; 25: 1365-75
71. Committee of Principal Investigators, World Health Organization. WHO cooperative trial on primary prevention of ischaemic heart disease using clofibrate to lower serum cholesterol: mortality follow-up. Lancet 1980; 2: 379-85
72. Coronary Drug Project Research Group. Clofibrate and niacin in coronary heart disease. Journal of the American Medical Association 1975; 231: 360-81
73. Canner PL, Berge KG, Wenger NK, et al. Fifteen year mortality in Coronary Drug Project patients: long-term benefit with niacin. Journal of the American College of Cardiology 1986; 8: 1245-55
74. Cashin-Hemphill L, Mack WJ, Pogoda JM, et al. Beneficial effects of colestipol-niacin on coronary atherosclerosis: a 4-year follow-up. Journal of the American Medical Association 1990; 264: 3013-7
75. Pedersen TR, Kjekshus J, Berg K, et al. Cholesterol lowering and the use of healthcare resources. Circulation 1996; 93: 1796-802
76. Pharoah PDP, Hollingworth W. Cost effectiveness of lowering cholesterol concentration with statins in patients with and without pre-existing coronary heart disease:

life table method applied to health authority population. British Medical Journal 1996; 312: 1443-6
77. Kannel WB, Cupples A. Epidemiology and risk profile of cardiac failure. Cardiovascular Drugs and Therapy 1988; 2 (Suppl. 1): 387-95
78. Dargie HJ, McMurray JJV. Diagnosis and management of heart failure. British Medical Journal 1994; 308: 321-8
79. Gaasch WH. Diagnosis and treatment of heart failure based on left ventricular systolic and diastolic dysfunction. Journal of the American Medical Association 1994; 271: 1276-80
80. Sutton GC. Epidemiologic aspects of heart failure. American Heart Journal 1990; 120: 1538-40
81. Grossman W. Diastolic dysfunction in congestive heart failure. New England Journal of Medicine 1991; 325: 1557-61
82. Setaro JF, Soufer R, Remetz MS, et al. Long-term outcome in patients with congestive heart failure and intact systolic left ventricular performance. American Journal of Cardiology 1992; 69: 1212-6
83. Swedberg K, Eneroth P, Kjekshus J, et al. Hormones regulating cardiovascular function in patients with severe congestive heart failure and their relation to mortality. Circulation 1990; 82: 1730-6
84. Kaye DM, Lefkovits J, Jennings GL, et al. Adverse consequences of high sympathetic nervous activity in the failing human heart. Journal of the American College of Cardiology 1995; 26: 1257-63
85. Krum H, Gu A, Wilshire-Clement M, et al. Changes in plasma endothelin-1 levels reflect clinical responses to beta-blockade in chronic heart failure. American Heart Journal 1996; 131: 337-41
86. Cohn JN, Mashiro I, Levine TB, et al. Role of vasconstrictor mechanisms in the control of left ventricular performance of the normal and damaged heart. American Journal of Cardiology 1979; 44: 1019-22
87. McCarthy M. Is there more to heart failure than a bad pump? Lancet 1996; 347: 110
88. Wilcox CS. Diuretics. In: Brenner BM, Rector Jr FC, editors. The kidney. 4th ed. Philadelphia: WB Saunders Co, 1991: 2133-47
89. Grantham JJ, Chonko AM. The physiologic basis and clinical use of diuretics. In: Brenner BM, Stein JH, editors. Contemporary issues in nephrology: sodium and water homeostasis. New York: Churchill Livingstone, 1978: 178-211
90. Brater DC. Clinical pharmacology of loop diuretics. Drugs 1991; 42: 14-22
91. Cody RJ, Kubo SH, Pickworth KK. Diuretic treatment for the sodium retention of congestive heart failure. Archives of Internal Medicine 1994; 154: 1905-14
92. Lant A. Diuretics: clinical pharmacology and therapeutic use (part 1). Drugs 1985; 29: 57-87
93. Lant A. Diuretics: clinical pharmacology and therapeutic use (part 2). Drugs 1985; 29: 162-88
94. Cutter RE, Blair AD. Clinical pharmacokinetics of furosemide. Clinical Pharmacokinetics 1979; 4: 279-96
95. Ellison DH. The physiologic basis of diuretic synergism: its role in treating diuretic resistance. Annals of Internal Medicine 1991; 114: 886-94
96. Wollam GL, Tarazi RC, Bravo EL, et al. Diuretic potency of combined hydrocholorothiazide and furosemide therapy in patients with azotemia. American Journal of Medicine 1982; 72: 929-38
97. Moses AM, Miller M. Drug-induced dilutional hyponatremia. New England Journal of Medicine 1974; 2911: 1234
98. Oster JR, Epstein M, Smoller S. Combined therapy with thiazide-type and loop diuretic agents for resistant sodium retention. Annals of Internal Medicine 1983; 99: 405-6
99. Myers MG, Kearns PM, Kennedy DS, et al. Postural hypotension and diuretic therapy in the elderly. Canadian Medical Association Journal 1988; 119: 581
100. Ikram H, Chan W, Espiner EA, et al. Haemodynamic and hormone responses to acute and chronic furosemide therapy in congestive heart failure. Clinical Science 1980; 59: 443-9
101. Robinson HN, Morison WL, Hood AF. Thiazide diuretic therapy and chronic photosensitivity. Archives of Dermatology 1985; 121: 522
102. Van der Linden W, Ritter B, Edlund G. Acute cholecystitis and thiazides. British Medical Journal 1984; 289: 654
103. Medical Research Council Working Party on Mild to Moderate Hypertension. Adverse reactions to bendrofluazide and propranolol for the treatment of mild hypertension. Lancet 1981; 2: 539
104. Ramsay LE, Yeo WW. Antihypertensive and adverse biochemical effects of bendrofluazide. British Medical Journal 1990; 301: 240
105. Gallagher KL, Jones JK. Furosemide-induced ototoxicity. Annals of Internal Medicine 1979; 91: 744
106. Dukes MNG, editor. Diuretics. In: Meyler's side effects of drugs. Amsterdam: Elsevier, 1988
107. Greenblatt DJ, Koch-Weser J. Adverse reactions to spironolactone. Journal of the American Medical Association 1973; 225: 40
108. Dyckner T, Wester PO. Plasma and skeletal muscle electrolytes in patients on long-term diuretic therapy for arterial hypertension and/or congestive heart failure. Acta Medica Scandinavica 1987; 222: 231-6
109. Tannen R. Diuretic-induced hypokalemia. Kidney International 1985; 28: 988-1000
110. Zalin AM, Hutchinson CE, John M, et al. Hyponatraemia during treatment with chlorpropamide and Moduretic (amiloride plus hydrochlorothiazide). British Medical Journal 1984; 289: 659
111. Crowe M, Wollner L, Griffiths RA. Hypercalaemia following vitamin D and thiazide therapy in the elderly. Practitioner 1984; 228: 312
112. Reyes AJ, Leary WP. Cardiovascular toxicity of diuretics related to magnesium depletion. Human Toxicology 1984; 3: 351
113. Kaplan NM, Carnegie A, Raskin P, et al. Potassium supplementation in hypertensive patients with diuretic-induced hypokalaemia. New England Journal of Medicine 1985; 312: 746
114. Semple PF. Drug-induced gout. Scottish Medical Journal 1973; 18: 239
115. Weinberger MH. Antihypertensive therapy and lipids: evidence, mechanisms and implications. Archives of Internal Medicine 1985; 145: 1102
116. Williams RL, Davies RO, Berman RS, et al. Hydrochlorothiazide pharmacokinetics and pharmacological effect: the influence of indomethacin. Journal of Clinical Pharmacology 1982; 22: 32
117. Watkins J, Abbott EC, Hansby CN, et al. Attenuation of the hypotensive effect of propranolol and thiazide diuretics by indomethacin. British Medical Journal 1980; 281: 702
118. Materson BJ. Diuretic-associated hypokalaemia. Archives of Internal Medicine 1966; 145: 1966
119. Ramsay LE. Interactions that matter. II. Diuretics and antihypertensive drugs. Prescribers' Journal 1984; 24: 60

120. Johnston CI. Angiotensin converting enzyme inhibitors. In: Doyle AE, editor. Handbook of hypertension. Vol. 5: clinical pharmacology of antihypertensive drugs. 2nd ed. Amsterdam: Elsevier, 1984: 272-311
121. Ader R, Chatterjee K, Ports T, et al. Immediate and sustained haemodynamic and clinical improvement in chronic heart failure by an oral angiotensin converting enzyme inhibitor. Circulation 1980; 61: 931-7
122. Heel RC, Brogden RN, Speight TM, et al. Captopril: a preliminary review of its pharmacological properties and therapeutic efficacy. Drugs 1980; 20: 409-52
123. Singhvi SM, Duchin KL, Morrison RA, et al. Disposition of fosinopril sodium in healthy subjects. British Journal of Clinical Pharmacology 1988; 25: 9-15
124. Hui KK, Duchin KL, Kripalani KJ, et al. Pharmacokinetics of fosinopril in patients with various degrees of renal function. Clinical Pharmacology and Therapeutics 1991; 49: 457-67
125. Murdoch D, McTavish D. Fosinopril: a review of its pharmacodynamic and pharmacokinetic properties, and therapeutic potential in essential hypertension. Drugs 1992; 43: 123-40
126. Noble S, Sorkin EM. Spirapril: a preliminary review of its pharmacology and therapeutic efficacy in the treatment of hypertension. Drugs 1995; 49: 750-66
127. Wiseman LR, McTavish D. Trandolapril: a review of its pharmacodynamic and pharmacokinetic properties, and therapeutic use in essential hypertension. Drugs 1994; 48: 71-90
128. The SOLVD Investigators. Effect of enalapril on survival in patients with reduced left ventricular ejection fractions and congestive heart failure. New England Journal of Medicine 1991; 325: 293-302
129. The Acute Infarction Ramipril Efficacy (AIRE) Study Investigators. Effect of ramipril on mortality and morbidity of survivors of acute myocardial infarction with clinical evidence of heart failure. Lancet 1993; 342: 821-8
130. Baker DW, Konstam MA, Bottorff M, et al. Management of heart failure. I. Pharmacologic treatment. Journal of the American Medical Association 1994; 272: 1361-6
131. Hasford J, Bussman WD, Delius W, et al. First dose hypotension with enalapril and prazosin in congestive heart failure. International Journal of Cardiology 1991; 31: 287-94
132. Cleland JG, Dargie HJ. Heart failure, renal function, and angiotensin converting enzyme inhibitors. Kidney International 1987; 31: 220-8
133. Packer M. Identification of risk factors predisposing to the development of functional renal insufficiency during treatment with converting-enzyme inhibitors in chronic heart failure. Cardiology 1989; 76: 50-5
134. The CONSENSUS Trial Study Group. Effects of enalapril on mortality in severe congestive heart failure. New England Journal of Medicine 1987; 316: 1429-35
135. Oster JR, Matterson BJ. Renal and electrolyte complications of congestive heart failure and effects of therapy with angiotensin-converting enzyme inhibitors. Archives of Internal Medicine 1992; 152: 704-10
136. Gibson GR. Enalapril-induced cough. Archives of Internal Medicine 1989; 149: 2701-3
137. Lunde H, Hedner T, Samuelsson O, et al. Dyspnoea, asthma and bronchospasm in relation to treatment with angiotensin converting enzyme inhibitors. British Medical Journal 1994; 308: 18-21
138. Overlack A. ACE inhibitor-induced cough and bronchospasm: incidence, mechanisms and management. Drug Safety 1996; 15: 72-8
139. Shotan A, Widerhorn J, Hurst A, et al. Risks of angiotensin-converting enzyme inhibition during pregnancy: experimental and clinical evidence, potential mechanisms and recommendations for use. American Journal of Medicine 1994; 96: 451-6
140. Slater EE, Merrill DD, Guess HA, et al. Clinical profile of angioedema associated with angiotensin converting-enzyme inhibition. Journal of the American Medical Association 1988; 260: 967-70
141. Gorlin R, for the Digoxin Intervention Group (DIG) Investigators. Final results of the DIG study. Presented at the American College of Cardiology 45th Annual Scientific Sessions, Orlando, FL, 1996
142. Thomas R, Gray P, Andrews J. Digitalis: its mode of action, receptor and structure-activity relationships. Advances in Drug Research 1990; 19: 313-562
143. Smith TW. Digoxin in heart failure. New England Journal of Medicine 1993; 329: 51-3
144. McGarry SJ, Williams AJ. Digoxin activates sarcoplasmic reticulum $Ca^{2+}$ release channels: a possible role in cardiac inotropy. British Journal of Pharmacology 1993; 108: 1043-50
145. Blatt CM, Marsh JD, Smith TW. Extracardiac effects of digitalis. In: Smith TW, editor. Digitalis glycosides. Orlando: Grune & Stratton, 1986: 209-16
146. Ferguson DW, Berg WY, Sanders JS, et al. Sympathoinhibitory responses to digitalis glycosides in heart failure patients. Direct evidence from sympathetic neural recordings. Circulation 1989; 80: 65-77
147. Wettrell G, Andersson KE. Cardiovascular drugs II: digoxin. Therapeutic Drug Monitoring 1986; 8: 129
148. Smith TW, Antman EM, Friedman PL, et al. Digitalis glycosides: mechanisms and manifestations of toxicity. Progress in Cardiovascular Diseases 1984; 26: 413
149. Taggart AJ, McDevitt DG. Digitalis - its place in modern therapy. Drugs 1980; 20: 398
150. Aronson JK. Clinical pharmacokinetics of digoxin 1980. Clinical Pharmacokinetics 1980; 5: 137
151. Lindenbaum J, Rudd DG, Butler BP, et al. Inactivation of digoxin by the gut flora: reversal by antibiotic therapy. New England Journal of Medicine 1981; 305: 789
152. Abernethy DR, Greenblatt DJ, Smith TW. Digoxin disposition in obesity: clinical pharmacokinetic investigation. American Heart Journal 1981; 102: 740
153. Mahdyoon H, Battilana G, Rosman H, et al. The evolving pattern of digoxin intoxication: observations at a large urban hospital from 1980 to 1988. American Heart Journal 1990; 120: 1189-94
154. Smith TW, Haber E. Digitalis (part four). New England Journal of Medicine 1973; 289: 1125
155. Spiegel A, Marchinski FE. Time courses for reversal of digoxin toxicity with digoxin specific antibody fragments. American Heart Journal 1985; 109: 1397
156. Marcus FI. Pharmacokinetic interactions between digoxin and other drugs. Journal of the American College of Cardiology 1985; 5 (Suppl. A): 82A-90A
157. Bussey HI. The influence of quinidine and other agents on digitalis glycosides. American Heart Journal 1982; 104: 289
158. Klein HO, Lang R, Segni EDI, et al. Verapamil-digoxin interaction. New England Journal of Medicine 1980; 303: 160
159. Aronson JK. Cardiac glycosides and drugs used in dysrhythmias. In: Dukes MNG, editor. Meyler's side ef-

fects of drugs. Annual 10. Amsterdam: Elsevier, 1986: 142

160. Lawrence JR. Antianginal and β-adrenoceptor blocking drugs. In: Dukes MNG, editor. Meyler's side effects of drugs. Annual 10. Amsterdam: Elsevier, 1986: 142
161. Parmley WW. Factors causing arrhythmias in chronic congestive heart failure. American Heart Journal 1987; 114: 1267
162. Channavasin P, Seiwell R, Brater DC. Pharmacokinetic-dynamic analysis of the indomethacin frusemide interaction in man. Journal of Pharmacology and Experimental Therapeutics 1980; 215: 77-81
163. Coats AJS, Adamopoulos S, Radaelli A, et al. Controlled trial of physical training in chronic heart failure. Exercise performance, hemodynamics and autonomic function. Circulation 1992; 85: 2119-31
164. Dracup K, Baker DW, Dunbar SB, et al. Management of heart failure. II. Counselling, education and lifestyle modifications. Journal of the American Medical Association 1994; 272: 1442-6
165. The SOLVD Investigators. Effect of enalapril on mortality and the development of heart failure in asymptomatic patients with reduced left ventricular ejection fractions. New England Journal of Medicine 1992; 327: 685-91
166. Paratt JR. Cardioprotection by angiotensin converting enzyme inhibitors - the experimental evidence. Cardiovascular Research 1994; 28: 183-9
167. Lewis EJ, Lawrence G, Hunsicker LG, et al. The effect of angiotensin-converting enzyme inhibition on diabetic nephropathy. New England Journal of Medicine 1993; 329: 1456-62
168. Pfeffer MA, Braunwald E, Moye LA, et al. Effect of captopril on mortality and morbidity in patients with left ventricular dysfunction after myocardial infarction. New England Journal of Medicine 1992; 327: 669-77
169. Kober L, Torp-Perdersen C, Carlsen JE, et al. A clinical trial of the angiotensin-converting enzyme inhibitor trandolapril in patients with left ventricular dysfunction after myocardial infarction. New England Journal of Medicine 1995; 333: 1670-6
170. ISIS-4 Collaborative Group. Fourth international study of infarct survival: protocol for a large simple study of the effects of oral mononitrate, of oral captopril, and of intravenous magnesium. American Journal of Cardiology 1991; 68: 87D-100D
171. Pfeffer MA. ACE inhibition in acute myocardial infarction. New England Journal of Medicine 1995; 332: 118-20
172. Reid JL, MacFadyan RJ, Squire IB, et al. Blood pressure response to the first dose of angiotensin converting enzyme inhibitors in congestive heart failure. American Journal of Cardiology 1993; 71: 57E-60E
173. Packer M, Gheorghiade M, Yough JB, et al. Withdrawal of digoxin from patients with chronic heart failure treated with angiotensin-converting enzyme inhibitors: RADIANCE study. New England Journal of Medicine 1993; 329: 1-7
174. Jaeschke R, Oxman AD, Guyatt GH. To what extent do congestive heart failure patients in sinus rhythm benefit from digoxin therapy? A systematic overview and meta-analysis. American Journal of Medicine 1990; 88: 279-86
175. Opie LH. Digitalis and sympathomimetic stimulants. Lancet 1980; 1: 912
176. Aronson JK. Indications for the measurements of plasma digoxin concentrations. Drugs 1983; 26: 230
177. Beta Blocker Heart Attack Trial Research Group. A randomized trial of propranolol in patients with acute myocardial infarction: I. Mortality result. Journal of the American Medical Association 1982; 247: 1707-14
178. Eichhorn EJ, Sobotka P. Novel approaches to congestive heart failure: use of beta-adrenergic blockade. Coronary Artery Disease 1994; 5: 101-6
179. CIBIS Investigators and Committees. A randomized trial of beta-blockade in heart failure: the Cardiac Insufficiency Bisoprolol Study (CIBIS). Circulation 1994; 90: 1765-73
180. Waagstein F, Bristow MR, Swedberg K, et al. Beneficial effects of metoprolol in idiopathic dilated cardiomyopathy. Lancet 1993; 342: 1441-6
181. Packer M, Colucci WS, Sackner-Bernstein J, et al. Prospective randomized evaluation of carvedilol on symptoms and exercise tolerance in chronic heart failure: results of the PRECISE trial. Circulation 1995; 92: 1-143
182. Curfman GD. Inotropic therapy for heart failure - an unfulfilled promise. New England Journal of Medicine 1991; 325: 1509-10
183. The German and Austrian Xamoterol Study Group. Double-blind placebo-controlled comparison of digoxin and xamoterol in chronic heart failure. Lancet 1988; 1: 489-93
184. DiBianco R, Shabetai R, Kostuk W, et al. A comparison of oral milrinone, digoxin, and their combination in the treatment of patients with chronic heart failure. New England Journal of Medicine 1989; 320: 677-83
185. Packer M, Carver JR, Rodeheffer RJ, et al. Effect or oral milrinone on mortality in severe chronic heart failure. New England Journal of Medicine 1991; 325: 1468-75
186. Tango M, Lyngborg K, Mehlsen J, et al. Xamoterol in severe congestive heart failure: long term oral treatment, a double blind randomised study. International Journal of Cardiology 1992; 34: 63-8
187. Cruickshank JM. Phosphodiesterase III inhibitors: long-term risks and short-term benefits. Cardiovascular Drugs and Therapy 1993; 7: 655-60
188. Gottlieb SS. New approaches to managing congestive heart failure. Current Opinion in Cardiology 1995; 10: 282-7
189. Feldman AM, Bristow MR, Parmley WW, et al. (Vesnarinone Study Group). Effects of vesnarinone on morbidity and mortality in patients with heart failure. New England Journal of Medicine 1993; 329: 149-55
190. Remme WJ, Kruijssen DA, van Hoogenhuyze DC, et al. Hemodynamic, neurohumoral, and myocardial energetic effects of pimobendan, a novel calcium-sensitizing compound, in patients with mild to moderate heart failure. Journal of Cardiovascular Pharmacology 1994; 24: 730-9
191. Cohn J. Treatment of moderate heart failure: V-HeFT-III. (Abstract). Presented at the American Heart Association's 68th Scientific Sessions, Anaheim CA, 1995
192. Packer M, O'Connor CM, Ghali LK, Prospective Randomized Amlodipine Survival Evaluation Study Group. Effect of amlodipine on morbidity and mortality in severe chronic heart failure. New England Journal of Medicine 1996; 335: 1107-14
193. The Cardiac Arrhythmia Suppression Trial Investigators. Preliminary report: effect of encainide and flecainide on mortality in a randomized trial of arrhythmia suppression after myocardial infarction. New England Journal of Medicine 1989; 321: 406-12

194. The Cardiac Arrhythmia Suppression Trial-II Investigators. Effect of the antiarrhythmic agent moricizine on survival after myocardial infarction: the Cardiac Arrhythmia Suppression Trial-II. New England Journal of Medicine 1992; 327: 227-33
195. Doval HC, Nul DR, Grancelli HO, et al. Randomised trial of low-dose amiodarone in severe congestive heart failure. Lancet 1994; 344: 493-8
196. Singh SN, Fletcher RD, Fisher SG, et al. Amiodarone in patients with congestive heart failure and asymptomatic ventricular arrhythmia. Survival Trial of Antiarrhythmic Therapy in Congestive Heart Failure. New England Journal of Medicine 1995; 333: 77-82
197. Hart W, Rhodes G, McMurray J. The cost effectiveness of enalapril in the treatment of chronic heart failure. British Journal of Medical Economics 1993; 6: 91-8
198. Paul SD, Kuntz KM, Fagle KA. Costs and effectiveness of angiotensin converting enzyme inhibition in patients with congestive heart failure. Archives of Internal Medicine 1994; 154: 1143-9
199. McMurray J, Davie A. The pharmacoeconomics of ACE inhibitors in chronic heart failure. PharmacoEconomics 1996; 3: 188-97
200. Uretsky BF, Young JB, Shahidi FE, et al. Randomized study assessing the effect of digoxin withdrawal in patients with mild to moderate congestive heart failure: results of the PROVED trial. Journal of the American College of Cardiology 1993; 22: 955-62
201. Fowler MB, Gilbert EM, Cohn JN, et al. Effects of carvedilol on cardiovascular hospitalizations in patients with chronic heart failure. Journal of the American College of Cardiology 1996; 27 (Suppl. A): 169
202. Van der Werf T. In: Cardiovascular pathophysiology. Oxford: Oxford University Press, 1980: 45
203. Mehta JL. Endothelium, coronary vasodilatation, and organic nitrates. American Heart Journal 1995; 129: 382-91
204. Abrams J. Use of nitrates in ischaemic heart disease. Current Problems in Cardiology 1992; 17: 481-54
205. Thadani U, Whitsett T. Relationship of pharmacokinetic and pharmacodynamic properties of the organic nitrates. Clinical Pharmacokinetics 1988; 15: 32-43
206. Harrison DG, Bates JN. The nitrovasodilators - new ideas about old drugs. Circulation 1993; 87: 1461-7
207. Lacoste LL, Theroux P, Lidon RM, et al. Antithrombotic properties of transdermal nitroglycerin in stable angina pectoris. American Journal of Cardiology 1994; 73: 1058-62
208. Elkayam U. Tolerance to organic nitrates: evidence, mechanisms, clinical relevance, and strategies for prevention. Annals of Internal Medicine 1991; 114: 667-77
209. Harrison DB, Freiman PC, Armstrong ML, et al. Alterations of vascular reactivity in atherosclerosis. Circulation Research 1987; 61: 1174
210. Luscher TF, Noll G. The pathogenesis of cardiovascular disease; role of the endothelium as a target and mediator. Atherosclerosis 1995; 118 (Suppl.): S81-90
211. Siber S. Nitrates: why and how should they be used today? Current status of the clinical usefulness of nitroglycerin, isosorbide dinitrate and isosorbide-5-mononitrate. European Journal of Clinical Pharmacology 1990; 38 (Suppl. 1): S35-S51
212. Chasseaud LF. Newer aspects of the pharmacokinetics of organic nitrates. Zeitschrift fur Kardiologie 1983; 72: 20-3
213. Nyberg G. Clinical experience with Imdur in angina pectoris: a review. European Journal of Clinical Pharmacology 1990; 38: S65-8
214. Todd PA, Goa KL, Langtry HD. Transdermal nitroglycerin (glyceryl trinitrate): a review of its pharmacology and therapeutic use. Drugs 1990; 40: 880-902
215. Bogaert MG. Clinical pharmacokinetics of glyceryl trinitrate following the use of systemic and topical preparations. Clinical Pharmacokinetics 1987; 12: 1-11
216. Jugdutt BI. Nitrates in myocardial infarction. Cardiovascular Drugs and Therapy 1994; 4: 635-46
217. Abrams J. Glyceryl trinitrate (nitroglycerin) and the organic nitrates: choosing the method of administration. Drugs 1987; 34: 391-403
218. Elkayam U, Mehra A, Shotan A, et al. Possible mechanisms of nitrate tolerance. American Journal of Cardiology 1972; 70: 49G-54G
219. Kelly KL. Beta-blockers in hypertension: a review. American Journal of Hospital Pharmacy 1976; 22: 1284-90
220. Wadworth AN, Murdoch D, Brogden RN. Atenolol: a reappraisal of its pharmacological properties and therapeutic use in cardiovascular disorders. Drugs 1991; 42: 468-510
221. Benfield P, Clissold SP, Brogden RN. Metoprolol: an updated review of its pharmacodynamic and pharmacokinetic properties and therapeutic efficacy in hypertension, ischaemic heart disease and related cardiovascular disorders. Drugs 1986; 31: 376-429
222. Goa KL, Benfield P, Sorkin EM. Labetalol: a reappraisal of its pharmacological properties and therapeutic use in hypertension and ischaemic heart disease. Drugs 1989; 37: 583-627
223. Fitzgerald JD. Do partial agonist beta-blockers have improved clinical utility? Cardiovascular Drugs and Therapy 1993; 7: 303-10
224. Aellig WH. Pindolol, a β-adrenoceptor blocking drug with partial agonist activity: clinical pharmacological considerations. British Journal of Clinical Pharmacology 1982; 13: 187S
225. Milne RJ, Buckley MM-T. Celiprolol: an updated review of its pharmacodynamic and pharmacokinetic properties and therapeutic efficacy in cardiovascular disease. Drugs 1991; 41: 941-69
226. Patel MK, Chan P, Betteridge LJ. Inhibition of vascular smooth muscle cell proliferation by the novel multiple-action antihypertensive agent carvedilol. Journal of Cardiovascular Pharmacology 1995; 25: 652-7
227. Yue TL, Cheng HY, Lysko PG, et al. Carvedilol, a new vasodilator and beta adrenoceptor antagonist is an antioxidant and free radical scavenger. Journal of Pharmacology and Experimental Therapeutics 1992; 263: 92-8
228. Nagakawa Y, Akedo Y, Kaku S, et al. Effects of carvedilol on common carotid arterial flow, peripheral hemodynamics and hemorheological variables in hypertension. European Journal of Clinical Pharmacology 1990; 38 (Suppl. 2): 115-9
229. Das Gupta P, Jain D, Lahiri A, et al. Long-term efficacy and safety of carvedilol, a new beta-blocking agent with vasodilating properties, in patients with chronic ischaemic heart disease. Drug Investigation 1992; 4: 263-72
230. Nahrendorf W, Rading A, Steinig G, et al. A comparison of carvedilol with a combination of propranolol and isosorbide dinitrate in the chronic treatment of stable angina. Journal of Cardiovascular Pharmacology 1992; 19: 114-6

231. Brooks AM, Gillis WE. Ocular β-blockers in glaucoma management: clinical pharmacological aspects. Drugs and Aging 1992; 2: 208-21
232. Lish PM, Weikel JH, Dungan KW. Pharmacological and toxicological properties of 2 β-adrenergic receptor antagonists. Journal of Pharmacology and Experimental Therapeutics 1965; 149: 161-73
233. Johnsson G, Regardh CG. Clinical pharmacokinetics of β-adrenoceptor blocking drugs. Clinical Pharmacokinetics 1976; 1: 233-63
234. van Zwieten PA. Antihypertensive drugs interacting with α- and β-adrenoceptors: a review of basic pharmacology. Drugs 1988; 35 (Suppl. 6): 6-19
235. Lipworth BJ, Irvine NA, McDevitt DG. The effects of time and dose on the relative $\beta_1$- and $\beta_2$-adrenoceptor antagonism of betaxolol and atenolol. British Journal of Clinical Pharmacology 1991; 31: 154-9
236. Heel RC, Brogden RN, Speight TM, et al. Atenolol: a review of its pharmacological properties and therapeutic efficacy in angina pectoris and hypertension. Drugs 1979; 17: 425-60
237. Cohn JN. The management of chronic heart failure. New England Journal of Medicine 1996; 335: 490-8
238. Aarons RD, Nies AS, Gal J, et al. Elevation of β-adrenergic receptor density in human lymphocytes after propranolol administration. Journal of Clinical Investigation 1980; 65: 949
239. Miller RR, Olson HG, Amsterdam FA, et al. Propranolol-withdrawal rebound phenomenon. New England Journal of Medicine 1975; 293: 416
240. Frishman WH, Christodoulou J, Weskler B, et al. Abrupt propranolol withdrawal in angina pectoris: effects on platelet aggregation and exercise tolerance. American Heart Journal 1978; 95: 169-79
241. Maling TJB, Dollery CT. Changes in blood pressure, heart rate and plasma noradrenaline concentration after sudden withdrawal of propranolol. British Medical Journal 1979; 2: 366
242. Feleke E, Lyngstrum O, Rastam L, et al. Complaints of cold extremities among patients on antihypertensive treatment. Acta Medica Scandinavica 1989; 213: 381
243. Belton P, Carmody M, Donohoe M, et al. Propranolol-associated hypoglycaemia in nondiabetics. Journal of the Irish Medical Association 1980; 73: 173
244. Barnett AH, Leslie D, Watkins PJ. Can insulin-treated diabetics be given beta-adrenergic blocking drugs? British Medical Journal 1980; 280: 976-8
245. Scheen AJ, Lefebvre PJ. Antihyperglycaemic agents: drug interactions of clinical importance. Drug Safety 1995; 12: 32-45
246. Kasiske BL, Ma JZ, Kalil RSN, et al. Effects of antihypertensive therapy on serum lipids. Annals of Internal Medicine 1995; 122: 133-41
247. Cruickshank JM. Beta-blockers, bradycardia and adverse effects. Acta Therapeutica 1981; 7: 309
248. Dahlof C, Dimenas E. Side effects of β-blocker treatments as related to the central nervous system. American Journal of the Medical Sciences 1990; 299: 236-44
249. McAinsh J, Cruickshank JM. Beta-blockers and central nervous system side effects. Pharmacology and Therapeutics 1990; 46: 163-97
250. Stevenson JG, Umstead GS. Sexual dysfunction due to antihypertensive agents. Drug Intelligence and Clinical Pharmacy 1984; 18: 113-21
251. Braunwald E. Mechanism of action of calcium channel-blocking agents. New England Journal of Medicine 1982; 302: 1618-27
252. Henry PD. Mechanisms of action of calcium antagonists in cardiac and smooth muscle. In: Stone PH, Antman EM, editors. Calcium channel blocking agents in the treatment of cardiovascular disorders. Mount Kisco, NY: Futura, 1983: 107-54
253. Mitchell LB, Schraeder JS, Mason JW. Comparative clinical electrophysiologic effects of diltiazem, verapamil and nifedipine: a review. American Journal of Cardiology 1982; 49: 629-35
254. Fabiato A. Appraisal of the physiological relevance of two hypotheses for the mechanism of calcium release from the mammalian cardiac sarcoplasmic reticulum: calcium-induced release versus charge-coupled release. Molecular and Cellular Biochemistry 1989; 89: 135-40
255. Soward AL, Vanhaleweyk GLJ, Serruys PW. The haemodynamic effects of nifedipine, verapamil and diltiazem in patients with coronary artery disease. Drugs 1986; 282: 948
256. Hollingshead LM, Faulds D, Fitton A. Bepridil: a review of its pharmacological properties and therapeutic use in stable angina pectoris. Drugs 1992; 44: 835-57
257. Echizen H, Eichelbaum M. Clinical pharmacokinetics of verapamil, nifedipine and diltiazem. Clinical Pharmacokinetics 1986; 11: 425-9
258. Schwartz JB, Capili H, Wainer IW. Verapamil stereoisomers during racemic verapamil administration: effects of aging and comparisons to administration of individual stereoisomers. Clinical Pharmacology and Therapeutics 1994; 56: 368-76
259. Brogden RN, McTavish D. Nifedipine gastrointestinal therapeutic system (GITS): a review of its pharmacodynamic and therapeutic properties and therapeutic efficacy in the hypertension and angina pectoris. Drugs 1995; 50: 495-512
260. Todd PA, Faulds D. Felodipine: a review of the pharmacology and therapeutic uses of the extended release formulation in cardiovascular disorders. Drugs 1992; 44: 251-77
261. Murdoch D, Heel RC. Amlodipine: a review of its pharmacodynamic and pharmacokinetic properties, and therapeutic use in cardiovascular disease. Drugs 1991; 41: 478-505
262. Opie L. Calcium antagonists: side effects. In: Clinical use of calcium channel antagonists. 2nd ed. Boston: Kluwer Academic Publishers, 1990: 316-8
263. Opie LH. Calcium channel antagonists. Part IV. Side effects and contraindications, drug interactions and combinations. Cardiovascular Drugs and Therapy 1988; 2: 177-89
264. Singh BN, Nademanee K, Baky SH. Calcium antagonists. Clinical use in the treatment of arrhythmias. Drugs 1983; 25: 125-53
265. Harper R, Whitford E, Middlebrook K, et al. Verapamil in patients with Wolff-Parkinson-White-syndrome - a potential hazard? New Zealand Journal of Medicine 1981; 11: 456
266. Jacob AS, Neilsen DH, Gianelly RE. Fatal ventricular fibrillation following verapamil in Wolff-Parkinson-White-syndrome with atrial fibrillation. Annals of Emergency Medicine 1985; 14: 159
267. Wachter RM. Symptomatic hypotension induced by nifedipine in the acute treatment of severe hypertension. Archives of Internal Medicine 1987; 147: 556
268. Krebs R. Adverse reactions with calcium antagonists. Hypertension 1983; 5 (Suppl. II): II125-9

269. Piepho RW, Culbertson VL, Rhodes RS. Drug interactions with the calcium entry blockers. Circulation 1987; 75 (Suppl. V): V181-94
270. Brooks N, Cattell M, Pidgeon J, et al. Unpredictable response to nifedipine in severe cardiac failure. British Medical Journal 1980; 281: 1324
271. Vaughan-Neil EF, Snell NJC, Bevan G. Hypotension after verapamil. British Medical Journal 1972; 2: 529
272. Carruthers SG, Freeman DJ, Bailey DG. Synergistic adverse haemodynamic interaction between oral verapamil and propranolol. Clinical Pharmacology and Therapeutics 1989; 46: 469-77
273. Kieval J, Kirsten EB, Kessler KM, et al. The effects of intravenous verapamil on haemodynamic status of patients with coronary artery disease receiving propranolol. Circulation 1982; 65: 653-9
274. Pedersen K, Dorph-Pedersen A, Hvidt S, et al. The long term effect of verapamil on plasma digoxin concentration and renal digoxin clearance in healthy subjects. European Journal of Clinical Pharmacology 1982; 22: 23
275. Bailey DG, Arnold JM, Spence JD. Grapefruit juice and drugs. How significant is the interaction? Clinical Pharmacokinetics 1994; 26: 91-8
276. Marcus WL. Lithium: a review of its pharmacokinetics, health effects, and toxicology. Journal of Environmental Pathology, Toxicology and Oncology 1994; 13: 73-9
277. Ward ME, Musa MN, Bailey L. Clinical pharmacokinetics of lithium. Journal of Clinical Pharmacology 1994; 34: 280-5
278. Horowitz JD, Button IK, Wing L. Is perhexiline essential for the optimal management of angina pectoris? Australian and New Zealand Journal of Medicine 1995; 25: 111-3
279. Horowitz JD, Sia STB, Macdonald PS, et al. Perhexiline maleate treatment of severe angina pectoris - correlations with pharmacokinetics. International Journal of Cardiology 1986; 13: 219-29
280. Shah RR, Oates NS, Idle JR, et al. Impaired oxidation of debrisoquine in patients with perhexiline neuropathy. British Medical Journal 1982; 284: 295-9
281. Frampton J, Buckley M, Fitton A. Nicorandil: a review of its pharmacology and therapeutic efficacy in angina pectoris. Drugs 1992; 44: 625-55
282. Gorlin R. Treatment of chronic stable angina pectoris. American Journal of Cardiology 1992; 70: 26G-31G
283. Abrams J. Silent myocardial ischaemia: role of nitrate therapy. Int Med Spec 1988; 9: 51-69
284. Antalczy Z, Kekes E. Antianginal effects of atenolol and pindolol in patients with stable effort angina pectoris. Journal of Drug Development 1989; 2: 21-6
285. Subramanian VB, Lahiri A, Paramasivan R, et al. Verapamil in chronic stable angina. Lancet 1980; 1: 841-4
286. Danish Study Group on Verapamil in Myocardial Infarction. Effect of verapamil on mortality and major events after acute myocardial infarction. The Danish Verapamil Infarction Trial II (DAVIT-II). American Journal of Cardiology 1990; 66: 779-85
287. Sorkin EM, Clissold SP, Brogden RN. Nifedipine: a review of its pharmacodynamic and pharmacokinetic properties, and therapeutic efficacy in ischaemic heart disease, hypertension and related cardiovascular disorders. Drugs 1985; 30: 181-96
288. Furberg CD, Psaty BM, Meyer JV. Nifedipine: dose-related increase in mortality in patients with coronary heart disease. Circulation 1995; 92: 1326-31
289. Markham A, Brogden RN. Diltiazem: a review of its pharmacology and therapeutic use in older patients. Drugs & Aging 1993; 3: 363-90
290. The Multicenter Diltiazem Postinfarction Trial Research Group. The effect of diltiazem on mortality and reinfarction after myocardial infarction. New England Journal of Medicine 1988; 319: 385-92
291. Falk E. Morphologic features of unstable atherothrombotic plaques underlying acute coronary syndromes. American Journal of Cardiology 1989; 63: 114E-20E
292. Braunwald E. Unstable angina: a classification. Circulation 1989; 80: 410-4
293. Freeman MR, Langer A, Wilson RF, et al. Thrombolysis in unstable angina: randomised double-blind trial of t-PA and placebo. Circulation 1992; 1985: 150-7
294. McMurray J, Rankin A. Cardiology. I. Treatment of myocardial infarction, unstable angina, and angina pectoris. British Medical Journal 1994; 309: 1343-50
295. Antiplatelet Trialist's Collaboration. Collaborative overview of randomised trial of antiplatelet therapy. I. Prevention of death, myocardial infarction, and stroke by prolonged antiplatelet therapy in various categories of patients. British Medical Journal 1994; 308: 81-106
296. RISC Group. Risk of myocardial infarction and death during treatment with low dose aspirin and intravenous heparin in men with unstable coronary artery disease. Lancet 1990; 336: 827-30
297. Lefkovits J, Plow EF, Topol EJ. Platelet glycoprotein IIb/IIIa receptors in cardiovascular medicine. New England Journal of Medicine 1995; 332: 1553-9
298. Theroux P, Kouz S, Roy L, et al. Platelet membrane receptor glycoprotein IIb/IIIa antagonism in unstable angina: the Canadian Lamifiban Study. Circulation 1996; 94: 899-905
299. Kereiakes DJ, Runyon JP, Kielman NS, et al. Differential dose-response to oral xemilofiban after antecedent intravenous abciximab administration for complex coronary intervention. Circulation 1996; 94: 906-10
300. Topol EJ, Califf RM, Welsman HF, et al. on behalf of the EPIC Investigators. Randomized trial of coronary intervention with antibody against IIb/IIIa integrin for reduction of clinical restenosis: results at six months. Lancet 1994; 343: 881-6
301. Lincoff AM, Tcheng JE, Miller DP, et al. Marked enhancement of clinical efficacy of platelet GP IIb/IIIa blockade with c7E3 Fab (abciximab) linked to reduction in bleeding complications: outcome in the EPILOG and EPIC trials. Presented at the American Heart Association's 69th Scientific Sessions. Circulation 1996; 94 (8 Suppl.): Abstract No. 2185
302. Braunwald E, Mark DB, Jones RH, et al. Unstable angina: diagnosis and management. Clinical Practice Guideline Number 10. AHCPR Publication No. 94-0602, May 1994
303. Theroux P, Waters D, Qui S, et al. Aspirin versus heparin to prevent myocardial infarction during the acute phase of unstable angina. Circulation 1993; 88: 2045-8
304. Theroux P, Waters D, Lam J, et al. Reactivation of unstable angina after the discontinuation of heparin. New England Journal of Medicine 1992; 327: 141-5
305. Gruppo Italiano per lo Studio della Sopravvivenza nell'Infarto Miocardico (GISSI-3). Effects of lisinopril and transdermal glyceryl trinitrate singly and together on 6-week mortality and ventricular

function after acute myocardial infarction. Archives of Internal Medicine 1993; 153: 345-53
306. ISIS-4 (Fourth International Study of Infarct Survival) Collaborative Group. ISIS-4: a randomised factorial trial assessing early oral captopril, oral mononitrate, and intravenous magnesium sulphate in 58,050 patients with suspected acute myocardial infarction. Lancet 1995; 345: 669-85
307. Figueras J, Lindon R, Cortadellas J. Rebound myocardial ischaemia following abrupt interruption of intravenous nitroglycerin infusion in patients with unstable angina at rest. European Heart Journal 1991; 12: 405-11
308. Yusuf S, Wittes J, Friedman L. Overview of results of randomised clinical trials in heart disease. II. Unstable angina, heart failure, primary prevention with aspirin, and risk factor modification. Journal of the American Medical Association 1988; 260: 2259-63
309. Balsano F, Rizzon P, Violi F, et al. Antiplatelet treatment with ticlopidine in unstable angina. A controlled multicentre clinical trial. The Studio della Ticlopidina nell'Angina Instabile Group. Circulation 1990; 82: 17-26
310. McTavish D, Faulds D, Goa KL. Ticlopidine: an updated review of its pharmacology and therapeutic use in platelet-dependent disorders. Drugs 1990; 40: 239-59
311. Schror K. Antiplatelet drugs: a comparative review. Drugs 1995; 50: 7-28
312. Lubsen J, Tijssen JG. Efficacy of nifedipine and metoprolol in the early treatment of unstable angina in the coronary care unit; findings from the Holland Interuniversity/Nifedipine/Metoprolol Trial (HINT). American Journal of Cardiology 1987; 60: 18A-25A
313. Muller JE, Turi ZG, Pearle DL, et al. Nifedipine and conventional therapy for unstable angina pectoris: a randomised double-blind comparison. Circulation 1984; 69: 728-39
314. Fuster V, Badimon L, Badimon JJ, et al. The pathogenesis of coronary artery disease and the acute coronary syndromes (first of two parts). New England Journal of Medicine 1992; 326: 242-50
315. Rogers WJ. Contemporary management of acute myocardial infarction. American Journal of Medicine 1995; 99: 195-206
316. Pfeffer MA, Braunwald E. Ventricular remodelling after myocardial infarction. Experimental observations and clinical implications. Circulation 1990; 81: 1161-72
317. Williams DO, Amsterdam EA, Mason DT. Haemodynamic effects of nitroglycerin in acute myocardial infarction. Decrease in ventricular pre-load at the expense of cardiac output. Circulation 1975; 51: 421
318. Task Force IV. Pharmacologic interventions. American Journal of Cardiology 1982; 50: 393
319. ISIS-2 (Second International Study of Infarct Survival) Collaborative Group. ISIS-2: randomised trial of intravenous streptokinase, oral aspirin, both or neither among 17,187 cases of suspected acute myocardial infarction. Lancet 1988; 2: 349-60
320. Roux S, Christeller S, Ludin E. Effects of aspirin on coronary reocclusion and recurrent ischaemia after thrombolysis: a meta-analysis. Journal of the American College of Cardiology 1992; 19: 671-7
321. Fibrinolytic Therapy Trialists' (FTT) Collaborative Group. Indications for fibrinolytic therapy in suspected acute myocardial infarction: collaborative overview of early mortality and major morbidity results from all randomised trials of more than 1,000 patients. Lancet 1994; 343: 311-22
322. The GUSTO Investigators. An international randomised trial comparing four thrombolytic strategies for acute myocardial infarction. New England Journal of Medicine 1993; 329: 673-82
323. Battershill PE, Benfield P, Goa KL. Streptokinase: a review of its pharmacology and therapeutic efficacy in acute myocardial infarction in older patients. Drugs and Aging 1994; 4: 63-86
324. Brogden RN, Speight TM, Avery GS. Streptokinase: a review of its clinical pharmacology, mechanism of action and therapeutic uses. Drugs 1973; 5: 357-445
325. Mueller H. Different fibrinolytic potencies of two forms of recombitant tissue type plasminogen activator. NHLBI Thrombolysis in Myocardial Infarction Trial. Clinical Research 1986; 34: 631A
326. Ferres H, Hibbs M, Smith RAG. Deacylation studies in vitro on anisoylated plasminogen streptokinase activator complex. Drugs 1987; 33 (Suppl. 3): 80-2
327. Mathey DG, Schofer J, Bleifeld W, et al. Coronary thrombolysis with intravenous urokinase in patients with acute myocardial infarction. American Journal of Medicine 1987; 83 (Suppl. 2A): 26
328. Verstraete M, Lijnen HR. Novel thrombolytic agents. Cardiovascular Drugs and Therapy 1994; 8: 801-12
329. Simoons ML, Maggioni AP, Knatterud G, et al. Individual risk assessment for intercranial haemorrhage during thrombolytic therapy. Lancet 1993; 342: 1523-8
330. Sleight P. Is there an age limit for thrombolytic therapy? American Journal of Cardiology 1993; 72: 30G-33G
331. Gruppo Italiano per lo Studio della Streptochinasi nell' Infarto Miocardico (GISSI). Effectiveness of intravenous thrombolytic treatment in acute myocardial infarction. Lancet 1986; 1: 397-402
332. Volpi A, Cavalli A, Santoro E, et al. Italiano per lo Studio della Streptochinasi nell' Infarto Miocardico, Milan. Incidence and prognosis of secondary ventricular fibrillation in acute myocardial infarction. Evidence for a protective effect of thrombolytic therapy. Circulation 1990; 82: 1279-88
333. Ridker PM, Herbert PR, Fuster V, et al. Are both aspirin and heparin justified as adjuncts to thrombolytic therapy for acute myocardial infarction? Lancet 1993; 341: 1574-7
334. Cairns J, Armstrong PW, Belenkie I, et al. Maximising the benefits of thrombolytic therapy for acute myocardial infarction [editorial]. Canadian Medical Association Journal 1995; 152: 819-22
335. Hirsh J, Raschke R, Warkentin TE, et al. Heparin: mechanism of action, pharmacokinetics, dosing considerations, monitoring, efficacy and safety. Chest 1995; 108: 258S-75S
336. Markwardt F. The development of hirudin as an antithrombotic drug. Thrombosis Research 1994; 74: 1-23
337. Antman EM, for the TIMI 9A Investigators. Hirudin in acute myocardial infarction: safety report from the Thrombolysis and Thrombin Inhibition in Myocardial Infarction (TIMI) 9A trial. Circulation 1994; 90: 1624-30
338. Global Use of Strategies to Open Occluded Coronary Arteries (GUSTO) IIa Investigators. Randomized trial of intravenous heparin versus recombinant hirudin for acute coronary syndromes. Circulation 1994; 90: 1631-7
339. Antman EM, for the TIMI 9B Investigators. Hirudin in acute myocardial infarction: Thrombolysis and Thrombin Inhibition in Myocardial Infarction (TIMI) 9B trial. Circulation 1996; 94: 911-21

340. Yusuf S, Sleight P, Held P, et al. Routine medical management of acute myocardial infarction. Lessons from overviews of recent randomised controlled trials. Circulation 1990; 82 (Suppl. 3): II-117-34
341. Yusuf S, Wittes J, Friedman L. Overview of results of randomised clinical trials in heart disease. I. Treatments following myocardial infarction. Journal of the American Medical Association 1988; 260: 2088-93
342. Roberts R, Rogers WJ, Mueller HS, et al. Immediate versus deferred beta-blockade following thrombolytic therapy in patients with acute myocardial infarction. Results of the Thrombolysis in Myocardial Infarction (TIMI) II-B Study. Circulation 1991; 83: 422-37
343. Held PH, Yusuf S. Calcium antagonists in the treatment of ischaemic heart disease: myocardial infarction. Coronary Artery Disease 1994; 5: 21-6
344. Woods KL, Fletcher S, Roff C, et al. Intravenous magnesium sulphate in suspected acute myocardial infarction: results of the second Leicester Intravenous Magnesium Intervention Trial (LIMIT-2). Lancet 1992; 339: 1553-8
345. Beta-blocker Heart Attack Study Group. A randomised trial of propranolol in patients with acute myocardial infarction. Journal of the American Medical Association 1981; 246: 207-304
346. Herlitz J, Elmfeldt D, Holmberg S, et al. The Goteborg metoprolol trial: mortality and causes of death. American Journal of Cardiology 1984; 53: 9D
347. Pedersen TR, and the Norwegian Multicenter Study Group. Timolol-induced reduction in mortality and reinfarction in patients surviving acute myocardial infarction. New England Journal of Medicine 1981; 304: 801-7
348. Chadda K, Goldstein S, Byington R, et al. Effect of propranolol after acute myocardial infarction in patients with congestive heart failure. Circulation 1986; 73: 503-10
349. May GS, Eberlein KA, Furberg CD, et al. Secondary prevention after myocardial infarction: a review of long-term trials. Progress in Cardiovascular Diseases 1982; 24: 331
350. Sleight P. Calcium antagonists during and after myocardial infarction. Drugs 1996; 51: 216-25
351. Jafri SM, Zarowitz B, Goldstein S, et al. The role of antiplatelet therapy in acute coronary syndromes and for secondary prevention following a myocardial infarction. Progress in Cardiovascular Diseases 1993; 36: 75-84
352. Herbert JM, Frechel D, Vallee E, et al. Clopidogrel, a novel antiplatelet and antithrombotic agent. Cardiovascular Drug Reviews 1993; 11: 180-8
353. CAPRIE Steering Committee. A randomized, blinded, trial of clopidogrel versus aspirin in patients at risk of ischaemic events (CAPRIE). Lancet 1996; 348: 1329-39
354. The SAVE Investigators. Effect of captopril on mortality and morbidity in patients with left ventricular dysfunction after myocardial infarction. Results of the survival and ventricular enlargement trial. New England Journal of Medicine 1992; 327: 669-77
355. Lonn EM, Yusuf S, Jha P, et al. Emerging role of angiotensin-converting enzyme inhibitors in cardiac and vascular protection. Circulation 1994; 90: 2056-69
356. Harris PJ. Management of the post-infarct patient. Australian Prescriber 1996; 19: 8-10
357. Pfeffer MA, Sacks FM, Moye LA, et al. Cholesterol and recurrent events: a secondary prevention trial for normolipidemic patients. CARE Investigators. American Journal of Cardiology 1995; 76: 98C-106C
358. Epstein AE, Hallstrom AP, Rogers WJ, et al. Mortality following ventricular arrhythmia suppression by encainide, flecainide, and moricizine after myocardial infarction. The original design concept for the Cardiac Arrhythmia Suppression Trial (CAST). Journal of the American Medical Association 1993; 270: 2451-5
359. Flapan AD. Management of patients after their first myocardial infarction. British Medical Journal 1994; 309: 1129-34
360. Roden DM. Risks and benefits of antiarrhythmic drug therapy. New England Journal of Medicine 1994; 331: 785-91
361. Camm AJ, Kautzner J. Assessment of arrhythmias after myocardial infarction in the post-CAST era. Canadian Journal of Cardiology 1996; 12 (Suppl. B): 9B-19B
362. Waldo AL, Wit AL. Mechanisms of cardiac arrhythmias. Lancet 1993; 341: 1189-93
363. Wit AL, Cranefield PF. Reentrant excitation as a cause of cardiac arrhythmias. American Journal of Physiology 1978; 49: 1-15
364. Hoffman BF, Cranefield PF. The physiological basis of cardiac arrhythmias. American Journal of Physiology 1978; 235: H1-17
365. Hoffman BF, Rosen MR. Cellular mechanisms for cardiac arrhythmias. Circulation Research 1981; 49: 1-15
366. Vaughan Williams EM. Classifying antiarrhythmic actions: by facts or speculation. Journal of Clinical Pharmacology 1992; 32: 964-77
367. Leon AR, Merlino JD. Quinidine: its value and danger. Heart Disease and Stroke 1993; 2: 407-13
368. Morganroth J, Goin JE. Quinidine-related mortality in the short-to-medium-term treatment of ventricular arrhythmias. A meta-analysis. Circulation 1991; 84: 1977-83
369. Coplen SE, Antman EM, Berlin JA, et al. Efficacy and safety of quinidine therapy for maintenance of sinus rhythm after cardioversion: a meta-analysis of randomized control trials. Circulation 1992; 82: 1106-16
370. Harrison DC, Meffin PJ, Winkle RA. Clinical pharmacokinetics of antiarrhythmic drugs. Progress in Cardiovascular Diseases 1977; 20: 217
371. Nielsen F, Rosholm JU, Brosen K. Lack of relationship between quinidine pharmacokinetics and the sparteine oxidation polymorphism. European Journal of Clinical Pharmacology 1995; 48: 501-4
372. Salerno DM. Quinidine: worse than adverse? Circulation 1991; 84: 2196-8
373. Hoffman BF, Rosen MR, Wit AL. Electrophysiology and pharmacology of cardiac arrhythmias. VII: cardiac effects of quinidine and procainamide. American Heart Journal 1975; 89: 804-8
374. Podrid PJ. Oral antiarrhythmic drugs used for atrial fibrillation. In: Falk RH, Podrid PJ, editors. Atrial fibrillation: mechanisms and management. New York: Raven Press, 1992: 127-233
375. Leahey EB, Reiffel JA, Drusin RE, et al. Interaction between quinidine and digoxin. Journal of the American Medical Association 1978; 240: 533-4
376. Ellenbogen KA, Wood MA, Stambler BS. Procainamide: a perspective on its value and danger. Heart Disease and Stroke 1993; 2(6): 473-6
377. Harron DWG, Brogden RN. Acecainide (N-acetylprocainamide): a review of its pharmacodynamic and pharmacokinetic properties, and therapeu-

tic potential in cardiac arrhythmias. Drugs 1990; 39: 720-40

378. Kluger J, Drayer D, Reidenberg M, et al. The clinical pharmacology and antiarrhythmic efficacy of acetylprocainamide in patients with arrhythmias. American Journal of Cardiology 1980; 45: 1250
379. Roden DM, Reele SB, Higgins SB, et al. Antiarrhythmic efficacy, pharmacokinetics and safety of N-acetylprocainamide. American Journal of Cardiology 1980; 46: 463
380. Schwartz JB, Keefe D, Harrison DC. Adverse effects of antiarrhythmic drugs. Drugs 1981; 21: 23
381. Lahita R, Kluger J, Drayer DE, et al. Antibodies to nuclear antigens in patients treated with procainamide or acetylprocainamide. New England Journal of Medicine 1979; 301: 1382
382. Morady F, Schienman MM, Desai J. Disopyramide. Annals of Internal Medicine 1982; 96: 337-43
383. Lie KI, Wellens HJ, van Capelle FJ, et al. Lidocaine in the prevention of primary ventricular fibrillation. New England Journal of Medicine 1974; 291: 1324-6
384. McMahon S, Collins R, Peto R, et al. Effects of prophylactic lidocaine in suspected acute myocardial infarction. An overview of results from randomised control trials. Journal of the American Medical Association 1988; 260: 1910-6
385. Nies AS, Shand DG, Wilkinson GR. Altered hepatic blood flow and drug disposition. Clinical Pharmacokinetics 1976; 1: 135-55
386. Thompson PD, Melmon KL, Richardson JA, et al. Lidocaine pharmacokinetics in advanced heart failure, liver disease and renal failure in humans. Annals of Internal Medicine 1973; 73: 499-508
387. LeLorier J, Grenon D, Latour Y, et al. Pharmacokinetics of lidocaine after prolonged intravenous infusions in uncomplicated myocardial infarction. Annals of Internal Medicine 1977; 87: 700-6
388. Campbell RWF. Mexiletine. New England Journal of Medicine 1987; 316: 29-34
389. Podrid PJ, Lown B. Mexiletine for ventricular arrhythmias. American Journal of Cardiology 1981; 47: 895-902
390. Roden DM, Woosley RL. Tocainide. New England Journal of Medicine 1986; 315: 41-5
391. Lalka D, Meyer MB, Duce BR, et al. Kinetics of the oral antiarrhythmic lignocaine congener, tocainide. Clinical Pharmacology and Therapeutics 1976; 19: 757-66
392. Maloney JD, Nissen RG, McColgan JM. Open clinical studies at a referral centre: chronic maintenance tocainide therapy in patients with recurrent sustained ventricular tachycardia refractory to conventional antiarrhythmic agents. American Heart Journal 1980; 100: 1023-30
393. Nestico PF, Morganroth J, Horowitz LN. New antiarrhythmic drugs. Drugs 1988; 35: 286-319
394. Oliphant LD, Goddard M. Tocainide associated neutropenia and lupus-like syndrome. Chest 1988; 94: 427-8
395. Bryson HM, Palmer KJ, Langtry HD, et al. Propafenone: a reappraisal of its pharmacology, pharmacokinetics and therapeutic use in cardiac arrhythmias. Drugs 1993; 45: 85-130
396. Fitton A, Buckley MM-T. Moricizine: a review of its pharmacological properties, and therapeutic efficacy in cardiac arrhythmias. Drugs 1990; 40: 138-67
397. Ikeda N, Singh BN, Davis LD, et al. Effects of flecainide on the electrophysiologic properties of isolated canine and rabbit myocardial fibres. Journal of the American College of Cardiology 1985; 5: 303-10
398. Gross AS, Mikus G, Fischer C, et al. Stereoselective disposition of flecainide in relation to sparteine/debrisoquine metaboliser phenotype. British Journal of Clinical Pharmacology 1989; 28: 555-66
399. Kroemer HK, Turgeon J, Parker RA, et al. Flecainide enantiomers: disposition in human subjects and electrophysiologic actions in vitro. Clinical Pharmacology and Therapeutics 1989; 46: 584-90
400. Henthorn RW, Waldo AL, Anderson JL, et al. Flecainide acetate prevents recurrence of symptomatic paroxysmal supraventricular tachycardia. Circulation 1991; 83: 119-25
401. Roden DM, Woosley RL. Flecainide. New England Journal of Medicine 1986; 315: 36-41
402. Buxton AE. Antiarrhythmic drugs: good for premature ventricular complexes but bad for patients? Annals of Internal Medicine 1992; 116: 420-2
403. Anderson JL. Reassessment of benefit-risk ratio and treatment algorithms for antiarrhythmic drug therapy after the Cardiac Arrhythmia Suppression Trial. Journal of Clinical Pharmacology 1990; 30: 981-9
404. Grant AO. Propafenone: an effective agent for the management of supraventricular arrhythmias. Journal of Cardiovascular Electrophysiology 1996; 7: 353-64
405. Hii JTY, Duff HJ, Burgess ED. Clinical pharmacokinetics of propafenone. Clinical Pharmacokinetics 1991; 21: 1-10
406. Funck-Brentano C, Kroemer HK, Lee JT. Propafenone. New England Journal of Medicine 1990; 322: 518-25
407. Hohnloser SH, Woosley RL. Sotalol. New England Journal of Medicine 1994; 331: 31-8
408. Fitton A, Sorkin EM. Sotalol: an updated review of its pharmacological properties and therapeutic use in cardiac arrhythmias. Drugs 1993; 46: 678-719
409. Advani SV, Singh BN. Pharmacodynamic, pharmacokinetic and antiarrhythmic properties of d-sotalol, the dextroisomer of sotalol. Drugs 1995; 49: 664-79
410. Campbell TJ. Proarrhythmic actions of antiarrhythmic drugs: a review. Australian and New Zealand Journal of Medicine 1990; 20: 275-82
411. Campbell TJ. Proarrhythmic complications of sotalol. Australian and New Zealand Journal of Medicine 1996; 26: 147-8
412. Waldo AL, Camm AJ, deRuyter H, et al. Effect of d-sotalol on mortality in patients with left ventricular dysfunction after recent and remote myocardial infarction. Lancet 1996; 348: 7-12
413. Mason JW. Amiodarone. New England Journal of Medicine 1987; 316: 455-66
414. Heger JJ, Prystowsky EN, Jackman WM, et al. Amiodarone. New England Journal of Medicine 1982; 305: 359
415. Latini R, Tognoni G, Kates RE. Clinical pharmacokinetics of amiodarone. Clinical Pharmacokinetics 1984; 9: 136
416. Harris L, Roncucci R, editors. In: Amiodarone: pharmacology, pharmacokinetics, toxicology, clinical effects. Paris: Med Sci Int., 1986
417. Podrid PJ. Amiodarone: reevaluation of an old drug. Annals of Internal Medicine 1995; 122: 689-700
418. Grant AO. On the mechanism of action of antiarrhythmic agents. American Heart Journal 1992; 123: 1130-6
419. Magro SA, Lawrence EC, Wheeler SH, et al. Amiodarone pulmonary toxicity: prospective evaluation of serial pulmonary function tests. Journal of the American College of Cardiology 1988; 12: 781-8

420. Nademanee K, Singh BN, Callahan B. Amiodarone, thyroid hormone indexes, and altered thyroid function: long-term serial effects in patients with cardiac arrhythmias. American Journal of Cardiology 1986; 58: 981-6
421. Harris L, McKenna WJ, Rowland E, et al. Side-effects of amiodarone therapy. Circulation 1983; 67: 45-51
422. Charness ME, Morady F, Scheinman MM. Frequent neurologic toxicity associated with amiodarone therapy. Neurology 1984; 34: 669
423. Ingram DV. Ocular effects in long-term amiodarone therapy. American Heart Journal 1983; 51: 1231
424. McKenna WJ, Harris L, Rowland E, et al. Amiodarone therapy during pregnancy. American Journal of Cardiology 1983; 51: 1231
425. Marcus FI. Drug interactions with amiodarone. American Heart Journal 1983; 106: 924-30
426. Koch-Weser J. Bretylium. New England Journal of Medicine 1979; 300: 473
427. Rapeport WG. Clinical pharmacokinetics of bretylium. Clinical Pharmacokinetics 1985; 10: 248
428. Lerman BB, Belardinelli L. Cardiac electrophysiology of adenosine: basic and clinical concepts. Circulation 1991; 83: 1499-509
429. Faulds D, Chrisp P, Buckley MT. Adenosine: an evaluation of its use in cardiac diagnostic procedures, and in the treatment of paroxysmal supraventricular tachycardia. Drugs 1991; 41: 596-624
430. Reid PG, Fraser AG, Watt AH, et al. Acute haemodynamic effects of intravenous infusion of adenosine in conscious man. European Heart Journal 1990; 74: 203-8
431. Murgatroyd FD, Camm AJ. Atrial arrhythmia. Lancet 1993; 341: 1317-22
432. Kannel WB, Abbott RD, Savage DD, et al. Epidemiologic features of atrial fibrillation: the Framingham Study. New England Journal of Medicine 1982; 306: 1018-22
433. Kopecky SL, Gersh BJ, McGoon MD, et al. The natural history of lone atrial fibrillation: a population based study over three decades. New England Journal of Medicine 1987; 317: 669-74
434. Olsson SB. Atrial fibrillation: new aspects on mechanism and treatment. Journal of Internal Medicine 1996; 239: 3-15
435. Schlepper M. Identification of patients with atrial fibrillation at risk for thromboembolism. In: Olsson SB, Allessie MA, Campbell RWF, editors. Atrial fibrillation: mechanisms and therapeutic strategies. Armonk, NY: Futura Publishing Co, 1994: 15-24
436. Stroke Prevention in Atrial Fibrillation Investigators. Stroke Prevention in Atrial Fibrillation Study: final results. Circulation 1991; 84: 527-39
437. Godtfredson J. The role of aspirin and oral anticoagulant therapy in chronic atrial fibrillation. In: Olsson SB, Allessie MA, Campbell RWF, editors. Atrial fibrillation: mechanisms and therapeutic strategies. Armonk, NY: Futura Publishing Co, 1994: 25-35
438. Ganz LI, Friedman PL. Supraventricular tachycardia. New England Journal of Medicine 1995; 332: 162-73
439. Moss AJ. Asymptomatic ventricular arrhythmias in healthy persons: smoke or smoke screen? Annals of Internal Medicine 1992; 117: 1053-4
440. Bikkina M, Larson MG, Levy D. Prognostic implications of asymptomatic ventricular arrhythmias: The Framingham Heart Study. Annals of Internal Medicine 1992; 117: 990-6
441. Campbell RWF. Ventricular ectopic beats and non-sustained ventricular tachycardia. Lancet 1993; 342: 314
442. Shenasa M, Borggrefe M, Haverkamp W, et al. Ventricular tachycardia. Lancet 1993; 341: 1512-9
443. Jackman WM, Friday KJ, Anderson JL, et al. The long QT syndromes: a critical review, new clinical observations and a unifying hypothesis. Progress in Cardiovascular Diseases 1988; 31: 115-72
444. Cranefield PF, Aronson RS. Torsade de pointes and early after depolarizations. Cardiovascular Drugs and Therapy 1991; 5: 531-7
445. Tan JL, Hou CJY, Lauer MR, et al. Electrophysiologic mechanisms of the long QT interval syndromes and torsade de pointes. Annals of Internal Medicine 1995; 122: 701-14
446. Roden DM. Long QT syndrome and torsade de pointes: basic and clinical aspects. In: El-Sherif N, Samet P, editors. Cardiac pacing and electrophysiology. Philadelphia: WB Saunders, 1991: 265-84
447. Tzivoni D, Vanai S, Schuger C, et al. Treatment of torsade de pointes with magnesium sulfate. Circulation 1988; 77: 392-7
448. Ben-David J, Zipes DP. Torsade de pointes and proarrhythmia. Lancet 1993; 341: 1578-82
449. O'Nunain S, Ruskin J. Cardiac arrest. Lancet 1993; 342: 1641-7
450. Marwick C. FDA gives calcium channel blockers clean bill of health but warns of short-acting nifedipine hazard. Journal of the American Medical Association 1996; 275: 423-4
451. Steiner JA. Antihypertensive drugs. In: Dukes MNG, editor. Meyler's side effects of drugs. Amsterdam: Elsevier, 1988: 402
452. McDevitt DG, MacConachie AM. Anti-anginal and beta-blocking drugs. In: Dukes MNG, editor. Meyler's side effects of drugs. Amsterdam: Elsevier, 1988: 367-8
453. Silberstein SD, Young WB. Safety and efficacy of ergotamine tartrate and dihydroergotamine in the treatment of migraine and status migrainosus. Neurology 1995; 45: 577-84
454. Lange RA, Willard JE. The cardiovascular effects of cocaine. Heart Disease and Stroke 1993; 2: 136-41
455. Isner JM, Estes III NAM, Thompson PD, et al. Acute cardiac events temporally related to cocaine abuse. New England Journal of Medicine 1986; 315: 1438-43
456. Plosker GL, McTavish D. Sumatriptan: a reappraisal of its pharmacology and therapeutic efficacy in the acute treatment of migraine and cluster headache. Drugs 1994; 47: 622-51
457. Robben NC, Pippas AW, Moore JO. The syndrome of 5-fluorouracil cardiotoxicity: an elusive cardiopathy. Cancer 1993; 71: 493-509
458. Von Hoff DD, Rozencweig M, Piccart M. The cardiotoxicity of anticancer agents. Seminars in Oncology 1982; 9: 23-33
459. Chazan R, Karwat K, Tyminska K, et al. Cardiac arrhythmias as a result of intravenous infusion of theophylline in patients with airway obstruction. International Journal of Clinical Pharmacology and Therapeutics 1995; 33: 170-5
460. Tan HL, Hou CJY, Lauer MR, et al. Electrophysiologic mechanisms of the long QT interval syndromes and torsade de pointes. Annals of Internal Medicine 1995; 122: 701-14
461. Davies AJ, Harindra V, McEwan A, et al. Cardiotoxic effect with convulsions in terfenadine overdose. British Medical Journal 1989; 298: 325

462. Wysowski DK, Bacsanyi J. Cisapride and fatal arrhythmias. (Letter). New England Journal of Medicine 1996; 335: 290-1
463. Tester-Daldenp CBM. Antiprotozoal drugs. In: Dukes MNG, editor. Meyler's side effects of drugs. Amsterdam: Elsevier, 1988: 594
464. Serafimovski N, Thorball N, Asmussen I, et al. Tricyclic antidepressant poisoning with special reference to cardiac complications. Acta Anaesthesiologica Scandinavica 1975; 19 (Suppl. 57): 55-63
465. D'Arcy PF, Griffin JP. Cardiac dysfunction. In: Iatrogenic diseases. London: Oxford University Press, 1972
466. Mullick FG, McAllister HA. Myocarditis associated with methyldopa therapy. Journal of the American Medical Association 1977; 237: 1699
467. Marquez-Julio A, Uldall PR. Pericardial effusions associated with minoxidil. Lancet 1977; 2: 816
468. Chung EK, Dean HM. Diseases of the heart and vascular system due to drugs. In: Meyler & Peck (editors) Drug-induced diseases. Amsterdam: Excerpta Medica, 1972; 345
469. Brogden RN, Heel RC, Speight TM, et al. Prazosin: a review of its pharmacological properties and therapeutic efficacy. Drugs 1977; 14: 163
470. Stannard M, Sloman G. Haemodynamic effects of propranolol. British Medical Journal 1967; 1: 700
471. Shafer N. Hypotension due to nitroglycerin combined with alcohol. New England Journal of Medicine 1965; 273: 1169
472. Moir DC, Dingwall-Fordyce I, Weir RD. A follow-up study of cardiac patients receiving amitriptyline. European Journal of Clinical Pharmacology 1973; 6: 98
473. Brogden RN, Speight TM, Avery GS. Levodopa: a review of its pharmacological properties and therapeutic uses with particular reference to Parkinsonism. Drugs 1971; 2: 262

Chapter 21

# Hypertensive Disease

*A.A.J. O'Brien* and *C.J. Bulpitt*

## Synopsis of Important Principles

1) The aims of antihypertensive therapy are to relieve or forestall symptoms, to prevent complications, and to prolong life.

2) Before drug treatment is started, causes of secondary hypertension should be looked for, and factors which tend to raise blood pressure, eliminated.

3) Similarly, care must be taken to determine the sustained level of blood pressure.

4) The primary aim of treatment is to find for each patient a drug or combination of drugs that is effective and has no adverse effects. Therapy should be individualised rather than blindly following a sequential list of drugs.

5) Very high blood pressure, when accompanied by symptoms, should be treated without delay. However, the lowering of blood pressure should be gradual.

6) The treatment of hypertension is not just a matter of prescribing drugs; quality of life and compliance issues must also be taken into account.

7) The cost benefit/cost effectiveness of drug therapy must be taken into account when treating patients over long periods.

The treatment of hypertension is preventive medicine in its most sophisticated form, with large potential benefits but concomitant problems. These problems stem from a number of factors: the sheer number of potential patients (up to 15% of the adult population when elderly individuals are included), the large number and complicated nature of available drugs, the sensitive end-point of therapy (a narrow range of blood pressure at which both the patient and doctor are satisfied), and the cost effectiveness or otherwise of long term therapy.

## 1. Clinical Pharmacological Considerations: Pathogenetic Factors in Hypertension

Only in a relatively small percentage of cases can a specific cause for hypertension can be found, e.g. primary renal or renovascular disease or an endocrine tumour. The majority (95%) of hypertensive patients differ in the balance of factors which contribute to their raised blood pressure, and consequently the term 'essential hypertension' should not be applied to this group as if it were a single entity. Strong evidence for this is the large interindividual differences in plasma renin and aldosterone values which are known to have a regulatory role on blood pressure.[1]

High plasma renin concentrations in relation to salt intake are found in accelerated and renovascular hypertension and in relatively young patients with essential hypertension. In the presence of high plasma renin levels, aldosterone levels will also be high. However, 20 to 30% of patients with essential hypertension have low plasma renin levels. In a minority of such cases, hypertension is due to a primary increase in mineralocorticoid secretion, but in most cases of 'low renin hypertension' this is not so.

The role of atrial natriuretic factor (ANF) in holding blood pressure down is uncertain; this peptide causes vasodilatation and natriuresis and thus opposes the effects of the renin-angiotensin system.[2] It also attenuates the aldosterone response to angiotensin II.[3] In a proportion of younger patients there is evidence for a correlation between plasma catecholamines and hypertension.[4] Lifestyle also plays a role in the pathogenesis of essential hypertension: obesity is a known causative factor in hypertension,[5] as is alcohol when taken in quantities exceeding 3 drinks a day.[6] A vegetarian[7] or low-fat diet[8] lowers blood pressure and an ultralow-fat, low-salt, low-animal protein diet has been found to be very effective in doing so.[9]

The relationship between salt intake and hypertension is still uncertain.[10] Interpopulation studies have shown a highly significant correlation between sodium intake (or excretion) and blood pressure; intrapopulation studies have shown this correlation in Japanese, Korean and Kenyan populations but, in general, not in Western populations. Nevertheless, the argument is not whether reducing salt intake reduces blood pressure but whether it does so to a clinically relevant extent. Salt restriction studies in hypertensive individuals have been encouraging and salt restriction leads to an enhanced effect of β-adrenoceptor blockers, ACE (angiotensin-converting enzyme) inhibitors and diuretics.

A high potassium intake probably protects to some extent against hypertension.[11] This effect appears greater with higher initial pressures,[12] but might be confounded by other dietary and social factors that show a degree of covariance with potassium.[13] The question of whether exercise has a major blood pressure-lowering effect is unclear, although its contribution to weight control and overall reduction in cardiovascular risk is accepted.[14,15] Similarly, the effect on blood pressure of removing stress by relaxation remains unclear.

Finally, some individuals may have a genetic predisposition to the development of hypertension; but so far, the nature of this has remained obscure. Regardless of genetic susceptibility, hypertension is uncommon in the absence of one or more of the following: bodyweight excess, regular alcohol consumption, physical inactivity and certain dietary habits.[16]

## 2. General Principles of Treatment

### 2.1 Rationale for Lowering Blood Pressure

High blood pressure carries with it an increased risk of cardiovascular disease and renal damage.[17] Treatment of hypertension leads to a significant reduction in cardiovascular mortality and morbidity.[18] The absolute benefit depends on age, gender, race and the severity of hypertension. In mild to moderate hypertension, stroke incidence will be reduced by 1/1000 per year in younger individuals and up to 1/100 per year in those aged 70 years. The corresponding figures for cardiac events are 0.3/1000 per year in middle-aged and 1/100 per year in elderly populations.[19,20]

**Table I.** Principal aims of treatment of hypertension (after Pardell[21])

| |
|---|
| • Attainment of good blood pressure control in the community |
| • Reduction of cardiovascular morbidity and mortality |
| • Prevention of arteriosclerosis |
| • Control of other vascular risk factors |
| • Avoidance of progression to more severe stages of hypertension |
| • Reversal of target-organ damage |

The principal aims of treatment of hypertension are outlined in table I.

### 2.2 Factors Influencing Prognosis

Patients with underlying *renal disease* generally have a worse prognosis than those with 'essential' hypertension. The combination of *obesity* and hypertension carries a worse prognosis from the cardiac point of view.[22] On the other hand, it has been observed that lean hypertensive patients have a higher mortality than obese patients with hypertension.[23]

In patients with *moderate* hypertension there is evidence that cardiovascular complications are reduced with antihypertensive therapy.[24] However, in *mild* hypertension, the situation is less clear.[25] Several trials have demonstrated benefit from antihypertensive therapy in patients with diastolic pressures of 95mm Hg or more, but there is no definite evidence to justify treating people with diastolic pressures in the range 90 to 94mm Hg.[19] The consensus regarding systolic blood pressure, such as it is, suggests treatment for sustained levels >160mm Hg.[26]

In patients with *accelerated* hypertension, the prognosis is dramatically improved with antihypertensive therapy. If untreated, expectation of life is less than 1 year.

### 2.3 Initiation of Treatment

#### *2.3.1 Investigations Prior to Starting Treatment*

Prior to starting treatment, secondary causes of hypertension should be identified such as renal failure (via serum creatinine determination) and hyperaldosteronism (serum potassium). Cardiovascular risk status should be determined from an electrocardiogram, and fasting blood lipids and glucose should also be measured. A chest radiograph indicating heart failure will suggest diuretic ± ACE inhibitor treatment, while a high serum uric acid concentration and a low peak expiratory flow rate (PEFR) will exclude diuretic and β-blocker therapy, respectively.

#### *2.3.2 Pharmacological or Nonpharmacological Treatment?*

Nonpharmacological treatment is to be preferred but unfortunately, is rarely sufficient to achieve reasonable goal blood pressures in patients with established sustained hypertension. The exception is the obese person who consumes too much alcohol. If such individuals lose weight and reduce their alcohol intake, hypertension may be controlled.

#### *2.3.3 Nonpharmacological Measures*

**Cessation of Smoking**

Smoking should be discouraged. It raises blood pressure acutely[27] and may be a factor in making hypertension proceed to the accelerated phase.[28] Cigarette smoking is a major factor in arterial complications in hypertensive patients.[29]

**Reduction of Obesity**

In a large study conducted in the US (Chicago), there was a 7-fold difference in the prevalence of hypertension between the heaviest and lightest individuals.[30] This effect of obesity was independent of all other factors studied but additive to effects of alcohol consumption. While there are practical problems in achieving adequate weight reduction in an obese patient, the results may be comparable to those achieved with drug therapy.[31]

**Reduction in Alcohol Consumption**

Alcohol abuse plays a role in the maintenance and progression of hypertension.[32] Alcohol consumption should therefore be reduced if it is greater than 3 drinks per day. In heavy drinkers, abstinence can lead to impressive reductions in blood pressure.[33]

## 3. Clinical Pharmacology of Drugs Used in Treatment of Hypertension

This section is limited to antihypertensives in common use in the 1990s. The main sites of action of these drugs are shown in figure 1.

### 3.1 Diuretics

Diuretics used in the treatment of hypertension include:

- ***Benzothiadiazines (thiazides)*** such as chlorothiazide, hydrochlorothiazide bendroflumethiazide (bendrofluazide), hydroflumethiazide, methyclothiazide, cyclopenthiazide and polythiazide.

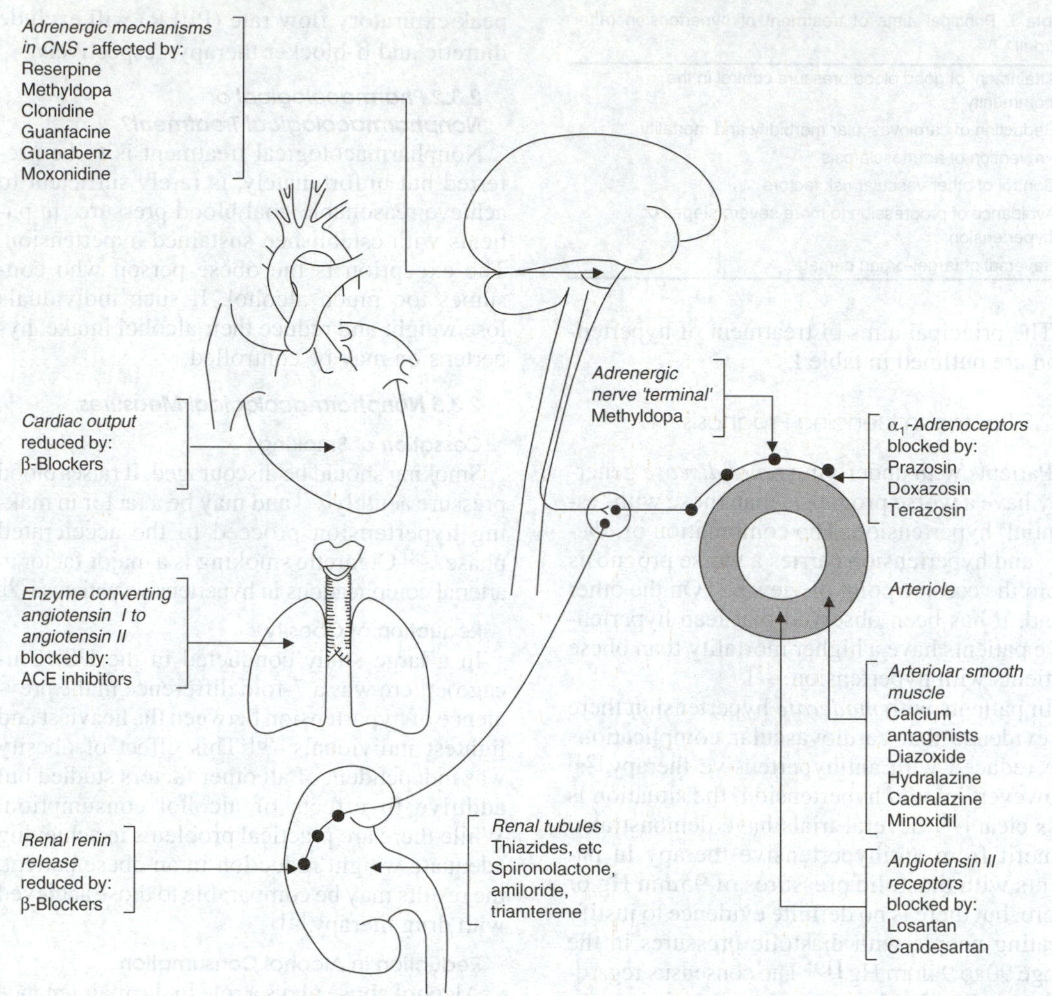


**Fig. 1.** Main sites of action of antihypertensive drugs.

- ***Heterocyclic (thiazide-like)*** agents such as chlorthalidone, clorexolone, quinethazone, metolazone, mefruside, clopamide, indapamide and xipamide.
- ***Loop diuretics*** such as furosemide (frusemide), bumetanide, piretanide, torasemide,[34] ethacrynic acid.
- ***Potassium-sparing diuretics*** such as spironolactone, amiloride and triamterene.

For further discussion of the clinical pharmacology of diuretics, see also chapter 24 (section 5.1) and reviews by Brater[35] and Lant.[36]

#### 3.1.1 Mechanism/Site of Action

The enhanced natriuresis (sodium excretion) achieved by diuretics leads to a reduction in plasma volume and cardiac output. These changes may be offset by reflex activation of the renin-angiotensin system. However, the antihypertensive effect seems to override this reaction. Long term studies have indicated that diuretic therapy is associated with a reduction in systemic vascular resistance, although the mechanism of this effect is unclear. An effect on prostaglandins and reduced arteriolar responsiveness to neuroendocrine vasoconstrictor stimuli have been cited as possible explanations.[37]

The loop diuretics act by inhibiting active chloride transport in the thick ascending limb of the loop of Henle. The benzothiadiazines (thiazides) and related heterocyclic compounds act on the early distal tubule while the potassium-sparing diuretics act at the late distal tubule (see further chapter 24; sect. 5.1).

### 3.1.2 Pharmacodynamic Properties

#### Thiazide and Thiazide-Like Diuretics

The thiazide and thiazide-like diuretics reach their active site in the early distal tubule of the nephron via the probenecid-sensitive organic acid secretory pathway. Their natriuretic effect is less than that of the loop diuretics – 10% *versus* 20% of filtered sodium excreted – and their exact molecular basis of action remains unspecified.[36] A major development in the last 5 years has been the reappraisal of the dose-response relationship of thiazides. It is now recognised that this relationship is of sigmoid shape with a plateau response at doses of 25mg for hydrochlorothiazide and 0.5mg for metolazone.[38,39] Above these threshold doses, hypokalaemia and other adverse effects increase exponentially.

#### Loop Diuretics

The loop diuretics, like the thiazides, are highly protein bound; consequently, they reach their active site by tubular secretion rather than glomerular filtration. After secretion they travel with the tubular fluid to the loop of Henle, where they exert their effect by inhibiting the chloride-sodium/potassium pump. This nephron site usually reabsorbs 20% of filtered sodium and at maximal doses, the loop diuretics cause excretion of 20% of filtered sodium. Because they act at the luminal side of the tubule, it is the luminal rather than the plasma concentration that correlates with natriuretic activity. This correlation is characterised by a sigmoid concentration-response curve. Each loop diuretic has the same maximal response and similar shaped curves; they differ only in potency, bumetanide being 10 times more potent than torasemide and 50 times more potent than furosemide.

#### Potassium-Sparing Diuretics

*Spironolactone*, which structurally resembles aldosterone, acts by competing with the mineralocorticoid for the corresponding receptor protein in the distal nephron. *Triamterene* and *amiloride* act at the cortical collecting duct of the distal tubule and their potassium-sparing effect is mediated by reversing the negatively orientated potential difference in this part of the nephron, thus preventing secretion of positively charged potassium ions. Like spironolactone, these agents have only a modest saluretic effect – 5% *versus* the loop diuretics' 20% fractional sodium excretion (i.e. sodium excretion as a percentage of the sodium filtered).

There is currently no consensus on the dose equivalence of the 3 available potassium-sparing agents.[40]

### 3.1.3 Pharmacokinetic Characteristics

#### Thiazide and Thiazide-Like Diuretics

A major difference between the various thiazide and thiazide-like agents lies in the time-course of their passage through the body. Whereas the plasma half-life of bendroflumethiazide is 3 hours, that of hydrochlorothiazide is 10 to 12 hours and that of the related heterocyclic compound indapamide is 15 to 25 hours. These differences probably relate to enhanced lipid solubility of the latter compounds with consequent larger volumes of distribution.

For other pharmacokinetic parameters of the thiazide and thiazide-like diuretics, see appendix A.

#### Loop Diuretics

The pharmacokinetic characteristics of drugs of this class are broadly similar, although furosemide is somewhat less bioavailable (65%) and torasemide has a slightly longer half-life (2 to 4 hours) than the other drugs. In patients with renal insufficiency, the clearance of loop diuretics is reduced to a fifth of that of individuals with normal renal function.[35] The maximal fractional excretion of sodium is maintained at 20%, but the rate of sodium excretion diminishes, simply because there is less sodium being filtered at the glomerulus. In patients with hepatic insufficiency, the pharmacokinetics of loop diuretics are unchanged but their pharmacodynamic responses are altered, with the result that the fractional excretion of sodium is decreased. The mechanism of this effect is unknown.

In patients with congestive cardiac failure, the absorption of furosemide is much slower than that of bumetanide and torasemide.[41]

#### Potassium-Sparing Diuretics

The oral bioavailability of spironolactone is >70%; following absorption, it is extensively metabolised, principally to canrenone which is pharmacologically active. Amiloride and triamterene have oral bioavailabilities of about 50%. Amiloride is mainly excreted unchanged in the urine, while triamterene is extensively metabolised, some of its metabolites having pharmacological activity (see also chapter 19; sect. 10.2.3).[42]

### 3.1.4 Clinical Effectiveness

Diuretics are effective antihypertensive agents that make a major contribution to reducing cardiovascular mortality. There have been many large multicentre trials in hypertension in which diuretics have been used as first-line treatment over periods of 25 years. The principal drugs used in these studies have been the thiazides hydrochlorothiazide, chlorothiazide and bendroflumethiazide, chlorthalidone, and the potassium-sparing agents amiloride, triamterene and spironolactone. None of these trials has shown any trend that might indicate a different effect of the various diuretics used, and all have produced positive results. In studies comparing diuretics and β-blockers, the results suggest that overall, the two types of drugs have similar effects in protecting against cardiovascular events,[43] although one trial[44] found that diuretics were more effective than a β-blocker (atenolol) in preventing myocardial infarction in elderly patients.

#### 3.1.5 Tolerability and Drug Interactions Potential

The UK Medical Research Council (MRC) trial in hypertension, which was the most comprehensive placebo-controlled study, demonstrated that the most notable adverse effect of bendroflumethiazide was impotence, which resulted in 19.6 withdrawals from the drug per 1000 patient-years.[45] This was surprising, although a similar incidence has been seen with methyldopa. Other adverse effects resulting in drug withdrawals, for which incidences were significantly different from placebo, were:

- In men, gout 12.2; impaired glucose tolerance 9.4; lethargy 6.9; nausea, dizziness or headache 8.6; and constipation 1.6 withdrawals per 1000 patient-years
- In women, impaired glucose tolerance 6.0; lethargy 2.1; nausea, dizziness or headache 16.3; and constipation 2.1 withdrawals per 1000 patient-years.

The MRC study used 10mg bendroflumethiazide per day. In a study that compared the effectiveness and safety of daily doses of 1.25, 2.5, 5.0 and 10mg bendroflumethiazide,[46] the reduction in blood pressure (%) was fairly similar in all four groups, but more importantly, the incidence of adverse effects was clearly dose-related. Similar dose-response and dose-related adverse effect findings have been found with other thiazide diuretics. Thus, previous views of the tolerability of diuretics were based on use of excessive doses.[47]

The most dangerous adverse effect of the potassium-sparing diuretics is hyperkalaemia. This is especially likely to occur in the presence of deteriorating renal function and for this reason elderly patients are at special risk.[48] Gynaecomastia is a prominent adverse effect with spironolactone, and this drug is no longer considered a first-line agent for treatment of hypertension.

Two of the most common adverse effects of diuretics are mild hypovolaemia, which can occur with any type of diuretic, and mild hypokalaemia with potassium-losing agents. The occurrence of the latter is dose-dependent and can be corrected by use of potassium supplements, although concomitant use of a potassium-sparing diuretic is preferable because these drugs also reduce the associated magnesium loss.[47] While elevated low density lipoprotein (LDL) cholesterol levels have been reported in some studies with diuretics, cholesterol elevations have again been shown to be dose-dependent – no effect being seen with bendroflumethiazide 2.5mg daily[46] – and long term studies have generally indicated that lipid changes are minor.[47]

***Drug interactions:*** the antihypertensive effect of thiazide diuretics is inhibited by nonsteroidal anti-inflammatory drugs (NSAIDs), with the possible exception of sulindac, which appears not to inhibit renal prostaglandin synthesis. NSAIDs are also known to decrease the creatinine clearance of patients taking triamterene by up to 72%.[49] The increased incidence of cardiac arrhythmias due to digoxin as a result of diuretic-induced hypokalaemia is well known. The interaction of thiazide diuretics and lithium leading to lithium toxicity is due to the increased proximal tubular reabsorption of lithium (see also appendix B).

Combinations of ACE inhibitors and potassium-sparing diuretics can result in dangerous hyperkalaemia, especially in patients with impaired renal function.

### 3.2 β-Adrenoceptor Blocking Drugs (β-Blockers)

The available β-blockers are listed in table II. Although they possess generally similar antihypertensive effectiveness, the β-blockers vary in their subsidiary pharmacodynamic effects and in their pharmacokinetic properties, and these differences, along with their acquisition costs, facilitate their selection in individual patients.

**Table II.** Pharmacodynamic and pharmacokinetic properties of some commonly used β-adrenoceptor blocking drugs

| Drug | β-Adrenoceptor blockade[a] | | Vasodilator activity | Partial agonist activity[b] | First-pass metabolism | Pharmacokinetic parameters | | | | Principal route(s) of elimination | Lipid solubility[c] |
|---|---|---|---|---|---|---|---|---|---|---|---|
| | $\beta_1$ | $\beta_2$ | | | | F (%) | $t_{1/2}$ (h) | Vd (L) | PB (%) | | |
| Acebutolol | + | 0 | 0 | + | Yes | 40 | 7 | 84 | 20 | Renal/hepatic | + |
| Alprenolol | + | + | 0 | ++ | Yes | 10 | 2.5 | 77 | 76 | Hepatic | +++ |
| Atenolol | + | 0 | 0 | 0 | No | 50-60 | 6-9 | 77 | <5 | Renal | ± |
| Betaxolol | + | 0 | 0 | 0 | No | 80-89 | 18 | 578 | 50 | Hepatic/renal | ++ |
| Bevantolol | + | 0 | 0 | 0 | Yes | 60 | 2 | 105 | 95 | Hepatic | ++ |
| Bisoprolol | + | 0 | 0 | 0 | Yes (10%) | 90 | 10 | 210 | 30 | Hepatic/renal | ++ |
| Bopindolol | + | + | 0 | ++ | ? Yes | 70 | 8-10 | 202 | | Hepatic | |
| Carteolol | + | + | 0 | ++ | Yes (15%) | 83 | 5-7 | 280 | 15 | Renal/hepatic | ± |
| Carvedilol | + | ± | +[d] | 0 | Yes | 25 | 5.8 | 105-140 | ≥95 | Hepatic | +++ |
| Celiprolol | + | 0 | +[e] | + | No | 30-70 | 4-5 | | 25 | Renal | + |
| Esmolol[f] | + | 0 | 0 | 0 | | | 0.15 | 238 | 56 | Blood esterase hydrolysis | + |
| Labetalol | + | + | +[g] | 0 | Yes | 10-80 | 3-5 | 490 | 50 | Hepatic | ++± |
| Metoprolol | + | 0 | 0 | 0 | Yes | 40-50 | 3-4 | 385 | 8-12 | Hepatic | ++ |
| Nadolol | + | + | 0 | 0 | No | 25-30 | 14-24 | 133 | 28 | Renal | ± |
| Oxprenolol | + | + | 0 | ++ | Yes | 25-60 | 2.2 | 91 | 92 | Hepatic | ++ |
| Penbutolol | + | + | 0 | + | No | 100 | 26 | | >95 | Hepatic | ++ |
| Pindolol | + | + | 0 | +++ | No | 100 | 2.5 | 84 | 50 | Renal/hepatic | + |
| Propranolol | + | + | 0 | 0 | Yes | 30 | 3-6 | 196 | 93 | Hepatic | +++ |
| Sotalol | + | + | 0 | 0 | No | >60 | 7.5 | 91 | <1 | Renal | ± |
| Timolol | + | + | 0 | ± | No | 60-75 | 3-5 | 119 | 60 | Hepatic/renal | ++ |

a Relative selectivity for $\beta_1$- and $\beta_2$-adrenoceptors. Although selectivity is not absolute, agents with relative selectivity for $\beta_1$-adrenoceptors are termed 'cardioselective'; those without this property are termed 'nonselective'.

b Intrinsic sympathomimetic activity (+ = mild; ++ = moderate; +++ = marked).

c Based on octanol/water partition coefficient (± = very low; + = low; ++ = moderate; +++ = high).

d Vasodilator activity results from $\alpha_1$-adrenoceptor blockade and possibly a direct peripheral vasodilator effect.

e Vasodilator activity results primarily from a $\beta_2$-agonist effect and direct vasodilator activity; a weak $\alpha_2$-adrenoceptor antagonist effect may also be involved.

f Administered by intravenous infusion only.

g Vasodilator activity results from $\alpha_1$-adrenoceptor blockade.

*Abbreviations:* Vd = apparent volume of distribution; $t_{1/2}$ = elimination half-life; F = oral bioavailability; PB = protein binding.

### 3.2.1 Mechanism/Site of Action

β-Blockers inhibit catecholamine binding at β-adrenoceptor sites. Although there is no consensus as to the precise mechanism whereby they exert their antihypertensive effect, some or all of the following physiological effects may be involved:

- Reduction in cardiac output
- A central nervous system effect
- Inhibition of renin
- Reduction in venous return and plasma volume
- Reduction in peripheral vascular resistance
- Resetting of baroreceptor levels
- Reduction in noradrenaline (norepinephrine) release
- Prevention of the pressor response to catecholamines with exercise and stress.[50]

### 3.2.2 Pharmacodynamic Properties

The pharmacodynamic properties of commonly used β-blockers are shown in table II. Relative selectivity for $\beta_1$-adrenoceptors is a useful attribute, although such selectivity is not absolute and consequently the effect of relatively $\beta_1$-selective agents in patients with chronic obstructive airways disease is unpredictable. For this reason, all β-blockers are contraindicated in patients with asthma. Relatively $\beta_1$-selective agents may however, be more appropriate in diabetic patients, as they are less likely to aggravate hypoglycaemia;[51] they may also be preferable in patients with peripheral vascular disease, as they do not block peripheral $\beta_2$-mediated vasodilatation.[52] At higher doses of these drugs, however, there is evidence that $\beta_2$-blocking effects are unmasked.[53]

β-Blockers with partial agonist (intrinsic sympathomimetic) activity are shown in table II, but it is doubtful whether this effect or any 'membrane-stabilising' activity are relevant clinically.[52] Some β-blockers have vasodilatory activity, e.g. labetalol (due to $\alpha_1$-adrenoceptor blockade), carvedilol (due to $\alpha_1$-adrenoceptor blockade and possibly a direct peripheral effect), and celiprolol (due primarily to a weak $\beta_2$-agonist effect). This has theoretical importance in enhancing the antihypertensive effect and reducing certain adverse effects such as cold extremities. However, postural hypotension may be a problem if the vasodilatation is too marked.

The effects of β-blockers on lipids are discussed in section 3.2.5.

#### 3.2.3 Pharmacokinetic Characteristics

The pharmacokinetic characteristics and lipid solubilities of the β-blockers are shown in table II. As a general rule, the more lipid soluble agents are eliminated by hepatic metabolism and require a dosage reduction in patients with cirrhosis, whereas the more water soluble agents are mainly eliminated by renal excretion and require dosage reduction in patients with renal insufficiency. Some β-blockers (e.g. pindolol, timolol, acebutolol, betaxolol, bisoprolol and carteolol) are partly metabolised and partly excreted unchanged.

For further information on dosage adjustments of β-blockers in renal and hepatic disease, see appendices D and F, respectively.

#### 3.2.4 Clinical Effectiveness

The clinical effectiveness of β-blockers as antihypertensives is well established [for reviews of individual agents, see Frishman et al.[54] (bevantolol); Singh et al.[55] (sotalol); Goa et al.[56] (labetalol); Lancaster & Sorkin[57] (bisoprolol); Dunn & Spencer[58] and Milne & Buckley[59] (celiprolol); Wadworth et al.[60] (atenolol); Harron et al.[61] (bopindolol); McTavish et al.[62] (carvedilol); Peters & Benfield[63] (metoprolol)]. Which patients should receive β-blockers is largely determined by the presence of concomitant disease. A comparison of drug-disease considerations for the β-blockers as compared with other antihypertensive drugs is shown in table III. β-Blockers are contraindicated in patients with congestive heart failure and asthma and are best avoided in patients with chronic obstructive pulmonary disease. However, this reservation may be outweighed by benefit where angina coexists. Similarly, in diabetic patients, aggravation of hypoglycaemia may be offset by benefit in coexisting angina. In patients with peripheral vascular disease, β-blockers have generally shown no benefit or a worsening of symptoms, although drugs with vasodilator activity such as celiprolol and labetalol have been found to produce decreases in peripheral vascular resistance.[64,65]

There appear to be some ethnic differences in clinical responsiveness to β-blockers, Black patients being less responsive than White patients.[66] Similarly, β-blockers appear less beneficial in elderly patients and consequently should not be considered first-line therapy in this age group.[67] The introduction of controlled-release preparations, e.g. of metoprolol, is an interesting recent development[68] as these formulations allow sustained β-blockade over a 24-hour period and minimise the loss of $\beta_1$-selectivity seen at higher doses. Propranolol has shown some adverse effects on quality of life,[69-71] but atenolol is comparable in this respect to captopril, enalapril, cilazapril and verapamil.[71-75]

#### 3.2.5 Tolerability and Drug Interactions Potential

Adverse cardiac effects of β-blockers include, bradycardia, heart failure and, following their abrupt withdrawal, worsening angina and even infarction. Peripheral vascular effects are more likely with drugs not possessing vasodilator activity or relative $\beta_1$-selectivity and include Raynaud's phenomenon, cold extremities and even gangrene, particularly in elderly patients, who show less ability to tolerate β-blockers. Bronchospasm is an important adverse effect but is usually confined to patients with a history of asthma or, more rarely, those with a history of chronic obstructive airways disease. The risk of this adverse effect is lower but still present with the relatively $\beta_1$-selective agents.

Nightmares, vivid dreams and even hallucinations can occur with the more lipophilic β-blockers such as propranolol and oxprenolol. These may sometimes be avoided by using a less lipophilic β-blocker such as atenolol or timolol and by avoiding evening administration.

**Table III.** Comparison of the clinical effects of β-blockers with those of other antihypertensive drugs

| Feature | β-Blockers | Thiazide diuretics | ACE inhibitors | Calcium antagonists | $\alpha_1$-Blockers |
|---|---|---|---|---|---|
| Efficacy in coexisting disease states: | | | | | |
| Angina pectoris | ✓ | x | x | ✓ | x |
| CHF/LVF | x | ✓[a] | ✓ | x | ✓ |
| Supraventricular arrhythmias | ✓ | x | x | ✓[b] | x |
| Raynaud's phenomenon | x | x | x | ✓ | ✓ |
| Asthma | x | ✓ | ✓ | ✓ | ✓ |
| Effect on heart rate | ↓ | ↔ | ↔ | ↔ or ↑ | ↔ |
| Effect on total peripheral resistance | ↑, ↓[c] | ↔ | ↓ | ↓ | ↓ |
| Effect on left ventricular hypertrophy | ↓ | ↔ or ↑ | ↓ | ↓ | ↓ |
| Effect on serum lipids | Generally adverse[d] | Adverse | Neutral/ favourable | Favourable | Favourable |
| Effect on glycaemic control | Generally adverse[e] | Adverse | None | Generally none | None |

a A loop diuretic such as furosemide, piretanide or torasemide may be more suitable if CHF/LVF is predominant.

b Some agents only (e.g. verapamil).

c β-Blockers initially cause a reflex increase in total peripheral resistance followed by a decrease towards or slightly below pretreatment levels with long term use. However, β-blockers with vasodilator activity (see table II) cause a reduction in total peripheral resistance.

d Not all β-blockers have adverse effects on the serum lipid profile; some agents (e.g. carvedilol, celiprolol, labetalol, pindolol) have no clinically significant adverse effects on serum lipids.

e β-Blockers may mask some of the warning signs of hypoglycaemic episodes. Some, though not all, β-blockers may also adversely affect carbohydrate metabolism.

*Abbreviations and symbols:* ACE = angiotensin-converting enzyme; CHF = congestive heart failure; LVF = left ventricular failure; ✓ = used in this indication; x = not indicated; ↑ = increased; ↓ = decreased; ↔ = no significant effect.

Significantly, treatment with β-blockers (particularly propranolol) can result in an increased incidence of sexual dysfunction and physical symptoms which decrease the patient's quality of life.[69] For a review of the adverse effects of β-blockers, see Lewis and Lofthouse.[76]

***Effects on plasma lipids:*** there is concern about the propensity of some (though not all) β-blockers to adversely affect plasma lipids, and in part this may explain the decrease in popularity of β-blockers as antihypertensive agents (as it may theoretically reduce their ability to decrease the risk of coronary artery disease long term). Nonselective β-blockers without partial agonist activity appear to cause a definite increase in very-low density lipoprotein (VLDL) cholesterol and triglycerides, and a decrease in high density lipoprotein (HDL) cholesterol.[77] With atenolol, the effect is less clear, some authors noting an adverse effect on lipoprotein profiles[78] while others have not.[79] Drugs that appear to have little or no adverse effect on plasma lipids include carvedilol, celiprolol, labetalol and pindolol.

***Drug interactions:*** pharmacokinetic drug interactions are seen more commonly with the lipophilic/hepatically metabolised β-blockers (e.g. alprenolol, metoprolol, oxprenolol, propranolol). Thus, cimetidine may cause an increase in plasma concentrations of these β-blockers, whereas rifampicin and phenobarbital, because of enzyme induction, may cause a decrease. Lipophilic β-blockers may cause an increase in plasma concentrations of chlorpromazine, theophylline and warfarin as a result of their effect on hepatic enzyme activity.[80]

Drugs that may cause pharmacodynamic interactions with β-blockers include NSAIDs (reduced antihypertensive effect of β-blockers), prazosin (enhanced first-dose hypotensive effect of prazosin), and verapamil and diltiazem (enhanced depression of myocardial function and atrioventricular conduction).

## 3.3 $\alpha_1$-Adrenoceptor Blockers

### 3.3.1 Mechanism/Site of Action

The quinazoline derivatives, which are selective for postjunctional $\alpha_1$-adrenoceptors, act by causing a decrease in peripheral resistance.[81] Prazosin,[82] doxazosin[83] and terazosin[84] are the most important members of this group in widespread clinical use.

**Table IV.** Key properties of some commonly used $\alpha_1$-adrenoceptor blocking drugs

| Drug | Relative potency[a] | Pharmacokinetic parameters | | | | | | Principal route of elimination |
|---|---|---|---|---|---|---|---|---|
| | | F (%) | $t_{1/2}$ (h) | CL (L/h) | Vd (L) | PB (%) | | |
| Doxazosin | 0.5 | 65 | 5.6[b] | 7.3 | 98 | >98 | | Hepatic |
| Prazosin | 1 | 57 | 3 | 10 | 35 | 94 | | Hepatic |
| Terazosin | 0.1 | 82 | 12 | 3.3 | 21 | 90 | | Hepatic |

a Prazosin = 1.

b At steady-state.

*Abbreviations:* F = oral bioavailability; CL = total plasma clearance; $t_{1/2}$ = elimination half-life; Vd = apparent volume of distribution; PB = protein binding.

### *3.3.2 Pharmacodynamic Properties*

Doxazosin is about one-half as potent as prazosin as a postsynaptic $\alpha_1$-adrenoceptor inhibitor in animal studies[85] while terazosin is about a tenth as potent (table IV).[86] None of these agents has appreciable activity as an inhibitor at the $\alpha_2$-adrenoceptor. All act by decreasing total peripheral resistance, but because of their limited effect at the $\alpha_2$-adrenoceptor, they cause only a small reflex increase in heart rate and cardiac output.

The concentration-effect relationship is complex for these agents but is definitely not linear; the maximum plasma concentration ($C_{max}$) for doxazosin occurs 2 to 3 hours after administration, whereas the maximum antihypertensive effect occurs at 5 to 6 hours.[87] However, using an integrated pharmacokinetic-pharmacodynamic analysis, drug concentrations in a peripheral 'effect' compartment have been correlated with reductions in blood pressure and $\alpha_1$-adrenoceptor activity.[88]

Doxazosin and prazosin increase plasma renin minimally,[89] whereas terazosin seems to have a greater effect.[90] Unlike other antihypertensive agents, the $\alpha_1$-blockers tend to have a favourable effect on plasma lipids, prazosin increasing HDL-cholesterol by up to 6%,[91] terazosin by up to 20%,[92] and doxazosin by up to 13%.[93]

### *3.3.3 Pharmacokinetic Characteristics*

Pharmacokinetic parameters for the α-blockers are shown in table IV. Whereas prazosin has a short elimination half-life of 2.5 hours and consequently a relatively short duration of action requiring 2 to 3 doses per day,[94] the elimination half-lives of doxazosin and terazosin are considerably longer at 13 to 16 and 12 hours, respectively, which allows once-daily administration of these agents. Elimination of all three drugs is mainly by hepatic metabolism (to inactive metabolites which are excreted via the biliary route). Neither renal insufficiency nor age appears to affect the pharmacokinetics of the $\alpha_1$-blockers.

### *3.3.4 Clinical Effectiveness*

In a comparative trial of once-daily terazosin and twice-daily prazosin, there was no significant difference between the blood pressure changes induced by either agent and both were superior to placebo.[91] However, a statistically significant increase in pulse rate over baseline of 4 beats/min was seen with terazosin. In an 18-week study comparing terazosin and doxazosin, the reductions in blood pressure were similar for both drugs.[95]

In a comparison between terazosin and hydrochlorothiazide, the reduction in supine diastolic pressure was significantly greater with the latter.[96] In two trials, doxazosin had similar effectiveness to hydrochlorothiazide[93,97] but was less effective in a third trial.[98]

### *3.3.5 Tolerability and Drug Interactions Potential*

The adverse effect profile is similar for all 3 agents, consisting mainly of postural dizziness and headache, with a slightly increased incidence of nasal congestion with terazosin in comparison with prazosin.[91,99] Verapamil decreases the first-pass metabolism of prazosin and increases its oral bioavailability and peak plasma concentrations, thereby enhancing its antihypertensive effect; the available data suggest that this is a result of a pharmacokinetic interaction between the two drugs,[100] although a pharmacodynamic interaction at vascular smooth muscle may also occur.[101] Cimetidine causes an increase in plasma concentrations of all the $\alpha_1$-blockers and a dose adjustment may be required when these agents are used concomitantly.

Overall, terazosin and doxazosin have proved more popular than prazosin because of their longer half-lives, which allow once or twice daily administration and hence better compliance, and also a perceived lesser incidence of 'first-dose' postural hypotension, which may reflect more careful dose titration. They have comparable effectiveness to β-blockers and diuretics and their effect on plasma lipids is a theoretical advantage. However, their effect on mortality from stroke and myocardial infarction has not been assessed, nor have many quality-of-life studies been carried out.[102] Consequently, the $\alpha_1$-blockers are not widely regarded as first-line therapy in hypertension at the present time.

## 3.4 Calcium Antagonists

The calcium antagonists available for the treatment of hypertension are shown in table V. Within this group, there are three distinct chemical classes:

- ***Phenylalkylamines*** such as verapamil[104] and gallopamil.[105]
- ***Benzothiazepines*** such as diltiazem.[106]
- ***Dihydropyridines*** such as nifedipine,[107,108] felodipine,[109,110] amlodipine,[111] isradipine,[112,113] lacidipine,[114] nicardipine,[115,116] nisoldipine,[117] nitrendipine,[118] and nilvadipine.[119]

### 3.4.1 Mechanism/Site of Action

The calcium antagonists act by blocking the entry of calcium ions into cells during the depolarised phase of the action potential.[120] Consequently, they reduce the amount of calcium ions available for excitation-contraction. Vascular smooth muscle is most sensitive to such blockade. There are two types of calcium channels: potential-mediated and receptor-mediated. The dihydropyridines (e.g. nifedipine) block the former while the phenylalkylamines (e.g. verapamil) block the latter. The benzothiazepines (e.g. diltiazem) seem to have an intermediate action.

### 3.4.2 Pharmacodynamic Properties

Unlike the three prototype agents verapamil, diltiazem and nifedipine, the newer calcium antagonists act at low plasma concentrations, thus making it difficult to carry out concentration-effect studies. Furthermore, as a class, they are subject to considerable intra- and inter-individual variability following a given dose. However, correlations (probably linear) have been shown between plasma concentrations and the blood pressure lowering effect for most agents.[103,121-123]

### 3.4.3 Pharmacokinetic Characteristics

Pharmacokinetic parameters for the available calcium antagonists are shown in table V. In general, the newer agents resemble the three prototype drugs (verapamil, diltiazem, nifedipine) in their pharmacokinetic characteristics, all being subject to substantial first-pass metabolism (leading to low and variable bioavailabilities) and are principally eliminated by hepatic metabolism, the fraction eliminated unchanged by the kidney being very small. However, the newer agents tend to have longer elimination half-lives and may be suitable for twice- or even once-daily administration; the two agents with the longest elimination half-lives are amlodipine and lacidipine (34h and 18.7h, respectively), both of which are given once daily. Nevertheless, controlled-release formulations of a number of agents are now available (e.g. nifedipine, verapamil, diltiazem, felodipine, nicardipine, isradipine) and these formulations permit once- or twice-daily administration of these drugs. The advantages of the controlled-release preparations are lower $C_{max} : C_{min}$ ratios (i.e. lower peak : trough plasma concentration ratios), lower $C_{max}$ values, and a slower rate of increase in plasma concentrations in comparison with conventional formulations, producing fewer fluctuations in blood pressure and a lower tendency for concentration-related adverse effects.[103]

In elderly patients, a reduction in intrinsic clearance and in hepatic blood flow leads to decreased clearance and increased plasma concentrations of calcium antagonists (table V). Similarly, clearance is decreased in patients with cirrhosis, resulting in higher plasma concentrations and greater peak blood pressure decreases. However, renal impairment has little effect on the clearance or plasma concentrations of these drugs.[103] Because calcium antagonists undergo hepatic metabolism, enzyme-inducing drugs would be expected to influence their kinetics.[124]

### 3.4.4 Clinical Effectiveness

The antihypertensive effectiveness of the calcium antagonists is well established, both for conventional and controlled-release formulations. In the Veterans Administration Cooperative Study Group on Antihypertensive Agents, in which 1292 men were randomised to mono-

**Table V.** Pharmacokinetic properties of some currently available calcium antagonists (after Kelly & O'Malley[103])

| Drug | Class[a] | Pharmacokinetic parameters | | | | | Influence of old age and disease states on elimination | | |
|---|---|---|---|---|---|---|---|---|---|
| | | F (%) | $t_{1/2}$ (h) | CL (L/h) | Vd (L) | PB (%) | old age | renal disease | hepatic disease |
| Amlodipine | D | 64 | 34 | 21.5 | 1470 | 95 | CL$\downarrow$, $t_{1/2}\uparrow$ | CL$\leftrightarrow$, $t_{1/2}\leftrightarrow$ | CL$\downarrow$, $t_{1/2}\uparrow$ |
| Diltiazem | B | 39 | 5.7 | 60 | 315 | 80-86 | CL$\downarrow$, $t_{1/2}\uparrow$ | CL$\leftrightarrow$, $t_{1/2}\leftrightarrow$ | CL$\downarrow$ |
| Felodipine | D | 16 | 11.4 | 69 | 679 | 99 | CL$\downarrow$, $t_{1/2}\uparrow$ | CL$\leftrightarrow$, $t_{1/2}\leftrightarrow$ | CL$\downarrow$ |
| Gallopamil | P | 22.6[b] | 2.5-5.5 | 66-72 | 145 | 93 | | | CL$\downarrow$, $t_{1/2}\uparrow$ |
| Isradipine | D | 19 | 8.4 | 40 | 203[c] | 96 | $t_{1/2}\uparrow$ | CL$\leftrightarrow$, $t_{1/2}\leftrightarrow$ | CL$\downarrow$ |
| Lacidipine | D | 18.5 | 18.7[c] | | 573 | >90 | | | |
| Nicardipine | D | 15-40[d] | 1 | 42 | 52.5 | >98 | | $t_{1/2}\leftrightarrow$ | CL$\downarrow$, $t_{1/2}\uparrow$ |
| Nifedipine | D | 45 | 3.4 | 37 | 98 | >96 | | | CL$\downarrow$, $t_{1/2}\uparrow$ |
| Nilvadipine | D | 14-19 | 14 | 76 | 1680 | 98 | | | CL$\downarrow$ |
| Nisoldipine | D | 4 | 15.4 | 50 | 245 | 99 | $t_{1/2}\uparrow$ | CL$\leftrightarrow$, $t_{1/2}\leftrightarrow$ | CL$\downarrow$ |
| Nitrendipine | D | 16 | 8.6 | 80 | 378 | 99 | $t_{1/2}\leftrightarrow$ | CL$\leftrightarrow$, $t_{1/2}\uparrow$ or $\leftrightarrow$ | CL$\downarrow$, $t_{1/2}\uparrow$ |
| Verapamil | P | 24 | 5.7[b] | 52 | 308 | 90 | CL$\downarrow$, $t_{1/2}\uparrow$ | | CL$\downarrow$, $t_{1/2}\uparrow$ |

a Chemical class (D = dihydropyridine; B = benzothiazepine; P = phenylalkylamine).

b With repeated administration.

c At steady-state.

d Dose-dependent.

*Abbreviations and symbols:* F = oral bioavailability; CL = total plasma clearance; $t_{1/2}$ = elimination half-life; Vd = apparent volume of distribution; PB = protein binding; $\downarrow$ = tends to decrease; $\uparrow$ = tends to increase; $\leftrightarrow$ = no change.

therapy with controlled-release diltiazem, clonidine, atenolol, hydrochlorothiazide, prazosin, captopril or placebo, controlled-release diltiazem achieved the highest response rates both in the titration period of up to 8 weeks and the maintenance phase of 1 year.[125] Diltiazem was also the most effective treatment in both older and younger Black patients. The latter may be a class effect, as it is also seen with sustained-release nifedipine and sustained-release verapamil.[126,127] Satisfactory effectiveness in elderly patients has also been demonstrated with nicardipine, diltiazem, felodipine, nilvadipine, sustained-release nifedipine, and sustained-release verapamil. Decreases in left ventricular hypertrophy have been seen with nicardipine and felodipine.[128,129] Whether regression of left ventricular hypertrophy in hypertensive patients has a beneficial effect on cardiac morbidity and mortality is still controversial.[130] Isradipine was found to be superior to atenolol for the treatment of hypertension in one study.[131]

With regard to heart rate, both diltiazem and verapamil tend to cause a decrease, isradipine causes a slight increase, and the other calcium antagonists are neutral in their effect. Sustained-release nicardipine has been observed to improve quality of life in elderly patients,[116] while sustained-release nifedipine had a deleterious effect on symptoms, psychological well-being and subjective cognitive function in elderly patients in contrast to sustained-release verapamil.[132]

### 3.4.5 Tolerability and Drug Interactions Potential

Adverse effects with the calcium antagonists appear to some extent to be class-related, the most common being headaches, flushing, ankle oedema and palpitations precipitated by the vasodilator properties of these drugs. Adverse effects are also dose-related, and tolerance to them develops with time. Interestingly, in a study with isradipine, tolerance to the adverse effects with time developed to the lower and not the higher dose.[133] Adverse effects with sustained-release nifedipine have led to higher treatment cessation rates than observed with isradipine, spironolactone, enalapril and metoprolol.[108] In general, vasodilatation-related adverse effects are less common with the sustained-release formulations, although this has not been seen with felodipine.[134] With verapamil, constipation is commonly experienced and can be a problem.

Meta-analyses of trials examining the use of immediate-release nifedipine in post-myocardial infarction patients have suggested an increased risk of mortality of 16%.[135,136] This drug, and possibly other calcium antagonists are therefore not recommended following a myocardial infarction. In addition, a recent case control study has suggested an increased mortality from immediate-release nifedipine in the treatment of hypertension.[137] However, a case control study cannot be conclusive in this situation as the presence of severe or complicated hypertension may have led to the use of a calcium antagonist. Consequently, the evidence against the use of any calcium antagonist in hypertensive patients who have not sustained a myocardial infarction is very weak.

***Drug interactions:*** calcium antagonists raise plasma digoxin concentrations when these agents are administered concomitantly, and this is a potentially serious interaction. They also raise plasma concentrations of lipophilic β-blockers and may cause potentially serious cardiac depression, as seen with sustained-release nifedipine and propranolol. Alcohol raises plasma nifedipine concentration while cimetidine raises plasma concentrations of all the calcium antagonists with which it has been studied, and its concomitant use may necessitate dosage adjustment. Both verapamil and nifedipine have been found to prolong the activity of neuromuscular blocking agents and this may be a class effect.

Theophylline concentrations are also increased by some calcium antagonists, and theophylline concentrations should be monitored. Diltiazem has been shown to increase cyclosporin concentrations, which has implications for renal transplant recipients in whom lower doses of cyclosporin can be given.[138]

### 3.5 Angiotensin-Converting Enzyme (ACE) Inhibitors

The currently available ACE inhibitors are shown in table VI. The first agents of this class to become available were captopril[141] and enalapril.[142,143] Subsequently, a number of others have been released including benazepril,[144] cilazapril,[145] fosinopril,[146,147] lisinopril,[148] perindopril,[149] quinapril,[150] ramipril,[151] spirapril,[152] trandolapril,[153] moexipril, zofenopril and delapril.

#### 3.5.1 Mechanism/Site of Action

ACE inhibitors competitively inhibit the action of the angiotensin-converting enzyme,[154] which catalyses the formation of the highly potent vasoconstrictor angiotensin II[155] and the destruction of the potent vasodilator bradykinin.[156] However, their main pharmacological and clinical effects are mediated through the inhibition of angiotensin II formation, as there are enzymes other than ACE that catalyse the de-

**Table VI.** Pharmacokinetic properties of ACE inhibitors (after Burnier & Biollaz;[139] Leonetti & Cuspardi[140])

| Drug | Prodrug | Pharmacokinetic parameters[a] | | | | Principal route(s) of elimination |
|---|---|---|---|---|---|---|
| | | $t_{max}$ (h) | $t_{1/2}$ (h) | Vd (L) | PB (%) | |
| Benazepril | Yes | 1.5 | 2-3 (22)[b] | 8.4 | >95 | Renal |
| Captopril | No | 1.0 | 2.0 | 49[c] | 30 | Renal |
| Cilazapril | Yes | 3.0 | 2 (40-50)[b] | 35 | | Renal |
| Delapril | Yes | 1.0 | 1.5 | | | Renal/hepatic |
| Enalapril | Yes | 3-4 | 5 (35)[b] | | 50 | Renal |
| Fosinopril | Yes | 3.0 | 2-4 (12)[b] | 10.5 | 95 | Hepatic/renal |
| Lisinopril | No | 6.0 | 12 (30)[b] | 124 | <1 | Renal |
| Moexipril | Yes | 1-4 | 2 | | 72 | Hepatic/renal |
| Perindopril | Yes | 3-4 | 4-5 (25)[b] | 15.4 | <30 | Renal/hepatic |
| Quinapril | Yes | 2.0 | 2-3 | | 97 | Renal |
| Ramipril | Yes | 3.0 | 3.0 (110)[b] | 90 | 56 | Renal/hepatic |
| Spirapril | Yes | 2-3 | 2 (30-40) | | | Renal/hepatic |
| Trandolapril | Yes | 4-6 | 16-24 | | 94 | Renal/hepatic |
| Zofenopril | Yes | 1.0 | 5.5 | 91 | 75-86 | Renal/hepatic |

a Values shown are for active metabolite if compound is a prodrug.

b Terminal phase elimination half-life.

c At steady-state.

*Abbreviations and symbols:* $t_{max}$ = time to peak plasma concentration (after oral administration); $t_{1/2}$ = elimination half-life; Vd = apparent volume of distribution; PB = protein binding; ACE = angiotensin-converting enzyme.

struction of bradykinin. The antihypertensive effect of the ACE inhibitors is due to a reduction in total peripheral resistance, an effect that is intensified in sodium-depleted states.[157]

### 3.5.2 Pharmacodynamic Properties

In terms of potency, enalapril is twice as potent as captopril, lisinopril is 7 times as potent, and ramipril and cilazapril 10 times as potent. In concentration-effect studies with ACE inhibitors, drug concentration–ACE inhibition effect plots have indicated that the binding to ACE is saturable. There is a nonlinear (exponential) relationship between plasma drug concentrations and angiotensin II concentrations[158] and also a complex correlation between ACE inhibition and blood pressure.[159]

With enalapril, there is a very close correlation between the first dose and long term blood pressure response, which may provide a simple method of response prediction.[160] However, this correlation does not hold for other ACE inhibitors. Although levels of angiotensin I rise with ACE inhibition, this rise does not seem to lead to the development of tolerance to these drugs.

For a review of the pharmacodynamics of the ACE inhibitors, see Belz et al.[161]

### 3.5.3 Pharmacokinetic Characteristics

Pharmacokinetic parameters for the ACE inhibitors are shown in table VI. Except for captopril and lisinopril, all are prodrugs and are converted to their pharmacologically active forms in the liver. Bioavailability varies between 25 and 80% for those drugs for which data are available (see appendix A). Food slows the absorption of captopril, cilazapril and perindopril with modest short term effects on intensity of ACE inhibition. Most ACE inhibitors are eliminated via the kidneys, with only minor amounts eliminated via hepatic metabolism. Thus, dosages of ACE inhibitors usually need to be reduced in renal failure in proportion to the reduction in creatinine clearance (see appendix D). However, some ACE inhibitors such as fosinopril, spirapril and trandolapril are eliminated by both the kidneys and liver, and when one route of elimination is reduced, there is an increase in the fractional elimination via the alternative route. With these drugs, dosage adjustments may not be needed in patients with renal impairment, except perhaps where renal function is markedly reduced.[140]

Many ACE inhibitors show polyphasic elimination kinetics, and terminal phase elimination half-lives for the various drugs are shown in table VI. Although the half-life corresponds to the elimination of ACE-bound drug and reflects the affinity and strength of binding to ACE, it does not always parallel the duration of antihypertensive activity; some drugs need to be given twice daily to maintain 24-hours' blood pressure control whereas others can be administered once daily.[140] For most ACE inhibitors, plasma concentrations and area under the plasma concentrations-time curve (AUC) are higher in elderly patients and consequently caution in initial dose selection in this age group is recommended.[162]

### 3.5.4 Clinical Effectiveness

When administered in effective dosages, all the ACE inhibitors produce a clinically relevant reduction in blood pressure in hypertensive patients. Several generalisations can be made:

- They are effective antihypertensives both as monotherapy and in combination
- An increased antihypertensive response is seen when ACE inhibitors are combined with diuretics
- Tolerance to the antihypertensive effect does not occur over time
- They are beneficial in diabetic patients because of their anti-proteinuric effect
- They are well tolerated in elderly patients.

Unlike other antihypertensives, the ACE inhibitors do not interfere with normal haemodynamic reactions to stress and exercise. A low sodium intake enhances their antihypertensive effect.

Although the ACE inhibitors appear equally effective in lowering blood pressure, there are some differences among them in terms of their effectiveness in Black patients. The antihypertensive response appears to be lower with lisinopril, benazepril, enalapril and captopril in Black patients than in White patients,[163-166] but equivalent for fosinopril and quinapril.[167,168] The lower response to enalapril is, however, eliminated with the addition of a diuretic.

Quality of life is well maintained with ACE inhibitors:

- Captopril has proved equivalent to atenolol and verapamil[72,73,75] and equivalent to enalapril and atenolol, all of which were superior to propranolol[169]
- Enalapril was equivalent to atenolol[71] and to verapamil, but superior to atenolol and a diuretic in a nonrandomised trial[170]

• Cilazapril was equivalent to atenolol and superior to sustained-release nifedipine.[74]

There have been relatively few trials of ACE inhibitors in severe hypertension, although ramipril either alone or in combination achieved satisfactory control in 18 of 20 of such patients in one trial.[171]

Although acute renal failure secondary to ACE inhibitor therapy in patients with bilateral renal artery stenosis has been rightly highlighted, long term treatment has been shown to improve renal function or arrest its deterioration in patients with essential hypertension, moderate to severe renal impairment and no renal artery stenosis.[172]

For further discussion of the use of ACE inhibitors in endocrine hypertension, see chapter 19 (section 10.2.4).

#### 3.5.5 Tolerability and Drug Interactions Potential

Adverse effects with ACE inhibitors are common to the whole class. The most frequent adverse effect is cough, which occurs in about 20% of patients,[73] while dizziness, headache, fatigue and musculoskeletal pain occur in less than 10%. First-dose and orthostatic hypotension are other class-specific effects, though they are reportedly less frequent with quinapril.[150] The first-dose hypotensive effect is exacerbated by volume depletion due either to disease or to prior diuretic therapy.[173] Interestingly, if a patient is intolerant of one ACE inhibitor, there is some evidence that he or she can successfully be switched to another.[174]

Angioneurotic oedema is a serious, although rare, adverse reaction. Some evidence suggests that ACE inhibitors suppress erythropoietin production in patients with chronic renal failure or in renal transplant recipients;[175] haemoglobin concentrations have decreased by 10 to 15% as a consequence. This does not occur, however, in patients with normal renal function. White cell counts are reduced but stay within normal limits with captopril in hypertensive patients without renal failure.[75]

Perinatal renal failure, oligohydramnios, delayed fetal growth and decreased fetal survival have been described when women received enalapril or captopril during pregnancy (see also chapters 2 and 18).[176,177] These must be considered class effects, and consequently ACE inhibitor use during pregnancy should be avoided.

***Drug interactions*** are unusual with ACE inhibitors. Concomitant administration of nonsteroidal anti-inflammatory drugs (NSAIDs) may attenuate the antihypertensive effect of ACE inhibitors. On the credit side, concomitant administration of ACE inhibitors with diuretics has been shown to improve the metabolic adverse effect profile of diuretics. However, administration with potassium-sparing diuretics should be avoided because of an increased risk of hyperkalaemia.

### 3.6 Drugs with a Central Action

The most commonly used agents of this class are methyldopa, clonidine,[178] and moxonidine.[179] Despite its age, methyldopa is still used either as add-on therapy in refractory hypertension or as maintenance therapy in hypertension in pregnancy (see further section 8 and chapter 18; sect. 3.3). Two older centrally-acting drugs which are less commonly used nowadays are guanabenz[180] and guanfacine.[181]

#### 3.6.1 Mechanism/Site of Action

***Methyldopa*** acts mainly by dampening down sympathetic outflow from the central nervous system but may also block adrenergic nerve terminals on the arteriole.

For ***clonidine***, the proposed mechanisms of action are multiple;[182] its antihypertensive effect is mainly due to stimulation of central postsynaptic $\alpha_2$-adrenoceptors, but it may also interfere with the peripheral regulation of noradrenaline via its partial agonist activity at presynaptic $\alpha_2$-adrenoceptors. Clonidine also suppresses plasma renin activity, the mechanism of which is uncertain. ***Moxonidine*** is structurally related to clonidine but has a different pharmacological profile. It is a selective high-affinity imidazoline $I_1$ receptor agonist with 600-fold greater affinity for this site than $\alpha_2$-receptors.[179]

#### 3.6.2 Pharmacodynamic Properties

***Methyldopa*** reduces blood pressure without causing much change in heart rate or cardiac output. The minimum effective dose is 125mg twice daily with a maximum daily dose of 3g. At 1.5g per day there does seem to be a plateau dose-response, with dose-related adverse effects becoming very prominent beyond this dose.

***Clonidine:*** after a 0.2mg oral dose of clonidine, renal, hepatic and limb blood flow are unaltered, while heart rate decreases by 10%, mean systemic pressure by 14%, and pulmonary capillary wedge pressure by 27%. Systemic vascular resistance is reduced slightly, but with 0.4mg orally it is reduced by 21%. The effect is dose-related and the antihypertensive effect is directly related to plasma clonidine concentrations. Rebound hypertension can occur on abrupt cessation of high-dose oral clonidine; however, this is not seen with transdermal clonidine which provides therapeutically effective concentrations at a constant rate over 7 days. Plasma concentrations of clonidine are similar for both the oral and transdermal forms. The maximum blood pressure lowering effect of the transdermal formulation is comparatively delayed, taking 2 or more days.[178]

***Moxonidine:*** binding at central imidazoline receptors correlates with the degree of blood pressure reduction. Like clonidine, moxonidine also causes a reduction in plasma noradrenaline (norepinephrine) and renin concentrations. Efficacy is dose-related in a linear fashion and is mediated through a reduction in systemic vascular resistance.[179]

#### 3.6.3 Pharmacokinetic Characteristics

***Methyldopa*** is incompletely absorbed, and its bioavailability varies between 8 and 62%.[183] Extrarenal clearance of the drug is 50% of total body clearance. Following oral administration, 25 to 50% of the total dose is excreted as acid-labile conjugates, mainly methyldopa-*O*-sulfate, which has some antihypertensive activity. Methyldopa accumulates in renal insufficiency, and dosage reduction is required (see appendix D). It is excreted in breast milk in small amounts.[184]

***Clonidine:*** oral absorption of this drug is rapid and its bioavailability by this route is up to 95%. The pharmacokinetics of clonidine are nonlinear with an elimination half-life of 6 to 13 hours. In contrast, transdermal clonidine gives similar mean plasma concentrations to the oral formulation but without the peak and trough characteristics of the latter. Around 50% of a clonidine dose is eliminated unchanged in the urine. Following oral administration, plasma concentrations are increased in patients with renal failure and in elderly patients. However, once-weekly application of the transdermal formulation controls blood pressure in patients with renal failure without concomitant increases in plasma concentrations. The transdermal formulation is well tolerated in elderly patients, in whom dose adjustment is not required.

***Moxonidine:*** the oral bioavailability of this drug is 88%, and peak plasma concentrations occur at 1 hour after administration; food has no effect on its absorption. Although the half-life of moxonidine is between 2 and 3 hours, the duration of its antihypertensive effect is up to 12 hours, signifying either slower clearance of drug from the central site of action or delayed decreases in noradrenaline concentrations. As 67% of an administered dose is cleared renally, dose reductions are required in patients with renal insufficiency and in elderly individuals.[179]

#### 3.6.4 Clinical Effectiveness

***Methyldopa:*** the clinical effectiveness of methyldopa in comparison with diuretics and β-blockers has been demonstrated (both as monotherapy and in combination), and it has also been shown to reduce left ventricular hypertrophy.[185] However, trials comparing it with the newer ACE inhibitors, calcium antagonists and newer α-blockers are lacking. Methyldopa has proved clinically useful as add-on therapy in refractory hypertension, which is its main current use. It is still the mainstay of maintenance antihypertensive therapy in pregnancy (see section 8 and also chapter 18; sect. 3.3).[186]

***Clonidine:*** transdermal clonidine has proved as effective as oral clonidine in open comparative clinical trials, and it was comparable to propranolol in a double-blind trial.[187] The use of oral clonidine has largely fallen into abeyance because of its adverse effects, but the once-weekly administration of schedule of the transdermal formulation may offer advantages in terms of patient convenience.

***Moxonidine:*** in noncomparative studies with this agent, systolic blood pressure was reduced by up to 30mm Hg and diastolic by up to 20mm Hg in patients with mild to moderate hypertension; the dose used was 0.2 to 0.4mg daily for up to 1 year. Unlike oral clonidine, rebound hypertension was not seen on drug withdrawal. In comparative trials, moxonidine 0.2mg once or twice daily has proved equivalent to clonidine, atenolol, sustained-release nifedipine, captopril and hydrochlorothiazide in terms of effectiveness.[179]

#### 3.6.5 Tolerability and Drug Interactions Potential

***Methyldopa:*** adverse effects are prominent (>15%) especially at the beginning of therapy; they are generally dose-related and include lassitude, somnolence, depression and sexual dysfunction. Autoimmune haemolytic anaemia, hepatic dysfunction, drug fever and antinuclear antibody formation, while rare and infrequent causes of clinical problems, do require vigilance.

Concomitant iron therapy reduces the absorption of methyldopa by up to 73%, probably by chelation.[188] Iron salts also seem to inhibit the excretion of the drug, with accumulation of the sulfate metabolite. This may be clinically significant, especially in pregnancy where the two drugs are commonly used together; in one study[188] concomitant administration led to an enhanced antihypertensive effect. Unlike the older adrenergic neuron blocking drugs (e.g. guanethidine, debrisoquine, bethanidine), a reduction in antihypertensive effect of methyldopa does not occur when it is given with tricyclic antidepressants, as its main action is central and, moreover, it would rarely be used in a depressed patient because of its own depressant effects. In one of the first quality-of-life studies performed,[69] 27% of patients taking methyldopa discontinued treatment (19% because of adverse effects), compared with 23% for propranolol (13% because of adverse effects) and 15% for captopril (8% because of adverse effects). The adverse effect of methyldopa on quality of life appeared to be due to its central actions.

***Clonidine:*** with oral administration, adverse effects include dry mouth (33% of patients), drowsiness (20%), dizziness (15%), nausea (7%) and impotence (6%). Adverse effects are less with the transdermal formulation but in a double-blind comparison with propranolol,[187] the incidence of drowsiness was 20% and dry mouth 26%.

***Moxonidine:*** the adverse effects of this drug include dry mouth (15%), tiredness (5.6%) and headache (1.2%). Significantly, sedation does not appear to occur.[179] Moxonidine appears to have fewer adverse effects than clonidine.

## 3.7 Direct-Acting Vasodilators

Drugs of this class include hydralazine, cadralazine and minoxidil.

### 3.7.1 Mechanism/Site of Action

Hydralazine lowers blood pressure by reducing peripheral vascular resistance as a result of arterial smooth muscle relaxation. Similarly, cadralazine acts by decreasing peripheral vascular resistance by an unspecified action on arteriolar smooth muscle.

Minoxidil acts by activating potassium channels. It is a powerful vasodilator acting directly on vascular smooth muscle.

### 3.7.2 Pharmacokinetic Characteristics

***Hydralazine:*** an important pharmacokinetic characteristic of hydralazine is that its elimination is subject to acetylation polymorphism, some individuals (50% of Caucasians) being classified as slow acetylators and others as rapid acetylators. Plasma concentrations of the drug are higher in slow acetylators; bioavailability is 35% in slow and 10% in rapid acetylators. Hydralazine is extensively metabolised, less than 10% of the drug being excreted unchanged. Despite this, its plasma concentrations are elevated in patients with renal insufficiency.

***Cadralazine*** is rapidly absorbed, and its bioavailability is 95%. Unlike hydralazine, cadralazine undergoes only limited metabolism; 80% of the drug is recovered unchanged in the urine. Consequently, dose reduction is necessary in elderly patients and those with renal failure.

***Minoxidil*** is mainly eliminated by hepatic metabolism, less than 12% being excreted in the urine as unchanged drug. Its plasma half-life is 3 to 4 hours, although its duration of effect may last up to 72 hours, perhaps because of its high affinity for vascular smooth muscle.

### 3.7.3 Clinical Effectiveness

In terms of antihypertensive effectiveness, ***hydralazine*** has proved comparable to diuretics, β-blockers and centrally-acting antihypertensives. ***Cadralazine*** has not been studied in large numbers of patients and comparative studies are few. However, in noncomparative studies, cadralazine 10 to 30 mg/day has reduced systolic and diastolic blood pressure by up to 16mm Hg. Also, combination therapy of cadralazine with a diuretic or a β-blocker was superior to β-blocker monotherapy. From the available comparative studies, cadralazine appears comparable in effectiveness to hydralazine and prazosin.[189]

***Minoxidil*** is particularly effective in patients who are resistant to standard antihypertensive therapy,[190] although comparative studies with modern antihypertensive therapy have not been performed.

### 3.7.4 Tolerability and Drug Interactions Potential

***Hydralazine:*** adverse effects are typical of a direct-acting vasodilator and include headache, asthenia, dizziness, oedema and flushing in more than 10% of patients. Concomitant administration of a β-blocker reduces the incidence of these adverse effects. Much importance has been attached to the occurrence of a systemic lupus-like syndrome with high-dose hydralazine. However, the incidence of this syndrome has lessened with decreasing dosage, and the syndrome, which is rare anyway, does not usually produce clinical difficulties and resolves quickly with withdrawal of the drug.

***Cadralazine:*** adverse effects are vasodilator-related and include headache, flushing, asthenia and dizziness seemingly with lesser frequency than that seen with hydralazine. The lupus-like syndrome has not yet been reported with cadralazine.

***Minoxidil:*** the main limitation to the use of minoxidil as monotherapy is the high incidence (>30%) of vasodilator effects. In addition, hirsutism has been seen in a substantial number of patients. Consequently, minoxidil is reserved for refractory hypertension, mainly in men.

## 3.8 Newer Agents

Newer agents include the 'potassium channel opener' *pinacidil*,[191] the serotonin$_2$ (5-HT$_2$) antagonist *ketanserin*,[192] and the angiotensin II receptor antagonist *losartan*.[193]

### 3.8.1 Mechanism/Site of Action

***Pinacidil*** is a vasodilator belonging to a novel class of drugs known as potassium channel openers. When potassium channels are opened, potassium leaks from cells, resulting in a negative shift in the resting membrane potential. The cells hyperpolarise, which results in a decrease in intracellular calcium and relaxation of smooth muscle, particularly in the vasculature.

***Ketanserin*** is a serotonin (5-HT) antagonist that binds primarily to 5-HT$_2$ receptors, but also has weak $\alpha_1$-adrenoceptor antagonist activity. It may also have other actions such as depression of the renin-angiotensin-aldosterone system and sympathetic inhibition, but the relevance of these mechanisms to its antihypertensive effect is uncertain.[192]

***Losartan*** is the first of a new class of antihypertensive agents that act by blocking angiotensin II, subtype 1 (AT$_1$) receptors. These receptors, which are located primarily in vascular and cardiac tissue and also in the brain, kidney and adrenal gland, mediate the effects of angiotensin II (the primary mediator of the renin-angiotensin system) which is involved in blood pressure control via: (a) direct vasoconstriction of arteriolar smooth muscle; (b) release of aldosterone (and cortisol) from the adrenal cortex; and (c) a direct antinatriuretic effect on the kidney. Losartan, an orally active, nonpeptide compound, binds competitively and selectively to the AT$_1$ receptor, thereby blocking angiotensin II-induced physiological effects. It appears to have no clinically relevant affinity for other pharmacological receptors. The active metabolite of losartan, E3174, binds to the AT$_1$ receptor with 10-fold greater affinity than the parent compound, and is about 15 to 20 times more potent in inhibiting angiotensin II-induced pressor and contractile responses.[193]

### 3.8.2 Pharmacodynamic Properties

***Pinacidil:*** the primary haemodynamic effect of pinacidil is peripheral vasodilatation, which is dose-related over the range 10 to 37.5mg. The maximum antihypertensive effect is achieved 3 hours after oral administration with a return to basal blood pressure levels within 6 hours. A controlled-release formulation has been developed which lengthens the antihypertensive effect to 12 hours. Not surprisingly, following the reduction in peripheral vascular resistance, the renin-angiotensin system is activated, especially in the acute phase of treatment. There is a linear correlation between plasma pinacidil concentrations and the reduction in blood pressure.[191]

***Ketanserin*** causes a dose-related reduction in total peripheral resistance after oral or intravenous administration; mean blood pressure is decreased by 10%. It also improves renal blood flow and blood flow in obstructive arterial disease of the legs.[192] Ketanserin also inhibits serotonin-induced platelet aggregation. It does, however, cause QTc prolongation at dosages of 40mg or more, which has led to important clinical complications, especially in patients taking a diuretic concomitantly.[194]

***Losartan***: in patients with hypertension, once-daily administration of losartan decreases blood pressure throughout a 24-hour period without affecting the heart rate. Renal function appears to be preserved in hypertensive patients both with and without renal dysfunction, and an albumin-sparing effect (lowering of proteinuria) has been demonstrated in some studies, as has a uricosuric effect. No changes in lipid/lipoprotein or prostaglandin concentrations have been noted, and plasma noradrenaline concentrations and insulin sensitivity also appear to be unchanged.[193]

### 3.8.3 Pharmacokinetic Characteristics

***Pinacidil:*** following oral administration of the controlled-release capsule formulations, the bioavailability of pinacidil was found to be 57%. Elimination is primarily by hepatic metabolism, and occurs rapidly via the cytochrome P450 system. The elimination half-life of the drug is 1 to 3 hours, while that of its major metabolite (pinacidil-*N*-oxide) is 4 hours; this metabolite also has blood pressure-lowering activity but has only one-quarter of the potency of pinacidil. The clearance of both the parent compound and the major metabolite is reduced with increasing age and with decreasing renal function; liver disease also increases the elimination half-life of both pinacidil and the *N*-oxide metabolite.[191]

***Ketanserin:*** following oral administration, extensive first-pass metabolism of ketanserin occurs and its bioavailability is about 50%. Peak plasma concentrations are achieved in around 1 hour and increase linearly with dosage. Elimination of ketanserin is primarily by hepatic metabolism, the principal metabolite formed being ketanserinol; this metabolite does not directly contribute to the pharmacological effect of ketanserin, but its oxidative regeneration to the parent drug may contribute to the relatively long elimination half-life of ketanserin of 14 hours after single doses and 29 hours at steady-state. The first-pass metabolism of ketanserin is decreased in patients with cirrhosis, and a reduction in dosage may be needed in such patients.[192]

***Losartan***: the oral bioavailability of losartan administered as the potassium salt is about 33%, indicating considerable first-pass metabolism. In most patients, about 14% of an oral dose is metabolised via hepatic carboxylation to an active metabolite, E3174, but in a small proportion of patients (<1%), the enzymes responsible for metabolism to E3174 are deficient and less than 1% of a dose is converted. Blockade of the angiotensin II-induced pressor response appears to correlate more closely with plasma concentrations of the metabolite than with those of the parent drug. The volume of distribution is about 34L for losartan and 12L for E3174; both compounds are more than 98% protein bound in plasma and their kinetics are not influenced by multiple-dose administration. The terminal elimination half-life of E3174 is slightly longer than that of losartan (4 to 6h *vs* 2h, respectively). Less than 5% of an oral dose is excreted in the urine unchanged, and renal dysfunction does not appear to affect the pharmacokinetics of either losartan or E3174 to any clinically important extent. However, plasma concentrations of both compounds are increased in patients with hepatic dysfunction, necessitating dosage adjustment.[193]

#### 3.8.4 Clinical Effectiveness

***Pinacidil*** has been evaluated in both noncomparative and comparative clinical trials, some of which have lasted for more than 1 year. Compared with a placebo, it reduces systolic blood pressure by up to 19mm Hg and diastolic by up to 15mm Hg.[191] Pinacidil has proved comparable to diuretics, prazosin, methyldopa and β-blockers in terms of its effectiveness and it is mainly used in combination therapy for patients who have refractory hypertension. A favourable effect of pinacidil on plasma lipids has been demonstrated.[191]

***Ketanserin*** 40 to 80 mg/day has proved superior to placebo in the treatment of mild to moderate hypertension. In comparative studies, it has shown similar effectiveness to several β-blockers and diuretics, and it also compares favourably with nifedipine and captopril. The response to ketanserin is more pronounced in elderly patients. Because of its effect on platelets, several trials have studied its potential as a protector against atheromatous disease. A 23% decrease in cardiovascular events was reported with ketanserin.[194] However, it was also shown that high-dose ketanserin and concomitant thiazide diuretic therapy led to clinical bradycardia and heart block.

***Losartan***: in doses of 50 to 100mg once daily, losartan monotherapy has proved effective in lowering diastolic blood pressure by about 8 to 13mm Hg in patients with mild to moderate hypertension, and has shown equivalent effectiveness to enalapril, atenolol and extended-release felodipine (see review by Goa & Wagstaff[193]). The addition of a thiazide diuretic (hydrochlorothiazide) to losartan produces larger blood pressure reductions than occur with either drug alone. In a trial in patients with severe hypertension, 22% of those who began therapy with losartan 50 mg/day were able to continue with monotherapy at week 12, 30% required losartan plus hydrochlorothiazide 12.5 or 25 mg/day for control, while 46% required the addition of atenolol and/or a dihydropyridine calcium antagonist.[195] In elderly patients, blood pressure reductions with losartan were similar to those achieved with extended-release felodipine, and the response did not differ between patients older or younger than 75 years.[196]

Further data on the therapeutic use of losartan are required to establish its place in the therapeutic armamentarium. Pending acceptable long term effectiveness and safety results, it may find initial use in the management of patients with mild to severe hypertension who are unresponsive to, or intolerant of, their current therapy.[193]

#### 3.8.5 Tolerability and Drug Interactions Potential

***Pinacidil:*** the adverse effects of this drug are those of the direct-acting vasodilators, i.e. headache, oedema (reported in up to 33% of patients), hirsutism and dizziness. These adverse effects are dose-related. Concomitant administration of a thiazide diuretic decreases their severity and may allow therapy to continue; however, the withdrawal rate is still 10 to 20%. There have been several reports of the development of antinuclear antibodies during the course of treatment with pinacidil, but without significant sequelae. Although pinacidil has a novel mode of action, it behaves like a direct-acting vasodilator. In a quality-of-life comparison with nifedipine, no major difference was detected between the two drugs.[197]

***Ketanserin:*** the most common adverse effects of this drug, all in fewer than 10% of patients, are dizziness, tiredness, oedema and dry mouth. Prolongation of the QTc interval has also been reported; this adverse effect is dose-related at doses above 40mg twice daily and is worsened by hypokalaemia and concomitant antiarrhythmic agents. The QTc prolongation is likely to limit severely the clinical options for ketanserin as it cannot be given with a diuretic.

***Losartan*****:** adverse effects experienced most commonly with losartan have been dizziness, headache, asthenia/fatigue and cough. Other, less common, adverse effects reported include orthostatic effects and first-dose hypotension, and rarely, angio-oedema, migraine and taste loss. No significant pharmacokinetic interactions have been detected between losartan and cimetidine, ketoconazole, warfarin or digoxin.[193]

## 4. Optimum Treatment

This discussion is limited to 'essential' hypertension, hypertension in elderly patients, hypertensive emergencies, and hypertension in pregnancy. The treatment of endocrine and renal hypertension is discussed in chapters 19 (section 10) and 24 (sections 4 and 7.1.1), respectively.

### 4.1 Essential Hypertension

For much of this century, hypertension was regarded as an entity associated with the physiology of aging, with unknown associated risks and hence not of major concern to clinicians; indeed, it did not figure in the major medical textbooks. The initial trials of antihypertensive therapy conducted by the Veterans Administration Cooperative Study Group in the US were the first to show that an active drug-induced reduction of elevated blood pressure was associated with a significant decrease in cardiovascular morbidity. These observations were initially reported in severe hypertension (diastolic blood pressure 115 to 129mm Hg),[198] and subsequently extended to mild to moderate hypertension (diastolic blood pressure 90 to 114mm Hg).[199] The medical community and the pharmaceutical industry took notice, the former in developing a *stepped-care* approach to treatment, and the above in developing new, more effective and safer drugs. The stepped-care approach was endorsed in the US by the Report of the National Committee[200] and by the World Health Organization.[201] The essential guidelines of this approach were as follows:

1) Use of nonpharmacological measures (weight reduction, cessation of smoking, low salt intake and moderate physical exercise).

2) Commencement of antihypertensive therapy with low doses of either β-blockers or thiazide diuretics (except in cases of severe hypertension).

3) Increase the dose of thiazides and β-blockers as necessary.

4) Combine diuretic and β-blocker therapy if the above approach was unsuccessful.

5) Add a third drug (e.g. methyldopa, hydralazine or prazosin) if satisfactory blood pressure was not achieved.

6) Add another drug (e.g. minoxidil, bethanidine or debrisoquine) if the previous measures were unsuccessful.

The implementation of this approach in the developed world quickly bore fruit. The Hypertension Detection and Follow-up Program (HDFP) demonstrated that the stepped-care approach, which lowered diastolic blood pressure by 5mm Hg more than the comparison 'referred-care' group, resulted in a 45% reduction in stroke mortality but a less striking 25% re-

**Table VII.** Characteristics of some currently available antihypertensive drugs

| Drug | First choice | Avoid in | Precautions in elderly patients | Comments |
|---|---|---|---|---|
| Thiazide diuretics[a] | Most patients | Uncontrolled or unstable diabetes mellitus<br>Hypercalcaemia<br>Anuria | May increase plasma glucose and lipid levels and exacerbate or precipitate diabetes and gout.<br>Hypokalaemia (maintain serum potassium ≥3.7 mmol/L) may occur and risk of digoxin toxicity increased. Elderly are particularly susceptible to volume depletion.<br>NSAIDs reduce effectiveness | Initial dosage should be equivalent to bendroflumethiazide 2.5 mg/day. Adjust dosage or add potassium-sparing diuretic to maintain potassium levels |
| β-Blockers | Angina<br>Previous MI | Asthma<br>CHF<br>Conduction disturbances<br>Peripheral vascular disease<br>Marked bradycardia | Atenolol, carteolol, celiprolol, nadolol and sotalol are primarily eliminated by the kidney and may require dosage reduction.<br>NSAIDs reduce effectiveness | Increase dosage gradually, based on BP measurements (e.g. atenolol 25 or 50 mg/day) |
| ACE inhibitors | CHF (if thiazides contraindicated) and/or LVH | Renal artery stenosis (bilateral or to a single functioning kidney) | Reduce dosage in renal impairment (fosinopril, spirapril and trandolapril appear to be exceptions; see text, section 3.5.3).<br>Increased potassium levels with potassium-sparing diuretics.<br>NSAIDs may reduce effectiveness | Add to diuretic therapy with care – may precipitate sudden drop in BP |
| Calcium antagonists | Supraventricular arrhythmia (verapamil) or peripheral vascular disease.<br>Also useful in angina or LVH | *Verapamil, diltiazem:* coadministration with β-blockers | Risk of orthostatic hypotension.<br>Flushing, headache, pedal oedema and palpitations may be more of a problem in the elderly | Low dosages to begin with, possibly just once daily |
| $\alpha_1$-Blockers | None, but have favourable effects on plasma lipids | | Increased sensitivity to sympathetic effects which may lead to orthostatic hypotension. Give first dose in the evening before bedtime | Start with minimum dosage and titrate gradually |

a Therapy is most effective when coupled with salt restriction. Thiazides cause calcium retention which reduces the risk of hip fractures.

*Abbreviations:* ACE = angiotensin-converting enzyme; CHF = congestive heart failure; LVH = left ventricular hypertrophy; MI = myocardial infarction; BP = blood pressure.

duction in cardiovascular mortality.[202] However, the intensive intervention group also experienced a reduction in non-cardiovascular mortality and the referred-care group also received a form of stepped-care treatment, *albeit* less intensive. Nevertheless, this policy for the treatment of blood pressure was inaugurated and accepted in the 1980s.

Subsequently, several problems with the stepped-care approach began to appear in the late 1980s:

1) The Multiple Risk Factor Intervention Trial[203] observed an increased rate of sudden death in diuretic-treated hypertensive men who entered the study with electrocardiographic abnormalities. Furthermore, a retrospective analysis of the HDFP data demonstrated a similar increase.[204] Admittedly, these results were based on a subset analysis, but they did raise concerns about the traditional diuretic-first stepped-care approach. Although these concerns have been subsequently refuted,[205] they did point to a reappraisal of antihypertensive strategy in terms of long term as opposed to short term gain.

2) While many trials confirmed the favourable effect of the stepped-care approach on cerebrovascular mortality, they failed to show as favourable an effect on coronary heart disease mortality.[19,206,207]

3) The stepped-care approach relegated the newer antihypertensive drugs such as calcium antagonists and ACE inhibitors to the status of 'also-rans'. Indeed, for many years, drug regulators followed this example by forbidding the use of these drugs as first-line therapy.

4) The standard drugs were not always found suitable as the demographic patterns changed (e.g. an increase in the elderly population).

### Individualised Treatment Approach

For these reasons, the report of the Joint National Committee on Detection, Evaluation and Treatment of High Blood Pressure[208] recommended an *individualised approach* to antihypertensive therapy. Moreover, the idea of adding a second treatment to the first, rather than substituting the second for the first, was questioned. For similar reasons, the aims of antihypertensive treatment in the 1990s are more than that of mere blood pressure control. Rather, a decrease in fatal and non-fatal complications is the major goal. The prevention of arteriosclerosis, the detection and treatment of other risk factors such as hypercholesterolaemia (see further chapter 20), the avoidance of progression of hypertension to more severe stages, and the reversal of end-organ damage are the cardinal endpoints if these aims are to be achieved. Based on individual patient risk profiles and concomitant diseases, therapy must also be individualised.[209] The primacy of treating the patient not the disease, has been emphasised.

In the individualised approach, the importance of nonpharmacological intervention (see section 2.3.3) has not been supplanted, and these measures should be advised for all patients with raised blood pressure. If these measures are not successful in reducing the blood pressure to an acceptable level, then drug therapy should be considered. In using antihypertensive drugs, it must be remembered that adverse effects and deterioration in quality of life are the main reasons for withdrawal of and noncompliance with treatment.[210] As antihypertensives vary in their adverse effect profile and effect on quality of life, the drug should be matched to the patient. For example, verapamil should be avoided in the constipated elderly person, and β-blockers should be avoided in patients with cold extremities or those performing in athletic sports. Methods of improving patient education regarding their therapy must also be implemented.[211] The characteristics of the commonly used antihypertensive drugs that enable their selection and rational use in individual patients are shown in table VII.

In the new (individualised) treatment approach, the concept of attaining maximum dosage with individual drugs, which was the mainstay of the stepped-care approach, has also been revised.[212] While it is difficult to generalise, the trend now is to add another antihypertensive when the first drug either has shown an inadequate response or has produced adverse effects. The classic agents (i.e. diuretics and β-blockers) and the more recently introduced antihypertensives (e.g. calcium antagonists and ACE inhibitors) can be used in a variety of combinations. Diuretics have an additive antihypertensive effect with both β-blockers and ACE inhibitors. Furthermore, ACE inhibitors reverse some diuretic-induced adverse metabolic effects (see section 3.1.5) and may have a beneficial effect in patients with coronary artery disease (see further chapter 20). Combinations of drugs are necessary, as it should be remembered that at best, single drug antihypertensive therapy is effective in only 30 to 50% of patients.[213]

### Goal Blood Pressure

The optimum goal blood pressure is unknown as trials comparing randomisation to different levels of blood pressure have not been completed, although a trial designed to examine the issue of diastolic blood pressure control is currently in progress (HOT study). In the meantime, epidemiological studies and clinical trial data suggest the following:

1) The J-shaped increase in cardiac mortality at lower levels of diastolic pressure is due to sick patients dying rather than to over-enthusiastic treatment. In the Systolic Hypertension in the Elderly Program (SHEP) trial,[214] active treatment reduced diastolic pressure to an average of 68mm Hg and also *reduced* cardiac mortality. In the European Working Party on High Blood Pressure in the Elderly (EWPHE) trial,[20] the J-shaped increase was observed but with both the active treatment and placebo.

2) A reasonable goal *diastolic* blood pressure is 80 to 85mm Hg.

3) A reasonable goal *systolic* blood pressure is less than 150mm Hg, although 125mm Hg or less has been suggested.[215]

In achieving the goal blood pressure, first-line treatment should be with drugs known to be effective in reducing mortality – namely a diuretic (in a low dosage; see above) or a β-blocker. The combination of a diuretic and a β-blocker is well recognised to reduce mortality. Hence, the differences between the stepped-care and individualised regimens may be much less than anticipated.

## 4.2 Hypertension in Elderly Patients

Hypertension is the most common treatable disorder of aged patients. The prevalence of hypertension is higher in elderly patients than in the younger population, and the incidence of complications of hypertension such as stroke, congestive heart failure and coronary heart disease is also higher in the aged. Most importantly, treatment has been shown to reduce these complications. Data from the Framingham and other studies in untreated older men with mild and moderate systolic and diastolic hypertension have shown that the incidence of cardiovascular disease almost doubles in elderly as compared with younger men (figs 2 & 3); however, the increase is less striking for older women.[216]

One of the most important prognostic features of untreated hypertension is its tendency to progress. In the Framingham study, which followed patients over 26 years, the incidence of hypertension in the high-normal diastolic blood pressure group (85 to 89mm Hg) was twice that of the normal diastolic (<85mm Hg) group. The second most important predictor of progression was gain in bodyweight.[217] The incidence of coronary artery disease almost triples in patients with combined hypertension and high cholesterol levels.[218]

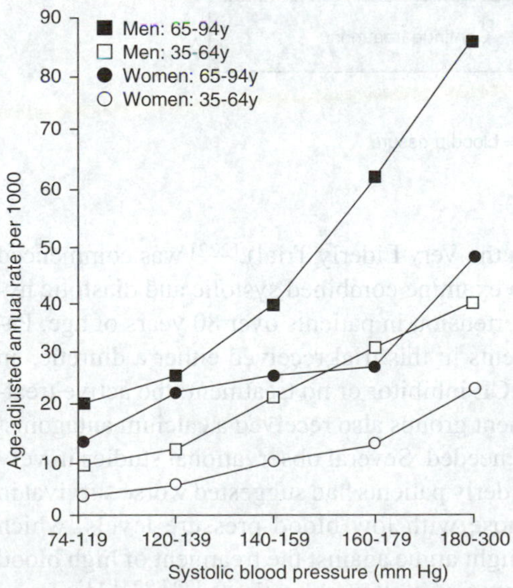


**Fig. 2.** Risk of cardiovascular disease by age, sex and systolic blood pressure from a 30-year follow-up in the Framingham Study (Vokonas et al.[216]) [after Freis[18]].

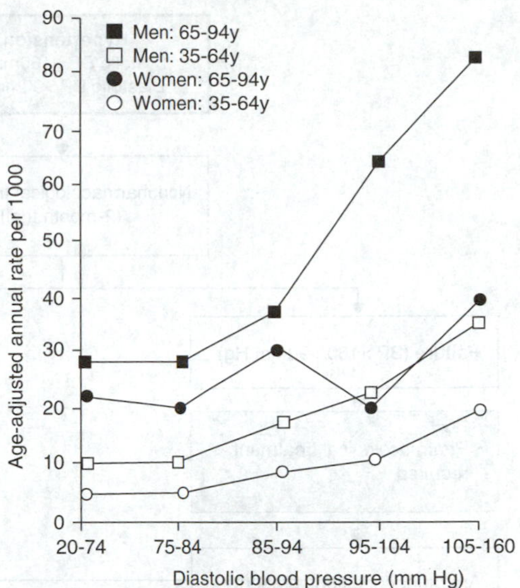


**Fig. 3.** Risk of cardiovascular disease by age, sex and diastolic blood pressure from a 30-year follow-up in the Framingham Study (Vokonas et al.[216]) [after Freis[18]].

Up to 1985, it was not considered appropriate to treat hypertension in elderly patients. The fear was that treatment would lead to hypotensive episodes that would in themselves predispose the patient to cardiovascular complications. This opinion ignored the findings of the Veterans Administration Cooperative Study Group on Antihypertensive Agents,[219] which had shown a remarkable 70% reduction in the incidence of stroke in a small number of treated hypertensive patients older than 60 years. Similarly, in 1981, the Management Committee of the Australian Therapeutic Trial in Hypertension[220] had shown that in a subgroup of treated patients between 60 and 69 years of age there was a 33% reduction in stroke and an 18% reduction in coronary artery disease compared with placebo recipients. Both these trials were in patients with diastolic hypertension.

Subsequently, the European Working Party trial (EWPHE) included elderly patients >60 years of age with both systolic and diastolic hypertension, and showed a reduction of 32% in stroke deaths and a 38% reduction in cardiac deaths.[20] In the STOP Hypertension trial,[221] which studied the use of β-blockers, a diuretic and placebo in patients aged 70 to 84 years with systolic and diastolic hypertension, the incidence of stroke was reduced by 45% in the active treatment groups but myocardial infarction by only 12%.

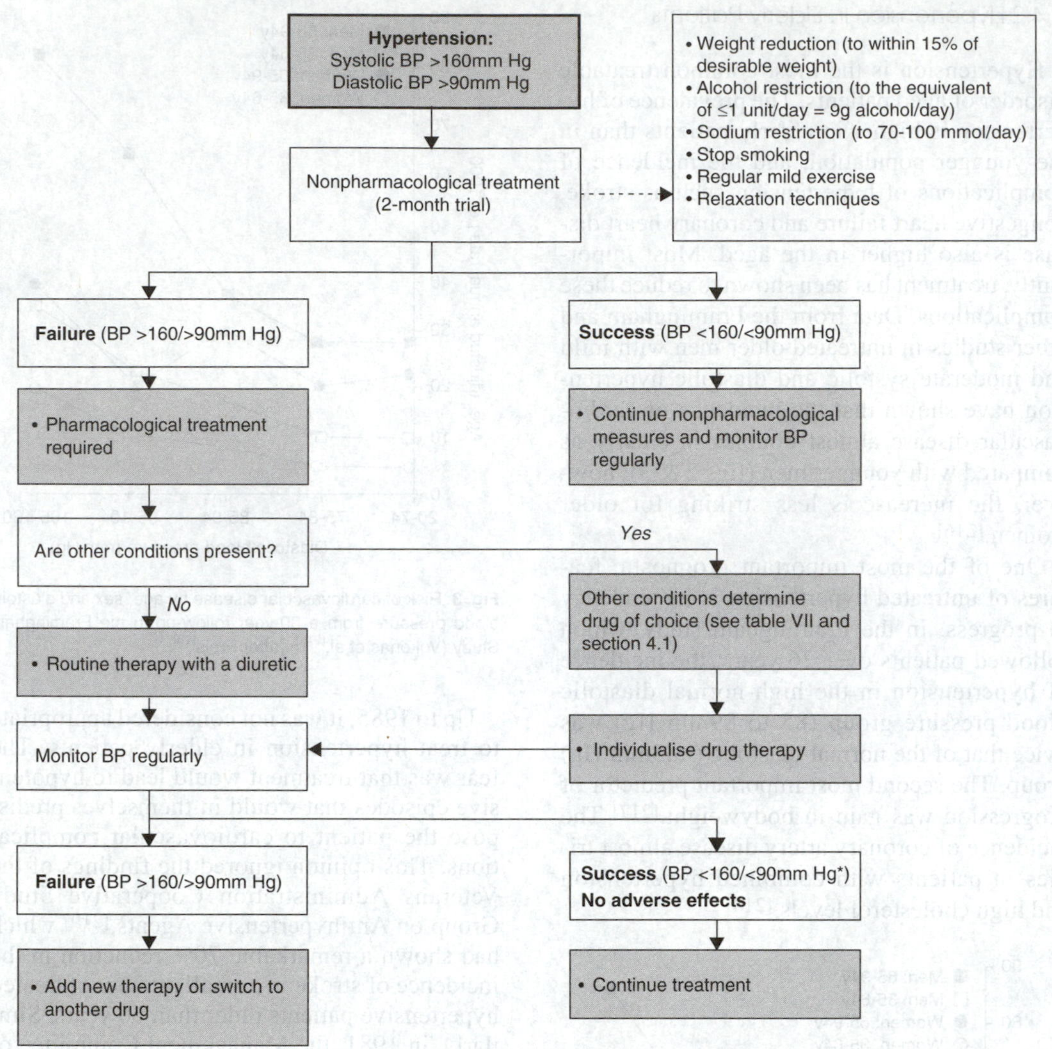


**Fig. 4.** Management of the older hypertensive patient. *Abbreviation:* BP = blood pressure.
***NB.** Success may also be defined as <150/<80mm Hg.

Another notable trial in elderly patients with systolic and often diastolic hypertension was the MRC Working Party trial[44] which compared groups aged 65 to 74 years randomised to either atenolol, or hydrochlorothiazide plus amiloride, or placebo. In this trial, stroke (31%) and coronary artery disease (44%) events were significantly reduced only in the diuretic group.

The Systolic Hypertension in the Elderly Program (SHEP) trial[214] considered isolated systolic hypertension in the >60 year age group. Treatment with chlorthalidone reduced the incidence of non-fatal strokes by 37% compared with placebo, and coronary artery disease by 25%. More recently, the HYVET (Hypertension in the Very Elderly Trial),[222] was commenced to examine combined systolic and diastolic hypertension in patients over 80 years of age. Patients in this trial received either a diuretic, an ACE inhibitor or no treatment; the active treatment groups also received a calcium antagonist if needed. Several observational studies in very elderly patients had suggested worse survival in those with low blood pressure levels, which might argue against the treatment of high blood pressure in very old patients.[223,224] However, low blood pressure is also a consequence of other diseases and probably reflects poor general health before death rather than increased risk *per se*.[225] The HYVET trial is expected to answer this question definitively.

### Treatment Approach

The approach to management of older hypertensive patients is shown in figure 4. While an individualised approach to therapy is recommended, several points can be made. ***Diuretics*** have performed well in the multicentre trials reviewed above. Earlier concerns regarding their safety have largely been refuted[205] and were probably related to inappropriate dose selection. Whichever diuretic is used, strict biochemical monitoring at least annually is advised.

***β-Blockers*** should probably not be considered first-line therapy in elderly patients, in view of the MRC Working Party trial.[44] Indeed, it has been shown that there is a reduced response to monotherapy with β-blockers compared with other antihypertensive drugs in this age group.[226] β-Blockers also reduce the capacity for adapting cardiac function in a situation where aging and cardiovascular disease secondary to hypertension already limit such capacity, i.e. cardiac failure is a particular risk.

***ACE inhibitors*** usually act best in a situation of high renin levels, but in elderly patients, renin levels are usually low. Despite this theoretical limitation, ACE inhibitors have been shown to be effective antihypertensive therapy in elderly patients (see also section 3.5). A combination of an ACE inhibitor and a diuretic is feasible, especially because of the ameliorating effect of ACE inhibitors on diuretic-induced adverse metabolic effects.[149] The initial dose of ACE inhibitor should be lower than in younger patients because plasma concentrations of ACE inhibitors are higher in elderly patients.[162] Clinicians should also beware of enhanced first-dose hypotension in patients who are already on a diuretic[227] and treatment should be initiated under medical supervision, usually in hospital.

Acute renal failure is always a possibility in patients with bilateral renal artery stenosis or those with severe renal atheromatous disease. Consequently, renal function should be monitored during ACE inhibitor therapy in elderly individuals.

***α1-Blockers and calcium antagonists:*** there is no reason why α1-blockers cannot be used, as they are well tolerated and have the added advantage of a beneficial effect in patients with concomitant prostatic hyperplasia. Similarly, calcium antagonists are probably also satisfactory in elderly patients. Nicardipine has been shown to be both effective and well tolerated in elderly patients,[116] but increased adverse effects and subjective cognitive dysfunction have been noted with sustained-release nifedipine.[132]

Treatment of hypertension in elderly patients is discussed further in chapter 4 (section 4.1.2).

**Table VIII.** Conditions that may present as hypertensive emergencies (after Garcia & Vidt[228])

| |
|---|
| **Severe hypertension associated with:** |
| Hypertensive encephalopathy |
| Phaeochromocytoma crisis |
| Drug-induced catecholamine excess: |
| • Rebound hypertension following abrupt withdrawal of clonidine |
| • Food and drug interactions with nonselective monoamine oxidase inhibitors |
| • Amphetamine overdose |
| Pre-eclampsia and eclampsia |
| Malignant hypertension |
| Severe burns |
| Vasculitis and acute glomerulonephritis |
| Severe head injury |
| **Moderate to severe hypertension complicated by:** |
| Acute congestive heart failure |
| Acute coronary insufficiency |
| Acute aortic dissection |
| Hypertensive intracranial haemorrhage |
| Acute atherothrombotic cerebral infarction |
| Postcoronary bypass procedure |
| Postoperative bleeding in vascular suture sites |

## 4.3 Hypertensive Emergencies

A true hypertensive emergency is a life-threatening condition that requires prompt reduction of blood pressure within minutes to 1 hour.[228] It is not just the severity of the raised blood pressure that causes concern, but also the immediate threat to the integrity of the cardiovascular system and the potential for vascular damage based on the patient's clinical status. Conditions that may present as hypertensive emergencies are shown in table VIII.

### Treatment Approach

The patient should be transferred to the intensive care unit. Insertion of a Swan Ganz catheter will help in fine-tuning management. It is important to note that blood pressure must not be lowered too quickly.

Initial treatment measures and the commonly used drugs in hypertensive emergencies are shown in table IX. Sodium nitroprusside should be used only in a true emergency, as the risk of toxicity from its metabolite thiocyanate (e.g.

**Table IX.** Initial management of hypertensive crises (after Garcia & Vidt[228])

**1. Transfer to an intensive care unit**

**2. Evaluation of:**

a) Plasma catecholamines or urine for vanilmandelic acid (VMA)

b) Creatinine clearance

c) Urinalysis

d) Chest radiograph

e) Electrocardiograph

**3. Initiation of drug therapy:** commence before results of the above tests are available. Drugs that may be used include:

a) Sodium nitroprusside[a] (by IV infusion; 0.5-6 μg/kg/min)

b) Hydralazine (5-10mg by intermittent IV injection; or 200 μg/min by IV infusion)

c) Labetalol (20-50mg by intermittent IV injection every 15 min; or 0.5-2 mg/min by IV infusion)

d) Nifedipine (5-10mg orally)

e) Phentolamine[b] (2-5mg IV)

f) Captopril (25mg orally)

a Drug of choice in fulminant hypertension with evolving neurological symptoms and signs.

b A nonselective $\alpha_1$- and $\alpha_2$-adrenoceptor blocker; it is not generally used for hypertensive emergencies but is useful for the treatment of hyperadrenergic crises (e.g. phaeochromocytoma; see further chapter 19, sect. 10.2.1).

*Abbreviation:* IV = intravenous.

nausea, disorientation and psychosis) is increased if the nitroprusside infusion is given for more than 24 hours. Diazoxide is less commonly used nowadays but if it is given, plasma glucose concentrations should be monitored as hyperglycaemia may occur with this drug.

Hypotension should be avoided and a drug that may have particular benefits should be chosen. Calcium antagonists are well tolerated, while an ACE inhibitor is useful if there is concomitant heart failure.

## 4.4 Hypertension in Pregnancy

Hypertension complicates 10% of all pregnancies. It falls into four categories: (1) pre-eclampsia/eclampsia; (2) chronic hypertension of whatever cause; (3) pre-eclampsia/eclampsia superimposed on chronic or renal hypertension; and (4) late (gestational) hypertension.[229] Pre-eclampsia, the association of hypertension, proteinuria and oedema, accounts for more than 50% of all hypertensive disorders during pregnancy and is a major cause of fetal and maternal morbidity and mortality.

Increased vascular resistance is the primary cause of pre-eclampsia. An altered prostacyclin to thromboxane $A_2$ ratio in the uteroplacental bed favours local platelet activation and vasoconstriction, leading to placental insufficiency and fetal distress. This finding led to the hope that low-dose *aspirin* (acetylsalicylic acid) might be effective in preventing pre-eclampsia by inhibiting excessive thromboxane $A_2$ production, and some earlier studies suggested that it may be beneficial in reducing the risk of pregnancy-induced hypertension and improving maternal and neonatal outcomes.[230] However, a recent multicentre trial[231] has not supported the routine use of aspirin for this purpose as it produced only a nonsignificant 12% reduction in the risk of pre-eclampsia in the mothers, with no useful effect on intrauterine growth retardation, stillbirths or neonatal deaths (see further chapter 18; sect. 3.3.1).

Two points are not contested: that hypertension of any severity should be treated and that a patient already receiving antihypertensive treatment should continue with it (provided it is nonteratogenic) if she becomes pregnant. Such a policy improves the outcome for both the mother and fetus.[232]

### Choice of Drug

In *severe pre-eclampsia* it is best to use drugs that are well tried and safe, both for the mother and fetus. Currently, hydralazine is the drug of choice in this situation.[233] Nifedipine has also been used successfully in severe pre-eclampsia,[234] while labetalol, and, as a last resort, sodium nitroprusside can be used in a hypertensive emergency situation.

For the treatment of *chronic hypertension*, methyldopa remains the treatment of choice.[229] Hydralazine, β-blockers and diuretics have also been used safely. However, ACE inhibitors may be fetotoxic and their use cannot be recommended. For all newer drugs, caution is mandatory and risk-benefit considerations must always be taken into account (see also chapter 2).

The management of hypertension in pregnancy is discussed further in chapter 18 (section 3.3).

## 4.5 Clinical Outcome and Economic Considerations

As health resources are not unlimited, we need to know the costs and benefits of antihypertensive treatment and how they compare with those of other treatments. Three main methods are used to assess the economic impact of therapy: cost-effectiveness analysis, cost-utility analysis and cost-benefit analysis. Table X shows how they are calculated.[235] The costs are divided into direct costs (i.e. the financial costs of medical care) and the indirect costs of productivity losses or illness, as measured by loss of earnings. An indirect benefit occurs when a treatment programme results in increased earnings.

The analyses can be expanded so that direct costs include lifetime costs of antihypertensive drugs plus costs of treating their adverse effects plus costs of treating any illness unrelated to hypertension in the extra years of life gained by treatment.[236] Others have excluded the last costs on the grounds that they are not incurred directly by antihypertensive treatment.[237,238] The financial benefits mainly consist of savings in healthcare costs due to reduced morbidity. One utility measure consists of quality of life-adjusted years of survival (i.e. quality-adjusted life-years; QALYs) gained from an extension to life, improved quality of life from prevention of morbidity, and a reduced quality of life from adverse effects.

#### Cost Effectiveness or Cost Utility of Antihypertensive Treatment

Some cost-effectiveness studies have considered the cost effectiveness of antihypertensive treatment in general, while others have compared different antihypertensive treatments.

Weinstein and Stason[236] considered both sexes and different ages, gains in years of life from saving events (0.5 to 1.5 years), and losses of 1% per annum in QALYs from adverse effects. They also used discounting (see chapter 10) and the costs of treating adverse effects. However, they made certain assumptions that we now know are not true – that the fraction of benefit (FOB) to be achieved for coronary heart disease (CHD) would be 100%; that this FOB would decrease with age; and that compliance would be 100%. These assumptions led to the conclusion that moderate to severe hypertension should be treated in young men and older women. Older men and younger women and everyone with mild hypertension yielded very high cost-effectiveness ratios of US$11,000 to US$50,000 per QALY gained. The recommendations from this study cannot be supported as we now know that the fraction of benefit for CHD cannot be higher than 50%. Fraction of benefit does not vary with age and 100% compliance is rarely or never achieved.

**Table X.** Methods of making cost-benefit, cost-effectiveness and cost-ulility analyses (after Bulpitt & Fletcher[235])

**Assumptions:**
- Costs are direct (C1) or indirect (C2)
- Economic benefit is direct (B1) or indirect (B2)
- Health effects of blood pressure reduction or life-years gained are E
- Utility units or quality-of-life adjusted units of survival (e.g. QALYs) are U

**Then:**

| | |
|---|---|
| Cost-benefit analysis | = B1 + B2 – C1 – C2 |
| Cost-effectiveness analysis | = (C1 + C2 – B1 – B2) / E |
| Cost-utility analysis | = (C1 + C2 – B1 – B2) / U |

*Abbreviation:* QALYs = quality-adjusted life-years.

Littenberg et al.[239] calculated the cost effectiveness of both screening and treating hypertension. They reported an acceptable cost effectiveness per QALY gained of US$8,000 to US$44,000, costs being 3 times higher at age 20 than age 60 and 1.5 times higher in women than in men. However, disease event rates were assumed (without treatment) to be the same at all ages and in both sexes, as was the percentage reduction in all-cause mortality. Moreover, quality of life due to treatment was not considered.

Kawachi and Malcolm[237] did take the above problem into account and calculated that the cost-utility ratios decreased with age, the degree of untreated hypertension and being male. The costs per QALY were £7,700 (sterling) for diuretic therapy given to a man aged 60 years with a diastolic pressure of 90mm Hg. The corresponding figure for a woman was £18,000. On this basis, the authors recommended drug treatment only for a diastolic pressure of 100mm Hg and over.

Johannesson and Jönnson[240] recognised 6 main problem areas: the epidemiological data (reliability), the fraction of benefit, the outcome measure (QALYs), the costs to be included, the discounting of effects, and the duration of treatment. They considered life-long treatment *versus* treatment during a certain period and concluded that results were very sensitive to assumptions concerning quality of life, but that the cost per life-year gained was less for men than women and decreased until age 75 years, thereafter increasing.

#### Comparisons of Antihypertensive Treatments

The cost effectiveness of treatment with atenolol and doxazosin was compared by Lindgren and Persson.[241] The fraction of benefit was assumed to be 100%; and the two drugs were assumed to be the same in terms of effectiveness, cost and adverse effects. Clearly, these

**Table XI.** Clinical outcome and economic considerations in selection of antihypertensive therapy

| Drug class | Clinical outcome considerations (effectiveness/safety profile, QOL, patient benefits) | Economic considerations | |
|---|---|---|---|
| | | direct acquisition costs (per day) | potential economic benefits |
| Diuretics | Good benefit/risk<br>Decreased mortality | Very low | High |
| β-Adrenoceptor blockers (β-blockers) | QOL good[a]<br>Decreased mortality[b] | Low | High (except in elderly) |
| Calcium antagonists | Effect on mortality unproven<br>QOL variable | High | Unknown |
| ACE inhibitors | Effective in CHF<br>QOL good | High | Unknown |
| $\alpha_1$-Adrenoceptor blockers ($\alpha_1$-blockers) | Second-line therapy<br>No mortality data<br>QOL data sparse | High | Unknown |
| Central $\alpha_2$-adrenoceptor agonists | Incidence of adverse effects relatively high | Low | Unknown |
| Hydralazine | Increased adverse effects | Low | Unknown |
| Minoxidil | Increased adverse effects | Low | Unknown |

a With newer relatively $\beta_1$-specific agents.

b In the elderly, mortality is decreased when given in combination with a diuretic.

*Abbreviations:* CHF = congestive heart failure; QOL = quality of life; ACE = angiotensin-converting enzyme.

assumptions cannot be supported and their conclusion that doxazosin is more cost effective must therefore be considered unproven.

Another study[238] compared the cost effectiveness of propranolol, nifedipine, prazosin and captopril, and concluded that propranolol was the most cost-effective agent. However, different quality-of-life values were not taken into account when comparing propranolol and nifedipine, although they were when comparing propranolol and captopril.

Johannesson and Fagerberg[242] performed a cost-effectiveness analysis for dietary *versus* drug treatment for obese men with hypertension. They relied on increases in HDL-cholesterol being translated into a reduction in CHD risk and assumed that the expected benefits from cholesterol intervention measures in epidemiological data would be translated into benefits from drug treatment. However, this may not be valid with antihypertensive treatment, as the benefits from such treatment on CHD mortality are less than half those expected.[243,244]

Johannesson et al.[245] considered the results of the Metoprolol Atherosclerosis Prevention in Hypertensives (MAPHY) trial,[246] where metoprolol was associated with a better survival rate than a diuretic. However, the MAPHY study was part of a larger study, the Heart Attack Primary Prevention in Hypertension (HAPPHY) trial, where the number of patients was larger and a different β-blocker (atenolol) was also used.[247] The overall results of the main trial did not favour β-blocker usage, but a subgroup analysis (the MAPHY study) showed a benefit for metoprolol. The non-discounted and 5% discounted gain from using metoprolol rather than a diuretic was 0.2 life-years. Although metoprolol is more expensive than a diuretic, the savings in costs from coronary events observed in this trial were such that the costs involved with metoprolol were less. However, this result is applicable only to the results of the subgroup in the MAPHY trial and an analysis based on the larger HAPPHY trial would not show a benefit for β-blockers (metoprolol and atenolol) over a diuretic. Moreover, the β-blocker treatment was associated with more adverse effects than the diuretics.

The major difficulty in cost-effectiveness analysis has been in determining the life-years gained. Extrapolation from epidemiological studies has not provided the correct denominator. Moreover, a simple measure of cost effectiveness does not take into account the quality of life during treatment and this is essential when considering the antihypertensives used in the past. The clinician must consider both the quantity and quality of life; and quality of life can be measured by collecting standard data on many aspects of well-being (physical and psychological) and activity. However, an overall score such as the Health Status Index (HSI), which is used in calculating QALYs, may be reasonable in a hierarchical sense but does not necessarily allow us to compare, say, hip replacement (no effect on survival) with antihypertensive treatment (less effect on quality of life). The numerical results will depend heavily on what is included in any assessment and the weightings given to various aspects of life.

There are sufficient problems with the current methodology to suggest we should not be using QALYs to determine treatment options.[248] Acceptance of this view does not imply that quality of life cannot be measured and compared within a double-blind randomised controlled trial. If such a trial contained an overall measure of quality of life (such as the Health Status Index), mortality as an outcome, and different treatments, then the trial would generate QALYs that could be used to decide on treatment options. Unfortunately, no trial has measured survival, costs and quality of life carefully enough to allow this comparison.

Despite these reservations we have attempted to correlate clinical outcome and economic considerations for the commonly used antihypertensives in table XI. Diuretics are currently the most cost-effective drugs. Overall, cost-effectiveness analysis tends to suggest that β-blockers and diuretics are to be preferred over ACE inhibitors, the cost per year of life saved having been estimated at US$10,900 for propranolol, US$16,400 for hydrochlorothiazide, and US$72,100 for captopril.[249] β-Blockers may thus reasonably be regarded as first-line therapy, provided that patient selection is appropriate. Tolerability considerations are also paramount in this assessment, since they may affect compliance.

## References


1. Laragh JH. Concept of anti-renin system therapy. American Journal of Medicine 1984; 77: 1
2. Laragh JH. Atrial natriuretic hormone, the renin-aldosterone axis and blood pressure-electrolyte homeostasis. New England Journal of Medicine 1985; 313: 1330
3. Anderson JV, Struthers AD, Payne NN, et al. Atrial natriuretic peptide inhibits the aldosterone response to angiotensin II in man. Clinical Science 1986; 70: 507
4. Goldstein DS, Lake CR. Plasma norepinephrine and epinephrine levels in essential hypertension. Federation Proceedings 1984; 43: 57
5. Dustan HP. Mechanisms of hypertension associated with obesity. Annals of Internal Medicine 1983; 98: 860
6. Friedman GD, Klatsky AL, Siegelaub AB. Alcohol intake and hypertension. Annals of Internal Medicine 1983; 98: 846
7. Rouse IL, Beilin LJ, Armstrong BK, et al. Blood pressure-lowering effect of a vegetarian diet: a controlled trial in normotensive subjects. Lancet 1983; 1: 5
8. Puska P, Lacono JM, Nissinen A, et al. Controlled randomised trial of the effect of dietary fat on blood pressure. Lancet 1983; 1: 1
9. Barnard RJ, Zifferblett SM, Rosenberg JM, et al. Effects of a high-complex carbohydrate diet and daily walking on blood pressure and medication status of hypertensive patients. Journal of Cardiovascular Rehabilitation 1983; 3: 839
10. Simpson FO. Blood pressure and sodium intake. In: Bulpitt CJ, editor. Handbook of hypertension, Vol 6: Epidemiology of hypertension. Amsterdam: Elsevier Scientific Publishers, 1985: 175
11. Editorial. Dietary potassium and hypertension. Lancet 1985; 1: 1308
12. Matlou SM, Isles CG, Higgs A, et al. Potassium supplementation in blacks with mild-moderate hypertension. Journal of Hypertension 1986; 4: 61
13. Reed D, McGee D, Yano K, et al. Diet, blood pressure and multicolinearity. Hypertension 1985; 7: 405
14. Beilin LJ. Diet and lifestyle in hypertension: changing perspectives. Journal of Cardiovascular Pharmacology 1990; 16 Suppl. 7: S62
15. Fagard RH. Physical fitness and blood pressure. Journal of Hypertension 1993; 11 Suppl. 2: S47
16. Beilin LJ. Epitaph to essential hypertension - a preventable disorder of known aetiology? Journal of Hypertension 1988; 6: 85
17. Kannel WB. Implications of the Framingham Study data for the treatment of hypertension: impact of other risk factors. In: Laragh JH et al., editors. Frontiers in hypertension research. New York: Springer Verlag, 1981: 17
18. Freis ED. Prognosis in elderly hypertensive patients. Drugs & Aging 1994; 4: 87
19. MRC Working Party. MRC trial of treatment of mild hypertension: principal results. British Medical Journal 1985; 291: 97
20. Amery A, Birkenhager W, Brixko R, et al. Mortality and morbidity results from the European Working Party on High Blood Pressure in the Elderly. Lancet 1985; 1: 1349
21. Pardell H, Armario P, Hernandez R. Progress in the 1980s and new directions in the 1990s with hypertension management: from the stepped-care approach to the individualised programme in hypertension treatment and control. Drugs 1992; 43: 1
22. Messerli FH. Obesity in hypertension: how innocent a bystander? American Journal of Medicine 1984; 77: 1077
23. Elliot P, Shipley MJ, Rose G. Are lean hypertensives at greater risk than obese hypertensives? Journal of Hypertension 1987; 5 Suppl. 5: S517
24. Shea S, Cook EF, Kannel WB, et al. Treatment of hypertension and its effect on cardiovascular risk factors: data from the Framingham Heart Study. Circulation 1985; 71: 22
25. Dollery CT. Management of hypertension: risk-benefit ratio. Journal of Hypertension 1984; 2 Suppl. 2: 9
26. Sever P, Beevers G, Bulpitt CJ, et al. Management guidelines in essential hypertension: report of the second working party of the British Hypertension Society. British Medical Journal 1993; 306: 983
27. Baer L, Radichevich I. Cigarette smoking in hypertensive patients. Blood pressure and endocrine responses. American Journal of Medicine 1985; 78: 564

28. Isles C, Brown JJ, Cumming AMM, et al. Excess smoking in malignant-phase hypertension. British Medical Journal 1979; 1: 579
29. Bulpitt CJ, Beilin LJ, Clifton P, et al. Risk factors for death in treated hypertensive patients. Lancet 1979; 2: 134
30. Pan W-H, Nanas S, Dyer A, et al. The role of weight in the positive association between age and blood pressure. American Journal of Epidemiology 1984; 124: 612
31. MacMahon SW, MacDonald GJ, Bernstein L, et al. Comparison of weight reduction with metoprolol in the treatment of hypertension in young overweight patients. Lancet 1985; 1: 1233
32. Regan TJ. Alcohol and the cardiovascular system. Journal of the American Medical Association 1990; 264: 377
33. Potter JF, Beevers DG. Pressure effect of alcohol in hypertension. Lancet 1984; 1: 119
34. Friedel HA, Buckley MM-T. Torasemide: a review of its pharmacological properties and therapeutic potential. Drugs 1991; 41: 81-103
35. Brater DC. Clinical pharmacology of loop diuretics in health and disease. European Heart Journal 1992; 13 Suppl. G: 10
36. Lant A. Diuretics. Clinical pharmacology and therapeutic use. (Part I). Drugs 1985; 29: 57
37. Van Zwieten PA. Comparative mechanisms of action of diuretic drugs in hypertension. European Heart Journal 1992; 13 Suppl. G: 2
38. Weinberger MH. Optimizing cardiovascular risk reduction during antihypertensive therapy. Hypertension 1990; 16: 201
39. Baldwin SP, Harless WT, Lacy CA, et al. A comparative study of the efficacy and side effects of metolazone 0.5 mg tablets vs triamterene 50 mg plus hydrochlorothiazide 25 mg in the treatment of mild hypertension. Advanced Therapeutics 1987; 4: 265
40. Saggar-Malik A, Cauppuccio FP. Potassium supplements and potassium-sparing diuretics. Drugs 1993; 46: 986
41. Brater DC, Day B, Burdette A, et al. Bumetanide and furosemide in heart failure. Kidney International 1984; 26: 183
42. Mutschler E, Gilfrich H, Knauf H, et al. Pharmacokinetics of triamterene. Clinical and Experimental Hypertension 1983; 5: 249
43. Hampton JR. Comparative efficacy of diuretics: benefit versus risk: results of clinical trials. European Heart Journal 1992; 13 Suppl. G: 85
44. MRC Working Party. MRC trial of treatment of hypertension in older adults. British Medical Journal 1992; 304: 405
45. MRC Working Party Report on Mild-Moderate Hypertension. Adverse reactions to bendrofluazide and propranolol for the treatment of mild hypertension. Lancet 1981; 2: 539
46. Carlsen JE, Kober L, Torp-Pedersen C, et al. Relation between dose of bendrofluazide, antihypertensive effect, and adverse biochemical effects. British Medical Journal 1990; 300: 975
47. Prichard BNC, Owens CWI, Woolf AS. Adverse reactions to diuretics. European Heart Journal 1992; 13 Suppl. G: 96
48. Jaffey L, Martin A. Malignant hyperkalaemia after amiloride/hydrochlorothiazide treatment. Lancet 1981; 2: 1272
49. Favre L, Glasson P, Vallotton MB. Reversible acute renal failure from combined triamterene and indomethacin. Annals of Internal Medicine 1982; 96: 317
50. Nadelmann J, Frishman WH. Clinical use of β-blockade in systemic hypertension. Drugs 1990; 39: 862
51. Brass EP. Effects of antihypertensive drugs on endocrine function. Drugs 1984; 27: 447
52. McDevitt DG. Clinical significance of cardioselectivity: state of the art. Drugs 1983; 25: 219
53. Lipworth BJ, Irvine NA, McDevitt DG. The effects of time and dose on the relative beta-1 and beta-2 adrenoceptor antagonism of betaxolol and atenolol. British Journal of Clinical Pharmacology 1991; 31: 154
54. Frishman WH, Goldberg RJ, Benfield P. Bevantolol: a preliminary review of its pharmacodynamic and pharmacokinetic properties, and therapeutic efficacy in hypertension and angina pectoris. Drugs 1988; 35: 1-21
55. Singh BN, Deedwania P, Nademanee K, et al. Sotalol: a review of its pharmacodynamic and pharmacokinetic properties and therapeutic use. Drugs 1987; 34: 311
56. Goa KL, Benfield P, Sorkin EM. Labetalol: a reappraisal of its pharmacology, pharmacokinetics and therapeutic use in hypertension and ischaemic heart disease. Drugs 1989; 37: 583
57. Lancaster SG, Sorkin EM. Bisoprolol: a preliminary review of its pharmacodynamic and pharmacokinetic properties and therapeutic use in hypertension and angina. Drugs 1988; 36: 256
58. Dunn CJ, Spencer CM. Celiprolol: an evaluation of its pharmacological properties and clinical efficacy in the management of hypertension and angina pectoris. Drugs & Aging 1995; 7: 394-411
59. Milne RJ, Buckley M-MT. Celiprolol: an updated review of its pharmacodynamic and pharmacokinetic properties and therapeutic efficacy in cardiovascular diseases. Drugs 1991; 41: 941
60. Wadworth AN, Murdoch D, Brogden RN. Atenolol: a reappraisal of its pharmacological properties and therapeutic use in cardiovascular disorders. Drugs 1991; 42: 468
61. Harron DWG, Goa KL, Langtry HD. Bopindolol: a review of its pharmacodynamic and pharmacokinetic properties and therapeutic efficacy. Drugs 1991; 41: 130-49
62. McTavish D, Campoli-Richards D, Sorkin EM. Carvedilol: a review of its pharmacodynamic and pharmacokinetic properties, and therapeutic efficacy. Drugs 1993; 45: 232-58
63. Peters DH, Benfield P. Metoprolol: a pharmacoeconomic and quality-of-life evaluation of its use in hypertension, post-myocardial infarction and dilated cardiomyopathy. PharmacoEconomics 1994; 6: 370-400
64. Otsuka K, Tsukiyama H. Haemodynamic effects of celiprolol, a β-1 selective β-adrenergic blocking agent with β-2 selective ISA in patients with essential hypertension. Rinsho Iyaku 1990; 6: 73
65. Fagard R, Lijnen P, Amery A. Response of the systemic pulmonary circulation to labetalol at rest and during exercise. British Journal of Pharmacology 1982; 13 Suppl. 1: 135
66. Seedat YK. Trial of atenolol and chlorthalidone for hypertension in Black South Africans. British Medical Journal 1980; 281: 1241
67. Buhler FR, Burkart F, Lutoid B, et al. Antihypertensive β-blocking action as related to renin and age: a pharmacological tool to identify pathogenic mechanisms in essential hypertension. American Journal of Cardiology 1975; 36: 653
68. Kendall MJ, Maxwell SRJ, Sandberg A, et al. Controlled release metoprolol: clinical pharmacokinetics and therapeutic implications. Drugs 1991; 41: 319

69. Croog SH, Levine S, Testa MA, et al. The effects of antihypertensive therapy on the quality of life. New England Journal of Medicine 1986; 314: 1657
70. Fletcher AE, Chester PC, Hawkins CMA, et al. The effects of verapamil and propranolol on quality of life in hypertension. Journal of Human Hypertension 1989; 3: 125
71. Herrick AL, Waller PC, Bernn KE, et al. Comparison of enalapril and atenolol in mild to moderate hypertension. American Journal of Medicine 1989; 86: 421
72. Croog SH, Kong BW, Levine S, et al. Hypertensive black men and women. Quality of life and effects of antihypertensive medications. Black Hypertension Quality of Life Multicentre Trial Group. Archives of Internal Medicine 1990; 150: 1733
73. Fletcher AE, Bulpitt CJ, Hawkins CM, et al. Quality of life on antihypertensive therapy: a randomised double-blind controlled trial of captopril and atenolol. Journal of Hypertension 1990; 8: 463
74. Fletcher AE, Bulpitt CJ, Chase DM, et al. Quality of life on 3 antihypertensive treatments: cilazapril, atenolol, nifedipine. Hypertension 1992; 19: 499
75. Palmer AJ, Fletcher AE, Rudge PJ, et al. Quality of life in hypertensives treated with atenolol or captopril: a double-blind crossover trial. Journal of Hypertension 1992; 10: 1409
76. Lewis RV, Lofthouse C. Adverse reactions with β-adrenoceptor blocking drugs: an update. Drug Safety 1993; 9: 272
77. Tanaka N, Sakaguchi S, Oshige K, et al. Effects of chronic administration of propranolol on lipoprotein composition. Metabolism: Clinical and Experimental 1976; 25: 1071
78. Fogari R, Zoppi A, Pasotti C, et al. Effects of different β-blockers on lipid metabolism in chronic therapy of hypertension. International Journal of Clinical Pharmacology Therapy and Toxicology 1988; 26: 597
79. Chiasmi-Pasha H, Taylor RJ, Barnes PC. Beta-blockers, lipids and coronary atherosclerosis. British Medical Journal 1988; 297: 1130
80. Lam YW, Shepherd AMM. Drug interactions in hypertensive patients. Pharmacokinetic, pharmacodynamic, and genetic considerations. Clinical Pharmacokinetics 1990; 18: 295
81. Lund-Johansen P, Omuik P, Haugland H. Acute and chronic haemodynamic effects of doxazosin in hypertension at rest and during exercise. British Journal of Clinical Pharmacology 1986; 21: 45S
82. Stanaszek WF, Kellerman D, Brogden RN, et al. Prazosin update: a review of its pharmacological properties and therapeutic use in hypertension and congestive heart failure. Drugs 1983; 25: 339-84
83. Young RA, Brogden RN. Doxazosin: a review of its pharmacodynamic and pharmacokinetic properties, and therapeutic efficacy in mild or moderate hypertension. Drugs 1988; 35: 525-41
84. Titmarsh S, Monk JP. Terazosin: a review of its pharmacodynamic and pharmacokinetic properties, and therapeutic efficacy in essential hypertension. Drugs 1987; 33: 461-77
85. Timmermanns PBMWM, Kwa HY, Karamat Ali F, et al. Prazosin and its analogues UK-18,596 and UK-33,274: a comparative study on cardiovascular effects and alpha-blocking activities. Archives Internationales de Pharmacodynamie et de Therapie 1980; 245: 218
86. Oates HF. A new prazosin analogue, Abbott-45975 (A-45795). New Zealand Medical Journal 1981; 94: 67
87. Elliot HL, Meredith PA, Sumner DJ, et al. A pharmacodynamic and pharmacokinetic assessment of a new alpha-adrenoceptor antagonist: doxazosin. British Journal of Clinical Pharmacology 1982; 13: 699
88. Donnelly R, Meredith PA, Elliot HL. Pharmacodynamic-pharmacokinetic relationships of α-adrenoceptor antagonists. Clinical Pharmacokinetics 1989; 17: 264
89. De Leeuw PW, Van Es PN, De Bos R, et al. Acute renal effects of doxazosin in man. British Journal of Clinical Pharmacology 1986; 21 Suppl. 1: 41S
90. Kondo K, Ohashi K, Ebihara A. The pharmacokinetics and pharmacological effects of terazosin, a new α-blocking agent, in normotensive volunteers. Japanese Journal of Clinical Pharmacology and Therapeutics 1983; 14: 147
91. Deger G, Cutler RE, Dietz AJ, et al. Comparison of the safety and efficacy of once daily terazosin versus twice daily prazosin for the treatment of mild to moderate hypertension. American Journal of Medicine 1986; 80 Suppl. 5B: 62
92. Pool JL, Nelson EB, Taylor AA, et al. Alpha-1 adrenergic blockade changes plasma lipids in man. Clinical Research 1982; 30: 213A
93. Trost BN, Weidman P, Riesen W, et al. Comparative effects of doxazosin and hydroclorothiazide on serum lipids and blood pressure in essential hypertension. American Journal of Cardiology 1987; 59: 99G
94. Bateman DN, Hobbs DC, Twomey TM, et al. Prazosin: pharmacokinetics and concentration-effect. European Journal of Clinical Pharmacology 1979; 16: 171
95. Hayduk K, Schneider HT. Antihypertensive effects of doxazosin in systemic hypertension and comparison with terazosin. American Journal of Cardiology 1987; 59: 95G
96. Ruoff G, Cohen A, Hollifield JW, et al. Comparative trials of terazosin with other antihypertensive agents. American Journal of Medicine 1986; 80 Suppl. 5B: 42
97. Hjortdahl P, Von Krogh H, Daee L, et al. A 24 week multicentre double-blind study of doxazosin and hydrochlorothiazide in patients with mild to moderate essential hypertension. Acta Medica Scandinavica 1987; 221: 427
98. Cox DA, Leader JP, Milwon JA, et al. The antihypertensive effects of doxazosin: a clinical overview. British Journal of Clinical Pharmacology 1986; 21 Suppl. 1: 83S
99. Torvik D, Madsbu HP. A multicentre twelve week double-blind comparison of doxazosin, prazosin and placebo in patients with mild to moderate hypertension. British Journal of Clinical Pharmacology 1980; 21: 69S
100. Pasanisi F, Elliott HL, Meredith PA, et al. Combined alpha-adrenoceptor antagonists and calcium channel blockers in normal subjects. Clinical Therapeutics and Pharmacology 1984; 36: 716
101. Meredith PA, Elliot HL, Pasanisi F, et al. Prazosin and verapamil: a pharmacokinetic and pharmacodynamic interaction. British Journal of Clinical Pharmacology 1986; 21: 85P
102. The Treatment of Mild Hypertension Research Group. Treatment of mild hypertension study. Archives of Internal Medicine 1991; 151: 1413
103. Kelly JG, O'Malley K. Clinical pharmacokinetics of calcium antagonists: an update. Clinical Pharmacokinetics 1992; 22: 416-33
104. McTavish D, Sorkin EM. Verapamil: an updated review of its pharmacodynamic and pharmacokinetic proper-

ties and therapeutic use in hypertension. Drugs 1989; 38: 19-76

105. Brogden RN, Benfield P. Gallopamil: a review of its pharmacodynamic and pharmacokinetic properties, and therapeutic potential in ischaemic heart disease. Drugs 1994; 47: 93-115
106. Buckley MM-T, Grant SM, Goa KL, et al. Diltiazem: a reappraisal of its pharmacological properties and therapeutic use. Drugs 1990; 39: 757-806
107. Sorkin EM, Clissold SP, Brogden RN. Nifedipine: a review of its pharmacodynamic and pharmacokinetic properties, and therapeutic efficacy in ischaemic heart disease, hypertension and related cardiovascular disorders. Drugs 1985; 30: 182-274
108. Murdoch D, Brogden RN. Sustained release nifedipine formulations: an appraisal of their current uses and prospective roles in the treatment of hypertension, ischaemic heart disease and peripheral vascular disorders. Drugs 1991; 41: 737-79
109. Saltial E, Ellrodt AG, Monk JP, et al. Felodipine: a review of its pharmacodynamic and pharmacokinetic properties, and therapeutic use in hypertension. Drugs 1988; 36: 387-428
110. Todd PA, Fauld D. Felodipine: a review of the pharmacology and therapeutic use of the extended release formulation in cardiovascular disorders. Drugs 1992; 44: 251-77
111. Murdoch D, Heel RC. Amlodipine: a review of its pharmacodynamic and pharmacokinetic properties, and therapeutic use in cardiovascular disease. Drugs 1991; 41: 478-505
112. Fitton A, Benfield P. Isradipine: a review of its pharmacodynamic and pharmacokinetic properties, and therapeutic use in cardiovascular disease. Drugs 1990; 40: 31-74
113. Brogden RC, Sorkin EM. Isradipine: an update of its pharmacodynamic and pharmacokinetic properties and therapeutic efficacy in the treatment of mild to moderate hypertension. Drugs 1995; 49: 618-49
114. Lee CR, Bryson HM. Lacidipine: a review of its pharmacodynamic and pharmacokinetic properties and therapeutic potential in the treatment of hypertension. Drugs 1994; 48: 274-96
115. Sorkin EM, Clissold SP. Nicardipine: a review of its pharmacodynamic and pharmacokinetic properties, and therapeutic efficacy, in the treatment of angina pectoris, hypertension and related cardiovascular disorders. Drugs 1987; 33: 296-345
116. Frampton JE, Sorkin EM. Nicardipine: a review of its pharmacology and therapeutic efficacy in older patients. Drugs & Aging 1993; 3: 165
117. Friedel HA, Sorkin EM. Nisoldipine: a preliminary review of its pharmacodynamic and pharmacokinetic properties, and therapeutic efficacy in the treatment of angina pectoris, hypertension and related cardiovascular disorders. Drugs 1988; 36: 682-731
118. Goa KL, Sorkin EM. Nitrendipine: a review of its pharmacodynamic and pharmacokinetic properties, and therapeutic efficacy in the treatment of hypertension. Drugs 1987; 33: 123-55
119. Brogden RN, McTavish D. Nilvadipine: a review of its pharmacodynamic and pharmacokinetic properties, therapeutic use in hypertension and potential in cerebrovascular disease and angina. Drugs & Aging 1995; 6: 150-71
120. Van Zwieten PA, Timmermanns PBMWM. Pharmacological basis of the antihypertensive action of calcium entry blockers. Journal of Cardiovascular Pharmacology 1985; 7 Suppl. 4: S11
121. Kleinbloesem CH, Van Brumelen P, Van de Linde JA, et al. Nifedipine: kinetics and dynamics in healthy subjects. Clinical Pharmacology and Therapeutics 1984; 35: 742
122. Meredith PA, Elliot HL, Ahmed JH, et al. Age and antihypertensive efficacy of verapamil: an integrated pharmacokinetic-pharmacodynamic approach. Journal of Hypertension 1987; 5 Suppl. 5: S57
123. Blychert E, Edgar B, Elmsfeldt D, et al. Plasma concentration versus effect relationship for felodipine. Journal of Cardiovascular Pharmacology 1990; 15 Suppl. 4: 557
124. Piepho RW, Culbertson VC, Rhodes RS. Drug interactions with the calcium entry blockers. Circulation 1987; 75 Suppl. V: V181
125. Materson BJ, Reda DJ, Cushman WC, et al. Single drug therapy for hypertension in men. A comparison of 6 antihypertensive agents with placebo. The Department of Veterans' Affairs Cooperative Study Group on Antihypertensive Agents. New England Journal of Medicine 1993; 328: 914
126. Oviasy VO, Obasohan AO. Use of nifedipine in the management of systemic hypertension in Nigerian patients. Current Therapeutic Research 1986; 39: 455
127. Cruickshank JK, Anderson NMcF, Wadsworth J, et al. Treating hypertension in black compared with white non-insulin dependent diabetics: a double-blind trial of verapamil and metoprolol. British Medical Journal 1988; 297: 1155
128. Dittrich HC, Adler J, Ong J, et al. Effects of sustained release nicardipine on regression of left ventricular hypertrophy. American Journal of Cardiology 1992; 69: 1559
129. Wetzchewald D, Klaus D, Garanin G, et al. Regression of left ventricular hypertrophy during long-term antihypertensive treatment: a comparison between felodipine and the combination of felodipine and metoprolol. Journal of International Medicine 1992; 231: 303
130. Lavie CJ, Ventura HO, Messerli FH. Regression of increased left ventricular mass by antihypertensives. Drugs 1991; 42: 945
131. Isradipine in Hypertension Study Group. A multicentre evaluation of the safety and efficacy of isradipine and atenolol in the treatment of hypertension. American Journal of Medicine 1989; Suppl. 4A: 119
132. Palmer A, Fletcher A, Hamilton G, et al. A comparison of verapamil and nifedipine on quality of life. British Journal of Clinical Pharmacology 1990; 30: 365
133. Sundstedt CD, Ruegg PC, Keller A, et al. A multicentre evaluation of the safety, tolerability and efficacy of isradipine in the treatment of essential hypertension. American Journal of Medicine 1989; 86 Suppl. 4A: 98
134. Hart W, Westberg B. Felodipine extended-release tablets once daily are equivalent to plain tablets twice daily in the treatment of hypertension. Journal of Cardiovascular Pharmacology 1990; 15 Suppl. 4: S65
135. Held PH, Yusuf S, Furberg C. Calcium channel blockers in acute myocardial infarction and unstable angina: an overview. British Medical Journal 1989; 299: 1187-92
136. Yusuf S, Held P, Furberg C. Update of effects of calcium antagonists in myocardial infarction or angina in light of the second Danish Verapamil Infarction Trial (DAVIT-II) and other recent studies. American Journal of Cardiology 1991; 67: 1295-7

137. Psaty BM, Heckbert SR, Koepsell TD, et al. The risk of myocardial infarction associated with antihypertensive drug therapies. Journal of the American Medical Association 1995; 274: 620-5
138. Wagner W, Phillip T, Heinemayer G, et al. Interaction of cyclosporin and calcium antagonists. Transplantation Proceedings 1989; 21: 1453
139. Burnier M, Biollaz J. Pharmacokinetic optimisation of angiotensin converting enzyme (ACE) inhibitor therapy. Clinical Pharmacokinetics 1992; 22: 375-84
140. Leonetti G, Cuspardi C. Choosing the right ACE inhibitor: a guide to selection. Drugs 1995; 49: 516-35
141. Heel RC, Brogden RN, Speight TM, et al. Captopril: a preliminary review of its pharmacological properties and therapeutic efficacy. Drugs 1980; 20: 409-45
142. Todd PA, Heel RC. Enalapril: a review of its pharmacodynamic and pharmacokinetic properties and therapeutic use in hypertension and congestive heart failure. Drugs 1986; 31: 198-248
143. Todd PA, Goa KL. Enalapril: a reappraisal of its pharmacology and therapeutic use in hypertension. Drugs 1992; 43: 346-81
144. Balfour JA, Goa KL. Benazepril: a review of its pharmacodynamic and pharmacokinetic properties, and therapeutic use in hypertension and chronic heart failure. Drugs 1991; 42: 511-39
145. Deget F, Brogden RN. Cilazapril: a review of its pharmacodynamic and pharmacokinetic properties, and therapeutic potential in cardiovascular disease. Drugs 1991; 41: 799-820
146. Murdoch D, McTavish D. Fosinopril: a review of its pharmacodynamic and pharmacokinetic properties, and therapeutic potential in essential hypertension. Drugs 1992; 43: 123-40
147. Wagstaff AJ, Davis R, McTavish D. Fosinopril: a reappraisal of its pharmacology and therapeutic efficacy in essential hypertension. Drugs 1996; 51: 777-91
148. Lancaster SG, Todd PA. Lisinopril: a preliminary review of its pharmacodynamic and pharmacokinetic properties and therapeutic use in hypertension and chronic heart failure. Drugs 1988; 35: 646-69
149. Todd PA, Fitton A. Perindopril: a review of its pharmacological properties and therapeutic use in cardiovascular disorders. Drugs 1991; 42: 90-114
150. Wadworth AN, Brogden RN. Quinapril: a review of its pharmacological properties and therapeutic efficacy in hypertension and chronic heart failure. Drugs 1991; 41: 378-99
151. Todd PA, Benfield P. Ramipril: a review of its pharmacological properties and therapeutic efficacy in cardiovascular disorders. Drugs 1990; 39: 110-35
152. Noble S, Sorkin EM. Spirapril: a preliminary review of its pharmacology and therapeutic efficacy in the treatment of hypertension. Drugs 1995; 49: 750-66
153. Wiseman LR, McTavish D. Trandolapril: a review of its pharmacodynamic and pharmacokinetic properties, and therapeutic use in essential hypertension. Drugs 1994; 48: 71-90
154. Ondetti MA, Cushman DW. Enzymes of the renin angiotensin system and their inhibition. Annual Review of Biochemistry 1982; 51: 283
155. Haber E, Carlson W. Renin-angiotensin system. In: Genest R, editor. Hypertension. 2nd ed. New York: McGraw Hill, 1983: 177
156. Douglas LW. Polypeptides: angiotensin, plasma kinins and others. In: Goodman & Gillman, editors. The pharmacological basis of therapeutics, 7th ed. New York: MacMillan, 1985: 639
157. Shoback DM, Williams GH, Swartz SL, et al. Time course and effect of sodium intake on vascular and hormonal responses to enalapril (MK-421) in normal subjects. Journal of Cardiovascular Pharmacology 1983; 5: 1010
158. Biollaz J, Schelling JL, Jacot-Des-Combes B, et al. Enalapril maleate and a lysine analogue (MK-521) in normal volunteers: relationship between plasma drug levels and the renin angiotensin system. British Journal of Clinical Pharmacology 1982; 14: 363
159. Johnston CL, Jackson B, McGraw B, et al. Relationship of antihypertensive effect of enalapril to serum MK-422 levels and angiotensin converting enzyme inhibition. Journal of Hypertension 1983; 1 Suppl. 1: 71
160. Meredith PA, Donnelly R, Elliott HL, et al. Prediction of the antihypertensive response to enalapril. Journal of Hypertension 1990; 8: 1085
161. Belz GG, Kirch W, Kleinbloesem CH. Angiotensin converting enzyme inhibitors: relationship between pharmacodynamics and pharmacokinetics. Clinical Pharmacokinetics 1988; 15: 295
162. Kelly JG, O'Malley K. Clinical pharmacokinetics of the newer ACE inhibitors: a review. Clinical Pharmacokinetics 1990; 19: 177
163. Pool JL, Gennari J, Goldstein R, et al. Controlled multicentre study of the antihypertensive effects of lisinopril, hydrochlorothiazide, and lisinopril plus hydrochlorothiazide in the treatment of 394 patients with mild to moderate essential hypertension. Journal of Cardiovascular Pharmacology 1987; 9 Suppl. 3: S36
164. Moser M, Abraham PA, Bennett WM, et al. The effects of benazepril, a new angiotensin-converting enzyme inhibitor, in mild-moderate essential hypertension: a multicentre study. Clinical Pharmacology and Therapeutics 1991; 49: 322
165. Gavras H. A multicentre trial of enalapril in the treatment of essential hypertension. Clinical Therapeutics 1986; 9: 24
166. Moser M, Cunn J. Response to captopril and hydrochlorothiazide in black patients with hypertension. Clinical Pharmacology and Therapeutics 1982; 32: 307
167. Goldstein RJ. A multicentre randomised, double-blind, parallel comparison of fosinopril sodium and enalapril maleate for the treatment of essential hypertension. Drug Investigation 1991; 3 Suppl. 4: 38
168. Schnaper HW. Comparison of the efficacy and safety of quinapril versus captopril in the treatment of moderate to severe hypertension. Angiology 1989; 40: 389
169. Steiner SS, Friedhoff AJ, Wilson BL, et al. Antihypertensive therapy and quality of life: a comparison of atenolol, captopril, enalapril and propranolol. Journal of Human Hypertension 1990; 4: 217
170. Stelmach WJ, Rush DR, Brucker PC, et al. Managing hypertension in family practice: a nationwide collaborative study of the use of four antihypertensives in the treatment of mild-to-moderate hypertension. Journal of the American Board of Family Practice 1989; 2: 172
171. Meisel S, Verho M, Rosenthal J. Ramipril (HOE 498) for the treatment of severe hypertension. International Symposium on ACE inhibitors, London, February 17-21, 1989
172. Bauer JH, Reams GP, Lal SM. Renal protective effect of strict blood pressure control with enalapril therapy. Archives of Internal Medicine 1987; 147: 1397
173. Baba T, Tomiyama T, Takebe K. Enhancement by an ACE inhibitor of first-dose hypotension caused by an

alpha-1 blocker. New England Journal of Medicine 1990; 322: 1237

174. Rucinska EJ, Small R, Mulcahy WS, et al. Tolerability of long term therapy with enalapril maleate in patients resistant to other therapies and intolerant to captopril. Medical Toxicology and Adverse Drug Experience 1989; 4: 144
175. Sizeland PCB, Bailey RR, Lynn KL, et al. Anemia with angiotensin-converting enzyme inhibition in renal transplant recipients. Journal of Cardiovascular Pharmacology 1990; 16 Suppl. 7: S117
176. Hanssens M, Keirse MJNC, Vankelecom F, et al. Fetal and neonatal effects of treatment with angiotensin-converting enzyme inhibitors in pregnancy. Obstetrics and Gynecology 1991; 78: 128
177. Kreft-Jais C, Plovin P-F, Tchobroutsky C, et al. Angiotensin-converting enzyme inhibitors during pregnancy: a survey of 22 patients given captopril and nine given enalapril. British Journal of Obstetrics and Gynaecology 1988; 95: 420
178. Langley MS, Heel RC. Transdermal clonidine: a preliminary review of its pharmacodynamic properties and therapeutic efficacy. Drugs 1988; 35: 123-42
179. Chrisp P, Faulds D. Moxonidine: a review of its pharmacology and therapeutic use in essential hypertension. Drugs 1992; 44: 993-1012
180. Holmes B, Brogden RN, Heel RC, et al. Guanabenz: a review of its pharmacodynamic properties and therapeutic efficacy in hypertension. Drugs 1983; 26: 212-29
181. Sorkin EM, Heel RC. Guanfacine: a review of its pharmacodynamic and pharmacokinetic properties, and therapeutic efficacy in the treatment of hypertension. Drugs 1986; 31: 301-36
182. Lowenthal DT, Matzek KM, MacGregor TM. Clinical pharmacokinetics of clonidine. Clinical Pharmacokinetics 1988; 14: 287
183. Myrhe E, Rugstad HE, Hansen T. Clinical pharmacokinetics of methyldopa. Clinical Pharmacokinetics 1982; 7: 221
184. White WB, Andreoli JW, Cohn RD. Alpha-methyldopa disposition in mothers with hypertension and in their breast-fed infants. Clinical Pharmacology and Therapeutics 1985; 37: 387
185. Tarazi RC, Fouad FM. Reversal of cardiac hypertrophy in humans. Hypertension 1984; 6: 11
186. Fletcher AE, Bulpitt CJ. A review of clinical trials in pregnancy. In: Rubin PC, editor. Hypertension in pregnancy. Amsterdam: Elsevier Science Publishers, 1988: 10: 186
187. Franklin SS, Tonkon MJ, Kirschenbaum MA, et al. Randomised, double-blind comparison of transdermal clonidine with oral propranolol. Journal of Cardiovascular Pharmacology 1987; 10 Suppl. 12: S244
188. Campbell N, Paddock V, Sundaram R. Alteration of methyldopa absorption, metabolism and blood pressure control caused by ferrous sulfate and ferrous gluconate. Clinical Pharmacology and Therapeutics 1988; 43: 381
189. McTavish D, Young RA, Clissold SP. Cadralazine: a review of its pharmacodynamic and pharmacokinetic properties and therapeutic potential in the treatment of hypertension. Drugs 1990; 40: 543
190. Campese VM. Minoxidil: a review of its pharmacological properties and therapeutic use. Drugs 1981; 22: 257
191. Friedel HA, Brogden RN. Pinacidil: a review of its pharmacodynamic and pharmacokinetic properties, and therapeutic potential in the treatment of hypertension. Drugs 1990; 39: 929-67
192. Brogden RN, Sorkin EM. Ketanserin: a review of its pharmacodynamic and pharmacokinetic properties, and therapeutic potential in hypertension and peripheral vascular disease. Drugs 1990; 40: 903-49
193. Goa KL, Wagstaff AJ. Losartan potassium: a review of its pharmacology, clinical efficacy and tolerability in the management of hypertension. Drugs 1996; 51: 820-45
194. PACK Claudication Substudy Investigators. Randomised placebo-controlled double-blind trial of ketanserin in claudicants. Changes in claudication distance and ankle systolic pressure. Circulation 1989; 80: 1544
195. Dunlay MC, Fitzpatrick V, Chrysant S, et al. Losartan potassium as initial therapy in patients with severe hypertension. Journal of Human Hypertension 1995; 9: 861-7
196. Chan JCN, Critchley JAJH, Lappe JT, et al. Randomised, double-blind, parallel study of the anti-hypertensive efficacy and safety of losartan potassium compared with felodipine ER in elderly patients with mild to moderate hypertension. Journal of Human Hypertension 1995; 9: 765-71
197. Fletcher AE, Battersby C, Adnitt P, et al. Quality of life on antihypertensive therapy: a double blind trial comparing quality of life on pinacidil and nifedipine in combination with a thiazide diuretic. Journal of Cardiovascular Pharmacology 1992; 20: 108
198. Veterans Administration Cooperative Study Group on Antihypertensive Agents. Effects of treatment on morbidity in hypertension. I. Results in patients with diastolic blood pressure averaging 115 through 129 mm Hg. Journal of the American Medical Association 1967; 202: 1028
199. Veterans Administration Cooperative Study Group on Antihypertensive Agents. Effects of treatment on morbidity in hypertension. II. Results in patients with diastolic blood pressure averaging 90 through 114 mm Hg. Journal of the American Medical Association 1970; 213: 1143
200. Report of the Joint National Committee on Detection, Evaluation and Treatment of High Blood Pressure. Journal of the American Medical Association 1977; 237: 1143
201. World Health Organization Expert Committee on Arterial Hypertension. Technical Report Series, No 628. Geneva: World Health Organization, 1978
202. Hypertension Detection and Follow-up Program Cooperative Group. Five year findings of the Hypertension Detection and Follow-up Program. I. Reduction in mortality in persons with high blood pressure including mild hypertension. Journal of the American Medical Association 1979; 242: 2562
203. Multiple Risk Factor Intervention Trial Research Group, MRFIT: risk factors and mortality results. Journal of the American Medical Association 1982; 248: 1465
204. Kuller LH, Hulley SB, Cohen JD, et al. Unexpected results of treating hypertension in men with electrocardiographic abnormalities: a critical analysis. Circulation 1986; 73: 1114
205. Freis ED. Critique of the clinical implications of diuretic-induced hypokalemia and elevated cholesterol level. Archives of Internal Medicine 1989; 149: 2640
206. Cutler JA, Furberg CD. Drug treatment trials in hypertension: a review. Preventive Medicine 1985; 14: 499

207. Toth PJ, Horowitz RI. Conflicting clinical trials and the uncertainty of treating mild hypertension. American Journal of Medicine 1983; 148: 1023
208. Report on the Joint National Committee on Detection, Evaluation and Treatment of High Blood Pressure (1988). Archives of Internal Medicine 1988; 148: 1023
209. Pardell H. Hypertension therapy: current and future strategies. Journal of International Medical Research 1988; 16 Suppl. 1: 2A
210. Reyes AJ, Alcocer L, Velasky M, editors. Risks conveyed by antihypertensive therapy. Progress in Pharmacology 1985; 6: 1
211. Grueniger UJ, Strasser T. editors. Educating the hypertensive patient. Journal of Human Hypertension 1990; 4 Suppl. 1: 1
212. Kaplan NM. Guidelines for the treatment of hypertension. American Journal of Hypertension 1989; 2: 75
213. Laragh JH. Nephron heterogeneity: clue to the pathogenesis of essential hypertension and effectiveness of angiotensin converting enzyme inhibitor treatment. American Journal of Medicine 1989; 87 (Suppl. 6B): 2-14
214. SHEP Cooperative Research Group. Prevention of stroke by antihypertensive treatment in older persons with isolated systolic hypertension. Final results of the Systolic Hypertension in the Elderly Progam (SHEP). Journal of the American Medical Association 1991; 265: 3255
215. Fletcher AE, Bulpitt CJ. How far should blood pressure be lowered? New England Journal of Medicine 1992; 326: 251-4
216. Vokonas DS, Kannel WB, Cupples LA. Epidemiology of risk of hypertension in the elderly. The Framingham Study. Journal of Hypertension 1988; 6: 535
217. Leitschuh M, Cupples LA, Kannel W, et al. High normal blood pressure progression to hypertension in the Framingham Heart Study. Hypertension 1991; 17: 22
218. Abbot RD, McGee D. The probability of developing certain cardiovascular diseases in eight years at specified values of some characteristics. Framingham Study section 37, NIH Publication, 1987: 2284
219. Veterans Administration Cooperative Study Group on Antihypertensive Agents. Effects of treatment on morbidity in hypertension. III. Influence of age, diastolic blood pressure and prior cardiovascular disease: further analysis of side effects. Circulation 1972; 45: 991
220. Management Committee of the Australian Therapeutic Trial in Hypertension. Treatment of mild hypertension in the elderly. Medical Journal of Australia 1981; 2: 398
221. Dahlof B, Lindholm LH, Hanson L, et al. Morbidity and mortality in the Swedish trial in old patients with hypertension. Lancet 1991; 338: 1281
222. Bulpitt CJ, Fletcher AE, Amery A, et al. The hypertension in the Very Elderly Trial (HYVET). Drugs & Aging 1994; 5: 171-83
223. Mattila K, Haavisto M, Rajala S, et al. Blood pressure and survival in the very old. British Medical Journal 1988; 296: 887
224. Langer RD, Ganiate TG, Barrett-Connor E. Paradoxical survival of elderly men with high blood pressure. British Medical Journal 1989; 298: 1356
225. Bulpitt CJ, Fletcher AE. Aging, blood pressure and mortality. Journal of Hypertension 1992; 10 Suppl. 7: S45
226. Lewis RV, McDevitt DG. Adverse reactions and interactions with β-adrenoceptor blocking drugs. Medical Toxicology and Adverse Drug Experience 1986; 1: 343
227. Di Bianco R. Adverse reactions with angiotensin converting enzyme (ACE) inhibitors. Medical Toxicology and Adverse Drug Experience 1986; 1: 122
228. Garcia Jr JY, Vidt DG. Current management of hypertensive emergencies. Drugs 1987; 34: 263
229. Remuzzi G, Riggenenti P. Prevention and treatment of pregnancy-associated hypertension: what have we learned in the last ten years? American Journal of Kidney Diseases 1991; 18: 285
230. Imperiale TF, Petrulis AS. A meta-analysis of low-dose aspirin for the prevention of pregnancy-induced hypertensive disease. Journal of the American Medical Association 1991; 266: 260-4
231. CLASP Collaborative Group. CLASP: a randomised trial of low-dose aspirin for the prevention of treatment of pre-eclampsia among 9364 pregnant women. Lancet 1994; 343: 619
232. Lubbe WF. Hypertension in pregnancy: pathophysiology and management. Drugs 1984; 28: 170
233. Silver HM. Acute hypertensive crisis in pregnancy. Medical Clinics of North America 1989; 73: 623
234. Seabe SJ, Moodley J, Becker P. Nicardipine in acute hypertensive emergencies in pregnancy. South African Medical Journal 1989; 76: 248
235. Bulpitt CJ, Fletcher AE. Cost-effectiveness of the treatment of hypertension. Clinical and Experimental Hypertension 1993; 15: 1131
236. Weinstein MD, Stason WB. Hypertension: a policy perspective. Cambridge, Mass: Harvard University Press, 1976
237. Kawachi I, Malcolm LA. The cost effectiveness of treating mild-moderate hypertension: a reappraisal. Journal of Hypertension 1991; 9: 199
238. Edelson JT, Weinstein MC, Tosteson AN, et al. Long term cost-effectiveness of various initial monotherapies for mild to moderate hypertension. Journal of the American Medical Association 1990; 263: 407
239. Littenberg B, Garber AM, Sox Jr HC. Screening for hypertension. Annals of Internal Medicine 1990; 112: 192
240. Johannesson M, Jönsson B. Cost-effectiveness analysis of hypertension treatment: a review of methodological issues. Health Policy 1991; 19: 55
241. Lindgren B, Persson U. The cost-effectiveness of a new antihypertensive drug, doxazosin. Current Therapeutic Research 1989; 45: 738
242. Johannesson M, Fagerberg B. A health-economic comparison of diet and drug treatment in obese men with mild hypertension. Journal of Hypertension 1992; 10: 1063
243. MacMahon S, Peto R, Cutler J, et al. Blood pressure, stroke and coronary heart disease. (Part I): Prolonged differences in blood pressure: prospective observational studies corrected for the regression dilution bias. Lancet 1990; 335: 765
244. Collins R, Peto R, MacMahon S, et al. Blood pressure, stroke and coronary heart disease. Part 2: short-term reductions in blood pressure: overview of randomised drug trials in their epidemiological context. Lancet 1990; 335: 837
245. Johannesson M, Wikstrand I, Jonsson B, et al. Cost-effectiveness of antihypertensive treatment: metoprolol versus thiazide diuretics. PharmacoEconomics 1993; 3: 36
246. Wikstrand J, Warnold I, Olsson G, et al. Primary prevention with metoprolol in patients with hypertension. Mortality results of the MAPHY

study. Journal of the American Medical Association 1988; 259: 1976

247. Heart Attack Primary Prevention in Hypertension Trial Research Group. Beta-blockers versus diuretics in hypertensive men: main results from the HAPPHY Trial. Hypertension 1987; 5: 561

248. Fletcher AE. Pressure to treat and pressure to cost: a review of cost-effectiveness analysis. Journal of Hypertension 1991; 9: 193

249. Stason WB. Opportunities to improve the cost-effectiveness of treatment for hypertension. Hypertension 1991; 18 Suppl. I: I161-6

Chapter 22

# Gastrointestinal and Hepatic Diseases

***D.W. Piper, D.J. de Carle, N.J. Talley, N.D. Gallagher, J.S. Wilson, L.W. Powell, D. Crawford, P.R. Gibson, T.C. Sorrell, J.E. Kellow*** and ***R.K. Roberts***

## Synopsis of Important Principles

1) Oral absorption of drugs can be affected by gastrointestinal disease. Abnormal drug responses due to altered drug kinetics can occur in severe liver disease with drugs eliminated by the liver, particularly those with a low therapeutic ratio. Liver disease may change responses to some drugs.

2) Management of gastro-oesophageal reflux disease has 3 phases: lifestyle changes, drug treatment, and, in non-responders, antireflux surgery. Drugs used include antacids ± alginate, antisecretory agents and prokinetic agents. $H_2$-Receptor antagonists and prokinetic agents may relieve symptoms but are less effective for healing, for which an acid pump inhibitor is preferred. Patients needing maintenance therapy may receive reduced dosages of antisecretory drugs.

3) Peptic ulcer is initially treated with antibacterials to eradicate *Helicobacter pylori*; this permits healing and decreases recurrence. Conventional antiulcer therapy (e.g. with $H_2$-receptor antagonists, acid pump inhibitors or cytoprotective agents) relieves symptoms and facilitates healing. Maintenance antiulcer agents may be needed in complicated (e.g. bleeding) or refractory ulcers, until eradication of *H. pylori* is confirmed. In NSAID-induced ulcers, NSAIDs should be stopped and *H. pylori* infection, if present, treated with antibacterial drugs.

4) 5-$HT_3$ receptor antagonists (ondansetron, granisetron, tropisetron) are of particular value, replacing older regimens in the management of nausea and vomiting due to cancer chemotherapy.

5) Treatment of intestinal malabsorption syndromes is aimed at eradicating the primary disease and its effects, or by diet or replacement therapy appropriate for the type of deficiency.

6) In acute pancreatitis, major objectives are relief of pain, avoidance of pancreatic stimulation, maintenance of intravascular volume, correction of electrolyte abnormalities, treatment of complications, and determining and treating the cause. In chronic pancreatitis, major objectives are pain control, elimination of causative factors, and correction of pancreatic enzyme deficiencies.

7) Management of most liver diseases involves a nutritious high protein diet and vitamin $K_1$ if the prothrombin index is low. Corticosteroids are valuable in chronic active hepatitis, while interferon-$\alpha$ helps some patients with chronic hepatitis B or C.

8) Acute ulcerative colitis or Crohn's disease must be managed promptly, the intensity of treatment depending on attack severity. Surgery is often needed in Crohn's disease.

9) Diarrhoea and constipation not due to organic disease can be controlled by symptomatic therapy. Persistent or severe bowel derangement must be fully investigated.

10) Irritable bowel syndrome requires reassurance, support, adequate dietary fibre, drugs to control constipation or diarrhoea, antispasmodics and/or tricyclic antidepressants for pain, and behavioural therapies.

11) Drugs can cause gastrointestinal or hepatic reactions. Diarrhoea is a common adverse effect. Antibiotic-induced diarrhoea must be investigated if more than trivial. Aspirin and ulcerogenic drugs may aggravate peptic ulcer; morphine or diuretics can precipitate coma in patients with cirrhosis.

In common with several other groups of diseases, major advances have been made in the management of gastrointestinal disease in the past decade. These advances have been at 3 levels:

1) The development of new diagnostic procedures such as endoscopy, ultrasound examination and computerised axial tomography (CAT) scanning.

2) The development of new drugs, especially new antisecretory drugs.

3) The assessment of therapeutic measures, both drug and nondrug, by the use of randomised clinical trials.

Provision of medical care is a large part of the cost to governmental agencies. Consequently, politicians are justifiably questioning whether treatment is cost effective. While mindful of the fact that the value of a life saved is difficult to assess in pecuniary terms, the cost effectiveness of treatment cannot be ignored.

Gastrointestinal and liver diseases are major causes of morbidity and mortality, and the therapeutic implications are vast. Cirrhosis of the liver, for example, remains the fourth most common cause of death in the US and probably elsewhere as well. It is clear that effective drugs may not provide demonstrable benefit in these diseases unless they are used appropriately, a process that involves both doctor and patient education.

## 1. Clinical Pharmacological Considerations

Physiological and biochemical perturbations occur in patients with hepatic or gastrointestinal disease and have the potential to affect pharmacodynamic or pharmacokinetic responses to drugs. The processes of absorption, first-pass metabolism, distribution, and elimination can separately or in concert influence the outcome of the drug-patient interaction.

### 1.1 Drug Absorption and Gastrointestinal Function

In certain circumstances, it is obvious that oral administration of a drug is unreliable, e.g. in repeated vomiting and intestinal obstruction. More subtle, but nonetheless significant, abnormalities of drug absorption may be related to conditions associated with an altered rate of gastric emptying, altered gastrointestinal transit and/or intestinal malabsorption syndrome.[1-4]

#### *1.1.1 Pathophysiological Factors*

Pathophysiological factors that affect drug absorption may be predominantly luminal, may occur within the mucosa of the gastrointestinal tract, or may be related to gastrointestinal motility disturbances. Changes can be viewed anatomically as gastric, small intestinal or colonic, either individually or in combination. In addition, other factors extraneous to these processes may modify drug effects, including the formulation of the medication itself.[5,6]

*Luminal factors* that can affect drug absorption include luminal pH, the presence or absence of food or other therapeutic substances, and the presence or absence of bacteria. The pH partition hypothesis was initially proposed to explain drug absorption. This suggests that, for example, weak acids such as aspirin (acetylsalicylic acid) should be absorbed more slowly in achlorhydric patients. However, the opposite effect has been observed, in that plasma salicylate concentrations are higher and peak concentrations of salicylates are reached more rapidly in these patients.[7] Thus, pH is not the only factor influencing absorption; blood flow, membrane permeability, the formulation of the compound and its physicochemical properties (e.g. polarity and degree of ionisation) are also important.[6,8]

*Bacteria* within gut lumen can also influence drug absorption. For example, in patients with abnormal bacterial flora, the amount of levodopa available for absorption is decreased.[9] The activity of sulfasalazine is reduced when colonic flora populations are diminished (e.g. due to concomitant administration of antibiotics). This is because colonic flora are required to split the azo bond and release the active constituent mesalazine. The same consideration applies to olsalazine as well.

#### *1.1.2 Influence of Gastrointestinal Motility*

The consequences of changes in gastric emptying or intestinal motility are often unpredictable. In patients with delayed gastric emptying and pyloric stenosis, the absorption of drugs such as paracetamol (acetaminophen) and aspirin may be markedly impaired.[10,11] This is particularly likely with enteric-coated or slow-release formulations.[12,13] The absorption of effervescent aspirin is delayed in patients during an attack of migraine and the degree of delay correlates well with the severity of headache and gastrointestinal symptoms. This delayed absorption appears to reflect the delay in gastric emptying during attacks of migraine, since aspirin absorption and relief of symptoms improve when the gastric emptying rate is increased following administration of intramuscular metoclopramide.[14]

Very rapid gastrointestinal transit, as in gastroenteritis, may decrease the rate of drug absorption. This effect is likely to be greatest for poorly soluble drugs (e.g. digoxin), and enteric-coated and slow-release formulations. The decreased drug absorption rate may be due to the reduced time available for absorption when gastrointestinal transit is very rapid and to impaired drug dissolution in the gut lumen.[15] A further example of this phenomenon is the influence of acute gastroenteritis on the absorption of norfloxacin. While total norfloxacin absorption is similar during the acute and convalescent stage of diarrhoeal illness, the time to reach maximal concentrations is higher when the drug is given during the acute phase.[16]

#### *1.1.3 Influence of Food and Antacids*

As a general principle, *food* does not usually interfere greatly with drug absorption.[17] The administration of drugs with food may in fact assist in obtaining therapeutic compliance. However, some studies have documented differences in drug absorption between the fasting and the fed state.[15,17-19] Drugs for which a clear interaction with food has been observed include isoniazid, rifampicin, penicillin, tetracyclines, and the antidiabetic agents, glipizide and glibenclamide (glyburide).

*Antacids* have a variable effect on drug absorption,[19,20] depending on the physicochemical and formulation characteristics of the particular drug. In general, for patients concurrently receiving antacids, it is advisable to administer other drugs at least half to one hour before antacid ingestion. For a listing of drugs whose absorption may be influenced to a clinically important extent by antacids, see appendix B.

#### *1.1.4 Intestinal Malabsorption Syndromes*

Frank malabsorption states, as in coeliac disease, might be expected to reduce absorption of drugs in the same way they decrease absorption of essential foodstuffs, vitamins and trace elements. However, the effect is inconsistent and depends on the degree of malabsorption, the treatment given, and the physicochemical and pharmacokinetic properties of the individual drug.[2,21] Absorption may be delayed (e.g. amoxicillin, lincomycin), decreased (e.g. phenoxymethylpenicillin, pivampicillin, thyroxine), increased (e.g. cotrimoxazole, fusidic acid, propranolol) or unchanged (e.g. indomethacin, aspirin, pivmecillinam). In untreated coeliac disease, the absorption of practolol (a water soluble drug) is delayed, whereas that of propranolol (a lipid soluble drug) is increased, with a resulting increase in the plasma concentration of unchanged drug.[22] On the other hand, in patients with coeliac disease in remission, plasma concentrations of propranolol are not increased.[23]

Absorption of some drugs is altered in Crohn's disease, but the effect is variable, as in coeliac disease, and is variously decreased (e.g. lincomycin), increased (e.g. clindamycin, cotrimoxazole, fusidic acid), slightly reduced (metronidazole) or unchanged (e.g. cefalexin, rifampicin).[24,25] The reasons for altered absorption of drugs in coeliac and Crohn's disease are not clear.[2] Increased plasma concentrations of propranolol in Crohn's disease are probably due to increased plasma protein binding and decreased clearance as a consequence of impaired hepatic function, rather than altered oral absorption.[26] The absorption of amoxicillin, ampicillin cefalexin, cotrimoxazole, lincomycin, clindamycin and rifampicin is, however, adequate in small bowel diverticulosis. Human immunodeficiency virus (HIV) infection and acquired immune deficiency syndrome (AIDS) are associated with gastrointestinal manifestations. AIDS gastropathy may cause ketoconazole malabsorption,[27] but fluconazole absorption does not appear to be affected.[28]

The absorption of digoxin is decreased in many malabsorption states due to mucosal disease, but does not seem to be altered in pancreatic disease.[29] While plasma concentrations of cefalexin and semisynthetic penicillins are markedly reduced in patients with cystic fibrosis, at least in the case of the penicillins this is due to increased renal clearance. Enteropathy associated with radiotherapy may also lead to impaired absorption of drugs.[30]

The extent of these changes in drug absorption and their significance in treating patients with malabsorption syndromes is difficult to predict. Drug absorption will likely vary depending on the drug administered and the clinical status of the patient. Thus, a change in treatment, such as introduction of a gluten-free diet in coeliac disease, may profoundly affect the ability of the intestinal mucosa to absorb certain drugs. For example, while phenoxymethylpenicillin (penicillin V) absorption is decreased in children with untreated coeliac disease, after 6 to 8 months of gluten-free diet, absorptive capacity is normal.[31]

Clinicians should, thus, be aware that dosage adjustments may be needed for some drugs, but this knowledge cannot be applied arbitrarily or to malabsorption syndromes in general. Suspicion of poor absorption of digoxin, for example, should call for more regular monitoring of plasma concentrations, with dosages adjusted accordingly. Reduced absorption of an orally administered antibiotic will lead to a decrease in the peak plasma concentration and potential therapeutic failure. Careful prescribing, with knowledge of pharmacokinetics and possible effects of a disease process, should prevent toxicity or therapeutic failure.

### 1.2 Drug Metabolism and Gastrointestinal Function

The bioavailability of some orally administered drugs is influenced by gut metabolism before absorption occurs, such that the amount of intact drug available for absorption is reduced. Losses may be substantial and can be influenced by gastric emptying or intestinal motility. Enterocytes are capable of a number of typical drug biotransformations, including acetylation and conjugation.[32] Hydralazine is subject to significant first-pass metabolism due to polymorphic acetylation within the gut mucosa and liver.[33] The pharmacokinetics of chlorpromazine are complex and demonstrate marked interpatient variability; some patients fail to absorb chlorpromazine,[34] apparently because of a pronounced capacity to metabolise the drug in the gut wall.[35,36]

Many factors influence the rate of gastric emptying and may alter the rate of absorption of orally administered drugs (table I).[1] Changes in gastric emptying rates or intestinal motility in most cases results only in a change in the rate of absorption. However, the extent of absorption of some drugs can be affected, e.g. those that are poorly soluble, erratically absorbed or metabolised in the gut.

### 1.3 Drug Distribution in Liver Disease

The distribution of a drug after administration depends in part on the nature of interactions between the drug and binding sites in tissues and blood. This in turn depends on the physicochemical properties of the drug and the composition of the body.

**Table I.** Rate of drug absorption: influence of associated conditions/disease or concomitant drug therapy

| Disorder/drug | Increased rate | Decreased rate |
|---|---|---|
| Gastric ulcer | | + |
| Duodenal ulcer | + | |
| Pyloric stenosis | | + |
| Migraine | | + |
| Myocardial infarction | | + |
| Labour | | + |
| Trauma and pain | | + |
| Anticholinergic drugs | | + |
| Tricyclic antidepressants | | + |
| Opioid analgesics | | + |
| Sodium bicarbonate | + | |
| Aluminium hydroxide | | + |
| Metoclopramide | + | |
| Domperidone | + | |
| Cisapride | + | |
| Erythromycin | + | |

Especially in places where nutrition is poor, liver disease alters body fat stores and total body water,[38] changing the distribution of predominantly water soluble or predominantly lipid soluble drugs.[39] Effects of the aging process and associated changes in body composition may be superimposed on changes associated with liver disease.

Changes in drug binding to blood constituents also occurs in liver disease. Albumin is quantitatively the most important protein responsible for binding of acidic drugs. Concentrations of albumin are often decreased in acute or chronic liver disease. The relative effects of qualitative changes in the albumin molecule or of increased concentrations of endogenous substances such as bilirubin and bile salts on binding are not known. However, reductions in binding of highly-bound acidic drugs (e.g. phenytoin) in liver disease is most marked when both hypoalbuminaemia and hyperbilirubinaemia are present.[40,41]

Some basic drugs bind to $\alpha_1$-acid glycoprotein, although concentrations of this protein do not appear to be altered in cirrhosis.[42] Whether changes in $\alpha_1$-acid glycoprotein concentrations occur in other liver diseases is not clear. Similarly, the influence of liver disease on plasma content of other binding proteins such as ligandin is not known. Tissue binding of drugs in liver disease may also be affected by changes in plasma or tissue pH, further influencing drug distribution.

Because of the interaction between drugs and various binding proteins, a drug circulating in blood will exist in both bound and unbound fractions, depending on the nature of the drug and the binding sites available. It is the unbound fraction of drug that is available for binding to tissue sites of action and for metabolism in the liver. The role of binding in hepatic elimination of drugs is discussed below.

## 1.4 Drug Elimination in Liver Disease

### *1.4.1 General Principles*

The total clearance of a drug by the body is the sum of its clearance by potential routes of elimination, including hepatic, renal and pulmonary elimination. When the major route of drug elimination is hepatic, liver disease can clearly influence the outcome of drug treatment. Before being excreted, many lipid soluble drugs are metabolised by mixed-function oxidases in the liver to more polar (water soluble) metabolites and often then conjugated by a variety of pathways, the most common of which is glucuronidation.

The effects of liver disease on hepatic metabolism of drugs are complex and difficult to predict (see also appendix F).[43-45] The nature and extent of organ damage varies depending on the type and stage of liver disease. Not all liver diseases produce the same patterns of change, at least while they are evolving, although many forms of chronic liver disease will ultimately lead to the typical clinical and histological picture of cirrhosis.

Often, there is reduced portal venous perfusion to a liver of reduced cell mass. Within the liver there may be intrahepatic shunts coursing through bands of thick fibrous tissue. The exposure to liver cells in regenerative nodules varies and where sinusoids and hepatocytes maintain some normal regular arrangement, sinusoidal membranes may be abnormal (capillarisation), with loss of fenestration and reduced permeability. There is also the potential for extrahepatic shunts to divert significant fractions of portal blood supply from the portal system to the systemic circulation. These factors, in concert, may lead to changes in drug disposition.[18,43,46]

Hepatic drug elimination may also be influenced by extraneous factors such as concomitant drug therapy, alcohol ingestion, nutritional status and associated organ dysfunction such as renal or cardiac impairment.

Hepatic function may fluctuate considerably over short periods of time. Thus, it is not surprising that it has been difficult to predict, using standard laboratory measurements of liver function, the appropriate dose of a given drug. Of all liver function tests, serum albumin concentration and vitamin K-corrected prothrombin time probably provide the best estimates of hepatic metabolic capacity.[47,48] Furthermore, even with normal hepatic function, there is considerable interindividual variation in hepatic drug metabolism. This variability may be even greater than that seen with liver disease.

The efficiency with which the liver can metabolise a drug has been termed the *intrinsic clearance* of that drug. Intrinsic clearance reflects the relationship between the rate of elimination of a drug by an organ and the unbound concentration of the drug in the absence of any limitation on drug delivery rate, e.g. due to blood flow to the organ.

The *extraction ratio* of the liver is a measure of the fraction of drug extracted by the liver on a single pass. For drugs eliminated by hepatic metabolism, there is a continuous spectrum of extraction ratios. Generally, drugs with an extraction ratio less than 0.3 are considered to have a *low hepatic clearance*. For these drugs, clearance is proportional to the concentration of unbound drug in the plasma. On the other hand, drugs with an extraction ratio greater than 0.7 have a *high hepatic clearance* that is greater than hepatic blood flow (≈90 L/h). For these drugs, the rate of hepatic elimination also depends on the rate of the delivery of the drug to the liver by hepatic blood flow, and the clearance of such drugs is considered to be 'flow-limited'.[49] Following oral administration, drugs with a high hepatic extraction ratio will undergo significant first-pass elimination by the liver. Thus, for a drug with an extraction ratio of 0.8, only 20% of the orally administered dose would reach the peripheral circulation after one pass through the liver (assuming complete absorption). Furthermore, for such drugs, small changes in the hepatic extraction ratio may lead to significant increases in bioavailability, due to reduced hepatic extraction and portal systemic shunts.[50,51]

Drugs shown to have an increased bioavailability in liver disease include propranolol,[52] pethidine (meperidine) and pentazocine,[51] labetalol[53] and clomethiazole (chlormethiazole).[54] With clomethiazole, a 10-fold increase in bioavailability can lead to a significant risk of toxicity in patients with advanced cirrhosis.

For drugs that are poorly extracted by the liver, changes in hepatic extraction produced by liver disease will not significantly affect bioavailability, assuming absorption is complete.

For further discussion of these concepts, see chapter 1 (section 5.4.3)

#### 1.4.2 Effect of Liver Disease on Elimination

From the discussion in section 1.4.1, it should be clear that liver disease has the capacity to influence the elimination of compounds with both high and low hepatic extraction ratios, although not necessarily to a similar degree.

While a detailed discussion of the effect of liver disease on the disposition of individual drugs is beyond the scope of this chapter, there are special instances that merit mention. The elimination of lidocaine (lignocaine) is critically dependent on hepatic blood flow and, since lidocaine has a low therapeutic ratio, relatively small increases in plasma concentration can lead to CNS toxicity. Clearance of lidocaine is markedly impaired in chronic active hepatitis and in cirrhosis.[55-57]

The elimination of morphine and other compounds with high hepatic extraction ratios is significantly reduced in patients with cirrhosis.[58,59] The hepatic elimination of theophylline, is reduced in cirrhosis, which is again of clinical significance because of the narrow therapeutic window of this agent.[60,61] However, as predicted from the discussion above, peak concentrations are not affected after an oral dose.[62]

There is some evidence that glucuronidation is relatively preserved in patients with liver disease, but there is controversy on this issue. A reasonable interpretation of the available data, however, is that glucuronidation of a compound does not necessarily guarantee preservation of hepatic elimination in the presence of acute or chronic liver disease. The effects of liver disease on variously conjugated, and particularly glucuronidated drugs have been examined in the literature.[45,46]

#### 1.4.3 Model or Marker Compounds as Predictors of Hepatic Functional Reserve

From the foregoing, it can be seen that it would be difficult to find a substrate that gives an accurate measure of hepatic function and predicts changes in drug elimination with deteriorating function, within a 'patient-friendly' test protocol. A number of attempts have been made over the years, but most have not led to clinically useful results. Drugs with both high and low hepatic clearance (predominantly bromsulphthalein, indocyanine green, lidocaine, propranolol) and drugs with a low hepatic clearance [phenazone (antipyrine), aminophenazone (aminopyrine), caffeine] have been used either alone or in combination, but generally without success.

Of all these substrates, phenazone has probably been studied most extensively. It can be given orally and is almost completely absorbed. It is solely metabolised by the liver and there is little protein binding. The reduction in phenazone clearance approximates the degree of liver disease, whether acute or chronic.[48,64] However, the correlation between phenazone clearance and the clearance of other therapeutic compounds is generally poor,[45] so that the use of phenazone clearance as a guide to drug dosage is limited.

It is not surprising, given the complexity of the liver and the variety of metabolic processes occurring there, that data are at times conflicting or confusing. However, general principles of rational prescribing in liver disease are emerging. If these are applied with thought and care, misadventure from inappropriate prescribing will be minimised (see further appendix F).

## 2. General Principles of Treatment

### 2.1 Accurate Diagnosis

For decades, the diagnosis of diseases of the hollow organs of the gastrointestinal tract was difficult. Symptoms were nonspecific and in many cases (e.g. coeliac disease) gross morphological changes were slight. However, fibreoptic endoscopy has enabled clinicians to inspect all the hollow organs internally and to photograph and biopsy any lesion seen.

### 2.2 Reassurance and Education of the Patient

When patients consult clinicians, they often fear life-threatening disease, unmindful of the fact that most diseases are minor and self-limiting. The nature of the disease should be explained to the patient, and the type of treatment and possible adverse effects discussed. Where applicable, patients should be reassured that life-threatening disease is absent. For some diseases, supportive literature of great value to the patient can explain in lay terms the disease process and its treatment.

### 2.3 Individualised Treatment

Treatment aims to relieve distressing symptoms and favourably alter the course of the disease. In some diseases, such as peptic ulcer, the healing process is so rapid that symptomatic treatment is rarely required. In individualising drug dosages, the patient's age, bodyweight and the presence of diseases of eliminating organs (e.g. liver, kidneys, etc.) must be taken into account.

### 2.4 Diet

Diet plays only a small role in the treatment of most gastrointestinal diseases. Exceptions are gluten enteropathy (coeliac disease, see section 6.2.1), where gluten exclusion is curative; irritable bowel syndrome where a high fibre diet is usually helpful; alactasia, where lactose exclusion may be dramatic; and diseases characterised by fluid retention, which require a low-salt diet. Diet plays no role in the treatment of peptic ulcer.

### 2.5 Supportive Measures and Rehabilitation of the Patient

As perinatal deaths and deaths due to infections have become more rare, and life has consequently been prolonged, it is essential for society to provide roles in the social structure for elderly people and patients with chronic diseases. On diagnosis, these aspects of disease management must be critically and constructively considered by the clinician, with the patient advised appropriately. Patients should be made aware of services provided by government and community support organisations.

## 3. Oesophageal Disease

### 3.1 Gastro-Oesophageal Reflux Disease and Reflux Oesophagitis

#### *3.1.1 Gastro-Oesophageal Reflux Disease (GORD)*

Symptomatic GORD is a relatively common disorder that may be mistaken for pulmonary or ischaemic heart disease by both patients and clinicians. GORD refers to the varied clinical manifestations of reflux of stomach and duodenal contents into the oesophagus. It is of a mild, intermittent or chronic nature in most patients. Heartburn is the most common manifestation and can vary from occasional mild burning after overeating to ever-present, severe discomfort that greatly limits patients' lifestyles.[65] Heartburn may be accompanied by regurgitation of gastric contents into the mouth or respiratory tree, leading in some cases to nocturnal wheezing, hoarseness, a need to clear the throat repeatedly and a sensation of deep pressure at the base of the neck.

GORD is multifactorial in origin, abnormal functioning of the lower oesophageal sphincter being the principal aetiological factor. Transient inappropriate lower oesophageal sphincter tone, such that the sphincter no longer provides a barrier against retrograde flow, is the prominent mechanism. Impaired efficiency of oesophageal clearance and/or gastric emptying are also implicated.[65] Anatomical derangement by hiatus hernia may also contribute. Symptoms may occur in the absence of endoscopically demonstrable oesophagitis.

**Optimum Treatment**

The management of GORD comprises 3 phases: lifestyle changes (phase I), drug treatment (phase II) and surgery (phase III). Approximately 60% of patients respond to phase I management and do not require more intensive treatment.[65] Figure 1 summarises the approach to treatment of GORD.

***Phase I*** measures aimed at preventing or minimising reflux include bodyweight reduction if the patient is obese, elevation of the bedhead by 15 to 20cm (6 to 8 inches), avoidance of bending, stooping and of wearing tight clothing, and abstinence from food or fluid for at least 2 hours before retiring.

***Drug treatment (phase II):*** drugs used in the medical management of GORD include:

- *Antacids with or without alginate* – which raise the pH of the refluxed gastric content and provide relief of symptoms
- *Drugs that prevent acid secretion* [e.g. the $H_2$-receptor antagonists and the acid (proton) pump inhibitors] – which decrease the volume of gastric fluid available for reflux and raise its pH
- *Prokinetic agents* (e.g. cisapride, metoclopramide and domperidone) – which act by increasing lower oesophageal sphincter tone and enhancing oesophageal motility.

The $H_2$-receptor antagonists include *cimetidine*, *ranitidine*,[66] *famotidine*,[67] *nizatidine*,[68] and *roxatidine*;[69] their clinical pharmacological properties are discussed in section 4.1.

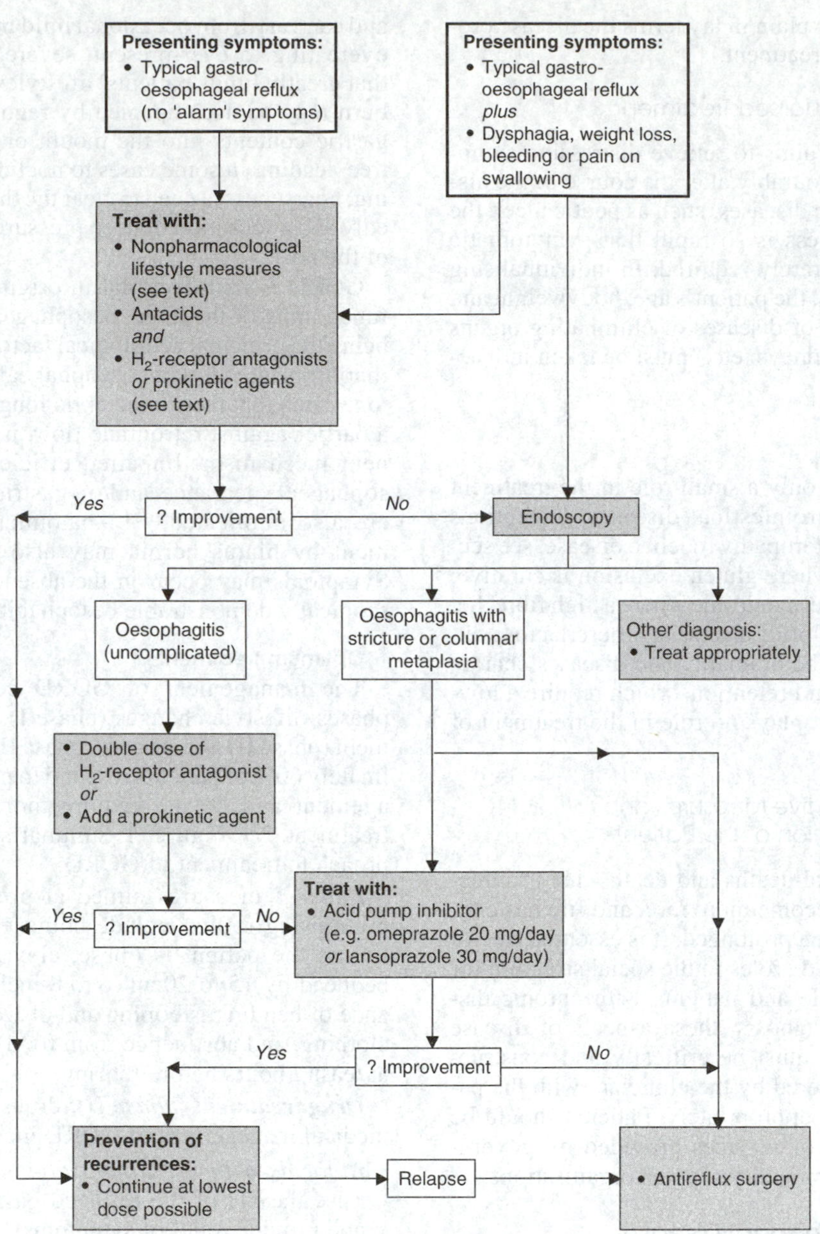


**Fig. 1.** Optimum treatment of gastro-oesophageal reflux.

When used in standard dosages, the $H_2$-receptor antagonists produce symptom relief in around 60% of patients with GORD.[70] However, they are less effective for healing of oesophagitis (see section 3.1.2), for which the acid pump inhibitors are generally preferred.

The prokinetic agent *cisapride*[71] diminishes gastro-oesophageal reflux by increasing the rate of gastric emptying (see also section 5.1.3). Cisapride may also increase the force of oesophageal contractions and, thus, improve oesophageal refluxate clearance. Its effectiveness in relieving reflux symptoms and healing of oesophagitis is comparable to that of the $H_2$-receptor antagonists, and when given in combination with $H_2$-receptor antagonists, healing rates in oesophagitis are higher than when given alone.[71] An advantage of this agent is that the underlying motility disorder is ameliorated. Cisapride also effectively prevents relapse during maintenance treatment.

Anticholinergic drugs, calcium antagonists and nitrates should be avoided in GORD patients, as they reduce the tone of the lower oesophageal sphincter and may delay gastric emptying and, consequently, increase reflux. Prolonged recumbency and nasogastric intubation should also be avoided (e.g. after surgical operations).

Oesophageal stricture, and columnar metaplasia in the distal oesophagus (Barrett's oesophagus), to which GORD may progress in severe cases, require more intensive therapy (see figure 1 and section 3.1.2). Respiratory disorders secondary to tracheobronchial aspiration, and bleeding are other infrequent complications of GORD.

Gastroparesis, a functional disorder of gastric emptying, is a common finding in patients with GORD (see section 11.2.2).[65]

### 3.1.2 Reflux Oesophagitis

Reflux oesophagitis is the pathological consequence of repeated reflux damage to the oesophageal mucosa. In patients with reflux oesophagitis, care should be taken to exclude other gastrointestinal diseases predisposing to reflux, particularly pyloric obstruction and gastroparesis (a functional disorder of gastric emptying; see section 11.2.2). Other disorders such as chronic duodenal ulcer can present with similar symptoms.

#### Optimum Treatment

The principles of treatment are to reduce gastro-oesophageal reflux by the methods described in section 3.1.1 and mitigate mucosal damage by raising the pH of the fluid that refluxes into the oesophagus.

*Antacids* may temporarily relieve heartburn; liquid preparations may facilitate oesophageal clearance of refluxed material. Some clinicians advocate use of an antacid/alginate preparation, which is said to produce a soft, viscous layer of antacid-containing foam that floats on the gastric content and enters the oesophagus whenever reflux occurs. However, there is little evidence that this preparation provides any more relief of symptoms than antacids alone.

Symptoms persist in most patients despite lifestyle changes (see section 3.1.1.) and antacids. In this situation, *$H_2$-receptor antagonists* and *cisapride* may provide symptomatic relief but are seldom associated with healing of oesophagitis.

Treatment with acid pump inhibitors such as *omeprazole*,[72] *lansoprazole*[73] and *pantoprazole*[74] given for 4 weeks produces rapid symptomatic relief and endoscopically proven healing of oesophagitis in around 80% of patients. Usual doses for healing of oesophagitis are omeprazole 20 to 40 mg/day, lansoprazole 30 mg/day and pantoprazole 40 mg/day. After cessation of acid pump inhibitor therapy, however, relapse occurs within 3 months in around 70% of patients and prolonged therapy is usually needed to maintain remission. For this purpose, reduced daily doses of an acid pump inhibitor (e.g. omeprazole 10 mg/day, lansoprazole 15 mg/day) may be sufficient. A recent study comparing five maintenance therapy regimens for reflux oesophagitis[75] showed that omeprazole (20 mg/day), given either alone or in combination with cisapride (10mg 3 times daily), was significantly more effective in preventing lesions or symptoms of oesophagitis over a period of 12 months than ranitidine alone (150mg 3 times daily) or cisapride alone, and that the combination of omeprazole and cisapride was more effective than ranitidine plus cisapride.

***Antireflux surgery:*** although adequate control of reflux oesophagitis can usually be achieved with acid pump inhibitors, in some patients, particularly the young and those with complications of oesophagitis, antireflux surgery may be considered as an alternative to prolonged drug therapy. A number of surgical procedures may be used, but Nissen fundoplication is the most common. Antireflux surgery may be performed laparoscopically and studies suggest that the early results of laparoscopic procedures are similar to those achieved with open operations. However, the long term outcome of laparoscopic antireflux surgery is not yet known.[76] A large para-oesophageal hernia is an indication for surgical correction because of the risk of gastric volvulus.[77]

### 3.1.3 Clinical Outcome and Economic Considerations

Although omeprazole has a higher daily acquisition cost than alternative agents, it has been shown to be more cost effective than ranitidine and cimetidine for initial healing of reflux oesophagitis, and also more cost effective than ranitidine in long term treatment.[78,79] In short term cost-effectiveness studies conducted in the UK, the cost of 4 weeks of treatment with omeprazole and ranitidine per endoscopically healed patient was £64 with omeprazole *versus* £93 with ranitidine; the corresponding figures for a patient freed of symptoms were £56 and £75.[78] In a longer term study, the cost-effectiveness advantage of omeprazole in reflux oesophagitis patients remained after 16 weeks, the cost per patient healed and symptom-free on omeprazole (20mg daily increased if necessary to 40mg daily) being £186 as compared with £442 for patients on ranitidine (300mg at night increased if necessary to 300mg twice daily).[79]

In a US study in patients with severe erosive oesophagitis (grade II and above), omeprazole has also been found to produce a superior clinical outcome at a comparable cost to a combination of ranitidine and metoclopramide.[80]

### 3.2 Oesophageal Spasm

Medical treatment of oesophageal spasm is aimed at improving retrosternal chest pain and dysphagia, and preventing bolus obstruction. Diffuse oesophageal spasm is a rare disorder that usually occurs as an isolated motility disturbance, although some features of oesophageal spasm may progress to typical achalasia (see section 3.3.1). When oesophagitis is present, it is not clear whether the motility disturbance is secondary to the oesophageal inflammation or if it leads to oesphagitis because of impaired oesophageal clearance. Several studies have shown that the motility disturbance persists when oesophagitis is healed with acid pump inhibitors, suggesting that the disturbance is the primary abnormality in some patients with oesophagitis.

#### Optimum Treatment

*Nitrate drugs* (isosorbide dinitrate, nitroglycerin),[81,82] *calcium antagonists* (verapamil, nifedipine, diltiazem)[83] and *hydralazine*[82] reduce the force of contractions and may be useful in patients with diffuse oesophageal spasm. Oral anticholinergics are of little value, but parenteral scopolamine butylbromide (hyoscine butylbromide) may be useful in patients with acute painful dysphagia.

### 3.3 Less Common Oesophageal Diseases

#### *3.3.1 Achalasia*

Achalasia is an uncommon disorder of oesophageal motility characterised by the failure of relaxation of the lower oesophageal sphincter and loss of peristaltic contractions in the body of the oesophagus. Pathologically, there is loss of intrinsic inhibitory nerves throughout the oesophagus and lower oesophageal sphincter. The cause of this loss of inhibitory nerves is not known. As the disease progresses, the oesophagus dilates and may assume a sigmoid shape. The cardinal symptoms of achalasia are *dysphagia* for both solids and liquids, *chest pain* which may be burning or gripping, and *regurgitation*. The chest pain may precede the onset of dysphagia. There may also be nocturnal cough and other symptoms of recurrent aspiration.

The diagnosis is usually established on clinical grounds and by barium swallow, which demonstrates delayed oesophageal emptying and smooth tapering at the lower end of the oesophagus with failure of oesophageal sphincter opening. In some patients, disordered contractions are seen in the distal oesophagus. Oesophageal dilatation is also usually present, except in young patients and those with short histories. The diagnosis should be confirmed by oesophageal motility studies. Upper gastrointestinal tract endoscopy shows a dilated oesophagus with retained food and fluid, but there is no mucosal abnormality and the endoscope passes easily into the stomach.

#### Optimum Treatment

Treatment of achalasia disorder is aimed at relieving dysphagia and preventing aspiration of food retained within the oesophagus. Pneumatic balloon dilatation is a simple procedure effective in 60 to 70% of patients and has a low (1 to 5%) risk of serious complications. Surgical cardiomyotomy (Heller's operation) is also highly effective in controlling symptoms and can be performed via either laparoscope or thoracoscope. Surgical myotomy is recommended in all patients when achalasia fails to respond to pneumatic dilatation, and may be considered as initial treatment. It is particularly recommended in young patients, who are known to respond less well to pneumatic dilatation.

While patients await definitive treatment or in those patients in whom such treatment is contraindicated, therapy with sublingual *isosorbide dinitrate* or *nifedipine* may partly relieve symptoms.

#### *3.3.2 Candidal Oesophagitis*

Candidal oesophagitis is an increasingly frequent complication of broad-spectrum antibiotics, corticosteroids and cytotoxic drug therapy. It is particularly common in patients using inhaled corticosteroid preparations and also occurs in patients immunocompromised for other reasons. Treatment is with orally administered antifungal agents such as *nystatin* or *amphotericin B* lozenges or oral drops. Systemic antifungal therapy with *ketoconazole* or *fluconazole* may occasionally be necessary.

#### 3.3.3 Viral (Herpes) Oesophagitis

Viral oesophagitis may cause severe retrosternal chest pain and dysphagia occurs in severely immunocompromised patients. Treatment with systemic antiviral agents (e.g. *aciclovir*) may be necessary.

#### 3.3.4 Bolus Obstruction

Food bolus obstruction usually occurs in patients with oesophageal strictures or rings and presents with acute aphagia. It may also be a manifestation of diffuse oesophageal spasm. Intravenous *scopolamine butylbromide* 20mg or intravenous *glucagon* 1mg may provide sufficient relaxation to permit passage of the bolus. Bolus obstruction may be associated with chest pain and/or marked anxiety. Intravenous *diazepam* 5mg and/or intravenous *opioids* (e.g. pethidine 50mg) may help in the treatment of acute bolus obstruction. Oesophagoscopic removal of the obstructing bolus is necessary if these measures fail.

## 4. Peptic Ulcer

Chronic peptic ulcer is a common disease with a prevalence of 3 to 5% and a lifetime incidence of 15 to 25%. Duodenal ulcers are more common than gastric ulcers and occur more often in males than females; both types occur more frequently in older individuals. Gastric ulcer is more frequently associated with use of nonsteroidal anti-inflammatory drugs (NSAIDs) than is duodenal ulcer.

Peptic ulceration refers to a breach in the gastric or proximal duodenal mucosa extending deep into the muscularis mucosa in an area exposed to acid-peptic digestion. Presenting signs and symptoms are nonspecific and include dyspepsia (commonly), night waking with pain, relief from ingestion of antacids, and (less frequently) nausea and/or vomiting. Symptoms often occur periodically.

#### Pathogenesis

Although the pathogenesis of this condition is incompletely understood, in recent years, substantial evidence has accrued that the bacterium *Helicobacter pylori* (formerly known as *Campylobacter pylori*) is implicated in causing gastritis and peptic ulcer disease.[84-89] Indeed, elimination of this organism is now an important focus in treatment of peptic ulcer.[90-93]

The association between *H. pylori* infection and both gastric and duodenal ulcer is very strong. *H. pylori* infection is apparent in 80% of patients with gastric ulcer (not due to NSAIDs) and 95% with duodenal ulcer. Furthermore, ulcer recurrence rates have been found to be markedly reduced if *H. pylori* is eradicated.[93] In a 7-year follow-up study, a recurrence of duodenal ulcer was found in 20% of patients who were *H. pylori*-positive as compared with only 3% of *H. pylori*-negative patients.[94]

An imbalance between aggressive luminal factors (acid, pepsin) and defensive mucosal factors (mucus, bicarbonate, blood flow) is also thought to be involved in the pathogenesis of peptic ulcer. Gastric acid secretion tends to be normal or low in patients with gastric ulcer, and normal or high in those with duodenal ulcer.

***NSAID-related ulcers:*** nonsteroidal anti-inflammatory drugs (including aspirin) cause a significant percentage of not only gastric but also duodenal ulcers, and if *H. pylori*-associated gastritis is present, an interaction between the two may be important in the pathogenesis of ulceration. However, present evidence indicates that eradication of *H. pylori* does not influence the healing or recurrence of NSAID-related ulcers, although individuals who are *H. pylori*-positive (especially those who smoke) appear more prone to develop gastric ulceration.[95]

### 4.1 Clinical Pharmacology of Antiulcer Drugs

Table II lists the modes of action and dosage regimens of drugs used to accelerate healing of peptic ulcers (other than antibacterial agents used to eradicate *H. pylori*). These agents can be grouped in separate classes according to their principal action:

- *Antacids and antisecretory drugs* (table II) – which act by elevation of the pH of gastric juice above the level at which pepsin is active, namely pH 5 (fig. 2).[96]
- *Cytoprotective drugs* – which have no effects on pH but act locally at the ulcer site to provide mucosal protection. These include bismuth compounds (e.g. colloidal bismuth subcitrate and bismuth subsalicylate) and sucralfate.
- *Drugs with both a cytoprotective and antisecretory action* – e.g. the prostaglandin de-

**Table II.** Principal characteristics of drugs (other than antibacterials) currently used to accelerate healing of peptic ulcers

| Drug | Mode of action | Dosage and duration of initial treatment | Maintenance dosage | Adverse effects/precautions | Comments |
|---|---|---|---|---|---|
| **Antisecretory drugs** | | | | | |
| *$H_2$-Receptor antagonists* | | | | | |
| Cimetidine | ↓ Gastric acid secretion | 400mg twice daily or 800mg at night (4-8 weeks) | 400mg at night | Headache, dizziness, skin rash, nausea, diarrhoea (uncommon). Rarely, impotence, gynaecomastia and mental confusion (high doses, renal or hepatic disease, elderly). Interferes with hepatic metabolism of some drugs, e.g. warfarin, phenytoin, oral antiarrhythmics, theophylline, certain benzodiazepines (especially in the elderly). Reduce dosage in renal or hepatic impairment (see appendices D and F) | Simple regimen (single daily dosage) |
| Ranitidine | ↓ Gastric acid secretion | 150mg twice daily or 300mg at night (4-8 weeks) | 150mg at bedtime | Headache, dizziness, nausea, diarrhoea, skin rash (rare). Reduce dosage in moderate to severe renal impairment (see appendix D) | Simple regimen (single daily dosage). Minimal interference with metabolism of other drugs (no major interactions reported) |
| Famotidine | ↓ Gastric acid secretion | 20mg twice daily or 40mg at night (4-8 weeks) | 20mg at night | Headache, dizziness, diarrhoea, constipation, skin rash (rare). Reduce dosage in moderate to severe renal impairment | Simple regimen (single daily dosage). Evidence suggests no interference with hepatic metabolism of other drugs |
| Nizatidine | ↓ Gastric acid secretion | 150mg twice daily or 300mg at night (4-8 weeks) | 150mg at night | Headache, somnolence, sweating, diarrhoea, urticaria (rare). Reduced dosage in moderate to severe renal impairment | Simple regimen (single daily dosage). Evidence suggests no interference with hepatic metabolism of other drugs |
| Roxatidine | ↓ Gastric acid secretion | 75mg twice daily or 150mg at night (4-8 weeks) | 75mg at night | Headache, dizziness, nausea, diarrhoea, constipation, skin rash (rare). Reduce dosage in moderate to severe renal impairment | Simple regimen (single daily dosage). Evidence suggests no interference with hepatic metabolism of other drugs |
| *Acid (proton) pump inhibitors* | | | | | |
| Omeprazole | ↓ Gastric acid secretion; suppression of *Helicobacter pylori* | 20-40mg once daily in the morning (2-8 weeks) | 10-20mg daily | Diarrhoea, headache, nausea, abdominal pain, dizziness (uncommon). Potential interference with metabolism of other drugs (e.g. warfarin, phenytoin, diazepam, cyclosporin) but few significant interactions reported. No dosage adjustment required in renal impairment | Simple regimen (single daily dosage). Prolonged duration of effect (greater antisecretory activity than $H_2$-receptor antagonists) |
| Lansoprazole | ↓ Gastric acid secretion; suppression of *Helicobacter pylori* | 15-30mg once daily (4-8 weeks) | | Diarrhoea, headache, nausea, abdominal pain, dizziness (uncommon). Potential interference with metabolism of other drugs but no significant interactions reported. No dosage adjustment required in renal impairment | Simple regimen (single daily dosage). Prolonged duration of effect (at least as potent as omeprazole) |
| Pantoprazole | ↓ Gastric acid secretion; suppression of *Helicobacter pylori* | 40mg once daily (2-8 weeks) | | Diarrhoea, headache, nausea (uncommon). No dosage adjustment required in renal impairment | Single regimen (single daily dosage). Prolonged duration of effect. No clinically significant interactions with other drugs reported |

**Table II.** *[Continued]*

| Drug | Mode of action | Dosage and duration of initial treatment | Maintenance dosage | Adverse effects/precautions | Comments |
|---|---|---|---|---|---|
| *Muscarinic $M_1$-receptor antagonist* | | | | | |
| Pirenzepine | ↓ Gastric acid secretion; ↑ Gastric blood flow and mucus secretion | 50mg twice daily or 100mg at night 0.5h before food (4-6 weeks) | 50mg at night | Dry mouth, visual disturbances (uncommon), skin rash (rare) | Simple regimen |
| **Cytoprotective drugs** | | | | | |
| Colloidal bismuth subcitrate (tripotassium dicitrato bismuthate) | Binds to ulcer surface providing barrier; inhibits *Helicobacter pylori* | 120mg 4 times daily or 240mg twice daily, 0.5h before food (4 to 8 weeks; followed by 60-day bismuth-free period) | | Renders motions black and discolours tongue and teeth. Caution in patients with a history of upper gastrointestinal bleeding and in long term therapy. Avoid in severe renal impairment | Frequent administration separate from meals a disadvantage. Inexpensive |
| Sucralfate | Adheres to ulcer surface providing barrier | 1g 4 times daily (1 hour before meals and at bedtime) or 2g twice daily on an empty stomach (8 weeks) | 1g twice daily | Constipation, nausea, headache, urticaria, dyspepsia. May interfere with absorption of some drugs (e.g. warfarin, phenytoin). Avoid in severe renal impairment | Frequent administration separate from meals a disadvantage |
| **Antisecretory and cytoprotective drugs** | | | | | |
| Misoprostol | ↓ Gastric acid secretion; ↑ mucosal blood flow and mucus secretion; cytoprotection | 200μg 4 times daily with food (4-8 weeks) | 400-800μg daily in divided doses[a] | Diarrhoea, nausea, dyspepsia, abdominal pain. Avoid pregnancy in females of childbearing age. No dosage adjustment required in renal impairment | Synthetic prostaglandin $E_1$ analogue. Useful in preventing NSAID-induced ulcers |
| Ranitidine bismuth citrate | ↓ Gastric acid secretion and binds to ulcer surface providing barrier; inhibits *Helicobacter pylori* | 400mg twice daily | | Renders motions black and discolours tongue and teeth; headache, diarrhoea, abdominal discomfort, skin rash (rare). Avoid in severe renal impairment | Simple regimen. 400mg ranitidine bismuth citrate is bioequivalent to 150mg ranitidine hydrochloride |
| **Antacids** | | | | | |
| Aluminium hydroxide gel-magnesium hydroxide suspension | ↓ Gastric acidity; binds or absorbs pepsin | *High-dose regimen:* 30ml 1h before and 3h after meals and at bedtime | | *Aluminium hydroxide:* constipation, phosphorus depletion (long term use). *Magnesium hydroxide:* diarrhoea, hypermagnesaemia in renal failure. Absorption of other drugs may be impaired (e.g. tetracyclines, isoniazid, chlorpromazine, digoxin) | Frequent administration separate from meals a disadvantage. Disturbance of bowel function in ≈50% of patients |

a Maintenance therapy for prevention of NSAID-induced ulcers only.

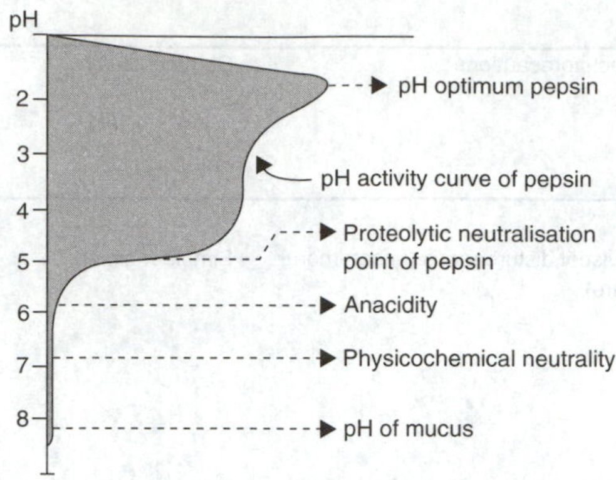


**Fig. 2.** Relationship of the pH of gastric juice to the end-points of titration and peptic activity (after Piper & Fenton[96]).

rivative misoprostol, and ranitidine bismuth citrate.

#### 4.1.1 Antacids

Antacids have been used for centuries in the treatment of dyspepsia. They act by elevating the pH of gastric juice to a level at which peptic digestion is impossible.[96] Aluminium hydroxide gel also acts by binding or adsorbing pepsin. Chemically, the antacids fall into 2 main groups:

1) Rapidly acting, highly potent compounds, such as sodium bicarbonate and calcium carbonate.

2) Less potent and less rapidly acting compounds such as aluminium and magnesium hydroxides.

Only the latter group has been shown in clinical trials to accelerate the healing of peptic ulcers. Initially, it was reported that an aluminium-magnesium hydroxide gel given in a dose of 1008 mmol neutralising capacity per day (as 30ml of 'Mylanta II' suspension before and after the 3 main meals and at bedtime) produced healing of duodenal ulcer.[97,98] Subsequently, other trials have shown that a daily dose of 200 mmol neutralising capacity, given in 6 to 8 doses daily, produces a healing rate in gastric and duodenal ulcer equivalent to that of cimetidine.[99-102]

Antacids have the disadvantages of causing disturbances of bowel function and electrolyte balance, and require frequent dosage. Their cost is comparable to that of other antiulcer drugs.

#### 4.1.2 Antisecretory Drugs

The currently available antisecretory drugs act through 1 of 3 mechanisms:

- Blockade of receptor sites, e.g. $H_2$-receptor antagonists and muscarinic $M_1$-receptor antagonists
- $H^+/K^+$-ATPase inhibition, e.g. substituted benzimidazoles such as omeprazole, lansoprazole and pantoprazole
- Inhibition of intracellular mechanisms involving calcium and/or cyclic-AMP metabolism, e.g. prostaglandin analogues.

##### $H_2$-Receptor Antagonists

It has been known for years that the final common pathway of all stimulants of acid secretion is mediated by histamine and that conventional antihistamines inhibit all the effects of histamine except those of gastric acid secretion. This led to the concept that there are 2 types of histamine receptors, designated $H_1$- and $H_2$-receptors, and that the latter are responsible for mediating the actions of histamine on gastric acid secretion. Consequently, an intensive research programme was undertaken to synthesise a compound that would inhibit the effect of histamine on gastric acid secretion.[103] This ultimately led to the development of cimetidine, which blocks parietal cell histamine $H_2$-receptor sites and, thus, effectively inhibits gastric acid secretion. More recently, newer agents with a similar locus of action have become available including, ranitidine, famotidine, nizatidine and roxatidine. Clinical trials have shown the $H_2$-receptor antagonists to accelerate the healing of both duodenal and gastric ulcers, and to be well tolerated.

Pharmacokinetic parameters for the available $H_2$-receptor antagonists are provided in appendix A. All drugs of this group are eliminated primarily by the kidney and hence their clearances are dependent on renal function. Consequently, in patients with renal impairment, dosage reduction of $H_2$-receptor antagonists is mandatory (see further appendix D). In patients undergoing dialysis procedures, no dosage supplementation is necessary as the drugs are removed in insignificant amounts.[104]

***Cimetidine*** is the most extensively studied member of this class. Given orally or intravenous, it effectively inhibits the secretion of gastric acid stimulated by histamine, food, pentagastrin, insulin and other secretagogues. The clinical effectiveness of cimetidine has been well established in the acceleration of healing of both duodenal and gastric ulcers, and in control of gastric hypersecretion and peptic ulceration in the Zollinger-Ellison syndrome.

Cimetidine is a potent inhibitor of the metabolism of numerous other drugs eliminated by the hepatic mixed-function oxidase system. It also binds to androgen receptors and may give rise to antiandrogenic adverse effects in some patients. Adverse reactions and interactions of cimetidine are discussed further in section 4.2.2.

***Ranitidine***[66] is a substituted aminoalkyl furan compound which does not contain an imidazole group (hitherto thought to be necessary for $H_2$-antagonism). Like cimetidine, it is a potent inhibitor of basal and stimulated gastric acid secretion, but differs from cimetidine in that:

- It is 5 to 8 times more active on a molar basis and has a more prolonged duration of action
- It has a lower affinity for androgen receptors
- It binds less strongly to cytochrome P450 and consequently exerts few (if any) significant effects on the metabolism of other concomitantly administered drugs (see section 4.2.2)
- Confusional states, which have been observed in some patients receiving cimetidine, have been reported only rarely with ranitidine.

In all clinical trials, ranitidine and cimetidine have shown similar effectiveness in accelerating healing of peptic ulcer. Ranitidine does appear to have some advantages over cimetidine in patients with Zollinger-Ellison syndrome and in those also receiving other drugs metabolised by the liver.

***Famotidine***[67] is structurally related to cimetidine and ranitidine, but differs in having a thiazole nucleus rather than an imidazole or furan ring. It is 20 times more potent than cimetidine on a weight-for-weight and 7.5 times more potent than ranitidine in inhibiting basal and pentagastrin-stimulated gastric acid secretion in humans. Unlike cimetidine, famotidine does not have antiandrogenic effects, and evidently does not influence the clearance of other drugs metabolised by the hepatic mixed-function oxidase system. It appears to be a well tolerated alternative to cimetidine and ranitidine for initial healing of peptic ulcers.

***Nizatidine***,[68] like ranitidine and famotidine, is also more active on a weight-for-weight basis than cimetidine in inhibiting basal and stimulated gastric acid secretion. It has proved as effective as ranitidine in increasing the rate of healing of both duodenal and gastric ulcers, and is well tolerated. Like famotidine, it does not have any antiandrogenic effects and does not alter the metabolism of other drugs.

***Roxatidine***[69] has an antisecretory potency which is about 3 to 6 times that of cimetidine and twice that of ranitidine. It is administered clinically as the acetate which is completely absorbed orally and rapidly converted to its active metabolite, roxatidine, by esterases in the small intestine, plasma and liver. Roxatidine has proved comparable in effectiveness to cimetidine and ranitidine in healing duodenal and gastric ulcers, and like famotidine and nizatidine, has no antiandrogenic effects and does not interfere with the metabolism of other drugs.

#### Anticholinergic (Antimuscarinic) Drugs

Anticholinergic drugs have a wide range of activities through their action on smooth muscle and exocrine secretory glands. Because of their effect on gastric acid secretion, they were previously widely used in the treatment of peptic ulcer. However, their acceptance was limited because clinical trials (using the crude non-endoscopic measures then available) failed to show a beneficial effect and because of their adverse effects, which include dry mouth, blurred vision and difficulty in micturition. Conventional anticholinergic drugs currently have no place in routine ulcer therapy.

***Pirenzepine:*** with the advent of this compound, interest in anticholinergic drug therapy was revived. Pirenzepine is a hydrophilic tricyclic compound which selectively blocks $M_1$-muscarinic receptors.[105-107] $M_1$-Receptors are located in gastrointestinal secretory glands and in the corpus striatum, whereas $M_2$-receptors are located in the heart, gastrointestinal and urinary tract smooth muscle, and in the cerebellum. At other sites, such as salivary and lacrimal glands, both $M_1$- and $M_2$-receptors have been identified.

Thus, due to selective $M_1$-blockade, pirenzepine inhibits gastric acid secretion with minimal effects on smooth muscle activity and saliva flow. Like the $H_2$-receptor antagonists, pirenzepine is principally eliminated by renal excretion. Trials using endoscopy have shown it to be effective in accelerating ulcer healing and in preventing duodenal ulcer recurrences.[105] However, its less dramatic effects on ulcer healing compared with $H_2$-receptor antagonists and its adverse effects, which include dry mouth, visual disturbances and diarrhoea, tend to render pirenzepine less acceptable to patients.

#### Acid (Proton) Pump Inhibitors

The final phase of acid secretion is mediated by an enzyme, hydrogen/potassium adenosine triphosphatase ($H^+/K^+$-ATPase), situated at the secretory membrane of the parietal cell. It is believed to be the 'acid pump' of the parietal cell. $H^+/K^+$-ATPase is bound and rendered inactive by benzimidazole drugs such as omeprazole, lansoprazole and pantoprazole.

***Omeprazole***[72] inhibits basal and stimulated gastric acid secretion. As an acid-inhibiting agent, it differs from $H_2$-receptor antagonists in that it possesses a greater potency and longer duration of action, the effect lasting more than 24 hours. Because of the marked inhibition of acid secretion, there is a hypergastrinaemic response. With high doses in rats (but not in other species), this has been reported to result in hyperplasia of the enterochromaffin-like cells of the stomach and, in some rats, carcinoid tumours. However, no premalignant changes have been observed in humans, and these changes in rats are considered to have no relevance to its use in humans.

Clinically, omeprazole produces more rapid healing of duodenal ulcers than the $H_2$-receptor antagonists, the response to omeprazole at 2 weeks being equivalent to that produced by cimetidine, ranitidine and famotidine at 4 weeks. It has also proved effective in patients with duodenal or gastric ulcers poorly responsive to $H_2$-receptor antagonists. When given as monotherapy, omeprazole appears to suppress, but does not eradicate, *H. pylori*; however, when given in combination with antibiotics such as clarithromycin and/or amoxicillin, good *H. pylori* eradication rates have been reported (see further section 4.3.2). Omeprazole is well tolerated both in short term and long term therapy, the most common adverse effects being diarrhoea, headache, nausea and abdominal pain.

***Lansoprazole***[73] has a similar mechanism of action to omeprazole, decreasing gastric acid secretion via its effect on the acid pump of the parietal cell. Like omeprazole, it produces more rapid healing of duodenal ulcers than the $H_2$-receptor antagonists, and has similar effectiveness to omeprazole in patients with ulcers refractory to $H_2$-receptor antagonists. Some studies have suggested that lansoprazole may have greater antimicrobial activity than omeprazole against *H. pylori*, although the clinical relevance of this finding is unclear. Combination therapy with antibacterial agents increases *H. pylori* eradication rates and healing of peptic ulcers compared with lansoprazole monotherapy. The drug is well tolerated, the incidence of adverse effects being similar to that of omeprazole.[73]

***Pantoprazole*** acts similarly to omeprazole and lansoprazole, causing irreversible inhibition of gastric acid pump ($H^+/K^+$-ATPase) function. It is chemically more stable than omeprazole and lansoprazole under neutral to mildly acidic conditions, but is rapidly converted to the active species under strongly acidic conditions. This pH-dependent activation profile appears to improve its selectivity against parietal cell $H^+/K^+$-ATPase, but whether this confers any advantage with regard to tolerability has not yet been proven. In short-term clinical studies, pantoprazole 40mg daily has proved superior to ranitidine 300mg daily and equivalent to omeprazole 20mg daily in accelerating the healing of gastric and duodenal ulcers. Preliminary results have also indicated that a combination (triple therapy) regimen of pantoprazole with clarithromycin and metronidazole is effective in eradicating *H. pylori* in duodenal ulcer patients.[74]

The acid pump inhibitors have similar pharmacokinetic properties, all three drugs being eliminated principally by hepatic metabolism (via the cytochrome P450 system), with negligible amounts of unchanged drug excreted in the urine. Although they all have short plasma half-lives, of the order of 0.7 to 1.3 hours, their antisecretory effects are prolonged for more than 24 hours, and once daily dosage schedules can be given. Unlike the $H_2$-receptor antagonists, no dosage adjustments are necessary in patients with renal impairment.[104]

### *4.1.3 Cytoprotective Agents*

#### Colloidal Bismuth Subcitrate (Tripotassium Dicitrato Bismuthate)

Colloidal bismuth subcitrate[108] has a selective coating affinity for the base of peptic ulcers, but not for normal gastric mucosa.[109-111] This property is not possessed by other bismuth compounds, and the mechanism of the formation of the bismuth layer is unclear.[109] On acidification of colloidal bismuth subcitrate to pH levels found in the stomach, two precipitates, bismuth oxychloride and bismuth citrate, cover the ulcer crater.[112]

Colloidal bismuth subcitrate has no antacid properties, but may be mildly antipeptic.[111,113] Although the precise mechanism of its antiulcer action is unknown, selective binding of the compound to the ulcer base appears to be an important property.[109] There are several mechanisms whereby the bismuth coat may heal ulcers:

1) The bismuth coat may provide passive protection against the action of acid and pepsin.

2) It may exert a local antipeptic effect.[111]

3) It may stimulate reparative processes – it has been observed that the microvilli of epithelial cells at the ulcer edge return more quickly to their normal height in patients treated with this agent than in those receiving cimetidine.[114]

4) Alternatively, it may act through as yet unknown mechanisms. Colloidal bismuth subcitrate is known to be bactericidal to *H. pylori* and, thus, may exert its antiulcer effect through a bactericidal action.

Bismuth undergoes systemic absorption to a minimal degree.[115] This absorption is of no relevance when colloidal bismuth subcitrate is used in the initial treatment of ulcer for 6 to 8 weeks, but long term use is not advised, since safety has not been established. Administration to patients with severe renal failure should also be avoided because of possible accumulation of bismuth and the associated risk of toxicity.[104]

For initial ulcer healing, 120mg of colloidal bismuth subcitrate should be taken 4 times daily or 240mg twice daily, half an hour before food. The duration of initial therapy is 4 to 8 weeks, followed by a 60-day bismuth-free period. The most common adverse effect of colloidal bismuth subcitrate therapy is blackening of the stools and less frequently, of the tongue (see further section 4.2.3).

#### Ranitidine Bismuth Citrate

This compound is formed from ranitidine hydrochloride and bismuth citrate, an oral dose of 400mg being bioequivalent to 150mg of ranitidine hydrochloride. It possesses both the mucosal protective and anti-*H. pylori* properties of the bismuth citrate component, and the antisecretory activity of ranitidine. In a clinical trial in peptic ulcer patients comparing 4 weeks of therapy with 3 different dose levels of ranitidine bismuth citrate (i.e. 200mg, 400mg and 800mg twice daily) with ranitidine 150mg twice daily, both the 400mg and 800mg twice daily regimens proved significantly more effective in healing ulcers and preventing recurrences than ranitidine alone, although there was no significant difference between the 200mg twice daily regimen and ranitidine alone.[116] The combination of ranitidine bismuth citrate with antibiotics (e.g. clarithromycin or amoxicillin) for eradication of *H. pylori* is currently under investigation. It appears to have an adverse effect profile similar to that of ranitidine, but like colloidal bismuth subcitrate, may cause blackening of the stools and tongue.

#### Sucralfate

Sucralfate is a basic aluminium salt of sulfated sucrose, structurally related to heparin, but without its anticoagulant effects.[117] It is viscous at acid pH, and forms a paste that selectively adheres to the ulcer base.[118-120] The adherent paste acts as a barrier to the diffusion of acid, pepsin and bile salts, and forms complexes with protein at the ulcer surface that resist peptic hydrolysis. The interaction of sucralfate polyanions with substrate proteins prevents the binding of pepsin to ulcer protein.[118,121,122]

Sucralfate has no antacid properties.[123,124] It is minimally absorbed, 0.5 to 2.2% of an oral dose being excreted in the urine over the first 4 hours postdose.[125] If the drug is taken an hour before meals, food does not reduce binding at the ulcer site.[125] Because of its aluminium content, mild constipation may occur.[126]

Sucralfate may also exert a cytoprotective effect through stimulation of local prostaglandin synthesis and release.[127] It has an effect on ulcer healing equivalent to that of cimetidine.[128] In long term maintenance treatment, the effectiveness of sucralfate in preventing duodenal ulcer recurrences has been demonstrated, but results in gastric ulcer recurrences permit no firm conclusion to be drawn.[117]

#### Prostaglandins

Prostaglandins are 20-carbon oxygenated fatty acids present in most tissues. They possess a wide diversity of effects on the gastrointestinal tract that include regulation of gastric acid secretion and protection of the gastric mucosa. With the discovery that naturally-occurring prostaglandins of the E series are potent inhibitors of basal and stimulated gastric acid secretion in humans, investigation of their influence on ulcer disease followed. However, the effects of these naturally-occurring agents are short-lived, as they are rapidly inactivated by enzymes in human tissues. Consequently, analogues of prostaglandins $E_1$ and $E_2$ that are resistant to normal enzymatic metabolism have been developed. These compounds inhibit histamine-, food- and pentagastrin-stimulated gastric acid secretion for up to 5 hours.

The exact cellular site of this antisecretory effect is not known.[129] However, as well as being antisecretory agents, the prostaglandins also exert a cytoprotective effect, which implies an ability to protect the mucosa from damage when exposed to noxious agents.[130] This effect is separate from the antisecretory effect and may involve:

1) Strengthening of the gastric mucosal barrier with a reduction in $H^+$ back-diffusion.

2) An increase in gastric and duodenal secretion of both mucus and bicarbonate.

3) An increase in gastric mucosal blood flow.

***Misoprostol:*** currently, this is the best-studied agent among the prostaglandin analogues. Misoprostol has been shown to produce a dose-related inhibition of gastric acid secretion in response to a variety of stimuli, and to have cytoprotective effects at dosages lower than those required to inhibit acid secretion. In therapeutic trials, misoprostol has been found effective in healing both duodenal and gastric ulcers, and is of comparable effectiveness to cimetidine. Whereas ranitidine is effective in preventing only duodenal ulcers in patients on NSAID therapy, misoprostol prevents both gastric and duodenal ulcers.[131] The main indications for its use appear to be in the prophylaxis of gastric and duodenal ulcer in NSAID users, and in the healing of established NSAID-induced gastric and duodenal ulcers.

For a review of the use of misoprostol in combination with diclofenac in patients at risk of NSAID-related gastrointestinal complications, see Davis et al.[131]

## 4.2 Tolerability and Drug Interactions Potential of Antiulcer Drugs

### *4.2.1 Antacids*

Adverse effects of antacids may be either local or systemic. Local effects include constipation, with aluminium-containing preparations, and an osmotic diarrhoea with magnesium-containing agents. Mixtures containing both aluminium hydroxide gel and magnesium hydroxide may cause either constipation or diarrhoea, but are intended to reduce the occurrence of either since they provide the proportion of magnesium and aluminium hydroxides needed to restore and maintain normal bowel function.

Systemic adverse effects due to magnesium or aluminium toxicity may occur in patients with renal failure. Calcium-containing antacids may cause hypercalcaemia and renal calculi, and sodium-containing antacids may cause fluid retention. The milk alkali syndrome can occur when sodium-containing antacids are ingested with large amounts of calcium, either as calcium carbonate or as milk.[132] Phosphorus depletion can occasionally produce an osteomalacia-like syndrome and may result from large and prolonged ingestion of aluminium hydroxide gels.[133,134]

A potential problem with the use of antacids is interference with the absorption of other concomitantly administered drugs, such as tetracyclines, isoniazid, quinidine, warfarin and digoxin.[19,20] Usually the interaction of drugs with antacids results in a 20% reduction in absorption of the concomitantly-administered drug; this is often of little clinical relevance. Antacids may slightly reduce the binding of sucralfate to the ulcer site,[125,135] but not to a clinically relevant extent.

### *4.2.2 Antisecretory Drugs*

#### $H_2$-Receptor Antagonists

Adverse effects are uncommon with the $H_2$-receptor antagonists. However, with cimetidine (principally), drug interactions with warfarin, phenytoin, theophylline, antiarrhythmics and some hypnosedatives are possible.

***Cimetidine:*** early experience with this drug indicated that nonspecific symptoms requiring withdrawal from clinical trials occurred in 2.1% of patients receiving cimetidine and 1.7% of those on placebo.[136] Adverse effects occur infrequently, and include headache, dizziness, skin rash, nausea and diarrhoea. Rarely, impotence, gynaecomastia or mental confusion may occur, the latter usually at high doses, in the presence of renal or hepatic disease or in the elderly. Dosages should be reduced in both renal and hepatic impairment.

Cimetidine binds to hepatic cytochrome P450, resulting in a stable cytochrome-substrate complex that prevents access of other drugs to the mixed-function oxidase system and denies their subsequent metabolism. Thus, cimetidine impairs the metabolism of phenytoin, warfarin, theophylline and other drugs oxidised by this system (e.g. quinidine, procainamide). However, it is not considered to be associated with any interaction of major clinical significance (i.e. well-documented and with potential to be harmful to the patient),[137] although interactions of moderate clinical significance (i.e. of lesser harmful potential and requiring more documentation) have been reported with acenocoumarol, alprazolam, β-blockers, calcium antagonists, carmustine, chlordiazepoxide, clonazepam, clorazepate, nordazepam (*N*-desmethyldiazepam), desipramine, diazepam, doxepin, halazepam, imipramine, ketoconazole, lidocaine, lorazepam, meperidine and opioid analgesics (for a review, see Piper[138]).

***Ranitidine:*** as with cimetidine, ranitidine therapy may occasionally be associated with headache, dizziness, skin rash, nausea, or diarrhoea. Dosages should be reduced in moderate to severe renal impairment.

Ranitidine binds only weakly to cytochrome P450 enzymes, and is not considered to be associated with any major interactions,[137] although moderate interactions with a number of drugs (e.g. enoxacin, ketoconazole, nifedipine and nitrendipine) have been described.

***Famotidine:*** in a postmarketing study of 6346 patients,[139] adverse effects occurred in 0.43% and abnormalities in laboratory tests in fewer than 1% of patients. Symptomatic adverse effects are similar to those of cimetidine and ranitidine (headache, dizziness, skin rash, constipation and diarrhoea). Mental confusion has been observed in elderly patients,[140] but famotidine has no antiandrogenic activity and does not alter hepatic glutathione concentrations or hepatic blood flow. No interactions of clinical significance have been identified with a range of drugs tested, including diazepam, phenytoin, procainamide, theophylline and warfarin.[141,142]

***Nizatidine and roxatidine*:** these drugs also have adverse effect profiles similar to those of cimetidine and ranitidine, the most commonly reported events being headache, diarrhoea, somnolence, sweating, diarrhoea and urticaria with nizatidine,[68] and headache, dizziness, diarrhoea, constipation, nausea and skin rash with roxatidine.[69] Neither drug has been reported to interfere with the hepatic metabolism of other drugs.

#### Anticholinergic Drugs (Pirenzepine)

The selective $M_1$-muscarinic receptor antagonist pirenzepine causes fewer anticholinergic effects than conventional anticholinergic drugs. This is because it inhibits basal and stimulated gastric acid secretion at doses lower than those required to affect cardiovascular, ocular and urinary function, salivation and gastrointestinal motility. In therapeutic trials, pirenzepine has generally been well tolerated, although dry mouth, blurred vision, constipation, diarrhoea and headache have occurred in some patients[105] and skin rashes have occurred rarely.

By inhibiting gastrointestinal motility, anticholinergic drugs can also alter the absorption of other orally administered drugs.[19]

#### Acid Pump Inhibitors

***Omeprazole:*** adverse effects occur infrequently with omeprazole and most commonly comprise gastrointestinal symptoms such as epigastric pain, dyspepsia, flatulence, diarrhoea, nausea and vomiting. In more than 19,000 patients treated with omeprazole in short term clinical trials, withdrawal of treatment because of adverse effects was necessary in fewer than 2% of patients.[72] The incidence of adverse events in comparative clinical trials was similar whether patients received omeprazole (1.1%), cimetidine (1.4%), ranitidine (0.8%) or placebo (4.0%).

Omeprazole is associated with few drug interactions of clinical significance. However, as it may interfere with the cytochrome P450 enzyme system, it has the potential to interfere with the metabolism of drugs such as diazepam, warfarin and, possibly, phenytoin and cyclosporin.[72]

***Lansoprazole and pantoprazole*:** tolerability data with these drugs indicate that their adverse effect profiles are similar to that of omeprazole. The most frequent adverse effects reported with lansoprazole in clinical trials have been diarrhoea, abdominal pain, nausea, headache and dizziness.[73] Although lansoprazole is a more selective inhibitor of the cytochrome P450 system than omeprazole, it appears to interact minimally with other drugs, and there have been no reports of clinically significant interactions.[73] With pantoprazole, the most frequent adverse effects reported have been diarrhoea, headache, dizziness and occasionally, pruritus and skin rash. As with lansoprazole, no clinically relevant drug interactions have been reported with pantoprazole.[74]

### 4.2.3 Cytoprotective Agents

#### Colloidal Bismuth Subcitrate

Adverse effects of colloidal bismuth subcitrate include discolouration of the tongue and teeth and blackening of stools. The drug should be taken separately from other medicines as they could theoretically interfere with its binding to the ulcer. Colloidal bismuth subcitrate should be administered with caution in patients with a history of upper gastrointestinal bleeding (as the blackening of the stools produced by bismuth can be confused with melaena), and in long term therapy (because of the possibility of toxicity resulting from gastrointestinal absorption of bismuth).

#### Sucralfate

Adverse effects of sucralfate include headache, constipation, gastric discomfort or dyspepsia, and urticaria. The drug should be taken separately from other medicines, and administered with caution in patients with renal impairment and in long term therapy.

Antacids may slightly reduce the binding of sucralfate to the ulcer site,[125,135] but not to a clinically relevant extent. There is evidence that the absorption of phenytoin and warfarin may be impaired by concomitantly-administered sucralfate.[135,144]

#### Misoprostol

Adverse effects of misoprostol are, in general, those expected of a prostaglandin analogue. They include colic or abdominal pain, nausea, dyspepsia, diarrhoea, headache and, in women, miscarriage and uterine bleeding. If colic and diarrhoea appear, the dosage should be reduced by a third or a half and the medication continued. Because of its stimulant effect on uterine tone, misoprostol is contraindicated in pregnant women.[143]

## 4.3 Optimum Treatment

### *4.3.1 Diagnosis*

Clinical history alone is inadequate to confirm a diagnosis of peptic ulcer and endoscopy or barium meal x-rays are mandatory. Endoscopy is desirable, particularly when gastric ulcer or other gastric abnormality is apparent on x-ray (where biopsy must exclude malignancy), to determine *H. pylori* status, monitor healing and confirm *H. pylori* eradication.[90] The differential diagnosis includes gastro-oesophageal reflux disease (see section 3.2.1), gastric cancer or lymphoma, and functional (nonulcer) dyspepsia.

Once a full clinical assessment is made, a decision can be taken whether to reassure the patient and provide symptomatic therapy in the interim (usually antacids), or to investigate and provide further treatment.

#### Confirmation of *Helicobacter pylori* Infection

Therapy for eradication of *H. pylori* should be linked to a verified diagnosis of peptic ulcer. Table III summarises the currently accepted indications for *H. pylori* eradication.

*H. pylori* is most easily detected at the time of the initial diagnostic endoscopy, where antral and sometimes gastric body biopsies can be taken for a rapid urease test (90 to 95% sensitive, 98% specific) and/or histology (98% sensitivity and specificity). Although culture of the bacterium is confirmative, it lacks the sensitivity of the simpler tests, is expensive and is usually reserved for research studies.[95] The *breath test* using $^{13}$C- or $^{14}$C-labelled urea is noninvasive, easy to perform and relatively inexpensive. While it is highly reliable in detecting *H. pylori*, it does not make the important link between the bacterium and actual peptic ulceration. However, it is an excellent test to confirm the presence of *H. pylori* where ulceration has previously been demonstrated, and to confirm eradication at least 4 weeks after the completion of therapy.

Serology (and more recently, saliva) can also be used to confirm *H. pylori* infection. Like the breath test, it currently has little value on its own in the absence of a diagnosis of peptic ulceration. Serology takes at least 3 to 6 months to show a significant reduction in serial titres, so it is not useful to confirm successful eradication.

### *4.3.2 Initial Treatment*

The aim of treatment in the short term is to relieve symptoms, accelerate ulcer healing and prevent complications, particularly haemorrhage, and in the long term to minimise the risk of ulcer recurrence. Patients should be advised to stop smoking and the ingestion of aspirin and nonsteroidal anti-inflammatory drugs (NSAIDs) should be ceased unless good reasons exist for their use (see further below). Diet is dictated by the patient's desires and does not influence the healing rate. There is no need for the patient to alter his or her normal work and social life. Sedation confers no benefit.

The need for compliance with treatment to ensure its success and the importance of taking medication at the recommended times should be emphasised.

**Table III. Summary of indications for *Helicobacter pylori* eradication**

1. Primary treatment of proven duodenal ulcer
2. Primary treatment of endoscopically proven benign gastric ulcer
3. NSAID-associated ulcers only if *H. pylori*-positive
4. Patients with peptic ulcers who would previously have been started on maintenance therapy
5. Prevention of peptic ulcer complications

**Table IV.** Some regimens that have been used for eradication of *Helicobacter pylori* (after Soll et al.,[93] Rauws & van der Hulst,[95] Markham & McTavish[146])

| Regimens | Dosage | Duration of therapy | *H. pylori* eradication rate |
|---|---|---|---|
| **Dual therapy regimens** | | | |
| Omeprazole + | 20mg bid (or 40mg od) | 14d | 55-87.5% |
| Clarithromycin | 500mg bid-tid | | |
| Omeprazole + | 20mg bid | 14d | 50-80% |
| Amoxicillin | 1g bid | | |
| **Triple therapy regimens** | | | |
| Colloidal bismuth subcitrate[a] + | 120mg qid | 14d | 80-90% |
| Tetracycline (or amoxicillin) + | 500mg qid | | |
| Metronidazole | 400mg tid (or 250mg qid) | | |
| [*standard triple therapy regimen*] | | | |
| Omeprazole + | 20mg bid | 7d | 87-91% |
| Clarithromycin + | 500mg bid | | |
| Metronidazole[b] | 400 tid (or 500mg bid) | | |
| Omeprazole + | 20mg bid | 7d | 86-91% |
| Clarithromycin + | 500mg bid | | |
| Amoxicillin | 1g bid | | |
| Ranitidine + | 300mg nocte[c] | 12d | 89% |
| Amoxicillin + | 750mg tid | | |
| Metronidazole | 500mg tid | | |

a In the US, bismuth subsalicylate is used (2 × 262mg tablets qid).

b Tinidazole (500mg bid) may be used as an alternative to metronidazole.

c Ranitidine therapy continued for 6-10 weeks.

*Abbreviations:* od = once daily; bid = twice daily; tid = 3 times daily; qid = 4 times daily; nocte = at night.

**Eradication of *H. pylori***

Therapy for eradication of *H. pylori* is now recognised as first-line treatment for both duodenal and gastric ulcer, including NSAID-induced ulcers where *H. pylori* is detected. Multiple-drug regimens are required to achieve this, one being a mucosal protective agent (e.g. colloidal bismuth subcitrate) or an antisecretory drug (e.g. an acid pump inhibitor or an $H_2$-receptor antagonist), and the others antibacterial agents effective against the bacterium *in vivo* (e.g. amoxicillin, tetracycline, metronidazole, tinidazole or clarithromycin).

Multiple agents have been studied in various combination regimens, some of which are shown in table IV. Although *H. pylori* is sensitive to many antibiotics *in vitro*, in practice it has proved difficult to eradicate with a single antibiotic, perhaps because the organism resides in the highly acidic milieu of the stomach where rapid removal of the administered antibiotics may occur, giving rise to variable correlations between *in vitro* and *in vivo* antibacterial activity.[92] Consequently, regimens involving the use of a single antibiotic with an antisecretory or mucosal protective drug ('dual therapy' regimens) have provided variable eradication rates that are generally lower than those involving the use of two antibiotics (i.e. 'triple therapy' regimens) [table IV]. Resistance to antibiotics, in particular to nitroimidazoles such as metronidazole and the macrolide drug clarithromycin, is an increasing problem,[93] and is an important cause of treatment failure. This underlines the importance of using regimens comprising at least two antibiotics despite the increased cost, lower tolerability and potentially lower patient compliance rates that such regimens may entail in comparison with 'dual therapy' regimens comprising one antibiotic.

Currently, the recommended regimens for eradication of *H. pylori* (defined as absence of detectable organisms at least 4 weeks after completion of therapy) are 'triple therapy' regimens such as those shown in table IV. These regimens produce good *H. pylori* eradication rates, shorten the treatment period required, and decrease failures due to antibiotic resistance.[93] The widely used *standard triple therapy* regimen involves the use of colloidal bismuth subcitrate (or bismuth subsalicylate in the US), tetracycline (or amoxicillin) and metronidazole (or tinidazole) given for 2 weeks, and has been reported to achieve cure rates of 85 to 90%. More recently, regimens involving the use of omeprazole and two antibiotics (e.g. clarithromycin + metronidazole; or clarithromycin + amoxicillin) have been shown to provide *H. pylori* cure rates of 85 to 90% with 1 weeks' treatment,[93] while a 12-day regimen of ranitidine, amoxicillin and metronidazole has been reported to provide an 89% cure rate.[86]

The ideal drug combination for eradication of *H. pylori* is still evolving and a number of alternative regimens to those shown in table IV have been proposed. As trials are reported, the recommended regimens and their duration of administration may change. The effectiveness of *H. pylori* eradication regimens is dependent on several factors including nitroimidazole/macrolide drug resistance patterns, patient tolerability, and patient compliance with the regimen. All the antibiotics presently advocated may cause adverse effects (e.g. diarrhoea and skin rash with amoxicillin; nausea, a metallic taste and alcohol intolerance with metronidazole; nausea and diarrhoea with clarithromycin), and amoxicillin should be avoided in those with penicillin hypersensitivity. In using the presently advocated regimens, patients should be educated about the importance of compliance and the anticipated adverse effects.

**Conventional Antiulcer Therapy**

Cure of *H. pylori* infection enhances ulcer healing and dramatically reduces the recurrence rate. The 1-week regimens comprising omeprazole (or colloidal bismuth subcitrate) and two antibiotics heal peptic ulcers as effectively as 4 weeks of omeprazole monotherapy.[93] However, conventional antiulcer drug therapy (see table II), e.g. with an antisecretory drug, colloidal bismuth subcitrate or sucralfate, may need to be continued to provide symptom relief and facilitate ulcer healing. For uncomplicated ulcers, continued antiulcer therapy beyond the initial *H. pylori* eradication treatment is probably not needed; however, for complicated, large or refractory ulcers, antiulcer therapy should be continued until successful cure of *H. pylori* has been confirmed. The duration of such therapy is not firmly established, but may need to be 4 to 8 weeks or longer in refractory cases.

Large ulcers (>15mm), especially gastric ulcers, may take 12 weeks to heal. In most cases, the cause of slow healing is not obvious, but ulcer size is a factor. The use of acid pump inhibitors is warranted in this relatively small subgroup. Longer treatment is also preferred for smokers, patients at particular risk (e.g. due to complications, age, other illnesses) and those with a previous history of rapid recurrence or slow healing.

Endoscopic confirmation of healing of gastric or persistent ulcers and reassessment of the *H. pylori* status should be made at the end of the initial treatment period. If the ulcer is unhealed, antiulcer therapy should be continued for 3 to 4 weeks or longer. Slow healing may indicate noncompliance with treatment, a gastrinoma, or missed cancer in the case of gastric ulcer. Slow healing is mostly due to unknown factors; in the case of gastric ulcers, a large ulcer is the usual cause. Prolongation of therapy usually produces healing (see further section 4.3.3 below).

Endoscopic confirmation of healing is not necessary in duodenal ulcer patients if symptomatic relief is obtained, unless there is a specific indication for it.

#### *4.3.3 Treatment of Refractory Ulcers*

The available evidence indicates that eradication of *H. pylori* infection, when present, is likely to facilitate ulcer healing and alter the natural history of refractory ulcers.[93] In patients who fail to heal on the regimens outlined above, a detailed clinical evaluation, including endoscopic assessment, is mandatory to elucidate whether other disorders that form the differential diagnosis of peptic ulcer (see section 4.3.1) are present. Factors that may delay ulcer healing include failure to eradicate *H. pylori*, NSAID/aspirin use, poor patient compliance with the recommended therapy, cigarette smoking, or acid hypersecretory conditions (e.g. gastrinoma).[93] Therapeutic options include maximal acid inhibition with the use of a higher dose of an acid pump inhibitor (e.g. omeprazole 40mg daily), alternative antibiotic regimens for treatment of persistent *H. pylori* infection, exclusion of NSAIDs, and admission to hospital for consideration of surgery (see section 4.3.5).

#### *4.3.4 Treatment of Ulcer Recurrences*

Previously, peptic ulcer relapse presented a greater therapeutic challenge than initial healing of the ulcer, and relapse rates for duodenal ulcer were as high as 80% within 1 year. However, with successful eradication of *H. pylori*, relapse rates have been greatly diminished, although cure of *H. pylori* does not totally eliminate ulcer recurrence. In one study, a recurrence rate of only 3% was described over a period of 7 years in patients who remained *H. pylori*-negative.[94] Persisting *H. pylori* infection is the major determinant of ulcer recurrence, and as many as 85% of patients who remain *H. pylori*-positive may experience a recurrence.

Recurrent ulcers usually respond to repeat treatment; if this occurs within 1 year, an alternative antibiotic regimen should be considered. *H. pylori* status should be checked to confirm eradication.

#### Maintenance Therapy

In the subset of patients with *H. pylori*-negative ulcers and those in whom antibiotic therapy has failed to eradicate the organism, conventional maintenance therapy may be considered. Other patients in whom maintenance therapy may be considered include those with a prior history of frequent recurrences (2 or more per year) or ulcer complications (e.g. bleeding or perforation), those living in areas remote from sophisticated medical care, or if the patient is a smoker or is receiving NSAID therapy.

Maintenance therapy involves the daily administration of those drugs that have been shown in well controlled clinical trials to be effective in preventing ulcer recurrences and thereby freeing the patient of the risk of complications, e.g. the $H_2$-receptor antagonists *cimetidine* or *ranitidine*, or *sucralfate* (for dosages, see table II). With such treatment, a reduction in the recurrence rate of 50% can sometimes be achieved. The duration of maintenance therapy varies with the individual, but continuation for 3 to 4 years may be necessary in patients with prior complications. Maintenance therapy is generally ceased after 4 years. If the patient remains well, the ulcer is considered to have 'burnt out'.

If dyspeptic symptoms recur during maintenance therapy, endoscopy should be performed; if no ulcer is present, a diagnosis of functional (nonulcer) dyspepsia may be made (see section 11.2.1) and maintenance therapy continued. However, if the ulcer is found to have recurred, 1 of 2 courses of action may be followed:

- If the duration of the remission was short, surgery is advised (see section 4.3.5)
- If the duration of the remission was several years, the ulcer may be treated again in a similar manner to that used in the initial healing (see section 4.3.2) and maintenance therapy recommenced.

### 4.3.5 Role of Surgery

Because *H. pylori* treatment has yielded such a degree of clinical success, the indications for surgery are now few. Surgery is usually reserved for patients with complications, with frequent recurrences in which *H. pylori* cannot be eradicated, those unsuitable for maintenance treatment, and individuals in whom medical treatment fails, as indicated by ulcer recurrence despite healing and maintenance therapy with an acid pump inhibitor for one year.

### 4.3.6 Special Considerations in Treatment

#### NSAID-Related Ulcers

NSAID-related ulcers differ from idiopathic ulcers in that they are often painless, are common in the elderly (especially women), prone to complication, and often respond poorly to medical treatment.

NSAID therapy should be ceased if at all possible, and *H. pylori* if present should be treated as outlined above (see section 4.3.2). If it is not possible to avoid NSAID use, concomitant treatment with *misoprostol* (see section 4.1.3) can be given to accelerate healing and reduce recurrence of both gastric and duodenal ulcers. $H_2$-Receptor antagonists provide useful treatment for duodenal ulcer, but are of uncertain benefit in gastric ulcer. Omeprazole is likely to be of benefit in these patients, but there are few data and treatment is expensive (see section 4.4).

#### Elderly Patients

There is no clear demarcation between ulcers in the elderly and those in younger age groups. However, among the elderly:

1) Complications are more frequent, and ulcers are often asymptomatic.

2) Exposure to NSAIDs is more common, due to the painful syndromes of aging.

3) Old age may slow ulcer healing.[147]

4) Adverse reactions to antiulcer drugs occur more frequently, because of patients' impaired renal and liver function.

5) The dose of antiulcer drugs is often poorly defined since most clinical trials exclude the elderly.

Therapy should aim at safe, simple regimens, with careful attention to possible interactions and complications. Contrary to some initial views, age is not a contraindication to *H. pylori* eradication therapy. However, the regimens used and their associated adverse effects necessitate individualised attention and careful monitoring. The benefits of effective short term treatment should be set against the disadvantages of possible maintenance treatment, which could complicate and compromise other drug treatment.

#### Children

Peptic ulcer occurs rarely in children and may be confused with other causes of duodenal pathology (e.g. Crohn's disease). Prolonged and critical clinical assessment should precede initiation of any treatment. Children should receive treatment as for adults and the emphasis should be on eradication of *H. pylori*. However, tetracycline is best avoided in this age group because of the likelihood of tooth discolouration.

#### Gastrinoma

Fewer than 1% of duodenal ulcers are of known endocrine origin. The best studied of these arise from a gastrinoma, or gastrin-secreting tumour (Zollinger-Ellison syndrome). This rare syndrome should be considered if:

- Symptoms are severe and respond poorly to medical or surgical treatment.
- Ulcers are large or multiple and situated distal to the first part of the duodenum.
- Reflux oesophagitis, diarrhoea and steatorrhoea are present (not in all cases).
- Ulcers recur following surgery.

The diagnosis is based on a consistent clinical syndrome, markedly elevated serum gastrin concentration and elevated basal acid output. Provocative tests are available in cases of doubt.

Specialist referral is required for these patients. Treatment is with surgery if practicable, but most patients have metastases (usually hepatic) when diagnosed. Omeprazole is effective in controlling the acid hypersecretion associated with these tumours.

### *4.3.7 Treatment of Complications of Peptic Ulcer*

#### Acute Upper Gastrointestinal Haemorrhage

In patients with acute upper gastrointestinal haemorrhage, admission to an intensive care ward of a major hospital is mandatory. As soon as the patient is resuscitated, endoscopy should be performed. Blood transfusion is indicated if the haemoglobin is less than 90 g/L, blood pressure is less than 110mm Hg systolic or the pulse rate is over 110 beats/min. Continuous gastric aspiration is performed to detect recurrent or continuous bleeding.

Surgery is indicated if the patient is over 60 years of age, has a chronic ulcer and bleeds continuously or recurrently after admission, or where there is evidence of large vessel bleeding as indicated by:

1) A reduction in central venous pressure exceeding 5cm $H_2O$ or in blood pressure exceeding 50mm Hg over 15 minutes.

2) A bleeding rate of at least 600 ml/h as estimated by blood transfusion requirements to maintain normal blood pressure and central venous pressure.

3) Protracted bleeding requiring transfusion of more than 2L blood in 24 hours or signs of recent haemorrhage at endoscopy.

$H_2$-Receptor antagonists and other antiulcer drugs play no role in the initial management of acute upper gastrointestinal bleeding. Discharge of the patient from hospital is usually possible after 5 to 7 days, after which the ulcer should be treated along conventional lines (see section 4.3.2).

#### Perforation

About 10% of ulcers perforate. Clinically, a perforated ulcer is one of the most dramatic events in medicine. The preferred treatment is surgery.

The diagnosis of perforated ulcer is essentially clinical. Plain abdominal x-ray and serum amylase determinations are essential investigations in the first hour. Serum amylase levels, if elevated, suggest pancreatitis. Air under the diaphragm indicates a perforated viscus, and a lateral and anteroposterior erect x-ray are essential. Nevertheless, 10 to 20% of perforations are not associated with air under the diaphragm. The ultimate decision regarding surgery must therefore be a value judgement. Delay in treatment may have a marked adverse impact on survival.

#### Gastric Outlet Obstruction

This can result from a prepyloric gastric ulcer or a duodenal ulcer. Obstruction is due to a combination of oedema, spasm and fibrosis. Gastric stasis with vomiting results, and dehydration and electrolyte depletion follow. Gastric outlet obstruction can be diagnosed by giving barium sulfate 20 or 30ml and taking a plain x-ray of the abdomen 2 to 4 hours later. This simple test enables obstruction resulting from organic disease to be demarcated from other causes of vomiting and progress of the obstruction to be assessed.

The initial treatment is medical, including gastric suction and fluid and electrolyte replacement. Attempts may be made to relieve spasm and oedema by maintaining the pH of gastric contents near neutral. This involves intravenous administration of *ranitidine* or *cimetidine* and

4-hourly administration of *antacids* (preferably calcium carbonate 4g), with the suction tube clamped for 2 hours after each dose. Anticholinergic drugs are best discontinued because a delay in gastric emptying may accentuate symptoms of obstruction. If after 48 hours there is no significant relief of obstruction, surgery is advised.

#### Hourglass Deformity

This radiological appearance may result from spasm or fibrosis associated with body ulcer. If it is due to spasm, the deformity will disappear in a few days with effective antiulcer treatment (see section 4.3.2). If it is due to fibrosis, it is the end result of recurrent attacks of ulceration with resultant scarring. Diagnosis is initially radiological, but subsequent endoscopy with biopsy is required.

## 4.4 Clinical Outcome and Economic Considerations

### *4.4.1 Cost Effectiveness of Helicobacter pylori Eradication*

A substantial body of evidence has now accumulated demonstrating that eradication of *H. pylori* is not only the most clinically efficacious, but is also usually the most cost-effective strategy in managing peptic ulcer.

Currently, it is recommended that antibacterial therapy should be given to all patients with documented duodenal and gastric ulcers associated with *H. pylori* infection.[92,93] A decision-analysis model[148] has provided further economic support for this recommendation. The aim of this cost-effectiveness analysis, conducted from a third-party payer perspective, was to compare costs and outcomes associated with a variety of strategies for the long term management of duodenal ulcer. Three global treatment strategies were considered:

1) *Strategy A:* heal with ranitidine, then wait until the first recurrence before continuing 1 of 4 treatments, i.e. ranitidine alone, omeprazole alone, omeprazole plus amoxicillin, or ranitidine plus standard triple therapy.

2) *Strategy B:* heal, then commence ranitidine maintenance therapy.

3) *Strategy C:* heal, then commence *H. pylori* eradication using standard triple therapy for 8 weeks or omeprazole 20mg twice daily and amoxicillin 1g twice daily for 14 days.

Meta-analysis of published randomised trials was used to estimate probabilities for endoscopically-confirmed ulcer recurrence, while an expert panel estimated resource usage associated with ulcer recurrence. The costs per symptomatic ulcer recurrence (in 1993 Canadian dollars) were \$329, \$341, \$456 and \$445 for the respective regimens in *strategy A* (treatment after recurrence), \$386 for ranitidine maintenance therapy *(strategy B)*, \$272 for omeprazole plus amoxicillin and \$253 for standard triple therapy *(strategy C)*.

Thus, it is clearly much less costly to treat uncomplicated duodenal ulcer associated with *H. pylori* by eradicating the infection than by continuing the previously conventional practice of intermittent or continuous maintenance therapy with $H_2$-receptor antagonists. Moreover, the cost savings are conservative estimates only, since the analysis did not include complicated ulcers or indirect costs (such as lost work time, visits to clinicians, etc.), and covered only 1 year.[149]

This study corroborated the findings of earlier studies, that eradication of *H. pylori* is the most cost-effective strategy in treating duodenal ulcers, compared with either $H_2$-receptor antagonists or omeprazole.[150,151] Others[152] have confirmed that, while *H. pylori* eradication results in higher initial costs, the low relapse rate that ensues reduces expected future costs; the investment in *H. pylori* eradication (using omeprazole and appropriate antibacterials) paid off within 1 year compared with maintenance treatment, and within 3 years compared with intermittent treatment.

Thus, at present, it appears clinically prudent and economically sound to treat all patients with peptic ulcer associated with *H. pylori* infection using a regimen including antibacterials (see section 4.3.2).

### *4.4.2 Cost Effectiveness of Misoprostol Prophylaxis for NSAID-Induced Gastropathy*

Misoprostol is effective in preventing NSAID-induced gastric ulcers, but taking account of the relatively high acquisition costs of the agent, together with the widespread use of NSAIDs, the cost of implementing prophylaxis in *all* NSAID users has been considered unjustifiable. However, the available evidence indicates that misoprostol prophylaxis is cost effective when given to elderly or high-risk patients receiving NSAIDs, including those with a history of gastric ulcer and those with an ulcerative complication rate exceeding 1.2%.[145]

## 5. Nausea and Vomiting

Nausea is a symptom, and refers to a desire to vomit; it is often accompanied by upper abdominal discomfort. Typically, nausea precedes or accompanies vomiting. Vomiting should be distinguished from acid regurgitation occurring in gastro-oesophageal reflux disease (see section 3), and from rumination, which is the spontaneous regurgitation of food with reswallowing.

There are many causes of nausea and vomiting,[153,154] but in women of child-bearing age, pregnancy must always be considered. Patients may be subdivided into those with acute and chronic symptoms. A patient with acute nausea and vomiting who is not toxic or dehydrated most likely has gastroenteritis that will spontaneously; clear liquids with or without an antiemetic should be given. If there is also acute abdominal pain, a major surgical condition such as acute appendicitis, cholecystitis or perforation must be considered. Patients who are febrile and dehydrated with nausea and vomiting may have bowel obstruction. The presence of feculent vomiting usually suggests distal small bowel obstruction or a gastrocolonic fistula.

Chronic nausea and vomiting may be the result of metabolic disease (e.g. uncontrolled diabetes mellitus, renal failure, hypercalcaemia) or gastric disease (e.g. peptic ulcer with or without gastric outlet obstruction, gastric cancer, gastroparesis, alcoholic gastritis). If there is a history of spontaneous vomiting in the absence of nausea, then raised intracranial pressure should be considered in the differential diagnosis.

Projectile vomiting refers to very forceful vomiting that may occur with CNS diseases that increase intracranial pressure. Labyrinthine disorders such as acute labyrinthitis or Ménière's disease may induce vertigo with nausea and vomiting. Nausea and vomiting can also occur with bulimia. Patients with psychogenic vomiting are unaware of any association between their vomiting and emotional state.

Antiemetics should not be used without a diagnosis having first been made.

### 5.1 Clinical Pharmacology of Drugs Used in Treatment

Nausea and vomiting can be inhibited by drugs acting at one or more of the following sites:

1) The vomiting centre, e.g. muscarinic receptor antagonists, histamine $H_1$-receptor antagonists.

2) The chemoreceptor trigger zone (CTZ) in the fourth ventricle, e.g. phenothiazines, butyrophenones, metoclopramide, domperidone.

3) Other sites in the CNS, e.g. cannabinoids, benzodiazepines.

4) Peripherally, e.g. $serotonin_3$ ($5\text{-}HT_3$)-receptor antagonists, cisapride (a $serotonin_4$-agonist), corticosteroids.

The indications and principal adverse effects of the major antiemetic drugs currently in use are shown in table V.

#### *5.1.1 Metoclopramide*

This phenothiazine derivative is an antagonist at dopamine $D_2$-receptors in the CTZ and peripherally. It also has $serotonin_3$ ($5\text{-}HT_3$)-receptor antagonist activity at high doses. It is effective in relieving nausea and vomiting due to a variety of diseases (except motion sickness and labyrinthine disorders). Metoclopramide accelerates gastric emptying by increasing the frequency and depth of antral contractions, and coordinating motor activity between the antrum and duodenum.

***Pharmacokinetic characteristics:*** following oral administration, metoclopramide undergoes variable first-pass metabolism (oral bioavailability 30 to 100%). The drug is eliminated by both hepatic metabolism (principally sulfate conjugation) and renal excretion (80% of an oral dose is recovered in the urine within 24 hours, either as unchanged drug or as the sulfate and glucuronide conjugates). In patients with severe renal failure, the elimination half-life (normally 4 to 6 hours) is prolonged to around 14 hours and therefore a reduced dose should be given.

***Clinical use:*** metoclopramide should be administered 15 to 30 minutes before meals. It can be given orally, intramuscularly or by suppository. The usual adult dose is 10mg 3 or 4 times daily. In children, a dose of 0.1 mg/kg/day to a maximum of 0.5 mg/kg/day can be given.

***Tolerability:*** adverse effects of metoclopramide include drowsiness, particularly at high doses, and restlessness (occurring in 20% of patients). Acute dystonic reactions occur in about 1% of cases and are more common in younger persons. Other neurological effects include muscle spasms, confusion, tremor and Parkinsonian features. Tardive dyskinesia can occur rarely, particularly in the elderly, and is irreversible in some patients. Hyperprolactinaemia associated with the use of metoclopramide can

**Table V. Indications and principal adverse effects of commonly used antiemetic drugs**

| Drugs | Major indications (type of nausea and vomiting) | Principal adverse effects | Relative cost |
|---|---|---|---|
| **Phenothiazines** | | | |
| Chlorpromazine<br>Prochlorperazine<br>Trifluoperazine<br>Perphenazine | Migraine<br>Ménière's disease<br>Chemotherapy- and radiotherapy-induced emesis | Sedation, extrapyramidal effects, hypotension, dry mouth | + |
| **Anticholinergics** | | | |
| Atropine<br>Scopolamine (hyoscine) | Motion sickness | Dry mouth, blurred vision, urinary and faecal retention. Avoid in glaucoma | + |
| **Antihistamines** | | | |
| Cyclizine<br>Dimenhydrinate<br>Promethazine<br>Meclozine | Motion sickness<br>Ménière's disease | Drowsiness | + |
| **Serotonin$_3$ (5-HT$_3$) receptor antagonists** | | | |
| Ondansetron<br>Granisetron<br>Tropisetron | Chemotherapy- and radiotherapy-induced emesis<br>Postoperative nausea and vomiting<br>Migraine | Constipation, headache, occasional disturbance of liver enzymes, sedation | +++ |
| **Prokinetic agents** | | | |
| Cisapride | Postoperative nausea and vomiting<br>Chemotherapy- and radiotherapy-induced emesis | Abdominal cramping, diarrhoea | ++ |
| Domperidone | (metoclopramide) | Extrapyramidal effects, sedation | - |
| Metoclopramide | Functional dyspepsia | | |
| **Corticosteroids** | | | |
| Dexamethasone | Chemotherapy-induced emesis | Cushing's syndrome, mood changes, insomnia, pruritus | + |

*Symbols:* + = low; ++ = medium; +++ = high.

cause menstrual irregularity, galactorrhoea and breast tenderness.

### 5.1.2 Domperidone

This drug is a dopamine $D_2$-receptor antagonist with antiemetic properties approximately equivalent to those of metoclopramide. However, domperidone does not cross the blood-brain barrier and seldom results in extrapyramidal effects or drowsiness. Like metoclopramide, domperidone is useful in controlling nausea and vomiting from a wide variety of causes.

Domperidone has a low systemic bioavailability (13 to 17%) due to first-pass hepatic and bowel wall metabolism. The drug is principally eliminated by metabolism and its elimination half-life is 7.5 hours in healthy individuals.

In acute vomiting, parenteral doses of domperidone should not exceed 1 mg/kg in adults or in children. The drug can also be given orally in a dose of 10 to 20mg 3 or 4 times daily. In children, the usual oral dose is 0.6 mg/kg 3 or 4 times daily.

### 5.1.3 Cisapride

This substituted benzamide is a serotonin$_4$ (5-HT$_4$) agonist that by indirect mechanisms facilitates acetylcholine release from the myenteric plexus. It does not cross the blood-brain barrier and has no extrapyramidal effects. Cisapride may cause transient diarrhoea or abdominal cramps. The usual oral dose in adults is 10 to 20mg 4 times daily. Cisapride is a prokinetic agent that accelerates gastric, small bowel and colonic transit. It is most useful in the treatment of nausea in the absence of vomiting.[155,156]

For a review of the clinical pharmacology of cisapride, see Wiseman and Faulds.[71]

### 5.1.4 Serotonin$_3$ (5-HT$_3$) Receptor Antagonists

This class of drugs prevents nausea and vomiting after chemotherapy and radiotherapy. They probably act by blocking the actions of serotonin [5-hydroxytryptamine (5-HT)] on vagal afferent pathways.[157,158] 5-HT$_3$ receptors have been identified in the brain (including in the area postrema) and, thus, central blockade effects may also be relevant. Ondansetron, granisetron, and tropisetron have been most extensively studied, but a number of other compounds are under development.[159-161]

***Ondansetron*** is 70-fold more active at peripheral 5-$HT_3$ receptors than metoclopramide.[157] The most frequent adverse effects are constipation (as the drug slows colonic transit), headaches, dizziness and drowsiness.[162] Ondansetron reaches its peak plasma concentration 1 to 1.5 hours after oral administration and has an elimination half-life of 3 hours; it undergoes predominantly hepatic metabolism. While dosage adjustment is not necessary in renal failure or in the elderly, high doses should be avoided in moderate or severe liver disease.

***Granisetron*** acts similarly via selective antagonism of 5-$HT_3$ receptors both peripherally and centrally.[161] Like ondansetron, it is administered intravenously and orally. Peak plasma concentrations are reached in around 1.5 to 2 hours following oral administration, and its elimination half-life in healthy volunteers is 3 to 4 hours; however, in cancer patients, a longer half-life of between 9 and 12 hours has been reported. The major route of elimination is via hepatic metabolism, with less than 20% of a dose being recovered unchanged in the urine. No dosage adjustments are necessary in the elderly or in renal impairment. The most common adverse effect of granisetron is headache, while other less common events include constipation, diarrhoea, asthenia and somnolence.[161]

***Tropisetron*** also has a high affinity for 5-$HT_3$ receptors, with some (weak) antagonist activity at 5-$HT_4$ receptors as well.[159] Its pharmacokinetic characteristics are similar to those of ondansetron and granisetron, elimination being predominantly by hepatic metabolism. However, due to polymorphism in its metabolism, some patients eliminate the drug faster than others; the elimination half-life of tropisetron following intravenous and oral administration is 7.3 and 8.6 hours, respectively, in extensive metabolisers, and 30.3 and 41.9 hours, respectively, in poor metabolisers. No dosage adjustments are needed in the latter or in patients with impaired renal function, since any accumulation during short term administration of the drug is unlikely to be clinically significant. As with granisetron, the most frequently reported adverse effect has been headache, while constipation, diarrhoea and fatigue have also occurred.[159]

#### *5.1.5 Antihistamines and Anticholinergics*

Histamine $H_1$-receptor antagonists (e.g. cyclizine, dimenhydrinate, meclozine and promethazine) are most useful for controlling nausea and vomiting due to vestibular disturbances (see further chapter 14). Antihistamines do not act on the CTZ and therefore are not usually of value in controlling other causes of nausea and vomiting.[163]

Muscarinic receptor antagonists (e.g. scopolamine, atropine) are effective predominantly in the prevention of motion sickness (by blocking the central afferent pathway vomiting reflex), but cause dry mouth, blurred vision and drowsiness. Selective muscarinic receptor antagonists may avoid these adverse effects.[163]

#### *5.1.6 Psychotropic Agents*

Phenothiazines (e.g. chlorpromazine) principally act on the CTZ and may reduce most types of nausea and vomiting, except motion sickness. However, they commonly produce adverse effects such as sedation, hypotension and extrapyramidal effects (e.g. dyskinesia and dystonia). Butyrophenones (e.g. haloperidol) are potent $D_2$-receptor antagonists. They are useful in postoperative vomiting and in helping to control anticipatory nausea and vomiting in patients receiving chemotherapy.

Psychogenic vomiting may respond to tricyclic antidepressants in some cases.

#### *5.1.7 Other Agents*

Cannabinoids (e.g. Δ-tetrahydrocannabinol) are effective in cancer chemotherapy-induced nausea and vomiting. Adverse effects include dysphoria, sedation, dry mouth and hypotension.

Corticosteroids are useful in chemotherapy-induced vomiting, possibly because they inhibit prostaglandin synthesis. Benzodiazepines (e.g. lorazepam) have some efficacy in chemotherapy-induced vomiting through their sedative, amnesic or anxiolytic action.

Erythromycin is a prokinetic agent that acts on motilin receptors in smooth muscle. However, its value in the treatment of vomiting is not established.[164,165] Pyridoxine in high doses is of uncertain effectiveness but has been used for radiation sickness, pregnancy-induced vomiting, and Ménière's disease.

### 5.2 Optimum Treatment of Nausea and Vomiting in Cancer Therapy

An approach to the prevention and control of nausea and vomiting in cancer patients receiv-

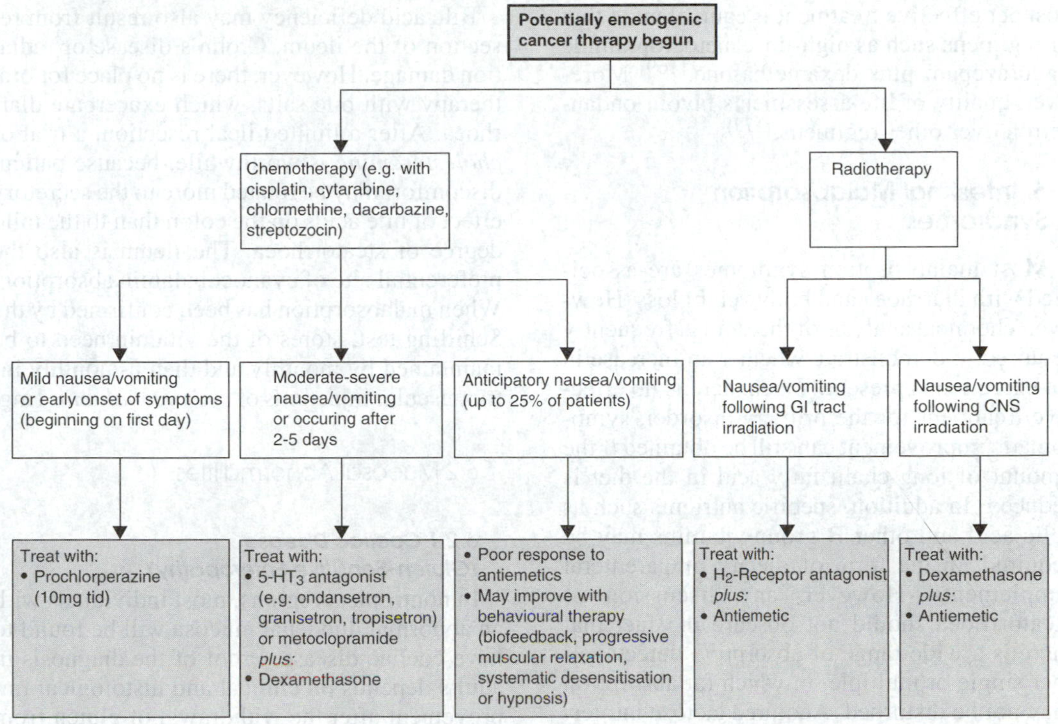


**Fig. 3.** Management of nausea and vomiting in cancer patients receiving chemotherapy or radiotherapy (after Levine[166]). *Abbreviations:* tid = 3 times daily; CNS = central nervous system; GI = gastrointestinal; 5-$HT_3$ = serotonin$_3$.

ing chemotherapy or radiotherapy is shown in figure 3. The severity of nausea and vomiting in these patients is related to the breakdown of neurotransmitters, particularly serotonin. Over two-thirds of patients receiving chemotherapy will develop significant nausea and vomiting. Drugs particularly likely to induce emesis include cisplatin, cytarabine, chlormethine, dacarbazine, streptozocin and, to a lesser extent, cyclophosphamide.

Radiotherapy can also induce nausea and vomiting, which is related to the field size and the site of the tumour. Direct radiation damage of the gut may induce effects such as inflammatory reactions that result in nausea and vomiting. Radiation of cerebral tumours is also commonly associated with vomiting.

For regimens that usually induce mild to moderate nausea and vomiting, *phenothiazines* such as prochlorperazine (10mg 3 times daily) are usually helpful. In patients who are to receive chemotherapy programmes that induce moderate to severe nausea and vomiting, the *5-$HT_3$-receptor antagonists* such as ondansetron, granisetron and tropisetron are of particular value. These agents are beginning to replace older regimens using high-dose metoclopramide, and are given with or without the addition of corticosteroids.[157,167]

*Ondansetron* (8 to 32mg) should be administered as a single intravenous dose for patients scheduled to receive very emetogenic chemotherapy. A dose of 8mg orally or intravenously is useful for high-dose radiotherapy or moderately emetogenic chemotherapy, either immediately or 1 or 2 hours prior to treatment. If this does not control the problem, ondansetron plus dexamethasone given 12-hourly has been shown to be significantly more effective than ondansetron alone.

Up to one-quarter of patients receiving chemotherapy will have anticipatory nausea and vomiting, which, once established, responds poorly to antiemetics. There may be improvement following behavioural therapy (biofeedback, progressive muscular relaxation, systematic desensitisation, or hypnosis).[168]

### 5.3 Clinical Outcome and Economic Considerations

Cost-effectiveness analyses suggest that, despite the higher initial cost of ondansetron, the cost per effective treatment is equivalent to that of regimens such as high-dose metoclopramide or lorazepam plus dexamethasone.[169] Moreover, quality of life assessments favour ondansetron over other regimens.[170]

## 6. Intestinal Malabsorption Syndromes

Most malabsorption syndromes are associated with diarrhoea and bodyweight loss. However, chemical analysis of the stool is frequently required to demonstrate whether an increase in fat excretion is present. When there is no effective treatment for the primary disorder, symptomatic improvement can still be obtained if the amount of long-chain fatty acid in the diet is reduced. In addition, specific nutrients such as folic acid and other B group vitamins may be required, in the form of dietary or parenteral supplements. However, any discussion of steatorrhoea should not obscure the fact that there is a wide range of absorptive defects, either single or multiple, in which fat absorption may not be disturbed. Acquired lactose intolerance, which is present in much of the world's population, is a clear example.

### 6.1 Luminal Abnormalities

#### *6.1.1 Pancreatic Exocrine Insufficiency*

Malabsorption of fat and protein does not occur until the output of pancreatic lipases and proteases is reduced by 90%. Pancreatic enzyme replacement is then required, and proves beneficial for conditions such as chronic pancreatitis (see section 7.2.2) and cystic fibrosis.

#### *6.1.2 Bile Acid Disturbances*

Bacterial overgrowth in the small intestine may reduce the quantities of conjugated acids required for effective solubilisation of triglyceride breakdown products. Contamination may arise from motility disorders, such as scleroderma or from the presence of a cul-de-sac, as, for example, with diverticulosis or a surgically created blind loop.

**Optimum Treatment**

Treatment is usually initiated with *metronidazole* 200mg 3 times daily for 2 to 4 weeks. Where improvement is poorly sustained, intermittent courses may be needed. *Tetracycline* or *cotrimoxazole* may also be helpful. Bacteria may compete for dietary cyanocobalamin (vitamin $B_{12}$) and produce a megaloblastic anaemia requiring treatment with injections of the vitamin.

Bile acid deficiency may also result from resection of the ileum, Crohn's disease or radiation damage. However, there is no place for oral therapy with bile salts, which exacerbate diarrhoea. After a limited ileal resection, a trial of *cholestyramine* is worthwhile, because patient discomfort may be related more to the secretory effect of bile acids on the colon than to the mild degree of steatorrhoea. The ileum is also the preferential site of cyanocobalamin absorption. When malabsorption has been confirmed by the Schilling test, stores of the vitamin need to be maintained by monthly and then 6-monthly intramuscular injections of *cyanocobalamin* 1mg.

### 6.2 Mucosal Abnormalities

#### *6.2.1 Coeliac Disease (Gluten-Sensitive Enteropathy)*

In nontropical regions, most individuals with an abnormal duodenal mucosa will be found to have coeliac disease. Proof of the diagnosis in adults depends on clinical and histological improvement after the withdrawal of gluten from the diet. An association with malignancy forms the basis of the recommendation that a strict gluten-free diet be followed for life.[171] The diet excludes food containing wheat, rye, barley and, in some cases, oats, and provides rice and corn as alternatives. Where a dietitian is not available, the list of foods and advice about the preparation of meals provided by support groups is very helpful, especially for parents of young children.

**Optimum Treatment**

Patients are now usually diagnosed at earlier stages of the illness, and respond quickly to the diet without the need for supplementation with iron, folic acid, calcium or fat soluble vitamins. Patients responding poorly to dietary measures usually benefit from a short course of *prednisone* 30 mg/day, but the diet should first be reviewed to establish that gluten restriction has been successful. A small number of unresponsive individuals will prove to have a lymphoma.

#### *6.2.2 Giardiasis*

This is a short-lived diarrhoeal illness (see also section 10.2.2), but a number of individuals develop chronic malabsorption. The protozoan may only be recognisable in duodenal biopsies or mucosal smears. Treatment with *metronidazole* 200mg 3 times daily for 7 days is usually curative.

#### 6.2.3 Tropical Sprue

This coliform-linked illness produces gastrointestinal symptoms in the early stages, but thereafter nutritional deficiencies appear. In the acute phase, *folic acid* 5 mg/day is indicated. *Cyanocobalamin* injections may be needed once the disease becomes chronic. Oral *tetracycline* 250mg 4 times daily, for a least a month, restores mucosal integrity in the long term.

#### 6.2.4 Disaccharidase Intolerance

The primary disorder results from an exaggerated decline in lactase concentrations in early or late childhood. Osmotic diarrhoea and other features can be controlled by reducing lactose intake in the form of milk and dairy products. Calcium intake needs to be maintained. Low-lactose milk may also be available.

Secondary lactose intolerance due to mucosal damage in coeliac disease or as a sequel to viral enteritis may require dietary restriction of lactose for a short period.

#### 6.2.5 Whipple's Disease

The causative organism in this condition has now been identified as *Tropheryma whippeli*. Treatment should be life-long, on the assumption that all affected persons have CNS involvement. A good response should be obtained with a combination of benzylpenicillin (penicillin G) 1.2MU and streptomycin 1g daily for 2 weeks, followed by maintenance therapy for 6 to 12 months with either tetracycline 1g plus cotrimoxazole 480mg twice daily, or phenoxymethylpenicillin 250mg 4 times daily.

Foamy macrophages in the lamina propria, which stain with the periodic acid Schiff reagent, resemble the acid-fast macrophages present in *Mycobacterium avium-intracellulare* infection in patients with AIDS.

#### 6.2.6 Malabsorption in Acquired Immune Deficiency Syndrome (AIDS)

Malabsorption may occur as a results of infections other than *M. avium-intracellulare*. Cryptosporidiosis, microsporidiosis and *Isospora belli* infection are examples. Intestinal lymphoma is sometimes a contributing factor. The various treatments available are frequently unsuccessful. A lactose-free, low-fat diet with calorie-rich fluid supplements may be well tolerated in early stages. The importance of maintaining adequate nutrition is identified in guidelines by the US National Task Force on Nutrition in AIDS.[172]

#### 6.2.7 Intestinal Lymphoma and Immunoproliferative Small Intestinal Disease (IPSID)

Tetracycline therapy of IPSID in the early prelymphomatous stage may result in a cure. In the late stages, chemotherapy combined with radiotherapy may be beneficial. Clinical status is improved by due attention to the variety of nutritional disorders that are frequently present. The same general principles apply in the treatment of T cell lymphoma, which is more common in Western nations. Occasionally, local resection of the small intestine may be necessary for complications such as bleeding or obstruction.

#### 6.2.8 Massive Intestinal Resection: Short Bowel Syndrome

In patients with extensive small bowel resection, diarrhoea is an early feature. Dehydration and electrolyte deficiencies, including hypocalcaemia and hypomagnesaemia, are to be anticipated. After several weeks, the effects of malabsorption become prominent, but with adequate support a stage is reached when the effect of treatment coupled with the adaptive response of the remaining intestine is sufficient to maintain nutrition.

##### Optimum Treatment

Enteral or polymeric formulas may need to become a routine part of daily living. Intermittent feeding through a fine nasogastric tube may help to overcome the effect of hyperosmolarity on stool volumes.[173]

### 6.3 Intestinal Lymphatic Obstruction

This is a troublesome disorder when it presents as a primary lymphatic abnormality in young children. Malabsorption of fat and fat soluble vitamins is compounded by the discharge of lymph into the intestinal lumen.

##### Optimum Treatment

Surgery is rarely feasible, and treatment is designed to diminish lymph flow and intralymphatic pressure by reducing dietary long-chain fatty acid triglycerides. Medium-chain triglycerides in powder or oil forms provide a substitute that directs C8 to C10 fatty acids into the portal vein. A high protein intake is desirable. Tetany may be a feature, but responds to calcium, magnesium and cholecalciferol (vitamin $D_3$) supplements. The treatment of secondary lymphatic obstruction is that of the underlying condition (e.g. lymphoma, Whipple's disease).

## 7. Pancreatic Disease

Pancreatitis is classified as either acute or chronic. Patients with *acute pancreatitis* typically present with constant abdominal pain and raised pancreatic enzymes due to inflammation of the pancreas. The disease ranges from a mild self-limiting disorder to severe (often fatal) necrotising pancreatitis. Complete recovery of pancreatic function is usually obtained. This distinguishes it from *chronic pancreatitis*, in which ongoing inflammation causes irreversible morphological changes, often with chronic pain and evidence of permanent loss of pancreatic exocrine and/or endocrine function.

The distinction between acute and chronic pancreatitis is often difficult to make in the initial stages, as acute pancreatitis can recur, and chronic pancreatitis often presents initially as an acute episode. This rarely causes clinical problems in managing the patient (see section 7.2), since a flare of chronic pancreatitis is managed similarly to acute pancreatitis.

***Causes and pathogenesis:*** in Western society the most common cause of acute pancreatitis is gallstone disease. The passage of a stone from the gallbladder to the duodenum appears to result in pancreatic ductular hypertension, with subsequent initiation of pancreatic autodigestion.[174] Biliary sludge and microlithiasis can also cause pancreatitis.[175] Alcohol abuse is the most common cause of chronic pancreatitis. This is probably due to chronic toxic effects of alcohol on pancreatic acinar cells.[176] Other causes of acute and chronic pancreatitis are listed in table VI.

**Table VI.** Associations of acute and chronic pancreatitis

| Common | Uncommon |
|---|---|
| **Acute pancreatitis** | |
| Gallstones | Hypertriglyceridaemia |
| Alcohol abuse | Hyperparathyroidism |
| Unknown cause | Trauma |
| | Endoscopic cholangiopancreatography |
| | Drugs (see table VII) |
| | Infections (mumps, *Mycoplasma* spp., Coxsackie virus, Echo virus) |
| | Connective tissue disorders with vasculitis |
| | Pancreas divisum |
| | Obstruction of ampulla of Vater |
| | Pancreatic carcinoma |
| | Penetrating duodenal ulcer |
| **Chronic pancreatitis** | |
| Alcohol abuse | Abdominal trauma |
| Idiopathic factors | Unknown inherited factors |
| Cystic fibrosis | Schwachman's syndrome |
| Protein calorie malnutrition | Hypertriglyceridaemia |
| | Hyperparathyroidism |
| | Haemochromatosis |
| | Prolonged parenteral hyperalimentation |

**Table VII.** Drugs associated with acute pancreatitis

| | |
|---|---|
| Thiazide diuretics | Sulfonamides |
| Furosemide (frusemide) | Tetracycline |
| Estrogens | Pentamidine |
| Azathioprine | Procainamide |
| Asparaginase | Nitrofurantoin |
| Mercaptopurine | Didanosine (dideoxyinosine) |
| Methyldopa | Valproic acid |

Up to 30% of cases of pancreatitis are idiopathic. A number of drugs have been associated with the development of acute pancreatitis, and some of the more commonly associated agents are listed in table VII.[177] Thus, a careful drug history should be taken in patients with unexplained pancreatitis.

### 7.1 Clinical Pharmacology of Drugs Used in Treatment

Although a variety of drugs have been considered for the treatment of acute and chronic pancreatitis, most have not proven to be of benefit in controlled trials.

The mainstays of treatment for acute pancreatitis are opioid analgesia (NB. not with morphine), intravenous fluids and electrolyte replacement, blood transfusions, antibiotics for infective complications, and possibly oxygen supplementation and inotropic support for critically ill patients.

Pancreatic insufficiency associated with chronic pancreatitis is managed by pancreatic enzyme replacement therapy, possibly accompanied by an $H_2$-receptor antagonist or acid pump inhibitor (e.g. omeprazole) to protect the enzymes against gastric acid digestion (see section 4.1.1 for a discussion on the clinical pharmacology of these drugs). The pain of chronic pancreatitis is difficult to manage pharmacologically, with opioid analgesics being most commonly used. High-dose pancreatic replacement therapy may also be of benefit.

### 7.2 Optimum Treatment

Appreciation of the optimum treatment of acute and chronic pancreatitis depends on an understanding of the disease states, their known causes and possible complications.

### 7.2.1 Acute Pancreatitis

Patients with suspected acute pancreatitis should be admitted to hospital. The principles of management include:

- Pain relief
- Avoidance of pancreatic stimulation ('resting' the pancreas)
- Maintenance of intravascular volume and correction of serum electrolyte abnormalities
- Detecting the presence of complications
- Determining the cause and removing or treating it.

#### Pain Relief

Pain relief usually requires the administration of opioid analgesics. Morphine should be avoided because of its spasmogenic effect on the sphincter of Oddi. Pethidine (meperidine) exerts less effect on sphincteric tone[178] and is generally the analgesic of choice for severe pancreatic pain. In terms of sphincteric effects, pentazocine is also considered a drug of choice[179] but is little used.

#### Avoidance of Pancreatic Stimulation

The pancreas is best 'rested' by fasting the patient and administering fluids intravenously. In mild pancreatitis, this may be all that is necessary. With more severe pancreatitis, nasogastric suction may be instituted. This will help alleviate the symptoms of nausea and vomiting, and may reduce pancreatic stimulation further by aspirating gastric acid.

Although 'resting the pancreas' is conceptually attractive, the pancreas probably secretes little when acutely inflamed. Randomised prospective clinical trials of nasogastric suction, atropine, glucagon, calcitonin, cimetidine and somatostatin (which may reduce pancreatic secretion) have uniformly failed to show benefit in acute pancreatitis.[180] In fact, anticholinergic drugs may exacerbate small intestinal ileus and cause tachycardia. Nonetheless, too early refeeding of a convalescent patient may produce relapse.

Despite considerable evidence that acute pancreatitis is an autodigestive disease, trials of enzyme inhibitors (particularly antiproteases, including aprotinin) have been disappointing.[180] Similarly, controlled trials of antibiotics in uncomplicated acute pancreatitis have failed to demonstrate benefit, although these drugs are indicated if the patient develops cholangitis, a pancreatic abscess or an infected pseudocyst (persistent, localised collection of pancreatic secretion and necrotic tissue, surrounded by fibrous tissue and lined by granulation tissue – differing from a true cyst, which has an epithelial lining).

Use of *somatostatin* and its longer-acting analogue *octreotide* in acute pancreatitis warrants particular note. Because of their inhibitory effects on pancreatic secretion, pancreatic uses have been suggested for these peptides. They probably hasten resolution of pancreatic fistulae and pancreatic ascites, and possibly of pseudocysts, but there have been no controlled trials. Somewhat disappointingly, 4 controlled trials (involving a total of 375 patients) failed to demonstrate a benefit in acute pancreatitis.[181]

The value of these agents in minimising pain and pancreatitis following endoscopic retrograde cholangiopancreatography (ERCP) has been subject to clinical debate. A large double-blind controlled trial failed to demonstrate any beneficial effect of *octreotide*.[182] In fact, failure of duct cannulation was higher in the treatment group, and the investigators suggested that any potential benefit of octreotide in suppressing pancreatic secretion may be offset by its effect on the sphincter of Oddi, i.e. increasing basal tone and frequency of phasic contractions. More encouraging are the data from 2 large multicentre European trials, suggesting that peri- and postoperative octreotide reduces the local complication rate of major pancreatic surgery.[183,184]

#### Maintenance of Intravascular Volume, Correction of Serum Electrolyte Abnormalities and Detection and Treatment of Complications

In acute pancreatitis, massive retroperitoneal exudation and haemorrhage may occur, contributing to shock, renal failure and subsequent mortality. In recent times, recognition of the existence of this intra-abdominal fluid sequestration and improvements in intensive care have led to an improvement in mortality in this condition.

In all patients with acute pancreatitis, careful attention should be paid to blood pressure, urine output, blood volume, haemoglobin concentrations, haematocrit, and serum creatinine and electrolyte concentrations. Blood glucose, calcium and magnesium concentrations should be estimated daily. Patients with severe or predicted severe disease should be managed in an intensive care unit (ICU).

Recent advances in the treatment of acute pancreatitis include early identification of patients with a worse prognosis and early endoscopic cholangiography in gallstone pancreatitis. Advances in intensive care mean that critically ill patients can be more successfully supported through their illness. It is, thus, important to recognise early the subgroup of patients with acute pancreatitis who are at risk of becoming critically ill. These patients may benefit from early transfer to an ICU for close monitoring, and for early identification and treatment of complications. Complications include cardiovascular collapse, respiratory distress, renal failure, and local complications such as pancreatic abscess, peripancreatic fluid collections and pseudocysts.

Well validated prognostic criteria have been developed and an example is shown in table VIII.[185] Close observation, frequent examination and attention to the biochemical indices listed in the table increases the chance that critically ill patients will be identified before their condition deteriorates irretrievably.

Two well controlled studies have shown that, in patients with predicted severe gallstone pancreatitis, early endoscopic cholangiography and removal of common bile duct stones via endoscopic sphincterotomy reduces morbidity and mortality.[186,187]

Surgery for acute pancreatitis is indicated when there is a pancreatic abscess or nonresolving pseudocyst. Surgery may also be performed if there is doubt about the diagnosis. Computed tomography (CT) scanning is the most reliable method of detecting necrotic tissue and fluid collections. Radiologically-guided fine-needle aspiration is necessary to distinguish infected tissue from sterile necrosis. While sterile collections and necrotic tissue may resolve spontaneously, the mortality from infected pancreatic tissue (pancreatic abscess) approaches 100% without surgery. Surgery involves drainage of collections and debridement of devitalised and necrotic tissue. This reduces the mortality of patients with pancreatic abscesses to approximately 30%.

**Table VIII.** Poor prognostic factors in acute pancreatitis (within 48h of diagnosis) [after Imrie et al.[185]]

| |
|---|
| Age >55 years |
| White cell count >15 x $10^9$/L |
| Blood sugar >10 mmol/L (in nondiabetic patients) |
| Urea >16 mmol/L (after rehydration) |
| $PaO_2$ <60mm Hg |
| Serum calcium <2.0 mmol/L |
| Lactate dehydrogenase >600 IU/L |
| Aspartate or alanine aminotransferase >100 IU/L |
| Albumin <32 g/L |

#### Determining and Treating the Cause

Every patient with acute pancreatitis must have an ultrasound examination to check for cholelithiasis. After recovery from gallstone pancreatitis, a cholecystectomy will prevent further attacks.

In addition, patients with acute pancreatitis should be screened for hypertriglyceridaemia and hypercalcaemia. These reversible causes of pancreatitis may result in recurrent attacks if undetected. Serum triglycerides and calcium should be measured when the patient has recovered from the acute attack, as acute pancreatitis *per se* can cause transient elevation of serum triglycerides and depression of serum calcium. Drug-induced pancreatitis is rare, but a careful drug history should be taken.

### *7.2.2 Chronic Pancreatitis*

Patients with chronic pancreatitis require treatment for chronic pain and pancreatic insufficiency. In those with alcoholic pancreatitis, total abstinence is paramount but rarely achieved. Continued drinking indicates a poor prognosis and likely treatment failure.

#### Treatment of Pain

The pathophysiology of pain in chronic pancreatitis is poorly understood, but may be related to episodes of acute pancreatic inflammation, the presence of a pseudocyst, obstruction of the pancreatic duct, obstruction of the common bile duct or perineural inflammation. Elevated pancreatic ductal and interstitial pressures are frequently found and their reduction often correlates with the relief of pain.

In the evaluation of pancreatic pain, imaging by CT scan and endoscopic pancreatography is essential. CT scans reveal the size and shape of the gland and may show a dilated pancreatic duct, intraductal calculi or pseudocysts. Endoscopic pancreatography is particularly valuable in delineating pancreatic duct size and may reveal calculi, strictures, pseudocysts, and associated common bile duct strictures.

The presence of pancreatic proteases in the duodenum has been shown to inhibit pancreatic secretion via a negative feedback loop.[188] The discovery of this phenomenon led to the use of oral *pancreatic enzyme replacement therapy* (even in the absence of pancreatic insufficiency) to treat pancreatic pain. Several small trials of this therapy have shown some benefit,[188,189] but in our experience, this treatment has been disappointing. The somatostatin analogue *octreotide* may have a role in the management of pancreatic pain and is currently undergoing controlled trials.

Surgery can provide good pain relief in carefully selected patients. Those with pseudocysts often benefit from surgical drainage. Patients with refractory pancreatic pain and a dilated main pancreatic duct (>8mm) often obtain relief of pain by pancreaticojejunostomy to decompress the duct. Pancreatic duct strictures and isolated areas of pancreatitis may be treated by resection of the head of the pancreas (Whipple's procedure) or the distal portion of the pancreas. However, these operations are often unsuccessful because of undiagnosed disease in the remainder of the gland. Overall, some 80% of patients will obtain complete or partial pain relief from pancreaticojejunostomy, although up to 20% will develop recurrence of pain during follow-up.

#### Treatment of Pancreatic Enzyme Insufficiency

Steatorrhoea due to pancreatic insufficiency is treated with pancreatic enzyme supplements. As long as adequate lipase is provided (at least 600U per tablet or capsule) these should reverse the steatorrhoea of chronic pancreatitis. In practice, 6 to 8 tablets of a potent enzyme preparation or 3 capsules of an enteric-coated preparation, per meal, satisfactorily reduce steatorrhoea in most patients. Addition of an $H_2$-receptor antagonist or acid pump inhibitor (e.g. omeprazole) raises gastric pH and prevents inactivation of the lipase by gastric acid. Diabetes mellitus is treated in the standard manner, but can often be extremely 'brittle'.

Treatment of acute exacerbations of chronic pancreatitis follows the principles of treatment for acute pancreatitis (see section 7.2.1).

### 7.3 Clinical Outcome and Economic Considerations

Most attacks of acute pancreatitis are mild and resolve with conservative therapy, i.e. fasting the patient and the administration of intravenous fluids. More severe disease often requires admission to an ICU and the cost of management of these cases often rivals that of liver transplantation. Even in patients who have survived severe acute pancreatitis, recovery of glandular function is the rule. Prevention of further attacks of acute pancreatitis depend on detection and correction of causative factors.

Chronic pancreatitis has a poorer outcome. Patients often continue to drink and become addicted to opioid analgesics, becoming invalids unable to maintain employment. Death generally ensues within about 10 years from complications of pancreatic disease or other alcohol-induced organ damage.

## 8. Liver Disease

### 8.1 Acute Hepatitis

#### *8.1.1 Acute Viral Hepatitis*

Although viral hepatitis is becoming increasingly common and important, there is currently no effective curative drug therapy available. Treatment is therefore symptomatic.

#### Optimum Treatment

Most patients prefer bedrest to ease symptoms of weakness and lethargy. Diet should be nutritious. Low fat diets may mitigate upper gastrointestinal symptoms and produce less nausea, but have no specific therapeutic benefit. Alcohol should be avoided.

Acute viral hepatitis infrequently progresses to fulminant liver failure and up to 10% of urgent liver transplantations are performed for fulminant viral hepatitis. Thus, it is wise to regard all cases as potentially fatal until progressive clinical and biochemical improvement is obvious. Attending clinicians should have a low threshold for admission to hospital and referral to a liver transplant centre. Other reasons for hospital admission, apart from such severe illness, include diagnostic and socioeconomic reasons. Hospitalised patients can be nursed in open wards provided that the principles of good personal hygiene are followed by patients and staff; special care must be taken with the handling of blood products.

Acute hepatitis A virus infection can sometimes result in a severe, cholestatic illness. Cholestyramine and antihistamines may reduce pruritus in this clinical setting. Corticosteroids may have a role in the management of cholestatic viral hepatitis secondary to hepatitis A. However, they should not be used in other forms of viral hepatitis, in which they do not alter the degree of necrosis or the rate of healing. Furthermore, corticosteroid-related adverse effects may develop even with short term use. Corticosteroids have not been shown to be of value in fulminant viral hepatitis. Patients may resume normal activity when they feel well and serum bilirubin is normal. Mild elevation of serum transaminases should not be regarded as a contraindication to mobilisation.

***Antiviral therapy:*** while some patients with acute viral hepatitis develop fulminant hepatic failure or chronic hepatitis, most will make a complete recovery. At present, the treatment of patients with acute viral hepatitis with interferon-α (or any other antiviral agent) cannot be recommended, as there is no evidence that such therapy speeds healing or prevents the development of chronic disease.

***Vaccination:*** active immunisation with vaccines directed against hepatitis A and hepatitis B is now possible. The development of these vaccines represents one of the most significant advances in medicine in the past decade.

*Hepatitis B vaccines* were initially derived from plasma and consisted of purified, inactivated surface antigen. In recent years, however, recombinant yeast vaccines have been developed. Three injections of the recombinant vaccine given in a dose of 10mg intramuscularly initially and at 1 and 6 months induces a prolonged antibody response in over 90% of individuals. The duration of protection is uncertain. However, further booster vaccination should be considered after 5 to 7 years. In areas of low prevalence, persons at high risk (e.g. healthcare workers, laboratory personnel, residents of institutions of the mentally handicapped, sexual and household contacts) should be considered for vaccination. Recent evidence indicates that targeting high risk groups in Western societies is unsuccessful. It is likely that universal childhood vaccination programmes will commence in affluent societies.

Simultaneous administration of *hepatitis B immune serum globulin* (HBIG) and hepatitis B vaccine should be given whenever immediate protection against hepatitis B is required, e.g. for infants of HBeAg-negative carrier mothers, or following percutaneous or needlestick exposure.

Immune globulin given before or shortly after exposure to hepatitis A virus is protective against clinical illness. *Hepatitis A vaccine* is effective in preventing infection in the pre-exposure setting. Travel to countries where hepatitis A is endemic is a common indication for hepatitis A vaccination. Other factors associated with an increased risk of hepatitis A infection include attendance at a daycare centres, institutional care, and unsafe sexual practices. Vaccination should be considered in any individual at risk of exposure to hepatitis A virus.

It should be emphasised that, despite the advent of vaccination, the control of viral hepatitis still lies mainly in good sanitation and hygiene, particularly at a personal level, together with adequate screening of blood and blood products before their administration. All excreta of patients with hepatitis A should be considered infectious, at least in the early stages of the disease.

#### *8.1.2 Acute Alcoholic Hepatitis*

The short term prognosis in patients with alcoholic hepatitis is related to the severity of the liver injury. In those patients with severe hepatic dysfunction, the short term mortality rate has been reported to be as high as 35%.[190]

##### Optimum Treatment

The principles of medical management focus on the need for abstinence from alcohol, an adequate nutrient intake, and the treatment of complications such as portal hypertension and hepatic encephalopathy. Various drug regimens have been tested, including corticosteroids, colchicine, penicillamine and propylthiouracil. Of these, corticosteroids have received most attention and there is evidence that they reduce mortality in patients with severe hepatic dysfunction.[191] These potential benefits must be balanced against the risks of sepsis and hyperglycaemia.

Every effort should be made to convince the patient of the importance of complete abstinence from alcohol. Expert psychiatric assistance may be helpful.

### 8.2 Chronic Hepatitis

#### *8.2.1 Chronic Viral Hepatitis*

Drug therapy for chronic hepatitis is evolving rapidly. The only widely available drug at present (interferon-α) has limited effectiveness and significant adverse effects. Its use should therefore be confined to specialist centres.

##### Optimum Treatment

*Interferon-α* therapy results in a sustained loss of viral replication in around 40% of patients with chronic HBeAg-positive hepatitis B. Such treatment is indicated in patients with HBsAg in serum together with HBV-DNA and/or HBeAg and raised transaminases. Factors predictive of a response to interferon-α therapy include high concentrations of transaminases, low concentrations of HBV-DNA, short duration of disease, and female gender.[192,193]

Adverse effects of interferon-α therapy are common and include an influenza-like syndrome (that diminishes with subsequent injections), bone marrow suppression, psychological changes (including depression and irritability), bacterial infections and autoimmune disorders.

Interferon-α is widely used in the therapy of chronic hepatitis C. Current evidence indicates that in around 50% of patients with chronic hepatitis C, transaminase concentrations normalise with interferon-α treatment. However, the response is not sustained in about 50% of apparent responders.[194]

#### 8.2.2 Autoimmune Hepatitis

Autoimmune hepatitis (previously called chronic active hepatitis) is characterised by the presence of the histological features of chronic hepatitis and autoantibodies such as anti–smooth muscle antibody, antinuclear antibody or liver-kidney microsomal antibody. Diagnosis must be confirmed by liver histology, serology, and exclusion of other known causes of persisting liver inflammation and piecemeal necrosis, e.g. Wilson's disease, various drugs and viral hepatitis.

##### Optimum Treatment

The first goal of treatment is to suppress hepatic inflammation and prevent cirrhosis. The second is to maintain remission once disease activity is controlled.

Treatment should commence with *pred nisolone* or *prednisone* 20mg 3 times daily. Although prednisone is known to be converted in the liver to its active form prednisolone, this biotransformation appears not to be significantly impaired in patients with active disease, in that serum prednisolone concentrations are similar regardless of which drug is given.[195] However, in severe disease, the metabolism of both drugs may be impaired and comparatively high serum concentrations of prednisolone are attained after modest doses, giving rise to significant adverse effects. This large dose of prednisone or prednisolone should be reduced when there is clinical or biochemical evidence of improvement. About 20% of patients fail to respond, deteriorate and develop hepatocellular failure.[196] In such patients, a trial of higher prednisolone dosages (50 to 60 mg/day) is worth considering, but is usually ineffective. Liver transplantation is a potential therapeutic option in these unresponsive patients.

The dose of prednisolone (or prednisone) for maintenance therapy is usually 10 to 15 mg/day, but is variable and may be as low as 2.5 mg/day. *Azathioprine* is often used as a steroid-sparing agent,[197] reducing the dose of prednisolone required to maintain remission to around 5 mg/day. Azathioprine alone may maintain remission in some patients, but appears unable to induce remission. Azathioprine should be commenced at 25 to 50 mg/day. If there are no adverse effects, the dose can be increased to around 100 mg/day. Complications of azathioprine include bone marrow suppression, cholestatic jaundice and pancreatitis.

Corticosteroids, with or without azathioprine, have been shown to induce remission and prolong life in autoimmune chronic hepatitis. Therapy usually has to be continued for 2 years or more. Withdrawal of drug therapy is often associated with relapse and should only be performed under strict surveillance.

### 8.3 Cirrhosis

#### 8.3.1 Compensated Cirrhosis

All patients should be advised to follow an adequate diet and to abstain from alcohol, and should be regularly reviewed for signs of hepatocellular failure. Long term care includes control of ascites, avoidance of drugs that may induce coma, and prompt treatment of infection and variceal bleeding.

#### 8.3.2 Decompensated Cirrhosis

In patients with alcoholic cirrhosis, permanent abstinence from alcohol is the most important aspect of treatment. Patients who are able to abstain completely may show remarkable improvement over time. Overall, 5-year survival rates vary from 40 to 56% among patients who continue drinking, whereas those who abstain have a survival rate of 60 to 86%. The diet should be as nutritious as possible. A high protein diet is recommended, provided that there is no evidence of hepatic precoma or coma. If the prothrombin time is high, oral vitamin $K_1$ (phytomenadione) should be given.

Liver transplantation is now an established therapy for end-stage liver disease. In general, transplantation should be performed when the prognosis of the untreated disease outweighs the risks of the operation. One-year survival rates reported from most centres approach 80%. Thus, current opinion is that transplantation should occur before the complications of chronic liver disease, such as malnutrition and renal failure, significantly increase the operative risk.

#### 8.3.3 Hepatic Encephalopathy

Hepatic encephalopathy is often precipitated by gastrointestinal haemorrhage, electrolyte disturbances arising from aggressive diuresis, sepsis, or excessive doses of analgesics, sedatives or hypnotics.

##### Optimum Treatment

Any precipitating factor should be treated. Oral *lactulose* and/or *neomycin* may be of benefit. Lactulose acts by acidifying the colonic contents and reducing the absorption of ammonia and possibly other toxins.[198,199] The dose of lactulose can be progressively increased until the desired effect is obtained. However, diarrhoea and dehydration may result and dose reduction may be required. In most cases, the desired faecal pH can be obtained, with 2 to 3 soft formed, but not liquid, bowel motions per day. The effect of neomycin is probably related to a reduction in numbers of urease-producing intestinal bacteria.

In patients with chronic portal-systemic encephalopathy, the protein content of the diet, and oral neomycin and/or lactulose dosages may be varied to meet the individual needs of the patient. The amount of neomycin absorbed is usually small, but care must be taken to avoid adverse effects, especially deafness. In established coma, intravenous glucose is used to prevent hypoglycaemia, minimise protein catabolism and provide calories. There is some evidence that branched-chain amino acids may confer some benefit in high-grade hepatic coma. However, in practice, they are rarely used.

#### 8.3.4 Cirrhotic Oedema and Ascites

The major recent advance in this condition has been the demonstration that therapeutic paracentesis in association with the use of plasma expanders, is safe and effective. This means that such patients can frequently be treated as outpatients. Potassium-sparing diuretics still have an important place in therapy.

##### Optimum Treatment

The goal of medical therapy is to mobilise peritoneal fluid by establishing a net negative sodium balance. Dietary intake of sodium should be reduced to 1 to 1.5 g/day [40 to 60 mmol (mEq) per day]. As patients are often unaware that they are taking excess sodium, a list of sodium-containing foods, medicines, etc. should be provided. In around 20% of patients, this measure alone results in significant mobilisation of ascites.

In the remaining cases, diuretic therapy is required to increase urinary sodium and water excretion. When diuretic treatment is considered, the aim is to produce a slow diuresis, gauged by a bodyweight loss of about 0.5kg daily. Dietary sodium restriction must be maintained in patients treated with diuretics, as it reduces diuretic requirements. Loop diuretics, usually furosemide (frusemide) and distally acting diuretics (in particular, spironolactone) are commonly used. A useful starting regimen is *spironolactone* 50 to 100 mg/day. There is often an interval of 2 to 4 days between the commencement of this drug and the initiation of the diuretic response. If there is no response after 5 days' therapy, the spironolactone dosage can be increased in a step-wise fashion. Alternatively, *furosemide* may be added and the dosage increased to 160 mg/day. Dosages of spironolactone up to 1000 mg/day have been used; however, patients unresponsive to furosemide 160 mg/day, spironolactone 400 mg/day and severe salt restriction are usually considered to have diuretic-resistant ascites. The reason why diuretic resistance occurs is poorly understood but it may relate to increasing hyperaldosteronism and other defects of the renin-angiotensin system.

Restricted water intake is only required when hyponatraemia develops. Complications of diuretic therapy include electrolyte disturbances, intravascular volume depletion with azotaemia, and hepatic encephalopathy. A specific adverse effect of spironolactone is gynaecomastia. Substitution of spironolactone by *amiloride* is a useful measure in this situation.

Therapeutic paracentesis, in association with the use of plasma expanders, is now regarded as a well tolerated, effective and rapid treatment of ascites in patients with cirrhosis. There is evidence that treatment of ascites by paracentesis is associated with fewer adverse effects and a shorter duration of hospital stay than with diuretic therapy. In the absence of severe renal or liver failure, large-volume paracentesis is probably the treatment of choice in patients with cirrhosis and tense ascites.

#### 8.3.5 Portal Hypertension and Variceal Haemorrhage

Spectacular advances in management have occurred in this area recently, particularly with respect to drug therapy of acute variceal bleeding, variceal obliteration, and the prevention of first variceal haemorrhage.

#### Optimum Treatment

Therapy is aimed at correcting hypovolaemic shock and achieving haemostasis at the bleeding site. A central venous line should be placed. After restoring blood pressure to normal values by infusing plasma volume expanders, whole blood or preferably packed red cells are transfused to maintain the haematocrit at around 30%. Airway aspiration should be avoided, especially in patients with impaired consciousness. This requires aspiration of the gastric contents and frequent gastric lavage through an indwelling nasogastric tube.

As soon as the patient is stabilised, emergency endoscopy must be performed to establish the precise site of bleeding. Patients frequently bleed from lesions other than varices, such as gastric erosions, peptic ulcers and so-called portal hypertensive gastropathy.[200]

***Oesophageal balloon tamponade:*** this is an effective way to achieve temporary control of variceal haemorrhage, and is best achieved by means of the Sengstaken-Blakemore tube. Tamponade is highly effective, the control of bleeding ranging from 85 to 95% in experienced centres. The 2 main disadvantages of this form of therapy are:

1) Its effects are limited to the period during which the balloons are inflated (24 hours).

2) There is a high rate of complications, some of which may be lethal.

The most frequent severe complication is aspiration pneumonia, occurring in over 10% of patients.

***Pharmacological therapy:*** if safe and effective agents were available, drug treatment would be the optimum therapy for variceal bleeding. Drug therapy is based on the use of agents that may decrease pressure and blood flow at the oesophageal varices. This can be achieved either by the use of splanchnic vasoconstrictors [vasopressin, glypressin (terlipressin) or somatostatin] that decrease portal-collateral blood flow, or by drugs that decrease vascular resistance at the intrahepatic and portal-collateral circulation [nitroglycerin (glyceryl trinitrate)], or by combination therapy.

*Vasopressin:* this agent has been used for many years to treat variceal haemorrhage, but its use is still controversial. Adverse effects of vasopressin derive from systemic vasoconstriction. These effects may result in serious complications, such as myocardial ischaemia or infarction, arrhythmias, mesenteric ischaemia, limb ischaemia and cerebrovascular accidents. Vasopressin is, thus, no longer recommended as monotherapy, since when given alone, it produces complications in 32 to 65% of patients, and may be lethal in some cases.[200,201]

*Combination of vasopressin and nitroglycerin:* this drug combination enhances the reduction in portal pressure while attenuating the systemic adverse effects of vasopressin.[202] In 3 randomised controlled trials that compared vasopressin alone with vasopressin plus nitroglycerin (given sublingually, intravenously or via transdermal continuous-release preparations), the combination of vasopressin and nitroglycerin was more effective in controlling bleeding than vasopressin alone.[201] In addition, the combination of transdermal nitroglycerin (*vs* placebo) with intravenous vasopressin significantly reduced transfusion requirements, the need for balloon tamponade and the requirement for emergency surgery.[203] In 2 of these trials, adverse effects were significantly reduced in patients receiving the combined regimen. These results indicate that vasopressin should always be used with nitroglycerin.[201]

*Glypressin:* this drug is a synthetic vasopressin derivative with prolonged duration of activity that permits administration as intravenous injections of 2mg every 4 hours until a bleeding-free period of 24 to 48 hours is achieved. The effects of glypressin differ from those of vasopressin, not only in its much longer duration of activity, but also in that glypressin causes fewer adverse effects and does not enhance fibrinolysis.

The clinical effectiveness of glypressin has been assessed in 3 placebo-controlled trials.[204] Pooled estimates showed a significant reduction in failure to control bleeding and in mortality. Glypressin controlled bleeding in 79% of cases. It must be emphasised that this is the only drug treatment that deals with variceal bleeding and reduces mortality. It is simpler, more effective and safer than vasopressin.

*Somatostatin* causes selective splanchnic vasoconstriction and thereby decreases portal and collateral blood flow and portal pressure. This is probably due to inhibition of the release of splanchnic vasodilatory peptides such as glucagon.[205] Bolus injections of somatostatin cause marked and rapid reductions in portal pressure and azygous blood flow. These changes are greater than those produced by continuous infusion. Thus, a recommended dosage is 3 bolus injections during the first hours of therapy and on rebleeding during treatment.

The usual bolus dose is 250mg, with a continuous infusion of 250 mg/h given thereafter. When successful, therapy is maintained for 2 to 5 days.

*Octreotide* is a cyclic octapeptide analogue of somatostatin, with a longer duration of activity. It has been shown to reduce portal pressure in animals, a finding not confirmed in patients with cirrhosis. The effect of octreotide on variceal pressure is unpredictable, with some increases in intravariceal pressure reported. Similarly, the effectiveness of octreotide in variceal haemorrhage has not been adequately assessed so far.[201] Results of initial studies suggest octreotide may be effective, but the small sample sizes, different schedules of octreotide treatment and ill-defined end-points of the available trials do not permit recommendation of octreotide in the treatment of acute variceal bleeding, outside the context of randomised clinical trials.

***Emergency sclerotherapy:*** this has become widely used as a first-line treatment, since it provides the possibility of starting long term therapy at the time of the initial endoscopy. It is performed either at diagnostic endoscopy or after bleeding has been controlled by the use of drugs or balloon tamponade. However, it can be a difficult procedure when there is active bleeding and is associated with a significant risk of airway aspiration and pneumonia, especially in encephalopathic patients.

Emergency sclerotherapy is also associated with a considerable risk of other significant complications. Mucosal ulceration at the site of injections is observed in up to 80% of patients and may cause rebleeding in up to 20%. Other major complications include oesophageal stricture, perforation and mediastinitis. The overall rate of serious complications is 10 to 20%, with an overall mortality of 2 to 5%. Available data suggest that emergency sclerotherapy produces a better outcome than balloon tamponade and vasopressin, but not better than somatostatin, although it is too early to draw definite conclusions. Emergency surgery is superior to emergency sclerotherapy in controlling bleeding and reducing rebleeding (particularly in patients whose condition is severe and unresponsive to medical treatment or balloon tamponade), but mortality rates are equal.

***Endoscopic banding ligation of varices:*** this technique has recently been developed to treat oesophageal varices and acute variceal bleeding.[201] The technique is not difficult for skilled endoscopists. However, an outer sheath is often necessary for repeated intubation, since the endoscope may only bear a single band, and each session requires several bands. The procedure takes more time and requires deeper sedation than sclerotherapy, increasing the risk of airway aspiration during acute bleeding. No controlled trials in acute variceal bleeding have been reported so far, although banding and emergency sclerotherapy in comparative randomised controlled trials had a similar effectiveness in patients treated early in the bleeding episode.[200,201]

***Emergency surgery:*** this is used less now than several years ago. In many centres, surgery is used as second-line treatment when all else fails to control bleeding. Surgery should never be delayed after failure of medical or endoscopic therapy, because of an increased mortality risk. As a practical guideline, a third sclerotherapy session should never be allowed. Conventional surgery carries a high risk in Child-Puch class C patients, who are best managed by transjugular intrahepatic portosystemic stent shunts (TIPS). Patients in good condition probably do better with portocaval, mesocaval or splenorenal shunts, which have less tendency to occlude. Post-shunt encephalopathy is, however, a frequent problem with these operations.[200]

#### Prevention of First Haemorrhage

The aim of prophylactic therapy is to prevent variceal bleeding and bleeding related deaths. Prophylactic medical therapy may have a major effect on the natural history of cirrhosis. Long term therapy is based on the use of drugs lowering portal pressure, endoscopic sclerotherapy or banding ligation, and portal decompressive surgery.

***β-Adrenoceptor blockers:*** propranolol lowers portal pressure by decreasing portal and collateral blood flow. This is the result of a decrease in cardiac output and of splanchnic vasoconstriction due to $\beta_2$-adrenoceptor blockade. The reduction in portal pressure is moderate, but there is a marked reduction in azygous blood flow.[206] Propranolol should be used at maximally tolerated doses. Dosage adjustment is made by step-wise increases, carefully considering clinical tolerability, heart rate and arterial blood pressure. In general, a decrease in heart rate of 25% (but not to <55 beats/min) is considered adequate.

Adverse effects of β-blockers occur in <15% of patients and are usually minor, necessitating withdrawal of therapy in fewer than half. The effect of therapy is limited to the time of drug administration. There is now enough evidence to recommend β-blocker therapy in all patients with varices without bleeding or contraindications to these drugs.[200]

**Prevention of Recurrent Variceal Bleeding**

Portacaval or distal splenorenal shunt surgery dramatically reduces the risk of rebleeding, but increases the risk of hepatic encephalopathy. Sclerotherapy also reduces the rebleeding rate, although gastric varices or portal hypertensive gastropathy are frequent sequelae. The risk of rebleeding is also reduced by long term β-blockade with propranolol in most, but not all, patients.

## 8.4 Special Types of Cirrhosis

### *8.4.1 Haemochromatosis*

An effective oral iron-chelating agent is not yet available but is eagerly awaited in view of the high prevalence of this disease and the importance of maintaining normal iron stores. Meanwhile, regular venesection remains the cornerstone of therapy, although *deferoxamine* (desferrioxamine) given parenterally is useful in specific circumstances.

**Optimum Treatment**

Treatment of haemochromatosis is by regular venesection, commencing initially with weekly phlebotomy of 500 to 1000ml to mobilise iron stores. One unit of blood contains around 250mg of iron and about 25g of iron must be removed. Thus, weekly phlebotomy may continue for up to 2 to 3 years. The adequacy of therapy may be evaluated at any time by measurement of serum ferritin concentrations, which reflect iron stores more accurately than serum iron and transferrin saturation.[207] Chelating agents such as *deferoxamine* are less effective. However, they can be used as a substitute for iron removal when anaemia or hypoproteinaemia are severe enough to preclude phlebotomy, or when venous access is difficult.[208]

### *8.4.2 Primary Biliary Cirrhosis and Primary Sclerosing Cholangitis*

Effective drug therapy for these diseases is still awaited. Despite numerous drug trials, only *ursodeoxycholic acid* appears to be effective in improving liver function and possibly prolonging life. Liver transplantation is still a major facet of therapy.

**Optimum Treatment**

Medical therapy is directed towards arresting progression of the underlying histological lesion and treating systemic complications of prolonged cholestasis. A number of drugs have been used in clinical trials to treat the hepatobiliary lesions, including penicillamine, azathioprine, chlorambucil, cyclosporin, prednisolone and colchicine. To date, none of these agents has consistently prolonged survival or arrested progression of the underlying disease. Recently, *ursodeoxycholic acid* has been advocated as a potential treatment for primary biliary cirrhosis. Current evidence (including several international collaborative trials) indicates that the administration of ursodeoxycholic acid is associated with beneficial biochemical effects and may reduce the probability of liver transplantation and death.[209-211]

Pruritus and bone disease are among the most frequent complications of cholestasis. *Cholestyramine* is the mainstay of therapy for pruritus. Unfortunately it has an unpleasant taste and may cause diarrhoea and abdominal discomfort. Cholestyramine can also affect the absorption of other medications and should not be administered concomitantly with important medical therapies. In some instances, pruritus is not controlled by cholestyramine in which case *antihistamines* may be of benefit. The mechanism of their effect is uncertain, but probably relates to sedative properties. Other potential therapies for pruritus include rifampicin and opioid receptor antagonists.

Osteopenia is a more frequent complication of cholestatic liver disease than osteomalacia. The increased risk of fractures, particularly after liver transplantation, is an important cause of morbidity. A calcium intake of around 1 to 1.5 g/day is recommended and should start early in the disease process. Estrogen replacement and cholecalciferol therapy in cholestatic liver disease are controversial and currently under review.

## 8.5 Gallstones

Gallstone disease (cholelithiasis), is a common problem in Western countries. Gallstones may be composed largely of cholesterol, bile pigments or a combination of both.

**Optimum Treatment**

Treatment for most types is by surgery, but selected patients with cholesterol gallstones can be successfully treated with the naturally-occurring primary bile salt, *chenodeoxycholic (chenic) acid*, although there is still debate as to the optimum dosage of this agent. Lithotripsy is an attractive therapeutic option if surgery carries a high degree of risk. Laparoscopic cholecystectomy is now widely practised and is associated with a reduced duration of hospitalisation. Indeed, the widespread application of this procedure and its reduced risks have rendered drug therapy (chenodeoxycholic acid and ursodeoxycholic acid) virtually obsolete.

## 9. Inflammatory Bowel Disease

Inflammatory bowel disease is a collective term for diseases that are clinicopathologically divided into 2 groups: ulcerative colitis and Crohn's disease. The divergent patterns of clinical and laboratory features between patients with Crohn's disease and those with ulcerative colitis provide compelling evidence that these 2 categories do represent different diseases.[212]

### 9.1 Clinical Pharmacology of Drugs Used in Treatment

#### *9.1.1 Mesalazine (Mesalamine) Analogues*

After more than 50 years since its introduction, *sulfasalazine* remains central to therapeutic strategies for ulcerative colitis and, to a lesser extent, Crohn's disease. Orally administered sulfasalazine is almost entirely delivered to the colonic lumen because it is poorly absorbed in the small intestine. The absorbed fraction is redelivered to the intestinal lumen via enterohepatic recirculation. Colonic bacteria cleave the azo bond, splitting sulfasalazine into its 2 components, mesalazine (5-aminosalicylic acid, mesalamine) which is the moiety responsible for the therapeutic effect[213] and sulfapyridine.

*Mesalazine*[214] is taken up by the colonic epithelium where it is largely acetylated,[215] while the fraction reaching the portal blood is also actively acetylated by the liver. Therefore, serum mesalazine concentrations are very low. Mesalazine must be delivered topically at high concentrations for clinical effectiveness. Thus, serum concentrations appear to reflect small bowel exposure to mesalazine, while faecal concentrations reflect colonic delivery and likely effectiveness. The sulfapyridine component of sulfasalazine acts as a carrier molecule, but is readily absorbed and is responsible for 80 to 90% of the adverse effects complicating sulfasalazine therapy, necessitating its termination in 10% of patients.

Alternative carrier molecules or delivery systems for mesalazine have been developed. The characteristics of these new formulations are outlined in table IX. Mesalazine linked via an azo bond to either another mesalazine molecule (to produce olsalazine) or to 4-aminobenzoyl-β-alanine (to produce balsalazide) exhibits similar pharmacokinetic characteristics to those of sulfasalazine. *Olsalazine*[216] has been extensively evaluated; it has the disadvantage of inducing net intestinal secretion and may cause diarrhoea in up to 15% of patients. This is usually avoided by its graded introduction over 7 to 10 days. Olsalazine is split by bacteria less effectively if gut transit time is markedly shortened, although this has little relevance to ulcerative colitis.

Three commercially available oral formulations of mesalazine, a slow-release preparation and 2 with pH-dependent coating, produce high concentrations of mesalazine in the colonic lumen. Serum mesalazine concentrations are at least 10-fold lower than with uncoated mesalazine, but are higher than those seen with azo drugs, due predominantly to small intestinal release of mesalazine. Luminal concentrations in the ileum, although high, are less than 20% of those found in the colon (table IX).

The formulation dictates where the drug is released in the intestine. Coated mesalazine may have potential effectiveness for small intestinal mucosal inflammation, although the higher serum concentrations obtained raise concern over nephrotoxicity, which has been reported.[218] Both azo prodrugs and coated mesalazine are well tolerated and have been successfully used in 80 to 90% of patients intolerant of sulfasalazine.

***Clinical use:*** all the preparations included in table IX have demonstrated effectiveness in mildly to moderately active ulcerative colitis, with similar effectiveness apparent in maintenance of remission (2- to 4-fold reduction in relapse rate during 12 months' therapy). Their effectiveness in Crohn's disease is less clear, and is subject to continuing evaluation. Sulfasalazine has demonstrated effectiveness in active Crohn's colitis, but uncertain benefits in ileitis, and has generally not proven useful as maintenance therapy. Coated mesalazine preparations may be effective in active Crohn's disease, predominantly in patients with ileitis, and

**Table IX.** Comparative properties of mesalazine-delivering drugs

| Property | Sulfasalazine | Olsalazine | Balsalazide | Mesalazine (mesalamine) | | |
|---|---|---|---|---|---|---|
| | | | | 'Asacol' | 'Claversal'/ 'Salofalk'/ 'Mesasal' | 'Pentasa' |
| Delivery system | Azo bond | Azo bond | Azo bond | 'Eudragit L100' coating (pH ±6) | 'Eudragit S' coating (pH ±7) | Slow-release (ethyl cellulose coated microgranules) |
| Sites of release | Colon | Colon | Colon | Terminal ileum, colon | Mid jejunum, ileum, colon | Duodenum, jejunum, ileum, colon |
| Excretion in urine (%) | 22-24 | 22[a] | 35[b] | 31[a] | 54[a] | 36[a] |
| Excretion in faeces (%) | 38-45 | 53[a] | 46[b] | 44[a] | 44[a] | 38[a] |
| Serum mesalazine concentration (μmol/L) | ≤2.5[b] | 2.4[a] | <2.0[b] | 13.7[a] | 6.4[a] | 2.6[a] |
| Faecal dialysate mesalazine concentration (mmol/L) | 10[b] | 23.7[a] | | 22.8[a] | 15.0[a] | 12.6[a] |
| Ileal mesalazine concentration (mmol/L) | Not detectable | Not detectable | | 1.8 | 3.4 | 2.0 |
| **Clinical effectiveness** | | | | | | |
| *Ulcerative colitis:* | | | | | | |
| • Relapse | Yes | Yes | Yes | Yes | Yes | Yes |
| • Remission | Yes | Yes | Yes | Yes | Yes | Yes |
| *Crohn's disease:* | | | | | | |
| • Relapse | Yes (colitis) ± (ileitis) | No | No | No | ± | Yes (4 g/day) |
| • Remission | No | No | No | Yes (ileitis) | Yes (ileitis) | Yes (ileitis) |
| **Adverse effects** | | | | | | |
| *Dose-related*[c] | Up to 20-30% of patients: nausea, vomiting, headaches, dizziness, oligospermia, macrocytosis, folate deficiency, Heinz body haemolytic anaemia | Diarrhoea (up to 15%) | | Nausea, vomiting, headaches, dizziness, rash (uncommon) | | |
| *Hypersensitivity/ idiosyncratic* | Rash, serum sickness-like illness, autoimmune haemolytic anaemia, agranulocytosis, aplastic anaemia, pancreatitis, pulmonary fibrosis, hepatic injury, exacerbation of colitis | Nausea, vomiting, headaches, dizziness (uncommon) | | Nephrotoxicity, hair loss, pericarditis, pancreatitis, asthma, exacerbation of colitis (all rare) | | |

a Based on crossover comparative study of olsalazine and coated mesalazine 2 g/day.[339]
b Based on studies delivering sulfasalazine or balsalazide ≈1 g/day.[217]
c Many effects avoidable by gradual introduction of the drug.

only when large doses are used (e.g. slow-release mesalazine 4 g/day).[219]

The most promising use for coated mesalazine preparations appears to be in ileal or ileocolic Crohn's disease in remission, where all 3 preparations have demonstrated 25 to 50% reductions in the rate of relapse during 1 to 2 years of therapy.[220-223] A therapeutic response is especially likely if the drug is started soon after ileal resection or within 3 months of achieving drug-induced remission.

***Rectal administration:*** local delivery of mesalazine has also been achieved via the rectal route. Sulfasalazine enemas and suppositories have the disadvantage of a bright yellow colour that may stain underwear, while mesalazine enemas are unstable, requiring the addition of antioxidants. Mesalazine enemas or suppositories appear to be at least as effective as corticosteroid enemas in inducing remission in active left-sided ulcerative colitis or proctitis, respectively.[224-226]

Mesalazine enemas are also effective in >75% of patients with distal colitis resistant to conventional therapy, although achieving remission may take up to 3 months. Locally administered mesalazine (used every 2 or 3 nights) also prevents relapse in patients with distal disease.[227,228]

The mechanism of action of mesalazine in these conditions is unclear, but a variety of *in vitro* and *in vivo* effects have been shown. Mesalazine affects eicosanoid synthesis via both lipoxygenase and cyclo-oxygenase pathways; impairs neutrophil function and natural killer activity, and synthesis of interleukin-1 and platelet-activating factor; inhibits antibody synthesis; scavenges reactive oxygen metabolites; and influences short-chain fatty acid oxidation and other processes in epithelial cells.[229]

#### *9.1.2 Corticosteroids*

Corticosteroids are the principal drugs used for inducing remission in both ulcerative colitis and Crohn's disease. They are effective whether given by intravenous, oral or rectal routes. However, their use in maintaining remission has not been proven and is considerably limited by toxicity. Prednisolone or prednisone and hydrocortisone are the most commonly used agents. The mechanisms underlying their effectiveness involve anti-inflammatory and immunosuppressive effects, and direct effects on absorption of sodium by the colonic epithelium.

The toxicity of corticosteroids is predictable, dependent on dosage and duration of treatment, and is a major limitation to longer term treatment. Systemic corticosteroid effects can be minimised by targeting locally active drug to the affected mucosa, resulting in high mucosal and low systemic concentrations.[230] This can be further enhanced by using corticosteroids with low systemic availability, due either to poor absorption (e.g. prednisolone sodium metasulfobenzoate) or high first-pass hepatic and/or extrahepatic extraction (e.g. budesonide, tixocortol pivalate). These 'high clearance' drugs administered rectally have effectiveness similar to or superior to that of rectal prednisolone in distal ulcerative colitis.[231]

For oral 'local' therapy, drugs that are readily absorbed must be coated to ensure release at the targeted intestinal region. Budesonide is well absorbed and has high local effectiveness. Preliminary studies have shown that, when coated with 'Eudragit' to achieve delivery to the ileum and colon, oral budesonide has effectiveness similar to prednisolone for ileitis, with minimal systemic effects.[232] Alternatively, a very poorly absorbed corticosteroid with high local effectiveness (e.g. fluticasone propionate) may be used. Results of initial clinical studies using fluticasone propionate in ulcerative colitis have been disappointing, but the drug appears more promising in Crohn's disease. Table X lists the characteristics of corticosteroids for topical use in inflammatory bowel disease (via rectal or oral administration).

For further discussion of the clinical pharmacological properties of corticosteroids, see chapter 19 (section 7.1.1).

#### *9.1.3 Immunomodulating Drugs*

##### Azathioprine and Mercaptopurine

The only immunosuppressive drugs with an established place in treatment of inflammatory bowel disease are azathioprine and its metabolite, mercaptopurine (table XI). The effectiveness of these drugs in both ulcerative colitis and Crohn's disease, given in conjunction with corticosteroids, has been demonstrated for active disease,[233-236] and as monotherapy for long term maintenance.[237,238] They are indicated for corticosteroid-dependent, corticosteroid-refractory or fistulating disease, or where relapses are frequent. The major concern about their use is toxicity. However, although reported adverse effects are numerous, they occur infrequently, and more than 80% of patients can tolerate the drugs in long term use without adverse effects (in contrast to 100% incidence of adverse effects with long term corticosteroids).

Although the development of neoplasia is well described in patients with renal allografts taking azathioprine, several large studies have failed to demonstrate an increased risk of neoplasia in patients with inflammatory bowel disease treated with azathioprine or mercaptopurine.[239-242] However, this issue will continue to be closely scrutinised.

##### Cyclosporin and Methotrexate

Three immunosuppressive agents are receiving increasing attention, and are compared with

**Table X.** Comparison of corticosteroids for topical use (either via rectal or oral administration) in inflammatory bowel disease

| Property | Hydrocortisone acetate | Prednisolone 21-phosphate | Prednisolone sodium metasulfobenz oate | Tixocortol pivalate | Budesonide | Beclomethasone dipropionate | Fluticasone propionate |
|---|---|---|---|---|---|---|---|
| Absorption | +++ | +++ | + | + | +++ | + | 0/+ |
| Bioavailability | +++ | ++++ | | + | + | + | 0/+ |
| First-pass hepatic metabolism | ++ | + | | +++[a] | +++ | +++ | +++ |
| Preparations available | Foam | Enema | Oral ('Eudragit'-coated) Enema | Enema | Oral ('Eudragit'-coated) Enema | Enema | Oral |
| Daily dosage | 80-178mg | 20mg | *Oral:* 20mg *Rectal:* 20mg | 250mg | *Oral:* 9mg *Rectal:* 1-4mg | 1-2mg | 20mg |
| **Systemic adverse effects:** | | | | | | | |
| Rectal | ++ | +++ | 0 | 0 | 0 | 0 | |
| Oral | | | 0 | | 0/+ | | 0 |
| **Clinical effectiveness:** | | | | | | | |
| Distal ulcerative colitis | +++ | +++ | +++ | +++ | +++ | +++ | 0/+ |
| Crohn's disease | | | | | +++ *(acute ileitis)* [oral] ++ *(maintenance for ileitis)* [oral] | | ? ++ |
| Other features | | | Enemas give higher rectal tissue concentrations than for prednisolone | | Water solubility and high topical potency highly suited to retarded oral formulation | Low water solubility less suited to retarded oral formulation | |

a Also extrahepatic metabolism.

azathioprine in table XI. Cyclosporin has the disadvantages of toxicity and a higher cost, and has been associated with disappointing long term results, despite encouraging results in acute management of active, corticosteroid-resistant disease.[243] Methotrexate shows promise, with tolerability superior to cyclosporin,[244,245] but further clinical trial results are awaited. The current role for these agents remains uncertain.

#### 9.1.4 Antibiotics

*Metronidazole* has proved effective in Crohn's colitis,[246,247] and in healing perineal disease.[248,249] Long term treatment is often required because of early relapse following cessation of therapy, but is poorly tolerated by many patients. Two other antibiotics, *tinidazole* and *ciprofloxacin*, have been used and are compared with metronidazole in table XII. Claims of effectiveness and superior tolerability are mainly based on anecdotal reports and personal experience.

Metronidazole is of no benefit in uncomplicated ulcerative colitis of any severity.[250,251] Oral tobramycin appears to improve the responsiveness of ulcerative colitis to corticosteroids,[252] but has no benefit in maintaining remission.[253] Other antibiotic regimens have been evaluated in inflammatory bowel disease, including antituberculous therapy for Crohn's disease, without good evidence of effectiveness.

### 9.2 Optimum Treatment

#### 9.2.1 Ulcerative Colitis

The aims of treatment in ulcerative colitis are to induce and maintain clinical, endoscopic and histological remission. These aims can be achieved in >80% of patients, and treatment effectiveness is simply assessed by history, sig-

**Table XI.** Non–corticosteroid immunomodulating drugs used in the treatment of inflammatory bowel disease

| Property | Azathioprine/mercaptopurine | Methotrexate | Cyclosporin |
|---|---|---|---|
| Mode of action | Cytostatic for T and B cells<br>Anti-inflammatory | Antimetabolite (cytostatic)<br>Anti-inflammatory | Inhibits lymphocyte activation |
| Onset of action | Slow (maximal 3-6 months) | Intermediate (2-10 weeks) | Rapid (5-14 days) |
| Usual dosage (route) | 1.5-2.5 mg/kg/day (oral) | 25 mg/wk (intramuscular)<br>15 mg/wk (oral) | 4-6 mg/kg/day (intravenous)<br>4-8 mg/kg/day (oral) |
| Clinical effectiveness: | | | |
| • Active disease (with corticosteroids) | ++ | ? +/++ | +++ |
| • Maintenance | ++ | ? +/++ | 0/+ |
| • Fistula | ++ | ? | ++ |
| Tolerability[a] | +++ | ++ | + |
| Adverse effects | Nausea, vomiting, leucopenia, pancreatitis, fever, rash, cholestasis, diarrhoea, arthralgia, ?neoplasia | Nausea, vomiting, diarrhoea, rash, pneumonitis, abnormal liver function tests, leucopenia, stomatitis, alopecia, ?neoplasia | Renal impairment, hypertension, hypertrichosis, gingival hypertrophy, seizures, hepatic injury, infections, ?neoplasia |
| Safety in pregnancy | Probably acceptable | Not recommended (teratogenic) | Not recommended |
| Important drug interactions | Allopurinol (reduce dose by 65%) | | Diltiazem (reduce dose by 50%)<br>Avoid nephrotoxic drugs<br>Multiple interactions (see further chapter 28 and appendix B) |
| Monitoring after start of therapy | Haematological examination, liver function tests at 2, 4, 8 and 12 weeks then every 3-6 months | | Blood pressure, renal function, liver function tests, plasma cyclosporin concentration |

a +++ = best tolerated; + = least tolerated.

moidoscopy and rectal biopsy. The general principles of treatment are:

1. To control an acute attack as rapidly as possible
2. To induce remission
3. To prevent relapse
4. To treat complications.

An essential adjunct of drug therapy is patient education about the relapsing nature of the disease, the importance of early treatment of a relapse and treatment options available. Education and general patient support is greatly facilitated by referral to self-help groups. Management and follow-up are best performed by a specialist clinician or in a specialist clinic, since a relationship built on mutual trust between clinician and patient is essential for this life-long disease.

Disease severity dictates the aggressiveness of treatment. Severity is judged by the number of stools/day, amount of blood present in stools, degree of pain or tenderness, and presence or absence of constitutional disturbance, and is confirmed by sigmoidoscopic and histological findings. For example, *severe disease* is associated with more than 6 bloody stools/day, abdominal pain and tenderness, fever, tachycardia, malaise and bodyweight loss. *Mild disease* is characterised by <4 stools/day containing little or no blood, while abdominal examination is unremarkable and constitutional symptoms are absent.

### Severe Attacks

These demand urgent admission to hospital and immediate intensive medical treatment. Fluid and electrolyte losses are replaced intravenously and potassium chloride supplementation is often required. Anaemia should be corrected by blood transfusion to maintain haemoglobin concentrations at >90 g/L. Complications of concern are perforation and toxic megacolon, which require careful monitoring and daily or alternate daily abdominal x-ray, and may be heralded by increasing abdominal pain and tenderness, and general deterioration.

*Intravenous corticosteroids* are administered (e.g. hydrocortisone sodium succinate 100mg every 6 to 8 hours or prednisolone 21-phosphate 20mg every 8 hours). Intrarectal hydrocortisone may be given via a drip infusion (e.g. 100mg in 150ml of warm saline), but is seldom used in practice. *Antibiotics* exert no significant effect on colitis itself, but should be used if specifically indicated. Benefits of fasting the patient are unproven,[254] but restriction of water by mouth is indicated in very ill patients, or if surgery is considered imminent. A low residue diet supplemented by high protein drinks is otherwise most appropriate.

Around 70 to 80% of patients will respond to intensive therapy within 5 days and can then be changed to oral *prednisolone* 40 to 60 mg/day after this period. Response is shown by normalisation of systemic signs (tachycardia, fever), reduction in frequency of bowel actions and blood loss, resolution of tenderness or pain, and a reduction in inflammatory indices such as erythrocyte sedimentation rate or C-reactive protein. If the condition remains stable, a further 5 days' intravenous corticosteroid therapy is warranted. If the patient's condition deteriorates during intensive therapy or has not improved after 10 days, colectomy is indicated.

Toxic megacolon requires close monitoring (vital signs, tenderness, radiology) and administration of intravenous antibiotics (metronidazole plus either a third-generation cefalosporin or aminoglycoside with amoxicillin). Deterioration or failure to respond within 24 to 48 hours are indications for urgent colectomy.

Responsiveness to the intensive regimen outlined above may be improved by adding other agents. Oral *tobramycin* 120mg 3 times daily for 7 days significantly improved response in one trial.[252] Intravenous *cyclosporin* 4 mg/kg/day led to significant improvement in 3 of 4 patients refractory to 10 days' treatment with intravenous corticosteroids.[255] Neither agent, however, is currently used in routine practice.

### Moderately Severe Attacks

Admission to hospital is usually only necessary if there is no response to oral therapy. *Corticosteroids* should be given orally at moderately high doses (e.g. prednisolone 40 to 60 mg/day) with dose tapering over 6 to 8 weeks (e.g. by weekly dose reduction). Adjunctive topical corticosteroid therapy with enemas or rectal foam may also be used. *Sulfasalazine* (or other mesalazine-delivering drugs) should be introduced after 2 weeks, initially in low doses, but escalating to maintenance dosages.

For patients unwilling to take corticosteroids, *sulfasalazine* is efficacious (but less so than corticosteroids) and should be used at doses of 3 to 4 g/day (in 3 or 4 divided doses). If the patient cannot tolerate sulfasalazine, then *olsalazine* or 'Eudragit'-coated *mesalazine* is used. Mesalazine enemas can be added to oral therapy. Failure to respond is an indication for hospital admission and intensive intravenous therapy.

### Mild Attacks

Ulcerative colitis of mild severity is usually, though not exclusively, associated with distal disease and should be treated with local therapy with either *corticosteroids* twice daily for 2 weeks and then daily for 2 weeks, or *mesalazine* 1 to 4g once or twice daily for 4 weeks. Whether an enema, foam or suppository formulation is used depends on the extent of the disease (e.g. enema for more extensive disease, suppository when limited to the rectum) and patient preference (e.g. foams are easier to retain than enemas). If there is only a partial response to this treatment, the duration of therapy can be extended.

If the response is poor, a combination of local mesalazine and corticosteroids can be used. Alternatively, a course of oral corticosteroids (e.g. prednisolone starting at 20 mg/day) may be required. Failure to respond after 2 to 4 weeks demands more intensive therapy (as outlined above) and for the diagnosis to be checked (especially regarding an infective cause or non-inflammatory bowel disease such as solitary rectal ulcer syndrome).

**Table XII.** Antibiotics used in the treatment of Crohn's disease

| Property | Metronidazole | Tinidazole | Ciprofloxacin |
|---|---|---|---|
| Spectrum of activity | Anaerobic bacteria<br>Some protozoa | Anaerobic bacteria<br>Some protozoa | Broad spectrum<br>Anaerobic and aerobic bacteria |
| Usual daily dosage | 1-2g | 1g | 1g |
| Doses/day | 3 | 2 | 2 |
| Clinical effectiveness: | | | |
| • Ileitis | 0 | ? | ? |
| • Colitis | ++ (controlled trials) | ++ (anecdotal) | ? |
| • Perineal disease | +++ (large series) | +++ (anecdotal) | +++ (anecdotal) |
| Tolerability[a] | + | ++ | +++ |
| Adverse effects | Metallic taste, nausea, vomiting, peripheral neuropathy | Metallic taste, nausea, vomiting, peripheral neuropathy | Nausea, vomiting, rash, fever |

a +++ = best tolerated; + = least tolerated.

#### Chronically Active Disease

Prolonged use of corticosteroids with systemic activity (given orally or rectally) should be avoided where remission cannot be satisfactorily achieved (e.g. when relapse occurs during dosage tapering or when only a partial response can be achieved). For extensive disease, continuous low-dose or alternate-day corticosteroid therapy may be tried, but it is preferable to introduce an immunomodulating agent, particularly azathioprine or mercaptopurine. These drugs are administered at a dose of 1.5 to 2.5 mg/kg/day, but will not have maximal effects for 3 to 6 months.[234,241] More refractory disease may require a trial of cyclosporin or methotrexate.

Resistant distal colitis is problematic, especially since colectomy is a harsh approach to disease affecting only the rectum or the rectum and sigmoid colon. The diagnosis should be reassessed (e.g. solitary rectal ulcer syndrome and Crohn's colitis distinguished), the possibility of hypersensitivity to mesalazine enemas must be considered, and the presence of constipation proximal to the inflamed segment should be evaluated by plain abdominal x-ray. Constipation is treated with bulking agents and/or osmotic laxatives. Its successful relief is often associated with an enhanced response of the proctitis to therapy.[256]

In more extensive disease, *azathioprine* or *mercaptopurine* may induce remission in some patients. *Cyclosporin* enemas have proven disappointing.[257] However, new therapies associated with minimal or no adverse effects have been of benefit in resistant distal colitis. Enemas of *butyrate* (80 mmol/L, pH 7.4 in 60ml) or combinations of *short-chain fatty acids* given twice daily for 4 to 6 weeks are effective as monotherapy,[258,259] but may be best used as adjuncts to mesalazine or corticosteroids. No commercial preparation is available, but it can easily be made up by a pharmacist.

Enemas of *local anaesthetics*,[260] *sucralfate*[261] or *colloidal bismuth subcitrate*[262] appear to be effective and well tolerated. However, suitable formulations are not available at present. Fish oil supplementation has some benefit,[263,264] but is an unattractive option.

Other approaches include the use of *nicotine* patches, despite common adverse effects and only mild effectiveness.[265] Subcutaneous *heparin* 10,000U twice daily appears promising,[266] but awaits controlled clinical evaluation. *Sodium cromoglycate* (cromolyn sodium) may be effective in patients with proctitis and eosinophilic infiltration, but the response to date has been disappointing.[267] The initial promise shown by *zileuton* in inhibiting 5-lipoxygenase was not confirmed in a controlled trial.[268]

#### Prevention of Relapse

Mesalazine-delivering drugs (table IX) sharply reduce the relapse rate, and should be administered to all patients with extensive disease and those with more than trivial distal disease. Duration of therapy should be indefinite; effectiveness does not diminish with time. The choice of mesalazine-delivering drug is controversial, but *sulfasalazine* 1g twice daily may be tried first (see also section 9.5.1). Potential reversible hypospermia with this agent should be discussed with male patients. For those hypersensitive to or not initially tolerating sulfasalazine, *olsalazine* 1g twice daily or coated *mesalazine* may be used (see sections 9.1.1 and 9.5.1). Maintenance therapy with mesalazine enemas 1 to 4g daily or on alternate days in patients with distal disease is also efficacious.

When mesalazine-delivering drugs are ineffective or poorly tolerated and relapses are frequent, *azathioprine* 2.0 to 2.5 mg/kg daily should be introduced, concurrently with a course of oral corticosteroids, for active disease. If the clinical course suggests that azathioprine is of benefit, therapy should continue for 24 months. The dosage can usually be successfully reduced to 1.5 mg/kg/day or less after 6 months' remission, but this should be done cautiously (e.g. by 25 mg/day every 3 months). Azathioprine withdrawal may be attempted after that time. For patients who relapse after its withdrawal, long term azathioprine is indicated.

Other strategies to prevent relapse have been investigated. Low-dose corticosteroids and long term oral tobramycin are not effective, but low-dose *metronidazole* 0.6 g/day may be as effective as sulfasalazine 2 g/day.[269] Addition of sulfhydryl-containing agents, allopurinol or dimethyl sulfoxide to sulfasalazine appears to be superior to sulfasalazine alone.[270,271] Dietary modifications (such as milk-free or high fibre diets) are generally ineffective. Broad-spectrum antibiotics should be used only if definitely indicated and extreme care should be taken regarding personal hygiene and food intake when travelling to other countries. In patients for whom emotional factors may contribute to relapses, strategies designed to improve the patient's ability to cope with stress may be worthwhile.

#### Extraintestinal Manifestations and Complications

Extraintestinal manifestations related to disease activity, such as uveitis, erythema nodosum, pyoderma gangrenosum, arthritis and mouth ulcers, usually respond to therapy for colitis. Specific therapy may be needed. Deep venous thrombosis can be treated with *heparin*, although colonic bleeding may increase. Associated conditions unrelated to disease activity (ankylosing spondylitis, primary sclerosing cholangitis) should be managed on their own merits.

Patients with extensive colitis of longer than 8 years' duration have an elevated risk of colorectal carcinoma. Current preventive measures principally consist of colonoscopic surveillance. Chemopreventive strategies have yet to be evaluated.

##### Pouchitis

Pouchitis complicates up to 30% of ileal-anal (pouch) reservoirs in patients with ulcerative colitis. It is clinically characterised by abdominal cramping, watery diarrhoea, urgency, incontinence, malaise and fever. Oral *metronidazole* 400 to 500mg 3 times daily for 14 days is usually effective, although no controlled trials have been conducted. When disease is refractory or antibiotics are poorly tolerated, oral sulfasalazine, mesalazine enemas, or local or systemic corticosteroids may be used. Rectal glutamine suppositories show promise as a nontoxic therapy.[272]

#### Avoiding Problems in Treatment

It is essential to build patient confidence in the therapy being used. To facilitate this, drug selection and dosage should be optimal. Patients should be given realistic expectations of likely drug effectiveness and alerted to possible adverse effects and their management. In patients with distal colitis who are unable to retain enemas for more than 30 (or preferably 60) minutes, corticosteroid or mesalazine enemas are not optimal therapy and oral or intravenous treatment should be initiated. Enemas may be introduced when disease activity and ability to retain an enema improve.

Mesalazine-delivering drugs should always be introduced at a low dose (e.g. 1 tablet/capsule daily) and increased by a further tablet/capsule every 2 to 4 days until the optimal dosage is reached. This strategy is especially important to minimise nausea and headaches with sulfasalazine and avoid diarrhoea with olsalazine, and may also improve tolerability of coated mesalazine. Use of enteric-coated sulfasalazine may reduce nausea.

Most adverse effects of sulfasalazine occur within 2 to 3 months of starting the drug. Monitoring of blood haemoglobin, blood film and liver function tests are recommended over that time (e.g. after 2, 6 and 12 weeks). Due to concern over nephrotoxicity of coated mesalazine, monitoring renal function and urinary sediment has been advocated, but is seldom practised. The cost effectiveness of repeated investigations to detect a rare idiosyncratic complication is debatable, and it is uncertain whether such surveillance will detect early nephrotoxicity.

More than short term use of corticosteroids should be avoided if possible. Corticosteroid dosages should be increased until the disease is controlled or adverse effects appear. Likewise, an inadequate initial dosage should also be avoided. A clear plan of management, in terms of the timing and indications for the use of adjunctive drug therapy or of surgery, should be clearly formulated for the individual patient. If azathioprine or mercaptopurine are to be used, patients must be prepared for a 3- or even 6-month delay for optimal effectiveness and for relatively long term therapy (2 years or more) if this treatment is efficacious. However, the drug should not be continued in the absence of objective signs of effectiveness. Adverse effects usually occur within 3 months of starting therapy, and monitoring of haemoglobin, white cell count, blood film and liver function tests at 2, 4, 8 and 12 weeks, and then 3-monthly, is recommended. Patients should also be warned of the potential significance of severe epigastric pain (i.e. pancreatitis).

### 9.2.2 Crohn's Disease

Crohn's disease contrasts with ulcerative colitis in that it is characterised by a poor correlation of symptoms to pathological findings, its involvement anywhere in the gastrointestinal tract (though usually in the distal small bowel or colon), a poorer response to medical therapy and the frequent need for surgery. However, like ulcerative colitis, long term management by a specialised gastroenterological team, including physicians and surgeons, is paramount for optimal care. Patient education and support (e.g. self-help groups) are also important adjuncts to management.

The major aim of therapy is to achieve clinical rather than histopathological remission, because of the relative ineffectiveness of therapy in achieving true remission and the difficulty in histopathologically assessing a patchy disease that may be out of the reach of biopsy forceps. Additional goals include the maintenance of nutrition, prevention of complications and avoidance of major adverse effects. Therapeutic strategies, duration of treatment and timing of surgery vary according to the distribution and severity of the disease and, to a lesser extent, the nature of the disease process (e.g. fistulating *vs* stenosing disease).

**Small Bowel Disease**

Small intestinal involvement (with or without colonic disease) occurs in about 70% of patients with Crohn's disease. In these patients, ileal disease is responsible for most clinical manifestations, which generally form 1 of 3 patterns, each with differing therapeutic challenges:

1) Chronic diarrhoea, pain or weight loss is usually associated with chronically active disease and requires a careful balance between risks and benefits of drugs used, as well as careful attention to nutrition.

2) Recurrent small intestinal obstruction secondary to ileal stenosis is generally less responsive to medical therapy. Early surgery is desirable if medical therapy has failed.

3) Fistulating 'septic' disease is often associated with abscess formation, and corticosteroid therapy may present a risk. Immunomodulating therapy often plays a more prominent role.

For the induction of remission of active disease, *corticosteroids* are the most effective and rapidly-acting therapy. They may be administered intravenously in very sick patients, using a regimen identical to that for ulcerative colitis (see section 9.2.1), or orally (e.g. prednisolone 40 to 60 mg/day). Dosage reduction is more gradual than in ulcerative colitis and the duration of a successful course of therapy is typically about 3 months.

For patients presenting with a tender mass in the right iliac fossa, corticosteroids can be safely used in hospital, with careful monitoring.[273] Failure of the mass to improve over a few days or evidence of abscess on imaging should prompt appropriate surgical intervention. The use of corticosteroids with potent topical activity and low systemic availability (e.g. 'Eudragit'-coated budesonide) is a promising approach to the therapy of ileitis (see further section 9.1.2).

*Sulfasalazine* and coated *mesalazine* have shown effectiveness in patients with ileitis, but both require relatively high doses (3 to 4g daily). These drugs may be used for milder disease presentations, when corticosteroids are refused or as an adjunct to corticosteroids. Mesalazine in the form of individually-coated microgranules ('Pentasa') is released throughout the small bowel and may be the most suitable formulation for more proximal small bowel involvement.

*Immunomodulating drugs* are also effective, but their use as remission-inducing agents is largely restricted to patients with corticosteroid-dependent, corticosteroid-refractory or fistulating disease. Azathioprine or mercaptopurine (2 to 2.5 mg/kg/day) are introduced together with corticosteroids and benefit about two-thirds of patients treated. More than half of patients with active fistulae have a good response to these drugs.

Oral *cyclosporin* 5 to 7.5 mg/kg/day has enhanced effectiveness if used in conjunction with corticosteroids, but its use long term in chronically active disease has been disappointing.[274] Cyclosporin may, however, play a role in fistulous disease where standard medical therapy has failed.[275,276] The use of *methotrexate* has permitted dose reduction or complete withdrawal of corticosteroids in uncontrolled studies. Therapy was initiated intramuscularly at 25 mg/week, changing to oral therapy after several weeks[244] or to low-dose oral therapy (15 mg/week).[245]

*Antibiotics,* either broad-spectrum or metronidazole alone, have little to offer as remission-inducing therapy, but are often used for specific indications. Remission can alternatively be induced nonpharmacologically by the use of elemental or polymeric diets as the sole source of nutrition; therapy is usually given for 6 weeks. These are at least as efficacious as prednisolone, but suffer from problems of palatability and consequent poor patient acceptance. Taste can be considerably improved by refrigerating or freezing the diets.

***Prevention of relapse:*** in patients with ileal Crohn's disease in remission, this is less satisfactory than for ulcerative colitis. Oral coated *mesalazine* 1.5 to 2.4 g/day has some effectiveness in preventing recurrent ileal disease, particularly following 'curative' ileal resection. In view of its safety profile (relative lack of adverse effects), it should probably be used in this subgroup of patients. Its effectiveness is, however, less clear in patients in whom remission was induced by corticosteroid therapy and the use of coated mesalazine in such patients cannot currently be recommended.

Low-dose prednisolone has no role in maintenance, but oral 'Eudragit'-coated *budesonide* has shown some promise, with mean time to relapse reduced in patients with corticosteroid-induced remission.[277] *Azathioprine* and *mercaptopurine*[234,237] may also be effective as maintenance therapy and their long term use is often necessary. The use of exclusion diets following induction of remission with elemental or polymeric diets has met with mixed success, and they are probably not worthwhile.[278]

The effective use of symptomatic therapy is important in reducing the need for corticosteroids or other immunomodulating therapy. For diarrhoea secondary to bile salt malabsorption following ileal resection, *cholestyramine* (usual dose 4 to 8g with meals, although smaller or less frequent doses may be sufficient) is effective in reducing stool volume. Antimotility agents for chronic diarrhoea may be used. *Loperamide* 4 to 12 mg/day in divided doses is the preferred agent, because it has similar effectiveness to codeine phosphate 30 to 60 mg/day or diphenoxylate 7.5 to 10 mg/day, a longer half-life, and lacks anticholinergic or opioid effects.

Antispasmodics may ease abdominal cramps, paracetamol may be helpful for pain, and antibiotics such as tetracycline and/or metronidazole may be useful if bacterial overgrowth occurs secondary to small intestinal stasis. Appropriate nutritional management is of paramount importance (see section 9.2.2).

#### Crohn's Colitis

Crohn's colitis can manifest clinically across a wide spectrum, from trivial symptoms to fulminating colitis with a risk of toxic megacolon. Treatment should be tailored to the severity of the clinical manifestations. Corticosteroids are the most effective therapeutic modality for quickly controlling symptoms and are used as outlined above for ileal disease. Enemas may be used for distal disease. Although controlled trials have failed to show a benefit, low-dose *prednisolone* (<15 mg/day) is effective in maintaining clinical remission in a small proportion of patients. The use of alternate-day therapy may improve tolerability while maintaining effectiveness.

*Sulfasalazine* 3 to 4 g/day is also effective and is useful as first-line therapy in mild to moderately symptomatic patients, or together with corticosteroids. It has not been shown which component of sulfasalazine is the active moiety in Crohn's disease, but mesalazine-delivering drugs have also been shown to have some effectiveness in Crohn's colitis. The benefit of mesalazine-delivering drugs or sulfasalazine as a maintenance therapy is not proven, but these are commonly used. Oral *metronidazole* (1 to 2 g/day, in 3 divided doses) has proven effectiveness, but relapses tend to occur early after its withdrawal and adverse effects may be troublesome. In patients for whom metronidazole is beneficial but long term tolerability is poor, a trial of oral *tinidazole* 0.5g twice daily may be useful, since it appears to be as efficacious with fewer adverse effects (although no controlled trials have been conducted).

*Immunomodulating drugs*, in dosages similar to those for ileal disease (see above), should be considered for chronically active disease causing more than trivial symptoms, or where symptomatic control can only be achieved with prednisolone 15 mg/day or greater. The use of diet as a primary therapy for Crohn's colitis is unproven, although nutritional repletion in a sick patient is an important adjunct.

Colonic strictures, which require careful exclusion of carcinoma, respond poorly to drug therapy. If symptomatic, endoscopic balloon dilatation provides a nonsurgical alternative.

#### Perineal Disease

Perineal Crohn's disease can range from trivial skin tags to perianal fistula and abscess formation, which may necessitate aggressive medical and surgical therapy. It is usually associated with disease of the large bowel, especially the rectum, but rarely may be associated only with small intestinal disease. The principles of therapy are institution of adequate local care, control of diarrhoea, judicious use of surgery and use of systemic drugs with the aim of treating both the colonic disease and chronic inflammatory disease of the perineum itself.

*Sulfasalazine, metronidazole* or *corticosteroids* alone may be effective. However, patients with refractory disease may require bowel rest and moderate to high doses of metronidazole (1 to 2g daily) for several weeks, in addition to anti-inflammatory and immunomodulating therapy.[248] Relapse often occurs soon after cessation of metronidazole,[249] necessitating its indefinite use, but long term tolerability is often poor. Tinidazole 0.5g twice daily and ciprofloxacin 500mg twice daily are alternatives that appear, on anecdotal evidence, to be both efficacious and better tolerated.

#### Proximal Gastrointestinal Disease

Histopathological evidence of gastroduodenal involvement is not uncommon, but oesophageal disease is rare. It is usually associated with more distal disease. Clinical manifestations, apparent in a minority of patients, comprise epigastric pain, symptoms of delayed gastric emptying, haematemesis and melaena. Empirical therapy with acid reduction (i.e. an $H_2$-receptor antagonist or acid pump inhibitor) or sucralfate may be of benefit for the peptic ulcer–like symptoms. The underlying disease process should be treated as for ileocolonic disease, except for the use of mesalazine drugs, the delivery of which bypasses the oesophagus, stomach and duodenum.

Oral involvement is common and manifests as aphthous ulcers. These are usually associated with active disease elsewhere and will generally resolve with successful treatment of intestinal disease. However, mouth ulcers are painful and major aphthous ulcers can be slow to heal and result in scarring. Specific therapy includes corticosteroid or local anaesthetic ointments (see further chapter 16).

#### Nutritional Management

Dietary modifications are indicated under certain conditions, including a role in primary therapy, as has already been noted.

***When oral intake must be restricted:*** total parenteral nutrition is indicated when, for example, a small bowel fistula or very severe perineal disease require that the patient take nothing by mouth.

***To correct poor nutrition:*** protein and energy malnutrition frequently complicate active disease because of reduced intake, increased utilisation, and increased loss of protein and other nutrients from the bowel. High protein foods should be favoured and the energy intake should be increased, by, for example, more frequent meals and supplementation with milk-based drinks or commercial supplements. When these manoeuvres are impracticable or when they fail, supplemental tube feeding or parenteral nutrition may be necessary. Vitamin and mineral supplements are often needed in active disease, but when the disease is quiescent, they should generally only be used for proven deficiency. Patients with cyanocobalamin malabsorption require intramuscular replacement therapy.

***To reduce symptoms:*** symptoms can be avoided by removing dairy foods in a minority of patients with lactase deficiency, and by restricting fat intake in patients with fat malabsorption. Low-fat diets, however, may be deceptively low in energy content. Dietary supplements may be necessary, with low-fat commercial products or medium-chain triglyceride oil 20 to 30g daily used in cooking or as part of a commercially available supplement.

***To avoid complications:*** patients with small bowel stenotic lesions should avoid foods containing skins, seeds or other poorly digestible components, to avoid obstruction. In patients with fat malabsorption and an intact large bowel, there is an increased risk of developing renal oxalate stones. Restriction of foods high in oxalate such as chocolate, nuts, berry fruits, spinach and tea is worthwhile, but more severe restrictions are usually not helpful and may be harmful.

Calcium supplementation may be beneficial in patients on moderate doses of long term corticosteroids (e.g. prednisolone 15 mg/day or more), because of reduced calcium absorption and increased risk of osteoporosis. The use of cholestyramine impairs absorption of fat soluble vitamins and attention to this may be important.

#### Avoiding Problems in Treatment

Issues outlined for ulcerative colitis (section 9.2.1) are also relevant for Crohn's disease. Adverse effects are a major problem, because of the nature of the drugs used and their relative inefficacy in healing the underlying disease process. A careful balance between symptoms and adverse effects must be maintained. Symptomatic treatment may reduce the need for more aggressive therapy. Similarly, careful attention should be paid to nutrition, since correction of malnutrition not only improves the quality of life, but may also enhance responsiveness to therapy.[279]

Prolonged use of corticosteroids with systemic action should be avoided where possible by the use of adjunctive immunomodulating therapy or the judicious use of surgery. This especially applies to children and adolescents because of the cosmetic changes and growth-retarding effects of corticosteroids, and to patients with osteopenia or diabetes mellitus.

Metronidazole is associated with several adverse effects and tolerability may improve if patients are warned about the likelihood of nausea, metallic taste and, especially, alcohol intolerance. Where long term treatment is likely (e.g. for perineal disease), tolerability may be enhanced by starting with low dosages (e.g. 800 mg/day), which can then be increased until an adequate response is obtained.

### *9.2.3 Microscopic Colitis*

Microscopic colitis, comprising both lymphocytic and collagenous colitis, represents one or more disorders of unknown causation and uncertain natural history. It mainly afflicts middle-aged and elderly patients, and presents as waxing and waning watery diarrhoea. Histopathological features are characteristic and diagnostic. There are no controlled trials on which therapeutic decisions can be based, but several reports of treatment experience provide some guidance.

Symptomatic treatment with *bulking agents* (see section 11.1.3) or *antimotility/antidiarrhoeal drugs* (see section 11.1.4) may be sufficient. Consideration must be given to associated disorders such as coeliac disease (indicating a trial of gluten-free diet; see section 6.2.1) or thyroid disease. *Sulfasalazine* 3 to 4 g/day is often effective and, in responders, a maintenance dose of 2 g/day may be given long term. When sulfasalazine is not tolerated, olsalazine or a coated mesalazine preparation can be used, although olsalazine may tend to aggravate the diarrhoea.

If mesalazine-delivering drugs provide insufficient symptom relief, oral *corticosteroid* therapy (e.g. prednisolone 20 to 30 mg/day), with or without a corticosteroid enema, may be of benefit. Following a 2- to 3-month dose-tapering course, consideration can be given to maintenance corticosteroid therapy, but there are no data on which the dosage or duration of therapy can be based. There have been some reports of the effectiveness of *metronidazole*, but immunomodulating drugs have not been systematically studied in this condition.

## 9.3 Inflammatory Bowel Disease in Children and Adolescents

The principles of drug treatment are the same as for adults, except that drug dosages must be modified (see table XIII). Three issues are, however, peculiar to children.

#### Physical Growth and Development

Growth failure is a serious problem, affecting one-third of patients with Crohn's disease and a smaller proportion of those with ulcerative colitis.[280] Although prolonged use of corticosteroids is associated with growth impairment, the major contributing factor is undernutrition, mainly caused by an inadequate intake of protein and energy. Growth retardation can be improved by optimal medical and surgical therapy, but attention to nutritional intake (130 to 150% of the Recommended Daily Allowance for height and weight) is of paramount importance. Monitoring of growth is also essential. High protein, high energy milk-based drinks or commercial supplements are useful, but may not be sufficient alone, due to the volumes needed and their taste. Nocturnal tube feeding has been successfully used and parenteral nutrition may be required.

#### Minimising the Adverse Effects of Drugs

Cosmetic changes and growth suppression are the major adverse effects of corticosteroids in children. Attempts should be made to minimise both by avoiding more than short courses with, for example, earlier use of immunosuppressive therapy, alternate-day therapy, or primary therapy with an elemental diet.[280]

#### Psychosocial Development

Chronic illness has a variable and unpredictable impact on emotional and social development. It is essential that the patient and immediate family are well educated about the disease, its treatment, its prognosis and everyday impact on schooling, sport, etc. A good relationship based on mutual trust must be developed between the gastroenterologist and the patient and family. Self-help groups play an essential role in providing information, advice

**Table XIII.** Recommended dosages of drugs used for inflammatory bowel disease in children

| Drug | Dosage |
|---|---|
| Sulfasalazine | 40-60 mg/kg/day (relapse)<br>20-30 mg/kg/day (maintenance) |
| Olsalazine | 10-15 mg/kg/day |
| Mesalazine coated formulations | 20 mg/kg/day |
| Prednisolone (oral) | 1-2 mg/kg/day (initial dose) |
| Prednisolone (enema) | 20 mg/day |
| Prednisolone (suppository) | 5mg once or twice daily |
| Hydrocortisone foam | 125mg once or twice daily |
| Azathioprine | Same as adults (1.5-2.5 mg/kg/day) |
| Metronidazole | 15 mg/kg/day |

**Table XIV.** Choice of mesalazine analogue for long term (lifetime) maintenance treatment for ulcerative colitis based on clinical outcome and economic considerations

| Property | Sulfasalazine | Olsalazine | Mesalazine (coated formulations) |
|---|---|---|---|
| Clinical effectiveness | +++ | +++ | +++ (? < olsalazine for distal colitis) |
| Pharmacokinetic characteristics | Better delivery of mesalazine to colon | Better delivery of mesalazine to colon | Higher serum concentrations of mesalazine |
| Doses/day | 2 | 2 | 3 |
| Short term tolerability | 10% intolerant | Diarrhoea (avoidable in most) | Intolerance uncommon |
| Long term safety | Unequivocally safe (>50 years' experience), but reversible male infertility | Safe (<15 years' experience) | Safe (<15 years' experience), some concern regarding nephrotoxicity (rare) |
| Safety in pregnancy | Established | Unknown | Unknown |
| Relative cost | + | +++ | ++++ |

and support. The need to take drugs at school should be avoided by sensible dosage schedules.

### 9.4 Inflammatory Bowel Disease in Pregnancy

Since inflammatory bowel disease predominates in child-bearing age groups, the issues associated with pregnancy are very important. Several large studies in patients with ulcerative colitis and Crohn's disease have been reported, with similar general conclusions being drawn. Patients with severe, active disease carry reduced fertility (females only) and there is a slight but statistically significant increase in the risk of death *in utero*, spontaneous abortion or premature delivery. Quiescent or mildly active disease is, however, associated with normal fertility and pregnancy outcome. Relapse rates during or after pregnancy are not increased.

**Optimum Treatment**

Of the drugs used, neither sulfasalazine nor corticosteroids are associated with fetal abnormalities, fetal loss[281] or ill-effects during breast feeding. Thus, they can be considered safe to use. Azathioprine doses of 2 mg/kg/day or less have not been associated with fetal abnormalities in patients with renal allografts[282] or inflammatory bowel disease.[283,284] Metronidazole has proved teratogenic in experimental animals (see further chapter 2), and should be used only in severe perineal disease. The safety of olsalazine or coated mesalazine (although likely) has not been confirmed.

With these considerations in mind, recommendations to patients regarding pregnancy and inflammatory bowel disease can be made. Ideally, pregnancy should be planned when the disease is inactive. Sulfasalazine maintenance therapy should be continued during pregnancy, although the risk associated with the use of newer mesalazine-delivering drugs is currently ill-defined. A decision regarding azathioprine must be made by the patient, weighing up the potential risks of the drug to the fetus *vs* those of a flair of the disease. If azathioprine is to be withdrawn, conception should not be contemplated for at least 6 months. Relapse usually occurs many months after withdrawal, because of the long offset of the action of the drug.

Relapse during pregnancy or active disease at conception should be treated as in the non-pregnant patient, except for the avoidance of metronidazole and other antibiotics (at least in the first trimester and postpartum period). Surgery for severe unresponsive colitis, toxic megacolon, intestinal obstruction or gastrointestinal bleeding can be performed without added risk to the fetus.

### 9.5 Clinical Outcome and Economic Considerations in Inflammatory Bowel Disease

#### *9.5.1 Choice of Mesalazine Analogues in Ulcerative Colitis*

The discovery of mesalazine as the active moiety of sulfasalazine and later development of mesalazine-delivering drugs without sulfapyridine as a carrier molecule has led to a dilemma about which drugs to use. This is especially the case since they appear generally to have equivalent effectiveness and are better tolerated than sulfasalazine in the short term. Table XIV provides an analysis of factors influencing drug selection.

Differences in cost, pharmacological characteristics and long term safety offset the advantage of better short term tolerability with coated mesalazine. Sulfasalazine remains first-line therapy in patients with no record of sensitivity

**Table XV.** Choice of local treatment for active distal ulcerative colitis

| Feature | Corticosteroid | Mesalazine (coated formulations) | Sulfasalazine |
|---|---|---|---|
| Clinical effectiveness | +++ | +++ | +++ |
| Relative cost | + | ++++ | +± |
| Unfavourable features | Systemic corticosteroid effects (usually minimal) | Antioxidants necessary for stability of formulation; local irritation, pruritus, exacerbation of colitis | Yellow staining of underwear; sulfonamide hypersensitivity |

to sulfonamides. The choice of second-line therapy is more controversial, but olsalazine may be preferable on the basis of its pharmacokinetics and safety and possibly, for distal colitis, its effectiveness.

### *9.5.2 Choice of Local Treatment for Distal Ulcerative Colitis*

The effectiveness, excellent tolerability and safety of mesalazine enemas or suppositories makes them a tempting first-line therapy for active distal ulcerative colitis, instead of rectally administered corticosteroids. However, mesalazine is considerably more expensive and, as shown in table XV, the added cost probably offsets the reduced adverse effects and improved effectiveness. Since about 80% of patients with corticosteroid-resistant distal colitis are responsive to mesalazine enemas, they may be best held in reserve for corticosteroid-resistant disease.

### *9.5.3 Long Term Maintenance Treatment*

Long term (life-long) treatment with sulfasalazine or other mesalazine-delivering drugs in patients with extensive or total colitis is essential. In patients with distal colitis, and particularly proctitis, symptoms are usually a nuisance rather than life-threatening, and are usually responsive to therapy. For patients who suffer trivial symptoms during a relapse, the use of continuous maintenance therapy is questionable and may not be cost effective. However, in patients with more than trivial symptoms or in whom relapses are frequent, continuous maintenance therapy is justified (table XVI).

Long term maintenance therapy in Crohn's disease is more controversial (table XVI). Patients with Crohn's colitis are often treated long term with mesalazine-delivering drugs, usually for ongoing suppression of the disease rather than true relapse prevention. In patients with ileitis, coated mesalazine appears to reduce the relapse rate by at least 50% after a curative ileal resection. The potential economic and quality of life benefits of such treatment outweigh the direct costs of the drug itself.

When remission is induced by drug therapy, the efficacy of coated mesalazine is less convincing and its use cannot be economically justified on present data. Azathioprine or mercaptopurine are efficacious in the subgroup of patients with Crohn's disease or ulcerative colitis who have attained remission with the drugs. The moderate direct cost and the potential (though rare and doubtful) long term adverse effects (e.g. neoplasia) of the drugs are out-

**Table XVI.** Clinical outcome and economic considerations in the selection of maintenance treatment of ulcerative colitis and Crohn's disease

| | Ulcerative colitis | | Crohn's ileitis | | Crohn's disease or ulcerative colitis |
|---|---|---|---|---|---|
| | extensive/total | proctitis/ proctosigmoiditis | post-ileal resection | drug-induced remission | |
| Drug therapy | Sulfasalazine Olsalazine/coated mesalazine | Sulfasalazine Olsalazine/coated mesalazine | Coated mesalazine | Coated mesalazine | Azathioprine/ mercaptopurine |
| Relative clinical outcome | +++ | ++ | ++ | + | ++ |
| Economic factors: | | | | | |
| • Relative cost (direct/acquisition) | +/++ | +/++ | ++ | ++ | ++ |
| • Potential indirect cost savings | +++ | + | + | + | ++ |
| Requirement for treatment | Therapy essential | Therapy only if symptoms more than trivial, or frequent relapse | Therapy should be instituted soon after surgery | Therapy cannot be justified | Therapy justified only where clear benefit of drug in inducing remission |

weighed by quality of life and indirect economic benefits in this subgroup of patients.

#### 9.5.4 Choice of Corticosteroids for Topical Use

The emerging family of topically-active corticosteroids with apparent clinical effectiveness but low systemic availability and minimal systemic effects (e.g. budesonide, beclomethasone dipropionate) will almost certainly be more expensive than low clearance corticosteroids such as prednisolone or hydrocortisone. If similar effectiveness of high and low clearance corticosteroids is confirmed in further controlled trials, a new problem regarding the choice of the most suitable preparation will emerge. The short term use of oral prednisolone (e.g. 4 to 6 weeks in ulcerative colitis) is associated with predictable adverse effects which are, in general, tolerable except in patients with specific relative contraindications, such as diabetes mellitus or osteoporosis. In this situation, the expense of high clearance (low systemic availability) corticosteroids is not justified.

In contrast, adverse effects associated with more prolonged corticosteroid therapy (especially cosmetic changes, osteoporosis and osteonecrosis) are unacceptable if an alternative medication without such effects is available. Thus, topically-active corticosteroids can be justified on economic and clinical outcome criteria in patients with Crohn's disease or chronically active ulcerative colitis.

In using corticosteroid enemas, systemic effects do occur, but are considerably less frequent than with equivalent oral doses. It is, therefore, only in long term use or in patients with relative contraindications to corticosteroid use that corticosteroid enemas with low systemic availability might be economically justified.

#### 9.5.5 Use of Cyclosporin

Cyclosporin has an impressive initial response rate in patients with corticosteroid-resistant Crohn's disease or severe ulcerative colitis and it has a rapid onset of action. However, as shown in table XVII, clinical outcomes in the longer term, associated morbidity and considerable economic cost indicate only a limited place for cyclosporin in routine clinical practice.

**Table XVII.** Advantages and disadvantages of cyclosporin treatment for corticosteroid-resistant Crohn's disease and ulcerative colitis

| Advantages | Disadvantages |
|---|---|
| • Initial response rate high (>75%) | • Relapses during therapy common (≈40%) |
| • Rapid onset of action | • Relapse following therapy common (≈50%) |
| • Prevents colectomy in 50% of patients with severe ulcerative colitis | • Erratic oral absorption<br>• Adverse effects considerable<br>• Economic cost high (daily cost >100-fold prednisolone; 35-fold metronidazole; 20-fold sulfasalazine; 4-fold azathioprine)<br>• Cost of monitoring serum concentrations |

#### 9.5.6 Choice of Antibiotics for Crohn's Colitis or Perineal Disease

Although intolerance of metronidazole (especially at a dosage >1g daily), limits its use, it has undoubted effectiveness in both Crohn's colitis and perineal disease, is the most extensively studied antibiotic for those indications and is relatively inexpensive. It remains first-line therapy for this condition. The alternatives, tinidazole and ciprofloxacin, are more expensive and their use has not been reported in large series or in controlled trials. Consequently, despite their superior tolerability *versus* metronidazole, they should probably remain second-line therapy.

### 9.6 Diverticular Disease

#### 9.6.1 Asymptomatic/Uncomplicated Disease

In most asymptomatic patients with uncomplicated diverticular disease (diverticulosis), the aim of treatment is to prevent development of symptomatic or complicated disease. Because of the putative role of a low fibre diet and raised intracolonic pressure in pathogenesis, a diet high in insoluble fibre (especially unprocessed wheat bran) is recommended.

#### 9.6.2 Symptomatic Disease

Symptomatic diverticular disease may present with intermittent abdominal pain, constipation, diarrhoea or bleeding, and may be associated with tenderness over the sigmoid colon.

##### Optimum Treatment

A high fibre diet may be useful in relieving pain and associated symptoms. This is best achieved with unprocessed wheat bran (10 to 25 g/day) taken in divided portions with meals and introduced in small quantities, with a graded increase to optimal amounts over several weeks. Too rapid introduction of bran will result in bloating and abdominal discomfort, and leads to the loss of patient confidence.

For those who cannot tolerate wheat bran or who find it unpalatable, commercial fibre products containing psyllium or ispaghula may be used. These preparations are often better tolerated, but are much more expensive and, for a lifelong condition, less than satisfactory for long term use. Antispasmodics such as *mebeverine* may relieve cramping abdominal pain.[285]

In patients with diarrhoea, *antimotility agents* (e.g. loperamide) may be useful, although these drugs are theoretically contraindicated because of the possibility of a further increase in colonic pressure. Patients with acutely painful episodes, associated with troublesome constipation not responding to fibre supplementation, may respond to an osmotic laxative such as magnesium sulfate (Epsom salts). The overall response to these measures, however, is often limited.

***Diverticulitis*** is the most frequent complication of diverticular disease, manifesting when focal inflammation in the wall of the diverticulum extends to peridiverticular regions. Usually, only localised inflammation results, but free perforation into the peritoneal cavity or fistula formation into adjacent organs can occur. Characteristic findings are localised abdominal pain, altered bowel habits, left iliac fossa tenderness with or without a mass, fever and leucocytosis. Hospitalisation is often required but medical therapy is successful in around 70 to 85% of patients.

Patients should be placed on either a low residue diet or nil orally (depending on the severity of the illness) and antibiotics should be administered. These should cover both anaerobic and aerobic Gram-negative organisms characteristic of the large bowel flora. A suitable regimen usually comprises a combination of intravenous *amoxicillin* 2g every 12 hours, *gentamicin* 4 to 5 mg/kg/day in 2 divided doses, and *metronidazole* 500mg every 12 hours intravenously or 1g suppository every 12 hours.

For analgesia in the acute stage, *pethidine* (meperidine) is preferred to morphine because the latter can raise intraluminal pressure in the sigmoid colon and cause dilatation of the diverticula.[286] Surgery is indicated if the condition does not settle, or if other complications (e.g. widespread peritonitis, fistulae, abscess) develop. Following recovery, patients should again be placed on a high fibre diet, to prevent further symptoms and complications.

Diverticular disease is present in more than 50% of elderly patients presenting with Crohn's disease involving the rectum and sigmoid colon. Diagnostic differentiation of complicated diverticular disease from Crohn's disease can be difficult. Furthermore, medical and surgical management of the 2 conditions are different. Where the diagnosis is uncertain, it is most appropriate to use intravenous fluids and nil orally, together with antibiotics, for presumed diverticulitis; corticosteroids for colitis; and to monitor closely for signs of perforation. Attention to nutrition (e.g. total parenteral nutrition) is of particular importance if a response is delayed.

## 10. Gastrointestinal Infections

### 10.1 Clinical Pharmacology of Drugs Used in Treatment

#### 10.1.1 Drugs Used in Acute Infectious Diarrhoea

Micro-organisms are the most common cause of acute diarrhoea worldwide. The extent of morbidity is influenced by the pathogen, the age, nutritional state and enteric defences of the host, and the rapidity with which appropriate management is instituted.

*Fluid and electrolyte replacement* is the cornerstone of therapy. Specific *antimicrobial therapy* is required where there is significant systemic toxicity, dysentery, evidence of severe inflammatory disease of the bowel wall (e.g. blood, toxic megacolon, impending perforation), malabsorption syndrome or failure to respond to other measures. The clinical pharmacology of selected antibacterial and antiprotozoal agents is summarised in table XVIII.

*Antidiarrhoeal drugs* have little place in the management of acute infectious diarrhoea, although in some circumstances antimotility agents such as diphenoxylate/atropine, loperamide and codeine phosphate may be useful in providing symptomatic relief (see further section 10.2.1). The clinical pharmacology of these drugs is discussed in section 11.1.4.

#### 10.1.2 Drugs Used in Intestinal Helminthic Infections

Gastrointestinal parasitisation with helminths is extremely common. Disease manifestations are proportional to the adult worm burden. Gastrointestinal symptoms are frequently minor and abdominal pain is more common than diarrhoea. The principal aim of treatment is to reduce the worm burden below the level of clinical significance.

The clinical pharmacology of anthelmintic drugs is less well defined than that of antiprotozoan and antibacterial drugs. The properties of some commonly used drugs are summarised in table XIX.

## 10.2 Optimum Treatment

### 10.2.1 Acute Infectious Diarrhoea

#### Infantile Gastroenteritis

Most cases of gastroenteritis in infants are due to viruses, especially rotavirus. Treatment must be initiated promptly, with particular attention being paid to fluid and electrolyte balance.

***Methods of rehydration:*** where possible, breast feeding should be continued since, even in the face of the lactose intolerance often associated with viral gastroenteritis, breast milk is better tolerated than proprietary formulae that have lower lactose concentrations. In mild cases, oral rehydration is appropriate initially. Within 24 hours, reintroduction of frequent, small feeds consisting of diluted milk or formula and/or bland, low-lactose solids (e.g. cereal, potato, rice) should begin. These are intended to prevent malnutrition or worsening malnutrition, which has a significant adverse influence on outcome. Lactose-containing feeds need only be reduced again if there is clinical evidence of lactose intolerance.

***Oral rehydration solutions (ORS):*** these solutions are based on the World Health Organization formula, (i.e. $Na^+$ 90 mmol/L; $K^+$ 20 mmol/L; $Cl^-$ 80 mmol/L; $HCO_3^-$ 30 mmol/L; glucose 110 mmol/L) and are suitable for moderately dehydrated infants. There is no evidence

**Table XVIII.** Properties of selected antimicrobial agents used to treat acute infectious diarrhoea

| Property | Erythromycin base | Doxycycline | Cotrimoxazole [trimethoprim (T) + sulfamethoxazole (S)] | Norfloxacin | Ciprofloxacin | Metronidazole |
|---|---|---|---|---|---|---|
| Antimicrobial spectrum[a] (selected) | *Campylobacter jejuni* | *Vibrio cholerae*<br>*Yersinia enterocolitica*<br>[ETEC] | [ETEC]<br>[*Shigella* spp.]<br>*Salmonella* spp.<br>*Yersinia enterocolitica*<br>[*Vibrio cholerae*] | ETEC<br>*Shigella* spp.<br>*Salmonella* spp.<br>[*Yersinia enterocolitica*] | ETEC<br>*Shigella* spp.<br>*Salmonella* spp.<br>[*Yersinia enterocolitica*]<br>[*C. jejuni*] | *Clostridium difficile*<br>Protozoa:<br>*Giardia intestinalis*<br>*Entamoeba histolytica* |
| Route of administration | Oral | Oral | Oral | Oral | Oral | Oral |
| Usual daily dosage | 250mg 4 × daily | 100mg once daily | S: 800mg 2 × daily<br>T: 160mg 2 × daily | 400mg 2 × daily | 500mg 2 × daily | 500mg 3 × daily |
| **Clinical effectiveness:**[b] | | | | | | |
| *C. jejuni* | +++ (see text) | +++ (see text) | | | +++ (see text) | |
| *V. cholerae* | | ++++ | +++ | see text | see text | |
| ETEC | | ++ | ++++ (see text) | ++++ | ++++ | |
| *Shigella* spp. | | | ++++ (see text) | ++++ | ++++ | |
| *Salmonella* spp. | | +++ | ++++ (see text) | ++++ | ++++ | |
| *Y. enterocolitica* | | | +++ | +++ (see text) | +++ (see text) | |
| *C. difficile* | | | | | | ++++ (see text) |
| Protozoa | | ++ (see text) | | | | ++++ |
| **Adverse effects:** | | | | | | |
| Gastrointestinal | +++ | +++ | ++ | + | + | + (see text) |
| Hypersensitivity reactions, esp. rash | + | ++ | ++ | + | + | + |
| Neurotoxicity | +[c] | | | | | |
| Staining of teeth in children | | +++ | | | + | + |
| Haematological | | | + | | | |

a Brackets indicate significant drug resistance in some countries or not the treatment of first choice.

b Clinical effectiveness is shown for drugs considered to be the main therapeutic options.

c Dose-related, reversible ototoxicity (rare).

*Abbreviation:* ETEC = enterotoxigenic *Escherichia coli.*

**Table XIX.** Properties of drugs used to treat some intestinal helminthic infections

| Property | Praziquantel | Pyrantel pamoate | Mebendazole | Albendazole | Thiabendazole |
|---|---|---|---|---|---|
| Spectrum of activity | Cestodes (tapeworms): *Taenia saginata* *Taenia solium* *Diphyllobothrium latum* *Hymenolepsis nana* | *Enterobius vermicularis* (threadworm, pinworm) *Ascaris lumbricoides* (roundworm) Hookworms (*Ancyclostoma duodenale, Necator americanus*) | *Ascaris lumbricoides* Hookworms *Trichuris trichuria* (whipworm) *Enterobius vermicularis* | *Strongyloides stercoralis* *Ascaris lumbricoides* Hookworms *Trichuris trichuria* *Enterobius vermicularis* | *Strongyloides stercoralis* *Trichinella spiralis* |
| Route of administration | Oral | Oral | Oral | Oral | Oral |
| Usual dosage | 10 mg/kg (*Taenia*) 10 mg/kg (*H. nana*) 25 mg/kg (*D. latum*) [single dose] | 11 mg/kg 20 mg/kg (hookworm) [single dose] | 100mg (*E. vermicularis*) [single dose] | 400mg [single dose] *S. stercoralis*: 200mg twice daily for 3 days | 25 mg/kg twice daily for 3 days |
| **Clinical effectiveness:** | | | | | |
| Tapeworms | ++++ | | | ++ (see text) | |
| *Enterobius vermicularis* (threadworm, pinworm) | | ++++ | ++++ | ++++ | ++++ (2nd-line; toxic) |
| *Ascaris lumbricoides* (roundworm) | | ++++ | ++++ | ++++ | +++ (2nd-line; toxic) |
| Hookworms | | +++ | ++++ | ++++ | +++ (2nd-line; toxic) |
| *Strongyloides stercoralis* | | | ++ (see text) | ++ (see text) | +++ |
| *Trichuris trichuria* | | | +++ | +++ | ++ |
| **Adverse effects:** | | | | | |
| Gastrointestinal | ++ | + | + | + | +++ |
| Neurological | ++ | + | + | + | +++ |
| Pruritus | + | + | + | | |
| Hypersensitivity | | | | | + |

that hypernatraemia is a problem with this formula (a matter of previous concern[287]). The use of glucose-supplemented oral rehydration solutions does not reduce the volume of diarrhoea and carries some osmotic penalty. In contrast, solutions containing polypeptides or polysaccharides (e.g. mashed potato or rice, wheat, sorghum, maize or millet flour) provide additional substrates and have decreased osmolality. They have the advantage of lessening diarrhoeal loss and improving nutrition.

***Intravenous rehydration:*** this is necessary in severely dehydrated or shocked infants, and in the presence of continued vomiting or abdominal distension.

***Other therapy:*** antidiarrhoeal agents and antiemetics should be avoided in infantile gastroenteritis. Antimicrobial therapy is indicated in those cases, often associated with epidemic diarrhoea in nurseries, caused by enteropathogenic *Escherichia coli* (EPEC), and in cases due to other specific pathogens.

**Acute Diarrhoea in Children and Adults**

This may be caused by a range of viruses, bacteria and protozoa, via direct effects on the enteric mucosal cells or via the production of enterotoxins or cytotoxins. Therapy depends on the severity of the illness.

***Rehydration:*** mild cases respond to rest and oral fluids containing glucose and electrolytes. Moderate dehydration can be corrected with ORS. In severe diarrhoea or dehydration associated with bodyweight loss of >10% in 24 hours, intravenous replacement of fluid and electrolytes is essential.

***Other therapy:*** the use of *antimotility drugs* such as diphenoxylate 2.5 to 5mg every 6 to 8 hours, loperamide 4mg followed by 2mg after each unformed stool, or codeine phosphate 15

**Table XX.** Antiprotozoal drugs used in the treatment of amoebiasis

| Drug | Site of action | Dosage (oral unless stated otherwise) | |
|---|---|---|---|
| | | adults | children |
| Metronidazole | All tissues | 750-800mg q8h for 10 days | 50 mg/kg/day in 3 divided doses for 10 days |
| Tinidazole | All tissues | 800mg q8h for 5 days *or* 2g once daily for 3 days | 50-60 mg/kg/day (maximum 60mg) once daily for 3 days |
| Emetine hydrochloride | All tissues | 1 mg/kg/day IM (maximum 60mg) for 10 days | 1 mg/kg/day IM (maximum 60mg) for 10 days |
| Dehydroemetine | All tissues | 1-1.5 mg/kg/day IM (maximum 90mg) for 10 days | 1.25 mg/kg/day IM (maximum 90mg) for 10 days |
| Tetracycline | Bowel wall only | 250mg q6h for 10 days | Avoid |
| Chloroquine (base) | Liver only | 300mg q12h for 1 day, then 150mg q12h for 20 days | 10 mg/kg/day in 2 divided doses for 21 days |
| Diloxanide furoate | Intestinal lumen | 500mg q8h for 10 days | 20-25 mg/kg/day in 3 divided doses for 10 days |
| Di-iodohydroxyquinoline | Intestinal lumen | 600-650mg q8h for 7 days | 40 mg/kg/day in 3 divided doses for 21 days |
| Paromomycin | Intestinal lumen | 500mg q8h for 7 days | 30 mg/kg/day in 3 divided doses for 7 days |

*Abbreviation:* IM = intramuscular.

to 30mg every 6 hours, may provide symptomatic relief. However, diphenoxylate and loperamide are potentially hazardous in children because of their adverse effects and in cases of severe diarrhoea, they may cause excessive fluid trapping in the bowel. In infections caused by enteroinvasive bacteria (e.g. *Shigella* or *Salmonella* spp.), their use may be associated with a delay in clearance of the pathogen from the bowel and consequent prolongation of the illness.[288]

*Antispasmodic drugs* (e.g. scopolamine butylbromide) may also help in the relief of pain and abdominal cramps. However, therapeutic doses are associated with anticholinergic adverse effects, most often dry mouth and blurred vision. Use of antimotility and antispasmodic drugs should be avoided in patients with high fever, systemic toxicity, bloody, mucoid stools or antibiotic-associated colitis, because of the potential complication of toxic megacolon. The use of kaolin-pectin and other *adsorbents* results in stools of increased form, but effectiveness in reducing fluid and electrolyte loss has not been demonstrated for these agents.

***Antimicrobial therapy:*** routine use of antimicrobial agents should be avoided. Not only can these drugs fail to limit the course of infection, but also their use may prolong the carrier state, increase the risk of subsequent relapse, and contribute to the emergence of drug resistance. However, specific antimicrobial therapy is indicated in severe disease and in the following syndromes: cholera, invasive amoebiasis, *Shigella* dysentery and enteroinvasive (enteropathogenic) *E. coli* infections in infants (see following sections and tables XIX and XX for drug selection).

### Shigellosis

Appropriate antibiotic treatment decreases the severity and duration of dysentery caused by *Shigella* spp., and hastens elimination of the pathogen. Coupled with the facts that humans are the natural reservoir of infection, and that transmission occurs by direct contact (faecal-oral spread), there is a strong rationale for treating all patients with shigellosis. The value of this approach has been offset in several developing countries by the emergence of antibiotic resistance; in these endemic areas, antibiotics are best reserved for severe infection.

***Choice and duration of therapy:*** ampicillin and doxycycline are no longer suitable for treatment of shigellosis, but are effective against sensitive strains. *Cotrimoxazole* (trimethoprim/sulfamethoxazole) is the preferred drug in areas where resistance is not a problem (usual dosage, trimethoprim 160mg plus sulfamethoxazole 800mg twice daily for 5 days in adults, and trimethoprim 5 mg/kg and sulfamethoxazole 25 mg/kg twice daily for 5 days in children). Clinically important resistance has been reported in several regions, including Bangladesh, Central America, Saudi Arabia and Thailand, and in travellers returning to developed countries from these areas.

Quinolone drugs are useful alternatives, although resistance to nalidixic acid is increasing amongst isolates of *Shigella dysenteriae*, especially from Bangladesh. Five-day courses of *nalidixic acid* (1g 4 times daily in adults and 55 mg/kg/day in 4 divided doses in children), *norfloxacin* (400mg twice daily in adults) or *ciprofloxacin* (500mg twice daily in adults) are curative. Therapy with the latter 2 agents is expensive, and they are not approved for use in children because they have been found to cause arthropathy in certain species of immature animals, but they are effective against strains resistant to nalidixic acid.

Third-generation cefalosporins such as *ceftriaxone* 1 g/day intravenously for 5 days in adults and 50 mg/kg/day in children) are effective alternatives[289] but are expensive. *Pivmecillinam* (amdinocillin), an oral β-lactam that is less expensive than the new quinolones and third-generation cefalosporins, has proved useful in Bangladesh for strains of *S. dysenteriae* I resistant to ampicillin, cotrimoxazole and nalidixic acid.

In all cases, *in vitro* sensitivity tests should be performed, since resistance patterns vary both geographically and with time.

#### Salmonella Enteritis

Antibacterial drugs are not beneficial in uncomplicated enterocolitis and may prolong the carrier state, probably by suppression of the normal intestinal flora. However, they are indicated in patients with high fever, systemic toxicity, bacteraemia or metastatic infection, and in infected patients with underlying diseases likely to be associated with systemic Salmonella infection, e.g. AIDS, renal transplantation, malignancies, haemodialysis, post-splenectomy and haemoglobinopathies.[290] The convalescent carrier state is not an indication for antimicrobial therapy.

***Choice and duration of therapy:*** in patients with proven or suspected bacteraemia, initial intravenous therapy with *ampicillin* 4 to 6 g/day is appropriate for sensitive *Salmonella* strains. *Chloramphenicol* 1g 3 times daily for 2 weeks is a suitable alternative and is well absorbed orally, and the regimen may be continued longer if the initial response is slow. *Cotrimoxazole* is an effective oral alternative in cases of significant toxicity, with or without positive blood cultures. The dosage regimen for adults is trimethoprim 160mg and sulfamethoxazole 800mg twice daily for 1 to 2 weeks, depending on whether blood cultures are positive. In the presence of metastatic infection, 4 to 6 weeks' therapy is required.

Some authorities suggest that relapse rates are sufficiently high that when older antibiotics are used, all treatment should be given intravenously. Parenteral therapy with third-generation cefalosporins or oral therapy with newer quinolones are useful alternative regimens in the presence of resistance to less expensive agents.

The duration of therapy may need to be prolonged in patients with AIDS, in whom relapses occur more frequently after conventional therapy than in normal hosts. In this group, cotrimoxazole is associated with an increased incidence of adverse drug reactions (in particular, severe skin rashes), and alternative therapies may be preferred. Since bone marrow function is frequently depressed in patients with AIDS, use of chloramphenicol is best avoided because of its potential to cause marrow toxicity.

#### Campylobacter Enteritis

Antimicrobial therapy is seldom beneficial in this condition, as symptoms have often settled before the organism has been identified, the convalescent state is rarely prolonged, and faecal-oral contact plays only a minor role in the spread of infection.[291] Treatment is indicated in patients with severe, acute ileitis, systemic toxicity or persistent, bloody diarrhoea.

***Choice and duration of therapy:*** a 5- to 7-day course of *erythromycin stearate* 1 g/day in 2 or 4 divided doses (adult dose) is the first-line treatment. Erythromycin base is a suitable alternative. A tetracycline (e.g. *doxycycline* 200mg immediately, then 100 mg/day) or *quinolone* drug (using dosages as for shigellosis) are also effective. The need to treat septicaemic illness with drugs other than erythromycin has not been established. Gentamicin 4 to 5 mg/kg/day, ceftriaxone 1 g/day or chloramphenicol 3 g/day (in adults) are effective; the choice between them should be made on the basis of *in vitro* sensitivity testing. Therapy is not usually required for more than 7 days.

Gastrointestinal intolerance of erythromycin may be a problem, especially in children. Dose-related, reversible, ototoxicity occurs rarely (see table XVIII).

#### Enteritis due to Other Bacteria

Gastroenteritis caused by *Vibrio parahaemolyticus*, *Bacillus cereus*, *Yersinia enterocolitica* and *Aeromonas* spp. generally requires supportive therapy only. Antibiotics are indicated in severe yersiniosis.

***Choice and duration of therapy:*** in patients with yersiniosis, intravenous *gentamicin* 5 mg/kg/day or oral or intravenous *chloramphenicol* 50 mg/kg/day have been used most commonly. As *Yersinia* is an intracellular pathogen, the duration of therapy should be at least 2 weeks. Cotrimoxazole, doxycycline and ciprofloxacin have also been used successfully.

*Yersinia* bacteraemia/septicaemia is most likely to occur in patients with iron-overload syndromes, cirrhosis or diabetes mellitus, and in the elderly. The choice of antimicrobial therapy should be based on *in vitro* sensitivity testing.

### Acute Food Poisoning

Toxin-mediated food poisoning caused by *Staphylococcus aureus*, *Bacillus cereus* and *Clostridium perfringens* should be managed symptomatically with appropriate replacement of fluid and electrolytes (see above). Antibacterial therapy is not indicated.

### Cholera

Antibiotics hasten the eradication of *Vibrio cholerae* from the faeces, and shorten the duration of diarrhoea.

***Choice and duration of therapy:*** *tetracycline* is the drug of choice in both classical and El Tor cholera, at a dosage of 250mg every 6 hours for 4 days. *Furazolidone* 5 mg/kg/day in 4 divided doses (half-doses in children) for 3 days is also effective. *Chloramphenicol* 500mg 4 times daily for 7 days or 75 mg/kg/day in 4 divided doses for 3 days) and *cotrimoxazole* (in the dosages used for salmonellosis) are slightly less effective, but are worth using when other drugs are not available.[292] *Norfloxacin* and *ciprofloxacin* are effective *in vitro* and may be superior to cotrimoxazole.

If alternative antibiotics are not available, the 4-day course of tetracycline 500mg 4 times daily should be given to children despite the (probably small) risk of teeth staining. Parenteral antibiotics have no advantage over oral agents. Antibiotic resistance is an increasing problem, particularly in East Africa, and sensitivity of prevalent cholera strains should be checked periodically.

### Enteritis due to Enterotoxigenic *Escherichia coli*

This pathogen is responsible for much of the diarrhoea suffered by visitors to tropical or subtropical countries.[63,293] The illness is usually self-limiting (see following section for further discussion).

### Travellers' Diarrhoea

Around 40% of travellers from highly industrialised countries develop acute diarrhoea within 2 weeks of arrival in developing countries in the tropics or subtropics. The risk declines after this time as exposure to the prevalent pathogens is followed by the development of immunity. Despite some regional and seasonal variation, the predominant pathogens include enterotoxigenic *E. coli*, *Shigella* spp., *Salmonella enteritidis*, *Campylobacter jejuni* and *Giardia lamblia*. Less common causes include non-cholera *Vibrio* spp. (especially in Asia), *Aeromonas* or *Plesiomonas* spp., *Cryptosporidium parvum*, and viruses.[294]

Infection is acquired by ingestion of contaminated food or beverages; attention to hygiene, and avoidance of contaminated water and improperly prepared foodstuffs are the basis of prevention. Prophylactic antibiotics, though effective in reducing diarrhoea in controlled clinical trials, are best avoided because of potential toxicity, possible development of resistance, and cost. In selected cases, such as when even short term illness will destroy the primary reason for the trip, antimicrobial prophylaxis using half the recommended therapeutic dose is appropriate, e.g. *cotrimoxazole* 960 mg/day, *norfloxacin* 400 mg/day, or *ciprofloxacin* 500 mg/day.[295] The duration of prophylactic therapy should not exceed 3 weeks.

***Choice and duration of therapy:*** in patients with acute, large-volume, watery diarrhoea, or a febrile or dysenteric syndrome, bacteria are the most likely cause. When empirical antimicrobial therapy is deemed necessary, a 3-day course of *cotrimoxazole* (960mg twice daily) plus *loperamide* (2mg after each unformed stool to a total of 8mg) is effective in over 90% of travellers to areas where there is little evidence of trimethoprim resistance amongst enteropathogens, and *Campylobacter jejuni* is an infrequent pathogen (e.g. Mexico). In most regions of South America, Africa and Southern Asia, trimethoprim resistance is common, and a 2- to 3-day course of a quinolone drug (e.g. *norfloxacin* 400mg twice daily or *ciprofloxacin* 500mg twice daily) plus *loperamide* is recommended.

*Furazolidone* (100mg 4 times daily in adults, 8 mg/kg 4 times daily in children, for 5 days), although less effective than cotrimoxazole or ciprofloxacin in reducing the duration of diarrhoea, has useful activity against *Shigella* spp., *Salmonella* spp., enterotoxigenic *E. coli* and trimethoprim-resistant bacteria, as well as *Giardia* spp. Furazolidone may be preferred for the traveller staying in remote areas for prolonged periods, who is likely to be exposed to bacterial and protozoal pathogens,[295] and it has the advantage of being available as a paediatric suspension. In patients with diarrhoea persisting longer than 2 weeks, especially when associated with bloating or flatulence, *Giardia lamblia* is the likely pathogen and *tinidazole* or *metronidazole* is the first-line treatment.

The use of loperamide should be avoided in patients with dysentery. In patients who do not improve while receiving antimicrobial therapy, investigations should be undertaken for amoebiasis, a resistant bacterial pathogen, or noninfectious causes of diarrhoea.

#### Antibiotic-Associated Diarrhoea

Diarrhoea is a relatively frequent complication of antimicrobial therapy. Most often there is no associated colitis and patients respond to cessation of the implicated antimicrobial agent. The mechanism of diarrhoea is thought to be an antibiotic-associated alteration in the normal bacterial flora of the bowel.

Antibiotic-associated colitis, with or without pseudomembrane formation, occurs as a result of production of an enterotoxin (toxin A) and a cytotoxin (toxin B) by the anaerobic bacterium *Clostridium difficile*. It is most often induced by broad-spectrum antimicrobial agents that have a major impact on colonic bacterial flora and allow overgrowth of *C. difficile*. These include clindamycin, ampicillin (or amoxicillin) and cefalosporins. Only bacitracin has been exempt from causing antibiotic-associated colitis. Disease is most frequent and severe in elderly debilitated, seriously ill patients. Although most cases arise 4 to 9 days after starting the antibiotic, diarrhoea may be noted as soon as 2 days after initiation and as long as 6 weeks after cessation of therapy.

Mild cases respond to appropriate fluid and electrolyte replacement and withdrawal of the offending antimicrobial agent. Symptomatic therapy with *cholestyramine* has been used to bind *C. difficile* toxin, but does not eliminate the organism. Specific antimicrobial therapy is required in persistent or severe illness.

***Choice and duration of therapy:*** oral *metronidazole* 500mg 3 times daily or *vancomycin* 250mg 4 times daily for 10 days are the first-line therapies. Metronidazole is less expensive than oral vancomycin and is preferred in hospital settings where vancomycin-resistant enterococci have emerged as important pathogens. Bacitracin given orally affords equivalent symptomatic relief; however, it is less successful in eradicating the pathogen[296] and in any case is not readily available in oral formulations. In patients intolerant of oral therapy, intravenous metronidazole can be given.

Relapses with the same organism follow the end of therapy in 5 to 50% of cases, irrespective of the initial antimicrobial agent selected.[297] Therapy with the same or an alternative drug should be prolonged to 14 days to treat the first relapse. A further relapse may respond to an increased dose of vancomycin (500mg 4 times daily), with or without the addition of oral rifampicin (600mg twice daily).[298]

Antimotility drugs should be avoided, since they appear to be ineffective, may prolong the course of the illness, and have been associated with the development of toxic megacolon. Case clusters of *C. difficile*-associated colitis have been reported in hospitalised patients as a result of cross-infection. Careful attention should be paid to handwashing and cleaning of potentially contaminated surfaces. If possible, hospitalised patients with diarrhoea should be isolated, especially in wards housing severely ill or immunocompromised patients. In patients with toxic megacolon, broad-spectrum intravenous therapy (e.g. ampicillin plus metronidazole and an aminoglycoside) is required for associated bacteraemia of bowel origin. Surgery may be life-saving in this circumstance.

### *10.2.2 Protozoal Infections*

#### Giardiasis

In this condition, nitroimidazole drugs are the treatment of choice. *Tinidazole* in a single dose of 1.5 to 2.0g in adults and 50 mg/kg in children is a convenient, effective treatment for small bowel infection due to *G. lamblia*. Doses of 150mg twice daily for 7 days in adults (2.5 mg/kg twice daily for 7 days in children) are of equal effectiveness and may cause fewer adverse effects. Alternatively, *metronidazole* 2g once daily for 3 days or 200 to 250mg every 8 hours for 7 to 10 days in adults (35 to 40 mg/kg once daily for 3 days or 5 mg/kg 3 times daily for 7 to 10 days in children), or *ornidazole* in a single dose of 1.5g in adults (50 mg/kg in children) are equally effective. Symptoms should resolve within 1 to 2 weeks. Retreatment is sometimes necessary. Persistent symptoms may respond to a low-lactose diet and avoidance of alcohol, herbs and spices.

*Mepacrine* (quinacrine) 100mg every 8 hours for 7 days in adults (5 mg/kg/day in 3 divided doses for 5 days in children) is also effective in giardiasis. However, its use is associated with significant adverse effects, particularly in young children, e.g. gastrointestinal upset, headache, dizziness, toxic psychosis and, rarely, severe rash or yellowing of the skin.[299]

Among the nitroimidazoles, dizziness appears most likely to occur with ornidazole.[300] A metallic taste disturbance may be associated with treatment with any of these agents. Concentration and short term memory may be impaired with the high-dose regimens, so patients should be cautioned against driving cars or operating dangerous machinery while on therapy.

#### Amoebiasis

Drug therapy in amoebiasis is directed to the eradication of *Entamoeba histolytica* from the bowel, prevention of spread to other tissues, and eradication of invasive amoebae. Dosages of drugs used in the treatment of amoebiasis are summarised in table XX. The drug and regimen of choice varies with the site and severity of amoebic infestation.

***Patients with mild to moderate dysentery or amoebic granuloma:*** oral *metronidazole* or *tinidazole* provide rapid control of symptoms and a parasitological cure rate of about 90%. Follow-up therapy with a luminal amoebicide such as *diloxanide furoate,* (alternatives are *di-iodohydroxyquinoline* or *paromomycin*) is desirable. These latter drugs are more effective than the nitroimidazoles in eradicating *E. histolytica* from the bowel of patients with nondysenteric infection and from asymptomatic cyst passers. Nitroimidazole courses shorter than those recommended in table XX significantly increase the risk of relapse. An alternative regimen of tetracycline followed by diloxanide furoate is almost as effective.[301]

***Patients with severe dysentery:*** these patients require hospitalisation for fluid and electrolyte replacement, attention to diet and drug therapy. The amoebicidal drugs of choice are *metronidazole* (initially intravenous, if necessary) and *tinidazole*. Alternative regimens include oral *tetracycline* plus *chloroquine* followed by *diloxanide furoate*, or intramuscular *emetine* (or dehydroemetine) followed by *diloxanide furoate*.

In fulminating infection, gastric suction should be instituted. Intramuscular emetine (or dehydroemetine) may be added to intravenous metronidazole during the first 3 days of therapy in these patients; chloroquine is rarely necessary. Diloxanide furoate should be given subsequently. In addition to drugs effective against *E. histolytica*, appropriate intravenous antibiotics are required to combat sepsis arising from the bowel. Surgery is indicated in the presence of toxic megacolon unresponsive to treatment within 48 to 72 hours, perforation or uncontrolled bleeding.

***Patients with nondysenteric (chronic) intestinal amoebiasis:*** the syndrome of chronic, intermittent diarrhoea, passage of mucus, abdominal pain, flatulence and bodyweight loss should be treated as for mild to moderate dysentery. This syndrome must be distinguished from postinfectious irritable bowel syndrome and the rare sequel of postdysenteric colitis, neither of which respond to antiamoebic therapy.

***Asymptomatic intestinal carriers (cyst passers):*** there is controversy regarding the use of specific therapy in patients with no evidence of invasive disease, especially in endemic areas or in subpopulations at high risk of reinfection. At present, potentially invasive and/or highly transmissible strains of *E. histolytica* cannot be identified accurately. In nonendemic areas, treatment with *diloxanide furoate*, *di-iodohydroxyquinoline* or *paromomycin* can be recommended. Metronidazole and tinidazole are less effective in this context.[302]

***Patients with amoebic liver abscess:*** *metronidazole* is the treatment of choice in patients with liver abscess, to be followed by a course of diloxanide furoate or di-iodohydroxyquinoline to eliminate luminal infestation. An alternative regimen is intramuscular *emetine* or *dehydroemetine*, combined with *chloroquine*, and followed by diloxanide furoate or di-iodohydroxyquinoline. *Tinidazole* alone as a single daily dose of 2g (50 mg/kg for children) for 2 or 3 days has shown a high cure rate and appears superior to metronidazole as a single daily dose short-course regimen.[303,304] When the abscess is associated with clinical dysentery, metronidazole or tinidazole, as for mild cases of amoebic dysentery, are the most appropriate agents.

If the liver abscess is large or pointing, needle aspiration is indicated. When the abscess is in the left lobe, open drainage is indicated. Corticosteroids appear to be a precipitating factor in some cases of amoebic liver abscess and the possibility of amoebiasis should be considered in patients who develop diarrhoea or fever during treatment with corticosteroids.[305,306]

The adverse effects nitroimidazole drugs are discussed in the section on giardiasis. The emetine-containing drugs are potentially cardiotoxic and are contraindicated in patients with cardiovascular disease, dehydroemetine probably being less cardiotoxic than emetine. Patients receiving either drug should remain sedentary and under observation during therapy. Other adverse effects include nausea, vomiting, diarrhoea, dizziness and weakness.

Adverse effects of diloxanide furoate are mild and include flatulence and abdominal discomfort. Di-iodohydroxyquinoline interferes with tests of thyroid function and may cause diarrhoea and rash. It has also been reported to cause optic atrophy, but not when used in the recommended dosages.[301] Paromomycin may produce nausea, abdominal cramps and diarrhoea.

#### Other Protozoal Infections

***Coccidian parasites*** that cause prolonged, often severe, watery diarrhoea and abdominal symptoms in patients with AIDS include *Cryptosporidium parvum*, *Isospora belli* and *Cyclospora* spp. There is no specific therapy for cryptosporidiosis. Isospora infections can be controlled by a course of *cotrimoxazole* (960mg 4 times daily for 10 days, followed by 960mg twice daily for 3 weeks). Up to 50% of patients will relapse and require maintenance therapy, although the optimal dosage regimen has not been defined. Patients with AIDS may not tolerate high doses of cotrimoxazole. Prolonged therapy with *sulfadiazine* plus *pyrimethamine* has been successful and *furazolidone* may be useful. Based on limited data, patients with *Cyclospora* infection may respond to cotrimoxazole.[307]

***Microsporidia*** are obligate intracellular parasites that cause chronic diarrhoea and bodyweight loss in patients with advanced AIDS. Malabsorption is a prominent feature. The most common pathogens are *Enterocytozoon bieneusi* and *Septata intestinalis*. There is limited anecdotal evidence that symptoms can be reduced in some patients by the use of *metronidazole* (250 to 500mg 3 times daily for 10 to 14 days or according to symptomatic responses). *Albendazole* (200 to 400mg twice daily) may be of value, especially in infection due to *Septata intestinalis*, but its effectiveness is unproven.[308]

### *10.2.3 Helminthic Infections*

The principal aim of anthelmintic therapy is to reduce the worm burden below the level of clinical significance. In temperate climates where reinfection is unlikely, most infections can be virtually eliminated very economically. In rural tropical areas, multiple infestations are common and the use of broad-spectrum anthelmintics is important for helminth control. However, in heavy infestation, selective treatment for the appropriate helminth is preferable.

#### Choice of Anthelmintic Drug

The choice of drug is dictated by cost, availability, effectiveness and toxicity. Drug regimens and practical hints regarding therapy of specific infections are provided in table XXI. The relative effectiveness and toxicity of the commonly used agents are summarised in table XIX.

#### Treatment of Common Helminthic Infections

***Enterobiasis*** (threadworm, pinworm infection): *Enterobius vermicularis* is the only intestinal nematode transmitted directly from person to person. Good personal hygiene, including washing the hands after defaecation and before handling food, is essential. Food should be kept covered. Affected individuals should wash the perianal area thoroughly every morning. Bedcovers should be changed each day without shaking, to minimise the dissemination of eggs. When there is more than 1 child in the household, all family members should be treated at the same time.

***Hookworm infection:*** human disease is usually due to *Ancyclostoma duodenale* or *Necator americanus*. The benzimidazole drugs *(mebendazole* and *albendazole)* or *pyrantel pamoate* are preferred because of their activity against both species, which obviates the need for precise identification of the causative agent.[309] *Bephenium hydroxynaphthoate* is more effective against *A. duodenale* than *N. americanus*. If used to treat the latter, up to 5 doses are required to reduce the worm burden by 50%.[309]

Infection with *N. americanus* can be treated with *tetrachloroethylene* taken on an empty stomach, provided that alcohol and fats are avoided for 24 hours before and after treatment. Heavy infections may require repeated treatment at 4-day intervals. Tetrachloroethylene

**Table XXI.** Treatment of some intestinal helminthic infections

| Infection | Drug(s) of choice | Dosage | Principal adverse effects/notes |
|---|---|---|---|
| *Ascaris lumbricoides* (roundworm) | Mebendazole | 100mg twice daily for 3 days for patients >2 years | Mild diarrhoea, abdominal pain |
| | Albendazole | *Adults and children* >2 years: 400mg single dose | |
| | Pyrantel pamoate | 11 mg/kg single dose (maximum 1g) | Headache, dizziness, vomiting, abdominal pain, diarrhoea (usually mild, in ≈20% of patients) |
| | Levamisole | *Adults:* 150mg single dose<br>*Children:* 50mg/20kg bodyweight single dose | Mild, transient pyrexia, nausea, vomiting, abdominal pain, dizziness, headache in ≈1% of patients |
| | Piperazine | *Adults:* 75 mg/kg, maximum 4g (equivalent hydrate) single dose<br>*Children:* 120 mg/kg (maximum 4g) single dose<br>*NB:* Effectiveness improved by second dose after 24h | Occasional nausea, vomiting, diarrhoea. Neurological effects are rare and mainly occur in children, renal failure, overdosage or underlying neurological disorder (ataxia is the most frequent sign)<br>Largely superseded |
| *Enterobius vermicularis* (threadworm, pinworm) | Pyrantel pamoate | 11 mg/kg single dose | All family members may need treatment with these drugs. Single doses may need to be repeated weekly for up to 6 weeks |
| | Mebendazole | 100mg single dose | |
| | Albendazole | As for *A. lumbricoides* (see above) | |
| | Piperazine hydrate | 1 × 50-75 mg/kg dose/day for 7 days | See above (second-line therapy) |
| | Vipyrnium (pyrvinium) pamoate | 5 mg/kg (maximum 350mg) single dose | Nausea and vomiting; stains clothing (second-line therapy) |
| Hookworm *(Ancylostoma duodenale* and *Necator americanus)* | Mebendazole | As for *A. lumbricoides* (see above) | See above |
| | Albendazole | *Adults and children >2 years:* 400mg single dose or 200 mg/day for 3 days | *Single dose:* 80% reduction in egg count; *3-day regimen:* 100% cure |
| | Pyrantel pamoate | 11 mg/kg single dose (maximum 1g) | For heavy infestation with *N. americanus* (>4000 eggs/g faeces), 11 mg/kg may be given for up to 3 consecutive days |
| | Bephenium hydroxynaphthoate | *Adults:* 5g (2.5g base) single dose<br>*Children (<2 years):* 2.5g (1.25g base) single dose | Nausea, vomiting, diarrhoea infrequent with single doses<br>Not very effective against *N. americanus* (see text; section 10.2.3) |
| | Tetrachloroethylene | 0.12 ml/kg (maximum 5ml) single dose | Dizziness, nausea, vomiting, abdominal cramps, diarrhoea<br>Patients should rest for 1h postdose. Use for *N. americanus* only (see text) |
| *Strongyloides stercoralis* (dwarf threadworm) | Thiabendazole | 25 mg/kg (maximum 3g) twice daily for 3 days | Tablets must be chewed thoroughly or a suspension used.<br>Treatment course 5-14 days if hyperinfection syndrome or patient with AIDS (see table XIX and text for adverse effects) |
| | Albendazole | *Adults and children >2 years:* 200mg twice daily for 3 days | See text |
| | Mebendazole | 200mg twice daily for 4 days | See text |
| *Trichuris trichuria* (whipworm) | Mebendazole | As for *A. lumbricoides* (see above) | |
| | Albendazole | As for *A. lumbricoides* (see above) | |
| Tapeworms<br>*Taenia saginata*<br>*Taenia solium* | Niclosamide | *Adults:* 2g single dose<br>*Children:* 11-34kg, 1g; >34kg, 1.5g single dose | Tablets must be chewed thoroughly after light meal. Causes mild colic and diarrhoea (see text) |
| *Diphyllobothrium latum*<br>*Hymenolepsis nana* | Praziquantel | 10 mg/kg single dose (25 mg/kg for *D. latum;* 15 mg/kg for *H. nana*) | Tablets should not be chewed.<br>Dizziness, drowsiness, gastrointestinal disturbance (dose-related). See text |

**Table XXI.** *[Continued]*

| Infection | Drug(s) of choice | Dosage | Principal adverse effects/notes |
|---|---|---|---|
| Tapeworms *(continued)* | Dichlorophen | *Adults:* 75 mg/kg (maximum 6g) daily for 2 days<br>*Children:* 2-4g daily for 2 days | Useful for *T. saginata, T. solium* only. Causes nausea, vomiting, colic, diarrhoea. Avoid alcohol during treatment and avoid use in liver disease |
| | Paromomycin | *Adults:* 1g every 15 min for 4 doses<br>*Children:* 11 mg/kg every 15 min for 4 doses | Not very effective for *D. latum, H. nana.* Nausea, vomiting, abdominal pain, diarrhoea reduced if drug taken after meals |

should not be given to patients with concomitant ascariasis, since it may stimulate migration of the ascaris. Although it is an inexpensive drug, its use has been greatly curtailed because of this potential. Anaemia caused by hookworm infection is most easily corrected with ferrous sulfate 200mg 3 times daily. Treatment should be continued for 3 months after the haemoglobin has returned to 120 g/L.

***Strongyloidiasis*** (dwarf threadworm infection): this is the only worm that can multiply within the host and, thus, perpetuate the infection. Since larval stages migrate through the tissues in cases of autoinfection, curative drugs must be active in the bowel lumen and in the tissues. *Thiabendazole* is considered the treatment of choice, but its use is associated with significant adverse effects in up to 50% of cases. Nausea, vomiting and dizziness are common; rash, bradycardia, hypotension and olfactory disturbances occur occasionally. High doses of mebendazole and albendazole eliminate the worm from the bowel in more than 80% of cases. Albendazole has the advantage of having an increased bioavailability and higher serum concentrations of active metabolites.

***Trichinosis:*** the initial (intestinal) phase occurs within the first week after ingestion of contaminated meat and is associated with the development of the adult worms. *Thiabendazole* 25 mg/kg twice daily for 5 days, *mebendazole* 100mg twice daily for 3 days, or *pyrantel pamoate* 11 mg/kg/day for 4 days will eliminate worms from the intestine. The second (muscle) stage of infection responds primarily to bedrest plus drugs to control the inflammatory and allergic effects of larval migration into muscle, heart and nervous system. *Prednisone* 40 to 60 mg/day should be taken until fever and allergic manifestations subside. Antipyretics and analgesics may replace corticosteroids in less severe cases. Thiabendazole has been used in severe cases, but its use is controversial, since by destroying tissue larvae and liberating antigens, systemic allergic or hypersensitivity reactions may be exacerbated. Although unproven, mebendazole may be an advantage because of its poor bioavailability, and doses of 5 mg/kg/day for 2 weeks are commonly recommended.

***Tapeworm infection:*** therapeutic options, effectiveness and adverse effects are summarised in tables XIX and XXI. Drowsiness occurs frequently with *praziquantel* therapy and is due to its structural similarity to benzodiazepines. Patients should avoid driving, operating machinery or performing other tasks requiring mental alertness. The use of praziquantel in patients with concomitant bowel infection with *Taenia solium* and active cerebral cysticercosis may provoke an acute cerebral inflammatory reaction, with features such as headaches, seizures and focal neurological signs. This reaction can be controlled by corticosteroids. *Albendazole* 800 mg/day for 2 weeks is equally effective therapy of neurocysticercosis.

There is a theoretical risk of cysticercosis following treatment of *T. solium* with niclosamide, praziquantel, dichlorophen and paromomycin, which have no effect on the eggs of the parasite. Although no cases of this complication have been reported, many advise that treatment of *T. solium* be followed 2 hours later by purgation with magnesium sulfate 15 to 30g to expel mature worm segments before the eggs are released. Post-treatment stool examination should be performed after 1 and 3 months.

## 10.3 Clinical Outcome and Economic Considerations

### *10.3.1 Acute Enteritis/Enterocolitis*

In most cases of acute enteritis, antimicrobial therapy offers few benefits and may be detrimental. The cost of the available antibiotics varies from low to high and there would be no savings expected in indirect costs. In seriously ill patients or those with certain infections (e.g. cholera, Shigella dysentery, amoebiasis), and in enteropathogenic (enteroinvasive) *E. coli* infection of infants, the balance between the effect of antimicrobial therapy on clinical outcome, and indirect cost savings in terms of other management options, shifts in favour of giving antimicrobial therapy. Assessment of cost-effectiveness relationships of different antimicrobial agents varies with the extent of drug resistance in the population being studied.

Treatment of invasive amoebiasis provides an example of the effect of illness severity on cost-effectiveness analysis for different antimicrobial therapies. *E. histolytica* is sensitive to metronidazole, tinidazole, tetracycline, emetine and dehydroemetine. To treat invasive infection, the nitroimidazoles (metronidazole and tinidazole) have the most favourable effectiveness/safety profile, followed by tetracycline and then emetine-containing drugs, except in patients with fulminating disease. In the latter group, the therapeutic advantage and indirect cost savings of combining an emetine-containing drug with intravenous metronidazole offsets the toxicity due to the former, and tetracycline becomes relatively less effective in terms of its effectiveness/safety profile.

The influence of antimicrobial sensitivity patterns on the cost-effectiveness ratio of different antimicrobial drugs is illustrated by the treatment of Shigella dysentery, summarised in table XXII.

#### *10.3.2 Helminthic Infections*

The broad-spectrum agents mebendazole, albendazole and pyrantel pamoate exhibit similar high effectiveness/safety and indirect cost-saving profiles. However, the benzimidazoles (mebendazole and albendazole) are more expensive than pyrantel pamoate. Bephenium hydroxynaphthoate and tetrachloroethylene, which are alternative drugs used in the treatment of hookworm (see table XXI), have a moderate effectiveness/safety outcome (since they are associated with significant toxicity), but are relatively inexpensive.

Although thiabendazole is considered the treatment of choice for strongyloidiasis, the balance of effectiveness/safety is comparable to that of albendazole, which is less toxic but more expensive and less widely available.

Of the drugs listed in table XXI for the treatment of taeniasis, niclosamide and praziquantel offer equal, major therapeutic benefit. Niclosamide has a higher incidence of adverse effects, but they are mild. Praziquantel is more expensive. Dichlorophen and paromomycin are inferior in their effectiveness/safety profiles, but are relatively inexpensive.

## 11. Functional Gastrointestinal Disease

The functional gastrointestinal disorders account for the largest proportion of consultations for digestive symptoms and can be subdivided into a number of distinct clinical syndromes.[310] The most common of these disorders are functional dyspepsia and gastroparesis, irritable bowel syndrome, functional constipation and functional diarrhoea. A largely nondrug approach to the management of these disorders should be undertaken. Indeed, only a proportion of patients in each of these categories will require drug therapy, and even then, the duration of therapy should be limited to short periods.

**Table XXII. Clinical outcome and economic considerations in selection of drugs for treatment of *Shigella* dysentery**

| Parameter | Cotrimoxazole [trimethoprim + sulfamethoxazole] | Nalidixic acid | Fluoroquinolones | Third-generation cefalosporins | Pivmecillinam |
|---|---|---|---|---|---|
| **Clinical effectiveness:** | | | | | |
| Drug-sensitive strains | +++ | +++ | +++ | +++ | +++ |
| Drug-resistant strains | None | None | NA | NA | NA |
| **Tolerability:** | | | | | |
| Adults | +++ | +++ | +++ | +++ | +++ |
| Children | +++ | +++ | +[a] | +++ | +++ |
| **Overall benefit:** | | | | | |
| Drug-sensitive strains | +++ | +++ | +++ | +++ | +++ |
| Drug-resistant strains | None | None | NA | NA | NA |
| **Relative cost** (direct/acquisition) | + | + | +++ | +++ | ++ |
| **Indirect cost savings** | +++ | +++ | +++ | +++ | +++ |

a Not approved for use in children because of potential (not proven) toxic effects on immature cartilage (see text).
*Abbreviation:* NA = not applicable.

A wide variety of medications and drug classes are used to treat functional gastrointestinal disorders, reflecting the often empirical nature of therapy.

## 11.1 Clinical Pharmacology of Drugs Used in Treatment

### *11.1.1 Drugs Used in Functional Dyspepsia*

For functional dyspepsia, the drugs used include prokinetic agents, antisecretory drugs, cytoprotective agents, and antacids. The clinical pharmacological properties of the prokinetic drugs (i.e. metoclopramide, domperidone and cisapride) are discussed in section 5.1, and those of the antisecretory drugs, cytoprotective agents and antacids in section 4.1. The prokinetic drugs stimulate and/or coordinate disturbed upper gastrointestinal motility, particularly improving delayed gastric emptying. Among these agents, *cisapride* has a relatively wide spectrum of activity within the gastrointestinal tract, reducing prolonged small bowel and probably colonic transit times.

Another class of drugs, the *motilin agonists*, is currently under study. The prototype in this class of drugs, i.e. erythromycin, and newer erythromycin analogues, accelerate gastric emptying, and can modify antropyloric and small bowel motor activity, especially when given intravenously.

### *11.1.2 Drugs Used in Irritable Bowel Syndrome*

In irritable bowel syndrome, drug use is targeted towards the predominant symptom, usually abdominal pain, diarrhoea or constipation. Laxatives and antidiarrhoeal agents may be useful. Drugs used for abdominal pain include simple analgesics, anticholinergic agents and low doses of tricyclic antidepressants.

***Anticholinergic/antispasmodic*** drugs are used to reduce intestinal smooth muscle contraction, particularly to reduce meal-stimulated colonic motor activity. A large number of anticholinergic drugs are available, and their precise mechanisms of action are not well understood. Available agents include atropine and other belladonna alkaloids, scopolamine (hyoscine) butylbromide, dicyclomine, penthienate methobromide and propantheline bromide. Individual responses to these agents vary considerably when used for irritable bowel syndrome. They are usually given orally 3 to 4 times daily, but anticholinergic effects, such as dry mouth, blurred vision, restlessness, insomnia, urinary hesitancy and constipation, can be dose-limiting.

***Mebeverine*** is a non-anticholinergic (papaverine-like) antispasmodic, the mechanism of action of which is not clearly elucidated, but may involve calcium channel blockade. ***Peppermint oil***, which is available in enteric-coated capsules, may also have an antispasmodic action. Few reliable data regarding the comparative effectiveness of these medications in irritable bowel syndrome are available.

### *11.1.3 Drugs Used in Functional Constipation*

For functional constipation, dietary fibre supplementation and laxative agents are most commonly prescribed (table XXIII).

#### Bulk Producers

Dietary fibre (i.e. complex polysaccharides and other polymers including cellulose, hemicelluloses, gum, mucilages, pectins and lignins) is thought to result in softer, bulkier stools while retaining water and decreasing transit time. An increased stool weight may also result from the stimulation of colonic bacterial proliferation. The increased stool mass in turn leads to faster transit and reduced water absorption by the colonic mucosa.

Unprocessed wheat bran is a cheap and convenient source of dietary fibre. Weight-for-weight, fibre from unprocessed bran produces almost double the stool weight achieved with carrot, cabbage, apple or guar gum fibre. It is not necessary to take bran in tablet form or high fibre granules, although these preparations may be more palatable for some patients. Several semisynthetic bulk laxatives are available, such as those containing psyllium, hydrophilic mucilloid, ispaghula and sterculia gum. These preparations are effective, convenient and widely used.

#### Laxatives

Laxatives can be classified according to their mode of action, although some probably act via more than 1 mechanism. *Stimulants* such as bisacodyl, senna, phenolphthalein, danthron and ricinoleic acid stimulate intestinal peristalsis and cause intraluminal accumulation of water. *Osmotic agents* such as lactulose and magnesium sulfate are poorly absorbed and act by drawing water into the gut lumen by an osmotic effect.

*Wetting agents:* stool softeners, e.g. dioctyl sodium sulfosuccinate (docusate sodium) work predominantly as detergents to hydrate the stool, but also cause increased accumulation of

**Table XXIII.** Medications used in the management of constipation

| Agent | Relative potency | Usual dose | Principal adverse effects/notes[a] |
|---|---|---|---|
| **Bulk producers[b,c]** | | | |
| Mucilaginous seeds, gums, ispaghula ('Fybogel') | + | 5-10g | All somewhat difficult to swallow; slow acting. May cause initial flatulence and abdominal discomfort. Ensure adequate fluid intake and avoid in faecal impaction and possible intestinal obstruction |
| Sterculia ('Normacol') | + | 5-10g | |
| Psyllium ('Metamucil','Agiofibe') | + | 7g | |
| Unprocessed bran | + | 1-4g | |
| Methylcellulose | + | 3-6g | |
| **Colonic stimulants or irritants** | | | |
| Senna[b] | ++ | 0.25-2g | Skin eruptions; changes in bowel ganglia. Adjust dose to individual requirements and smallest effective dose |
| Danthron | + | 75-150mg | Skin eruptions; avoid in breast-feeding mothers |
| Bisacodyl (oral and rectal) | +++ | 5-15mg | Abdominal cramps. Enteric-coated tablets take 6h or more to exert effect |
| Phenolphthalein | ++ | 50-250mg | Skin eruptions (infrequent); syncope; hypersensitivity (infrequent) |
| **Osmotic agents** | | | |
| Magnesium sulfate | ++ | 5-15g | Hypermagnesaemia in impaired renal function |
| Lactulose[c] | + | 15-30ml | Abdominal cramps; diarrhoea (excessive dosage) |
| Small volume enemas (phosphate; citrate) | ++++ | 100-130ml | Mucosal irritation may interfere with interpretation of sigmoidoscopic findings |
| **Wetting agents (stool softeners)** | | | |
| Sodium dioctyl sulfosuccinate (docusate sodium; oral[b] and rectal) | + | 30-100mg | Slow action; anorexia, vomiting, diarrhoea. May facilitate absorption of other normally unabsorbed laxatives and should not be used with such drugs |
| **Others** | | | |
| Microdose enemas (sodium citrate, surface active agents, glycerol) | +++ | 5ml | |

a Habitual use of any purgative can cause severe potassium loss and accompanying muscle weakness and also impairment of homeostasis in the elderly.
b Drugs most commonly used in clinical practice.
c Suitable for long term use in some circumstances (see text).

water in the intestine. Because these agents can disrupt the intestinal epithelium, they should be used with care in the presence of other medications. Mineral oil (liquid paraffin) has no advantage over other laxatives, is associated with significant adverse effects (lipoid pneumonia, anal incontinence, pruritus ani) and is no longer used routinely. Laxatives can also be administered rectally as a suppository or enema, e.g. glycerol (glycerin), saline or bisacodyl.

### 11.1.4 Drugs Used in Functional Diarrhoea

For functional diarrhoea, antidiarrhoeal agents are useful in moderate to severe cases.

***General adsorbents*** (e.g. kaolin, chalk, aluminium hydroxide, pectin, activated charcoal) are widely used for symptomatic control of diarrhoea, but there is little evidence that they are effective.

***Opioid antidiarrhoeal drugs*** include morphine, codeine phosphate, diphenoxylate and loperamide. The antidiarrhoeal effect of these agents is generally attributed to their action on intestinal and colonic motor activity to prolong transit time. They have also been shown to inhibit intestinal secretion and/or to increase fluid and electrolyte absorption. With the exception of loperamide, the central analgesic properties of these agents contribute to their adverse effects and preclude their use in patients with liver failure. Codeine phosphate should not be used long term because of the risk of dependence.

Diphenoxylate is a derivative of pethidine and, like codeine, has opioid activity. Although a possibility with high doses, habituation has not been reported with usual therapeutic dosages. Diphenoxylate is combined with atropine to discourage excessive self-medication.

Loperamide is a butyramide derivative with structural similarities to diphenoxylate, but without opioid activity at normal therapeutic doses. It has a more rapid onset and prolonged duration of action than diphenoxylate or codeine phosphate. In addition to its antimotility and antisecretory effects, loperamide increases anal sphincter tone and improves continence in patients with diarrhoea.

## 11.2 Optimum Treatment

### 11.2.1 Functional Dyspepsia

According to current definitions, patients with functional dyspepsia have no structural or biochemical explanation for their symptoms. Patients who in addition have symptoms compatible with irritable bowel syndrome (see section 11.2.3) or gastro-oesophageal reflux disease (see section 3.1.1) are excluded. A working definition of functional dyspepsia is chronic or recurrent abdominal pain or discomfort, with a duration of >1 month and with symptoms present >25% of the time.[310] The prevalence of functional dyspepsia is around 20% among patients with dyspepsia and no endoscopic evidence of peptic ulcer, reflux oesophagitis, gastric carcinoma or other organic disease. It is always important to consider whether the patient's other medications may be associated with dyspeptic symptoms.

The pathophysiology of functional dyspepsia is poorly understood. Factors that have been implicated are:

1) Abnormal upper gastrointestinal motility with antral hypomotility, delayed gastric emptying and antroduodenal incoordination.

2) Abnormal visceral perception, where there is an enhanced sensitivity to gastric distension.

3) Increased mucosal sensitivity to gastric acid.

4) *H. pylori*-associated chronic active gastritis.

5) Psychosocial factors such as chronic difficulties/stress.

#### General Measures

Management of functional dyspepsia is based on reassurance about the absence of serious disease and an explanation of the possible factors producing symptoms. Patients should be advised to avoid foods that aggravate their symptoms, such as coffee and alcohol, and to avoid medications that may provoke symptoms. A reduced-fat diet may be beneficial, as fat alters gastric motor function more profoundly than other dietary constituents. For postprandial symptoms, a decrease in meal size, with more frequent meals, should be tried.

The presence of anxiety, depression and/or excessive chronic stress should be explored and addressed from the outset with simple forms of counselling. Untreated anxiety or depression may impair the response to other forms of therapy. An explanation of the ways in which stress can affect upper gut function is often valuable and can be used to emphasise the recurrent or episodic nature of the symptoms.

#### Drug Therapy

If symptoms are affecting quality of life significantly, drug therapy should be considered. Medical therapy can usually provide at least partial relief of symptoms. This may be related to the high placebo treatment effect (up to 60% for functional dyspepsia). The subgrouping of patients with functional dyspepsia into specific symptom clusters, such as 'motility-like' dyspepsia, has not proven useful in identifying differential responses to therapy. Consequently, rational guidelines for selecting candidates for therapy are lacking. Nevertheless, empirical treatment based on these symptom clusters is commonly undertaken.

***Prokinetic drugs*** (see section 11.1.1): each of the drugs in this group has been shown to be effective in improving symptoms in functional dyspepsia. Most studies have been with *cisapride*, which has produced good to excellent global symptomatic responses in 60 to 90% of patients (superior to placebo). Although there are few comparative data for the 3 prokinetic agents, on current evidence the first choice especially for 'motility-like' dyspepsia should be cisapride 5 to 10mg 3 times daily, taken half an hour before meals. Treatment should be continued in most cases for 1 month before assessing effectiveness. If there is no improvement, another prokinetic agent (e.g. *domperidone* or *metoclopramide*) or a motilin agonist (e.g. *erythromycin* 125mg 2 or 3 times daily for a 2- to 4-week trial period) could be given. Combination prokinetic therapy is currently under study and macrolide compounds related to erythromycin but without antibacterial properties are being developed as prokinetic agents.

***Antisecretory agents*** (see section 4.1.2): trials with these drugs, in particular $H_2$-receptor antagonists, indicate that they are modestly superior to placebo in functional dyspepsia. Patients with 'ulcer-like' dyspepsia are most likely

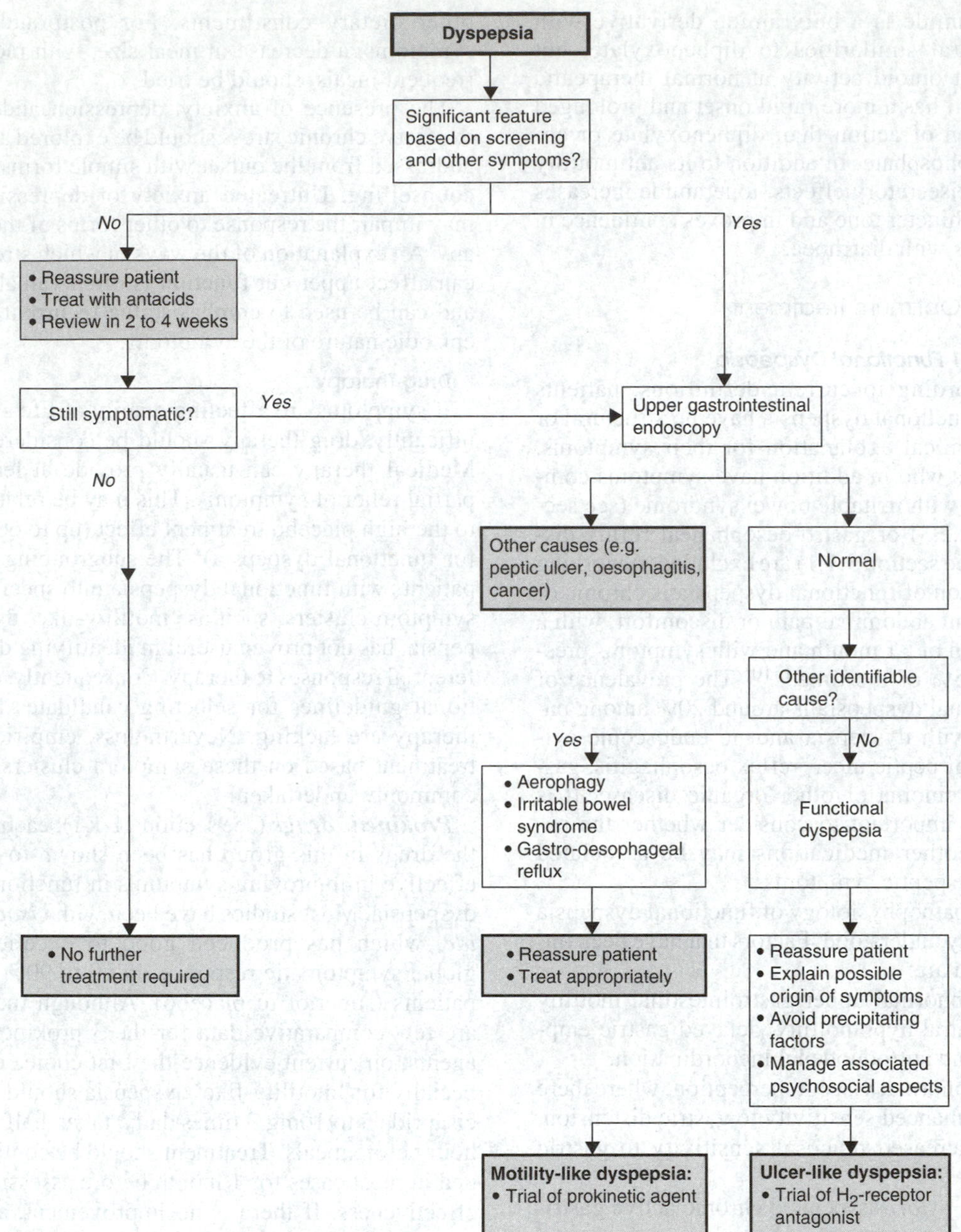


**Fig. 4.** Management of dyspepsia.

to respond. It is, thus, reasonable to suggest that antisecretory drugs should provide first-line treatment for this symptom cluster. If there is no improvement, a prokinetic agent can be tried. Further study of the role of sucralfate in functional dyspepsia is required.

The principles of managing dyspepsia are outlined in figure 4.

### *11.2.2 Gastroparesis*

In patients with severe chronic dyspepsia, the presence of gastroparesis should also be suspected. Gastroparesis is a functional disorder of gastric emptying, characterised by gastric stasis and atony, with chronic postprandial nausea and vomiting, occurring in the absence of mechanical pyloric or duodenal obstruction. It is believed to be an important factor in the development of upper gastrointestinal symptoms in some patients with chronic dyspepsia. At its worst, the patient experiences severe postprandial nausea and vomiting, with bodyweight loss developing over time. However, less severe symptoms such as early satiety, bloating, fullness and dyspepsia may also be clinical manifestations.

Dietary measures and a gradual recovery of contractile function usually result in symptomatic improvement. Treatment with *cisapride* results in sustained improvement of gastric emptying during long term management. Surgery is sometimes recommended in cases resistant to medical therapy, but its long term effectiveness is not established and in some cases, symptoms do not improve or may even be exacerbated by operative intervention.

### 11.2.3 Irritable Bowel Syndrome

Irritable bowel syndrome (IBS) can be defined as continuous or recurrent abdominal pain associated with defaecation or a change in bowel habit, and disordered defaecation and distension, in the absence of demonstrable organic disease.[310] The diagnosis depends on positive clinical features and the exclusion of organic disease. Most patients are under 40 years of age, but IBS occurs at any age, and predominantly in women, the ratio of females to males being 2 : 1. The pathophysiology of IBS, like functional dyspepsia, is poorly understood. Factors affecting gastrointestinal sensorimotor function that have been implicated include:

1) Abnormal gastrointestinal motor activity, especially in the small and large intestine, associated with disordered gut transit.

2) Abnormal visceral perception, in which 'up-regulation' of sensory afferent pathways appears to account for a heightened perception of normal gut sensations and may trigger disordered gut motility.

3) Dietary factors, whereby certain foods may cause diarrhoea by idiosyncratic, nonimmunological mechanisms.

4) Psychosocial factors, such as chronic stress, and abnormal illness behaviour.

5) Post-infective factors, whereby an acute attack of infectious diarrhoea may cause subtle damage to the enteric nervous system.

#### General/Dietary Measures

The most important aspect of therapy in IBS is a good clinician/patient relationship. The clinician must provide reassurance and support for a chronic or recurrent disorder, while at the same time addressing factors specific to each patient and modifying treatment approaches according to variations in symptom patterns. The clinician should emphasise to each patient that IBS is a genuine clinical entity in which the intestine is hypersensitive to various stimuli such as food and mental stress, and both luminal and central factors may interact to produce symptoms.

Most patients should have a trial of adequate dietary fibre supplementation. This can be achieved by including more fibre-rich foods in the diet, or by the use of semisynthetic bulking supplements. Well controlled trials of such treatment show that significant improvement occurs in patients with predominant constipation, but patients with an irregular bowel habit, and even those with predominant diarrhoea, may gain benefit.

Bran should be introduced at a dosage such as 1 tablespoon (15ml) twice daily with meals. The dosage can then be varied according to the response. The propensity for bran to provoke abdominal pain and distension should be mentioned and the patient advised to reduce the dose if these occur. At least 3 months' treatment may be necessary to assess effectiveness.

Semisynthetic bulking agents may be more effective than unprocessed bran, but are more expensive. As well as decreasing constipation, it has been suggested that they improve the overall well-being of patients, relative to placebo. In practice, there is little to choose between bran and the semisynthetic bulking agents, although the greater palatability of the latter may enhance acceptance by patients. If the patient's symptoms have not diminished after 3 months with one type of fibre, another type should be introduced for a similar trial period, since patients differ in their responses to different types of fibre.

Other dietary manipulation is also often indicated, particularly when a history of food-related exacerbation of symptoms is obtained. Fatty foods slow transit through the gut and may exacerbate symptoms of bloating and constipation. Excessive ingestion of carbohydrates (e.g. fructose, sorbitol or other complex carbohydrates) may provoke flatulence and diarrhoea. A diary kept for several weeks may assist the clinician and patient to identify such foods, although a delay between ingestion and the onset of symptoms may make identification of offending items difficult.

#### Drug Therapy

For dominant predictable symptoms, a trial of drug therapy, especially for short term relief, may be warranted.

For patients with ***predominant diarrhoea***, an antidiarrhoeal agent such as *loperamide* can be used prophylactically, or on an intermittent basis. In this setting, 2 to 4mg (1 or 2 capsules) daily during exacerbations is often all that is required. *Aluminium hydroxide* is a relatively inexpensive mild constipating agent that may have a role in patients with concomitant upper gastrointestinal symptoms.

For patients with ***predominant constipation***, if bulking agents are insufficient, *osmotic laxatives* such as magnesium salts or lactulose are often effective. The dose should be titrated carefully over a period of time before effectiveness is assessed. Long term use of stimulant laxatives such as senna should be actively discouraged, as neurogenic bowel paralysis may result, producing an intestinal pseudo-obstruction syndrome ('cathartic colon').

For patients with ***predominant pain***, especially if it occurs postprandially and predictably, *antispasmodic agents* can be tried. Unfortunately, no drug of proven effectiveness is currently available, and the high placebo response rate should be borne in mind. Dosages should be varied according to symptoms and the timing of administration adjusted to coincide with periods when symptoms are worst (e.g. postprandially, morning or evening). Patients should continue a high fibre diet during therapy with these agents, to enhance their effectiveness. Continuation of therapy for up to 3 months may be required before assessing the response. If no improvement occurs with one agent, it is reasonable to undertake a trial of another agent from this same group.

*Tricyclic antidepressants* can be useful in patients with more resistant predominant pain, even in the absence of clinical depressive symptoms. The mechanism of their action in this arena is poorly understood, but may involve both central analgesia and an anticholinergic action on the gut, in addition to relief of any depression. They should be given at doses lower than standard antidepressant doses (e.g. amitriptyline 10 to 25mg at night) and the patient should be encouraged to continue treatment for several months before effectiveness is assessed. Nocturnal administration minimises daytime drowsiness.

#### Other Treatment

In motivated patients, especially those with identifiable psychosocial stressors, various behavioural treatments are reported to be beneficial. These include stress management programmes and relaxation classes, progressive muscular relaxation, or brief psychotherapy. Combinations of psychological interventions and medical treatment appear to produce significant symptomatic improvement in some patients with IBS, especially those with intermittent abdominal pain and a shorter history of symptoms.

Hypnotherapy has also been shown to be beneficial in patients with refractory IBS, although any long term effect is yet to be substantiated. The mechanism of its effect is speculative, but it probably reduces stress levels and increases coping ability. Hypnotherapy may also modify gut sensitivity or alter contractile activity.

The management of IBS is summarised in figure 5.

### *11.2.4 Functional Constipation*

Constipation may be defined as a stool frequency of fewer than 3 per week, but a variety of other descriptions, especially the passage of hard or scybalous stools with excessive straining, are also used. The differential diagnosis of constipation includes intracolonic lesions such as colorectal carcinoma, metabolic causes such as hypothyroidism, drug-induced constipation, psychological disorders such as depression, and functional constipation.

A large number of drugs can cause or provoke constipation and include opioid-containing analgesic preparations and antitussives, certain antacids such as aluminium hydroxide, ferrous sulfate, verapamil, tricyclic antidepressants and anti-Parkinsonian drugs (especially when taken with antipsychotic agents with anticholinergic activity, such as chlorpromazine). Chemotherapeutic agents such as the vinca alkaloids (vincristine and vinblastine) may also cause constipation, which is exacerbated when patients also require opioid analgesics.

According to a recent international definition, functional constipation is defined as the presence, for at least 3 months, of 2 or more of the following: straining, hard stools, incomplete evacuation (each occurring on more than 25% of occasions), in association with 2 or fewer bowel actions per week.[310] Abdominal pain need not be present, and there should be no episodes of loose stools. This definition is used

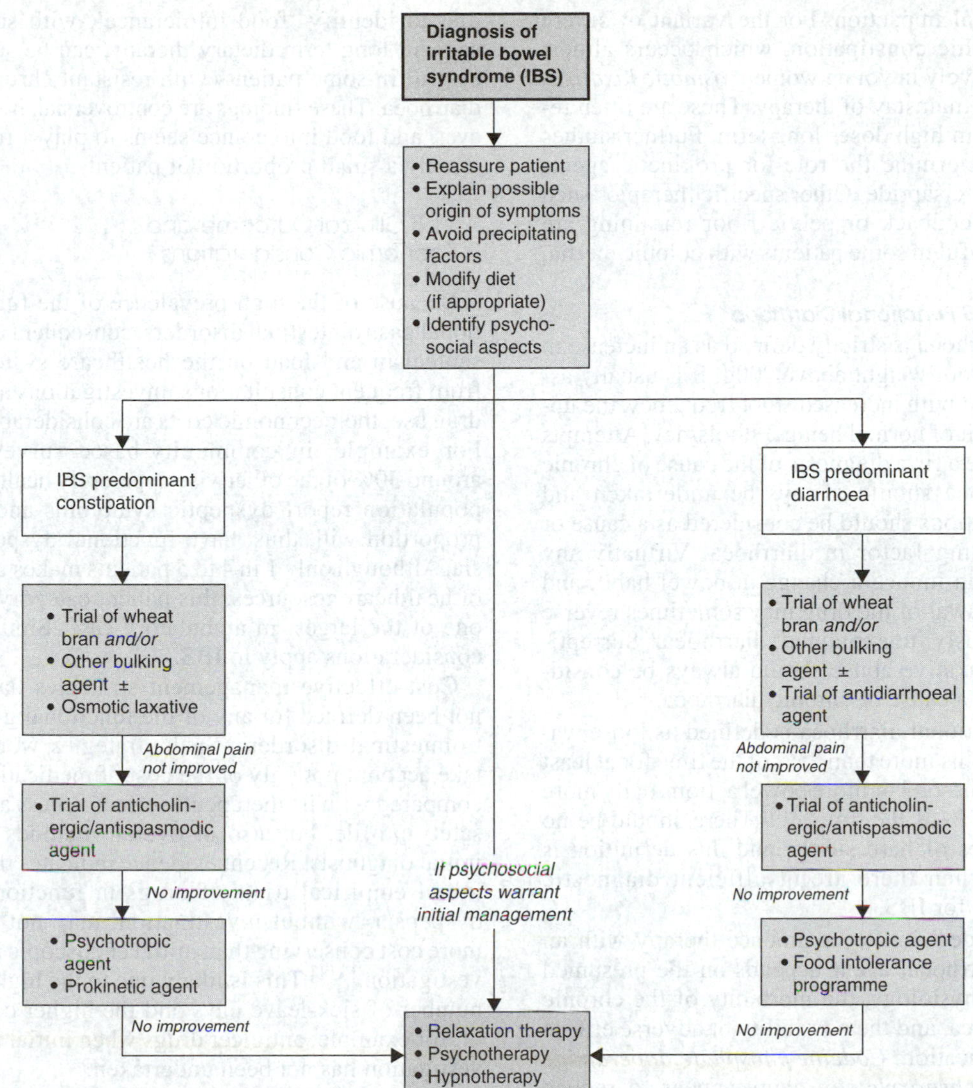


**Fig. 5.** Management of irritable bowel syndrome.

when there are insufficient criteria for IBS. The pathophysiology of functional constipation appears to involve a disorder of colonic motility. In some cases, a delay in colonic transit and/or disordered anorectal function can be objectively demonstrated.

Appropriate treatment of any primary condition is essential and may be sufficient to manage the constipation. Usually, constipation is best treated by simple measures such as ensuring an adequate intake of dietary fibre and fluid, encouragement of physical activity and ensuring the urge to defaecate is regularly heeded. Laxative preparations have little place in the long term management of simple constipation, unless all dietary measures have failed. Laxatives are, however, indicated in specific instances or disorders associated with constipation, such as disease or injury to the spinal cord, painful disorders of the anorectum, immobilisation such as after surgery or after myocardial infarction, or when constipating medications cannot be avoided, e.g. opioid analgesics in patients with malignancy. The response to different preparations varies from patient to patient. The dose should therefore be titrated to produce 1 or 2 soft formed stools daily.

*Suppositories* or *enema* preparations are useful in obstetrics, in the preparation of the large bowel for endoscopy, radiology or surgery, and in faecal impaction. For the variant of severe idiopathic constipation, which occurs almost exclusively in young women, *osmotic laxatives* are the mainstay of therapy. These are often required in high doses long term. Further studies may determine the role for prokinetic agents such as cisapride. Other specific therapies such as biofeedback or pelvic floor retraining are successful in some patients with colonic inertia.

#### 11.2.5 Functional Diarrhoea

Diarrhoea is strictly defined as an increase in daily stool weight above 200g. It is usually associated with increased stool frequency, the upper limit of normal being 3 stools/day. Attempts to make a firm diagnosis of the cause of chronic diarrhoea should always be undertaken and medications should be considered as a cause or provoking factor in diarrhoea. Virtually any drug can induce a change in bowel habit, and withdrawal of the drug may sometimes reverse previously unexplained diarrhoea. Surreptitious laxative abuse should always be considered as a cause of chronic diarrhoea.

Functional diarrhoea is defined as loose watery stools more than 75% of the time for at least 3 months, or 3 or more bowel actions daily more than 25% of the time.[310] There should be no episodes of hard stools, and this definition is used when there are insufficient diagnostic criteria for IBS.

The decision to commence therapy with an antidiarrhoeal agent depends on the presumed pathophysiology, the morbidity of the chronic diarrhoea, and the possibility of adverse effects of medication. *Codeine phosphate, loperamide* and *diphenoxylate/atropine* appear to reduce stool frequency to a similar extent, although the latter may be the least effective in producing a solid stool and relieving urgency and incontinence. Adverse effects are least common with loperamide. For these reasons, loperamide is usually the preferred agent for chronic diarrhoea. In patients in whom high doses of loperamide (up to 16 mg/day) have not been successful, a trial of *cholestyramine* can be employed. Theoretically, this will identify patients with idiopathic bile acid malabsorption, by preventing the secretory effect of bile salts on the colonic mucosa.

If available, the radiolabelled bile acid ($^{75}$Se-HCAT) test can lead to a more positive diagnosis of this condition, but its true prevalence in this group of patients is unknown. There are also some data indicating that an elimination diet to identify 'food intolerance', with subsequent long term dietary therapy, can be successful in some patients with resistant chronic diarrhoea. These findings are controversial, however, and food intolerance seems to play a role in only a small proportion of patients.

### 11.3 Clinical Outcome and Economic Considerations

Because of the high prevalence of the functional gastrointestinal disorders, consequent absenteeism and load on the healthcare system from frequent consultations, investigations and drug use, their economic costs are considerable. For example, in community-based surveys, around 30% of the otherwise apparently healthy population report dyspeptic symptoms and a proportion will, thus, have functional dyspepsia. Although only 1 in 4 to 5 patients makes use of healthcare resources, this patient category is one of the largest in ambulatory care. Similar considerations apply to IBS.

Cost-effective management strategies have not been defined for any of the functional gastrointestinal disorders. Such strategies would take account not only of the cost of medication compared with its therapeutic effectiveness and safety profile, but also of overall methods of initial diagnosis. Recent evidence indicates that initial empirical trials of drugs in functional dyspepsia, without investigation, may not be more cost conserving than initial endoscopic investigation.[311] This is likely due to the higher number of sick-leave days and the higher cost of, for example, antiulcer drugs when initial investigation has not been undertaken.

The use of drugs in functional gastrointestinal disorders is extensive,[312] despite the fact that most studies in functional dyspepsia[156] and IBS[313] have been methodologically flawed, and no drug is of proven benefit. Moreover, many of these drugs have significant adverse effects and an initial placebo effect may influence patients to continue drugs indefinitely even if they are ineffective. These considerations apply to all drug classes. Clearly, well controlled prospective studies in large patient populations are needed to obtain adequate cost-effectiveness data.

## 12. Use of Drugs in the Presence of Associated Gastrointestinal and Hepatic Disease

Abnormal drug responses can sometimes occur in patients with gastrointestinal or liver disease, because of the effects of drugs on gastrointestinal or liver pathology, and also occasionally because of altered pharmacokinetics (see section 1).

## 12.1 Peptic Ulcer

The chief risk of peptic ulcer in terms of the use of other drugs relates to the use of NSAIDs. Figure 6 provides data on the relative risks associated with NSAIDs in both gastric and duodenal ulcer. A 10-fold greater prevalence of gastric ulcer, peptic ulcer or both has been shown in patients receiving NSAIDs long term than would be expected in the general population. However, it is usually impossible to decide whether NSAID-associated ulcer is a new lesion or an exacerbation of a pre-existing ulcer.

Treatment of analgesic-associated ulcers involves a review of the need for analgesic drugs, the use of paracetamol for pain relief, and the replacement of other antiulcer drugs with misoprostol.

## 12.2 Nausea and Vomiting

Direct gastric irritants that may induce or exacerbate nausea include iron preparations and NSAIDs. Many other drugs may induce nausea with or without vomiting, usually in the absence of pain. One drug that commonly induces nausea is erythromycin. Drugs that have central emetic effects include digoxin, morphine and some chemotherapeutic agents. Other drugs such as salicylates, aminophylline and ipecac stimulate the medullary vomiting centre.

Before an extensive diagnostic evaluation for nausea and vomiting is undertaken, it is important to discontinue potentially offending drugs, wherever possible. If a drug cannot be stopped, monitoring its plasma concentration may be helpful diagnostically in certain situations, e.g. with digoxin or theophylline.

## 12.3 Pancreatitis

During an acute attack of pancreatitis, pancreatic stimulation should be avoided. This is generally achieved by fasting the patient. The use of any drug that can result in pancreatic stimulation (e.g. cholecystokinin, its analogue sincalide, or cholinergic drugs) should be avoided, as should anticholinergic drugs, as they may exacerbate associated ileus. During a prolonged severe attack of acute pancreatitis, parenteral hyperalimentation may be of value in providing nutritional support for the patient while minimising pancreatic stimulation.

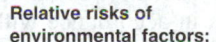


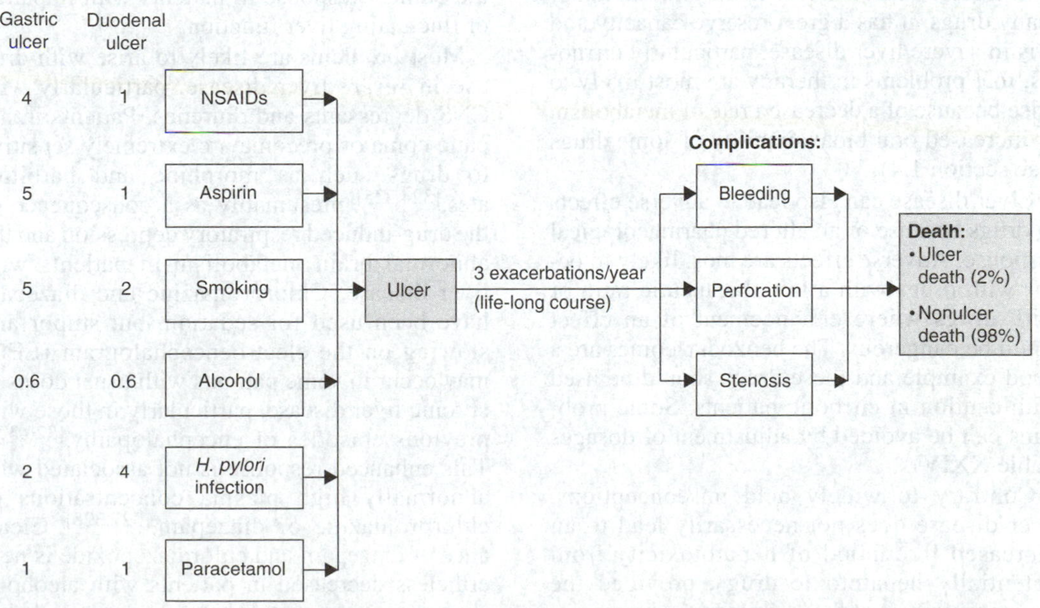


**Fig. 6.** Natural history of chronic peptic ulcer and the relative risks associated with environmental factors in gastric and duodenal ulcer. *Abbreviations:* NSAID = nonsteroidal anti-inflammatory drug; *H. pylori* = *Helicobacter pylori.*

Opioid analgesics such as morphine increase the tone of the sphincter of Oddi and theoretically can exacerbate the severity of an attack by increasing pressure in the pancreatic ductular system (see section 7.2.1). Naturally, if drug-induced pancreatitis is suspected (e.g. with azathioprine), the offending agent should be withdrawn.

In chronic pancreatitis, pain relief often requires strong analgesics and there is considerable potential for dependence, particularly in patients already addicted to alcohol. Patients are best managed in a multidisciplinary pain clinic. Exocrine insufficiency will result in malabsorption of fat soluble drugs and vitamins unless adequate enzyme replacement therapy is given.

### 12.4 Liver Diseases

When drugs are used in a patient with liver disease, any problem which is likely to arise depends very largely on the nature and severity of the liver disease itself and on the pharmacological action and pharmacokinetic properties of the particular drug. While an accurate assessment of the severity of liver disease is essential, unlike renal disease, there is no simple test of liver function that enables the therapeutic regimen to be easily adjusted for all drugs that are mainly eliminated by hepatic metabolism (see section 1.4 and also appendix F). Although the liver has an important role in the elimination of many drugs, it has a great reserve capacity and it is in severe liver disease, particularly cirrhosis, that problems in therapy are most likely to arise because of a decreased rate of metabolism or increased oral bioavailability of some drugs (see section 1.4).

Liver disease can also lead to adverse effects of drugs because of an altered pharmacological response. Adverse effects are most likely to occur with drugs with a low therapeutic ratio or with drugs where enhancement of an effect could be dangerous. The benzodiazepines are a good example and these drugs should be used with caution in cirrhotic patients. Some problems can be avoided by adjustment of dosages (table XXIV).

Contrary to widely held misconceptions, liver disease does not necessarily lead to an increased likelihood of hepatotoxicity from potentially hepatotoxic drugs, provided the hepatotoxicity is of the idiosyncratic, hypersensitivity type. If hepatotoxicity is dose-related, this does not apply. For example, patients with impaired liver function are much more likely to sustain liver damage from pyrazinamide and rifampicin than tuberculosis patients with normal liver function, and dosages should be reduced accordingly.[321,322] Potentially hepatotoxic drugs should only be used in liver disease if the benefits outweigh the risks. Such patients already have a reduced hepatic reserve and are not only at greater risk of further hepatic damage (i.e. independently of the type of damage induced by the drugs), but use of potentially hepatotoxic drugs may confuse patient management if it depends on biochemical monitoring.

The following guidelines are suggested when use of drugs is considered in patients with liver disease:[323]

1) As in all therapeutic decisions, evaluate the possible benefit to risks. If the risks outweigh the benefits, do not prescribe the drug.

2) If possible, select drugs that have no potential for hepatotoxicity.

3) If possible, select drugs that are mainly eliminated unchanged by the kidney.

4) Avoid drugs that have an effect on the central nervous system.

5) Start treatment with small doses and increase cautiously.

6) Clinical and laboratory observations, including estimations of plasma drug concentrations where feasible, provide the best means for adjusting dosage regimens in accordance with the clinical response in patients with impaired or fluctuating liver function.

Most problems are likely to arise with drug use in *severe* liver disease, particularly with CNS depressants and diuretics. Patients in hepatic coma or precoma are extremely sensitive to drugs such as morphine and barbiturates,[324,325] presumably as a consequence of the drug-induced respiratory depression and the abnormal brain metabolism in patients with liver disease. Chlorpromazine and diazepam have been used for sedation, but stupor and slowing on the electroencephalogram (EEG) may occur in some patients with usual doses in chronic liver disease, particularly in those with previous episodes of encephalopathy.[326,327] This enhanced response is not associated with abnormally high plasma concentrations of chlorpromazine or diazepam.[327,328] Clearance of diazepam and chlordiazepoxide is nevertheless decreased in patients with alcoholic cirrhosis. Oxazepam or lorazepam are probably the safest drugs for sedation in liver disease. Unlike diazepam and chlordiazepoxide, they do

**Table XXIV.** Examples of altered drug responses in severe liver disease[a]

| Drug | Notes |
|---|---|
| Morphine<br>Barbiturates<br>Chlorpromazine<br>Monoamine oxidase inhibitors | May precipitate encephalopathy in those with hepatic precoma. Due to altered brain sensitivity, respiratory depression |
| Diuretics | Overvigorous diuretic therapy can precipitate encephalopathy in those with cirrhotic oedema and ascites. Due to excessive potassium loss |
| Oral anticoagulants | Enhanced response due to reduced absorption of vitamin K in obstructive jaundice or decreased production of vitamin K-dependent clotting factors in hepatitis, cirrhosis (see also chapter 26) |
| Oral antidiabetic drugs | Increased risk of symptomatic hypoglycaemia with sulphonylureas and of lactic acidosis with biguanides (see also chapter 19) |
| Theophylline | Increased risk of toxicity if usual doses used. Due to impaired hepatic metabolism[60,61] |
| Clomethiazole (chlormethiazole) | Increased risk of toxicity if usual doses used. Due to impaired hepatic metabolism and increased oral bioavailability |
| Chloramphenicol | Increased risk of haematological toxicity; most likely in presence of both ascites and jaundice. Due to impaired hepatic metabolism (conjugation) of drug[340] |
| Pyrazinamide<br>Rifampicin | Increased risk of hepatic toxicity in patients with impaired liver function if usual doses used[314] |
| Ergotamine | Ergot poisoning has occurred in presence of acute viral hepatitis,[315] and in association with drug-induced jaundice.[316] Due to impaired hepatic metabolism |
| Phenytoin | Increased risk of CNS toxicity in some patients with usual dosages,[317] particularly if liver disease associated with renal impairment. Due to impaired hepatic metabolism and/or delayed clearance. Probably dependent on dose used |
| Lidocaine (lignocaine) | Increased risk of severe CNS toxicity.[318] Due to impaired hepatic elimination |
| Niridazole | Increased incidence of adverse CNS effects in bilharziasis patients with liver complications.[319] Due to development of portal systemic shunts and increased bioavailability |
| Tubocurarine<br>Pancuronium<br>Suxamethonium (succinylcholine) | Decreased plasma cholinesterase levels due to liver cell damage may prolong activity of suxamethonium and decrease activity of nondepolarising relaxants (e.g. tubocurarine, pancuronium). However, with pancuronium, while a high initial dose is required for adequate relaxation, clearance is delayed with risk of prolonged activity if repeated doses are excessive (see also chapter 12) |
| Vitamin D | Failure of conventional vitamin D therapy in primary biliary cirrhosis due to impaired hepatic hydroxylation of vitamin D.[320] Calcifediol (25-hydroxyvitamin $D_3$) is the preferred form of vitamin D in liver disease |

a See also discussion in section 12.4 and appendix F.

not form active metabolites and are not likely to accumulate with repeat doses in liver disease, but they should still be given with care and in smaller doses because of possible increased cerebral sensitivity.

Clomethiazole is widely used for delirium tremens in patients with alcoholic cirrhosis, but prolonged sedation and intoxication may occur if its dosage is not reduced. This is especially important when clomethiazole is given orally, as its bioavailability is increased markedly due to reduced hepatic first-pass metabolism.[54]

Morphine should never be given to patients with liver disease who have a history of hepatic encephalopathy or who have evidence of jaundice or ascites. Nor should it be given to patients with liver disease complicated by gastrointestinal bleeding.[324] Overvigorous diuretic treatment of patients with cirrhotic oedema and ascites can precipitate hepatic coma, particularly in those with prior hepatic encephalopathy.[329-331] Monoamine oxidase inhibitors are also prone to precipitate hepatic precoma in patients with cirrhosis.[332] Small doses of a nonsedating tricyclic drug such as protriptyline may be used if an antidepressant is indicated.

Ergot poisoning, which is dramatically demonstrable, is common in the presence of acute liver disease (e.g. acute viral hepatitis) because of a reduced rate of elimination.[315] Other abnormal drug responses due to alteration of pharmacokinetic processes are shown in table XXIV. Oral anticoagulants should be avoided in liver disease (due to depression of vitamin K-dependent clotting factor synthesis) and in biliary obstruction (due to impaired vitamin K absorption). In these situations, there is an increased and variable response to oral anticoagulants (see chapter 26; sect. 3.1.5).

Oral contraceptives should not be prescribed in the presence of cholestatic hepatobiliary disease of any type (see chapter 18; sect. 10.2).

However, they are probably safe in acute viral hepatitis,[333] and also in those with a past history of liver disease, provided there is no history of cholestasis or pruritus during pregnancy or following use of estrogens,[334] although the risk of cholestasis developing during use of oral contraceptives (usually in the first few cycles) in such patients may have been exaggerated, at least with some formulations,[335] and is probably most likely in those populations (e.g. Chile, parts of Scandinavia) where genetic factors seem to predispose to cholestasis of pregnancy and oral contraceptive-related jaundice.[336,337] Both are probably caused by estrogens, but progestagens (particularly 19-nortestosterone derivatives) may be occasionally responsible and may also have an additive effect with the estrogen.[337] The widespread use of low-dose estrogen-containing formulations has probably contributed to a reduction in the incidence of oral contraceptive-related jaundice.

## 12.5 Inflammatory Bowel Disease

### *12.5.1 Drugs that May Precipitate Relapse*

NSAIDs can precipitate intestinal inflammation, but can also exacerbate intestinal inflammation in patients with inflammatory bowel disease.[338] The mechanisms underlying this observation are only partly understood, but include inhibition of synthesis of anti-inflammatory eicosanoids such as prostaglandin $E_2$ and enhancement of epithelial permeability to luminal macromolecules. NSAIDs are, however, not absolutely contraindicated and decisions regarding their use in patients with inflammatory bowel disease should be made by balancing the likely effectiveness of the drug against the risk of exacerbating the condition.

Antibiotics, particularly those with a broad spectrum of activity, may precipitate relapse of colitis, if their use is associated with *Clostridium difficile* infection or other causes of antibiotic-induced colitis. Patients with ulcerative colitis are less likely to recover spontaneously from antibiotic-induced colitis and often require corticosteroid therapy. However, this complication is unpredictable and the decision to use antibiotics should be made on the merits of the infection being treated, and not on the basis of the presence or absence of inflammatory bowel disease.

The use of oral contraceptives has been tenuously associated with development of colitis (of possibly ischaemic origin), but any association with ulcerative colitis or Crohn's disease remains uncertain. Chenodeoxycholic acid frequently induces diarrhoea and is metabolised by colonic bacteria to lithocholic acid, which is toxic to plasma membranes. For both of these reasons, it should not be used in patients with inflammatory bowel disease.

Other drugs that have, rarely, been associated with the development of colitis or enteritis include auranofin, retinoids and flucytosine. There are no guidelines on their use in patients with inflammatory bowel disease, but, if indicated, they should be used with careful attention to disease activity.

### *12.5.2 Drugs that May Precipitate Complications*

Opioids and anticholinergic drugs should be avoided in patients with severe colitis, because of the risk of precipitating toxic megacolon. In patients with stenotic small intestinal regions in Crohn's disease, drugs that disperse poorly should be avoided, particularly if high concentrations are toxic to tissues, because they might cause acute obstruction or exacerbation of the local inflammatory process. Slow-release potassium chloride preparations are of particular importance in this regard.

The use of anticoagulants (especially heparin) in patients with inflammatory bowel disease may be associated with increased gastrointestinal bleeding. However, other than in exceptional circumstances, decisions regarding their use should not be adversely influenced by the presence of active inflammatory bowel disease.

### *12.5.3 Drugs that Potentially Interfere with Nutritional Intake*

Malnutrition is common in seriously ill patients with inflammatory bowel disease and drugs that potentially interfere with the intake of food should be avoided. Oral iron therapy is frequently associated with nausea and is not recommended in seriously ill patients. If iron repletion is considered necessary in the short term, parenteral iron therapy is preferred. Oral iron therapy can be instituted when the patient has shown considerable improvement in disease activity.

The choice of antibiotics for intercurrent infection or to treat complications of inflammatory bowel disease, should also be considered carefully. For example, erythromycin therapy is frequently associated with nausea and should be avoided (see also section 12.3).

### 12.6 Functional Gastrointestinal Disease

Among patients with functional dyspepsia, it is usually only in those with delayed gastric emptying (idiopathic gastroparesis) that alterations in absorption of other drugs may occur. Likewise, in both irritable bowel syndrome and functional diarrhoea, it is among patients with abnormally rapid small bowel transit that absorption of other drugs, especially enteric-coated or slow-release formulations, may theoretically be affected. However, these considerations do not normally constitute a significant clinical problem.

#### Further Reading

Lynn RB, Friedman, LS. Irritable bowel syndrome. New England Journal Medicine 1993; 329: 1940-5

Snape Jr WJ, editor. Pathogenesis of functional bowel disease. New York: Plenum Publishing Corporation, 1989

Smout AJPM, Akkermanns LMA. Normal and disturbed motility of the gastrointestinal tract. Petersfield: Wrightson Biomedical Publishing, 1992

#### References


1. Nimmo WS. Drugs, diseases and altered gastric emptying. Clinical Pharmacokinetics 1976; 1: 189
2. Parsons RL. Drug absorption in gastrointestinal disease with particular reference to malabsorption syndromes. Clinical Pharmacokinetics 1977; 2: 45
3. Gubbins PO, Bertch KE. Drug absorption in gastrointestinal disease and surgery. Pharmacotherapy 1989; 9: 285-95
4. Gubbins PO, Bertch KE. Drug absorption in gastrointestinal disease and surgery: clinical pharmacokinetic and therapeutic implications. Clinical Pharmacokinetics 1991; 21: 431-47
5. Kaplan SA. Absorption screening and new drug development. In: Prescott LF, Nimmo J, editors. Drug absorption: proceedings of the Edinburgh International Conference. Auckland: Adis Press, 1979: 144-56
6. Robinson DH, Narducci WA, Veda T, et al. In: Dipiro et al., editors. Pharmacotherapy: a pathophysiological approach. Amsterdam: Elsevier Science Publishing Co., 1989: 15-34
7. Pottage A, Nimmo J, Prescott LF. The absorption of aspirin and paracetamol in patients with achlorhydria. Journal of Pharmacy and Pharmacology 1974; 26: 144
8. Schultz NJ. Principles of drug therapy. Journal of Enterostomal Therapy 1987; 14: 212-5
9. Goldman P, Peppercorn MA, Goldin BR. Drugs metabolised by intestinal microflora. In: Morselli et al., editors. Drug interactions. New York: Raven Press, 1974: 91
10. Heading RC, Nimmo J, Prescott LF, et al. The dependence of paracetamol absorption on the rate of gastric emptying. British Journal of Pharmacology 1973; 47: 415
11. Nimmo J, Heading RC, Tothill P, et al. Pharmacological modification of gastric emptying: effects of propantheline and metoclopramide on paracetamol absorption. British Medical Journal 1973; 1: 587
12. Harris FC. Pyloric stenosis: hold-up of enteric coated aspirin tablets. British Journal of Surgery 1973; 60: 979
13. Leonards JR, Levy G. Absorption and metabolism of aspirin administered in enteric-coated tablets. Journal of the American Medical Association 1965; 193: 99
14. Volans GN. Migraine and drug absorption. Clinical Pharmacokinetics 1978; 3: 313
15. Prescott LF. Gastrointestinal absorption of drugs. Medical Clinics of North America 1974; 48: 907
16. Bergan T, Lolekha S, Cheong MD, et al. Consequences of diarrhoeal disease on the pharmacokinetics of norfloxacin. Scandinavian Journal of Infectious Diseases 1988; 56: 11-3
17. Melander A. Influence of food on the bioavailability of drugs. Clinical Pharmacokinetics 1978; 3: 337
18. McLean AJ, Melander A. The influence of food on oral drug usage. Current Therapeutics 1983; 24(9): 51
19. Welling PG. Interactions affecting drug absorption. Clinical Pharmacokinetics 1984; 9: 404
20. Hurwitz A. Antacid therapy and drug kinetics. Clinical Pharmacokinetics 1977; 2: 269
21. Parsons RL, Kaye CM, Raymond K. Pharmacokinetics of salicylate and indomethacin in coeliac disease. European Journal of Clinical Pharmacology 1977; 11: 473
22. Parsons RL, Kaye CM, Raymond K, et al. Absorption of propranolol and practolol in coeliac disease. Gut 1976; 17: 139
23. Schneider RE, Babb J, Bishop H, et al. Plasma levels of propranolol in treated patients with coeliac disease and patients with Crohn's disease. British Medical Journal 1976; 2: 794
24. Parsons RL, Paddock GM, Hossack GA, et al. Antibiotic absorption in Crohn's disease. In: Williams & Geddes, editors. Chemotherapy, Vol. 4, Pharmacology of antibiotics. New York: Plenum Press, 1976: 219
25. Melander A, Kahlmeter G, Kamme C, et al. Bioavailability of metronidazole in fasting and non-fasting healthy subjects and in patients with Crohn's disease. European Journal of Clinical Pharmacology 1977; 12: 69
26. Routledge PA, Shand DG. Clinical pharmacokinetics of propranolol. Clinical Pharmacokinetics 1979; 4: 73
27. Lake-Bakaar G, Tom W, Lake-Bakaar D, et al. Gastropathy and ketoconazole malabsorption in the acquired immunodeficiency syndrome (AIDS). Annals of Internal Medicine 1988; 109: 471-3
28. Drew RH, Perfect JR, Gallis HA. Use of fluconazole in a patient with documented malabsorption of ketoconazole. Clinical Pharmacy 1988; 7: 622-3
29. Heizer WD, Smith TW, Goldfinger SE. Absorption of digoxin in patients with malabsorption syndromes. New England Journal of Medicine 1971; 285: 257
30. Sokol GH, Greenblatt DJ, Lloyd BL, et al. Effect of abdominal radiation therapy on drug absorption in humans. Journal of Clinical Pharmacology 1978; 18: 388
31. Bolme P, Eriksson M, Stintzing G. The gastrointestinal absorption of penicillin V in children with suspected coeliac disease. Acta Paediatrica Scandinavica 1977; 66: 573
32. Hartiala K. Metabolism of hormones, drugs and other substances by the gut. Physiological Reviews 1973; 53: 496
33. Talseth T. Clinical pharmacokinetics of hydralazine. Clinical Pharmacokinetics 1977; 2: 317
34. Rivera-Calimlim L, Castaneda L, Lasagna L. Effects of mode of management of plasma chlorpromazine in psychiatric patients. Clinical Pharmacology and Therapeutics 1973; 14: 978

35. Curry SH, D'Mello A, Mould GP. Destruction of chlorpromazine during absorption in the rat in vitro and in vivo. British Journal of Pharmacology 1971; 42: 403
36. Dahl SG, Strandgord RE. Pharmacokinetics of chlorpromazine after single and chronic dosage. Clinical Pharmacology and Therapeutics 1977; 21: 437
37. Levitt MD. Lack of clinical significance of the interaction between $H_2$-receptor antagonists and ethanol. Alimentary Pharmacology and Therapeutics 1993; 7: 131-8
38. Crawford DH, Shepherd RW, Halliday JW, et al. Body composition in nonalcoholic cirrhosis: the effect of disease etiology and severity on nutritional compartments. Gastroenterology 1994; 106: 1611-7
39. Hoyumpa HM, Schenker S. Major drug interactions: effects of liver disease, alcohol and malnutrition. Annual Review of Medicine 1982; 33: 113
40. Hooper WD, Bochner F, Eadie MJ, et al. Plasma protein binding of diphenylhydantoin: effects of sex hormones, renal and hepatic disease. Clinical Pharmacology and Therapeutics 1974; 15: 276
41. Olsen GD, Bennett WM, Porter GA. Morphine and phenytoin binding to plasma proteins in renal and hepatic failure. Clinical Pharmacology and Therapeutics 1975; 17: 677
42. Piafsky KM, Borgå O, Odar-Cederlöff I, et al. Increased plasma protein binding of propranolol and chlorpromazine mediated by disease-induced elevations of plasma $\alpha_1$-acid glycoprotein. New England Journal of Medicine 1978; 299: 1435
43. Wilkinson GR, Schenker S. Drug disposition and liver disease. Drug Metabolism Reviews 1975; 4: 139
44. Wilkinson GR, Schenker S. Effect of liver disease on drug disposition in man. Biochemical Pharmacology 1976; 25: 2675
45. McLean AJ, Morgan DJ. Clinical pharmacokinetics in patients with liver disease. Clinical Pharmacokinetics 1991; 21: 42-69 and 1995; 29: 370-91
46. Bass NM, Williams RL. Guide to drug dosage in hepatic disease. Clinical Pharmacokinetics 1988; 15: 396-420
47. Branch RA, Herbert CM, Read AE. Determinants of serum antipyrine half-lives in patients with liver disease. Gut 1973; 14: 569
48. Farrell GC, Cooksley WGE, Hart P, et al. Drug metabolism in liver disease. Identification of patients with impaired hepatic drug metabolism. Gastroenterology 1978; 75: 580
49. Nies AS, Shand DG, Wilkinson GR. Altered hepatic blood flow and drug disposition. Clinical Pharmacokinetics 1976; 1: 135
50. Gugler R, Lain P, Azarnoff DL. Effect of portacaval shunt on the disposition of drugs with and without first-pass effect. Journal of Pharmacology and Experimental Therapeutics 1975; 195: 416
51. Neal EA, Meffin PJ, Gregory PB, et al. Enhanced bioavailability and decreased clearance of analgesics in patients with cirrhosis. Gastroenterology 1979; 77: 55
52. Wood AJJ, Kornhauser DM, Wilkinson GR, et al. The influence of cirrhosis on steady-state blood concentrations of unbound propranolol after oral administration. Clinical Pharmacokinetics 1978; 3: 478
53. Homeida M, Jackson L, Roberts CJC. Decreased first pass metabolism of labetalol in chronic liver disease. British Medical Journal 1978; 2: 1048
54. Pentikainen PJ, Neuvonen PJ, Tarpila S, et al. Effect of cirrhosis of the liver on the pharmacokinetics of chlormethiazole. British Medical Journal 1978; 2: 861
55. Adjepon-Yamoah KK, Nimmo J, Prescott LF. Gross impairment of hepatic drug metabolism in a patient with chronic liver disease. British Medical Journal 1974; 4: 387
56. Thomson PD, Melmon KL, Richardson JA, et al. Lidocaine pharmacokinetics in advanced heart failure, liver disease, and renal failure in humans. Annals of Internal Medicine 1973; 78: 499
57. Huet PM, Villeneuve JP. Determinants of drug disposition in patients with cirrhosis. Hepatology 1983; 3: 913-8
58. Crotty B, Watson KJ, Desmond PV, et al. Hepatic extraction of morphine is impaired in cirrhosis. European Journal of Clinical Pharmacology 1989; 36: 501-6
59. Hasselstrom J, Eriksson S, Persson A, et al. The metabolism and bioavailability of morphine in patients with severe liver cirrhosis. British Journal of Clinical Pharmacology 1990; 29: 289-97
60. Mangione A, Imhoff TE, Lee RV, et al. Pharmacokinetics of theophylline in hepatic disease. Chest 1978; 73: 616
61. Piafsky KM, Sitar DS, Rango RE, et al. Theophylline disposition in patients with hepatic cirrhosis. New England Journal of Medicine 1977; 296: 1495
62. Colli A, Buccino G, Cocciolo M, et al. Disposition of a flow-limited drug (lidocaine) and a metabolic capacity-limited drug (theophylline) in liver cirrhosis. Clinical Pharmacology and Therapeutics 1988; 44: 642-9
63. Gorbach SL. Travellers' diarrhea. New England Journal of Medicine 1982; 307: 881
64. Villeneuve JP, Thibeault MJ, Ampelas M, et al. Drug disposition in patients with HBsAg-positive chronic liver disease. Digestive Diseases and Sciences 1987; 32: 710-4
65. Tytgat GNJ, editor. Gastro-oesophageal reflux and gastric stasis: pathophysiology, diagnosis and therapy. Chester: Adis International Limited, 1991
66. Grant SM, Langtry HD, Brogden RN. Ranitidine: an updated review of its pharmacodynamic and pharmacokinetic properties and therapeutic use in peptic ulcer disease and other allied diseases. Drugs 1989; 37: 801-70
67. Langtry HD, Grant SM, Goa KL. Famotidine: an updated review of its pharmacodynamic and pharmacokinetic properties, and therapeutic use in peptic ulcer disease and other allied diseases. Drugs 1989; 38: 551-90
68. Price AH, Brogden RN. Nizatidine: a preliminary review of its pharmacodynamic and pharmacokinetic properties, and its therapeutic use in peptic ulcer disease. Drugs 1988; 36: 521-39
69. Murdoch D, McTavish D. Roxatidine acetate: a review of its pharmacodynamic and pharmacokinetic properties, and its therapeutic potential in peptic ulcer disease and related disorders. Drugs 1991; 42: 240-60
70. DeVault KR, Castell MO. Guidelines for the diagnosis and treatment of gastroesophageal reflux disease. Archives of Internal Medicine 1995; 155: 2165
71. Wiseman LR, Faulds D. Cisapride: an updated review of its pharmacology and therapeutic efficacy as a prokinetic agent in gastrointestinal motility disorders. Drugs 1994; 47: 116-52
72. Wilde MI, McTavish D. Omeprazole: an update of its pharmacology and therapeutic use in acid-related disorders. Drugs 1994; 48: 9-132
73. Spencer CM, Faulds D. Lansoprazole: a reappraisal of its pharmacodynamic and pharmacokinetic proper-

ties, and its therapeutic efficacy in acid-related disorders. Drugs 1994; 48: 404-30

74. Fitton A, Wiseman L. Pantoprazole: a review of its pharmacological properties and therapeutic use in acid-related disorders. Drugs 1996; 51: 460-82
75. Vigneri S, Termini R, Leandro G, et al. A comparison of five maintenance therapies for reflux esophagitis. New England Journal of Medicine 1995; 333: 1106-10
76. Hinder RA, Filipi CJ, Wetscher G, et al. Laparoscopic Nissen fundoplication is an effective treatment for gastroesophageal reflux disease. Annals of Surgery 1994; 200: 472
77. Skinner DB, Belsey RHR. Surgical management of esophageal reflux and hiatus hernia: long term results with 1030 patients. Journal of Thoracic Cardiovascular Surgery 1967; 53: 33
78. Bate CM, Richardson PDI. Clinical and economic factors in the selection of drugs for gastroesophageal reflux disease. PharmacoEconomics 1993; 3: 94-9
79. Green JRB, Bate CM, Copeman MB, et al. A comparison of the cost-effectiveness of omeprazole and ranitidine in reflux oesophagitis. British Journal of Medical Economics 1995; 8: 157-69
80. Bloom BS, Hillman AL, LaMont B, et al. Omeprazole or ranitidine plus metoclopramide for patients with severe erosive oesophagitis: a cost-effective analysis. PharmacoEconomics 1995; 8: 343-9
81. Orlando RC, Bozymski EM. Clinical and manometric effects of nitroglycerin in diffuse esophageal speasm. New England Journal of Medicine 1973; 289: 23
82. Mellow MH. Effect of isosorbide and hydralazine in painful primary esophageal motility disorders. Gastroenterology 1982; 83: 364
83. Short TP, Thomas E. An overview of the role of calcium antagonists in the treatment of achalasia and diffuse oesophageal spasm. Drugs 1992; 43: 177-84
84. Coghlan JG, Gilligan D, Humphries H, et al. *Campylobacter pylori* and recurrence of duodenal ulcers: a 12-month follow-up study. Lancet 1987; 2: 1109-11
85. Graham DY, Lew GM, Klein PD, et al. Effect of treatment of *Helicobacter pylori* infection on the long-term recurrence of gastric or duodenal ulcer. Annals of Internal Medicine 1992; 116: 705-8
86. Hentschel E, Brandstatter G, Dragosics B, et al. Effect of ranitidine and amoxicillin plus metronidazole on the eradication of *Helicobacter pylori* and the recurrence of duodenal ulcer. New England Journal of Medicine 1993; 328: 308-12
87. Marshall BJ, Warren JR. Unidentified curved bacilli in the stomach of patients with gastritis and peptic ulceration. Lancet 1984; 1: 1311-4
88. Marshall BJ, Goodwin CS, Warren JR, et al. Prospective double-blind trial of duodenal ulcer relapse after eradication of *Campylobacter pylori*. Lancet 1988; 2: 1437-41
89. Warren JR. Unidentified curved bacilli on gastric epithelium in active chronic gastritis. Lancet 1983; 1: 1273
90. Barbezat GO. The current status of *Helicobacter pylori* as a pathogen in upper gastrointestinal tract. New Zealand Medical Journal 1994; 107: 478-80
91. Marshall BJ. *Helicobacter pylori*. American Journal of Gastroenterology 1994; 89: S116-28
92. NIH Consensus Development Panel on *Helicobacter pylori* in peptic ulcer disease: *Helicobacter pylori* in peptic ulcer disease. Journal of the American Medical Association 1994; 272: 65-9
93. Soll AH, for the Practice Parameters Committee of the American College of Gastroenterology. Medical treatment of peptic ulcer disease. Practice guidelines. Journal of the American Medical Association 1996; 275: 622-9
94. Forbes GM, Glaser ME, Cullen FJE, et al. Duodenal ulcer treated with *Helicobacter pylori* eradication: seven year follow-up. Lancet 1994; 343: 258-60
95. Rauws EAJ, van der Hulst RWM. Current guidelines for the eradication of *Helicobacter pylori* in peptic ulcer disease. Drugs 1995; 50: 984-90
96. Piper DW, Fenton BH. pH Stability and activity curves of pepsin with special reference to their clinical importance. Gut 1965; 6: 506
97. Peterson WL, Sturdevant RAL, Frankl HD, et al. Healing of duodenal ulcer with an antacid regimen. New England Journal of Medicine 1977; 297: 341
98. Ippoliti AF, Sturdevant RAL, Isenberg JI, et al. Cimetidine versus intensive antiacid therapy for duodenal ulcer. Gastroenterology 1978; 74: 393
99. Berstad A, Rydning A, Aadland E, et al. Controlled trial of duodenal ulcer healing with antacid tablets. Scandinavian Journal of Gastroenterology 1982; 17: 953
100. Kumar N, Viz JL, Karol A. Controlled therapeutic trial to determine the optimum dose of antacids in duodenal ulcer. Gut 1984; 25: 1199
101. Lam SK. Antacids: the past, present and future. In: Bailliere's Clinical gastroenterology. Peptic ulceration. Balliere Tindall/WB Saunders, 1988: 641-54
102. Rydning A, Weberg R, Lange O, et al. Healing of benign gastric ulcer with low-dose antacids and fiber diet. Gastroenterology 1986; 91: 56
103. Duncan WAM, Parsons ME. Reminiscences of the development of cimetidine. Gastroenterology 1980; 78: 620
104. Gladziwa U, Klotz U. Pharmacokinetic optimisation of the treatment of peptic ulcer in patients with renal failure. Clinical Pharmacokinetics 1994; 27: 393-408
105. Carmine AA, Brogden RN. Pirenzepine: a review of its pharmacodynamic and pharmacokinetic properties and therapeutic efficacy in peptic ulcer disease and other allied diseases. Drugs 1985; 30: 85
106. Sewing KF. Clinical and pharmacological properties of pirenzepine. In: Bianci Porro & Bardhan, editors. Peptic ulcer disease: advances in pathogenesis and treatment. New York: Raven Press, 1982; 87: 44
107. Walan A. Clinical results with pirenzepine. In: Bianchi Porro & Bardhan, editors. Peptic ulcer disease: advances in pathogenesis and treatment. New York: Raven Press, 1982: 133
108. Brogden RN, Pinder RM, Sawyer PR, et al. Tripotassium dicitrato bismuthate: a report of its pharmacological properties and therapeutic efficacy in peptic ulcer. Drugs 1976; 12: 401
109. Koo J, Ho J, Lam SK, et al. Colloidal bismuth in the treatment of experimental gastric ulcer. Mechanism of action. I. Histochemical study. Proceedings of the IVth International Conference for Experimental Ulcer, Tokyo, Oct 1980: 18-9
110. Lee SP, Lim TH, Pybus J, et al. Tissue distribution of orally administered bismuth in the rat. Clinical and Experimental Pharmacology and Physiology 1980; 7: 319
111. Wieriks J. Pharmacological properties of colloidal bismuth subcitrate (CBS, De-Nol). Scandinavian Journal of Gastroenterology 1982; 17 Suppl. 80: 11
112. Williams DR. Analytical and computer simulation studies of a colloidal bismuth citrate system used as ulcer treatment. Journal of Inorganic Nuclear Chemistry 1977; 39: 711

113. Bateson PR. The effect of bismuth carbonate and other antiacids on the activity of pepsin. Medicine 1954; 8: 370
114. Moshal MG, Gregory MA, Pillary C, et al. Does the duodenal cell ever return to normal? A comparison between treatment with cimetidine and De-Nol. Scandinavian Journal of Gastroenterology 1979; 14 Suppl. 54: 48
115. Lee SP, Nicholson GI. Studies on the absorption and excretion of tripotassium dicitrato bismuthate in man. Research Communications in Chemical Pathology and Pharmacology 1981; 34: 359
116. Bardhan KD, Dekkers CPM, Lam SK, et al. GR122311X (ranitidine bismuth citrate), a new drug for the treatment of duodenal ulcer. Alimentary Pharmacology and Therapeutics 1995; 9: 497-506
117. Brogden RN, Heel RC, Speight TM, et al. Sulcralfate: a review of its pharmacological properties and therapeutic use in peptic ulcer disease. Drugs 1984; 27: 194
118. Nagashima R. Development of characteristics of sucralfate. Journal of Clinical Gastroenterology 1981; 3 Suppl. 2: 103
119. Nagashima R, Hirano T. Selective binding of sucralfate to ulcer lesion. I. Experiments in rats with acetic acid-induced gastric ulcer receiving unlabelled sucralfate. Arzneimittel-Forschung 1980; 30: 80
120. Steiner K, Bühring KU, Faro HP. Sucralfate: pharmacokinetics, metabolism and selective binding to experimental gastric and duodenal ulcers in animals. Arzneimittel-Forschung 1982; 32: 512
121. Nakazawa S, Nagashima R, Samloff IM. Selective binding of sucralfate to gastric ulcer in man. Digestive Diseases and Sciences 1981; 26: 297
122. Samloff IM. Inhibition of peptic aggression by sucralfate: the view from the ulcer crater. Scandinavian Journal of Gastroenterology 1983; 18 Suppl. 834: 7
123. Borella LE, Seethaler K, Lippman W. Sucralfate: antipeptic, anti-ulcer activities and antagonism of gastric emptying. Arzneimittel-Forschung 1979; 29: 793
124. McGraw BP, Hesterlec EJ, Lanza FL, et al. In vitro and in vivo evaluations of a tableted antacid and sucralfate, a new anti-ulcer agent. American Journal of Gastroenterology 1981; 76: 412
125. Giesing D, Lonsaan R, Runsen D, et al. Absorption of sucralfate in man. Gastroenterology 1980; 82: 1066
126. Ishimori A. Safety experience with sucralfate in Japan. Journal of Clinical Gastroenterology 1981; 3 Suppl. 2: 169
127. Hollander D, Tarnawski A, Gergely H, et al. Sucralfate protection of gastric mucosa against alcohol-induced necrosis: a prostaglandin mediated process? (abstract). Gastroenterology 1983; 84: 1190
128. Piper DW, Stiel D. Site protective agents for peptic ulcer: when should they be used? Current Therapeutics 1986; 27(4): 13
129. Sontag SJ. Prostaglandins in peptic ulcer disease: an overview of current status and future directions. Drugs 1986; 32: 445
130. Robert A. Cytoprotection by prostaglandins. Gastroenterology 1979; 91: 761
131. Davis R, Yarker YE, Goa KL. Diclofenac/misoprostol: a review of its pharmacology and therapeutic efficacy in painful inflammatory conditions. Drugs & Aging 1995; 7: 372-93
132. Texter EC, Laureta HC. The milk alkali syndrome. American Journal of Digestive Diseases 1966; 11: 413
133. Lotz M, Ney R, Barter FC. Osteomalacia and debility resulting from phosphorus depletion. Transactions of the Association of American Physicians 1964; 77: 281
134. Lotz M, Zisman E, Barter FC. Evidence for a phosphorus depletion syndrome in man. New England Journal of Medicine 1968; 278: 409
135. Lacz JP, Groschang AG, Giesing DH, et al. The effect of sucralfate on drug absorption in dogs [abstract]. Gastroenterology 1982; 82: 1108
136. McGuigan JE. A consideration of the adverse effects of cimetidine. Gastroenterology 1981; 80: 181-92
137. Hansten PD, Horn JR. Drug interactions. 6th ed. Philadelphia: Lea & Febiger, 1989
138. Piper DW. A comparative overview of the adverse effects of antiulcer drugs. Drug Safety 1995; 12: 120-38
139. Saigenti K, Fukutomi H, Nakazawa S. Famotidine: post marketing clinical experience. Scandinavian Journal of Gastroenterology 1987; 22 Suppl. 134: 34-40
140. Dal Negro R, Torco P, Romani C, et al. Famotidine teofill in a enterfer enza farmaco cinetica cimetidino simile. Italian Journal of Chest Diseases 1988; 42: 185-6
141. Humphries TJ. Famotidine: a notable lack of drug interactions. Scandinavian Journal of Gastroenterology 1987; Suppl. 134: 55-60
142. Lauritsen K, Laursen LS, Rash-Madsen T. Clinical pharmacokinetics of drugs used in the treatment of gastrointestinal diseases. Part I. Clinical Pharmacokinetics 1990; 19: 11-31
143. Monk JP, Clissold SP. Misoprostol: a preliminary review of its pharmacodynamic and pharmacokinetic properties and therapeutic efficacy in the treatment of peptic ulcer disease. Drugs 1987; 33: 1
144. Mungall D, Talbert RL, Phillips C, et al. Sucralfate and warfarin [letter]. Annals of Internal Medicine 1983; 98: 557
145. Barradell LB, Whittington R, Benfield P. Misoprostol: pharmacoeconomics of its use as prophylaxis against gastroduodenal damage induced by nonsteroidal anti-inflammatory drugs. PharmacoEconomics 1993; 2: 140-70
146. Markham A, McTavish D. Clarithromycin and omeprazole as *Helicobacter pylori* eradication therapy in patients with *H. pylori*-associated gastric disorders. Drugs 1996; 51: 161-78
147. Herrmann RP, Piper DW. Factors influencing the healing rate of chronic gastric ulcer. American Journal of Digestive Diseases 1973; 18: 1-6
148. O'Brien B, Goeree R, Mohamed AH, et al. Cost effectiveness of *Helicobacter pylori* eradication for the long-term management of duodenal ulcer in Canada. Archives of Internal Medicine 1995; 155: 1958-64
149. Fennerty MB. 'Cure' of *Helicobacter pylori*: clinically indicated and economically wise! Archives of Internal Medicine 1995; 155: 1929-31
150. Bell GD, Powell KU, Bolton G. Clinical and pharmacoeconomic evaluation of management strategies for duodenal ulcer disease. British Journal of Medical Economics 1993; 6: 45-58
151. Imperiale TF, Speroff T, Cebul RD. A cost comparison of alternative treatments for duodenal ulcer in the *H. pylori* era. American Journal of Gastroenterology 1993; 88: 1509
152. Unge P, Jonsson B, Stalhammar N-O. The cost effectiveness of *Helicobacter pylori* eradication versus maintenance and episodic treatment in duodenal ulcer patients in Sweden. PharmacoEconomics 1995; 8: 410-27

153. Hanson JS, McCallum RW. The diagnosis and management of nausea and vomiting: a review. American Journal of Gastroenterology 1985; 80: 210-8
154. Malagelada J-R, Camilleri M. Unexplained vomiting: a diagnostic challenge. Annals of Internal Medicine 1984; 101: 211-8
155. McCallum RW. Cisapride: a new class of prokinetic agent. American Journal of Gastroenterology 1991; 86: 135-49
156. Talley NJ. Drug treatment of functional dyspepsia. Scandinavian Journal of Gastroenterology 1991; 26 Suppl. 1982: 47
157. Markham A, Sorkin EM. Ondansetron: an update of its therapeutic use in chemotherapy-induced and postoperative nausea and vomiting. Drugs 1993; 45: 931-52
158. Talley NJ. 5-Hydroxytryptamine agonists and antagonists in the modulation of gastrointestinal motility and sensation: clinical implications. Alimentary Pharmacology and Therapeutics 1992; 6: 273-89
159. Lee CR, Plosker GL, McTavish D. Tropisetron: a review of its pharmacodynamic and pharmacokinetic properties, and therapeutic potential as an antiemetic. Drugs 1993; 46: 925-43
160. Plosker GL, Goa KL. Granisetron: a review of its pharmacological properties and therapeutic use as an antiemetic. Drugs 1991; 42: 805-24
161. Yarker YE, McTavish D. Granisetron: an update of its therapeutic use in nausea and vomiting induced by antineoplastic therapy. Drugs 1994; 48: 761-93
162. Talley NJ, Phillips SF, Haddad A, et al. GR 38032F (ondansetron), a selective 5HT3 antagonist, slows colonic transit in healthy man. Digestive Diseases and Sciences 1990; 35: 477-80
163. Mitchelson F. Pharmacological agents affecting emesis: a review (Pts 1 & 2). Drugs 1992; 43: 295-315 & 443-63
164. Janssens J, Peeters TL, Vantrappen G, et al. Improvement of gastric emptying in diabetic gastroparesis by erythromycin. New England Journal of Medicine 1990; 322: 1028-31
165. Peeters TL. Erythromycin and other macrolides as prokinetic agents. Gastroenterology 1993; 105: 1886-99
166. Levine JS. Decision making in gastroenterology. St Louis: Mosby, 1992: 77
167. Marty M, Pouillart P, Scholl S, et al. Comparison of the 5-hydroxytryptamine$_3$ (serotonin) antagonist ondansetron (GR 38032F) with high-dose metoclopramide in the control of cisplatin-induced emesis. New England Journal of Medicine 1990; 322: 816-21
168. Morrow GR, Morrell C. Behavioral treatment for the anticipatory nausea and vomiting induced by cancer chemotherapy. New England Journal of Medicine 1982; 307: 1476-80
169. Plosker GL, Milne RJ. Ondansetron: a pharmacoeconomic and quality-of-life evaluation of its antiemetic activity in patients receiving cancer chemotherapy. PharmacoEconomics 1992; 2: 285-304
170. Soukop M, McQuade B, Hunter E, et al. Ondansetron compared with metoclopramide in the control of emesis and quality of life during repeated chemotherapy for breast cancer. Oncology 1992; 49: 295-304
171. Holmes GRT, Prior R, Lane MR, et al. Malignancy in coeliac disease: effect of a gluten free diet. Gut 1989; 30: 333
172. Winnick M. Guidelines on nutritional support in AIDS. Nutrition 1989; 5: 390
173. Brasitus TA, Sitrin MD. Short bowel syndrome. In: Yamada T, et al., editors. Textbook of Gastroenterology. Philadelphia: Lippincott, 1991: 1541
174. Bettinger JR, Grendell JH. Intracellular events in the pathogenesis of acute pancreatitis. Pancreas 1991; 6: S2
175. Lee SP, Nicholls JF, Park HZ. Biliary sludge as a cause of acute pancreatitis. New England Journal of Medicine 1992; 326: 589
176. Wilson JS, Korsten MA, Thomas MC, et al. The drinker's pancreas: enhanced synthesis of zymogens, secretory block and lysosomal fragility in the pathogenesis of alcoholic pancreatitis. International Journal of Pancreatology 1990; 6: 343
177. Mallory A, Kern F. Drug-induced pancreatitis: a critical review. Gastroenterology 1980; 78: 813
178. Kjellgren K. The influence of morphine and pethidine in combination with levallorphan on biliary duct pressure after cholecystectomy. British Journal of Anaesthesia 1960; 32: 2-6
179. Economou G, Ward-McQuaid JN. A crossover comparison of the effect of morphine, pethidine, pentazocine and phenazocine on biliary pressure. Gut 1971; 12: 218-21
180. Leach SD, Gorelick FS, Modlin IM. New perspectives on acute pancreatitis. Scandinavian Journal of Gastroenterology 1992; 27 Suppl. 192: 29
181. McKay CJ, Imrie CW, Baxter JN. Somatostatin and somatostatin analogues - are they indicated in the management of acute pancreatitis? Gut 1993; 1622
182. Binmoeller KF, Harris AG, Dumas R, et al. Does the somatostatin analogue octreotide protect against ERCP induced pancreatitis? Gut 1992; 133: 1129
183. Buchler M, Friess H, Klempa I. Role of octreotide in the prevention of postoperative complications following pancreatic resection. American Journal of Surgery 1992; 163: 125
184. Bassi C, Falconi M, Lombardi D, et al. Prophylaxis of complications after pancreatic surgery; results of a multicenter trial in Italy. Digestion 1994; 55 Suppl. 1: 41
185. Imrie CW, Benjamin IS, Ferguson JC, et al. A single-centre double-blind trial of Trasylol therapy in primary acute pancreatitis. British Journal of Surgery 1978; 65: 337-41
186. Neoptolemos JP, London NJ, James D, et al. Controlled trial of urgent endoscopic retrograde cholangiopancreatography and endoscopic sphincterotomy versus conservative treatment for acute pancreatitis due to gallstones. Lancet 1988; 29: 979
187. Fan ST, Lai ECS, Mok FPT, et al. Early treatment of acute biliary pancreatitis by endoscopic papillotomy. New England Journal of Medicine 1993; 328: 228
188. Slaff J, Jacobson D, Tillman CR, et al. Protease specific suppression of pancreatic exocrine secretion. Gastroenterology 1984; 87: 44
189. Isaksson F, Ihse I. Pain reduction by an oral pancreatic enzyme preparation in chronic pancreatitis. Digestive Diseases and Sciences 1983; 28: 97
190. Pares A, Caballeria J, Breguera M, et al. Histological course of alcoholic hepatitis: influence of abstinence, sex and extent of liver damage. Journal of Hepatology 1986; 2: 33-42
191. Ramonde MJ, Poynard T, Rueff B, et al. A randomised trial of prednisolone in patients with severe alcoholic hepatitis. New England Journal of Medicine 1992; 326: 507-12
192. Perillo RP, Regenstein FG, Peters MG, et al. Prednisone withdrawal followed by recombinant alpha interferon

in the treatment of chronic hepatitis B: a randomised, controlled trial. Annals of Internal Medicine 1988; 109: 95-100

193. Scullard GH, Pollard RB, Smith JI, et al. Antiviral treatment of chronic hepatitis B virus infection: changes in viral markers with interferon combined with adenine arabinoside. Journal of Infectious Diseases 1987; 143: 772-83
194. Davis GL, Balart LA, Schiff ER, et al. Treatment of chronic hepatitis C with recombinant interferon alpha. A multicentre, randomised, controlled trial. New England Journal of Medicine 1989; 321: 1501-6
195. Uribe M, Summerskill WHJ, Go VLW. Comparative serum prednisone and prednisolone concentrations following administration to patients with chronic active liver disease. Clinical Pharmacokinetics 1982; 7: 452
196. Schalm SW, Ammon HV, Summerskill WHJ. Failure of customary treatment of chronic active liver disease: causes and management. Annals of Clinical Research 1976; 8: 221
197. Stellon AJ, Hegarty JE, Portmann B, et al. Randomised controlled trial of azathioprine withdrawal in autoimmune chronic active hepatitis. Lancet 1985; 1: 668
198. Avery GS, Davies E, Brogden RN. Lactulose: a review of its therapeutic and pharmacological properties with particular reference to ammonia metabolism and its mode of action in portal systemic encephalopathy. Drugs 1972; 4: 7
199. Conn HO, Leevy CM, Vlahcevic ZR, et al. Comparison of lactulose and neomycin in the treatment of chronic portal systemic encephalopathy. Gastroenterology 1977; 72: 573
200. Burroughs AK, Bosch J. Clinical manifestations and management of bleeding episodes in cirrhotics. In: McIntyre N, Behamou JP, Bircher J, et al. editors. Oxford textbook of clinical hepatology. Oxford: Oxford University Press, 1991
201. Bosch J, D'Amico G, Luca A, et al. Drug therapy for variceal haemorrhage. Portal hypertension: pathophysiology and treatment, IASL Meeting, May 1994. Oxford: Blackwell Scientific Publications, 1994: 108-23
202. Groszmann RJ, Kravetz D, Bosch J, et al. Nitroglycerin improves the hemodynamic response to vasopressin in portal hypertension. Hepatology 1982; 2: 762
203. Bosch J, Groszmann RJ, Garcia-Pagan JC, et al. Association of transdermal nitroglycerin to vasopressin infusion in the treatment of variceal haemorrhage: a placebo controlled clinical trial. Hepatology 1989; 10: 962-8
204. Bosch J, Bruix J, Mas A, et al. Rolling review: the treatment of major complications of cirrhosis. Alimentary Pharmacology and Therapeutics 1994; 8: 639-57
205. Pizcueta MP, Garcia-Pagan JC, Fernandez M, et al. Glucagon hinders the effects of somatostatin on portal hypertension. Gastroenterology 1991; 101: 1710-5
206. Bosch J, Mastai R, Kravetz D, et al. Effects of propranolol on azygous venous blood flow and hepatic and systemic hemodynamics in cirrhosis. Hepatology 1984; 4: 1200-5
207. Bassett ML, Halliday JW, Powell LW. HLA typing in idiopathic hemochromatosis: distinction between homozygotes and heterozygotes with biochemical expression. Hepatology 1981; 1: 120
208. Isselbacher KJ, Braunwald E, Wilson JD, et al., editors. Harrison's principles of internal medicine. 14th ed. New York: McGraw-Hill, 1996
209. Lindor KD, Dickson ER, Baldus WP, et al. Ursodeoxycholic acid in the treatment of primary biliary cirrhosis. Gastroenterology 1994; 106: 1284-90
210. Poupon RE, Poupon R, Balkau B. Ursodiol for the long-term treatment of primary biliary cirrhosis. New England Journal of Medicine 1994; 330: 1342-7
211. Heathcote EJ, Cauch-Duder K, Walker V, et al. The Canadian multicenter double-blind randomized controlled trial of ursodeoxycholic acid in primary biliary cirrhosis. Hepatology 1994; 19: 1149-56
212. Gibson PR. Inflammatory bowel disease: current concepts in pathogenesis and therapy. Clinical Immunology and Immunopathology 1994; 2: 134-60
213. Azad Khan AK, Piris J, Truelove SC. An experiment to determine the active therapeutic moiety of sulphasalazine. Lancet 1977; 2: 892
214. Brogden RN, Sorkin EM. Mesalazine: a review of its pharmacodynamic and pharmacokinetic properties, and therapeutic potential in chronic inflammatory bowel disease. Drugs 1989; 38: 500-23
215. Ireland A, Priddle JD, Jewell DP. Acetylation of 5-aminosalicylic acid by isolated human colonic epithelial cells. Clinical Science 1990; 78: 105
216. Wadworth AN, Fitton A. Olsalazine: a review of its pharmacodynamic and pharmacokinetic properties, and therapeutic potential in inflammatory bowel disease. Drugs 1991; 41: 647-64
217. Chan RP, Pope DJ, Gilbert AP, et al. Studies of two novel sulfasalazine analogs, ipsalazide and balsalazide. Digestive Diseases and Sciences 1983; 28: 609
218. Committee on Safety of Medicines. Nephrotoxicity associated with mesalazine (Asacol). Current problems 30. London: Committee on Safety of Medicines, 1990
219. Singleton JW, Hanauer SB, Gitnick GL, et al. Mesalamine capsules for the treatment of active Crohn's disease: results of a 16-week trial. Gastroenterology 1993; 104: 1293
220. International Mesalazine Study Group. Coated oral 5-aminosalicylic acid versus placebo in maintaining remission of ulcerative Crohn's disease. Alimentary Pharmacology and Therapeutics 1990; 4: 55
221. Brignola C, Iannone P, Pasqualis C, et al. Placebo controlled trial of oral 5-ASA in relapse prevention of Crohn's disease. Digestive Diseases and Sciences 1992; 37: 29
222. Prantera C, Pallone F, Brunetti G, et al. Oral 5-aminosalicylic acid (Asacol) in the maintenance treatment of Crohn's disease. Gastroenterology 1992; 103: 363
223. Gendre JP, Mary JY, Florent C, et al. Oral mesalamine (Pentasa) as maintenance treatment in Crohn's disease: a multicenter placebo-controlled study. Gastroenterology 1993; 104: 435
224. Campieri M, Lanfranchi GA, Bazzochi G, et al. Treatment of ulcerative colitis with high-dose 5-aminosalicylic acid enemas. Lancet 1981; 2: 270
225. Danish 5-ASA Group. Topical 5-aminosalicylic acid versus prednisolone in ulcerative proctosigmoiditis. A randomised, double-blind multicentre trial. Digestive Diseases and Sciences 1987; 32: 598
226. Sutherland LR, Martin F, Greer S, et al. 5-Aminosalicylic acid enema in the treatment of distal ulcerative colitis, proctosigmoiditis, and proctitis. Gastroenterology 1987; 92: 1894
227. Biddle WL, Greenberger J, Swan T, et al. 5-Aminosalicylic acid enemas: effective agent in maintaining remission in left-sided ulcerative colitis. Gastroenterology 1988; 94: 1075

228. D'Arienzo A, Panarese A, Darmiento FP, et al. 5-Aminosalicylic acid suppositories in the maintenance of remission in idiopathic proctitis or proctosigmoiditis: a double-blind placebo-controlled clinical trial. American Journal of Gastroenterology 1990; 85: 1079
229. Ireland A, Jewell DP. Mechanism of action of 5-aminosalicylic acid and its derivatives. Clinical Science 1990; 78: 119
230. Brattsand R. Overview of newer glucocorticosteriod preparations for inflammatory bowel disease. Canadian Journal of Gastroenterology 1990; 4: 407
231. Gilvarry JM, O'Morain CA. New treatments in inflammatory bowel disease. European Journal of Gastroenterology and Hepatology 1993; 5: 893
232. Rutgeerts P, Lofberg R, Malchow H, et al. Budesonide versus prednisolone for the treatment of active ileocecal Crohn's disease: a European multicenter trial. Gastroenterology 1993; 104: A772
233. Rosenberg JL, Wall AJ, Levin B, et al. A controlled trial of azathioprine in the management of chronic ulcerative colitis. Gastroenterology 1975; 69: 96
234. Present DH, Korelitz BI, Wisch N, et al. Treatment of Crohn's disease with 6-mercaptopurine: a long term randomised double blind study. New England Journal of Medicine 1980; 302: 981
235. Kirk AP, Lennard-Jones JE. Controlled trial of azathioprine in chronic ulcerative colitis. British Medical Journal 1982; 284: 1291
236. Ewe K, Press AG, Singe CC, et al. Azathioprine combined with prednisolone or monotherapy with prednisolone in active Crohn's disease. Gastroenterology 1993; 2: 367
237. O'Donoghue DP, Dawson AM, Powell-Tuck J, et al. Double-blind withdrawal trial of azathioprine as maintenance treatment for Crohn's disease. Lancet 1978; 2: 955
238. Hawthorne AB, Logan RF, Hawkey CJ, et al. Randomised controlled trial of azathioprine withdrawal in ulcerative colitis. British Medical Journal 1992; 305: 20
239. Kinlen LJ. Incidence of cancer in lupoid arthritis and other disorders after immunosuppressive treatment. American Journal of Medicine 1985; 78: 44
240. Present DH, Meltzer SJ, Krumholz MP, et al. 6-Mercaptopurine in the management of inflammatory bowel disease: short- and long-term toxicity. Annals of Internal Medicine 1989; 111: 641
241. O'Brien JJ, Bayless TM, Bayless JA. Use of azathioprine or 6-mercaptopurine in the treatment of Crohn's disease. Gastroenterology 1991; 101: 39
242. Connell WR, Kamm MA, Dickson M, et al. Long-term neoplasia risk after azathioprine treatment in inflammatory bowel disease. Lancet 1994; 343: 1249
243. Guslandi M, Tittobello A. Cyclosporin for Crohn's disease? Drugs 1992; 43: 440
244. Kozarek RA, Patterson DJ, Gelfand MD, et al. Methotrexate induces clinical and histological remission in patients with refractory inflammatory bowel disease. Annals of Internal Medicine 1989; 110: 353
245. Baron TH, Truss CD, Elson CO. Low-dose methotrexate in refractory inflammatory bowel disease. Digestive Diseases and Sciences 1993; 38: 1851
246. Blichfeldt P, Bloomhoff JP, Myhre E, et al. Metronidazole in Crohn's disease. A double-blind cross-over clinical trial. Scandinavian Journal of Gastroenterology 1978; 13: 123
247. Sutherland L, Singleton J, Sessions J, et al. Double blind, placebo controlled trial of metronidazole in Crohn's disease. Gut 1991; 32: 1071
248. Bernstein LH, Frank MS, Brandt LT, et al. Healing of perineal Crohn's disease with metronidazole. Gastroenterology 1980; 79: 357
249. Brandt LJ, Bernstein LH, Boley SJ, et al. Metronidazole therapy for perineal Crohn's disease. A follow-up study. Gastroenterology 1982; 83: 383
250. Chapman RW, Selby WS, Jewell DP. Controlled trial of metronidazole as an adjunct to corticosteroids in severe ulcerative colitis. Gut 1986; 27: 1210
251. Gilat T, Sussa A, Leichtman MD, et al. A comparative study of metronidazole and sulfasalazine in active, not severe, ulcerative colitis. Journal of Clinical Gastroenterology 1987; 9: 415
252. Burke DA, Axon ATR, Clayden SA, et al. The efficacy of tobramycin in the treatment of ulcerative colitis. Alimentary Pharmacology and Therapeutics 1990; 4: 123
253. Lobo AJ, Burke DA, Sobala GM, et al. Oral tobramycin in ulcerative colitis: effect on maintenance of remission. Alimentary Pharmacology and Therapeutics 1993; 7: 155
254. McIntyre PB, Powell-Tuck J, Woods SR, et al. Controlled trial of bowel rest in the treatment of severe acute colitis. Gut 1986; 27: 481
255. Lichtiger S, Present DH. Preliminary report: cyclosporin in treatment of severe ulcerative colitis. Lancet 1990; 336: 16
256. Allison MC, Vallance R. Prevalence of proximal faecal stasis in active ulcerative colitis. Gut 1991; 32: 179
257. Sandborn WJ, Tremaine WJ, Schroeder KW, et al. A placebo-controlled trial of cyclosporine enemas for mildly to moderately active left-sided ulcerative colitis. Gastroenterology 1994; 106: 1429
258. Scheppach W, Sommer H, Kirchner T, et al. Effect of butyrate enemas on the colonic mucosa in distal ulcerative colitis. Gastroenterology 1992; 103: 51
259. Breuer RI, Buto SK, Christ ML, et al. Rectal irrigation with short-chain fatty acids for distal ulcerative colitis. Preliminary report. Digestive Diseases and Sciences 1991; 36: 185
260. Bjorck S, Dahlstrom A, Johansson L, et al. Treatment of mucosa with local anaesthetics in ulcerative colitis. Agents and Actions 1972; Special No. C60
261. Riley SA, Gupta I, Mani V. A comparison of sucralfate and prednisolone enemas in the treatment of active distal ulcerative colitis. Scandinavian Journal of Gastroenterology 1989; 24: 1014
262. Pullan RD, Ganesh S, Mani V, et al. Comparison of bismuth citrate and 5-aminosalicylic acid enemas in distal ulcerative colitis: a controlled trial. Gut 1993; 34: 676
263. Aslan A, Triadafilopoulos G. Fish oil fatty acid supplementation in active ulcerative colitis: a double-blind, placebo-controlled, crossover study. American Journal of Gastroenterology 1992; 87: 432
264. Stenson WF, Cort D, Rodgers J, et al. Dietary supplementation with fish oil in ulcerative colitis. Annals of Internal Medicine 1992; 116: 609
265. Pullan RD, Rhodes J, Ganesh S, et al. Transdermal nicotine for active ulcerative colitis. New England Journal of Medicine 1994; 330: 811
266. Williams A. Heparin and inflammatory bowel disease [letter]. Lancet 1991; 337: 622

267. Binder V, Elsborg L, Greibe J, et al. Disodium cromoglycate in the treatment of ulcerative colitis and Crohn's disease. Gut 1981; 22: 55
268. Peppercorn M, Das K, Elson C, et al. Zileuton, a 5-lipoxygenase inhibitor, in the treatment of active ulcerative colitis: a double-blind, placebo-controlled trial. Gastroenterology 1994; 106: A751
269. Gilat T, Leichtman G, Delpre G, et al. A comparison of metronidazole and sulfasalazine in the maintenance of remission in patients with ulcerative colitis. Journal of Clinical Gastroenterology 1989; 11: 392
270. Salim AS. Role of oxygen-derived free radical scavengers in the management of recurrent attacks of ulcerative colitis: a new approach. Journal of Laboratory and Clinical Medicine 1992; 119: 710
271. Salim AS. Role of sulphydryl-containing agents in the management of recurrent attacks of ulcerative colitis: a new approach. Pharmacology 1992; 45: 307
272. Wischmeyer P, Pemberton JH, Phillips SF. Chronic pouchitis after ileal pouch-anal anastomosis: responses to butyrate and glutamine suppositories in a pilot study. Mayo Clinic Proceedings 1993; 68: 978
273. Felder JB, Adler DJ, Korelitz BI. The safety of corticosteroid therapy in Crohn's disease with an abdominal mass. American Journal of Gastroenterology 1991; 86: 1450
274. Brynskow J, Freund L, Rasmussen SN, et al. Final report on a placebo-controlled, double-blind, randomised, multicentre trial of cyclosporin treatment in active chronic Crohn's disease. Scandinavian Journal of Gastroenterology 1991; 26: 689
275. Hanauer SB, Smith MB. Rapid closure of Crohn's disease fistulas with continuous intravenous cyclosporin A. American Journal of Gastroenterology 1993; 88: 646
276. Present DH, Lichtiger S. Efficacy of cyclosporine in treatment of fistula of Crohn's disease. Digestive Diseases and Sciences 1994; 39: 374
277. Lofberg R, Rutgeerts P, Lalchow H, et al. Budesonide CIR for maintenance of remission in ileocaecal Crohn's disease: a European multicenter placebo controlled trial for 12 months. Gastroenterology 1994; 106: A722
278. Pearson M, Teahon K, Levi AJ, et al. Food intolerance and Crohn's disease. Gut 1993; 6: 783
279. Harries AD, Danis V, Heatley RV, et al. Controlled trial of supplemented oral nutrition in Crohn's disease. Lancet 1983; 1: 887
280. Seidman EG, Roy CC, Weber AM, et al. Nutritional therapy of Crohn's disease in childhood. Digestive Diseases and Sciences 1987; 32: 82S
281. Mogadam M, Dobbins WO, Korelitz BI, et al. Pregnancy in inflammatory bowel disease: effect of sulfasalazine and corticosteroids on fetal outcome. Gastroenterology 1981; 80: 72
282. Davidson JM, Lindheimer MD. Pregnancy in women with renal allografts. Seminars in Nephrology 1984; 4: 240
283. Goldstein FJ. Immunosuppressant therapy for inflammatory bowel disease. Journal of Clinical Gastroenterology 1987; 9: 654
284. Alstead EM, Ritchie JK, Lennard-Jones JE, et al. Safety of azathioprine in pregnancy in inflammatory bowel disease. Gastroenterology 1990; 99: 730
285. Srivastava GS, Smith AN, Painter NS. Sterculia, bulk-forming agent with smooth-muscle relaxant, versus bran in diverticular disease. British Medical Journal 1976; 1: 315
286. Painter NS, Truelove SC. The intraluminal pressure patterns in diverticulosis of the colon. Gut 1964; 5: 201
287. Sack DA. Use of oral rehydration therapy in acute watery diarrhoea: a practical guide. Drugs 1991; 41: 566
288. DuPont HL, Hornick RB. Adverse effect of Lomotil therapy in shigellosis. Journal of the American Medical Association 1973; 226: 1525
289. Lima AAM, Lima NL. Epidemiology, therapy and prevention of infection with *Shigella* organisms and *Clostridium difficile*. Current Opinion in Infectious Diseases 1993; 6: 63
290. Maloney WJ, Guerrant RL. Epidemiology, therapy, and prevention of infection with *Salmonella* organisms. Current Opinion in Infectious Diseases 1992; 5: 74
291. Mandal BK, Ellis ME, Dunbar EM, et al. Double-blind placebo-controlled trial of erythromycin in the treatment of clinical Campylobacter infection. Journal of Antimicrobial Chemotherapy 1984; 13: 619
292. Nalin DR, Morris Jr JG. Cholera and other vibrioses. In: Strickland GT, editor. Hunter's tropical medicine. 7th ed. Philadelphia: W.B. Saunders, 1991
293. Gracey M. Travellers' diarrhoea: is drug therapy for prophylaxis and treatment of real benefit? Drugs 1984; 27: 1
294. Okhuysen PC, Ericsson CD. Traveler's diarrhea: prevention and treatment. Medical Clinics of North America 1992; 76: 1357
295. DuPont HL. Travellers' diarrhoea: which antimicrobial? Drugs 1993; 45: 910
296. Dudley MN, McLaughlin JC, Carrington G, et al. Oral bacitracin vs vancomycin therapy for *Clostridium difficile*-induced diarrhea: a randomized double-blind trial. Archives of Internal Medicine 1986; 146: 1101
297. Andrèjak M, Schmit J-L, Tondriaux A. The clinical significance of antibiotic-associated pseudomembranous colitis in the 1990s. Drug Safety 1991; 6: 339
298. Buggy BP, Fekety R, Silva J. Therapy of relapsing *Clostridium difficile*-associated diarrhea and colitis with the combination of vancomycin and rifampicin. Journal of Clinical Gastroenterology 1987; 9: 155
299. Wolfe MS. Giardiasis. New England Journal of Medicine 1978; 298: 319
300. Jokipii L, Jokipii AMM. Treatment of giardiasis: comparative evaluation of ornidazole and tinidazole as a single oral dose. Gastroenterology 1982; 83: 399
301. Wolfe MS. The treatment of intestinal protozoal infections. Medical Clinics of North America 1982; 66: 707
302. Spillman R, Ayala SC, de Sanchez CE. Double-blind test of metronidazole and tinidazole in the treatment of asymptomatic *Entamoeba histolytica* and *Entamoeba hartmanni* carriers. American Journal of Tropical Medicine and Hygiene 1976; 25: 549
303. Bakshi JS, Ghiara JM, Nanivadekar AS. How does tinidazole compare with metronidazole? A summary report of Indian trials in amoebiasis and giardiasis. Drugs 1978; 15 Suppl. 1: 33
304. Islam N, Hasan K. Tinidazole and metronidazole in hepatic amoebiasis. Drugs 1978; 15 Suppl. 1: 26
305. El-Hennaway M, Abd-Rabbo H. Hazards of cortisone therapy in hepatic amoebiasis. Journal of Tropical Medicine and Hygiene 1978; 81: 71
306. Stuiver PC, Goud ThJLM. Corticosteroids and liver amoebiasis. British Medical Journal 1978; 2: 394
307. Wurtz R. *Cyclospora*: a newly identified intestinal pathogen of humans. Clinical Infectious Diseases 1994; 18: 620

308. Asmuth DM, DeGirolami PC, Federman M, et al. Clinical features of microsporidiosis in patients with AIDS. Clinical Infectious Diseases 1994; 18: 819
309. Bell DR. Anthelminthic drug therapy. In: Reeves & Geddes, editors. Recent advances in infection. London: Churchill Livingstone, 1982: 179
310. Drossman DA, Thompson WG, Talley NJ, et al. Identification of subgroups of functional gastrointestinal disorders. Gastroenterology International 1990; 3: 159
311. Goulston KJ, Dent OF, Mant A, et al. Use of $H_2$-receptor antagonists in patients with dyspepsia and heartburn: a cost comparison. Medical Journal of Australia 1991; 155: 20
312. Loof L, Adami HO, Agenas I, et al. The diagnosis and therapy survey October 1978 - March 1983, health care consumption and current drug therapy in Sweden with respect to the clinical diagnosis of gastritis. Scandinavian Journal of Gastroenterology 1985; 20 Suppl. 109: 35
313. Klein KB. Controlled treatment trials in the irritable bowel syndrome: a critique. Gastroenterology 1988; 95: 232
314. Di Piazza S, Cottone M, Craxi A, et al. Severe rifampicin-associated liver failure in patients with compensated cirrhosis. Lancet 1978; 1: 774
315. Whelton MJ, Allaway A, Stewart A, et al. Ergot poisoning in acute hepatic necrosis. Gut 1968; 9: 287
316. Hayton AC. Precipitation of acute ergotism by triacetyloleandomycin. New Zealand Medical Journal 1969; 69: 42
317. Kutt H, Winters W, Scherman R, et al. Diphenylhydantoin and phenobarbital toxicity. Archives of Neurology 1964; 11: 649
318. Selden R, Sasahara AA. Central nervous system toxicity induced by lidocaine: report of a case in a patient with liver disease. Journal of the American Medical Association 1967; 202: 908
319. Faigle JW. Blood levels of a schistosomicide in relation to liver function and side-effects. Acta Pharmacologica et Toxicologica 1971; 29 (Suppl. 3): 233
320. Wagonfeld JB, Nemchausky BA, Bolt M, et al. Comparison of vitamin D and 25-hydroxy-vitamin D in the therapy of primary biliary cirrhosis. Lancet 1976; 2: 391
321. Acocella G. Clinical pharmacokinetics of rifampicin. Clinical Pharmacokinetics 1978; 3: 108
322. Knop P, Kindler V, Austerhoff A. Plasma levels of rifampicin and isoniazid and serum levels of aminotransferases in combined tuberculostatic treatment. Deutsche Medizinische Wochenschrift 1977; 102: 1913
323. James I. Prescribing in patients with liver disease. British Journal of Hospital Medicine 1975; 13 (Suppl. 1): 67
324. Laidlaw J, Read AE, Sherlock S. Morphine tolerance in hepatic cirrhosis. Gastroenterology 1961; 40: 389
325. Sessions JT, Minkel HP, Bullard JC, et al. The effect of barbiturates in patients with liver disease. Journal of Clinical Investigation 1954; 33: 1116
326. Read AE, Laidlaw J, McCarthy CF. Effects of chlorpromazine in patients with hepatic disease. British Medical Journal 1969; 3: 497
327. Branch RA, Morgan MH, James J, et al. Intravenous administration of diazepam in patients with chronic liver disease. Gut 1976; 17: 975
328. Maxwell JD, Carrella M, Parkes JD, et al. Plasma disappearance and cerebral effects of chlorpromazine in cirrhosis. Clinical Science 1972; 43: 143
329. Sherlock S, Senewiratne B, Scott A, et al. Complications of diuretic therapy in hepatic cirrhosis. Lancet 1966; 1: 1049
330. Naranjo CA, Gonzalez G, Pontigo E, et al. Adverse reaction to furosemide in liver cirrhosis. Clinical Pharmacology and Therapeutics 1978; 23: 123
331. Naranjo CA, Pontigo E, Valdenegro C, et al. Furosemide-induced adverse reactions in cirrhosis of the liver. Clinical Pharmacology and Therapeutics 1979; 25: 154
332. Morgan MH, Read AE. Antidepressants and liver disease. Gut 1972; 13: 697
333. Schweitzer IL, Weiner JM, McPeak CM, et al. Oral contraceptives in acute viral hepatitis. Journal of the American Medical Association 1975; 233: 979
334. Mowat AP, Arias IM. Liver function and oral contraceptives. Journal of Reproductive Medicine 1969; 3: 19
335. Rannevik G, Jeppsson S, Kullander S. Effect of oral contraceptives on the liver in women with recurrent cholestasis (hepatosis) during previous pregnancies. Journal of Obstetrics and Gynaecology of the British Commonwealth 1972; 79: 1128
336. Dalen E, Westerholm D. Occurrence of hepatic impairment in women jaundiced by oral contraceptives and in their mothers and sisters. Acta Medica Scandinavica 1974; 195: 459
337. Thompson RPH, Williams R. Developments in jaundice. Postgraduate Medical Journal 1969; 45: 196
338. Bjarnason I, Hallyar J, Macpherson AJ, et al. Side effects of nonsteroidal anti-inflammatory drugs on the small and large intestine in humans. Gastroenterology 1993; 104: 1832
339. Staerk Laursen L, Stokholm M, Bukhave K, et al. Disposition of 5-aminosalicylic acid by olsalazine and three mesalazine preparations in patients with ulcerative colitis: comparison of intraluminal colonic concentrations, serum values, and urinary excretion. Gut 1990; 31: 1271
340. Surland LG, Weisberger AS. Chloramphenicol toxicity in liver and renal disease. Archives of Internal Medicine 1963; 112: 161

Chapter 23

# Respiratory Diseases

*J.G. Douglas, J.S. Legge, J.A.R. Friend* and *J.C. Petrie*

## Synopsis of Important Principles

1) Management of respiratory disease involves attainment and preservation of normal pulmonary function. For airways obstruction, this includes bronchodilatation, removal of retained secretions, treatment of infection and correction of abnormal ventilation. In restrictive ventilatory disorders, it involves suppression of interstitial inflammation and prevention of fibrosis.

2) Bronchial asthma is a common chronic respiratory disorder. Drug treatment aims to achieve and maintain the best possible pulmonary function. This requires the appropriate use of regular prophylactic medication and inhaled bronchodilators. It is vital that inhaler technique is efficient. Good patient education is paramount in achieving optimal control of symptoms.

3) Severe acute asthma occurs when worsening symptoms of dyspnoea, wheeze and chest tightness are not relieved by bronchodilator therapy. Patients prone to acute episodes should start themselves on oral corticosteroids and know when to seek urgent medical help. A peak flow meter may be of value in confirming deterioration in pulmonary function.

4) Management of respiratory failure relies on measurement of arterial blood gas tensions and delivery of an appropriate oxygen concentration. Patients with hypercapnic respiratory failure require careful monitoring, and may need respiratory stimulants and assisted ventilation.

5) Community-acquired pneumonia is most commonly caused by *Streptococcus pneumoniae*. Initial drug treatment should usually contain a penicillin, plus a macrolide to cover other common organisms such as *Mycoplasma pneumoniae*.

6) Bronchiectasis, a common disorder in which the bronchi are colonised by organisms such as *Haemophilus influenzae*, is treated with postural drainage and appropriate antibacterial therapy.

7) Children with cystic fibrosis now live into adulthood, largely due to advances in the management of associated suppurative lung disorders and of Pseudomonas and staphylococcal respiratory infections. Gene therapy and lung transplantation may further improve survival.

8) The prevalence of pulmonary tuberculosis is rising, in association with AIDS in Africa and Southeast Asia. Multiresistant organisms have been reported in the eastern US. Six months of a 3- or 4-drug regimen is considered curative in immunocompetent patients, but atypical organisms should always be considered in those with HIV.

9) The lung is a common site for opportunistic infection in patients with HIV infection. Effective treatment for pneumonias due to *Pneumocystis carinii* or cytomegalovirus (CMV) is available. Prophylaxis against these conditions should be considered for patients with severe immunodeficiency.

10) Thromboembolic diseases are common. While heparin is the mainstay of treatment, thrombolytic therapy should be given to patients with a severely compromised circulation and hypotension. After an acute episode, oral anticoagulant therapy (usually with warfarin) should be given for >12 weeks.

11) Many drugs used for nonrespiratory conditions can adversely affect lung function in patients with respiratory disease, e.g. aspirin and β-blockers in asthma; opioids and anxiolytics in ventilatory failure.

Diseases of the respiratory system are a major cause of mortality and morbidity throughout the world. In the UK, 7% of all acute hospital admissions and approximately 17% of all deaths are due to lung disease. Over 5 million people in the UK have a respiratory disease which is associated with the loss of 50 million working days each year, at an estimated cost of over £2000 million to the British economy. Asthma has become one of the most common chronic disorders at all ages in the Western world and in 1993, 11% of all drug prescription costs in the UK were for asthma medications. Despite modern antibiotics, pneumonia remains a major cause of mortality, causing 10 times as many deaths in the UK as all other infectious diseases combined and 4 times as many deaths as asthma in those aged 16 to 50 years. In the US, pneumonia ranks 5th among the 15 leading causes of death and in developing countries, it is the most common cause of hospitalisation in both children and adults. In addition, the prevalence of pulmonary tuberculosis is rising, with more deaths throughout the world in 1995 than any other year this century. The return of pulmonary tuberculosis, particularly in Africa and South-east Asia, has been associated with HIV infection which, in the Western world, is often complicated by opportunistic lung infections, especially *Pneumocystis carinii* pneumonia.

Respiratory disease, therefore, poses a major challenge throughout the world which is being addressed by the development of newer therapeutic agents, and in the case of asthma, newer forms of drug delivery to the lung. This chapter describes the modern management of common respiratory disorders, focusing on clinical outcomes and economic factors in the selection and use of drugs.

## 1. Clinical Pharmacological Considerations

Drug treatment of airways obstruction reflects the importance of increased understanding of molecular biology underlying the inflammatory response to allergens in susceptible individuals.[1] Muscular responses are now believed to be a consequence of the epithelial inflammatory process, rather than being the primary element in asthma.[2] Several important agents alter these responses.

### 1.1 Immune System Mediators

Allergen challenge in susceptible individuals results in the production of mediators by mast cells, basophils and eosinophils. Mast cells and basophils release histamine and synthesise mediators such as leukotrienes $C_4$ and $D_4$, which result in bronchoconstriction, increased capillary permeability and increased bronchial mucus secretion. The cells also produce cytokines such as interleukin (IL)-4 and IL-5. T cell activation and specific cytokine production, particularly IL-5, activate eosinophils and immunoglobulin E (IgE) production. Eosinophils also produce cytokines, including IL-5. They also contain basic proteins which damage respiratory epithelial cells at concentrations found in the sputum in asthmatic patients, and produce platelet activating factor (PAF) and leukotriene $C_4$, which provoke bronchoconstriction and airway oedema.

IgE binds to receptors on the surface of mast cells and basophils. Allergens that reach the cell surface and crosslink two or more IgE molecules in the cell membrane trigger the release of the mediators.[3,4]

Corticosteroids bind to and disrupt the activity of transcription factors involved in the production of cytokines. They also have direct inhibitory effects on macrophages, T cells, eosinophils and airway epithelial cells (for a review, see Barnes[5])[see also chapter 28; sect. 3.4].

### 1.2 Neural Influences

The dominant bronchoconstrictor pathway is cholinergic. There are no adrenergic nerves in the airway. In asthmatic patients, exaggerated bronchoconstrictor responses may reflect reduced $M_2$ inhibitory preganglionic muscarinic receptors.

Circulating catecholamines may influence bronchoconstriction via presynaptic α- and β-adrenoceptors. The role of neuropeptides is not yet defined.

### 1.3 Role of β-Adrenoceptors

β-Adrenoceptors are widely distributed. In the lung, 80% of β-adrenoceptors are of the $\beta_2$ subtype. $\beta_2$-Adrenoceptors are also present on mast cells, neutrophils, eosinophils, lymphocytes and alveolar macrophages. Drugs that act as $\beta_2$-agonists relax bronchial smooth muscle, increase mucociliary clearance and inhibit the release of mediators.

Selective β2-agonists activate the enzyme adenyl cyclase through a G protein mechanism to increase the intracellular production of cyclic-adenosine monophosphate (cyclic-AMP) from adenosine triphosphate (ATP). Cyclic-AMP causes bronchodilatation by activating protein kinase A, causing relaxation of smooth muscle in the bronchial wall.[6]

## 2. General Principles of Treatment

The clinician must first establish the diagnosis and then assess the severity of the illness to determine the correct management. Most patients are treated in the community, but those with more acute symptoms requiring intensive management and investigation, such as severe acute asthma or respiratory failure, must be identified and referred urgently to hospital.

Assessment of the severity of respiratory disease depends on a careful history and full clinical examination. Simple pulmonary function tests, such as measurement of peak flow rate or spirometry are now widely available. Most clinicians will also have access to facilities for chest radiology and sputum culture. Measurement of arterial (or, in children, arterialised) blood gas tensions and acid-base status is important, particularly for patients hospitalised with acute illness.

The main aims of management in respiratory disease are to treat:

- Reductions in airway calibre
- Respiratory infections
- Disorders of ventilation and control of respiration.

Disorders of ventilation and control of respiration are discussed in section 5.

### 2.1 Treatment of Reduced Airway Calibre

Environmental factors that may contribute to airway narrowing include cigarette smoke, atmospheric pollution, cold air, fog, smog, exposure to substances at work, various allergens and bronchial infections. These factors can cause acute episodes of wheeze, breathlessness and sputum production in susceptible individuals and, if at all possible, should be removed, avoided or treated. Expectoration of sputum can be eased by liberal fluid intake and efficient physiotherapy including postural drainage. Abnormal sputum production can cause airway obstruction, but other factors, such as bronchoconstriction, are also important and interfere with the clearing of retained secretions.

Selective β2-adrenoceptor agonists, which are commonly given by aerosol inhalation, are first-line therapy to achieve bronchodilatation. However, it is not rational to prescribe bronchodilator drugs unless there is evidence that a component of the airways obstruction is reversible. The effect of bronchodilator drugs should be assessed by peak flow rate or spirometry and show an improvement by 15% or more from baseline with treatment.

### 2.2 Treatment of Respiratory Infection

Bacterial infection of the respiratory tract must be recognised early and treated promptly and effectively. Treatment, preferably with bactericidal drugs, can be started before laboratory sensitivity reports are available. The choice of drug depends on a clear understanding of the likely pathogens. For instance, in exacerbations of chronic bronchitis, *Streptococcus pneumoniae* and *Haemophilus influenzae* are likely organisms, while in pneumonia associated with HIV infection, *Pneumocystis carinii*, cytomegalovirus (CMV) and fungal or mycobacterial infection must be considered. Before any antimicrobial drug is prescribed, it must be established that there is no contraindication and that the patient has never previously shown hypersensitivity.

If symptoms or fever fail to respond to initial therapy within 48 hours, an alternative agent should be substituted, if possible based on the results of sputum or blood culture and sensitivity, or other positive findings. Treatment is usually continued until the patient has been afebrile for 36 to 48 hours and the sputum has become mucoid. Any patient who shows slow resolution of fever should be carefully investigated to exclude underlying pathology, particularly bronchial carcinoma, pulmonary infarction, postpneumonic effusion and pulmonary tuberculosis. In the absence of other pathology, the possibility of drug fever should always be considered.

## 3. Bronchial Asthma

Bronchial asthma is characterised by variable dyspnoea due to widespread narrowing of intrapulmonary airways which changes in severity over short periods of time either spontaneously or as a result of treatment. This airway narrowing causes the typical symptoms of cough, wheeze, chest tightness and dyspnoea, which are often worst at night.

There is believed to be a persisting overactive inflammatory response to a variety of trigger stimuli (allergens, irritants, exercise, cold air) – also known as bronchial hyper-reactivity or hyper-responsiveness. The recognition of the importance of inflammation and inflammatory mediator release underlies the change in approach to asthma treatment. Specifically, there is now more emphasis on anti-inflammatory measures as prophylaxis and less on crisis management with bronchodilators.

Evidence of inflammation in asthma includes the presence in bronchial biopsies of an inflammatory cellular response, plasma exudation, oedema, shedding of epithelium, mucus plugging of the airways, increased deposition of collagen beneath the basement membrane, and smooth muscle hypertrophy.[7,8]

Causes of asthma have not been completely elucidated, but include influences from environment and genetic inheritance. Its prevalence is increasing, alarmingly so in children, rising from 4% in 1964 to 10% in 1989 in the UK for instance.[9-11]

Asthma is often characterised as 'extrinsic' or 'intrinsic', although the distinction between the two is usually of little value in deciding on therapy or prognosis. *Extrinsic asthma* patients have early onset asthma, are atopic (often with associated hay fever or eczema), produce skin sensitising antibodies of the IgE class, and have reactive skin prick tests. Asthma reactions may be immediate (within minutes of exposure) or delayed (up to 12 hours later). *Intrinsic asthma* starts in later life, skin prick tests are negative, and IgE concentrations are normal. However, there is no difference in histological findings on bronchial biopsies, and both groups have blood and sputum eosinophilia.

The clinical features of asthma vary greatly in different patients and consist of anything from mild, easily controlled attacks through to severe life-threatening episodes or chronic semi-invalidism. Some patients have severe variable or 'brittle' asthma with acute catastrophic attacks; others experience symptoms entirely at night or waken with low morning peak expiratory flow rates ('morning dippers'). Others have chronic, largely irreversible airway obstruction. In a general practice study, nocturnal wakening occurred once a week in 74% and every night in 39% of patients with asthma.[12]

**Table I.** Therapeutic agents used in asthma

| Bronchodilators | Anti-inflammatory drugs |
|---|---|
| $\beta_2$-Agonist drugs | Corticosteroids (inhaled, systemic) |
| Anticholinergic drugs | Sodium cromoglycate (cromolyn sodium) |
| Methylxanthines | Nedocromil |
| | Ketotifen |

### 3.1 Clinical Pharmacology of Drugs Used in Treatment

The general classes of drugs used in asthma are shown in table I.

#### *3.1.1 Bronchodilators*

**$\beta_2$-Adrenoceptor Agonists**

$\beta_2$-Adrenoceptor agonists (table II) are classified as short- or intermediate-acting, with an onset of action within 10 minutes and a duration of effect 3 to 6 hours (shorter in the case of rimiterol), and long-acting (e.g. salmeterol, formoterol) with a duration effect of more than 12 hours. They are usually given by inhalation, most commonly by metered-dose inhaler. Only about 10% of the inhaled dose is deposited in the intrapulmonary airways, even with good inhaler technique. Poor inhaler technique with metered-dose inhalers is encountered in up to 50% of patients. Using dry powder devices and large volume spacers improves drug deposition to about 30%.

Metered-dose inhalers also contain surfactant and a propellant, hitherto a chlorofluorocarbon, now being replaced by more environmentally friendly propellants. Dry powder devices usually include lactose powder as a vehicle for particle transport to the lungs.

Short/intermediate-acting $\beta_2$-agonist drugs may also be given by nebuliser as a wet aerosol and with some agents orally, intravenously, intramuscularly or subcutaneously as well (table II). The inhaled route is preferred to minimise $\beta_1$-adrenoceptor effects that follow significant drug concentrations in the blood from parenteral administration, i.e. tremor, cramps, tachycardia, hypokalaemia.

***Clinical use:*** short/intermediate-acting $\beta_2$-agonists may be used in all patients with asthma, from the mildest to the most severe. Recent controversy over the use of these well established agents was stimulated by reports from New Zealand and Canada[13,14] implicating one drug (fenoterol) in asthma mortality statistics from these countries. The ensuing debate has stressed the importance of patients not being over-reliant on bronchodilators at the expense

**Table II.** Commonly used $\beta_2$-agonist bronchodilators[a]

| Drug | Dosage (adults) | Adverse effects |
|---|---|---|
| **Short-acting** (1.5-3 hours) | | *All drugs:* tremor, cramps, tachycardia. Hypokalaemia (may be potentiated by methylxanthines, corticosteroids, diuretics, hypoxia – caution and monitor in these situations). Caution in thyrotoxicosis |
| Rimiterol | MDI: 200-400μg | |
| **Intermediate-acting** (3-6 hours) | | |
| Bitolterol[b] | MDI: 370-740μg | |
| Fenoterol | MDI: 100-200μg<br>Neb: 5mg | |
| Isoetharine | MDI: 340-680μg | |
| Orciprenaline (metaproterenol) | MDI: 750-1500μg[c]<br>PO: 20mg (tid-qid) | |
| Pirbuterol | MDI: 200-400μg<br>PO: 15mg (tid-qid) | |
| Reproterol | MDI: 500-1000μg | |
| Salbutamol (albuterol) | MDI: 100-200μg<br>DPD: 200-400μg<br>Neb: 2.5-5mg<br>PO: 2-8mg (tid-qid); 8mg SR (bid) | |
| Terbutaline | MDI: 250-500μg[d]<br>DPD: 500μg<br>Neb: 5-10mg<br>PO: 2.5-5mg (tid); 7.5mg SR (bid) | |
| Tulobuterol | PO: 2mg (bid-tid) | |
| **Long-acting** (>12 hours) | | |
| Bambuterol[e] | PO: 10-20mg (od) | |
| Formoterol | MDI: 12-24μg (bid) | |
| Salmeterol | MDI: 50μg (bid)<br>DPD: 50μg (bid) | As above plus headache |

a Activity primarily at $\beta_2$-adrenoceptors, although some activity at $\beta_1$-adrenoceptors may occur at high doses.
b Ester prodrug of colterol (hydrolysed predominantly by lung esterases to colterol).
c In the US, 650-1300μg.
d In the US, 200-400μg.
e Lipophilic ester prodrug of terbutaline (metabolised by oxidation and hydrolysis to terbutaline over a prolonged period).
*Abbreviations:* DPD = dry powder device; MDI = metered-dose inhaler; Neb = nebuliser; PO = oral; SR = sustained-release formulation; od = once daily; bid = twice daily; tid = 3 times daily; qid = 4 times daily.

of inhaled or oral corticosteroids for chronic disease management and crises, respectively. The UK Committee on the Safety of Medicines did not find that short/intermediate-acting bronchodilators were intrinsically dangerous.[15] Although there is some evidence that regular use of these agents without corticosteroids increases bronchial hyper-reactivity and may increase asthma severity,[16,17] retrospective studies of fatal asthma cases have usually found evidence of underuse of corticosteroids, inadequate assessment of severity, poor education of patients about their condition, and no objective measurements of airway obstruction.[18]

Long-acting $\beta_2$-agonist drugs (e.g. salmeterol[19] and formoterol[20]) have a sustained bronchodilator effect for up to 15 hours and are used in more severe asthma, coadministered with inhaled corticosteroids in twice-daily regimens where the inhaled corticosteroid is insufficient to control symptoms. They are particularly useful in persisting nocturnal asthma, in patients with morning dipping of peak flow, and in exercise-induced asthma.

*Oral therapy* with $\beta_2$-agonist drugs is generally much less effective than by inhalation (the latter route providing better, quicker and more prolonged bronchodilatation with a much smaller dose), and is attended by many more adverse effects. Sustained-release oral preparations of salbutamol (4 or 8mg) and terbutaline (7.5mg) and the long-acting drug bambuterol (10 or 20mg) may be useful for patients who have nocturnal asthma despite inhaled treatment or for those who cannot master the inhalation of bronchoactive substances.

### Anticholinergic Drugs

In asthmatic patients, anticholinergic agents act on airway obstruction mediated by cholinergic/muscarinic receptors in the parasympathetic nervous system. Ipratropium bromide has a 6-hour duration of action, while oxitropium bromide has a longer duration of action of 12 hours. These drugs are administered by metered-dose aerosol, breath-actuated and dry powder devices. Ipratropium can also be given by nebuliser in a wet aerosol. Neither drug is given orally or parenterally (table III).

***Clinical use:*** anticholinergic drugs are less useful in the management of asthmatic airway obstruction than $\beta_2$-agonist drugs, but may be useful in acute severe asthma when given by nebuliser with $\beta_2$-agonists, where they produce more bronchodilatation than the $\beta_2$-agonist agent used alone.[21] Anticholinergic drugs can also be tried with other measures when control of chronic asthma with $\beta_2$-agonists and high-dose inhaled corticosteroids is insufficient.

In theory, the anticholinergic agents might be expected to be associated with atropine-like adverse effects such as dry mouth, constipation, urinary retention and tachycardia. In practice, the only potentially dangerous unwanted effect is pupillary dilatation in patients predisposed to glaucoma. This is most likely to happen when direct absorption occurs in the course of ipratropium administration by wet aerosol using a face mask. Use of a mouthpiece instead of a mask obviates the problem.

### Methylxanthines

Theophylline and its derivatives (e.g. aminophylline, the ethylenediamine salt) are useful bronchodilators, but have drawbacks. They cannot be given by inhalation and thus can only reach the target organ (the bronchi) via the circulation when given orally, intravenously or (increasingly rarely) rectally. They were thought to act mainly by inhibiting the intracellular enzyme phosphodiesterase, which breaks down cyclic-AMP (thought to be essential for bronchodilatation). However, antagonism of adenosine receptors has also been postulated as

a mode of action, and they have been shown to

a mode of action, and they have been shown to have weak anti-inflammatory actions.

Aminophylline is given intravenously in acute severe asthma, usually when other measures (nebulised $\beta_2$-agonists, anticholinergics and intravenous corticosteroids) have not proved effective. Care is required in this situation, particularly if the patient has received an oral theophylline preparation, since theophylline has a narrow therapeutic index.

***Clinical use:*** the methylxanthines are used orally to supplement the effect of $\beta_2$-agonists and inhaled corticosteroids in chronic asthma. They are available in sustained-release oral preparations which may be taken twice daily, or in some cases once daily before bedtime. Methylxanthines are often poorly tolerated because of gastrointestinal side effects, insomnia and irritability. They can be very useful in some patients with poorly controlled nocturnal asthma, improving their night symptoms and early morning peak flow rates.

Intravenous aminophylline is given in acute severe asthma in a bolus dose of 5 to 6 mg/kg over 15 to 30 minutes, ideally by slow infusion. It is not first-line therapy but is given where there has been a poor response to nebulised $\beta_2$-agonists and intravenous hydrocortisone. Aminophylline should be used with caution and patients should have their heart rate and rhythm monitored during administration. The bolus dose of aminophylline can be followed by up to 0.5 to 0.9 mg/kg/h by continuous infusion, continuing the monitoring of heart rate and rhythm, peak flow rate and blood gas tensions.

There is wide interindividual variation in metabolism and many situations alter the clearance of methylxanthines (table IV). The dose of theophylline should therefore be individualised to maintain serum concentrations within the therapeutic range (10 to 20 mg/L). Therapeutic effects are often obtained with blood concentrations below this range and it is common to experience adverse effects with blood concentrations well within that range and even below

**Table III.** Anticholinergic drugs used to treat respiratory conditions

| Drug | Pharmacological activity | Dose | Duration of action (hours) | Adverse effect |
|---|---|---|---|---|
| Ipratropium bromide | Anticholinergic (antimuscarinic) | MDI: 10-40μg<br>Neb: 250-500μg | 6 | Pupillary dilatation with Neb route and face mask (caution if glaucoma present) |
| Oxitropium bromide | Anticholinergic (antimuscarinic) | MDI: 100-200μg | 12 | As for ipratropium |

*Abbreviations:* MDI = metered-dose inhaler; Neb = nebuliser.

**Table IV.** Principal clinical pharmacological characteristics of theophylline and related drugs

**Preparations**

Theophylline sometimes given as a salt, e.g. choline theophyllinate (oxtriphylline) or in a combined preparation

Anhydrous theophylline content varies between products[a]

Completeness of absorption is related to formulation (e.g. enteric-coated and some sustained-release preparations not completely or reliably absorbed, rectal absorption erratic)

**Elimination**

Hepatic metabolism (demethylation, oxidation); marked interindividual variation in elimination

a) *Factors **decreasing** theophylline clearance:*

- Special populations (premature neonates, age >50y, obese)
- Dietary methylxanthines (e.g. heavy coffee intake)
- Disease (hepatic cirrhosis, congestive heart failure, acute pulmonary oedema, chronic obstructive pulmonary disease with cor pulmonale, pneumonia, acute febrile episodes)
- Drugs (troleandomycin, erythromycin, cimetidine, high-dose allopurinol, oral contraceptives, influenza vaccines, ciprofloxacin, nortriptyline, diltiazem, nifedipine, verapamil, mexiletine, β-adrenoceptor antagonists)

b) *Factors **increasing** theophylline clearance:*

- Age (children 1 to 16y)
- Heavy cigarette smoking (>10 per day)
- Marijuana
- High carbohydrate, low protein diet
- Enzyme-inducing drugs (e.g. phenobarbital, phenytoin, carbamazepine, rifampicin, isoniazid)

**Principal adverse effects**

May be reduced by monitoring serum concentrations (keep <20 mg/L)

Nausea, gastric irritation, cardiovascular effects including arrhythmias, excitation, insomnia, nightmares, convulsions

Rectal theophylline causes irritation

a For aminophylline, the anhydrous theophylline content varies from 78 and 84% (i.e. 1.27g aminophylline is approximately equivalent to 1g theophylline). For choline theophyllinate (oxtriphylline), it is around 64% (i.e. 1.57g choline theophyllinate is approximately equivalent to 1g theophylline).

it. Such adverse effects commonly limit the usefulness of these important agents.

The methylxanthines are associated with a number of important drug interactions, and adjustment of their dosages may be necessary when certain commonly used antibiotics and other drugs are given concomitantly (see further appendix B).

#### Assessment of the Effect of Bronchodilator Drugs

The effectiveness of all bronchodilator drugs should be assessed objectively to avoid unnecessary (and sometimes expensive) prescription of drugs and aids to inhalation including spacers, dry powder inhalers and nebulisers.

Measurement of peak expiratory flow rate (PEFR) and/or forced expiratory volume in 1 second ($FEV_1$) before and after administration of $\beta_2$-agonists, anticholinergics and methylxanthines is easy to perform in the clinic or consulting room and should not be omitted (to avoid prescribing inappropriate and potentially expensive medicines). Monitoring peak flow rates twice daily before and after $\beta_2$-agonists or anticholinergics may be performed at home; morning peak flow rates are useful in assessing the effect of oral methylxanthines, particularly if taken once daily before bedtime. In the situation of home monitoring, it is important to know the patient's predicted peak expiratory flow rate, personal best peak expiratory flow rate (often achieved after a short course of high-dose corticosteroids), and the variability or amplitude of peak flow rates looking at the percentage change about the mean value. Such amplitude is never more than 8% in normal individuals but is frequently and characteristically over 20% in patients with symptomatic asthma. The greater the variability of peak flow rate, the more unstable and dangerous the condition.

In acute severe asthma, arterial blood gases and peak expiratory flow rates should be measured and the response to bronchodilator therapy carefully monitored.

### *3.1.2 Anti-Inflammatory Drugs*

#### Sodium Cromoglycate and Nedocromil Sodium

*Sodium cromoglycate (cromolyn sodium)* is believed to act stabilising the membranes of mast cells and preventing the release of preformed inflammatory mediators. It is of value in children, some young adults with exercise-induced asthma, and where there is reluctance to accept inhaled corticosteroids. It is used only by inhalation, is well tolerated and has no adverse effects. It may be given by metered-dose inhaler, dry powder inhaler or nebuliser.

Since sodium cromoglycate is a prophylactic agent, the patient should be in the best possible state before therapy is started. The drug is usually taken 4 times daily, an instruction that reduces compliance in many patients.

*Nedocromil sodium* is a similar inhalational drug that has various inhibitory effects on mediator release from mast cells, eosinophils and other inflammatory cells (see also chapter 28; section 3.4.1). Some studies have shown nedocromil to have a corticosteroid-sparing effect (for a review, see Gonzalez and Brogden).[22] Like sodium cromoglycate, it is generally less useful than inhaled corticosteroids, must be given 4 times daily, and is relatively expensive.

Inhaled corticosteroids are usually preferred to these anti-inflammatory drugs, as they are almost invariably more efficacious and less expensive.

#### Inhaled Corticosteroids

Asthmatic patients requiring the use of inhaled, short/intermediate-acting $\beta_2$-agonists on more than 3 days a week, or who waken at night with asthma, should have inhaled corticosteroid therapy. Topically active inhaled corticosteroids include *beclomethasone dipropionate, budesonide, fluticasone propionate* and *triamcinolone acetonide*. They are prophylactic agents that are usually administered twice daily and must be taken regularly. They are not appropriate for use in an acute attack.

***Clinical use:*** inhaled corticosteroids are the most useful anti-inflammatory agents for asthma, giving good control and at the same time avoiding the adverse effects of oral corticosteroids or at least minimising the dose of oral corticosteroid needed for control. This treatment reduces inflammatory cells in bronchoalveolar lavage fluid from asthmatic patients and decreases airway hyper-responsiveness to nonspecific stimuli and antigen.

A wide dosage schedule is possible; for example, beclomethasone dipropionate is provided in a range of metered-dose inhalers containing 50, 100, 200 or 250 μg/puff,[1] allowing convenient administration of up to 2000μg daily. Such high doses can improve the overall control and enable the reduction of oral corticosteroid dosages in patients with severe asthma not well controlled by usual inhaled doses.

With budesonide, the usual dose is 200 to 400 μg/day (as with beclomethasone dipropionate), although up to 1600μg daily may be required in some cases (table V). There is little to choose between beclomethasone dipropionate and budesonide in terms of clinical effectiveness or adverse effects.[23] Studies have shown that twice-daily administration is just as good as administration every 6 hours.[24] Fluticasone propionate appears to have greater topical activity than the other inhaled corticosteroids and is possibly less bioavailable.[25] The dose range of this agent is from 100 to 2000 μg/day (for a review of its use in asthma, see Holliday et al.[26]).

All of these corticosteroids can be given by metered-dose inhaler and dry powder device. A breath-actuated inhaler is available with beclomethasone dipropionate at different strengths. Budesonide and fluticasone propionate can be given by nebuliser.

Careful patient instruction and education are essential. The best technique and device to obtain maximum airway deposition is important and patients must understand that treatment is prophylactic only and must be taken regularly. Reassurance about freedom from adverse effects is often necessary and needs to be repeated.

***Tolerability:*** oropharyngeal candidiasis occurs in 10% of patients using corticosteroid inhalers, but this adverse effect can be minimised by using large volume spacer devices[27] and gargling after use; this is aimed at reducing oropharyngeal deposition. In troublesome cases of candidiasis, nystatin lozenges or oral fluconazole therapy may be necessary (see further chapter 16; sect. 5.1). Occasionally, dysphonia (presenting as hoarseness) from a localised vocal cord adductor muscle myopathy, can develop.[28] It is dose-related and reversible.[27]

Inhaled corticosteroid daily dosages in excess of beclomethasone dipropionate 2000μg and budesonide 1600μg can result in biochemical evidence of hypothalamic-pituitary-adrenal (HPA) axis suppression. This is rarely manifest clinically and patients using an inhaled corticoste-

1. In the US, beclomethasone dipropionate 50 μg/metered-dose inhaler is stated to deliver 42 μg/metered-dose, since 8μg of the standard 50μg dose delivered by the valve is lodged on the inside of the inhaler device with each actuation.

**Table V.** Corticosteroid drugs used in asthma

| Drug | Route of administration | Dosage (adults) | Principal adverse effects/notes[a] |
|---|---|---|---|
| Beclomethasone dipropionate[b] | Inhaled | 100-200μg puff twice daily. *Severe cases:* up to 1000μg twice daily | *Surface active topical corticosteroids:* oropharyngeal candidiasis, hoarseness and sore throat are the most common adverse effects. |
| Budesonide | Inhaled | 200-400μg (1 to 2 puffs) twice daily. *Severe cases:* up to 1600μg daily (high-dose therapy). *Nebuliser:* 0.5 to 1 mg twice daily | Symptomatic oropharyngeal candidiasis most likely at doses >800 μg/day. Activity may diminish as obstruction increases. Adverse systemic effects of exogenous corticosteroids reduced at therapeutic doses of aerosols. Care during changeover from oral to aerosol therapy. Requirements for $\beta_2$-agonists may diminish |
| Fluticasone propionate | Inhaled | 50-1000μg twice daily | |
| Prednisolone/ prednisone[c] | Oral | 30 to 60 mg/day reducing to <10 mg/day in 1-3 divided doses | Prednisone metabolised to biologically active prednisolone in liver. Adverse effects (see chapter 19; sect. 7.1.1) are clinically important, especially at >7.5 mg/day. Enzyme inducers (e.g. barbiturates, rifampicin) may reduce effectiveness. Substitution by inhaled corticosteroids desirable but care needed |
| Hydrocortisone sodium succinate | Intravenous | 3 to 4 mg/kg loading dose, then 3 mg/kg every 6h | For adverse effects, see chapter 19 (section 7.1.1) |
| Tetracosactide (tetracosactrin) | Intramuscular | 0.5 to 1.0mg alternate days; titrate to response | For adverse effects, see chapter 19 (section 7.1.1). Less growth stunting not proven. Allergic reaction hazardous. Supervision for at least 30 minutes essential |

a Use corticosteroids with care in patients with active or quiescent tuberculosis.

b In the US, beclomethasone dipropionate 50 μg/metered-dose inhaler is stated to deliver 42 μg/metered dose, since 8μg of the standard 50μg dose delivered by the valve is lodged on the inside of the inhaler device with each actuation.

c The clinical pharmacological properties of systemic corticosteroids are discussed further in chapter 19 (section 7.1.1). Other corticosteroids that may be used include methylprednisolone, triamcinolone, betamethasone and dexamethasone.

roid who have acute severe asthma and are admitted to hospital are able to produce normal amounts of adrenal corticosteroids in response to the stress of severe asthma and hospital admission.

The effect of inhaled corticosteroids on bone growth in children has occasioned recent debate. The general consensus is that poorly controlled asthma is more inhibitory to normal bone growth than are inhaled corticosteroids at normal therapeutic doses.[29]

Large doses of inhaled corticosteroids in adults can result in skin thinning and purpura, a possibly increased incidence of cataract formation, and some biochemical evidence of increased bone resorption.[30]

***Assessment of the therapeutic effect*** of inhaled corticosteroid involves symptom assessment (particularly asthma at night, early in the morning and on exercise), the degree of use of relief or rescue short/intermediate-acting $\beta_2$-agonist inhalers, and objective measurements of morning and evening PEFR.

The effect of inhaled corticosteroids should be apparent within 1 to 2 weeks, rising to a peak effect at 4 to 6 weeks. If the patient is still symptomatic with peak flow rates significantly below predicted, the inhaled corticosteroid dose should be increased at that point.

#### Oral Corticosteroids

Short courses of high-dose oral corticosteroids (e.g. 30 to 40mg daily of prednisolone) are indicated in acute severe asthma or in asthmatic patients at risk of developing that state. They may be taken for 1 to 3 weeks and are not associated with many of the unwanted effects of long term oral corticosteroid therapy. Once the condition has restabilised, oral corticosteroids may be stopped abruptly or stepped down. Either way, adrenal function may take some days or weeks to return to normal.

Tapering courses of corticosteroids have been given in the belief that they cause less adrenal suppression but there is little difference in this outcome between tapering courses and abruptly stopping a short, high-dose course; in addition, the tapering course is probably less effective in terms of the peak flow rate achieved. Short courses of corticosteroids may cause fluid retention in the elderly, euphoria and insomnia in some patients. They must be used with caution in diabetics and those with coexisting or previous peptic ulceration (in this situation they should be coadministered with an $H_2$-receptor antagonist). Short courses of corticosteroids should be given as often as necessary but if required frequently (more than 2-monthly) then control is clearly poor and other problems should be explored such as compliance, inhaler technique, consideration of other delivery systems, and environmental or occupational factors.

Some patients require long term low-dose maintenance oral corticosteroids, although they are much fewer in number with the advent of inhaled corticosteroids and other steroid-sparing agents. Where possible, the oral daily dose should not exceed prednisolone 7.5mg, since below this dosage level, there is relatively less HPA axis suppression.

The clinical pharmacology or corticosteroids is discussed further in chapter 19 (section 7.1.1).

#### 3.1.3 Other Drugs

##### Leukotriene Antagonists and Synthesis Inhibitors

Leukotriene receptor antagonists (e.g. *ibudilast, pranlukast, zafirlukast*) and synthesis inhibitors (e.g. *zileuton*) are under development. These agents provide a potential new approach to inhibit the pro-inflammatory properties of leukotrienes. Their place in chronic asthma therapy is not yet established but in short term studies, improvements have been reported in respiratory function and asthma symptoms with some reduction in the rate of $\beta_2$-agonist use and the requirement for rescue corticosteroids.

##### Antihistamine/Antiallergic Drugs

Antihistamines ($H_1$-receptor antagonists) are of little or no value in asthma except for the treatment of concomitant upper airway problems, i.e. hay fever or vasomotor rhinitis commonly experienced by asthmatic patients.

*Ketotifen* is an orally administered antihistaminic agent with anti-inflammatory effects similar to those of sodium cromoglycate. Trials in adults have been disappointing and, although more beneficial in children, absolute improvement in lung function is usually no more than slight. This, together with the long run-in period necessary and initial drowsiness, especially in older children and adults, has resulted in a lack of widespread acceptance of this agent. For a review of its clinical pharmacological properties, see Grant et al.[31]

##### Antibiotics

Antibiotics have no place in asthma management unless there is proven bacterial infection, e.g. bronchitis with fever and frankly purulent sputum, or pneumonia.

### 3.2 Optimum Treatment

Concern about the rising prevalence of asthma in developed countries with increased morbidity and significant mortality, has led to several consensus documents on the management of asthma.[32-35]

#### 3.2.1 Chronic Asthma

The British Thoracic Society guidelines recommend a stepwise approach to management, treatment being appropriate to the severity of the condition in individual patients at different times in their illness. The aims of management include accurate diagnosis, abolition of symptoms and achievement of best possible function, reducing the risk of severe attacks and minimising absence from school or work. Common to all steps is recognition and avoidance (where possible) of causative or precipitating factors such as occupational hazards, drugs (e.g. β-blockers, aspirin, etc.), allergens and exposure to everyday pollutants, aerosols and irritants like cigarette smoke.

Management requires careful education of the patient about the nature of asthma, the drugs used for prevention and relief of symptoms, and advice, both spoken and written, about how to adjust treatment in the light of changes in symptoms or objective measurements such as PEFR. At all stages of asthma severity, it is permissible to use short courses of *oral corticosteroids* to regain control, e.g. when:

- Symptoms and PEFR worsen day by day
- The PEFR falls below 60% of the patient's best
- Sleep disturbance from asthma becomes a problem
- Morning symptoms persist until midday
- Emergency injection or nebulised treatment has been needed.

The stepwise approach to management recommended in the International Consensus Report[35] is shown in figure 1. Patients with chronic asthma are introduced to treatment at whatever level is considered appropriate by their clinician and the treatment stepped up or down as appropriate. Many believe in optimising the patient's condition with a short course of a corticosteroid at the outset, in the belief that

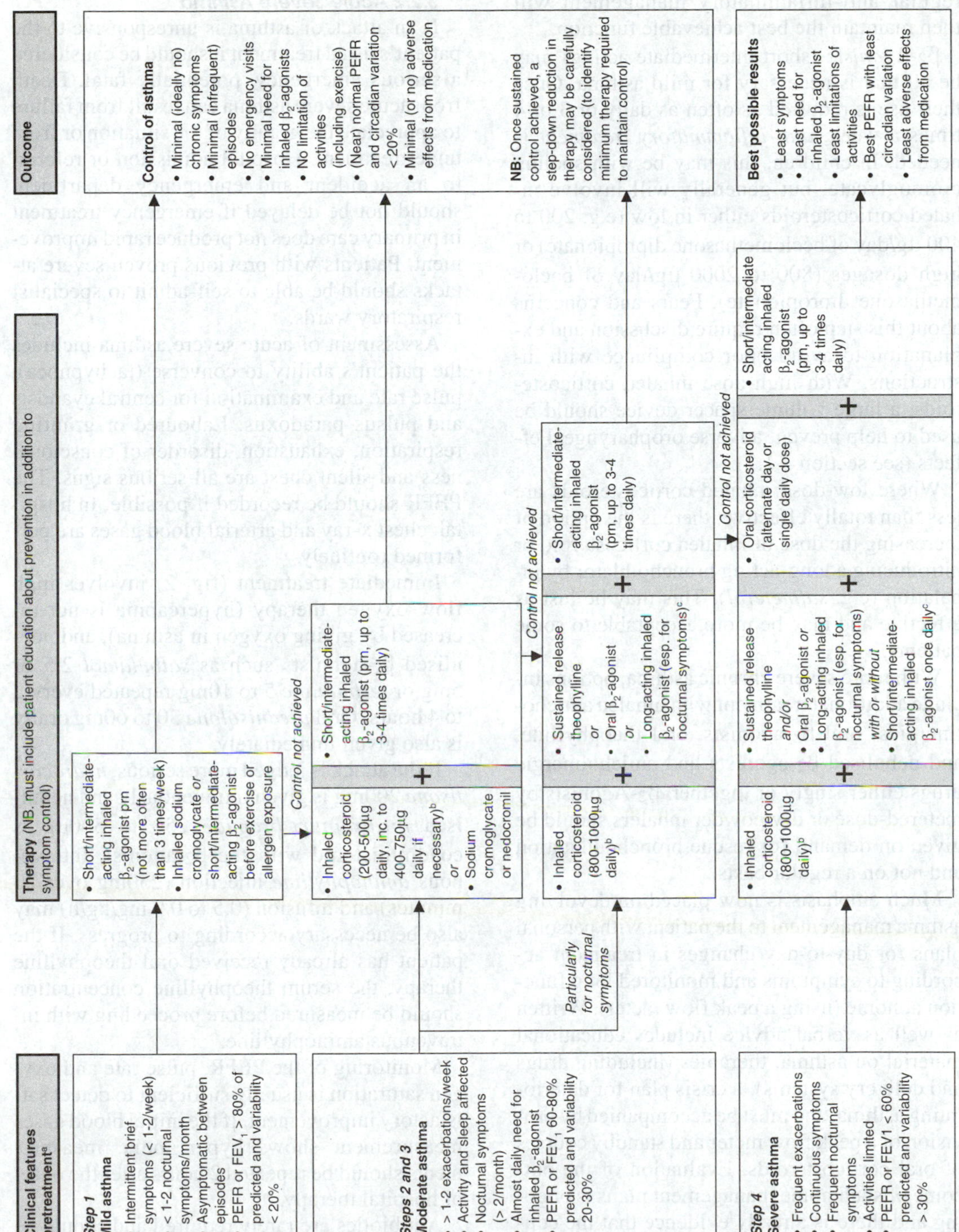


**Fig. 1.** Stepwise approach to management of chronic asthma (after International Consensus Report[35]).
a) One or more features may be present; assign patient to most severe grade in which any feature is present.
b) Inhaled corticosteroid dose refers to beclomethasone dipropionate.
c) Inhaled anticholinergic (e.g. ipratropium bromide or oxitropium bromide) may also be considered.
*Abbreviations:* PEFR = peak expiratory flow rate; $FEV_1$ = forced expiratory volume in 1 second.

regular anti-inflammatory management will then maintain the best achievable function.

$\beta_2$-*Agonists* (short/intermediate-acting) may be all that is necessary for mild asthma. Once their use is required as often as daily or 3 or 4 times a week, *anti-inflammatory treatment* is needed. In children, this may be with sodium cromoglycate, but generally will involve inhaled corticosteroids either in low (e.g. 200 to 400 μg/day of beclomethasone dipropionate) or high dosages (800 to 2000 μg/day of beclomethasone dipropionate). Fears and concerns about this step often require discussion and explanation to avoid poor compliance with instructions. With high-dose inhaled corticosteroids, a large volume spacer device should be used to help prevent adverse oropharyngeal effects (see section 3.1.2).

Where low-dose inhaled corticosteroids are less than totally effective, there is the option of increasing the dose of inhaled corticosteroid or introducing a long-acting bronchodilator by inhalation (e.g. *salmeterol*). This may be just as effective and may be more acceptable to some patients.

With more severe chronic asthma, options include additional treatment with inhaled anticholinergics, oral $\beta_2$-agonists, oral theophylline, and nebulised $\beta_2$-agonists and anticholinergic drugs either singly or together. $\beta_2$-Agonists by metered-dose or dry powder inhalers should be given on demand for rescue bronchodilatation and not on a regular basis.

Much emphasis is now placed on devolving asthma management to the patient with personal plans for day-to-day changes in treatment according to symptoms and monitored lung function at home (using a peak flow meter). Written as well as verbal advice includes educational material on asthma, therapies (including drugs and delivery systems), a crisis plan for deteriorating asthma, and must be accompanied by provision of a peak flow meter and standby courses of oral corticosteroids. Evaluation of the outcome of such home management plans is ongoing and there is already evidence that the education of asthma sufferers has an effect on hospital admission rates with acute severe asthma.

The establishment of asthma clinics in primary care often run by trained asthma nurses is another initiative likely to result in improved general asthma control.

#### *3.2.2 Acute Severe Asthma*

If an attack of asthma is unresponsive to the patient's usual treatment it should be considered a serious emergency, potentially fatal. Death from acute severe asthma can result from failure to appreciate the gravity of the situation or from undertreatment. Hospital admission or referral to an accident and emergency department should not be delayed if emergency treatment in primary care does not produce rapid improvement. Patients with previous proven severe attacks should be able to self-admit to specialist respiratory wards.

Assessment of acute severe asthma includes the patient's ability to converse (tachypnoea), pulse rate and examination for central cyanosis and pulsus paradoxus. Laboured or grunting respiration, exhaustion, disorder of consciousness and silent chest are all serious signs. The PEFR should be recorded if possible. In hospital, chest x-ray and arterial blood gases are performed routinely.

Immediate treatment (fig. 2) involves high flow oxygen therapy (hypercapnia is not increased by giving oxygen in asthma), and nebulised $\beta_2$-agonists such as *salbutamol* 2.5 or 5mg or *terbutaline* 5 to 10mg repeated every 2 to 4 hours. Oral *prednisolone* 30 to 60mg orally is also given immediately.

If the attack is judged more serious, *hydrocortisone* 200mg is given intravenously and nebulised *ipratropium bromide* 250 to 500μg is coadministered with the $\beta_2$-agonist. Intravenous *aminophylline* injection (250mg over 20 minutes) and infusion (0.5 to 0.9 mg/kg/h) may also be necessary according to progress. If the patient has already received oral theophylline therapy, the serum theophylline concentration should be measured before proceeding with intravenous aminophylline.

Monitoring of the PEFR, pulse rate and oxygen saturation is usually sufficient to detect satisfactory improvement. If the initial blood gases measurement shows hypercapnia, measurements should be repeated 2 hours after the onset of hospital therapy.

Antibiotics are rarely required and should be reserved for situations where there is specific evidence of infection. Sedation is absolutely contraindicated.

Intermittent positive-pressure ventilation (IPPV) is not often required; indications include progressive exhaustion, failing respiratory efforts, coma, respiratory arrest, or a $paCO_2$ that

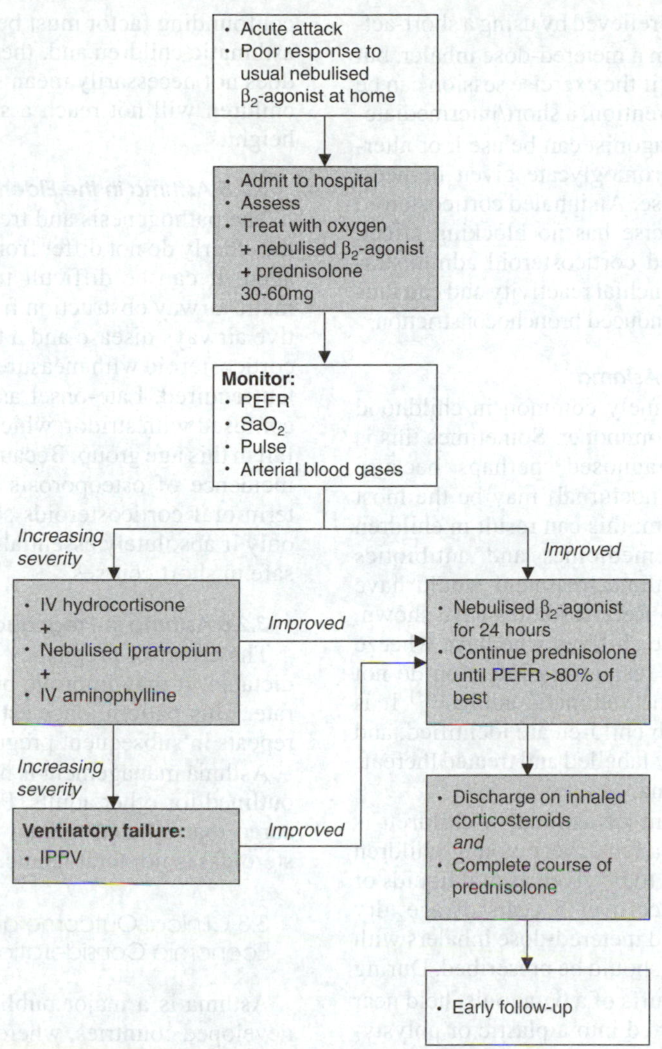


**Fig. 2.** Management of acute severe asthma. *Abbreviations:* PEFR = peak expiratory flow rate; $SaO_2$ = arterial oxygen saturation; IPPV = intermittent positive-pressure ventilation; IV = intravenous.

exceeds 6 kPa and is rising despite intensive medical treatment.

Once the patient has recovered, the reason for deterioration and loss of control must be explored and advice given to avoid further episodes. Inhaler technique must be checked and, if unsatisfactory, training given or a more suitable device found. All patients must be discharged on an anti-inflammatory regimen (inhaled corticosteroid) with rapid review in primary care (in <1 week) and within 4 weeks at a specialist chest clinic. Clear instructions about the duration of the course of oral prednisolone must be given. The PEFR should have reached 75% of predicted or best possible values before discharge and should show less than 20% variability. Provision of a peak flow meter and a self-management plan is usually appropriate at this stage.

For a review of the treatment of acute asthma, see McFadden and Hejal.[36]

### 3.2.3 Exercise-Induced Asthma

Airflow limitation after exercise is common in asthma, e.g. after 5 to 10 minutes running on the flat, more often when the air is dry and cold. The phenomenon is thought to arise from airway cooling and evaporation of moisture from the bronchial mucosa, influencing bronchial hyper-reactivity already present. It most often affects children and young adults (possibly because they are more likely to indulge in exercise).

An attack can be relieved by using a short-acting $\beta_2$-agonist from a metered-dose inhaler, but is better prevented if the exercise session can be predicted. For prevention, a short/intermediate- or long-acting $\beta_2$-agonist can be used, or alternatively sodium cromoglycate given immediately before exercise. An inhaled corticosteroid given before exercise has no blocking effect, but regular inhaled corticosteroid administration influences bronchial reactivity and can thus diminish exercise-induced bronchoconstriction.

#### 3.2.4 Childhood Asthma

Asthma is extremely common in childhood and is becoming commoner. Sometimes this is not accurately diagnosed, perhaps because cough (especially nocturnal) may be the most prominent symptom; this can result in children receiving cough medicines and antibiotics where specific asthma treatment would have been indicated.[37] Recent studies have shown, however, that some children who have wheeze in the presence of respiratory infection do not grow up to become asthmatic adults.[38] It is important that such children are identified, and not inappropriately labelled and treated thereafter as having asthma.

The management of asthma in children is similar to that in adults. Very young children require their drugs to be given as oral liquids or nebulisers, but once over 5 years of age, dry powder devices and metered-dose inhalers with or without spacers should be prescribed. During attacks, multiple puffs of a $\beta_2$-agonist held near the mouth or inserted into a plastic or polystyrene cup held over the face can be very effective.

Oral bronchodilators such as theophylline are often well tolerated by children and can be useful. Sodium cromoglycate is used more in children than adults, but the modern mainstay of anti-inflammatory treatment (as in adults) is inhaled corticosteroids in a dose sufficient to give good control. There are legitimate concerns over possible inhibition of bone growth, so the minimum dose controlling symptoms should be used. Oral prednisolone (which definitely does suppress growth) should be avoided as far as possible.

A stepwise approach to childhood asthma, as in adults, is followed and similar monitoring performed, with the important addition of height and weight, which are plotted carefully on percentile charts. Growth in children is influenced greatly by the onset of puberty, which is frequently delayed by asthma. This important confounding factor must be borne in mind with asthmatic children and, therefore, small stature does not necessarily mean stunting or that such children will not reach a satisfactory eventual height.

#### 3.2.5 Asthma in the Elderly

The pathogenesis and treatment of asthma in the elderly do not differ from that in the middle-aged. It can be difficult to differentiate asthmatic airway obstruction from chronic obstructive airways disease and a therapeutic trial of a corticosteroid with measurement of PEFR is often required. Late-onset asthma should not be confused with stridor, which is a diagnostic pitfall in this age group. Because of the widespread incidence of osteoporosis in the elderly, long term oral corticosteroids should be prescribed only if absolutely essential. They are relatively safe in short courses.

#### 3.2.6 Asthma in Pregnancy

The effect of pregnancy on asthma is unpredictable; it may improve but may also deteriorate. This pattern, once established, frequently repeats in subsequent pregnancies.

Asthma management is no different from that outlined for other adults. Patients may be reassured that inhaled therapy (especially corticosteroids) is not teratogenic.

### 3.3 Clinical Outcome and Economic Considerations

Asthma is a major public health problem in developed countries, where it consumes a large and increasing share of scarce health resources. While much is known about asthma morbidity, there is very little information relating to the cost and economic efficiency of current asthma management. Although the true total expenditure on asthma is unknown, current estimates suggests that it is high.[39,40] In the US, the total healthcare cost of asthma has been estimated at $US6200 million in 1992 or around 1% of all healthcare costs.

In the UK, the 1990 Action Asthma Project[41] showed that the average net ingredient cost for medication was £7.28. In 1988, around 27 million prescriptions were issued for asthma medications, implying an overall cost in primary care including dispensing fees paid to pharmacists of £228 million in the UK. In 1985, it was estimated that asthma accounted for 16.2 hospital discharges (or deaths) per 100,000 population, with a mean duration of stay of 4.9

**Table VI.** Estimated costs of asthma in the UK in 1988

| Factor | Cost (£ million) |
|---|---|
| Primary care: | |
| • Consultations | 19.4 |
| • Prescribed medicines | 228.0 |
| Hospital inpatients | 57.6 |
| Hospital outpatients | 6.9 |
| **Total** | 311.9 |

days. Translating this to 1988 prices, this is equivalent to an average cost of £127.14/day or a total of £57.6 million. Estimates of outpatient referral costs are difficult, but suggest that around 3% of asthmatic patients may be referred each year, which together with patients referred after hospital admission can be extrapolated to an overall outpatient cost of £6.9 million in 1988. Drawing these figures together suggests that the cost of asthma in the UK in 1988 was around £312 million (table VI).

Prevention of asthma through a greater understanding of its causes and triggers is the long term goal of management. The therapeutic aim should be to maintain best lung function by optimal drug therapy. Economic considerations and drug selection should include an assessment of differing routes of administration, since inhaled therapy is usually highly effective and is associated with minimal adverse effects. There are now a wide range of inhalation devices, ranging from the metered-dose inhaler through the new multidose dry powder devices to nebulised therapy. This makes the complexity of drug selection in asthma almost unique in therapeutics.

The optimal bronchodilator is a $\beta_2$-agonist by inhalation, since this will give immediate relief at low doses with minimal adverse effects. Ability to use the inhaler efficiently is an important factor in deciding which device and hence which drug to choose. It has been estimated that as many as half of adult patients and a greater proportion of children gain little benefit from using metered-dose inhalers because of poor technique.[42]

A formal cost-benefit analysis of the different inhaler devices has yet to be published, but there is evidence comparing nebulised $\beta_2$-agonist therapy with metered-dose inhalers. While nebulisers can deliver large doses of the $\beta_2$-agonist and avoid difficulties with inhaler technique, 2 randomised studies in the US of hospital patients with asthma and obstructive airways disease suggest that, after the acute illness, a $\beta_2$-agonist by metered-dose inhaler is as effective as by nebuliser and is associated with a 4-fold reduction in cost with no extension of hospital stay.[43,44]

Sodium cromoglycate is one of the few anti-asthma drugs that has been the subject of a cost-effectiveness analysis.[45] In a retrospective analysis, hospital service use by 27 asthmatic children treated with sodium cromoglycate was compared with that of 26 children treated with other drugs. Over 3.5 years, the cost of emergency room visits and hospitalisation was considerably less than in those taking sodium cromoglycate, while the total cost of asthma medication in the 2 groups was almost identical.

Although no formal cost-effectiveness study has been performed, the evidence that inhaled corticosteroids reduce asthma morbidity is overwhelming. In a UK randomised trial in general practice, acute attacks of asthma in 160 patients were virtually abolished by the introduction of inhaled corticosteroid therapy.[46] A prospective study of over 300 patients in California compared asthma specialist and generalist care.[47] After 6 months, emergency room visits were reduced by 50% in patients receiving specialist care. This difference was associated with a marked increase in the use of prophylactic medications, particularly inhaled corticosteroids. Compliance with preventative treatment is of paramount importance and effective inhaler technique, as with $\beta_2$-agonist bronchodilators, is relevant in drug selection.

Theophylline is an alternative bronchodilator, but is not available as an aerosol and hence the onset of action in the oral form is slow. Although it is relatively inexpensive, serum concentrations of theophylline must be monitored because of its potential toxicity, and this adds to the cost of treatment. It is important to undertake serum concentration monitoring when the pharmacokinetics of theophylline are likely to be altered, such as during acute febrile episodes or when intravenous aminophylline is to be given to patients already on long term oral theophylline.

## 4. Bronchitis

### 4.1 Acute Bronchitis

Acute bronchitis is usually preceded by a viral upper respiratory tract infection, especially influenza, parainfluenza, rhinovirus and, in children, respiratory syncytial virus. In infants and young children, acute bronchitis or bronchiolitis is often especially severe and requires hospital treatment. Because of the dimensions of infants' airways, any narrowing results in wheezing and may lead on to patchy atelectasis and bacterial pneumonia.

#### Optimum Treatment

The treatment of acute viral bronchitis is essentially symptomatic: bedrest until afebrile, liberal fluid intake to maintain hydration and facilitate expectoration, aspirin or paracetamol (acetaminophen) for myalgic symptoms, and an antibiotic only if the sputum is purulent.

## 4.2 Chronic Bronchitis

This common disease is usually the result of smoking cigarettes, although people in occupations exposed to dust may be affected. The condition starts with bronchial irritation that leads to mucus gland hypertrophy and increased sputum production. The patient has a productive cough, usually in the morning ('smoker's cough'). If present daily for 3 consecutive months in 2 consecutive winters, this mucus hypersecretion is called *chronic simple bronchitis*.

Continued smoking leads, in some but not all individuals, to chronic obstructive bronchitis, where the patient develops chest tightness, wheezing and breathlessness in addition to the chronic productive cough. Respiratory function measurements show diffuse small airway obstruction from bronchial scarring, inflammation and retained secretions. The condition is also complicated by centilobular emphysema that increases airway obstruction by loss of elastic retractile forces on the airways. The condition is also known as *chronic obstructive pulmonary disease* (COPD) or *chronic obstructive airways disease* (COAD).

What determines progression from simple mucus hypersecretion to chronic obstructive bronchitis is not clear except in the rare variety of familial emphysema associated with $\alpha_1$-antitrypsin deficiency. The rate of progression and decline of the $FEV_1$ can be slowed by stopping smoking.

### 4.2.1 Optimum Treatment

Advice and support over smoking cessation is vital. Patients should receive annual influenza vaccination just before the onset of winter.

#### Infection

Antibiotics are best prescribed for infective exacerbations of chronic bronchitis and not used prophylactically or intermittently. The latter tactic rarely prevents exacerbations and only encourages growth of resistant organisms, making subsequent therapy more difficult.

In the presence of infection, with fever and purulent sputum, broad-spectrum agents such as *amoxicillin* or a *macrolide antibiotic* (e.g. erythromycin, clarithromycin, azithromycin, roxithromycin) should be effective for infection acquired in the community. The usual pathogens are *S. pneumoniae* and *H. influenzae,* and sometimes *Moraxella catarrhalis.* In the event of a poor response or if the infection is hospital-acquired, it should be assumed that the organism is β-lactam resistant and amoxicillin/-clavulanic acid combination or a macrolide or quinolone drug should be used. With severe infections in hospitalised patients, a parenteral antibiotic such as intravenous amoxicillin/clavulanic acid or a cefalosporin (e.g. cefuroxine or cefotaxime) may be used.

The dosages and principal adverse effects of these antibiotics are discussed in section 6.

#### Sputum Retention

Expectoration of sputum is helpful in relieving airway obstruction and is helped by liberal fluid intake, physiotherapy and postural drainage. It is often assisted by nebulising bronchodilators, which have been shown to increase mucociliary clearance, a host defence mechanism known to be impaired by cigarette smoking.

#### Airways Obstruction

The relief of airways obstruction by *$\beta_2$-agonist* and *methylxanthine* bronchodilators in chronic obstructive bronchitis is much less dramatic than in the treatment of asthma, largely because of irreversible airway damage and emphysema. There is evidence that *anticholinergic drugs* such as ipratropium bromide given by inhalation may be more effective than $\beta_2$-agonists in this condition.[48]

Inhaled drugs are given by metered-dose inhaler, breath-actuated devices or dry powder, as in asthma (see section 3). Often much larger doses of these agents are needed than in asthma, and these are best achieved via nebuliser administration. It is important to establish that there is an objective benefit before prescribing this to patients on a domiciliary basis.

*Corticosteroids* are often given in an attempt to relieve dyspnoea and wheeze. It is vitally important that a proper trial with objective measurements of $FEV_1$ or PEFR is conducted to prove that the airway obstruction is truly diminished. Some patients with chronic obstructive pulmonary disease will exhibit an increase in $FEV_1$ of 10% or more with oral corticosteroids, especially if they can also be shown to have eosinophilia. Such patients may benefit from continuing an inhaled corticosteroid. However, patients with emphysema do not usually respond to corticosteroids and are at risk of adverse effects such as osteoporosis if they are committed to long term oral therapy in the mistaken belief that it is helping their airway obstruction.

## 5. Respiratory Failure

The early recognition of respiratory failure depends on the measurement of arterial blood gas tensions. There are 2 types of respiratory failure:

1) Hypoxaemic normocapnic respiratory failure – i.e. hypoxaemia ($paO_2$ 8 kPa or 16mm Hg or less) *without* carbon dioxide retention.

2) Hypoxaemic hypercapnic respiratory failure – i.e. hypoxaemia *with* carbon dioxide retention ($paCO_2$ 6.7 kPa or 50mm Hg or more), which is often known as ventilatory failure.

In *hypoxaemic normocapnic respiratory failure*, the most frequent functional abnormality is an increase in the ventilation-perfusion imbalance in the lung, in which the level of alveolar ventilation is normal or even increased. In general, disorders responsible for this type of failure affect the interstitium of the lung, e.g. pulmonary infarction, pneumonia, fibrosing alveolitis, pulmonary oedema and adult respiratory distress syndrome.

In *hypoxaemic hypercapnic (ventilatory) respiratory failure*, there is a reduction in the level of alveolar ventilation that leads to carbon dioxide retention. There is also usually a ventilation-perfusion imbalance. This type of respiratory failure occurs in:

1) Airways obstruction, such as emphysema or very severe asthma.

2) Respiratory muscle disorders, such as myasthenia gravis or Guillain-Barré syndrome.

3) Thoracic skeletal deformities, such as kyphoscoliosis or chest wall injuries.

4) Central depression of respiration by drugs such as opioids or by encephalitis or brain stem disorders.

The use of hypnotics and sedatives in patients with chronic airways obstruction may also precipitate ventilatory failure.[49]

### 5.1 Clinical Features/Diagnosis

Hypoxaemia without carbon dioxide retention is usually associated with distressing breathlessness. The patient is often alert, anxious and active. Confusion only occurs with severe hypoxaemia. Central cyanosis is an unreliable sign and only indicates gross hypoxaemia.

The clinical features of carbon dioxide retention are usually only seen when the development of hypercapnia has been rapid and associated with respiratory acidosis. Vasodilatation, causing warm extremities and retinal vein engorgement and papilloedema, muscle twitching and a flapping hand tremor may then become evident.

### 5.2 Optimum Treatment

The principles of treatment of both types of respiratory failure involve treatment of the underlying cause and correction of hypoxaemia.

#### *5.2.1 Hypoxaemic Normocapnic Respiratory Failure*

Oxygen can be administered in high concentrations since patients without carbon dioxide retention have normal central carbon dioxide responsiveness and there is no risk of precipitating respiratory acidosis. In practice, oxygen should be given in a concentration of 35% or more.

#### *5.2.2 Hypoxaemic Hypercapnic Respiratory Failure*

Oxygen therapy in patients with carbon dioxide retention is potentially dangerous since, once carbon dioxide responsiveness is lost, patients depend on an 'hypoxic drive' to stimulate ventilation. Thus, administration of high concentrations of oxygen in this situation can impair ventilation and worsen carbon dioxide retention. Masks that deliver low concentrations of oxygen, i.e. 24 or 28% via Venturi-type masks, should be used and the effects of treatment monitored by arterial blood gas analysis.

If controlled oxygen therapy is required for long periods, most patients will prefer the use of nasal cannulae; with a flow rate of 2 L/min, inspired oxygen concentration is usually 25 to 30%. It may not be possible to achieve $paO_2$ concentrations of 7 kPa (50mm Hg) without precipitating high $paCO_2$ concentrations. In such cases, a lower $paO_2$ concentration must be accepted, but below 5 kPa (30mm Hg) tissue damage is likely.

#### 5.2.3 Role of Long Term Oxygen Therapy

Two multicentre controlled clinical trials have shown that long term oxygen therapy improves survival in chronic stable hypoxaemia associated with chronic obstructive pulmonary disease. A UK study showed an improvement in outcome in patients who received oxygen for 15 hours/day, compared with no oxygen.[50] A US study showed markedly improved survival with continuous ambulatory oxygen therapy, compared with only nocturnal oxygen therapy from a stationary system.[51] Taken together, these 2 studies showed that in selected patients with chronic stable hypoxaemia, survival without oxygen was poor. Survival was better with oxygen given 12 to 15 hours per day and best in patients who could receive oxygen on an ambulatory basis for nearly 20 hours per day.

In general, oxygen is prescribed for patients with a chronic stable oxygen tension of <7.3 kPa (55mm Hg), which corresponds to an oxygen saturation of 88%. Patients with higher concentrations of oxygen tension and saturation, but with evidence of pulmonary hypertension, cor pulmonale or secondary polycythaemia are also candidates for long term continuous oxygen. Improved exercise tolerance and better mental function with oxygen are additional indications for long term continuous oxygen therapy.

Developments in oxygen therapy include the transtracheal route of delivery.[52] This offers improved comfort in patients with nasal congestion or other problems with the nasal cannulae, such as painful ears. A reduced flow rate of less than 50% and cosmetic advantages make this form of therapy attractive in selected individuals (for a review, see Tarpy and Celli).[53]

##### Clinical Outcome and Economic Considerations with Oxygen Therapy

Long term oxygen therapy is now available to patients with chronic airways obstruction and significant hypoxaemia. While oxygen delivery by large or small cylinders, liquid oxygen or oxygen concentrators are all considered to be equally effective, a UK study of the total cost per patient showed that oxygen concentrators with a service support system were the least costly form of treatment.[54] In contrast, small domiciliary oxygen cylinders were the most expensive and least convenient alternative.

#### 5.2.4 Role of Respiratory Stimulants

In some patients with ventilatory failure, the level of alveolar ventilation may be temporarily increased by respiratory stimulant drugs.[55] These drugs may increase the sensitivity of the respiratory centre to carbon dioxide or act less specifically as central nervous system stimulants.

##### Doxapram

Doxapram was the first drug to have a specific respiratory stimulating effect via an action on the carotid bodies, although it also stimulates neural tissue, generally at higher concentrations.[56] It is given by intravenous infusion in a dose titrated to achieve adequate stimulation of ventilation, usually 1 to 4 mg/min. Doxapram is indicated for acute ventilatory failure with carbon dioxide retention when the patient is becoming drowsy or when respiration has been suppressed by sedatives or drug overdosage. It has a narrow therapeutic range and there is frequent interindividual variation in response. Great care must be taken in patients with epilepsy, severe coronary artery disease or those taking monoamine oxidase inhibitors.

#### 5.2.5 Role of Pulmonary Vasodilators

Several pulmonary vasodilators have been given to patients with severe hypoxaemia and cor pulmonale in the belief that reduction of pulmonary hypertension and pulmonary vascular resistance will be beneficial. Several of these drugs, including prazosin, sodium nitroprusside, nifedipine, hydralazine and captopril, have been tried in long term studies for up to 1 year. Mean pulmonary artery pressure decreases and cardiac output increases, indicating a large reduction in pulmonary vascular resistance. Arterial blood gas tensions show little change. Overall, pulmonary vasodilators have not been shown to prolong survival in chronic airways obstruction and at present have an uncertain place in clinical management.[57]

#### 5.2.6 Role of α-Antiprotease

Human blood-derived α-antiprotease is becoming available for replacement therapy in patients with $\alpha_1$-antitrypsin deficiency and emphysema.[58] Weekly or monthly infusions raise the concentration of circulating antiprotease to around 800 mg/L, a level believed to be protective. Use of the inhaled route for delivery may offer economic and practical advantages.[59]

#### 5.2.7 Role of Assisted Ventilation

Assisted positive-pressure ventilation may be used in suitable patients. This tides the patient over acute episodes until the precipitating factors (infection, sputum retention, airway obstruction and central venous system depression) are treated. Assisted ventilation is indicated only in patients whose respiratory function was adequate for a reasonable quality of life before the acute episode. Respiratory invalids in terminal illness should not be ventilated, because it may be impossible to wean the patient off the respirator.

## 6. Pneumonia

Pneumonia is defined as a lower respiratory tract infection with alveolar involvement, causing consolidation, either very patchy (lobular or bronchopneumonia) or uniformly in a more defined area (e.g. segmental or lobar pneumonia). Since consolidation is present, pneumonia is normally accompanied by shadowing on the chest x-ray, whereas purely bronchial infection (bronchitis) does not result in x-ray changes.

### 6.1 Clinical Features/Aetiology

#### *6.1.1 Community-Acquired Pneumonia*

Pneumonia developing in adult patients in the community include specific pneumonias due to bacterial organisms such as *Streptococcus pneumoniae* (60 to 75%), *Haemophilus influenzae* (4 to 5%), *Legionella pneumophila* (2 to 5%), *Staphylococcus aureus* (1 to 5%); *Mycoplasma pneumoniae* (5 to 18%), *Chlamydia* spp. (2 to 3%), and viral or rickettsial infections (up to 20%). Such pneumonias occur in patients with previously normal lungs or pre-existing lung disease (such as chronic bronchitis), elderly patients, or those with diabetes mellitus. Rarely, pneumonia may be acquired by transmission from animals; examples include Q fever (caused by *Coxiella burnetii* which is usually passed from animals such as sheep and deer to those who work in abattoirs or are in contact with animal blood); pneumonic plague (caused by *Yersinia pestis* carried to humans from rodents by fleas, and subsequently by human-to-human transmission); anthrax (*Bacillus anthracis* from infected animal materials); and tularaemia (*Francisella tularensis* from tick bites).

#### *6.1.2 Hospital-Acquired Pneumonia (Nosocomial Pneumonia)*

Such pneumonias arise in patients after admission to hospital, and are usually caused by aerobic Gram-negative bacteria such as *Escherichia coli*, *Pseudomonas* spp., *Acinetobacter* spp., *Serratia marcescens* and *Klebsiella* spp.; or by staphylococci and anaerobes, probably by colonisation of the upper respiratory tract and subsequent aspiration of secretions in patients with impaired defences as a result of illness or surgical trauma.

#### *6.1.3 Aspiration and Anaerobic Pneumonias*

Aspiration pneumonia acquired in the community commonly occurs with aspiration during episodes of impaired consciousness, such as during alcohol intoxication, or when there is dysphagia or vomiting. In over 50% of cases, the infecting organisms are a mixture of anaerobes, such as *Bacteroides* spp., *Fusobacterium* spp., and Gram-positive anaerobic cocci (e.g. peptococci) derived from the teeth and upper respiratory passages. In hospital-acquired aspiration pneumonias, such as those following general anaesthesia with aspiration of gastric contents, the organisms are more likely to be Gram-negative aerobic enterobacteriaciae such as *E. coli*, and *Pseudomonas aeruginosa*.

#### *6.1.4 Pneumonias in Immunocompromised Patients*

Patients with the acquired immune deficiency syndrome (AIDS) are at risk of infection with *Pneumocystis carinii* (up to 80%), CMV (15%), mycobacteria (both *M. avium-intracellulare* 4% and *M. tuberculosis* 4% and much higher in Africa), fungi (e.g. *Cryptococcus neoformans*), pyogenic organisms, and *Legionella pneumophila*. Immunocompromised patients without AIDS, such as those receiving cytotoxic chemotherapy for leukaemias, lymphomas or other malignancies, and those on organ-transplant immunosuppression, are prone to infection with Gram-positive and Gram-negative bacteria, mycobacteria, *Nocardia asteroides*, fungi (including *Aspergillus* and *C. neoformans*), cytomegalovirus (CMV), and *P. carinii*.

### 6.2 Optimum Treatment

#### *6.2.1 Community-Acquired Pneumonia*

Detailed guidelines for the management of community-acquired pneumonia have been published in the US by the American Thoracic Society[60] and in the UK by the British Thoracic Society.[33,34] Pneumonia should be regarded as severe and life-threatening in those with a respiratory rate over 30 breaths/minute, hypotension or confusion, and in elderly patients and those with underlying disease. Raised blood urea, marked hypoxaemia ($pO_2$ less than

**Table VII.** Antimicrobial therapy recommended by the American Thoracic Society (ATS)[60] and British Thoracic Society (BTS)[33,34] for treatment of pneumonia

| BTS guidelines | ATS guidelines |
|---|---|
| *1. Tolerant of penicillin:*<br>• Amoxicillin 500mg q8h PO<br>• Ampicillin 500mg q6h IV<br>• Benzylpenicillin (penicillin G) 1.2g q6h IV | *1. Aged up to 60 years:*<br>• Erythromycin or other macrolide; possibly tetracycline |
| *2. Penicillin hypersensitivity:*<br>• Erythromycin 500mg q6h PO *or*<br>• Cefuroxime or cefotaxime IV | *2. Aged >60 years or requiring hospitalisation:*<br>• 2nd/3rd Generation cefalosporin *or*<br>• β-Lactam/β-lactamase inhibitor ± macrolide |

*Abbreviations:* PO = oral; IV = intravenous.

8 kPa) and leucopenia are also adverse findings. If a number of these features are present, there will be a need for active supportive therapy, usually involving transfer to an intensive care unit.

Initial investigations should include Gram staining and culture of sputum, blood culture, and arterial blood gas analysis, blood count and white cell count, as well as chest x-ray. Serum may sometimes be positive for pneumococcal antigen. Further clues to the causative organism may be obtained from transtracheal aspiration, bronchoalveolar lavage, or other invasive techniques such as sampling by protected specimen brushing of the airways, although the merits of such techniques are a matter for debate.[61,62]

In most cases, antibiotic therapy must be started before the pathogen can be identified, and in uncomplicated pneumonia where the cause is unknown, or where no special clinical features suggest a particular pathogen.

Table VII shows the antimicrobial therapy recommended in the American and British Thoracic Societies' guidelines. In the case of more severe pneumonias demonstrating the features associated with a poorer prognosis noted above, the antibiotic therapy recommended is shown in table VIII.

### 6.2.2 Antibiotic Therapy for Specific Pneumonias

#### Pneumococcal Pneumonia (*Streptococcus pneumoniae*)

*S. pneumoniae* remains the most common cause of community-acquired pneumonia in the general population; some individuals are particularly susceptible to pneumococcal infection, such as those with sickle-cell anaemia and post-splenectomy patients. Such individuals should be protected by vaccination with pneumococcal vaccine. Pneumococci are usually susceptible to penicillins, macrolides and second-generation cefalosporins, which can be given in the doses recommended in tables VII and VIII. However, antibiotic-resistant strains of *S. pneumoniae* are increasing in several countries. For example, up to 7% of strains are resistant to penicillin in the US, over 30% are resistant to penicillin in Hungary, 31% are resistant to erythromycin in Uruguay, and resistance to cefalosporins has also been reported. A knowledge of local resistance patterns is essential. All isolates should be tested for resistance so that antibiotic therapy is appropriate.[63]

In most cases, treatment brings about a rapid reduction in fever, followed by gradual resolution of the physical signs over a few days. Radiological clearing of the pneumonia usually takes about 2 weeks, but may take up to 10 weeks, especially in the elderly or in those with underlying lung disease, such as chronic bronchitis. If clinical improvement does not occur, the pneumonia may be due to organisms that are insensitive to the agent first used, or the diagnosis of pneumonia may be incorrect. The patient may have a condition that simulates pneumonia, such as pulmonary infarction, or the pneumonia may be secondary to some underlying pathology, such as carcinoma of the bronchus.

#### Staphylococcal Pneumonia (*Staphylococcus aureus*)

Staphylococcal pneumonia may be a primary infection, or may occur as a complication of influenza, particularly in major epidemics of influenza. It is a severe pneumonia, with a mortality rate of about 30%. The appearance of penicillinase-producing strains requires that staphylococcal pneumonia be treated with β-lactamase-resistant penicillins, such as fluclox-

**Table VIII.** Antimicrobial therapy recommended by the American Thoracic Society (ATS)[60] and British Thoracic Society (BTS)[33,34] for severe pneumonia with poor prognosis

| BTS guidelines | ATS guidelines |
|---|---|
| • Erythromycin 1g q6h IV + 2nd/3rd generation cefalosporin (e.g. cefuroxime 1.5g or cefotaxime 2g q8h IV)<br>*or*<br>• Ampicillin 1g + flucloxacillin 2g + erythromycin 1g (in combination) q6h IV | • Macrolide + 3rd generation cefalosporin with antipseudomonal activity<br>*or*<br>• Other antibiotic with similar activity (e.g. imipenem/cilastatin or ciprofloxacin) |

*Abbreviation:* IV = intravenous.

acillin. Doses of up to flucloxacillin 2g 4 times daily intravenously may be required in severe cases; the addition of fusidic acid (0.5 to 1g 3 times daily) or an aminoglycoside may bring added benefits.

More recently, methicillin-resistant strains of *S. aureus* have posed particular problems in some hospitals; for such organisms, vancomycin is first-line treatment.

### Gram-Negative Pneumonias

*H. influenzae*, a common pathogen in infective exacerbations of chronic bronchitis, is also increasingly recognised as a cause of adult community-acquired pneumonia. More than 10% of strains are now capable of producing β-lactamase, so ampicillin is no longer the antibiotic of choice in many areas. Recommended antibiotics include the amoxicillin/clavulanic acid combination, a second- or third-generation cefalosporin such as cefotaxime, ciprofloxacin, or cotrimoxazole (trimethoprim/sulfamethoxazole).

Nosocomial infections with organisms such as *Pseudomonas aeruginosa*, *Acinetobacter* spp., *Klebsiella pneumoniae*, *Enterobacter* spp., *Proteus* spp., *S. marcescens* and *E. coli* are best treated following careful assessment of antibiotic sensitivity, but treatment may be started with a third-generation cefalosporin such as ceftazidime in combination with an aminoglycoside such as gentamicin, tobramycin or netilmicin. Subsequent therapy, once antibiotic sensitivity is known, may include agents such as the quinolones (e.g. ciprofloxacin), monobactams (e.g. aztreonam), and carbapenems (e.g. imipenem).

### Legionnaire's Disease (*Legionella pneumophila*)

This is a severe pneumonia with many potential complications and a mortality rate of around 15%. Sporadic community-acquired cases may account for 2% of all community-acquired pneumonias, but outbreaks have also occurred, often being attributed to contamination of water in air conditioning systems with evaporative condensers, or water fittings in showers and sinks. A number of outbreaks have occurred in hospitals and other public buildings.

Erythromycin administered in high doses (1g every 6 hours intravenously or orally) is first-line treatment. In severe cases and those not responding adequately to erythromycin alone, the addition of rifampicin is recommended. Ciprofloxacin is a further option.

### Other Bacterial Pneumonias (Zoonoses)

Pneumonic plague (*Yersinia pestis*) responds to tetracyclines and chloramphenicol, and also to streptomycin. Anthrax pneumonia (*B. anthracis*) responds to penicillin, and tularaemia to gentamicin and streptomycin.

### Mycoplasmal, Chlamydial and *Coxiella* Pneumonias

The so-called atypical pneumonias due to *Mycoplasma pneumoniae, Chlamydia psittaci* and *Coxiella burnetii* (the causative agent of Q fever) differ from common bacterial pneumonias in having an influenza-like presentation, often with generalised symptoms, and in responding to tetracyclines and macrolides rather than penicillins.

Mycoplasma pneumonia may be suspected in epidemic years, which occur every 4 to 5 years, and by a persistent cough that often induces retching. Infection with *C. psittaci* is usually contracted from infected birds, though person-to-person transmission has been suggested in the TWAR strain. *C. burnetii* infection is usually contracted by patients, such as abattoir workers or shepherds, who are exposed to the blood of infected animals.

*M. pneumoniae* infection responds to erythromycin or the tetracyclines, although even with treatment, the course of the illness may be prolonged for up to 6 or 8 weeks. Tetracyclines are also first-line treatment for *C. psittaci* and *C. burnetii* infection.

### *Pneumocystis carinii* Pneumonia

This form of pneumonia occurs in patients with AIDS, those immunosuppressed by cytotoxic chemotherapy for lymphomas or leukaemias, and those receiving immunosuppressive therapy after organ transplantation. The treatment of *Pneumocystis carinii* pneumonia (PCP) is discussed in section 10.1.

### Aspiration Pneumonias

Since these infections often involve either Gram-negative bacilli or anaerobes, and often both, it is best to use an aminopenicillin such as amoxicillin or ampicillin plus metronidazole (400mg 3 times daily orally or 500mg 3 times daily intravenously). Clindamycin (up to 450mg 3 times daily orally or intravenously) is another option.

During the treatment of any pneumonia, general support will be required with adequate hydration, intravenously if necessary, and pain relief for pleuritic pain. Hypoxia requires well-controlled oxygen therapy, although only in patients with pre-existing chronic bronchitis is there any major risk of hypercapnia and ventilatory failure. Oxygen should, therefore, be given at concentrations that permit the maintenance of arterial $paO_2$ >8 kPa wherever possible. The presence of serious prognostic signs (see section 6.2.1) demands transfer to an intensive therapy unit and consideration of ventilatory support.

#### 6.2.3 Failure to Respond to Treatment

A poor response to therapy requires review of the diagnosis and examination for conditions such as pulmonary embolism, pulmonary eosinophilia or pulmonary oedema. Alternatively, the causative organism may not be sensitive to the antibiotic therapy, either because of antibiotic resistance or if the infection has not been correctly identified. For instance, atypical pneumonias will not respond to penicillins, and tuberculosis will only respond to specific antituberculous therapy (see section 9).

Some pneumonias may continue to cause fever and clinical or radiological persistence because they have been complicated by parapneumonic effusion, empyema or a lung abscess. Pleural effusions should be aspirated, and empyemas require repeated aspiration or formal surgical drainage. Lung abscesses are primarily seen in infection with staphylococci, *Klebsiella* and anaerobes, although the possibility of tuberculosis should always be considered. Appropriate antibiotic therapy, coupled with physiotherapy, will usually heal an abscess, but occasionally surgical resection may be required. Persistent fever in pneumonia may also result from drug hypersensitivity. Finally, pneumonias may fail to clear if there is bronchial obstruction, as by a tumour or foreign body; other underlying diseases such as chronic bronchitis or cardiac failure may be associated with slower resolution.

Radiological abnormalities take longer to resolve than clinical signs and may persist for many weeks. In more severe pneumococcal pneumonia associated with bacteraemia or antigenaemia, less than 50% of x-rays were normal at 8 weeks. Chlamydial and mycoplasmal pneumonias clear more quickly, Legionnaire's pneumonia more slowly.[64] In any instance where radiological resolution is further delayed, investigation including bronchoscopy is mandatory to exclude underlying pathology such as bronchial neoplasms. If there is a persistence of the symptomatology and clinical signs, less common pathogens such as *M. tuberculosis* must be excluded.

## 7. Bronchiectasis

The term bronchiectasis describes abnormal dilatation of the bronchi, usually resulting from bronchial infection associated with obstruction. It may result when a severe infection, often in childhood (e.g. whooping cough or adenovirus infection) or in adulthood (e.g. a pneumonic infection), damages the airway walls. Patients with defects of bronchial defences (e.g. deficiencies of immunoglobulins or ciliary abnormalities) or abnormal bronchial mucus, as in cystic fibrosis, also develop bronchiectasis.

Bronchiectasis may be localised to 1 or more of the segmental and subsegmental bronchi, especially after localised bronchial obstructive episodes, but may also be much more generalised, particularly when there is a constitutional cause, as in cystic fibrosis. The diagnosis is suspected from a history of chronic sputum production, with recurrent purulence of the sputum. Haemoptysis may occur (particularly during infective episodes) and pleuritic pain over affected segments is not unusual. The diagnosis may be confirmed by fine-section (high resolution) computerised tomography (CT) scanning. Formal bronchography is now rarely indicated.

#### Optimum Treatment

Management of established bronchiectasis is largely medical; surgical resection of affected segments is only rarely indicated.

Medical treatment of bronchiectasis consists of regular postural drainage, continued by the patient on a lifelong basis using the forced expiratory technique and postural drainage. It appears that percussive techniques, requiring the help of a physiotherapist or relative, are of less value.[65] Regular sputum samples should be cultured. The most important pathogens are *H. influenzae* and *S. pneumoniae*. All patients should be given a reserve supply of antibacterial drugs at home and instructed to submit a sputum sample for culture as soon as infection threatens, then start antibiotic therapy. Antibiotics with particularly good penetration in bronchiectatic sputum include doxycycline and high-dose amoxicillin (i.e. 3g twice daily). Other agents that may be considered, particularly if β-lactamase-producing *H. influenzae* is present, include amoxicillin/clavulanic acid or ciprofloxacin. Such treatments may need to be prolonged for 10 to 14 days to minimise early relapse. Antibacterial chemotherapy is not indicated when the sputum is mucoid.

Immunisation against influenza should be offered each autumn. Infection in the sinuses and teeth should be eradicated, if possible. Other associated conditions should be considered and treated where possible, e.g. hypogammaglobulinaemia. In addition to energetic treatment for retained bronchial secretions, any associated reversible airway obstruction can be treated with bronchodilators (see section 3.1.1). There may be particular advantages in giving a bronchodilator by inhalation 15 minutes before postural drainage. Should symptoms continue unabated despite good antibiotic therapy and regular assiduous postural drainage, surgical resection of the affected segments may be considered, but only if the bronchiectasis is truly localised to a well defined area where surgical resection can be undertaken without serious loss of lung function.

## 8. Cystic Fibrosis

Cystic fibrosis is an inherited autosomal recessive disorder and affects around 1 in 2000 live births. The fundamental defect has been identified at a locus on chromosome 7, 7q31. This cystic fibrosis gene, which can arise from a variety of mutations, produces the cystic fibrosis transmembrane conductance regulator (CFTR), a 1480-amino acid protein that functions as a small conductance chloride channel in epithelial membranes, altering the composition of epithelial secretions and accounting for the viscid secretions in airways, pancreas, and bile ducts. These viscid secretions account for abnormalities of function in these tissues, resulting in bronchiectasis in all cystic fibrosis patients, malabsorption from pancreatic exocrine dysfunction in most patients, and biliary cirrhosis in some.

Abnormalities in the sodium content of sweat gland secretions, with abnormally high sodium concentrations, form the basis of the main diagnostic test for the condition and have practical importance in hot climatic conditions, since sodium depletion can arise from the unusual sodium loss of sweating in cystic fibrosis patients.

### 8.1 Optimum Treatment of Respiratory Disease in Cystic Fibrosis

Viscid bronchial secretions are often accompanied by bronchial infection and obstruction and compound the tendency to bronchiectasis. The infections most commonly occurring in the earlier years of the clinical course of cystic fibrosis are due to *S. aureus* and *H. influenzae*.

Treatment with flucloxacillin, in some cases with the addition of fusidic acid, is recommended for staphylococcal infection, using higher than average doses for longer periods, e.g. oral flucloxacillin 500mg or 1g every 6 hours for 14 days. So-called prophylactic use of continuous antistaphylococcal agents have been advocated by some, but may accelerate the development of colonisation of the respiratory tract with *Pseudomonas aeruginosa*.

*H. influenzae* infections are becoming increasingly resistant to amoxicillin, and are best treated with amoxicillin/clavulanic acid, or macrolides. The newer macrolide agents such as azithromycin and clarithromycin show particular promise, as they are better tolerated than erythromycin, though more costly.

Eventually, most patients with cystic fibrosis become infected with *P. aeruginosa,* and become permanently colonised by the organism. Although initially, these organisms may be sensitive to oral ciprofloxacin (in high doses of 750mg twice daily for >14 days), antibiotic resistance to ciprofloxacin usually develops and other agents, only available for parenteral use, are then required for exacerbations of infection. It is usual to give an aminoglycoside (e.g. gentamicin, tobramycin, amikacin or netilmicin) together with an antibiotic from one of the groups shown in table IX, depending on antibiotic sensitivity testing. While most centres treat infectious exacerbations in cystic fibrosis as and when they arise, some centres have advocated a policy of regular 2-week courses of antibiotics every 3 months, irrespective of symptoms.[66]

Although all these antibiotics are given intravenously, it is now common for trained patients to self-administer the drugs at home through a previously placed intravenous cannula, or via a fully-implanted vascular port system, allowing more normal life to continue outside hospital.

#### *8.1.1 Role of Nebulised Antibiotic Therapy*

Between exacerbations, regular treatment with nebulised, inhaled antipseudomonal agents can reduce the frequency of exacerbations and the rate of decline of lung function. Appropriate agents include carbenicillin and gentamicin used together,[67] or an aminoglycoside alone, or colistin sulfomethate.[68,69]

**Table IX.** Antipseudomonal antibiotics used in cystic fibrosis

| Antibiotic class | Drug and dosage (adults) |
|---|---|
| Aminoglycosides | *Gentamicin:* 5 mg/kg/day divided q8h |
| | *Tobramycin:* 5 mg/kg/day divided q6-8h |
| | *Amikacin:* 15 mg/kg/day divided q12h |
| | *Netilmicin:* 6.5 mg/kg/day divided q8h |
| Carboxypenicillins | *Carbenicillin:* 400-600 mg/kg/day in 4-6 doses |
| | *Ticarcillin:* 15-20 g/day divided q6h |
| Ureidopenicillins | *Piperacillin:* 100-150 mg/kg/day in divided doses (up to 300 mg/kg/day if severe) |
| | *Azlocillin:* 2-5g q8h |
| Third-generation cefalosporins | *Ceftazidime:* 1-3g q8h |
| | *Cefsulodin:* 1-4 g/day divided q6-12h |
| Monocyclic β-lactams | *Aztreonam:* 1g q8h or 2g q12h (2g q8h in severe infections) |
| Carbapenems | *Imipenem/cilastatin:* 1-2 g/day (imipenem) in divided doses; higher in severe infections |

#### 8.1.2 Patients with Antibiotic-Resistant Gram-Negative Infections

Cystic fibrosis patients with *Pseudomonas* infections can develop antibiotic-resistant strains of organisms, including variants of *P. aeruginosa, P. maltophilia, P. fluorescens,* and others. In addition, an organism previously known as *P. cepacia*, but now named *Burkholderia cepacia*, has become an important pathogen in cystic fibrosis patients. This organism, previously known as a plant pathogen responsible for a form of rot in onions, appears in different strains, some of which are so-called epidemic strains which can be transmitted between patients, and which are associated with a more rapid downhill clinical course in the lung disease of cystic fibrosis. Other strains appear as non-epidemic strains, and are, in general, not as harmful to their host. However, segregation of patients with *B. cepacia* from other cystic fibrosis patients is now recommended.[70]

Antibiotic treatment of such resistant strains must be guided by laboratory resistance testing, but treatment is often very difficult, and eradication virtually impossible. Combinations including intravenous *ceftazidime* and either oral *cotrimoxazole* or intravenous *tobramycin* have been used, but there are no controlled studies to define the best management.[71]

#### 8.1.3 Role of Bronchodilators and Mucolytic Agents

As with other forms of bronchiectasis, bronchodilator therapy before physiotherapy and postural drainage is of value in increasing the amount of secretion expectorated.

Mucolytic agents have also been used, but until the development of *dornase-alfa* (DNase; recombinant human deoxyribonuclease-1)[72] there had been little evidence from controlled trials to suggest benefit. Dornase-alfa destroys the increased amounts of DNA produced from inflammatory leucocytes in respiratory secretions in cystic fibrosis. It appears to reduce sputum viscosity and the frequency of infections, and improve lung function if given by nebuliser on a daily basis to patients with cystic fibrosis.[73,74] The mean improvement in the $FEV_1$ was 5% over a 48-week period. This therapy offers a significant, if not dramatic, improvement for some but not all patients with cystic fibrosis, although longer term effects remain to be investigated.

#### 8.1.4 Future Treatment Possibilities: Gene Therapy

Identification of the locus of the cystic fibrosis gene raises the possibility of therapy to replace the abnormal gene in affected secretory cells. Early studies using virus particles or liposomes as the vehicle are underway, using a nebulised aerosol to deliver the gene to the respiratory mucosa. Secretory function of the cells can be restored to normal by such techniques for the duration of the survival of the treated cells, but the treatment must be repeated every few weeks as these cells are replaced with cells from the cystic fibrosis-affected germ cell line, if the replacing cells are to function normally. It is likely that more satisfactory vehicles for gene therapy will be developed in future.

### 8.2 Nutritional Management

Most patients with cystic fibrosis have some pancreatic insufficiency and about 8% also develop diabetes mellitus. The diet should be high in calories (at least 125% of the predicted required calorie intake) and protein, and unrestricted in fat. *Pancreatic enzyme preparations* should be taken with food in a dose large enough to ensure normal stool consistency and optimal absorption, and *vitamin supplements* should also be given, especially of retinol, calciferol and tocopherol (vitamins A, D and E). The aim should be to achieve a body mass index (weight in kg divided by height$^2$ in meters) of at least 20 in adult patients.

For further reading on recent advances in the management of cystic fibrosis, see Wilmott and Fielder.[75]

## 9. Pulmonary Tuberculosis

Pulmonary tuberculosis remains a major and increasing world problem. The World Health Organization (WHO) estimates that the number of new cases of tuberculosis will rise from 7.5 million in 1990 to 10.2 million by the year 2000, and the number of tuberculosis deaths will increase from 2.5 million in 1990 to 3.5 million in 2000, amounting to a quarter of all preventable deaths. The increase in tuberculosis has occurred both in developed and developing countries. In Africa, the increase in tuberculosis infection has occurred at the same time as a dramatic and overwhelming increase in human immunodeficiency virus (HIV) infection, so that in some parts of Africa, up to 80% of tuberculosis patients are HIV positive; an estimated 3.5 million Africans have dual infection with tuberculosis and HIV.[76] This association may result from HIV infection leading to reactivation of previously acquired but dormant tuberculosis infection, or to an increased susceptibility to acquire tuberculosis when immunosuppressed by HIV infection. There has also been a steep increase in the prevalence of tuberculosis in some areas of the US, especially in New York, perhaps partially because of HIV infection, but also because of inner-city social deprivation and the absence of adequate primary health care facilities and community control measures. A further concern arises from increasing prevalence of tuberculosis infection with organisms resistant to many of the standard antituberculosis agents.[77,78]

Prompt diagnosis and effective treatment of pulmonary tuberculosis reduces the danger to the patient and lessens the risk of further spread in the community. The presenting features classically include general symptoms such as weight loss, malaise and fevers ('night sweats'), and respiratory symptoms such as cough, sputum and haemoptysis. Less typical presentations may include unexplained fever, pleural pain or effusion, or symptoms resulting from involvement of other organs.

Although patients can usually be managed outside hospital, particularly if the home circumstances are satisfactory, it is sometimes preferable to start treatment in hospital, particularly if there is severe infection, poor social circumstances or uncertain cooperation. It may also be necessary to start treatment in hospital if there are vulnerable contacts at home or if the patient may have drug-resistant bacteria, hypersensitivity to drugs or associated disease of other organs.

The aim of treatment is to cure the patient by eradicating infection with an effective drug regimen that is continued for a course of the full recommended duration. This means prescribing a regimen adequate for the disease and acceptable to the patient and making sure that the patient takes it to the end of the course. In tuberculosis, more than any other disease, failure of the patient to complete the course of therapy is the commonest cause of treatment failure with regimens that are otherwise potentially 100% effective, so the clinician should aim for the best rapport and understanding to achieve full cooperation.

### 9.1 Clinical Pharmacology of Drugs Used in Treatment

The principal drugs used to treat tuberculosis are shown in table X. For reviews of the pharmacokinetics and adverse effects of these and other antituberculosis drugs, see Holdiness[79-82] and Girling.[83]

#### *9.1.1 Major Antituberculosis Drugs*

**Isoniazid**

Isoniazid (INH) is the hydrazide of isonicotinic acid, and is bactericidal to growing tubercle bacilli by interfering with cell wall synthesis. It is invaluable as a first-line drug in combination therapy with rifampicin and pyrazinamide. It is also used as a single agent in chemoprophylaxis to prevent tuberculosis infection in susceptible people in contact with tuberculosis (primary chemoprophylaxis) and to prevent activation in those with dormant infection (secondary chemoprophylaxis). As with other antituberculosis drugs, isoniazid should *never* be used as a single agent to treat active tuberculosis, because of the high risk of inducing drug-resistant organisms. If in doubt, secondary chemoprophylaxis should be given with 2 or more effective drugs.

***Pharmacokinetic characteristics:*** isoniazid is well and rapidly absorbed after oral administration on an empty stomach (peak concentration attained in 1 to 2 hours), although more slowly in the presence of food. The distribution of isoniazid is extensive, including cerebrospinal fluid, with negligible protein binding, and it persists in caseous material. Metabolism is by acetylation and hydroxylation. Patients who are 'slow' acetylators (see chapter 1; sect. 5.2.1) have higher concentrations of the drug which

**Table X.** Drugs used to treat tuberculosis

| Drug and dosage | Notes | Principal adverse effects/precautions/contraindications |
|---|---|---|
| **Isoniazid** (H)<br>*Adults:* 300mg; or 5 mg/kg/day<br>*Children:* 10 mg/kg/day | • Take 30 mins before food<br>• Bactericidal in high doses<br>• Active against intracellular organisms<br>• Reduce dose in slow acetylators<br>• Twice weekly intermittent therapy uses 15 mg/kg plus pyridoxine 10mg | • **Adverse effects:** few at doses <350 mg/day Hypersensitivity reactions rare (fever, rash, lymphadenopathy). Slow acetylators (see chapter 1; sect. 5.2.1) have greater incidence of some effects, esp. peripheral neuropathy (pyridoxine responsive).<br>Optic neuritis is rare, occasional liver disturbance; ataxia, euphoria, convulsions, tinnitus, insomnia and muscle twitching. Occasional hyperglycaemia, gynaecomastia, pellagra-like state, dryness of mouth, epigastric discomfort, urinary retention.<br>• **Caution** in convulsive disorders, renal and hepatic dysfunction, alcoholism, breast-feeding<br>• **Contraindications:** manic states, porphyria, drug-induced liver disease<br>• **Potential interactions** with diazepam, carbamazepine, ethosuximide and phenytoin in slow acetylators; antacids (e.g. aluminium hydroxide) reduce absorption |
| **Rifampicin** (R)<br>*Adults:* 450 to 600 mg/day<br>*Children:* 10 mg/kg/day | • Take 30 mins before food<br>• Bactericidal<br>• Reduce dose in hepatobiliary disease<br>• Twice weekly intermittent therapy uses <15 mg/kg | • **Adverse effects:** gastrointestinal disturbances; transient elevations of bilirubin and hepatic enzymes; orange-red urine and possibly staining saliva, tears, etc.; jaundice and skin rashes can occur.<br>• With intermittent therapy, a flu-like syndrome with chills, fever and aches may occur. Rare shock, breathlessness, haemolytic anaemia, acute renal failure, thrombocytopenia purpura, eosinophilia, leucopenia.<br>• **Contraindications:** porphyria, hepatic disease.<br>• **Potential interactions:** rifampicin induces liver enzymes; hastens metabolism of oral contraceptives (use additional methods of contraception); other interactions may reduce the effects of antiepileptics, anticoagulants and oral antidiabetic drugs, diazepam, β-blockers, cyclosporin, calcium antagonists, antiarrhythmics (disopyramide, mexiletine), tricyclic antidepressants, cimetidine, thyroxine, methylxanthines; absorption of rifampicin is reduced by antacids. |
| **Pyrazinamide** (Z)<br>*Adults:* 1.5-2 g/day<br>*Children:* 35 mg/kg/day | Bactericidal, especially in acid pH | • **Adverse effects:** gastrointestinal disturbance, hepatotoxicity; fever, nausea, vomiting, jaundice, liver failure; liver function should be monitored during therapy; can precipitate gout, arthralgia, urticaria, sideroblastic anaemia.<br>• **Contraindications:** porphyria, liver disease.<br>• **Caution** in diabetes, gout, impaired renal function.<br>• **Potential interactions:** antagonises uricosuric effect of sulfinpyrazone and probenecid |
| **Ethambutol** (E)<br>*Adults:* 15-25 mg/kg/day<br>*Children ≥ 6 years:* 15-25 mg/kg/day | • Bacteriostatic<br>• Reduce dose in renal failure; avoid in severe renal failure unless no alternative<br>• Absorption not reduced by food<br>• For intermittent therapy, 30 mg/kg 3 times/week, or 45 mg/kg 2 times/week | • **Adverse effects:** optic neuropathy, red/green colour-blindness, peripheral neuropathy (optic effects more common with higher doses); test visual acuity before starting therapy and recheck regularly; warn patients to report any visual change<br>• **Contraindications:** poor vision, young children <6y. Reduce dose in renal impairment |
| **Streptomycin** (S)<br>*Adults:* 1 g/day<br>*Children:* 20-40 mg/kg/day | • Reduced dose in patients >40y and <50kg<br>• Intramuscular injection (an aminoglycoside)<br>• Bactericidal in combination with pyrazinamide<br>• Useful in some fully supervised intermittent regimens | • **Adverse effects:** as for aminoglycosides; ototoxicity (especially disorders of balance), renal damage, skin rashes, fevers; paraesthesiae around mouth.<br>• **Caution:** renal disease (reduce dose and monitor blood levels to prevent ototoxicity) |
| **Thioacetazone** (T)<br>150 mg/day | • Bacteriostatic<br>• Well absorbed<br>• Inexpensive | • **Adverse effects:** nausea, vomiting and diarrhoea in up to 20% of patients; bone marrow depression, vertigo, ataxia, occasional liver toxicity, exfoliative dermatitis |

**Table X.** *[Continued]*

| Drug and dosage | Notes | Principal adverse effects/precautions/contraindications |
|---|---|---|
| **Ethionamide** (and prothionamide) 500-750 mg/day | • Chemically related to isoniazid, but usually highly effective in isoniazid-resistant infections<br>• Bactericidal<br>• Crosses CSF and placenta | • **Adverse effects:** frequent gastrointestinal adverse effects, liver toxicity; rarely, hypotension, hypoglycaemia, alopecia, convulsions, neuropathy.<br>Prothionamide may be better tolerated than ethionamide |
| **Cycloserine**<br>*Adults:* 10 mg/kg/day<br>*Children:* 10-20 mg/kg/day | • Bactericidal<br>• Well absorbed<br>• Crosses CSF and placenta | • **Adverse effects:** frequent CNS effects (drowsiness, vertigo, disorientation, confusion, coma, psychosis, personality changes in up to 50%) |
| **Capreomycin** (also kanamycin, amikacin)<br>1 g/day | • Reduce dose if >40y or in renal impairment<br>• Intramuscular injection<br>• Similar activity to streptomycin, but may be effective in streptomycin-resistant infections | • **Adverse effects:** as for aminoglycosides, but may have higher incidence of 8th auditory nerve toxicity than streptomycin |
| **Clofazimine**<br>100-200 mg/day | • Riminophenazine compound, mainly used in leprosy, now used in drug-resistant tuberculosis and atypical mycobacterial infections.<br>• Half-life 70 days; crystallises in many organs, including fatty tissues; not found in CSF or brain | • **Adverse effects:** brown discolouration of the skin |
| **Quinolones** (ciprofloxacin 1-1.5 g/day; ofloxacin 400 mg/day) | • Value in drug-resistant tuberculosis and in infections with mycobacteria other than tuberculosis being explored | • **Adverse effects:** generally well tolerated, apart from some gastrointestinal adverse effects in about 5% of patients |

appears to increase the frequency of some adverse effects. Conversely, 'rapid acetylators' are less likely to be effectively treated with intermittent regimens that involve once-weekly doses, although they respond equally as well as slow acetylators to twice-weekly bactericidal and sterilising regimens. The elimination half-life of isoniazid (0.75 to 1.8h in rapid acetylators or 2 to 4.5h in slow acetylators) is prolonged in acute or chronic liver disease and in neonates (up to 19.8 hours), but is not significantly altered in renal dysfunction.[79]

***Clinical use:*** the recommended dose of isoniazid is 3 to 5 mg/kg/day, but children tolerate much higher doses (up to 20 mg/kg/day). Twice-weekly (and in slow acetylators, once-weekly) regimens (usually combined with pyridoxine to reduce or reverse neurological and haematological adverse reactions) are also used (table X). The dose should be reduced or therapy stopped in hepatic insufficiency.

***Tolerability:*** adverse reactions to isoniazid are infrequent if the above recommendations are followed; the benefits usually outweigh the risks of therapy. However, at higher dosages (>6 mg/kg/day), peripheral neuropathy, particularly in slow acetylators, occurs. This can usually be prevented and treated with the use of pyridoxine supplements. Isoniazid-induced hepatic injury is also well recognised. This reaction appears to be associated with a metabolite of isoniazid, monoacetylhydrazine, via the formation of a reactive intermediate. Increasing age, slow acetylation and alcohol (ethanol) consumption appear to be risk factors for isoniazid-induced hepatotoxicity. The onset of the hepatotoxic reaction is variable (1 week to many months) and its severity varies from a mild reversible reaction (elevation of transaminases in 10 to 20% of patients) to severe hepatitis with considerable morbidity and some mortality.[84,85]

#### Rifampicin (Rifampin)

Rifampicin is a first-line bactericidal antituberculosis agent that probably acts through inhibition of RNA-polymerase. It is a semisynthetic antibiotic, available in both oral and intravenous formulations, which, along with pyrazinamide, has the ability to kill so-called 'persisters' (mycobacteria that lie dormant, often within cells or caseous material).

***Pharmacokinetic characteristics:*** absorption of rifampicin is rapid and nearly complete (peak concentrations are attained within 2 to 4 hours) following oral administration on an empty stomach. The presence of food causes marked variations in serum concentrations. Concurrent isoniazid administration (e.g. in combination formulations) does not affect its absorption. At rifampicin doses above 300 to 450mg, the excretory capacity of the liver is saturated and further dosage increases lead to high serum concentrations. In plasma, rifampicin is bound is to albumin (weak, reversible, approximately 80%). Distribution is extensive and patients should be warned about probable red-brown colouration of body fluids (e.g. urine, sweat, tears, faeces, etc.).[86,87]

Metabolism of rifampicin is principally by deacetylation. The deacetylated metabolite is active and accounts for most of the biliary antibacterial activity. Rifampicin stimulates its own metabolism as well as being a potent inducer of hepatic drug metabolising enzymes of certain other drugs, leading to clinically important adverse drug interactions (table X). Rifampicin does not affect isoniazid acetylation. Its elimination half-life ranges from 2.3 to 5.1 hours after initial doses, but decreases to 2 to 3 hours after repeated administration, due to increased hepatic metabolism.[79] The excretion of rifampicin is both biliary and renal, and modifications in dosage are required in patients with hepatobiliary or hepatorenal insufficiency.

***Tolerability:*** adverse reactions to rifampicin are infrequent if attention is paid to recommended dosage levels, dose intervals, associated disease and concurrent drug therapy.[83] Interpretation of cause and effect relationships (e.g. hepatic dysfunction) is complicated by the fact that rifampicin is usually combined with isoniazid, which has important adverse reactions of its own (see above).

#### Rifabutin

Rifabutin is a newer rifamycin derivative that may be effective in the treatment of some rifampicin-resistant mycobacterial infections. The main role for this drug at present is in the treatment of pulmonary tuberculosis where the organisms are rifampicin-resistant, in whom 30% of isolations show a response to regimens containing rifabutin. In addition, rifabutin has proved valuable in infections with *Mycobacterium avium* complex, particularly where this infection occurs in AIDS patients.[88]

***Pharmacokinetic characteristics:*** rifabutin has a relatively low bioavailability following oral administration (about 20% after single doses of 300 to 1200mg), and is largely eliminated by metabolism, the percentage of unchanged drug appearing in the urine being about 8 to 9% of an administered dose. With long term administration, rifabutin induces its own metabolism (and the metabolism of other drugs); its elimination half-life varies between individuals but is relatively long, ranging from 32 to 67 hours.[89,90] Although the pharmacokinetics of rifabutin are influenced to some extent by hepatic and renal impairment, dosage alteration is probably only required in patients with severe renal or hepatic dysfunction.

***Clinical use:*** in newly diagnosed tuberculosis patients, rifabutin-containing regimens (i.e. combinations with 2 other antimycobacterial drugs) have demonstrated similar effectiveness to regimens containing rifampicin. In patients with multidrug-resistant tuberculosis, rifabutin combinations with other antimycobacterial drugs have been reported to produce overall response rates (i.e. negative sputum cultures) of about 33%.[89]

***Tolerability and drug interactions potential:*** adverse effects with rifabutin are uncommon at the usually recommended dose of 300 mg/day but become more common as the total daily dose approaches 1g.[90] The dose-limiting toxicity consists of a polyarthralgia/arthritis syndrome, possibly complicated by uveitis. Other adverse effects include discolouration of the urine, eructation and taste perversion, nausea/vomiting, and skin rash.

As with rifampicin, rifabutin has the potential to interact with other drugs metabolised in the liver since it induces drug metabolising enzymes; however, its enzyme-inducing properties appear to be less than those of rifampicin.[89]

#### Pyrazinamide

Pyrazinamide is especially bactericidal to mycobacteria multiplying intracellularly at low pH levels. Its inclusion in the first 2 months of a treatment regimen can reduce later relapse rates and allow a shorter duration of therapy.

Pyrazinamide is well absorbed after oral administration and eliminated principally by hepatic metabolism (half-life 9 to 10 hours). Only about 3% of an oral dose is excreted unchanged in the urine in the first 24 hours.[79] As with isoniazid, pyrazinamide penetrates well into cerebrospinal fluid[80] and is, thus, especially useful in tuberculous meningitis. The drug commonly causes nausea, flushing and arthralgia.[83] Hepatotoxic reactions have also occurred (table X) and may limit the duration of therapy.

#### *9.1.2 Supportive Antituberculosis Drugs*

**Ethambutol**

Ethambutol is an essentially bacteriostatic drug that seems to inhibit mycobacterial cell wall synthesis. It is well absorbed after oral administration (75 to 80%), with peak plasma concentrations occurring at 2 hours. Ethambutol is distributed to most body fluids, is 40% protein bound and does not cross the blood-brain barrier; even in meningitis, CNS transmission is variable. Hepatic metabolism is less than with isoniazid or rifampicin. The drug is mainly excreted unchanged in the urine, so it can be used safely in liver disease, but in renal insufficiency the dose must be modified (table X).

Adverse reactions with ethambutol are infrequent at recommended doses. The most important reaction is the occurrence of dose-related retrobulbar neuritis and the drug should be immediately withdrawn if visual symptoms occur.[83] Fortunately, most patients with retrobulbar neuritis recover normal vision if ethambutol is stopped at the first symptoms. However, it is recommended that all patients started on ethambutol have regular checks of visual acuity, and be firmly warned of the possibility of and need to report promptly any visual impairment.

**Streptomycin**

Streptomycin is an aminoglycoside that must be given by injection, usually intramuscularly. It is widely distributed in the tissues, but does not cross well into the cerebrospinal fluid. As with other aminoglycosides, high blood concentrations of streptomycin cause eighth cranial nerve damage, particularly vestibular toxicity, and drug rashes are common. The drug is 90% excreted in the urine, so particular care is required in patients with renal impairment.

In the treatment of active pulmonary tuberculosis, initial therapy should include a minimum of 3 of the above drugs, because of the ready development of resistance to a single drug. If resistance is suspected, 4 or more drugs should be used as initial therapy.

***Thioacetazone***

Thioacetazone is a relatively weak antituberculosis agent, but is of value as a companion drug to isoniazid in prevention of the development of isoniazid resistance. It also has the advantage, in developing countries, of being relatively inexpensive. There are considerable ethnic differences in tolerance to thioacetazone as it is poorly tolerated (with nausea, vomiting, and cutaneous reactions) by Europeans and Chinese, but well tolerated by Africans, although tolerance is much impaired in those with HIV infection. Thioacetazone must be used as a daily therapy.[91]

### 9.2 Optimum Treatment

Detailed recommendations for the treatment of tuberculosis have been published,[92-94] and are regularly updated. There is wide agreement that treatment should consist of an initial intensive phase, usually of 2 months, followed by a longer continuation phase of 4 to 16 months, depending on the drugs used.

#### *9.2.1 Initial Intensive Treatment*

Once specimens of sputum have been obtained for culture, treatment should be started with *at least* 3 drugs to which the organism is likely to be sensitive. Multidrug therapy is more effective and reduces infectivity and the development of resistant strains of *M. tuberculosis*. The 3 most commonly used first-line drugs are isoniazid, rifampicin, and pyrazinamide, which should be taken before food. The choice of initial therapy may, however, be influenced by factors such as cost, availability, convenience and toxicity, and by pre-existing liver disease, renal disease or pregnancy. In these circumstances, alternative drugs may be required, but in any case a minimum of 3 drugs must be used.

The initial 3-drug regimen should be continued for at least 8 weeks and ideally until sensitivity of the organism has been established (usually 8 to 12 weeks, although new techniques sometimes allow earlier results). The importance of adequate patient instruction and surveillance of compliance cannot be overemphasised.

#### *9.2.2 Continuation Treatment*

Once the sensitivity of the organism to antituberculosis drugs has been established, therapy is continued with the 2 most appropriate drugs until completion of the recommended course.[33,34,95] The usual drugs included in the continuation regimen are rifampicin and isoniazid and, using these drugs, only a further 4 months of treatment is required. The 6-month regimen of isoniazid and rifampicin, supplemented for the first 2 months by pyrazinamide (the so-called 2HRZ/4HR regimen) is as effective as the previously favoured 9-month regimen of isoniazid and rifampicin supplemented for the first 2 months by ethambutol (2EHR/7HR regimen).[96] If for reason of cost or toxicity, one of these first-line drugs cannot be used, a reserve drug should be substituted and the course of therapy extended to 18 months, especially if rifampicin is not included. In African countries, an 8-month regimen of initial isoniazid, rifampicin and pyrazinamide can be followed by 6 months of isoniazid and thioacetazone (150mg daily).

During continuation therapy, patients should be reviewed at regular intervals to monitor clinical and bacteriological progress and assess compliance with drug therapy. In patients suspected of irregular compliance, a *supervised* daily or intermittent (twice weekly) regimen should be introduced, in which a clinic or practice nurse watches while the medication is administered.

#### 9.2.3 Intermittent Treatment Regimens

Intermittent therapy, given twice or 3 times weekly, permits greater supervision of treatment and may be more convenient and less expensive, particularly in developing countries. A wide variety of effective intermittent regimens have been devised, with a daily initial phase followed by twice- or 3-times-weekly continuation therapy. Some 3-times-weekly regimens have proven to be effective even without an initial daily phase of treatment. To be effective, the individual doses may need to be higher than those used in daily therapy, at the risk of inducing adverse effects. For a 3-times-weekly regimen, the dose of rifampicin can be similar to the daily dose; isoniazid can be given in doses of 200 to 400mg 3 times weekly according to bodyweight, along with rifampicin.

After an 8-week daily initial regimen with isoniazid, rifampicin and pyrazinamide, 4 months of 3-times-weekly rifampicin and isoniazid is an effective continuation regimen. An alternative regimen consists of twice-weekly streptomycin 0.75g or 1g according to bodyweight, plus isoniazid 15 mg/kg twice weekly, along with pyridoxine 10mg to prevent isoniazid-induced peripheral neuropathy with the higher isoniazid doses. However, with this regimen, the continuation phase must last 16 months after the initial phase of daily treatment.

Rifampicin can be used in twice-weekly regimens, but there is a higher risk of adverse reactions (especially chills and flu-like symptoms), which may be ameliorated by reducing the dose to <15 mg/kg twice weekly. For details of other regimens, including intermittent regimens, see Crofton et al.[91] and Davies.[97]

#### 9.2.4 Treatment During Pregnancy

The transplacental pharmacokinetics of antituberculosis drugs have been reviewed by Holdiness.[82] In general, active tuberculosis in pregnancy should be treated observing the usual principles of treating with at least 2 drugs, and giving a course of the full effective duration. In general, isoniazid, ethambutol and rifampicin seem to reasonably safe in pregnancy, even though placental transmission occurs. There is no clear evidence of a teratogenic effect of these 3 antituberculosis drugs, although caution is advised in using rifampicin in the first trimester. Streptomycin also crosses the placenta, but carries the risk of ototoxicity in up to 1 in 6 fetuses exposed, so is best avoided. Little is known about other drugs in pregnancy, although some, such as thiacetazone and pyrazinamide are poorly tolerated. Ethionamide is teratogenic and is contraindicated.

A standard regimen with isoniazid, pyrazinamide and rifampicin can be used in pregnancy, substituting ethambutol if any of the first 3 drugs prove unsuitable or poorly tolerated.

#### 9.2.5 Treatment in Renal Disease

Ethambutol is largely excreted by the kidneys, whereas isoniazid, rifampicin and pyrazinamide are mainly metabolised or excreted through the biliary system. Consequently, rifampicin can be given in normal doses to patients with renal failure, but the other drugs may have to be given in reduced dosage, particularly in severe renal failure, and pyridoxine should be given to prevent isoniazid neuropathy. In renal failure, the dosage of ethambutol should be reduced but the drug is best avoided in severe renal failure, particularly if the glomerular filtration rate is less than 50 ml/min (3 L/h), because of the increased risks of visual field defects and colour-blindness.

With pyrazinamide, caution is required because of its tendency to precipitate gout. Streptomycin should only be given if essential, and at reduced dosage with blood concentration monitoring. For patients on renal dialysis, ethambutol and streptomycin can be given immediately after each dialysis treatment.

#### 9.2.6 Treatment in Liver Disease

Isoniazid, rifampicin, ethionamide and pyrazinamide can all be hepatotoxic, although they are not necessarily all toxic in the same patient. Patients with hepatic failure can be treated with ethambutol, streptomycin and isoniazid, with careful monitoring of liver function tests, although if the patient can tolerate rifampicin, there are considerable advantages in shortening the treatment course. Clearly, great caution and regular liver function monitoring (i.e. of transaminases) are required.

#### 9.2.7 Treatment in Children

Children with active tuberculosis can be treated with the standard initial regimen of isoniazid, rifampicin, and pyrazinamide. Ethambutol is best avoided because children may not be able to report visual adverse effects. In most children, the bacillary load in the tuberculous lesions may be small and pyrazinamide can be omitted if there is no likelihood of drug-resistant organisms, but it will in that case be necessary to continue therapy with isoniazid and rifampicin for 9 months.

### 9.3 Difficult Treatment Problems in Mycobacterial Infection

#### 9.3.1 Drug-Resistant Tuberculosis

Tubercle bacilli have a spontaneous tendency to mutate, causing resistance to antimicrobial drugs. Patients treated with a single antituberculosis drug can rapidly develop strains resistant to that drug; hence, the essential principle that all patients be treated with at least 2 drugs to which the organism is sensitive. Unfortunately, through improperly prescribed therapy, erratic drug ingestion, inadequate dosage, incomplete therapy or a combination of these defects in therapy, there have been steep increases in the frequency of tubercle bacilli resistant to multiple antituberculosis drugs in many areas of the world, both in developing countries and also in developed areas such as New York city.[77] Many patients have a history of previous therapy for tuberculosis, and can therefore be classified as having developed secondarily drug resistant organisms, but there is increasing concern that these organisms are passed on to other individuals, who then demonstrate primary drug resistance, with HIV-positive individuals being particularly susceptible.

A variety of regimens have been suggested to treat patients with multiple resistance to such drugs as isoniazid, rifampicin and pyrazinamide, employing second-line agents such as capreomycin, streptomycin, or amikacin by injection, with ethionamide, cycloserine, and ciprofloxacin as oral preparations. It is always wise in such patients to treat with as many drugs as possible to which the organisms are sensitive, within the limits of the patient's drug tolerance. Such patients should be treated by specialist clinicians (for details, see Iseman).[98]

#### 9.3.2 Non-Tuberculosis Mycobacteria

These infections, sometimes called 'atypical' mycobacterial infections, include groups such as *M. avium-intracellulare, M. kansasii, M. malmoense*. Such organisms often demonstrate resistance to standard antituberculosis agents under laboratory testing, but may not invariably prove resistant *in vivo*. Again, it is necessary to employ multiple drugs including second-line agents. These infections are best treated by specialists.

#### 9.3.3 Control and Prevention of Tuberculosis

Tuberculosis cannot be controlled without a comprehensive programme that includes expeditious diagnosis and effective treatment of all active cases, checking of close contacts and preventive measures in the community. UK recommendations[99] include procedures for the segregation of tuberculosis patients, contacts and hospital staff, and the use of Bacille-Calmette-Guerin (BCG) vaccination in defined circumstances. US[94] and WHO[93] recommendations are also available. Although BCG vaccination has been an important measure in Europe and developing countries for several decades, it has not achieved worldwide support, particularly in the US. However, selective vaccination of groups at risk is now being proposed.[100]

### 9.4 Clinical Outcome and Economic Considerations

Developing countries, in particular, are handicapped by shortages of funds, not only for the purchase of antituberculosis drugs, but also for essential measures to control tuberculosis in a community and for training of medical personnel. The cost of antituberculosis drugs clearly has a major influence on the effectiveness of a tuberculosis control programme.[93] Tables XI and XII indicate the comparative costs of individual drugs, together with costs of complete courses of combined drug therapy.

For reviews of current and potential treatment of tuberculosis, see Houston and Fanning,[101]

**Table XI.** Costs of drugs for 2 months of treatment at average adult doses (derived from WHO Guidelines,[93] using UNICEF prices)

| Drug | Daily dose | Cost ($US) |
|---|---|---|
| Isoniazid | 300mg | 0.43 |
| Rifampicin | 600mg | 11.00 |
| Pyrazinamide | 1500mg | 6.44 |
| Streptomycin | 1g | 16.30 (plus injection costs) |
| Ethambutol | 1g | 3.50 |

International Union Against Tuberculosis,[102] and Crofton et al.[91]

## 10. HIV Infection and Lung Disease

HIV infection results in an increasingly severe defect of immune function. The lung is a common site for the opportunistic infections that characterise AIDS.

### 10.1 *Pneumocystis carinii* Pneumonia

In Europe and North America, *P. carinii* pneumonia (PCP) is the most common opportunistic pathogen in AIDS. 85% of all patients with AIDS will have 1 or more episode of PCP (in Africa, PCP is unusual, but tuberculosis is commonly found). *P. carinii* has a greater degree of homology with fungi than with protozoa,[103] but it is paradoxical that, as yet, antifungal drugs have been ineffective. Serological evidence suggests that this organism is prevalent in the environment. Several studies suggest that infection is most likely to occur through reinfection rather than reactivation after long term pulmonary carriage.[104,105]

PCP usually starts insidiously with an irritating cough and breathlessness. There is often a background of fatigue, weight loss and fever, as well as other signs of HIV infection such as oral candidiasis. Sputum production is unusual and lung crackles are rare. The diagnosis is most often made on typical clinical picture in a patient known to be HIV antibody positive. Examination of induced sputum obtained after nebulising hypertonic saline may be helpful in demonstrating the characteristic cysts of *P. carinii]*[106] but definitive diagnosis may require bronchoscopy with bronchoalveolar lavage using monoclonal antibodies specific for *P. carinii*[107]

#### Optimum Treatment

Antimicrobial therapy for PCP is summarised in table XIII. First-line treatment is with high-dose cotrimoxazole. The response to treatment given for 3 weeks is generally excellent and mortality in patients with a first episode of PCP is less than 10%. It may be useful to stratify PCP into *mild* (minor perihilar shadowing on chest radiograph with normal resting $paO_2$), *moderate* (diffuse interstitial shadowing with mild hypoxaemia), and *severe* (extensive shadowing and $paO_2$ <8 kPa) since only intravenous high-dose cotrimoxazole and intravenous pentamidine are effective in more severe cases. There is little difference in outcome between intravenous cotrimoxazole and intravenous pentamidine;[108] however, the approximate cost of a 3-week course of intravenous cotrimoxazole is £200 as compared with £330 for intravenous pentamidine. Oral therapy should be reserved for those with PCP of mild to moderate severity.[109]

In severe PCP, anti-*Pneumocystis* treatment may cause an initial rapid acceleration of intrapulmonary inflammation, leading to a reduction in arterial oxygenation and possibly death in the first 5 days of treatment. Adjunctive treatment with corticosteroids (oral prednisolone or intravenous methylprednisolone) reduces the likelihood of death, respiratory failure or deterioration in oxygenation in patients with moderate to severe PCP.[110] In the UK, the regimen most commonly used is intravenous methylprednisolone 1 mg/day for 3 consecutive days.

In the first few years of the AIDS epidemic, patients with severe progressive PCP and respiratory failure had a very poor prognosis with

**Table XII.** Costs of commonly used regimens of antituberculosis therapy (derived from WHO Guidelines,[93] using UNICEF prices)

| Regimen[a] | Cost ($US)[b] |
|---|---|
| *Initial phase:* | |
| 2HRZ | 25 |
| 2HRZS | 44 |
| 2HRZE | 29 |
| $2H_3R_3Z_3$ | 11 |
| *Continuation phase:* | |
| 4HR | 31 |
| 6HT | 2 |
| $4H_3R_3$ | 13 |
| 6HE | 11 |

a H = isoniazid; R = rifampicin; Z = pyrazinamide; S = streptomycin; E = ethambutol; T = thioacetazone. Large numerals indicate duration of therapy in months; small subscript numerals indicate doses per week and where no subscript is listed, daily therapy is indicated.

b Costs are total drug costs for the period of treatment shown.

**Table XIII. Antimicrobial therapy for *Pneumocystis carinii* pneumonia**

| Drug | Dosage (adults) | Comments |
|---|---|---|
| Cotrimoxazole (trimethoprim/sulfamethoxazole) | 20/100 mg/kg/day PO | • First-line therapy<br>• Usually given initially IV<br>• Adverse effects common, especially nausea, skin rashes, myelotoxicity |
| Pentamidine | 4 mg/kg/day IV | • Ineffective orally<br>• Severe adverse effects, especially hypoglycaemia, pancreatitis, nephrotoxicity, hepatotoxicity |
| Dapsone + trimethoprim | 100 mg/day + 20 mg/kg/day | • Usually given orally<br>• Useful in sulfonamide hypersensitivity<br>• Less effective in severe pneumonia |
| Clindamycin + primaquine | 600mg 4 times daily IV + 15 mg/day PO | • May be as effective as cotrimoxazole |
| Piritrexim | 250 mg/m$^2$ twice daily or 150 mg/kg twice daily PO | • Oral antifolate drug<br>• Causes bone marrow suppression |
| Eflornithine | 400 mg/kg/day IV | • Less effective than cotrimoxazole |
| Trimetrexate | 30-60 mg/m$^2$/day IV | • Need to give calcium folinate<br>• Adverse effects include bone marrow suppression |
| Atovaquone | 750mg 3 times daily PO | • Less toxic than cotrimoxazole |

*Abbreviations:* IV = intravenous; PO = oral.

survival rates to hospital discharge of 1 to 14%. Nowadays, however, with improvements in primary and secondary prophylaxis for PCP, and the addition of corticosteroid therapy, survival rates for severe PCP have improved to around 35%, which has resulted in increased referral to intensive care units.[111]

PCP tends to recur in patients with immunosuppression due to AIDS, so all patients should be offered secondary prophylaxis. Primary prophylaxis against PCP should also be offered to HIV antibody positive patients with CD4 lymphocyte counts of <200 cells/µl and perhaps to those with unexplained persistent fever and intractable oral candidiasis. Agents available for prophylaxis of PCP in AIDS are shown in the table XIV. In a study of secondary prophylaxis in 310 patients with AIDS who were also receiving zidovudine, the relapse rate of PCP appeared to be higher in those receiving nebulised pentamidine, while overall mortality was similar to those taking oral cotrimoxazole.[112]

### 10.2 Bacterial Pneumonia

HIV-infected individuals have an increased incidence of bacterial pneumonia and bacteraemia. One study has shown an annual rate of pneumococcal pneumonia of 18 per 1000 HIV infected patients, as compared with 3 to 4 per 1000 in the general population.[113] The increased susceptibility to capsulated organisms such as *S. pneumonia* and *H. influenzae* in AIDS patients is thought to relate to the inability to mount normal antibody responses. In view of this, the US Centers for Disease Control (CDC) recommends that all HIV infected individuals over 2 years of age be immunised with pneumococcal polyvalent vaccines,[114] although there are no current data to support this policy.

#### Optimum Treatment

Most bacterial infections respond to appropriate antibiotics (see section 6.2.2), although there is a tendency to relapse following treatment.

### 10.3 Cytomegalovirus Pneumonitis

Cytomegalovirus (CMV) is a major opportunistic pathogen in AIDS, causing choroidoretinitis, colitis, hepatitis, adrenalitis, radiculitis and oesophagitis. While it is frequently isolated from saliva, sputum and bronchoalveolar lavage fluid in immunocompromised patients with HIV infection, true pneumonitis due to CMV is now considered rare. This is in contrast to transplant recipients in whom CMV can cause fatal pneumonitis. CMV infection is almost universal in homosexual HIV seropositive patients, but if CMV pneumonitis is diagnosed, it is usually after exclusion of other causes of pulmonary involvement.

#### Optimum Treatment

CMV infection responds to a 2-week course of intravenous ganciclovir[115] or foscarnet,[116] which are probably equally effective. Long term prophylaxis, usually with intravenous ganci-

**Table XIV. Prophylactic therapy against *Pneumocystis carinii* infection in AIDS patients**

| Drug | Dosage (adults) | Comment |
|---|---|---|
| Cotrimoxazole (trimethoprim/sulfamethoxazole) | 960 mg/day PO | • Adverse effects common, especially skin rashes, nausea, myelotoxicity |
| Pentamidine | 300 mg/month nebulised | • Needs high output nebuliser<br>• Causes bronchospasm; pretreat with nebulised salbutamol |
| Dapsone | 25mg qid PO | • Adverse effects include anaemia<br>• Toxic effects may be additive to zidovudine |
| Pyrimethamine + sulfadoxine | 25mg + 500mg once weekly PO | • Sulfonamide hypersensitivity<br>• Adverse effects include Stevens-Johnson syndrome (rarely) |

*Abbreviations:* PO = oral; qid = 4 times daily.

clovir through an indwelling intravenous line, is usually then necessary (see also chapter 32; sect. 3.2).

### 10.4 Tuberculosis and Atypical Mycobacterial Infection

Both tuberculosis and atypical mycobacterial infection are being seen with increasing frequency in HIV seropositive individuals (for treatment of *M. tuberculosis* infection, see section 9). Disseminated infection with an atypical mycobacterium such as *M. avium-intracellulare* is common in the terminal phase of AIDS. These organisms are often resistant to many first-line antituberculosis drugs *in vitro* and are difficult to treat.

#### Optimum Treatment

A 4-drug regimen consisting of rifampicin, ethambutol, amikacin and ciprofloxacin has been suggested for *M. avium-intracellulare* infection[117] and it is likely that treatment will have to be continued long term. It has also been suggested that primary prophylaxis against *M. avium-intracellulare* infection using rifabutin should be considered for patients with HIV and evidence of immunosuppression as this drug has demonstrated clinical effectiveness against *M. avium-intracellulare* infection in AIDS patients.[118]

## 11. Thromboembolic Disease

Pulmonary infarction follows embolisation to the peripheral branches of the pulmonary arteries. Emboli are often multiple, involving the lower zones more frequently than the upper parts of the lungs, and only some cause infarction. There is often a recent history of illness, trauma, anaesthesia or other factors known to predispose to deep venous thrombosis. The characteristic symptom is sudden breathlessness, which is later associated with pleuritic chest pain and haemoptysis if infarction occurs.

The clinical diagnosis is often difficult, but important findings are a history of predisposing factors, an obvious deep venous thrombosis, haemoptysis and a pleural rub. The chest radiograph is frequently normal and an electrocardiograph rarely helpful, but may show right axis deviation, right bundle branch block or an S-wave in lead I, and Q-wave and inverted T-wave in lead III. Isotope ventilation/perfusion lung scans are often helpful and demonstrate normal ventilation, but reduced perfusion, in the area of the embolus. Although a typically abnormal scan in a patient with a normal chest radiograph is considered diagnostic, isotope scans are more difficult to interpret in the presence of an abnormal chest radiograph such as in advanced obstructive airways disease. In difficult cases, pulmonary angiography with computerised digital subtraction techniques may be necessary. The diagnosis/initial management of acute pulmonary thromboembolism is shown (fig. 3).

#### Optimum Treatment

Therapy is urgent and potentially lifesaving. A scheme for treating acute pulmonary thromboembolism is shown (fig. 4). Heparin is the mainstay of treatment, both before the diagnosis has been established (fig. 3) and for all patients who do not have severe circulatory embarrassment. There is little to choose between continuous infusion or intermittent intravenous boluses of heparin, although haemorrhage may be slightly more common with the latter procedure.[119] Careful control of the level of anticoagulation may be easier with heparin if given by continuous infusion. The activated partial thromboplastin time (APTT) or prothrombin time should be maintained at 1.5 to 2.0 times their control value, which is equivalent to a

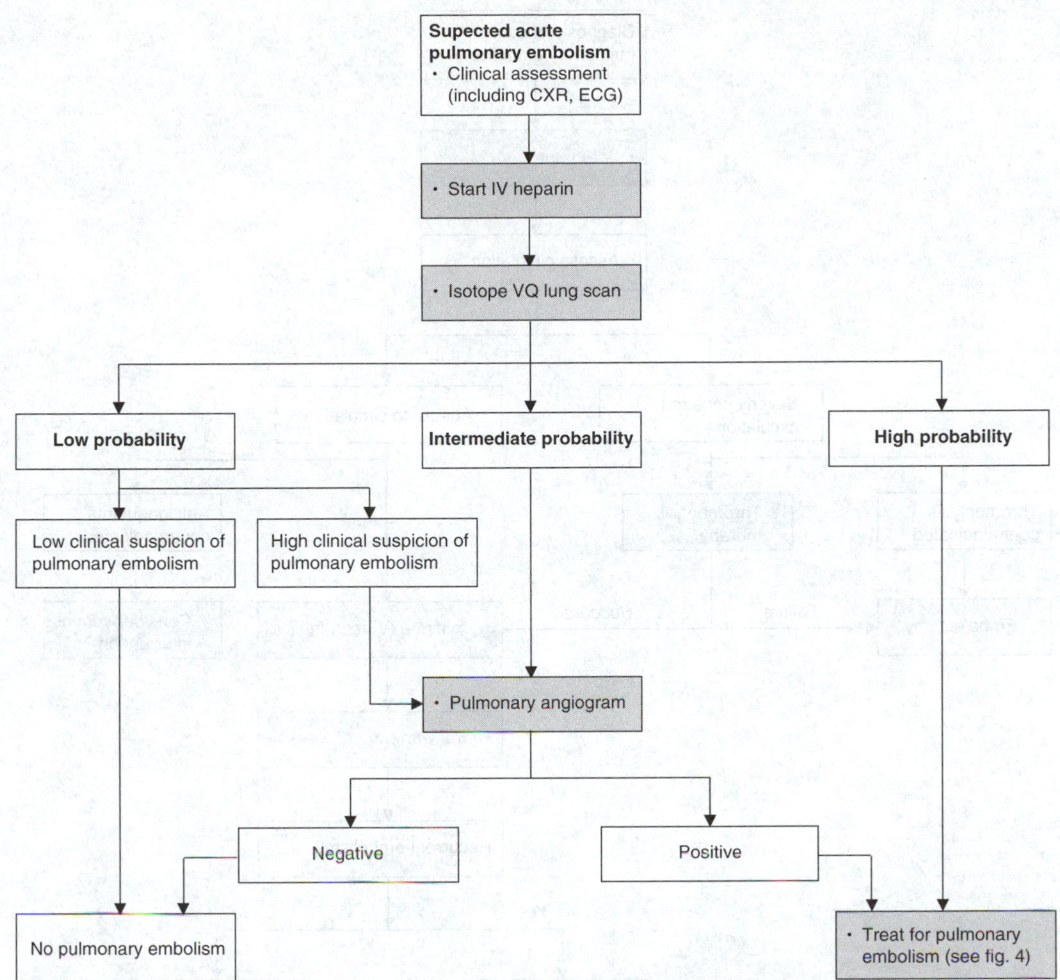


**Fig. 3.** Diagnosis/initial management of acute pulmonary thromboembolism. *Abbreviations:* CXR = chest x-ray; ECG = electrocardiogram; VQ = ventilation/perfusion ratio; IV = intravenous.

plasma heparin concentration of 0.3 to 0.4 U/ml. Heparin activity may vary throughout the day, so tests should be performed at the same time of day.[120] The dose of heparin is empirical, but most studies suggest that it should be 480 to 600 U/kg/day, with an initial dose of 10,000U. The appropriate duration of treatment is also unknown, but for a major thromboembolic episode should be >1 week, because this is the minimum time that it takes for a thrombus already present to become adherent to vein walls. Haemorrhagic complications occur in up to 20% of patients, but are serious in only 4 to 7%.[121]

Several trials have compared *thrombolytic agents* (see chapter 26; sect. 3.1.6) with heparin. The unequivocal conclusion of these studies is that pulmonary emboli clear more rapidly with the former.[122,123] However, the trials showed no differences in mortality, and consequently thrombolytic drugs are probably best reserved for patients in the acute phase and with evidence of a severely compromised circulation with hypotension, impaired peripheral circulation, oliguria and severe hypoxaemia. The duration of thrombolytic treatment is not established, but often marked improvement has occurred after 12 to 24 hours. Heparin should then be given after a pause of 4 hours and without a loading dose. Pulmonary embolectomy is now rarely required because of the excellent results of treatment with heparin and/or thrombolytic agents.

*Oral anticoagulants* have no role in the immediate treatment of pulmonary thromboembolism, but their effectiveness in preventing recurrences is well established, even though the

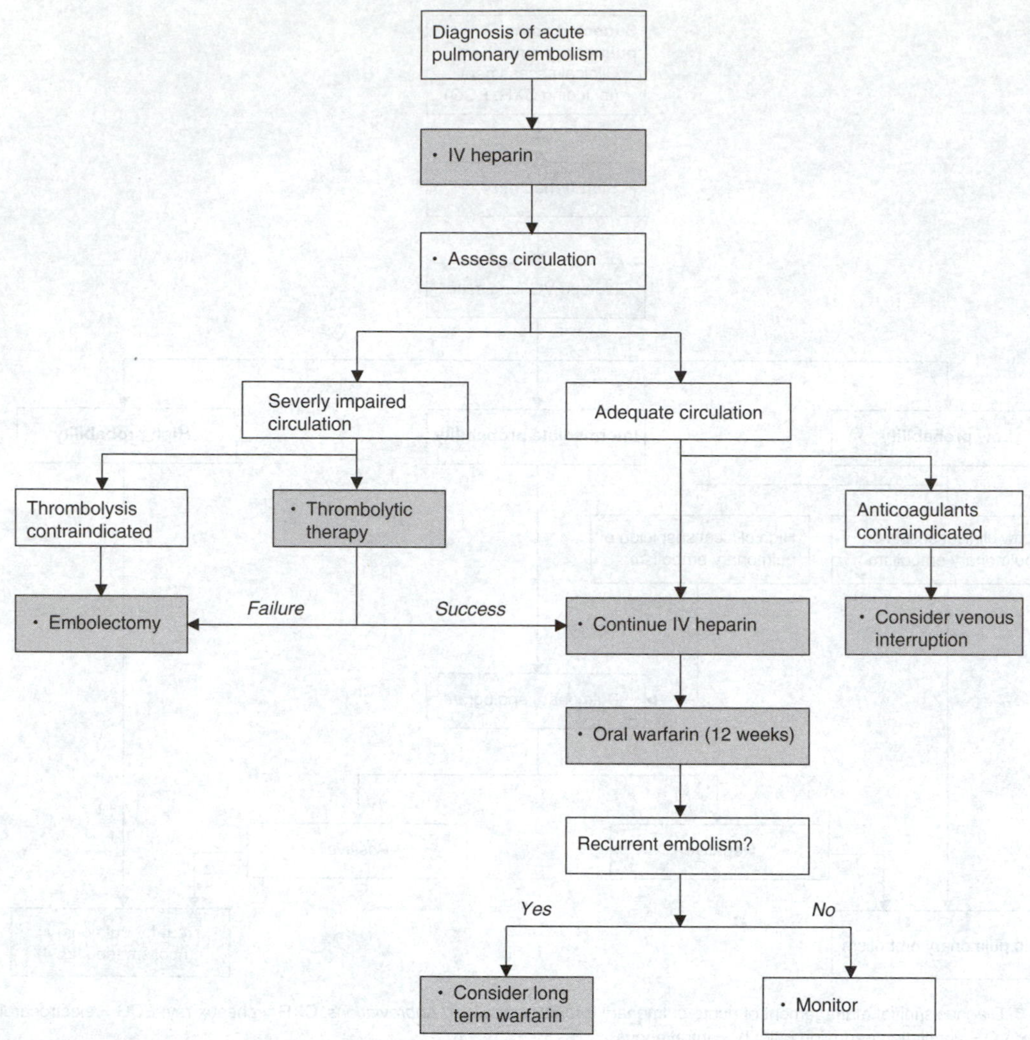


**Fig. 4.** Treatment of acute pulmonary thromboembolism. *Abbreviation:* IV = intravenous.

duration of treatment is uncertain. Several studies suggests that they should be given for at least 12 weeks after a major thromboembolic episode.[124,125] The dosage is usually controlled so as to achieve an international normalised ratio (INR; see chapter 26, sect. 3.1.5) of approximately 3, but less intense anticoagulation may also provide effective prophylaxis.[124] The risk of haemorrhage is always present and with long term therapy, the cumulative risk is not inconsiderable. Other adverse effects are rare, but there is a wide range of interactions with other drugs, among the most common being concurrent prescription of broad-spectrum antibiotics that can lead to over-anticoagulation.

## 12. Sarcoidosis

Sarcoidosis is a disease of unknown causation, characterised by involvement of more than 1 organ or tissue by noncaseating epithelioid cell granulomas that proceed either to resolution or fibrosis. It has a worldwide distribution, but may be less common in tropical than temperate areas. The highest incidence is in young adults, and females develop sarcoidosis more commonly than males.

The clinical course of sarcoidosis follows 2 principal patterns, a subacute or a chronic form. *Subacute sarcoidosis* usually presents with bilateral hilar lymphadenopathy with or without erythema nodosum and only occasionally affects other organs such as the eyes (uveal tract), nerves, salivary glands, heart, bones, spleen and liver. The Kveim skin test biopsy is positive in approximately 80% of patients with hilar lymphadenopathy and biopsy of tissue (e.g. lymph node) may show noncaseating granulomata. CT scan of the thorax usually confirms hilar and mediastinal lymph node enlargement, while pulmonary function is usually normal. In the subacute form of the disease, the prognosis is usually good and in 80% of patients, pulmonary changes disappear within 2 years.

For the 10 to 20% of patients with *chronic sarcoidosis*, the onset is more insidious. The initial presentation is with fever, cough and breathlessness. The chest radiograph shows bilateral mid-zone shadowing, possibly with cavitation and bulla formation. Pulmonary function tests show a restrictive ventilatory defect with low gas transfer measurements and the Kveim skin test biopsy is positive in only 40% of patients. Extrapulmonary manifestations may include small papules, plaques or subcutaneous nodules, lupus pernio, uveitis in up to 25%, hypercalciuria and renal stone formation, lymphadenopathy, myocarditis and bone cysts. Patients with chronic pulmonary sarcoidosis may progress to respiratory failure, while chronic extrapulmonary sarcoidosis often responds poorly to treatment.

#### Optimum Treatment

Most patients with subacute sarcoidosis and bilateral hilar lymphadenopathy recover spontaneously and therefore require no treatment. Anti-inflammatory analgesics such as aspirin or indomethacin are useful to treat the pain associated with erythema nodosum and musculoskeletal discomfort. There is some controversy about the indications for corticosteroids in the subacute phase of the illness as it is often self-limiting. Nevertheless, corticosteroids are indicated if uveitis, nervous system involvement or hypercalcaemia develop.

In chronic sarcoidosis, indications for corticosteroids include:

1) Active ocular sarcoidosis.

2) Persisting pulmonary symptoms and signs without improvement over a 3-month period, and evidence of progressive deterioration of lung function.

3) Severe endobronchial involvement with persistent cough and wheeze.

4) Persistent hypercalcaemia or hypercalciuria.

5) Involvement of the central nervous system.

6) Myocardial sarcoidosis.

7) Disfiguring facial lesions.

8) Persistent hepatomegaly or splenomegaly.

9) Lacrimal and salivary gland enlargement.

Most patients respond to prednisolone 20 to 40 mg/day, but occasionally higher doses are required to control ocular, cardiac or neurological involvement.[126,127] Alternative immunosuppressive agents (methotrexate, chloroquine, azathioprine or cyclosporin) may be used for severe chronic sarcoidosis, particularly skin involvement,[128] but there is no evidence that these agents are superior to oral corticosteroids. Single lung transplantation has been performed for end-stage pulmonary disease.

## 13. Interstitial Lung Diseases

The interstitial lung diseases are a heterogenous group of disorders classified together because of common clinical, radiological and physiological features. This discussion is restricted to *cryptogenic fibrosing alveolitis* (often known as idiopathic pulmonary fibrosis in the US), *extrinsic allergic alveolitis*, and *connective tissue disorders*.

### 13.1 Cryptogenic Fibrosing Alveolitis

Cryptogenic fibrosing alveolitis can occur at any age, but most often affects patients over 55 years and seems commoner in males. Clinical manifestations include progressive breathlessness on exertion, nonproductive cough, fine later inspiratory crackles at the lung bases, and usually finger clubbing. The chest radiograph typically reveals diffuse interstitial infiltrates, most often predominantly at the lung bases. Pulmonary function tests show a restrictive ventilatory defect with low gas transfer measurements and often arterial oxygen desaturation on exercise. A pathological diagnosis may require open lung biopsy, which demonstrates pulmonary fibrosis with variable degrees of cellular infiltration and cystic change in advanced disease. The clinical course is variable, with a mean survival of 4 to 6 years from diagnosis.

#### Optimum Treatment

On the basis that cryptogenic fibrosing alveolitis is an inflammatory disease with concurrent remodelling of the lung by fibrosis, the natural choice of treatment has been oral corticosteroids. However, the response to treatment is extremely variable and difficult to quantify. In a retrospective analysis of 127 patients treated with oral corticosteroids and followed for 4 years, only 17% showed an objective response to treatment.[129] Treatment is usually started with high-dose prednisolone (e.g. 1 mg/kg up to 80 mg/day) which should be continued for 6 to 8 weeks. After this, the dose is then slowly reduced to a maintenance level which is acceptable in terms of adverse effects but keeps the disease process under control. Factors that predict a good response to corticosteroids include:

- Less dyspnoea
- Less radiological abnormality
- Higher arterial oxygen concentration
- An excess of lymphocytes on bronchoalveolar lavage
- A more cellular lung biopsy.

Relapse on a moderate dose of an oral corticosteroid is an indication to consider a combination including an immunosuppressant.

Two combinations can be tried: low-dose prednisolone (20mg on alternate days); plus cyclophosphamide (up to 125mg daily)[130] *or* azathioprine (up to 150mg daily).[131]

Penicillamine prevents collagen cross-linking and therefore may be beneficial, but studies in fibrosing alveolitis have reported a high rate of adverse effects, particularly nephrotic syndrome.[132] Both colchicine[133] and cyclosporin[134] have been tried in the treatment of cryptogenic fibrosing alveolitis but the results have been disappointing. Newer drugs such as interferon-α (which blocks collagen gene transcription) may prove to be of value but have not yet been evaluated.

### 13.2 Extrinsic Allergic Alveolitis

Extrinsic allergic alveolitis is caused by repeated inhalation of finely dispersed organic dusts. This produces diffuse patchy interstitial and alveolar infiltrates in the lung after the formation of antigen-antibody complexes (Arthus reaction). Farmer's lung, from exposure to mouldy hay containing fungal spores, is the classic form. In urban areas, humidifier fever, due to fungal contamination of water in humidifiers and air conditioners, and bird fancier's lung are more common. The disorder presents in 2 forms. An acute reaction may occur after heavy exposure, typically 4 to 6 hours previously, which is characterised by abrupt onset, fever, chills, malaise, nausea, cough and dyspnoea without wheezing. These symptoms settle over hours to days and may be associated with diffuse fine crackles throughout the chest and fleeting interstitial shadows in the mid and upper lung zones on the chest radiograph. The second form of the disease is insidious, with gradually worsening breathlessness that results from repeated episodes of antigen exposure. These patients may present with pulmonary fibrosis that can progress to respiratory failure.

The diagnosis of extrinsic allergic alveolitis is important, as it is a reversible condition in the early stages after removal of the antigen. Precipitating antibodies indicate that immune reactivity has occurred, but do not prove causation because similar responses will occur in exposed but unaffected individuals. A negative precipitin test makes the diagnosis less likely, but can occur in about 10% of cases. Diagnosis of the chronic form usually requires open lung biopsy, which may show granulomatous pneumonitis, pulmonary fibrosis and the development of 'honeycomb' lung.

#### Optimum Treatment

Treatment is firstly to stop exposure to the antigen, which is usually sufficient in acute cases. However, when chronic exposure has led to persistent radiological interstitial shadowing and restrictive pulmonary function tests, treatment with corticosteroids is necessary.

### 13.3 Connective Tissue Disorders

Interstitial lung disease associated with connective tissue disorders usually occurs after connective tissue disease has been recognised. The most common form of pulmonary involvement is a chronic interstitial pattern indistinguishable from cryptogenic fibrosing alveolitis. Although rheumatoid disease has a female predominance, pulmonary involvement is more common in men. Interstitial lung disease occurs in up to 20% of cases of rheumatoid disease and is usually slowly progressive. It is also found in association with progressive systemic sclerosis, polymyositis and with Sjögren's syndrome, but is uncommon in systemic lupus erythematosus.

#### Optimum Treatment

As with cryptogenic fibrosing alveolitis (see section 13.1), corticosteroids can be tried, with varying success.

## 14. Use of Drugs in the Presence of Associated Respiratory Disease

Drugs used in the treatment of nonrespiratory disease may have pulmonary effects and adversely affect lung function in those with respiratory disease. These should be predictable, as rational drug therapy depends on the knowledge of the spectrum of activity of the drugs prescribed. Alternatively, the respiratory disease itself or drugs being used to treat respiratory illnesses may modify the response to other drugs or alter their pharmacokinetic behaviour in the body.

### 14.1 Problems Due to the Mode of Action of Drugs

Factors that influence bronchial secretion and airway calibre include cholinergic and adrenergic mechanisms. *β-Adrenoceptor blocking drugs* are widely used in the treatment of cardiac arrhythmias, angina pectoris, glaucoma (topically) and hypertension. They may precipitate or intensify airway obstruction in susceptible patients. No β-adrenoceptor blocking drug is completely safe in patients with asthma; even relatively $\beta_1$-selective blockers must be used with care, as their effect on lung function is unpredictable[90] and bronchoconstriction may still occur.[135] Indeed, it is advisable to give a test dose and measure the effect on PEFR. Some advocate that a relatively $\beta_1$-selective drug should only be used in patients with airway obstruction if it can be given in low dosages and in combination with full dosage of a $\beta_2$-agonist bronchodilator.[136]

*Dinoprost* (prostaglandin $F_{2\alpha}$) is being increasingly used to induce labour and abortion. This drug and *aspirin* and other *nonsteroidal anti-inflammatory drugs* may also precipitate airway obstruction in susceptible individuals.

*Cholinergic (parasympathomimetic) drugs* are widely used in therapeutics, e.g. carbachol in stimulating bladder emptying. In susceptible patients, such drugs may precipitate airway obstruction and increase tracheobronchial secretion. Many other commonly used drugs (atropine, tricyclic antidepressants, antipsychotics, antihistamines and anti-Parkinsonian drugs) have anticholinergic (parasympathomimetic blocking) properties, and the effects of these agents on airway calibre and bronchial secretion are variable.

### 14.2 Altered Response Due to Altered Tissue Sensitivity or Pharmacokinetics

Pulmonary disease or secondary complications may modify the response to drugs or affect their pharmacokinetic behaviour in the body. Patients with severe respiratory disease, particularly when accompanied by hypoxia, may have increased myocardial sensitivity to the action of digoxin.[137,138] These patients are seriously ill and are already prone to arrhythmias that may be more easily provoked by digoxin. Although digoxin toxicity in this situation occurs at lower than usual serum concentrations[139] and a reduced volume of distribution and renal clearance of digoxin have been demonstrated in cor pulmonale,[140,141] control of the ventilatory dysfunction appears of as much importance as digoxin dosage in this situation. Smaller doses of digoxin are recommended except when it is necessary to control a ventricular response with atrial fibrillation.[140]

The hypoxic state may also alter hepatic microsomal drug metabolising enzyme activity. While the clinical significance of this observation is unclear, it may explain the increased metabolic clearance of cortisol noted in corticosteroid recipients with severe attacks of asthma.[142] This finding drew attention to the need for very large doses of corticosteroids to achieve adequate plasma cortisol concentrations and a good clinical response in a severe attack of asthma. Similarly, drugs such as rifampicin and phenobarbital can, by their own hepatic microsomal enzyme-inducing activity, contribute to the increased metabolic clearance of cortisol in corticosteroid-treated asthmatic patients, with consequent reductions in therapeutic effectiveness of the corticosteroid.

Theophylline can be effective in airways obstruction but the intersubject variation in hepatic drug metabolism is considerable. Smoking and a high protein diet can increase theophylline clearance, while acute pulmonary oedema[141,143] and certain antibiotics notably erythromycin and ciprofloxacin can reduce clearance. In these situations, theophylline dosages should be modified accordingly.

### 14.3 Oxygen Therapy and Sedatives

The dangers of oxygen therapy and of sedative opioid and antianxiety drugs in patients with hypercapnia have been emphasised in section 5. In addition, hyperbaric oxygen therapy (at 2 atmospheres) may lead to convulsions and, when oxygen is given in atmospheric pressure at concentrations of 50% or more for more than 12 hours, it may be followed by adverse pulmonary effects including intra-alveolar oedema and atelectasis and eventually by irreversible pulmonary fibrosis.

## References


1. Barnes PJ. Molecular biology of receptors: implications for lung disease. Thorax 1990; 45: 482-8
2. Frew AJ, Holgate ST. Clinical pharmacology of asthma: implications for treatment. Drugs 1993; 46: 847-62
3. Holgate ST, Church MK, editors. Allergy. London: Gower Medical Publishing, 1993
4. Robinson DS, Durham SR, Kay AB. Cytokines in asthma. Thorax 1993; 48: 845-54
5. Barnes PJ. Inhaled glucocorticoids for asthma. New England Journal of Medicine 1995; 332: 868-75
6. Nelson HS. β-Adrenergic bronchodilators. New England Journal of Medicine 1995; 333: 499-506
7. Beasley R, Roche W, Roberts JA, et al. Cellular events in the bronchi in mild asthma and after bronchial provocation. American Review of Respiratory Disease 1989; 139: 806-17
8. Jeffery BK, Godfrey RW, Adelroth E, et al. Effect of treatment on airway inflammation and thickening of basement membrane reticular collagen in asthma: a quantitative light and electron microscopic study. American Review of Respiratory Disease 1992; 145: 890-9
9. Ninan T, Russell G. Respiratory symptoms and atopy in Aberdeen school children: evidence from two surveys 25 years apart. British Medical Journal 1992; 304: 873-5
10. Burney BGJ, Chinn S, Rona RJ. Has the prevalence of asthma increased in children? Evidence from the national study of health and growth 1973-86. British Medical Journal 1990; 300: 1306-10
11. Burney P. Epidemiology of asthma. In: Clark TJ, Godfrey S, Lee T, editors. Asthma. 3rd ed. London: Chapman and Hall, 1992
12. Turner-Warwick M. Nocturnal asthma: a study in general practice. Journal of the Royal College of General Practitioners 1989; 39: 239
13. Grainger J, Woodman K, Pearce N, et al. Prescribed fenoterol and death from asthma in New Zealand 1981-87; a further case controlled study. Thorax 1991; 46: 101-11
14. Spitzer WO, Suissa S, Ernst P, et al. The use of beta agonists and the risk of death or near death from asthma. New England Journal of Medicine 1992; 326: 501-6
15. Committee on the Safety of Medicines. Report of the Beta Agonist Working Party. London: Medicines Control Agency, 1992
16. Sears MR, Taylor DR, Print CJ, et al. Regular inhaled β agonist in bronchial asthma. Lancet 1990; 336: 1391-6
17. Tattersfield AE. Effect of β-agonists and anticholinergic drugs on bronchial reactivity. American Review of Respiratory Disease 1987; 136: 645-85
18. British Thoracic Association. Death from asthma in two regions of England. British Medical Journal 1982; 285: 1251-5
19. Brogden RN, Faulds D. Salmeterol xinafoate: a review of its pharmacological properties and therapeutic potential in reversible obstructive airways disease. Drugs 1991; 42: 895-912
20. Faulds D, Hollingshead LM, Goa KL. Formoterol: a review of its pharmacological properties and therapeutic potential in reversible obstructive airways disease. Drugs 1991; 42: 115-37
21. Ward MJ, Fentem PH, Roderick-Smith WH, et al. Ipratropium bromide in acute asthma. British Medical Journal 1981; 282: 598
22. Gonzalez JP, Brogden RN. Nedocromil sodium: a preliminary review of its pharmacodynamic and pharmacokinetic properties, and therapeutic efficacy in the treatment of reversible obstructive airways disease. Drugs 1987; 34: 560-77
23. Rafferty P, Tucker LG, Fram MH, et al. Comparison of budesonide and beclomethasone dipropionate in patients with severe chronic asthma: assessment of relative prednisolone sparing effect. British Journal of Diseases of the Chest 1985; 79: 244-50
24. Boyd G, Abdallah S, Clark R. Twice or four times daily beclomethasone dipropionate in mild asthma. Clinical Allergy 1985; 15: 383-9
25. Grove A, Allam C, McFarelane LC, et al. A comparison of the systemic bioavailability of inhaled budesonide and fluticasone propionate in normal subjects. British Journal of Clinical Pharmacology 1994; 38: 527-32
26. Holliday SM, Faulds D, Sorkin EM. Inhaled fluticasone propionate: a review of its pharmacodynamic and pharmacokinetic properties, and therapeutic use in asthma. Drugs 1994; 47: 318-31
27. Toogood JH, Baskerville J, Jennings B, et al. Use of spacers to facilitate inhaled corticosteroid treatment of asthma. American Review of Respiratory Disease 1984; 129: 723-9
28. Williams AJ, Baghat MS, Stableforth DE, et al. Dysphonia caused by inhaled steroids: recognition of the characteristic laryngeal abnormality. Thorax 1983; 38: 813-21
29. Russell G, Ninan T, Carter P, et al. Effect of inhaled corticosteroids on HPA function and growth in children. Research and Clinical Forums 1989; 11: 77-86
30. Jennings BH, Anderson JE, Johnassen SA. Assessment of systemic effects of inhaled corticosteroids: comparison of the effects of inhaled budesonide and oral prednisolone on adrenal function and markers of bone turnover. European Journal of Clinical Pharmacology 1991; 40: 77-82
31. Grant SM, Goa KL, Fitton A, et al. Ketotifen: a review of its pharmacodynamic and pharmacokinetic properties, and therapeutic use in asthma and allergic disorders. Drugs 1990; 40: 412-48
32. British Thoracic Society. Research Unit of the Royal College of Physicians of London, Kings Fund Centre, National Campaign: Guidelines for the Management of Asthma in Adults: II Acute severe asthma. British Medical Journal 1990; 301: 797-800
33. British Thoracic Society. British Paediatric Association Research Unit, Royal College of Physicians of London, Kings Fund Centre, National Asthma Campaign, Royal College of General Practitioners, General Practitioners in Asthma Group, British Association of Accident and Emergency Medicine, British Paediatric Respiratory Group: guidelines on the management of asthma. Thorax 1993; 48: S1-S24
34. British Thoracic Society. Guidelines for the management of community-acquired pneumonia in adults admitted to hospital. British Journal of Hospital Medicine 1993; 49: 346
35. International Consensus Report on the Diagnosis of Management of Asthma. Clinical and Experimental Allergy 1992; Suppl. 22: 1-72
36. McFadden ER, Hejal R. Asthma. Lancet 1995; 345: 1215-9

37. Speight ANP, Lee DA, Hey EN. Underdiagnosis and undertreatment of asthma in childhood. British Medical Journal 1983; 286: 1253
38. Godden DJ, Ross S, Abdalla M, et al. Outcome of wheeze in childhood. American Journal of Respiratory and Critical Care Medicine 1994; 149: 106-12
39. Mellis CM, Peak JK, Bauman AE, et al. The cost of asthma in New South Wales. Medical Journal of Australia 1991; 155: 522
40. Weiss KB, Gergen PJ, Hodgson TA. An economic evaluation of asthma in the United States. New England Journal of Medicine 1992; 326: 862
41. Clark TJH, editor. The occurrence and cost of asthma. Worthington: Cambridge Medical Publications, 1990
42. Crompton GK. New inhalation devices. European Journal of Respiratory Diseases 1988; 1: 679
43. Jasper AC, Mohseiifar Z, Kahan S, et al. Cost-benefit comparison of aerosol bronchodilator delivery methods in hospitalised patients. Chest 1987; 91: 614
44. Summer W, Elston R, Thorpe L, et al. Aerosol bronchodilator delivery methods: relative impact on pulmonary function and cost of respiratory care. Archives of Internal Medicine 1989; 149: 618
45. Ross RN, Morris M, Sakawitz SR, et al. Cost-effectiveness of including cromolyn sodium in the treatment program for asthma: a retrospective case-record study. Clinical Therapeutics 1989; 10: 188
46. Horn CR, Clark TJH, Cochrane GM. Can the morbidity of asthma be reduced by high dose inhaled therapy? A prospective study. Respiratory Medicine 1990; 84: 61
47. Zeigler RS, Heller S, Mellon MH, et al. Facilitated referral to asthma specialist reduces relapse in asthma emergency room visits. Journal of Allergy and Clinical Immunology 1991; 87: 1160
48. Braun SR, Levy SF. Comparison of ipratropium bromide and albuterol in chronic obstructive pulmonary disease: a three center study. American Journal of Medicine 1991; 91: 285
49. Gaddie J, Palmer KNV, Petrie JC, et al. Effect of nitrazepam in chronic obstructive bronchitis. British Medical Journal 1972; 2: 688
50. Medical Research Council Working Party. Long term domiciliary oxygen therapy in chronic hypoxic cor pulmonale complicating chronic bronchitis and emphysema. Lancet 1981; 1: 681
51. Nocturnal Oxygen Therapy Trial Group. Continuous or nocturnal oxygen therapy in hypoxaemic chronic obstructive lung disease: a clinical trial. Annals of Internal Medicine 1980; 93: 391
52. Christopher KL, Spoffard BT, Petrun MD, et al. A programme for transtracheal oxygen delivery. Annals of Internal Medicine 1987; 107: 802
53. Tarpy SP, Celli BR. Long term oxygen therapy. New England Journal of Medicine 1995; 333: 710-4
54. Lowson KV, Drummond MF, Bishop JM. Costing new services long-term domiciliary oxygen therapy. Lancet 1981; 2: 1146
55. Franz DN. Central nervous system stimulants. In: Goodman & Gilman (editors) The pharmacological basis of therapeutics. New York: Macmillan, 1975
56. Hirsch WH, Wang SC. Selective respiratory stimulating action of doxapram compared to pentylenetetrazol. Journal of Pharmacology and Experimental Therapeutics 1974; 189: 1
57. White KF, Flenley DC. Can pulmonary vasodilators improve survival in cor pulmonale due to hypoxic chronic bronchitis and emphysema? Thorax 1988; 43: 1
58. Hubbard RC, Chrystal RG. Alpha-1-antitrypsin augmentation therapy for alpha-1-antitrypsin deficiency. American Journal of Medicine 1988; 84: 52
59. Snider GL. Chronic obstructive pulmonary disease: a definition and implications of structural determinants of airflow obstruction for epidemiology. American Review of Respiratory Disease 1989; 140: 83
60. American Thoracic Society: guidelines for the initial management of adults with community-acquired pneumonia: diagnosis, assessment of severity, and initial antimicrobial therapy. American Review of Respiratory Disease 1993; 148: 141
61. Niederman MS, Torres A, Summer W. Invasive diagnostic testing is not needed routinely to manage ventilator-associated pneumonia. American Journal of Respiratory and Critical Care Medicine 1994; 150: 565
62. Chastre J, Fagon JY. Invasive diagnostic testing should be routinely used to manage ventilated patients with suspected pneumonia. American Journal of Respiratory and Critical Care Medicine 1994; 150: 570
63. Friedland IR, McCracken GH. Management of infections caused by antibiotic-resistant *Streptococcus pneumoniae*. New England Journal of Medicine 1992; 331: 377
64. Macfarlane JT, Millar AC, Smith WHR, et al. Comparative radiographic features of acquired Legionnaires' disease, pneumococcal pneumonia, and psittacosis. Thorax 1984; 39: 28
65. Sutton P. Chest physiotherapy: time for reappraisal. British Journal of Diseases of the Chest 1988; 82: 127
66. Szaff M, Hoiby N, Flensborg EW. Frequent antibiotic therapy improves survival of cystic fibrosis patients with Pseudomonas chest infection. Acta Paediatrica Scandinavica 1983; 72: 651
67. Hodson ME, Penketh ARL, Batten JC. Aerosol carbenicillin and gentamicin treatment of *Pseudomonas aeruginosa* infection in patients with cystic fibrosis. Lancet 1981; 2: 1137
68. Littlewood JM, Miller MG, Chonheim AT, et al. Nebulised colomycin for early pseudomonas colonisation in cystic fibrosis. Lancet 1985; 1: 865
69. Smith AL, Ramsey B. Aerosol administration of antibiotics. Respiration 1995: 62 (Suppl. 1): 19-24
70. Govan JRW, Nelson JW. Microbiology of lung infection in cystic fibrosis. British Medical Bulletin 1992; 48: 912-30
71. Hoiby N. Microbiology in cystic fibrosis. In: Hodson ME, Geddes DM, editors. Cystic fibrosis. London: Chapman & Hall, 1995
72. Bryson HM, Sorkin EM. Dornase alfa: a review of its pharmacological properties and therapeutic potential in cystic fibrosis. Drugs 1994; 48: 894-906
73. Ranasinha C, Assoufi B, Shak S, et al. Efficacy and safety of short-term administration of aerosolised recombinant human DNase 1 in adults with stable stage cystic fibrosis. Lancet 1993; 342: 199
74. Ramsay B, for the Pulmozyme (rhDNase) Study Group. A summary of the results of the phase III multicenter clinical trial: aerosol administration of recombinant DNase reduces the risk of respiratory tract infections and improves pulmonary function in patients with cystic fibrosis. Dallas, Texas: North American Cystic Fibrosis Conference, 1993: 152-3
75. Wilmott RW, Fielder MA. Recent advances in the treatment of cystic fibrosis. Paediatric Clinics of North America 1994; 41: 431-51

76. Sudre P, ten Dam G, Kochi A. Tuberculosis: a global overview of the situation today. Bulletin of the World Health Organization 1992; 70 (2): 149-59
77. Frieden TR, Sterling T, Pablos Mendez A, et al. The emergence of drug-resistant tuberculosis in New York City. New England Journal of Medicine 1993; 328: 521
78. Porter J, MacAdam K, editors. Tuberculosis: back to the future. London School of Hygiene and Tropical Medicine Public Health Forum. 3rd ed. Chichester: John Wiley & Sons, 1994
79. Holdiness MR. Clinical pharmacokinetics of the antituberculosis drugs. Clinical Pharmacokinetics 1984; 9: 511
80. Holdiness MR. Cerebrospinal fluid pharmacokinetics of the antituberculosis drugs. Clinical Pharmacokinetics 1985; 10: 532
81. Holdiness MR. Neurological manifestations and toxicities of the antituberculosis drugs. Medical Toxicology and Adverse Drug Experience 1987; 2: 33
82. Holdiness MR. Transplacental pharmacokinetics of the antituberculosis drugs. Clinical Pharmacokinetics 1987; 13: 125
83. Girling DJ. Adverse effects of antituberculosis drugs. Drugs 1982; 23: 56
84. Jordan TJ, Lewitt EM, Reichman LB. Isoniazid prevention therapy for tuberculosis. American Review of Respiratory Disease 1991; 144: 1357-60
85. Schaberg T. The dark side of antituberculosis therapy: adverse events involving liver function. European Respiratory Journal 1995; 8: 1247-9
86. Winstanley PA. The clinical pharmacology of antituberculous drugs. In: Davies PDO, editor. Clinical tuberculosis. London: Chapman & Hall, 1994
87. Davidson PT, Hanh Quoc Le. Drug treatment of tuberculosis – 1992. Drugs 1992; 43: 651-73
88. Olliaro P, Dolfi L, Morelli P, et al. Rifabutin for prevention and treatment of mycobacterial diseases: a review of microbiology, clinical pharmacology, efficacy, and tolerability data. European Respiratory Review 1995; 5: 77-83
89. Brogden RN, Fitton A. Rifabutin: a review of its antimicrobial activity, pharmacokinetic properties and therapeutic efficacy. Drugs 1994; 47: 983-1009
90. Skinner MH, Blaschke T. Clinical pharmacokinetics of rifabutin. Clinical Pharmacokinetics 1995; 28: 115-25
91. Crofton J, Horne N, Miller F, editors. Clinical tuberculosis. London: Macmillan Education Ltd, 1992
92. Joint Tuberculosis Committee of the British Thoracic Society. Chemotherapy and management of tuberculosis in the United Kingdom: recommendations. Thorax 1990; 45: 403
93. World Health Organisation. Treatment of tuberculosis: guidelines for national programmes. Geneva: World Health Organization, 1993
94. American Thoracic Society. Control of tuberculosis in the United States. American Review of Respiratory Disease 1992; 146: 1623
95. British Thoracic Association. A controlled trial of six months chemotherapy in pulmonary tuberculosis. First report: results during chemotherapy. British Journal of Diseases of the Chest 1981; 75: 141
96. British Thoracic Society. A controlled trial of six months chemotherapy in pulmonary tuberculosis: results during the 36 months after the end of chemotherapy and beyond. British Journal of Diseases of the Chest 1984; 78: 330
97. Davies PDO, editor. Clinical tuberculosis. London: Chapman and Hall Medical, 1994
98. Iseman MD. Treatment of multidrug-resistant tuberculosis. New England Journal of Medicine 1993; 329: 784
99. Subcommittee of the Joint Tuberculosis Committee of the British Thoracic Society. Control and prevention of tuberculosis in Britain: an updated code of practice. British Medical Journal 1990; 300: 995
100. Koch-Weser D. BCG vaccination: can it contribute to tuberculosis control? Chest 1993; 103: 1641
101. Houston S, Fanning A. Current and potential treatment of tuberculosis. Drugs 1994; 48: 689-708
102. International Union against Tuberculosis. Tuberculosis guide for low income countries. 3rd ed. Paris: International Union against Tuberculosis, 1994
103. Sinclair K, Wakefield AE, Banerji S, et al. *Pneumocystis carinii* organisms derived from rat and human hosts are genetically distinct. Molecular and Biochemical Parasitology 1991; 45: 183
104. Wakefield AE, Guiver L, Miller RF, et al. Amplification of induced sputum samples for diagnosis of *Pneumocystis carinii* pneumonia. Lancet 1991; 337: 1378
105. Peters SE, Wakefield AE, Sinclair K, et al. A search for *Pneumocystis carinii* in post mortem lungs in DNA amplification. Journal of Pathology 1992; 166: 195
106. Leigh TR, Parsan P, Hume C, et al. Sputum induction for the diagnosis of *Pneumocystis carinii* pneumonia. Lancet 1990; 2: 205
107. Ng VL, Yajko DM, McPhaul LW. Evaluation of an indirect fluorescent antibody stain for the detection of *Pneumocystis carinii* in respiratory specimens. Journal of Clinical Microbiology 1990; 28: 975
108. Sattler F, Cowan R, Neilsen DM, et al. Trimethoprim-sulfamethoxazole compared with pentamidine for treatment of *Pneumocystis carinii* pneumonia in the acquired immunodeficiency syndrome: a prospective non-cross-over study. Annals of Internal Medicine 1988; 109: 280
109. Medina I, Mills I, Leoung G, et al. Oral therapy for *Pneumocystis carinii* pneumonia in the acquired immune deficiency syndrome. New England Journal of Medicine 1990; 323: 776
110. Gagnon S, Boota AM, Fischl MA, et al. Corticosteroids as adjunctive therapy for severe *Pneumocystis carinii* pneumonia in the acquired immunodeficiency syndrome. New England Journal of Medicine 1990; 323: 1444
111. Jeffrey AA, Bullen C, Miller RF. Intensive care management of *Pneumocystis carinii* pneumonia. Care of the Critically Ill 1993; 9: 258-60
112. Schneider NME, Hoepelman AIM, Efftinick J, et al. A controlled trial of aerosolised pentamidine or trimethoprim-sulphamethoxazole as primary prophylaxis against *Pneumocystis carinii* pneumonia in patients with human immunodeficiency virus. New England Journal of Medicine 1992; 327: 1836-41
113. Chaisson RE. Bacterial pneumonia in patients with human immunodeficiency virus infection. Seminars in Respiratory Infections 1989; 4: 133
114. Immunisation Practices Advisory Committee, Centres for Disease Control. Pneumococcal polysaccharide vaccines. Morbidity and Mortality Weekly Report 1989; 38: 64
115. Collaborative DHPG Treatment Study Group. Treatment of serious cytomegalovirus infections with 9-(1,3-dihydroxy-2-propoxymethyl) guanine in patients with AIDS and other immunodeficiencies. New England Journal of Medicine 1986; 314: 801

116. Farthing C, Anderson MG, Ellis ME, et al. Treatment of cytomegalovirus pneumonitis with foscarnet (trisodium phosphanoformate) in patients with AIDS. Journal of Medical Virology 1987; 22: 157
117. Murray JF, Mills J. Pulmonary infectious complications of human immunodeficiency virus infection. American Review of Respiratory Disease 1990; 141: 1356
118. US Public Health Service Task Force on Prophylaxis and Therapy for Mycobacterium Avium Complex. New England Journal of Medicine 1993; 329: 898
119. Hall RJC. Difficulties in the treatment of acute pulmonary embolism. Thorax 1985; 40: 729
120. Decousus HA, Croze M, Levi FA. Changes in anticoagulant effect of heparin infused at a constant rate. British Medical Journal 1985; 290: 341
121. Levine MN, Goldhaber SZ, Gore JM, et al. Haemorrhagic complications of anticoagulant treatment. Chest 1995; 108 (Suppl. 4): 276-90
122. Goldhaber SZ, Vaughan DE, Markis JE. Acute pulmonary embolism treated with tissue plasminogen activator. Lancet 1986; 2: 886
123. Verstraete M, Miller GAH, Bounameaux H. Intravenous and intrapulmonary recombinant tissue type plasminogen activator (r-tPA) in the treatment of acute massive pulmonary embolism. Circulation 1988; 77: 353
124. Hull R, Delmore T, Genton E. Warfarin sodium versus low-dose heparin in the long-term treatment of venous thrombosis. New England Journal of Medicine 1979; 301: 855
125. Lagerstedt CI, Olsson CG. Need for long-term anticoagulant therapy in symptomatic calf-vein thrombosis. Lancet 1985; 2: 515
126. Sharma OP. Pulmonary sarcoidosis and corticosteroids. American Review of Respiratory Disease 1993; 147: 1598-600
127. Hunninghake GW, Gilbert S, Pueringer R. Outcome of the treatment of sarcoidosis. American Journal of Respiratory and Critical Care Medicine 1994; 149: 893-8
128. Zic JA, Horowitz DH, Arzubiaga C, et al. Treatment of cutaneous sarcoidosis with chloroquine. Archives of Dermatology 1991; 127: 1034-40
129. Turner-Warwick M, Burrows B, Johnson A. Cryptogenic fibrosing alveolitis: response to corticosteroid treatment and its effect on survival. Thorax 1989; 35: 593-9
130. Johnson MA, Kwan S, Snell NJC, et al. Randomised controlled trial comparing prednisolone alone with cyclophosphamide and low dose prednisolone in combination in cryptogenic fibrosing alveolitis. Thorax 1989; 44: 280
131. Raghu G, DePaso WJ, Cain K. Azathioprine combined with prednisolone in the treatment of idiopathic pulmonary fibrosis: a prospective double-blind randomised, placebo-controlled trial. American Review of Respiratory Disease 1991; 144: 291-5
132. Meier-Sydow J, Rust M, Kronenberger H, et al. Survival of patients with idiopathic pulmonary fibrosis following treatment with azathioprine, d-penicillamine or prednisolone: a 10 year follow-up. Chest 1990; 94: 18S
133. Rennard SI, Bitterman PB, Ozaki T, et al. Colchicine suppresses the release of fibroblast growth factors from alveolar macrophages. American Review of Respiratory Disease 1988; 137: 181-5
134. Moolman JA, Bardin PG, Rossouw DJ, et al. Cyclosporin as treatment for interstitial lung disease of unknown aetiology. Thorax 1991; 46: 592-5
135. McDevitt DG. β-Adrenoceptor antagonists and respiratory function. British Journal of Clinical Pharmacology 1978; 5: 97
136. Formgren H. The effect of metoprolol and practolol on lung function and blood pressure in hypertensive asthmatics. British Journal of Clinical Pharmacology 1976; 3: 1007
137. Hargreave FE. Digitalis and cor pulmonale. British Medical Journal 1971; 2: 713
138. Baum CL, Dick MM, Blum A, et al. Factors involved in digitalis sensitivity in chronic pulmonary insufficiency. American Heart Journal 1959; 57: 460
139. Paciaroni E, Fosch F, Vittori N, et al. Le digoxinemia nei soggetti con cuore pulmonare cronico. Giornale di Gerontologia 1974; 22: 832
140. Doherty JE, Kane JJ, Phillips JR, et al. Digitalis in pulmonary heart disease (cor pulmonale). Drugs 1977; 13: 142
141. du Souich P, McLean AJ, Lalka D, et al. Pulmonary disease and drug kinetics. Clinical Pharmacokinetics 1977; 3: 257
142. Dwyer J, Lazarus L, Hickie JB. A study of cortisol metabolism in patients with chronic asthma. Australasian Annals of Medicine 1967; 16: 297
143. Ogilvie RI. Clinical pharmacokinetics of theophylline. Clinical Pharmacokinetics 1978; 3: 2767

Chapter 24

# Renal Diseases

*J.A.J.H. Critchley, T.Y.K. Chan* and *A.D. Cumming*

## Synopsis of Important Principles

1) Ideally, drugs used in renal disease should be therapeutically effective and not cause a deterioration in renal function.

2) Kidney disorders alter the chemical composition of body fluids and hence the pharmacokinetic properties of many drugs. Thus, standard regimens of some drugs may be inappropriate and need to be adjusted if adverse effects are to be avoided in patients with renal failure.

3) The clinical significance of a reduction in glomerular filtration rate, decreased drug clearance and increased half-life depends on the relative importance of renal excretion and metabolism as a mode of elimination, and on the therapeutic ratio of the drug.

4) Dosages of drugs that are mainly excreted in active form by the kidney (i.e. as unchanged drug or active metabolites) may need to be modified to avoid accumulation – by giving the usual dose at increased intervals or a reduced dose at the usual intervals.

5) Chronic renal failure is accompanied by many changes in homeostatic mechanisms which in turn alter the response to drugs. There is an increased incidence of adverse effects in such patients.

6) Many drugs can cause or exacerbate renal disease and sometimes permanently.

7) In renal failure, potentially toxic drugs should only be used if there is a specific indication for their use and if therapy can be monitored appropriately.

8) Many cases of renal failure are due to identifiable and treatable causes, and these should always be sought. Supportive treatment of disordered renal function is directed towards replacement of substances inappropriately lost, and at reducing the dietary intake of those substances that are retained. Factors that place an added load on renal function should be avoided. Extracellular fluid volume and blood pressure should be optimised and infection controlled.

9) Asymptomatic urinary tract infections in adults with normal renal tracts probably do not require antibacterial therapy. However, they should be treated in pregnant women and in infants and children.

10) Corticosteroids and/or immunosuppressive drugs are of value in certain specific types of glomerulonephritis.

11) Renal replacement therapy by dialysis or transplantation involves particular problems in drug selection and dosage.

12) The early detection and prevention, or at least delay, of diabetic and/or hypertensive nephropathies is one of the greatest challenges facing renal medicine today.

The relationship between the kidney and the action of drugs is important from 2 different points of view. The kidney is the major excretory organ for many drugs and their metabolites. Changes in renal function therefore exert a profound effect on the rate of excretion of these drugs or their metabolites and thus on the intensity and duration of their action. In addition, a number of drugs act directly on the kidney and are capable of altering glomerular and tubular function.

## 1. Clinical Pharmacological Considerations

Diseases of the kidney can modify the relationship between drug dose and clinical effect in many ways. Accordingly, standard dosage regimens are often inappropriate and require adjustment if adverse and toxic reactions are to be avoided (see also appendix D). Effects on absorption, volume of distribution and elimination of drugs alter plasma concentrations and drug concentrations at their sites of action (i.e. drug receptors). Monitoring the plasma concentrations of a drug (see chapter 5) may not be sufficient for optimum therapeutic management, since changes in plasma protein binding and in drug receptor sensitivity affect the relationship between plasma concentration and pharmacological response. The accumulation of active metabolites not measured by the assay for the parent drug is another hazard. Although renal impairment primarily affects drug and metabolite excretion, other aspects of pharmacokinetics and pharmacodynamics may also be affected.

The increased incidence of adverse drug reactions in patients with renal failure emphasises the need to understand the pharmacokinetic factors involved. Special considerations should also be given to patients on renal replacement therapies, which may significantly affect the pharmacokinetics of some drugs. Theoretically, for all drugs that are affected by renal impairment, changes in dose and dose interval need to be considered. However, in practice, dose adjustment is usually only necessary for those drugs with a narrow therapeutic index and with adverse effects related to drug or metabolite accumulation.

For reviews of pharmacokinetic and pharmacodynamic factors and the principles of drug prescribing in patients with renal failure, see Bennett,[1] Carmichael[2] and Cove-Smith.[3]

### 1.1 Absorption and Bioavailability of Drugs in Renal Diseases

Few studies have been done on the oral absorption of drugs by patients with renal diseases. In chronic renal failure, increased gastric ammonia production occurs concurrently with urea accumulation and hydrolysis. Ammonia buffers hydrochloric acid, causing an increase in gastric pH. Consequently, there may be reduced absorption of drugs such as cloxacillin, ferrous sulfate, folic acid, pindolol and chlorpropamide,[1] but these changes are unlikely to be clinically important.

Like other antacids and adsorbents, aluminium hydroxide, which can be used as a phosphate binding agent in patients with chronic renal failure, may bind several drugs including phenytoin, iron, aspirin (acetylsalicylic acid), phenothiazines, quinolones, tetracyclines, rifampicin and ketoconazole[4] and therefore should not be administered simultaneously with these agents.

D-Xylose absorption is used to measure proximal small intestinal absorption and is reduced in renal failure.[5] However, despite most drug absorption normally occurring in the proximal small intestine, malabsorption of drugs in renal failure does not appear to be a problem. This is presumably due to therapeutic drug doses being relatively small in comparison with the intestinal absorptive capacity, even when the latter is reduced by renal failure.

It is not known whether the homeostatic changes associated with renal disease affect the absorption of drugs from intramuscular or subcutaneous injection sites. In patients with acute renal failure who are critically ill with shock or hypotension, absorption from these sites is certainly impaired due to reduced tissue perfusion.

### 1.2 Distribution of Drugs in Renal Diseases

The activity of most drugs is related to the available drug concentration at receptor sites. While in most instances this is not measurable, it is usually related to the plasma concentration of unbound (free) drug. The latter is a function of the total amount of drug in the body, its volume of distribution and the extent of protein binding. The total amount of drug in the body depends on the dose administered, and on the bioavailability and total body clearance.

Renal failure is accompanied by raised plasma concentrations of acidic compounds (e.g. free fatty acids, indoxyl sulfate) that compete for binding sites on albumin and other plasma proteins.[6,7] Hydrogen ion concentration (pH) changes resulting from acidosis and alterations in the molecular configuration of albumin can also reduce protein binding. Protein binding is reduced in renal failure for drugs such as theophylline, phenytoin, methotrexate, diazepam, prazosin, furosemide (frusemide), warfarin, barbiturates, clofibrate, morphine, salicylates and dicloxacillin.[2] The plasma albumin concentration is low in patients with nephrotic syndrome, and may also be decreased in cachectic patients and elderly patients, thus reducing the capacity for protein binding.

For basic drugs such as propranolol, quinidine and desipramine, which are more avidly bound to $\alpha_1$-acid glycoprotein in plasma than to albumin, binding to $\alpha_1$-acid glycoprotein can actually increase in renal failure.

Few of the changes in pharmacokinetics that are caused by altered protein binding are of clinical significance.[7] Phenytoin therapy is an important exception. Routine measurement of the plasma phenytoin concentration includes both bound and unbound drug. Since protein binding is reduced in proportion to the reduction in glomerular filtration rate (GFR), the therapeutic range based on *total* plasma concentrations has to be lowered to avoid toxicity. For more detailed discussion of these issues, see chapter 1, section 5.4.2 and chapter 5, section 1.6.3.

Digoxin tissue binding and consequently its volume of distribution is reduced in renal failure and a smaller loading dose is needed. The effect of reduced digoxin clearance as GFR decreases is even more important. A lower maintenance dose is required. Monitoring plasma concentrations is helpful, as well as assessing dosage in terms of the therapeutic response such as the ventricular rate in atrial fibrillation.

The volume of distribution of drugs may be altered in renal failure because of increases in extracellular fluid volume and alterations in protein/tissue binding as well as in the proportion of fat and muscle in the body.

Important changes in total body clearance and in the relationship between plasma concentration and clinical effect occurring as a result of changes in distribution predominantly concern those drugs that are highly albumin-bound with relatively low distribution volumes and low hepatic extraction ratios. These are usually acidic drugs such as warfarin, phenytoin, furosemide, phenylbutazone and salicylic acid. However, it should be noted that the changes in total body clearance with such drugs occurring as a result of changes in distribution do not necessarily mean that the unbound drug concentration will be altered.

### 1.3 Metabolism of Drugs in Renal Diseases

Most drugs are excreted by the kidney either as the original compound or after metabolism in the liver to more water-soluble metabolites. Renal failure reduces the nonrenal clearance of drugs such as aciclovir and captopril. However, this alteration in clearance is minor when compared with the accumulation of active metabolites that have therapeutic or adverse effects. Examples are the metabolites of allopurinol, glibenclamide, morphine, pethidine (meperidine) and procainamide.

The clearances of most drugs metabolised by microsomal oxidation (a major pathway of metabolism for many drugs) have been found to be within their normal ranges in most patients with renal failure (e.g. tolbutamide, quinidine).[8] Similarly, glucuronide conjugation, another major pathway, sulfate conjugation and *O*-methylation also proceed normally. For agents with metabolites usually eliminated by the kidney, accumulated inactive glucuronide conjugates in renal failure may undergo biliary excretion with subsequent bacterial or systemic deconjugation and the release of active drug. This recycling has been demonstrated with oxazepam, lorazepam and paracetamol but probably occurs to some extent with most drugs undergoing glucuronide conjugation with biliary excretion.

### 1.4 Renal Excretion of Drugs

The kidney handles drugs and their metabolites by glomerular filtration, active reabsorption and/or secretion by the tubules and passive diffusion. All these processes will be influenced by changes in renal blood flow, the greatest effect being on drugs with high renal extraction ratios such as the penicillins and sulfate and glucuronide conjugates.

Renal clearance of drugs can be expressed as follows:[9]

$$CL_R = (f_u \cdot GFR) + \text{secretion} - \text{reabsorption}$$

where $CL_R$ is renal clearance and $f_u$ is the fraction of unbound drug (available for filtration). Where there is no active tubular transport, renal clearance of a drug is proportional to GFR.

#### 1.4.1 Filtration at the Glomerulus

The amount of drug filtered depends on its plasma concentration, the degree of drug protein binding and the GFR. Compounds with a molecular weight below 60,000D are filtered to a variable extent (depending on molecular size) unless they are protein bound, in which case only the unbound portion is filtered. The amount of a drug filtered increases linearly with its unbound concentration.

Decreased functional nephron mass, as reflected in the GFR and hence the creatinine clearance, results in diminished drug excretion and prolongation of the plasma half-lives of predominantly renally eliminated drugs. The clinical significance depends on the relative importance of renal excretion as a mode of elimination and the therapeutic ratio of the drug. For example, ampicillin is excreted mainly by glomerular filtration, but the therapeutic ratio of the drug is so great that no modification of the dosage schedule need be made. Moreover, ampicillin is excreted in the bile and excretion by this route becomes more important as the GFR decreases. On the other hand, gentamicin and other aminoglycosides and digoxin, which have a low therapeutic ratio, require dosage modification when the GFR is reduced.

#### 1.4.2 Renal Tubular Secretion

This involves active transport of the drug from peritubular capillary blood into the renal tubular cells and then out into the tubular lumen. For low extraction ratio drugs, protein binding does not influence the rate of tubular secretion; however, for high extraction ratio drugs, i.e. when tubular secretion clearance approaches renal blood flow, then a decrease in protein binding will reduce drug delivery and the unbound drug clearance will be decreased.

There are 2 major pathways for tubular excretion, i.e. that for weak organic acids (e.g. penicillins, cefalosporins, sulfonamides, furosemide, thiazides, salicylates, probenecid) and that for weak bases (e.g. amiloride, procainamide, quinidine, ranitidine). These pathways are not substrate specific. Some drugs may interact to inhibit the tubular excretion of others (e.g. probenecid with the penicillins, some cefalosporins, furosemide and chlorothiazide; salicylate with methotrexate). The organic acids accumulating in renal failure will compete with drugs that are secreted by the weak acid pathway. In the case of furosemide, this is a factor in the greatly increased dosage often required to initiate a diuresis in patients with substantial renal impairment in comparison with those with normal renal function (250 to 1000mg intravenously *vs* 20 to 80mg intravenously).

Competition between organic bases is usually not important clinically. However, one example is the decrease in procainamide clearance by ranitidine. Creatinine is a base and is excreted by renal tubular secretion as well as by glomerular filtration. Thus, basic drugs such as cimetidine and trimethoprim may reduce creatinine clearance in a dose-dependent manner, although the actual glomerular filtration rate is not altered; this phenomenon should not be mistaken for nephrotoxicity. In the case of digoxin, the secretory component of its elimination by the distal nephron can be reduced by amiloride, spironolactone, verapamil and quinidine, thus raising plasma digoxin concentrations and possibly resulting in toxicity.

#### 1.4.3 Passive Diffusion

Weak acids and bases are more readily reabsorbed from the renal tubules in their non-polar (lipid soluble) forms than when they are ionised (water soluble). Excretion of weak acids and bases can therefore be modified by altering the urinary pH and consequently the non-ionised fraction.

Forced alkaline diuresis is traditionally employed to increase renal salicylic acid elimination following significant aspirin poisoning. However, alkalinising the urine (to pH >8) is far more important than diuresis.[10] Phenobarbital elimination can also be enhanced by urinary alkalinisation but this is rarely clinically necessary, particularly now that intestinal dialysis with multiple-dose activated charcoal has proven effectiveness. For further discussion of this topic, see chapter 8, sect. 6.2.

### 1.5 Drug Response in the Presence of Uraemia

Uraemia is accompanied by many changes in homeostatic mechanisms that in turn alter the response to drugs. The following are examples of this:[11,12]

1) The brain may be more sensitive than usual to the central nervous system (CNS) depressant effects of sedatives, hypnotics, and opioid analgesics. A possible explanation for the increased sensitivity to these drugs and to other drugs in uraemia is that the blood-brain barrier is less effective. However, renal failure has to be quite advanced for this to be significant.

2) In renal failure, the control of body fluid volume may be disturbed. If for any reason patients are hypovolaemic, especially after diuretic therapy, they become very sensitive to antihypertensive agents, particularly α-adrenoceptor antagonists, angiotensin-converting enzyme (ACE) inhibitors and angiotensin II receptor antagonists (e.g. losartan).

3) Any impairment in coagulation renders the individual more sensitive to anticoagulants. Aspirin and other NSAIDs are more liable to produce significant gastrointestinal bleeding.

4) Drugs that cause sodium retention (e.g. NSAIDs) may exacerbate fluid overload, and heart failure.

5) Renal failure is often accompanied by hyperkalaemia, which may be particularly severe when patients are given potassium-sparing diuretics, potassium supplements, ACE inhibitors or angiotensin II receptor antagonists.

6) Sodium and potassium metabolism are abnormal so the use of digoxin may be associated with an increased risk of adverse reactions.

7) Acidosis may also affect the response to drugs, in particular by altering the tissue penetration of drugs such as weak acids.

8) Patients in renal failure may be more sensitive to the effects of acetylcholinesterase inhibitors such as neostigmine, because of reduced cholinesterase activity.

Apart from the increased risk of enhanced effects due to the accumulation of renally excreted drugs or active metabolites in uraemia, the kidneys themselves have an increased susceptibility to the nephrotoxic effects of drugs. Clinicians must therefore be wary of drug-induced renal deterioration being mistakenly attributed to the natural history of the underlying renal disorder.

### 1.6 Renal Function, Age and Drugs

Renal blood flow in the neonate is low due to high renal vascular resistance; glomerular filtration is low and proximal tubular transport mechanisms are immature (see also chapter 3; sect. 2.4.2). Thus, overall renal function is less than that predicted in terms of bodyweight. In addition, hepatic metabolism is also reduced. Renal vascular resistance decreases rapidly in the first few months of life and tubular transport mechanisms, which are inducible, quickly develop.

At the other end of our life span, renal function diminishes with age. Thus, dosages of drugs that are mainly eliminated by the kidneys may need to be reduced in elderly patients (see further chapter 4).

## 2. General Principles of Drug Prescribing in Patients with Renal Failure

Prescribing for patients with renal failure requires knowledge of the metabolism and activity of the drug, its duration of action, and the method of excretion. The following guidelines, which in some cases are applicable to any therapeutic situation, are particularly important in renal failure:[3]

- Use drugs only if there is a definite indication
- Choose a drug that has no or minimal nephrotoxicity
- Use recommended dosage regimens for renal failure; if these are not available, estimate a 'safe' dose and a suitable interval between doses
- Use plasma concentration measurements to adjust the dose wherever possible
- Avoid prolonged courses of potentially toxic drugs
- Monitor the patient carefully for evidence of clinical effectiveness and toxicity of drugs.

### 2.1 Modification of Dosage Regimen

Since drugs that are mainly excreted in active form by the kidney have a prolonged half-life when given to patients with renal failure, accumulation occurs with resulting toxicity if the normal dosage regimen is not modified. The level of renal function below which the dosage regimen of a drug must be modified depends on whether the drug is eliminated entirely by renal excretion or is at least partly metabolised, and on how toxic the drug is. There are 2 approaches to this problem: (1) either the standard dose can be given but at extended intervals; or (2) a reduced dose is given at the usual intervals. However, the loading dose should normally be kept the same as for a patient with unimpaired renal function (fig. 1).

For many drugs with minor or no dose-related adverse effects, very precise modifications of the dosage regimen are unnecessary and a simple scheme for dose reduction is sufficient.[4] Some widely used guides can be imprecise, simply stating 'reduce dosage',[4] so it is recommended that an unchanged loading dose is given followed by half the usual adult maintenance dose. This recommendation is straightforward for dispensing and compliance. However, for

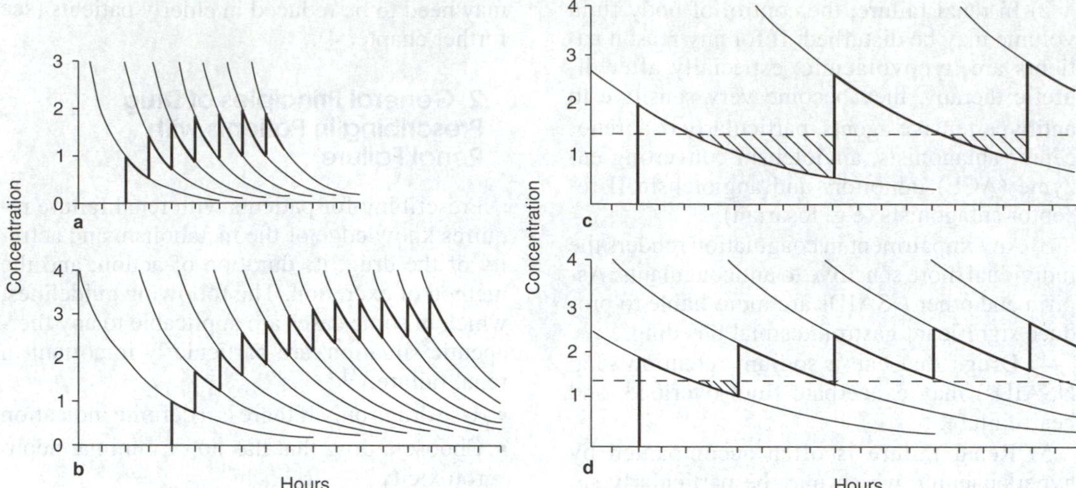


**Fig. 1.** Steady-state concentrations on different drug regimens and effect of dosage modification in renal failure.

a) *Normal renal function:* the thin lines are identical curves showing the reduction in concentration of an agent having a half-life of 1 hour. The thick line shows the effect of repeating the same dose every half-life. After about 4 half-lives, the concentration reaches steady-state and oscillates between 1 and 2 times that produced by the first dose.

b) *Impaired capacity to excrete drug:* the thin lines are identical curves showing the reduction in concentration of an agent having a half-life of 2 hours in the patient. The thick line shows the effect of the same regimen as that used in *panel a*. Steady-state is again reached after about 4 half-lives (i.e. about 8 hours), but the concentration oscillates between about 2.5 to 3.5 times that produced by the first dose.

c) *Renal failure – reduction in dosage frequency:* hypothetical example in which the thin lines represent a fall in concentration of an agent with a half-life of 8 hours in the patient (the normal half-life is 4 hours). The thick line shows the effect of doses given every 8 hours. Assuming that the agent is an antibiotic and that the dotted line represents the minimum inhibitory concentration (MIC) of the micro-organism, this method of administration in renal failure may result in prolonged periods of subinhibitory concentrations (represented by shaded portion).

d) *Renal failure – reduced dosage at normal intervals:* same hypothetical example as in *panel c*, except that here the thick line shows the effect of giving the same loading dose as in *panel c*, followed by maintenance doses half this size at the normal interval of 4 hours. With this method of administration, the likelihood that subinhibitory concentrations may result is lessened, but there is a greater risk of accumulation and toxicity (after O'Grady[13]).

more toxic drugs with a small safety margin, dosage regimens based on the GFR should be used. For those drugs where both effectiveness and toxicity are closely related to plasma concentrations, recommended regimens should serve only as a guide for the commencement of treatment. Subsequent dosages must be adjusted according to the clinical response with careful monitoring for signs of toxicity and, preferably, plasma concentrations should be measured.

If an antibiotic is given in the normal dosage, but at extended intervals, to a patient with renal failure, there may be considerable periods when subinhibitory concentrations of the antibiotic are present (fig. 1). On the other hand, more frequent doses of the antibiotic engender a greater risk of accumulation and toxicity. Frequent measurements of plasma concentrations of certain antibiotics (e.g. vancomycin and gentamicin) are therefore necessary (see further chapter 5, sect. 4.8).

The time taken to reach 90% of the steady-state concentration for a drug given in repeated doses, is 3.3 times the half-life of the drug. Thus, in clinical situations where the steady-state 'plateau' concentration is important for full therapeutic effect, and when a reduced dose with a normal dose interval regimen has been selected, a loading dose should be given. For example, if gentamicin 15mg 8-hourly is given to attain a steady-state peak concentration of 8 mg/L in a patient with a GFR of less than 0.3 L/h (5 ml/min), it will take 80 hours to reach 90% of the equilibrium concentration. Therefore a single loading dose of 80mg should be given that will give a peak concentration around 8 mg/L within 2 hours. If the alternative approach of using standard doses with extended dose intervals is used, then 80mg should be given every 48 to 72 hours. However, plasma concentrations will then be less than 4 mg/L for periods up to 24 hours. This is clearly too long, as many strains of *Pseudomonas aeruginosa* are resistant to concentrations of less than 4 mg/L. Nevertheless, the bactericidal action of aminoglycosides is peak concentration-dependent, and this should be borne in mind when designing dosage schedules.

For further discussion on dosage modifications in renal failure, see section 11 and also appendix D.

### 2.2 Drug Dosage in Patients During Renal Replacement Therapy

The extent to which a drug is removed from the body during dialysis is determined by factors relating to the characteristics of the drug, the patient, and (for haemodialysis) the equipment.[14] The larger the drug molecule, the lower its clearance by dialysis. The dialysis of a drug with molecular weight <500D depends on the effective membrane surface area and the rate of flow of blood and dialysate. For drugs with molecular weights >500D, only the membrane surface area is important. Poorly water-soluble drugs are poorly dialysed, as are highly protein-bound drugs, since the rate of transfer across the dialysis membrane depends on the concentration gradient between unbound drug in the plasma and drug in the dialysis fluid. If a drug is extensively bound to body tissues (e.g. digoxin), little of the total body drug load may be removed.

Clearance of a drug by the body's normal mechanisms is usually proportional to bodyweight, but dialysis clearance is dependent on the equipment. The lighter the patient, the greater will be the contribution of dialysis to the overall clearance.

For guidelines on drug dosages in patients being treated with continuous dialysis procedures and continuous ambulatory peritoneal dialysis, see reviews by Keller et al.,[15] Maher,[16] and Reetze-Bonorden et al.[17]

## 3. Urinary Tract Infection

Urinary tract infection (UTI) refers to the presence of micro-organisms in the urinary tract, including the bladder, prostate, collecting systems and kidneys. Most commonly, UTIs are caused by bacteria, although occasionally fungi and viruses are involved.

UTI remains one of the most common infections seen in clinical practice. Nearly 50% of all women have symptoms of UTI at some stage during their lives.[18] In addition, UTIs, including catheter-related bacteriuria, constitute the most common nosocomial bacterial infections, with an average infection rate of 13 cases per 1000 hospital discharges.[19] In institutionalised elderly patients, the prevalence of asymptomatic bacteriuria approaches 20 to 50% in women and 5 to 20% in men.[20]

Medical treatment of UTI rests on antibiotics.[21] An appropriate drug must be bactericidal and must cover the usual spectrum of enterobacteria that are the usual infecting organisms. Its pharmacology should include: (1) high penetration and hence adequate concentrations in renal tissue; (2) a predominant urinary excretion profile; and (3) if able to be given orally, rapid absorption and attainment of peak serum concentrations. Several classes of antibiotics fulfil these specifications: the aminoglycosides, aminopenicillins, ureidopenicillins, monobactams, carbapenems, cefalosporins, quinolones and trimethoprim (with or without sulfonamides) [see also chapter 31; sect. 1].

### 3.1 Optimum Treatment

#### *3.1.1 Urinary Tract Infection in Adults*

In patients to be prescribed antibiotics, every effort should be made to identify the infecting organism and determine its sensitivity pattern to antibacterial agents. A pretreatment urine culture is indicated in anyone who has a presumptive upper UTI or who has atypical symptoms. Urine cultures are also indicated if one of the following complicating factors is present:

- Male gender
- Presentation to an emergency department
- Hospital-acquired infection
- Pregnancy
- Indwelling urinary catheter
- Recent urinary tract instrumentation
- Functional or anatomical abnormality of the urinary tract
- Recent antimicrobial drug use
- Presence of symptoms for >7 days
- Diabetes mellitus
- Immunosuppression.[22]

Nearly 90% of community-acquired UTI in women are due to *Escherichia coli*; other Gram-negative bacteria such as *Proteus mirabilis* and *Klebsiella* spp. are less frequently responsible.[23] Saprophytic staphylococci account for 10% of UTI in sexually active women, and enterococci are occasionally isolated. *E. coli* is responsible for only half of hospital-acquired infections; *Pseudomonas aeruginosa*, *Proteus* spp., *Klebsiella* spp., *Serratia*, *Enterobacter*, enterococci, staphylococci, yeasts and many other organisms account for the remainder. Gram-positive organisms are cultured in about 40% of elderly men with UTI, whereas enterobacteria (*E. coli*, *Klebsiella* spp., *Proteus* spp.) account for over 90% of isolates in elderly women.[20] Anaerobic bacteria are rare, and are usually associated with obstruction.

#### Acute Uncomplicated Cystitis in Women

Acute cystitis has traditionally been treated with 7- to 14-day regimens of oral antibiotics. However, it is now well established that shorter regimens are highly effective, and have the advantages of improved compliance, lower cost and a lower incidence of adverse effects.[22,24-27] Some of the more commonly used single-dose and 3- or 7-day regimens for acute cystitis are shown in table I.

***Single-dose regimens*** should be used only in reliable patients in whom post-treatment follow-up can be ensured, and in whom symptoms have been present for less than 10 days. They should not be used if upper UTI or urological abnormalities are suspected, or there is a past history of UTI due to antibiotic-resistant organisms.

The high prevalence of ampicillin-resistant bacteria is a problem. Moreover, neither ampicillin nor amoxicillin effectively eradicates carriage of *E. coli* in vaginal and faecal reservoirs, leading to a higher reinfection rate. Higher cure rates and lower relapse rates have generally been observed with *trimethoprim* and *cotrimoxazole* (trimethoprim/sulfamethoxazole) than with β-lactams, presumably because the former maintain higher urinary concentrations for longer. However, there is concern regarding the incidence of severe allergic reactions to sulfamethoxazole-containing combinations. Trimethoprim alone appears to be equally effective and without this risk.

**Table I.** Oral antibiotic regimens for acute uncomplicated cystitis

| Antibiotics | Single dose regimens | 3-day/7-day regimens |
|---|---|---|
| Trimethoprim[a] | 400mg | 100mg q12h |
| Norfloxacin[a] | 800mg | 400mg q12h |
| Ciprofloxacin[a] | 500mg | 250mg q12h |
| Ofloxacin[a] | | 100-200mg q12h |
| Nitrofurantoin[a] | | 50mg q8h |
| Nalidixic acid[a] | | 500mg q8h |
| Amoxicillin | 3g | 500mg q8h |
| Amoxicillin/clavulanic acid | | 500mg q8h |
| Cefalexin | | 500mg q6h |
| Cefradine | | 250mg q8h |
| Cefaclor | | 250mg q8h |

a Current first-line agents.

***Multiple-dose regimens:*** three days of therapy retains the lower incidence of adverse effects from single-day therapy, with improved effectiveness. Longer periods of therapy are reserved for infections in patients with known or suspected complicating factors (see above). Some clinicians favour the use of cotrimoxazole 960mg (trimethoprim 160mg/ sulfamethoxazole 800mg) twice daily for 3 days as first-line therapy for empirical treatment of acute uncomplicated cystitis in women[22] but trimethoprim alone in a dosage of 100mg twice daily for 3 days is preferable due to the risk of allergic reactions with sulfamethoxazole. An alternative regimen is nitrofurantoin 100mg 4 times daily. Ampicillin and amoxicillin are not recommended because of the high incidence of ampicillin-resistance and relatively high failure rates. First-generation cefalosporins (e.g. cefalexin, cefradine) are infrequently used as they have also been associated with high failure rates. Although the quinolones (e.g. norfloxacin, ciprofloxacin, ofloxacin) are highly effective and well tolerated, they are also more expensive, and should be reserved for recurrent or antibiotic-resistant infections.

A 7-day regimen (instead of a 3-day regimen) should be considered in women with acute uncomplicated cystitis if one of the following factors is present: diabetes, symptoms for >7 days, recent UTI, use of a diaphragm, and age >65 years.[26]

In women whose symptoms do not resolve by the end of treatment and in those whose symptoms recur within 2 weeks, a urine culture and antimicrobial susceptibility testing should be obtained. In the former situation, treatment with a 7-day regimen using another agent is indicated.[22] The approach to the latter situation is the same as for sporadic infections.

#### Acute Uncomplicated Pyelonephritis in Women

Acute pyelonephritis should be treated promptly and vigorously and may require parenteral antibiotics in a hospital setting. Broad-spectrum regimens usually have to be prescribed empirically until the results of blood and urine cultures become available.

Women with acute pyelonephritis who are able to take fluids orally, are not pregnant or diabetic, and have no complicating factors may

**Table II.** Oral antibiotic regimens for mild to moderate acute uncomplicated pyelonephritis (given for 10 to 14 days)

| Antibiotics | Dosage |
|---|---|
| Trimethoprim[a] | 200mg q12h |
| Amoxicillin/clavulanic acid | 500mg q8h |
| Ciprofloxacin[a] | 500mg q12h |
| Norfloxacin[a] | 400mg q12h |
| Ofloxacin[a] | 200-300mg q12h |

a Current first-line agents.

be treated at home with oral antibiotics.[28] Oral regimens for use in mild to moderate acute uncomplicated pyelonephritis are shown in table II.[22] Ampicillin and amoxicillin should not be used as initial therapy since 20 to 30% of *E. coli* isolates are now resistant to these agents *in vitro*. The duration of treatment should be of the order of 10 to 14 days.[21,26]

***Indications for admission to hospital***, generally for parenteral therapy, include inability to take oral fluids or medications, severe illness with high fever, severe pain and marked debility, and presence of complicating factors. The choice of drugs should be between *aminoglycosides, quinolones*, and *second-* or *third-generation cefalosporins* (see table III).[22,24,27,29] Initial treatment of acute pyelonephritis with aminopenicillins (with the exception of amoxicillin/clavulanic acid) and cotrimoxazole is not recommended due to the high frequency of resistance. Aminoglycosides are inexpensive and effective against most Gram-negative organisms, but plasma concentrations must be carefully monitored to avoid toxicity. An advantage of drugs such as *ciprofloxacin* or *amoxicillin/clavulanic acid* is that the patient can be conveniently switched from parenteral to oral formulations when the clinical situation allows this. However, amoxicillin/clavulanic acid is not universally accepted because of the possible development of resistant strains, and because it can induce diarrhoea.[21]

Parenteral therapy can generally be tailored within 48 hours, based on susceptibility data, to the least toxic and expensive regimen. Oral treatment (e.g. with *trimethoprim, norfloxacin, ofloxacin* or *ciprofloxacin*) is indicated 48 hours after the fever has settled and when the patient has improved symptomatically. Oral therapy is usually given for a further 2 weeks. It is noteworthy that many quinolones accumulate in the body, and after ending treatment, significant urinary excretion continues for several days.[30] This means that 10 days of treatment with these drugs may result in about 15 days of antimicrobial urinary concentrations.

### Complicated Urinary Tract Infections

Complicated UTIs are those that occur in patients with a functionally, metabolically or anatomically abnormal urinary tract or that are caused by pathogens that are resistant to antibiotics. Complicated UTIs of mild to moderate severity without nausea and vomiting can be managed on an outpatient basis. An oral *quinolone* (see table II) should be given for 10 to 14 days.[26]

Patients with severe illness should be hospitalised and treated with parenteral antibiotics until resolution of the fever (see table III). Subsequently, oral therapy (e.g. trimethoprim, norfloxacin, ofloxacin, ciprofloxacin) should be given for 14 to 21 days.[26]

### Catheter-Associated Urinary Tract Infection

Prevention remains the best way to reduce the morbidity, mortality and costs of catheter-associated infection. Effective strategies include sterile insertion and care of the catheter, prompt removal, and the use of a closed collecting system. Prophylactic antibiotics may be useful in patients at high risk who are undergoing short term catheterisation (e.g. patients undergoing urological or gynaecological surgery, or surgery involving a foreign body) [see section 3.2]. Intermittent catheterisation has resulted in lower rates of bacteriuria than long term indwelling catheterisation.

Symptomatic episodes of infection should be treated with antibiotics, as recommended for complicated UTIs (see above).

Prophylactic antibiotics are not effective in patients with long term indwelling catheters. Likewise, treating episodes of asymptomatic bacteriuria does not reduce the complications from bacteriuria in these patients.

**Table III.** Intravenous antibiotic regimens for severe urinary tract infection

| Antibiotics | Dosage |
|---|---|
| Cotrimoxazole | 960mg q12h |
| Ceftriaxone | 1-2g q24h |
| Gentamicin (± ampicillin) | 1 mg/kg q8h (1g q6h) |
| Ciprofloxacin | 200-400mg q12h |
| Ofloxacin | 200-400mg q12h |
| Aztreonam[a] | 1g q8-12h |
| Ticarcillin/clavulanic acid[a] | 3.2g q8h |
| Imipenem/cilastatin[a] | 250/500mg q6-8h |

a Initial therapy for complicated urinary tract infections.

#### Urinary Tract Infection in Pregnancy

The overall prevalence of bacteriuria in pregnancy is estimated to be 4 to 7%.[31] The risk of acquiring bacteriuria during pregnancy increases as pregnancy progresses. If left untreated, about 20 to 40% of patients with bacteriuria later develop UTI or acute pyelonephritis. Many complications of pregnancy have been attributed to UTI during gestation, including preterm labour, low birthweight, and growth retardation.

Microbiological findings during gestation are similar to those seen in nonpregnant women.[31] *Ureaplasma urealyticum* and *Gardnerella vaginalis* can both be isolated from the bladder urine of an additional 10 to 15% of pregnant women, raising the overall rate of bacteriuria. However, it is unclear if these organisms play a significant pathogenic role.

Since 20 to 40% of pregnant women with asymptomatic bacteriuria will later develop UTI, and there is no way to predict the course of any individual, all patients should be treated.[31] Single-dose therapy has not yet proved to be adequate. Therefore, the current recommendation is for a 7- to 14-day course of a relatively nontoxic drug such as *ampicillin, amoxicillin, cefalexin*, or *nitrofurantoin*.[27,31] Tetracyclines are contraindicated because of their deposition into fetal teeth and bones. Sulfonamides should also be avoided in late pregnancy because of the risk of kernicterus in the neonate (see chapter 2, sect. 7.5.2). Treatment should be followed by a repeat urine culture to confirm clearance of the organism.

Acute pyelonephritis in pregnancy should be managed by hospitalisation and parenteral antibiotics, generally a *cefalosporin* or an extended-spectrum *penicillin*.[25] Aminoglycosides should be used only in patients with severe infection and for the shortest possible time. Quinolones should be avoided as they have been associated with arthropathy in animal studies.

#### Uncomplicated Urinary Tract Infection in Adult Men

Most UTIs in males occur in neonates, infants or elderly patients, and are associated with urological abnormalities.[32] UTIs in men aged between 15 and 55 years are very uncommon and should prompt a thorough search for the cause. Two risk factors associated with UTI in otherwise healthy adult males are homosexuality and intercourse with an infected female partner.[22] The aetiological agents are similar to those in women, although the relative prevalence differs. *E. coli* accounts for fewer than half of such infections, and *S. saprophyticus* is found only rarely. Other Enterobacteriaceae and Gram-positive organisms are more common than in women. All these pathogens tend to have the same antibiotic sensitivities as those in women.

Any of the agents discussed previously for uncomplicated UTI in women can be used (see tables I, II and III), with the exception of nitrofurantoin, which does not achieve good tissue concentrations. Single doses or short courses of antimicrobials should not be used, and treatment for 14 days is recommended.

#### Urinary Tract Infection in Elderly Patients

Bacteriuria occurs commonly in debilitated elderly patients, probably due to perineal soiling, incomplete bladder emptying and catheterisation.[27] The typical signs of UTI may be altered or absent. In general, asymptomatic bacteriuria is benign, and should not be treated in view of the high rate of reinfection or relapse and the high rate of adverse reactions to drugs in this population.

Elderly women with typical symptoms of lower UTI should be treated with 3 days of therapy (see table I). Some clinicians recommend *trimethoprim* or *quinolones* as the initial choice because of the increasing resistance of *E. coli* isolates to other agents.[20] Relapse when therapy is stopped suggests upper urinary tract infection, and symptomatic patients should be retreated for 14 days. Lack of symptomatic response suggests antibiotic resistance. Elderly men should receive 7 to 10 days of therapy.

Elderly patients with upper urinary tract infections are more likely to have bacteraemia and hypotension than younger patients. Hospitalisation for parenteral antibiotic therapy is often needed (see table III). Elderly patients are also more susceptible to the adverse effects of antibiotics than younger patients. Dosages should be chosen with care and plasma drug concentrations, where appropriate, monitored. Aminoglycosides should be used with caution, and should normally be reserved for severe Gram-negative infections. Multiple antibiotic-resistant organisms may be more common in hospital or with institutionally-acquired pyelonephritis; initial therapy should cover organisms such as *Pseudomonas aeruginosa*.

### *3.1.2 Urinary Tract Infection in Children*

Asymptomatic bacteriuria occurs more frequently than symptomatic UTI at all ages during childhood.[33] Overall, the prevalence of asymptomatic bacteriuria is approximately 1 to

2% in children aged 5 to 10 years. Asymptomatic bacteriuria has been associated with upper urinary tract damage in children examined in follow-up studies. Approximately 1% of boys and 3% of girls will experience a symptomatic UTI before the 11th year of life. It has been suggested that circumcised boys are 10 to 39 times more likely than uncircumcised boys to have UTI during the first year of life.[33]

Recurrence of UTI is common in childhood.[33] About 25% of neonates with UTI will experience a recurrence. In older children, the recurrence rate after the first UTI is approximately 30%, but increases to 60 to 75% after the second or third infections. Approximately 32% of boys and 40% of girls with a UTI will have a recurrence, which may be asymptomatic. The usual signs and symptoms of UTI in adults may not be as obvious in children, so the clinician must have a high index of suspicion.

#### Infants

Infants with UTI are at particular risk of developing serious sequelae, including septicaemic shock. Also, as the infection may be the result of haematogenous spread to the kidney, these infants are best treated in hospital with parenteral antibiotics.[34] Recommended initial therapy includes *ampicillin* plus *gentamicin*, or a *cefalosporin*. If the infant has improved clinically (3 to 5 days after the fever has settled) and the urine culture becomes sterile, antibiotics may then be given orally to complete a 10- to 14-day course. A 2- to 3-week course may be required in ill patients and in those with genitourinary abnormalities.

#### Children Over 6 to 12 Months of Age

Children over 6 to 12 months of age with normal urinary tracts who are not toxic may be treated as outpatients with oral antibiotics. Initial therapy can be started with *ampicillin, amoxicillin, amoxicillin/clavulanic acid* or *trimethoprim*.[34] A repeat urine culture should be obtained after 48 hours of treatment. Antibiotics should be given for 7 to 10 days as shorter courses are associated with a higher recurrence rate.

Children over 6 to 12 months of age who appear toxic or who have an abnormal urinary tract or who have undergone recent instrumentation should be treated aggressively with intravenous antibiotics. Initial therapy is usually with ampicillin or gentamicin. Intravenous therapy should be continued well into the period of clinical improvement, with subsequent oral antibiotics chosen on the basis of sensitivity testing and given for the remainder of a 2- to 3-week course.[34]

### 3.2 Antimicrobial Prophylaxis in Urinary Tract Infection

Antimicrobial prophylaxis has been recommended for women with recurrent UTI, which is a particular problem in sexually active females as well as after acute pyelonephritis in pregnancy, before instrumentation of the urinary tract, for short term urinary catheterisation, and before extracorporeal shock wave lithotripsy (ESWL).[27]

Continuous prophylaxis, postcoital prophylaxis or intermittent treatment have all been shown to be effective in reducing relapse rates.[22] Prophylaxis is generally indicated in women who experience 2 or more symptomatic UTIs over a 6-month period or 3 or more over a 12-month period after any existing infection has been eradicated. Many women may also benefit from completely emptying their bladders by double micturition, particularly after intercourse, and from applying an antiseptic cream to the periurethral area before intercourse.[35]

Prophylactic antibiotic regimens for women with recurrent UTI have been reviewed by Bailey[35] and Hooton & Stamm.[22] *Nitrofurantoin* 50mg, *trimethoprim* 100mg or *norfloxacin* 200mg taken at bedtime should initially be continued for 3 to 6 months. Some clinicians advocate prophylactic treatment for 2 or more years in women who continue to have symptomatic UTIs. For women who wish to continue prophylaxis, it may be just as effective to give a dose on alternate nights, or on 3 nights a week.

Postcoital prophylaxis is more efficient and acceptable than continuous prophylaxis in women whose UTIs clearly relate to sexual intercourse.[22] *Cotrimoxazole* 240mg or 480mg, *nitrofurantoin* 50mg or 100mg, *cinoxacin* 250mg, and *cefalexin* 250mg are all highly effective when used in this way. *Nitrofurantoin* is the ideal agent for prophylactic use in pregnancy.[35]

### 3.3 Prostatitis

Inflammations and infections of the prostate gland rarely affect prepubertal boys but are common in adult men. In the US, 25% of visits for genitourinary symptoms in men are due to prostatitis. Presenting symptoms may be urinary, pelvic, testicular or genital. Based on bacterial culture of urine collections and prostatic fluid and microbiological examination of the prostatic fluid, 4 types are recognised:[36-38] acute bacterial prostatitis, chronic bacterial prostatitis, nonbacterial prostatitis, and prostatodynia.

#### *3.3.1 Acute and Chronic Bacterial Prostatitis*

Acute bacterial prostatitis is an abrupt febrile illness with marked urinary and constitutional signs and symptoms. Urine culture will identify the pathogen as there will be heavy overflow of prostatic fluid and pathogens into the urine. Massage of the prostate is not recommended during the acute stage as bacteraemia may follow. Bacteria causing acute prostatitis are commonly *Escherichia coli* and other Enterobacteriaceae, while in hospital cases, *Pseudomonas* spp., enterococci and *Staphylococcus aureus* may be involved.

Chronic bacterial prostatitis is usually a relapsing infection with varying clinical symptoms including frequency, dysuria, urgency, nocturia and perineal, testicular and low back pain. A history of recurrent UTI is usually present and the symptoms are due to the pathogen persisting in the prostatic tissue despite treatment. The organisms responsible are generally Gram-negative bacteria.

**Optimum Treatment**

The main principle of treatment of bacterial prostatitis is to use a prolonged course of high-dose antibiotics for at least 14 to 28 days. *Trimethoprim* achieves high concentrations in prostatic fluid, but the clinical success rate of cotrimoxazole (trimethoprim plus sulfamethoxazole) is only about 30 to 40%. The *quinolones* diffuse readily into the prostate and the clinical results with these drugs, particularly *ofloxacin*, are good.

*Erythromycin* (for appropriate pathogens) and the *tetracyclines* are successful as long term suppressive treatments. *Azithromycin* achieves high prostatic fluid concentrations and may be useful against susceptible organisms.

Culture of urethral, bladder and prostatic urine and prostatic fluid (Stamey test) should be repeated to confirm eradication. Patients not cured by medical therapy can usually be managed satisfactorily by use of continuous suppressive therapy using low-dose antibiotics. Preferred regimens include cotrimoxazole 480mg daily or nitrofurantoin 100mg once or twice daily.[38]

#### *3.3.2 Nonbacterial Prostatitis*

This is an inflammatory condition where all bacteriological studies are negative. It does not usually have a history of recurrent UTI but symptoms may be similar to chronic bacterial prostatitis. In many instances, the inflammation may be chemical in origin due to intraprostatic reflux of urine. The role of *Chlamydia trachomatis* and other nonbacterial agents has been much debated.

As the cause of nonbacterial prostatitis is unknown, effective clinical management is often difficult to achieve. The main treatment plan is to control symptoms and to relieve anxiety and concerns.

#### *3.3.3 Prostatodynia*

In this condition, patients have symptoms referrable to the prostate but no abnormality in the prostate, prostatic fluid or evidence of infection. Prostatodynia may be associated with stress, emotional tension or sexual difficulties, and there may be bladder neck or urethral spasm. The typical patient has symptoms of abnormal urinary flow, and a wide range of pain or discomfort in the perineum, groin, testicles and particularly the penis and urethra. $\alpha_1$-Adrenoceptor antagonists such as *prazosin* may be useful.

## 4. Renal Disease and Hypertension

The kidney is both villain and victim in hypertension.[39] The kidney, even when histologically normal, is believed to play an important role in the pathogenesis of essential hypertension (see also chapter 21). Underlying primary renal parenchymal disease (e.g. diabetic nephropathy, glomerulonephritis, polycystic kidney disease, reflux nephropathy, chronic renal failure of any cause) or abnormalities of the renal arteries can cause secondary hypertension (see below). On the other hand, the kidney may suffer the brunt of hypertension, particularly in malignant hypertension or in the setting of underlying primary renal disease and chronic renal insufficiency (see section 7).

### 4.1 Hypertension as a Risk Factor for Renal Disease

It has long been recognised that malignant or accelerated hypertension can cause renal failure.[40,41] In the era before the availability of effective antihypertensive drug therapy, approximately 90% of patients with malignant hypertension died within 12 months of their initial presentation. The vast majority died from renal failure, and their prognosis was closely related to the level of renal function at the time of initial presentation. The advent of effective antihypertensive drugs makes it possible to reduce not only blood pressure but also the risk of renal failure and other sequelae of malignant hypertension.

Even if not all uncomplicated mild to moderate essential hypertension causes end-stage renal disease, the specific subsets of patients at increased risk are uncertain.[40] However, it has been suggested that the higher incidence of end-stage renal diseases in Black compared with White patients in the US may be the consequence of a higher risk of progressive hypertensive nephrosclerosis among Black patients.[42]

## 4.2 Hypertension in Diabetic Nephropathy

Up to 40% of patients with insulin-dependent diabetes mellitus (IDDM) or non-insulin-dependent diabetes mellitus (NIDDM) will develop nephropathy leading to end-stage renal disease (ESRD)[43-45] [see also chapter 19; sect. 3.4.3]. In non-Caucasian populations such as North American Blacks and Hong Kong Chinese, NIDDM is reaching epidemic proportions. Studies in Hong Kong in 1990 revealed a prevalence of NIDDM of over 10% in individuals aged 65 years or above, and more recent surveys have indicated that this proportion may have doubled, especially in women.[46] Abnormal albuminuria predicts renal impairment and mortality in Chinese NIDDM patients.[47] Our studies have revealed that 50% of Chinese patients with NIDDM have hypertension,[48,49] and a simlar proportion appear to have dyslipidaemia. All these risk factors for renal disease are treatable.

#### Optimum Treatment

*ACE inhibitors* [and probably angiotensin II receptor antagonists (e.g. losartan)[50]] have specific favourable effects on the development of both hypertensive and diabetic nephropathies. A US trial in IDDM patients with nephropathy revealed a near 50% reduction in the risks of progressive renal insufficiency and the combined end-point of death, dialysis and transplantation in patients receiving *captopril* therapy as compared with those with blood pressure control alone.[51] A recent economic analysis of this study has highlighted the potential importance of the preventive treatment of diabetic nephropathy in terms of both healthcare and humanitarian costs.[52] The results may be even more impressive if treatment is begun at the microalbuminuria stage (i.e. urinary protein excretion rates of 30 to 300 mg/day) rather than when patients are excreting over 500mg of urinary protein daily, as was the case in earlier trials.[53] This early detection and prevention (or at least delay) of diabetic and/or hypertensive nephropathies is one of the greatest challenges facing renal medicine today.

## 4.3 Hypertension in Glomerulonephritis and Nephrotic Syndrome

### *4.3.1 Glomerulonephritis*

Glomerulonephritis refers to a group of immune diseases of the kidney involving damage to the glomeruli. It is often asymptomatic, being diagnosed after the incidental finding of urinary proteinuria with blood and tubular casts (in the absence of infection). However, it can present with frank haematuria, hypertension, oedema, or varying degrees of chronic or even acute renal failure. Various types are described such as IgA nephropathy, minimal change and membranous nephropathies, focal glomerulosclerosis, membranoproliferative (mesangiocapillary) glomerulonephritis, and idiopathic crescentic glomerulonephritis. These conditions cannot be reliably differentiated clinically and a renal biopsy is therefore essential to identify treatable pathology.

#### Optimum Treatment

Associated hypertension should be treated assiduously as this has been shown to minimise the rate of progression of renal failure. A sitting blood pressure of <140/90mm Hg is a satisfactory goal, and it is essential to encourage good drug compliance. *ACE inhibitors* (introduced at the lowest dose to avoid initial hypotensive complications) are the current treatment of choice as they have additional 'renal protective' actions independent of their blood pressure-lowering effect. Lipid abnormalities, if present, should be treated with lipid-lowering drugs such as the *HMG CoA reductase inhibitors* (e.g. lovastatin, simvastatin or pravastatin), while potentially nephrotoxic agents such as NSAIDs should be scrupulously avoided.

***Other treatment:*** no specific treatment has been shown to be effective in IgA nephropathy or in mesangiocapillary glomerulonephritis. Postinfectious proliferative glomerulonephritis usually resolves spontaneously. In membranous nephropathy, a finite course (3 to 6 months depending on the response) of *corticosteroids* and *azathioprine* or *cyclophosphamide* has been shown to reduce the probability of progressive renal failure, and will improve renal function and proteinuria in some cases. Similar benefit has been described in focal glomerulosclerosis

**Table IV.** Common types of glomerulonephritis, their clinical features and response to therapy

| Condition | Typical clinical picture | Prognosis for renal function | Treatment | Associated conditions/notes |
|---|---|---|---|---|
| Minimal change nephropathy | Proteinuria; rapid onset of nephrotic syndrome; heavy (>10 g/day), selective proteinuria | No risk | Corticosteroids for 8 weeks; relapses common | Lymphoma (rare)<br>SLE (rare) |
| Focal and segmental glomerulosclerosis (FSGS) | Proteinuria with variable selectivity; nephrotic syndrome | Very bad | None; does not respond to corticosteroids | |
| Membranous nephropathy | Proteinuria (any severity); often insidious onset of nephrotic syndrome; nonselective proteinuria | 30% recover, 30% static, 40% get worse (odds improved by treatment) | Corticosteroids and immunosuppressive agents (azathioprine or cyclophosphamide) for 8 weeks or until maximal benefit seen | Tumours<br>Drugs (gold, penicillamine)<br>Malaria<br>Hepatitis B antigenaemia<br>SLE |
| Mesangiocapillary glomerulonephritis (previously membranoproliferative glomerulonephritis) | Proteinuria and haematuria; often nephrotic syndrome; often renal failure | Poor | None proven to be effective | Complement abnormalities (alternate pathway activation, C3 nephritic factor) |
| Mesangial proliferative glomerulonephritis | Chronic microscopic haematuria or recurrent naked eye haematuria (Berger's disease); sometimes minor proteinuria | 10% progress to renal failure | None | Most common type of IgA nephropathy |
| Focal segmental proliferative glomerulonephritis | Proteinuria and haematuria; sometimes nephrotic syndrome; sometimes renal failure | Good, especially if part of CTD | Corticosteroids<br>Immunosuppressive agents (if part of CTD) | Connective tissue diseases (SLE, polyarteritis, Henöch-Schonlein, etc.) |
| Diffuse endocapillary proliferative glomerulonephritis | 'Nephritic syndrome' (oliguria, haematuria, minor proteinuria, hypertension, puffy face; usually postinfectious) | Good | Eradication of infection | Any infection (streptococci, viruses, endocarditis, etc.)<br>SLE |
| Crescentic glomerulonephritis | Rapid onset of renal failure; often oligoanuric; very little blood or protein in urine; often lung pathology also (watch for lung haemorrhage) | Poor | Corticosteroids<br>Immunosuppressive agents<br>Plasma exchange | ANCA-associated syndromes (Wegener's, microscopic polyarteritis)<br>Anti-GBM disease (Goodpasture's syndrome) |
| Hereditary nephritis (Alport's syndrome) | Haematuria; minor proteinuria; renal failure in males | Poor in males | None | X-linked type 4 collagen gene mutations<br>Deafness<br>Lens abnormalities |
| Thin basement membrane disease | Asymptomatic haematuria (diagnosed by electron microscopy) | Good | None | Probably a milder variant of Alport's syndrome |
| Loin pain-haematuria syndrome | Loin pain, often severe and chronic; microscopic or macroscopic haematuria | No risk | Very difficult (short courses of NSAIDs or stronger analgesics; sometimes corticosteroids) | C3 complement in renal blood vessel walls; kidneys otherwise normal |

*Abbreviations:* ANCA = antineutrophil cytoplasmic antibody; CTD = connective tissue disease; GBM = glomerular basement membrane; NSAIDs = nonsteroidal anti-inflammatory drugs; SLE = systemic lupus erythematosus.

in some series, but the data overall are less convincing. Focal and segmental proliferative glomerulonephritis and crescentic glomerulonephritis are both often associated with systemic connective tissue disorders and, as such, are responsive to immunosuppression as above, sometimes with the addition of plasmapheresis therapy. The common types of glomerulonephritis, their clinical features and response to therapy are shown in table IV.

Any associated urinary tract infection should be promptly treated and prophylaxis considered, as untreated infections can contribute to the deterioration in renal function. However, the management of glomerulonephritis should be left to specialists. For reviews on its management, see Mason & Pusey[54] and Keller & Schwarz.[55]

#### 4.3.2 Nephrotic Syndrome

The primary pathology in the nephrotic syndrome is a glomerular capillary leak resulting in heavy proteinuria (>3 g/24h). The consequent protein loss results in hypoalbuminaemia (<30 g/L) and dependent oedema. Coexisting hypertension is common and hyperlipidaemia is usually associated. Causes of the glomerular leak include diabetes mellitus, systemic lupus erythematosus (SLE), and glomerulonephritis such as from minimal change or membranous nephropathies or focal glomerulosclerosis. Drugs such as gold and penicillamine and exposure to toxins such as heavy metals can also be responsible. Diagnosis usually depends on renal biopsy findings making specialist referral advisable.

##### Optimum Treatment

Hypertension, if present, should be treated aggressively. *ACE inhibitors* have the additional benefit of their 'renal protective' actions, but calcium antagonists have the disadvantage of tending to exacerbate the peripheral oedema of the nephrotic syndrome.

***Other treatment:*** therapeutic options for the capillary lesion are often limited to immunosuppressive drugs (as for glomerulonephritis, see section 4.3.1), but treatable causes do occur and should be identified. The most common form in children is minimal change (idiopathic) nephrotic syndrome which responds well to intensive, prolonged *prednisolone* therapy starting with 60 mg/m$^2$/day and continuing with stepwise reductions for at least 8 weeks. Although early prolonged therapy reduces the chance of relapse, this is still to be expected in up to two-thirds of cases. The relapse rate in adults is even higher. Relapses usually respond to further courses of immunosuppressive therapy but corticosteroid-induced adverse effects are a problem, particularly in children. *Cyclophosphamide, chlorambucil* and long term *cyclosporin* are useful, especially in patients with unacceptable corticosteroid-induced adverse effects or those who are corticosteroid-resistant but, of course, have their own adverse effects.

Other management is directed towards optimising sodium and water balance. Restriction of sodium intake is essential. In hospitalised patients, a 60 mmol sodium/day diet can be ordered with moderate fluid restriction (e.g 1 L/day), followed by a 'no added salt and salty food avoidance' diet (approximately 100 mmol sodium/day) on discharge. High protein diets are no longer recommended and some dietary protein restriction in the acute phase is probably desirable.

*Loop diuretics* (e.g. furosemide or bumetanide) are useful in treatment, with doses of 40 to 80mg furosemide daily or every other day being sufficient. Unlike the situation in uraemia, where very high doses may be required due to competition with accumulated organic acids, etc. (see section 5.1.2), diuretic resistance in this condition is usually due to excessive dietary sodium intake (i.e. >180 mmol/day) which can be revealed by measuring the 24-hour urinary sodium output. Another common cause of diuretic failure is relative hypovolaemia due to the hypoalbuminaemia. Despite the ongoing capillary leak, this can be transiently relieved by albumin infusions following which intravenous loop diuretics regain their effectiveness.

The secondary hyperaldosteronism that may occur with loop diuretics can itself enhance sodium retention. In this situation, *spironolactone* may have a role but is relatively contraindicated if uraemia is present (due to the risk of hyperkalaemia). *HMG CoA reductase inhibitors* are usually effective in treating the associated hyperlipidaemia. A hypercoagulable state is also associated with the nephrotic syndrome and patients may benefit from prophylactic low-dose *aspirin* or, in the acute hospital phase, from low-dose *heparin*. Bed rest itself should not be forgotten as an important adjunct to mobilising peripheral oedema and promoting sodium excretion.

Any concurrent urinary tract infection should be effectively treated and prophylaxis attempted, especially in severe refractory cases of the nephrotic syndrome. For more detailed accounts of management of the nephrotic syndrome, see reviews by Brodehl,[56] Melvin & Bennett,[57] and Ponticelli & Passerini.[58]

### 4.4 Renovascular Hypertension

Renovascular hypertension refers to hypertension resulting from renal ischaemia. Although a variety of pathological lesions may cause renovascular hypertension, the most common lesion is stenosis of the renal artery caused by atherosclerosis or fibromuscular dysplasia.[59] It has been estimated that less than 0.5% of the total hypertensive population has renovascular hypertension.[60] However, at clinical centres with a special interest in hypertensive disorders, the prevalence is 2 to 4%. The prevalence is much higher in patients with accelerated or malignant hypertension and in those with severe hypertension and renal failure. For further discussion on screening tests, clinical features and management of renal artery stenosis, see reviews by McGrath & Clarke,[61] Nolan & Schrier,[62] Ram,[59] and Stansby et al.[63]

The principal cause of renal artery stenosis is atheromatous narrowing of one or both renal arteries. Atherosclerotic renal artery stenosis occurs in older individuals, the incidence peaking in the 6th decade. Men are affected twice as often as women. It is often associated with diffuse atherosclerotic disease of the aorta, coronary arteries, cerebral arteries and peripheral arteries. The site of the stenosis is usually at the origin of the renal arteries and it can present with chronic renal failure or acute renal failure after starting ACE inhibitors. Patients often remain asymptomatic until the second renal artery occludes.

Fibromuscular dysplasias affecting the main renal artery account for one-third of cases of renal artery stenosis. The most common form is medial fibroplasia, which is typically seen in young to middle-aged women. The risk of progression to total arterial occlusion is small. The other variants include perimedial fibroplasia, intimal fibroplasia, and periarterial fibroplasia. These 3 lesions are more severely stenotic and are associated with a substantial risk of progression to complete occlusion.

#### Optimum Treatment

The major objectives in the management of renal artery stenosis are adequate control of blood pressure and preservation of renal function. There has been no prospective controlled trial of medical therapy *versus* angioplasty and surgical revascularisation.

***Medical therapy:*** in most patients with unilateral renal artery stenosis and normal renal function, this will be a short term measure before angioplasty or surgery is undertaken. In patients with diffuse atherosclerotic disease, conservative treatment is appropriate as long as the blood pressure is controlled and renal function remains stable. *Calcium antagonists* (see chapter 21; sect. 3.4) are acceptable first-line therapy but ACE inhibitors should be used with caution, as glomerular filtration may be dependent on angiotensin II–dependent post-glomerular arteriolar constriction. Patients with either poor blood pressure control or deteriorating renal function should be considered for surgical revascularisation or angioplasty.

The key problem with ACE inhibitors in this setting is in patients with bilateral renal artery stenosis or unilateral renal artery stenosis with only one functioning kidney, because of the substantial risk of acute renal failure.

***Angioplasty:*** percutaneous transluminal renal angioplasty is the treatment of choice in patients with fibromuscular dysplasia. The technical success rate is 90% and cure of hypertension is obtained in 60%. Although hypertension secondary to medial fibroplasia can often be managed medically, cure of hypertension with angioplasty would obviate the need for life-long antihypertensive drugs in these young patients. Intimal fibroplasia and perimedial fibroplasia often progress to ischaemic atrophy; thus early angioplasty is indicated to preserve renal function.

## 5. Oedema and Other Conditions Requiring Diuretic Therapy

### 5.1 Clinical Pharmacology of Diuretics

Diuretics have been widely used for more than 40 years, particularly in the treatment of oedema and hypertension. Their major renal effects are to increase the excretion of sodium and water. In this section, an overview of the action and clinical use of diuretics is provided, with emphasis on their use in various renal diseases. The use of diuretics in the management of heart failure, hypertension and liver cirrhosis with ascites is discussed in chapters 20, 21 and 22, respectively. Other indications for diuretic therapy are discussed briefly in section 5.3 (below).

#### *5.1.1 Mechanism/Sites of Action*

Diuretics are traditionally classified according to their main site of action in the nephron. Each nephron segment has a relatively characteristic variety of transport proteins or channels by which filtered sodium enters the cells (table V). These transport systems are inhibited by particular types of diuretics, and it is this relationship that determines the site of action of a diuretic (fig. 2) [see also reviews by Greger & Heidland[65] and Rose[64]].

***Carbonic anhydrase inhibitors:*** acetazolamide is the carbonic anhydrase inhibitor currently

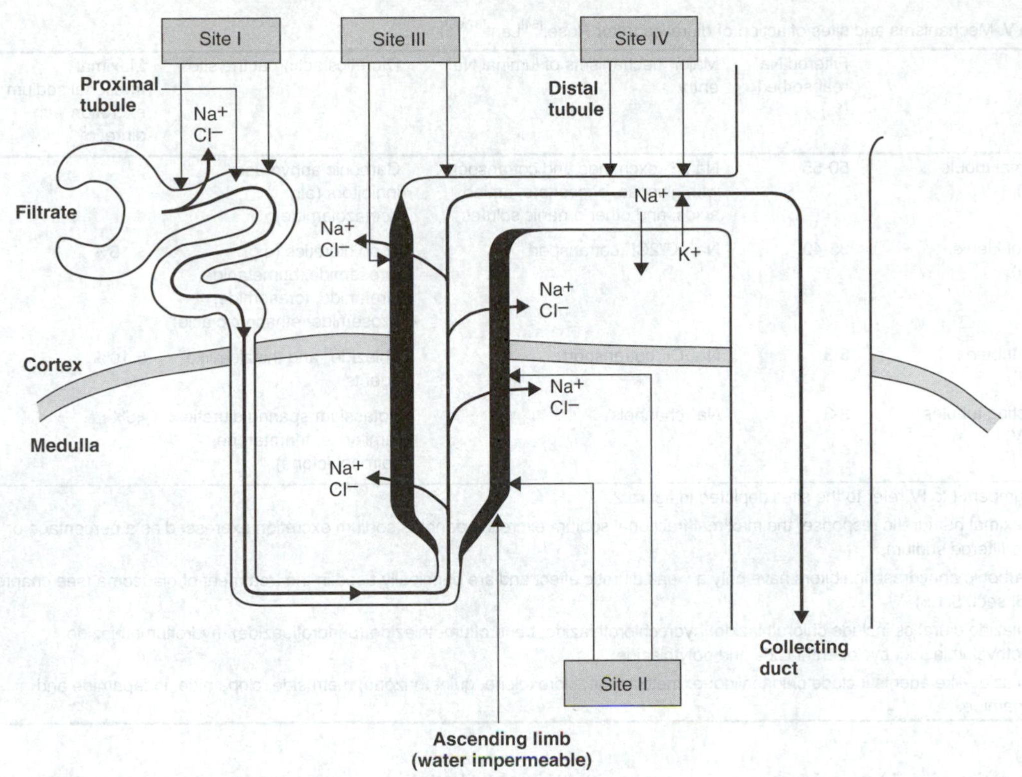


**Fig. 2.** The nephron, depicting sites of diuretic action on sodium and chloride reabsorption. Site I = proximal tubule; Site II = thick ascending limb of Henle's loop; Site III = early distal tubule (cortical diluting segment); Site IV = distal tubule $Na^+$-$K^+$/$H^+$ exchange site (after Davies & Wilson[66] and Lant[67,68]). See table V for diuretics acting at the different sites.

in use as a diuretic. It decreases sodium bicarbonate and sodium chloride absorption by the proximal tubule. The diuresis produced by this agent tends to be small and self-limited for 2 reasons: (1) most of the excess sodium delivered out of the proximal tubule can be reabsorbed in the more distal segments; and (2) the diuretic action is progressively diminished by the metabolic acidosis that results from the loss of bicarbonate in the urine.

***Osmotic diuretics:*** mannitol is the only osmotic diuretic used clinically. It is freely filtered at the glomerulus and poorly absorbed by the tubule. Hence, its tubular concentration increases as water is reabsorbed. The presence of mannitol in the tubule lumen inhibits the reabsorption of sodium chloride and water throughout the nephron.

***Loop diuretics*** (table V): these drugs act in the medullary aspect of the ascending limb of the loop of Henle. The diuresis and natriuresis produced by these drugs is profound: up to 20 or 30% of the filtered sodium load may be excreted. They also increase potassium excretion (kaliuresis).

***Thiazide and thiazide-like diuretics*** (table IV) act on the cortical distal tubule. Their natriuretic and diuretic effects are of smaller magnitude than those of loop diuretics, but they still produce a substantial increase in distal tubule sodium chloride load and hence cause kaliuresis.

***Potassium-sparing diuretics*** act on the collecting tubules. Amiloride and triamterene directly inhibit the luminal channels, whereas spironolactone does this indirectly by competing with aldosterone for its receptor. The net effect is a mild increase in the excretion of sodium and a reduction in that of potassium.

### 5.1.2 Pharmacodynamic and Pharmacokinetic Characteristics

The pharmacodynamic and pharmacokinetic characteristics of diuretics are discussed in chapter 21 (sections 3.1.2 and 3.1.3), and their pharmacokinetic parameters are listed in appendix A.

The clinical response to a diuretic is related to a variety of factors including its site of action

**Table V.** Mechanisms and sites of action of diuretics (after Rose;[64] Lant[67,68])

| Site[a] | Filtered $Na^+$ reabsorbed (%) | Major mechanisms of luminal $Na^+$ entry | Diuretics acting at the site | Maximal fractional sodium excretion with diuretic[b] |
|---|---|---|---|---|
| Proximal tubule (site I) | 50-55 | $Na^+/H^+$ exchange and cotransport with glucose, phosphate, amino acids, and other organic solutes | Carbonic anhydrase inhibitors (e.g. acetazolamide)[c] | ...[c] |
| Loop of Henle (site II) | 35-40 | $Na^+/K^+/2Cl^-$ cotransport | Loop diuretics (e.g. furosemide, bumetanide, piretanide, torasemide, azosemide, ethacrynic acid) | > 15% |
| Distal tubule (site III) | 5-8 | $Na^+/Cl^-$ cotransport | Thiazide[d] and thiazide-like[e] agents | 5-10% |
| Collecting tubules (site IV) | 2-3 | $Na^+$ channels | Potassium-sparing diuretics (amiloride, triamterene, spironolactone) | <5% |

a Numbers I to IV refer to the sites depicted in figure 2.
b Maximal natriuretic response; the maximal fractional sodium excretion denotes sodium excretion expressed as a percentage of the filtered sodium.
c Carbonic anhydrase inhibitors have only a weak diuretic effect and are principally used in the treatment of glaucoma (see chapter 15; sect. 5.1.5).
d Thiazide diuretics include chlorothiazide, hydrochlorothiazide, bendroflumethiazide (bendrofluazide), hydroflumethiazide, methyclothiazide, cyclopenthiazide and polythiazide.
e Thiazide-like agents include chlorthalidone, metolazone, clorexolone, quinethazone, mefruside, clopamide, indapamide and xipamide.

(see section 5.1.1), the duration of its effect, the rate of excretion, dietary sodium intake, the activity of counter-regulatory sodium-retaining mechanisms (such as the renin-angiotensin-aldosterone system and the sympathetic nervous system), and the dose administered.[64] The principal pharmacodynamic and pharmacokinetic determinants of the diuretic response are shown in table VI, along with the mechanisms by which certain disease states may exert an influence.

***Diuretic resistance:*** conditions that may give rise to diuretic resistance include chronic renal failure, the nephrotic syndrome, congestive heart failure (CHF), and cirrhosis. In CHF, the time-course of absorption of loop diuretics such as furosemide and bumetanide is slowed to such an extent that the time to maximum plasma concentrations ($t_{max}$) and peak excretion rates are considerably delayed, which can significantly influence the onset, magnitude and/or duration of any subsequent diuresis; in addition, the dose-response relationship is distinctly altered in CHF, such that very large doses of loop diuretics may generate only a blunted response. However, it should be remembered that the most common reason for diuretic resistance in clinical practice is poor compliance.

In the nephrotic syndrome, the mechanisms by which the response to diuretics is altered include increases in the steady-state volume of distribution and non-renal clearance, and increased intratubular binding to albumin (see review by Sica & Gehr[69]). It should be noted that disease-related changes in the pharmacokinetics of diuretics are generally of minor importance in comparison with altered pharmacodynamics, and only infrequently account for true diuretic resistance.[69] However, pharmacokinetic factors underlie the diuretic resistance observed in patients with renal failure.[74] Diminished renal blood flow and sodium filtration and accumulated organic acids which compete for tubular secretion of the diuretic (limiting its access to its intraluminal sites of action) all contribute to diuretic resistance in these patients. Generally, a larger dose of the diuretic can overcome this problem by forcing more diuretic into the luminal fluid by simple mass action.

For reviews of the clinical pharmacology of diuretics, see Beermann & Grind,[70] Ponto & Schoenwald,[71,72] Greger & Heidland,[65] Saggar-Malik & Cappuccio,[73] Swan[74] and Sica & Gehr.[69]

### 5.1.3 Clinical Use/Effectiveness

#### Osmotic Diuretics

Osmotic diuretics may expand the blood volume acutely and precipitate heart failure. *Man-*

*nitol* is used in the treatment of cerebral oedema and renal failure (see sections 5.2.2, 6.1.1, and also chapter 29; section 6.1).

#### Thiazide and Thiazide-Like Diuretics

The thiazides and related compounds are moderately strong diuretics. They act within 1 to 2 hours of oral administration and most have a duration of action of 12 to 24 hours. In the management of hypertension (see also chapter 21; sect. 3), low-dose thiazide diuretic therapy (e.g. *bendroflumethiazide* 2.5mg daily) exerts a near-maximal blood pressure-lowering effect without many biochemical changes such as adverse lipid profiles or elevations in fasting blood glucose. However, effective doses for treating heart failure and oedema are usually higher than this.

*Chlorthalidone,* a thiazide-like compound, has a longer duration of action than the thiazides, and may be effective when given on alternate days. *Xipamide* resembles chlorthalidone structurally, and is mainly used as an antihypertensive. It exerts its renal effect on the distal convoluted tubule. However, the pattern of adverse effects with regard to disturbances in electrolyte balance is similar to that of the thiazides.

*Indapamide* is also chemically related to chlorthalidone, but is stated to cause fewer metabolic disturbances (although in our experience it may cause severe hyponatraemia). *Metolazone* is particularly effective when combined with a loop diuretic, even in renal failure.

**Table VI.** Pharmacodynamic and pharmacokinetic determinants of the response to diuretics (after Sica & Gehr[69])

**Pharmacodynamic factors** (modifiers of dose-response relationship)

a) Excessive sodium intake

b) Underlying disease compensatory mechanisms (e.g. in decompensated CHF, giving rise to blunted responses to loop diuretics)

c) Post-diuretic sodium retention ('braking phenomenon' – due to counterbalancing hormonal, neurological, haemodynamic and physical changes that stimulate sodium and water reabsorption at sites proximal and distal to the site of diuretic action)

d) Distal tubule cellular hypertrophy (increasing sodium reabsorptive capacity; e.g. following long term loop diuretic therapy)

e) Intratubular albumin binding of diuretic (e.g. in the nephrotic syndrome)

**Pharmacokinetic factors**

a) Amount of drug reaching the urine:
- Dose administered
- Bioavailability
- Tubular secretory capacity for organic acids (dependent on protein binding and renal blood flow)
- Extrarenal diuretic clearance

b) Time course of drug delivery:
- Rate of absorption (delayed in CHF for loop diuretics)
- Tubular secretory capacity (decreased in uraemia due to competition between endogenous organic acids and diuretic)

*Abbreviation*: CHF = congestive heart failure.

#### Loop Diuretics

The loop diuretics exert a more powerful effect than the thiazides and care is needed to avoid dehydration and hypovolaemia. Significant hypokalaemia may also develop with these drugs.

Both *furosemide* (frusemide) and *bumetanide* act within 1 hour of oral administration and their diuresis is complete within 6 hours; after intravenous administration, their peak effects occur within 30 minutes. The diuresis with these drugs is dose-related. Very large doses (e.g. furosemide 160 to 200mg or bumetanide 8 to 10mg by intravenous infusion) may be needed in severe chronic renal failure (GFR < 20 ml/min); however, with such doses, both drugs can cause deafness and bumetanide can cause myalgia.

*Ethacrynic acid* is now rarely used. Gastrointestinal adverse effects are more severe and deafness due to ototoxic plasma concentrations may occur in renal failure, especially when given intravenously. *Azosemide* resembles furosemide chemically in its mode of action and is essentially equipotent to furosemide on a weight basis. *Piretanide* also has some structural resemblance to furosemide, and its diuretic potency is intermediate between that of furosemide and bumetanide. *Torasemide*[75] is at least twice as potent as furosemide on a weight basis and has a longer duration of action, allowing once-daily administration.

#### Potassium-Sparing Diuretics

*Amiloride* and *triamterene* on their own are weak diuretics. They cause retention of potassium and are therefore used as an alternative to potassium supplements with thiazide or loop diuretics. However, hyponatraemia is more common with such combinations.

*Spironolactone* potentiates the thiazide and loop diuretics by antagonising aldosterone. It is of particular value in oedema due to liver cirrhosis, and is also used in primary aldosteronism (see chapter 19; sect. 10.3). Potassium supplements must *not* be given together with the

**Table VII.** Adverse effects of diuretics

| |
|---|
| **Thiazides, thiazide-like and loop diuretics:** |
| Hyponatraemia |
| Hypovolaemia |
| Hypokalaemia and alkalosis |
| Hyperuricaemia and gout |
| Hypomagnesaemia |
| Glucose intolerance (more likely with thiazides) |
| Hypercholesterolaemia |
| Raised blood urea |
| Rashes |
| *Thiazides:* |
| Reversible impotence |
| Hypercalcaemia |
| Neutropenia |
| Thrombocytopenia |
| *Loop diuretics:* |
| Gastrointestinal disturbances (more severe with ethacrynic acid) |
| Bone marrow depression |
| Pancreatitis (with large parenteral doses) |
| Ototoxicity (usually with large parenteral doses and rapid administration and in renal impairment) |
| Myalgia (bumetanide) |
| **Potassium-sparing diuretics:** |
| Hyperkalaemia |
| Hyponatraemia (particularly severe when combined with thiazides) |
| Gastrointestinal disturbances |
| *Spironolactone:* painful gynaecomastia (particularly in cirrhosis); possible carcinogenicity (use should be confined to cirrhosis/ascites) |

potassium-sparing diuretics or to patients with renal failure.

#### *5.1.4 Tolerability and Drug Interactions Potential*

The common adverse effects of diuretics are listed in table VII (see also reviews by Freis,[76] Greger & Heidland[65] and Saggar-Malik & Cappuccio[73]).

***Diuretic-induced hyponatraemia*** is frequently observed in patients with congestive heart failure, in elderly patients, and after volume contraction. The pathogenetic factors include excessive urinary sodium loss in the presence of a low sodium intake, impaired free water excretion, inappropriate secretion of antidiuretic hormone (ADH), unrestricted intake of hypotonic fluid, and combination diuretic therapy (e.g. thiazide or loop diuretics given with a potassium-sparing diuretic). The management of these patients involves withdrawal of the diuretic, restriction of fluid intake (to less than 1 L/day) and, if necessary, sodium and potassium repletion.

***Hypokalaemia*** (plasma potassium concentration <3.5 mmol/L) develops in 30 to 50% of diuretic-treated patients. In general, long-acting diuretics cause more severe hypokalaemia, but potassium depletion is less pronounced with the short-acting loop diuretics. The decrease in plasma potassium is generally proportional to the dose, and hypokalaemia may be aggravated by very low or very high sodium intakes. It should be noted that plasma potassium concentrations do not closely reflect intracellular potassium stores. Replacement for potassium loss is especially necessary in:

1) Patients taking digoxin or antiarrhythmic drugs, where potassium depletion may induce arrhythmias.

2) Patients with secondary hyperaldosteronism, e.g. renal artery stenosis, cirrhosis of the liver, nephrotic syndrome, or severe heart failure.

3) Patients with excessive faecal potassium loss, e.g. chronic diarrhoea.

4) Elderly patients, since their dietary potassium intakes are often inadequate.

Potassium supplements do not appear to be required with the small dosages of diuretics used in hypertensive patients. However, diuretic-induced hypokalaemia may potentiate arrhythmias due to ischaemic heart disease, left ventricular hypertrophy or acute myocardial infarction. Other diuretic-induced electrolyte disturbances, such as magnesium depletion, may contribute to the occurrence of arrhythmias.

The first-line measure for prevention of hypokalaemia is to use low-dose diuretic therapy. Current evidence recommends giving potassium supplements to all patients whose serum potassium concentrations decrease to below 3 mmol/L and to certain subgroups of patients whose concentrations are 3.0 to 3.5 mmol/L (e.g. those taking digoxin or drugs that prolong the QT interval and those with a history of arrhythmias, severe heart disease, chronic liver disease, and elderly patients with a poor diet). However, prescribed potassium supplements are often not effective, having little effect on plasma potassium concentrations and this may be due to poor compliance. In this regard, advice to elderly patients to eat more fruit is usually ineffective as even a high potassium-containing fruit such as a banana only contains about 5 to 8 mmol of potassium. It is naive to expect most patients in urbanised communities to regularly buy and eat half a kilogram of bananas every day! Potassium-sparing diuretics have both a potassium- and magnesium-sparing effect. Concomitant use of ACE inhibitors may prevent hypokalaemia but these drugs should only be used with great care with potassium-sparing diuretics.

***Impaired glucose tolerance:*** the appearance of impaired glucose tolerance and worsening of diabetes is common during long term diuretic therapy. Impaired glucose tolerance is found more frequently in patients with non–insulin-dependent diabetes, in elderly patients, in patients with essential hypertension and/or dyslipidaemia, and when thiazides are combined with β-blockers. It is particularly frequent following the use of long-acting diuretics, but may also occur after the use of moderate or high doses of loop diuretics. The main mechanisms underlying diuretic-induced glucose intolerance include reduced insulin sensitivity of muscle and other tissues and, in those with hypokalaemia, inhibition of insulin secretion. The diabetogenic effects of diuretics appear to be reversible. Again, care should be taken to use the lowest effective diuretic dose.[77]

***Lipid changes:*** potassium-depleting diuretics may cause unfavourable alterations in blood lipids within the first few months. However, long term studies with the thiazides have shown either no change in cholesterol or a slight decrease compared with baseline. It should be noted that these clinical trials used considerably larger doses of diuretics than are used today.[76]

***Drug interactions:*** the potential interactions of diuretics with other drugs are discussed in chapter 21 (sect. 3.1.5) and also in appendix B.

## 5.2 Optimum Use of Diuretics in Treatment of Resistant Oedema and Acute and Chronic Renal Failure

### 5.2.1 Resistant Oedema

Some patients (e.g. those with nephrotic syndrome or congestive heart failure) are resistant to even high-dose intravenous therapy with loop diuretics given several times daily. Diuretic resistance is particularly common in patients with renal failure, due to both pharmacokinetic and pharmacodynamic factors[74] [see also section 5.1.2]. Possible treatment approaches to such patients include the following:[64]

1) A 24-hour urine collection should be obtained to estimate sodium excretion. If sodium excretion exceeds 100 mmol/day and adequate diuresis is occurring, a factor contributing to the persistent oedema will be excess sodium intake, which should be reduced with dietary control.

2) Combination therapy can be given with a *loop diuretic* and a *thiazide diuretic*, and, if necessary, a *potassium-sparing diuretic* to minimise potassium losses. This regimen has the advantage of inhibiting sodium reabsorption at multiple sites. However, some patients have an exaggerated response; thus, careful monitoring of the diuresis, renal function and serum electrolytes is essential.

3) Careful use of an *ACE inhibitor* or *angiotensin II receptor antagonist*, introduced at a low dosage, can dramatically potentiate thiazide-induced diuresis. However, first-dose hypotension is a potential problem due to diuretic-induced prior activation of the renin-angiotensin system, the latter being responsible for the attenuated diuretic efficacy.

4) Assumption of a supine or legs-elevated position enhances venous return and maximises cardiac output, and hence improves renal function and diuretic responsiveness. Elastic stockings can also help mobilise resistant tissue oedema, but great care must be taken to avoid venous occlusion.

5) In patients with severe hypoalbuminaemia (serum albumin <20 g/L), infusion of albumin has been shown to increase the diuretic response.[78] However, the effect of this therapy is limited in nephrotic syndrome since the albumin is lost rapidly in the urine.

### 5.2.2 Acute Renal Failure

Traditionally, high doses of *loop diuretics* or *mannitol* are used both to prevent oliguric acute renal failure (ARF), and to convert it into a milder non-oliguric form (see also section 6.1.3). The latter is easier to manage and is believed to have a better prognosis. However, it is still uncertain whether loop diuretics given at high dosages can alter the clinical course of oliguric ARF.[79]

### 5.2.3 Chronic Renal Failure

Most patients with severe chronic renal failure [glomerular filtration rate <0.6 L/h (<10 ml/min)] have increased total body sodium and water. Fluid overload is the major cause of hypertension in these patients and predisposes patients to cardiac failure and pulmonary oedema (see also section 7). High doses of loop diuretics can be useful. The increased urine volume, even if relatively small, may enable patients to increase their daily oral fluid intake and improve their quality of life.

### 5.3 Other Indications for Diuretics

#### 5.3.1 Carbonic Anhydrase Inhibitors

*Glaucoma* is the most common indication for the use of carbonic anhydrase inhibitors, which reduce intraocular pressure by inhibiting fluid secretion into the anterior chamber (see further chapter 15; sect. 5.1.5). However, treatment may be complicated by metabolic acidosis and hypokalaemia.

Acetazolamide-induced urinary bicarbonate excretion may be beneficial in acute urate and pigment nephropathy. Alkalinisation of the tubule fluid increases renal clearance of weak acids such as barbiturates and salicylic acid but is not useful in the management of overdosage. The effect of acetazolamide may be increased by additional bicarbonate administration (see section 1.4.3).

The symptoms of acute mountain sickness may be treated or attenuated by acetazolamide as it helps balance the central effect of the respiratory alkalosis induced by hypoxic hyperventilation. Hyperphosphataemia due to acute phosphate load (chemotherapy, abuse of phosphate-containing laxatives, rhabdomyolysis) can also be treated with acetazolamide (due to its phosphaturic effects), and it has been reported to be useful in periodic paralysis due to hyperkalaemia as well as hypokalaemia.

#### 5.3.2 Thiazide and Thiazide-Like Diuretics

The thiazide diuretics (and indapamide) reduce urinary calcium excretion and stone formation in hypercalciuric or normocalciuric patients. In patients with diabetes insipidus (pituitary and renal type), polyuria and polydipsia can be reduced by the thiazides and dietary sodium restriction. The beneficial effect appears to be due to a reduction in glomerular filtration rate, reduced extracellular volume, and inhibition of the diluting effect of the distal tubule.

Thiazides may also be useful in type II renal tubular acidosis, which is due to proximal tubule bicarbonate wasting. Their beneficial effect is probably related to a reduced glomerular filtration rate and increased proximal tubule bicarbonate reabsorption.

#### 5.3.3 Loop Diuretics

As well as inhibiting reabsorption of sodium chloride, loop diuretics also inhibit magnesium and calcium reabsorption in the thick ascending limb of the loop of Henle, and may reduce plasma calcium in hypercalcaemic patients. However, they should only be given after adequate volume and sodium repletion. Otherwise, volume depletion will increase proximal tubule calcium reabsorption.

Loop diuretics are also beneficial in distal (type I) renal tubular acidosis and in hyperkalaemic (type IV) renal tubular acidosis.

For further discussion of the clinical uses of diuretics, see review by Greger & Heidland.[65]

## 6. Acute Renal Failure

Acute renal failure (ARF) is a syndrome, not a disease. For therapeutic purposes, ARF may be conveniently classified as: (a) prerenal renal failure; (b) intrinsic ARF (acute tubular necrosis); and (c) postrenal renal failure (urinary obstruction). Both prerenal and postrenal renal failure are potentially reversible, and prompt recognition and treatment are essential.

### 6.1 Optimum Treatment

#### 6.1.1 Initial Management of Prerenal Renal Failure

The first principle of therapy in this condition is to identify causes of the deterioration in renal function that are potentially susceptible to remedial therapy.[80] If the events leading to a decrease in renal perfusion pressure and/or an increase in renal vascular resistance are reversed before irreversible damage is done, the renal failure can be corrected rapidly. Such an improvement in renal function may involve increasing the extracellular volume, enhancing cardiac output, or treating bacteraemia.

In oliguric patients in whom prerenal factors have been corrected, it is common clinical practice to give either a *loop diuretic* or *mannitol* in an attempt to enhance urine flow.[81] In patients who remain oliguric despite the use of diuretics, low-dose *dopamine* (1 to 3 μg/kg/min) may increase renal blood flow and allow diuretics to act. It is thought that there is an early phase of renal failure during which the correction of prerenal factors and establishment of urine flow can prevent an oliguric state.[81] Morbidity and mortality are lower in non-oliguric than oliguric ARF (see section 6.1.3).

#### 6.1.2 Initial Management of Postrenal Renal Failure

Once urinary retention such as that due to prostatic hypertrophy is excluded, the cause of postrenal renal failure may be determined by an ultrasonogram of the kidneys. Computerised axial tomography may reveal additional information, especially if extrinsic ureteric compression is suspected, but should not be allowed to delay treatment. If a patient has uraemic symptoms or advanced renal failure on biochemical testing, immediate relief of obstruction by percutaneous antegrade nephrostomy should be considered. Successful drainage of one or both sides will restore kidney function unless there is permanent damage due to long-standing obstruction or a second source of renal pathology is present. If the percutaneous antegrade approach is not feasible, retrograde ureteric cannulation by cystoscopy is advisable and dialysis treatment may be necessary to render the patient fit for this procedure.

### *6.1.3 Treatment of Acute Renal Failure*

Once the diagnosis of intrinsic ARF is made by exclusion, little specific therapy is available. However, percutaneous renal biopsy should be considered, not to establish a diagnosis of acute tubular necrosis or cortical necrosis, but to rule out suspected rapidly progressive glomerulonephritis that may present as ARF.[82]

#### Induction of Diuresis

The rationale for the induction of diuresis is to minimise the severity of tubular lesions, shorten the length of the oliguric phase, and to facilitate fluid and electrolyte management.[83] The incidence of hyperkalaemia, congestive heart failure and other severe complications may be reduced. Both the mortality and morbidity are lower in non-oliguric than in oliguric ARF. However, it is not known whether diuretic-induced non-oliguric ARF will have similarly low morbidity and mortality as spontaneous non-oliguric ARF.

Induction of diuresis may be achieved by the continuous intravenous infusion of *furosemide* (20 mg/h) together with low-dose *dopamine* (1 to 3 μg/kg/min).[82] The response to this infusion may be monitored by the hourly urine output and urinary electrolyte concentrations. A prompt and increasing natriuresis [urinary sodium >60 mmol/L in a single (spot) urine specimen], accompanied by a diuresis suggests a positive response. Conversely, if the urinary output is not increased within 6 to 12 hours of infusion, a later diuretic response is unlikely, and the infusion should be discontinued to prevent further fluid overload.

#### Dietary Measures

The therapeutic goals of dietary management in ARF are to minimise sodium and fluid overload, to avoid protein catabolism, and to maintain adequate nutrition.[80-82]

Total fluid intake should normally match the daily urine output plus an extra 500ml for insensible losses through perspiration, etc., but greater fluid intake should be allowed for any additional fluid losses due to fever, vomiting or diarrhoea. The daily sodium intake should be reduced to about 100 mmol. Daily monitoring of fluid balance and bodyweight allow assessment of volume status. Measurement of the plasma sodium concentration also provides a guide to water administration. A decrease in plasma sodium indicates a relative excess of total body water, while an abnormally high sodium concentration indicates a relative deficiency of body water compared with total body sodium.

Protein intake should be of high biological value and restricted to 0.6 g/kg bodyweight or 1.0 g/kg if dialysis treatment is being given. To minimise catabolism, patients should receive a high calorie diet, mostly in the form of carbohydrate (100 g/day) and supplied in the diet or administered intravenously as hypertonic dextrose solution. Since parenteral hyperalimentation may be associated with significant complications, this form of nutrition should be reserved for catabolic patients in whom the enteral route of alimentation is not satisfactory.

#### Treatment of Metabolic Acidosis, Hyperkalaemia, Hyperphosphataemia and Hyperuricaemia

The mild metabolic acidosis associated with ARF in general need not be treated unless the plasma bicarbonate concentration decreases to below 15 mmol/L.[81] The rapid correction of metabolic acidosis by acute alkali administration may decrease the ionised calcium concentration and precipitate tetany.

Mild elevations of plasma potassium (<6.0 mmol/L) can best be treated by withdrawal of all sources of potassium and by close laboratory monitoring.[81] However, if the plasma potassium concentration is above 6.0 mmol/L and particularly if any electrocardiographic (ECG) changes appear, active therapy should be given. Emergency therapy includes intravenous administration of calcium (10 to 20ml of 10% calcium gluconate over 2 min with ECG monitoring) and hypertonic dextrose (50ml of 50% dextrose over 5 min). Intravenous insulin is not usually required but the plasma glucose concentration must be monitored and small doses of soluble (regular) insulin given if significant hyperglycaemia occurs. Any significant accompanying metabolic acidosis should be corrected with 1.26% sodium bicarbonate (e.g. 500ml over 2 hours). *Calcium polystyrene sulfonate* resin should be given at the same time to remove excess potassium from the body. This can be given orally (15g 3 to 4 times daily) or rectally as an enema (30g in methylcellulose solution, retained for 9 hours if possible). For refractory hyperkalaemia, haemodialysis may be necessary.

Hypocalcaemia is usually asymptomatic and rarely requires treatment. Hyperphosphataemia should be controlled with oral phosphate binding agents, such as calcium carbonate or aluminium hydroxide, taken with food. Calcium carbonate (500 to 1000mg 3 times daily) is preferred because of potential aluminium toxicity, but plasma calcium concentrations must be monitored as a high calcium-phosphate product may cause soft tissue calcification.

Unless acute uric acid nephropathy is a diagnostic consideration, the secondary hyperuricaemia of ARF is usually not treated. Clinical gout rarely complicates ARF.

#### Dialysis Management

In patients with ARF, *haemodialysis* and *peritoneal dialysis* reduce the mortality due to renal failure. However, over the last 10 to 15 years, the availability of *continuous haemofiltration* techniques has led to further improvements in prognosis.[84]

Mandatory indications for immediate introduction of renal replacement therapy are the presence of uraemic complications (vomiting, encephalopathy, pericarditis, bleeding), hyperkalaemia, fluid overload, and acidosis leading to circulatory compromise. Usually, renal replacement therapy is begun when the blood urea reaches 25 to 30 mmol/L and the plasma creatinine 500 to 700 μmol/L, unless there is clear evidence that spontaneous recovery is occurring. The aim is to prevent the morbidity and mortality associated with renal failure.

Dialysis treatment should be started gradually to avoid the symptoms of the 'disequilibrium syndrome' (muscle cramps, headaches, mental obtundation, and convulsions).[80] This complication is more commonly seen with haemodialysis than peritoneal dialysis.

The choice of peritoneal dialysis *versus* haemodialysis in the treatment of ARF depends primarily on the capacity to prevent uraemic symptoms. In some catabolic states, even the continuous use of peritoneal dialysis is inadequate to prevent renal failure. After 36 to 48 hours of continuous peritoneal dialysis, the risk of peritonitis increases. The persistent elevation of the diaphragm and the immobilisation associated with continuous peritoneal dialysis predispose patients to respiratory complications, including atelectasis and pneumonia.

The need for heparinisation with haemodialysis may exacerbate any bleeding tendency or bleeding already present. In addition, cardiovascular consequences are more pronounced with haemodialysis. Haemodialysis cannot be used if arterial perfusion pressure is inadequate.

Continuous haemofiltration or haemodialysis can be performed either via an arteriovenous-driven circulation (continuous arteriovenous haemofiltration, CAVH, and continuous arteriovenous haemodiafiltration, CAVHD) or by a pump-driven circulation (continuous venovenous haemofiltration, CVVH, and continuous venovenous haemodiafiltration, CVVHD) [for a review, see Ronco[85]]. The advantages over intermittent haemodialysis are the continuous, slow fluid removal, which reduces the likelihood of dialysis hypotension and osmolar-shift symptoms, and the reduced technical demand for both equipment and personnel. Disadvantages include the need for continuous heparinisation, arterial access, and strict monitoring of volume status. One of the advantages of CAVHD and CVVHD over CAVH and CVVH is that uraemic symptoms are better controlled. CAVHD and CVVHD are normally required if serum urea concentrations are persistently high (e.g. 40 mmol/L or more).

#### Other Therapies

Various pharmacological agents have been used in an attempt to mitigate further cellular damage or enhance cellular recovery in acute tubular necrosis.[82,83] Among these, *pentoxifylline,* which enhances red blood cell deformability, may increase microcirculatory blood flow. However, the only pharmacological agent of proven benefit in ARF is *mannitol*, which acts as an osmotic diuretic and a possible free radical scavenger. It can be used prophylactically for high risk patients (e.g. aortic surgery in patients with renovascular disease), or to establish diuresis in early or incipient renal failure. It is of particular value in patients with acute muscle injury or rhabdomyolysis and myoglobinuria. 100 to 200ml of 20% mannitol are given intravenously and repeated as indicated to establish urine flow.

**Table VIII.** Intercurrent events that may accelerate the rate of loss of renal function in patients with chronic renal failure

| |
|---|
| Hypovolaemia (e.g. vomiting and diarrhoea) |
| Infection (e.g. systemic or urinary tract) |
| Heart failure |
| Drugs (e.g. nonsteroidal anti-inflammatory drugs) |
| Urinary tract obstruction |
| Severe hypertension |
| Hypotension (e.g. volume depletion or drug-induced) |
| Metabolic disturbances (e.g. hypercalcaemia, hyperuricaemia) |
| Pregnancy |

Urinary alkalinisation with intravenous sodium bicarbonate has been recommended to increase urate solubility and protect the kidneys in rhabdomyolysis but the evidence for its effectiveness is equivocal. In anuric patients, care is needed to avoid circulatory overload and pulmonary oedema.

## 7. Chronic Renal Failure

Where possible, it is most important to establish the cause of chronic renal failure and treat the underlying disease.[86] Some causes, such as obstruction and hypertension, are reversible and appropriate treatment may delay progression to end-stage renal failure, or stabilise renal function. In some conditions (e.g. focal glomerulosclerosis, polycystic kidneys), a prognosis for the likelihood and rate of development of end-stage renal failure can be given. If transplantation is contemplated, the risk of recurrent disease in the graft can be assessed (e.g. in patients with antiglomerular basement membrane disease). Diagnosis of a hereditary disease (e.g. Alport's syndrome) may benefit other family members by early diagnosis, treatment and genetic counselling.

Common causes of end-stage renal failure include glomerulonephritis, diabetes mellitus, hypertension, renovascular disease, pyelonephritis, reflux nephropathy and adult polycystic disease. In most cases, however, no specific therapy is possible and the aim is to provide optimum conditions in which the diseased kidneys may function.

### 7.1 Optimum Treatment

The correct management of patients with renal impairment is important in order to prevent further deterioration in renal function and prevent or treat the complications of renal failure.[87] Renal function should be closely monitored, e.g. by reciprocal plots of serum creatinine over time.

Irrespective of the cause of chronic renal failure, several intercurrent events (table VIII) may lead to either a transient or a permanent loss of renal function.[88] Their early detection and correction may slow the progression of renal failure.

#### *7.1.1 Prevention of the Decline in Renal Function*

Progression of chronic renal disease is mediated by several risk factors that operate either alone or in combination, including systemic hypertension, proteinuria, hyperlipidaemia, high protein or phosphate intake, and conditions that promote clotting or infiltration of the renal parenchyma by immune cells. Therapeutic interventions to minimise the potentially deleterious effect of one or more of these factors may halt or slow the decline in renal function. Increasingly convincing evidence suggests that dietary protein restriction and *ACE inhibitor* therapy can effectively slow the progression of both diabetic and nondiabetic renal diseases. For further discussion on the pathogenesis of progressive renal disease and therapeutic interventions to prevent progression, see reviews by Pedrini et al.,[89] Becker et al.,[90] Bourgoignie,[91] Curtis,[92] Jacobson,[93] Klahr et al.[94] and Ter Wee & Donker.[95]

**Management of Systemic Hypertension**

Hypertension is very common in patients with chronic renal disease. One major cause is hypervolaemia due to chronic sodium and water retention. Other contributory factors include inappropriate activation of the renin-angiotensin system and excessive activity in the sympathetic nervous system, and possibly disturbance of normal endothelial vasoconstrictor and vasodilator functions.[96]

Effective blood pressure control is an essential part of the management of advanced renal failure. The development of hypertension accelerates the progression of renal dysfunction and the consequent worsening of renal failure in turn predisposes to increased hypertension. Cardiovascular complications are an important cause of death in patients with renal failure. It is likely that severe, poorly controlled hypertension is a major risk factor for their development.

The optimum target blood pressure in patients with chronic renal failure is not known, but it has been suggested that blood pressure should be reduced to 130/85mm Hg or less to provide adequate protection of renal function.[97] In any patient, excessive blood pressure control, which may lead to deterioration in renal function, or postural hypotension should be avoided.

Most antihypertensive drugs can be used safely in patients with renal failure, but reduction in the dosage of drugs predominantly eliminated by the kidney is usually required.[29] A combination of antihypertensive drugs is often required for good blood pressure control.

***Diuretics:*** larger doses of diuretics than normal are often required as part of the treatment regimen to overcome the volume expansion that occurs in chronic renal failure. Thiazide diuretics become less effective as renal function declines and are virtually ineffective once the serum creatinine exceeds 300 μmol/L. The kidney remains responsive to loop diuretics but high doses (e.g. 160 to 500mg furosemide daily orally) may be required (see section 1.4.2). *Metolazone,* although a thiazide-like diuretic, remains effective when used as an adjunct to loop diuretics in resistant cases. When used with care, diuretics can usefully potentiate ACE inhibitor therapy. However, potassium-sparing diuretics should be avoided, especially with ACE inhibitors, as they may cause life-threatening hyperkalaemia.

***ACE inhibitors and angiotensin II receptor antagonists:*** provided that sodium retention is adequately treated with diuretic therapy or dialysis, *ACE inhibitors* (see chapter 21; sect. 3.5) are effective antihypertensive drugs in patients with chronic renal failure (CRF).[98] Furthermore, there are theoretical arguments in favour of using these drugs in patients with CRF, in view of their potentially beneficial effects on the progression of renal disease as well as the serum lipid profile [reduction in total cholesterol, low-density lipoprotein (LDL) cholesterol and plasma lipoprotein(a) concentrations] and their ability to reduce proteinuria.[99] The ACE inhibitors are first-line treatment in cases where there has been loss of nephrons such as after an episode of glomerulonephritis, and they reduce glomerular capillary pressure by dilatation of the efferent arterioles. However, ACE inhibitor therapy should be initiated with great care in a stepwise manner, starting with a low dose, and renal function should be monitored very closely (initially by plasma urea and creatinine measurements before and 1 and 3 weeks after starting treatment). Early experience when relatively high-dose therapy was abruptly initiated was discouraging, with sudden declines in renal function being encountered.

With some exceptions (e.g. fosinopril, spirapril and trandolapril), elimination of ACE inhibitors is principally renal and significant accumulation can occur in renal failure. Their doses should therefore be kept as low as possible in patients with significant renal impairment. Therapy should be monitored closely for elevations in plasma creatinine and potassium, the latter occurring due to the reduction in circulating aldosterone. A further note of caution is that ACE inhibitors can worsen anaemia by decreasing erythropoietin levels.[100] Furthermore, when there is haemodynamically significant renal artery stenosis, ACE inhibitors can be expected to cause an abrupt and profound reduction in glomerular function.

In patients with diabetic nephropathy, ACE inhibitors can decrease proteinuria and preserve the glomerular filtration rate (see also section 4.2 above);[101] these effects appear to occur independently of changes in systemic blood pressure. In patients with non-diabetic nephropathies, it is not clear whether ACE inhibitors are superior to other antihypertensive drugs with regard to renal protection, and if so to what extent this is due to better blood pressure control or a specific effect.[98,102] However, on a patient-by-patient basis, a trial of ACE inhibitor therapy is clearly indicated in hypertensive patients whose renal injury is progressing despite vigorous antihypertensive therapy. In those patients whose blood pressure is unresponsive to ACE inhibitors, the addition of calcium antagonists is an effective strategy.

The experience with the new angiotensin II receptor antagonist, *losartan*, which selectively blocks the $AT_1$ receptor, is encouraging and it appears to have all the beneficial actions of the ACE inhibitors without some of the adverse effects (see chapter 21, section 3.8 for further discussion of its clinical pharmacological properties). Thus, cough, which can be a particularly irritating adverse effect of ACE inhibition, especially in Chinese patients, does not appear to be increased in incidence with losartan. This is presumably because the accumulation of bradykinin and other kinins which occurs with the ACE inhibitors (due to kininase inhibition) does not occur with losartan. However, some investigators have argued that this lack of effect on kinins is a disadvantage as their vasodilator and other actions are considered beneficial, especially in the case of ramipril. Theoretically, negative feed-back control mechanisms result in elevated angiotensin II concentrations with the selective $AT_1$ antagonism produced by losartan, but increased $AT_2$ stimulation does not appear to be a problem and probably reduces with time. Furthermore, it is alleged by some to be beneficial.

*β-Adrenoceptor blockers:* the antihypertensive action of the β-blockers (see chapter 21; sect. 3.2) may be specifically augmented by their inhibitory effects on renin secretion. Thus, small doses of β-blockers may help to control renal renin release in high-renin hypertension. Atenolol is eliminated by renal excretion; a maximum dosage of 50mg daily should be used if the GFR is <2.1 L/h (<35 ml/min; serum creatinine 300 to 600 μmol/L) and 25mg daily when it is <0.9 L/h (<15 ml/min; >600 μmol/L). Metoprolol, on the other hand, is substantially eliminated by the liver and dosage reduction is not necessary as any accumulation of its metabolites does not appear to be clinically important.

***Calcium antagonists:*** the effectiveness of the calcium antagonists (see chapter 21; sect. 3.4) is maintained as GFR decreases, presumably due to their direct effect on vascular smooth muscle, and they can be very useful antihypertensive agents in renal failure. Therapy with slow-release formulations of nifedipine (*NB.* avoid immediate-release formulations; see chapter 21, sect. 3.3.5) is usually effective, with 10mg twice daily (rather than 20mg twice daily) often being sufficient. It should be noted that some calcium antagonists (e.g. diltiazem, nicardipine, verapamil) interfere with cyclosporin metabolism, leading to increased plasma concentrations and toxicity in transplant recipients receiving this drug unless its dosage is reduced (see further section 10.1.2).

Calcium antagonists induce dilatation of preglomerular vessels resulting in potential increases in glomerular capillary pressure. They have been shown to have renoprotective effects in several experimental models of renal disease[103] but to date, it has not been ascertained whether they manifest renoprotective properties in human renal diseases independent of their blood pressure-lowering effects.[102]

***Other drugs:*** the value of vasodilators such as *hydralazine* and *minoxidil* may be limited by adverse effects including fluid retention, reflex sympathetic activation and, in the case of minoxidil, hypertrichosis. *Methyldopa* commonly causes sedation. The *$\alpha_1$-adrenoceptor antagonists* (prazosin, doxazosin and terazosin) are effective and may be particularly useful in resistant hypertension.

The importance of considering poor drug compliance should be stressed when treating resistant cases of hypertension and the possibility of excessive sodium chloride intake should be borne in mind.

#### Restriction of Dietary Protein and Phosphate Intake

Patients with CRF who adopt a protein-restricted diet have fewer uraemic symptoms than those on a normal diet. Protein restriction may also slow the progression of renal failure in patients with a variety of common renal diseases.[90] It is thus essential to undertake a dietary assessment in all patients to ensure that dietary protein intake is not excessive (i.e. >1 g/kg/day). However, it must be recognised that patients on a low protein diet also have a reduced phosphate intake and modification of the consumption of dietary constituents such as lipids, potassium and sodium.

The results of the largest randomised controlled study, the Modification of Diet in Renal Diseases (MDRD) study, suggest that the progression of renal diseases in humans is only minimally slowed by dietary protein restriction to 0.58 g/kg/day in those with moderate renal insufficiency or to 0.28 g/kg/day supplemented by a keto acid-amino acid mixture in those with more severe renal insufficiency.[104] In this study, it is possible that dietary therapy would have been more effective if it had been started earlier. However, the authors of 2 meta-analyses based on the pooling of results of 10 studies from a survey of the literature between 1966 to 1994, concluded that dietary protein restriction significantly delays the progression of both diabetic and nondiabetic renal disease.[89] The data were more convincing for the latter, but for both types of disease, a daily protein intake of 0.6 g/kg of bodyweight with adequate high biological value protein and calorie intake was recommended. Particularly in diabetic patients, complex carbohydrates should be used to replace lost calories and nutritional status assessed periodically in view of the potentially harmful systemic effects of protein restriction.

Dietary phosphate restriction is required to prevent hyperparathyroidism and bone disease in patients with CRF. It has been assumed that renal tissue injury in hyperphosphataemia results from calcium-phosphate deposition. A low-protein diet may also affect progression of renal disease by decreasing the amount of phosphate in the diet. Whether dietary phosphate and protein restrictions have a synergistic effect is not known. Furthermore, phosphate-rich diets in CRF patients are frequently associated with increased pruritus that is at least attenuated by strict adherence to dietary phosphate restriction. The reason for this relationship is obscure.

#### Treatment of Proteinuria

Severe proteinuria is either a sign of more severe and progressive renal disease or helps to accelerate the original disease.[88] Drugs that reduce proteinuria might have a beneficial effect on the progression of renal disease. Treatment aiming at decreasing the degree of proteinuria in renal patients would also be appropriate, since many features of the nephrotic syndrome (hypoalbuminaemia, oedema, hyperlipidaemia) are related to protein loss in the urine. Among the few therapeutic options that are available,[88,102] *ACE inhibitors* are the most promising. Evidence suggests that their effect is maximal in the absence of sodium and water overload. Aggressive *diuretic therapy* may also be required, while monitoring renal function carefully. Thus, some of the effects of ACE inhibitors on progression of renal failure relate not only to control of blood pressure but also to diminished proteinuria. The antiproteinuric actions of ACE inhibitors, independent of their beneficial effects in controlling hypertension, have now been demonstrated in both nondiabetic and diabetic renal disease.

Although most of the evidence for the latter is from studies in patients in Europe and the US with insulin-dependent diabetes mellitus (IDDM), there is now good evidence of the effectiveness of ACE inhibitors in non–insulin-dependent diabetes mellitus (NIDDM).[105] This is of considerable socioeconomic importance in the Asian world as NIDDM is by far the most common form of diabetes in Asia, and in the more affluent regions is reaching epidemic proportions. In Hong Kong and Singapore, it will eventually affect at least 10% of the population with half of those afflicted having co-existing hypertension. NIDDM is thus the most common cause of renal failure in these regions. Consequently, the importance of the potential role of *ACE inhibitors* and possibly angiotensin II receptor antagonists such as *losartan* in reducing the burden of NIDDM-related CRF is considerable. However, in our experience, ACE inhibitors are relatively ineffective as sole antihypertensive agents in Chinese patients with NIDDM as compared with Chinese nondiabetic hypertensive patients. Whether this applies to other ethnic groups remains to be seen.

Although combination therapy with an ACE inhibitor and a diuretic usually effectively controls blood pressure, alarming increases in plasma creatinine have been reported with this regimen in NIDDM patients.[105] Thus, the combination of choice for effective blood pressure control with maximal antiproteinuric effect appears to be an *ACE inhibitor* with a *calcium antagonist*. When planning such long term prophylactic therapy, it is essential to aid compliance by choosing simple once-daily regimens. However, it is then important to consider each agent's peak-trough ratio so as to give as complete a 24-hour activity profile as possible.

#### Treatment of Hyperlipidaemia

An increasing body of experimental evidence indicates that abnormal lipid metabolism contributes to progressive renal insufficiency,[95] and conversely, pharmacological treatment of hyperlipidaemia reduces glomerular injury. Treatment of hyperlipidaemia in renal patients is also appropriate to reduce cardiovascular mortality and morbidity.

The major lipid abnormality in patients with renal insufficiency is hypertriglyceridaemia, with increases in very-low-density (VLDL) and intermediate-density lipoproteins.[88] These patients may be treated with dietary manipulation, exercise and fibrate drugs (e.g. *bezafibrate* and *gemfibrozil*). The daily dose of fibrates should be halved in patients with more than mild renal impairment (GFR 10 to 20 ml/min) since renal excretion is an important component of their elimination. Due to a fairly flat dose-response relationship, this reduction in dosage often has little effect on their effectiveness, even in individuals with normal renal function.

In the nephrotic syndrome, total plasma cholesterol, triglyceride, VLDL and LDL concentration are elevated.[106] Although high-density lipoprotein (HDL) concentrations may be normal, HDL subtypes are abnormally distributed. The principles of treatment are similar to those in other populations and include diet, and the use of lipid-lowering drugs. Five classes of drugs seem effective in the treatment of primary hypercholesterolaemia.[107] These include nicotinic acid, the HMG CoA (3-hydroxy-3-

methylglutaryl coenzyme A) reductase inhibitors, fibrates, probucol, and bile acid sequestrants (see also chapter 20; sect. 4.2). Adverse effects and palatability considerations, with the need to encourage compliance, favour use of the HMG CoA reductase inhibitors for long term treatment.

Dyslipoproteinaemia with alterations in apolipoprotein profiles and lipoprotein composition is also prevalent in normolipidaemic patients with renal failure.[108]

#### Other Therapies

Antiplatelet agents and anticoagulants have also been used in an attempt to slow the rate of deterioration of renal function in a range of renal diseases.[88] However, there is no convincing evidence of their effectiveness.

### 7.1.2 Prevention and Treatment of Complications of Chronic Renal Failure

Complications commonly seen in patients with chronic renal failure include fluid and electrolyte disturbances, systemic acidosis, hypertension (see section 7.1.1), nausea and vomiting, renal osteodystrophy, pruritus, anaemia, bleeding diathesis and hypercoagulability, hyperlipidaemia (see section 7.1.2) and infections.

#### Fluid and Electrolyte Disturbances and Metabolic Acidosis

Fluid and electrolyte disturbances are common in advanced renal failure.[109] Because of an inability to dilute or concentrate urine, if water intake is restricted, the patient will develop hypernatraemia; if water intake is excessive, hyponatraemia may occur.

The ability to regulate sodium balance is usually fairly well maintained, but the obligatory loss increases with renal failure and sometimes a sodium-depleting state is seen (usually in patients with medullary cystic disease, polycystic kidney disease or interstitial nephritis). However, if an excess of sodium and water is given, pulmonary oedema and cardiac failure develop. On the other hand, insufficient intake causes postural hypotension and aggravates renal failure.

In the absence of an endogenous or exogenous potassium load, hyperkalaemia rarely occurs in patients who have a GFR >10 ml/min. Other causes include drug use (e.g. potassium-sparing diuretics, ACE inhibitors, NSAIDs) and hyporeninaemic hypoaldosteronism (e.g. due to diabetes mellitus or NSAID use).

Hypokalaemia may also occur in patients with CRF. Factors responsible include poor dietary potassium intake, diuretic therapy, hyperaldosteronism secondary to volume depletion or malignant hypertension, and renal tubular defects.

Systemic acidosis may contribute to increased serum potassium concentrations as well as dyspnoea, lethargy, and renal osteodystrophy. It may be treated with sodium bicarbonate (600 to 1200mg 2 or 3 times daily) when venous bicarbonate concentrations decrease to below 20 mmol/L.

#### Nausea and Vomiting

Nausea and vomiting due to uraemia (azotaemia) may be partly alleviated by protein restriction and low-dose *metoclopramide* or newer antiemetics such as *domperidone* and *cisapride* (see further chapter 22; sect. 5.1). Early dialysis should be considered if these measures are unsuccessful.

#### Renal Osteodystrophy

Chronic renal failure results in a complex disturbance of calcium and phosphate metabolism,[110] with secondary hyperparathyroidism, soft tissue and vascular calcification, osteomalacia, and the risk of aluminium deposition in bone and other soft tissues, especially the brain.

Both reduced renal 1α-hydroxylation of 25-hydroxycholecalciferol (lowering intestinal calcium absorption) and hyperphosphataemia result in hypocalcaemia and increased secretion of parathyroid hormone. Hyperphosphataemia also increases the risk of metastatic calcification. Two other major factors in renal bone disease are vitamin D deficiency and aluminium deposition at the interface between osteoid and mineralised bone, which inhibits the normal bone deposition of calcium. For further discussion on the pathogenesis and management of bone disease in uraemic patients with or without dialysis therapy, see reviews by Coburn,[111] Cronin,[112] Delmez,[113] Gower,[110] Ritz et al.[114] and Winchester et al.[115]

***Hyperphosphataemia*** can be controlled by dietary restriction and the use of oral phosphate-binding agents. *Aluminium-containing compounds* can result in significant absorption of aluminium, especially if given for long periods, and they have now largely been replaced by *calcium carbonate* or other calcium salts, which also help to raise the serum calcium concentration and combat acidosis. Some patients receiving calcium salts may develop hypercalcaemia, requiring a reduction in dose. Magnesium hydroxide should be avoided as it is a less efficient phosphate binder and may lead to hypermagnesaemia. For further discussion on the use of calcium and magnesium salts, see review by Schaefer.[116]

***Hypocalcaemia*** in chronic renal failure is rarely symptomatic and is treated to reduce the tendency to parathyroid bone disease. Serum calcium can be maintained in the normal range through the use of synthetic vitamin D analogues, such as *alfacalcidol* (1α-hydroxycholecalciferol) or *calcitriol* (1α,25-dihydroxycholecalciferol). Calcium supplements are rarely used unless the diet is very deficient. Frequent monitoring of the serum calcium concentration is essential for the early detection of hypercalcaemia.

Aluminium in the blood may be derived from the water supply to the dialysis machine, or from aluminium-containing salts given orally for phosphate binding. Prevention is obviously the desirable objective. Aluminium intoxication can be treated with the chelating agent *deferoxamine* (desferrioxamine) and avoidance of further exposure to aluminium. For details on the diagnosis and treatment of aluminium intoxication, see reviews by Boelaert & de Locht[117] and De Broe et al.[118,119]

#### Pruritus

Pruritus is a problem common to all patients with chronic renal failure. Its pathophysiology in renal failure is unclear, but itching appears to be less severe with better dialysis.[120] It is important that other causes such as allergic diseases and scabies first be excluded. For reasons that are obscure, strict adherence to dietary phosphate and protein restrictions may reduce pruritus.

The treatment of uraemic pruritus is difficult. Tepid baths, cooling of the skin, cholestyramine, intensive dialysis, phototherapy with ultraviolet B (UVB) light, and acupuncture have all been tried.[121] In patients with severe hyperparathyroidism, parathyroidectomy can be followed by an improvement of pruritus, accompanied by a decrease in calcium content of the skin.

#### Anaemia

Anaemia affects over 90% of patients with end-stage renal failure. It is a major contributing factor to many of the debilitating symptoms experienced by these patients, and contributes to the increased mortality and morbidity. Anaemia in renal failure is due to decreased erythropoietin production, decreased red blood cell survival, and a decreased response to erythropoietin.

Long term dialysis may improve the degree of anaemia but does not correct it in the majority of patients. In many patients, the prolongation of life and inevitable blood losses associated with being repeatedly connected to a haemodialysis system results in the need for frequent transfusions of blood products, with all the associated risks.

***Epoetin:*** the availability of epoetin (recombinant human erythropoietin) since 1989 has dramatically changed the approach to treatment of anaemia in renal failure (for reviews, see Bergstrom;[122] Eschbach;[123] Faulds & Sorkin;[124] Dunn & Markham;[125] Korbet;[126] Tabbara;[127] Winearls[129]). The indications for epoetin treatment in patients with chronic renal failure include: blood transfusion dependence, angina or heart failure aggravated by anaemia, haemoglobin concentration <8 g/dl, livelihood threatened by anaemia, and transfusions withheld to reduce sensitisation to transplantation antigens. The latter is a complex phenomenon as some evidence suggests that multiple previous blood transfusions reduce the chance of rejection of a transplanted kidney. Sensitisation is common in parous women, who should not be transfused prior to transplantation.

Epoetin may be given intravenously or subcutaneously. The latter route has a more favourable pharmacokinetic profile, allowing maintenance on a lower dose (see further chapter 26; sect. 5.1.2). The most important adverse effects of epoetin are a consequence of rapid changes in haematocrit, including the development or exacerbation of hypertension, generalised tonic-clonic seizures, headaches, and clotting of vascular access sites. Some patients develop troublesome hyperkalaemia. Transient 'flu-like' symptoms with chills and bone aches have been reported, primarily in relation to the first few intravenous injections. Some patients may find subcutaneous injections painful. One of the main problems with epoetin is its cost, especially as therapy, once started, tends to be lifelong.

#### Haemostasis and Thrombosis

Both a bleeding diathesis and a hypercoagulable state may be caused by renal abnormalities. The bleeding diathesis generally results in mucosal bleeding and increased blood loss with surgery. The hypercoagulability leads to thrombotic events, such as pulmonary embolism and renal vein thrombosis. For further discussion of the pathophysiology and management of these complications, see reviews by Eberst & Berkowitz[130] and Rabelink et al.[131]

The bleeding tendency seen in renal disease tends to be related to the degree and duration of renal failure. Possible contributory factors include uraemic retention products, anaemia, platelet dysfunction, deficiency of coagulation factors, and thrombocytopenia.

Some improvement in platelet function will occur after each dialysis, but this improvement only lasts 1 to 2 days. Peritoneal dialysis appears to be superior to haemodialysis in this regard as the haemodialysis process itself offsets some of the benefits of dialysis. Haemostatic disadvantages with haemodialysis include activation of the coagulation cascade, the use of heparin, and modifications of the fibrinolytic system and the natural inhibitors of coagulation. Correction of anaemia may improve haemostasis because platelet function improves when the haematocrit is increased. During acute bleeding episodes, patients should be transfused to a haematocrit of 25% and given *desmopressin* (DDAVP) 0.3 μg/kg subcutaneously or intravenously (onset of action 1 to 2 hours). *Conjugated estrogens* given intravenously for 5 days (onset of action 6 hours to several days) or orally for about 7 days has also been shown to be effective. In patients with life-threatening bleeding, transfusions of platelets and cryoprecipitates will have an immediate beneficial effect.

Pathogenic mechanisms contributing to the hypercoagulability associated with the nephrotic syndrome include decreases in antithrombin III, protein C and protein S, and increases in platelet aggregation and clotting factors. A high incidence (approaching 30%) of thromboembolic events is seen in such patients. There is no way to reverse completely such a predisposition in an individual patient. Once a diagnosis of thromboembolic disease is confirmed, systemic anticoagulant therapy should be initiated with *heparin*, followed by oral *warfarin*. The optimal duration of anticoagulant therapy is not clearly established.

#### Infections

It is widely accepted that patients with renal failure have an increased risk of infection.[132-134] Impaired humoral and cell-mediated immunity, nutritional deficiencies, iron overload and the administration of immunosuppressive drugs are some of the contributory factors. Infections in patients who are on maintenance haemodialysis or on continuous ambulatory peritoneal dialysis (CAPD) are mainly related to vascular and peritoneal access (see section 7.2).

Precautions to avoid blood-borne spread, regular serological testing and immunisation against hepatitis B have resulted in a significant decrease in prevalence and incidence of this infection in haemodialysis units.[135] However, haemodialysis patients remain highly susceptible to other blood-borne infections such as hepatitis C and, in some countries, human immunodeficiency virus.[136]

## 7.2 Renal Replacement Therapy in Chronic Renal Failure

Patients with end-stage renal disease will die unless renal replacement by dialysis and/or transplantation (see section 9) is instituted. The facilities available vary enormously between countries. The US National Institute of Health Consensus Development Conference on Morbidity and Mortality of Dialysis emphasised the importance of the early and continued involvement of a multidisciplinary renal team before and after dialysis therapy is instituted, and of treating all the cardiovascular risk factors in such patients.[137]

Dialysis involves the transfer of solutes from a solution of high to one of low concentration, across a semipermeable membrane without free mixing of fluid. In haemodialysis, the blood, in an extracorporeal circulation, is exposed to dialysis fluid separated by an artificial membrane. In peritoneal dialysis, the semipermeable membrane of the peritoneum is used by introducing dialysis fluid into the peritoneal cavity. For further details on both techniques, see reviews by Michael,[138] Gokal & Mallick[139] and Jameson & Wiegmann.[140]

### *7.2.1 Haemodialysis*

The most reliable form of vascular access is the arteriovenous fistula, created by joining the radial artery to an adjacent vein. An arteriovenous prosthesis is used when an arteriovenous fistula cannot be created.

Exposure of blood to dialysis membranes initiates the clotting cascade, and heparin is used routinely to prevent occlusion of the dialyser; however, bleeding is a possible complication of the use of heparin. Patients receiving chronic haemodialysis are treated in hospitals or units where they attend for outpatient treatment. Most patients require 9 to 15 hours of haemodialysis each week in 2 or 3 sessions. Patients can be trained to carry out haemodialysis with the aid of a helper at home. Shorter, higher efficiency dialysis is used in the US; however, less time on dialysis has to be balanced against possibly increased disequilibrium symptoms.

Dietary restrictions of protein, sodium, potassium, phosphate and water intake are required.

#### *7.2.2 Peritoneal Dialysis*

Intermittent peritoneal dialysis, which consists of 2 or 3 sessions of rapid exchange peritoneal dialysis per week, is conducted in hospital using an automatic fluid cycler. However, unless there is significant renal function or more than 40 hours of dialysis each week, dialysis may be inadequate.

In many countries, continuous ambulatory peritoneal dialysis (CAPD) now accounts for more than half of all patients on dialysis. After insertion of the permanently placed silastic (Tenckhoff) catheter, patients can be trained over a period of 7 to 10 days to perform their daily exchanges of dialysis fluid themselves. Usually, 3 to 4 exchanges of 2L of fluid are required every 24 hours. The effectiveness of the dialysis can be altered by changing the volume and frequency of the exchanges while more fluid can be removed from the patient by increasing the concentration of glucose in the peritoneal exchange fluid. A relatively high dietary protein intake (1 g/kg/day) is recommended to compensate for protein losses via the dialysis fluid. Dietary restrictions on sodium, water and phosphate intake are also required.

Peritonitis remains a major complication in CAPD. It may present as a turbid dialysis effluent with or without abdominal pain and fever. About 60% of episodes are due to Gram-positive organisms (predominantly *Staphylococcus epidermidis*), 20% to Gram-negative organisms, and 5% to fungi; no organisms are isolated in the remaining 15%.[139] Most patients can be treated with intraperitoneal antibiotics at home. Commonly used agents include vancomycin, ceftazidime, aminoglycosides and imipenem/cilastatin, which are added to the dialysis fluids.

Other problems associated with CAPD include catheter-related problems, infections of the exit site and catheter track, sclerosing peritonitis, loss of ultrafiltration, hyperglycaemia and hypertriglyceridaemia due to frequent use of hypertonic dialysis bags, and hydrothorax.

## 8. Benign Prostatic Hyperplasia

Benign prostatic hyperplasia (BPH) is a common condition in elderly men. About 50% of men by the age of 60 years show histological evidence of BPH and by age 80 years, this increases to nearly 100%.[141]

BPH is a heterogeneous disease that often becomes symptomatic from the 5th decade of life. Poor stream and bladder emptying, terminal dribbling, increased abdominal and intravesical pressure during voiding, and hesitancy are referred to as obstructive symptoms of BPH.[142] Urge, nocturia and increased diuria are called the irritative symptoms of BPH. However, the symptoms of BPH often vary. Other features include urinary tract infections, haematuria, acute urinary retention and chronic renal failure.

The pathogenesis of BPH is not yet fully understood, but the 2 major aetiological factors appear to be ageing and androgenic activity.[143] It is believed that ageing of the testes provides the hormonal environment and growth factors that induce hyperplasia. The accumulation of dihydrotestosterone, which is the major metabolite of testosterone within the prostate, may be primarily responsible. An alternative hypothesis postulates a synergistic effect between androgens and estrogens.[143]

Treatment options in BPH include surgical procedures (see section 8.2) and drug treatment with androgen-suppressing agents or $\alpha_1$-adrenoceptor antagonists.

### 8.1 Clinical Pharmacology of Drugs Used in Treatment

Bladder neck obstruction due to BPH is believed to be the result of 2 components: (1) a static component from the presence of an obstructive bulk of tissue; and (2) a dynamic component resulting from contraction of smooth muscle fibres rich in α-adrenoceptors in the bladder neck area, prostate and prostatic capsule.[143,144] The drug treatment of BPH may therefore be divided into 2 groups: mass reduction by hormonal drugs and functional effects provided primarily by the $\alpha_1$-adrenoceptor blockers.

#### *8.1.1 Androgen-Suppressing Drugs*

As androgen deprivation is known to induce prostatic shrinkage, therapy has been directed towards blocking the action of androgens or suppressing their production within the prostate. Drugs that exert androgen-suppressing properties include the *GnRH (gonadorelin) agonists* (e.g. buserelin, goserelin, leuprorelin, nafarelin), *progestagens* (e.g. megestrol acetate), *antiandrogens* (e.g. flutamide), and the *5α-reductase inhibitor* finasteride. However, with the exception of the latter, for which good clinical trial data are available, studies investigating the effectiveness of androgen-suppressing therapy in BPH have generally suffered from weaknesses such as too few patients, lack of follow-up, and no evaluation of the patients' quality of life and sexual function. In addition, the adverse effects of GnRH agonists (e.g. impotence, flushing, gynaecomastia), progestagens (decreased libido and impotence), and flutamide (e.g. breast pain and gynaecomastia) have limited the use of these agents in treatment of BPH.[142] With finasteride, however, sexual dysfunction appears to occur in only a small percentage of patients, and this agent now has an established place in the management of BPH (see further below). For further discussion on GnRH agonists and antiandrogens, and their role in testicular disorders, see chapter 19 (section 8).

**Finasteride**

By inhibiting 5α-reductase, an enzyme largely confined to the prostate that converts testosterone to its more active form dihydrotestosterone, finasteride reduces prostatic dihydrotestosterone levels and hence prostate size. It is a 4-azasteroid compound with specific 5α-reductase blocking activity, and does not exert androgenic, antiandrogenic or other steroid hormone-related effects. At therapeutic doses (5mg daily), the use of finasteride in men with symptomatic BPH has been associated with significant improvements in peak urinary flow rates and reductions in urological symptoms, although the maximal effects of the drug may take some time to manifest. Some studies have suggested that 6 months of therapy may be required to achieve maximal prostatic shrinkage and the full extent of other beneficial effects.[145]

Finasteride is rapidly and well absorbed when given orally (bioavailability approximately 80%), and is widely distributed in the body (apparent volume of distribution 76L). It is extensively metabolised by oxidative mechanisms, and the metabolites are mainly eliminated via biliary excretion in the faeces and to a slightly lesser extent by renal excretion. The elimination half-life is 4.8 to 6.0 hours, but is slightly longer in elderly subjects (7.8 to 9.1 hours). Finasteride is well tolerated, and sexual dysfunction (decreased libido, ejaculation disorders and impotence) has occurred in only a small proportion of patients (2.2 to 3.4% *versus* 0.8 to 1.6% with placebo) [see review by Peters & Sorkin[145]]. No clinically significant drug interactions have been observed with agents such as digoxin, propranolol, aminophylline, warfarin or glibenclamide (glyburide).

#### *8.1.2 $\alpha_1$-Adrenoceptor Antagonists*

$\alpha_1$-Adrenoceptor antagonists investigated in the treatment of BPH have included *prazosin, doxazosin, terazosin, alfuzosin* and *tamsulosin* (for reviews, see Jonler et al.,[142] Fulton et al.[146] and Wilde et al.[147,148]). These drugs act by selectively antagonising $\alpha_1$-adrenoceptor-mediated contraction of the prostate, prostatic capsule, bladder base and proximal urethra, thereby reducing the tone of these structures. Consequently, urethral pressure and resistance, bladder outlet resistance, bladder instability and symptoms associated with BPH are reduced. Almost all studies evaluating the $\alpha_1$-adrenoceptor antagonists in patients with BPH have concluded that they improve both symptoms and urinary flow rates (increased by ≈50%). Prazosin and alfuzosin have relatively short elimination half-lives (3 and 4.8 hours, respectively) and need to be administered 2 or 3 times daily, while terazosin, doxazosin and tamsulosin have longer half-lives (8 to 13 hours, 16 to 22 hours, and 9 to 11 hours, respectively) and are able to be given once daily.

The $\alpha_1$-adrenoceptor antagonists have a more rapid onset of effect in BPH than finasteride and generally improve urinary symptoms and peak flow rates within 2 to 4 weeks. However, their beneficial effects have to be balanced against a small but significant incidence of adverse effects such as dizziness, tiredness and headache. As with finasteride, not all patients respond to therapy with the $\alpha_1$-adrenoceptor antagonists, and currently there is no noninvasive parameter that will predict treatment responders.[142,149]

### 8.2 Optimum Treatment

The aim of treatment in BPH is to restore the patient's voiding pattern and improve quality of life. Although surgical transurethral resection of the prostate (TURP) is well established as the standard treatment for BPH, this operation is not without complications such as postoperative haemorrhage, infection, urethral stricture, bladder neck contracture, retrograde ejaculation, and need for re-operation.[144] Alternatives to TURP include mechanical treatment by dilating the prostatic urethra with a balloon or implanting a stent into the prostatic urethra, and pharmacological treatment.

Patients suitable for drug treatment are those with mild to moderate symptoms of BPH and contraindications or no strong indications for surgery. Currently, there is no way of predicting a response to treatment with either $\alpha_1$-adrenoceptor antagonists or finasteride. Both drug classes have been documented as clinically effective (see section 8.1), and the response to the two classes appears to be of similar magnitude in terms of symptom control and objective improvements. Although the $\alpha_1$-adrenoceptor antagonists have a more rapid onset of effect, adverse events with these drugs are more frequently encountered than with finasteride.[149]

Drug therapy must be taken indefinitely to maintain the clinical benefit and will therefore be costly over a patient's lifetime. Trials evaluating the long term efficacy of drug therapy, its cost-effectiveness in comparison with other procedures, and its impact on the patients' quality of life are in progress, as are studies evaluating the effects of a combination of $\alpha_1$-adrenoceptor blockade and $5\alpha$-reductase inhibition. However, the results are not yet available.

## 9. Renal Transplantation

Successful renal transplantation is the goal of treatment for most patients with end-stage renal failure. Contraindications to renal transplantation primarily relate to the ability of the patient to withstand the surgical procedure and tolerate immunosuppression, and include:

- Severe cardiac or respiratory disease
- Peripheral vascular disease severe enough to preclude successful anastomosis of the donor artery to the iliac vessels
- Chronic or recurrent bacterial or viral infection
- Inadequate bladder function (in some cases this may be overcome by a urinary diversion procedure or by self-catheterisation)
- Malignancy
- Repeated failed transplants (if due to rejection) – usually associated with a high titre of preformed cytotoxic antibodies.

Age *per se* is not an absolute contraindication, but in most centres it is unusual to offer transplantation to patients over 70 years of age.

### 9.1 Optimum Drug Treatment of Transplant Recipients

#### 9.1.1 Perioperative Treatment

Most centres give prophylactic antibiotics (e.g. *flucloxacillin, amoxicillin*, or *ceftazidime*) at the time of surgery. If the donor is positive for antibodies to cytomegalovirus and the recipient negative, prophylactic *aciclovir* should be given.

Young Rhesus (Rh)-negative female recipients with an Rh-positive donor should be given *anti-D immunoglobulin* with the induction of anaesthesia. Any fluid deficit should be corrected prior to surgery, usually via a central venous catheter.

#### 9.1.2 Corticosteroid Therapy

It is usual to give *methylprednisolone* 500mg intravenously at the end of the operation and again 24 hours later. Thereafter, treatment with oral *prednisolone* 20mg (as enteric-coated tablets) daily may be given, reducing to 10mg daily over 18 to 20 weeks if good graft function is established.

#### 9.1.3 Immunosuppressive Therapy

The principal choices for immunosuppressive therapy after transplantation include:

- Monotherapy with cyclosporin
- Dual therapy with cyclosporin and prednisolone
- Triple therapy with cyclosporin, prednisolone and azathioprine.

Some centres use antibodies such as *polyclonal antilymphocyte globulin* or *muromonab-CD3* (OKT3) routinely as initial therapy, but such treatment is expensive and is not of proven benefit in comparison with more conventional regimens. Antibody therapy is also sometimes used in transplant recipients with poor tissue matching (e.g. more than one mismatch at the HLA-DR locus).

The choice of immunosuppressant regimen depends on the degree of tissue matching between the donor and recipient, previous transplantation and/or sensitisation of the recipient, and in some cases, concerns about corticosteroid-induced adverse effects. *Triple therapy* is commonly used in patients with 2 previous immunological graft failures, and also in paediatric transplant recipients. It can also be used as an upgrade of therapy after rejection in patients who received dual or monotherapy. *Dual therapy* is used in patients with at least one mismatch at the HLA-DR locus, or one previous immunological graft failure. Other patients can be treated with cyclosporin monotherapy.

Patients receiving triple therapy or antibody regimens should be given cotrimoxazole as prophylaxis for *Pneumocystis carinii* pneumonia (see further chapter 23; sect. 10.1).

#### Clinical Use of Cyclosporin

The clinical pharmacology of this agent is discussed in detail in chapter 28 (sect. 2.1.3). Its introduction in the 1980s as a routine immunosuppressant for renal transplantation was a major advance, and it has improved 5-year graft survival rates in most centres by 20 to 30%. Most patients are able to take it orally the morning after transplantation, but if not, it can be given intravenously. The initial dosage of cyclosporin is 4 to 5 mg/kg intravenously or 8 to 10 mg/kg/day orally. Target blood concentrations, measured as trough levels, are 200 to 350 μg/L in the initial post-transplant period.

#### Other Immunosuppressive Drugs

***Azathioprine:*** this agent may be given orally (in a dosage of 1 to 2 mg/kg/day) as part of triple therapy regimens. However, leucopenia is a common adverse effect and its occurrence should prompt a reduction in dosage. Azathioprine should not be given together with allopurinol as its metabolism is inhibited by the latter drug.

***Tacrolimus*** (FK 506): at present, this drug is used for renal transplantation primarily as rescue therapy for severe rejection episodes unresponsive to corticosteroids and/or antilymphocyte globulin, and in patients who, for whatever reason, cannot tolerate cyclosporin (for further information on the adverse effects of cyclosporin, see chapter 28; sect. 2.1.3). The usual dosage of tacrolimus is 0.15 mg/kg twice daily, which should be adjusted to achieve plasma concentrations of 5 to 15 μg/L. Although the nephrotoxic potential of tacrolimus is similar to that of cyclosporin, an advantage of tacrolimus, particularly in women, is that it does not cause hirsutism (for further information on the clinical pharmacology of tacrolimus, see chapter 28; sect. 2.1.3).

***Mycophenolate mofetil:*** this agent appears to exert a potent immunosuppressant effect in renal transplant recipients, but at present, its use is largely confined to clinical trials, and its precise role is not yet clear.

#### *9.1.4 Maintenance Therapy*

Because of the long term nephrotoxicity of cyclosporin (see further section 10.1 below), blood concentrations should be kept as low as possible (around 100 μg/L). Many centres limit the use of cyclosporin to the first 6 to 12 months of transplantation, and convert to *azathioprine* at that stage. There is a small but significant incidence of graft loss from rejection at the time of conversion, but this can be minimised by an increase in the corticosteroid dosage to cover the conversion period. The maintenance corticosteroid dosage is usually 7.5 to 10mg prednisolone daily.

#### *9.1.5 Treatment of Rejection*

***Acute rejection*** is treated by short term use of high-dose corticosteroids, either orally (e.g. prednisolone 200mg daily for 3 days) or intravenously (e.g. methylprednisolone 1g daily for 3 days). These regimens can be repeated 2 or 3 times if graft function fails to respond. Monitoring of acute rejection by renal biopsy is usual.

In resistant cases, either polyclonal antilymphocyte globulin, or an anti-T cell monoclonal antibody such as muromonab-CD3 (OKT3) can be used. Administration of muromonab-CD3 leads to a rapid (<1 hour) depletion of circulating T-lymphocytes, and has been shown to reverse approximately 50% of corticosteroid-resistant acute rejection episodes. Its use is limited to one or at most two doses, because of the formation of anti-idiotype antibodies. *Plasmapheresis* has also been used successfully for resistant rejection episodes.

***Chronic rejection*** is the major cause of graft failure after the initial period, and no specific therapy has been shown to reverse it.

#### *9.1.6 Clinical Outcomes*

For cadaver donor transplantation, 5-year graft survival rates of the order of 80% are now usual, and for living donors, the 5-year graft survival rates are 90 to 95%.

## 10. Drug-Induced Renal Diseases

The susceptibility of the kidney to the toxic effects of drugs stems from its unique physiological characteristics.[150] It receives 20 to 25% of the cardiac output and provides the final common pathway for the excretion of most drugs and their metabolites. Thus, the kidney is subjected to particularly high concentrations of

**Table IX.** Drugs reported to cause nephrotoxicity: underlying mechanisms

**Direct toxicity**

a) *Biochemical:*

- Analgesics (e.g. phenacetin, NSAIDs)
- Antimicrobials (e.g. aminoglycosides, sulfonamides, cefalosporins, amphotericin B)
- Radiographic contrast media
- Heavy metals (e.g. mercury, lead, iron)
- Solvents (e.g. carbon tetrachloride, ethylene glycol)
- Cyclosporin
- Cisplatin

b) *Immunological:*

- Penicillins, sulfonamides, isoniazid, hydralazine, procainamide, phenytoin, probenecid, penicillamine, gold compounds

**Indirect toxicity**

- Vitamin D and calcium supplements (via calcium deposition)
- Uricosurics and cytotoxics (via urate deposition)
- Excessive diuretic and laxative use (via sodium and potassium depletion)
- ACE inhibitors (via loss of glomerular filtration pressure)
- Tetracyclines (via hypercatabolism)

potentially toxic substances. Furthermore, the kidney has high metabolic demands and is therefore more susceptible to toxic injury.

The incidence of drug-induced renal disease remains uncertain. Reports suggest that 5 to 20% of cases of acute renal failure can be directly attributed to drugs and chemicals,[3] but minor degrees of damage and chronic damage may not be recognised. The possibility that drugs may be responsible should be considered in every patient presenting with a renal problem.

A large number of drugs may induce renal lesions (see reviews by Cove-Smith,[3] Fillastre & Godin,[151] Hoitsma et al.,[152] Koren,[150] and Mathew[153]). In the following sections, the various forms of drug-related nephrotoxicity are classified according to their clinical (and sometimes histological) presentation.

## 10.1 Drug-Induced Acute Renal Failure

Drug-induced acute renal failure (ARF) may be due to prerenal causes (volume depletion, renal artery occlusion, etc.), intrinsic renal involvement (acute interstitial nephritis, acute tubular necrosis), or postrenal causes (obstruction to urinary flow). The underlying mechanism is usually direct biochemical or immunological toxicity. However, some drugs have indirect toxic effects such as via hypercalcaemia or volume depletion (table IX).

### *10.1.1 Prerenal Renal Failure*

Water and electrolyte loss occurs with excessive use of *diuretics* and laxatives. Diuretic therapy is an important cause of renal impairment in elderly patients, but severe renal failure seldom occurs. However, the latter can be precipitated by the concurrent use of NSAIDs (see also below) in patients, particularly the elderly, who have been rendered hypovolaemic by diuretic therapy.

Factors that reduce the volume and pressure of blood delivered to the glomerulus may cause prerenal renal failure. In the glomerulus, the tone of the afferent arteriole is largely controlled by vasodilatory prostaglandins,[153] while the efferent arteriole is largely under the control of the renin-angiotensin system. When the blood flow to the kidney is reduced (e.g. in hypovolaemia), activation of these 2 systems will help to control the filtration pressure across an individual glomerulus. *Nonsteroidal anti-inflammatory drugs* (NSAIDs) inhibit the formation of prostaglandins through inhibition of cyclo-oxygenase enzymes. In conditions in which the overall blood flow to the kidney is reduced, prostaglandins can modulate the vasoconstrictor action of angiotensin II. The administration of NSAIDs to these patients can lead to renal failure, which is usually reversible after stopping the treatment.

*ACE inhibitors* can cause an abrupt reduction in the glomerular filtration rate through inhibition of angiotensin II synthesis if filtration pressure is maintained by vasoconstriction of the postglomerular efferent arteriole. This is likely to be the case in bilateral renal artery stenosis, hypovolaemia and cardiac failure.

In general, patients with hypovolaemia, cardiac failure, pre-existing renal disease, renal vascular disease and sodium depletion, patients on diuretic or cyclosporin therapy, and elderly patients are particularly at risk of NSAID- or ACE inhibitor-induced acute renal failure.

Acute renal dysfunction with *cyclosporin* is dose-related and reversible. It induces vasoconstriction of the afferent glomerular arteriole. An increased risk of ARF can be expected when cyclosporin is combined with an NSAID, ACE inhibitor or other nephrotoxic drug. Cyclosporin may also cause tubular damage (see section 10.1.2). Toxicity is associated with increases in plasma creatinine and, particularly, potassium.

*Tetracyclines* can precipitate acute renal failure through causing hypercatabolism.

### 10.1.2 Acute Tubular Necrosis

Acute tubular necrosis (ATN) is the most common form of drug nephrotoxicity. Tubular lesions are due to a direct toxic action on the tubule, and it is the proximal tubule that is primarily affected.

*Aminoglycoside antibiotics:* all aminoglycosides in current use are nephrotoxic to a greater or lesser degree.[151-153] About 50% of the cases of drug-induced, hospital-acquired ARF are related to the use of aminoglycosides, and 6 to 26% of patients treated with gentamicin develop renal insufficiency.[152,154] Aminoglycosides accumulate in high concentrations in the proximal tubules and disappear slowly from this site on drug withdrawal.

Early signs of aminoglycoside nephrotoxicity are due to tubular damage and altered proximal tubular transport, e.g. increased excretion of brush border and lysosomal enzymes, low molecular weight proteins, amino acids and glucose. These defects resolve if the drug is stopped. Aminoglycosides may also cause changes in permeability to potassium and magnesium, resulting in severe wasting of these elements. Polyuria may also be seen initially. Renal failure (generally non-oliguric) may develop 7 to 10 days after the start of the treatment. Recovery from ATN will occur once the aminoglycoside is withdrawn, although full recovery may take some time because of drug accumulation.

The occurrence of renal failure is related to the duration and the total dosage of aminoglycosides given. More frequent administration with high trough plasma concentrations will increase the risk of toxicity. Other risk factors include advanced age, pre-existing renal or liver disease, volume depletion, potassium or magnesium depletion, hypotension, Gram-negative sepsis, and the concomitant use of other nephrotoxic drugs. The risk of aminoglycoside nephrotoxicity can be minimised with cautious dosage selection, use of a long dosage interval regimen, and a short overall course. Electrolyte and volume depletion should be avoided, and renal function and plasma drug concentrations measured frequently.

Once-daily administration of aminoglycosides appears to be associated with decreased nephrotoxicity.[155,156] However, definitive recommendations await further clinical evaluation in appropriate patient groups.[155] Some have suggested that modified once-daily dosing, where the dose interval is determined by the individual's renal clearance (hence avoiding subtherapeutic trough concentrations or drug accumulation) is a better approach.[157]

*Cefaloridine* and *cefalothin*, the first 2 cefalosporins introduced into clinical practice, are also nephrotoxic. However, with other cefalosporins, renal damage has been found only rarely,[151] although renal function should still be monitored during their use.

*Vancomycin:* in the early 1970s, a high rate of vancomycin-induced nephrotoxicity was encountered which was subsequently attributed to impurities in the formulation. Currently, about 5% of patients given vancomycin and 35% of patients given vancomycin together with aminoglycosides exhibit nephrotoxicity as evidenced by an increase in plasma creatinine concentrations.[150] Vancomycin plasma concentrations should be routinely monitored during therapy.

*Amphotericin B* is an important antifungal drug, but impairment of renal function develops in up to 80% of patients treated with it.[152,153] Toxicity is dose-related and predictable with total doses >5g. Clinically, the initial phase is characterised by defects in urinary concentrating ability causing polyuria, distal renal tubular acidosis and sometimes inability to retain magnesium. Within 2 weeks of starting treatment, a reduction of the GFR by about 40% is observed. Renal function usually improves after the drug is stopped, but irreversible damage may occur. Risk factors for the development of renal insufficiency include the total dose and average dose, concomitant administration of other nephrotoxic drugs, and pre-existing renal impairment. Renal damage may be minimised by concomitant sodium loading (300 mmol/day).

*Radiocontrast agents:* the incidence of nephrotoxicity due to radiocontrast agents varies from 0.6% in patients with normal renal function, to 80 to 90% in elderly patients and those with diabetes, arteriosclerosis, and chronic renal failure (and possibly those with hypovolaemia).[151,152] In most cases, renal impairment is mild, with an increase in serum creatinine occurring in the first few days after administration of the agent. Permanent impairment of renal function may occur in up to 33% of patients with severe pre-existing renal insufficiency. Several mechanisms may be involved, including direct toxicity to renal tubular cells, intense vasoconstriction and intravascular effects with aggregation of blood cells.

*Cyclosporin* can damage the nephron at various levels including the arteriole, glomerulus and proximal tubule.[150,152] Clinically, patients develop fluid retention, oedema and hypertension; in general, a slow increase in serum creatinine, hyperkalaemia and sometimes metabolic acidosis occurs. Renal function improves after the dosage is reduced or the drug stopped. However, there have been reports of irreversible nephrotoxicity.

An important risk factor for the development of renal insufficiency with cyclosporin is a high average daily dose. In the early days when dosages were as high as 17.5 mg/kg, nephrotoxicity was found in nearly all patients. Much lower dosages are used nowadays. Other risk factors for cyclosporin nephrotoxicity are drug interactions resulting in an increase in plasma cyclosporin concentrations (see appendix B), and concurrent use of other nephrotoxic drugs.[152] The azole antifungal drugs (ketoconazole, itraconazole), diltiazem, corticosteroids, sex hormones and some macrolide antibiotics (e.g. erythromycin) increase plasma cyclosporin concentrations by inhibiting its hepatic metabolism. These interactions may cause potentially fatal nephrotoxicity but some (e.g. ketoconazole and diltiazem) are now being exploited in an attempt to reduce the dosage requirements for cyclosporin due to its very high cost (see further chapter 7; sect. 2.3.4). However, with the inevitable problems of ensuring reliable compliance, the feasibility of utilising an interaction for this purpose long term must be drawn into question.

*Anticancer drugs:* a large number of anticancer drugs are capable of causing serious renal damage. These include cisplatin, nitrosoureas [e.g. carmustine (BCNU), semustine (CCNU)] and methotrexate.[150,151]

*Paracetamol* in therapeutic doses is not nephrotoxic. However, following paracetamol overdosage, patients may develop renal failure as well as hepatic failure, and occasionally present with acute renal failure alone. This toxicity is due to the formation of excessive amounts of a highly reactive alkylating intermediate (*N*-acetyl-*p*-benzoquinonimine; NABQI) by cytochrome P450 microsomal enzymes. The usually protective stores of reduced glutathione become saturated and the NABQI binds covalently to intracellular macromolecules in a manner similar to that which causes the liver damage.[158]

#### 10.1.3 Acute Interstitial Nephritis

More than 70 drugs have been implicated in causing acute interstitial nephritis, of which the most common are *antibiotics* and *NSAIDs*.[150,151,153] The mechanisms by which drugs cause this condition are not clear. The histological picture is dominated by a diffuse or patchy mononuclear cell infiltrate with a large eosinophilic component, and there may be evidence of tubular damage and interstitial oedema.

Clinically, acute deterioration in renal function occurs within 15 days (range 2 to 44 days) after drug exposure. Signs of allergic reactions (fever, rash, arthralgia, eosinophilia) are common. Eosinophils can be detected in the urine in up to 100% of patients. Two-thirds of patients become oliguric, and proteinuria (usually <1 g/day), erythrocyturia and sterile leucocyturia are common.

After the offending drug is withdrawn, spontaneous resolution usually occurs, although recovery may sometimes take many months. Noncomparative studies suggest that corticosteroids promote recovery. A reasonable approach is to give corticosteroids if there is no sign of spontaneous recovery 10 days after drug withdrawal.

#### 10.1.4 Obstructive Nephropathy

A variety of drugs and their metabolites may be deposited in the renal tubule, causing obstruction of urine flow and secondary damage to the tubular epithelium.[150,152,153]

The first *sulfonamides* formed crystalline aggregates due to their poor solubility. Although the currently used sulfonamides are substantially more soluble, a high urine output and urinary alkalinisation decrease the likelihood of sulfonamide deposition. Cellular debris from tubular cells damaged by *aminoglycosides* may also cause intratubular obstruction.

Acute renal failure can also result from intratubular precipitation of urate, as in acute uric acid nephropathy. This occurs after administration of *cytotoxic drugs* to patients with leukaemia or lymphoma. Rapid lysis of tumour cells leads to overproduction of uric acid. This complication can be avoided by pretreatment with allopurinol and adequate hydration and urinary alkalinisation.

*Methotrexate* is almost entirely eliminated through the kidneys by both filtration and tubular secretion. Like the sulfonamides, the solubility of this drug is pH-dependent, and acute renal dysfunction can be largely prevented by appropriate hydration and alkalinisation of the urine.

*Aciclovir* given by intravenous bolus may cause intratubular obstruction and acute renal failure. This complication can be largely, but not completely, avoided by administering the appropriate dosage slowly with adequate hydration.[153] Acute renal failure has not been observed with oral aciclovir.

Crystalluria may occur in patients treated with *ciprofloxacin*. However, it is not clear if crystalluria is the cause of ARF occasionally associated with ciprofloxacin therapy.[159] By ensuring adequate fluid intake and avoiding excessive alkalinity of urine, this complication is less likely to develop.

Drugs that promote the formation of renal calculi can potentially cause an obstructive nephropathy. Excessive ingestion of calcium-containing antacids and over-enthusiastic consumption of vitamins (i.e. vitamin D and calcium) may result in renal stones. Triamterene has been found as a component of renal stones but there is no evidence that stone formation is increased in patients taking this drug. Attacks of renal colic should always be followed up, as calculi of about 4 to 5mm cross-sectional diameter can become lodged in the ureter. The colic may subside, leading to an asymptomatic hydronephrosis with subsequent renal destruction.

## 10.2 Drug-Induced Chronic Renal Failure

Several drugs that cause acute renal failure can cause chronic renal failure when administered for a prolonged period.

### 10.2.1 Analgesic Nephropathy

The most common form of drug-induced chronic renal failure is analgesic nephropathy.[153] Analgesic nephropathy manifested as a chronic interstitial nephritis and papillary necrosis is seen in patients, mainly women, who consume large quantities of analgesics, usually over many years. These patients often suffer from chronic headache or low back pain. Caucasian women living in relatively hot climates such as Australia and South Africa appear to be particularly at risk while in the past, European 'production line' factory workers were actively encouraged to take analgesics, particularly phenacetin. In these situations, relative dehydration may have been a predisposing factor.

The precise mechanism of analgesic nephropathy is unclear, but probably relates to a combination of injury produced by toxic metabolites and medullary ischaemia. *Phenacetin* is metabolised to paracetamol but in view of the very low toxicity of the latter in therapeutic doses, this pathway is unlikely to be responsible for phenacetin's toxicity. *Aspirin* and *NSAIDs* inhibit prostaglandin synthesis in the kidney. Loss of the vasodilator prostaglandins decreases renal blood flow and causes ischaemic injury to the inner medulla and papillary necrosis. Aspirin may also deplete reduced glutathione directly. Other analgesics including *phenazone* (antipyrine) and *aminophenazone* (amidopyrine) have also been implicated but are no longer generally available in many countries.

Most cases are caused by long term consumption of a combination of analgesics or phenacetin. Although there is little doubt that single agents (paracetamol, aspirin, NSAIDs) can themselves produce papillary necrosis and renal dysfunction, the magnitude of the problem is small compared with overall usage. However, since patients often intentionally or unintentionally underestimate their consumption of analgesics, diagnosis requires a high index of suspicion and a careful history. Many patients also have adverse gastrointestinal reactions to these drugs.

Patients with analgesic nephropathy usually present with a slow progressive decline in renal function with acute episodes of deterioration related to the passage of papillae and urinary obstruction. During these episodes, patients can have flank pain, pyuria, haematuria, and necrotic papillary tissue in the urine. Sodium loss, a tendency to metabolic acidosis and hypertension are other characteristic features.

Patients with analgesic nephropathy often have stabilised renal function once they cease drug consumption. These patients are also at increased risk of developing transitional cell carcinoma of the urinary collecting system and bladder – a risk that may continue even after cessation of analgesic use. Retroperitoneal fibrosis has also been reported with analgesic abuse.[160]

### 10.2.2 Chronic Interstitial Nephritis

*Cyclosporin* may cause chronic interstitial nephritis and chronic renal failure, possibly consequent to renal vasoconstriction and chronic ischaemia. Chronic interstitial nephritis, histologically characterised by fibrosis, is also associated with *lithium, cisplatin* and *aminoglycosides*.[152]

## 10.3 Drug-Induced Proteinuria and Nephrotic Syndrome

Drug-induced glomerulonephritis usually presents as proteinuria or a full nephrotic syndrome.[151-153] Membranous glomerulonephritis is the most frequent type of lesion encountered. The precise mechanisms of damage have not been identified, but there are 3 main hypotheses. Firstly, the drugs could act as haptens and induce antibodies against glomerular components. Secondly, the drugs could bind to the glomerular antigens and modify them, becoming the target of antibodies. Thirdly, the drugs may have an immunomodulatory effect, thus causing an autoimmune disease. Several drugs may cause more than one type of histological change. In this section, they are classified according to the most frequently occurring pattern.

### *10.3.1 Membranous Glomerulonephritis*

Membranous glomerulonephritis and the nephrotic syndrome have been most frequently reported with *gold salts* and *penicillamine*. Proteinuria and nephrotic syndrome may occur in 6 to 17% and 2.6 to 5.3%, respectively, of patients receiving gold salts for rheumatoid arthritis. About 90% of patients with a gold-induced nephrotic syndrome have membranous glomerulonephritis, while the remainder have minimal glomerular change. Renal function is usually not impaired and proteinuria disappears slowly over 6 to 12 months after the drug is stopped. Patients with rheumatoid arthritis who have HLA-B8 or DRW3 antigens have an increased risk of proteinuria. The oral route of gold administration is less frequently associated with this problem. Reintroduction of gold is not recommended, although re-exposure does not always lead to recurrence.

With penicillamine use in rheumatoid arthritis, about 7 to 20% of patients develop proteinuria, usually 6 to 12 months after drug exposure. Membranous glomerulonephritis is found in 85% of patients with nephrotic syndrome. Proteinuria does not appear to be dose-related, but will subside within 6 to 12 months of drug withdrawal. Recurrence of proteinuria with penicillamine rechallenge is frequent. There appears to be a genetic predisposition to nephrotoxicity. Patients who developed proteinuria when treated with gold are at higher risk when subsequently treated with penicillamine. The frequency of penicillamine-induced proteinuria is higher in HLA-DRW3 positive patients. Whether this drug should be withdrawn once proteinuria occurs is not clear from current data. A good policy might be to continue the drug (perhaps at a lower dosage), provided that renal function tests remain normal, oedema is absent and proteinuria does not exceed 2 g/day. However, the drug should clearly be discontinued when proteinuria exceeds 3 g/day. Penicillamine has also been described as a cause of rapidly progressive glomerulonephritis resembling Goodpasture's syndrome and a lupus-like syndrome.

Like penicillamine, *captopril* contains a sulfhydryl group. The overall incidence of proteinuria in patients treated with high doses of this drug is 1%. With doses under 150 mg/day, this complication appears to be uncommon.

### *10.3.2 Minimal Change Glomerulonephritis*

*NSAIDs* can cause a third form of renal disease, i.e. minimal change nephrotic syndrome. Most reports have concerned fenoprofen. Patients with renal failure and elderly patients on diuretics seem especially prone to develop this complication. Renal function usually improves after the drug is stopped. Prednisolone may hasten recovery, although, despite corticosteroids, progression to chronic renal failure has been described. Recurrence of the syndrome after re-exposure to the same or to another NSAID has been reported.

There are rare reports of *lithium* causing the nephrotic syndrome. It occurs after several months and disappears rapidly following withdrawal of the drug. Minimal glomerular changes are usually found in these patients. Lithium-induced nephrogenic diabetes insipidus is discussed in section 10.5.2.

## 10.4 Drug-Induced Lupus-Like Syndrome

The incidence of a lupus-like syndrome with *hydralazine* is 10 to 20%, but renal involvement seldom occurs;[3] patients with HLA-DR4 are more likely to develop hydralazine-associated lupus.

*Procainamide* may cause a lupus-like syndrome in up to 30% of patients on long term therapy, but again, renal involvement is uncommon.

Other drugs that have been associated with a lupus-like syndrome include *isoniazid, methyl-*

*dopa, phenytoin, chlorpromazine,* and *penicillamine*.

### 10.5 Miscellaneous Drug-Induced Conditions

#### *10.5.1 Renal Vasculitis*

Although the extrarenal features of drug-induced vasculitis are common, its renal manifestations are infrequently seen. Angiitis involving the small vessels and capable of inducing acute renal failure has mainly been described during treatment with *penicillin* and *sulfonamides*.[151] Renal involvement is characterised by proteinuria, microscopic haematuria, hypertension, and elevated serum creatinine. Corticosteroids in high doses may be beneficial.

#### *10.5.2 Nephrogenic Diabetes Insipidus*

Nephrogenic diabetes insipidus occurs in up to 50% of patients taking *lithium* and is directly related to dosage. The concentration defect is due to both reduced proximal tubular resorption and a defect in chloride and water handling in the ascending limb of the distal tubule.

## 11. Use of Drugs in the Presence of Associated Renal Failure

As discussed in sections 1 and 2, the presence of renal failure presents a complex situation which can modify both the pharmacokinetic behaviour of and the response to drugs. There will be accumulation of those drugs or active metabolites that are mainly eliminated by the kidneys. Moreover, as discussed in section 10, some drugs may themselves aggravate renal dysfunction. Thus, dosage modification of such drugs is required if toxic effects are to be avoided. This is particularly important for drugs eliminated mainly by the kidney that have a low therapeutic ratio. For these drugs, careful monitoring of patients for toxicity should be undertaken and plasma concentrations should be measured to guide continuing therapy.

In this section, only brief guidelines on dosage modification in renal failure are given.[2,4] For further information, see appendix D and also individual drug monographs.

### 11.1 Antimicrobial Agents

With the exception of the aminoglycosides and vancomycin, most antimicrobial drugs have a wide therapeutic index and little or no dosage adjustment is normally made until the GFR is below 1.2 L/h (<20 ml/min). Drugs that are removed by dialysis (see review by Reetze-Bonorden et al.[17]) should be administered after dialysis or a supplemental dose should be given at that time.

***Aminoglycoside antibiotics*** (e.g. gentamicin, tobramycin, netilmicin, amikacin) require dosage adjustment in even mild renal impairment. Their use may worsen renal impairment and cause ototoxicity (see further chapter 14; sect. 8.1.1). Several factors make such toxicity more likely. These include prior or prolonged treatment, hypovolaemia, dehydration, concomitant use of loop diuretics, hypokalaemia, hypomagnesaemia and obstructive jaundice.[154,161] A combination of reduction in dosage and in frequency of administration with frequent peak and trough plasma concentration measurements are required. Once-daily administration appears to reduce the renal toxicity of these drugs (see further section 10.1.2).

***Vancomycin*** is both nephrotoxic and ototoxic (see further chapter 31; sect. 8.10) and plasma concentrations of this drug should be monitored. Since it is not dialysed (except at extremely high flow rates), after a single intravenous infusion, therapeutic concentrations can be maintained for 5 days in patients with end-stage renal failure on dialysis.

***Tetracyclines:*** with the exception of minocycline and doxycycline, the tetracyclines are renally excreted and are moreover, antianabolic, causing a concentration-related increase in blood urea with further deterioration in renal function. Thus, they should not be used in patients with renal failure. However, minocycline and doxycycline can be used if necessary.

***Antituberculosis drugs:*** normal daily doses of isoniazid, rifampicin and pyrazinamide may be given in renal impairment;[162] with isoniazid, pyridoxine should be given concomitantly to prevent peripheral neuropathy. However, streptomycin and ethambutol should be avoided where possible. The major toxicity associated with streptomycin is vestibular. Clearly, if this drug is required, a reduced dose should be given 2 or 3 times weekly for the first 2 months and the plasma concentration must be monitored. Ethambutol is particularly likely to cause optic neuritis where excessive dosages are used or the patient's renal function is impaired. A reduced dose given intermittently should therefore be used. If patients develop any visual changes, they should be warned to discontinue therapy immediately and to seek medical advice promptly. It has been recommended that for the treatment of renally impaired patients with tuberculosis, a fourth drug should be given. Here, streptomycin rather than ethambutol should be used.[162]

***Amphotericin B*** is nephrotoxic (see also chapter 31; sect. 6.1.1) and should only be used in patients with renal failure if there is no alternative. Plasma concentrations and renal function should be closely monitored. Its protein binding to lipoproteins is reduced in renal failure and thus low plasma concentrations of amphotericin B need to be interpreted accordingly.

***Antiviral drugs:*** aciclovir (given for the treatment of herpes and cytomegalovirus infections) and ganciclovir (for treatment of cytomegalovirus infection) are both eliminated by the kidney. Dosage reduction of these agents is necessary in the presence of renal failure, as accumulation can lead to CNS toxicity and unconsciousness.

### 11.2 Analgesics

***Opioid analgesics:*** responses to opioids are affected by renal failure and retention of metabolites can produce adverse effects. Dosage reduction and close observation for respiratory depression and other adverse effects are therefore necessary. Diamorphine (heroin) is metabolised to morphine and then to morphine-3-glucuronide and morphine-6-glucuronide. These metabolites accumulate and cause prolonged analgesia and respiratory depression. Pethidine (meperidine) is converted to norpethidine (normeperidine), which also accumulates and can cause seizures. Weaker opioids (e.g. dextropropoxyphene, dihydrocodeine and codeine) also have the potential to cause severe respiratory depression in some patients, due to active metabolite accumulation.

***Nonsteroidal anti-inflammatory drugs:*** all NSAIDs have the disadvantage of directly causing gastrointestinal bleeding and increasing the bleeding tendency in uraemic renal failure. They may also cause further deterioration in renal function as well as hyperkalaemia, and sodium and water retention.

### 11.3 Antianxiety Drugs, Hypnotics and Antipsychotics

Patients with advanced renal failure may be particularly sensitive to the CNS depressant effects of these drugs. It is therefore advisable to start treatment with a smaller than normal dose.

### 11.4 Lithium and Antidepressants

Lithium should be avoided if possible or the dose reduced with careful monitoring of plasma concentrations (see chapter 5, sect. 4.6; and chapter 30; sect. 4). However, the tricyclics and newer antidepressants can be prescribed in normal dosages.

### 11.5 Cardiovascular Drugs

***β-Adrenoceptor antagonists*** (β-blockers) should be started in low doses. These drugs may reduce renal blood flow and adversely affect renal function in patients with severe impairment. Dosage adjustments are particularly necessary for those β-blockers mainly eliminated by renal excretion (e.g. atenolol, celiprolol, nadolol, sotalol).

***Calcium antagonists*** are principally eliminated by hepatic metabolism and can all be used in usual dosages in patients with renal impairment.

***ACE inhibitors:*** starting doses of these drugs should be low, and the dose increased slowly with careful monitoring of plasma potassium and creatinine. Most ACE inhibitors are eliminated principally by the kidneys and their maintenance doses should be reduced. However, some drugs (e.g. fosinopril, spirapril, trandolapril) are eliminated by both renal excretion and hepatic metabolism, and dosage adjustments for these agents only appear necessary where renal function is markedly reduced (see also chapter 21; sect. 3.5.3).

***Digoxin:*** maintenance doses of digoxin should be reduced in severe renal failure and plasma concentrations monitored with particular care.

### 11.6 Insulin and Oral Antidiabetic Drugs

***Insulin*** requirements decrease with declining renal function, probably as a consequence of reduced elimination of insulin by the kidney. Dosage reduction is often required in renal failure. There is also a state of insulin resistance in uraemia due to a post-receptor defect.[163] This is corrected by dialysis. The decrease in insulin requirements is variable, depending on which effect predominates – a longer half-life or reduced insulin action. The compensatory response to hypoglycaemia may also be impaired in uraemic patients.

***Oral antidiabetic drugs:*** chlorpropamide has an extended half-life of >36 hours and should be avoided in renal impairment, as the risk of severe and prolonged hypoglycaemia is greatly increased. Prolonged hypoglycaemia can also occur with glibenclamide, probably due to the accumulation of an active metabolite in renal impairment that binds tightly to pancreatic β-cells.[164] Metformin is contraindicated in patients with renal failure because of the risk of lactic acidosis.

Glipizide appears to be the oral antidiabetic drug of choice in patients with renal impairment because of its shorter duration of action and its method of elimination (hepatic metabolism to an inactive metabolite) [see also chapter 19; sect. 3.2.1].

### 11.7 Gastrointestinal Drugs

***Antiulcer drugs:*** cimetidine is predominantly eliminated by hepatic metabolism but metabolites accumulate if renal impairment is severe. Ranitidine is eliminated by both the liver and kidneys. The dosage of both drugs should be reduced if severe renal impairment is present; both can occasionally cause confusion. However, no dosage adjustment appears necessary with omeprazole.

***Antacids:*** some antacid preparations (e.g. magnesium trisilicate mixtures) may have a high sodium content. The use of aluminium-containing compounds such as aluminium hydroxide or sucralfate in patients with severe renal impairment or those on dialysis may increase the risk of aluminium toxicity. These drugs should therefore be avoided (see section 7.1.2).

### 11.8 Antigout Drugs

***Allopurinol*** is metabolised to oxypurinol, which accumulates in renal impairment and may be responsible for some of the drug's adverse effects, including rashes, bone marrow depression and gastrointestinal upset. Rashes can be particularly severe with potentially fatal toxic epidermolysis, and the maximum daily dose should be reduced to 100mg in patients with more than mild renal impairment.

***Colchicine*** has been largely superseded by NSAIDs for the treatment of acute gout but a short course may be useful in some patients (see further chapter 25; sect. 13.2). In excessive doses, colchicine can cause profuse diarrhoea, gastrointestinal haemorrhage, rashes and renal impairment. Its dosage should therefore be reduced if renal impairment is present.

## References

1. Bennett WM. Drug therapy in renal failure: dosing guidelines for adults. Parts I and II. Annals of Internal Medicine 1980; 93: 62
2. Carmichael DJS. Handling of drugs in kidney disease. In: Cameron S, Davidson AM, Grunfeld J-P, et al., editors. Oxford textbook of clinical nephrology. Vol. 1. Oxford: Oxford University Press, 1992: 159
3. Cove-Smith R. Drugs and the kidney. Medicine International (Quarterly edition) 1991; 4: 3539
4. British Medical Association and Royal Pharmaceutical Society of Great Britain. British National Formulary No. 23, 1993
5. Craig RM, Murphy P, Gibson TP, et al. Kinetic analysis of D-xylose absorption in normal subjects and in patients with chronic renal failure. Journal of Laboratory and Clinical Medicine 1983; 101: 496-506
6. Tillement JP, Lhoste F, Guidicelli JF. Diseases and drug protein binding. In: Gibaldi M, Prescott L, editors. Handbook of clinical pharmacokinetics. Balgowlah: Adis Health Science Press, 1983: 57-69
7. Reidenberg MM. The binding of drugs to plasma proteins from patients with poor renal function. In: Gibaldi M, Prescott L, editors. Handbook of clinical pharmacokinetics. Balgowlah: Adis Health Science Press, 1983: 89-95
8. Reidenberg MM, Drayer DE. Drug therapy in renal failure. Annual Review of Pharmacology and Toxicology 1980; 20: 45
9. Gibaldi M. Biopharmaceutics and clinical pharmacokinetics. Philadelphia: Lea and Febiger, 1984
10. Prescott LF, Balali-Mood M, Critchley JAJH, et al. Diuresis or alkalisation for salicylate poisoning. British Medical Journal 1982; 285: 1383
11. Aronson JK, Grahame-Smith DG, Firth JD. Drugs and the kidney and the drug therapy of renal, urinary tract, and prostatic disorders. In: Aronson JK, Grahame-Smith DG, editors. Oxford textbook of clinical pharmacology and drug therapy. 2nd ed. Oxford: Oxford University Press, 1993: 343
12. Critchley JAJH, Robson JS. Renal diseases. In: Speight TM, editor. Avery's drug treatment: principles and practice of clinical pharmacology and therapeutics. 3rd ed. Auckland: Adis Press, 1987
13. O'Grady F. Antibiotics and renal failure. British Medical Bulletin 1971; 27: 142
14. Grahame-Smith DG, Aronson JK, Firth JD. Drugs and the kidney and the drug therapy of renal, urinary tract, and prostatic disorders. In: Grahame-Smith DG, Aronson JK, editors. Oxford textbook of clinical pharmacology and drug therapy. 2nd ed. Oxford: Oxford University Press, 1992
15. Keller E, Reetze P, Schollmeyer P. Drug therapy in patients undergoing continuous ambulatory peritoneal dialysis: clinical pharmacokinetic considerations. Clinical Pharmacokinetics 1990; 18: 104
16. Maher JF. Influence of continuous ambulatory peritoneal dialysis on elimination of drugs. Peritoneal Dialysis Bulletin 1987; 7: 159
17. Reetze-Bonorden P, Bohler J, Keller E. Drug dosage in patients during continuous renal replacement therapy: pharmacokinetic and therapeutic considerations. Clinical Pharmacokinetics 1993; 24: 362
18. Topley N, Williams JD. Urinary tract infections in adults. Medicine International (Quarterly edition) 1991; 4: 3604, 1001
19. Javis WR, White JW, Munn VP, et al. Nosocomial infection surveillance, 1983. MMWR Morbidity and Mortality Weekly Report 1983; 33 (2SS): 9SS
20. Baldassarre JS, Kaye D. Special problems of urinary tract infection in the elderly. Medical Clinics of North America 1991; 75: 375

21. Meyrier A, Guibert J. Diagnosis and drug treatment of acute pyelonephritis. Drugs 1992; 44: 356
22. Hooton TM, Stamm WE. Management of acute uncomplicated urinary tract infection in adults. Medical Clinics of North America 1991; 75: 338
23. Rubin RH, Tolkoff-Rubin NE, Cotran RS. Urinary tract infection, pyelonephritis and reflux nephropathy. In: Brenner BM, Rector FC, editors. The kidney. Vol. 2. Philadelphia: WB Saunders, 1991: 1369
24. Bailey RR. Urinary tract infections in adults: part 1 - curative regimens of treatment. New Zealand Medical Journal 1992; 105: 224
25. Stamm WE, Turck M. Urinary tract infections and pyelonephritis. In: Wilson JD, Braunwald E, Isselbacher KJ, et al., editors. Harrison's principles of internal medicine. New York: McGraw-Hill, 1991: 538
26. Stamm WE, Hooton TM. Management of urinary tract infections in adults. New England Journal of Medicine 1993; 329: 1328
27. Wilkie ME, Almond MK, Marsh FP. Diagnosis and management of urinary tract infection in adults. British Medical Journal 1992; 305: 1137
28. Patton JP, Nash DB, Abrutyn E. Urinary tract infection: economic considerations. Medical Clinics of North America 1991; 75: 495
29. British Medical Association and Royal Pharmaceutical Association of Great Britain. British National Formulary No. 27, 1994
30. Norrby SR. Treatment of urinary tract infections with quinolone antimicrobial agents. In: Wolfson JS, Hooper DC, editors. Quinolone antimicrobial agents. Washington DC: American Society for Microbiology, 1989: 107-23
31. Andriole VT, Patterson TF. Epidemiology, natural history, and management of urinary tract infections in pregnancy. Medical Clinics of North America 1991; 75: 359
32. Gower PE. Urinary tract infections in men. British Medical Journal 1989; 298: 1595
33. Stull TL, LiPuma JJ. Epidemiology and natural history of urinary tract infections in children. Medical Clinics of North America 1991; 75: 287
34. Sherbotie JR, Cornfeld D. Management of urinary tract infection in children. Medical Clinics of North America 1991; 75: 327
35. Bailey RR. Urinary tract infections in adults: part 2 - prophylactic regimens of treatment. New Zealand Medical Journal 1992; 105: 247
36. Aagaard J, Madsen PO. Diagnostic and therapeutic problems in prostatitis: therapeutic position of ofloxacin. Drugs and Aging 1992; 2: 196
37. Leigh DA. Prostatitis: an increasing clinical problem for diagnosis and management. Journal of Antimicrobial Chemotherapy 1993; 32 Suppl. A: 1
38. Meares EM. Prostatitis. Medical Clinics of North America 1991; 75: 405
39. Klahr S. The kidney and hypertension: villain and victim. New England Journal of Medicine 1989; 320: 731
40. Weisstuch JM, Dworkin LD. Does essential hypertension cause end-stage renal disease? Kidney International 1992; 41 Suppl. 36: S33
41. Whelton PK, Klag MJ. Hypertension as a risk factor for renal disease: review of clinical and epidemiological evidence. Hypertension 1989; 13 Suppl. 5: I19
42. Relman AS. Race and end-stage renal disease. New England Journal of Medicine 1982; 306: 1290
43. The National Institutes of Health, the National Institute of Diabetes and Digestive and Kidney Diseases, Division of Kidney, Urologic, and Hematologic Diseases. United States Renal Data System, 1993 Annual Data Report, March 1993; 55-67
44. Anderson AR, Christiansen JS, Andersen J, et al. Diabetic nephropathy in type I (insulin-dependent) diabetes: an epidemiological study. Diabetologia 1983; 25: 497-501
45. Tuttle KR, Stein JH, DeFronzo RA. The natural history of diabetic nephropathy. Seminars in Nephrology 1990; 10: 184-93
46. Cockram CS, Woo J, Lau E, et al. The prevalence of diabetes mellitus and impaired glucose tolerance among Hong Kong Chinese adults of working age. Diabetes Research and Clinical Practice 1993; 21: 67-73
47. Chan JCN, Cheung CK, Cheung MYF, et al. Abnormal albuminuria as a predictor of mortality and renal impairment in Chinese patients with NIDDM. Diabetes Care 1995; 18: 1013-16
48. Lau GSN, Chan JCN, Chu PLM, et al. Use of antidiabetic and antihypertensive drugs in hospitals and outpatient settings in Hong Kong. Annals of Pharmacotherapy 1996; 30: 232-7
49. Chan TYK, Lee KKC, Chan AWK, et al. Utilization of antidiabetic drugs in Hong Kong: relation to the common occurrence of antidiabetic drug-induced hypoglycemia amongst acute medical admissions and the relative prevalence of NIDDM. International Journal of Clinical Pharmacology and Therapeutics 1996; 34: 43-6
50. Chan JCN, Critchley JAJH, Tomlinson B, et al. Antihypertensive and anti-albuminuric effects of losartan potassium and felodipine in Chinese elderly hypertensive patients with or without non-insulin-dependent diabetes mellitus. American Journal of Nephrology 1997; 17: 72-80
51. Lewis EJ, Hunsicker LG, Bain RP, et al. for the Collaborative Study Group. The effect of angiotensin-converting-enzyme inhibition on diabetic nephropathy. New England Journal of Medicine 1993; 329: 1456-62
52. Rodby RA, Lewis EJ, Firth LM, for the Collaborative Study Group. An economic analysis of captopril in the treatment of diabetic nephropathy. Diabetes Care 1996; 19: 1051-61
53. Viberti G, Mogesen CE, Groop LC, et al. for the European Microalbuminuria Study Group. Effect of captopril on progression to clinical proteinuria in patients with insulin-dependent diabetes mellitus and microalbuminuria. Journal of the American Medical Association 1994; 271: 275-9
54. Mason PD, Pusey CD. Glomerulonephritis: diagnosis and treatment. British Medical Journal 1994; 309: 1557-63
55. Keller F Schwarz A. Fundamental concepts and immunosuppressive treatment in the various forms of glomerulonephritis. Renal Failure 1995; 17: 1-11
56. Brodehl J. Management of nephrotic syndrome in children. Clinical Immunotherapeutics 1996; 5: 175-92
57. Melvin T, Bennett W. Management of nephrotic syndrome in childhood. Drugs 1991; 42: 30-51
58. Ponticelli C, Passerini P. Conventional treatment of idiopathic nephrotic syndrome and membranous nephropathy in adults. Clinical Nephrology 1991; 35 (Suppl. 1): S16-S21
59. Ram CVS. Current concepts in renovascular hypertension. American Journal of the Medical Sciences 1992; 304: 53
60. Working Group on Renovascular Hypertension. Detection, evaluation and treatment of renovascular hypertension: final report. Archives of Internal Medicine 1987; 147: 820
61. McGrath BP, Clarke K. Renal artery stenosis: current diagnosis and treatment. Medical Journal of Australia 1993; 158: 343
62. Nolan CR, Schrier RW. The kidney in hypertension. In: Schrier RW, editor. Renal and electrolyte disorders. 4th ed. Boston: Little Brown and Company, 1992: 447
63. Stansby G, Hamilton G, Scoble J. Atherosclerotic renal artery stenosis. British Journal of Hospital Medicine 1993; 49: 388
64. Rose BD. Diuretics. Kidney International 1991; 39: 336
65. Greger R, Heidland A. Action and clinical use of diuretics. In: Cameron S, Davison AM, Grunfeld J-P, et al., editors.

Oxford textbook of clinical nephrology. Oxford: Oxford University Press, 1992: 197
66. Davies DL, Wilson GM. Diuretics: mechanism of action and clinical application. Drugs 1975; 9: 170
67. Lant A. Diuretics: clinical pharmacology and therapeutic use (part I). Drugs 1985; 29: 57-81
68. Lant A. Diuretics: clinical pharmacology and therapeutic use (part II). Drugs 1985; 29: 162-88
69. Sica DA, Gehr TWB. Diuretic combinations in refractory oedema states: pharmacokinetic-pharmacodynamic relationships. Clinical Pharmacokinetics 1996; 30: 229-49
70. Beerman B, Grind M. Clinical pharmacokinetics and some newer diuretics. Clinical Pharmacokinetics 1987; 13: 254
71. Ponto LLB, Schoenwald RD. Furosemide (frusemide): a pharmacokinetic/pharmacodynamic review (part 1). Clinical Pharmacokinetics 1990; 18: 381
72. Ponto LLB, Schoenwald RD. Furosemide (frusemide): a pharmacokinetic/pharmacodynamic review (part 2). Clinical Pharmacokinetics 1990; 18: 460
73. Saggar-Malik A, Cappuccio FP. Potassium supplements and potassium-sparing diuretics: a review and guide to appropriate use. Drugs 1993; 46: 986
74. Swan SK. Diuretic strategies in patients with renal failure. Drugs 1994; 48: 380
75. Friedel HA, Buckley MMT. Torasemide: a review of its pharmacological properties and therapeutic potential. Drugs 1991; 41: 81
76. Freis ED. Adverse effects of diuretics. Drug Safety 1992; 7: 364
77. Chan JCN, Cockram CS, Critchley JAJH. Drug-induced disorders of glucose metabolism: mechanisms and management. Drug Safety 1996; 15: 135-57
78. Puschett JB, Greenberg A. Treatment of oedematous states. In: Suki WN, Massry SG, editors. Therapy of renal diseases and related disorders. Boston: Martinus Nijhoff Publishing, 1984: 3-45
79. Russo D, Memoli BB, Andreucci VE. The place of loop diuretics in the treatment of acute and chronic renal failure. Clinical Nephrology 1992; 38 Suppl. 1: S69
80. Conger JD, Briner VA, Schrier RW. Acute renal failure: pathogenesis, diagnosis, and management. In: Schrier RW, editor. Renal and electrolyte disorders. 4th ed. Boston: Little, Brown and Company, 1992: 495
81. Anderson RJ, Schrier RW. Acute renal failure. In: Wilson JD, et al. editors. Harrison's principles of internal medicine. 12th ed., Vol. 2. New York: McGraw-Hill, 1991: 1145
82. Mandal AK, Visweswaran RK, Kaldas NR. Treatment considerations in acute renal failure. Drugs 1992; 44: 567
83. Finn WF. Diagnosis and management of acute tubular necrosis. Medical Clinics of North America 1990; 74: 873
84. Firth JD. Renal replacement therapy on the intensive care unit. Quarterly Journal of Medicine 1993; 86: 75
85. Ronco C. Continuous renal replacement therapies for the treatment of acute renal failure in intensive care patients. Clinical Nephrology 1993; 40: 187
86. Williams DG. The common causes of chronic renal failure. Medicine International (Quarterly edition) 1991; 4: 3563
87. Walls J. Chronic renal failure: conservative management. Medicine International (Quarterly edition) 1991; 4: 3565
88. Klahr S. Chronic renal failure: management. Lancet 1991; 338: 423
89. Pedrini MT, Levey AS, Lau J, et al. The effects of dietary protein restriction on the progression of diabetic and nondiabetic renal diseases: a meta-analysis. Annals of Internal Medicine 1996; 124: 627-32
90. Becker GJ, Whitworth JA, Ihle BU, et al. Prevention of progression in non-diabetic chronic renal failure. Kidney International 1994; 45 Suppl. 45: S167
91. Bourgoignie JI. Progression of renal disease: current concepts and therapeutic approaches. Kidney International 1992; 41 Suppl. 36: S61
92. Curtis JR. Interventions in chronic renal failure. British Medical Journal 1990; 301: 622
93. Jacobson HR. Chronic renal failure: pathophysiology. Lancet 1991; 338: 419
94. Klahr S, Schreiner G, Ichikawa I. The progression of renal disease. New England Journal of Medicine 1988; 318: 1657
95. Ter Wee PM, Donker AJM. Clinical strategies for arresting progression of renal disease. Kidney International 1992; 42 Suppl. 38: S114
96. Lipkin G, Raine A. Hypertension and renal disease. Practitioner 1993; 237: 173
97. Joint National Committee on Detection, Evaluation and Treatment of High Blood Pressure. The Fifth Report of the Joint National Committee of Detection, Evaluation, and Treatment of High Blood Pressure. Archives of Internal Medicine 1993; 153: 154
98. Aurell M. ACE inhibition: antihypertensive treatment of choice in progressive chronic renal failure? Nephrology Dialysis Transplantation 1993; 8: 680
99. Keilani T, Schlueter WA, Levin ML, et al. Improvement of lipid abnormalities associated with proteinuria using fosinopril as angiotensin-converting enzyme inhibitor. American Journal of Medicine 1993; 118: 246
100. Graafland AD, Doorenbos CJ, van Sasse JC. Enalapril-induced anaemia in two kidney transplant recipients. Transplant International 1992; 5: 51-3
101. Kasiske BL, Kalil RSN, Ma JZ, et al. Effect of antihypertensive therapy on the kidney in patients with diabetes: a meta regression analysis. Annals of Internal Medicine 1993; 118: 129-38
102. Ter Wee TM, Donker AJM. Pharmacologic manipulation of glomerular function. Kidney International 1994; 45: 417
103. Epstein M. Calcium antagonists and renal protection. Annals of Internal Medicine 1992; 152: 1573-84
104. Klahr S, Levey AS, Beck GJ, et al. The effects of dietary protein restriction and blood-pressure control on the progression of chronic renal disease. New England Journal of Medicine 1994; 330: 877
105. Chan JCN, Cockram CS, Nicholls MG, et al. Comparison of enalapril and nifedipine in treating non-insulin dependent diabetes associated with hypertension: one year analysis. British Medical Journal 1992; 305: 981-8
106. Wheeler DC, Bernard DB. Lipid abnormalities in the nephrotic syndrome: causes, consequences, and treatment. American Journal of Kidney Diseases 1994; 23: 331-46
107. Grundy SM. Management of hyperlipidaemia of kidney disease. Kidney International 1990; 37: 847
108. Attman P-O. Hyperlipoproteinaemia in renal failure: pathogenesis and perspectives for intervention. Nephrology Dialysis Transplantation 1993; 8: 294
109. Alfrey AC, Chan L. Chronic renal failure: manifestations and pathogenesis. In: Schrier RW, editor. Renal and electrolyte disorders. 4th ed. Boston: Little, Brown and Company, 1992: 539
110. Gower P. Prevention of bone disease in chronic renal failure. Prescribers' Journal 1992; 32: 245
111. Coburn JW. Mineral metabolism and renal bone disease: effects of CAPD versus haemodialysis. Kidney International 1993; 43 Suppl. 40: S92
112. Cronin RE. Bone disease in kidney failure: diagnosis and management. American Journal of the Medical Sciences 1993; 306: 192
113. Delmez JA. Long-term complications of dialysis: pathogenetic factors with special reference to bone. Kidney International 1993; 43 Suppl. 41: S116
114. Ritz E, Matthias S, Seidel A, et al. Disturbed calcium metabolism in renal failure: pathogenesis and therapeutic strategies. Kidney International 1992; 42 Suppl. 38: S37

115. Winchester JF, Rotellar C, Goggins M, et al. Calcium and phosphate balance in dialysis patients. Kidney International 1993; 41 Suppl.: S174-8
116. Schaefer K. Alternative phosphate binders: an update. Nephrology Dialysis Transplantation 1993; 1: 35
117. Boelaert JR, de Locht M. Side-effects of desferrioxamine in dialysis patients. Dialysis and Transplantation 1993; 8 Suppl. 1: 43
118. De Broe ME, D'Haese PC, Couttenye MM, et al. New insights and strategies in the diagnosis and treatment of aluminium overload in dialysis patients. Nephrology Dialysis Transplantation 1993; 8 Suppl. 1: 680
119. De Broe ME, D'Haese PC, Drueke TB, et al. Diagnosis and treatment of aluminium overload in end-stage renal failure patients. Nephrology Dialysis Transplantation 1993; 8 Suppl. 1: 1
120. Masi CM, Cohen EP. Dialysis efficacy and itching in renal failure. Nephron 1992; 62: 257
121. Ponticelli C, Bencini PL. Uremic pruritus: a review. Nephron 1992; 60: 1
122. Bergstrom J. New aspects of erythropoietin treatment. Journal of Internal Medicine 1993; 233: 445
123. Eschbach JW. Erythropoietin: the promise and the facts. Kidney International 1994; 45 Suppl. 44: S70
124. Faulds D, Sorkin EM. Epoetin (recombinant human erythropoietin): a review of its pharmacodynamic and pharmacokinetic properties and therapeutic potential in anaemia and the stimulation of erythropoiesis. Drugs 1989; 38: 863-99
125. Dunn CJ, Markham A. Epoetin beta: a review of its pharmacological and clinical use in the management of anaemia associated with chronic renal failure. Drugs 1996; 51: 299-318
126. Korbet SM. Anemia and erythropoietin in hemodialysis and continuous ambulatory peritoneal dialysis. Kidney International 1993; 43 Suppl. 40: S111
127. Tabbara IA. Erythropoietin: biology and clinical applications. Archives of Internal Medicine 1993; 153: 298
128. Temple RM. Use of epoetin in the management of renal anaemia. Hospital Update 1994; p.166
129. Winearls C. Treatment of anaemia in renal failure. Prescribers' Journal 1992; 32: 238
130. Eberst ME, Berkowitz LR. Hemostasis in renal disease: pathophysiology and management. American Journal of Medicine 1994; 96: 168
131. Rabelink TJ, Zwaginga JJ, Koomans HA, et al. Thrombosis and hemostasis in renal disease. Kidney International 1994; 46: 287
132. Haag-Weber M, Horl WH. Uremia and infection: mechanisms of impaired cellular host defence. Nephron 1993; 63: 125
133. Kessler M, Hoen B, Mayeux D, et al. Bacteremia in patients on chronic hemodialysis. Nephron 1993; 64: 95
134. Khan IH, Catto GRD. Long-term complications of dialysis: infection. Kidney International 1993; 43 Suppl. 41: S143
135. Johnson DW, Fleming SJ. The use of vaccines in renal failure. Clinical Pharmacokinetics 1992; 22: 434
136. Petrosillo N, Puro V, Ippolito G. Prevalence of human immunodeficiency virus, hepatitis B virus and hepatitis C virus among dialysis patients. Nephron 1994; 64: 636
137. Consensus Development Conference Panel. Morbidity and mortality of renal dialysis: an NIH consensus conference statement. Annals of Internal Medicine 1994; 121: 62
138. Michael J. Chronic renal failure: end-stage management. Medicine International (Quarterly edition) 1991; 4: 3569
139. Gokal R, Mallick N. Continuous ambulatory peritoneal dialysis. Prescribers' Journal 1992; 32: 251
140. Jameson MD, Wiegmann TB. Principles, uses and complications of hemodialysis. Medical Clinics of North America 1991; 74: 945
141. Isaacs JT. Importance of the natural history of benign prostatic hypertrophy in the evaluation of pharmacological intervention. Prostate 1990; 3 Suppl.: 1
142. Jonler M, Riehmann M, Bruskewitz RC. Benign prostatic hypertrophy: current pharmacological treatment. Drugs 1994; 47: 66
143. Pascual J, Woodhouse K. Pharmacological treatment of benign prostatic hypertrophy. British Journal of Clinical Practice 1994; 48: 137
144. Chisholm GD, Khan MS. Benign prostatic hyperplasia. Practitioner 1992; 236: 325
145. Peters DH, Sorkin EM. Finasteride: a review of its potential in the treatment of benign prostatic hyperplasia. Drugs 1993; 1: 177
146. Fulton B, Wagstaff AJ, Sorkin EM. Doxazosin: an update of its clinical pharmacology and therapeutic applications in hypertension and benign prostatic hyperplasia. Drugs 1995; 49: 295-320
147. Wilde MI, Fitton A, McTavish D. Alfuzosin: a review of its pharmacodynamic and pharmacokinetic properties, and therapeutic potential in benign prostatic hyperplasia. Drugs 1993; 45: 410
148. Wilde MI, Fitton A, Sorkin EM. Terazosin: a review of its pharmacodynamic and pharmacokinetic properties, and therapeutic potential in benign prostatic hyperplasia. Drugs and Aging 1993; 3: 258
149. Anderson JT. $\alpha_1$-Blockers *vs* 5$\alpha$-reductase inhibitors in benign prostatic hyperplasia: a comparative review. Drugs and Aging 1995; 6: 388-96
150. Koren G. The nephrotoxic potential of drugs and chemicals: pharmacological basis and clinical relevance. Medical Toxicology 1989; 4: 59
151. Fillastre J-P, Godin M. Drug-induced nephropathies. In: Cameron S, Davidson AM, Grunfeld J-P, et al., editors. Oxford textbook of clinical nephrology. Vol. 1. Oxford: Oxford University Press, 1992: 159
152. Hoitsma AJ, Wetzels JFM, Koene RAP. Drug-induced nephropathy: aetiology, clinical features and management. Drug Safety 1991; 6: 131
153. Mathew TH. Drug-induced renal disease. Medical Journal of Australia 1992; 156: 724
154. Humes HD. Aminoglycoside nephrotoxicity. Kidney International 1988; 33: 900
155. Levison ME. New dosing regimens for aminoglycoside antibiotics. Annals of Internal Medicine 1992; 117: 693-4
156. Walker R. Aminoglycoside nephrotoxicity: recent developments. New Zealand Medical Journal 1994; 107: 54-5
157. McLean AJ, Ioannides-Demos LL, Spicer WJ, et al. Aminoglycoside dosing: one, two or three times a day? Medical Journal of Australia 1996; 164: 39-42
158. Chan TYK, Critchley JAJH, Chan AYW. Renal failure is common in Chinese patients with paracetamol (acetaminophen) poisoning. Veterinary and Human Toxicology 1995; 37: 154-6
159. Paton JH, Reeves DS. Clinical features and management of adverse effects of quinolone antibacterials. Drug Safety 1991; 6: 8
160. Critchley JAJH, Smith MF, Prescott LF. Distalgesic abuse and retroperitoneal fibrosis. British Journal of Urology 1985; 57: 486
161. Desai TK, Tsang TK. Aminoglycoside nephrotoxicity in obstructive jaundice. American Journal of Medicine 1988; 85: 47
162. Ellard GA. Chemotherapy of tuberculosis for patients with renal impairment. Nephron 1993; 64: 169
163. Mak RHK, De Fronzo RA. Glucose and insulin metabolism in uremia. Nephron 1992; 61: 377
164. Hellman B, Sehlin J, Taljedal IB. Glibenclamide is exceptional among hypoglycaemic agents in accumulating progressively in $\beta$-cell rich pancreatic islets. Acta Endocrinologica 1984; 105: 385

Chapter 25

# Rheumatic Disorders

*P.M. Brooks*

## Synopsis of Important Principles

1) Management of the rheumatic disorders is aimed at relief of pain, stiffness and joint swelling, maintenance of morale, of joint function and general health and well-being, control of anxiety and depression, correction of any metabolic abnormalities, and prevention of deformities and disability.

2) Drugs are used as part of a total management programme comprising patient education, specific advice on general and local rest and exercise, splintage, occupational and physiotherapy, and surgery where indicated.

3) Patients must appreciate and understand the rationale and the techniques of their own treatment since, for much of their lives, they are their own physician and therapist, and their daily ration of drugs, though controlled by the doctor, must be varied by themselves in the light of daily needs, toxic reactions and other factors.

4) Inflammation is the basis of rheumatoid arthritis and most other rheumatic disorders, but there is no agent available that can with certainty stop this inflammation progressing to erosion and destruction of joint tissues, without causing dangerous or unpleasant adverse effects.

5) Disease-modifying antirheumatic drugs (DMARDs) together with analgesics and nonsteroidal anti-inflammatory drugs (NSAIDs) are the basis of drug therapy in rheumatoid arthritis. As NSAIDs only alleviate symptoms, DMARDs such as methotrexate, chloroquine, hydroxychloroquine, gold, penicillamine and sulfasalazine should be considered at an early stage in the course of the disease and continued until lasting remission or evidence of toxicity has set in. If the disease is not controlled or intolerable adverse effects occur, DMARD therapy can be serially changed to another agent used either alone or in combination.

6) Prophylactic measures are the most desirable means of management of osteoporosis. Adequate amounts of calcium, mobility and outdoor exercises are the basis of prevention. In patients with established osteoporosis, treatment options include bone antiresorbing agents (e.g. calcium, vitamin D, estrogens, calcitonin and bisphosphonates) and drugs that stimulate bone formation (e.g. sodium fluoride, anabolic steroids).

7) Management of gout is directed at early treatment of the acute attack, prevention of subsequent attacks, and dissolution of tophaceous deposits by reducing plasma urate concentrations to normal and maintaining them there. Asymptomatic hyperuricaemia is sometimes due to reversible causes and only very rarely requires treatment. Reduction of intake of food and alcohol with weight reduction is often necessary.

8) A large number of drugs in common usage can cause aches and pains in muscles, bones, and joints, and some may precipitate gout (e.g. thiazide diuretics) or exacerbate arthritis. Drug-induced systemic lupus erythematosus (e.g. due to hydralazine or procainamide) and the bone complications of corticosteroids and long term antiepileptic drug therapy are among the most important problems.

Rheumatic diseases cause a significant burden to society in both developed and underdeveloped countries. They are a common cause of presentation to a general practitioner and the cost of these diseases in both direct and indirect terms is enormous. They are a major cause of long term disability and there is increasing evidence that the inflammatory rheumatic diseases such as the vasculitides, systemic lupus erythematosus and rheumatoid arthritis significantly shorten lifespan.[1] The major forms of rheumatic disease are shown in table I. The therapeutic issues involved in the management of rheumatic diseases cover a wide spectrum, not only because of the high prevalence of the disease in the community but also because rheumatic diseases often affect young people and the duration of their disability is significant.

## 1. Clinical Pharmacological Considerations and General Principles of Treatment

The study of the rheumatic disorders is essentially a study of 'long pain'.[2] This brings with it all the attendant problems of managing chronic disease with persisting symptoms and progressive disability. Pain must be managed comprehensively as must the associated patient responses of anxiety, depression and despair.

**Table I.** Classification of rheumatoid diseases

| Class | Diseases |
|---|---|
| Soft tissue | Fibrositis<br>Strains, sprains<br>Tissue and tendon injuries<br>Fibrositis (fibromyalgia syndrome) |
| Regenerative disease | Osteoarthritis |
| Crystal arthropathies | Gout<br>Calcium pyrophosphate<br>Calcium hydroxyapatite |
| Inflammatory poly- or oligoarthritis | Rheumatoid arthritis<br>Spondyloarthropathies:<br>• ankylosing spondylitis<br>• psoriatic<br>• reactive<br>• associated with inflammatory bowel disease |
| Vasculitides | Polyarteritis nodosa<br>Wegener's<br>Churg-Strauss<br>Temporal arteritis/polymyalgia rheumatica |
| Systemic connective tissue disease | Systemic lupus erythematosus<br>Progressive systemic sclerosis/CREST<br>Polydermatomyositis |

*Abbreviation:* CREST = calcinosis, Raynaud's phenomenon, oesophageal dysfunction, sclerodactyly, telangiectasia.

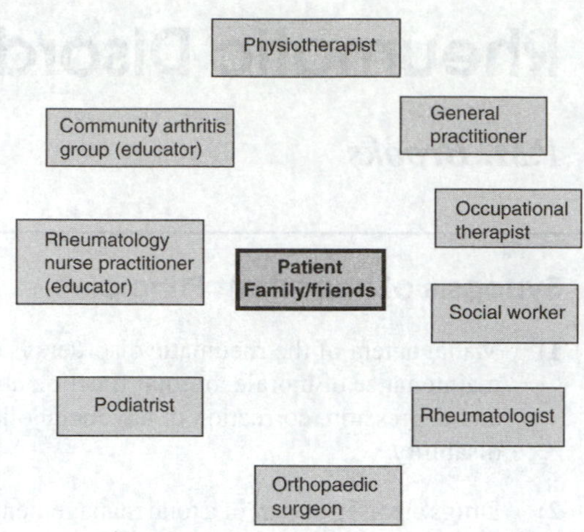


**Fig. 1.** Healthcare team involved in the management of rheumatoid arthritis.

Multidisciplinary management is very important in the rheumatic diseases, each individual in the team (including the patient and the patient's family) playing an important role. Pain is usually not alleviated completely, but any small decrease provided by an individual intervention may mean the difference between the patient coping or not. The various individuals involved in the team management of rheumatic diseases are shown in figure 1.

The patient and the patient's pain must remain the focus of attention but will need to be supported by physical therapies, advice regarding activities of daily living (including appropriate rest, splinting, support or orthoses for painful feet), education delivered by medical practitioners and nurses (possibly rheumatologically trained) or community groups, and surgical support for joint replacement and other techniques. Management of the multidisciplinary team can become a difficulty in itself, but is usually coordinated by the rheumatologist and the general practitioner, who must maintain the confidence of the patient over a long period of time. The patient's family and friends, including the employer, also play an important role.

### 1.1 Aims of Treatment

Since the causes of most rheumatic diseases are unknown, treatment is aimed at relief of pain and control of inflammation, slowing the disease process while maintaining good general health. The aim of therapy in the management of rheumatic disorders, therefore, is to:

- Relieve pain and enable more normal function at work, home and rest
- Relieve stiffness and swelling, thus maintaining function and mobility, and preventing contractures and deformities
- Maintain and promote general health, well-being and normal nutrition, and prevent and treat anaemia
- Prevent and control depression and anxiety, and maintain morale and normal mental health
- Correct any metabolic abnormalities.

These goals are approached by judicious use of drugs as part of a total management programme that includes patient education, specific advice on general and local rest and exercise, splinting, occupational and physiotherapy, podiatry and surgery delivered by the individuals depicted in figure 1.

### 1.2 Clinical Pharmacological Factors and Drug Selection

Drugs available to treat rheumatic disorders include analgesics, nonsteroidal anti-inflammatory drugs (NSAIDs), the so-called disease-modifying antirheumatic drugs (DMARDs) [also called slow-acting antirheumatic drugs (SAARDs)], corticosteroids, and drugs that may elevate mood and promote general well-being. To this list must now be added newer immunomodulating agents that, although in an early phase of clinical development, have enormous potential for the treatment (and possible control) of many inflammatory rheumatic conditions (table II) [see also chapter 28; sect. 3.3].

All these drugs must be used judiciously and for appropriate reasons, to relieve pain and inflammation in each patient. There are no fixed rules and trial and error must be applied in most cases, with patients often knowing what suits them best.[3] Some general guidelines, however, can be given regarding clinical pharmacological factors that influence the selection and use of these drugs.

#### *1.2.1 The Nature of the Disease*

Where a powerful anti-inflammatory action is required, as in the treatment of acute gout, severe active rheumatoid arthritis or reactive arthritis, anti-inflammatory agents such as an NSAID in high dosage are required. With regenerative non-inflammatory conditions such as osteoarthritis, which cause intermittent pain, rapid-acting, simple analgesics such as paracetamol (acetaminophen) are more appropriate. However, if this does not control the pain or if there is evidence of an inflammatory component, NSAIDs may be required intermittently.

**Table II.** Drugs used in the management of rheumatic disorders

| | |
|---|---|
| **Analgesics without anti-inflammatory activity** | |
| *Mild analgesics:* | *Opioids* (rarely used): |
| • Paracetamol (acetaminophen) | • Morphine |
| • Codeine | • Pethidine (meperidine) |
| • Dextropropoxyphene | |
| **Nonsteroidal anti-inflammatory drugs (NSAIDs)** | |
| *Salicylates:* | *Oxicams:* |
| • Aspirin | • Ampiroxicam |
| • Benorilate (benorylate) | • Droxicam |
| • Choline magnesium salicylate | • Lornoxicam |
| | • Meloxicam |
| • Diflunisal | • Piroxicam (and piroxicam-β-cyclodextrin) |
| • Salsalate | |
| *Benzene acetic acid derivatives:* | • Tenoxicam |
| | *Indole/indene derivatives:* |
| • Aceclofenac | • Acemetacin |
| • Bromfenac | • Indomethacin |
| • Diclofenac | • Sulindac |
| *Propionic acid derivatives:* | *Pyrazolones:* |
| • Carprofen | • Azapropazone |
| • Fenbufen | • Oxyphenbutazone |
| • Fenoprofen | • Phenylbutazone |
| • Flurbiprofen | *Fenamates:* |
| • Ibuprofen | • Meclofenamate sodium |
| • Ketoprofen | *Others:* |
| • Naproxen | • Etodolac |
| • Oxaprozin | • Nabumetone |
| • Pirprofen | • Nimesulide |
| • Tiaprofenic acid | • Tolmetin |
| • Zaltoprofen | |
| **Corticosteroids** | |
| • Prednisolone, prednisone | |
| • Methylprednisolone | |
| **Disease-modifying antirheumatic drugs (DMARDs)** | |
| • Gold compounds (auranofin, aurothiomalate sodium, aurothioglucose) | |
| • Penicillamine | |
| • Antimalarials (chloroquine, hydroxychloroquine) | |
| • Sulfasalazine | |
| • Methotrexate | |
| • Azathioprine | |
| • Cyclophosphamide | |
| • Chlorambucil | |
| • Cyclosporin | |
| *Cytokine modulator:* | |
| • Tenidap[a] | |
| **Other immunomodulators** | |
| • Anti-TNF-α (anti-tumour necrosis factor-α) | |
| • Anti-CD4 monoclonal antibody | |
| **Antidepressants and anxiolytics** | |
| • Selective serotonin reuptake inhibitors (SSRIs) | |
| • Benzodiazepines | |

a Tenidap also exerts NSAID-like anti-inflammatory activity via inhibition of cyclo-oxygenase.

#### 1.2.2 Stage of the Disease

NSAIDs will only relieve symptoms and, therefore, in chronic diseases such as rheumatoid arthritis or seronegative spondyloarthritis, disease-modifying antirheumatic drugs should be commenced when the diagnosis has been confirmed. There is increasing evidence that these drugs will slow progression of the disease, particularly if they are used early.[4]

#### 1.2.3 Patient Preferences

Patients are often the best judge of what drug provides the greatest relief from symptoms with minimum adverse effects. However, they need to be provided with appropriate information about the adverse effects of continuing active disease and of drug therapy.

#### 1.2.4 Presence of Complications

Some patients, particularly those with a recent history of peptic ulcer, tolerate anti-inflammatory drugs poorly. Appropriate alternative agents should be selected or prophylaxis with antiulcer preparations given (e.g. misoprostol; see further chapter 22; sect 4.1.3). Simple analgesic drugs may be substituted for NSAIDs but, if NSAIDs are required, then use of a suppository formulation may be appropriate.

#### 1.2.5 Coexisting Disease States

Many patients with rheumatic diseases are elderly and have cardiac, renal or hepatic disease. Particular care must be taken with these patients since many NSAIDs and disease-modifying antirheumatic drugs cause fluid retention and exacerbate cardiac failure, or interfere with renal or hepatic function.

#### 1.2.6 Clinically Important Drug Interactions

Interactions may occur between various drugs a patient may be taking. For example, most NSAIDs modify the dosage requirements of lithium and attenuate the effects of antihypertensive agents, and may potentiate the effects of other drugs such as oral anticoagulants. The major interactions with NSAIDs are shown in table III.

Interactions involving the disease-modifying antirheumatic drugs appear to be of less clinical significance, although with *methotrexate*, considerable caution is required if this drug is used in combination with NSAIDs since the latter may reduce the renal clearance of methotrexate and thereby increase its plasma concentrations and the risk of toxicity. However, this does not usually occur with the low dosage (up to 25mg weekly) of methotrexate normally used in rheumatic disease. Serious haematological toxicity can occur with methotrexate if it is administered with other folate antagonists such as cotrimoxazole (trimethoprim/sulfamethoxazole) and other sulfonamides, and such combinations should be avoided. Methotrexate has, however, been successfully combined with sulfasazaline without significant toxicity. The combined cytokine/cyclo-oxygenase modulator *tenidap* appears to have a similar drug interaction profile to that of the NSAIDs[5] [see also review by Munro & Sturrock[6] for further discussion on potential drug interactions with DMARDs].

### 1.3 General Education and Instruction of the Patient

Patient education has become an important part of the management of chronic disease. This is particularly so in the rheumatic diseases where patients need to feel that they are in control of their disease and can use a variety of strategies for reducing pain. They need to know about the disease, what it will do and, probably more importantly, what it will not do. They need to appreciate that some rheumatic diseases cause chronic disability, making early treatment (particularly in rheumatoid arthritis) essential if disability is to be reduced. They should also be advised on the management of their lives at home and at work, and instructed in the art of rest, relaxation and exercise. Time must be made during the consultation for patients to ask questions about their condition and to discuss their own and their families' futures. They may receive different forms of physiotherapy, including nonspecific and specific exercises, and may be given advice regarding splints.

It is essential that all patients are counselled about their drugs and particularly about potential adverse effects. Patients receiving drugs such as gold and penicillamine can be instructed to test their own urine for evidence of proteinuria and haematuria and to be involved in monitoring their own treatment.

Patients with rheumatic diseases live with their condition for long periods of time. They often know and understand their disease much better than their doctor does, but they still need to be given appropriate advice and support, and be shown that there is always something that can be done.

## 2. Rheumatic Fever

Acute rheumatic fever (ARF) is an inflammatory disease presenting as a delayed response to

**Table III.** Interactions of nonsteroidal anti-inflammatory drugs (NSAIDs) with other drugs (after Brooks & Day[14])

| Drug affected | NSAIDs implicated | Effect | Management/implications for therapy |
|---|---|---|---|
| **Pharmacokinetic interactions** | | | |
| *NSAIDs affecting other drugs:* | | | |
| Warfarin | Phenylbutazone, oxyphenbutazone<br>Azapropazone | Inhibition of metabolism of *S*-warfarin, increasing anticoagulant effect | Avoid these NSAIDs if possible, or monitor closely |
| Lithium | Probably all (except possibly sulindac and aspirin) | Inhibition of renal excretion of lithium and risk of toxicity | Use sulindac or aspirin if an NSAID must be used. Monitor lithium concentration carefully and make appropriate dose reduction |
| Oral antidiabetic agents | Phenylbutazone, oxyphenbutazone<br>Azapropazone | Inhibition of metabolism of sulphonylurea drugs, prolonging their half-lives and increasing the risk of hypoglycaemia | Avoid these NSAIDs if possible; if not, monitor blood glucose closely |
| Phenytoin | Phenylbutazone, oxyphenbutazone | Inhibition of metabolism of phenytoin, increasing plasma phenytoin concentration and risk of toxicity | Avoid these NSAIDs if possible; if not, intensify therapeutic drug monitoring |
| | Others | Reduction of total phenytoin concentration for the same unbound (active) concentration [via displacement from plasma protein binding sites] | Interpret total plasma concentration of phenytoin carefully; measuring the unbound concentration may be helpful |
| Methotrexate (high nonrheumatological dosage) | Probably all | Reduced clearance of methotrexate (by unknown mechanism), increasing plasma methotrexate concentration and risk of toxicity | Coadministration is contraindicated. Use of NSAIDs between cycles of chemotherapy is probably safe. Interaction not seen with rheumatological dosages of methotrexate |
| Valproic acid | Aspirin | Inhibition of valproic acid metabolism, increasing plasma valproic acid concentration | Avoid aspirin; monitor plasma valproic acid concentration closely if an NSAID is used |
| Digoxin | All | Potential reduction in renal function (esp. in very young and very old patients), reducing digoxin clearance and increasing plasma digoxin concentration and risk of toxicity (no interaction if renal function is normal) | Avoid NSAIDs if possible; if not, measure plasma digoxin and creatinine concentrations frequently |
| Aminoglycosides | All | Reduction in renal function in susceptible persons, lowering aminoglycoside clearance and increasing plasma aminoglycoside concentrations | Monitor plasma aminoglycoside concentrations closely and adjust the dosage accordingly |
| *Other drugs affecting NSAIDs:* | | | |
| Antacids | Indomethacin | Variable effects of different preparations; rate and extent of absorption of indomethacin reduced by aluminium-containing antacids, but increased by sodium bicarbonate | No action required unless interaction results in poor response to the NSAID; dosage may need to be increased. Rate of absorption of other NSAIDs can be slowed by antacids |
| Probenecid | Probably all | Reduction in metabolism and renal clearance of NSAIDs and acyl glucuronide metabolites, which are hydrolysed back to parent drug | |
| Barbiturates | Phenylbutazone, possibly others | Increased metabolic clearance of NSAID | May require higher doses of phenylbutazone |
| Cholestyramine | Naproxen and probably others | Binding of NSAIDs to cholestyramine in gut, reducing rate (and possibly extent) of absorption | No action required; separate administration times by 4h; may need larger than expected doses of NSAID |
| Metoclopramide | Aspirin and others | Increased rate and extent of absorption of aspirin in patients with migraine | |

[Continued over]

Table III. *[Continued]*

| Drug affected | NSAIDs implicated | Effect | Management/implications for therapy |
|---|---|---|---|
| **Pharmacodynamic interactions** | | | |
| *NSAID affecting other drugs:* | | | |
| β-Blockers<br>Diuretics<br>ACE inhibitors | Indomethacin<br>Others (except possibly sulindac) | Reduction in antihypertensive effect, probably related to inhibition of prostaglandin synthesis in kidneys (via retention of salt and water) and blood vessels, increasing vasconstriction | Avoid NSAIDs in patients treated for hypertension, if possible. Check blood pressure repeatedly after starting NSAID; additional antihypertensive therapy may be needed |
| Diuretics | Indomethacin<br>Others (except possibly sulindac) | Reduction in natriuretic effects; may exacerbate congestive cardiac failure | Avoid NSAID use in patients with cardiac failure, if possible; if not, use sulindac and monitor for clinical signs of fluid retention |
| Anticoagulants | All | Damage to mucosa of gastrointestinal tract and inhibition of platelet aggregation, both increasing risk of gastrointestinal bleeding | Avoid all NSAIDs, if possible |
| Antidiabetic agents | Salicylates (high-dose) | Hypoglycaemic effects (unknown mechanism) | Monitor blood glucose level |
| *Combination with increased risk of toxicity:* | | | |
| Diuretics (in general) | All | Combination associated with increased risk of haemodynamic renal failure | Avoid combination if possible |
| Triamterene | Indomethacin | Potentiation of nephrotoxicity, even when renal function is normal | Combination contraindicated |
| Potassium-sparing diuretics | All | Potassium retention and hyperkalaemia | Avoid combination; monitor plasma potassium level |

pharyngeal infection with group A streptococci. The major clinical features are those of arthritis and carditis with major and minor clinical manifestations making up the Jones' criteria for diagnosis (table IV).[7] Although developed countries report a steady decline in the incidence of this disease, it is still seen in countries where poor hygiene and overcrowding are social problems.[8] Between 1 and 3% of children with known untreated epidemic exudative pharyngitis and a positive culture for *Streptococcus pyogenes* will develop acute rheumatic fever[9] and the most important preventive measure is early diagnosis and effective treatment with penicillin for at least 10 days.

## 2.1 Optimum Treatment

The principles of management of rheumatic fever include:

- Early diagnosis and application of the Jones' criteria (table IV)
- Salicylate therapy for the control of joint inflammation and fever
- Corticosteroids if severe carditis is present
- Bedrest if carditis is present (until signs of acute inflammation have decreased and remain low)
- Antibacterial therapy to eradicate possible *S. pyogenes* infection from the throat (10 days of oral phenoxymethylpenicillin or erythromycin or a single intramuscular dose of benzathine benzylpenicillin)
- Control of chorea symptoms (e.g. with haloperidol, carbamazepine, phenobarbital or valproic acid)
- Prevention of recurrent attacks by continuous penicillin prophylaxis (for 10 years or until age 21 years, whichever is longer); erythromycin prophylaxis may be given in penicillin-allergic patients
- Primary prevention of rheumatic fever by adequate treatment of pharyngeal infection by group A β-haemolytic streptococci.[10]

### Acute Attacks

In the treatment of an acute attack, bedrest is the rule for as long as there is evidence of disease activity but, in the absence of carditis, strict bedrest is unnecessary after other acute symptoms have abated. Any β-haemolytic streptococcal carrier state, whether confirmed or not by throat culture, is treated by full doses of penicillin for 10 days, e.g. *benzylpenicillin* (penicillin G) 1MU by intramuscular injection daily or oral *phenoxymethylpenicillin* (penicillin V) 250mg (young children) to 500mg every 6 hours. *Erythromycin* (250mg 4 times daily for 10 days) can be used in penicillin-allergic patients.

*Aspirin* has a profound effect on the clinical manifestations of rheumatic fever and is given in a dose of 100 to 130 mg/kg of bodyweight daily. The total dosage can vary from 2 g/day in children to 8 g/day in adults, and is usually only required for 1 to 2 weeks. Serum salicylate concentrations of 1.8 mmol/L (25 mg/100ml) or more are usually required in adults and should be greater in children. Concentrations of about 1.8 to 2.5 mmol/L (25 to 35 mg/100ml) give maximum symptomatic control. Salicylates appear to have no effect on the disease process or its eventual outcome, even when given in larger amounts. However, symptoms are relieved, although salicylates may precipitate heart failure and must be used carefully if carditis is present.

*Corticosteroids* may be indicated in severely ill patients, although there is no evidence that corticosteroids will decrease the severity or prevent the development of residual heart disease. If congestive cardiac failure occurs, treatment with digitalis and diuretics may be required.

**Prevention of Recurrences**

The prevention of rheumatic fever recurrence is based essentially on the elimination of streptococcal infection. This can be achieved by an intramuscular injection of 1 to 1.5 MU *benzathine benzylpenicillin* every month. Oral *phenoxymethylpenicillin* 250mg twice daily 1 hour before food is probably slightly less effective and is only suitable for cooperative patients in whom compliance can be assured. *Erythromycin* 125mg twice daily can be used in cases of penicillin hypersensitivity. This preventive treatment is given to all children who have had rheumatic fever and/or evidence of rheumatic carditis. Such prophylaxis should be carried out throughout childhood.

Though options vary thereafter, prophylaxis for life is considered necessary by many investigators for patients with rheumatic carditis. The risk, though less, still remains in late middle life. Crowded living conditions such as in army barracks, schools, hospitals, and disadvantaged groups carry extra risk and it is wise to continue prophylaxis throughout such periods of greater exposure. In general, only special risk groups or patients with carditis need continued preventive therapy after 25 years of age. The major risk is in childhood and early adolescence. Should streptococcal infection occur despite the prophylactic regimen, a full therapeutic dosage of penicillin (or erythromycin in penicillin-hypersensitive individuals) should be given for a minimum of 10 days. Where valvular damage has occurred, prophylactic antibiotics to prevent bacterial endocarditis should be given to cover operations on teeth and tonsils, and instrumentation of the urogenital tract.

## 3. Rheumatoid Arthritis

Rheumatoid arthritis is a chronic inflammatory arthritis of variable expression. It may present as an acute polyarthritis or as fleeting joint pains progressing over a period of months. Rheumatoid arthritis has a worldwide distribution, with an incidence of approximately 1% of

**Table IV.** Revised Jones criteria for diagnosis of acute rheumatic fever. The presence of 2 major or 1 major and 2 minor manifestations, plus evidence of a preceding streptococcal infection, indicates a high probability of rheumatic fever[a]

| Major manifestations | Minor manifestations |
|---|---|
| Carditis | *Clinical:* |
| Polyarthritis | Fever |
| Chorea | Arthralgia |
| Erythema marginatum | Previous rheumatic fever or rheumatic heart disease |
| Subcutaneous nodules | Prolonged pulse rate interval |
| | *Laboratory:* |
| | Acute-phase reactants |
| | Abnormal erythrocyte sedimentation rate |
| | C-reactive protein |
| | Leucocytosis |

*Previous infection is indicated by:*[b]

- Increased antistreptolysin O or other streptococcal antibody
- Positive throat culture for group A streptococci
- Recent scarlet fever

a These recommendations of the American Heart Association are approved by the World Health Organization Study Group so long as the following rheumatic fever entities are dealt with separately and exempted from fulfilling the Jones Criteria: pure chorea, late onset carditis, and rheumatic recurrence.

b Manifestations with a long latent period, such as chorea and late onset carditis, are exempted from this last requirement.

the population. The expression of the disease varies across the world, with a lower incidence of vasculitis and extra-articular manifestations in tropical countries. It is now appreciated that patients with rheumatic disease presenting to tertiary referral centres have significant morbidity and mortality, and have a reduction in life expectancy similar to that of patients with 3-vessel coronary artery disease or Hodgkin's disease.[11] We also know that joint erosions occur within the first 2 years of rheumatoid arthritis and cartilage damage will, therefore, manifest at a much earlier stage. This demands that patients with rheumatoid arthritis be treated aggressively from the time of diagnosis. Pain relief must be provided with analgesic and anti-inflammatory agents, but disease-modifying antirheumatic drugs must also be used at this early stage.

## 3.1 Clinical Pharmacology of Drugs Used in Treatment

### *3.1.1 Analgesics*

Although NSAIDs (see section 3.1.2) will provide some analgesic effect, the addition of regular paracetamol (acetaminophen) can lead to a significant reduction in NSAID requirements.[12] Analgesics such as paracetamol can be used prophylactically before performing necessary tasks that produce pain and can be added to an NSAID regimen. Other analgesics such as codeine, dihydrocodeine and dextropropoxyphene are sometimes used, but tend to have a greater potential for causing constipation (for further discussion of the clinical pharmacology of analgesics, see chapter 12. sect. 7.1). It has been suggested that low doses of NSAIDs are also analgesic without having an anti-inflammatory component and this may be the case for doses of salicylates <2 g/day.[13]

When analgesics are employed in patients with rheumatoid arthritis, they should be used to reduce baseline requirements for NSAIDs.

### *3.1.2 Nonsteroidal Anti-Inflammatory Drugs (NSAIDs)*

NSAIDs are used extremely widely in the community for a variety of musculoskeletal conditions and still provide the mainstay of therapy for inflammatory forms of arthritis. However, while they provide good symptomatic relief in rheumatoid arthritis, there is no evidence that they alter disease progression.

NSAIDs are also being used increasingly in non-rheumatic conditions including acute and chronic pain, biliary and ureteric colic, dysmenorrhoea and potentially for cancer and Alzheimer's disease. They make up one of the largest groups of pharmaceutical agents sold around the world, and upwards of 20% of those aged over 65 years as well as 20% of persons admitted to hospital are taking these drugs.[14]

#### Mechanism/Site of Action

The major mechanism of action of NSAIDs is the inhibition of cyclo-oxygenase activity and, therefore, the synthesis of prostaglandins.[15] Recent data suggest that the cyclo-oxygenase enzymes can be divided into two isoforms – a constitutive enzyme (COX-1), which is responsible for maintaining normal function particularly of the gastrointestinal and renal tracts, and an inducible form (COX-2), which is found at inflammatory sites and in the brain.[16] The majority of NSAIDs currently available are nonselective inhibitors, although some (e.g. meloxicam, nimesulide) are much more specific for COX-2 and may have the advantage of reduced gastrotoxicity.[17-19]

Cyclo-oxygenase inhibition by NSAIDs may have secondary effects including the inhibition of neutrophil activation, leukotriene production and T and B cell proliferation.[20] NSAIDs also interfere with a variety of membrane-associated processes including the activity of NADPH oxidase in neutrophils and the activity of phospholipase C in macrophages. A variety of non-prostaglandin processes are also effected, including activity of enzymes such as phospholipase C, the synthesis of proteoglycans by chondrocytes, transmembrane ion fluxes and cell-cell binding. Some of these effects are concentration-dependent, and are seen within the range found in joint tissues with standard dosages so that variations in dosage and pharmacokinetics may explain some of the variability in response to NSAIDs. The principle processes influenced by NSAIDs are shown in table V.

The differential effects of various NSAIDs on neutrophil activation and aggregation and on lipoxygenase pathway inhibition are exemplified in table VI. Similar differences between NSAIDs can be found with respect to oxygen radical regeneration and chemotaxis. These *in vitro* differences have been corroborated *ex vivo* in small numbers of patients with rheumatoid arthritis.[20]

#### Pharmacodynamic Properties

The anti-inflammatory actions of naproxen, carprofen and ibuprofen are linear in relation to

**Table V.** Processes influenced by nonsteroidal anti-inflammatory drugs (NSAIDs)

| |
|---|
| Prostaglandin production |
| Leukotriene synthesis |
| Superoxide generation |
| Lysosomal enzyme release |
| Neutrophil aggregation and adhesion |
| Cell-membrane functions: |
| • Enzyme activity (NADPH oxidase, phospholipase C) |
| • Transmembrane anion transport |
| • Oxidative phosphorylation |
| • Uptake of arachidonic acid |
| Lymphocyte function |
| Rheumatoid factor production |
| Cartilage metabolism |

the dose or plasma concentration in patients with rheumatoid arthritis. However, relationships between plasma concentrations and the toxicity of NSAIDs in humans have not been demonstrated, with the exception of the linear relationship between plasma concentrations of salicylate and ototoxicity,[21] and a relationship between NSAID dosage and gastrointestinal bleeding.[22,23]

Circadian rhythms have been demonstrated for both drug activity and inflammation and there may be preferable times for the administration of even sustained-release preparations. Flurbiprofen given at bedtime and in the morning has been shown to provide more relief than treatment regimens that included a morning and noon dose or a noon and evening dose.[24]

A number of other factors relating to clinician prescribing behaviour and the patient's previous experience or expectations with NSAIDs can also determine the response.

### Pharmacokinetic Characteristics

NSAIDs can be divided into 2 general groups with regard to plasma half-life - those with a short half-life (less than 4 hours) and those with longer half-lives (12 hours or more). Interestingly, even short half-life drugs such as ibuprofen have been shown to produce equivalent disease control with a twice-daily administration regimen as opposed to a 4-times-daily regimen. This is because the pharmacokinetics of NSAIDs within synovial fluid (and probably synovial tissue) tend to decrease the differences between drugs with long and short plasma half-lives. The mean total drug concentration (bound plus unbound) in synovial fluid within a dosage interval is approximately 60% of the mean concentration in plasma over that period regardless of the elimination half-life, and this concentration varies little between patients.[25] Synovial fluid concentrations of long half-life NSAIDs tend to parallel plasma concentrations, while the synovial fluid concentrations of NSAIDs with a shorter half-life are initially lower, but often remain higher than plasma concentrations beyond the equilibration points.[14]

Most NSAIDs are extensively bound (>98%) to albumin. Protein binding is saturable in the usual therapeutic dosage range for some NSAIDs, including naproxen, phenylbutazone and ibuprofen, so that an increasing daily dosage leads to a less than proportional increase in steady-state trough concentrations, with unbound concentrations increasing in proportion to the dose. Unbound concentrations of naproxen are higher in elderly patients and those with active rheumatoid arthritis.[26]

The disposition of some NSAIDs is complicated by the fact that they exist as 2 optical isomers or enantiomers[27] (see also chapter 1, sect. 3.2.1). Naproxen is marketed as the active *S*-enantiomer, but other aryl propionic acids such as ibuprofen, ketoprofen and flurbiprofen are available as equal mixtures of the inactive

**Table VI.** Differences in mechanisms of action among various nonsteroidal anti-inflammatory drugs (NSAIDs). All values are percentages over or under control, after treatment with the given NSAID (after Furst[20])

| Mechanism | Indomethacin | Piroxicam | Salicylate | Aspirin | Ibuprofen |
|---|---|---|---|---|---|
| $LTB_4$-induced PMN aggregation[a] | –43 | –70 | –50 | –50 | - |
| Lysozyme release[b] | –47 | –85 | - | - | –60 |
| FMLP-induced superoxide generation[b] | - | –60 | - | - | –5 |
| FMLP-induced increase in cyclic-AMP[c] | 123 | NS | 124 | 118 | - |
| Inhibition of calcium uptake[c] | –50 | –20 | –21 | - | - |
| Arachidonic acid-induced platelet aggregation | - | - | Minimal | –100 | - |

a Reflects polymorphonuclear cell (PMN) aggregation.
b Reflects PMN function and activation.
c Reflects PMN chemotaxis.
*Abbreviations and symbols:* $LTB_4$ = leukotriene $B_4$; NS = not significant; PMN = polymorphonuclear cell; FMLP = *N*-formyl-methionyl-leucylphenylalanine.

**Table VII.** Factors contributing to interindividual variability in response to nonsteroidal anti-inflammatory drugs (NSAIDs)

| Factor | Relevance for response variability |
|---|---|
| **Physicochemical properties of NSAIDs:** | |
| Lipid solubility | More lipid-soluble NSAIDs may have greater anti-inflammatory activity, analgesia and CNS toxicity |
| Synovial fluid pH | Variable depending on pathology; interacts with NSAID $pK_a$ to influence NSAID uptake into joints |
| Prodrug (e.g. sulindac) | May be less nephrotoxic than other NSAIDs due to its unique metabolic activation/inactivation |
| **Pharmacokinetic factors:** | |
| Genetic | Polymorphic oxidation (e.g. piroxicam) and enantiomers (e.g. ibuprofen) may affect the active plasma concentration |
| Environmental | Diet, smoking, physical activity and circadian rhythms may variably influence NSAID metabolism |
| Renal disease or age-related decline in renal function | A variable reduction occurs in the clearance of renally excreted NSAIDs and in the clearance of NSAIDs metabolised to acyl glucuronides |
| **Pharmacodynamic factors:** | |
| Polymorphonuclear cell function | NSAIDs differ in their effects on aggregation, lysosomal enzyme release, free radical production and membrane viscosity |
| Arachidonic acid and cartilage metabolism | NSAIDs have various effects on these processes |
| Immune function | Inhibition of rheumatoid synovial tissue synthesis of rheumatoid factor |
| **Physician prescribing behaviour and patient expectations:** | |
| Concurrent use of >1 NSAID | Prevalence of concurrent use of multiple NSAIDs varies across countries and may differentially affect the risk of adverse reactions |
| Placebo response | More likely in educated professionals, single women and women working outside the home |

*R*- and active *S*-enantiomers. A unique unidirectional conversion of aryl propionic acid NSAIDs from the *R* to the *S* form occurs to a variable degree *in vivo*, depending on the drug and the recipient. For example, the *R* form of fenoprofen is converted almost totally to the *S* form, whereas little if any *R*-ketoprofen or *R*-flurbiprofen is converted to the *S* form. Recently, it has been demonstrated[28] that *S*-ibuprofen accounts for most of analgesic efficacy of ibuprofen in hip and knee osteoarthritis, while the *R* component adds little to correlations between the plasma concentration and clinical response.

Most NSAIDs, with the notable exception of azapropazone, are extensively metabolised by the liver. The drug is either inactivated (e.g. ibuprofen, diclofenac) or activated (e.g. sulindac, nabumetone or aspirin). NSAIDs such as indomethacin and sulindac undergo extensive enterohepatic recycling and many drugs are glucuronidated in the liver, making them more soluble for renal excretion. Some NSAIDs are partly excreted unchanged in the urine, and the clearance of ketoprofen, fenoprofen, naproxen and carprofen is decreased to a variable degree in patients with renal failure or those taking probenecid. This is because the acyl glucuronide metabolites of these agents are retained and hydrolysed to reform the parent compound.

Lipid solubility is also an important determinant of distribution and lipid-soluble drugs such as indomethacin, although having potent anti-inflammatory activity, cause a significant incidence of CNS adverse effects.

### Clinical Effectiveness

It is often said that all NSAIDs are similar with respect to effectiveness. Although this statement is generally true when dealing with populations of patients with rheumatoid arthritis, it is clearly not true for each individual. A number of factors influence the variability in response to NSAIDs (table VII). The origin of this variability between individuals in responsiveness and for patient preferences for different NSAIDs is still not clear, and its study is complicated by the fluctuations in intensity of symptoms in rheumatoid arthritis.

### Tolerability and Drug Interactions Potential

NSAIDs are one of the most common causes of adverse drug reactions reported to drug regulatory authorities. The most common adverse effects are those affecting the gastrointestinal system, but renal toxicity, skin reactions, blood dyscrasias and headaches can also occur.[29]

The common adverse effects noted with NSAIDs are shown in table VIII. As prostaglandins play an important role in maintaining normal gastrointestinal and renal physiology, it is not surprising that these drugs interfere with the normal functioning of these organs. NSAIDs are associated with gastric erosion, peptic ulceration and haemorrhage, as well as producing inflammation in the small and large intestine.[30] Nonspecific colitis has also been described.

Estimates for the absolute risk of developing a serious gastrointestinal adverse event varies from approximately 2 cases per 10,000 person months of prescription to a 7-fold risk in the increase of hospitalisation in patients with rheumatoid arthritis.[31] Recently, there have been a series of studies which for the first time suggest a hierarchy of NSAIDs with respect to the risk of serious upper gastrointestinal adverse effects.[23,32,33]

***Prophylaxis of NSAID-induced ulcers:*** the prostaglandin analogue *misoprostol* decreases the incidence of gastric ulcers by between 50 and 90% when used with NSAIDs for a 3- to 12-month period. The cost-effectiveness of misoprostol prophylaxis is dependent on a number of factors, including the ulcer occurrence rate, the high outpatient and inpatient hospital costs, and the relatively low cost of misoprostol (of the order of $US90 or less for 3 months).[34] $H_2$-Receptor antagonists such as cimetidine or ranitidine and the mucosal protective agent sucralfate do not seem to prevent NSAID-induced gastric ulcers. Although $H_2$-antagonists are useful in preventing duodenal ulcers, most NSAID-induced ulcers occur in the stomach. Precisely which patients should receive prophylaxis is still debated, but people over 65 years of age, with a previous history of peptic ulceration and severe rheumatoid arthritis requiring an NSAID should probably be given prophylaxis.

**Table VIII.** Adverse effects of nonsteroidal anti-inflammatory drugs (NSAIDs)

| System | Effect |
|---|---|
| Gastrointestinal | Peptic ulceration |
| | Oesophagitis and strictures |
| | Small and large bowel ulceration |
| | Colitis |
| Renal | Reversible acute renal failure |
| | Fluid and electrolyte disturbances |
| | Chronic renal failure and interstitial fibrosis |
| | Interstitial nephritis |
| | Nephrotic syndrome |
| | Cystitis |
| Cardiovascular | Exacerbation of hypertension |
| | Exacerbation of congestive cardiac failure |
| | Exacerbation of angina |
| Hepatic | Transaminitis |
| | Fulminant hepatic failure (rare) |
| Central nervous system | Headache |
| | Drowsiness |
| | Confusion and behaviour disturbance |
| | Aseptic meningitis |
| Haematological | Thrombocytopenia |
| | Haemolytic anaemia |
| | Agranulocytosis and aplastic anaemia |
| Other | Exacerbation of asthma in patients with nasal polyposis |
| | Skin rash |

Patients who develop peptic ulceration while taking an NSAID should be treated as follows: if an analgesic such as paracetamol can be substituted for the NSAID or if corticosteroids can be given for a short period of time, the ulcer is likely to heal more rapidly. The ulcer should be treated with an $H_2$-antagonist, sucralfate or an acid (proton) pump inhibitor such as omeprazole.[35] If *Helicobacter pylori* is present, antibiotics (e.g. clarithromycin or amoxicillin plus metronidazole) should also be given (see further chapter 22; sect. 4.3.6).

***NSAID-induced renal impairment:*** NSAIDs have been associated with reversible impairment of glomerular filtration, acute renal failure, oedema, interstitial nephritis, capillary necrosis, chronic renal failure or hyperkalaemia.[36] They are particularly likely to decrease glomerular filtration in patients with hypovolaemic states due to salt depletion or hypoalbuminaemia and in those with pre-existing renal impairment due to age, atherosclerosis, hypertensive renal disease or other intrinsic renal disease. There is general agreement that no NSAID can be prescribed with absolute safety with respect to renal adverse effects. There does, however, seem to be some selectivity in the type of renal reaction produced by NSAIDs, interstitial nephritis, for example, being seen most commonly with some drugs while interstitial cystitis has been reported with tiaprofenic acid.

***Drug interactions:*** the most common drug interactions that may occur with NSAIDs are shown in table III. Only a limited number of these, however, are clinically significant. They include a decrease in lithium clearance with most NSAIDs and interference with the activity of diuretics, β-adrenoceptor blockers and ACE inhibitors. Elderly patients should always have their blood pressure checked and should be reviewed for any signs of fluid retention or congestive cardiac failure when they are commenced on an NSAID, whether they are taking antihypertensive or heart failure medications or not. Although the use of NSAIDs and warfarin is not absolutely contraindicated, assuming that there are no other serious risks of bleeding, the prothrombin time must be very carefully monitored whenever NSAIDs are added to warfarin treatment.

#### NSAID Selection and Clinical Use

The choice of NSAID in an individual patient will be determined by the previous experiences of the clinician and the patient, the selection remaining, in part, more of an art than a science. Dosages should be increased to the recommended maximum over 1 to 2 weeks and, if results are disappointing, an alternative NSAID should be tried. The dosage of the NSAID can be titrated against symptoms by the patient and concurrent use of on demand or regular analgesics such as paracetamol may reduce the NSAID requirement. Dosages of some commonly used NSAIDs are shown in table IX.

### 3.1.3 Drugs that May Affect the Rheumatoid Disease Process

Disease-modifying (or slow-acting) antirheumatic drugs such as corticosteroids,[37] methotrexate, gold and sulfasalazine[38,39] do slow the erosion rate in patients with rheumatoid arthritis. Unfortunately, patients tolerate these drugs only for a relatively short period of time, with the majority having to cease them within 5 years of commencement due to either the development of toxicity or a subsequent failure of treatment following initial control.[40]

The properties of the disease-modifying antirheumatic drugs (DMARDs) and their mechanisms of action are listed in tables IX and X. We now know that if patients with rheumatoid arthritis are going to develop joint erosions, they will do so within the first 2 years of the disease. This makes it very important that DMARDs are initiated as early as possible in the course of the disease. Most rheumatologists will now prescribe DMARDs at the time of diagnosis of rheumatoid arthritis. Given the range of drugs available, it is important to consider their individual mechanisms of action, spectra of adverse effects and to know how to choose an agent for a particular patient, and how to monitor effectiveness and toxicity[38] [table XI].

For reviews of the clinical pharmacology and therapeutic use of DMARDs, see Brooks,[38] Gardner & Furst,[41] and Wilke et al.[42]

#### Antimalarials (Chloroquine and Hydroxychloroquine)

Hydroxychloroquine and chloroquine have been used to treat rheumatoid arthritis since the 1950s. These drugs bind strongly to DNA, inhibit lymphocyte function, stabilise lysosomal membranes, and reduce chemotaxis, phagocytosis and superoxide production by polymorphonuclear leucocytes. They also reduce the production and release of interleukin-1.

***Pharmacokinetic characteristics:*** both drugs have extremely long elimination half-lives of about 40 days and it may take 3 to 4 months before steady-state plasma concentrations are reached, thus providing a partial explanation for their delayed effect. A therapeutic plasma concentration range for chloroquine in rheumatoid arthritis of between 0.7 and 2.1 g/L has been suggested,[43] although recent data indicate that most patients with rheumatoid arthritis treated with hydroxychloroquine do not achieve that concentration.[44] This may have important implications, since antimalarials are considered to be relatively weak (though safe) antirheumatic drugs. The explanation for this relative lack of efficacy may be that patients are not achieving adequate tissue concentrations. On the other hand, if doses of antimalarials are increased, there may be an increase in toxicity.

***Tolerability:*** the adverse effects of the antimalarial drugs include skin rashes, leucopenia, peripheral neuropathy and ocular effects. Acute but transient deterioration in vision with poor focusing may occur at the start of therapy and haziness of vision, photophobia and haloes around lights may occur with prolonged use. Permanent visual disturbance is extremely rare if the maintenance dose of chloroquine or hydroxychloroquine is held at 200 and 250mg per day, respectively. However, it is standard practice in most countries to advise fundoscopy and visual field charting at 4- to 6-month intervals, although no studies to validate this practice have been carried out. Other screening procedures such as the use of an Amsler grid (a chart enabling patients to simply check their retinal fields) and retinal photography may also provide a simple and less expensive way of detecting early retinal changes.[38] If any signs of retinal toxicity due to antimalarial drugs occur, they should be stopped immediately and not restarted.

#### Gold Compounds

The gold compounds used in rheumatoid arthritis comprise 2 major groups – the water-sol-

**Table IX.** Clinical pharmacological properties of analgesic and anti-inflammatory drugs used in rheumatic disorders

| Drug | Dosage[a] (daily) | Elimination[b] | Adverse effects and precautions |
|---|---|---|---|
| **Analgesics** | | | |
| Aspirin (acetylsalicylic acid) | 1-2 g/day | Hepatic metabolism and renal excretion of free salicylate | Gastric irritation, occult bleeding |
| Paracetamol (acetaminophen) | 0.5-1g q4-6h | Hepatic metabolism and renal excretion (3% unchanged) | Hepatic necrosis (overdosage) |
| Codeine | 30mg q4h | Hepatic metabolism and renal excretion (<17% unchanged) | Constipation, nausea, vomiting, dizziness |
| Dihydrocodeine | 30-60mg q4-6h | Hepatic metabolism | As for codeine (less constipating and more effective); use with caution in asthma and in patients with impaired liver function; mild sedative effect useful for pain at night; can be given by injection |
| Dextropropoxyphene (propoxyphene) | 65mg q6h | Hepatic metabolism and renal excretion (<10% unchanged) | Nausea, vomiting, dizziness, respiratory depression (overdosage); may be combined with aspirin or paracetamol |
| Pentazocine | 50-75mg q4h | Hepatic metabolism and renal excretion (<5-23% unchanged) | Nausea, vomiting, dizziness, hallucinations; low abuse potential; can also be given by injection |
| Nefopam | 60mg q8h | Hepatic metabolism (<5% excreted in urine unchanged) | Nausea, sweating, dry mouth, drowsiness, dizziness; can also be given by injection |
| Buprenorphine | 0.2-0.4mg sublingually q6-8h | Hepatic metabolism; ≈70% excreted in faeces, remainder in urine | Drowsiness, dizziness, nausea, euphoria; can also be given by injection |
| **Anti-inflammatory analgesics (NSAIDs)** | | | |
| *Salicylates:* | | | |
| Aspirin | 4g or more (enteric coated 1g qid) | Dose-related hepatic metabolism and renal excretion of free salicylate (pH dependent) | Tinnitus, nausea, gastric irritation (exacerbation of peptic ulcer), haematemesis, melaena, asthma sensitivity reactions (rare); use of antacids decreases plasma concentrations (and effectiveness) by hastening renal excretion |
| Benorilate | 4-8g (2-3 divided doses) | Hydrolysed to aspirin and paracetamol (see above) | As for aspirin and paracetamol (see above) |
| Choline magnesium trisalicylate | 2-3g (2 divided doses) | As for aspirin (see above) | As for aspirin but less frequent |
| Diflunisal | 0.5-1g (2 divided doses) | Glucuronide conjugation and renal excretion | As for aspirin but less frequent |
| Salsalate | 2-4g (3-4 divided doses) | As for aspirin | As for aspirin but less frequent |
| *Benzene acetic acid derivatives:* | | | |
| Diclofenac | 75-150mg (1-3 divided doses with food) | Hepatic metabolism | Gastrointestinal disturbances, headache, dizziness |
| *Propionic acid derivatives:* | | | |
| Carprofen | 300mg (2 divided doses with food) | Hepatic metabolism (≈5% excreted in urine unchanged) | Gastrointestinal intolerance, rashes, headaches, drowsiness |
| Fenbufen | 900mg (2 divided doses with food) | Hepatic metabolism to active metabolites (≈4% excreted in urine unchanged) | Gastrointestinal intolerance, headaches, dizziness, rashes (uncommon) |
| Fenoprofen | 1200-2400mg (2 divided doses with food) | Hepatic metabolism | Gastrointestinal disturbances (usually well tolerated); headache and skin rash (uncommon) |
| Flurbiprofen | 150-300mg (2 divided doses with food) | Hepatic metabolism and renal excretion (20-25% unchanged) | Gastrointestinal intolerance, headache, skin rash |
| Ibuprofen | 1200-2400mg (2-4 divided doses with food) | Hepatic metabolism | Gastrointestinal disturbances (usually well tolerated); headache and skin rash (uncommon) |

*[Continued over]*

**Table IX.** *[Continued]*

| Drug | Dosage[a] (daily) | Elimination[b] | Adverse effects and precautions |
|---|---|---|---|
| Ketoprofen | 100-200mg (2 divided doses with food) | Hepatic metabolism | As for ibuprofen |
| Naproxen | 500-1000mg (2 divided doses with food) | Hepatic metabolism and renal excretion (10% unchanged drug) | As for ibuprofen |
| Oxaprozin | 1200mg (od with food) | Hepatic metabolism (slow elimination rate) | Gastrointestinal intolerance, rashes, headaches |
| Pirprofen | 600-800mg (2 divided doses) | Hepatic metabolism (1-5% excreted in urine unchanged) | Gastrointestinal intolerance, rashes, headaches, dizziness |
| Tiaprofenic acid | 600mg (2-3 divided doses with food) | Hepatic metabolism | Gastrointestinal intolerance, rashes, headaches, drowsiness (uncommon) |
| *Oxicams:* | | | |
| Lornoxicam | 8-16mg (2-3 divided doses) | Hepatic metabolism | Gastrointestinal intolerance, dizziness |
| Meloxicam | 7.5-15mg od | Hepatic metabolism | Gastrointestinal intolerance |
| Piroxicam | 10-20mg (od with food) | Hepatic metabolism (2-5% excreted in urine unchanged); undergoes enterohepatic circulation | Gastrointestinal intolerance, rashes, peripheral oedema |
| Tenoxicam | 10-20mg od | Hepatic metabolism | Gastrointestinal intolerance, rashes |
| *Indole/indene derivatives:* | | | |
| Acemetacin | 120-180mg (2-3 divided doses) | Hepatic metabolism and renal excretion (major metabolite is indomethacin) | As for indomethacin (see below) |
| Indomethacin | 25-150mg (1-3 divided doses with food) plus 75-100mg at night (for night pain) | Hepatic metabolism, enterohepatic circulation via bile and renal excretion (glomerular filtration and tubular secretion; 10-20% unchanged) | Gastrointestinal intolerance; headaches and unpleasant cerebral sensations (dose-related); anaemia; psychotic disturbances (rare); use with care in patients with impaired biliary function |
| Sulindac | 200-600mg (2 divided doses after food) | Metabolised to active sulfide and inactive sulfone metabolites; excreted in urine (sulfone metabolite and unchanged drug) and faeces (active sulfide metabolite); undergoes enterohepatic circulation | Gastrointestinal intolerance, headache, dizziness |
| *Pyrazolones:* | | | |
| Azapropazone | 1200mg (2-4 divided doses with food) | Renal excretion of unchanged drug (60%); little hepatic metabolism | Gastrointestinal intolerance, skin rash; reduce dose in patients with impaired renal function |
| Oxyphenbutazone[c] | 200-400mg (single daily dose) | Slow hepatic metabolism and very slow excretion | As for phenylbutazone (see below) |
| Phenylbutazone[c] | 200-400mg (single daily dose) | Slow and extensive hepatic metabolism and very slow renal excretion of active metabolites (in plasma, oxyphenbutazone ≈14%; compound with uricosuric properties ≈ 14%) | Gastrointestinal intolerance; fluid retention (may precipitate heart failure in elderly); skin reactions, hypersensitivity (serum-sickness type), ulcerative stomatitis (stop drug if sore throat or other oral lesions); haematological complications (more common in women over 65 years); goitre and myxoedema (occasionally seen). Avoid in patients with severe liver disease |
| *Fenamates:* | | | |
| Meclofenamate sodium | 200-400mg (2 divided doses with food) | Hepatic metabolism | Gastrointestinal disturbances (esp. diarrhoea); rashes, headache, dizziness |
| *Others:* | | | |
| Etodolac | 200mg bid | Hepatic metabolism and renal excretion (<20% unchanged) | Gastrointestinal intolerance, headache, dizziness, rashes |

**Table IX.** *[Continued]*

| Drug | Dosage[a] (daily) | Elimination[b] | Adverse effects and precautions |
|---|---|---|---|
| Nabumetone | 1000mg (od at night with food) | Hepatic metabolism (principal active metabolite is 6-methoxy-2-naphthylacetic acid) | Gastrointestinal intolerance (mild), headache, dizziness |
| Nimesulide | 100-400mg (2 divided doses) | Hepatic metabolism and excretion of metabolites in urine and faeces | Gastrointestinal disturbances, dizziness, headache, rashes, pruritus |
| Tolmetin | 1200-1800mg (2-4 divided doses with food) | Hepatic metabolism and renal excretion (up to 17% unchanged) | Gastrointestinal intolerance, headache, dizziness |
| **Drugs that affect the disease process** (these drugs should probably be started only in consultation with a specialist) | | | |
| Sodium aurothiomalate | 10mg IM; increase to 50 mg/week max. Reduce dose or increase intervals (to every 2-4 weeks) once ESR decreases and clinical improvement achieved (usually when around 400-700mg given) | Extremely slow renal excretion (60-90%; during weekly therapy patient remains in positive gold balance with progressive increase in body stores; increased fraction of dose excreted during monthly maintenance therapy, negative balance) and also faecal excretion (10-40%) | Blood dyscrasias, including aplastic anaemia (may occur with little warning, despite normal blood counts); fever, skin reactions including exfoliative dermatitis, mouth ulcers (stop drug immediately); haemorrhage from platelet deficiencies (give dimercaprol); proteinuria, haematuria, pulmonary reactions. *Discontinue gold immediately if toxic symptoms are reported or if abnormalities appear in blood count: monitor white cells and platelets before each injection.* |
| Auranofin | 6mg (od with food) | Faecal (≈88% of dose) and renal excretion (≈12%) | Diarrhoea; other complications as for injectable gold (see above) but less common |
| Chloroquine | 200mg (sulfate) or 250mg (phosphate) od | Some hepatic metabolism and slow renal excretion of unchanged drug (50-70%) and metabolites; faecal excretion (≈10% unchanged) | Skin rashes, hair discolouration; leucopenia; peripheral neuropathy; ocular reactions which may be permanent; reduce dose in renal failure |
| Penicillamine | 125mg (base) increased gradually to 750mg daily; only rarely to 1g or more | Some hepatic metabolism and rapid renal excretion of unchanged drug | Gastrointestinal disturbances; loss of taste; skin reactions; haematological complications (thrombocytopenia, leucopenia, aplastic anaemia); proteinuria, haematuria, nephrotic syndrome; myasthenia-like syndrome. |
| Azathioprine | 1-2.5 mg/kg (2-3 divided doses) | Conversion to free mercaptopurine; some hepatic metabolism; renal excretion of metabolites and unchanged drug (10%) | Haematological complications (bone marrow suppression with leucopenia, thrombocytopenia, aplastic anaemia); gastrointestinal disturbances; reduce dose in renal failure; use only in specialist centres in severe, active and progressive disease (see text; section 3.1.3) |
| Cyclophosphamide | 1-1.5 mg/kg (2-3 divided doses) | Hepatic bioactivation and renal excretion of active metabolites and <20% unchanged drug; faecal excretion (17-30% unchanged) after oral administration | Haematological complications (bone marrow suppression with leucopenia, thrombocytopenia); alopecia; haemorrhagic cystitis; nausea, vomiting; ovarian (amenorrhoea) and testicular (azoospermia) toxicity; reduce dose in renal failure; use only in specialist centres in severe, active and progressive disease with risk to life (see text; section 3.1.3) |
| Methotrexate | 7.5-25 mg/week PO or 10-15 mg/week IM | Mainly renal excretion | Bone marrow suppression, liver toxicity, cirrhosis, pneumonitis, anaphylactic reactions |
| Tenidap[d] | 120mg od | Hepatic metabolism (elimination increased after multiple oral doses, possibly due to induction of its own metabolism) | Gastrointestinal intolerance, headache, asthenia, dizziness, rash; proteinuria (mild, non-progressive and reversible) |

*[Continued over]*

**Table IX.** *[Continued]*

| Drug | Dosage[a] (daily) | Elimination[b] | Adverse effects and precautions |
|---|---|---|---|
| **Corticosteroids** | | | |
| Prednisolone, prednisone, methylprednisolone | 2.5mg q8h (>7.5 mg/day suppresses HPA axis); 5mg at night (for pain and stiffness); higher doses permitted for certain conditions (giant cell arteritis, active SLE, etc.) | Hepatic metabolism | Electrolyte disturbances; gastrointestinal irritation; metabolic disturbances; osteoporosis and vertebral crush fractures, Cushingoid features, HPA axis suppression (excessive dosage); growth retardation (children) |
| Dexamethasone | 0.25mg q12h | Hepatic metabolism | As for prednisolone |
| Betamethasone | 0.25mg q12h | Hepatic metabolism | As for prednisolone |
| Corticotrophin depot gel | IM daily at lowest effective dose (usually 10-20 U/day) | Hepatic metabolism | Corticotrophin or tetracosactide may be used in hospital to control acute inflammatory episodes |
| Tetracosactide depot | Daily or alternate days at lowest effective dose (usually 0.1-0.2mg; max. 1 mg/week) | | |

a Oral unless specified otherwise.

b Significant impairment of renal function often necessitates a change of dosage (reduce dose or intervals for drugs largely excreted unchanged or as active metabolites; see appendix D). Severe liver disease often necessitates a change of dosage of drugs with significant hepatic metabolism (see appendix F).

c Now withdrawn from general use in many countries.

d Tenidap exerts both NSAID-like anti-inflammatory activity and cytokine modulatory properties (inhibition of the production of pro-inflammatory cytokines, including interleukins-1 and -6 and tumour necrosis factor-α).

*Abbreviations and symbols:* bid = twice daily; od = once daily; qid = 4 times daily; IM = intramuscular; PO = oral; HPA = hypothalamic-pituitary-adrenal; SLE = systemic lupus erythematosus.

uble thiolates (*sodium aurothiomalate* and *aurothioglucose*) and the lipid-soluble phosphine derivative *auranofin*. Although their mechanism of action is not completely understood, gold compounds are known to modify the activity of monocytes and lymphocytes, and auranofin seems to have a particular effect on polymorphonuclear leucocytes. Sodium aurothiomalate and aurothioglucose are given intramuscularly while auranofin is given orally.

***Pharmacokinetic characteristics:*** metabolites of gold circulate in the blood bound primarily to plasma proteins, but significant concentrations of gold are also found within erythrocytes.[45] The injectable gold compounds are rapidly absorbed after intramuscular injection, with the more oily aurothioglucose showing slightly delayed maximum plasma gold concentrations. Gold is eliminated slowly from the body and has been found in tissues over 20 years after the last dose. Approximately 25% of auranofin is absorbed following oral administration, the major route of elimination for this compound being the faeces. Both intramuscular gold salts and auranofin are widely distributed throughout the body and there is some evidence to suggest they are concentrated within inflammatory tissues, particularly in macrophages.

***Clinical effectiveness:*** the major clinical trials involving gold compounds have shown that gold is more effective than placebo (*clinical end-points:* tender and swollen joint count; visual analogue score of pain; patient and physician global assessment; and functional index), although changes in end-points in these clinical trials were relatively modest.[46] The optimum dosage of the injectable gold compounds has not yet been clearly established. Dosages as low as 10 mg/week appear to be no different from

**Table X.** Mechanism of action of disease-modifying antirheumatic drugs (DMARDs)

| Agents | Mechanism |
|---|---|
| Antimalarials | Inhibition of lysosomal enzymes |
| • Chloroquine<br>• Hydroxychloroquine | Inhibit PMN and lymphocyte responses *(in vitro)* |
| | Inhibit IL-1 release *(in vivo)* |
| | ? Cartilage protection *(in vitro)* |
| Sulfasalazine | Inhibits PMN migration |
| | Reduces lymphocyte responses |
| | Inhibits angiogenesis |
| Gold | Inhibits PMN function |
| | Inhibition of T and B cell activity |
| | Inhibits macrophage activation *(in vitro)* |
| Penicillamine | Inhibits neovascularisation *(in vitro)* |
| | Inhibits PMN myeloperoxidase |
| | Scavenges free radicals |
| | Inhibits T-cell function |
| | Impairs antigen presentation |
| Corticosteroids | Increase lipocortin levels leading to inhibition of phospholipase $A_2$ |
| | Reduce cytokine production |
| | Inhibit $F_c$ receptor expression |
| | Suppress lymphocyte function |
| | Redistribute circulating leucocytes |
| Methotrexate | Decreases thymidylate synthetase activity and subsequent DNA synthesis |
| | Diminishes PMN chemotaxis |
| Azathioprine | Interferes with DNA synthesis |
| | Inhibits lymphocyte proliferation |
| Cyclophosphamide | Cross-links DNA leading to cell death |
| | Decreases circulating T and B cells |
| Chlorambucil | Similar to cyclophosphamide |
| Cyclosporin | Blocks synthesis/release of IL-1 and IL-2 |

*Abbreviations:* IL = interleukin; PMN = polymorphonuclear cell.

50 mg/week, which in turn is as effective as 150 mg/week. Gold injections are usually started with a test dose of 10mg intramuscularly (to ensure that the patient has not developed an acute allergic reaction), followed by between 10 and 50 mg/week until a dose of approximately 1g has been given or the patient has shown a significant response. After a response, the frequency of injections is decreased, but gold therapy should be continued unless adverse effects occur. Unfortunately, 3 to 5 years after the start of gold treatment, most patients have to stop treatment because of lack of effectivenes or adverse effects.[40] From the available data, the following points can be made:

- Dosages in the range of 10 to 50mg (weekly/monthly) for 1 to 2 years are more effective than placebo.
- A dose-response relationship in the range of 10 to 150 mg/week has not been established.
- A clinical response (i.e. a significant decrease in pain and in the number of tender swollen joints together with an improvement in function) occurs in 10 to 35% of patients, peaking at 12 months, but only half of these patients maintain this response after 12 months; long term remissions are rare.
- Gold compounds retard the development of joint erosions, which, as stated above, occur in the majority of patients with rheumatoid arthritis within 2 years of developing the disease. The clinical relevance of erosions is that they indicate severe disease which will invariably result in significant disability. Once erosions have occurred, there is little evidence that they disappear.
- Even when the dosage is reduced to maintenance levels, only ≈20% of patients continue treatment after 4 years.
- As the incidence of toxicity declines, terminations of therapy due to loss of effectiveness continue to rise.

**Table XI.** Guidelines for monitoring of therapy with disease-modifying antirheumatic drugs (DMARDs)

| Drug | Parameters to monitor |
|---|---|
| Antimalarials (chloroquine and hydroxychloroquine) | Regular visual assessment (fundoscopy, visual field evaluation or use of Amsler grid) |
| Sulfasalazine | FBC fortnightly for 3 mos, then every 1 to 3 months |
| Gold compounds: | |
| • Injectable | FBC, urinalysis before each injection initially, then before every 2nd or 3rd injection. Urinalysis monitored by patient |
| • Oral | FBC, urinalysis q2-4wks |
| Penicillamine | FBC and urinalysis q2wks when starting or changing dose, then urinalysis q4wks |
| Methotrexate | FBC, LFTs q2wks, then q1-3mos |
| Cyclophosphamide | FBC and urinalysis q4wks after initial weekly tests |
| Azathioprine | FBC q1-2wks initially, then q1-3mos; LFTs q1-3mos |
| Chlorambucil | FBC q4wks initially, then q3mos |
| Cyclosporin | FBC, serum creatinine, BP q1wk, then q2-4wks on maintenance therapy |

*Abbreviations:* BP = blood pressure; FBC = full blood count; LFTs = liver function tests.

• Injectable gold compounds are more efficacious than auranofin, but are associated with a higher incidence of adverse reactions.

***Tolerability:*** adverse effects with gold compounds are important as these are a major reason for discontinuation of therapy. Auranofin has fewer serious adverse effects, although diarrhoea with this drug is dose-related and mucocutaneous reactions, proteinuria and thrombocytopenia are also seen. The major adverse effects of injectable gold compounds include skin rashes, proteinuria, blood dyscrasias and the rare problems of enterocolitis, peripheral neuropathy, pneumonia and bronchiolitis obliterans. In most clinical studies, up to 20% of patients have to stop gold treatment because of adverse effects, while 40% of patients may experience adverse reactions. Mild psoriatic skin rashes and transient proteinuria are common, but some patients go on to develop severe exfoliative dermatitis or membranous glomerulonephritis. Eosinophilia is common in patients with rheumatoid arthritis, but has been described in up to 50% of patients receiving gold and does not seem to correlate well with toxicity.

The most severe adverse reactions with gold salts are neutropenia or aplastic anaemia. A significant number of patients who develop blood dyscrasias while taking gold treatment show a progressive reduction in leucocyte or platelet counts before aplastic anaemia occurs. This emphasises the importance of careful and continuing evaluation of blood parameters (table XI). There are, however, some cases where the changes in blood parameters can be precipitous and occur without warning. Aplastic anaemia has a high mortality rate, but this can be reduced by aggressive treatment with high-dose corticosteroids, a chelating agent [dimercaprol (BAL)] and bone marrow transplantation.[47]

***Monitoring of gold treatment*** is important since adverse events must be identified as early as possible to prevent severe or even fatal sequelae. Although there is a wide variation in the practice of rheumatologists regarding monitoring strategies, most check the full blood count before each injection, at least for the first 3 months. Urine should be tested before each injection for evidence of proteinuria and haematuria and the patient can often be taught to monitor this themselves. With careful monitoring, gold treatment can be extremely effective and relatively safe in the management of rheumatoid arthritis.

**Penicillamine**

Penicillamine has been used in the treatment of rheumatoid arthritis for over 20 years but its use has been decreasing recently because of the advent of other DMARDs. It has 3 functional groups, an amino, a carboxyl and a sulfhydryl group which determine its pharmacokinetics and biological activity. Penicillamine forms disulfides through oxidation and acts as a metal chelator; these chemical reactions modulate macrophage, granulocyte and oxygen radical production. It may influence mediator production and may protect joint tissues from oxygen radical damage.[48]

***Pharmacokinetic characteristics:*** peak plasma concentrations of penicillamine occur between 1.5 and 4 hours after oral administration and the terminal elimination half-life of the drug has been estimated at 1 to 7.5 hours. Penicillamine binds strongly to tissues and to plasma albumin.

***Clinical effectiveness:*** using the same assessment criteria described above (i.e. tender and swollen joint count, visual analogue score of pain, patient and physician global assessment, and functional index) penicillamine has been shown to be significantly more effective than placebo in doses between 600 and 1500 mg/day, but few patients are now treated with more than 750 mg/day. Response rates are usually of the order of 50% by 6 months, but one-quarter of patients will withdraw during this time due to adverse effects. The effectiveness and toxicity of penicillamine in rheumatoid arthritis has been compared with other DMARDs, but many of the clinical trials have been of insufficient power to detect differences between the treatment groups. Penicillamine does, however, appear to be slightly more efficacious than hydroxychloroquine and auranofin. Whether penicillamine retards joint erosions in rheumatoid arthritis is not clear, but this end-point may be missed if studies are not continued into the second year.

***Tolerability:*** penicillamine produces a wide range of adverse effects similar to those of intramuscular gold. There are certain differences seen with penicillamine such as the occurrence of bullous pemphigoid and autoimmune disturbances with induction of antinuclear antibodies, systemic lupus erythematosus, myasthenia gravis, Goodpasture's syndrome and dermatopolymyositis. Patients developing adverse reactions may exhibit poor sulfoxidation status,[49] and there is a suggested association with the HLA antigens DR3 and B8.

Penicillamine should be initiated at a low dosage (125 to 250 mg/day) and the dosage then increased from 500 to 750 mg/day over a period of a few months. Careful monitoring of patients for the development of skin rashes and renal and haematological adverse effects with regular full blood counts and urinalyses must be carried out. If thrombocytopenia and proteinuria occur, penicillamine may be continued at a lower dosage as long as the abnormalities revert rapidly to normal. Once the disease has been controlled, the dosage of penicillamine may be reduced, but it is usual that when the drug is stopped, an exacerbation of rheumatoid arthritis occurs.[50]

#### Sulfasalazine

Sulfasalazine was first developed in the 1930s as an antibacterial agent and subsequently established a place in the management of inflammatory bowel disease.[51] Over the past decade, it has come to play an important role in the management of inflammatory arthritis, particularly rheumatoid arthritis. It has multiple actions including inhibition of synovial angiogenesis and suppression of lymphocyte and polymorphonucleocyte function.

***Pharmacokinetic characteristics:*** sulfasalazine is poorly absorbed from the gut, with delivery of most of the dose into the large bowel, where it is split by colonic bacteria into mesalazine (5-aminosalicylic acid, 5-ASA) and sulfapyridine. Most of the mesalazine is excreted unchanged in the faeces while sulfapyridine is absorbed and metabolised in the liver. The active component of sulfasalazine in rheumatoid arthritis appears to be sulfapyridine, and this agent is significantly more toxic than the parent drug.[52]

***Clinical effectiveness:*** significant benefit of sulfasalazine over placebo with some slowing of erosion rates has been demonstrated in controlled clinical trials. Sulfasalazine seems to have similar effectiveness to gold and penicillamine. Although up to 50% of patients develop adverse effects, less than half of these will need to stop treatment.

***Tolerability:*** adverse effects of sulfasalazine include skin rashes, nausea and abdominal pain, hepatic enzyme abnormalities, central nervous system disturbances and blood dyscrasias, particularly in those patients who have glucose-6-phosphate dehydrogenase (G6PD) deficiency. Gastric adverse effects can be reduced by enteric coating of the drug. Bodily secretions also commonly become discoloured and patients wearing plastic contact lenses should be warned that these may become tinged yellow.[38] In a large study,[53] most of the potentially serious adverse effects seemed to occur within the first 4 months of sulfasalazine treatment and the frequency of blood monitoring can be reduced after that time. Oligospermia is a common accompaniment of sulfasalazine therapy and, although these changes revert to normal on ceasing treatment, this must be discussed with the patient. It is recommended that full blood counts and liver function tests be monitored each fortnight for the first 3 months and then at 6-week to 3-month intervals thereafter.

For a review of the clinical pharmacology and therapeutic use of sulfasalazine in rheumatoid arthritis, see Rains et al.[54]

#### Methotrexate

Weekly oral or intramuscular doses of methotrexate are rapidly becoming the most commonly prescribed DMARD regimen. Methotrexate is a folic acid analogue that inhibits dihydrofolate reductase and impairs DNA synthesis.[55] It reduces lymphocyte proliferation and rheumatoid factor production, interferes with polymorphonucleocyte chemotaxis and may influence cytokine production.

***Pharmacokinetic characteristics:*** at the dosages used in rheumatoid arthritis (5 to 25 mg/week), the mean oral absorption time of methotrexate is ≈1.2 hours, and its bioavailability is 70%. The parent compound and its metabolites circulate bound to serum albumin and accumulate in the liver as polyglutamates. Methotrexate is eliminated from the body by renal excretion and also by biliary/faecal excretion.

***Clinical effectiveness:*** in doses of 7.5 to 25 mg/week, methotrexate has proved more effective than placebo and equally or slightly more effective than azathioprine, injectable gold, auranofin, penicillamine and hydroxychloroquine. A meta-analysis[56] has shown that patients on methotrexate have a 26% reduction in pain that occurs relatively quickly (in 1 to 2 months) and reaches a maximum in 6 months. Other studies have shown that patients will remain on methotrexate for longer than on other DMARDs.[57] Recently, carefully conducted studies have suggested that methotrexate can slow erosion rates in rheumatoid arthritis.[39]

***Tolerability:*** a major concern with methotrexate is its adverse effects. Anorexia and nausea, particularly in the 24 hours after a dose, are relatively common and can be reduced or eliminated by coadministration of folic acid (5mg daily or weekly) or calcium folinate without affecting the anti-inflammatory effects of the drug. Transient, mild elevation of liver enzymes occur in up to 60% of patients, but do not correlate with the development of hepatic fibrosis. Hypersensitivity reactions, including rashes, fever and pneumonitis, have been reported. The true incidence of pneumonitis is not known, but it is seen in less than 5% of cases.

The foremost concern with methotrexate is the development of hepatic fibrosis and cirrhosis. The incidence of severe liver disease is about 1 per 1000 methotrexate patients.[58,59] Risk factors for hepatic fibrosis include a previous history of liver disease. Patients must therefore be monitored carefully while receiving treatment. Alcohol intake should be kept to a minimum and the patient warned not to take antibiotics that are folate antagonists (e.g. cotrimoxazole or trimethoprim) and to report any infections or persistent cough.

For reviews of the clinical pharmacology and therapeutic use of methotrexate, see Markham & Faulds[60] and Bannwarth et al.[61]

#### Corticosteroids

Corticosteroids have played an important role in the management of rheumatic disorders since the late 1940s. The mechanism of action of these drugs in rheumatoid arthritis has been reviewed by George & Kirwan.[37] Corticosteroids diffuse across cell membranes and bind to specific cytoplasmic receptors that then undergo conformational change before moving into the nucleus to become attached to chromosomal DNA. Here, they modify the synthesis of messenger RNA, an action that can occur relatively quickly and lead to the detection of most cellular responses within 2 hours of drug administration. A major protein induced by corticosteroids is lipocortin, which inhibits phospholipase $A_2$, thus reducing the conversion of membrane phospholipids to arachidonic acid. This leads to a decrease in prostaglandin and leukotriene production. Corticosteroids also inhibit a wide variety of cytokines including interleukins, interferons and tumour necrosis factor (see also chapter 28; sect. 3.3). For a discussion on their pharmacodynamic and pharmacokinetic properties, see chapter 19 (section 7.1.1).

Corticosteroids can be used in the treatment of inflammatory joint disease in the following situations:

- As continuous oral background therapy (preferably in doses of no more than 10 mg/day of prednisolone)
- In short courses of rapidly decreasing doses for disease flares
- In large oral pulses (up to 1g prednisolone)
- As intra-articular or intralesional injections
- As intravenous pulses during a flare
- As induction treatment at the time of commencement of other disease-modifying antirheumatic drugs.

***Clinical effectiveness:*** corticosteroids are more effective than placebo and NSAIDs for the management of pain and stiffness in inflammatory joint disease. A recent study has shown that 7.5mg prednisolone daily significantly reduces the ocurrence and progression of erosions in patients with early rheumatoid arthritis (less than 2 years of disease).[62] Patients treated with a combination of low-dose corticosteroids (<7.5 mg/day of prednisolone) and exercise had a more favourable outcome than patients treated without corticosteroids (i.e. with usual antirheumatic therapies).[63]

***Tolerability:*** the adverse effects of long term corticosteroids are well recognised (see further chapter 19; sect. 7.1.1), but low doses (<7.5 mg/day of prednisolone) do not by themselves seem to be a risk factor for the development of peptic ulcers or significant osteoporosis. Nevertheless, corticosteroids taken in association with NSAIDs are associated with a higher incidence of gastric ulceration and should be avoided if possible. Prednisolone or prednisone are usually the first choice of oral corticosteroids because they can be given as 1mg tablets that allow for small dosage adjustments.

***Intra-articular instillation*** of corticosteroids (e.g. triamcinolone acetonide, methylprednisolone acetate or betamethasone sodium phosphate/acetate) into a swollen joint after aspiration of fluid avoids the undesirable systemic effects of corticosteroids and is often followed not only by an improvement in the joint itself, but also in a generalised systemic effect for at least the next week.[64] The dose of corticosteroid injected depends on the size of the joint and varies from 10 to 80mg of methylprednisolone acetate or equivalent. Intra-articular corticosteroid injection should always be performed under strict aseptic technique and is contraindicated if there is any evidence of infection in or around the joint. Patients should be instructed to return at once if the joint becomes worse, because of the possibility of infection. Injections into weight-bearing joints should not be repeated more than 3 to 4 times a year and, if patients require them more often, this is an indication that other measures should be taken to control disease activity.

#### Azathioprine, Cyclophosphamide and Chlorambucil

These drugs are still used occasionally to manage severe rheumatoid disease, but all have substantial long term toxicity, especially an increased risk of neoplasia. Patients treated with azathioprine have an increased rate of lymphoproliferative disorders and other malignancies.[65] Cyclophosphamide can produce haemorrhagic cystitis and may lead to substantial immunosuppression, with the attendant risks of infection, suppression of gonadal function and neoplasia. If cyclophosphamide is to be given, it should probably be administered as intermittent pulse therapy rather than continuous daily treatment, since pulses reduce the total dose of cyclophosphamide and hence the potential for malignant disease.

Chlorambucil is occasionally used in doses of 0.1 to 0.2 mg/kg/day, but adverse effects are significant, with a significantly increased risk of the development of leukaemia.[66]

#### Cyclosporin

This immunomodulating agent inhibits the production of both interleukin-1 and interleukin-2, which are important mediators in rheumatoid arthritis. Although shown to be more effective than placebo and similar in effectiveness to penicillamine and azathioprine, there is a relatively high incidence of renal toxicity with this drug. The renal toxicity is dose-related and, in most patients receiving up to 4 mg/kg/day, increases in serum creatinine can be controlled by dosage adjustment. Cyclosporin requires intensive monitoring, but may be useful in patients resistant to other forms of treatment.[67]

For a review of the clinical pharmacology and therapeutic use of cyclosporin, see Faulds et al.[68]

### *3.1.4 New Approaches*

A number of newer immunomodulating agents are now being tested in patients with rheumatoid arthritis, including monoclonal antibodies to particular T cell subsets, cytokines, and cytokine inhibitors. Noncomparative studies of a number of these agents have suggested that short term benefits occur, but longer and properly controlled trials are awaited.[38]

#### Tenidap

This drug is the first of a new class of compounds with anti-inflammatory and immunomodulatory activity. As well as inhibiting cyclooxygenase (in common with NSAIDs), it also reduces the production of certain proinflammatory cytokines including interleukins-1 and -6 and tumour necrosis factor-$\alpha$ (TNF-$\alpha$). It is well absorbed when given orally (bioavailability 82 to 89%) and eliminated relatively slowly, with a half-life of 25 hours and clearance of 0.25 to 0.3 L/h. Preliminary clinical studies in rheumatoid arthritis patients have suggested that tenidap is more effective in producing improvement in various disease activity parameters than NSAIDs, and is at least as effective as NSAIDs plus DMARDs such as hydroxychloroquine or auranofin,[69] though its place in therapy has yet to be established. Tenidap appears to have similar tolerability to the NSAIDs, but may cause proteinuria more commonly (generally mild and reversible on discontinuation of treatment).[70]

#### Combination DMARD Regimens

Although combinations of DMARDs are often used to treat rheumatoid arthritis, the few randomised, double-blind studies of combination therapy have failed to demonstrate any significant benefit of the combination over the drugs used singly. It does, however, seem logical that DMARDs with different mechanisms of action and different adverse effect profiles could be used in smaller than normal dosages to provide added effectiveness without added toxicity. Further studies are required to confirm this.[42]

## 3.2 Optimum Treatment

It is now accepted that there is little to choose between the various NSAIDs in the management of rheumatoid arthritis, although variability in response to these agents might lead to significant individual preferences (see section 3.1.2 above). Recent data on toxicity does, however, suggest that there may be a hierarchy with drugs such as ibuprofen, naproxen and diclofenac being better tolerated by the stomach.

Once a patient is diagnosed with rheumatoid arthritis, a DMARD should be started immediately. It has been suggested[71] that the treatment of rheumatoid arthritis be put on a much more scientific footing, with 6 principles proposed to establish this strategy:

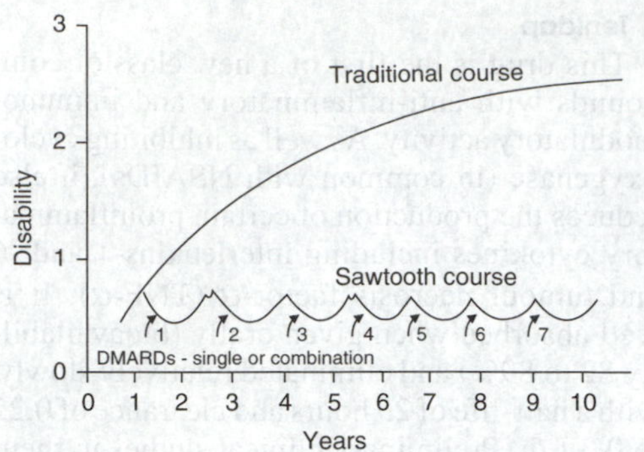


**Fig. 2.** Strategy for the treatment of rheumatoid arthritis (after Fries[71]). The numbered arrows 1-7 indicate a change or addition of a disease-modifying antirheumatic drug (DMARD).

1) Early use of DMARDs before joint damage occurs.

2) One or multiple DMARDs used continuously throughout the disease.

3) Disability and outcome measures regularly monitored so that disease progression can be serially plotted.

4) Goals for treatment should be set *a priori:* aim to reduce the ESR by 30%, the number of swollen joints by 30%, and to decrease disability within a set time period, i.e. 4 to 6 months, otherwise treatment will need to be changed.

5) DMARD therapy is serially changed to new agents used alone or in combination at each decision point.

6) Analgesics and NSAIDs are used as adjunctive therapy to relieve symptoms.

This approach is summarised in figure 2, which shows where regular review of activity of the disease and treatment should be carried out. Recent meta-analyses of placebo-controlled and comparative studies of methotrexate, injectable gold, penicillamine, sulfasalazine, auranofin and antimalarial drugs for both effectiveness and toxicity have provided interesting comparative data (summarised in figure 3).[72] These data showed that auranofin was significantly less effective than methotrexate, injectable gold, penicillamine or sulfasalazine, and slightly but not significantly less effective than antimalarials. 30% of patients dropped out of the studies and in half of these the reason was an adverse drug effect. Injectable gold had the highest rate of toxicity, while antimalarials and auranofin had the lowest (fig. 4).[72]

Most patients who respond to a DMARD will do so within 6 months and if they do not respond, it is important to either change the DMARD or add another one to try to suppress disease activity. With close monitoring of both clinical effectiveness and adverse reactions,

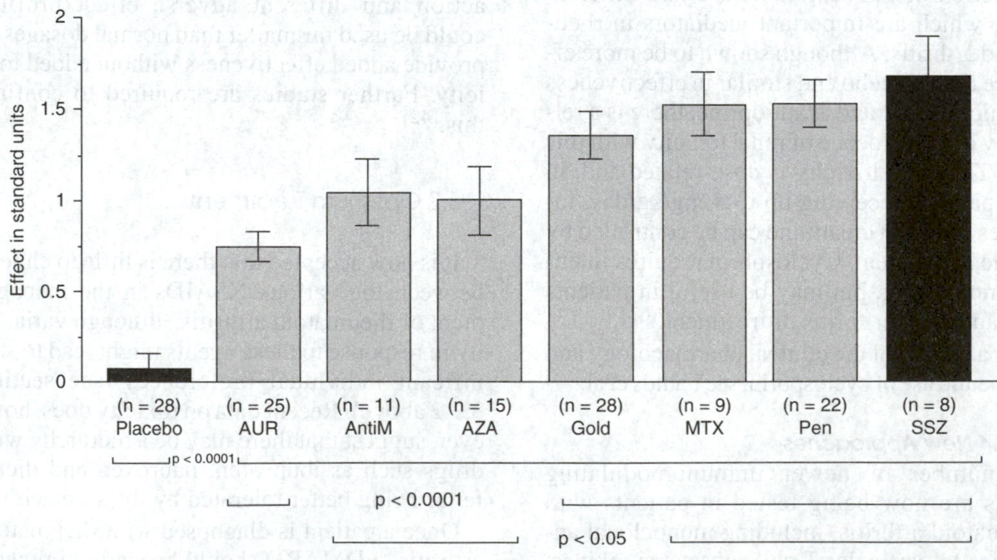


**Fig. 3.** Effect of various treatments on a composite figure representing grip strength (adjusted for disease duration and trial length), the number of tender joints (adjusted for initial count and blinding), and erythrocyte sedimentation rate. *Abbreviations:* AUR = auranofin; AntiM = antimalarials; AZA = azathioprine; Gold = injectable gold; MTX = methotrexate; Pen = penicillamine; SSZ = sulfasalazine (after Felson et al.;[72] with permission).

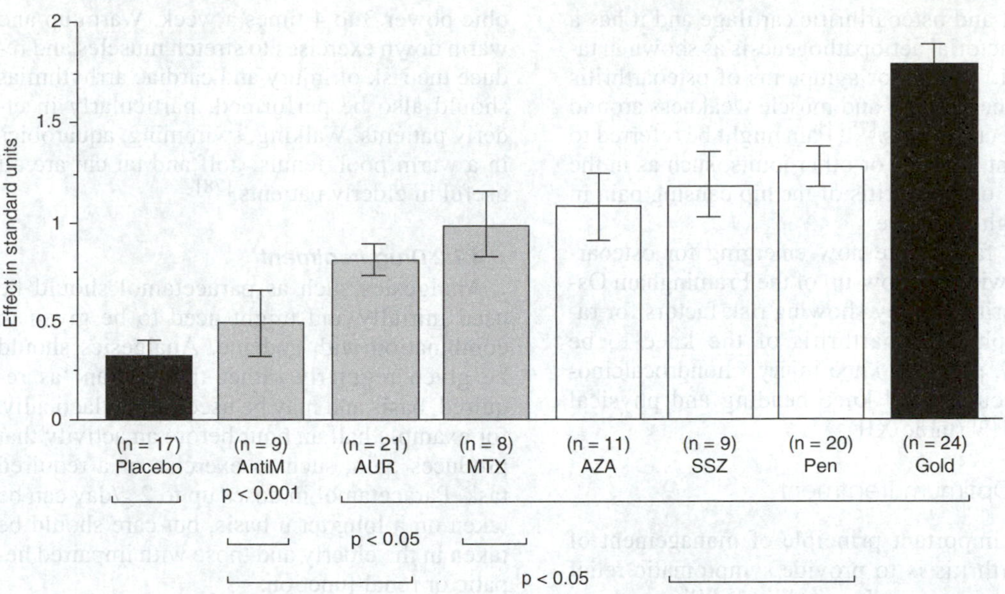


**Fig. 4.** Toxicity of various treatments, assessed using a modified Fries index, adjusted for length of study and disease duration. The Fries index is a composite index of toxicity, which includes symptoms, abnormal investigations (liver function tests or full blood counts) and admissions to hospital. *Abbreviations:* AUR = auranofin; AntiM = antimalarials; AZA = azathioprine; Gold = injectable gold; MTX = methotrexate; Pen = penicillamine; SSZ = sulfasalazine (after Felson et al.;[72] with permission).

significant benefits can be achieved in most patients with rheumatoid arthritis by DMARD treatment without producing major adverse events. Although DMARDs do not always provide the 'answer', clinicians can still help patients significantly and, by defining the questions to be answered, help design future trials that will significantly benefit patients.

### 3.3 Management of Specific Problems in Rheumatoid Arthritis

#### *3.3.1 Pain Control at Night*

Adequate sleep is important for patients with rheumatoid arthritis. Relatively large dosages of nonsteroidal anti-inflammatory drugs, either orally or by suppository, can be supplemented with analgesic agents such as paracetamol or paracetamol with codeine. Small doses of antidepressant drugs may also help for short periods of time, together with simple advice such as having a hot shower or bath and avoiding drinking coffee or tea before retiring.

#### *3.3.2 Treatment of Acutely Swollen Joints*

These should be aspirated and sepsis excluded. Intra-articular corticosteroids (see section 3.1.3) might be helpful and, if the effusion is resistant to this, radioactive synovectomy with yttrium or dysprosium could be considered. However, recent meta-analyses of the use of radionuclide synovectomy have not been encouraging.[73] Arthroscopic synovectomy has been used for relatively large joints such as in the shoulder and may help in the short term.

## 4. Osteoarthritis

Osteoarthritis occurs in most people and is probably the most common joint disorder in the world. Radiographic evidence of osteoarthritis occurs in most people over 65 years of age and the disease is a major cause of work disability and morbidity. Epidemiological studies are difficult to interpret because radiological changes are not always symptomatic. What is clear is that osteoarthritis is not just an associate of aging.[74] Marked differences occur between

**Table XII.** Factors associated with the development of osteoarthritis

| |
|---|
| Body build (obese) |
| Heredity |
| Osteoporosis |
| Hypermobility |
| Smoking |
| Other diseases (particularly inflammatory joint disease) |
| Mechanical factors |
| Trauma-joint shape |
| Repetitive use |

normal and osteoarthritic cartilage and it has a multifactorial aetiopathogenesis as shown in table XII. The major symptoms of osteoarthritis are pain, stiffness and muscle weakness around the affected joints.[75] Pain might be referred to adjacent muscles or other joints, such as in the case of osteoarthritis of the hip causing pain in the thigh and knee.

Risk factors are now emerging for osteoarthritis with a follow-up of the Framingham Osteoarthritis Survey showing risk factors for radiographic osteoarthritis of the knee to be obesity, previous knee injury, chondrocalcinosis, occupational knee bending and physical labour[76] (table XII).

### 4.1 Optimum Treatment

The important principle of management of osteoarthritis is to provide symptomatic relief by reducing pain, increasing mobility and improving the patient's quality of life. The management of osteoarthritis can be divided into nondrug therapy and pharmacological options. Nondrug treatments include patient education, joint protection, splinting, physiotherapy, occupational therapy, footwear and walking aids, and surgery, including joint replacement. Pharmacological options include the use of analgesics, nonsteroidal anti-inflammatory drugs, local corticosteroid injections, radiochemical synovectomy, use of so-called chondroprotective agents (these drugs are still relatively experimental but some, such as hyaluronic acid, have been shown to be of some short term benefit in osteoarthritis of the knee), and antidepressants or other drugs used in the relief of chronic pain.

#### *4.1.1 Physio/Hydrotherapy and Exercise*

Physiotherapy and hydrotherapy play an important role in the maintenance of function and in reduction of pain. Treatment needs to be tailored to each patient, should be simple and involve exercises that the patient can perform on a regular basis at home once they have been taught by the physiotherapist.

A recent survey of clinical trials of nonmedicinal and noninvasive therapies for osteoarthritis of the hip and knee demonstrated that exercise reduced pain and improved function in patients with osteoarthritis of the knee.[77] Specific exercises may be directed to certain joints, but a general exercise programme should be designed to provide at least 20 to 30 minutes of activity at approximately 60% of maximum aerobic power 3 to 4 times a week. Warm up and warm down exercises to stretch muscles and reduce the risk of injury and cardiac arrhythmias should also be performed, particularly in elderly patients. Walking, swimming, aquarobics in a warm pool, tennis, golf and tai chi are all useful in elderly patients.[78]

#### *4.1.2 Drug Treatment*

Analgesics such as paracetamol should be used initially and might need to be given in combination with codeine. Analgesics should be given regularly rather than on an 'as required' basis and may be used prophylactically, for example half an hour before an activity that produces pain, such as exercise or a required task. Paracetamol in doses up to 2 g/day can be taken on a long term basis, but care should be taken in the elderly and those with impaired hepatic or renal function.

Nonsteroidal anti-inflammatory drugs (NSAIDs; see section 3.1.2 and table IX) may be required in situations where inflammatory episodes of osteoarthritis are superimposed on the general disease or where analgesics are not sufficient to reduce pain and improve function. Elderly patients may tolerate NSAIDs less well than younger patients, and the dosages should be reduced accordingly in the elderly and care taken to observe renal and cardiac function. In two recent 2-year comparative studies of NSAIDs (naproxen and sustained-release diclofenac) in the treatment of osteoarthritis of the knee,[79,80] significant numbers of patients previously controlled on NSAIDs were able to continue on paracetamol alone for the duration of the study. In a short term study comparing an anti-inflammatory dose of ibuprofen (2.4 g/day), an analgesic dose of ibuprofen (1.2 g/day) and paracetamol (4 g/day), no significant differences were found between the treatments in terms of disability or pain on walking.[81] In a study in which patients were repeatedly randomised to receive paracetamol or diclofenac, symptoms were adequately controlled by paracetamol alone in approximately 30% of patients.[82]

Considerable attention has been paid recently to the complications of NSAIDs, particularly their adverse gastrointestinal effects. In NSAID users, there is a significant increase in the risk of peptic ulceration and the relative risk of developing gastrointestinal bleeding or perforation is 3 to 4 times that in the normal population. Given this increased incidence of adverse effects, particularly in the elderly, NSAIDs should only be used when analgesics and other measures have failed. When NSAIDs are used, they should be used for short periods of time (<1 to 2 months) and attempts continually made to withdraw treatment and reintroduce or increase the dosage of analgesic drugs.

#### 4.1.3 Surgical Management

Advances in surgery, with the refinement of hip and knee replacements, have meant that many patients previously destined for a life of continuing pain can now be restored to almost normal function. Joint replacement should virtually eliminate pain and significantly increase mobility and independence in most patients with severe joint disease. In major orthopaedic surgical units, the failure rate for hip and knee prostheses should be less than 5% at 10 years, although some patients will continue to have a degree of pain when weight bearing. There are few, if any, situations where this operation should not at least be considered. Spinal anaesthesia negates the requirement for a general anaesthetic, but preoperative assessment of bodyweight reduction and an exercise programme can improve the outcome.

## 5. Ankylosing Spondylitis and Other Seronegative Arthropathies

These forms of inflammatory arthritis are associated with both peripheral and axial (spinal) disease (table XIII). Stiffness of the spine and joint pain are the major features. Treatment is directed at maintaining posture with an active exercise programme, reducing inflammation with nonsteroidal anti-inflammatory drugs and considering the use of second-line drugs such as sulfasalazine. Associated features of the seronegative spondyloarthropathies such as iritis, urethritis and enteritis associated with reactive arthritis may also need to be treated.

**Table XIII.** Forms of inflammatory arthritis associated with peripheral and axial disease

| |
|---|
| Spondyloarthropathies |
| Ankylosing spondylitis |
| Psoriatic arthritis |
| Reactive arthritis |
| Post-dystenteric |
| Post-NSU |
| Inflammatory bowel disease |

*Abbreviation:* NSU = nonspecific urethritis.

### 5.1 Optimum Treatment

#### 5.1.1 Ankylosing Spondylitis

Night pain and early morning stiffness are often the most distressing features of ankylosing spondylitis. To combat early morning stiffness and nocturnal pain, a large dose of an NSAID taken at night may be appropriate. NSAIDs should be taken regularly throughout the day, sometimes with the use of sustained-release preparations at night and a rapid-release dosage form of the same drug early in the morning. All NSAIDs have been used in the management of ankylosing spondylitis, although traditionally phenybutazone and indomethacin have been the first-line treatments. Corticosteroids may sometimes be required, but are generally not useful. Local corticosteroid injections (see section 3.1.3) can be used for peripheral joint disease or for the local treatment of enthesopathies.

Recently, *sulfasalazine* in doses of up to 2 g/day has shown benefits in some patients with ankylosing spondylitis, psoriatic arthritis and reactive arthritis. This drug seems to be more effective on peripheral manifestations of spondyloarthropathies, although some studies suggest benefits on the actual disease as well.[83,84]

The most important management issue in patients with ankylosing spondylitis is to institute a continuous exercise programme, stressing extension exercises with regular hydrotherapy. Inflammation of the eye should be reviewed rapidly and in most cases will respond to topical treatment with corticosteroid eye drops and mydriatics.

#### 5.1.2 Psoriatic Arthritis

NSAIDs form the mainstay of treatment for psoriatic arthritis, but in significant disease methotrexate, corticosteroids and sulfasalazine can be used. Methotrexate should be used in single weekly doses of 7.5 to 15mg and the patient monitored for hepatotoxicity.[85] Intramuscular gold and auranofin have also been used to suppress disease activity in psoriatic arthritis without making the skin rash worse.

Retinoids may be required for the management of skin rash (see further chapter 17; sect. 6.1.2) and more recently cyclosporin has been used to some effect in severe psoriasis and psoriatic arthritis.[86]

#### 5.1.3 Enteropathic Arthropathies

The arthritis of Crohn's disease and ulcerative colitis tend to improve when the gut disease is under control (see chapter 22; sect. 9.2.2).

The arthritic symptoms can be treated with NSAIDs, although these agents can sometimes exacerbate the gastrointestinal symptoms.

#### 5.1.4 Reactive Arthritis

Reactive arthritis refers to an inflammatory oligoarthropathy (less than 5 joints involved) which commonly occurs in patients who are HLA B27 positive following an acute bowel infection or nonspecific urethritis.[87,88] Arthritic symptoms must be treated with NSAIDs or local injections of corticosteroids. Sulfasalazine has been used in persistent cases.

## 6. Polymyalgia Rheumatica

Polymyalgia rheumatica is a clinical syndrome of middle aged or elderly patients, characterised by pain and stiffness in the neck, shoulders and pelvic girdle, and often accompanied by constitutional symptoms. It may be associated with giant cell arteritis involving the temporal or other arteries.

### 6.1 Optimum Treatment

*Corticosteroids* are usually dramatically effective in polymyalgia rheumatica, even in small doses (20 mg/day of prednisolone or prednisone). Few studies have reviewed initial corticosteroid doses but high- and low-dose regimens have been compared over the first 2 months of treatment,[89] with a significantly higher proportion of patients relapsing after initial treatment with prednisolone 10 to 20 mg/day.[89] Patients should be commenced on prednisolone 20 mg/day and if a dramatic response does not occur, the diagnosis should be re-evaluated. Once a response has occurred, the prednisolone or prednisone dosage can be reduced by 1mg/day every 2 to 4 weeks depending on symptoms and the erythrocyte sedimentation rate (ESR). Analgesics may also be given as required, but an effective dose of corticosteroids is essential.

The disease may persist for 2 to 6 years and prednisolone/prednisone will have to be continued in the lowest effective dose throughout this period. Although NSAIDs are useful in milder cases, prednisolone or prednisone remain the first-line treatment.

#### Giant Cell Arteritis

If the disease pattern is more that of giant cell arteritis with evidence of disease affecting other arteries of the body, including the temporal arteries, higher doses of prednisolone or prednisone (60 mg/day) should be used. If the temporal symptoms persist, there is a danger of blindness, with involvement of branches of the ophthalmic arteries. There should be no delay in initiation of therapy as complete loss of vision may occur.

It is not unusual for the polymyalgic pattern of the disease to progress to giant cell arteritis if therapy is interrupted or discontinued prematurely. When high doses of prednisolone or prednisone have to be maintained for long periods of time, corticosteroid-sparing drugs such as azathioprine or methotrexate may be used.

Synovitis involving the hands and knees may also occur in association with polymyalgia rheumatica and it is possible that some cases of polymyalgia rheumatica in the elderly are due to seronegative arthritis (see section 5). A similar syndrome is seen on occasions with malignant disease and also with rheumatoid arthritis and this can cause diagnostic confusion.

## 7. Soft Tissue Lesions

Patients with soft tissue lesions of the musculoskeletal system commonly present to general practitioners. They are best treated by initial rest (for a short period of time) followed by a graded exercise programme. If it is an acute sports injury and severe injury has been excluded, then the principle of ‘RICE’ should be used, i.e.

- Rest
- Ice
- Compression
- Elevation.

Early return to activity is to be encouraged. NSAIDs may influence the acute inflammatory phase, but analgesics are often just as effective. Local NSAID application by gel or cream formulations (e.g. of benzydamine, diclofenac, felbinac, ibuprofen, ketoprofen or piroxicam) may be useful.[90,91] Most chronic soft tissue lesions such as shoulder capsulitis take many months to settle, if at all. Ruptures of the shoulder joint capsule may respond to surgical correction, and corticosteroid injections associated with gentle exercises may be helpful.

Other soft tissue lesions may occasionally respond to injection of the painful areas with corticosteroids or local anaesthetics. Although this is common practice, clinical trials rarely demonstrate benefit. *Tennis* or *golfer's elbow* will often respond to local corticosteroid injections but it is important to follow these up with gentle stretching exercises and advice regarding grips for the racquet or golf club. Rubefacients are commonly used and may be of benefit along with transdermal NSAIDs (see above). Soft tissue musculoskeletal pain may also be referred from degenerative disease in adjacent joints and such cases are helped by analgesics, physiotherapy and NSAIDs.

## 8. Fibromyalgia Syndrome

Fibromyalgia syndrome occurs in up to 2% of people presenting to general practitioners and is characterised by chronic, diffuse, musculoskeletal pain and tender points in the absence of evidence of inflammation.[92,93] Most patients are women, with a peak age between 30 and 50 years.[94] Associated features include fatigue, sleep disturbances, stiffness, paraesthesia, headache, depression and anxiety. These patients often have associated irritable bowel syndrome and Raynaud's-like symptoms. For classification, patients must have pain for at least 3 months involving both sides of the upper and lower body and pain in at least 11 of 18 tender points on digital examination.[57] Underlying diseases such as inflammatory rheumatic disease and hypothyroidism should be excluded. A recent population study from England demonstrated a significant incidence of tender points in the normal population, throwing some doubt on the concept of fibromyalgia as a separate entity.[95]

### 8.1 Optimum Treatment

Treatment is difficult, but low doses of tricyclic antidepressants such as *amitriptyline* and the centrally-acting muscle relaxant *cyclobenzaprine* have been shown to be more effective than placebo in controlled trials. NSAIDs are not usually of great benefit, but analgesics can help. The most important factor in treatment is education of the patient and the development of a graded exercise programme.[96,97]

## 9. Low Back Pain

Most people will develop back pain at some point during their lives and, while most episodes improve within 8 weeks, a small percentage of patients have chronic low back pain that costs the community billions of dollars annually.[98-100]

Back pain has many causes and it is important to exclude serious disease such as neoplasia. In most cases, the exact source of the pain cannot be identified and overinvestigation at an early stage may encourage illness behaviour. Patients should be continually reminded that the vast majority of individuals improve over a 2- to 3-week period.

### 9.1 Optimum Treatment

For people with acute back pain and no neurological abnormalities, bedrest should be no longer than 2 days, with a graded exercise programme started once the pain has settled.[101] Physical treatments include icepacks, heat and use of a transdermal electrical nerve stimulation (TENS) machine.

Analgesics are the mainstay of treatment and, although strong (opioid) analgesics may be required in the first 24 to 48 hours, most patients can be managed with paracetamol or paracetamol/codeine combinations. NSAIDs may provide additional relief and are more effective than placebo in relieving low back pain. Muscle relaxants do not usually provide any additional relief, although they may be used sparingly with drugs such as tricyclic antidepressants to manage patients with chronic back pain. Facet joint injections and epidural corticosteroids may be used in patients not responding to conservative management, but few properly controlled studies of this treatment have been carried out.

The most important aspect of the management of low back pain is to provide a continuing exercise programme, particularly concentrating on abdominal muscles and encouraging activities such as swimming. Exercises must be individualised to each patient and persisted with for long periods of time. The general management of back pain requires a positive and confident therapeutic attitude and must take into account all the methods of treatment available and their use where appropriate, e.g. drugs, physical therapy (intermittent traction, manipulation and mobilisation), isometric exercises, heat and cold, back supports, epidural analgesia, rest and occasionally surgery. Back care education is most important, with instructions on carrying and lifting techniques.[102]

## 10. Juvenile Chronic Arthritis

Juvenile chronic arthritis is the most commonly diagnosed rheumatic disease in children and is an important cause of disability and blindness.[103] The criteria for diagnosis include arthritis occurring before the age of 16 years, excluding other forms of juvenile arthritis. After 6 months of disease, 3 major subsets can be identified that are useful in determining prognosis:

- Pauciarticular (4 or fewer joints)
- Polyarticular onset (5 or more joints)
- Systemic onset with fever and arthritis.[104]

## 10.1 Optimum Treatment

Therapy in juvenile chronic arthritis should provide pain relief, preserve joint function, and maintain normal growth and psychosocial development.[105] One of the most important factors is to manage the multidisciplinary team involved in the care of a young person with arthritis.

Medical treatment involves the use of NSAIDs, corticosteroids and disease-modifying antirheumatic drugs. *Aspirin* is an effective NSAID, both for pain and for systemic features, but must be used extremely carefully in childhood because of the risks of intoxication. Drowsiness and hyperventilation are 2 of the earliest signs of aspirin intoxication in young children who may later complain of tinnitus or deafness, the margin between tinnitus and acidosis being very small. The dosage of aspirin in juvenile chronic arthritis is of the order of 80 mg/kg/day in divided doses. The dose can be modified according to the therapeutic response and plasma concentration (2 to 2.5 mg/L). Larger dosages may be required in certain patients (up to 130 mg/kg/day). An association between aspirin administration and the development of Reye's syndrome characterised by encephalopathy and fatty degeneration has been reported. Because of this, salicylates should be stopped in any sick child who is vomiting or who may have a viral illness.[106]

If a child does not respond to salicylates after a sufficient trial (≈50% do), a number of NSAIDs can be substituted, e.g.:

- *Tolmetin* 25 mg/kg/day (in 4 divided doses)
- *Naproxen* 10 to 15 mg/kg/day (in divided doses)
- *Ibuprofen* 20 to 35 mg/kg/day (in divided doses)
- *Diclofenac* 2 to 3 mg/kg/day (in divided doses)
- *Sulindac* 6 mg/kg/day (in divided doses)
- *Indomethacin* 2.5 mg/kg/day (in divided doses).

A range of disease-modifying antirheumatic drugs (DMARDs) similar to that used in adult rheumatoid arthritis (see section 3.1.3) is available for children not responding adequately to NSAIDs alone. This includes antimalarials, gold (intramuscular and oral), penicillamine and sulfasalazine. Gold therapy is often beneficial in patients with severe persistent disease activity and enables reductions in corticosteroid dosages. The dose of *sodium aurothiomalate* is about 1 mg/kg/week until objective improvement occurs, when the frequency of injections can be reduced. *Auranofin* 0.15 to 0.2 mg/kg/day is also beneficial in some children. However, gold compounds should be used carefully, if at all, in patients with active systemic disease as there may be an increased risk of toxicity.[107]

*Penicillamine* may be given to children in doses of 10 mg/kg/day and should be taken on an empty stomach to avoid chelation by metals contained in food. As with gold salts, very close monitoring is necessary.

*Hydroxychloroquine* is also useful in the management of juvenile chronic arthritis in doses of around 7 mg/kg/day. This may be difficult to achieve with the 200mg tablet size but the total weekly dose may be divided irregularly over the week as an alternative. Regular ophthalmological examinations must be carried out and this is difficult with particularly young children.

*Sulfasalazine* has a relatively rapid onset of action (6 to 8 weeks) and can be used in maintenance doses of 40 to 60 mg/kg/day in divided doses.

In patients failing to respond to the above treatments, *methotrexate* 10 mg/m$^2$/week has been used.[108] Risk factors for toxicity that are commonly seen in adults such as diabetes, obesity and alcoholism are rarely found in children, but liver function tests should be monitored regularly.

*Corticosteroids* are occasionally indicated in children with chronic arthritis who have life-threatening complications of their disease. Prednisolone is a first-line treatment in dosages of 0.5 to 1.0 mg/kg/day as a single daily dose or in divided doses. Methylprednisolone has sometimes been used as pulse therapy in a dosage of 10 to 30 mg/kg/pulse (usually given 3 times). Intra-articular corticosteroids can be used as in adult disease, but the major problem with corticosteroids is that of adverse events. Children rapidly develop Cushingoid features even while receiving comparatively small dosages, and osteoporosis with vertebral collapse and stunting of growth may be even more marked than that seen in untreated patients.

Corticosteroid eye drops may be required for chronic uveitis, but this treatment should be supervised by an ophthalmologist since blindness may occur as a result (see further chapter 15; sect. 6). Intravenous human gammaglobulin and cyclosporin have also been used in patients with severe juvenile arthritis, but should be reserved for those whose disease is resistant to other treatments.[109]

## 11. Other Rheumatic Conditions

### 11.1 Connective Tissue Diseases of Immunological Origin

Connective tissue diseases of immunological origin include systemic lupus erythematosus, polyarteritis nodosa, progressive systemic sclerosis, polymyositis and dermatomyositis. These are generalised systemic connective tissue diseases and require careful diagnosis and management.

#### *11.1.1 Systemic Lupus Erythematosus*

Systemic lupus erythematosus (SLE) is a chronic rheumatic disease with exacerbations and remissions of clinical activity. Management must be directed at treating the acute exacerbations of the disease and developing strategies to minimise progressive damage.[110]

Many patients with systemic disease can be controlled with *NSAIDs*, although care must be taken with these since adverse reactions to NSAIDs, particularly involving the kidneys and the central nervous system, may be confused with manifestations of the disease. *Antimalarial drugs* (chloroquine, hydroxychloroquine) are used extensively for the cutaneous and musculoskeletal manifestation of SLE. Recent studies have suggested that the disease (including systemic features) may flare when antimalarials are ceased.[111]

*Corticosteroids* are required for most systemic features of the disease, an initial dose of prednisolone 45 to 60 mg/day usually being sufficient.[112] Although renal biopsies should be performed to diagnose lupus nephritis, they are not usually prognostically helpful. However, if early diffuse proliferative glomerulonephritis is found, immunosuppressive therapy should be started immediately. Approximately 20% of patients with mesangial proliferation will develop more serious glomerulonephritis, and corticosteroid therapy and other treatments may not prevent this progression.[113]

Corticosteroids are also associated with significant morbidity in the long term and their dosage should be kept to a minimum with the use of NSAIDs, antimalarial agents and immunosuppressive drugs.

In patients with severe lupus glomerulonephritis, a regimen including cyclophosphamide is more effective in preserving renal function than corticosteroids alone[114] and is probably more effective than treatment with corticosteroids and azathioprine.[115] Cyclophosphamide given as a monthly high-dose intravenous pulse is as effective and less toxic than a lower daily oral dose.[116] The potential for toxicity with cyclophosphamide is substantial, but the drug can be extremely effective when given intravenously for haematological, central nervous system and vascular manifestations of severe lupus. Adverse effects include damage to gonadal tissue (leading to ovarian failure and azoospermia), haemorrhagic cystitis and bladder fibrosis, and the subsequent development of malignancy. Mesna (2-mercaptoethane-sulfonate), which binds acrolein, the toxic metabolite responsible for acute cystitis, should be given to patients receiving intravenous pulse therapy with cyclophosphamide.[117]

Clinicians managing patients with SLE must be ever watchful for symptoms which might indicate a flare of disease and must monitor patients long term for exacerbations of the disease and adverse effects of treatment.[110]

#### *11.1.2 Polyarteritis Nodosa*

Treatment of polyarteritis nodosa depends on the extent of disease involvement. Patients who have limited and nonprogressive disease may be treated with corticosteroids alone while those with extensive systemic features and evidence of progression despite corticosteroids require a cytotoxic agent as well.

The initial management of polyarteritis requires doses of prednisolone 40 to 60 mg/day and there is no place for alternate-day therapy.[118] Once the disease is under control, as indicated by normalisation of the erythrocyte sedimentation rate and improvement in clinical features, the prednisolone dosage can be reduced slowly, but long term maintenance at low dosages is usually required. Cytotoxic drugs such as cyclophosphamide or chlorambucil should be considered if the disease is very aggressive from the outset, or if corticosteroids at an acceptable dosage do not control disease activity.

#### 11.1.3 Progressive Systemic Sclerosis

Over the past decade, significant changes have occurred in the management of progressive systemic sclerosis. NSAIDs may control the arthralgia of finger joints associated with the disease. Hand care and instruction of finger exercises is most important to preserve function in and prevent injury to the hands. Raynaud's phenomena (with or without underlying systemic connective tissue disease) should be treated aggressively by recommending abstinence from smoking and avoidance of exposure to cold. Drugs such as *nifedipine* (30 to 90 mg/day) are useful.[119] Other calcium antagonists and occlusive dressings are useful for digital ulcers. Prostaglandin infusions or sympathectomy may be necessary for acute ischaemia, and antibiotics and adequate pain control are useful for gangrenous infected ulcers, with or without surgical debridement.[120]

Many other drugs have been recommended for progressive systemic sclerosis but only *penicillamine* has been shown to improve 5-year survival rates in patients with progressive systemic disease.[121,122] These studies show not only improvement in the skin features but also improved survival suggesting decreased systemic disease. *Corticosteroids* may be used for complications such as pulmonary involvement or pericarditis and gastrointestinal disturbances are usually treated with $H_2$-receptor antagonists or acid (proton) pump inhibitors.

Of major importance is the use of ACE inhibitors in the prevention and management of renal dysfunction.[123] Blood pressure should be monitored carefully in patients with progressive systemic sclerosis, and ACE inhibitors and other aggressive treatment for hypertension started as soon as the blood pressure rises.[124]

#### 11.1.4 Polymyositis and Dermatomyositis

*Corticosteroids* remain the mainstay of treatment for these conditions.[125] It is important to obtain an objective assessment of muscle involvement by muscle biopsy and then start prednisolone (40 to 80 mg/day in adults or 1 to 2 mg/kg/day in children) for 4 to 6 weeks until maximum benefit or remission of the disease has been achieved. Thereafter, the dose can be reduced slowly, depending on clinical features and muscle enzymes.

When the disease does not respond to adequate corticosteroid doses, other immunosuppressive drugs should be considered.[126] *Methotrexate* has been used orally or intravenously in doses up to 50 mg/week and *azathioprine, cyclophosphamide* and *cyclosporin* have been used in resistant cases. *Hydroxychloroquine* may be helpful in suppressing the dermatological features of dermatomyositis and also in improving muscle strength.

### 11.2 Infective Arthritis

Infective arthritis may be caused by bacteria, viruses or fungi. In some cases of infective arthritis, the disease is due to the presence of organisms within the joint tissues but in others there may be a cross reaction between the joint tissues and the infective agent. In viraemic states, such as rubella, mumps or infectious mononucleosis, no therapy other than analgesics or nonsteroidal anti-inflammatory drugs is usually necessary, since the condition rapidly subsides. Occasionally a short course of corticosteroids may be required to suppress inflammation.

*Septic arthritis* associated with bacteria such as gonococci, staphylococci or streptococci requires urgent diagnosis and treatment. Joint aspiration and washout, usually with surgical drainage and appropriate antibiotics, must be started immediately. Joint tissues and, in particular, cartilage will be destroyed by septic synovial fluid extremely rapidly. Early diagnosis and treatment is essential, because delay in therapy is associated with a high mortality and morbidity.[127] Septic arthritis or bursitis may arise following superficial skin infections.

*Lyme disease* is now being reported much more frequently around the world. This disease is a multisystem tick-borne disorder caused by the spirochaete *Borrelia burgdorferi*. Clinical manifestations of Lyme disease include an erythematous macule (erythema migrans) followed by a general systemic upset which may include arthralgias, myalgias and headache and then, in some cases, the development of chronic neurological manifestations, cardiac involvement and a migratory polyarthritis. Chronic musculoskeletal and neurological disease can occur. After serological or clinical diagnosis, doxycycline or amoxicillin may be given for 10 to 30 days and if severe or chronic disease persists, intravenous antibiotics such as ceftriaxone or benzylpenicillin (penicillin G) for up to 14 days may be required.[128]

Rheumatoid joints are more susceptible to infection from the bloodstream than normal joints. A sudden flare in a single joint in a patient with an inflammatory polyarthritis should suggest trauma or infection rather than an exacerbation of rheumatoid disease.[129]

## 12. Bone Disorders

### 12.1 Malignant Bone Diseases

Multiple myeloma, metastatic carcinoma, sarcoma and a number of malignant diseases may directly affect bones or joints or be indirectly associated with arthritis, such as the hypertrophic pulmonary osteoarthropathy associated with bronchial carcinoma.

Malignant deposits cause pain in bone and joints, but are usually metastatic and life expectancy is extremely limited. In such cases, pain relief is the standard treatment, in association with treatment of the underlying disease. *NSAIDs* are helpful in the management of bone pain due to secondary carcinoma. *Analgesics* may also be required. Paracetamol, with or without codeine, may be helpful but, if the pain is severe, then slow-release morphine preparations may be beneficial in doses that relieve the pain. Analgesics should be taken regularly in this situation and not 'on demand' (see further chapter 12; sect. 7.2). In certain situations, bone pain may respond to localised radiotherapy.

### 12.2 Osteoporosis

Osteoporosis is a reduction in the amount of bone tissue per unit volume of bone, resulting in skeletal weakness and subsequent fracture, often following minimal trauma.[130] Primary prevention of osteoporosis may be assisted by optimising peak adult bone mass through adequate dietary intake of calcium and regular weight-bearing exercise.

Bone density increases in both men and women from early childhood to a peak in the late teens or early adulthood. This peak bone mass appears to be determined largely by genetic factors, but is also influenced by environmental and lifestyle issues. With increasing age, both men and women start to lose bone gradually, although in women there is also a rapid phase of bone loss immediately after the menopause (fig. 5). Bone loss appears to be less rapid after 65 years of age, but even in older people with established osteoporosis, bone loss may continue.

Fracture risk in later life is directly related to bone density and, because of this, prevention of osteoporosis may be considered in the following terms:

- Maximisation of peak bone mass

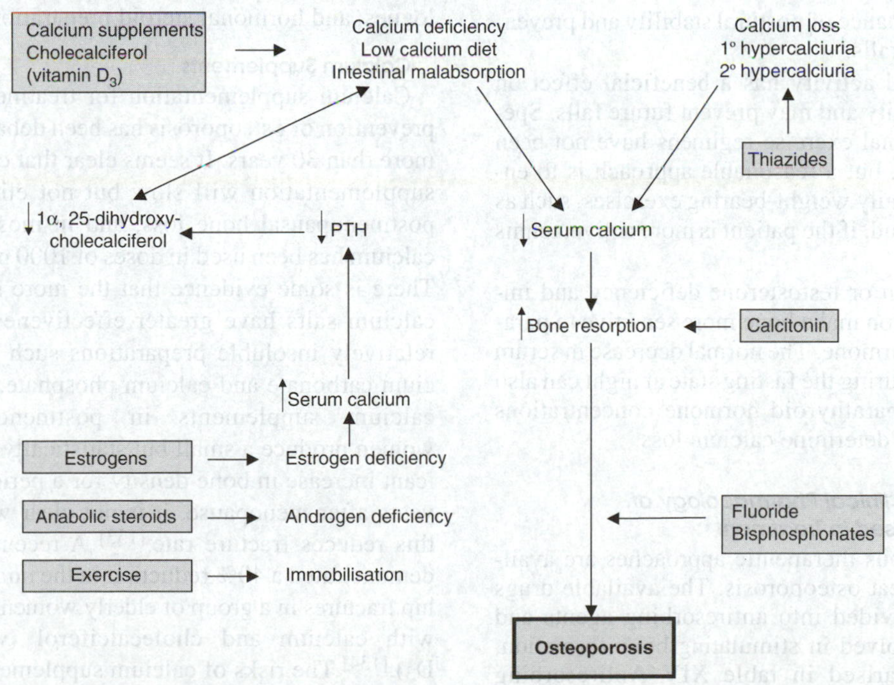


**Fig. 5.** Pathophysiology of osteoporosis and mechanisms/sites of action of drugs used in treatment. *Abbreviation:* PTH = parathyroid hormone.

**Table XIV.** Osteoporosis therapy (after Dequeker[131])

| Drug | Effect on bone | | Indication | | Comments/adverse effects |
|---|---|---|---|---|---|
| | cortical | trabecular | prevention | therapy | |
| **Antiresorbing agents:** | | | | | |
| Calcium | + | + | + | + | Take at bedtime |
| Thiazides | + | + | + | + | Useful in hypercalciuria and patients with hypertension |
| Vitamin D | + | + | + | + | May cause hypercalcaemia and hypercalciuria |
| Estrogens | + | + | ++ | +? | Compliance low<br>Annual mammography required<br>?Biopsy of endometrium |
| Calcitonin | − | + | +? | + | Pain relief<br>Temporarily active |
| Bisphosphonates | − | + | +? | + | May affect bone quality (brittle) |
| **Formation stimulating agents:** | | | | | |
| Sodium fluoride | − | +++ | − | + | *Adverse effects:* gastrointestinal, articular, ?bone quality |
| Anabolic steroids | ++ | + | − | ++ | Positive effect on muscle mass in the very elderly<br>Virilisation manageable |
| Vitamin D analogues | − | + (+) | − | + | Corticosteroid-induced osteoporosis |
| Hormonal steroid preparations (estrogen/progestagen or androgen) | + | ++ | + | + | ?Lipid profile changes<br>Good compliance |

- Avoidance or modification of lifestyle and environmental factors that cause bone loss
- Use of treatments, e.g. estrogens, to prevent postmenopausal bone loss
- Maintenance of postural stability and prevention of falls.

Physical activity has a beneficial effect on bone density and may prevent future falls. Specific optimal exercise regimens have not been identified, but a reasonable approach is to encourage daily weight-bearing exercises, such as walking and, if the patient is more active, tennis and golf.

Estrogen or testosterone deficiency and immobilisation make bone more sensitive to parathyroid hormone. The normal decrease in serum calcium during the fasting state at night can also increase parathyroid hormone concentrations and, thus, determine calcium loss.

#### *12.2.1 Clinical Pharmacology of Drugs Used in Treatment*

Numerous therapeutic approaches are available to treat osteoporosis. The available drugs can be divided into antiresorbing agents and those involved in stimulating bone formation, as summarised in table XIV. Antiresorbing agents are primarily considered to prevent further bone loss and include calcium, estrogens, calcitonin, bisphosphonates, thiazide diuretics and vitamin D.[132] Drugs that stimulate bone formation include sodium fluoride, anabolic steroids, cholecalciferol (vitamin $D_3$) analogues, and hormonal steroid preparations.

##### Calcium Supplements

Calcium supplementation for treatment and prevention of osteoporosis has been debated for more than 30 years. It seems clear that calcium supplementation will slow but not eliminate postmenopausal bone loss, and in most trials calcium has been used in doses of 1000 mg/day. There is some evidence that the more soluble calcium salts have greater effectiveness than relatively insoluble preparations such as calcium carbonate and calcium phosphate. While calcium supplements in postmenopausal women produce a small but statistically significant increase in bone density for a period of 5 years after menopause, it is not clear whether this reduces fracture rate.[133] A recent study demonstrated a 40% reduction in the number of hip fractures in a group of elderly women treated with calcium and cholecalciferol (vitamin $D_3$).[134] The risks of calcium supplementation are small, the main concern being the possibility of increasing the risk of renal calculi.

**Calcitonin**

Calcitonin is a 32-amino acid peptide hormone that decreases bone resorption through a direct action on osteoclasts. It also decreases renal tubular reabsorption of calcium and has an analgesic effect, the mechanism of which appears to be independent of its action on osteoclastic bone resorption and is possibly mediated via β-endorphins. Several forms of calcitonin have been produced for therapeutic use, including porcine, salmon and human preparations, the most active in terms of its hypocalcaemic activity being salmon calcitonin. The salmon preparation also has a lower metabolic clearance than the mammalian forms, although all have short elimination half-lives. As proteolytic digestion prevents their oral administration, the majority of clinical studies in patients with bone diseases characterised by excessive bone resorption such as osteoporosis, Paget's disease (see section 12.4) and malignant and hyperparathyroid hypercalcaemia have been with parenteral (subcutaneous or intramuscular) administration.[135]

Recently, however, calcitonin formulations administered by other routes have been developed, and amongst these, an intranasal formulation of salmon calcitonin appears to be the most promising and provides a more convenient means of administering the drug. Following intranasal administration, salmon calcitonin is rapidly absorbed with peak plasma plasma concentrations obtained in 15 to 60 minutes. In comparison with intramuscular administration, intranasal salmon calcitonin results in relatively low peak plasma concentrations but a more sustained (≥4 hours) hypercalcitoninaemia. In terms of the acute biochemical response, the relative biological activity of the intranasal formulation is 25 to 50% of the parenteral preparation, an intranasal dose of 100U being bioequivalent to a subcutaneous dose of 50U.[136]

In patients with osteoporosis, parenterally administered calcitonin stabilises and increases indices of cortical and trabecular bone mass and total body calcium, although the routine use of calcitonin administered by this route has been limited by poor patient compliance and tolerability.[137] Studies with intranasal salmon calcitonin have shown this preparation to slow bone loss in postmenopausal women and provide small increases in bone mass in patients with established osteoporosis.[136]

***Tolerability***: the most commonly encountered adverse effects of parenteral calcitonin therapy are nausea, vomiting, facial flushing, rashes and a local inflammatory reaction at the injection site. The severity of these adverse effects appears to be dose-related and they can often be attenuated by reduction of the dose.[137] With intranasal salmon calcitonin, transient local reactions such as stinging, tingling, sneezing, rhinitis, mucosal erythema and rarely, bleeding have occurred, as well as mild systemic effects such as flushing, itching, nausea and dizziness.[136]

**Bisphosphonates**

The bisphosphonates are analogues of pyrophosphate (an endogenous regulator of bone turnover) but instead of the P-O-P (phosphorus-oxygen-phosphorus) structure of pyrophosphate, they have a P-C-P (phosphorus-carbon-

**Table XV.** Bisphosphonates used in the treatment of osteoporosis and Paget's disease (after Rosen & Kessenich[139])

| Drug | Route of administration | Oral bioavailability (%) | Dosage osteoporosis | Dosage Paget's disease | Clinical effectiveness osteoporosis | Clinical effectiveness Paget's disease |
|---|---|---|---|---|---|---|
| Alendronate | PO/IV | 1-10 | 10 mg/day PO | 40 mg/day PO for 6 mos *or* 5-10mg IV over 4h q3-12 mos | +++ | ++ |
| Etidronate | PO/IV | 1-10 | 400 mg/day PO for 14d every 3 mos | 5 mg/kg/day PO for 6 mos | +++/– | ++ |
| Pamidronate | IV | 1-10 | 150 mg/day PO[a] | 30mg IV over 4h weekly for 6 wks | ++/– | +++ (IV) |
| Tiludronate | PO | 1-10 | 50-400 mg/day PO for 7d per month, or daily | 400 mg/day PO for 6 mos | +++ | + |

a An oral dosage form of pamidronate is not yet generally available.

*Abbreviations and symbols:* IV = intravenous; PO = oral; + = some evidence of effectiveness; ++ = positive benefits and minimal risk; ++/– = positive benefits and some adverse effects; +++ = very positive benefits; +++/– very positive benefits and some adverse effects.

phosphorus) structure which renders them resistant to enzymatic hydrolysis by skeletal phosphatases. As a class, these drugs exhibit strong affinity for hydroxyapatite crystal of bone. Numerous bisphosphonates have been synthesised, and a number have been studied in metabolic bone diseases, including the first-generation agent *etidronate*, the second-generation agents *pamidronate* and *tiludronate*, and the newer third-generation agent *alendronate*.

The bisphosphonates act by inhibiting osteoclast-mediated bone resorption, although the mechanisms by which they exert this activity are not clearly defined. They also inhibit calcium phosphate formation and dissolution, and inhibit normal and ectopic mineralisation through a physicochemical inhibition of crystal growth. As the bisphosphonates do not undergo enzymatic degradation by skeletal phosphatases, they are bone-avid agents and persist in the skeleton for prolonged periods.[138,139]

The available drugs of this class (table XV) differ widely in their antiresorptive potencies, which may be attributable to differing biochemical effects at the cellular level. The newer bisphosphonates such as alendronate and pamidronate have structures that convey high potency, thereby improving the margin between doses that inhibit osteoclast-mediated bone resorption and doses that inhibit bone mineralisation. For example, alendronate has a margin of 125 to 1000 between the dose that inhibits resorption and the dose that inhibits mineralisation.[138] With the less potent drug etidronate, the dose that inhibits resorption is close to that which impairs normal mineralisation. However, etidronate is given cyclically in doses of 400mg per day for 14 days every 3 months (with calcium 500mg per day administered in the intervening period), and with this regimen, adverse effects on mineralisation (which may lead to the development of osteomalacia) have not been described in therapy lasting up to 3 years, although it remains a potential concern with longer term treatment.[140,141]

***Pharmacokinetic characteristics***: the bisphosphonates, as a class, are poorly absorbed from the gastrointestinal tract, and their oral bioavailabilities range from only 1 to 10%. Their plasma half-lives are short (0.25 to 2 hours) as the drugs are cleared rapidly from the circulation, and around 50 to 75% of an absorbed dose is excreted in the urine – the values varying with the different agents and administration regimens. However, between 20 and 60% of an absorbed dose is taken up into the skeleton, where in contrast to the circulation, the half-life is very long. Skeletal turnover of the bisphosphonates occurs only during active bone resorption, and therefore it is likely that the drugs remain in the skeleton for prolonged periods and their bone half-lives may be several years.[139-141]

***Tolerability***: the bisphosphonates are generally well tolerated drugs, although gastrointestinal problems (e.g. dyspepsia, nausea, vomiting, diarrhoea, gastritis, oesophagitis, abdominal pain) may occur in some patients and some severe reactions have been reported. These adverse effects are dose-related, and appear less common with the lower doses used in the treatment of osteoporosis. Other adverse effects reported include hypocalcaemia (which is rarely a clinical problem and is prevented by ensuring an adequate calcium and vitamin D intake), occasional skin reactions, and with pamidronate, a transient self-limiting pyrexia and a few instances of reversible iritis.[140,141]

**Estrogens**

The available estrogens and their clinical pharmacological properties are discussed in chapter 18 (section 11.4), along with the benefits and risks of their use in hormone replacement therapy (HRT). Their clinical use in postmenopausal osteoporosis is discussed below.

### 12.2.2 Optimum Treatment

*Calcium supplements* at night (1000mg as effervescent or other tablets) and vitamin D in small doses (1000 U/day of vitamin D or its analogues), if adequate exposure to sunlight is not possible, are given to raise the serum calcium concentrations.[131,142]

*Estrogens* can be prescribed for women with postmenopausal osteoporosis within 20 years of menopause. Bone loss can be prevented in perimenopausal women by use of hormone replacement therapy (HRT) and there is now evidence that bone density can be increased in women well into the postmenopausal period. Combination estrogen and progestagen regimens are recommended to produce amenorrhoea which is much more acceptable to elderly women. Adverse effects of this therapy include breast tenderness, which may be reduced by using very small doses of estrogen (e.g. conjugated estrogens 0.3 mg/day). For most women the normal minimum effective dose is conjugated estrogens 0.625 mg/day and in women with an intact uterus, cyclical progestagens should also be prescribed (e.g. medroxyprogesterone acetate 5 to 10 mg/day for the first 14 days of each calendar month while conjugated estrogens are taken continuously). Patients on HRT should undergo a yearly mammogram and frequent breast examination and any vaginal bleeding should be investigated thoroughly.[143] Estrogens may also be administered transdermally (e.g. as estradiol patches) in women who are intolerant of oral estrogen therapy.[144,145]

*Calcitonin* (see section 12.2.1) has been shown to be modestly effective in the treatment of osteoporosis for periods of up to 2 years. *Bisphosphonates* (see section 12.2.1 and table XV) are effective inhibitors of osteoclastic bone resorption, and recent studies have demonstrated that not only do they produce a progressive increase in bone mineral density at all skeletal sites, but that treatment is associated with a significant reduction in the proportion of women reporting new vertebral fractures.[146]

*Vitamin D* or its analogues are recommended if there is evidence of calcium malabsorption. Doses of 10,000 U/day vitamin D or 0.5 μg/day *calcitriol* (1α,25-dihydroxycholecalciferol) are useful in corticosteroid-induced osteoporosis, renal bone dystrophy and menopausal osteoporosis, although hypercalcaemia and hypercalciuria may occur.

Although *sodium fluoride* has been used for a long time in osteoporosis and there is clear evidence that it increases bone density, there are concerns as to whether it increases skeletal fragility. Recent studies have suggested that fluoride may have a beneficial effect in reducing the fracture rate.[147]

*Thiazide diuretics* should be used in osteoporotic patients with hypercalcaemia and in those with hypertension. There are some data to suggest that the use of thiazide diuretics is associated with a reduction of approximately one-third in the risk of hip fractures.[148]

Bone densitometry should be performed in selected patients who are suitable for therapy and should influence patients' decisions about therapy. New methods for measuring bone mineral density such as DEXA (dual energy x-ray absorptiometry) can be applied to both actual and peripheral sites with high precision. Measurements should be made at more than one site and patients followed carefully.[149]

#### *12.2.3 Clinical Outcome and Economic Considerations*

Osteoporosis represents a major health problem and is estimated to afflict at least 25% of postmenopausal Caucasian women in the western world. In the US, nearly 1.3 million fractures each year are attributable to osteoporosis (including 250,000 hip, 250,000 wrist and 500,000 vertebral fractures), and the costs of treating these fractures has been estimated to be as high as US$10 billion per year.[150] For hip fractures, the lifetime risk has been estimated to be 15% in Caucasian women and 5% in Caucasian men, although considerable interregional differences exist. The risk in Black women is considerably smaller and the sex difference in the rate of hip fractures is also less pronounced in Black people.[151]

Fractures arising as a result of decreased bone mass and disrupted bone structure are associated with a marked increase in morbidity in postmenopausal women, and in both morbidity and mortality in elderly people of either sex.[151] In addition to the direct costs of treating osteoporotic fractures, their impact on the quality of life in the elderly is also an important consideration since they often lead to long term immobility and dependency on others. As the population continues to age, the personal and social costs of osteoporosis can be expected to rise, unless comprehensive and effective prevention and treatment programmes are implemented. The currently available therapies for treating established osteoporosis (see sections 12.2.1 and 12.2.2) are effective in reducing pain and disability but because they primarily slow the rate of bone loss and permit replacement of only a small portion of lost bone mass, it may already be too late to avert the costs of treating the consequences of osteoporosis over the next 15 to 20 years.[150] This underlines the importance of prevention which may be achieved by various strategies to increase bone mass (e.g. health recommendations on calcium intake and increasing physical activity) directed at the whole population and especially those considered to be at high risk of osteoporosis.

In postmenopausal women, preventive measures assume particular importance since the reduction in estrogen levels associated with the menopause is an important contributory factor to bone mineral loss. There is a sharp acceleration of bone loss during the 5 years following the menopause, with the greatest losses occurring in the first 2 years. In this scenario, screening procedures to identify women most likely to benefit from pharmacological measures to reduce postmenopausal bone loss are a critical component of the overall cost of prevention, and it is clear that the cost-effectiveness of such therapy would be improved if an effective model for identifying women at high risk was found.[151] Currently, the use of bone mineral density measurements appears to provide the most accurate, reproducible means of stratifying patients according to their fracture risk, and advancements in the use of such technology is enhancing our ability to detect high risk individuals.

Among the various pharmacological measures for prevention in postmenopausal women, the use of estrogens with or without progestagens (i.e. hormone replacement therapy; HRT) has been the most studied intervention in pharmacoeconomic studies. The available cost-benefit, cost-effectiveness and cost-utility studies have indicated that HRT appears to be most economically useful in the prevention of osteoporotic fracture if used in women who have undergone hysterectomy and those identified as being at high risk, and long term therapy (≥10 years) has usually proved more cost-effective than shorter term (5 years) treatment. Moreover, the cost-effectiveness of HRT is substantially improved when adjusted for quality of life, and, in general, the cost per quality-adjusted life year (QALY) with HRT was found to be comparable to that of other health interventions relevant to the older adult population (see review by Whittington & Faulds[144]). HRT has the added benefit of reducing menopausal symptoms and also cardiovascular risk (see also chapter 18; sect. 11.4 for further discussion of the benefits and risks of HRT).

At present, pharmacoeconomic data on other drug therapies for osteoporosis are not available.

## 12.3 Osteomalacia

Vitamin D deficiency is relatively rare in developed countries, especially those where there is an abundance of sunlight. Nevertheless, abnormalities of vitamin D metabolism occur in patients with renal disease and malabsorption syndromes, and sometimes as a consequence of antiepileptic drug therapy. Patients may complain of bone pain or muscular weakness.

### 12.3.1 Optimum Treatment

When the diagnosis is equivocal, a diagnostic trial of *vitamin D* replacement in dosages of 1500 to 3000 IU/day will produce a brisk rise in serum phosphate if the diagnosis is correct. Failure to respond to physiological vitamin D replacement indicates a vitamin D-resistant cause. *Calcitriol* 2 to 6 μg/day may be required to treat severe vitamin D-resistant disease and this dosage can be reduced over 3 to 4 months to maintenance levels of 0.5 to 1.25 μg/day. *Calcium supplements* are useful when the initial mineral deficit is large. Long term *phosphate supplements* are advisable in X-linked hypophosphataemia and are mandatory in adult-onset hypophosphataemic osteomalacia.[152]

## 12.4 Paget's Disease of Bone

Paget's disease of bone affects about 4% of the population over the age of 40 years. There is evidence of family clustering and the disease appears to be rare in the Middle East, China, Japan, Scandinavia and among those of Black African descent. Isolated areas of the skeleton undergo increased bone resorption with subsequent deposition of bone, and are disorganised, enlarged and structurally weak.[153,154] Paget's disease may be entirely asymptomatic, in which case no treatment is necessary, but in other cases it causes significant pain and disability. Such painful episodes may be associated with small, often incomplete, bony fractures.

### 12.4.1 Optimum Treatment

*Analgesics* may be required during the painful episodes and *NSAIDs* may also be used. Current clinical recommendations for treatment have been outlined[155] and include use of the *bisphosphonates* and *calcitonin* (see section 12.2.1 for a discussion on the clinical pharmacology of these agents).

#### Calcitonin

Both human and salmon calcitonin can relieve pain and suppress bone turnover, but may be associated with unpleasant adverse effects. These are less frequent when the drug is given intranasally. Remission in patients treated with calcitonin is incomplete and the condition may relapse despite continuation of therapy. Adverse effects usually occur within a few minutes of an injection, may last for an hour and are generally mild and include gastrointestinal irritation (nausea, vomiting, abdominal pain and diarrhoea), flushing of the face, tingling of the extremities, rashes and pain at the site of injection. The adverse effects are dose-related and are more marked after intramuscular injections that produce higher peak concentrations than after subcutaneous injections. The optimum dosage of salmon calcitonin is 50 to 100U (0.5mg in the case of human calcitonin) given 3 to 7 times a week.[135,156,157]

#### Bisphosphonates

The future treatment of Paget's disease lies in the second- and third-generation bisphosphonates (e.g. tiludronate and alendronate; see table XV) which are potent inhibitors of bone resorption. The first-generation compound etidronate can be given in a dose of 5 mg/kg/day for 6 months and then discontinued. Remissions appear to last longer than after calcitonin, but there is a risk of causing defective bone mineralisation that may result in the development of traumatic long bone fractures. Combinations of calcitonin and etidronate in conventional dosages seem to provide an additive suppressant effect on bone turnover and may be indicated for more active disease.[135,158,159]

More potent second- and third-generation bisphosphonates are now available and can be given intravenously on an intermittent basis. The best studied of these is *pamidronate*, which is given in a single 30mg infusion at weekly intervals for 6 weeks. Oral administration of pamidronate can lead to gastrointestinal irritation; hence, the parenteral route is recommended.[160]

Paget's disease can now be well controlled, although active disease tends to recur. All patients in their eighth decade should be treated when symptomatic and younger patients in their fifth decade should be treated aggressively. Whether this aggressive approach can reduce the serious complication of osteogenic sarcoma is as yet unproven.

## 13. Gout

Gout is a clinical syndrome caused by an inflammatory response to crystals of monosodium urate monohydrate that develop as a consequence of hyperuricaemia. Hyperuricaemia may be produced by overproduction or underexcretion of uric acid (fig. 6). Risk factors for gout include obesity, hypertension, alcohol consumption, and occupational and environmental exposure to lead.[162] Precipitation of urate crystals into joints, renal tubules and other tissues may result in acute arthritis, renal (uric acid) calculi and tophi. Renal calculi occur in some patients and they precede an acute attack of gout, whereas tophi are usually late manifestations of gouty arthritis. Treatment of gout falls under 3 main headings: (1) treatment of the acute attack; (2) prevention of acute and recurrent episodes of gout; and (3) dissolution of tophaceous deposits. The management of asymptomatic hyperuricaemia must also be considered.

### 13.1 Clinical Pharmacology of Drugs Used in Treatment

#### *13.1.1 Acute Gout*

Drugs used in the treatment of acute attacks of gout include the *nonsteroidal anti-inflammatory drugs* (NSAIDs; see section 3.1.2 for a discussion of their clinical pharmacology) and *colchicine*. The latter is less commonly used nowadays due to its unpleasant adverse effects, but may be useful when the NSAIDs are contraindicated or as an adjunct to NSAIDs in resistant cases.

***Colchicine*** appears to act by inhibiting the motility of leucocytes and their action in mediating urate crystal-induced inflammation. The drug also exerts antimitotic activity. Colchicine is rapidly absorbed after oral administration and peak plasma concentrations are reached within 2 hours. It is partially metabolised in the liver, and both the metabolites and unchanged drug are excreted in the bile with some being reabsorbed in the intestine; most of the drug is excreted in the faeces, although some (10 to 20%) is also eliminated in the urine. Although it often provides effective relief of acute gouty attacks, the usefulness of colchicine is limited by its gastrointestinal adverse effects which include diarrhoea, abdominal cramps, nausea and vomiting; if these adverse effects occur, treatment should be stopped to avoid more serious toxicity. Colchicine may also be given intravenously, but may cause thrombophlebitis (rarely) and local irritation if extravasation occurs.

#### *13.1.2 Recurrent Gout (Urate-Lowering Drugs)*

In patients with persistent hyperuricaemia experiencing recurrent attacks of gout, the drugs used for prophylaxis include the xanthine oxidase inhibitor *allopurinol*, and the uricosuric agents *probenecid, sulfinpyrazone* and *benzbromarone*. Allopurinol reduces the formation of uric acid, while the uricosuric agents increase the renal excretion of urate by inhibiting its tubular reabsorption. The latter drugs are now rel-

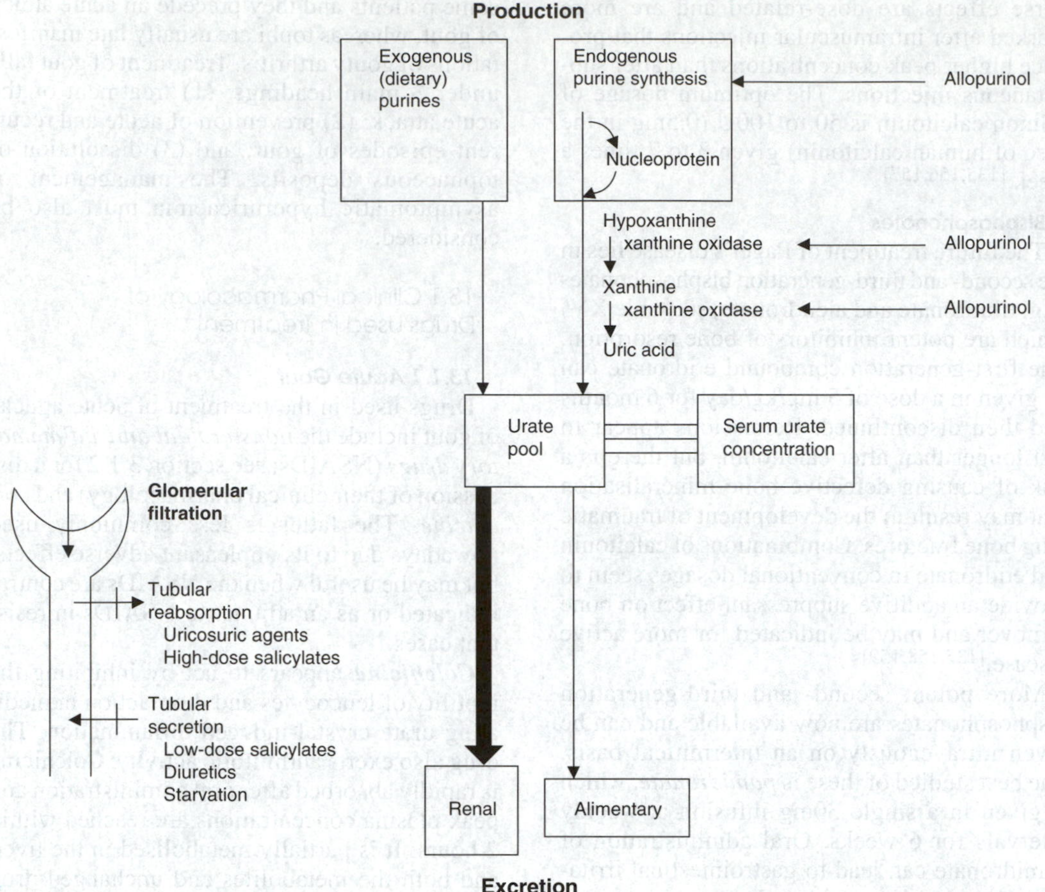


**Fig. 6.** Schematic representation of the urate pool (a balance between urate production and excretion) and its modification by urate-altering drugs (after Emmerson;[161] with permission).

atively uncommonly used to control hyperuricaemia and are usually reserved for patients who are intolerant of allopurinol; however, they may be preferred in patients who are 'underexcretors' of uric acid (< 800mg per day) provided tophi or joint damage are not present. The uricosurics are contraindicated in patients with uric acid calculi, and are relatively ineffective when the glomerular filtration rate is less than 50 ml/min (3 L/h).

#### Probenecid

Probenecid is readily absorbed orally and extensively protein bound but has a relatively short half-life of 6 to 12 hours. The dosage of probenecid should be increased slowly and a liberal fluid intake encouraged. Probenecid is usually well tolerated in doses up to 2 g/day, although mild gastrointestinal disturbances and skin rashes are seen and, rarely, hepatic necrosis and aplastic anaemia may occur.

#### Sulfinpyrazone

Sulfinpyrazone is also readily absorbed when given orally and has a half-life of approximately 4 hours. As well as promoting uric acid excretion, it has potent antiplatelet activity, reducing the tendency to thrombosis in atrioventricular shunts and mechanical intravascular devices.[161] It is sometimes more effective than probenecid in patients with renal insufficiency. Initial doses are 50mg twice daily, increasing to 400 to 600 mg/day. Adverse reactions include anorexia, nausea, vomiting, abdominal pain and, rarely, bone marrow suppression and skin rash.

#### Allopurinol

Allopurinol acts by competitive inhibition of the enzyme xanthine oxidase, which is instrumental in the conversion of the purine metabolite hypoxanthine to xanthine and its subsequent conversion to uric acid. Allopurinol is well absorbed orally and has a plasma half-life of between 40 minutes and 2 hours. Most of a dose of allopurinol is rapidly metabolised to its active metabolite oxypurinol, which has a much longer half-life (14 to 28 hours) and is largely excreted unchanged by the kidney. For this reason allopurinol can be given on a once-daily basis,[163] but dosage adjustments should be made when there is evidence of renal impairment[164] (see further appendix D).

In contrast to uricosuric agents, allopurinol causes a decrease in uric acid excretion and a corresponding increase in the concentrations of urinary (and plasma) hypoxanthine and xanthine. Changes in plasma uric acid concentrations may precipitate acute attacks of gout, but uric acid crystal and stone formation in the urinary tract are not a complication of this form of treatment. In addition to its effect on xanthine oxidase, allopurinol also reduces *de novo* purine synthesis. Allopurinol should be started at 100 mg/day and increased to 300 mg/day to reduce plasma urate concentrations to less than 0.4 μmol/L.

***Tolerability:*** 25% of patients are unable to tolerate allopurinol because of adverse reactions, which include hepatitis, nausea, vomiting, skin rashes and occasionally hypersensitivity vasculitis. Toxic epidermal necrosis may occur and can be fatal if not recognised early. Allopurinol sensitivity is more common in patients with renal dysfunction. Drug interactions have been noted between allopurinol and azathioprine, mercaptopurine, cyclophosphamide, ampicillin, warfarin, thiazide diuretics and theophylline (see further appendix B).

## 13.2 Optimum Treatment

### 13.2.1 Acute Attacks of Gout

In the treatment of an acute attack, a rapid-acting and effective anti-inflammatory agent is required to relieve pain as soon as possible.[165] Whichever drug is used, it is essential that treatment is started as soon as possible after the onset of symptoms. Many patients develop premonitory signs and symptoms, and treatment is best commenced at this stage. The essential aim of treatment is for the patient to find, by trial and error, the drug that suits him/her best and take it in an adequate dosage as soon as possible. Although *indomethacin* is probably the most popular NSAID for the treatment of acute gout, any NSAID can be effective, particularly when used in adequate dosage.

*Colchicine* is also useful, but frequently causes diarrhoea when given in adequate doses. A 1mg dose of colchicine should be taken immediately, followed by 0.5mg every 1 to 2 hours until diarrhoea has occurred or a total dose of 6mg has been given.[166] Colchicine may also be given intravenously, but should not exceed 2 to 3mg in a single dose. Great care should be taken to prevent extravasation. The dosage of colchicine should be reduced in elderly patients.

Only in cases where the above drugs have been ineffective or are contraindicated (e.g. in the postoperative state) should other drugs be considered. *Corticosteroids* can be given by the intra-articular route or alternatively *corticotrophin* 40 to 80IU may be given intramuscularly.[167] Oral corticosteroids have also been used in doses of 20 to 50 mg/day (of prednisolone) for 3 days, but are rarely necessary.

### 13.2.2 Prevention of Acute Episodes

Once an attack of acute gout has subsided, patients should be counselled on reducing risk factors such as obesity and should be advised to avoid rich foods and to abstain from excessive alcohol intake. Other drug treatments should be reviewed and alternatives found for thiazide diuretics and aspirin. Urate-lowering drugs should be reserved for patients with hyperuricaemia and recurrent attacks of gout, chronic tophaceous gout or where there is evidence of renal stones or decreased renal function. Whenever any drug that lowers plasma urate is introduced, there is the risk of precipitating an acute attack of gout. Prophylaxis with either an NSAID or colchicine 0.5mg 2 or 3 times daily should therefore be given for the first 2 months. It has recently been argued that colchicine is a less expensive and less toxic alternative to NSAIDs for prophylactic therapy.[168]

#### Persistent Hyperuricaemia

In normal circumstances, most uric acid is filtered by the glomerulus and then reabsorbed in the proximal tubule. The proximal tubule also secretes uric acid in humans. Small doses of uricosuric agents (including NSAIDs) decrease the excretion of uric acid by inhibiting tubular secretory, but not absorptive, mechanisms. Higher doses of NSAIDs, however, depress the resorption of uric acid in the renal tubules and lead to increased excretion and a reduction in plasma urate levels. Allopurinol, on the other

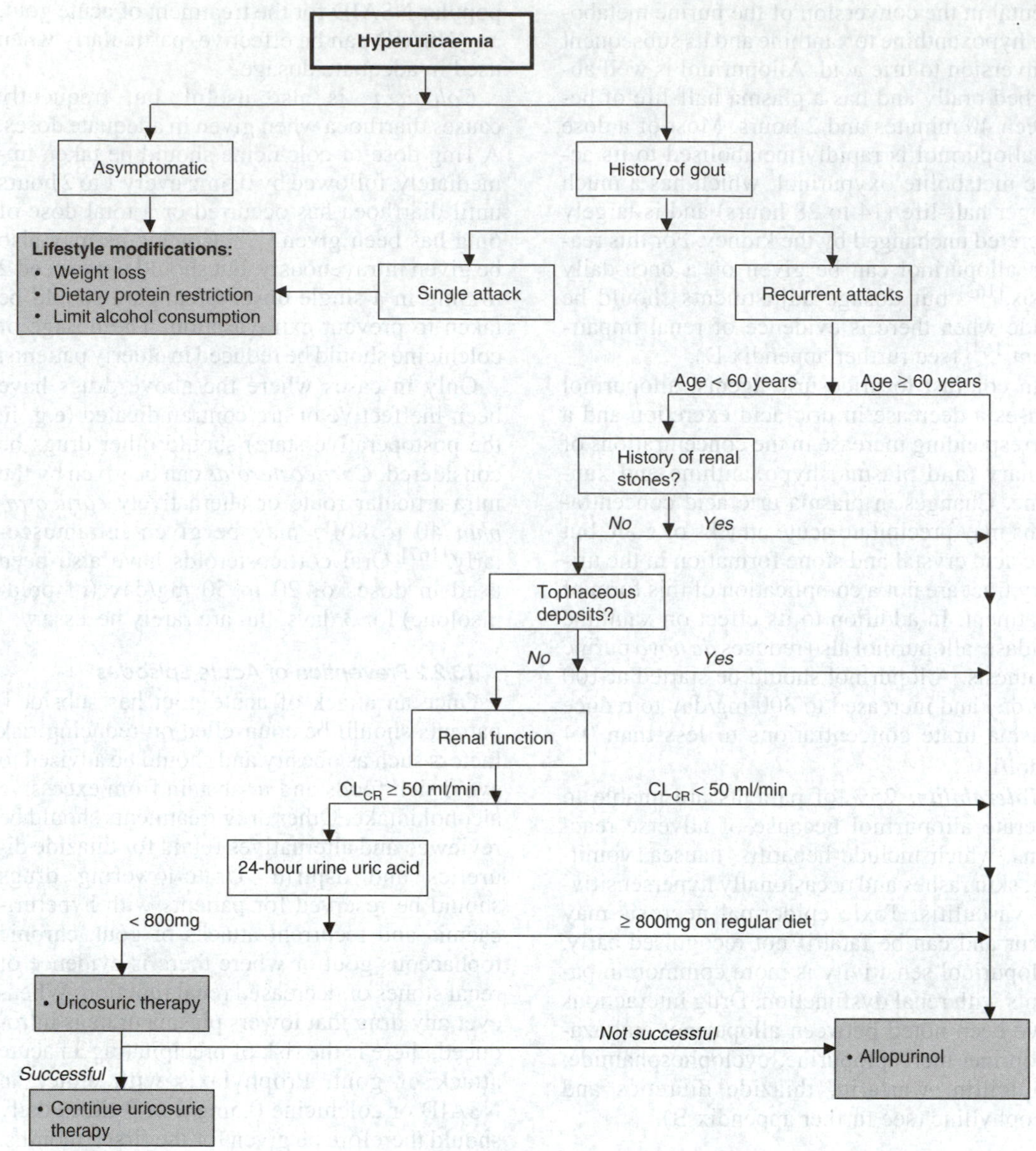


**Fig. 7.** Management of hyperuricaemia. *Abbreviation:* $CL_{CR}$ = creatinine clearance.

hand, reduces the production of uric acid by inhibiting the conversion of hypoxanthine to xanthine and xanthine to uric acid. Xanthines are very soluble and are excreted in the urine. A guide to the management of hyperuricaemia is shown in figure 7.

#### Clinical Use of Urate-Lowering Drugs

Whenever allopurinol or uricosuric agents are used, it must be made clear to patients that they might have to continue these drugs for a significant period of time, if not for the rest of their lives. It is very important not to stop and start these treatments, as this might precipitate attacks of gout. Patients should be aware of the adverse effects of the proposed therapy and the importance of compliance with the treatment programme. The introduction of urate-lowering therapy should be postponed until at least 2 weeks after an attack of gout has resolved and, whenever one of these drugs is instituted, prophylaxis with colchicine 0.5mg twice daily or an NSAID should be given for a 2-month period to prevent attacks of acute gout.

The urate-lowering agents should be introduced at a low dose (allopurinol 50 to 100 mg/day, probenecid 500 mg/day, sulfinpyrazone 100 mg/day) and titrated upwards until the plasma urate concentration is less than 0.4 mmol/L. Such a titration strategy allows the plasma uric acid level to be optimised without committing the patient to excessive drug dosages. Allopurinol can be given in a once-daily dosage of 100 to 600 mg/day, although most patients will not require more than 300 mg/day. Whenever a uricosuric agent is chosen, the urine should be adequately alkalinised and a liberal oral intake of fluid encouraged during the induction phase.

If recurrent attacks of gout occur, urate-lowering drugs should not be discontinued. Instead, they should be continued throughout the period of acute inflammation and, if necessary, the dosage subsequently increased (following resolution) to one that maintains the plasma urate concentration below 0.4 mmol/L. Plasma uric acid concentrations should be checked after the introduction of urate-lowering therapy, after any subsequent dosage adjustment, and periodically thereafter, since it is a measure not only of the effectiveness of such treatment, but also of compliance.

#### *13.2.3 Asymptomatic Hyperuricaemia*

Asymptomatic hyperuricaemia has long been considered an area of therapeutic controversy. Recent risk-benefit analyses have confirmed that, with one exception (patients receiving chemotherapy for lymphoproliferative and myeloproliferative disorders), this condition should *not* be treated.[46,169] This is because many of the conditions previously thought to be related to hyperuricaemia, i.e. hypertension and coronary artery disease, are now known not to be causally related, while renal disease, including stone formation, appears to be related to the level of hypouricosuria rather than hyperuricaemia. Although plasma urate concentrations >0.53 mmol/L carry an increased risk, hyperuricaemia may exist for many years before the first attack of arthritis occurs and it is not possible to identify which hyperuricaemic individual will subsequently develop gout.

Although acute gout is painful, it is usually not dangerous and attacks are self-limiting. There may be an argument for use of allopurinol in asymptomatic patients with hyperuricaemia who have a very high plasma urate (>0.55 mmol/L) or urinary uric acid excretion (>5 mmol/24h). Allopurinol therapy may be indicated in this group of patients to reduce the risk of urolithiasis. The key elements in the management of hyperuricaemic states are shown in figure 7.

#### *13.2.4 Acute Crystal Deposition Disease (Pseudogout)*

Pseudogout from the deposition of calcium pyrophosphate dehydrate or calcium hydroxyapatite may present as an acute or chronic arthritis, particularly in elderly people. The acute inflammatory response resembles gout, but usually involves the knee joint rather than the big toe. Colchicine may not be effective, but *NSAIDs* or *intra-articular corticosteroid injections* can resolve the attacks.

Pyrophosphate crystal deposition can be distinguished from urate crystals by polarised-like microscopy of synovial fluid, while crystals of calcium hydroxyapatite may be demonstrated by alizarine red stain, electron microscopy or x-ray powder diffraction.

## 14. Rheumatic Disease in Pregnancy: Drug Treatment Considerations

Pregnancy can modify the expression of some rheumatic diseases such as rheumatoid arthritis, though some patients are still likely to require treatment with a range of medications, including analgesics, NSAIDs and specific antirheumatic drugs. It is wise to discontinue any drugs that can be removed during pregnancy, but it is also important to maintain control of the underlying disease. Analgesics such as paracetamol and codeine can be taken during pregnancy (and lactation). However, NSAIDs may cause closure of a patent ductus arteriosus and suppress labour (see chapter 2, sect. 7.1.2), while salicylates may prolong gestation, increase the length of labour and increase the risk of pre- and post-partum haemorrhage, as well as predisposing premature infants to intracranial haemorrhage. NSAIDs do not seem to be associated with teratogenicity, but their use should be restricted in the late phases of pregnancy.

Gold compounds, antimalarial drugs and sulfasalazine can be continued during pregnancy, but although penicillamine is usually continued in patients with Wilson's disease, safer alternatives are probably available to treat rheumatic diseases. Although corticosteroids have been associated with cleft palate formation in animals, there is no clear evidence of teratogenicity in humans. The dosage of corticosteroids should be kept to a minimum, especially during the first trimester of pregnancy, but the primary disease for which corticosteroids are taken is usually far more likely to affect the pregnancy than the drug treatment. Cytotoxic agents such as chlorambucil, cyclophosphamide and methotrexate should all be ceased before pregnancy, as they are clearly teratogenic when used during the first trimester.

Although most NSAIDs are excreted in breast milk, their concentrations are extremely low. If an NSAID is to be used during lactation, the drug of choice is one with a short half-life taken at such a time as to produce low plasma concentrations at the time of breast feeding. Antimalarials, sulfasalazine and corticosteroids are all secreted into breast milk in small amounts, as are methotrexate and azathioprine. Because of the small amounts, these drugs are probably not harmful when taken during lactation. Conversely, cyclophosphamide is found in significant quanti-

**Table XVI.** Rheumatic diseases and disorders of bone induced by drugs (after Hart[170])

| Condition | Examples | Comments |
|---|---|---|
| Systemic lupus erythematosus-like syndrome | Procainamide<br>Hydralazine<br>Isoniazid<br>Phenytoin<br>Chlorpromazine<br>Quinidine | Development may depend on genetic susceptibility (especially slow acetylator status) |
| Arthritis, arthralgia | Drug hypersensitivity | Generalised skin reactions; 'serum sickness'-type reaction |
| | Sulfonamides | Manifestation of a polyarteritis |
| | Corticosteroids | Symptoms of arteritis if dose or preparation changed |
| | Oral contraceptives | Aches and pain, myalgia in calves on walking; arthritis of hands |
| | Isoniazid<br>Pyrazinamide<br>Ethionamide | Joint swelling common with pyrazinamide + isoniazid |
| | Rubella vaccine<br>Quinidine | More common in females |
| Muscle pain, cramps | Clofibrate | Excessive dosage in nephrotic syndrome |
| | Corticosteroids<br>Oral contraceptives<br>Estrogens | Fluid retention |
| | Diuretics<br>Lipid-lowering drugs (HMG CoA reductase inhibitors) | Sodium and potassium depletion |
| | Suxamethonium (succinylcholine) | Delayed muscle pains common |
| Acute gout | Diuretics<br>Pyrazinamide | Thiazides, furosemide (frusemide), etc. raise urate |
| | Cytotoxic drugs (esp. leukaemia) | Increased breakdown of nucleoprotein and urate overproduction |
| Haemarthrosis | Anticoagulants | Misdiagnosed as acute gout |
| Osteoporosis | Corticosteroids | Especially in high doses and in partly immobilised females >50 years |
| | Heparin | Long term high doses |
| | Methotrexate | Prepubertal children on long term treatment |
| Osteomalacia | Antiepileptic drugs | Long term high-dose therapy in institutionalised children |
| | Non-absorbable antacids | Long term therapy and activation of condition at time of partial gastrectomy |
| | Bisphosphonates | Inhibit mineralisation of bone |
| | Fluoride | If used alone in osteoporosis (and not combined with calcium + vitamin D) |
| Aseptic necrosis | Corticosteroids | Unpredictable and not duration or dose-related |
| Tooth discolouration | Tetracyclines | |
| Inhibition of bone growth | Tetracyclines | Premature neonates or use in pregnancy. Reversible if short courses given |
| | Corticosteroids | Use in children |
| Osteosclerosis Fluorosis | Fluorides | Excessive dosage |

ties in human breast milk and is contraindicated during lactation (see further appendix C).

## 15. Drug-Induced Rheumatic and Bone Disorders

A large number of drugs may cause aches and pains in muscles, bones and joints (table XVI).[170]

### 15.1 Systemic Lupus Erythematosus-Like Syndromes

Systemic lupus erythematosus-like syndromes associated with clinical features and positive antinuclear antibodies may be associated with a number of drugs. When compared with non-drug lupus, the disease is associated with more fever, rashes and pleuropulmonary involvement and is usually less severe and tends to disappear completely within weeks of stopping the causative agent. In some cases, the disease persists and requires treatment with corticosteroids.

The drugs most often involved include procainamide, hydralazine, sulfasalazine, propylthiouracil, β-adrenoceptor blockers and quinidine. Patients who develop hydralazine-, isoniazid- or procainamide-related lupus are more likely to exhibit low activity of hepatic acetylation enzymes.[171]

### 15.2 Arthritis and Arthralgia

Arthralgia may accompany a variety of generalised skin reactions caused by drugs and may be a feature of the serum sickness reaction associated with antibiotics or barbiturates. Myalgia and arthralgia have been reported with oral contraceptives and quinidine. Antituberculosis drugs such as isoniazid, pyrazinamide and ethionamide can also cause arthritis and arthralgia.

Vaccinations (in particular rubella or influenza vaccines) have also been reported to be associated with arthralgia and arthritis.

### 15.3 Muscle Pain and Cramps

**Table XVII.** Major drug-induced generalised myopathies

| Painless myopathies | Painful myopathies |
|---|---|
| **Without neuropathy:**<br>• Corticosteroids<br>• β-Adrenoceptor blockers<br>**With neuropathy:**<br>• Colchicine<br>• Chloroquine and hydroxychloroquine<br>**With abnormal neuromuscular transmission (myasthenic syndromes):**<br>• Penicillamine, pyritinol (pyrithioxine)<br>• Chloroquine<br>• Antibiotics<br>• β-Adrenoceptor blockers | **Without neuropathy**<br>a) Polymyositis:<br>• Penicillamine, tiopronin, pyritinol (pyrithioxine)<br>• Cimetidine<br>• Penicillin, sulfonamides<br>• Phenylbutazone, niflumic acid<br>• Propylthiouracil<br>• Zidovudine<br>• Cocaine<br>b) Other painful myopathies:<br>• Quinolones, nalidixic acid<br>• Clofibrate, 'statins' (HMG CoA reductase inhibitors)<br>• Cyclosporin<br>• Enalapril<br>• Emetine<br>• Carbimazole<br>• Etretinate<br>• Ipecac<br>• Minoxidil<br>• ε-Aminocaproic acid<br>• Metoprolol<br>**With neuropathy:**<br>• Tryptophan (eosinophilia-myalgia syndrome)<br>• Vincristine<br>• Amiodarone<br>• Drugs causing hypokalaemia and phosphate deficiency |

Myalgia, with or without cramps, may be an early symptom of a drug-induced polyneuropathy or a myopathy. The major drug-induced myopathies are shown in table XVII and can be divided into painless or painful myopathies with or without a neuropathy. Acute and severe drug-induced myopathies are seen in association with rhabdomyolysis (caused by alcohol, heroin), malignant hyperpyrexia (associated with anaesthetic agents or muscle relaxants) or myotonic syndrome [seen with suxamethonium (succinylcholine)]. The major symptoms of drug-induced myopathies are proximal muscle weakness, increased muscle enzyme concentrations, and electromyographic and histological changes. Discontinuation of the causative agent will eliminate the problem. Several criteria have been described for reporting drug-induced myopathy,[172] and include:

- Lack of pre-existing muscle symptoms
- A symptom-free period following the beginning of treatment
- Lack of another cause
- Complete or incomplete resolution after withdrawal of treatment.

It is recommended that re-challenge not be performed because of the risk of recurrence.

### 15.4 Acute Gout

Drugs that increase plasma urate, such as the thiazide diuretics, nicotinic acid and cytotoxic agents, may precipitate acute gout. Drugs that alter plasma urate concentrations, such as uricosuric agents or allopurinol, may also precipitate acute attacks of gout if prophylaxis with colchicine or low-dose NSAIDs is not given initially.

### 15.5 Bone Disorders

Pain may arise from osteoporotic crush fractures and from osteomalacia. Osteoporosis has been reported with long term treatment with heparin and in children with acute leukaemia treated with methotrexate. Corticosteroid therapy may lead to osteoporosis or to osteonecrosis. Although corticosteroid-induced osteoporosis is extremely unusual if dosages of less than 7.5mg of prednisolone daily are given, some form of prophylaxis with calcium and vitamin D supplements, hormone replacement therapy, calcitonin or bisphosphonates may need to be considered if higher prednisolone dosages are given long term.[173] Corticosteroid-induced asepsis necrosis, which usually affects the femoral head (bilaterally), does not seem to correlate with the duration of treatment or dosage and has been reported following intravenous pulse corticosteroid therapy as well as continuous therapy.

### 15.6 Scleroderma or Scleroderma-Like Lesions

Scleroderma or scleroderma-like lesions have been reported with bleomycin, pentazocine, cocaine, appetite suppressants such as the amphetamines, and also with penicillamine.[174] Tryptophan may also give rise to a scleroderma-like disease with the eosinophilia-myalgia syndrome.

Fluoride therapy can be associated with arthralgias or stress fracture of bone, as can the retinoids.

## 16. Use of Drugs in the Presence of Associated Rheumatic Disease

Arthritis may be exacerbated by certain drugs.[175] Total dose infusion of iron dextran may produce an acute exacerbation of rheumatoid arthritis, but may also produce a mild arthralgia in those without rheumatic disease. Oral contraceptives may appear to cause an exacerbation of pre-existing rheumatoid disease, though this occurrence is very rare. There have also been reports of dramatic worsening of the condition of patients with systemic lupus erythematosus while they were taking oral contraceptives, with improvement when these were withdrawn.[176] Thiazide diuretics may precipitate an attack of gout in a hyperuricaemic individual (see section 15.4), as may various other diuretics or cytotoxic drugs or radiotherapy given for leukaemia, $^{32}P$ for polycythemia, pyrazinamide for tuberculosis, or nicotinic acid for hyperlipidaemias.

A full preoperative assessment, and in patients who have recently had or who are still taking large doses of corticosteroids, pre- and postoperative cover with hydrocortisone sodium succinate is essential in the anaesthetic management of the patient with rheumatoid arthritis.[177]

Certain other drugs given concurrently, especially oral anticoagulants, may interact with some nonsteroidal anti-inflammatory agents used in rheumatic diseases, particularly aspirin and phenylbutazone (table III) but clinically important reactions seem to be relatively uncommon, perhaps because problem combinations are avoided. Nevertheless, fatalities have occurred (see also chapter 7 and chapter 26). This also seems to be so in gout. The xanthine oxidase inhibitor allopurinol is a special case. Mercaptopurine and azathioprine (which is converted in the body to mercaptopurine) are metabolised by xanthine oxidase and the dose of these drugs must be reduced to 33% of usual when allopurinol is used to combat the increased nucleoprotein breakdown and consequent urate overproduction which can follow cytotoxic chemotherapy. The incidence of ampicillin rashes appears to be higher in hyperuricaemic patients treated with allopurinol.[178]

NSAIDs, via inhibition of renal prostaglandin biosynthesis, have been implicated in causing a variety of clinical renal syndromes, including acute renal failure (for which patients with pre-existing renal disease or compromised renal function appear at greatest risk), sodium and water retention, hyponatraemia, hyperkalaemia and rarely, interstitial nephritis and papillary necrosis of the kidney.[36] Patients receiving diuretic therapy may be at increased risk of NSAID-induced renal failure. Additionally, NSAIDs may inhibit the natriuretic response to diuretics, with resultant deleterious effects in patients with heart failure and other forms of oedema, and may also attenuate the blood pressure-lowering effect of various antihypertensive drugs, including β-adrenoceptor blockers and thiazide diuretics, and control of blood pressure may be lost.[179] The latter effect has mainly been reported with indomethacin; however, the possibility of clinically significant interactions occurring with other NSAIDs (albeit to a lesser extent with some drugs, e.g. sulindac[179-181]) should be borne in mind.

Severe and in some cases fatal toxicity has been observed in patients given high-dose methotrexate therapy together with NSAIDs such as ketoprofen, azapropazone and diclofenac.[182,183] The mechanism of this interaction may be inhibition of methotrexate renal excretion, perhaps by interference with its active renal tubular secretion, although an adverse effect of NSAIDs on renal function may also be involved.

## References


1. Vandenbourke JP, Hazevoet HM, Cass A. Survival and death in rheumatoid arthritis: a 25 year prospective follow-up. Journal of Rheumatology 1984; 11: 158-61
2. Hart FD. Rheumatic disorders. In: Speight TM, editor. Avery's drug treatment. 3rd ed. Auckland: Adis Press, 1987: 910-57
3. Huskisson EC, Hart FD. Pain threshold and arthritis. British Medical Journal 1972; 4: 193
4. Brooks PM. Clinical management of rheumatoid arthritis. Lancet 1993; 341: 286-90
5. Miles SM, Bird HA. Clinical significance of drug interactions with antirheumatic agents. Clinical Immunotherapeutics 1996; 5: 205-13
6. Munro RAL, Sturrock RD. Slow-acting antirheumatic drugs: drug interactions of clinical significance. Drug Safety 1995; 13: 25-30
7. Stollerman GH, Markowitz M, Taranta A, et al. Jones criteria (revised) for guidance in the diagnosis of rheumatic fever. Circulation 1965; 32: 66
8. Amigo M-C, Martinez-Lavin M, Reyes PA. Acute rheumatic fever. Rheumatic Clinics of North America 1993; 19: 333
9. Markowitz M, Cordis L, editors. Rheumatic fever. Philadelphia: W. Saunders & Co., 1972
10. Lennon D. Rheumatic fever. In: Speight T, Sutherland J (editors). New Ethicals Disease Index. 3rd ed. Auckland: Adis International, 1995: 370-4
11. Pincus T. Disappointing long-term outcomes despite successful short-term clinical trials. Journal of Clinical Epidemiology 1988; 41: 1037-41
12. Seideman P, Melander A. Equianalgesic effects of paracetamol and indomethacin in rheumatoid arthritis. British Journal of Rheumatology 1988; 27: 117
13. Boardman PL, Hart FD. Clinical measurement of anti-inflammatory effects of salicylates in rheumatoid arthritis. British Medical Journal 1967; 4: 264
14. Brooks PM, Day RO. Non-steroidal anti-inflammatory drugs: differences and similarities. New England Journal of Medicine 1991; 324: 1716-25
15. Vane JR. Inhibition of prostaglandin synthesis as a mechanism of action of aspirin-like drugs. Nature (New Biology) 1971; 231: 232
16. Frölich JC. Prostaglandin endoperoxide synthetase isoenzymes - clinical relevance of selective inhibition. Annals of the Rheumatic Diseases 1995; 54: 942-3
17. Richardson CE, Emery P. New cyclooxygenase and cytokine inhibitors. Balliere's Clinical Rheumatology 1995; 9: 731-58
18. Bennett A, Tavares IA. NSAIDs, Cox-2 inhibitors and the gut. Lancet 1995; 346: 1105
19. Vane JR. NSAIDs, Cox-2 inhibitors and the gut. Lancet 1995; 346: 1105-6
20. Furst DE. Are there differences among non-steroidal anti-inflammatory drugs? Comparing acetylated salicylates, non-acetylated salicylates, and non-acetylated nonsteroidal antiinflammatory drugs. Arthritis and Rheumatism 1994; 37: 1-9
21. Day RO, Graham GG, Bieri D, et al. Concentration-response relationships for salicylate-induced ototoxicity in normal volunteers. British Journal of Clinical Pharmacology 1989; 28: 695
22. Carson JL, Strom BL, Sopper KA, et al. The association of non-steroidal anti-inflammatory drugs with upper gastrointestinal tract bleeding. Archives of Internal Medicine 1987; 147: 85
23. Langman MJS, Weil J, Wainwright P, et al. Risks of bleeding peptic ulcer associated with individual non-steroidal anti-inflammatory drugs. Lancet 1994; 343: 1075
24. Pownall R, Pickvane NJ. The optimal interval between flurbuprofen doses scheduling for circadian rhythms in RA. British Journal of Clinical Practice 1987; 4: 689
25. Day RO, Graham GG, Williams KM. Pharmacokinetics of non-steroidal anti-inflammatory drugs. Balliere's Clinical Rheumatology 1988; 2: 363-93
26. Day RO, Furst DE, Dromgoole SH, et al. Relationships of serum naproxen concentrations to efficacy in rheumatoid arthritis. Clinical Pharmacology and Therapeutics 1982; 31: 733-4
27. Lee EJD, Williams K, Day R, et al. Stereoselective disposition of ibuprofen enantiomers in man. British Journal of Clinical Pharmacology 1985; 19: 669
28. Bradley JD, Rudy AC, Katz BP, et al. Correlations of serum concentrations of ibuprofen stereoisomers with clinical response in the treatment of hip and knee osteoarthritis. Journal of Rheumatology 1992; 19: 130
29. O'Brien WM, Bagby GF. Rare adverse reactions to non-steroidal anti-inflammatory drugs. Journal of Rheumatology 1985; 12: 13, 347, 562, 785
30. Bjarnasson I, Hayllar J, MacPherson AJ, et al. Side effects of non-steroidal drugs on the small and large intestine in humans. Gastroenterology 1993; 104: 1832
31. Langman MJS. Epidemiologic evidence on the association between peptic ulceration and anti-inflammatory drug use. Gastroenterology 1989; 96 Suppl. 2: 640
32. Fries JF, Williams CA, Bloch DA. The relative toxicity of non-steroidal anti-inflammatory drugs. Arthritis and Rheumatism 1991; 34: 1353
33. Garcia-Rodriguez LA, Jick H. Risks of upper gastrointestinal bleeding and perforation associated with individual non-steroidal anti-inflammatory drugs. Lancet 1994; 343: 769
34. Gabriel SE, Jaakkimainen RL, Bombardier C. The cost effectiveness of misoprostol for non-steroidal anti-inflammatory drug associated adverse gastrointestinal events. Arthritis and Rheumatism 1993; 36: 447
35. Brooks PM, Yeomans ND. Non-steroidal anti-inflammatory drug gastropathy: is it preventable? Australian and New Zealand Journal of Medicine 1992; 22: 685
36. Clive DM, Stoff JS. Renal syndromes associated with non-steroidal anti-inflammatory drugs. New England Journal of Medicine 1984; 310: 563
37. George E, Kirwan JR. Corticosteroid therapy in rheumatoid arthritis. Baillière's Clinical Rheumatology 1990; 4: 621

38. Brooks PM. The use of suppressive agents for the treatment of rheumatoid arthritis. Australian and New Zealand Journal of Medicine 1993; 23: 193
39. Girgis L, Conaghan PG, Brooks PM. Disease-modifying anti-rheumatic drugs including methotrexate, sulphasalazine, gold, antimalarials and penicillamine. Current Opinion in Rheumatology 1994; 6: 252
40. Wolfe F, Hawley DJ, Cathey MA. Termination of slow acting anti-rheumatic therapy in rheumatoid arthritis: a 14 year prospective evaluation of 1017 consecutive starts. Journal of Rheumatology 1990; 17: 994
41. Gardner G, Furst DE. Disease-modifying antirheumatic drugs: potential effects in older patients. Drugs and Aging 1995; 7: 420-37
42. Wilke WS, Sweeney TJ, Calabrese LH. Early aggressive therapy for rheumatoid arthritis: concerns, descriptions and estimate of outcome. Seminars in Arthritis and Rheumatism 1993; 23 Suppl. 26
43. Frisk-Holmberg M, Bergquist Y, Dotieij-Nyberg B. Chloroquine serum concentrations and side effects: evidence for dose dependent kinetics. Clinical Pharmacology and Therapeutics 1979; 25: 345
44. Tett S, Cutler D, Day RO. Antimalarials in rheumatic diseases. Baillière's Clinical Rheumatology 1990; 4: 467
45. Champion GD, Graham GG, Ziegler JB. The gold complexes. Baillière's Clinical Rheumatology 1990; 4: 490
46. Campion EW, Glynn RJ, De Labry LO. Asymptomatic hyperuricaemia: risks and consequences in the normative ageing study. American Journal of Medicine 1987; 82: 321
47. Adachi JD, Bensen WG, Kassam Y, et al. Gold induced thrombocytopenia - 12 cases and a review of the literature. Seminars in Arthritis and Rheumatism 1987; 16: 287-93
48. Joyce DA. D-penicillamine. Baillière's Clinical Rheumatology 1990; 4: 553
49. Emery P. Sulphoxidation ability and thiol status in rheumatoid arthritis patients. British Journal of Rheumatology 1987; 26: 163-5
50. Ahern MJ, Hall NO, Case N, et al. D-penicilliamine withdrawal in rheumatoid arthritis. Annals of the Rheumatic Diseases 1984; 84: 213
51. Porter DR, Capell HA. The use of sulphasalazine as a disease modifying anti-rheumatic drug. Baillière's Clinical Rheumatology 1990; 4: 535
52. Taggart AJ, Neumann VC, Hill J, et al. 5-Aminosalicylic acid or sulphapyridine: which is the active moiety of sulphasalazine in rheumatoid arthritis? Drugs 1986; 32 Suppl. 1: 27
53. Donovan S, Hawley S, MacCarthy J, et al. Tolerability of enteric coated sulphasalazine in rheumatoid arthritis: results of a co-operative clinical study. British Journal of Rheumatology 1990; 29: 201
54. Rains CP, Noble S, Faulds D. Sulfasalazine: a review of its pharmacological properties and therapeutic efficacy in the treatment of rheumatoid arthritis. Drugs 1995; 50: 137-56
55. Songsiride N, Furst DE. Methotrexate: a rapidly acting drug. Baillière's Clinical Rheumatology 1990; 4: 575
56. Tugwell P, Bennett K, Gent M. Methotrexate in rheumatoid arthritis. Annals of Internal Medicine 1987; 107: 358
57. Wolfe F, Smythe HA, Yunus MB, et al. The American College of Rheumatology 1990 criteria for the classification of fibromyalgia: report of the multicentre criteria committee. Arthritis and Rheumatism 1990; 33: 160
58. Walker AM, Funch D, Dreyer NA, et al. Determinants of serious liver disease among patients receiving low dose methotrexate for rheumatoid arthritis. Arthritis and Rheumatism 1993; 36: 329
59. Kevat S, Ahern M, Hall P. Hepatotoxicity of methotrexate in rheumatoid diseases. Medical Toxicology and Adverse Drug Experience 1988; 3: 197
60. Markham A, Faulds D. Methotrexate: a review of its pharmacodynamic and pharmacokinetic properties, and therapeutic efficacy in rheumatoid arthritis and other immunoregulatory disorders. Clinical Immunotherapeutics 1994; 1: 217-44
61. Bannwarth B, Péhourcq F, Schaeverbeke T, et al. Clinical pharmacokinetics of low-dose pulse methotrexate in rheumatoid arthritis. Clinical Pharmacokinetics 1996; 30: 194-210
62. Kirwan JR, Arthritis and Rheumatism Council Low Dose Glucocorticoid Study Group. The effect of glucocorticoids on joint destruction in rheumatoid arthritis. New England Journal of Medicine 1995; 333: 142-6
63. Millon R, Poole P, Kellgren JH, et al. Long term study of management of rheumatoid arthritis. Lancet 1984; 1: 812
64. Bird HA. Intra-articular and intralesional therapy. In: Klippel JH, Dieppe PA, editors. Rheumatology. St Louis: Mosby, 1994: 8.16.1
65. Matteson EL, Hickey AR, Maguire L, et al. Occurrence of neoplasia in patients with rheumatoid arthritis enrolled in a DMARD registry. Journal of Rheumatology 1991; 10: 809
66. Luqmani RA, Palmer RG, Bacon PA. Azathioprine, cyclophosphamide and chlorambucil. Baillière's Clinical Rheumatology 1990; 4: 595
67. McCune WJ, Friedman AW. Immunosuppressive therapy for rheumatic disease. Current Opinion in Rheumatology 1993; 5: 282
68. Faulds D, Goa KL, Benfield P. Cyclosporin: a review of its pharmacodynamic and pharmacokinetic properties, and therapeutic use in immunoregulatory disorders. Drugs 1993; 45: 953-1040
69. Faulds D, Irvine S. Tenidap. Clinical Immunotherapeutics 1996; 5: 161-7
70. Breedveld F. Tenidap: a novel cytokine-modulating antirheumatic drug for the treatment of rheumatoid arthritis. Scandinavian Journal of Rheumatology 1994; 23 (Suppl. 100): 31-44
71. Fries JF. Re-evaluating the therapeutic approach to rheumatoid arthritis: the 'sawtooth' strategy. Journal of Rheumatology 1990; 17 Suppl. 22: 12-15
72. Felson DT, Anderson JJ, Meenan RF. The comparative efficacy and toxicity of second-line drugs in rheumatoid arthritis: results of two meta-analyses. Arthritis and Rheumatism 1990; 33: 1449-61
73. Jones G. Yttrium synovectomy: a meta-analysis of the literature. Australian and New Zealand Journal of Medicine 1993; 23: 272-5
74. Brooks PM, March LM. New insights into osteoarthritis. Medical Journal of Australia 1995; 163: 367-9
75. Cooper C. Osteoarthritis - epidemiology. In: Klippel JH, Dieppe PA, editors. Rheumatology. St. Louis: Mosby, 1994: 7.3.1
76. Felson DJ. The epidemiology of knee osteoarthritis: the results from the Framingham Osteoarthritis Study. Seminars in Arthritis and Rheumatism 1990; 20: 42
77. Puett DW, Griffin MR. Published trials of non-medical and non-invasive therapies for hip and knee osteoarthritis. Annals of Internal Medicine 1994; 121: 134

78. National Health and Medical Research Council. Musculoskeletal disorders in the older person. Canberra: Australian Government Printing Service, 1994
79. Williams HJ, Ward JR, Egger MJ, et al. Comparison of naproxen and acetaminophen in a two-year study of treatment of osteoarthritis of the knee. Arthritis and Rheumatism 1993; 36: 1196
80. Dieppe P, Cushnagan J, Jasini MK, et al. A two year placebo-controlled trial of non-steroidal anti-inflammatory therapy in osteoarthritis of the knee joint. British Journal of Rheumatology 1993; 32: 595
81. Bradley JD, Brandt KD, Katz BP, et al. Comparison of an anti-inflammatory dose of ibuprofen, an analgesic dose of ibuprofen and acetaminophen in the treatment of patients with osteoarthritis of the knee. New England Journal of Medicine 1991; 325: 87
82. March LM, Irwig LM, Schwarz JM, et al. N-of-1 trials comparing a non-steroidal anti-inflammatory drug and paracetamol on osteoarthritis. British Medical Journal 1994; 309: 1041
83. Ferraz MB, Tugwell P, Goldsmith CH, et al. Meta-analysis of sulfasalazine in ankylosing spondylitis. Journal of Rheumatology 1990; 17: 1482
84. Dougados M, van der Linden S, Leirisalo-Repo M, et al. Sulfasalazine in the treatment of spondylarthropathy: a randomised, multicentre, double-blind, placebo-controlled study. Arthritis and Rheumatism 1995; 38: 618-27
85. Espinoza LR, Zakraoui L, Espinola CG, et al. Psoriatic arthritis: clinical response and side effects to methotrexate therapy. Journal of Rheumatology 1992; 12: 872
86. Espinoza LR, Cuellar MC. Psoriatic arthritis. In: Klippel JH, Dieppe PA, editors. Rheumatology. St Louis: Mosby, 1994: 333
87. Edmonds J. Spondylarthropathies. Medical Journal of Australia 1996; in press
88. Rahman MU, Hudson AP, Schumacher Jr HR. Chlamydia and Reiter's syndrome (reactive arthritis). Rheumatic Disease Clinics of North America 1992; 18: 67-79
89. Kyle V, Hazleman BL. Treatment of polymyalgia rheumatica and giant cell arteritis: steroid regimes in the first two months. Annals of the Rheumatic Diseases 1989; 48: 658
90. McLatchie GR, McDonald M. Soft tissue trauma - a randomised trial of the topical application of felbinac - a new NSAID. British Journal of Clinical Practice 1989; 43: 277-80
91. Evans JMM, MacDonald TM. Tolerability of topical NSAIDs in the elderly: do they really convey a safety advantage? Drugs and Aging 1996; 9: 101-8
92. McCain GA. A cost effective approach to the diagnosis and treatment of fibromyalgia. Rheumatic Disease Clinics of North America 1996; 22: 323-49
93. Bennett RM. Beyond fibromyalgia: ideas on etiology and treatment. Journal of Rheumatology 1989; 16 Suppl. 19: 185
94. Goldenberg DL. Fibromyalgia syndrome, an emerging but controversial condition. Journal of the American Medical Association 1987; 257: 2782-7
95. Croft P, Schullum J, Silman A. Population study of tender point counts and pain as evidence of fibromyalgia. British Medical Journal 1994; 309: 696
96. McCain GA, Bell DA, May FM, et al. A controlled study of the effects of supervised cardiovascular training programme on the manifestations of primary fibromyalgia. Arthritis and Rheumatism 1988; 31: 1135
97. Bennett RM. Multidisciplinary groups programmes to treat fibromyalgia patients. Rheumatic Disease Clinics of North America 1996; 22: 351-68
98. Dixon AStJ. Progress and problems in back pain research. Rheumatology and Rehabilitation 1973; 12: 165
99. Borenstein DG, Weisel SW, editors. Low back pain: medical diagnosis and comprehensive management. Philadelphia: Saunders, 1989
100. Frymoyer JW, Cats-Baric WL. An overview of the incidence and costs of low back pain. Orthopedic Clinics of North America 1991; 22: 263
101. Deyo RA, Diehl AH, Rosenthal M. How many days of bed rest for acute low back pain? A randomised clinical trial. New England Journal of Medicine 1986; 315: 1064
102. Borenstein DG. Low back pain. In: Klippel JH, Dieppe PA, editors. Rheumatology. St Louis: Mosby, 1994: 5: 4.1
103. White P. Juvenile chronic arthritis clinical features. In: Klippel JH, Dieppe PA, editors. Rheumatology. St Louis: Mosby, 1994: 3.17.1
104. Cassidy JT, Levinson JE. Brass JC, et al. A study of the classification criteria for the diagnosis of juvenile chronic arthritis. Arthritis and Rheumatism 1986; 29: 274
105. Cassidy JT. Juvenile chronic arthritis management. In: Klippel JH, Dieppe PA, editors. Rheumatology. St. Louis: Mosby, 1994: 3.20.1
106. Committee on Infectious Diseases. Report of the Committee on Infectious Diseases. 20th ed. Elk Grove, Illinois: American Academy of Pediatrics, 1986: 210
107. Manners PJ, Ansell BM. Slow acting antirheumatic drug use in systemic onset juvenile chronic arthritis. Pediatrics 1986; 77: 99
108. Kyzmina N, et al. Methotrexate in resistant juvenile rheumatoid arthritis. Results of the USA-USSR double-blind, placebo-controlled trial. New England Journal of Medicine 1992; 326: 1043
109. Athreya BH, Cassidy JD. Current status of the medical treatment of children with juvenile rheumatoid arthritis. Rheumatic Disease Clinics of North America 1991; 17: 871-99
110. Klippel J. SLE management. In: Klippel JH, Dieppe PA, editors. Rheumatology. St Louis: Mosby, 1994: 6.1
111. Canadian Hydroxychloroquine Study Group. A randomised study of the effect of withdrawing hydroxychloroquine sulphate in systemic lupus erythematosus. New England Journal of Medicine 1991; 324: 150
112. Mills JA. Systemic lupus erythematosus. New England Journal of Medicine 1994; 330: 1871
113. Fessler BJ, Boumpas DT. Severe major organ involvement in systemic lupus erythematosus - diagnosis and management. Rheumatic Disease Clinics of North America 1995; 21: 81-98
114. Steinberg AD, Steinberg SC. Long term preservation of renal function in patients with lupus nephritis receiving treatment that includes cyclophosphamide versus those treated with prednisolone alone. Arthritis and Rheumatism 1991; 34: 945
115. Austin III HA, Klippel JH, Balow JE, et al. Therapy for lupus nephritis: controlled trial of prednisolone and cytotoxic drugs. New England Journal of Medicine 1986; 314: 614
116. Boumpas DT, Austin III HA, Vaughan EM, et al. Controlled trial of pulse methyl prednisolone versus two regimens of pulse cyclophosphamide in severe lupus nephritis. Lancet 1992; 340: 741

117. Hows JM, Mehta A, Ward L. Comparison of mesna with forced diuresis to prevent cyclophosphamide-induced haemorrhagic status in marrow transplantation - a prospective randomised study. British Journal of Cancer 1984; 50: 735-56
118. Conn DL. Polyarteritis. In: Klippel JH, Dieppe PA, editors. Rheumatology. St Louis: Mosby, 1994: 6.17.1
119. Rodeeheffer RJ, Rommer JA, Wigley F, et al. Controlled double-blind trial of nifedipine in the treatment of Raynaud's phenomenon. New England Journal of Medicine 1983; 308: 880
120. Steen VD. Problems with the diagnosis of Raynaud's phenomenon. In: Klippel JH, Dieppe PA, editors. Rheumatology. St Louis: Mosby, 1994: 6.11.1
121. Steen VD, Medsger TAJ, Rodnan GP. D-penicillamine therapy in progressive systemic sclerosis (scleroderma). Annals of Internal Medicine 1984; 97: 652
122. Jimenez SA, Sigal SH. A 15 year prospective study of treatment of rapidly progressive systemic sclerosis with d-penicillamine. Rheumatology 1991; 18: 1496
123. Steen VD, Medsger Jr TA, Osial Jr TA, et al. Factors predicting the development of renal involvement in progressive systemic sclerosis. American Journal of Medicine 1984; 76: 779
124. Steen VD, Constantino JP, Shapiro AP, et al. Outcome or renal crisis in systemic sclerosis: relation to angiotensin converting enzyme (ACE) inhibitors. Annals of Internal Medicine 1990; 113: 352
125. Oddis CV, Medsger T. Current management of polymyositis and dermatomyositis. Drugs 1989; 37: 382
126. Kagen LJ. Inflammatory muscle disease management. In: Klippel JH, Dieppe PA, editors. Rheumatology. St Louis: Mosby, 1994: 14.1
127. Hart FD. Infective arthropathies. In: Hart FD, editor. Drug treatment of rheumatic diseases. 2nd ed. Sydney: Adis Press, 1982: 177
128. Kalish R. Lyme disease. Rheumatic Disease Clinics of North America 1993; 19: 399-426
129. Mitchell WS, Brooks PM, Stevenson RD, et al. Septic arthritis in patients with rheumatoid disease: a still undiagnosed complication. Journal of Rheumatology 1976; 3: 124
130. Ellerington MC, Stevenson JC. Prevention of osteoporosis. Drugs and Aging 1992; 2: 508
131. Dequeker J. Management of osteoporosis. In: Klippel JH, Dieppe PA, editors. Rheumatology. St Louis: Mosby, 1994: 7.34.1
132. Riggs BL, Melton III LJ. Drug therapy: the prevention and treatment of osteoporosis. New England Journal of Medicine 1992; 327: 620
133. Reid IR. Benefits, risks and costs of calcium supplements in postmenopausal women. PharmacoEconomics 1994; 5: 1-4
134. Chapuy MC, Arlot ME, Duboeuf F, et al. Vitamin $D_3$ and calcium to prevent hip fractures in elderly women. New England Journal of Medicine 1992; 327: 1637-42
135. Gennari C, Nuti R, Agnusdei D, et al. Management of osteoporosis and Paget's disease: an appraisal of the risks and benefits of drug treatment. Drug Safety 1994; 11: 179-95
136. Clissold SP, Fitton A, Chrisp P. Intranasal salmon calcitonin: a review of its pharmacological properties and potential utility in metabolic done disorders associated with aging. Drugs and Aging 1991; 1: 405-23
137. Gennari C, Agnusdei D. Calcitonins and osteoporosis. British Journal of Clinical Practice 1994; 84: 196-9
138. Patel S, Lyons AR, Hosking DJ. Drugs used in the treatment of metabolic bone disease: clinical pharmacology and therapeutic use. Drugs 1993; 46: 594-617
139. Rosen CJ, Kessenich CR. Comparative clinical pharmacology and therapeutic use of bisphosphonates in metabolic bone diseases. Drugs 1996; 51: 537-51
140. Johansen A, Stone M, Rawlinson F. Bisphosphonates and the treatment of bone disease in the elderly. Drugs and Aging 1996; 8: 113-26
141. Adami S, Zamberlan N. Adverse effects of bisphosphonates: a comparative review. Drug Safety 1996; 14: 158-70
142. Mundy GR, Raisz LG. Drugs for disorders of bone. Drugs 1974; 8: 250
143. Mundy GR. Bone agents. In: Klippel JH, Dieppe PA, editors. Rheumatology. St Louis: Mosby, 1994: 8.17.1
144. Whittington R, Faulds D. Hormone replacement therapy: Part II. A pharmacoeconomic appraisal of its role in the prevention of postmenopausal osteoporosis and ischaemic heart disease. PharmacoEconomics 1994; 5: 513-54
145. Reid IR. Osteoporosis: prevention and treatment. New Ethicals 1996; 33(2): 27-33
146. Liberman UA, Weiss SR, Bröll J, et al. Effect of oral alendronate on bone mineral density and the incidence of fractures in postmeopausal osteoporosis. New England Journal of Medicine 1995; 333: 1437-43
147. Seeman H, Tsalamandris C, Bass S, et al. Present and future of osteoporosis therapy. Bone 1995; 17: 23S-9S
148. La Croix AZ, Weinpahl J, White LR, et al. Thiazide diuretic agents and the incidence of hip fracture. New England Journal of Medicine 1990; 322: 286
149. Sambrook P, Eisman J. Diagnosis and treatment of osteoporosis. Current Opinion in Rheumatology 1993; 5: 346
150. Abbott TA, Lawrence BJ, Wallach S. Osteoporosis: the need for comprehensive treatment guidelines. Clinical Therapeutics 1996; 18: 127
151. Rungby J, Hermann AP, Mosekilde L. Epidemiology of osteoporosis: implications for drug therapy. Drugs and Aging 1995; 6: 470-8
152. Stamp TCB. Rickets and osteomalacia. In: Klippel JH, Dieppe PA, editors. Rheumatology. St Louis: Mosby, 1994: 7.35.1
153. Altman RD. Paget's disease of bone (osteitis deformans). Bulletin on the Rheumatic Diseases 1984; 34: 1
154. Nagant de Deuxchaisnes C. Paget's disease of bone. In: Klippel JH, Dieppe PA, editors. Rheumatology. St Louis: Mosby, 1994: 7.3.1
155. Hosking DJ. Advances in the management of Paget's disease of bone. Drugs 1990; 40: 829
156. Singer FR. Clinical efficacy of salmon calcitonin in Paget's disease. Calcified Tissue International 1991; 49 (Suppl. 2): S7-S8
157. Evans RA, Sommers NM, Dunstan CR, et al. Treatment of Paget's disease of bone with a combination of intranasal salmon calcitonin and oral calcium and thiazide. Calcified Tissue International 1991; 49: 164-7
158. Russell RGG, Smith R, Preston C, et al. Diphosphonates in Paget's disease. Lancet 1974; 1: 894-8
159. Reginster JY, Lecart MP, Deroisy R. Treatment of Paget's disease of bone with high oral doses of tiludronate given during a 5-day course of therapy. Journal of Bone and Mineral Research 1990; 5 (Suppl. 2): 170
160. Gallagher SJ. Paget's disease of bone. Current Opinion in Rheumatology 1993; 5: 351

161. Emmerson BT. Antihyperuricaemics. In: Klippel JH, Dieppe PA, editors. Rheumatology. St Louis: Mosby, 1994: 8.15.1
162. Star VL, Hochberg M. Gout: prevention and management. Current Therapeutics 1994; 35: 51
163. Brewis I, Ellis RM, Scott JT. Single daily dose of allopurinol. Annals of the Rheumatic Diseases 1975; 34: 256
164. Hande KR, Noone RM, Stone WJ. Severe allopurinol toxicity: description and guidelines for prevention in patients with renal insufficiency. American Journal of Medicine 1984; 76: 47
165. Hart FD. Inflammatory disease and its control in rheumatic disorders. British Medical Journal 1975; 4: 191
166. Wallace SL, Singer JZ. Therapy of gout. Rheumatic Disease Clinics of North America 1988; 14: 441
167. Groff GD, Franck WA, Raddatz DA. Systemic steroid therapy for acute gout: a clinical trial and review of the literature. Seminars in Arthritis and Rheumatism 1990; 19: 329
168. Kot TV, Day RO, Brooks PM. Preventing acute gout when starting allopurinol therapy: colchicine or NSAIDs? Medical Journal of Australia 1993; 159: 182
169. Liang MH, Fries JF. Asymptomatic hyperuricaemia: the case for conservative management. Annals of Internal Medicine 1978; 88: 666
170. Hart FD. Drug-induced arthritis. Current Medical Research and Opinion 1974; 2: 505
171. Alarçon-Segovia D, Kraus A. Drug-related lupus syndromes and their relationship to spontaneously occurring systemic lupus erythematosus. Baillière's Clinical Rheumatology 1991; 5: 1
172. Le Quintrec J-S, Le Quintrec J-L. Drug induced myopathies. Baillière's Clinical Rheumatology 1991; 5: 21
173. Geusens P, Dequeker J. Locomotor side-effects of corticosteroids. Baillière's Clinical Rheumatology 1991; 5: 99
174. Bourgeois P, Aeschlimann A. Drug-induced scleroderma. Baillière's Clinical Rheumatology 1991; 5: 13
175. Hart FD. Drug-induced arthritis and arthralgia. Drugs 1984; 28: 347
176. Chapel TA, Burns RE. Oral contraceptives and exacerbation of lupus erythematosus. American Journal of Obstetrics and Gynecology 1971; 110: 336
177. Jenkins LC, McGraw RW. Anaesthetic management of the patient with rheumatoid arthritis. Canadian Anaesthetists' Society Journal 1969; 16: 407
178. Boston Collaborative Drug Surveillance Program. Excess of ampicillin rashes associated with allopurinol and hyperuricaemia. New England Journal of Medicine 1972; 286: 505
179. Webster J. Interactions of NSAIDs with diuretics and β-blockers; mechanisms and clinical implications. Drugs 1985; 30: 32
180. Koopmans PP, Kateman WGPM. Effects of indomethacin and sulindac on hydrochlorothiazide kinetics. Clinical Pharmacology and Therapeutics 1985; 37: 625
181. Koopmans PP, Thien TH, Thomas CMG. The effects of sulindac and indomethacin on the antihypertensive and diuretic action of hydrochlorothiazide in patients with mild to moderate essential hypertension. British Journal of Clinical Pharmacology 1986; 21: 417
182. Daly H, Boyle J, Roberts C, et al. Interaction between methotrexate and non-steroidal anti-inflammatory drugs. Lancet 1986; 1: 557
183. Thyss A, Milano G, Kubar J, et al. Clinical and pharmacokinetic evidence of a lift threatening interactions between methotrexate and ketoprofen. Lancet 1986; 1: 256

Chapter 26

# Haematological Disorders

*M. Verstraete, R. Verhaeghe, K. Peerlinck* and *M.A. Boogaerts*

## Synopsis of Important Principles

1) The basic aim of antithrombotic and thrombolytic drug therapy in thromboembolic disorders is to reduce morbidity and mortality. In some situations (e.g. myocardial infarction), the therapeutic gain of thrombolytic drugs is considerable while that of antithrombotic drugs is small but real. In others (e.g. massive life-threatening pulmonary embolism), thrombolytic drugs, while being highly effective, sometimes may not be able to be given soon enough or may not act quickly enough.

2) The benefit from antithrombotic drugs in the treatment of thrombosis and embolism is now as well documented in the arterial as the venous circulation. Anticoagulant therapy is primarily prophylactic and can only prevent deposition of a thrombus or limit its extension and fragmentation (embolisation). Thrombolytic drugs, if given early enough, can hasten the lysis of preformed thrombi. Agents affecting platelet function, particularly aspirin (acetylsalicylic acid) and ticlopidine are of potential use in attempts to prevent thrombus formation in the arterial and apparently also the venous circulation.

3) Despite the availability of effective prophylactic therapy (mainly heparin and oral anticoagulants) for venous thrombosis, considerable emphasis must still be placed on the recognition of thrombosis-prone patients, and on early diagnosis and prompt treatment of established deep vein thrombosis.

4) Effective and safe use of the currently available oral anticoagulant drugs (coumarins) depends on careful regulation of the intensity of pharmacological response, the margin between adequate therapy and haemorrhage being relatively narrow. Dosages vary from patient to patient and depend not only on individual differences in the rate of elimination, but also on the numerous factors affecting vitamin K availability or clotting factor synthesis, which can influence the response or increase the risk of complications.

5) The treatment of a patient with a defect of the haemostatic mechanism is very specific and is determined by the type of abnormality and its pathogenesis. Accurate diagnosis is essential. In every anaemic patient, a correct diagnosis must precede the use of haematinics, with identification and elimination, if possible, of any underlying cause. There is no place for 'shot gun' therapy.

6) Some drugs can increase the risk of haematological complications when used in patients with disorders of the blood – for example, aspirin in those with bleeding disorders or in those on anticoagulants, and cotrimoxazole (trimethoprim/sulfamethoxazole) in those with megaloblastic anaemia.

7) The haematopoietic system is particularly sensitive to the action of drugs and many drugs are regularly associated with idiosyncratic haematological reactions in susceptible individuals. Bleeding disorders and coagulation disturbances are not infrequently caused by drugs.

Disorders of the blood are of major importance in therapeutics. This is not only because of the high morbidity and mortality associated with conditions like thromboembolic occlusive vascular disease and blood dyscrasias such as aplastic anaemia, but also because they illustrate well the application of clinical pharmacological principles to individualisation of therapy. This is not only because the blood is an easily sampled tissue and individualised therapy is necessary for effective treatment, but also because excessive drug effects on the blood can be disastrous.

## 1. Clinical Pharmacological Considerations

Drugs used in haematological diseases include agents for the management of haemorrhagic disease, anaemias and white cell disorders, and drugs for the prevention and treatment of thromboembolic disorders. An understanding of the pathophysiology of haemostasis is fundamental to the individualised therapy of both haemorrhagic disease and thromboembolic disorders, and an awareness of the clinical pharmacological factors that can modify the response of antithrombotic drugs is essential in the control of anticoagulant therapy. Similar considerations apply for the haematopoietic system.

### 1.1 Haemostasis and Coagulation

#### *1.1.1 Role of the Vessel Wall and the Endothelium*

**The Vessel Wall**

The first event in haemostasis in response to vascular injury is contraction of smooth muscle cells. The vast majority of vessels are capillaries where smooth muscle cells are absent and haemostasis depends on direct sealing. On the other hand, breaks in arterioles and venules depend on vascular contraction, which is soon followed by local perivascular and intravascular activation of platelets and coagulation components.

**The Endothelium**

One of the unsolved mysteries of haemostasis and thrombosis is why platelets do not, or hardly ever, adhere to normal (unstimulated) endothelial cells *in vivo*. One answer is that both platelets and the endothelium have a negative charge and thus would be mutually repulsive. This negativity could also prevent the contact phase of the intrinsic coagulation system. The negative electrical charge of endothelial cells is due to a pronounced glycocalyx, consisting of glycoprotein-β and proteoglycans of which heparan sulfate (a heparin-like substance that binds antithrombin III) is the most important.[1,2] Stimulated or injured endothelial cells lose their negative surface charge.

Normal endothelial cells are much more than a semipermeable barrier between the blood and the vascular smooth muscle. They can be re-

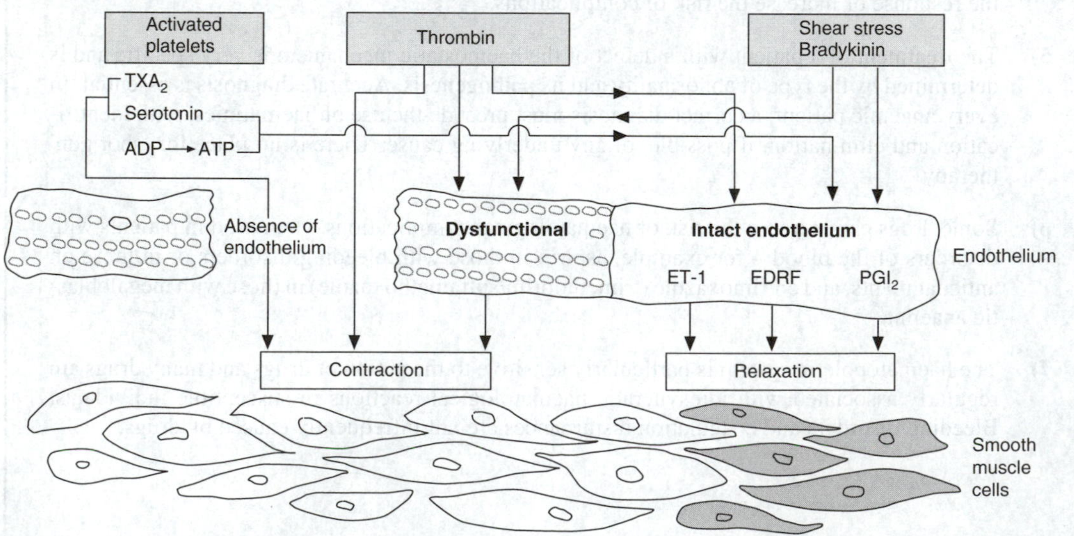


**Fig. 1.** Effect of platelet components, thrombin and other factors on normal and dysfunctional endothelium and its indirect impact on smooth muscle cells. *Abbreviations:* ADP = adenosine diphosphate; ATP = adenosine triphosphate; EDRF = endothelium-derived relaxing factor (nitric oxide, NO); ET-1 = endothelin-1; $PGI_2$ = prostaglandin $I_2$ (prostacyclin); $TXA_2$ = thromboxane $A_2$.

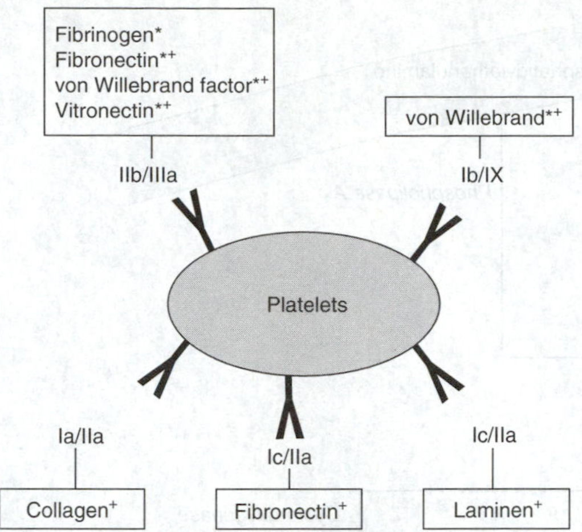


**Fig. 2.** Stimulated platelets express on their membrane different glycoprotein receptors (integrins) which bind to ligands present in plasma (*) or in endothelial basement membranes (+).

garded as a highly active metabolic and endocrine organ that plays a major role in maintaining a proper balance between the formation of haemostatic plugs and the avoidance of intraluminal thrombi.

Endothelial cells inactivate vasoactive substances and have an important function on vasomotor tone.[3,4] For instance, carrier mechanisms in their cell membranes specifically transport serotonin, adenosine and adenine nucleotides into the cell where they are metabolised. Angiotensin-converting enzyme (ACE) on the outer surface of the cell inactivates bradykinin, a potent vasodilator. Perhaps a more crucial function is the synthesis of active substances which intervene in important physiological and pathological processes (fig. 1).[5,6]

The production of prostacyclin [prostaglandin (PG) $I_2$] by endothelial cells is stimulated by contact with activated platelets or leucocytes, by stretching of the arterial wall (pulsatile pressure), and by some drugs. Prostacyclin has strong antiplatelet and vasodilator properties and thus acts as the biological antipole of thromboxane $A_2$. A direct link between impaired biosynthesis of prostacyclin in the vessel wall and thrombosis or atherosclerosis is suggested by the decreased capacity of the endothelium to generate prostacyclin with age, with heavy smoking, and in atherosclerosis or diabetes. Endothelium-derived relaxing factor (EDRF or nitric oxide)[7] is formed from L-arginine by an oxidation pathway that requires several cofactors. EDRF relaxes smooth muscle cells through stimulation of guanylate cyclase which in turn generates cyclic guanosine monophosphate (cyclic-GMP).[8] By the same mechanism, it also potently inhibits adhesion and aggregation of platelets. There is a clear synergism between prostacyclin and EDRF in preventing platelet activation. EDRF is effective only in the immediate vicinity of its site of release because haemoglobin inactivates almost immediately any EDRF that enters the blood stream. Deficient EDRF production has been suggested to contribute to the pathogenesis of complications of atherosclerosis and diabetes.

Endothelin-1[9] is a 21-residue peptide that is slowly released from endothelial cells by various stimuli, and acts as a local hormone to induce a strong contraction of the underlying smooth muscle. Cleavage of a larger propeptide ('big' endothelin) by a putative endopeptidase (endothelin-converting enzyme) produces the active peptide. Its possible role in physiological conditions and in several diseases is currently under intense scrutiny. Synthesis of platelet-activating factor (PAF),[10] a strong stimulator of platelet aggregation, may be activated by thrombin that is locally generated if a breach in the endothelial lining occurs. Thrombin is normally captured by thrombomodulin, a transmembranous protein that serves as an endothelial receptor for thrombin.[11,12] In the complex that is formed, thrombin loses its procoagulant activity and expresses its anticoagulant role by activating protein C.

Thus, apart from a metabolic function with respect to vasoactive substances, the primary role of the endothelium is in maintaining the patency of blood vessels and the fluidity of blood. However, the endothelium also has the potential to enhance and amplify the formation of a haemostatic plug initiated by a local endothelial lesion.

#### *1.1.2 Role of Platelets*

Under normal conditions, platelets are quiescent and circulate freely in the blood as they do not attach to a normally functioning endothelium. Vessel injury however, exposes subendothelial tissue with its various elements to which platelets can adhere.[13-16] Collagen and fibronectin interact readily with platelets, particularly with their membrane glycoproteins Ia and Ic/IIa (fig. 2). Several adhesive proteins such as von Willebrand factor strengthen the initial bonds. Adhered platelets lose their discoid shape, form pseudopods and spread out over the

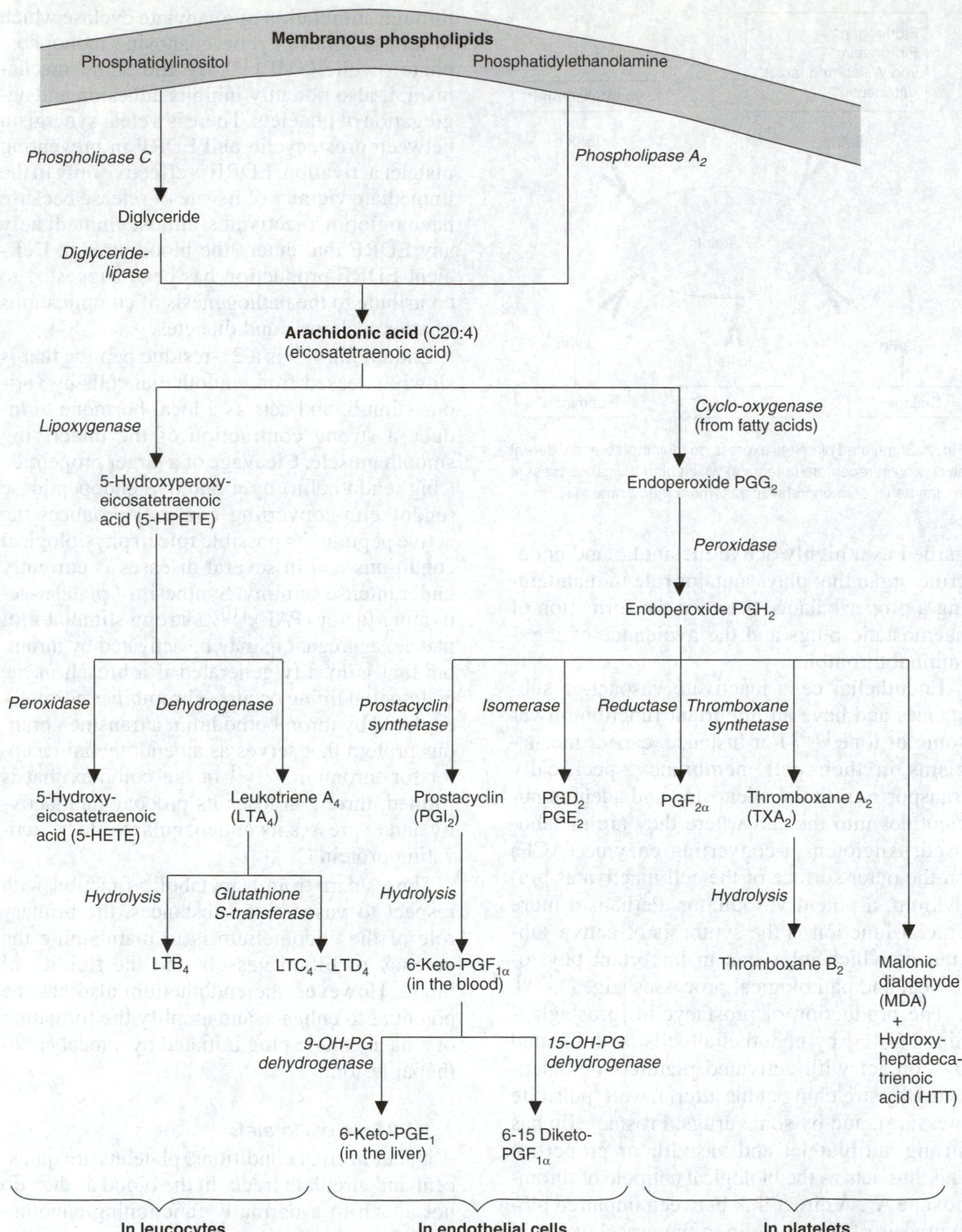


**Fig. 3.** Cytoplasmic formation of arachidonic acid and its lipoxygenase- and cyclo-oxygenase–dependent metabolism. *Abbreviations:* LT = leukotriene; PG = prostaglandin.

injured surface. Through the action of activators such as collagen and eventually thrombin and noradrenaline (norepinephrine), the adhered platelets soon become activated whereby platelet receptors are expressed and several mediators released.[17] Phospholipase C acts on platelet membrane phosphatidylinositol, hydrolysis of which leads to the release of calcium from the dense tubular system (fig. 3). Calcium in turn activates a protein kinase that phosphorylates intraplatelet regulatory proteins; activation of the actin-myosin system results in platelet contraction with release of adenosine diphosphate (ADP) and serotonin from the platelet dense granules, and also of thromboxane $A_2$.[18,19] These potent inducers of platelet aggregation are able to recruit additional circulating platelets which in turn adhere to and transform the initial monolayer of platelets into an aggregate. The platelet glycoproteins IIb-IIIa on the platelet membrane undergo a conformational change in the activation process, so that they can interact with plasma fibrinogen and other adhesive proteins such as fibronectin and endothelial thrombospondin, which serve to link platelets together into a tighter aggregate.

In addition, phospholipase $A_2$ acts on phosphatidylcholine to release arachidonic acid from the platelet membrane. Arachidonic acid is converted to proaggregating prostaglandin endoperoxide intermediates (prostaglandins $G_2$ and $H_2$) by cyclo-oxygenase. Thromboxane $A_2$ is then formed by the action of thromboxane synthetase on prostaglandin $H_2$; this further promotes platelet activation, thrombus growth and local vasoconstriction. On the other hand, the vascular endothelial cells synthesise prostacyclin ($PGI_2$) starting from arachidonic acid or from platelet-derived prostaglandin $G_2$. Prostacyclin stimulates adenylate cyclase and leads to an increased level of cyclic adenosine monophosphate (cyclic-AMP) in the platelet. Cyclic-AMP, in turn, inhibits the discharge of calcium from the dense tubular system and thus prevents platelet aggregation and secretion. Phosphodiesterase enhances the breakdown of cyclic-AMP. Arachidonic acid also serves as a substrate for the formation of leukotrienes, a pathway that is mediated by lipoxygenase in the leucocytes.

Thus, eicosanoids derived from arachidonic acid in platelets, endothelial cells and leucocytes provide short-acting biological mediators that not only further promote platelet activation and local vasoconstriction but also platelet inhibition and vasodilatation and, as well, intervene in local immune-mediated reactions.

### *1.1.3 The Coagulation Pathway*

Activated platelets rearrange their surface lipoproteins so that phospholipids on which coagulation factors can concentrate are now exposed to the blood stream. Thus, activated platelets, which lose their electronegativity in the process, markedly accelerate the formation of thrombin. Thrombin occupies a central position in the coagulation process. It is formed as the end-result of a chain of reactions which transform in sequence a number of coagulation factors present as precursors (zymogens) in plasma into activated factors. The reactions mainly occur on the membrane of activated platelets and other stimulated cells and tissue factor (a membrane protein which is exposed to the blood, e.g. after trauma) on which coagulation factors bind. Because of the low concentration of these factors in plasma and because of the abundant presence of circulating inhibitors, the interaction and subsequent transformation proceeds only slowly in a fluid phase.

Coagulation factors are activated one by one, mainly through limited proteolysis. Most activated factors are serine proteases: they split arginyl bonds in their specific substrate which then become another activated coagulation factor (waterfall or cascade sequence of events). Factors VIII and V, on the other hand, do not split bonds in other proteins but rather form complexes with activated factors IX and X (IXa, Xa), respectively, to stimulate the activity of the latter 2 enzymes. They can therefore be considered as regulatory proteins which influence the reaction rate.

The traditional coagulation scheme distinguishes an *'intrinsic'* from an *'extrinsic'* activation pathway.

#### Intrinsic Pathway

All factors participating in the intrinsic pathway are present in circulating blood and the reaction sequence is initiated by contact of platelets and/or coagulation components with subendothelial tissue; in addition, antigen-antibody complexes and activated platelets may serve this purpose as do foreign surfaces, e.g. during extracorporeal circulation or renal dialysis. This initial contact phase involves the interaction of factor XII (Hageman factor), prekallikrein and high molecular weight kininogen. However, the precise mechanism of the initial firing spark triggering the contact activation remains elusive.

Factor XII circulates in plasma and has a great affinity for negatively charged surfaces. Upon adsorption, bound factor XII exerts traces of biological activity. In terms of the mechanism of this phenomenon, conformational changes of the molecule with exposure of the enzyme site have been postulated (fig. 4).[20,21] The actual activation of factor XII is facilitated by kallikrein. Prekallikrein and high molecular weight kininogen circulate in plasma as equimolar complexes and are also readily absorbed to negatively charged surfaces. Traces of activated factor XII (i.e. XIIa) presumably generate traces of kallikrein from prekallikrein. Kallikrein then activates factor XII more rapidly, which in turn generates more kallikrein and the reciprocal activation of these 2 surface-bound molecules continues until the substrates are locally exhausted. Factor XIIa then proceeds to activate the next factor of the coagulation cascade, factor XI, from its zymogen form to its enzymatic constellation. Factor XI also circulates in plasma complexed with high molecular weight kininogen; the latter protein thus serves as a helper protein or cofactor carrying factors XII and XI in the blood and 'delivering' them to activated (negatively charged) surfaces in the activation reaction of factor XII and factor XI (fig. 5).

Factor XI is bound to the surfaces by high molecular weight kininogen and upon activation, interacts with factor IX in a calcium-dependent 2-step reaction. Each light chain of factor XIa contains a catalytic site, while its heavy chain has the binding site for factor IX. Binding of calcium ion to factor IX (a vitamin K-dependent protein) induces a conformational change in the molecule that facilitates its binding to the heavy chain of factor XIa which is essential for the optimal rate of factor IX activation.

Platelets are also important in the intrinsic system as they contain high molecular weight kininogen which can be expressed when the platelets are stimulated, as they indeed are on foreign surfaces. Activated factor IX, thrombin-modified factor VIII, negatively charged phospholipid (e.g. activated platelets) and calcium ions form a complex termed 'tenase' complex because it activates factor X (fig. 5).

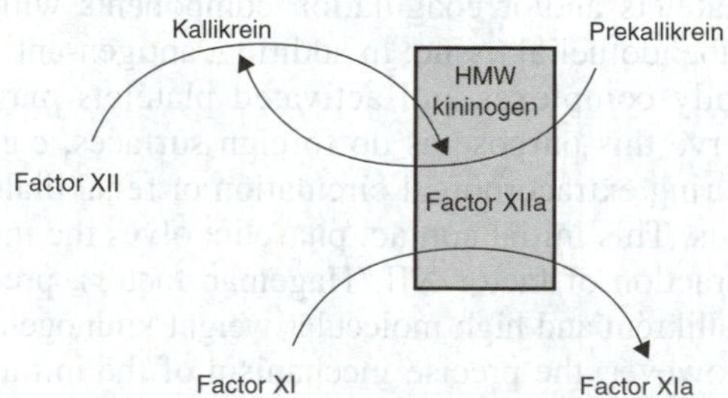


**Fig. 4.** The contact phase of the intrinsic activation pathway. The initial event *in vitro* is the adsorption of factor XII to negatively charged surfaces where it undergoes a conformational change to expose its active site. Factor XII converts prekallikrein to kallikrein. Additional factor XIIa and kallikrein are then generated by reciprocal activation. Factor XIIa also activates factor XI. Both prekallikrein and factor XI bind to a cofactor, high molecular weight (HMW) kininogen, which serves to anchor them to the charged surface.

#### Extrinsic Pathway

In the extrinsic system, membrane-bound tissue factor starts off the chain of events by forming a complex with factor VII in the presence of calcium ions (fig. 5). The molecular structure of tissue factor is well known; it is present on cell surfaces as a dimer composed of two identical subunits with interacting enzyme binding sites.[22-25] Factor VII is a single-chain protein which, in this form, already has some enzymatic activity and can complex with tissue factor. However, by cleavage of an Arg-Ile bond, the molecule of factor VII splits into a light chain and a heavy chain (containing the active site), linked by 2 disulfide bonds. This activation increases the coagulant activity of factor VII about 100-fold. The tissue factor-factor VIIa complex then combines with the substrate (factor X) producing a further conformational change in factor VIIa so that it binds even more tightly to tissue factor, precluding dissociation of factor VIIa from tissue factor. The tissue factor-factor VIIa complex primarily activates factor X but also factors XI and IX, which interconnect the 2 activation pathways. It should be noted that phospholipids of the platelet membrane in conjunction with factor Xa, can also activate factor VII, another bridge between the intrinsic and extrinsic pathways.

That factor VII is essential to ensure normal haemostasis is underlined by the bleeding condition of patients with severe congenital factor VII deficiency.

### The Coagulation Pathway in Common: The Formation of Prothrombinase (the Enzyme Converting Prothrombin to Thrombin)

Factor X stands at the crossroad of the extrinsic and intrinsic activation pathways. This means that factor X can be activated either by the tenase complex or by the tissue factor-factor VIIa complex. In both instances, activation of factor X results from the cleavage of a single peptide bond between Arg and Ile in the zymogen (fig. 5).[24] This is brought about by the enzymatic activity residing in factor IXa which is part of the tenase complex (factor IXa-factor VIIIa phospholipid). The presence of proteolytically modified factor VIII (albeit by thrombin, factor

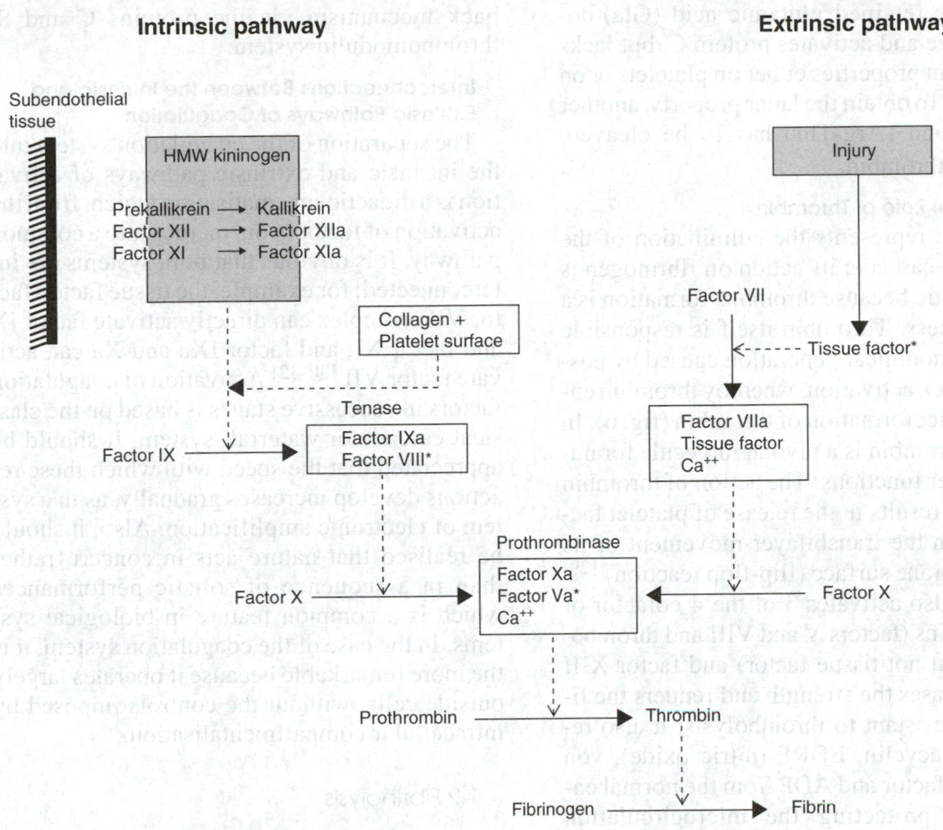


**Fig. 5.** Mechanisms of clotting factors interactions. Coagulation is initiated by either an intrinsic or extrinsic pathway. In the intrinsic pathway, negatively charged surfaces initiate the contact activation and the phospholipid is furnished by platelets. In the extrinsic system, the phospholipid portion of tissue thromboplastin functions in conjunction with factor VIIa on the activation of factor X. From factor Xa on, both pathways converge upon a common path. Omitted from the diagram are inhibitors of the various steps, the augmentation of action of each pathway by activated factors, and the interaction between the intrinsic and extrinsic systems. An asterisk (*) denotes proteins which are cofactors (helper proteins). *Abbreviation:* HMW = high molecular weight.

Xa or factor IXa) enhances 10,000-fold the rate of activation of factor X by factor IXa. Factor VIII is thus a helper protein (a cofactor) which, to exert its function, binds to phospholipid vesicles, provided phosphatidylserine is available on the platelet membrane.[26] In fact, there are specific binding sites available on activated platelets for factor VIII (binding domains in its light subunit) which are distinct from the binding sites for factor V expressed during stimulation of platelets.

To be fully active, factor Xa has to form a stoichiometric 1 : 1 complex with factor Va; the latter molecule enhances the activation of prothrombin by factor Xa 300,000-fold). Normal plasma contains factor V in trace amounts and in an inactive state; its activation requires 3 specific enzymatic cleavages which can be brought about by thrombin or less efficiently by factor Xa.[27] The association of factor Va with factor Xa on a phospholipid membrane termed 'prothrombinase' has been reported to position the active site at a proper distance above the membrane for optimal enzymatic activity.[28] Factor Va increases the turnover 1000-fold which means that the number of thrombin molecules generated by the enzyme upon saturation by the substrate is multiplied by a factor of approximately 1000. In contrast to the vitamin K-dependent coagulation factors (prothrombin, factors VII, IX, X, proteins C and S), factor Va does not bind to phospholipids via calcium bridges but penetrates into the lipid bilayer.

#### Effect of Prothrombinase on Prothrombin

Prothrombinase initially cleaves the Arg-Ile bond in the prothrombin molecule producing the intermediate meizothrombin.[27] This intermediate molecule remains membrane-bound through the retained glutamic acid (Gla)-domain linkage and activates protein C, but lacks procoagulant properties either on platelets or on fibrinogen. To obtain the latter property, another arginine bond (Arg-Thr) has to be cleaved, yielding α-thrombin.

### The Pivotal Role of Thrombin

Thrombin represents the culmination of the coagulation cascade; its action on fibrinogen is most dramatic because thrombus formation is a visible process. Thrombin itself is responsible for its own nonlinear generation caused by positive feedback activation, whereby thrombin enhances the neoformation of thrombin (fig. 6). In addition, thrombin is a pivotal molecule for numerous other functions. The action of thrombin on platelets results in the release of platelet factor V and in the transbilayer movement of its inner membrane surface (flip-flop reaction).[29] Thrombin also activates 3 of the 4 cofactor or helper proteins (factors V and VIII and thrombomodulin, but not tissue factor) and factor XIII which increases the strength and renders the fibrin more resistant to thrombolysis; it also releases prostacyclin, EDRF (nitric oxide), von Willebrand factor and ADP from the normal endothelium, protecting the microcirculation against thrombosis. Furthermore, thrombin inhibits its own production by a negative feedback mechanism via the proteins C and S-thrombomodulin system.

### Interconnections Between the Intrinsic and Extrinsic Pathways of Coagulation

The separation of the coagulation system into the intrinsic and extrinsic pathways of activation is a didactic schematisation which, from the activation of factor X on, merges into a common pathway. It is obvious that both systems are interconnected; for example, the tissue factor-factor VIIa complex can directly activate factor IX and factor XI; and factor IXa and Xa can activate factor VII.[30-32] Activation of coagulation factors in successive stages is based on the classical cascade or waterfall system. It should be appreciated that the speed with which these reactions develop increases gradually, as in a system of electronic amplification. Also, it should be realised that nature acts in concert, rather than in a sequence of solistic performances which is a common feature in biological systems. In the case of the coagulation system, it is the more remarkable because it operates largely outside cells, without the controls imposed by intracellular compartmentalisation.

## 1.2 Fibrinolysis

Fibrin is primarily cleared from the circulation by the fibrinolytic system which acts as an

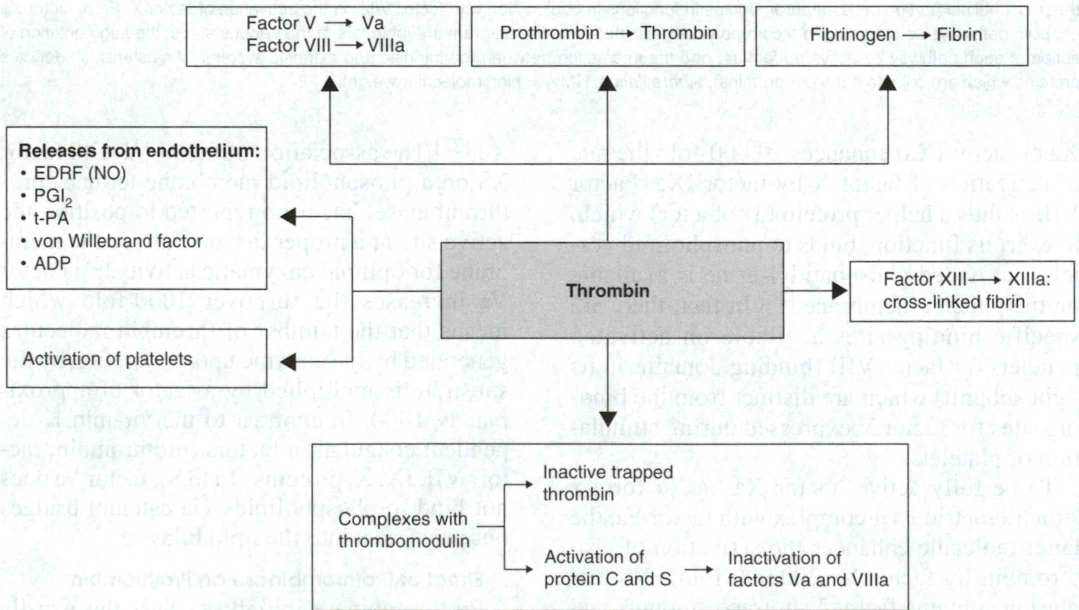


**Fig. 6.** Thrombin is the pivotal enzyme in coagulation, being responsible for positive feedback activation, rapid activation of platelets and endothelial cells and, indirectly via thrombomodulin, for its inactivation. *Abbreviations:* ADP = adenosine diphosphate; EDRF = endothelium-derived relaxing factor (nitric oxide, NO); $PGI_2$ = prostaglandin $I_2$ (prostacyclin); t-PA = tissue-type plasminogen activator.

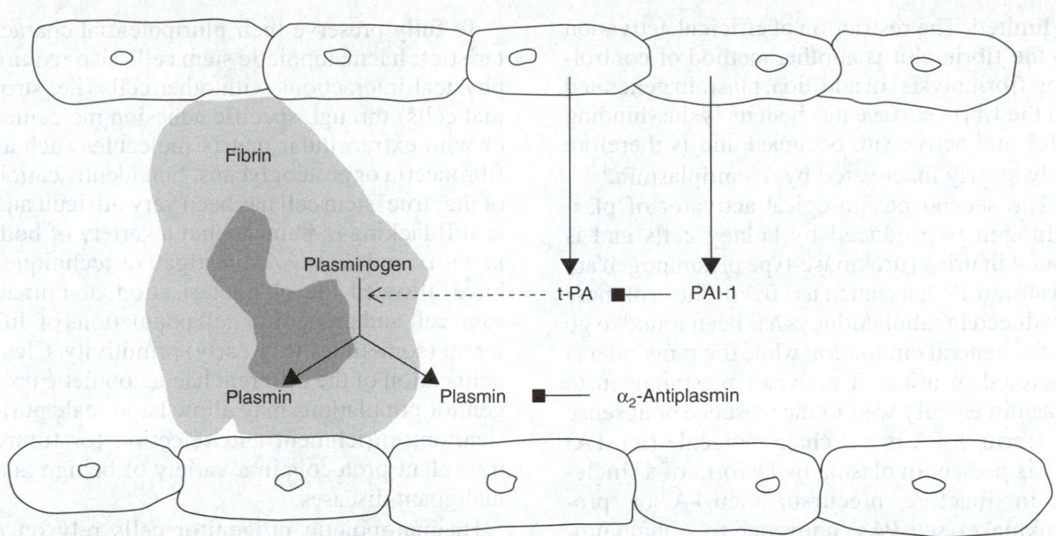


**Fig. 7.** Tissue-type plasminogen activator (t-PA) is released by the stimulated endothelium and has a greater affinity for fibrin than for circulating plasminogen. Plasminogen activator inhibitor-1 (PAI-1) neutralises only free t-PA in the circulation; similarly, plasmin bound to fibrin is not neutralised by circulating $\alpha_2$-antiplasmin in contrast to circulating plasmin. The broken arrow denotes activation and the continuous arrows transformation.

antithrombotic defence mechanism, albeit at a rather slow pace. Plasmin is the effector enzyme of the system; it is formed from an inactive precursor, plasminogen, under the action of plasminogen activator. Physiological fibrinolysis is regulated by specific molecular interactions between plasminogen activators and their inhibitors, plasminogen, and plasmin and its inhibitors, as well as by the interaction of these molecules with fibrin and with cellular and extracellular binding sites.[33-35] The liver metabolises and eliminates most of the components of the fibrinolytic system and contributes to modulating their plasma levels.

Human plasminogen is a glycoprotein with amino terminal glutamic acid in its native form (Glu-plasminogen), but native plasminogen is easily converted by limited plasmic digestion to modified forms with amino terminal lysine, valine or methionine, commonly designated as Lys-plasminogen.[36] Plasminogen is converted to plasmin by cleavage of a single peptide bond.

Plasmin is a 2-chain molecule. The heavy chain contains structures which mediate the interaction with fibrin and antiplasmin, the so-called lysine binding sites, which may play a crucial role in the endogenous regulation of fibrinolysis. The active site contains serine and is located on the light chain.

### Plasminogen Activators

The most important physiological activator is tissue-type plasminogen activator (t-PA). It is continuously synthesised and secreted by endothelial cells as a 1-chain molecule that is converted to a 2-chain molecule in the presence of plasmin or kallikrein, but the activity of both forms is roughly comparable. Control of the release of t-PA represents an initial method of regulating the fibrinolytic activity of blood. However, an increase in the plasma concentration of t-PA (e.g. as induced by physical exercise) produces only a slight increase in plasmin activity which is rapidly neutralised by circulating $\alpha_2$-antiplasmin.

t-PA has a low affinity for plasminogen in the absence of fibrin, but the presence of a fibrin surface strikingly enhances (1000-fold) the activation rate of plasminogen. This increased affinity results from surface assembly of plasminogen and plasminogen activator on the fibrin clot. Plasminogen binds specifically but weakly with fibrin through the structures called 'lysine binding sites'. t-PA also has a specific affinity for fibrin and the presence of t-PA enhances the binding of plasminogen to fibrin (fig. 7). Thus, fibrin essentially increases the local plasminogen concentration and facilitates the interaction between t-PA and its substrate. Efficient activation of plasminogen by t-PA is therefore limited to the fibrin surface while activation in plasma is limited. The restriction of efficient activation to the fibrin clot is another method of controlling fibrinolysis. In addition, plasmin generated on the fibrin surface has both its lysine-binding sites and active site occupied and is therefore only slowly inactivated by $\alpha_2$-antiplasmin.[36]

The second physiological activator of plasminogen is produced by kidney cells and is found in urine (urokinase-type plasminogen activator, u-PA); as much as 90% of the urokinase produced in rabbit kidneys has been found to go to the general circulation while the remainder is excreted in urine. It activates plasminogen to plasmin equally well in the presence or absence of fibrin. u-PA is a 2-chain molecule (tcu-PA) but is present in plasma in the form of a single-chain inactive precursor (scu-PA or pro-urokinase). scu-PA is converted to 2-chain urokinase by hydrolysis of a single peptide bond in the presence of plasmin.[37-39]

#### Inhibitors of Plasminogen Activators

Further regulation of fibrinolytic activity occurs at the level of the interaction of plasminogen activators with specific inhibitors.[40-44] Plasminogen activator inhibitor-1 (PAI-1) is synthesised in endothelial cells and is also found in platelets from where it is released during aggregation. Interaction of t-PA with PAI-1 results in decreased activity of the activator, but t-PA bound to fibrin is largely protected from inactivation. Clinical studies support a role for an elevated plasma concentration of PAI-1 in the genesis of thrombotic events. A second inhibitor, PAI-2, is only detected in pregnant women.[45]

### 1.3 Haematopoiesis

Mature blood cells – erythrocytes, leucocytes and thrombocytes (platelets) – are derived from a relatively small number of so-called pluripotent haematopoietic progenitor cells, which are characterised by full self-renewal potential, extensive proliferative and repopulating ability, and a capacity to differentiate into all haematopoietic lineages (fig. 8). These haematopoietic functions are regulated by a network of more than 20 fully characterised growth and differentiation or inhibitory factors – called variably colony-stimulating factors (CSFs), growth factors, interleukins (ILs) or cytokines – of which the majority have been molecularly cloned and purified to homogeneity. Many of these factors have already been successfully used in clinical indications.

To fully preserve their pluripotential characteristics, haematopoietic stem cells also require physical interactions with other cells (i.e. stromal cells) through specific adhesion molecules or with extracellular matrix molecules such as fibronectin or proteoglycans. Full identification of the 'true' stem cell has been very difficult and is still lacking in humans, but a variety of both *in vitro* and *in vivo* investigative techniques have allowed the characterisation of human stem cell and progenitor cell populations of different (sometimes very early) primitivity. Clear delineation of the different haematopoietic progenitor populations may allow large scale purification, enrichment and selection for future transplant protocols in a variety of benign and malignant diseases.

Haematopoietic progenitor cells rely on a complex network of growth factors and cytokines for their survival (prevention of programmed cell death), proliferation and differentiation. From many recent studies, it has become apparent that combinations of growth factors are often necessary for optimal effects and that both synergistic and antagonistic reactions may be encountered. When embarking on clinical studies, it should be remembered that most growth factors can exert powerful functional effects on mature cells (e.g. macrophages, endothelial cells, granulocytes, etc.), often leading to significant adverse effects.

*In vitro* proliferation of haematopoietic progenitors in serum- and stroma-free conditions requires repeated addition of a 'soup' of growth factors, among which the following are thought to be important: G-CSF (granulocyte colony-stimulating factor), GM-CSF (granulocyte macrophage colony-stimulating factor), IL-1, IL-3, IL-6, IL-11, stem cell factor, and erythropoietin (EPO). Combinations of at least 3 and often more of these cytokines are needed for optimal growth.[46] Already, clinical trials using these *in vitro* expanded progenitors are underway.[47] Optimisation of *in vitro* culture systems, e.g. with other stromal factors, allowing the use of less (expensive) growth factors may further improve their clinical applicability.

Some cytokines have been shown to negatively influence progenitor cell proliferation and differentiation. Transforming growth factor-β (TGF-β) and macrophage inflammatory protein (MIP)-1α suppress the proliferation of CD34+ cells *in vitro*.[48] However, both stimulatory and inhibitory effects may be seen, depending on the cell type considered (e.g. more

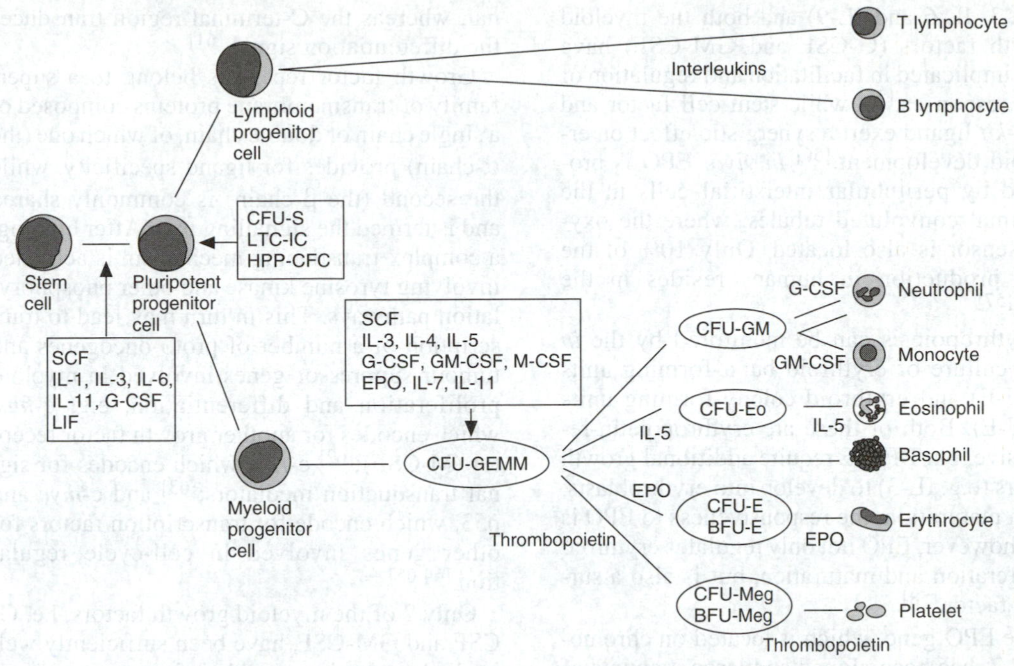


**Fig. 8.** Regulation of haematopoiesis. *Abbreviations:* BFU-E = burst-forming unit – erythrocyte; BFU-Meg = burst-forming unit – megakaryocyte; CFU-GEMM = colony-forming unit – granulocyte, erythrocyte, macrophage, megakaryocyte; CFU-GM = colony-forming unit – granulocyte, macrophage; CFU-E = colony-forming unit – erythrocyte; CFU-Eo = colony-forming unit – eosinophil; CFU-Meg = colony-forming unit – megakaryocyte; CFU-S = colony-forming unit – spleen; EPO = erythropoietin; G-CSF = granulocyte colony-stimulating factor; GM-CSF = granulocyte macrophage colony-stimulating factor; HPP-CFC = high-proliferative potential colony-forming cells; IL = interleukin; LIF = leukaemia inhibitory factor; LTC-IC = long term culture-initiating cells; M-CSF = macrophage colony-stimulating factor; SCF = stem cell factor.

or less differentiated). MIP-1α can thus be used to prevent primitive multipotent stem cells going into cycle and synthesising DNA, thereby making them less vulnerable to cycle-specific cytotoxic agents or allowing selective enrichment of long term repopulating cells.[49]

The receptor molecules for many growth factors, e.g. G-CSF, GM-CSF, IL-3, IL-4, IL-5, IL-6 and IL-7, share structural features of the extracellular domain and are grouped in the haematopoietin receptor superfamily.[50] It is well known that the high-affinity GM-CSF and IL-3 receptors share a common β-chain leading to cross-competition between these growth factors.[51] The receptors for human haematopoietic growth factors are strictly regulated, their absolute numbers on stem cells being low, but they increase during cellular differentiation. Up- and down-regulation can be provoked by their own growth factors or by others.

Soluble versions of many haematopoietic factor receptors have been described.[52] These can act as antagonists by their ability to competitively bind to the same ligands as their cellular counterparts; alternatively, they may potentiate the action of growth factors by preventing their binding to secondary targets or by slowing their clearance from the circulation. Growth factor receptors are also present on many malignant cells, opening therapeutic perspectives, e.g. to induce cycling and make leukaemic cells more vulnerable to cycle-specific cytotoxic agents,[53] and use of growth factor-toxin fusion proteins.[54] Alternatively, broad spectrum use of growth factors may promote tumour cell growth, accelerate tumour progression and impair survival.

Finally, mutations in cellular growth factor receptors can be involved in the primary pathogenesis of, for example, human leukaemia, by inducing unlimited proliferation, by suppressing p53 activity, or by interfering with normal programmed cell death.[53]

#### *1.3.1 Erythropoiesis and Erythropoietin*

Erythropoiesis is dependent on a number of humoral and cell-associated factors, of which erythropoietin (EPO) is certainly the most important. However, some of the interleukins (IL-

1, IL-3, IL-6 and IL-9) and both the myeloid growth factors (G-CSF and GM-CSF) have been implicated in facilitation and regulation of EPO responses,[55] while stem cell factor and the c-*kit* ligand exert a synergistic effect on erythroid development.[56] *In vivo,* EPO is produced by peritubular interstitial cells in the proximal convoluted tubules, where the oxygen-sensor is also located. Only 10% of the EPO production in humans resides in the liver.[57]

Erythropoiesis can be monitored by the *in vitro* culture of erythroid burst-forming units (BFU-E) and erythroid colony-forming units (CFU-E). Both of these are erythropoietin-responsive, but BFU-E require additional growth factors (e.g. IL-3) to develop into erythroblasts. Upon maturation, the responsiveness to EPO is lost; however, EPO not only regulates erythroid proliferation and maturation, but is also a survival factor.[58]

The EPO gene, which is located on chromosome 7, has been cloned and large amounts of recombinant human erythropoietin (rHuEPO; epoetin) have become available for clinical use (see further section 5.1.2).

#### *1.3.2 Myelopoiesis and Myeloid Growth Factors*

Myelopoiesis or the complex process by which multipotent haematopoietic progenitors develop into mature granulocytes, monocytes and macrophages, is tightly regulated by a wide variety of both external and internal stimuli. At least 5 different growth factors have been shown to interfere with the progression of myeloid progenitors through the successive stages of commitment to the granulocyte-macrophage lineage and with the terminal differentiation of lineage restricted progenitors into mature cells, i.e. IL-3, IL-6, GM-CSF, M-CSF and G-CSF.[59] These growth factors all share the capacity to activate multiple functions in their target cells, including mitogenesis and proliferation, inhibition of programmed cell death (apoptosis) and survival, enzyme expression and differentiation, stimulation of cellular function and host defence.[60] Possibly the same growth factors may exert widely different actions by using different receptor subunits or regions, by activating different signal transduction mechanisms, or by encountering different receptor densities. It has recently been recognised that the *N*-terminal region of the G-CSF receptor transduces the proliferation signal, whereas the C-terminal region transduces the differentiation signal.[61]

Growth factor receptors belong to a superfamily of transmembrane proteins composed of a single chain or double chain, of which one (the α-chain) provides for ligand specificity, while the second (the β-chain) is commonly shared and is termed the signalling part. After binding, a complex transducing mechanism is activated involving tyrosine kinase and other phosphorylation pathways. This in turn may lead to transcription of a number of proto-oncogenes and tumour suppressor genes involved in myeloid proliferation and differentiation, e.g. c-*fms*, which encodes for another growth factor receptor (M-CSF);[62] c-*ras*, which encodes for signal transduction mediators;[63] and c-*myc* and p53, which encode for transcription factors for other genes involved in cell-cycle regulation.[64,65]

Only 2 of the myeloid growth factors, i.e. G-CSF and GM-CSF, have been sufficiently well studied to provide reliable information on their clinical use (see further section 5.1.3). Clinical trials with IL-3, IL-6 and with the hybrid GM-CSF/IL-3 molecule PIXY 321 are now underway.

#### *1.3.3 Thrombopoiesis and Thrombopoietin*

Megakaryocyte development and thrombopoiesis have long remained enigmatic. The early stages of megakaryocyte production have been studied *in vitro* by the evaluation of the burst-forming unit – megakaryocyte (BFU-Meg) and the colony-forming unit – megakaryocyte (CFU-Meg). The terminal differentiation of megakaryocytes involves increasing cell ploidy, while platelet formation depends on the invagination of the megakaryocyte plasma membrane, formation of the so-called demarcation membrane system, and platelet shedding.[66]

The site(s) of megakaryocytopoiesis have not been completely elucidated. Recent studies have pointed to the lungs as well as to the bone marrow as primary production sites.[67,68]

Megakaryocytopoiesis is regulated at 2 levels: firstly, at the progenitor level by broad-spectrum cytokines such as IL-3 and IL-6;[69] and secondly, at the more mature stages by *thrombopoietin*.[70-72] The MPL-receptor – encoded by the viral myeloproliferative leukaemia proto-oncogene (v-*mpl*) – had long been predicted to be involved in megakaryocytopoiesis.[73] Upon cloning, its ligand was subsequently shown to support megakaryocyte colony formation, to increase megakaryocyte size and ploidy, and to induce the expression of megakaryocyte differentiation markers. It was therefore termed *thrombopoietin*.[71]

Thrombopoietin is produced by bone marrow stroma but also in the liver. Clinical studies in humans are underway.

## 2. General Principles of Treatment

Rational treatment of haematological disorders is based on an accurate diagnosis, individualisation of therapy, and with antithrombotic drugs, on an awareness of the many factors that can modify the response to therapy or increase the risk of complications.

1) ***Correct diagnosis:*** effective treatment of haemorrhagic disorders and anaemias requires accurate diagnosis so that highly specific treatment can be given or the causative factor removed or treated (see sections 3, 4, 5 and 6).

2) ***Early diagnosis:*** in thromboembolic disorders, screening techniques are important to identify patients at high risk of, for example, postoperative deep vein thrombosis (see section 3.2.1). Early and accurate diagnosis is also vital to the success of treatment in pulmonary embolism (see section 3.2.1), while early detection of drug-induced blood dyscrasias can be crucial to the chances of success of initial therapy (e.g. in drug-induced aplastic anaemia) or recovery (e.g. phenothiazine-induced agranulocytosis).

3) ***Early and empirical therapy:*** in severe haematological disorders with significant early mortality, empirical therapy might be warranted (e.g. corticosteroids in severe acute haemolysis, platelet pheresis and corticosteroids in idiopathic thrombocytopenic purpura, antibiotics in aplastic anaemia).

4) ***Prevention:*** since aplastic anaemia and severe episodes of acute haemolytic anaemia carry a poor prognosis and there is no effective treatment, drugs that are known to cause these reactions should not be used for trivial indications or in patients known to be at risk (see sections 5.2.2 and 5.2.3).

5) ***Basic aims of therapy:*** the basic premise of antithrombotic therapy in thromboembolic disorders is to reduce or prevent morbidity and mortality. In some cases, the therapeutic gains are real but small (e.g. anticoagulants in myocardial infarction; see section 3.2.1), while in others they are significant (e.g. prevention of acute major pulmonary embolism).

6) ***Individualised therapy:*** in thromboembolic disorders, effective and safe therapy with oral anticoagulants depends on careful regulation of the intensity of the pharmacological response. The margin between adequate therapy and undue haemorrhage is relatively narrow, varies from patient to patient, and depends not only on dosage, but also on the numerous factors that can influence the response or increase the risk of complications (see section 3.1.5).

7) ***Patient cooperation:*** in thromboembolic disorders, because of the ever present risk of haemorrhage and the importance of tight anticoagulant control for effective but safe therapy, patients should be educated in the aims and expectations of treatment and made aware of those factors that may alter their response to anticoagulants.

Anticoagulants should not be used for inadequately established indications if full cooperation and supervision of the patient cannot be achieved. Long term therapy should not be given to patients who cannot understand instructions about therapy, particularly dosage, or who do not attend regularly for control of dosage. Patients should be given written instructions about the nature of therapy, the dangers of abnormal bleeding or symptoms of recurring thromboembolism, the times to contact their clinician, the danger of relying on memory for the frequency and size of the dose, the value of keeping a diary of the amount of anticoagulant drug and all other medication actually taken, and the need to record any authorised changes in therapy.

Patients who genuinely require replacement therapy for deficiency anaemias should be encouraged to take their medication as prescribed; many patients with iron deficiency anaemia do not take or do not complete their course of iron tablets. Patients receiving drugs that regularly cause idiosyncratic blood dyscrasias should always be instructed about warning symptoms and the need to report these, particularly any unusual minor bleeding.

## 3. Thromboembolic Disorders

The high morbidity and mortality from thromboembolic occlusive vascular disease has prompted the continuing search for effective methods for its prevention and treatment.

## 3.1 Clinical Pharmacology of Drugs Used in Prevention/Treatment

### 3.1.1 Antiplatelet Agents

#### Aspirin (Acetylsalicylic Acid)

***Mechanism/site of action:*** the effect of aspirin in haemostasis appears to be primarily related to the permanent inactivation of 2 isoenzymes of prostaglandin G/H synthetase which converts arachidonic acid to endoperoxides (fig. 3). Isoenzyme type 1 is present in most tissues and in platelets and is involved in the synthesis of the prostaglandins and thromboxane that participate in maintaining cellular functions such as regulating interactions between platelets and endothelium.[74] The second isoenzyme of prostaglandin synthetase, type 2, is expressed only after cell activation in response to growth factor and mediators of inflammation.[75] Aspirin selectively acetylates the hydroxyl group of a single serine residue at position 52 within the polypeptide chain of the isoenzyme type 1, causing the irreversible loss of its cyclo-oxygenase activity. As platelets are anucleated cells they cannot synthesise new proteins and the thromboxane defect induced by aspirin is permanent during their life span (around 8 to 10 days). This explains the apparent paradox of how a drug with a half-life of 20 minutes in the systemic circulation can be fully effective as an antiplatelet agent when administered once daily.

The second isoenzyme is also acetylated by aspirin and as a result it converts arachidonic acid to 15-hydroxyeicosatetraenoic acid instead of prostaglandin $G_2$.[76]

***Pharmacodynamic properties:*** information on the pharmacodynamics of aspirin is based on measurement of serum thromboxane $B_2$ ($TXB_2$) as a reflection of thrombin-induced platelet thromboxane $A_2$ ($TXA_2$) production during whole blood clotting. This method evaluates the capacity of platelets to synthesise $TXB_2$ in response to virtually maximal stimulation and does not reflect the actual production rate of $TXB_2$ *in vivo*, which is several orders of magnitude lower.[77] Platelet $TXB_2$ generation during arachidonate-induced aggregation is inhibited by 95% with 50mg and by 99% with aspirin 324 mg/day administered for 21 days.[78] This inhibitory effect is rapid, occurring even before the appearance of the drug in the systemic circulation, probably as a result of the acetylation of platelet prostaglandin G/H synthetase in the portal circulation. Thus, the antiplatelet effect of aspirin is unrelated to its systemic availability; controlled-release and dermal preparations with reduced availability have been shown to minimise the extraplatelet effects of aspirin.[79,80]

Because of the permanent nature of the inactivation of prostaglandin synthetase in platelets, the inhibitory effect of repeated daily aspirin doses of less than 100mg is cumulative.[81] The rate at which the maximal effect is obtained can be accelerated by administering a single loading dose, e.g. 200 to 300mg (which achieves maximal inhibition at 30 minutes post-dose), followed by a daily maintenance dose of 50 to 100mg. However, patients with unstable coronary artery disease have enhanced platelet activity and might need a higher initial dose of aspirin compared with healthy persons to obtain the same platelet inhibitory effect.

***Pharmacokinetic characteristics:*** aspirin is rapidly absorbed in the stomach and upper small intestine, reaching appreciable plasma concentrations in 20 minutes. This results primarily by passive diffusion of the non-dissociated lipid-soluble aspirin across gastrointestinal membranes. The bioavailability of regular aspirin tablets is of the order of 40 to 50% after doses ranging from 20 to 1300mg. However, considerably lower bioavailability has been reported for enteric-coated tablets and sustained release microencapsulated preparations.[79,82]

Following absorption, aspirin is rapidly hydrolysed to salicylate in the liver but also in plasma, the lungs and erythrocytes. The plasma half-life of aspirin is approximately 20 minutes.

***Clinical use:*** the clinical benefit of aspirin in preventing occlusive vascular events appears similar at a wide dosage range varying from as low as 75 mg/day to as high as 1500 mg/day.[83] However, high aspirin doses are clearly associated with an increased incidence of adverse gastrointestinal effects, including erosive gastritis or ulceration, bleeding, epigastric distress, nausea, vomiting and constipation. Thus, the present recommendation of a single loading dose of 200 to 300mg followed by a daily dose of 75 to 100mg is based on findings that this dose is as clinically effective as higher doses but is safer than higher doses.[84]

***Tolerability:*** the occurrence of adverse reactions has been well documented in studies involving the repeated daily administration of aspirin (i.e. 3 or 4 times daily) for long periods of time. These include both mild and serious (i.e. bleeding, ulcer or both) gastrointestinal events, a moderate increase in blood pressure, and slightly elevated serum creatinine concentrations.

The British TIA Aspirin Trial provided a unique opportunity for comparing the incidence of adverse effects in patients treated with 300mg *versus* 1200mg daily for approximately 4 years.[85] In essence, 1200 mg/day was tolerated less well than 300 mg/day, which was tolerated less well than placebo. A definite dose-response effect emerged for upper gastrointestinal symptoms (indigestion, nausea, heartburn, vomiting) and gastrointestinal bleeding (1.6, 2.6 and 4.7% in the placebo, 300mg and 1200mg groups, respectively), but not for constipation (2.3, 5.6 and 6%, respectively).

As far as adverse renal and haemodynamic effects are concerned, these are unlikely to occur with a single daily administration of 300 to 325mg of aspirin because of limited and reversible suppression of renal cyclo-oxygenase activity. Thus, there seems to be no rationale and no existing information to discourage the use of aspirin as an antiplatelet agent for patients with mild impairment of renal function or essential hypertension. However, episodes of bronchial asthma can occur in patients with aspirin hypersensitivity, even in response to a single 30mg dose; this may reflect the involvement of platelets in this adverse reaction.

Considerations regarding the relative risk : benefit ratio of long term antiplatelet therapy with aspirin clearly relate to patients who are at definite risk of occlusive vascular events, such as those with a prior history of such events studied in the published clinical trials. However, for apparently healthy individuals without atherosclerotic risk factors or a positive family history, it is possible that any small benefit derived from aspirin might be outweighed by a small increase in cerebral or other serious haemorrhagic events.[86]

#### Dipyridamole

Dipyridamole is a pyrimidopyrimidine compound with pharmacological properties similar to those of papaverine.

***Mechanism/site of action:*** although it has been in clinical use for some time, the precise mechanism of action of dipyridamole remains obscure. Three mechanisms by which intracellular platelet cyclic adenosine monophosphate (cyclic-AMP) is increased by the drug have been proposed. At high concentrations, dipyridamole inhibits phosphodiesterase, which reduces the breakdown of cyclic-AMP; it also activates the enzyme adenylate cyclase by a prostacyclin-mediated effect on the platelet membrane.[87] At more physiological concentrations, dipyridamole increases plasma adenosine concentrations by inhibiting its uptake from the vascular endothelium and erythrocytes,[88] thereby enhancing platelet adenylate cyclase activity.

There is some evidence that dipyridamole prevents thrombosis on prosthetic surfaces in animals, but not in animal models of arterial stenosis or injury. In humans, moderately high doses of dipyridamole (300 to 450mg) have only a weak effect on platelet aggregation.[87] Nevertheless, dipyridamole prolongs the shortened survival time of platelets in patients with arterial thromboembolism, prosthetic heart valves, and prosthetic grafts.

***Pharmacokinetic characteristics:*** the oral absorption of dipyridamole is highly variable, with peak plasma concentrations varying up to 15-fold, and is decreased by food or a high gastric pH. In plasma, the drug is strongly bound to both albumin and $\alpha_1$-acid glycoprotein. Elimination is primarily by biliary excretion as a glucuronide conjugate. At steady-state, the elimination half-life of dipyridamole is approximately 10 hours; some enterohepatic recirculation occurs.[87]

***Clinical uses:*** in clinical practice, dipyridamole is usually administered in combination with oral anticoagulants or aspirin. However, most clinical trials in survivors of myocardial infarction or stroke and in those undergoing coronary angioplasty or coronary artery bypass surgery have not been able to document an advantage of the combination of aspirin and dipyridamole over aspirin alone.[89]

The antithrombotic effects of dipyridamole are more evident on prosthetic than on biological surfaces.[90] Patients with prosthetic mechanical heart valves are at continuous risk of thromboembolism despite adequate anticoagulation. For those at the highest risk, the addition of a platelet inhibitor to an oral anticoagulant regiment has been advocated. Most studies have shown that adding dipyridamole reduces the incidence of embolism in such patients, without increasing the risk of bleeding.

***Tolerability:*** the main adverse effects of dipyridamole are epigastric discomfort and nausea, which occur in up to 10% of patients, are dose-related, and often subside with continued use. Dipyridamole does not exacerbate gastroduodenal ulcers and does not increase the bleeding risk, even when combined with an anticoagulant. Because dipyridamole, in contrast to aspirin, does not increase perioperative bleeding in patients undergoing coronary artery bypass surgery, its use for 2 days before surgery is not associated with bleeding risks.[87]

#### Ticlopidine and Clopidogrel

Ticlopidine is a thienopyridine derivative which is structurally different from other antiplatelet agents. Clopidogrel is a chemical analogue of ticlopidine which is approximately 6 times as active in tests of inhibition of *ex vivo*-induced aggregation of human platelets. Both drugs can be considered as prodrugs since they require metabolic activation in the liver to express their activity.

***Mechanism/site of action:*** the active forms of ticlopidine and clopidogrel interact rapidly and irreversibly with platelets at a site located at a very early stage in the signal transduction following ADP interaction with the platelet receptor.[91-93] The most probable hypothesis is that they alter the platelet membrane and block the interaction between fibrinogen and its membrane glycoprotein receptor IIb-IIIa.

Inhibition of platelet aggregation induced by arachidonic acid, collagen, thrombin, adrenaline (epinephrine), serotonin and platelet-activating factor-acether (PAF-acether) has also been observed with ticlopidine in volunteers and patients, but is probably an indirect result of the drug blocking the amplification of aggregation by ADP released following low concentrations of these agonists.[93] Both ticlopidine (250mg twice daily) and clopidogrel (75mg twice daily) prolong the bleeding time, their maximal effects being seen 5 to 6 days after repeated oral administration. In comparison, the lag time before maximal inhibition of platelet aggregation occurs is 3 to 5 days. Both effects return to baseline levels simultaneously after 4 to 8 days when ticlopidine or clopidogrel treatment is discontinued.

***Pharmacodynamic properties:*** in animal studies, the administration of ticlopidine in doses of 30 to 40 mg/kg/day orally for 3 days produces concentration-dependent inhibition of platelet aggregation in response to thrombin, ADP or collagen. In humans, the *ex vivo* inhibition of ADP-induced platelet aggregation appears to be proportional to ticlopidine dosage, reaching a maximum effect at 500 mg/day.

Neither ticlopidine nor clopidogrel have an effect on phospholipase $A_2$ activity or on thromboxane and prostacyclin synthesis. Also, both drugs have no direct effect on cyclic-AMP phosphodiesterase nor on adenylate cyclase. Ticlopidine does not affect leucocyte adhesion and migration or procoagulant activity, but does cause a mild reduction of fibrinogen concentrations and seems to increase erythrocyte deformability in diabetic and atherosclerotic patients.

***Pharmacokinetic characteristics:*** following oral administration, about 80 to 90% of a ticlopidine dose is absorbed. Ticlopidine is rapidly and extensively metabolised and several metabolites have been isolated. Its elimination half-life is 7.9 hours after a single dose but this is extended to 96 hours after administration of 250mg twice daily for 14 days.[93]

Clopidogrel is also rapidly absorbed after oral administration and is extensively metabolised, the principal metabolite being the carboxylic acid derivative. After single-dose oral administration of clopidogrel, the elimination half-life of the carboxylic acid metabolite is 7.7 hours.[94]

***Tolerability:*** the most commonly reported adverse effects of ticlopidine and clopidogrel are gastrointestinal disturbances. These may include diarrhoea, nausea, vomiting, anorexia or epigastric pain but usually do not require withdrawal of treatment. The symptoms disappear if treatment is given with food. Diarrhoea is the most frequent of these symptoms, affecting about 20% of patients receiving ticlopidine. Epistaxis, ecchymoses and menorrhagia have been reported in less than 10% of patients, but these are generally not serious and do not require withdrawal of treatment.

Other adverse effects reported with ticlopidine include skin reactions (urticaria, pruritus, erythema), liver dysfunction and haematological effects. Leucopenia, thrombocytopenia, agranulocytosis and pancytopenia have been reported in about 1% of patients in large clinical studies. These disturbances usually appear early in treatment and are reversible on discontinuation of therapy. However, these blood dyscrasias may pose a severe hazard if not identified immediately; therefore, close monitoring is recommended for at least the first 12 weeks of ticlopidine administration.

#### Dextran

Dextran is a polysaccharide produced by the bacterium *Leuconostoc mesenteroides* by fermentation of saccharose. Two types of dextran polymer have been used clinically – dextran 70 (mean molecular weight 70,000D) and dextran 40 (mean molecular weight 40,000D).

Dextran is mainly used as a plasma expander, a property based on its colloid osmotic (oncotic) effect. As its clinical use was sometimes associated with haemorrhage, dextran has been studied as a possible antithrombotic agent. Experiments in animal models of thrombosis revealed that dextrans, regardless of their molecular size, reduce the adhesiveness and aggregation of platelets. These effects are maximal at 4 to 6 hours after the infusion, and are synchronous with a reduction of von Willebrand factor.[95]

***Clinical use:*** intravenous administration of dextran 40 in a volume of 500ml over 4 to 6 hours commencing at the time of operation and then daily for 2 to 5 days postoperatively has proved effective in the prevention of deep vein thrombosis in general surgical patients at moderate thrombotic risk and in patients undergoing hip surgery.[96] Data supporting the role of dextran as an antithrombotic agent on foreign materials (arterial stents and grafts) are also emerging.

***Tolerability:*** dextran is well tolerated by most patients, but its use may be complicated by volume overload in those with impaired cardiac function, particularly in the elderly with unrecognised cardiac failure. Furthermore, dextran has been associated with a low but disturbing incidence (0.6%) of anaphylactoid reactions. These can be prevented by blocking the reactive sites of antibodies to dextran with small dextran fragments (molecular weight 1000D), the so-called hapten inhibitors.[97] In hip surgery patients, dextran has been associated with excessive bleeding but only when given in doses greater than 500ml during the operation.

#### Prostaglandin $E_1$, Prostacyclin ($PGI_2$) and Synthetic Analogues

Prostaglandin $E_1$ and prostacyclin are powerful systemic vasodilators and inhibitors of platelet aggregation by virtue of their ability to increase platelet cyclic-AMP.[98] However, the clinical use of prostacyclin has been limited by its instability at neutral pH and its propensity to cause significant systemic hypotension at the doses required for platelet inhibition. Moreover, its duration of action is very short, the pharmacological effects disappearing in 30 minutes.

***Iloprost***, a new synthetic prostacyclin analogue for intravenous use, is chemically stable at neutral pH. In an *in vitro* comparison with equimolar concentrations of prostaglandin $E_1$ and prostacyclin, iloprost was found to be more potent in increasing the concentrations of cyclic-AMP and inhibiting platelet aggregation by various agonists, particularly thrombin.[99,100] An oral preparation of iloprost is currently in clinical development.

*Limaprost, ciprostene, taprosten* and *beraprost* are other synthetic analogues of prostacyclin being developed, as is *alprostadil* ($PGE_1$). Clinically stable analogues of prostacyclin and $PGE_1$ may be effective for temporary control of platelet activity in the management of thromboembolic disorders. These compounds now are undergoing extensive clinical testing.

#### Glycoprotein IIb/IIIa Antagonists

The heterodimer GPIIb/IIIa complex is a member of the integrin superfamily of receptors which mediates such apparently diverse phenomena as platelet aggregation, platelet adhesion to collagen, fibroblast adhesion to fibronectin and vitronectin, and leucocyte binding to endothelial cells and matrix proteins.

The first platelet GPIIb/IIIa antagonists to be developed were murine monoclonal antibodies.[101] These antibodies completely inhibited platelet aggregation *in vitro,* and, in animal models of angioplasty injury and thrombolysis, prevented thrombosis and augmented the activity of thrombolytic agents.[102,103] Because of concerns about their immunogenicity, the derivative product, chimeric monoclonal c7E3 Fab (abciximab), was created via genetic recombination. This new hybrid molecule consists of the mouse-derived variable regions from the original molecule linked to the constant region derived from human immunoglobulin IgG.

***Abciximab:*** data from a dose-escalation study[104] and a pilot therapeutic trial[105] suggested an abciximab dosage regimen which was evaluated in patients undergoing percutaneous transluminal coronary angioplasty (PTCA).[106,107] Compared with placebo, an abciximab bolus of 0.25 mg/kg followed by an infusion of 10 μg/kg/h for 124 hours in 708 patients resulted in a 35% reduction in the rate of the primary end-points (death, nonfatal myocardial infarction, unplanned surgical revascularisation, unplanned repeat PTCA, stent or balloon pump for refractory ischaemia). However, bleeding episodes and transfusions were more frequent in abciximab recipients.[106] At 6 months, the absolute difference between the placebo and abciximab groups in patients with a major ischaemic event or elective revascularisation was 8.1%.[107]

The effectiveness of abciximab has also been tested in patients with unstable angina unresponsive to heparin, aspirin and nitrate therapy who were undergoing PTCA. This placebo-controlled pilot study in 60 patients showed a substantial reduction in major clinical events (death, myocardial infarction, urgent invasive intervention for recurrent ischaemia).[108] Subsequently, a large multicentre trial in 1400 patients with refractory unstable angina was terminated prematurely after inclusion of 1050 patients because a significant difference in the primary composite end-point was obtained in patients treated for 24 hours with abciximab compared with placebo.

***Integrelin:*** this synthetic cyclic heptapeptide antagonist of GPIIb/IIIa displays antithrombotic effects in several animal models of thrombosis. In a randomised, double-blind, placebo-controlled study,[109] complete inhibition of platelet aggregation was observed at infusion rates between 1.0 and 1.5 μg/kg/min; the half-life of integrelin was found to be 50 to 60 minutes. The bleeding time returned to baseline values within 30 minutes and platelet aggregation was normal within 2 to 4 hours following cessation of drug infusion. A randomised multicentre trial to evaluate the effectiveness of integrelin in preventing coronary thrombosis is now underway.

***Other agents:*** in recent years, a series of synthetic nonpeptide GPIIb/IIIa antagonists have been developed. They include *fradafiban*,[110] *lamifiban*,[111,112] and *tirofiban*.[113,114] Clinical trials evaluating the effectiveness of these agents are also underway.

#### 3.1.2 Thrombin Inhibitors

An emerging strategy in antithrombotic therapy involves the synthesis of peptides that specifically block thrombin-mediated activation.[115,116] A number of these agents have been studied, including hirudin, hirulog, argatroban and inogatran.

##### Hirudin

Natural hirudin is a single-chain, carbohydrate-free polypeptide containing 3 intramolecular disulfide bridges and a sulfated tyrosine residue. Hirudin was initially isolated from the salivary glands of the leech *Hirudo medicinalis*, but has recently been synthesised by recombinant DNA technology using *Escherichia coli* and yeast. With both methods, hirudin is expressed as desulfatohirudin lacking the sulfate residue on tyrosine 63. The importance of the latter is controversial since the anticoagulant activity of natural and recombinant hirudin appears to be similar.[117]

Unlike heparin, which requires endogenous cofactors for activity (mainly antithrombin III and to a much lesser extent heparin cofactor II), hirudin does not need a cofactor for its anticoagulant activity and therefore is still active in states of deficiency of these proteins or when their activity is inhibited. Hirudin is a specific inhibitor of thrombin to which it binds near the active centre at the substrate recognition site with extraordinary tightness. In addition, there are extensive close contacts between hirudin and thrombin over an extended area of the molecule, forming a highly stable noncovalent complex. All known functions of thrombin are inhibited.

The plasma half-life of hirudin in healthy young volunteers is 50 to 65 minutes,[118,119] but in older patients it is extended to 2 to 3 hours[120] which is consistent with the half-life of its effect on the activated partial thromboplastin time (APTT) of about 2 to 3 hours; 62 to 77% of the APTT plateau value was seen within 30 minutes of starting hirudin infusions and was directly related to dose.

In early clinical trials comparing hirudin with heparin in patients undergoing PTCA, fewer early cardiac events were seen in patients receiving hirudin,[121,122] though hirudin had no apparent advantage with longer-term follow-up.[121] Three large phase III trials of high-dose hirudin (i.e. 0.6 mg/kg bolus followed by 0.2 mg/kg/h[123,124] or 0.4 mg/kg followed by 0.15 mg/kg/h[125]) *vs* heparin in patients with acute myocardial infarction or unstable angina were subsequently begun, but a high bleeding risk with hirudin, particularly of haemorrhagic stroke, became apparent in these investigations. In view of these results, and the observation that hirudin at 0.1 mg/kg/h appears to be as efficacious as higher doses of hirudin, both in unstable angina[107] and acute myocardial infarction,[126] 2 of these studies (i.e. the GUSTO-IIb and TIMI-9B studies) were restarted at lower hirudin dosages of 0.1 mg/kg bolus followed by 0.1 mg/kg/h, with target APTT times to avoid values >100 seconds which are clearly associated with an increased risk of intracerebral haemorrhage. Down-titration of hirudin and adjustment to an APTT prolongation of 2 to 3 times baseline may take better advantage of the lower anticoagulant to antithrombotic ratio of hirudin compared with heparin, which was clearly established in preclinical studies.

#### Hirulog

Hirulog is a bifunctional 20-amino acid peptide designed on the structure of hirudin; it combines a fragment of the C-terminus of hirudin which interacts with the anion binding site of thrombin, with an *N*-terminus fragment which interacts with the catalytic site. The hirulog-thrombin complex is only transient as thrombin can slowly cleave the Pro-Arg bond in the *N*-terminus extension, and this metabolic cleavage contributes to its short half-life of effect on the APTT of about 40 minutes. A good correlation between plasma hirulog concentrations and the APTT has been noted in a dose-finding study,[127] with no major haematoma or thrombotic complications at the doses tested (0.05 and 0.15 mg/kg boluses, followed by infusions of 0.2 and 0.6 mg/kg/h, respectively).

Pilot studies have evaluated hirulog in patients undergoing elective angioplasty[128] and as an adjunct to thrombolysis with streptokinase in patients with acute myocardial infarction.[129] In the latter study, hirulog provided superior results to heparin in terms of TIMI grade 2 and 3 flow rates at 90 and 120 minutes, with fewer bleeding complications. Further studies to evaluate its clinical effectiveness are ongoing.

### *3.1.3 Defibrotide*

Defibrotide is the sodium salt of a single-strand polydeoxyribonucleotide of mean molecular weight 15 to 30kD with a defined ratio of purine to pyrimidine bases of >0.85. It is prepared by controlled depolymerisation of deoxyribonucleic acid (DNA) obtained from mammalian organs. For a review of its pharmacological and therapeutic properties, see Palmer and Goa.[130]

#### Mechanism/Site of Action

Defibrotide appears to stimulate prostaglandin $I_2$ and $E_2$ production and to increase the function of tissue plasminogen activator, while decreasing that of plasminogen activator inhibitor.[131-134] Although it is largely devoid of anticoagulant properties, animal studies have provided some evidence that it has *in vivo* anti-ischaemic, antiatherosclerotic and antithrombotic effects, and it has been evaluated clinically in the treatment of a number of vascular disorders and as a prophylactic agent against postoperative deep vein thrombosis.

#### Pharmacokinetic Characteristics

Investigation of the pharmacokinetic behaviour of defibrotide is difficult because the drug is degraded in the body to a number of products and the identity of the active derivative is unclear. To date, most pharmacokinetic data have been determined by following the fate of the carbohydrate moiety of the drug, 6-deoxyribose as a marker of the parent compound.[130]

Intravenous injection of defibrotide 0.5 to 16 mg/kg in healthy volunteers results in a dose-dependent increase in plasma 6-deoxyribose concentrations. The drug is absorbed after oral administration, the amount absorbed being around 50 to 70% of the dose (which is consistent with the finding that oral administration produces fibrinolytic effects that are approximately 50% of these achieved with the same dose given parenterally). There is no accumulation of defibrotide after repeated administration.[130]

Elimination of defibrotide follows different kinetic models depending on the dose, with a 1-compartment model being the most appropriate following administration of low doses, and a 2-compartment model better suited following high doses. The elimination half-life is short and increases with dose, with values of between 9.8 and 27.1 minutes after intravenous doses of 0.5 to 16 mg/kg.[135,136]

#### Clinical Use

Defibrotide is available in intravenous, intramuscular and oral formulations. In all studies of its use for prevention of deep vein thrombosis in surgical patients, the intravenous or intramuscular routes were used. The intravenous or oral dosage of defibrotide has commonly been between 400 and 1200 mg/day, with 800 mg/day the most frequently used.

#### Tolerability

Defibrotide appears to be well tolerated with a global incidence of adverse events reported to range from <1 to 9%, including allergic reactions, fever and gastrointestinal disturbances.

### *3.1.4 Heparin and Low Molecular Weight (LMW) Fractions*

Heparin consists of a simple chain constructed of repeating disaccharide units, all of which contain glucosamine and uronic acid; the latter may be glucuronic acid or iduronic acid. The iduronic acid residues and possibly the glucuronic acid residues are sulfated to a varying degree. Because of its large number of acid groups, heparin is a strong acid. A combination of chemical properties is required for coagulation inhibiting activity: free carboxyl groups, *O*-sulfate ester groups from hexuronic acid, and sulfamino groups on glucosamine.[137-139]

**Mechanism/Site of Action**

Heparin exerts the main part of its anticoagulant action via a plasma protein called antithrombin III. The active serine centre of thrombin and other serine coagulation enzymes (factors Xa, IXa, XIa and XIIa) is inhibited by an arginine reactive centre on the antithrombin III molecule. This process is, however, a slow one. Direct binding of heparin to lysine sites on the antithrombin III molecule is responsible for a 1000-fold acceleration of thrombin-antithrombin III complex formation. After the covalent binding of antithrombin III to the active serine centre of coagulation enzymes, heparin then dissociates from the ternary complex and can be reutilised. The remaining antithrombin III-thrombin complexes are removed by the endothelial system.

A 3-way complex is thus required in which heparin, antithrombin III, and thrombin bind to each other for maximal heparin-enhanced inhibition of thrombin by antithrombin III. The site on the heparin molecule that binds to antithrombin III has been shown to contain a unique glucosamine unit and to have a pentasaccharide sequence.[138,140-144]

In pharmaceutical grade heparin, most anticoagulant activity is accounted for by a small functional fraction of the molecules, i.e. the one-third with high affinity to antithrombin III. The remaining molecules have only a limited anticoagulant effect at therapeutic concentrations but may still increase bleeding in experimental animals,[145] inhibit the activation of prothrombin by factor Xa,[146,147] or potentiate the action of high-affinity, low molecular weight fractions.[148] Furthermore, heparin molecules with low affinity for antithrombin III appear to inhibit hyperplasia of vascular smooth muscle,[149,150] the activation of lipoprotein lipase,[151] the suppression of aldosterone secretion, and the induction of platelet aggregation.[152] At concentrations higher than therapeutic levels, heparin and heparin-like mucopolysaccharides have an additional effect by catalysing the inhibition of thrombin by a second plasma protein, heparin cofactor II.[153] The latter anticoagulant is specific for thrombin.

***Low molecular weight heparins:*** these preparations are obtained by chemical or enzymatic depolymerisation of unfractionated commercial grade heparin and have mean molecular weights ranging between <4000 and about 6500D. As well as differing in molecular size, the available low molecular weight heparins also differ in their affinity for antithrombin III and in various other characteristics (table I).[154-157] Fragments below 16 to 20 monosaccharide units per heparin molecule (molecular weight <5000D), although containing the essential pentasaccharide binding sequence to antithrombin III, are not long enough to also bind to thrombin; they therefore inhibit only factor Xa.[158] Even a synthetic pentasaccharide containing only 5 monosaccharide units (about 1700D) contains the domain that binds to antithrombin III and possesses a high specific activity *in vitro* against factor Xa but little activity against thrombin.[143] Heparin preparations weighing more than 5000D maintain their inhibitory property against factor Xa but gain, with increasing chain length, a progressively stronger inhibitory capacity against thrombin.

The unexpected discovery that heparins of low molecular weight essentially lack the ability to prolong clotting time (indicating no thrombin inhibition) but are still capable of potentiating the inhibition of factor Xa, raised the hope of a dissociation of the antithrombotic property (antifactor Xa) from the anticoagulant property (inhibition of thrombin), which then would reduce the haemorrhage-inducing effect of unfractionated heparin. According to this hypothesis, a low molecular weight heparin with high antifactor Xa activity and little effect on the APTT would exert an antithrombotic effect without causing bleeding. Animal experiments have shown that an antifactor Xa activity is a prerequisite, but is not sufficient in itself for a thrombosis-preventing effect: heparin molecules large enough to retain some thrombin-blocking action are also necessary. Thus, some other factors, possibly including a molecular weight-dependent vascular wall interaction, must also contribute to the antithrombotic effect.[159-164]

An advantage of low molecular weight heparins is that they interact less with platelets, von Willebrand factor and endothelial cells than high molecular weight heparin. Therefore, reduced bleeding may be related more to a decreased effect on platelets than to the reduced antithrombin property of low molecular weight heparins.

**Table I.** Characteristics of commercial low molecular weight (LMW) heparins and their recommended dosages in the prevention of deep venous thrombosis (DVT)

| Generic name (brand name) | MW (range) [daltons] | Plasma half-life[a] (h) | Anti-Xa activity (U/mg)[b] | Anti-IIa activity (U/mg) | Bioavailability[c] (%) | Dosage in prevention of DVT | |
|---|---|---|---|---|---|---|---|
| | | | | | | general surgery and other conditions of moderate thrombotic risk | orthopaedic surgery and other conditions of high thrombotic risk |
| Dalteparin sodium ('Fragmin') | 6000 (3000-9000) | IV: 1.8-2.3 SC: 3.8 | 160 | 60 | 87 | 2500 anti-Xa IU once daily SC | 5000 anti-Xa IU once daily SC |
| Enoxaparin sodium ('Lovenox'; 'Clexane') | 4500 (3000-8000) | IV: 2.8-4.0 SC: 4.6-5.9 | 90-110 | 20-40 | 91 | 20mg once daily SC | 40mg once daily or 30mg twice daily SC |
| Nadroparin calcium ('Fraxiparin') | 4500 (2000-8000) | IV: 2.7-2.16 SC: 3.35-3.79 | 98[d] | 45 | 98 | 3075 anti-Xa IU (0.3ml) once daily SC | 60 anti-Xa IU/kg once daily SC |
| Parnaparin sodium ('Fluxum'; 'Alphaparin') | 4500 (2000-8000) | IV: 1.2-1.61 SC: 1.95-5.68 | 90 | 40 | 100 | 3200 anti-Xa IU once daily SC | 6400 anti-Xa IU once daily SC |
| Reviparin sodium ('Clivarine') | 3900 (3500-4500) | IV: 2.6 SC: 3.3 | 120 | 30 | 90 | 2500 anti-Xa units[f] once daily SC | 5000 anti-Xa units[g] once or twice daily SC |
| Tinzaparin sodium ('Logiparin'; 'Innohep') | 4500 (3400-5600) | IV: 1.85 SC: 2.9 | 90 | 45 | 84 | 3500 anti-Xa IU once daily SC | 50 anti-Xa IU/kg once daily SC |
| Danaparoid sodium[e] ('Lomoparin'; 'Orgaran') | 5500 | IV: 24 SC: 24 | 14 | <0.5 | 100 | 750 anti-Xa IU twice daily SC | 750 anti-Xa IU twice daily SC |
| Ardeparin sodium ('Normiflo') | 6000 (2000-15,000) | IV: 3.3 SC: 2.5-3.3 | 122 | 60 | 88-97 | | 50 anti-Xa IU/kg twice daily |

a Plasma half-life in healthy volunteers measured as anti-factor Xa activity.
b Assessed against the First International Standard for Low Molecular Weight Heparins.
c Bioavailability based on anti-factor Xa activity.
d Institute Choay Units (ICU) converted to International Standard Units (1 ICU is equivalent to 0.41 Units First International Standard for Low Molecular Weight Heparins).
e Danaparoid sodium is a low molecular weight heparinoid. It is a polydisperse mixture comprising sulfate glycosaminoglycuronides derived from porcine intestinal mucosa containing heparan sulfate, dermatan sulfate, and a minor amount of chondroitin sulfate.
f Corresponds to 1750IU.
g Corresponds to 3500IU.

*Abbreviations:* IV = intravenous; SC = subcutaneous; MW = molecular weight.

**Pharmacokinetic Characteristics**

Heparin is not absorbed when given orally and must be given parenterally. After intravenous injection of unfractionated heparin, there is a rapid elimination phase due to equilibration, followed by a more gradual disappearance.[165,166] The disappearance of the anticoagulant activity of unfractionated heparin is compatible with a model based on the combination of a saturable mechanism (most probably rapid uptake by the endothelium and desulfatation by mononuclear phagocytosis) and an unsaturable/linear mechanism (most probably elimination by the kidney).[167,168] The faster disappearance of the thrombin inhibitor activity (i.e. antifactor IIa activity) than the antifactor Xa activity during the initial elimination phase suggests an earlier elimination of large molecules having a high antifactor IIa : antifactor Xa ratio. Thus, in practice, the dose-response relationship of unfractionated heparin is not linear and increases disproportionately in intensity and duration as the dose increases. After bolus injection of doses of 25 U/kg, the half-life of heparin is approximately 30 minutes *versus* 60 minutes after a bolus dose of 75 U/kg.

Heparin is partially degraded in the liver and is partially eliminated by the kidneys in unchanged form. Elimination might be prolonged after larger doses in patients with chronic renal failure or severe liver disease,[169] but the clinical importance of any alteration in clearance is not known. However, variability in clearance between patients is sufficiently marked to make laboratory control of dosage desirable.

The available low molecular weight heparins (see table I) are all readily adsorbed from subcutaneous tissue. They do not bind to endothelial cells (in culture) and are eliminated from the blood more slowly than unfractionated heparin. These properties are probably responsible for their plasma half-lives being 2- to 4-fold longer than that of unfractionated heparin.

#### Clinical Use

Heparin, as with other anticoagulant drugs, should not be used in unreliable outpatients, or in patients in whom there is a definite risk of haemorrhage that cannot be avoided by careful adjustment of dosage, particularly when the bleeding could occur in certain tissues (e.g. eyes, brain, central nervous system). Arterial hypertension inadequately responding to antihypertensive treatment is an absolute contraindication. The presence of a haemostatic defect obviously contraindicates the initiation of full-dose heparin.

***Dosage and administration:*** intravenous heparin may be given by continuous infusion or by intermittent injection. Major bleeding is considerably less frequent with continuous infusion.[170] Moreover, continuous infusions reduce the dosage of the drug. However, it is uncertain how intense the anticoagulant effect of heparin must be to prevent thrombosis, as is the relationship of the degree of effect to bleeding complications.[171]

When given by continuous intravenous infusion, the standard dosage of unfractionated heparin is a loading dose of 5000U (sometimes 10,000U) given as bolus, followed by 15 to 20 U/kg/h in normal saline or 5% dextrose with an automatic infusion pump. The rate of the infusion is subsequently regulated to keep the activated partial thromboplastin time (APTT) at about twice the baseline level.

When given intermittently, the usual dose of standard unfractionated heparin is 10,000U at 6-hour intervals or 15,000U at 8-hour intervals. Some clinicians use 5000 to 10,000U every 4 hours. Intermittent injection is preferred by some because laboratory monitoring can be ignored. However, failure to monitor the appropriate coagulation parameters increases the risk of bleeding. There is a wide variation between individuals in the anticoagulant response to a given dose of heparin or in the dose required to produce a particular anticoagulant response.[171]

Concentrated aqueous unfractionated heparin usually contains between 20,000 and 25,000 U/ml and is given subcutaneously in a skinfold raised from the abdominal wall. The full dose of this form of heparin is 20,000 to 30,000 U/24h, administered in 1 or 2 injections. In 'low-dose' regimens, 5000U of concentrated heparin is given subcutaneously 8- or 12-hourly for prophylaxis of deep venous thrombosis. In most cases, it causes only slight, if any, prolongation of clotting times and no clinically significant bleeding, except in a few cases after major orthopaedic surgery when 5000U is given 8-hourly.[172]

Recommended dosages for the various low molecular weight (LMW) heparins in the prevention of deep venous thrombosis are shown in table I. The LMW heparins each have a distinct profile of pharmacological effects in both *in vitro* and *in vivo* tests and thus different antithrombotic/bleeding properties. The recommended dosages therefore differ for each preparation.

***Monitoring procedure:*** the response of all antithrombotic drugs can be measured reasonably well; therefore, therapy can be governed by appropriate laboratory control of the desired anticoagulant effect, but it is not always required. Some monitoring is desirable with continuous infusion of heparin. However, monitoring is not essential with short term, intravenous administration or with long term subcutaneous administration. Some suggested desirable ranges of clotting tests and dose adjustment protocols are given in table II. A heparin dose adjustment nomogram has been developed for a specific APTT reagent for which the therapeutic range is 1.9 to 2.7 times control (based on a heparin concentration of 0.2 to 0.4 U/ml plasma);[173] This nomogram is not applicable to all APTT systems but can be adapted to other systems by the local laboratory.[174]

#### Tolerability and Drug Interactions Potential

Bleeding is the most frequent complication of heparin and is a direct extension of its therapeu-

**Table II.** Protocol for heparin dose adjustment. Starting dose of 5000U intravenous bolus followed by 32,000U per 24h as a continuous infusion (40 U/ml). The first APTT is performed 6h after the bolus injection. Dosage adjustments are made according to protocol and APTT and repeated as indicated in the far right column. Therapeutic range of 60 to 85 sec is equivalent to a heparin level of 0.2 to 0.4 U/ml by protamine titration or 0.35 to 0.7 U/ml as an anti-factor Xa heparin level. Therapeutic range will vary with responsiveness of the APTT reagent to heparin (after Hirsh & Fuster[175])

| APTT[a] (sec) | Repeat bolus dose (U) | Stop infusion (min) | Change in rate (dose) of infusion, ml/h[b] (U per 24h) | Time of next APTT |
|---|---|---|---|---|
| <50 | 5000 | 0 | +3 (+2880) | 6h |
| 50-59 | 0 | 0 | +3 (+2880) | 6h |
| 60-85 | 0 | 0 | 0 (0) | Next morning |
| 86-95 | 0 | 0 | −2 (−1920) | Next morning |
| 96-120 | 0 | 30 | −2 (−1920) | 6h |
| >120 | 0 | 60 | −4 (−3840) | 6h |

a APTT obtained with Dade Actin F8 reagent.

b 40 U/ml solution.

*Abbreviations:* APTT = activated partial thromboplastin time; U = unit.

tic action. Spontaneous bleeding is most likely in patients over 60 years of age (3-fold greater risk), in the presence of underlying morbidity (4-fold greater risk), in heavy drinkers (7-fold greater risk), in women (2-fold greater risk), and in patients with a blood urea nitrogen value over 50 mg/dl (1.5-fold greater risk).[176]

There is a consensus that with unfractionated heparin, the average incidence of major bleeding is 7% among patients given continuous intravenous heparin infusions, and 14% when intermittent intravenous injections are given. Postoperative or post-traumatic bleeding is more common than spontaneous bleeding.[171] Other complications are uncommon, but osteoporosis can occur with full doses continued for 6 months or more. Thrombocytopenia has been recognised with increasing frequency with both unfractionated heparin and low molecular weight heparins.[177,178]

***Drug interactions:*** a large number of drugs inhibit platelet aggregation, and so prudence is obligatory if they are given concomitantly with heparin. This is particularly true for aspirin and ticlopidine.

Because of the formation of relatively insoluble complexes, heparin should not be mixed in the infusion fluid with most antibiotics and a number of psychotropic drugs.

### *3.1.5 Oral Anticoagulants*

There are 2 types of vitamin K antagonist anticoagulants – the *coumarins* (dicoumarol, warfarin, acenocoumarol, phenprocoumon) and *indanediones* (phenindione); however, the latter group is associated with an excess of non-haemorrhagic toxicity. Among the coumarins, the most popular drug is warfarin because of its high bioavailability and predictable onset and duration of action. This agent will therefore be emphasised in this section as the prototype oral anticoagulant. For comprehensive reviews of the coumarin compounds and their clinical use, see Hirsh[164] and Hirsh & Fuster.[175]

#### Mechanism/Site of Action

The essential chemical characteristic of warfarin is an intact 4-hydroxycoumarin nucleus with a substituent in the 3 position. Along with other coumarins, it has an asymmetric carbon atom in the substituent group at the 3 position of the coumarin nucleus, which means that the clinically available preparations are racemic mixtures composed of 2 optical isomers.[179]

Warfarin acts as an anticoagulant by inhibiting carboxylation of acid glutamate residues (glu) to acid γ-carboxyglutamates (gla) residues of vitamin K-dependent proteins. Gla residues in the amino terminal region of some coagulation zymogens are a prerequisite for their $Ca^{++}$-dependent binding to their cofactors on negatively charged phospholipid surfaces. These gla residues are formed during a post-translational modification, in which the enzyme γ-glutamyl-carboxylase and vitamin K are of vital importance. During this reaction, vitamin K-hydroquinone is oxidised to an inactive vitamin K epoxide. Vitamin K epoxide reductase then recycles vitamin K epoxide to the hydroquinone form. Coumarins inhibit the action of the dithiol-dependent epoxide reductase and thus prevent the conversion back into biologically active vitamin K-hydroquinone.[180-183]

In consequence, coumarins depress the synthesis of 6 vitamin K-dependent coagulation zymogens: prothrombin (factor II), factors VII, IX and X, and proteins C and S. The latter 2 proteins are endogenous inhibitors of coagulation by inactivating factors Va and VIIIa (see fig. 6). Oral anticoagulants are therefore indirect-acting drugs and all require a delay before their action is seen. The delay in onset of their effect depends on the clearance from the circulation of the coagulation factors whose synthesis is inhibited, and on the extent of this inhibition, which in turn depends on the induction dose.

**Pharmacokinetic Characteristics**

All oral anticoagulants, with the exception of dicoumarol (bishydroxycoumarin), are completely absorbed when given orally. They are highly protein bound, mainly to plasma albumin, and distribution volumes are low (see appendix A). However, there are major pharmacokinetic and pharmacodynamic differences between the available oral anticoagulants (table III). They are extensively metabolised by the enzymes of the hepatic reticulum, and genetically determined individual variations in enzymatic activity lead to marked differences in clearance between individuals. Other drugs can also influence the activity of these drug metabolising enzymes. Along with variation in vitamin K availability and clotting factor turnover, these differences in clearance cause marked variability in the dose requirements of oral anticoagulants in individual patients; 10- or even 20-fold differences being common.[184-186] The slow clearance of some of the coumarins means that there will be a slow approach to a new steady-state plasma concentration after a dosage change. Rare instances of abnormal sensitivity to warfarin apparently due to a defect in metabolism have occurred,[187] as have rare instances of resistance due to a genetically determined defect in hepatic receptor site affinity for vitamin K and warfarin.[188]

Dicoumarol and ethylbiscoumacetate have 2 coumarin ring systems and both have dose-dependent elimination half-lives, which increase with increasing doses. This does not occur with the other coumarins which are single ring compounds. The dose-dependent elimination of dicoumarol and ethylbiscoumacetate means that small dose increases of these drugs may result in disproportionately larger increases in plasma concentrations, making initial anticoagulant control and subsequent dose adjustment more difficult (see further chapter 1; sect. 2.2.8) and thus increasing the risk of bleeding episodes.

The ring system of the coumarins also influences the pathways of metabolism due to differences in kinetics of the optical isomers (enantiomers) of the single ring compounds. Warfarin is a racemic mixture of roughly equal amounts of 2 isomers, *R* and *S* warfarin.[189] The 2 major metabolites of warfarin are *R*(+)-warfarin and *S*(–)-warfarin, the latter having approximately 5 times the anticoagulant potency of *R* warfarin. The isomers are also metabolised at different rates and by different pathways, which has potentially important implications for pharmacokinetic interactions with certain other drugs (see table IV). Thus, amiodarone inhibits the clearance of both isomers, while phenylbutazone and sulfonamides inhibit the clearance of the more rapidly eliminated *S* iso-

**Table III.** Pharmacokinetic properties of some oral anticoagulants (after Kelly & O'Malley[185])

| Drug | Absorption | Protein binding (%) | Half-life (h) | Maintenance dose (mg/24h) | Time to produce therapeutic levels (h) | Duration of effect | Important excretion in breastmilk | Placental transfer |
|---|---|---|---|---|---|---|---|---|
| **Coumarin analogues** | | | | | | | | |
| Dicoumarol (bishydroxycoumarin) | Poor and erratic | >99 | 24-100 | 24-150 | 36-72 | Long | No | Yes |
| Ethylbiscoumacetate | Good | 90 | 2-5[a] | 150-900 | 8-36 | Short | ? | Yes |
| Phenprocoumon[b] | Good | >99 | 65-170 | 0.75-6 | 30-48 | Long | No | Yes |
| Warfarin[b] | Good | ≥99 | 35-45 | 2.5-25 | 36-48 | Intermediate | No | Yes |
| **Indanediones** | | | | | | | | |
| Phenindione | Good | 90 | 5-10 | 25-200 | 36-48 | Intermediate | Yes | Yes |

a Dose-dependent.

b Phenprocoumon and warfarin are administered as racemic mixtures of their *S*(–) and *R*(+) enantiomers, the biological activities and pharmacokinetic properties of which differ. With both drugs, the *S*(–) enantiomer has greater anticoagulant potency than the *R*(+) enantiomer. In the case of warfarin, the more potent *S*(–) enantiomer is cleared more rapidly from the circulation than the *R*(+) enantiomer, while for phenprocoumon the reverse is true.

**Table IV.** Factors which can alter the usual dose of oral anticoagulants (after O'Reilly & Aggeler[179])

| Condition | Mechanism |
|---|---|
| **Increased responsiveness**[a] | |
| Obstructive jaundice<br>Biliary fistula (particularly in patients with associated pancreatitis) | These disorders hinder delivery of bile to the small bowel, reduce absorption of the lipid soluble vitamin K and may also inhibit biliary excretion |
| Steatorrhoea | Reduced absorption of vitamin K |
| Periods of starvation | Reduced dietary intake of vitamin K |
| Liver disease<br>Acute viral hepatitis | Decreased production of vitamin K-dependent clotting factors |
| Onset of congestive heart failure | Increased response to anticoagulant as hepatic congestion develops (i.e. decreased clotting factor synthesis) with decreased responsiveness on relief of the congestion by diuretics (i.e. increased clotting factor synthesis) |
| Hyperthyroidism<br>Fever<br>Bleeding tendency (many conditions) | Increased rate of decay of vitamin K-dependent clotting factors |
| Other drugs | Some drugs (i.e. 17α-alkylated anabolic steroids) may cause liver dysfunction and increase the response to oral anticoagulants. Others do so by affecting platelet function (e.g. aspirin) or by pharmacokinetic mechanisms (see table V) |
| **Decreased responsiveness** | |
| Nephrotic syndrome | Decreased protein binding and marked increase in plasma clearance of warfarin. Dosage requirements increased |
| Hereditary resistance (autosomal dominant) | Marked increase in affinity for vitamin K and anticoagulant (warfarin) at its receptor site. Major increase in dose requirements |

a In many of these conditions, the increased response is variable, and the clinical significance difficult to predict.

mer of warfarin but do not affect (or may even induce) the metabolism of the less active *R* isomer. Metronidazole also inhibits metabolism of the more potent *S* isomer of warfarin, as do sulfinpyrazone and cotrimoxazole (trimethoprim/sulfamethoxazole); cimetidine and omeprazole selectively inhibit the metabolism of the *R* isomer and therefore have only a limited effect on the prothrombin time.[164,190]

Other single ring coumarins also have optical isomers with differences in potency and pharmacokinetic properties, the *S*(–) isomer of phenprocoumon being around 2 times more potent and having a lower plasma clearance than the *R*(+) isomer. The potency, degree of protein binding and clearance of the racemic mixture, as used clinically, is between that of the 2 enantiomers.[191] In the case of acenocoumarol (nicoumalone), the reverse activity has been reported, the *R*(+) isomer being more potent than the *S*(–) isomer, presumably because of its much lower plasma clearance.[192]

***Influence of protein binding:*** protein binding of all the coumarins has an important influence on their elimination from the body, since with acidic drugs that are highly albumin bound and have a low hepatic extraction ratio (i.e. capacity-limited metabolism), there is a correlation between the free (unbound) drug in the plasma and hepatic clearance (see chapter 1; sect. 5.4.2). Thus, an increase in the free fraction of a coumarin such as warfarin will result in an increased total drug clearance, as more drug is available for metabolism, but there will be no change in unbound clearance. Differences in extent of protein binding of coumarins also exist between individuals and are an important contribution to interindividual variations in rate of elimination. It should be noted, however, that a decrease in binding of coumarins as a consequence of displacement by other drugs from its specific binding site on albumin (see chapter 1; sect. 3.2.3), or in uraemia, largely as a consequence of the presence of an endogenous binding inhibitor, does not lead to an enhanced drug effect.[193] As a consequence of redistribution of the displaced drug throughout the body and increased total drug clearance, the concentration of unbound drug in plasma remains the same (see also chapter 1, sect. 3.2.3 and chapter 5, sect. 1.6.3), although before the new steady-state is established, there may be a significant *temporary* increase in the plasma concentration of unbound drug. The total drug concentration falls to a new steady-state level but the unbound drug concentration returns to the predisplacement level. Since the anticoagulant response is related to the unbound drug concentration, any increased effect is only transient.[190]

***Secretion in breastmilk:*** warfarin, dicoumarol and phenprocoumon are not secreted in breastmilk (see further appendix C). In contrast, phenindione can be detected in breastmilk and has caused bleeding problems in breast-fed infants undergoing surgery.[194]

***Concentration-effect relationships:*** the relationship between plasma concentrations of oral anticoagulants and their pharmacological effect is complex. Their primary effect is due to inhibition of the synthesis of vitamin K-dependent clotting factors (see above) and the observed effect is a function of both the synthesis rate of clotting factors and their degradation rates. There is therefore no simple correlation between the plasma concentration and anticoagulant effect. Individual differences in vitamin K activity at the hepatic receptor site or in receptor affinity for the oral anticoagulant may also affect the plasma concentration-effect relationship, since patients with a similar rate of elimination and plasma concentration of dicoumarol have widely different concentrations of plasma prothrombin. For these reasons, plasma concentration estimation is of no value for monitoring routine therapeutic use of oral anticoagulants, but is useful to prove its surreptitious intake. For reviews of the clinical pharmacokinetics of coumarin anticoagulants, see Bachmann & Shapiro;[193] Kelly & O'Malley;[185] Verstraete & Vermylen;[195] Shetty et al.;[186] Hirsh;[164] and Verstraete & Wessler.[196]

#### Clinical Use

***Choice of oral anticoagulant:*** selection of a particular oral anticoagulant is generally based on adverse effects (indanedione compounds can cause serious and even fatal sensitivity reactions) and personal experience (where familiarity with a coumarin compound is probably more important than its duration of action), but pharmacokinetic considerations should also be taken into account (table III). Dicoumarol (bishydroxycoumarin) is poorly and erratically absorbed. Ethylbiscoumacetate has a short duration of effect (1 day) and phenprocoumon a prolonged one (5 days); with ethylbiscoumacetate, a 'see-saw' effect on prothrombin times occurs but this can be avoided by use of phenprocoumon and to some extent warfarin. It should be noted that new orally active antithrombotic agents are in clinical development which do not belong to this class of vitamin K antagonists.

The pharmacokinetic properties of some compounds such as dicoumarol also influence the type and likelihood of interactions with other drugs. Its absorption is increased by drugs which decrease the gastric emptying rate or intestinal transit, and dicoumarol is capable of inhibiting the metabolism of drugs as phenytoin, tolbutamide and chlorpropamide (table IV).

***Factors affecting the response to oral anticoagulants:*** many factors, particularly those which alter the amount of vitamin K available at the site of synthesis or which alter the plasma concentration of the anticoagulant, can influence the response to oral anticoagulants (table IV). For reviews see O'Reilly & Aggeler;[179] Breckenridge;[184] Kelly & O'Malley;[185] Shetty et al.;[186] and Hirsh.[164] Enhancement of the response to warfarin in liver disease appears to be largely associated with altered clotting factor synthesis.

The risk of anticoagulant-induced bleeding is increased in patients in poor general health and in the elderly, in whom dosage requirements of warfarin are also less than in younger patients (see also chapter 4; sect. 4.1.10).[197,198] The onset of congestive heart failure or a deterioration in cardiac status is a frequent cause of increased responsiveness to oral anticoagulants (as a consequence of cardiac congestion and slower metabolism of the drugs). An increased response is also seen in hepatic disease (including active viral hepatitis), in hyperthyroidism, following surgery, and in the postcardiotomy syndrome. Periods of starvation, conditions impairing bile delivery to the bowel (e.g. obstructive jaundice, biliary fistula), gastrointestinal disturbances (e.g. steatorrhoea) and fever due to infections of any sort, also lead to a reduction in oral anticoagulant dose requirements (table IV).

***Monitoring oral anticoagulant therapy:*** modifications of the Quick prothrombin time are the most widely used tests to monitor warfarin therapy. The lack of standardisation of the prothrombin time assay, particularly of the nature and reproducibility of the thromboplastic reagent, has led to striking discrepancies, which have been further compounded by the variety of ways in which the data are expressed for clinical use. This variability has led not only to confusion among clinicians, but also to different intensities of treatment.

To decrease the problems related to lack of standardisation, a system of reporting results based on thromboplastin standards has been developed. One primary standard, the World Health Organization international reference thromboplastin, and 3 secondary standards, a rabbit brain, a human brain, and an ox brain (Thrombotest®) preparation, have been cali-

**Table V.** Recommended target international normalised ratio (INR) values in the prevention/treatment of various thromboembolic disorders

| Indication | Target INR values | | | |
|---|---|---|---|---|
| | Leuven Conference 1985[201] | British Society of Haematology 1990[202] | Consensus ACCP 1992[203] | Consensus ACCP 1995[204] |
| Prevention of DVT: | | | | |
| a) In general surgery | 1.5-2.5 | 2.0-2.5 | 2.0-3.0 | 1.5 |
| b) In orthopaedic surgery | 2.0-3.0 | 2.0-3.0 | 2.0-3.0 | 2.0-3.0 |
| Treatment of DVT | 2.0-4.0 | 2.0-3.0 | 2.0-3.0 | 2.0-3.0 |
| Treatment of pulmonary embolism | 2.0-4.0 | 2.0-3.0 | 2.0-3.0 | 2.0-3.0 |
| Recurrent DVT or pulmonary embolism | 2.0-4.0 | 3.0-4.5 | 2.0-3.0 | 2.0-3.0 |
| Prevention of myocardial infarction | 2.0-3.0 | 2.0-3.0 | 2.0-3.0 | 2.0-3.0 |
| Mechanical prosthetic heart valves | 3.0-4.5 | 3.0-4.5 | 2.5-3.5 | 2.0-3.0 |
| Recurrent arterial embolism | 3.0-4.0 | 3.0-4.5 | 3.0-4.5 | 2.5-3.5 |

*Abbreviations:* ACCP = American College of Chest Physicians; DVT = deep venous thrombosis.

brated against each other and assigned international normalised ratios (INR).[164,199,200] With this accomplished, any commercial thromboplastin reagent can be calibrated against a related reference standard, and the calibration curve employed to translate a given reporting method to the international normalised ratios. INR ranges that should be aimed for in prevention/treatment of various thromboembolic disorders are given in table V and section 3.2. Maintenance of good anticoagulant control is important to avoid thrombosis and bleeding. The dose required to bring the INR into the target range differs with the drugs used (see table III), the sensitivity of the patient, and the use of interacting drugs. Based on the INRs obtained in the first 7 days, computerised programs have been developed which give satisfactory control compared with empirical dosage adjustment by experienced clinicians in the target range 2.0 to 3.0 but significantly better control with more intensive therapy (INR 3.0 to 3.5) than empirical dosage adjustment.

#### Tolerability and Drug Interactions Potential

The risk of bleeding is by far the most common problem in oral anticoagulant therapy, and intracerebral haemorrhage is the most feared bleeding site (major or fatal bleeding 0.3 to 2% per year).[205] The rate of clinically important bleeding is directly related to the intensity of anticoagulation. This rate is ≤1 per 1000 days at risk in patients with INR values kept at levels within the range 1.5 to 3, but increases to 5 to 10 per 1000 days at risk with INRs of 3 to 5 and exceeds 50 when the INRs are over 5 (for reviews, see Harrington et al.,[206] Caron & Libersa[207] and Hirsh[208]).

Coumarin drugs constitute a risk throughout pregnancy because of reports of embryopathy in women taking warfarin between the 6th and 12th week of pregnancy; moreover, central nervous system and ocular fetal abnormalities may occur with administration at any time during pregnancy.[209] Therefore, when pregnancy is an immediate possibility, consideration should be given to substituting heparin for the oral anticoagulant and continuing with heparin if pregnancy is confirmed.[210-212]

Coumarin-induced *necrosis of the skin and subcutaneous tissues* is a rare but striking complication of warfarin therapy and is not to be confused with simple haemorrhage. The lesion appears within 3 to 10 days of drug administration, usually in the lower half of the body. It occurs particularly in women and in areas of abundant subcutaneous fat, such as the buttocks, breasts, thighs and abdomen. Beginning as an erythematous patch, frank haemorrhagic necrosis may develop within 24 hours. No explanation for this toxic reaction has been established, although it may be related to protein C depression in many instances. In patients with protein C or S deficiency, heparin should always be given at the initiation of oral anticoagulant therapy.[212,213]

***Reversal of oral anticoagulant toxicity:*** natural vitamin $K_1$ (phytomenadione) given parenterally in doses of 0.5 to 10mg effectively reverses a moderately excessive anticoagulant effect. Some correction of the prothrombin time is noted within 6 hours of its administration, with full correction usually within 24 hours. If the patient is to remain on warfarin, the dose of vitamin $K_1$ should preferably be limited to 0.5 to 1mg. Higher amounts, up to 10mg, may be

**Table VI.** Interactions of drugs with coumarin compounds (after Caron & Libersa[207]) [see also appendix B]

| Drugs | Effects on anticoagulant response | Mechanism | Clinical relevance |
|---|---|---|---|
| β-Adrenoceptor antagonists (β-blockers) | None | | |
| Alclofenac | None | | |
| Allopurinol | Potentiation | Inhibition of metabolism | Adjustment of dosage |
| Aminoglutethimide | Reduction possible | Induction of microsomal enzymes | Adjustment of dosage |
| Aminoglycoside antibiotics | Potentiation possible | ? Decreased availability of vitamin K | Monitoring of prothrombin time |
| *p*-Aminosalicylic acid (PAS) | Potentiation possible | Unknown | ? |
| Amiodarone | Potentiation | Reduced warfarin and acenocoumarol metabolism | Adjustment of dosage |
| Anabolic steroids and androgens (C17-alkylated) | Potentiation | ? Inhibition of metabolism | Adjustment of dosage |
| Antacids containing magnesium | Potentiation possible (only documented for dicoumarol) | Increased absorption | No practical importance |
| Antithyroid drugs [propylthiouracil, thiamazole (methimazole), carbimazole] | Reduction | Attenuation of increased catabolism of vitamin K-dependent clotting factors | Adjustment of dosage |
| Ascorbic acid | None | | |
| Aspirin (acetylsalicylic acid) | Potentiation (at doses >1.5 g/day) | ? Pharmacodynamic potentiation (due to antiplatelet effect of aspirin) | Avoid concurrent use; may also cause thrombocytopathy and gastric erosion; ulcerogenic |
| Azapropazone | Potentiation | ? Stereoselective inhibition of warfarin metabolism | Avoid concurrent use; may also cause gastric erosion |
| Barbiturates | Reduction | Induction of microsomal enzymes | Adjustment of dosage |
| Benfluorex | None | | |
| Benziodarone | Potentiation | Unknown | Adjustment of dosage |
| Benzodiazepines | None | | |
| Benzydamine | None | | |
| Bumetanide | None | | |
| Carbamazepine | Reduction | Induction of microsomal enzymes | Adjustment of dosage |
| Cefalosporins [cefoperazone, cefamandole, cefotetan, latamoxef (moxalactam)] | Potentiation possible | Inhibition of hepatic vitamin K-dependent clotting factors | Monitoring of prothromin time |
| Chloral hydrate | Minor potentiation during initial phase of anticoagulant therapy, not during maintenance therapy | ? | No practical importance |
| Chloramphenicol | Potentiation | Unknown | Adjustment of dosage |
| Chlorthalidone | (Pseudo) reduction | Haemoconcentration | No practical importance |
| Cholestyramine | Reduction | Decreased absorption and interruption of enterohepatic circulation | Adjustment of dosage; separate dosage of both drugs with as long a time interval as possible |
| Cimetidine | Potentiation (not documented for phenprocoumon) | Stereoselective inhibition of warfarin metabolism | Adjustment of dosage |
| Clofibrate | Potentiation | Unknown | Adjustment of dosage |
| Colestipol | None | | |
| Corticosteroids | Variable | | No practical importance |
| Cotrimoxazole (trimethoprim/sulfamethoxazole) | Potentiation | Stereoselective inhibition of warfarin metabolism | Adjustment of dosage |
| Cyclophosphamide | Reduction possible | Unknown | ? |
| Cyclosporin | Reduction possible | Unknown | Adjustment of dosage |
| Danazol | Potentiation | Unknown | Adjustment of dosage |

**Table VI.** *[Continued]*

| Drugs | Effects on anticoagulant response | Mechanism | Clinical relevance |
|---|---|---|---|
| Dichloralphenazone | Reduction | Induction of microsomal enzymes | Adjustment of dosage |
| Diclofenac | None | | |
| Diflunisal | Potentiation possible | ? Pharmacodynamic potentiation (due to antiplatelet effect of diflunisal) | Avoid concurrent use; may also cause thrombocytopathy and gastric erosion |
| Diltiazem | None | | |
| Dipyridamole | None | | |
| Disopyramide | None | | |
| Disulfiram | Potentiation | Inhibition of warfarin metabolism | Adjustment of dosage |
| Erythromycin | Potentiation possible | Inhibition of warfarin metabolism | Monitoring of prothrombin time |
| Ethachlorvynol | Reduction | Unknown | Adjustment of dosage |
| Ethacrynic acid | Potentiation possible | Unknown | ? |
| Fenbufen | None | | |
| Feprazone | Potentiation | Stereoselective inhibition of warfarin metabolism | Avoid concurrent use; also ulcerogenic |
| Floctafenine | Minor potentiation | Unknown | Monitoring of prothrombin time |
| Fluconazole | Potentiation possible | Inhibition of warfarin metabolism | Monitoring of prothrombin time |
| Fluoroquinolones (ciprofloxacin, enoxacin, ? norfloxacin) | Potentiation possible | Inhibition of warfarin metabolism | Monitoring of prothrombin time |
| Fluoxetine | Potentiation possible | Unknown | Monitoring of prothrombin time |
| Flurbiprofen | Potentiation possible | ? Pharmacodynamic potentiation (due to antiplatelet effect of flurbiprofen) | Monitoring of prothrombin time |
| Furosemide (frusemide) | None | | |
| Fluvoxamine | Potentiation possible | Unknown | Monitoring of prothrombin time |
| Gemfibrozil | Potentiation | Unknown | Adjustment of dosage |
| Glafenine | Minor potentiation | Unknown | Monitoring of prothrombin time |
| Glucagon | Potentiation | Unknown | Avoid concurrent use |
| Glutethimide | Reduction | Induction of microsomal enzymes | Adjustment of dosage |
| Griseofulvin | Reduction | ? Increased metabolism | Adjustment of dosage |
| Halofenate | Potentiation | Unknown | ? |
| Haloperidol | Reduction possible | Unknown | ? |
| Ibuprofen | None | | |
| Indomethacin | None | | |
| Influenza vaccine | Potentiation possible | Unknown | ? |
| Isoniazid | Potentiation possible | Unknown | ? |
| Itraconazole | Potentiation possible | Inhibition of warfarin metabolism | Monitoring of prothrombin time |
| Ketoconazole | Potentiation possible | Inhibition of warfarin metabolism | Monitoring of prothrombin time |
| Lovastatin | Potentiation possible | Unknown | Monitoring of prothrombin time |
| Maprotiline | None | | |
| Mefenamic acid | Potentiation possible | ? | No clinical importance |
| Meprobamate | None | | |
| Mercaptopurine | Reduction | Unknown | Adjustment of dosage |
| Methaqualone | None | | |
| Methylphenidate | None | | |
| Metronidazole | Potentiation | Stereoselective inhibition of warfarin metabolism | Adjustment of dosage |
| Mianserin | None | | |

*[Continued over]*

Table VI. *[Continued]*

| Drugs | Effects on anticoagulant response | Mechanism | Clinical relevance |
|---|---|---|---|
| Miconazole | Potentiation possible even with topical applications | Inhibition of warfarin metabolism | Avoid concurrent use |
| Nafcillin | Reduction possible | Unknown | ? |
| Nalidixic acid | Potentiation possible | | ? |
| Naproxen | None | | May cause gastric erosion |
| Nutritional preparations | Reduction | Increased availability of vitamin K | Adjustment of dosage |
| Oral contraceptives | Variable | Unknown | No practical importance |
| Oxametacin | Potentiation | Unknown | Monitoring of prothrombin time |
| Omeprazole | Potentiation | Stereoselective inhibition of warfarin metabolism | Monitoring of prothrombin time |
| Oxolamine | Potentiation possible | Unknown | Adjustment of dosage |
| Oxyphenbutazone | Potentiation | Stereoselective inhibition of warfarin metabolism | Avoid concurrent use; also ulcerogenic |
| Paracetamol (acetaminophen) | Potentiation possible | Unknown | No practical importance |
| Penicillin | None | | |
| Phenylbutazone | Potentiation | Stereoselective inhibition of warfarin metabolism | Avoid concurrent use; also ulcerogenic |
| Phenyramidol | Potentiation | Inhibition of metabolism | Adjustment of dosage |
| Phenytoin | Reduction (effect of warfarin may be increased initially) | Induction of microsomal enzymes | Adjustment of dosage |
| Piracetam | Potentiation possible | | ? |
| Piroxicam | Potentiation | ? Pharmacodynamic potentiation (due to antiplatelet effect of piroxicam) | Monitoring of prothrombin time |
| Prolintane | None | | |
| Propafenone | Potentiation | Inhibition of warfarin metabolism | Monitoring of prothrombin time |
| Psyllium colloid | None | | |
| Quinidine | Potentiation possible | Unknown | Monitoring of prothrombin time |
| Ranitidine | Possible potentiation (at high dosages) | Unknown | Monitoring of prothrombin time |
| Rifampicin | Reduction | Induction of microsomal enzymes | Adjustment of dosage |
| Spironolactone | (Pseudo) reduction | Haemoconcentration | No practical importance |
| Sucralfate | Reduction possible | ? Inhibition of absorption | ? |
| Sulfinpyrazone | Potentiation possible (not documented with phenprocoumon) | Stereoselective inhibition of warfarin metabolism | Adjustment of dosage |
| Sulfonamides | Potentiation possible | Stereoselective inhibition of warfarin metabolism | ? |
| Sulphonylureas | None | | |
| Sulindac | Potentiation possible | ? Pharmacodynamic potentiation (due to antiplatelet effect of sulindac) | Monitoring of prothrombin time |
| Suloctidil | None | | |
| Tamoxifen | Potentiation possible | Unknown | Adjustment of dosage |
| Tetracyclines | Potentiation possible | Decreased availability of vitamin K | Monitoring of prothrombin time |
| Thiazides | None | | |
| Thyroid hormones | Potentiation | Increased catabolism of vitamin K-dependent clotting factors | Adjustment of dosage |
| Tocopherol (vitamin E) | Potentiation possible | Unknown | ? |
| Tolmetin | None | | May cause gastric erosion |
| Tricyclic antidepressants | None | | |

indicated if the patient is not to be maintained on therapy after the haemorrhage is controlled. Large doses of vitamin $K_1$ may subsequently make the patient resistant to warfarin for many days, preventing effective anticoagulant therapy for that period.

Vitamin $K_1$ may be administered intravenously, subcutaneously, or orally. Water-soluble vitamin $K_1$ derivatives are distinctly less effective than the natural vitamin.

***Drug interactions with oral anticoagulants:*** drug interactions are a particular problem with this group of drugs since they may be used for prolonged periods and, because of the nature of the diseases for which they are given, numerous other drugs are often given concurrently. A number of agents have the potential to modify the response to coumarin anticoagulants, and drugs inhibiting platelet function such as aspirin, ticlopidine, large doses of penicillins, nonsteroidal anti-inflammatory drugs and latamoxef (moxalactam) have the potential to increase the risk of bleeding. Changes of other drug therapy in patients on anticoagulants should therefore be kept to a minimum and, with certain drugs, should only be made under careful laboratory control.

Although the potential for interaction is considerable, in practice, clinically harmful interactions are not very common and predictable effects are largely confined to a few drugs such as phenylbutazone, oxyphenbutazone, clofibrate, allopurinol, cimetidine and danazol (which potentiate the anticoagulant effect), and barbiturates, rifampicin, aminoglutethimide, griseofulvin and cholestyramine (which reduce the anticoagulant effect) [see table VI].[196] Nevertheless, several fatalities have resulted from severe bleeding and, conversely, many patients taking potentially interacting drugs may not achieve desirable anticoagulant control if seen only irregularly. Moreover, some coumarin anticoagulants (notably dicoumarol) can affect the metabolism of other drugs such as phenytoin (see chapter 29; sect. 4.1.4), tolbutamide and chlorpropamide.

***Mechanisms of interaction and time-course of interaction effect:*** there are many possible mechanisms for interaction. These include:

1) Interference with clotting factor synthesis (e.g. anabolic steroids, quinidine).

2) Alteration of vitamin K availability (oral broad-spectrum antibiotics, ion exchange resins, colestipol, oil laxatives).

3) Interference with the rate of decay of clotting factors (e.g. thyroid drugs).

4) Interference with absorption (e.g. cholestyramine, alkalinising agents, antacids).

5) Enhancement of coumarin metabolism (e.g. barbiturates, rifampicin, griseofulvin, carbamazepine).

6) Inhibition of coumarin metabolism (e.g. phenylbutazone, metronidazole, cotrimoxazole, sulfinpyrazone, cimetidine, omeprazole, amiodarone, chloramphenicol).

*The time-course of onset and also the extent of the interaction effect* vary considerably among patients and depend on the mechanism involved, as well as the specific drug, its dose, and duration of administration. As discussed above, the importance of protein binding displacement as a mechanism of altered drug effects is minimal. With repeated daily doses of a displacing drug, any potentiation of the hypoprothrombinaemic effect is only likely to be transient; the time required for the subsequent return to previous values is complex and depends on several factors, particularly the rate of elimination of the individual coumarin and the displacing drug.

*Enhancement of metabolism interactions (enzyme induction):* the inducibility of hepatic microsomal enzymes varies considerably among individuals and is in part genetically determined; it is also dependent on the specific inducing drug, its dosage and the duration of exposure. An enzyme-inducing drug (e.g. a barbiturate) introduced to a stable regimen might accelerate coumarin metabolism with a single dose, but up to 3 weeks may be required for maximum induction to be reached.[214,215] On withdrawal of the inducing drug, return to the original rate of coumarin metabolism takes place gradually over several weeks. Even with careful monitoring, optimum anticoagulant control may be difficult with potent enzyme-inducing drugs and consequently they should be avoided and alternatives used.

*Inhibition of metabolism interactions:* in contrast to hepatic microsomal enzyme induction, interference with coumarin metabolism may become apparent within hours of administration of the inhibiting drug. When such a drug (e.g. phenylbutazone) is given to a patient stabilised on long term anticoagulant therapy, the maintenance dose of the coumarin drug must be reduced to avoid excessive hypoprothrombinaemia and bleeding. However, the extent of enhancement cannot be predicted and dose adjustment must

**Table VII.** The vitamin K content of some common foods and beverages

| <1.0 μg/100g | 1-10 μg/100g | 10-50 μg/100g | 50-100 μg/100g | >100 μg/100g |
|---|---|---|---|---|
| Canned pears | Peanut oil | Sunflower oil | Olive oil | Soya bean oil |
| Banana | Corn oil | Sesame oil | Liver (beef) | Rape seed oil |
| Orange | Safflower oil | Vegetable oil | Cauliflower | Broccoli |
| Apple (no peel) | Apple (with peel) | Pumpkin | Asparagus | Cabbage |
| Potatoes | Blueberries | Mustard | Watercress | Spinach |
| Onions | Cranberries | Cheese | | Lettuce |
| Black tea | Tomatoes | Butter | | Brussels sprouts |
| Orange juice | Sweet potatoes | Liver (pork, chicken) | | Turnip greens |
| Apple juice | Squash | Eggs | | Kale |
| Grapefruit juice | Whole wheat flour | Green beans | | Chewing tobacco |
| Lemonade | Corn | Peas | | |
| Ginger ale | Carrots | Oats | | |
| Cola | Peaches | | | |
| Vinegar | Corn flakes cereal | | | |
| Lemon extract | 'Rice Krispies' cereal | | | |
| Vanilla extract | | | | |
| Almond extract | | | | |
| Brewed coffee | | | | |
| Honey | | | | |
| Salt | | | | |
| Sugar | | | | |
| Peanut butter | | | | |
| White flour | | | | |
| Egg white | | | | |
| White rice | | | | |
| Brown rice | | | | |
| White pasta | | | | |
| Chicken breast | | | | |
| Lean pork | | | | |
| Lean ground beef | | | | |

be made on the basis of results of careful monitoring of the prothrombin time.

***Avoiding interactions:*** adverse clinical events due to interactions with coumarin anticoagulants can be prevented by following a few simple rules:[216]

1) Before prescribing, review all medications the patient is taking and instruct him/her not to change or add to their intake of medication, either prescribed or self-prescribed, without first communicating with their doctor.

2) Drug therapy should always be kept as simple as possible and restricted to those drugs genuinely indicated and of proven benefit.

3) Occasional use of predictable interacting drugs (see table VI) should be avoided and alternatives prescribed. The patient should also be informed about foods and beverages with a high vitamin K content (table VII) as fluctuating levels of dietary vitamin K modify the sensitivity to oral anticoagulants.

4) Changes of drug therapy should be kept to a minimum. If changes are necessary and involve known interacting drugs, some alteration in coumarin dosage can be anticipated, but dose adjustment should only be made on the basis of results of close monitoring of anticoagulant control over a period of some weeks after the change. The time-course and extent of interaction can vary considerably among individual patients (see above).

### 3.1.6 Thrombolytic Agents

Five plasminogen activators are available for thrombolytic therapy: *streptokinase, anistreplase* (anisoylated plasminogen-streptokinase activator complex, APSAC), *saruplase* (single-chain urokinase-type plasminogen activator, scu-PA, prourokinase), *urokinase* (2-chain urokinase-type plasminogen activator, tcu-PA), and *alteplase* (tissue-type plasminogen activator, t-PA).

#### Streptokinase and Anistreplase (Anisoylated Plasminogen-Streptokinase Activator Complex; APSAC)

Streptokinase is produced by several strains of β-haemolytic streptococci. It consists of a single polypeptide chain with a molecular weight of 47,000 to 50,000D and contains 414 amino acids.[217] Streptokinase has no active site and thus cannot directly cleave peptide bonds, but it activates plasminogen to plasmin indirectly following the formation of an equimolar complex with plasminogen. The active site residues in the plasmin(ogen)-streptokinase complex are the same as those in the plasmin molecule. However, plasmin is unable to activate plasminogen, while the plasmin(ogen)-streptokinase complex, in contrast to plasmin, is not inhibited by $\alpha_2$-antiplasmin.

Anistreplase (APSAC) was developed with the aim of controlling the enzymatic activity of the plasmin(ogen)-streptokinase complex by a specific reversible chemical protection of its catalytic centre (i.e. by titration with a *p*-anisoyl group).[218] Anisteplase is an equimolar non-covalent complex between human Lys-plasminogen and streptokinase, containing the titrated catalytic centre and the lysine-binding sites of plasminogen. Reversible acylation of the catalytic centre does not affect the weak fibrin-binding capacity of the plasminogen moiety in the complex. Deacylation of anistreplase, which regenerates the catalytic centre, occurs both in the circulation and at the fibrin surface.

***Mechanism/site of action:*** *streptokinase* activates plasminogen to plasmin indirectly, following a 3-step mechanism.[219] In the first step, streptokinase forms an equimolar complex with plasminogen. This complex undergoes a conformational change resulting in the exposure of an active site in the plasminogen moiety. In the second step, this active site catalyses the activation of plasminogen to plasmin. In the third step, plasminogen-streptokinase molecules are converted to a plasmin-streptokinase complex. The activation of native plasminogen by the plasminogen-streptokinase complex is enhanced 6.5-fold in the presence of fibrin and 2-fold in the presence of fibrinogen.[220] The plasminogen activating potential of the plasminogen-streptokinase complex is 2- to 3-fold higher than that of the plasmin-streptokinase complex. Conversion of the equimolar plasminogen-streptokinase complex to the plasmin-streptokinase complex occurs rapidly by proteolytic cleavage of both the plasminogen and the streptokinase moieties. In plasminogen, the $Arg^{560}$-$Val^{561}$ and the $Lys^{77}$-$Lys^{78}$ peptide bonds are cleaved,[221] while 4 modified forms of streptokinase differing in molecular weight by 4000 to 5000D have been observed depending on the species origin of the plasminogen. In the presence of human plasminogen, streptokinase is degraded to a major proteolytic derivative with a molecular weight of 36,000D.[222]

*Anistreplase* binds to fibrin via the lysine-binding sites of plasminogen. Deacylation of anistreplase uncovers the catalytic centre in the complex, which converts plasminogen to plasmin. Deacylation of anistreplase does, however, occur both in the circulation and at the fibrin surface. *In vitro*, the catalytic efficiency of the preformed streptokinase-plasminogen complex (deacylated anistreplase) for plasminogen activation is enhanced 8-fold by the presence of fibrin.[223]

***Pharmacokinetic characteristics:*** *streptokinase* disappears from the circulation with a half-life of approximately 20 minutes. The level of antistreptokinase antibodies, which may result from previous infections with β-haemolytic streptococci, varies widely amongst individuals. Since streptokinase is inactivated by interaction with these antibodies, sufficient streptokinase must be infused to neutralise the antibodies. A few days after streptokinase administration, the antistreptokinase titre rises rapidly to 50 to 100 times the preinfusion value and remains high for 4 to 6 months, during which time renewed treatment is impracticable.

In patients, with acute myocardial infarction treated with anistreplase (30U intravenously over 2 to 15 minutes), half-lives of fibrinolytic activity of 90 to 112 minutes have been reported.[224,225] Patients with high streptokinase antibody titres show very little response to low doses of anistreplase. In some healthy volunteers, administration of anistreplase caused an up to 60-fold increase in the streptokinase antibody titre after 2 to 3 weeks, which was still high after 3 months.[226]

*Anistreplase* has been found to have a first-order deacylation half-life of about 105 minutes in human plasma and whole blood, a value which closely approaches its plasma elimination half-life in humans.[226,227]

***Clinical use:*** an initial dose of *streptokinase* which is adequate to neutralise the plasma levels of antistreptococcal antibodies must be given; the streptokinase-antibody complex thus formed is rapidly cleared from the circulation. The initial dose for an individual patient can be either determined by the streptokinase resistance test (i.e. titration *in vitro* of the streptokinase dose required to lyse a clot induced in the patient's plasma in a given time), or a standard initial intravenous dose ranging from 500,000 to 750,000U can be given over a period of 10 to 30 minutes, followed by a continuous intravenous maintenance dose of 100,000U hourly for

1 or more days. Such a fixed dosage regimen produces a satisfactory thrombolytic effect in the vast majority of patients.[228]

High-dose (1.5MU), short term (15 to 20 min infusion) streptokinase treatment is now routinely used in patients with acute myocardial infarction. Transient hypotension has been reported in up to 10% of patients in some trials[229,230] but this is usually aborted by cessation of the infusion.

The recommended dose of *anistreplase* in patients with acute myocardial infarction is 30U (30mg, containing approximately 1.25MU streptokinase) given as a bolus injection.[231] Comparative studies indicate that the efficacy of anistreplase in coronary thrombolysis (angiographic patency) is comparable or somewhat higher than that of intravenous streptokinase, but lower than that of intracoronary streptokinase.[232]

***Tolerability:*** *streptokinase* is antigenic in humans and thus is able to provoke serious anaphylactic reactions (urticaria, bronchospasm, angio-oedema). However, in practice, major allergic reactions are relatively rare. Shivering, pyrexia or rashes appear in 10% of patients during or shortly after streptokinase infusion. Furthermore, streptokinase infusion, if repeated between 5 days and 6 months following the initial infusion, may be clinically ineffective as a result of a high titre of circulating antibodies.

Bleeding is the most common complication of streptokinase. Minor bleeding (not requiring transfusion) occurs in 3 to 4% of patients in the absence of invasive procedures.[229,230] These are usually related to puncture or injection sites but microscopic haematuria and blood-streaked sputum or vomit are also noted. Significant or major bleeding (requiring transfusion) occurs in approximately 1% of patients.[229] Heparin and/or aspirin treatment may also enhance the frequency of bleeding, as do invasive catheter approaches. The most serious complication is cerebral bleeding which is reported at an incidence of 0.1 to 0.5%, while ischaemic stroke during thrombolytic treatment of myocardial infarction occurs in approximately 0.8% of patients. In large clinical trials conducted with streptokinase, there has been an excess of early cerebral bleeding with streptokinase treatment, but the overall risk of stroke is similar in streptokinase and placebo-treated patients.[230] The occurrence of bleeding with streptokinase in comparison with alteplase (t-PA) is discussed in more detail below.

Bleeding complication rates with *anistreplase* have been found to vary widely, depending on the nature of the study (invasive or non-invasive). In a comparative study of anistreplase with streptokinase, bleeding and blood loss were more pronounced in the anistreplase group than in the intracoronary streptokinase group.[233] In trials comparing anistreplase (30U) with intravenously infused streptokinase (1.5MU over 60 min), the same drop in fibrinogen concentration and the same incidence of adverse events were noted.

In the largest available study with anistreplase, the angiographically documented reocclusion frequency, between 90 minutes and 24 hours after treatment, was 8% in a subgroup of patients treated; however, about a third of the patients had undergone additional interventional procedures.[233]

#### Saruplase and Urokinase

Saruplase is the generic name for non-glycosylated human recombinant scu-PA (single-chain urokinase-type plasminogen activator) obtained from *Escherichia coli.* scu-PA is a single chain glycoprotein with a molecular weight of 54,000D and containing 411 amino acids. Upon limited hydrolysis by plasmin or kallikrein of the $Lys^{158}$-$Ile^{159}$ peptide bond, the molecule is converted to a 2-chain derivative (tcu-PA, urokinase).[234] The amino terminal chain contains a region homologous to human epidermal growth factor (residues 9 to 45) and 1 kringle region (residues 45 to 134). The catalytic centre is located in the proteinase domain (residues 159 to 411) and is composed of $His^{204}$, $Asp^{255}$ and $Ser^{356}$. A low molecular weight 2-chain urokinase (MW 33,000D) can be generated by hydrolysis of the $Lys^{135}$-$Lys^{136}$ peptide bond with plasmin. A low molecular weight scu-PA (MW 32,000D) can be obtained by specific hydrolysis of the $Glu^{143}$-$Leu^{144}$ peptide bond in scu-PA.[235]

scu-PA has a very low reactivity towards low molecular weight synthetic substrates or active site inhibitors that are very reactive towards tcu-PA (2-chain urokinase-type plasminogen activator). In mixtures of purified scu-PA and plasminogen, both tcu-PA and plasmin are quickly generated, suggesting that scu-PA has intrinsic plasminogen-activating activity. The magnitude of this intrinsic activity is, however, still controversial.[236,237]

***Mechanism/site of action:*** tcu-PA (urokinase) has no fibrin-specificity and activates fibrin-bound and circulating plasminogen relatively indiscriminately, resulting in extensive plasminogen activation and depletion of $\alpha_2$-antiplasmin.[238] In contrast, scu-PA has a significant fibrin-specificity. Several hypotheses for the mechanism of plasminogen activation and fibrin-specificity of clot lysis with scu-PA in a plasma milieu have been proposed. One hypothesis claims that scu-PA is inactive towards circulating native plasminogen (Glu-plasminogen) but active towards conformationally altered plasminogen (Lys-plasminogen) bound to partially digested fibrin.[38] A second hypothesis proposes that scu-PA is a genuine proenzyme with negligible activity towards plasminogen;[236] fibrinolysis with scu-PA would thus depend entirely on generation of tcu-PA. Alternatively, scu-PA is claimed to have some intrinsic plasminogen-activating potential which is counteracted by a competitive inhibitory mechanism in plasma, that is reversed by fibrin. Studies in human plasma *in vitro* have suggested that conversion of scu-PA to tcu-PA during clot lysis constitutes a primary positive feedback system, whereas binding of plasminogen to fibrin or predigestion of fibrin by plasmin results in relatively minor additional acceleration of fibrinolysis.[239]

The observation that plasmin-resistant mutants of scu-PA have only a 3- to 5-fold lower *in vivo* thrombolytic potency as compared with wild-type scu-PA,[240] suggests that for *in vivo* thrombolysis, conversion of scu-PA to tcu-PA may play a less important role.

***Pharmacokinetic characteristics:*** in animal studies with recombinant and natural scu-PA and tcu-PA, the plasma disappearance of u-PA was adequately represented by a 2-compartment model composed of a central (intravascular) and a peripheral (interstitial) compartment, with clearance occurring from the central compartment. The turnover in blood of all urokinase species occurred with an initial half-life of about 3 minutes. The main mechanism of removal of urokinase from the blood appears to be hepatic clearance of the molecule; experimental hepatectomy markedly prolonged the initial half-life of scu-PA (from 3 to 20 min up to 30 min).

The rapid clearance of urokinase is apparently not mediated via carbohydrate receptors nor via reaction with plasma protease inhibitors, and the amino terminal kringle-containing portion of the molecule does not seem to be involved.[241] Following intravenous infusion of natural scu-PA in patients with acute myocardial infarction,[242] a biphasic disappearance rate was observed with an initial half-life in plasma (post-infusion) of about 4 minutes. This short half-life suggests that the maintenance of a therapeutic concentration of the agent in plasma may require its continuous infusion.

***Clinical use:*** *saruplase* (recombinant scu-PA) has been used clinically as a preparation containing 160,000 U/mg. The dose used successfully in patients with acute myocardial infarction was 20mg given as a bolus and 60mg over the next 60 minutes, immediately followed by an intravenous heparin infusion (20 U/kg/h) for 72 hours.[243] In this direct double-blind comparison between intravenous saruplase (80mg over 60 min) and streptokinase (1.5MU over 60 min), a somewhat smaller reduction in circulating fibrinogen levels was observed in patients treated with saruplase. The transfusion requirement was significantly less in the saruplase group in comparison with the streptokinase group (4 *vs* 11%), and the same was true of bleeding episodes (14 *vs* 25%). Reocclusion rates at 24 to 36 hours with both saruplase and streptokinase were low.

In patients with acute myocardial infarction, the dose of *urokinase* (tcu-PA) is 2MU, given as a bolus or 3MU administered over 90 minutes. For acute major pulmonary embolism, an initial intravenous dose of 4400 U/kg bodyweight over 10 minutes followed by the same maintenance dose per kg hourly has been used clinically for over a decade. More recently, a bolus dose in the right atrium of 15,000 U/kg bodyweight has been recommended in this indication, and an intravenous infusion of 3MU urokinase over 2 hours (1MU over 10 min and 2MU over the next 110 min) has also been successfully applied.

***Tolerability:*** purified urokinase preparations are non-antigenic, non-pyrogenic and their use is usually associated with a milder coagulation defect than with streptokinase, but with a similar incidence of bleeding as that observed in streptokinase-treated patients.

#### Alteplase (Tissue-Type Plasminogen Activator)

Alteplase is the generic name for recombinant human tissue-type plasminogen activator (rt-PA). Human t-PA is a serine proteinase with a molecular weight of about 70,000D, composed of 1 polypeptide chain containing 527 amino acids.[244] Limited plasma hydrolysis of the $Arg^{275}$-$Ile^{276}$ peptide bond converts the molecule to a 2-chain activator held together by 1 interchain disulfide bond. The t-PA molecule contains 4 domains:

1) A 47-residue long (residues 4 to 50) amino terminal region which are homologous with the finger domains mediating the fibrin-affinity of fibronectin.

2) Residues 50 to 87 which is homologous with human epidermal growth factor.

3) Two regions comprising residues 87 to 176 and 176 to 262 which share a high degree of homology with the 5 kringles of plasminogen.

4) A serine proteinase domain (residues 276 to 527) with the active site residues $His^{322}$, $Asp^{371}$ and $Ser^{478}$.

***Mechanism/site of action:*** t-PA is a poor enzyme in the absence of fibrin, but the presence of fibrin strikingly enhances the activation rate of plasminogen by at least 2 orders of magnitude.[245] The kinetic data support a mechanism in which fibrin provides a surface to which t-PA and plasminogen adsorb in a sequential and ordered way, yielding a cyclic ternary complex. Fibrin essentially increases the local plasminogen concentration by creating an additional interaction between t-PA and its substrate. The high affinity of t-PA for plasminogen in the presence of fibrin thus allows efficient activation on the fibrin clot, while plasminogen activation by t-PA in plasma is a comparatively inefficient process. Plasmin formed on the fibrin surface has both its lysine-binding sites and active site occupied and is thus only slowly inactivated by $\alpha_2$-antiplasmin; in contrast, free plasmin, when formed, is rapidly inhibited by $\alpha_2$-antiplasmin.[246]

It has been proposed that initial binding of t-PA to fibrin is governed by the finger domain, and that partial degradation of fibrin results in enhanced binding of t-PA via kringle 2 to newly exposed COOH-terminal lysine residues.[247] Early fibrin digestion by plasmin may accelerate fibrinolysis by increasing the binding of both t-PA and plasminogen. The fibrinolytic process mediated by t-PA thus seems to be triggered by and confined to fibrin.

***Pharmacokinetic characteristics:*** in several animal species, the disappearance of t-PA from the circulation was found to be rapid (initial half-life of 1 to 4 min). The predominant role of the liver in clearance was confirmed by the observation that the half-life of t-PA is very long in rabbits with a functional hepatectomy.[248] Two different recognition systems for removal of t-PA by hepatocytes and by endothelial cells in the liver have been described.[249]

The initial half-life of alteplase (recombinant t-PA) following infusion in patients or in healthy volunteers is 6 minutes and the terminal elimination phase half-life 64 minutes.[250,251]

***Clinical use:*** the presently recommended dose of alteplase for the treatment of acute myocardial infarction is 100mg, administered as 60mg in the first hour (of which 6 to 10mg is administered as a bolus over the first 2 minutes), 20mg over the second hour, and 20mg over the third hour. More recently, it was proposed to give the same total dose of 100mg but 'front loaded', i.e. starting with a bolus of 15mg, followed by 50mg in the next 30 minutes, and the remaining 35mg in the following 60 minutes.[252] A 15mg intravenous bolus of alteplase, followed by 0.75 mg/kg over 30 minutes (not exceeding 50mg), and then 0.5 mg/kg over 60 minutes (not exceeding 35mg) was used in the large GUSTO trial.[253] The rationale for use of the front loaded dosage regimen of alteplase is based on the observation that the effectiveness and speed of the drug in inducing lysis of experimental thrombi and emboli in animals is increased by using high concentrations infused over a short interval.[254] As the thrombolytic effect of alteplase persists beyond its clearance from the circulation (due to its enhanced binding to fibrin in the thrombus), it was considered logical to test the rapid infusion of high doses of alteplase or even the administration of boluses in patients.

For catheter-directed local thrombolysis with alteplase in patients with recent peripheral arterial occlusion, a dose of 0.05 to 0.1 mg/kg/h over an 8-hour period is usually recommended.[232]

***Tolerability:*** alteplase does not appear to be immunogenic and no serious or life-threatening allergic reactions have been reported. Bleeding complications in association with thrombolytic therapy are most probably due to the combined actions of the thrombolytic agents on blood coagulation components, on the vessel wall, and on the haemostatic plug. In addition, the demographic characteristics of the patient and adjunctive anticoagulant or antiplatelet therapy may contribute to a bleeding tendency. In 4 clinical trials comparing streptokinase with alteplase, the frequency of bleeding complications was comparable in 2 trials,[255,256] and less frequent with alteplase than with streptokinase in the other 2.[250,257] Thus, the markedly higher fibrin-selectivity of alteplase has not resulted in a proportional reduction of haemorrhagic complications.

A major recent concern with the use of alteplase has been the occurrence of intracerebral bleeding. In the TIMI-II trial, the frequency of intracranial haemorrhage in 2952 patients treated with 100mg alteplase in combination with heparin and aspirin was 0.5%.[255] In the GUSTO-1 trial, haemorrhagic stroke occurred in 0.72% of the 10,268 patients treated with front loaded alteplase (100mg) and in 0.54% of 10,314 those treated with streptokinase; all patients also received intravenous heparin and aspirin.[253] The possibility of intracerebral bleeding due to thrombolytic therapy remains a serious concern.[258-261]

### 3.2 Optimum Prevention/Treatment of Thromboembolic Disorders

#### *3.2.1 Clinical Indications for Antithrombotic Agents*

Research over the last 2 decades has revealed the importance of platelet activation and thrombus formation in the physiopathology of ischaemic events in the heart, brain and peripheral arterial territories. This section is limited to the use of antithrombotic agents for the primary and secondary prevention of arterial thromboembolism and the treatment of deep venous thrombosis and pulmonary embolism. The key clinical trials on which current recommendations are based are reviewed.

##### Prevention of First Myocardial Infarction and Stroke in Healthy Men

Only 2 randomised primary prevention trials have addressed this issue.[262,263] In the US Physicians' Health Study which included 22,071 healthy male doctors aged 40 to 84 years who were followed up for 4.8 years, aspirin 325mg on alternate days significantly reduced the incidence of a first nonfatal myocardial infarction from about 0.44 to 0.24% per year and the incidence of fatal myocardial infarction by 44%.[262] However, this effect was limited to individuals over 50 years of age. Total cardiovascular deaths in the aspirin and placebo groups were identical as a result of a slightly increased incidence of stroke (in particular haemorrhagic stroke) and 'sudden death' in the aspirin group. Moreover, low-dose aspirin did not alter the incidence or delay the onset of confirmed angina pectoris.[264] This study also revealed that long term administration of aspirin reduces the need for peripheral arterial surgery.[265]

In the British Primary Prevention Trial conducted in 5139 male physicians, two-thirds of whom were randomly assigned to aspirin 500mg daily while one-third were instructed to avoid it (no placebo was used), the incidence of nonfatal myocardial infarction or stroke after 6 years of follow-up was similar in the 2 groups.[263] Deaths due to myocardial infarction or stroke did not differ between the 2 groups; the nonsignificant 10% reduction in total mortality was mainly due to a nonsignificant 15% reduction in nonvascular death rates in the aspirin group. Even though the incidence of transient ischaemic attacks was lower in the aspirin group, that of disabling stroke was higher. There was no difference in the event rate of definite nonfatal myocardial infarction between the 2 treatment groups but 3 times as many 'possible' nonfatal myocardial infarctions were reported in aspirin-treated patients. Nonfatal strokes were also more frequent in the aspirin group, a difference which for disabling stroke reached a level of statistical significance.

Both these primary prevention trials were conducted in a health conscious group of male physicians who had already eliminated as many risk factors as possible, and this may explain the exceptionally low cardiovascular mortality rate among participants, which was only 15% of that expected for a general population of White American males with the same age distribution over a similar period. Also, in the British trial, there were only 137 vascular deaths despite 6 years of follow-up of over 5000 patients. Thus extrapolation of the findings of the 2 trials to the overall male population is hazardous.[266]

The finding that the advantage offered by aspirin in preventing myocardial infarction and stroke is of the same magnitude whether risk factors for these cardiovascular events are present or not[267] is important for clinical practice. As the incidence of cardiovascular events is considerably higher in patients who smoke, and in those with diabetes, hypercholesterolaemia, and hypertension, the absolute impact of aspirin will be greater in high-risk groups. Thus, the decision to prescribe aspirin for the primary prevention of stroke and myocardial infarction must remain an individual judgement, balancing the cardiovascular benefit and the well-recognised hazard of gastrointestinal discomfort and bleeding, and the risk of haemorrhagic stroke. Considerable caution should be exercised before the widespread use of aspirin at any age and at any dose for primary prevention is advocated. Therefore, it is important to target aspirin to asymptomatic patients over 50 years of age with a parental history and personal high-risk factors for coronary and cerebral artery disease.

#### Prevention of First Myocardial Infarction and Stroke in Healthy Women

As the American and British doctors' trials (see above) were limited to males, extrapolation of the results to women may not be appropriate. The results of 4 observational studies of the effect of aspirin on cardiovascular disease in healthy women are contradictory. Although 3 of the studies were very large, their limitations in terms of evaluation of a moderate benefit are obvious and can only be solved by randomised placebo-controlled trials of adequate sample size.

#### Primary Prevention of Myocardial Infarction and Stroke in Patients With Mild or Moderate Arterial Hypertension

The efficacy of antithrombotic drugs in this setting is unproven. Patients with hypertension, even when mild or borderline, cannot be considered healthy, and the combined results of 9 major prospective studies of the association of diastolic blood pressure with stroke and coronary heart disease have indicated positive, continuous, and apparently independent associations, with no significant heterogeneity of effect between the different studies.[268,269] Reducing the diastolic blood pressure by 5 to 10mm Hg over a few years in patients who have had a transient ischaemic attack appears to reduce subsequent strokes by 40 to 50%. In 14 randomised trials of antihypertensive drugs (chiefly diuretics or β-blockers) without confounding factors, pooling of the results revealed a highly significant odds reduction in fatal and in nonfatal stroke of 42%.[270] However, the proportional reductions in nonfatal (14%) and fatal (11%) myocardial infarction were much less and only significant for nonfatal myocardial infarction.

Thus, antihypertensive treatment (see further chapter 21), particularly with diuretics, appears to provide the best protection against stroke in patients with mild or moderate hypertension, but it is considerably less effective in reducing the incidence of myocardial infarction in the same time frame. The efficacy of a combination of low-dose aspirin with antihypertensive drugs in the primary prevention of stroke and myocardial infarction is currently being tested in patients with moderate hypertension.

#### Primary Prevention of Myocardial Infarction in Patients With Diabetic Retinopathy

The available data indicate that aspirin may reduce the risk of myocardial infarction in diabetic patients. In a total of 3711 patients with a clinical diagnosis of diabetes mellitus who were randomly assigned to either aspirin (325mg twice daily) or placebo over a follow-up period of 4 to 9 years, the aspirin and placebo groups had, respectively, 18 and 19% mortality rates.[271] However, the incidence of myocardial infarction at 5 years was 9% in the aspirin group and 12% in the placebo group, a difference of borderline statistical significance. Stroke incidence was about 4% in each group. The reduction in myocardial infarction in the aspirin group was slightly greater for men than for women (relative risk 0.74 *vs* 0.91), while women taking aspirin had a slightly greater relative risk for stroke than men (1.31 *vs* 1.07).

Thus, although the data do not clearly show a beneficial effect on mortality, aspirin may be a reasonable prophylactic therapy for diabetic patients at increased risk for cardiovascular disease.

#### Primary Prevention in Patients With Stable Angina

On the basis of present knowledge, aspirin is probably effective in preventing myocardial infarction in patients with stable angina. In a 5-year study in which 370 patients with stable coronary heart disease were randomly allocated to aspirin (975 mg/day) and dipyridamole (225 mg/day) or to placebo,[272] treated patients had significantly fewer infarcts (5.3 *vs* 12.1%) and a significantly lower incidence of new coronary lesions at repeat angiography (23 *vs* 45%). Similarly, in a subgroup analysis of the US Physician's Health study in 333 patients with a history of chronic stable angina but without previous myocardial infarction, stroke or transient ischaemic attack, aspirin administration was associated with a significant 50% reduction in nonfatal first myocardial infarction over a 5-year period.[273] All fatal myocardial infarctions occurred in the control group (zero *vs* 4). However, of the 13 strokes which were not fatal, 11 occurred in the aspirin group.

More recently, a Swedish trial conducted over a period of 50 months in 2035 patients who were receiving sotalol for control of angina symptoms, showed that aspirin (75 mg/day) plus sotalol administration was associated with a significant 34% reduction in primary outcome events (myocardial infarction and sudden death) in comparison with placebo plus sotalol. The reduction in secondary outcome events (vascular events, vascular death, all-cause mortality, stroke) ranged from 22 to 32%.

#### Prevention of Myocardial Infarction and Vascular Death in Patients with Unstable Angina

Aspirin and ticlopidine reduce the incidence of death and nonfatal myocardial infarction by about 50% over a 3- to 24-month period in patients with unstable angina. This conclusion is based on an analysis of the results of large trials in patients admitted to a coronary care unit on different doses of aspirin (75 mg/day;[274] 324 mg/day;[275,276] 325mg 4 times daily[277]) or on ticlopidine.[278]

In 4 randomised trials of combined full-dose heparin plus aspirin treatment *versus* either drug alone and placebo in the acute stage of unstable angina,[279-282] the combination provided the greatest reduction in myocardial infarction and death. For instance, in 1 trial,[279] there was a significant reduction of cardiac death or myocardial infarction from 11.9% in the control group to 3.3% with aspirin alone and 1.6% when aspirin and heparin were combined.

Thus, patients with unstable angina should be admitted to a coronary care unit and receive either aspirin (160 to 325mg daily) or ticlopidine (250mg twice daily) which should be continued on a long term basis. Heparin administered at full doses for 7 days should be added in more severe cases; however, this combination may be safer with a reduced daily aspirin dose of 75mg. The rebound phenomena observed when heparin is discontinued can be prevented by aspirin.[283]

#### Secondary Prevention of Myocardial Infarction

***Anticoagulants:*** numerous trials have been conducted to test the hypothesis that oral anticoagulant therapy prevents coronary rethrombosis, reinfarction and death, but have failed to demonstrate unequivocally that the potential benefit exceeds the risk of bleeding. An analysis of acceptable short-term randomised trials showed a case-fatality rate of 15.4% for patients receiving anticoagulants and 20% for untreated patients, i.e. a reduction of 21% which was not convincing;[284] reanalysis of the same data yielded a similar mortality reduction.[285] However, a revival of interest followed the Dutch Sixty Plus Study which assessed the risk of discontinuation of long term anticoagulant therapy in patients over 60 years of age who had been given anticoagulants for a least 6 months after a proven infarct.[286] At 2 years of follow-up, the mortality rate was significantly lower at 7.6% in the group maintained on anticoagulants *versus* 13.4% in the placebo group, while the incidence of nonfatal reinfarction was 4.1% *versus* 8.4%. Major extracranial and intracranial bleeding were more frequent in patients receiving anticoagulants.[286] However, it should be noted that this study did not assess the value of initiation of anticoagulants.

Two major studies have assessed the efficacy of anticoagulants initiated up to 6 weeks after a myocardial infarction. In the large Norwegian Warfarin Re-Infarction Study (WARIS)[218] in which 1214 patients were randomised 27 days (mean) after myocardial infarction to receive either warfarin (anticoagulation sustained in the INR range of 2.8 to 4.8) or placebo, the risk reduction was 24% for total mortality, 34% for nonfatal reinfarction, and 55% for stroke after 37 months. Serious bleeding occurred in 0.6% of the patients receiving anticoagulants per year compared with zero percent in the placebo group.

In the recent Anticoagulants in the Secondary Prevention of Events in Coronary Thrombosis (ASPECT) trial, 3404 hospital survivors of myocardial infarction were randomly assigned to a coumarin drug or placebo within 6 weeks after discharge.[287] The target INR was 2.4 to 4.8, and the mean follow-up period was 37 months (range 6 to 76 months). In patients receiving anticoagulants, the occurrence of death was reduced by 10%, while recurrent myocardial infarction was reduced by 53% and cerebrovascular events by 40%. Thus, long term oral anticoagulant treatment after myocardial infarction in low-risk patients has a limited effect on mortality but substantially reduces the incidence of cerebrovascular events and recurrent myocardial infarction.

***Antiplatelet agents:*** several trials have been conducted with antiplatelet agents (mainly aspirin) in survivors of myocardial infarction, but no one study has reached the conventional level of statistical significance, probably because of the small number of patients included in each trial. However, in a meta-analysis of the results of 175 randomised trials involving a total of about 100,000 patients with either myocardial infarction (two-thirds) or stroke (one-third), there was a 32% reduction in nonfatal myocardial infarction, a 25% decrease in nonfatal stroke, a 17% reduction in vascular death, and a 16% reduction in any death.[288] The benefit lasted for at least 2 years and was similar in patients with a cardiac disease, in those with a history of cerebrovascular disease, and in both men and women. Over a 2-year period, the typical patient had a 7% risk of death from vascular disease and a further 7% risk of a major nonfatal vascular myocardial infarction or stroke. In none of these studies was a combination of aspirin and dipyridamole significantly superior to aspirin alone. Moreover, there was no evidence that a high dose of aspirin (900 to 1500mg daily) is more efficacious than a low dose of 300mg daily.

In comparison with aspirin, the decrease in vascular mortality achieved with long term oral anticoagulants is somewhat less (10 to 24% with anticoagulants *vs* 23% with aspirin), but the risk of bleeding is far greater with oral anticoagulants and convenience, simplicity and lower cost all favour aspirin. It is a reasonable assumption that suppression of platelet function simultaneously with inhibition of fibrin formation may be more effective than either therapy on its own, and the concurrent use of low-dose aspirin and low-intensity oral anticoagulants is presently being tested in the primary prevention of ischaemic heart disease.[289]

Thus, on the basis of present evidence, all patients with myocardial infarction should receive antithrombotic protection. If thrombolytic therapy is instituted, non–enteric-coated aspirin (100 to 325mg) should be given immediately and intravenous heparin administered conjointly with alteplase (and probably also with other thrombolytic drugs) and maintained for at least 48 hours. If no thrombolytic treatment is given, all patients should be given aspirin immediately and patients at increased risk for severe left ventricular dysfunction, congestive heart failure, large anterior infarction and atrial fibrillation should receive in addition therapeutic doses of heparin for 1 week, followed by oral coumarin drugs (INR 2 to 4) for at least 3 months and indefinitely if atrial fibrillation persists.[290]

Regardless of whether thrombolytic drugs are given or not, all patients should continue on aspirin indefinitely, preferably an enteric-coated form to reduce adverse gastric effects.

#### Prevention of Systemic Embolism in Patients With or at Risk of Left Ventricular Thrombi

Stroke attributable to cerebral embolism occurs in 1 to 3% of all patients with acute myocardial infarction, including 2 to 6% of those with anterior infarction and 10 to 20% of those with extensive anteroseptal infarction and apical dyskinesis.[291] Clinical evidence of cerebral embolism is found in about 10% of acute myocardial infarction patients with echocardiographically evident mural thrombi, and the risk continues during the first 3 months of the acute phase. Numerous studies have been conducted with heparin followed by oral anticoagulants and, in general, thrombus formation detected by echocardiography has been reduced by more than 50% with anticoagulant therapy, which also decreased the incidence of cerebral embolism from 3 to 1% when compared with controls.[290] Thus, in patients with a higher embolic risk, e.g. those with a large akinetic myocardial zone, oral anticoagulant therapy should be maintained for 3 months or longer.[290] If unfractionated heparin is used first, 12,500U should be given subcutaneously every 12 hours in the first 10 to 16 days.[292]

Other studies have shown that patients with dilated cardiomyopathy have a reduced incidence of systemic embolism when treated with oral anticoagulants at moderate intensity (INR 2.0 to 3.0).[293]

#### Prevention of Acute Occlusions and Recurrent Stenosis in Percutaneous Transluminal Coronary Angioplasty (PTCA)

After PTCA, acute occlusions occur in 4 to 10% and recurrent stenosis in 30 to 40% of patients within 6 months.[294] In 7 well-conducted studies, *aspirin* alone or in association with dipyridamole has been found to prevent early reocclusion after PTCA.[295] The incidence of Q-wave myocardial infarction was 1.6% in treated patients in the first week after PTCA compared with 6.9% in the placebo group. In a study comparing ticlopidine (250mg 3 times daily), aspirin (325mg twice daily) combined with dipyridamole (75mg 3 times daily), and placebo, ischaemic complications occurred in 1.8, 5.4 and 13.6% of patients, respectively.[296]

Two randomised, double-blind studies with *abciximab*, a monoclonal antibody that binds to platelet glycoprotein IIb/IIIa receptors, have shown that ischaemic complications of PTCA and atherectomy are significantly reduced by this agent in the first month[106] and also at 6 months;[297] however, this was at the cost of increased bleeding during hospitalisation. For further discussion of the use of abciximab, see review by Faulds and Sorkin.[298]

Numerous antithrombotic drugs, including oral anticoagulants, short term heparin, aspirin and dipyridamole, nifedipine, ticlopidine and a thromboxane receptor blocker have proved ineffective in reducing the rate of restenosis after coronary angioplasty.[299-301] The same conclusion also holds for hirudin administered during 3 days after PTCA in patients with unstable angina; although significantly fewer early cardiac events occurred with hirudin than with heparin, no reduction in restenosis at 6 months of follow-up was observed.[121]

#### Prevention of Graft Occlusion After Aortocoronary Bypass Surgery

Provided prophylaxis was commenced before or at least 6 hours after surgery, the combined use of aspirin (1000 mg/day) and dipyridamole (225 mg/day) was found to significantly reduce graft occlusion rates after aortocoronary bypass surgery from 25 to 11%; moreover, this benefit was maintained in the first year.[302,303] In other studies, aspirin alone at daily doses of 100mg,[304] 150mg,[305] 324mg[306] or 1000mg[307] and ticlopidine alone (500 mg/day)[308,309] significantly increased graft patency, provided therapy was started before or at surgery.

Four antithrombotic treatments were compared in 1 placebo-controlled randomised trial: aspirin 325mg as a single daily dose, aspirin 325mg 3 times daily, the combination of aspirin 325mg and dipyridamole 75mg 3 times daily, and sulfinpyrazone 267mg 3 times daily, with treatment starting 12 to 48 hours before surgery.[310] The angiographic patency rate in the first 60 postoperative days was higher in those patients taking aspirin when compared with those receiving placebo, but there was no difference between the lower (325mg daily) or higher (975mg daily) aspirin dose. However, it should be noted that aspirin given 12 hours before surgery was associated with a greater blood loss and a higher number of early reoperations.

Thus, it appears that antiplatelet therapy is mandatory for prevention of early vein graft occlusion. Preoperative administration of aspirin increases intraoperative bleeding and does not seem to be more beneficial than aspirin started within a few hours of surgery. Although preoperative dipyridamole does not increase intraoperative bleeding, its advantage over postoperative aspirin has not been investigated. Ticlopidine is also effective, but its relative benefit and safety compared with aspirin after coronary bypass surgery still needs to be assessed.

The appropriate duration of antiplatelet therapy after surgery is still controversial but is at least 1 year.

#### Prevention of Embolic Complications in Patients With Heart Valve Replacement

The main long term complications of heart valve replacement are valve failure, myocardial infarction, prosthetic endocarditis and thromboembolism. The latter problem exists for all older and newer synthetic heart valves and bioprosthetic valves, but to a different degree.

The present recommendation for patients with mechanical heart valves is to start with intravenous heparin (about 600 U/h) 4 to 6 hours after surgery, adjusting the dose to maintain the partial thromboplastin time at the upper limit of normal. This infusion is continued until chest tubes are removed and then subcutaneous unfractionated heparin (12,500U twice daily) is substituted, this dose being adjusted to increase the partial thromboplastin time to 1.5 to 2 times the normal level. After a few days, aspirin (500 mg/day) and oral anticoagulants should be started and the INR maintained at between 3.0 and 4.5.

At this level of anticoagulation, bleeding is not uncommon and it would be important to know whether a lower level of anticoagulation (e.g. INR 2.5 to 3.5) would be as effective, but with a reduced bleeding incidence. A trial in which all patients with mechanical prosthetic valves were randomised to receive oral anticoagulation at an INR range of either 2.0 to 3.0 or 3.0 to 4.5 showed that protection from embolism was equal in the 2 treatment groups but at the cost of more bleeding at the higher dose range.[311] In a Canadian study comparing warfarin with or without aspirin (100 mg/day) after heart valve replacement in which all patients were targeted to an INR range of 3.0 to 4.5, those in the combined treatment group had significantly fewer major emboli (1.9% per year *versus* 8.5% per year) and had no major bleeding complications.[312]

Patients with newer bioprosthetic valves in a mitral position should be treated for the first 3 months with oral anticoagulants at an INR range of 2.0 to 3.0. This lower level of anticoagulation is based on a randomised study of patients with a bioprosthetic valve in the mitral position, which showed that a less intensive oral anticoagulant regimen (INR 2.0 to 3.0) gave the same protection from thromboembolism (1.2%) as more intensive anticoagulation (INR 3.0 to 4.5) but with significantly less bleeding (5.7% *vs* 20.6%).[313] After 3 months, these patients can then discontinue coumarin drugs and switch to aspirin, but only in the absence of atrial fibrillation, a large left atrium, or a history of previous systemic thromboembolism.

#### Primary and Secondary Prevention of Arterial Thromboembolism in Patients with Valvular Atrial Fibrillation

Atrial fibrillation is nearly always associated with mitral valve disease, and the incidence of thromboembolism in mitral valve disease is 5.5 per 100 patient-years without anticoagulation.[314] In 1 study, 33% of thromboemboli occurred within the first month and 66% within 12 months of the onset of atrial fibrillation.[315] Recurrent thromboemboli in patients with valvular heart disease occur at approximately 10% per year and in 30 to 75% of patients, often within the first 6 months after the initial event.[316] Mortality from recurrent emboli in patients with mitral stenosis may be as high as 42%.

Thus, primary and secondary prevention of arterial embolism in such high-risk patients should be at a higher level of anticoagulation (INR 3.0 to 4.5), which can reduce the risk of thromboembolism from 5.5 to 1 per 100 patient-years.[314] The addition of aspirin can be considered in these high-risk patients. For all other patients with valvular heart disease and atrial fibrillation who are at medium risk, an INR between 2.0 and 3.0 will suffice.

#### Primary and Secondary Prevention in Patients With Nonrheumatic Atrial Fibrillation

Nonrheumatic atrial fibrillation is found in about 15% of all stroke patients and is the most common source of cardiogenic embolism to the brain. Among these patients, the risk of embolism is around 5 to 10% per year. The stroke recurrence rate varies between 2 and 15% in the first year, and 5% yearly thereafter, with a mortality rate of 5% per year.[317] This incidence is about 5 to 7 times that in a general population of comparable age and gender.

In the primary prevention of cerebral embolism in nonrheumatic atrial fibrillation, the superiority of oral anticoagulant therapy (INR 1.5 to 3.5) over placebo was demonstrated in 5 prospective trials which showed that the annual incidence of stroke was reduced from 5% to about 2%.[318] An even lower intensity of anticoagulation (INR 1.2 to 1.5) significantly reduced the annual incidence of cerebral infarction from 4.3% (placebo group) to 0.9% (warfarin group).[319] Aspirin is also effective, particularly in patients under the age of 75 years of age who are free of clinical and echographic risk factors.[320,321]

In a study of the secondary prevention of stroke in patients with nonrheumatic atrial fibrillation, in which patients with a recent transient ischaemic attack or minor stroke were randomised to open anticoagulant therapy (target INR 2.5 to 4.0) or double-blind treatment with either aspirin (300mg) or placebo, the annual rate of outcome events over a mean follow-up period of 2.3 years was 8% in patients assigned to anticoagulants, 15% in aspirin-treated patients and 19% in placebo patients.[322] Anticoagulant therapy was significantly more effective than aspirin. The incidence of major bleeding was low, both on anticoagulants (2.8% per year) and on aspirin (0.9% per year). Thus, patients with nonrheumatic atrial fibrillation and recent neurological symptoms should be treated with oral anticoagulants.

#### Secondary Prevention of Transient Ischaemic Attacks

A meta-analysis of 7 controlled studies with antiplatelet agents in patients with transient ischaemic attacks showed a significant risk reduction of 40 to 90% in recurrent transient ischaemic attacks, stroke or death.[323] In 2 of these trials, the combination of dipyridamole and aspirin did not prove superior to aspirin alone. A more recent, broader meta-analysis of antiplatelet therapy in survivors of a transient ischaemic attack, stroke, unstable angina or myocardial infarction showed that the incidence of nonfatal stroke was reduced by 25%, that of nonfatal myocardial infarction by 25%, and that of vascular mortality by 17%.[287]

A trial comparing ticlopidine (500mg daily) with aspirin (1300mg daily) in 3069 patients with a transient ischaemic attack or very minor and rapidly regressive stroke revealed a 3-year risk reduction in fatal and nonfatal stroke for ticlopidine in comparison with aspirin of 21%.[324] However, ticlopidine was associated with more adverse effects.

Thus, aspirin and ticlopidine appear to be efficacious in reducing fatal and nonfatal stroke in patients who have had a transient ischaemic attack. Anticoagulant therapy is an option in patients who continue to have symptoms despite antiplatelet therapy.[325]

#### Secondary Prevention of Ischaemic Stroke

Survivors of thromboembolic stroke have a 25% risk of recurrence of stroke, myocardial infarction or vascular death over the ensuing 2 years.[326] Secondary prevention is therefore important in these patients. At least 10 clinical studies of aspirin in patients with transient ischaemic attack or minor stroke have been reported,[327] in all but 2 of which, a statistically significant benefit of aspirin was demonstrated. A meta-analysis of trials of antiplatelet therapy in patients with transient ischaemic attacks, minor or major stroke, unstable angina, or myocardial infarction suggests that antiplatelet drugs reduce vascular mortality by 15% and nonfatal events, such as myocardial infarction and stroke, by 22%.[288,328] The dose of aspirin used in most trials ranged from 325 to 1300 mg/day. In studies with lower doses, a Swedish trial comparing aspirin 75 mg/day *versus* placebo revealed a significant 18% decrease in stroke or death with aspirin,[329] while a Dutch trial found no differences in the primary endpoints of vascular deaths, stroke or myocardial infarction between aspirin doses of 30 and 283 mg/day.[330] Although no definite data are available to indicate whether a low (50mg), medium (300mg) or high (1000mg) dose of aspirin is to be preferred in terms of efficacy, the higher dose is associated with more adverse effects.

In the second European Stroke Prevention Study, dipyridamole (sustained-release, 200mg twice daily) and aspirin (25mg twice daily) was studied in a factorial and blinded design in 6602 survivors of an ischaemic cerebrovascular accident. There was little effect on total mortality with either drug, or their combination. However, a significant risk reduction for strokes with aspirin and dipyridamole compared with placebo was noted (18% and 16%, respectively). The combination of the two drugs yielded a significant risk reduction for stroke recurrence of 37%, indicating an additive effect.

A 3-year study comparing ticlopidine (250mg twice daily) with placebo in 1072 patients who had suffered a thromboembolic stroke between 1 week and 4 months before selection showed a risk reduction with ticlopidine of 24% for stroke, myocardial infarction or vascular death.[331]

Thus, in patients with completed stroke, treatment with aspirin or ticlopidine is effective for prevention of vascular death, further stroke and, in some studies, myocardial infarction as well. The usefulness of anticoagulant therapy in atherothrombotic stroke remains questionable and is only recommended for patients with embolic stroke from a cardiac source.

#### Prevention of Disease Progression and Thrombotic Complications in Patients with Obliterative Disease in Limb Arteries

Since thrombosis of atherosclerotic arteries is only the final step in a long process, long term oral anticoagulant therapy is unlikely to represent a major advance in the pharmacological prevention of progression of peripheral arterial occlusive disease. In a placebo-controlled study of the value of oral anticoagulants in patients with intermittent claudication, no benefit in terms of total mortality was found, although there was a lower incidence of vascular events (peripheral, cerebrovascular, cardiovascular) in patients receiving anticoagulants.[332]

There is angiographic evidence that aspirin and ticlopidine retard the progression of atherosclerosis and the occurrence of its thrombotic complications in the legs of patients with obstructive arterial disease.[333] A meta-analysis of 4 placebo-controlled trials with ticlopidine in patients with claudication showed not only a decreased incidence of vascular events with this drug, but also an improvement in walking distance. A decreased mortality and less cardiovascular complications in claudicating patients treated with ticlopidine was reported in another study.[334]

#### Prevention of Postoperative Deep Venous Thrombosis

The incidence of postoperative proximal deep venous thrombosis (DVT) in the limbs and pelvis is estimated to be 0.4% in low-risk patients (uncomplicated surgery in patients under 40 years of age with no other risk factors for venous thromboembolism), 2 to 8% in moderately high-risk patients (surgery in patients over 40 years of age lasting at least 30 minutes), and 10 to 20% in high-risk patients (major surgery in patients over 40 years of age plus previous DVT, pulmonary embolism, or any orthopaedic surgery) [table VIII].[335]

Leg elevation, early ambulation, and graduated compression stockings can provide effective prevention in low-risk patients. *'Miniheparin'* prevention is a term applied to subcutaneous administration of a fixed dose of 5000U of concentrated heparin (20,000 to 25,000 U/ml) every 8 to 12 hours. Numerous well-conducted trials with objective diagnostic end-points have established the efficacy of *'miniheparin'* therapy in the prevention of DVT and pulmonary

**Table VIII.** Risk categories of deep vein thrombosis in surgical patients

| Patients | Risk of calf vein thrombosis | Risk of proximal vein thrombosis | Risk of fatal pulmonary embolism |
|---|---|---|---|
| **High risk:** | 40-80% | 10-20% | 1-5% |
| • General and urological surgery in patients >40 years with recent history of DVT or PE | | | |
| • Extensive pelvic or abdominal surgery for malignant disease | | | |
| • Major orthopaedic surgery of lower limbs | | | |
| • Gynaecological patients >40 years with history of DVT, PE or with cancer | | | |
| **Moderate risk:** | 10-40% | 2-8% | 0.1-0.7% |
| • General surgery in patients >40 years lasting >30 minutes and patients <40 years on oral contraceptives | | | |
| **Low risk** | <10% | <0.4% | <0.01% |
| • Uncomplicated surgery in patients <40 years without additional risk factors | | | |
| • Minor surgery (<30 minutes) in patients without additional risk factors | | | |

*Abbreviations:* DVT = deep venous thrombosis; PE = pulmonary embolism.

embolism in patients at medium thrombotic risk.[164] For this purpose, the first dose of heparin is usually given 2 hours before surgery. An injection of unfractionated heparin every 8 hours is associated with a slightly higher but still acceptable rate of bleeding complications compared with a scheme of injections given at 12-hourly intervals. With antiplatelet therapy, an odds reduction of 39% with aspirin has been reported in a meta-analysis.[288]

In high-risk patients, including those with fractures or undergoing elective operations of the hip, open urological operations, gynaecological malignancy, and major amputation, a fixed dose of 5000U heparin given at 8-hourly intervals is not sufficient. In such patients, the dose of subcutaneous heparin should be monitored in order to maintain the APTT at around 50 to 70 seconds, which improves prophylaxis but not at the cost of increased postoperative bleeding. The addition of *dihydroergotamine* 0.5mg to each 5000U of unfractionated heparin results in greater antithrombotic protection, and this is also the case in patients undergoing traumatic or elective orthopaedic surgery, even if the dose is reduced to 2500U.[336] Dihydroergotamine increases the sympathetic tone in veins and the venous flow rates in the legs and pelvis region. The greater efficacy of the combination of heparin and dihydroergotamine compared with heparin alone could therefore be due to an accelerated venous return, although there are other possible explanations. The use of dihydroergotamine may, however, occasionally result in leg ischaemia due to arterial spasm, especially in patients with major trauma, obstructive arterial disease and during pregnancy. In these patients, the risk outweighs the potential benefit.

In recent years, a number of clinical trials have established that *low molecular weight (LMW) heparins* given subcutaneously once or twice daily offer better protection against distal and proximal DVT and pulmonary embolism than subcutaneous unfractionated heparin in orthopaedic surgery[337] and in other patients at high thrombotic risk.[163] Dosages of the various LMW heparins are given in table I.

Antithrombotic prophylaxis is usually discontinued at hospital discharge, although the thromboembolic risk persists for some weeks. In a double-blind study conducted in patients discharged 14 days after total hip replacement with a normal bilateral phlebogram, a second phlebogram 3 weeks later revealed a 19% incidence of deep venous thrombosis in patients receiving a placebo and a 7% incidence in patients on continued low molecular weight heparin (40mg enoxaparin twice daily), a significant reduction of 63%.[338]

*Oral anticoagulants* are effective in preventing venous thrombosis after hip surgery and major gynaecological surgery when used at a targeted INR of 2.0 to 3.0, both when started before surgery or on the first postoperative day.[339,340] The bleeding risk is relatively small with this low-intensity treatment but warfarin treatment is more complicated than fixed-dose low molecular weight heparin.[175]

*Hirudin:* a recent double-blind trial with recombinant hirudin *versus* unfractionated heparin indicated that hirudin is significantly more effective in reducing proximal deep vein thrombosis after elective hip surgery than heparin.[341]

#### Prevention of Deep Venous Thrombosis During Pregnancy

Women who may become pregnant and who need prolonged oral anticoagulant therapy should be placed on minidoses of heparin. This is because of the teratogenic effects of warfarin (and other coumarin derivatives) which should not be given during the first trimester. Also, from week 36 onwards, unfractionated heparin or LMW heparin should again be used for prophylaxis since they do not cross the placenta. The dose of subcutaneous heparin should be adjusted and given 12-hourly until term. The dose of LMW heparin may differ among the various forms.[211]

#### Prevention of Deep Venous Thrombosis in Bedridden Patients

Low-dose heparin prophylaxis is often recommended for patients with severe heart failure as well as for paralysed patients. Compared with placebo, low molecular weight heparins produce a relative risk reduction in positive fibrinogen leg scanning of 40 to 86%; this effect is not associated with an increased incidence of bleeding.

#### Treatment of Established Deep Venous Thrombosis

Heparin is the initial and essential treatment for all recent proximal vein thromboses not treated with thrombolytic agents. The treatment of calf vein thrombosis is controversial because only 20% extend into proximal venous segments and they are rarely associated with major pulmonary embolism (provided they remain confined to the calf). Proximal extension of calf vein thrombosis can be investigated with non-invasive tests. If this monitoring is unavailable, all venous thromboses, irrespective of their site, should be treated with heparin. A bolus injection of 5000U of unfractionated heparin is given initially, followed by a constant maintenance infusion of approximately 30,000U per 24 hours. A more optimal method is to adapt the dosage to bodyweight (i.e. 15 to 20U heparin/kg/h). If administered subcutaneously, the usual dose is 17,500U every 12 hours. The APTT at 6 hours should be between 1.5 and 2.5 times control.

Based on several randomised and objectively documented clinical trials, it appears that a fixed dose of unfractionated heparin, administered by the subcutaneous route, is at least as effective and safe as a continuous intravenous infusion of unfractionated heparin for the initial treatment of established deep venous thrombosis.[342] The time honoured practice of using a 7- to 10-day course of heparin with a 4- to 5-day overlap with oral anticoagulants has now been superseded by a short course of heparin (4 to 5 days).[343] Low molecular weight (LMW) heparins have also been given intravenously, and seem to be as effective as unfractionated heparin. LMW heparins have been used safely and effectively to treat patients with proximal deep vein thromboses both in hospital and at home.[344-346]

To prevent a recurrence of venous thrombosis, oral anticoagulants are usually given for 3 to 6 months or longer in those with persisting risk factors. A practical alternative is adjusted-dose prophylaxis with subcutaneous unfractionated heparin.[343] This preventive measure is associated with a lower risk of bleeding than oral anticoagulation given at doses producing an INR of 3.0 to 4.5.

#### Treatment of Acute Pulmonary Embolism

For acute pulmonary embolism, an initial bolus injection of 10,000 to 20,000U unfractionated heparin followed by 30,000 to 40,000U per 24 hours should be given as soon as the diagnosis is suspected. For medium-sized pulmonary emboli without haemodynamic disturbance, this is the treatment of choice, supplemented by investigation of the peripheral veins.[347] Prior to discharge, the patient should be switched to oral anticoagulants for 3 to 6 months to prevent further embolism.

For patients with a massive embolus and lasting haemodynamic effects, the choice is between surgical embolectomy and thrombolytic therapy (see section 3.2.2 below). While awaiting surgery, thrombolytic and anticoagulant treatment should be started, especially in patients with underlying cardiac or respiratory disease.

### *3.2.2 Clinical Indications for Thrombolytic Agents*

#### Treatment of Acute Myocardial Infarction

A collaborative overview of placebo-controlled trials of intravenous thrombolytic therapy, encompassing more than 60,000 patients[348] has clearly shown that thrombolytic therapy is beneficial in all patients with suspected myocardial infarction admitted to hospital within 12 hours of the onset of symptoms and ST segment elevations or bundle branch block on the electrocardiogram. Overall mortality rates at 5 weeks were significantly lower at 10.1% in the thrombolysis group *versus* 13.0% in the control group, an absolute difference of 2.9%.

The equal outcome reported with different thrombolytic agents (i.e. streptokinase, alteplase and anistreplase) in the GISSI-2[349] and ISIS-3[350] trials, despite the differences between these agents in speed of coronary recanalisation, appeared to challenge the importance of early reperfusion as the principal mechanism by which thrombolytic agents produce their effects. However, the results of the GUSTO-1 trial[253,351] have resolved many uncertainties. In this multicentre trial, standard treatment (1.5MU streptokinase over 60 minutes plus aspirin and fixed-dose subcutaneous heparin) was compared with 3 more aggressive strategies:

1) 'Front loaded' weight-adjusted alteplase (≤100mg over 90 minutes plus concomitant intravenous heparin and aspirin).

2) 1.5MU streptokinase over 60 minutes plus concomitant intravenous heparin and aspirin.

3) Combination therapy with weight-adjusted alteplase (≤90mg over 60 minutes) plus streptokinase (1.0MU over 60 minutes) plus concomitant intravenous heparin and aspirin.

In the 3 arms in which intravenous heparin was used, the infusion rates were adjusted to keep the activated partial thromboplastin time (APTT) between 60 to 85 seconds. A 30-day mortality rate of 6.3% was observed with front loaded alteplase as compared with 7.2% for streptokinase plus subcutaneous heparin, 7.4% for streptokinase plus intravenous heparin, and 7.0% for the thrombolytic drug combination plus intravenous heparin. This represented a significant 14% reduction in mortality for front loaded alteplase as compared with the 2 streptokinase-only strategies. This survival benefit for the front loaded alteplase regimen was consistently observed across different subgroups and seemed to be related to the faster recanalisation of the infarct-related vessel, as shown in the GUSTO angiographic substudy confirming the link between early reperfusion and survival.[351]

Since no significant difference in clinical outcome was observed between the 2 streptokinase-only arms in GUSTO and since neither the GISSI-2 nor ISIS-3 trials showed any additional benefit when heparin was added to streptokinase plus aspirin, there appears to be no need to give concomitant heparin if streptokinase is chosen as the thrombolytic agent.

In a recent study with *reteplase*, a variant of t-PA with a longer half-life, the same mortality at 35 days was obtained as with streptokinase (9.0% *versus* 9.5%), with a stroke rate of 1.2% and 1.0%, respectively.[352]

#### Treatment of Peripheral Arterial Occlusions

Removal of the occluding fibrin mass with a Fogarty catheter, usually under local anaesthesia, is the first and fastest therapeutic approach in acute arterial thromboembolic occlusion. However, the short and long term success rate of thromboembolectomy in an atherosclerotic artery is considerably lower than that for an arterial embolus in a healthy artery. Moreover, embolectomy with a Fogarty catheter is less often successful in arteries distal to the popliteal artery or when treatment is delayed for 24 hours. If active removal of the occlusion by means of a Fogarty catheter fails or is not feasible, thrombolytic therapy may be considered.

***Systemic administration of thrombolytic drugs:*** the ability of thrombolytic drugs to restore blood flow in acutely occluded leg arteries seems to depend on the delay between the acute event and the initiation of treatment. Intravenous streptokinase (500,000U loading dose over 15 minutes followed by 100,000 U/h) and urokinase (4400 U/kg over 10 minutes followed by 4400 U/kg/h for 12 to 24 hours) clear 70 to 80% of occlusions treated within 12 hours and 25 to 60% when the treatment is delayed for up to 3 to 5 days. Iliac or femoral artery occlusions older than 3 months have a much lower success rate.[299,353] More recently, short-term ultra-high streptokinase treatment has been advocated in acute and chronic peripheral arterial occlusion. Over a period of 6 hours, 9MU streptokinase is infused intravenously and the same 6-hour infusion is repeated on subsequent days until satisfactory recanalisation is obtained. In a clinical trial, the success rate of this treatment was between 50 and 60% with the best results in femoral artery occlusions. The treatment was well tolerated, although 5 cerebral haemorrhages were encountered in 585 patients.[354]

Overall, however, these results are not very encouraging and most clinicians have abandoned systemic thrombolysis in favour of local catheter-directed infusion of thrombolytic agents (see below).

***Local or regional intra-arterial administration of thrombolytic drugs:*** with this technique, as in percutaneous transluminal coronary angioplasty (PTCA), a suitable catheter is introduced into the occluded vessel for local delivery of the thrombolytic agent. The catheter is inserted close to the proximal part of the occluding thrombus; a more aggressive technique is to perforate the thrombus with the guide wire or to push the tip of the catheter into the thrombus.

Several therapeutic regimens have been tried, but basically they fall into 1 of 2 types:

1) Repeated intrathrombotic 'pulsed' injections, e.g. 1000 to 3000U streptokinase delivered into the thrombus every 5 to 15 minutes. Between infiltrations, the catheter is advanced step by step under fluoroscopy with or without a guide wire. The procedure is continued until the thrombus is completely infiltrated and the open distal lumen is reached.[355] The mechanical effect of the catheter movement may add to the thrombolytic effect.

2) Continuous infusion of streptokinase 5000 U/h administered with the aid of an arterial infusion pump.[356] This regimen has proved more popular. In some centres, an initial bolus injection of 20,000U or an initial rapid infusion of 2000 U/min for 20 minutes has been given.[357] The duration of treatment is determined by the individual patient's response. For a recent thrombus, an infusion of limited duration (up to a few hours) may suffice to obtain complete lysis, but an extended occlusion occasionally requires several days to clear. Apart from clinical evaluation and noninvasive testing, progression of clot lysis is followed by fluoroscopy or angiography via the catheter every 12 to 24 hours or earlier if rapid clearance is anticipated. As soon as evidence for partial clot lysis is obtained, the catheter can be advanced into the proximal edge of the remaining clot and the infusion is continued. Thrombolytic treatment is considered to have failed, and is normally stopped, if no lysis is observed after 24 to 48 hours.

A frequently used dosage scheme for the local delivery of urokinase is 240,000 U/h for 1 to 2 hours, reduced to 120,000 U/h for the next 1 to 2 hours, and then 60,000 U/h until completion.[358] Local alteplase is often given in a dose of 0.05 mg/kg/h for 4 to 8 hours.

***Intraoperative use of thrombolytic agents:*** urgent surgical bypass is the conventional treatment in many cases of extensive thrombosis of a distal artery, but the operations are long and complex. In cases of incomplete operative thromboembolectomy or of surgical bypass with thrombotic occlusion of runoff vessels, thrombolysis may be an excellent conjunctive therapy.[359] A short infusion of a thrombolytic drug given intraoperatively has proved safe and effective in restoring patency. The technique entails instilling 100,000U of streptokinase into the distal vessels over 30 minutes. The streptokinase is mixed in 60ml isotonic saline and infused through a catheter with a syringe driver set at 99 ml/h and the arterial inflow clamped. Alternatively, the streptokinase may be mixed in 100ml isotonic saline and given in five 20ml boluses at 5-minute intervals. In cases of femoropopliteal bypass, the proximal anastomosis can be completed while the infusion is still running. The technique can be used during explorations of either the femoral or popliteal artery. When used after failed femoral embolectomy, it has the advantage of avoiding the need for direct popliteal artery exploration.

There is little alteration in coagulation, and bleeding is unusual even if fasciotomy is subsequently necessary. Other thrombolytic agents such as urokinase and alteplase may be used, and indeed lysis may be faster with the latter drug.[360]

### Treatment of Acute Ischaemic Stroke

An analysis of 6 randomised trials of thrombolysis in acute ischaemic stroke conducted prior to 1992 yielded contradictory results. However, if 2 trials conducted without CT scanning before inclusion are excluded, the results point to a 37% reduction in the odds of death (not significant) and a significant reduction of 56% in the odds of death or deterioration after thrombolytic treatment. There is no evidence for an excess risk of haemorrhagic transformation of the cerebral ischaemic infarct or of severe oedema formation.[317]

The recent trial of the National Institute of Neurological Disorders and Stroke (NINDS) rt-PA Stroke Study Group[361] is an important step forward in the treatment of stroke. Patients with symptoms of cerebral ischaemia in the area of the anterior or posterior circulation were randomly assigned to receive intravenous alteplase or placebo if they arrived at the hospital within 3 hours of the onset of symptoms. The alteplase group had significant improvement in neurological outcome at 3 months, including residual neurological deficit as scored on the National Institute of Health stroke scale (NIHSS) and 3 measures of disability of functional outcome (the modified Rankin scale, Barthel index, and Glasgow outcome scale), with no net change in mortality.

Measures of activities of daily living are useful in describing the functional status of a patient, whereas mortality may be a less useful outcome in studies of stroke. The NINDS study and the European Cooperative Acute Stroke Study (ECASS)[362] – another randomised, placebo-controlled trial of intravenous alteplase in ischaemic stroke in which patients were treated within 6 hours of the onset of symptoms – highlight 2 approaches to the assessment of outcomes and the question of their validity. Both studies assessed the efficacy of thrombolytic treatment with outcome measures not yet validated in either study. The Barthel index has a U-shaped distribution among patients with stroke, with values ranging from zero (complete disability or death) to 100 (complete independence). The investigators in the NINDS study dichotomised all outcomes and focused their analysis on the number or patients with minimal or no disability, whereas in the ECASS analysis, shifts in median scores were examined. In the intention-to-treat analysis, the ECASS investigators found no benefit of alteplase in median scores on the Barthel index or the modified Rankin scale.

In a subsequent analysis in which 109 patients with protocol violations were excluded, the alteplase group had an improvement of 1 unit in the median score and an absolute increase of 11.7% in the number of patients with Rankin scores of zero or 1 (indicating a more favourable outcome). This mirrors the improvement of 11 to 12% in the number of patients with the best outcomes on each test in the NINDS study. However, the ECASS results are more difficult to interpret. For instance, it is not clear what a shift of 1 unit in the median score may mean for the individual patient. Also, these scales have not yet been completely validated for use in patients with acute stroke.

#### Treatment of Retinal Artery or Vein Occlusion

A thromboembolic occlusion of the central retinal artery is abrupt; thus the duration of occlusion can easily be determined as is the case in ischaemic stroke. However, treatment with thrombolytic drugs, even when started within a few hours of the onset of visual symptoms, has yielded poor results.[363,364]

#### Treatment of Lower Limb Deep Venous Thrombosis

In deep venous thrombosis of the legs, thrombolytic therapy is more effective than heparin in producing thrombus clearance, particularly in patients with symptoms of less than 7 days' duration and with more extensive involvement. In an analysis of 9 studies involving 297 patients, substantial phlebographic improvement was noted in 45% treated with streptokinase, and 61% showed either substantial or partial improvement. In contrast, only 5% of patients treated with heparin alone showed substantial improvement and 25% substantial or partial improvement.[365] A meta-analysis of 6 randomised trials of streptokinase and heparin treatment showed that a reduction in clot mass was achieved 3.7 times more often by thrombolytic therapy than by heparin but the major bleeding rate was 2.9 times greater. Similar degrees of lysis are obtained with the use of alteplase or urokinase.[366] Responsiveness to thrombolysis may be influenced by age and extent of thrombus, degree of venous obstruction, and local concentration of the thrombolytic agent.

The usual dose of streptokinase for the treatment of deep venous thrombosis is a loading dose of 250,000U administered over 10 minutes followed by a maintenance dose of 100,000 MU/h for up to 4 to 6 days. Alternatively, daily intermittent infusions of 1.5 MU/h for 6 hours may be used.[367] The regimen for urokinase is an initial loading dose of 4400 U/kg over 10 minutes followed by 4400 U/kg/h for several days, but the optimum dose of urokinase is not yet established as similar results were obtained with 4 different regimens varying from 1500 to 4000 U/kg/h given over 2 to 7 days.[368]

Uncertainty also prevails over the optimum dosage regimen of alteplase. A dose of 0.5 mg/kg over 4 hours results in significant lysis in 50% of patients; in contrast, high-dose (50 to 100mg in 4 to 8 hours) infusions over 1 to 2 days have yielded limited success.[369-371] A continuous infusion of alteplase in low dosages (0.25 *vs* 0.5 mg/kg/24h) over 3 to 7 days has also given disappointing results.[372]

#### Treatment of Acute Pulmonary Embolism

***Acute massive pulmonary embolism with life-threatening haemodynamic impairment:*** in a limited number of cases with acute massive pulmonary emboli and hypotension or shock, death does not occur within the first hours and vigorous treatment should be started immediately. If the unconscious cyanotic patient develops cardiac arrest, heart massage and artificial respiration will be required to save his/her life. Immediate thrombolytic therapy with urokinase 30,000 U/kg, streptokinase 3MU or alteplase 50mg should be administered over 10 minutes into a peripheral vein while the patient is transferred for pulmonary embolectomy.[373,374] Vasopressor agents such as adrenaline (epinephrine) should be given simultaneously. The clinical response may be rapid and dramatic. Most patients who can tolerate a 50% occlusion of the pulmonary artery are able to survive with aggressive medical therapy, including thrombolysis. Nevertheless, some continue to deteriorate, particularly those with previously compromised heart or lung pathology despite thrombolysis, respiratory support and inotropic drugs. In these patients, pulmonary embolectomy under total cardiopulmonary bypass should be performed urgently. The use of a membrane oxygenator may improve the outcome in some patients.

***Rapidly evolving major pulmonary embolism of haemodynamic importance:*** in patients with major acute pulmonary embolism associated with serious haemodynamic disturbance, thrombolytic therapy can be life-saving. The initial study demonstrating the effectiveness of intravenous alteplase in treating patients with major pulmonary embolism and compromised haemodynamics[375] was followed by a subsequent study indicating that direct infusion of alteplase into the pulmonary artery does not offer a significant benefit over the systemic intravenous route and that a prolonged infusion of alteplase over 7 hours (100mg) is superior to a single infusion of 50mg over 2 hours.[376] A comparison of urokinase (4400 U/kg as a bolus, followed by 4400 U/kg/h over 12 hours) *versus* alteplase (10mg as a bolus, followed by 90mg over 2 hours) followed by heparin showed that at 2 hours, total pulmonary resistance was decreased significantly less in the urokinase group (18 ± 22%) than in the alteplase group (36 ± 17%).[377] Continuous monitoring of pulmonary artery mean pressure, cardiac index and total pulmonary resistance revealed that these variables improved faster in the alteplase group with consistently significant intergroup differences from 30 minutes up to 3 to 4 hours. After 12 hours, the reduction of the angiographic severity score was 30 ± 25% with urokinase compared with 24 ± 18% with alteplase.

An accelerated infusion of urokinase (1MU bolus followed by 3MU over 2 hours) has similar efficacy and safety to 100mg alteplase administered over 2 hours.[378]

#### Treatment of Occluded Arteriovenous Fistulae or Hickman Catheters

In patients with occluded arteriovenous fistulae or occluded Hickman catheters, a local infusion of a thrombolytic agent is usually sufficient to clear the thrombotic obstruction. Doses of 5000 to 10,000 U/h streptokinase or up to 20,000 U/h urokinase are the usual regimens used for this indication.

## 3.3 Clinical Outcome and Economic Considerations

### *3.3.1 Nonrheumatic Atrial Fibrillation*

Long term therapy with warfarin in this condition is superior to aspirin in patients over the age of 75 years and in those with concomitant risk factors for thromboembolic events (hypertension, congestive heart failure, previous thromboembolic event);[379] however, the risk of intracranial bleeding in older patients is greater with warfarin. In patients less than 75 years of age and with no risk factors, aspirin and warfarin are comparable. Treating a patient with warfarin costs US$840 more than no anticoaguation, but yields an additional 0.49 quality-adjusted life expectancy resulting in a marginal cost utility of roughly US$1700/QALY (quality-adjusted life year).[380] Aspirin is the least expensive strategy, with an average discounted lifetime cost of US$8500, yet it is more effective than no anticoagulant therapy. Over a lifetime, oral anticoagulant therapy costs on average US$2200 more than aspirin but results in an average gain of only 0.12 QALYs.[381]

### *3.3.2 Valvular Heart Disease*

In this condition, cost utility for a 35-year-old woman with mitral stenosis and atrial fibrillation has been analysed. Assuming a life expectancy of 32 years (*versus* 41 years without mitral stenosis) and emboli and bleeding rates of 4.7% and 0.05%, respectively, without anticoagulant therapy, and 1.7% and 4.5%, respectively with anticoagulant therapy, cost utility was US$3100/QALY (undiscounted) and US$4200/ QALY discounted. It was also US$3100/QALY with an assumption of 2% bleeding with anticoagulants. With previous emboli, events were assumed to occur at a rate of 9.5%/year, and cost utility was US$1800/QALY. For the same patient, with mitral stenosis and normal sinus rhythm (emboli 1.4% year), cost utility was much higher, i.e. US$174,100/QALY.[382] When the risk of emboli decreased to below 2% per year, cost utility soared, but when the risk decreased to below 1.3%, results did not, according to this analysis, justify its use – a finding with implications for mitral stenosis and normal sinus rhythm and for mitral valve prolapse where the embolism rate is at very low levels.[383,384]

#### 3.3.3 Ischaemic Stroke Prevention

A statistical overview conducted by the Antiplatelet Trialists' Collaboration of randomised clinical trials of antiplatelet therapy in the prevention of stroke showed that allocation to antiplatelet therapy was associated with a 27% reduction in the relative odds of stroke, and a 15% reduction in the relative odds of vascular death in patients presenting with prior stroke, transient ischaemic attacks (TIAs), unstable angina or myocardial infarction.[288,328] The data from these overviews have been used to calculate the cost effectiveness of antiplatelet therapy in secondary prevention of stroke in patients with acute myocardial infarction, unstable angina, prior stroke/TIA, and prior myocardial infarction. Direct medical costs were considered from a UK perspective and included the costs of therapy, adverse effects and nonfatal strokes prevented, while effectiveness was measured in terms of life-years free of vascular death or stroke. Cost-effectiveness ratios ranged from £240 to £3000 (1991 prices) per year of life gained over a treatment period of 2 years. Antiplatelet therapy would therefore seem to be a very cost effective means of preventing stroke in high-risk individuals.[385]

#### 3.3.4 Acute Myocardial Infarction

To save 1 year of life in patients with acute myocardial infarction, the costs of thrombolytic therapy using intravenous streptokinase, alteplase (rt-PA) or anistreplase under standard restricted indications criteria, has been found to vary from £1000 to £1700 in the UK, SEK3090 to SEK9660 in Scandinavia, and US$3500 to $800,000 in the US, depending on the time delay in starting treatment after pain onset, infarct size, thrombolytic agent used, study methodology, clinical events considered in cost counting, and the discount rate applied.[386] Economic assessments confirm that thrombolytic treatment of the elderly (>70 years) is as cost effective as treatment of younger patients and that both early and late thrombolytic therapy (given 6 to 12 hours after infarction) are beneficial and cost effective. However, there are major logistical problems with prehospital thrombolysis, which despite great initial enthusiasm, is unlikely to be cost effective in saving lives unless savings in time are greater than 1 hour.

The superiority of alteplase, particularly when administered in an accelerated manner, in achieving more rapid coronary artery patency than streptokinase, anistreplase and urokinase has been reported in a number of clinical trials. On the basis of survival data from the GUSTO trial, the cost-effectiveness value for the routine use of the accelerated regimen of alteplase rather than streptokinase is US$32,678 per year of life saved.[387] Cumulative 1-year costs for hospital services, thrombolytic agents and physician fees were higher after treatment with alteplase than streptokinase but alteplase recipients also had a significantly lower mortality rate than patients who received streptokinase. No difference in patient quality of life was evident on the basis of treatment with either drug 1 year after treatment. Alteplase was more cost effective in patients with anterior rather than inferior infarctions and in older rather than in younger patients.

#### 3.3.5 Prevention of Deep Venous Thrombosis

Prevention of deep venous thrombosis with low-dose, unfractionated heparin is relatively inexpensive and the advantage of subcutaneous injections over intravenous infusions of unfractionated heparin are obvious. The practical convenience of a single subcutaneous injection of a low molecular weight (LMW) heparin for the prevention (and also treatment) of deep venous thrombosis has to be taken into consideration. The clinical effectiveness of LMW heparins, and their low bleeding incidences and safety without laboratory monitoring have to be balanced against their higher cost compared with unfractionated heparin.

## 4. Bleeding Disorders

Effective treatment of the numerous bleeding disorders depends on accurate diagnosis. A haemorrhagic tendency can be due to an abnormality of any of the 3 major components of the haemostatic mechanism – vascular defects, platelet abnormality or clotting factor deficiency – and can be congenital or acquired. Bleeding following surgery or trauma is most often directly attributable to injury of blood vessels and is not, or only to a very small extent, influenced by systemic treatment with drugs. The treatment of a patient with a defect of the haemostatic mechanism is very specific and is determined by the nature of the defect and its pathogenesis.[388] A precise diagnosis is therefore essential; however, the variety of causes of abnormal bleeding requires a large range of laboratory procedures.

### 4.1 Clinical Pharmacology of Drugs Used in Treatment

Many agents are available for the treatment of specific types of bleeding, but none of these is a haemostatic substance in the strict sense of the term. For instance, ascorbic acid (vitamin C) is a most effective drug in the treatment of scurvy, a bleeding disorder which in most countries is limited to extreme dietary deficiency (e.g. bottle-fed infants and elderly men living alone), but it is of no value in all the other bleeding disorders for which it is prescribed. The same holds true for the practice of giving vitamin K to patients with a normal prothrombin level. However, when topical measures are not feasible or are inadequate, and no specific treatment is available, synthetic haemostatic drugs may be used, usually with more hope than certainty of efficacy.[389,390]

#### 4.1.1 Antifibrinolytic Drugs

A few types of blood loss can be controlled by drugs that inhibit the fibrinolytic enzyme system. Synthetic inhibitors of fibrinolysis include *ε-aminocaproic acid (EACA), tranexamic acid* and *p-aminomethyl benzoic acid (PAMBA)*. The antifibrinolytic effect of these synthetic compounds is related to a reversible complex formation with a modified plasminogen and the associated conformational changes of this proenzyme. Tranexamic acid is about 10 times more potent than ε-aminocaproic acid and it persists longer in the tissues. These drugs are also inhibitors of C1 esterase, which is deficient in patients with familial angio-oedema, who have spontaneous attacks (see chapter 17; sect. 10.4), and their use has enabled these patients to undergo dental and general surgery. For a review of the use of fibrinolysis inhibitors, see Verstraete.[391]

*Aprotinin,* a polypeptide isolated and purified from bovine lung and liver, inhibits serine proteases including plasmin and kallikrein, the proteinase which liberates vasoactive peptides from the $\alpha_2$-globulin fraction of plasma. The inhibitory effect of aprotinin is due to formation of aprotinin-proteinase complexes by the active site of the enzyme. In contrast to the above synthetic fibrinolysis inhibitors, aprotinin also has anticoagulant and vasoactive properties. In prospective controlled trials in patients undergoing repeat open heart surgery, 5 million KIU (kallikrein inhibitor units) of aprotinin (700mg) given intravenously from the start of anaesthesia to the end of the procedure has been shown to reduce the mean drainage blood loss by an average of 81%, the mean haemoglobin loss by 89%, and the blood transfusion requirement by 91% (for reviews, see Royston,[392] Lemmer et al.,[393] Green et al.[394] and Levy et al.[395]). Similar blood-saving results with aprotinin have been obtained in liver transplantation[396] and in lung transplantation.[397]

#### 4.1.2 Desmopressin (DDAVP)

This synthetic vasopressin analogue (1-desamino-8-D-arginine vasopressin) causes a 2- to 4-fold rise in factor VIII activity when given to patients with mild haemophilia A or von Willebrand's disease, and its use prior to minor surgical procedures may avoid the need for blood products. The usual dose of desmopressin is 0.3 to 0.4 μg/kg given intravenously over 15 to 30 minutes. Its effects tend to diminish with repeated administration given more frequently than every 48 hours; fluid intake may need to be adjusted to decrease the potential occurrence of fluid overload.

### 4.2 Optimum Treatment

#### 4.2.1 Congenital Bleeding Disorders

This discussion of the treatment of congenital bleeding disorders is confined to the use of drugs, including blood components, and does not deal with general measures for the prevention of bleeding.[398] Patients with a marked deficiency of a specific clotting factor tend to have delayed but persistent bleeding, even after minor injury. The aim of replacement therapy is to raise the concentration of the deficient clotting factor activity in the patient's blood to a level that will bring about haemostasis and to maintain this level until healing of the injury is adequately advanced. Additional administration of fibrinolytic inhibitors such as ε-aminocaproic acid and tranexamic acid can significantly reduce the severity of bleeding,[389] while desmopressin is an effective nontransfusional form of treatment for patients with mild haemophilia A and von Willebrand's disease.[399]

**Table IX.** Levels of factor VIII in the blood and doses of factor VIII (given as factor VIII concentrate) for treatment of various complications of haemophilia

| Complication | Level of factor VIII desirable in patient's blood immediately after transfusion | Factor VIII dose (U/kg)[a] | Duration of therapy |
|---|---|---|---|
| Spontaneous bleeding<br>Early haemarthrosis | 5-20 (0-5)[b] | 10-15 | 1-2 doses |
| Dangerous haematomas<br>Multiple dental extraction | 20-40 (5-10) | 15-30 | *Haematoma:* daily for 2-4 days; immobilise limb<br>*Dental extraction:* single dose on morning of procedure plus intravenous ε-aminocaproic acid 0.1 g/kg over 24h and also 0.1 g/kg orally 6-hourly for 7 to 10 days. For tranexamic acid: 25 mg/kg intravenously over the first day and 25 mg/kg orally 6-hourly for 7 to 10 days |
| Major surgery<br>Serious accidents | 80-100 (20-25) | 50-70 | Preoperative dose, followed by 12-hourly infusions of 30 U/kg for 6 to 10 days, then daily until wound healing well advanced |

a A unit of factor VIII is the amount of factor VIII present in 1ml of fresh average normal citrated plasma.

b The figures in parentheses are the approximate levels to which the patient's factor VIII will have fallen in 24 hours after transfusion.

### Classical Haemophilia (Haemophilia A)

Administration of human plasma or concentrates of factor VIII (AHF) is the only effective treatment of major bleeding in classical haemophilia.

Factor VIII can be purified from human plasma or it can be produced by genetic engineering.[400] The development of cryoprecipitate in the 1960s, obtained by rapid freezing and subsequent thawing of plasma, marked a turning point in haemophilia treatment: it made possible effective on-demand treatment of bleeding episodes, but was also the starting point for the development of more purified concentrates manufactured using conventional or immunoaffinity chromatography. In the 1980s, several methods to prevent the transmission of blood-borne viral infections were developed (for a review, see Kasper et al.[401]). The first study of the use of recombinant factor VIII for the treatment of haemophilia A was undertaken in 1989.[256] Since then, recombinant concentrates have proved to be safe and effective. Following transfusion, the half-life of factor VIII in the blood of a haemophiliac is about 12 hours.

Early spontaneous haemarthrosis and intramuscular haematoma will be controlled by increasing the concentration of factor VIII to 15-20% of normal, and this can be achieved with a dose of 10 to 15U of factor VIII per kg bodyweight (table IX). Severe haematomas and haemarthrosis may require factor VIII concentrations of about 20 to 30%, while concentrations of over 40% of normal are required in haemophilic patients who are to undergo major surgery (for reviews, see Mannucci;[402] and Nilson et al.[403]).

Minor surgical procedures such as dental extraction can be performed with minimal requirement of factor VIII replacement therapy, provided fibrinolytic inhibitors such as ε-aminocaproic acid (EACA) or tranexamic acid are also given both *during* (EACA 100 mg/kg/day or tranexamic acid 25mg/kg/day intravenously) and *after* the procedure (EACA 100 mg/kg 6-hourly orally or tranexamic acid 25 mg/kg 6-hourly orally) [table IX]. Tranexamic acid administration has reduced the need for factor VIII or IX concentrates by 80%, thereby avoiding the potential hazards inherent to blood products. Because of the possible complication of intrarenal obstruction, fibrinolysis inhibitors should not be given in the presence of haematuria.

A rise in factor VIII concentrations high enough to provide normal haemostasis during dental procedures or operations has been obtained with desmopressin in cases of mild haemophilia type A.[404]

Some patients with haemophilia A develop a high titre of neutralising IgG antibodies, which makes them unresponsive to treatment with normal factor VIII concentrates. Treatment of bleeding episodes in these patients requires specific treatment, i.e. porcine factor VIII,[405] large doses of concentrates of the vitamin K-dependent clotting factors that 'by-pass' the inhibitor,[406] and recombinant activated factor VII (rFVIIa).[407]

#### Christmas Disease (Haemophilia B)

The general principles of replacement of factor IX in haemophilia B are the same as for that of factor VIII in haemophilia A. The same level of the missing coagulation factor is required for haemostasis in similar clinical situations (see table IX).

The first factor IX concentrates developed for clinical use contained other vitamin K-dependent clotting factors (prothrombin, factor VII and factor X) and are often referred to as 'prothrombin complex concentrates' (PCCs). However, a rather high incidence of thrombotic complications was noted, especially in patients receiving large, repeated doses of PCCs. More recently, purified factor IX concentrates have become available, which seem to be free of thromboembolic complications (for a review, see Thompson[408]).

The half-life of factor IX in the blood is 18 to 36 hours but the *in vivo* recovery is less complete than after factor VIII administration in haemophilia A, a finding that has still not been satisfactory explained. It is assumed that because of its smaller molecular weight, factor IX is distributed throughout the intravascular and extravascular fluid spaces (which are 2 to 7 times larger than the plasma volume), whereas factor VIII is largely retained within the circulation.

As in classical haemophilia, the amount of factor IX required by transfusion in dental surgery can be reduced by the concomitant use of ε-aminocaproic acid.

#### von Willebrand's Disease

This disease is a heterogeneous bleeding disorder that results from a quantitative or qualitative defect of the von Willebrand factor (vWF). This large, multimeric protein is required for the normal adhesion of platelets to the vessel wall, and it is a carrier and stabilising protein for factor VIII. Due to this latter function, a decrease in vWF is accompanied by a proportionally low factor VIII concentration. The inheritance pattern is generally autosomal dominant (the gene for vWF has been located on chromosome 12); some of the most severe forms are inherited in an autosomal recessive way (for a review, see Ginsburg and Bowie[409]).

The treatment of choice in most types of von Willebrand's disease is desmopressin, provided its effect has been verified by giving a test infusion. Patients unresponsive to desmopressin or requiring long term correction of haemostasis can be treated with cryoprecipitate, or more recently with virus-inactivated plasma concentrates specifically enriched in von Willebrand factor (for a review, see Rodeghiero et al.[410]).

#### Congenital Afibrinogenaemia

Effective haemostasis in this condition is usually obtained by raising the concentration of fibrinogen to 100mg per 100ml plasma. This level is easily obtained with 4g of commercial fibrinogen preparations. The half-life of fibrinogen in the blood is about 4 days so that injection of 1 or 2g every second day is usually satisfactory (table X).

#### Congenital Deficiency of Factors II, VII and X

These somewhat rare hereditary deficiencies do not respond to the administration of even large doses of vitamin K. Stored blood contains factors II, VII and X and is therefore convenient for the treatment of these patients. The same dose regimen as in classical haemophilia is used because the half-life of factor VII is also short (4 to 6 hours; the corresponding value for factor X is about 40 hours and for factor II 3 to 5 days).

**Table X.** Stability of blood factors in stored plasma and their dosages in the treatment of congenital bleeding disorders (note that recommended dosages are not available for some congenital deficiency states)

| Congenital deficiency | Half-life of deficient factor (hours) | Assumed haemostatic level in plasma | Stability in plasma | Recommended initial dose | Maintenance dose |
|---|---|---|---|---|---|
| Factor I (fibrinogen) | 96-120 | 100mg/100ml | Yes | 4 g/L | 1-2g every 2nd day |
| Factor II (prothrombin) | 72-120 | 40% | Yes | | |
| Factor V | 12-36 | 20% | No | 20ml plasma/kg | 10 ml/kg every 12h |
| Factor VII | 4-6 | 20% | Yes | 25 U/kg | 10 U/kg every 12h |
| Factor VIII | 10-12 | 30% | No | 15 U/kg | 10 U/kg |
| Factor IX | 18-36 | 30% | Yes | | |
| Factor X | 16-72 | 20% | Yes | | |
| Factor XI | 60-84 | ? | | | |
| Factor XIII | 96-168 | 1% | Yes | | |

#### Congenital Factor V Deficiency

The hereditary deficiency of factor V or parahaemophilia requires fresh frozen plasma, as factor V is unstable upon storage, even at 4°C. The same doses are used as in classical haemophilia, but because the half-life of factor V is 12 to 36 hours, only 1 infusion daily is required.

### *4.2.2 Acquired Defects of Coagulation*

In contrast to the common congenital haemorrhagic states, acquired disorders are due to multiple clotting factor deficiency.

#### Prothrombin Complex Deficiency

The 3 distinguishable causes of prothrombin complex deficiencies are:

1) Severe liver disease, which primarily affects factor V but factors II, VII, IX and X may also be low.

2) Vitamin K deficiency, characterised by a reduction of factors II, VII, IX, X and proteins C and S.

3) Excessive utilisation of factor V and to a lesser extent of factors II and X.

In the presence of liver disease, a poor response to vitamin K is obtained and replacement therapy with fresh plasma is required, because of the lability of factor V in stored plasma and because factor V is often decreased in patients with liver disease. The administration of a fibrinogen preparation or a prothrombin complex may be required if surgery is contemplated.

Major vitamin K deficiency may be caused by interference with the flow of bile salts in the gastrointestinal tract (e.g. obstructive jaundice, biliary fistula), any conditions with impaired absorption from the intestine following extensive surgical resection of the intestinal tract, dietary deprivation (e.g. with some enteral feeding preparations), sterilisation of the intestinal tract, and therapeutic or surreptitious intake of oral anticoagulants. In adults, vitamin K 5 mg/day given orally raises and maintains a normal prothrombin time. In patients with obstructive jaundice or biliary fistula, oral treatment should be confined to water-soluble vitamin K (i.e. not phytomenadione).

In all situations, any vitamin K preparation will be adequate if given parenterally. With normal liver function, safe therapeutic concentrations are obtained in 4 to 6 hours with parenteral administration. In patients receiving oral anticoagulant therapy, a dose of 5 to 10mg is usually sufficient, depending on the intensity of anticoagulation, but if haemorrhage is actually present, 10 to 25mg should be given parenterally and repeated every 12 hours for the first 2 days if a coumarin drug of prolonged action has been used. If the patient is to remain on warfarin, the dose of vitamin $K_1$ should preferably be limited to 0.5 to 1mg.

The daily vitamin K requirement of infants of mothers not receiving oral anticoagulants is 25μg, because there is no bacterial synthesis during the neonatal period. Cow's milk contains approximately 6μg vitamin K per 100ml but normal human milk only 1 to 5μg per 100ml. Parenteral administration of phytomenadione 1mg is usually sufficient, but may be repeated after 6 hours. Excessive amounts, especially of water-soluble vitamin K analogues, can produce haemolytic anaemia with its consequences, particularly in premature infants.

#### Disseminated Intravascular Coagulation

Disseminated intravascular coagulation (DIC), the defibrination syndrome or consumption coagulopathy all refer to a complication which may occur in many diseases but is not a disease in itself. DIC is defined as demonstrable *in vivo* conversion of fibrinogen to fibrin, exclusive of local arterial or venous thrombosis in major vessels. A heterogeneous group of rare conditions (table XI) can lead to an acute process, with production of a severe haemorrhagic state, or a subacute or chronic form with mild or no bleeding features. In both situations, very small vessel obstructions by fibrin and/or platelets, tissue necrosis, and single or multiple organ dysfunction may occur. The intravascular presence of fibrin normally stimulates secondary development of local fibrinolytic activity but may, on very rare occasions, be accompanied by an increase in systemic fibrinolytic enzyme activity. The correct diagnosis is often difficult to make in time because the pattern of abnormalities may be continually changing and may even have disappeared by the time of blood sampling. Useful clues are a low platelet count, decreased levels of factor V, fibrinogen and plasminogen, associated with fibrin degradation products X and Y which cause prolongation of the thrombin time.

Treatment must first be directed at termination of the underlying disease (e.g. antibiotics in sepsis, emptying of the uterus in abruptio placentae and dead fetus syndrome) and this may be the only therapy necessary in chronic defibrination states. In acute defibrination, supportive therapy (expansion of blood volume, if depleted, control of acidosis and electrolyte

**Table XI.** Conditions leading to intravascular coagulation

| Acute | Subacute | Chronic |
|---|---|---|
| Abruptio placentae | Septic abortion | *Falciparum* malaria |
| Amniotic fluid embolism | Toxaemia of pregnancy | Cirrhosis (decompensated) |
| Haemolytic transfusion | Acute leukaemia | Dead fetus (>3 weeks) |
| Purpura fulminans | Rhabdomyosarcoma | Congenital haemangioma |
| Septicaemia (Gram-negative) | Carcinomatosis (including lung, prostate) | (Kasabach-Merritt syndrome) |
| Snake bite | Neuroblastoma | Hydatidiform mole |
| Waterhouse-Friderichsen syndrome | Haemolytic-uraemic syndrome | Aortic aneurysm |
| Lung surgery | (Gasser syndrome) | |
| Some allergic reactions | Eclampsia | |
| Burns | Sickle cell disease | |
| Heat stroke | | |
| Acute promyelocytic leukaemia | | |
| Dengue fever | | |
| Psittacosis | | |
| Some viral and rickettsial infections | | |
| Rocky mountain spotted fever | | |
| Fat embolism | | |
| Head injury | | |
| Trauma (massive) | | |

imbalance) is the first step. In cases of bleeding with serious anaemia, fresh whole blood is indicated with replacement of depleted coagulation factors and of platelets. The administration of coagulation factor concentrates is a double-edged weapon and should be used with caution in active, uncontrolled DIC.

The use of heparin in DIC is controversial. Heparin probably has no effect on the progress of DIC when it complicates septicaemia or endotoxinaemia. In other patients with DIC, heparin administered either subcutaneously or intravenously may be highly effective. In small groups of patients, fulminant DIC has been successfully treated with antithrombin III concentrates (for reviews, see Bick;[411] and Rubin & Colman[412]).

#### Transfusion-Induced Bleeding

Massive transfusion of citrated blood can cause hypocalcaemia and induce cardiac standstill, especially in patients in prolonged shock. Citrate overdosage is rare because the liver can metabolise 0.03 to 0.04 mmol/kg/min, which allows the safe transfusion of 2L of citrated blood in 20 minutes. If more than 10 units of blood or plasma per hour are administered, 0.25g calcium chloride should be administered after each unit. If bleeding occurs, this is not because of hypocalcaemia but due to massive transfusion of stored blood low in platelets and factors V and VIII. When more than 10 units of blood are required on the same day, 1 of every 3 units should be less than 6 hours old.

#### Uraemia

The cause of the bleeding tendency observed in uraemic patients is unclear and there is no satisfactory treatment. High levels of prostacyclin-like activity, capable of inhibiting platelet aggregation generated by the vessel wall, have been found in uraemic patients with a prolonged bleeding and normal platelet count.[413] Desmopressin has been found to reduce the bleeding time in uraemia.[399]

### *4.2.3 Platelet Disorders*

#### Idiopathic Thrombocytopenia (ITP)

ITP results from the presence of antiplatelet autoantibodies, usually of the IgG class, which coat platelets and lead to their removal from the circulation by splenic and hepatic macrophages.

The mainstays of treatment for ITP are corticosteroids in a dose equivalent to prednisone 1 to 2 mg/kg/day. Patients who relapse after the withdrawal of corticosteroids or who are unresponsive to them are usually offered a splenectomy. Intravenous immunoglobulins are nearly as effective as corticosteroids; however, their efficacy is often short-lived and the treatment extremely costly. Consequently, their use is generally restricted to providing cover during a brief period of high bleeding risk, e.g. surgery, delivery, cerebral bleeding. The usual dose of polyvalent IgG is 0.4 g/kg daily for 5 consecutive days (for reviews, see Verstraete & Perez-Requejo;[414] and Imbach et al.[415]).

Other treatments used in ITP patients refractory to corticosteroids/splenectomy include vincristine, immunosuppressive agents and pulsed high-dose dexamethasone.[416,417]

#### Neonatal Thrombocytopenic Purpura

This condition occurs not infrequently in neonates and infants of mothers who have idiopathic thrombocytopenia or disseminated lupus erythematosus. Agglutinins crossing the placenta have been demonstrated. Isoimmune neonatal thrombocytopenic purpura due to incompatible platelet groups is another rather rare cause of severe bleeding and is a self-limiting condition.

The management of thrombocytopenia associated with disseminated lupus erythematosus is the same as for idiopathic thrombocytopenia (see above).

#### Thrombocythaemia

This condition can be associated with myeloproliferative disorders or may be primary.

***Essential thrombocytosis:*** the primary symptoms of this condition are thrombosis and hyperviscosity. Antiaggregating agents, e.g. aspirin, are needed in the prevention of thromboembolic complications. In some instances, overt bleeding may occur, caused by qualitative platelet defects. Antiaggregating agents are then contraindicated. Suppression of platelet production by hydroxycarbamide (hydroxyurea) or busulfan are the usual treatments, with more hesitation for the latter in view of the risk of secondary leukaemia. For this reason, radioactive phosphorus has also been abandoned.

*Anagrelide,* a cyclic-AMP phosphodiesterase inhibitor inhibits the production of platelets by megakaryocytes; if ongoing trials confirm the lack of leukaemogenic and mutagenic potential, anagrelide may become the agent of choice in the treatment of thrombocythaemia (for a review, see Spencer and Brogden[418]).

#### Other Functional Platelet Disorders

Various haemorrhagic congenital bleeding disorders have been ascribed to defective platelet function in the presence of adequate numbers of platelets. Hereditary disorders of platelet function may be due to disorders of connective tissue with which platelets interact, disorders of plasma proteins necessary for this interaction, or a defect of the platelets themselves.

Acquired disorders of platelet function can be associated with other conditions (e.g. myeloproliferative or renal diseases, fibrin degradation products) or occur after intake of drugs that affect platelet function (e.g. aspirin and other nonsteroidal anti-inflammatory agents, antihistamines, penicillins, etc.). This defect can be counteracted only by administration of fresh, normal platelet concentrates.

## 5. Anaemias

Anaemias can be conveniently classified as follows:

1) Anaemias due to deficiency of factors essential for normal blood formation: iron, vitamin $B_{12}$, folic acid.

2) Anaemias due to excessive blood destruction: haemolytic anaemias, either due to intrinsic congenital abnormalities, or extrinsic acquired causes.

3) Anaemias due to a primary haematopoietic defect in the bone marrow, e.g. aplastic anaemia.

4) Anaemias of uncertain origin, e.g. anaemia of chronic disease (ACD), rheumatoid arthritis, disseminated malignancy, chronic infection, etc.

Success in the treatment of patients with anaemia depends on a correct diagnosis with early identification and elimination, if possible, of any underlying cause. While the aetiology of many anaemias still remains unknown, most of the commonly occurring anaemias arise as a result of blood loss or nutritional and toxic causes. The hereditary anaemias are an ever increasing cause of morbidity.

### 5.1 Clinical Pharmacology of Drugs Used in Treatment

#### *5.1.1 Iron Preparations*

The total body iron has been estimated at about 3.8g in adult males *versus* 2.5 to 3.0g in adult females. The majority of this iron is present in haemoglobin (approximately 2.5g), the rest being storage iron in ferritin and haemosiderin (0.1 to 1.0g), myoglobin (130mg), and tissue enzymes (8mg), and transferrin bound iron (5mg).[419]

The basal physiological losses of iron from the body (mainly from the skin and the gastrointestinal tract) have been estimated at 15 μg/kg/day, or about 1mg in an adult male and 0.8mg in an adult female.[420] Menstrual iron losses may increase the latter figure by 0.5 to 1.5 mg/day. In pregnancy, iron is needed to cover the basal losses of the mother (240mg), the increase in her red cell mass (500mg), and the requirements of the fetus and placenta (300mg), i.e. a total of 1000mg.[421] Therefore, pregnant women require an average daily intake of at least 3 to 4 mg iron.

Iron is poorly absorbed from food, about 10% being taken up, but this varies depending on whether iron deficiency is present (in which case absorption rises to 25%), and with the form in which iron is presented to the duodenum and jejunum (haem iron is 20 to 40% absorbed).[422]

Ingested iron must be reduced to the ferrous form in the stomach and intestine before it is absorbed. Absorption is greatest in the upper part of the small intestine and duodenum and progressively less in the distal segments. The total amount absorbed is proportional to the amount ingested. Simple reduced forms of iron like ferrous sulfate or gluconate are commonly used. An average tablet of ferrous sulfate contains 200mg iron, of which 63mg is elemental iron and of which an iron deficient patient will absorb up to 25%, i.e. 16mg. This will allow the production of about 16ml of red cells. While a maximally stimulated marrow may require up to 50 to 80mg of iron per day for optimal haemoglobin output, as much iron as can be tolerated should be administered.

#### Clinical Use

The main iron preparations (sulfate, gluconate, fumarate, succinate) produce similar effects.[423] A tablet of 300mg ferrous gluconate contains 35mg of elemental iron, a tablet of 200mg ferrous succinate 70mg, and a tablet of 200mg ferrous fumarate 65mg. By keeping iron in the ferrous form, reducing agents like ascorbic acid (vitamin C) promote iron absorption and are often added to the commercial preparations. Selection of one or the other compound will be mainly based on the prescriber's preference and the patient's taste (table XII). Sustained release iron preparations offer no real advantage over conventional preparations,[424] other than a reduced frequency of administration.

For parenteral administration, iron dextran is the most widely available form. Iron sorbitol or dextriferron preparations are less commonly used.

#### Tolerability and Drug Interactions Potential

All oral iron preparations produce some adverse effects, principally gastrointestinal discomfort. To improve tolerability, it may be advisable to give iron with meals, although this may result in diminished absorption of iron and necessitate an increase in the daily dosage. Plant phytates, phosphates and tannic acid (tea) can form insoluble complexes with iron. Iron medication should not be given simultaneously with tetracyclines, as there is a mutual decrease in absorption of both drugs; however, this effect is no longer apparent when the drugs are given about 3 hours apart.[427,428]

Following intramuscular administration, local reactions are not uncommon. Permanent subcutaneous staining may occur and persist for over 2 years, and sarcomas have been reported following protracted treatment.

Systemic reactions to iron dextran may be life-threatening. In less than 1% of patients treated by either the intramuscular or intravenous route, a severe anaphylactic reaction may occur. This reaction is not dose-dependent. Treatment with adrenaline (epinephrine), methylprednisolone, ventilatory assistance, etc. is not uniformly successful.

#### Iron Toxicity and Overload

Acute iron toxicity, mainly in children, can occur after accidental intake of oral iron preparations (as little as ferrous sulfate 1g may be fatal in a young child) and needs urgent treatment, including intensive intragastric and systemic administration of iron chelators.

Excessive dosage of iron salts or of haemoglobin iron in polytransfused patients can result in iron overload and secondary haemochromatosis. Moreover, 10% of the Western Caucasian population is heterozygous for the haemochromatosis gene, which may increase the chances of tissue damage by excess iron.[429] A higher iron status may also confer an increased risk for the development of ischaemic heart disease and cancer.[430] This has much to do with the capacity of iron to catalyse the formation of highly toxic oxygen radicals, which may provoke lipid peroxidation and cellular damage. Consequently, it is prudent to avoid prescribing iron for patients with adequate or near adequate iron stores. Male blood donors should therefore not be given iron supplements routinely, although menstruating female blood donors may still benefit. From a public health perspective, it is not wise to promote iron fortified food products.

***Treatment:*** if iron overload is present (e.g. in polytransfused thalassaemic patients), life-expectancy can be considerably prolonged by the administration of iron chelators.[431,432] *Deferoxamine* (desferrioxamine) is a highly efficient, but very expensive and only parenterally effective agent used in the treatment of iron overload. Prior to the age of 3 years, long term administration of deferoxamine may lead to growth retardation.[433] Daily subcutaneous administra-

**Table XII.** Iron content and dosage of some oral and parenteral iron preparations (after Beal[425,426])

| Preparation | Iron content[a] | Daily adult dose[b] | Adverse effects |
|---|---|---|---|
| **Oral preparations – conventional** | | | |
| Sodium iron edetate, 190 mg/5ml | 27.5 mg/5ml | 5-10ml tid | Nausea, diarrhoea and/or constipation |
| Ferrous gluconate, 300mg | 35mg | 1-2 tid | |
| Ferrous succinate, 106 mg/5ml | 37 mg/5ml | 5-10ml tid | |
| Ferrous glycine sulfate, 282 mg/10ml | 50 mg/10ml | 5-10ml tid | |
| Ferrous sulfate, 300mg | 60mg | 1-2 tid | |
| Ferrous fumarate, 200mg | 65mg | 1-2 tid | |
| **Oral preparations – sustained release** | | | |
| Ferrous glycine sulfate | 100mg | 1-2 od | As above |
| Ferrous sulfate, dried | 47mg | 1-2 od | |
| | 100mg | 1-2 od | |
| | 105mg | 1-2 od | |
| **Parenteral preparations** | | | |
| Dextriferron | 20 mg/ml | 1.5-5ml slow IV (not for IM use) | *Intravenous:* venous spasm; systemic chills, fever, nausea; chest, lumbar and loin pain |
| Iron dextran | 50 mg/ml | 2-5ml deep IM; also by IV infusion | *Intramuscular:* local pain and inflammation; skin staining (if administration not correct); systemic reactions; metallic taste |
| Iron polymaltose | 50 mg/ml | 2-5ml deep IM; also by IV infusion | |
| Iron sorbitol (iron sorbitol citric acid complex) | 50 mg/ml | 2-5ml deep IM (not for IV use) | |

a As elemental iron per tablet, capsule or specified volume of liquid.

b The daily therapeutic adult dose for optimum haemoglobin response is usually in the range 180 to 270mg elemental iron. The daily prophylactic dose (e.g. in pregnancy) is about 60 to 100mg elemental iron.

***Parenteral dosage*** can be calculated by a formula based on the severity of the anaemia and size of the patient. One formula which has been used to calculate the approximate total amount is:

Total ml to be injected = body weight in kg × haemoglobin deficiency (100% – actual concentration) × 0.0132.

An empirical intramuscular dosage is to give an initial 1ml trial dose, followed by 2 to 5ml daily into alternate buttocks. In practice, a course of 1.5 to 3g elemental iron will be required.

*Abbreviations:* od = once daily; tid = 3 times daily; IV = intravenous; IM = intramuscular; SC = subcutaneous.

tion should therefore not exceed 20 to 30 mg/kg. In older patients, dosages as high as 50 mg/kg may be needed to maintain negative iron balances; supplementary ascorbic acid (vitamin C) will help mobilise iron from its stores. In the past, deferoxamine was given overnight by subcutaneous administration over 10 to 12 hours. However, much better results have been obtained with continuous intravenous ambulatory administration through implantable venous access ports.[434]

The most serious adverse effects encountered with deferoxamine include hypotension, renal insufficiency, visual and auditory neurotoxicity, cataract, growth retardation and opportunistic infections.[435] Many of these are dose-related.

Orally active iron chelating agents have long been looked for and one of the most effective is the L1 chelator *deferiprone* (1,2-dimethyl-3-hydroxypyrid-4-one). Large scale clinical trials are underway to assess its long term safety and efficacy.[436] Adverse effects thus far noted include drug-associated arthralgias, joint effusions and acute reversible agranulocytosis. The latter may be entirely dose-dependent.

### *5.1.2 Epoetin (Recombinant Human Erythropoietin; rHuEPO)*

Human erythropoietin (EPO) is a glycoprotein composed of 165 amino acids and is heavily glycosylated. Its biological activity depends on this glycosylation, while the removal of sialic acid results in its rapid inactivation by the liver and clearance from the circulation.[437]

The physiological action of EPO is initiated by binding to its receptor on the cell surface, followed by receptor-mediated endocytosis.[438] Three forms of EPO receptor genes have been isolated, leading to receptor chains of different length, differing cytoplasmic and extracellular domains, and different capability to prevent programmed cell death.[439] The number of EPO receptors on the cell surface increases with increasing maturation. The EPO-induced signal transduction involves both tyrosine and serine-threonine phosphorylation.[440]

#### Pharmacokinetic Characteristics

The pharmacokinetic profile of epoetin administered subcutaneously is different from that when given intravenously. The half-life of epoetin after intravenous infusion is around 5 hours *versus* more than 20 hours after subcutaneous injection, with elevated concentrations of epoetin remaining in the serum at 48 hours. Hence the now classical dosage schemes of 3 doses per week for most indications.[269]

In haemodialysis patients, the median dose of epoetin required to maintain a target haematocrit of more that 35% is 75 U/kg intravenously 3 times a week. However, some patients may require double that dose, depending on the steady-state plasma EPO concentrations.[441] Dose changes within intervals shorter than 4 weeks are not recommended, because the response cannot be evaluated over a shorter time. If dosages greater than 150 U/kg are needed, risk factors for resistance to epoetin should be assessed (e.g. iron deficiency, aluminium overload, infection, bleeding, tumour, hypersplenism, etc.).

In the treatment of cancer-related anaemia or of anaemia secondary to chronic infections, much higher doses of epoetin may be needed, e.g. 200 U/kg 3 times a week. The response to epoetin may be predicted according to the endogenous EPO concentrations (e.g. the observed over predicted ratio of EPO concentrations), the early reticulocyte response at 2 weeks, ferritin levels, etc.

For reviews of epoetin, see Faulds & Sorkin[442] and Dunn & Markham.[443]

#### Clinical Use

The anaemic states in which epoetin has been successfully used are listed in table XIII. The effect of epoetin on erythropoiesis is not immediate, since it may take several days to weeks for the EPO-responsive erythroid precursors to mature in the bone marrow and to be released as reticulocytes. Improvements in haematocrits may take 4 weeks to appear, and hence iron supplements may be necessary initially.[444]

Epoetin therapy in responsive conditions leads to a dramatic increase in quality of life, with better exercise tolerance, sense of well-being, improved appetite, decreased depression, decreased cold intolerance, etc. However, epoetin therapy is unlikely to be cost effective when prescribed indiscriminately.

#### Tolerability

Common adverse effects of epoetin administration include flu-like symptoms (fever, arthralgias, myalgias), headache, hypertension, seizures, conjunctival injection, arteriovenous fistula or shunt thrombosis.[445]

Possible mechanisms of increasing resistance to epoetin administration may relate to deficiencies of iron, folate or vitamin $B_{12}$ in inflammatory conditions (infections, malignancies, postoperatively) or in aluminium overload, osteitis fibrosa, significant haemolysis, etc.[446]

### *5.1.3 Colony-Stimulating Factors (CSFs)*

The commercially available CSF preparations are listed in table XIV.

The recombinant human colony-stimulating factors (rHuCSFs) are indistinguishable from their natural counterparts in terms of amino acid composition, peptide separation on HPLC, and clinical effects. Although G-CSF and GM-CSF in their natural forms are glycosylated proteins, the recombinant products seem to be active both in deglycosylated (*Escherichia coli*-derived) and moderately (CHO cell-derived) or heavily (yeast-derived) glycosylated forms. Glycosylation *per se* does not seem to be essential for biological activity,[447] but glycosylation may offer advantages with regard to *in vitro* stability or resistance to protease degradation in human serum.[448] *Lenograstim,* a glycosylated G-CSF, produces more and larger neutrophil colonies *in vitro* than its non-glycosylated counterpart, *filgrastim*.[449] Glycosylated GM-CSF, when subcutaneously injected in normal volunteers, has a longer plasma half-life, greater neutrophil-stimulating activity, induces less leukotriene production and has fewer adverse effects than the non-glycosylated form.[450]

#### Pharmacokinetic Characteristics

Pharmacokinetic studies have shown a rapid clearance of CSFs after bolus intravenous injections. Protracted plasma concentrations can be

**Table XIII.** Clinical indications for epoetin (rHuEPO) administration

| |
|---|
| Chronic renal failure and haemodialysis |
| Bone marrow transplantation |
| Cancer-related anaemia |
| Multiple myeloma |
| Acquired immune deficiency syndrome (AIDS) |
| Neonatal anaemia |
| Myelodysplastic syndromes |
| Rheumatoid arthritis |
| Autologous blood donation |

**Table XIV.** Commercially available haematopoietic colony-stimulating factors (CSFs)

| Native molecule | Generic name | Synthesis | Form |
|---|---|---|---|
| G-CSF (granulocyte colony-stimulating factor) | Filgrastim | Bacteria | Non-glycosylated |
| | Lenograstim | CHO cells | Glycosylated |
| GM-CSF (granulocyte macrophage colony-stimulating factor) | Molgramostim | Bacteria | Non-glycosylated |
| | Sargramostim | Yeast | Glycosylated |

*Abbreviation:* CHO = Chinese hamster ovary.

expected after subcutaneous injection or with continuous intravenous infusions.[451] Peak plasma concentrations are proportional to dose regardless of the route of administration. The peak plasma concentrations of G-CSF are maintained for 30 to 60 minutes after short intravenous infusions (30 minutes), and the terminal plasma elimination half-life ranges from 0.75 to 7.2 hours following doses of up to 60 μg/kg. With GM-CSF, the terminal elimination phase half-life after short intravenous infusions of doses of 3 to 30 μg/kg ranges from 0.6 to 9.1 hours. After single subcutaneous doses of G-CSF, plasma concentrations are higher than 10 μg/L for 10 to 16 hours. With subcutaneous boluses of GM-CSF, plasma concentrations exceeding 1 μg/L are maintained for 8 to 24 hours.[60]

### Clinical Use

The haematological and biochemical effects of the *in vivo* administration of colony-stimulating factors are summarised in table XV.

The optimum dosages of the CSFs have not been clearly defined. Recommended doses from a number of studies with G-CSF range from as low as 50 μg/m$^2$ (e.g. in myelodysplasia) to 500 μg/m$^2$ (e.g. in collection of peripheral blood progenitors cells). With *lenograstim,* doses greater than 5 μg/kg/day have been found to provide no overt additional benefit, leading to the recommendation that for routine administration (e.g. in neutropenia and post–bone marrow transplantation) the dosage should be 150 μg/m$^2$/day.[452] With *filgrastim,* the optimum dose is 5 μg/kg/day. G-CSF has not been shown to have any dose-limiting adverse effects.[453]

For GM-CSF, the recommended daily dose is 250 μg/m$^2$.[454] Dose-finding studies have clearly demonstrated excessive toxicity with daily dosages above 16 μg/kg, at least when non-glycosylated *molgramostim* is used. However, the glycosylated product, *sargramostim,* has been clinically used without too much toxicity in doses ranging from 500 to 750 μg/m$^2$/day. Sargramostim has a greater molecular weight than molgramostim and a potentially lower specific activity with possibly different receptor binding characteristics. Direct comparisons of glycosylated *versus* non-glycosylated products are therefore difficult.

The rational use of CSF preparations in clinical practice has been the subject of much debate. In order to maximise patient benefit while minimising costs, the development of guidelines for the use of these expensive drugs is essential.

Myeloid growth factors can be used in 3 ways:[455]

1) *Interventional,* i.e. therapeutic, to treat neutropenic infections, correct quantitative bone marrow deficiency states, modulate antimicrobial or antitumour host defence systems,

**Table XV.** Haematological and biochemical effects of the administration of granulocyte and granulocyte macrophage colony-stimulating factors (G-CSF and GM-CSF) [after Lieschke & Burgess[60]]

| Tissue/function | Effects |
|---|---|
| Peripheral blood | Increase in neutrophils with left shift (excess immature forms) |
| | Transient immediate leucopenia |
| | Transient mild decrease in platelets |
| | Increase in circulating haematopoietic progenitors |
| | Altered granulocyte morphology |
| | Increase in monocytes and eosinophils (only GM-CSF) |
| Bone marrow | Increase in cellularity and erythroid: myeloid ratio |
| | Increase in cycling progenitors |
| | Increase in eosinophil precursors |
| Leucocyte function | Priming of superoxide production |
| | Decreased chemotactic response (GM-CSF more than G-CSF) |
| | Increased expression of adhesive surface markers (e.g. CD11b) [GM-CSF more than G-CSF] |
| | Increased monocyte cytotoxicity, TNF and interferon production (GM-CSF) |
| Serum biochemistry | Increase in lactate dehydrogenase |
| | Increase in alkaline phosphatase |
| | Increase in uric acid |
| | Increase in lysozyme (G-CSF) |
| | Increase in cobalamin (GM-CSF) |
| | Decrease in albumin (GM-CSF) |
| | Decrease in cholesterol |

*Abbreviation:* TNF = tumour necrosis factor.

and improve the harvest of haematopoietic progenitor cells (table XVI).

2) *Prophylactic,* i.e. to prevent infections post-chemotherapy, post-bone marrow transplantation or in immunodeficiency states [e.g. human immunodeficiency virus (HIV) infection or chronic lymphocytic leukaemia].

3) *Pre-emptive,* i.e. in secondary prophylaxis for markedly neutropenic patients who have experienced infections in previous neutropenic episodes or who are at extremely high risk of becoming infected (e.g. heavy fungal colonisation).

In no instance can the use of myeloid growth factors be advocated in low-risk patients, for short-term neutropenia, or for broad-spectrum indiscriminate prophylaxis. A European Working Party[456] and the American Society of Clinical Oncology[457] have elaborated clinical practice guidelines based on the published evidence. On this basis, the following specific indications for G-CSF and GM-CSF were advanced:

- Alleviation of congenital neutropenia
- Mobilisation of peripheral blood progenitor cells for autotransfusion
- Encouragement of engraftment following bone marrow transplantation
- Supportive therapy for continuation of ganciclovir in certain patients with AIDS, where a switch to foscarnet is contraindicated or where excessive toxicity to foscarnet develops.
- Prevention of infections in high-risk neutropenia, i.e. prolonged (projected duration of more than 5 to 7 days) and marked (less than $0.5 \times 10^9$/L) or after documented febrile neutropenia in a prior chemotherapy cycle.

The use of colony-stimulating factors in myeloid malignancies or for the purpose of dose intensification in solid tumours has not been universally accepted. For reviews of the pharmacology and therapeutic use of G-CSF and GM-CSF, see Hollingshead & Goa,[458] Frampton et al.[459] and Grant & Heel.[454]

### Tolerability

The human recombinant colony-stimulating factors G-CSF and GM-CSF have generally been well tolerated in clinical use.[453] However, some adverse effects may be encountered (table XVII).

Although few well-conducted randomised studies are available, the toxicity of GM-CSF seems to be more pronounced than that of G-CSF. Dose-independent toxicity includes fever and bone pain, varying in incidence from 20% (G-CSF) to 50% (GM-CSF).[460,461] These symptoms are easily controlled and/or prevented with paracetamol (acetaminophen).

**Table XVI.** Interventional (therapeutic) uses of myeloid growth factors

| |
|---|
| 1. **Modulation of haematopoiesis in bone marrow failure states** |
| Aplastic anaemia |
| Myelodysplasia |
| Diamond-Blackfan anaemia |
| Congenital neutropenia (Kostmann syndrome) |
| Cyclic neutropenia |
| Drug-induced agranulocytosis |
| Felty's syndrome |
| Graft failure |
| 2. **Modulation of haematopoiesis in dysfunctional bone marrow states** |
| Myelodysplasia (maturation induction) |
| AIDS |
| Anaemia of cancer |
| Post-bone marrow transplantation |
| 3. **Replacement therapy of inadequate levels of endogenous cytokines** |
| Chronic renal failure |
| 4. **Antitumour activity** |
| Priming effect, S-phase induction, cycling |
| Differentiation induction, e.g. with retinoids |
| Biochemical upgrade, e.g. nucleoside phosphorylation |
| Modulation of cellular cytotoxicity, e.g. IL-2, LAK, rHuG-CSF-ADCC |
| 5. **Primary immunomodulation** |
| IL-2 post-remission induction in leukaemia |
| IL-2 receptor antibodies for graft *versus* host disease |
| IL-1 receptor antibodies for graft *versus* host disease |
| IL-4 in multiple myeloma |
| 6. **Direct growth factor antagonism** |
| Anti-IL-6 in Castleman syndrome |
| IL-6 toxin conjugates in myeloma |
| 7. **Stimulation of defective host defence** |
| Congenital granulocyte dysfunction |
| Acquired granulocyte dysfunction, e.g. myelodysplasia, sepsis, burns, neonates |
| 8. **Treatment of infectious diseases** |
| Neutropenia (chemotherapy and non-chemotherapy related) |
| Antiretroviral therapy support |
| Anti-CMV therapy support |
| 9. **Harvest of haematopoietic progenitor cells (blood/marrow)** |
| Chemotherapy + rHuG-CSF/GM-CSF/IL-3 |
| rHuG-CSF, GM-CSF/IL-3 |
| 10. ***In vitro* expansion of haematopoietic progenitor cells with cocktails of growth factors** |
| (IL-1/IL-3/IL-6/rHuG-CSF/GM-CSF/SCF/EPO) |

*Abbreviations:* ADCC = antibody-dependent cellular cytotoxicity; AIDS = acquired immune deficiency syndrome; CMV = cytomegalovirus; EPO = epoetin; rHuG-CSF = recombinant human granulocyte colony-stimulating factor; GM-CSF = granulocyte macrophage colony-stimulating factor; IL = interleukin; LAK = lymphokine-activated killer; SCF = stem cell factor.

**Table XVII.** Adverse effects of granulocyte and granulocyte macrophage colony-stimulating factors (G-CSF and GM-CSF)

| Adverse effect | G-CSF | GM-CSF |
|---|---|---|
| Fever | Rare | Common |
| Bone pain | Common (dose-related) | Common |
| Myalgia | Rare | Common |
| Splenomegaly | Rare (long term use) | Rare |
| Oedema | None | Common (dose-related) |
| Capillary leak (pleuritis, ascites) | None | Common (dose-related) |
| Thrombosis (catheter, pulmonary) | None | Rare |
| Injection site reactions | Rare | Common |
| Allergic reactions | Rare | Common |
| Decreased platelets | Rare | Rare |
| Neutralising antibodies | Rare | Rare |

Dose-dependent toxicity is especially seen with GM-CSF. This is illustrated by the common association of the capillary leak syndrome (hypoalbuminaemia, pleuritis, pericarditis, peripheral oedema and dramatic weight gain) with doses of GM-CSF above 16 to 32 μg/kg. The production of secondary mediators, such as IL-1 and tumour necrosis factor (TNF), may be responsible for this effect.[462] The so-called 'first pass' effect, which is seen only with non-glycosylated GM-CSF (molgramostim), is characterised by hypotension, flushing, tachycardia, musculoskeletal pain, dyspnoea, rigors and nausea.[463] Allergic reactions (either locally at the injection site or systemically) with skin rash and pruritus are rather uncommon. More disturbing is the occasional thrombocytopenia after both G-CSF and GM-CSF, although generally, no clinical bleeding is observed.[464]

Long term administration of G-CSF to patients with congenital neutropenia has rarely been associated with splenomegaly and mild alopecia.[465] Laboratory abnormalities are mostly related to increased myeloid turnover and include increased lactate dehydrogenase, alkaline phosphatase and uric acid concentrations, and decreased cholesterol and albumin (GM-CSF). Neutralising antibodies to G-CSF have not been reported, but may be seen in as many as 4% of patients treated with glycosylated GM-CSF (sargramostim).[466]

Indirect toxicity of the colony-stimulating factors may relate to the potential stimulation of clonogenic tumour cells bearing specific growth factor receptors. This is a major concern when growth factors are used in patients with myeloid leukaemias and myelodysplasia.[467] At present, there is no evidence that CSFs promote leukaemic cell growth *in vivo* when given to patients with acute myeloid leukaemia in complete remission. However, in patients with high-risk myelodysplasia some leukaemic transformations have been reported.[468] Initial concerns about a possible stem cell exhaustion effect or about biased stem cell commitment have not been substantiated by any clinical study.[453]

## 5.2 Optimum Treatment

### 5.2.1 Deficiency Anaemias

Appropriate treatment is extremely rewarding in these conditions. However, an early correct diagnosis is essential. Iron deficiency anaemia may be due to blood loss from a malignant gastrointestinal lesion, survival in which depends largely on early recognition.

There is no place for blind treatment of anaemia without a thorough search for an underlying cause. This is not only wasteful, but may also delay or mask the correct diagnosis. The treatment of deficiency anaemias consists of the administration of the deficient substance and there is no justification for 'shotgun' treatment with mixtures of haematinics.[425,426]

#### Iron Deficiency Anaemias

Iron body stores can be adequately estimated by the measurement of serum iron concentration, the saturation of the iron transporter molecule transferrin, and the concentration of the iron storage molecule ferritin. A saturation of transferrin below 10% and a ferritin concentration below 12 μg/L are strong indicators of iron deficiency. However, transferrin and ferritin are largely influenced by concomitant conditions, e.g. infections, so that sometimes a bone marrow examination needs to be performed to adequately assess iron stores. Immunoassays that can detect the soluble truncated form of the transferrin receptor in human serum will soon be routinely available and will allow rapid detection of true iron deficiency. An increase in receptor concentrations provides a sensitive and quantitative measure of tissue iron deficiency and will allow the differential diagnosis of anaemia of chronic diseases.[469]

Iron deficiency anaemia is characteristically hypochromic and microcytic, and sometimes leucopenia and/or leucocyte dysfunction may be present. It may be accompanied by increased infectivity, and if active bleeding continues, the platelet count may be increased.

Iron deficiency is of course a sign of an underlying disease. Although severe iron deficiency has virtually been eliminated from the Western world, mild or subclinical iron deficiency persists, especially in certain population groups, and may have serious clinical and economic consequences.[470] One of the most targeted groups in this respect have been neonates and infants, in whom prevention of iron deficiency remains a high priority.

***Causes:*** in adults, the major cause of iron deficiency is blood loss, with inadequate dietary intake (e.g. in vegetarians) remaining a rare finding. In Third World countries, however, nutritional deficiency may be omnipresent. Iron deficiency anaemia in early pregnancy is associated with premature delivery and low birth weight,[471] but the advisability of routine iron supplements during pregnancy has been questioned.[472]

Malabsorption of iron is rare but may occur in coeliac disease and post-gastrectomy. In females, obstetric and gynaecological causes may be prevalent; in males, gastrointestinal loss due to malignancy, angiodysplasia or extensive haemorrhoids may be found. Unusual causes include urinary iron loss after intravascular haemolysis (e.g. marathon runners, march haemoglobinuria), but haematuria *per se* can only rarely be blamed as the sole cause of deficiency.

***Clinical work-up:*** in cases of confirmed iron deficiency, a thorough clinical workup is always needed (see fig. 9)

***Iron therapy:*** although adequate therapy may be given orally or parenterally, the treatment of choice in iron deficient anaemia is oral iron given in an adequate dosage and for a sufficient length of time to restore the body iron stores to normal. Oral iron therapy is usually effective and has none of the dangers of the parenteral administration of iron (see section 5.1.1). Gastrointestinal intolerance of oral iron preparations has often been given as a reason for preference of parenteral administration, but this is not rational. Although gastric discomfort, diarrhoea or constipation can occur when oral treatment is started (and their psychological impact may be reinforced by the black discolouration of the stools), the importance of these complaints has been grossly exaggerated.[422]

Iron therapy should aim at quickly restoring the deficit and haemoglobin concentrations, i.e. within 10 to 12 weeks, after which lower dosage therapy to replenish iron body stores is usually necessary. The reticulocyte response should initially be monitored closely to assess true iron absorption. Later, ferritin concentrations can be followed to evaluate continuous malabsorption and/or continuous losses, and to assess the need for maintenance therapy. It should be noted that as patients often feel better very rapidly, iron therapy may be interrupted prematurely.

*Parenteral iron administration* should be limited to:

1) Genuine and severe gastrointestinal intolerance or clearly demonstrable malabsorption (as in coeliac disease, postgastrectomy patients, ulcerative colitis and Crohn's disease).

2) Chronic and intractable blood loss which cannot be corrected with oral iron because of the large quantities needed and poor compliance.

3) Instances where self-medication with iron is unreliable.

In view of the significantly greater hazards with parenteral therapy (see section 5.1.1), all indications for its use must be carefully considered.

The parenteral iron dosage can be calculated by a variety of formulae, one of which is given in table XII. A quick way of estimating the number of injections of iron dextran needed is: 1 ampoule of 250mg iron dextran (5ml) per gram of haemoglobin missing.

***Blood transfusion*** is not a suitable form of treatment for iron deficiency anaemia, but in some emergency conditions where acute problems with oxygen supply to the tissues exist, rapid correction of haemoglobin concentrations may be necessary.

#### Vitamin $B_{12}$ Deficiency Anaemia

Vitamin $B_{12}$ (cyanocobalamin) deficiency is due mainly to defective absorption. In pernicious anaemia, the main form of megaloblastic anaemia in Caucasians, defective absorption of vitamin $B_{12}$ results from the absence or inactivation of intrinsic factor, which is normally secreted by the gastric mucosa. More than 50% of patients with pernicious anaemia have intrinsic factor antibodies and/or related autoimmune

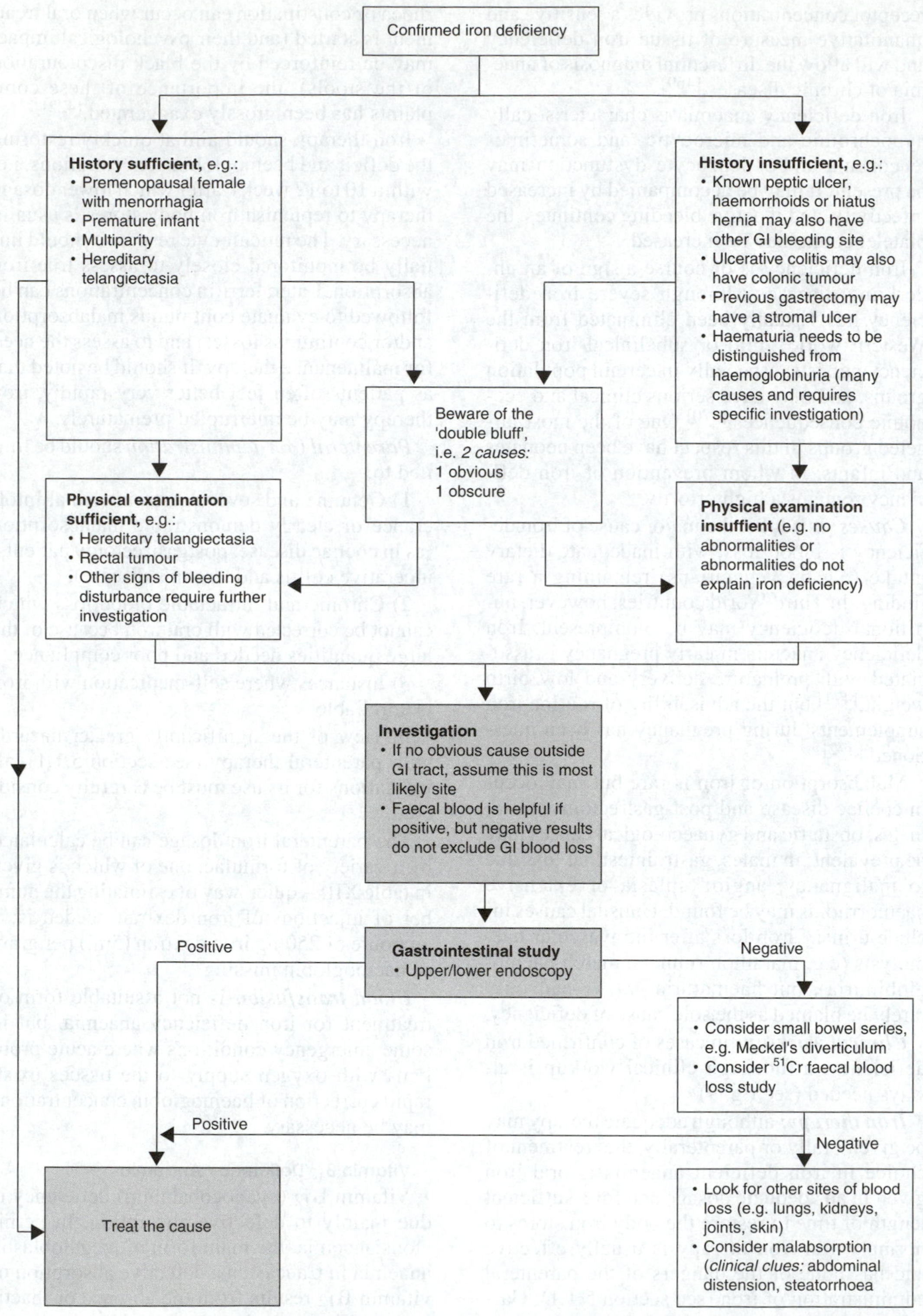


**Fig. 9.** Summary of the investigation and clinical workup of iron deficiency (after Arthur & Isbister[422]).

diseases. Atrophic gastritis is a hallmark of the disease.[473] Patients with pernicious anaemia have a greatly increased risk for gastric cancer and for carcinoid syndrome,[474] and yearly gastroscopic evaluation remains mandatory.

Other mechanisms can also result in inadequate vitamin $B_{12}$ absorption, e.g. extensive gastrointestinal surgery, pathology of the terminal ileum, fish tapeworm infestation, etc. Dietary causes of poor vitamin $B_{12}$ intake may be found in strict vegetarians. Disorders of DNA synthesis in tissues with a high mitotic rate and disturbances of the nervous system are the main abnormalities observed in Vitamin $B_{12}$ deficiency.

Recently, renewed interest has emerged in the so-called 'subtle cobalamin deficiency'. Although serum cobalamin concentrations fall as people age, the incidence of abnormally low serum concentrations has been estimated to be between 5 and 20% of the elderly population.[474] However, most of these patients do not show overt megaloblastic anaemia nor abnormal Schilling tests. Metabolic studies have shown that borderline low cobalamin concentrations are often accompanied by abnormal metabolite concentrations (methylmalonic acid and homocysteine). Even with a normal serum cobalamin, metabolite abnormalities may be present.[475] Whether this has any clinical significance is not known, but some elderly patients do show neurological abnormalities which can be corrected with vitamin $B_{12}$ therapy. Low cobalamin concentrations have also been found in dementia and multiple sclerosis, while raised homocysteine concentrations have been associated with increased thrombogenesis.[79,476]

***Vitamin $B_{12}$ therapy:*** intramuscular or subcutaneous administration of vitamin $B_{12}$ is the treatment of choice. Although *hydroxocobalamin* has some clear advantages (effectiveness in lower doses and at longer dose intervals), *cyanocobalamin* given in a sufficient amount and at appropriate intervals gives satisfactory results. Treatment is aimed at achieving a haematological remission and at restoring body stores of vitamin $B_{12}$. The dose regimen therefore should take into account an initial need to replace vitamin $B_{12}$ stores and a subsequent daily maintenance need of 1 to 2μg. If the response to vitamin $B_{12}$ is poor or absent, it is likely that the megaloblastic anaemia is due to folate deficiency (see below).

Several different initial dosage regimens of vitamin $B_{12}$ are in use. They include intramuscular or subcutaneous administration of 1000 μg/day for 7 days, followed by 1000 μg/week for 4 weeks and if pernicious anaemia is present, 1000μg per month lifelong. Causal therapy should of course be attempted. Adverse effects with vitamin $B_{12}$ injections are rare but include occasional allergic responses and very rarely, anaphylactic reactions. Patients should be carefully monitored during the first days of therapy when the sudden reversal of inefficient to highly efficient erythropoiesis may dramatically decrease potassium concentrations, with consequent life-threatening hypokalaemia.

*Blood transfusion* in megaloblastic anaemia should be avoided, except when life-threatening anaemic complications are present and it is not possible to wait for a response to vitamin $B_{12}$ injections.

#### Folate Deficiency Anaemia

Folate deficiency states are relatively frequent and result mainly from several coexisting causes, such as inadequate dietary intake, poor absorption, increased requirements or loss, and the use of drugs that interfere with folate metabolism (e.g. methotrexate therapy) or absorption (e.g. phenytoin). The daily folic acid requirements for an adult are about 0.1 to 0.2mg. Folate deficiency anaemia may rapidly follow a deficient intake while body stores are low.

Low concentrations of folate (and cobalamin and pyridoxine) may be associated with hyperhomocysteinaemia,[477] which is associated with an increased risk for stroke, coronary disease and peripheral vascular disease. Local cellular depletion of folate may also be a risk factor for carcinogenesis, as has been suggested in smokers.[478] Furthermore, it has been shown that the risk of births with neural tube defects can be halved by the mother taking folic acid 0.4 mg/day during the periconceptional period.[479] This has led to renewed calls for folate supplements to be administered to all women of reproductive age and certainly in early pregnancy. Fortification of food with folate has also been advocated.

In patients with folate deficiency anaemia, oral treatment with *folic acid* will give satisfactory results, even in patients suffering from malabsorption. Daily oral doses of 5mg may be needed for a short time, after which more physiological daily doses of 0.5mg may be continued. Large doses of folic acid may precipitate neurological deficits when erroneously given to patients with vitamin $B_{12}$ deficiency.

Parenteral administration of *folinic acid* may be useful for patients treated with high doses of folic acid antagonists (i.e. 'Leucovorin' rescue in high-dose methotrexate therapy) or in intravenous nutrition protocols.

Folic acid may be administered to patients with increased bone marrow strain, such as postchemotherapy, chronic haemolysis (congenital haemoglobinopathies or acquired), extensive blood loss, post-bone marrow transplantation, etc. Daily intakes above 2mg should be avoided.

#### *5.2.2 Haemolytic Anaemias*

In haemolytic anaemias there is evidence of excessive blood destruction. These anaemias may be caused by an intrinsic red cell defect, either at the membrane, the haemoglobin chains or the enzymatic machinery, or by an extrinsic acquired mechanism, such as autoimmune phenomena, drugs, infections, etc. In the latter forms, therapy will often be restricted to treatment or removal of the underlying cause. Preventive measures are clearly of importance in the acquired or 'extrinsic' haemolytic anaemias.

##### Hereditary Spherocytosis

Hereditary spherocytosis is the most common form of congenital haemolytic anaemia among white Caucasians. It is due to the formation of more fragile spherocytic red cells, caused by a loss of membrane lipids leading to a reduction in the surface-volume ratio. The loss of lipids results from a deficient coverage of the bilayer by the spectrin deficiency. In most cases, the reduction in spectrin content is secondary to a defective attachment of spectrin to ankyrin. Genetic lesions in the ankyrin genes have been demonstrated.[480,481]

Spherocytes display an increased osmotic fragility and autohaemolysis, accounting for the chronic haemolysis *in vivo*. The clinical picture varies from very mild to very severe, with acute haemolytic crisis and life-threatening anaemia. Parvoviruses may cause severe aplastic crises.

Treatment centres around whether or not to perform splenectomy, which invariably alleviates the symptoms and diminishes haemolysis. Most patients with spherocytosis lead perfectly normal lives, but it is probably best to perform splenectomy early in the disease to avoid later complications (aplastic or haemolytic crises) and when no cholecystolithiasis has developed. Splenectomy should be postponed until at least 14 years of age, as postsplenectomy infections may be life-threatening in early childhood. Presplenectomy immunisation against pneumococcal infection should be performed, and in high-risk (younger) patients, penicillin prophylaxis presplenectomy and monthly benzathine benzylpenicillin injections thereafter may be warranted.

Severe haemolytic and aplastic crises are symptomatically treated by blood transfusion. *Epoetin* and *colony-stimulating factors* (CSFs) may be useful in prolonged aplasia.

##### Haemoglobinopathies

The haemoglobinopathies may be caused either by mutations (or deletions) in or around the globin genes, leading to deficient globin chain production and abnormal synthesis of the globin moiety of haemoglobin (thalassaemias) – either by mutations in the coding sequences of the globin gene, or alterations of the protein structure and physicochemical properties of the globin chain (sickle cell anaemia).

***Thalassaemias:*** these haemoglobinopathies are commonly encountered in people of Mediterranean or Southeast Asian origin. Depending on the number of genes involved and on the homo/heterozygosity, the clinical picture of the disease ranges from *thalassaemia minor* with only minor symptoms and normal life-expectancy, and *thalassaemia intermedia* with haemolytic symptoms in stress conditions, to *thalassaemia major* with major symptomatology and premature death. Some homozygous deletions are incompatible with life (hydrops fetalis).

Haemolysis and ineffective erythropoiesis lead to chronic anaemia with marked marrow hyperplasia, resulting in characteristic bone deformities, hepatosplenomegaly, icterus and retarded growth. Increased iron turnover with increased iron absorption, together with chronic transfusions lead rapidly to iron overload, which may be the direct cause of death.[482]

Thalassaemia minor does not require treatment. For symptomatic thalassaemic patients, modern management permits a near normal quality and extended quantity of life. In patients with thalassaemia major, hypertransfusion programmes have been designed to keep haemoglobin concentrations around 12 g/dl in order to avoid bone deformities and growth retardation. A *conditio sine qua non* for these programmes is adequate iron chelation to avoid organ damage by haemochromatosis. *Deferoxamine* in average doses of 30 to 50 mg/kg/day subcutaneously or intravenously should be administered.[431] Splenectomy is only carried out if transfusion requirements exceed the chelatable iron burden.

Bone marrow transplantation has become a realistic option for patients with severe thalassaemia major.[483] In patients with bad prognostic factors (hepatomegaly, portal fibrosis, poor quality of chelation therapy), the event-free survival ranges between 60 and 90%. However, sudden cardiac tamponade is a major risk post-transplant and remains unexplained.[484]

A number of drugs (e.g. hydroxycarbamide, azacytidine, butyrate, cytarabine) are presently being evaluated for their therapeutic efficacy in augmenting the synthesis of fetal haemoglobin, which may compensate for the unbalanced $\alpha$/non-$\alpha$ globin chain ratio in $\beta$-thalassaemia. Although these attempts have been less successful in thalassaemia than in sickle cell disease, some patients may benefit from hydroxycarbamide therapy.[485] Intravenous infusion of the short-chain fatty acid arginine butyrate modestly increased haemoglobin concentrations in children with homozygous thalassaemia.[486]

Other potential therapies include epoetin which has been shown to increase haemoglobin concentrations in patients with thalassaemia intermedia.[487] Finally, gene therapy using retroviral vectors may open exciting perspectives in the treatment of these disorders.

***Sickle cell anaemia:*** a single base pair substitution in the $\beta$-globin gene leads to the production of the sickle $\beta$ chain, which under the influence of deoxygenation, forms the sickle cell haemoglobin polymer. Associated events are an impaired deformability of the sickle red cell, an increased adhesion of red cells to the endothelium, the entrapment of cells in the microvasculature, and infarctisation.

Sickle cell anaemia occurs mainly in Negroid populations, but also in some Mediterranean, Indian and Arabic populations. Only homozygous sickle cell patients are symptomatic. However, the phenotypic expression of the disease is highly heterogeneous, leading to a wide variety in clinical syndromes. The coinheritance of $\alpha$-thalassaemia usually leads to a less severe form of the disease.

Classically, sickle cell symptomatology is dominated by painful vaso-occlusive crises,[488] which may sometimes be complicated by stroke, priapism, pulmonary vaso-occlusive disease, and acute chest syndrome (respiratory distress, fever, pain). Often, these crises are provoked by intercurrent infections.

Symptomatic treatment includes pain management with morphine, orally or intravenously. Patient-controlled analgesia (see chapter 12; sect. 7.2.1) has been tried with good success.[489] Acute haemodilution with glucose infusions can sometimes be helpful, while prevention or prompt treatment of infections can prevent sickle cell crises. Intensive, long term transfusions can reduce the frequency of thrombotic complications in children,[490] and keeping the concentration of haemoglobin S at around or below 50% can prevent sickle cell stroke recurrence. Exchange transfusions may be used in acute complications such as stroke or priapism.[491] Folic acid and other haematinics can also be used when indicated.

Newer approaches to the management of sickle cell disease include attempts to increase haemoglobin F concentrations with agents such as hydroxycarbamide or butyrate. Preliminary data[492] indicate that *hydroxycarbamide* in dosages up to 1000 mg/day can raise haemoglobin F concentrations in most patients, possibly leading to diminished symptomatology. However, larger randomised trials are needed to prove the validity of this approach.

*Epoetin* can be used to increase haemoglobin concentrations (with or without hydroxycarbamide) in sickle cell patients.[493] However, cost : benefit ratios should be carefully considered before embarking on long term epoetin treatment.

Bone marrow transplantation has already been successfully used both in the US and Europe.[494] The majority of patients become asymptomatic and splenic function is restored. However, the selection of candidates for transplant remains difficult in view of the dangers involved with the procedure. Gene therapy offers exciting perspectives, but has not yet entered the clinical arena.

#### Glucose-6-Phosphate Dehydrogenase (G6PD) Deficiency

Glucose-6-phosphate dehydrogenase deficiency is a common hereditary defect of red cells in African, Black and Oriental populations, and in Sephardic Jews, Northwest Indians, and some Mediterranean and Asian peoples. The red cells lack a critical enzyme in oxidant defence and are extremely vulnerable to oxidant stress (i.e. the generation of reactive oxygen species, e.g. superoxide, hydrogen peroxide, hydroxyl radicals leading to oxidation of membrane phospholipids, red cell leakage and haemolysis). Many factors, including fava beans, certain drugs (table XVIII), infections and metabolic disturbances such as diabetic ketoacidosis can precipitate acute intravascular haemolysis, haemoglobinuria, renal blockade and sometimes death.[495]

Since there is no effective treatment, it is important that patients are screened before being given drugs known to provoke haemolysis. Transfusion is rarely necessary, although exchange transfusion has been tried in hyperacute situations. Maintenance of a good urine flow during the haemolytic crisis is crucial. Tocopherol (vitamin E) may be given as antioxidant prophylaxis.

### Acquired Haemolytic Anaemias

Acquired haemolysis may be due to immunological, physical, chemical or microbiological agents.

***Immune haemolytic anaemia:*** most of the immune-mediated haemolytic anaemias are autoimmune in origin. Alloimmune haemolysis may be encountered in transfusion medicine.

Autoimmune haemolytic anaemia, either by warm or cold type autoantibodies, may be idiopathic or caused by underlying malignant (lymphoma), systemic (lupus) or infectious (viral) conditions, or by various drugs (table XIX). Where possible, the underlying cause should be corrected. However, if this is not possible or if urgent intervention is needed, *corticosteroids* (e.g. methylprednisolone 64 mg/day orally or 1000mg intravenously for 3 days) form the cornerstone of therapy. Corticosteroids should be given for at least 6 to 8 weeks before their failure can be documented. Splenectomy may then become necessary. Transfusion is rarely indicated and may be complicated by increased haemolysis. If life-threatening conditions are present, premedication with high-dose corticosteroids (methylprednisolone 1000mg intravenously) before transfusion and very close clinical monitoring of the patient is necessary.

In cold agglutinin syndromes, corticosteroids are less effective. Transfusions should always be given through blood warming devices and patients should be kept warm. Plasmapheresis may be useful, but care should be given to prewarm all components used during the procedure.

If corticosteroids and splenectomy fail to control the disease, immunosuppressive drugs can be used (e.g. azathioprine and mercaptopurine).[496] High doses of intravenous gammaglobulins have also been advocated in refractory immune-mediated haemolysis.[497] However, the excessive cost of these infusions precludes their routine use. Danazol may be a useful addition to the therapeutic armamentarium in refractory patients.[498]

***Haemolysis caused by mechanical damage:*** march haemoglobinuria and other sport-related haemolytic anaemias are rare. Adaptation of the shoes to the conditions and increased fluid intake are usually sufficient.

***Haemolysis caused by chemicals or physical agents:*** heat and cold may provoke acute haemolysis. In such cases, preventive measures to avoid exposure are warranted. Lead may cause low-grade haemolysis and in cases of poisoning, chelation therapy with edetic acid (EDTA) is necessary. Chlorates and nitrites are oxidative agents which may cause haemolysis upon accidental ingestion. Therapy is purely symptomatic.

***Haemolysis due to infections with microorganisms:*** malaria parasites are probably the world's most common cause of haemolytic anaemia. Viruses mostly mediate haemolysis through immune reactions, while Gram-negative bacteria may provoke intravascular haemolysis with massive haemoglobinuria. *Clostridium welchii* infection (e.g. in septic abortion) is a well known cause of life-threatening intravascular haemolysis.

**Table XVIII.** Drugs that can and cannot be safely given in the presence of glucose-6-phosphate dehydrogenase (G6PD) deficiency

| |
|---|
| **1. Drugs associated with severe haemolysis in G6PD deficiency:** |
| Primaquine and other antimalarials |
| Aminophenazone |
| Nalidixic acid |
| Nitrofurantoin |
| Sulfonamides (sulfapyridine, sulfamethoxazole) |
| Quinine, quinidine |
| Sulfones (dapsone) |
| **2. Drugs that can safely be given in G6PD deficiency:** |
| Aspirin (acetylsalicylic acid)) |
| Ascorbic acid |
| Chloramphenicol |
| Colchicine |
| Diphenhydramine |
| Isoniazid |
| Phenytoin |
| Probenecid |
| Pyrimethamine |
| Trimethoprim |
| Vitamin K |

**Table XIX.** Drugs possibly associated with immune haemolytic anaemia

| Mechanism | Drugs |
|---|---|
| Hapten mechanism | Penicillin (high doses) |
| | Cefalosporins (high doses) |
| | Tetracyclines |
| Immune complex mechanism ('innocent bystander') | Quinine |
| | Quinidine |
| | Stibophen |
| | Chlorpropamide |
| | Rifampicin |
| Autoantibody mechanism | Methyldopa |
| | Mefenamic acid |
| Nonspecific protein absorption | Cefalothin |
| Unknown | Chlorpromazine |
| | Isoniazid |
| | Melphalan |
| | Paracetamol (acetaminophen) |
| | Thiazides |
| | Ibuprofen |
| | Triamterene |
| | Erythromycin |

Treatment of the underlying cause is of course preferable, wherever possible, and symptomatic treatment may be given when clinically indicated.

#### *5.2.3 Aplastic Anaemia*

Aplastic anaemia is a heterogeneous disorder with often a grim prognosis. The primary defect lies more often with the haematopoietic stem cell than with the stroma.[499] The precise nature of the injury to the haematopoietic progenitors remains enigmatic. Aplastic anaemia progenitors are still responsive to growth factors (e.g. stem cell factor[500]), but responses appear to be more blunted in patients than in healthy controls. Aplastic marrow stroma also produces similar or even higher amounts of endogenous growth factors and cytokines.[501] However, recent data have renewed interest in excessive production of interferons as a direct cause of haematopoietic progenitor suppression.[502] In addition, an immune-mediated suppression (possibly T cell mediated) has strongly been suggested by many *in vitro* studies and by the successes of immunosuppressive therapy.

Clinically, the aetiology of aplastic anaemia often remains idiopathic, but postinfective (e.g. viral hepatitis, parvovirus) cases have been well documented. In many other cases drugs, chemicals (e.g. benzene) and radiation have been incriminated. The most frequently implicated drugs are chloramphenicol, phenylbutazone and oxyphenbutazone, sulfonamides and gold (table XX). In many cases, 2 forms of bone marrow suppression by drugs can be discerned, i.e. a dose-related usually transient one, and a dose-independent, idiosyncratic and irreversible aplasia. The latter can occur some weeks to months after ingestion of the drug. Following chloramphenicol ingestion, the risk of severe aplastic anaemia has been calculated to be between 1 : 24,000 and 1 : 40,000.[503] Both a genetically-determined hypersensitivity of the bone marrow progenitors and an impaired or abnormal metabolism of some drugs in some patients, may play a role in the pathogenesis.

Prevention is clearly very important. Drugs that have been implicated in the aetiopathogenesis of aplastic anaemia should be avoided and alternatives used. If blood counts decrease, immediate withdrawal of all drugs is indicated.

From a clinical viewpoint, aplastic anaemia has been subdivided into very severe, severe and minor aplastic cases, depending on the degree of myelosuppression (as illustrated by granulocyte and platelets counts, the reticulocyte index and bone marrow histology). Therapeutic strategies largely depend on this grading system. In non-severe cases, a 'wait and see' attitude can be adopted, while in very severe cases, immediate highly interventional measures must be taken. Management in such cases centres around 3 questions:

1) Who should receive a bone marrow transplant?

2) Which is the most effective form of immunosuppression?

3) What role do growth factors play?

Formerly, aplastic anaemia patients were often treated with androgens (e.g. oxymetholone 2 mg/kg/day) or with corticosteroids (methylprednisolone 1 to 3 mg/kg/day with progressive tapering); however, these regimens are now reserved for older patients with not very severe aplastic indices. In children and younger adults (<30 years) with very severe aplastic anaemia who have a fully matched HLA-identical sibling, *allogeneic bone marrow transplantation* (BMT) remains the treatment of choice. The available data indicate that in such cases, a 5-year survival of 69% can be expected.[504] Conditioning of the transplants with total body irradiation has not proved to be beneficial (due to a rising incidence of secondary tumours), while cyclosporin prevention of graft-*versus*-host disease has yielded the best results. Adverse risk factors include the use of parous or transfused female donors, the presence of pretransplant infections, polytransfusion and age.

**Table XX.** Chemical agents associated with the development of aplastic anaemia

| |
|---|
| Benzene; trinitrotoluene |
| Insecticides |
| Anticancer agents |
| Analgesics |
| • phenylbutazone |
| • oxyphenbutazone |
| Antimicrobial agents |
| • chloramphenicol |
| • mepacrine |
| • sulfafurazole (sulfisoxazole) |
| Antiepileptic drugs |
| • mephenytoin |
| • trimethadione (troxidone) |
| • carbamazepine |
| Gold compounds |
| Psychotropic agents |
| • meprobamate |
| • chlorpromazine |

Non-related HLA-identical donors may also be used, but survival may be significantly less than in the sibling situation (50%).[505] For very young patients with a grim prognosis, unrelated or minor mismatched BMT remains a valuable option.[506]

*Immunosuppressive treatment* has progressed considerably over recent years and is the treatment of choice for younger patients without a bone marrow donor or for patients with severe (as opposed to very severe) aplastic anaemia. In a comparison of cyclosporin with antithymocyte globulin (ATG), cyclosporin proved to be at least as effective and possibly better than ATG in inducing clinical and haematological remissions.[507] The actuarial 5-year survival rate with immunosuppression is around 60%, which compares favourably with the more hazardous transplant procedure. Combinations of cyclosporin with ATG upfront or with growth factors may further improve survival figures.[508]

*Growth factors and cytokines* have become increasingly important in the supportive care of aplastic anaemia patients. G-CSF induces transient but significant increases in granulocyte counts, which may be extremely helpful in combatting neutropenic sepsis or in bridging the period between therapies.[509] However, considerable concern has arisen after the report that growth factors may lead to, enhance, or promote clonal evolution of aplasia to myelodysplasia.[510] Clonal disorders – either premalignant or malignant – may occur much more frequently in aplastic anaemia than was expected previously. Long term follow-up points to an incidence of between 25 and 40% of paroxysmal nocturnal haemoglobinuria, myelodysplasia and leukaemia, mostly in patients treated with immunosuppressive therapy.[511] Using sensitive techniques, aplastic anaemia can often be shown to be a clonal disorder itself, even before treatment.[512]

*Supportive care* of patients with aplastic anaemia, directed towards the control of bleeding and infection, remains crucial. Early empirical or prophylactic antimicrobial, antiviral and antifungal agents and red cell and platelet transfusions may be life-saving. Menorrhagia in female patients should be controlled with progestagens; mucosal bleeding may respond to fibrinolysis inhibitors such as tranexamic acid.

#### Fanconi's Anaemia or Congenital Aplastic Anaemia

The Fanconi gene has recently been cloned.[298] In many patients with Fanconi's anaemia, leukaemia or myelodysplasia will develop. Bone marrow transplantation remains the choice treatment, leading to a 5-year survival rate of 65%.[513] Low-dose cyclophosphamide and irradiation are superior to other conditioning regimens.

Growth factors can transiently improve neutrophil counts. Androgens should be used with caution, because of the possibility of clonal evolution.

#### Pure Red Cell Aplasia

The congenital form of pure red cell aplasia (Diamond Blackfan anaemia) responds poorly to classical treatments such as androgens and/or corticosteroids. Iron overload, secondary to polytransfusions, carries a grave prognosis. While bone marrow transplantation may offer cure for the few patients who have a compatible sibling donor, growth factors such as interleukin-3, with or without epoetin, and especially stem cell factor may offer new hopes for the future.[514]

Acquired pure red cell aplasia is often associated with immune disorders, lymphoma and/or thymoma. Some drugs have also been incriminated (e.g. gold salts). Treatment of the causal condition by corticosteroids, thymectomy or drug withdrawal may lead to sustained remissions. However, in refractory cases, occasional successes have been reported with plasmapheresis. Cyclosporin has now been proven to be effective as rescue treatment in resistant cases.[515]

#### Human Parvovirus B19-related Aplasia

Human parvovirus B19 may be the cause of aplastic crises in chronic haemolytic anaemias or in immunocompromised patients.[516] Pure red cell aplasia may also be encountered following infections in otherwise normal children. Spontaneous remissions are not infrequent.

Supportive measures are important. In chronic cases, corticosteroids and/or cyclosporin may be used.

#### 5.2.4 Anaemias of Uncertain Origin and Chronic Disorders

Secondary anaemias may accompany chronic infectious or inflammatory conditions, systemic diseases or neoplastic disorders. They are believed to be caused by a diffuse immune activation against chronic antigenaemia, leading to the production of a variety of cytokines (i.e. interleukin-1, tumour necrosis factor, interferon-α and interferon-γ, and transforming growth factor-β). Most of these cytokines exert an inhibitory action on bone marrow erythroid colony-forming units. This leads to a reduction in reticulocyte production and the appearance of normocytic normochromic anaemia. Moreover, the physiological response of the kidneys to the lower haematocrit is blunted and less erythropoietin than expected is produced. This may also be an effect of inappropriate interleukin-1 secretion.[517]

*Epoetin* has therefore been used in the treatment of secondary anaemias. In rheumatoid arthritis, high dosages of epoetin (i.e. more than 100 U/kg 3 times weekly) can lead to significant increases and normalisation of haematocrit.[518] In patients with the acquired immune deficiency syndrome (AIDS), who have serum erythropoietin concentrations below 500 U/L, treatment with epoetin (100 to 200 U/kg 3 times weekly) can increase the haematocrit by at least 4% and significantly reduces red cell transfusion requirements.[519]

Similar doses of epoetin administered to patients with active multiple myeloma not only improve haemoglobin concentrations, but also increase the quality of life and the general sense of well-being.[520] Other forms of cancer tend to respond at least as favourably to prolonged treatment with epoetin.[521] When using pharmacological doses of epoetin, cost : benefit ratios must be considered. Mere 'cosmetics of the numbers' should be avoided and improved quality of life must remain the primary goal.

### 5.3 Clinical Outcome and Economic Considerations

Anaemia is a relatively common medical problem, with a rather minor impact on survival, but often major impairment on the quality of life of patients. Effective therapy is mostly available, the cost of which may vary from a few dollars for iron supplementation to thousands of dollars for epoetin therapy. In the current cost conscious environment, cost-effectiveness and cost-benefit ratios are becoming increasingly important. In the anaemia of chronic renal failure and dialysis, the impact of epoetin therapy on quality of life has been enormous, including a potential for return to full employment, reduced need for hospitalisation and an improved general sense of well-being. However, compared with blood transfusions, the acquisition cost of epoetin is very great. Cost-effectiveness analyses to date have indicated that the expense of epoetin warrants its use in only severely incapacitated and transfusion-dependent patients.[522]

Low dosage regimens of epoetin can be expected to improve its cost benefit. Lowering the target haematocrit levels, preferential use of the subcutaneous route, and varying the frequency of administration, will lead to considerable cost savings, while maintaining clinical benefit. Median dosages of 75 U/kg weekly may be equally effective as the previously recommended 150 U/kg. Moreover, the risks of allogeneic transfusions – the alternative option – including transmission of infectious disease and immediate and delayed transfusion reactions, should not be underestimated. The adverse effects of transfusions easily outscore those of epoetin therapy. Much depends on what society is willing to pay for these benefits in a small group of patients.[523]

The economic problem is even more complex in the treatment of the anaemia of cancer. Epoetin has been shown to be an effective drug in patients with multiple myeloma, lymphoproliferative disorders and various solid tumours under chemotherapeutic treatment. Clinical benefits include a reduction in the number of blood units transfused and an improvement in the quality of life of responding patients. However, the anaemia of cancer is multifactorial in origin and the effects of any therapy may be masked by the underlying disease or its complications. For rational use, good predictors of response are urgently needed. Ludwig et al.[524]

found that after 2 weeks of treatment, serum erythropoietin (<100 mU/ml) and change in haemoglobin (>0.5 g/dl) taken together were a powerful predictor or responsiveness to epoetin treatment. Others have substituted or supplemented the initial erythropoietin concentration as the most powerful predictor by use of the O/P (observed over predicted) ratio, i.e. a comparison of the patient's serum erythropoietin concentration and the reference serum erythropoietin threshold values for that degree of anaemia.[525]

An O/P ratio of <0.9 together with a serum erythropoietin concentration below 50 mU/ml will predict a positive response with an overall accuracy of 90%.[526] Preliminary data suggest that the use of circulating transferrin receptor values may even further increase the predictive power of this model.

Economic analysis of new treatment regimens will have to be repeated and kept up to date with changing patient risk categories and changing societal views.

## 6. Neutropenia and Agranuloyctosis

Blood neutrophil counts 2 standard deviations below normal are termed neutropenia, while agranulocytosis literally means zero granulocytes, but is often used to indicate very low neutrophil counts (i.e. below $0.5 \times 10^9$/L).

### 6.1 Optimum Treatment

#### *6.1.1 Congenital Neutropenias*

Among these rare disorders, Kostmann's syndrome and cyclic neutropenia are the most frequently encountered. Many more cases are termed chronic idiopathic neutropenia, often accompanied by functional defects of granulocytes (e.g. Chediak-Higashi, Schwachman-Diamond, etc.).

While in the most severe cases, bone marrow transplantation may offer a chance for cure, myeloid growth factors may significantly improve the quality of life in these patients.[465] Even low doses of G-CSF are capable of increasing neutrophil counts above infection levels. However, long term administration of these growth factors may, in some cases, lead to osteopenia and splenomegaly.

#### *6.1.2 Immune Neutropenia*

Antineutrophil antibodies can be found in a variety of immune disorders, e.g. rheumatoid arthritis, lupus erythematosus, Felty syndrome, etc. Treatment of these neutropenias is causal.

#### *6.1.3 Drug-Induced Agranulocytosis*

Agranulocytosis is a rare but potentially serious adverse event of drug administration. It can be expected as a normal consequence of the treatment with chemotherapeutic drugs, but it may also appear as an idiosyncratic reaction to very small amounts of a multitude of drugs (table XXI).[527]

The pathogenesis is not fully understood. Both a peripheral 'immune' type and a central 'toxic' type can be recognised. Mostly antineutrophil antibodies (drug-dependent or drug-induced autoantibodies) are involved, leading to peripheral destruction, but sometimes direct toxic effects on the bone marrow may be seen.[528] No direct genetic or environmental susceptibility factors have yet been identified, although subtle inherited metabolic abnormalities in drug clearance or disposition may be present.

The immune type of agranulocytosis is characterised by a sudden onset of chills, fever, bone aches and collapse shortly after the ingestion of a small amount of drug in a previously sensitised individual. The peripheral blood shows an abrupt disappearance of all mature granulocytes, and antigranulocyte antibodies can be demonstrated. Complete recovery can be expected within 5 to 7 days after stopping the drug, but subsequent administration of even very small amounts of the drug will precipitate a recurrence. Drugs that can cause agranulocytosis via this immune mechanism include pyrazolones such as aminophenazone (amidopyrine) and dipyrone, penicillins (high doses), phenytoin, propylthiouracil, quinidine and other antiarrhythmics, tolbutamide, and $H_2$-receptor antagonists. Antibodies may be directed against the drug itself or against drug-induced membrane alterations. Drugs may also induce the formation of autoantibodies, and sometimes a drug-induced lupus-like syndrome is involved.

The toxic type of drug-induced agranulocytosis is characterised by a rather slow onset, with a decrease in granulocytes after a certain latency period or after ingestion of cumulative dosages. Infectious symptoms may soon appear and are often accompanied by severe mucositis and infections of the throat and upper airways. Retreatment with the same drug will not necessarily induce a sudden relapse, but this may be likely when a certain threshold or cumulative

**Table XXI.** Drugs associated with agranulocytosis

**1. Predictable**

Cytostatics, antimetabolites, alkylating agents
Benzene, toluene, ethanol
Irradiation
High-dose chloramphenicol, thiamphenicol, cotrimoxazole (trimethoprim/sulfamethoxazole), rifampicin

**2. Idiosyncratic**

*Analgesics and anti-inflammatory drugs:*
Aminophenazone (aminopyrine) and combinations
Phenazone (antipyrine)
Dipyrone and combinations
Phenylbutazone, oxyphenbutazone
Indomethacin, ibuprofen and similar drugs

*Antihistamines:*
Thenalidine

*Antimicrobial drugs:*
Penicillins (high-dose)
Antimalarial drugs
Cefalosporins
Tetracyclines
Sulfonamides
Cotrimoxazole
Metronidazole
Clindamycin
Rifampicin
Isoniazid
Antiviral drugs
Antifungal drugs
Chloramphenicol, thiamphenicol

*Antithyroid drugs:*
Propylthiouracil
Thiamazole (methimazole)

*Cardiovascular drugs:*
Quinidine
Aprindine
Procainamide
Propranolol and other β-blockers
Tocainide
Captopril
Nifedipine
Methyldopa

*Antidiabetic drugs:*
Tolbutamide
Carbutamide
Chlorpropamide

*Antiepileptic drugs:*
Phenytoin, mephenytoin
Carbamazepine
Ethosuximide
Valproic acid (sodium valproate)
Trimethadione (troxidone)

*Antipsychotics, antidepressants, anxiolytics:*
Phenothiazines (especially chlorpromazine)
Haloperidol
Imipramine
Meprobamate
Chlordiazepoxide
Diazepam
Mianserin
Perazine

*Antirheumatics:*
Gold
Penicillamine
Levamisole
All anti-inflammatory drugs

*Diuretics:*
Chlorothiazide and related drugs
Ethacrynic acid
Triamterene

*Gastrointestinal drugs:*
Cimetidine, ranitidine, omeprazole
Sulfapyridine

*Others:*
Allopurinol
Levodopa
Dapsone
Ticlopidine

dose is exceeded. Prototype drugs for this type of agranulocytosis are the phenothiazines, especially chlorpromazine. Tricyclic antidepressants and anxiolytic drugs may also provoke bone marrow depression.

For a number of drugs evidence exists for both an immune-mediated and a toxic mechanism.[528]

Prevention of the (re)development of drug-induced agranulocytosis is crucial in susceptible patients. Lists of potentially causative drugs should be distributed to patients and clinicians. In treating drug-induced agranulocytosis, immediate withdrawal of the offending drug is very important because the prognosis may be dependent on the total dose of drug administered. Early empirical antibiotic treatment, institution of prophylactic gut decontamination and antifungal agents, protective isolation, etc. may be urgently needed. Neither corticosteroids nor immunoglobulins are of any proven value.

Treatment with colony-stimulating factors (CSFs) can be rapidly instituted to accelerate granulocyte recovery, but it is difficult to prove that they change the natural course of the disease and that survival will eventually be improved.[529]

## 7. Use of Drugs in the Presence of Associated Haematological Disorders

Drugs used in the treatment of non-haematological disease may have adverse haematological effects and cause serious toxicity in patients with blood diseases. A knowledge of the spectrum of activity of the drugs prescribed is obviously essential for their safe use. Alternatively, the haematological disease itself may influence the response to other drugs. Interactions with certain groups of drugs used in haematological disorders can also be important.

### 7.1 Thromboembolic Disorders

Many drugs have the potential to modify the response to oral coumarin anticoagulants and although clinically harmful effects are not common, fatalities from severe bleeding have occurred. Predictably interacting drugs such as phenylbutazone and enzyme-inducing drugs such as barbiturates should be avoided. Most adverse interactions may be prevented if a few simple precautions are followed (see section 3.1.5).[216] Oral contraceptives of the combined estrogen-progestagen type, especially high-dose preparations, should be avoided in those with thrombotic lesions or a thrombotic tendency of any kind (see also chapter 18; sect. 10.2).

### 7.2 Bleeding Disorders

Ingestion of usual therapeutic dosages of aspirin produces a marked prolongation of bleeding time in some patients with haemophilia A or B, or with von Willebrand's disease (see section 3.1.1 and 4.2.1). Aspirin and other drugs that affect platelet function (see section 3.1.1) should be avoided in those with functional platelet disorders, and also in the presence of even a mild haemostatic defect, e.g. a history of even slightly prolonged bleeding after tooth extraction. Paracetamol (acetaminophen) is a suitable alternative analgesic. Fibrinolysis inhibitors such as ε-aminocaproic acid and tranexamic acid can lead to temporary kidney blockade if used in patients with haematuria.[530]

### 7.3 Anaemias

In patients with iron deficiency anaemia, simultaneous administration of oral iron preparations (ferrous sulfate, fumarate, succinate) and oral tetracyclines can markedly inhibit the absorption of the tetracycline. Iron absorption (from supplements but not food) is inhibited as well. If such combined therapy is indicated, the interaction can be avoided (except in the case of doxycycline and minocycline) by giving the drugs 3 hours apart.[427] Anaemias can also affect the rate of elimination of some drugs.

Patients with megaloblastic anaemia given cotrimoxazole not only show a poor response to specific haematinic therapy, but the antifolate effect of the drug can also increase the severity of the megaloblastic changes and cause significant haematopoietic depression.[531] In patients with pernicious anaemia and achlorhydria, the absorption of drugs such as cefalexin can be impaired in some patients, but the clinical significance of this is far from clear.

Individuals with inherited abnormalities of erythrocyte (e.g. G6PD deficiency) or haemoglobin (haemoglobin H, Zurich) function are particularly susceptible to oxidising agents (e.g. nitrites) and certain other drugs. Such drugs also cause an increase in methaemoglobinaemia in those with hereditary methaemoglobinaemia.

## References

1. Rosenberg RD, Rosenberg JS. Natural anticoagulant mechanisms. Journal of Clinical Investigation 1984; 74: 1-6
2. Marcum JA, Rosenberg JS, Bauer KA, et al. The heparin-antithrombin mechanism and vessel wall function. In: Gimbrone MA, editor. Vascular endothelium in hemostasis and thrombosis. Edinburgh: Churchill Livingstone, 1986: 70-98
3. Vane JR, Anggard EE, Botting RM. Regulatory functions of the vascular endothelium. New England Journal of Medicine 1990; 323: 27-36
4. Jaffe EA. Endothelial cell structure and function. In: Hoffman R, Benz EJ, Shattil SJ, et al., editors. Hematology: basic principles and practice. New York: Churchill Livingstone, 1991: 1198-212
5. Weksler BB, Jaffe EA. Prostacyclin and endothelium. In: Gimbrone MA, editor. Vascular endothelium in hemostasis and thrombosis. Edinburgh: Churchill Livingstone, 1986: 40-56
6. Gimbrone MA. Vascular endothelium: nature's blood container. In: Fimbrone A, editor. Vascular endothelium in hemostasis and thrombosis. Edinburgh: Churchill Livingstone, 1986: 1-13
7. Radomski MW, Moncada S. Regulation of nitric oxide in the vascular system. Thrombosis and Haemostasis 1993; 70: 36-9
8. Furchgott RF, Vanhoutte PM. Endothelium-deriving relaxing and contracting factors. FASEB Journal 1989; 3: 2007-18

9. Rubanyl GM, editor. Endothelin. New York: Oxford University Press, 1992
10. Hanahan DJ. Platelet-activating factor; a biologically active phosphoglyceride. Annual Review of Biochemistry 1986; 55: 483-509
11. Esmon CT. Regulation of protein C activation by components of the endothelium surface in vascular endothelium. In: Gimbrone MA, editor. Vascular endothelium in hemostasis and thrombosis. Edinburgh: Churchill Livingstone, 1986: 99-119
12. Esmon CT. The roles of protein C and thrombomodulin in the regulation of blood coagulation. Journal of Biological Chemistry 1989; 264: 4743-6
13. Fressinaud E, Baruch D, Rothschild C, et al. Platelet von Willebrand factor: evidence for its involvement in platelet adhesion to collagen. Blood 1987; 70: 1214-7
14. Baumgartner HR, Haudenschild C. Adhesion of platelets to subendothelium. Annals of the New York Academy of Sciences 1972; 201: 22-36
15. Harker LA. Pathogenesis of thrombosis. In: Williams WJ, editor. Hematology. 4th ed. New York: McGraw-Hill, 1990: 1559-69
16. Ruoslahti E. Integrins. Journal of Clinical Investigation 1991; 87: 1-5
17. Kieffer N, Philips DR. Platelet membrane glycoproteins: functions in cellular interactions. Annual Review of Cell Biology 1990; 6: 329-57
18. Lapetina EG. The signal transduction induced by thrombin in human platelets. FEBS Letters 1990; 268: 400-4
19. Rhee SG. Inositol phospholipid-specific phospholipase C: interaction of the τ1 isoform with tyrosine kinase. Trends in Biochemical Sciences 1991; 16: 297-301
20. Ratnofff OD, Saito H. Interactions among Hageman factor, plasma prekallikrein, high molecular weight kininogen, and plasma thromboplastin antecedent. Proceedings of the National Academy of Sciences USA 1979; 76: 958-61
21. Cochrane CG, Griffin JH. The biochemistry and pathophysiology of the contact system of plasma. Advances in Immunology 1982; 32: 242-306
22. Silverberg SA, Nemerson Y, Zur M, et al. Kinetics of the activation of bovine coagulation factor X by components of the extrinsic pathway. Kinetic behavior of two-chain factor VII in the presence of tissue factor. Journal of Biological Chemistry 1977; 252: 8481-8
23. Nemerson Y. Tissue factor of hemostasis. Blood 1988; 71: 1-8
24. Mann KG, Jenny RJ, Krishnaswamy S. Cofactor proteins in the assembly and expression of blood clotting enzyme complexes. Annual Review of Biochemistry 1988; 57: 915-56
25. Edgington TS, Mackman M, Brand K, et al. The structural biology of expression and function of tissue factor. Thrombosis and Haemostasis 1991; 66: 67-79
26. Gilbert GE, Furie BC, Furie B. Binding of human factor VIII to phospholipid vesicles. Journal of Biological Chemistry 1990; 265: 815-22
27. Newcomb TF, Hoshida M. Factor V and thrombin. Scandinavian Journal of Clinical and Laboratory Investigation 1965; 17 Suppl. 84: 61-9
28. Husten EJ, Esmon CT, Johnson AE. The active site of blood coagulation factor Xa. Its distance from the phospholipid surface and its conformational sensitivity to components of the prothrombinase complex. Journal of Biological Chemistry 1987; 262: 12953-61
29. Bevers EM, Comfurius P, van Rijn JLML, et al. Generation of prothrombin-converting activity and the exposure of phosphatidylserine at the outer surface of platelets. European Journal of Biochemistry 1982; 122: 429-36
30. Zur M, Nemerson Y. Kinetics of factor IX activation via the extrinsic pathway. Journal of Biological Chemistry 1980; 255: 5703-7
31. Jesty J, Silverberg SA. Kinetics of the tissue factor-dependent activation of coagulation factors IX and X in a bovine system. Journal of Biological Chemistry 1979; 254: 12337-45
32. Marlar RA, Griffin JH. Alternative pathways of thromboplastin-dependent activation of human factor X plasma. Annals of the New York Academy of Sciences 1981; 370: 325-35
33. Collen D. On the regulation and control of fibrinolysis. Thrombosis and Haemostasis 1980; 43: 77-89
34. Lijnen HR, Collen D. Molecular mechanisms of thrombolytic therapy. Haemostasis 1986; 16 Suppl. 3: 3-15
35. Collen D, Lijnen HR. Basic and clinical aspects of fibrinolysis and thrombolysis. Blood 1991; 78: 3114-24
36. Castellino FJ. Structure-function relationships of human plasminogen and plasmin. In: Tissue-type plasminogen activator (t-PA): physiological and clinical aspects. Boca Raton: CRC Press, 1988: 145-70
37. Holmes WE, Pennica D, Haber M, et al. Cloning and expression of the gene for pro-urokinase in Escherichia coli. Biotechnology 1985; 3: 923-9
38. Pannell R, Gurewich V. Pro-urokinase: a study of its stability in plasma and of a mechanism for its selective fibrinolytic effect. Blood 1986; 67: 1215-23
39. Lijnen HR, Stump DC, Collen D. Single-chain urokinase-type plasminogen activator: mechanism of action and thrombolytic properties. Seminars in Thrombosis and Hemostasis 1987; 13: 152-9
40. Lijnen HR, Zamarron C, Blaber M, et al. Activation of plasminogen by pro-urokinase. I. Mechanism. Journal of Biological Chemistry 1986; 261: 1253-8
41. Erickson LA, Ginsberg MH, Loskutoff DJ. Detection and partial characterization of an inhibitor of plasminogen activator in human platelets. Journal of Clinical Investigation 1984; 74: 1465-72
42. Pannell R, Black J, Gurewich V. Complementary modes of action of tissue-type plasminogen activator and pro-urokinase by which their synergistic effect on clot lysis may be explained. Journal of Clinical Investigation 1988; 81: 853-9
43. Kruithof EKO, Tran-Thang C, Ransijn A, et al. Demonstration of a fast-acting inhibitor of plasminogen activators in human plasma. Blood 1984; 64: 907-13
44. Verheijen JH, Chang GTG, Kluft C. Evidence for the occurrence of a fast acting inhibitor of tissue-type plasminogen activator in human plasma. Thrombosis and Haemostasis 1984; 51: 392-5
45. Astedt B, Lecander I, Ny T. The placental type plasminogen activator inhibitor, PAI-2. Fibrinolysis 1987; 1: 203-8
46. Lemoli RM, Fogli M, Fortuna A, et al. Interleukin-11 stimulates the proliferation of human hematopoietic CD34+ and CD34+CD-33-DR-cells and synergizes with stem cell factor, interleukin-3, and granulocyte-macrophage colony-stimulating factor. Experimental Hematology 1993; 21: 1668-72
47. Muench MO, Firpo MT, Moore MAS. Bone marrow transplantation with interleukin-1 plus kit-ligand ex vivo expanded bone marrow accelerates hematopoietic reconstitution in mice without the loss of stem

cell lineage and proliferative potential. Blood 1993; 81: 3463-73
48. Lu L, Xiao M, Grigsby S, et al. Comparative effects of suppressive cytokines on isolated single CD34+++ stem/progenitor cells from human bone marrow and umbilical cord blood plated with and without serum. Experimental Hematology 1993; 21: 1442-6
49. Verfaillie CM, Catanzarro PM, Li WN. Macrophage inflammatory protein 1α, interleukin 3 and diffusible marrow stromal factors maintain hematopoietic stem cells for a least eight weeks in vitro. Journal of Experimental Medicine 1994; 179: 643-9
50. Bazan JF. Structural design and molecular evolution of a cytokine receptor superfamily. Proceedings of the National Academy of Sciences of the United States of America 1990; 87: 6934
51. Budel LM, Elbaz O, Hoogerbrugge H, et al. Common binding structure for granulocyte macrophage colony-stimulating factor and interleukin-3 on human acute myeloid leukemia cells and monocytes. Blood 1990; 75: 1439
52. Gearing DP, Ziegler SF. The hematopoietic growth factor receptor family. Current Opinion in Hematology 1993: 19-25
53. Löwenberg B, Touw IP. Hematopoietic growth factors and their receptors in acute leukemia. Blood 1993; 81: 281-92
54. Pastan I, FitzGerald D. Recombinant toxins for cancer treatment. Science 1991; 254: 1173
55. Tsukada J, Misago M, Kikuchi M, et al. Interactions between recombinant human erythropoietin and serum factor(s) on murine megakaryocyte colony formation. Blood 1992; 80: 37-45
56. Ohneda O, Yanai N, Obinata M. Combined action of c-kit and erythropoietin on erythroid progenitor cells. Development 1992; 114: 243-52
57. Lacombe C, Da Silva JL, Bruneval P. Peritubular cells are the site of erythropoietin synthesis in the murine hypoxic kidney. Journal of Clinical Investigation 1988; 81: 620-3
58. Spivak JL, Pham TH, Issacs MA, et al. Erythropoietin is both a mitogen and a survival factor. Blood 1991; 77: 1228-33
59. Metcalf D. The molecular control of cell division differentiation, commitment and maturation of hematopoietic cells. Nature 1989; 339: 27-30
60. Lieschke GJ, Burgess AW. Granulocyte colony-stimulating factor and granulocyte-macrophage colony-stimulating factor (Part II). New England Journal of Medicine 1992; 327: 99-106
61. Fukunaga R, Ishizaka-Ikeda E, Nagata S. Growth and differentiation signals mediated by different regions in the cytoplasmic domain of granulocyte colony-stimulating factor receptor. Cell 1993; 74: 1079-87
62. McArthur GA, Rohrschneider LR, Johnson GR. Induced expression of C-FMS in normal hematopoietic cells shows evidence for both conservation and lineage restriction of signal transduction in response to macrophage colony-stimulating factor. Blood 1994; 83: 972-81
63. Hibi S, Lohler J, Friel J, et al. Induction of monocytic differentiation and tumorigenicity by v-Ha-ras in differentiation-arrested hematopoietic cells. Blood 1993; 81: 1841-8
64. Dand CV. c-myc Oncoprotein function. Biochimica et Biophysica Acta 1991; 1072: 103-3
65. Kastan MB, Radin AI, Kuerbitz SJ, et al. Levels of p53 protein increase with maturation in human hematopoietic cells. Cancer Research 1991; 51: 4279-84
66. Gewirtz AM. Developmental biology of megakaryocytes and platelets. Current Opinion in Hematology 1993: 256-64
67. Tong M, Seth P, Pennington DG. Proplatelets and stress platelets. Blood 1987; 69: 522-8
68. Trowbridge EA. Pulmonary platelet production: a physical analogue of mitosis. Blood Cells 1988; 13: 451-65
69. Carrington PA, Hill RJ, Stenberg PE, et al. Multiple in vivo effects of interleukin 3 and interleukin 6 on murine megakaryocytopoiesis. Blood 1991; 77: 34-41
70. Lok S, Kauhansky K, Holly RD, et al. Cloning and expression of murine thrombopoietin cDNA and stimulation of platelet production in vivo. Nature 1994; 369: 565-8
71. Bartley RD, Bogenberger J, Hunt P, et al. Identification and cloning of a megakaryocyte growth and development factor that is a ligand for the cytokine receptor Mpl. Cell 1994; 77: 1117-24
72. Kaushansky K, Lok S, Holly RD, et al. Promotion of megakaryocyte progenitor expansion and differentiation by the c-Mpl ligand thrombopoietin. Nature 1994; 369: 568-71
73. Methia N, Louache F, Vainchenker W, et al. Oligodeoxynucleotides antisense to proto-oncogene c-Mpl specifically inhibit in vitro megakaryocytopoiesis. Blood 1993; 82: 1395-401
74. Smith WL. Prostanoid biosynthesis and mechanism of action. American Journal of Physiology 1992; 263: F181-91
75. Xie WL, Chipman JG, Robertson DL, et al. Expression of a mitogen-responsive gene encoding prostaglandin synthase is regulated by mRNA splicing. Proceedings of the National Academy of Sciences USA 1991; 88: 2692-6
76. Meade EA, Smith WL, De Witt DL. Differential inhibition of prostaglandin endoperoxide synthase (cyclooxygenase) isozymes by aspirin and other non-steroidal anti-inflammatory drugs. Journal of Biological Chemistry 1993; 268: 6610-4
77. Patrono C, Ciabattoni G, Pugliese F, et al. Estimated rate of thromboxane secretion into the circulation of normal humans. Journal of Clinical Investigation 1986; 77: 590-4
78. De Caterina R, Giannessi D, Boem A, et al. Equal antiplatelet effects of aspirin 50 or 324 mg/day in patients after acute myocardial infarction. Thrombosis and Haemostasis 1985; 54: 528-32
79. Clarke RJ, Mayo G, Price P, et al. Suppression of thromboxane $A_2$ but not of systemic prostacyclin by controlled-release aspirin. New England Journal of Medicine 1991; 325: 1137-41
80. Keimowitz RM, Pulvermacher G, Mayo G, et al. Transdermal modification of platelet function: a dermal aspirin preparation selectively inhibits platelet cyclooxygenase and preserves prostacyclin biosynthesis. Circulation 1993; 88: 556-61
81. Patrono C, Ciabattoni G, Patrignani P, et al. Clinical pharmacology of platelet cyclooxygenase inhibition. Circulation 1985; 72: 1177-84
82. Pedersen AK, FitzGerald GA. Dose-related kinetics of aspirin: presystemic acetylation of platelet cyclooxygenase. New England Journal of Medicine 1984; 311: 1206-1

83. Fuster V, Ip JH, Jang IK, et al. Antithrombotic therapy in cardiac disease. In: Parmley WW, Chatterjee K, editors. Cardiology. Philadelphia: JB Lippincott, 1993
84. Patrono C. Aspirin as an antiplatelet drug. New England Journal of Medicine 1994; 330: 1287-94
85. UK-TIA Study Group. United Kingdom transient ischaemic attack (UK-TIA) aspirin trial: interim results. British Medical Journal 1988; 296: 316-20
86. Willard JE, Lange RA, Hillis LD. The use of aspirin in ischemic heart disease. New England Journal of Medicine 1992; 327: 175-81
87. FitzGerald GA. Dipyridamole. New England Journal of Medicine 1987; 316: 1247-57
88. Gresele P, Arnout J, Deckmyn H, et al. Mechanisms of the antiplatelet action of dipyridamole in whole blood: modulation of adenosine concentration and activity. Thrombosis and Haemostasis 1986; 44: 12-8
89. Stein B, Fuster V. Clinical pharmacology of platelet inhibitors. In: Fuster V, Verstraete M, editors. Thrombosis in cardiovascular disorders. Philadelphia: WB Saunders, 1992: 99-120
90. Hanson SR, Harker LA, Bjornsson TD. Effect of platelet modifying drugs on arterial thromboembolism in baboons: aspirin potentiates the antithrombotic effects of dipyridamole and sulfinpyrazone by mechanisms independent of platelet cyclo-oxygenase inhibition. Journal of Clinical Investigation 1985; 79: 159
91. Saltiel E, Ward A. Ticlopidine: a review of its pharmacodynamic and pharmacokinetic properties, and therapeutic efficacy in platelet-dependent disease states. Drugs 1987; 34: 222-62
92. Gachet C, Stierle A, Cazenave JP, et al. The thienopyridine PCR4099 selectively inhibits ADP-induced platelet aggregation and fibrinogen binding without modifying the membrane glycoprotein IIb-IIIa complex in rat and in man. Biochemical Pharmacology 1990; 40: 229-38
93. McTavish D, Faulds D, Goa KL. Ticlopidine: an updated review of its pharmacology and therapeutic use in platelet-dependent disorders. Drugs 1990; 40: 238-59
94. Herbert JM, Frehel D, Vallee E, et al. Clopidogrel, a novel antiplatelet and antithrombotic agent. Cardiovascular Drug Reviews 1993; 11: 180-98
95. Aberg M, Hedner U, Bergentz SE. The antithrombotic effect of dextran. Scandinavian Journal of Haematology 1979; Suppl. 34: 61-8
96. Ljungström KG. The antithrombotic efficacy of dextran. Acta Chirurgica Scandinavica 1988; Suppl. 543: 26-30
97. Renck H, Ljungström K-G, Hedin H, et al. Prevention of dextran-induced anaphylactic reactions by hapten inhibition. III. A Scandinavian multicenter study on the effects of 20 ml dextran 1, 15%, administered before dextran 70 or dextran 40. Acta Chirurgica Scandinavica 1983; 149: 355-60
98. Moncada S, Vane JR. Arachidonic acid metabolites and the interaction between platelets and blood vessel walls. New England Journal of Medicine 1979; 300: 1142-7
99. Fisher CA, Kappa JR, Sinha AK, et al. Comparisons of equimolar concentrations of iloprost, prostacyclin, and prostaglandin $E_1$ on human platelet function. Journal of Laboratory and Clinical Medicine 1987; 109: 184-90
100. Grant SM, Goa KL. Iloprost: a review of its pharmacodynamic and pharmacokinetic properties, and therapeutic potential in peripheral vascular disease, myocardial ischaemia and extracorporeal circulation procedures. Drugs 1992; 43: 889-924
101. Coller BS. A new murine monoclonal antibody reports inactivation-dependent change in the conformation and/or microenvironment of the platelet glycoprotein IIb/IIIa complex. Journal of Clinical Investigation 1985; 76: 101-8
102. Hanson SR, Pareti FI, Fuggeri ZM, et al. Effects of monoclonal antibodies against the platelet glycoprotein IIb/IIIa complex on thrombosis and hemostasis in the baboon. Journal of Clinical Investigation 1988; 81: 149-58
103. Gold HK, Coller BS, Yasuda T, et al. Rapid and sustained coronary artery recanalization with combined bolus injection of recombinant tissue-type plasminogen activator and monoclonal anti-platelet GPIIb/IIIa antibody in a dog model. Circulation 1988; 77: 670-7
104. Tcheng JE, Ellis SG, George BS, et al. Pharmacodynamics of chimeric glycoprotein IIb/IIIa integrin antiplatelet antibody Fab 7E3 in high-risk coronary angioplasty. Circulation 1994; 90: 1757-64
105. Kleiman NS, Ohman E, Califf RM, et al. Profound inhibition of platelet aggregation with monoclonal antibody 73E Fab after thrombolytic therapy. Results of the Thrombolysis and Angioplasty in Myocardial Infarction (TAMI) 8 Pilot Study. Journal of the American College of Cardiology 1993; 22: 381-9
106. The EPIC Investigators. Use of a monoclonal antibody directed against the platelet glycoprotein IIb/IIIa receptor in high-risk coronary angioplasty. New England Journal of Medicine 1994; 330: 956-61
107. Topol EJ, Fuster V, Harrington RA. Recombinant hirudin for unstable angina pectoris. Circulation 1994; 89: 1557-66
108. Simoons ML, de Boer MJ, Van den Brand M, et al. Randomized trial of IIb/IIIa platelet receptor blocker in refractory unstable angina. Circulation 1994; 89: 596-603
109. Charo IF, Scarborough RM, du Mée CP, et al. Pharmacodynamics of the GPIIb/IIIa antagonist integrelin: phase I clinical studies in normal healthy volunteers (Abstract). Circulation 1992; 86: 260
110. Narjes H, Weisenberger H, Muller TH, et al. Tolerability and platelet fibrinogen receptor occupancy (FRO) after oral treatment with BIBU 104 XX in healthy volunteers (Abstract). Thrombosis and Haemostasis 1995; 73: 1315
111. Takiguchi Y, Asai F, Wada K, et al. Comparison of antithrombotic effects of GPIIb/IIIa receptor antagonist and $TXA_2$ receptor antagonist in the guinea-pig thrombosis model: possible role of $TXA_2$ in reocclusion after thrombolysis. Thrombosis and Haemostasis 1995; 73: 683-8
112. Théroux P, Kouz S, Knudtson ML, et al. A randomised double-blind controlled trial with the nor peptidic platelet GPI IIb/IIIa antagonist RO 44-9833 in unstable angina (Abstract). Circulation 1994; 232, Part 2
113. Barrett JS, Murphy G, Peerlinck K, et al. Pharmacokinetics and pharmacodynamics of MK-383, a selective non-peptide platelet glycoprotein IIb-IIIa receptor antagonist in healthy men. Clinical Pharmacology and Therapeutics 1994; 56: 377-88
114. Peerlinck K, De Lepeleire I, Goldberg M, et al. MK-383 (L-700,462), a selective nonpeptide platelet glycoprotein IIb/IIIa antagonist, is active in man. Circulation 1993; 88: 1512-7
115. Hanson SR, Harker LA. Interruption of acute platelet-dependent thrombosis by the synthetic antithrombin

p-phenylalanyl-L-proly-L-arginyl chloromethyl ketone. Proceedings of the National Academy of Sciences USA 1988; 85: 3184-8
116. Maraganore JM. Thrombin, thrombin inhibitors, and the arterial thrombotic process. Thrombosis and Haemostasis 1993; 70: 208-11
117. Stringer KA, Lindenfeld JA. Hirudins: antithrombin anticoagulants. Annals of Pharmacotherapy 1992; 26: 1535-40
118. Markwardt F, Nowak G, Stürzebecher J, et al. Pharmacokinetics and anticoagulant effect of hirudin in man. Thrombosis and Haemostasis 1984; 52: 160-3
119. Bichler J, Fichtl B, Siebeck M, et al. Pharmacokinetics and pharmacodynamics of hirudin in man after single subcutaneous and intravenous bolus administration. Arzneimittel-Forschung Drug Research 1988; 38: 704-10
120. Zoldhelyi P, Webster MWI, Fuster V, et al. Recombinant hirudin in patients with chronic, stable coronary artery disease: safety, half-life and effect on coagulation parameters. Circulation 1993; 88: 2015-2
121. Serruys PW, Herrman JPR, Simon R, et al. For the HELVETICA Investigators. A comparison of hirudin with heparin in the prevention of restenosis after coronary angioplasty. New England Journal of Medicine 1995; 333: 757-63
122. van den Bos AA, Deckers JW, Heyndrickx GR, et al. Safety and efficacy of recombinant hirudin (CGP 39393) versus heparin in patients with stable angina undergoing coronary angioplasty. Circulation 1993; 88: 2058-66
123. Antman E, for the TIMI-9A Investigators. Hirudin in myocardial infarction. Safety report from the thrombolysis and thrombin inhibition in myocardial infarction (TIMI-9A) trial. Circulation 1994; 90: 1624-30
124. The GUSTO IIa Investigators. Randomized trial of intravenous heparin versus recombinant hirudin for acute coronary syndromes. Circulation 1994; 90: 1631-7
125. Neuhaus KL, von Essen R, Tebbe U, et al. Safety observations from the pilot phase of the randomized r-hirudin for improvement of thrombolysis (HIT-III) study. Circulation 1994; 90: 1638-42
126. Cannon CP, McCabe CH, Henry TD, et al. A pilot trial of recombinant desulfatohirudin compared with heparin in conjunction with tissue-type plasminogen activator and aspirin for acute myocardial infarction: results of the Thrombolysis in Myocardial Infarction (TIMI) 5 trial. Journal of the American College of Cardiology 1994; 23: 993-1003
127. Cannon CP, Maraganore JM, Loscalzo J, et al. Anticoagulant effect of hirulog, a novel thrombin inhibitor, in patients with coronary artery disease. American Journal of Cardiology 1993; 71: 778-82
128. Topol EJ, Bonan R, Jewitt D, et al. Use of a direct antithrombin, hirulog, in place of heparin during coronary angioplasty. Circulation 1993; 87: 1622-9
129. Lidon RM, Théroux P, Lesprance J, et al. A pilot, early angiographic patency study using a direct thrombin inhibitor as adjunctive therapy to streptokinase in acute myocardial infarction. Circulation 1994; 89: 1567-72
130. Palmer KJ, Goa KL. Defibrotide: a review of its pharmacodynamic and pharmacokinetic properties, and therapeutic values in vascular disorders. Drugs 1993; 45: 259-94
131. Niada R, Mantovani M, Prino G, et al. Antithrombotic activity of a polydeoxyribonucleotide substance extracted from mammalian organs: a possible link with prostaglandin. Thrombosis Research 1981; 23: 233-46
132. Niada R, Mantovani M, Prino G, et al. $PGI_2$-generation and antithrombotic activity of orally administered defibrotide. Pharmacological Research Communications 1982; 14: 949-57
133. Niada R, Porta R, Pescador R, et al. Cardioprotective effects of defibrotide in acute myocardial infarction in the cat. Thrombosis Research 1985; 38: 71-81
134. Niada R, Pescador R, Porta R, et al. Defibrotide is antithrombotic and thrombolytic against rabbit venous thrombosis. Haemostasis 1986; 16 Suppl. 1: 3-8
135. Noseda G, Fragiacomo C, Ferrari D. Pharmacokinetics of defibrotide in healthy volunteers. Haemostasis 1986; 16 Suppl. 1: 26-30
136. Viano L, Colangelo D, Silvestro L, et al. The pharmacokinetics of defibrotide (125-I) in humans. [in Italian]. Medical Praxis 1992; 13: 1-4
137. Lindahl U, Höök M, Backström G, et al. Structure and biosynthesis of heparin-like polysaccharides. Federation Proceedings 1977; 36: 19-24
138. Lindahl U, Backström G, Thunberg L, et al. Structure of the antithrombotic binding site of heparin. Proceedings of the National Academy of Sciences of the United States of America 1979; 76: 3198-202
139. Barrowcliffe TW, Johnson EA, Thomas DP. Low molecular weight heparin. Chichester: John Wiley, 1992
140. Lindahl U, Kjellén L. Heparin or heparin sulfate: what is the difference? Thrombosis and Haemostasis 1991; 66: 44-8
141. Casu B, Oreste P, Torti G, et al. The structure of heparin oligosaccharide fragments with high anti-(factor Xa) activity containing the minimal antithrombin III-binding sequence. Biochemical Journal 1981; 197: 599-609
142. Choay J, Lormeau JC, Petitou M, et al. Structural studies on biologically active hexasaccharide obtained from heparin. Annals of the New York Academy of Sciences 1981; 270: 644-9
143. Choay J, Petitou M, Lormeau JC, et al. Structure-activity relationship in heparin: a synthetic pentasaccharide with high affinity for antithrombin III and eliciting high anti-factor Xa activity. Biochimica et Biophysica Acta - Research Communications 1983; 116: 492-9
144. Rosenberg RD, Lam L. Correlation between structure and function of heparin. Proceedings of the National Academy of Sciences USA 1979; 76: 1218-22
145. Ockelford P, Carter CJ, Cerskus A, et al. Comparison of the in vivo hemorrhagic and antithrombotic effects of a low antithrombin III affinity heparin fraction. Thrombosis Research 1982; 27: 679-90
146. Walker FJ, Esmon CT. Interactions between heparin and factor Xa, inhibition of prothrombin activation. Biochimica et Biophysica Acta 1979; 585: 405-15
147. Ofosu FA, Blajchman MA, Hirsh J. The inhibition by heparin of the intrinsic pathway activation of factor X in the absence of antithrombin III. Thrombosis Research 1980; 20: 391-403
148. Barrowcliffe TW, Merton RE, Havercroft SJ, et al. Low affinity heparin potentiates the action of high affinity heparin oligosaccharides. Thrombosis Research 1984; 34: 124-33
149. Rosenberg RD, Reilly C, Fritze L. Atherogenic regulation by heparin-like molecules. Annals of the New York Academy of Sciences 1985; 454: 270-8
150. Caplice NM, West MJ, Campbell GR, et al. Inhibition of human vascular smooth muscle cell growth by heparin. Lancet 1994; 344: 97-8

151. Bengtsson-Olivecrona G, Olivecrona T. Binding of active and inactive forms of lipoprotein lipase to heparin: effects of pH. Biochemical Journal 1985; 226: 409-13
152. Zucker MB. Heparin and platelet function. Federation Proceedings 1977; 36: 47-9
153. Tollefsen DM, Blank MK. Detection of a new heparin-dependent inhibitor of thrombin in human plasma. Journal of Clinical Investigation 1981; 68: 589-96
154. Hoppensteadt D, Walenga JM, Fareed J. Low molecular weight heparins. An objective overview. Drugs & Aging 1992; 2: 406-22
155. Barradell LB, Buckley MM. Nadroparin calcium: a review of its pharmacology and clinical applications in the prevention and treatment of thromboembolic disorders. Drugs 1992; 44: 858-8
156. Buckley MM, Sorkin EM. Enoxaparin: a review of its pharmacology and clinical applications in the prevention and treatment of thromboembolic disorders. Drugs 1992; 44: 465-97
157. Frampton JE, Faulds D. Parnaparin: a review of its pharmacology, and clinical application in the prevention and treatment of thromboembolic and other vascular disorders. Drugs 1994; 47: 652-76
158. Oosta GM, Gardner WT, Beeler DL, et al. Multiple functional domains of the heparin molecule. Proceedings of the National Academy of Sciences USA 1981; 78: 829-33
159. Holmer E, Mattson C, Nilsson S. Anticoagulant and antithrombotic effects of heparin and low molecular weight heparin fragments in rabbits. Thrombosis Research 1982; 25: 475-85
160. Thomas DP, Merton RE, Barrowcliffe TW, et al. Effects of heparin oligosaccharides with high affinity for antithrombin III in experimental venous thrombosis. Thrombosis and Haemostasis 1982; 47: 244-8
161. Ockelford P, Carter CJ, Mitchell L, et al. Discordance between the anti-Xa activity and the antithrombotic activity of an ultra-low molecular-weight heparin fraction. Thrombosis Research 1982; 28: 401-9
162. Ofosu FA, Blajchman MA, Modi GJ, et al. The importance of thrombin inhibition for the expression of the anticoagulant activities of heparin, dermatan sulphate, low molecular weight heparin and pentosan sulphate. British Journal of Haematology 1985; 60: 695-704
163. Hirsh J, Levine MN. Low molecular weight heparin. Blood 1992; 79: 1-17
164. Hirsh J. Oral anticoagulant drugs. New England Journal of Medicine 1991; 324: 1865-75
165. Olsson P, Lagergren H, Ek S. The elimination from plasma of intravenous heparin: an experimental study on dogs and humans. Acta Medica Scandinavica 1963; 173: 619-30
166. Kandrotas RJ. Heparin pharmacokinetics and pharmacodynamics. Clinical Pharmacokinetics 1992; 22: 359-74
167. de Swart CAM, Nymeyer B, Roelofs JMN, et al. Kinetics of intravenously administered heparin in normal humans. Blood 1982; 60: 1251-8
168. Simon TL, Hyers TIM, Gaston JP, et al. Heparin pharmacokinetics. Increased requirements in pulmonary embolism. British Journal of Haematology 1978; 39: 111-20
169. Teien AN. Heparin elimination in patients with liver cirrhosis. Thrombosis and Haemostasis 1977; 38: 701-6
170. Salzman EW, Hirsh J. Prevention of venous thromboembolism. In: Colman RW, Hirsh J, Marder VJ, et al., editors. Haemostasis and thrombosis. 3rd ed. Philadelphia: JB Lippincott, 1987: 1331-45
171. Basu D, Gallus A, Hirsh J, et al. A prospective study of the value of monitoring heparin treatment with the activated partial thromboplastin time. New England Journal of Medicine 1972; 287: 324-7
172. Hyers TM. Heparin therapy. Regimens and treatment considerations. Drugs 1992; 44: 738-49
173. Cruickshank MK, Levine MN, Hirsh J, et al. A standard heparin nomogram for the management of heparin therapy. Archives of Internal Medicine 1991; 151: 333-7
174. Brill-Edwards P, Ginsberg JS, Johnston M, et al. Establishing a therapeutic range of heparin therapy. Annals of Internal Medicine 1993; 119: 104-9
175. Hirsh J, Fuster V. Guide to anticoagulant therapy. Part 1: heparin. Part 2: oral anticoagulants. Circulation 1994; 89: 1449-68 and 1469-80
176. Levine MN, Hirsh J, Kelton JG. Heparin-induced bleeding. In: Lane DA, Lindahl U, editors. Heparin: chemical and biological properties. London: Edward Arnold, 1989: 517-32
177. Warkentin TE, Kelton JG. Heparin-induced thrombocytopenia. Annual Review of Medicine 1989; 40: 31-44
178. Chong BH, Ismail F, Cade J, et al. Heparin-induced thrombocytopenia: studies with a low molecular weight heparin Org 10172. Blood 1989; 73: 1592-6
179. O'Reilly RA, Aggeler PM. Determinants of the response to oral anticoagulant drugs in man. Pharmacology Reviews 1970; 22: 35-96
180. Stenflo J, Ferlund P, Egan W, et al. Vitamin K dependent modifications of glutamic acid residues in prothrombin. Proceedings of the National Academy of Sciences USA 1974; 71: 2730-3
181. Nelsestuen GL, Zytkoviez TH, Howard JB. The mode of action of vitamin K: identification of τ-carboxyglutamic acid as a component of prothrombin. Journal of Biological Chemistry 1974; 249: 6347-50
182. Furie B, Furie BC. Molecular basis of vitamin K-dependent τ-carboxylation. Blood 1990; 75: 1753-62
183. Vermeer C, Hamulyák K. Pathophysiology of vitamin K-deficiency and oral anticoagulants. Thrombosis and Haemostasis 1991; 66: 153-9
184. Breckenridge AM. Interindividual differences in the response to oral anticoagulants. Drugs 1977; 14: 367-75
185. Kelly JG, O'Malley K. Clinical pharmacokinetics of oral anticoagulants. Clinical Pharmacokinetics 1979; 4: 1-15
186. Shetty HGM, Fennerty AG, Routledge PA. Clinical pharmacokinetic considerations in the control of oral anticoagulant therapy. Clinical Pharmacokinetics 1989; 16: 238-53
187. Bochner F, Hooper WD, Eadie MJ, et al. Decreased capacity to metabolize diphenylhydantoin in a patient with hypersensitivity to warfarin. Australian and New Zealand Journal of Medicine 1975; 5: 462
188. O'Reilly RA, Sahud MA, Aggeler PM. Impact of aspirin and chlorthalidone on the pharmacodynamics of oral anticoagulant drugs in man. Annals of the New York Academy of Sciences 1971; 179: 173-86
189. Lewis RG, Trager WF, Chan KK, et al. Warfarin: stereochemical aspects of its metabolism and the interaction with phenylbutazone. Journal of Clinical Investigation 1974; 53: 1607-7
190. Serlin MJ, Breckenridge AM. Drug interactions with warfarin. Drugs 1983; 25: 610-20

191. Jahnchen E, Meinertz T, Gilfrich HJ, et al. The enantiomers of phenprocoumon: pharmacodynamic and pharmacokinetic studies. Clinical Pharmacology and Therapeutics 1976; 20: 342
192. Godbillon J, Richard J, Gerardin A, et al. Pharmacokinetics of the enantiomers of acenocoumarol in man. British Journal of Clinical Pharmacology 1981; 12: 621-9
193. Bachman K, Shapiro R. Protein binding of coumarin anticoagulants in disease states. Clinical Pharmacokinetics 1977; 2: 110-26
194. Goguel M, Noël G, Gillet JY, et al. Thérapeutique anticoagulante et allaitment. Revue Francaise Gynécologie 1970; 65: 409
195. Verstraete M, Vermylen J. Thrombosis. Oxford-New York: Pergamon Press, 1984: 229
196. Verstraete M, Wessler S. Drug interference with heparin and oral anticoagulants. In: Fuster V, Verstraete M, editors. Thrombosis in cardiovascular disorders. Philadelphia: WB Saunders, 1992: 141-6
197. Shepherd AMM, Hewick DS, Moreland TA, et al. Age as a determinant of sensitivity to warfarin. British Journal of Clinical Pharmacology 1977; 4: 315
198. Husted S, Andreasen F. The influence of age on the response to anticoagulants. British Journal of Clinical Pharmacology 1977; 4: 559
199. Hermans J, van den Besselaar, Loeliger EA, et al. A collaborative calibration study of reference materials for thromboplastins. Thrombosis and Haemostasis 1983; 50: 712-3
200. Le DT, Weibert RT, Sevilla BK, et al. The international normalized ratio (INR) for monitoring warfarin therapy: reliability and relation to other monitoring methods. Annals of Internal Medicine 1994; 120: 552-8
201. Loeliger EA, Poller L, Samama M, et al. Questions and answers on prothrombin time standardization in oral anticoagulant control. Thrombosis and Haemostasis 1985; 54: 515-7
202. British Society of Haematology. Guidelines on oral anticoagulation: second edition. Journal of Clinical Pathology 1990; 43: 177-83
203. Dalen JE, Hirsh J. editors. Third ACCP Consensus Conference on antithrombotic therapy. Chest 1995; 108: 305S-311S
204. Dalen JE, Hirsh J. editors. Fourth ACCP Consensus Conference on antithrombotic therapy. Chest 1995; 108 (Suppl. 4): 225S-522S
205. Hylek EM, Singer DE. Risk factors for intracranial hemorrhage in outpatients taking warfarin. Annals of Internal Medicine 1994; 120: 897-902
206. Harrington R, Ansell J. Risk-benefit assessment of anticoagulant therapy. Drug Safety 1991; 6: 54-69
207. Caron J, Libersa C. Drugs affecting blood clotting fibrinolysis and haemostasis. In: Dukes MNG, editor. Meyler's side effects of drugs. Amsterdam: Excerpta Medica, 1992: 878-927
208. Hirsh J. Oral anticoagulant therapy. Urgent need for standardization. Circulation 1992; 86: 1332-5
209. Hall JG, Pauli RM, Wilson KM. Maternal and fetal sequelae of anticoagulation during pregnancy. American Journal of Medicine 1980; 68: 122-40
210. Salazar E, Zajarias A, Gutierrez N, et al. The problem of cardiac valve prostheses, anticoagulants and pregnancy. Circulation 1984; 70 Suppl. 1: 169-77
211. Ginsberg JS, Hirsh J. Use of antithrombotic agents during pregnancy. Chest 1995; 108 305S-311S
212. Pineo GF, Hull RD. Adverse effects of coumarin anticoagulants. Drug Safety 1993; 9: 263-71
213. Comp PC. Coumarin-induced skin necrosis: incidence, mechanisms, management and avoidance. Drug Safety 1993; 8: 128-35
214. Breckenridge A, Orme M, Davis L, et al. Dose dependent enzyme induction. Clinical Pharmacology and Therapeutics 1973; 14: 514-20
215. Breckenridge A. Oral anticoagulants: the totem and the taboo. British Medical Journal 1976; 1: 419-23
216. Koch-Weser J. Drug interactions in cardiovascular therapy. American Heart Journal 1975; 90: 93-116
217. Jackson KW, Tang J. Complete amino acid sequence of streptokinase and its homology with serine proteases. Biochemistry 1982; 21: 6620-5
218. Smith P, Dupe RJ, English PD, et al. Fibrinolysis with acyl-enzymes: a new approach to thrombolytic therapy. Nature (London) 1981; 290: 505-8
219. Reddy KNN. Mechanism of activation of human plasminogen by streptokinase. In: Kline DL, Reddy KNN, editors. Fibrinolysis. Boca Raton: CRC Press, 1980: 71-94
220. Markus G, Evers JL, Hobika GH. Comparison of some properties of native (Glu) and modified (Lys) human plasminogen. Journal of Biological Chemistry 1978; 253: 733-9
221. Bajaj SP, Castellion FJ. Activation of human plasminogen by equimolar levels of streptokinase. Journal of Biological Chemistry 1977; 252: 492-8
222. Markus G, Evers JL, Hobika GH. Activator activities of the transient forms of the human plasminogen-streptokinase complex during its proteolytic conversion to the stable activator complex. Journal of Biological Chemistry 1976; 251: 6495-504
223. Fears R. The effect of heparin and fibrin on the enzymatic efficiencies of thrombolytics in vitro. Drugs 1987; 33 Suppl. 3: 69-74
224. Been M, de Bono DP, Muir AL, et al. Clinical effects and kinetic properties of intravenous APSAC - anisoylated plasminogen-streptokinase activator complex (BRL 26921) in acute myocardial infarction. International Journal of Cardiology 1986; 11: 53-61
225. Nunn B, Esmail A, Fears R, et al. Pharmacokinetic properties of anisoylated plasminogen streptokinase activator complex and other thrombolytic agents in animals and in humans. Drugs 1987; 33 Suppl. 3: 88-92
226. Staniforth DH, Smith RAG, Hibbs M. Streptokinase and anisoylated streptokinase plasminogen complex. Their action on haemostasis in human volunteers. European Journal of Clinical Pharmacology 1983; 24: 751-6
227. Ferres H, Hibbs M, Smith RAG. Deacylation studies in vitro on anisoylated plasminogen streptokinase activator complex. Drugs 1987; 33 Suppl. 3: 80-2
228. Verstraete M, Vermylen J, Amery A, et al. Thrombolytic therapy with streptokinase using a standard dosage scheme. British Medical Journal 1966; 5485: 454-6
229. Goa KL, Henwood JM, Stolz JF, et al. Intravenous streptokinase: a reappraisal of its therapeutic use in acute myocardial infarction. Drugs 1990; 39: 693-719
230. Battershill PE, Benfield P, Goa KL. Streptokinase: a review of its pharmacology and therapeutic efficacy in acute myocardial infarction in older patients. Drugs & Aging 1994; 4: 63-86
231. Monk JP, Heel RC. Anisoylated plasminogen streptokinase activator complex (APSAC): a review of its mechanism of action, clinical pharmacology and therapeutic use in acute myocardial infarction. Drugs 1987; 34: 25-49

232. Verstraete M. Thrombolytic treatment in acute myocardial infarction. Circulation 1990; 82 Suppl. 3: II96-II109
233. Anderson JL, Rothbart RL, Hackworthy RA, et al. Multicenter reperfusion trial of intravenous anisoylated plasminogen streptokinase activator complex (APSAC) in acute myocardial infarction: controlled comparison with intracoronary streptokinase. Journal of the American College of Cardiology 1988; 11: 1153-63
234. Günzler WA, Steffens GJ, Otting F, et al. Structural relationship between human high and low molecular mass urokinase. Hoppe-Seylers Zeitschrift für Physiologische Chemie 1982; 363: 133-41
235. Stump DC, Lijnen HR, Collen D. Purification and characterization of a novel low molecular weight form of single-chain urokinase-type plasminogen activator. Journal of Biological Chemistry 1986; 261: 17120-6
236. Husain SS. Single-chain urokinase-type plasminogen activator does not possess measurable intrinsic amidolytic or plasminogen activator activities. Biochemistry 1991; 30: 5797-805
237. Manchanda N, Schwartz BS. Single chain urokinase. Augmentation of enzymatic activity upon binding to monocytes. Journal of Biological Chemistry 1991; 266: 14580-4
238. Collen D, Lijnen HR. Fibrinolysis: thrombolytic agents, mechanisms, and new developments. In: Hacke et al., editors. Thrombolytic therapy in acute ischemic stroke. Berlin: Springer-Verlag, 1991: 9-23
239. Lijnen HR, Van Hoef B, De Cock F, et al. The mechanism of plasminogen activation and fibrin dissolution by single chain urokinase-type plasminogen activator in a plasma milieu in vitro. Blood 1989; 73: 1864-72
240. Collen D, Mao J, Stassen JM, et al. Thrombolytic properties of Lys-158 mutants of recombinant single chain urokinase-type plasminogen activator in rabbits with jugular vein thrombosis. Journal of Vascular Medicine and Biology 1989; 1: 46-9
241. Stump DC, Kieckens L, De Cock F, et al. Pharmacokinetics of single-chain forms of urokinase-type plasminogen activator. Journal of Pharmacology and Experimental Therapeutics 1987; 242: 245-50
242. Van de Werf F, Nobuhara M, Collen D. Coronary thrombolysis with human single-chain, urokinase-type plasminogen activator (pro-urokinase) in patients with acute myocardial infarction. Annals of Internal Medicine 1986; 104: 345-8
243. PRIMI Trial Study Group. Randomised double-blind trial of recombinant pro-urokinase against streptokinase in acute myocardial infarction. Lancet 1989; 1: 863-8
244. Pennica D, Holmes WE, Kohr WJ, et al. Cloning and expression of human tissue-type plasminogen activator cDNA in E. coli. Nature (London) 1983; 301: 214-21
245. Hoylaerts M, Rijken DC, Lijnen HR, et al. Kinetics of the activation of plasminogen by human tissue plasminogen activator. Role of fibrin. Journal of Biological Chemistry 1982; 257: 2912-9
246. Wiman B, Collen D. On the kinetics of the reaction between human antiplasmin and plasmin. European Journal of Biochemistry 1978; 84: 573-8
247. van Zonneveld AJ, Veerman H, Pannekoek H. On the interaction of the finger and the kringle-2 domain of tissue-type plasminogen activator with fibrin. Journal of Biological Chemistry 1986; 261: 14214-8
248. Korninger C, Stassen JM, Collen D. Turnover of human extrinsic (tissue-type) plasminogen activator in rabbits. Thrombosis and Haemostasis 1981; 46: 658-61
249. Rijken DC, Emeis JJ. Clearance of the heavy and light polypeptide chains of human tissue-type plasminogen activator in rats. Biochemical Journal 1986; 238: 643-6
250. Verstraete M, Bounameaux H, De Cock F, et al. Pharmacokinetics and systemic fibrinogenolytic effects of recombinant human tissue-type plasminogen activator (rt-PA) in humans. Journal of Pharmacology and Experimental Therapy 1985; 235: 506-12
251. Verstraete M, Su CAPF, Tanswell P, et al. Pharmacokinetics and effects on fibrinolytic and coagulation parameters of two doses of recombinant tissue-type plasminogen activator in healthy volunteers. Thrombosis and Haemostasis 1986; 56: 1-5
252. Neuhaus KL, Feuerer W, Jeep-Tebbe S, et al. Improved thrombolysis with a modified dose regimen of recombinant tissue-type plasminogen activator. Journal of the American College of Cardiology 1989; 14: 1566-9
253. The GUSTO Investigators. An international randomized trial comparing four thrombolytic strategies for acute myocardial infarction. New England Journal of Medicine 1993; 329: 673-82
254. Agnelli G, Buchanan MR, Fernandez F, et al. Sustained thrombolysis with DNA-recombinant tissue type plasminogen activator in rabbits. Blood 1985; 66: 399-401
255. The TIMI Study Group. Comparison of invasive and conservative strategies after treatment with intravenous tissue plasminogen activator in acute myocardial infarction. Results of the thrombolysis in myocardial infarction (TIMI) phase II trial. New England Journal of Medicine 1989; 320: 618-27
256. White GC, McMillan CW, Kingdon HS, et al. Use of recombinant antihemophilic factor in the treatment of two patients with classic hemophilia. New England Journal of Medicine 1989; 320: 166-70
257. Magnani B, for the PAIMS Investigators. Plasminogen Activator Italian Multicenter Study (PAIMS). Comparison of intravenous recombinant single-chain human tissue-type plasminogen activator (rt-PA) with intravenous streptokinase in acute myocardial infarction. Journal of the American College of Cardiology 1989; 13: 19-26
258. Horton R. t-PA fast by GUSTO. Lancet 1993; 341: 1188
259. Lee KL, Califf RM, Simes J, et al. Holding GUSTO up to the light. Annals of Internal Medicine 1994; 120: 876-1
260. Ridker PM, O'Donnell C, Marder VJ, et al. Large-scale trials of thrombolytic therapy for acute myocardial infarction: GISSI-2, ISIS-3, and GUSTO-1. Annals of Internal Medicine 1993; 119: 530-2
261. Farkouh ME, Lang JD, Sackett DL. Thrombolytic agents: the science of the art of choosing the better treatment. Annals of Internal Medicine 1994; 120: 886-8
262. The Steering Committee of the Physician's Health Study Research Group. Preliminary report: findings from the aspirin component on the ongoing Physician's Health Study. New England Journal of Medicine 1988; 318: 262-4
263. Peto R, Gray R, Collins R, et al. Randomised trial of prophylactic daily aspirin in British male doctors. British Medical Journal 1988; 296: 313-6
264. Manson JE, Grobbee DE, Stampfer MJ, et al. Aspirin in the primary prevention of angina pectoris in a ran-

domized trial of United States physicians. American Journal of Medicine 1990; 89: 772-6

265. Goldhaber SZ, Manson JA, Stampfer MJ, et al. Low-dose aspirin and subsequent peripheral arterial surgery in the Physician's Health Study. Lancet 1992; 340: 143-5
266. Verstraete M. Primary prevention of myocardial infarction and stroke with aspirin. Nutrition Metabolism and Cardiovascular Diseases 1993; 3: 145-50
267. The Steering Committee of the Physician's Health Study Research Group. Final report on the aspirin component of the ongoing Physician's Health study. New England Journal of Medicine 1989; 321: 129-35
268. MacMahon S, Cutler JA, Furberg CD, et al. The effects of drug treatment for hypertension on morbidity and mortality from cardiovascular disease: a review of the randomized controlled trials. Progress in Cardiovascular Diseases 1986; 29 Suppl. 1: 99-118
269. MacMahon S, Peto R, Cutler J, et al. Blood pressure, stroke, and coronary heart disease. Part I. Prolonged differences in blood pressure: prospective observational studies corrected for the regression dilution bias. Lancet 1990; 335: 765-4
270. Collins R, Peto R, MacMahon S, et al. Blood pressure, stroke and coronary heart disease. Part 2. Short-term reductions in blood pressure: overview of randomised drug trials in their epidemiological context. Lancet 1990; 335: 827-38
271. Early Treatment Diabetic Retinopathy Study Investigators. Aspirin effects on mortality and morbidity in patients with diabetes mellitus. Journal of the American Medical Association 1992; 268: 1292-300
272. Chesebro JH, Opie LH, Fuster V, et al. The recent trials for aspirin in the prevention of cardiovascular mortality. Cardiovascular Drugs and Therapy 1989; 3: 353-4
273. Ridker PM, Manson JE, Gaziano JM, et al. Low-dose aspirin therapy for chronic stable angina. A randomised, placebo-controlled clinical trial. Annals of Internal Medicine 1991; 114: 835-9
274. Lewis Jr HD, Davis JW, Archibald DG, et al. Protective effects of aspirin against acute myocardial infarction and death in men with unstable angina. New England Journal of Medicine 1983; 309: 396-403
275. Cairns JA, Gent M, Singer J, et al. Aspirin, sulfinpyrazone, or both in unstable angina. New England Journal of Medicine 1985; 313: 1369-75
276. Cairns JA, Lewis Jr HD, Meade TW, et al. Antithrombotic agents in coronary artery disease. Chest 1995; 108: 352S-60S
277. Wallentin LC, Research Group on Instability in Coronary Artery Disease in Southeast Sweden. Aspirin after an episode of unstable coronary artery disease: long-term effect on the risk for myocardial infarction, occurrence of severe angina and the need for revascularization. Journal of the American College of Cardiology 1991; 18: 1587-93
278. Balsano F, Rizzon P, Violi F, et al. Antiplatelet treatment with ticlopidine in unstable angina: a controlled multicenter clinical trial. Circulation 1990; 82: 17-26
279. Théroux P, Quimet H, McCans J, et al. Aspirin, heparin, or both to treat acute unstable angina. New England Journal of Medicine 1988; 319: 1105-11
280. The RISC Group. The risk of myocardial infarction and death during treatment with low dose aspirin and intravenous heparin in men during unstable coronary artery disease. Lancet 1990; 336: 827-30
281. Neri Serneri GG, Gensini GF, Poggesi L, et al. Effect of heparin, aspirin, or alteplase in reduction of myocardial ischaemia in refractory unstable angina. Lancet 1990; 335: 615-8
282. Cohen M, Adams PC, Hawkins L, et al. Usefulness of antithrombotic therapy in resting angina pectoris or non-Q wave myocardial infarction in preventing death and myocardial infarction: a pilot study from the Antithrombotic Therapy in Acute Coronary Syndromes Study Group. American Journal of Cardiology 1990; 66: 1287-92
283. Théroux P, Waters D, Lam J, et al. Reactivation of unstable angina after the discontinuation of heparin. New England Journal of Medicine 1992; 327: 141-5
284. Chalmers TC, Matta RJ, Smith H, et al. Evidence favoring the use of anticoagulants in the hospital phase of acute myocardial infarction. New England Journal of Medicine 1977; 297: 1091-6
285. Yusuf S, Wittes J, Friedman L. Overview of results of randomized clinical trials in heart disease. I. Treatments following myocardial infarction. Journal of the American Medical Association 1988; 260: 2088-93
286. Sixty Plus Reinfarction Study Research Group. A double-blind trial to assess long-term oral anticoagulant therapy in elderly patients after myocardial infarction. Lancet 1980; 2: 989-4
287. Anticoagulants in the Secondary Prevention of Events in Coronary Thrombosis (ASPECT) Research Group. The effect of long-term oral anticoagulant treatment on mortality and cardiovascular morbidity after myocardial infarction. Lancet 1994; 343: 499-503
288. Antiplatelet Trialists' Collaboration. Collaborative overview of randomised trials of antiplatelet therapy. British Medical Journal 1994; 308: 81-106, 159-68, 235-46
289. Meade TW. Low-dose warfarin and low-dose aspirin in the primary prevention of ischemic heart disease. American Journal of Cardiology 1990; 65: 7C-11C
290. Halperin JL, Petersen P. Thrombosis in cardiac chambers: ventricular dysfunction and atrial fibrillation. In: Fuster V, Verstraete M, editors. Thrombosis in cardiovascular disease. Philadelphia: WB Saunders, 1992: 215-36
291. Visser CA, Kan G, Meltzer RS, et al. Long-term follow-up of left ventricular thrombus after acute myocardial infarction: a two-dimensional echocardiographic study in 96 patients. Chest 1984; 86: 532-6
292. Turpie AGG, Robinson JG, Doyle DG, et al. Comparison of high-dose with low-dose subcutaneous heparin in the prevention of left ventricular mural thrombosis in patients with acute transmural anterior myocardial infarction. New England Journal of Medicine 1989; 320: 352-7
293. Fuster V, Gersh BJ, Giuliani ER, et al. The natural history of idiopathic dilated cardiomyopathy. American Journal of Cardiology 1981; 47: 525-31
294. Badimon JJ, Ip J, Badimon L, et al. Thrombosis and accelerated atherosclerosis in coronary bypass surgery and restenosis after percutaneous transluminal coronary angioplasty: implications for therapy. Coronary Artery Disease 1990; 1: 170-9
295. Stein PD, Dalen JE, Goldman S, et al. Antithrombotic therapy in patients with saphenous vein and internal mammary artery bypass grafts following transluminal coronary angioplasty. Chest 1995; 108: 424S-430S
296. White CW, Knudsen M, Schmidt D, et al. Neither ticlopidine nor aspirin-dipyridamole prevents restenosis post PTCA: results from a randomized placebo-controlled multicenter trial. Circulation 1987; 76 Suppl. 4: 213

297. Topol EJ, Califf RM, Weisman HF, et al. on behalf of the EPIC Investigators. Randomised trial of coronary intervention with antibody against platelet GPIIb/IIIa integrin for reduction of clinical restenosis: results at six months. Lancet 1994; 343: 881-6
298. Strathdee CA, Gavish H, Shannon WR, et al. Cloning of cDNAs for Fanconi's anaemia by functional complementation. Nature 1992; 356: 763-
299. Verstraete M. Risk factors, interventions and therapeutic agents in the prevention of atherosclerosis-related ischaemic diseases. Drugs 1991; 42 Suppl. 5: 22-38
300. Herrman JPR, Hermans WRM, Vos J, et al. Pharmacological approaches to the prevention of restenosis following angioplasty. The search for the holy grail. Part II. Drugs 1993; 46: 18-52, 249-62
301. Ryan TJ, Bauman WB, Kennedy JW, et al. Guidelines for percutaneous transluminal coronary angioplasty: a report of the American Heart Association/American College of Cardiology Task Force on assessment of diagnostic and therapeutic cardiovascular procedures (Committee on Percutaneous Transluminal Coronary Angioplasty). Circulation 1993; 88: 2987-3007
302. Chesebro JH, Clements IP, Fuster V, et al. A platelet-inhibitor drug trial in coronary artery bypass operations. Benefit of perioperative dipyridamole and aspirin therapy on early postoperative vein-graft patency. New England Journal of Medicine 1982; 307: 73-8
303. Chesebro JH, Fuster V, Elveback R, et al. Effect of dipyridamole and aspirin on late vein-graft patency after coronary bypass operations. New England Journal of Medicine 1984; 310: 209-14
304. Lorenz RL, Schacky CV, Weber M, et al. Improved aortocoronary bypass patency by low-dose aspirin (100mg daily). Lancet 1984; 1: 1261-4
305. Sanz G, Pajaron A, Alegria E, et al. Prevention of early aortocoronary bypass occlusion by low-dose aspirin and dipyridamole. Circulation 1990; 82: 765-3
306. Gavaghan TP, Gebski V, Baron DW. Immediate postoperative aspirin improves vein graft patency early and late after coronary artery bypass graft surgery. A placebo-controlled, randomized study. Circulation 1991; 83: 1526-33
307. Brown BG, Cukingham RA, DeRouen T, et al. Improved graft-patency on patients treated with platelet-inhibiting therapy following coronary bypass surgery. Circulation 1985; 72: 138-46
308. Limet R, David JL, Magotteaux P, et al. Prevention of aorto-coronary bypass graft occlusion: beneficial effect of ticlopidine on early and late patency rates of venous-coronary bypass grafts: a double-blind study. Journal of Thoracic and Cardiovascular Surgery 1987; 94: 773-83
309. Chevigné M, David JL, Rigo P, et al. Double-blind clinical trial of ticlopidine versus placebo in peripheral atherosclerotic disease of the legs. Angiologie 1988; Suppl. 7: 14-20
310. Goldman S, Copeland J, Moritz T, et al. Saphenous vein graft patency 1 year after coronary artery bypass surgery and effects of antiplatelet therapy. Circulation 1989; 80: 1190-7
311. Altman R, Rouvier J, Gurfinkel E, et al. Comparison of two levels of anticoagulant therapy in patients with substitute heart valves. Journal of Thoracic and Cardiovascular Surgery 1991; 101: 427-31
312. Turpie AGG, Gent CM, Laupacis A, et al. A comparison of aspirin with placebo in patients treated with warfarin after heart-valve replacement. New England Journal of Medicine 1993; 329: 524-9
313. Turpie AGG, Gunstensen J, Hirsh J, et al. Randomised comparison of two intensities of oral anticoagulant therapy after tissue heart valve replacement. Lancet 1988; 1: 1242-5
314. Laupacis A, Albers GW, Dalen JE, et al. Antithrombotic therapy in atrial fibrillation. Chest 1995; 108: 352S-360S
315. Szekely P. Systemic embolism and anticoagulant prophylaxis in rheumatic heart disease. British Medical Journal 1964; 1: 1209-12
316. Chesebro JH, Fuster V, Halperin JL. Atrial fibrillation-risk marker for stroke. New England Journal of Medicine 1990; 323: 1556-8
317. Cerebral Embolism Task Force. Cardiogenic brain embolism, second report. Archives of Neurology 1989; 46: 727-43
318. Petersen P. Thrombo-embolic complications in atrial fibrillation. Stroke 1990; 21: 4-13
319. Ezekowitz MD, Bridgers SL, James KE, et al. Warfarin in the prevention of stroke associated with non-rheumatic atrial fibrillation. New England Journal of Medicine 1992; 327: 1406-2
320. The Stroke Prevention in Atrial Fibrillation Investigators. The stroke prevention in atrial fibrillation: final results. Circulation 1991; 84: 527-39
321. Matchar DB, McCrory DC, Barnett HJM, et al. Medical treatment for stroke prevention. Annals of Internal Medicine 1994; 121: 41-53
322. European Atrial Fibrillation Trial Study Group. Secondary prevention in non-rheumatic atrial fibrillation after transient ischaemic attack or minor stroke. Lancet 1993; 342: 1255-62
323. Sherman DG, Dyken Jr ML, Gent M, et al. Antithrombotic therapy for cerebrovascular disorders: an update. Chest 1995; 108: 444S-456S
324. Hass WK, Easton JD, Adams HP, et al. A randomized trial comparing ticlopidine hydrochloride with aspirin for the prevention of stroke in high-risk patients. New England Journal of Medicine 1989; 321: 501-7
325. Feinberg WM, Albers GW, Barnett HJM, et al. Guidelines for the management of transient ischemic attacks. From the ad hoc Committee on Guidelines for the Management of Transient Ischemic Attacks of the Stroke Council of the American Heart Association. Circulation 1994; 89: 2950-65
326. Gent M, Blakely JA, Hachinski V, et al. A secondary prevention, randomized trial of suloctidil in patients with a recent history of thromboembolic stroke. Stroke 1985; 16: 416-24
327. Sherman DG, Dyken Jr ML, Fisher M, et al. Antithrombotic therapy for cerebrovascular disorders. Chest 1992; 102 Suppl.: 529S-37S
328. Antiplatelet Trialists' Collaboration. Secondary prevention of vascular disease by prolonged antiplatelet treatment. British Medical Journal 1988; 296: 320-1
329. The SALT Collaborative Group. Swedish Aspirin Low-dose Trial (SALT) of 75mg aspirin as secondary prophylaxis after cerebrovascular ischemic events. Lancet 1991; 338: 1345-9
330. The Dutch TIA Trial Study Group. A comparison of two doses of aspirin (30mg vs 283mg a day) in patients after a transient-ischemic attack or minor ischemic stroke. New England Journal of Medicine 1991; 325: 1261-6
331. Gent M, Blakely JA, Easton JD, et al. The Canadian American Ticlopidine Study (CATS) in thromboembolic stroke. Lancet 1989; 1: 1215-20

332. de Smit P, van Urk H. The effect of long-term treatment with oral anticoagulants in patients with peripheral vascular disease. In: Tilsner V, Matthias FR, editors. Arterielle Verschlusskrankheit und Blutgerinnung. Editiones 'Roche', 1987: 211-7
333. Stiegler H, Hess H, Mietaschk A, et al. Einfluss von Ticlopidin auf die periphere oblitierende Arteriopathie. Deutsche Medizinische Wochenschrift 1984; 109: 1240-3
334. Janzon L, Bergqvist D, Boberg J, et al. Prevention of myocardial infarction and stroke in patients with intermittent claudication: effects of ticlopidine. Swedish Multicenter Study. Journal of Internal Medicine 1990; 227: 301-8
335. Gallus AS, Jackman J, Tillett J, et al. Safety and efficacy of warfarin started early after submassive venous thrombosis or pulmonary embolism. Lancet 1994; 341: 1293-6
336. Gent M, Roberts SS. A meta-analysis of the studies of dihydroergotamine plus heparin in the prophylaxis of deep vein thrombosis. Chest 1986; Suppl. 89: 369S-400S
337. Nurmohamed MT, Rosendaal FR, Büller HR, et al. Low-molecular-weight heparin versus standard heparin in general and orthopaedic surgery: a meta-analysis. Lancet 1992; 340: 152-6
338. Planes A, Vochelle N, Darmon J-Y, et al. Efficacy and safety of post-discharge administration of enoxaparin in the prevention of deep venous thrombosis after total hip replacement: a prospective randomised double-blind placebo controlled trial. Drugs 1996; 52 Suppl.: in press
339. Powers PJ, Gent M, Jay RM, et al. A randomized trial of less intense postoperative warfarin or aspirin therapy in the prevention of venous thromboembolism after surgery for fractured hip. Archives of Internal Medicine 1989; 149: 771-4
340. Francis CW, Marder VJ, Evarts CM, et al. Two-step warfarin therapy: prevention of postoperative venous thrombosis without excessive bleeding. Journal of the American Medical Association 1983; 249: 374-8
341. Eriksson BI, Ekman S, Kalebo P, et al. Prevention of deep-vein thrombosis after total hip replacement: direct thrombin inhibition with recombinant hirudin, CGP 39393. Lancet 1996; 347: 635
342. Hommes DW, Bura A, Mazzolai L, et al. Subcutaneous heparin compared with continuous intravenous heparin administration in the initial treatment of deep vein thrombosis. A meta-analysis. Annals of Internal Medicine 1992; 116: 279-84
343. Hull R, Raskob GE, Rosenbloom D, et al. Heparin for 5 days as compared with 10 days in the initial treatment of proximal venous thrombosis. New England Journal of Medicine 1990; 322: 1260-4
344. Levine M, Gent M, Hirsh J, et al. A comparison of low-molecular weight heparin administered primarily at home with unfractionated heparin administered in the hospital for proximal deep vein thrombosis. New England Journal of Medicine 1996; 334: 677-81
345. Schafer AI. Low-molecular weight heparin – an opportunity for home treatment of venous thrombosis. New England Journal of Medicine 1996; 334: 724-5
346. Hull RD, Pineo GF, Brant RF. Effect of low molecular weight heparin versus warfarin sodium on mortality in long-term treatment of proximal deep vein thrombosis. Clinical and Applied Thrombosis – Haemostasis 1996; 2: S4-S11
347. Clagett GP, Anderson Jr FA, Heit J, et al. Prevention of venous thromboembolism. Chest 1995; 108: 312S-334S
348. Fibrinolytic Therapy Trialists' (FTT) Collaborative Group. Indications for fibrinolytic therapy in suspected acute myocardial infarction: collaborative overview of mortality and major morbidity results from all randomised trials of more than 1000 patients. Lancet 1994; 343: 311-22
349. The International Study Group. In-hospital mortality and clinical course of 20 891 patients with suspected acute myocardial infarction randomised between alteplase and streptokinase with or without heparin. Lancet 1990; 336: 71-5
350. ISIS-3 (Third International Study of Infarct Survival) Collaborative Group. A randomised trial of streptokinase vs tissue plasminogen activator vs anistreplase and of aspirin plus heparin vs aspirin alone among 41 299 cases of suspected acute myocardial infarction. Lancet 1992; 339: 753-60
351. The GUSTO Angiographic Investigators. The comparative effects of plasminogen activator, streptokinase, or both on coronary artery patency, ventricular function, and survival after acute myocardial infarction. New England Journal of Medicine 1993; 329: 1615-22
352. International Joint Efficacy Comparison of Thrombolytics Trialists. Randomised, double-blind comparison of reteplase double-bolus administration with streptokinase in acute myocardial infarction (INJECT): trial to investigate equivalence. Lancet 1995; 346: 329-36
353. Martin M, Schoop W, Zeitler E. Streptokinase in chronic arterial occlusive disease. Journal of the American Medical Association 1970; 211: 1169-73
354. Martin M, Fiebach BJ. Short-term ultrahigh streptokinase treatment of chronic arterial occlusions and acute deep venous thromboses. Seminars in Thrombosis and Hemostasis 1991; 17: 21-38
355. Hess H, Ingrisch H, Mietaschk A, et al. Local low-dose thrombolytic therapy of peripheral arterial occlusions. New England Journal of Medicine 1982; 307: 1627-30
356. Graor RA, Risius B, Young JR, et al. Low-dose streptokinase for selective thrombolysis: systemic effects and complications. Radiology 1984; 152: 35-9
357. Mori KW, Bookstein JJ, Heeney DJ, et al. Selective streptokinase infusion: clinical and laboratory correlates. Radiology 1983; 148: 677-82
358. McNamara TO, Fischer JR. Thrombolysis of peripheral arterial and graft occlusions: improved results using high-dose urokinase. American Journal of Roentgenology 1985; 144: 769-5
359. Comerota AJ, White JV, Grosch JD. Intraoperative intra-arterial thrombolytic therapy for salvage of limbs in patients with distal arterial thrombosis. Surgery Gynecology and Obstetrics 1989; 169: 283-9
360. Earnshaw JJ, Beard JD. Intraoperative use of thrombolytic agents. Should be available in every hospital treating acute limb ischaemia. British Medical Journal 1993; 307: 638-9
361. National Institute of Neurological Disorders and Stroke rt-PA Stroke Study Group. Tissue plasminogen activator for acute ischemic stroke. New England Journal of Medicine 1995; 333: 1581-7
362. Hacke W, Kaste M, Fieschi C, et al. Intravenous thrombolysis with recombinant tissue plasminogen activator for acute hemispheric stroke: the European Coop-

erative Stroke Study (ECASS). Journal of the American Medical Association 1995; 274: 1017-25
363. Brogden RN, Speight TM, Avery GS. Streptokinase: a review of its clinical pharmacology, mechanism of action and therapeutic uses. Drugs 1973; 5: 357-445
364. Kwaan H. Thrombo-embolic disorders of the eye in thrombolytic therapy. In: Comerota AJ, editor. Thrombolytic therapy. New York: Grune and Stratton, 1988: 163
365. Francis CW, Marder VJ. Fibrinolytic therapy for venous thrombosis. Progress in Cardiovascular Diseases 1991; 34: 193-204
366. Goldhaber SZ, Buring JE, Lipnick RJ, et al. Pooled analysis of randomized trials of streptokinase and heparin in phlebographically documented acute deep venous thrombosis. American Journal of Medicine 1984; 76: 393-7
367. Theiss W, Baumann G, Klein G. Fibrinolytische Behandlung tiefer Venenthrombosen mit Streptokinase in ultrahoher Dosierung. Deutsche Medizinische Wochenschrift 1987; 122: 668-74
368. D'Angelo A, Mannucci PA. Outcome of treatment of deep-vein thrombosis with urokinase: relationship to dosage, duration of therapy, age of the thrombus and laboratory changes. Thrombosis and Haemostasis 1984; 51: 236-9
369. Verhaeghe R, Besse P, Bounameaux H, et al. Multicentre pilot study of the efficacy and safety of systemic rt-PA administration in the treatment of deep vein thrombosis of the lower extremities and or pelvis. Thrombosis Research 1989; 55: 5-11
370. Goldhaber SZ, Meyerovitz MF, Green D, et al. Randomized controlled trial of tissue plasminogen activator in proximal deep venous thrombosis. American Journal of Medicine 1990; 88: 235-40
371. Turpie AGG, Levine MM, Hirsh J, et al. Tissue plasminogen activator (rt-PA) vs heparin in deep vein thrombosis. Results of a randomized trial. Chest 1990; 97 Suppl. 4: 172S-5S
372. Bounameaux H, Banga JD, Bluhmki E, et al. Double-blind, randomized comparison of systemic continuous infusion of 0.25 versus 0.50 mg/kg/24 h of alteplase over 3 to 7 days for treatment of deep venous thrombosis in heparinized patients: results of the European Thrombolysis with rt-PA in Venous Thrombosis (ETTT) Trial. Thrombosis and Haemostasis 1992; 67: 306-9
373. Prewitt RM. Principles of thrombolysis in pulmonary embolism. Chest 1991; 99 Suppl. 4: 157S-64S
374. Mitchell JP, Trulock EP. Tissue-plasminogen activator for pulmonary embolism resulting in shock: two case reports and discussion of the literature. American Journal of Medicine 1991; 90: 255-60
375. Goldhaber SZ, Vaughan DE, Markis JE, et al. Acute pulmonary embolism treated with tissue plasminogen activator. Lancet 1986; 2: 886-9
376. Verstraete M, Miller GAH, Bounameaux H, et al. Intravenous and intrapulmonary recombinant tissue-type plasminogen activator in the treatment of acute massive pulmonary embolism. Circulation 1988; 77: 353-60
377. Meyer G, Sors H, Charbonnier B, et al. The effect of intravenous urokinase versus alteplase on total pulmonary resistance in acute massive pulmonary embolism. A European multicenter double-blind trial. Journal of the American College of Cardiology 1992; 19: 239-45
378. Goldhaber SZ, Kessler CM, Heit JR, et al. Recombinant tissue-type plasminogen activator versus a novel dosing regimen of urokinase in acute pulmonary embolism: a randomized controlled multicenter trial. Journal of the American College of Cardiology 1992; 20: 24-30
379. Phillips BG, Bauman JL. Prescribing trends and pharmacoeconomic considerations in the treatment of arrhythmias. Focus on atrial fibrillation and flutter. PharmacoEconomics 1995; 7: 521-33
380. Eckman MH, Beshansky JR, Durand-Zaleski I, et al. Anticoagulation for noncardiac procedures in patients with prosthetic heart valves. Journal of the American Medical Association 1990; 263: 1513-21
381. Eckman MH, Levine HJ, Pauker SG. Making decisions about antithrombotic therapy in heart disease. Decision analytic and cost-effectiveness issues. Chest 1995; 108: 457S-70S
382. Eckman MH, Levine HJ, Pauker SG. Decision analytic and cost-effectiveness issues concerning anticoagulant prophylaxis in heart disease. Chest 1992; 102: 538S-49S
383. Eckman MH, Levine HJ, Pauker SG. Effect of laboratory variation in the prothrombin time ratio on the results of oral anticoagulant therapy. New England Journal of Medicine 1993; 329: 696-702
384. Kupersmith J, Holmes-Rovner M, Hogan A, et al. Cost-effectiveness in heart disease, Part II: preventive therapies. Progress in Cardiovascular Diseases 1995; 37: 243-71
385. Dundabin D. Cost-effective intervention in stroke. PharmacoEconomics 1992; 2: 468-99
386. Woo KS, White HD. Pharmacoeconomic aspects of treatment of acute myocardial infarction with thrombolytic agents. PharmacoEconomics 1993; 3: 192-204
387. Gillis JC, Wagstaff AJ, Goa KL. Alteplase: a reappraisal of its pharmacological properties and therapeutic use in acute myocardial infarction. Drugs 1995; 50: 102-36
388. Forbes CD, Davidson JF. Management of coagulation defects. Clinics in Haematology 1973; 2: 101
389. Verstraete M. Haemostatic drugs. A critical appraisal. The Hague: Martinus Nijhoff, 1977: 155
390. Verstraete M. Haemostatic drugs. In: Bloom D et al., editors. Haemostasis and thrombosis. Edinburgh: Churchill Livingstone, 1994: 1057-74
391. Verstraete M. Clinical application of inhibitors of fibrinolysis. Drugs 1985; 29: 236-61
392. Royston D. High-dose aprotinin therapy: a review of the first five years' experience. Journal of Cardiothoracic and Vascular Anesthesia 1992; 6: 76-100
393. Lemmer JH, Stanford W, Bonney SL, et al. Aprotinin for coronary bypass operation: efficacy, safety, and influence on early saphenous vein graft potency. Journal of Thoracic and Cardiovascular Surgery 1994; 107: 543-53
394. Green D, Sanders J, Eiken M, et al. Recombinant aprotinin in coronary artery bypass graft operations. Journal of Thoracic and Cardiovascular Surgery 1995; 110: 963-70
395. Levy JH, Pifarre R, Schaff HV, et al. A multicentre, double-blind, placebo-controlled trial of aprotinin for reducing blood loss and the requirement for donor-blood transfusion in patients undergoing repeat coronary artery bypass grafting. Circulation 1995; 92: 2236-44
396. Mallett SV, Cox D, Burroughs AK, et al. Aprotinin and reduction of blood loss and transfusion requirements in orthoptic liver transplantation. Lancet 1990; 336: 886-7

397. Jaquiss RDB. Use of aprotinin in pediatric lung transplantation. Journal of Heart and Lung Transplantation 1995; 14: 302-7

398. Seremetis SV, Aledort LM. Congenital bleeding disorders: rational treatment options. Drugs 1993; 45: 541-7

399. Mannucci PM, Remuzzi G, Pusineri F, et al. Desamino 8-D-arginine vasopressin shortens the bleeding time in uremia. New England Journal of Medicine 1983; 308: 8-12

400. Kaufman RJ, Wasley LC, Dorner AJ. Synthesis, processing, and secretion of recombinant human factor VIII expressed in mammalian cells. Journal of Biological Chemistry 1988; 263: 6352-2

401. Kasper CK, Lusher JM. Recent evolution of clotting factor concentrates for hemophilia A and B. Transfusion 1993; 33: 422-34

402. Mannucci PM. Modern treatment of hemophilia: from the shadow towards the light. Thrombosis and Haemostasis 1993; 70: 17-23

403. Nilson IM, Berntrop E, Freeburghaus C. Treatment of patients with factor VIII and IX inhibitors. Thrombosis and Haemostasis 1993; 70: 56-9

404. de la Fuente B, Kasper CK, Rickles FR, et al. Response of patients with mild and moderate hemophilia A and von Willebrand's disease to treatment with desmopressin. Annals of Internal Medicine 1985; 103: 6-14

405. Brettler DB, Forsberg AD, Levine PH, et al. The use of porcine factor VIII concentrate (Hyate:C) in the treatment of patients with inhibitor antibodies to factor VIII: a multicenter US experience. Archives of Internal Medicine 1989; 149: 1381-5

406. Lusher JM, Shapiro SS, Palascak JE, et al. Efficacy of prothrombin complex concentrates in hemophiliacs with antibodies to factor VIII. A multicenter trial. New England Journal of Medicine 1980; 303: 421-5

407. Hedner U, Glazer S, Pingel K, et al. Successful use of recombinant factor VIIa in a patient with severe haemophilia A during synovectomy. Lancet 1988; 2: 1193

408. Thompson AR. Factor IX concentrates for clinical use. Seminars in Thrombosis and Hemostasis 1993; 19: 25-36

409. Ginsberg D, Bowie EJW. Molecular genetics of von Willebrand disease. Blood 1992; 79: 2507-19

410. Rodeghiero FCF, Castaman G, Meyer D, et al. Replacement therapy with virus inactivated plasma concentrates in von Willebrand disease. Vox Sanguinis 1992; 62: 193-9

411. Bick RL. Disseminated intravascular coagulation. Hematology Oncology Clinics of North America 1992; 6: 1259-85

412. Rubin RN, Colman RW. Disseminated intravascular coagulation: approach to treatment. Drugs 1992; 44: 963-71

413. Remuzzi G, Cavenaghi AE, Mecca G. Prostacyclin-like activity and bleeding in renal failure. Lancet 1977; 2: 1195

414. Verstraete M, Perez-Requejo JL. Intravenous immunoglobulins in the treatment of chronic idiopathic thrombocytopenia In: Poller, editor. Recent advances in blood coagulation, No. 4. Edinburgh: Churchill Livingstone, 1985: 215

415. Imbach P, Berchtold W, Hirt A, et al. Intravenous immunoglobulin versus oral corticosteroids in acute immune thrombocytopenic purpura in childhood. Lancet 1985; 2: 464

416. Warkentin TE, Kelton JG. Current concepts in the treatment of immune thrombocytopenia. Drugs 1990; 40: 531-42

417. Anderson JC. Response of resistant idiopathic thrombocytopenic purpura to pulsed high-dose dexamethasone therapy. New England Journal of Medicine 1994; 330: 1560-4

418. Spencer CM, Brogden RN. Anagrelide: a review of its pharmacodynamic and pharmacokinetic properties, and therapeutic potential in the treatment of thrombocythaemia. Drugs 1994; 47: 809-22

419. Finch CA, Huebers H. Perspectives in iron metabolism. New England Journal of Medicine 1982; 306: 1520-1

420. Charlton RW, Fatti LP, Lynch SR, et al. Equilibration of tracer radioiron with body iron. Clinical Science 1980; 58: 93-100

421. World Health Organization. Requirements of ascorbic acid, vitamin D, vitamin B12, folate and iron. WHO Technical Report, Series 452, 1970

422. Arthur CK, Isbister JP. Iron deficiency, misunderstood, misdiagnosed and mistreated. Drugs 1987; 33: 171-82

423. Brise H, Hallberg L. A method for comparative studies on iron absorption in man using two radio iron isotopes. Acta Medica Scandinavica 1962; 171 Suppl. 376: 7-9

424. Elwood PC, Williams G. A comparative trial of slow-release and conventional iron preparations. Practitioner 1970; 204: 812-5

425. Beal RW. Haematinics I. Pathophysiological and clinical aspects. Drugs 1971; 2: 190-207

426. Beal RW. Haematinics II. Clinical pharmacological and therapeutic aspects. Drugs 1971; 2: 207-21

427. Neuvonen PJ. Interactions with the absorption of tetracyclines. Drugs 1976; 11: 45-61

428. Harju E. Clinical pharmacokinetics of iron preparations. Clinical Pharmacokinetics 1989; 17: 69-89

429. Edwards CQ, Griffen LM, Goldgar D, et al. Prevalence of hemochromatosis among 11,065 presumably healthy blood donors. New England Journal of Medicine 1988; 318: 1355-62

430. Lauffer RB. Iron balance: the new 'Iron-Lite' health plan that restores your inner vitality. New York: St Martin's Press, 1991

431. Berkovitch M, Collins AF, Papadouris D, et al. Need for early, low-dose chelation therapy in young children with transfused homozygous beta-thalassemia. Blood 1993; 82: 359

432. Brittenham GM, Griffith PM, Nienhuis AW, et al. Efficacy of deferoxamine in preventing complications or iron overload in patients with thalassemia major. New England Journal of Medicine 1994; 331: 567-73

433. De Virgillis S, Congia M, Frau F, et al. Deferoxamine-induced growth retardation in patients with thalassemia major. Pediatrics 1988; 113: 661-9

434. Olivieri NF, Berriman AM, Tyler BJ, et al. Continuous intravenous administration of deferoxamine in adults with severe iron overload. American Journal of Hematology 1992; 41: 61-3

435. Bentur Y, McGuigan M, Koren G. Deferoxamine (desferrioxamine): new toxicities for an old drug. Drug Safety 1991; 6: 37-46

436. Al-Refaie FN, Wonke B, Hoffbrand AV, et al. Efficacy and possible adverse effects of the oral iron chelator 1,2-dimethyl-3-hydroxypyrid-4-one (L1) in thalassemia major. Blood 1992; 80: 592-9

437. Higuchi M, Oh-Eda M, Kuboniwa H, et al. Role of sugar chains in the expression of the biological activity of human erythropoietin. Journal of Biological Chemistry 1992; 267: 7703-9

438. Jones SS, D'Andrea AD, Hains LL, et al. Human erythropoietin receptor, cloning, expression, and biologic characterization. Blood 1990; 76: 31-5
439. Nakamura Y, Komastu N, Nakuchi H. A truncated erythropoietin receptor that fails to prevent programmed cell death of erythroid cells. Science 1992; 257: 1138-41
440. Spivak JL, Fisher J, Isaacs MA, et al. Protein kinases and phosphatases are involved in erythropoietin-mediated signal transduction. Experimental Hematology 1992; 20: 500-4
441. Gimenez LF, Scheel P. Clinical application of recombinant erythropoietin in renal dialysis patients. Hematology Oncology Clinics of North America 1994; 8: 913-26
442. Faulds D, Sorkin EM. Epoetin (recombinant human erythropoietin): a review of its pharmacodynamic and pharmacokinetic properties and therapeutic potential in anaemia and the stimulation of erythropoiesis. Drugs 1989; 38: 863-99
443. Dunn CJ, Markham A. Epoetin beta: a review of its pharmacological properties and clinical use in the management of anaemia associated with chronic renal failure. Drugs 1996; 51: 299-318
444. Eschbach JW, Abduladi MH, Browne JK, et al. Recombinant human erythropoietin in anemic patients with end-stage renal disease: results of phase 3 multicenter clinical trial. Annals of Internal Medicine 1989; 111: 992-1000
445. Winearls CG, Pippard MJ, Downing MR, et al. Effects of human erythropoietin derived from recombinant DNA on the anaemia of patients maintained by chronic haemodialysis. Lancet 1986; 2: 1175-8
446. Drueke TB. Resistance to recombinant human erythropoietin in hemodialysis patients. American Journal of Nephrology 1990; 105: 34-9
447. Metcalf D. The molecular biology and functions of the granulocyte-macrophage colony stimulating factors. Blood 1986; 67: 257-67
448. Oh-eda M, Hasegawa M, Hattori K, et al. O-linked sugar chain of human granulocyte colony stimulating factor protects it against polymerization and denaturation allowing it to retain its biological activity. Journal of Biological Chemistry 1990; 265: 11432-5
449. Nissen C, Dalle Carbonare V, Moser Y. Comparison of the biological potency of glycosylated versus nonglycosylated rG-CSF. Drug Investigation 1994; 7: 346-52
450. Denzlinger S, Tetzlosf W, Gerhartz H, et al. Differential activation of the endogenous leukotriene biosynthesis by two different preparations of granulocyte-macrophage colony stimulating factor in health volunteers. Blood 1993; 81: 2007-13
451. Cebon J, Dempsey P, Fox R, et al. Pharmacokinetics of human granulocyte-macrophage colony-stimulating factor using a sensitive immunoassay. Blood 1988; 72: 1340-7
452. Linch DC, Scarffe H, Proctor S, et al. Randomised vehicle-controlled dose-finding study of glycosylated recombinant human granulocyte colony-stimulating factor after bone marrow transplantation. Bone Marrow Transplantation 1993; 11: 307-11
453. Schriber JR, Negrin RS. Use and toxicity of the colony-stimulating factors. Drug Safety 1993; 6: 457-68
454. Grant SM, Heel RC. Recombinant granulocyte-macrophage colony-stimulating factor (rGM-CSF): a review of its pharmacological properties and prospective role in management of myelosuppression. Drugs 1992; 43: 516-60
455. Boogaerts MA. Growth factors in haematology: prophylactic versus interventional use. European Journal of Cancer 1994; 30A: 238-43
456. Boogaerts M, Cavalli F, Cortés-Funes H, et al. Granulocyte growth factors: achieving a consensus. Annals of Oncology 1995; 6: 237-44
457. American Society of Clinical Oncology. Recommendations for the use of hematopoietic colony-stimulating factors: evidence-based, clinical practice guidelines. Journal of Clinical Oncology 1994; 12: 2471-508
458. Hollingshead LM, Goa KL. Recombinant granulocyte colony-stimulating factor (rG-CSF): a review of its pharmacological properties and prospective role in neutropenic conditions. Drugs 1991; 42: 300-30
459. Frampton JE, Lee CR, Faulds D. Filgrastim: a review of its pharmacological properties and therapeutic efficacy in neutropenia. Drugs 1994; 48: 731-60
460. Crawford J, Ozer H, Stoller R, et al. Reduction by granulocyte colony-stimulating factor of fever and neutropenia induced by chemotherapy in patients with small-cell lung cancer. New England Journal of Medicine 1991; 315: 164-70
461. Powles R, Smith C, Milan S, et al. Human recombinant GM-CSF in allogeneic bone marrow transplantation for leukaemia: double-blind placebo-controlled trial. Lancet 1990; 2: 1417-20
462. Brandt SJ, Peters WP, Atwater SK, et al. Effect of recombinant human granulocyte-macrophage colony-stimulating factor on hematopoietic reconstitution after high-dose chemotherapy and autologous bone marrow transplantation. New England Journal of Medicine 1988; 318: 869-76
463. Lieschke G, Cebon J, Morstyn G. Characterization of the clinical effects after the first dose of bacterially synthesized recombinant human granulocyte-macrophage colony stimulating factor. Blood 1989; 74: 2634-43
464. Lindemann A, Herrmann F, Oster W, et al. Hematologic effects of recombinant human granulocyte colony stimulating factor in patients with malignancy. Blood 1989; 74: 2644-51
465. Welte K, Zeidler C, Reiter A, et al. Differential effects of granulocyte-macrophage colony-stimulating factor and granulocyte colony-stimulating factor in children with severe congenital neutropenia. Blood 1990; 75: 1056-63
466. Herrman F, Schultz G, Lindermann A, et al. Hematopoietic responses in patients with advanced malignancy treated with recombinant human granulocyte-macrophage colony stimulating factor. Journal of Clinical Oncology 1989; 7: 159-67
467. Vellenga E, Young DC, Wagner K, et al. The effect of GM-CSF and G-CSF in promoting growth of clonogenic cells in acute myeloblastic leukemia. Blood 1987; 69: 1771-6
468. Ganser A, Volkers B, Greher J, et al. Recombinant human granulocyte-macrophage colony-stimulating factor in patients with myelodysplastic syndromes: a phase I/II trial. Blood 1989; 76: 31-7
469. Cook JD, Skikne BS, Baynes RD. Serum transferrin receptor. Annual Review of Medicine 1993; 44: 63-74
470. Oski FA. Iron deficiency in infancy and childhood. New England Journal of Medicine 1993; 329: 190-3
471. Scholl TO, Hediger ML. Anemia and iron-deficiency anemia: compilation of data on pregnancy outcome.

American Journal of Clinical Nutrition 1994; 59: 492S-501S
472. US Preventive Services Task Force. Routine iron supplementation during pregnancy. Journal of the American Medical Association 1993; 270: 2846-54
473. Carmel R. Pernicious anemia: definitions, expressions and the long-term consequences of atrophic gastritis. In: Holt PR, Russell RM, editors. Chronic gastritis and hypochlorhydria in the elderly. Boca Raton: CRC Press, 1993: 99-114
474. Hsing AW, Hansson LE, McLaughlin JK, et al. Pernicious anemia and subsequent cancer: a population-based cohort study. Cancer 1993; 71: 745-50
475. Pennypacker LC, Allen RH, Kelly JP, et al. Prevalence of cobalamin deficiency in elderly outpatients. Journal of the American Geriatrics Society 1992; 40: 1197-204
476. Clarke R, Daly L, Robinson K, et al. Hyperhomocysteinemia: an independent risk factor for vascular disease. New England Journal of Medicine 1991; 324: 1149-55
477. Ubbink JB, Vermaak WJH, Van der Merwe A, et al. Vitamin B12, vitamin B6 and folate nutritional status in men with hyperhomocysteinemia. American Journal of Clinical Nutrition 1993; 57: 47-53
478. Piyathilake CJ, Hine RJ, Dasanayake AP, et al. Effects of smoking on folate levels in buccal mucosal cells. International Journal of Cancer 1992; 52: 566-9
479. Czeizel AD, Dudas I. Prevention of the first occurrence of neural-tube defects by periconceptional vitamin supplementation. New England Journal of Medicine 1992; 327: 1832-5
480. Lux SE, Tse WT, Menninger JC, et al. Hereditary spherocytosis associated with deletion of human erythrocyte ankyrin gene on chromosome 8. Nature 1990; 345: 736-9
481. Costa FF, Agre P, Watkins PC, et al. Linkage of dominant hereditary spherocytosis to the gene for the erythrocyte membrane-skeleton protein ankyrin. New England Journal of Medicine 1990; 323: 1046-50
482. Weatherall DJ, Clegg JG. The thalassemia syndromes. Oxford: Blackwell Scientific Publications, 1981: 744
483. Lucarelli G, Galimberti M, Polchi P, et al. Bone marrow transplantation in children and adults with thalassemia. Bone Marrow Transplantation 1991; 7: 72
484. Angelucci E, Mariotti E, Lucarelli G, et al. Sudden cardiac tamponade after chemotherapy for marrow transplantation in thalassemia. Lancet 1992; 339: 287-9
485. Fucharoen S, Siritanaratkul N, Winichagoon P, et al. Hydroxyurea increases HbF levels and improves the effectiveness of erythropoiesis in β-thalassemia/HbE disease. Blood 1993; 82: 357
486. Sher GD, Entsush B, Ginder G, et al. Intravenous infusions of arginine butyrate increases τ-globin mRNA expression and F-reticulocytes in patients (PTS) with homozygous β-thalassemia and sickle cell disease. Blood 1993; 82: 312
487. Rachmilewitz EA, Goldfarb A, Dover G. Administration of erythropoietin to patients with beta-thalassemia intermedia: a preliminary trial. Blood 1991; 78: 1145-7
488. Platt OS, Thorington BD, Brambilla DJ, et al. Pain in sickle cell disease: rates and risk factors. New England Journal of Medicine 1991; 325: 11-6
489. Shapiro BS, Cohen DE, Howe CJ. Patient-controlled analgesia for sickle-cell related pain. Journal of Pain and Symptom Management 1993; 8: 22-8
490. Miller ST, Jensen D, Rao SP. Less intensive long-term transfusion therapy for sickle cell anemia and cerebrovascular accident. Journal of Pediatrics 1992; 120: 54-7
491. Cohen AR, Martin MB, Siber JH, et al. A modified transfusion program for prevention of stroke in sickle cell disease. Blood 1992; 79: 1657-61
492. Charache S, Dover GJ, Moore RD, et al. Hydroxyurea: effects on hemoglobin F production in patients with sickle cell anemia. Blood 1992; 79: 2555-65
493. Steinberg MH. Erythropoietin in anemia of renal failure in sickle cell disease. New England Journal of Medicine 1991; 324: 1369-70
494. Vermylen C, Cornu G. Bone marrow transplantation in sickle cell anaemia. Blood Reviews 1993; 7: 1-3
495. Beutler E. Abnormalities of the hexose monophosphate shunt. Seminars in Hematology 1971; 8: 311
496. Panceri R, Fraschini D, Tornotti G, et al. A successful use of high-dose cyclophosphamide in a child with severe autoimmune hemolytic anemia. Haematologica 1992; 77: 76-8
497. Blanchette VS, Kirby MA, Turner C. Role of intravenous immunoglobulin G in autoimmune hematologic disorders. Seminars in Hematology 1992; 29: 72-82
498. Pignon JM, Poirson E, Rochant H. Danazol in autoimmune haemolytic anaemia. British Journal of Haematology 1993; 83: 343-5
499. Marsh JCW, Chang J, Testa NG, et al. In vitro assessment of marrow 'stem cell' and stromal function in aplastic anemia. British Journal of Haematology 1991; 78: 258-67
500. Wodnar-Filipowicz A, Tichelli A, Zsebo KM, et al. Stem cell factor stimulates the in vitro growth of bone marrow cells from aplastic anemia patients. Blood 1992; 79: 3196-202
501. Gibson FM, Scopes J, Gordon-Smith EC. Aplastic anemia stromal cells produce greater colony stimulating activity than normal stromal cells. Experimental Hematology 1991; 19: 261
502. Nakao S, Yamaguchi M, Shiobara S, et al. Interferon gamma gene expression in unstimulated bone marrow mononuclear cells predicts a good response to cyclosporin therapy in aplastic anemia. Blood 1992; 79: 2532-5
503. Clarke WTW. Fatal aplastic anemia and chloramphenicol. Canadian Medical Association Journal 1967; 97: 815-9
504. Gluckman E, Horowitz MM, Champlin RE, et al. Bone marrow transplantation for severe aplastic anemia: influence of conditioning in graft versus host disease prophylaxis regimens on outcome. Blood 1992; 79: 269-75
505. Hows J, Szydlo R, Anasetti C, et al. Unrelated donor marrow transplants for severe acquired aplastic anemia. Bone Marrow Transplantation 1992; 10 Suppl. 1: 102-6
506. Ash RC, Horowitz MM, Gakle RP, et al. Bone marrow transplantation from related donors other than HLA-identical siblings: effect of T cell depletion. Bone Marrow Transplantation 1991; 7: 443-52
507. Gluckman E, Esperou-Bourdeau H, Baruchel A, et al. Multicentre randomised study comparing cyclosporine-A alone and antithymocyte globulin with prednisone for treatment of severe aplastic anemia. Blood 1992; 79: 2540-6
508. Bertrand Y, Amri F, Capdeville R, et al. The successful treatment of two cases of severe aplastic anaemia with

granulocyte-colony stimulating factor and cyclosporine-A. British Journal of Haematology 1991; 79: 648-52

509. Kojima S, Fukuda M, Miyajima Y, et al. Treatment of aplastic anemia in children with recombinant human granulocyte colony-stimulating factor. Blood 1991; 77: 937-41
510. Kojima S, Tsuchida M, Matsuyama T. Myelodysplasia and leukemia after treatment of aplastic anemia with G-CSF. New England Journal of Medicine 1992; 326: 1294-5
511. De Planque MM, Bacigalupo A, Wursch A, et al. Long term follow up of severe aplastic anaemia patients treated with antithymocyte globulin. British Journal of Haematology 1989; 73: 121-6
512. Young NS. The problem of clonality in aplastic anaemia: Dr. Damashek's riddle restated. Blood 1992; 79: 1385-92
513. Flowers ME, Doney KC, Storb R, et al. Marrow transplantation for Fanconi anemia with or without leukemic transformation: an update of the Seattle experience. Bone Marrow Transplantation 1992; 9: 167-73
514. Dunbar CE, Smith DA, Kimble J, et al. Treatment of Diamond-Blackfan anaemia with haematopoietic growth factors, granulocyte-macrophage colony-stimulating factor and interleukin 3: sustained remission following IL-3. British Journal of Haematology 1991; 79: 316-21
515. Raghavachar A. Pure red cell aplasia: review of treatment and proposal for a treatment strategy. Blut 1990; 61: 47-50
516. Young N. Hematologic and hematopoietic consequences of B19 parvovirus infection. Seminars in Hematology 1988; 25: 159-72
517. Baer AN, Dessypris EN, Goldwasser E, et al. Blunted erythropoietin response to anaemia in rheumatoid arthritis. British Journal of Haematology 1987; 66: 559-64
518. Pincus T, Olsen NJ, Russell IJ, et al. Multicenter study of recombinant human erythropoietin in correction of anemia in rheumatoid arthritis. American Journal of Medicine 1990; 89: 161-8
519. Henry DA, Beall GN, Benson CA, et al. Recombinant human erythropoietin in the treatment of anemia associated with human immunodeficiency virus (HIV) infection and zidovudine therapy: overview of four clinical trials. Annals of Internal Medicine 1992; 117: 739-48
520. Ludwig H, Fritz E, Kotzmann H, et al. Erythropoietin treatment of anemia associated with multiple myeloma. New England Journal of Medicine 1990; 322: 1693-9
521. Abels RI. Use of recombinant human erythropoietin in the treatment of anemia in patients who have cancer. Seminars in Oncology 1992; 19 Suppl. 8: 29-35
522. Whittington R, Barradell LB, Benfield P. Epoetin: a pharmacoeconomic review of its use in chronic renal failure and its effects on quality of life. PharmacoEconomics 1993; 3: 45-82
523. Denton T, Diamond GA, Matloff JM, et al. Anemia therapy: individual benefit and societal cost. Seminars in Oncology 1994; 21 Suppl. 3: 29-35
524. Ludwig H, Fritz E, Leitgeb C, et al. Prediction of response to erythropoietin treatment in chronic anaemia of cancer. Blood 1994; 84: 1056-63
525. Beguin Y, Clemons G, Pootrakul P, et al. Quantitative assessment of erythropoiesis and functional classification of anemia based on measurements of serum transferrin receptor and erythropoietin. Blood 1993; 81: 1067-76
526. Barosi G, Cazzola M, De Vincentiis A, et al. Guidelines for the use of recombinant human erythropoietin. Haematologica 1994; 79: 526-33
527. Heimpel H. Drug-induced agranulocytosis. Medical Toxicology and Adverse Drug Experience 1988; 3: 449-62
528. Boogaerts MA, Peters M, Peersman C, et al. Mechanisms of aprindine induced agranulocytosis: direct toxicity on CFU-GM and CFU-GEMM. Scandinavian Journal of Haematology 1984; 32: 175-8
529. Demuynck H, Zachee P, Verhoef G, et al. Risks of rh G-CSF treatment for drug-induced agranulocytosis. Annals of Hematology 1995; 70: 143-7
530. van Itterbeek H, Vermylen J, Verstraete M. High obstruction of urine flow as a complication of the treatment with fibrinolysis inhibitors of haematuria in haemophiliacs. Acta Haematologica 1968; 39: 237-42
531. Chanarin I, England JM. Toxicity of trimethoprim-sulphamethoxazole in patients with megaloblastic haemopoiesis. British Medical Journal 1972; 1: 651-3

Chapter 27

# Malignant Diseases

*F.M. Muggia* and *D.D. Von Hoff*

## Synopsis of Important Principles

1) Cancer prevention and treatment rely on an understanding of tumour biology and aetiology. Once invasive cancer is present, surgery, radiotherapy, chemotherapy and treatment with biological response modifiers all have their specific role in the general strategy employed against malignant diseases.

2) Cancer prevention relies on surveillance of high-risk individuals, early identification of premalignant changes and, to an increasing degree, on the introduction of chemopreventive measures.

3) Treatment of invasive cancer is based on the principles of local control and the use of drug therapy for systemic dissemination to the cancer.

4) Most cytotoxic agents are not specific for tumour cells and affect all cells of the patient, especially rapidly proliferating tissues such as the bone marrow, lymphoid system, oral and gastrointestinal epithelium, skin and hair roots, germinal epithelium of the gonads and embryonic structures. Anticancer drugs can also be carcinogenic.

5) The final outcome of administration of an anticancer drug is determined by the dynamic interplay of drug, tumour cell and patient characteristics. Some drugs may exert their effects via modulation of the immune system, or other modifications of biological responses of the host to the tumour.

6) For the most responsive tumours, combination chemotherapy is more effective than single agent therapy. Combinations include drugs with differing actions that are active when used alone against the specific tumour type, and given in nearly full doses.

7) Dose-intensity may be maximised by appropriate dose-scheduling, specific cytokines, reconstitution of bone marrow through the use of progenitor cells, and protection against toxicity to individual organ systems.

8) Dose-intensity strategies, including the use of autologous or allogeneic bone marrow reconstitution, have achieved their most impressive results in the treatment of acute leukaemias, Hodgkin's disease, non-Hodgkin's lymphomas and germ cell tumours.

9) In most solid tumours, chemotherapy has been useful as an adjuvant to surgery and radiotherapy of localised tumours that are at high risk of relapse or dissemination. This principle has been successfully applied in childhood solid tumours, and breast and colorectal cancer. Chemotherapy simultaneous with radiation, or preceding local measures has recently yielded superior results in other solid tumours, including lung cancer.

Improved understanding of the biology and genetic origins of cancer has brought about major changes in the prevention, diagnosis and therapeutic approaches directed to individuals at risk of developing cancer or afflicted with a specific neoplastic disease.

#### Cancer Biology

While cancer has always been considered a problem of uncontrolled growth,[1] insights into other important processes have triggered new forms of therapeutic interventions. For example, the process of *metastasis* has been characterised at anatomical, biochemical and molecular levels: tumour cell invasion, motility, attachment to basement membranes, extravasation and neovascularisation occur through activation of specific enzymatic pathways, and elaboration of growth factors under the control of oncogenes.[2] Another focus has been *differentiation*, which followed the recognition of the reciprocal relationship between differentiation and proliferation signals. *Immunological surveillance*, and modifiers of the immune response or of immunological interactions of immune cells with cancer cells, have also been the subject of extensive study, with some concepts integrated into clinical testing.[3]

Finally, much has been learned about *proliferation* and cell death. Several key steps in the cell cycle have been identified that may be deranged in cancer cells such that important transition points are inappropriately regulated, allowing these cells to proceed to pathways causing *apoptosis* (programmed cell death) or abnormal cell division.[4] Apoptosis has been investigated as an important physiological mechanism, and it has also been shown to be the end result of chemotherapeutic drug action.[5]

#### Genetic Change and Predisposition

Studies of familial cancer syndromes in relation to molecular changes in the genome have unravelled several important aspects of cancer genetics and carcinogenesis. Following an analysis of the differences between familial and sporadic retinoblastoma in 1971,[6] it was hypothesised that the familial disease, which is often bilateral and multicentric, is a result of a transmitted genetic abnormality in one chromosome (maternal or paternal), and a subsequent acquired abnormality (the second hit in the '2-hit' hypothesis) in the corresponding normal allele. The sporadic form, on the other hand, which as a rule is unilateral, depends on the unlikely occurrence of 2 hits on the 'retinoblastoma' gene. A decade later, the retinoblastoma (RB) gene was localised to chromosome 13q, and became the first of the 'tumour suppressor' genes to be identified.

The study of familial cancers has been intensified by techniques including the loss of heterozygosity that would similarly imply localisation of other tumour suppressor genes at sites of common chromosomal deletions. The gene of the p53 protein is localised to chromosome 17q13 and appears to have a central role in the regulation of proliferation.[7,8] Germ line mutations in the p53 gene have been identified in the Li-Fraumeni syndrome, which confers genetic predisposition to a wide variety of carcinomas and sarcomas.[9,10] Acquired mutations in the p53 protein have been described in a wide variety of other malignancies.[11]

Other recurrent chromosomal abnormalities have been fully or partially characterised as being related to the familial occurrence of certain cancers: abnormalities in 3p and lung cancer, 11p and Wilms' tumour,[12] 17q where the BRCA1 gene is located[13] and breast cancer, 18q and colon cancer are among those that have received the most attention. More recently, susceptibility to colon cancer has been linked with a familial susceptibility to increasing misrepair of tandem repeats of 2 bases.[14] This insight will have an effect on the identification of high-risk individuals and, in future, on programmes of cancer diagnosis and prevention.

#### Carcinogenesis and Cancer Prevention

Cancer induction is related to genetic damage that may originate either in inherited abnormal genes, inadequate mechanisms to repair damage, or environmental endogenous or exogenous carcinogenic influences. Major advances are being made in the identification of inherited abnormalities, but the effects on clinical practice have not yet been widespread. On the other hand, the epidemiology of certain cancers has provided clues to their origin in relation to hormonal influences. Estrogen-driven cancers include breast and endometrial cancers, with progesterone exerting a major modulatory effect on endometrial growth by inducing differentiation, whereas it enhances proliferation of the breast lobules. Ovarian epithelial growth may be stimulated by ovulation, but hormonal influences on cancer are less well characterised. Prostate cancer, on the other hand, is an androgen-driven tumour.[15] These concepts have stimulated interest in cancer prevention: medical castration

**Table I.** Pharmacokinetic characteristics of some commonly used anticancer drugs

| Drug | Route(s) of administration | Predominant route of elimination[a,b] | Notes[c] |
|---|---|---|---|
| Altretamine | PO | Hepatic metabolism to several metabolites (some of which are excreted in urine) | Variable plasma concentrations (due to variable first-pass metabolism); $t_{½β}$ 2.3-13.7h |
| L-Asparaginase (colaspase) | IV | Slow sequestration by reticuloendothelial system | As a bacterial protein, it can induce an antibody response that influences plasma clearance (much interindividual variation in elimination) |
| Azacitidine | IV | Rapid hepatic metabolism (possible spontaneous decomposition); excretion in urine | Plasma concentration of parent drug remains higher for longer periods with continuous infusion than after IV boluses |
| Bleomycin | IV, IM | Renal excretion (60% unchanged in urine); inactivation by intracellular aminopeptidase | Elimination markedly prolonged in renal impairment; use extreme caution in patients currently receiving nephrotoxic drugs (e.g. high-dose methotrexate, aminoglycosides) |
| Busulfan | PO | Hepatic metabolism (metabolites inactive) | |
| Carboplatin | IV | Renal excretion (50-75% of total platinum administered is excreted in urine in first 24h) | Not extensively protein bound (unlike cisplatin), but bound fraction increases with time. Half-life of unbound platinum ≈ 6h Clearance reduced in renal impairment |
| Carmustine (BCNU) | IV | Hepatic metabolism (metabolites active); renal excretion of metabolites | Readily penetrates CSF |
| Chlorambucil | PO | Hepatic metabolism | |
| Chlormethine (mustine, nitrogen mustard, mechlorethamine) | IV | Very rapid chemical transformation to inactive drug in body fluids | Rapid degradation allows protection of a given tissue from drug action by interrupting bloodflow for a few minutes after administration |
| Cisplatin | IV | Renal excretion; some nonenzymatic metabolism to inactive metabolites | Extensively protein bound (time-dependent; bound fraction increases to ≥90% over 2-4h); half-life of unbound (active) form <1h |
| Cyclophosphamide | IV, PO | Hepatic metabolism (microsomal bioactivation); renal excretion of active metabolites and up to 20% unchanged drug | Well absorbed orally; active metabolites ≈50% protein bound, parent drug 12-14% bound; bioactivation and elimination enhanced by enzyme-inducing agents but influence on therapeutic activity not clear; delayed elimination of active metabolites in renal impairment; active metabolites cause chemical cystitis |
| Cytarabine (cytosine arabinoside) | IV, SC | Hepatic metabolism (partly activated by kinases and partly inactivated by deamination); renal metabolism (deamination); and renal excretion of active drug | Continuous infusion or short dosage interval needed due to rapid elimination ($t_{½β}$ ≈ 0.5-3h); penetrates CSF to some extent |
| Dacarbazine | IV | Hepatic metabolism and renal excretion (≈50% unchanged, ≈50% active metabolite in urine) | Chemically transformed by light, with uncertain effect on activity |
| Dactinomycin (actinomycin D) | IV | Biliary (50-90%) and renal excretion (up to 20%) of unchanged drug | |
| Daunorubicin (daunomycin) | IV | Hepatic metabolism (active metabolite); biliary and renal excretion (≈25% unchanged and active metabolite in urine) | High hepatic clearance; reduce dose in liver disease to avoid severe toxicity |
| Doxorubicin | IV | Hepatic metabolism and biliary excretion (active metabolite and unchanged drug); <15% excreted in urine | High hepatic clearance; reduce dose in liver disease to avoid severe toxicity |
| Epirubicin* | IV | Hepatic metabolism (to several metabolites) and biliary excretion; ≈ 11-15% excreted in urine as unchanged drug and metabolites | * 4' epimer of doxorubicin. Terminal phase $t_{½}$ 15-45h. Clearance reduced in liver dysfunction and plasma concentrations increased |

*[Continued over]*

**Table I.** *[Continued]*

| Drug | Route(s) of administration | Predominant route of elimination[a,b] | Notes[c] |
|---|---|---|---|
| Estramustine phosphate | PO, IV | Hepatic metabolism (to active metabolites) and excretion in bile | Oral bioavailability ≈ 44% (reflecting incomplete absorption). NB. absorption is impaired by calcium ions<br>Half-lives of metabolites are longer than parent drug |
| Etoposide (VP 16-213) | IV, PO | Renal (20-45% unchanged) and biliary (≈6%) excretion; some hepatic metabolism | Oral bioavailability ≈30-50%; >94% protein bound; $t_{½β}$ ≈6h |
| Fludarabine | IV | Dephosphorylation to F-Ara-A which is largely excreted in the urine (mean 60%) | Wide variability in $t_{½β}$ (6.9-33.5h). Clearance of F-Ara-A is reduced in renal impairment |
| Fluorouracil (5-fluorouracil, 5-FU) | IV | Hepatic metabolism (initial pathway saturable) and renal excretion (10-15% unchanged) | Oral bioavailability variable due to high first-pass metabolism; readily penetrates CSF; intracellular bioactivation and catabolism |
| Floxuridine (fluorodeoxyuridine) | IV | Hepatic metabolism | Greater first-pass metabolism than with fluorouracil renders it suitable for regional use |
| Hydroxycarbamide (hydroxyurea) | PO | Hepatic and renal metabolism to urea | |
| Idarubicin | IV | Hepatic metabolism (to idarubicinol); <5% excreted in urine as either parent drug or metabolite | Oral bioavailability ≈ 30%; $t_{½β}$ 6-35h (idarubicinol 8-73h) |
| Ifosfamide* | IV | Hepatic metabolism (to active metabolites); metabolic pathway appears route-dependent (differs with IV and oral administration) | * Administered with mesna to reduce urothelial toxicity (haemorrhagic cystitis). Oral bioavailability of ifosfamide 100% |
| Lomustine (CCNU) | PO | Hepatic metabolism (metabolites active); renal excretion of metabolites | Well absorbed orally; readily penetrates CSF |
| Melphalan | PO, IV | Some hepatic metabolism (extent unknown) and renal excretion (?% unchanged) | Oral bioavailability variable |
| Mercaptopurine | PO | Hepatic metabolism (xanthine oxidase); faecal excretion (50%) after oral dose; renal excretion (20% unchanged) after IV dose | Incomplete oral bioavailability; concurrent allopurinol (xanthine oxidase inhibitor) therapy requires reduction of oral dose by about one-third |
| Methotrexate | IV, IM, PO | Renal excretion (up to 90% unchanged); excretion parallels creatinine clearance; ≈30% of oral dose metabolised by gut bacteria during absorption; some hepatic metabolism (10% in urine as 7-hydroxy metabolite with low doses; up to 30-40% with high doses) | Saturable oral absorption (large doses ≈10 mg/kg or 80 mg/m$^2$ not completely absorbed); up to 70% protein bound, primarily to albumin; marked accumulation in renal impairment; renal clearance decreased by weak organic acids (e.g. salicylates, NSAIDs) |
| Mitomycin (mitomycin C) | IV | ≈30% unchanged in urine; insufficient data on remaining portion | Oral bioavailability variable |
| Mitoxantrone | IV | Hepatobiliary and renal excretion (≈7% unchanged in urine) | Slow elimination ($t_{½β}$ ≈37h); delayed elimination in liver impairment and ascites |
| Paclitaxel | IV | Hepatic metabolism (to several metabolites) and biliary excretion; <5% excreted unchanged in urine | Wide variability in half-life (4.3-49.8h) |
| Procarbazine | PO | Hepatic metabolism (metabolites inactive) | |
| Teniposide (VM 26) | IV | Hepatic metabolism; less biliary and renal excretion than etoposide | >99% protein bound; $t_{½β}$ ≈9-10h |
| Thioguanine | PO, IV | Hepatic metabolism (metabolite inactive) | |
| Thiotepa | IV, IM | Hepatic metabolism (metabolites inactive) | IM absorption variable |
| Vinblastine | IV | Hepatic metabolism, biliary and renal excretion (≈20% unchanged in urine) | Extensive binding to tissues |

**Table I.** *[Continued]*

| Drug | Route(s) of administration | Predominant route of elimination[a,b] | Notes[c] |
|---|---|---|---|
| Vincristine | IV | Hepatic metabolism, biliary excretion (≈40% unchanged in faeces) | Extensive binding to tissues |
| Vinorelbine | IV, PO | Hepatic metabolism and biliary excretion (activity of principal metabolite unknown) | Oral bioavailability 24-40%; $t_{½β}$ 40-45h |

a Amounts given as unchanged drug relate to percentage of an administered dose.

b Dosages of drugs excreted in significant quantities as unchanged drug or active metabolite (e.g. bleomycin, carboplatin, cisplatin, cyclophosphamide, cytarabine, dacarbazine, etoposide, fludarabine, methotrexate, mitomycin, carmustine, lomustine) may need to be reduced if renal function is impaired (see appendix D). Dosages of drugs subject to significant hepatobiliary elimination (e.g. dactinomycin, cyclophosphamide, cytarabine, daunorubicin, doxorubicin, epirubicin, fluorouracil, mitoxantrone, paclitaxel, vinblastine, vincristine, vinorelbine) may need to be reduced in liver or hepatobiliary diseases (see appendix F).

c For other pharmacokinetic data, see appendix A.

*Abbreviations and symbols:* IV = intravenous; IM = intramuscular; PO = oral; SC = subcutaneous; $t_{½β}$ = elimination half-life.

and add-back low-dose estrogens have resulted in beneficial effects and improvement in mammographic changes in women with strong family histories of breast cancer.[16] The antiestrogen tamoxifen has also been used in breast cancer 'chemoprevention' trials.[17]

Identification of environmental carcinogens has been aided by the introduction of biochemical and molecular biology techniques. Mutations in p53 protein in hepatocellular cancer and in bladder cancers have been related to aflatoxin and cigarette smoking, respectively. Genetic influences may also be responsible for susceptibility to carcinogen-induced cancer. For example, slow acetylators have lower susceptibility to smoking-induced bladder cancer than fast acetylators.[18] This may explain some of the differences in bladder cancer susceptibility between Oriental and Caucasian populations. Other carcinogenic influences may be from physical agents, such as exposure to ultraviolet light leading to enhanced susceptibility to melanoma. Genetic influences may also play a role in such susceptibility since immune surveillance may differ among different HLA haplotypes.

Finally, exposure to anticarcinogens such as the antioxidant vitamins retinol, ascorbic acid and tocopherol (vitamins A, C and E, respectively) have been considered to lessen the effects of adverse environmental factors. However, clinical trials have not yet borne this out. Chemopreventive agents may be increasingly tested if these factors are better understood.[19]

## 1. Clinical Pharmacological Considerations

### 1.1 General Considerations

Important variables in patients that must be considered during treatment with anticancer drugs include clearance, which is dependent on renal function (for drugs such as cisplatin, bleomycin, etoposide or methotrexate) and liver function (for agents such as doxorubicin or vincristine) [see table I]. Variations from normal volume of distribution values may be found (e.g. due to ascites or pleural effusion) for agents such as methotrexate. In addition, drug interactions that may result from use of concomitant medications (such as phenytoin, which enhances methotrexate toxicity) are also an important consideration (for potentially important interactions, see review by Loadman and Bibby[20] and also appendix B). The clinician must consider these aspects before designing a treatment regimen.

For each anticancer drug, major considerations also include the dosage and administration schedule. Many agents have entirely different toxicity profiles depending on the schedule of administration used. For example, the dose-limiting toxicity of fluorouracil (5-FU) given as a bolus every week is myelosuppression. However, when fluorouracil is given as a continuous infusion over several weeks, the dose-limiting toxicity is mucositis or erythrodysaesthesias (hand-foot syndrome).[21]

**Table II.** Anticancer drugs classified by mechanism of action and most common indication(s)

| Drug/classification | Most common cancer indication(s) |
|---|---|
| **Antimetabolites** | |
| *Pyrimidine antagonists:* | |
| Cytarabine | AML |
| Floxuridine (fluorodeoxyuridine, FUDR) | Regional use |
| Fluorouracil | Gastrointestinal, breast |
| Tegafur (ftorafur) | Gastrointestinal |
| *Purine antagonists:* | |
| Cladribine (chlorodeoxyadenosine) | Hairy cell leukaemia |
| Fludarabine | CLL |
| Mercaptopurine | ALL |
| Pentostatin | Hairy cell leukaemia |
| Thioguanine | ALL |
| *Folate antagonist:* | |
| Methotrexate | Breast, ALL, head and neck lymphoma, trophoblastic disease |
| *Alkylating agents:* | |
| Altretamine (hexamethylamine) | Ovarian |
| Busulfan | CML |
| Carboplatin | Ovarian |
| Carmustine | Brain tumours, multiple myeloma, lymphoma |
| Chlorambucil | CLL |
| Chlormethine (mustine, nitrogen mustard, mechlorethamine) | Hodgkin's disease |
| Cisplatin | Testicular, ovarian, bladder, cervix, non-small cell lung |
| Cyclophosphamide | Breast, lymphoma, rhabdomyosarcoma, neuroblastoma, sarcoma |
| Darcarbazine (DTIC) | Melanoma, sarcoma, Hodgkin's disease |
| Ifosfamide | Testicular, sarcoma |
| Lomustine | Brain tumours, lymphoma |
| Melphalan | Multiple myeloma |
| Mitomycin (mitomycin C) | Stomach, pancreas, breast |
| Procarbazine | Hodgkin's, disease |
| Streptozocin | Islet cell tumour of pancreas, carcinoid tumour |
| Thiotepa | Superficial bladder, breast, ovarian |
| **Topoisomerase II inhibitors** | |
| Etoposide | Testicular, small cell lung, lymphoma |
| Teniposide | AML in children |
| **DNA intercalating agents** | |
| Bleomycin | Lymphoma, testicular |
| Dactinomycin (actinomycin D) | Wilms', rhabdomyosarcoma, trophoblastic tumours |
| Daunorubicin | AML, ALL |
| Doxorubicin | Breast, bladder, soft tissue, osteogenic and Ewing's sarcoma, lymphoma, AML, ALL, neuroblastoma, gastric, thyroid, myeloma, prostate |
| Epirubicin | Breast, bladder, small and non-small cell lung, ovarian, gastric, prostate, lymphoma, hepatocellular |
| Idarubicin | Acute non-lymphocytic leukaemia |
| Mitoxantrone | AML, lymphoma, breast |
| **Tubulin interactive agents** | |
| Paclitaxel | Ovarian, breast, non-small cell lung, head and neck |
| Vincristine | AML, ALL, lymphoma, rhabdomyosarcoma, neuroblastoma |
| Vinblastine | Lymphoma, testicular, breast |
| Vinorelbine (navelbine) | Non-small cell lung, breast |

**Table II.** *[Continued]*

| Drug/classification | Most common cancer indication(s) |
|---|---|
| **Hormonal agents** | |
| *Antihormonal agents:* | |
| Aminoglutethimide (antiadrenal; aromatase inhibitor) | Breast, adrenal |
| Fadrozole (aromatase inhibitor) | Breast |
| Flutamide (antiandrogen) | Prostate |
| Formestane (aromatase inhibitor) | Breast |
| Mitotane (antiadrenal) | Adrenal |
| Tamoxifen (antiestrogen) | Breast |
| Toremifene (antiestrogen) | Breast |
| *Gonadotrophin-releasing hormone (GnRH) agonists:* | |
| Buserelin | Prostate |
| Goserelin | Prostate |
| Leuprorelin (leuprolide) | Prostate |
| Triptorelin | Prostate |
| *Estrogens:* | |
| Ethinylestradiol | Prostate, breast |
| Stilbestrol (diethystilbestrol) | Prostate, breast |
| *Androgens:* | |
| Fluoxymesterone | Breast |
| Methyltestosterone | Breast |
| *Progestagens:* | |
| Megestrol | Endometrial, breast |
| Medroxyprogesterone | Endometrial, renal cell, breast |
| *Adrenal corticosteroids:* | |
| Dexamethasone | ALL, CLL |
| Hydrocortisone | Lymphoma |
| Prednisone | Prostate |
| **Miscellaneous** | |
| L-Asparaginase | ALL |
| Estramustine phosphate[a] | Prostate |
| Hydroxycarbamide (hydroxyurea) | CML, cervical (with XRT) |
| Interferon-α | Hairy cell leukaemia, AIDS-associated Kaposi's sarcoma |
| Interleukin-2 | Renal cell |

a May act via intercalation with tubulin.

*Abbreviations:* AML = acute myeloid leukaemia; CLL = chronic lymphocytic leukaemia; CML = chronic myeloid leukaemia; ALL = acute lymphocytic leukaemia; XRT = radiation therapy; AIDS = acquired immune deficiency syndrome.

## 1.2 Classification and Clinical Pharmacological Properties of Commonly Used Anticancer Drugs

Table I lists anticancer drugs alphabetically and shows their predominant routes of elimination and pharmacokinetic characteristics. Anticancer drugs are generally classified by their mechanism of action, even though their precise effects on tumour viability and growth are often not known. Table II lists anticancer drugs according to their mechanism of action and shows their most common indications. Not included in this table are newer biological compounds, other than interferon-α and interleukin-2 which represent the first examples of the use of pharmacological doses of endogenous products synthesised or modified in part by bioengineering (e.g. recombinant technologies) [see further chapter 28; sect. 3.6.3].[22] Precautions in using anticancer drugs and toxicity encountered at usual doses and routes of administration are shown in table III.

**Table III.** Toxicity, precautions and dosages of some commonly used anticancer drugs

| Drug | Major toxicity | | Some precautions | Dosage and route of administration |
|---|---|---|---|---|
| | acute | delayed | | |
| **Alkylating agents** | | | | |
| Altretamine (hexamethyl-amine) | Nausea and vomiting | Bone marrow depression; CNS depression; peripheral neuritis | | 260 $mg/m^2$/day × 2-3 weeks |
| Busulfan | Nausea and vomiting; diarrhoea | Bone marrow depression; pulmonary fibrosis; hyperpigmentation of skin; alopecia; gynaecomastia; impotence, sterility | | 2-10 mg/day PO × 2-3 wks; maintenance 1-3 mg/day |
| Chlorambucil | | Bone marrow depression; sterility; secondary malignancy | | 0.1-0.2 mg/kg/day (higher in intermittent schedules); reduce PO dose if bone marrow depression is severe; only 2-4 mg/day may be needed in chronic lymphocytic leukaemia |
| Chlormethine (mustine, mechlorethamine, nitrogen mustard) | Mild nausea | Bone marrow depression; alopecia | Unstable (use immediately after reconstitution); strong local irritant: administer through a running IV infusion; protect eyes and skin of person administering the drug | 0.4 mg/kg IV in 1 or 2 divided doses |
| Cyclophospha-mide | Nausea and vomiting | Bone marrow depression; alopecia; haemorrhagic cystitis; possible secondary malignancy; sterility (may be temporary); pulmonary fibrosis; hyperpigmentation | Maintain adequate fluid intake to avoid cystitis | 500-1500 $mg/m^2$ as single IV dose; 60-120 $mg/m^2$/day PO; reduce dose if severe leucopenia develops |
| Melphalan (L-phenylalanine mustard) | Severe nausea and vomiting, local reactions, phlebitis | Bone marrow depression (especially platelets); secondary malignancy | Check platelets before each dose | 0.2 mg/kg/day PO × 4 q6wks (myeloma); or 0.1 mg/kg/day PO × 2-3 wks; maintenance 2-4 mg/day when bone marrow has recovered |
| Thiotepa (triethylene thiophosphora-mide) | Nausea and vomiting; local pain | Bone marrow depression; anorexia | | 0.2 mg/kg/day IV × 5. Also given IM or IC |
| **Antimetabolites** | | | | |
| Azacitidine | Nausea and vomiting: diarrhoea; fever | Leucopenia (may be prolonged); thrombocytopenia; hepatic damage; unrelated to dosage | Change infusion solution every 3-4h to avoid loss of potency | 150-300 $mg/m^2$/day IV × 5; or 150-200 $mg/m^2$ 2 ×/wk × 2-8 wks |
| Cytarabine (cytosine arabinoside) | Nausea and vomiting; diarrhoea | Bone marrow depression; megaloblastosis; oral ulceration; hepatic damage, CNS toxicity (high doses) | Use with special caution in hepatic disease | *Leukaemia:* 3 mg/kg/day IV × 1-3 wks; or 2.5 mg/kg q12h IV × 1-3 wks with thioguanine; or IT 20-30 $mg/m^2$ |
| Fluorouracil (5-FU) | Nausea and vomiting; diarrhoea; may precipitate angina | Oral and gastrointestinal ulceration; stomatitis; bone marrow depression; neurological defects, usually cerebellar; pigmentation; alopecia; dermatitis | Decrease dose in hepatic or renal dysfunction, or after adrenalectomy; contraindicated in poor nutritional states. Reduce dose if given with calcium folinate (leucovorin) | *Initial therapy:* 12 mg/kg/day IV × 4, then 6 mg/kg every other day × 4 or until toxicity. *Maintenance:* 12-15 mg/kg/wk IV (max. dose 1g). Also given by infusion (1 $g/m^2$/day × 5d or 28d infusion (300 $mg/m^2$/day) |

**Table III.** *[Continued]*

| Drug | Major toxicity | | Some precautions | Dosage and route of administration |
|---|---|---|---|---|
| | acute | delayed | | |
| Mercaptopurine (6-MP) | Occasional nausea and vomiting, usually well tolerated | Bone marrow depression; hepatic damage | Allopurinol potentiates oral mercaptopurine if given to prevent hyperuricaemia, so dosage of mercaptopurine should be reduced to ≤ one-third of usual | 2.5 mg/kg/day PO |
| Methotrexate | Nausea; diarrhoea | Oral and gastrointestinal ulceration; bone marrow depression; hepatic toxicity including cirrhosis; renal toxicity; pulmonary infiltration; osteoporosis | Normal renal function should be present and urine output must be maintained. Adjust dosage to creatinine clearance in renal dysfunction and in elderly | *Choriocarcinoma:* 10-30 mg/day PO or IM × 5 *Acute leukaemia maintenance:* child, 1.25-5 mg/day PO; adult, 5-10 mg/day PO; or both, 30 mg/m$^2$ IM or PO 3 ×/wk *Meningeal leukaemia:* 0.2-0.4 mg/kg IT, or 2 mg/m$^2$ × 3d via IVT port *Head and neck:* 40 mg/m$^2$/wk IV; 50 mg/day IA with calcium folinate |
| Thioguanine (6-TG) | Occasional nausea and vomiting, usually well tolerated | Bone marrow depression; possible hepatic damage | Lower doses in renal or hepatic dysfunction | 100 mg/m$^2$ PO q12h × 8d, often combined with cytarabine |
| **Natural compounds (plant alkaloids and antibiotics)** | | | | |
| Bleomycin | Nausea and vomiting; fever | Pneumonitis and pulmonary fibrosis; cutaneous reactions; stomatitis; alopecia; anorexia (may be prolonged) | Possible anaphylactic reactions in patients with lymphoma – two 2U test doses recommended; use extreme caution in renal or pulmonary disease; do not exceed total dosage of 400U | 10-20 U/m$^2$ IV or IM 1-2 ×/wk; start with 5U for first 2 doses in lymphoma |
| Dactinomycin (actinomycin D) | Nausea and vomiting; diarrhoea; local reaction and phlebitis | Stomatitis; oral ulceration; alopecia; folliculitis; bone marrow depression | Administer through running IV infusion; use special caution in hepatic disease | 15-40 μg/kg/wk IV × 3-5 wks in adults; 15 μg/kg/day IV × 5 in children |
| Daunorubicin (daunomycin) | Nausea and vomiting; fever, red urine (not haematuria) | Bone marrow depression; cardiotoxicity; alopecia | Administer through running IV infusion; avoid in heart disease | 1 mg/kg/day IV × 5; or 30-60 mg/m$^2$/day IV × 3; or 30-60 mg/m$^2$/wk IV |
| Doxorubicin | Nausea and vomiting; red urine (not haematuria); severe local tissue damage at infiltration site; diarrhoea | Bone marrow depression; cardiotoxicity (may be irreversible); alopecia; stomatitis; hepatic damage; cutaneous toxicity; renal damage | Administer through running IV infusion; special caution in heart disease; reduce dose in hepatic dysfunction; do not exceed total dosage of 550 mg/m$^2$ | 60-90 mg/m$^2$ IV q3wks; or 20-30 mg/m$^2$/wk IV |
| Etoposide (VP 16-213) | Nausea and vomiting | Bone marrow depression; alopecia | Rare anaphylactic reactions | 150 mg/m$^2$/day PO × 3-5 |
| Mitomycin | Nausea and vomiting; local reaction if extravasation; fever | Bone marrow depression (cumulative); stomatitis; renal and pulmonary toxicity; alopecia | Administer through running IV infusion (acts as alkylating agent) | 0.05 mg/kg/day IV × 6d, then every other day until 50mg total dose |

*[Continued over]*

**Table III.** *[Continued]*

| Drug | Major toxicity | | Some precautions | Dosage and route of administration |
|---|---|---|---|---|
| | acute | delayed | | |
| Streptozocin (streptozotocin) | Nausea and vomiting; local pain | Renal damage | Slow infusion rate to prevent local pain; contraindicated in renal disease; proteinuria used to monitor toxicity; do not repeat dose until renal function recovers | 1 g/m$^2$/wk × 5-6 wks |
| Teniposide (VM 26) | Nausea and vomiting | Bone marrow depression; alopecia | Rare anaphylactic reactions | 100 mg/m$^2$/wk IV |
| Vinblastine | Nausea and vomiting; local reaction and phlebitis | Bone marrow depression; alopecia; stomatitis; loss of deep tendon reflexes | Administer through running IV infusion or inject with great care to prevent extravasation | 0.10-0.15 mg/kg/wk IV |
| Vincristine | Local reaction if extravasation | Peripheral neuropathy; neuritic pain; alopecia; bone marrow depression (leucopenia); constipation leading to paralytic ileus; sterility | Administer though running IV infusion or inject with great care to prevent extravasation; omit or decrease dose if reflexes diminish or paraesthesiae appear; patients with underlying neurological problems may be more susceptible to neurotoxicity; prophylactic laxatives may be helpful | 0.4-1.4 mg/m$^2$/wk IV in adults; 2 mg/m$^2$/wk in children |
| Vinorelbine | Nausea and vomiting; local reactions | Bone marrow depression; neutropenia; peripheral neuropathy | | 30 mg/m$^2$/wk IV |
| **Other synthetic agents** | | | | |
| Amsacrine (m-AMSA) | Nausea, vomiting; diarrhoea; pain or phlebitis; ventricular fibrillation (when hypokalaemia present); convulsions | Bone marrow depression; hepatic damage; stomatitis; alopecia | Monitor serum potassium | *Leukaemia:* 100 mg/m$^2$ IV × 3d |
| L-Asparaginase (colaspase) | Nausea, fever, possible anaphylaxis; abdominal pain; diabetes leading to coma | Hepatic damage; pancreatitis; CNS depression; coagulation defects | Keep adrenaline (epinephrine) available; rise in BUN and ammonia is not evidence of toxicity. Do not repeat courses without testing for hypersensitivity | 10-500 IU/kg/day IV × 2-20; or 100-500 IU/kg IM 3 ×/wk |
| Carmustine (BCNU) | Nausea and vomiting; local phlebitis | Delayed leucopenia and thrombocytopenia (may be prolonged); secondary malignancy; renal damage; pulmonary fibrosis | Slow infusion rate to prevent local pain | 75-100 mg/m$^2$/day IV × 2; repeat course in 6-8 wks |
| Cisplatin (cis-platinum) | Nausea and vomiting; acute renal failure | Bone marrow depression; renal damage; ototoxicity | Maintain adequate fluid intake; lower dose in renal dysfunction; do not repeat until baseline renal function recovers | 75-100 mg/m$^2$ IV once or 20 mg/m$^2$/day IV × 5; repeat course in 3-4 wks |
| Dacarbazine (DTIC; DIC) | Severe nausea and vomiting | Bone marrow depression; flu-like syndrome; alopecia; renal impairment; liver damage | | 150-250 mg/m$^2$/day IV × 5; or 950-1200 mg/m$^2$ IV once |

**Table III.** *[Continued]*

| Drug | Major toxicity | | Some precautions | Dosage and route of administration |
|---|---|---|---|---|
| | acute | delayed | | |
| Estramustine phosphate | Nausea, vomiting, phlebitis, urticaria | Thrombocytopenia (rare); gynaecomastia (rare) or breast tenderness | Control early nausea and vomiting with phenothiazines; avoid administration with calcium-containing foods or drugs (as oral absorption markedly impaired) | 600-1000 mg/day PO |
| Hydroxycarbamide (hydroxyurea) | Mild nausea and vomiting | Bone marrow depression; hyperkeratosis and hyperpigmentation; stomatitis | Decrease dose in renal dysfunction | 80 mg/kg q3d PO; or 20-30 mg/kg/day |
| Lomustine (CCNU) | Nausea and vomiting | Delayed (4-6 wks) leucopenia and thrombocytopenia (may be prolonged); stomatitis; alopecia; secondary malignancy; renal damage; pulmonary fibrosis | | 130 mg/m$^2$ PO; repeat in 6-8 wks |
| Mitotane (ortho-p'-DDD) | Nausea and vomiting; diarrhoea | CNS toxicity; mental depression; visual disturbances; dermatitis; adrenal insufficiency | Use low dose initially with gradual build-up to maximum tolerated dose (usually 8-10 g/day); discontinue after shock or severe trauma; lower dose in hepatic disease | 8-10 g/day PO in 3-4 divided doses; tolerated dose varies (from 2-16 g/day); accumulation in fat requires dose reductions after several wks |
| Mitoxantrone | Nausea and vomiting | Bone marrow depression; cardiotoxicity | | 16 mg/m$^2$ IV q3wks |
| Procarbazine | Nausea and vomiting; CNS depression | Bone marrow depression; stomatitis; dermatitis | Decrease dose in patients on CNS depressants (phenothiazines, barbiturates); mental disturbances or disulfiram-like reaction may occur with alcohol (ethanol); acts as mild MAO inhibitor – avoid sympathomimetic drugs and foods with high tyramine or dopamine content | 50-300 mg/day PO with slow build-up in dose |
| **Hormones** | | | | |
| Fluoxymesterone | | Fluid retention; masculinisation; cholestatic jaundice; hypercalcaemia | Contraindicated in prostate cancer; immobilised patients are likely to develop hypercalcaemia; use with caution in cardiac, hepatic, or renal disease | 20-30 mg/day PO |
| Medroxyprogesterone acetate | Orally: nausea (rare); IM: local pain, abscess at site of injection | Fluid retention; hypercalcaemia | Use with care in hepatic dysfunction | 400-800 mg/wk IM or PO |
| Megestrol acetate | | Weight gain; hypercalcaemia | | 40mg qid PO |
| Prednisone or prednisolone | | Hyperadrenocorticism (see also chapter 19; sect. 7.1.1) | | 40-100 mg/day PO of prednisone or equivalent; use lower maintenance doses, if possible |

*[Continued over]*

Table III. *[Continued]*

| Drug | Major toxicity: acute | Major toxicity: delayed | Some precautions | Dosage and route of administration |
|---|---|---|---|---|
| Stilbestrol (diethylstilbestrol, DES) | Nausea and vomiting; cramps | Fluid retention; hypercalcaemia; feminisation; uterine bleeding; during pregnancy, may cause vaginal carcinoma in offspring; increased frequency of vascular accidents | Use low doses in prostate cancer; do not use in premenopausal breast cancer; serum calcium can rise rapidly in breast cancer shortly after start of therapy, especially with bone disease | *Prostate cancer:* up to 1 mg/day PO |
| Testosterone propionate | | Fluid retention; masculinisation; hypercalcaemia | Contraindicated in cancer of prostate and hepatic disease; immobilised patients are likely to develop hypercalcaemia | 50-100mg IM 3 ×/wk |
| **Other hormonal agents** | | | | |
| Aminoglutethimide | Drowsiness; nausea; dizziness | Skin rash; hypothyroidism (rare); fever | Begin at one-quarter of usual dose; induces its own metabolism and that of other drugs. Must be given with replacement hydrocortisone | 250-1000 mg/day PO with oral hydrocortisone 40 mg/day |
| Tamoxifen | Nausea and vomiting | Hot flushes; pruritus vulvae; vaginal bleeding; hypercalcaemia; ocular toxicity (with excessive doses); endometrial polyps and cancer | Can induce ovulation – use with mechanical contraceptive in premenopausal patients | 10mg bid PO |

*Abbreviations and symbols:* PO = oral; IV = intravenous; IT = intrathecal; IM = intramuscular; IC = intracavitary; IVT = intraventricular; IA = intra-arterial; BUN = blood urea nitrogen; bid = twice daily; qid = 4 times daily.

## 1.3 Application of Clinical Pharmacological Knowledge to Specific Therapeutic Use Situations

Although plasma concentrations are measured in the development of all anticancer drugs, to date, there are only a few agents for which there are plasma concentration considerations when planning routine therapy.

### *1.3.1 Methotrexate, Teniposide and Cytarabine Therapy*

Studies in children with acute lymphoblastic leukaemia have examined prospectively the outcome and toxicity from 'targeted systemic exposure' [in which drug dosages are individualised to achieve target steady-state plasma concentrations or AUC (area under the plasma concentration-time curve) values] in comparison with conventional dosage methods. The conventional reinduction dosage after a standard 6-drug induction treatment plus maintenance mercaptopurine and methotrexate consisted of 5 pulses of moderately high-dose methotrexate infusion (1.5 g/m$^2$) alternating with teniposide (200 mg/m$^2$) plus cytarabine (300 mg/m$^2$) given daily for 5 days every 6 weeks. The experimental arm consisted of pharmacokinetically guided use of these 3 induction drugs with an aim towards achieving a steady-state methotrexate concentration of 16 μmol/L and target AUC values of teniposide and cytarabine. Clearance predictions were based on measurements at 1 and 6 hours after methotrexate, 1 and 3 hours after cytarabine, and 1, 3, 8 and 20 hours after teniposide. The results showed that severe toxicity was less in the patients randomised to targeted systemic exposure dosage adjustments.[23]

#### High-Dose Methotrexate

Use of high-dose methotrexate may pose a considerable danger of lethal toxicity. Plasma concentrations of methotrexate may be used to determine how long to continue hydration, alkalinisation of the urine and 'rescue' therapy with calcium folinate (leucovorin calcium). These measures must be continued until plasma concentrations of methotrexate are $<5 \times 10^{-7}$ mol/L.

### *1.3.2 Carboplatin Therapy*

The Calvert formula is based on the concept that the dose equals the area under the plasma concentration-time curve (AUC) multiplied by clearance. This formula can be adapted to use a target AUC to determine the dosage of carboplatin:[24]

Dose (mg, *not* mg/m$^2$) = target AUC (mg/ml • min) × [glomerular filtration rate (ml/min) + 25]

The target AUC is 7 mg/ml • min when carboplatin is used alone in adults, and is 4.5 to 5 mg/ml • min when carboplatin is used in combination therapy or for patients who receive carboplatin after other treatments that limit bone marrow reserves. This approach for estimating carboplatin dosages has been successful in achieving maximum antitumour effects with acceptable levels of toxicity (thrombocytopenia), whereas using conventional (per square metre) dosages may lead to excessive toxicity in elderly individuals with poor renal function and underdosage of young patients who might have glomerular filtrations rates in excess of 150 ml/min.

#### 1.3.3 Fluorouracil Therapy (Avoidance of Toxicity in Patients With Enzyme Deficiencies)

In patients receiving fluorouracil it has been recognised for some time that there are occasional individuals (about 1% of patients) who experience *severe* or even lethal toxicity. It is now known that some of these patients have a deficiency in the rate-limiting enzyme in pyrimidine metabolism, dihydropyrimidine dehydrogenase.[25] Tests to identify patients with this enzyme deficiency should help avoid this severe and sometimes lethal toxicity.

It is anticipated that in the future, we will be better able to phenotype patients for other metabolising enzymes to help avoid or minimise the toxicity of anticancer drugs.

### 1.4 Principles of Combination Chemotherapy

It is well known that most effective (e.g. curative) chemotherapy regimens use drugs given in combination, and efforts have been made to develop mathematical models for optimising regimens.[26] The most important principles for developing combinations of chemotherapeutic regimens are:

1) Each single agent should have activity against the disease.

2) The agents should have different mechanisms of action.

3) The agents should have non-overlapping toxicity profiles.

4) The regimen should combine cell cycle specific and cell cycle nonspecific agents.

Common combination regimens are discussed under several of the clinical entities described in section 4.

### 1.5 Development of New Agents

It is clear that to combat widely disseminated malignancy in patients or to eradicate even small numbers of tumour cells in distant sites, more effective anticancer agents are needed. The development of new anticancer drugs is crucial to making progress against the disease. The development of a new agent takes a total of about 14 years. The time from discovery until the first trial in patients takes about 7 years. The rest of the development time is consumed by clinical development tasks. The 4 phases of clinical drug development are outlined in table IV.

The most recent development in clinical trials with new anticancer drugs has been the introduction of a method called the *continual reassessment method* in the conduct of phase I trials. In the usual conduct of phase I trials, the first 3 patients are treated at a dose of one-tenth the murine lethal dose required to kill 10% of animals ($LD_{10}$). Dose escalation then proceeds either by using a modified Fibonacci search scheme [dose levels = n (starting dose), 2n, 3.3n, 5n, 7n.., etc.] or by doubling the dose at each level. The continual reassessment method uses only 1 patient (instead of 3) at each dose level. This means fewer patients are exposed to ineffective dosages. Of course, when toxicity is noted, additional patients are entered at that

**Table IV.** Stages in new anticancer drug development

| Phase | Objectives and population/patients studied |
|---|---|
| Phase I | Dose escalation study to achieve maximally tolerated dose and determine toxicity (patients with advanced refractory malignancies for which there is no treatment of high priority) |
| Phase II | Effectiveness study in which a uniform population of patients with a specific type of tumour (e.g. breast cancer) is given the drug to determine the percentage of patients whose tumours have ≥50% shrinkage in the total area of their tumour *(partial response)* or a complete disappearance of their tumour *(complete response)* |
| Phase III | New drug is compared in a randomised controlled trial to a standard agent, or the drug is added to a standard combination chemotherapy regimen |
| Phase IV | Drug is introduced into general medical practice |

**Table V.** Newer anticancer agents in of development that have already demonstrated substantial clinical antitumour activity

| Agent | Mechanism of action | Dose-limiting toxicity | Tumour types in which responses noted |
|---|---|---|---|
| Irinotecan (CPT-11) | Topoisomerase I inhibitor | Diarrhoea, neutropenia | Colon, non-small cell lung, lung, gastric, breast, cervix, lymphoma |
| Raltitrexed (ZD 1694) | Thymidylate synthesis inhibitor | Myelosuppression, elevation of transaminases | Colorectal, non-small cell lung |
| Topotecan | Topoisomerase I inhibitor | Neutropenia/ thrombocytopenia | Small cell lung, non-small cell lung, ovarian, sarcoma, glioma |
| Docetaxel (taxotere) | Tubulin interactive agent | Neutropenia, cumulative fluid retention | Breast, ovary, non-small cell lung, cholangiocarcinoma, pancreas |
| Mitoguazone (methyl-glyoxal-bisguanyl-hydrazone, MGBG) | Polyamine biosynthesis inhibitor | Perioral numbness with administration | AIDS-associated non-Hodgkin's lymphoma |
| Gemcitabine | Antimetabolite (ribonucleotide reductase inhibitor) | Myelosuppression, flu-like syndrome | Pancreas, non-small cell lung |

dose level.[27] This and other new dose escalation techniques will both accelerate new agent development and allow more patients to receive higher, more effective doses of the new agents.

Another important development is the use of AUC targeting (determined from preclinical pharmacokinetic data) to guide the selection of the first dose of anticancer agents and subsequent escalation. However, not all drugs are suitable for such an approach if the animal species differ substantially in their handling of the drug.[28]

Table V lists some new agents undergoing phase I, II and/or early phase III clinical trials. These agents are noteworthy because they have already demonstrated clinical activity even though it is relatively early in their development. Not included in the table are important new formulations of standard drugs, such as etoposide phosphate developed to improve the bioavailability of etoposide, and liposomal preparations encapsulating doxorubicin or daunorubicin.

The most noteworthy of these newer agents is irinotecan (CPT-11), which gives a remarkable 25% response rate in patients with colon cancer refractory to fluorouracil.[29] Raltitrexed (ZD 1694) has also been documented to have activity in patients with advanced colorectal cancer. The activity of topotecan in patients with small cell lung cancer and the activity of gemcitabine in patients with advanced pancreatic cancer are also of interest,[30] as is the finding that the polyamine biosynthesis inhibitor mitoguazone (methyl-glyoxal-bisguanyl-hydrazone, MGBG) has very substantial activity in patients with AIDS-associated non-Hodgkin's lymphoma who have progressed on prior chemotherapy regimens. This activity has been noted as incurring essentially no toxicity in these patients.[31]

Other new agents that may be brought into clinical trials in the near future include the retinoblastoma (RB) protein (used to restore the RB gene suppressor protein), and farnesyl transferase inhibitors (used to suppress the functioning of mutated ras).

Thus, there are a number of new agents with substantial clinical activity against some of the more refractory types of malignancies in patients. As these agents are folded into combination chemotherapy regimens, there is no doubt they will have an effect on these malignancies.

## 2. General Principles of Treatment

Drug therapy of cancer evolved initially for neoplasms such as lymphomas and leukaemias, in which local modalities played little or no role in eradicating or controlling the disease. Beginning in 1945, chlormethine (mechlorethamine, mustine) or 'nitrogen mustard' was tested and found to have antitumour activity against 'lymphosarcomas'.[32] Three years later, aminopterin was introduced by Farber as a treatment for childhood leukaemia.[33]

Interest in anticancer drug development prompted the US government to start a chemotherapy programme at the National Cancer Institute in 1952. A screening programme evolved that was based on the ability to prolong the lifespan of mice inoculated intraperitoneally with a defined number of leukaemic cells. A number of principles of cancer treatment were subsequently established by Skipper and Schabel at the Southern Research Institute, on the basis of on their observations in these leukaemic mice and on solid tumour models, as interest shifted to establish the role of systemic therapies in the treatment of common cancers in humans.[34]

Up to the late 1950s, there was little consideration of a role for drugs as a supplement to surgery or radiation in the treatment of cancer, and the experience with drugs in the advanced cancers of adults was to prove increasingly disappointing. An exception was the endocrine-based treatment applied as palliation to hormone-dependent cancers originating in the prostate and the breast – already pioneered in the 1940s by Huggins and others.[35]

Currently, the role of drugs in the treatment of cancer has become much more complex, and in addition to conventional *cytotoxic agents*, there has been widespread testing of *biological response modifiers* that exploit immune mechanisms and cytokine-mediated changes in host or tumour status. More recently, these 2 approaches have been combined to increase targeting to tumour cells. Finally, although the conventional role of drugs is in the systemic treatment of cancer, examples of their action in complementing or enhancing local control are increasing. Specific drug classes such as *radiosensitisers* have been introduced to enhance the actions of radiation.

### 2.1 Basis of Cytotoxic Chemotherapy

Cytotoxic chemotherapy follows the principles of fractional cell kill and dose-intensity. Concepts of drug resistance from bacterial systems were used to elaborate combination chemotherapy principles that supported the introduction of multidrug regimens initially in leukaemias, then in Hodgkin's disease and non-Hodgkin's lymphomas, and subsequently in childhood tumours and breast cancer. In these latter 2 instances, therapeutic results proved encouraging enough to lead to a planned introduction of drugs and combinations in multimodality approaches (i.e. combined with initial surgery and radiation). The success of these approaches in Wilms' tumour was the forerunner of breast cancer adjuvant programmes.

### 2.2 Adjuvant Therapy

Adjuvant therapy of cancer became an important new development and has been an established treatment modality since the 1970s. Its basis follows naturally from the fractional cell kill hypothesis, and emphasises the importance of low tumour burden for successful drug treatment. Since the kinetics of experimental tumour cell killing approximates a first-order geometric process, it is often expressed in logarithmic terms. Repetitive administration is required to eradicate tumour burdens in clinical settings. Moreover, tumour cell heterogeity and variations in susceptibility to drugs must be taken into account. Accordingly, a number of additions and modifications of the fractional cell kill hypothesis, such as the Goldie-Coldman (early use of combinations in sequence to avoid mutations) and Norton-Simon hypotheses (late intensification of treatment crossover to eradicate a cell population intrinsically resistant to the first treatment), were subsequently introduced and used in the design of clinical protocols with varying success.[36]

Some success in the adjuvant treatment of various malignancies led to more radical departures in treatment strategies. Intervention with chemotherapy administered before the local modality has been called *neoadjuvant*, or primary or preoperative chemotherapy. This strategy has yielded impressive results in osteosarcoma of the extremities, with the response of the primary tumour after chemotherapy being assessed at the time of limb salvage surgery. The degree of necrosis achieved with chemotherapy bears a close relationship to outcome.

### 2.3 Simultaneous Radiation and Chemotherapy

With our increasing attention to causes of drug resistance, attention has shifted somewhat to simultaneous radiation and chemotherapy as the initial treatment, either by itself or followed by surgical intervention. Such a treatment strategy is now preferred in conditions where radiation is an effective primary modality for locally advanced disease, and also in situations where both local control and control of distant metastases need to improve, such as in advanced cancers of the head and neck or uterine cervix.

### 2.4 Reversal or Modulation of Drug Resistance

Drug resistance has been extensively characterised during the past 2 decades, and its study represents an important bridge between the laboratory and the clinic. Therapeutic strategies attempting to reverse or modulate drug resistance factors have been introduced into clinical studies. For further in this area, see Ling,[37] Los and Muggia,[38] and Fisher et al.[39]

Specific abnormalities associated with resistance to antimetabolites have been characterised *in vitro*, but their relationship to clinically observed resistance is not obvious. For example, resistance to methotrexate, the classical inhibitor of the enzyme dihydrofolate reductase, has been related to overexpression of the target enzyme, enzymatic forms with lesser affinity for methotrexate, and decreases in intracellular transport.[40] For cisplatin, resistance has been related to decreased intracellular uptake, increased intracellular detoxification, increased tolerability of DNA-platinum adducts, and increased DNA-repair.[41]

A major area of research was introduced in the mid-1970s with the recognition of a cell membrane glycoprotein, the overexpression of which mediated multidrug resistance to natural products. Subsequently, extensive characterisation of this P-170 glycoprotein (Pgp) has taken place, indicating that it is one of a family of ATP-binding cassette proteins which is encoded in humans by the MDR1 gene. Reversal of resistance to anthracyclines, vinca alkaloids, taxanes, epipodophyllotoxins, and other natural products that are substrates of this efflux pump, has been achieved through exposure to a variety of compounds, starting with the demonstration that verapamil achieves this reversal *in vitro*. One feature of drug-resistance reversing agents is their cytotoxicity for cells that overexpress Pgp. Another feature is their ability to increase intracellular concentrations of the cytotoxic drug that is a substrate for Pgp-mediated efflux; the list of drugs achieving this reversal *in vitro* is extensive.[39]

The physiological role of Pgp, which is also expressed in normal tissues such as gastrointestinal tract epithelia, the renal tubule, the adrenal cortex, and certain vascular endothelia (including the placenta), is unknown. However, a role in protecting against xenobiotics, and in the selective uptake and secretion of steroids is likely. This distribution may be important in determining toxicity to cytotoxic drugs and the selectivity of these agents.

More recently, MDR-related proteins (MRPs) conferring resistance by similar mechanisms in certain cell lines and tumours arising in lung and brain tumours have been described.[42] Although clinical trials to date have not employed treatment selection based on the presence or absence of MDR1-Pgp expression in tumours, there is evidence that such expression confers an adverse prognosis to neuroblastomas and to acute leukaemias, and that susceptibility of previously-treated breast cancer to paclitaxel is inversely correlated to such expression.[43,44]

## 2.5 Biochemical Modulation

Biochemical modulation is a strategy that involves changing the susceptibility of tumour cells to anticancer drugs, through biochemical pathways that may be accentuated or selectively altered in cancer cells. The most widespread use of biochemical modulation as a therapeutic strategy involves the use of calcium folinate (leucovorin) to increase intracellular folate cofactors and, thus, enhance the binding of fluorodeoxyuridylate (FdUMP) to the target enzyme thymidylate synthase. This enhanced binding leads to increased cytotoxicity of fluorouracil and floxuridine (fluorodeoxyuridine, FUDR) and, in some schedules using these compounds, to a shift in dose-limiting toxicity to mucositis rather than myelosuppression.[45] This shift results in an enhanced therapeutic index for the combination as opposed to higher doses of fluorouracil (see further section 4.2.2).

## 2.6 Toxicity Protection

Toxicity protection is the converse strategy, whereby normal tissue toxicity is selectively diminished by a protective agent.[46] Several agents have been shown to achieve such selectivity, e.g.:

- *Thiols* effectively decrease the renal toxicity of cisplatin. Sodium thiosulfate confers protection, allowing high doses of cisplatin to be used intraperitoneally[47] without incurring renal toxicity. However, the therapeutic benefit obtained from such dose escalation and toxicity neutralisation is uncertain.
- *Aminophosphothiols* (substrates of alkaline phosphatase) selectively protect against the marrow toxicity of platinum compounds and alkylating agents. Amifostine has been shown to allow timely treatment with cisplatin and cyclophosphamide in patients with ovarian cancer, incurring significantly less cumulative myelosuppression and its complications, and less renal toxicity. This was accomplished without any reduction in efficacy.[48]
- *Chelating agents* such as dexrazoxane selectively protect against the cardiomyopathy of anthracyclines. An indication for dexrazoxane has been its use whenever retreatment with doxorubicin is contemplated after patients have already received 300 mg/m$^2$ cumulative

**Table VI.** Examples of cytoprotective agents

| Drug/strategy | Mechanism | Protected tissue/toxic drug |
|---|---|---|
| Dexrazoxane | Chelation<br>↓ Free radicals | Cardiac muscle (doxorubicin) |
| Amifostine | Thiol quench<br>↓ Free radicals<br>↓ Alkylation | Bone marrow (platinums)<br>Radiation<br>Alkylating agents |
| Calcium folinate (leucovorin) | Differential rescue<br>Differential transport | Bone marrow (methotrexate)<br>Gastrointestinal tract |
| Mesna | ↓ Acrolein | Bladder (oxazaphosphorines) |
| MDR1 transduction | ↑ P-170 glycoprotein (Pgp) | Bone marrow (natural products) |
| Oxonic acid | ↓ Phosphorylation of fluoropyrimidines | Gastrointestinal tract |

doses.[49] Other indications are likely in childhood leukaemias and other childhood tumours, in view of the greater susceptibility of children to manifest late cardiac failure secondary to anthracyclines even at cumulative doses not exceeding 180 mg/m$^2$.[50]

Examples of cytoprotective agents are shown in table VI.[51]

### 2.7 Combination Chemotherapy

Combination chemotherapy has been the mainstay of cancer treatment since the 1960s, having been initially patterned after antimicrobial chemotherapy and based on preventing the emergence of drug resistance. Empirical principles for building effective combinations have evolved and rely on the use of drugs that as monotherapy are active against a particular tumour type, on combining drugs with different mechanisms of action (and resistance) in minimising overlapping toxicity, and on the administration of doses in combination that are only minimally reduced from the usually effective doses (see also section 1.4 above).

Initially, little attention was paid to the sequence of these drugs. More recently, studies of combinations have explored the importance of sequencing: this has assumed considerable importance with the introduction of taxanes and topoisomerase-acting drugs. For example, it is apparent that paclitaxel preceding cisplatin results in better tolerability, and perhaps improved therapeutic effects. Conversely, doxorubicin or cyclophosphamide should precede paclitaxel for improved tolerability. With topoisomerase-acting drugs, sequencing of topoisomerase-I and -II inhibitors yields better results than simultaneous administration.[52] Experimental correlates suggest topoisomerase I inhibition leads to upregulation of topoisomerase II.[53]

### 2.8 Combinations of Chemotherapy and Biological Response Modifiers

Combinations of chemotherapy and biological agents may represent an important avenue for future therapeutic strategies. Monoclonal antibodies to growth factor receptors potentiate the effect of cytotoxic drugs.[54] Cytokines such as interleukin-1 and tumour necrosis factor (TNF) have enhanced effects when combined with cytotoxic drugs against tumour cell lines and experimental animal tumour models. Conversely, small doses of cyclophosphamide, presumably acting by decreasing suppressor lymphocytes, have been used to potentiate the antitumour effects of interleukin-2.[55]

### 2.9 Gene Therapy

An emerging treatment that has predominantly local potential so far, but may eventually be applied systemically is that of gene therapy.[56] Vectors introducing genes into local cancers to reverse the neoplastic changes (or to render them susceptible to antiviral drugs such as ganciclovir) may be considered complex engineered 'drugs' as well as totally new strategies in the treatment of cancer that await clinical verification.

### 2.10 Difficulties in Developing Future Strategies for Therapeutic Enhancement

Difficulties in developing improved therapeutic strategies from laboratory observations include:

1) Rigorous determinations of dose-responses for the individual drugs and their combinations, which are required to understand whether a combination results in synergy, additivity or antagonism; and

2) Separating enhanced cytotoxicity against tumours from enhanced toxicity to normal tissues.

It is likely that any therapeutic enhancement will be demonstrable *in vitro* and apply to a specific set of circumstances, and not to all tumour types necessarily.

## 3. Factors Affecting Choice of Chemotherapy Regimen

Drug treatment of cancer must take into account the following:

1) The general sensitivity of the tumour to chemotherapy.

2) Specific sensitivity of a tumour to individual agents.

3) The likelihood of response and clinical improvement *versus* serious toxicity (assessment of therapeutic index).

4) Whether chemotherapy is to be used in the setting of advanced disease as a single method of therapy (modality), in a combined modality setting (e.g. with radiation therapy for regional disease), or in an adjuvant setting after potentially curative surgery.

Since acute leukaemia, lymphomas, paediatric solid tumours, breast and ovarian cancer, testicular cancer, and small cell lung cancer are sensitive to chemotherapy, the choice of anticancer drug treatment is generally an appropriate one, even if the disease leaves the patient bedridden. In tumours in which chemotherapy has resulted in low response rates (e.g. melanoma, renal, pancreatic, colorectal cancer), routine drug treatment is not recommended by many oncologists. This is especially true for non-ambulatory patients who have only a minimal possibility of achieving benefit. Whether to treat the ambulatory patient with dissemination of one of these cancers depends on several factors, including the patient's own informed desire for treatment, the availability of adequate facilities, and the possibility of contributing to an eventual solution through involvement in a research protocol. In some instances, new treatments such as paclitaxel for non-small cell lung cancer may be the preferred option. This drug has had reproducible antitumour activity in phase II trials, a favourable 1-year survival, and has easily been combined with full doses of carboplatin.

To determine the sensitivity of a tumour to chemotherapeutic agents is a long sought goal. The estrogen receptor content of a mammary tumour has been helpful in determining whether endocrine therapy should be employed.[57] Effects of chemotherapeutic agents on clonability of human tumour cells *in vitro* as predictive assays fall short of routine clinical usefulness.[58] Polmerase chain reaction (PCR) technologies to quantify target enzymes[59] or to identify causes of drug resistance[60] offer new methods for predictive tests. In addition, immunocytochemistry has emerged as a powerful indicator of tumour behaviour including responsiveness to drugs: p53 mutations identify prognostic subsets of bladder cancer[61] and are also associated with radiation and drug resistance.

### 3.1 Drug Selection in Combination Chemotherapy Regimens

Potential circumvention of resistance to treatment is probably the most important factor prompting studies of combination anticancer regimens attempting to prevent drug resistance by rapidly alternating therapies (Goldie-Coldman hypothesis, see section 2.2). However, these approaches to overcoming resistance are now generally regarded as too simplistic, since pathways leading to resistance are often shared by seemingly unrelated drugs.[36]

Other reasons for combinations include biochemical rationales (e.g. drugs producing biochemical changes at multiple sites by sequential, concurrent or complementary blockade; or toxicity protection enhancing selectivity) and cytokinetic approaches. However, use of one drug to alter the tumour cell cycle and enhance cell killing by another drug (e.g. using estrogens to induce breast cancer cells into cycle and render them susceptible to antimetabolites) remains of unproven benefit.

The most successful approach to combination chemotherapy remains empirical and has involved the use of drugs known to be active as monotherapy against the particular tumour. In line with this, tumours successfully treated with combinations have generally been those regarded as 'drug sensitive', i.e amenable to treatment by several drugs that act by different mechanisms (see section 1.4). In haematological malignancies, such combinations remain the standard treatment approaches. When several choices of drugs are available within a class of agents, drug selection is guided by the type of dose-limiting toxicity likely to be produced by other agents employed in the combination. Selections made in this manner have allowed anticancer agents to be used in combination at nearly full tolerated dosages.

Another facet of successful combination chemotherapy has been the application of intermittent treatment schedules, which permit treatment of greater intensity. One theoretical advantage of this is that if the combination exerts a more highly selective killing effect on tumour cells, an interval of 2 to 3 weeks between courses is usually sufficient to allow recovery of the normal tissues to their pretreatment condition. An additional advantage of intermittent scheduling is the potential recovery of the patient's immune system between exposures to chemotherapy. The dose rate (commonly referred to as dose intensity) has been deemed important in optimising results,[62] and cytokines to enhance marrow recovery have permitted exploration of enhanced dose rates of combinations of drugs with dose-limiting neutropenia. Continuous infusion schedules and administration of drug orally, coupled with the ability to sequentially administer very high doses of a drug with support of peripheral blood progenitor cells, have heightened awareness of the importance of the dose schedule with anticancer drugs and led to questioning of dogmas of combination chemotherapy, implying a therapeutic advantage when drugs are given together vis-a-vis use of sequential cycles of single drugs.[63]

### 3.2 Drug Selection in Combined Modality Treatment

Surgical and radiotherapeutic interventions are successful only if metastatic spread from the primary tumour has not yet occurred. Since many malignant tumours in humans have metastasised before being clinically recognised, they may be beyond the reach of surgical and radiotherapeutic treatment when they initially present. Metastatic tumour cell foci of $10^8$ or fewer cells, particularly if widely disseminated, are generally undetectable and therefore a target for chemotherapy, and this has been the basis of adjuvant therapy of solid tumours such as breast cancer and colon cancer.

Chemotherapy preceding local modalities (i.e. *neoadjuvant chemotherapy*) has been advocated in some conditions.[64-66] Clinical experience in several circumstances indicates a better response to neoadjuvant chemotherapy of the primary tumour than when treatment is given after surgery and/or radiation. By using chemotherapy first, there is a gain in time of onset of systemic treatment of micrometastases, thus avoiding the spontaneous development of resistance. In addition, the response of the primary tumour to chemotherapy may be used in planning subsequent treatments. However, potential disadvantages of this approach include promoting resistance to a local therapy such as radiation, and obscuring or prompting modification or surgical procedures and findings.

When radiation therapy and chemotherapy are combined, the situation is more complicated than with surgery and drugs. Drugs can kill tumour cells that radiation cannot kill and, thus, function as an adjuvant to radiation cell kill. In addition, drugs can sensitise cells to the killing effect of radiation, thereby increasing the therapeutic ratio for radiation through a sensitisation effect.[67] These approaches may, however, be limited by both acute and chronic toxicity and by undefined cross-resistance.

***Chronic toxicity of combined radiation and chemotherapy:*** this can be viewed from 3 conceptual aspects (table VII). Firstly, many drugs can cause chronic organ damage; e.g. the cardiac toxicity of doxorubicin, the pulmonary toxicity of bleomycin, the renal toxicity of cisplatin and mitomycin, the bladder toxicity of cyclophosphamide, and the leucoencephalopathy of methotrexate.[68] Secondly, immunosuppression is an adverse effect of both radiation and cytotoxic chemotherapy. Combined radiation and cytotoxic drugs may lead to a synergism of immunosuppressive effects with resultant chronic adverse effects of infection, increased incidence of failure of the metastatic disease to respond, or the development of second primary neoplasms.

Finally, radiation therapy and most cytotoxic chemotherapy regimens are carcinogenic in potential.[69] When the 2 modalities are used together, there is the risk that an enhancement of their carcinogenic effects will occur. Studies in patients with Hodgkin's disease are most indic-

**Table VII.** Chronic toxicity of combined radiation therapy and chemotherapy

| |
|---|
| **Organ and tissue damage:** |
| Heart |
| Lung |
| Central nervous system |
| Kidney |
| Liver |
| Gonads |
| Mucous membranes |
| Hair roots |
| Bladder |
| **Immunosuppression** |
| **Carcinogenicity** |

ative of the heightened risk for acute leukaemias and second epithelial or mesenchymal malignancies to appear in the radiation field.[70]

## 4. Optimum Treatment Approaches for Specific Cancers

### 4.1 Breast Cancer

Breast cancer is a disease of major importance in developed countries where the lifespan of women routinely reaches the eighth decade, and early menarche and deferred pregnancy are the rule. Recent estimates indicate that 1 in 8 women are at risk of developing breast cancer during their lifetime.[71] Some of this increase in incidence may be accounted for by its detection at early microinvasive stages accompanying *in situ* cancer detected principally through mammographic screening. It has been persuasively argued that breast cancer demographics reflect the role of estrogens and other hormones in inducing proliferation of mammary tissues, with a logarithmic increase beginning a few years after menarche, and a diminishing slope with menopause or any other factor interfering with such hormonal effects.[72] In addition, the basis of a high genetic risk attributable to individuals in certain families is being identified at the gene level, and several candidates for explaining breast cancer susceptibility are emerging. While this provides hope for preventive intervention in the most seriously afflicted families, most women diagnosed with breast cancer are not expected to have specific genetic abnormalities. Moreover, while administration of hormones to postmenopausal women raises concerns of enhancing the risk of breast cancer, such risk must be viewed against the background of potential benefits in averting cardiovascular disease and osteoporosis (see further chapter 18; sect. 11.4).

Increasingly, breast cancer is being diagnosed through the use of mammography, which often identifies calcifications associated with ductal carcinoma *in situ* (DCIS), and is not infrequently accompanied by microinvasion. At diagnosis, the disease is further defined by surgicopathological staging using TNM (tumour-node-metastasis) classifications (for an explanation of breast cancer staging, see table VIII). However, this may be modified by omitting axillary lymph node dissection in groups at very low risk for dissemination. Breast-preserving surgery, supplemented by radiation to the breast has replaced mastectomy in most instances where tumours are small, with good aesthetic results expected without compromising surgical principles of adequate margins of resection.[71] A number of established prognostic factors in addition to stage have been identified, and DNA ploidy, tumour S-phase, other markers of proliferation, presence of the Her2/neu growth factor receptor, and oncogene mutations, among many others, are under investigation both for prognosis and prediction of response to systemic therapy.[73-75]

#### 4.1.1 Chemoprevention

With the ability to identify factors responsible for the development of breast cancer, interest in prevention of this common malignant disease

**Table VIII.** Breast cancer TNM (tumour-node-metastasis) staging

| | |
|---|---|
| **Primary tumour** | |
| TX | Primary tumour cannot be assessed |
| T0 | No evidence of primary tumour |
| Tis | Carcinoma *in situ*: intraductal carcinoma, lobular carcinoma *in situ*, or Paget's disease of the nipple with no tumour |
| T1 | Tumour 2cm or less in greatest diameter |
| T1a | 0.5cm or less in greatest diameter |
| T1b | More than 0.5cm but not more than 1cm in greatest diameter |
| T1c | More than 1cm but not more than 2cm in greatest diameter |
| T2 | Tumour more than 2cm but not more than 5cm in greatest diameter |
| T3 | Tumour more than 5cm in greatest diameter |
| T4 | Tumour of any size with direct extension into chest wall of skin |
| T4a | Extension to chest wall |
| T4b | Oedema (excluding peau d'orange or ulceration of the skin of the breast or satellite skin nodules confined to the same breast) |
| T4c | Both (T4a and T4b) |
| T4d | Inflammatory carcinoma (clinicopathological entity characterised by diffuse brawny induration of the skin of the breast with a crypsipeloid edge, usually without an underlying palpable mass) |
| **Regional lymph nodes** | |
| NX | Regional lymph nodes cannot be assessed (e.g. previously removed) |
| N0 | No regional lymph node metastasis |
| N1 | Metastasis to movable ipsilateral axillary lymph node(s) |
| N2 | Metastasis to ipsilateral axillary lymph node(s) fixed to one another or to other structures |
| N3 | Metastasis to ipsilateral internal mammary node(s) |
| **Distant metastasis** | |
| MX | Presence of distant metastasis cannot be assessed |
| M0 | No distant metastasis |
| M1 | Distant metastasis [includes metastasis to ipsilateral supraclavicular lymph node(s)] |

has been mounting.[17,76] Use of an antiestrogen drug (e.g. tamoxifen) as a preventive is controversial at present, in terms of risk-benefit ratios, in the absence of results from randomised trials.[77,78] Such trials have, however, sharpened our awareness of risks to patient populations, not only of breast cancer, but also of important causes of mortality such as cardiovascular disease. Trials with micronutrients, or manipulations of dietary fat have also been instituted on a relatively small scale, mainly to define their feasibility.[79] The largest study planned, that of the Woman's Health Initiative in the US, attempts to define the effects and risks of hormone replacement therapy and anti-osteoporosis measures on vital health issues of women, including breast cancer.

#### 4.1.2 Integrative Approach to Treatment at Diagnosis

Breast cancer has been the most compelling example of the effect of chemotherapy on the survival of patients first diagnosed with a common adult cancer – an achievement of surgical adjuvant studies during the past 3 decades. These studies unequivocally show that combination chemotherapy regimens or, in some instances, antiestrogen (tamoxifen) therapy, improves relapse-free survival and often the overall survival of patients undergoing surgery who have been found to have positive lymph nodes, or negative lymph nodes with otherwise adverse prognostic features (tumour >2cm, S-phase >6%, negative hormone receptors).[80] The results from adjuvant tamoxifen in large meta-analyses indicate from 10 to 30% reduction in mortality with an overall 17% reduction in the annual hazard. At 10 years, the survival rates for adjuvant tamoxifen were 50.4% in node-positive women and 74.5% in node-negative women. This contrasts with 42.2% and 71.0%, respectively, in untreated controls.[81] For adjuvant chemotherapy, the 10-year survival rates were 51.3% compared with 45.5% for untreated controls (a 13% reduction in mortality).

Although modest and often disputed because of the added cost and morbidity of chemotherapy, these trials have revolutionised our approaches to this common cancer. [71,82,83]

Clinical trials are now exploring the addition of *paclitaxel*, issues of dose-intensity short of autologous bone marrow or stem cell support,[84] sequencing or combinations of hormones and cytotoxic agents, and the use of primary or neoadjuvant chemotherapy. Despite the achievements, it is imperative that trials be structured to further improve these modest results. In locally advanced disease and inflammatory breast cancer, efforts to improve results both in terms of local control and appearance of distal metastases utilising some of these strategies continue to be urgent.

**Table IX.** Cytotoxic chemotherapy of breast cancer

| |
|---|
| **1. Established first-line combination regimens:** |
| CAF: oral cyclophosphamide + doxorubicin + fluorouracil |
| FAC: IV cyclophosphamide + doxorubicin + fluorouracil |
| AC: doxorubicin + cyclophosphamide |
| CMF: cyclophosphamide + methotrexate + fluorouracil |
| **2. Investigational regimens:** |
| Doxorubicin or epirubicin followed by paclitaxel |
| **3. Salvage regimens[a]:** |
| Docetaxel, paclitaxel |
| Mitoxantrone + fluorouracil + calcium folinate |
| Mitomycin + vinblastine |
| **4. Other drugs undergoing research:** |
| Ifosfamide |
| Pirarubicin |
| Vinorelbine |
| Edatrexate |
| Idarubicin |
| Piroxantrone |
| Iodoxorubicin |

a Beyond the 'first-line' setting.

#### 4.1.3 Drug Treatment for Evident (Metastatic) Disease

In the late 1960s, combination chemotherapy for breast cancer was widely introduced as the results of studies with the 'Cooper' 5-drug regimen (weekly CMFVP, i.e. *cyclophosphamide, methotrexate, fluorouracil, vincristine, prednisone*) and with CMFP (*cyclophosphamide, methotrexate, fluorouracil, prednisone*) from the US National Cancer Institute became known. Since the 1970s, *doxorubicin* has been increasingly used either as part of the first treatment regimen [i.e. the in CAF (oral *cyclophosphamide* plus *doxorubicin* plus *fluorouracil*) and FAC (*intravenous cyclophosphamide* plus *doxorubicin* plus *fluorouracil*) regimens] for metastatic disease, or by itself following failure of the initial treatment. Table IX lists the cytotoxic chemotherapy regimens commonly employed to treat breast cancer.

Although objective responses have exceeded those obtained following hormonal therapy, effects on survival, duration of response and associated morbidity have remained inferior to endocrine manipulations. Consequently, efforts have concentrated on:

1) Refining the selection of patients for endocrine *versus* cytotoxic chemotherapy.

2) Improving results from current regimens through dose-intensification – including use of cytokines, and marrow reconstitution techniques.

3) Identification of new regimens and active drugs.

4) Learning about predictive correlates of response and resistance, and their modulation.

Some hope exists that newly introduced drugs (e.g. the taxanes) together with doxorubicin will demonstrate superior results to those previously achieved. Biological response modifiers and immunotherapies including tumour vaccines have also undergone trials in advanced breast cancer, but no persuasive evidence of consistent activity is currently available. Over the years, new hormonal agents have been introduced, while current cytotoxic drug regimens are widely testing the incorporation of taxanes, with both *paclitaxel* and *docetaxel* showing substantial activity in doxorubicin-resistant patients.[85] Table IX indicates those agents currently of interest in the treatment of breast cancer. Drugs that do not form part of the initial therapy are used after failure of other drugs. However, response rates in this 'salvage' or 'beyond the first-line' setting are usually disappointing.[86]

***Endocrine manipulation:*** historically, this preceded the interest in cytotoxic drugs and but has recaptured wide attention with the identification of hormone receptors on breast cancer and the introduction of antiestrogen drugs such as *tamoxifen*.[87,88] Ancillary measures such as control of hypercalcaemia and/or bone destruction with bisphosphonates (e.g. *pamidronate*) are helpful adjuncts.[89] Tumour markers may be helpful in follow-up.[90] More recently, the relationship of hormone dependence and independence to the elaboration of autocrine, juxtacrine and paracrine growth factors have expanded our understanding of drug mechanisms, as well as identifying causes of resistance. Undoubtedly, the next decade will witness an expansion of our abilities to exploit such knowledge therapeutically.

## 4.2 Colorectal Cancer

Colorectal cancer occupies an important place among adult solid tumours, because its combined incidence in men and women makes it the most common non-skin malignancy, and the key role of early detection in improving the results of treatment. Molecular oncology has provided strong support for the origin of cancer from adenomatous polyps, and for an accumulation of genetic abnormalities leading from polyps to invasive carcinoma and metastases.[91] Dietary factors and micronutrients including intake of fibre and calcium have been under intensive study, but clinical application of dietary concepts are difficult. Many of these concepts derive from epidemiological clues, including the connection of colorectal cancer with a high intake of fat and calories, and the shifting incidence from fewer left-sided to more right-sided colon cancer in the last 4 decades.[76]

When the disease is diagnosed in the invasive stages, surgery with adequate margins is required. Prognosis depends on the extent of penetration of the tumour into the muscular layers and beyond, together with the presence or absence of regional lymph nodes. The presence of distant metastases leads to a pattern of relentless progression and development of symptomatic disease manifestations, particularly in the liver. It is in the patients at risk of local and distant relapse, as in breast cancer, that adjuvant therapy has been proven to be beneficial following trials performed by cooperative groups in the US.[92] This adjuvant therapy has consisted of fluorouracil in combination with levamisole, and studies combining fluorouracil with calcium folinate are ongoing.

### 4.2.1 Prevention

Epidemiological studies have pointed to high fat content and red meat as important dietary causative factors in polyp formation and susceptibility to cancer. Studies have also suggested that a deficiency in calcium is associated with an increased risk.[93] Therefore, studies have been initiated to determine the role of low fat diets and higher intakes of calcium in decreasing cancer risk. Using polyp formation as a surrogate end-point, patients with adenomatous polyps have been followed after random assignment to dietary intervention or to no intervention. Conclusive results are not available, but periodic screening and resection of polyps may be beneficial.[94]

### 4.2.2 Treatment

*Fluorouracil* has been successful when used in the surgical adjuvant setting in colon cancer. Increases in disease-free-survival and in survival of patients with positive lymph nodes in resected specimens have been confirmed in patients receiving adjuvant therapy *versus* those followed in an observation arm.[92] The risk of recurrence was decreased by 41% and the rate by 33% with adjuvant therapy. Similarly, in rectal cancer, studies of fluorouracil combined with postoperative radiation have demonstrated an analogous prolongation of overall survival and disease-free survival.[95] Moreover, the local recurrence rate was reduced to 8%.[96] Not only is fluorouracil suitable for adjuvant therapy because of its therapeutic index and ability to yield enhanced results with radiation, but it also has antitumour activity unsurpassed by other drugs. The effect of fluorouracil and other fluorinated pyrimidines (e.g. *floxuridine*) in advanced colorectal cancer, however, is marginal at best, with only exceptional complete regressions of tumour being observed. In disseminated disease studies, the median duration of response is always <1 year and the median survival varies between 1 year and 18 months.[97]

Because of poor results in phase II studies of new agents, and insight into the biochemical target of fluorouracil, interest in the 1980s shifted towards biochemical modulation (see section 2.5) as a means of enhancing thymidylate synthase inhibition. Administration of *calcium folinate* (leucovorin) enhances cytotoxicity *in vitro* and also yields increased response rates in patients with advanced colorectal cancer.[98] A number of trials have confirmed this last observation, but with no clear effects on survival with the exception of studies where the control arm used an inadequate dose of fluorouracil. Explorations of whether high or low doses of calcium folinate are required for this enhanced clinical effect are inconclusive.[99] Even low doses of calcium folinate are able to shift the toxic manifestations to greater stomatitis, and less myelosuppression. Therefore, calcium folinate is able to enhance antitumour drug effects in a manner that is different than administering a greater amount of drug.

The fluorouracil schedule is another variable in achieving this enhanced toxicity: weekly administration requires a 20-fold greater dosage of calcium folinate for biochemical modulation. It has been postulated that in an adjuvant setting, this combination will yield results superior to fluorouracil alone. Indeed, significant improvement in survival has been reported in situations where adjuvant therapy in the 1960s had been negative (see review by Muggia and Groshen).[100]

***Locoregional administration:*** an important use of fluoropyrimidines is locoregional administration (e.g. infusions into the hepatic artery for liver metastases, intraperitoneal administration) for the palliation of either intrahepatic or intraperitoneal metastases. *Floxuridine* has been given by the intra-arterial or the intraperitoneal routes because of its greater solubility and potency, as well as favourable pharmacology (better hepatic extraction than its parent). Use of the intra-arterial route has been complicated by the development of biliary sclerosis, which may be prevented by some dose schedules and the use of corticosteroids. A review of randomised trials has indicated no significant improvement in survival, but response rates were improved in all trials.[101]

In the 1990s, drugs have appeared that hold some promise of activity against colorectal cancer, although their role has not yet been defined. These include the topoisomerase I inhibitor *irinotecan*[52] and the quinazoline antifolate drug (also targeting thymidylate synthase) *ralitrexed* (see table V). A number of other modulators of fluoropyrimidine action such as *hydroxycarbamide* (hydroxyurea), *interferons*, *sparfosic acid* (PALA) and others are also undergoing testing in clinical and laboratory studies.

### 4.3 Lung Cancer

With the widespread use of cigarette smoking, this neoplasm has become a major public health problem and the most common cause of cancer deaths in most countries. The increasing incidence over the past few decades has been paralleled by an increasing cause of mortality in men as noted from registry data in the US. During the past decade, presumably reflecting changing smoking patterns, the rising incidence curve has begun to flatten in men, but has continued to increase in women, where this cancer has overtaken breast cancer as a cause of cancer deaths. Treatment has been unable to alter these grim statistics and has played only a minor role, except when diagnosis at early stages allows curative surgical resections to be performed.[102] Unfortunately, more than half of lung cancers show evidence of dissemination at the time of diagnosis. There are ongoing efforts to understand the complex biology of lung neoplasms, identify individuals at high risk, prevent the disease (in particular, via smoking cessation), and to promote early diagnosis and treatment.

Lung cancer has a heterogeneous histology, and is usually subdivided into small cell and non-small cell types. Although small cell lung cancers share neuroendocrine markers and morphologies, unified hypotheses view small and non-small cell lung cancers as sharing a common precursor and subsequent diverging differentiation patterns. It is, therefore, not unusual that mixed histological types are identified within one individual. Nevertheless, differences in biology and treatment have assisted in the development of treatment strategies for small cell and common non-small cell histologies (i.e. adenocarcinoma, large cell anaplastic carcinoma, squamous cell cancer).

It is likely that new biological markers will replace partial reliance on histological characterisations. For example, mutations in the k-ras oncogene have been documented among most patients with adenocarcinoma and such mutations confer a poorer prognosis.[103] At present, however, the initial treatment decisions rely on appropriate staging and whether small cell lung cancer has been identified. If a diagnosis of small cell lung cancer is made on the basis of bronchoscopy specimens or bronchial washings, this should trigger a search for metastases at distant sites (marrow, liver, adrenals, retroperitoneum, brain) and a plan to incorporate local therapy around primarily systemic treatment. Diagnostic staging procedures have undergone major changes, with refinements in fibreoptic bronchoscopy, computed tomography or magnetic resonance imaging assessments of the thorax, abdomen, bone and CNS, mediastinoscopy to verify the status of regional nodes, and fine-needle aspiration verification in a wide variety of sites.[104] Under experimentation, in a disease with a propensity to haematogenous dissemination, are diagnostic techniques such as positron emission tomography (PET) scanning, immunoscintigraphy, and polymerase chain reaction (PCR) methods to detect mutation in various body fluids and blood.

#### 4.3.1 Prevention

Major efforts are ongoing to curb smoking addiction, and to minimise 'second-hand' smoke exposure that may also contribute to cancer causation in susceptible individuals. Although government health agencies recognise the importance of such efforts, they must compete with advertising campaigns of cigarette companies that are designed to lure the young towards habituation. For individuals in whom a damaged respiratory tract is thought to be a forerunner of malignancy, attention has turned to the identification and reversion of premalignant changes. Such studies have been emphasised over screening for cancer, in view of the absence of any effects of cytological and radiographical screening of smoking populations performed during the late 1970s.

The use of monoclonal antibody staining to aid in the identification of small numbers of tumour cells in the sputum is now the subject of a prospective study in high risk individuals (already curatively resected for lung cancer). Chemopreventive measures have included consideration of free radical scavengers and antioxidants (such as carotenoids). However, a large study from Finland in a group of heavily smoking individuals, concluded that neither carotenoids (β-carotene) nor tocopherol (vitamin E) conferred protection, and may have enhanced the risk of developing cancer.[105,106]

At present, early diagnosis and surveillance of high-risk groups, i.e. people who smoke, those with family histories of lung cancer, occupational exposures to asbestos, pneumoconioses, and uranium mining, and those with previously diagnosed cancers of the aerodigestive passages are the focus of preventive efforts. In the head and neck area, premalignant lesions have reverted to normal through the use of *isotretinoin*,[107] and similar studies are being performed in patients who have already had a curative resection for lung cancer since their risk of second primary neoplasms is considerable.

#### 4.3.2 Treatment

Some therapies commonly used for lung cancers are listed in table X.

##### Non-Small Cell Lung Cancer

In non-small cell lung cancer, the focus of therapeutic research has been on a combined modality for regional disease: the staging classification was revised in 1986 to subclassify stage III patients into those potentially amenable to surgery and to radiation, and separate them from those with stage IV disease.[108] Randomised trials have now unequivocally established the value of drug regimens preceding or given concomitantly with local measures. For example, in 60 patients with stage IIIA non-small cell lung cancer randomised to either surgery or to *mitomycin*, *ifosfamide* and *cisplatin* for 3 cycles before surgery, the median survival was 8 months for surgery alone *versus* 26 months for the combined group ($p < 0.001$).[109]

**Table X.** Drugs commonly used for the treatment of lung, head and neck cancers

| Drugs currently preferred | Alternative drugs or regimens | Other drugs with activity |
|---|---|---|
| **Non-small cell lung cancer:** | | |
| Carboplatin or cisplatin + paclitaxel | Docetaxel<br>Vinorelbine + cisplatin<br>Cisplatin + etoposide<br>Cisplatin + vinblastine or vindesine | Gemcitabine[a] |
| **Small cell lung cancer:** | | |
| Cisplatin + etoposide<br>Carboplatin + etoposide | CAV: cyclophosphamide + doxorubicin + vincristine | Paclitaxel<br>Etoposide (oral)<br>Carmustine<br>Lomustine |
| **Head and neck cancers:** | | |
| Cisplatin + fluorouracil<br>PFL: cisplatin + fluorouracil + calcium folinate (leucovorin) | Methotrexate<br>Paclitaxel | Epirubicin<br>Doxorubicin<br>Ifosfamide<br>Carboplatin<br>Bleomycin<br>Hydroxycarbamide (hydroxyurea) |

a Available only for investigational use in the US.

Results are also promising for combined drugs and radiation before surgery, or without surgery in inoperable disease. These advances belie the cynicism that prevailed because of the initial detrimental effects of treatment given as an adjuvant to surgery and the minimal effects on survival of combination chemotherapy on stage IV disease.

Drug therapy of non-small cell lung cancer has become firmly established from the following additional considerations:

1) The responsiveness noted in early stage trials exceeds the response rates seen in stage IV, and includes pathological complete responses.

2) Clinical trials have documented survival advantages of drug treatment *versus* best supportive care.

3) Prospects for more effective drug therapy are combinations of platinum compounds with new drugs with specific activity such as the taxanes (*paclitaxel, docetaxel*), drugs affecting topoisomerase I (*irinotecan*), newer vinca alkaloids (*vinorelbine*), and antimetabolites with solid tumour activity (*gemcitabine*).[110,111]

### Small Cell Lung Cancer

In small cell lung cancer, prospects for major advances from combination chemotherapies developed in the 1970s gave way to a sobering realisation that development of resistance, early metastatic spread to the CNS and long term complications, including CNS damage and non-small cell lung cancer, were obstacles to therapeutic advantages of empirical intensification of these treatment strategies. On the other hand, clinical trials suggested that early eradication of disease was possible through aggressive chemotherapy and radiation therapy delivery, particularly to patients with disease classified as being 'limited' to the hemithorax. A Canadian clinical trial documented advantages in survival and reduced frequency of CNS metastases from early radiation therapy in these combined approaches, consistent with the hypothesis that drug resistance in unsuspected uncontrolled primary sites leads to metastases.[112] French investigators championing this aggressive combined approach have achieved a 43% 2-year survival in a cohort receiving high-dose cisplatin and cyclophosphamide *versus* 26% in those randomised to lower doses.[113,114] Prophylactic brain irradiation in these patients is being increasingly questioned because of its morbidity, but lower doses may be effective and should be considered in selected instances.

In 'extensive' small cell lung cancer, the impasse over a median survival hardly exceeding 1 year, despite its initial responsiveness, has given way to identification of patients who may benefit from combined modalities and those more suitably palliated by sequential treatment regimens. Also identified are drugs that may provide additionally effective tools over the action of cisplatin or carboplatin, etoposide (and its analogue teniposide), cyclophosphamide, doxorubicin (and its analogue epirubicin), and vinca alkaloids. An understanding of drug resistance in relation to tumour biology and exposure to drugs and radiation will help devise strategies of the future.[115] High-dose chemotherapy with bone marrow reconstitution has been tested, but is not yet a promising strategy.

## 4.4 Ovarian Cancer

Drug treatment occupies a central role in the management of this disease which had been increasing in incidence in Western countries, attributed in part to deferral of pregnancy and early menarche. However, its incidence may now be decreasing due to the widespread use of oral contraceptives, which prevent ovulation and lead to a diminished risk in women who take them. By contrast with breast adenocarcinoma, which it superficially resembles, ovarian cancer tends to remain localised within the peritoneal cavity, and its growth is influenced by a different set of growth factors. However, a common genetic origin has been identified in some families who carry a gene (BRCA 1) localised to the long arm of chromosome 17, and confers dominant susceptibility to breast and ovarian cancers in women.[116] Moreover, both in ovarian cancer and in breast cancer, the presence of the Her2/neu oncogene that codes for a membrane growth factor receptor of the epidermal growth factor receptor family confirms a poor prognosis.[74] Prevention and treatment approaches have begun to test hypotheses emanating from tumour biology.

### 4.4.1 Prevention

Screening and prophylactic oophorectomy have been instituted in patients with hereditary predisposition. The value of screening even in high risk groups has not been established and routine use of tumour markers such as the CA-125 and transvaginal ultrasonography is considered experimental. Future directions will likely focus on genotyping and on prevention since identification of this malignancy at early stages remains elusive. Preventive measures have included prophylactic castration, but induction of a 'medical menopause' by GnRH (gonadotrophin- releasing hormone) agonists and add-back low-dose estrogens must be tested in women at high risk who do not wish to become pregnant.

### 4.4.2 Treatment

All but 5% of patients with epithelial ovarian cancer require chemotherapy to improve on surgical salvage because even in stage I (disease confined to the ovary), certain tumour characteristics are associated with a risk of peritoneal, lymph node and, to a lesser extent, distant metastases. Systemic chemotherapy in the past decade has been platinum-based (i.e. *cisplatin* or *carboplatin*) together with other drugs, usually *alkylating agents* and *doxorubicin*. More recently, the addition of *paclitaxel* to cisplatin has yielded superior results in randomised trials including women with advanced disease.[117] Although these improvements have altered the dismal prognosis in stages III and IV, with a median survival of 1 year prevalent 3 decades ago, the long term outlook remains problematic for most of these patients. Only in patients with no gross residual disease after initial surgical debulking does the median survival exceed 5 years.

Accordingly, trials are ongoing with new therapeutic modalities, including intraperitoneal administration of established drugs,[51,118] the introduction of biological therapy and gene therapy, high-dose chemotherapy with bone marrow reconstitution, and cytotoxic agents not previously applied in ovarian cancer (e.g. irinotecan, long infusions of topotecan, vinorelbine, gemcitabine, raltitrexed, edatrexate). As in breast cancer, identification of biochemical correlates of response and strategies of biochemical modulation, resistance reversal, cytoprotection and others are under investigation. With the prominent role of *paclitaxel* (first established in this disease), interest in identifying P-glycoprotein positivity and, therefore, overexpression of the MDR1 gene has captured the attention of clinicians.[119]

## 4.5 Prostate Cancer

This cancer is emerging as the most important cancer in men, with a similar frequency of clinical presentations as breast cancer in women. Complicating these statistics is the known frequency of prostate cancers as an incidental finding at necropsy. A vast number of these carcinomas may have no clinical significance, as would the finding of *in situ* tumours of the breast. However, in the prostate, the diagnostic problem is more complicated and the epidemiology of these *in situ* tumours has not been defined. Moreover, in populations in places such as Japan, the percentage of clinical presentations is substantially lower than in the US. In the US, marked differences in incidence occur among various ethnic subsets. For example, Blacks have a very high incidence, with an earlier age of onset than Caucasians, who, in turn, have a higher incidence than Asians.[15] These differences have been attributed to variations in androgen concentrations and in their metabolic degradation.

Androgen deprivation has been central in therapeutic strategies since the 1940s and the work of Huggins at the University of Chicago.[35] It is likely that androgens play a role in tumour progression and eventually in the emergence of androgen-independent cells. Tumour markers such as acid phosphatase (of historical interest) and prostate specific antigen (PSA) are dependent in part on androgens for their expression. Prostate specific antigen has assumed a very important role in the early diagnosis of this cancer, but its role in screening has not been established and is being investigated.

Prostate specific antigen bears a relationship to the stage of disease. It is nearly always elevated in stages denoting regional extension and those indicating dissemination (usually to retroperitoneal or even more distant lymph nodes) and bone, where osteoblastic metastases are typically recognised.[120]

#### 4.5.1 Prevention

It was hoped that screening for prostate specific antigen could lead to early detection of this cancer. However, it is apparent that while this test is more sensitive than others, most abnormalities already indicate clinical disease, with some correlation between the magnitude of the elevation and the size of the primary tumour or the presence of extraprostatic extension.[121] The focus on epidemiological clues has encouraged preventive trials through modulation of androgens.

The introduction of the 5α-reductase inhibitor *finasteride*, which inhibits the activation of testosterone to its active intracellular metabolite 5-dihydrotestosterone, permitted large scale testing of chemoprevention through androgen modulation.[122] The US National Cancer Institute is sponsoring trials of finasteride as prevention of prostate cancer in men over 55 years. This compound has a good toxicity profile, the incidence of problems with libido being $<2\%$.

Other longer range preventive measures will undoubtedly require a better understanding of causative factors responsible for the wide variation in disease incidence. One clue under investigation is the possibility that antiandrogenic factors such as genistein, present in tofu, may be responsible for the lower rate of tumour progression in Japanese men.

#### 4.5.2 Treatment

Androgen deprivation 'orchiectomy' was introduced by Huggins and has been central to treatment. Estrogens were subsequently substituted as a medical method to achieve the same goals. A better appreciation of adverse effects and the adverse effect of estrogens on survival in relation to cardiovascular complications, shifted the treatment of advanced disease back to orchiectomy. Awareness of the importance of adrenal androgens led to exploration of 'secondary' ablation via hypophysectomy or surgically or medically induced adrenal suppression. However, the effect of secondary hormonal manipulations after failure of castration or estrogen therapy has been modest.

Although it has not lived up to the initial expectations, the concept of 'total androgen blockade' confirmed partly by group studies[123] has stimulated a new generation of treatment approaches based on elimination of both testicular and adrenal androgen from the outset. The availability of antiandrogens such as *flutamide*, *cyproterone* or *bicalutamide* (casodex), and inhibitors of pituitary gonadotrophins (GnRH agonists or antagonists) [see further chapter 19; sect. 8.2] has allowed trials of this hypothesis on a wide scale. A 6-month (from 29 to 35 months) increase in the median survival was seen in patients receiving the combination of flutamide with leuprorelin *vs* leuprorelin alone. The ability to achieve castration or total androgen blockade through medical means has also stimulated testing androgen deprivation as an adjunct to surgery or radiation for bulky disease confined to the gland. This has become standard practice when dealing with very large tumours confined to the prostate in patients undergoing radiation, but more data must be obtained to assess its therapeutic benefit.

Adrenal suppression has been achieved by *aminoglutethimide*, *ketoconazole* and *glucocorticoids*. *Progestagens* in high doses, particularly when combined with low-dose estrogen, can also interfere with androgen action.[124] More recently, understanding of growth factor regulation stimulated trials of *suramin*, with responses seen in patients who presumably had tumours that had become androgen-independent.[125] Subsequently, it became apparent that some of these responses occurred in the setting of flutamide withdrawal,[126] and such therapeutic benefit is reminiscent of the benefit observed generally for several months after withdrawal of estrogens in patients with breast cancer. Since retinoid-binding proteins may be hormonally regulated, the study of compounds that alter such proteins has opened new lines of investigation.

Cytotoxic chemotherapy has played a relatively minor role in prostate cancer. *Estramustine phosphate* is a complex moiety linking a bis-chloroethyl group via a carbamate bond to estradiol. Its activity against prostate cancer could in part be accounted for by its metabolism to estrogens (estrone and estradiol), but more recently is attributed to its ability to interact with microtubular-associated proteins. Combinations of estramustine phosphate and chemotherapeutic agents acting on the mitotic spindle have been tested experimentally and clinically.[127] The use of *vinblastine* or *paclitaxel* with estramustine has produced some encouraging results, and *doxorubicin* has also shown some activity. The survival of patients on these ototoxic therapies may be improved by continued androgen ablation.[124]

### 4.6 Other Adult Solid Tumours

#### 4.6.1 Germ Cell Tumours

Both testicular and extragonadal germ cell tumours have usually been curable since the introduction of *cisplatin*. This drug is more effective than carboplatin and is usually given in combination with *etoposide* and *bleomycin*. Testicular seminomas, when small, are treated with radiation to lymph node bearing areas after excision.[128,129]

#### 4.6.2 Gastric Cancer

This cancer has major importance in certain countries. Although its incidence had been decreasing in developed countries, presumably as a result of the advent of refrigeration (leading to decreased salting of food and other unknown factors related to storage), in recent years there has been some increase in cancers arising in the proximal stomach (oesophageal cardiac junction). In addition, the aetiological role of *Helicobacter pylori* is being studied.[130]

Emphasis on treatment before surgery has provided renewed interest in chemotherapy, which has had relatively minor effectiveness in advanced stages, and as an adjuvant.[51] Regimens have included *fluorouracil* plus *cisplatin; etoposide* plus both *doxorubicin* and *cisplatin*; and *etoposide* plus both *calcium folinate* and *fluorouracil*, among others. All these regimens have demonstrated considerable activity against these potentially resectable tumours, although only a small percentage show pathologically complete responses. Superior results in excess of 3 years median survival have been obtained using a neoadjuvant approach complemented by postoperative intraperitoneal therapy with *floxuridine*,[131] and randomised trials comparing this approach with surgery are ongoing. *Paclitaxel* is another agent of potential interest in this disease.

#### 4.6.3 Oesophageal Cancer

Combining *cisplatin* and *fluorouracil* has proven more effective in oesophageal cancer than radiation alone.[132] The chemotherapy-radiation arm has up to 25% long term survivors, compared with less than 10% for radiation alone. This again has stimulated integration of additional drugs into treatment approaches, despite the relatively few effects of chemotherapy in advanced metastatic disease. Among drugs with antitumour activity, against both the squamous and adenocarcinoma histologies, is *paclitaxel*.

#### 4.6.4 Head and Neck Cancers

Except for nasopharyngeal cancers, which are dependent on radiation therapy, other sites of origin are treated principally with surgery alone or with surgery plus radiation.[133] The role of chemotherapy on locally advanced tumours has been explored on a wide scale during the past 2 decades, but it has defied definition. In some trials, the results of radiation and chemotherapy have proven superior to radiation alone,[134] and in laryngeal cancer have led to sparing of laryngectomy in a substantial number of patients without compromising survival.[135] Drugs of major interest are *cisplatin, carboplatin, fluorouracil, methotrexate, bleomycin,* and more recently *paclitaxel* (table X). In the poorly differentiated nasopharyngeal cancer, *doxorubicin* or *epirubicin* have shown substantial activity.

#### 4.6.5 Cancer of the Uterine Cervix

In cervical cancer, some analogy may be made with squamous cell cancers, in that combined modality therapy has received major attention, but its effects remain largely undefined. An exception is the use of *hydroxycarbamide* (hydroxyurea) or *cisplatin* and *fluorouracil* in locally advanced stages, given together with conventional radiation.[136] Studies by the Gynecologic Oncology Group have shown only modest advantages (up to 10%) in medical survival rates over radiation alone. In recurrent or disseminated disease, the effect of chemotherapy is modest and combinations of drugs have uncertain advantages over cisplatin alone.

*Paclitaxel* has modest activity, but additional trials are anticipated in view of the interest in this compound and its analogue *docetaxel* as a possible radiosensitiser. Biological agents, such as *interferon-α* and *isotretinoin* (cis-retinoic acid), have also been noted to have antiproliferative effects in localised stages.[137] *In situ* changes have yielded to retinoids.[138]

#### 4.6.6 Carcinoma of the Uterine Corpus

The aetiology of this carcinoma is clearly related to increased estrogen stimulation unopposed by progesterone.[17] More recently, antiestrogens with weak estrogenic effects such as tamoxifen have also been incriminated as a causative factor.[139] A minority of these tumours has hormone receptors and may respond to progestational agents; these tumours are predominantly well differentiated pulmonary metastases occurring several years after initial diagnosis and have been related to tobacco smoking.[140]

Chemotherapy has been primarily based on *doxorubicin*, but tumours giving rise to metastases at distant sites are biologically more aggressive and the effect on survival has been modest to date. Combined modality approaches in patients with tumours at risk of metastases have not proven effective. However, additional drugs such as *cisplatin, carboplatin* and *paclitaxel* may eventually lead to more effective regimens.[141]

#### 4.6.7 Bladder and Other Urothelial Cancer

This transitional cell cancer goes through a well delineated preinvasive stage and the biological characteristics of the invasive stages are being studied in a manner analogous to what has taken place in colon cancer. Mutations of the p53 protein are frequent and define a poor prognostic subset.[61]

Surgery is the treatment for invasive bladder cancer. The quality of life of patients undergoing total cystectomy has much improved through the use of continence pouches which can be intermittently catheterised by the patient, as opposed to the need to carry bags over ileo-cutaneous stomas. Combination chemotherapy regimens such as M-VAC (*methotrexate, vinblastine, doxorubicin*, and *cisplatin*) are more effective than single agents and are being tested for their effects in the neoadjuvant setting. In a trial of 246 patients, significantly more complete responses (13 *vs* 3%) occurred after M-VAC than cisplatin, and median survival for all patients was 12.5 months, versus 8.5 months for cisplatin alone. *Paclitaxel* and *gallium nitrate* have also shown efficacy.[142,143]

#### 4.6.8 Bone and Soft Tissue Sarcomas

Chemotherapy has played a major role in bone sarcomas, providing an excellent demonstration of the value of preoperative treatment.[144] In soft tissue tumours, the effect of chemotherapy is more limited in adults,[145] as opposed to the certain effect on the survival of children with these tumours (table XI). Regimens indicate a vast amount of experimentation based on *doxorubicin, ifosfamide* and frequently *dacarbazine*. In bone sarcomas, *cisplatin* plays a considerable role and high-dose *methotrexate* with *calcium folinate* rescue also has antitumour activity. Biological features such as p53 are also under study.[146,147]).

#### 4.6.9 Malignant Melanoma

This malignancy has assumed increasingly greater importance because of its greater frequency in relation to sun exposure in susceptible fair-skinned populations. The behaviour of these cutaneous tumours after they assume a certain thickness is highly unpredictable. Once lymph node metastases occur, disseminated disease will eventually appear in most nodes and become biologically more aggressive with time.

Systemic treatment has been generally disappointing, although greater susceptibility to both biological response modifiers and to chemotherapy is noted in the less aggressive tumours. *Interferon-α* and *interleukin-2* have shown some effectiveness, with responses of up to 30% and occasional (5%) lasting complete responses. Trials in the adjuvant setting have recently demonstrated the efficacy of intensive interferon-α. Chemotherapy has relied principally on *cisplatin, carmustine* and *dacarbazine* alone or in combination.[148] Tamoxifen was shown to enhance the antitumour effect of dacarbazine in a randomised trial, but the improvement in median survival was quite modest (from 28 to 48 weeks).[149] The effect of tamoxifen was not seen in another subsequent trial.[150]

#### 4.6.10 Renal Cancer

This cancer has also shown relatively little response to chemotherapy, presumably because multidrug resistance is common because of the association with P-glycoprotein overexpression. The same biological response modifiers (interleukin-2 and interferon-α) may show some

**Table XI.** Drugs commonly used to treat major types of cancer

| Cancer type | Drugs currently preferred | Alternative or secondary drugs | Other drugs with reported activity |
|---|---|---|---|
| **Haematological malignancies:** | | | |
| Acute lymphocytic leukaemia | *Induction:* vincristine + prednisone<br>Prophylaxis of CNS disease with IT methotrexate ± radiotherapy<br>*Maintenance:* combination chemotherapy with methotrexate + mercaptopurine, or other combinations | Daunorubicin<br>Doxorubicin<br>L-Asparaginase<br>Cyclophosphamide<br>Cytarabine | Thioguanine<br>Teniposide |
| Acute granulocytic leukaemia | Doxorubicin or daunorubicin + cytarabine *or*<br>Cytarabine + thioguanine *or*<br>Cytarabine, vincristine + prednisone | Amsacrine<br>Mitoxantrone | Azacitidine[a]<br>Mercaptopurine<br>Etoposide |
| Acute myelomonocytic or monocytic leukaemia | Doxorubicin or daunorubicin + cytarabine *or*<br>Cytarabine + thioguanine *or*<br>Cytarabine, vincristine + prednisone | | Etoposide |
| Chronic granulocytic leukaemia | Hydroxycarbamide (hydroxyurea), interferon-α | Busulfan | Mercaptopurine<br>Plicamycin (mithramycin) |
| Chronic lymphocytic leukaemia | Chlorambucil or cyclophosphamide | Prednisone | |
| Multiple myeloma | Melphalan or cyclophosphamide + prednisone | Doxorubicin<br>vincristine | VAD: Vincristine + doxorubicin + dexamethasone |
| Hodgkin's disease | ABVD (doxorubicin, bleomycin, vinblastine, dacarbazine) | MOPP [chlormethine (mustine), vincristine, procarbazine, prednisone] | Lomustine<br>Carmustine<br>Chlorambucil<br>Thiotepa<br>Etoposide |
| Low grade (nodular) lymphomas | CVP (cyclophosphamide, vincristine, prednisone) | Fludarabine | Lomustine<br>Carmustine<br>Interferon-α |
| High grade (e.g. diffuse histiocytic) lymphomas | CHOP (cyclophosphamide, doxorubicin, vincristine, prednisone) *or*<br>M-BACOD (methotrexate + bleomycin, doxorubicin, cyclophosphamide, vincristine, dexamethasone) | Etoposide<br>Mitoxantrone<br>Ifosfamide<br>Cytarabine<br>Cisplatin | Lomustine<br>Carmustine |
| Burkitt's tumour | Cyclophosphamide | Carmustine | Methotrexate |
| Mycosis fungoides | Methotrexate | Chlormethine (mustine, mechlorethamine) | Vinblastine<br>Cyclophosphamide |
| **Paediatric solid tumours, brain tumours, germ cell tumours and sarcomas:** | | | |
| Wilm's tumour | Dactinomycin (actinomycin D) + vincristine | Doxorubicin | Cyclophosphamide |
| Ewing's sarcoma | Cyclophosphamide + doxorubicin + vincristine | Dactinomycin[b] | |
| Embryonal rhabdomyosarcoma | Doxorubicin<br>Cyclophosphamide<br>Vincristine alternating with cisplatin + etoposide | Dactinomycin | Thiotepa<br>Methotrexate |
| Retinoblastoma | Cyclophosphamide | Carboplatin | |

**Table XI.** *[Continued]*

| Cancer type | Drugs currently preferred | Alternative or secondary drugs | Other drugs with reported activity |
|---|---|---|---|
| Neuroblastoma | Cyclophosphamide or vincristine | Doxorubicin | Etoposide<br>Cisplatin or carboplatin<br>Vinblastine<br>Prednisone |
| Osteogenic sarcoma | Doxorubicin + cisplatin | Cisplatin or high-dose methotrexate + folinic acid 'rescue' | Melphalan<br>Mitomycin |
| **Solid tumours:** | | | |
| Adrenocortical carcinoma | Mitotane | | |
| Bladder | Cisplatin or doxorubicin<br>Thiotepa bladder instillation where indicated | Methotrexate<br>Vinblastine<br>Mitomycin bladder instillation | Fluorouracil<br>Cyclophosphamide |
| Breast | CMF ± P (cyclophosphamide, methotrexate, fluorouracil, prednisone) *or*<br>Doxorubicin<br>Cyclophosphamide (see also table VIII) | Doxorubicin + vincristine if CMF ± P used as primary, otherwise combination or single agent regimen of preferred drugs not previously used (including vincristine) | Vinblastine<br>Thiotepa<br>Melphalan<br>Mitomycin |
| | *Additive* (where hormones indicated): stilbestrol, testolactone, tamoxifen, megestrol, depending on menopausal and tumour hormone receptor status | Depending on response to initial treatment and location of recurrent disease | Ethinylestradiol<br>Fluoxymesterone |
| Bronchogenic carcinoma small cell or 'oat cell' | Doxorubicin<br>+ cyclophosphamide<br>+ vincristine *or*<br>Cyclophosphamide + lomustine + methotrexate | Etoposide + cisplatin | Procarbazine<br>Altretamine[a] |
| Squamous cell, large cell anaplastic, and adenocarcinoma[c] | Cisplatin + vinblastine *or*<br>Cisplatin + etoposide | Doxorubicin *or*<br>Cyclophosphamide *or*<br>Methotrexate | Mitomycin |
| Cervix squamous cell | Cisplatin | Bleomycin<br>Mitomycin (also given with cisplatin in primary treatment) | Methotrexate<br>Fluorouracil<br>Vincristine<br>Cyclophosphamide<br>Doxorubicin |
| Colon carcinoma | Fluorouracil | Semustine *or*<br>Mitomycin | Tegafur[a] (ftorafur) |
| Endometrial carcinoma | Megestrol *or*<br>Medroxyprogesterone | Doxorubicin | Fluorouracil[b]<br>Cyclophosphamide |
| Gastric adenocarcinoma | FAM (fluorouracil, doxorubicin, mitomycin) *or*<br>Fluorouracil + semustine | Semustine or mitomycin if not used in primary combination | Tegafur[a] |
| Head and neck squamous cell | Cisplatin + bleomycin or methotrexate or fluorouracil | Single agent not used in primary treatment | Vinblastine |
| Hepatocellular carcinoma, primary[c] | Doxorubicin | Fluorouracil[b]; etoposide, cisplatin (intra-arterial) | Tegafur[a] |
| Malignant insulinoma or islet cell carcinoma | Streptozocin + doxorubicin or fluorouracil | Dacarbazine | |
| Malignant melanoma | Dacarbazine or semustine | Cisplatin | Hydroxycarbamide |
| Ovary | Cisplatin + cyclophosphamide ± doxorubicin | Doxorubicin *or* altretamine (depending on primary treatment) | Fluorouracil<br>Chlorambucil<br>Thiotepa<br>Melphalan |
| Pancreatic adenocarcinoma[c] | Fluorouracil | Mitomycin<br>Doxorubicin | Tegafur[a] |
| Prostate | Stilbestrol | Cyclophosphamide<br>Doxorubicin | Estramustine |

*[Continued over]*

**Table XI.** *[Continued]*

| Cancer type | Drugs currently preferred | Alternative or secondary drugs | Other drugs with reported activity |
|---|---|---|---|
| Sarcomas, miscellaneous | Doxorubicin + dacarbazine[b] | Cyclophosphamide<br>Vincristine | Methotrexate<br>Ifosfamide[a] |
| Testicular | Vinblastine + ifosfamide + cisplatin *or*<br>Etoposide + bleomycin + cisplatin | Melphalan (seminoma only)<br>Doxorubicin<br>Bleomycin | |
| Brain neoplasms, primary | Carmustine *or*<br>Lomustine | PCV [procarbazine[d] + lomustine (CCNU) + vincristine]<br>Teniposide + carmustine | Plicamycin (mithramycin)[b] |
| Choriocarcinoma (testicular, ovarian or gestational) | Methotrexate *or*<br>Dactinomycin (gestational only)<br>Etoposide + cisplatin | Vinblastine<br>Chlorambucil | |
| Renal cell[c] | Medroxyprogesterone | Vinblastine | Interferon-α |

a Available only for investigational use in the US.
b Not approved for this indication by the US FDA for oligodendrogliomas.
c Chemotherapy considered ineffective by some authorities.
d For oligoendrogliomas.
*Abbreviation:* IT = intrathecal.

effectiveness, although long term remissions are rare. Chemotherapeutic agents have been ineffective, even if some responses have been reported with *floxuridine* in circadian or infusion regimens, and rarely with *vinblastine*.

#### 4.6.11 Central Nervous System (CNS) Tumours

Primary tumours of the brain include both lymphomas and malignant gliomas. The sensitivity of primary lymphomas to treatment is similar to that of lymphomas arising from nodal sites. Gliomas in adults are generally of a higher grade than in paediatric age groups, and occur in supratentorial locations. Treatment consists of radiation, with *nitrosoureas* playing a small secondary role. Oligodendrogliomas have recently been identified to be chemosensitive to several drugs, with reproducibly good results having been achieved with procarbazine, lomustine (CCNU), and vincristine (PCV).[151]

#### 4.6.12 Endocrine and Miscellaneous Cancers

##### Thyroid Cancer

Thyroid cancers in persons <50 years of age are generally associated with prolonged survival, even when presenting with metastatic disease. Anaplastic carcinomas arising in older patients require aggressive local and systemic treatment, but survival is dismal. Whenever possible, thyroidectomy followed by radioiodine has been the conventional approach. Thyroid suppression may delay and inhibit tumour progression. Chemotherapy with *cisplatin* and *doxorubicin* is occasionally effective.

##### Islet Cell Cancers and Carcinoids

Islet cell cancers and carcinoids are associated with important systemic syndromes reflecting the overproduction of endocrine products; in addition, tumour manifestations related to liver involvement are not infrequent. Systemic or locally directed (via hepatic artery) infusion of chemotherapy may be effective, as is chemoembolisation. Drugs such as *streptozocin, doxorubicin, dacarbazine, fluorouracil,* and *cisplatin* have been commonly used.[92,152,153]

##### Hepatocellular Cancer

Hepatocellular cancer is important because of its high frequency in persons originating from areas where hepatitis is endemic. Its treatment consists of surgical resection whenever possible, and this approach has been increasingly used. Chemotherapy, however, has been disappointing.

##### Neuroendocrine Tumours

Neuroendocrine tumours occur at various sites, but are also of unknown primary origin. Tumours of unknown primary origin have a prognosis that varies with places of involvement and site of disease at diagnosis, with the neuroendocrine histology or the presence of markers such as β-human chorionic gonadotrophin or α-fetoprotein carrying a chance of complete response to chemotherapy based on cisplatin.

## 4.7 Childhood Solid Tumours

### *4.7.1 Wilms' Tumour*

Combined modality treatment has become well established in this disease of the first years of life. Initially, radiation and *dactinomycin* (actinomycin D) conveyed benefit. Subsequent trials have focused on neoadjuvant approaches, eliminating the use of radiation and its deleterious long term effects on growth, and adding other drugs such as the *vinca alkaloids* and *doxorubicin*. Nearly all paediatric patients may now be cured through such combined modalities, but the results in adults and in some histological subtypes continue to be less favourable.[154]

### *4.7.2 Neuroblastoma*

This tumour also occurs in a similar age group, but shows less chemocurability. Biological characteristics of poor prognosis have been linked to stage and age at presentation, and the presence of amplification of the myc oncogene. Strategies in these poor prognosis tumours include high-dose chemotherapy with cytokine and bone marrow/stem cell support.[155]

### *4.7.3 Rhabdomyosarcoma*

Cooperative group trials in Europe and US have systematically established the role of chemotherapy as part of combined modality treatment in various sites of disease. Prognostic factors have been well characterised, with parameningeal tumours having the worst outlook.[156] Chemotherapy with *doxorubicin, ifosfamide,* and *vincristine* plays an increasing role in sparing young children from disfiguring surgery or growth retarding radiation. Long term cures in over 80% of patients with less morbidity are increasingly being achieved. Poor prognosis is related to overexpression of MDR 1 gene.[157]

### *4.7.3 Other Tumours*

#### Ewing's Sarcoma and Peripheral Neuroectodermal Tumour (PNET)

These tumours are considered together because chromosomal changes have indicated a common genetic origin (an 11,22 translocation). Combined chemotherapy, surgery and radiation offer the only possibilities for cure.

#### Retinoblastoma

Study of the genetics of this disease of infancy was instrumental in identifying the RB gene in chromosome 11 that was an essential step in understanding tumour suppressor genes. Treatment consists of surgery with other modalities playing a role in advanced or recurrent disease.

#### CNS Tumours

Medulloblastomas are tumours with a propensity for meningeal spread. They are radiosensitive and chemosensitive, although chemotherapy is not fully integrated into its front-line management. Gliomas of childhood are an important cause of morbidity, but have a better prognosis than in adults.

## 4.8 Haematological Malignancies

### *4.8.1 Hodgkin's Disease*

Combination chemotherapy in Hodgkin's disease (table XI) became firmly established following the demonstration of its curative potential in the late 1960s and early 1970s.[158] Long term sequelae of chemotherapy have also been studied in these patients, and include effects on fertility, chronic organ dysfunction (lungs, heart, bone marrow), and, most importantly, secondary malignancies including both acute leukaemias and some solid tumours. For all these complications, the combination of radiation and chemotherapy accounts for an enhanced risk over that with chemotherapy alone. Combinations of *doxorubicin, bleomycin, vinblastine*, and *dacarbazine* (ABVD) are more effective and less toxic than the initial combination of *chlormethine* (mustine), *vincristine* (Oncovin) *procarbazine*, and *prednisone* (MOPP), with a long term survival of 84% versus 64% for MOPP.[159] Other potentially less toxic combinations deserve testing. However, most current clinical trials are confined to salvage settings, since many years of follow-up are required to demonstrate improvement over standard therapies in the setting of initial treatment.

### *4.8.2 Non-Hodgkin's Lymphomas*

This term includes a broad range of conditions that vary greatly in prognosis and to some extent in treatment approaches.[160] Recognition of the variable course these conditions may have is reflected in part in the classifications that describe them: low grade, intermediate grade, and high grade lymphomas.

In general, low grade lymphomas are sensitive to *anthracycline* drugs, but *interferon-α* has also been shown to play a role. Intermediate grade lymphomas, particularly the more common diffuse histiocytic type, are curable by combination chemotherapies including *doxorubicin, vinca alkaloids, etoposide, bleomycin*, and the antimetabolites *cytarabine* and *methotrexate*.

Randomised studies have shown the effectiveness of CHOP [*cyclophosphamide, doxorubicin* (hydroxydaunorubicin), *vincristine* (Oncovin), and *prednisone*] to be comparable to that of other combinations appearing a decade later. Recent efforts at subclassifying these tumours continues, since tumour biology is now better understood through the study of cell surface markers, chromosomal translocations, oncogenes and clonal identification. Improvements in understanding of tumour biology is being applied in high-dose strategies developed for patients where sensitivity to chemotherapy persists. The long term survivors in these unselected series may vary from 40 to 60% of patients.[161]

#### 4.8.3 Chronic Lymphocytic Leukaemia

For many years, treatment of this chronic leukaemia did not substantially change and relied primarily on remissions induced by alkylating agents. More recently, nucleoside analogues [fludarabine, pentostatin and cladribine (chlorodeoxyadenosine)] have provided other effective tools, with responses approaching the 60% initial response rates of chlorambucil and prednisone, and perhaps better therapeutic indices resulting.[162,163] Unfortunately, cross-resistance may exist between fludarabine, pentostatin and cladribine.

#### 4.8.4 Myeloproliferative Diseases

The treatment of chronic myeloid leukaemia (CML) has undergone evolution with the introduction of *interferon*-$\alpha$[164] and the verification of karyotypic complete remission (i.e. absence of the Philadelphia chromosome, which would indicate that all cells that could give rise to recurrent CML have been eradicated). Another strategy that has enjoyed some success is high-dose chemotherapy and autologous bone marrow support during complete response. Such manoeuvres may delay or avoid the otherwise inexorable development of the accelerated phase. At this stage, sensitivity to *busulfan* and *hydroxycarbamide* (hydroxyurea) decreases, with only brief remissions obtained with antimetabolites and vinca alkaloids used in acute leukaemia.

Other myeloproliferative disorders, including polycythaemia vera are often treated with *hydroxycarbamide* and less often with alkylating agents. Acute leukaemia represents a common fatal complication.

#### 4.8.5 Acute Myeloid Leukaemias

The French-American classification is commonly used to group these leukaemias into 7 different types, and has been well integrated into biological and karyotypical characteristics. The M2 or promyelocytic type has assumed special importance because of its sensitivity to *all-trans retinoic acid*, an example of a differentiation therapy. This biological effect may be related to the chromosomal break point at the retinoic acid receptor-$\alpha$. Anthracyclines also induce durable complete responses in this leukaemia.

Other myeloid leukaemias are treated with combinations of *cytarabine* and DNA intercalating drugs, such as *anthracyclines* or *mitoxantrone*. An unfavourable prognosis is conveyed by advanced age, pronounced leucocytosis and identifiable causative factors, such as prior radiation or chemotherapy. Autologous and allogeneic bone marrow transplantation have shown favourable results in selected cohorts.

#### 4.8.6 Acute Lymphocytic Leukaemias

These are the predominant leukaemias in childhood, and historically represent the first targets for curative chemotherapeutic strategies. Complete responses were first obtained with the antifolates such as *methotrexate* and eventually regimens relied on *vincristine* plus *prednisone*, and consolidation with *mercaptopurine* and *methotrexate*.[33] Intrathecal methotrexate is used prophylactically to avoid meningeal disease. Most children fall into favourable prognostic categories, achieving an 80% event-free survival at 4 years.[165] Patients at high risk for relapse or not achieving complete response may have their treatment further consolidated with *teniposide, anthracyclines* and *cytarabine*. Adults have a poorer outlook, but may achieve up to 60% event-free survival with aggressive chemotherapy.[166]

#### 4.8.7 Multiple Myeloma

Osteolytic bone disease, paraproteinaemia and plasma cells in the bone marrow, and many morphological abnormalities constitute the hallmarks of this disease. Treatment has consisted almost uniformly of the alkylating agent *melphalan*, with higher doses given by the intravenous route leading to more durable remissions and median survival between 2 and 3 years. Recently, combinations with *vincristine* and *doxorubicin* have been used with some increase in complete responses, but median survival continues to fall short of 4 years.[167]

However, the patients do not achieve more than partial declines in paraprotein and eventually succumb to complications, including renal failure, hypercalcaemia, infection and haematological failure. Again, high-dose marrow-ablative regimens have also been tried with only preliminary evidence of promising effectiveness. Bisphosphonates have been shown to prolong survival in recent randomised trials.[168]

## 5. Clinical Outcome and Economic Considerations

The expansion in drug treatment of cancer and in supportive care measures has brought with it concerns over the cost-effectiveness of applying treatment in a wide range of circumstances. Concerns are greatest when treatment is not curative, must be maintained for long periods of time, and when expensive investigative approaches are introduced, but a favourable outcome is achievable in only a minority of patients. Debates on costs will, hopefully, not inhibit the type of clinical investigations that have provided the foundation for currently successful approaches. Clearly, in any universally applied cost-containment effort, provisions must be made to encourage participation in clinical trials as a means to seek solutions for difficult dilemmas of cost escalation with less than adequate documentation of results.

Cost-effectiveness analyses in oncology have been concerned primarily with:

1) Supportive care measures during conventional chemotherapy.

2) Conventional chemotherapy in situations deemed of ‘borderline’ value.

3) Adjuvant chemotherapy in situations where benefit may be confined in a small subset of patients (e.g. node-negative breast cancer).

4) High-dose chemotherapy with autologous bone marrow support.

### 5.1 Cost-Effectiveness of Chemotherapy and Supportive Care in Advanced Cancer

Reluctance to pay for cancer treatments that have not been approved by government agencies has brought this issue into sharp focus. Although many treatments have often exhibited varying degrees of antitumour activity, some totally negative results and uncertain effects on survival abound in patients with dire prognoses. The ethical dilemma becomes greater as the expense escalates.

Trials comparing best supportive care (BSC) *versus* conventional chemotherapy for advanced *non-small cell lung cancer* – a situation where effectiveness has been the subject of debates – have been carried out, including assessment of economic effects and quality of life.[169] In this situation, a small, statistically significant improvement in median survival (8 and 12.8 weeks, respectively) in patients receiving chemotherapy was demonstrated to be cost effective when compared with best supportive care. The cost incurred during the treatment of 50 patients with advanced *breast cancer* has also been retrospectively analysed. This study from an oncology unit in the UK concluded that with a median and mean duration of disease of 17 months and 27 months, respectively (range 7 days to 12 years), the mean cost per patient was £7620. Inpatient days averaged 32 and represented 56% of all costs, and most of the time (>80%) was spent on the care of serious illnesses rather than being treatment associated.[169]

A more expensive example of both treatment and accompanying supportive care costs is acute leukaemia of adults. Not only are diagnostic costs greater, but attempts at chemotherapy induction could dramatically increase costs. A retrospective analysis of 2 studies indicated that costs per patient were related to how promptly complete remission could be achieved. If complete remission took 2 courses, the costs went from US$16,000 to >US$37,000.[170] Therefore, any innovation that brings about an improvement in the rate of complete remissions, either through better selection or new drugs, could decrease costs dramatically.

Another chemotherapy responsive disease such as *small cell lung cancer* has also been the subject of investigation, with conclusions that costs were mostly associated with hospitalisation for palliation and disease progression.[171] This disease has also been the target of analysis of hospitalisations due to treatment and avoidance of complications through cytokines such as *granulocyte colony-stimulating factor* (G-CSF).[123] A similar analysis has been performed for the cytoprotector *amifostine* in patients with advanced ovarian cancer treated with cisplatin plus cyclophosphamide.[48] The cumulative number of days in the hospital for complications did not exceed 10 for the amifostine group but exceeded 80 by the sixth course of therapy without amfostine.[48]

Analyses of the economic benefits of *antiemetics* have also been attempted. Routine administration of these compounds has escalated costs of chemotherapy and comparisons of costly, more effective treatments with cheaper, less effective regimens have been carried out.[172] Costs were nearly the same in both groups of a prospective study if 'rescue' costs are included. This study clearly highlighted the dangers of basing decisions 'purely on the narrow basis of drug costs alone' leading to 'inefficient use of resources'.[173]

Several analyses of cost effectiveness have been made among various subsets of patients treated for *early breast cancer* but with no evident disease. Age over 70 years is associated with a considerable increase in costs when taking into account effects on active life expectancy.[174] Quality-months were used as an end-point to assess cost effectiveness in women with node-negative breast cancer. Another example in cost effectiveness applicable to the setting of adjuvant colorectal cancer was provided over the debate on levamisole costs in humans relative to costs of veterinary use. The issue may be moot, since recent adjuvant studies indicate that calcium folinate (leucovorin) may replace levamisole without a loss of efficacy.

An extreme situation concerning potential benefit *versus* costs is faced in treating *metastatic renal cell carcinoma*. All measures in the treatment of this disease have been considered investigational.[175] Recently, however interleukin-2 was approved for its treatment in the US. This treatment is expensive and only benefits a minority of patients. Other investigational approaches clearly need to be studied and must be considered 'best available therapy'. A continued commitment of society's resources to clinical trials is, therefore, required to make further progress.

On the other hand, some authorities have cautioned against the adoption of the technological imperative. For example, 'because we can now insert Infusaid pumps for infusion of hepatic metastases does not mean that we should do so without a rational evaluation of the benefit to the patient'.[176] In this example, patients with colon cancer and liver metastases were found to derive a limited (and in some trials non-significant) prolongation of life compared with systemic therapy. Newer treatments such as chemoembolisation and cryotherapy have since been introduced for this clinical problem, re-emphasising the need for cost and quality of life analyses before widespread uncritical adoption.

### 5.2 Cost Effectiveness of High-Dose Chemotherapy with Bone Marrow Support

High-dose chemotherapy with marrow support represents the ultimate example of drug costs and 'technological imperatives'. Certain rules have emerged for successful medical applications. There must be:

1) A known chemosensitive tumour.

2) Drugs amenable to escalation without incurring nonhaematological toxicity.

3) A fit host without pre-existing diminished end-organ (e.g. pulmonary, renal, cardiac) reserve.

In one cost-effectiveness study in the US, the higher costs from bone marrow transplantation per life-year became nearly equivalent to those from conventional chemotherapy because of the better rate of disease-free survival in the former group.[177] Recent analyses have also been carried out in Hodgkin's disease and non-Hodgkin's lymphoma treated with various degrees of marrow support and/or cytokines.[178,179] The more rapid bone marrow support recovery in these and in subsequent studies from the use of cytokines and peripheral blood progenitor cells (CD34+ cells) have resulted in drastic reductions in costs in such high-dose settings. However, extending these procedures to conditions not adequately meeting requirements for obtaining patient benefit remains problematic. Clinical trials are attempting to resolve these issues in a somewhat less sensitive and more common tumour type such as metastatic breast cancer. Decision analyses with a review of costs within individual units may identify ways to substantially cut costs or alter eligibility criteria.

These and other cost analyses of oncological treatments have been performed during the last decade. The results have not been used (and correctly so, because of the exploratory nature of such retrospective analyses) to set policy, but to highlight the issues involved. As described, they vary greatly among the therapeutic areas covered. Understanding the issues may result in cost-saving measures including better selection of patients likely to benefit. Patient benefit must not be viewed as stationary data and is preferably assessed through prospective clinical trials. Quality of life issues are best studied in this setting comparing 2 treatment strategies. Selection of the appropriate end-points is the key to such analyses and is very much dependent on the clinical situation. Drug costs are generally only a small facet of cost-effectiveness estimates, but are the ones most easily targeted by governmental agencies and controlled by private institutions.

## 6. Use of Drugs in the Presence of Associated Malignant Disease

The most commonly used drugs given together with anticancer agents are antiemetics and analgesics. In general, these drugs show little tendency to give rise to problematic interactions. With the exception of aminoglycosides, antibiotics are also generally free of problems. The aminoglycosides may give rise to acute renal failure when given in conjunction with cisplatin, and cisplatin may lead to renal insufficiency even weeks after the patient has received aminoglycosides.

Phenytoin has been notorious in giving rise to exfoliative dermatitis in the setting of brain irradiation. Thiazides and loop diuretics may compound electrolyte abnormalities associated with the administration of cisplatin (particularly in a daily 5-day schedule) and the hydration that is required.

Patients with sensitive tumours – such as lymphomas or leukaemias – and large tumour burdens may have life-threatening and even fatal complications from sudden lysis of cells and an extra load of potassium, phosphate, urates and lactic acid (tumour lysis syndrome).

In experimental studies, the presence of a tumour has been shown to modify the metabolic capacity of the host, resulting in alterations in the distribution, elimination and consequent pharmacological activity of drugs administered.[180] However, the implications of these findings in humans need further study. Interactions can occur between anticancer drugs and other classes of drugs, and between different anticancer drugs (see appendix B and review by Loadman and Bibby[20]). The latter may be additive, synergistic or antagonistic, and may occur due to modifications of the distribution and elimination of other anticancer drugs, or through non-pharmacokinetic mechanisms.[180]

Drugs that may cause anaemia, leucopenia or thrombocytopenia (see chapter 26; sect. 5 and 6), and immunosuppressive agents are best avoided in cancer patients, who tend to be cytopenic and immunosuppressed as a result of their disease or its treatment.

## References


1. Nowell PC. The clonal evolution of tumor cell populations. Science 1976; 194: 23-8
2. Aaronson SA. Growth factors and cancer. Science 1991; 254: 1146-53
3. Roselli M, Guadagni F, Buonomo O, et al. Systemic administration of recombinant interferon alfa in carcinoma patients upregulates the expression of the carcinoma-associated antigens tumor-associated glycoprotein-72 and carcinoembryonic antigen. Journal of Clinical Oncology 1996; 14: 2031-42
4. Hunter T, Pines J. Cyclins and cancer. Cell 1991; 66: 1071-4
5. Eastman A. Activation of programmed and unprogrammed cell death. Toxicology and Applied Pharmacology 1993; 121: 160-4
6. Knudson AG. Mutation and cancer: statistical study of retinoblastoma. Proceedings of the National Academy of Science of the USA 1971; 68: 820
7. Wong M, Gruber J. Viral interactions with the p53 gene in human cancer: NCI Workshop. Journal of the National Cancer Institute 1994; 86: 177-82
8. Harris CC. p53: at the crossroads of molecular carcinogenesis and risk assessment. Science 1993; 262: 1980-1
9. Li F, Fraumeni J. Prospective study of a family cancer syndrome. Journal of the American Medical Association 1982; 247: 1692-4
10. Weichselbaum RR, Beckett M, Diamond A. Some retinoblastomas, osteosarcomas, and soft tissue sarcomas may share a common etiology. Proceedings of the National Academy of Science USA 1988; 85: 2106-9
11. Hollstein M, Sidransky D, Vogelstein B, et al. p53 mutations in human cancer. Science 1991; 253: 49-53
12. Coppes MJ et al. Genetic events in the development of Wilms' tumor. New England Journal of Medicine 1994; 331: 586
13. Collins FC. BRCA1: lots of mutations, lots of dilemmas. New England Journal of Medicine 1996; 334: 186-8;Miki Y, Sensen J, et al. A strong candidate for the breast and ovarian cancer susceptibility gene BRCA1. Science 1994; 266: 66-71
14. Ionov Y, Peinado MA, Malkhosyan S, et al. Ubiquitous somatic mutations in simple repeated sequences reveal a new mechanism for carcinogenesis. Nature 1993; 363: 558-61
15. Ross RK, Bernstein L, Shimuzu H, et al. Evidence for reduced 5-alpha-reductase activity in Japanese compared to US White and Black males: implications for prostate cancer risk. Lancet 1992; 339: 887-9
16. Spicer D, Ursin G, Parisky YR, et al. Changes in mammographic densities induced by a hormonal contraceptive designed to reduced breast cancer risk. Journal of the National Cancer Institute 1994; 86: 431-6
17. Henderson BE, Pike MC. Hormonal chemoprevention of cancer in women. Science 1993; 259: 633-8
18. Yu MC, Skipper PL, Taghizadeh K, et al. Acetylator phenotype, aminobiphenyl-hemoglobin adduct levels and bladder cancer risk in White, Black and Asian men in Los Angeles, California. Journal of the National Cancer Institute 1994; 86: 712-6
19. Sporn MB. Chemoprevention of cancer. Lancet 1993; 342: 1211-3
20. Loadman PM, Bibby MC. Pharmacokinetic drug interactions with anticancer drugs. Clinical Pharmacokinetics 1994; 26: 486-500
21. DelaFlor-Weiss E, Uziely B, Muggia FM. Protracted drug infusions in cancer treatment: an appraisal of

5-fluorouracil, doxorubicin, and platinums. Annals of Oncology 1993; 4: 723-33
22. Borden EC. Interferons expanding therapeutic roles. New England Journal of Medicine 1992; 326: 1491
23. Evans WE, Rodman JH, Relling MV, et al. Concept of maximum tolerated systemic exposure and its application to phase I-II studies of anticancer drugs. Medical Pediatric Oncology 1991; 19: 153-9
24. Calvert AH, Gumbrell LA, et al. Carboplatin dosing; prospective evaluations of a simple formula based on renal function. Journal of Clinical Oncology 1989; 7: 1748-56
25. Lu Z, Zhang R, Diasio RB. Dihydropyrimidine dehydrogenase activity in human peripheral blood mononuclear cells and liver: population characteristics, newly identified deficient patients, and clinical implications in 5-fluorouracil chemotherapy. Cancer Research 1993; 53: 5433-8
26. Simon R, Korn EL. Selecting drug combinations based on total equivalent dose (dose intensity). Journal of the National Cancer Institute 1990; 82: 1469-76
27. O'Quigley J, Pepe M, Fisher L. Continual reassessment method: a practical design for phase I clinical trials in cancer. Biometrics 1990; 46: 33-48
28. Newell DR. Pharmacologically based phase I trials in cancer chemotherapy. In: Muggia FM, Speyer JL (editors). New drug therapy. Hematology/Oncology Clinics of North America. Philadelphia: WB Saunders, 1994: 257-75
29. Shimada Y, Yoshino M, Wakui A, et al. A late phase II study of CPT-11, a new camptothecin derivative, in metastatic colorectal cancer. Journal of Clinical Oncology 1993; 11: 909-13
30. Casper ES, Green MR, Kelsen DP, et al. Phase II trial of gemcitabine (2,2'-difluorodeoxycytidine) in patients with adenocarcinoma of the pancreas. Investigational New Drugs 1991; 12: 29-34
31. Rizzo J, Levine A, Weiss G, et al. Pharmacokinetics of MGBG (methylglyoxal(bis)guanylhydrazone) in patients with AIDS-related non-Hodgkin's lymphoma [abstract]. Proceedings of the American Society of Clinical Oncology 1994; 13: 149
32. Sartorelli AC. Some approaches to the therapeutic exploitation of metabolic sites of vulnerability of neoplastic cells. Cancer Research 1969; 29: 2292
33. Farber S. Chemotherapy in the treatment of leukemia and Wilms' tumor. Journal of the American Medical Association 1966; 198: 826
34. Schabel Jr FM, Griswold Jr DP, Laster WR, et al. Quantitative evaluation of anticancer agent activity in experimental animals. Pharmacology and Therapeutics 1977; 1: 411-35
35. Huggins C, Bergenstal DM. Inhibition of human mammary and prostatic cancer by adrenalectomy. Cancer Research 1952; 12: 134
36. Norton L, Simon R. The Norton-Simon hypothesis revisited. Cancer Treatment Reports 1986; 70: 163-9
37. Ling V. P-glycoprotein and resistance to anticancer drugs. Cancer 1992; 69; 2603-9
38. Los G, Muggia FM. Platinum resistance: experimental and clinical status. Hematology/Oncology Clinical of North America 1994; 8: 411-429
39. Fisher GA, Lum BL, Sikio BI. The reversal of multidrug resistance. In: Muggia FM, editor. Concepts, mechanisms and new targets for chemotherapy. Boston: Kluwer Academic Publishers, 1995
40. Bertino JR. Karnofsky Memorial Lecture: ode to methotrexate. Journal of Clinical Oncology 1993; 11: 15
41. Los G, Muggia FM. Platinum resistance: experimental and clinical status In: Muggia & Speyer, editors. New drug therapy; Hematology-Oncology Clinics of North America. Philadelphia: Saunders, 1994
42. Cole SPC, Bhardwaj G, Gerlach GH, et al. Overexpression of a transporter gene in multidrug-resistant human lung cancer cell line. Science 1992; 258: 1650
43. Saha S, Hoddinott M, Arora M, et al. Therapeutic implications of a chemoresistance assay for management of solid tumors [abstract]. Proceedings of the American Society of Clinical Oncology 1995; 14: 183
44. Rowinsky EK, Donehower RC. Drug therapy: paclitaxel. New England Journal of Medicine 1995; 332: 1004-14
45. Aschele C, Sobrero A, Faberen MA, et al. Novel mechanisms of resistance to 5-fluorouracil in human colon cancer (HCT-8) sublines following exposure to two different clinically relevant dose schedules. Cancer Research 1992; 52: 1855-64
46. Muggia FM. How to improve survival after diagnosis of gastric cancer? It's back to the drawing board. Journal of Clinical Oncology 1994; 11: 1437-9
47. Shea M, Koziol JA, Howell SB. Kinetics of thiosulfate, a cisplatin neutraliser. Clinical Pharmacology and Therapeutics 1989; 35: 419-25
48. Kemp G, Rose P, Lurain J, et al. Pretreatment for protection against cyclophosphamide-induced and cisplatin-induced toxicities: results of a randomised controlled trial in patients with advanced ovarian cancer. Journal of Clinical Oncology 1996; 14: 2101-12
49. Speyer JL, Green MD, Zeleniuch-Jacquotte A, et al. ICRF-187 permits longer treatment with doxorubicin in women with breast cancer. Journal of Clinical Oncology 1992; 10: 117-22
50. Steinherz LJ, Graham T, Hurwitz R, et al. Guidelines for cardiac monitoring of children during and after anthracycline therapy: report of the cardiology committee of the Children's Cancer Study Group. Pediatrics 1992; 89: 942-9
51. Muggia FM. Cytoprotection: concepts and challenges. Supportive Care 1994; 2: 377
52. Burris HA, Fields SM. Topoisomerase I inhibitors: an overview of camptothecin analogs. In: Muggia & Speyer, editors. New drug therapy; Hematology-Oncology Clinics of North America. Philadelphia: Saunders, 1994
53. Bertrand R, O'Conor PM, Kerrigan D, et al. Sequential administration of campothecin and etoposide circumvents the antagonistic cytotoxicity of simultaneous drug administration in slowly growing human carcinoma HT-29 cells. European Journal of Cancer 1992; 28A: 743-8
54. Baselga J, Norton L, Masui H, et al. Antitumor effects of doxorubicin in combination with antiepidermal growth factor receptor. Journal of the National Cancer Institute 1993; 85: 1327
55. Mitchell MS. Chemotherapy in combination with biomodulation: a 5-year experience with cyclophosphamide and interleukin-2. Semininars in Oncology 1992; 19 Suppl. 4: 80
56. Kotani H, Newton PB, Zhang S, et al. Improved methods of retroviral vector transduction and production for gene therapy. Human Gene Therapy 1994; 5: 19
57. McGuire WL. Hormone receptors. Their role in predicting prognosis and response to endocrine therapy. Seminars in Oncology 1978; 5: 428

58. Wiesenthal LM, Lippman ME. Clonogenic and non-clonogenic in vitro chemosensitivity assays. Cancer Treatment Reports 1985; 69: 615
59. Horikoshi T, Daneberg KD, Stadlbauer TH, et al. Quantitation of thymidylate synthase, dihydrofolate reductase, and dt-diaphorase gene expression in human tumors using the polymerase chain reaction. Cancer Research 1992; 52: 108-16
60. Chaudhary PM, Roninson IB. Induction of multidrug resistance in human cells by transient exposure to different chemotherapeutic drugs. Journal of the National Cancer Institute 1993; 85: 632-9
61. Esrig D, Elmajian D, Groshen S, et al. Accumulation of nuclear p53 and tumour progression in bladder cancer. New England Journal of Medicine 1994; 331: 1259-64
62. Hryniuk WM, Bush H. The importance of dose intensity in chemotherapy of metastatic breast cancer. Journal of Clinical Oncology 1984; 2: 1281
63. Crown J, Kritz A, et al. Rapid administration of multiple cycles of high-dose myelosuppressive chemotherapy in patients with metastatic breast cancer. Cancer Research 1993; 11: 1194-9
64. Frei III E. Clinical Cancer Research: embattled species. Cancer 1982; 50: 1797
65. Muggia FM, Blum RH, Foreman JD. Role of chemotherapy in the treatment of lung cancer: evolving strategies for non-small cell histologies. International Journal of Radiation Oncology and Biological Physics 1984; 10: 137
66. Wagener DTT, Biljham GH, Smeets JBE, et al., editors. Primary chemotherapy in cancer medicine. Progress in clinical and biological research. v. 201. New York: Alan R Liss, 1985
67. Elkind MM. Some principles for rational cell based development of combined radiation-drug therapy. Frontiers of Radiation Therapy and Oncology 1969; 4: 76
68. Ziegler JL, Muggia FM. Long term sequelae of cancer chemotherapy. In: Mathé G, Muggia FM, editors. Recent results of Cancer Research. v. 74. Berlin: Springer-Verlag, 1980
69. Sieber SM, Adamson RH. Toxicity of antineoplastic agents in man. Chromosomal aberrations, effects, congenital malformations and carcinogenic potential. Advances in Cancer Research 1975; 22: 57
70. Coleman CN, Williams CJ, Flint A, et al. Hematologic neoplasia in patients treated for Hodgkin's disease. New England Journal of Medicine 1977; 297: 1249
71. Harris JR, Veronesi U. Breast cancer. New England Journal of Medicine 1992; 327: 319, 390, 473
72. Pike MC. Age-related factors in cancer of the breast, ovary and endometrium. Journal of Chronic Diseases 1987; 40: 59
73. Slamon DJ, Clark GM, Wong SG. Correlation of relapse and survival with amplification of the HER-2/neu oncogene. Science 1987; 235: 177-82
74. Slamon DJ, Godolphin W, Jones LA, et al. Studies of the HER-2/neu proto-oncogene in human breast and ovarian cancer. Science 1989; 244: 707-12
75. Muss HB, Wood WC. c-erbB-2 expression and response to adjuvuant therapy in women with node-positive early breast cancer. New England Journal of Medicine 1994; 330: 1260
76. Henderson BE, Ross RK, Pike MC. Toward the primary prevention of cancer. Science 1991; 254: 1131-8
77. Friedman MA, Trimble EL, Abrams JS. Tamoxifen: trials, tribulations, and trade-offs. Journal of the National Cancer Institute 1994; 86: 478-9
78. Davidson NE. Tamoxifen: panacea or Pandora's box. New England Journal of Medicine 1992; 326: 885
79. Hunter DJ, Manson JE, Colditz GA, et al. A prospective study of the intake of vitamins C, E, and A and the risk of breast cancer. New England Journal of Medicine 1993; 329: 234-40
80. Fisher B, Redmond C, Fisher ER. Systemic adjuvant therapy in treatment of primary operable breast cancer: National Surgical Adjuvant Breast and Bowel Project experience. NCI Monograms 1986; 1: 35-46
81. Early Breast Cancer Trialists' Collaborative Group. Systemic treatment of early breast cancer by hormonal, cytotoxic, or immune therapy: 133 randomized trials involving 31,000 recurrences and 24,000 deaths among 75,000 women. Lancet 1992; 339: 1-15, 71-85
82. Wood WC. Dose and dose intensity of adjuvant chemotherapy for stage II node positive breast carcinoma. New England Journal of Medicine 1994; 330: 1253
83. Budman DR, Koizud AH, Cooper AR, et al. Dose and dose intensity of adjuvant chemotherapy for stage II node-positive breast carcinoma. New England Journal of Medicine 1994; 330: 1253-9
84. Hillner BE, Smith TJ, Desch CE. Efficacy and cost-effectiveness of autologous bone marrow transplantation in metastatic breast cancer. Journal of the American Medical Association 1992; 267: 2055-61
85. Seidman AD, Reichman BS, Crown JPA, et al. Paclitaxel as second and subsequent therapy for metastatic breast cancer: activity independent of prior anthracycline response. Journal of Clinical Oncology 1993; 11: 1943-51
86. Muggia FM. Search for the optimal treatment of ovarian cancer: heavy metals 'belly baths' and yew trees. Journal of Clinical Oncology 1992; 10: 683-5
87. Jensen EV, De Sombre ER, Jungblut PW. Estrogen receptors in hormone responsive tissues and tumors. In: Wissler et al., editors. Endogenous factors influencing host-tumor balance. Chicago: University Press, 1967
88. Heel RC, Brogden RN, Speight TM, et al. Tamoxifen: a review of its pharmacological properties and therapeutic use in breast cancer. Drugs 1978; 16: 1
89. Lipton A. The role of pamidronate. Annals of Oncology 1994; 5 Suppl. 7: 25
90. Hayes DF, Zurawski Jr VR, Kufe DW. Comparison of circulating CA 15-3 and carcinoembryonic antigen levels in patients with breast cancer. Journal of Clinical Oncology 1986; 4: 1542-50
91. Fearon ER, Vogelstein B. A genetic model for colorectal tumorigenesis. Cell 1990; 61: 759-67
92. Moertel CG, Fleming T, Macdonald J, et al. Levamisole and fluorouracil for adjuvant therapy of resected colon carcinoma. New England Journal of Medicine 1990; 322: 352-8
93. DeCosse JJ, Miller HH, Lesser ML. Effect of wheat fiber and vitamins C and E on rectal polyps in patients with familial adenomatous polyposis. Journal of the National Cancer Institute 1989; 81: 1290-7
94. Winawer SJ, Zauber AG, Ho MN, et al. Prevention of colorectal cancer by colonoscopic polypectomy. New England Journal of Medicine 1993; 329: 1977-81
95. Krook JE, Moertel CG, Gunderson L, et al. Effective surgical adjuvant therapy for high risk rectal carcinoma. New England Journal of Medicine 1991; 324: 709
96. Moertel CG. Chemotherapy for colorectal cancer. New England Journal of Medicine 1994; 330: 1136-42

97. Saltz L. Drug treatment of colorectal cancer: current results. Drugs 1991; 42: 616-27
98. Poon MA, O'Connell MJ, Moertel CG, et al. Biochemical modulation of fluorouracil: evidence of significant improvement of survival and quality of life in patients with advanced colorectal carcinoma. Journal of Clinical Oncology 1989; 7: 1407-7
99. Leichman CG, Fleming T, Muggia FM, et al. Phase II study of 5-FU and its modulation in advanced colorectal cancer. Journal of Clinical Oncology 1995; 13
100. Muggia FM, Groshen S. Adjuvant therapy of colon cancer: lessons while looking for breakthroughs. Annals of Oncology 1991; 2: 641-4
101. Kemeny N, Daly J, Reichman B, et al. Intrahepatic infusion of fluorodeoxyuridine in patients with liver metastases from colorectal carcinoma. Annals of Internal Medicine 1987; 107: 459-65
102. Minna JD, Ihde DC, Glatsein EJ. Lung cancer: scalpels, beams, drugs and probes. New England Journal of Medicine 1986; 315: 1411
103. Rodenhuis S, Slebos RJ, Boot AJM, et al. Incidence and possible clinical significance of K-ras oncogene activation in adenocarcinoma of the human lung. Cancer Research 1988; 48: 5738-41
104. Abrams J, Doyle LA, Aisner J. Staging, prognostic features, and special considerations in small cell lung cancer. Seminars in Oncology 1988; 15: 261-77
105. Alpha-Tocopherol, Beta Carotene Cancer Prevention Study Group. The effect of vitamin E and beta carotene on the incidence of lung cancer and other cancers in male smokers. New England Journal of Medicine 1994; 330: 1029-35
106. Marantz PR. Beta carotene, vitamin E, and lung cancer. New England Journal of Medicine 1994; 331: 611
107. Hong WK, Lippman S, Itri LM, et al. Prevention of second primary tumors with isotretinoin in squamous cell carcinoma of the head and neck. New England Journal of Medicine 1990; 323: 795-801
108. Mountain CF. Prognostic implications of the international staging system for lung cancer. Seminars in Oncology 1988; 15: 236-45
109. Rosell R, et al. Randomized trial comparing preoperative chemotherapy plus surgery with surgery alone in patients with non-small cell lung cancer. New England Journal of Medicine 1994; 330: 153.
110. Le Chevalier T, Brisgnad D, Douillard J-Y, et al. Randomized study of vinorelbine and cisplatin versus vindesine and cisplatin versus vinorelbine alone in advanced non-small-cell lung cancer: results of a European multicentre trial including 612 patients. Journal of Clinical Oncology 1994; 12: 360-7
111. van Zandwijk N, Rodenhuis S, Mooi W. New treatment opportunities in non-small cell lung cancer. Lung Cancer Ireland 1993; 9 Suppl. 2: S109-16
112. Murray N, Coy P, Pater JL, et al. Importance of timing for thoracic irradiation in the combined modality treatment of limited-stage small-cell lung cancer. Journal of Clinical Oncology 1993; 11: 336
113. Arriagada R. Initial chemotherapeutic doses and survival in patients with limited small-cell lung cancer. New England Journal of Medicine 1993; 329: 1848
114. Pignon J-P. Meta-analysis of thoracic radiotherapy for small-cell lung cancer. New England Journal of Medicine 1992; 327: 1618
115. Johnson DH, Turrisi AT, Chang AY, et al. Alternating chemotherapy and twice-daily thoracic radiotherapy in limited-stage small-cell lung cancer. A pilot study of the Eastern Cooperative Oncology Group. Journal of Clinical Oncology 1993; 11: 879
116. Weber BL. Susceptibility genes for breast cancer. New England Journal of Medicine 1994; 331: 1523
117. McGuire WL, Hoskins WJ, Brady MF, et al. A phase III trial comparing cisplatin/Cytoxan and cisplatin/Taxol in advanced ovarian cancer. Proceedings of the American Society of Clinical Oncology 1993; 12: 255 (Abstract No. 808)
118. Muggia FM. Managing breast cancer in an outpatient setting. Breast Cancer Research Treat 1992; 21: 27-34
119. Sikic BI. Modulation of multidrug resistance at the threshhold. Journal of Clinical Oncology 1993; 10: 679-82
120. Catalona WJ. Management of cancer of the prostate. New England Journal of Medicine 1994; 331: 996
121. Lange PH. Early detection of prostate cancer? Journal of the National Cancer Institute 1991; 83: 1199
122. Gormley GJ. Effect of finasteride in men with benign prostatic hyperplasia. New England Journal of Medicine 1992; 327: 1185
123. Crawford ED, Eisenberger MA, McLeod DG, et al. A controlled trial of leuprolide with and without flutamide in prostatic carcinoma. New England Journal of Medicine 1989; 321: 419-24
124. Geller J, Albert J, Vik J. Advantages of total androgen blockade in the treatment of advanced prostate cancer. Seminars in Oncology 1988; 15: 53-61
125. Myers CE, Cooper M, Stein C, et al. Suramin: a novel growth factor antagonist with activity in hormone-refractory metastatic prostate cancer. Journal of Clinical Oncology 1992; 10: 881
126. Scher HJ, Kelly WK. The flutamide withdrawal syndrome: its impact on clinical trials in hormone-refractory prostatic cancer. Journal of Clinical Oncology 1993; 11: 1566
127. Hudes GR, Greenberg R, Krigel RL, et al. Phase II study of estramustine and vinblastine, two microtubule inhibitors, in hormone-refractory prostate cancer. Journal of Clinical Oncology 1992; 10: 1754-61
128. Einhorn LH. Testicular cancer as a model for a curable neoplasm. Cancer Research 1981; 4: 3275
129. Motzer RJ, Bosl GJ. High-dose chemotherapy for resistant germ cell tumors: recent advances and further directions. Journal of the National Cancer Institute 1992; 84: 1703-9
130. Parsonnet J, Friedman GD, Vandersteen DP, et al. Helicobacter pylori infection and the risk of gastric carcinoma. New England Journal of Medicine 1991; 325: 1127-31
131. Leichman L, Silberman H, Leichman CG, et al. Preoperative systemic chemotherapy followed by adjuvant postoperative intraperitoneal therapy for gastric cancer: a University of Southern California pilot program. Journal of Clinical Oncology 1992; 10: 1933-42
132. Herskovic A. Combined chemotherapy and radiotherapy compared with radiotherapy alone in patients with cancer of the esophagus. New England Journal of Medicine 1992; 326: 1593
133. Dimery IW, Hong WK. Overview of combined modality therapies for head and neck cancer. Journal of the National Cancer Institute 1993; 85: 95-111
134. Merlano M, Vitali V, Rosso R, et al. Treatment of advanced squamous cell carcinoma of the head and neck with alternating chemotherapy and radiotherapy. New England Journal of Medicine 1992; 327: 1115-21

135. Hong WK, Wolf GT. Recent advances in head and neck cancer - larynx preservation and cancer chemoprevention: the Seventeenth Annual Richard and Hinda Rosenthal Lecture. Cancer Research 1993; 53: 5113-20
136. Stehman FB, Bundy BN. Carcinoma of the cervix treated with chemotherapy and radiation therapy: cooperative studies in the Gynecology Oncology Group. Cancer 1993; Suppl. 71: 1697-701
137. Lippman SM, Kavanagh JJ, Paredes-Espinoza M, et al. 13-cis-Retinoic acid plus interferon-α 2a in locally advanced squamous cell carcinoma of the cervix. Journal of the National Cancer Institute 1993; 85: 499-500
138. Meyskens Jr FL, Surwit E, Moon TE, et al. Enhancement of regression of cervical intraepithelial neoplasia II (moderate dysplasia) with topically applied all-trans-retinoic acid: a randomized trial. Journal of the National Cancer Institute 1994; 86: 539-43
139. Fisher B, Costantino JP, Redmond CK, et al. Endometrial cancer in tamoxifen-treated breast cancer patients: findings from the National Surgical Adjuvant Breast and Bowel Project (NSABP) B-14. Journal of the National Cancer Institute 1994; 86: 527-37
140. Ross RK, Paganini-Hill A, Landolph J, et al. Analgesics, cigarette smoking and other risk factors for cancer of the renal pelvis and ureter. Cancer Research 1989; 49: 1045-8
141. Muggia FM, Muderspach L. Platinum compounds in cervical and endometrial cancers: focus on carboplatin. Seminars in Oncology 1994; 21 Suppl. 2: 35-41
142. Seidman AD, Scher HI, Heinemann MH, et al. Continuous infusion gallium nitrate for patients with advanced refractory urothelial tract tumors. Cancer 1991; 68: 2561-5
143. Roth BJ, Dreicer R, Einhorn LH, et al. Significant activity of paclitaxel in advanced, transitional cell carcinoma of the urothelium: a phase II trial of the Eastern Cooperative Oncology Group. Journal of Clinical Oncology 1994; 12: 2264-76
144. Rosen G, Caparros B, Huvos AG, et al. Preoperative chemotherapy for osteogenic sarcoma. Selection of postoperative adjuvant chemotherapy based on the response of the primary tumor to preoperative chemotherapy. Cancer 1982; 49: 1221
145. Gottlieb JA, Baker LH, Quagliana JM, et al. Chemotherapy of sarcomas with a combination of adriamycin and dimethyl triazeno imidazole carboxamide. Cancer 1972; 30: 1632
146. Drobnjak M, Latres E, Pollack D, et al. Prognostic implications of p53 nuclear overexpression and high proliferation index of Ki-67 in adult soft-tissue sarcomas. Journal of the National Cancer Institute 1994; 86: 549
147. Oliner JD, Kinzler KW, Meltzer PS, et al. Amplification of a gene encoding a p53-associated protein in human sarcomas. Nature 1992; 358: 80-3
148. McClay E, Albright KD, Jones JA, et al. Modulation of cisplatin resistance in human malignant melanoma cells. Cancer Research 1992; 52: 6790
149. Cocconi G. Treatment of metastatic malignant melanoma with dacarbazine plus tamoxifen. New England Journal of Medicine 1992; 327: 516
150. Rusthoven JJ, Quirt IC, Iscoe NA, et al. Randomized, double-blind, placebo-controlled trial comparing the response rates of carmustine, dacarbazine and cisplatin with and without tamoxifen in patients with metastatic melanoma. Journal of Clinical Oncology 1996; 14: 2083-90
151. Peterson K, Cairncross JG. Oligodendroglioma. Cancer Investigation 1996; 14: 243-51
152. Moertel CG, Johnson M, McKusick MA, et al. The management of patients with advanced carcinoid tumors and islet cell carcinomas. Annals of Internal Medicine 1994; 120: 302-9
153. Moertel CG, Hanley JA, Johnson LA. Streptozotocin alone compared with streptozotocin plus fluorouracil in the treatment of advanced islet cell carcinoma. New England Journal of Medicine 1980; 303: 1189
154. Tournade MF, Commougue C, Voute PA, et al. Results of the 6th International Society of Pediatric Oncology Wilms' tumour trial and study – a risk-adapted approach in Wilms' tumor. Journal of Clinical Oncology 1993; 11: 1014-23
155. Brodeur GM, Seeger RC, Barrett A, et al. International criteria for diagnosis, staging and response to treatment in patients with neuroblastoma. Journal of Clinical Oncology 1988; 6: 1874
156. Maurer HM, Beltangady M, Gehon EA, et al. The Intergroup Rhabdomyosarcoma Study I: a final report. Cancer 1988; 61: 209
157. Chan HSL, DeBoer G, Thorner PS, et al. Multidrug resistance: clinical opportunities in diagnosis and circumvention. Hematology-Oncology Clinics of North America 1994; 8: 383-410
158. DeVita VT, Lewis BJ, Rozencweig M, et al. The chemotherapy of Hodgkin's disease: past experiences and future directions. Cancer 1978; 42: 979
159. Bonadonna G, Valagussa P, Santoro A. Alternating non-cross-resistant combination chemotherapy with ABVD or MOPP in stage IV Hodgkin's disease: a report of eight year results. Annals of Internal Medicine 1985; 104: 739-46
160. DeVita Jr VT, Canellos GP, Chabner B, et al. Advanced diffuse histiocytic lymphoma, a potentially curable disease. Results with combination chemotherapy. Lancet 1975; 1: 248
161. Philip T. Proceedings of the American Society of Clinical Oncology 1995; 14: 390
162. O'Brien S, Kantarjian H, Beran M, et al. Results of fludarabine and prednisone therapy in 264 patients with chronic lymphocytic leukaemia with multivariate analysis-derived prognostic model for response to treatment. Blood 1993; 82: 1695-1700
163. Tallman MS, Hakinion D, Zanzig C, et al. Cladribine in the treatment of relapsed or refractory CLL. Journal of Clinical Oncology 1995; 13: 983-8
164. Talpaz M, Kantarjian H, Kuzrock R, et al. Interferon-alpha produces sustained cytogenic responses in chronic myelogenous leukemia. Annals of Internal Medicine 1991; 114: 532-8
165. Miller D, Coccia P, Bleyer WA, et al. Early response to induction therapy as a predictor of disease-free survival and late-recurrence of childhood acute lymphoblastic leukemia: a report from CCSG. Journal of Clinical Oncology 1989: 7: 1807-15
166. Hoelzer D. Treatment of acute lymphoblastic leukemia. Seminars in Hematology 1994; 31: 1-15
167. Boccadoro M, Marmont F, Tribalto M, et al. Multiple myeloma: VMCP/VBAP alternating combination chemotherapy is not superior to melphalan and prednisone even in high-risk patients. Journal of Clinical Oncology 1991; 9: 444-8
168. Berenson JR, Lichtenstein A, Porter L, et al. Pamidronate disodium reduces the occurrence of skeletal-re-

lated events (SRE) in advanced multiple myeloma (MM). Blood 1994; 84 Suppl.: 386a

169. Richards MA, Braysher S, Gregory WM, et al. Advanced breast cancer: use of resources and cost implications. British Journal of Cancer 1993; 67: 856-60
170. Marie J-P, Wdowik T, Bisserbe S, et al. Cost of complete remission induction in acute myeloblastic leukemia: evaluation of the cost-effectiveness of a new drug. Leukemia 1992; 6: 720-2
171. Goodwin PJ, Feld R, Evans WK, et al. Cost-effectiveness of cancer chemotherapy: an economic evaluation of a randomized trial in small-cell lung cancer. Journal of Clinical Oncology 1988; 6: 1534-47
172. Cunningham D, Gore M, Davidson N, et al. The real cost of emesis – an economic analysis of ondansetron vs metoclopramide in controlling emesis in patients receiving chemotherapy for cancer. European Journal of Cancer 1993; 29A: 303-6
173. Goddard M. The real costs of emesis. European Journal of Cancer 1993; 29A: 297-8
174. Desch CE, Hillner BE, Smith TJ, et al. Should the elderly receive chemotherapy for node-negative breast cancer? A cost-effectiveness analysis examining total and active life expectancy outcomes. Journal of Clinical Oncology 1993; 111: 777-82
175. Gilewski T, Vogelzang N. Cost-effectiveness and reimbursement issues in renal cell carcinoma. Seminars in Oncology 1989; 16 Suppl. 1: 20-6
176. Macdonald EA. Cost-effectiveness of cancer chemotherapy: risk/benefit ratio, socio-economic and ethical considerations. Cancer Treatment Reviews 1987; 14: 345-50
177. Welch HG, Larson EB. Cost effectiveness of bone marrow transplantation in acute nonlymphocytic leukemia. New England Journal of Medicine 1989; 321: 807-12
178. Gulati S, Bennett C, Toia M, et al. Role of granulocyte-macrophage colony stimulating factor (GM-CSF) after autologous bone marrow transplantation for Hodgkin's disease. Anti-Cancer Drugs 1993; 4 Suppl. 1: 13-16
179. Zagonel V, Babare R, Merola MC, et al. Cost-benefit of granulocyte colony-stimulating factor administration in older patients with non-Hodgkin's lymphoma treated with combination chemotherapy. Annals of Oncology 1994; 5 Suppl. 2: S127-32
180. Garattini S, Donelli MG, Spreafico F. Specific problems in cancer chemotherapy - drug interaction. In: Proceedings of the 5th International Congress of Pharmacology, San Francisco, Vol. 3. Basel: Karger, 1973: 393

Chapter 28

# Immune System Disorders

*C.C. McCombs* and *R.D. deShazo*

## Synopsis of Important Principles

1) Although there are many diseases for which immune responses are clearly central to their pathogenesis, the initiating factors and control mechanisms are, more often than not, poorly understood.

2) Elucidation of some of the mechanisms involved in immune responses has, nevertheless, allowed an increasingly rational approach to the development of agents that modulate these responses. Many therapeutic agents are available to either suppress or enhance immune responsiveness.

3) Since many immune system disorders are chronic and debilitating, there is a propensity to 'try out' available agents, but the risks are often high and difficult to quantify, especially in the absence of controlled clinical trials.

4) The risk : benefit ratio of any proposed immunomodulatory therapy must be carefully considered for each patient. The potential adverse effects of immunomodulating agents necessitate close patient monitoring.

5) Aggressive immunosuppressive therapy requires good patient compliance and clinician vigilance to avoid serious problems. Disease flares need to be recognised and treated promptly.

6) Localised immunological or inflammatory processes should be treated with localised therapy when possible.

7) In using combinations of immunomodulatory drugs, selecting those with complementary actions and non-overlapping adverse effects can allow the use of lower doses of each, which may reduce the risk of adverse effects while improving efficacy.

8) Treatment of immune system disorders, and therapeutic manipulation of immune responses, will continue to be one of the fastest moving areas of medical research. Future advances will be based upon extensions of current successes, and upon the development of entirely novel strategies as the underlying mechanisms of immunity and immune disorders become better understood.

The importance of the immune system in the maintenance of health is evident from the devastating consequences of either primary immunodeficiencies or acquired immunodeficiency syndrome (AIDS), while lesser degrees of immune dysfunction may increase susceptibility to many infections and possibly to cancer. On the other hand, many clinical disorders, including autoimmune and inflammatory diseases, are characterised by aberrant immune reactivity. Transplantation of organ allografts also requires suppression of undesirable immunological responses to maintain the graft.

In the past three decades, significant advances have been made in the treatment of disorders characterised by either depressed or exaggerated immunity. Many therapeutic agents are available to either suppress or enhance immune responsiveness. An understanding of the mechanisms of action and pharmacological properties of immunotherapeutic agents will aid clinicians in appropriately employing these therapies.

## 1. Biology of the Immune Response and Targets for Pharmacological Intervention

In the last decade, knowledge of the mechanisms involved in immune responses has advanced at a phenomenal rate. Elucidating these mechanisms at a molecular level has allowed an increasingly rational approach to the discovery and development of drugs or agents that modulate immune responses. Most of the immunosuppressive drugs that have been in clinical usage for a long time were discovered by empiric processes. In the 1980s, a more rational approach developed, whereby extensive drug screening by *in vitro* studies was undertaken. For example, drugs potentially useful in organ transplantation were sought by screening for xenobiotics capable of suppressing mixed lymphocyte responses, an *in vitro* correlate of allograft reactions. The potent immunosuppressive drug tacrolimus (FK 506) was discovered through just such a screening programme.

As the mechanisms underlying immune responses were elucidated at a molecular level, more sophisticated drug discovery efforts have become possible. For instance, as cell surface receptors involved in signal transduction were identified, and their genes cloned, the development of agonists or antagonists to these receptors was able to proceed using cell lines transfected with the relevant genes. Identification of the specific molecular moieties of immunomodulatory drugs that mediate their pharmacological actions has also allowed rational drug design based on structure-activity relationships. Analogues of cyclosporin have been developed using this approach. The following overview of the biology of the immune response identifies some of the current and potential targets for pharmacological intervention.

### 1.1 Targets for Modulation of the Immune Response

#### Initial Interaction of the Immune System with Foreign Antigens

The earliest steps in the immune response involve antigen uptake, processing and presentation. Cells capable of these functions are collectively called 'antigen-presenting cells' (APCs), and include dendritic cells, monocytes, macrophages, and B lymphocytes. These cells take up proteins recognised as foreign, process them into peptide fragments, and present the peptides bound to HLA (human leucocyte antigen) molecules on their cell surfaces. At least one soluble mediator, interleukin-1 (IL-1) is produced by antigen-presenting cells, and enhances lymphocyte triggering.

A number of immunostimulating agents are believed to act at the stage of antigen processing and presentation, as do agents such as glucocorticosteroids and gusperimus (deoxyspergualin). Vaccines and adjuvants influence the immune response from the initial steps, introducing an antigen in a milieu designed to stimulate antigen presentation and recognition. Potential strategies for antigen-specific immunosuppression could act at this stage. For example, it has been suggested that peptides could be designed to occupy the antigen binding groove of HLA molecules, so as to inhibit binding of epitopes (antigenic determinants) involved in autoimmune responses.

#### T Cell Engagement and Signal Transduction

In a typical T cell-dependent immune response, the antigenic peptide, which is bound to the HLA molecule, interacts with an antigen-specific T cell receptor on the surface of a CD4+ T lymphocyte (a T helper cell). T cell receptors, or associated CD3 molecules, are the targets of a number of immunosuppressive monoclonal antibodies. These antibodies are thought to act by either physically blocking the antigen receptor, or by down regulation of the receptors on the lymphocyte surface. Engagement of the T cell receptor by peptide on the HLA molecule triggers a cascade of events, termed *signal transduction*, which results in the transcription of specific genes involved in T cell activation.

Several immunosuppressive drugs are known to act by inhibiting signal transduction. Cyclosporin and tacrolimus both inhibit the activity of *calcineurin*, a key enzyme in the signal transduction pathway. Signal transduction from antigen-specific T cell receptors alone, however, is not sufficient to functionally activate a CD4+ T lymphocyte. A 'costimulatory' signal is also required, and several receptor-ligand pairs capable of delivering such a signal from an antigen-presenting cell to a T lymphocyte have been identified. Antibodies to either the receptor or ligand of such pairs are under investigation as another route to preventing functional T cell activation. Blocking the transmission of a costimulatory signal is a very promising pharmacological target, as there is evidence that the interaction of antigen with the antigen-specific T cell receptor in the absence of a costimulatory signal can lead to a state of unresponsiveness or anergy.

#### T Cell Activation

In response to antigen and a costimulatory signal, T cell activation proceeds with the transcription of multiple genes, leading to the synthesis of cytokines, including interleukin-2 (IL-2), and increased expression of cell surface receptors for IL-2. The binding of IL-2 to IL-2 receptors is a central event leading to T cell proliferation and clonal expansion. This reaction is also a target for pharmacological interventions. Antibodies specific for the IL-2 receptor target activated T cells, and are useful in allograft antirejection therapy. IL-2 itself has been investigated for several clinical applications employing its ability to promote T cell activation and proliferation.

#### Cell Proliferation and Differentiation

The proliferation of T cells, B cells and other cell lineages involved in immune response is the target of nearly all drugs termed *cytotoxic agents*. Proliferation is often a necessary precursor of differentiation, so *antiproliferative agents* also act by preventing differentiation of cells at many points in the immune response. An understanding of the nucleic acid synthesis pathways in lymphocytes has allowed the development of cytotoxic agents that are relatively selective for lymphocytes.

#### Cell Recruitment and Trafficking

After antigen presentation and recognition, numerous events recruiting additional cells into the response and driving cell differentiation take place, largely coordinated by the production of cytokines. These events lead to the functional activation of the various effector cells responsible for immunological effects. B lymphocytes differentiate into plasma cells and produce the antibodies that are the basis of the humoral immune response. Cytotoxic T lymphocytes, primarily of the CD8+ subset, are among the principal effector cells of cell-mediated immune responses. Additional types of cells, not antigen-specific, that are involved in allergic and inflammatory reactions include neutrophils, eosinophils, basophils, and activated macrophages. The steps in the differentiation of each of these effector cell types are potential targets for pharmacological intervention. The xenobiotic immunosuppressive drug gusperimus (deoxyspergualin) is thought to act, at least in part, by affecting cell maturation, although the mechanism of the effect is, at this time, unknown.

Yet another aspect of the immune response that has potential for pharmacological intervention involves the role of 'adhesion molecules'. These comprise a diverse family of ligands and receptors that mediate cell-cell interactions, including the migration or 'trafficking' of cells to sites of inflammatory and immune reactions.

This brief overview of the biology of the immune response provides a basis for discussion of the pharmacology and clinical use of the principle immunomodulatory agents currently available.

## 2. Clinical Pharmacology of Immunomodulating Agents

### 2.1 Immunosuppressive Agents

#### *2.1.1 Cytotoxic Drugs*

Immunosuppressive drugs that act predominantly by interfering with some aspect of DNA synthesis and hence cell proliferation are commonly called cytotoxic drugs. Alternative terms are cytostatic, antiproliferative, or antimetabolic drugs. Their toxicity for rapidly dividing cells has given them a role in cancer chemotherapy, and in most cases they were developed for their antineoplastic effect and continue to be used for that purpose. Ironically, most are themselves potentially carcinogenic.

**Table I.** Important actions of various cytotoxic drugs

| Drug | Chemical class | Intracellular action | Cell types affected | Adverse effects |
|---|---|---|---|---|
| Azathioprine | Purine analogue | Inhibition of inosine monophosphate dehydrogenase, phosphoribosyl pyrophosphate amido transferase, and adenylosuccinate synthetase | All rapidly proliferating cells: T cells > B cells | Myelosuppression<br>Hepatotoxicity<br>Alopecia<br>Gastrointestinal intolerance<br>Infections<br>Malignancy |
| Cyclophosphamide | Nitrogen mustard derivative | Alkylating agent; crosslinks nucleic acid, preventing replication | All rapidly proliferating cells: B cells and monocyte lineage > T cells | Myelosuppression<br>Haemorrhagic cystitis<br>Alopecia<br>Gastrointestinal intolerance<br>Infections<br>Malignancy |
| Methotrexate | Folic acid antagonist | Inhibits dihydrofolate reductase and hence reduction of folic acid to tetrahydrofolic acid, and inhibits the synthesis of purines | All rapidly proliferating cells | Hepatotoxicity<br>Myelosuppression<br>Gastrointestinal effects, including bleeding<br>Pulmonary toxicity |
| Mizoribine | Imidazole nucleoside | Selectively inhibits inosine monophosphate dehydrogenase and hence *de novo* guanine ribonucleotide synthesis; depletes cells of guanine ribonucleotides | Lymphocyte and monocyte lineage > other proliferating cells | Gastrointestinal intolerance<br>Infections |
| Mycophenolate mofetil | Prodrug of mycophenolic acid | Selectively inhibits inosine monophosphate dehydrogenase and hence *de novo* guanine ribonucleotide synthesis | Lymphocyte and monocyte lineage > other proliferating cells | Gastrointestinal intolerance<br>Infections |
| Brequinar sodium | Antimetabolite (enzyme inhibitor) | Inhibits dihydro-orotate dehydrogenase and citidine deaminase; disrupts *de novo* pyrimidine synthesis | Lymphocyte and monocyte lineage > other proliferating cells | Gastrointestinal intolerance<br>Infections |

#### Mechanism/Site of Action

The earliest cytotoxic drugs used for immunosuppression, including *azathioprine*, *cyclophosphamide*, and *methotrexate*, have a broad spectrum of toxicity for proliferating cells. Newer agents, such as *mizoribine*, *mycophenolate mofetil* and *brequinar sodium* have a mechanism of action that is more selective for cells of the immune system.

The mechanisms of action of 6 cytotoxic drugs used for immunosuppression are compared in table I. Five of the six act, at least in part, by inhibiting nucleic acid synthesis at a metabolic level. The broad spectrum of action of azathioprine is due to the disruption of both the *de novo* and salvage pathways of purine synthesis. This affects the ability of all proliferating cells to generate precursors of DNA synthesis. A metabolite of azathioprine is incorporated into DNA, which may also interfere with DNA replication and function. Methotrexate also has a broad spectrum of action, as products of folate metabolism participate in biochemical reactions that result in the synthesis of DNA, RNA and various protein molecules. In addition to its effect as a competitive inhibitor of dihydrofolate reductase, methotrexate may inhibit a number of other enzymes involved in *de novo* purine biosynthesis, transmethylation of proteins, and neutrophil adherence and chemotaxis.[1]

Recently, immunosuppressive agents have been developed that selectively inhibit the *de novo* pathway of purine synthesis, rather than the salvage pathway. Lymphocytes are more dependent on the *de novo* pathway than are most other types of cells, so selectively disrupting *de novo* purine synthesis affects lymphoid cells more than other proliferating cells that can utilise the salvage pathway. Mycophenolate mofetil and mizoribine both inhibit inosine monophosphate dehydrogenase, a key enzyme in the *de novo* synthesis pathway.[2,3] Brequinar sodium inhibits *de novo* pyrimidine synthesis, and achieves a greater effect on lymphoid cells than myeloid cells through disruption of the pyrimidine as opposed to purine pathway. This mechanism of action is distinct from other immunosuppressive agents, and appears to result in a more pronounced effect on antibody synthesis than is seen with inhibitors of the purine synthesis pathway.[4]

The mechanism of action of cyclophosphamide differs markedly from the cytotoxic drugs discussed above. Cyclophosphamide is converted in the liver to active metabolites which act as alkylating agents. Alkylation of nucleic acids results in crosslinking that interferes with DNA replication and transcription. This results in a potent toxic effect on cells in the mitotic phase.

#### Pharmacodynamic Properties

The immunosuppression of cytotoxic drugs is due, at least in part, to interference with those stages of the immune response that require proliferation. This includes clonal expansion of T and B lymphocytes; in many cases, preventing replication also blocks differentiation and acquisition of an effector phenotype. The antiproliferative effect of cytotoxic drugs also inhibits the development of lymphocytes and monocytes from stem cells and precursors, thus limiting the number of cells available for an immune response.

Cytotoxic drugs often have additional immunological effects that appear to be independent of their antiproliferative action. For example, mycophenolate mofetil interferes with glycosylation of adhesion molecules, apparently because the depletion of guanosine triphosphate (GTP) inhibits the transfer of fucose and mannose to glycoproteins.[5] Methotrexate inhibits enzymes in addition to dihydrofolate reductase, and one consequence is the accumulation and enhanced release of adenosine, a potent inhibitor of neutrophil adherence.[6] Thus, cytotoxic drugs act at multiple stages of the immune response.

The major pharmacodynamic characteristics that provide the basis for selecting one cytotoxic drug over another are their intrinsic activity, risk of adverse effects, and clinical effectiveness. They are fairly similar in terms of their effects on immune responses, although cyclophosphamide is considered to affect B cell responses more than T cells, while the opposite is true for azathioprine. Brequinar sodium appears to suppress antibody synthesis more than other drugs in this class.

#### Pharmacokinetic Characteristics

Cytotoxic drugs may be administered orally, intramuscularly, or intravenously. They are often given in an intermittent or bolus dosage schedule. Compared with other immunosuppressive drugs, their clinical effects and toxicities may not become apparent for days to weeks after therapy is begun; thus they are sometimes termed 'slow-acting' agents. The cytotoxic drugs that have been in use for some time – azathioprine, cyclophosphamide and methotrexate – are often used in standardised dosages. This is feasible because of their wide therapeutic range and low pharmacokinetic variability. The pharmacokinetic characteristics of azathioprine, cyclophosphamide and methotrexate are discussed further in chapters 25 and 27, and their pharmacokinetic parameters are listed in appendix A (see under antineoplastic and immunosuppressive drugs).

*Brequinar sodium* has high oral bioavailability but exhibits a nonlinear (dose-dependent) pharmacokinetic profile. It appears to be eliminated mainly by hepatic metabolism, and has an elimination half-life varying from 1.5 to 8.2 hours.[7] *Mycophenolate mofetil* is also well absorbed after oral administration and is rapidly hydrolysed to the active moiety, mycophenolic acid.[8] Elimination occurs by conjugation to a glucuronide form which is excreted in the urine; its half-life after oral administration is around 11.6 hours.[9]

Following oral administration, *mizoribine* is converted to the active 5' phosphate form by intracellular phosphorylation. In patients with normal renal function, its elimination half-life is 4.7 hours. In the presence of renal dysfunction, the half-life is significantly prolonged, and the increase in plasma concentration is correlated with the degree of renal dysfunction.[10]

#### Clinical Effectiveness

All of the cytotoxic drugs discussed in this section have proven highly efficacious for the prevention or treatment of allograft rejection. They are usually used in combination regimens, which allows the use of reduced dosages of each agent (e.g. cyclophosphamide and corticosteroids) and achieves better efficacy with fewer adverse effects.[11] The cytotoxic drugs are not usually combined with each other, but there may be a rationale for combining brequinar sodium, which disrupts pyrimidine synthesis, with mycophenolate mofetil or mizoribine.[12,13] There has been less clinical experience with the newer, more lymphocyte-selective cytotoxic agents, but they appear to have reduced toxicity compared with azathioprine and cyclophosphamide.

Cyclophosphamide is the agent most commonly used to ablate lymphoid elements in patients who are to receive bone marrow transplants. Azathioprine, cyclophosphamide and methotrexate are used in the treatment of immune-mediated disorders, including severe, active and progressive rheumatoid arthritis.[14] Recent studies have demonstrated that methotrexate has a significantly better efficacy/toxicity profile than azathioprine, cyclophosphamide, or most other 'second-line' agents for the treatment of rheumatoid arthritis.[15-18]

The newer, more lymphocyte-selective agents, mizoribine, mycophenolate mofetil, and brequinar sodium, have had only limited use in autoimmune disorders to date, but their reduced toxicity compared with azathioprine and cyclophosphamide suggests that they may be substituted for these agents in the future. Brequinar sodium suppresses IL-4-induced synthesis of IgE *in vitro* in a dose-dependent manner, suggesting a possible role for this agent in the therapy of allergic disorders.[19]

**Tolerability and Drug Interactions Potential**

*Myelosuppression* is a relatively common, dose-related adverse effect of both azathioprine and cyclophosphamide.[20] In the case of azathioprine, leucopenia is most frequently observed, with thrombocytopenia, macrocytic anaemia and red blood cell aplasia occurring less frequently. Up to 50% of transplant recipients receiving azathioprine experience some degree of haematological toxicity. Bone marrow suppression with cyclophosphamide usually involves neutropenia or thrombocytopenia. Careful monitoring of complete blood counts in patients receiving these agents is therefore essential. As would be expected from the more lymphocyte-selective action of mizoribine, mycophenolate mofetil and brequinar sodium, myelosuppression has not been a problem in the early clinical experience with these agents.

*Hepatotoxicity*, both acute and chronic, is a significant adverse effect when azathioprine or methotrexate are used in higher dosages. Liver function tests, and sometimes liver biopsies, are advised for monitoring the effects of these drugs. However, with the lower doses used in the treatment of rheumatoid arthritis, hepatotoxicity is less common. Less than 1% of patients receiving azathioprine for rheumatoid arthritis experience hepatotoxicity.[21] Guidelines for monitoring hepatotoxicity in rheumatoid arthritis patients receiving methotrexate have recently been formulated.[22] When used for rheumatoid arthritis, the most common adverse effect of methotrexate is gastrointestinal intolerance. With high-dose methotrexate used in cancer chemotherapy, the adverse effects of the drug can often be ameliorated by concomitant or subsequent 'rescue' by folic acid or folinic acid (Leucovorin) administration, but trials of these agents to reduce the adverse effects of methotrexate in patients with rheumatoid arthritis have yielded inconsistent results. However, some studies have suggested that gastrointestinal intolerance to methotrexate may be reduced without reducing clinical efficacy, when folic acid or folinic acid is given along with the methotrexate.[23,24]

In several trials of the more lymphocyte-specific cytotoxic drugs, hepatotoxicity and nephrotoxicity were not observed. Gastrointestinal intolerance and infections may be the most common adverse effects of mizoribine, mycophenolate mofetil, and brequinar sodium. A further advantage of these agents may be that inhibition of the enzymes in the *de novo* purine and pyrimidine pathways is rapidly reversible.[25]

*Other adverse effects:* as well as myelosuppression, both cyclophosphamide and azathioprine are associated with alopecia, gastrointestinal intolerance, infections, and possibly an increased risk of malignancy. In addition, haemorrhagic cystitis occurs in up to 20% of patients on long term cyclophosphamide therapy. This can often be prevented or ameliorated by concurrent administration of *mesna*, a synthetic sulfhydryl compound that chemically interacts with the urotoxic metabolites of cyclophosphamide. Long term, high-dose cyclophosphamide therapy also carries a risk of developing severe, sometimes fatal interstitial pulmonary fibrosis.

*Drug interactions:* one of the few clinically significant adverse drug interactions involving cytotoxic drugs is the combination of methotrexate with NSAIDs or salicylates (see also appendix B). These combinations can markedly increase the serum concentrations of methotrexate, and should be avoided.

### 2.1.2 Corticosteroids

Corticosteroids are naturally occurring hormones produced by the adrenal cortex, or are synthetic analogues of these hormones. Natural corticosteroids play a role in the endocrine regulation of virtually all functional systems of the body. Their multiple effects give them the broadest, most comprehensive range of actions of any of the immunosuppressive/anti-inflammatory agents. Their potent activities have revolutionised the treatment of immune-mediated disorders, and they are clinically indispensable in the treatment of a wide variety of conditions, including allergic and autoimmune disorders, transplant rejection, and the treatment of certain malignant neoplasms. Of all of the immunomodulating drugs, corticosteroids also have the broadest range of unwanted effects; indeed, their potential for serious, and even catastrophic adverse effects is the limiting factor in their use. Safe and effective use of corticosteroids requires clinical judgement and a knowledge of their physiological and pharmacological properties.

#### Mechanism/Site of Action

Corticosteroids are traditionally classified as *mineralocorticoids* or *glucocorticoids*, based on their primary pharmacological activity. Mineralocorticoid properties affect homeostasis of fluids and electrolytes, and are often essential for the effective treatment of adrenocortical insufficiency. The anti-inflammatory and immunosuppressive actions that make corticosteroids useful as immunomodulating agents are considered glucocorticoid effects, and the agents that are clinically useful in immune-mediated disorders are all generally classified as glucocorticoids or glucocorticosteroids.

***Intracellular actions:*** the initial steps underlying the mechanisms of action of glucocorticosteroids are now understood.[26] Following their entry into cells they bind to intracellular glucocorticoid receptors. These receptors, encoded by a cDNA that was first cloned in 1985,[27] are ubiquitously distributed among cell types. The ubiquity of the receptor accounts for the multiple effects of the glucocorticosteroids, although the subsequent effect of receptor binding differs by cell type and even the state of activation or differentiation of the cell. The glucocorticosteroid, bound to the receptor, is transported into the nucleus to an 'acceptor site'. This complex modulates the transcription of specific genes, and the post-transcriptional expression of some genes, that account for the multiple effects of glucocorticosteroids.

***Physiological actions:*** the physiological actions of the glucocorticosteroids that render them useful in the management of immune-mediated disorders include effects on cell trafficking, cell recruitment, inhibition of antigen-specific immune responses, and lytic effects on lymphocytes. These effects are dose-related, and are increasingly being defined at a molecular level. Understanding the mechanisms of the various actions of glucocorticosteroids may allow development of new immunosuppressive agents and treatment strategies that replicate the desirable actions of the steroids while avoiding their unwanted effects.

Systemically administered glucocorticosteroids increase the numbers of neutrophils, while decreasing the numbers of peripheral blood lymphocytes, eosinophils and monocytes.[28] The characteristic neutrophilia is multifactorial, and involves increased mobilisation of neutrophils from bone marrow reserves, prolongation of their circulating half-life, and decreased migration into inflammatory sites. The last action is perhaps one of the major mechanisms whereby glucocorticosteroids exert their anti-inflammatory effects. The accumulation of neutrophils and other inflammatory cells in inflammatory loci is decreased due to steroid-induced changes in both the membranes of the inflammatory cells and in the vascular endothelial cells, such that cellular adherence and transmigration are inhibited. Glucocorticosteroids decrease the numbers of circulating lymphocytes, monocytes and eosinophils by affecting the distribution of cells between the intravascular and extravascular recirculating pools. The molecular basis of these effects involves modulation of adhesion molecules and their receptors.[29] As discussed below (section 4), other approaches to directly modulating adhesion molecules are currently being investigated in the hope of selectively replicating this particular action of glucocorticosteroids.

Glucocorticosteroids also affect recruitment of cells into sites of immune and inflammatory responses by inhibiting intercellular messages, including the production of and response to chemotactic factors. The production of and response to intercellular hormones termed *cytokines* and *lymphokines* are also affected. Some of the actions of glucocorticosteroids thought to be central to their anti-inflammatory and immunosuppressive actions include inhibition of macrophage and T lymphocyte interactions by blocking the release of IL-1, IL-6 and tumour necrosis factor-alpha (TNF-$\alpha$). The functions of T lymphocytes, especially of T cells of the CD4 (helper/inducer) subclass, in the development of cell-mediated immunity and provision of T cell help for antibody responses are also decreased by the blockade of lymphokine expression. Both the production and action of IL-2, a lymphokine central to the proliferation and function of CD4 (helper) T cells, are inhibited by glucocorticosteroids.

As the complex cascade of cytokine and lymphokines involved in immune responses is progressively revealed, more sites of glucocorticosteroid actions are identified, further accounting for the multiple effects of these immunomodulating agents. The relationship between drug concentration and effect on cellular function is complex, but in general it can be stated that T lymphocytes of the CD8 subclass (cytotoxic and suppressor T cells) are less readily affected by glucocorticosteroids than are cells of the CD4 subclass, and B lymphocytes are less affected than T lymphocytes. With high concentrations of glucocorticosteroids, however, virtually all lymphocyte functions can be affected.

Under some circumstances, glucocorticosteroids lead to the death of T lymphocytes. Normal human peripheral blood T cells are far more resistant to steroid-induced cell death than the equivalent cells of rodents, in which the mechanism of steroid-induced lysis has been extensively studied. However, abnormal human lymphocytes, including some neoplastic cells, can be much more susceptible, and this sensitivity is exploited in the treatment of some lymphoid malignancies, as discussed in section 3.6.

It has recently been appreciated that glucocorticosteroids may induce programmed cell death, or apoptosis, in lymphocytes in conjunction with certain sequences of lymphocyte activating events. This may represent yet another physiological role for glucocorticosteroids in the regulation of immune responses, and another mechanism of action underlying their therapeutic effects.

#### Pharmacodynamic Properties

Separation of corticosteroids into glucocorticoids and mineralocorticoids is not absolute; most agents have both types of activity to some extent. Their relative activities, however, provide some basis for selection among various drugs. The naturally occurring glucocorticoids, hydrocortisone (cortisol) and cortisone, have clinically important mineralocorticoid activity in addition to their glucocorticoid activity. Of the synthetic agents, prednisone and prednisolone have approximately half the mineralocorticoid activity of the natural hormones, while betamethasone, dexamethasone, meprednisone, methylprednisolone, paramethasone and triamcinolone have considerably less mineralocorticoid activity.[21] Structure-activity relationships that would allow development of analogues differing in their specific glucocorticoid effects have not yet been elucidated. The available glucocorticosteroids, therefore, differ from each other principally in terms of potency and half-life (see chapter 19, sect. 7.1.1).

Since both the therapeutic effects and adverse effects of glucocorticosteroids are dose-related, a major strategy for achieving clinical efficacy with reduced systemic adverse effects is targeting the drug to the site of inflammation. This is possible through the use of topical and local dosage forms, including inhaled preparations for asthma, nasal sprays for rhinitis, suppositories and enemas for inflammatory bowel disease, topical formulations for skin conditions, and intra-articular injections for joint inflammation.

Unwanted effects, including suppression of the hypothalamic-pituitary- adrenal (HPA) axis, are also related to the duration of exposure to pharmacological concentrations of glucocorticosteroids. When using these agents systemically for acute indications, the therapeutic objective should be to use the lowest dose, for the shortest duration, that will achieve clinical efficacy. If the dosage and/or duration of treatment have been such that suppression of the HPA-axis is likely, it is imperative that the dose of the glucocorticosteroid is reduced gradually, i.e. tapered, rather than withdrawn abruptly. Following long term therapy with systemic glucocorticosteroids, one suggested protocol for tapering is to decrease the dosage by the equivalent of 2.5 to 5mg prednisone every 3 to 7 days until the physiological dose of approximately 5mg prednisone is reached. If the patient's condition worsens during withdrawal, it may be necessary to increase the dose and resume tapering more gradually.[21]

Another strategy to avoid or reduce adverse effects when using oral glucocorticosteroids is to use a treatment regimen that avoids continuous exposure to pharmacological doses. It has been empirically determined that a single daily dose produces fewer adverse effects than divided doses, and that alternate-day therapy is better still for minimising adrenal suppression, protein catabolism, and other adverse effects.[26,30,31] In alternate-day therapy, a single dose is administered every other day, and is given in the morning to simulate the natural circadian rhythm of corticosteroid secretion (see also chapter 19; sect. 7.1.1).

A further extension of the principle of intermittent administration is the use of pulse therapy. This involves the intravenous infusion of a large bolus of drug, such as methylprednisolone 1g, over the course of 30 minutes or so. Several alternate-day pulses are then administered, followed by a resting phase of around 6 weeks.[32] Pulse therapy with glucocorticosteroids was first used for organ transplant rejection, and later for the treatment of other renal diseases such as the nephritis of systemic lupus erythematosus. Pulsed methylprednisolone is also used in the treatment of rheumatoid arthritis.[33]

Still another treatment strategy to achieve clinical efficacy with the minimum dose of glucocorticosteroids is to use, in addition, a drug from another class of immunosuppressive agents with a mechanism of action that complements that of the glucocorticosteroids. Cytotoxic drugs, in combination with glucocorticosteroids, have been most frequently used as 'steroid-sparing' agents. Other types of immune modulating agents such as the antirheumatic drugs hydroxychloroquine, gold salts, and sulfasalazine are also used in combination therapy to reduce the required dose of glucocorticosteroids. A steroid-sparing strategy used in the treatment of organ transplant rejection has been the combination of cyclosporin and glucocorticosteroids, and often the inclusion of additional immunosuppressive agents in triple or quadruple drug regimens.

#### Pharmacokinetic Characteristics

***Absorption:*** orally administered glucocorticosteroids are readily absorbed, although there is some interindividual variability. Absorption following intramuscular administration depends upon the chemical form of the drug. Those administered in freely soluble forms such as the sodium phosphate or sodium succinate salts are rapidly absorbed, while those administered in poorly soluble forms such as the acetate, acetonide, diacetate, hexacetonide or tebutate, are absorbed slowly but completely. Following topical administration, absorption varies markedly with different formulations, as stratum corneum penetration is influenced by the molecular structure of the compound. Substitution of 16- or 17-hydroxy groups with side chains such as acetonide, propionate, or valerate increases the compound's lipophilicity and penetration. Stratum corneum penetration is also markedly influenced by the vehicle, the condition of the skin, and the use of occlusive dressings (see further chapter 17; sect. 1.4 and 6.1.1).

***Distribution/elimination:*** once absorbed, the various glucocorticosteroids differ in the extent to which they are bound to plasma proteins, and in their rates of metabolism and excretion. Typical pharmacokinetic parameters for the more commonly used glucocorticosteroids are given in appendix A. Both linear and non-linear kinetics are found with this class of drugs; in terms of protein binding, concentration-dependent binding to plasma transcortin has been described for prednisolone.[34] The pharmacokinetics of the glucocorticosteroids are known to be influenced by concomitant administration of drugs that induce hepatic enzymes, and by the presence of hepatic disease (see further appendix F). In patients with hypoalbuminaemia, a higher percentage of glucocorticosteroids will be present in the unbound form, although the unbound concentrations of the drugs will be unaltered in this situation [as distinct from the bound (inactive) drug concentrations, which will be decreased].

Beyond these factors known to influence the pharmacokinetics of glucocorticosteroids, the variability of plasma drug concentrations in individual patients given similar doses of these drugs indicates that clinicians need to individualise and carefully monitor glucocorticosteroid therapy for each patient.

#### Clinical Effectiveness

In many clinical situations, glucocorticosteroids are clearly the most clinically efficacious therapeutic agents available. Since the adverse effects of these drugs are numerous and potentially severe, the risk : benefit ratio must be carefully assessed when considering their use.

As short term use of glucocorticosteroids poses far less risk than long term use, therapy with these drugs is often justified in acute situations. These include serious flares of any of the immune-mediated diseases, when relatively high doses may be required to bring the acute exacerbation under control, with the expectation that the dosage can then be tapered and a less toxic therapy substituted. Despite their known adverse effects, the use of glucocortico-

**Table II.** Serious adverse effects of systemic glucocorticosteroid therapy

| |
|---|
| Hypothalamic-pituitary-adrenal (HPA) axis suppression |
| Glucose intolerance |
| Fluid retention |
| Weight gain |
| Growth retardation in children |
| Osteoporosis |
| Aseptic necrosis of bone |
| Glaucoma |
| Cataracts |
| Hypertension |
| Muscle wasting, pain or weakness |
| Increased susceptibility to infection: |
| • Severe or fatal course (especially varicella and measles) |
| • Reactivation of tuberculosis |
| Diabetes mellitus |
| Psychological disturbances |
| Peptic ulcer disease |

steroids in potentially life-threatening situations such as the nephrotic syndrome or organ transplant rejection is often indispensable in view of their clinical efficacy.

Long term therapy with glucocorticosteroids carries the greatest risk of serious adverse effects, and in most cases the use of these agents should be avoided if treatment with less toxic agents can achieve the same effects. The remarkable clinical efficacy of the glucocorticosteroids, has, however, spurred the development of safer dosage forms and therapy regimens that can in some cases confer an acceptable risk : benefit ratio for even long term treatment. The principal strategies are discussed above and include the use of topical or local dosage forms, alternate-day administration schedules, and combination therapy that includes glucocorticosteroids in relatively low doses. Specific uses of glucocorticosteroids are discussed in section 3 below, and in other chapters.

**Tolerability and Drug Interactions Potential**

In general, the adverse effects of the glucocorticosteroids parallel their therapeutic effects, and are similar for the various agents in this class when equipotent doses are compared. Table II lists the adverse effects that may result from systemic therapy or, rarely, from systemic absorption of topical glucocorticosteroids. Depending upon the dose and duration of therapy, it may be necessary to monitor patients with periodic evaluations of height, weight, chest and spinal radiographs or bone densitometry for osteoporosis, haematopoietic parameters, glucose tolerance, ocular effects, and blood pressure.

Some of the adverse effects of glucocorticosteroids may be prevented or effectively treated. Recently, it has been appreciated that bone loss during high-dose glucocorticosteroid therapy is greatest during the first 6 to 12 months of treatment. Concomitant treatment with calcitonin, calcitriol, or bisphosphonate drugs should be considered for patients at high risk of osteoporosis.[35] All patients on long term glucocorticosteroid therapy should supplement their calcium intake. Those who are potentially immunosuppressed by their steroid regimen should be cautioned about their susceptibility to infection. In the case of exposure to varicella or measles, administration of varicella-zoster immune globulin (VZIG) or immune globulin, respectively, may be indicated. Patients undergoing surgery may require additional glucocorticosteroid coverage because their normal response to stress has been blunted by HPA axis suppression.

Clinically significant interactions between glucocorticosteroids and other drugs are listed in appendix B and are discussed further in chapter 19 (sect. 7.1.1). It should be noted that diabetic patients receiving glucocorticosteroids may require modifications of their antidiabetic medications, due to the hyperglycaemic effect of steroids. Drug interactions may modulate the effects of a given dose of glucocorticosteroids, but this is seldom a critical factor in their use. The clinical use of glucocorticosteroids is not standardised; the drug regimen must always be tailored to the individual patient and the condition under treatment.

#### *2.1.3 Xenobiotic Immunosuppressants (Cyclosporin, Tacrolimus, Gusperimus, Rapamycin)*

Xenobiotic agents are substances derived from one organism (usually bacteria or fungi) that can be used therapeutically in another type of organism (usually humans or other mammals). The term xenobiotic immunosuppressants has come into vogue to classify cyclosporin, tacrolimus (FK 506), rapamycin, and a number of newer compounds. These agents are structurally and functionally diverse, and their commonality derives from their discovery in systematic screening surveys of fermentation products, following the spectacular clinical and financial success of cyclosporin.

Three of the newest xenobiotic immunosuppressants, mizoribine, mycophenolate mofetil, and brequinar sodium, act primarily through interference with DNA synthesis. Because their mechanisms of action are similar to those of the cytotoxic drugs azathioprine, cyclophosphamide, chlorambucil and methotrexate, these agents were discussed in section 2.1.1 above. This section deals with cyclosporin, tacrolimus, gusperimus (deoxyspergualin) and rapamycin, the latter only briefly as it is not yet available for clinical use.

**Mechanism/Site of Action**

*Cyclosporin (cyclosporin A)* is a neutral, lipophilic cyclic undecapeptide isolated in 1971 from a fungus, *Tolypocladium inflatum gams*. It was found to block both *in vitro* and *in vivo* immune responses. Its subsequent development as an immunosuppressive drug revolutionised organ transplantation, making transplantation of new types of organs and of mismatched organs feasible for the first time. Its intrinsic activity and relatively immunologically selective action have extended its use into the management of a variety of immune-mediated conditions.[36]

The success of cyclosporin prompted drug screening of microbiological products in a deliberate attempt to identify other xenobiotics with similar actions, and this led to the discovery of *tacrolimus* (FK 506) in 1985.[37] Tacrolimus is quite different structurally from cyclosporin, being a hydrophobic macrocyclic lactone, and is approximately 100-fold more potent than cyclosporin. However, despite their structural dissimilarity, the mechanisms of action of cyclosporin and tacrolimus are quite similar, and their biological effects are nearly identical.[25] Both drugs bind to intracellular proteins that have been termed immunophilins.[38] Cyclosporin binds to a group of immunophilins called cyclophilins, which are structurally dissimilar to the immunophilins bound by tacrolimus – the so-called FK binding proteins. In each case, however, the resulting complex binds to *calcineurin*, which is now believed to be a key enzyme in the T cell transduction cascade following T cell receptor stimulation.[39,40] The final molecular link between the complexes containing both the drug and calcineurin, and the inhibition of the early steps of T cell activation may be a T cell specific transcription factor (NFAT) which is required for transcription of IL-2.[41,42] This sequence of events provides an explanation for the major biological effects of cyclosporin and tacrolimus, and the relative specificity of their actions for T lymphocytes. However, these drugs appear to have additional actions, that may be mediated through other mechanisms; for example, the inhibition by cyclosporin of extracellular immunophilins with chemotactic activity may also account for some of its immunomodulatory effects.[43]

*Rapamycin* is another macrocyclic lactone, and its close structural resemblance to tacrolimus suggests that its immunosuppressive effect may be mediated by a similar mechanism of action. Indeed, rapamycin binds to the same cytoplasmic immunophilins as tacrolimus, i.e. the FK binding proteins, but the resulting complex does not block calcineurin activity. Although the molecular bases of the intracellular actions of rapamycin are not yet clear, this drug appears to block T cell activation at a later stage than cyclosporin and tacrolimus. For example, rapamycin does not inhibit the transcription of IL-2, but does inhibit the response of lymphocytes and other cells to this and other cytokines, including IL-1, IL-6, and interferon-γ. Rapamycin also inhibits the proliferation of smooth muscle cells in blood vessel walls and the consequent intimal thickening.[44]

*Gusperimus (deoxyspergualin)* is a synthetic analogue of spergualin, a xenobiotic isolated from a soil bacterium in Japan.[45] It is quite different, both structurally and functionally, from cyclosporin, tacrolimus, and rapamycin. The molecular basis of its mechanism of action has only recently begun to be elucidated. Gusperimus binds to two heat shock proteins (HSPs), HSP 70 and HSP 90. These proteins are thought to be involved in immune responses in a number of ways, including antigen processing, interaction with glucocorticoid receptors, and the post-translational processing of proteins that would be expected to include mediators of immunological and inflammatory events.[46]

**Pharmacodynamic Properties**

*Cyclosporin* and *tacrolimus* inhibit both cell-mediated and humoral immune responses, primarily by blocking the early events in the activation of T lymphocytes via the T cell receptor. The inhibition of signal transduction by these drugs prevents the transcription of a set of lymphokines and thus inhibits most of the functions of T cells in the induction of immune responses. Most of the effects of these drugs on the functions of other cells appear to be secondary to their actions on T lymphocytes. Rapamycin blocks many of the activities of T lymphocytes by interfering in somewhat later events in T cell activation, and has effects on other immune cells, including B lymphocytes, as well. *Gusperimus (deoxyspergualin)* may act both at a very early stage of the immune response, affecting antigen processing and presentation, and at a very late stage, affecting the differentiation of effector cells such as cytotoxic T cells and the maturation of B lymphocytes to plasma cells.[47]

Understanding the biological effects of these xenobiotic immunosuppressants has allowed prediction of drug combinations that would provide additive or even synergistic effects, and preclinical studies and clinical experience have confirmed these expectations. Cyclosporin and tacrolimus, having essentially identical biological effects, offer no advantage when used in combination. Either drug can be combined advantageously with rapamycin or with gusperimus. By combining drugs with complementary actions and non-overlapping adverse effects, it is possible to use lower doses of each and achieve clinical efficacy with less toxicity.[25]

#### Pharmacokinetic Characteristics

Both cyclosporin and tacrolimus have a narrow therapeutic window. It would therefore seem desirable to control drug concentrations closely and to define a therapeutic but nontoxic range of concentrations. Both of these objectives have proven extremely difficult. Oral absorption, tissue distribution, and elimination of both cyclosporin and tacrolimus are variable, leading to wide fluctuations in plasma drug concentrations between individuals receiving the same dosage.[48] Even determining the drug concentration is complex, being dependent both on the assay used and the biological fluid (blood, plasma or serum) sampled. However, a number of clinically relevant observations have emerged.

*Cyclosporin* is rapidly distributed between blood cells (60 to 70%) and plasma, and has a large volume of distribution [280 to 560L (4 to 8 L/kg)]. It is principally eliminated by metabolism, which occurs predominantly in the liver, although some presystemic metabolism in the gastrointestinal mucosa also occurs and this may be a major contributor to the variability of oral cyclosporin absorption. More than 30 metabolites have been observed, most having only 10 to 20% of the immunosuppressive activity of the parent drug. Cyclosporin exhibits a linear elimination profile with wide interindividual variability in clearance (26.6 to 210 L/h); its apparent half-life in blood is about 19 hours. The majority of an oral dose (90%) is excreted in the bile (<1% unchanged), with only 6% excreted in the urine (<0.1% unchanged).[49]

*Tacrolimus* undergoes extensive tissue distribution and also has a large volume of distribution [1295L (18.5 L/kg)]. In the vascular compartment, plasma drug concentrations are approximately 10 to 30 times lower than whole blood concentrations. Tacrolimus is extensively metabolised in the liver, and less than 1% of the drug is excreted unchanged in the bile and urine. As with cyclosporin, there is wide interindividual variability in its plasma clearance (range 87 to 269 L/h, mean 143 L/h), while the half-life ranges from 5.5 to 16.6 hours (mean 8.7h).[50]

The pharmacokinetics of both cyclosporin and tacrolimus are significantly affected by liver function, but less so by renal function. Their pharmacokinetics are also markedly affected by the age of the patient. To achieve the same therapeutic blood levels, paediatric patients require higher oral doses of tacrolimus on a mg/kg basis than do adults.[51] The same is also true of cyclosporin, for which patients over age 40 or 45 years require lower doses due to decreased clearance.[48]

*Gusperimus (deoxyspergualin)* must be given parenterally, because only 5% of the drug is systemically available when given orally. However, it is hoped that chemical modifications will subsequently allow it to be given orally. Pharmacokinetic studies have indicated that its clearance is rapid, with an elimination half-life of 2.5 hours following intravenous administration. The identified metabolites of gusperimus do not appear to have immunosuppressive activity.[52]

#### Clinical Effectiveness

***Organ transplant rejection:*** the primary use of *cyclosporin* and *tacrolimus* has been in antirejection therapy, and their use ushered in a new era of organ transplant success. The use of cyclosporin brought 1-year cadaver kidney success rates from approximately 50% to over 75%. Both of these xenobiotics have been more efficacious in preventing acute rejection than chronic rejection. Long term outcomes for organ recipients have also improved because these drugs have allowed the use of reduced doses of corticosteroids. Neither drug is commonly used as monotherapy, but rather as part of a regimen involving two, three or four immunosuppressive agents in an effort to improve therapeutic effect while minimising adverse effects.

Although cyclosporin and tacrolimus are very similar in their clinical effects, slight differences (seldom confirmed in comparative trials) have led to some preferences in their applications for organ transplants, e.g. tacrolimus may be associated with somewhat better results than cyclosporin when used for liver transplantation. While the two agents have comparable adverse effects in most respects, the incidence of infectious complications, hypertension and hypercholesterolaemia may be lower with tacrolimus. For comprehensive discussions on the clinical use of cyclosporin and tacrolimus, see reviews by Faulds et al.[49] and Peters et al.,[50] respectively.

*Gusperimus (deoxyspergualin)* has only recently come into clinical use for organ transplantation, but early results suggest that it may be less toxic than cyclosporin or tacrolimus. The novel mechanism of action of gusperimus suggests that it may beneficially be combined with other agents to treat acute graft rejection, and it may be able to rescue grafts that are undergoing rejection on other therapy.[52-54] However, its use for maintenance therapy will not be feasible until an oral dosage form is developed. Preliminary clinical experience using gusperimus to prevent rejection of transplanted allogeneic or xenogeneic pancreatic islet cells suggests that it may have unique clinical efficacy in this situation, where neither cyclosporin nor tacrolimus is particularly effective.[55,56] The ability of gusperimus to inhibit the initial antigen processing and antigen presentation events in the induction of immune responses, may be used to advantage by administering the drug along with xenogeneic monoclonal antibodies, such as muromonab-CD3 (OKT3) to prevent or reduce the development of host immune responses to these foreign proteins.[46]

***Other immune-mediated disorders:*** in addition to their use in transplantation, the xenobiotic immunosuppressants appear to have great potential in the treatment of a wide variety of immune-mediated disorders. When used in the treatment of autoimmune diseases, lower doses of these drugs are used than are required for suppressing graft rejection, so the toxicity of cyclosporin and tacrolimus is not as problematic or limiting as it is in antirejection therapy.

By far the greatest experience with the use of xenobiotic immunosuppressants in autoimmune disorders has been gained with the use of *cyclosporin*.[57] This agent has established value in the treatment of Behçet's syndrome, psoriasis, atopic dermatitis, and rheumatoid arthritis. In addition, it may also be effective in the treatment of asthma, systemic lupus erythematosus, and inflammatory bowel disease. Table III summarises the current literature on the efficacy of cyclosporin in immune-mediated disorders.

*Tacrolimus* has only recently been used in autoimmune disorders. Early clinical experience suggests that, like cyclosporin, tacrolimus may be effective in the treatment of psoriasis, uveitis, and probably other immune-mediated disorders.[58-61]

Preclinical studies have shown that *gusperimus (deoxyspergualin)* is effective in a variety of animal models of autoimmune disease. Its ability to block late stages of the immune response and to suppress established immune responses, along with the relative absence of serious toxicity, suggests that this is a promising candidate for immunomodulation in autoimmune disorders. The available parenteral form of gusperimus has been used in Europe in small scale clinical trials for treatment of systemic lupus erythematosus, polyarteritis, nephritis, and multiple sclerosis.[52]

#### Tolerability and Drug Interactions Potential

***Adverse effects:*** the most frequent and clinically important adverse effect of cyclosporin is nephrotoxicity, which is usually manifested as increased serum creatinine or blood urea nitrogen (BUN) levels. Renal toxicity appears to be dose-related and may be associated with high trough concentrations of the drug. It is usually reversible.[21] Nephrotoxicity may occur in 25 to 38% of patients receiving the drug for antirejection therapy, but is less common when cyclosporin is used in lower doses for treatment of autoimmune disorders, particularly if the dose used is less than 5 mg/kg/day.[62] Tacrolimus, when used at therapeutically equivalent doses, causes nephrotoxicity similar to that caused by cyclosporin in terms of frequency, severity, morphology and clinical presentation.[50]

Other major adverse effects of cyclosporin and tacrolimus include hepatotoxicity, neurotoxicity, hypertension, and increased susceptibility to infection. However, some clinical strategies can help to prevent or manage the adverse effects of cyclosporin and probably tacrolimus as well (see section 3.1.3 below). For the most part, the incidence and severity of the complications are comparable for the two drugs, although there is some evidence that hypertension[63] and infections[50] are less of a problem with tacrolimus. Another difference between the adverse effects of these two xenobiotics is that hirsutism and gingival hyperplasia occur in response to cyclosporin but not tacrolimus.

In comparison with cyclosporin and tacrolimus, gusperimus (deoxyspergualin) may have a lower incidence of adverse effects. Neurological symptoms, including numbness, and gastrointestinal disturbances are among the most common reactions. Evidence of bone marrow suppression, including leucopenia, thrombocytopenia and anaemia, has been reported when gusperimus was used to treat episodes of graft rejection.[54]

***Drug interactions:*** more than 10 years of clinical experience with cyclosporin, with monitoring of its blood concentrations for safety and efficacy, has allowed the accumulation of a considerable body of information concerning potential interactions between cyclosporin and other drugs (table IV). Concurrent use of agents known or suspected of potentiating the nephrotoxicity of cyclosporin should be avoided. However, the effects of agents that may increase or decrease cyclosporin blood concentrations are usually manageable if cyclosporin concentrations are monitored. In this respect, it is es-

**Table III.** Summary of therapeutic efficacy of cyclosporin in immunoregulatory disorders. In most cases, oral therapy was administered for patients refractory to standard therapies (after Faulds et al.[49])

| Immunoregulatory disorder | Efficacy rating[a] | | |
|---|---|---|---|
| | good/excellent | moderate | equivocal/none |
| Ophthalmological disorders | Behçet's syndrome[1]<br>Vernal conjunctivitis[1] | Endogenous uveitis[3] | |
| Dermatological disorders | Psoriasis vulgaris[1]<br>Palmoplantar pustulosis[3]<br>Atopic dermatitis[3]<br>Pyoderma gangrenosum[4] | Lichen planus[3]<br>Alopecia areata[3]<br>Bullous disorders[5] | Allergic contact dermatitis[4] |
| Haematological disorders | Primary aplastic anaemia[1b] | | |
| Gastrointestinal disorders | | Crohn's disease[2c]<br>Ulcerative colitis[3]<br>Other bowel disorders[5] | Crohn's disease[1d] |
| Liver disorders | Primary biliary cirrhosis[2e] | Autoimmune chronic active hepatitis[5] | Viral chronic active hepatitis[4] |
| Neurological disorders | Subarachnoid haemorrhage neurological deficit[3] | Myasthenia gravis[3] | Amyotrophic lateral sclerosis[2]<br>Multiple sclerosis[2] |
| Nephrotic syndrome | Minimal change nephrotic syndrome[3] | Focal segmental glomerular sclerosis[2]<br>Membranous nephropathy[4] | |
| Rheumatoid arthritis | Rheumatoid arthritis[1] | Juvenile rheumatoid arthritis[4] | |
| Diabetes mellitus | | | Type 1 diabetes mellitus[1] |
| Other immunoregulatory disorders | Polymyositis/ dermatomyositis[4] | Asthma[3]<br>Sclerosis[5]<br>Systemic lupus erythematosus[5] | Sjögren's syndrome[3]<br>Pulmonary fibrosis[5] |

a Good/excellent = similar or better than standard therapy and/or most patients responding. Moderate = some patients responding. Equivocal/none = no response or worsening disease, or initial response but relapse with continued therapy (diabetes mellitus).
b Patients who are not candidates for bone marrow transplantation.
c Short term treatment of active disease.
d Long term maintenance therapy, particularly of disease in remission.
e Particularly patients with less advanced disease.
1 Large (≥ 30 patients per treatment arm) controlled comparison(s) with standard therapy.
2 Large (≥ 30 patients per treatment arm) controlled comparison(s) with placebo.
3 Small comparative trial(s).
4 Noncomparative trial(s).
5 Anecedotal reports (case reports/series).

**Table IV.** Interactions between cyclosporin and other agents (after Faulds et al.[49])

| Drug class | Interaction: known | suspected/possible | controversial |
|---|---|---|---|
| **Increased trough blood cyclosporin concentrations** | | | |
| Antimicrobials | Erythromycin<br>Josamycin<br>Ketoconazole | Amikacin<br>Fluconazole<br>Itraconazole<br>Metronidazole<br>Norfloxacin<br>Roxithromycin<br>Ticarcillin<br>Tobramycin | Doxycycline<br>Imipenem/cilastatin |
| Calcium antagonists | Diltiazem<br>Nicardipine<br>Verapamil | | |
| Corticosteroids | | Methylprednisolone | Prednisolone |
| $H_2$-Receptor antagonists | | Cimetidine<br>Ranitidine | |
| Oral anticoagulants | | Warfarin | |
| Sex hormones | | Danazol/norethisterone<br>Levonorgestrel<br>Methyltestosterone | |
| Other | | Amiodarone<br>Alcohol (ethanol)<br>Metoclopramide<br>Sulindac | Acetazolamide<br>Omeprazole |
| **Decreased trough blood cyclosporin concentration** | | | |
| Antiepileptics | Carbamazepine<br>Phenobarbital<br>Phenytoin | Primidone | Valproic acid |
| Antimicrobials | Rifampicin (rifampin) | Pyrazinamide<br>Sulfadiazine<br>Sulfadimidine (IV) | Isoniazid<br>Nafcillin |
| Other | | Dipyrone<br>Metoprolol<br>Octreotide<br>Sulfinpyrazone | |
| **Enhanced cyclosporin nephrotoxicity** | | | |
| Antimicrobials | Amphotericin B<br>Gentamicin<br>Tobramycin<br>Trimethoprim | Aciclovir<br>Ceftazidime<br>Ciprofloxacin<br>Cotrimoxazole (trimethoprim-sulfamethoxazole) | Ganciclovir<br>Latamoxef |
| Diuretics | | Furosemide<br>Metolazone | |
| Nonsteroidal anti- inflammatory drugs (NSAIDs) | | Diclofenac<br>Indomethacin | |
| Other | Colchicine<br>Digoxin<br>Melphalan | Disopyramide<br>Doxorubicin | |

*Abbreviation:* IV = intravenous.

pecially important to monitor the effects on cyclosporin concentrations when such agents are added or deleted from a therapeutic regimen. The increase in serum concentration of cyclosporin with coadministration of diltiazem has been used to reduce the cost of cyclosporin therapy. Cost savings of 14 to 48% have been obtained in transplant pharmacotherapy.[64-66]

Information about drug interactions with gusperimus is not yet available. On the principle that concurrent use of immunosuppressive drugs with overlapping toxicities should be avoided, it is probable that combining gusperimus with other agents capable of causing bone marrow suppression would be inadvisable.

### *2.1.4 Antibodies*

Antibodies are powerful tools that can be used to modulate the immune response either up or down. The use of antibodies to augment or substitute for an immune response by the recipient is discussed below.

When used for immunosuppressive purposes, two broad categories of effects can be distinguished. The most common type of therapeutic application seeks to use the antigen-specificity of immunoglobulins to selectively target specific cell types or specific soluble factors in order to modulate the immune system in a very selective way. The therapeutic effect naturally depends on the distribution and function of the antigens to which the antibodies are directed. The second type of therapeutic application, however, does not depend upon antigen specificity, but rather uses whole immunoglobulin preparations to effect a broad immunosuppression, through a mechanism that is not well understood.

While the therapeutic effect of antibodies is, in most applications, related to their antigen specificity, the major adverse effects are often related to the type of antibody. Remarkable strides in antibody 'engineering' are producing new types of antibodies with fewer adverse effects and more marked desired effects. Thus, the clinical usefulness of antibodies is likely to increase dramatically in the near future. On the other hand, the requirement for parenteral administration will continue to be a limiting factor.

#### Mechanism/Site of Action

***Immunosuppressive actions of antibodies directed against cellular antigens:*** the mode of action of antibodies to the Rhesus (Rh) factor, which are administered to an Rh-negative mother before and during birth to prevent an immunological response to red blood cells of her Rh-positive fetus, is unique in that it prevents sensitisation to the Rh antigen. The exact mechanism is uncertain, but likely involves physical covering of the antigenic epitopes, rapid clearance of the opsonised red cells, and direct lysis of the erythrocytes, thus preventing immune recognition of the Rh antigen.

Antibodies directed against antigens on the recipient's immune cells can have immunosuppressive effects through several different mechanisms. Rapid clearance of the opsonised (antibody-coated) cells by the reticuloendothelial system is thought to be a major mechanism underlying the effects of murine monoclonal antibodies against human T cells.[67] For instance, intravenous administration of monoclonal antibodies to the CD3 T cell antigen can result in total disappearance of CD3-bearing cells within one hour.

In addition to opsonisation, however, other mechanisms can lead to cell removal or immunological nonresponsiveness. Another important mechanism thought to underlie the immunosuppressive effects of anti-CD3 antibodies is modulation of the CD3-T cell receptor complex. This complex, which is essential for antigen recognition, is internalised or shed from the cell surface when bound by anti-CD3 antibodies.[68] In addition, antibodies can lyse cells by complement fixation or antibody-mediated cellular cytotoxicity. Antibody binding to receptors may block signal transduction or, conversely, lead to signal transduction. In the latter case, however, the effect can still be immunosuppressive. It is now appreciated, for example, that engagement of the T cell antigen receptor, in the absence of appropriate secondary signals, can lead to apoptosis or programmed cell death.[69]

***Immunosuppressive actions of antibodies directed against soluble factors:*** antibodies against soluble factors such as cytokines have at least two mechanisms of action. They block the action of the soluble factors by preventing their binding to receptors. They also promote rapid clearance of the bound factors through the usual mechanisms for clearing antigen-antibody complexes.

***Immunosuppressive actions of nonspecific immunoglobulin preparations:*** the mechanism by which intravenously administered immunoglobulin preparations are effective in suppressing immune-mediated disorders is not clear. In the case of idiopathic thrombocytopenic purpura, autoimmune neutropenia or autoimmune haemolytic anaemia, the large doses of immunoglobulins administered may effectively block Fc receptors in the reticuloendothelial system and prevent uptake of opsonised cells. In the case of other disorders of an autoimmune or unknown aetiology, other mechanisms of action have been postulated. The exogenous immunoglobulins may contain naturally-occurring anti-idiotype antibodies which could neutralise pathogenic autoantibodies. Anti-idiotype antibodies or other mechanisms may also reduce production of pathogenic antibodies by a feedback inhibition mechanism.

#### Pharmacokinetic Characteristics

All currently available antibody preparations must be administered parenterally. Their half-lives in the circulation depend in part on the presence of their target antigen. Antibodies that react with and coat cellular elements are removed as the opsonised cells are removed by the reticuloendothelial system. Similarly, antibodies that bind to soluble factors are removed as immune complexes. After the target antigens are depleted, however, the half-lives of the antibodies are measured in days.

#### Clinical Effectiveness

The antigen specificity of antibodies makes them uniquely capable of selectively modulating the immune system. Their therapeutic potential is currently limited, however, by the need for parenteral administration and the development of sensitisation in the recipient.

The major clinical application of antibodies as immunosuppressive agents is in the prevention or treatment of graft rejection. While the current clinical use is dominated by *equine antithymocyte globulin* (ATG) and murine monoclonal antibodies to the CD3 component of the T cell antigen receptor (*muromonab-CD3; OKT3*), antibodies to many other target molecules are in clinical or preclinical development. Table V lists some of these and illustrates the specificity of antibodies that can be exploited for defined manipulation of the immune response. Antibodies to soluble factors, including cytokines and toxins associated with infectious organisms and venoms are also coming into increasing clinical use.

The effectiveness of monoclonal antibodies can be increased by various modifications. The Fc portion can be altered to increase or decrease complement binding and hence cytotoxicity. A variety of toxins such as ricin-A have been conjugated to antibodies to promote destruction of their target cells.

#### Tolerability and Drug Interactions Potential

An unusual and clinically important pharmacodynamic phenomenon occurs with the use of many antibodies directed against T cells. Almost all patients treated with anti-CD3 antibodies for organ graft rejection develop an acute symptom complex following the first, and sometimes the second, injection of antibody.[68] This phenomenon is called the 'first-dose effect' and can include fever, chills, tremor, chest tightness, dyspnoea and wheezing. Patients with fluid overload may develop a capillary leak-type pulmonary oedema. The syndrome is thought to be due to the release of cytokines by T lymphocytes, and can be ameliorated by the concomitant administration of corticosteroids.

Beyond the first-dose effect, most of the adverse effects associated with the administration of antibodies occur after repeated doses, and are primarily related to the development of an immune response to the antibodies. For this reason, currently used antibodies have the highest therapeutic index when used in a short term dosage schedule. In transplantation medicine, for example, they are used as 'induction' therapy, or for treatment of acute rejection, rather than being used for maintenance therapy. Sensitisation is expected to be far less of a problem with 'humanised' or truly human monoclonal antibodies, and the clinical use of therapeutic antibodies will consequently broaden as such preparations become commercially available.

Drug interactions with antibody therapy have received little attention, except for the effects of concurrent drug administration on the 'first-dose effect', or the possibility of delaying or reducing sensitisation to the antibodies by concurrent use of other immunosuppressive agents.

A major factor limiting the use of otherwise highly efficacious antibody therapy at this time is sensitisation to the antibodies themselves. This is most problematic in the case of heterologous polyclonal antibodies, which are now seldom used except for indications where only short term administration is required, such as neutralisation of snake or other venoms. Rat or murine monoclonal antibodies induce sensitisation in the majority of patients in whom they are administered more than once.

At least three strategies to engineer antibodies to prevent immune recognition have proven effective. The first strategy developed was creation of chimeric antibody molecules combining the antigen-combining site of a rat or mouse antibody with the constant region from human antibodies. The construct is made by fusing portions of disparate genes and transfection into myeloma cells for expression. The immunogenicity of such chimeric antibodies is reduced but not eliminated, as many recipient antibodies are directed against the antigen-combining site. An example of a chimeric antibody in clinical use is *abciximab (c7E3 Fab)*, an antibody with antithrombotic activity. Following a 12-hour infusion of abciximab during coronary angioplasty or directional atherectomy, about 6% of recipients develop antichimeric immune responses.[71]

**Table V.** Monoclonal antibodies useful or potentially useful as immunosuppressive agents

| Antibody | Target antigen | Efficacy |
|---|---|---|
| **Antibodies with broad specificity against T cells** | | |
| Anti-CD3 (muromonab-CD3; OKT3) | CD3 is present on all T cells, and is associated with the T cell receptor | Antibodies to CD3 have become a mainstay in the treatment of transplant rejection |
| Anti-CD6 | The target antigen, CD6 (formerly called T-12) is present on 95% of T cells and some B cells | Early clinical studies (between 1982 and 1986) demonstrated efficacy equivalent to high-dose corticosteroids and little first-dose effect (see text; sect. 2.1.4) |
| Anti-CD45 (LM-CD45) | This antigen is widely distributed on lymphocytes and other leucocytes, and is thought to be involved in cellular activation | Antibodies, or combinations of antibodies to CD45, with cytolytic function have been used both for grafted organ pretreatment and for graft rejection |
| Anti-TCR | The T cell receptor is physically associated with CD3 on the surface of T lymphocytes, and is specific for T cells | In early clinical trials, the efficacy of anti-TCR mouse monoclonal antibodies was similar to anti-CD3 antibodies, but showed less propensity for causing a first-dose effect |
| Anti-CD5 | CD5 is an antigen with costimulatory properties and is found on most T cells and a subset of B cells | A toxin-conjugated monclonal antibody to CD5 has shown clinical efficacy in trials involving graft-*vs*-host disease, rheumatoid arthritis and systemic lupus erythematosus |
| Anti-ICAM-1 (enlimomab) | ICAM-1, a molecule expressed on many peripheral blood mononuclear cells, follicular dendritic cells, and endothelial cells, interacts with LFA-1 on T cells to provide a costimulatory signal for cell activation. Alternative targets would be LFA-1 itself, or the related ligand/ receptor partners CTLA-4/B7 | In preclinical and early clinical trials, anti-ICAM-1 was effective in preventing and treating graft rejection. Early clinical results have also been promising in the treatment of autoimmune disorders |
| **Antibodies against subsets of T cells** | | |
| Anti-CD4 | CD4 is a marker for 'helper' T cells, or those that recognise antigen in the context of HLA-class II molecules. Antigen recognition by CD4+ T cells is a prerequisite for the development of host humoral and cell-mediated immune responses | Certain monoclonal antibodies against CD4 prolong graft rejection in animal models. Clinical trials of anti-CD4 antibodies in rheumatoid arthritis have shown significant, though transient, clinical improvement[14,70] |
| Anti-CD8 | CD8 is a marker for cytotoxic/suppressor T cells, or those that recognise antigen in the context of HLA class I molecules | In a small clinical trial, anti-CD8 antibodies were able to reverse steroid-resistant graft rejection in a majority of patients |
| **Antibodies directed against activated T cells** | | |
| Anti-IL-2 receptor | Activation of T cells induced the expression of the IL-2 receptor. Interaction of the receptor with IL-2 leads to cell proliferation and differentiation | Antibodies against epitopes on the several transmembrane polypeptide chains that comprise the receptor have shown efficacy in the prevention, but not the reversal, of graft rejection. Recipient immune responses that developed did not interfere with the subsequent use of an anti-CD3 antibody |

*Abbreviations:* HLA = human leucocyte antigen; ICAM = intercellular adhesion molecule; IL = interleukin; LFA = leucocyte function associated antigen; TCR = T cell receptor.

A more extensive type of genetic engineering is termed 'humanising' the antibodies. By recombination and sometimes by site-directed mutagenesis, the hypervariable portions of the antigen-recognition site, or individual residues therein, are combined with human antibody components to create an antibody of a desired specificity that is largely human in its amino acid sequence. Several humanised antibodies have been tested in clinical trials. They generally have significantly longer half-lives than murine monoclonals and induce sensitisation only after long term use or in a minority of recipients.[72-77]

The ultimate strategy to avoid recipient sensitisation is to use fully human antibodies. Human monoclonal antibodies can be derived from Epstein-Barr virus transformed human B cells or certain other approaches. A recent breakthrough that may assure a reliable source of fully human antibodies is the development of transgenic mice that produce human antibodies. Elements of human heavy- and light-chain loci are inserted into the genome of mice whose production of endogenous antibodies has been disrupted by genetic 'knock out' techniques. These mice can be immunised to produce a variety of antibody specificities and to generate hybridomas for monoclonal antibody production.[78,79] Overcoming the sensitisation problem will greatly extend the clinical usefulness of therapeutic antibodies.

### *2.1.5 Cytokines*

#### Role of Cytokines in Immune Responses

Cytokines are chemical mediators of communication between cells, especially the cells of the immune, haematological, and endothelial systems. They are proteins or glycoproteins that are secreted by one cell type and recognised by means of specific receptors on cells of the same or of other cell types. In general, they instruct cells bearing specific receptors to alter their proliferation, differentiation, effector function, or rate of migration.

There are now more than 60 identified cytokines, and it is no longer possible to describe their individual functions succinctly. Table VI groups many of the known cytokines into families. Since most cytokines mediate immune responses in a positive way, their direct pharmacological use has principally been in the context of augmenting immunity, as discussed in section 2.2.1. Interest in exploiting cytokine networks for anti-inflammatory or immunosuppressive effects has primarily focused on the development of antagonists of pro-inflammatory cytokines. A few of the known cytokines, such as IL-10, IL-13, and interferon-beta-1 (IFN-β1) can be directly used, or their production increased, to achieve a down-regulation of immune responses.

#### Strategies to Exploit Cytokine Modulation for Anti-Inflammatory or Immunosuppressive Effects

A number of highly effective immunosuppressive drugs are known to work, at least in part, by blocking the production of or response to cytokines. Corticosteroids (see section 2.1.2) block the release of IL-1, IL-6, tumour necrosis factor-alpha (TNF-α), and other lymphokines and chemotactic factors. Cyclosporin and tacrolimus (see section 2.1.3) inhibit the transcription of IL-2, IL-3, IL-4, IFN-γ, TNF-α, and GM-CSF (granulocyte macrophage colony-stimulating factor) by activated T cells.[80] Rapamycin has been shown to block the response to IL-1, IL-2, IL-3, IL-4 and IL-6.[80,81]

Major efforts are now underway to rationally design agents to inhibit the expression or effects

**Table VI.** Cytokine families

| Family | General function | Members |
|---|---|---|
| Interleukins | Immunomodulatory and growth regulating functions | IL-1α, IL-1β, IL-2, IL-3, IL-4, IL-5, IL-6, IL-7, IL-8, IL-9, IL-10, IL-11, IL-12, IL-13, IL-14, IL-15 |
| Colony-stimulating factors | Growth and differentiating factors for haematopoietic cells | G-CSF, GM-CSF, M-CSF, EPO |
| Interferons | Antiviral and immunomodulatory actions | IFN-α, IFN-β, IFN-γ |
| Chemokines | Chemoattractant and growth regulatory factors | GRO-α, GRO-β, GRO-γ, MIP-1α, MIP-1β, MCP-1, MCP-2, MCP-3, RANTES |
| Growth factors | Affect connective tissue functions; TNFs have immunomodulatory actions | TGF-β1, TGF-β2, TGF-β1.2, TGF-β3, TGF-β5, EGF, HB-EGF, TGF-α, FGF acidic, FGF basic, β-ECGF, FGF-4, FGF-5, FGF-6, FGF-7, PDGF-AA, PDGF-BB, PDGF-AB, TNF-α, TNF-β |

*Abbreviations:* ECGF = endothelial cell growth factor; EGF = epidermal growth factor; EPO = erythropoietin; FGF = fibroblast growth factor; G-CSF = granulocyte colony-stimulating factor; GM-CSF = granulocyte macrophage colony-stimulating factor; GRO = growth regulated oncogene (a cytokine now recognised in α, β and γ subtypes); HB-EGF = heparin-binding epidermal growth factor-like growth factor; IFN = interferon; IL = interleukin; MCP = monocyte chemotactic protein; M-CSF = macrophage colony-stimulating factor; MIP = macrophage inflammatory protein; PDGF = platelet-derived growth factor; RANTES = regulated on activation, normal T cell expressed, and secreted; TGF = transforming growth factor; TNF = tumour necrosis factor.

of specific pro-inflammatory cytokines. At least four strategies are being explored:

1) Monoclonal antibodies to cytokines.

2) Receptor antagonism.

3) Blockade of target cell signalling pathways.

4) Biosynthesis inhibition.

Only a few examples of these strategies are given here, although this is an area of pharmaceutical development that is growing explosively.

***Monoclonal antibodies to cytokines*** have already been studied clinically. For example, antibodies to TNF-α and IL-6 have given good results in phase II clinical trials for rheumatoid arthritis.[82] However, while anti-cytokine antibodies can produce anti-inflammatory and immunosuppressive effects, they must be administered parenterally and can lead to sensitisation, as discussed in section 2.1.4.

***Blockade of cytokine receptors*** is being pursued by the use of soluble forms of cytokine receptors, or specific antagonists of receptors. Soluble ligand binding portions of receptors for IL-1 and for tumour necrosis factors are in early clinical trials for inflammatory disorders. The discovery of naturally occurring receptor antagonists has opened another pathway to the blockade of cytokine receptors. IL-1 (which is actually a general term for two proteins, IL-1α and IL-1β, that bind to the same receptor) has long been considered an attractive target for intervention in inflammatory conditions. An endogenous antagonist to the IL-1 receptor, termed IL-1ra (for receptor antagonist) has been found to be effective in animal models of inflammation, and is now being tested in sepsis and rheumatoid arthritis.

***Blockade of target cell signalling pathways:*** pharmaceutical efforts directed at disruption of signal transduction from cytokine receptors to the cell nucleus are still in the early stages of development. Since signal transduction mechanisms may be similar for a number of cytokines, this may be a less selective approach. One promising agent is *lisofylline*, a small molecular inhibitor of phosphatidic acid, an intermediary molecule in the signal transduction pathway of several pro-inflammatory cytokines. Lisofylline has exhibited protective effects in animal models of lung and kidney ischemia/reperfusion, IL-8-induced lung injury and endotoxic shock. Phase II clinical trials are now underway.

***Inhibiting the biosynthesis of cytokines*** is being approached at several levels, including gene transcription, translation, and post-translational processing. Cyclosporin and tacrolimus prevent cytokine transcription by a series of events culminating in the inhibition of a T cell-specific nuclear transcription factor, NFAT. As gene transcription is increasingly elucidated, screening assays for specific cytokine transcription inhibitors can be developed. Agents that disrupt translation of RNA transcripts from cytokine genes are also under development. The bicyclic imidazoles represent a novel class of inhibitors of the synthesis of a number of pro-inflammatory cytokines, and appear to act primarily at the translation level.[83] Translation can also be disrupted with some specificity by the use of a catalytic form of RNA, termed ribozymes, with the capacity to cleave nucleic acids at specific sites.

Post-translational modification is the target of still another approach, the development of convertase inhibitors. For example, both IL-1β and TNF-α are initially synthesised in an inactive form that is subsequently altered by a specific converting enzyme to yield the active form of the cytokine. Interleukin-1β converting enzyme, or ICE, has been considered an attractive target for pharmacological intervention since its cloning in 1992.[84] Elucidation of the crystal structure of ICE has now provided a molecular framework for the design of inhibitors.[85]

A few of the known cytokines have effects that down-regulate immunity, and may therefore be used directly for anti-inflammatory and immunosuppressive purposes. Interleukin-10 (IL-10) inhibits the production of the pro-inflammatory cytokines IL-1, IL-6, IL-8, GM-CSF, TNF-α, and macrophage inflammatory protein-1α (MIP-1α) by activated macrophages. IL-10 also acts directly on T cells to inhibit production of IL-2 and TNF-α by these cells. IL-13 suppresses the cytotoxic function of activated macrophages and the production of pro-inflammatory cytokines.[86] Interferon-β1b increases suppressor T cell function, inhibits production of IFN-γ, TNF-β and other cytokines. It has recently been approved for the treatment of relapsing/remitting multiple sclerosis;[87,88] its clinical efficacy in this condition when administered subcutaneously has been demonstrated in a multicentre, randomised, double-blind, placebo-controlled trial conducted in the US and Canada.[89-91] The frequency of attacks was decreased by one-third, and serious attacks by a half. These clinical observations were buttressed by a serial magnetic resonance imaging (MRI) study which showed significantly greater accumulating disease burden in the placebo arm than in the INF-β1b arm of the trial.[90]

### 2.2 Immunostimulating Agents

Immunologists have long sought ways to enhance the body's immunological defences against external invasion by micro-organisms or internally arising disorders such as cancer. Immune deficiencies, both congenital and acquired, create urgent needs for restoration of immune functions. Recent advances in understanding immune responses have led to unprecedented opportunities for developing effective therapies for enhancing and restoring critical functions of the immune system.

*Vaccines* were the first and remain the most successful of all attempts to enhance immune responses. All of the currently available vaccines are used to prevent rather than treat disorders, and are outside the scope of this chapter. Attempts to develop therapeutic vaccines are discussed in the sections on AIDS (section 3.2), cancers (section 3.6), and future trends in clinical immunology (section 4).

In general, the development of immunostimulatory agents has lagged behind the development of immunosuppressive agents. This may be due in part to the frequent lack of correlation between immune enhancement *in vitro* and *in vivo*, and the absence of animal models for some of the clinical conditions in which immunostimulation would be desirable. Nonetheless, a large number of immunostimulatory agents, affecting almost all aspects of the immune response, are in clinical use (table VII). The major categories of immunostimulating agents are briefly reviewed below.

#### *2.2.1 Cytokines and Cytokine Modulating Agents*

**Clinical Applications and Effectiveness**

The principal cytokines that have been used clinically to date include colony-stimulating factors, interferons, interleukins (primarily IL-2), and a number of cytokines involved in macrophage and granulocyte activation. Some chemical agents with immunostimulatory activity modulate cytokine production.

***Colony-stimulating factors (CSFs)***, particularly G (granulocyte)-CSF and GM (granulocyte-macrophage)-CSF, have proven clinically useful in inducing granulocyte production following chemotherapy with cytotoxic anticancer drugs (see also chapter 26; sect. 5.1.3).[93] G-CSF has also been used with some success in patients with AIDS, whose bone marrow is often suppressed both by the disease and by the therapy used for it. Severe agranulocytosis will likely be an indication for the use of CSFs in the future. The costs of these cytokines, however, will discourage their use for drug-induced myelosuppression that may reasonably be reversed by drug withdrawal or dose reduction. At least 17 distinct haemopoietic regulators have so far been cloned and expressed in recombinant form. All have clinical potential and many are in clinical or preclinical trials.[94]

***Interferons (IFNs)*** were first studied for their direct antiviral activity, but they also affect many cell-mediated immune responses, and many of their clinically useful effects may be mediated through immune modulation. Interferons are used in the treatment of a variety of cancers, with the success of IFN-α in the treatment of hairy cell leukaemia being especially notable. Other approved uses of IFN-α include AIDS-related Kaposi's sarcoma and prevention of infection in persons with chronic granulomatous disease,[95] and it has been used experimentally in allergic disorders.[96] Interferons have also been used successfully in a number of infectious diseases, and IFN-α is currently licensed for the treatment of papilloma virus and hepatitis C infections. The ability of interferons to enhance cell-mediated immunity, as well as their direct antiviral action, may account for their efficacy in promoting viral clearance.

***Interleukins (ILs)*** [see also section 2.1.5 above] are a diverse family of intercellular mediators produced by leucocytes. To date, the only interleukin that has been fully accepted into clinical use has been IL-2. The ability of IL-2 to generate cytotoxic immune responses against malignant cells has led to the testing of this cytokine as a therapeutic agent in many types of cancer. Good responses in a few patients have been observed in several forms of cancer, but tumour regression has been consistently observed only in renal cell carcinoma and malignant melanoma.[97,98] IL-3, an interleukin that modulates macrophage functions and regulates haematopoiesis, is in phase III trials for a number of indications; potential clinical uses include stimulation of haematopoiesis after bone marrow transplantation, in conjunction

**Table VII.** Facets of the immune response. Possible sites of action for immunostimulation (after Drews;[92] with permission of the author and publisher)

| Site of action | Possible mechanism of action | Known substances |
|---|---|---|
| Antigen presentation | Absorption and processing of antigen<br>Expression of MHC antigens | Constituents of microbial cell walls<br>Interferons |
| Antigen recognition | Improvement of intracellular signal transmission by optimising current reactions | |
| Lymphocyte activation | Expression of interleukin-2 receptors<br>Synthesis of interleukin-2 and other lymphokines | Interferon-γ ?<br>Interleukin-1 |
| Clonal expansion | Action of interleukin-2; amplification of T helper functions | Interleukin-2 |
| Recruitment of T precursor cells | Thymus-dependent function<br>Thymus hormones?<br>Dendritic cells of thymus? | Thymosin fraction 5<br>Thymosin-$\alpha_1$ |
| Induction of cytotoxic T-lymphocytes | Thymus-dependent<br>IL-1 and IL-2-dependent | ? Inosine pranobex (isoprinosine)<br>Thymosins<br>THF, STF and other thymic hormones<br>Interleukin-2 |
| Enhancement of non-specific but specifically controllable effector mechanisms | Activation of macrophages (phagocytosis, Fc and C3b receptors, MHC complex, secretory functions)<br>Recruitment of monocytes and macrophages | Microbial antigens<br>Interferons (interferon-γ)<br>? Levamisole, ? bestatin<br>M-CSF<br>GM-CSF |
| NK cells | Recruitment and activation of NK cells | Interferons (interferon-γ)<br>Interleukin-2 |
| Granulocytes | Activation and recruitment | ? Neutrophil activation inhibitory factor (NAF)<br>GM-CSF |

*Abbreviations:* G-CSF = granulocyte colony-stimulating factor; GM-CSF = granulocyte macrophage colony-stimulating factor; IL= interleukin; M-CSF = macrophage colony-stimulating factor; MHC = major histocompatability complex; NAF = neutrophil activation inhibitory factor; NK = natural killer; STF = serum thymic factor; THF = thymic humoral factor.

with chemotherapy, and in patients with AIDS. Other interleukins appear to have great potential for enhancing specific aspects of immune responsiveness, and clinical applications of these and other cytokines are under intensive investigation.

### Mechanism/Site of Action

*Colony-stimulating factors (CSFs)* control the development of pluripotential bone marrow stem cells into mature blood cells. A number of the *interleukins* also act as haemopoietic regulators. Colony-stimulating factors typically have four distinct effects on responsive cell populations:

1) They are necessary for the survival of cells.
2) They stimulate proliferation.
3) They control differentiation.
4) They activate the differentiated cells.[92]

These actions are mediated through binding to specific receptors on the target cells, followed by a cascade of cytoplasmic and nuclear events.[94] Colony-stimulating factors may either control the development of a specific cell type (e.g. G-CSF induces granulocytes) or may be pluripotent (e.g. GM-CSF induces both granulocytes and monocytes).

*Interferons* are pleiotropic cytokines with multiple immunomodulatory actions.[99] The interferons are of two types, with multiple subtypes. Type I interferons, which are secreted by nucleated cells after viral infections, include α and β interferons. There are at least 20 subtypes of IFN-α. Type II interferons, also called γ or immune interferons, are the product of activated lymphocytes, primarily T cells of the $T_H1$ subset, and are generally more potent than the type I interferons.[100] Interferons regulate the expression of important cell surface molecules involved in immune responses, and have antiviral, antitumour, antiproliferative and other immunomodulatory effects. The cellular effects are mediated by the binding of interferons to specific receptors, that are widely distributed on haematological, endothelial, immunological and other cells, and induce differing effects in specific cell types. At least some of the intracellular actions of interferons are mediated by protein kinases, and involve inhibition or disruption of RNA translation. The up-regulation of major histocompatibility (MHC) class II genes by IFN-γ has recently been shown to be attributable to the induction by IFN-γ of the MHC class II transactivator gene CIITA.[101]

Thus, a major immunomodulatory action of IFN-γ has been traced, beginning with the initial kinase-mediated phosphorylation of the p91 protein,[102] and continuing through the induction of a gene- and tissue-specific coactivator intermediary, to up-regulation of a major class of cell surface molecules involved in immune responses. In general, it can be said that interferons inhibit the further differentiation of cells, while enhancing the expression of differentiated function already present.[103]

*Interleukin-2* has numerous mechanisms of action that can result in immune stimulation. All are initially mediated by the binding of IL-2 to specific cell surface receptors. Interleukin-2 has an autocrine action on T lymphocytes, in that its release by activated T cells induces further T cell proliferation and activation. It also activates natural killer (NK) cells, lymphokine-activated killer (LAK) cells and macrophages, and promotes B cell growth.[100]

#### Pharmacodynamic and Pharmacokinetic Characteristics

The pharmacodynamics and pharmacokinetics of *interleukins* and *interferons* have been extensively reviewed.[104,105] In general, cytokines are produced and act locally, and their action at remote sites is prevented by an array of inhibitors and catabolic mechanisms. As a result, they have very short half-lives, lasting only minutes in the circulation. The half-lives of recombinant cytokines produced in prokaryotic organisms are usually even shorter than those of the natural products. Recombinant cytokines can also be immunogenic, provoking antibodies that interfere with the desired effects.[106]

Cytokines are larger molecules than most drugs, most being 14,000 to 40,000D. Each cytokine has multiple biological functions, giving rise to many unwanted effects when the cytokine is given systemically. It is hoped that structure-activity studies will allow the development of smaller agonists or antagonists of cytokines, with more defined biological effects and less susceptibility to inhibitors.

#### Tolerability and Drug Interactions Potential

*Colony-stimulating factors:* compared with interferons and interleukins, colony-stimulating factors are relatively free of serious systemic toxic effects. They are not given shortly before or after the administration of cytotoxic chemotherapy, because by inducing the proliferation of myeloid cells, they render them more sensitive to the cytotoxic drugs. For example, *filgrastim*, a recombinant G-CSF, should not be given sooner than 24 hours after a dose, nor sooner than 24 hours before administration of cytotoxic chemotherapy. In general, other drug interactions have not been observed in phase II and III trials. Colony-stimulating factors should not be used in the presence of any malignancy with myeloid characteristics, because of the possibility that they might promote tumour growth.

*Interferons:* the adverse effects associated with therapeutic use of interferons are qualitatively similar for the various types and subtypes. Acute effects include influenza-like symptoms of fever, chills, myalgias, arthralgias, headache and diaphoresis. These symptoms can sometimes be prevented or ameliorated by the concurrent administration of paracetamol (acetaminophen) or a prostaglandin synthetase inhibitor.[104,106] Long term effects include fatigue, anorexia, and weight loss. Additional rare but serious effects have been observed when high doses of interferons have been used. For example, doses of IFN-γ1b in excess of 250 $\mu g/m^2$/day may result in neutropenia and elevated hepatic enzymes, exacerbate cardiac disease, or cause mental impairment, gait disturbance, and dizziness, especially in patients with compromised central nervous system function or seizure disorders.

*Interleukins and tumour necrosis factor:* toxic systemic effects have been a major limiting factor in exploiting the diverse immunomodulating effects of interleukins. The adverse effects are somewhat specific for the various lymphokines, and can be severe or even fatal. For example, IL-2 causes a syndrome of capillary leakage with cardiorespiratory effects, and tumour necrosis factor can cause disseminated intravascular coagulation.[105]

If toxic and therapeutic effects are mediated by different parts of the cytokine molecules, it may be possible to dissociate them by rational drug design. Alternatively, if it were possible to administer cytokines at the specific site for the desired effect, this would mimic their natural pharmacodynamic actions, i.e. they would be released and act in a paracrine manner only in restricted microenvironments.

**Table VIII.** Clinical studies with thymic hormones (after Chirigos;[108] Dechant & Bryson[107])

| Hormone | Clinical condition | Results |
|---|---|---|
| Thymostimulin | Post-surgical infection prophylaxis in immunocompromised patients | ↓ Postoperative infection rate |
| | Cancer | ↓ Chemotherapy-associated myelosuppression |
| | Human immunodeficiency virus infection | ↓ Treatment-associated myelosuppression |
| | Viral hepatitis (acute and chronic) | Clinical improvement |
| Thymic humoral factor | Varicella/zoster in immunocompromised patients | Recovery from infections that might otherwise be fatal |
| Thymosin fraction 5 | Primary immunodeficiencies | ↑ T cells, clinical improvement |
| | Lung cancer (nonresectable small cell) | Prolonged survival |
| Thymosin-$\alpha_1$ | Lung cancer (non-oat cell) | Prolonged disease-free interval, and ↑ survival |
| Thymulin | Rheumatoid arthritis, Di George's syndrome, ataxia, telangiectasia | Clinical improvement, ↑ cell-mediated immunity |
| Thymopentin | Di George's syndrome | Clinical improvement, ↑ cell-mediated immunity |
| | Rheumatoid arthritis | Clinical improvement, ↓ relapses |
| | Recurrent herpes | |

### *2.2.2 Thymic Hormones*

#### Clinical Applications and Effectiveness

The thymus is the site of T lymphocyte maturation and initial differentiation, and also produces soluble factors that may act at a distance to effect the further maturation and functional competence of T cells. These soluble factors, termed thymic hormones, appear to have clinical potential. They are likely to be useful in patients with primary or secondary immunodeficiencies to induce differentiation and maturation of nonfunctional precursor cells into immunologically competent T lymphocytes. By augmenting T cell-mediated aspects of the immune response, they may enhance the responses of immunocompromised and possibly of immunologically normal individuals to infections or, in some instances, to malignancies. Many small scale studies or case reports on the clinical use of thymic hormones have been published, but few controlled clinical trials have been conducted. These have usually reported modestly successful results, and a number of clinical trials of thymic hormones are summarised in table VIII. The greatest clinical experience has been amassed with *thymostimulin* (see review by Dechant & Bryson[107]).

Many problems remain to be resolved before any of the thymic hormones come into routine clinical use. Most of the thymic hormones listed in table VIII are extracted from calf thymus, and only partially purified. Most consist of a mixture of peptides, and can be recognised as foreign antigens by the immune system of the recipient. Identification and purification of the active moieties will facilitate their use as pharmaceutical agents.

#### Mechanism/Site of Action

Thymic hormones have been shown to modulate prothymocyte differentiation and T lymphocyte function in various assays, both *in vitro* and *in vivo*. Few direct comparisons of the different preparations have been made to permit assessment of differences in their action. Their precise mechanisms of action are poorly defined, but probably involve induction of cell surface markers and lymphokine production.

#### Pharmacodynamic and Pharmacokinetic Characteristics

Thymic hormones have generally been administered intramuscularly, in daily or less frequent doses. Elucidation of their pharmacokinetics is hampered by lack of assays clearly related to the active moieties and by the presence of endogenous thymic hormones in most patients. However, their catabolism and elimination is expected to be similar to that of other peptides.

#### Tolerability and Drug Interactions Potential

Allergic reactions, especially to the less purified preparations, are not uncommon, and severe anaphylactic responses have been documented. Initiation or exacerbation of autoimmunity seems possible, and has been suspected in some patients with severe reactions. Thymic hormones should therefore not be administered to patients with atopy or autoimmune disorders. The use of these agents in any disease is experimental and they should only be administered under strictly controlled circumstances.

### *2.2.3 Bacterial and Fungal Products*

A variety of products derived from bacteria or fungi, as well as some preparations of intact bacteria, have been found to augment immune responses. Table IX lists some that are actively being tested in animal models and, in some cases, in clinical trials.

***Bacterial products:*** the bacillus of Calmette-Guérin (BCG) is an attenuated strain of *Mycobacterium bovis* that has been known for many years to be an immunostimulant. It is approved for intravesical use for bladder carcinoma, and has been used experimentally for the treatment of many cancers. It is a live bacterium, and can cause disseminated infection in immunocompromised patients.

A small molecular weight derivative of mycobacteria, *muramyl dipeptide*, has attracted considerable interest for its immunostimulating effects, especially when combined with IFN-γ.[92] Antitumour effects and protection against infections have been documented in many animal models. Muramyl dipeptide is also under clinical investigation as a vaccine adjuvant.[109]

*Picibanil*, a lyophilisate of penicillin-treated *Streptococcus pyogenes* A3su, has been launched in Japan as an anticancer immunostimulant. Indications for its use include gastrointestinal, lung, and head and neck cancers.

***Fungal products:*** a number of fungi have yielded immunostimulatory products, such as β-1, 3-D-glucans. Two such preparations, *krestin* and *lentinan*, have proved to have clinically useful antitumour effects, particularly in the treatment of stomach cancer.[96] The mechanism of action and clinical efficacy of lentinan have been reviewed by Suzuki et al.[110]

**Table IX.** Bacterial and fungal products with immunostimulatory properties

| |
|---|
| **Intact bacteria** |
| Bacille Calmette-Guérin (BCG) |
| *Corynebacterium parvum* |
| *Brucella abortus* |
| *Bordetella pertussis* |
| *Nocardia* sp. |
| *Pseudomonas aeruginosa* |
| **Bacterial products** |
| Muramyl dipeptide *(M. smegmatis)* and analogues |
| MER (BCG) |
| Biostim *(Klebsiella pneumoniae)* |
| ERB *(Listeria monocytogenes, Salmonella typhimurium)* |
| Peptidoglycans (Gram-negative bacteria) |
| Picibanil *(Staphylococcus pyogenes)* |
| **Fungal products** |
| Lentinan *(Lentinus edodes)* |
| Bestatin (ubenimex) *[Streptomyces olivoreticuli]* |
| *p*-Hydroxybestatin (metabolite of bestatin) |
| Krestin *(Coriolus versicolor)* or other β1, 3-D-glucans (various fungi) |

The main clinical applications being targeted in the development of immunostimulants derived from bacteria and fungi are cancers and infectious diseases, especially upper respiratory infections in children and adults.[111] While their clinical application in infectious diseases is almost entirely experimental, the clinical efficacy of bacterial and fungal immunostimulants in the treatment of some cancers has gained clinical acceptance.

The mechanisms of action of bacterial and fungal products are largely undefined, but activation of macrophages and stimulation of cytokine expression are likely to be involved. Bacterial and fungal immunostimulatory products often have adverse effects that have been associated with the release of cytokines. These include the influenza-like symptoms of chills, fever, headache and malaise that are also seen with the administration of many therapeutic antibodies directed against T cells.[112]

The immune augmentation resulting from the systemic administration of bacterial and fungal immunostimulants is nonspecific, and it is reasonable to assume that undesirable immune responses may be similarly enhanced.[112] One approach to employing immunomodulators in a more selective manner is to combine them with a specific antigen. A cancer vaccine composed of tumour antigens coupled to BCG is an example of this approach, and has recently proven efficacious in metastatic melanoma.[113]

#### *2.2.4 Synthetic Immunostimulating Agents*

Although some of the bacterial and fungal products listed in table IX, e.g. muramyl dipeptide and bestatin, have now been synthesised, this section focuses on a diverse group of synthetic drugs that are usually considered separately. Table X lists some synthetic immunostimulants that are at various stages of clinical development or approval. The first three agents listed are discussed in a little more detail below.

##### Levamisole

Levamisole, the levoisomer of tetramisole, is an anthelmintic drug that has been studied for its immunostimulatory properties for over 20 years. Levamisole is able to restore depressed or deficient immune responses, while normal response are usually unchanged. T cell functions are enhanced, and phagocytosis, chemo-

**Table X.** Synthetic immunostimulants

| |
|---|
| Levamisole |
| Inosine pranobex (isoprinosine) |
| Cimetidine |
| Tuftsin |
| Ditiocarb sodium (diethyldithiocarbamate) |
| Azimexon |
| Ciamexon |
| Methyl inosine monophosphate (MIMP) |
| Bropirimine |
| Forphenicin |

taxis and effector functions of macrophages and polymorphonuclear cells are increased.

Based upon extensive experience in animal models indicating that levamisole can augment resistance to infections, numerous small scale clinical trials have assessed its potential for preventing or treating human infectious diseases. Although there is some evidence that prophylactic treatment with levamisole may reduce the frequency and duration of upper respiratory infections in children, it has not come into accepted clinical usage for this or any other infectious condition.

Although extensive testing of levamisole in immune-mediated disorders has revealed some efficacy, its clinical acceptance has been limited by the risk of severe granulocytopenia, which is a well established adverse effect of the drug. Levamisole has been used to maintain corticosteroid-free remission in children with steroid-responsive but dependent nephrotic syndrome.[114] It also promotes healing of mucosal ulcers in Behçet's syndrome, and has demonstrated clinical efficacy in rheumatoid arthritis, but the frequency of drug-induced agranulocytosis has deterred clinicians from adopting this therapy in light of available alternatives.

In the US, the only approved use of levamisole is for adjunctive therapy, in combination with fluorouracil, in patients with resected Duke's stage C colon cancer (see section 3.6). Clinical trials in patients with other forms of cancer have yielded conflicting results.[92]

In addition to rare but serious cases of agranulocytosis, other adverse effects seen with levamisole include the influenza-like symptoms that are associated with cytokine release, and occasional exacerbations of immune-mediated disorders.[112]

#### Inosine Pranobex

Inosine pranobex (isoprinosine) is a T cell stimulant that appears to have antiviral effects as well. It may be useful for some acute and chronic viral infections (see chapter 32; sect. 2.19), but has not been approved for such use in the US.[96]

#### Cimetidine

Cimetidine is an $H_2$-receptor blocking antihistamine that appears to decrease the actions of suppressor T cells, and thus enhances immunity, especially cell-mediated immunity. It may be useful in the treatment of common variable hypogammaglobulinaemia.[115]

## 3. Clinical Application of Immunomodulatory Agents in Selected Immune Systems Disorders

### 3.1 Organ Transplantation

#### *3.1.1 Role of Immunomodulation in Therapy*

Transplantation of an organ from one individual to another, except in the case of identical twins, triggers a rejection process that represents an iatrogenic immune-mediated disorder. The triggering event is clear-cut, and the target antigens well defined, so in many ways graft rejection serves as a paradigm for organ-specific autoimmune diseases.

Prevention and treatment of graft rejection require rigorous, long term suppression of the immune system sufficient to prevent graft rejection, while attempting to preserve an adequate response capability of warding off infections and malignancy. Transplantation medicine has been the proving ground for nearly all immunosuppressive drugs in the pharmacological armamentarium. Drug discovery efforts for immunosuppressive agents are usually directed towards transplantation as the initial clinical application, because:

- The immune responses to be manipulated have good *in vitro* correlates, most notably mixed lymphocyte responses; and
- Experimental organ transplantation in animals is well suited for preclinical testing.

#### *3.1.2 Choice of Therapy*

Organ rejection is classically divided into three phases that differ in mechanism and, to some extent, in therapy required. These are hyperacute, acute, and chronic rejection.

#### Hyperacute Rejection

Hyperacute rejection occurs at the time of transplantation, and is usually apparent within the first 30 to 60 minutes following revascularisation of the transplanted organ. It is mediated by preformed antibodies against donor antigens, and should not occur if the pretransplant lymphocytotoxic antibody crossmatching between donor lymphocytes and recipient serum is negative. Once it occurs, however, the only course is to remove the transplanted organ.

**Acute Rejection**

Acute rejection is caused by a cell-mediated immune response by the recipient's immune system to the foreign histocompatibility antigens of the engrafted organ. Therapeutic intervention can be directed at any of several stages of the immune response. It is in the prevention and treatment of graft rejection that the utility of a multidrug regimen, manipulating several aspects of the immune response simultaneously, has most clearly established the value of combination therapy. Routine maintenance of graft tolerance, as practised by most transplant centres, uses triple or quadruple drug therapy.

Such protocols typically include a xenobiotic immunosuppressive agent such as cyclosporin or tacrolimus, a cytotoxic agent to block proliferative stages of the immune response, corticosteroids for their multiple immunosuppressive effects, and often some use of anti-T cell antibodies as well.

*Cyclosporin* or *tacrolimus* is the mainstay of antirejection therapy today. The introduction of cyclosporin in the 1970s revolutionised transplantation, boosting cadaver kidney 1-year success rates from 50% to 70% or more, and making transplantation of new types of organs feasible. Tacrolimus, which has very similar efficacy and a somewhat more favourable adverse effects profile, is being substituted for cyclosporin in many transplant centres. A recent European multicentre randomised trial comparing the two xenobiotics found fewer rejection episodes in the first year following liver transplantation, and less requirement for concurrent immunosuppression when tacrolimus rather than cyclosporin was the primary immunosuppressive agent.[116]

Cytotoxic agents, particularly *azathioprine*, were among the first drugs to be used for antirejection therapy. Azathioprine continues to be used in most protocols, but newer and more lymphocyte-selective agents such as mycophenolate mofetil, mizoribine, and brequinar sodium are rapidly gaining acceptance.

*Corticosteroids* are almost invariably involved in multidrug regimens, as their broad spectrum of activity, affecting monocytes, T cells, B cells, and polymorphonuclear leucocytes, has proven to be nearly indispensable clinically. Nonetheless, there has recently been considerable interest among transplant clinicians in 'weaning' recipients off corticosteroids, or using minimal doses, because in the long term, adverse effects attributable to these agents are among the most troublesome complications of immunosuppressive regimens.[117]

*Immunosuppressive antibodies*, especially antibodies directed against T lymphocytes, are widely used as antirejection therapy. Long term use of xenogeneic antibodies is not feasible, due to the development of sensitisation in the host, so their use is limited to acute situations. In renal transplantation, *antilymphocyte antibodies* are often administered just prior to transplantation and in the first week or two following surgery. This allows the use of cyclosporin, which has nephrotoxic effects, to be postponed until renal function has been established. Antilymphocyte antibodies are commonly used to treat acute rejection episodes, with efficacy that is often similar to that of high-dose corticosteroids. 'Steroid-resistant' rejection may respond to treatment with immunosuppressive antibodies.[118,119]

Acute rejection episodes resistant to other therapy have shown good responses to the new cytotoxic agent *mycophenolate mofetil* in both renal and liver transplants.[120,121] The new xenobiotic *gusperimus* (deoxyspergualin) has also been used in Japan to treat refractory episodes of acute rejection.[122,123]

The type of transplantation procedure also contributes to variability in immunosuppressive regimens favoured by different centres. A recent survey of transplant programme directors showed that pancreas transplant programmes were most likely to consider the use of immunosuppressive antibodies important or essential in their protocols.[124] Maintenance regimens involving only two drugs, either cyclosporin and corticosteroids or cyclosporin and azathioprine, were most likely to be used in renal transplantation.

As additional new immunosuppressive drugs are developed, an almost unlimited number of protocols are likely to come into clinical use. Selection of specific combinations of immunosuppressive agents to be tested in controlled trials is likely to be increasingly rational, rather than empiric, based upon knowledge of their mechanisms of action. The general principle now seems well established that synergistic effects can be obtained by combining drugs with complementary actions and non-overlapping adverse effects.

#### Chronic Rejection

This type of rejection is the least well understood. It is the leading cause of graft failure in the period beyond six months post-transplant, and is usually identified by declining function of the engrafted organ. Antibody-mediated immune responses are believed to play a role and, in particular, anti-HLA antibodies are significantly more common in patients experiencing chronic rejection than in those with stable graft function.[125] Likewise, the beneficial effect of HLA matching is even more evident in terms of 5- or 10-year graft survival than it is at 1 year post-transplant.[126] This has led to the suggestion that improved suppression of B lymphocyte responses may prevent chronic rejection.[127]

Although chronic rejection appears relatively unresponsive to conventional immunosuppressive therapy employed for graft maintenance or treatment of acute rejection, some of the newer immunosuppressive agents may be more effective in preventing or treating chronic rejection. In particular, *mycophenolate mofetil* has shown promising results in long term maintenance of renal allografts.[128] Studies in an experimental model of chronic rejection have demonstrated the efficacy of mycophenolate mofetil, alone, or in combination with brequinar sodium.[129]

### 3.1.3 Avoiding Problems in Treatment

Adverse effects of immunosuppressive therapy used in organ transplantation are of two types. There are specific adverse effects associated with the use of various agents, and more general consequences of immunosuppression such as increased infections and malignancies.

***Specific adverse effects*** of immunosuppressive drugs, and strategies for their prevention and management have been reviewed by Rossi et al.[20] In general, myelosuppression is managed by dose reduction or withdrawal. Management of the adverse effects of corticosteroids involves use of alternate-day and dosage reduction protocols. The nephrotoxicity associated with cyclosporin is often treated with prostaglandin analogues, calcium antagonists, pentoxifylline and thromboxane antagonists. Dose reduction of cyclosporin may also be in order, although this is an area of current controversy.[130,131] The first dose or two of immunosuppressive anti-T cell antibodies are often followed by a syndrome termed the 'first dose effect', which can be ameliorated by concurrent treatment with diphenhydramine, low-dose corticosteroids and paracetamol (acetaminophen).

***Other (general) consequences of immunosuppression:*** the more general effect of immunosuppression, i.e. increased susceptibility to infection, is usually managed by prophylactic measures and aggressive treatment of infections. Prophylactic measures include vaccination against hepatitis B and pneumococci, and perioperative and postoperative antibiotics, often including 'second generation' cefalosporins, cotrimoxazole (trimethoprim/sulfamethoxazole), aciclovir, and nystatin.[11]

An increased incidence of malignancy is a well-recognised risk of organ transplantation, and is probably related both to the chronic immune stimulation resulting from the graft and to the carcinogenic potential of many immunosuppressive agents. As comparative data are accumulated concerning the relative carcinogenicity of immunosuppressive drugs, selection of safer agents is expected to reduce the risk of malignancy following organ transplantation.

## 3.2 Acquired Immunodeficiency Syndrome (AIDS)

### 3.2.1 Role of Immunomodulation in Therapy

One of the more active areas of medical research today is the search for effective therapies for human immunodeficiency virus (HIV) infection. While the major therapeutic approach to AIDS currently relies on antiretroviral agents (see chapter 32; sect. 2 and 3.1), it is likely that successful treatment of HIV infection will require the addition of immune-based therapies to modify the course of the disease. In addition, there is a clear role for immunomodulation in the prevention or treatment of opportunistic infections. Identification of successful therapeutic strategies involving immunomodulation is critically dependent on gaining and applying an understanding of the immunobiology of HIV infection.

#### Immunobiology of HIV Infection

The HIV virus infects cells of the immune system, including T cells, macrophages, and dendritic cells, and can replicate or remain dormant, depending upon circumstances that are not entirely understood. An oligoclonal expansion of CD8+ T cells appears to be one of the earliest events in the immune response of infected patients, and correlates with a decrease in plasma viraemia.[132] This suggests that HIV-specific cytotoxic T lymphocytes may be initially effective in holding the virus in check.[133] There is evidence that the virus preferentially replicates in activated T cells, and because of this, some strategies to enhance immune responses have proven counter- productive. Paradoxically, some types of immunosuppressive drugs may have a therapeutic role in containing the infection, especially during the latent stage.

After a variable period of time, HIV infection causes progressive immune deficiency, with depletion of CD4+ ('helper') T lymphocytes being the most marked feature. Some individuals have remained clinically asymptomatic for more than a decade after HIV infection, and studies of these long term survivors may elucidate mechanisms that can hold the virus in check. It appears likely that viral containment is mediated by some aspect of the immune response, with current evidence suggesting that cell-mediated immunity, rather than humoral immunity, may be the more effective response.

The exact mechanism of T cell depletion in HIV infection is the subject of intensive investigation, as a possible target for immune intervention. The depletion is not simply accounted for by viral lysis, and some form of apoptosis, or programmed cell death, is thought to be involved.

Another paradigm under investigation is based upon observations that the cytokine profile during HIV infection shifts from a preponderance of cytokines characteristic of one subset of CD4 T cells, termed T helper 1 ($T_H1$) cells, to that characteristic of another subset, T helper 2 ($T_H2$) cells. The cause of this shift is not clear, but may correlate with loss of control of the infection, and disease progression.[134]

#### Immunomodulating Strategies

As the immunodeficiency progresses, HIV infected individuals become increasingly susceptible to opportunistic infections and cancer, and these conditions are often the immediate cause of death. At this point, various strategies to boost the immune response and prevent or treat infections offer the greatest potential for extending the life of AIDS patients. Furthermore, some of the antiviral agents used for HIV infection have myelosuppressive effects themselves, and immunomodulation to offset this effect may play a critical role in preventing opportunistic infections.

Current efforts to use immunomodulation to treat aspects of HIV infection have principally focused on the use of cytokines, adoptive immunotherapy (i.e. the transfer of bone marrow or peripheral blood lymphocytes from another individual), and the development of a therapeutic vaccine. Determination of the clinical efficacy of any type of therapy in HIV infection has been very difficult. The slow and variable course of the illness has prompted the use of surrogate markers of disease progression, such as CD4+ T cell counts or p24 antigenaemia. However, these markers do not reliably correlate with clinical progression or outcome (see also chapter 32; sect. 3.1).

### *3.2.2 Therapeutic Potential of Cytokines in HIV Infection*

Of the many cytokines that have been examined as possibly therapeutic in patients with HIV infection, colony-stimulating factors, interferons, and interleukins 2 and 12 have received the most attention.

#### Colony-Stimulating Factors (CSFs)

Both granulocyte colony-stimulating factor (G-CSF) and granulocyte macrophage colony-stimulating factor (GM-CSF) have been evaluated in clinical trials in patients with HIV infection. They are usually used as adjunctive therapy with zidovudine or interferon-α, both of which have myelosuppression as a prominent adverse effect. These CSFs are effective in ameliorating treatment-induced neutropenia, and are likely to have an important supportive role in helping patients tolerate anti-HIV agents and other therapy.[135] For example, in patients with AIDS and cytomegalovirus (CMV) retinitis who developed unacceptable leucopenia in response to ganciclovir therapy, concurrent treatment with GM-CSF has been found to raise neutrophil counts into the normal range, allow continued treatment with ganciclovir, and prevent progression of the retinitis.[136] Several studies have shown GM-CSF to improve leucopenia that would have prevented treatment with antiviral agents and leucopenia associated with such therapy (for a review see Grant and Heel[137]).

#### Interferons (IFNs)

Both IFN-α and IFN-γ have been assessed as possible therapy in HIV infection. The consensus appears to be that IFN-γ is ineffective, and that IFN-α is only clearly efficacious when used as a treatment for Kaposi's sarcoma. IFN-α is, in fact, approved for the treatment of Kaposi's sarcoma in AIDS patients, and is most effective in patients whose CD4+ T cell counts have not fallen below 400 cells/μl. A review of clinical trials of IFN-α is epidemic Kaposi's sarcoma has indicated that the clinical features of the condition most likely to be associated with a good response (in terms of tumour regression) are absence of a prior history of opportunistic infections, absence of systemic 'B' symptoms (fever, weight loss, night sweats), and relative preservation of immune function.[138] The observed correlation between clinical response and immune competence suggests that IFN-α acts through immune modulation, rather than through a direct antiviral or antiproliferative effect.[139] The use of IFN-α for HIV infection in the absence of Kaposi's sarcoma, especially in combination with other agents, is still under evaluation.

Adverse effects, including neutropenia, thrombocytopenia, and transaminase elevations have been limiting factors. Concurrent use of G-CSF has been recommended to offset the myelosuppression seen with IFN-α.

**Interleukins**

The interleukin that has received the most attention in HIV infection is IL-2. This cytokine has the ability to expand CD4+ T cell populations both *in vitro* and *in vivo*. Thus, it was logical to hope that exogenous IL-2 could forestall the decrease of CD4+ T cells that accompanies the decline of immunocompetence in HIV infection. However, trials of the cytokine, alone or in combination with other drugs, have proved very disappointing. This appears to be an instance where immune augmentation favours the spread of the HIV virus, which preferentially infects activated T cells and uses many of the same regulatory elements for replication as the cells it infects.[139,140]

#### *3.2.3 Adoptive Immunotherapy in HIV Infection*

Adoptive immunotherapy has been tried in HIV infection for two separate purposes. Firstly, transfer of antibody or immunocompetent cells to prevent or treat opportunistic infections utilises established protocols that have proven effective in patients with primary immunodeficiencies or drug-induced immunosuppression. Attempts to reconstitute the immune system of AIDS patients by bone marrow transplantation from HLA-identical siblings not infected with HIV have led to only transient immunological improvement. Recently, two large trials of intravenous immunoglobulins in children with HIV infection have demonstrated successful prophylaxis of bacterial infections in these patients.[141]

The second application of adoptive immunotherapy is intended to combat or contain the HIV infection itself. A number of strategies employing *in vitro* expansion of cytotoxic T cells specific for HIV antigens are now under investigation.

#### *3.2.4 Potential Role of Therapeutic Vaccination*

The long and slowly progressive course of HIV infection presents an opportunity to modulate the course of the disease by post-infection vaccination. The objective of such therapeutic vaccination would be to potentiate immune responses that would contain the infection and maintain clinical latency. Perhaps the greatest obstacle to implementing such a strategy is lack of understanding concerning the immunological correlates of non-progression of HIV disease.

Several different approaches to development of a therapeutic vaccine are being actively pursued, and have recently been reviewed.[142] Current understanding of the immunopathogenesis of HIV disease suggests several immunological objectives for therapeutic vaccination. Antigenic variation of HIV poses a major problem for vaccine development, and thus target antigens should be selected from among the most conserved and stable antigenic epitopes. Antibodies induced in response to vaccination should have virus-neutralising properties; the induction of non-neutralising antibodies should be avoided to decrease the possibility of antibody-dependent enhancement. Cell-mediated immunity may be more effective than humoral immunity for containing the infection. Strategies to maximise the cell-mediated immune response should be employed, such as selection of relevant epitopes, and use of vectors or adjuvants designed to elicit T cell responses.

### 3.3 Rheumatoid Arthritis

#### *3.3.1 Role of Immunomodulation in Therapy*

Rheumatoid arthritis is clearly an immune-mediated disorder, and almost all of the drugs used for its treatment have anti-inflammatory or immunosuppressive effects (see also chapter 25).[143] Rheumatoid arthritis is a chronic, progressive disorder characterised by inflamma-

**Table XI.** 'Second-line' drugs for the treatment of rheumatoid arthritis (after Kavanaugh & Lipsky[143])

| Drug | Mechanism of action | Common adverse effects |
|---|---|---|
| **Disease-modifying antirheumatic drugs (DMARDs)** | | |
| Injectable gold (aurothioglucose, sodium aurothiomalate) | Inhibits macrophage function and angiogenesis; inhibits the activity of protein kinase C | Mucocutaneous eruptions, proteinuria, thrombocytopenia |
| Oral gold (auranofin) | Inhibits function of macrophages and polymorphonuclear leucocytes | Diarrhoea, mucocutaneous eruptions |
| Antimalarials (hydroxychloroquine) | Inhibits cytokine secretion, lysosomal enzymes and macrophage function | Rash, visual disturbances |
| Penicillamine | Inhibits helper T cell function and angiogenesis | Mucocutaneous eruptions, proteinuria, thrombocytopenia |
| Sulfasalazine | Inhibits B cell responses, angiogenesis and G-protein-mediated signal transduction | Nausea, anorexia, rash |
| Methotrexate | Inhibits dihydrofolate reductase and chemotaxis; anti-inflammatory effect via induction of adenosine release | Mucocutaneous eruptions, bone marrow suppression, nausea, hepatic abnormalities |
| Tenidap | Inhibits cyclo-oxygenase, interleukins-1 and -6 and tissue necrosis factor-α | Mild reversible proteinuria |
| **Systemic immunosuppressive agents** | | |
| Azathioprine | Inhibits DNA synthesis and cellular proliferation | Bone marrow suppression, nausea, hepatic abnormalities |
| Cyclophosphamide | Crosslinks DNA and inhibits cellular proliferation | Nausea, emesis, bone marrow suppression, ovarian failure, haemorrhagic cystitis, increased risk of cancer |
| Cyclosporin | Inhibits synthesis of T cell cytokines (especially interleukin-2) | Hypertension, renal insufficiency |

tion of the joint spaces and surrounding structures. The events or agents responsible for the initiation of this autoimmune disorder are unknown, but the inappropriate immune response results in progressive damage to the joints.[144] Rheumatoid arthritis is a very heterogeneous disorder in terms of its course. There is no 'correct' way to treat rheumatoid arthritis and each treatment programme must be individualised.[145]

The drugs that are used to treat rheumatoid arthritis can be divided into three groups:

1) Nonsteroidal anti-inflammatory drugs (NSAIDs).

2) Corticosteroids.

3) A large and heterogeneous group of agents that are commonly termed 'second-line' drugs, because they traditionally have not been used as the first choice drugs to treat patients with rheumatoid arthritis.

'Second-line' drugs include the cytotoxic drugs discussed in section 2.1.1, immunosuppressive xenobiotics (section 2.1.4) and a variety of other agents whose anti-inflammatory or immunomodulating mechanisms are not well understood, including gold compounds, antimalarials, penicillamine, and sulfasalazine.[146] Table XI summarises the actions and adverse effects of the commonly used second-line drugs. The views of rheumatologists regarding the relative place of these three groups of drugs in the treatment of rheumatoid arthritis represents a rapidly evolving and somewhat controversial aspect of rheumatology practice. In the traditional approach to therapy, termed the 'pyramid' model, salicylates and nonsteroidal anti-inflammatory drugs were used for initial treatment, and more aggressive forms of therapy only used later, when disease progression became evident. Recently, however, this treatment paradigm has been challenged and alternative approaches have been proposed. These alternative strategies have in common the early use of more aggressive forms of therapy. The rationale for this change is the recognition that progression of disease may be most rapid in the first few years, and that the traditional conservative approach to treatment may allow substantial damage to occur[147] (see further chapter 25; sect. 3.2).

#### *3.3.2 Choice of Therapy*

Rheumatoid arthritis is considered an incurable, lifelong condition, but the intensity of disease activity fluctuates markedly over time, and therapy must be appropriately adjusted in response to the variable disease course. Therapeutic choices would be very much simplified if it were possible to predict the course of disease activity in individual patients. Considerable effort has gone into identifying prognostic factors that may predict rapid progression or development of severe disease.[148] Nonetheless, it remains largely a matter of clinical judgement how best to structure the therapy for an individual patient.

#### Nonsteroidal Anti-Inflammatory Drugs (NSAIDs)

There are a large number of NSAIDs already available for use in rheumatoid arthritis, and many more are under development. Although there are some differences in efficacy and to a lesser extent in toxicity, the choice between them is largely empirical. The best drug for a given patient is usually determined by trial and error, with clinicians switching a patient from one NSAID to another, after a reasonable trial, because of lack of efficacy, adverse effects, or both.[149]

Gastrointestinal toxicity is the major cause of NSAID-induced morbidity and mortality. Risk factors for serious adverse gastrointestinal effects include increased patient age, increased dosage, use of more than one NSAID, a history of peptic ulcer, and use of corticosteroids. A number of preventive and therapeutic strategies to prevent ulceration caused by NSAIDs have been devised (see further chapter 25; sect. 3.1.2).[150]

#### Corticosteroids

Corticosteroids in varying doses and regimens continue to play a role in managing rheumatoid arthritis.[32] Low-dose therapy with 5 to 7.5mg prednisone as a single morning dose may provide relief from inflammation in patients in whom NSAIDs have been ineffective. Older patients in particular may have a better clinical response with fewer serious adverse effects to corticosteroids than to NSAIDs.[145] High doses of corticosteroids are used to control disease flares, but must be tapered appropriately.

Intra-articular injections of corticosteroids can be highly efficacious in patients with a single or a few painful joints. Corticosteroids used in this way often have extended durations of action, and few adverse effects (see also chapter 25; sect. 3.1.3).[151]

#### 'Second-Line' Agents

The diverse group of drugs called 'second-line' agents (table XI) are now used earlier in the course of rheumatoid arthritis, because of the possibility that they may alter the course of joint destruction. Recent studies have attempted to compare the relative efficacy and toxicity of these agents, either via large multicentre studies or meta-analyses of smaller comparative studies.[15,146,152,153] Although there continues to be a role for each of these agents, *methotrexate* appears to be, overall, the most effective and best tolerated of these drugs.[17,154]

Newer agents with better efficacy/toxicity profiles are continually being sought. Evidence that T lymphocytes are critical in the pathogenesis of rheumatoid arthritis has led to therapies targeting T cells. *Cyclosporin* is effective, but nephrotoxicity limits its use.[145] Trials of monoclonal antibodies directed against T lymphocytes, particularly CD4+ or 'helper' T cells, have yielded promising results, but are limited by the drawbacks of current therapeutic antibodies.[70] Early trials of the new cytotoxic drug *mycophenolate mofetil* in patients with severe rheumatoid arthritis refractory to other treatments demonstrated sustained improvements in the majority of patients, with few limiting adverse effects,[9] and this drug would appear to offer benefits over other cytotoxic drugs used in rheumatoid arthritis.[155]

Among the more promising experimental therapies are agents that modulate cytokine functions.[14] One such drug is *tenidap*, a new anti-inflammatory antirheumatic drug that is chemically unrelated to NSAIDs (see also chapter 25; sect. 3.1.4). Tenidap is a cyclo-oxygenase inhibitor that also inhibits production of cytokines, including IL-1, IL-6, and TNF-$\alpha$, with consequent decreases acute phase proteins and erythrocyte sedimentation rate (ESR). These changes correlate with clinical efficacy, which has been superior to that of selected NSAIDs in clinical trials.[156-160]

An intriguing recent finding was a double-blind trial of oral administration of *collagen* in an attempt to induce antigen-specific tolerance to this potentially important autoantigen. A few patients experienced complete remission, with many more showing some benefit.[161] As our understanding of the pathogenesis of rheumatoid arthritis improves, it is likely that more specific forms of therapy can be developed.[162]

### *3.3.3 Avoiding Problems in Treatment*

All immunomodulating drugs are capable of eliciting adverse effects and this is the principal reason that otherwise effective therapies are discontinued in rheumatoid arthritis. Close patient monitoring is required in the treatment of this disorder, and strategies to prevent toxicity should be employed whenever they are available. Gastrointestinal erosions induced by NSAIDs may be prevented by oral administration of a prostaglandin $E_1$ analogue (misoprostol) or the acid (proton) pump inhibitor omeprazole.[150] Osteoporosis associated with corticosteroids can be reduced by calcium supplementation, plus calcitonin, bisphosphonates, or possibly calcitriol (1α,25-dihydroxyvitamin $D_3$) [see also chapter 25; sect. 12.2].

Close monitoring of patients receiving methotrexate can reduce the risk of unrecognised serious liver disease.[22] Agents that have myelosuppression as an adverse effect, such as the cytotoxic drugs, require frequent monitoring of complete blood cell counts to avoid serious adverse effects. In all cases, use of the lowest effective dose of a potentially toxic drug is a sound strategy.

#### *3.3.4 Clinical Outcome and Economic Considerations*

Measurement of disease activity is typically used to assess the response to therapy. Joint tenderness, grip strength, and the quantification of acute phase reactants such as serum C-reactive protein and the erythrocyte sedimentation rate are the most commonly used measures. Global functional assessments and health assessment questionnaires are also widely used. Radiographic changes are a critical indicator of disease progression, but the sensitivity of radiographs may not allow detection of progression except over a period of years. Assessment of long term outcomes are essential for selecting optimum treatment strategies and are under study (see further chapter 25).

In considering the economics of therapy for rheumatoid arthritis, more than the acquisition cost of the drugs must be considered. The cost of ineffective therapy, with resulting disability and loss of productivity, is very high. The cost of monitoring patients for adverse effects, and treating these adverse effects, must be factored into the cost of drug usage. Although cost should not be a primary factor in the choice of treatment, some comments on the comparative expense of some therapeutic agents may be in order. Among the NSAIDs, newer drugs may be considerably more expensive than older ones, while being marginally better, if at all. A few therapies, such as intravenous immunoglobulin and cyclosporin have had limited use due to their relatively high cost. Calculation of true cost-effectiveness ratios for drug treatments will require more information on how therapies affect the long term course of rheumatoid arthritis.

### 3.4 Asthma and Rhinitis

#### *3.4.1 Role of Immunomodulation in Therapy*

Although the pathogenesis of allergic rhinitis and asthma is incompletely understood, there is a growing consensus that these immunological diseases are ultimately mediated by T lymphocytes. This conclusion has resulted from a series of histopathological and lavage studies demonstrating complex patterns of mucosal inflammation in experimental and clinical disease where chronic allergen exposure occurs. Nasal and bronchial biopsies show a mixed cellular infiltrate of T lymphocytes, monocytes, and a denser accumulation of degranulated eosinophils.[163,164] Deposition of eosinophil proteins, such as major basic protein, is also present in the context of desquamated mucosal epithelium. Special histopathological stains show accumulations of a degranulated mast cells in these reactions.

Detection and quantification of mediators of hypersensitivity and cytokines from human allergic reactions have been possible using fluids from nasal and bronchoalveolar lavage of patients with experimental asthma and rhinitis.[163,165,166] The interactions between lymphocytes, mast cells, mediators, and cytokines in these reactions are complex and are the subject of intensive study (fig. 1). Taken together, these data support the hypothesis that asthma, with or without an identifiable allergen, and allergic rhinitis are driven by activated CD4+ (helper-inducer) T cells which release IL-3, IL-5, and GM-CSF. These cytokines facilitate the accumulation and activation of eosinophils in the respiratory mucosa.

**Timing of Allergic Reactions**

Allergic responses have traditionally been called 'immediate hypersensitivity reactions', a term reflecting the original understanding of IgE-mediated clinical responses as those which occur within 2 hours of allergen exposure. Such reactions are associated with the release of preformed mediators of immediate sensitivity from mast cells, and the generation of arachidonic acid metabolites including prostaglandins, leukotrienes and hydroxyeicosatetraenoic acid (HETE) [fig. 2]. These events lead to the clinical manifestations associated with anaphylaxis, including bronchospasm, myocardial toxicity, vasodilatation, and increased vascular perme-

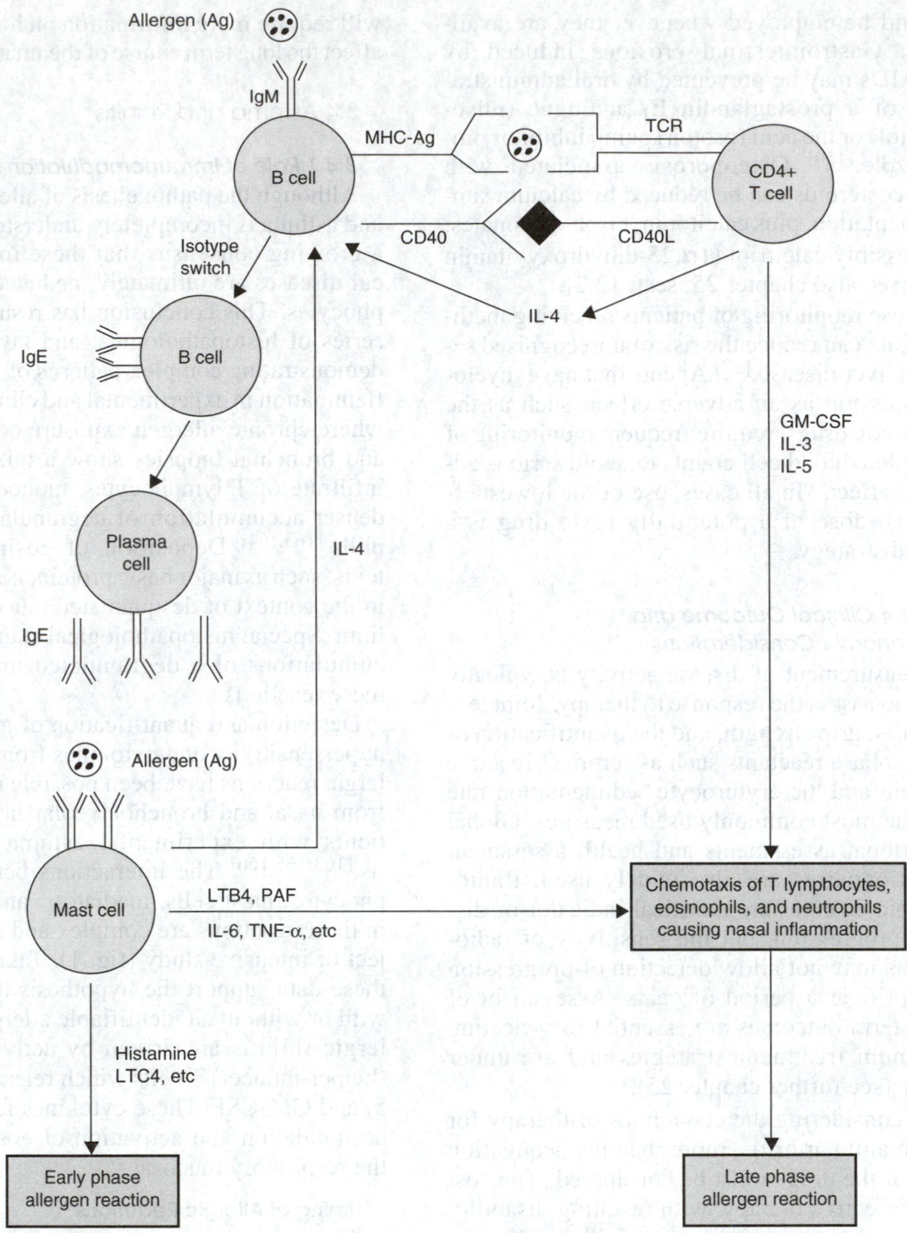


**Fig. 1.** Pathophysiology of allergic rhinitis and asthma. Allergen is presented to $T_H2$ helper T lymphocytes by antigen-presenting cells (such as macrophages or B lymphocytes) in the context of major histocompatibility protein (MHC). In atopic individuals, this leads to the production of cytokines including IL-4, GM-CSF, IL-3, and IL-5. The IL-4 from these $T_H2$ lymphocytes induces B cell isotype switching to IgE. This isotype switch requires contact-dependent help from T cells via the interaction of the CD40 molecule on B cells and the CD40 ligand (CD40L) on T cells. B cells that produce allergen-specific IgE mature into plasma cells that produce IgE, which binds to mast cells in the nasal mucosa. When inhaled allergens bridge IgE molecules on mast cells, mast cell degranulation occurs releasing preformed mediators. These mediators induce the *early phase* nasal reaction, characterised by rhinorrhoea, sneezing, itching, and nasal obstruction. A second release of mast cell mediators may occur 2 to 6 hours later, leading to a recurrence of symptoms. This *late phase* reaction is associated with an inflammatory response in the respiratory tract and the ongoing symptoms. Inflammation is promoted by the release of mast cell chemotactic factors such as LTB4 and cytokines from mast cells and $T_H2$ lymphocytes. These cytokines promote eosinophil differentiation, activation, and survival. *Abbreviations:* GM-CSF = granulocyte macrophage colony-stimulating factor; IL = interleukin; LT = leukotriene; MHC = major histocompatibility protein; PAF = platelet-activating factor; TNF = tumour necrosis factor; TCR = T cell receptor.

ability manifested by urticaria, angio-oedema and hypotension. However, recent studies of allergic reactions suggest that the term immediate hypersensitivity may be a misnomer, since allergic responses are frequently biphasic in nature with a late phase reaction occurring 4 to 12 hours after the immediate phase. Late phase reactions occur in approximately 50% of experimentally-induced allergic responses and, in contrast to immediate reactions, which are generally acellular in nature, contain the eosinophil-rich mixed cellular infiltrate associated with the chronic allergic responses discussed above.

From a clinical standpoint, late phase reactions are resistant to treatment with antihistamines and bronchodilators, which are often effective in attenuating the symptoms associated with immediate reactions.[167]

#### Immunomodulatory Therapy of Asthma and Rhinitis

Several sets of guidelines for the treatment of asthma have been published.[168] The principles used to develop these guidelines apply to the treatment of rhinitis as well. In general, treatment has moved toward preventing or treating the mucosal inflammatory reaction rather than attempting to reverse the consequences of the reaction once it has occurred.[169] Table XII lists some of the principal immunomodulatory agents used in the treatment of asthma and allergic rhinitis.

***Corticosteroids:*** the use of inhaled (topical) corticosteroids by metered dose inhalers (e.g. beclomethasone dipropionate, budesonide, fluticasone propionate, flunisolide, dexamethasone sodium phosphate and triamcinolone acetonide) is a mainstay in the treatment of chronic allergic asthma and rhinitis (see further chapter 23; sect. 3.2 and chapter 14; sect. 2.4). These agents directly inhibit the phospholipase $A_2$ enzyme which is responsible for the production of prostaglandin and leukotriene mediators from lipid membrane constituents. These mediators are essential to allergic inflammation. In doses frequently adequate to control mild to moderately severe asthma or rhinitis, few if any of the adverse effects associated with oral corticosteroid therapy occur.

***Sodium cromoglycate (cromolyn sodium) and nedocromil sodium*** (table XIII): these agents are related and have a multiplicity of desirable anti-inflammatory effects on mediator release from mast cells and on inflammatory cells (including eosinophils). The specific site of action responsible for their clinical efficacy is unknown. They block both the immediate and late phase experimental allergic reaction whereas low doses of corticosteroids block only the late phase reaction. In contrast to inhaled corticosteroids, they have few if any adverse effects, even at full doses, and are therefore especially attractive for use in children.

***Antihistamines:*** the 'second generation' histamine $H_1$-receptor antagonists have a variety of anti-inflammatory and immunomodulatory effects *in vitro* over and above antagonism of the effect of histamine on the $H_1$ receptor seen with the 'first generation' agents (table XIV).[170] Although these agents are effective and have few adverse effects in allergic rhinitis, their efficacy in asthma is minimal in comparison with that of the corticosteroids, nedocromil sodium, sodium cromoglycate, or agents with no significant anti-inflammatory effects including bronchodilators such as the $\beta_2$-agonists, theophylline and ipratropium bromide. This experience

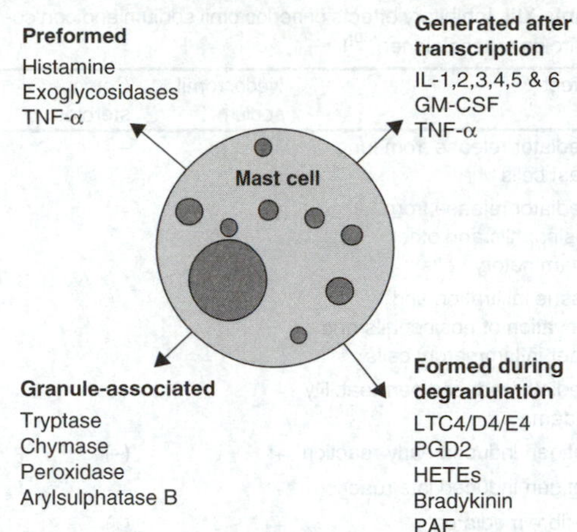


**Fig. 2.** Mast cell mediators. *Abbreviations:* TNF = tumour necrosis factor; IL = interleukin; GM-CSF = granulocyte macrophage colony-stimulating factor; PG = prostaglandin; PAF = platelet-activating factor; HETE = hydroxyeicosatetraenoic acid.

**Table XII.** Immunomodulatory agents used in asthma and/or rhinitis

| |
|---|
| Corticosteroids |
| Sodium cromoglycate (cromolyn sodium) |
| Nedocromil sodium |
| Newer $H_1$ antihistamines |
| Arachidonic acid pathway inhibitors or competitors (e.g. zileuton, zafirlukast, pobilukast, ibudilast, pranlukast) |
| Allergen immunotherapy |
| Methotrexate |
| Gold salts |
| Cyclosporin |

**Table XIII.** Inhibitory effects of nedocromil sodium and corticosteroids (after Salonen[30])

| Effect | Nedocromil sodium | Corticosteroids |
|---|---|---|
| Mediator release from lung mast cells | ++ | – |
| Mediator release from eosinophils and other inflammatory cells | + | + |
| Tissue infiltration and activation of eosinophils and other inflammatory cells | + | +++ |
| Mediator-induced permeability oedema | + | ++ |
| Antigen-induced early reaction | + | (–) |
| Antigen-induced late reaction | + | ++ |
| 'C-fibre mediated' bronchoconstriction and symptoms (bradykinin, $SO_2$, metabisulfite) | ++ | (+) |
| Bronchial hyperresponsiveness | + | + |

*Key:* +++ = marked inhibitory effect; ++ = moderate inhibitory effect; + = mild inhibitory effect.

has reinforced the dictum that *in vitro* pharmacological activities may not be predictive of antiallergic activities.

***Methotrexate*** and ***gold salts*** have been reported to have steroid-sparing effects in severe asthma, but data to support these effects are limited, unclear and controversial.[172,173] ***Cyclosporin*** also appears to have steroid-sparing effects in severe asthma[174] but because of the considerable adverse effects associated with all three of these drugs, their use in allergic disease should be considered experimental and, except in exceptional cases, should be used only under strictly controlled circumstances.[175]

***5-Lipoxygenase inhibitors and leukotriene (LT) antagonists:*** metabolism of arachidonic acid by 5-lipoxygenase leads to the formation of biologically active lipid leukotrienes. Leukotrienes have the capacity to modulate the vascular and cellular aspects of inflammation, as well as producing direct effects on airway smooth muscle and mucous secretion. The peptidoleukotrienes, LTC4, LTD4, and LTE4, formerly called slow-reacting substances of anaphylaxis (SRS-A), induce wheal and flare reactions when injected intradermally and are 100 times more potent than histamine as bronchoconstrictors. Peptidoleukotrienes are the predominant 5-lipoxygenase products of mast cells, while LTB4 is the predominant product in polymorphonuclear leucocytes. LTB4 is chemotactic for neutrophils, eosinophils, monocytes, and lymphocytes, stimulates adherence of neutrophils to the endothelium, and induces a neutrophil-rich inflammatory response when injected into the skin.

A number of 5-lipoxygenase inhibitors are currently under investigation. There are four main categories of these drugs: redox inhibitors, hydroxamates and *N*-hydroxyureas, nonredox inhibitors of 5-lipoxygenase, and inhibitors of the translocation of the lipoxygenase enzyme to the cell membrane.[176] Clinical trials with 5-lipoxygenase inhibitors (e.g. *zileuton*) and antagonists of the peptidoleukotrienes (e.g. *zafirlukast*, *pobilukast*, *pranlukast* and *ibudilast*) are currently underway in asthma.[177]

### Allergen Immunotherapy

Allergen immunotherapy uses the stepwise, subcutaneous administration of increasing doses of extracts containing the glycoprotein constituents of pollen, insects, animals, and mould spore allergens. It is used only in highly selected individuals with allergen-specific serum IgE and symptoms on exposure to these substances. Controlled clinical studies using purified, characterised allergens have clearly

**Table XIV.** Some pharmacological effects of 'second-generation' $H_1$ antihistamines in addition to binding to the $H_1$ receptor (after Rihoux[171])

| Effect | Drug(s) for which effect noted |
|---|---|
| Inhibition of histamine release from mast cells and basophils *in vitro* | Oxatomide<br>Azelastine<br>Terfenadine<br>Loratadine |
| Inhibition of LTC4 release from various cells *in vitro* | Azatadine<br>Terfenadine<br>Loratadine |
| LTC4, LTD4 antagonism | Azelastine |
| PAF antagonism | Azelastine |
| *In vitro* inhibition of fMLP, PAF, C5a, LTB4 and IL-8- induced eosinophilia | Cetirizine |
| *In vitro* inhibition of calcium mobilisation | Oxatomide<br>Azelastine<br>Loratadine<br>Terfenadine |
| *In vitro* potentiation of $\beta_2$-response | Cetirizine |
| *In vivo* inhibition of antigen-induced eosinophil accumulation in atopics | Cetirizine |
| *In vivo* inhibition of antigen-induced late histamine release in atopics | Cetirizine |
| *In vivo* inhibition of antigen-induced mediators (histamine, kinins, $PGD_2$, LTC4) release in nasal fluid of atopics | Azatadine<br>Terfenadine<br>Loratadine<br>Cetirizine |

*Abbreviations:* IL = interleukin; LT = leukotriene; PAF = platelet-activating factor; fMLP = *N*-formylmethionyl chemotactic factor; PG = prostaglandin.

demonstrated the efficacy of allergen immunotherapy in the treatment of allergic rhinitis and insect venom allergy in association with a number of immunological changes reflecting its immunomodulatory effects.[178] These changes include decreased production of allergen-specific IgE, increased production of allergen specific IgG, decreased release of inflammatory mediators, down-regulation of eosinophils, and a switch from the release of IL-4 and IL-5 by allergen exposed lymphocytes to production of IFN-γ. This change in lymphocyte cytokine profile is associated with a switch from IgE to IgG production in response to allergen. Clinically, these immunological changes are manifested by inhibition of both the immediate and late phase allergic reaction which occur even before rises in allergen specific IgG are noted. However, the efficacy of allergen immunotherapy in asthma has been more difficult to demonstrate.

The use of high-dose purified allergen extracts by primary care clinicians without special training in allergic diseases has been associated with reports of fatal anaphylaxis to allergen immunotherapy and the limitation of its use in Europe. In contrast, the cautious use of allergen immunotherapy by allergists elsewhere continues to have a role in the treatment of patients with severe allergic disease unresponsive to medical therapy or requiring multiple medications.

#### 3.4.2 Choice of Therapy

Previous concerns about the use of $H_1$ antihistamines in asthmatic patients appears unwarranted. The use of long-acting, nonsedative antihistamines in patients with multiple organ system allergic disease, e.g. combinations of allergic rhinitis, conjunctivitis, atopic dermatitis and asthma, is efficacious, well tolerated, and cost-effective. Allergen immunotherapy in such patients is also a cost-effective option. In patients with only seasonal allergic rhinitis, 'as required' therapy (i.e. weeks at a time) with intranasal corticosteroids, intranasal sodium cromoglycate, or systemic or intranasal antihistamines is usually efficacious.

For individuals with symptoms of asthma a few times per week only, 'as required' therapy with inhaled short-acting $\beta_2$-agonist bronchodilators is used. More frequent symptoms are associated with underlying airways inflammation and associated nonspecific bronchial hyperreactivity, and require anti-inflammatory therapy, either with inhaled sodium cromoglycate, nedocromil sodium or corticosteroids (see further chapter 23; sect. 3.2). If symptoms are not totally relieved, 'as required' short-acting $\beta_2$-agonist bronchodilator therapy may be used as an adjunct. The role of long-acting $\beta_2$-agonists (e.g. salmeterol) in such patients is unclear, as is the role of theophylline. Inhaled ipratropium bromide has limited utility in the treatment of asthma, although it is clearly beneficial as a bronchodilator in chronic bronchitis (see further chapter 23; sect. 4.2.1).

#### 3.4.3 Avoiding Problems in Treatment

The concurrent use of the long-acting nonsedating antihistamines terfenadine or astemizole with either macrolide antibiotics such as erythromycin or imidazole antifungal agents such as ketoconazole has been associated with reports of the difficult to treat ventricular arrhythmia, torsades de pointes. Nedocromil sodium and sodium cromoglycate have no clinically significant drug interactions or toxicities and idiosyncratic reactions are very rare. Inhalation of aerosol corticosteroids, especially in high doses, may be associated with growth retardation in children and with oral thrush, fungal laryngitis, or even fungal oesophagitis, the attendant symptoms of which include hoarseness and dysphagia. These problems can usually be avoided by training in inhalation technique with the use of spacers, and washing the oropharynx after inhalation.

Allergen immunotherapy may be associated with local dermal reactions at the injection site or frank anaphylaxis. These complications can be decreased, though but not totally eliminated, by careful dose titration using standard techniques applied by specialists trained in this method of treatment.

#### 3.4.4 Clinical Outcome and Economic Considerations

Although a host of new medications for asthma have become available and have been associated with a proportionate overall increase in expenditure for asthma treatment, a worldwide epidemic of asthma deaths has occurred over the last 10 years.[179] At one point, this appeared related to the use of long-acting inhaled β-agonists, but more recent studies suggest that an increase in the prevalence and the severity of asthma may be a more correct explanation.

In an individual patient, the cost of medications for allergy treatment is a major consideration. In the US, the concomitant use of a long-acting antihistamine and an inhaled corticosteroid costs over $60 per month. Therefore, it is important that the first step in treatment of all allergic conditions is identification of the allergen responsible for the problem (if possible) and the avoidance of that allergen. The use of medications, immunomodulators or otherwise, is the next step. The costs of allergen immunotherapy have been assessed and this form of therapy is considered cost effective.[180]

## 3.5 Inflammatory Bowel Disease

The two major conditions that comprise inflammatory bowel disease (IBD) are ulcerative colitis and Crohn's disease, both inflammatory disorders of unknown cause. Certain clinical features are used to separate the two conditions (see chapter 22; sect. 9 and also review by Podolsky[181,182]), although the validity of the diagnostic classification remains uncertain.

In assessing patients with a likely diagnosis of inflammatory bowel disease, attempts should be made to exclude infectious aetiologies since organisms such as *Campylobacter jejuni* and *Yersinia enterocolitica*, among others, can produce similar syndromes of abdominal pain and bloody diarrhoea.

### 3.5.1 Immune Mechanisms in Pathogenesis

Immune mechanisms appear to be involved in these diseases, since a number of extraintestinal manifestations, including arthritis and cholangitis, occur and the diseases respond to a variety of immunosuppressive agents.[183] The predominant hypothesis suggests an immune response to bacterial cell wall products or toxins leading to the production of cytokines and ongoing inflammation. Patients with inflammatory bowel disease have humoral antibodies to colonic cells, bacterial antigens and *Escherichia coli*, lipopolysaccharides, and foreign proteins such as cow's milk protein. Recently, antineutrophil cytoplasmic antibody (ANCA) has been demonstrated in 70% of patients with ulcerative colitis but not in those with Crohn's disease. Serum levels of soluble IL-2 receptor correlated with disease activity.

An antibody specific for the 40kD tropomyosin antigen is expressed on the apical membrane of colonocytes and biliary epithelium in 50% of patients with active ulcerative colitis.[184] The presence of antigen in association with complement activation products suggests a mechanism for epithelial damage. There is limited evidence for T cell-mediated immune mechanisms in ulcerative colitis.

In Crohn's disease, collections of macrophages and lymphocytes form distinctive microgranulomas. Fibrinoid occlusive lesions are present in small arteries, even in areas where epithelial ulceration is not present. There is also evidence of diffuse mucosal T cell activation, while immunostaining shows an increased density of IgM-positive plasma cells diffusely throughout the gastrointestinal tract.

In ulcerative colitis, the inflammatory reaction primarily involves the colonic mucosa. The inflammation is uniform and continuous with no intervening areas of normal mucosa. The rectum is involved in 95% of cases and the inflammation extends proximally in a continuous fashion. Minimal involvement of a few centimetres of the terminal ileum, termed backwash ileitis, sometimes occurs. A neutrophil-rich inflammatory reaction involves surface mucosal cells and crypt epithelium that progresses to epithelial damage, loss of surface epithelial cells, and multiple ulcerations. Neutrophil infiltration of crypts results in characteristic small crypt abscesses.

In Crohn's disease, unlike ulcerative colitis, deeper layers of the bowel beneath the submucosa are involved. The disease is often discontinuous and severely involved segments of bowel are separated from each other by skip lesions of apparently normal bowel. The colon and the rectum may be spared in approximately 50% of patients with Crohn's disease. Since Crohn's disease is a transmural inflammatory process, and involves the serosal mesentery, fistula and abscess formation occur.

### 3.5.2 Role of Immunomodulation in Therapy

The medical management of ulcerative colitis and Crohn's disease are similar and depend on the severity of the disease (see further chapter 22; sect. 9). Corticosteroids are first-line therapy in bringing acute disease under control, although in subacute disease 5-aminosalicylic acid compounds may be used (table XV). More often, the two drug groups are used simultaneously and corticosteroid dosages are tapered as the disease goes into remission. In chronic or refractory disease, azathioprine or its metabolite mercaptopurine may be employed. The use of methotrexate, cyclosporin, 5-lipoxygenase pathway inhibitors, butyrate enemas, hydroxychloroquine and superoxide dismutase are all experimental therapies under evaluation.

**Table XV.** Oral 5-aminosalicylic acid preparations used in inflammatory bowel disease (after Geier & Miner[185])

| Drug | Release mechanism | % Renal excretion | Clinical use |
|---|---|---|---|
| Sulfasalazine | Colonic bacterial cleavage of diazo bond | 23.9 (16.6-32.6) | Active UC and CD; remission maintenance in UC |
| Olsalazine sodium | Colonic bacterial cleavage of diazo bond | 27 (19-41) | Active UC; remission maintenance in UC |
| Mesalazine (mesalamine) | Coated with Eudragit-S, release at pH7[a] | 20 | Active UC, ? CD; remission maintenance in UC |
| | Coated with Eudragit-L, release at pH6[b] | ≈37 | Active UC, ? CD; remission maintenance in UC |
| | pH and time-released[c] | 28 | Active UC and CD; remission maintenance in UC |

a 'Asacol'.
b 'Claversal'; 'Salofalk'.
c 'Pentasa'.
*Abbreviations:* CD = Crohn's disease; UC = ulcerative colitis.

Proctocolectomy, when necessary, is curative for patients with ulcerative colitis. In contrast, the high likelihood of recurrence makes surgery less appealing for patients with Crohn's disease.

### 5-Aminosalicylic Acid Preparations

*Sulfasalazine* is a congener of sulfapyridine and 5-aminosalicylic acid (5-ASA) and remains a highly valued agent for the management of mild to moderately severe ulcerative colitis and large bowel involvement of Crohn's disease. Recent studies have shown that sulfasalazine has several actions that attenuate inflammation of the bowel. It is a potent inhibitor of both prostaglandin synthetase and 5-lipoxygenase leading to the reduced production of prostaglandins and leukotrienes. The latter may be especially important in inflammatory bowel disease as chemoattractant compounds that also activate neutrophils. Sulfasalazine also appears to block the chemotactic activity of formylated bacterial peptides, and acts as a scavenger of oxygen free radicals.

Sulfasalazine reduces both the frequency and severity of recurrent ulcerative colitis and is effective in the acute phase, but not maintenance therapy, of Crohn's disease. Around 20% of patients receiving sulfasalazine develop hypersensitivity reactions associated with rash, arthritis, pericarditis, pancreatitis and/or pleuritis. In addition, sulfasalazine has been found to cause reversible infertility in men.

The therapeutic activity of sulfasalazine is attributable to its 5-aminosalicylic acid component, whereas hypersensitivity and intolerance is induced by the sulfapyridine moiety.[186] However, the sulfapyridine moiety is necessary to prevent absorption of the drug in the proximal gastrointestinal tract, which would make the 5-aminosalicylic acid unavailable to the colonic mucosa. When sulfasalazine reaches the colon, it is cleaved by the action of bacterial azoreductase to liberate 5-aminosalicylic acid. These observations stimulated efforts to circumvent the need for the sulfapyridine and led to the availability of effective alternative 5-aminosalicylic acid preparations. Topical 5-aminosalicylic acid enemas are effective in distal proctocolitis but are expensive and associated with a high rate of disease recurrence. In many patients treated with topical 5-aminosalicylic acid, the dosage may be tapered and maintenance therapy on alternate nights considered.[182]

A number of orally active 5-aminosalicylic acid preparations have been developed. Several use newer methods of drug delivery; for example, *mesalazine (mesalamine)* has the active agent (5-ASA) encapsulated in a pH-sensitive, slow release matrix. Others use conjugates to compounds other than sulfapyridine. In the case of *olsalazine*, 5-aminosalicylic acid is conjugated to itself to form a dimer that is hydrolysed by bacterial azoreductase. In general, the newer 5-ASA drugs offer little additional benefit to sulfasalazine (in those patients who can tolerate the latter) but are more expensive.

### Corticosteroids

Corticosteroids continue to be highly useful in patients with moderate to severe ulcerative colitis or Crohn's disease, especially Crohn's disease with small intestinal involvement. Their inhibitory effects on the production of pro-inflammatory cytokines and arachidonic acid metabolism appear to explain their effects. Corticosteroids have not been demonstrated to affect recurrence in patients with either ulcerative colitis or Crohn's disease in remission, and their use is tempered by an awareness of potential complications, including abscess formation in patients with Crohn's disease.

Topical hydrocortisone and prednisolone sodium phosphate are the mainstays of therapy for distal proctocolitis. In recent years, topical preparations with increased potency, including beclomethasone dipropionate, budesonide and tixocortol pivalate have proved equally effective to topical hydrocortisone or prednisolone. These newer agents are less likely to produce systemic steroid effects because of their extensive first-pass metabolism in the liver. This property allows the safe delivery of higher, more effective doses of the corticosteroids to the affected areas of the distal colon.

#### Cytotoxic Immunosuppressive Drugs

*Azathioprine* and its active metabolite *mercaptopurine* have a clear role as immunosuppressive agents in the management of inflammatory bowel disease. A specific regimen involving the use of mercaptopurine has been found to be useful in refractory Crohn's disease.[187] In contrast to sulfasalazine and corticosteroids, mercaptopurine appears to diminish the likelihood and severity of flares in patients with Crohn's disease in remission. Although few data are available, mercaptopurine and azathioprine also appear to be effective in minimising the requirements for corticosteroids in patients with refractory ulcerative colitis.

The use of mercaptopurine or azathioprine is associated with pancreatitis in about 5% of patients. Bone marrow suppression occurs in 2% of patients, but malignancy does not appear to be a problem at the doses used. Thus, azathioprine or mercaptopurine appear useful in patients with refractory disease who are not acutely ill.

The usefulness of *methotrexate* in doses of 25mg per week or less in refractory Crohn's disease or ulcerative colitis appears promising but should be considered experimental. *Cyclosporin* has also been evaluated extensively and is apparently active in Crohn's disease, although the response to it is not sustained when the drug is withdrawn. This is especially problematic because of its serious adverse effects when used long term. In patients who are severely ill with ulcerative colitis, relatively short term therapy with cyclosporin may offer a reasonable alternative to surgery. The drug may need to be given intravenously at first to ensure adequate absorption. Studies to determine the utility of low-dose cyclosporin and prednisone in inflammatory bowel disease are currently underway.

#### Metronidazole

Metronidazole, which has both immunomodulatory and antibacterial effects, is often effective in high doses in improving recalcitrant perineal fistulas in Crohn's disease.[188] However, it has dose-related neurological toxicity which often limits its use and fistulas often reemerge after the drug has been discontinued. Metronidazole is sometimes useful in the treatment of Crohn's disease confined to the large bowel, although it does not appear effective in ulcerative colitis.

#### Other Immunomodulating Agents

A number of 5-lipoxygenase inhibitors (including FPL 62064 and CMI 392) are undergoing clinical trials in inflammatory bowel disease, as is hydroxychloroquine sulfate. Levamisole, oral sodium cromoglycate, n-3 fatty acids, and nonsteroidal anti-inflammatory drugs have not proved effective.

## 3.6 Cancers

### 3.6.1 Role of Immunomodulation in Cancer Therapy

It is well established that immunosuppressed patients, such as organ graft recipients, have an increased incidence of malignancies. An early theory to explain this phenomenon coined the phase 'immune surveillance', and postulated that the immune system plays a central role in eliminating malignant cells, a capacity that is deficient in immunosuppressed patients, and possibly also in normal patients who develop cancers. The immune surveillance hypothesis has become less compelling as mechanisms underlying malignant transformation have been elucidated, but it is clear that most cancer patients do mount a measurable cell-mediated immune response to their tumours. That immune responses to tumours can be enhanced, or immune-based therapy designed, to reduce tumour burdens, treat metastases, or prevent recurrences remains a very attractive proposition. Many forms of cancer immunotherapy are effective in animal models, and some therapies have now proven effective in the treatment of human cancers as well.

### 3.6.2 Immune Responses to Human Tumours (Cell-Mediated Immunity)

An important element of cell-mediated immunity to cancer is directed against glycoproteins on tumour cell surface antigens on allografted organs. T lymphocytes of the CD4 (helper/inducer) subset recognise tumour antigens associated with HLA class II molecules on antigen presenting cells, while cytotoxic T cells (primarily of the CD8 subset) recognise antigens on HLA class I molecules. Thus, many cytotoxic T cells are ordinarily restricted to responding to antigens that are associated with HLA molecules on the tumour cell surface.

At least three additional aspects of cell-mediated immunity are not HLA restricted. Activated macrophages and natural killer (NK) cells can lyse some kinds of malignant cells without the requirement for HLA-associated tumour antigens. T lymphocytes can be activated by interleukin-2 to generate 'lymphokine-activated killers', or LAK cells, which acquire cytotoxic activity that is not HLA restricted.

Antibodies are produced against antigens expressed on tumour cells. Antibodies bound to tumour cells can be lytic either by complement fixation or the involvement of cells bearing receptors for the Fc portion of antibodies – an effector mechanism termed antibody-dependent cellular cytotoxicity.

### 3.6.3 Cancer Immunotherapy

#### Immunostimulants

A number of bacteria or bacterial products have been administered with the objective of enhancing cell-mediated immune responses to tumour antigens. The mycobacterium bacille Calmette-Guérin (BCG) has been the most studied of the intact bacteria, and has induced regression of human melanomas and superficial bladder carcinomas when injected into the tumour site. Systemic administration of bacteria or bacterial products has generally not been effective, although the adjuvant effects of such agents have been employed in the development of cancer vaccines (see below). Chemically-defined immunostimulants have also been employed in cancer therapy. The most successful application to date is the use of *fluorouracil* and *levamisole* in patients with resected Duke's C colon cancer.[189-191]

#### Cancer Vaccines

Numerous attempts have been made to actively immunise cancer patients against their tumours by the vaccine-like use of tumour cells or antigens plus an adjuvant. Some therapeutic cancer vaccines have proven effective in reducing tumour burden, treating metastases, or preventing tumour recurrence, e.g. a vaccine composed of glycosylated lipids specific to tumour cell membranes linked to BCG, which reduces the rate of cancer recurrence and increases survival in patients with metastatic melanoma.[113]

Other cancer vaccines have proven efficacious in melanoma and colonic carcinoma, two forms of cancer that may be particularly immunogenic.[192]

#### Monoclonal Antibodies

The exquisite specificity of monoclonal antibodies has been exploited in several approaches to developing highly selective forms of immunotherapy for cancers. Unmodified antibodies can help eliminate tumour cells by opsonisation, complement-mediated lysis, or antibody-dependent cellular cytotoxicity. Antibodies have also been modified to deliver toxins or radioisotopes to tumour cells. Antibodies that are specific for tumour cell receptors through which growth signals are received may inhibit tumour growth, while antibodies to other receptors may be capable of inducing apoptosis. Yet another approach (discussed below under adoptive cellular immunotherapy) uses monoclonal antibodies to target cytotoxic cells to malignant cells.

In clinical trials, some remissions have been achieved using monoclonal antibodies for immunotherapy of non-Hodgkin's lymphoma, but the problems associated with the clinical use of nonhuman antibodies have limited this therapeutic approach.[193]

The monoclonal antibody 17-1A is a murine monoclonal antibody which acts against the tumour-associated antigens CO17-1A expressed in colorectal cancer cells. It is presently undergoing clinical trials.

#### Adoptive Cellular Immunotherapy

Adoptive transfer of LAK cells plus interleukin-2 can mediate tumour regression in animal tumour models, and has resulted in objective responses in some patients with renal cell carcinoma, melanoma, colorectal cancer, and B cell lymphoma. Attempts to improve on this approach have included the use of tumour-infiltrating lymphocytes (TILs) as the starting population for lymphokine activation, and genetically engineering lymphocytes to constitutively express interleukin-2.

*In vitro* sensitisation of a patient's lymphocytes to tumour antigens has met with some success, but it is also clear that many human tumours do not express antigens in association with HLA molecules that can trigger HLA-restricted cell-mediated immunity. A promising strategy to overcome this problem employs bispecific antibodies, with one binding arm specific for a tumour antigen and the other binding arm specific for the T cell receptor on effector cells.[194]

Although clinical results with adoptive cellular immunotherapy for cancer have been modestly successful at best, this form of immunotherapy is still regarded as very promising and novel approaches are being actively developed.[195]

**Biological Response Modifiers**

Natural biological substances that have a regulatory role in immune responses, including interleukin-2 and interferons, have shown therapeutic efficacy against a number of tumours. Tumour regression is frequently achieved when *interleukin-2* is used as therapy of renal cell carcinoma or melanoma.[97,98] *Interferon-α* is effective against a number of tumours, with hairy cell leukaemia and Kaposi's sarcoma in AIDS patients being especially notable.

*Tumour necrosis factor-α (TNF-α)* is a cytokine produced by macrophages and natural killer cells in response to inflammatory stimuli. It increases macrophage and neutrophil cytotoxicity and regulates the production of other cytokines. Despite a variety of toxic effects, it has shown promise in the treatment of malignant glioma, malignant melanoma and some solid tumours.

A novel approach to chemotherapy came from the observation that children with the adenosine deaminase deficient form of severe combined immunodeficiency disease (SCID) have dysfunctional lymphocytes caused by the accumulation of natural deoxyadenosine antimetabolites such as *cladribine (2-chloro-2'-deoxyadenosine)*. This lymphotoxin is now undergoing clinical trials for the treatment of chronic lymphocytic leukaemia, low-grade non-Hodgkin's lymphoma, and transplant rejection.

## 3.7 Infectious Diseases

### *3.7.1 Role of Immunoaugmentation in Therapy*

Most clinical applications for immunomodulators are applications for immunosuppression rather than immunoaugmentation. Although recombinant technologies have made available many biological response modifiers with the ability to up-regulate immune responses, the pro-inflammatory nature of most of these agents used *in vivo* has required extraordinary caution in their clinical use. For instance, attempts to use recombinant interleukin-2 (IL-2) resulted in a life-threatening, generalised, capillary leak syndrome during initial trials.[196] This experience must be contrasted, however, with the striking reduction in infections with polysaccharide encapsulated organisms in patients with congenital and acquired hypogammaglobulinaemia treated with high doses of intravenous gamma globulin.[197]

A large number of agents with the potential for immunoaugmentation are now available (table XVI), and many recent reviews of present and possible uses have been published.[198] Several examples of their application in infectious diseases are especially informative. For instance, a number of these agents have and are continuing to undergo trials in the treatment of HIV-1 infection and its complications and are discussed in section 3.2 (above). In general, the most successful application of immunoaugmentative therapy in infectious diseases has been with interferons.

### *3.7.2 Interferons (IFNs)*

Interferons are of two types: type I (α and β) interferons are secreted by all nucleated cells after viral infection. Type II (γ or immune) interferon is the product of lymphocytes stimulated by antigens or mitogens. IFN-α is produced by most cells, but especially virally infected leucocytes. IFN-β is produced by fibroblasts, among other cells, and IFN-γ is produced by T lymphocytes. Interferons have antiviral and cell differentiation effects, and are potent inducers of natural killer cell activity. They appear to have the ability to act synergistically with antiviral drugs.

Several clinical trials have found IFN-α to be effective in treating anogenital warts caused by human papilloma viruses. However, the infectious disease where interferons have had the greatest impact is the treatment of viral hepatitis. A number of clinical trials with IFN-α have been carried out in patients with hepatitis A, B, C, and delta infections.[199,200]

**Hepatitis B and C**

Controlled studies have established that patients with biopsy proven chronic hepatitis B respond to treatment. For instance, a 16-week course of 5 million units per day of IFN-α subcutaneously or 10 million units 3 times per

**Table XVI.** Some immunomodulators with evidence of clinical potential in infectious diseases

| Category | Examples |
|---|---|
| Bacterial and fungal products | Glucan<br>Muramyl peptides<br>BCG (Bacille Calmette-Guérin ) |
| Interleukins (IL) | IL-1α, IL-1β<br>IL-2<br>IL-6<br>IL-7<br>IL-8<br>IL-12 |
| Colony-stimulating factors | GM-CSF<br>G-CSF<br>M-CSF |
| Tumour necrosis factor (TNF) | TNF-α |
| Interferons (IFNs) | IFN-α<br>IFN-β<br>IFN-γ |
| Monoclonal antibodies | Edobacomab (E5)<br>Sevirumab<br>Tuvirumab |
| Thymic hormones | Thymosin $B_1$<br>Thymopoietin |
| Pharmacological agents | Levamisole<br>Inosine pranobex (isoprinosine)<br>Cimetidine |
| Adoptive immunotherapy | Immunoglobulin<br>Immune cell transfusions (untreated or treated with immunomodulators) |
| Leucocyte extracts | Transfer factor |

*Abbreviations:* GM-CSF = granulocyte macrophage colony-stimulating factor; G-CSF = granulocyte colony-stimulating factor; M-CSF = macrophage colony-stimulating factor.

week resulted in seroconversion from HBeAg and HBV DNA positivity to non-replicative status (anti-HBe detectable) in association with improvement in liver histology. Approximately 10% of these patients no longer had HBsAg present in the serum. With continued treatment, up to 70% of patients lose serologic markers for the infection. Interestingly, successful therapy is accompanied by acute elevation in serum aminotransferase levels. This is believed to result from the immunostimulatory effect of interferon leading to increased cell-mediated immunity against virally infected hepatocytes. Other potential complications of therapy with IFN-α include influenza-like symptoms, bone marrow suppression, emotional lability and autoimmune thyroiditis.

In adults, chronic hepatitis is much less common with hepatitis B than with hepatitis C infection where it reaches 50%. Since corticosteroids are not effective in the treatment of either infection, patients with chronic hepatitis C, like those with hepatitis B, are candidates for IFN-α. Doses of 3 to 5 million units 3 times per week are associated with improvement or normalisation of liver aminotransferase levels in 50% of individuals, but 50% of responding patients relapse even after 6 months of therapy. This leaves a sustained response rate to IFN-α in hepatitis C of 25%. Neither larger doses nor longer term therapy affects the rate of relapse. Interestingly, the elevation of liver enzymes noted after starting IFN-α therapy in hepatitis B does not occur with hepatitis C treatment.

**Other Infections**

IFN-α has also been studied with encouraging results in the treatment of adenovirus, cytomegalovirus, herpes simplex virus types 1 and 2, varicella, and herpes zoster infections.[100]

#### *3.7.3 Monoclonal Antibodies*

*Edobacomab* (E5) is an IgM murine monoclonal antibody directed at the lipid A moiety of the endotoxins of Gram-negative bacteria. It is currently undergoing clinical trials for the treatment of Gram-negative sepsis with the intention of reducing circulating endotoxin levels. A similar monoclonal antibody, *nebacumab,* was withdrawn from the market after its second clinical trial showed increased mortality in patients receiving it.

*Sevirumab* is a monoclonal antibody directed at an envelope glycoprotein of cytomegalovirus. It has shown promise as adjunctive therapy in the treatment of CMV retinitis in HIV seropositive patients.

*Tuvirumab* is a human monoclonal antibody directed against hepatitis B virus surface antigen. It is undergoing clinical trials for patients with persistent hepatitis B antigen seropositive hepatitis.

### 3.8 Renal Disease

Many renal diseases have an immunological aetiology or an immunopathogenic component. This is often evident by histological examination, which reveals deposition of antibodies and complement in the kidney. In some cases, an immunopathogenesis is deduced from the observation that the condition responds to immunosuppressive therapy. Table XVII lists some of the renal disorders that have an immunological basis.

#### *3.8.1 Role of Immunomodulation in Therapy*

Immunosuppressive therapy for immune-mediated renal disease has generally been empirically determined but can, to some extent, be related to the immunopathological mechanisms involved. Three types of mechanisms that can induce renal parenchymal damage have been demonstrated:

1) Circulating antigens and antibodies can form immune complexes that are deposited in the kidney.

2) Antibodies to antigens present in the kidney, e.g. antibodies to glomerular basement antigens, can react with *in situ* antigens.

These two antibody-mediated mechanisms appear to predominate in glomerular injury.

3) Cell-mediated immunity, which appears to predominate in interstitial damage and transplant rejection.

Recent studies have also established a role for macrophages as mediators of glomerular injury.

Currently, the immunosuppressive agents most commonly used in the treatment of renal disease are the corticosteroids and cytotoxic drugs, often in combination.

#### Corticosteroids

Relatively high doses of corticosteroids are required, possibly because only at higher doses are B cells affected. Of course, at these doses, the multiple effects of corticosteroids become evident. In terms of therapeutic effects, this means that T lymphocytes, cells of the monocyte-macrophage lineage, and other inflammatory cells are also affected. The many adverse effects of corticosteroids are potentially serious problems when high doses are used, and most treatment protocols involving the use of corticosteroids attempt to reduce their adverse effects by employing alternate-day regimens or pulse therapy. For example, two protocols that have been used for the treatment of acute interstitial nephritis are either 120mg prednisone every alternate day, or 0.5 to 1g prednisone given intravenously every alternate day for a total of three pulses.[201]

**Table XVII.** Immune-mediated renal diseases

| |
|---|
| **Primary renal diseases** |
| IgA nephropathy |
| Idiopathic rapidly progressive glomerulonephritis |
| Acute post-streptococcal glomerulonephritis |
| Membranoproliferative glomerulonephritis |
| Acute interstitial nephritis |
| Idiopathic nephrotic syndrome |
| **Systemic disorders** |
| Systemic lupus erythematosus |
| Infection-related glomerulonephritis |
| Cryoglobulinaemia |
| Goodpasture's syndrome |
| Subacute bacterial endocarditis |
| 'Shunt' nephritis |
| *Vasculitic disease:* |
| Wegener's granulomatosis |
| Hypersensitivity vasculitis |
| Polyarteritis nodosa |
| Henoch-Schönlein purpura |

#### Cytotoxic Drugs

When cytotoxic drugs are used, the most commonly employed agents are *cyclophosphamide* or *chlorambucil*. The greater efficacy of these drugs as opposed to azathioprine may be due to their greater effect on B cells. To the extent that this is true, it is possible that some of the newer immunosuppressive drugs that have significant effects on B cells, such as *brequinar sodium* and *gusperimus (deoxyspergualin)*, will also be found to be efficacious in renal diseases with an antibody-mediated immunopathology. *Cyclophosphamide* is often used in the form of high-dose pulse therapy, especially in the treatment of the nephritis of systemic lupus erythematosus.[202]

Cytotoxic drugs are often used in combination with corticosteroids, and the efficacy of combination therapy has been demonstrated in a number of renal disorders.

## 4. Future Trends in Clinical Immunology

It can safely be predicted that treatment of immune system disorders, and therapeutic manipulation of immune responses, will continue to be one of the fastest moving areas of medical research. Future advances will be based both upon extensions of current successes, and upon the development of entirely novel strategies.

Many therapeutic advances can be clearly envisioned, and have been alluded to in the foregoing sections. Antibody-based therapeutics will become much more useful as the technology shifts to the production of humanised or even fully human monoclonal antibodies. As the molecular mechanisms involved in immune responses are increasingly elucidated, new targets for therapeutic intervention will become evident. For example, *adhesion molecules* that mediate the intercellular interactions governing the recruitment of inflammatory cells into extravascular sites, are attracting a lot of interest as pharmacological targets (table XVIII). The same types of modalities that are being developed to modulate cytokine actions will be ap-

**Table XVIII.** Adhesion molecules

| Adhesion molecule family | General function | Members | Ligand |
|---|---|---|---|
| Selectin family | Act in the initial phases of adhesion of circulating leucocytes onto vascular endothelium | E-, P-, & L-selectins | Sialylated, fucosylated tetrasaccharides |
| Immunoglobulin superfamily | Firm adhesion of leucocytes to endothelium following selectin-mediated adhesion; cell-cell interactions of lymphocytes | ICAM-1, 2, 3<br>VCAM-1<br>MadCAM-1<br>PECAM-1 | LFA-1, Mac-1<br>VLA-4<br>$\beta$-$\alpha$4, L-selectin<br>PECAM-1 |
| Integrins | Interact with ICAMs in activation and cytotoxic functions of lymphocytes | | |
| $\beta_1$ family | | VLA-4, $\beta$,$\alpha$4 | VCAM-1, fibronectin |
| $\beta_2$ family | | LFA-1, $\beta_2\alpha_L$<br>Mac-1 $\beta_2\alpha_M$<br>p150 95, $\beta_2\alpha_x$ | ICAM-1, -2, -3<br>ICAM-1, fibrinogen, C3bi<br>C3bi |

*Abbreviations:* ICAM = intercellular adhesion molecule; LFA = leucocyte function associated antigen; Mac-1 = macrophage integrin-1; MadCAM = mucosal addressin cell adhesion molecule; PECAM = platelet endothelial cell adhesion molecule; VCAM = vascular cell adhesion molecule; VLA = very late antigen.

plied to adhesion molecules as well – i.e. blockade of the receptors and their ligands, interference with signal transduction, or inhibition of their biosynthesis. Inflammatory diseases and transplant rejection are among the clinical applications for which anti-adhesion molecule therapies are most promising.[203,204]

Drug discovery efforts focusing on selected aspects of the immune response that can be manipulated for specific therapeutic goals are certain to yield new drugs for the immunopharmacological armamentarium. For example, a promising new drug with a novel mechanism of action is SKF 105686. This immunomodulatory azaspirane derivative acts by inducing suppressor cells, and is effective in animal models of graft rejection.[205] New cyclosporin analogues are also in various stages of development, while rapamycin appears to act synergistically in combination with cyclosporin or tacrolimus.[37] Identifying *synergistic drug combinations* is part of a trend that is already well established, using complementary combinations of immunomodulatory drugs. Combinations are selected based upon an understanding of their mechanisms of action, and can improve the therapeutic window for potent immunosuppressive protocols.

Safer and more effective use of immunomodulatory agents will also be achieved by *improved delivery mechanisms*. The advantages of treating localised inflammatory processes with localised therapy has been amply demonstrated by the development of topical, inhaled and intra-articular dosage form of corticosteroids. It is abundantly clear that our ability to manipulate cytokines would be more efficacious if the modulating agents could be targeted to the sites of cytokine activity, and the same would be true of modulating adhesion molecules.

A major goal for future immunotherapy is to develop additional methods for antigen-specific manipulation of the immune response. This would allow specific immune responses to be regulated up or down, without affecting the rest of the immune system. Antigen specificity has always been a feature of vaccines, which probably have done more to improve human health than any other medical advance. Researchers are taking a renewed look at the possibility that *therapeutic vaccines* may boost immunity in a chronically infected host above that achieved naturally in response to the infection. Current efforts to develop therapeutic vaccines are focused on HIV infection, herpes, leprosy, leishmaniasis, tuberculosis, and hepatitis B.[206]

Another type of vaccine, termed a *T cell vaccine*, has demonstrated potential to abrogate pathological immune responses in diseases mediated by cytotoxic T cells.[207] In animal models of autoimmunity, T cell vaccines can be used either prophylactically or therapeutically. The vaccine may consist of either whole (usually cloned) T cells whose immunopathogenic activity has been abrogated in some way, or T cell receptors specific for the autoantigen. The immune response engendered by these cells or receptors is capable of preventing or abrogating the cell-mediated immune response in which they are involved. Other approaches to achieving antigen-specific T cell tolerance attempt to modify epitopes of antigens recognised by T cells so that they will block, but not trigger, T cell receptors, or to present the antigen in a 'tolerising' protocol.

A novel and intriguing approach to treating immune-mediated diseases by inducing antigen-specific tolerance has recently emerged. Immunologists have known for some time that feeding an antigen to animals often induces a systemic inability to respond immunologically to that antigen, termed oral tolerance. Now clinical trials in human autoimmune diseases suggest that this immune mechanism may be exploited clinically.[208] This adds new impetus to the search to identify the specific antigens involved in the pathological immune responses in autoimmune and inflammatory diseases.

It can be anticipated that most future advances in immunopharmacology will be the result of research on the underlying mechanisms of immunity and of immune disorders. Progress in this field dramatically illustrates the interdependence of basic and clinical research.

## Further Reading

Allison AC, Lafferty KJ, Fliri H, editors. Immunosuppressive and anti-inflammatory drugs. Annals of the New York Academy of Sciences, Vol. 696. New York: New York Academy of Sciences, 1993

Drews J. Immunopharmacology: principles and perspectives. Berlin: Springer-Verlag, 1990

Frank MM, Austen KF, Claman HN, et al. editors. Samter's immunologic diseases. 5th ed. Boston: Little, Brown & Co., 1994

Oppenheim JJ, Rosio J, Gearing ASH, editors. Clinical applications of cytokines: role in diagnosis, pathogenesis and therapy. Oxford: Oxford University Press, 1993

St Georgiev V, Yamaguchi H, editors. Immunomodulating drugs. Annals of the New York Academy of Sciences, Vol. 685. New York: New York Academy of Sciences, 1993

Thomson AW, Starzl TE, editors. Immunosuppressive drugs: developments in anti-rejection therapy. Boston: Little, Brown & Co., 1994

## References

1. Kremer JM. The mechanism of action of methotrexate in rheumatoid arthritis: the search continues. Journal of Rheumatology 1994; 21: 1-5
2. Turka LA, Dayton J, Sinclair G, et al. Guanine ribonucleotide depletion inhibits T cell activation: mechanism of action of the immunosuppressive drug mizoribine. Journal of Clinical Investigation 1991; 87: 940-8
3. Allison AC, Eugui EM. Immunosuppressive and other effects of mycophenolic acid and an ester prodrug mycophenolate mofetil. Immunological Reviews 1993; 136: 5-28
4. Makowka L, Sher LS, Cramer DV. The development of brequinar as an immunosuppressive drug for transplantation. Immunological Reviews 1993; 136: 51-70
5. Allison AC, Kowalski WJ, Muller CJ, et al. Mechanisms of action of mycophenolic acid. Annals of the New York Academy of Sciences 1993; 696: 63-86
6. Cronstein BN, Eberle MA, Gruber HE, et al. Methotrexate inhibits neutrophil function by stimulating adenosine release from connective tissue cells. Proceedings of the National Academy of Sciences of the United States of America 1991; 88: 241-5
7. De Forni M, Chabat GG, Armand J-P, et al. Phase I and pharmacokinetic study of brequinar (DUP 785; NSC 368390) in cancer patients. European Journal of Cancer 1993; 29A: 983-8
8. Allison AC, Eugui EM. Mycophenolate mofetil, a rationally designed immunosuppressive drug. Clinical Transplantation 1993; 7: 96-112
9. Goldblum R. Therapy of rheumatoid arthritis with mycophenolate mofetil. Clinical and Experimental Rheumatology 1993; 11 Suppl. 8: S117-9
10. Zaoui P, Serre-Debeauvais F, Bayle F, et al. Clinical use of mizoribine (Bredinin) and pharmacologic monitoring assessment in renal transplantation. Transplantation Proceedings 1995; 27: 1064-5
11. Barry JM. Immunosuppressive drugs in renal transplantation: a review of the regimens. Drugs 1992; 44: 554-66
12. Allison AC, Eugui EM. Inhibitors of de novo purine and pyrimidine synthesis as immunosuppressive drugs. Transplantation Proceedings 1993; 25 Suppl. 2: 8-18
13. Allison AC, Kowalski WJ, Muller CJ, et al. Mycophenolic acid and brequinar, inhibitors of purine and pyrimidine synthesis, block and glycosylation of adhesion molecules. Transplantation Proceedings 1993; 25 Suppl. 2: 67-70
14. Luqmani R, Gordon C, Bacon P. Clinical pharmacology and modification of autoimmunity and inflammation in rheumatoid disease. Drugs 1994; 47: 259-85
15. Felson DT, Anderson JJ, Meenan RF. Use of short-term efficacy/toxicity trade-offs to select second-line drugs in rheumatoid arthritis: a metaanalysis of published clinical trials. Arthritis and Rheumatism 1992; 35: 1117-25
16. Alarcon GS, Lopez-Mendez A, Walter J, et al. Radiographic evidence of disease progression in methotrexate treated and nonmethotrexate disease modifying antirheumatic drug treated rheumatoid arthritis patients: a meta-analysis. Journal of Rheumatology 1992; 19: 1868-72
17. Schnabel A, Gross WL. Low-dose methotrexate in rheumatic diseases - efficacy, side effects, and risk factors for side effects. Seminars in Arthritis and Rheumatism 1994; 23: 310-27
18. Markham A, Faulds D. Methotrexate: a review of its pharmacodynamic and pharmacokinetic properties, and therapeutic efficacy in rheumatoid arthritis and other immunoregulatory disorders. Clinical Immunotherapeutics 1994; 1: 217-44
19. Chang C-C, Aversa G, Punnonen J, et al. Brequinar sodium, mycophenolic acid, and cyclosporin A inhibit different stages of IL-4- or IL-13-induced human IgG4 and IgE production in vitro. Annals of the New York Academy of Sciences 1993; 696: 108-22
20. Rossi SJ, Schroeder TJ, Hariharan S, et al. Prevention and management of the adverse effects associated with immunosuppressive therapy. Drug Safety 1993; 9: 104-31

21. McEvoy GK, editor. American Hospital Formulary Service 1994: drug information. Bethesda, MD: American Society of Hospital Pharmacists, Inc., 1994
22. Kremer JM, Alarcon GS, Lightfoot RW, et al. Methotrexate for rheumatoid arthritis: suggested guidelines for monitoring liver toxicity. Arthritis and Rheumatism 1994; 37: 316-28
23. Morgan SL, Alarcon GS, Krumdieck CL. Folic acid supplementation during methotrexate therapy: it makes sense. Journal of Rheumatology 1993; 20: 929-30
24. Weinblatt ME, Maier AL, Coblyn JS. Low dose leucovorin does not interfere with the efficacy of methotrexate in rheumatoid arthritis: an 8 week randomized placebo controlled trial. Journal of Rheumatology 1993; 20: 950-2
25. Morris RE. Immunopharmacology of new xenobiotic immunosuppressive molecules. Seminars in Nephrology 1992; 12: 304-14
26. Boumpas DT, Chrousos GP, Wilder RL, et al. NIH conference: glucocorticoid therapy for immune-mediated diseases: basic and clinical correlates. Annals of Internal Medicine 1993; 119: 1198-208
27. Hollenberg SM, Weinberger C, Ong ES, et al. Primary structure and expression of a functional human glucocorticoid receptor cDNA. Nature 1985; 318: 635-41
28. Parillo JE, Fauci AS. Mechanisms of glucocorticoid action on immune processes. Annual Review of Pharmacology and Toxicology 1979; 19: 179-201
29. Cronstein BN, Kimmel SC, Levin RI, et al. A mechanism for the anti-inflammatory effects of corticosteroids: the glucocorticoid receptor regulates leukocyte adhesion to endothelial cells and expression of endothelial-leukocyte adhesion molecule 1. Proceedings of the National Academy of Sciences of the United States of America 1992; 89: 9991-5
30. Fauci AS, Dale DC, Balow JE. Glucocorticosteroid therapy: mechanisms of action and clinical considerations. Annals of Internal Medicine 1976; 84: 305-15
31. Lewis GP, Jusko WJ, Burke CW, et al. Boston Collaborative Drug Surveillance Program. Prednisone side-effects and serum protein levels: a collaborative study. Lancet 1971; 2: 778-80
32. Kirwan JR. Systemic corticosteroids in rheumatology. In: Kippel JH, Dieppe PA, editors. Rheumatology. St. Louis: Mosby, 1994
33. Smith MD, Ahern MJ, Roberts-Thompson PJ. Pulse methylprednisolone therapy in rheumatoid arthritis: unproved therapy, unjustified therapy or effective adjunctive treatment? Annals of the Rheumatic Diseases 1990; 49: 265-7
34. Jusko WJ, Ludwig EA. Corticosteroid pharmacokinetics and pharmacodynamics. In: Evans, et al., editors. Applied pharmacodynamics: principles of drug monitoring. Spokane, WA: Applied Therapeutics Inc., 1992
35. Sambrook P, Birmingham J, Kelly P, et al. Prevention of corticosteroid osteoporosis: a comparison of calcium, calcitriol and calcitonin. New England Journal of Medicine 1993; 328: 1747-82
36. Keown PA. Emerging indications for the use of cyclosporin in organ transplantation and autoimmunity. Drugs 1990; 40: 315-25
37. Morris RE. In vivo immunopharmacology of the macrolides FK 506 and rapamycin: toward the era of rational immunosuppressive drug discovery, development and use. Transplantation Proceedings 1991; 23: 2722-4
38. Soldin SJ, Murthy JN, Donnelly JG, et al. Immunophilin receptors for immunosuppressive drugs. Therapeutic Drug Monitoring 1993; 15: 468-71
39. Wiederrecht G, Lam E, Hung S, et al. The mechanism of action of FK-506 and cyclosporin A. Annals of the New York Academy of Sciences 1993; 696: 9-19
40. Clipstone NA, Crabtree GR. Calcineurin is a key signalling enzyme in T lymphocyte activation and the target of the immunosuppressive drugs cyclosporin A and FK 506. Annals of the New York Academy of Sciences 1993; 696: 20-30
41. Thomson AW, Starzl TE. New immunosuppressive drugs: mechanistic insights and potential therapeutic advances. Immunological Reviews 1993; 136: 71-98
42. Liu J. FK 506 and cyclosporin, molecular probes for studying intracellular signal transduction. Immunology Today 1993; 14: 290-5
43. Erlanger BF. Why cyclosporin is an effective drug. Immunology Today 1993; 14: 369
44. Gregory CR, Huie P, Billingham ME, et al. Rapamycin inhibits arterial intimal thickening caused by both alloimmune and mechanical injury. Transplantation 1993; 55: 1409-18
45. Takeuchi T, Iinuma H, Kunimoto S, et al. A new antitumor antibiotic, spergualin: isolation and antitumor activity. Journal of Antibiotics 1981; 34: 1619
46. Tepper MA. Deoxyspergualin: mechanism of action studies of a novel immunosuppressive drug. Annals of the New York Academy of Sciences 1993; 696: 123-32
47. Tepper MA, Nadler S, Mazzucco C, et al. 15-Deoxyspergualin, a novel immunosuppressive drug: studies of the mechanism of action. Annals of the New York Academy of Sciences 1993; 685: 136-47
48. Fahr A. Cyclosporin clinical pharmacokinetics. Clinical Pharmacokinetics 1993; 24: 472-95
49. Faulds D, Goa KL, Benfield P. Cyclosporin: a review of its pharmacodynamic and pharmacokinetic properties, and its use in immunoregulatory disorders. Drugs 1993; 45: 953-1040
50. Peters DH, Fitton A, Plosker GL, et al. Tacrolimus: a review of its pharmacology, and therapeutic potential in hepatic and renal transplantation. Drugs 1993; 46: 746-94
51. McDiarmid SV, Colonna JO, Shaked A, et al. Differences in oral FK 506 dose requirements between adult and pediatric liver transplantation patients. Transplantation 1993; 55: 1328-32
52. Thomas FT, Tepper MA, Thomas JM, et al. 15-Deoxyspergualin: a novel immunosuppressive drug with clinical potential. Annals of the New York Academy of Sciences 1993; 685: 175-92
53. Okobu M, Tamura K, Kamata K, et al. 15-Deoxyspergualin 'rescue therapy' for methylprednisolone-resistant rejection of renal transplants as compared with anti-T cell monoclonal antibody (OKT3). Transplantation 1993; 55: 505-8
54. Amemiya H. Deoxyspergualin: clinical trials in renal graft rejection. Annals of the New York Academy of Sciences 1993; 685: 196-201
55. Gores P, Najarian JS, Stephanian E, et al. Insulin independence in type 1 diabetes after transplantation of unpurified islets from single donor with 15-deoxyspergualin. Lancet 1993; 341: 19-20
56. Groth CG. Deoxyspergualin in allogenic kidney and xenogeneic islet transplantation. Early clinical trials. Annals of the New York Academy of Sciences 1993; 685: 193-5

57. Kahan BD. editor. Cyclosporine: applications in autoimmune diseases. Orlando: Grune & Stratton, Inc., 1988
58. Jegasothy BV, Ackerman CD, Todo S, et al. Tacrolimus (FK 506) - a new therapeutic agent for severe recalcitrant psoriasis. Archives of Dermatology 1992; 128: 781-5
59. Lemster B, Rilo HR, Carroll PB, et al. FK 506 inhibits cytokine gene expression and adhesion molecule expression in psoriatic skin lesions. Annals of the New York Academy of Sciences 1993; 696: 250-6
60. Whitcup SM, Nussenblatt RB. Treatment of autoimmune uveitis. Annals of the New York Academy of Sciences 1993; 696: 307-18
61. Thomson AW, Carroll PB, McCauley J, et al. FK 506: a novel immunosuppressant for treatment of autoimmune disease. Springer Seminars in Immunopathology 1993; 14: 323-44
62. Feutren G, Mihatsch MJ, International Kidney Biopsy Registry of Cyclosporin in Autoimmune Diseases. Risk factors for cyclosporine-induced nephropathy in patients with autoimmune diseases. New England Journal of Medicine 1992; 326: 1654-60
63. Textor SC, Wiesner R, Wilson DJ. Systemic and renal hemodynamic differences between FK 506 and cyclosporine in liver transplant recipients. Transplantation 1993; 55: 1332-9
64. Valantine H, Keogh A, McIntosh N, et al. Cost containment: coadministration of diltiazem with cyclosporine after heart transplantation. Journal of Heart and Lung Transplantation 1992; 11: 1-7
65. Smith CL, Hampton EM, Pederson JA, et al. Clinical and medicoeconomic impact of the cyclosporine-diltiazem interaction in renal transplant recipients. Pharmacotherapy 1994; 14: 471-81
66. Patton PR, Brunson ME, Pfaff WW, et al. A preliminary report of diltiazem and ketoconazole: their cyclosporine-sparing effect and impact on transplant outcome. Transplantation 1994; 57: 889-92
67. Todd PA, Brogden RN. Muromonab CD3: a review of its pharmacology and therapeutic potential. Drugs 1989; 37: 871-99
68. O'Connell PJ, Corpier CL, Steel A, et al. Monoclonal antibody therapy. In: Thomson AW, Catto GRD, editors. Immunology of renal transplantation. London: Edward Arnold, 1993
69. Critchfield JM, Racke MK, Zuniga-Pflucker JC, et al. T cell depletion in high antigen dose therapy of autoimmune encephalomyelitis. Science 1994; 263: 1139
70. Lipsky P. Immunopathogenesis and treatment of rheumatoid arthritis. Journal of Rheumatology 1992; 19 Suppl. 32: 92-4
71. Faulds D, Sorkin EM. A review of its pharmacology and therapeutic potential in ischaemic heart disease. Drugs 1994; 48: 583-98
72. Friend PJ, Rebello P, Oliveira D, et al. Successful treatment of renal allograft rejection with a humanized antilymphocyte monoclonal antibody. Transplantation Proceedings 1995; 27: 869-70
73. Anasetti C, Hansen JA, Waldmann TA, et al. Treatment of acute graft-versus-host disease with humanized anti-Tac: an antibody that binds to the interleukin-2 receptor. Blood 1994; 84: 1320-7
74. Caron PC, Jurcic JG, Scot AM, et al. A phase IB trial of humanized monoclonal antibody M195 (anti-CD33) in myeloid leukemia: specific targeting without immunogenicity. Blood 1994; 83: 1760-8
75. Caron PC, Schwartz MA, Co MS, et al. Murine and humanized constructs of monoclonal antibody M195 (anti-CD33) for the therapy of acute myelogenous leukemia. Cancer 1994; 73: 1049-56
76. Winter G, Harris WJ. Humanized antibodies. Immunology Today 1993; 14: 243-6
77. Isaacs JD, Watts RA, Hazleman BL, et al. Humanised monoclonal antibody therapy for rheumatoid arthritis. Lancet 1992; 340: 748-52
78. Green LL, Hardy MC, Maynard-Currie CE, et al. Antigen-specific human monoclonal antibodies from mice engineered with human Ig heavy and light chain YACs. Nature Genetics 1994; 7: 13-21
79. Lonberg N, Taylor LD, Harding FA, et al. Antigen-specific human antibodies from mice comprising four distinct genetic modifications. Nature 1994; 368: 856-9
80. Quesniaux VFJ. Immunosuppressants: tools to investigate the physiological role of cytokines. Bioessays 1993; 15: 731-9
81. Dumont FJ, Staruch MJ, Koprak SL, et al. Distinct mechanisms of suppression of murine T cell activation by the related macrolides FK 506 and rapamycin. Journal of Immunotherapy 1990; 144: 251
82. DeKeyser F, Elewaut D, Malfait A, et al. Monoclonal antibody therapy in rheumatoid arthritis. Clinical Immunotherapeutics 1994; 1: 148-56
83. Lee JC, Badger AM, Griswold DE, et al. Bicyclic imidazoles as a novel class of cytokine biosynthesis inhibitors. Annals of the New York Academy of Sciences 1993; 696: 149-70
84. Thornberry NA. Key mediator takes shape. Nature 1994; 370: 251-2
85. Wilson KP, Black J-AF, Thomson JA, et al. Structure and mechanism of interleukin-1β converting enzyme. Nature 1994; 370: 270-5
86. Zurawaski G, deVries JE. Interleukin 13, an interleukin 4-like cytokine that acts on monocytes and B cells, but not on T cells. Immunology Today 1994; 15: 19-26
87. Faulds D, Benfield P. Interferon beta-1b in multiple sclerosis: an initial review of its rationale for use and therapeutic potential. Clinical Immunotherapeutics 1994; 1: 79-87
88. Kinkel RP, Goodkin DE. Immunotherapy for multiple sclerosis: a review of the clinical experience. Clinical Immunotherapeutics 1994; 1: 117-34
89. Arnason BGW. Interferon-beta in multiple sclerosis. Neurology 1993; 43: 641-3
90. Paty DW, Li DKB, The UBC MS/MRI Study Group and The IFNB Multiple Sclerosis Study Group. Interferon beta-1b is effective in relapsing-remitting multiple sclerosis. II. MRI analysis results of a multicenter, randomized, double-blind, placebo-controlled trial. Neurology 1993; 43: 662-7
91. The IFNB Multiple Sclerosis Study Group. Interferon-beta-1b is effective in relapsing-remitting multiple sclerosis. I. Clinical results of a multicenter, randomized, double-blind, placebo-controlled trial. Neurology 1993; 43 655-61
92. Drews J. Immunopharmacology: principles and perspectives. Berlin: Springer-Verlag, 1990
93. Ariad S, Geffen D. Role of colony-stimulating factors during high dosage chemotherapy. Clinical Immunotherapeutics 1994; 1: 449-59
94. Metcalf D. The hemopoietic regulators - an embarrassment of riches. Bioessays 1992; 14: 799-805
95. Todd PA, Goa KL. Interferon gamma-1b: a review of its pharmacology and therapeutic potential in chronic granulomatous disease. Drugs 1992; 43: 111-22

96. Hadden JW, Smith DL. Immunopharmacology: immunomodulation and immunotherapy. Journal of the American Medical Association 1992; 268: 2964-9
97. Rosenberg SA, Yang JC, Topalian SL, et al. Treatment of 283 consecutive patients with metastatic melanoma or renal cell carcinoma using high-dose bolus interleukin 2. Journal of the American Medical Association 1994; 271: 907-13
98. Oleksowicz L, Sparano J, O'Boyle K, et al. Interleukins in cancer therapy. Clinical Immunotherapeutics 1994; 1: 271-81
99. Volz MA, Kirkpatrick CH. Interferons 1992: how much of the promise has been realized? Drugs 1992; 43: 285-94
100. Warren RP, Sidwell RW. The potential role of cytokines in the treatment of viral infections. Clinical Immunotherapeutics 1994; 1: 15-30
101. Steimle V, Siegrist C-A, Mottel A, et al. Regulation of MHC class II expression by interferon-τ mediated by the transactivator gene CIITA. Science 1994; 265: 106-9
102. Shuai K, Stark GR, Kerr IM, et al. A single phosphotyrosine residue of stat 91 required for gene activation by interferon-gamma. Science 1993; 261: 1744
103. Moore M, Dawson MM. Interferons. In: Dale MM, Foreman JC, editors. Textbook of immunopharmacology. Oxford: Blackwell Scientific Publications, 1989
104. Wills RJ. Clinical pharmacokinetics of interferons. Clinical Pharmacokinetics 1990; 19: 390-9
105. Bocci V. Interleukins: clinical pharmacokinetics and practical implications. Clinical Pharmacokinetics 1991; 21: 274-84
106. Pope BL. Immunopharmacology: a new frontier. Canadian Journal of Physiology and Pharmacology 1989; 67: 537-45
107. Dechant KL, Bryson HM. Thymostimulin: a review of its pharmacology and prospective role in immunotherapy. Clinical Immunotherapeutics 1994; 1: 378-98
108. Chirigos MA. Immunomodulators: current and future development and application. Thymus 1992; 1a Suppl. 1: S7-S20
109. St Georgiev V. Immunomodulating drugs: major advances in research and development. Annals of the New York Academy of Sciences 1993; 685: 1-10
110. Suzuki M, Takatsuki F, Maeda YY, et al. Rationale for development and therapeutic potential. Clinical Immunotherapeutics 1994; 121-33
111. Revillard JP. Overall evaluation of immunomodulators. Developmental Biological Standards 1992; 77: 233-9
112. Descotes J. Immunotoxicology of immunomodulators. Developmental Biology 1992; 77: 99-102
113. Livingston PA, Wong GY, Adluri S, et al. Improved survival in stage III melanoma patients with GM2 antibodies: a randomized trial of adjuvant vaccination with GM2 ganglioside. Journal of Clinical Oncology 1994; 12: 1036-44
114. AMA Division of Drugs and Toxicology. Immunomodulating agents. Drug Evaluations Annual 1993; 1994: 1903
115. White WB, Ballow M. Modulation of suppressor cell activity by cimetidine in patients with common variable hypogammaglobulinemia. New England Journal of Medicine 1985; 312: 198-202
116. European FK 506 Multicentre Liver Study Group. Randomized trial comparing tacrolimus (FK 506) and cyclosporine in prevention of liver allograft rejection. Lancet 1994; 344: 423-8
117. Hricik DE, Almawi WY, Strom TB. Trends in the use of glucocorticoids in renal transplantation. Transplantation 1994; 57: 979-89
118. D'Alessandro AM, Pirsch JD, Stratta RJ, et al. OKT3 salvage therapy in a quadruple immunosuppressive protocol in cadaveric renal transplantation. Transplantation 1989; 47: 297
119. Tvedegaard E, Olgaard K. Orthoclone OKT3 as rescue treatment for steroid-resistant and recurrent acute rejection in clinical renal transplantation. Transplantation Proceedings 1990; 22: 217
120. Sollinger HW, Belzer FO, Deierhoi MH, et al. RS-61443 (mycophenolate mofetil): a multicenter study for refractory kidney transplant rejection. Annals of Surgery 1992; 216: 513-8
121. Klintmalm GB, Ascher NL, Busuttil RW, et al. RS-61443 for treatment-resistant human liver rejection. Transplantation Proceedings 1993; 25: 697
122. Amemiya H, Suzuki S, Kazuo O, et al. A novel rescue drug, 15-deoxyspergualin. Transplantation 1990; 49: 337
123. Suzuki S. Deoxyspergualin: mode of action and effects on graft rejection. In: Thompson AW, Starzl TE, editors. Immunosuppressive drugs: developments in anti-rejection therapy. London: Edward Arnold, 1994
124. Evans RW, Manninen DL, Dong FB, et al. Immunosuppressive therapy as a determinant of transplantation outcomes. Transplantation 1993; 55: 1297-305
125. Sucia-Foca N, Reed E, d'Agati VD, et al. Soluble HLA antigens, anti-HLA antibodies and anti-idiotypic antibodies in the circulation of renal transplant recipients. Transplantation 1991; 51: 593-601
126. Opelz G, Schwartz V, Engelmann A, et al. Long-term impact of HLA matching on kidney graft survival in cyclosporine-treated recipients. Transplantation Proceedings 1991; 23: 373-5
127. Nield GN, Rudge CJ. Acute and chronic rejection. In: Thomson AW, Catto GRD, editors. Immunology of renal transplantation. London: Edward Arnold, 1993
128. Laskow DA, Deirhoi MH, Hudson SL, et al. The incidence of subsequent acute rejection following the treatment of refractory renal allograft rejection with mycophenolate mofetil (RS611443). Transplantation 1994; 57: 640-3
129. Hullett DA, Sollinger HW. Mycophenolate mofetil and brequinar sodium: new immunosuppressive agents. Transplantation Proceedings 1993; 25: 45-7
130. Burke Jr JF, Pirsch JD, Ramos EL, et al. Long-term efficacy and safety of cyclosporine in renal-transplant recipients. New England Journal of Medicine 1994; 331: 358-63
131. Luke RG. New issues in therapy after renal transplantation. New England Journal of Medicine 1994; 331: 393-4
132. Pantaleo G, Demarest JF, Soudeyns H, et al. Major expansion of CD8+ T cells with a predominant Vβ usage during the primary immune response to HIV. Nature 1994; 370: 463-7
133. Koup RA, Ho DD. Shutting down HIV. Nature 1994; 370: 416
134. Mosmann TR. Cytokine patterns during the progression to AIDS. Science 1994; 265: 193-4
135. Groopman JE. Antiretroviral therapy and immunomodulators in patients with AIDS. American Journal of Medicine 1991; 90 Suppl. 4A: 185-215
136. Grossberg HS, Bonnem EM, Buhles Jr WC. GM-CSF with ganciclovir for the treatment of CMV retinitis

in AIDS. New England Journal of Medicine 1989; 320: 1560

137. Grant SM, Heel RC. Recombinant granulocyte-macrophage colony-stimulating factor (rGM-CSF): review of its pharmacological properties and prospective role in the management of myelosuppression. Drugs 1992; 43: 516-60
138. Krown SE. The role of interferon in the therapy of epidemic Kaposis sarcoma. Seminars in Oncology 1987; 14 Suppl. 3: 27-33
139. Sneller MC, Lane HC. Immunologic approaches to the therapy of HIV-1 infection. Annals of the New York Academy of Sciences 1993; 685: 687-96
140. Green WC. The molecular biology of human immunodeficiency virus type 1 infection. New England Journal of Medicine 1991; 324: 308-17
141. Mofenson LM. Prevention of infections in children with human immunodeficiency virus infection. Clinical Immunotherapeutics 1994; 1: 258-70
142. Cease KB, Berzofsky JA. Toward a vaccine for AIDS: the emergence of immunobiology-based vaccine development. Annual Reviews in Immunology 1994; 12: 923-89
143. Kavanaugh AF, Lipsky PE. Immunological aspects of rheumatic diseases: implications for treatment. Clinical Immunotherapeutics 1994; 1: 209-16
144. Harris ED. Rheumatoid arthritis: pathology and implications for therapy. New England Journal of Medicine 1990; 322: 1277-89
145. Slotkoff AT, Katz P. Approach to the patient with rheumatoid arthritis. Advances in Internal Medicine 1994; 39: 197-240
146. Cash JM, Klippel JH. Second-line drug therapy for rheumatoid arthritis. New England Journal of Medicine 1994; 330: 1368-75
147. Pincus T. Is control of rheumatoid arthritis using available therapies a realistic goal? Rheumatology 1994; 8: 3-4
148. McQueen FM, Tan PLJ. Predicting disease severity in rheumatoid arthritis. New Zealand Medical Journal 1994; 107: 122-4
149. Kantor TG. Current nonsteroidal anti-inflammatory drug applications for rheumatic diseases. Primary Care 1993; 20: 955-63
150. Hollander D. Gastrointestinal complications of nonsteroidal anti-inflammatory drugs: prophylactic and therapeutic strategies. American Journal of Medicine 1994; 96: 274-80
151. McCarthy GM, McCarty DJ. Intrasynovial corticosteroid therapy. Bulletin on the Rheumatic Diseases 1994; 43 (3): 2-4
152. Fries JF, Williams CA, Ramey D, et al. The relative toxicity of disease-modifying antirheumatic drugs. Arthritis and Rheumatism 1993; 36: 297-306
153. Morand EF, McCloud PI. Life table analysis of 879 treatment episodes with slow acting antirheumatic drugs in community rheumatology practice. Journal of Rheumatology 1992; 19: 704-8
154. Kremer JM, Phelps CT. Long-term prospective study of the use of methotrexate in the treatment of rheumatoid arthritis: update after a mean of 90 months. Arthritis and Rheumatism 1992; 35: 138-45
155. Allison AC, Eugui EM. Immunosuppressive and other anti-rheumatic activities of mycophenolate mofetil. Variability in response to anti-rheumatic drugs. Agents and Actions 1993; 44 Suppl.: 165-88
156. Kraska AR, et al. Tenidap vs piroxicam vs piroxicam plus hydroxychloroquine in rheumatoid arthritis: a 24-week interim analysis. Clinical Rheumatology 1994; 13: 355
157. Kirby DS, et al. Tenidap vs naproxen in the treatment of rheumatoid arthritis (RA). Clinical Rheumatology 1994; 13: 354
158. Leeming MRG, et al. A double-blind randomized comparison of tenidap versus auranofin plus diclofenac in early rheumatoid arthritis (RA). Clinical Rheumatology 1994; 13: 355
159. Pluck ND, et al. A 56-week study of tenidap vs diclofenac in rheumatoid arthritis. Arthritis and Rheumatism 1994; 37: 336
160. Littman BH, et al. In vivo reduction of RA synovial tissue metalloproteinase mRNA levels by tenidap. Arthritis and Rheumatism 1995; 38: 29-37
161. Trentham DE, Dynesius-Trentham RA, Orav EJ, et al. Effects of oral administration of collagen on rheumatoid arthritis. Science 1993; 261: 1727-30
162. Harris ED. Excitement in the synovium: the rapid evolution of understanding of rheumatoid arthritis and expectations for therapy. Journal of Rheumatology 1992; 19 Suppl. 32: 3-5
163. Naclerio RM. Allergic rhinitis. New England Journal of Medicine 1991; 325: 860-9
164. Bochner BS, Undem BJ, Lichenstein LM. Immunological aspects of allergic asthma. Annual Reviews in Immunology 1994; 12: 295-335
165. Smith DL, deShazo RD. Bronchoalveolar lavage in asthma: an update and perspective. American Review of Respiratory Disease 1993; 148: 523-32
166. Katz MF, Beer DJ. T lymphocytes and cytokine networks in asthma: clinical and therapeutic implications. Advances in Internal Medicine 1993; 38: 189-222
167. Pipkorn U, Proud D, Lichtenstein LM, et al. Inhibition of mediator release in allergic rhinitis by pretreatment with topical glucocorticosteroids. New England Journal of Medicine 1987; 316: 1506-10
168. International Consensus Report on Diagnosis and Treatment of Asthma. European Respiratory Journal 5: 601-41, 1992
169. Corrigan CJ. Immunological aspects of asthma: implications for future treatment. Clinical Immunotherapeutics 1994; 1: 31-42
170. Church MK. The actions of antihistamines in allergic disease. In: Langer SZ, Church MK, Vargaftig BB, et al., editors. New developments in the therapy of allergic disorders and asthma. Karger (Basel): International Academy for Biomedical Drug Research, 1993; 6: 107-114
171. Rihoux JP. H1 antihistamines as broad-spectrum drugs for the treatment of various allergic disorders. In: Langer SZ, Church MK, Vargaftig BB, et al., editors. New developments in the therapy of allergic disorders and asthma. Karger (Basel): International Academy for Biomedical Drug Research, 1993; 6: 55-9
172. Coffey MJ, Sanders G, Eschenbacher WL, et al. The role of methotrexate in the management of steroid dependent asthma. Chest 1994; 105: 117-21
173. Muranaka M, Nakajima K, Suzaki S. Bronchial responsiveness to acetylcholine in patients with bronchial asthma after long-term treatment with gold salt. Journal of Allergy and Clinical Immunology 1981; 67: 350-6
174. Calderon E, Lockey RF, Bukantz SC, et al. Is there a role for cyclosporine in asthma? Journal of Allergy and Clinical Immunology 1992; 89: 629-36
175. Ruhl R, Halpern GM, Gershwin ME. Unconventional approaches to drug therapy in severe asthma. Allergologia et Immunopathologia 1993; 21: 53-60

176. McMillan RM. Inhibitors of leukotriene synthesis and actions: asthma drugs of the near future? In: Langer SZ, Church MK, Vargaftig BB, et al., editors. New developments in the therapy of allergic disorders and asthma. Karger (Basel): International Academy for Biomedical Drug Research, 1993; 6: 71-85
177. Israel E, Rubin P, Kemp JP, et al. The effect of inhibition of 5-lipoxygenase by zileuton in mild-to-moderate asthma. Annals of Internal Medicine 1993; 119: 1059-66
178. Creticos PS. Immunotherapy with allergens. Journal of the American Medical Association 1992; 268: 2834-9
179. McFadden ER. Evolving concepts in the pathogenesis and management of asthma. Advances in Internal Medicine 1994; 39: 357-94
180. Creticos PS, Reed CE, Norman PS, et al. The NIAID cooperative study of the role of immunotherapy in ragweed-induced adult asthma: 3rd year clinical endpoints; cost-effectiveness. Journal of Allergy and Clinical Immunology 1993; 91: 227
181. Podolsky DK. Inflammatory bowel disease. New England Journal of Medicine 1991; 325: 928-37
182. Podolsky DK. Inflammatory bowel disease. New England Journal of Medicine 1991; 325: 1008-16
183. Gibson PR. Inflammatory bowel disease: current concepts in pathogenesis and therapy. Clinical Immunotherapeutics 1994; 2: 134-60
184. Takahasi T, Shah HS, Wise LS, et al. Circulating antibodies against human colonic extract enriched with a 40kDa protein in patients with ulcerative colitis. Gut 1990; 31: 1016-20
185. Geier DL, Miner Jr PB. Treatment of inflammatory bowel disease. American Journal of Medicine 1992; 93: 199-208
186. Khan AK, Pires J, Trulove SC. An experiment to determine the active therapeutic moiety of sulfasalazine. Lancet 1977; 2: 892-963
187. Present DH, Korelitz BI, Wisch N, et al. Treatment of Crohn's disease with 6-mercaptopurine: a long term, randomized, double-blind study. New England Journal of Medicine 1980; 302: 981-7
188. Hanauer SB. Inflammatory bowel disease revisited: newer drugs. Scandinavian Journal of Gastroenterology 1990; 25 Suppl. 175: 97-106
189. Laurie JA, Moertel CG, Fleming TR, et al. Surgical adjuvant therapy of large bowel carcinoma: an evaluation of levamisole and the combination of levamisole and fluorouracil. Journal of Clinical Oncology 1989; 7: 1447-56
190. Moertel CG, Fleming TR, MacDonald JS, et al. Levamisole and fluorouracil for adjuvant therapy of resected colon carcinoma. New England Journal of Medicine 1990; 322: 352-8
191. Margolin KA. Immunotherapy of colorectal cancer. Clinical Immunotherapeutics 1994; 2: 42-52
192. Schlag PM, Milleck J, Liebrich W. Progress with tumour vaccines. Clinical Immunotherapeutics 1994; 2: 23-31
193. Lee LH, Lim SH. Monoclonal antibodies in the treatment of non-Hodgkin's lymphoma. Clinical Immunotherapeutics 1994; 2: 109-20
194. Beun GDM, van de Velde CJH, Fleuren GJ. T-cell based cancer immunotherapy: direct or redirected tumor-cell recognition? Immunology Today 1994; 15: 11-5
195. Whiteside TL, Herberman RB. Adoptive immunotherapy of cancer: current concepts and future prospects. Clinical Immunotherapeutics 1994; 2: 13-22
196. Oldham RK. Therapy with interleukin-2 and tumor-derived activated lymphocytes. Immuno Series 1994; 61: 251-71
197. Hall PD. Immunomodulation with intravenous immunoglobulin. Pharmacotherapy 1993; 13: 564-73
198. Clark JW. Biological response modifiers. Cancer Chemotherapy and Biological Response Modifiers 1993; 14: 207-26
199. Hoofnagle JH. Interferon therapy of viral hepatitis. In: Baron S, editor. Interferon: principles and medical applications. Galveston: University of Texas Medical Branch, 1992
200. Perrillo RP, Schiff ER, Davis GL, et al. A randomized, controlled trial of interferon alpha-2b alone and after prednisone withdrawal for the treatment of chronic hepatitis B. New England Journal of Medicine 1990; 323: 295-301
201. Appel GB, Levine MI. Acute interstitial nephritis. In: Lichtenstein LM, Fauci AS, editors. Current therapy in allergy, immunology and rheumatology. Toronto: BC Decker Inc., 1988
202. Appel GB, Valeri A. The course and treatment of lupus nephritis. Annual Review of Medicine 1994; 45: 525-37
203. Cronstein BN. Adhesion molecules in inflammation. Current research and new therapeutic targets. Clinical Immunotherapeutics 1994; 1: 323-6
204. Kavanaugh AF, Davis LS, Nichols LA, et al. Treatment of refractory rheumatoid arthritis with a monoclonal antibody to intercellular adhesion molecule 1. Arthritis and Rheumatism 1994; 37: 992-9
205. Schmidbauer G, Hancock WW, Badger AM, et al. SK&F 105685 treatment induces suppressor cell activity and modulates cell adhesion properties in rat recipients of cardiac allografts. Transplantation Proceedings 1993; 25: 758-60
206. Cohen J. Vaccines get a new twist. Sciences 1994; 264: 503-5
207. Mor F, Cohen IR. T cell vaccines for autoimmunine diseases. Annals of the New York Academy of Sciences 1993; 685: 784-7
208. Weiner HL, Friedman A, Miller A, et al. Oral tolerance: immunologic mechanisms and treatment of animal and human organ-specific autoimmune diseases by oral administration of autoantigens. Annual Review of Immunology 1994: 809-37

Chapter 29

# Neurological Diseases

*M.J. Eadie*

## Synopsis of Important Principles

1) Much drug treatment of neurological disease is symptomatic. Most drugs correct neurological dysfunction by acting on synaptic mechanisms: fewer act on nerve impulse conduction. To reach their sites of action, such drugs must first cross the blood-brain barrier.

2) Optimum drug treatment depends on: (a) a correct diagnosis; (b) an understanding of the relevant disease mechanisms; (c) administration of drugs that will correct the disordered mechanisms; (d) individualising drug dosage, guided by knowledge of the drug's pharmacokinetic characteristics; and (e) ensuring that the disadvantages of therapy (i.e. its adverse effects) never become greater than its advantages.

3) Drug therapy of migraine is directed at relieving individual attacks, and in some instances at preventing attacks.

4) Successful drug therapy of epilepsy depends on using a drug, or drugs, appropriate for the patient's seizure type. The drug should be given in a dosage sufficient to control all seizures without causing disadvantageous effects. Plasma drug concentration monitoring may assist in determining the optimum dose.

5) Osmotically active agents and corticosteroids are used to reduce raised intracranial pressure.

6) Dopaminergic agents, particularly levodopa, have revolutionised the treatment of Parkinsonism, but late-stage treatment difficulties are an increasing problem.

7) Various neurological autoimmune disorders, e.g. myasthenia gravis, polymyositis, Guillain-Barré syndrome, may respond to high-dose corticosteroids and other immunosuppressive therapy.

8) Exacerbations of multiple sclerosis respond to high-dose corticosteroids. Interferon-β1b therapy may slow the progression of relapsing-remitting varieties of the disease.

9) Drug therapy offers little benefit in many forms of cerebral vascular disease, but antiplatelet therapy (e.g. with aspirin or ticlopidine) may help in stroke prevention.

10) Certain drugs prescribed for the treatment of coexisting disorders may aggravate neurological disease.

Many disorders of nervous system function have unknown or uncertain causes. If they have known causes, these may be untreatable. Therefore, much drug therapy in neurological diseases is necessarily symptomatic, and is intended to relieve manifestations of the disorder rather than correct its underlying cause.

In general, drug treatment of neurological disease is aimed at:

- Reversing the pathogenesis of the underlying disease process; or
- Altering axon conduction or synaptic (or myoneural junction) neurotransmission to correct abnormal neural function.

There is much greater scope for modifying synaptic function than for altering axon conduction. Therefore, most symptomatic treatment in neurology involves applied synaptic pharmacology. The pharmacology of the glia is virtually unexplored.

## 1. Clinical Pharmacological Considerations

Drugs that act within the nervous system undergo the same processes of absorption, distribution and elimination as drugs that act elsewhere in the body, although there are some peculiar features of drug entry into the brain that have important therapeutic implications.

### 1.1 Pharmacodynamic Considerations

Nearly all drug action within the nervous system is mediated via specific receptors, and growing knowledge of receptor pharmacology is rapidly outstripping its clinical application. Numerous additional receptor subtypes are currently being identified but as yet, the various molecules that are known to act as specific ligands at these receptors have not been studied in human disease. Moreover, drugs long established in human therapeutics are sometimes being shown to act via these newly recognised receptors, rather than by, or in addition to, their traditional receptors [e.g. ergotamine at serotonin$_1$ (5-HT$_1$) rather than at noradrenaline receptors, amantadine at excitatory amino acid receptors rather than on dopaminergic mechanism]. The neuropharmacological concepts of 5 to 10 years ago have not yet been fully reconciled with the exploding knowledge of receptor function.

### 1.2 Pharmacokinetic Considerations

The distribution of neurological drugs throughout the body follows the principles which govern the distribution of drugs in general (see chapter 1). However, unlike the situation for many other organs, there is considerable impediment to the movement of drugs between the blood and the parenchyma of the nervous system. This so-called 'blood-brain barrier' appears to result from the unusual tightness of the junctions between cerebral capillary endothelial cells.

The passive transfer of molecules through the blood-brain barrier is mostly determined by the lipid solubility of the substances in question. Relatively polar drug molecules that pass through the capillary endothelium elsewhere in the body may not enter the brain from the bloodstream, except in a few special regions (the area postrema in the floor of the fourth ventricle, the anterior perforated substance, parts of the hypothalamus and the pineal). Certain molecules pass through the barrier by active carrier-mediated transport (e.g. levodopa). The blood-brain barrier may prevent polar synaptic neurotransmitter molecules (e.g. monoamines, acetylcholine) released at one site in the brain from entering the capillary circulation and being transported in it to enter neural tissue elsewhere and there alter synaptic function inappropriately. Circulating catecholamines and indole alkylamines formed outside the central nervous system, which could serve as neurotransmitters if they entered the brain, are also excluded by the blood-brain barrier.

The blood-brain barrier also prevents certain drugs that act elsewhere in the body from entering the brain. This may sometimes offer therapeutic advantages. For example, certain quaternary ammonium anticholinergic agents that are too polar to cross the blood-brain barrier can be used when a peripheral anticholinergic action is required but an action on the central nervous system is undesirable. Similarly, the blood-brain barrier excludes some inhibitors of the enzyme L-aromatic amino acid decarboxylase (dopa-decarboxylase). If these inhibitors (e.g. carbidopa and benserazide) are given with the amino acid L-dihydroxyphenylalanine (levodopa), the amino acid will not be wastefully decarboxylated to dopamine outside the brain. However, levodopa can still be converted to dopamine (its pharmacologically active metabolite) within the brain, where the decarboxylase is not inhibited (see section 7.1). Certain diseases may impair the integrity of the barrier, permitting greater penetration of some drugs; if this happens, the effects of these drugs on neural function may be increased. Thus in uraemia, penicillin may enter the brain in sufficient quantities to cause convulsions.

Drug entry into the cerebrospinal fluid (CSF) is often thought to be determined purely by the blood-brain barrier effect. This may be so for drugs that enter the CSF mainly from the brain parenchyma, but there is likely to be at least some drug entry into the CSF from capillaries on the dural surface of the pia-arachnoid membranes in direct contact with the fluid over the cerebral and spinal cord surfaces. This entry may contribute to the concentrations of some drugs in the CSF. Furthermore, the choroid plexus cells have a mechanism which actively transports certain acid substances from the CSF into the bloodstream, and this may reduce the concentration of acid drugs (e.g. penicillins) in the CSF.

## 2. General Principles of Treatment

Despite the contemporary explosion in neuropharmacological knowledge, for the practising clinician, the aim of therapy of neurological disorders remains unchanged, namely to relieve the condition being treated without producing unacceptable adverse effects, and to do this as economically as possible. To achieve this aim, the clinician requires a correct diagnosis of the disorder, an understanding of its probable natural history, an appreciation of its likely effects on all aspects of the quality of life of the patient, his or her family and the community, and an awareness of the potential benefits that therapy can offer, as well as its possible undesirable consequences. In the light of this knowledge, the clinician should attempt to achieve the best compromise possible between the benefits and disadvantages of treatment.

Clinically, headache and epilepsy are the two most commonly encountered neurological disorders. However, many other neurological conditions, some reasonably common, some relatively rare, are treatable and also warrant consideration.

## 3. Headaches and Cranial Neuralgias

Numerous types of headache have been recognised in a classification produced in 1988 by the International Headache Society.[1] This revised the earlier classification of the Ad Hoc Committee of the American Neurological Association.[2] The 3 most common headache varieties seen in clinical practice are tension headache, migraine and its variants, and mixed migraine-tension headache.

### 3.1 Tension (Contraction) Headache

Conventionally, tension (contraction) headache has been considered to be due to excessive sustained contraction of the posterior cervical muscles exerting painful traction on the epicranial aponeurosis. The excessive semispinalis muscle contraction sometimes causes secondary compression neuralgia of the greater occipital nerves. The postulated excessive muscle contraction has not been well established electromyographically, although it occurs in some cases.[3] There is a growing view that vascular factors are often involved in the pathogenesis, thus relating the condition to migraine. Indeed, some consider episodic tension headache to really be migraine.[4] Excessive neck muscle contraction may result from local neck disease or injury (e.g. whiplash injury), but it often arises in reaction to other types of head pain, including that of migraine, so that the two headache mechanisms become intertangled. This often makes it difficult to determine the true mechanisms of action of various treatments in relieving tension headache.

#### Optimum Treatment

When tension headache is not complicated by migraine, e.g. after whiplash injury, simple analgesics (e.g. aspirin and paracetamol) generally fail to relieve the pain. The use of strong (opioid) analgesics is most undesirable in this situation because a continued demand for their use may lead to drug dependence. Generally, physical methods, e.g. heat and massage applied to the neck muscles and physiotherapy, provide the most satisfactory and lasting relief. However, these treatments may have to be used frequently over days or weeks. A centrally-acting skeletal muscle relaxant such as *diazepam* (2 to 5mg or more) once or twice daily may help. In addition, the disorder that initiated the tension headache mechanism should be treated if it continues to be active. If this is not done, the methods mentioned above will probably fail to provide lasting relief, although they may produce short term benefit. Since migraine often underlies otherwise idiopathic tension headache, it may be necessary to diagnose its presence and treat it (see section 3.2) before the tension headache will finally subside.

Measures such as the injection of corticosteroids or local anaesthetics into the cervical muscles near their insertion into the occiput or near the greater occipital nerves, or even surgical division of these nerves, have been used in recalcitrant tension headache. Although such procedures may relieve secondary occipital neuralgia, they generally fail in the longer term, probably because they do not deal with the underlying disorder which maintains the tension headache mechanism.

## 3.2 Migraine

Migraine is a very common disorder. Its mechanisms remain controversial; it seems likely that some migraine attacks are initiated via cerebral mechanisms, but it is possible that migraine headache results from involvement of a final common pathway activated by a number of separate mechanisms, not all of which are cerebral. If the attack involves an aura, some believe that cerebral vasospasm, not necessarily restricted to a single cerebral artery, is responsible. The alternative explanation is that there is a spreading regional disturbance of cerebral function, akin to the spreading depression of Leão, an experimental animal phenomenon.[5] Locally altered brain metabolism associated with this spreading depression of cerebral cortical activity causes a secondary reduction in local blood flow.

Clinically, the aura of migraine behaves as a semi-independent variable in relation to the headache. For some years, the latter was thought to be produced by scalp vasodilatation plus chemically mediated sensitisation of perivascular pain nerve endings. More recently, it has been suggested that similar pial or dural artery dilatation may be responsible and that reduced serotonergic activity in the descending spinal nucleus of the trigeminal nerve may amplify afferent trigeminal nociceptive impulses. However, there is no direct evidence for this latter mechanism. The pial or dural artery dilatation may result from centrally mediated activation of peptidergic fibres running with facial nerve branches.[6] Later in the migraine attack, as mentioned above (section 3.1), the vascular headache can activate secondary tension headache.

Whatever the mechanism of migraine headache, there is considerable evidence that altered serotonin (5-hydroxytryptamine; 5-HT) biology is involved. Prior to attacks, platelets have been shown to form microaggregates and release their serotonin content (possibly contributing to vasoconstriction), while nearly all drugs effective in treating or preventing migraine act on serotonergic mechanisms, in various ways. A number of subtypes of serotonin receptor are now known to exist, though their definitive classification is not yet settled and their relation to human migraine not fully elucidated.[7,8]

### *3.2.1 Clinical Pharmacology of Drugs Used in Treatment*

#### Drugs Used in Acute Migraine Attacks

Drugs used for treating acute migraine attacks include the simple analgesics aspirin and paracetamol, the ergot alkaloids ergotamine and dihydroergotamine, sumatriptan, and various other agents (table I) such as nonsteroidal anti-inflammatory drugs and the antiemetic/gastric motility enhancers metoclopramide and domperidone (table I and fig. 1).

***Mechanism/site of action:*** the ergot alkaloids *ergotamine and dihydroergotamine* were formerly regarded as α-adrenoceptor agonists with some dopaminergic properties, but are now known to be agonists at vascular 5-$HT_1$-like receptors (and brain 5-$HT_{1D}$ receptors) as well. Ergotamine appears to relieve migraine headache by inducing scalp and/or dural artery constriction, although it may also act centrally to impair pain impulse transmission in the trigeminal nucleus. It would be expected to be most useful in the earlier stages of migraine before tension headache has come to dominate the pain production mechanism.

*Sumatriptan*[9] is also a serotonergic agent and was originally developed as an alternative to ergotamine. It appears to be a specific agonist at brain 5-$HT_{1D}$ receptors and vascular 5-$HT_1$-like receptors, but lacks other pharmacological activity. It does not cross the intact blood-brain barrier, and hence is unlikely to have a cerebral action *in vivo*. Sumatriptan probably relieves migraine via similar vascular actions to ergotamine.

***Pharmacokinetic characteristics:*** *ergotamine* has a low oral bioavailability (<5%) due to poor absorption or, more probably, high presystemic clearance.[10,11] It is usually administered orally but because of its low bioavailability, delayed absorption and possible loss from the body as a result of vomiting during migraine

**Table I.** Characteristics of the principal drugs used to treat acute migraine attacks

| Feature | Ergotamine | Dihydroergotamine | Sumatriptan |
|---|---|---|---|
| **Mechanism/site of action** | Agonist at vascular 5-$HT_1$-like and brain 5-$HT_{1A}$, 5-$HT_{1B}$, 5-$HT_{1D}$ receptors<br>Antagonist at 5-$HT_{1C}$ and 5-$HT_2$ receptors<br>Potent agonist at $\alpha_1$- and $\alpha_2$-adrenoceptors and weaker agonist at $\beta$-adrenoceptors<br>Agonist at $D_1$, $D_2$ receptors | Agonist at vascular 5-$HT_1$-like and brain 5-$HT_{1A}$, 5-$HT_{1B}$, 5-$HT_{1D}$ receptors<br>Antagonist at 5-$HT_{1C}$ and 5-$HT_2$ receptors<br>Potent agonist at $\alpha_1$- and $\alpha_2$-adrenoceptors and weaker agonist at $\beta$-adrenoceptors<br>Agonist at $D_1$, $D_2$ receptors | Agonist at vascular 5-$HT_1$-like and brain 5-$HT_{1A}$, 5-$HT_{1B}$, 5-$HT_{1D}$, 5-$HT_{1X}$ receptors, but does not enter brain *in vivo* |
| **Pharmacokinetic characteristics:** | | | |
| Bioavailability (F) | 1-2% (oral); 5% (rectal); 47% (IM) | Low (oral) | 14% (oral); 96% (SC) |
| Half-life | 3.35h (? active metabolites more slowly eliminated) | Short | 2.0h |
| Clearance (CL) | 45 L/h<br>[CL/F: 2800 L/h] | | 72 L/h |
| Principal route of elimination | Hepatic metabolism | Hepatic metabolism | Hepatic metabolism |
| **Clinical effectiveness** | Moderate orally; better rectally | Poor orally; fairly good intravenously | Superior to ergotamine orally; very effective subcutaneously |
| **Adverse effects** | Nausea, vomiting, leg pain, peripheral and central vasospastic phenomena, ? rebound headache on frequent use | Nausea, vomiting, leg pain, peripheral and central vasospastic phenomena | Nausea, vomiting, taste disturbance, facial flushing, sensations of pressure, fairly frequent chest and shoulder discomfort, injection site pain/redness, myocardial ischaemia |
| **Drug interactions** | Increased risk of peripheral vasospastic phenomena with erythromycin and troleandomycin | | Possible myocardial ischaemia if used within 24 hours of ergotamine. No interactions with propranolol, pizotifen, flunarazine, alcohol |

*Abbreviations:* IM = intramuscular; SC = subcutaneous; 5-HT = 5-hydroxytryptamine (serotonin).

attacks, the drug is also administered sublingually, rectally (as a suppository), by inhalation, and by intramuscular or intravenous injection. Following sublingual administration, it is poorly absorbed[12] and when given by inhalation, much of an inhaled dose probably reaches the alimentary tract rather than the lungs. However, ergotamine is absorbed more efficiently when given by inhalation than when swallowed.[13] Although mean peak plasma ergotamine concentrations after inhalation are about 4 times greater than after oral tablet administration, the conventional initial dose of 2 inhalations (each of 0.36mg) is almost certainly too small to produce effective plasma ergotamine concentrations. Two doses of 6 inhalations (2.16mg) were used in one study in patients with cluster headache.[13] Rectally administered ergotamine sometimes proves more effective in migraine than orally administered drug. Since part of the rectal venous blood flow drains into the systemic rather than the portal circulation, this may contribute to the slightly higher bioavailability and sometimes greater efficacy of rectal ergotamine.

Intramuscular ergotamine has a much higher bioavailability (≈47%), though there is considerable interindividual variation.[11] Consequently, the intramuscular dose is smaller than the oral or rectal dose (0.25mg *versus* 1 or 2mg). In aqueous solution, ergotamine isomerises to its epimer ergotaminine, which is relatively inactive pharmacologically. By the time the preparation is several days old, the actual ergotamine dose in the ampoules is about 50% of the nominal content. Ergotamine has a fairly short half-life (3.35h; table I), but may be metabolised to biologically active metabolites which persist longer in the body.

In general, *dihydroergotamine* behaves like a weaker version of ergotamine, and also has a low oral bioavailability. It has been given intranasally with some success in treating migraine attacks.[14]

*Sumatriptan* is given orally (bioavailability ≈14%) or by subcutaneous injection (bioavail-

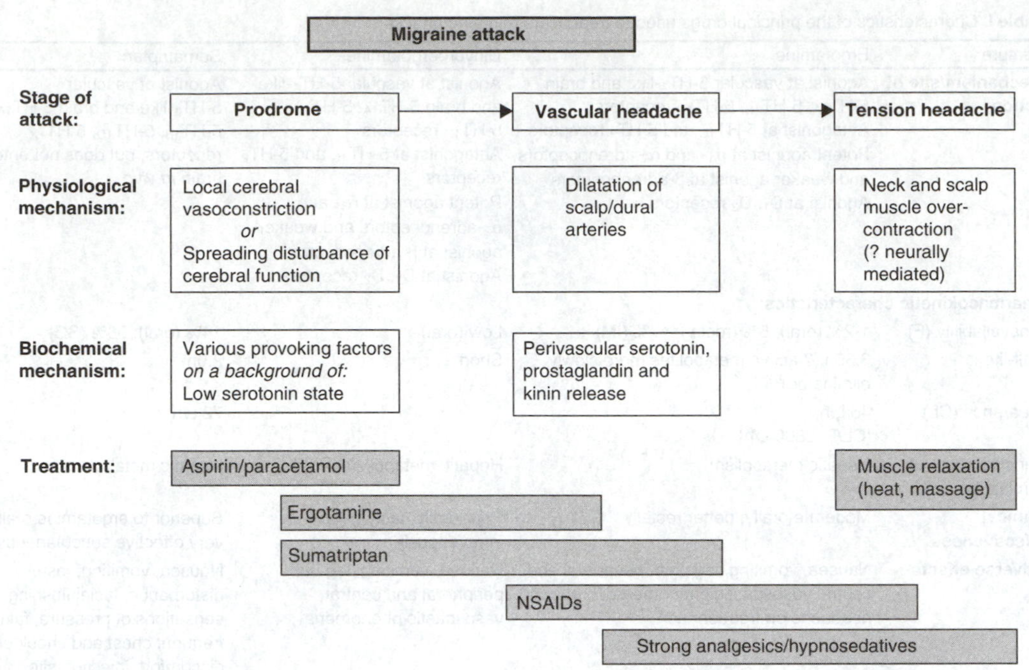


**Fig. 1.** Physiological and biochemical mechanisms involved at different stages of a migraine attack, and their treatment.

ability ≈96%). It also has a short half-life (≈2h) but unlike ergotamine, has no known active metabolites.

***Clinical effectiveness:*** *ergotamine* is an old drug whose reputation in treating migraine rests on clinical opinion rather than on controlled clinical trials. However, the efficacy of *sumatriptan* given both orally and subcutaneously has been well demonstrated in controlled studies.[9] Orally, 100mg sumatriptan appears more effective than 2mg ergotamine, but it has the disadvantage of being very expensive. Its relatively short half-life means that a significant proportion of patients require a second dose during a single migraine attack to maintain pain relief.

***Tolerability and drug interactions potential:*** *sumatriptan* has fewer adverse peripheral vasoconstrictive effects than ergotamine, and is less likely to cause nausea. However, it has been associated with upper chest and shoulder region discomfort, and occasional instances of proven coronary artery pain. It appears hazardous to give sumatriptan within 24 hours of ergotamine intake, because of the risk of myocardial ischaemia.

*Ergotamine* is often combined with caffeine and various sedative and/or antiemetic agents in marketed preparations intended for oral or rectal use. Caffeine may enhance ergotamine absorption (though this has not been demonstrated conclusively) and may have some direct antimigraine action; antiemetics may help the many migraine sufferers who experience nausea during attacks. However, such fixed-dose combinations often cause annoying and sometimes unacceptable adverse effects which arise more from the other components than from the ergotamine. Rather than using fixed-dose combination preparations, it is often more satisfactory to prescribe ergotamine and an antiemetic agent separately, each in appropriate dosage. Frequent ergotamine intake may lead to ergotamine-withdrawal headaches, though many reported instances seem to have involved use of an ergotamine-caffeine combination, and caffeine-withdrawal headache is known to exist (see section 15.1).

### Drugs Used in Migraine Prevention

With the exception of methysergide, all drugs used in migraine prevention have major uses in other areas of medicine.

***Methysergide:*** this drug is an antagonist at $5\text{-HT}_{1A}$, $5\text{-HT}_{1C}$, $5\text{-HT}_{1X}$, $5\text{-HT}_{1Y}$ and $5\text{-HT}_2$ receptors.[7] Its plasma half-life is approximately 0.8 hours and its oral bioavailability approximately 13%.[15] It has been suggested that part of the antimigraine action of methysergide may reside in its *N*-demethylated metabolite, methylergometrine,[16] which has activity at 5-$HT_{1C}$ and dopamine receptors[17] and a plasma half-life of about 3 hours.[15]

Methysergide was the first agent established as a migraine preventative by modern clinical trial techniques and it remains probably the most effective prophylactic agent available. However, as its adverse effects are more severe than those of the other commonly used migraine preventatives, it tends not to be used unless other agents have failed. The adverse effects of methysergide include anorexia, nausea, hypotension, hypertension, vasospastic manifestations, hair loss, and periureteric, retroperitoneal, pleural, pericardial and cardiac valvular fibrosis. The usual initial oral dose of methysergide is 1 or 2mg twice daily, with 1 or 2mg dosage increments every 3 or 4 weeks thereafter. Doses of 4 to 8 mg/day are often effective. Methysergide should not be used continuously for more than 6 months without a break in therapy for at least 4 weeks. This practice is believed to minimise the risk of fibrosis.

***β-Adrenoceptor antagonists (β-blockers):*** *propranolol* is the most commonly used β-blocker for migraine prevention and is moderately effective.[18,19] In the study of Stensrud and Sjaastad,[20] it was more effective than placebo in 64% of patients. However, it is not certain that the preventative effect of propranolol depends on its β-blocking action. The drug is also known to bind to 5-$HT_{1B}$, 5-$HT_{1C}$, and 5-$HT_2$ receptors and to prevent serotonin uptake by nerve terminals and platelets, and thus its antimigraine effects may depend more on these actions than on β-adrenoceptor antagonism. Except in patients with asthma, propranolol has relatively few serious adverse effects. Therapy is usually begun in low oral doses, e.g. 20mg 2 or 3 times daily, with dosage increments every 2 or 3 weeks until either the migraine attacks become significantly less frequent and/or easier to relieve, or adverse effects (often feelings of weakness or lassitude) preclude any further dosage increase.

A number of other β-blockers have also been used in migraine prevention, including pindolol,[21] *atenolol*,[22] *metoprolol*,[23] and *timolol*.[24] Pindolol has not proved successful in all trials,[25] while oxprenolol[26] and alprenolol[27] have proved unsuccessful.

***Antiserotonin/antihistamine drugs:*** three agents in this class *(cyproheptadine, pizotifen* and *methdilazine)*, which have both antihistamine and antiserotonin (5-$HT_2$ antagonist) properties, sometimes prove useful in preventing migraine.[28,29] These drugs also have other potentially relevant pharmacological actions: methdilazine and cyproheptadine are bradykinin antagonists; cyproheptadine exerts calcium channel blocking activity;[30] and all 3 have anticholinergic effects. They are relatively safe, their main adverse effects being appetite stimulation and weight gain. This may be minimised by warning patients at the commencement of therapy to restrict their food intake, thus avoiding lapsing into overeating. Treatment with these agents is usually begun with 4mg of cyproheptadine or methdilazine or 0.5mg of pizotifen given orally 2 or 3 times daily. The dosage is then increased every 3 or 4 weeks until a satisfactory response occurs or adverse effects become unacceptable.

***Amitriptyline:*** this tricyclic antidepressant has proved a moderately efficient migraine preventative in controlled clinical trials,[31,32] being more effective than placebo in 70 to 80% of patients. Amitriptyline blocks amine neurotransmitter reuptake into nerve terminals, and may interfere with the uptake of serotonin by platelets. It also binds to 5-$HT_{1B}$ and 5-$HT_2$ receptors. The antimigraine effect of amitriptyline appears independent of its mood elevating action. For migraine prevention, a dose of 50 to 100mg is given once daily in the evening. Amitriptyline has anticholinergic activity (resulting in dry mouth and blurred vision) and sedative effects, but these are usually not particularly troublesome at the doses used in migraine prophylaxis, particularly if the drug is introduced into therapy gradually.

The role of other tricyclic antidepressants in migraine prophylaxis is not as well established.

***Calcium antagonists:*** regular intake of calcium antagonist drugs is useful to prevent migraine. The best documented agent appears to be *flunarizine*,[33,34] the usual dose of which is 10mg given once daily in the evening.[35] *Verapamil*,[36] *nimodipine*,[37] *diltiazem*[38] and *nifedipine*[39] have also proved useful. These agents affect calcium-related cytoplasmic mechanisms in many tissues, but it is not known whether their migraine-preventing effects depend on impairing neurotransmitter release from synaptic vesicles or serotonin release from platelets, or whether they simply reduce the tendency to spasm of arterial and arteriolar smooth muscle.

***Antiepileptic drugs:*** clinical experience has shown that *phenytoin* is sometimes useful in preventing childhood migraine. In adult migraine, phenytoin appears to be consistently useful only in migraine with a prodrome comprising a hemisensory disturbance, dysphasia or manifestations consistent with reversible brain stem ischaemia, e.g. severe rotational vertigo. Its mechanism of action in migraine prevention is obscure. The effective dose of phenytoin, and its therapeutic concentrations in plasma, appear to be lower than those required to control epilepsy (see section 4.1).

There have also been reports of successful migraine prophylaxis with *valproic acid (sodium valproate)*.[40]

***Clonidine:*** early clinical reports suggested that this central $\alpha_2$-adrenoceptor agonist was a useful migraine preventative. However, in the majority of subsequent controlled clinical trials it has failed to produce statistically significant benefit. The recommended dose of clonidine for migraine prevention is 25 to 50μg 2 or 3 times daily, which is lower than that used for treating hypertension.

***Monoamine oxidase (MAO) inhibitors:*** the nonselective MAO inhibitor *phenelzine* has been reported to be effective in preventing migraine.[41] However, many would consider these drugs as a last resort in migraine prevention. The usual dietary restrictions recommended in association with nonselective MAO inhibitor intake are mandatory.

***Ergotamine:*** oral administration of ergotamine 1mg 2 or 3 times daily sometimes appears to help prevent migraine. However, such therapy is not often recommended, largely because of the fear that continued ergotamine administration will cause ergotamine-withdrawal headache on ceasing treatment. If this occurs, it may be mistakenly treated by increased ergotamine intake.

#### 3.2.2 Optimum Treatment

Many persons with migraine manage their own attacks adequately by using measures such as bed rest and simple analgesics, and require no formal medical treatment. When patients do seek treatment for migraine, their management entails:

- Treatment of acute attacks; and
- Prevention of attacks, if the attacks are frequent enough or are inadequately relieved by treatment taken early in their course.

##### Treatment of Acute Attacks

Patients with milder migraine sometimes find that *aspirin*, particularly if taken early in an attack, affords satisfactory relief. In adults, 600mg aspirin orally may be as effective as larger doses; a migraine aura, which allows early recognition that a headache is imminent, improves the prospect of success with aspirin.[42] However, the presence of gastric stasis, which tends to occur in migraine attacks, may delay aspirin absorption and reduce its efficacy. This can be circumvented by early administration of the dopamine antagonist/antiemetic drug *metoclopramide*. Unlike certain other antiemetics (e.g. thiethylperazine[43]), metoclopramide increases alimentary tract peristalsis. Given intramuscularly in a dose of 10mg[44] or orally in a similar dose,[45] it increases the speed of aspirin absorption during migraine attacks.

If aspirin fails or is not tolerated, *paracetamol* and various *nonsteroidal anti-inflammatory drugs*, e.g. naproxen[46] or diclofenac,[47] may be effective. Rectally administered ketoprofen proved more effective than oral ergotamine in one study.[48]

Other agents that may be tried include the calcium antagonist *nifedipine*, which has been used in the aura phase to abort migraine but has failed in some trials.[49] *Domperidone*, a dopamine antagonist which (unlike metoclopramide) does not cross the blood-brain barrier, may be used orally to diminish the nausea of migraine. A combination of domperidone 20mg orally with paracetamol has proved effective in shortening the duration of migraine attacks.[50]

***Treatment of severe attacks:*** if the above treatments prove ineffective, ergotamine, dihydroergotamine or sumatriptan may be used during the vascular headache phase of migraine. *Ergotamine* is often prescribed as a 1 or 2mg oral dose taken as early as possible in the attack, the dose being repeated hourly or half-hourly as required to achieve pain relief. The recommended ergotamine dose is limited to 6mg in an individual attack, and 8 to 10mg in a single week. Clinically, it is uncommon to find a patient whose migraine attack benefits from the second or subsequent oral dose of ergotamine when the initial dose has failed. In view of the low and variable oral bioavailability of ergotamine, and the fact that the drug is most likely to work during the early vasodilatation phase of migraine, it seems sensible to find by trial and error a single effective initial oral dose of ergotamine for each individual. Thereafter, this dose should be taken as early as possible in that patient's attacks, and not repeated in a given attack. The clinician's chief concern in prescribing ergotamine is that the drug will produce vasospastic tissue injury. Exceptional patients are exquisitely sensitive to ergotamine in this regard, and it should be prescribed very cautiously in individuals with known arterial disease. However, the vast majority of patients tolerate more ergotamine than the recommended prescribing limit without developing toxicity. It has sometimes been suggested that ergotamine should not be used for migraine in which there is clinical evidence of cerebral vasoconstriction (i.e. an aura) although, fortunately, ergotamine does not constrict intracranial arteries.[51]

Oral *sumatriptan* (100mg) has proved more effective than oral ergotamine (2mg plus caffeine 200mg) in relieving migraine[52] but, because of its greater cost, it is likely to be used mainly when ergotamine has been unsatisfactory in the past. The usual oral dose (100mg) may provide fairly rapid headache relief, though the pain may recur some hours later and require a further dose. A subcutaneous injection of sumatriptan (6mg) is more effective than oral administration, and avoids the problem of impaired absorption due to altered alimentary tract motility.

***Attacks not responding to other treatment:*** if a migraine attack does not settle, the tension headache mechanism may come to dominate the pathogenesis of the pain. The measures discussed in section 3.1 for tension headache may then be instituted. Simple analgesics (aspirin, paracetamol and various nonsteroidal anti-inflammatory drugs) given orally or rectally or, as a last resort, strong (opioid) analgesics may be used to provide symptomatic pain relief at any stage in migraine attacks. However, sedation with parenteral diazepam or chlorpromazine may be a safer alternative, as this avoids the risk of setting the patient on the path to opioid dependence if migraine attacks occur frequently. The need for a clinician to administer strong analgesics parenterally more than once or twice a year to a patient with migraine indicates that more needs to be done to improve the management of the patient's disorder, and that preventative therapy should be considered.

The treatment of an acute migraine attack is summarised in figure 1.

#### Migraine Prevention

In occasional patients, migraine occurs reasonably predictably in certain circumstances, e.g. exertion at sport, menstruation, long car journeys. If these situations cannot be avoided, one or two small oral doses of aspirin or ergotamine, taken a short time before the provoking circumstances, may prevent the expected attack. However, the duration of action of sumatriptan may be too short for such use.

Unfortunately, most migraine attacks occur unpredictably, or develop because of factors which are present much or all of the time, e.g. work situations. If any factor responsible for attacks can be identified, e.g. oral contraceptive use, that factor should be removed from the patient's life situation, if possible, before long term migraine preventative therapy is considered.

When individual attacks of migraine cannot be relieved speedily and satisfactorily by the agents discussed above, or the attacks interfere significantly with the sufferer's life and occur more frequently than once or twice a month, and causative factors cannot be identified and removed, continuous preventative drug therapy with one of the regimens discussed in section 3.2.1 is indicated. The order in which such agents might be used clinically, if no contraindication exists, is β-adrenoceptor blockers first, then antiserotonin/antihistamine drugs, amitriptyline, calcium antagonists, methysergide, phenytoin, and monoamine oxidase inhibitors.

In the dosage regimens for preventative drugs suggested above (section 3.2.1), there has been little emphasis on pharmacokinetic considerations. The main reason for this is a lack of pharmacokinetic information for many of these agents. Even when such information is available, there is still the impression that the maximum protection against migraine from a given drug dose may not develop until well after steady-state has been attained. This is the reason for suggesting that the dose of migraine preventative drugs should not be increased more often than every 3 or 4 weeks. In this way, unnecessarily high dosages with their attendant adverse effects may be avoided.

### *3.2.3 Clinical Outcome and Economic Considerations*

Migraine occurs frequently in the population and causes considerable morbidity with loss of time from work and inefficiency at work. The current treatments for more severe attacks are not particularly satisfactory, and the most effective agent, sumatriptan, has the disadvantage of being very expensive *versus* the other drugs. However, the very considerable economic cost of migraine to the community does need to be taken into account in selecting appropriate treatment.

Although none of the agents used for migraine prevention is costly, preventative therapy rarely stops all migraine attacks. It is much more realistic to hope that the treatment will decrease the frequency of attacks to a more acceptable level, and make individual attacks milder and more responsive to interval therapy. Once such a response has been maintained for 2 or 3 months in a patient, it is often possible to reduce the dosage of the migraine preventative drug gradually over the course of several months, without loss of benefit.

### 3.3 Cluster Headache (Migrainous Neuralgia)

Although this disorder has obvious affinities to migraine, it is a discrete entity with highly characteristic clinical features.[53] Its pathogenesis is not well established, although it has been thought to depend on severe spasm in one internal carotid artery just within the skull, perhaps followed by painful dilatation of arteries of the forehead on the same side. The biochemical basis is unclear.

#### Optimum Treatment

***Acute attacks*** of cluster headache can be relieved by subcutaneous injection of *sumatriptan* 6mg, but further injections will be needed in subsequent attacks, and several may be required each 24 hours. Early in an attack several inhalations of pure oxygen are sometimes helpful, presumably by producing vasoconstriction.[54] Otherwise, it is often difficult to relieve the pain of individual attacks except by the injection of strong analgesics, an inadvisable policy when the attacks occur several times a day.

***Prevention of attacks:*** treatment in cluster headache is usually directed at preventing attacks, which occur 2 to 8 (or more) times a day, often regularly and with a predictable timing.

*Ergotamine,* injected intramuscularly in a dose of 0.25mg (or later 0.5mg if necessary) 2 or 3 times a day, has been the traditional therapy for cluster headache. It is continued until the patient is free from all attacks for 5 days. Treatment is then ceased, as the cluster of attacks has probably passed. Ergotamine is also effective for prophylaxis when taken orally.[55] The initial oral dose is 1mg 3 times daily, but the drug may have to be given up to 4 times daily, perhaps in a total daily dose of 6 to 8mg, before the attacks will cease. The dosage may be increased every 2 or 3 days, as determined by the clinical response. Such ergotamine intakes may appear excessive, relative to the usually recommended maximum dosage; however, these doses rarely cause serious adverse effects, and failure of inadequate therapy to control the pain of cluster headache within a reasonably short period can lead to insistent demands for strong analgesics.

*Other agents:* should regular oral ergotamine fail to prevent attacks of cluster headache, or not be tolerated, other agents such as *verapamil* (40mg 3 times daily or later in higher dosage) may bring the situation under control.[56] *Pizotifen* and *methysergide* have also been used, but are not as effective as ergotamine in preventing attacks. *Prednisone* or *prednisolone* given orally in doses of 40 to 60mg daily may also control cluster headache,[57] the corticosteroid dose being tapered off once the attacks have disappeared for several days.

In chronic variants of cluster headache, *lithium carbonate* may bring the attacks under control.[58,59] As with its use in bipolar affective disorder (see chapter 30; sect. 4.1), the plasma lithium concentration should be maintained between 0.8 and 1.2 mmol/L.[60] As clinical benefit with lithium may develop slowly over days or weeks, lithium therapy is not very useful early in clusters, or in short clusters. It is therefore used mainly when other treatments have failed and the cluster has persisted for several weeks or longer. Oral sumatriptan does not appear to be effective in preventing cluster headache, probably because of its duration of action is too brief.

It is important to control cluster headache episodes as quickly as possible, not only to spare the patient suffering, but also because the longer the delay before potentially effective treatment is prescribed, the more difficult it is to stop the attacks. Thus, early correct diagnosis of the disorder is essential. Prophylactic treatment is usually continued for about a week after the last attack, and then withdrawn progressively. Further therapy is not needed until the next cluster occurs. The various prophylactic therapies discussed above are relatively inexpensive, but treatment of individual attacks with subcutaneous sumatriptan injections given several times a day is very costly.

### 3.4 Chronic Paroxysmal Hemicrania

This disorder is characterised by multiple episodes of head pain similar to that of cluster headache, but more brief, and sometimes provoked by neck movement. It responds to oral indomethacin 25mg 3 times daily, and probably to other nonsteroidal anti-inflammatory agents as well.

### 3.5 Cranial Neuralgias (Particularly Trigeminal Neuralgia)

Neuralgic pain may occur in the territories of various branches of the trigeminal nerve and the upper cervical nerve roots. Many of the neuralgias arise from mechanical compression of the relevant nerves. There is increasing evidence that idiopathic trigeminal neuralgia (tic douloureux) is often caused by intracranial compression of the trigeminal root by branches of the anterior inferior cerebellar artery or neighbouring vessels.

**Optimum Treatment**

The cause of cranial neuralgia should always be sought and, where practicable, corrected. The pain may be treated symptomatically, with drugs. Various forms of surgical treatment may be used if medical treatment proves unsatisfactory.

*Carbamazepine* (see also section 4.1) is of specific benefit in trigeminal neuralgia.[61] The initial dosage should be low, e.g. 100 to 200mg twice daily for the first 4 to 7 days, to allow autoinduction of its metabolism (see chapter 1; sect. 3.3) to occur and to minimise the sedation which often manifests if the drug is given in full dosage from the outset. To reduce the chance of unnecessarily high intake, the carbamazepine dosage should be increased no more often than every 4 to 5 days, in increments of 100 or 200mg daily, until either the attacks of pain are fully controlled or unacceptable adverse effects, mainly drowsiness, ataxia and blurred vision, supervene. Carbamazepine doses of the order of 2000 mg/day may occasionally be necessary to prevent attacks. These doses may be tolerated if achieved gradually.

It has been suggested that after the pain of trigeminal neuralgia is controlled by carbamazepine, treatment should be ceased in the hope that the attacks will not recur for a time. However, this policy may ultimately lead to the pain becoming refractory to the maximum tolerated carbamazepine dosage. If carbamazepine therapy is continued, not necessarily in full dosage, during the remissions that occur early in the course of trigeminal neuralgia, the risk of its later becoming refractory appears lessened. Although the carbamazepine dosage is determined by the clinical response, the target plasma concentration that correlates with therapeutic benefit appears similar to the threshold for epilepsy control, i.e. 5 mg/L.

If carbamazepine therapy proves unsatisfactory, there are several alternatives. *Phenytoin* has proved useful, but is less effective than carbamazepine. *Clonazepam* is probably more effective than phenytoin,[62] while *baclofen* (see section 8.1.1) has been reported to be useful in some patients.[63] The initial dosages of the antiepileptic drugs are similar to those used in epilepsy (see section 4.1), their final dosages being determined by the clinical response. Baclofen is given initially in a dosage of 10mg 3 times daily, increasing to 60 to 75 mg/day.

Should all drug therapy fail, various surgical measures are available.

### 3.6 Other Painful Neuropathies

Similar drug therapies have been used for certain painful neuralgias and neuropathies. *Glossopharyngeal neuralgia* responds to carbamazepine, administered as for trigeminal neuralgia.[64] Carbamazepine may also ease the lightning pains of *tabes dorsalis*[65] and certain painful *peripheral polyneuropathies*.[66] In these disorders, tricyclic antidepressants such as imipramine and amitriptyline may sometimes be of benefit, and sodium channel blockers such as mexiletine and tocainide may help.

#### *3.6.1 Postherpetic Neuralgia*

The *tricyclic antidepressants* and *carbamazepine* are used for the pain of chronic postherpetic neuralgia, although they are often not of great benefit. There appears to be no known reliable specific drug therapy for this condition. A variety of measures may help different individuals, e.g. local use of cold sprays, local anaesthetic ointments, local procaine infiltration, and percussing the painful margins of the herpetic scars. Benefit appears slowly and is incomplete, raising suspicion that the underlying condition may simply be resolving spontaneously (see also chapter 32; sect. 3.4.2).

In acute herpes zoster, several treatments have been used to decrease pain and to diminish the risk of subsequent postherpetic neuralgia, e.g. corticosteroids, cyanocobalamin (vitamin $B_{12}$) and amantadine.[67] However, there is little convincing evidence for their efficacy.

#### *3.6.2 Painful Radiculopathy*

Painful radiculopathy from compression of lumbar roots by spinal disc protrusions or arachnoid adhesions has sometimes been treated with carbamazepine or tricyclic antidepressants (usually without major benefit) when surgery is not possible. Local intrathecal or extradural injection of corticosteroids, e.g. methylprednisolone acetate, has also been used. Such measures may help some patients, but there is no convincing evidence that they are useful in the majority of affected individuals, or that local corticosteroid administration is more effective than systemic corticosteroid therapy. Repeated intrathecal corticosteroid injections may cause a progressive spinal arachnoiditis. Some consider that intraspinal corticosteroid therapy has no place in contemporary therapeutics.[68]

## 4. Epileptic Seizures

In recent years, clinical pharmacological knowledge in this area has expanded considerably and has had a major influence on the drug treatment of epilepsy. Recently, several newer antiepileptic drugs have become available, including vigabatrin,[69] lamotrigine,[70] gabapentin,[71,72] and oxcarbazepine.[73] The definitive place of these drugs in therapy is not yet established. [For reviews on the management of epilepsy and the drugs used in its treatment, see Eadie and Tyrer;[74] Levy et al.[75] and Ressor & Kutt[76]].

### 4.1 Clinical Pharmacology of Drugs Used in Treatment

#### *4.1.1 Mechanism/Site of Action*

Numerous biochemical actions of the antiepileptic drugs are known. Many of these actions occur at concentrations not relevant to human therapeutics and will not be considered in detail. The antiepileptic drugs tend to limit the spread of epileptogenic activity rather than prevent its initiation. They appear to have 3 main mechanisms of action:[77]

1) Phenytoin, carbamazepine and possibly lamotrigine inhibit voltage-dependent $Na^+$ channels in axonal cell membranes. This selectively impairs the conduction of rapid trains of impulses (as occur during epileptic seizures) without impeding axon traffic at more physiological rates.

2) Ethosuximide and valproic acid inhibit 'T' type $Ca^{++}$ channels in thalamic neurons, thus interfering with neuronal function in one of the neural circuits involved in absence seizures.[78]

3) Various antiepileptic drugs enhance $Cl^-$ entry into postsynaptic neurons and thus inhibit these neurons. Phenobarbital acts directly on the $Cl^-$ channel, vigabatrin and probably valproic acid inhibit the degradation of γ-aminobutyric acid (GABA), thus increasing its postsynaptic effect in opening $Cl^-$ channels, while benzodiazepine antiepileptic drugs facilitate the effect of GABA on $Cl^-$ channels.

Various mechanisms of action have been proposed for gabapentin including activity at an as yet unidentified receptor linked to the L-'system' amino acid transporter protein; however, it may also inhibit the degradation of GABA and/or increase its synthesis rate[71] or otherwise alter brain amino acid concentration or metabolism.[79]

#### *4.1.2 Pharmacokinetic Characteristics*

The pharmacokinetic characteristics of commonly used antiepileptic drugs and representative values for their pharmacokinetic parameters are shown in table II. The following points are of clinical importance:

1) Hepatic metabolism of phenytoin is saturable within the therapeutic range of plasma concentrations; the elimination of this drug is better described by Michaelis-Menten (nonlinear) kinetics than by first-order (linear) ones (see chapter 1; sect. 2.2.8). Steady-state plasma phenytoin concentrations rise more than expected as its dose is increased in the individual

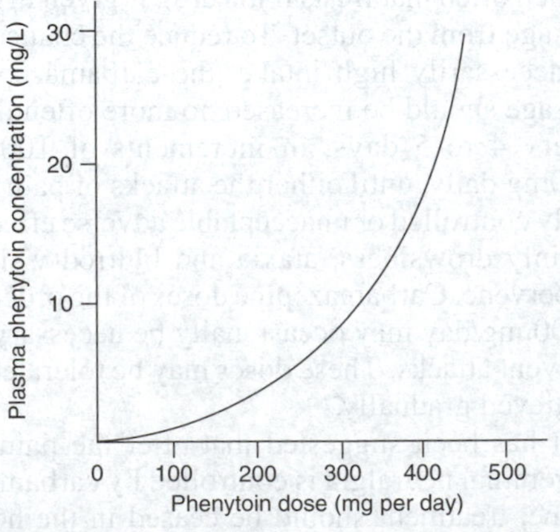


**Fig. 2.** Effects of dose increments on steady-state plasma concentrations of phenytoin in the individual patient.

**Table II.** Pharmacokinetic characteristics of antiepileptic drugs

| Drug | Nature | Protein binding (%) | Vd (L) [per 70kg] | Half-life (h) | Clearance (L/h) | Percentage in body fluid relative to plasma | | | Route of elimination | Active metabolites | Comments |
|---|---|---|---|---|---|---|---|---|---|---|---|
| | | | | | | CSF | saliva | breast milk | | | |
| Phenytoin[a] | Acid | 87-93 | 35-70 | ≈20-30* | | 10 | 10-12 | 18 | Hepatic metabolism (saturable under therapeutic conditions) | No | *Half-life is concentration-dependent; some brands have reduced oral bioavailability |
| Phenobarbital | Acid | 50-60 | 35-70 | 48-120 | 0.2-0.4 | 43-47 | 43 | 46 | Mainly hepatic metabolism; 25% excreted unchanged in urine | No | Half-life shorter in children |
| Methylphen-obarbital | Acid | | 364*<br>119** | 7.5*<br>70** | 33*<br>1.2** | | | | Hepatic metabolism | Yes (phenobarbital) | **R*-enantiomer<br>***S*-enantiomer |
| Primidone | Neutral | ≈20 | 42 | 6-12 | 2.5-3.6 | 80 | 85-97 | 81 | Hepatic metabolism and renal excretion (15-66% excreted unchanged in urine) | Yes (phenobarbital; phenylethyl-malonamide) | Metabolites determine much of the drug's activity |
| Carbamazepine | Neutral | 70-80 | 56-98 | 10-20 | 3.5 | 20 | 19-33 | 39 | Hepatic metabolism | Yes (carbamazepine 10, 11-epoxide) | Autoinduction of metabolism occurs (half-life and clearance values shown are after repeat doses) |
| Oxcarbazepine | | 40* | 49-56* | 8* | | | | | Hepatic metabolism | Yes (10, 11-dihydro-10-OH-carbamaze-pine) | *Activity depends largely on principal metabolite (data shown are for metabolite) |
| Valproic acid | Acid | ≈90 | 10.5 | 8-15 | 0.5-2.1 | 7.6-25 | 0.4-4.5 | 8 | Hepatic metabolism | Yes (2-en-valproic acid) | Concentration-dependent protein binding |
| Ethosuximide | Acid | 0 | 47 | 52-56* | 0.7-0.9 | 100 | 96 | 96 | Hepatic metabolism | No | *Half-life is shorter in children (≈30h) |
| Diazepam | Base | 97-99 | 49-329 | 24-48 | 2.1 | 2-3 | 1.7 | 10-15 | Hepatic metabolism | Yes (nordazepam) | Nordazepam (*N*-desmethyl-diazepam) has a half-life of 50-120h |
| Nitrazepam | Base | ≈90 | 168 | 18-34 | 4.9 | 8-16 | | | Hepatic metabolism | No | |
| Clonazepam | Base | ≈80 | 105-308 | 20-60* | 6.3 | | | | Hepatic metabolism | No | *Half-life is shorter in children (≈22-33h) |
| Clobazam | Base | 85-89 | | 10-30 | | | | | Hepatic metabolism | Yes (desmethyl-clobazam) | Action partly due to metabolite (half-life 36-48h) |
| Vigabatrin | Amino acid | 0 | 56 | 7 | 5.6 | ≈10 | 0 | | Renal excretion (unmetabolised) | No | Activity depends on *S*-enantiomer but data are for racemate |
| Lamotrigine | Base | ≈55 | 63-91 | ≈24 | 1.5-2.5 | | | | Hepatic metabolism | No | Some autoinduction of metabolism occurs with continued administration |
| Gabapentin | Amino acid | 0 | 49-63 | 5-7 | 5.5-9.0 | 9-14 | | | Renal excretion (unmetabolised) | No | Absorption kinetics are dose-dependent |

a Elimination of phenytoin is dose-dependent and is best described by Michaelis-Menten kinetics (see section 4.1.2). Representative parameters are Km = 5.7 mg/L (adults), 3.2 mg/L (children < 15 years); and $V_{max}$ = 6.5 mg/kg/day (adults), 11.7 mg/kg/day (children <15 years) [see also appendix G].

*Abbreviations:* Vd = apparent volume of distribution; $V_{max}$ = maximum rate of metabolism; Km = concentration at which rate of metabolism is one-half maximum (Michaelis-Menten constant); CSF = cerebrospinal fluid.

patient (fig. 2). If the phenytoin dose is increased in expectation that the plasma phenytoin concentration will rise proportionately, there is a substantial risk of the patient becoming overdosed.

The elimination characteristics of phenobarbital and ethosuximide appear to be adequately described by first-order (linear) kinetics but the relationships between their steady-state plasma concentrations and dosages in the individual show similar nonlinearities to phenytoin, although to a lesser degree. In contrast, steady-state plasma carbamazepine concentrations in the individual patient may rise less than would be expected as the dosage of this drug is increased in patients receiving carbamazepine monotherapy, due to autoinduction of its metabolism with repeated administration. The clinician needs to consider these empirically established concentration-dose relationships when adjusting the dosage of antiepileptic drugs.

2) With the exception of valproic acid, gabapentin and vigabatrin, plasma half-lives of the antiepileptic drugs are generally long enough (18 to 24 hours, or longer) to permit their administration twice or even once a day without excessive fluctuation in steady-state plasma concentrations. Primidone has a relatively short plasma half-life (6 to 12 hours), but both its active metabolites, phenobarbital and phenylethylmalonamide (PEMA), have substantially longer half-lives (see table II). The derived phenobarbital achieves higher steady-state plasma and tissue concentrations than primidone itself. Hence the overall antiepileptic effect arising from primidone administration remains virtually static over a dosage interval, even if the drug is taken only once a day.

3) Although its half-life is relatively short, vigabatrin acts irreversibly as an inhibitor of GABA transaminase. Hence its effects outlive its presence in the body after a single drug dose

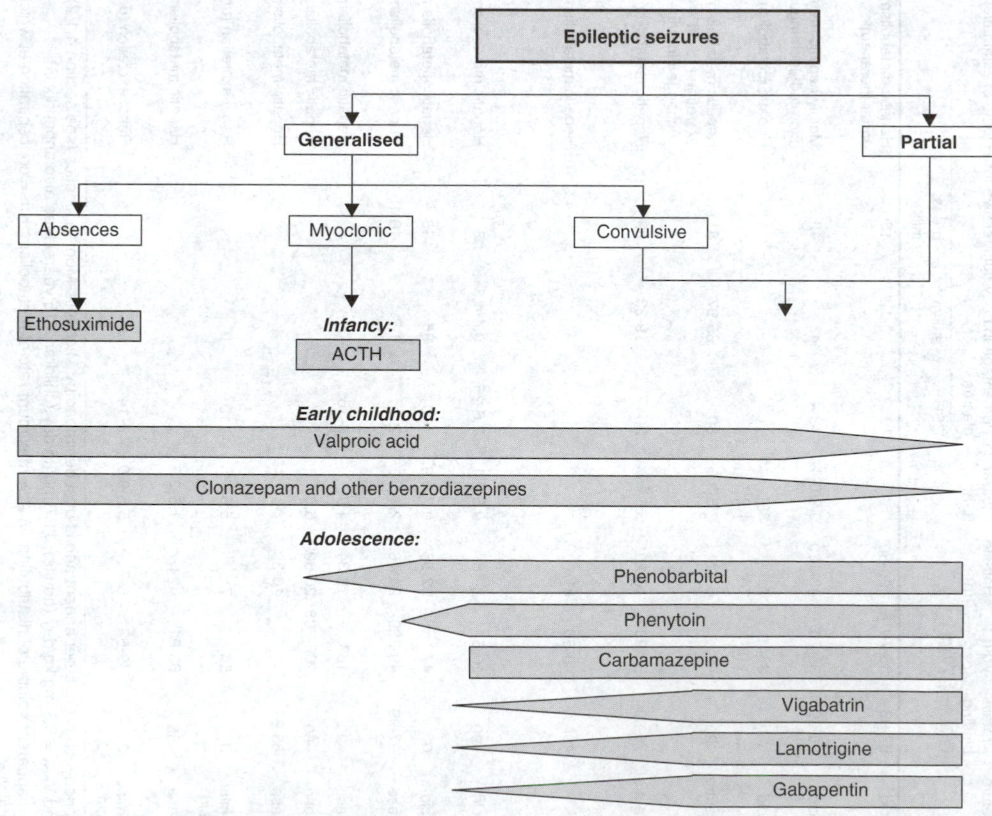


**Fig. 3.** Correlation between types of human epileptic seizure and effective antiepileptic drugs. Where the boxes around the drug names taper, efficacy is less definite. Seizure types are classified according to the International League Against Epilepsy (1989). In generalised epilepsy, the seizures behave as if the function of the entire cerebrum becomes disturbed from the outset, so that consciousness is impaired abruptly from the start of the attack, and any motor events that occur are bilateral. In partial epilepsy, clinical and electroencephalographic manifestations suggest that the seizure begins locally in some region of the cerebrum, although the epileptic discharge may subsequently become secondarily generalised in at least some seizures, with bilateral convulsing then occurring.

**Table III.** Average doses and therapeutic plasma concentration ranges for the commonly used antiepileptic drugs

| Drug | Therapeutic plasma concentration range (predose steady-state concentrations of total drug) | | | Typical dose (mg/kg/day)[a] |
|---|---|---|---|---|
| | mg/L (μg/ml) | μmol/L | comment | |
| Phenytoin | 10-20 | 40-80 | Widely accepted | 6 (adults)<br>11 (children) |
| Phenobarbital | 10-25 or<br>10-35 | 45-110 or<br>45-160 | Upper limit rather indefinite | 4.5 (<5y)<br>3 (5-14y)<br>2.5 (15-40y)<br>2.0 (>40y) |
| Methylphenobarbital | As for phenobarbital | | | 7.5 (<15y)<br>6.5 (15-40y)<br>4.0 (>40y) |
| Primidone | 5-11 | | Simultaneous phenobarbital concentrations may be a better guide | 10 |
| Carbamazepine | 6-12 | 25-50 | | 8-20 |
| Ethosuximide | 40-100 | 300-700 | Often little toxicity below 150 mg/L | 30 |
| Clonazepam | 0.025-0.075 | 0.08-0.24 | Not very useful clinically | 0.15 |
| Valproic acid | 50-100 | 350-700 | Whether there is a range is controversial | 15-25 |
| Vigabatrin | ? | ? | Acts irreversibly so little correlation between plasma concentration and effect likely | 30-60 |
| Lamotrigine | ≈2 | ? | Tentative | 2-4 |
| Gabapentin | ? | ? | Monitoring of plasma concentrations appears unnecessary | 8.5-25 |

a Mean dose or dose range likely to achieve a therapeutic range of plasma drug concentrations at steady-state.

and do not necessarily parallel its plasma concentrations.

4) Overdosage manifestations (particularly for carbamazepine)[80] are most likely to appear at the time when peak plasma drug concentrations are reached after each dose. To avoid unnecessarily high concentrations, dosages should not be increased until there has been time for steady-state conditions to apply after the most recent dose increment (i.e. after 4 to 5 half-lives of the drug).

5) With the exception of vigabatrin and gabapentin which are predominantly eliminated by renal excretion, and primidone which shows significant renal excretion of unchanged drug, the antiepileptic drugs are cleared mainly by metabolism.[81] Hence their dosages may need to be reduced in the presence of liver dysfunction, but usually not in renal insufficiency, except for vigabatrin and gabapentin (see also appendix D). However, in renal disease, altered plasma protein binding may change the relationship between free (unbound) drug and total drug in plasma. This is important in interpreting total drug concentrations measured in plasma (see further chapter 5; sect. 1.6.3).

6) Gabapentin and vigabatrin do not undergo appreciable hepatic biotransformation and both drugs are largely excreted in the urine unchanged. Moreover, neither drug binds to plasma proteins to any significant extent, and these properties lessen the probability of interactions with other antiepileptic drugs (see also section 4.1.4). As would be expected, however, the dosages of gabapentin and vigabatrin need to be reduced in patients with renal dysfunction.

For a review of the pharmacokinetics of newer antiepileptic drugs, see Bialer.[82]

#### *4.1.3 Clinical Effectiveness and Therapeutic Ranges of Plasma Concentrations*

Various antiepileptic drugs are more effective in certain types of seizure disorder than in others. The indications for the various agents are shown in figure 3.

The therapeutic ranges of plasma concentrations for the commonly used antiepileptic drugs are shown in table III, along with the doses likely to achieve these concentrations in the average patient. These therapeutic ranges refer to predose steady-state concentrations of total (plasma protein bound plus unbound) drug; they apply for the treated population, but not necessarily for each individual member of it. The therapeutic range of concentrations of a drug may differ for different types of epileptic seizure, to an extent depending on whether partial seizures become secondarily generalised.[83,84]

**Table IV.** Common and/or important adverse effects of antiepileptic drugs

| Affected tissue | Pattern of disturbance | Drug(s) responsible |
|---|---|---|
| Skin | Rashes | Carbamazepine, phenytoin, lamotrigine |
| | Facial coarsening | Phenytoin |
| | Hair loss (scalp) | Valproic acid |
| | Hirsutism | Phenytoin |
| Gums | Hypertrophy | Phenytoin |
| Gastrointestinal system | Abdominal discomfort, nausea, vomiting | Phenytoin, ethosuximide, valproic acid |
| | Hepatic injury | Valproic acid, phenytoin, phenobarbital (rarely), carbamazepine |
| | Pancreatitis | Valproic acid (rarely) |
| Nervous system | Sedation | All antiepileptic drugs |
| | Paradoxical irritability and hyperkinesis | Barbiturates, clonazepam |
| | Nystagmus, ataxia, diplopia | Mainly phenytoin, but also barbiturates, carbamazepine, oxarbazepine, gabapentin, ? lamotrigine |
| | Dyskinesia | Phenytoin, carbamazepine, barbiturates |
| | Tremor | Valproic acid |
| | Intellectual dulling | All antiepileptic drugs |
| | Worsening epilepsy | Overdosage with phenytoin or carbamazepine |
| | Peripheral neuropathy | Phenytoin, carbamazepine, barbiturates |
| Bone/cardiovascular system | Osteomalacia and hypocalcaemia | Phenytoin, barbiturates, cabamazepine |
| | Hypotension | Phenytoin (intravenous) |
| | Presence of antinuclear antibodies | Phenytoin, ethosuximide |
| | Leucopenia | Phenytoin, carbamazepine, ethosuximide |
| | Folate depletion manifestations | Barbiturates, phenytoin, carbamazepine |
| | Thrombocytopenia and altered platelet function | Valproic acid |
| | Pseudolymphoma syndrome | Phenytoin |
| Endocrine | Hyperglycaemia | Phenytoin |
| | Thyroiditis | Phenytoin |
| | Hyponatraemia | Oxcarbazepine, carbamazepine |
| Respiratory | Decreased lung diffusion capacity | Phenytoin |
| | Increased bronchial secretion | Clonazepam, nitrazepam |
| Renal | Nephritis | Phenytoin |
| | Crystalluria | Primidone |
| Muscle | Myopathy | Phenytoin |
| Fetus (teratogenesis) | Facial clefts, congenital heart lesions | Phenytoin, phenobarbital, primidone, carbamazepine |
| | Spina bifida | Carbamazepine, valproic acid |

Overall, the ranges shown in table III provide a useful guide to antiepileptic therapy for most, though not all patients. Some patients cannot tolerate plasma antiepileptic drug concentrations that are within, or even below, the therapeutic range. Others tolerate plasma concentrations well above the range, and achieve control of seizures only at these levels. In contrast, seizures in other patients may be fully controlled with plasma drug concentrations below the lower limit of the therapeutic range (see also chapter 5; sect. 4.3). Although the levels are an aid to therapy, achieving plasma antiepileptic drug concentrations in the therapeutic range should never be regarded as the main criterion of adequate drug treatment of epilepsy.

#### *4.1.4 Tolerability and Drug Interactions Potential*

The antiepileptic drugs have many known adverse effects, the more important of which are listed in table IV. All have sedative properties, which determine many of their unwanted effects. Some of the drugs have peculiar individual adverse effects, for example gum hypertrophy, hirsutism and lymphadenopathy with phenytoin, hyponatraemia and hypo-osmolality for carbamazepine and oxcarbazepine, and liver failure and pancreatitis with valproic acid. Lamotrigine was originally developed as an antifolate agent, but does not appear to alter serum folate levels.[85]

A considerable number of interactions are known between antiepileptic drugs used in combination, and between antiepileptic agents and other drugs taken concurrently. [For reviews, see Perucca & Richens;[86] Perucca;[87] Eadie;[88] Patsalos & Duncan.[89]] Some of the more important or more frequent interactions are shown in tables V and VI. The benzodiazepine antiepileptic drugs are involved in relatively few interactions. Phenytoin, because of its saturable elimination capacity at therapeutic concentrations, is particularly vulnerable to interactions which inhibit its metabolism. Conversely, the newer (renally excreted) agents gabapentin and vigabatrin are involved in few interactions with other antiepileptic drugs, although vigabatrin may lower plasma concentrations of phenytoin (via mechanisms that have not yet been elucidated).

Not all of the interactions listed in tables V and VI occur consistently, possibly because some involve the algebraic sum of 2 processes:

a) An induction of drug-metabolising capacity by one drug causing diminished plasma concentrations of another; and

b) Competition for the induced metabolic pathway between 2 drugs raising the plasma concentrations of both.

An interaction resulting in raised plasma concentrations of an antiepileptic drug is often first suspected when toxicity develops in a patient who has been taking the antiepileptic drug in constant dosage for some time. Falling antiepileptic drug concentrations due to an interaction are less likely to be suspected until control of epilepsy deteriorates or plasma drug concentrations are measured.

## 4.2 Optimum Treatment

Before prescribing drug therapy for a patient who presents with definite epileptic seizures, several important issues should be considered:

1) Whether the seizures are due to a disorder which requires treatment in its own right, e.g. a cerebral tumour.

2) Whether there is a significant risk that further seizures will occur and, if so, how great a problem the seizures will be for the patient. If prolonged drug therapy is indicated, both patient and clinician should be satisfied that the treatment offers real advantages, taking into consideration the patient's physical, psychological and social circumstances, and their interplay.

3) What type, or types, of epileptic seizure the patient has. Particular types of seizures, or seizure syndromes, are best treated with particular antiepileptic drugs (for selection, see figure 3).

4) Whether the therapy is intended merely to suppress the more obvious and troublesome manifestations of the seizures, or whether it is to cure the disorder by fully controlling seizures for so long that the underlying tendency subsides. Such cure is likely only when the seizures are due to non-progressive cerebral disease or inherited neural instability. Clinicians increasingly believe that, wherever realistic, the initial aim of antiepileptic drug therapy should be cure of the disorder; suppression of the more troublesome manifestations of epilepsy is usually an inferior alternative.

### *4.2.1 General Principles of Drug Treatment*

After a decision has been made to treat a patient's epilepsy, and the aims of the treatment have been defined for that individual, the following principles should be applied:

- The least toxic drug appropriate for the patient's type of seizure disorder should be prescribed.
- When seizures have occurred frequently, the dosage of the drug should be adjusted until full seizure control is attained or further dosage increase produces troublesome adverse effects. Each dosage increase should not occur until there has been enough time for steady-state conditions to apply at the current dosage.
- When it is too early to know the natural history of the patient's epilepsy, or when seizures have occurred only at long intervals, the initial antiepileptic drug dosage should produce plasma drug concentrations in the therapeutic range for the patient's type of seizures, without causing serious adverse effects (see table IV). Thereafter, dosage should be adjusted in relation to the clinical response, as described above. With every dosage adjustment, the clinician should avoid allowing the disadvantages of therapy to outweigh its benefits.
- If full seizure control cannot be achieved with the maximum tolerated dose of the first drug used, a second appropriate drug should be substituted progressively, and its dose adjusted as for the first drug. The substitution of one antiepileptic drug for another, particularly if the original drug has been used in full or reasonably full dosage, may be associated with increased seizures. This may occur because the new drug is not as effective as the

**Table V.** Pharmacokinetic interactions affecting antiepileptic drugs (after Eadie;[88] Patsalos & Duncan[89]). *Note:* Not all these interactions occur consistently

| Drug | Plasma concentration change | Drugs causing the interaction: antiepileptic drugs | Drugs causing the interaction: other drugs |
|---|---|---|---|
| Phenytoin | Raised | Clobazam, ?clonazepam, ?diazepam, ?ethosuximide, methsuximide, phenobarbital[a], sulthiame, valproic acid | Allopurinol, amiodarone, chloramphenicol, chlordiazepoxide, chlorpheniramine, chlorpromazine, cimetidine, clofibrate, cyclosporin, dextropropoxyphene, dicoumarol, diltiazem, disulfiram, fluconazole, haloperidol, imipramine, isoniazid[b], ?methylphenidate, miconazole, omeprazole, phenylbutazone, prochlorperazine, sulfonamides, tolbutamide, warfarin |
| | Lowered | Carbamazepine, phenobarbital, ?primidone, valproic acid[c], vigabatrin | Alcohol (long term use), activated charcoal, ?antacids, calcium sulfate, cisplatin, diazoxide, digoxin, folate, methotrexate, nitrofurantoin, oxacillin, pyridoxine, rifampicin, sucralfate, theophylline, vinblastine |
| Phenobarbital | Raised | Methsuximide, phenytoin, sulthiame, valproic acid | ?Furosemide |
| | Lowered | ?Vigabatrin | Activated charcoal, chloramphenicol, dicoumarol, ?folate, thioridazine, urinary alkalinising agents |
| Carbamazepine | Raised | ?Clonazepam<br>Lamotrigine and valproic acid raise carbamazepine-10,11-epoxide concentrations | Cimetidine, clarithromycin, dextropropoxyphene, danazol, diltiazem, erythromycin, fluoxetine, isoniazid, nicotinamide, omeprazole, troleandomycin (triacetyloleandomycin), verapamil, viloxazine |
| | Lowered | Phenobarbital, phenytoin, primidone | Activated charcoal |
| Oxcarbazapine | Lowered | | Verapamil (lowers concentrations of 10, 11-dihydro-10-hydroxy metabolite) |
| Primidone | Raised | ?Clonazepam, valproic acid | Isoniazid, nicotinamide |
| | Lowered | Carbamazepine, phenytoin[d], vigabatrin | ?Acetazolamide |
| Ethosuximide | Raised | Methylphenobarbital, valproic acid | Isoniazid |
| | Lowered | Carbamazepine | |
| Diazepam | Raised | Valproic acid | Halothane |
| | Lowered | | Alcohol (continued use) |
| Valproic acid | Raised | | Salicylates, isoniazid |
| | Lowered | Carbamazepine, phenobarbital, phenytoin | Antacids, chlorpromazine, cisplatin, doxorubicin, naproxen |
| Lamotrigine | Raised | Valproic acid | |
| | Lowered | Carbamazepine, phenobarbital, phenytoin | |

a Phenobarbital may either stimulate or inhibit the metabolism of phenytoin, and the overall result of the interaction is unpredictable but of small magnitude.

b Particularly in slow acetylators of isoniazid.

c Valproic acid has been reported to both increase and decease total plasma concentrations of phenytoin; however, the free drug concentration may increase in spite of the uncertain change in total concentration. Measurement of free drug concentrations may therefore be helpful clinically.

d Phenytoin may increase the metabolism of primidone, resulting in higher concentrations of derived phenobarbital.

original one, or because its initial dosage is too low. Because of this, it is sometimes safer to add the second drug to the first, intending to discontinue the first drug later. However, if the combination proves successful and does not cause adverse effects, both clinician and patient may prefer to persist with it rather than risk loss of seizure control.

- If maximum tolerated doses of 2 drugs fail to provide control, another potentially suitable drug should be substituted for the more toxic or apparently less effective of the pair of drugs being used.
- If, and when, full seizure control is attained, the successful therapy should be continued in full dosage for several years in the hope that the underlying epileptic tendency will die out. During this period of therapy, plasma drug concentrations should be monitored at intervals, partly to encourage compliance

with therapy. When the patient has been free from seizures for several years, and preferably when all paroxysmal activity has disappeared from the electroencephalogram (EEG), antiepileptic drug therapy may be withdrawn progressively over many weeks or months. This withdrawal is best carried out at a time when the patient's life is relatively free from stress. The risk of relapse is greatest in the first year or two after dosage reduction begins.

- If, and when, it becomes apparent that full seizure control cannot be achieved with all appropriate available therapy, or can be achieved only with an unacceptable level of adverse drug effects, doses should be adjusted downward to keep both seizures and adverse effects as untroublesome as possible. By this time, the possibility of epilepsy surgery should have been considered.

#### 4.2.2 Treatment of the More Common Seizure Types

In the following discussion, epileptic seizures are categorised in terms of the classification of the Commission on Classification and Terminology of the International League against Epilepsy.[90]

##### Generalised (Onset) Epilepsy

1. ***Absence seizures***

Absence seizures (petit mal) usually present in children over 5 years of age and occur many times a day. The clinical response can easily be used to guide therapy. Ethosuximide, clonazepam and valproic acid/sodium valproate are effective in treatment of absences.

*Ethosuximide:* the usual initial ethosuximide dose is at least 250mg twice daily. The dosage is then increased by 250 mg/day every 7 to 10 days until the attacks cease or adverse effects begin to trouble the patient. Ethosuximide need not be taken more often than twice a day; once daily intake is pharmacokinetically feasible, but patients may be reluctant to take the whole daily dose at one time because of its bulk. Patients with absence seizures often experience, or subsequently develop, bilateral tonic-clonic (grand mal) fits. Ethosuximide does not prevent these. Therefore, an antiepileptic drug effective against generalised convulsive seizures, e.g. phenytoin, carbamazepine or a barbiturate, is often prescribed together with ethosuximide from the outset. If this is done, it is better to establish the patient on the agent effective against generalised convulsive seizures first, and then add ethosuximide.

*Clonazepam and valproic acid:* unlike ethosuximide, clonazepam and valproic acid protect against the tonic-clonic seizures of generalised epilepsy as well as against absences. Clonazepam causes relatively few adverse effects but it is difficult to judge its initial dose clinically. In children, it may be wise to commence therapy with 0.25mg twice daily, and let the patient

**Table VI.** Pharmacokinetic interactions involving an effect of antiepileptic agents on other classes of drugs or on biological substances (after Eadie;[88] Patsalos & Duncan[89])

| Antiepileptic drug | Drug or biological substance affected | |
|---|---|---|
| | increased plasma concentration | decreased plasma concentration/effect |
| Phenytoin | Caeruloplasmin, copper, γ-glutamyl transpeptidase, sex hormone binding globulin (women), warfarin | Chloramphenicol, ?cortisol, cyclosporin, dexamethasone, dicoumarol, digitoxin, doxycycline, folate, furosemide, immunoglobulins A, M & G, lidocaine, methadone, nortriptyline, oral contraceptives, pethidine, praziquantel, prednisolone, pyridoxine, theophylline, thyroxine |
| Phenobarbital (primidone, methylphenobarbital) | Immunoglobulins A & B | Bile salts, bilirubin, chloramphenicol, cholesterol, chlorpromazine, cimetidine, cortisol and other corticosteroids, cyclosporin, dicoumarol, digitoxin, doxycycline, felodipine, folate, griseofulvin, haloperidol, lidocaine, methadone, misonidazole, nimodipine, nortriptyline, oral contraceptives, paracetamol, pethidine, phenylbutazone, serum lipids, warfarin, theophylline |
| Carbamazepine | | β-Adrenoceptor blockers, dexamethasone, doxycycline, felodipine, fentanyl, haloperidol, oral contraceptives, praziquantel, warfarin (and other oral anticoagulants) |
| Oxcarbazepine | | Felodipine, oral contraceptives |
| Valproic acid | Diazepam, nimodipine | |
| Ethosuximide | | Pyridoxine |
| Diazepam | Testosterone | |

halve this dose if drowsiness occurs. The dosage is then increased gradually every 4 to 7 days until seizures cease. Clonazepam need be taken only twice a day, and once daily intake may be satisfactory. The effective dose in absence seizures is often between 0.5 and 4.0 mg/day. Very low initial doses and gradual dosage build-up minimise the problems of sedation and aggressiveness, which may occur early in the course of therapy and cause some patients to abandon the treatment.

Valproic acid is easier to use than clonazepam or ethosuximide and is at least as effective. Were it not for the occasional, unpredictable, and sometimes lethal hepatotoxicity[91] and pancreatic damage associated with its use, it would probably be the agent of choice for absence seizures. For the age group in which absence seizures are likely to begin, the initial valproic acid dose might be 200mg 3 times daily, with dosage increases as often as every 2 or 3 days until the absences cease.

For refractory absence seizures, any two of the above agents can be combined. Even when absences are completely controlled, antiepileptic drug therapy is usually continued until the patient reaches the mid-teenage years. At this stage, provided paroxysmal activity has disappeared from the EEG, drug dosage is reduced progressively over some months, in the hope that the underlying epileptic tendency has subsided.

2. ***Myoclonic seizures***

The epileptic syndromes characterised by myoclonic seizures, and their treatments, vary according to the patient's age at the onset of the seizures.

*In infancy:* myoclonic seizures beginning in infancy typically present between the ages of 6 and 18 months with the clinical syndrome of infantile spasms (hypsarrhythmia, West's syndrome). In this condition, frequent myoclonic jerks are associated with intellectual deterioration and, later, other patterns of seizure. *Clonazepam* and *valproic acid* may reduce the frequency of the seizures. However, apart from the very rare pyridoxine-dependent variety of the syndrome, the only treatments that may control the disorder completely, i.e. both the seizures and the mental retardation, are *corticotrophin* and *adrenal corticosteroids*, e.g. prednisolone. There is some evidence that corticotrophin is more effective than the adrenal corticosteroids. Corticotrophin 20IU, or later 40IU, is given daily by injection, or prednisolone 5 to 10mg 4 times daily is given orally. The response, if it occurs, usually appears within a few days. If the higher corticotrophin doses fail, the disorder will probably prove refractory to all therapy, as it does in some 50% of sufferers. The mechanism of action of corticotrophin and corticosteroids in the disorder is uncertain, although it has been suggested that corticotrophin may have a neurotransmitter or neuromodulator role.[92]

*In early childhood:* when myoclonic seizures begin in childhood, they are usually frequent and severe, with recurrent drop attacks during which injury may occur (the Lennox-Gastaut syndrome: myoclonic-astatic seizures). Corticotrophin and corticosteroids are not useful but *clonazepam* or its congener *nitrazepam* may be of some benefit. However, the most effective generally available agent is *valproic acid.* In so severe a form of epilepsy, the hazards of valproic acid toxicity are more acceptable than in absence seizures. Initial valproic acid dosages are as suggested above for absence seizures, although final doses may be higher, the dosage limit often being determined by the advent of toxicity rather than control of seizures.

Among the newer agents, lamotrigine has shown some efficacy when used as 'add-on' therapy in the Lennox-Gastaut syndrome[70] and is currently being evaluated further.

*In adolescence:* the later in life myoclonic seizures begin, the milder the disorder usually proves, and the easier it is to treat. In adolescence, a characteristic syndrome (the Janz syndrome) occurs, typically with repeated myoclonic jerks in the hour or so after waking, sometimes mounting into a bilateral tonic-clonic convulsive seizure, the situation being worsened by lack of sleep. *Valproic acid* and *clonazepam* are effective, as are the *barbiturate* antiepileptic drugs (phenobarbital, methylphenobarbital, primidone). Dosages of the latter drugs are given below. Despite the greater effectiveness and often lesser toxicity of valproic acid in this syndrome, the risk of associated hepatotoxicity, albeit very small, and of teratogenicity if given during pregnancy (low risk of spina bifida[93]) can lead to other drugs being preferred.

3. ***Tonic, clonic, tonic-clonic (convulsive; grand mal) seizures***

Generalised epilepsy may be manifest as bilateral convulsive seizures only. Other sufferers from generalised epilepsy may have absence or myoclonic seizures as well as convulsive attacks. *Clonazepam* and *valproic acid* will prevent these convulsive seizures, although somewhat higher total daily doses than those cited above may be necessary, particularly in older children and adults. The convulsive seizures of generalised epilepsy can also be controlled by *phenytoin*, *carbamazepine* and the *barbiturate* antiepileptic drugs. These older agents and *valproic acid* are more or less equally effective for such seizures. However, the main use of the barbiturate antiepileptic drugs and of phenytoin and carbamazepine is in the seizures of partial epilepsy, and they are discussed below in relation to this entity.

**Partial Seizures (Whether or Not Secondarily Generalised)**

*Phenytoin* and *carbamazepine* appear to be equally effective for these seizures, with *phenobarbital* a little less so[94] and there is increasing evidence for the efficacy of valproic acid.[95] *Clonazepam* is also useful, although perhaps not as effective as the other agents. Until recently, phenytoin was probably the preferred agent for partial seizures but a view has developed that its adverse effects are less acceptable than those of carbamazepine, which many have come to regard as the agent of first choice for this type of seizure. The barbiturates are considered too sedative for general use. Each of these antiepileptic drugs has its advantages and its disadvantages; if used carefully, they are of considerable value, and usually relatively free from serious adverse effects.

Partial seizures may occur rather infrequently, and initially it may be impractical to use the clinical response as a guide to drug dosage. Rather, it may be necessary to prescribe an appropriate antiepileptic drug in an initial dose which will achieve a therapeutic plasma concentration range of the agent (or, in the case of methylphenobarbital and primidone, of the biologically active metabolite phenobarbital). Thereafter, dosage adjustments can be made on the basis of the clinical response, aiming to stop all seizures without causing adverse effects.

*Phenytoin* in a dose of approximately 5 to 6 mg/kg/day in adults, or 10 to 11 mg/kg/day in children, has a reasonable chance of achieving the desired range of plasma drug concentrations. The full dose may be given from the outset, since phenytoin usually has relatively little sedative effect. The difficulty with phenytoin therapy occurs when dose increments are made, particularly if the consequences of the nonlinear elimination kinetics of the drug are not remembered (see section 4.1.1).

With *carbamazepine,* there is considerable interindividual variation in steady-state plasma concentrations relative to dose, but 8 to 10 mg/kg/day often suffices to achieve the therapeutic range of plasma drug concentrations. However, such a dose may cause troublesome and even unacceptable drowsiness at first and it is often better to commence carbamazepine therapy with half the expected definitive dose, allowing 2 to 4 weeks for both autoinduction of drug metabolism[96] and a measure of tolerance to the sedative effect to develop before the dosage is increased to produce the therapeutic range of plasma drug concentrations.

The newer analogue *oxcarbazepine* has proved as effective as carbamazepine in partial seizures and may be slightly less sedating; patients developing skin rashes with carbamazepine may be able to tolerate oxcarbazepine.[73] If a *barbiturate antiepileptic drug* is used, it should be introduced gradually over several weeks to minimise the problems of drowsiness early in therapy. This is particularly so for primidone, since even a single 125mg or 250mg initial dose may cause severe drowsiness lasting for 1 or 2 days. The phenobarbital dose required is of the order of 2.5 mg/kg/day in young adults; it is lower in the elderly and higher in children (see table III). The dose of methylphenobarbital is about twice that of phenobarbital, while the dose of primidone in adults is around 10 mg/kg/day. As methylphenobarbital and primidone are both biotransformed to phenobarbital, there is little point in combining two or more of the barbiturate antiepileptic drugs.

*Newer agents:* vigabatrin, gabapentin and lamotrigine have all proved effective for partial seizures, but their definitive places in therapy have yet to be established. They have often been used as 'add-on' treatment when other agents have failed. For adults, the effective vigabatrin dose is likely to be 2 to 4g daily, the drug being introduced gradually with 0.5g increments no more often than every few days or once a week, as indicated by the clinical response. For gabapentin, the usual dosage range is 600 to 1800mg daily in 3 divided doses, beginning with 300g once daily initially and increasing gradually until seizures cease or adverse effects occur. Lamotrigine is also introduced gradually, with 50 or 100mg increments no more often than every few days, to 200 to 400mg daily if lower doses do not control seizures or cause adverse effects. Lower doses (e.g. 25mg every second day at first) are used when lamotrigine is prescribed concurrently with valproic acid, because the clearance of lamotrigine is reduced by valproic acid.

The subsequent management of partial seizures follows the principles set out above. Such seizures are sometimes difficult to control fully, and patients may receive antiepileptic drug combinations in an attempt to suppress all attacks. However, the use of combinations may cause pharmacokinetic interactions between the drugs (see table V). This possibility should be kept in mind when interpreting plasma concentration data and the clinical picture.

#### Febrile Convulsions in Infancy

All epileptic seizures that occur during fever in infants are not necessarily benign febrile convulsions, although a significant number are (see also chapter 3; sect. 4.3.2). Benign febrile convulsions are brief bilateral tonic-clonic seizures which occur as the body temperature rises in infants who have no non-febrile seizures, no neurological abnormality and normal interictal EEGs.

One or two such seizures carry a very good long term prognosis and are better left untreated.[97,98] However, treatment should be offered if they recur frequently or if a prolonged seizure (with the risk of anoxic brain damage) has occurred. The drugs of established efficacy in this situation are *phenobarbital* and *valproic acid.* The sedative properties of the former, which often causes irritability in the infant, are clearly undesirable, and plasma phenobarbital concentrations above 15 mg/L are required to prevent further attacks.[99] Valproic acid is as effective and lessens the problem of sedation. However, its use exposes healthy infants with relatively small risks of on-going non-febrile epilepsy to the very occasional but very serious hazard of drug-associated hepatotoxicity. Phenytoin, at 'therapeutic' plasma concentrations,[100,101] and carbamazepine[102] are ineffective.

If benign febrile seizures are to be treated by continuous antiepileptic drug prophylaxis, one can use an unproven agent such as clonazepam, run the risks associated with valproic acid, or introduce phenobarbital or methylphenobarbital in a very low dose, for example 7.5 or 15 mg/day, respectively, and slowly increase the dose at fortnightly intervals (phenobarbital has a shorter half-life in infants than in adults; see table III) until plasma phenobarbital concentrations of at least 15mg/L (but not much more) are attained. Parents need to understand that such a cautious, progressive introduction of phenobarbital is necessary to reduce the behavioural problems that arise if the infant becomes sedated. Prophylaxis of febrile convulsions is usually continued until the child is 4 or 5 years of age, has had no febrile convulsions for 12 months or longer, and has experienced no other epileptic manifestation.

As an alternative to continuous prophylaxis, strategically timed interval administration of *diazepam* (rectally or intramuscularly) at the onset of fever in predisposed infants has had some success in preventing febrile convulsions.[98]

#### Epileptic Seizures in Pregnancy and Lactation

Antiepileptic therapy may become less effective in pregnancy because the drugs are cleared more rapidly from the body so that their plasma and tissue concentrations fall relative to pre-pregnancy values.[103,104] Hence, doses may have to be increased to maintain seizure control. However, administration of antiepileptic drugs during pregnancy carries a roughly doubled or trebled risk of the mother having a child with a congenital malformation[105] (see also chapter 2; sect. 7.1.5). The risk is higher if multiple antiepileptic drugs, particularly valproic acid with carbamazepine, are used.[106] Nevertheless, apart from valproic acid and carbamazepine (low risks of spina bifida), and phenytoin (risk of minor deformities of the terminal phalanges), it is unclear whether antiepileptic drugs really cause the reported malformations or whether the malformations are associated with maternal epilepsy which happens to receive drug treatment. Many neurologists are now wary about prescribing valproic acid during pregnancy; however, most consider that, on balance, the advantages of careful use of the other antiepileptic drugs during pregnancy outweigh the disadvantages.

If seizure control is to be maintained during pregnancy, plasma antiepileptic drug concentrations should be measured at least once each month, and drug doses adjusted to maintain the concentrations at pre-pregnancy values. In labour, the mother should be given an injection of vitamin K in case induction of hepatic metabolising capacity by the antiepileptic drug causes a coagulation factor deficiency in the neonate.[107] In the puerperium, plasma antiepileptic drug concentrations may need to be monitored as often as weekly or fortnightly, since the plasma clearances of the drugs will fall to prepregnancy values anywhere between 1 week and 6 months after childbirth. If the drug dose is not reduced as the levels rise, the mother may develop signs of toxicity.

With such precautions, antiepileptic drug therapy need not contraindicate breast feeding. The neonate has probably been exposed to higher circulating drug concentrations *in utero* than those which will occur from drug intake in maternal milk. However, phenobarbital concentrations in nursing neonates may reach levels approaching or even exceeding those of the mother; to avoid toxicity problems, plasma phenobarbital concentrations in the fully breast-fed infant should be monitored if the mother's plasma concentration of the drug is high.[108]

#### Status Epilepticus (and Other Situations Requiring Rapid Seizure Control)

In urgent situations one can usually accept some temporary overdosage of the patient, and some sedation, to control seizures, although vital functions should not be impaired by the treatment. If the sufferer is conscious between seizures and can swallow, appropriate therapy for the patient's type of seizure (fig. 3) may be given by mouth. In a previously untreated patient, an oral loading dose of 2 to 2.5 times the expected daily maintenance antiepileptic drug dose may be given, preferably subdivided into 2 or 3 portions taken over 2 or 3 hours (to decrease the risk of gastric irritation and vomiting). If the patient is already receiving an antiepileptic drug, a 'topping up' dose can be given. The size of this dose, although lower than that recommended above, is a matter for clinical judgement but is preferably guided by plasma drug concentration measurement; 12 to 24 hours after the loading dose, maintenance therapy should commence with the expected antiepileptic drug dose required for this purpose. The clinical state and plasma drug concentration should be followed for several days in case further dosage adjustments are needed.

When the patient is unconscious (or, if conscious, cannot swallow), the clinician must ascertain the cause of this, and remedy it, if possible. Status epilepticus and serial seizures are often caused by omitting antiepileptic drug doses, but they can be due to diseases requiring urgent treatment (e.g. meningitis). While the cause of the status is being determined, and perhaps treated in its own right, parenteral antiepileptic drug therapy is necessary to suppress the seizures. Some antiepileptic agents (e.g. carbamazepine, primidone) are not available in injectable form. With others, drug absorption from intramuscular administration sites may be undesirably slow, e.g. diazepam,[109] or unacceptably slow, e.g. phenytoin.[110] Thus, intravenous drug administration is nearly always preferable. Some antiepileptic drugs, notably phenytoin, are very poorly soluble in water and may precipitate out of aqueous solutions in drip bottles. Their administration is more reliable if they are injected into the tubing of an intravenous drip that is already running.

Certain drugs have antiepileptic properties but are too sedative for use as long term maintenance therapy. Such drugs may be helpful in status epilepticus, and in impending status. They are given intravenously, under close clinical and preferably EEG monitoring, in a dosage sufficient to stop the seizures without impairing vital functions. Care should be taken to maintain airway patency; sufficient fluid and, in more protracted situations, nutritional intake should be ensured. The drugs listed below are recommended; the dosages shown are initial intravenous doses for previously untreated patients, though in each case the dosage must be adapted to meet the individual clinical situation:

- *Diazepam* 0.15 mg/kg over 5 minutes; or *clonazepam* 0.025 to 0.05 mg/kg over 5 minutes; or *midazolam* 0.1 mg/kg at a rate of 2 mg/min.[111]
- *Sodium phenytoin* 15 mg/kg given over 4 to 6 hours (to minimise any hypotensive effect of the amount of phenytoin solvent that must be injected).
- *Clomethiazole (chlormethiazole)* [0.8% solution] given at a rate of 4 ml/min until seizure control is obtained or adverse effects (e.g. sedation or respiratory depression) preclude any further administration.

Of these agents, midazolam and clomethiazole have the shortest half-lives (approximately 2 and 4 hours, respectively) and are therefore the least likely to cause persisting depression of vital functions if an overdose is given. Phenobarbital (injected as its sodium salt) has an undesirably long half-life for easy use in these circumstances; sodium valproate (valproic acid) injection, though effective,[112] is not widely available.

If the above measures fail, the patient with status epilepticus may have to be anaesthetised with thiopental, paralysed with skeletal muscle relaxants, and managed with assisted respiration in an intensive care unit.

If the patient with status epilepticus has already received antiepileptic drugs, lower initial dosages than those shown above should be infused. The paramount consideration is to achieve seizure control, and this determines subsequent management. When the seizures have been controlled, and the patient's level of consciousness permits oral therapy, maintenance antiepileptic drug therapy along the lines previously discussed can be instituted.

## 5. Other Paroxysmal Disturbances of Brain Function

### 5.1 Narcolepsy

The pathological drowsiness of narcolepsy may be relieved by the central stimulants dexamphetamine and (in milder instances) methylphenidate.

*Dexamphetamine* causes catecholamine release from axon terminals centrally and peripherally. It has a plasma half-life of 7 to 14 hours at urinary pH <6.6,[113] but the half-life increases as urinary pH rises. The initial dose should be kept as low as possible, e.g. 2.5mg morning and midday, and increased only as necessary to keep the patient normally alert. If possible, dexamphetamine intake in the afternoons and evenings should be avoided to minimise interference with nocturnal sleep and to diminish the temptation to use the drug to cram more and more activities into an increasingly long day, thereby risking dependence. In this regard, dexamphetamine doses above 10mg twice daily, or increasing dosage requirements after a period of satisfactory steady dosage, should cause concern.

### 5.2 Cataplexy

This disorder occurs only in association with narcolepsy. Treatment of the narcolepsy with dexamphetamine often fails to control cataplexy. However, agents such as imipramine or clomipramine may prevent cataplectic drop attacks.

## 6. Raised Intracranial Pressure

Several disease processes may raise the intracranial pressure, including neoplasms, haematomas, abscesses, areas of cerebral oedema, and obstruction of the CSF circulation (hydrocephalus). Raised intracranial pressure often causes headache, and sometimes vomiting and drowsiness. These symptoms are best managed by curing the cause of the raised pressure, if practicable. The intracranial pressure can be lowered by medical measures, namely cerebral dehydrating agents or high-dose corticosteroids. Diuretics, particularly furosemide (frusemide), have sometimes been used. In neurosurgical units, barbiturate-induced coma is also used to reduce raised intracranial pressure. The pharmacokinetics of the relevant agents have been reviewed by Heinemeyer.[114]

### 6.1 Clinical Pharmacology of Drugs Used in Treatment

#### *6.1.1 Osmotic Dehydrating Agents*

*Mannitol* and *glycerol* are the main osmotic dehydrating agents currently used. Both are low molecular weight polyhydric alcohols. Glycerol is adequately absorbed from the alimentary tract, but mannitol is not. Mannitol is eliminated mainly unchanged in the urine, whereas glycerol is extensively metabolised, providing a source of cellular energy. Mannitol has a plasma half-life of 1.1 hours while that of glycerol is 0.5 hours.

Osmotic dehydrating agents act by causing the osmotic transfer of water from the brain to the vascular compartment. This osmotic effect depends on the agent raising the plasma osmolality, and yet itself being transferred across the blood-brain barrier too slowly to raise the osmotic pressure within the brain before it is cleared from the body (by diuresis). If the blood-brain barrier is defective, as it may be in and around tumours or areas of infarction or infection, the osmotic dehydrating agent may enter the diseased area more readily than the surrounding normal brain. Should this happen, water may be transferred osmotically from normal to diseased brain, increasing its volume. This offsets the advantage of shrinking the rest of the organ. Because of this, osmotic dehydrating agents are generally infused rapidly and, if clinical benefit does not appear quickly, the therapy is terminated, or repeated only with considerable caution.

#### *6.1.2 Corticosteroids (Dexamethasone, Prednisone, Prednisolone)*

In contrast to the water-transferring mode of action of the osmotic dehydrating agents, high-dose corticosteroids restore the integrity of the blood-brain barrier, and are useful mainly when raised intracranial pressure is associated with loss of blood-brain barrier integrity. This may not always be the case in obstructive hydrocephalus, although it probably is, to some degree, in most other circumstances in which the intracranial pressure is raised. The effect of corticosteroids usually requires 12 to 36 hours to become obvious clinically.

The corticosteroids are eliminated mainly by metabolism; they have plasma half-lives of about 2 to 3 hours and are given at least 3 or 4 times per day to lower raised intracranial pressure. Given orally, they may be incompletely bioavailable, particularly if hepatic microsomal enzyme-inducing agents such as phenytoin or barbiturate antiepileptic drugs are prescribed, e.g. if a glioma causes seizures as well as raised intracranial pressure. Coadministered phenytoin can reduce the bioavailability of oral dexamethasone to about 25% of its normal value;[115] patients with cerebral tumours may die because conventional oral corticosteroid doses are insufficient when phenytoin is prescribed.

The clinical pharmacology of the corticosteroids is discussed in more detail in chapter 19.

## 6.2 Optimum Treatment

As the osmotic dehydrating agents and corticosteroids reduce intracranial pressure by different mechanisms, it is logical to use them together. The dehydrating agents produce early benefit while corticosteroids maintain the benefit after 12 hours or more.

### *6.2.1 Use of Osmotic Dehydrating Agents*

Mannitol volumes of 200 to 500ml (10 or 20% aqueous solution) are infused intravenously over 1 to 2 hours, while intravenous glycerol in 0.45 or 0.9% saline is given over a relatively short period at a rate below 1.5 ml/min. Excessive dosages of the latter can cause haemolysis. Plasma glycerol concentrations of 1 to 3 g/L (10 to 30 Osm/L) are required to lower intracranial pressure.[116] Glycerol can also be given orally in a dose of at least 1 ml/kg/day to control chronically raised intracranial pressure, as in benign intracranial hypertension. However, patients often find the sweet taste intolerable.

Intravenous mannitol and glycerol produce an osmotic diuresis as well as brain dehydration, although the brain dehydration does not depend on the diuresis.

### *6.2.2 Use of High-Dose Corticosteroids*

High-dose corticosteroids, mainly dexamethasone, prednisone and prednisolone, can be given intravenously, intramuscularly or orally to reduce intracranial pressure. The doses used are 12 to 24 mg/day for dexamethasone, and 100 to 200 mg/day for prednisone or prednisolone. The minimum effective corticosteroid dose for this purpose is not known, but the situation is generally such that the hazards of underdosage nearly always exceed those of overdosage.

The expected adverse effects of corticosteroid therapy may be seen. Hyperchlorhydria and peptic ulceration are particular hazards since the disease that raises the intracranial pressure may also disturb hypothalamic function, causing a Cushing's ulcer. Thus, oral antacids or oral or parenteral cimetidine or ranitidine are often given with the corticosteroids. Neither antacids[117] nor cimetidine[118] alter the bioavailability of prednisolone.

After control of raised intracranial pressure is achieved with corticosteroids, their dosage should be reduced to the minimum that maintains a clinically satisfactory situation. Making one dosage interval each day as long as 8 to 12 hours may avoid adrenal suppression. When dexamethasone is used, suppressed endogenous plasma cortisol concentrations often rise again once plasma dexamethasone concentrations become unmeasurable, or nearly unmeasurable, after each dose.[119]

### *6.2.3 Other Therapy*

***Diuretics:*** intravenous furosemide has been used to reduce intracranial pressure quickly by producing a rapid diuresis, with consequent water shifts from brain to plasma. Cerebrospinal fluid production may also lessen.[120] However, the efficiency of this approach is uncertain.

***Barbiturate-induced coma:*** especially where intracranial pressure monitoring and intensive care facilities are available, intracranial hypertension may be controlled by an intravenous bolus of 3 to 5 mg/kg of phenobarbital followed by 1 to 3 mg/kg/h until the pressure becomes normal.[121] Pentobarbital is an alternative.[122]

## 6.3 Clinical Outcome and Economic Considerations

The above relatively inexpensive pharmacological measures may relieve the symptoms of intracranial hypertension, purchase time for surgical treatment, and make surgery technically easier. Corticosteroids can also be used long term, if no curative procedure is possible, but their adverse effects can then be severe.

## 7. Involuntary Movement Disorders

Disorders of involuntary (i.e. associated or automatic) movement are of two main clinical types:

1) Those characterised by a decrease in normally occurring involuntary movements.

2) Those characterised by excessive and abnormal involuntary movements.

The former appear associated with deficient dopaminergic neurotransmission in the corpus striatum, while some, but not all, of the latter are associated with relatively excessive dopaminergic activation of postsynaptic striatal neurons. Some related clinical syndromes feature both paucity of involuntary movement and the presence of abnormal involuntary movements, e.g. rigidity, bradykinesia, loss of arm swinging, and immobile facies, yet the characteristic resting tremor of Parkinsonism, which is the most common involuntary movement disorder.

### 7.1 Parkinsonism

Contemporary Parkinsonism is nearly always idiopathic, or else drug-induced (e.g. due to phenothiazines, particularly those with aliphatic side chains, and other antipsychotic agents). The pathogenesis of idiopathic Parkinsonism depends on a progressive degeneration of pars compacta substantia nigra neurons which have dopaminergic synapses on striatal neurons. In drug-induced Parkinsonism, phenothiazines and related drugs block postsynaptic dopamine receptors on striatal neurons, while other causal agents such as reserpine or tetrabenazine deplete the dopamine stores of presynaptic nigrostriatal axon terminals. The striatal dopamine depletion state explains Parkinsonian rigidity, bradykinesia and paucity of associated movement. However, it does not easily explain other manifestations of idiopathic Parkinsonism, e.g. the tremor.

Detailed knowledge of the neurotransmitter circuitry of the basal ganglia has expanded greatly in recent years. Basal ganglia function appears to be mediated via neocortical → subcortical → neocortical circuits.[123] The relevant neurotransmitter anatomy is summarised in figure 4. In the more direct circuit, the initial synapse is in the striatum, the second in either the inner globus pallidus or the pars reticularis of the substantia nigra, and the third in the thalamus, from which the fourth neuron projects back to the neocortex. The final neocortical output influences motor function via the ordinary

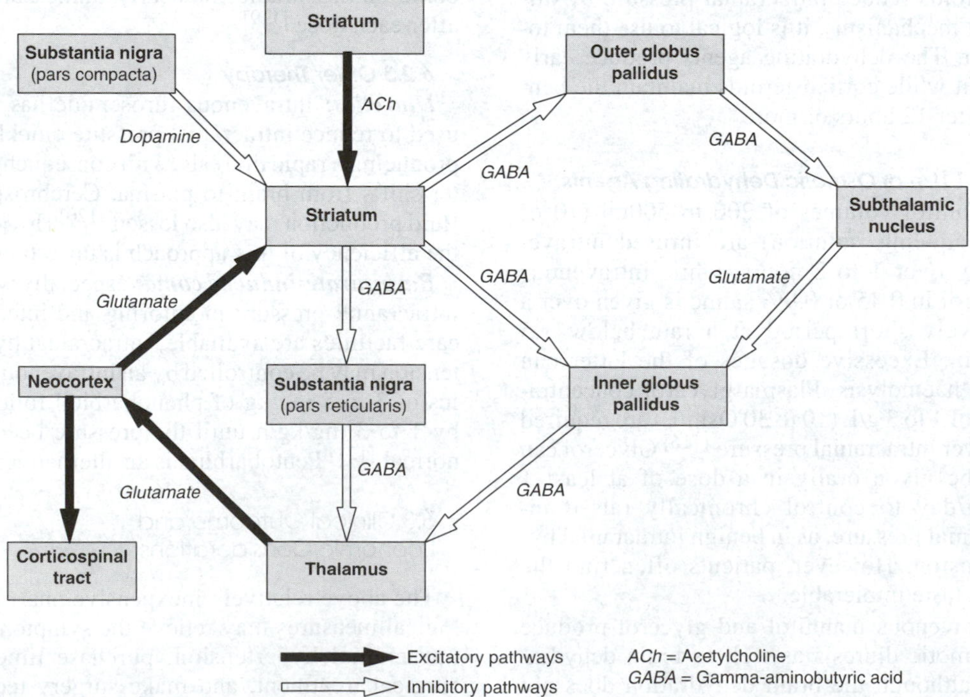


**Fig. 4.** Neural circuits involved in basal ganglia motor function.

corticospinal motor system. There is also a more indirect neocortical → subcortical → neocortical loop which has its first synapse in the striatum, its second in the outer layer of the globus pallidus, its third in the subthalamic nucleus, its fourth in the inner globus pallidus, and its fifth in the thalamus, from which there is a projection back to the neocortex. These circuits are modulated at the striatal level by a dopaminergic input from the pars compacta of the substantia nigra. Impairment of this nigrostriatal input explains most of the manifestations of Parkinsonism.

There may also be some modulation of striatal activity by cholinergic interneurons. A further cholinergic pathway of possible relevance to Parkinsonism arises in neurons of the nucleus basalis, immediately medial to the inner part of the globus pallidus, and projects diffusely to the cerebral cortex. Its degeneration may be responsible for the dementia that sometimes occurs in late stage idiopathic Parkinsonism.[124]

At least 5 types of dopamine receptor are now known.[125] Their roles in the pathogenesis of Parkinsonism are still being explored.

***The treatment possibilities in Parkinsonism*** are to:

- Restore dopaminergic neurotransmission in the nigrostriatal pathway
- Adjust GABA-mediated effects on the ventrolateral nucleus of the thalamus
- Inhibit the relative excess of cholinergic neurotransmission within the striatum
- Dampen down the relatively excessive glutaminergic neurotransmission in the neural circuits.

Unfortunately, drugs that have anticholinergic effects in the striatum will decrease cholinergic neurotransmission in the degenerating pathway from the nucleus basalis to the cerebral cortex. This may worsen memory failure in Parkinsonism. Attempts to alter GABA-mediated events in the substantia nigra and thalamus seem to have little influence on Parkinsonism. The best therapeutic approach is to enhance striatal dopaminergic neurotransmission. This relieves Parkinsonian rigidity, bradykinesia and loss of associated movements more effectively than it helps tremor. Agents influencing glutaminergic neurotransmission often have unacceptable adverse effects, though amantadine, a low affinity *N*-methyl-D-aspartate (NMDA) channel blocker,[126] has weak but useful anti-Parkinsonian actions. The agents currently used or being tested in the treatment of Parkinsonism are:

- Dopamine agonists
- The dopamine precursor levodopa
- Agents which delay dopamine degradation, e.g. monoamine oxidase type B or catechol-*O*-methyl transferase inhibitors (though the latter are still at clinical trial stage)
- Centrally-acting anticholinergic agents
- Excitatory amino acid receptor antagonists.

### *7.1.1 Clinical Pharmacology of Drugs Used in Treatment*

#### Dopamine Agonists

The principal agents in this category are *amantadine*,[127] *bromocriptine*[128] and *pergolide*,[129] though recent evidence suggests that at least part of the anti-Parkinsonian action of amantadine may depend on blockade of glutaminergic neurotransmission in the pathway from the subthalamic nucleus to the globus pallidus.[126] Their clinical pharmacological properties are summarised in table VII.

Amantadine was originally developed as an antiviral agent for influenza $A_2$ and during clinical trials was found to benefit Parkinsonism. Bromocriptine and pergolide are ergot peptide alkaloids. The relationships between the plasma concentrations and effects of these agents have not been investigated in detail, partly because of the assay difficulties that have prevented their pharmacokinetics being defined in detail.

***Clinical effectiveness:*** amantadine is modestly effective in relieving Parkinsonian rigidity and bradykinesia, but often loses some of its effect after a few months. This may really represent maintenance of a constant level of effect while the underlying disorder worsens with time. Pergolide is probably a little more effective than bromocriptine, and seems to have a longer duration of effect. Both of these drugs are considerably more effective than amantadine and are nearly as effective as levodopa in the average patient if high enough dosages can be tolerated.

***Tolerability:*** amantadine has relatively few serious adverse effects, though if it is the sole anti-Parkinsonian drug used and its intake is ceased abruptly, severe Parkinsonian rigidity can develop some 24 hours later. In the doses necessary to control moderate or severe Parkinsonism as monotherapy (30 to 60mg daily), bromocriptine may produce more severe mental changes than levodopa (confusion, hallucina-

**Table VII.** Characteristics of the principal anti-Parkinsonian drugs (after Cedarbaum[130])

| Feature | Bromocriptine | Pergolide | Amantadine | Selegiline | Levodopa |
|---|---|---|---|---|---|
| **Mechanism/site of action** | $D_1$ partial antagonist<br>$D_2$ agonist | $D_1$ agonist (weak)<br>$D_2$ agonist | Increased dopamine synthesis and release<br>Weak NMDA receptor antagonist | $MAO_B$ inhibition raises synaptic dopamine concentrations | Metabolism to dopamine in nigrostriatal neurons |
| **Pharmacodynamic properties/plasma concentration-effect relationship** | Little correlation between plasma concentration and effect | Longer duration of action than bromocriptine<br>Plasma concentration-effect relationship unknown | Plasma concentration-effect relationship unknown | Irreversible inhibition, hence no close plasma concentration-effect correlation | Used with decarboxylase inhibitors (e.g. benserazide, carbidopa) to prevent peripheral dopamine effects; some plasma concentration-effect correlation but enters brain by active transport |
| **Pharmacokinetic characteristics:** | | | | | |
| Bioavailability (oral) | 6% | ? | 55-90% | | 15-30% without decarboxylase inhibitor; higher with inhibitor |
| Half-life | 3h | 27h | 18-45h in Parkinson's disease age group (longer in renal insufficiency) | 0.15h | 1.3h without decarboxylase inhibitor; 2.2h with inhibitor |
| Clearance | 55 L/h | ? | 28 L/h (IV) | | 35 L/h without decarboxylase inhibitor; 21 L/h with inhibitor |
| Principal route of elimination | Hepatic metabolism | Hepatic metabolism | Renal excretion (≈10% metabolised) | Hepatic metabolism | Hepatic metabolism |
| **Clinical effectiveness** | Nearly as effective as levodopa if high enough doses can be tolerated | Possibly a little more effective than bromocriptine | Useful in milder Parkinsonism (effect may not be sustained) | Prolongs levodopa effects by ≈0.5h; ?favourably affects natural history of Parkinsonism | Overall, the most effective and most satisfactory therapy |
| **Adverse effects/ interactions** | Confusion, hallucinations, paranoid ideation, nausea, postural hypotension, dyskinesias, retroperitoneal/ pulmonary fibrosis | Dyskinesia, nausea, dizziness, hallucinations, rhinitis, confusion, constipation, somnolence, postural hypotension | Few serious adverse effects (dependent oedema, livedo reticularis, hypotension, hallucinations, confusion).<br>Hydrochlorothi-azide-triamterene decreases renal excretion | *Monotherapy:* dry mouth, altered liver enzymes<br>*Selegiline + levodopa:* enhanced levodopa-type effects<br>Avoid concomitant use of fluoxetine and pethidine (due to possible interactions) | Dyskinesias, late-stage treatment problems.<br>*If no decarboxylase inhibitor given:* nausea, vomiting.<br>Pyridoxine blocks effect of levodopa if no decarboxylase inhibitor given |

*Abbreviations:* IV = intravenous; MAO = monoamine oxidase; NMDA = *N*-methyl-D-aspartate.

tions and paranoid ideation). Pergolide has similar adverse effects.

#### Levodopa (L-Dopa)

The advent of levodopa therapy some 30 years ago revolutionised the treatment of Parkinsonism, and illustrated the potential of neurotransmitter replacement to reverse the manifestations of neurological disease.

***Mechanism/site of action:*** when it first became available, levodopa was administered alone. Dopamine cannot cross the blood-brain barrier but its amino acid metabolic precursor levodopa (L-dopa; L-dihydroxyphenylalanine) is actively transported across the barrier, utilising the specific uptake mechanism for aromatic amino acids. Dopamine is then formed from the dopa (fig. 5) within surviving nigrostriatal neurons, and released near enough to dopamine receptors on striatal neurons to correct the consequences of local dopamine depletion. Monoaminergic neurons often release their neurotransmitters over their axon terminals in a scattered 'shotgun blast' fashion, rather than in a precisely directed point-to-point manner into a particular synaptic cleft.[131] This transmitter release pattern permits dopamine replacement therapy to work in Parkinsonism, if enough nigrostriatal dopaminergic neurons survive.

Most patients given levodopa alone develop manifestations of excessive circulating dopamine (mainly nausea and vomiting) due to extracerebral conversion of levodopa to dopamine. This peripherally formed dopamine can cross the blood-brain barrier (where it is unusually permeable) in the region of the medullary vomiting centre, the area postrema in the floor of the fourth ventricle. Much of the levodopa dose is in fact 'wasted' in futile peripheral metabolism to dopamine. However, giving levodopa with a dopa-decarboxylase inhibitor (e.g. carbidopa or benserazide) which does not cross the blood-brain barrier avoids these difficulties. The decarboxylation of levodopa to dopamine outside the central nervous system is inhibited but dopamine can still form from levodopa within the brain (fig. 6). Use of dopa-decarboxylase inhibitors therefore allows substantially lower levodopa doses to be used, and permits a

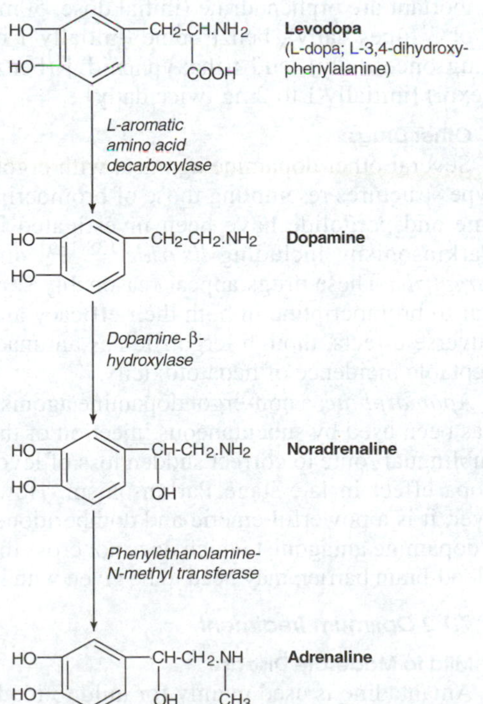


**Fig. 5.** Steps in the biotransformation of levodopa to adrenaline.

more rapid build-up to the optimum levodopa dose in each patient. Levodopa is now almost always used in combination with one or other of the peripheral dopa-decarboxylase inhibitors carbidopa or benserazide, in a single dosage form.

***Pharmacodynamic properties:*** in Parkinsonism, levodopa relieves rigidity and bradykinesia, restores associated movements, and often makes it difficult or impossible to recognise the presence of the disorder in milder cases. However, it offers relatively little benefit for Parkinsonian tremor. Levodopa enters the brain by active transport, and the relationship between its simultaneous plasma and brain concentrations may be altered by the plasma amino acid concentration, which increases after a high protein meal.

***Pharmacokinetic characteristics:*** levodopa conversion to dopamine is catalysed by the enzyme L-aromatic amino acid decarboxylase (dopa-decarboxylase) which is found in the brain and many other tissues, including the stomach, intestinal wall, liver, kidneys and heart. Levodopa is absorbed by an active transport mechanism in the small intestine. Before it is absorbed from the intestinal tract into the systemic circulation, much of an oral dose is converted to dopamine by dopa-decarboxylase in the stomach and small intestine walls, unless a decarboxylase inhibitor is present. The bioavailability of levodopa is very variable and highly dependent on the gastric emptying rate. Conditions which delay gastric emptying such as hyperacidity reduce the amount of levodopa available for absorption.

The bioavailability of controlled release oral formulations of levodopa (with a decarboxylase inhibitor) is lower than that of conventional rapid release formulations, and thus higher daily dosages of levodopa are usually needed if one of the controlled release formulations is used. These preparations have the advantage of decreasing fluctuations in levodopa plasma concentrations and allowing less frequent administration; clinically, however, they have not always proved useful in smoothing out late-stage fluctuations in the response to levodopa (see further section 7.1.2).

Carbidopa (plasma half-life 2 hours) and benserazide (plasma half-life less than 2 hours) have relatively little pharmacological effect if taken alone. They prolong the plasma half-life of levodopa (plasma half-life around 1 hour) by some 30 minutes.[132]

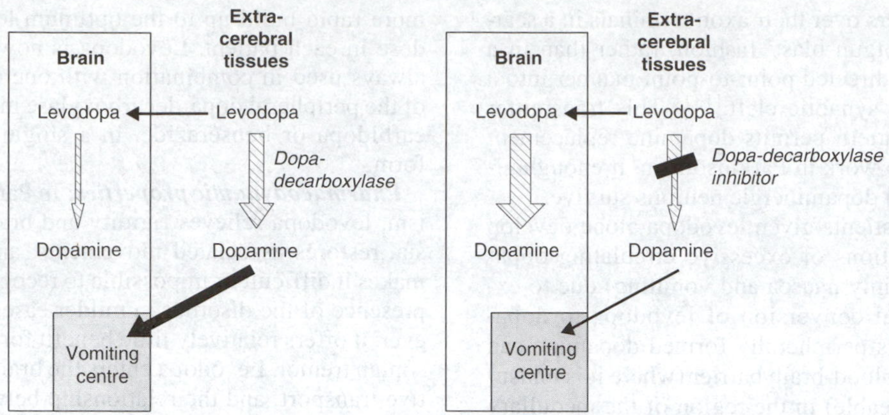


**Fig. 6.** The effects of dopa-decarboxylase inhibition on dopamine concentrations in the brain, and in the vomiting centre.

***Clinical effectiveness and tolerability:*** levodopa is the most effective therapy currently available for relieving the manifestations of Parkinsonism, particularly the rigidity and the bradykinesia.

The adverse effects of levodopa are discussed below (section 7.1.2) in relation to treatment of the disorder.

#### Selegiline

Selegiline (L-deprenyl),[133] a selective inhibitor of type B monoamine oxidase, prolongs the half-life of dopamine and thus benefits Parkinsonism; it may also elevate mood.[134] The prolongation of levodopa action achieved by this approach is used to reduce the early 'wearing-off' effect in levodopa therapy. However, selegiline appears ineffective in patients with advanced disease with severe levodopa 'on-off' swings.[135]

There has been considerable recent interest in the possibility that selegiline, if used early in the course of Parkinsonism, will delay the progression of the disorder,[136] but the matter remains controversial. There is no direct pathological evidence that the disease process is retarded; its alleged effect could arise from longer persistence of endogenous cerebral dopamine.

#### Centrally-Acting Anticholinergics (e.g. Benztropine, Orphenadrine, Trihexyphenidyl)

Prior to the availability of amantadine and levodopa, the drug therapy of Parkinsonism revolved around a number of acetylcholine antagonists which acted at central muscarinic receptors. These agents relieved Parkinsonian rigidity, and possibly tremor to some extent, but they did not improve bradykinesia or restore the impoverished associated movements. They also produced troublesome adverse effects, e.g. dry mouth, blurred vision, constipation, urinary retention, confusion and hallucinations. Compared with levodopa, the centrally-acting anticholinergics were ineffective and more toxic. They are now little used in Parkinsonism, serving merely as adjuvants to levodopa, although they may be used to reduce tremor and decrease the drooling of saliva. Certain anticholinergics, e.g. benztropine, have dopaminergic actions.[137]

Among the agents still available, the more important are orphenadrine (initial dose, 50mg 2 or 3 times daily), benztropine (initially 1 or 2mg once daily), and trihexyphenidyl (benzhexol) [initially 1 to 2mg twice daily].

#### Other Drugs

Several other dopamine agonists with ergot-type structures resembling those of bromocriptine and pergolide have been investigated in Parkinsonism, including *lisuride*[138,139] and *lergotrile*. These drugs appear reasonably similar to bromocriptine in both their efficacy and adverse effects, though lergotrile has an unacceptable incidence of hepatotoxicity.

*Apomorphine,* a non-ergot dopamine agonist, has been used by subcutaneous injection or the sublingual route to correct sudden loss of levodopa effect in late-stage Parkinsonism. However, it is a powerful emetic and domperidone, a dopamine antagonist which does not cross the blood-brain barrier, may need to be given with it.

### *7.1.2 Optimum Treatment*

#### Mild to Moderate Disease

Amantadine is used mainly for mild to moderate Parkinsonism. The initial dose is 100mg twice daily, increased progressively to 100mg 4 times daily if the clinical situation warrants higher dosage, particularly in younger patients.

#### More Severe Symptoms

Levodopa-decarboxylase inhibitor combinations are used if amantadine proves inadequate in milder Parkinsonism, and from the outset in more severe disease. These agents are the mainstay of treatment for the typical case. Levodopa is usually given (combined with benserazide or carbidopa) in an initial dose of 100mg 3 or 4 times daily. Thereafter, the dosage is increased up to once or twice weekly to obtain an optimum clinical response. In early disease, almost full normality can be restored, at least for a time.

As the levodopa dosage is increased, manifestations of excessive striatal dopamine activity may appear. Parkinsonian patients often consider that their treatment is optimum at the stage when these manifestations (commonly choreic movements) begin to appear; by then, rigidity is well relieved and movement feels free. However, their relatives may be concerned at the dyskinetic movements.

#### Long Term Management of Levodopa-Treated Patients

After Parkinsonism has been treated with levodopa for several years, or longer, peculiar motor disturbances often develop. There is some evidence that these late-stage treatment problems occur earlier in patients whose disorder has previously been very fully corrected, or even overcorrected, with levodopa.[140] Consequently, it may be preferable to keep most Parkinsonian patients slightly underdosed with levodopa,[141] although little is gained by delaying the introduction of the drug.[142] Late-stage levodopa treatment difficulties take various forms:[143]

***Overdosage manifestations*** (choreiform dyskinesias) develop at the time of the expected peak effect from a previously satisfactory drug dose, but localised dystonias (often in one leg) may occur when a minimum effect would be likely, e.g. on waking after a night's sleep many hours after the most recent levodopa dose.

***End-of-dose deterioration ('wearing-off' effect):*** some late-stage disturbances seem related to altered levodopa pharmacokinetics, e.g. the more or less predictable 'wearing-off' response that occurs after some years of therapy (characterised by earlier fading of treatment effects during each dosage interval). This may be helped for a time by shortening the levodopa dosage interval and reducing the size of individual doses. This process becomes increasingly cumbersome to the patient, and decreasingly effective. In such circumstances, the more protracted dopaminergic actions of *bromocriptine* or *pergolide* may help prolong the dopaminergic effects, although these agents are not always successful in practice and may cause unacceptable adverse effects. Controlled release levodopa-decarboxylase inhibitor preparations may be helpful in controlling end-of-dose deterioration by prolonging the action of each drug dose,[144] but in practice they have proved a little disappointing. Another approach is to attempt to prolong the duration of the dopaminergic effect of each levodopa dose by the use of selegiline, which should slow the metabolic degradation of dopamine.

***Other late-stage response fluctuations:*** the late-stage levodopa-treated patient may also oscillate between choreic dyskinesia and Parkinsonian immobility within a single 4- or 6-hour dosage interval, or may develop sudden periods of intense Parkinsonian rigidity, which after some minutes disperses spontaneously (the so-called 'on-off' phenomenon). In a few patients these late-stage fluctuations in motor function have been smoothed out by continuous intravenous infusion of levodopa, with a decarboxylase inhibitor,[145,146] or by taking the combination in solution every half hour.[147]

Various pharmacokinetic explanations have been proposed for these peculiar late-stage treatment problems. However, levodopa enters the brain by active transport rather than by the process of passive diffusion that usually applies for drugs; consequently, plasma and brain levodopa concentrations may not always parallel each other. Certain late-stage treatment difficulties during levodopa therapy may be better explained by adaptive postsynaptic dopamine receptor changes in the striatum, perhaps in response to a progressively decreasing number of nigrostriatal axon terminals releasing dopamine. The surviving axon terminals may also become unable to retain dopamine once it is formed, resulting in oscillation between levodopa intake-related apparent overdosage and subsequent underdosage.[148]

***Use of 'drug holidays':*** a 'drug holiday' from levodopa may help temporarily in late-stage treatment failure, but not permanently.[149] During 'drug holidays' patients take no levodopa for 2 or 3 weeks. They develop severe rigidity and immobility, and need to be hospitalised to receive physiotherapy and nursing care and to have their dietary and fluid intakes maintained. When levodopa therapy is resumed, the previous late-stage treatment problems are said to no longer occur, at least for several months, but then reappear. Although there was some enthusiasm for this approach at one time, it is now little used.

#### Role of Bromocriptine and Related Dopamine Agonists

Bromocriptine is still finding a definitive place in the treatment of Parkinsonism. In milder Parkinsonism, instead of next using levodopa, bromocriptine (5 to 20 mg/day) can be substituted for amantadine when the latter drug has proved inadequate. As the Parkinsonism progresses with time, the bromocriptine dose may have to be increased to maintain acceptable control. By the time no more bromocriptine can be tolerated or no further benefit can be obtained from it, levodopa often confers no additional advantage.[150] Late complications of bromocriptine therapy are less frequent than those of levodopa therapy.[150,151]

Overall, bromocriptine is more expensive and probably less effective than levodopa in treating Parkinsonism. However, bromocriptine combined with levodopa can improve the 'wearing-off' phenomenon often seen with the latter drug, and may occasionally benefit patients with unpredictable response swings ('on-off' phenomena);[135] it is rarely, if ever, effective in patients who do not respond to a potentially adequate dosage of levodopa. There is a growing belief that bromocriptine-levodopa combinations used from the outset of therapy may provide the best control of Parkinsonism currently possible, delaying the onset of later-stage treatment failure and decreasing mortality.[152]

Other dopamine agonists such as pergolide and lisuride may be used in the same manner as bromocriptine. These agents may be useful if the adverse effects of bromocriptine preclude its use.

#### Management of Resting and Intention Tremor

Some Parkinsonian patients have an element of action (intention) tremor, as well as true Parkinsonian resting tremor. No drug therapy is particularly effective for the resting tremor of Parkinsonism (which is best controlled by stereotaxic thalamotomy, though few patients would contemplate such surgery). The intention tremor element resembles essential tremor (see section 7.6) and may be helped by the drugs used for this disorder, e.g. propranolol.

### *7.1.3 Clinical Outcome and Economic Considerations*

Dopaminergic therapy has transformed the outlook for Parkinsonism. The agents used are relatively expensive (bromocriptine and pergolide more so than levodopa), but they can restore the sufferer to reasonably normal mobility for some years. Subsequently, however, the later-stage levodopa treatment failure manifestations, and our inability to remedy them, constitute a sad limitation of current therapeutics. In addition to these problems, other difficulties may also arise during dopaminergic therapy, particularly dementia and paranoid hallucinations, which are an increasing problem in elderly Parkinsonian patients. To some extent, this problem may be a consequence of the longer survival of such patients. Their increased mobility resulting from levodopa therapy may make the behaviour disturbance associated with their thought disorder more apparent. Therapy with levodopa or a dopamine agonist tends to increase the hallucinations and behavioural changes. Although phenothiazine or butyrophenone antipsychotic drugs quieten the disturbed behaviour, these drugs, being centrally-active dopamine antagonists, worsen the Parkinsonism. However, the $D_4$ receptor antagonist clozapine can improve the hallucinations without affecting the Parkinsonism,[153] but it may cause agranulocytosis. In practice, it often proves necessary to reduce or withdraw the dopaminergic therapy, allowing the patient to exhibit more acceptable behaviour at the cost of more limited mobility.

Attempts to correct Parkinsonian dementia by trying to restore the deficient acetylcholinergic innervation of the neocortex resulting from degeneration of the nucleus basalis, by use of acetylcholine precursors (e.g. choline, lecithin) or anticholinesterases (e.g. physostigmine), have produced little clinically useful benefit.

## 7.2 Chorea

Chorea, mainly either rheumatic or due to Huntington's disease, is functionally, and in terms of biochemical pathogenesis, the converse of Parkinsonism. In Huntington's disease, in which the structural pathology is well established, loss of striatal neurons allows the normal numbers of incoming nigrostriatal axon terminals to deliver a relative excess of dopamine around the surviving neurons. Levodopa overdosage in Parkinsonism also produces choreiform dyskinesia.

#### Optimum Treatment

Since chorea appears to be a consequence of striatal synaptic dopamine excess, it appears logical to control it by:

1) Depleting nigrostriatal axon terminals of dopamine stores by giving drugs which prevent amine neurotransmitter retention in storage granules in axon terminals; *or*

2) Blocking postsynaptic dopamine receptors on surviving striatal neurons.

Both therapeutic approaches are successful, provided adequate drug dosages are used.

***Dopamine depletion:*** *tetrabenazine* (initially 25mg 2 or 3 times daily in adults, increased as necessary) and *reserpine* are the available neurotransmitter depleting agents. Tetrabenazine is preferred because it has a stronger central action relative to its peripheral one. Tetrabenazine has a plasma half-life of about 24 hours; it has sedative properties, tends to cause depression of mood, and occasionally produces episodes of distressing dysphagia.

***Dopamine receptor blockade:*** *phenothiazines,* and also *haloperidol* and *pimozide,* are the main dopamine receptor antagonists used. *Thioridazine* (a phenothiazine with a piperidine side chain) has less tendency to produce dystonia than the phenothiazines with piperazine side chains (see also chapter 30; sect. 3.1.5). It may be used in an initial dose of 25mg twice daily for an adult, with 25mg dose increments every 4 to 7 days (the drug being given twice daily) until the choreic movements settle, or drowsiness rules out any further dose increase. This treatment does not correct the dementia of Huntington's disease. The dosage of the dopamine antagonist should be kept as low as possible, while still restraining the disordered movements. In Huntington's disease, the treatment will continue for the remainder of the patient's life.

In Sydenham's chorea, attempts may be made to reduce the dosage every 1 or 2 weeks, knowing that the movement disorder will ultimately die out.

### 7.3 Hemiballismus

This disorder is a severe unilateral chorea, caused by a vascular lesion involving the subthalamic nucleus on the opposite side. The dyskinesia responds to the pharmacological measures used for chorea (see section 7.2). The movement disorder nearly always dies out as time passes, and it is usually possible to withdraw therapy after some weeks or months.

### 7.4 Dystonia

The term 'dystonia' embraces a number of dyskinesias in which relatively slow repetitive changes in muscle tone cause a pattern of twisting involuntary movements sometimes more conspicuous in the axial structures than in the limbs. It includes some instances of the movement disorder formerly called 'athetosis'. The biochemical pathogenesis of dystonia is not adequately understood, although it appears related in some way to disordered dopaminergic function. Thus, temporary acute dystonic reactions, commonly involving the head, neck and external eye muscles, occasionally follow a single dose of a phenothiazine or related drug (e.g. prochlorperazine given for vomiting). Various forms of dystonia may be improved by centrally-acting anticholinergic [e.g. trihexyphenidyl (benzhexol)] or dopaminergic agents (e.g. bromocriptine or levodopa), and worsened by cholinergics and dopamine antagonists.[154] Dystonia may occur in biochemical disorders such as Wilson's disease, in the genetic disorder (autosomal dominant inheritance) dystonia musculorum deformans (torsion spasm), and in idiopathic spasmodic torticollis.

#### Optimum Treatment

Acute drug-induced dystonia can be corrected by intravenously administered *benztropine* (0.5mg) or *diazepam* (5 to 10mg); sometimes a second injection some hours later may be required before the dystonic tendency finally settles. The dystonia of Wilson's disease may be relieved, or prevented, by treating the underlying disorder of copper metabolism with *penicillamine* (see section 13.4).

There is no consistently effective drug therapy for the other varieties of dystonia. Dopaminergic agents (e.g. levodopa) may produce limited and temporary benefit. There are reports of dystonia musculorum deformans being relieved by high doses of *diazepam* (100 mg/day)[155] or *carbamazepine*.[156] High-dose *trihexyphenidyl* (ultimately 30 mg/day) produced sustained benefit in some 70% of a series of 31 patients with torsion dystonia.[157]

Localised dystonias, e.g. spasmodic torticollis, may be relieved for some weeks or months by locally injected *botulinum A toxin*. The injection may be repeated as necessary. Two preparations are currently commercially available but their dosage units are not equivalent.[158] Overdosage results in a degree of botulism (see section 8.3).

### 7.5 Myoclonus

Myoclonus (shock-like involuntary muscle jerks) is a symptom with several known causes[159] and various clinical expressions. Some types of myoclonus respond to drug therapy.

#### Optimum Treatment

Certain antiepileptic drugs, including *valproic acid* and *clonazepam,* help epileptic myoclonus (see section 4.1).

Postanoxic intention myoclonus appears related to cerebral serotonin depletion and can be controlled by raising the brain serotonin level in a manner analogous to that used to raise brain dopamine levels. The serotonin precursors *tryptophan* or *5-hydroxytryptophan* are given orally together with a peripheral L-aromatic amino acid decarboxylase inhibitor (carbidopa or benserazide) to prevent wasteful extracerebral metabolism of the amino acid. *Clonazepam,* which alters serotonergic neurotransmission, is also useful.

Palatal myoclonus, related to lesions involving the olives, also seems to depend on central serotonin depletion. It may respond to the measures mentioned above, and to *carbamazepine.* Facial myoclonus (hemifacial spasm) may be treated with locally injected *botulinum A toxin* or by microsurgical decompression of the facial nerve in the posterior fossa.

### 7.6 Essential Tremor

The rhythmic, repetitive involuntary movements of relatively constant amplitude that constitute tremor have various established clinical patterns, and several known causes. Essential (senile) tremor, comprising an intention tremor of the upper limbs, sometimes with a vertical or transverse tremor of the head, is the only tremor syndrome for which drug therapy offers much benefit. Temporary relief produced by drinking a small amount of ethanol is almost diagnostic. Essential tremor often does not warrant treatment: all the patient requires is to understand the disorder and its outlook, and to be reassured that the diagnosis is not Parkinsonism.

#### Optimum Treatment

When treatment is indicated, β-adrenoceptor antagonists (β-blockers) lacking partial agonist (intrinsic sympathomimetic) activity are useful. *Propranolol* is the agent usually employed, but *timolol,*[160] *metoprolol*[161] and *sotalol*[162] are also effective. Some patients use β-blockers intermittently, to ease the tremor only when in particular social situations. Others prefer to suppress the tremor continuously. Such patients may be given propranolol in doses of up to 240 or 320 mg/day, although 20 to 40mg 3 times daily may suffice.

*Primidone* may also control essential tremor,[163] and methylphenobarbital has sometimes proved effective when propranolol is not tolerated.

### 7.7 Gilles de la Tourette Syndrome and Paroxysmal Choreoathetosis

The uncommon Gilles de la Tourette syndrome, with its tics, involuntary vocalisations, and coprolalia, can be helped by *haloperidol.*[159] The paroxysms of choreiform movement in the rare disorder paroxysmal choreoathetosis can be prevented by *phenytoin.*[164]

***Tardive dyskinesia*** is discussed in chapter 30 (sect. 3.1.5).

## 8. Disorders Affecting Voluntary Movement

No drug treatment is available for paralysis due to upper or lower motor neuron lesions. However, drugs may decrease the spasticity that often occurs in upper motor neuron lesions. Also, certain disorders of neurotransmitter function at myoneural junctions respond to drug therapy (e.g. myasthenia, botulism), as does myotonia.

### 8.1 Spasticity

Spasticity in upper motor neuron lesions is often but not always associated with weakness. Relief of spasticity may make voluntary movement easier and may release power previously masked by increased tone.

#### *8.1.1 Clinical Pharmacology of Drugs Used in Treatment*

The 3 main antispasticity drugs are baclofen, dantrolene and diazepam. Their properties are compared in table VIII.

***Baclofen*** [β-(*p*-chlorophenyl)-γ-aminobutyrate] was developed as a GABA analogue but has

**Table VIII.** Characteristics of antispasticity drugs

| Feature | Baclofen | Dantrolene | Diazepam |
|---|---|---|---|
| **Mechanism/site of action** | $GABA_B$ agonist in CNS | Impairs $Ca^{++}$-mediated myofibril contraction in muscle | Increases $GABA_A$-mediated inhibition in CNS |
| **Duration of pharmacodynamic effect** | 4-8h | 8-12h | Effect wears off over >24h |
| **Pharmacokinetic characteristics:** | | | |
| Bioavailability (oral) | High (also given intrathecally) | ≈20% | High |
| Half-life | 2.5-6h | ≈9h | 24-48h<br>Metabolite (nordazepam) has a longer $t_{½}$ (50-120h) |
| Principal route of elimination | Renal excretion (70% excreted in urine unchanged) | Hepatic metabolism | Hepatic metabolism |
| **Clinical effectiveness** | Effective in spasticity due to spinal cord disease | Relieves spasticity of spinal or cerebral origin; useful in malignant hyperthermia | Modest relief of spasticity |
| **Adverse effects** | Hallucinations, confusion, weakness in overdosage, drowsiness, nausea, vertigo, headache, diarrhoea, increase in epileptic seizures | Weakness, dizziness, drowsiness. Hepatotoxicity has occurred with long term use (monitor liver function tests periodically) | Often too sedative in effective doses |

*Abbreviations:* GABA = γ-aminobutyric acid; CNS = central nervous system.

proved to be a specific agonist at $GABA_B$ receptors, without effect at $GABA_A$ receptors. Given in doses of 10 to 25mg or more 3 times daily, it can relieve spasticity, particularly that resulting from spinal cord disease, and reduces the frequency and severity of painful flexor or extensor spasms. It can be infused intrathecally or epidurally if oral therapy fails,[165] although the infusion system is expensive.

***Dantrolene*** relieves spasticity by a direct action on muscle, inhibiting $Ca^{++}$-mediated myofibril contraction. It is effective in spasticity associated with stroke, cerebral palsy, spinal cord injury and multiple sclerosis, but the price of decreased spasticity is often increased weakness. Therefore, dantrolene is used mainly in bedfast patients who would not be disadvantaged by decreased muscle power. Hepatoxic reactions of an idiosyncratic or hypersensitivity type have been reported occasionally with long term use of dantrolene.

***Diazepam*** in doses sufficient to relieve spasticity is likely to produce troublesome or unacceptable sedation. This offsets the advantage of its low cost.

#### *8.1.2 Optimum Treatment*

Spasticity may convert a paralysed leg into a rigid crutch, which permits weight bearing and walking after a fashion. Reducing such spasticity pharmacologically may therefore make locomotion impossible. On the other hand, spasticity may sometimes limit the delivery of available power. In such cases, relief of spasticity can enhance mobility. Treatment of spasticity with agents such as baclofen or dantrolene offers benefit when:

a) The patient cannot walk, and spasticity, or flexor spasms, causes pain or deformity; and

b) Spasticity, rather than weakness, interferes with walking and running, as may occur in spinal multiple sclerosis.[166,167]

Some years ago, there was a vogue for treating lower limb spasticity with intrathecally administered phenol, which tended to produce selective damage of gamma efferent fibres in motor nerve roots. The procedure is now little used.

### 8.2 Myasthenia Gravis

Myasthenia gravis results from thymic autoantibody production against the (nicotinic) acetylcholine receptors of skeletal muscle, destroying some and competitively blocking others.[168,169] Consequently, acetylcholine released from nerve terminals has less chance of initiating and maintaining skeletal muscle contraction, resulting in muscle weakness and fatigue, with temporary recovery following rest.

The logical possibilities for treatment of myasthenia gravis are:

1) Removal of the source of antibody production (i.e. the thymus) surgically or, if this is not feasible, its destruction by irradiation.

2) Removal of circulating antibodies by plasmapheresis.[170] Each treatment produces benefit lasting for several days, and the procedure can be repeated. It is used mainly in severe or resistant cases to obtain temporary respite until other measures have time to work.

3) Prevention of antibody formation by using high-dose corticosteroids or other immunosuppressive agents (e.g. azathioprine, cyclosporin[171]). Benefit may take days or weeks to appear, and corticosteroids may make the disorder worse initially.

4) Increasing acetylcholine concentrations in the myoneural junction, thus allowing the neurotransmitter to compete more successfully against the antibody for subjunctional nicotinic acetylcholine receptors. This aim may be achieved by inhibiting the enzyme acetylcholinesterase, which catalyses the hydrolysis of acetylcholine and thus terminates its action.

#### 8.2.1 Clinical Pharmacology of Drugs Used in Treatment

Apart from the anticholinesterases, the various drugs used in myasthenia gravis have uses in other areas of medicine and their clinical pharmacological properties are discussed in other chapters (e.g. corticosteroids in chapter 19 and immunosuppressive drugs in chapter 28).

##### Anticholinesterase Agents

The main anticholinesterase drugs used are:

- ***Edrophonium*** (plasma half-life 1.8 hours[172]), which has a very brief duration of action during the α phase of its distribution when it is given intravenously as a diagnostic agent
- ***Neostigmine*** (plasma half-life 1 to 1.5 hours[173]), which has a duration of action of 3 to 4 hours following oral administration in conventional dosage
- ***Pyridostigmine*** (plasma half-life 1 to 4 hours[174]), which has a duration of action of around 4 hours following oral administration
- ***Ambenonium,*** which has a duration of action of 4 to 6 hours following oral administration
- ***Distigmine,*** which has a much longer duration of action than the other drugs of this class. Maximum inhibition of cholinesterase occurs 9 hours after a single intramuscular dose of 0.5mg and persists for about 24 hours.

The anticholinesterase drugs are poorly bioavailable orally (neostigmine ≈2%, pyridostigmine ≈7.6%[174]), possibly because of presystemic elimination. They increase the effect of acetylcholine at nicotinic receptors on skeletal muscle and at muscarinic receptors on the alimentary tract, bladder and other parasympathetic sites, causing cramping abdominal pain and sometimes defecation. These muscarinic adverse effects can be selectively antagonised by atropine, or by quaternary ammonium anticholinergics which do not cross the blood-brain barrier (e.g. propantheline 15mg 3 times daily).

Anticholinesterase overdosage causes weakness from depolarisation blockade of neuromuscular transmission. This weakness can be confused with myasthenic weakness. It requires entirely different therapy, namely ceasing anticholinesterase intake until strength recovers. Overdosage also causes excessive sweating and miosis (unless these are concealed by the administration of anticholinergics).

#### 8.2.2 Optimum Treatment

##### Initial Therapy

Treatment of myasthenia gravis usually commences with anticholinesterase drugs. In adults, *pyridostigmine* in a dosage of 60mg 3 times daily may be given initially. If benefit is insufficient at the time of the expected peak effect (1 to 2 hours after intake), the size of each dose can be increased; if the benefit does not last long enough, the dosage interval can be shortened. Cautious intravenous test injections of edrophonium may be given at the time of expected maximum effect, and also just before the next pyridostigmine dose, to assess how much more improvement is possible at these times.

When treating generalised myasthenia, priority is given to controlling myasthenic weakness in the biologically most important muscles. Different anticholinesterase doses may be needed to control myasthenia in different muscle groups. Thus, patients may complain of diplopia, but there is little sense in producing cholinergic paresis of the respiratory muscles to relieve the visual disturbance.

Myasthenia gravis is often most difficult to control in the first year or two of its course, while the disease is reaching its maximum severity. During this stage, much careful dosage adjustment may be necessary. Later, management is often easier. The various approaches to treatment discussed above can be applied in combination. Reduction in anticholinesterase dosage to avoid cholinergic weakness may be necessary when other measures (e.g. corticosteroid therapy) are implemented. Severe and brittle myasthenic patients may have to be managed for a time in an intensive care unit, with facilities for assisted respiration.

If anticholinesterase drugs prove insufficient, *corticosteroids* or other *immunosuppressive* agents (e.g. azathioprine or cyclosporin) may be added. High-dose corticosteroids may be given as a single oral bolus dose every second morning, e.g. 100mg prednisone or prednisolone, or 8 to 12mg dexamethasone. This method of administration usually controls the disorder and reduces the need for anticholinesterase therapy (see above). It also minimises the adverse effects that are likely to develop when corticosteroids are given several times a day over long periods.

#### Other Treatment Measures

Thymectomy may be considered in patients with generalised myasthenia, while plasmapheresis may be used to help the patient through particularly difficult periods.

These policies have generally served patients well. However, as intermittent bolus administration minimises the adverse effects of corticosteroids, it has been argued that therapy should begin with corticosteroids, since this represents a more fundamental attack on the disease process. Furthermore, there is some evidence that long term anticholinesterase therapy may cause damage in the end-plate region.[175] Despite these arguments, one hesitates to abandon well tried and usually successful therapeutic practices.

Certain drugs make myasthenia worse, and should be avoided (see section 15). Penicillamine therapy, for example, may cause reversible myasthenia.

### 8.3 Botulism and the Eaton-Lambert Myasthenic Syndrome

The weakness in both these disorders is due to failure to release sufficient stored acetylcholine from axon terminals at myoneural junctions. In botulism, this is due to botulinum toxin; in the Eaton-Lambert syndrome, it is due to circulating antibodies, produced in 50% of cases by neoplasms elsewhere in the body. Certain agents, e.g. guanidine and germine diacetate, can enhance acetylcholine release and improve muscle strength. 4-Aminopyridine may also be useful.[176]

There may also be some response to anticholinesterase therapy. Plasmapheresis can be used to remove circulating antibodies.

### 8.4 Tetanus

The muscular hypertonus and spasms of tetanus result from the action of tetanus toxin on spinal and bulbar interneurons. Management, in principle, comprises removing the source of the toxin, administering tetanus antitoxin intravenously, and producing skeletal muscle relaxation, or if necessary paralysis (with assisted respiration), until the effects of the toxin wear off.

### 8.5 Myotonia

Myotonic inability to achieve quick relaxation of contracted voluntary muscle depends on altered chloride ion conductance and perhaps $Na^+$ channel function in muscle fibres. In myotonic dystrophy, the main problem is nearly always weakness rather than myotonia, and little may be gained by treating the latter. In myotonia congenita, the myotonia may interfere enough with physical activity to warrant treatment.

#### Optimum Treatment

Quinine, procainamide, prednisone (or other corticosteroid), and phenytoin will lessen myotonia. Baclofen[177] and taurine[178] may also be useful. *Phenytoin* is probably the safest agent for long term use, although its efficacy is questionable. *Quinine sulfate* 300mg 2 to 4 times daily is reasonably effective; it may occasionally cause thrombocytopenia and agranulocytosis and in overdosage, manifestations of cinchonism may develop. *Procainamide* 250mg 4 times daily is also useful but its adverse effects are perhaps less acceptable than those of quinine. They include fever, arthralgia, itching, skin rashes, anorexia, nausea, vomiting, psychosis, cardiac arrhythmia and agranulocytosis. Slow acetylators may develop systemic lupus erythematosus (see chapter 6; sect. 4.2.1).

Corticosteroids, even in minimal effective dosage, may be associated with the usual adverse effects of this group of drugs when used for prolonged periods.

### 8.6 Hypokalaemic (Familial) Periodic Paralysis and Paramyotonia Congenita

The attacks of paralysis in hypokalaemic periodic paralysis may be relieved by giving potassium. Acetazolamide (250mg 3 or 4 times daily) may help prevent attacks.[179]

The manifestations of paramyotonia congenita depend on abnormality of the muscle membrane $Na^+$ channel. Acetazolamide therapy,[180] and potassium-losing diuretics (e.g. thiazides) are useful in treatment.

## 9. Immunological Disorders of the Nervous System

Autoantibody formation directed at various tissue elements in the central and peripheral nervous systems, at the motor end-plate of skeletal muscle, at muscle itself, and at the vascular supply of the nervous system, may cause various neuroimmunological disorders. These disorders and the site at which they occur include:

1) Central nervous system myelin – acute disseminated encephalomyelitis.

2) Peripheral nervous system myelin – Guillain-Barré polyneuropathy and chronic inflammatory demyelinating polyneuropathy.

3) Motor end-plates – myasthenia gravis (see section 8.2).

4) Skeletal muscle – polymyositis.

5) Various vascular elements – polyarteritis nodosa, systemic lupus erythematosus, temporal (giant cell) arteritis, all of which can cause ischaemic neural injury.

The autoantibody production can occur as a single self-limited episode, a series of such episodes, or can persist. All the above neuroimmunological disorders are managed in essentially similar ways.

### Optimum Treatment

The principles involved in treatment of these immunological disorders have already been outlined under myasthenia gravis (see section 8.2). Abnormal antibody production is suppressed with corticosteroids or immunosuppressive drugs. Acute crises are dealt with by removing circulating antibodies by plasmapheresis. Local inflammatory manifestations are managed by appropriate drug treatment.

***Corticosteroids*** are the mainstay of treatment in these disorders. The method of administration depends on whether an anti-inflammatory or an immunosuppressive action is most desired. For an anti-inflammatory action, continuous or reasonably continuous high corticosteroid concentrations seem desirable. For immunosuppression, pulses of high corticosteroid concentrations every 48 hours appear to be adequate. Pulsed corticosteroid administration substantially reduces glucocorticoid-type adverse effects, and the risk of adrenal suppression.

In the acute phase of the above disorders, when both an anti-inflammatory and immunosuppressive effect are useful, corticosteroids are given in high dosages 3 or 4 times a day (e.g. dexamethasone 4 to 8mg 3 times daily, or prednisolone 25 to 50mg 4 times daily). Benefit takes at least 24 hours to appear. In the acute phase, the earlier the treatment, the faster the benefit. Several studies failed to show benefit from corticosteroids in the Guillain-Barré syndrome, but the doses used were probably too low for an optimum response. In adults, at least 100 mg/day of prednisolone (or prednisone) often seems necessary. There is a current vogue for treating the Guillain-Barré syndrome by plasmapheresis, with reasonable success. The possibility of successful high-dose corticosteroid, or intravenous gammaglobulin therapy,[181] should not be forgotten.

Once the acute phase has been controlled, those disorders involving continuing or intermittent autoantibody production (e.g. chronic inflammatory demyelinating polyneuropathy, polymyositis) may need sustained immunosuppression. This may be achieved with the lowest effective daily corticosteroid dose. Alternate daily bolus corticosteroids, initially in high doses but later in the minimum clinically effective dose, may be advantageous. Some clinicians prefer to achieve immunosuppression with agents such as azathioprine or cyclophosphamide, since these drugs offer a 'steroid-sparing' effect. Such agents should certainly be tried if corticosteroids fail, or are not tolerated, but there is a risk of later secondary malignancy from cyclophosphamide.

## 10. Multiple Sclerosis

The pathogenesis of multiple sclerosis is incompletely understood, although an autoimmune process may be involved. Many treatments have been advocated, but few have stood the test of time or survived the scrutiny of properly designed controlled clinical trials.[182]

### Optimum Treatment

***Acute exacerbations:*** it is now accepted that high-dose corticosteroids shorten the duration and reduce the disability from acute exacerbations of the disease.[183] Bolus methylprednisolone, e.g. 500mg intravenously daily for 5 days, with reducing dosage over the next week or two, is sometimes used. Other corticosteroids in equivalent dosage, orally or parenterally, might be as effective.

***Prevention of exacerbations/disease progression:*** attempts to prevent further exacerbations of multiple sclerosis by an immunosuppressive regimen given by intermittent bolus or by continuous high-dose corticosteroids appear of little avail. *Azathioprine* may offer minor benefit, but the overall risk-benefit ratio of this agent is unfavourable.[184] Recent studies have suggested that *interferon-β1b* may slow the progression of the disease,[185] although such therapy is very expensive.

Certain symptoms of multiple sclerosis may be amenable to drug therapy. Spasticity can be treated as outlined in section 8.1, while peripherally acting anticholinergics (e.g. propantheline) may help urgency of micturition and mild degrees of urinary incontinence. The management of sphincter disturbances is discussed further in chapter 4 (section 4.6).

## 11. Degenerative Vascular Diseases

Hypertensive and atheromatous arterial diseases are major causes of neurological disability. The management of hypertension and atheroma is discussed in chapters 21 and 20, respectively. The treatment of their neurological consequences is discussed below.

Primary prevention of stroke may be attempted by correcting or eliminating various stroke risk factors, e.g. hypertension, diabetes, hypercholesterolaemia, cigarette smoking. The risk of stroke in non-valvular atrial fibrillation is lessened by anticoagulation and also by antiplatelet therapy.[186]

### 11.1 Established Stroke

Cerebral haemorrhage, cerebral infarction from arterial thrombosis or embolism, or ischaemia arising from arterial spasm (in subarachnoid haemorrhage) may cause permanent neurological deficits.

#### *11.1.1 Intracranial Haemorrhage*

No curative medical treatment is available for intracranial haemorrhage. If necessary, intracranial pressure may be reduced by the measures discussed earlier (see section 6). Reduction of reactionary arterial hypertension may be undesirable unless the heart is becoming overloaded, as it may cause further neuronal injury due to diminished brain perfusion. Surgical evacuation of an intracerebral haematoma is sometimes feasible.

#### *11.1.2 Cerebral Infarction*

Drug treatment has little to offer in acute cerebral infarction, unless there is ischaemic cerebral swelling, which may be treated by medical measures for reducing raised intracranial pressure (see section 6). Routinely administered corticosteroids do not improve the prognosis in ischaemic stroke,[187] but may be of use in the occasional patient who develops significant ischaemic brain swelling. Cerebral ischaemia is believed to cause excitotoxic neuronal death mediated by glutamate activation of NMDA (*N*-methyl-D-aspartate)-type excitatory amino acid receptors, with subsequent $Ca^{++}$ influx into neurons. Therefore, NMDA receptor antagonists, and calcium antagonists such as nimodipine, are being tested in acute cerebral ischaemia, but their place in therapeutics is unclear. Thrombolytic therapy with streptokinase or alteplase (recombinant tissue-type plasminogen activator; rt-PA) is also under trial in acute ischaemic stroke, in the hope that it will produce benefit akin to that in coronary artery occlusion (see chapter 26 sect. 3.2.2).

If cerebral infarction is due to cardiogenic emboli, prophylactic anticoagulation (heparin, later warfarin) may be used unless CT scan of the brain shows haemorrhagic infarction. Therapy is continued until echocardiography shows there has been no residual endocardial clot for several weeks, or longer. If possible, atrial fibrillation should be reversed.

### 11.2 Progressing Stroke

Cerebral arterial disease occasionally presents as a progressive focal neurological deficit over a time-course of several days. If the diagnosis is established and surgical correction of the underlying thrombus is not possible, anticoagulation is recommended as long as CT scanning shows no intracranial bleeding. In this situation, rapid reduction of a mildly or moderately raised systemic blood pressure may critically compromise the cerebral circulation.

### 11.3 Arterial Spasm in Subarachnoid Haemorrhage

There have been numerous attempts to find effective drug therapy for arterial spasm following subarachnoid haemorrhage. The calcium antagonist nimodipine,[188] administered intravenously soon after the ictus, improves the neurological outcome. It is uncertain whether the benefit is due to overcoming arterial spasm or protecting neurons against excitotoxic cell death.

Antifibrinolytic agents, for example ε-aminocaproic acid, have been used to reduce the risk of rebleeding from ruptured aneurysms but their efficacy is disputed.[189]

### 11.4 Hypertensive Encephalopathy

Now that hypertension is usually treated effectively, hypertensive encephalopathy has become quite uncommon. The disorder may present as a progressing stroke. Therapy has traditionally involved rapid blood pressure reduction, although it would also seem logical to reduce the intracranial pressure by the measures for cerebral oedema discussed earlier (see section 6). For management of hypertensive crises, see chapter 21 (section 4.3).

### 11.5 Transient Ischaemic Attacks (TIAs)

Transient cerebral ischaemic attacks are usually due to the release of platelet emboli, clots or other debris from atheromatous ulcers in the walls of the great arteries of the neck. Less often, they are caused by episodes of hypotension when there is a critical degree of arterial narrowing. Management in the two situations differs. If the attacks are due to embolism, the treatment possibilities are:

- Aspirin or ticlopidine to help prevent platelet aggregation (see below)
- Anticoagulation (e.g. with warfarin)
- Surgical repair of the site of origin of the emboli.

If the attacks are of haemodynamic origin, the possibilities are:

1) Correction of any hypotension, including iatrogenic hypotension, and of any cardiac arrhythmia which could reduce blood pressure.

2) Surgical replacement of the stenotic segment of the artery.

Of these possibilities, only antiplatelet therapy is considered here. The preferred therapeutic approach in each individual may demand some nicety of judgement. Individual transient ischaemic attacks are themselves relatively harmless, but their occurrence is associated with an increased risk of stroke and of death from myocardial infarction.

#### Clinical Use of Antiplatelet Agents in Treatment

Aspirin and ticlopidine[190] are the principal antiplatelet agents used. Their properties are compared in table IX.

***Aspirin*** appears to offer some protection against thrombotic and embolic events in various parts of the arterial circulation, including transient ischaemic attacks, where it reduces the risk of stroke.[191] Its antiplatelet action depends on acetylating, and thus irreversibly inhibiting, the enzyme cyclo-oxygenase, which catalyses thromboxane $A_2$ formation in platelets, and prostacyclin formation in endothelial cells (fig. 7). Cyclo-oxygenase inhibition prevents thromboxane-mediated platelet aggregation, but simultaneously prevents the anti-aggregatory effect of prostacyclin formed in endothelial cells. After a single aspirin dose, the former is inhibited for the life span of the platelet, whereas the latter is inhibited only for some hours, since endothelial cells, but not platelets, can synthesise new enzyme. Furthermore, platelet thromboxane $A_2$ formation may be more sensitive to inhibition by aspirin than endothelial cell prostacyclin synthesis,[192] which could in part explain why a low aspirin dose (e.g. 325mg or less taken once daily) appears to be as effective or more effective in protecting against platelet-mediated vascular events than higher doses.

Pharmacokinetic factors may provide an alternative explanation. When aspirin is administered orally it undergoes substantial hydrolysis to salicylic acid (which is devoid of inhibitory activity against cyclo-oxygenase) in the gut wall and the liver before entering the systemic circulation. Consequently, when low aspirin doses are administered, higher concentrations of aspirin will be available for the inhibition of platelets passing through the gut capillaries during absorption than are available to systemic vascular endothelial cells. With continued administration, this results in cumulative presystemic acetylation of platelet cyclo-oxygenase and thus inhibition of thromboxane $A_2$ formation.[193]

As yet, the minimal effective dose of aspirin in clinical practice has not been conclusively established, but seems likely to be in the range 50 to 100 mg/day. Certainly, the lower the dose, the fewer and less serious the adverse effects of the drug.

***Ticlopidine*** given in a dose of 250mg twice daily inhibits platelet aggregation without affecting cyclo-oxygenase activity or endothelial cell function. It therefore has theoretical advantages over aspirin, and has proved more effective in some trials of stroke prevention.[194] However, it is substantially more expensive,

**Table IX.** Characteristics of the principal antiplatelet drugs

| Feature | Aspirin (acetylsalicylic acid) | Ticlopidine |
|---|---|---|
| **Mechanism/site of action** | Platelet aggregation inhibited by irreversibly blocking platelet thromboxane $A_2$ formation, but facilitated by inhibiting endothelial cell prostacyclin production (NB. prostacyclin production is restored more rapidly than thromboxane $A_2$ production; see also text, section 11.5) | Platelet aggregation inhibited by blocking platelet fibrinogen receptors and altering ADP binding; no effects in endothelial cells |
| **Duration of pharmacodynamic effect** | Single-dose effect lasts for life span of platelets then present in body; endothelial cell action shorter | Antiplatelet effect lasts >72h |
| **Pharmacokinetic characteristics:** | | |
| Bioavailability (oral) | Varies with absorption characteristics of preparation used | 80-90% |
| Half-life | 12-20 min | 96h (at steady-state) |
| Principal route of elimination | Gut wall/hepatic metabolism | Hepatic metabolism |
| **Clinical effectiveness** | Protects against platelet-mediated vascular events, e.g. TIA, stroke | Superior to aspirin in clinical trials |
| **Adverse effects/interactions** | Gastrointestinal intolerance (minimal with low doses), hypersensitivity reactions, bleeding episodes (uncommon). Additive effect with warfarin | Diarrhoea, rash, neutropenia (monitor blood counts for first 3 months), bleeding episodes (uncommon). Additive effect with warfarin, heparin |
| **Relative cost** (per day) | ± | +++ |

*Abbreviation and symbols:* +++ = high; ± = very low, TIA = transient ischaemic attack; ADP = adenosine diphosphate.

and can cause neutropenia; patients receiving ticlopidine should therefore have their neutrophil counts checked regularly during the first 3 months of treatment.

***Dipyridamole*** has also been used for its antiplatelet effect, usually in combination with aspirin. However, when used alone, there is no convincing evidence that it helps prevent stroke or transient ischaemic attacks.

## 12. Infections of the Central Nervous System

Central nervous system infection, mainly meningitis and cerebral abscess, is uncommon in contemporary Western society. Nevertheless, many different organisms may cause such infection.[195] Only the principles of treatment are discussed below; specific infections are covered in chapter 31.

The general principles of treatment of CNS infection are:

1) Identification of the causative organism, and then provision of specific antimicrobial therapy, remembering that certain antibiotics do not enter the CSF and brain.

2) Use of drug therapy to reduce the intracranial pressure (see section 6) if the infection has caused cerebral swelling, and treatment of any local inflammatory mass.

3) Maintenance of the patient's general condition, fluid and nutritional requirements, and relief of troublesome symptoms such as headache or fever.

## 13. Metabolic Disorders of the Nervous System

Several metabolic (often deficiency or toxic) disorders of the nervous system are amenable to drug therapy.

### 13.1 Thiamine Deficiency

Thiamine deficiency, often in alcoholics, causes peripheral neuropathy and the Wernicke-Korsakoff syndrome. Management comprises the removal of causative factors and the administration of thiamine, initially intravenously (50 to 100mg daily), and subsequently intramuscularly or orally in similar dosage. Fatal coma may occur if intravenous glucose is given before thiamine is injected, as the glucose load then cannot be metabolised.

### 13.2 Cyanocobalamin (Vitamin $B_{12}$) Deficiency

The neurological disorder caused by vitamin $B_{12}$ deficiency (subacute combined degeneration) is treated with hydroxocobalamin 1000μg injected daily for 5 days to replenish tissue stores. Then, after 2 or 3 weekly injections of

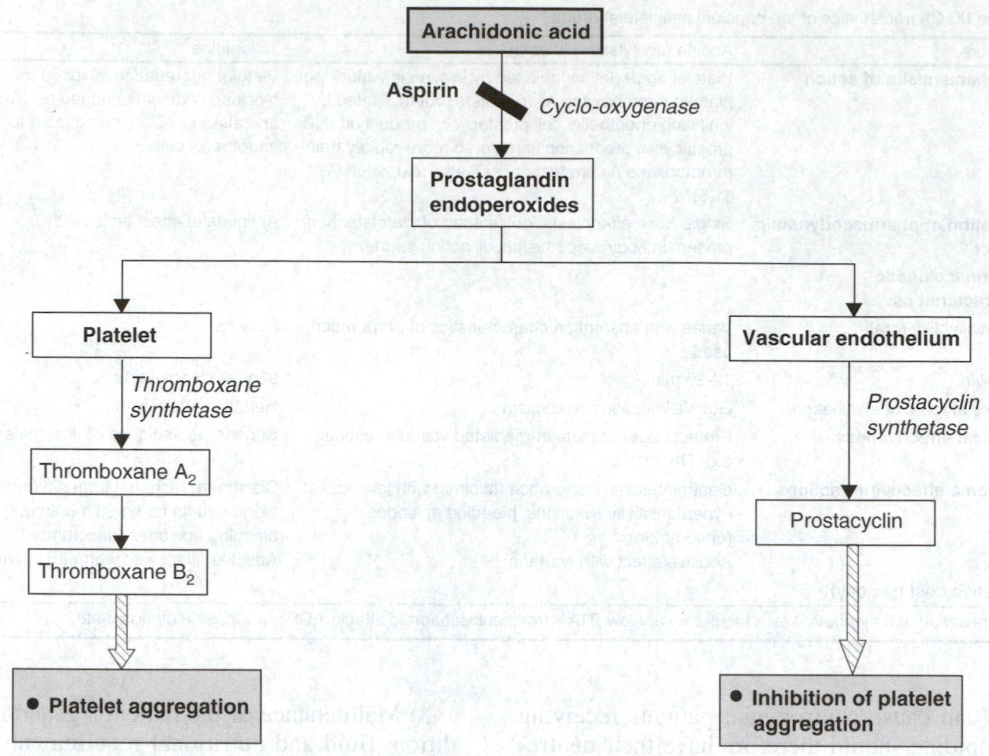


**Fig. 7.** Effects of aspirin inhibition of cyclo-oxygenase on the synthesis of thromboxane $A_2$ in platelets and prostacyclin in vascular endothelial cells.

100μg, lifelong maintenance therapy is begun (100μg every second month).

### 13.3 Folate Deficiency

Folate deficiency may occasionally cause a neurological disorder resembling subacute combined degeneration.[196] Serum folate concentrations are often low in patients taking antiepileptic drugs long term (mainly phenytoin, carbamazepine and phenobarbital); however, it is not established that such folate depletion causes symptoms.

Folic acid 5mg is given orally 2 or 3 times daily to correct deficiency states. The maintenance dose is 0.5mg 2 or 3 times daily.

### 13.4 Wilson's Disease

The caeruloplasmin deficiency of Wilson's disease results in copper, which is transported in the circulation loosely bound to albumin, becoming detached from this protein and binding to, and damaging, various tissue molecules. Once the diagnosis is made, preferably before neurological manifestations have appeared, attempts may be made to chelate the accumulating tissue copper so that it can subsequently be excreted in urine in a biologically inert form. Such treatment (see below) should prevent further symptomatic deterioration, and may allow some recovery.

#### Optimum Treatment

*Penicillamine* is the first line of therapy in Wilson's disease. This drug is a chelating agent with a plasma half-life of 1.66 to 3.15 hours[197] and is given orally in a dose of 250mg 3 or 4 times daily. Treatment continues for the remainder of the patient's life. The dosage should be adjusted to maintain satisfactory biochemical indices of liver function, and the optimum achievable neurological status. Penicillamine is nephrotoxic (necessitating renal function monitoring) and occasionally causes polymyositis, optic neuritis, lupus erythematosus, acute sensitivity reactions and reversible myasthenia.

*Dimercaprol* (BAL) is also useful in Wilson's disease. This drug is administered by deep intramuscular injection in a dose of 2.5 mg/kg/day. The patient's urine should be made alkaline to prevent heavy metal chelates breaking down again at an acid pH.

*Trientine* (triethylenetetramine) has been reported to be safe and effective in Wilson's disease sufferers who cannot tolerate penicillamine.[198] *Potassium sulfate* (40mg) may be added to meals to reduce dietary copper absorption.

### 13.5 Heavy Metal Poisoning

Poisoning with certain heavy metals, e.g. arsenic, lead and mercury, may cause peripheral neuropathy and other forms of nervous system damage. Exposure to the causative agent should be ceased, and the chelating agents used for Wilson's disease (see section 13.4) should be given to remove the metal from the body. *Sodium calcium edetate* may also be used for this purpose.

### 13.6 Cerebral Neoplasms

As far as possible, cerebral neoplasms, benign or malignant, are treated surgically. Since surgical removal of gliomas is almost always incomplete, attempts should be made to eradicate the residual tumour burden with radiotherapy and chemotherapy. However, the possibilities of chemotherapy are limited by the blood-brain barrier restricting the entry of many agents. Nitrosoureas are the principal antineoplastic drugs used. There have been trials of combination chemotherapy, but the outcomes have not been particularly encouraging.[199] Chemotherapy is discussed further in chapter 27.

Raised intracranial pressure due to the tumour is dealt with in section 6.

## 14. Miscellaneous Neurological Disorders

### 14.1 Bell's Palsy

Oral corticosteroids, e.g. prednisone or prednisolone 60 mg/day, improve the recovery of idiopathic facial nerve palsy.[200] Physiotherapy and electrical stimulation of the facial nerve are of no value.

Most cases of Bell's palsy recover spontaneously. Therefore, corticosteroids should be used when the facial paresis is complete, or nearly complete and should be given early. This treatment should be continued in full doses for some 10 days, and thereafter in reducing doses over the next 2 weeks. Corticosteroids probably reduce oedema around the facial nerve in the facial canal.

### 14.2 Diabetic Cranial Neuritis, Amyotrophy and Peripheral Neuropathy

Elderly patients with mild diabetes mellitus, or merely prediabetic glucose tolerance curves, sometimes develop painful paresis of one of the cranial nerves innervating the external eye muscles, but the causal role of the diabetes is doubtful. Similar persons may develop painful weakness and wasting of one, or later of both, quadriceps muscles due to a femoral neuropathy – so-called 'diabetic amyotrophy'.

Despite the comparatively mild diabetic state, it is usually necessary to treat diabetic amyotrophy with *soluble insulin,* adjusting the dose to keep the blood glucose concentration within physiological limits.[201] If the disorder is diagnosed and treated fairly early, the pain often begins to ease after a few days, and then power and muscle bulk begin to recover. Once recovery is reasonably complete, oral antidiabetic agents, or diet alone, can be substituted (see further chapter 19; sect. 3).

There has been recent interest in using *aldose reductase inhibitors* to prevent, and treat, diabetic peripheral neuropathy. However, the outcomes are not yet clear.

## 15. Use of Drugs in the Presence of Associated Neurological Disease

Occasionally, drugs taken for unrelated conditions may relieve coincidental neurological disorders. Thus, corticosteroids given for asthma may temporarily relieve manifestations of raised intracranial pressure or polymyositis; benzodiazepines given as tranquillisers may decrease the frequency of epileptic seizures; and quinine taken as a component of a 'tonic' may mask myotonia. However, various neurological disorders may be worsened by drugs given for other conditions. Some clinically relevant examples are discussed below.

### 15.1 Headache

Drugs such as reserpine and nitroglycerin (glyceryl trinitrate) may activate migraine, although if their administration is continued, they may later prevent it.[202] Continued ergotamine administration may lead to what is regarded as ergotamine-withdrawal headache, but this may really be caffeine-withdrawal headache because caffeine is present in many oral ergotamine preparations.[203]

Estrogens, when prescribed unopposed by progestagens for various gynaecological disorders, may activate migraine in a dose-related fashion.

### 15.2 Epilepsy

Phenothiazines and both tricyclic and tetracyclic antidepressants (particularly maprotiline[204]) may activate seizures in patients with epilepsy. Theophylline, when given in high dosages for asthma, may also increase seizure frequency.

### 15.3 Raised Intracranial Pressure

Various hypnosedatives and opioid analgesics may further elevate raised intracranial pressure, at least in part by depressing respiration.

### 15.4 Involuntary Movement Disorders

Certain antiemetic agents that are dopamine antagonists, e.g. prochlorperazine, may make Parkinsonism worse if they are prescribed for nausea. Sympathomimetic agents (e.g. dexamphetamine, ephedrine) may temporarily aggravate essential tremor.

### 15.5 Disorders Affecting Voluntary Movement

Many drugs can cause peripheral neuropathy[205] and, if given to patients with peripheral neuropathy, may increase its severity.

Aminoglycoside antibiotics (gentamicin, tobramycin, netilmicin, sisomicin, kanamycin, amikacin and streptomycin), polymixin B and colistin sulfomethate interfere with neuromuscular transmission in myasthenia gravis, while quinidine, quinine, procainamide, lidocaine (lignocaine), propranolol, chlorpromazine and phenytoin worsen myasthenia by actions on cell membranes.[206]

Patients with pseudocholinesterase deficiency develop prolonged paralysis after conventional doses of the neuromuscular blocking agent suxamethonium (succinylcholine), which they cannot inactivate.

Patients with myotonia may sometimes develop life-threatening myotonic laryngeal spasm if given a depolarising neuromuscular blocking agent (e.g. suxamethonium) prior to endotracheal intubation. Non-depolarising (competitive) blocking agents (e.g. tubocurarine) are safer in this situation.

Some patients with inherited overt or subclinical myopathies may develop the malignant hyperpyrexia syndrome when given certain inhalational anaesthetics, particularly halothane.

### 15.6 Cerebral Vascular Disease

Hypotension resulting from excessive pharmacological reduction of blood pressure may cause ischaemic neural injury, particularly if there is atheromatous stenosis of cerebral arteries.

## Further Reading

Cooper JR, Bloom FE, Roth RH. The biochemical basis of neuropharmacology. 6th ed. New York: Oxford University Press, 1991

Dam M, Gram L, editors. Comprehensive epileptology. New York: Raven Press, 1991

Eadie MJ, editor. Drug therapy in neurology. Edinburgh: Churchill-Livingstone, 1992

Lance JW. Mechanism and management of headache, 5th ed. London: Butterworth-Heinemann, 1993

## References

1. International Headache Society Headache Classification Committee. The classification and diagnostic criteria for headache disorders, cranial neuralgias, and facial pain. Cephalalgia 1988; 8 Suppl. 7: 9
2. Ad Hoc Committee. Classification of headache. Archives of Neurology 1962; 6: 173
3. Boquet J, Moore N, Boismare F. Hemicrania and lateralized cervicoscapular muscular hypertonicity. In: Critchley et al., editors. Headache: physiopathological and clinical concepts. Advances in Neurology 1982; 33: 401
4. Daroff RB. New headache classification. Neurology 1988; 38: 1138
5. Leao AAP, Morrison RS. Propagation of spreading cortical depression. Journal of Neurophysiology 1945; 8: 33
6. Moskowitz MA, Reinhardt Jr JF, Romero J, et al. Neurotransmitters and the fifth cranial nerve: is there a relation to the headache phase of migraine? Lancet 1979; 2: 883
7. Saxena PR, Ferrari MD. From serotonin receptor classification to the antimigraine drug sumatriptan. Cephalalgia 1992; 12: 187
8. Zifa E, Fillion G. 5-Hydroxytryptamine receptors. Pharmacological Reviews 1992; 44: 402
9. Dechant KL, Clissold SP. Sumatriptan: a review of its pharmacodynamic and pharmacokinetic properties, and therapeutic efficacy in acute treatment of migraine and cluster headache. Drugs 1992; 43: 776
10. Eadie MJ. Ergotamine pharmacokinetics in man [editorial]. Cephalalgia 1983; 3: 135
11. Perrin VL. Clinical pharmacokinetics of ergotamine in migraine and cluster headache. Clinical Pharmacokinetics 1985; 10: 334
12. Sutherland JM, Hooper WD, Eadie MJ, et al. Buccal absorption of ergotamine. Journal of Neurology, Neurosurgery and Psychiatry 1974; 37: 1116
13. Waldenlind E, Ekbom K, Krabbe AAE, et al. Ergotamine for cluster headache. A pharmacokinetic study. Acta Neurologica Scandinavica 1982; 65 Suppl. 90: 83
14. Ziegler D, Ford R, Kriegler J, et al. Dihydroergotamine nasal spray for the acute treatment of migraine. Neurology 1994; 44: 447
15. Tfelt-Hansen P, Pedersen HR. Migraine prophylaxis with $5\text{-HT}_2$ partial agonists and antagonists. In: Olesen J, Saxena PR, editors. 5-Hydroxytryptamine mechanisms in primary headache. New York: Raven Press, 1992: 305
16. Müller-Schweinitzer E, Tapparelli C. Methylergometrine, an active metabolite of methysergide. Cephalalgia 1986; 6: 35
17. Fozard J. $5\text{-HT}_{1C}$ receptor agonism as an initiating event in migraine. In: Olsen J, Saxena PR, editors. 5-Hydroxy-

tryptamine in primary headache. New York: Raven Press, 1992: 200
18. Ludvigsson J. Propranolol used in prophylaxis of migraine in children. Acta Neurologica Scandinavica 1974; 50: 109
19. Wideroe TE, Vigander T. Propranolol in the treatment of migraine. British Medical Journal 1974; 2: 699
20. Stensrud P, Sjaastad O. Short-term clinical trial of propranolol in racemic form (Inderal), d-propranolol and placebo in migraine. Acta Neurologica Scandinavica 1976; 53: 233
21. Anthony M, Lance JW, Somerville B. A comparative trial of pindolol, clonidine and carbamazepine in the interval therapy of migraine. Medical Journal of Australia 1972; 1: 1343
22. Stensrud P, Sjaastad O. Comparative trial of Tenormin (atenolol) and Inderal (propranolol) in migraine. Headache 1980; 20: 206
23. Olsson J-E, Behring HC, Forssman B, et al. Metoprolol and propranolol in migraine prophylaxis: a double-blind multicentre study. Acta Neurologica Scandinavica 1984; 70: 160
24. Biggs RS, Millac PA. Timolol in migraine prophylaxis. Headache 1979; 19: 379
25. Ekbom K, Lundberg PO. Clinical trial of LB46, an adrenergic beta receptor blocking agent in migraine prophylaxis. Headache 1975; 12: 15
26. Ekbom K, Zetterman M. Oxprenolol in the treatment of migraine. Acta Neurologica Scandinavica 1977; 56: 181
27. Ekbom K. Alprenolol for migraine prophylaxis. Headache 1975; 15: 129
28. Lance JW, Anthony M, Somerville B. Comparative trial of serotonin antagonists in the management of migraine. British Medical Journal 1970; 2: 327
29. Speight TM, Avery GS. Pizotifen (BC-105): a review of its pharmacological properties and its therapeutic efficacy in vascular headaches. Drugs 1972; 3: 159
30. Peroutka SJ, Banghart SB, Allen GS. Selectivity of calcium channel antagonists for intracerebral versus peripheral vascular smooth muscle. Headache 1983; 23: 138
31. Couch JR, Hassanein RS. Amitriptyline in migraine prophylaxis. Archives of Neurology 1979; 36: 695
32. Gomersall JD, Stuart A. Amitriptyline in migraine prophylaxis. Change in pattern of attacks during a controlled clinical trial. Journal of Neurology, Neurosurgery and Psychiatry 1973; 36: 684
33. Amery WK. Flunarazine, a calcium channel blocker: a new prophylactic drug in migraine. Headache 1983; 23: 70
34. Louis P, Spierings ELH. Comparison of flunarizine (Sibelium(R)) and pizotifen (Sandomigran(R)) in migraine treatment: a double-blind study. Cephalalgia 1982; 2: 197
35. Holmes B, Brogden RN, Heel RC, et al. Flunarizine: a review of its pharmacodynamic and pharmacokinetic properties and therapeutic use. Drugs 1984; 27: 6
36. Solomon GM, Steel JG, Spaccavento LJ. Migraine prophylaxis with verapamil - a preliminary report. Headache 1983; 23: 139
37. Gelmers HJ. Nimodipine: a new calcium antagonist, in the prophylaxis of migraine. Headache 1983; 23: 106
38. Smith R, Schwartz A. Diltiazem prophylaxis in refractory migraine. New England Journal of Medicine 1984; 310: 1327
39. Kahan A, Weber S, Amor B, et al. Nifedipine in the treatment of migraine in patients with Raynaud's phenomenon. New England Journal of Medicine 1983; 308: 1102
40. Raskin NH. Acute and prophylactic treatment of migraine: practical approaches and pharmacologic rationale. Neurology 1993; 43 Suppl. 3: S39
41. Anthony M, Lance JW. Monoamine oxidase inhibition in the treatment of migraine. Archives of Neurology 1969; 21: 263
42. Ross-Lee LM, Eadie MJ, Tyrer JH. Aspirin treatment of migraine attacks: clinical observations. Cephalalgia 1982; 2: 71
43. Wainscott G, Kaspi T, Volans GN. The influence of thiethylperazine on the absorption of effervescent aspirin in migraine. British Journal of Clinical Pharmacology 1976; 3: 1015
44. Volans GN. The effect of metoclopramide on the absorption of effervescent aspirin in migraine. British Journal of Clinical Pharmacology 1975; 2: 57
45. Ross-Lee LM, Eadie MJ, Heazlewood V, et al. Aspirin pharmacokinetics in migraine. The effect of metoclopramide. European Journal of Clinical Pharmacology 1983; 24: 777
46. Pradalier A, Pancurel G, Dordain G, et al. Acute migraine attack therapy: comparison of naproxen sodium and an ergotamine tartrate compound. Cephalalgia 1985; 5: 107
47. Dahlöf C, Björkman R. Diclofenac-K (50 and 100 mg) and placebo in acute treatment of migraine. Cephalalgia 1993; 13: 117
48. Kangasniemi P, Kaaja R. Ketoprofen and ergotamine in acute migraine. Journal of Internal Medicine 1992; 231: 551-4
49. Hoffert MJ, Scholz MJ, Kanter R. A double-blind controlled study of nifedipine as an abortive treatment in acute attacks of migraine with aura. Cephalalgia 1992; 12: 323
50. MacGregor EA, Wilkinson M, Bancroft K. Domperidone plus paracetamol in the treatment of migraine. Cephalalgia 1993; 13: 124
51. Raskin NH. Pharmacology of migraine. Annual Review of Pharmacology and Toxicology 1981; 21: 463
52. Tfelt-Hansen P. Sumatriptan for the treatment of migraine attack - a review of controlled clinical trials. Cephalalgia 1993; 13: 238
53. Symonds CP. A particular variety of headache. Brain 1956; 79: 217
54. Kudrow L. Response of cluster headache attacks to oxygen inhalation. Headache 1981; 21: 1
55. Sutherland JM, Eadie MJ. Cluster headache. Research and Clinical Studies in Headache 1972; 3: 92
56. Solomon SS, Lipton RB, Newman LC. Prophylactic therapy of cluster headache. Clinical Neuropharmacology 1991; 14: 116
57. Couch JR, Ziegler DJ. Prednisone therapy for cluster headache. Headache 1978; 18: 219
58. Ekbom K. Lithium for cluster headache: review of the literature and preliminary results of long-term treatment. Headache 1981; 21: 132
59. Pearce JMS. Chronic migrainous neuralgia. A variant of cluster headache. Brain 1980; 103: 149
60. Klimek A, Azulc-Kuberska J, Kawiorski S. Lithium therapy in cluster headache. European Neurology 1979; 18: 267
61. Blom S. Trigeminal neuralgia: its treatment with a new anticonvulsant (G-32883). Lancet 1962; 1: 839
62. Court JE, Kase CS. Treatment of tic douloureux with a new anticonvulsant (clonazepam). Journal of Neurology, Neurosurgery and Psychiatry 1976; 39: 297
63. Fromm GH, Terrence CF, Chattha AS, et al. Baclofen in trigeminal neuralgia. Its effect on the spinal trigeminal nucleus. A pilot study. Archives of Neurology 1980; 37: 768
64. Ekbom K, Weserberg CE. Carbamazepine in glossopharyngeal neuralgia. Archives of Neurology 1966; 14: 595
65. Ekbom K. Carbamazepine in the treatment of tabetic lightning pains. Archives of Neurology 1972; 26: 374
66. Chakrabarti AK, Samantaray SK. Diabetic peripheral neuropathy: nerve conduction studies before, during and after carbamazepine therapy. Australian and New Zealand Journal of Medicine 1976; 6: 565
67. Galbraith AW. Treatment of acute herpes zoster with amantadine hydrochloride (Symmetrel). British Medical Journal 1973; 4: 493
68. Bernat JL. Intraspinal steroid therapy. Neurology 1981; 31: 168

69. Grant SM, Heel RC. Vigabatrin: a review of its pharmacodynamic and pharmacokinetic properties, and therapeutic potential in epilepsy and disorders of motor control. Drugs 1991; 41: 889
70. Goa KL, Ross SR, Chrisp P. Lamotrigine: a review of its pharmacological properties and clinical potential in epilepsy. Drugs 1993; 46: 152
71. Goa KL, Sorkin EM. Gabapentin: a review of its pharmacological properties and clinical potential in epilepsy. Drugs 1993; 46: 409
72. Schmidt B. Potential antiepileptic drugs. Gabapentin. In: Levy RH, Mattson R, Meldrum B, et al., editors. Antiepileptic drugs. 3rd ed. New York: Raven Press, 1989: 925
73. Grant SM, Faulds D. Oxcarbazepine: a review of its pharmacology and therapeutic potential in epilepsy, trigeminal neuralgia and affective disorders. Drugs 1992; 43: 873
74. Eadie MJ, Tyrer JH. Anticonvulsant therapy. Pharmacological basis and practice. 3rd ed. Edinburgh: Churchill-Livingstone, 1989
75. Levy RH, Mattson R, Meldrum B, et al., editors. Antiepileptic drugs. 3rd ed. New York: Raven Press, 1989
76. Ressor Jr SR, Kutt H, editors. The medical treatment of epilepsy. New York: Marcel Dekker, 1992
77. Rogawski MA, Porter RJ. Antiepileptic drugs: pharmacological mechanisms and clinical efficacy with consideration of promising developmental stage compounds. Pharmacological Reviews 1990; 42: 223
78. Snead III OC. Basic mechanisms of generalized absence seizures. Annals of Neurology 1995; 37: 146
79. Taylor CP. Emerging perspectives on the mechanism of action of gababentin. Neurology 1994; 44 Suppl. 5: S10
80. Hoppener RJ, Kuyer A, Meijer JWA, et al. Correlations between daily fluctuations of carbamazepine serum levels and intermittent side effects. Epilepsia 1980; 21: 341
81. Eadie MJ. Metabolism of anticonvulsant drugs. Reviews on Drug Metabolism and Drug Interactions 1981; 3: 317
82. Bialer M. Comparative pharmacokinetics of the newer antiepileptic drugs. Clinical Pharmacokinetics 1993; 24: 441
83. Schmidt D, Haenel F. Therapeutic plasma levels of phenytoin, phenobarbital and carbamazepine: individual variation in relation to seizure frequency and type. Neurology 1984; 34: 1252
84. Turnbull DM, Rawlins MD, Weightman F, et al. 'Therapeutic' serum concentration of phenytoin: the influence of seizure type. Journal of Neurology, Neurosurgery and Psychiatry 1984; 47: 231
85. Sander JWAS, Patsalos PN. An assessment of serum and red blood cell folate concentrations in patients with epilepsy on lamotrigine therapy. Epilepsy Research 1992; 13: 89
86. Perucca E, Richens A. Anticonvulsant drug interactions. In: Tyrer JH, editor. The treatment of epilepsy. Lancaster: MTP Press, 1980: 95
87. Perucca E. Pharmacokinetic interactions with antiepileptic drugs. Clinical Pharmacokinetics 1982; 7: 57
88. Eadie MJ. Anticonvulsant drugs: an update. Drugs 1984; 27: 328
89. Patsalos PN, Duncan JS. Antiepileptic drugs: a review of clinically significant drug interactions. Drug Safety 1993; 9: 156
90. Commission on Classification and Terminology of the International League Against Epilepsy: Proposal for revised classification of epilepsies and epileptic syndromes. Epilepsia 1989; 30: 389
91. Zimmerman HJ, Ishak KG. Valproate-induced hepatic injury. Analysis of 23 fatal cases. Hepatology 1982; 2: 591
92. Farwell J, Milstein J, Opheim K, et al. Adrenocorticotrophic hormone controls infantile spasms independently of cortisol stimulation. Epilepsia 1984; 25: 605
93. Omtzigt JGC, Los FJ, Grobbee DE, et al. The risk of spina bifida aperta after first-trimester exposure to valproate in a prenatal cohort. Neurology 1992; 42 Suppl. 5: 119
94. Mattson RH, Cramer JA, Collins JF, et al. Comparison of carbamazepine, phenobarbital, phenytoin and primidone in partial and secondarily generalised tonic-clonic seizures. New England Journal of Medicine 1985; 313: 145
95. Richens A, Davidson DLW, Cartlidge NEF, et al. A multicentre comparative trial of sodium valproate and carbamazepine in adult onset epilepsy. Journal of Neurology, Neurosurgery and Psychiatry 1994; 57: 682
96. Eichelbaum M, Tomson T, Tybring G, et al. Carbamazepine metabolism in man: induction and pharmacogenetic aspects. Clinical Pharmacokinetics 1985; 10: 80
97. Hirtz DG, Nelson KB. The natural history of febrile seizures. Annual Review of Medicine 1983; 34: 453
98. Wolf SM. Controversies in the treatment of febrile convulsions. Neurology 1979; 29: 287
99. Faero O, Kastrup KW, Lykkegaard Neilsen E, et al. Successful prophylaxis of febrile convulsions with phenobarbital. Epilepsia 1972; 13: 279
100. Bacon CJ, Hierons AM, Mucklow JC, et al. Placebo controlled study of phenobarbitone and phenytoin in the prophylaxis of febrile convulsions. Lancet 1981; 2: 600
101. Melchior JC, Buchthal F, Lennox-Buchthal MA. The ineffectiveness of diphenylhydantoin in preventing febrile convulsions in the age of greatest risk, under three years. Epilepsia 1971; 12: 55
102. Camfield PR, Camfield CS, Tibbles JA. Carbamazepine does not prevent febrile seizures in phenobarbital failures. Neurology 1982; 32: 288
103. Dam M, Christiansen J, Munck O, et al. Antiepileptic drugs: metabolism in pregnancy. Clinical Pharmacokinetics 1979; 4: 53
104. Lander CM, Smith MT, Chalk JB, et al. Bioavailability and pharmacokinetics of phenytoin during pregnancy. European Journal of Clinical Pharmacology 1984; 27: 105
105. Delgardo-Escueta AV, Janz D. Consensus guidelines: preconception counselling, management, and care of the pregnant woman with epilepsy. Neurology 1992; 42 Suppl. 5: 149
106. Kaneko S, Otani K, Kondo T, et al. Malformations in infants of mothers with epilepsy receiving antiepileptic drugs. Neurology 1992; 42 Suppl. 5: 68
107. Solomon GE, Hilgartner MW, Kutt H. Coagulation defect caused by diphenylhydantoin. Neurology 1972; 22: 1165
108. Nau H, Kunz W, Egger H-J, et al. Anticonvulsants during pregnancy and lactation: transplacental, maternal and neonatal pharmacokinetics. Clinical Pharmacokinetics 1982; 7: 508
109. Hillestad L, Hansen T, Melsom H, et al. Diazepam metabolism in normal man. 1. Serum concentrations and clinical effects after intravenous, intramuscular and oral administration. Clinical Pharmacology and Therapeutics 1974; 16: 479
110. Kostenbauder HB, Rapp RP, McGovern JP, et al. Bioavailability and single dose pharmacokinetics of intramuscular phenytoin. Clinical Pharmacology and Therapeutics 1975; 18: 449
111. Galvin GM, Jelnick GA. Successful treatment of 75 patients in status epilepticus with intravenous midazolam. Emergency Medicine 1992; 4: 11
112. Giroud M, Gras D, Escousse A, et al. Use of injectable valproic acid in status epilepticus. Drug Investigation 1993; 5: 154
113. Anggard E, Johnsson LE, Hogmark AL, et al. Amphetamine metabolism in amphetamine psychosis. Clinical Pharmacology and Therapeutics 1973; 14: 870
114. Heinemeyer G. Clinical pharmacokinetic considerations in the treatment of increased intracranial pressure. Clinical Pharmacokinetics 1987; 13: 1

115. Chalk JB, Ridgeway K, Brophy TRO'R, et al. Phenytoin impairs the bioavailability of dexamethasone in neurological and neurosurgical patients. Journal of Neurology, Neurosurgery and Psychiatry 1984; 47: 1087
116. Pitlick WH, Pirikitakuhir P, Painter MJ, et al. Effects of glycerol and hyperosmolality on intracranial pressure. Clinical Pharmacology and Therapeutics 1982; 31: 466
117. Lee DAH, Taylor GM, Walker JG, et al. The effect of concurrent administration of antacids on prednisolone absorption. British Journal of Clinical Pharmacology 1979; 8: 92
118. Morrison PJ, Rogers HJ, Bradbook ID, et al. Concurrent administration of cimetidine and enteric-coated prednisolone: effect on plasma level of prednisolone. British Journal of Clinical Pharmacology 1980; 1: 87
119. Brophy TRO'R, Chalk JB, Ridgeway K, et al. Cortisol production during high dose dexamethasone therapy in neurological and neurosurgical patients. Journal of Neurology, Neurosurgery and Psychiatry 1984; 47: 1081
120. Sahar A, Tsipstein E. Effects of mannitol and furosemide on the rate of formation of cerebro-spinal fluid. Experimental Neurology 1978; 60: 584
121. Rea CL, Rockswold GL. Barbiturate therapy in uncontrolled intracranial hypertension. Neurosurgery 1983; 12: 401
122. Rockoff MA, Marshall LF, Shapiro HM. High-dose barbiturate therapy in humans: a clinical review of patients. Annals of Neurology 1979; 6: 194
123. Kopin IJ. The pharmacology of Parkinson's disease therapy: an update. Annual Review of Pharmacology and Toxicology 1993; 32: 281
124. Rossor MN. Parkinson's disease and Alzheimer's disease as disorders of the isodendritic core. British Medical Journal 1981; 283: 1588
125. Civelli O, Bunzow JR, Grandy DK. Molecular diversity of dopamine receptors. Annual Review of Pharmacology and Toxicology 1993; 32: 281
126. Greenberg DA. Glutamate and Parkinson's disease. Annals of Neurology 1994; 35: 639
127. Akoi FY, Sitar DS. Clinical pharmacokinetics of amantadine hydrochloride. Clinical Pharmacokinetics 1988; 14: 35
128. Parkes JD. Bromocriptine in the treatment of Parkinsonism. Drugs 1979; 17: 365
129. Langtry HD, Clissold SP. Pergolide: a review of its pharmacological properties and therapeutic potential in Parkinson's disease. Drugs 1990; 39: 491
130. Cedarbaum JE. Clinical pharmacokinetics of anti-Parkinsonian drugs. Clinical Pharmacokinetics 1987; 13: 141
131. Iversen LI. Neurotransmitters and CNS disease. Introduction. Lancet 1982; 2: 914
132. Nutt JG, Fellman JH. Pharmacokinetics of levodopa. Clinical Neuropharmacology 1984; 7: 35
133. Chrisp P, Mammen GJ, Sorkin EM. Selegiline: a review of its pharmacology, symptomatic benefits and protective potential in Parkinson's disease. Drugs & Aging 1991; 1: 228
134. Eisler T, Teravainen H, Nelson R, et al. Deprenyl in Parkinson's disease. Neurology 1981; 31: 19
135. Quinn NP. Anti-Parkinsonian drugs today. Drugs 1984; 28: 236
136. Parkinson Study Group. DATATOP: a multicentre controlled clinical trial in early Parkinson's disease. Archives of Neurology 1989; 46: 1052
137. McKillop D, Bradford HF. Comparative effects of benztropine and nomifensine on dopamine uptake and release from striatal synaptosomes. Biochemical Pharmacology 1981; 30: 2753
138. Laihinen A, Rinne UK, Suchy I. Comparison of lisuride and bromocriptine in the treatment of advanced Parkinson's disease. Acta Neurologica Scandinavica 1992; 86: 593
139. Lieberman AN, Goldstein M, Leibowitz M, et al. Lisuride combined with levodopa in advanced Parkinson's disease. Neurology 1981; 1: 1466
140. Lesser RP, Fahn S, Snider SR, et al. Analysis of the clinical problems in Parkinsonism and the complications of long-term levodopa therapy. Neurology 1979; 29: 1253
141. Rajput AH, Stern W, Laverty WH. Chronic low-dose levodopa therapy in Parkinson's disease: an argument for delaying levodopa therapy. Neurology 1984; 34: 991
142. Muenter MD. Should levodopa therapy be started early or late? Canadian Journal of Neurological Sciences 1984; 11: 195
143. Marsden CD, Parkes JD, Quinn N. Fluctuations of disability in Parkinson's disease - clinical aspects. In: Marsden CD, Fahn S, editors. Movement disorders. London: Butterworth Scientific, 1982: 96
144. LeWitt PA. Clinical studies with and pharmacokinetic considerations of sustained-release levodopa. Neurology 1992; 42 Suppl. 1: 29
145. Quinn N, Marsden CD, Parkes JD. Complicated response fluctuations in Parkinson's disease: response to intravenous infusion of levodopa. Lancet 1982; 2: 412
146. Quinn N, Parkes JD, Marsden CD. Control of on/off phenomenon by continuous intravenous infusion of levodopa. Neurology 1984; 34: 1131
147. Kurth MC, Tetrud JW, Irwin I, et al. Oral levodopa/carbidopa solution versus tablets in Parkinson's patient with severe fluctuations: a pilot study. Neurology 1993; 43: 1036
148. Wooten GF. Progress in understanding the pathophysiology of treatment-related fluctuations in Parkinson's disease. Annals of Neurology 1988; 24: 363
149. Koller WC, Weiner WJ, Perlik S, et al. Complications of chronic levodopa therapy: long term efficacy of drug holiday. Neurology 1981; 31: 473
150. Lees AJ, Stern GM. Sustained bromocriptine therapy in previously untouched Parkinson's disease. Journal of Neurology, Neurosurgery and Psychiatry 1981; 44: 1020
151. Rascol A, Guiraud B, Montastruc JL, et al. Long-term treatment of Parkinson's disease with bromocriptine. Journal of Neurology, Neurosurgery and Psychiatry 1979; 42: 143
152. Przuntek H, Welzel D, Blümner E, et al. Bromocriptine lessens the incidence of mortality in L-dopa-treated parkinsonian patients: PRADO study discontinued. European Journal of Clinical Pharmacology 1992; 43: 357
153. Friedman JH, Lannon MC. Clozapine in the treatment of psychosis in Parkinson's disease. Neurology 1989; 39: 1219
154. Stahl SM, Berger PA. Bromocriptine, physostigmine, and neurotransmitter mechanisms in the dystonias. Neurology 1982; 32: 889
155. Ziegler DK. Prolonged relief of dystonic movements with diazepam. Neurology 1981; 31: 1457
156. Garg BP. Dystonia musculorum deformans. Implications of therapeutic response to levodopa and carbamazepine. Archives of Neurology 1982; 39: 376
157. Burke RE, Fahn S, Marsden D. Torsion-dystonia: a double-blind, prospective trial of high-dosage trihexphenidyl. Neurology 1986; 36: 160
158. Morris JGL. Involuntary movement disorders. In: Eadie MJ, editor. Drug therapy in neurology. Edinburgh: Churchill-Livingstone, 1992: 291
159. Marsden CD, Fahn S. Problems in dyskinesias. In: Marsden CD, Fahn S, editors. Movement disorders. London: Butterworth Scientific, 1982: 191
160. Dietrichson P, Espen E. Effects of timolol and atenolol on benign essential tremor: placebo-controlled studies based on quantitative tremor recording. Journal of Neurology, Neurosurgery and Psychiatry 1981; 44: 677
161. Calzetti S, Findley LJ, Gresty MA, et al. Metoprolol and propranolol in essential tremor: a double blind controlled study. Journal of Neurology, Neurosurgery and Psychiatry 1981; 44: 814
162. Leigh PN, Jefferson D, Twomey A, et al. Beta-adrenoceptor mechanisms in essential tremor; a double-blind placebo controlled trial of metoprolol, sotalol and atenolol. Jour-

nal of Neurology, Neurosurgery and Psychiatry 1983; 46: 710

163. Chakrabarti A, Pearce JMS. Essential tremor: response to primidone. Journal of Neurology, Neurosurgery and Psychiatry 1981; 44: 650
164. Sweet RD. The pharmacology of athetosis. In: Barbeau, editor. Disorders of movement. Lancaster: MTP Press, 1981: 43
165. Penn RD, Savory SM, Corcos D, et al. Intrathecal baclofen for severe spinal spasticity. New England Journal of Medicine 1989; 320: 1517
166. Davidoff RA. Pharmacology of spasticity. Neurology 1978; 28: 46
167. Young RR, Delwaide PJ. Drug therapy. Spasticity. New England Journal of Medicine 1981; 304: 96
168. Lindstom J, Dau P. Biology of myasthenia gravis. Annual Review of Pharmacology and Toxicology 1980; 20: 337
169. Havard CWH, Scadding GK. Myasthenia gravis: pathogenesis and current concepts in management. Drugs 1983; 26: 174
170. Kornfeld P, Ambinder EP, Mittag T, et al. Plasmapheresis in refractory generalised myasthenia gravis. Archives of Neurology 1981; 38: 478
171. Shah A, Lisak RP. Immunopharmacologic therapy in myasthenia gravis. Clinical Neuropharmacology 1993; 16: 97
172. Morris RB, Cronnelly R, Miller RD, et al. Pharmacokinetics of edrophonium and neostigmine when antagonising d-tubocurarine neuromuscular blockade in man. Anaesthesiology 1981; 54: 399
173. Solomani SM, Chan K, Dehghan A, et al. Kinetics and metabolism of intramuscular neostigmine in myasthenia gravis. Clinical Pharmacology and Therapeutics 1980; 28: 64
174. Aquilonius S-M, Eckemas S-A, Hartvig P, et al. Clinical pharmacology of pyridostigmine and neostigmine in patients with myasthenia gravis. Journal of Neurology, Neurosurgery and Psychiatry 1983; 46: 929
175. Newsom-Davis J. Myasthenia. In: Crow, editor. Disorders of neurohumoral transmission. London: Academic Press, 1982: 7
176. Murray NMF, Newsom-Davis J. Treatment with oral 4-aminopyridine in disorders of neuromuscular transmission. Neurology 1981; 31: 265
177. Karli P, Bergstom L. Effect of baclofen on myotonia. Lancet 1974; 1: 1285
178. Durelli L, Mutani R, Fassio F. The treatment of myotonia: evaluation of chronic oral taurine therapy. Neurology 1993; 33: 599
179. Jarrell MA, Greer M, Maren TH. The effect of acidosis in hypokalemic periodic paralysis. Archives of Neurology 1976; 33: 791
180. McArdle BJ. Adynamia episodica hereditaria and its treatment. Brain 1962; 85: 121
181. Dyck PJ. Intravenous immunoglobulin in chronic inflammatory demyelinating polyneuropathy and in neuropathy associated with IgM monoclonal gammopathy of uncertain significance. Neurology 1990; 40: 327
182. Noseworthy JH. Therapeutics of multiple sclerosis. Clinical Neuropharmacology 1991; 14: 49
183. Milligan NM, Newcombe R, Compston DAS. A double-blind controlled trial of high dose methylprednisolone in patients with multiple sclerosis: 1. Clinical effects. Journal of Neurology, Neurosurgery and Psychiatry 1987; 50: 511
184. British and Dutch Multiple Sclerosis Azathioprine Trial Group. Double-blind masked trial of azathioprine in multiple sclerosis. Lancet 1988; 2: 179
185. The IFNB Multiple Sclerosis Study Group. Interferon beta-1b is effective in relapsing-remitting multiple sclerosis. Neurology 1993; 43: 655
186. Sila CA. Prophylaxis and treatment of stroke. The state of the art in 1993. Drugs 1993; 45: 329
187. Anderson DC, Cranford RE. Corticosteroids in ischemic stroke. Stroke 1979; 10: 68
188. Wadworth AN, McTavish D. Nimodipine: a review of its pharmacological properties, and therapeutic efficacy in cerebral disorders. Drugs & Aging 1992; 2: 262
189. Adams Jr HP. Current status of antifibrinolytic therapy for treatment of patients with aneurysmal subarachnoid hemorrhage. Stroke 1982; 13: 256
190. McTavish D, Faulds D, Goa KL. Ticlopidine: an updated review of its pharmacology and therapeutic use in platelet-related disorders. Drugs 1990; 40: 238
191. Ramirez-Lassepas M. Platelet inhibitors for TIAS. A review of prospective drug trial results. Postgraduate Medicine 1984; 75: 52
192. De Gaetano G, Cerletti C, Beriele V. Pharmacology of anti-platelet drugs and clinical trials on thrombosis prevention: a difficult link. Lancet 1982; 2: 974
193. Pedersen AK, FitzGerald GA. Dose-related kinetics of aspirin. Presystemic acetylation of platelet cyclo-oxygenase. New England Journal of Medicine 1984; 311: 1206
194. Hass WK, Easton JD, Adams Jr HP, et al. A randomized trial comparing ticlopidine hydrochloride with aspirin for the prevention of stroke in high risk patients. New England Journal of Medicine 1989; 321: 501
195. Sorrell TC, Gilbert GL. Infections. In: Eadie MJ, editor. Drug therapy in neurology. Edinburgh: Churchill-Livingstone, 1992: 421
196. Manzoor M, Runcie R. Folate-responsive neuropathy: report of 10 cases. British Medical Journal 1976; 1: 1176
197. Bergstom RF, Kay DR, Harkcom TM, et al. Penicillamine kinetics in normal subjects. Clinical Pharmacology and Therapeutics 1981; 30: 404
198. Walshe JM. Treatment of Wilson's disease with trientine (triethylene tetramine) dihydrochloride. Lancet 1982; 1: 643
199. Kaye AH. Neoplasia. In: Eadie MJ, editor. Drug therapy in neurology. Edinburgh: Churchill-Livingstone, 1992: 401
200. Taverner D, Kemble F, Cohen SB. Prognosis and treatment of idiopathic facial (Bell's) palsy. British Medical Journal 1957; 4: 581
201. Garland H. Diabetic amyotrophy. In: Williams, editor. Modern trends in neurology. 2nd Series. London: Butterworth, 1957: 229
202. Nattero G, Lisino F, Brandi G, et al. Reserpine for migraine prophylaxis. Headache 1976; 15: 279
203. Hanington E. Diet and migraine. Journal of Human Nutrition and Dietetics 1980; 34: 175
204. Bryan GE, Marsh EE, Jabbari B, et al. Incidence of seizures in patients receiving tricyclic and tetracyclic antidepressants. Annals of Neurology 1983; 14: 153
205. Olesen LL, Jensen TS. Presentation and management of drug-induced peripheral neuropathy. Drug Safety 1991; 6: 302
206. Lane RJM, Mastalgia FL. Drug-induced myopathies in man. Lancet 1978; 2: 562

Chapter 30

# Psychiatric Disorders

*M. Lader*

## Synopsis of Important Principles

1) Psychotropic drugs comprise several classes of agent, each with a distinct pharmacology. The biochemical effects of these compounds are known in some detail but how these relate to their therapeutic properties often remains obscure. However, most of the adverse effects of psychotropic drugs are explicable in terms of their pharmacological actions.

2) Accordingly, the use of psychotropic drugs is empirical rather than rational. These drugs are not generally curative, but accelerate recovery and prevent or postpone relapse in the course of schizophrenic, manic-depressive and depressive disorders, and provide short term adjunctive symptomatic relief in anxiety and insomnia.

3) The antipsychotic drugs, lithium and the antidepressants are powerful compounds and should be reserved for use in major psychiatric conditions. The anxiolytics and hypnotics, with a few exceptions, have a dependence-inducing liability and should only be used short term or intermittently. They should never be used for trivial indications or in lieu of sympathetic supportive therapy.

4) Drug treatment is not indicated for everyone who complains of depression, anxiety, tension or poor sleep. Excessive reliance on medication may prove counter-productive in suppressing the patient's own coping mechanisms.

5) Most classes of psychotropic drugs have been known for several decades and many compounds are available in each class. The clinician should learn to use a few psychotropic drugs well. On the other hand, the last few years have seen the introduction of newer, more selective compounds and the clinician should not be over-conservative in ignoring them.

6) Individual variability in response is quite marked with most psychotropic drugs. Initial dosage must be cautious, especially in the elderly, but the dosage should then be increased until a clinical response occurs, adverse effects become intolerable, or the generally accepted safe maximum level is reached.

7) With some drugs such as the antidepressants and antipsychotics, it is better to treat for a little longer than is strictly necessary rather than to terminate the course of treatment prematurely and risk relapse. Some agents, such as lithium, may be continued indefinitely. With others, e.g. the anxiolytics and hypnotics, the duration should be minimised.

8) Poor compliance is a major problem with psychotropic drugs and stems from their numerous and often severe adverse effects, which may mimic symptoms of the condition for which they are prescribed. In addition, the psychopathology or personality of the patient may be antagonistic to drug usage. Simple psychotherapeutic measures such as support, reassurance and information about possible adverse effects are essential to gain the confidence of the patient and to maximise compliance and cooperation.

The modern era of psychopharmacology started in the 1950s with the introduction of chlorpromazine (the first antipsychotic drug) and lithium, and later in that decade, the two major groups of antidepressants, the tricyclics and the monoamine oxidase inhibitors. Soon after, the benzodiazepines were introduced as anxiolytics and hypnotics, and for a while were the most successful commercially of all drug groups. The efficacy of psychotropic drugs, although often partial, led to a revival of interest in the biological aspects of psychiatry, which in many countries had been eclipsed by psychoanalytic theory and practice. Sometimes, however, the pendulum swung too far and uncritical espousal of the utility of psychotropic drugs led to their overuse, with consequent concern by both medical and lay people. The safety of these compounds was also overestimated in many instances.

The introduction of antipsychotic drugs coincided with a more liberal attitude to the mentally ill in many countries. This has resulted in a return of these psychotic people to the community, all too often with inadequate or inexpert supervision. Many psychiatric hospitals have closed or contracted to a fraction of their previous size. Often when a patient relapses in the community, readmission proves difficult or he/she has to be discharged prematurely. Antipsychotic medication is known to postpone if not prevent relapse and to shorten the acute episode when it does occur. Compliance, however, is poor because of unwanted effects such as sedation and restlessness. The usual way to improve compliance has been to use injectable depot preparations and these have made community care much more practicable. More recently, antipsychotic drugs have been introduced with better adverse effect profiles, although improved compliance has not yet been demonstrated. The advent of clozapine, with its improved efficacy, has been a major influence in encouraging the development of new antipsychotic drugs, but so far it remains unique as a therapy in specialist practice.

The antidepressant field has also undergone major changes in the past decade. The earlier drugs, which were discovered largely by accident, have multiple actions. In contrast, the newer drugs are more selective; although their efficacy is no greater, their adverse effect profiles are generally much less complicated and severe. For example, the reversible and selective inhibitors of type A monoamine oxidase (MAO-A) can be prescribed without real dietary precautions. Again, however, the improved adverse effect profile has not been shown to result in better compliance, although this is widely assumed to be the case.

Concern about the long term dependence potential of the benzodiazepines has led to the development of several new types of antianxiety drug, mostly acting via serotonin [5-hydroxytryptamine (5-HT)] mechanisms,[1] e.g. buspirone which has had limited success in a market dominated by the benzodiazepines. However, the trend has been to limit the prescription of antianxiety medication in general and to explore the use of non-pharmacological methods of treatment. In the case of hypnotics, no pharmacological alternatives to the benzodiazepines have appeared, although chemically distinct compounds with some advantages have been marketed. The widespread and long term use of hypnotic drugs remains a source of concern.

Recently, dementia has excited much research interest. The demographics of most Western countries predict an aging population with an increasing burden of demented individuals. Although various compounds have been available to treat behavioural and cognitive deficits symptomatically, none has proved to have really useful clinical effectiveness. Many newer compounds are being researched intensively and some are at the point of marketing.

Other indications for which drug therapy is now playing a bigger role include obsessive-compulsive disorder, the eating disorders and some sleep disorders.

## 1. Clinical Pharmacological Considerations

### 1.1 Pharmacodynamic Considerations

#### *1.1.1 Nomenclature*

The usual way to classify psychotropic drugs is in terms of their main indication, although the severity of the indication may be difficult to measure.[2] Thus, agents used to treat psychosis are 'antipsychotics'; those used to treat depression are 'antidepressants'; and those used to treat anxiety are 'antianxiety drugs'. Older terms are still extant, e.g. hypnotic or sedative for anti-insomnia drugs, and neuroleptic or ataraxic for antipsychotic drugs. This still leaves many classes for which clumsy terms exist. Lithium is classified as a 'mood-stabilising agent', but there is no accepted term for a drug that treats bulimia nervosa.

The alternative method, to classify according to biochemical action, is inappropriate, as many therapeutic effects may ensue. For example, a drug that binds to benzodiazepine receptors may be an antianxiety agent, an hypnotic, muscle relaxant, antiepileptic, or an anaesthetic.

#### 1.1.2 Multiple Actions of Psychotropic Drugs

Most psychotropic drug classes were discovered by accident in the search for other types of compound (the principle of serendipity). Also, as most are over 30 years old, they were developed before techniques of receptor binding allowed the selection of specific types of compound.[3] Thus, most psychotropic compounds have multiple actions resulting from effects on several receptor systems. In addition, these receptor systems, e.g. dopamine or serotonin (5-HT), have multiple actions in the brain. Thus, serotonin is involved in the regulation of mood, appetite, temperature, etc.[4]

Because of this, many psychotropic drugs have multiple therapeutic actions and also complex adverse effect profiles. Differences among classes are translated into complex therapeutic choices, and this may often have to be on a patient-by-patient basis. Thus, one patient suffering from schizophrenia may dislike feeling sedated; another may be upset by the feeling of restlessness (akathisia) which an antipsychotic drug may induce. A depressed patient may be greatly inconvenienced by constipation which his/her tricyclic antidepressant may exacerbate; another may tolerate this but be concerned by impaired sexual functioning. Knowledge of 3 or 4 drugs within each class is important so that the best-tolerated medication can be prescribed. Occasionally, more esoteric choices may be necessary; for example, the patient with recent myocardial infarction needs the least cardiotoxic drug.

Some unwanted effects are common to several groups of drugs. The most notable is sedation, which occurs with most antipsychotics, antidepressants, antianxiety drugs, and with hypnotics the next morning. The sedation is associated with psychomotor and cognitive impairment, memory in particular often being disrupted in subtle ways. When patients are treated in hospital, sedation is unimportant or even welcomed by the patient and his/her attendants. Nowadays, patients treated in the community are often attempting to keep at work, and sedation is unacceptable. Usually, a non-sedative alternative can be found.

The multiple actions of psychotropic drugs can be turned to advantage. For example, the tricyclic antidepressants can be used to treat premature ejaculation. The prolactin-elevating properties of some antipsychotic drugs are useful in women with infertility secondary to hypoprolactinaemia. Even the sedative actions of antipsychotic drugs have been used to tranquillise non-psychotic but agitated patients – hence the formerly used term 'major tranquilliser'.

### 1.2 Pharmacokinetic Considerations

The pharmacokinetic characteristics of each class of psychotropic drugs are outlined in subsequent sections (i.e. sections 3 to 6). Only the general principles pertaining to psychotropic drugs are discussed here.

To exert an effect, psychotropic drugs must enter the brain. To do this they must be lipophilic in order to cross the blood-brain barrier. In general, most psychotropic drugs are highly lipophilic and this has several important consequences.

**Absorption**

Psychotropic drugs are usually rapidly and completely absorbed from the gastrointestinal tract when given orally, but after intramuscular injection, their absorption may not be particularly rapid because the drug can be taken up by the surrounding muscular tissue. With oral administration, the usual considerations concerning the degree of ionisation of the drug pertain (see chapter 1); psychotropic drugs may be acidic, but are more usually alkaline, and sometimes amphoteric. Absorption is typically from the upper intestine and can be slowed by the presence of food.

**Distribution**

After absorption, some psychotropic drugs penetrate rapidly into the brain but may show significant redistribution (e.g. to a lipid compartment) which governs the duration of action; diazepam is an example of a drug whose initial effects appear to be reduced by this process. Being lipophilic, most psychotropic drugs have a large apparent volume of distribution.

**Elimination**

Because they are lipophilic, psychotropic drugs (with the exception of lithium) cannot be excreted by the kidney. Thus, metabolism is necessary to convert them to compounds that are more polar and water soluble.[5] The metabolic processes involved can be either phase I (oxidation, etc.) and/or phase II (conjugation) reactions; the metabolites formed are then excreted in the urine. Compounds that undergo phase I metabolic reactions tend to have longer half-lives in the elderly and in those with hepatic dysfunction. Drugs that undergo only phase II reactions are much less affected and are generally to be preferred in such patients (although the conjugated metabolites of drugs that undergo phase II metabolism may accumulate in the elderly because of decreased renal function in this age group). Drug interactions also tend to be less marked with these drugs than with those that undergo phase I metabolic reactions.

## 2. General Principles of Treatment

Some general principles of treatment are relevant to psychotropic drugs, although they are not unique to this class of drugs.

1) ***Diagnosis and assessment of the response to treatment:*** the diagnosis of psychiatric illness is less precise compared with most other branches of medicine.[6] Consequently, drug treatments are generally directed towards symptoms or syndromes and rarely towards disorders. Also, the boundary between normality and pathology is often unclear, arbitrary or highly subjective, and the clinician must avoid attempting to treat normal worry and misery, or eccentric behaviour, with powerful psychotropic drugs.

The therapeutic effect of psychotropic drugs is to suppress symptoms until either natural remission occurs or the treatment is discontinued. Often, it is difficult to discern when remission has occurred and a cautious trial of discontinuation with a tapering dosage may be needed. In some cases, indefinite treatment may be needed, unless the risks of inducing dependence outweigh the continuing therapeutic benefit.

2) ***Maintenance or prophylactic therapy?*** Many psychiatric conditions are intermittent rather than chronic, or are characterised by acute episodes superimposed on a background of low-grade morbidity. It is therefore important to distinguish between maintenance therapy and prophylactic therapy. In the former, the treatment is directed towards preventing the recrudescence of symptoms in the current episode. In the latter, the treatment is aimed to prevent further episodes after a symptom-free ('well') period.

3) ***Multiple therapeutic effects of psychotropic drugs:*** because of the imprecise nature of psychiatric nosology, the non-specificity of many drugs, and the complexities of brain function, psychotropic drugs have several therapeutic actions (see also section 1.1.2).

4) ***Establishing the optimum dosage:*** the dosages of psychotropic drugs vary widely from patient to patient. With older drugs, doses tended to be increased until adverse effects occurred. For example, it was hypothesised at one time that an antipsychotic drug could not exert any useful therapeutic effect until incipient extrapyramidal movement disorders were induced. With newer drugs, however, standardised dosages are generally appropriate, but because adverse effects no longer provide an end-point, dosages have to be established directly in terms of the clinical response.

Some psychotropic drugs show a delay in onset of action. Sometimes this is real, e.g. with MAO inhibitors, but for others it is more apparent than real, as the clinical response is gradual and special care is needed to detect the first signs of improvement. Nevertheless, the time scales imposed delay establishment of an appropriate dosage. When injectable depot antipsychotic drugs are used, the process may stretch out into months.

5) ***Duration of treatment:*** this depends on many factors, the most important being the natural history of the treated condition. With antipsychotic and antidepressant medication, the trend is to lengthen treatment, as it has become apparent that schizophrenic episodes and depressive illnesses follow a fairly long time-course. With prophylactic treatment, life-long drug usage may be needed.

6) ***Drug selection and use in specific patient groups:*** the young, the elderly and the physically ill need special considerations in terms of choice of drug, dosage and duration of treatment. Often data are incomplete in these groups. Sometimes they are completely lacking for children and scanty for the physically ill. Even where drugs are mainly used in the elderly, such as hypnotics, data are insufficient, at least with respect to toxicity.

7) ***Concomitant use of non-pharmacological treatments:*** psychological treatment methods are playing an increasingly important role in the management of the mentally ill. This trend has accelerated recently, as the deficiencies of psychotropic drug treatment have been documented. Unfortunately, many of the tech-

niques used have been inadequately evaluated, and some of the more esoteric have no efficacy data to support their use. Despite this, some areas of therapy have accrued a worthwhile body of data. The more mature areas, e.g. management of anxious patients, are now concentrating on the relative indications for drug and non-drug treatments, and how they can be best combined.

Finally, it must be constantly borne in mind that psychiatrists in many countries work under supervisory and legal restraints not imposed on clinicians in other areas of medicine. It is even more important, therefore, that they learn to use psychotropic drugs wisely and well.

## 3. Psychosis and Schizophrenia

Psychosis is a mental disorder characterised by loss of touch with reality. Hallucinations, delusions and thought disorder are common features. The psychosis can be organic or functional. Organic psychoses result from detectable brain abnormalities such as trauma and vascular insufficiency. These psychoses often include clouding of consciousness, confusion and delirium.

The most important of the common psychoses is schizophrenia. It is, however, a spectrum of mental disorders and it is becoming increasingly evident that many sufferers have detectable brain changes such as expanded ventricles. Schizophrenia was originally thought to include a progressive deterioration of mental functions with thought disorder, emotional blunting, hallucinations and delusions. However, most patients have acute psychotic episodes, recover at least partially in between, and the course is by no means one of inevitable deterioration. It is important to emphasise that the diagnosis of schizophrenia is a value judgement on the part of the involved professionals and for some patients, disagreements may occur.

The symptoms of schizophrenia are thought disorder in which the train of thought may stop or alien thoughts are reported. The patient may believe his/her thoughts are being broadcast to the world. Hallucinatory voices are very common and may talk to the patient or talk about him/her in the third person. Visual hallucinations, sensations of heat, cold, pain and sexual feelings may be complained of. Emotional disorders include secondary depression, anxiety, elation or perplexity. Emotional responses may be flattened or incongruous. The patient may become hostile, aggressive and destructive. Very occasionally, the patient may become emotionless and empty or even enter a catatonic stupor. In the later stages of schizophrenia, the symptoms become very negative with social withdrawal, lack of motivation and deterioration in personal care. However, in some patients, the clinical picture is dominated by these features from the start.

About 1% of adults suffer from schizophrenia and there is an increased representation of the lower social classes. There is a definite genetic loading. Schizophrenia is associated with social isolation and sufferers drift down the social scale. There is a major load on carers, and the medical and social services. Despite the advent of antipsychotic medication, the long term prognosis has not really improved.[7]

### 3.1 Clinical Pharmacology of Drugs Used in Treatment

Antipsychotic drugs were among the first of the modern psychotropic drugs to be introduced, starting with chlorpromazine in the early 1950s. These drugs have also been called 'neuroleptics' as an acknowledgment of their readiness to induce movement disorders, and 'major tranquillisers' by virtue of their ability to control violently disturbed behaviour of whatever aetiology. However, their main utility and use is in treating the acute symptoms of schizophrenic disorder and preventing further relapse.

The main chemical groups of antipsychotic drugs are:

1) The phenothiazines (aliphatic, piperidine and piperazine subtypes).

2) The thioxanthenes.

3) The butyrophenones.

4) The substituted benzamides.

All affect dopamine mechanisms, but typically many other CNS systems are also affected and their adverse effects may be numerous and often complex. They are all available for use in oral dosage forms and some also as injections, both in regular and depot formulations.

The antipsychotic drugs have been the subject of criticism by various healthcare groups as being relatively ineffective and yet having many adverse effects. Indeed, about a third of psychotic patients respond poorly, and many others suffer severe adverse effects. Despite this, these drugs can be invaluable in many cases and have radically altered the management of psychotic disorders.

**Table I.** Simplified classification of the dopamine receptors

| | $D_1$ group | | $D_2$ group | | |
|---|---|---|---|---|---|
| | $D_1$ | $D_5$ | $D_2$ | $D_3$ | $D_4$ |
| Agonists | SKF 38393 | Dopamine | Bromocriptine | Dopamine | Dopamine |
| Antagonists | α-Flupenthixol | SCH-23390 | Haloperidol Sulpiride | Sulpiride | Clozapine |
| Distribution | Striatum | Hypothalamus | Striatum | Olfactory tubercle | Frontal cortex |
| Chromosomal localisation of gene | 5q 33-35 | 4p 15.1-15.3 | 11q 22-23 | 3q 13.3 | 11p 15.5 |

#### 3.1.1 Mechanism/Site of Action

The pharmacology of the antipsychotic drugs is complex because they interact with numerous transmitter systems in the brain and also in the periphery. The first true antipsychotic drug, chlorpromazine, was discovered by accident in the search for a better antihistamine. Many others followed and it quickly became apparent that all could induce extrapyramidal symptoms, particularly Parkinsonism. This eventually focused interest on dopaminergic systems in the brain. It was postulated that antipsychotic drugs antagonise dopamine at its receptors in the brain and induce extrapyramidal effects by blocking receptors in the basal ganglia (globus pallidus and corpus striatum). The site of action of the antipsychotic effect was presumed to be in the mesolimbic and cortical areas. Other effects of dopamine receptor blockade are inhibition of the vomiting centre, stimulation of prolactin release, and reduction of growth hormone levels.

The localisation and binding of various antipsychotic drugs can be measured in animal brain using radioactive compounds. This can also be done in humans using positron emission tomography (PET) or single photon emission tomography (SPET). Close correspondence is seen between receptor affinity and clinical potency. Furthermore, in humans, extrapyramidal effects are only seen when the drug occupancy in the basal ganglia exceeds about 75%. Antipsychotic effects may, however, be seen at lower occupancy levels. Conversely, unresponsive patients may still have evidence of dopamine receptor blockade.

Most studies of antipsychotic drug action have concentrated on the dopamine $D_2$ receptor. The atypical antipsychotic drug clozapine exhibits much lower $D_2$ occupancy (38 to 63% of receptors bound) than typical antipsychotics, but also binds to $D_1$ receptors.[8] Other actions implicated in antipsychotic drug activity include blockade of other dopamine receptor subtypes ($D_4$, $D_3$, $D_5$). This area is evolving rapidly as the techniques of molecular biology are applied.[9] The current classification of dopamine receptors is summarised in table I.

#### 3.1.2 Pharmacodynamic Properties

Antipsychotic drugs also bind to many other receptors but vary greatly in their relative affinities. Most bind to 5-$HT_2$ (serotonin$_2$) receptors. Chlorpromazine has such an effect as does clozapine. Indeed, the latter's unique efficacy in treatment-resistant depression has been attributed to this property (among other hypotheses). Risperidone binds even more strongly to 5-$HT_2$ receptors than to $D_2$ receptors.[10] It may be that therapeutic effects on so-called 'negative' symptoms of schizophrenia (withdrawal, lack of motivation, etc.) are related to this effect, whereas efficacy against 'positive' symptoms (overactivity, hallucinations, delusions) reflects dopamine receptor blockade.

Antipsychotic drugs also have variable anticholinergic activity, which for some, such as thioridazine, is quite marked. This effect underlies such adverse effects as dry mouth, constipation and blurring of vision. Anticholinergic drugs are used routinely to treat extrapyramidal symptoms and their anticholinergic effects may add to those of the antipsychotic drug itself to cause severe adverse effects, even to the point of, for example, paralytic ileus. One potentially serious effect of excessive anticholinergic activity is a toxic confusional psychosis which can obfuscate the underlying functional psychosis.

In addition, antipsychotic drugs bind to α-adrenoceptors to varying extents and this can cause postural hypotension, often to a quite troublesome degree. They also bind to histaminic receptors ($H_1$) in the brain and can therefore induce unpleasant sedation. Some antipsychotic drugs are less sedative than others, while some such as trifluoperazine have the reputation of being alerting or activating. They are not true stimulants but the extrapyramidal adverse effect of akathisia can sometimes be mistaken for cerebral stimulation.

### Time-Course of Clinical and Biochemical Effects

The clinical effects of antipsychotic drugs may take several weeks to develop. Some of the clinical and biochemical effects of antipsychotic drugs wane with continuous administration whereas others persist. For example, drowsiness lessens over a week or two and drug-induced Parkinsonism usually disappears within a few months. However, the elevation in serum prolactin tends to persist along with the clinical effect.

### Lack of Suitable Experimental Models to Evaluate Antipsychotic Activity

Although a large body of data has accumulated concerning the pharmacology of antipsychotic drugs in animals, there is no convincing animal model of psychosis in general, or schizophrenia in particular. The early models were sensitive to the extrapyramidal effects of the drugs and this led to a whole series of compounds being screened in this way, but all inevitably produced extrapyramidal symptoms.

In normal humans, a wide range of drug effects can be detected but often, secondary effects such as sedation are mostly clearly seen.[11] Consequently, normal individuals can only tolerate low doses of these drugs, which limits the value of such studies. Again, however, no models for functional psychosis can be mimicked or induced in normal individuals, despite uncritical vogues in the past for using LSD- or phencyclidine-induced states.

## 3.1.3 Pharmacokinetic Characteristics

### Chlorpromazine

Among the antipsychotics, chlorpromazine has been studied most extensively because it

**Table II.** Pharmacokinetic characteristics of some antipsychotic drugs (after Hollister[12])

| Drug | Plasma half-life (h) | Route of elimination | Comments |
|---|---|---|---|
| Chlorpromazine | 16-30 | Hepatic metabolism with enterohepatic recirculation; very little renal excretion of unchanged drug. Possible metabolism in gut wall. Many metabolites possible (some active, others inactive) | Oral absorption variable. Effective plasma concentrations decreased in presence of delayed gastric emptying and by use of drugs that decrease gastrointestinal motility |
| Thioridazine | 26-36 | Hepatic metabolism (active metabolite); little renal excretion of unchanged drug | |
| Perphenazine | ≈21 | Hepatic metabolism, possibly enterohepatic recirculation; some renal excretion of unchanged drug | Significant first-pass metabolism after oral administration |
| Fluphenazine | ≈33 | Hepatic metabolism; many metabolites | Significant first-pass metabolism after oral administration. Injectable enanthate and decanoate preparations have apparent half-lives of 3.5-4 days and 6.8-9.6 days, respectively |
| Thiothixene | ≈34 | Hepatic metabolism; some renal excretion of unchanged drug | |
| Haloperidol | 10-22 | Hepatic metabolism | Reduced metabolite may exert some activity. Injectable decanoate preparation has an apparent half-life of 21 days |
| Pimozide | ≈29 | Hepatic metabolism | |
| Loxapine | 3-4 | Hepatic metabolism (active metabolites) | Active metabolites have longer half-lives than parent drug. One metabolite (amoxapine) exerts antidepressant activity |
| Sulpiride | 5-8 | Mainly renal excretion | Oral absorption variable; bioavailability is low (≈27%), probably due to incomplete absorption |
| Tiapride | 3-5 | Mainly renal excretion | Oral bioavailability ≈75% |
| Bromperidol | 22-24 | Hepatic metabolism (inactive metabolites) | Significant first-pass metabolism after oral administration. Injectable decanoate preparation has an apparent half-life of 3 weeks |
| Clozapine | 9-17 | Hepatic metabolism (? active metabolites) | |
| Risperidone | 2.5 | Hepatic metabolism | Active metabolite, 9-hydroxyrisperidone has a long half-life (>24h) |

was the first drug of its class and a large amount of data has accumulated. Its metabolism is exceedingly complex as over 160 metabolites have been postulated and many have been identified. Plasma concentrations of chlorpromazine (table II) reach their peak after oral administration at between 2 and 4 hours. Some patients absorb the drug poorly, giving low plasma concentrations. Bioavailability after oral administration varies from about 33 to 66% and may reflect metabolism in the gut wall. Delayed gastric emptying and gut motility may therefore impair absorption. Intramuscular administration, although often painful, almost always provides prompt and probably total systemic availability of the drug, with measurable plasma concentrations evident in 15 minutes and plasma concentrations 3 to 4 times higher than those with the same dose given orally. Intramuscular injection is therefore appropriate in emergency situations.

The disappearance of chlorpromazine from the plasma follows the typical biphasic course of a highly lipophilic compound. An early rapid redistribution phase with a half-life of about 2 hours is followed by a slow elimination phase with a half-life averaging 16 hours, but with wide interindividual variability. Chlorpromazine is highly protein bound (over 98%) and is localised in tissues to a marked extent (reflected in its large apparent volume of distribution of around 30 L/kg).

Plasma concentrations of chlorpromazine vary greatly between patients, up to 50-fold in some studies. This is attributed to several influences including both the rate and pattern of metabolism. Steady-state plasma concentrations are maintained throughout the day following single daily dosage, but can vary over time, often lessening, as chlorpromazine can induce its own metabolism.[12]

#### Other Phenothiazines

*Thioridazine* also undergoes complex metabolism and has one active metabolite, mesoridazine. Thioridazine is a long-acting compound with a plasma half-life of around 30 hours, a high level of protein binding (over 96%) and a large apparent volume of distribution (18 L/kg).

*Perphenazine* is eliminated somewhat faster than chlorpromazine but also has a large apparent volume of distribution. Like chlorpromazine, it undergoes extensive first-pass metabolism and plasma concentrations show wide interindividual variability. *Fluphenazine* undergoes similar metabolism but its plasma half-life is longer than that of perphenazine (see table II).

#### Haloperidol

Haloperidol is extensively used worldwide and its pharmacokinetics have been evaluated in detail. Its bioavailability after oral administration varies between 50 and 90%. Following intramuscular injection, haloperidol is rapidly absorbed, with peak plasma concentrations reached in about 20 minutes. Steady-state plasma concentrations do not vary greatly between patients after intramuscular injection, but after oral administration may vary up to 30-fold between individuals. The metabolism of haloperidol is not as complex as that of the phenothiazines but, nevertheless, many metabolites have been identified. Its plasma half-life is 10 to 22 hours and the apparent volume of distribution 17 to 30 L/kg.

Attempts have been made to relate the clinical response to plasma haloperidol concentrations.[13] Although claims of such a relationship have been made, the correlation is too weak to be clinically useful.

Haloperidol is also available as an intravenous preparation, which is used in the management of acutely disturbed patients, and as a depot intramuscular formulation for long term maintenance therapy.[14] Haloperidol solutions are odourless, colourless and tasteless, and have been administered clandestinely, for example, to captors in siege situations.

#### Clozapine

This drug is a dibenzodiazepine with a unique clinical profile. It shows wide interpatient variability in pharmacokinetic parameters such as time to peak plasma concentrations (1.1 to 3.6h), plasma half-life (9.1 to 17.4h), and apparent volume of distribution (1.6 to 7.3 L/kg).[15] Clozapine is metabolised to demethyl and *N*-oxide derivatives, the pharmacological activity of which is reported to be much lower than that of the parent compound. No correlation between plasma concentrations and clinical response has yet been established.[15]

#### Sulpiride and Risperidone

*Sulpiride*, a substituted benzamide compound, is absorbed slowly, with a relatively low bioavailability of less than 33%. It enters the brain slowly and is mainly excreted unchanged in the urine, its plasma half-life being about 5 hours.

*Risperidone* is a benzisoxazole derivative which is rapidly absorbed from the gastrointes-

**Table III.** Characteristics of the depot antipsychotic drugs (after Davis et al.[17])

| Drug | Ester | Vehicle | Dosage (mg) [interval (weeks)] | $t_{max}$ (days) | Apparent half-life (days) | |
|---|---|---|---|---|---|---|
| | | | | | single dose | multiple dose |
| Fluphenazine | Decanoate | Sesame oil | 12.5-100 [2-5] | 0.3-1.5 | 6-9 | 14 |
| | Enanthate | Sesame oil | 12.5-100 [1-4] | 2-3 | 3.5-4.0 | |
| Haloperidol | Decanoate | Sesame oil | 20-400 [4] | 3-9 | | 21 |
| Flupenthixol | Decanoate or palmitate | Low viscosity vegetable oil | 10-50 [2-4] | 7 | 8 | 17 |
| Zuclopenthixol [cis(Z)-clopenthixol] | Decanoate | Low viscosity vegetable oil | 50-600 [1-4] | 4-7 | | 19 |
| Pipothiazine | Palmitate | Low viscosity vegetable oil | 50-200 [4] | 10 | | 14-21 |
| Bromperidol | Decanoate | Sesame oil | 40-300 [4] | 3-9 | | 21 |
| Perphenazine | Enanthate | Sesame oil | 25-200 [2] | 2-3 | | 4-6 |
| Fluspirilene | | Aqueous solution of microcrystals | 2-6 [1] | 2 | 7 | |

*Abbreviation:* $t_{max}$ = time to reach peak plasma concentration.

tinal tract. It is also rapidly metabolised (plasma half-life 2.5 hours), but has a longer-acting active metabolite, 9-hydroxyrisperidone, which has a plasma half-life of around 20 hours. The oxidative metabolism of risperidone is subject to genetic polymorphism, and in poor metabolisers, the half-life of the drug is extended to around 16 hours.[16]

#### Depot Preparations

Several long-acting depot preparations are now available. Their advantage is that they avoid the problem of non-compliance with oral medication (which can be high and variable). Some of the available preparations are listed in table III. Their duration of action varies from 1 to 4 weeks, depending on the drug and formulation. With the exception of fluspirilene, which is not bound to a carrier to achieve delayed release, the depot antipsychotics are administered in esterified form in an oily vehicle (table III). Following deep intramuscular injection in this form, the drug is slowly absorbed and then rapidly cleaved by plasma esterases, releasing the active drug. The apparent half-life lengthens with repeated injections, probably because of continuing absorption from multiple injection sites.

### *3.1.4 Clinical Effectiveness*

The antipsychotic drugs have multiple uses:

1) Quietening disturbed patients with various diagnoses, including acute schizophrenia, mania and organic brain disease.

2) Treating the acute symptoms of schizophrenia, either in the initial episode or on relapse.

3) Providing maintenance therapy to lessen symptoms and abnormal behaviour in chronic schizophrenic patients in the community or in mental hospitals.

4) Treating anxiety (in low dosages).

In practice, these uses overlap; for example, a schizophrenic patient maintained on a depot preparation may start to relapse and need additional oral drugs.

#### 'Tranquillisation'

Acutely psychotic patients present a danger to themselves and to others, and thus require swift, safe and effective treatment which facilitates subsequent evaluation and longer term management. Rapid tranquillisation usually requires the administration of parenteral antipsychotic drugs, often combined with a benzodiazepine.[18] For example, one survey[19] found the combination of intravenous haloperidol 10mg with intravenous diazepam 10mg to be effective. However, in a quarter of the incidents monitored, a second injection was needed. The effects of the injection are to quieten the patient without excessive sedation.

#### Acute Schizophrenia

Most schizophrenics break down in a less dramatic fashion, with increasing psychotic symptoms, bizarre behaviour, and failure to function in the family, socially and at work. Many patients can still be managed at home or in their hostel but hospital admission may be indicated to facilitate a full medical and social assessment, minimise the risk of suicide, and lessen the stresses on the individual by providing temporary asylum. It is also useful in allowing institution or modification of therapy with careful monitoring. For example, oral medication may need to be switched to intramuscular depot medication if poor compliance is suspected as a factor in the relapse.

The efficacy of antipsychotic drugs in the management of the acute schizophrenic patient has been established in a multitude of clinical trials.[20] However, in most patients, the exacerbation in their symptoms tends to remit spontaneously, so the effect of the medication is to accelerate that trend, not initiate it. The symptoms that are helped include delusions, hallucinations, belligerence, thinking disorders and paranoid ideas.[21] All of these are termed 'positive' symptoms. The so-called 'negative' symptoms such as inertia, social withdrawal and lack of motivation are affected to a lesser extent, and in some patients hardly at all. In general, only about two-thirds of patients respond adequately, the rest being dubbed 'treatment-resistant schizophrenics' (see further below).

The efficacy of the antipsychotic drugs must be set into the context of non-pharmacological management undertaken concomitantly. In an analysis of the results of over 100 trials comparing various treatments,[22] hospitalisation with usual ward care was the minimal treatment. Psychotherapy conveyed no additional benefits while social intervention did not have much effect unless it was combined with drug treatment, the latter being by far the most efficacious part of management.

High doses of antipsychotic drugs have been advocated in treating acute schizophrenia. However, this carries with it the burden of increased adverse effects and concern has been mounting that such dosage is associated with an increased risk of sudden unexpected death.[23] As the evidence for enhanced efficacy of high doses is meagre, the consensus is that high doses should not be used indiscriminately but only in patients who have failed to respond to conventional doses. Even then, careful dose escalation is essential with adequate time being given for equilibration after each rise in dose.[24]

Evidence is accruing that patients who are started late in the episode on antipsychotic medication have a poorer outcome than those whose treatment is prompt and vigorous. This may reflect the insidious onset of illness in the former, a factor known to have a poor prognostic import. However, despite all the adverse effects of antipsychotic drug therapy, it still remains the single most efficacious component of the management of the acute schizophrenic patient.

#### Maintenance Therapy

This term is used to describe the long term treatment with antipsychotic drugs of patients living in the community with family or friends or in a hostel. Some may be inmates of a long-stay psychiatric ward. The antipsychotic drugs suppress symptoms such as hallucinations, render delusions less insistent, and also help to prevent acute relapses.

The efficacy of maintenance therapy can be evaluated in terms of both symptom severity and frequency and also postponement of relapse. Patients taking drugs are much less likely to relapse than those not on medication or on placebo. As a rough guide, maintenance therapy, carefully administered and monitored, should double the interval between relapses. As each relapse lessens the social and occupational performance of the patient, as well as inducing symptomatic distress, this degree of efficacy is important.[17]

As with acute symptoms, however, a minority of patients seem resistant to maintenance therapy, their rate of relapse not slowing or even continuing to accelerate. Part of this difficulty relates to poor compliance, although this is complex.[25] Thus, failure to take medication may reflect worsening of the condition rather than *vice versa*.

Whatever the mechanisms, undoubted benefits accrue from using depot maintenance therapy. When using depot medication (with supplementation as needed for incipient relapse), together with psychosocial rehabilitation, a substantial reduction in the number of relapses occurs. Instead of having 10 or more relapses over a lifetime, the patient may suffer only 2 or 3. Consequently, they can be maintained in the community, hold down a job, and function in family and society.

***Duration of therapy:*** most data concerning the optimum duration of treatment do not go beyond a few years. Clinical experience would suggest that once a firm diagnosis of schizophrenia is made, treatment should be for life. If the psychosis is atypical, for example, with marked affective features, then a review every 5 years or so may be warranted.

***Intermittent therapy*** is an alternative approach that has been evaluated.[26] This involves a strategy in which drugs are withheld or administered at a low dose. The patient is closely monitored and at the first sign of relapse, full dosages are instituted. The aim is to lessen the adverse effects of medication, which are linked to social impairment, depression and dysphoria. However, it is not always easy to detect the early signs of relapse, and the patient may then prove more difficult to treat, eventually taking more rather than less medication. Thus, intermittent therapy is only indicated in patients who refuse maintenance therapy.

The interactions between drug and non-drug factors in maintenance therapy are complex. Factors which help prevent relapse include a sympathetic and supportive family and friends, and avoidance, wherever possible, of adverse life stresses. In patients in such circumstances, antipsychotic drug therapy has a less important role to play than in those not so protected, where the drugs may prove crucial.

#### Drug-Resistant Schizophrenia

The definition of drug-resistant schizophrenia varies but about 30% of schizophrenics diagnosed and treated by psychiatrists show little or no response, and a further 30 to 40% show only a partial response. A response may refer to amelioration of acute symptoms or prevention of relapse, but often treatment-resistant schizophrenic patients show a combination of both, with continuing symptoms fluctuating in intensity. A few pursue an inexorably deteriorating course despite all attempts at treatment. Early onset, poor premorbid work and social adjustment, and a negative symptom profile predict poor outcome. Males do worse than females.

***Non-compliance*** is an important factor with over a third of day-patients and a half of outpatients failing to comply within 6 weeks of discharge from hospital.[27] The main reason for this is the troublesome nature of adverse effects, particularly akathisia and sedation. Others include anticholinergic and endocrine symptoms, as well as weight gain. Many schizophrenics become depressed and this may result in a sense of futility and a rejection of all medication. Some refuse medication because of their delusional beliefs.

The evaluation of compliance is not easy but it is important to do so to avoid repeatedly changing medications, none of which are taken. Plasma concentration estimations may be helpful but are often not widely available, and their interpretation is problematic. Patients may sometimes take a few doses of their tablets just before attending the clinic.

***Use of clozapine:*** this drug has proved effective in some patients with treatment-resistant schizophrenia. Clozapine is an 'atypical' antipsychotic with a complex pharmacology.[15] It was first evaluated in the late 1960s and early 1970s and found to be an effective antipsychotic agent.[28] Even then, its efficacy rates suggested that it was better than standard drugs. Symptomatic improvement was obtained in 50 to 80% of patients and seemed longer lasting than with standard drugs. Then in 1975, reports were received from Finland of agranulocytosis, including 8 fatalities. The development of the drug was stopped forthwith. However, it remained available in some countries, notably Germany, and clinicians became increasingly convinced of its superior efficacy.

Because of the risk of blood dyscrasias, it was evident that the use of clozapine could only be justified if regular blood monitoring was carried out and if the indication was severe. In treatment-resistant schizophrenics, clozapine has demonstrated significant superiority over chlorpromazine in terms of improving most rating scale items.[29] This was particularly marked for the 'negative' symptoms (see above) which hardly responded to chlorpromazine. The superiority of clozapine was still increasing at 6 weeks and longer term trials have suggested continued efficacy. Even so, between a third and a half of patients remain refractory to clozapine. Claims for enhanced efficacy for other atypical antipsychotic drugs such as risperidone are so far unestablished.[16,30]

### 3.1.5 Tolerability and Drug Interactions Potential

The adverse effects of antipsychotic drugs have been extensively documented (see table IV for comparative data on the most commonly occurring adverse effects). However, their importance is often under-appreciated. The choice of medication is usually dictated by the tolerability of the individual patient, rather than by any differences in efficacy (with the notable exception of clozapine). Adverse effects are often overlooked, or their significance to the patient devalued. However, the clinician does this at his/her peril because of their effects on compliance.

Adverse effects can be divided into two broad categories, those predictable from the drug's pharmacology and those resulting from an allergic or idiosyncratic response. Dopamine blocking effects underlie some adverse effects; blockade of other receptors most of the remainder.[32]

#### Extrapyramidal Syndromes

The extrapyramidal syndromes comprise a range of reactions, mostly well-defined but occasionally atypical. They are caused by most antipsychotic drugs, though clozapine and sulpiride have very little tendency to do so. Some

**Table IV.** Doses and adverse effects of some commonly used antipsychotic drugs (after Menkes[31])

| Class/agent | Dose equivalents (mg/day)[a] | Adverse effects | | | |
|---|---|---|---|---|---|
| | | sedative | extra-pyramidal | postural hypotension | anticholinergic |
| **Phenothiazines** | | | | | |
| *Aliphatic:* | | | | | |
| Chlorpromazine | 100 | +++ | + | +++ | ++/+++ |
| Methotrimeprazine | 25 | +++ | + | +++ | ++ |
| *Piperidine:* | | | | | |
| Pericyazine | 6 | ++ | +/++ | ++ | ++ |
| Pipothiazine[b] | 6 | + | ++ | + | + |
| Thioridazine | 100 | +++ | ± | +++ | +++ |
| *Piperazine:* | | | | | |
| Fluphenazine[b] | 3 | ± | +++ | + | + |
| Perphenazine | 8 | + | ++ | + | + |
| Prochlorperazine | 16 | +/++ | +++ | + | + |
| Trifluoperazine | 5 | ± | +++ | + | + |
| **Thioxanthenes** | | | | | |
| Flupenthixol[b] | 6 | ± | ++ | + | + |
| Thiothixene | 4 | ± | ++ | + | + |
| **Butyrophenones** | | | | | |
| Droperidol | 5 | ++ | ++ | ++ | + |
| Haloperidol[b] | 3 | ± | +++ | + | + |
| **Diphenylbutylpiperidines** | | | | | |
| Fluspirilene[c] | 1 | ± | ++ | + | + |
| Pimozide | 2 | ± | ++ | + | + |
| **Azepines** | | | | | |
| Loxapine | 10 | + | ++ | + | + |
| Clozapine | 60 | +++ | ± | +++ | +++ |
| **Benzamides** | | | | | |
| Sulpiride | 100 | + | ± | ± | ± |
| Tiapride | 100 | + | ± | ± | ± |
| **Benzisoxazoles** | | | | | |
| Risperidone | 2 | + | ± | ++ | + |

a Dose equivalents are expressed as oral mg/day amounts equivalent clinically to chlorpromazine 100mg. Long acting or depot intramuscular doses may be estimated by multiplying the daily dose x days between injections (see below) × 1/5 to allow for increased bioavailability.

b Available as depot intramuscular formulations. Fluphenazine and flupenthixol decanoates are usually given 2- to 4-weekly, and haloperidol decanoate and pipothiazine palmitate 4-weekly.

c Available as a long-acting intramuscular formulation (usually given weekly).

*Symbols:* ± = rare or negligible; + = occasional or mild; ++ = common or moderate; +++ = frequent or severe.

reactions occur early in treatment, some – the 'tardive' conditions – late in treatment.

*Acute dystonia* usually develops 24 to 48 hours after first exposure to the drug or to a dosage increase, or about 72 hours after the injection of a depot preparation. The symptoms can last several hours if untreated. The condition particularly affects young males. It usually involves the tongue, lips and jaw but the trunk and limbs may be affected. It may be misdiagnosed as tetanus or 'hysteria'. Parenteral anti-Parkinsonian medication (e.g. benztropine) is indicated in such cases.

*Akathisia* is a subjective sense of restlessness ('innere unruhe') together with ceaseless movements of the hands or feet, repeatedly standing up or pacing. It may be misdiagnosed as a sign of increasing agitation and the drug dosage increased, thereby worsening the condition. Anti-Parkinsonian drugs are ineffective but a benzodiazepine or a β-adrenoceptor blocking drug may help.

*Parkinsonism* is the most common extrapyramidal symptom. The mildest form is bradykinesia. Akinesia may supervene, together with rigidity, stooped posture, festinant gait, coarse tremor, hypersalivation and seborrhoea. It is more common in the elderly and in women, and may be mistaken for apathy, depression or dementia. It usually manifests in the first month or two of treatment but may be delayed. Anti-Parkinsonian drugs [e.g. benztropine or trihexyphenidyl (benzhexol)] are traditionally used to treat the condition but there is no evidence that they prevent the syndrome developing. Furthermore, drug-induced Parkinsonism tends to lessen after a few months. The anti-Parkinsonian medication has appreciable anticholinergic effects, is dangerous in overdose, and has an abuse potential because of its euphoriant effects. Consequently, its use is best minimised and confined to treating patients inconvenienced by Parkinsonian adverse effects whose dosage of antipsychotic drug cannot be safely lowered.

#### Neuroleptic Malignant Syndrome

The neuroleptic malignant syndrome (NMS) is the most dangerous neuromuscular adverse effect, with an incidence between 0.2% and 1% of patients treated with antipsychotic medication.[33] However, milder cases may go unrecognised.[34] The clinical features comprise hyperthermia, muscle rigidity, autonomic instability and impairment of consciousness. Symptoms of autonomic instability include labile hypertension, tachycardia, vasoconstriction and sweating. The severe hyperthermia proves fatal in about 20% of cases. The mechanism of the reaction is unclear but probably involves the dopaminergic systems in the striatum and hypothalamus.

Treatment of the neuroleptic malignant syndrome must be prompt and vigorous, with reversal of the hyperthermia by use of cooling blankets, etc., reversal of dehydration, and general support. Specific measures that have been advocated include the dopamine agonists amantadine and bromocriptine, and the antispasticity drug dantrolene. The optimum treatment remains to be established.

#### Tardive Dystonia and Dyskinesia

Long term extrapyramidal effects comprise tardive dystonia and tardive dyskinesia. The former is a comparatively rare disorder with a prevalence of about 2%. It tends to manifest itself as a craniofacial syndrome but the ankle may be affected with sustained spasm. Tardive dystonia affects younger patients and is even more difficult to treat than tardive dyskinesia.

***Tardive dyskinesia*** is fairly common with an estimated incidence of 15 to 20%.[32] It supervenes months or years after starting antipsychotic medication, and in about 50% of cases is irreversible. It comprises choreoathetoid movements, usually of the mouth and face, but may also affect the limbs and trunk. It can occur spontaneously in the elderly who have never taken antipsychotic drugs, but the prevalence in those who have taken drugs proves that most cases are drug-related.

Risk factors for tardive dyskinesia include increasing age, organic brain disease, 'negative' symptomatology, prior Parkinsonism and alcohol abuse. However, the cumulative dosage of antipsychotic medication is believed to be an important determinant and the condition may mostly reflect higher doses and/or duration of use. Tardive dyskinesia is probably heterogeneous: some cases have an insidious onset, others an acute one, and the course is very variable. Subsyndromes have been described, e.g. orofacial and limb types, the former being easier to manage.

Aetiological theories have become increasingly complex. The earliest was that dopamine receptor supersensitivity developed but more recently the GABA ($\gamma$-aminobutyric acid) system has been implicated. It is difficult to give rational guidelines for preventing tardive dyskinesia, other than the obvious ones of minimising dosage and duration of antipsychotic medication. Depot injections are more likely to be associated with tardive dyskinesia than oral medication, but this presumably reflects enhanced compliance.

Treatment of the established condition comprises reduction of dosage where possible. Many specific therapies have been tried including dopamine-depleting agents such as tetrabenazine, benzodiazepines used as general relaxants, and lithium. Clozapine is atypical in rarely producing either acute or long term extrapyramidal symptoms, and is currently being assessed as a treatment for severe cases of tardive dyskinesia.

#### Tardive Akathisia

Tardive akathisia is sometimes seen both in patients on long term antipsychotic medication and after withdrawal of medication. It is as yet incompletely characterised.

#### Other Adverse Effects

Other adverse effects of the antipsychotic drugs affect many body systems (table IV). Among their endocrine and metabolic effects, weight gain can be marked and unacceptable to the patient. It reflects increased appetite and decreased activity, and may impair compliance. The secretion of prolactin is increased by antipsychotic drugs due to dopaminergic blockade. Galactorrhoea (often with amenorrhoea) may be seen in women, and loss of libido in men. Bone density may decrease in women with the risk of osteoporosis. Growth hormone levels may also be lowered but this does not appear to be clinically relevant, even in children.

Autonomic effects attributable to the drugs' anticholinergic properties include dry mouth, blurred vision, difficulty in micturition, and constipation. Their sympatholytic effects comprise orthostatic hypotension with reflex tachycardia and delayed ejaculation. Priapism is a rare but potentially serious effect.

Psychological effects are common, almost inevitable, and often complex.[35] Coordination, attention and memory may all be impaired.[36] Subjective sedation is often marked and usually wears off but some patients continue to complain of feeling detached, unaware – 'like a zombie'.[37] This has been termed the 'neuroleptic-induced deficit syndrome' (NIDS).[38] Depression is common in schizophrenic patients and they may attribute this to their medication. It is difficult to distinguish depression from drug-induced akinesia and a trial of therapy with an anti-Parkinsonian drug may be helpful.

Serious adverse effects include blood dyscrasias, cholestatic jaundice, rashes and cardiac irregularities. The incidence of granulocytopenia with most antipsychotic drugs is less than 1 in 1000. However, it may be as high as 2 to 3% with clozapine, necessitating weekly blood monitoring for the first 18 weeks of treatment, and at least once-monthly monitoring thereafter. By this means, progression to agranulocytosis with possible fatalities can be prevented in almost all cases. Clozapine is also more likely than other antipsychotics to induce epileptic attacks. This adverse event is strongly dose-related, the risk being 5% above 600 mg/day.

#### Withdrawal Reactions

Withdrawal of antipsychotic medication is usually uneventful but may be followed by the emergence of a withdrawal dyskinesia or even a rebound psychosis. Both eventually subside.

#### Overdosage Effects

Intentional overdoses with psychotropic drugs are very common. Schizophrenic patients are at high risk of suicide, about 10 to 12% ending their lives this way.[39] Some take an overdose of their antipsychotic or anti-Parkinsonian medication. The first signs of overdosage are drowsiness, then agitation or confusion. Dystonias, twitching or fits may be seen, hypotension is marked, and cardiac arrhythmias may occur. Anticholinergic effects may also be marked, especially with chlorpromazine and thioridazine.

Treatment is essentially symptomatic with maintenance of body temperature. Dialysis is of little use but gastric emptying may be delayed and gastric lavage may be appropriate. Early and continued treatment with activated charcoal is helpful. Hypotension is difficult to treat because of the autonomic blockade. Specific antidotes are not available; although physostigmine has been advocated, it is probably more trouble than it is worth.

#### Drug Interactions

The phenothiazines interact with several groups of compounds. They increase the central nervous system depressant effects of alcohol, opioid analgesics, anxiolytics and sedatives. The absorption of chlorpromazine may be impaired by some antacids. The phenothiazines can also interact with fluoxetine and tiapride and produce an increased incidence of extrapyramidal effects. The combination of lithium and antipsychotic drugs such as haloperidol has given rise to concerns over extrapyramidal effects and careful monitoring of the serum lithium concentration should be undertaken.

Clozapine is another compound that may interact with fluoxetine, resulting in increased plasma clozapine and norclozapine concentrations (see also appendix B).

## 3.2 Optimum Treatment

### *3.2.1 Acutely Disturbed Patients*

Drug treatment is needed when behavioural methods of management have failed. The combination of an antipsychotic drug with a benzodiazepine, both given parenterally, is generally preferred to larger doses of either alone. The choice of drugs is not standard, but haloperidol (or droperidol) among the antipsychotic drugs, and diazepam or lorazepam among the benzodiazepines are popular. Intravenous administration is preferable to intramuscular injection as it produces a more rapid effect – an important consideration when the patient is aggressive and requires the force of several nurses to restrain him or her. In such cases, the tension in the attendants may be transmitted to the patient, setting up a vicious circle.

An antipsychotic drug whose effect spans the gap between emergency tranquillisation and the treatment of acute schizophrenia is *zuclopenthixol acetate*. This drug is given by intramuscular injection (in a vegetable oil vehicle) and its effects last for about 3 days.

The dosage of the antipsychotic drug must be chosen carefully. Factors to take into account include the age, sex, weight and body build of the patient, whether oral medication is being taken, and previous responses to emergency medication. Patients at higher risk of adverse reactions (including even sudden death) are the aged, obese, heavy users of alcohol and tobacco, and those with a history of heart disease. Dehydration and electrolyte imbalance are also dangerous. Previous electrocardiograms (ECGs) should be checked but it is usually impractical to attempt an ECG at the time. However, when the patient has settled, it is wise to obtain an ECG to establish a baseline. Both before and after the injection, it is necessary to carry out regular checks on pulse, blood pressure, temperature and the state of hydration. A switch to oral therapy should be attempted as soon as possible.

### 3.2.2 Acute Schizophrenia

Both for this situation and for the prevention of relapse, a range of considerations govern the choice of drug, its dosage regimen, and concomitant treatment measures (fig. 1). There is no evidence to suggest that any one drug is more efficacious than another, with the exception of clozapine in otherwise treatment-resistant schizophrenic patients. The other major proviso is that the depot formulations of a drug are usually more effective than oral formulations.

The most relevant differences among antipsychotic drugs relate to their unwanted effects. Thioridazine (like clozapine, sulpiride, and risperidone) is almost devoid of extrapyramidal effects but has marked autonomic effects. Haloperidol and high-potency phenothiazines such as fluphenazine have the reverse profile. Chlorpromazine appears to have the worst of both worlds. Patients vary in their tolerance to the various adverse effects, some finding extrapyramidal symptoms quite unacceptable, others avoiding autonomic effects or sedation. Thus, some trial and error may be needed to establish the patient on his/her preferred medication. The clinician should become experienced in the use of a few agents with varying profiles in the adverse effect continuum. In this respect, it should be noted that some of the newer drugs have atypical profiles. For example, the substituted benzamides sulpiride and tiapride have a low incidence of extrapyramidal adverse effects with few autonomic effects; however, they do raise prolactin levels substantially.

#### Mode of Administration

The mode of administration depends on likely patient compliance. Depot injections are relatively expensive, inflexible and often resented by patients. They may improve the response in compliers with oral medication who are rapid metabolisers but this is still unclear. Patients well maintained on oral medication should not be switched to depot preparations just for the sake of convenience.

#### Dosage Selection

The correct dosage is that which adequately controls the patient's symptoms and behaviour with minimal adverse effects. As psychotic illnesses fluctuate in severity, regular monitoring and adjustment of dosage is good practice. High doses are not justified routinely, although a few patients do seem to do best on doses beyond the usual range. This must be established in each case. Once-daily dosage should be aimed at to optimise compliance but this must be balanced against the possibility of milder adverse effects if the daily dose is divided.

The dosage regimen of depot antipsychotic drugs is complex to establish, as both amount and dosage interval need independent manipulation. Again, a few patients seem to respond only to colossal doses.

#### Other Considerations

An acutely psychotic patient may improve spontaneously on admission to hospital or with the intervention of a crisis team, as stresses and life events are dealt with. Most, however, require adequate medication to combat the symptoms. The patient is often frightened at the bizarre things which are happening in his/her mind, and sedation as well as antipsychotic medication may be a temporary expedient.

The mainstay of treatment is, nevertheless, antipsychotic medication in adequate dosage, together with experienced and sympathetic nursing. A supportive framework of care is essential and a locked ward may provide much-

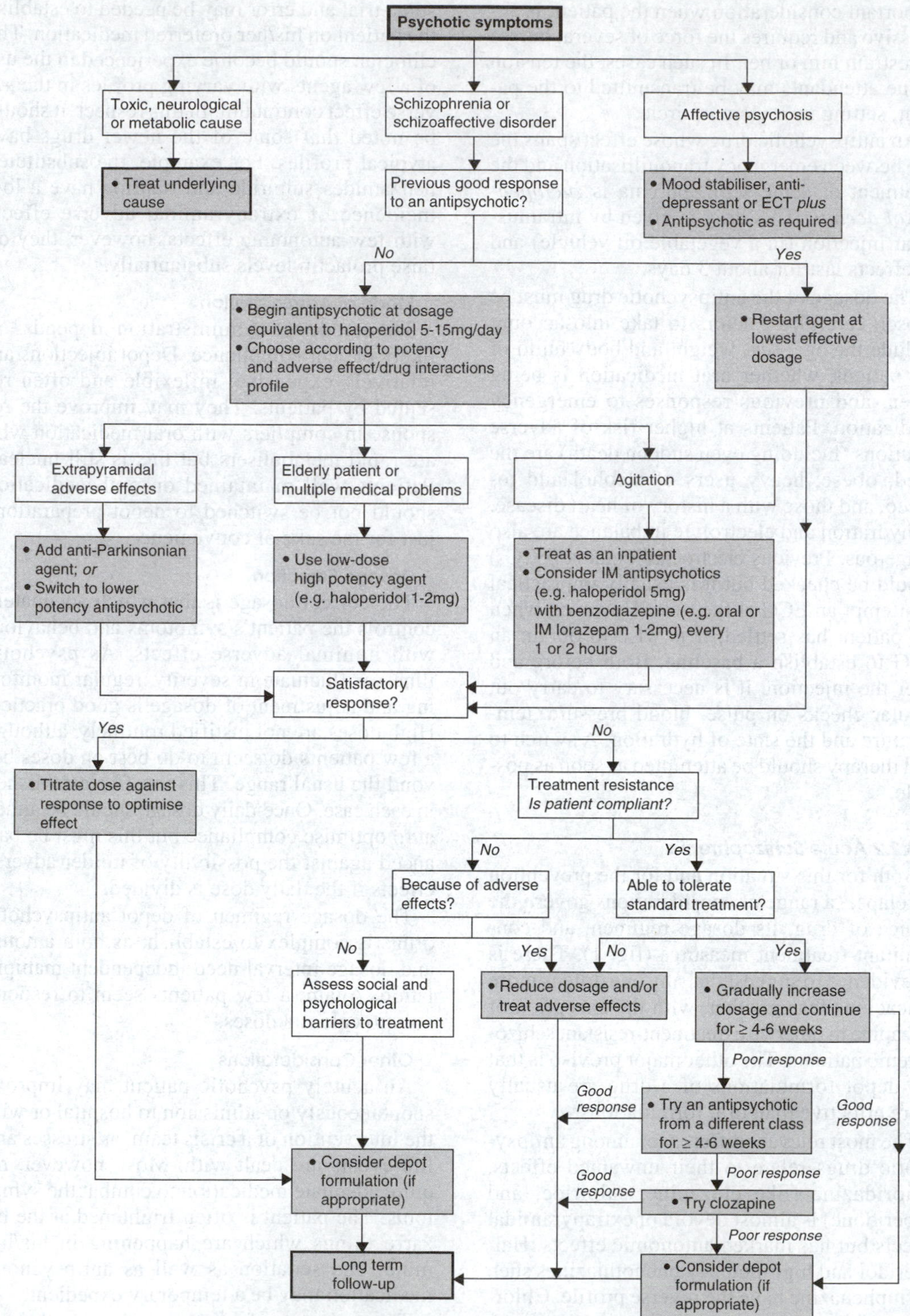


**Fig. 1.** Optimum treatment of psychotic disorders. *Abbreviation:* ECT = electroconvulsive therapy.

needed security for the patient. There is often sensory overload as defence mechanisms break down, and antipsychotic drugs help prevent this sensory bombardment. The drug choice and dosage is as outlined above; liquid formulations may be advisable to prevent hiding of tablets in the mouth with subsequent spitting out. Anti-Parkinsonian medication should only be used if extrapyramidal symptoms are intolerable and dosage reduction impractical.

It is important to persist with medication and not to switch therapy prematurely. In this regard, careful monitoring of the psychopathology will uncover signs of incipient response such as lessening of intensity of hallucinations and delusions, more social contacts, and less impulsive behaviour. Once improvement occurs, the dosage should be cautiously reduced.

#### 3.2.3 Prevention of Relapse

One in four patients meeting the diagnostic criteria for schizophrenia recover quickly, but 10% become severely disabled despite treatment and require residential care. The remaining 60 to 70% endure persisting symptoms and social problems, and are helped by a combination of antipsychotic medication and social support. Most can survive in the community with regular supervision. Tardive dyskinesia may also emerge, further worsening the prognosis.

The treatment of 'negative' symptoms of schizophrenia is a major problem for the clinician. There is controversy as to whether and to what extent these symptoms respond to antipsychotic medication.[40] The evidence is strongest for clozapine which is the drug of choice for patients with negative symptoms or treatment-resistant schizophrenia. Other medications that have been suggested include risperidone and some antidepressants such as fluoxetine.

As well as maintenance drug therapy (see section 3.1.4), psychological interventions aimed at modifying both the patient's behaviour and the attitudes of those around him/her are helpful. However, a tight-rope has to be walked between overstimulation with stress-induced relapses, and understimulation with 'institutionalisation', even in the patient's own home. In some countries, community mental health teams have been set up to optimise the management of these patients, including supervising medication and helping find suitable accommodation and work. Each patient is assigned a 'key worker' who takes on the main role. General practitioners are also becoming increasingly involved.

#### 3.2.4 Treatment-Resistant Patients

Such patients need careful assessment to review the diagnosis, gauge compliance and evaluate psychosocial factors. Adverse effects should be minimised and treated. High dosages of antipsychotic drugs may be justified but should be embarked on cautiously. Adjunctive treatments such as benzodiazepines, antidepressants and lithium may be helpful.

Otherwise, the use of *clozapine* should be considered (see also section 3.1.4). Up to 50% of patients will respond to this agent, some dramatically. Despite the adverse effects and the tedium of haematological monitoring, many patients are prepared to continue on clozapine because they feel so much better. However, its use is best left to specialists with extensive clinical experience of the drug and the logistics of its prescription.

#### 3.2.5 Special Patient Groups

##### Pregnant and Lactating Women

Antipsychotic drugs undergo placental transfer and should only be used if the benefits outweigh the risks – as they usually do in a schizophrenic mother. The drugs also pass into breast milk, and while little can be expected to be delivered to the infant (see appendix C), because their potential effects on the infant are unknown, breast feeding should be discouraged.

##### Elderly Patients

Adverse effects are more common in the elderly, particularly tardive dyskinesia and postural hypotension. Nevertheless, antipsychotic drugs are used routinely in the elderly to treat agitation, e.g. tiapride in agitation associated with dementia.[41] Low doses of high-potency agents are preferred for this purpose, e.g. haloperidol 1 to 2 mg/day.

##### Children and Adolescents

Psychotic disorders in these age groups may be serious and unresponsive to medication. High-dose medication is usually unjustified and may worsen behavioural disturbances associated with brain damage. In those with learning disabilities, the detection of adverse effects that are distressing the patient may be difficult (see also section 10.4).[42]

### 3.3 Clinical Outcome and Economic Considerations

The assessment of clinical outcome is complex. Among the many outcome variables are behavioural measures such as combativeness, retardation and agitation, social variables such as occupational and residential status, administrative factors such as time spent in hospital, and psychopathological factors such as symptom type and severity. Some of these assessment criteria may not be compatible with others. Thus, patients with 'negative' symptoms may be least discontented lying on their beds at home listening to music, but their families may find this social withdrawal worrying, and society may regard such patients as unproductive economically.

The economics of the treatment of schizophrenia are difficult to quantify.[43] The cost of an illness which has a lifetime expectancy rate of 1% and is typically chronic and severe is manifestly very high, both in terms of direct health costs and indirect costs relating to the lack of productivity to the economy. The advent of clozapine therapy, which is expensive compared with standard treatment, has generated considerable interest in terms of its long term economic benefits in treatment-resistant schizophrenia.[44,45] One study in the US estimated the total costs of severely ill schizophrenic patients to be around US$50,000 per year, made up mostly of the cost of repeated hospital admissions. During clozapine treatment, costs dropped steadily to about $13,000 per year in the treatment responders but remained high in those who dropped out of treatment. Taking all patients into consideration, responders and non-responders, about US$9000 was saved per year per patient.[46]

If the costs of these patients before treatment ($50,000 per year) are multiplied by the estimated point prevalence of schizophrenia (0.2% to 0.5%), the economic burden of the illness on society is apparent.

## 4. Bipolar Disorder

Affective disorders can involve episodes of depression only (unipolar), or episodes of depression and hypomania/mania (bipolar disorder). The features of the depressive episodes are similar to those in major depressive illness (see section 5). The symptoms of mania are of persistently elevated mood, ranging from exuberant cheerfulness to unruly high spirits. The patient resents control or persuasion and may be irritable or even sad and weeping at times. The behaviour is outside normal parameters and may become outrageous.

Patients are also overactive with a host of projects being started but not completed. Speech is garrulous and sprinkled with puns and illusions. It may become 'flight of ideas' with the train of thought being obscured. The patient's ideas are grandiose and may become delusional. The overactivity can lead to loss of weight and physical exhaustion. Financial disaster may sometimes occur before any intervention can be made.

Bipolar illness has strong genetic influences and biochemical changes (particularly involving serotonin) have been documented. It is a recurrent disorder and episodes tend to get more frequent and sometimes merge into chronic mania. The risk of suicide is high.

### 4.1 Clinical Pharmacology of Drugs Used in Treatment

#### *4.1.1 Lithium*

Lithium was introduced into medicine in the mid-19th century and in 1871 was recommended for the acute treatment of mania and depression. Soon after, it was advocated for the prevention of periodic depression. The rediscovery of these therapeutic properties was made first by Cade in 1949 and then promoted by Schou from the mid 1960s. Throughout its therapeutic history, lithium has been dogged by the reputation of being toxic.

**Mechanism/Site of Action**

The exact mode of action of lithium in stabilising mood disturbances is uncertain, both because the biology of affective disorders is unclear and because the actions of lithium, as a simple cation, are complex. Lithium cannot substitute for sodium in the sodium pump, and cannot maintain membrane potentials. At therapeutic concentrations, it inhibits the calcium-dependent release of noradrenaline (norepinephrine) and dopamine but enhances the release of serotonin.

Lithium also inhibits the hydrolysis of inositol phosphate in the brain, thereby reducing the cellular content of this second messenger family. Depletion of these phosphatidylinositides may lessen the sensitivity of neurones to endogenous neurotransmitters.

**Table V.** Pharmacokinetic characteristics of mood-stabilising drugs (after Hollister[12])

| Drug | Plasma half-life (h) | Route of elimination | Comments |
|---|---|---|---|
| Lithium | 8-35 | Renal excretion | Renal excretion dependent on sodium balance and urine volume. Elimination delayed in the elderly. Patients exhibiting long half-lives (>20h) presumably reflect delayed clearance due to impaired renal function or decreased sodium balance |
| Carbamazepine | 10-20* | Hepatic metabolism (active metabolites); little renal excretion of unchanged drug (2-3%) | *Induces its own metabolism (half-life shown is after repeat doses). Ratio of active 10,11-epoxide metabolite to parent drug shows 5-fold interindividual variability (0.1-0.5) |

### Pharmacodynamic Properties

Lithium is almost devoid of psychotropic activity in normal volunteers. Subjective well-being is decreased and cognitive performance, particularly some memory functions, may be impaired on formal laboratory testing. This parallels the reports of poor memory in some patients.

The effects of lithium on various body systems are more obvious. It antagonises the renal response to antidiuretic hormone, thus producing a diuresis. Thyroid function is also impaired and weight gain is common. Hand tremor is aggravated, and ECG changes such as low or inverted T-waves have been recorded.

### Pharmacokinetic Characteristics

Lithium has relatively simple pharmacokinetic properties (table V). Being a metallic cation, it is not metabolised, nor is it bound to plasma proteins. Its apparent volume of distribution approximates to body water volume (0.8 L/kg), but high concentrations are present in thyroid tissue, bones and white matter of the brain. It penetrates into the brain and cerebrospinal fluid (CSF) fairly slowly, and the equilibrium concentration there is about half that in the plasma.[47] Subsequently, lithium is eliminated by the kidneys rather like sodium. Thus, it is filtered through the glomeruli and reabsorbed in the proximal (but not distal) tubules.

The pharmacokinetics of lithium depend on the formulation used. Sustained-release formulations have become standard medication as they smooth out the peaks in plasma concentrations; however, they vary widely in their absorption characteristics. Thus, after taking an aqueous solution, peak plasma concentrations are attained in about 30 minutes but after a sustained-release preparation, peak concentrations are not achieved until 3 to 6 hours. The plasma half-life of lithium ranges from 8 to 35 hours, with a mean of 24 hours. The renal clearance of lithium is correlated with creatinine clearance.

Lithium is the only drug used in psychiatry whose plasma concentration is monitored routinely. However, the standard 12-hour postdose plasma concentration is an aid to management and dose adjustment and not a substitute for it. The therapeutic range for treatment of mania is 0.8 to 1.2 mmol/L, and for prophylaxis of affective disorder, 0.5 to 0.8 mmol/L (see table VI). Concentrations above these may be associated with toxicity but lower concentrations do not automatically guarantee safety.

### Clinical Effectiveness

***Treatment of mania:*** the first clinical use of lithium was in the treatment of mania and its lesser form, hypomania.[48] Lithium is as effective as antipsychotic drugs in the management of hypomanic patients, but it is less effective in the more severe forms of mania, especially in deluded patients. Part of the problem relates to the delay of about a week before lithium attains its full efficacy. Therefore, it is customary to combine lithium with an antipsychotic drug, traditionally haloperidol, in the initial phases of treatment. If the patient is very disturbed, high doses of antipsychotic drugs are needed. Because of possible neurotoxic interactions with lithium, it may be wise to delay its use until

**Table VI.** Correlation of lithium plasma concentrations with toxicity

| Feature | Plasma concentration 12 hours postdose (mmol/L) |
|---|---|
| *Therapeutic range:* | |
| prophylaxis | 0.5-0.8 |
| treatment | 0.8-1.2 |
| Impending toxcity[a] | 1.5-2.4 |
| Mild clinical toxicity[a] | 2.5-3.4 |
| Severe, life-threatening toxicity[a] | > 3.5 |

a *Toxic symptoms:* Grade I – tremor, nausea, vomiting, drowsiness; Grade II – impaired consciousness, twitching, tremor; Grade III – semi-coma, muteness, convulsions. *Sequelae:* renal impairment; cerebellar damage – ataxia, dysarthria.

dosages can be reduced. When the patient has settled, the antipsychotic medication can be tapered off and the patient maintained on lithium.

Controlled trials demonstrating the efficacy of lithium in this indication are surprisingly sparse but about 75% of patients show an adequate response in due course. Non-responders are often characterised by rapid swings in mood.

***Treatment of acute depression:*** lithium has also been used in the treatment of acute phases of depression, whether bipolar, unipolar or schizoaffective in natural history. However, efficacy data are difficult to interpret because of differences in diagnostic criteria. About 50% of depressed bipolar patients will show a good response but few unipolar depressed patients do so. Lithium has also been used with some success in combination with tricyclic and other antidepressants in refractory patients.

***Prophylaxis:*** the main use of lithium is to prevent manic and depressive episodes in bipolar patients and also depressive episodes in unipolar sufferers.[47] As a rule, lithium therapy should be considered when a patient has a new distinct manic or depressive episode within 3 to 4 years of the last one. Some would also consider lithium if the patient has suffered one attack of depression and one of mania (thus establishing the diagnosis of bipolar disorder) or after three episodes of depression. However, the total clinical picture must be taken into account.

A large number of controlled clinical trials now attest to the efficacy of lithium in lessening the frequency or preventing affective disturbances in patients with bipolar disorder. However, the response rate is not complete, about a third of patients deriving little or no benefit, or suffering intolerable adverse effects. Even among those who respond, fewer than 50% show total cessation of episodes. In most cases, the episodes, particularly the manic ones, become less severe or muted and the patient is much less likely to need hospital admission. Depressive episodes are less clearly suppressed.

Special lithium clinics have been set up in many countries to provide prophylactic therapy for patients with recurrent affective disorder. Over the years, patients who have apparently done well tend to accumulate in such clinics, whereas poor responders tend to drift away and failures are placed on other treatment. Thus, efficacy data for patients treated in lithium clinics must be assessed on an 'intent-to-treat' rather than a 'survivor' basis. Long term data are also essential, as short term data (e.g. up to 2 years) may reflect natural remission of a relapsing condition rather than any therapeutic effect.

The use of lithium in the prophylaxis of recurrent unipolar depression is less widely accepted. A meta-analysis of the published data showed a definite therapeutic effect for lithium in reducing the frequency of relapse.[49] However, tricyclic antidepressants have also been shown to be effective in preventing recurrent episodes of unipolar depression, and while there is some controversy as to whether they are more or less effective than lithium, many clinicians perceive tricyclic antidepressants as being safer and therefore preferable (see section 5.1.4). This is particularly so if the patient has shown a good response to an antidepressant drug and tolerated it well in a previous episode. However, if ECT was needed in a previous episode or if lithium augmentation was required, then lithium is probably the treatment of choice for prophylaxis.

***Other indications:*** lithium has also been evaluated in a range of psychiatric conditions usually characterised by periodicity, poor impulse control or aggression.[47] It has been tried in children with conduct disorders or episodic assaultative behaviour, with apparently good effect. Lithium has been used much less in adults with behavioural disturbances. Some schizophrenic patients with episodic affective disturbances may be helped by lithium therapy administered usually as an adjunct to antipsychotic drugs. Another condition in which lithium has been tried fairly extensively is alcoholism; however, results are unimpressive except in a few patients whose alcohol-related problems seem secondary to mood swings.

Lithium has also been tried in a range of non-psychiatric conditions including cluster headaches, migraine and Ménière's disease (see also chapters 14 and 29).

### Tolerability and Drug Interactions Potential

The therapeutic index of lithium is narrow and adverse effects are common. Early adverse effects which may lessen include nausea, often associated with loose bowel movements, and fine tremor of the fingers and hands. Polyuria occurs as a result of reduced renal concentrating ability. This is closely dose-related and not often seen with the lower serum concentrations currently favoured. Although there was alarm in the 1970s concerning possible glomerular toxicity, long term data have suggested that lithium (except in repeated overdosage) does not lead to renal impairment.

Weight gain can be a problem, with most patients gaining a few kilograms during the first year or two. Higher initial weight, higher doses and concomitant antidepressant therapy predispose to weight gain. The mechanism of the weight gain is unclear but may reflect the excessive intake of calorie-containing fluids to assuage the thirst secondary to polyuria. Hypothyroidism can be induced by long term lithium treatment, together with a mild goitre. Treatment with thyroxine is indicated, usually until the increase in thyroid-stimulating hormone has been reversed.

Other adverse effects include impairment of concentration and memory, a metallic taste in the mouth, and mild pretibial oedema. Lithium may also induce or exacerbate psoriasis or acneiform eruptions.

***Lithium intoxication*** is by far the most serious complication of lithium treatment (table VI). Diarrhoea, vomiting, increased tremor, dysarthria, weakness (especially of the lower jaw), drowsiness and ataxia all indicate that the safe limit is being exceeded (grade I toxicity). More severe effects (grade II) include coarse tremor, twitching, fasciculation in the limbs, hands and face, drowsiness, impaired concentration, unsteadiness, loss of memory, mild disorientation and dizziness. Finally, restlessness, confusion, nystagmus, and delirium (grade III toxicity) herald coma with muscle hypertonia, oliguria and epileptic fits.

A plasma lithium concentration over 1.5 mmol/L indicates impending toxicity. With concentrations in excess of 2.5 mmol/L, signs of toxicity are usually present, and over 3.5 mmol/L, life is threatened. With more severe states, a vicious circle is set up with reduction in renal function leading to toxicity which, in turn, causes further shut-down of the kidneys. Toxicity may be initiated by a primary kidney disorder, the addition of a diuretic for hypertension, dehydration due to fever, vomiting, salt-poor diets and heavy sweating. In severe intoxication, haemodialysis is essential, as permanent neurological damage is more likely the longer plasma lithium concentrations are elevated. Sequelae include cerebellar and basal ganglia damage and reduced renal function.

It is generally accepted that lithium may induce cardiac abnormalities in the fetus, so it should be withdrawn if a woman wishes to become or has become pregnant. If lithium must be continued, frequent monitoring is needed. As lithium is secreted in breast milk, breast-feeding is best avoided.

***Drug interactions:*** lithium clearance is reduced by long term diuretic therapy and combined treatment needs very careful monitoring. Similarly, nonsteroidal anti-inflammatory drugs (NSAIDs) may also reduce lithium clearance to some extent, leading to increased plasma concentrations. As lithium may prolong the action of neuromuscular blocking agents (e.g. pancuronium), it should be withdrawn at least three days prior to elective surgery.

#### 4.1.2 Other Mood-Stabilising Drugs

Other drugs with mood-stabilising activity that may be used in patients who fail to achieve an adequate response to lithium include the antiepileptics carbamazepine and valproic acid (sodium valproate), clonidine,[50] and calcium antagonists.[51] The clinical pharmacological properties of these drugs are discussed in other chapters (see chapters 21 and 29).

### 4.2 Optimum Treatment

Lithium is used to treat the acute episodes and also to prevent episodes, both depressive and manic. However, it seems better at preventing the manic episodes. The confidence of the patient must be won as long term compliance is essential to a successful outcome.

#### 4.2.1 Lithium Therapy

When the decision has been taken to initiate lithium treatment in patients with bipolar disorders, it is necessary to evaluate renal function with serum creatinine and clearance measurements and serum electrolyte analysis. Thyroid function should also be measured, and an ECG recorded in patients over 50 years of age. Fluctuating kidney disease (such as active glomerulonephritis), heart disease and disturbed electrolyte balance are contraindications to lithium treatment. Fad diets, particularly low sodium ones, also pose a danger (since lithium clearance is reduced by sodium depletion), and patients must normalise their food and drink intake.

Long term prophylactic administration of lithium requires the full cooperation of the patient, who should be informed of the likely benefits and possible adverse effects and should be instructed in how to detect early signs of lithium intoxication. In the first week or two, a low dose of lithium (e.g. 300 to 400mg lithium carbonate, or 6 to 8 mmol) should be given and the patient's plasma concentration (at 12 hours postdose) monitored after 1 week. The dosage should then be adjusted to provide a plasma concentration of about 0.5 mmol/L. The dosage and plasma concentration are roughly linearly correlated. Elderly patients may only tolerate plasma concentrations around 0.3 to 0.4 mmol/L, whereas young adults may need levels over 0.8 mmol/L for symptomatic control. Fine-tuning can be easily carried out and even small changes in dosage may avoid troublesome adverse effects and/or improve the therapeutic effect.

Few data are available concerning the optimum duration of lithium therapy. For the acute episode of mania, 6 months is about the average, provided symptoms have remitted. Most patients taking lithium prophylactically will need to continue therapy indefinitely. Even if discontinuation is attempted, it should be done gradually, as manic relapse is likely.[52]

#### 4.2.2 Other Therapy

Other medications have been tried in the management of bipolar disorder. During acute episodes, antipsychotic drugs may be needed for hypomanic behaviour and antidepressants for depressive illness. Often the patient ends up on both.

For the prevention of episodes, *carbamazepine* has been used as an alternative to lithium but tends to be somewhat less effective, except in rapidly cycling patients. This agent has been used in combination with lithium. Increasingly, *valproic acid* (sodium valproate) is also being used.

## 5. Depressive Illness

Depressive disorder covers a range of illnesses from severe retardation to mild episodes of lowered mood. The middle range of depression includes major depressive disorder which is a common condition. It can occur on its own (unipolar disorder), or with episodes of mania and hypomania (bipolar disorder).

The symptoms of depression are primarily lowered mood with sustained dejection. It is qualitatively different from normal unhappiness. There is loss of reactivity to external circumstances and patients appear miserable, frowning and tearful. All appears gloomy and hopeless to them and no future can be envisaged at all. Patients are often worse in the mornings and they are often anxious as well. Memory is poor and attention ill-sustained.

Many patients with depressive illness suffer from morbid guilt and can be retarded with inhibition of movement and speech. Paranoid delusions may develop and some patients have intractable hypochondriacal complaints. There is loss of appetite and weight, disturbance of sleep, typically with early morning wakening, and lowered or absent sexual libido. Suicidal thoughts or intent are common in the moderate or severe grades of depression, and are most dangerous when retardation is slight.

About 5 to 10% of the population suffer from depression at any one time, depending on the criteria used. Many escape detection and remain untreated. Women are twice as likely as men to suffer from depression, and the condition can occur at any age. Genetic influences are marked in the more severe forms.

### 5.1 Clinical Pharmacology of Drugs Used in Treatment

The drugs used to treat depressive illness are termed 'antidepressants'. Other less frequently used terms include 'antidepressives', 'mood elevators' and 'thymoleptics'. The main groups of antidepressants in clinical use are the 'tricyclics', a few of which do not have three-ringed chemical structures, the monoamine oxidase inhibitors (MAOIs), the selective serotonin reuptake inhibitors (SSRIs), and the reversible inhibitors of monoamine oxidase type A (RIMAs).

The first antidepressants, introduced in the late 1950s, were the tricyclic agent imipramine, and the MAOI iproniazid. Several members of each class were introduced in subsequent years but it was 20 years before the advent of compounds with significant differences in basic and clinical pharmacology. In the past 10 years, the availability of the SSRIs and the first RIMA has led to a reappraisal of the risk : benefit ratio of the older tricyclic and MAOI compounds and also to the evaluation of comparative costs.

#### 5.1.1 Mechanism/Site of Action

Over the past 40 years or so, many studies using a variety of techniques have suggested that depressive disorders are associated with some malfunctioning of nervous function in parts of the brain involved in the organisation and integration of emotional responses. In parallel, studies on antidepressant drug action have elucidated the major effects that these drugs have on the neurons in these areas of the brain. These two sets of data were collated and gave rise to the monoamine theory of depression which implicates serotonin and/or noradrenaline (norepinephrine) in the brain.

The biochemical mechanisms of effect of antidepressants have been elucidated in some detail. Thus, almost all drugs increase the availability of monoamine neurotransmitters in the synaptic cleft. The tricyclic antidepressants do this by preventing the reuptake of serotonin (5-HT) and/or noradrenaline from the synaptic cleft into the presynaptic neuron. The MAOIs prevent rapid breakdown of the neurotransmitters.

While the availability of monoamines occurs rapidly, the clinical response to antidepressants is a more gradual process. This has led to revision and elaboration of the simple monoamine theories to incorporate adaptational changes in receptors upon which serotonin, noradrenaline, dopamine and perhaps GABA act. For example, cortical β-adrenoceptors undergo decreased functional activity and density; cortical 5-$HT_2$ receptors react in a similar way; and dopaminergic autoreceptors decrease in density with antidepressant treatment. Furthermore, these various amine systems interact: antidepressants that act selectively on serotonin systems decrease the functional activity of the noradrenergic system as well. Conversely, destruction of the serotonin system in animals largely prevents the decrease in function of cortical β-receptors that follows long term antidepressant treatment.

Dopamine turnover can also be influenced by serotonin function. Correlations have been found between concentrations of serotonin and dopamine metabolites in the CSF. Stimulation of serotonin neurons in the central brainstem raphé nuclei results in reduced firing of dopaminergic neurons in the substantia nigra.

Another system which may be involved is the pituitary-adrenal axis. Hypercortisolism occurs commonly in depression. Glucocorticoid receptors may be abnormal in depression, and antidepressants may act to lessen or reverse this malfunction.

Nevertheless, it is still unclear how the biochemical changes induced by the various groups of antidepressants are translated into clinical activity. The reason why about a third of depressed patients fail to respond to medication is not precisely known. No clear differences between these individuals and responders have been found with respect to either pre-existing biochemical patterns or to changes effected by the antidepressants. Also, irrespective of the acute specificity of antidepressants, in the longer term they all result in similar biochemical effects.

### *5.1.2 Pharmacodynamic Properties*

#### Tricyclic Antidepressants

The tricyclic and related antidepressants produce slow-wave activity (theta frequencies) in the electroencephalogram (EEG). They may activate epilepsy and this can be quite a marked effect with some members of this class such as maprotiline. REM sleep is suppressed. Sedation is common with some antidepressants, perhaps because of secondary effects such as blockade of histaminic receptors, and may be marked. Memory disturbances have also been described and reflect both sedation and specific effects in blocking cholinergic pathways. Other anticholinergic effects of the tricyclic antidepressants include blurring of vision, slowing of gastrointestinal function and impairment of bladder function. Potentiation of noradrenaline can be demonstrated but indirectly-acting sympathomimetics such as tyramine have less effect because their uptake into presynaptic noradrenergic neurons is blocked.

Mood changes cannot be demonstrated in normal individuals, in contrast to stimulants such as the amphetamines. However, some ostensibly normal volunteers have quite high depression ratings and these people are capable of showing an antidepressant response.

#### Selective Serotonin Reuptake Inhibitors (SSRIs)

The SSRIs (e.g. citalopram,[53] fluoxetine,[54] fluvoxamine,[55] paroxetine,[56] sertraline[57]) have rather different pharmacodynamic profiles because they are much more selective than the tricyclic antidepressants, not only with respect to monoamine uptake but also because of their reduced affinity for other receptors such as muscarinic receptors. These drugs produce little or no sedation, but may be somewhat alerting and induce insomnia. EEG changes are, however, similar to those of the tricyclic antidepressants. Again, REM sleep is reduced but deep (slow-wave) sleep is enhanced. The SSRIs are devoid of significant effects on psychomotor or cognitive function, and they do not potentiate the effects of alcohol, a property of most tricyclic antidepressants.

The SSRIs have definite effects on feeding behaviour, lessening food intake in animals and appetite in humans. Unlike the tricyclic antidepressants, cardiovascular effects are minimal.

Animal studies have shown that whereas the tricyclic drugs produce tachycardia, myocardial depression and cardiac irregularities, the SSRIs have little effect except at high doses. In humans, the SSRIs have no effect on the ECG, heart rate or blood pressure. Adverse effects of these drugs are discussed in section 5.1.5.

#### Monoamine Oxidase Inhibitors (MAOIs)

Repeated doses of an MAOI (e.g. phenelzine, tranylcypromine, isocarboxazid) can cause overactivity in animals, together with sympathomimetic effects such as mydriasis and vasoconstriction. Phenelzine is rather sedative whereas tranylcypromine tends to be alerting and even amphetamine-like at high dose. The main cardiovascular effect of the MAOIs is marked postural hypotension, which may limit the dosage attained clinically. The mechanism of this effect is not clear.

#### Reversible Inhibitors of MAO Type A (RIMAs)

Moclobemide, the first RIMA to become available, is almost devoid of cardiovascular effects. It has no effect on psychomotor or cognitive function and it has much less anticholinergic activity than its predecessors, the MAOIs.

### 5.1.3 Pharmacokinetic Characteristics

#### Tricyclic Antidepressants

The tricyclic drugs are rapidly absorbed, and are detectable in the plasma a few minutes after oral administration.[58] The bioavailability of orally administered imipramine ranges between 30 and 75%, while that of nortriptyline is between 55 and 80%. Distribution is rapid, with the drugs readily crossing the blood-brain barrier; concentrations are highest in the liver, adrenal glands, lung, brain and heart. Plasma protein binding is generally high, as are the apparent volumes of distribution (see appendix A).

Elimination mainly occurs via hepatic metabolism (table VII). Side-chain transformations are the most important metabolic step. The initial step with tertiary amines such as imipramine and amitriptyline is demethylation with the formation of active secondary amine metabolites, desipramine and nortriptyline, respectively. Sometimes, as with clomipramine, the metabolite attains higher steady-state plasma concentrations than the parent compound.[59] Ring hydroxylation is another important step and this leads to the formation of conjugated compounds, usually glucuronides. The ring hydroxylated compounds tend to be rather inactive pharmacologically, but may be present in fairly high concentrations.

As with the phenothiazines, the plasma half-lives of the tricyclic drugs show marked inter-individual variability. The range is 6 to 20 hours for imipramine and 15 to 90 hours for nortriptyline. The elderly and patients with hepatic impairment exhibit reduced metabolism (and hence prolonged half-lives), which may be associated with elevated steady-state plasma concentrations.[58] For example, mean steady-state concentrations of imipramine in the elderly are around 84 μg/L as compared with 32 μg/L in younger individuals; the corresponding values for desipramine are 57 *vs* 21 μg/L.[60]

Steady-state concentrations are usually attained within 1 to 4 weeks, depending on the drug and the characteristics of the patient. However, it is customary to initiate antidepressant treatment with half the usual dosage so several weeks may elapse before equilibrium at full dosage is achieved. The steady-state plasma concentrations reached vary widely. Thus, values for nortriptyline have been reported to vary from 48 to 238 μg/L, for imipramine from 6 to 356 μg/L, and for the active metabolite desipramine (after imipramine administration) from 28 to 659 μg/L.

***Correlation of plasma concentrations with clinical response:*** much effort has gone into attempts to relate the clinical response to plasma concentrations of the tricyclic antidepressants.[61] The drug that has been most systematically studied is nortriptyline. Patients with plasma concentrations below about 50 μg/L show little or no clinical response. At the other extreme, i.e. above about 150 μg/L, the response is also poor. Thus, the concept of a 'therapeutic window' lying between these two regions has been applied to nortriptyline. However, the presence of possibly active metabolites complicates matters. Desipramine appears to have a similar therapeutic range, but with the tertiary amines the therapeutic window is less obvious, even when the active metabolite is taken into account. A combined concentration of greater than 200 μg/L is believed to be therapeutic; for amitriptyline and protriptyline, the therapeutic ranges are 80 to 200 μg/L and 70 to 170 μg/L, respectively.

Although some advocate routine plasma monitoring of the tricyclics for efficacy, most find such estimations of more use in checking compliance or in investigating serious adverse

**Table VII.** Pharmacokinetic characteristics of some antidepressants (after Hollister[12])

| Drug | Plasma half-life (h) | Route of elimination | Comments |
|---|---|---|---|
| **Tricyclic and 'atypical' agents** | | | |
| Amitriptyline | 32-40 | Hepatic metabolism (active metabolite) | Active metabolite (nortriptyline) may accumulate and eventually attain greater concentrations than parent drug |
| Imipramine | 6-20 | Hepatic metabolism and renal excretion of active metabolite and small amounts of unchanged drug | Active metabolite (desipramine) may accumulate and eventually attain greater concentrations than parent drug. Subject to significant hepatic first-pass metabolism after oral administration. Plasma half-life prolonged in the elderly |
| Nortriptyline | 15-90 | Hepatic metabolism | Significant first-pass hepatic metabolism after oral administration |
| Desipramine | 12-54 | Hepatic metabolism | |
| Clomipramine | 17-28 | Hepatic metabolism | Probable significant hepatic first-pass metabolism after oral administration |
| Doxepin | 8-25 | Hepatic metabolism; little renal excretion of unchanged drug | Significant hepatic first-pass metabolism after oral administration |
| Dothiepin (dosulepin) | 20-25 | Hepatic metabolism (active metabolites) | Probable significant hepatic first-pass metabolism after oral administration |
| Trimipramine | 24 | Hepatic metabolism | Significant hepatic first-pass metabolism after oral administration |
| Lofepramine | Short* | Hepatic metabolism (active metabolites) | Extensive first-pass metabolism after oral administration (bioavailability <10%)<br>*Principal active metabolite (desipramine) has a long half-life (12-54h) |
| Maprotiline | 27-58 | Hepatic metabolism (active metabolites) | |
| Mianserin | 8-19 | Hepatic metabolism; renal excretion of small amount of unchanged drug (4-7%) | |
| Viloxazine | 2-3 | Hepatic metabolism; some renal excretion of unchanged drug (12-15%) | |
| Amoxapine | ≈8* | Hepatic metabolism (active metabolites); little renal excretion of unchanged drug (≈3%) | *Half-life shown is for parent drug. Principal active metabolite (8-hydroxyamoxapine) has a longer half-life (≈30h) |
| Trazodone | 4-8 | Hepatic metabolism; little renal excretion of unchanged drug (<1%) | Plasma half-life prolonged in the elderly (6-16h) |
| Nefazodone | 3-7* | Hepatic metabolism (active metabolites) | Extensive first-pass metabolism after oral administration (bioavailability ≈20%)<br>*Half-life shown is for parent drug. The primary active metabolite (hydroxynefazodone) has equivalent activity to the parent drug and a similar half-life. Other less active metabolites identified include m-CPP (also similar half-life to parent drug) and triazole dione (longer half-life, 11-13.5h) |
| Venlafaxine | 4* | Hepatic metabolism (active metabolite); little renal excretion of unchanged drug (4.7%) | Extensive first-pass metabolism after oral administration<br>*Half-life shown is for parent drug. The major active metabolite (*O*-demethylvenlafaxine) has a longer half-life (10h) |
| **Selective serotonin reuptake inhibitors (SSRIs)** | | | |
| Fluoxetine | 1-4 days | Hepatic metabolism (both active and inactive metabolites); little renal excretion of unchanged drug (≈2.5%) | Considerable interindividual variability in rate of elimination. Active *N*-demethyl metabolite (norfluoxetine) has a longer plasma half-life than parent drug (7-15 days) |
| Fluvoxamine | ≈15 | Hepatic metabolism (inactive metabolites) | |
| Paroxetine | ≈24 | Hepatic metabolism (inactive metabolites) | Considerable interindividual variability in rate of metabolism |
| Sertraline | ≈24 | Hepatic metabolism (inactive metabolites) | Slowly absorbed |
| Citalopram | ≈33 | Hepatic metabolism | Demethylated metabolite probably inactive *in vivo* |
| **Reversible monoamine oxidase (type A) inhibitors [RIMAs]** | | | |
| Moclobemide | 1-2 | Hepatic metabolism | Half-life increases on repeated administration |

effects. Monitoring is, however, routine in overdosage.

#### Selective Serotonin Reuptake Inhibitors (SSRIs)

The SSRIs are well absorbed with high oral bioavailability.[62] As with the tricyclics, they have large apparent volumes of distribution, are highly bound to plasma proteins, and are extensively metabolised in the liver and largely excreted in the urine as inactive, conjugated metabolites. The plasma half-lives of the available SSRIs vary from about 15 hours for fluvoxamine, 21 hours for paroxetine, 26 hours for sertraline, and 84 hours for fluoxetine.

The metabolism of fluoxetine is quite complex. Firstly, it forms a metabolite (norfluoxetine) with a half-life ranging from 77 to 235 hours. This means that the time taken to reach steady-state concentrations after starting treatment and to decline from plateau levels to zero on discontinuation is several weeks. This has important implications when it is decided to stop the drug and institute another, particularly a MAOI. Secondly, the kinetics of fluoxetine are nonlinear, with higher doses associated with disproportionately high plasma concentrations. Also, after long term administration, the half-life of fluoxetine becomes even more prolonged, probably because it inhibits its own metabolism.[62] The drug's nonlinear kinetics may be due to partial saturation of first-pass metabolism. Despite these complications, fluoxetine does not show an unduly delayed onset of action. Furthermore, like the other SSRIs, it is well tolerated, even by the elderly. However, some drug interactions do occur (see section 5.1.5), due to its effects on the liver microsomal CYP2D6 system. As with fluoxetine, paroxetine may also show some nonlinear characteristics.

Extensive studies have failed to establish any useful relationship between plasma concentrations of the SSRIs and their therapeutic effects. However, high plasma fluoxetine/norfluoxetine ratios in the plasma may be indicative of a good response.

#### Monoamine Oxidase Inhibitors (MAOIs)

The pharmacokinetics of the older irreversible MAOIs are of little practical importance because the kinetics of drug action are primarily dependent on the irreversible inhibition of MAO and synthesis of new enzyme activity which is independent of drug concentration. Thus, even though brain levels of the drugs are no longer detectable in animal studies, MAO activity remains low for several days until new enzyme is synthesised. Isocarboxazid, phenelzine and nialamide are rapidly absorbed and metabolised in the liver. The metabolism of phenelzine includes acetylation by liver acetyl transferase and this is genetically determined. It has been suggested that slow acetylators may have a better clinical response and more adverse effects than rapid acetylators, but this has never been established. However, there is some evidence to suggest that the degree of inhibition of MAO, as monitored by blood platelet MAO activity or by amine metabolites in the urine, is related to the clinical response to nonselective MAOIs. At least 85% inhibition of MAO activity seems to be needed.

Tranylcypromine is structurally similar to amphetamine and is rapidly absorbed and excreted.

#### Moclobemide

Moclobemide is a reversible inhibitor of MAO type A and therefore its plasma concentrations determine its effects.[63] It is virtually completely absorbed from the gastrointestinal tract, and undergoes extensive but saturable first-pass metabolism in the liver, resulting in a bioavailability of 45 to 60% after single doses but about 85% after repeated administration. Moclobemide has a large apparent volume of distribution (1.1 to 1.4 L/kg). Its elimination follows first-order kinetics with several metabolites being formed, most of which are largely inactive. Multiple doses result in a reduction in the drug's hepatic clearance, suggesting autoinhibition or metabolite-mediated inhibition of its metabolism.

### *5.1.4 Clinical Effectiveness*

#### Tricyclic Antidepressants

The efficacy of the tricyclic antidepressants has been established over 30 years of both clinical experience and many controlled clinical trials. More recently, tricyclics such as imipramine and amitriptyline have been used as active comparators in placebo-controlled evaluations of new compounds. The early clinical observations concurred in regarding the main indication for the tricyclics as being 'endogenous' depression, i.e. disorder characterised by biological features such as poor sleep and appetite together with features such as guilt, self-blame and marked diurnal variation.

The tricyclic drugs show efficacy across the midrange of the spectrum of severity. Thus, very severely depressed patients with delusions or even hallucinations may respond poorly, as may patients with very mild illnesses. However, they are effective even in patients undergoing major life-stresses and should be tried even when the depression appears understandable. Controlled trials have confirmed the early clinical impression that the tricyclics are indicated for patients with moderate and severe depressions where, irrespective of cause, there is a persistent picture of the depressive syndrome – i.e. symptoms additional to the depressed mood itself such as pessimistic thoughts, suicidal feelings, sleep and appetite disturbance, severe impairment of energy, interest, motivation, drive, or concentration; and impaired capacity to function.[64]

The tricyclic antidepressants have consistently been shown to be superior to placebo in the treatment of depressed patients of the type described above, the major depressive disorder of the American Psychiatric Association's diagnostic schema (DSM-III-R). Overall, about two-thirds of depressed patients show an adequate response but, as about a third respond to placebo alone, fewer than 50% actually benefit from tricyclic treatment, at least in the initial treatment phase. The placebo response contains two independent components. Firstly, depression tends to be an episodic condition so some of these patients are actually undergoing natural remission. Secondly, there is a genuine placebo response in some patients. The latter is facilitated by general support, reassurance and counselling, and by simple manipulation of the patient's situation. For example, a young mother can be helped by placement of a child in a nursery a few hours a week, enabling her to do the shopping unencumbered. These nonspecific factors have resulted in an increasing placebo response rate in controlled trials, making it more difficult for the efficacy of antidepressants, new and old, to be demonstrated at acceptable levels of significance.

***Onset of clinical response:*** it is generally considered that there is a delay of 2 to 4 weeks before the effects of the tricyclic drugs become apparent. The explanation for this is both pharmacokinetic and pharmacodynamic. Pharmacokinetically, most of the tricyclics have long plasma half-lives and treatment needs to be initiated with half the usual therapeutic dose to minimise adverse effects; this results in therapeutic plasma concentrations only being attained after a delay of 2 weeks or more. The second hypothesis is that the therapeutic response is based on secondary changes in receptor function in the brain, which are slow to occur. In fact, the delay in onset is mostly an artefact of pooling data. Thus, placebo and drug responders show a steady improvement from quite early on but this is obscured by the third of patients who show no response at all. Consequently, the attainment of significance is postponed. If, however, the data from the eventual responders alone are analysed in detail, the response is not delayed.[65]

***Response rates of different depressive features:*** the various features of the depressive disorder respond at different rates. One detailed study[65] showed that sad affect, lack of interest, hopelessness and helplessness, suicidal thinking, and somatic dysfunction recovered rapidly. An intermediate rate was seen for low self-esteem, sleep disturbances, cognitive slowing, impulsivity, emotional blunting, self-criticism, anhedonia, and subjective memory complaints. Guilt, anger, indecision, hostility, diminished libido, and anxiety remitted slowly. Several studies have attempted to characterise those patients most likely to respond, but results have not been very consistent. A favourable outcome is associated with few previous episodes, insidious onset, brief duration of present episode, and lack of precipitating causes. Patients with appetite disturbance and weight loss, early wakening and psychomotor slowing often do well. Conversely, patients with hypochondriacal or histrionic features usually do poorly on tricyclic antidepressants.

#### Selective Serotonin Reuptake Inhibitors (SSRIs)

The SSRIs have undergone fairly extensive evaluation, not only for depression but also for panic and obsessive-compulsive disorders and for eating disorders such as bulimia nervosa.[66]

The overall efficacy of the SSRIs in depression has been established in numerous controlled trials, many of which have incorporated a tricyclic comparator as well as placebo.[67] The majority of these studies have indicated the superiority of SSRIs to placebo, and most suggest that their efficacy is similar to that of the tricyclic drugs. In a meta-analysis of 63 randomised controlled trials involving SSRIs and tricyclic and related antidepressants,[68] no differences in efficacy were found between the various drugs in terms of Hamilton depression (HAM-D) rating scale scores. On the standard 17-item scale, the average baseline score was about 24 points, i.e. moderate depression. No differential predictors of efficacy were detected, i.e. there was no evidence that one type of patient responded preferentially to one or other type of antidepressant.

Few trials, as yet, have evaluated the efficacy of SSRIs in the prevention of relapse and recurrence of depression. However, initial studies suggest general efficacy in these longer term uses. Sertraline has undergone a trial in this respect and is available in some countries for these extended indications.[57]

*Clomipramine* (a tricyclic agent with potent serotonin reuptake inhibitory activity[69]) has been extensively evaluated in the treatment of obsessive-compulsive disorder. Very consistent data have emerged.[70] The placebo response in obsessive-compulsive disorder is less than 10%, reflecting both the chronicity of the condition with little tendency to natural remission, and a true lack of responsivity to placebo. This contrasts with an efficacy rate for clomipramine akin to or even higher than that in depression. The response is also quite prompt. The improvement in obsessive ruminations and/or compulsive rituals is not dependent on improvement in coexisting depressive affect but seems to be a primary effect. Preliminary studies with the newer SSRIs in obsessive-compulsive disorder have also been encouraging.

The SSRIs have also been used in patients with comorbid anxiety and depression. With paroxetine, efficacy on both these affects has been established in controlled trials. Clinical usage is also extending into management of panic disorder, generalised anxiety disorder and post-traumatic stress disorder, especially when long term treatment seems likely.

Fluoxetine has been assessed for its efficacy in regularising food intake, particularly in bulimia nervosa (see further section 9.1). Its efficacy in this condition has been established, the frequency and severity of the episodes being substantially reduced.

#### 'Atypical' Antidepressants

Other antidepressants, which are neither tricyclic nor SSRIs, include mianserin, trazodone and its congener nefazodone,[71] and venlafaxine.[72,73] These drugs act in different ways but are all as effective as the standard tricyclic antidepressants.

*Mianserin* has been available for many years but has not achieved uniform success. Rarely, it has caused blood dyscrasias in the elderly and monitoring is recommended in some countries. Mianserin is an $\alpha_2$-adrenoceptor antagonist and also affects serotonin reuptake. *Venlafaxine* impairs the transport of both serotonin and noradrenaline.[73] It has good efficacy and may be appropriate for treatment-resistant depressives. However, it has definite adverse effects, especially at high doses, and the blood pressure should be monitored during treatment. *Nefazodone* has some serotonin reuptake inhibitory effects but is a powerful 5-$HT_2$ antagonist. It is the only antidepressant that improves the structure of sleep and may be appropriate for the depressed insomniac.

*Maprotiline* is sometimes called 'atypical' but is a bridged tricyclic compound that acts via selective blockade of noradrenaline reuptake.

#### Monoamine Oxidase Inhibitors (MAOIs)

The MAOIs have long been eclipsed by other antidepressants because of their unfavourable dietary and drug interactions. Their efficacy has also been questioned. In non-selected groups of depressed patients, MAOIs such as phenelzine and tranylcypromine usually prove superior to placebo but may fall short of the efficacy of the tricyclic drugs. However, some trials have suggested that larger doses of MAOIs are associated with a better response, e.g. 60mg rather than 30mg phenelzine per day. The response is often delayed with MAOIs, sometimes up to 6 weeks.

Many attempts have been made to select patients particularly likely to respond to MAOIs. Early clinical surveys identified such favourable prognostic indicators as 'anxiety hysteria', 'atypical depression', 'hypochondriacal depression', and so on. However, controlled trials have suggested that depressed patients with comorbid phobic anxiety and panics respond well; indeed, some studies indicate that these patients do better on MAOIs than on tricyclic antidepressants.

#### Reversible Inhibitors of MAO Type A (RIMAs)

The efficacy of MAO inhibition in the treatment of depression is being re-examined because of the advent of the RIMAs. The first drug of this group, moclobemide, has been extensively evaluated; in doses up to 600 mg/day, it has proved superior to placebo on short term (up to 6 weeks) administration to patients with major depressive disorder. Using a halving of the Hamilton rating scale score as the criterion of response, 60 to 70% of patients on moclobemide have achieved this, as compared with 30%

on placebo. The drug has proved effective in all types of depression, with psychomotor retardation and depressed mood itself being most responsive. In most but not all comparative trials, moclobemide has proved equivalent to standard tricyclic drugs,[74] with a similar onset of action time.

#### Other Antidepressants

As well as the usual antidepressants listed above, a variety of other compounds have been claimed to have antidepressant properties or have been developed for this purpose. The best established is *tryptophan* (L-tryptophan), the amino acid precursor of serotonin.[75] Few controlled data are available but doses of about 3 g/day have been shown to have an antidepressant efficacy similar to that of amitriptyline. However, tryptophan has been largely advocated as an adjunct to other antidepressant drugs in the management of severe and treatment-resistant depression. A presumed contaminant of tryptophan was implicated in a serious eosinophilia-myalgia syndrome, and it was temporarily withdrawn from most markets.[75] Another naturally occurring compound for which antidepressant effects have been reported is *ademetionine* (S-adenosyl-L-methionine).[76]

Drugs with other indications that have been tried with varying success in the treatment of depression include antipsychotics in low dosage (e.g. flupenthixol and sulpiride), benzodiazepines (alprazolam), and antiepileptic agents (carbamazepine and phenytoin). Of these, the efficacy of sulpiride is perhaps the best established, but it is more convincingly established for mixed anxiety-depression syndromes than for major depressive disorder. Nevertheless, the use of antipsychotic drugs of the 'activating' type in low doses as antidepressants is widespread in some countries.

### *5.1.5 Tolerability and Drug Interactions Potential*

#### Tricyclic and Related Antidepressants

The adverse effects of the tricyclics may be so unpleasant as to compromise the patient's compliance, either in terms of stopping medication entirely or in failing to attain an adequate dose. Because of the different types of receptors affected by these drugs, adverse effects involve many body systems.

A common adverse effect of many, but not all, tricyclic antidepressants is *drowsiness* and *torpor* (table VIII). This appears rapidly, within a dose or two, but usually wanes after the first week. Amitriptyline, trimipramine, doxepin, dothiepin, clomipramine, mianserin and trazodone are the most sedative; imipramine, nortriptyline, lofepramine and desipramine have much less effect, whereas protriptyline is rather stimulant. Thinking, attention, concentration and especially memory are all impaired and may add to the deficits in mental functioning associated with the depressive disorder itself. The elderly are particularly affected or may become confused; they may also suffer a tremor or even mild extrapyramidal symptoms. Almost all the tricyclics and related drugs lower the convulsive threshold, maprotiline particularly so.[78] As with all antidepressant therapy, patients with a bipolar diathesis may swing into hypomania.[79] The abrupt withdrawal of a tricyclic is occasionally followed by an akathisia-like syndrome with muscular aches, nausea and vomiting.

*Cardiovascular effects:* postural hypotension, secondary to α-adrenoceptor blockade, may occur, particularly in the elderly, the young and the physically debilitated, as may reflex tachycardia. Changes in cardiac conduction resemble those of the phenothiazines with lengthened QT interval and inverted T-waves. Tricyclic antidepressants have membrane stabilising activity and may cause prolongation of atrioventricular (AV) conduction. Cardiac arrhythmias can ensue and have been blamed for sudden deaths in depressed patients with a history of cardiac disease treated with these drugs. Although, the precise role of the tricyclics is unclear, they should be withheld from such patients now that safer alternatives are available. In this respect, some of the newer compounds such as lofepramine seem less cardiotoxic.[80]

*Anticholinergic effects* on the gastrointestinal tract include reduced gut motility, with severe constipation ('obstipation'). Achalasia of the oesophagus and relaxation of the sphincter may result in a hiatus hernia. However, acid formation in the stomach is reduced, so that peptic ulcers may be healed. Anticholinergic activity also results in increased bladder sphincter tone, with the risk of urinary retention in elderly males with an enlarged prostate. Another effect is delayed ejaculation, which can be exploited therapeutically to treat premature ejaculation. Trazodone has such marked α-adrenoceptor blocking properties that occasional cases of priapism have been reported.

Weight gain is often a problem, part of which is a reversal of weight loss earlier in the illness and part a drug-related increase in hunger. Ef-

**Table VIII.** Major adverse effect profile of some commonly used antidepressants (after Menkes[77])

| Class/agent | Adverse effects | | |
|---|---|---|---|
| | sedative | anticholinergic | postural hypotension |
| **Tricyclics** | | | |
| Amitriptyline | +++ | +++ | ++ |
| Clomipramine | ++ | ++ | + |
| Desipramine | + | + | +/++ |
| Dothiepin | +++ | ++ | ++ |
| Doxepin | +++ | ++ | ++ |
| Imipramine | ++ | ++ | ++ |
| Nortriptyline | + | +/++ | ± |
| Protriptyline | ± | +++ | + |
| Trimipramine | +++ | ++ | ++ |
| **Atypical agents** | | | |
| Amoxapine | + | + | + |
| Maprotiline | ++ | ± | + |
| Mianserin | ++ | ± | + |
| Trazodone | +++ | ++ | + |
| **Selective serotonin reuptake inhibitors (SSRIs)** | | | |
| Fluvoxamine | ± | ± | ± |
| Fluoxetine | ± | ± | ± |
| Paroxetine | ± | ± | ± |
| Sertraline | ± | ± | ± |
| Citalopram | ± | ± | ± |
| **MAO inhibitors** (nonselective) | | | |
| Phenelzine | ± | ± | ++ |
| Tranylcypromine | ± | ± | ++ |
| **Reversible MAO type A inhibitors** | | | |
| Moclobemide | ± | ± | + |

*Symbols:* ± = rare or negligible; + = uncommon; ++ = common or moderate; +++ = frequent or severe.

fects on the pituitary-gonadal axis include menstrual irregularities, breast enlargement and milk secretion in women, and impotence, gynaecomastia and testicular swelling in men.

Other adverse effects include loss of accommodation in the eye with blurring of vision. Intraocular pressure rises, which is a danger for patients with incipient glaucoma. Paradoxically, hyperhidrosis can also occur. Some compounds may affect liver function tests or cause allergic reactions including rashes, urticaria and oedema. Blood dyscrasias may occur rarely (e.g. agranulocytosis with mianserin in the elderly).

None of the tricyclic drugs is known to be teratogenic but the general principle of avoiding medication in pregnancy wherever possible still applies. Secretion into breast milk varies among the different drugs but it is probably best to avoid breast-feeding, as there is no information on the effects of these agents on the developing human brain.

***Overdosage:*** this is a major problem with most of the tricyclics, lofepramine being the most noticeable exception. These drugs are prescribed for depression, a major feature of which is often suicidal ideas or intent. A dose of a tricyclic drug above 600mg poses a distinct hazard, particularly in children, the elderly and the frail. Doses over 2.5g are likely to prove fatal. As the typical dose is 150 mg/day, this represents only about 2 weeks' supply.

On overdosage, symptoms usually appear within 4 hours and comprise dry mouth, blurred vision, dilated pupils, extrapyramidal signs, and either drowsiness or excitement, depending on the particular tricyclic. The cardiovascular effects range from tachycardia to major arrhythmias and are often life-threatening. The ECG shows QRS and ST segment prolongation with various types of conduction defects, including bundle branch block. The elderly, and those with cardiac or respiratory pathology are most at risk. The convulsive threshold is lowered and up to 20% of patients develop fits. The cause of death is generally cardiac failure secondary to arrhythmias and anoxaemia. Occasionally, patients die in status epilepticus. Toxic effects on the heart are potentiated by central depressants such as alcohol, barbiturates and the benzodiazepines, but these drugs may also protect against convulsions. Treatment is supportive and symptomatic, with phenytoin indicated if the patient convulses. Respiratory function must be maintained and carefully monitored, as anoxaemia results in increased cardiac irritability.

***Drug interactions:*** the tricyclic antidepressants are involved in numerous interactions with other drugs. Their central sedative effects are potentiated by other CNS sedatives, particularly alcohol, and patients must be warned to avoid alcohol when on antidepressant therapy. The stimulant effects of amphetamine and other sympathomimetics are also potentiated. At high tricyclic antidepressant doses, antipsychotic drugs can be potentiated due to competition for metabolism in the liver. Marked anticholinergic effects may ensue.

Some older antihypertensive drugs such as debrisoquine and guanethidine are antagonised by tricyclic antidepressants, as their uptake into noradrenergic neurons is blocked and control of hypertension may be lost. Conversely, the tricyclics may potentiate the proarrhythmic effects of antiarrhythmic drugs such as quinidine and also digoxin. Thyroid hormones are also mildly potentiated.

#### Selective Serotonin Reuptake Inhibitors (SSRIs)

The SSRIs have a distinctly different activity profile from the tricyclic drugs. The most frequently reported adverse effects are nausea and vomiting, anxiety, insomnia, sweating, headaches and dry mouth.[55] Gastrointestinal effects are reported by about a third of patients but are generally mild and transient, and clearly dose-related. The nausea can, however, be troublesome in some patients and lead to cessation of treatment. Weight gain does not occur; rather, loss of weight is seen but this is generally only of note in patients who are initially overweight. Sexual problems are probably common but under-reported; the most common are anorgasmia in women and delayed ejaculation in men. Urticarial rashes have also been reported.

Toxicity in overdose is much less than with the tricyclic drugs. However, concerns have been voiced about the possible increased risk of suicide in patients taking SSRIs. It has been postulated that antidepressants may 'redistribute' the suicide risk, attenuating the risk in some patients who respond well, while enhancing the risk in some who respond poorly.[81] Although the SSRIs and fluoxetine in particular have been implicated in increasing the risk,[82] some data suggest that the SSRIs reduce suicidal ideation more effectively than the tricyclics, and they are certainly much safer in overdose. Thus, both the US FDA and the Committee on Safety in Medicine in the UK concluded that there was no evidence of such a risk.

A related claim is that fluoxetine can increase hostility and aggression. Again, however, epidemiological data do not support this association; depressed individuals are capable of violent acts by virtue of their psychopathology alone. Another putative adverse effect of the SSRIs is akathisia and agitation, which may be particularly distressing. All the SSRIs and paroxetine in particular may occasionally give rise to extrapyramidal symptoms, including tardive dyskinesia.

***Drug interactions:*** the potential for drug interactions varies among the SSRIs. The most serious interaction is with the MAOIs, with which enhancement of serotonergic effects with hyperpyrexia, tremor, myoclonic jerks and convulsions may occur. Several weeks must elapse after stopping fluoxetine before an MAOI can be instituted. The toxic effects of lithium may also be potentiated.

Fluvoxamine inhibits the metabolism of several drugs including propranolol, theophylline and carbamazepine, and the demethylation of tricyclic antidepressants. Likewise, fluoxetine inhibits the hydroxylation of tricyclic drugs,[62] and also the metabolism of carbamazepine and diazepam. However, sertraline and paroxetine appear to have few drug-drug interactions.[56,57]

#### Monoamine Oxidase Inhibitors (MAOIs)

The adverse effects of the MAOIs have been extensively studied because of their interesting pharmacological mechanisms. Orthostatic hypotension is a common and troublesome dose-related effect, often limiting the maximum attainable dosage of the MAOI. An unexplained adverse effect is oedema of the legs, feet or hands which often persists until the drug is discontinued. Restlessness and insomnia may occur and schizophrenic patients may suffer a reactivation of their psychotic symptoms. Bipolar patients may become hypomanic. Some patients complain of twitches in the limbs or paraesthesias of the extremities.

The early MAOIs (e.g. isocarboxazid, nialamide and phenelzine), being hydrazine derivatives, have been reported to cause liver damage, often fatal. Autonomic adverse effects include dry mouth, constipation, hesitancy of urination and dysuria, and blurring of vision. Changes in libido and delayed ejaculation have been reported, as have rashes and leucopenia.

***Dietary and drug interactions:*** the most dangerous adverse effects of the MAOIs are those involving dietary and drug interactions.[83] MAO inhibition prevents the breakdown of exogenous amines such as tyramine in the gut wall and liver and also increases body stores of noradrenaline. The amines reach the systemic circulation and release noradrenaline, producing a potentially dangerous hypertensive crisis. Symptoms comprise severe throbbing headache, and death from intracranial haemorrhage may follow the rupture of an aneurysm. The hypertensive crisis needs urgent, vigorous treatment. Symptomatic, supportive management must be instituted with monitoring of vital signs. Pharmacological intervention is with α-adrenoceptor blocking drugs, e.g. phentolamine 2.5 to 5mg intravenously. If unavailable, chlorpromazine 50mg may be administered intramuscularly instead.

The list of foods implicated in such reactions has grown inordinately, but only a few are really important. They include aged cheeses, smoked or pickled meats, meat or yeast extracts, fava and broad beans. Less important are high-protein foods such as pâté, chopped liver and meat salads.

Interactions with indirect-acting sympathomimetic amine drugs are actually more dangerous. These drugs stimulate the release of noradrenaline from nerve endings; they include ephedrine, pseudoephedrine and phenylpropanolamine, all common constituents of cough and cold remedies. Similarly, amphetamines may also interact dangerously, as may pethidine (and possibly other opioid analgesics). The combination of MAOIs with tricyclic antidepressants can be hazardous, the more dangerous ones being the drugs that block serotonin reuptake such as clomipramine. SSRIs also pose a potential hazard in combination with the MAOIs (see above).

***Overdosage*** with the MAOIs is characterised by headache, chest pain, hyperactivity and later nausea, vomiting, confusion, hyperthermia and dilated pupils. Profound hypotension is a harbinger of death. Treatment is supportive, no antidotes being available.

**Reversible Inhibitors of MAO Type A (RIMAs)**

Much of the above discussion does not apply to the RIMA, moclobemide.[63] In fact, the available evidence from clinical trials shows only one adverse effect to be more common with moclobemide than placebo, i.e. nausea which occurs in about 10% of patients receiving moclobemide compared with 5% of placebo-treated patients. It is largely devoid of the anticholinergic effects seen with the older MAOIs and tricyclic antidepressants. In addition, postural hypotension is not a problem, and oedema has not been reported. There is little or no central excitation, nor any sedation. Weight gain is undocumented and the drug is well-tolerated by the elderly. Limited experience with moclobemide suggests it is considerably safer in overdosage than its predecessors.

Particular attention has been paid to possible dietary and drug interactions with moclobemide. Potentiation of intravenously administered tyramine is less than 2-fold. When tyramine is given orally, thus mimicking the clinical situation, sensitivity to it is increased up to 7-fold in volunteers taking moclobemide. However, this potentiation is much less if tyramine is administered in conjunction with food. This degree of potentiation is of little clinical importance, as the patient would have to ingest 300g of strong fermented cheese or 100g of yeast extract before hypertension occurred. Therefore, provided moclobemide is given immediately after meals, dietary restrictions are largely unnecessary. Sympathomimetic amines should, however, still be avoided.[63]

## 5.2 Optimum Treatment

### *5.2.1 Primary Management*

When a depressive disorder has been diagnosed, it should be appraised both in terms of the present state and in terms of that patient's medical and psychiatric history, and social circumstances (fig. 2). Non-pharmacological treatments are important particularly in primary care of mildly ill patients. They comprise a wide range of strategies including counselling, cognitive therapy and interpersonal psychotherapy, and specialist intervention. Social support and help with particular difficulties may prevent the condition becoming intransigent to treatment. If drug treatment is deemed necessary, the patient should be told about the benefits and drawbacks of drugs, in particular that antidepressants may have unpleasant adverse effects but are not dependence-inducing. Admission to hospital will be necessary if the patient is actively suicidal or is deeply depressed yet denies such intent. Some patients are particularly at risk, e.g. recently widowed socially isolated older men.

#### Drug Selection Considerations

The choice of antidepressant is not an easy one and the popularity of various members of this class varies enormously between countries. For example, in the UK, dothiepin and lofepramine are the most frequently prescribed agents[80,84] yet in other countries, these drugs are unavailable or relatively unused. In many countries, cost is an overriding factor and the tricyclics, being mostly out of patent, are generally much less expensive than the newer SSRIs.

The greatest debate revolves around whether the tricyclics are still the drugs of first choice or whether their adverse effects and toxicity in overdose have rendered them obsolescent in this capacity. My view is that the older tricyclics are no longer acceptable as drugs of first choice, despite their proven (if limited) efficacy and low cost. However, the newer agent lofepramine (where available) is an appropriate choice, as it is much better tolerated than its predecessors, safer in overdosage and intermediate in cost. Where it is not available, or where suicide is a risk, and cost considerations are not paramount, then an SSRI is the treatment of first choice. In patients who need to maintain full alertness, most tricyclic drugs are inappropriate.

The above debate is further complicated by the advent of moclobemide. Whereas MAOIs have hitherto been eschewed or relegated to third or fourth choice, the tolerability of this agent makes it acceptable as a first choice for some patients, particularly those with coexisting phobic anxiety. Further on, the introduction of yet newer compounds such as nefazodone and venlafaxine will make the choice even more difficult to establish.

***Special patient groups:*** there are, of course, considerations pertinent to special groups. Patients with cardiac pathology should avoid tricyclic antidepressants, while those with migraine should avoid SSRIs. Patients with epilepsy pose particular difficulties, as very few antidepressants are free of being epileptogenic. However, viloxazine is one of these.

If the patient has had antidepressants previously, this can help in the choice of drug. Some patients welcome a little sedation to lessen their anxiety and agitation, whereas others prefer a slight stimulant effect. Some find the nausea and insomnia of the SSRIs much less tolerable than the dry mouth and constipation of a tricyclic drug.

#### Establishing the Optimum Dosage

The dosage of an antidepressant is usually arrived at by trial and error in each patient's case. About half the usual dosage of a tricyclic drug is used initially, or even less in the elderly and frail. The dosage is then increased weekly until adverse effects become too marked or clinical improvement manifests. Final dosages in the US are typically 50% higher than elsewhere. With the SSRIs, less dosage adjustment is needed, many patients staying on the same dose throughout. Gastrointestinal symptoms usually limit the final dose attained.

Divided doses are generally used but many patients prefer to take the bulk of the dose at night, particularly of a sedative tricyclic drug, which then acts as an hypnotic. Trazodone, which is very sedative, was favoured for this purpose in the US. However, tricyclic drugs should not be given in excessive single doses in the elderly or those with cardiovascular conditions.

#### Prediction of Response and Relapse

Although as a general rule, the patients with 'biological' features tend to respond best, it is not possible to predict this with accuracy. However, if no response whatsoever can be detected after 2 weeks' therapy at adequate dosage, the likelihood of response is low. The dexamethasone suppression test has been used in this context as it detects patients whose pituitary-adrenal function has been disrupted. It is not a worthwhile predictor of response but can predict who will relapse if treatment is discontinued prematurely.

#### Duration of Treatment

More emphasis is now placed on longer term treatment with antidepressants. After successful treatment of the acute episode, further management can be divided into two phases. The first is the *continuation phase*, which lasts up to 6 months after resolution of depressive symptoms. Several quite large-scale trials have shown that patients maintained on their tricyclic drugs have relapse rates of 20% or less, whereas

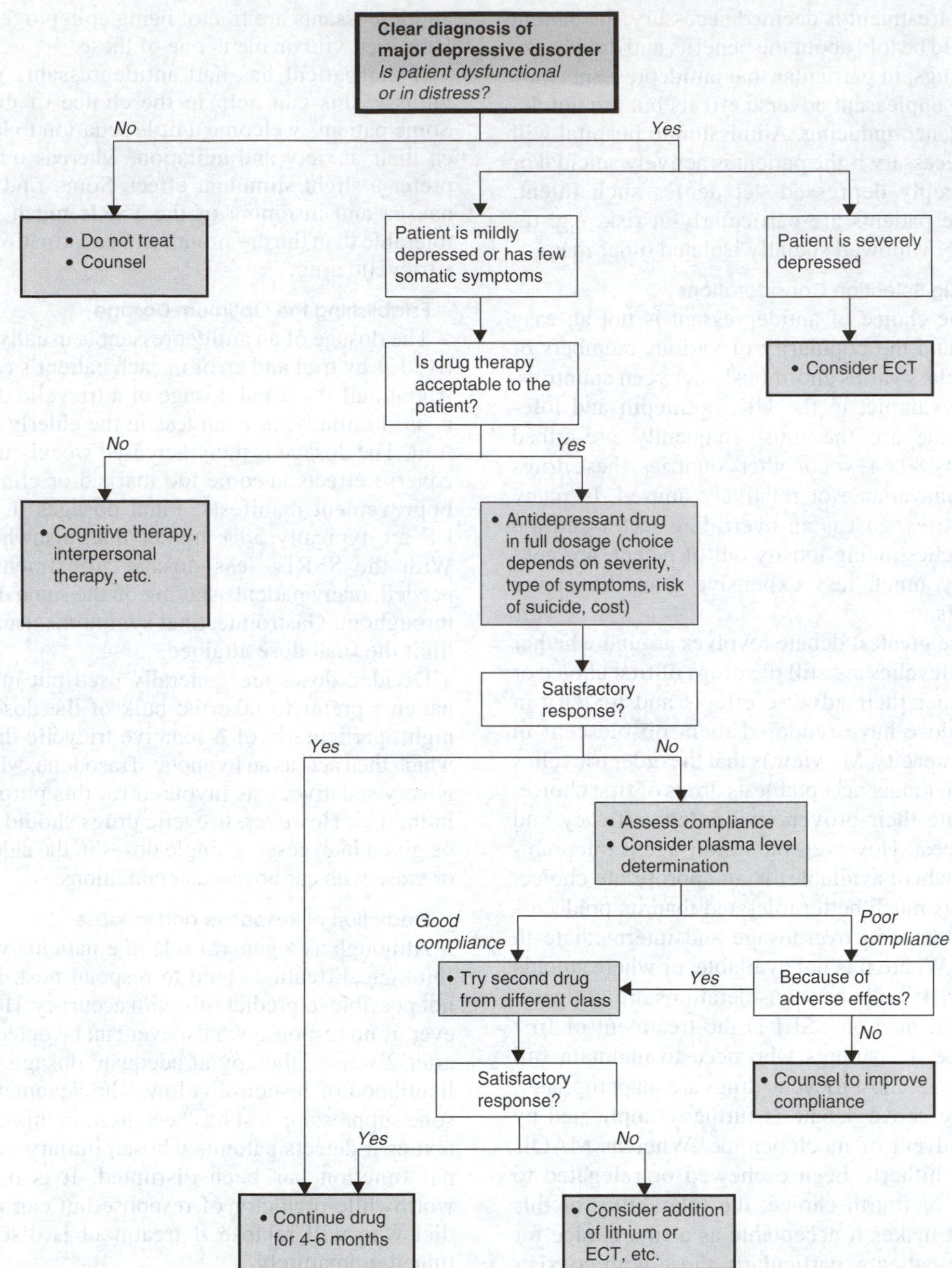


**Fig. 2.** Optimum treatment of major depressive disorder. *Abbreviation:* ECT = electroconvulsive therapy.

those switched to placebo relapse at a rate of over 50%. Continued medication is therefore routinely indicated. It was once customary to halve the therapeutic dose for the maintenance phase but it is now deemed necessary to maintain the full dosage throughout this period.

Some patients need particular attention because they are more likely to relapse. They include patients with a history of previous episodes of depressive illness, patients recovering from a severe disorder who still have residual symptoms, those who lack social support, and those with chronic social problems such as the long term unemployed or those with marital or family disharmony.

The second phase is *prevention of further episodes (prophylaxis).* This is usually taken quite arbitrarily to commence 4 months after resolution of the previous episode. However, the natural history of depressive disorders varies quite widely; some patients have short episodes, others more protracted periods of ill-health. Prophylaxis should be considered when there have been recurrent episodes of severe depression (unipolar disorder) or of manic-depressive illness (bipolar disorder). Lithium is also indicated in both conditions (see section 4.1.1) but many clinicians prefer an antidepressant as an alternative in unipolar disorder. The total duration of prophylaxis is a matter for clinical judgement and experience but 5 years is probably the minimum. The appropriate dosage has not been established but the need for efficacy must be balanced against the minimisation of adverse effects with improved compliance.

#### 5.2.2 Refractory Depression

About a third of patients with major depressive disorder fail to respond adequately to their initial medication.[85] No firm criteria for such treatment resistance have been identified but psychiatrists recognise the phenomenon as particularly common in specialist practice. Sometimes, the problem can be tackled by counselling to improve compliance and/or by an increase in dosage, e.g. where plasma drug concentrations are insufficient. Pharmacokinetic monitoring can be helpful in this situation.

For many patients, however, the condition seems refractory to what is usually adequate treatment. In such cases, the first stratagem is to review the diagnosis and auxiliary factors. Organic factors may perpetuate the depression; for example, hepatitis, viral pneumonia, infective mononucleosis and brucellosis may be associated with a subsequent chronic depression. Neoplasia, particularly of the pancreas, is another cause, as are hypothyroidism and pituitary/adrenal dysfunction. Neurological conditions associated with depression include early dementia, Parkinsonism, space-occupying lesions, temporal lobe epilepsy and multiple sclerosis. A particularly refractory form of depression may be induced by drugs such as antihypertensive agents and corticosteroids. Abuse of alcohol or other drugs such as amphetamine and appetite suppressants is another factor. Psychosocial causes, especially with life events of loss, can contribute greatly to the chronicity of a depression.

The practical management of these patients depends on their previous history and antidepressant drug use, combined with the personal, and sometimes idiosyncratic, experience of the clinician. Initially, a series of antidepressants may be tried which typically should include a tricyclic drug, (often clomipramine), an SSRI, and an MAOI, each given in maximal tolerated dosage for at least 8 weeks. ECT may also be considered for the more seriously and psychotically ill.[86] As the next step, various combinations may be tried, such as adding lithium to a tricyclic antidepressant.[87] Some clinicians combine a tricyclic and an SSRI on an empirical basis. A few will combine a tricyclic (usually trimipramine) with an MAOI, but such heroics are best left to those experienced in their use.

Antipsychotic medication may be added and sometimes a benzodiazepine if the patient is very anxious. Triple or even higher-order combinations may then be resorted to. However, it is sometimes most profitable to try withdrawing all medication for a while, carefully monitoring the patient, and later reinstituting it in a stepwise manner. Support may be afforded by day-hospital attendance.

### 5.3 Clinical Outcome and Economic Considerations

As discussed above (section 5.1.4), the antidepressants produce a clinical response in about two-thirds of patients in the short term and higher than this as other treatments are tried. Depression is a serious and agonising condition, with the attendant risk of suicide.[88]

The economics of depression include consideration of the direct costs of treatment and indirect costs to society. Estimates of these vary so widely as to raise serious doubts about the validity of the methods used.[89] Three studies based on primary care in the UK estimated direct annual costs of £271 million, £333 million, and £416 million whereas a US study (on just over 4 times the population) computed a figure of US$2100 million (= £329 million for UK). Indirect costs varied widely from £271 million to £2973 million in the UK, and to $14,200 million in the US.

A more recent study[90] estimated the direct annual costs in the US of medical, psychiatric and pharmacological care to be US$12.4 billion; mortality costs arising from depression-related suicides were estimated at US$7.5 billion, and morbidity costs associated with depression in the workplace at US$23.8 billion – a total of US$43.7 billion. The pharmaceutical costs broke down (in 1990) to US$890 million for antidepressants, with US$190 million spent on anxiolytics, US$25 million on antipsychotics, and the remaining US$70 million on other drugs. Thus, the pharmacological component of treating depression is less than 10% of the total estimated costs.

Recently, with advent of the SSRIs and moclobemide, questions have been asked as to whether these compounds are worth the increased cost in comparison with the less expensive tricyclics. Since the efficacy of all antidepressant drugs is very similar, the debate has crystallised around the different and better tolerated adverse effect profile of the SSRIs *versus* the tricyclics and their undoubted lesser toxicity in overdose. A meta-analysis of comparative efficacy studies has looked at comparative drop-out rates using these as an operational criterion for overall efficacy and tolerability.[68] There were no differences in drop-outs due to lack of efficacy but a slightly higher proportion of patients dropped out because of adverse effects in the tricyclic group (18.8%) than in the SSRI group (15.4%). This is probably an underestimate of the difference because these trials involve a comparison of a new SSRI (with which the investigators have had little experience) with a tricyclic agent which the investigators are usually familiar with and can more easily optimise the dosage.

The context in which the medication is given is also an important consideration. In primary care, most depressions are mild to moderate, and remit spontaneously.[91] If a mildly ill patient experiences adverse effects and becomes noncompliant, no great harm is done provided he/she is not suicidal. In secondary care clinics, depressive disorders are usually more severe and chronic and compliance becomes much more important. Despite this, few data have accrued to determine whether the better adverse effect profile of the SSRIs is reflected in higher compliance rates.

The economic considerations must also take into account the suicide aspects. About 50% of all suicides are committed by depressed individuals, and suicide accounts for over 1% of all deaths. The cost of a successful suicide, apart from the family's anguish, is the loss to society of what is often a very productive individual. However, unsuccessful suicides place a significant cost on healthcare services. Intensive care is generally needed after a determined attempt with a tricyclic drug and the cost can run into several thousand dollars equivalent. The greatly reduced toxicity in overdose of the SSRIs must result in at least partial savings in this context.

Finally, it should be noted that the newer antidepressants are not really expensive in comparison with newer drugs in other areas of medicine. It is just that the older drugs, being available as generics, are very inexpensive.

## 6. Anxiety Disorders and Insomnia

The anxiety disorders comprise several conditions, all characterised by anxiety which may be constant or episodic (panic attacks). Anxiety is an unpleasant emotional state directed towards the future with inexplicable threat and constant disquiet. Bodily changes are almost inevitable and include palpitations, overbreathing, chest pain, dryness of the mouth, churning in the stomach and muscle tension. Psychological symptoms include irritability, poor memory and insomnia. In the generalised anxiety disorder, the emotion is persistent, and is more common in women than men. Panics may be superimposed on the generalised anxiety or may occur unpredictably. There is a strong onset of fear of impending doom and the patient may fear he/she is going to die, go insane or lose control.

Panics can occur on their own but most commonly in association with phobic situations; these situations or events are then avoided. In agoraphobia, the fear is of leaving home, of open spaces or of crowded shops. In social phobia, the fears are of possible public exposure or eating in restaurants, or of performance situations, e.g. speaking in public. Specific phobias include fear of animals such as cats or dogs, or insects or heights. Post-traumatic disorder is a condition which comes on after either a single overwhelming stress or a chronic episode of severe stress. As well as anxiety symptoms, sleep is disturbed and there may be flashback experiences.

Insomnia is a complex disorder which can be transient, short-lived or chronic. In transient and short-lived insomnia, situational factors are important such as jetlag or acute stress. In chronic insomnia, the condition may be secondary to anxiety or depression or to other psychiatric conditions. It may be caused by physical conditions such as pain, or drugs such as caffeine. Nocturnal routines may be disrupted or there may be specific causes of insomnia such as restless leg syndrome or obstructive sleep apnoea.

## 6.1 Clinical Pharmacology of Drugs Used in Treatment

The term 'sedative' originally meant anxiety-allaying or calming. Now, however, it has come to mean feelings of drowsiness or torpor, a state originally called 'oversedation'. The term 'tranquilliser' was introduced to try and distance newer compounds such as the benzodiazepines from the older barbiturates, and this term is sometimes qualified by the adjectives 'minor' to mean sedatives and 'major' to denote antipsychotics. The word 'anxiolytic', despite its dubious etymology, is quite popular and is shorter than 'antianxiety agent'. Drugs used to treat insomnia are usually termed 'hypnotics'.

This area of therapeutics is dominated by the benzodiazepine group of compounds, the barbiturates and other older agents such as meprobamate, methaqualone, glutethimide and chloral hydrate having been rendered mostly obsolescent. Recently however, several compounds acting on serotonin (5-HT) mechanisms have been developed. Also, drugs with primary indications in other areas, such as psychosis and depression, have found some usage as anxiolytics.

### *6.1.1 Mechanism/Site of Action*

#### Benzodiazepines

It is only about 15 years since the mechanism of action of the benzodiazepines was clearly attributed to actions on receptors involving γ-aminobutyric acid (GABA), the inhibitory neurotransmitter.[92] Since then, our knowledge of these drugs has burgeoned to the point where they are now the best understood of all the major psychotropic drugs. In turn, this provides a rational basis for the optimisation of their risk : benefit profiles and for their clinical use.[93]

GABA is the most abundant, important CNS transmitter. The $GABA_A$ receptors are controllable ion channels which permit the passage of chloride ions into the neuron, hyperpolarising it and thereby inducing inhibition. There are various target sites on neuronal $GABA_A$ receptors to which benzodiazepines bind. Other sites bind the barbiturates, convulsants (such as picrotoxin), anaesthetics, and neurosteroids. The benzodiazepine site is unique in that it can mediate opposite pharmacological effects by reducing or increasing GABAergic neurotransmission, depending on the ligand. These modulatory effects are limited in intensity, never surpassing the extremes of physiological GABA function. In addition to agonism (benzodiazepines), and inverse agonism (e.g. some β-carbolines), antagonism can occur, as with *flumazenil*. The antagonist can block the actions of both agonists and inverse agonists without having any intrinsic activity.

Using electrophysiological techniques, the benzodiazepines have been shown to have GABA-potentiating actions in various parts of the CNS. These regions include the spinal cord, the hippocampus and the cerebellar and cerebral cortices. At all of these sites, the effects of the benzodiazepines are to increase inhibition, thereby dampening down neuronal activity. This translates clinically into muscle relaxant, anxiolytic, hypnotic and antiepileptic activity.

The $GABA_A$ ion channel unit consists of several subunits, each one of which can be of different types. Thus, the possible number of different types of unit is very high, probably several hundred. Many of these different isoforms have been identified and expressed using molecular pharmacological techniques. Benzodiazepine and related drugs vary in their affinities for the various types of ion channel unit. This opens up the possibility of developing drugs much more selective for one type than another, with perhaps differing pharmacological properties. Thus, it is conceivable that an anxiolytic drug could be developed without sedative or dependence-inducing properties.

The benzodiazepines vary in their degree of agonism, most being full agonists, others such as clonazepam being partial agonists. Again, the possibility of partial agonists having useful therapeutic actions without major adverse actions is being explored. Finally, the two phenomena can be combined, with a compound being a full agonist at one type of receptor, and a partial agonist at another.

#### Non-Benzodiazepine Agents

Two non-benzodiazepine hypnotics have been introduced. However, both these compounds act on the GABA system. *Zopiclone* is a cyclopyrrolone which binds close to the benzodiazepine receptor. *Zolpidem* is an imidazopyradine compound which binds selectively to some benzodiazepine receptors.

Drugs which seem to act by lessening serotonin activity have been developed as anxiolytics. *Buspirone* is a partial 5-$HT_{1A}$ agonist which is used as an anxiolytic agent. It appears to lessen serotonin activity by a presynaptic action. Blockade of 5-$HT_2$ (and perhaps 5-$HT_3$) receptors also has an anxiolytic but not an hypnotic effect.

### *6.1.2 Pharmacodynamic Properties*

#### CNS Effects

A wide range of animal models has been used to screen for putative anxiolytic compounds.[92] Some of these models are based on reactions to non-painful stressors such as light and dark and their effects on exploration or social interactions of one animal with another. Other models are based on reactions to painful stimuli or to taste aversion. Another depends on fear-potentiated startle. In general, these tests are quite efficient at detecting anxiolytics of the benzodiazepine type, but less good at detecting anxiolytics acting on serotonin mechanisms.

In normal humans, the depressant effects of single high doses of the benzodiazepines can be easily detected. At lower doses, it is more difficult to discern any psychomotor or cognitive effects. With repeated dosage, two processes occur which render prediction of effects difficult. Firstly, cumulation may occur, especially with benzodiazepines with long plasma half-lives. Secondly, tolerance may supervene, tending to cancel out the build-up in drug effects. In patients, the situation is even more complex. The anxiety or insomnia itself may be associated with a decrement in psychomotor and cognitive performance. Improvement in the condition with drug therapy will be attended by an improvement in functioning, and this may counteract any direct depressant effect of the medication. Hypnotic drugs, by definition, are expected to produce sedation but that sedation should not persist to the next day. Moreover, hypnotics are used primarily by elderly people who may rise in the night, so excessive sedation can be dangerous.

The benzodiazepines have characteristic effects on the EEG, causing a marked increase in fast-wave (beta) activity. The typical effects of benzodiazepines on sleep and the sleep EEG include the reduction of slow-wave sleep and REM sleep and the prolongation of REM sleep latency. Slow-wave amplitude is reduced by benzodiazepines. The withdrawal of the benzodiazepine is attended by a reversal or even rebound of these effects. Clinical changes occur in parallel with rebound anxiety and insomnia.

#### Other Effects

Outside the CNS, the benzodiazepines have relatively few effects. Respiration is hardly affected by benzodiazepines, hypnotic doses having no significant clinical effect except in individuals whose respiratory function is already compromised, such as patients with obstructive sleep apnoea. However, higher doses, like those given as premedication or preanaesthetic, are capable of lowering ventilation and may cause $CO_2$ narcosis in patients with chronic obstructive respiratory disease. Benzodiazepines tend to lower blood pressure to a minor degree but more by a central sedative action than by affecting cardiovascular mechanisms. Coronary blood flow is increased.

The gastrointestinal tract is affected in a similar way. Benzodiazepine-induced sedation is associated with a decrease in gastric secretion and motility, especially at night. Endocrine effects include a rise in prolactin levels.

### *6.1.3 Pharmacokinetic Characteristics*

#### Benzodiazepines

The pharmacokinetic characteristics of individual benzodiazepines are shown in table IX. In general, the benzodiazepines are highly lipid-soluble compounds and are therefore rapidly and completely absorbed after oral administration, penetrate the brain readily, and are metabolised and/or conjugated in the liver to more polar compounds that are excreted in the urine.[94] Absorption is usually erratic after intramuscular injection, lorazepam being an exception. Intravenous preparations are rapidly effective but problems have been encountered in formulating some benzodiazepines for intravenous use because of their insolubility in water.

As with most psychotropic drugs, there is considerable interindividual variability in pharmacokinetic parameters for each drug. Also, concentration-effect relationships, although demonstrable within each patient, are not clearly established between patients.[95] Consequently, monitoring of plasma concentrations is unhelpful when faced by an unresponsive patient, except as a rough indicator of compliance.

Two aspects of the pharmacokinetics of the benzodiazepines are germane to the clinician. Firstly, the *speed of onset* is important both when dealing with acute anxiety and with insomnia. With the former, the sufferer wants prompt relief; with the latter, time to onset of sleep should be minimised to prevent a mounting wave of anxiety about lying awake. Some benzodiazepines enter the brain very rapidly, diazepam being an example. Others such as oxazepam are much slower in doing so, being less lipophilic. Lorazepam enters the brain fairly rapidly but temazepam, despite its popularity as an hypnotic, is somewhat slower. The formulation also affects the onset of action, liquid preparations being more rapidly absorbed.

As with some barbiturates, *redistribution* is also an important factor in determining the duration of effect. Some benzodiazepines such as diazepam and flunitrazepam have short durations of action (less than 6 hours) after single doses, despite being slowly metabolised.

The *metabolism* of the benzodiazepines is often quite complex with pharmacologically active metabolites being quite common. In the case of diazepam, the major metabolic route is via demethylation to the long-acting active metabolite nordazepam (*N*-desmethyldiazepam); this compound is in fact marketed as an anxiolytic in some countries. A lesser metabolic route is by hydroxylation to temazepam, which is used widely as an hypnotic. This is then demethylated to oxazepam, an anxiolytic compound. Furthermore, hydroxylation of nordazepam also results in oxazepam. Other benzodiazepines which largely end up in this chain include chlordiazepoxide, medazepam and clorazepate. Once an hydroxyl group is attached to the heterocyclic ring, conjugation can take place. Thus, benzodiazepines can be divided into those that are metabolised solely by conjugation, such as lorazepam, temazepam and oxazepam, and those that undergo phase I metabolic processes first. Because nordazepam (*N*-desmethyldiazepam) has a very long plasma half-life, compounds metabolised to it tend to accumulate and be long-acting.

As phase I (metabolism) but not phase II (conjugation) processes are age-dependent, the duration of action of some benzodiazepines (e.g. diazepam) is increased in the elderly, whereas others benzodiazepines (e.g. lorazepam and oxazepam) are largely unaffected. Consequently, the latter drugs are preferred for sedating patients with liver dysfunction.

*Diazepam* has been the most widely studied of the benzodiazepines, reflecting its widespread usage. It is rapidly absorbed with peak plasma concentrations occurring at around 1 hour. Discernible effects may occur as soon as 15 minutes after oral administration. Diazepam is highly plasma protein bound (97 to 99%) and has an apparent volume of distribution of about 1 L/kg, or somewhat higher in the elderly. The redistribution phase determines the duration of action after single doses but diazepam is slowly eliminated with a plasma half-life of 24 to 48 hours in young adults. In the elderly, this may be doubled, and accumulation may occur.[96,97] The major active metabolite nordazepam (*N*-desmethyldiazepam) has a longer plasma half-life of 50 to 150 hours, and thus marked accumulation can occur. In the elderly, half-lives over 200 hours have been recorded and psychotropic effects can persist for weeks. Because of marked interindividual variation, the effects of a constant dose will vary greatly and this accounts for the dosage ranges being arrived at empirically in clinical practice.

*Chlordiazepoxide*, *halazepam* and *medazepam* are also partly metabolised to nordazepam (*N*-desmethyldiazepam) and, accordingly, are long-acting compounds. *Clorazepate* is a prodrug for nordazepam, being converted to the latter in an acid medium such as the stomach or on absorption.

*Lorazepam* is more slowly absorbed than diazepam, with peak plasma concentrations occurring at around 2 hours. It has a large apparent volume of distribution and is highly bound (over 90%) to plasma proteins. The plasma half-life varies between 8 and 24 hours, but is only weakly age-related and not markedly prolonged in patients with hepatic impairment. Some studies have suggested a second peak of activity at around 6 hours after administration. This may be due to reabsorption and breakdown of the conjugated glucuronide which is excreted into the gut via the biliary tract.

Three other widely-used drugs have similar pharmacokinetic characteristics to lorazepam. *Oxazepam* is rather slowly absorbed rendering it inappropriate as a treatment for insomnia. Its plasma half-life is 6 to 24 hours. Because it undergoes only conjugation in the liver, it can be safely given (initially in cautious dosage) to patients with hepatic impairment. Conversely, its elimination is prolonged in uraemic patients. *Temazepam* is very similar but is used as an hypnotic, usually in a formulation which permits rapid availability in the gut. It has a plasma half-life of 8 to 16 hours and tends not to accumulate, although residual effects the next day are detectable after high doses. *Lormetazepam,* the chlorinated derivative of temazepam, has a similar half-life of 8 to 16 hours but is much more potent.

**Table IX.** Pharmacokinetic characteristics of some antianxiety drugs and hypnotics (after Hollister[12])

| Drug | Plasma half-life (h) | Route of elimination | Comments |
|---|---|---|---|
| **Benzodiazepines** | | | |
| Chlordiazepoxide | 5-30 | Hepatic metabolism (active metabolites) | Plasma clearance decreased in the elderly and in severe liver disease.<br>Active metabolites (demethyl-chlordiazepoxide, demoxepam) metabolised more slowly than parent drug and can accumulate on repeated dosage |
| Diazepam | 24-48 | Hepatic metabolism (active metabolites) | Plasma half-life is age dependent: 20h at age 20, 90h at age 80 but owing to change in distribution volume, plasma clearance not altered in elderly.<br>Severe liver disease decreases plasma clearance.<br>Active metabolites are nordazepam (*N*-desmethyldiazepam, major metabolite), oxazepam and temazepam.<br>Nordazepam (*N*-desmethyldiazepam) is metabolised more slowly than parent drug and can accumulate on repeated dosage |
| Bromazepam | 8-19 | Hepatic metabolism | |
| Clobazam | ≈50* | Hepatic metabolism (active metabolites) | *Half-life shown is for parent drug and active metabolites |
| Halazepam | 35 | Hepatic metabolism (active metabolites) | Major active metabolite is nordazepam (*N*-desmethyldiazepam), which is metabolised more slowly than parent drug (half-life ≈58h) |
| Ketazolam | ≈1.5* | Hepatic metabolism (active metabolites) | *Plasma half-life short; rapidly metabolised to active compounds with longer half-lives, including diazepam |
| Medazepam | ≈1-2* | Hepatic metabolism (active metabolites) | *Plasma half-life short; rapidly metabolised to active compounds with longer half-lives, including diazepam |
| Prazepam | ≈78* | Hepatic metabolism (active metabolites) | *Half-life shown is for parent drug and active metabolites |
| Flunitrazepam | ≈13-19 | Hepatic metabolism (active metabolites); possible metabolism in gut wall | Plasma half-life of active metabolites about 25-30h |
| Flurazepam | 47-100* | Hepatic metabolism (active metabolites) | *Plasma half-life very short. Value shown is for principal active metabolite (dealkylflurazepam), which can accumulate on repeated dosage |
| Nitrazepam | 18-34 | Hepatic metabolism (? activity of metabolites) | Acetylation of amine metabolite subject to genetic polymorphism |
| Quazepam | 41 | Hepatic metabolism (active metabolites) | Major active metabolites have longer plasma half-lives than the parent drug |
| Alprazolam | 10-12 | Hepatic metabolism (some active metabolites) | Principal active metabolite (α-hydroxyalprazolam) does not attain appreciable plasma concentrations |
| Oxazepam | 6-25 | Hepatic metabolism to inactive glucuronide | Plasma half-life not affected by severe liver disease or in the elderly |
| Lorazepam | 8-25 | Hepatic metabolism to inactive glucuronide | Plasma half-life not affected by severe liver disease but clearance is slightly reduced in the elderly |
| Loprazolam | 6-8 | Hepatic metabolism (active metabolites) | Active piperazine-*N*-oxide metabolite has a similar half-life to parent drug |
| Lormetazepam | 9-15 | Hepatic metabolism (largely to inactive glucuronides) | |
| Midazolam | 2-5 | Hepatic metabolism (active metabolites) | Principal active metabolite (α-hydroxymidazolam) has a very short plasma half-life.<br>Probable significant hepatic first-pass metabolism |
| Temazepam | 8-13 | Hepatic metabolism (primarily to inactive metabolites; oxazepam is a minor metabolite) | |
| Triazolam | 2-5 | Hepatic metabolism (? activity of metabolites); small amounts excreted unchanged in urine | Probable significant first-pass hepatic metabolism after oral administration |
| Brotizolam | 4-7 | Hepatic metabolism (active metabolites) | Principal active metabolite (1-methyl-hydroxy-brotizolam) rapidly eliminated |

**Table IX.** *[Continued]*

| Drug | Plasma half-life (h) | Route of elimination | Comments |
|---|---|---|---|
| **Barbiturates** | | | |
| Pentobarbital | 22-30 | Hepatic metabolism and renal excretion of unchanged drug (20%) | Induces hepatic drug metabolising enzymes |
| Phenobarbital | 48-144 | Hepatic metabolism and renal excretion of unchanged drug (27-50%) | Induces hepatic drug metabolising enzymes<br>Clearance greater in alkaline urine |
| **Others** | | | |
| Meprobamate | 6-17 | Hepatic metabolism and renal excretion of unchanged drug (8-19%) | Induces hepatic drug metabolising enzymes |
| Methaqualone | 20-60 | Hepatic metabolism, about 2% excreted unchanged in urine | Induces hepatic drug metabolising enzymes |
| Glutethimide | 5-22 | Hepatic metabolism (active metabolite); enterohepatic recirculation; <2% excreted unchanged in urine | Active metabolite 4-hydroxyglutethimide accumulates on overdosage and is eliminated more slowly than parent drug.<br>Oral absorption erratic.<br>Induces hepatic drug metabolising enzymes |
| Chloral hydrate | 7-10* | Hepatic metabolism (active metabolite) | *Plasma half-life very short; value shown is for active metabolite trichloroethanol; second major metabolite trichloroacetic acid has a half-life of 4-5 days |
| Clomethiazole (chlormethiazole) | 3-9 | Hepatic metabolism (active metabolites) | Significant first-pass hepatic metabolism after oral administration.<br>Bioavailability increased and clearance decreased in the elderly and in cirrhosis |
| Buspirone | 2-8 | Hepatic metabolism (active metabolites); little renal excretion of unchanged drug | Metabolites rapidly eliminated |
| Zopiclone | 4-5 | Hepatic metabolism (active and inactive metabolites); little renal excretion of unchanged drug (≈4%) | Metabolites rapidly eliminated (similar plasma half-lives to parent drug) |
| Zolpidem | 1.5-2.4 | Hepatic metabolism (no active metabolites) | |

*Nitrazepam* is a widely-used hypnotic in some countries. It is long-acting with a plasma half-life of 18 to 36 hours, and therefore accumulates, particularly in the elderly. *Flunitrazepam* is a more potent, fluorinated analogue, which is also long-acting. However, the longest-acting of all the benzodiazepine hypnotics is *flurazepam*. Although the parent compound has a short half-life, the main active metabolite, *N*-dealkylflurazepam, has a half-life of 50 to 100 hours, and thus resembles nordazepam (*N*-desmethyldiazepam). *Quazepam* is also largely converted to long-acting metabolites.[98]

*Alprazolam* is a triazolo-derivative of high potency which is widely used to treat anxiety and panic. It has a plasma half-life of around 12 hours, with many metabolites, some active but probably of no clinical importance.[99] A related compound, *triazolam*, is a very short-acting hypnotic with a half-life of 2 to 5 hours and therefore does not accumulate when given once-nightly.[100] *Midazolam* is a water-soluble compound that also has a very short plasma half-life (around 2 to 5h); this drug is also used as an anaesthetic and for sedation prior to diagnostic or surgical procedures.

**Non-Benzodiazepine Agents**

*Buspirone* is rapidly absorbed but has a low bioavailability. It is extensively metabolised and one metabolite, although present in low concentrations, may affect noradrenergic rather than serotonin mechanisms. The plasma half-life of buspirone is around 2 to 8 hours, necessitating divided daily administration.

The non-benzodiazepine hypnotics *zopiclone* and *zolpidem* are also rapidly absorbed, and both are eliminated by hepatic metabolism. Zopiclone, which has a plasma half-life of about 5 hours, is extensively metabolised to a number of metabolites, including one which has pharmacological activity; however, the metabolite has a similar plasma half-life to the parent drug.[101] Zolpidem has 3 major metabolites, though all are pharmacologically inactive; its plasma half-life is shorter than that of zopiclone and ranges from 1.5 to 2.4 hours.[102]

#### 6.1.4 Clinical Effectiveness

##### Generalised Anxiety Disorder

The efficacy of the benzodiazepines as short term antianxiety compounds is well established. However, this efficacy is somewhat limited. In a meta-analysis of 81 controlled trials in anxiety disorders conducted up to the mid-1980s, two-thirds of which involved benzodiazepines, the overall effect was found to be modest (about one effect-size) and about 50% of it was attributable to nonspecific and placebo effects.[103] Prospective studies have identified various factors as being predictive of above average outcome. These include being female, older, higher social class, having somatic symptoms and no histrionic traits. Belief that medication can help also improves the outcome.

***Short term efficacy:*** the onset of action of benzodiazepines is prompt, relief often being felt after a few doses. Diazepam has a particularly quick effect and is useful to relieve acute anxiety attacks short of panic. The benzodiazepines vary somewhat in efficacy, although with such modest overall efficacy, these differences do not often reach significant levels. The clinical impression is that diazepam, lorazepam and alprazolam are more effective than chlordiazepoxide and oxazepam.

Buspirone has a more gradual onset of action and may take 2 to 3 weeks before full symptom relief occurs. Another problem is reduced efficacy in patients with recent exposure to a benzodiazepine. A direct switch is inadvisable because buspirone will not suppress benzodiazepine rebound or withdrawal effects.

***Longer term efficacy:*** anxiety disorders tend to be chronic and/or fluctuating conditions. Thus, the longer term efficacy of antianxiety medication is more difficult to demonstrate. When patients maintained long-term on a benzodiazepine are switched to placebo, rebound or more severe withdrawal effects may obscure the picture, the increased anxiety being misinterpreted as a return of the original anxiety. However, some patients show an increase in anxiety which is identical in characteristics to their underlying disorder, and not closely related to the cessation of active treatment. As a rough estimate, about a third of patients withdrawing from long term (over 1 year) benzodiazepine treatment will show a withdrawal syndrome, a third will suffer a relapse, and a third will suffer neither. However, different patient samples have different characteristics. The best predictor of chronicity is obviously the duration of previous illness. Newly presenting patients with a short history tend not to need long term drug treatment, as natural remission is likely.

***Efficacy versus non-pharmacological measures:*** the efficacy of non-pharmacological treatments of anxiety disorders has been compared directly with that of drug treatment in a meta-analysis of a few studies.[104] In a comparison of 5 treatments (diazepam, dothiepin, placebo, cognitive and behaviour therapy, and self-help treatment) given for 6 to 10 weeks in patients with generalised anxiety disorder, panic disorder and dysthymic disorder (mild depression), the diazepam-treated group showed significantly less improvement than the non-drug and antidepressant groups, with a consistent trend to a worse outcome even than the placebo group.[105] Manifestly, the characteristics of various types of patients differ from one study to another. Even within a study, the type of patient is important. The closer the patient meets the rigorous criteria for undoubted generalised anxiety disorder, and the more severe and more chronic the anxiety, the better will be the response to a benzodiazepine, at least in the short term and probably in the long term.

##### Panic Disorder

The treatment of panic disorder has become a focus of interest. It had long been held that benzodiazepines were not effective in panic disorder, either in preventing or treating the attacks. However, the advent of *alprazolam* led to a reappraisal of the efficacy of benzodiazepines in panic disorder. Early studies suggested that high doses of alprazolam (2 to 6 times the usual anxiolytic dose) could suppress panic attacks quite effectively. Consequently, some large-scale studies were mounted to examine this more closely.[106,107] These showed good efficacy for alprazolam in suppressing both predictable panic attacks (i.e. going into a phobic situation) and unpredictable (spontaneous) panic attacks. Anticipatory anxiety was also reduced. However, placebo responses were often quite high, as with generalised anxiety disorder patients. At first it was not clear whether alprazolam had unique efficacy in panic disorder, or whether most or all benzodiazepines are capable of suppressing panics when given in sufficiently high dosage. More recent studies have suggested that other benzodiazepines such as diazepam, lorazepam and clonazepam are also effective.

Comparisons of the efficacy of alprazolam with that of antidepressants such as imipramine in suppressing panic attacks have shown that although the benzodiazepine is better tolerated, patients who tolerate the adverse effects respond equally well to the two treatments.[107,108] However, on discontinuation of treatment, rebound appears to occur in patients who received alprazolam and within a month of withdrawal, they appeared to be worse than those who received imipramine, often requiring resumption of medication.

Non-pharmacological treatments are also being developed to help patients with panic disorder. As well as relaxation and anxiety management techniques, cognitive therapy is being adapted to this purpose and preliminary data suggest useful efficacy, at least in less severely handicapped patients. The approach postulates that patients with panic attacks are oversensitive to normal bodily cues such as a missed heart beat. These perceptions are elaborated into a 'catastrophic' misinterpretation of impending bodily harm which triggers off a vicious circle, culminating in a panic attack. Therapy aims to intervene in this cycle by teaching the patient to reinterpret his/her bodily sensations in a less threatening manner.

#### Insomnia

Almost uniquely in psychopharmacology, the efficacy of hypnotic medication can be accurately assessed using EEG and other recordings – the so-called 'polysomnogram'.[109] Procedures in sleep laboratories are now fairly standard, although debate continues on the more subtle points of analysis of sleep recordings.

In general, the objective efficacy of benzodiazepine hypnotics falls into two types. Firstly, the drug can shorten the latent period between 'lights out' and the onset of the early stage of sleep (sleep latency). These benzodiazepines tend to be rapidly absorbed and penetrate the brain quickly. Secondly, the drug can alter the duration of sleep, both in total (total sleep time) and in reducing wakefulness during the night. These agents tend to be medium-acting in duration (or even long-acting). In addition, the structure of sleep is altered, with slow-wave sleep being curtailed. Some newer hypnotics such as zopiclone and zolpidem, which act like benzodiazepines but are chemically dissimilar, have much less effect on sleep architecture and, in low dose, may even increase slow-wave sleep.[101,102,110]

Insomnia is a subjective complaint and therefore the efficacy of an hypnotic drug must be assessed using subjective ratings of quality and duration of sleep. Unfortunately, the correlation between the objective and subjective measures is often poor, particularly in chronic insomnia. Furthermore, subjective ratings are imprecise so that efficacy is hard to establish to acceptable statistical levels. Also, insomnia fluctuates markedly from night to night so that efficacy in short term administration (a night or two) may be unconvincing.

Consistent data suggest that sleep laboratory measures of hypnotic effect revert to pretreatment values within 1 to 4 weeks of administration of an hypnotic on a nightly basis.[111] Efficacy is better preserved if the drug is given intermittently. Despite this, subjective reports of efficacy may suggest that the patient remains satisfied with the therapeutic effect. This may be largely an artefact of the subjective nature of the ratings. In a study of 40 middle-aged, chronic insomniacs on medication, the patients estimated that they had slept for an average of 72 minutes more than the sleep recordings indicated.[112] When the recordings were repeated the next night without the patients being medicated, sleep was underestimated by an average of 61 minutes. Thus, the efficacy of the medication appeared to be 2 hours better in prolonging sleep time than it actually was. This apparent efficacy overestimation may be attributable to the effects of the benzodiazepine in suppressing the patient's recall the next day of having woken in the night, i.e. an 'amnesiogenic effect'.

As with the other indications, the use of benzodiazepines is being challenged by the development of non-pharmacological techniques. The simplest is *sleep hygiene*, where the patient is given advice about how to optimise his/her sleeping arrangements, to avoid caffeine and alcohol, and to reserve the bedroom for sleep so that the conditioned reflexes associated with sleep routines are reinforced. More elaborate psychological techniques involve relaxation, stimulus control, cognitive therapy, etc. but few studies have evaluated these methods systematically.

### 6.1.5 Tolerability and Drug Interactions Potential

#### Adverse Effects of Benzodiazepines

The benzodiazepines have well-known subjective effects which have been documented in detail in controlled trials. During the first week of treatment, about a third of patients treated with a benzodiazepine anxiolytic report drowsiness, tiredness or a feeling of heaviness; this compares with about 10% on placebo. The effects are most marked at or just before the time of maximum blood concentration, i.e. 1 to 2 hours after each dose, but usually diminish after a few days of continuing treatment. The degree of sedation is strongly dose-dependent and varies from one agent to another, diazepam being more sedative than clobazam. Older patients are more sensitive to the sedative effects, partly because of altered pharmacokinetics (increased volume of distribution), and partly because of increased tissue and end-organ sensitivity.[113] Longer-acting hypnotics such as flurazepam and nitrazepam are more likely to produce residual effects the next day, usually a subjective feeling of hangover.

***Paradoxical excitation:*** a less predictable but nevertheless fairly common effect is a paradoxical increase in anxiety or the induction of feelings of hostility and aggression. Occasionally, this may result in antisocial behaviour such as shop-lifting, sexual indiscretions or assault, or in emotional lability such as uncontrollable weeping. Often the feelings and impulses bewilder the sufferer, who fails to attribute them to the medication and fears he/she is losing control. It is unclear how frequent these reactions are; the more severe ones result in forensic complications and give rise to public concern. Less severe reactions affect fewer than 5% of those given a benzodiazepine for anxiety, panic or insomnia. However, concern about such reactions with triazolam led to its removal from the UK market and to reappraisal elsewhere.

***Effects on depression:*** benzodiazepines have complex effects on depression.[114] They are not really antidepressants but can induce some euphoria which may temporarily combat the lowering of mood. They can relieve the anxiety comorbid with or secondary to a depressive illness, thereby uncovering the depression; this may be misinterpreted as a depressogenic effect. A paradoxical reaction which can include depressive feelings may also occur.

***Effects on cognitive function:*** the memory-impairing effects of the benzodiazepines are welcomed by patients given premedication. However, amnesic episodes may also occur occasionally in patients receiving antianxiety and hypnotic benzodiazepine therapy. Definite and fairly specific cognitive deficits can be quantified in both normal volunteers and patients given a benzodiazepine.[115] The drugs act to disrupt the consolidation process whereby semantic material is transferred from short term to long term memory stores. Thus, a patient can recall material immediately but may not later. Tolerance of this effect is less than with psychomotor impairments.

These deleterious effects seen on laboratory tests carry over into real-life situations. For example, simulated driving and driving on a test-track or in real life are impaired after administration of a benzodiazepine. Epidemiological data suggest, however, that benzodiazepines play a much lesser role in traffic accidents than does alcohol. Accidents are most likely during the first month of treatment.

***Other adverse effects*** include vertigo, dizziness, dysarthria and ataxia, all dose-related and more common in the elderly. Incoordination may lead to falls with risk of fracture. In addition, rash, weight gain, impairment of sexual function, menstrual irregularities, and rarely blood dyscrasias may occur. Claims that benzodiazepines are teratogenic have not been confirmed. As the benzodiazepines are secreted in small amounts in breast milk, the suckling child may become floppy and listless.

#### Adverse Effects of Buspirone

Buspirone has an adverse effect profile dissimilar to that of the benzodiazepines. The most common adverse effect is dizziness, and others include nausea and headache. However, sedation is not a problem, nor are paradoxical reactions.

### Dependence and Abuse of Antianxiety/Hypnotic Drugs

Over the last 15 years, increased concern has been expressed that the extensive long term usage of the benzodiazepines stems not from efficacy but from a state of dependency. Numerous studies have established that a state of physical dependence can develop, even in patients taking normal therapeutic doses, as manifested by a withdrawal syndrome despite tapering of the dosage. Even short term usage can be followed by rebound.

***Rebound*** has been most carefully studied following the discontinuation of hypnotic benzodiazepines. Thus, some patients suffer a night or two of worsened sleep as estimated on subjective reports, and confirmed by polysomnogram.[116] Sleep latency is prolonged, total sleep time is curtailed, and nocturnal awakenings are more frequent and prolonged. Dosage is an important determinant but duration of usage is not usually relevant, as rebound can occur after only a few nights.[117] Short-acting hypnotics such as triazolam are more likely to be associated with rebound than medium-duration compounds, and rebound is virtually undetectable after stopping a long-acting benzodiazepine. The clinical relevance of rebound is unclear[118] but it might well result in resumption of medication with prolonged use.

***Withdrawal syndromes:*** the hallmark of dependence is the detection of a characteristic withdrawal syndrome. With the benzodiazepines, this is characterised by anxiety, insomnia, shakiness, tremor, nausea, loss of appetite, impaired concentration, lethargy and dysphoria. Perceptual changes include hyperacusis, photophobia, paraesthesias and a feeling of constantly moving. The symptoms are time-locked to final cessation, supervening within 48 hours of stopping medium-duration compounds and 5 to 10 days after stopping long-acting benzodiazepines. The symptoms usually subside over a few weeks but may persist longer.[119]

*Influence of dose and duration of use:* patients on high doses are much more likely to manifest a withdrawal syndrome than those on lower doses, although the syndrome may be no more severe. Duration of use also determines the likelihood of a withdrawal reaction; patients taking a benzodiazepine for 6 months to a year have about a 1 in 3 chance, but the probability is almost 100% beyond 5 years.

Patients attempting to discontinue short- and medium-acting benzodiazepines have more severe but usually shorter reactions than those stopping long-acting compounds. However, more resume medication because they cannot tolerate the symptoms. Some benzodiazepines such as lorazepam and alprazolam have the reputation of presenting particular withdrawal problems. Success rates vary greatly depending mainly on the type of patient and whether they have attempted withdrawal previously.[120] Sustained abstinence is achieved in only about 50% of patients experiencing withdrawal symptoms. Depressed patients usually fail to withdraw successfully and some patients become clinically depressed on withdrawal. Physical dependence can develop in infants *in utero* and neonatal withdrawal syndromes have been recorded.

***High-dose dependence*** is fairly uncommon among benzodiazepine users, in contrast to the previous situation with the barbiturates. It is unclear why some patients escalate their dose while most do not. Previous problems with other sedatives or with alcohol are an ominous prognosticator, and benzodiazepines should not be prescribed for such patients.

***Abuse potential:*** the benzodiazepines were originally thought to have a low abuse potential but it is now clear that they pose a considerable and increasing addiction problem worldwide. They are used as part of polydrug abuse to induce euphoria or to potentiate opioid actions. Cocaine and amphetamine users take benzodiazepines to cushion the crashdown from the 'high'. However, benzodiazepines are being used increasingly as primary addictive drugs.[121] About half the users inject them. Temazepam is popular for this purpose in the UK, but worldwide, flunitrazepam, often taken intranasally, is a bigger problem. Combined abuse of benzodiazepines and alcohol is very common.

***Buspirone:*** unlike the benzodiazepines, buspirone is rarely associated with dependence or abuse.

### Drug Interactions

A wide range of CNS depressants potentiate, and in turn are potentiated by, the benzodiazepines. Alcohol is the most notable example, the potentiation often resulting in disinhibition, hostility and amnesia for the events. The interactions are quite complex in the clinical situation. Potentiation may occur but often the effects are merely additive. In some instances, interactions cannot be detected and it may be that tolerance developed during treatment with a benzodiazepine is transferred to alcohol, the combination having less than expected effects.

### Overdosage

Overdosage with a benzodiazepine is quite common, especially among young women. However, deaths are uncommon, although they can occur, especially in the young, the old, the frail and those with existing respiratory pathology.[122] Their combination with other CNS depressants is hazardous. In most cases, the patient falls asleep but is still rousable. The sleep or light coma lasts up to 48 hours, depending on the amount taken and the plasma half-life of the drug ingested. The light coma can be reversed by giving an intravenous injection of the benzodiazepine antagonist *flumazenil.*

## 6.2 Optimum Treatment

### Generalised Anxiety Disorder

Anxiety can be a self-limiting condition which needs treatment when it becomes subjectively intolerable or unrealistic, or interferes with normal function. However, reduction of anxiety is also a helpful part of management when the symptoms occur in the context of real problems such as unemployment, marital breakdown, bereavement, or physical disease. Some patients suffer more protracted syndromes with chronic anxiety punctuated by episodes of severe and disabling anxiety. Pharmacological and psychological treatment can be used alone or in combination.[123] However, with drug treatments given alone, patients may become passive participants and this may provide no incentive for them to learn methods of coping with anxiety in other ways.

Most patients suffering from anxiety are treated in a primary care setting. A few quite brief sessions of support, reassurance and counselling may suffice for all but the most chronic and severe patients.[124] Patients already taking a benzodiazepine need particularly careful initial assessment. Reassurance should be directed towards explanation of the symptom mechanisms but should not be diffuse and bland. The particular problem underlying the anxiety should be identified and an active problem-solving approach encouraged.[125] Patients with more complicated or resistant problems may benefit from more formal psychological therapy but the availability of appropriate expertise varies widely.

Patients who are severely disabled by acute anxiety will need a brief course of treatment with an antianxiety drug (fig. 3). Otherwise, other forms of treatment including behavioural methods and psychotherapy are unlikely to succeed. The selection of appropriate drug treatment depends on the individual needs of the patient and likely duration of therapy. The benzodiazepines are still the first choice when a rapid antianxiety effect is needed. However, the clinician must tell the patient that the supply will be restricted to one or two small prescriptions, and should emphasise that the benzodiazepine is an aid to management and not its mainstay. The patient must be warned that the performance of skilled tasks such as driving may be affected, as may intellectual performance and memory, and that the medication must not be combined with alcohol. The dose and duration of treatment must be the minimum effective level to relieve symptoms adequately.

If depression coexists, an *antidepressant* (see section 5.1) is the best choice. However, a brief course of benzodiazepines can be helpful in such patients to relieve symptoms until the antidepressant becomes fully effective. In general, however, polypharmacy should be avoided. Antidepressants are also indicated when the anxiety is chronic or episodic.[126] Most patients tolerate SSRIs better than the tricyclic drugs. For very severe anxiety, *clomipramine* may be the drug of choice.

*Buspirone* is suitable for the short term management of moderate to severe anxiety when a rapid onset of effect is not essential, and also for the treatment of anxious patients with histories of dependence on CNS depressants.

The risks of using benzodiazepines intermittently and infrequently to control situational anxiety are probably small. An alternative is to use a β-adrenoceptor blocker, especially when somatic symptoms such as palpitations and tremor predominate.[127]

***Duration of treatment:*** this varies widely depending on the natural history of the patient's type of syndrome. However, the duration of treatment for a particular episode should take into account the progress, or lack of it, in the general management of the anxiety. It is, nevertheless, economic of time in the long run to mobilise resources to teach the patient anxiety-management techniques for coping with episodes of anxiety, rather than to expect symptomatic relief with a benzodiazepine each time.

***Avoidance of problems*** largely revolves around minimising the duration of benzodiazepine treatment to less than a month. Nevertheless, a few patients respond well only to a benzodiazepine or are intolerant of antidepressants. It may then be better to maintain them long term on their benzodiazepine of choice, despite the risk of dependence.

### Panic Disorder

The management of this condition is similar to that of generalised anxiety disorder, although the emphases are rather different.[128] The main controversy concerns the use of alprazolam in high dosage over long periods of time. Such usage is quite common in the US but elsewhere, the risk of dependence is generally regarded as too high to justify its use except when other measures have failed. Accordingly, the preferred drug treatment is an antidepressant. The

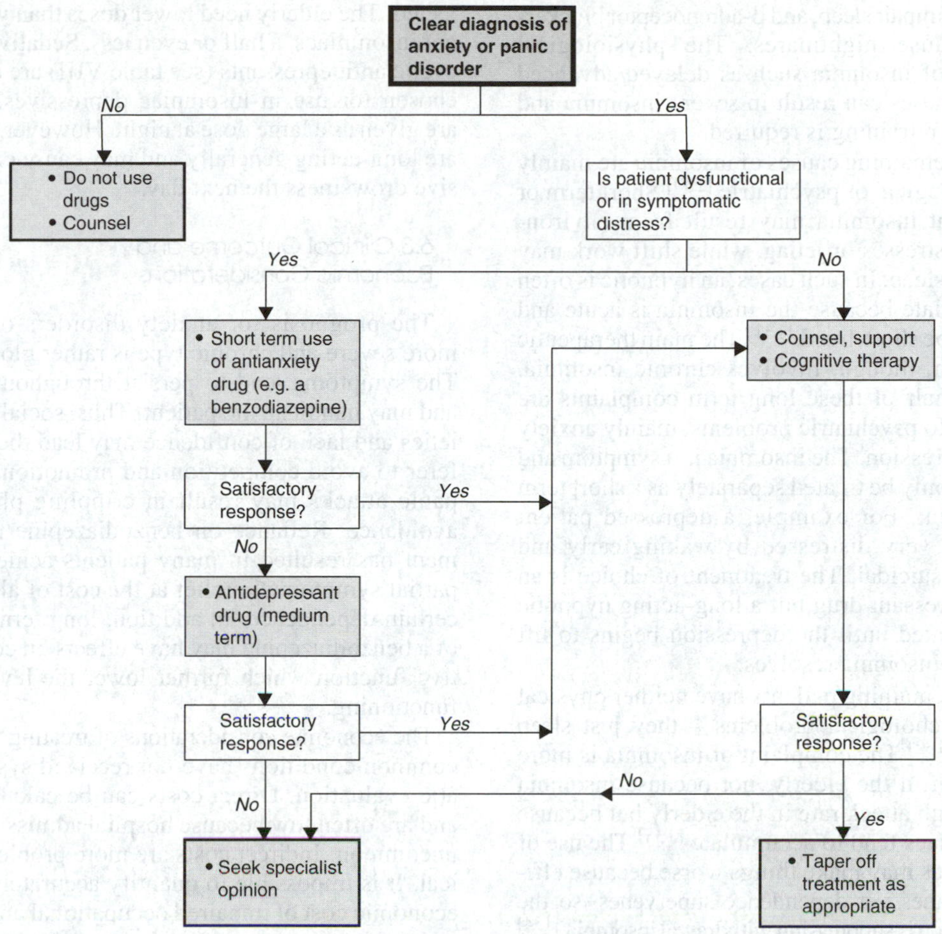


**Fig. 3.** Optimum treatment of anxiety disorders.

trend is towards using an antidepressant with effects primarily on serotonin mechanisms, such as clomipramine or a selective serotonin reuptake inhibitor (SSRI).[129]

Panic attacks can be largely suppressed by such treatment. In the early stages, however, anxiety and panic increase transiently. The initial dosage must be cautious and the patient warned about this possibility. Eventually, full dosage can be attained and the panics will subside. However, they will recur if the medication is withdrawn before non-pharmacological interventions have become effective. Management is similar to that for generalised anxiety disorder but psychological treatments such as cognitive therapy are only just becoming available.

The treatment of the actual panic attack should be conservative. Patients should be reassured that they are in no physical danger during the attack and should be instructed to mobilise any anxiety-coping responses they have been taught. They should also be instructed not to flee from any anxiety-provoking situation. Giving large doses of a benzodiazepine is only justifiable if the patient is severely distressed.

Panic attacks may occur spontaneously or in specific situations. Phobic avoidance may develop secondary to the panics and will require behavioural treatment.

#### Insomnia

About a third of the adult population complain at times of poor sleep, the incidence rising with age. Any physical causes need assessment and treatment in their own right, and hypnotic drugs are only indicated if treatment of the primary cause is unsatisfactory. Pharmacological causes of insomnia can be identified and advice should be given about avoiding caffeine in the evenings and keeping alcohol intake to a modicum. Various stimulants and sympathomimetics may impair sleep, and β-adrenoceptor blockers may cause nightmares. The physiological causes of insomnia such as delayed/advanced sleep phases can result in severe insomnia and gradual retraining is required.

The remaining causes of insomnia are mainly psychological or psychiatric.[130] Short term or transient insomnia may result from environmental stresses or jetlag, while shift work may disrupt sleep. In such cases, an hypnotic is often appropriate because the insomnia is acute and should be short-lived.[131] The main therapeutic problem, though, involves chronic insomnia. About half of these long term complaints are related to psychiatric problems, mainly anxiety and depression. The insomnia is a symptom and should only be treated separately as a short term expedient. For example, a depressed patient may be very distressed by waking early and feeling suicidal. The treatment of choice is an antidepressant drug but a long-acting hypnotic is indicated until the depression begins to lift and the insomnia resolves.

The remaining patients have neither physical nor psychological problems – they just sleep poorly.[132] The complaint of insomnia is more common in the elderly, not because insomnia has a high attack rate in the elderly but because insomniacs tend to accumulate.[133] The use of hypnotics may make things worse because efficacy wanes yet dependence supervenes, so the medication is suppressing withdrawal insomnia.[134]

More and more, it is becoming recognised that hypnotic drugs should be avoided in these patients or used intermittently. Thus, the patient can be advised about *sleep hygiene,* in particular, to reinforce the body's natural circadian rhythms, even if this means not lying in bed at the weekend. Daytime naps should also be avoided, and unreal expectations about sleep should be corrected. Hypnotic medication should be reserved for the patient who has developed secondary anxieties and phobias about not sleeping (fig. 4). No more than 2 to 3 doses of an hypnotic per week should be prescribed. The patient can be instructed to go to bed, but to get up and go elsewhere to read if he/she has not fallen asleep in 30 minutes. If this fails a couple of times, then the hypnotic can be taken.

Patients must be warned about possible daytime drowsiness with hypnotic use. The lowest possible dose should be used and a short-acting benzodiazepine drug such as *temazepam* or *lormetazepam,* or a similar newer compound such as *zopiclone* or *zolpidem*, should be selected. The elderly need lower doses than younger insomniacs, a half or even less. Sedative tricyclic antidepressants (see table VIII) are often chosen for use in insomniac depressives, and are given as a large dose at night. However, they are long-acting generally and may cause excessive drowsiness the next day.

### 6.3 Clinical Outcome and Economic Considerations

The prognosis for anxiety disorders of the more severe and chronic type is rather gloomy. The symptoms tend to persist throughout life and may handicap the patient. Thus, social anxieties and lack of confidence may lead the sufferer to avoid competition and promotion, and panic attacks may result in crippling phobic avoidance. Reliance on benzodiazepine treatment has resulted in many patients achieving partial symptomatic relief at the cost of almost certain dependence. In addition, long term use of a benzodiazepine may have effects on cognitive function which further lower the level of functioning.

The economic considerations of treating these common conditions have not received systematic evaluation. Direct costs can be calculated and are often low because hospital admission is uncommon. Indirect costs are more problematical. It is impossible to quantify accurately the economic cost of impaired occupational and social performance resulting from anxiety, panic and insomnia. They are certainly not trivial conditions which is the perception of many healthcare providers and even some clinicians.

## 7. Other Anxiety Disorders

### 7.1 Obsessive-Compulsive Disorder

Obsessive-compulsive disorder (OCD) is generally classified with the anxiety disorders, although anxiety is not always a marked feature. Both the obsessive ruminations and the compulsive rituals are responsive to *clomipramine* (see section 5.1), but full doses are usually needed.[135] The effects of the more selective serotonin reuptake inhibitors (SSRIs) are currently being assessed but preliminary data suggest they are also effective.[136] The response to antidepressant therapy is not dependent on an antidepressant response of any co-morbid depressive affect (fig. 5). The onset of improvement of the obsessive-compulsive symptoms is often quite rapid and very noticeable in compar-

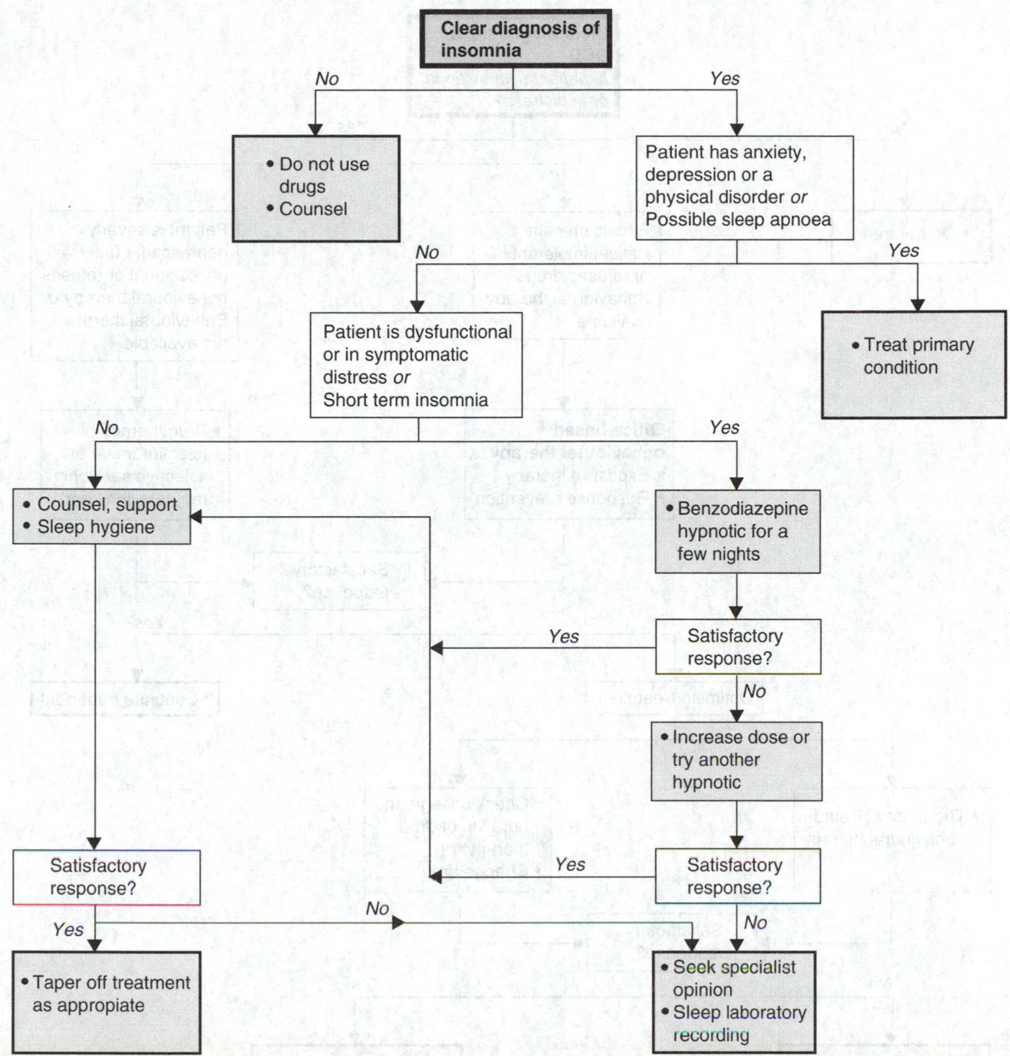


**Fig. 4.** Optimum treatment of insomnia.

ative trials because of the low placebo response (less than 10%).

### 7.2 Post-Traumatic Stress Disorder

The treatment of post-traumatic stress disorder is still unclear. Benzodiazepines, antidepressants and other drugs have been used. Psychological treatments are also being tried. It is evident, however, that treatment needs to be fairly long term in order to effect an improvement.[137]

## 8. Other Sleep Disorders

Although insomnia is by far the most common sleep disorder, several other conditions can be helped by drug therapy.

### 8.1 Somnambulism and Night Terrors

Somnambulism is fairly common in children but usually disappears as they mature. Benzodiazepines have been tried with mixed results. They have also been claimed to reduce the frequency of night terrors in adults.

### 8.2 Obstructive Sleep Apnoea

Obstructive sleep apnoea is a condition in which the sufferer, typically a middle-aged obese male, obstructs his respiratory passages as his pharyngeal muscles lose tone during sleep. The patient becomes apnoeic and the rise in $CO_2$ tension results in a gasping inspiration which disturbs his sleep, up to several hundred times per night. The patient is tired and hyper-

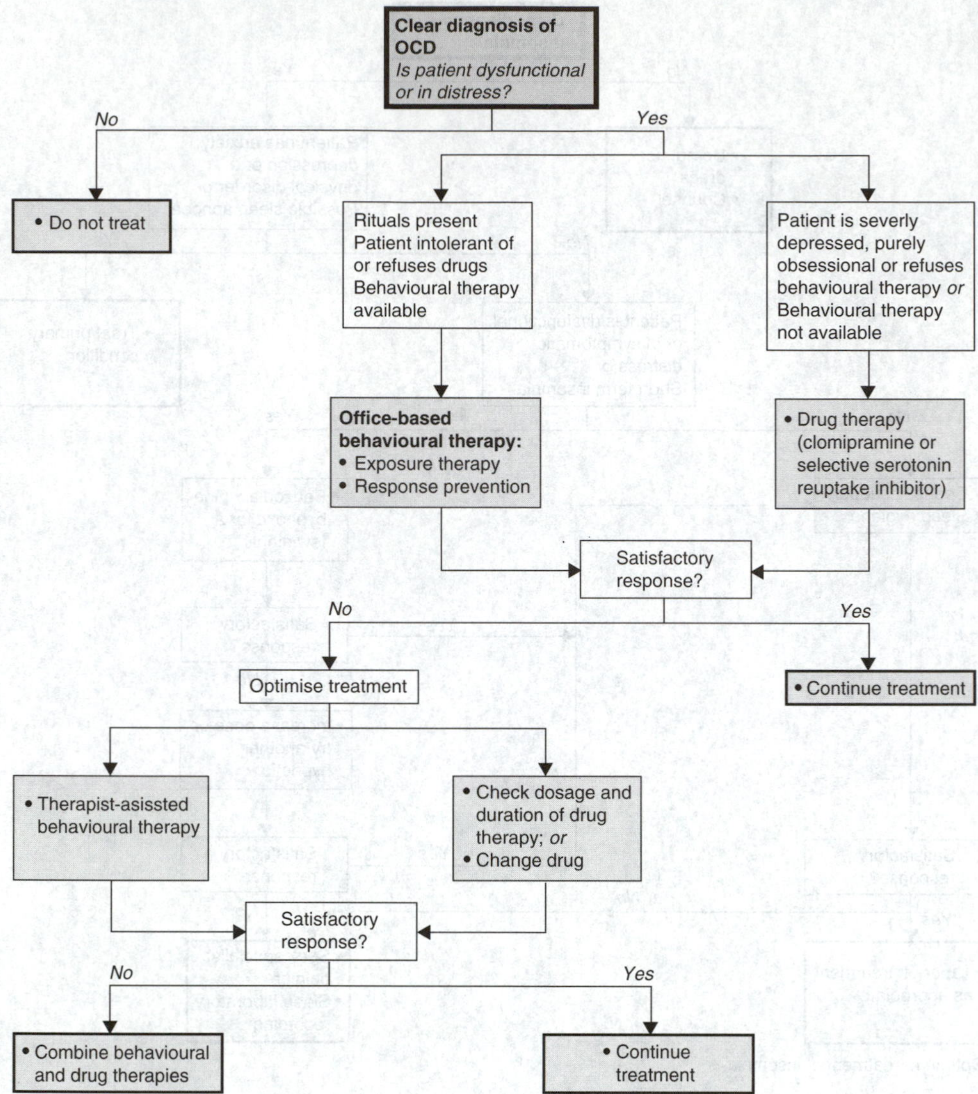


**Fig. 5.** Optimum treatment of obsessive-compulsive disorders (OCD).

somniac the next day. The history given by the bed-partner is typical – very loud snoring and gasping for breath intermittently.

Hypnosedatives are contraindicated in patients with this disorders, the treatment of choice being positive-pressure aids to respiration.

### 8.3 Narcolepsy

Narcolepsy is another hypersomnia which can be disabling. The patient suffers bouts of irresistible sleepiness several times a day, often accompanied by cataplectic attacks of profound muscle weakness, in which the patient falls to the ground. The attacks are sometimes provoked by laughter or other emotion. Another feature is sleep paralysis and waking nightmares.

Treatment of narcolepsy is difficult but stimulants such as *dexamphetamine* remain widely used (see also chapter 29; sect. 5.1). The dosage may need to be high but patients do not seem to develop a state of dependence. SSRIs may also help some patients.

### 8.4 Nocturnal Enuresis

Children and adults may suffer the embarrassment of nocturnal enuresis. The primary treatment is behavioural, such as use of a pad and buzzer, together with sympathetic support and encouragement. *Imipramine* can suppress the enuresis and may be useful as a temporary expedient.

## 9. Eating Disorders

### 9.1 Bulimia Nervosa

Bulimia nervosa is characterised by recurrent uncontrolled bouts of overeating, together with extreme measures to reverse the weight gain. These measures include self-induced vomiting, overuse of laxatives or diuretics, or excessively stringent dieting regimens between the binges.

Antidepressants are effective in lessening the abnormal dietary behaviour. Some of this efficacy relates to an improvement in the mood. However, the SSRIs appear to have a direct regulating effect on the dietary behaviour and are probably the treatment of choice, along with education and support measures. Other treatments that have been advocated include the MAOIs, antiepileptic drugs, benzodiazepines, lithium, fenfluramine, and opioid antagonists.[138]

### 9.2 Anorexia Nervosa

Anorexia nervosa is a condition with marked fear of obesity, dieting and self-induced vomiting, with a weight loss of at least 15% of original bodyweight and amenorrhoea in women. It can coexist or alternate with bulimia.

There are no specific treatments for anorexia nervosa, and the best results appear to follow pragmatic combinations of management approaches. Education and support are vital. Various drugs have been tried, but generally with scant success.[138]

## 10. Psychological Disorders of Childhood

This heading covers a range of disorders, some of which have their equivalent in adult life, but some of which are peculiar to childhood. Thus, stress in the family or at school may manifest itself as a symptomatic disorder with anxiety and depression, or as a behavioural disturbance such as truancy or delinquency. Primary development disorders include autism and the hyperkinetic syndrome. Brain damage due to epilepsy sustained perinatally may be apparent as behavioural disturbances, and these may be exhibited quite frequently by children with severe learning difficulties.

### 10.1 Important Considerations in Administering Psychotropic Drugs to Children

Drug therapy poses additional problems in children.[139] Even more than in adults, drug therapy should be part of general management, with carefully selected and applied social, educational and vocational measures. In particular, the family dynamics need exploration and perhaps correction. Drugs should not be used in acute stress or adjustment reactions where the cause is obvious such as a change at home or school, or a physical illness. Nor should drugs be used to placate the family or as a token of the 'medicalisation' of a psychological maladjustment.

If drugs are given, children and their parents must be warned about the limitations of efficacy and possible adverse effects. The latter are difficult to assess in children and need great experience to detect in children with severe learning disabilities, especially those without speech. Doses must be flexible and variable but older children can often tolerate and may need full adult dosages.

### 10.2 Hyperkinetic Syndrome

The hyperkinetic syndrome, also known as 'minimal brain dysfunction syndrome' or 'attention deficit hyperactivity disorder' is an ill-defined behavioural syndrome with short attention span, distractibility, emotional lability, aggressiveness and hyperactivity in a child with normal intelligence but failure to learn. Boys are much more frequently diagnosed than girls but the apparent prevalence varies several-fold from country to country, and even state to state within the US. Minor neurological signs may be detected and the more severely affected children may show antisocial problems in adult life.

#### Optimum Treatment

Stimulant drugs are still used quite widely to treat hyperkinetic syndrome, *amphetamine, methylphenidate* and *pemoline* each having their advocates.[140] The dosages of these drugs must be arrived at by trial and error and kept as low as possible. The frequency of administration also needs some experimentation to maintain adequate symptom cover. The efficacy of stimulants in this condition is more convincing the more abnormal the child's behaviour. Sometimes, intermittent therapy can be resorted to, e.g. medication only during school terms.

Adverse effects with stimulant drugs are not usually a problem, although transient anorexia and insomnia have been reported. Growth retardation is common and persists for as long as medication is continued. Regular monitoring of weight and height is therefore obligatory. The longer term effects of stimulant medication on psychological development are largely unknown.

Other drugs that have been tried in hyperkinetic syndrome include antipsychotics and antidepressants.[141] In general, their effects are unpredictable, although a few children do well. Benzodiazepines should be avoided, as they are disinhibiting and may make the behaviour worse.

### 10.3 Depression in Children

Childhood depression is now believed to be a fairly common condition, especially in older children. Drug treatment may be necessary, especially where biological features such as appetite and sleep loss are apparent, as well as behavioural problems and symptomatic distress. Therapy should be instituted cautiously with the dosage being increased as necessary.

### 10.4 Psychoses in Children

Severe psychotic illnesses are seen in children. In younger children, these tend to be associated with the syndrome of childhood autism[142] but in older children, early-onset schizophrenia is occasionally encountered.

Antipsychotic drugs are usually prescribed for persons with mental retardation and behavioural disorders, but their efficacy is unpredictable and highly variable.[42] Benzodiazepines are only occasionally helpful but β-adrenoceptor blockers such as propranolol may lessen aggressive behaviour. Psychological techniques to improve abnormal and unacceptable behaviour are being developed and show promise.

### 10.5 Movement Disorders

Some movement disorders are more common in children. The most dramatic is Gilles de la Tourette's syndrome with tics, dystonias and explosive utterances or even swearing. It has all the hallmarks of an organic disease. Antipsychotic drugs acting strongly on $D_2$ receptors, e.g. haloperidol and pimozide, are usually tried and can be quite successful. However, drug-induced movement disorders may then complicate the clinical picture.

## 11. Psychological Disorders in the Elderly

The elderly are prone to develop acute organic syndromes such as delirium, with a fluctuating level of awareness, confusion, tremor, visual hallucinations and sleep disturbances. A wide range of conditions can lead to this state, infections and brain damage being the most common. The treatment is of the underlying condition, together with experienced nursing in a controlled environment. Antipsychotic medication may help.

### 11.1 Dementias

Dementia in the elderly can be of several types. Most patients will show changes of the Alzheimer's type, i.e. similar to those seen in younger patients with Alzheimer's disease.[143] The neuropathological changes in this condition include shrinkage of the brain, particularly the cerebral cortex, and the presence in the brain of amyloid-like plaques and neurofibrillary tangles. Finding these post-mortem establishes the diagnosis. The disorder itself is marked by impairment of short term memory, decreased alertness, failing judgement and eventually total disorientation. Changes in personality are evidenced by emotional lability, irritability, decreased motivation and initiative and self-neglect. The onset is insidious; the course of the disease is progressive but variable in rate, and reversible causes of intellectual deterioration such as hypothyroidism must be excluded. In England in 1990-91, it was estimated that the cost of Alzheimer's disease exceeded £1 billion.[144]

Multi-infarct dementia is also common and may occur in the same patient suffering from dementia of the Alzheimer's type. However, the progression is more stepwise and focal neurological deficits can usually be elicited. Other forms of dementia include Loewy-body dementia and rarities such as Pick's disease and Creutzfeldt-Jakob disease. The last is believed to involve a transmissible agent.

#### Optimum Treatment

Most symptomatic control of dementia involves the use of antipsychotic or antidepressant drugs.[145,146] Doses must be very low and carefully increased. Benzodiazepines may elicit a paradoxical reaction but are sometimes worth trying, particularly in correcting abnormal sleep rhythms.

Although various drugs are available to treat dementia, their efficacy is generally marginal and their adverse effects often troublesome. Various nutritional and hormonal approaches have been used, as have vasodilators which enjoyed an undeserved vogue.[147] A number of metabolic enhancers that act, at least *in vitro* or in animal models, to protect the brain against a variety of insults (e.g. anoxia) have been developed. *Ergoloid mesylates* (codergocrine mesylate) has been used in medical practice for over 30 years, mainly to the disappointment of the prescribing clinician.[148] Indeed, it probably did more to maintain the morale of the patient's carers, who felt 'something was being done', than to improve the clinical state of the patient. *Piracetam, oxiracetam* and related compounds, which have been dubbed 'nootropic agents', have also been used,[149] but the evidence for their efficacy is unconvincing both statistically and in terms of useful and practical clinical improvement.[150]

Research into the neuropathology of Alzheimer's disease has shown multiple deficits involving several neurotransmitter systems. However, the most important appears to be acetylcholine, and its involvement in memory processes is consistent with this. Various cholinomimetics have therefore been tried including cholinesterase inhibitors (e.g. physostigmine) and cholinergic agonists (e.g. nicotine), but most such approaches have shown minor effects, falling short of clinical practicability and usefulness. Only one drug has so far come through clinical testing, i.e. *tacrine* (tetrahydroaminoacridine, THA), a cholinesterase inhibitor. Definite clinical improvement has been seen with this agent, but only in a subgroup of patients, the identity of whom cannot be detected in advance. In addition, tacrine can be hepatotoxic so the risk : benefit ratio has to be carefully evaluated in each patient.[151] Other compounds of this type but with an enhanced safety profile are currently being developed.[152]

### 11.2 Depression in the Elderly

Depression is a common condition in the elderly and may masquerade as a dementing process (depressive pseudodementia). A trial of therapy with an antidepressant may be needed to distinguish between the two. The elderly need cautious introduction of treatment with slow dosage escalation. They may be more tolerant of newer tricyclics like lofepramine or an SSRI than the older tricyclic antidepressants.

## 12. Alcohol and Substance Abuse

### 12.1 Acute Alcohol Poisoning

Acute alcohol poisoning is a dangerous condition which needs expert supportive treatment to prevent respiratory depression. Acute alcohol withdrawal or 'delirium tremens' is a condition with appreciable mortality.[153] The syndrome varies from minor shakes to hyperthermic tremors with severe behavioural disturbances. The condition is a severe abrupt discontinuation syndrome.

#### Optimum Treatment

The treatment of acute alcohol poisoning involves two steps: firstly, the substitution of medication cross-tolerant to alcohol, and secondly the gradual and controlled withdrawal of the medication. In addition, large doses of B complex vitamins are essential to prevent neurological complications (Wernicke's encephalopathy).

Large doses of substitute medication are needed and must be established fairly empirically. For example, doses of *chlordiazepoxide* over 500mg or of *diazepam* over 100mg may be needed to suppress delirium. In some countries, *clomethiazole* (chlormethiazole) is available and this drug may be preferred. Diazepam and clomethiazole have more anticonvulsant activity than chlordiazepoxide. All these compounds substitute for the alcohol and can themselves become the addictive substance. In patients prone to fits, phenytoin may be added, and propranolol may help the tremor.

Withdrawal of the substituted medication must be instituted immediately and tapering of dosage effected fairly rapidly. This can usually be accomplished in a week (range 4 to 10 days). Once withdrawal has been attained (drying-out) attention can be turned to treating the alcohol problems. Various approaches have been used, some of which have almost an evangelical flavour to them. Nevertheless, many patients achieve and maintain abstinence, but these individuals tend to have a better than average prognosis anyway, e.g. are married, employed and have no coexisting psychiatric morbidity such as depression.

### 12.2 Chronic Alcoholism

The use of alcohol-sensitising drugs (e.g. *disulfiram* or *calcium carbimide*) as deterrent therapy remains controversial, some specialists using them routinely, others regarding them as ineffective or, worse, hazardous. Most experience has been obtained with disulfiram. This drug inhibits the liver enzyme aldehyde dehydrogenase which catalyses the breakdown of the alcohol metabolite acetaldehyde to acetic acid. The accumulation of acetaldehyde leads to a strong unpleasant reaction with flushing, rapid pulse, hypotension, nausea and vomiting. Disulfiram has to be taken on a daily basis and a test dose of alcohol may be given to demonstrate the unpleasant effects of drinking. Regular assessment and support is necessary.

The use of disulfiram may just tip the balance in the well-motivated alcoholic, but it can also prove hazardous if drinking is resumed impulsively.

### 12.3 Opioid Abuse

Abuse of opioids is endemic in many parts of the world, most stemming from illicit 'street' supplies. As with alcohol, treatment involves aiding withdrawal from opioids and then trying to maintain abstinence.

#### Optimum Treatment

Withdrawal of opioids involves substitution of an equivalent opioid, usually *methadone,* and then controlled tapering of the substitute. The dose of methadone needed is a matter of experience but most addicts exaggerate their usage, either deliberately or in ignorance of how much their illicit diamorphine ('heroin') has been diluted ('cut'). Indeed, fatalities occur when an unusually pure form of heroin appears on the street and addicts overdose with it. *Clonidine,* an $\alpha_2$-adrenoceptor agonist, may also help in opioid withdrawal by lessening the irritability and discomfort.

The maintenance treatment of opioid addicts has become standard. The rationale is that by giving addicts adequate doses of a substitute opioid, compulsive use of illicit drugs, mainly heroin, will be lessened or even obviated. In addition, the antisocial activities sustaining the habit will be rendered unnecessary. The most usual form of substitution is to prescribe oral *methadone.* It has a plasma half-life of about 24 hours and can be given once daily, usually as a liquid formulation and under supervision. Although evidence of effectiveness has accumulated, it is not compelling and methadone maintenance is not universally accepted, either on medical or on moral grounds.

Recently, a long-acting homologue of methadone has become available, i.e. *levacetylmethadol* (LAAM), which can be given less frequently than oral methadone. Another approach has been to give an opioid antagonist such as *naltrexone* to block the effects of heroin and other opioids.[154] Often, this drug has to be given under some element of compulsion, such as a court order. It is only useful as part of a multidisciplinary treatment programme which includes individual and group psychotherapy, and a graded reintroduction into the wider social context and away from the drug subculture.[155]

### 12.4 Nicotine Addiction

Nicotine is the drug of addiction carrying the highest mortality and morbidity. It is estimated that 300 people per day die prematurely in the UK as a result of the depredations of cigarette smoking. This addiction has a pharmacological component and a behavioural component, and individuals vary in their mix of these factors.[156] For those who are physically addicted, separation of these components and treatment of each in turn may encourage abstinence.

A further complication is that cigarette smoking provides a background level of nicotine which builds up over the day. Superimposed on this are peaks corresponding to each cigarette.[157] Therefore, in treating the condition, drug delivery systems are needed to substitute the nicotine in both ways.

#### Optimum Treatment

Nicotine-containing chewing gums were the first treatment approach to be used but their pharmacokinetic characteristics are such that they do not closely replicate either the background levels of nicotine or the peaks. Transdermal nicotine patches have been introduced and these can maintain a fairly constant background level.[158] The problem of reproducing the peaks is being addressed by developing nasal and inhalational nicotine sprays.[159]

Despite these pharmacological elaborations, the most effective method of encouraging patients to stop smoking is to mobilise the resources of primary care practitioners. Such treatment is also cost effective.[160]

## 13. Use of Drugs in the Presence of Associated Psychiatric Disorders

Some drugs can precipitate or worsen psychiatric conditions. Examples include corticosteroids, amphetamines, and levodopa. Indeed, amphetamine-induced psychosis has been used as a model of paranoid schizophrenia.

Potentiation of the effects of psychotropic drugs can also occur. In particular, alcohol can potentiate central depressants and result in grossly abnormal paradoxical reactions. Other drug interactions involving psychotropic drugs are discussed in sections 4.1, 5.1 and 6.1, and also in appendix B.

### Further Reading

Addington D, Addington J. The psychopharmacology of schizophrenia. Royal College of Psychiatrists 1993; 163, Suppl. 22

Angrist B, Schulz SC, editors. The neuroleptic-non-responsive patient: characterization and treatment. Washington DC: American Psychiatric Press, 1990

Ashton H. Brain function and psychotropic drugs. Oxford: Oxford University Press, 1992

British Journal of Psychiatry. Clozapine - the atypical antipsychotic. British Journal of Psychiatry 1992; 160, Suppl. 17

Schizophrenia. Current concepts and therapeutic prospects. Clinician 1993; 11 (4)

Feighner JP, Boyer WF. Selective serotonin re-uptake inhibitors. Perspectives in Psychiatry, Vol. 1. Chichester: Wiley, 1991

Jönsson B, Rosenbaum J, editors. Health economics of depression. Chichester: Wiley, 1993

Journal of Clinical Psychiatry. The use of benzodiazepine hypnotics: a scientific examination of a clinical controversy. Journal of Clinical Psychiatry 1992; 53 Suppl. Dec

Journal of Clinical Psychiatry. Current issues in drug therapy of depression. Journal of Clinical Psychiatry 1993; 54 Suppl. Aug

Journal of Clinical Psychiatry. Clinical crossfire: pharmacokinetics and psychiatric drugs. Journal of Clinical Psychiatry 1993; 54 Suppl. Sept

Kane JM, Lieberman JA, editors. Adverse effects of psychotropic drugs. New York: Guilford Press, 1992

Lader M, editor. The psychopharmacology of addiction. British Association for Psychopharmacology, Monograph No. 10. Oxford: Oxford University Press, 1988

Lader M, Herrington R. Biological treatments in psychiatry. 2nd ed. Oxford: Oxford University Press, 1996

Mendlewicz J, Racagni G, editors. Target receptors for anxiolytics and hypnotics: from molecular pharmacology to therapeutics. International Academy for Biomedical and Drug Research, Vol. 3. Basel: Karger, 1992

Miller NS, editor. Comprehensive handbook of drug and alcohol addiction. New York: Marcel Dekker, 1991

Montgomery SA. Anxiety and depression. Petersfield, Hants: Wrightson Biomedical Publishing, 1990

Montgomery SA. Psychopharmacology of panic. British Association for Psychopharmacology, Monograph No. 12. Oxford: Oxford University Press, 1993

Montgomery S, Rouillon F, editors. Long-term treatment of depression. Perspectives in Psychiatry, Vol. 3. Chichester: Wiley, 1992

Sandler M, Coppen A, Harnett S, editors. 5-Hydroxytryptamine in psychiatry. A spectrum of ideas. Oxford: Oxford University Press, 1992

Sloan EP, Shapiro CM, editors. Insomnia in the medically ill and behavioural treatment approaches to insomnia. Journal of Psychosomatic Research 1993; 37 Suppl. 1

Task Force Report of the American Psychiatric Association. Benzodiazepine dependence, toxicity and abuse. Washington DC: APA, 1990

Van Praag HM, Lecrubier Y. New perspectives on the treatment of depression. Drugs 1992; 43, Suppl. 2

### References

1. Barrett JE, Vanover KE. 5-HT receptors as targets for the development of novel anxiolytic drugs: models, mechanisms and future directions. Psychopharmacology 1993; 112: 1
2. Bech P, Malt UF, Dencker SJ, et al., editors. Scales for assessment of diagnosis and severity of mental disorders. Acta Psychiatrica Scandinavica 1993; 87 Suppl. 372
3. Fuller RW. Basic advances in serotonin pharmacology. Journal of Clinical Psychiatry 1992; 53: 36
4. Harrington MA, Zhong P, Garlow SJ, et al. Molecular biology of serotonin receptors. Journal of Clinical Psychiatry 1992; 53 Suppl.: 8-27
5. Caccia S, Garattini S. Formation of active metabolites of psychotropic drugs. An updated review of their significance. Clinical Pharmacokinetics 1990; 18: 434
6. Sanderson WC, Barlow DH. A description of patients diagnosed with DSM-III-R generalized anxiety disorder. Journal of Nervous and Mental Disease 1990; 178: 588-91
7. Hegarty JD, Baldessarini RJ, Tohen M, et al. One hundred years of schizophrenia: a meta-analysis of the outcome literature. American Journal of Psychiatry 1994; 151: 1409
8. Pilowsky LS, Costa DC, Ell PJ, et al. Clozapine, single photon emission tomography, and the D2 dopamine receptor blockade hypothesis of schizophrenia. Lancet 1992; 340: 199
9. Seeman P, Guan H-C, van Tol HHM. Dopamine D4 receptors elevated in schizophrenia. Nature 1993; 365: 441
10. Bench CJ, Lammertsma AA, Dolan RJ, et al. Dose dependent occupancy of central dopamine $D_2$ receptors by the novel neuroleptic CP-88,059-01: a study using positron emission tomography and $^{11}$C-raclopride. Psychopharmacology 1993; 112: 308
11. King DJ. The effect of neuroleptics on cognitive and psychomotor function. British Journal of Psychiatry 1990; 157: 799

12. Hollister LE. Psychiatric disorders. In: Speight TM, editor. Drug treatment: principles and practice of clinical pharmacology and therapeutics. 3rd ed. Auckland: Adis Press, 1987: 1137-206
13. Balant-Gorgia AE, Balant L. Antipsychotic drugs. Clinical pharmacokinetics of potential candidates for plasma concentration monitoring. Clinical Pharmacokinetics 1987; 13: 65
14. Beresford R, Ward A. Haloperidol decanoate: a preliminary review of its pharmacodynamic and pharmacokinetic properties and therapeutic use in psychosis. Drugs 1987; 33: 31
15. Jann MW, Grimsley SR, Gray EC, et al. Pharmacokinetics and pharmacodynamics of clozapine. Clinical Pharmacokinetics 1993; 24: 161
16. Grant S, Fitton A. Risperidone: a review of its pharmacology and therapeutic potential in the treatment of schizophrenia. Drugs 1994; 48: 253-73
17. Davis JM, Metalon L, Watanabe MD, et al. Depot antipsychotic drugs: place in therapy. Drugs 1994; 47: 741-73
18. Lingjærde O. Benzodiazepines in the treatment of schizophrenia: an updated survey. Acta Psychiatrica Scandinavica 1991; 84: 453
19. Pilowsky LS, Ring H, Shine PJ, et al. Rapid tranquillisation. A survey of emergency prescribing in a general psychiatric hospital. British Journal of Psychiatry 1992; 160: 831
20. Farmer AE, McGuffin P. The pathogenesis and management of schizophrenia. Drugs 1988; 35: 177
21. Schwartz JT, Brotman AW. A clinical guide to antipsychotic drugs. Drugs 1992; 44: 981
22. Quality Assurance Project. Treatment outlines for the management of schizophrenia. Australian and New Zealand Journal of Psychiatry 1984; 18: 19
23. Brown RP, Kocsis JH. Sudden death and antipsychotic drugs. Hospital and Community Psychiatry 1984; 35: 486
24. Hirsch SR, Barnes TRE. Clinical use of high-dose neuroleptics. British Journal of Psychiatry 1994; 164: 94
25. Weiden PJ, Dixon L, Frances A, et al. Neuroleptic noncompliance in schizophrenia. In: Tamminger CA, Schulz SC, editors. Advances in neuropsychiatry and psychopharmacology. Vol. 1. New York: Raven Press, 1991: 185
26. Jolley AG, Hirsch SR. Continuous versus intermittent neuroleptic therapy in schizophrenia. Drug Safety 1993; 8: 331
27. Farmer AE, Blewett A. Drug treatment of resistant schizophrenia. Limitations and recommendations. Drugs 1993; 45: 374
28. Fitton A, Heel RC. Clozapine: a review of its pharmacological properties, and therapeutic use in schizophrenia. Drugs 1990; 40: 722
29. Kane J, Honigfeld G, Singer J, et al. Clozapine for the treatment-resistant schizophrenic. Archives of General Psychiatry 1988; 45: 789
30. Kerwin RW. The new atypical antipsychotics. A lack of extrapyramidal side-effects and new routes in schizophrenia research. British Journal of Psychiatry 1994; 164: 141
31. Menkes DB. Schizophrenia. In: Speight TM, editor. Disease index, 3rd edition. Auckland: Adis International, 1993: 636-40
32. Bristow MF, Hirsch SR. Pitfalls and problems of the long term use of neuroleptic drugs in schizophrenia. Drug Safety 1993; 8: 136
33. Harpe C, Stoudemire A. Aetiology and treatment of neuroleptic malignant syndrome. Medical Toxicology and Adverse Drug Experience 1987; 2: 166
34. Bristow MF, Kohen D. How 'malignant' is the neuroleptic malignant syndrome? British Medical Journal 1993; 307: 1223
35. Spohn H, Strauss ME. Relation of neuroleptic and anticholinergic medication to cognitive functions in schizophrenia. Journal of Abnormal Psychology 1989; 98: 367
36. Cassens G, Inglis AK, Appelbaum PS, et al. Neuroleptics: effects on neuropsychological function in chronic schizophrenic patients. Schizophrenia Bulletin 1990; 16: 477
37. Windgassen K. Treatment with neuroleptics: the patient's perspective. Acta Psychiatrica Scandinavica 1992; 86: 405
38. Lader M, Lewander T. The neuroleptic-induced deficit syndrome. Acta Psychiatrica Scandinavica 1994; 89 Suppl. 380
39. Allebeck P. Schizophrenia: a life-shortening disease. Schizophrenia Bulletin 1989; 15: 81
40. Coffey I. Options for the treatment of negative symptoms of schizophrenia. CNS Drugs 1994; 1: 107
41. Steele JW, Faulds D, Sorkin EM. Tiapride: a review of its pharmacodynamic and pharmacokinetic properties and therapeutic potential in geriatric agitation. Drugs & Aging 1993; 3: 460
42. Baumeister AA, Todd ME, Sevin JA. Efficacy and specificity of pharmacological therapies for behavioural disorders in persons with mental retardation. Clinical Neuropharmacology 1993; 16: 271
43. Awad AG, Voruganti LNP, Heslegrave RJ. The aims of antipsychotic medication: what are they and are they being achieved? CNS Drugs 1995; 4: 8
44. Fitton A, Benfield P. Clozapine: an appraisal of its pharmacoeconomic benefits in the treatment of schizophrenia. PharmacoEconomics 1993; 4: 131-56
45. Frankenburg FR. Is clozapine worth its cost? PharmacoEconomics 1993; 4: 311
46. Meltzer HY, Cola P, Way L, et al. Cost effectiveness of clozapine in neuroleptic-resistant schizophrenia. American Journal of Psychiatry 1993; 150: 1630
47. Jefferson JW, Greist JH. Lithium in psychiatry: a review. CNS Drugs 1994; 1: 448-64
48. Peet M, Pratt JP. Lithium: current status in psychiatric disorders. Drugs 1993; 46: 7
49. Souza FGM, Goodwin GM. Lithium treatment and prophylaxis in unipolar depression: a meta-analysis. British Journal of Psychiatry 1991; 158: 666
50. Shaw DM. Drug alternatives to lithium in manic-depressive disorders. Drugs 1988; 36: 249
51. Höschl C. Do calcium antagonists have a place in the treatment of mood disorders? Drugs 1991; 42: 721
52. Goodwin GM. Recurrence of mania after lithium withdrawal. Implications for the use of lithium in the treatment of bipolar affective disorder. British Journal of Psychiatry 1994; 164: 149
53. Milne RJ, Goa KL. Citalopram: a review of its pharmacodynamic and pharmacokinetic properties, and therapeutic potential in depressive illness. Drugs 1991; 41: 450
54. Harris MG, Benfield P. Fluoxetine: a review of its pharmacodynamic and pharmacokinetic properties, and therapeutic use in older patients with depressive illness. Drugs & Aging 1995; 6: 64-84
55. Wilde MI, Plosker CL, Benfield P. Fluvoxamine: an updated review of its pharmacology, and therapeutic use in depressive illness. Drugs 1993; 46: 895
56. Dechant KL, Clissold SP. Paroxetine: a review of its pharmacodynamic and pharmacokinetic properties, and therapeutic potential in depressive illness. Drugs 1991; 41: 225
57. Murdoch D, McTavish D. Sertraline: a review of its pharmacodynamic and pharmacokinetic properties, and therapeutic potential in depression and obsessive-compulsive disorder. Drugs 1992; 44: 604
58. Sallee FR, Pollock BG. Clinical pharmacokinetics of imipramine and desipramine. Clinical Pharmacokinetics 1990; 18: 346-64
59. Balant-Gorgia AE, Gex-Fabry M, Balant LP. Clinical pharmacokinetics of clomipramine. Clinical Pharmacokinetics 1991; 20: 447
60. Norman TR. Pharmacokinetic aspects of antidepressant treatment in the elderly. Progress in Neuro-Psychopharmacology and Biological Psychiatry 1993; 17: 329

61. Furlanut M, Benetell P, Spina E. Pharmacokinetic optimisation of tricyclic antidepressant therapy. Clinical Pharmacokinetics 1993; 24: 301
62. Van Harten J. Clinical pharmacokinetics of selective serotonin reuptake inhibitors. Clinical Pharmacokinetics 1993; 24: 203-220
63. Fitton A, Faulds D, Goa KL. Moclobemide: a review of its pharmacological properties and therapeutic use in depressive illness. Drugs 1992; 43: 561
64. Paykel ES, Priest RG. Recognition and management of depression in general practice: consensus statement. British Medical Journal 1992; 305: 1198
65. Lader M, Lang RA, Wilson GD. Patterns of improvement in depressed in-patients. Oxford: Oxford University Press, 1987
66. Palmer KJ, Benfield P. Fluvoxamine: an overview of its pharmacological properties and review of its therapeutic potential in non-depressive disorders. CNS Drugs 1994; 1: 57
67. Rudorfer MV, Potter WZ. Antidepressants: a comparative review of the clinical pharmacology and therapeutic use of the 'newer' versus the 'older' drugs. Drugs 1989; 37: 713
68. Song F, Freemantle N, Sheldon TA, et al. Selective serotonin reuptake inhibitors: meta-analysis of efficacy and acceptability. British Medical Journal 1993; 306: 683
69. McTavish D, Benfield P. Clomipramine: an overview of its pharmacological properties and a review of its therapeutic use in obsessive compulsive disorder and panic disorder. Drugs 1990; 39: 136
70. Clomipramine Collaborative Study Group. Clomipramine in the treatment of patients with obsessive-compulsive disorder. Archives of General Psychiatry 1991; 48: 730
71. Whittington R, McTavish D. Nefazodone: a review of its pharmacological properties and therapeutic potential in depressive illness. Drugs 1995; 50: in press
72. Workman EA, Short DD. Atypical antidepressants versus imipramine in the treatment of major depression: a meta-analysis. Journal of Clinical Psychiatry 1993; 54: 5
73. Holliday SM, Benfield P. Venlafaxine: a review of its pharmacology and therapeutic potential in depression. Drugs 1995; 49: 280-94
74. Danish University Antidepressant Group. Moclobeminde: a reversible MAO-A-inhibitor showing weaker antidepressant effect than clomipramine in a controlled multicenter study. Journal of Affective Disorders 1993; 28: 105
75. Kaufman LD, Philen RM. Tryptophan: current status and future trends for oral administration. Drug Safety 1993; 8: 89
76. Friedel HA, Goa KL, Benfield P. S-Adenosyl-L-methionine: a review of its pharmacological properties and therapeutic potential in liver dysfunction and affective disorders in relation to its physiological role in cell metabolism. Drugs 1989; 38: 389
77. Menkes DB. Depressive illness. In: Speight TM, editor. Disease index. 3rd ed. Auckland: Adis International, 1993: 185-90
78. Rosenstein CL, Nelson JC, Jacobs SC. Seizures associated with antidepressants: a review. Journal of Clinical Psychiatry 1993; 54: 289
79. Sulzer DL, Cummings JL. Drug induced mania - causative agents, clinical characteristics and management. A retrospective analysis of the literature. Medical Toxicology and Adverse Drug Experience 1989; 4: 127
80. Lancaster SG, Gonzalez JP. Lofepramine: a review of its pharmacodynamic and pharmacokinetic properties, and therapeutic efficacy in depressive illness. Drugs 1989; 37: 123
81. Teicher MH, Glod CA, Cole JO. Antidepressant drugs and the emergence of suicidal tendencies. Drug Safety 1993; 8: 186
82. Power AC, Cowen PJ. Fluoxetine and suicidal behaviour. Some clinical and theoretical aspects of a controversy. British Journal of Psychiatry 1992; 161: 735
83. Lippman SB, Nash K. Monoamine oxidase inhibitor update. Potential adverse food and drug interactions. Drug Safety 1990; 5: 195
84. Lancaster SG, Gonzalez JP. Dothiepin: a review of its pharmacodynamic and pharmacokinetic properties, and therapeutic efficacy in depressive illness. Drugs 1989; 38: 123
85. Guscott R, Grof P. The clinical meaning of refractory depression: a review for the clinician. American Journal of Psychiatry 1991; 148: 695
86. Janicak PG, Davis JM, Gibbons RD, et al. Efficacy of ECT: a meta-analysis. American Journal of Psychiatry 1985; 142: 297
87. Schöpf J. Treatment of depressions resistant to tricyclic antidepressant related drugs or MAO-inhibitors by lithium addiction: review of the literature. Pharmacopsychiatry 1989; 22: 174
88. Coryell W, Scheftner W, Keller M, et al. The enduring psychosocial consequences of mania and depression. American Journal of Psychiatry 1993; 150: 720
89. Weich S. The economics of depression. Focus on Depression, November 1993: 4
90. Greenberg PE, Stiglin LE, Finkelstein SN, et al. The economic burden of depression in 1990. Journal of Clinical Psychiatry 1993; 54: 405
91. Ormel J, Oldehinkel T, Brilman E, et al. Outcome of depression and anxiety in primary care. Archives of General Psychiatry 1993; 50: 759
92. Haefely W. Pharmacology of anxiety. European Neuropsychopharmacology 1991; 1: 89
93. Lader M. Benzodiazepines: a risk-benefit profile. CNS Drugs 1994; 1: 377-87
94. Meier PJ, Ziegler WH, Neftel K. Benzodiazepines - Praxis und Probleme ihrer Anwendung. Schweizerische Medizinische Wochenschrift 1988; 118: 381
95. Colburn WA, Jack ML. Relationships between CSF drug concentrations, receptor binding characteristics, and pharmacokinetic and pharmacodynamic properties of selected 1,4-substituted benzodiazepines. Clinical Pharmacokinetics 1987; 13: 179
96. Greenblatt DJ, Harmatz JS, Shader RI. Clinical pharmacokinetics of anxiolytics and hypnotics in the elderly. Therapeutic considerations (Part I). Clinical Pharmacokinetics 1991; 21: 165
97. Greenblatt DJ, Harmatz JS, Shader RI. Clinical pharmacokinetics of anxiolytics and hypnotics in the elderly. Therapeutic considerations (Part II). Clinical Pharmacokinetics 1991; 21: 262
98. Ankier S, Goa KL. Quazepam: a preliminary review of its pharmacodynamic and pharmacokinetic properties, and therapeutic efficacy in insomnia. Drugs 1988; 35: 42
99. Greenblatt DJ, Wright CE. Clinical pharmacokinetics of alprazolam. Therapeutic implications. Clinical Pharmacokinetics 1993; 24: 453
100. Garzone PD, Kroboth PD. Pharmacokinetics of the newer benzodiazepines. Clinical Pharmacokinetics 1989; 16: 337
101. Goa KL, Heel RC. Zopiclone: a review of its pharmacodynamic and pharmacokinetic properties and therapeutic efficacy as an hypnotic. Drugs 1986; 32: 48
102. Langtry HD, Benfield P. Zolpidem: a review of its pharmacodynamic and pharmacokinetic properties and therapeutic potential. Drugs 1990; 40: 291
103. The Quality Asurance Project. Treatment outlines for the management of anxiety states. Australian and New Zealand Journal of Psychiatry 1985; 19: 138-51
104. Durham RC, Allan T. Psychological treatment of generalised anxiety disorder. A review of the clinical significance of results in outcome studies since 1980. British Journal of Psychiatry 1993; 163: 19

105. Tyrer P, Seivewright N, Murphy S, et al. The Nottingham study of neurotic disorder: comparison of drug and psychological treatments. Lancet 1988; 2: 236
106. Ballenger JC, Burrows GD, DuPont RL, et al. Alprazolam in panic disorder and agoraphobia: results from a multicenter trial. Archives of General Psychiatry 1988; 45: 413-22
107. Cross-National Collaborative Panic Study, Second Phase Investigators. Drug treatment of panic disorder. Comparative efficacy of alprazolam, imipramine, and placebo. British Journal of Psychiatry 1992; 160: 191-202
108. Wilkinson G, Balestrieri M, Ruggeri M, et al. Meta-analysis of double-blind placebo-controlled trials of antidepressants and benzodiazepines for patients with panic disorders. Psychological Medicine 1991; 21: 991
109. Borbély AA, Åkerstedt T, Benoit O, et al. Hypnotics and sleep physiology: a consensus report. European Archives of Psychiatry and Clinical Neuroscience 1991; 241: 13
110. Wadworth A, McTavish D. Zopiclone: a review of its pharmacological properties and therapeutic efficacy as an hypnotic. Drugs & Aging 1993; 3: 441
111. Vela-Bueno A, Kales A. Benzodiazepine hypnotics in the multidimensional treatment of insomnia. Drugs of Today 1986; 22: 271-81
112. Schneider-Helmert D. Why low-dose benzodiazepine-dependent insomniacs can't escape their sleeping pills. Acta Psychiatrica Scandinavica 1988; 78: 706
113. Kruse WH-H. Problems and pitfalls in the use of benzodiazepines in the elderly. Drug Safety 1990; 5: 328
114. Tiller JWG, Schweitzer I. Benzodiazepines. Depressants or antidepressants? Drugs 1992; 44: 165
115. Ghoneim MM, Mewaldt SP. Benzodiazepines and human memory: a review. Anesthesiology 1990; 72: 926
116. Lader M. Rebound insomnia and newer hypnotics. Psychopharmacology 1992; 108: 248
117. Merlotti L, Roehrs T, Zorick F, et al. Rebound insomnia: duration of use and individual differences. Journal of Clinical Psychopharmacology 1991; 11: 368
118. Roehrs T, Merlotti L, Zorick F, et al. Rebound insomnia and hypnotic self administration. Psychopharmacology 1992; 107: 480
119. Tyrer P. The benzodiazepine post-withdrawal syndrome. Stress Medicine 1991; 7: 1
120. Marriott S, Tyrer P. Benzodiazepine dependence. Avoidance and withdrawal. Drug Safety 1993; 9: 93
121. Ruben SM, Morrison CL. Temazepam misuse in a group of injecting drug users. British Journal of Addiction 1992; 87: 1387
122. Serfaty M, Masterton G. Fatal poisonings attributed to benzodiazepines in Britain during the 1980s. British Journal of Psychiatry 1993; 163: 386
123. Fineberg N, Drummond LM. Anxiety disorders: drug treatment or behavioural cognitive psychotherapy? CNS Drugs 1995; 3: 448
124. Consensus Conference. Clinical practice. Guidelines for the management of patients with generalised anxiety. Psychiatric Bulletin 1992; 16: 560
125. King MB. Counselling services in general practice. The need for evaluation. Psychiatric Bulletin 1994; 18: 65
126. Rickels K, Downing R, Schweizer E, et al. Antidepressants for the treatment of generalized anxiety disorder. Archives of General Psychiatry 1993; 50: 884
127. Tyrer P. Current status of β-blocking drugs in the treatment of anxiety disorders. Drugs 1988; 36: 773
128. Levin AP, Liebowitz MR. Drug treatment of phobias. Efficacy and optimum use. Drugs 1987; 34: 504
129. Boyer W. Serotonin uptake inhibitors are superior to imipramine and alprazolam in alleviating panic attacks: a meta-analysis. International Clinical Psychopharmacology 1995; 10: 45
130. Benca RM, Obermeyer WH, Thisted RA, et al. Sleep and psychiatric disorders. A meta-analysis. Archives of General Psychiatry 1992; 49: 651
131. Consensus Conference. Drugs and insomnia. The use of medications to promote sleep. Journal of the American Medical Association 1984; 251: 2410
132. Lader M, editor. The medical management of insomnia in general practice. Round Table Series No. 28. London: Royal Society of Medicine, 1992
133. Prinz PN, Vitiello MV, Raskind MA, et al. Geriatrics: sleep disorders and aging. New England Journal of Medicine 1990; 323: 520
134. Morgan K. Hypnotics in the elderly. What cause for concern? Drugs 1990; 40: 688
135. Zohar J, Zohar-Kadouch RC, Kindler S. Current concepts in the pharmacological treatment of obsessive-compulsive disorder. Drugs 1992; 43: 210
136. Fulton B, McTavish D. Fluoxetine: an overview of its pharmacodynamic and pharmacokinetic properties and review of its therapeutic efficacy in obsessive-compulsive disorder. CNS Drugs 1995; 3: 305
137. Choy T, de Bosset F. Post-traumatic stress disorder: an overview. Canadian Journal of Psychiatry 1992; 37: 578
138. Kennedy SH, Goldbloom DS. Current perspectives on drug therapies for anorexia nervosa and bulimia nervosa. Drugs 1991; 41: 367
139. Kaplan CA, Hussain S. Use of drugs in child and adolescent psychiatry. British Journal of Psychiatry 1995; 166: 291
140. Brown CS, Cooke SC. Attention deficit hyperactivity disorder. Clinical features and treatment options. CNS Drugs 1994; 1: 95
141. Simeon JG, Wiggins DM. Pharmacotherapy of attention-deficit hyperactivity. Canadian Journal of Psychiatry 1993; 38: 443
142. Gordon CT, State RC, Nelson JE, et al. A double-blind comparison of clomipramine, desipramine, and placebo in the treatment of autistic disorder. Archives of General Psychiatry 1993; 50: 441
143. Rossor M. Alzheimer's disease. British Medical Journal 1993; 307: 779
144. Gray A, Fenn P. Alzheimer's disease: the burden of the illness in England. Health Trends 1993; 25: 31
145. Schneider LS, Sobin PB. Non-neuroleptic treatment of behavioural symptoms and agitation in Alzheimer's disease and other dementias. Psychopharmacology Bulletin 1992; 28: 71
146. Schneider LS. A meta analysis of controlled trials of neuroleptic treatment in dementia. Journal of the American Geriatrics Society 1990; 38: 553
147. Hermann CK. Dementia. A costly problem. PharmacoEconomics 1992; 2: 444
148. Wadworth AN, Chrisp P. Co-dergocrine mesylate: a review of its pharmacodynamic and pharmacokinetic properties and therapeutic use in age-related cognitive decline. Drugs & Aging 1992; 2: 153
149. Vernon MW, Sorkin EM. Piracetam: an overview of its pharmacological properties and a review of its therapeutic use in senile cognitive disorders. Drugs & Aging 1991; 1: 17
150. Nicholson CD. Pharmacology of nootropics and metabolically active compounds in relation to their use in dementia. Psychopharmacology 1990; 101: 147
151. Davis KL, Powchik P. Tacrine. Lancet 1995; 345: 625-30
152. Allen NHP, Burns A. The treatment of Alzheimer's disease. Journal of Psychopharmacology 1995; 9: 43
153. Adinoff B, Bone GHA, Linnoila M. Acute ethanol poisoning and the ethanol withdrawal syndrome. Medical Toxicology and Adverse Drug Experience 1988; 3: 172
154. Gonzalez JP, Brogden RN. Naltrexone: a review of its pharmacodynamic and pharmacokinetic properties and thera-

peutic efficacy in the management of opioid dependence. Drugs 1988; 35: 192
155. Ginzburg HM, MacDonald MG. The role of naltrexone in the management of drug abuse. Medical Toxicology and Adverse Drug Experience 1987; 2: 83
156. Benowitz NL. Nicotine replacement therapy. What has been accomplished - can we do better? Drugs 1993; 45: 157
157. Schneider NG. Nicotine therapy in smoking cessation. Pharmacokinetic considerations. Clinical Pharmacokinetics 1992; 23: 169
158. Palmer KJ, Buckley MM, Faulds D. Transdermal nicotine: a review of its pharmacodynamic and pharmacokinetic properties, and therapeutic efficacy as an aid to smoking cessation. Drugs 1992; 44: 498
159. Glassman AH, Covey LS. Future trends in the pharmacological treatment of smoking cessation. Drugs 1990; 40: 1
160. Cohen DR, Fowler GH. Economic implications of smoking cessation therapies. A review of economic appraisals. PharmacoEconomics 1993; 4: 331

Chapter 31

# Infectious Diseases (Bacterial and Fungal): Principles and Practice of Antimicrobial Therapy

*R.N. Jones, M.A. Pfaller* and *M.G. Cormican*

## Synopsis of Important Principles

1) Successful chemotherapy of bacterial and fungal infections requires an accurate bacteriological as well as clinical diagnosis.

2) The clinical diagnosis alone may enable suitable treatment to be started. Subsequent skilled laboratory guidance is required in making a proper choice of antimicrobial agent.

3) The site of infection is an important factor to take into account; for example, if this is in the urinary or biliary tract or the meninges, a drug must be chosen which attains adequate concentrations in these areas.

4) A combination of two agents may be advisable to obtain the widest cover immediately. Once a specific pathogen has been identified, treatment should be reviewed. Synergistic activity could result from combination therapy.

5) Antimicrobial drug dosages often require reduction at the two extremes of life. They also often need to be reduced in renal disease, since drugs eliminated by this route may accumulate to hazardous concentrations. Dosages may also require modification in the presence of severe hepatic disease.

6) Factors such as convenience or ease of administration, relative incidence of troublesome adverse effects, emerging resistance, and cost influence the choice of antimicrobial agents in modern chemotherapy.

The origins of effective antimicrobial chemotherapy can be traced to ancient China (>2500 years ago) and to Greece at the time of Hypocrates where antimicrobial qualities of mouldy soybean curds, fermented beverages, spices and inorganic salts were recognised. However, it was not until relatively modern times that specific compounds or naturally-occurring substances were characterised and applied to the chemotherapy of specific infectious pathogens. The most important examples have been the use of heavy metals (arsenic, bismuth) to treat syphilis, the discovery of sulfonamides in the 1930s, and ultimately the recognition of β-lactams (penicillins, cefalosporins) and aminoglycosides (streptomycin) derived from specific fungal species. The latter events in the 1940-1950 period represent the true beginning of the antimicrobial chemotherapy era as we know it today.

The general principles of antimicrobial chemotherapy can be applied equally to antibacterial, antifungal, antiviral and antiparasitic therapy. Important concepts include:

1) Recognition of the infection-causing pathogen or knowledge of the most likely pathogen derived from information about the infection site and other factors.

2) Laboratory based data enabling pathogen identification and susceptibility to therapeutic agents.

3) Assessment of host factors that may influence therapy such as immune status, organ function, age, sex, travel history, etc.

Specifically, the first key action by the clinician should be the provision of a specimen for accurate identification of the offending pathogen or pathogens. Until the organism is recognised, empirical drug choices can be applied on the basis of knowledge of various micro-organism frequencies indexed by site of infection, hospital *versus* outpatient presentations, age, symptoms, local epidemiology and prior experience. The specimen quality is essential, necessitating appropriately timed sampling (blood cultures and adequate volumes during febrile episodes), direct samples of body fluids or swabs where aspirates are not practical, midstream clean-catch urine or catheter samples, and the use of appropriate transport reagents to maximise the culture of fastidious species.

The next step in the initial process is good laboratory practice that includes rapid determination of organism morphology via stained samples to provide early direction of chemotherapy. This is followed by plating on appropriate media or the use of various newer technologies [rapid diagnostic tests and molecular methods such as polymerase chain reaction (PCR) and gene probes].

After the organism is isolated, susceptibility tests (usually standardised or commercial systems validated against reference methods) are performed. These procedures require only a few hours or up to 24 hours to achieve accurate results. Rapid results for some severely ill patients (blood stream infections, nosocomial pneumonia, immunocompromised patients) has been beneficial in lowering morbidity and mortality, and thus reducing overall hospital costs in this patient subset,[1] but only if the rapid method is accurate for the tested species. Laboratories should select standardised methods that allow intra- and interlaboratory comparisons of results and the highest probability of accuracy and reproducibility.

Lastly, host factors must be assessed and the therapy selected. The choice of therapeutic agent or agents could remain empirical if symptoms continue in the face of a sterile or non-contributing culture, or if the organism cultured or discovered by non-culture techniques does not have susceptibility test results. In such cases, prior knowledge or locally derived epidemiology data become paramount. When susceptibility information is available, the therapy may be directed and a modification of the initial empirical regimen may be appropriate.

The dogma of infection chemotherapy has dictated that clinicians:

- Use effective agents
- Avoid use of ineffective agents
- Use the narrowest spectrum antimicrobial to which the organism has been demonstrated susceptible
- Use combinations where appropriate to achieve enhanced (synergistic) inhibition
- Monitor for toxicity or appropriate therapeutic concentrations when using some drug classes (e.g. aminoglycosides, chloramphenicol, glycopeptides, etc.)
- Sustain therapy until a stable clinical response has been achieved (usually ≈5 days).

However, several of these principles have been challenged by changing practices of antimicrobial chemotherapy. For example, narrow-spectrum agents may be less cost effective and prone to compromised outcomes due to copathogenicity. For instance, benzylpenicillin (penicillin G) or phenoxymethylpenicillin (penicillin V) for streptococcal pharyngitis may be destroyed by β-lactamases produced by normal upper airways flora. Similarly, use of plasma concentration monitoring and selection of less toxic drugs appear to be changing now that once-daily aminoglycoside regimens have been introduced.[2]

Determination of susceptibility patterns to commonly used antimicrobials has become critical in antimicrobial chemotherapy as the number of drug-resistant species increases. Important resistance problems include:

- Methicillin (and oxacillin)-resistant staphylococci
- Penicillin-resistant *Streptococcus pneumoniae* and other streptococci
- Glycopeptide-resistant enterococci
- Multiresistant non-enteric Gram-negative bacilli (*Pseudomonas aeruginosa*, *Stenotrophomonas maltophilia*, *Acinetobacter* spp.)
- *Enterobacter* and *Citrobacter* species resistant to third-generation cefalosporins
- *Escherichia coli* and *Klebsiella* spp. producing extended-spectrum β-lactamases
- Penicillin-resistant *Neisseria* spp. (via altered penicillin binding proteins and β-lactamase production)
- Ampicillin-resistant *Haemophilus* spp.
- Anaerobes that have become more resistant to clindamycin, cefamycins and newer cefalosporins.

The appropriate use of antimicrobial chemotherapy seeks to minimise the emergence of resistance and the cost of morbidity associated with treatment failures or persistent disease. Local surveillance of resistance rates should help guide appropriate empirical antimicrobial chemotherapy. The education of primary care providers to be more selective in the use of these agents will be most effective in extending the clinical utility of contemporary drugs.

## 1. Clinical Pharmacological Considerations

### 1.1 Classification and Mechanisms of Action of Antimicrobial Agents

The number of antimicrobial agents available is continually increasing as a result of new drug discoveries and synthetic modifications of existing structures. The clinically usable drugs have escalated markedly to hundreds of agents on a worldwide basis. Most of these compounds belong to a relatively small group of drugs or classes that should be considered by clinicians when prescribing drugs for infection chemotherapy or prophylaxis. Each class of antimicrobial agents has a mechanism of action that often sets it apart from other groups.

The recent past has witnessed the development of pharmacodynamics as applied to antimicrobial agents. This science of understanding drug effects is based on studies of antimicrobial activity (i.e. potency measured by microbiologists as minimum inhibitory concentrations in mg/L or μg/ml) and drug concentrations (usually measured in serum or at the site of infection). The principles of pharmacodynamics[3] focus on the type of bactericidal action for each drug, e.g. concentration- or time-dependent killing (table I).

The widely used β-lactam antimicrobials are *time-dependent* in their antimicrobial action; thus, unbound serum drug concentrations must remain above the minimum inhibitory concentration (MIC) of the infecting pathogen for at least 25 to 50% of the dosage interval to achieve success, as measured by a minimal (inhibitory) or maximal (bactericidal) effect. The proportion of the dosage interval required can vary with the species involved, shorter times being needed for staphylococci and longer times for inhibition of streptococci and Gram-negative bacilli.

*Concentration-dependent* antimicrobial effects have been observed for the aminoglycosides and quinolones (table I), whereby a maximal effect can be achieved by a drug concentration above the recorded MIC. The effect can

**Table I.** Prediction of important pharmacodynamic parameters of antimicrobials

| Drug class | Property | Parameter |
|---|---|---|
| Cefalosporins and penicillins | Time-dependent killing and short or no PAE | Time during which concentrations exceed MIC |
| Aminoglycosides and quinolones | Concentration-dependent killing and prolonged PAE | $C_{max}$/MIC or AUC/MIC ratios |

*Abbreviations:* AUC = area under the plasma concentration-time curve; $C_{max}$ = peak plasma concentration; MIC = minimum inhibitory concentration; PAE = postantibiotic effect.

be enhanced by elevating the peak concentration achieved, if possible within the safety profile (toxicity limits) of the individual therapeutic agent. Concentration-dependent killing and drug effects related to the area under the concentration-time curve (AUC) or the AUC above the inhibitory concentration (AUIC) have been linked for some compounds studied such as the newer quinolones.

The concept of postantibiotic effect (PAE) has also been incorporated into pharmacodynamics, wherein the PAE measured *in vitro* and *in vivo* (in animal models) adds to the understanding of the time-concentration dependency relationship. Understanding these therapeutic principles of infection chemotherapy may markedly alter dosage schedules to maximise treatment outcomes. For example, the β-lactams generally have no PAE against Gram-negative bacilli, whereas the aminoglycosides have a PAE of 1 to 2 hours.

This section summarises the mechanism of action, spectrum of activity, basic pharmacokinetics and therapeutic use of commonly used antimicrobial agents. For a review of mechanisms of action and emerging resistance patterns, see 'The Microbial Wars'[4] and 'Frontiers in Biotechnology'.[5]

#### 1.1.1 β-Lactams and β-Lactam/β-Lactamase Inhibitor Combinations

This group of antimicrobial agents has become the most widely used therapeutic class because of its varied antimicrobial spectrum and its safety. The chemical structures of the various agents are listed in figure 1 and include penicillins, mecillinam, β-lactamase inhibitors (clavulanic acid, sulfones), carbapenems, cefalosporins, cefamycins, oxacephems, carbacephems and monobactams.

The common structural component is the β-lactam ring, which can be fused to a 5- or 6-member ring or remain monocyclic (as in the monobactams, e.g. aztreonam). The amide bond active site interacts with penicillin binding protein (PBPs; enzymes necessary for cell wall synthesis) of bacteria to prevent peptidoglycan cell wall formation and leads to a bacteriostatic and often bactericidal effect. The target PBPs can differ for these compounds in the β-lactam class and only a few (2 or 3) are considered essential to a bacterial species, i.e. lethal PBPs. When the β-lactam drug bonds to these enzymes, bacterial morphological changes or specific lytic actions are produced. Examples for

**Table II.** Classification of currently used penicillins

| Group | Drugs |
|---|---|
| • Benzylpenicillin (penicillin G) and long-acting parenteral formulations | Benzylpenicillin<br>Benzathine benzylpenicillin |
| • Orally-absorbed narrow-spectrum penicillins | Phenoxymethylpenicillin (penicillin V)<br>Phenethicillin |
| • Penicillinase-resistant penicillins | Isoxazoyl penicillins (cloxacillin, dicloxacillin, flucloxacillin, oxacillin)<br>Methicillin<br>Nafcillin |
| • Extended-spectrum penicillins (active against some Gram-negative bacilli) | Aminopenicillins (ampicillin, amoxicillin)<br>Mecillinam (amdinocillin) |
| • *Pseudomonas*-active penicillins | Acylureidopenicillins (apalcillin, azlocillin, mezlocillin, piperacillin)<br>Carboxypenicillins (carbenicillin, ticarcillin) |
| • Gram-negative β-lactamase-resistant penicillins | Temocillin |

Enterobacteriaceae include bacteriolytic effects with bonding to PBP 1a and 1b (cefazolin, cefuroxime, cefotaxime, etc.), to PBP 2 causing spheroplast formation (mecillinam), and filament formation by action against PBP 3 (cefalexin, some third-generation cefalosporins, monobactams). Many newer broad-spectrum β-lactams bind with clinically useful affinity to more than one PBP, enhancing overall potency.

##### Penicillins

The penicillins have their origin with the discovery by Fleming in 1929 of an antimicrobial substance produced by *Penicillium notatum*.[6] The active substance was isolated in 1941 under the direction of Florey and Chain, leading to its use in the second World War and in civilian clinical cases in the UK and US. Modified production was achieved (*Penicillin chrysogenum* source) and isolation of the penicillin nucleus (6-aminopenicillanic acid) allowed semisynthetic high volume production of numerous penicillin subclasses (table II).[7] The principal breakthrough penicillin drugs have been the penicillinase-resistant penicillins (isoxazolyl penicillins, methicillin, nafcillin), orally administered penicillins (phenoxymethylpenicillin, phenethicillin), extended-spectrum penicillins (aminopenicillins, mecillinam), *Pseudomonas*-active extended-spectrum penicillins (acylureidopenicillins, carboxypenicillins) and the Gram-negative β-lactamase-resistant penicillins (temocillin). The antimicrobial activity of each class differs markedly and their application to

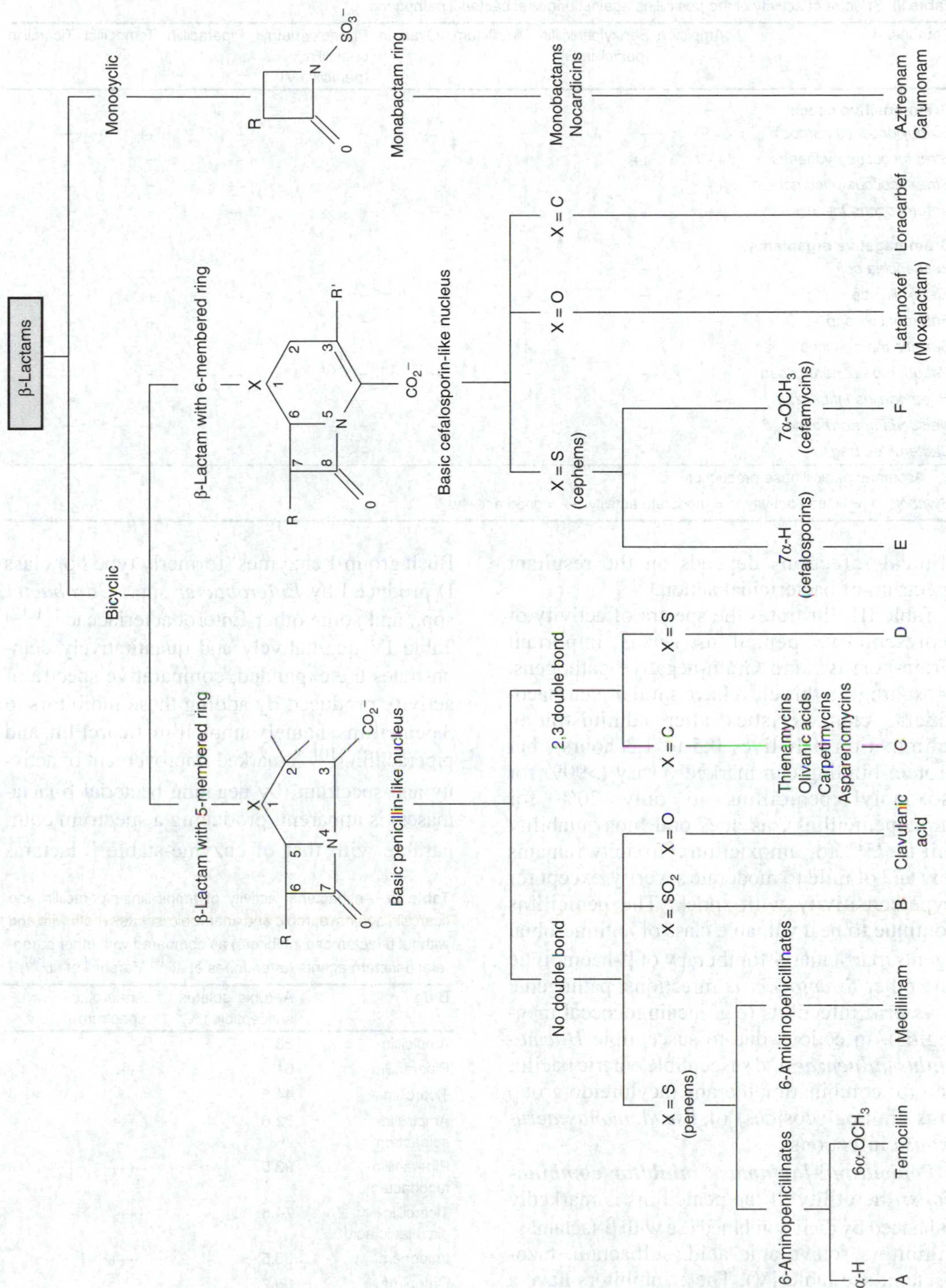


**Fig. 1.** Classification of the clinically available β-lactam antimicrobial agents. *Symbols:* A = penicillins (e.g. see table I); B = sulfones [e.g. sulbactam (β-lactamase inhibitor used with ampicillin), tazobactam (β-lactamase inhibitor used with piperacillin)]; C = carbapenems (e.g. imipenem, meropenem); D = penems [e.g. SCH 29482; SCH 34343; faropenem, RO-481220 (inhibitor)]; E = cefalosporins (see table VI); F = cefamycins (see table VI).

**Table III.** Spectra of activity of the penicillins against principal bacterial pathogens

| Pathogen | Ampicillin | Benzylpenicillin (penicillin G) | Mecillinam | Oxacillin | Phenoxymethyl-penicillin (penicillin V) | Piperacillin | Temocillin | Ticarcillin |
|---|---|---|---|---|---|---|---|---|
| **Gram-positive cocci:** | | | | | | | | |
| *Staphylococcus aureus*[a] | – | – | – | ++ | – | – | ++ | – |
| *Streptococcus pyogenes* | ++ | ++ | + | + | ++ | ++ | – | + |
| *Streptococcus pneumoniae* | ++ | ++ | + | + | ++ | ++ | – | + |
| *Enterococcus faecalis* | ++ | + | – | – | + | ++ | – | – |
| **Gram-negative organisms:** | | | | | | | | |
| *Escherichia coli* | + | – | + | – | – | + | ++ | + |
| *Klebsiella* spp. | – | – | + | – | – | ++ | ++ | – |
| *Enterobacter* spp. | – | – | + | – | – | + | + | + |
| *Serratia marcescens* | – | – | + | – | – | ++ | + | ++ |
| *Pseudomonas aeruginosa* | – | – | – | – | – | ++ | – | ++ |
| *Haemophilus influenzae* | + | – | – | – | – | + | + | + |
| *Neisseria gonorrhoeae* | + | + | + | – | – | + | + | – |
| *Bacteroides fragilis* | – | – | – | – | – | ++ | – | + |

a Assumes penicillinase production.

*Symbols:* – = limited activity; + = moderate activity; ++ = good activity.

clinical infections depends on the resultant spectrum of bactericidal action.[8]

Table III illustrates the spectra of activity of representative penicillins *versus* important Gram-positive and Gram-negative pathogens. Most drugs in this class have similar pharmacokinetic characteristics after administration (elimination half-lives 0.5 to 1.3 hours), but protein binding can markedly vary (>90% for isoxazolyl penicillins to only 20% for aminopenicillins), as does oral bioavailability (nil to 75% for amoxicillin). Toxicity remains low and of mild to moderate severity, except for hypersensitivity with shock. The penicillins continue to be a valuable class of antimicrobial agents, particularly for therapy of β-haemolytic and other *Streptococcus* infections, pathogenic *Neisseria* infections (e.g. meningococcal meningitis), infections due to susceptible *Haemophilus influenzae* and susceptible enteric bacilli, and for combination therapy (acylureido group plus aminoglycosides) of *Pseudomonas aeruginosa* infections.

***Penicillin/β-lactamase inhibitor combinations:*** the utility of the penicillins is markedly enhanced by their combined use with β-lactamase inhibitors (clavulanic acid, sulbactam, tazobactam; see table IV). These inhibitors have a greater affinity for the bacterial β-lactamases than the active penicillin co-drug, and generally act as irreversible 'suicide' inhibitors of intracellular and extracellular β-lactamase. However, their spectrum of activity does not include Bush group 1 enzymes (formerly type I or class I) produced by *Enterobacter* spp., *Citrobacter* spp., and some other Enterobacteriaceae.[11,12] Table IV qualitatively and quantitatively demonstrates the expanded, comparative spectra of activity produced by adding these inhibitors to 3 penicillins, namely ampicillin, ticarcillin, and piperacillin.[10] A marked improvement of activity and spectrum (by negating bacterial β-lactamases) is apparent, producing a spectrum comparable with that of enzyme-stable β-lactams

**Table IV.** Antibacterial activity of ampicillin, piperacillin and ticarcillin against aerobic and anaerobic isolates (both with and without β-lactamase inhibitors) as compared with other parenteral β-lactam agents (after Jones et al.;[9] Marshall et al.[10])

| Drug | Aerobic isolates susceptible (%)[a] | Anaerobic spectrum |
|---|---|---|
| Ampicillin | 33.3 | – |
| Piperacillin | 61.0 | +++ |
| Ticarcillin | 44.5 | ++ |
| Ampicillin-sulbactam | 72.6 | ++++ |
| Piperacillin-tazobactam | 93.5 | ++++ |
| Ticarcillin-clavulanic acid | 74.5 | ++++ |
| Imipenem | 93.5 | ++++ |
| Cefepime | 86.7 | – |
| Ceftazidime | 79.4 | – |
| Ceftriaxone | 74.0 | + |

a 1994 data.

*Symbols:* – = <50% of isolates; + = 50-75%; ++ = 76-85%; +++ = 86-95%; ++++ = >95%.

such as the carbapenems (imipenem) and newer cefalosporins.

Amoxicillin/clavulanic acid is available for use by both oral and parenteral routes, while combinations of ampicillin/sulbactam, ticarcillin/clavulanic acid and piperacillin/tazobactam are used only parenterally. The pharmacokinetic characteristics are well matched for each of these combinations (elimination half-lives, 1 hour) and dosages of the inhibitors are comparable with those of the penicillins, although the ratio of penicillin to inhibitor ranges from 30 to 1 for ticarcillin/clavulanic acid to 2 to 1 for amoxicillin/clavulanic acid and ampicillin/sulbactam. Adverse effects mirror those of the active penicillin co-drug. Excellent clinical trial results have been achieved, particularly for therapy of mixed flora infections caused by aerobic and anaerobic species and in the empirical treatment of serious infections in seriously ill patients (e.g. neutropenic fever, post-trauma or postsurgical sepsis, nosocomial pneumonia, etc.).[11,12]

**Cefalosporins**

The cefalosporin class began with the research of Giuseppe Brotzu following the discovery of a fungus (*Cephalosporium acremonium*) in sea water near a sewage outlet in Sardinia. Subsequently, Abraham in Oxford identified and isolated cefalosporin C from among several substances produced by the fungus.[13] With this discovery and that of 7-aminocephalosporanic acid, semisynthetic modifications rapidly emerged, leading to the initial clinical compounds, cefaloridine, cefalexin, cefalothin and cefaloglycin. Early modifications of the cephem ring structure (fig. 1) led to drugs with acceptable activity against penicillinase-producing staphylococci, various *Streptococcus* spp., and *E. coli*, *Klebsiella* spp., and *Proteus mirabilis* among the enteric bacilli (table V).

The mechanism of action of the cefalosporins was found to be similar to that of other β-lactams. These drugs exert their antimicrobial action by binding to target PBPs located within

**Table V.** Spectra of activity of cefalosporins against principal bacterial pathogens

| Pathogen | First-generation agents | | Second-generation agents | | | Third-generation agents | | | Fourth-generation agent |
|---|---|---|---|---|---|---|---|---|---|
| | Cefalexin | Cefazolin | Cefaclor | Cefuroxime | Cefoxitin | Cefpodoxime proxetil | Cefotaxime | Ceftazidime | Cefepime |
| **Gram-positive cocci:** | | | | | | | | | |
| *Staphylococcus aureus* | ++ | ++ | ++ | ++ | + | + | ++ | + | ++ |
| *Streptococcus pyogenes* | ++ | ++ | ++ | ++ | ++ | ++ | ++ | + | ++ |
| *Streptococcus pneumoniae* | + | ++ | ++ | ++ | + | + | ++ | + | ++ |
| *Enterococcus faecalis* | – | – | – | – | – | – | – | – | – |
| **Gram-negative organisms:** | | | | | | | | | |
| *Escherichia coli* | ++ | ++ | ++ | ++ | ++ | ++ | ++ | ++ | ++ |
| *Klebsiella* spp. | ++ | ++ | ++ | ++ | ++ | ++ | ++ | ++ | ++ |
| *Enterobacter* spp. | – | – | – | – | – | + | + | + | ++ |
| *Serratia marcescens* | – | – | – | – | + | + | ++ | ++ | ++ |
| *Haemophilus influenzae* | + | + | + | + | + | ++ | ++ | ++ | ++ |
| *Neisseria gonorrhoeae* | – | – | – | + | + | ++ | ++ | + | ++ |
| *Acinetobacter* spp. | – | – | – | – | – | – | – | + | + |
| *Pseudomonas aeruginosa* | – | – | – | – | – | – | + | ++ | ++ |
| *Stenotrophomonas maltophilia* | – | – | – | – | – | – | – | + | + |
| *Bacteroides fragilis* | – | – | – | – | ++ | – | + | – | – |

*Symbols:* – = limited activity; + = moderate activity; ++ = good activity.

the cell, on the cell membrane. The PBPs are carboxypeptidases, endopeptidases and transpeptidases that cross-link the peptidoglycan polymers. Generally, in Enterobacteriaceae (the most studied organisms), PBP 1a, 1b, 2 and 3 are considered critical (lethal PBPs) and PBP 4, 5 and 6 are not required for cell survival.

The pharmacokinetic characteristics of the cefalosporins vary considerably (see appendix A for a compilation of their pharmacokinetic parameters). These drugs must be considered individually and selected on the basis of their spectrum of activity (table V) and route of administration (table VI). The widely used 'generations' classification of cefalosporins is shown in table VI.

***Tolerability:*** adverse reactions of clinical importance have occasionally been identified although, as a class, the cefalosporins are generally well tolerated. The usual adverse effects are minor and include local effects (nausea and vomiting with oral agents; thrombophlebitis with intravenous drugs), β-lactam cross-allergenicity (rare *vs* penicillins, probably ≈1%),[14] positive Coombs' tests without haemolytic anaemia, nephrotoxicity (rare since the cefaloridine era), diarrhoea (increased with drugs having high hepatic elimination, e.g. cefoperazone and ceftriaxone), disulfiram-like intolerance of alcohol (drugs that have a 3-thiomethyltetrazole side chain, e.g. cefamandole, cefoperazone, latamoxef), biliary sludging (ceftriaxone), bilirubin encephalopathy (ceftriaxone), and hypoprothrombinaemia (vitamin K-depleted patients receiving cephems with a 3-thiomethyltetrazole side chain). Latamoxef (moxalactam) has been less commonly used since 1987 because of its tendency to cause haematological adverse effects.[15]

Newer cefalosporins have become the most used agents in developed countries because of their wide spectra of activity (β-lactamase stable) and overall safety. The spectra of activity of representative oral and parenteral cefalosporins are listed in table V.[16] An expanded spectrum of use has been achieved with each generation of parenteral cefalosporins. The second-generation cefamycins (cefoxitin, cefmetazole, cefotetan) are more active *in vitro* and *in vivo* against anaerobic bacteria, especially *Bacteroides fragilis* group isolates. Considerable experience has accumulated over the past 15 years with the third-generation compounds (very β-lactamase stable), and the fourth-generation drugs are now seeking a therapeutic role.

**Table VI.** Generations classification of cefalosporins by route of administration

| Generation | Route of administration: oral | parenteral |
|---|---|---|
| First | Cefalexin[a] | Cefalothin |
| | Cefradine | Cefapirin |
| | Cefadroxil | Cefazolin[a] |
| Second | Cefaclor[a] | Cefamandole |
| | Cefprozil | Cefonicid |
| | Loracarbef[b] | Ceforanide |
| | Cefuroxime axetil | Cefuroxime[a] |
| | | Cefoxitin[a,c] |
| | | Cefmetazole[c] |
| | | Cefotetan[c] |
| Third | Cefixime | Cefotaxime[a] |
| | Cefpodoxime proxetil[a] | Ceftizoxime |
| | | Ceftriaxone |
| | Cefetamet | Cefmenoxime |
| | Ceftibuten | Cefodizime |
| | | Latamoxef (moxalactam)[d] |
| | | Cefoperazone[e] |
| | | Cefpiramide[e] |
| | | Ceftazidime[a,e] |
| Fourth | | Cefepime[a] |
| | | Cefpirome |
| | | Cefclidin |

a Spectrum of activity shown in table V.
b A 1-carbacephem.
c Cefamycin structures.
d 1-Oxacephem with similar spectrum to the 5 agents listed above it.
e Possess expanded activity against *Pseudomonas aeruginosa*.

At present, the third-generation cefalosporins (e.g. cefotaxime, ceftriaxone, ceftazidime) have established first-line utility,[17,18] and other newer drugs (e.g. cefpirome, cefepime, carbapenems, monobactams) may be used for specific indications, resistant strains and in some specialty care units, especially if their pharmacokinetic and safety profiles are acceptable.[19,20] Older compounds in this class (e.g. cefazolin, cefuroxime, cefotetan) have a greater role in single- or limited-dose perioperative prophylaxis (see further section 7).

The spectrum of activity of each 'generation' of orally administered cefalosporins does not equal that of corresponding parenteral drugs. As a rule, a more limited bioavailability and reduced PBP target site affinity decreases the spectrum of activity of third-generation oral cephems against many Gram-positive cocci (*Staphylococcus* spp., penicillin-resistant pneumococci), *Pseudomonas* and anaerobic bacteria.[21-23]

#### Monobactams

The monobactams (fig. 1) have a unique chemical structure and a more limited spectrum of antimicrobial activity. Their mechanism of action is comparable to that of other β-lactams, but the PBP 3 target site is preferred. The adverse effect profile of *aztreonam* is similar to that of the third-generation cefalosporins, with the exception that aztreonam does not share cross-allergenicity with the penicillins, cefalosporins or carbapenems.[24] Its antimicrobial activity includes Enterobacteriaceae with a spectrum equivalent to that of cefotaxime, ceftriaxone or ceftizoxime. Most *P. aeruginosa* strains are inhibited at up to 16 mg/L and the activity is excellent (MIC values up to 1 mg/L) against pathogenic *Neisseria* spp. and *H. influenzae*. Some β-haemolytic streptococci may be susceptible to aztreonam, but all other Gram-positive cocci and anaerobes must be considered aztreonam-resistant.

Aztreonam is a well tolerated agent with a spectrum of activity equivalent to that of the aminoglycosides and has been used in combination therapy (usually with drugs active against Gram-positive cocci and anaerobes) at 8-hour dosage intervals (elimination half-life 1.6 hours). The rates of enhanced killing (synergy), however, have not been found to be comparable with those of aminoglycoside/β-lactam regimens. Aztreonam requires a co-drug (clindamycin, erythromycin, metronidazole, penicillinase-resistant penicillins, vancomycin) for activity against clinically important Gram-positive and anaerobic bacteria to allow empirical therapy. Against susceptible Gram-negative pathogens, aztreonam has achieved success in the treatment of pneumonia, blood stream infections, cutaneous infections and urinary tract infections.

#### Carbapenems

Carbapenems (e.g. imipenem, meropenem) were first described in 1979 as a product of *Streptomyces cattleya*.[25] The compound was first named thienamycin and the chemically stabilised, *N*-forminidoyl thienamycin was called *imipenem* (fig. 1). These drugs are very stable to β-lactamase hydrolysis and have activity against nearly all important bacterial species (except *Enterococcus faecium*, *S. maltophilia*, oxacillin-resistant staphylococci and *Pseudomonas (Burkholderia) cepacia*).[26,27]

Some strains of *P. aeruginosa* (≈10%) are resistant to imipenem, and carbapenem-hydrolysing enzymes have been recently described in Europe and Japan, usually among enteric bacilli and *Bacteroides* spp. Imipenem is metabolised in the body (intrarenally) by peptidases to potentially nephrotoxic products. Coadministration with a specific peptidase inhibitor, cilastatin, allows more extended imipenem dosage intervals, less toxicity and higher active drug concentrations in renal tissues and urine. The elimination half-life of imipenem is 1 hour and organisms with an MIC of up to 4 mg/L are considered susceptible (peak plasma concentration 10 to 13 mg/L). Its greatest use has been in the treatment of infections resistant to other β-lactam agents (e.g. caused by cefalosporin-resistant Enterobacteriaceae), empirical treatment of serious infections in immunocompromised patients, and treatment of patients with a high likelihood of mixed aerobic and anaerobic infections. In these situations, imipenem offers cost-effective therapy by minimising the need for costly and/or toxic combinations.[27-29]

*Meropenem* has a spectrum of activity essentially identical to that of imipenem, but with greater activity against Gram-negative organisms.[30] However, meropenem is generally less active against Gram-positive cocci.[31] Meropenem does not require a peptidase inhibitor co-drug and does not need to be administered any more frequently than 8-hourly. The occurrence of seizures with meropenem appears to be less than that with imepenem. Meropenem has been used for meningitis in several patient populations.[30,32]

### *1.1.2 Aminoglycosides and Aminocyclitols*

This older class of antimicrobials began with the discovery of streptomycin, derived from *Streptomyces griseus* in 1943. This was followed by neomycin in 1949 (of *Streptomyces fradiae* origin) and kanamycin in 1957. More recent and still more effective aminoglycosides include: gentamicin, tobramycin, amikacin, netilmicin,[33] sisomicin, isepamicin,[34,35] dibekacin, and the aminocyclitols spectinomycin, trospectomycin. The '-micin' suffix indicates either a compound originating from *Micromonospora* species or a semisynthetic derivative while, the '-mycin' suffix indicates a compound derived from *Streptomyces* spp.

Most compounds have a basic streptidine (streptomycin) or 2-deoxystreptamine core

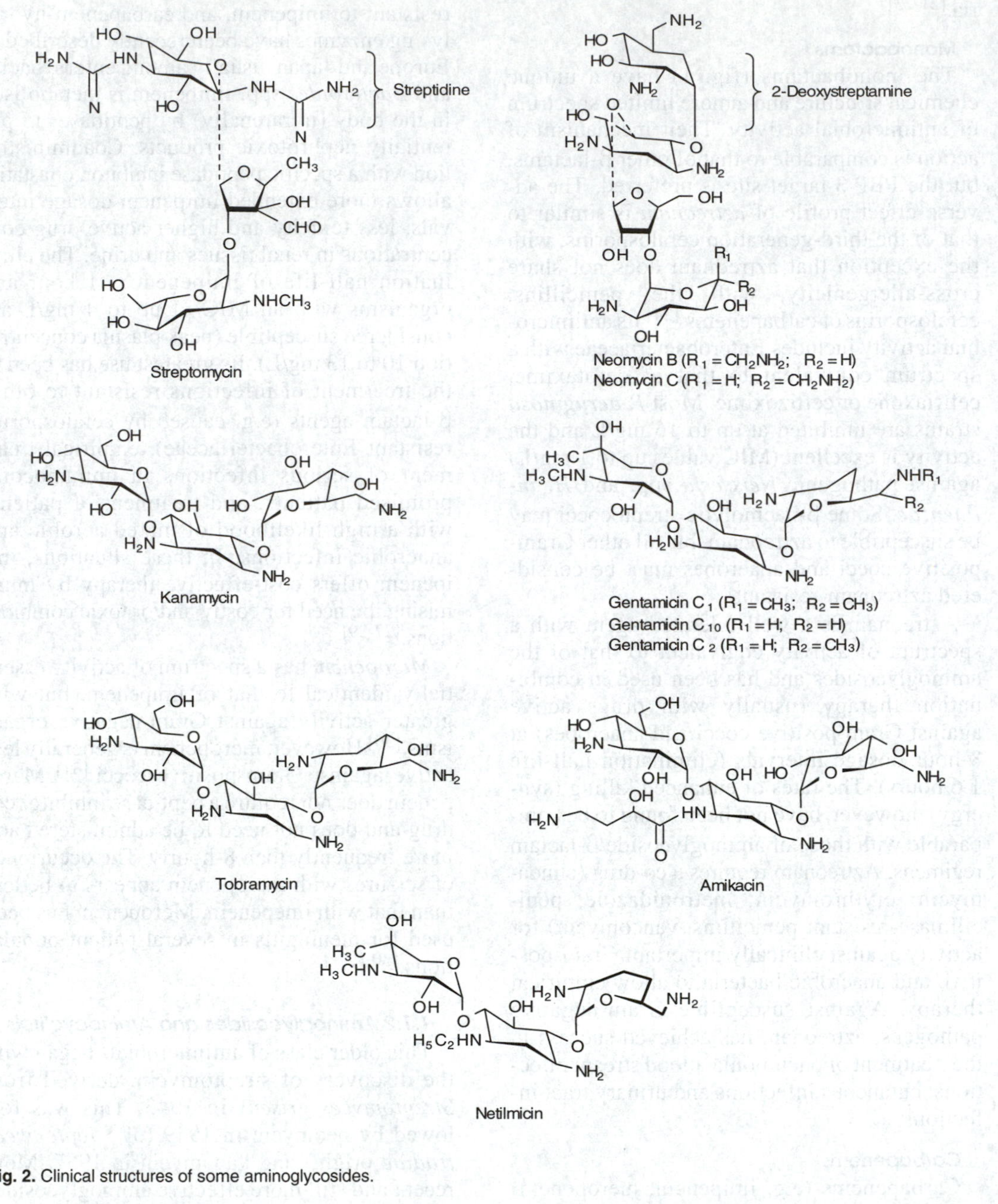

Streptidine
Streptomycin
2-Deoxystreptamine
Neomycin B ($R_1 = CH_2NH_2$; $R_2 = H$)
Neomycin C ($R_1 = H$; $R_2 = CH_2NH_2$)
Kanamycin
Gentamicin $C_1$ ($R_1 = CH_3$; $R_2 = CH_3$)
Gentamicin $C_{1a}$ ($R_1 = H$; $R_2 = H$)
Gentamicin $C_2$ ($R_1 = H$; $R_2 = CH_3$)
Tobramycin
Amikacin
Netilmicin

**Fig. 2.** Clinical structures of some aminoglycosides.

aminocyclitol structure, with modifications in aminosugars attached by glycosidic bonds (fig. 2). These drugs have a complex mechanism of action that is still being explored. Their excellent bactericidal action cannot be totally explained by the impaired protein synthesis produced by aminoglycosides. This action induces the production of genetic miscoded proteins (inaccurate codon-anticodon recognition), and impairs total protein synthesis and disrupts polysomal function. Other secondary effects have also been postulated to explain the rapid lethal action of these drugs. The spectrum of activity of the entire class is focused against Gram-negative aerobic bacilli (Enterobacteriaceae, *Pseudomonas* spp.), some staphylococci, and mycobacteria. Their use in combination with cell-wall active agents produces synergistic bactericidal effects against streptococci and enterococci which do not possess high-level ribosomal/inactivity enzyme resistance against the most commonly used aminoglycosides (gentamicin, streptomycin).

***Tolerability:*** renal and inner ear toxicity is not uncommon with the aminoglycosides and is directly linked to sustained high *in vivo* concentrations. Neuromuscular paralysis can also be a problem following rapid absorption from the pleural space or abdominal cavity and after bolus infusions. This concentration-dependent toxicity has been controlled by therapeutic drug monitoring programmes and recent modifications in dosage to once-daily regimens [fig. 3].[2,34,36,37] Adjustments in dosage must be considered in patients with compromised renal function. The pharmacokinetic characteristics are remarkably similar for all drugs, but concentrations associated with toxicity may vary. Members of this class are generally well absorbed from intramuscular sites of injection, distributed widely in the body tissue, and are suitable for topical, intrathecal and irrigation use.

Resistance among certain bacterial species has various mechanisms (e.g. inactivating enzymes, altered targets, poor cellular permeability, etc.). More complex and multiple mechanisms of resistance have necessitated the development of broader spectrum, enzyme-stable drugs such as *isepamicin*.[9,38] Isepamicin[38] and other newer aminoglycosides generally remain active against most pathogens and Gram-negative bacilli. Enhanced (synergistic or additive) activity can usually be achieved by combination therapy with broad-spectrum cell wall-active drugs (e.g. piperacillin, ceftazidime, cefotaxime, aztreonam, imipenem, etc.). Among the currently available aminoglycosides, amikacin and isepamicin have the widest spectrum of activity.[35]

*Spectinomycin* is an aminocyclitol that originated from *Streptomyces spectabilis*. It contains no aminosugar or glycosidic bond. Its mechanism of action is similar to that of the aminoglycosides, but its spectrum of activity is more narrow and it is also less active. Spectinomycin is most often used to treat sexually transmitted diseases in areas where resistance to the penicillins and tetracyclines remain high. Spectinomycin and its derivative *trospectomycin* are active against *Neisseria gonorrhoeae* at a single dose of 2g intramuscularly. *Ureaplasma urealyticum* and *Gardnerella vaginalis* are only marginally inhibited.

### *1.1.3 Tetracyclines*

The tetracyclines are biosynthetic broad-spectrum antimicrobial agents that have continued to generate developmental interest in the 1990s.[39] Their mechanism of action is via blockade of binding of t-RNA-amino acid complexes to the organism ribosome (30S subunit). This action is generally bacteriostatic, but these agents inhibit a wide variety of species including Gram-positive and Gram-negative bacteria, Chlamydia, Mycoplasmas and the rickettsiae.

Earlier compounds (tetracycline, chlortetracycline, oxytetracycline) were followed by improved second-generation agents such as doxycycline and minocycline. The latter possess greater spectra of activity and/or potency as

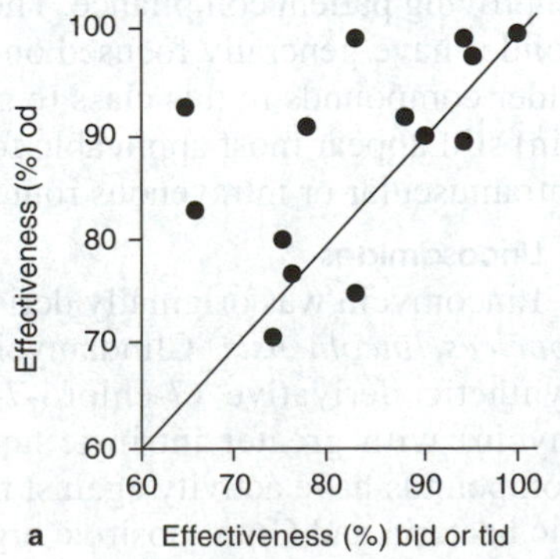


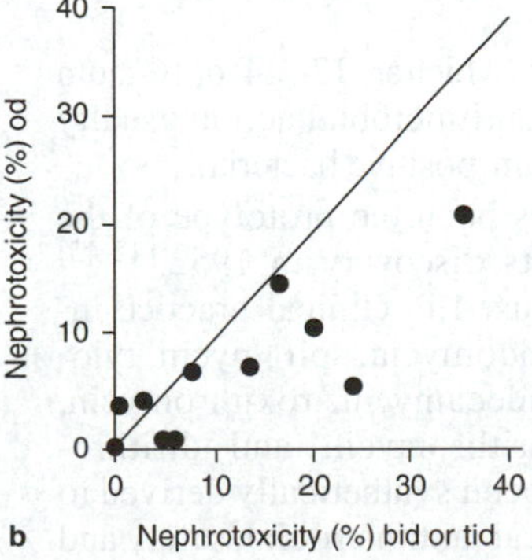


**Fig. 3.** Percentage effectiveness (a) and percentage nephrotoxicity (b) for once-daily (od) *versus* twice-daily (bid) or 3-times-daily (tid) administration of aminoglycosides in reported clinical trials (after Craig;[34] with permission). The diagonal lines indicate equivalent effectiveness and nephrotoxicity, respectively. While these trials have generally shown no statistically significant differences in effectiveness between the once-daily and multiple-daily dosage regimens, most studies favour once-daily administration in terms of the incidence of nephrotoxicity.

well as improved pharmacokinetic characteristics. They have a greater volume of distribution due to increased lipophilicity (minocycline partition coefficient 39 > doxycycline 0.63 > tetracycline 0.10). In addition, their bioavailabilities and elimination half-lives are also greater (half-lives >15 hours) allowing once- or twice-daily dosage regimens. Doxycycline and minocycline remain active against many tetracycline-resistant staphylococci and are also more effective against *Acinetobacter* spp. and some anaerobes. Doxycycline is effective against many isolates of vancomycin-resistant *Enterococcus* spp.

The most recent tetracycline derivatives are the glycylcyclines which are *N,N*-dimethylglycylamino-(DMG) modifications of 9-aminominocycline and oxytetracycline. These chemical changes broaden the spectrum of activity, especially against Gram-positive cocci resistant to contemporary antimicrobial agents, by overcoming nearly all known resistance mechanisms for this class.[40,41] However, some unexpected toxicity has been observed and further investigation of the glycylcyclines will await ongoing molecular modification.

#### *1.1.4 Macrolides, Lincosamides and Streptogramins*

##### Macrolides

The macrolides are part of a group of 4 macrocyclic antimicrobial agents comprising:

1) Macrolactams or ansomycins.

2) Polyenes (which exhibit antifungal activity; see section 6.1.1).

3) Macrocyclic lactams such as the avermectins (which exhibit potent antiparasitic activity).

4) True macrolides (which are 12-, 14- or 16-atom structures with an antimicrobial action usually directed against Gram-positive bacteria).

*Erythromycin* has been the prototype of the macrolides since its discovery in 1952.[42-45] Other compounds used in clinical practice include triacetyloleandomycin, spiramycin, tylosin, josamycin, midecamycin, roxithromycin, azithromycin, clarithromycin and dirithromycin. Most have been synthetically derived to improve the chemical, antimicrobial, safety and pharmacokinetic features of the basic erythromycin molecule.[44,46] These structures vary from 14 to 16 atoms (lactone ring) to which are attached (via glycosidic bonds) 1 or more sugars. The lactone ring can also be modified (with added hydroxyl or alkyl groups) to stabilise these structures to chemical alteration.

The antimicrobial spectra of the macrolides generally include Gram-positive cocci such as *Staphylococcus aureus*, coagulase-negative staphylococci, β-haemolytic streptococci, other *Streptococcus* spp. and some enterococci.[46] Additional activity has been documented against *H. influenzae*, some pathogenic *Neisseria* spp., *Bordetella* spp., *Corynebacterium* spp., *Chlamydia*, *Mycoplasma*, *Rickettsia* and *Legionella* spp. Many of these Gram-negative macrolide-susceptible species are considered cell-associated pathogens and macrolide drugs are generally concentrated (>5-fold) in phagocytic cells.[47]

*Azithromycin* (a 15-member macrolide or azilide) has more potent Gram-negative activity, a higher volume of distribution and a long tissue/serum half-life.[48,49] *Clarithromycin* (a 14-member macrolide) also has improved pharmacokinetic features (longer half-life and greater tissue penetration), and enhanced activity against *H. influenzae* and some cell-associated pathogens. The 14-hydroxy metabolite of clarithromycin is also very active against key pathogens (*H. influenzae*, *Legionella pneumophila*).[46,50]

*Roxithromycin* (also a 14-member macrolide) has activity comparable to that of erythromycin, and its pharmacokinetic characteristics (elevated serum concentrations) favour its application to some respiratory tract infections.[51]

All of these newer compounds appear to have tolerability and safety profiles equal or superior to that of erythromycin. Furthermore, they can be administered once or twice daily, potentially improving patient compliance. The newer macrolides have generally focused on oral use, but older compounds in this class (e.g. erythromycin) still appear most applicable for therapy by intramuscular or intravenous routes.

##### Lincosamides

Lincomycin was originally derived by *Streptomyces lincolnensis*. Clindamycin is a semisynthetic derivative (7-chloro-7-deoxylincomycin) with greater intrinsic activity. These compounds have activity against many anaerobic bacteria and Gram-positive organisms such as *Staphylococcus* spp. and streptococci (though not enterococci). They share certain biological properties with the macrolides and streptogramins (e.g. there is some degree of cross-resistance), depending on the species tested.[52,53]

A similar mechanism of action to that of the macrolides has been described, with binding to the 50S ribosome blocking protein synthesis. Lincomycin is administered orally as the hydrochloride, and clindamycin as the phosphate or palmitate. Their bioavailabilities are acceptable and both are hydrolysed *in vivo* to the active drug.

**Streptogramins**

The streptogramins are a large group of cyclic peptides naturally produced by some species of *Streptomyces*.[54] Each drug in the class is a combination of at least 2 unrelated molecules (group A and group B). These molecules are polyunsaturated macrolactones (group A) and cyclic hexadepsipeptides (group B), both capable of inhibiting protein synthesis by acting at the peptidyltransferase domain of the 50S ribosomal subunit, thus blocking 2 peptide chain elongation steps and interfering with the positioning of the peptidyl-tRNA. The streptogramin combinations are often synergistic and provide a wide spectrum of activity against Gram-positive organisms and some species of Gram-negative cocci and bacilli. The combinations also may reduce the likelihood of emerging resistance.

Included among the streptogramins are dalfopristin/quinupristin (derivatives of pristinamycin $I_A$ and $II_B$, respectively, which together comprise RP-59500), pristinamycin $I_A/II_A$ (produced by *Streptomyces pristinaespiralis*), and virginiamycin $S_1$ (produced by *Streptomyces virginiae*). Group B streptogramins share cross-resistance with plasmid-borne macrolide/lincosamide-resistant strains of Gram-positive cocci. The currently available agents are administered orally and are insoluble in water (i.e. incompatible with intravenous use) preventing therapy of serious hospital-associated infections.

The synergy of the group A and B streptogramin components expands the spectrum of activity of these compounds to include macrolide- or lincosamide-resistant staphylococci or streptococci, *Moraxella (Branhamella) catarrhalis*, *Listeria monocytogenes*, *B. fragilis*, *Clostridium* spp., *Legionella* spp., and some pathogenic *Neisseria* spp. Furthermore, their bacteriostatic action is enhanced to be rapidly bactericidal against many emerging resistant species, e.g. penicillin-resistant pneumococci, vancomycin-resistant *E. faecium*, and methicillin-resistant staphylococci. A postantibiotic effect (PAE) against staphylococci has been documented. Resistance to streptogramin combinations appears rare and currently limited to enzymes that destroy the individual components (streptogramin A acetylase and B hydrolase).[52,53]

Newer drugs of this class (dalfopristin/quinupristin) are intended for parenteral therapy of severe Gram-positive infections. Peak plasma concentrations of dalfopristin/quinupristin ranging from 0.95 to 24.2 mg/L are achieved after infusion of doses of 1.4 to 29.4 mg/kg. Oral pristinamycin achieves a concentration of 1.5 mg/L after a 2g dose,[54] but its activity against the more important Gram-positive species is 2- to 4-fold less than with the parenteral formulation. With these characteristics, this class may become more valuable in the therapy of infections due to organisms currently resistant to other classes of antimicrobial agents.

#### *1.1.5 Quinolones*

No single class of orally administered antimicrobial agents has had such a dramatic impact on infection chemotherapy as the quinolones (also known as 4-quinolones or fluoroquinolones).[55] Earlier members of this class included nalidixic acid (the prototypical compound), pipemidic acid, oxolinic acid, cinoxacin, flumequine, norfloxacin and others. All of these drugs had their primary role in the therapy of Gram-negative urinary tract infections. With the subsequent introduction of pefloxacin, enoxacin, ciprofloxacin,[56] ofloxacin,[57] sparfloxacin, lomefloxacin,[58] fleroxacin and others, the class enjoys a spectrum of activity allowing therapy of all types of community-acquired and many nosocomial infections. Furthermore, several compounds (e.g. ciprofloxacin, ofloxacin, pefloxacin) are available as parenteral formulations which facilitates their greater use in hospitals as monotherapy or in combinations with β-lactams and other parenteral agents.

The quinolones originally grew out of research on an alkaloid derivative with usable activity, i.e. nalidixic acid. The number of analogues synthesised now approaches 10,000, and a number of these drugs have established clinical effectiveness against a wide range of mild to severe infections. The compounds with 2 structural components (breakthrough radicals), a 7-piperazine ring and halogen (usually fluorine) substitutions, form the most commonly used group of quinolones. Among these, ciprofloxacin, ofloxacin and pefloxacin are the most versatile (i.e. they are available as oral and parenteral forms) and possess the broadest spectrum.

In general, the quinolones act by inhibiting DNA gyrase. They are useful against Enterobacteriaceae, *P. aeruginosa*, oxacillin-susceptible staphylococci, many enterococci, and some streptococci. Anaerobic organisms are resistant, but investigational quinolones (e.g. clinafloxacin, grepafloxacin, levofloxacin, DU-6859a, trovafloxacin) are active against *B. fragilis* and other anaerobes. Newer compounds may also have enhanced activity against streptococci (especially pneumococci), ciprofloxacin-resistant staphylococci, and some difficult to treat Gram-negative bacilli (e.g. *S. maltophilia*).

Modifications of the quinolone structure have also allowed therapy of mycobacteria infections, including drug-resistant tuberculosis and leprosy,[59] chronic prostatitis secondary to *Chlamydia* spp.,[60] traveller's diarrhoea caused by drug-resistant bacilli,[61] chronic cutaneous infections caused by mixed flora in diabetic patients,[62] and infections previously requiring long term parenteral chemotherapy.

Orally administered quinolones have reasonably long elimination half-lives and acceptable bioavailability. As examples, pharmacokinetic parameters for ciprofloxacin are: bioavailability 50 to 70%, half-life 3 to 4 hours, and peak serum concentrations 1.51 to 2.91 mg/L after a 500mg dose.[63] Ofloxacin values are 95 to 100%, 5 to 8 hours and 2 to 3 mg/L, respectively, following a 400mg dose[64] (see appendix A for pharmacokinetic data on other drugs). Differences between the quinolones exist in their tolerability profiles, potential for interactions with methylxanthines (e.g. theophylline), polyvalent metal ion antacids, anticholinergics, $H_2$-receptor antagonists, and their overall safety. One compound, temafloxacin, was recalled from clinical use worldwide after the discovery of fatal adverse events (haemolytic anaemia, hypoglycaemia, anaphylaxis, rhabdomyolysis and electrocardiographic abnormalities). These life-threatening adverse effects were not recognised until the drug had been used clinically in hundreds of thousands of patients.[65]

Emerging resistance to the quinolones has already compromised their therapeutic role.[55,66-68] Resistance continues to be discovered in most areas of the world, driven by escalating oral quinolone use. The species most rapidly emerging as resistant to ciprofloxacin or ofloxacin are: methicillin-resistant staphylococci, *P. aeruginosa*, *Acinetobacter* spp., *Serratia* spp., *Providencia* spp., *Proteus vulgaris*, enterococci and some streptococci.

#### 1.1.6 Sulfonamides and Dihydrofolate Reductase Inhibitors (Trimethoprim-like Compounds)

The sulfonamides are among the oldest antimicrobial drugs available for contemporary use.[69] They have diverse oral bioavailabilities, but generally similar spectra of activity. The drug most commonly prescribed is sulfamethoxazole, which is used either alone or in combination with trimethoprim-like compounds.

Dihydrofolate reductase inhibitors (e.g. trimethoprim) evolved from the synthesis of pyrimidine and purine analogues that were to be used as nucleic acid antagonists. Some were identified as inhibitors of folic acid utilisation in bacteria, thus providing broad antimicrobial activity.[70] Trimethoprim, tetroxoprim and brodimoprim are used clinically either alone or in combination with sulfonamides.

***Cotrimoxazole:*** the combination of trimethoprim with the pharmacokinetically similar sulfonamide sulfamethoxazole was said to have synergistic antimicrobial activity,[71] a characteristic challenged shortly after its clinical introduction.[72] Cotrimoxazole has been widely used to treat common community-acquired infections (acute otitis media, urinary tract infections, sinusitis, etc.) and some severe infections such as toxoplasmosis and *Pneumocystis carinii* pneumonia. However, the trimethoprim component exhibits the dominant activity against most pathogens (excluding *P. carinii*) whereas the sulfonamide appears to be responsible for most of the reported adverse effects.

Trimethoprim, brodimoprim and various sulfonamides can be used individually to maximise cost containment, improve clinical outcomes, and minimise adverse effects. Brodimoprim has some advantages over trimethoprim, in particular:

1) Activity against Gram-negative anaerobic bacteria.

2) A higher volume of distribution (due to its greater lipophilicity).

3) A longer half-life (permitting once-daily administration).

4) Possibly reduced teratogenic potential.

Sulfonamides and dihydrofolate reductase inhibitors continue to be valuable and well tolerated agents in the therapy of susceptible pathogens, especially those causing respiratory and urinary tract infections.[70]

#### *1.1.7 Rifampicin*

This ansamycin antimicrobial agent was originally derived from rifampicin B. It is active against Gram-positive species and has documented therapeutic activity against many mycobacteria, especially *Mycobacterium tuberculosis*. This activity has led to its widespread use in the treatment of tuberculosis and as combination therapy for other mycobacterial infections (see further section 5.1.5 and chapter 23; sect. 9.1.1). Resistance to rifampicin, although rare in most mycobacteria, does emerge in the treatment of other bacteria. This makes combination regimens preferable when using rifampicin against staphylococci, enterococci or selected streptococci. Rifampicin with various co-drugs has proved effective in treating staphylococcal endocarditis or osteomyelitis and infections associated with intravascular devices or foreign bodies (e.g. orthopaedic appliances). However, antagonism has been reported with some co-drugs and *in vitro* kill curve studies can be helpful in selecting appropriate therapeutic combinations.

Rifampicin acts by inhibiting DNA-derived RNA polymerase, thus suppressing RNA synthesis. Its elimination half-life is sufficient to allow twice-daily or once-daily administration for most infections. Newer rifampicin and rifamycin derivatives (e.g. rifaximin, rifabutin, rifapentine) have improved activity against some nontuberculosis mycobacteria, and some can be used as topical or nonabsorbable agents for selected cutaneous, vaginal and enteric (hepatic encephalopathy, diarrhoea, diverticulitis) infections or prophylaxis before gastrointestinal surgery.[73]

#### *1.1.8 Chloramphenicol*

This broad-spectrum antimicrobial agent originally derived from *Streptomyces venezuelae* is a small molecule containing a dichloracetyl group. The current production of this drug is synthetic and various derivatives (e.g. florfenicol, thiamphenicol) have been introduced into human and veterinary practice. Its spectrum of activity is truly broad, with inhibitory (usually bacteriostatic) activity against Gram-positive cocci, Gram-negative cocci and bacilli, anaerobic bacteria, *Mycoplasma* spp., *Chlamydia* spp. and rickettsiae. It acts via an effect on protein synthesis by inhibiting the formation of peptide bonds. Chloramphenicol can be administered by all routes, but the palmitate formulation is required for oral use to maximise its absorption and toleration of the bitter taste, while parenteral formulations mainly contain the succinate salt. These formulations are readily metabolised *in vivo* to active chloramphenicol, but further metabolism produces predominantly inactive forms that are then excreted in the urine. *In vitro* testing is usually performed with the free base.

Modified derivatives of chloramphenicol such as thiamphenicol and florfenicol are described as being less toxic. These drugs have generally been used in the treatment of meningitis (as a co-drug with ampicillin), enteric fever, anaerobic infections and some sexually transmitted diseases.

#### *1.1.9 Fusidic Acid*

Fusidic acid is a fusidane originally described in 1962 as being derived from a strain of *Fusidium coccineum*. Its structure is steroid-like and is related to cefalosporin P and to helvolic acid. The drug is highly protein bound (95 to 97%). Its mechanism of action is via inhibition bacterial protein synthesis by interference with elongation factor G (translocase). Fusidic acid has a predominantly bacteriostatic action and its spectrum of activity includes Gram-positive species such as *S. aureus*, coagulase-negative staphylococci, *Clostridium* spp. and some *Corynebacterium* spp. Marginal activity has also been described against streptococci, *Neisseria* spp., some *Bacteroides* spp., *Nocardia* spp. and *Legionella pneumophila*.[74]

Fusidic acid is well absorbed after oral administration, but patients may experience nausea. Due to its relatively long elimination half-life (10 to 16 hours), it results in high and sustained serum concentrations that increase (accumulation ratio 3.6) on oral or parenteral administration. Mutation rates of fusidic acid resistance are high. The drug is metabolised *in vivo* to a microbiologically inactive form before excretion or concentration in the bile; jaundice and abnormal liver function tests have been reported in 40.7% of patients.[74] Combination therapy is recommended to treat strains of Gram-positive cocci resistant to other drug classes (e.g. β-lactams, glycopeptides, macrolides, tetracyclines, sulfonamides), and to treat methicillin-resistant staphylococci and multiresistant pneumococci. The effects of these combinations are usually additive or negligible but synergy is uncommon; combination therapy does not prevent emergence of fusidic acid-resistant strains.

#### *1.1.10 Glycopeptides*

This unique class of antimicrobial agents comprises soluble peptides of high molecular weight such as teicoplanin and vancomycin. The latter is the prototype drug for this class and was introduced in 1956 to treat serious Gram-positive infections. Initial toxicity and other adverse reactions (some secondary to formulation impurities) relegated vancomycin to a backup role until methicillin-resistant staphylococcal infections became highly prevalent in the early 1980s. Vancomycin is derived from *Streptomyces orientales* and exhibits activity against *Staphylococcus* spp., streptococci, *Enterococcus* spp., *Corynebacterium* spp. (including *Corynebacterium jeikeium*), *L. monocytogenes*, Gram-positive anaerobes (including *Clostridium difficile*), *Bacillus* spp., Actinomyces, some pathogenic *Neisseria* spp. and *Flavobacterium meningosepticum*. Its bactericidal activity is lower against enterococci and some isolates of this species, and against *Leuconostoc* and *Pediococcus* spp. Many lactobacilli are resistant to vancomycin and to other glycopeptides.

The glycopeptides act by inhibiting cell wall synthesis by preventing peptidoglycan formation through complexing at the D-alanyl-D-alanine terminus. A secondary action has been documented against protoplasts (via altered permeability) and by direct inhibition of RNA synthesis.

The adverse effects of vancomycin persist in the modern era of highly purified formulations. The 'red man' syndrome (see further section 8.10), oto- and nephrotoxicity, and local infusion site irritations are among the most commonly reported adverse effects. Some toxicity can be minimised by monitoring of serum concentrations and through the use of long infusion times (>60 minutes).

*Teicoplanin* and *daptomycin* (LY 146032) are newer compounds in this class, the latter being withdrawn from clinical trials due to serious toxicity. Teicoplanin is a mixture of 5 related compounds produced by *Actinoplanes teichomyceticus*, each with antimicrobial activity.[75,76] Its mechanism of action is similar to that of vancomycin and its spectrum of activity is also clinically similar. The most important differences are that vancomycin can be more active against some isolates of coagulase-negative staphylococci (*Staphylococcus haemolyticus*, *Staphylococcus epidermidis*) while teicoplanin is generally more active by weight and can be more active against some enterococci (*Van B* genotype). The tolerability and safety of teicoplanin are superior to that of vancomycin and it can be given intramuscularly. 'Red man' syndrome has not been reported with teicoplanin. Clinical success with appropriate dosages appears comparable to that with vancomycin when treating susceptible strains. Great care must be taken when treating serious Gram-positive infections such as endocarditis, to achieve adequate trough concentrations (at least 20 mg/L). A long elimination half-life (terminal phase 20 to 114 hours) allows once-daily intravenous administration following twice-daily loading doses.

Other compounds in this class (e.g. LY 333328; ramoplanin) are undergoing *in vitro* study in an effort to find drugs that will be effective against the emerging vancomycin- and teicoplanin-resistant Gram-positive cocci.

#### *1.1.11 Other Drugs*

Several other classes of antimicrobial agents are currently in use to treat significant infections or are under investigation. Examples include nitrofurantoin, fosfomycin, nitroimidazoles, and the newer oxazolidinones.

##### Nitrofurantoin

Nitrofurantoin has been used clinically to treat urinary tract infections since 1953. Serum concentrations allowing for therapy of systemic infections cannot be achieved with safe doses of nitrofurantoin, which has a half-life of 0.3 hours. This compound is a synthetic nitrofuran which acts against various enzymes produced by bacteria. Specific action sites on these enzymes have not been determined after more than 4 decades of use. Additional effects include immobilisation of human sperm and the arrest of spermatogenesis in various animal species. Its spectrum of activity (MICs up to 32 mg/L) includes most Enterobacteriaceae (not *Proteus* spp. or *Serratia marcescens*), staphylococci, *E. faecalis*, some pathogenic *Neisseria* spp., streptococci and corynebacteria. Nitrofurantoin concentrates in the urine (200 mg/L) via glomerular filtration, tubular secretion and reabsorption, and is more active at an alkaline pH. Toxicity (peripheral neuropathy, nausea, vomiting, allergic or immunological reactions such as pulmonary eosinophilia or infiltrates, cholestatic jaundice, etc.) is generally mild and reversible after withdrawal of the drug. The most commonly used formulation is the macrocrystalline form which provides an even and delayed absorption from the gastrointestinal tract, minimising concentration-related adverse effects.

#### Fosfomycin

Fosfomycin (phosphomycin) is L-(cis)-1,2-epoxypropylphosphonic acid produced by *S. fradiae*.[77] This drug acts by decreasing peptidoglycan synthesis via inhibition of a key transferase. Its activity is directed against many enteric bacilli and staphylococci, including methicillin-resistant *S. aureus* [MIC against 90% of strains ($MIC_{90}$) 4 to 8 mg/L]. Remarkable synergy has been reported against Gram-positive and Gram-negative (*P. aeruginosa*) pathogens when fosfomycin is combined with selected broad-spectrum β-lactams (e.g. cefotaxime, piperacillin, cefoperazone, cefsulodin). The addition of an aminoglycoside further enhances killing. However, resistance to fosfomycin emerges rapidly, making combination regimens advisable for moderate to severe infections.

Plasmid-mediated resistance (causing enzyme modification of the drug) has become prevalent in some geographic areas of high usage.[78] Recently, high single-dose fosfomycin therapy of urinary tract infections has achieved some clinical success.

#### Nitroimidazoles

The nitroimidazoles include several clinically effective drugs (e.g. metronidazole, benznidazole, misonidazole, nimorazole, ornidazole, tinidazole), among which metronidazole has become the most widely used compound. It was first used to treat *Trichomonas vaginalis* infection and subsequently for other parasitic diseases, amoebiasis and giardiasis. Subsequently, its activity against anaerobic bacteria was appreciated and metronidazole has become first-line therapy for severe infections caused by *Bacteroides* spp. and other anaerobes. The drug is highly bioavailable after oral and parenteral administration, is widely distributed in tissues, including the central nervous system, and metabolised *in vivo* to several forms, one of which (hydroxymetronidazole) has more potent antibacterial activity (by 2- to 10-fold) than the parent drug. The mechanism of action of metronidazole is not well characterised, but anaerobic conditions are required for maximal effects. A key component to its activity is the reduction of the nitro group that makes the imidazole a preferred electron acceptor (forming toxic intermediates and free radicals) which increases within pathogens by gradient diffusion.

The nitroimidazole drugs generally have long elimination half-lives (metronidazole 6 to 10 hours, ornidazole 14 hours, tinidazole 13 hours) and are primarily eliminated by hepatic metabolism. Initially, the recommended dose of metronidazole was 500mg every 6 hours, but contemporary practice dictates 500 to 750mg doses given once or twice daily. After intravenous administration, these regimens produce peak plasma concentrations of 4 to 20 mg/L[79] which greatly exceed MIC values of susceptible species. Interactions with other drugs (warfarin, phenytoin, lithium, rifampicin, etc.) and alcohol may be significant and cause severe adverse reactions. Metronidazole is generally well tolerated and remains a valuable drug in the treatment of anaerobic infections, infections due to susceptible parasites, and *C. difficile*-related pseudomembranous enterocolitis.

#### Oxazolidinones

The oxazolidinones are relatively new chemical entities first described in 1988. Recently, the chemical modification of previously toxic oxazolidinone structures[80] led to several compounds (e.g. U-100592, U-100766) active (MIC values up to 2 mg/L) against all Gram-positive cocci, especially those resistant to methicillin, glycopeptides, macrolides, tetracyclines, aminoglycosides, quinolones and sulfonamides. Their mechanism of action appears to be directed toward protein synthesis inhibition at the step preceding the interaction of fMet-tRNA and the 30S ribosome subunit with the initiator codon. They are bacteriostatic or slowly bactericidal [requiring at least 24 hours for at least 3 $log_{10}$ colony-forming units (CFU) killing]. Infection model results are promising, but human clinical trials are pending.

### 1.2 Routes of Administration

Antimicrobial agents may be administered systemically by enteral (oral, rectal) or parenteral (intravenous, intramuscular, intrathecal) routes, or applied locally to a specific site of infection. The route of administration of an antimicrobial agent depends on the properties of the agent (e.g. bioavailability, toxicity), type and severity of infection, and practical issues of access to and patient compliance with the specific routes (table VII). For many agents, formu-

**Table VII.** Routes of administration of commonly used antimicrobial drugs

| Intravenous only | Intravenous or intramuscular | Intramuscular only | Oral or parenteral | Usually oral only |
|---|---|---|---|---|
| Amphotericin B | Aminoglycosides | Spectinomycin | Amoxicillin | Azithromycin |
| Cefalothin | Aztreonam | | Amoxicillin/ clavulanic acid | Cefaclor |
| Imipenem/cilastatin | Benzylpenicillin (penicillin G) | | Ampicillin | Cefetamet |
| Miconazole | Carboxypenicillins[b] | | Cefradine | Cefixime |
| Ticarcillin/clavulanic acid | Most newer cefalosporins | | Chloramphenicol | Cefpodoxime proxetil |
| Vancomycin[a] | Teicoplanin | | Ciprofloxacin | Cefprozil |
| | Ureidopenicillins[c] | | Clindamycin | Ceftibuten |
| | | | Cotrimoxazole (trimethoprim/ sulfamethoxazole)[d] | Cefadroxil |
| | | | Erythromycin | Cefalexin |
| | | | Fusidic acid | Cinoxacin |
| | | | Mecillinam | Clarithromycin |
| | | | Metronidazole | Griseofulvin |
| | | | Ofloxacin | Itraconazole |
| | | | Rifampicin | Ketoconazole |
| | | | Sulfadimidine | Loracarbef |
| | | | Sulfadiazine | Most sulfonamides |
| | | | Trimethoprim | Naladixic acid |
| | | | | Nitrofurantoin |
| | | | | Norfloxacin |
| | | | | Phenoxymethylpenicillin (penicillin V) |
| | | | | Tetracyclines |

a Vancomycin is also given orally in the treatment of antibiotic-associated pseudomembranous colitis.
b Includes carbenicillin and ticarcillin.
c Includes mezlocillin, azlocillin and piperacillin.
d Special precautions necessary with intravenous administration.

lations permitting more than one route of administration are available and switching from one route (e.g. parenteral) to a more convenient and less expensive route (e.g. oral) during a course of therapy is an area of continuing interest.[81]

### *1.2.1 Intravenous Administration*

Intravenous administration is the primary route for parenteral administration of antimicrobial agents. The ability to establish and maintain peripheral or central venous access for administration permits maximum bioavailability (with the exception of chloramphenicol; see further section 1.2.3) without patient discomfort resulting from repeated skin puncture, while being convenient for healthcare providers. However, the maintenance of venous access for antimicrobial drug administration is not without risk of device-related infection and preparations for parenteral administration are generally more expensive than orally administered drugs, as well as involving greater labour costs.

It has been accepted practice for decades that a patient with a presenting illness necessitating intravenous therapy should receive a full course of parenteral antimicrobial therapy. With increasing pressure to reduce therapeutic costs, this concept is being re-evaluated and there is evidence that in many circumstances early switching to a less expensive (orally active) antimicrobial of a related class or with a similar spectrum of activity may be equally efficacious[81] (see also chapter 10; sect 6.2.5). As an additional measure to reduce overall costs, parenteral therapy, when necessary, is increasingly administered outside of the hospital setting.

Venous access permits administration of the relatively large volumes of fluid (50 to 500ml) used to administer many agents, including certain broad-spectrum penicillins and vancomycin.[82] These volumes may be required to solubilise relatively large doses of antimicrobials, e.g. the 2 to 4g doses of piperacillin commonly used. Relatively large volumes of fluid also facilitate controlled infusion and/or adequate dilution of acidic substances such as vancomycin hydrochloride.

The controlled administration of vancomycin is clearly important in reducing the risk of 'red man' syndrome. Likewise, amphotericin B, which has a central role in therapy of fungal infection, is an extremely toxic agent. Rapid administration is associated with fever and rigors, but these problems can be substantially reduced by administration of an infusion over 6 hours.

Controlled rates of intravenous administration are also of increasing importance as our understanding of the pharmacodynamics of antimicrobial therapy improves (see section 1.1 above). An established approach to therapy of Gram-negative septicaemia is the use of a combination of an aminoglycoside and a β-lactam agent such as an extended-spectrum cefalosporin (e.g. cefotaxime, ceftazidime) or a ureidopenicillin (e.g. mezlocillin, piperacillin). The concentration-dependent killing characteristics of the aminoglycosides support once-daily bolus or short (up to 30 minutes) intravenous infusions via maximal drug concentrations. Conversely, β-lactam agents reach maximal bactericidal activity at serum concentrations that do not greatly exceed the MIC and which can be reached with lower total daily doses administered by continuous intravenous infusion.[3,83]

When administering multiple agents (e.g. intravenous solutions, antimicrobials, other drugs) through a single intravenous line, it is critical to determine the compatibility of the agents. The only safe course is to assume that agents are incompatible unless clear data to the contrary are available from the product manufacturers or the hospital pharmacy. In addition, it is essential to ensure that agents administered by infusion are stable throughout the duration of infusion. A notable example is the need to protect amphotericin B from light exposure (degradation) during infusion.

#### *1.2.2 Intramuscular Administration*

The intramuscular route remains appropriate for single-dose or intermittent administration of an antimicrobial agent. The most commonly used site is the upper outer quadrant of the buttock, but any large muscle mass can be used. A hazard of buttock intramuscular injection is injury to the sciatic nerve; use of the upper outer quadrant is therefore essential to avoid this complication. In very obese patients, it may be difficult to ensure that the injection is administered into the vasculature-rich muscle and not into fat, where the rate of absorption is likely to be reduced.

Intramuscular injection can be painful, particularly if repeated administration is required. Absorption from the site of intramuscular injection is generally gradual, and dependent on blood flow to the site and on the formulation of the agent injected. Intramuscular administration in patients in shock is likely to result in markedly delayed absorption. In some cases (e.g. procaine penicillin) the drug is formulated to result in slow absorption enabling sustained concentrations of the drug.

An advantage of intramuscular injection is that it is robust in the sense that relatively little training is required and that no indwelling device is placed in the patient. It has a particular role in single-dose therapy of gonococcal infection (e.g. intramuscular third-generation cefalosporins) where follow-up may be problematical and compliance with multidose oral regimens is uncertain. It may also be useful (though perhaps not optimal) for parenteral therapy in emergencies and other circumstances where establishment and maintenance of intravenous access is not immediately practical.

While many antimicrobials for intravenous administration may also be administered by intramuscular injection (e.g. penicillin, some cefalosporins, aminoglycosides), this should never be assumed. For example, vancomycin is too acidic for intramuscular injection, intramuscular cefalothin is often painful compared with cefazolin, and the intramuscular route is not recommended for most quinolones.

#### *1.2.3 Oral and Rectal Administration*

The oral route is the most widely used and convenient method for administration of antimicrobial drugs. However, for metronidazole in particular, excellent blood concentrations can also be achieved following rectal administration. Oral (and rectal) preparations of antimicrobial agents are generally less expensive than corresponding parenteral formulations of the same drug or class, and are suitable for use in both hospital and community (clinic) settings.

Oral administration is not, however, without limitations. Even for drugs with excellent bioavailability after oral delivery, consideration should be given to the functional status of the individual patient's gastrointestinal tract. Conditions associated with vomiting, delayed gastric emptying, abnormal gastric acidity or dysfunction of the small intestine may result in inadequate absorption and poor serum concentrations of the antimicrobial drug.

For many antimicrobial drugs, bioavailability after oral administration is limited. Large polar molecules such as vancomycin, amphotericin B and aminoglycosides are not absorbed to a significant degree and oral administration of these agents is suitable only for luminal therapy of gastrointestinal infection. For many agents that are regularly administered by the oral route, bioavailability is only of the order of 20 to 30%; examples include phenoxymethylpenicillin and ampicillin. Such limited bioavailability has 2 potentially negative consequences:

1) Large doses may be needed to achieve adequate therapeutic blood concentrations.

2) Residual unabsorbed drug may alter the gastrointestinal flora, resulting in diarrhoea and the selection of antimicrobial-resistant strains.

Because of these adverse consequences, where agents of similar activity spectrum and cost are available, care should be taken to select drugs with optimal bioavailability. As an example, absorption of amoxicillin is 2- to 4-fold greater than that of ampicillin, making amoxicillin the preferred form for oral administration of an aminopenicillin.[84]

A similar and serious factor that complicates use of the oral route is unpredictable bioavailability. Itraconazole is an important, relatively new antifungal agent that can be administered only by the oral route. Bioavailability is extremely variable from patient to patient and depends critically on low gastric pH. Certain diseases such as the acquired immune deficiency syndrome (AIDS) or medications that reduce gastric acidity may result in a marked reduction in itraconazole blood concentrations. A similar degree of individual variability in absorption has been noted for some antimycobacterial agents in patients with AIDS. For such agents, measurement of blood concentrations may be warranted, particularly when there is a failure to respond to therapy.

Conversely, low gastric pH may result in inactivation of other antimicrobial agents, including methicillin and erythromycin base. In many cases this problem has been overcome by chemical modification of the molecule (e.g. nafcillin, cloxacillin and dicloxacillin are acid-stable penicillinase-resistant penicillins) or by formulations of the drug in a coating that protects the drug from gastric acidity (erythromycin).

Ingestion of food can affect bioavailability adversely after oral administration. Examples include phenoxymethylpenicillin, ampicillin and erythromycin, which are frequently dispensed with patient instructions to take the medication at specific intervals before meals. Clinicians should consider how realistic it is to anticipate proper compliance with such recommendations. For some antimicrobial classes, alternative agents that have overcome these problems may be available (amoxicillin, clarithromycin), although in some cases at a very substantial increase in cost.

Despite the problems posed by oral administration of many agents, oral therapy has distinct advantages for some antimicrobials. Chloramphenicol is unique in that blood concentrations after oral administration are higher than those achieved after intravenous administration. Chloramphenicol is administered by the oral route as crystalline chloramphenicol or as chloramphenicol palmitate. The latter is hydrolysed in the gastrointestinal tract to free chloramphenicol which is absorbed. The form of chloramphenicol for parenteral administration is chloramphenicol succinate. The latter is hydrolysed in the tissues; however, concentrations of free chloramphenicol are generally lower than those achieved following oral administration.[85]

The bioavailability of fusidic acid after oral administration approaches 90% for some formulations and is well tolerated, but parenteral administration should be by slow intravenous infusion because of the risk of venospasm and thrombosis. Thus, for both these agents, the oral route is generally preferred.

#### *1.2.4 Intrathecal Administration*

Intrathecal administration of antimicrobials is not commonly performed or recommended. When used, the basis for this approach is to bypass the blood-brain barrier, which markedly impedes diffusion of hydrophilic or large antimicrobial molecules from the plasma to the cerebral spinal fluid (CSF). Access of many agents to the CSF is improved during meningeal inflammation, but at best, CSF concentrations of many β-lactams may not exceed 10% of the simultaneously sampled (unbound) plasma concentration. The CSF concentration of penicillin is low because it is almost completely ionised and has a low lipid/water partition coefficient at physiological pH. In addition, the choroid plexus actively excretes penicillin which does enter the CSF. Benzylpenicillin is approximately 50% protein bound, and the concentration of benzylpenicillin in the CSF with intact meninges is of the order of 1% of the total serum concentration.

There is limited clinical experience for drugs administered by the intrathecal route and the hazards may be substantial. The emergence of penicillin- and extended-spectrum cefalosporin-resistant pneumococci may, however, compel clinicians to reconsider this route of administration to achieve effective concentrations of alternative drugs (e.g. glycopeptides) in the CSF.

#### *1.2.5 Topical Administration*

For specific types of localised infection or colonisation, direct application of antimicrobial agents to the site of infection may be effective. Local application of antimicrobials is no longer limited to topical application of antimicrobial or antiseptic creams to skin lesions, but is also important for treatment of vaginal infections (see chapter 18; sect. 13.1), infections of the external auditory meatus (see chapter 14; sect. 3.1), prophylaxis and therapy of chronic pulmonary infections (e.g. aerosolised aminoglycosides or pentamidine) [see chapter 23; sect. 8.1.1 and 10.1), and subconjunctival or intraocular administration (see chapter 15; sect. 3). Local application generally achieves high concentrations at the site of infection with minimal systemic absorption. In this way, it is possible to use antimicrobials that are too toxic for systemic use. A contemporary example is the use of mupirocin for eradication of nasal colonisation with oxacillin-resistant *S. aureus*.

In addition to limiting toxicity by reducing systemic absorption, local application may also reduce the costs of therapy and may result in high local concentrations. It is important to understand that the high local concentrations of antimicrobial agents achieved with topical application make it difficult to apply standard laboratory susceptibility test results to topical therapy in a meaningful way. The categorisation of bacteria as susceptible or resistant to a given antimicrobial is based on an established correlation between *in vitro* MIC results and the clinical response to systemic therapy with that antimicrobial in a large group of patients. Other factors taken into account are the pharmacokinetics of the antimicrobial agent when administered systemically. Clinical correlations between MIC results and topical therapy are not usually available and the local concentration of the antimicrobial is often much higher than can be achieved safely by systemic administration. It is possible therefore that organisms categorised as resistant for the purposes of systemic therapy may be treatable by topical application of the same agent, although an agent to which the infecting organism is fully susceptible should be chosen whenever possible.

Problems associated with local application include the potential for patient sensitisation to antimicrobials and the emergence of resistant organisms. For these reasons, topical application of β-lactams has been avoided and many clinicians prefer to confine the use of antimicrobials for topical therapy to those that are neither suitable or widely used for systemic disease (e.g. bacitracin, polymixin B). In addition, locally applied antimicrobials can be absorbed systemically and may accumulate to toxic concentrations in some circumstances. Application of antimicrobials to extensive areas of denuded skin or to the respiratory tract by aerosolisation may result in significant systemic absorption. This is particularly important where renal impairment or other factors may permit rapid accumulation of the agents to toxic concentrations.

## 2. Bacteriological Considerations

### 2.1 Diagnosis

Regardless of the clinical condition of the patient, rational antimicrobial therapy should be based on a presumptive diagnosis. Although immediate treatment may seem essential in a seriously ill febrile patient, administration of antimicrobial agents should ideally be delayed until appropriate diagnostic specimens are obtained. The patient may present with clinical signs of pneumonia, sepsis or meningitis; however, the clinical diagnosis alone may not be sufficient to enable the correct treatment to be chosen. Each of these conditions can have several different microbial causes and usually no single drug is effective against them all. A microbiological diagnosis is essential in these potentially life-threatening infections or when prolonged therapy may be required.

In the early stages of infection (from zero to 72 hours), the patient may be clinically unstable and the clinician is frequently uncertain as to the causative organism or even the site of infection. Under these circumstances, empirical therapy may be warranted and may include combination therapy with a β-lactam and an aminoglycoside or monotherapy with an expanded-spectrum cefalosporin.[86,87] Although such an approach may be successful, it would be an advance if clinicians were trained to also think microbiologically and to have, rather than a disease, a specific causative agent in mind when selecting therapy. Such an approach would allow the prescriber to begin therapy based on the susceptibility patterns of the locale or hospital unit. Later in the course of the infection, the treatment regimen may be simplified based on the susceptibility profile of the documented causative organism(s). Thus, combination therapy may be changed to monotherapy or a broad-spectrum agent may be changed to a narrower spectrum agent. Ideally, therapy should be consolidated to encompass the least costly, least toxic, yet effective alternative.

### 2.2 The Contribution of the Laboratory

Rational treatment of infectious diseases depends heavily on the clinical microbiology laboratory, to rapidly isolate and identify the causative agent and report susceptibility results for available antimicrobial agents. Although the performance of the laboratory in this regard is frequently taken for granted, there are several stages at which it can fail.

Proper collection of appropriate clinical specimens and prompt delivery to the laboratory, are essential in ensuring a timely and accurate microbiological diagnosis. Once delivered to the laboratory, the specimen must be examined and processed, preferably by experienced personnel, using laboratory procedures that are controlled and standardised in accordance with national or international guidelines. These efforts are aided by the provision of clinical information including pertinent exposures, clinical signs and symptoms, prior use of antibiotics, and suspected causative agents. Clinical judgement should always be used when interpreting laboratory findings, particularly when they appear to conflict with the available clinical evidence. When in doubt, specialist advice should be sought to aid interpretation of results of microbiological examinations.

Prompt identification of antimicrobial resistance depends on the proper selection, execution and interpretation of antimicrobial susceptibility tests. In the US, antimicrobial susceptibility testing procedures should be standardised in accordance with National Committee for Clinical Laboratory Standards (NCCLS) guidelines because of rigid regulatory controls. If standardised testing methods are employed, errors should be infrequent.

The antimicrobial susceptibility test panel should include agents relevant to the clinical needs of the medical staff, the patient population under consideration, and local resistance patterns. In general, the profile of susceptibility of an organism to a number of agents should be ascertained, since there is no guarantee that the infecting organism(s) will be susceptible to the first or alternative agents chosen. In some institutions, selective reporting of antibiotic susceptibilities is used as a means of controlling costs and influencing appropriate selection of antimicrobial agents.

As a rule, the more rapidly that antimicrobial susceptibility testing data can be provided, the less that empirical multidrug therapy should be required. Laboratory efforts to aid the selection of less costly but effective antimicrobial therapy have obvious benefits for both the individual patient as well as the institution as a whole.

### 2.3 Bacterial Resistance

Numerous mechanisms of bacterial resistance have emerged with some being responsible for growing public health threats worldwide.[4,5,88] The most common mechanisms of resistance are:

1) Enzymatic inactivation of the antimicrobial agents.

2) Impermeability of the bacterial membrane to the drug.

3) Altered target sites.

4) Altered target bacterial enzymes.

5) Increased production of the target enzymes.

6) Auxotrophs that could bypass the lethal or altered position in bacterial metabolism.

7) Efflux transport of antimicrobials to the outside of the organism (table VIII).

Some antimicrobials are affected by multiple mechanisms of resistance (e.g. β-lactams) and others by only one principal or known target (e.g. glycopeptides). Bacterial species may be intrinsically resistant to some drugs because of membrane barriers to drug access, naturally occurring enzymes, lack of target sites or very low affinity of the drug for the native targets of the species. Other organisms acquire new or novel genetic elements that allow them to escape the inhibitory or lethal effects of the antimicrobial agent.

In the past 50 years, the number of patient populations compromised by resistance to antimicrobial agents has increased in concert with escalated antimicrobial use, thus disturbing the human-microbial ecosystem toward greater genetic resistance.[4,5,89] The most important recent threats to infection chemotherapy[89,90] are:

a) Altered target sites among staphylococci (oxacillin resistance), *S. pneumoniae* (penicillin

**Table VIII.** Most frequent occurrences of various mechanisms of resistance among antimicrobial classes

| Antimicrobial agents | Mechanism of resistance | | | | | | |
|---|---|---|---|---|---|---|---|
| | enzyme activation | membrane permeability | altered target site | altered target enzyme | increased target enzyme | auxotrophic bypass | efflux |
| Aminoglycosides | ++ | + | ++ | − | − | − | − |
| β-Lactams | ++ | + | − | + | − | − | − |
| Chloramphenicol | ++ | + | + | − | − | − | + |
| Glycopeptides | − | − | ++ | − | − | − | − |
| Macrolides/ lincosamides | ++ | − | + | − | − | − | (+) |
| Rifampicin | − | − | − | ++ | − | − | − |
| Quinolones | − | + | − | ++ | − | − | + |
| Sulfonamides[a] | − | + | − | + | ++ | ++ | − |
| Tetracyclines | − | + | + | − | − | − | ++ |

a Includes trimethoprim-like dihydrofolate reductase inhibitors.

resistance)[91] and enterococci (ampicillin and vancomycin resistance).[92,93]

b) Inactivating enzymes among Enterobacteriaceae (extended-spectrum β-lactamases)[94-97] and other Gram-negative bacilli (aminoglycoside inactivating enzymes, with multiple types in one organism).[38]

c) Altered affinity enzyme targets responsible for quinolone resistance.[66] Resistance in related organisms, such as *M. tuberculosis*[98,99] and *Mycobacterium avium-intracellulare*, has also increased, although the recent rise in frequency of tuberculosis in developed nations seems to have been controlled (US CDC 1995 statistics).

The continued effectiveness of antimicrobial agents has always been compromised by their use or abuse. *The development of resistance is a natural consequence of advancing infection chemotherapy and can only be delayed or slowed by prudent use of the individual agents.* When resistance to a drug emerges, it becomes dependent on direct antimicrobial use pressure within a patient, ward, hospital, region or nation, or on spontaneously occurring genetic events within the rapidly growing bacterial world.

Excellent examples of each of these events have been documented since the beginning of the antimicrobial era in the 1930s and 1940s. Use-related evolution of resistance has been exemplified by the decades of β-lactam (penicillins and cefalosporins) selection leading to penicillin nonsusceptible pneumococci (<1% resistance in 1970 to >25% in 1995)[91,100] and the use of ceftazidime in some medical centres promoting the increased appearance of third-generation cefalosporin-resistant *Enterobacter* and *Citrobacter freundii* strains.[96] Spontaneous and rapid genetic events can be characterised by the β-lactamases derived from *E. coli* and other enteric bacilli that were transmitted to *H. influenzae* and *N. gonorrhoeae*. The rates of enzyme-producing penicillin-resistant isolates have steadily increased in most countries. This increase has resulted in the need to alter routine therapy of pathogens to β-lactamase-resistant agents such as third-generation cefalosporins or potent non-β-lactam drugs (quinolones, macrolides, etc.).

Resistance among some species has stabilised to a baseline level that can vary by geographical area. This phenomenon is influenced by numerous factors including:

- Drug use patterns
- Population (patient and organism) demographics
- Socioeconomic considerations
- Public health and sanitation quality
- Hospital practices of infection control and epidemiology
- Travel or passage of flora within or between populations
- The ability of clinicians and laboratories to recognise the emergence of drug-resistant strains.

Although resistance to antimicrobial agents has dramatically increased in the past 10 years, numerous drugs remain clinically active and the pharmaceutical industry continues to search for new and structurally novel agents to address the diminished utility of some antimicrobial classes via bacterial target site alteration. Furthermore, alternative or adjunctive vaccine prophylaxis will take on a greater role in infection chemotherapy, as exemplified by the success of *H. influenzae* serotype B and meningococcal vaccines.[88,101,102] Continued research, education and resistance surveillance appear to be key elements in the control of antimicrobial resistance in the future.[88]

### *2.3.1 Genetics of Antimicrobial Resistance*

Although the spontaneous rates of mutations to resistance have been low ($10^{-7}$ to $10^{-11}$), resistance by this genetic mechanism has occurred at an alarming speed as new antimicrobial agents have been introduced. In fact, the discovery of a penicillinase capable of destroying penicillin was observed before the actual introduction of penicillins into clinical use. Therefore, bacterial adjustments via genetic processes have been in place well before the antimicrobial era. As the genetic mechanism becomes established within a species or bacterial family, modifications by point mutations become easier or more frequent, particularly in response to existing drug-use pressures.

Mutations from existing plasmid or chromosomal genes are best demonstrated by the Enterobacteriaceae. Here, single amino acid changes in the coding gene for a plasmid-mediated enzyme can markedly alter substrate (penicillin or cefalosporin) specificity (tables IX and X). These β-lactamases have been classified into group 2b, and those capable of hydrolysing third-generation cefalosporins (extended-spectrum β-lactamases; ESβL) are designated 2b' or 2be.[94,97,103,104] Table X lists several mutations leading to greater resistance to newer cefalosporins, each group 2be enzyme derived from parent enzymes such as TEM-1, TEM-2 or SHV-1. The latter parent β-lactamases were incapable of significantly altering recently released β-lactam compounds such as cefotaxime or ceftazidime.[94,103,104]

Other mutations, generally in chromosomal-based genes, create overexpression of the enzyme secondary to alteration in regulatory or promoter genes (Bush group 1 enzymes). This hyperproduction of β-lactamases among some enteric bacilli also results in resistance to extended-spectrum cefalosporins and most penicillins. These enzymes are not inhibited by clinical β-lactamase inhibitors (clavulanic acid or sulfones).

Not uncommonly, resistance mechanisms can be observed in combination within a single strain (e.g. enzymatic drug interactivation, altered PBP targets) and diminished drug uptake by the bacterial cell. In contrast to the β-lactamases, the aminoglycoside inactivating enzymes (mediated by more than 30 genes) rarely undergo mutation, but unique genes are produced in response to the clinical pressure of new drug use. Efficient bifunctional aminoglycoside-modifying enzymes are produced by a fused gene that codes for an acetyltransferase and a phosphotransferase. This gene is widely distributed among Gram-positive species (enterococci and staphylococci) and some Gram-negative bacilli. Genetic codes for other enzymes capable of destroying antimicrobial agents have also been described: chloramphenicol acetyltransferases (CAT) producing resistance to chloramphenicol and closely related structural entities (e.g. fusidic acid); glutathione-*S*-transferase mediated resistance to fosfomycin; and *O*-phos-

**Table IX.** β-Lactamase classification (after Bush[94,103,104])

| Enzyme group | Preferred β-lactam substrate: penicillins | Preferred β-lactam substrate: cefalosporins | Inhibited by clavulanic acid (10 μmol/L) | Enzyme examples |
|---|---|---|---|---|
| 1 | | ✓ | No | Chromosomal β-lactamases of Gram-negative bacteria (Enterobacters, Citrobacters, etc.) |
| 2a | ✓ | | Yes | Gram-positive penicillins (*Staphylococcus* spp.) |
| 2b | ✓ | ✓ | Yes | TEM-1 and -2, SHV-1 (*Escherichia coli*) |
| 2b'(2be) | ✓ | ✓ | Yes | TEM-3 to TEM-12, SHV-2 to SHV-5, chromosomal K1 (*E. coli, Klebsiella* spp.) |
| 2b' (2br) | ✓ | | No | Inhibitor-resistant variants (*E. coli*) |
| 2c | ✓ (carboxypenicillins)[a] | | Yes | PSE-1, PSE-2, PSE-4 |
| 2d | ✓ (cloxacillin)[a] | | Yes | OXA-1, PSE-2 |
| 2e | | ✓ | Yes | *Proteus vulgaris* |
| 3 | ✓[b] | ✓[b] | No | *Bacillus cereus* II, *Stenotrophomonas maltophilia* L1 |
| 4 | ✓ | | No | *Pseudomonas (Burkholderia) cepacia* |

a Principal substrate within group.
b Variable substrate hydrolyses reported.

**Table X.** The position of gene mutations responsible for greater substrate affinity among extended-spectrum β-lactamases of the Bush[103] group 2b' or 2be (after Davies;[105] Philippon et al.[97])

| Enzyme | Amino acid by position | | | | | |
|---|---|---|---|---|---|---|
| | 39 | 104 | 164 | 205 | 238 | 240 |
| TEM-1[a] | Gln | Glu | Arg | Gln | Gly | Glu |
| TEM-12 (CAZ-3) | | | Ser | | | |
| TEM-10 | | | Ser | | | Lys |
| TEM-26 | | Lys | Ser | | | |
| TEM-2[a] | Lys | Glu | Arg | Gln | Gly | Glu |
| TEM-7 | Lys | | Ser | | | |
| TEM-11 | Lys | | His | | | |
| TEM-3 (CTX-1) | Lys | Lys | | | Ser | |
| SHV-1[a] | Gln | Asp | Arg | Arg | Gly | Glu |
| SHV-2 | | | | | Ser | |
| SHV-5 (CAZ-4) | | | | | Ser | Lys |

a Original or parent enzyme of plasmid origin.

phorylases or *O*-nucelotidyltranserases (rare) capable of inactivating macrolides and lincosamides.

The origin of the resistance genes is a complex DNA pool produced by antimicrobial-producing fungi or bacterial strains, antimicrobial-resistant strains, plants, unknown or unspeciated bacterial intermediates, and free DNA with resistance coding sequences. The *Streptomyces* (origin of many antimicrobial classes) possess self-protective mechanisms against many antimicrobials, therefore offering a genetic source of resistance DNA. In addition, mycobacteria and many enteric bacilli harbour cryptic enzyme genes (protein kinases, etc.) capable of modifications to resistance under the selective pressures of antimicrobial use in human medicine, veterinary practice, or in growth enhancement in animal husbandry. These situations would also promote genetic material movement between bacterial replicons and their hosts.

The phenomenon of antimicrobial resistance is not new, but studies of ancient strains suggest that most multiresistant strains have emerged in the past 50 years. This indicates that bacteria have access to the available resistance gene pool and have rapidly passed the characteristics to other species or between strains. The key structural elements appear to be transposons called 'integrons' that are capable of mobility and insertion into the genome of a wide variety of bacteria. These elements produce many of the currently identified resistance plasmids that carry resistance to contemporary antimicrobial agents.

*Gene transfer* among bacteria can be horizontal or vertical by 3 mechanisms:

1. Conjugation
2. Transduction
3. Transformation.

Clearly the most prevalent mechanism is conjugation, which can occur between closely-related or very different organisms (gene transfer between Gram-positive and Gram-negative species, or between aerobic and anaerobic bacteria). A sex factor (*ori* T)-dependent mating creates the potential for transfer of resistance genomes among virtually all bacterial species. This process can be enhanced either by species-specific bacterial proteins that can mobilise large resistance factor elements across cell barriers, or by the antimicrobials (e.g. tetracyclines) themselves. The latter finding is most troublesome because the use of one drug could promote the transfer of resistance genes relating to another drug.

The most important place of the ecological change to greater antimicrobial resistance remains unknown, but it could occur in nature (soil, environmental flora, etc.) or within human hosts (either as a response to therapy or within the endogenous flora in response to environmental antimicrobial pressures). Certainly, the only controllable environments are those associated with the therapeutic use of antimicrobial agents. Prudent antimicrobial use as human therapeutic agents and in animal care practices could minimise the rapidity of emergence and the spread of resistance genes. However, the resistance gene pool is vast, generally uncharacterised and ubiquitous within the DNA of our world.

### *2.3.2 Biochemical Mechanisms of Resistance*

Various mechanisms of microbial resistance to antimicrobial agents have been recognised (table VIII) and many have been well charac-

**Table XI.** Enzyme [AAC(6')-Ib and IIa] inactivation variations produced in two representative aminoglycosides by replacing 118-120 positive amino acids by a serine (after Miller et al.[38])

| Enzyme | Amino acid position | | MIC (μg/ml) | |
|---|---|---|---|---|
| | 119 | 120 | gentamicin | amikacin |
| AAC(6')-Ib | leu | leu | 0.25 | 16 |
| | Ser | | 4 | 2 |
| | | Ser | 0.25 | 0.25 |
| AAC(6')-IIa | Ser | Leu | 8 | 1 |
| | Leu | | 0.5 | 4 |

*Abbreviation:* MIC = minimum inhibitory concentration.

terised to the molecular level. Some of the principal causes of drug resistance are enzyme inactivation of drugs, membrane impermeability and altered sites of enzymes.

### Enzyme Inactivation of Drugs

This type of resistance may be the most common and certainly affects the clinical utility of the most frequently used class of antimicrobial agents – the β-lactams (penicillins, cefalosporins, monobactams, carbapenems). The enzymes produced by the organisms include aminoglycoside inactivating or modifying types and the β-lactamases. The genetic basis for their production is generally controlled by episomal genes; however, many enzymes are also controlled by the bacterial chromosomes. A wide variety of β-lactamases have been characterised and classified (see table IX).[94,103,104]

Some β-lactamases may exert their hydrolysing action external to the cell, examples being the penicillinases of *Staphylococcus* spp. Other β-lactamases are cellular-associated or cell-bound, and include most of those produced by Gram-negative bacilli. The latter enzymes are found in the periplasmic space, external to the target sites (PBPs) of β-lactam drugs. Although the amount of enzyme produced may be low by tests with conventional detection methods, the resistance produced can be highly efficient due to limited access of the drug to the periplasmic space. The best examples are strains of *Enterobacter* spp. and *Citrobacter freundii* that exhibit high MICs for newer cefalosporins such as ceftazidime, cefotaxime, ceftriaxone, and structurally similar β-lactams like aztreonam.

Modifications of the more common TEM-1 or -2 amino acid gene sequences have been associated with the ability to destroy third-generation cefalosporins (table X). Similarly, aminoglycoside-inactivating enzymes could arise from minor changes in the amino acid coding sequences.[38] Table XI lists the phenotypic susceptibility test results (MICs) for 2 representative aminoglycosides after the substitution of a serine in amino acid sequences coding for enzymes of the AAC(6') class. Such changes markedly alter the ability of the enzyme to destroy gentamicin and amikacin.

In some species, the existence of these enzymes appears to be an intrinsic trait, as demonstrated by SHV-mediated ampicillin resistance in *Klebsiella* spp., and Bush group 1 chromosomal-mediated β-lactamases in *Enterobacter aerogenes* and *E. cloacae* (ampicillin and cefazolin resistance). Yet other β-lactamases and aminoglycoside-inactivating enzymes are readily transferred among strains and species via plasmids or tranposons. Co-resistance produced by enzyme modification are not uncommonly transferred together. The presence of β-lactam molecules can induce bacteria to generate greater amounts of enzyme and the inducing power of β-lactams varies over a wide range. Similarly, the ability of β-lactamase inhibitors to bind the enzymes varies by group of enzymes as well as between species or between strains within the same species.

*In vitro* susceptibility tests have been designed to assess the clinically significant risk of enzyme destruction by individual strains.[106,107] However, some recently characterised extended-spectrum β-lactamases have lower affinity for cefalosporin substrates, thus producing false-susceptible or false-intermediate results. These flawed test results will vary by method, by the applied national susceptible breakpoint criteria used, and by the substrate antimicrobial agent tested. The destruction of the drug is an irreversible kinetic process, rendering the substrate molecule inactive against microbial species, e.g. hydrolysis of the β-lactam ring by β-lactamases.

Other antimicrobial agents modified by enzymes include: macrolides/lincosamides (nucleotidyl transferase), streptogramins (acetylase) and chloramphenicol (acetyltransferase).[54] Most are mediated by plasmid genetics and are becoming more prevalent in geographic areas of high clinical drug use.

### Membrane Impermeability

The action of antimicrobial agents is directly affected by the ability of the drug to reach the target site. Since the target sites are located within bacteria, penetration of the cell and/or cytoplasmic membrane is critical to the level of activity. The ability of a drug to enter the bacterial cell is influenced by its hydrophilic-hydrophobic characteristics, porin proteins, the drug concentration gradient, and active transport systems that can recognise the antimicrobial agent as a potential substrate. For β-lactams, the bacterial cell permeability barrier rarely produces significant resistance[108] because these antimicrobials travel into bacteria via water-filled porin channels. Loss of these channels (e.g. Omp F, C or D) can confer some degree of resistance to β-lactams, imipenem (Opr D), and some cross resistances to tetracyclines, chloramphenicol and quinolones (table VIII). Active efflux transport systems for siderophones such as pyoverdine, export several drug classes in *P. aeruginosa*.

In contrast, aminoglycoside-resistant (cross-resistant among all drugs in the class) strains of Gram-negative bacilli can be secondary to decreased drug uptake. The cationic aminoglycosides displace the surface divalent cations (calcium and magnesium) thus disrupting the bacterial membrane (greater permeability). The bacterial surface lipopolysaccharides (LPS) differ, accounting for differences in the measured efficiency of aminoglycosides *versus* pathogenic species. Some altered membrane proteins (H1, etc.) have been protective against aminoglycoside 'self-promoted uptake'.[108] Further, the bacterial electron transport system assists aminoglycoside entry into cells. However, species (anaerobes) or strains deficient of the transport system appear to be resistant.

Antimicrobials or chemical agents that alter cell membrane toward greater permeability (polymixins, edetic acid, chaotrophics, etc.) could be used in combination against strains with known barrier-mediated resistances that are unresponsive to established regimens.

#### Altered Target Sites or Enzymes

All major classes of antimicrobial agents have resistance mediated by this mechanism (table VIII). For the macrolide-lincosamide-streptogramin class, resistance is due to an erythromycin resistance methylase (*erm*) encoding an alternate (demethylated) adenine residue for the 23S RNA. Numerous genes have been described in Gram-positive and Gram-negative species that appear to be derived from a common genetic origin.

β-Lactam PBP target alterations responsible for resistance are diverse and complex. Examples include:

1) PBP 2 (transpeptidase) alterations by the *mec A* gene causing methicillin-resistant staphylococci.

2) PBP 2 altered by the *Fen A* gene in pathogenic *Neisseria* spp., usually mosaic genes derived from *N. flavescens*.

3) PBP 3, 4, and 5 modifications in β-lactam refractory, β-lactamase-negative *H. influenzae*.

4) PBP 1 and 2 alterations in cefamycin-resistant *Bacteroides fragilis*.

5) Variations in the PBP 2a, 2b, 2x, 1a, and 1b producing penicillin resistance (of varying degrees) in *S. pneumoniae*.

The latter resistant strains are due to mosaic encoding genes thought to be the result of transformational acquisition of sequences from viridans group streptococci (*S. mitis* and others) or by spontaneous mutations at key sites such as position 445. Resistance among pneumococci to newer, extended-spectrum cefalosporins is caused by mutations and subsequent alterations of the PBP 2x and 1a.

Other target site mediated resistance of clinical importance involves ribosomal proteins (streptomycin), dihydrofolate reductase (trimethoprim), and dihydropteroate synthetase (sulfonamides).

## 3. The Choice of Drug

The choice of the most appropriate antimicrobial agent for a specific infection requires broad clinical experience and knowledge of the *in vitro* and *in vivo* characteristics of the available agents. The decision must take into account the characteristics of the infection and host factors that may influence the likely causative agents and response to therapy (table XII). Ideally, therapeutic decision making will be supported by microbiological data including identification of the infecting agent and the results of antimicrobial susceptibility tests.

### 3.1 Causative Organism and Drug Susceptibility

In many instances of infectious diseases, initial therapy is based on informed clinical and microbiological guesswork. The initial clinical impression may be further refined by the results of rapid microscopic examination of clinical material (e.g. Gram-stain of material from the suspected site of infection). On the basis of such

Table XII. General principles and considerations relating to the choice and use of systemic antibacterial drugs

**Assessment:**
- If possible, determine nature of infection
- Assess severity of infection and withhold systemic drugs in trivial infections
- Obtain specimens for culture. This is mandatory in severe infections to confirm the provisional diagnosis. Choice of therapy may have to be made on clinical grounds based on experience and modified with the help of a microbiologist

**Causative organism:**
- Identify the organism. If a specific disease with a single microbial cause exists, clinical diagnosis alone may suffice
- Verify susceptibility. To what drug is the strain of organism most susceptible? In the absence of laboratory guidance, this requires knowledge of the antimicrobial spectrum of clinical activity and local knowledge of the frequency of resistance to drugs
- Interpretation of laboratory findings. Reports are not infallible; seek specialist advice if these conflict with clinical experience

**Drug characteristics:**
- Site of infection: does the drug attain adequate concentrations at the location of infection?
- Toxicity: use the less toxic drug if possible
- Single drug or combination: consider a combination if broad spectrum coverage is required
- Drug interaction or incompatibility with other therapy: review drug-drug interactions and adjust accordingly
- Cost

**Patient characteristics:**
- Age: reduce dosages at both extremes of life
- Renal disease: avoid some drugs; modify dosage of some others (see appendix D)
- Liver disease: avoid hepatotoxic drugs; modify dose of certain drugs in severe liver disease (see appendix F and review by Westphal & Brogard[109])
- Allergy: some patients have an increased risk of sensitisation reactions; avoid some drugs
- Other associated diseases may influence effectiveness or increase risk of toxicity with some drugs
- Pregnancy: avoid some drugs

**Choice among a class of drug:**
- Degree of antibacterial activity
- Efficiency of absorption: blood or tissue concentration attained; effect of food
- Convenience or ease of administration: does a particular derivative simplify administration or require less frequent dosage?
- Relative incidence of troublesome adverse effects
- Relative cost

a tentative diagnosis, therapy may be selected from a variety of options on the basis of knowledge of both the antimicrobial spectrum of available agents and the frequency of acquired resistance. In the absence of definitive antimicrobial susceptibility test results, a reasonable choice of initial therapy may be made using reference tables reflecting the current consensus regarding the range of antimicrobial activity of available agents (table XIII). To use such data wisely, it must be understood that the susceptibility pattern of many organisms can vary with the hospital, clinic or community in which they are isolated. Thus, local knowledge of the frequency of certain resistance patterns, whether in a hospital or an entire community, may be a helpful guide.

Specific laboratory testing of a documented causative agent is certainly preferred to the use of reference tables and may afford a broad choice of potentially effective antimicrobial agents. The choice of agent should take into consideration toxicity, the potential need for combination therapy, the accuracy of the diagnosis, and host factors, among others.

### 3.2 Toxicity

When 2 drugs offer an equal prospect of cure, the least toxic will naturally be preferred (see section 8). When the potentially more toxic agent is likely to be more effective, the choice is more difficult and demands balanced judgement.

### 3.3 Combination Therapy

Use of antimicrobial combinations is encountered most frequently in the early stages of an infectious process when the patient is clinically unstable and there is uncertainty as to the causative organism or the site of infection. Administration of 2 or more antimicrobials in this situation provides broad-spectrum coverage that can be modified when the causative organism is identified and results of *in vitro* susceptibility tests are available. In certain instances, combinations of agents may be chosen because the specific pathogen is known to be resistant to inhibition or killing by a single agent, but may be treated effectively by a multiple drugs. Infections in immunocompromised individuals and those with organisms such as *P. aeruginosa* or enterococci are examples of situations where antimicrobial combinations are known to be useful.[110,111]

The rationale for selecting specific combinations of antimicrobial agents vary. However, it generally includes the desire to achieve antimicrobial synergy (and avoid antagonism), prevent the emergence of resistance, decrease

**Table XIII.** Selection of antimicrobial agents for use in treating commonly isolated and/or important organisms

| Organism | First-line agent(s) | Second-line agent(s) | Other agent(s) |
|---|---|---|---|
| *Acinetobacter* spp. | Piperacillin<br>Ticarcillin | 3rd gen Cefalosporin<br>Imipenem<br>Quinolone | Aminoglycoside |
| *Actinomyces israelii* | Benzylpenicillin (penicillin G) | Tetracycline<br>3rd gen Cefalosporin | Imipenem |
| *Aeromonas hydrophila* | 3rd gen Cefalosporin<br>Quinolone | Aminoglycoside<br>Cotrimoxazole[a] | Imipenem |
| *Alcaligenes (Achromobacter)* spp. | Piperacillin<br>Ticarcillin | Cotrimoxazole<br>Quinolone<br>Ceftazidime | Imipenem |
| *Bacillus cereus* | Vancomycin<br>Clindamycin | Aminoglycoside<br>Quinolone | Imipenem |
| *Bacteroides* spp. | Metronidazole<br>β-LIC | Cefamycin<br>Clindamycin | Imipenem<br>Piperacillin<br>Ticarcillin |
| *Bordetella pertussis* | Macrolide | Cotrimoxazole | |
| *Borrelia burgdorferi* | Ceftriaxone<br>Cefotaxime<br>Doxycycline | Penicillin<br>Ampicillin | Clarithromycin<br>Azithromycin |
| *Brucella* spp. | Doxycycline + rifampicin or gentamicin | Cotrimoxazole + gentamicin | Chloramphenicol<br>Quinolone |
| *Calymmatobacterium granulomatis* | Doxycycline | Cotrimoxazole | |
| *Campylobacter fetus* | Imipenem | Aminoglycoside<br>Macrolide | Ampicillin<br>Chloramphenicol |
| *Campylobacter jejuni* | Quinolone | Macrolide | Clindamycin<br>Doxycycline |
| *Capnocytophaga* spp. | β-LIC | Clindamycin<br>Quinolone | Imipenem<br>3rd gen Cefalosporin |
| *Chlamydia pneumoniae* | Doxycycline | Macrolide | |
| *Chlamydia psittaci* | Tetracycline | Macrolide | |
| *Chlamydia trachomatis* | Tetracycline | Macrolide | Quinolone |
| *Citrobacter koseri (diversus)* | 3rd gen Cefalosporin<br>Aminoglycoside | Aztreonam<br>Quinolone | |
| *Citrobacter freundii* | 3rd gen Cefalosporin | Aminoglycoside<br>Imipenem<br>Aztreonam<br>Quinolone | |
| *Clostridium difficile* | Metronidazole (oral) | Vancomycin (oral) | Fusidic acid (oral)<br>Bacitracin (oral) |
| *Clostridium perfringens* | Benzylpenicillin + clindamycin | Macrolide<br>Tetracycline | Metronidazole<br>Cefamycin<br>Imipenem |
| *Clostridium tetani* | Benzylpenicillin<br>Cefamycin<br>Metronidazole | Tetracycline | Clindamycin<br>Imipenem |
| *Corynebacterium diphtheriae* | Penicillin | Macrolide | Clindamycin<br>Rifampicin |
| *Corynebacterium jeikeium* | Vancomycin | Quinolone | Penicillin + aminoglycoside |
| *Eikenella corrodens* | Benzylpenicillin<br>Amoxicillin | Macrolide | Cefamycin<br>Doxycycline<br>Imipenem |
| *Enterobacter* spp. | Aminoglycoside<br>Imipenem | 3rd gen Cefalosporin<br>Ticarcillin<br>Piperacillin | Aztreonam<br>Quinolone |
| *Enterococcus* spp. | Amoxicillin (add gentamicin if infective endocarditis) | Vancomycin (add gentamicin if infective endocarditis) | Nitrofurantoin (UTI only) |

*[Continued over]*

**Table XIII.** *[Continued]*

| Organism | First-line agent(s) | Second-line agent(s) | Other agent(s) |
|---|---|---|---|
| *Enterococcus faecium* or *E. faecalis*, ampicillin-resistant, high-concentration aminoglycoside- and vancomycin-resistant | No regimen of proven effectiveness. Consultation recommended if patient has endocarditis or other life-threatening infection | Chloramphenicol<br>Doxycycline<br>Rifampicin | Novobiocin<br>Quinolone |
| *Erysipelothrix rhusiopathiae* | Penicillin<br>Amoxicillin | 3rd gen Cefalosporin<br>Quinolone | Imipenem<br>Piperacillin<br>Ticarcillin |
| *Escherichia coli* | β-LIC<br>Trimethoprim (UTI) | 3rd gen Cefalosporin<br>Quinolone | Cotrimoxazole<br>Aminoglycosides<br>Imipenem<br>Piperacillin<br>Ticarcillin |
| *Fusobacterium* spp. | Penicillin | Metronidazole<br>Clindamycin | |
| *Gardnerella vaginalis* | Metronidazole | Amoxicillin | Clindamycin |
| *Haemophilus aphrophilus* | Penicillin + gentamicin | 3rd gen Cefalosporin<br>Gentamicin | |
| *Haemophilus ducreyi* | Azithromycin<br>3rd gen Cefalosporin | Quinolone<br>Macrolide | Cotrimoxazole<br>β-LIC |
| *Haemophilus influenzae* (meningitis, epiglottitis, other infections) | 3rd gen Cefalosporin<br>β-LIC | Amoxicillin<br>Cefuroxime<br>Cotrimoxazole<br>Macrolide | Chloramphenicol |
| *Helicobacter pylori* | Metronidazole + amoxicillin or tetracycline + bismuth subcitrate or subsalicylate | | |
| *Klebsiella* spp. | 2nd gen Cefalosporin<br>3rd gen Cefalosporin | Aminoglycoside<br>β-LIC<br>Quinolone | Aztreonam<br>Piperacillin<br>Ticarcillin<br>Imipenem |
| *Legionella pneumophila* | Macrolide ± rifampicin | Quinolone | |
| *Leptospira* spp. | Penicillin<br>Doxycycline | | |
| *Listeria monocytogenes* | Amoxicillin | Benzylpenicillin<br>Tetracycline | Cotrimoxazole<br>Macrolide |
| *Moraxella (Branhamella) catarrhalis* | β-LIC | Cotrimoxazole<br>Macrolide | Tetracycline<br>Quinolone |
| *Morganella* spp. | Aminoglycoside<br>3rd gen Cefalosporin | Imipenem | Quinolone<br>Aztreonam |
| *Mycobacterium tuberculosis* | Isoniazid<br>Rifampicin<br>Ethambutol<br>Pyrazinamide | Streptomycin<br>*p*-Aminosalicylic acid<br>Capreomycin | Quinolone |
| *Mycoplasma pneumoniae* | Macrolide | Tetracycline | |
| *Neisseria gonorrhoeae* | 3rd gen Cefalosporin | Spectinomycin<br>Quinolone | Azithromycin |
| *Neisseria meningitidis* | Benzylpenicillin<br>3rd gen Cefalosporin<br>Rifampicin (for contacts) | Imipenem<br>Minocycline (for contacts) | Doxycycline<br>Sulfonamide<br>Chloramphenicol<br>Quinolone (for contacts) |
| *Nocardia asteroides* | Cotrimoxazole | Minocycline<br>Amikacin | Imipenem<br>3rd gen Cefalosporin |
| *Pasteurella multocida* | Benzylpenicillin | Tetracycline<br>β-LIC | 3rd gen Cefalosporin<br>Quinolone |
| *Pleisomonas shigelloides* | Quinolone | Cotrimoxazole | β-LIC<br>3rd gen Cefalosporin<br>Imipenem |

**Table XIII.** *[Continued]*

| Organism | First-line agent(s) | Second-line agent(s) | Other agent(s) |
|---|---|---|---|
| *Pneumocystis carinii* | Cotrimoxazole | Pentamidine<br>Dapsone<br>Clindamycin + primaquine | Atovaquone |
| *Proteus mirabilis* | Ampicillin | 2nd gen Cefalosporin<br>Cotrimoxazole<br>β-LIC | 3rd gen Cefalosporin<br>Aminoglycoside |
| *Proteus vulgaris* | 3rd gen Cefalosporin<br>Aminoglycoside | Imipenem | Aztreonam |
| *Providencia* spp. | Aminoglycoside<br>3rd gen Cefalosporin | Imipenem<br>Cotrimoxazole<br>Quinolone | Aztreonam<br>Piperacillin<br>Ticarcillin |
| Pseudomonas aeruginosa | Ticarcillin<br>Piperacillin<br>Aminoglycoside | Ceftazidime<br>Imipenem | Aztreonam<br>Quinolone |
| *Pseudomonas (Burkholderia) cepacia* | Cotrimoxazole | Quinolone<br>Imipenem | Minocycline<br>Chloramphenicol |
| *Pseudomonas (Burkholderia) pseudomallei* | Cotrimoxazole | 3rd gen Cefalosporin | Imipenem<br>Quinolone |
| *Rhodococcus equi* | Vancomycin | Macrolide | Imipenem + rifampicin |
| *Salmonella typhi* | Azithromycin<br>Ceftriaxone<br>Cefoperazone | Cotrimoxazole<br>Ampicillin | Chloramphenicol<br>Quinolone |
| *Serratia marcescens* | Aminoglycoside<br>3rd gen Cefalosporin | Quinolone<br>Imipenem | Aztreonam |
| *Shigella* spp. | Cotrimoxazole<br>Quinolone | Ampicillin | 2nd or 3rd gen Cefalosporin |
| *Staphylococcus aureus:* | | | |
| • methicillin-susceptible | Oxacillin<br>Nafcillin | Cefalosporin<br>Macrolide | Quinolone<br>β-LIC<br>Clindamycin<br>Vancomycin<br>Imipenem |
| • methicillin-resistant | Vancomycin | Teicoplanin<br>Fusidic acid | |
| *Staphylococcus epidermidis* | Oxacillin<br>Nafcillin<br>Vancomycin | Cefalosporin | Cotrimoxazole<br>Rifampicin |
| *Staphylococcus saprophyticus* | Cotrimoxazole | Nitrofurantoin (UTI only) | |
| Stenotrophomonas (Xanthomonas) maltophilia | Cotrimoxazole | Ticarcillin/clavulanic acid<br>Minocycline | Quinolone<br>Ceftazidime<br>Cefoperazone |
| *Streptococcus* spp. (including *S. pneumoniae* Lancefield Group A, B, C, and G and *S. bovis*) | Benzylpenicillin<br>Vancomycin (penicillin-resistant) | Macrolide<br>3rd gen Cefalosporin | Rifampicin |
| *Toxoplasma gondii* | Pyrimethamine + sulfonamide (short-acting)[b] | | |
| *Vibrio cholerae* | Tetracycline<br>Quinolone | Cotrimoxazole | |
| *Yersinia enterocolitica* | Cotrimoxazole<br>3rd gen Cefalosporin | Aminoglycoside<br>Quinolone | |

a Cotrimoxazole = trimethoprim/sulfamethoxazole combination (1 : 5 ratio).

b Regimen should also include calcium folinate.

*Abbreviations:* UTI = urinary tract infection; β-LIC = β-lactam/β-lactamase inhibitor combinations; 2nd gen = second-generation; 3rd gen = third-generation; ***Quinolones*** = ciprofloxacin, ofloxacin, norfloxacin, enoxacin, pefloxacin, lomefloxacin, fleroxacin and sparfloxacin; ***2nd-generation cefalosporins*** = cefuroxime, cefamandole, cefaclor, cefprozil, loracarbef or cefamycins (see also table VI); ***3rd-generation cefalosporins*** = cefotaxime, ceftazidime and ceftriaxone (see also table VI); ***Cefamycins*** = cefmetazole, cefotetan and cefoxitin; **Aminoglycosides** = gentamicin, tobramycin, netilmicin and amikacin; ***Tetracyclines*** = tetracycline, doxycycline, minocycline and other derivatives; β-***Lactam***/β-***lactamase inhibitor combinations*** = amoxicillin/clavulanic acid, ampicillin/sulbactam, piperacillin/tazobactam, and ticarcillin/clavulanic acid; ***Macrolides*** = erythromycin, clarithromycin, azithromycin and roxithromycin.

dose-related toxicity and provide adequate coverage for polymicrobial infections.

#### Antimicrobial Synergy

One of the early applications of antibiotic combinations was the use of the synergistic combination of penicillin and streptomycin to achieve bactericidal activity in the treatment of enterococcal endocarditis.[112-114] The use of combinations of antibiotics to achieve greater bactericidal activity than either agent used alone continues to be the subject of considerable laboratory investigation and a matter of great clinical relevance. Mechanisms by which this synergistic antibacterial activity may be achieved include:

1) Serial or sequential inhibition of a common biochemical pathway, e.g. cotrimoxazole (trimethoprim-sulfamethoxazole).

2) Inhibition of protective bacterial enzymes, e.g. a β-lactamase inhibitor plus a β-lactamase susceptible penicillin.

3) Combinations of cell wall–active agents.

4) Use of cell wall–active agents to enhance the uptake of other antimicrobials, e.g. a β-lactam or glycopeptide plus an aminoglycoside.

The literature regarding antimicrobial synergism in the treatment of Gram-negative and Gram-positive infections is extensive.[115] However, aside from the well-documented value of synergistic combinations of β-lactams (penicillin or ampicillin) or glycopeptides (vancomycin) plus aminoglycosides to treat enterococcal endocarditis,[110] and of fixed combinations of trimethoprim-sulfamethoxazole (cotrimoxazole) in certain situations,[116] the importance of synergy under normal clinical circumstances has been grossly overrated. Certainly, advantages of synergistic antimicrobial combinations have been observed in treatment of Gram-negative infections, particularly those due to *P. aeruginosa*, but the advantages have been seen primarily in neutropenic patients.[111,117,118] The increased potency of several of the newer β-lactam antibiotics may in fact produce greater serum bactericidal activity when used as monotherapy than can be achieved with combinations of aminoglycosides and older β-lactams.[119] Recently, monotherapy with the broad-spectrum carbapenem imipenem was shown to be as effective and less nephrotoxic than an imipenem/netilmicin combination in the treatment of severe infections in non-neutropenic patients.[120]

One concern about the use of antimicrobial combinations is the fact that certain combinations of agents may yield antagonistic effects. One of the first reported[121] and most tragic examples of antimicrobial antagonism was that the addition of chlortetracycline markedly reduced the survival rate for children treated with penicillin for pneumococcal meningitis from 79 to 21%. Although there are few documented reports of clinically significant antagonism, it is possible that such adverse interactions are often not recognised in patients with complex presentations. Examples from contemporary practice show the potential for antagonistic interactions between β-lactam antibiotics used together against Gram-negative bacilli possessing inducible chromosomally mediated β-lactamases.[122]

#### Preventing the Emergence of Resistance

Combination therapy is occasionally used to prevent or delay the emergence of drug-resistant microbes during the course of therapy.[115] The rationale for this approach is that if the mechanisms of resistance to each of the antibiotics is different, then the chance that the infecting organism will become resistant to all the antibiotics used is theoretically very low. The best example of this approach is with mycobacteria, where simultaneous treatment with multiple drugs is standard practice and clearly reduces the risk of selection of resistant strains.[123] This approach is also relevant for specific antimicrobials such as rifampicin (staphylococci) and flucytosine (*Candida* spp. and cryptococci), agents to which organisms readily develop resistance if used alone.

Conventional wisdom also suggests that infections with *P. aeruginosa* should be treated with combination therapy both to provide a bactericidal regimen and to prevent the development of resistance. Several studies indicate that treatment of *P. aeruginosa* infections with a β-lactam plus an aminoglycoside can reduce the development of resistance to either agent.[124-126] However, the results of other studies do not support this conclusion. For example, the addition of netilmicin did not prevent the emergence of *P. aeruginosa* resistant to imipenem among non-neutropenic patients treated with either imipenem alone or with imipenem plus netilmicin.[120]

#### Decreasing Dose-Related Toxicity

Because important antimicrobial agents such as the aminoglycosides may have significant dose-related toxicity that limits their use, it is reasonable to attempt to avoid their toxicity by lowering the dose while using an additional agent, usually a β-lactam, to ensure a successful outcome. Although this is a useful theoretical concept, in practice it is usually difficult to lower the dose of an antimicrobial significantly without compromising activity. As newer agents with greater potency and less toxicity are developed, this approach may become unnecessary.

**Providing Coverage for Polymicrobial Infections**

Polymicrobial or mixed infections may be difficult to treat and carry a higher mortality than many infections due to a single pathogen.[127,128] Antimicrobial combinations may be used empirically to provide broad-spectrum coverage in infections that may be caused by multiple pathogens. In some mixed infections, it may be necessary to use agents that are active against each of the major pathogens present. However, the development of newer agents with potent activity against anaerobes as well as aerobic Gram-negative and Gram-positive bacteria permits successful monotherapy of many mixed infections. Frequently, in the case of mixed aerobic and anaerobic infections, treatment with a single agent directed against the aerobic component may be all that is necessary to ensure a successful outcome.[129] However, some investigators advocate adding anaerobic coverage, particularly in deep-seated abscesses that may be difficult to drain.[130] As indicated above (section 3.3), caution must be applied when using drug combinations, to avoid antimicrobial antagonism.

## 3.4 Reasons for Failure of Antimicrobial Therapy

It may be an unpleasant surprise to the clinician if an antimicrobial drug that is apparently effective *in vitro* fails to eradicate an infection. There is still a tendency for antimicrobials to be considered by some clinicians as 'wonder drugs', failure of which can be attributed to only one cause, namely resistance. These clinicians may fail to understand that the inherent artificiality of *in vitro* susceptibility testing systems may also account for lack of correlation between *in vitro* and *in vivo* results. *In vitro* susceptibility tests are generally designed to determine the activity of antimicrobial agents in a static test situation that is convenient for the laboratory and thus may have little if any relationship to the clinical situation.[131] On the other hand, the microbiologist may be surprised that an antimicrobial drug ever succeeded in curing an infection, bearing in mind how much the drug had been abused since its introduction.

It is remarkable that an overall cure rate of about 70% is now regarded as commonplace in such apparently disparate clinical situations as infections in granulocytopenic patients and recurrent urinary tract infections in otherwise completely healthy women (accompanied by close laboratory control). Clearly, there is more to the failure of antimicrobial therapy than mere resistance. In many instances, the actual capability of *in vitro* susceptibility testing to predict clinical effectiveness of antimicrobial therapy is vastly overrated by microbiologists and clinicians alike.[131] Numerous factors, including host-pathogen factors and factors intrinsic to the interaction between the antimicrobial agent and the organism, influence clinical outcomes. Several of these factors are examined here.

### *3.4.1 Inadequate Dosage*

The location of an infection must be considered when deciding on dosage. For example, consider 3 separate situations in each of which the causative agent is a fully susceptible strain of *S. pneumoniae*, for which benzylpenicillin has an MIC of 0.01 mg/L. Historically, lobar pneumonia caused by such a strain has responded well to a dose of 100,000U of benzylpenicillin (60mg). The same pneumococcus causing meningitis will require doses of 1MU (600mg), while pneumococcal endocarditis calls for a regimen involving doses of 10MU each (6g). In the latter 2 circumstances, treatment will need to be continued until a therapeutic effect is achieved.

Failure to appreciate the importance of the location may well result in underdosage and consequent treatment failure, despite a fully susceptible *in vitro* test result.

### *3.4.2 Incorrect Diagnosis*

A common cause of apparent failure of antimicrobial therapy is when a viral illness (e.g. upper or lower respiratory tract infection) is treated with antibacterial agents. The failure of the antimicrobial drug is often masked by the fact that many such diseases treated in this way are of short duration and may appear to respond temporarily to the administration of the drug. This may lead to a situation where patients expect to be given antimicrobial drugs for the common cold and complain bitterly if denied such treatment by conscientious clinicians.

Such inappropriate use of antibacterial agents is responsible in part for the growing problem of antimicrobial resistance worldwide.[100,132]

Another example of apparent antimicrobial drug failure is in the empirical treatment of febrile episodes of granulocytopenic patients. Many such episodes are either non-bacterial infections (the causative agents being viruses, fungi or parasites) or are not caused by microbes at all (e.g. drug reactions).

#### 3.4.3 Mechanical Factors

Mechanical factors may be of great importance in apparent failure of antimicrobial therapy. Examples include:

1) Accumulations of pus, as in the subphrenic abscess or a carbuncle.

2) The presence of a foreign body, which may be present by accident, such as a splinter, or by intention, such as a surgical stitch or implanted prosthetic device (e.g. valve, joint or catheter).

3) Obstruction, such as a staghorn calculus.

4) The highly mucoid growth of *P. aeruginosa* in cystic fibrotic lungs.

The existence of such factors will make it virtually impossible for an antimicrobial drug to sterilise a lesion. Removal of these factors, in some cases by surgical intervention, is often sufficient to clear the infecting organisms without recourse to antimicrobial drugs.

#### 3.4.4 Inadequate Duration of Treatment

An antimicrobial drug may fail because it has not been administered for a sufficient length of time. Strains of *Streptococcus pyogenes* causing pharyngitis are virtually all highly susceptible to benzylpenicillin, with an MIC of 0.01 mg/L or less. Eradication of the infection depends on the duration of treatment, not the size of the dose. Administration of benzylpenicillin or phenoxymethylpenicillin for 10 days is necessary to completely eradicate the streptococcus.

Premature withdrawal of therapy may be deliberate, as in the case of hypersensitivity or due to other adverse effects (see section 8). However, the usual problem is unintentional curtailment of treatment before all the infecting organisms have been eradicated. Deep-seated infections, such as tuberculosis, leprosy, osteomyelitis and endocarditis may need treatment for a period of months and relapse occurs if the treatment duration is too short. In such instances, premature cessation of therapy may contribute to the development of antimicrobial-resistant strains.[133]

#### 3.4.5 Use of an Inappropriate Antimicrobial Drug

There are 3 separate categories in this context. Firstly, there is the use of an antimicrobial drug to which the infecting bacteria are resistant by usual laboratory tests. Such usage has been shown to be highly deleterious in terms of cure rate in patients with serious infections such as septicaemia,[131,134] but it is noteworthy that even under such adverse conditions, some cures do occur. These must be attributed to the host defence mechanisms and/or correction of mechanical factors (see section 3.4.3). Urinary tract infections, on the other hand, may show high cure rates when so-called 'inappropriate' antimicrobial drugs are used. This is the result of inaccurate laboratory testing, which in this case fails to consider the very high concentrations of antibiotics that may be attained in the urine after conventional treatment (concentrations >100 mg/L of β-lactam agents are commonplace). Several studies have shown that it is the concentration of an antimicrobial drug in the urine rather than in the serum that determines the outcome of the treatment of infections of the lower urinary tract. The same may be true for infections of the upper urinary tract if the infection is restricted to the renal pelvis and medulla.

In addition, the emergence of resistance during the course of treatment is an unusual phenomenon under most clinical circumstances. It occurs with only a few antimicrobial drugs (e.g. streptomycin, fusidic acid, novobiocin, rifampicin and flucytosine) and is by no means a universal finding even with these agents. Recently, emergence of broad-spectrum β-lactam resistance among enteric Gram-negative organisms (*Enterobacter*, *Citrobacter* and *Serratia* species) exposed to newer cefalosporins (cefotaxime, ceftriaxone, ceftazidime, and cefoperazone) has been reported.[135] Despite the infrequent nature of these occurrences, it is a wise precaution to use these drugs in combination with a suitable co-drug and to be aware of inducible β-lactamases in many of the enteric Gram-negative organisms.

Secondly, an antimicrobial drug may be inappropriate not for microbiological, but for pharmacokinetic reasons. Examples here include nitrofurantoin used to treat staphylococcal pneumonia; fusidic acid or novobiocin used for staphylococcal urinary infections; vancomycin used for an infection of the biliary tree with *Enterococcus faecalis*. In all these cases, the laboratory report will indicate *in vitro* susceptibility of the organism to the antibiotic. However, such treatment will fail, as the microbiologically active form of the drug is not present at the site of infection. Nitrofurantoin attains microbiologically active concentrations only in the urine and not in the blood or tissues. Likewise, both fusidic acid and novobiocin are metabolised in the liver and are excreted almost exclusively in the bile and not in the urine, whereas vancomycin does not enter the bile at all.

The third category of inappropriate choice of antimicrobial drug is less clearcut, but is still important. The problem is that the *in vivo* response does not correlate with the result of *in vitro* susceptibility tests. The best example is that of *Salmonella typhi*. This organism appears susceptible *in vitro* to a wide range of antimicrobial drugs yet only a few (amoxicillin, ceftriaxone, chloramphenicol, cotrimoxazole) are effective treatments of typhoid fever. The precise reason for this discrepancy is not known, although it may be connected with the intracellular location of the infecting organism. Brucellosis, legionellosis and tuberculosis are other examples of diseases due to intracellular parasites that require a careful choice of appropriate antimicrobial agents.

#### *3.4.6 Host Factors*

Unquestionably the most important factor affecting the outcome of the treatment of infection is the status of the patient. Underlying good health combined with the possession of adequate defence mechanisms (humoral and cellular) make for an excellent chance of recovery from any infection. Patients with a rapidly fatal underlying disease state respond less well. A reduction in specific defence mechanisms is also a grave prognostic sign. Intensive combination therapy, preferably with agents known to have synergistic bactericidal activity against a specific pathogen, is important to minimise the risk of treatment failure in infected immunocompromised individuals.

## 4. Dosages of Antimicrobial Drugs

Many dosage regimens recommended by the manufacturers of antimicrobial drugs are purely arbitrary. When antimicrobial drugs were first introduced, little attention was given to their pharmacokinetic characteristics and the unit dose of a drug was arbitrarily selected as 1g. This practice was still popular in the early 1960s and its application almost led to the withdrawal of trimethoprim, gentamicin and polymixin as being too toxic for use.

The only way to establish the optimum dosage is to determine the dose-response curve. This is not an easy undertaking and one that some ethical committees might consider improper, since by definition, a stated goal of the study is to give at least one group of patients suboptimum therapy.

The frequency of dosage is somewhat easier to arrange in a logical manner. This is usually accomplished based on the half-life of the drug, but as table XIV shows, there are some inconsistencies. It should also be borne in mind that almost all data on half-lives of antimicrobial drugs have been obtained in healthy young ambulatory volunteers (often males only). Such values will almost certainly not be representative of either sick patients confined to bed, or of elderly or very young patients, in whom pharmacokinetic characteristics may be altered.

### 4.1 Dosages at Extremes of Age

Neonates, particularly if premature, have immature and therefore underactive livers and kidneys. This means that the rates of metabolism and/or excretion of antimicrobial drugs is decreased. Furthermore, the volume of distribution of many drugs is proportionally greater than in adults. Taking these differences into consideration means that it is not possible to extrapolate merely in terms of bodyweight from adult to child in determining drug dosage. Because of the reduced rate of elimination in very young patients, antimicrobial drugs remain in the body for longer than in adults. Drugs given in the form of an ester that require activation *in vivo* to generate the microbiologically active form, e.g. erythromycin estolate and chloramphenicol palmitate, may not be completely hydrolysed in this age group,[136] and may achieve inadequate antimicrobial concentrations. This may be counterbalanced in the case of chloramphenicol by decreased elimination of the drug due to the reduced rate of glucuronidation in neonates (for dosages of some commonly used drugs in neonates and children, see chapter 3; tables IV, V and VII).[136,137]

In elderly patients, elimination half-lives of drugs tend to rise despite a lack of apparent change in conventional measurements of renal function such as creatinine clearance. Reduced hepatic clearance of drugs and changes in extra-

**Table XIV.** Half-lives of some antibacterial drugs and their recommended dosage schedules

| Drug | Half-life (h) | Recommended doses/day |
|---|---|---|
| Nitrofurantoin | 1 | 4 |
| Penicillins and cefalosporins[a] | 1-2 | 3-4 |
| Nalidixic acid | 1.5 | 4 |
| Cinoxacin | 1.5-2 | 2 |
| Aminoglycosides | 2-3 | 3 |
| Chloramphenicol | 2-3 | 4 |
| Clindamycin | 2-3 | 4 |
| Norfloxacin | 3-4 | 2 |
| Erythromycin | 2-4 | 4 |
| Ciprofloxacin | 4-5 | 2 |
| Lincomycin | 4-6 | 3-4 |
| Fusidic acid | ≈6 | 3 |
| Tetracycline, chlortetracycline, oxytetracycline | 6-10 | 4 |
| Metronidazole | 6-10 | 3 |
| Trimethoprim | 11 | 2 |
| Minocycline | ≈15 | 2 |
| Doxycycline | 16-20 | 1 |

a Exceptions include ceftriaxone (half-life 7h), cefonicid (half-life 4-5h) and cefotetan (half-life 3-4h).

cellular water may lead to higher serum concentrations of antimicrobial drugs. Thus, overdosage may occasionally be a problem in elderly patients.[138]

## 4.2 Dosages in Pregnancy

Several major physiological changes occur during pregnancy (see further chapter 2; sect. 4), two of which would be expected to have an effect on the pharmacokinetics of antimicrobial agents:

1) An increase in total body water, and

2) An increase by 70% in the glomerular filtration rate.

Thus, lower peak concentrations and shorter elimination half-lives would be expected for many antimicrobial drugs in pregnancy. This has been shown to be true experimentally for several antimicrobial drugs.[139] It has been suggested that it may be necessary to double the dose of ampicillin needed to attain serum concentrations similar to those achieved in non-pregnant women.[140] However, this suggestion is theoretical and adjustment of the dosage has not been necessary in practice, since the antibiotic is already given in excess.

## 4.3 Dosages in Hepatic Disease

Hepatic disease may produce significant and highly variable effects on the pharmacokinetics of antimicrobial drugs. Antibiotic distribution may be altered by pathophysiological mechanisms such as modifications in the volume of distribution induced by decreased albumin synthesis or portal hypertension-related ascites.[109] Despite the frequency with which antibiotics are administered in patients with liver disease, few studies have been carried out on antimicrobial drug behaviour in this setting.[109,141]

Chloramphenicol, rifampicin, isoniazid and cefoperazone have been reported to have increased half-lives in patients with hepatic diseases and reductions in their dosages may be necessary (see further appendix F). These recommendations aside, it must be stressed that there is still no reliable tool to predict accurately in a quantitative fashion the pharmacokinetic and pharmacodynamic changes that liver disease may produce for a given drug in an individual patient.[109] The obvious practical solution to the problem is to monitor plasma concentrations at appropriate intervals if potentially toxic antimicrobial drugs are being used in patients with liver disease. Potentially hepatotoxic drugs should be avoided if possible.

## 4.4 Dosages in Renal Failure

Since most antimicrobial drugs in common usage are removed from the body predominantly by renal excretion, major dosage adjustments may need to be made in the case of renal failure (see appendix D). Exceptions are those drugs eliminated primarily by the liver, either by metabolism or biliary excretion, for which little or no dosage modification is required (e.g. cefoperazone, erythromycin, rifampicin, isoniazid, chloramphenicol, doxycycline and minocycline). However, dosage alterations are necessary for most penicillins, cefalosporins, aminoglycosides, trimethoprim, sulfonamides, polymixins, quinolones and vancomycin. In the case of the penicillins, if the creatinine clearance remains above 30 ml/min (1.8 L/h) the dosage need not be reduced.

Certain antibiotics should be avoided in patients with renal failure as they may contribute to acidosis, raise blood urea nitrogen (BUN) and phosphorous levels, and increase catabolism. These include the tetracyclines (with the exception of doxycycline, which is excreted into the intestine), nitrofurantoin and nalidixic acid.

There are no obvious guidelines to determine which antimicrobial drugs are removed by dialysis. For example, benzylpenicillin is removed by haemodialysis, but not by peritoneal dialysis, methicillin is removed by neither method and carbenicillin by both. For reviews, see Lee and Marbury,[142] Paton et al.,[143] St Peter et al.[144] and Reetze-Bonorden et al.[145]

## 5. Optimum Treatment of Diseases and Infections Caused by Specific Bacterial Pathogens

### 5.1 Infections Due to Specific Pathogens

Although Gram-negative organisms such as *Enterobacter* species and *P. aeruginosa* remain important causes of infection, the emergence of the Gram-positive cocci, mycobacteria and *Candida* species as prominent nosocomial and community-acquired pathogens is noteworthy. Over the past decade, there has been a reduction in the frequency of *E. coli* infections and an increase in infections due to staphylococci, enterococci and *Candida albicans*.[133,146] Serious infections due to *M. avium* and *M. intracellulare*, as well as *M. tuberculosis*, have become extremely common in association with the severe immunosuppression accompanying infection with human immunodeficiency virus (HIV) and among homeless persons.[147,148] In the past decade, the trend has been away from antimicrobial-susceptible species towards more resistant pathogens. Even among susceptible species, there has been a shift from the appearance of readily susceptible to more resistant strains.[133]

#### 5.1.1 Staphylococcal Infections

With the increase in infections due to staphylococci (both coagulase-negative as well as *S. aureus*) has come a growing appreciation of antibiotic resistance in these organisms. Over >90% of coagulase-negative staphylococci (CNS) and *S. aureus* causing infections are resistant to penicillin by virtue of β-lactamase production. Although many of these isolates are treatable with penicillinase-resistant penicillins such as oxacillin, methicillin or nafcillin, an increasing number are also resistant to these agents. So-called methicillin-resistant strains of *S. aureus* (MRSA) and coagulase-negative staphylococci (MRCNS) are resistant to methicillin and other penicillinase-resistant penicillins, cefalosporins, carbapenems and penems by virtue of a chromosomal gene (mec A) that encodes a new penicillin binding protein (PBP) with reduced affinity for β-lactam antibiotics (PBP 2a). In addition, MRSA and MRCNS are often resistant to erythromycin, clindamycin, aminoglycosides, tetracyclines, cotrimoxazole and chloramphenicol. Despite the generally excellent staphylococcal coverage afforded by quinolones, resistance to this class of compounds can also develop rapidly among staphylococci, particularly among methicillin-resistant isolates, if selective pressure is applied.

Current therapy of staphylococcal infections includes the use of a *penicillinase-resistant penicillin* for susceptible strains. Patients allergic to β-lactam drugs may be given *erythromycin* or *first-generation cefalosporins*. For serious infections with methicillin-resistant strains, use of a glycopeptide such as *vancomycin* or *teicoplanin* is recommended. Combinations of cell wall–active agents with an aminoglycoside, rifampicin or both have been used to treat endocarditis and other life-threatening infections.[149,150]

The continuing problems with MRSA infections and infections due to coagulase-negative staphylocci have resulted in a major increase in the use of *vancomycin*.[151] This increase includes extensive use of vancomycin in initial treatment of nosocomial fevers and other infections in which MRSA and coagulase-negative staphylococci are considered among the possible pathogens. It is alarming that this excessive use of vancomycin increases the selective pressure for development of glycopeptide resistance among staphylococci and other Gram-positive pathogens. Although infections due to vancomycin-resistant staphylococci appear to be rare, serious infections due to vancomycin-resistant *S. haemolyticus* have been documented.[152,153]

#### 5.1.2 Enterococcal Infections

Enterococci are important pathogens capable of causing local and systemic infection in hospitalised patients. Data from the US National Nosocomial Infection Surveillance System (NNIS) show that enterococci are now the third most frequent nosocomial bloodstream pathogen and second and third most common causes of nosocomial urinary tract and wound infections, respectively.[146] These infections carry considerable morbidity and mortality, e.g. a 31% mortality rate was directly attributed to enterococcal blood stream infection in one study.[154]

In contrast to the streptococci, enterococci are relatively resistant to many antibiotics, including penicillin and ampicillin, and are intrinsically resistant to cefalosporins, semisynthetic penicillinase-resistant penicillins, and low concentrations of clindamycin and aminoglycosides. The increasing resistance of enterococci to aminoglycosides, penicillins, and most recently, to vancomycin is further cause for concern.[93] Because they resist many antimicrobial agents, enterococci survive and even thrive in the hospital environment.

Since the 1950s, treatment of serious enterococcal infection has involved the use of a combination of *penicillin* and an *aminoglycoside*. Simple urinary tract or other non–life-threatening infections may be treated adequately with penicillin or ampicillin alone. However, more serious infections usually require cell wall–active agents such as penicillin, ampicillin or vancomycin, plus an aminoglycoside, to attain bactericidal activity and therapeutic success. The emergence of high-concentration (>2000 mg/L) resistance to aminoglycosides and of major resistance to penicillins due to a low-affinity PBPs or β-lactamase production has complicated treatment of enterococcal infections. Specifically, organisms with high concentration aminoglycoside resistance are completely unresponsive to aminoglycosides and synergistic bactericidal activity will not be achieved by the combination of an aminoglycoside and a penicillin. Infections with these organisms may be treated with *vancomycin* or *teicoplanin*, although bactericidal activity may not be achieved in the face of high-concentration aminoglycoside resistance.[155]

The difficulties posed in treating enterococcal infections were compounded in the late 1980s with the discovery of vancomycin resistance among clinical enterococcal isolates. Subsequent nosocomial outbreaks of infections due to vancomycin-resistant enterococci (VRE) have been reported throughout the US and other parts of the world.[133] From 1989 to 1993, the percentage of nosocomial enterococcal infections due to VRE in the US increased from 0.3 to 7.9%.[93] The increase has been most profound in intensive care units, where a 34-fold increase in incidence has been noted.[93] The fact that VRE emerged against a background of high-concentration resistance to penicillins and aminoglycosides presents a serious challenge for clinicians treating patients with infections due to these organisms. Treatment options are frequently limited to combinations of antimicrobials or experimental agents with unproven effectiveness.[93,155]

Several species of enterococci resistant to vancomycin have been described, including *E. faecalis*, *E. faecium*, *E. avium*, and *E. gallinarum*. The resistant strains may be divided into 3 classes, Van A, Van B and Van C, on the basis of the level of resistance to vancomycin and teicoplanin and whether the glycopeptide resistance is inducible. Van A strains show inducible high-concentration (>64 mg/L) resistance to both vancomycin and teicoplanin, whereas Van B strains show inducible moderate (16 to 32 mg/L) concentrations of resistance to vancomycin, but not to teicoplanin. Van C strains show constitutive low-concentration (8 to 16 mg/L) resistance to vancomycin only. The expression of resistance is associated with the synthesis of a new protein, Van A, that may produce vancomycin resistance by either target protection or target modification.[92]

Resistance to high concentrations, but not to low concentrations, of vancomycin is transferable to other enterococci as well as to other species, including streptococci and *L. monocytogenes*. The ability to detect vancomycin resistance varies with the susceptibility testing method used in the laboratory.[156] Generally, broth dilution methods are adequate to detect vancomycin resistance. Disk agar diffusion using previously recommended interpretive zone sizes can fail to detect resistance, but zone size interpretive criteria have recently been modified to improve detection.[157]

Given the prominence of enterococci as nosocomial pathogens, the development and spread of multidrug resistant (MDR) strains may well be the most serious nosocomial threat of the 1990s.[93,155] The potential for enterococci to be the reservoir for resistance genes for other organisms is well known. Surveillance for MDR strains of enterococci should be considered by clinical laboratories. Many laboratories are currently screening enterococci for β-lactamase in addition to doing agar or broth screens for high-concentration aminoglycoside and vancomycin resistance. The limitations of automated systems in detecting resistant enterococci, particularly vancomycin and high-concentration aminoglycoside resistant strains, must be appreciated. Appropriate manual methods may be necessary to optimise detection of these important nosocomial pathogens.[156]

#### 5.1.3 Streptococcal Infections

Streptococci remain important agents of both nosocomial and community-acquired infection.

Viridans group streptococci are important agents of subacute bacterial endocarditis and are recently emerging as important causes of nosocomial bloodstream infection in immunocompromised patients.[158] These organisms are generally considered to be highly susceptible to penicillin (MIC up to 0.25 mg/L). However, the significance of bacteraemia due to viridans streptococci and the emergence of resistance to penicillin among isolates causing bloodstream infections in neutropenic patients undergoing chemotherapy for haematological malignancies was described recently.[158] The resistant isolates appeared to be selected by the inclusion of penicillin in an antimicrobial prophylaxis regimen used at the institution in question.

Among the streptococci, *S. pneumoniae* remains a significant pathogen. The growing incidence of penicillin-resistant *S. pneumoniae* is of major concern worldwide.[100,159] Penicillin-resistant pneumococci are often also resistant to macrolides, cotrimoxazole and third-generation cefalosporins including cefotaxime and ceftriaxone. The increasing frequency of penicillin-resistant pneumococci in the US was underscored by a report from Tennessee where 29% of isolates from children with otitis media were found to be resistant to penicillin.[91] Likewise, 18.5% and 12.9% of pneumococcal isolates in Dallas, Texas were resistant to penicillin and to cefotaxime or ceftriaxone, respectively.[160] This resistance is significant clinically and there are numerous reports of failure of penicillin and third-generation cefalosporin therapy due to resistant pneumococcal strains.[161-163]

Selection of penicillin- and cefalosporin-resistant *S. pneumoniae* is thought to be due to the excessive use of penicillin and other β-lactam antibiotics in the community setting.[100,159] Although management strategies for infection with resistant pneumococci are still evolving, *vancomycin, rifampicin* and *imipenem* appear to be useful in patients with pneumococcal pneumonia or meningitis.[100,159,162]

Given the increasing incidence of penicillin-resistant *S. pneumoniae*, laboratories must perform *in vitro* testing using methods that are adequate to detect penicillin- and cefalosporin-resistant strains.[100] Screening tests using oxacillin disks to detect penicillin resistance are recommended.[106] Isolates resistant by the oxacillin screening test should be confirmed by MIC testing with standard methods.[107] Isolates of *S. pneumoniae* from patients with pneumococcal pneumonia or meningitis should be tested for susceptibility to the first-choice drug plus at least 3 alternative drugs (e.g. ceftriaxone or cefotaxime, vancomycin, imipenem, rifampicin and chloramphenicol).[100,159] Empirical therapy should be based on available epidemiological data showing patterns of resistance.

Despite an apparent increase in the frequency and severity of Group A streptococcal infections in the US and Europe, the susceptibility of *S. pyogenes* to *penicillin* has not changed appreciably over the years. Penicillin remains unquestionably the drug of choice for infection with this organism. Penicillin-allergic patients may be treated with *erythromycin* or one of the newer macrolides with good results.

Group B streptococci remain an important cause of serious infection among neonates. This organism tends to be less susceptible to penicillin than Group A strains. Combination therapy with *penicillin* or *ampicillin* plus *gentamicin* may be used to provide synergistic bactericidal activity in serious Group B streptococcal infections.

#### 5.1.4 Infections with Gram-Negative Bacilli

Gram-negative bacilli as a group are among the most frequent and important causes of nosocomial infections.[146] They are also the most common cause of community-acquired urinary tract infection. In the hospital setting, Gram-negative bacilli commonly colonise patients who are debilitated by surgery, disease or chemotherapy. Infection is most likely in individuals requiring catheterisation, prolonged hospital stays or treatment in an intensive care unit.

It is now recognised that many Gram-negative nosocomial pathogens have developed broad-spectrum resistance to the newer β-lactam antibiotics through small changes in the structure of the TEM-1, TEM-3 and SHV-1 β-lactamase enzymes that they already possess. These extended-spectrum β-lactamases (ESβLs) mediate resistance to the extended-spectrum penicillins as well as to cefotaxime, cefuroxime, ceftriaxone, ceftazidime and aztreonam. They are particularly common in isolates of *E. coli*, *Klebsiella*, *Citrobacter* and *Serratia* spp. Frequently located on a transmissible plasmid, they may present simultaneously with other resistance factors (e.g. aminoglycoside and quinolone resistance), resulting in pathogens with broad antibiotic resistance profiles.[95,133] Organisms containing ESβLs have been responsible for a number of nosocomial outbreaks, usually originating in an intensive care unit.[96,132] Dissemination of ESβL-related drug resistance is usually associated with extensive use of broad-spectrum cefalosporins and may involve spread of a single strain of bacteria or horizontal spread of a resistance plasmid or other resistance genes.

Particularly problematical are Gram-negative species such as *Enterobacter cloacae*, *Enterobacter aerogenes*, *Serratia* spp., *Providencia* spp., *C. freundii*, *Morganella morganii* and *P. aeruginosa*. These organisms possess an inducible chromosomal type I cefalosporinase, and while laboratory tests may indicate susceptibility, they are not truly susceptible to the newer cefalosporins (e.g. cefotaxime, ceftriaxone, ceftazidime, cefoperazone). They typically possess a cefalosporinase capable of inactivating all the cefalosporins and penicillins.[135] The enzyme is not normally expressed, but can be induced to high concentrations on exposure of the organism to newer cefalosporins, resulting in resistance to multiple β-lactam antibiotics.[135]

Unfortunately, many *in vitro* susceptibility assays used in the laboratory fail to detect these new forms of resistance before induction of the enzyme. Those assays that are particularly susceptible to these errors include microdilution methods in which a relatively low inoculum of organisms ($10^5$ CFU/ml) are tested and rapid (4 to 6 hours' incubation) automated or semiautomated methods. Testing organisms using a macrobroth dilution method (1 to 5ml total volume), agar disk diffusion method, or by microdilution with sufficient inoculum ($5 \times 10^5$ CFU/ml) and an incubation time of 18 to 24 hours may be needed to detect this form of resistance.

Many resistance factors, including β-lactamase, aminoglycoside and chloramphenicol resistance genes, can be carried on mobile genetic elements or transposons. Members of the Tr 21-related transposons are capable of transferring a wide variety of resistance factors from organism to organism and are likely responsible for the development of many multidrug resistant (MDR) Gram-negative bacilli that have been implicated in nosocomial outbreaks. These MDR strains appear to arise following specific antibiotic selection pressure in hospitals. As such, the proliferation and spread of MDR strains is common in intensive care units and transplantation units where third-generation cefalosporin use is highest.[132]

Treatment of Gram-negative infections in the face of such broad resistance is increasingly difficult.[133] In many cases, empirical combination therapy is needed to provide adequate antibacterial coverage, since no single agent is reliably effective. Given these difficulties, it is critical that the laboratory use adequate methods to detect and trace the presence of MDR Gram-negative bacilli within the hospital. This type of laboratory-based surveillance goes hand-in-hand with efforts to limit selective pressures contributing to development of MDR strains.

β-Lactam antibiotics that can be used in the treatment of Gram-negative infections despite the presence of various β-lactamases are listed in table XV.[95] It should be noted that while strains making ESβLs may remain susceptible to cefamycins and carbapenems, resistance to these agents may arise due to other mechanisms such as permeability barriers.[164]

#### 5.1.5 Mycobacterial Infections

Serious infections due to *Mycobacterium* species, including *M. tuberculosis*, *M. avium*, and *M. intracellulare* have become extremely common in association with severe immunosuppression in patients with HIV and among the homeless.[99] Notably, several outbreaks of infection due to multidrug-resistant strains of *M. tuberculosis* (MDR-TB) have been identified. These outbreaks have occurred in shelters for the homeless, in AIDS treatment facilities and domiciliaries, and in hospitals (nosocomial infections), and have been linked to previously undiagnosed infections with heavy organism burdens.[98,99,148] The problems have been compounded by the multidrug-resistant nature of the organisms, lack of appropriate isolation facilities and the inherent delay in the methods of microbiological diagnosis and susceptibility testing used in many hospital laboratories.[99,165]

Tuberculosis and non-tubercular mycobacterioses require different treatment protocols. For example, a localised granuloma due to *Mycobacterium marinum* may be self-limiting and require no treatment, whereas pulmonary disease due to resistant *M. tuberculosis* requires the use of multidrug regimens over an extended period of time.

Ineffective therapy is the chief cause of increasing resistance among mycobacteria. Therapy can be ineffective because multiple drugs are not used where appropriate or because a pa-

**Table XV.** Options for treatment of infections caused by β-lactam-resistant Gram-negative bacilli (after Jacoby & Medeiros;[95] with permission)

| Enzyme or mechanisms of resistance | Clinical isolates | β-Lactams affected | β-Lactams not affected |
|---|---|---|---|
| Common plasmid-mediated β-lactamase | Many Gram-negative organisms | Ampicillin<br>Azlocillin<br>Carbenicilin<br>Cefamandole<br>Cefalothin<br>Mezlocillin<br>Piperacillin<br>Ticarcillin | Cefotetan<br>Cefoxitin<br>Extended-spectrum cefalosporins<br>Latamoxef (moxalactam)<br>Carbapenems<br>Monobactams |
| Plasmid-mediated extended-spectrum β-lactamase in TEM or SHV family | *K. pneumoniae*<br>*E. coli*<br>*C. freundii*<br>*S. marcescens*<br>*E. cloacae* | All drugs listed above *plus*:<br>Aztreonam<br>Cefotaxime<br>Ceftazidime<br>Ceftizoxime<br>Ceftriaxone<br>Cefuroxime | Cefmetazole<br>Cefotetan<br>Cefoxitin<br>Imipenem<br>Meropenem<br>Latamoxef |
| Constitutive production of chromosomal β-lactamase | *E. cloacae*<br>*C. freundii*<br>*P. aeruginosa*<br>*S. marcescens* | All drugs listed above *plus*:<br>Cefmetazole<br>Cefotetan<br>Cefoxitin<br>Latamoxef | Imipenem<br>Meropenem |
| Plasmid-mediated extended-spectrum β-lactamase related to Amp C | *K. pneumoniae*<br>*E. coli* | All drugs listed above | Imipenem<br>Meropenem |
| Carbapenem-hydrolysing chromosomal β-lactamase | *S. maltophilia*<br>*B. fragilis*<br>*S. marcescens*<br>*E. cloacae* | Imipenem<br>Meropenem | Variable |
| Plasmid-mediated β-lactamase conferring carbapenem resistance | *P. aeruginosa* | All drugs listed above | Aztreonam<br>Piperacillin |

tient is non-compliant with the long course of therapy necessary to cure infections with *M. tuberculosis* and other mycobacteria. The presence of MDR-TB (resistant to at least isoniazid and rifampicin) is an additional barrier to effective therapy of tuberculosis.

Effective antituberculosis therapy (see also chapter 23; sect. 9.2) depends on the susceptibility of the isolate to available antimicrobial agents and on the state of the disease process. Resistance, especially to isoniazid and rifampicin, is increasing.[99] Variables associated with an increased predictability of resistance include prior antituberculosis therapy and the patient's original country of residence.[99] Increased incidence of resistance has been especially prominent in Asian and Hispanic populations.

Recently, the combination of *isoniazid* and *rifampicin* administered for only 9 months has been found to be efficacious in uncomplicated tuberculosis.[123] The use of *pyrazinamide* in combination with isoniazid and rifampicin for the first 2 months allows the course of therapy to be shortened to 6 months. This is in contrast to the 2-year course of therapy recommended previously.[123] HIV-positive individuals should be treated for a total of 9 months with isoniazid and rifampicin and for at least 6 months beyond culture conversion.

MDR-TB requires the use of additional agents.[99,123] Four or 5 drugs should be used initially, usually isoniazid, rifampicin, pyrazinamide and ethambutol with or without streptomycin. Newer agents that may be useful include the quinolones ofloxacin and ciprofloxacin, and β-lactam/β-lactamase inhibitor combinations. Isoniazid continues to be recommended as prophylaxis (6 months) for appropriate individuals with recent skin test conversion who are otherwise disease free. The optimal prophylactic regimen for individuals exposed to MDR-TB is unknown. Most experts recommend 2 drugs for 1 year: pyrazinamide plus ofloxacin or pyrazinamide plus rifampicin if the organism is susceptible to rifampicin.

The final choice of agents for treatment of infections due to *M. tuberculosis* may be aided by *in vitro* susceptibility studies.[123,165] These studies may be performed using the standard proportion method or the more rapid broth-based radiometric method. Unfortunately, at present, the radiometric method can only be used to study susceptibility to isoniazid, rifampicin, ethambutol and streptomycin.

Members of the *M. avium* complex (*M. avium* and *M. intracellulare*) are notoriously resistant to antimicrobial agents and often must be treated with regimens combining 4 or more agents.[147] Combinations of isoniazid, rifampicin and pyrazinamide with ethionamide, streptomycin, capreomycin or kanamycin are often used. Clofazimine and rifabutin have been disappointing in some regimens for persons with AIDS. Surgical intervention is often recommended for localised disease. The clinical usefulness of *in vitro* susceptibility studies of *M. avium* complex has not been established.

## 5.2 Specific Diseases

### 5.2.1 Sepsis Syndrome

It is estimated that there are up to 300,000 cases of sepsis per year in the US. The incidence of sepsis syndrome has increased from 73.6 to 175.9 per 100,000 persons discharged from hospital between 1979 and 1987.[166] Mortality from Gram-negative sepsis ranges from 20 to 50% and is significantly higher among the 40% of individuals who develop shock and organ failure.[167] Several factors account for these problems, including Gram-negative bacteria, new modes of transmission of pathogens and a susceptible hospital population. Sepsis cannot be restricted to infection with Gram-negative organisms. In recent years it has become clear that a wide variety of micro-organisms can cause septic shock, including Gram-positive cocci, Gram-negative cocci, Gram-negative bacilli, yeasts, viruses and protozoa.

Risk factors for the development of sepsis include immunosuppressive treatments, invasive devices or procedures, penetrating wounds or other trauma, intestinal ulceration and progressive clinical conditions such as malignancy, AIDS, diabetes and other chronic illnesses.[167,168] Therapy for some of these illnesses may provide a focus of infection that may lead to septic shock. Prolonged survival of individuals with chronic progressive diseases due to improved treatment of the primary disease has resulted in a large population of patients at risk for systemic infection with Gram-positive and Gram-negative bacteria or fungi.

Bacteraemia or fungaemia is not a requirement for the diagnosis of sepsis, sepsis syndrome or septic shock. The factor that appears to be necessary, irrespective of the infecting organism, is the ability of the micro-organism to interact with the host to initiate a cascade of endogenous mediators [e.g. tumour necrosis factor (TNF), interleukins (IL-1, IL-6, etc.), prostaglandins, platelet-activating factor (PAF)]. The physiological changes affected by these mediators result in a stereotypical presentation recognised clinically as a spectrum of conditions ranging from sepsis to septic shock and finally to multiple organ dysfunction.[167,168]

The management of septic shock should focus on vigorous fluid resuscitation, appropriate use of pressors and antimicrobial therapy.

#### Antimicrobial Therapy

The early administration of appropriate antimicrobial therapy is extremely important in the management of early sepsis.[167] Antimicrobial therapy alone will not reduce mortality once this illness has progressed to severe sepsis or multiorgan failure. However, appropriate antimicrobial therapy may reduce shock and mortality rates by as much as 50%.[167] Because the results of blood cultures and susceptibility tests may not be available for 48 to 72 hours and more than 50% of deaths occur in the first 48 hours of illness, empirical parenteral broad-spectrum antimicrobial therapy is required. Selection of anti-infective therapy should be based on the probable source of infection, Gram-stained smears of appropriate clinical material, and the immune status of the patient. The choice should reflect the current status of antimicrobial resistance patterns in the community and in the hospital.

Standard empirical therapy generally includes an *extended-spectrum cefalosporin* (cefotaxime, ceftizoxime, cefoperazone, ceftriaxone or ceftazidime) or an *antipseudomonal penicillin* combined with an *aminoglycoside*. For nosocomial infections in non-neutropenic patients, *an extended-spectrum cefalosporin, imipenem* or *aztreonam* alone may be adequate, thus avoiding the potential toxicity (ototoxicity and nephrotoxicity) of the aminoglycosides. Coverage for suspected *P. aeruginosa* infection usually includes a β-lactam plus an aminoglycoside. The synergistic bactericidal activity of β-lactam and aminoglycoside combinations has been shown to be important in the treatment of both *Klebsiella* and *P. aeruginosa* infections in immunocompromised patients.[111,117,118]

**Immunomodulation Approaches**

In recent years, a great deal of effort has been expended in designing strategies to modify the clinical course of sepsis by either neutralising the effects of bacterial endotoxin or interrupting the inflammatory cascade.[167,168] Several large studies of novel therapeutic interventions for sepsis, such as antibodies to endotoxin, TNF, IL-1 and PAF, have been undertaken.[167-169] Although none of the interventions has shown efficacy in prospectively designed study groups, these studies have improved our understanding of the epidemiological and physiological characteristics of sepsis.[170] Despite claims that retrospectively defined subgroups may benefit,[167,169] it is clear that dramatic improvement in survival among critically ill patients is unlikely to be achieved with therapy directed against a single component in the complex cascade of mediators that produce the clinical picture of sepsis. Combination therapies with agents that block more than one step in the cascade, such as IL-1 and TNF, may provide greater benefit than previously observed with inhibition of a single mediator.

Thus, although modulation of the inflammatory response in general and anticytokine therapy in particular hold great interest and promise for the treatment of sepsis, clinical benefits have not yet been consistently shown (see also chapter 28; sect. 3.7).

### 5.2.2 Infections in Immunocompromised Patients

Infection is a constant hazard in the immunocompromised host and is the cause of death in a high proportion of cases. Infection may be difficult to diagnose and the initial evaluation frequently does not reveal a specific site or microbial cause of infection. In view of the wide range of potential pathogens, initial therapy tends to be empirical and broad-spectrum antimicrobial agents should be started without delay because untreated sepsis in such patients is rapidly fatal. Treatment strategies must take into account the prominent role of enteric Gram-negative bacilli and *P. aeruginosa*.

Based on studies of 2 antibiotics exhibiting *in vitro* synergy against Gram-negative bloodstream isolates, particularly *P. aeruginosa* and *Klebsiella* species,[111,118] many infectious disease specialists recommend concurrent use of an *aminoglycoside* and either an *extended-spectrum penicillin* (e.g. mezlocillin, piperacillin or ticarcillin) or another broad-spectrum β-lactam such as *ceftazidime* or *imipenem*. Alternatively, monotherapy with agents such a *ceftazidime, imipenem* or *piperacillin/tazobactam* have been advocated, particularly in non-neutropenic patients.[120] The advantage of one approach over the other is unclear, but most likely will vary depending on the various patients and hospital settings.

Because of the importance of Gram-positive cocci as causative agents of infection in immunocompromised patients, some clinicians advocate the addition of *vancomycin* to the regimen if there is suspected line sepsis or a cutaneous source of infection. The empirical use of vancomycin without strong evidence of infection with a β-lactam-resistant Gram-positive organism should be discouraged. Vancomycin use may be a risk factor for colonisation and infection with vancomycin-resistant enterococci[93] and the empirical addition of vancomycin to the initial treatment regimen has not been shown to improve outcome among cancer patients with fever and granulocytopenia.[171]

After starting empirical therapy, clinical parameters, particularly temperature and haemodynamics, should be monitored closely. Antimicrobial therapy should be tailored to the organism once a specific diagnosis has been established. In severely neutropenic patients (white blood cell count <500 cells/μl), antimicrobial therapy should be continued until neutropenia is resolved, since there is a substantial risk of relapse if the antimicrobial drugs are stopped while neutropenia persists. Once neutropenia resolves, antimicrobial drugs should be stopped, but it is probably wise to stop them after 1 to 2 weeks despite persistent neutropenia in patients with negative blood cultures or other diagnostic studies. If there is no initial clinical response, antimicrobial therapy should be re-evaluated after 2 to 3 days and possibly adjusted to optimise the Gram-negative coverage or add Gram-positive coverage. If there is no clinical response after 3 to 7 days of appropriate antibacterial therapy, the possibility of a fungal infection must considered seriously. Use of empirical amphotericin B or a newer azole antifungal agent (fluconazole or itraconazole) may be appropriate (see further section 6), but the exact indications, choice of agent or duration of therapy remain uncertain at this time.

#### 5.2.3 Bacterial Meningitis

Acute meningitis is a major medical emergency where rapid diagnosis and the initiation of appropriate antimicrobial treatment at the earliest possible moment are essential. Failure to do this may result in the patient dying or suffering irreversible brain damage. Despite advances in diagnostic techniques and the introduction of newer antimicrobial agents and therapeutic modalities, bacterial meningitis remains an important infectious disease with significant morbidity and mortality.

Although *S. pneumoniae* and *Neisseria meningitidis* remain prominent causes of meningitis worldwide, in many areas, a substantial (≈85%) reduction in invasive *H. influenzae* disease has been observed since the introduction of vaccines in the mid-1980s.[101] Group B streptococci are now the most important cause of bacterial meningitis in neonates and *L. monocytogenes* is occasionally isolated from neonates and adults. Enteric Gram-negative bacilli can also cause meningitis, especially in newborn infants, patients >60 years of age, and in those who have had neurosurgery or have a compromised immune response. Meningitis due to *S. epidermidis* and other coagulase-negative staphylococci frequently complicates the placement of central nervous system shunts and is an increasingly common cause of nosocomial meningitis.

The diagnosis of meningitis rests on examination of the cerebrospinal fluid (CSF). There is a plethora of new tests including antigen detection, CSF lactate, C-reactive protein, limulus lysate assay, polymerase chain reaction (PCR) and tests for TNF and IL-1. However, the diagnosis of meningitis still rests on interpretation of traditional CSF parameters (opening pressure, protein, glucose and white blood cell count) and CSF Gram-stain.

The general approach to a patient with bacterial meningitis requires recognition of the problem, early identification of the pathogen, and rapid initiation of antimicrobial therapy.[172] Although specimens of CSF and blood should be obtained for laboratory examination and culture, antimicrobial drugs should not be withheld until laboratory studies are complete. If focal findings are present on neurological examination, a computed tomography (CT) scan may be warranted to rule out a mass lesion, because some processes, particularly brain abscess, may lead to serious consequences following lumbar puncture. The time from initial evaluation to onset of antimicrobial therapy with a bactericidal agent should not exceed 30 minutes. In addition to antimicrobial therapy, close observation and treatment of complications (e.g. shock, disseminated intravascular coagulation, or the syndrome of inappropriate antidiuretic hormone secretion) are mandatory.

To treat meningitis, pending results of cultures, most specialists recommend *cefotaxime* or *ceftriaxone* both in adults and in children over 3 months of age. *Benzylpenicillin* (penicillin G) is first-line therapy for penicillin-susceptible meningococcal or pneumococcal meningitis. However, the recent appearance of relatively resistant meningococci and pneumococci in many geographic areas has necessitated a change in this recommendation.[100] The finding of penicillin-resistant pneumococci with increased MIC values for third-generation cefalosporins has made the addition of *vancomycin* to the initial antimicrobial regimen necessary in some areas.[163]

Although rare in immunised populations, when *H. influenzae* occurs, it is best treated with a third-generation cefalosporin. Group B streptococci and *L. monocytogenes* may be treated effectively with *ampicillin* with or without *gentamicin*. For meningitis due to *P. aeruginosa*, concurrent use of *ceftazidime* and an *aminoglycoside* is recommended. Other aerobic Gram-negative bacilli may be treated effectively with a third-generation cefalosporin alone. Shunt infections due to coagulase-negative staphylococci require vancomycin with or without rifampicin.

In penicillin-allergic individuals, cefotaxime or ceftriaxone may be used, although some patients may also have allergic reactions to these agents. Alternatives to penicillins and cefalosporins are not entirely satisfactory, but include chloramphenicol, vancomycin with or without rifampicin (for Gram-positive organisms only), and cotrimoxazole (for *Listeria*).

The standard therapy for neonatal meningitis remains *ampicillin* plus an *aminoglycoside* (see further chapter 3; sect. 4.2.3 and table V). This regimen provides adequate coverage for aerobic Gram-negative bacilli, group B streptococci and *L. monocytogenes*. To avoid the problems with the administration of aminoglycosides, many experts now recommend *ampicillin* plus *cefotaxime* as initial therapy pending the results of culture and susceptibility tests.

Adjunctive therapy to improve survival and decrease neurological sequelae in patients with meningitis has received a great deal of attention in recent years. Current evidence suggests that the administration of dexamethasone is beneficial in children with purulent meningitis of presumed or proved *H. influenzae* origin.[173] The use of adjunctive corticosteroids in other age groups (neonates or adults) or in meningitis due to other causes remains controversial and cannot be recommended routinely at present.[174]

#### *5.2.4 Pneumonia*

Pneumonia remains an exceedingly important cause of morbidity, mortality and hospital admissions worldwide (see also chapter 23; sect. 6). In the US, more than 3 million cases of community-acquired pneumonia each year result in over 500,000 hospital admissions. Nosocomial pneumonia accounts for 15% of all hospital-acquired infections, has an associated mortality of 20 to 50% and on average adds ≈6 excess days to a hospital stay.[146] Overall, pneumonia ranks as the 6th leading cause of death in the US.

Clinical criteria for the diagnosis of pneumonia vary, but diagnosis is generally established by a combination of clinical, roentgenographic and laboratory evidence of infection. Most criteria include new onset of purulent sputum, new or progressive pulmonary infiltrate on x-ray, and culture of sputum or other respiratory secretions. In seriously ill or immunocompromised individuals, specimens may need to be obtained by transtracheal aspiration, bronchoalveolar lavage (BAL), protected specimen brush bronchoscopy or open lung biopsy. Unfortunately, a specific microbiological diagnosis is frequently elusive.

Among potential causes of community-acquired pneumonia, *S. pneumoniae* remains the most common cause of pneumonia leading to hospitalisation. Other agents causing community-acquired pneumonia include *Legionella* spp., *Mycoplasma* spp., *Chlamydia pneumoniae*, *H. influenzae* and *Moraxella catarrhalis*. Additionally, in the era of HIV infection, *P. carinii* and *M. tuberculosis* must also be considered as agents causing a community-acquired pneumonia-like illness in HIV-infected patients.

Approximately 50% of nosocomial pneumonias are caused by Gram-negative bacilli, 20% by Gram-positive cocci and 5% by fungi.[146] *P. aeruginosa*, *Klebsiella*, *Acinetobacter* and *Enterobacter* species are among the most common Gram-negative causes. Individuals with chronic pulmonary disease may develop infections due to *H. influenzae* or *M. catarrhalis*. Important Gram-positive pathogens include *S. pneumoniae* and *S. aureus*. Hospitalised immunocompromised patients are at risk of infections due to *Legionella* and *Aspergillus* spp.

Although penicillins remain useful in the treatment of many community-acquired infections, the emergence of resistant species limits the effectiveness of these agents. Most strains of *M. catarrhalis* and 15 to 20% of *H. influenzae* produce β-lactamase. Relative resistance to penicillin among *S. pneumoniae* further complicates the issue.

Initial therapy of community-acquired pneumonia should be based on the clinical presentation, degree of illness and results of the sputum Gram-stain and chest x-ray. Generally, pneumonia due to *S. pneumoniae* that presents in a typical fashion and is positive on Gram-stain will respond well to either a *penicillin* or a *second-generation cefalosporin*. Individuals with sputum Gram-stain results suggestive of *H. influenzae* or *M. catarrhalis* can be treated with a second- or third-generation *cefalosporin* or with *amoxicillin/clavulanic acid* or *cotrimoxazole*. If the clinical presentation is atypical and/or the sputum Gram-stain is unrevealing, *tetracycline* or *erythromycin* are generally effective. Quinolones are also effective against most community-acquired pathogens, but are not considered optimal due to lack of activity against *S. pneumoniae*. Two new macrolides, *azithromycin* and *clarithromycin*, offer broad-spectrum coverage against respiratory pathogens including *S. pneumoniae*, *H. influenzae* and *M. catarrhalis*. They are also active against *Mycoplasma pneumoniae*, *Chlamydia pneumoniae* and *Legionella pneumophila*.

As with other serious nosocomial infections, the initial treatment of nosocomial pneumonia requires a broad-spectrum approach including agents that will cover *P. aeruginosa*. Thus, an *antipseudomonal penicillin* or *broad-spectrum cefalosporin* plus an *aminoglycoside* is appropriate pending the results of culture and susceptibility testing. Pneumonia due to *S. aureus* should be treated with a *penicillinase-resistant penicillin* or with *vancomycin* if the organism is methicillin-resistant. Where *Legionella* is suspected, *erythromycin* should be added until cultures, DNA probe or antigen tests are completed. Finally, if the clinical setting is suggestive of a fungal cause, consideration must be given to specific antifungal therapy (see section 6). If possible, culture and histopathological evidence documenting fungal invasion should be obtained, but this frequently cannot occur, and presumptive therapy with amphotericin B must be initiated.

#### *5.2.5 Urinary Tract Infections*

Both asymptomatic and symptomatic urinary tract infections (UTI) are common clinical problems, accounting for up to 40% of all nosocomial infections and for more than 10 million office visits and 1 million hospital admissions annually in the US alone (see also chapter 24; sect. 3).[146,175] The most common causative agents include Enterobacteriaceae (particularly *E. coli*, *Klebsiella* spp. and *P. mirabilis*), *Staphylococcus saprophyticus* (young women) and enterococci. In complicated UTI, the range of possible causative agents is broader and includes *E. coli*, *Klebsiella*, *Proteus*, *Providencia*, *Morganella*, *Serratia* and *Pseudomonas* species, staphylococci, enterococci and *Candida* spp. (including *Torulopsis glabrata*). Bacterial resistance to the most commonly used antimicrobial drugs is increasing, so in both hospital and general practice patients, *in vitro* susceptibility testing has become more important in ensuring effective treatment. Over 25% of *E. coli* strains causing acute cystitis demonstrate *in vitro* resistance to sulfonamides, nitrofurantoin and amoxicillin. Resistance to trimethoprim and cotrimoxazole occurs in 5 to 15% of organisms and varies geographically, whereas resistance to the quinolones remains <5% in most regions in the US.[175]

##### Uncomplicated Infections

Many simple UTIs will respond to a short course (1 to 3 days) of antimicrobial therapy. Regimens of 7 days or longer offer little in terms of increased effectiveness and have significant disadvantages in terms of cost and adverse effects. Single-dose regimens (see chapter 24; sect. 3.1.1) are effective, have fewer adverse effects and cost less, but have higher early recurrence rates, especially with β-lactam drugs such as amoxicillin or oral cefalosporins. Three days of therapy with most antimicrobials appears optimal and offers decreased relapse rates without increased adverse effects.[175] The low rate of *in vitro* resistance coupled with favourable pharmacokinetics make *cotrimoxazole* and *quinolones* optimal choices for 3-day therapy of uncomplicated UTI.

##### Recurrent Infections

Recurrent infections (2 or more per year) occur in about 20 to 25% of women after the initial episode of acute uncomplicated UTI.[175] Management of recurrent UTI generally requires a full 7-day course of antimicrobial therapy with follow-up at 1 and 5 weeks after the end of treatment. In these circumstances, the choice of antibiotic therapy should be guided by *in vitro* susceptibility of the causative organism. In most cases, recurrent UTIs can be effectively prevented by antimicrobial prophylaxis. This can be administered in several ways: on a continuous daily or every other day (3 times weekly) basis, or after intercourse in women whose infections are temporally related to intercourse. Low doses of *trimethoprim* (100mg), *cotrimoxazole* (trimethoprim 40mg and sulfamethoxazole 200mg, i.e. half of a single strength tablet), *nitrofurantoin* (100mg) or *norfloxacin* (200mg) can be used (see also chapter 24; sect. 3.2).

##### Pyelonephritis

Treatment of acute pyelonephritis must often start with parenteral antimicrobial therapy because such patients often experience nausea and vomiting and up to 20% will have concomitant bacteraemia. Causative organisms include *E. coli* (80%), *S. saprophyticus*, enterococci, *Klebsiella* and *Proteus* spp. Because >30% of organisms causing acute uncomplicated pyelonephritis exhibit resistance to ampicillin and amoxicillin, these agents should not be used if results of *in vitro* susceptibility tests are not available. Initial selection of therapy should be based on a Gram-stain of urine. Gram-negative rods can be treated with a variety of regimens. For patients requiring initial parenteral therapy, *cotrimoxazole*, *ciprofloxacin*, *ofloxacin* or *gentamicin* can be used. In most cases, clinical improvement is noted after 48 to 72 hours and the remainder of 14 days of therapy can be given orally. Gram-positive cocci, usually enterococci, are rare causes of pyelonephritis, but require treatment with *ampicillin* and *gentamicin*.

##### Prostatitis

The management of prostatitis depends on isolation of the infecting organism because the cause may vary. Causative organisms include *E. coli*, other Enterobacteriaceae, *Pseudomonas* and enterococci. Prostatic infection can be confirmed by prostatic massage and culture of appropriate specimens including a first-void urine, midstream urine, prostatic expressate and postmassage expressate. Each organism isolated should be followed up.

Eradication of the infecting organism from the prostate usually requires prolonged therapy with an antimicrobial agent that penetrates the gland. *Cotrimoxazole* given for 6 to 12 weeks is successful in up to 70% of cases with susceptible organisms, but not all infecting strains are susceptible. The quinolones *ciprofloxacin* and *ofloxacin* penetrate well into prostatic tissue, have a broad antibacterial spectrum and may cure 70 to 80% of cases. Ciprofloxacin 500mg twice daily or ofloxacin 400mg twice daily can be given for 4 to 6 weeks. In exceptionally difficult cases, a modified radical prostatectomy may be performed to eradicate the source of infection. In less severe persistent infections, long term low-dose suppressive therapy can be given to prevent symptoms and urinary tract infection (cystitis).

## 6. Antifungal Chemotherapy

The emergence of fungal pathogens, such as *Candida* spp., *Cryptococcus neoformans* and *Aspergillus* spp., among others, as important agents of human infection has resulted in an increase in the use of systemic antifungal agents worldwide and the introduction of new antifungal agents with systemic activity (table XVI). Although the principles of antifungal chemotherapy are essentially the same as those for antibacterial therapy, it is useful to deal separately with antifungal therapy, given the major structural and biochemical differences that exist between fungi and bacteria. As a result of these differences, therapy of fungal infections involves a different strategy of microbial inhibition and completely different antimicrobial agents than those used for antibacterial therapy.[177]

A variety of systemically active antifungal agents are available, including representatives of polyene macrolides (amphotericin B, amphotericin B lipid complex, liposomal amphotericin B and amphotericin B cholesterol dispersion), azoles (miconazole, ketoconazole, fluconazole and itraconazole) and flucytosine, an inhibitor of pyrimidine synthesis (table XVI).

### 6.1 Systemic Antifungal Agents

#### *6.1.1 The Polyenes*

Amphotericin B remains the 'gold standard' for the treatment of life-threatening fungal infections. Amphotericin B and the liposomal and lipid complex formulations of amphotericin B

**Table XVI.** Established and investigational antifungal agents with systemic activity (after Pfaller;[173] with permission)

| Drug | Route | Mechanism | Comments |
|---|---|---|---|
| **Polyenes:** | | | |
| Amphotericin B | IV | Binds to ergosterol causing direct membrane damage | Established agent<br>Broad-spectrum activity<br>Toxic |
| Amphotericin B lipid complex | IV | As for amphotericin B | Investigational agent<br>Less toxic than amphotericin B |
| Liposomal amphotericin B | IV | As for amphotericin B | Investigational agent<br>Less toxic than amphotericin B |
| Amphotericin B cholesterol dispersion | IV | As for amphotericin B | Investigational agent<br>Less toxic than amphotericin B |
| **Azoles:** | | | |
| Miconazole | IV | Inhibition of membrane sterol synthesis | Toxic agent with modest activity against *Candida* and other yeasts<br>Active against *Pseudallescheria boydii* |
| Ketoconazole | PO | As for miconazole | Established agent with modest broad-spectrum activity |
| Fluconazole | PO, IV | As for miconazole | Triazole with broad-spectrum activity<br>Good central nervous system penetration<br>Good *in vivo* activity against *Candida* and *Cryptococcus neoformans* |
| Itraconazole | | As for miconazole | Triazole with broad-spectrum activity including *Aspergillus* spp.<br>Excellent *in vivo* activity against endemic mycoses |
| **Nucleic acid synthesis inhibitors:** | | | |
| Flucytosine | PO | Inhibition of DNA and RNA synthesis | Toxicity and resistance are problems<br>Used in combination with amphotericin B |

*Abbreviations:* IV = intravenous; PO = oral.

act by binding to ergosterol in the fungal cell membrane, causing loss of membrane integrity and osmotic instability. Changes in the membrane sterols have been correlated with the development of resistance to amphotericin B both *in vitro* and *in vivo*. Although amphotericin B resistance is rare, it has assumed clinical importance with certain species such as *Candida lusitaniae*, *Trichosporon beigelii* and *Pseudallescheria boydii*.

Amphotericin B is first-line therapy for aspergillosis, haematogenously disseminated candidiasis, cryptococcosis, and zygomycosis.[178,179] It is also a mainstay in the treatment of the endemic mycoses, coccidioidomycosis, histoplasmosis and blastomycosis (table XVII). Unfortunately, the therapeutic effectiveness of amphotericin B is limited, particularly in severely immunosuppressed patients. Although the drug is reasonably effective in treating candidaemia,[180] it has been generally ineffective in the treatment of infections due to *Aspergillus*, *Fusarium* and *Trichosporon* spp. Early or empirical amphotericin B therapy has been somewhat efficacious in preventing fungal infections in neutropenic patients[179,181] and high-dose amphotericin B therapy (0.7 to 1.5 mg/kg daily) may result in improved outcomes in patients with invasive aspergillosis.[182] Clearly, the recovery of the immune system, particularly the reversal of neutropenia, is a major factor in determining the outcome of fungal infections, irrespective of the antifungal agent used.

***Tolerability:*** a major hindrance in the use of amphotericin B clinically is the toxicity associated with its parenteral administration. Adverse effects of amphotericin B include nephrotoxicity, phlebitis, hypokalaemia, anaemia, headache, flushing, fever, chills, nausea and vomiting and, rarely, seizures and cardiac arrhythmias.[182] Efforts to minimise amphotericin B toxicity have been extensive and include administration of antipyretics and antihistamines, sodium repletion and avoidance of concurrent use of aminoglycosides, diuretics and cyclosporin.

Because of the severe and limiting toxicity associated with amphotericin B, several alternative formulations using liposomal or lipid complex delivery systems have been developed (table XVI).[183] Liposomal encapsulation, cholesterol dispersion and lipid complex delivery systems are designed to increase the therapeutic index of amphotericin B and to maximise the delivery of the drug in patients with deep-seated fungal infections, such as hepatosplenic candidiasis. These preparations all have selec-

**Table XVII.** Antifungal therapy for deep mycoses (after Pfaller;[173] with permission)

| Infection | First-line agents | Alternatives[a] |
|---|---|---|
| Aspergillosis | Amphotericin B (± flucytosine) | Itraconazole |
| Blastomycosis | Amphotericin B<br>Itraconazole[b] | Ketoconazole[b] |
| Candidiasis | Amphotericin B (± flucytosine) | Fluconazole<br>Itraconazole |
| Chromomycosis | Itraconazole | Flucytosine |
| Coccidioidomycosis | Amphotericin B | Ketoconazole[b]<br>Itraconazole[b]<br>Fluconazole[c]<br>Intrathecal amphotericin B[c] |
| Cryptococcosis | Amphotericin B (± flucytosine) | Fluconazole |
| Fusariosis | Amphotericin B | Itraconazole |
| Histoplasmosis | Amphotericin B<br>Itraconazole[d] | Ketoconazole[d]<br>Fluconazole[d] |
| Phaeohyphomycosis | Amphotericin B | Itraconazole |
| Pseudallescheriosis | Itraconazole | Miconazole or ketoconazole |
| Sporotrichosis | Itraconazole[e]<br>Amphotericin B[f] | Oral iodides[e] |
| Trichosporonosis | Amphotericin B | None established |
| Zygomycosis | Amphotericin B | None established |

a Limited data exist for most alternative agents.

b Indolent, nonmeningeal.

c Meningeal.

d Chronic pulmonary or indolent, nonmeningeal disseminated infection.

e Lymphocutaneous.

f Extracutaneous.

tive toxicity for fungal cells and theoretically increase the delivery of amphotericin B to the site of infection, while avoiding the toxicity of high doses of the drug. The available clinical data indicate that these formulations allow the administration of higher doses of amphotericin B (>2.5 mg/kg daily) with no increase in acute toxicity or evidence of dose-limiting nephrotoxicity.[178] Although preliminary data on the clinical effectiveness of these formulations is promising, they must be studied further in controlled, randomised clinical trials.

#### *6.1.2 The Azoles*

The azole class of antifungal compounds consists of an ever-increasing number of agents with systemic antifungal activity (table XVI). Azoles interact with cytochrome P450-dependent enzymes with resulting impairment of ergosterol synthesis and depletion of ergosterol in the fungal cell membrane. This results in the inhibition of fungal cell growth.

The imidazoles *miconazole* and *ketoconazole* are established broad-spectrum agents active against a variety of fungal pathogens including yeasts, dimorphic organisms, dermatophytes and opportunistic pathogens (table XVII). Although miconazole is active in infections due to *Candida* spp., *C. neoformans*, *Histoplasmas capsulatum*, *Paracoccidioides brasiliensis* and *Coccidioides immitis*, it is not an effective replacement for amphotericin B. Ketoconazole is used for some of the endemic mycoses and may be considered as a useful alternative to amphotericin B for non-meningeal blastomycosis and paracoccidioidomycosis, chronic cavitary histoplasmosis, disseminated histoplasmosis in non-immunosuppressed patients, and certain (non-meningeal) conditions of coccidioidomycosis (table XVII). Ketoconazole has not improved the management of serious fungal infections in immunosuppressed or neutropenic patients and should not be used to treat haematogenously disseminated or localised deep visceral fungal infections in these patients.

The triazoles *fluconazole* and *itraconazole* show promise as broad-spectrum, orally active, systemic antifungal agents.[184] Fluconazole is available in both oral and parenteral forms and has favourable pharmacokinetic characteristics, with >90% bioavailability, little protein or tissue binding, wide distribution throughout the body, and excretion largely unchanged via the kidneys. Fluconazole appears to be effective in the therapy of dermatomycoses; oral, vaginal, and oesophageal candidiasis; and for maintenance therapy in AIDS patients with cryptococcal meningitis. Recently, fluconazole has proven to be equivalent to amphotericin B in treating candidaemia in non-neutropenic patients.[180] It is also effective in the treatment of infections due to the endemic fungal pathogens (coccidioidomycosis, blastomycosis and histoplasmosis), but whether it is equal to other agents such as itraconazole is not yet established.

Fluconazole has little useful clinical activity against most filamentous fungi including *Aspergillus* spp. and the *Zygomycetes*. Reports of clinical resistance to fluconazole have begun to appear and include instances of superinfection with natively resistant species such as *Candida krusei* and decreased susceptibility to fluconazole among *C. albicans* isolates from AIDS patients with oropharyngeal candidiasis.[185,186] Development of resistance is encouraged by the widespread use of fluconazole for extended periods of time in highly immunosuppressed populations. At present, the clinical indications for fluconazole are limited in scope and include superficial yeast infections, treatment of candidaemia in non-neutropenic patients, and maintenance therapy in patients with cryptococcal meningitis.

Itraconazole is an orally active lipophilic triazole with acceptable bioavailability, high protein binding and good tissue distribution. It has been most completely assessed in endemic mycoses for its tolerability and effectiveness and may be considered the agent of choice for the treatment of blastomycosis, histoplasmosis, paracoccidioidomycosis, sporotrichosis and chromomycosis. Itraconazole is efficacious in selected cases of coccidioidomycosis and may be useful in the treatment of phaeohyphomycosis. It is also useful in the treatment of acute and chronic aspergillosis and has produced remissions in patients who were neutropenic or receiving continued immunosuppressive therapy.[187-189] The activity of itraconazole against *Aspergillus* species represents a potentially clinically important extension of the antifungal spectrum of the azoles. Further controlled trials will be necessary to clarify its use in various clinical settings.

***Tolerability:*** although the azoles are easier to administer and considerably less toxic than amphotericin B, there are certain adverse occurrences that may limit their use in selected individuals. While oral administration is usually considered an advantage for the azoles, the absorption of ketoconazole and itraconazole is dependent on an acidic environment and may be impaired in bone marrow transplant and AIDS patients and those receiving antacids and $H_2$-receptor antagonists. Parenteral administration of miconazole is frequently limited due to toxicity ascribed to the solvent (polyethoxylated castor oil), including anorexia, nausea, vomiting, headache, cardiac arrest and intense pruritus. Important dose-limiting toxicity of ketoconazole includes anorexia, nausea and vomiting, and, less commonly, hepatotoxicity and endocrinological abnormalities.

The triazoles, fluconazole and itraconazole, have less affinity for mammalian cytochromes than ketoconazole and, thus, produce less inhibition of corticosteroid synthesis and consequently fewer endocrinological abnormalities.

***Drug interactions:*** both ketoconazole and itraconazole are susceptible to agents that increase their hepatic metabolism. Rifampicin, phenytoin and isoniazid all reduce serum concentrations of ketoconazole, and rifampicin and phenytoin have the same effect on itraconazole. Conversely, serum concentrations of digoxin, terfenadine, astemizole, cyclosporin and phenytoin may be increased by concurrent administration of ketoconazole or itraconazole. Concurrent administration of ketoconazole or itraconazole with terfenadine or astemizole may result in life-threatening cardiac arrhythmias (ventricular tachycardia and ventricular fibrillation). Cyclosporin concentrations should be measured whenever that drug is used in conjunction with ketoconazole or itraconazole, and neither terfenadine nor astemizole should be used with these agents. Fluconazole is much less affected by such interactions. For further discussion on these drug interactions, see chapter 7 and appendix B.

#### *6.1.3 Flucytosine*

Flucytosine is a water-soluble fluorinated pyrimidine antimetabolite used orally (the parenteral form is investigational) in the treatment of systemic infections caused by susceptible pathogenic or opportunistic yeasts and fungi. This compound acts by being deaminated in the fungal cell to fluorouracil, which interferes with nucleic acid biosynthesis. The spectrum of susceptible fungal pathogens is narrow and includes *Candida* species, *C. neoformans* and some agents of chromoblastomycosis.

*In vitro* susceptibility testing with flucytosine is more important clinically than testing with either the polyenes or the azoles, because both primary and secondary resistance is observed. It is estimated that 5 to 10% of isolates of *C. neoformans* and *Candida* species are inherently resistant to flucytosine and that at least 5% of susceptible organisms develop resistance during therapy. For these reasons, flucytosine is almost never used alone in the treatment of serious fungal infections. Because the combination of flucytosine and amphotericin B has been shown to have synergistic antifungal activity *in vitro*, it has been used most commonly in the treatment of cryptococcosis and candidiasis. The clinical effectiveness of this combination has been documented in controlled clinical trials for cryptococcal meningitis, but not for other fungal infections.

***Tolerability:*** adverse effects associated with the use of flucytosine limit its clinical utility and include bone marrow suppression, and liver and gastrointestinal toxicity. The bone marrow toxicity is the most difficult to manage and is associated with serum flucytosine concentrations in excess of 100 mg/L. Because flucytosine is excreted almost exclusively by the kidney, it is recommended that both renal function and flucytosine serum concentrations be monitored frequently throughout administration of the drug to assure optimal antifungal therapy. The desired target concentration of flucytosine is 50 to 70 mg/L (peak level).

### 6.2 Combination Antifungal Therapy

Combinations of various antifungal agents have been investigated in efforts to achieve maximal fungicidal activity and minimise the toxicity associated with amphotericin B.[182] However, amphotericin B plus flucytosine is the only antifungal combination with documented clinical effectiveness. In addition to the treatment of cryptococcal meningitis, it has been suggested that survival of patients with *Candida tropicalis* fungaemia is improved when these patients are treated with amphotericin B plus flucytosine, as compared with historical controls treated with amphotericin B alone.[178] The use of this combination must be accompanied by an awareness that the nephrotoxicity associated with amphotericin B may make it difficult to control the serum concentration of flucytosine and avoid bone marrow toxicity.

Other combinations that have been studied include amphotericin B and rifampicin, amphotericin B and azoles, and azoles plus flucytosine. Although several of these combinations have been found to be additive or synergistic *in vitro*, documentation of their clinical effectiveness is currently anecdotal at best.

### 6.3 Antifungal Susceptibility Testing

The increase in fungal infections, increased availability and use of new and established antifungal agents, and the increased awareness of resistant fungal species have all resulted in greater attention to methods of *in vitro* susceptibility testing of antifungal agents. The rationale for performing antifungal susceptibility testing is the same as for antibacterial testing (see section 2.2), i.e. to provide the clinician with a reliable measure of the relative activity of the available antifungal agents and to provide a means of monitoring the development of resistance among a normally susceptible population of organisms.[190,191] As a result of these various clinical pressures, microbiology laboratories are now being asked to assume a greater role in the selection and monitoring of antifungal therapy.

In response to these demands, the National Committee for Clinical Laboratory Standards (NCCLS) in the US has established a subcommittee to develop a reference method for *in vitro* susceptibility testing of fungi as a means of standardising methodology used in clinical laboratories. Over the past decade, collaborative efforts by the NCCLS and other groups have resulted in development of a macrodilution reference method for susceptibility testing of yeast isolates that is reliable and promises to facilitate both research and clinical evaluation of antifungal agents.[192] Although the clinical relevance of *in vitro* antifungal susceptibility testing is not yet firmly established, it is readily apparent that such evidence is accumulating at a slow but steady pace.[185,193,194] Further work is necessary to refine test methods and evaluate the clinical relevance of fungal susceptibility test results for both immunocompromised and non-immunocompromised individuals with localised and disseminated infection.[191]

## 7. Prophylactic Use of Antimicrobial Drugs

There are few topics involving antimicrobial drugs that have engendered more confusion than that of prophylaxis. The principle of successful prophylaxis is simple: namely, to be aware of the potential pathogens to be guarded against and to use an antimicrobial agent appropriate for that purpose, and at the same time, to avoid drug toxicity. Examples of effective prophylaxis are:

- Antistreptococcal drugs in patients with rheumatic heart disease
- Agents active against *Clostridium perfringens* for above the knee amputations and hip replacement
- Metronidazole for protection against *Bacteroides* species in appendectomy with local peritonitis.

In these indications, prophylaxis is effective therapeutically and prevents complications. Because the drugs are used in low dosages for a short period, they are unlikely to have toxic effects.

The problem of inappropriate antimicrobial prophylaxis is a major one. About one-third of all hospital patients at any one time are receiving some sort of antimicrobial drug and in up to 60% of these cases, there is no evidence of an infection against which the prescribed drug would be effective. It must be assumed, therefore, that this represents prophylactic use. An example of irrational and ineffective prophylaxis is the wholesale use of broad-spectrum β-lactam agents in immunocompromised patients without fever or other evidence of infection. This practice seems often to be accompanied by colonisation (and sometimes infection) of the patient with resistant organisms such as R-factor–bearing *Klebsiella* or *Enterobacter* spp., enterococci or *Candida* spp. It would be logical to blame the practice for the continued increase in the incidence of antibiotic resistance in hospitals.

Prophylactic therapy should be limited to those procedures and patients in whom infection is a significant problem. Antimicrobial prophylaxis in surgery is now an established principle for clean-contaminated, contaminated and some clean operative procedures.[195] In general, *cefazolin* is the drug of choice for prevention of *S. aureus* as the major pathogen. In some institutions with *S. aureus* strains resistant to cefazolin, a second-generation cefalosporin such as *cefuroxime* or *cefamandole* may be useful. The rational usage of prophylactic antimicrobial therapy demands that the drug concentration should be high at the site of possible infection when the operation is carried out and that the duration of prophylactic therapy should be as short as possible. Several studies have documented considerable variation in the timing of antibiotics given for surgical prophylaxis, and timing of administration is now known to be important.

Antibiotic prophylaxis is most effective in preventing surgical wound infection if given in the 2 hours before the surgical incision.[195] If the timing of administration is correct, 1 day of antimicrobial prophylaxis is probably sufficient in most cases. When compounds with appropriate pharmacokinetics are used, 1- or 2-dose therapy should usually suffice.

## 8. Principal Adverse Effects of Antimicrobial Drugs

Considering that large doses of up to 20 g/day of some antimicrobial drugs may be given to sick patients, the incidence and nature of adverse effects is remarkably low. Skin rashes are the most common adverse effect caused by antimicrobial drugs. The less well absorbed oral compounds may cause diarrhoea or in a few cases pseudomembranous colitis. Some adverse effects associated with specific antimicrobial drugs or groups of drugs are discussed in this section.

### 8.1 β-Lactams

Common adverse effects of β-lactam agents include allergic reactions, diarrhoea, and drug fever. About 10% of the population give a history of skin rashes after having taken a penicillin, but in about one-half of these, there is no response on further challenge. The true overall incidence of penicillin allergy is therefore ≈5%. β-Lactam compounds combine with body proteins to form haptens that evoke the formation of antibodies. If these antibodies become fixed or are of the IgE type, allergy may ensue. All penicillins cross-react immunologically with each other because the antibody is directed against the penicilloyl moiety (common to all the penicillins) rather than to the side chain. Hence, a penicillin-allergic individual should not be given penicillin of any sort. Cefalosporins, on the other hand, give rise to side chain recognising antibodies and so cross-reactions are less common. However, about 8 to 10% of penicillin-allergic patients react to cefalosporins, so it would be prudent to avoid any β-lactam drug in a patient with proven allergy. Aztreonam, a monolactam, has only rare (≈ 1%) cross-reactivity with other β-lactams and can be used safely in patients allergic to penicillins or cefalosporins.[196]

Although allergy to β-lactam compounds usually manifests as a skin reaction, severe anaphylactic reactions, which can be fatal, may occur in previously sensitised individuals rechallenged with these agents. Fortunately, such events are quite rare. Skin testing is not a satisfactory method of screening for penicillin allergy since a minute challenge may cause a major anaphylactic reaction.

Most β-lactam antibiotics contain a relatively high proportion of sodium.[197] This should be borne in mind, especially when treating patients for whom an increased sodium load may have serious consequences. At high doses (usually >30 MU/day), benzylpenicillin and other β-lactams (ureidopenicillins, imipenem) can cause seizures due to central nervous system toxicity. Other infrequent adverse effects include pseudomembranous colitis, leucopenia, thrombocytopenia and Coombs-positive haemolytic anaemia.

Certain cefalosporins, including cefoperazone, cefamandole and latamoxef that contain an *N*-methylthiotetrazole side chain have been reported to cause a disulfiram-like reaction with alcohol, as well as bleeding episodes due to hypoprothrombinaemia.[198]

### 8.2 Aminoglycosides

The toxicity associated with aminoglycosides is considerable and includes nephrotoxicity and auditory or vestibular toxicity. The nephrotoxic potential varies among the different aminoglycosides, with neomycin being the most and streptomycin the least nephrotoxic. Aminoglycoside nephrotoxicity is usually not permanent and may be reversed once the drug is discontinued. The risk of nephrotoxicity is increased by factors such as hypotension, prolonged duration of therapy, pre-existing renal insufficiency and possibly excessive serum aminoglycoside concentrations.

All drugs in this group may produce ototoxicity in humans. The vestibular branch of the 8th cranial nerve is mainly affected by streptomycin, gentamicin and tobramycin, whereas the auditory branch is mainly affected by neomycin, kanamycin and amikacin (see also chapter 14; sect. 8.1.1). However, all of the aminoglycosides may affect both branches of the 8th cranial nerve. The ototoxicity is a result of selective destruction of the hair cells in the cochlea.

This adverse effect is frequently irreversible and is cumulative with repeated courses of the agent. Careful monitoring and dosage adjustment (see further chapter 5; sect. 4.8.1) reduces aminoglycoside-induced ototoxicity and nephrotoxicity to a low level.

Other minor adverse effects of aminoglycosides include local pain and allergic skin rashes. Contact dermatitis may occur in nurses, pharmacists or others who repeatedly handle streptomycin.

### 8.3 Quinolones

The most prominent adverse effect of the quinolone class of antimicrobials is gastrointestinal intolerance with nausea, vomiting, abdominal discomfort and diarrhoea occurring in up to 5% of patients. In contrast with the β-lactams and clindamycin, *C. difficile* colitis is rarely associated with the use of quinolones. Other reported adverse effects include headache, fatigue, insomnia, dizziness and agitation. High doses of quinolones in elderly patients may cause seizures, although this is rare.

Cutaneous manifestations of allergic reactions are uncommon, but include rash, urticaria, generalised pruritus and photosensitive eruptions. On rare occasions, quinolone therapy may cause abnormalities in laboratory tests. These changes include elevations in serum transaminases, eosinophilia and neutropenia.

Certain quinolones, particularly enoxacin, interfere with the hepatic clearance of drugs such as theophylline and other xanthines resulting in increased serum concentrations of these agents. Ofloxacin has been reported to augment the anticoagulant effects of warfarin.

Quinolones have been shown to produce irreversible cartilage erosion and skeletal abnormalities in young experimental animals. As a result, they are generally contraindicated in children and pregnant or nursing women.

### 8.4 Tetracyclines

Gastrointestinal disturbances are the most commonly observed adverse effects of the tetracyclines. These effects may be due to the local initiative properties of tetracyclines on the gastrointestinal mucosa or to alterations in the enteric flora, and include oesophageal ulcerations, epigastric distress, nausea, vomiting and diarrhoea. Pseudomembranous colitis can develop with prolonged use.

Allergic reactions are unusual, but may appear as urticaria, fixed drug eruptions, morbilliform rashes and anaphylaxis. Photosensitivity reactions may occur with all tetracycline analogues, but are particularly prominent with demeclocycline.

The tetracyclines are contraindicated in pregnant women because of their ability to cause liver damage, as well as discolouration of the primary dentition of their child. Tetracyclines should also be avoided in children below the age of 8 years as they may cause depression of bone growth, permanent discolouration of the teeth, and enamel hypoplasia when given during tooth and skeletal development.

Minocycline has been reported to cause lightheadedness, dizziness and vertigo. Benign intracranial hypertension (pseudotumour cerebri) has been associated with many tetracycline analogues.

### 8.5 Macrolides

Gastrointestinal adverse effects such as abdominal cramps, nausea, vomiting and diarrhoea are common with oral administration of erythromycin. These effects have been reported in 5% of patients receiving erythromycin propionate and 2% of those treated with the estolate. Cholestatic jaundice occurring in adults has been associated most frequently with the estolate form, but has also been reported with use of other forms of erythromycin. Gastrointestinal adverse effects are reportedly less frequently with the newer macrolides azithromycin and clarithromycin.

Hypersensitivity reactions occur in about 0.5% of patients exposed to erythromycin and include skin rashes, fever and eosinophilia. Erythromycin interferes with the hepatic metabolism of several drugs and may increase serum concentrations of concomitantly administered theophylline, cyclosporin and digoxin. Erythromycin may also increase the anticoagulant effect of warfarin.

### 8.6 Lincosamides

Pseudomembranous colitis is an unusual but well documented adverse reaction associated with the use of clindamycin and lincomycin. Although rare, its potential consequences are so serious that use of these compounds has been much reduced. This complication is not dose-related and may occur after oral or parenteral administration. Prompt cessation of the antibiotic, and administration of oral vancomycin, metronidazole or bacitracin therapy is effective in reversing this complication.

Other adverse effects associated with the lincosamides are rare and include skin rashes, fever and reversible elevation of serum transaminases.

### 8.7 Chloramphenicol

Bone marrow toxicity is the major complication of chloramphenicol use. The drug can cause aplastic anaemia and has been responsible for several hundred deaths. However, the true incidence of this idiosyncratic adverse effect is difficult to assess. A figure of between 1 in 24,000 and 1 in 40,000 patients treated has been estimated. This response is not dose-related, can occur weeks to months after the use of chloramphenicol and can develop after the use of oral, intravenous or even topical preparations. The precise mechanism of this effect is unknown. More commonly, reversible dose-related bone marrow suppression may occur as a result of a direct effect of the drug on haematopoiesis. Predisposing factors include high dosages (>4 g/day), prolonged therapy and excessive serum concentrations (>20 mg/L).

The 'grey baby syndrome' may occur in premature infants and neonates and is characterised by vomiting, abdominal distention, cyanosis, hypothermia and circulatory collapse. This toxicity is due to the immature hepatic function of neonates, which impairs hepatic inactivation of the drug. Since the recognition of this hazard and the observation that in many cases, administration of chloramphenicol served no useful purpose, the use of this agent in neonates has been largely discontinued and the 'grey baby syndrome' has virtually disappeared.

Chloramphenicol potentiates the action of warfarin, phenytoin and oral antidiabetic agents by competitive inhibition of hepatic microsomal enzymes. Allergic reactions are also seen, including skin rashes, drug fevers and anaphylaxis.

### 8.8 Sulfonamides and Trimethoprim

Skin reactions are the most common adverse effect observed with these compounds. Hypersensitivity reactions can occur as rashes, vasculitis, erythema multiforme and Stevens-Johnson syndrome. Skin reactions are much more common with sulfonamides than with trimethoprim. Sulfonamides may also cause nausea, vomiting, headache, fever, and at very high doses, crystalluria with tubular deposits of sulfonamide crystals. Bone marrow toxicity with anaemia, leucopenia and thrombocytopenia may also occur, usually in patients with pre-existing folate deficiency. Patients with AIDS have a much higher frequency (as much as 70%) of adverse reactions to these agents.[199]

### 8.9 Rifampicin

Antibody formation may occur after intermittent high-dose rifampicin therapy, i.e. >1g taken at weekly intervals. This is associated with the 'flu syndrome'. Induction of liver enzymes by rifampicin may result in reduced activity of other drugs metabolised by the liver, including oral anticoagulants, oral antidiabetic agents and oral contraceptives. Thus, dosage adjustments for these compounds may be necessary when rifampicin is taken.

### 8.10 Vancomycin

One of the most well known adverse effects of vancomycin administration is the tingling and flushing of the face, neck and thorax observed on rapid or bolus infusion of the drug. This phenomenon is known as the 'red man' or 'red neck' syndrome and is due to histamine release by basophils and mast cells. Other common adverse effects of vancomycin are fever, chills and phlebitis at the site of infusion. Hypersensitivity reactions can occur in up to 5% of individuals and include maculopapular diffuse erythematous skin rashes.

Although vancomycin is frequently thought of as nephrotoxic, nephrotoxicity is now rare with the availability of highly purified vancomycin preparations. Permanent auditory nerve damage and hearing loss may occur if serum vancomycin concentrations exceed 50 mg/L. There may be an increased risk of both ototoxicity and nephrotoxicity when vancomycin and aminoglycosides are used in combination.

## Further Reading

Greenwood D, editor. Antimicrobial chemotherapy. Oxford: Oxford University Press, 1989

Lorian V, editor. Antibiotics in laboratory medicine, 3rd ed. Baltimore: Williams & Wilkins, 1986

Mandell GL, Douglas RG, Dolin R, editors. Principles and practices of infectious disease, 4th ed. New York: Churchill Livingston, 1995

Murray PR, Baron EJ, Pfaller MA, et al. editors. Manual of clinical microbiology, 6th ed. Washington, DC: ASM Press, 1995

Pennington JE, editor. Respiratory infections, diagnosis, and management. New York: Raven Press, 1994

Sande MA, Root RK, editors. Treatment of serious infections in the 1990s. New York: Churchill Livingston, 1992

Sanford JP, Gilbert DN, Sande MA. Guide to antimicrobial therapy 1996 (a yearly pocket manual). Dallas: Antimicrobial Therapy, Inc., 1996

Wenzel RP, editor. Prevention and control of nosocomial infections, 2nd ed. Baltimore: Williams & Wilkins, 1993

## References

1. Doern GV. The clinical impact of same-day antimicrobial susceptibility testing. Clinical Microbiology Newsletter 1996; 18: 13
2. Blaser J, Konig C. Once-daily dosing of aminoglycosides. European Journal of Clinical Microbiology and Infectious Diseases 1995; 14: 1029
3. Craig WA. Interrelationship between pharmacokinetics and pharmacodynamics in determining dosage regimens for broad-spectrum cephalosporins. Diagnostic Microbiology and Infectious Disease 1995; 22: 89
4. Various authors. The microbial wars. Science 1992; 257: 1021, 1050-82
5. Various authors. Frontiers in biotechnology: resistance to antibiotics. Science 1994; 264: 360-70
6. Fleming A. On the antibacterial action of cultures of a penicillium, with special reference to their use in the isolation of *B. influenzae*. British Journal of Experimental Pathology 1929; 10: 226
7. Batchelor FR, Doyle FP, Naylor JHC. Synthesis of penicillin: 6-aminopenicillinic acid in penicillin fermentation. Nature 1959; 183: 257-60
8. Nathwani D, Wood MJ. Penicillins: a current review of their clinical pharmacology and therapeutic use. Drugs 1993; 45: 866
9. Jones RN, Pfaller MA, Fuchs PC, et al. Piperacillin/tazobactam (YTR 830) combination comparative antimicrobial activity against 5889 recent aerobic clinical isolates and 60 *Bacteroides fragilis* group strains. Diagnostic Microbiology and Infectious Disease 1989; 12: 489
10. Marshall SA, Aldridge KE, Allen SD, et al. Comparative antimicrobial activity of piperacillin-tazobactam tested against more than 5000 recent clinical isolates from five medical centers: a re-evaluation after five days. Diagnostic Microbiology and Infectious Disease 1995; 21: 153
11. Campoli-Richards DM, Brogden RN. Sulbactam/ampicillin: a review of its antibacterial activity, pharmacokinetic properties and therapeutic use. Drugs 1987; 33: 577
12. Todd PA, Benfield P. Amoxicillin/clavulanic acid: an update of its antibacterial activity, pharmacokinetic properties, and therapeutic use. Drugs 1990; 39: 264
13. Abraham EP, Loder PB. Cephalosporin. In: Flynn EH, editor. Cephalosporins and penicillins. New York: Academic Press, 1972
14. Saxon A, Beall GN, Rohn AS. Immediate hypersensitivity reaction to beta-lactam antibiotics. Annals of Internal Medicine 1987; 107: 204
15. Thompson JW, Jacobs RF. Adverse effects of newer cephalosporins: an update. Drug Safety 1993; 9: 132
16. Sader HS, Jones RN. Historical overview of the cephalosporin spectrum: four generations of structural evolution. Antimicrobial Newsletter 1992; 8: 75
17. Brogden RN, Ward A. Ceftriaxone: a reappraisal of its antibacterial activity and pharmacokinetic properties, and an update on its therapeutic use with particular reference to once-daily administration. Drugs 1988; 35: 604
18. Todd PA, Brogden RN. Cefotaxime: an update of its pharmacology and therapeutic use. Drugs 1990; 40: 608
19. Okamoto MP, Nakahiro RK, Chin A, et al. Cefepime clinical pharmacokinetics. Clinical Pharmacokinetics 1993; 25: 88
20. Rubinstein E, Labs R, Reeves A. A review of the adverse events profile of cefpirome. Drug Safety 1993; 9: 340
21. Brogden RN, Campoli-Richards DM. Cefixime: a review of its antibacterial activity, pharmacokinetic properties and therapeutic potential. Drugs 1989; 38: 524
22. Frampton JE, Brogden RN, Langtry HD, et al. Cefpodoxime proxetil: a review of its antibacterial activity, pharmacokinetic properties, and therapeutic potential. Drugs 1992; 44: 889-917
23. Bryson HM, Brogden RN. Cefetamet pivoxil: a review of its antibacterial activity, pharmacokinetic properties and therapeutic use. Drugs 1993; 45: 589
24. Saxon A, Swabb EA, Adkinson Jr NF. Investigation into the immunologic cross-reactivity of aztreonam with other beta-lactam antibiotics. American Journal of Medicine 1985; 78 Suppl. 2A: 19
25. Kahan JS, Kahan FM, Goegleman R. Thienamycin, a new beta-lactam antibiotic. Journal of Antibiotics 1979; 32: 1
26. Jones RN. Review of the in vitro spectrum of activity of imipenem. American Journal of Medicine 1985; 78 Suppl. A: 22
27. Balfour JA, Bryson HM, Brogden RN. Imipenem/cilastatin: an update of its antibacterial activity, pharmacokinetics, and therapeutic efficacy in the treatment of serious infections. Drugs 1996; 51: 99-136
28. Clissold SP, Todd PA, Campoli-Richards DM. Imipenem/cilastatin: a review of its antibacterial activity, pharmacokinetic properties, and therapeutic efficacy. Drugs 1987; 33: 183
29. Buckley MM, Brogden RN, Barradell LB, et al. Imipenem/cilastatin: a reappraisal of its antibacterial activity, pharmacokinetic properties, and therapeutic efficacy. Drugs 1992; 44: 408
30. Wiseman LR, Wagstaff AJ, Brogden RN, et al. Meropenem: a review of its antibacterial activity, pharmacokinetic properties and clinical efficacy. Drugs 1995; 50: 73
31. Jones RN, Barry AL, Thornsberry C. In vitro studies of meropenem. Journal of Antimicrobial Chemotherapy 1989; 24 Suppl. A: 9
32. DeSarro A, Ammendola D, Zappala M, et al. Relationship between structure and convulsant properties of some beta-lactam antibiotics following intracerebroventricular microinjection in rats. Antimicrobial Agents and Chemotherapy 1995; 39: 232
33. Campoli-Richards DM, Chaplin S, Sayce RJ, et al. Netilmicin: a review of its antibacterial activity, pharmacokinetic properties, and therapeutic use. Drugs 1989; 38: 703
34. Craig WA. Once-daily versus multiple-daily dosing of aminoglycosides. Journal of Chemotherapy 1995; 7 (Suppl. 2): 47
35. Jones RN. Isepamicin (SCH 21420, 1-*N*-HAPA gentamicin B): microbiological characteristics including

antimicrobial potency and spectrum of activity. Journal of Chemotherapy 1995; 7: 7

36. Bates RD, Nahata MC. Once-daily administration of aminoglycosides. Annals of Pharmacotherapy 1994; 28: 757-66
37. Rotschafer JC, Rybak MJ. Single daily dosing of aminoglycosides: a commentary. Annals of Pharmacotherapy 1994; 28: 797
38. Miller GH, Sabatelli FJ, Naples L, et al. The changing nature of aminoglycoside resistance mechanisms and the role of isepamicin: a new broad-spectrum aminoglycoside. Journal of Chemotherapy 1995; 7: 31
39. Chopra I, Hawkey PM, Hinton M. Tetracyclines, molecular and clinical aspects. Journal of Antimicrobial Chemotherapy 1992; 29: 245
40. Sum PE, Lee VJ, Testa RT, et al. Glycylcyclines. I: A new generation of potent antibacterial agents through modifications of 9-aminotetracyclines. Journal of Medicinal Chemistry 1994; 37: 184
41. Tally FT, Ellestad GA, Testa RT. Glycylcyclines: a new generation of tetracyclines. Journal of Antimicrobial Chemotherapy 1995; 35: 449
42. Washington JA, Wilson WR. Erythromycin: a microbial and clinical perspective after 30 years of clinical use (first of two parts). Mayo Clinic Proceedings 1985a; 60: 189
43. Washington JA, Wilson WR. Erythromycin: a microbial and clinical perspective after 30 years of clinical use (second of two parts). Mayo Clinic Proceedings 1985b; 60: 271
44. Fernandes PB. The macrolide revival: thirty-five years after erythromycin. Antimicrobial Newsletter 1987; 4: 25
45. Kirst HA. New macrolides: expanded horizons for an old class of antibiotics. Journal of Antimicrobial Chemotherapy 1991; 28: 787
46. Hardy DJ, Hensey DM, Beyer JM, et al. Comparative in vitro activities of new 14-, 15- and 16-membered macrolides. Antimicrobial Agents and Chemotherapy 1988; 32: 1710
47. Ishiguro M, Koga H, Kohno S, et al. Penetration of macrolides into human polymorphonuclear leukocytes. Journal of Antimicrobial Chemotherapy 1989; 24: 719
48. Peters DH, Frudel HA, McTavish D. Azithromycin: a review of its antimicrobial activity, pharmacokinetic properties, and clinical efficacy. Drugs 1992; 44: 750
49. Dunn CJ, Barradell LB. Azithromycin: a review of its pharmacological properties and use as 3-day therapy in respiratory tract infections. Drugs 1996; 51: 483-506
50. Peters DH, Clissold SP. Clarithromycin: a review of its antimicrobial activity, pharmacokinetic properties, and therapeutic potential. Drugs 1992; 44: 117
51. Young RA, Gonzalez JP, Sorkin EM. Roxithromycin: a review of its antimicrobial activity, pharmacokinetic properties, and clinical efficacy. Drugs 1989; 27: 8
52. LeClercq R, Courvalin P. Bacterial resistance to macrolide, lincosamide, and streptogramin antibiotics by target modification. Antimicrobial Agents and Chemotherapy 1991; 35: 1267
53. LeClercq R, Courvalin P. Intrinsic and unusual resistance to macrolide, lincosamide, and streptogramin antibiotics. Antimicrobial Agents and Chemotherapy 1991; 35: 1273
54. Pechere J-C. Streptogramins: a unique class of antibiotics. Drugs 1996; Suppl. 13
55. Wolfson JS, Hooper DC. The fluoroquinolones: clinical and laboratory considerations. Clinical Microbiology Newsletter 1992; 14: 1
56. Campoli-Richards DM, Monk JP, Price A, et al. Ciprofloxacin: a review of its antimicrobial activity, pharmacokinetic properties, and therapeutic use. Drugs 1988; 35: 373
57. Todd PA, Faulds D. Ofloxacin: a reappraisal of its antimicrobial activity, pharmacology, and therapeutic use. Drugs 1991; 42: 825
58. Wadworth AN, Goa KL. Lomefloxacin: a review of its antibacterial activity, pharmacokinetic properties, and therapeutic use. Drugs 1991; 42: 1018
59. Grosset JH, Ji BH, Guelpa-Lauras CC, et al. Clinical trial of pefloxacin and ofloxacin in the treatment of lepromatous leprosy. International Journal of Leprosy and other Mycobacterial Diseases 1990; 2: 281
60. Naber KG. The role of quinolones in the treatment of chronic bacterial prostatitis. Infection 1991; 3: S170
61. Wistrom J, Norrby R. Antibiotic prophylaxis of travellers' diarrhoea. Scandinavian Journal of Infectious Diseases 1990; 70: 111
62. Peterson LR, Lissack LM, Canter K, et al. Therapy of lower extremity infections with ciprofloxacin in patients with diabetes mellitus, peripheral vascular disease, or both. American Journal of Medicine 1989; 86: 801
63. Vance-Bryon K, Guay DRP, Rotschafer JC. Clinical pharmacokinetics of ciprofloxacin. Clinical Pharmacokinetics 1990; 19: 434
64. Lamp KC, Boaley EM, Rybak MJ. Ofloxacin clinical pharmacokinetics. Clinical Pharmacokinetics 1992; 22: 32
65. Finch RG. The withdrawal of temafloxacin: are there implications for other quinolones? Drug Safety 1993; 8: 9
66. Ball AP. Emergent resistance to ciprofloxacin amongst *Pseudomonas aeruginosa* and *Staphylococcus aureus*: clinical significance and therapeutic approaches. Journal of Antimicrobial Chemotherapy 1990; 26 Suppl. F: 165-79
67. Endtz HP, Ruijs GH, van Klingeren B, et al. Quinolone resistance in *Campylobacter* isolated from man and poultry following the introduction of fluoroquinolones in veterinary medicine. Journal of Antimicrobial Chemotherapy 1991; 2: 199
68. Truckis M, Hooper DC, Wolfson JS. Emerging resistance to fluoroquinolones in staphylococci: an alert. Annals of Internal Medicine 1991; 114: 424
69. Woods DD. The relation of p-aminobenzoic acid to the mechanism of action of sulphanilamide. British Journal of Experimental Pathology 1940; 21: 74
70. Periti P. Evolution of the bacterial dihydrofolate reductase inhibitors. Journal of Antimicrobial Chemotherapy 1995; 36: 887-90
71. Avery GS. Trimethoprim-sulphamethoxazole: a review. Drugs 1971; 1: 7-53
72. Brumfitt W, Hamilton-Miller JMT. Cotrimoxazole or trimethoprim alone? A viewpoint on their relative place in therapy. Drugs 1982; 24: 453
73. Gillis JC, Brogden RN. Rifaximin: a review of its antibacterial activity, pharmacokinetic properties and therapeutic potential in conditions mediated by gastrointestinal bacteria. Drugs 1995; 49: 467
74. Verbist L. The antimicrobial activity of fusidic acid. Journal of Antimicrobial Chemotherapy 1990; 25: 1
75. Campoli-Richards DM, Brogden RN, Faulds D. Teicoplanin: a review of its antibacterial activity,

pharmacokinetic properties and therapeutic potential. Drugs 1990; 40: 449

76. Rowland M. Clinical pharmacokinetics of teicoplanin. Clinical Pharmacokinetics 1990; 18: 184
77. Hendlin D, Stapley EO, Jackson M, et al. Phosphamycin, a new antibiotic produced by strains of Streptomyces. Science 1969; 166: 122
78. Llaneza J, Villar CJ, Sales JA, et al. Plasmid-mediated fosfomycin resistance is due to enzymatic modification of the antibiotic. Antimicrobial Agents and Chemotherapy 1985; 28: 163
79. Lau AH, Lam NP, Piscitelli SC, et al. Clinical pharmacokinetics of metronidazole and other nitroimidazole anti-infectives. Clinical Pharmacokinetics 1992; 23: 328
80. Jones RN, Johnson DM, Erwin ME. In vitro antimicrobial activities and spectra of U-100592 and U-100766, two novel fluorinated oxazolidinones. Antimicrobial Agents and Chemotherapy 1996; 40: 720-6
81. Ramirez JA. Switch therapy in community-acquired pneumonia. Diagnostic Microbiology and Infectious Disease 1995; 22: 219
82. Cunha BA. Vancomycin. Medical Clinics of North America 1995; 79: 817-31
83. Turnidge J. Pharmacodynamic (kinetic) considerations in the treatment of moderately severe infections with cefotaxime. Diagnostic Microbiology and Infectious Disease 1995; 22: 57
84. Mandell GL, Sande MA. Penicillins, cephalosporins and other beta-lactam antibiotics. In: Goodman-Gilman A, Goodman LS, Rall TW, et al., editors. Goodman and Gilmans The pharmacological basis of therapeutics, 7th ed. New York: McMillan, 1985; 1115-49
85. Jawetz E. Chloramphenicol and tetracycline. In: Katzung BG, editor. Basic and clinical pharmacology, 6th ed. London: Prentice Hall International 1995; 693-8
86. Quintiliani R, Cooper BW, Briceland LL, et al. Economic impact of streamlining antibiotic administration. American Journal of Medicine 1987; 82 Suppl. 4A: 391
87. Guay DRP. Sequential antimicrobial therapy: a realistic approach to cost containment? PharmacoEconomics 1993; 3: 341
88. American Society of Microbiology. Report of the ASM Task Force on antibiotic resistance. Antimicrobial Agents and Chemotherapy 1995; Suppl: 1-23
89. Tomasz A. Multiple-antibiotic-resistant pathogenic bacteria: a report of the Rockefeller University workshop. New England Journal of Medicine 1994; 330: 1247
90. Neu HC. The crisis in antibiotic resistance. Science 1992; 257: 1064
91. Centers for Disease Control. Drug-resistant *Streptococcus pneumoniae*: Kentucky and Tennessee, 1993. MMWR Morbidity and Mortality Weekly Report 1994; 43: 23
92. Arthur M, Courvalin P. Genetics and mechanisms of glycopeptide resistance in enterococci. Antimicrobial Agents and Chemotherapy 1993; 37: 1563
93. Centers for Disease Control and Prevention. Nosocomial enterococci resistant to vancomycin: United States 1989-1993. MMWR Morbidity and Mortality Weekly Report 1993; 42: 597
94. Bush K. Classification of beta-lactamases: groups 1, 2a, 2b and 2b'. Antimicrobial Agents and Chemotherapy 1989; 33: 264
95. Jacoby GA, Medeiros AA. More extended-spectrum β-lactamases. Antimicrobial Agents and Chemotherapy 1991; 35: 1697
96. Burwen DR, Banerjee SN, Gaynes RP, et al. Ceftazidime resistance among selected nosocomial Gram-negative bacilli in the United States. Journal of Infectious Diseases 1994; 170: 1622
97. Philippon A, Arlet G, Larange PH. Origin and impact of plasmid-mediated extended-spectrum beta-lactamases. European Journal of Clinical Microbiology and Infectious Diseases 1994; 13 Suppl. 1: S17
98. Beck-Sague C, Dooley SW, Hutton MD, et al. Hospital outbreak of multidrug-resistant *Mycobacterium tuberculosis* infections: factors in transmission to staff and HIV-infected patients. Journal of the American Medical Association 1992; 268: 1280
99. Centers for Disease Control. Meeting the challenge of multidrug-resistant tuberculosis: summary of a conference. MMWR Morbidity and Mortality Weekly Report 1992; 41 (RR-11): 49
100. Breiman RF, Butler JC, Tenover FC, et al. Emergence of drug-resistant pneumococcal infections in the United States. Journal of the American Medical Association 1994; 271: 1831
101. Shapiro ED. Infections caused by *Haemophilus influenzae* type b: the beginning of the end? Journal of the American Medical Society 1993; 269: 264
102. Jordens JR, Slack MPE. *Haemophilus influenzae*: then and now. European Journal of Clinical Microbiology and Infectious Diseases 1995; 14: 935-48
103. Bush K. Characterization of beta-lactamases. Antimicrobial Agents and Chemotherapy 1989; 33: 259
104. Bush K. Classification of beta-lactamases: groups 2c, 2d, 2e, 3 and 4. Antimicrobial Agents and Chemotherapy 1989b; 33: 271
105. Davies J. Inactivation of antibiotics and the dissemination of resistance genes. Science 1994; 264: 375
106. National Committee for Clinical Laboratory Standards. Performance standards for antimicrobial disk susceptibility tests: Approved Standard M2-A5. National Committee for Clinical Laboratory Standards, Villanova, PA, 1993
107. National Committee for Clinical Laboratory Standards. Methods for dilution antimicrobial susceptibility tests for bacteria that grow aerobically: Approved Standard M7-A3. National Committee for Clinical Laboratory Standards, Villanova, PA, 1993
108. Quintiliani R, Courvalin P. Mechanisms of resistance to antimicrobial agents. In: Murray PR, Baron EJ, Pfaller MA, et al., editors. Manual of clinical microbiology. 6th ed. Washington, DC: American Society of Microbiology, 1995: 1308-26
109. Westphal JF, Brogard JM. Clinical pharmacokinetics of newer bacterial agents in liver disease. Clinical Pharmacokinetics 1993; 24: 46
110. Weinstein AJ, Moellering Jr RC. Penicillin and gentamicin therapy for enterococcal infections. Journal of the American Medical Association 1973; 223: 1030
111. EORTC International Antimicrobial Therapy Cooperative Group. Ceftazidime combined with a short or long course of amikacin for empirical therapy of Gram-negative bacteremia in cancer patients with granulocytopenia. New England Journal of Medicine 1987; 317: 1692
112. Hunter TH. Use of streptomycin in treatment of bacterial endocarditis. American Journal of Medicine 1947; 2: 436
113. Hunter TH. The treatment of some bacterial infections of the heart and pericardium. Bulletin of the New York Academy of Medicine 1952; 28: 213

114. Jawetz E, Gunnison JB, Colman VR. The combined action of penicillin with streptomycin or Chloromycetin on enterococci in vitro. Science 1950; 111: 254
115. Eliopoulos GM, Moellering RC. Antimicrobial combinations. In: Lorian V, editor. Antibiotics in laboratory medicine. 3rd ed. Baltimore: Williams and Wilkins, 1991
116. Butler T, Linh NN, Arnold K, et al. Therapy of antimicrobial resistant typhoid fever. Antimicrobial Agents and Chemotherapy 1977; 11: 645
117. Anderson ET, Young LS, Hewitt WL. Antimicrobial synergism in the therapy of Gram-negative rod bacteremia. Chemotherapy 1978; 24: 45
118. De Jongh CA, Joshi JH, Thompson BW, et al. A double beta-lactam combination versus an aminoglycoside-containing regimen as empiric antibiotic therapy for febrile granulocytopenic cancer patients. American Journal of Medicine 1986; 80 Suppl. 5C: 101
119. Eliopoulos GM, Eliopoulos CT. Antibiotic combinations: should they be tested? Clinical Microbiology Reviews 1988; 1: 139
120. Cometta A, Baumgartner JD, Lew D, et al. Prospective randomized comparison of imipenem monotherapy with imipenem plus netilmicin for treatment of severe infections in non-neutropenic patients. Antimicrobial Agents and Chemotherapy 1994; 38: 1309
121. Lepper MH, Dowling HF. Treatment of pneumococcic meningitis with penicillin compared with penicillin plus Aureomycin: studies including observations on an apparent antagonism between penicillin and Aureomycin. Archives of Internal Medicine 1951; 88: 489
122. Sanders CC. Novel resistance selected by the new expanded-spectrum cephalosporins: a concern. Journal of Infectious Diseases 1983; 147: 585
123. Inderlied CB. Antimycobacterial agents: in vitro susceptibility testing, spectrums of activity, mechanisms of action and resistance and assays for activity in biological fluids. In: Lorian V, editor. Antibiotics in laboratory medicine. 3rd ed. Baltimore: Williams and Wilkins, 1991
124. Johnson DE, Thompson B. Efficacy of single-agent therapy with azlocillin, ticarcillin, and amikacin and beta-lactam/amikacin combinations for treatment of *Pseudomonas aeruginosa* bacteremia in granulocytopenic rats. American Journal of Medicine 1986; 80 Suppl. 5C: 53
125. McLaughlin FJ, Matthews Jr WJ, Strieder DJ, et al. Clinical and bacteriological responses to three antibiotic regimens for acute exacerbations of cystic fibrosis: ticarcillin-tobramycin, azlocillin-tobramycin, and azlocillin-placebo. Journal of Infectious Diseases 1983; 147: 559
126. Van Leatherem Y, Lagast H, Klastersky J. Serum bactericidal activity of ceftazidime and cefoperazone alone or in combination with amikacin against *Pseudomonas aeruginosa* and *Klebsiella pneumoniae*. Antimicrobial Agents and Chemotherapy 1983; 23: 435
127. Pittet D, Li N, Wenzel RP. Association of secondary and polymicrobial nosocomial bloodstream infections with higher mortality. European Journal of Clinical Microbiology and Infectious Diseases 1993; 12: 813
128. Weinstein MP, Reller LB, Murphy JR. Clinical importance of polymicrobial bacteremia. Diagnostic Microbiology and Infectious Disease 1986; 5: 185
129. Bartlett JG, Gorbach SL. Treatment of aspiration pneumonia and primary lung abscess: penicillin G vs clindamycin. Journal of the American Medical Association 1975; 234: 935
130. Levison ME, Mangura CT, Lorber B, et al. Clindamycin compared with penicillin for the treatment of anaerobic lung abscesses. Annals of Internal Medicine 1983; 98: 466
131. Stratton IV CW. In vitro testing: correlations between bacterial susceptibility, body fluid levels, and effectiveness of antibacterial therapy. In: Lorian V, editor. Antibiotics in laboratory medicine. 3rd ed. Baltimore: Williams and Wilkins, 1991
132. Tenover FC, Hughes JM. The challenge of emerging infectious diseases: development and spread of multiply-resistant bacterial pathogens. Journal of the American Medical Association 1996; 275: 300
133. Swartz MN. Hospital-acquired infections: diseases with increasingly limited therapies. Proceedings of the National Academy of Sciences USA 1994; 91: 2420
134. McCabe WR, Jackson GG. Gram-negative bacteremia II: clinical laboratory and therapeutic considerations. Archives of Internal Medicine 1962; 110: 856
135. Chow JW, Fine MJ, Shlaes DM, et al. *Enterobacter* bacteremia: clinical features and emergence of antibiotic resistance during therapy. Annals of Internal Medicine 1991; 115: 585
136. Morselli PL, Franco-Morselli R, Bossi L. Clinical pharmacokinetics in newborns and infants. Clinical Pharmacokinetics 1980; 5: 485
137. Yaffe SJ. Antimicrobial therapy and the neonate. Obstetrics and Gynecology 1981; 58 Suppl. 5: 85S
138. Meyers BR, Wilkinson P. Clinical pharmacokinetics of antibacterial drugs in the elderly: implications for selection and dosage. Clinical Pharmacokinetics 1989; 17: 385
139. Chow AW, Jeweson PJ. Pharmacokinetics and safety of antimicrobial agents during pregnancy. Reviews of Infectious Diseases 1985; 7: 28
140. Philipson A. Pharmacokinetics of antibiotics in pregnancy and labour. Clinical Pharmacokinetics 1979; 4: 297
141. Dooley JS, Hamilton-Miller JMT, Brumfitt W, et al. Antibiotics in the treatment of biliary infection. Gut 1984; 25: 988
142. Lee CC, Marbury TC. Drug therapy in patients undergoing haemodialysis: clinical pharmacokinetic considerations. Clinical Pharmacokinetics 1984; 9: 42
143. Paton TW, Cornish WR, Manuel MA, et al. Drug therapy in patients undergoing peritoneal dialysis: clinical pharmacokinetic considerations. Clinical Pharmacokinetics 1995; 10: 404
144. St Peter WL, Redic-Kill A, Halstenson CE. Clinical pharmacokinetics of antibiotics in patients with impaired renal function. Clinical Pharmacokinetics 1992; 22: 169-210
145. Reetze-Bonorden P, Böhler J, Keller E. Drug dosage in patients during continuous renal replacement therapy. Clinical Pharmacokinetics 1993; 24: 362-79
146. Emori TG, Gaynes RP. An overview of nosocomial infections, including the role of the microbiology laboratory. Clinical Microbiology Reviews 1993; 6: 428
147. Wolinsky E. Mycobacterial diseases other than tuberculosis. Clinical Infectious Diseases 1992; 15: 1
148. Barnes PF, Silva C, Otaya M. Testing for human immunodeficiency virus infection in patients with tuberculosis. American Journal of Respiratory and Critical Care Medicine 1996; 153: 1448-50
149. Karchmer AW. Staphylococcal endocarditis: laboratory and clinical basis for antibiotic therapy. American Journal of Medicine 1985; 78 Suppl. 6B: 116

150. Turnidge J, Grayson ML. Optimum treatment of staphylococcal infections. Drugs 1993; 45: 353

151. Ena J, Dick RW, Jones RN, et al. The epidemiology of intravenous vancomycin usage in a university hospital: a 10-year study. Journal of the American Medical Association 1993; 269: 598

152. Schwalbe RS, Stapleton JT, Gilligan PH. Emergence of vancomycin resistance in coagulase-negative staphylococci. New England Journal of Medicine 1987; 316: 927

153. Veach LA, Pfaller MA, Barrett M, et al. Vancomycin resistance in *Staphylococcus haemolyticus* causing colonization and blood stream infection. Journal of Clinical Microbiology 1990; 28: 2064

154. Landry SL, Kaiser DL, Wenzel RP. Hospital stay and mortality attributed to nosocomial enterococcal bacteremia: a controlled study. American Journal of Infection Control 1989; 17: 323

155. Moellering Jr RC. The *Enterococcus*: a classic example of the impact of antimicrobial resistance on therapeutic options. Journal of Antimicrobial Chemotherapy 1991; 28: 1

156. Tenover FC, Tokars J, Swenson J, et al. Ability to clinical laboratories to detect antimicrobial agent-resistant enterococci. Journal of Clinical Microbiology 1993; 31: 1695

157. Swenson JM, Ferraro MJ, Sahm DF, et al. New vancomycin disk diffusion breakpoints for enterococci. Journal of Clinical Microbiology 1992; 30: 2525

158. Bochud PY, Eggiman P, Calandra T, et al. Bacteremia due to viridans *Streptococcus* in neutropenic patients with cancer: clinical spectrum and risk factors. Clinical Infectious Diseases 1994; 18: 25

159. Jernigan DB, Cetron MS, Breiman RF. Minimizing the impact of drug-resistance *Streptococcus pneumoniae* (DRSP): a strategy from the DRSP working group. Journal of the American Medical Association 1996; 275: 206

160. Paris MM, Hickey SM, Uscher MI, et al. Effect of dexamethasone on therapy of experimental penicillin- and cephalosporin-resistant pneumococcal meningitis. Antimicrobial Agents and Chemotherapy 1994; 38: 1320

161. Bradley JS, Conner JD. Ceftriaxone failure in meningitis caused by *Streptococcus pneumoniae* with reduced susceptibility to beta-lactam antibiotics. Pediatric Infectious Disease Journal 1991; 10: 871

162. Friedland IR, Shelton S, Paris M, et al. Dilemmas in diagnosis and management of cephalosporin-resistant *Streptococccus penumoniae* meningitis. Pediatric Infectious Disease Journal 1993; 12: 196

163. John CC. Treatment failure with use of a third-generation cephalosporin for penicillin-resistant pneumococcal meningitis: case report and review. Clinical Infectious Diseases 1994; 18: 188

164. Nikaido H. Prevention of drug access to bacterial targets: permeability barriers and active efflux. Science 1994; 264: 382

165. Pfaller MA. Application of new technology to the detection, identification, and antimicrobial susceptibility testing of mycobacteria. American Journal of Clinical Pathology 1994; 101: 329

166. Geerdes HF, Ziegler D, Lode H, et al. Septicemia in 980 patients at a university hospital in Berlin: prospective studies during four selected years between 1979 and 1989. Clinical Infectious Diseases 1992; 15: 991

167. Bone RC. Gram-negative sepsis: a dilemma of modern medicine. Clinical Microbiology Reviews 1993; 6: 57

168. Glauser MP, Heumann D, Baumgartner JD, et al. Pathogenesis and potential strategies for prevention and treatment of septic shock: an update. Clinical Infectious Diseases 1994; 18 Suppl. 2: S205

169. Fisher Jr CJ, Dhainaut JFA, Opal SM, et al. Recombinant human interleukin 1 receptor antagonist in the treatment of patients with sepsis syndrome. Journal of the American Medical Association 1994; 271: 1836

170. Abraham E, Raffin TA. Sepsis therapy trials: continued disappointment or reason for hope? Journal of the American Medical Association 1994; 271: 1876

171. EORTC International Antimicrobial Therapy Cooperative Group and the National Cancer Institute of Canada - Clinical Trials Group. Vancomycin added to empirical combination antibiotic therapy for fever in granulocytopenic cancer patients. Journal of Infectious Diseases 1991; 163: 951

172. Tunkel AR, Wisplewey B, Scheld WM. Bacterial meningitis: recent advances in pathophysiology and treatment. Annals of Internal Medicine 1990; 12: 610

173. Odio CM, Faingezicht I, Paris M, et al. The beneficial effects of early dexamethasone administration in infants and children with bacterial meningitis. New England Journal of Medicine 1991; 324: 1525

174. Quagliarello V, Scheld WM. Bacterial meningitis: pathogenesis, pathophysiology, and progress. New England Journal of Medicine 1992; 327: 864

175. Stamm WE, Hooton TM. Management of urinary tract infections in adult. New England Journal of Medicine 1993; 329: 1328

176. Pfaller MA. Antifungal therapy. In: Scheld SM, editor. MKSAP in the subspecialty of infectious diseases. Philadelphia, PA: American College of Physicians, 1995

177. Georgopapadakou NH, Walsh TJ. Human mycoses: drugs and targets for emerging pathogens. Science 1994; 264: 371

178. Armstrong D. Treatment of opportunistic fungal infections. Clinical Infectious Diseases 1993; 16: 1

179. Sugar AM. Empiric treatment of fungal infections in the neutropenic host: review of the literature and guidelines for use. Archives of Internal Medicine 1990; 150: 2258

180. Rex JH, Bennett JE, Sugar AM, et al. A randomized trial comparing fluconazole with amphotericin B for the treatment of candidemia in patients without neutropenia. New England Journal of Medicine 1994; 331: 1325

181. Walsh TJ, Lee J, Lecciones J, et al. Empiric therapy with amphotericin B in febrile granulocytopenic patients. Reviews of Infectious Diseases 1991; 13: 496

182. Meyer RD. Current role of therapy with amphotericin B. Clinical Infectious Diseases 1992; 14 Suppl. 1: S148

183. Brajtburg J, Powderly WG, Kobayashi GS, et al. Amphotericin B: delivery systems. Antimicrobial Agents and Chemotherapy 1990; 34: 381

184. Bodey GP. Azole antifungal agents. Clinical Infectious Diseases 1992; 14 Suppl. 1: S161

185. Redding S, Smith J, Farinacci G, et al. Resistance of *Candida albicans* to fluconazole during treatment of oropharyngeal candidiasis in a patient with AIDS: documentation of in vitro susceptibility testing and DNA subtype analysis. Clinical Infectious Diseases 1994; 18: 240

186. Wingard JR, Merz WG, Rinaldi MG, et al. Increase in *Candida krusei* infection among patients with bone marrow transplantation and neutropenia treated pro-

phylactically with fluconazole. New England Journal of Medicine 1991; 325: 1274-7
187. Denning DW, Stepan DE, Blume KG, et al. Control of invasive pulmonary aspergillosis with oral itraconazole in a bone marrow transplant patient. Journal of Infection 1992; 24: 3
188. DuPont B. Itraconazole therapy in aspergillosis: study in 49 patients. Journal of the American Academy of Dermatology 1990; 23: 607
189. Sanchez C, Mauri E, Dalmau D, et al. Treatment of cerebral aspergillosis with itraconazole: do high doses improve the prognosis? Clinical Infectious Diseases 1995; 21: 1485
190. Pfaller MA, Rinaldi MG. Antifungal susceptibility testing: current state of technology, limitations, and standardization. Infectious Disease Clinics of North America 1993; 7: 435
191. Rex JH, Pfaller MA, Rinaldi MG, et al. Antifungal susceptibility testing. Clinical Microbiology Reviews 1993; 6: 367
192. National Committee for Clinical Laboratory Standards. Reference method for broth dilution antifungal susceptibility testing of yeasts: Tentative standard, M27-T. National Committee for Clinical Laboratory Standards, Wayne, PA, 1995
193. Cameron ML, Schell WA, Bruch S, et al. Correlation of in vitro fluconazole resistance of *Candida* isolates in relation to therapy and symptoms of individuals seropositive for human immunodeficiency virus type 1. Antimicrobial Agents and Chemotherapy 1993; 37: 2449
194. Troillet N, Durussel C, Bille J, et al. Correlation between in vitro susceptibility to *Candida albicans* and fluconazole-resistant oropharyngeal candidiasis in HIV-infected patients. European Journal of Clinical Microbiology and Infectious Diseases 1993; 12: 911
195. Classen DC, Evans RS, Pestotnik SL, et al. The timing of prophylactic administration of antibiotics and the risk of surgical wound infections. New England Journal of Medicine 1992; 326: 281
196. Adkinson Jr NF, Saxon A, Spence MR, et al. Cross-allergenicity and immunogenicity of aztreonam. Reviews of Infectious Diseases 1985; 7 Suppl. 4: S613
197. Baron DN, Hamilton-Miller JMT, Brumfitt W. Sodium content of injectable β-lactam antibiotics. Lancet 1984; 1: 1113
198. Norrby SR. Adverse reactions and interactions with newer cephalosporin and cephamycin antibiotics. Medical Toxicology and Adverse Drug Experience 1986; 1: 32
199. Gordin FM, Simon GL, Wofsy CB, et al. Adverse reactions to trimethoprim-sulfamethoxazole in patients with acquired immunodeficiency syndrome. Annals of Internal Medicine 1984; 100: 495

Chapter 32

# Viral Diseases

*B.G. Gazzard*

## Synopsis of Important Principles

1) Until more effective antiviral drugs are developed, prevention and symptomatic therapy will remain the mainstay of treatment of viral diseases.

2) For prevention, vaccines are used to provide active immunisation in individuals prior to exposure and for epidemiological control in the community. Vaccines for the prevention of poliomyelitis, measles, rubella, mumps, smallpox, hepatitis A and B, yellow fever, influenza and rabies are currently available.

3) The desirability of controlling a viral disease in the community is dependent on its health impact, and whether one attack of the disease confers long-lasting immunity.

4) The effectiveness of mass immunisation programmes is decreased if susceptible neonates are not vaccinated at the appropriate time.

5) For treatment of acute viral infections, early commencement of antiviral drug therapy is necessary as most replication occurs shortly after infection. Similarly, in chronic disease, where the viral load is low shortly after infection, early treatment is again more likely to be efficacious.

6) Prolonged single agent antiviral chemotherapy may lead to viral resistance, and where available, combinations should be considered.

7) Host factors, the natural history of the disease, and the benefit : risk ratio of drug therapy must all be considered before beginning treatment.

Many viral infections produce no accompanying illness or are mild self-limiting diseases that induce long-lasting specific immunity. However, some human viral infections may be extremely serious. While the pandemic of human immunodeficiency virus (HIV) infection is the most obvious example, viral infections are also known to be associated with human cancer (e.g. hepatoma, Burkitt's lymphoma and certain T-cell leukaemias) and to be the cause of other conditions of previously undetermined aetiology such as congestive cardiomyopathy.

The causative virus may be eliminated following infection or, alternatively, viral material may be incorporated in the human gene, producing true latency, and may be vertically transmitted. Productive replication may also occur at low levels over many years (e.g. hepatitis C).

## 1. General Principles of Treatment

### 1.1 Nonspecific Preventive Measures

Nonspecific measures for preventing viral infections apply to individuals as opposed to a community, and are the same as for nonviral infections. They are largely influenced by socioeconomic factors, among which adequate nutrition may be the most important. For example, the mortality from measles in Western countries a century ago was 15%, a figure which now applies only in developing nations.

### 1.2 Epidemiological Control of Virus Infection

A number of specific epidemiological measures can be used in attempts to control certain viral infections in a community, including:

1) *Quarantine measures:* these may rarely be used to inhibit the spread of highly lethal and infectious viruses (e.g. viral haemorrhagic fevers).

2) *Increasing herd immunity:* vaccination of a large proportion of a population not only protects individuals but also decreases the amount of virus in the community and thus reduces the exposure of unvaccinated groups. To be effective, such vaccine programmes need to be maintained to keep a critical mass immune and revaccination may be required if lifelong immunity is not produced.

3) *Environmental sanitary control:* appropriate environmental sanitary control, especially of water, food and sewage is an effective general approach, and can be readily applied in developed countries. However, while the lower rate of faecal transmission of viruses (e.g. of hepatitis A) in most developed countries would also be desirable in the developing world, it should be noted that early childhood acquisition of some infections may be relatively innocuous, whereas later transmission may be associated with more severe disease (e.g. polio).

4) *Establishment of early warning mechanisms:* these detect new viral activity and are successfully used, for example, in the management of influenza outbreaks. A global network of laboratory surveillance posts provides information about impending epidemics and allows the antigenic components of influenza vaccines to be modified. The value of such systems was demonstrated by the rapid recognition by the Centers for Disease Control in Atlanta, Georgia of an epidemic of a new syndrome of acquired immune deficiency occurring initially in a well defined population (homosexual males).

5) *Controlling the life cycle of zoonotic viruses:* the life cycle of zoonotic viruses can be controlled in some instances, e.g. by mosquito control, bird and bat elimination, and quarantine or rabies vaccination of animals.

### 1.3 Immunisation

The practice of immunisation dates back to at least the 6th century AD, when pledgets of cotton soaked in material obtained from smallpox lesions were placed in the nostrils of susceptible hosts. Vaccination has since led to the elimination of smallpox and to a reduced incidence of diseases such as polio, measles, mumps and rubella in many countries.

*Active immunisation* elicits a specific immune response following the administration of an immunogen, while *passive immunisation* utilises immunoglobulins in an attempt to modify the course of disease.

#### 1.3.1 Active Immunisation (Vaccination)

Before embarking upon vaccination either for the individual or to provide herd immunity, it is important to decide whether this is worthwhile according to the following criteria:

- The health impact of the disease and its complications should be greater than the adverse effects of vaccination.
- Vaccination should provide long term immunity; that following natural infection is usually life long.
- The vaccination programme should not render adults susceptible to infection, as this age group often suffer more serious adverse

effects from viral disease or from vaccination itself.[1]

The general indications and immunisation schedules for viral vaccines in adults are shown in table I.

#### Inactivated Virus Vaccines

The prototype of the inactivated viral vaccine is the Salk polio vaccine,[4] the introduction of which was associated with a dramatic drop in the incidence of polio. More recent studies have demonstrated the efficacy of inactivated influenza vaccines in the elderly, in those with chronic diseases, and in medical personnel who may potentially spread this disease to others at high risk of complications. The composition of the inactive influenza vaccine is reviewed yearly and changed according to prevalent viral subtypes.

Human diploid cell rabies vaccine and an inactivated vaccine have been shown to be efficacious in the prevention of rabies after exposure. However, these should be given in conjunction with human rabies immunoglobulin, as occasional failures of vaccination alone have been reported.

An inactivated hepatitis A vaccine is now available and is recommended as personal protection for travellers to regions of high endemicity.

#### Live Attenuated Virus Vaccines

The original live virus used for a vaccine is vaccinia, a close relative of variola, which confers nearly 100% protection against smallpox. The Sabin polio vaccine[5] was introduced in the US in 1962. However, as it can cause paralysis in both immunodeficient and, rarely, normal individuals (1 per 11.5 million recipients),[6] there has been debate over the relative advantages of live versus inactivated polio vaccine.[7]

Other live attenuated virus vaccines include measles, mumps, rubella, varicella, yellow fever and adeno-type viruses 4 and 7. A measles vaccine with a live attenuated strain has been available in the US since the 1960s and has been associated with a considerable reduction in the incidence of this potentially serious illness with its important sequelae, particularly middle ear infection. Although there have been recent increases in the frequency of infection, these have been associated with non-vaccination of preschool children and adults who did not mount a primary response to the vaccine, rather than evidence of waning immunity.[8] Mumps and rubella vaccines using live attenuated strains have been available in combination with measles [i.e. as measles, mumps and rubella virus vaccine (MMR vaccine)] since 1984.

#### Viral Subunit Vaccines

Hepatitis B vaccine[9] is a representative of this class, consisting of purified hepatitis B surface antigen (HBsAg). It is recommended for those at high risk of developing hepatitis B (e.g. homosexual men, intravenous drug users and certain healthcare workers) and in conjunction with hepatitis B immunoglobulin for those exposed to hepatitis B (e.g. infants born to seropositive mothers, sexual contacts and those with needlestick injuries). More controversially, universal vaccination for all neonates has been recommended by some in countries of both high and low endemicity. An alternative strategy is to vaccinate the offspring of hepatitis B infected mothers and to vaccinate other individuals in adolescence.

Although the initial hepatitis B vaccines were made from the plasma of hepatitis B carriers, more recently, subunit vaccines produced by recombinant DNA techniques have now been introduced.

#### HIV Vaccine Development

Much of the effort to combat the spread of AIDS has focused on the development of an effective vaccine.[10] However, there are a number of major problems associated with development of HIV vaccines:

1) Marked antigenic variation exists between strains of HIV in different geographical locations.

2) There is potential integration of HIV into the host gene, producing silent infection without antigenic expression.

3) HIV affects cells (antigen-presenting cells and CD4 cells) that are important in elaborating the immune response.

4) The important aspects of the immune response that a vaccine needs to elicit are not clear. Neutralising antibodies occur after infection but wane rapidly. Although vaccines may protect in animal models, they may not produce sufficiently high titres of antibodies active against a sufficiently broad spectrum of antigens in humans. Cytotoxic T lymphocyte responses to vaccines are perhaps more important, particularly as these can be induced against less variable parts of HIV (e.g. core antigen).

5) There is no satisfactory animal model in which to test vaccines. Chimpanzees, the only animal model that can be infected with HIV-1, do not develop disease. Other primates develop disease with Simian immunodeficiency virus

**Table I.** General indications and immunisation schedules for viral vaccines in adults (after Immunization Practices Advisory Committee;[2] American College of Physicians Task Force on Adult Immunization[3])

| Vaccine | Indications | Precautions and contraindications | Schedule | Adverse effects | Comments |
|---|---|---|---|---|---|
| **Inactivated virus vaccines** | | | | | |
| Hepatitis B (recombinant hepatitis surface antigen) | Healthcare workers and patients in contact with blood/blood products; homosexual and bisexual men; intravenous drug abusers; residents, immigrants and refugees from endemic areas; others in contact with carriers | None known; pregnancy is not a contraindication for women in whom the vaccine is otherwise indicated | *Primary:* 3 IM doses: 2nd dose 4 weeks after 1st; 3rd 5 months later or 4 doses 4 weeks apart and 4th dose 10 months after 3rd; no booster needed for 7 years | Mild soreness at injection site lasting 1-2 days (15-20%) | Booster (1 dose) produces prompt anamnestic response |
| Influenza | Persons at high risk of complications (i.e. >65 years old or having chronic illnesses); those who may transmit virus to people at high risk | Hypersensitivity to eggs (anaphylaxis or allergy); people who can eat eggs without incident can be vaccinated | 1 dose IM | Soreness at injection site for 1-2 days; fever, myalgia and malaise starting 6-12h after vaccination and lasting 1-2 days in antigen-naive patients; severe immediate hypersensitivity is very rare | Patients should be revaccinated every year. Occasional respiratory illnesses after vaccination usually are due to unrelated coincidental infection |
| Rabies | *Pre-exposure:* veterinarians, animal handlers, some laboratory workers, those living in or visiting (for >1mo) countries with endemic rabies; spelunkers<br>*Postexposure:* whenever significant exposure has occurred | Pregnancy is not a contraindication for women in whom the vaccine is otherwise indicated, pre-exposure vaccine should be given before pregnancy if possible | *Pre-exposure* - 3 IM doses days 0, 7 and 28; 1-dose boosters every 6-24 mos if needed, depending on exposure.<br>*Postexposure* - give unimmunised patients rabies immune globulin, then 5 vaccine doses IM days 0, 3, 7, 14 and 28; immunised patients: IM vaccine on days 0 and 3 | Mild local reactions in patients receiving 5 doses (25-50%); mild headache, nausea, abdominal pain, myalgias and dizziness (up to 20%); immune-complex-like syndrome 2-21 days after booster (6%); serious reactions are rare | Start postexposure prophylaxis with soap and water; pre-exposure prophylaxis does not eliminate need for postexposure prophylaxis; immunosuppression interferes with antibody response - give additional doses if needed |
| **Live attenuated virus vaccines** | | | | | |
| Measles | All adults born after 1956, without prior vaccination after 1st birthday, physician-diagnosed measles, or evidence of immunity; those who had killed vaccine alone or followed within 3 mos by live vaccine, or received vaccines of unknown types from 1963-67 | Do not immunise pregnant women, immunocompromised patients and those with anaphylactic reaction to neomycin or eggs; women should avoid becoming pregnant for 3 mos after vaccine | 1 dose SC (preferably as MMR); when 2 doses are needed, separate them by at least 1 mo | Fever >39.4°C between 5-12 days after vaccine and lasting 1-2 days (5-15%); transient rashes (5%); local reactions with low grade fever lasting 1-2 days in 40-55% of those who previously received killed vaccine | Vaccinate after recovery from severe febrile illness; allow 6-12 wks after administration of blood products containing antibody; measles vaccine can suppress tuberculin reactivity for 4-6 weeks |
| Mumps | All adults believed susceptible and without prior vaccination or physician-diagnosed mumps (those born before 1957 are considered immune) | Do not immunise pregnant women, immunocompromised patients and those with anaphylactic reactions to neomycin or eggs; women should avoid becoming pregnant for 3 mos after vaccine | 1 dose SC (preferably MMR) | Parotiditis and CNS dysfunction are reported rarely; brief and mild allergic reactions (rash, pruritus, purpura) to vaccine are uncommon | Allow 14 days before and 6-12 weeks after administration of blood products containing antibody |
| Rubella | All adults with no documentation of live vaccine after 1st birthday or evidence of immunity, especially young nonpregnant women of childbearing potential | Do not immunise pregnant women, immunocompromised patients and those with anaphylactic reactions to neomycin; women should avoid becoming pregnant for 3 mos after vaccine | 1 dose SC (preferably MMR); revaccination is not recommended | Joint pain may begin 3-25 days after vaccine and persist 1-11 days in up to 40% of nonimmune persons, which tends to be more severe in women; frank arthritis is infrequent | Allow 14 days before and 6-12 weeks after administration of blood products containing antibody; usually given with mumps and measles vaccines (MMR) |

**Table I.** *[Continued]*

| Vaccine | Indications | Precautions and contraindications | Schedule | Adverse effects | Comments |
|---|---|---|---|---|---|
| Yellow fever | Persons travelling or living in areas where infection occurs, laboratory staff who may be exposed to wild or vaccine strains | Do not give to immunosuppressed patients or those hypersensitive to eggs; avoid in pregnancy unless travel to endemic areas is essential | 1 dose SC 10 days before travel; revaccinate every 10 years | Mild headache, low grade fever 5-10 days after vaccine (2-5%) | Administer at least 3 weeks apart from cholera vaccine; can be given with immune globulin |
| **Live or inactivated virus vaccines** | | | | | |
| Polio | Previously unvaccinated adults at increased risk of exposure because of foreign travel or work as healthcare providers or laboratory personnel; travellers receiving less than a full primary course of either oral or inactivated vaccine should complete the course | *Oral:* immunocompromised patients and household contacts should receive inactivated vaccine if needed. *Inactivated:* avoid during pregnancy if possible, use oral vaccine in patients with anaphylaxis to neomycin | *Oral:* 3 PO doses - day 0, 6-8 weeks, then >6 weeks and preferably 8-12 mos after 2nd dose. *Inactivated:* 3 SC doses - day 0, 4-8 weeks, then >4 weeks and preferably 6-12 mos after 2nd dose | *Oral:* rare paralysis in recipients and their contacts. *Inactivated:* no serious reactions documented | Risk of oral polio vaccine-associated paralysis is higher in adults than children, so enhanced-potency inactivated vaccine is preferred in adults |

*Abbreviations:* PO = oral; SC = subcutaneous; IM = intramuscular; MMR = measles, mumps and rubella combination vaccine.

(SIV) or HIV-2, but it is not clear that vaccines effective in this model will protect humans.

6) Immunological mechanisms for prevention of infection via the genital tract, the most important route of HIV infection, are not well understood and most of the animal models have used parenteral challenge to assess potential vaccines.

Although inactivated whole SIV virus vaccines protect primates against subsequent challenge,[11] this is mainly because of antigenic stimulation from human cellular proteins present in the culture medium.[12] Subunit envelope vaccines have been developed which will protect the chimpanzee from HIV-1 challenge and some of these are now in phase I and phase II clinical trials (e.g. gp160 vaccine).

A live attenuated SIV virus (lacking the *nef* gene) has provided long term protection against subsequent high-dose SIV wild-type challenge.[13] Although there are likely to be continuing reservations about the use of attenuated vaccines in a fatal disease associated with incorporation of virus into host DNA, this should be considered further in the absence of other effective measures.

### Other Vaccine Developments

Newer vaccine developments include:

1) *Herpes simplex vaccines*[14]: a number of subunit glycoprotein vaccines are currently undergoing phase III clinical trials.

2) *Cytomegalovirus (CMV) vaccines:* a live attenuated strain of CMV that does not enter a latent phase (Towne) has been shown to protect seronegative recipients of seropositive renal transplants. Subunit vaccines are also under study.[15] Such vaccines would potentially be useful for neonates and immunocompromised individuals.

3) *Papilloma virus vaccines*[16]: attempts to prevent infection with papilloma virus, in particular human papilloma virus (HPV)-16, might be important in preventing a variety of subsequent carcinomas. Potential vaccines include live attenuated strains and protein subunit immunogens.

4) *Rotavirus vaccines:* although rotavirus is a major cause of acute gastrointestinal infection, vaccination is not an immediate prospect because of lack of evidence that antibody responses produce protection, and the need to select a wide variety of serotypes to potentially provide broad protection. Nevertheless, research is continuing with animal-human recom-

binant viruses, which are unharmful to man but whose envelope is identical to the pathogenic strain.

5) *Varicella vaccines:* in a small number of countries, the OKA attenuated strain vaccine, which provides detectable antibodies at 10 years in more than 90% of subjects with a 90% clinical protection rate, is now available. However, this vaccine produces a varicella-like illness in up to 10% of adults and concerns about the long term persistence of immunity have prevented its widespread licensure. Such a vaccine may have a role in immunocompromised patients, but concern about the use of a live attenuated strain in such individuals has prevented its wider use.

6) *Vaccines for travellers:* rabies vaccination should be considered for individuals such as veterinary surgeons who are at high risk when travelling. Hepatitis A is now recommended for all travellers, and measles should be considered for unvacccinated and unexposed individuals travelling to the developing world (where the prevalence of disease remains high). A live attenuated vaccine against yellow fever provides lifelong immunity for those travelling to endemic areas. Although a killed Japanese encephalitis vaccine is available, the high incidence of adverse effects has limited its use to visitors to rural endemic areas and those staying for prolonged periods.

7) *Oral vaccines:* a current area of considerable interest is the development of oral vaccines for a wide range of viral infections, the Sabin polio vaccine being the prototype. Newer uses for oral vaccines include stimulation of antibody and cell-mediated immune responses initiated in Peyer's patches of the gut.[17] Specialised M cells in the domes of these Peyer's patches transport particulate antigen to specialised B and T cell areas within the gut wall. Partial maturation of stimulated cells occurs in this area and is completed in regional lymph nodes.

Oral vaccination is difficult to achieve as the immunity produced is often evenescent, requiring multiple doses. Furthermore, repeated small exposure may induce specific non-responsiveness (tolerance) rather than immunity. Oral vaccination may be affected by intestinal transit and the preferential affinity of certain substances to M cells. Cholera toxin binding subunit (CLB) binds well and also enhances immune responses to oral vaccines in unknown ways. Simian immunodeficiency virus antigens have been combined with CLB, and oral and vaginal administration have produced immune responses. Other molecules that might also improve adhesion to M cells and hence enhance immunogenicity include a variety of polymers used to form microspheres and liposomes.

#### 1.3.2 Passive Immunisation

The use of immunoglobulins was shown to reduce the incidence of enteric disease in outbreaks of hepatitis as early as 1945.[18] Today, active vaccination of travellers to areas of high endemicity for hepatitis A is to be preferred as prophylaxis but the use of immunoglobulins following exposure should be continued in association with a vaccine programme. Similarly, hyperimmune gammaglobulin specifically prepared from individuals with high titres of anti-hepatitis B antibodies should be given to people exposed to hepatitis B, along with vaccination.

Immunoglobulin therapy given within 6 hours of exposure to varicella has also been shown to be efficacious in the prevention of illness in both normal and immunocompromised children.[19,20] It is recommended for those at high risk of complications, i.e. immunocompromised individuals, neonates of mothers who develop varicella within 5 days before or 14 days after delivery, and premature infants. However, its high cost and limited availability prevent it being recommended routinely for exposed susceptible adults.

### 1.4 Antiviral Chemotherapy

As viruses are intracellular organisms that utilise host systems to reproduce, antiviral drugs should interfere with viral synthetic pathways in preference to those of the host cell. Potential sites for the inhibitory action of antiviral drugs include sites of viral attachment, penetration and uncoating transcription, translation, replication, assembly and release (fig. 1).

Important general principles in using antiviral drugs include:

1) As many antiviral agents are prodrugs that act intracellularly, knowledge of their relevant pharmacodynamics is often extremely limited. Thus the attainment of particular plasma concentrations commensurate with their minimum inhibitory concentrations *in vitro* may not be pertinent.

2) For long term use in chronic infections, an antiviral drug should be well absorbed when given orally. However, intravenous administration of poorly absorbed agents may be acceptable for short periods in acute infections.

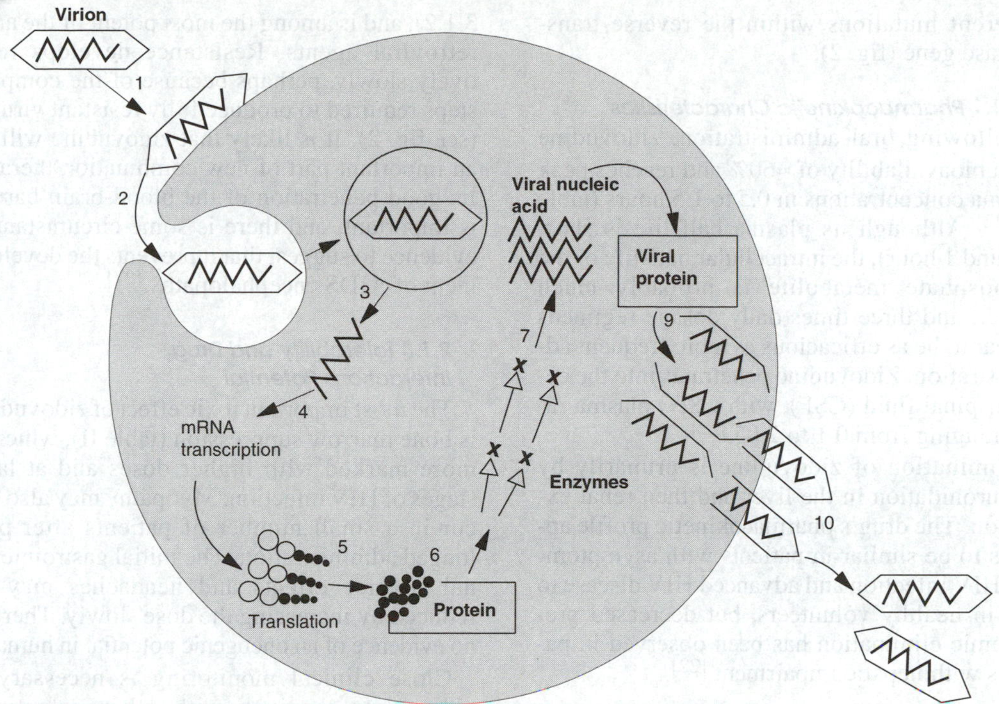


**Fig. 1.** Schematic representation of the multiplication cycle of viruses (and the inhibitory action of various antiviral drugs). 1. Attachment to cell surface. 2. Penetration into the cell (amantadine). 3. Uncoating of viral nucleic acid molecule (amantadine). 4. Transcription of viral messenger RNA (interferon). 5. Translation of proteins which depress synthesis of cell molecules (interferon). 6. Translation of enzymes required for viral nucleic acid replication. 7. Replication of the viral nucleic acid (idoxuridine, vidarabine and aciclovir). 8. Translation of virus proteins. 9. Assembly of new virions. 10. Release of more virions; can attack more cells (photodynamic inactivation).

3) Only agents that cross the blood-brain barrier should be administered to individuals with central nervous system (CNS) infections. This may be particularly important in the long term treatment of HIV infection.

4) The natural history of particular infections will determine the need for drug therapy; some viruses produce an immune response which causes most of the tissue damage, e.g. hepatitis B.

5) Host factors such as age, previous exposure and underlying immune competence affect the overall risk : benefit ratio.

6) Long term use of a single antiviral drug may be associated with the emergence of viruses with reduced sensitivity to the drug, due to either mutation or selection of naturally resistant strains. Although lack of development of resistance is a desirable property of an antiviral drug, this may be because the compound is relatively ineffective and so provides little selective pressure on the virus. In bacterial infections, the use of drug combinations has successfully combated the problem of resistance emerging; however, this strategy has not been widely applied to date in antiviral therapy.

## 2. Clinical Pharmacology of Antiviral Drugs

### 2.1 Zidovudine (AZT, ZDV)

Zidovudine, a dideoxy nucleoside analogue of thymidine which is active against HIV-1 and HIV-2, remains the mainstay of treatment in patients with HIV infection.[21,22] It is, in effect, a prodrug as it is phosphorylated intracellularly by cellular kinases to the active triphosphate form, the mechanism of action of which appears to involve inhibition of the incorporation of thymidine into viral DNA by reverse transcriptase (RT), thus terminating elongation of viral DNA chains. Zidovudine delays disease progression to AIDS and AIDS-related complex, reduces opportunistic infections, and increases survival in patients with advanced HIV infection. However, following long term exposure to the drug, viruses with reduced sensitivity can often be cultured from patients; this occurs to a lesser extent and less rapidly in those treated early in the course of the disease. Resistance appears to occur in a step-wise manner due to different mutations within the reverse transcriptase gene (fig. 2).

#### 2.1.1 Pharmacokinetic Characteristics

Following oral administration, zidovudine has a bioavailability of ≈60% and reaches peak plasma concentrations in 0.5 to 1.5 hours (table II).[22] Although its plasma half-life is short (around 1 hour), the intracellular half-life of the triphosphate metabolite is probably much longer, and three times daily dosage regimens appear to be as efficacious as more frequent administration. Zidovudine penetrates into the cerebrospinal fluid (CSF), with CSF : plasma ratios ranging from 0.1 to 2.05.[22]

Elimination of zidovudine is primarily by glucuronidation in the liver and then renal excretion. The drug's pharmacokinetic profile appears to be similar in patients with asymptomatic HIV infection and advanced HIV disease to that in healthy volunteers, but decreased presystemic elimination has been observed in patients with hepatic impairment.[22]

#### 2.1.2 Clinical Effectiveness

Zidovudine is the only drug shown to prolong survival in HIV infection (see further section 3.1.2), and is among the most potent of the antiretroviral agents. Resistance develops relatively slowly, perhaps because of the complex steps required to produce fully resistant viruses (see fig. 2). It is likely that zidovudine will be an important part of new combination therapy. Its good penetration of the blood-brain barrier is important, and there is some circumstantial evidence to suggest that it prevents the development of AIDS encephalopathy.[27]

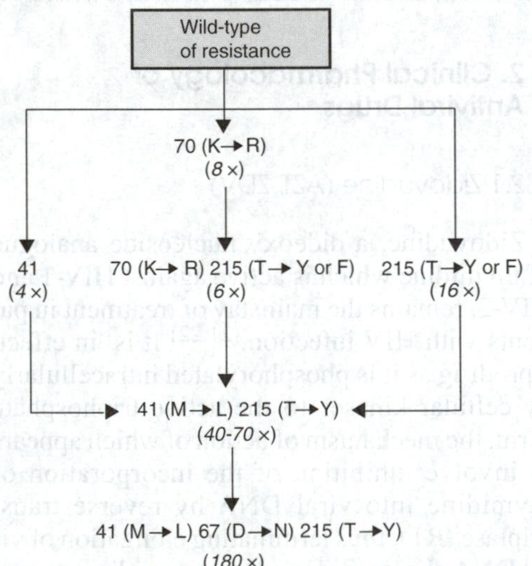


**Fig. 2.** Development of zidovudine resistance. Numbers represent the codon on reverse transcriptase with standard abbreviations for the amino acid changes. × indicates the degree of decrease in sensitivity compared with wild-type resistance (e.g. 4× denotes a 4-fold decrease). Single codon mutations at 70 and 41 tend to occur initially and this encourages the development of an additional mutation at 215. Subsequently, the 74 codon mutation tends to be lost and the combination of codon changes at 41, 67 and 215 becomes the dominant species and has the greatest *in vitro* resistance to zidovudine.

#### 2.1.3 Tolerability and Drug Interactions Potential

The most important toxic effect of zidovudine is bone marrow suppression (table II), which is more marked with higher doses and at later stages of HIV infection. Myopathy may also occur in a small number of patients after prolonged administration. The initial gastrointestinal adverse effects and headaches may be reduced by increasing the dose slowly. There is no evidence of an oncogenic potential in humans.

Close clinical monitoring is necessary if zidovudine is given with other potentially myelosuppressive drugs, particularly ganciclovir, the concomitant administration of which may be precluded due to the risk of neutropenia. A number of drugs including probenecid, valproic acid, methadone and trimethoprim have been reported to increase plasma concentrations of zidovudine (either via inhibition of its glucuronidation in the liver or interference with its renal tubular excretion or both), while rifampicin has been shown to decrease plasma zidovudine concentrations (presumably via its enzyme-inducing effect). However, no significant pharmacokinetic interaction between paracetamol and zidovudine has been demonstrated.[28]

### 2.2 Didanosine (Dideoxyinosine; ddI)

Didanosine, a dideoxy nucleoside analogue of adenine, acts on the reverse transcriptase of HIV-1, HIV-2 and zidovudine-resistant HIV-1 following intracellular phosphorylation.[29,30] *In vitro* synergism against HIV has been observed between didanosine and various other antiviral agents including zidovudine and ribavirin. The development of viruses resistant to didanosine has been less well studied than for zidovudine, but resistant strains do develop after long term therapy and are associated with mutations at codon 74 of the reverse transcriptase.

**Table II.** Pharmacokinetic parameters and adverse effects of antiviral drugs (after Morse et al.;[23] Morris;[24] Pue & Benet;[25] Dorr[26])

| Drug | F[a] (%) | $t_{1/2}$ (h) | CL (L/h) | Vd (L) [per 70kg] | PB (%) | $f_e$ (%) | CSF[b] (%) | Principal adverse effects |
|---|---|---|---|---|---|---|---|---|
| Aciclovir | 15-30 | 2-3 | 12-14 | 49 | 9-24 | 63 | 50 | Minor GI disturbances (oral); occasional reversible renal failure with IV use (reduce dosage in renal impairment) |
| Amantadine | 80 | 15-16 | 16.5 | 560 | | 80-90 | 50 | Restlessness, anxiety, insomnia, minor GI disturbances. Accumulation and toxicity more likely in renal impairment (reduce dosage; see appendix D) |
| Didanosine (ddI) | 20-40 | 0.5-2.0 | 48-56 | 53.2-84[c] | <5 | 35-60 | 21 | Headaches, restlessness, peripheral neuropathy. Pancreatitis (rare) |
| Famciclovir[d] | 77 | 2.0 | 38-42 | 105-126 | | 70 | | Headache, nausea, diarrhoea |
| Foscarnet | <10 | 3.3-6.8<br>88[e] | 5.3-12.8 | 91-357[c] | | 83-88 | 31-69 | Rashes, minor GI disturbances, anaemia; hypocalcaemia, seizures (rare).<br>Renal failure (reduce dosage in renal impairment) |
| Ganciclovir | 3-6 | 2-3 | 12-18 | 35-70[c] | 2 | 91 | 24-70 | Neutropenia, thrombocytopenia, confusion |
| Interferon-α | 80-100 (SC, IM) | 4-5[f] | ≈12 | 28[c] | | | | 'Flu-like' symptoms, GI disturbances, vertigo, confusion, paraesthesias, hypotension.<br>Leucopenia, thrombocytopenia, mild anaemia (reversible) |
| Lamivudine (3TC) | 82 | 2.5 | 24 | 91 | | 71 | | Headache, GI disturbances, neutropenia |
| Ribavirin | 20-50 | 20-50 | 14-21 | 21-42[c] | 0 | 24-35 | 73-113 | Headache, abdominal cramps, reversible anaemia, elevated serum bilirubin |
| Rimantadine | | 24-36 | 34-40 | 1400 | | 12 | | GI disturbances, headache, insomnia, light-headedness. Reduce dosage in renal impairment |
| Stavudine (d4T) | >80 | 0.8-1.6 | 32-42 | 56-77 | | 50-70 | 15 | Peripheral neuropathy; anaemia, elevated transaminases; insomnia, dizziness, GI disturbances (occasionally) |
| Vidarabine (Ara-A) | | 3.5[g] | 7[g] | | 20-30 | 1-3 | 30-100[g] | GI disturbances, painful extremities, paraesthesias, bone marrow depression.<br>Toxicity more likely in renal/hepatic impairment |
| Zalcitabine (ddC) | 70-80 | 1.2 | 14-21 | ≈35[c] | <4 | 75 | 9-37 | Peripheral neuropathy, mouth ulcers, rash.<br>Pancreatitis (rare) |
| Zidovudine (AZT, ZDV) | 63 | 0.9-1.4 | 70-126 | 112[c] | 7-38 | 14 | 15-135 | Anaemia, neutropenia, myopathy, headache, insomnia, vomiting, anorexia, asthenia |

a Oral bioavailability unless otherwise stated.
b CSF concentration as a percentage of that in plasma.
c Volume of distribution at steady-state ($Vd_{ss}$).
d Active drug is penciclovir.
e Terminal elimination phase half-life.
f Biological activity extends for 2 to 3 days after administration.
g Values shown are for metabolite, Ara-Hx.

*Abbreviations and symbols:* F = bioavailability; $t_{1/2}$ = plasma half-life; CL = total body clearance; Vd = apparent volume of distribution; PB = protein binding; $f_e$ = proportion excreted unchanged in the urine; CSF = cerebrospinal fluid.

#### 2.2.1 Pharmacokinetic Characteristics

Didanosine is acid-labile and is usually given with a buffer on an empty stomach. Under these conditions, its oral bioavailability has ranged from 20 to 40%. Like zidovudine, it has a short plasma half-life (0.5 to 2h; table II) but the intracellular half-life of its active metabolite is more than 12 hours, which has allowed twice daily dosage regimens to be developed.[30] Concentrations in the CSF are about 21% of plasma concentrations at 1 hour after intravenous infusion.

Didanosine undergoes extensive metabolism (to dideoxyadenosine triphosphate, uric acid and/or purine metabolites), but ≈35 to 60% is excreted in the urine unchanged. Its plasma half-life is increased ≈3-fold in renal failure.[30]

#### 2.2.2 Clinical Effectiveness

Direct comparisons of didanosine and zidovudine have indicated a similar overall clinical effectiveness. Although zidovudine appears marginally more effective in the first few weeks of therapy, subsequently switching to didanosine has proved marginally superior to continuing zidovudine.[31] Limited data indicate that didanosine and zidovudine combinations have enhanced effects on surrogate markers of HIV infection in comparison with either drug used alone (see also section 3.1.1).[32]

#### 2.2.3 Tolerability and Drug Interactions Potential

Unlike zidovudine, didanosine's haematological toxicity is minimal. Peripheral neuropathy and rare (but potentially fatal) pancreatitis are the major dose-limiting adverse effects of the drug. Didanosine should be withdrawn in patients with signs or symptoms of pancreatitis and should be used with care in those receiving treatment for *P. carinii* pneumonia who may be receiving other drugs (e.g. pentamidine and cotrimoxazole) that have been associated with the development of pancreatitis.[30]

Drugs whose absorption is affected by gastric acidity (e.g. ketoconazole and dapsone) should be given at least 2 hours before didanosine administration. Didanosine formulations containing magnesium and/or aluminium antacids (as buffers) may decrease the plasma concentrations of some quinolone and tetracycline antibiotics, which should not be administered within 2 hours of a didanosine dose.[30]

### 2.3 Zalcitabine (Dideoxycytidine; ddC)

Zalcitabine is an analogue of the nucleoside deoxycytidine which, when converted intracellularly to its active triphosphate metabolite, inhibits replication of HIV. Like zidovudine and didanosine, zalcitabine is believed to act by inhibiting reverse transcriptase and terminating viral DNA chains. It is active against HIV-1, HIV-2 and zidovudine-resistant variants, and it shows an additive to synergistic antiviral effect when combined with zidovudine. Zalcitabine-resistant HIV strains may be slower to develop than strains resistant to zidovudine.[33]

#### 2.3.1 Pharmacokinetic Characteristics

Zalcitabine has an oral bioavailability of 70 to 80% and achieves peak plasma concentrations 1 to 2 hours after administration. It penetrates the CSF to a lesser extent than zidovudine, with CSF concentrations being around 14 to 20% (range 9 to 37%) of simultaneous plasma concentrations. Zalcitabine is mainly eliminated by renal excretion and has a plasma half-life of 1.2 hours. This is prolonged in patients with renal impairment.[33]

#### 2.3.2 Clinical Effectiveness

Zalcitabine can affect surrogate markers of HIV infection (see section 3.1.1) but it appears less effective clinically than zidovudine,[34] and its main use is likely to be in combination therapy. Switching to or adding zalcitabine produced a small delay in clinical disease in individuals with CD4 counts above 150 cells/μl who had been taking long term zidovudine.[35]

#### 2.3.3 Tolerability and Drug Interactions Potential

The most important adverse effects of zalcitabine are peripheral neuropathy, stomatitis and rash. Pancreatitis is a serious but rare complication, affecting less than 1% of patients receiving the drug as monotherapy. Unlike zidovudine, haematological toxicity is rare with zalcitabine.[33]

The likelihood of peripheral neuropathy with zalcitabine may be increased by its coadministration with other drugs known to cause this adverse effect (e.g. dapsone, isoniazid, vincristine).

### 2.4 Stavudine (d4T)

Stavudine is a newer nucleoside analogue currently under investigation in HIV disease. It is a dideoxythymidine derivative that acts as an inhibitor of HIV reverse transcriptase, and is

**Table III.** Mutations in reverse transcriptase (numbers represent codon on reverse transcriptase)

| Drug/combination | Site of mutation |
|---|---|
| **1. Reverse transcriptase mutations seen *in vitro* when various drugs are administered:** | |
| Zidovudine | 41, 60, 67, 70, 215 |
| DDN/lamivudine | 65, 69, 74, 75, 184 |
| **2. *In vitro* combinations of mutations in reverse transcriptase that re-establish zidovudine sensitivity:** | |
| Didanosine + zidovudine | 74 + 215 |
| TIBO + zidovudine | 181 + 215 |
| NNA + zidovudine | 100 + 215 |
| Lamivudine/FTC + zidovudine | 184 + 215 |

*Abbreviations:* DDN = dideoxynucleoside analogues other than zidovudine; FTC = 5-fluoro congener of lamivudine (3TC); NNA = non-nucleoside analogue (see section 2.6); TIBO = tetrahydro-imidazo-benzodiazepin-2-(1,H)-one.

effective against both HIV-1 and HIV-2, including strains resistant to zidovudine. Stavudine has a relatively high oral bioavailability (>80%) and is mainly eliminated by renal excretion. Although its plasma half-life is short (0.8 to 1.6h), the active triphosphate form of the drug has an intracellular half-life of about 3.5 hours, which is similar to that of zidovudine triphosphate.[21,36]

Limited clinical data thus far available have shown that switching from zidovudine to stavudine is associated with an improvement in both clinical outcome and surrogate markers of HIV infection in comparison with continuing on zidovudine. Surrogate marker data indicate a very similar magnitude of effect of zidovudine or stavudine in individuals who had not previously received antiretroviral therapy.[37]

The principal dose-limiting adverse effect of stavudine appears to be peripheral neuropathy. Other adverse effects reported less commonly include anaemia and elevated transaminases.[21]

### 2.5 Lamivudine (3TC)

Lamivudine (2'-deoxy-3'-thiacytidine) is a nucleoside analogue structurally related to zalcitabine. Although it is a potent inhibitor of HIV-1 and HIV-2 *in vitro*, initial studies showed it to have little effect as a single agent on surrogate markers of HIV infection, except for transient reductions in HIV viral load, probably because of the rapid selection of resistant viruses. However, when coadministered with zidovudine, there may be a delay in the development of strains resistant to zidovudine, and viruses resistant to this drug may regain sensitivity to it (table III). Certainly, in patients who have never received antiretroviral agents, greater improvement in surrogate markers of HIV infection (CD4 count and viral load) occur than when zidovudine is given alone. Lamivudine is also currently under investigation for the treatment of hepatitis B infection.

Lamivudine has a high oral bioavailability (82%), and around 70% of an oral dose is excreted unchanged in the urine.[38] It appears to be well tolerated, although neutropenia has been reported rarely.

### 2.6 Non-Nucleoside Analogues (NNAs)

This group of antiviral compounds with diverse chemical structures are grouped together because they inhibit HIV-1 but not HIV-2 reverse transcriptase.[21] Although the oral bioavailability of some compounds is low, plasma concentrations exceeding the *in vitro* minimum inhibitory concentrations can be achieved because of the high sensitivity of HIV. However, resistance develops rapidly *in vivo* because of selection of a variety of mutations in the reverse transcriptase gene (table III). Despite this, there is continued interest in these classes of compound because they have few adverse effects, and plasma concentrations that exceed the minimum inhibitory concentrations for resistant strains can sometimes be achieved. Furthermore, some drugs restore the sensitivity of viruses previously resistant to zidovudine.

Compounds in this class include:

1) *TIBO [tetrahydro-imidazo-benzodiazepin-2(1,H)-one] and thione derivatives:* these compounds were the prototypes of the NNA group but they have to be given intravenously and were not found to be effective in small pilot studies.

2) *α-Anilinophenylacetamide derivatives:* these compounds can be given orally and their development is continuing.

3) *Pyridone derivatives:* no further clinical evaluation as sole therapy for HIV is planned for these drugs, but their evaluation in combination studies with zidovudine is continuing.

4) *Nevirapine:* this compound is the most extensively studied of the non-nucleoside analogues. High plasma concentrations can be achieved with oral administration, although the maximum dose may be limited by the occurrence of a drug rash. In a few patients, prolonged suppression of viral markers of HIV replication has been achieved, although resistant variants develop rapidly in most. In patients who had previously received zidovudine for a year or more, the addition of nevirapine has produced a slight improvement in surrogate markers of HIV infection.

At present, there is no evidence of sustained clinical benefit when these agents are administered alone. Data on the use of combinations of NNAs and dideoxynucleosides are very limited but do not suggest a major synergistic effect.

## 2.7 Protease Inhibitors

HIV contains a unique protease which becomes active at the time of viral budding and splits a large viral polypeptide derived from the *gag* gene into its constituent proteins. This protease has been successfully crystallised and its tertiary structure elucidated by crystallography.

Protease inhibitors that have marked anti-HIV effects have been developed by molecular modelling.[39] Noncompetitive inhibitors have not proved effective and most agents are competitive inhibitors that mimic the transitional states of the protease. These drugs have no activity against mammalian proteases. Although their oral bioavailability is low, sufficient drug is usually absorbed to produce plasma concentrations above *in vitro* minimum inhibitory levels; however, absorption into infected cells may be more difficult and some of the drugs bind strongly to plasma proteins, limiting their biological activity. Early clinical studies have sometimes demonstrated marked short term changes in surrogate markers of infection when protease inhibitors are used as single agents, although this is usually limited by the development of resistance. The available data on combination therapy with dideoxynucleoside analogues and protease inhibitors have suggested that such combinations are synergistic *in vitro*[40] and produce a moderate improvement in surrogate markers of HIV infection compared with the use of protease inhibitors alone. Those drugs continuing in development (e.g. *saquinavir, indinavir* and *ritonavir*) have no discernible toxicity.

## 2.8 Aciclovir

Aciclovir (hydroxyethoxymethyl-guanine) is an acyclic purine nucleoside analogue with high specific activity against certain herpes viruses.[41] This specificity is due to its phosphorylation to aciclovir monophosphate by a thymidine kinase which is present only in herpes-infected cells. Aciclovir monophosphate is subsequently phosphorylated to the di- and triphosphate forms predominantly by host cell kinases. Aciclovir triphosphate inhibits viral DNA polymerase and can act as a chain terminator when incorporated into viral DNA, although it has little effect on host cell DNA polymerase.[42-44]

Aciclovir is highly active against herpes simplex virus types 1 and 2 and varicella-zoster virus, but has much less activity against cytomegalovirus (CMV) and Epstein-Barr virus, which do not produce their own thymidine kinase. Resistant herpes virus mutants isolated from patients treated with aciclovir most commonly have deletion or alteration of the gene producing thymidine kinase. More rarely, changes in the DNA polymerase gene have occurred. Resistant mutants are less virulent in immunocompetent individuals but may cause serious disease in the immunosuppressed.

Aciclovir is widely used systemically and topically in the treatment of herpes simplex infections and herpes zoster (see sections 3.3 and 3.4) and has a good toxicity profile (table II). However, poor absorption following oral administration limits the plasma concentrations achieved, which remain below those that would be effective for the treatment of most CMV isolates and some varicella-zoster infections.

### 2.8.1 Pharmacokinetic Characteristics

The absorption of aciclovir following oral administration is slow and variable, and its bioavailability is around 15 to 30%. Transcutaneous penetration following topical administration varies with the preparation used, but around 30 to 50% of the drug reaches the basal epidermis in patients with cutaneous infections treated with the cream formulation. Similarly, substantial intraocular penetration has been observed with the ophthalmic ointment.[44]

Orally or intravenously administered aciclovir is distributed to a wide range of tissues; CSF concentrations are ≈50% of those in plasma. Aciclovir is principally eliminated by renal excretion, with 45 to 79% of an intravenous dose recovered in the urine unchanged. Its plasma half-life is around 2 to 3 hours in adults with normal renal function, but is greater in those with renal impairment (≈20h in end-phase renal failure), necessitating dosage reduction (see appendix D).

Aciclovir is readily haemodialysable, a single 6-hour course of haemodialysis reducing aciclovir plasma concentrations by 60%. The dialysis half-life is 5.7 hours, and the dialysis clearance 4.92 L/h (82 ml/min).[45]

#### 2.8.2 Clinical Effectiveness

Aciclovir has revolutionised the treatment of herpes simplex infections and has a modest effect in the treatment or prophylaxis of herpes zoster.[46] Its use in these infections is discussed further in sections 3.3 and 3.4.

#### 2.8.3 Tolerability

Aciclovir is well tolerated whether administered topically or systemically, adverse effects being mainly limited to mild local effects (e.g. rash) and gastrointestinal disturbances. Occasional instances of acute, usually reversible, renal failure have been reported, principally in patients receiving intravenous aciclovir in whom high plasma concentrations of the drug were present.

### 2.9 Valaciclovir

Valaciclovir, the L-valyl ester of aciclovir, is well absorbed after oral administration and is rapidly converted to the parent drug (aciclovir). Its bioavailability is 3 to 5 times greater than that of aciclovir,[47] providing higher plasma concentrations of aciclovir and permitting less frequent administration. Oral doses of valaciclovir 250mg given 4 times daily have been found to provide a similar AUC value (area under the plasma concentration-time curve) to that provided by aciclovir 800mg 5 times daily.[48]

Valaciclovir is likely to improve the management of herpes zoster, and it may produce sufficiently high plasma concentrations of aciclovir to make it an effective treatment for CMV infections, although this has yet to be established clinically. Its pharmacokinetic properties make it a potentially useful agent for the treatment of herpes simplex infection. The adverse effect profile of valaciclovir appears to be similar to that of aciclovir.

### 2.10 Penciclovir and Famciclovir

Penciclovir is a 9-hydroxyalkylguanosine derivative with similar activity to aciclovir against herpes simplex and varicella-zoster viruses. However, it has limited bioavailability when given orally and is only suitable for intravenous administration.

Famciclovir, the oral form of penciclovir, is extensively absorbed and rapidly metabolised to penciclovir; the systemic availability of penciclovir after oral famciclovir administration is around 77%. Like aciclovir, penciclovir is principally eliminated by renal excretion, and 60 to 70% of an oral dose is excreted unchanged in the urine.[25] The plasma half-life of penciclovir is around 2 hours, but the intracellular half-life of its active triphosphate form is much longer which may reduce the frequency of administration and/or the duration of therapy. In doses of 500mg or 750mg three times daily, famciclovir has proved effective in reducing healing time in patients with uncomplicated herpes zoster and in shortening the duration of virus shedding and the duration of pain,[49] and it has proved at least as effective in this respect as aciclovir 800mg five times daily.[50] It has also proved effective in recurrent genital herpes, doses of 125, 250 and 500mg twice daily shortening healing time and the duration of viral shedding.[51]

The advantages of these compounds over aciclovir are marginal.

### 2.11 Ganciclovir

Ganciclovir, like aciclovir, is a nucleoside analogue which is phosphorylated by viral kinases within cells and prevents replication of various herpes viruses. It has significant activity against cytomegalovirus (CMV) and is mainly used in the treatment of CMV infections.[52] A major drawback to its clinical use is its poor oral bioavailability (3 to 6%) and it is usually given intravenously. However, an oral formulation is available for maintenance treatment of CMV retinitis (see section 3.2.1).

Ganciclovir is primarily eliminated by renal excretion, with 91% of an administered dose being excreted unchanged within 24 hours; no metabolites have been identified. Compared with patients with normal renal function, those with renal dysfunction have a more prolonged plasma half-life and are more susceptible to the drug's haematological toxicity.[23]

Intravenous ganciclovir is the drug most commonly used in the initial treatment of CMV infection in immunocompromised patients. Its most important adverse effect is neutropenia, which is only partly dose-related.[24] The high risk of neutropenia in patients given ganciclovir and zidovudine together precludes the use of this combination in patients with HIV infection.

## 2.12 Foscarnet

A pyrophosphate analogue, foscarnet acts directly to inhibit viral DNA kinases and the reverse transcriptase of HIV. It is used to treat cytomegalovirus (CMV) infection and herpes simplex virus infections resistant to aciclovir in immunosuppressed individuals.[28,53]

### 2.12.1 Pharmacokinetic Characteristics

Foscarnet is poorly absorbed and is given intravenously in a 2 or 3 times daily dosage regimen. Its pharmacokinetic profile shows substantial interindividual variability. The drug is primarily eliminated by renal excretion with 83% of a cumulative intravenous dose being recovered unchanged in the urine within 36 hours, and 88% within a week. The elimination of foscarnet appears to be triphasic with two relatively short phases (half-lives of 0.5 to 1.4h and 3.3 to 6.8h, respectively) and a long term terminal phase (mean half-life 88h); sequestration of the drug into bone and its subsequent slow release is the likely cause of the latter phenomenon.[53]

### 2.12.2 Clinical Effectiveness

Although the use of foscarnet in CMV infection in late-stage AIDS patients has resulted in longer survival when compared with ganciclovir therapy, patients tolerate this drug less well and it is still mainly used in individuals who experience adverse reactions with ganciclovir or who have progressive CMV disease despite treatment with the latter. Foscarnet is also used in the treatment of herpes simplex infection resistant to aciclovir in immunocompromised individuals.

### 2.12.3 Tolerability

The most frequent dose-limiting adverse effect of foscarnet is a 2- to 3-fold increase in serum creatinine in about 45% of patients, the cause of which appears to be renal tubular necrosis. The incidence and severity of renal dysfunction is reduced by adjusting the dose of foscarnet in relation to the serum creatinine level, using intermittent rather than continuous infusions, providing adequate prehydration, and avoiding other potentially nephrotoxic drugs. Anaemia, hypercalcaemia and hyperphosphataemia are other adverse effects, although symptomatic hypocalcaemia has also been observed. Thrombophlebitis, diarrhoea and headache have been reported occasionally.[53]

The concomitant administration of foscarnet and intravenous pentamidine appears to be contraindicated because of additive renal toxicity and an increased risk of hypocalcaemia.[53]

**Table IV.** Clinical uses of interferon-α in viral diseases

| Disease | Response rate |
|---|---|
| Condyloma acuminata due to human papilloma virus (HPV)[94,95] | Moderate |
| Chronic active hepatitis B virus (HBV) infection[96] | High |
| Chronic active hepatitis C virus (HCV) infection[81] | Moderate-high |
| Rhinovirus infection[a] | High |
| Human immunodeficiency virus (HIV) infection[a] [97] | Low-moderate |

a Currently non-approved indications.

## 2.13 Interferon-α (IFN-α)

Interferons are produced naturally by the body in response to viruses and prevent subsequent infection for short periods. There are three main types: interferon-α, which is produced by a wide variety of cells in the body, interferon-β which is produced by fibroblasts, and interferon-γ which is produced by activated T cells.[54] Most clinical experience in antiviral chemotherapy has been obtained with two forms of interferon-α (IFN-α) produced by recombinant DNA techniques, i.e. IFN-α2a and IFN-α2b, and with a nonrecombinant form harvested from human white blood cells exposed to a virus *in vitro,* i.e. IFN-αN1.[26]

Interferons have complex immunomodulatory and antiviral effects partly mediated by stimulation of guanyl cyclase, which in turn stimulates cellular phosphorylating activity and indirectly inhibits viral replication. Interferons also directly inhibit viral replication by stimulating nuclear factors, and inhibit viral budding by affecting the cytoskeleton of the cell membrane.

Broad-spectrum antiviral activity has been demonstrated for both recombinant and naturally occurring IFN-α. Clinically, IFN-α has proved effective in some (though not all) studies in the treatment of human papilloma virus infection (condyloma acuminata) and in the treatment of chronic hepatitis B and C infection (table IV). Long term suppression of hepatitis B is commonly achieved with IFN-α therapy, but while hepatitis C is responsive to IFN-α in about 40% of patients, long term remissions are rare.[26] IFN-α also has some anti-HIV activity and causes significant regression of Kaposi's sarcoma in HIV seropositive patients with CD4 counts above 200 cells/μl.

IFN-α is administered subcutaneously. Although its elimination half-life is short (4 to 5h), its biological activity extends for 2 to 3 days after administration which facilitates daily or twice weekly administration. Clearance of IFN-α is mediated by catabolism in the renal tubules; no intact drug is excreted in the urine.[26]

IFN-α has an established role in the treatment of hepatitis B and Kaposi's sarcoma in HIV seropositive individuals with CD4 counts above 200 cells/μl; its role in the management of hepatitis C is less clear. While it may have beneficial effects on other virus infections and some tumours, the expense of interferon therapy and its adverse effects have led to only restricted clinical use.

The adverse effects of IFN-α are dose-related and include 'flu-like' symptoms, gastrointestinal disturbances, vertigo, confusion, and reversible leucopenia, thrombocytopenia and mild anaemia.[24]

### 2.14 Vidarabine (Adenine Arabinoside; Ara-A)

Vidarabine is a purine nucleoside analogue developed initially as an antineoplastic agent. It is phosphorylated intracellularly to the triphosphate form and is active against various viral DNA polymerases, including those of pox viruses and hepatitis B.

Vidarabine is available for intravenous infusion and as a topical ophthalmic preparation. Following intravenous administration, it is rapidly deaminated to a less active metabolite, arabinosylhypoxanthine (Ara-Hx), which reaches higher plasma concentrations than the parent drug. Both vidarabine and Ara-Hx are predominantly eliminated by the kidney, although Ara-Hx is also metabolised by xanthine oxidase to form xanthine arabinoside – a step which is inhibited by the xanthine oxidase inhibitor allopurinol with potential enhancement of toxicity. In patients with normal renal function, the plasma half-life of Ara-Hx is around 3.5 hours, but this is moderately increased in those with severe renal dysfunction requiring dosage reduction in order to avoid accumulation (see appendix D). Because of its low solubility, vidarabine must be administered by continuous intravenous infusion in large volumes of fluid over a period of 12 hours.[55]

Although vidarabine has been widely used in the treatment of hepatitis B, there is little place for it in present therapy. Its adverse effects include gastrointestinal disturbances, neurological toxicity and bone marrow suppression. Vidarabine is no longer the agent of first choice for the treatment of either aciclovir-resistant herpes virus infection or hepatitis B infection.

### 2.15 Amantadine and Rimantadine

Amantadine (1-adamantanamine hydrochloride) and its analogue rimantadine (methyl-1-adamantanamine hydrochloride) are symmetrical tricyclic amines that inhibit the multiplication of all subtypes of influenza A, although they have little activity against influenza B.[56] *In vitro* activity has also been observed against other viruses such as rubella, but only at concentrations not safely achieved clinically. Although their mechanism of action is unclear, these agents act at an early stage of viral infection, possibly by preventing the uncoating of viruses following cellular penetration or by interfering with RNA transcription. Resistance has been seen when influenza virus is grown in tissue culture in the presence of amantadine, and resistant clinical isolates have been reported.

Only limited pharmacokinetic data are available for amantadine and rimantadine (table II). Amantadine is well absorbed when given orally and has a bioavailability of around 80%. It is predominantly eliminated by renal excretion, with 80 to 90% of a single dose being recovered unchanged in the urine. In patients with normal renal function, the plasma half-life of amantadine is about 15 to 16 hours, but this is markedly prolonged in renal impairment (up to 144 hours in severe renal failure), requiring dosage reduction (see appendix D). Rimantadine has a longer half-life of around 24 to 36 hours.

Amantadine and rimantadine have only a limited role in the treatment of influenza (see further section 3.5), although there may be a place for the latter in serious respiratory syncytial virus infection (see section 3.7). The adverse effects of amantadine consist mainly of mild CNS symptoms and include insomnia, nervousness and difficulty in concentrating. Rimantadine reportedly has fewer adverse effects.[55]

2.16 Ribavirin

Ribavirin is a synthetic purine nucleoside analogue with activity against a wide variety of viruses including herpes viruses, respiratory syncytial virus (RSV), influenza A and B viruses, and HIV. It is administered orally and by aerosol. Following oral administration, ribavirin is well absorbed, though its bioavailability ranges from only 20 to 50% (mean ≈40%) due to first-pass metabolism. The drug accumulates in red blood cells, achieving concentrations that eventually exceed the plasma concentration by ≈50-fold. Ribavirin is eliminated by both metabolic and renal mechanisms; the primary metabolite is 1,2,4-triazole-3-carboxamide, the recovery of which in the urine accounts for ≈30% of an oral dose. The terminal elimination phase half-life of ribavirin ranges from about 20 to 50 hours, but small amounts persist in the plasma for as long as 4 weeks after administration.[23]

Ribavirin is primarily used in RSV infections, for which it is administered by aerosol, but it has also demonstrated activity and/or efficacy in the treatment of Lassa fever, influenza, and HIV infection. It is well tolerated when given by aerosol, the only adverse effects being rashes and conjunctivitis. With oral or intravenous administration, transient dose-dependent anaemia has occurred.[24]

2.17 Idoxuridine

Idoxuridine (5-iodo-2'-deoxyuridine) acts by inhibiting the uptake of thymidine into viral (and host) DNA, and has activity against herpes simplex virus, cytomegalovirus, adenovirus and varicella-zoster virus. Although it has been administered intravenously, it is now considered to be ineffective and too toxic to justify use by this route.[55] Consequently, idoxuridine is only used topically, principally in mucocutaneous herpes simplex infections and in herpes zoster.

2.18 Trifluridine

Trifluridine (trifluorothymidine; 5-trifluoromethyl-2'-deoxyuridine) is active against herpes simplex virus and is used as an ophthalmic preparation in the treatment of herpetic keratitis. It appears to act by inhibiting enzymes involved in DNA synthesis. Trifluridine seems to cause a similar incidence of toxicity to topically administered vidarabine (mainly transient burning or stinging and palpebral oedema), but less than that of idoxuridine.[55]

Trifluridine is poorly tolerated when given systemically due to bone marrow suppression.

2.19 Inosine Pranobex (Isoprinosine)

Inosine pranobex is a synthetic compound formed from the *p*-acetamido-benzoate salt of *N-N*-diethylamino-2-propranol and inosine. It exerts antiviral and antitumour activities *in vivo* which are secondary to an immunomodulatory effect (see further chapter 28; sect. 2.2.5). Beneficial clinical effects with oral administration have been reported in mucocutaneous herpes simplex infections, subacute sclerosing panencephalitis, influenza, varicella-zoster infection and type B viral hepatitis. Inosine pranobex is rapidly metabolised and has a short plasma half-life of about 50 minutes following an oral dose. The major excretion product of the inosine moiety is uric acid, while the *p*-acetamidobenzoic acid and *N-N*-diethylamino-2-propanol components are excreted in the urine both unchanged and as the glucuronidated and oxidised metabolites, respectively.

The only adverse effects associated with inosine pranobex therapy have been transient increases in serum and urinary uric acid and occasional transient nausea.[57]

## 3. Optimum Treatment of Specific Viral Infections

### 3.1 HIV Infection

HIV infects two immunologically competent cell types. Infection of macrophages which migrate to the central nervous system is associated in some individuals with the eventual development of dementia. Infection of macrophages with release of cytokines such as tumour necrosis factor (TNF) may also be important in the development of wasting. CD4 cell infection is associated with a loss of cellular immune function which takes place over 5 to 15 years, and is associated with the development of various opportunistic infections (see table V and section 3.1.3 below). The two tumours most commonly associated with AIDS, non-Hodgkin's lymphoma and Kaposi's sarcoma, are probably both associated with opportunistic viral infections (Epstein-Barr virus and a herpes virus).

Although the classification of diseases associated with HIV infection promulgated by the Centers for Disease Control (CDC) [table V] is an important epidemiological tool, it is cumbersome to use clinically but does serve to remind

**Table V.** Simplified Centers for Disease Control (CDC) classification of diseases associated with human immunodeficiency virus (HIV) infection (revised 1987)

**Group I:** Acute infection
**Group II:** Asymptomatic
**Group III:** Persistent generalised lymphadenopathy syndrome
**Group IV:**
- a) Constitutional disease (weight loss, fever, diarrhoea)
- b) Neurological disease (dementia, myelopathy, peripheral neuropathy)
- c) Infections
  - i) Serious opportunistic infections (see text; section 3.1.3)
  - ii) Less serious opportunistic infections (oral hairy leukoplakia, multidermatome herpes zoster, recurrent Salmonella infections, Nocardia infection, recurrent oral candidiasis)
- d) Tumours (invasive cervical cancer, primary cerebral lymphoma, Kaposi's sarcoma, non-Hodgkin's lymphoma)
- e) Other conditions (other opportunistic infections, neurological symptoms, and symptoms not listed elsewhere)

that in addition to major life-threatening diseases, a wide variety of minor opportunistic infections can occur which reduce the quality of life of affected individuals.

#### *3.1.1 Surrogate Markers of HIV Infection*

As the number of drugs potentially active against HIV is large, and they are likely to be used in combination, large scale clinical trials will be needed to show which combination of agents prolong survival. The potential efficacy of drugs or combinations that might result in clinical improvement in HIV disease is therefore tested initially by using surrogate markers. The two most popular have been a rise in CD4 count and a fall in HIV p24 antigen. Although both are valuable prognostic markers in the natural history of HIV infection, it has not been established that such changes in response to therapy can be related to improved survival or a delay in clinical events. Indeed, a large study has shown that this is not the case, perhaps because the changes were small.[58] The findings of this study therefore cast doubt on the validity of approving drugs for treating large numbers of patients on the basis of improvement in surrogate markers. Measurements of the amount of virus present in peripheral blood mononuclear cells and free in plasma may be more directly related to the underlying disease process, and are more likely to be effective surrogate markers for assessing treatment.

Although the development of a first or a new opportunistic infection in HIV-infected patients is regarded as a clinical end-point in large scale trials, only some of these may be predictive for improved survival.

#### *3.1.2 Drug Treatment*

A drug treatment plan for HIV disease is shown in figure 3. Zidovudine, didanosine and zalcitabine are available for the treatment of HIV infection in many countries. Zidovudine has been found to prolong life and reduce the incidence of opportunistic infections in individuals who have *symptomatic* HIV disease.[59,60] However, the extent of the improved survival is not clear but is perhaps 1 to 2 years. Most patients eventually succumb to progressive immune deficiency which might be related to the development of a virus with reduced sensitivity to the drug. The dosages of zidovudine currently used in clinical practice (i.e. 400 to 600 mg/day) have been compared in clinical trials with the higher doses formerly used (1.2 g/day); the survival and number of clinical events were similar but there was much less toxicity with the lower dosage.[61]

Didanosine appears to have similar efficacy to zidovudine in symptomatic disease,[31] but zalcitabine is less effective and is mainly used in combination with zidovudine to increase its antiviral effect.[34] Most clinicians starting with single agent therapy would use zidovudine first because its toxicity profile is well known and is more easily managed than that of didanosine, and there is also circumstantial evidence that it may reduce the frequency of AIDS dementia complex. There is little evidence that patients at late stages of the disease with low CD4 counts (less than 50/μl) and multiple opportunistic infections are helped by any drug, and toxicity is a major problem.

Controversy currently exists as to the best time to initiate therapy with antiretroviral agents. Although initial studies suggested that in asymptomatic patients with CD4 counts below 500 cells/μl, zidovudine therapy is associated with a delay in the development of opportunistic infections,[62] a larger study has failed to confirm that this difference is significant and also failed to show a survival advantage for long term use of zidovudine as sole therapy in this group.[58] Thus, some clinicians prefer not to administer antiviral treatment until patients develop symptomatic disease, while others consider that there is logic in using antiviral therapy early in the disease when the viral burden is lower and when toxicity to drugs is less. In these

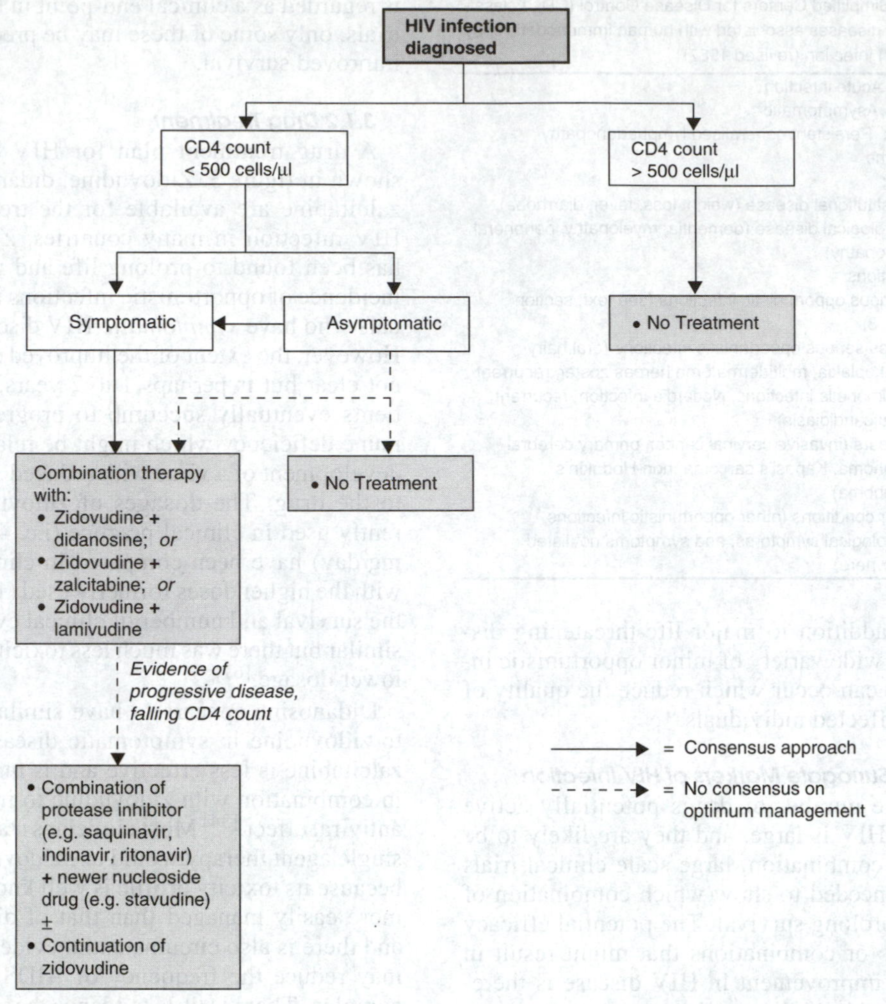


**Fig. 3.** Drug treatment of HIV disease.

patients, treatment often begins with *combinations* of more than one antiretroviral agent, and such an approach has been shown to provide greater clinical benefit than zidovudine monotherapy in two recent studies (Delta and ACTG 175 trials).[63] The Delta trial showed a survival benefit using either zidovudine/didanosine or zidovudine/zalcitabine combinations in antiretroviral naive patients as compared with zidovudine alone. In the ACTG 175 trial, similar results were achieved as assessed by a combined end point that included clinical events and a fall in the CD4 count of greater than 50%. However, in the latter trial, a didanosine monotherapy arm was also included, and this regimen appeared superior to zidovudine monotherapy, although the study did not have sufficient power to determine whether didanosine monotherapy was as effective as zidovudine/didanosine or zidovudine/zalcitabine combinations.

An alternative approach is to give one agent until there are clinical data to suggest waning effectiveness, and then change to an alternative drug. As yet, the combination and sequential approaches have not been compared in studies with appropriate clinical endpoints.

Combinations or sequential therapy utilise drugs targeted at different parts of the life cycle of HIV (divergent therapy) or alternatively, a number of drugs that inhibit HIV reverse transcriptase may be given together (convergent therapy). A concerted attack on HIV reverse transcriptase may delay the development of resistance, and this approach might be helpful even if resistance does develop. Thus, strains of HIV with reduced sensitivity to zidovudine remain sensitive to zalcitabine or didanosine. When individuals with strains with reduced sensitivity to zidovudine are given didanosine, lamivudine or a non-nucleoside analogue, these strains become phenotypically sensitive to zidovudine again, although they remain genotypically resistant. Another possibility with convergent therapy is that sufficient numbers of mutations can be introduced into HIV reverse transcriptase so that eventually, a non-viable virus may be produced.

Alternatively, a reverse transcriptase inhibitor may be combined with a drug acting post-transcriptionally, e.g. a protease inhibitor. Both can inhibit infection of new cells and prevent productive replication in already infected cells. This approach is currently being tested in phase III clinical trials.

The role of immunomodulating agents in therapy is discussed in chapter 28 (sect. 3.2.1).

### *3.1.3 Prevention and Treatment of Common Secondary Infections*

All opportunistic infections in patients with HIV disease are either latent within the body, having been controlled but not eradicated by the immune system, or are ubiquitous within the environment. In both instances, chemoprophylaxis can prevent their development in susceptible individuals (primary prophylaxis) or alternatively, once disease has developed, continuing therapy can prevent relapse (secondary prophylaxis). The need for prophylaxis is governed by the following factors:

- The course of the HIV disease and the intrinsic virulence of the organism. Whereas tuberculosis has an increased occurrence throughout the course of HIV disease, cytomegalovirus and *Mycobacterium avium intracellulare* infections are only seen in individuals with a CD4 count of less than 100 cells/μl.
- *For ubiquitous infections, the prevalence in the community*, e.g. cryptococcosis is relatively rare in the developed world and therefore primary prophylaxis is not usually given. For latent infections, the need for prophylaxis is governed by evidence of previous infection; thus 30% of individuals with positive toxoplasma serology and a CD4 count of less than 100 cells/μl will develop cerebral abscesses without prophylaxis, whereas in those with negative serology, only 0.3% will develop such a condition per year.
- *The health impact of the disease*. Tuberculosis disseminates widely both in HIV positive and negative individuals and therefore prophylaxis of tuberculosis would be expected to have a major health impact. On the other hand, oral and oesophageal candidal infections respond readily to treatment and so prophylaxis may not be necessary.
- *The adverse effects of treatment*. Unfortunately, those diseases with the highest health impact that are most desirable to avoid are also those in which treatment is most difficult, e.g. cytomegalovirus and *Mycobacterium avium intracellulare* infections, although recent advances in approaches to prophylaxis for both these infections (see below) give hope that much debility in late HIV infection can be avoided or delayed.

#### Treatment of Opportunistic Infections

**Pneumocystis carinii *pneumonia (PCP):*** *Pneumocystis carinii* still accounts for 60% of presenting AIDS illness, despite primary prophylaxis. Cotrimoxazole (trimethoprim-sulfamethoxazole) remains the treatment of choice, although other combinations inhibiting folic acid metabolism, including trimethoprim and dapsone, and primaquine and clindamycin are being increasingly used. Intravenous pentamidine is also effective therapy but produces serious toxicity, including renal failure and hypoglycaemia in a small proportion of patients.

***Tuberculosis:*** a major pandemic of tuberculosis across the developing world has been caused, at least in part, by immunosuppression due to HIV. Thus, 60% of individuals with tuberculosis in sub-Saharan Africa are HIV infected and the proportion of individuals on the India subcontinent with this dual infection is also rapidly increasing. Tuberculosis in this situation responds to standard therapy (see chapter 23; sect. 9), although in the US, multiple drug-resistant tuberculosis is a rapidly developing problem.

***Toxoplasmosis:*** the optimum treatment for toxoplasmosis is still pyrimethamine and sulfadiazine, although sensitivity to the latter is common, in which case a clindamycin/pyrimethamine combination may be used. Cotrimoxazole given primarily as prophylaxis for PCP also appears to be effective prophylaxis against toxoplasmosis, although it is not of value for treatment.

***Cryptococcosis:*** in seriously ill individuals with cryptococcal meningitis and disturbance of consciousness, amphotericin B improves survival in comparison with fluconazole. In other situations, fluconazole is equally effective. Recent studies have indicated that primary prophylaxis with fluconazole reduces the frequency of cryptococcosis, but the overall frequency of this infection may not be sufficient to justify this therapy.

***Cytomegalovirus infection:*** see section 3.2 (below).

***Mycobacterium avium intracellulare infection:*** the macrolides clarithromycin and azithromycin are the most effective single agents against this mycobacterium, but resistance develops rapidly when they are used alone. Combinations of these drugs with rifabutin and ethambutol have been shown to be synergistic *in vitro* and in experimental models *in vivo*, and probably produce symptomatic improvement and improved survival in infected HIV seropositive individuals.

## 3.2 Cytomegalovirus (CMV) Infection

CMV infection in the fetus or in the neonate produces potentially serious sequelae. Most adults develop either no disease or a mild self-limiting illness rather like glandular fever. The virus is not eradicated but becomes latent and may replicate if immunodeficiency occurs. CMV then produces widespread damage to many organs, particularly the gastrointestinal tract, lung and central nervous system.

The treatment of patients with CMV disease who are immunosuppressed because of transplantation or chemotherapy is usually relatively straightforward as the period of immunosuppression is short and the disease will be controlled as the immune system recovers. However, in AIDS patients, there is no prospect of immune recovery. CMV infection in these individuals is rare until the CD4 count has fallen below 50 cells/μl, but once infection is manifest, the treatment needs to be lifelong.

The drugs of choice for the treatment of CMV infections (*ganciclovir* and *foscarnet*) are both given intravenously twice daily, and are associated with major adverse effects and a long term risk of sepsis due to the need for central venous access. A more recently developed compound *cidofovir* (HPMPC), a cytosine analogue, is also active against CMV *in vitro* and has been shown to be effective *in vivo* in the initial treatment of CMV retinitis or in preventing recurrences in AIDS patients when given as an intravenous injection once weekly for 2 weeks and then every two weeks together with probenecid and hydration (to prevent nephrotoxicity).[64] Serious renal toxicity has occurred with cidofovir but this is presaged by the development of proteinuria, and if the drug is stopped at this stage, renal recovery occurs. Probenecid administration causes a rash in up to 25% of HIV seropositive patients but this disappears with continuing treatment.

### 3.2.1 CMV Retinitis

CMV retinitis, which virtually always leads to blindness if untreated, is treated equally effectively by either *ganciclovir* or *foscarnet*.[65] The retina is not restored to normal but further disease is prevented. Both drugs are given intravenously in high doses during the initial (induction) phase of treatment (ganciclovir 6 mg/kg twice daily and foscarnet 90 mg/kg twice daily), and the dose is then reduced during the maintenance phase (ganciclovir 6 mg/kg daily and foscarnet 90 to 120 mg/kg daily), which is associated with less toxicity. Recurrence, which is relatively common, may be due to either use of a low dose of the chosen antiviral drug or development of viral resistance. An increase in dosage or a switch to alternative therapy is usually effective in re-establishing remission.

In the treatment of HIV-related CMV retinitis, a modest survival advantage of about 6 months for the use of foscarnet as compared with ganciclovir has been demonstrated.[65] This may be due to the antiretroviral activity of foscarnet or the ability to continue zidovudine therapy with this drug (but not with ganciclovir). However, improved survival is only one factor to take into consideration when deciding which drug should be used for initial treatment. As ganciclovir is more readily tolerated by patients, its infusion times are shorter, prehydration to prevent renal damage is not required, and most patients with CMV retinitis are eventually exposed to both treatments anyway, it is perhaps reasonable to choose ganciclovir as initial therapy.

Although ganciclovir is poorly absorbed after oral administration, adequate blood concentrations to inhibit CMV replication are obtained if doses of 3 g/day are given. This regimen has proved acceptable to patients rather than having a long term indwelling catheter, and has been shown to be only marginally less effective than intravenous therapy.[66] It is likely that oral ganciclovir will be widely used, at least while cidofovir therapy is being further assessed.

#### 3.2.2 Prevention of CMV Infection in Immunocompromised Patients

Prophylaxis against CMV infection is difficult because the most effective drugs are only active intravenously. In patients undergoing transplantation, short term intravenous ganciclovir therapy reduces the incidence of subsequent CMV disease. It is possible that high-dose oral *aciclovir* (800mg five times daily) might achieve sufficient blood levels to inhibit some strains of CMV, and this therapy has been shown to reduce the incidence of subsequent CMV infection in CMV seronegative patients who were immunosuppressed following bone marrow transplantation or renal grafting and were given tissue from a CMV seropositive donor.[67] However, studies in AIDS patients with a low CD4 count given high-dose oral aciclovir therapy failed to show any significant benefit in the rate of subsequent development of CMV infection.[68]

Oral *ganciclovir* has also proved effective in primary prophylaxis in a group of HIV seropositive individuals with a CD4 count of less than 100 cells/μl.[69] However, concerns about cost, compliance and the potential development of resistance may limit its use for this indication.

### 3.3 Herpes Simplex Infection

Herpes simplex (types 1 and 2) is responsible for a wide variety of disease, including keratitis (a common cause of blindness), encephalitis and recurrent mucocutaneous infections. Immunocompromised patients such as transplant recipients and patients with AIDS are at special risk for developing serious disseminated and visceral disease. Currently, aciclovir and its analogue famciclovir are the drugs of choice. Other effective agents available include ganciclovir and foscarnet.

#### 3.3.1 Herpes Simplex Encephalitis

Herpes simplex encephalitis causes high mortality and leads to severe morbidity in adults. Intravenous *aciclovir* 10 mg/kg 8-hourly for 10 days has been shown to be more effective than vidarabine and is currently the treatment of choice.[70] As early treatment improves outcome, and clinical suspicion of the diagnosis is correct in only about 50% of cases, a definitive diagnostic test is required. It is hoped that polymerase chain reaction (PCR) technology may allow herpes simplex virus to be detected within the cerebrospinal fluid in a few hours, but for the present, brain biopsy remains the only certain test. The clinician is faced with the choice of either doing a brain biopsy, or more commonly, treating suspected herpes encephalitis with intravenous aciclovir.

#### 3.3.2 Genital, Labial and Oral Mucocutaneous Herpes Simplex Infections

A number of studies of acute herpes genitalis, labialis and oral mucocutaneous infections have demonstrated that the early administration of oral *aciclovir* (200mg 5 times daily) reduces the duration or viral shedding and accelerates healing of ulceration. Oral medication is more effective than topical ointments or creams. Recurrent herpes infections also respond to oral aciclovir, with self-medication at the first sign of an attack producing the most rapid improvement.[43]

Prophylaxis with aciclovir 200 or 400mg twice daily has been shown to reduce the frequency of recurrences by more than 70%, although herpes viruses resistant to aciclovir may be produced. In immunocompetent individuals, these viruses appear to be less virulent and if aciclovir is withdrawn, subsequent attacks tend to be with aciclovir-sensitive strains.

The treatment of genital herpes is discussed further in chapter 33 (sect. 5.2.1).

#### 3.3.3 Mucocutaneous Herpes Infections in AIDS Patients

The frequency of recurrent herpes simplex infection in AIDS patients is increased, particularly in those with low CD4 counts. Many patients are given long term prophylaxis with *aciclovir*, for which a dosage 400mg twice daily is usually given. However, aciclovir-resistant mutants of herpes simplex appear to be a particularly common problem and may cause serious disease in immunosuppressed patients. Intravenous *foscarnet* is superior to vidarabine in the management of such patients[71] but relapse occurs rapidly following treatment, and subsequent attacks in these patients may still be caused by resistant variants.

#### 3.3.4 Neonatal Herpes Simplex Infections

Neonates exhibit a variety of herpes simplex infections, including disease localised to the skin, eyes and mouth, CNS infection or disseminated disease. *Aciclovir* (10 mg/kg IV 8-hourly) is currently the treatment of choice for neonatal herpes simplex infections, having proved as effective as vidarabine in this age group.[43]

#### 3.3.5 Herpes Simplex Keratitis

Oral *aciclovir* is also the drug of choice for superficial herpes simplex keratitis (see also chapter 15; sect. 3.7). However, deep stromal disease may require intravenous therapy.

### 3.4 Varicella-Zoster Infection

Varicella-zoster infection usually causes a benign disease in healthy children but can cause severe manifestations in neonates, in immunocompromised children or susceptible healthy adults, and as reactivated disease (zoster) in adults, particularly immunocompromised individuals. Although a number of antiviral drugs have activity against varicella-zoster virus, the drug of choice is aciclovir or its analogue famciclovir.

#### 3.4.1 Acute Herpes Zoster (Shingles)

In acute herpes zoster in immunocompetent adults, early initiation of oral *aciclovir* (800mg five times daily) within 48 to 72 hours of the onset of rash accelerates the rate of cutaneous healing, reduces pain and the incidence of serious ocular complications, and reduces both the incidence and duration of subsequent postherpetic neuralgia.[43] Unlike herpes simplex, varicella-zoster virus infections require higher concentrations of aciclovir than can sometimes be achieved by oral administration, and intravenous aciclovir (10 mg/kg 8-hourly) may be necessary in some patients. In immunocompromised individuals with varicella-zoster infection, intravenous aciclovir has been shown to reduce the rate of visceral complications,[72] and to reduce pain and promote cutaneous healing.[73]

Recently, the aciclovir analogue *famciclovir* (250mg, 500mg or 750mg orally three times daily) has been shown to be as effective as aciclovir (800mg five times daily) in accelerating healing of cutaneous lesions and reducing the duration of pain,[50] and this drug may be used as an alternative in immunocompetent patients with acute herpes zoster. Although the less frequent administration regimen of famciclovir *versus* aciclovir (3 times daily *vs* 5 times daily) may be advantageous, it has not been demonstrated that famciclovir produces more rapid resolution of symptoms or is more effective in ameliorating postherpetic neuralgia. The same applies to *valaciclovir*, the L-valyl ester of aciclovir, which provides higher concentrations of the parent drug than can be achieved with aciclovir itself, and can be given in a twice daily regimen.

Other drugs that have been used in acute herpes zoster include intravenous vidarabine and topical idoxuridine. Intravenous *vidarabine* (10 mg/kg/day for 5 to 7 days) has proved effective in treating immunosuppressed individuals and use of this drug may be considered in combination with aciclovir when resistance to the latter develops during cutaneous or visceral dissemination of herpes zoster in severely immunosuppressed patients. Topical *idoxuridine* (40% in dimethyl sulfoxide applied over 4 days) has been reported to enhance resolution of skin lesions in uncomplicated herpes zoster and may be considered in the local treatment of immunocompetent patients.[74]

#### 3.4.2 Postherpetic Neuralgia

Approximately 10% of patients with herpes zoster experience prolonged neuralgia following resolution of the acute rash, of whom approximately one-third to one-half still have pain at 3 months and one-quarter to one-third still have pain at 1 year. The incidence of postherpetic neuralgia increases with age, and it is a substantial course of morbidity among the elderly.

*Tricyclic antidepressants* such as amitriptyline, nortriptyline, desipramine and maprotiline are currently the most effective agents for treatment of established postherpetic neuralgia. The sooner this therapy is started, the more likely it is to be effective in relieving pain. The usual dosage of these agents is 10 to 25mg at night initially, which is then increased weekly by a similar amount until a dose of 50 or 75mg at night (or more) is reached. This therapy should be continued for 3 months after the pain has disappeared and then gradually reduced.[75]

Topical agents such as lidocaine 5% ointment or gel, lidocaine/prilocaine eutectic mixture ('EMLA'), aspirin in chloroform (700mg in 30ml), and capsaicin 0.025% cream have been reported to provide some relief, but their benefit appears temporary and they are probably best used as adjuncts to tricyclic antidepressant therapy.[75] The evidence that short courses of systemic corticosteroids are of benefit in postherpetic neuralgia is inconclusive, and the case for using this treatment remains unproven.

### 3.5 Influenza

*Amantadine* inhibits all influenza A subtypes (but not B subtypes), and reduces the duration of symptoms by about a third if given within 48 hours of the onset of influenza A. Prophylaxis of contacts of influenza is effective, resulting in a 70% reduction of symptomatic illness. Although it has few adverse effects, amantadine has been shown to be teratogenic in rats and should not be given to potentially pregnant women. Resistance occurs rapidly; resistant strains remain pathogenic and spread of such viruses has been documented in epidemics. Amantadine is not widely used both because of the (incorrect) perception of influenza as a minor illness, and because of concern over its potential toxicity.[55]

***Influenza vaccination:*** pandemics of influenza arising in China have spread worldwide because of the development of novel haemagglutinin (H) or neuraminidase (N) antigen subtypes. These are likely to arise from genetic reassortment, stemming from recombinations occurring within animal reservoirs. Humans in the Far East live in close proximity with domestic pigs and ducks, allowing zoonotic spread to occur. Cases occurring in apparently immune people between pandemics are likely to arise through antigenic drift as a result of random point mutations. It was estimated that 29,000 excessive deaths occurred in England and Wales in the 1989-90 pandemic, and thus an effective vaccine would be very valuable.[76]

Current influenza subunit vaccines are well tolerated. Either disrupted viral particles are partially purified in organic solvents or highly purified surface haemagglutinin neuraminidase antigens are prepared. Commercial vaccines are trivalent containing two A antigen subunits and influenza B. Although serological responses decline over 3 to 6 months and are decreased in the elderly, vaccination does reduce disease severity and provides herd immunity in institutions (e.g. old peoples' homes) which limits disease spread. Current recommendations for immunisation include individuals of all ages but particularly the elderly with chronic respiratory, cardiac or renal disease, and those who have endocrine disease or are immunocompromised.

### 3.6 Respiratory Syncytial Virus (RSV) Infection

*Ribavirin* exhibits good activity against RSV, interfering with its replication at multiple sites with no evidence of the development of resistance. However, ribavirin is too toxic to use orally in the population most susceptible to RSV, and nebulised administration has been developed to provide topical treatment. Although nebulised ribavirin has been associated with shortening of the mechanical ventilation time and improvements in oxygenation, its effects are not dramatic (or cost-effective) for most patients. Therefore, ribavirin treatment is only recommended for patients with underlying immunosuppression with associated cardiac or pulmonary disease, those sufficiently unwell to be hospitalised, and for very young (less than 6 weeks old) infants.[77]

As RSV causes 91,000 hospitalisations and 4500 deaths in the US annually, an effective vaccine would be valuable. Unfortunately, natural immunity allows repeated infections and early experience with vaccines is not encouraging. A formalin-killed vaccine has resulted in the development of neutralising antibodies but many vaccinated children developed severe or fatal RSV infection subsequently.[78] This fits with the severe disease seen in children under 3 months of age who have received antibodies by passive maternal transfer. It is likely that the severe damage associated with some RSV infections is immunologically-mediated and there is experimental evidence that the vaccine produced an inappropriate $T_H2$ response and inhibited a $T_H1$ response which allowed subsequent infection to spread to the lungs.

Although subunit vaccines and attenuated vaccines are being developed, there continues to be considerable nervousness about their application to children because of the above experiences.

### 3.7 Rhinovirus Infection

Many different species of rhinovirus cause the common cold and as the dominant immunotype of each species appears 'hidden' from the immune system, control is unlikely to be obtained by vaccination.

Although interferon-α, β-serine and capsid binders inhibit viral replication of the majority of species, none produces a satisfactory effect prophylactically and they reduce symptoms and viral shedding to only a modest extent. The addition of ipratropium bromide and naproxen to nasal instillation of interferon-α may produce a greater symptomatic improvement.[79]

**Table VI.** Patient-related variables found to influence response to antiviral therapy in chronic hepatitis B

| Determinants of positive response | Determinants of negative response |
|---|---|
| Low pretherapy HBV DNA | High pretherapy HBV DNA |
| High pretherapy ALT | Low pretherapy ALT |
| Short duration of hepatitis | Long term, established infection |
| Acquisition in adulthood | Acquisition in infancy or childhood |
| Anti-delta negative | Anti-delta positive |
| HIV antibody negative | HIV antibody positive |
| Heterosexual lifestyle | ?Homosexual lifestyle |
| Active histology | Inactive histology or mild liver injury |
| | Male sex |

*Abbreviations:* ALT = alanine aminotransferase; HBV = hepatitis B virus; HIV = human immunodeficiency virus.

### 3.8 Hepatitis B Infection

Hepatitis B infection is associated with acute and chronic hepatitis, cirrhosis and an increased incidence of hepatoma. In the majority of patients with acute hepatitis B infection, viral replication ceases after a few weeks. However, in a small proportion (less than 10%), continuing viral replication, detected by core antigen (e) and/or hepatitis B DNA (HBV DNA) in the blood, is associated with an increased risk of chronic liver disease and cirrhosis. Cessation of replication is associated with loss of e antigen and HBV DNA from the circulation and the development of e antibodies.

Treatment of patients with chronic liver disease secondary to hepatitis B with either vidarabine or interferon-α is associated with a loss of plasma e antigen, and eventually e antibodies develop in about 40% of patients. This occurs after several weeks of treatment accompanied by a short hepatitic illness. Therapy must be continued for several months. *Interferon-α* is now the most commonly used drug (10mU 3 times per week) to treat chronic hepatitis B, although it is of limited value in a number of unfavourable circumstances (table VI), in established cirrhosis, and possibly in certain racial groups. Although this treatment reduces the extent of subsequent chronic liver disease, there is no evidence of a reduced incidence of hepatoma.[80]

*Lamivudine* also has activity against hepatitis B and appears to inhibit replication in some patients. However, it remains to be seen whether replication recommences after therapy is discontinued, and whether the suppression of replication influences chronic liver disease or hepatoma.

### 3.9 Hepatitis C Infection

An antibody test and polymerase chain reaction (PCR) tests can now detect hepatitis C virus, which is the most common cause of post-transfusion hepatitis. About 50% of individuals with hepatitis C infection develop chronic liver disease and there is also an increased incidence of hepatoma. *Interferon-α* in lower doses than those required to treat hepatitis B (2mU 3 times per week) appears to prevent replication of hepatitis C virus in about half the individuals who are treated, and to reduce the severity of ongoing liver damage.[81] However, viral replication recommences in about 50% of patients once the drug is discontinued.

## 4. Clinical Outcome and Economic Considerations

### 4.1 HIV Disease

#### *4.1.1 Key Issues in Estimating the Economic Impact*

As all antiretroviral drugs are expensive and the chief burden of HIV disease falls on impoverished nations, it is not surprising that a number of pharmacoeconomic analyses have been performed, all of which have been hampered by major problems:

1) Defining the direct costs of HIV disease care is difficult because of changing patterns of standard treatment, improvements in life expectancy and continuing decreases in the length of inpatient stay. Many new therapies directed against HIV or used in the treatment or prophylaxis of opportunistic infections are widely used in developed countries before knowledge of their long term effectiveness and quality of life benefits becomes available. For example, expensive treatment with inhaled pentamidine as prophylaxis for *Pneumocystis carinii* pneumonia was widely introduced prior to studies which showed the much less expensive agent cotrimoxazole to be as effective for disease prevention.[82] Despite these difficulties, a number of different estimates from various countries in the developed world have suggested that the annual treatment cost for an AIDS patient is around US$20,000, and it is estimated that the treatment of AIDS currently consumes 1% of the healthcare budget in the US and France.[83] Estimation of the costs of treatment in the de-

veloping world is much more difficult. One analysis, shown in table VII, estimated both high costs (with use of zidovudine and frequent clinic visits and palliative care for opportunistic infections) and low costs (minimum palliative care for opportunistic infections), and these costs were related to the gross national products of the countries concerned. Paradoxically, in many countries in sub-Saharan Africa, the group of patients most often infected with HIV are employed and the hospital is able to charge for admission, which indirectly enables less well provided groups to be cared for as well.[83]

2) The potential indirect costs of HIV diseases are also difficult to model. Unemployment benefits and loss of productive capacity are obvious examples of indirect costs but the impact in countries with already high unemployment rates is difficult to assess. The indirect economic costs in countries in sub-Saharan Africa, where the most productive members of the community are predominantly affected, may be much higher.

3) The degree and extent to which antiviral drugs prolong life in HIV-infected patients is unclear. The original placebo-controlled trial of zidovudine therapy in symptomatic disease[59] was prematurely terminated before the survival benefit could be calculated. However, the results of the Concorde study[58] indicate that early use of zidovudine in patients in an asymptomatic phase does not prolong life when compared with treatment of symptomatic disease only. Nevertheless, estimates of 1 to 2 years' improvement in survival with zidovudine are available from retrospective analyses. In terms of quality of life, only small studies have assessed the improvement in quality of life which may be obtained with zidovudine therapy. They indicate a small improvement, which is dissipated within 1 year of therapy. Studies using the lower, now routinely used doses of zidovudine which produce fewer adverse effects are not yet available.

4) The use of zidovudine or other antiretroviral agents in patients in an asymptomatic phase could prolong this period, which might produce more widely disseminated HIV infection. Alternatively, antiretroviral agents could reduce infectivity, thereby reducing spread of the disease. A recent study indicating a reduction in feto-maternal transmission with zidovudine[85] suggests that the latter view may be correct.

#### *4.1.2 Pharmacoeconomic Considerations in Using Zidovudine*

In AIDS patients treated with zidovudine, there is likely to be a reduction in a number of opportunistic infections and hospital admissions during the following year.[86] This has been analysed retrospectively in a small study of 7 pairs of patients, given either zidovudine or placebo (table VIII).[87] Most of the gain seen with zidovudine treatment was limited to the first 6 months of therapy, as the frequency of hospital visits and inpatient care rose rapidly in the second half of the year. Most of this 'saving' will, of course, be spent in subsequent years as the patients become ill.

In the treatment of asymptomatic disease, a number of pharmacoeconomic analyses have been performed using the initial US study of early intervention with zidovudine.[62] These analyses are now seriously flawed, as the promise of this initial study has not been realised and there is now known to be no progressive improvement either in AIDS-free time or survival. Moreover, the dosage of zidovudine used in one arm of this study was higher than that currently used, and the costs of zidovudine have also diminished quite significantly since this study

**Table VII.** Estimated costs of treating AIDS in selected developing countries (after Over & Piot[84])

| Country | GNP/person ($US)[a] | HIV-related treatment cost ($US)[a] | | Cost relative to GNP/person (%) | |
|---|---|---|---|---|---|
| | | low[b] | high[b] | low[b] | high[b] |
| Brazil | 2473 | 6000 | 12,000 | 243 | 485 |
| Mexico | 2076 | 3594[c] | 8033[c] | 173 | 387 |
| Tanzania | 118 | 111[c] | 673[c] | 94 | 570 |
| Zaire | 178 | 141[c] | 1689[c] | 79 | 949 |
| US | 19,840 | 60,000 | 90,000 | 302 | 454 |

a Given in 1988 US dollars.

b Low and high estimates correspond, respectively, to the most limited healthcare options (minimum palliative care for opportunistic infections) and most comprehensive healthcare options (use of zidovudine plus frequent clinic visits plus palliative care for opportunistic infections) within each country.

c Adjusted to 1988 costs using GNP implicit price deflator for 1985, 1986 and 1988 (US Bureau of Census 1991).

*Abbreviations:* GNP = gross national product; AIDS = acquired immune deficiency syndrome; HIV = human immunodeficiency virus.

**Table VIII.** Mean costs, charges and services attributed to 7 zidovudine recipients and 7 matched control patients with AIDS over a 12-month period (after Scitovsky et al.[88])

| Parameter | Zidovudine recipients | Controls |
|---|---|---|
| **Costs (US$):** | | |
| Inpatient services | 3003 | 32,544[a] |
| Outpatient services | 10,498 | 6761 |
| Zidovudine | 8000 | 0 |
| All other charges | 971 | 1828 |
| Total costs | 22,472 | 41,133 |
| **Services:** | | |
| Hospital admissions | 0.57 | 2.29 |
| Hospital days | 3.57 | 33.71 |
| Outpatients phsycians visits | 44.86 | 29.29 |

a Statistically significant difference from zidovudine group ($p < 0.05$).

was analysed. Nevertheless, other studies have shown that the early use of zidovudine may be associated with a delay in the development of the first opportunistic infection, and the approximate cost of buying 1 year of AIDS-free time (US$70,000) was similar in two independent analyses.[89,90] This cost is high because many asymptomatic patients who will not develop AIDS within the period of the study also have to be treated to prevent AIDS progression in the minority. Nevertheless, this cost falls within the same range as other preventive treatments in current use.

It has been estimated that it would cost US$1.093 billion to treat all the available HIV seropositive patients in the US with a CD4 count of less than 500 cells/μl, but this might save US$475 million in hospital costs in the first year.[89] These costs are sensitive to the costs of zidovudine and to its dosage, and the pharmacoeconomic analysis needs to be repeated using the drug's new costings and also the less optimistic projections provided by the Concorde Study.[58]

Seen within the context of the developing world, the treatment costs of zidovudine, both for AIDS care and HIV infection in symptomatic individuals, are unrealistic. Using a conservative estimate of the number of HIV infections in Latin America, the annual cost of treatment of all HIV seropositive individuals with zidovudine would be US$220 million, which should be viewed in the context of the total AIDS spending in the same region of only US$13 million.[84]

## 4.2 Non-HIV Viral Disease

As most non-HIV viral infections are self-limiting and do not require hospital admission, the economic benefits of antiviral drugs are limited, particularly as most are very expensive. However, the health impact of some infections (e.g. mucocutaneous herpes infection) is high and the use of drugs such as aciclovir is desirable. Similarly, the personal disability caused by CMV infection in immunocompromised patients is great, indicating the need for effective therapy.

Cost-utility analyses (CUA) or cost-benefit analyses (CBA) of viral vaccines are relatively few in number, in part because with many of the earlier life-threatening or severe infections like smallpox or polio, their value was self-evident. However, with expensive vaccines like hepatitis B or vaccination against diseases perceived, sometimes erroneously, to be less serious, cost-benefit analyses are more important. To be meaningful, such analyses need to consider marginal and intangible costs, as well as some method of discounting long term as compared with short term health gain. A sensitivity analysis is also important and it is clear that cost-utility or cost-benefit analysis will vary from country to country and from time to time. Changes in healthcare expectation and capacities will also have a major impact on long term costs. Thus, a cost-benefit analysis for hepatitis B is very different if newer treatments for cirrhosis, such as liver transplantation, are included in the cost analysis. Such analyses are very difficult to perform in developing countries where a number of factors have a major impact on vaccine efficiency,[91] including nutritionally induced immunosuppression, difficulty in transporting the vaccine while maintaining its potency, inexperience and lack of training of administering personnel, and strong religious and gender biases affecting vaccine acceptance.

### Measles

Since it is a severe disease, an effective vaccine has been clearly shown to be cost-effective in measles. Recent studies have mainly investigated revaccination strategies to control local outbreaks with variable results.

### Mumps

The benefit of mumps vaccination is less clear as the disease and its sequelae are less severe, but when indirect costs (including parental time off work) are included, a vaccine programme, in addition to decreasing mortality, does show a cost benefit.

### Hepatitis B

It is clear that if indirect costs (e.g. loss of earnings) are taken into account, vaccination against hepatitis B is cost effective for high risk groups.[8] Vaccination of neonates from hepatitis B positive mothers also reduces morbidity and mortality, but whether there is a cost benefit to vaccinating all neonates is controversial, partly because sophisticated studies have not been performed. Sensitivity analyses have indicated that vaccine cost, the discount rate (for long term health gain), and the prevalence of hepatitis B within a geographical area are important factors in determining cost benefit.

It is likely that universal neonatal vaccination is cost effective and appropriate for control in high and moderate prevalence regions. Although high-risk vaccination policies are cost effective, in low endemicity areas, an inability to reach sufficient numbers of these groups will mean that effective control of hepatitis B is unlikely and may indicate the need for expanded vaccination strategies.[92]

### Influenza

The cost benefit of influenza virus vaccination of the elderly has been clearly demonstrated.[93]

## References


1. Stuart-Harris C. The principles and practice of immunization. Practitioner 1975; 215: 285
2. Immunization Practices Advisory Committee. Update on adult immunization. Recommendations of the Immunization Practices Advisory Committee (ACIP). Morbidity and Mortality Weekly Report 1991; 40 (RR-12): 1-94
3. American College of Physicians Task Force on Adult Immunization IDS of A. Guide for adult immunization. 2nd ed. Philadelphia: American College of Physicians, 1990
4. Salk JE. Studies in human subjects on active immunization against poliomyelitis. I. A preliminary report of experiments in progress. Journal of the American Medical Association 1953; 151: 1081
5. Sabin AB. Oral poliomyelitis vaccine: history of its development and prospects for eradication of poliomyelitis. Journal of the American Medical Association 1964; 194: 49
6. Nightingale EO. Recommendations for a national policy on poliomyelitis vaccination. New England Journal of Medicine 1977; 297: 249
7. Melnick JLO. Advantages and disadvantages of killed and live poliomyelitis vaccines. Bulletin of the World Health Organization 1978; 56: 21
8. van den Oever R, de Graeve D, Hepp B, et al. Pharmacoeconomics of immunisation. Pharmacoeconomics 1993; 3: 286
9. Smuzness W, Stevens CE, Harley EJ, et al. Hepatitis B vaccine: demonstration of efficacy in a controlled clinical trial in a high-risk population in the United States. New England Journal of Medicine 1980; 303: 833
10. Norley SG, Vogel T, Kurth R. Anti-HIV vaccines: current status and future development. Drugs 1993; 46: 947
11. Murphey-Corb M, Martin LN, Davison-Fairburn B, et al. A formalin-inactivated whole SIV vaccine confers protection in macaques. Science 1989; 246: 1293-7
12. Stott EJ. Anti-cell antibody in macaques. Nature 1991; 353: 393
13. Desrosiers RC, Wyand NS, Kodama T, et al. Vaccine protection against simian immunodeficiency virus infection. Proceedings of the National Academy of Sciences of the United States of America 1989; 86: 6353
14. Burnstead DI, Stansbury LR. Herpes vaccine current status and future prospects. Clinical Immunotherapeutics 1994; 2: 325-30
15. Adler SP. Development and clinical status of cytomegalovirus vaccines. Clinical Immunotherapy 1994; 2: 1-6
16. Cason J. Papillomavirus vaccines: current status. Clinical Immunotherapy 1994; 1: 293-306
17. Shallaby SW. Development of oral vaccines to stimulate mucosal and systemic immunity: barriers and novel strategies. Clinical Immunology and Immunopathology 1995; 74: 127-34
18. Stokes J, Neele JR. The prevention and attenuation of infectious hepatitis by gamma globulin. Journal of the American Medical Association 1945; 127: 144
19. Brunell PA, Ross A, Miller LH, et al. Prevention of varicella by zoster immune globulin. New England Journal of Medicine 1969; 280: 1191
20. Brunell PA, Gershon AA, Hughes WT, et al. Prevention of varicella in high risk children: a collaborative study. Pediatrics 1972; 50: 718
21. Sandstrom E, Oberg B. Antiviral therapy in human immunodeficiency virus infections: current status (Pts I and II). Drugs 1993; 45: 488-508 and 637-53
22. Wilde MI, Langtry HD. Zidovudine: an update of its pharmacodynamic and pharmacokinetic properties, and therapeutic efficacy. Drugs 1993; 46: 515-78
23. Morse GD, Shelton MJ, O'Donnell AM. Comparative pharmacokinetics of antiviral nucleoside analogues. Clinical Pharmacokinetics 1993; 24: 101-23
24. Morris DJ. Adverse effects and drug interactions of clinical importance with antiviral drugs. Drug Safety 1994; 10: 281-91
25. Pue MA, Benet LZ. Pharmacokinetics of famciclovir in man. Antiviral Chemistry and Chemotherapy 1993; 4 Suppl. 1: 47-55
26. Dorr RT. Interferon-α in malignant and viral disease: a review. Drugs 1993; 45: 177-211
27. Portegies P. AIDS dementia complex: a review. Journal of Acquired Immune Deficiency Syndromes 1994; 7: 534-49
28. Jacobson MA, Dennis C, Polsky B, et al. A dose-ranging study of daily maintenance intravenous foscarnet therapy for cytomegalovirus retinitis in AIDS. Concise Communications JID, 1993: 168
29. Collier AC, Coombs RW, Fischl MA, et al. Combination therapy with zidovudine and didanosine compared with zidovudine alone in HIV-1 infection. Annals of Internal Medicine 1993; 119: 786-93
30. Faulds D, Brogden RN. Didanosine: a review of its antiviral activity, pharmacokinetic properties and therapeutic potential in human immunodeficiency virus infection. Drugs 1992; 44: 94-116
31. Kahn JD, Lagakos SW, Richman DD, et al. A controlled trial comparing zidovudine with didanozine in human immunodeficiency virus infection. New England Journal of Medicine 1992; 327: 581-7
32. Johnson VA, Merrill DP, Videler JA, et al. Two-drug combinations of zidovudine, didanosine and recombinant interferon-alpha inhibit replication of zidovudine resistant human immunodeficiency virus type 1 synergistically in vitro. Journal of Infectious Diseases 1991; 164: 646-55

33. Whittington R, Brogden RN. Zalcitabine: a review of its pharmacology and clinical potential in acquired immunodeficiency syndrome (AIDS). Drugs 1992; 44: 656
34. Remick S, Follansbee S, Olsen R, et al. Safety and tolerance of zalcitabine (ddc, HIVID) in a double-blind comparative trial (ACTG 114; N3300) [abstract]. International Conference on AIDS, Berlin 1993
35. Fischl MA, Stanley K, Collier AC, et al. Combination and monotherapy with zidovudine and zalcitabine in patients with advanced HIV disease. Annals of Internal Medicine 1995; 122: 24-32
36. Hitchcock MJM. 2',3'-Didehydro-2',3'-dideoxythymidine (D4T), an anti-HIV agent. Antiviral Chemistry and Chemotherapy 1991; 2: 125
37. Browne MJ, Mayer KH, Chafee SBD, et al. 2',3'-didehydro-3'-deoxythymidine (d4T) in patients with AIDS or AIDS-related complex: a phase I trial. Journal of Infectious Diseases 1993; 167: 21-9
38. Angel JB, Hussey EK, Hall ST, et al. Pharmacokinetics of 3TC (GR 109714X) administered with and without food to HIV-infected patients. Drug Investigation 1993; 6: 70-4
39. Norbeck DW, Kempf DJ. HIV protease inhibitors. Annual Reports in Medicinal Chemistry 1991; 26: 141
40. Craig JC, Duncan IB, Whittaker L. Antiviral synergy between inhibitors of HIV proteinase and reverse transcriptase. Antiviral Chemistry and Chemotherapy 1993; 4: 335-9
41. King DH, Galasso G, editors. Proceedings of a symposium on acyclovir sponsored by the Burroughs Wellcome Company and the National Institute of Allergy and Infectious Diseases. American Journal of Medicine 1982; 73 Suppl. 1A: 1
42. Weinberg A, Bate BJ, Masters HB, et al. In vitro activities of penciclovir and acyclovir against herpes simplex virus types 1 and 2. Antimicrobial Agents and Chemotherapy 1992; 36: 2037-8
43. Whitley RJ, Gnann JW. Acyclovir: a decade later. New England Journal of Medicine 1992; 327: 782
44. Wagstaff AJ, Faulds D, Goa KL. Acyclovir: a reappraisal of its antiviral activity, pharmacokinetic properties and therapeutic efficacy. Drugs 1994; 47: 153-205
45. O'Brien JJ, Campoli-Richards DM. Acyclovir: an updated review of antiviral activity, pharmacokinetic properties and therapeutic efficacy. Drugs 1989; 37: 233-309
46. Perren TJ, Powles RL, Easton D, et al. Prevention of herpes zoster in patients by long-term oral acyclovir after allogeneic bone marrow transplantation. American Journal of Medicine 1988; 85(2A): 99-101
47. Weller S, Blum MR, Smiley L. Phase I pharmacokinetics of the acyclovir prodrug, valacyclovir. Antiviral Research 1993; 20 Suppl. 1: 144
48. Beauchamp LM, Krenitsky TA. Acyclovir prodrugs: the road to valaciclovir. Drugs of the Future 1993; 18: 619-28
49. Tyring S, Barbarash R, Nahlik J, et al. and the Collaborative Famciclovir Herpes Zoster Clinical Study Group. Efficacy of famciclovir on herpes rash resolution and post-herpetic neuralgia. Antiviral Research 1994; 23 Suppl. 1: 73
50. Degreef H, et al. (Famciclovir Herpes Zoster Clinical Study Group). Famciclovir, a new oral antiherpes drug: results of the first controlled clinical study demonstrating its efficacy and safety in the treatment of uncomplicated herpes zoster in immunocompetent patients. International Journal of Antimicrobial Agents 1994; 4: 241-6
51. Sacks SL, Aoki FY, Diaz-Mitoma F, et al. Patient-initiated treatment of recurrent genital herpes with oral famciclovir: a Canadian multicenter, placebo-controlled, dose-ranging study [abstract]. 34th Interscience Conference on Antimicrobial Agents and Chemotherapy, Florida, 4-7 Oct. 1994
52. Faulds D, Heel RC. Ganciclovir: a review of its antiviral activity, pharmacokinetic properties and therapeutic efficacy in cytomegalovirus infections. Drugs 1990; 39: 597
53. Chrisp P, Clissold SP. Foscarnet: a review of its antiviral activity, pharmacokinetic properties and therapeutic use in immunocompromised patients for cytomegalovirus retinitis. Drugs 1991; 41: 104-29
54. Volz MA, Kirkpatrick CH. Interferons 1992. How much of the promise has been realised? Drugs 1992; 43: 285
55. Eisenberg M, Merigan TC. Viral diseases. In: Speight TM, editor. Drug treatment. 3rd ed. Auckland: Adis Press, 1987: 1236-51
56. Oxford JS, Galbraith A. Antiviral activity of amantadine: a review of laboratory and clinical data. Pharmacology and Therapeutics 1980; 11: 181
57. Campoli-Richards DM, Sorkin EM, Heel RC. Inosine pranobex: a preliminary review of its pharmacodynamic and pharmacokinetic properties, and therapeutic efficacy. Drugs 1986; 32: 383-424
58. Concorde Coordinating Committee. Concorde: MRC/ANRS randomised double-blind controlled trial of immediate and deferred zidovudine in symptom-free HIV infection. Lancet 1994; 343: 871-1
59. Fischl MA, Richman DD, Grieco MH, et al. The efficacy of azidothymidine (zidovudine) in the treatment of patients with AIDS and AIDS-related complex. New England Journal of Medicine 1987; 317: 185
60. Fischl MA, Richman DD, Hansen N, et al. The safety and efficacy of zidovudine (AZT) in the treatment of subjects with mildly symptomatic human immunodeficiency virus type 1 (HIV) infection. Annals of Internal Medicine 1990; 112: 727-37
61. Fischl MA, Parker CB, Pettinelli C, et al. A randomised controlled trial of a reduced daily dosage of zidovudine in patients with the acquired immunodeficiency syndrome. New England Journal of Medicine 1990; 323: 1009
62. Volberding PA, Lagakos SW, Koch MA, et al. Zidovudine in asymptomatic human immunodeficiency virus infection: a controlled trial in persons with fewer than 500 CD4-positive cells per cubic millimeter. New England Journal of Medicine 1990; 322: 941
63. Hirsch MS, Yeni P. A bend in the road – implications of ACTG 175 and Delta trials. Antiviral Therapy 1996; 1: 6-8
64. Lalezari J, Stagg R, Kuppermann B, et al. A phase II/III randomized study of immediate versus deferred intravenous cidofovir (HPMPC) for the treatment of peripheral CMV retinitis in patients with AIDS. 2nd National Conference on Human Retroviruses and Related Infections, LB18, 170, 1995
65. Jabs DA, et al. (Studies of Ocular Complications of AIDS Research Group, in Collaboration with the AIDS Clinical Trials Group). Mortality in patients with the acquired immunodeficiency syndrome treated with either foscarnet or ganciclovir for cytomegalovirus retinitis. New England Journal of Medicine 1992; 326: 213-20
66. Oral Ganciclovir European and Australian Cooperative Study Group. Intravenous versus oral ganciclovir: European/Australian comparative study of efficacy and safety in the prevention of cytomegalovirus retinitis recurrence in patients with AIDS. AIDS 1995; 9: 471-7
67. Balfour HH, Chace BA, Stapleton JT, et al. A randomised placebo controlled trial or oral acyclovir for the prevention of cytometalovirus disease in recipients of renal allografts. New England Journal of Medicine 1989; 320: 1381-7
68. Youle MS, Gazzard BG, Johnson MA, et al. The effects of high dose oral acyclovir on herpes virus disease and survival in patients with advanced HIV disease: a double blind placebo controlled study. AIDS 1994; 8: 641-9
69. Spector SA, McKinley G, Drew WL, et al. A randomised double-blind study of the efficacy and safety of oral

ganciclovir for the prevention of CMV disease in HIV infected persons [abstract]. Second National Conference on Human Retroviruses and Related Infections, Washington DC, Jan 1995
70. Whitley RJ. Herpes simplex virus infections of the central nervous system: encephalitis and neonatal herpes. Drugs 1991; 42: 406
71. Safrin S, Crumpacker C, Chatis P, et al. A controlled trial comparing foscarnet with vidarabine for acyclovir-resistant mucocutaneous herpes simplex in the acquired immunodeficiency syndrome. New England Journal of Medicine 1991; 325: 551
72. Prober CG, Kirk LE, Keeney RE. Acyclovir therapy of chicken pox in immunosuppressed children - a collaborative study. Journal of Pediatrics 1982; 101: 622
73. Shepp DH, Newton BA, Dandliker PS, et al. Oral acyclovir therapy for mucocutaneous herpes simplex virus infections in immunocompromised marrow transplant recipients. Annals of Internal Medicine 1985; 102: 783
74. Nikkels AF, Piérard GE. Recognition and treatment of shingles. Drugs 1994; 48: 528-48
75. Bowsher D. Post-herpetic neuralgia in older patients. Drugs & Aging 1994; 5: 411-8
76. Wiselka M. Influenza diagnosis: management and prophylaxis. British Medical Journal 1994; 308: 1341-5
77. American Academy of Pediatrics. Use of ribavirin in the treatment of respiratory syncitial infections. Pediatrics 1993; 92: 501-4
78. Murphy BR, Hall SL, Kulkarni AB, et al. An update on approaches to the development of respiratory syncytial virus (RSV) and parainfluenza virus type 3 (PIV3) vaccines. Virus Research 1994; 32: 13-36
79. Gwaltney J. Combined antiviral and antimediator therapy: treatment of rhinovirus colds. Journal of Infectious Diseases 1992; 166: 776-82
80. Eddleston WF, Dixon B. Interferons in the treatment of chronic virus infection of the liver. Macclesfield: Pennine Press, 1990
81. Hoofnagle JH, Mullen KD, Jones DB, et al. Treatment of chronic non-A-non-B hepatitis with recombinant human alpha interferon: a preliminary report. New England Journal of Medicine 1986; 315: 1575-8
82. Lynn LA, Schulman KA, Eisenberg J. The pharmacoeconomics of HIV disease. Pharmacoeconomics 1992; 1: 161
83. Winkenwerder W, Kessler AR, Stolec RM. Federal spending for illness caused by the human immunodeficiency virus. New England Journal of Medicine 1989; 320: 1598
84. Over M, Piot P. HIV infection and sexually transmitted diseases. In: Jamison DT, Mosley WH, editors. Disease control priorities in developing countries. New York: Oxford University Press, 1992
85. Cotton EM, Sperling RS, Gelber R, et al. (for the Pediatric AIDS Clinical Trials Group Protocol 076 Study Group). Reduction of maternal-infant transmission of human immunodeficiency virus type I with zidovudine treatment. New England Journal of Medicine 1994; 331: 1173-80
86. Langtry HD, Palmer KJ, Benfield P. Zidovudine: a review of pharmacoeconomic and quality-of-life considerations for its use in patients with human immunodeficiency virus. Pharmacoeconomics 1993; 3: 309
87. Scitovsky AA, Cline MW, Abrams DI. Effects of the use of AZT on the medical care costs of persons with AIDS in the first 12 months. Journal of Acquired Immune Deficiency Syndromes 1990; 3: 904-12
88. Scitovsky AA. The economic impact of the HIV epidemic in the United States. AIDS Updates 1991; 4: 1-13
89. Cheung TW, Fahs M, Sacks HS. Cost effectiveness analysis of early treatment of HIV disease with zidovudine (AZT) [abstract 4078]. 6th International Conference on AIDS, San Francisco, 1990
90. Schulman KA, Lynn LA, Glick HA, et al. Cost effectiveness of low-dose zidovudine therapy for asymptomatic patients with human immunodeficiency virus (HIV) infection. Annals of Internal Medicine 1991; 114: 798-802
91. Aryta SC. Human immunisation in developing countries: practical and theoretical problems and prospect. Vaccine 1994; 12: 1423-34
92. Holliday SM, Faulds D. Hepatitis B vaccine: a pharmacoeconomic evaluation of its use in the prevention of hepatitis B virus infection. Pharmacoeconomics 1994; 5: 141-71
93. Gradenstein JD, Hartzema AG, Guess AJ, et al. Community pharmacists as immunisation advocates - cost-effectiveness of a cue to influenza vaccination. Medical Care 1992; 30: 503-13
94. Gross G, Ikenberg H, Roussaki A, et al. Systemic treatment of condylomata acuminata with recombinant interferon-alpha-2a: low-dose superior to the high-dose regimen. Chemotherapy 1986; 32: 537-41
95. Condylomata International Collaborative Study Group. A comparison of interferon alfa-2a and podophyllin in the treatment of primary condylomata acuminata. Genitourinary Medicine 1991; 67: 394-9
96. Perrillo RP, Schiff ER, Davis GL, et al. A randomized controlled trial of interferon alfa-2b alone and after prednisolone withdrawal for the treatment of chronic hepatitis B. The Hepatitis Interventional Therapy Group. New England Journal of Medicine 1990; 323: 295-301
97. Lane HC, Davey V, Kovacs JA, et al. Interferon-alpha in patients with asymptomatic human immunodeficiency virus (HIV) infection: a randomized placebo-controlled trial. Annals of Internal Medicine 1990; 112: 805-11

Chapter 33

# Sexually Transmissible Diseases

*W.R. Bowie*

## Synopsis of Important Principles

1) The incidence of most sexually transmissible diseases (STDs) increased dramatically in the 1960s and 1970s, particularly gonorrhoea, non-gonococcal urethritis, pelvic inflammatory disease, genital herpes and genital warts. More recently, the incidence of acquired immune deficiency syndrome (AIDS) has been increasing steadily since its recognition in the 1980s. However, in many parts of the world where curative medications are available and multifaceted control programmes are in place, the incidence of the first three STDs has fallen significantly. In the case of the latter three viral infections, for which curative therapy is not available, rates have either not fallen as dramatically or have not fallen at all.

2) Most severe sequelae of STDs occur in women. Many sequelae only become apparent years after the initial, often asymptomatic infection. Important sequelae such as involuntary infertility and ectopic pregnancy secondary to tubal damage have significant effects on individuals and on population dynamics.

3) The presence of one genital pathogen often heralds the presence of others in the patient or partner(s). Concurrent infection with *Chlamydia trachomatis* is so frequent in those with proven or suspected gonococcal infection that a regimen active against *C. trachomatis* should be given in addition to other treatments that may be required.

4) Infection with sexually transmitted pathogens is often totally asymptomatic and may only be detected by screening, or suspected because of disease in a partner.

5) Effective control is aimed at seeking out cases and reducing the 'silent reservoir' of infection, thus preventing further spread of the disease. With all STDs, a basic principle is identification and treatment of the sexual partner(s) who may be asymptomatic (contact tracing).

6) Curative treatment means the use of a regimen which approaches a 100% cure rate for the causative organism(s) of the syndrome or infection being treated, and is given in a dose schedule that avoids or minimises noncompliance. Single-dose regimens, when effective, are always to be preferred.

7) In many cases, e.g. urethritis, cervicitis and pelvic inflammatory disease, syndromic management should be initiated prior to specific microbiological diagnosis of the cause in an attempt to decrease the risk of long term sequelae and the spread of infection.

8) The level of resistance of sexually transmitted pathogens to antimicrobial drugs varies geographically and over time, but has posed a major problem in the treatment of gonorrhoea and chancroid, and a lesser problem in the treatment of *Trichomonas vaginalis* infection.

9) Other key components of prevention of further spread of infection are education and other social awareness programmes (e.g. delay in initiation of coitus, decreasing the number of sexual partners, and use of barrier methods such as condoms), and post-treatment surveillance as appropriate for the condition treated.

10) Classical STDs facilitate the spread and acquisition of human immunodeficiency virus (HIV), and one important way of reducing its spread is to detect and treat STDs, particularly those associated with genital ulceration (mainly chancroid and syphilis).

After being considered nearly beaten in the early 1950s, sexually transmissible diseases (STDs) staged a phenomenal comeback, with some now epidemic or pandemic in most countries of the western world. The primary reasons for this are largely social, not medical. Popularisation of pre- and extramarital sex, sexual activity linked with prostitution or drug abuse, and the decline in popularity of the condom as a contraceptive with the advent of the 'pill' and intrauterine devices have probably facilitated the spread of the organisms concerned. In addition, in the past, control programmes usually focused primarily on gonorrhoea and syphilis, which are present worldwide, and chancroid, lymphogranuloma venereum, and granuloma inguinale, which are seen primarily in tropical countries. However, there are many other sexually transmissible pathogens, some of which are much more important in certain populations. For example, *Chlamydia trachomatis* is much more frequent and more important than gonorrhoea in many populations.

From a laboratory perspective it is easiest to focus on a specific microbiological diagnosis, but the clinician must usually manage a patient who presents with a group of symptoms or signs, i.e. a syndrome. Current management combines recognition and treatment of syndromes with variable degrees of microbiological support. The availability of microbiological support is especially important for the screening of infected individuals who would not normally be treated.

Table I lists the most important sexually transmissible pathogens according to whether they are spread primarily by sexual activity or have sexual transmission as but one means of spread. Many of the latter infections are seen primarily in homosexual or bisexual men. Table II lists the most important sexually transmissible syndromes, other less important but nevertheless frequently seen syndromes, and also the important sequelae of STDs, which are the major reasons why these diseases need to be controlled. This chapter discusses treatment of infections due to the major sexually transmissible pathogens, and the major sexually transmissible syndromes. Other syndromes and infections due to organisms that have sexual transmission as only one means of spread are discussed in other chapters. Human immunodeficiency virus (HIV) infection and acquired immune deficiency syndrome (AIDS) will be discussed in terms of their important interactions with STDs, and how they affect treatment and the response to treatment, but are mainly dealt with in other chapters (see chapter 32; sect. 3.1).

**Table I.** Sexually transmissible pathogens: degree of spread by sexual transmission

| Primarily spread by sexual activity | Sexual transmission as one means of spread |
|---|---|
| **Bacteria** | **Bacteria** |
| *Chlamydia trachomatis* | *Shigella* spp. |
| *Neisseria gonorrhoeae* | *Campylobacter* spp. |
| *Treponema pallidum* | ? *Yersinia* spp. |
| *Ureaplasma urealyticum* | ? *Salmonella* spp. |
| *Mycoplasma hominis* | Group B streptococci |
| *Haemophilus ducreyi* | *Gardnerella vaginalis* |
| *Calymmatobacterium granulomatis* | |
| **Viruses** | **Viruses** |
| Herpes simplex viruses types 1 and 2 | Hepatitis B virus |
| Genital wart (human papilloma) viruses | Hepatitis A virus |
| Molluscum contagiosum virus | Cytomegalovirus |
| Human immunodeficiency virus (HIV) | |
| **Protozoa** | **Protozoa** |
| *Trichomonas vaginalis* | *Entamoeba histolytica* |
| | *Giardia lamblia* |
| | **Ectoparasites** |
| | *Phthirus pubis* |
| | *Sarcoptes scabies* |
| | **Yeasts** |
| | *Candida* spp. |

## 1. Prevalence

The availability of accurate data on the prevalence of most STDs is compromised by the use of over-the-counter medications, variable utilisation of screening procedures and diagnostic testing, variability in diagnostic methodology and the definitions used for reporting, and major variability in the consistency of reporting.

Nevertheless, certain findings are noted repeatedly. The highest occurrence rates for most STDs are seen in 20- to 24-year-olds, 25- to 29-year-olds, and 15- to 19-year-olds.[1-4] Within these age groups, there are often dramatic differences according to gender and ethnicity[1,2] and the actual ranking of age groups varies between disease, gender, locale and markers like ethnicity. When corrected for those who are actually sexually active, rates of uncomplicated diseases and complications such as pelvic inflammatory disease (PID) are probably highest in those in their early teens, with a decrease with increasing age.[5] This is particularly unfortunate because younger individuals

**Table II.** Sexually transmissible syndromes and their consequences

| |
|---|
| **Most important syndromes** |
| Urethritis |
| Vulvovaginitis |
| Cervicitis |
| Epididymitis |
| Endometritis/salpingitis |
| Genital ulcers |
| Acquired immune deficiency syndrome (AIDS) |
| **Other syndromes** |
| Enteritis |
| Anorectal syndrome |
| Frequency-dysuria syndrome |
| Hepatitis |
| Balanoposthitis |
| Bartholinitis |
| Pharyngitis |
| **Important sequelae** |
| Involuntary infertility |
| Ectopic pregnancy |
| Cervical dysplasia and cancer |
| Reactive arthritis |
| Fetal consequences |
| Infection in infancy |
| Death (AIDS) |

are those who may be least concerned about symptoms, least likely to comply with treatment, least likely to try to get their partners treated, and almost totally unaware of the long term sequelae, which may not become apparent until they try to have a family.

Although reported age-specific rates have traditionally been higher for men, in the HIV era this pattern has changed so that for pathogens like *Chlamydia trachomatis*, reported disease rates are much higher in women.[4,6] Rates are higher for homosexual than heterosexual men, but female homosexuals have very low rates of STDs. Rates are also higher in single, divorced or separated individuals compared with married individuals, in urban compared with rural populations, and in those of lower socioeconomic status.[7,8]

There are marked differences in the prevalence of different pathogens in different geographical locations, and there have been dramatic changes in the prevalence of different STDs over time. In Africa, and many other less developed regions, the major STDs seen are gonorrhoea, syphilis and chancroid.[9-11] Rates of infection can be very high, and STDs, even excluding HIV infection, probably have a major impact on overall population dynamics.[12-15] Similar high frequencies of these pathogens may also be seen in inner city locations in other parts of the world, including the US.[7,8] However, in developed countries, the major genital infections are *C. trachomatis*, genital herpes, genital warts, and in some places gonorrhoea.

In countries with the resources and commitment to deliver more effective STD control, for those diseases for which effective treatments exist, disease rates have fallen, in some cases precipitously; this is particularly true for infection with *Neisseria gonorrhoeae*.[1-3,16] The decrease in incidence of gonorrhoea has been evident since the early 1970s in Nordic countries, and the 1980s in Canada and the US. However, overall rates are still much higher in the US than in most parts of Europe and Canada.

In the case of infectious syphilis, the incidence has fallen in developed countries, with the dramatic exception of the US, where rates increased in the late 1980s.[2,16] Reasons for the better control of this disease are thought to be the long incubation period, which enables more effective contact tracing, and the fortuitous use of penicillin in large dosages for all types of infections. However, in many less developed countries, and in inner city populations in some developed countries, syphilis remains a major problem, including being a cause of congenital disease and perinatal mortality.[2] In the US, much of the recent increase has been linked with drug abuse, particularly use of crack cocaine.[17,18]

Although the reported rates of infection with *C. trachomatis* are many times higher than with *N. gonorrhoeae*, the rates for this pathogen have also been falling. This has been documented in several countries or places and appears to be a real fall.[6,19-21] However, as with gonorrhoea, rates remain highest in 15- to 24-year-olds, the groups at greatest risk of long term complications.

Trichomoniasis shows an extremely varied world pattern, but its prevalence is also decreasing.[22,23] Also encouraging is the fact that rates of some complications are falling. This is most notable with pelvic inflammatory disease,[1,6,19,20,24] particularly in places where infection with gonorrhoea and *C. trachomatis* has decreased. However, late complications of pelvic inflammatory disease such as ectopic pregnancies have not yet shown a significant decrease,[25] which probably reflects the fact that complications like ectopic pregnancy or infertility on the basis of tubal damage may not become apparent until years after the initial infection. In some less developed countries, pelvic inflammatory disease remains a frequent complication.[11]

In contrast to the pathogens for which effective treatments are available, for those like herpes simplex virus,[1,26,27] human papilloma viruses[1] and HIV,[1,2,28,29] infection rates have not fallen as dramatically or, in the case of HIV, have continued to rise. Since they cannot be eradicated, each incident (new) case adds to the overall prevalence. However, in countries that have made a major effort in implementing better educational programmes to decrease unprotected sexual activity, there is now evidence that even viral infections like herpes are decreasing.[30]

For countries where the relative number of adolescents and young adults is decreasing, part of this apparent improvement is artifactual. This is one of the reasons that it is particularly important to look at age and gender specific rates. Where the changes are real, it is impossible to attribute the changes in prevalence to any one factor, but contributing factors probably include better means of detection, effective treatments, use of syndromic management, contact tracing, and a focus on preventive measures. The latter include deferral of onset of sexual activity, reduction in numbers of sexual partners, avoidance of riskier forms of sexual activity, and use of barrier methods to decrease the spread of pathogens. Fear of HIV has probably contributed to changes in all of these; nevertheless, the explanation for the much greater decrease in diseases for which curative treatment is available, in comparison with diseases like genital herpes and genital warts, is the availability of effective treatments.

## 2. General Principles of Treatment

Effective control of STDs is aimed at reducing the prevalence of infection by detecting and treating cases, identification and treatment of asymptomatic infection, detection and treatment of sexual contacts of these individuals, and efforts to decrease sexual activity that places individuals at risk of acquiring infection. This requires a multidisciplinary effort. It also means that the conditions should be recognised as deserving of treatment and prevention.[31] Access to effective treatments is a key element in these efforts.

### 2.1 Why Treat?

The main reason for treatment is to prevent the complications listed in table II. It is noteworthy that most of the complications of STDs other than AIDS arise in women. The major ones follow infections with *C. trachomatis, N. gonorrhoeae* and *Treponema pallidum*, all of which are treatable.

***Syphilis*** is a potentially lethal and crippling disease, especially in the fetus[32,33] and in those who later develop tertiary symptoms. ***N. gonorrhoeae*** and ***C. trachomatis*** infections can cause infertility,[11-14,34-39] ectopic pregnancy,[25,36,37,39,40] and chronic pelvic pain[37,39] in a sizeable proportion of infected women as a consequence of tubal inflammation. Infertility arises in 10 to 20% of women who are known to have had tubal infection, but it undoubtedly also occurs in many other women.[37-39] As many as two-thirds of women who are found to have tubal obstruction as a consequence of inflammation deny ever having had any symptoms suggestive of endometrial or tubal infection.[34,39] *N. gonorrhoeae* can also cause septicaemia with arthritis, particularly in females, and in infants born to mothers with gonorrhoea.[41] *C. trachomatis* causes reactive arthritis, including Reiter's syndrome,[42-44] and conjunctivitis and pneumonia in infants. *C. trachomatis*, *N. gonorrhoeae* and *T. pallidum* also contribute to adverse outcomes in pregnancy.[32,45,46] Although in some areas, urethral strictures are said to be frequent sequelae in men, physical complications in males are uncommon with both *C. trachomatis* and *N. gonorrhoeae* infections in developed countries. Urethritis in males may, however, be associated with significant psychological trauma and disruption of relationships.

***Vulvovaginitis*** in women is usually due to *Trichomonas vaginalis*, genital yeasts or bacterial vaginosis (see further section 5.1). These entities can frequently result in continuing discomfort and suffering both because of inadequate diagnosis and because of treatment failures. Though usually not associated with severe consequences, there is increasing evidence that in pregnancy, infection with *T. vaginalis* and bacterial vaginosis are associated with increased rates of premature rupture of membranes.[46-49]

***Genital herpes***, particularly in females, can be transiently crippling, necessitating hospital admission.[50,51] In many individuals, it is a recurrent and intractable condition associated with major psychosocial consequences.[52] Neonatal herpes occurs infrequently, but arises in approximately 50% of infants delivered vaginally to mothers with primary herpes simplex virus infection and 3% with recurrent herpes at delivery.[27,53] Without treatment, approximately 60% of infected neonates die of disseminated infection.[54] Treatment of neonatal infection with vidarabine greatly improved the outcome but long term morbidity was still frequent. Treatment with aciclovir is more effective, but does not prevent all sequelae.[27,54,55] An oncogenic role of herpes simplex virus in cervical cancer has also been suspected but current data more strongly associate human papilloma viruses with cervical cancer.[56]

***Genital warts*** result in numerous visits to clinicians for treatment, and are strongly associated with cervical dysplasia and malignancy.[56-58] Other viruses such as cytomegalovirus occur frequently and can cause pneumonitis or severe brain damage to the fetus *in utero*, as well as more subtle infections when infection is not clinically evident at birth and complications arise years later.[54]

***Hepatitis B*** is often acquired sexually,[59] including by heterosexual individuals, and there is evidence that concurrent syphilis increases the transmission of hepatitis B.[60] Hepatitis B is associated with short term risks of acute, fatal hepatitis, and long term complications of cirrhosis and hepatocellular carcinoma are associated with a chronic carrier state (see also chapter 32; sect. 3.8). The availability of hepatitis B vaccine now provides the first, effective vaccine for any sexually transmitted pathogen.[59]

Another reason to prevent STDs and to diagnose and treat them diligently is to decrease the associated economic costs, which are very large. Effective treatment can decrease these costs.[12,33,61-67]

## 2.2 Diagnosis

Accurate history-taking and diagnosis (clinical and laboratory) are essential for the proper treatment and control of the major STDs.

### 2.2.1 Clinical Diagnosis

The biggest obstacle to taking an accurate history is failure to consider the possibility that an individual may be at risk for an STD. This is particularly true for adolescent patients. Once considered, key elements of an optimal history are straightforward.

Clinical diagnosis requires direct examination of the genital region, with particular attention directed to sites of infection suggested by the history. In some cases, a total body examination is indicated (e.g. consideration of AIDS or syphilis). In all cases, the examination should be as thorough as possible. This is especially critical with male urethritis where recent voiding can remove discharge and impede detection of a polymorphonuclear leucocyte response.[68] A speculum examination and a bimanual examination are required for optimal evaluation of postpubertal women.

It is crucial to note that for almost all STDs, infection with serious pathogens like *C. trachomatis* and *N. gonorrhoeae* can be present without any objective evidence of disease.

### 2.2.2 Laboratory Diagnosis

When specimens are obtained for laboratory diagnosis, the sites chosen are critical. In women, for *N. gonorrhoeae* and *C. trachomatis* infections, the endocervix yields the highest number of positives, followed by the urethra. For detection of *N. gonorrhoeae*, anal culture is next in importance. The vaginal swab is used for detection of *T. vaginalis*, *Candida* species and bacterial vaginosis, but it should never be relied on to diagnose gonorrhoea in postpubertal women by Gram stain or routine culture. Urethritis in males is diagnosed by a Gram-stained smear of urethral discharge or endourethral material. These should be tested routinely for *N. gonorrhoeae*, both for diagnosis and, when indicated, for susceptibility to antimicrobials (which requires a cultured specimen). If the diagnosis of *C. trachomatis* infection is attempted in men, the optimal specimen is a deep (4cm) endourethral swab. Newer methodologies like polymerase chain reaction (PCR) allow use of urine as an alternative specimen for detection of *C. trachomatis*.[69]

Throat swabs for *N. gonorrhoeae* should be taken in those who have had orogenital contact. Pharyngeal gonorrhoea can be more difficult to cure than genital gonorrhoea, although this is less of a problem with newer antimicrobial agents.[70] Swabs from the throat, rectum and urethra should be obtained routinely in homosexual male patients.

For the diagnosis of genital lesions, specimens should be obtained from the lesion as early in the course of the disease as possible.[71,72] Especially for the diagnosis of herpes simplex virus, the specimen must be taken vigorously so that cells are obtained from the base of the lesion. With other genital lesions, if fluctuant lymph nodes are present, the material should be aseptically aspirated and Gram-stained and cultured (if cultures are available). Serology for syphilis is always indicated.

In infectious syphilis, a dark ground microscopic examination of serum squeezed from the suspected chancre, or any moist lesion, is the first effective diagnostic measure to be undertaken.[73] Pitfalls are lack of familiarity with the technique of setting up a dark ground microscope or preparing a proper dark ground slide, and the differentiation of *T. pallidum* from the commensal treponemes that are often present. Determinations from the dark ground examination of mouth lesions are especially unreliable. Standard and treponemal antibody serological tests are essential for diagnosis.

The specific microbiological diagnostic tests currently available are in a state of flux with the increased use of non-culture tests, especially for *N. gonorrhoeae* and *C. trachomatis*.[69] Different tests may also require use of different swabs, different media to be inoculated or even use of slides, and may also require different means and conditions of transportation to the laboratory. In general, serology is of little use for the management of specific individuals, with the major exception of those with syphilis. Serological tests for syphilis should be performed in all cases of STDs. When lymphogranuloma venereum is suspected, serological tests are usually beneficial.

Most individuals with an STD should also be offered diagnostic testing for HIV.

### 2.3 Management by Syndrome

There are situations where treatment may be recommended solely on the basis of a clinical impression of the presenting symptoms and signs, e.g. where a syndrome such as pelvic inflammatory disease is diagnosed in the absence of microbiological or laboratory confirmation. Diagnosis of a syndrome on the basis of presenting symptoms or signs, or in conjunction with simple laboratory tests such as a smear of secretions or direct assessment of urine or vaginal secretions, predicts the likely cause(s) and allows rationally directed therapy,[74] and can also circumvent the need for more expensive diagnostic testing. Diagnosis of a syndrome often allows initiation of therapy at the time the patient is first seen,[74,75] which is particularly important in those who might not return for a subsequent visit. This has been a problem even in those who have had a microbiological diagnosis established. A recent study of individuals who had *C. trachomatis* diagnosed but not initially treated found that only three-quarters returned for treatment, and half of these returned after 2 weeks, with some developing pelvic inflammatory disease in the interim.[76]

Syndromic management also allows earlier treatment of sexual partners and decreases concerns about missing infected individuals because of false-negative diagnostic tests. It accepts the idea of overtreatment and the use of antimicrobials which in many cases are not needed, but assumes that there is both little risk and also acceptable benefit for the patient, partners and overall control efforts.[77]

### 2.4 Use of Effective Treatment Regimens

The aim of treatment is to approach a 100% cure rate, not only to prevent further spread of disease, but also to limit (or even decrease) the development of 'relatively resistant' organisms due to failed treatment.[77-79] If administered appropriately and the treated individual is not reinfected, currently recommended regimens usually attain cure rates well in excess of 95%.

This goal can only be achieved if a drug or regimen that is highly active against the causative organism or potential causative organisms is used and if the treatment regimen minimises or avoids noncompliance by the patient. Single-dose curative regimens have been available for *N. gonorrhoeae*, *T. vaginalis* and early *T. pallidum* infection for years, and one is now available for *C. trachomatis*. However, single-dose regimens for gonorrhoea other than azithromycin will not eradicate concurrent *C. trachomatis* infection, which is present in 20% of heterosexual men and 40 to 50% of women with *N. gonorrhoeae*.[80] Thus, single-dose treatment directed only at *N. gonorrhoeae* will often fail to treat patients with gonorrhoea fully and may leave them and their partners at risk for significant sequelae.[81,82]

Traditionally, optimum treatment of most infections usually mandates the use of a regimen with as narrow a spectrum as possible. For diseases like syphilis, trichomoniasis and candidiasis, this approach remains preferable. However, this traditional approach to treatment is not appropriate for all STDs because:

1) Clinicians often manage patients with syndromes.

2) The syndromes may have numerous causes that cannot always be readily and specifically diagnosed when the patient is first seen.

3) Sexually transmissible pathogens frequently coexist.

4) Traditional specific treatment (especially that directed solely at *N. gonorrhoeae*) can leave patients at risk for significant sequelae.

5) The incidence of long term sequelae is increasing.

6) Drug resistance may develop.

Thus, for uncomplicated syndromes like urethritis and cervicitis, treatment should normally be directed at multiple pathogens, and no single drug treatment is entirely effective. For complicated diseases like salpingitis, even combination therapy as currently advocated does not totally cover all potential pathogens.

Use of syndromic management and regimens active against two or more pathogens does not lessen the importance of making accurate clinical and laboratory diagnoses. Nor does it detract from the lessons previously learned which showed that the routine use of regimens that attain close to 100% efficacy in treatment may ultimately decrease the prevalence of resistant organisms.[78] Indeed, the current combined approach may accomplish what single-dose treatments will no longer do.

#### 2.4.1 Cost, Compliance and Adverse Outcomes

When a drug regimen is chosen, there are concerns about toxicity, cost, compliance and the potential effect on the microbial environment. Toxicity is especially relevant because:

1) Patients with STDs often become reinfected and need multiple courses of treatment.

2) Infected women are usually of childbearing age and consequently could be pregnant.

3) Common knowledge of toxicity or adverse effects may dissuade potentially infected individuals from seeking medical attention, thus exacerbating the problem of management.

##### Cost Considerations

From a global perspective, drug costs contribute minimally to the overall costs of STD prevention and management,[62,63,83,84] yet when used in conjunction with other measures are a major means by which control can be facilitated. However, for the individual, and for the vast majority of programmes which have fixed budgets, the costs of antimicrobial agents, especially the more expensive regimens, can be a major problem. The marginal cost with use of an expensive regimen may be very high both in terms of cost per additional patient cured and in terms of other components of management programmes that have to be sacrificed because of reduction in the remaining available funds. Cost is a major limiting factor in all areas, especially in developing countries. The problem has been exacerbated as older, inexpensive medications like penicillins lose their efficacy, and newer more expensive agents are introduced. For those who must pay for their own medication, and in particular adolescent or nonworking patients for whom cost is a substantial burden, control efforts could potentially be impeded if prescriptions cannot be filled.

Formal cost-effectiveness studies could theoretically be very helpful in allowing decisions to be made. They could also be very helpful in assessing the cost effectiveness of more expensive regimens that have similar outcomes to less expensive agents in efficacy studies, but would be expected to have greater effectiveness because of single-dose administration or greatly reduced rates or severity of adverse drug effects. This is currently an issue with azithromycin, and whether programmes should use it rather than doxycycline to treat infection with *C. trachomatis* and associated syndromes.[62,63] However, these studies have assumed 100% compliance with single-dose therapies, ignoring the distinct possibility that if the medication is prescribed and must be filled by prescription, many will not be able or willing to fill them. This is a realistic concern. In a recent study where inner city women diagnosed with pelvic inflammatory disease were given prescriptions for doxycycline, 72 of 265 (27%) women who were contactable for follow-up by phone did not fill their prescriptions.[85] The most common reasons given were cost (50%), inconvenience (28%), and resolution of symptoms (20%).

##### Compliance Issues

Compliance is a major concern with recommended regimens, and is the major reason for the search for effective, single-dose regimens. Compliance with multidose therapy is an issue even in the artificial situation of efficacy studies and is likely to be much worse in the real world. In a recent study, there was only 63% compliance with a week of tetracycline or erythromycin therapy.[86] Compliance is better with once-daily administration than with multiple daily doses.[87] Particularly in core group populations, single agent, single-dose oral therapy should have major advantages for treatment of proven or presumptive infection and for control efforts, at least when it can be directly administered.

#### Toxicity Considerations

That STDs typically infect individuals who are otherwise well, and cause no or few symptoms, has several important implications for drug therapy. Firstly, many infected individuals will escape detection and hence will only be recognised as needing treatment because of screening evaluations, presentation with a concurrent infection correlated with an increased risk of another pathogen (e.g. *C. trachomatis* in someone with gonorrhoea[81,83,88]), or because of disease recognised in a sexual partner. Secondly, because they do not feel that they are ill, they may be less willing to take treatment, and if they do, may be more aware of adverse effects and less willing to continue treatment if adverse effects occur. Furthermore, because they are usually active and continue their activities of daily living, they may be more likely to notice new symptoms. A young, healthy, asymptomatic person is more likely to notice adverse effects than one who has symptoms that may be improved by therapy, or who is accustomed to taking medications or has experienced more severe disease in the past.[89]

Adverse effects are particularly important in treatment of STDs. Because for most STDs there are regimens that are very well tolerated, a new agent that, compared with the standard, has similar microbiological efficacy and no great advantages in terms of cost or ease of use but has a slightly worse adverse effect profile, has little usefulness for routine management.

#### Potential Effects on the Microbial Environment

Concerns about effects on the microbial environment are unique considerations with antimicrobials because although we treat one individual, this can have an effect on the bacteria in many other individuals around them. Even appropriate use of antimicrobials promotes the development of resistance in bacteria exposed to them and these bacteria reach the environment by multiple means besides sexual transmission. This poses a risk to all individuals. Undoubtedly, antimicrobial drug use for other diseases has played a significant role in the development of resistant isolates of *N. gonorrhoeae* and *Haemophilus ducreyi*. Similarly, the frequency of administration of antimicrobial drugs for the treatment of STDs must also contribute to this problem.

### 2.5 Contact Tracing

Effective management also means preventing the risk of reinfection of the index case by the partner(s). Contact tracing allows identification of potentially infected source(s) and secondary contacts, who are often asymptomatic, without the time, expense and lower yield of surveillance programmes. The optimal methods of doing this are still uncertain and are perhaps dependent upon the population involved.[90] Potential methods include follow-up by the initial health-care provider, notification by the patient, and use of mail, telephone or direct contact by specially trained individuals. In some settings, the index case may be given medication to provide to the contact.

Whatever method is used, to be successful, speed is essential and the partner(s) of index patients should be identified and treated as quickly as possible. This is especially important for infections like gonorrhoea that have short incubation periods, where further spread from infected contacts occurs before effective contact tracing can be achieved. Traditionally, the symptomless female consort of the male attending for treatment of gonorrhoea was the target. However, it is now clear that asymptomatic infection in males as well as females is a major problem both with gonorrhoea[91] and *C. trachomatis* infection.[92] Because of difficulty in obtaining specimens, particularly from males, but also the failure of diagnostic tests to detect everyone who is infected, contacts should almost always be treated whether or not they are symptomatic, and whatever the test result.

Contact tracing in syphilis, with its long incubation period, is critical for epidemiological control. Contacts of a proven case of infectious syphilis should be treated prophylactically during the incubation period. If a lesion is already present, a diagnosis should be made by serology and dark ground examination before treatment is given. However, if there is any concern that individuals will be lost to follow-up, they should be treated before results are available.

### 2.6 Post-Treatment Surveillance

Relapse of *N. gonorrhoeae* infection occurs most often during the week after treatment, whereas with *C. trachomatis*, clinically or microbiologically detectable relapse may take weeks to months. Because treatment regimens for these two pathogens are sufficiently efficacious, routine test-of-cure evaluations are not recommended in individuals who are believed to have taken their treatment, have not been re-exposed, and are or have become asymptomatic.[75] In this respect, test-of-cure evaluations for *C. trachomatis* are not cost effective.[93]

Because individuals who have acquired gonorrhoea or *C. trachomatis* infection once are at relatively high risk of becoming reinfected, a strong case can be made for rescreening them 3 to 6 months later.[94]

In the case of infectious syphilis, however, post-treatment surveillance is essential.

### 2.7 Screening

Even detection of all symptomatic individuals and their contacts will not identify all infected individuals. Screening, usually by a culture or direct non-culture technique, is required to detect others with unsuspected infection. For initial screening, particularly of adolescent males, use of tests to detect pyuria has been effective in some populations, allowing more selective use of more expensive techniques.[62,95-98]

The degree to which screening will be successful depends upon the degree of laboratory sophistication available, the limitations of the diagnostic tests, the available manpower, and access to patient populations. Non-culture diagnostic tests other than polymerase chain reaction (PCR) or ligase chain reaction (LCR) techniques are especially likely to have limitations in low prevalence situations, unless a second means of confirming the positive test is used. When screening is to be performed, cost benefit is usually greatest in younger sexually active women and in those with a history of previous or other concurrent STDs.[1,61,64,84,99-107]

## 3. Optimum Treatment of the Major Sexually Transmissible Diseases

### 3.1 Gonorrhoea

Antimicrobial agents are used to treat patients with proven or suspected gonorrhoea, patients with a syndrome compatible with the presence of *N. gonorrhoeae*, and contacts of these individuals. They are also used for ocular prophylaxis at birth.

Although the use of penicillin (or ampicillin or amoxicillin) would still be expected to cure some cases of *N. gonorrhoeae* infection in restricted geographic locations, there is no longer any role for the routine use of penicillins in the management of gonorrhoea or its complications. This is due to the rapid emergence of penicillinase-producing *N. gonorrhoeae* (PPNG) in many parts of the world, the emergence of chromosomally mediated resistance to *N. gonorrhoeae* (CMRNG), and the recognition of the prevalence and importance of concurrent infection with *C. trachomatis*.[70,81,82,88,108,109]

The development of resistance is not restricted to the penicillins. There is now sufficient resistance to the tetracyclines that reliance cannot be placed on these agents for treatment of *N. gonorrhoeae*. Many isolates are also resistant to spectinomycin, and there are now even reports of resistance to members of the newest class of agents used for treatment, the fluoroquinolones (e.g. with ciprofloxacin and ofloxacin).[110]

#### 3.1.1 Goals of Treatment

Whatever treatment is utilised, the goals should be to use a regimen that has an effectiveness against *N. gonorrhoeae* as close to 100% as possible. Based on calculations with penicillin, the antimicrobial agent must be present at a level 3 to 4 times the strain's minimum inhibitory concentration to penicillin for at least 7 to 10 hours.[111] Although multiple doses of other antimicrobial drugs may be needed as part of the treatment (especially against *C. trachomatis*), the treatment directed against uncomplicated *N. gonorrhoeae* infection should ideally be effective in a single dose, and active against *N. gonorrhoeae* at all body sites.[70,75,109] Both parenteral and oral regimens are available. Although many consider parenteral therapy to be more desirable because patient compliance can be guaranteed and absorption is likely to be more consistent than with oral therapy, the latter has the advantages of easier administration, greater patient acceptance, and usually lower cost per dose administered.

The choice of regimens depends on many factors, but most importantly on the local level of resistance to antimicrobials,[112] and whether the infection is complicated. No regimen with a less than 95% expected efficacy rate should be used. There is no role for treatment with penicillin or amoxicillin in areas where PPNG or CMRNG comprise more than a very small percentage of isolates.[112] Even in areas where isolates remain penicillin-sensitive, penicillin should not be used when the patient gives a history suggesting potential exposure to PPNG (e.g. travel to Southeast Asia, Africa, or even travel to large urban centres) or for treatment failures.

The drugs and doses given below are those recommended in the 1993 US Centers for Disease Control (CDC) STD treatment guidelines.[75] Numerous other regimens have been studied to various degrees,[70] but those listed were felt by an expert panel to be the best current choices as of the spring of 1993.

### 3.1.2 Treatment of Uncomplicated Gonococcal Infection in Adults and Adolescents

The recommended drugs of choice for the component of regimens active against *N. gonorrhoeae*[75] are:

- Ceftriaxone 125mg intramuscularly in a single dose
- Cefixime 400mg orally in a single dose
- Ciprofloxacin 500mg orally in a single dose
- Ofloxacin 400mg orally in a single dose.

All of these regimens appear to be effective at all body sites so that there is no longer a need to use different regimens for uncomplicated gonococcal infection at different body sites. There is, however, more experience with the ceftriaxone and ciprofloxacin regimens for treatment of pharyngeal gonorrhoea. All of these single-dose treatments should be given concurrently with a regimen active against *C. trachomatis* (see section 3.1.3).

Of the four regimens, only ceftriaxone is believed to have adequate efficacy against incubating syphilis. With the other three regimens, activity against syphilis is only provided by the adjunctive therapy given for *Chlamydia trachomatis*. However, the routine need for the chosen regimen to be active against incubating syphilis has been questioned.[113]

The dosage of ceftriaxone differs from the 1989 CDC recommendation in that it is half the previously recommended dose of 250mg.[114] The lower dose has been shown to have equivalent efficacy at a lower cost, and has not so far resulted in any apparent trend towards greater selection of cefalosporin-resistant isolates.[115] The dose of cefixime, at 400mg, is lower than that used in earlier studies, but appears to have equivalent efficacy to ceftriaxone.[116] Lower doses of cefixime are also usually effective,[117] but are not recommended. Similarly, ciprofloxacin 250mg orally is almost 100% effective and some advocate use of that dose.[118]

The cefalosporins are safe for use in pregnant women and in children, and the only significant contraindication to their use is prior cefalosporin allergy or a history of immediate hypersensitivity to the penicillins. Neither of the fluoroquinolones (ciprofloxacin or ofloxacin) should be used in pregnancy, in nursing mothers, or in those under 17 years of age.

***Other regimens:*** numerous other regimens have been used for treatment of *N. gonorrhoeae* infection and may continue to be effective.[70] However, none has any major advantages over the recommended regimens. Spectinomycin 2g intramuscularly in a single dose remains useful for treatment of individuals unable to tolerate either cefalosporins or fluoroquinolones, but has the disadvantages of being expensive, inactive against *T. pallidum*, unreliable for treatment of pharyngeal gonorrhoea, and has reduced activity against some strains of *N. gonorrhoeae*.[75]

Other injectable cefalosporins that could potentially be used include ceftizoxime 500mg intramuscularly in a single dose, cefotaxime 500mg intramuscularly in a single dose, cefotetan 1g intramuscularly in a single dose, and cefoxitin 2g intramuscularly in a single dose.[70,75] The most promising of these agents is ceftizoxime, but for none is there as much experience as with ceftriaxone.

There are also numerous other oral cefalosporins for which there is some, albeit insufficient, clinical experience, particularly with pharyngeal gonorrhoea. Examples include cefuroxime axetil 1g orally in a single dose and cefpodoxime 200mg orally in a single dose.[70,75] Alternative fluoroquinolones with no obvious advantage over ciprofloxacin and ofloxacin include enoxacin 400mg orally in a single dose, lomefloxacin 400mg orally in a single dose, and norfloxacin 800mg orally in a single dose.[70,75] Penicillins combined with a β-lactamase inhibitor (e.g. amoxicillin/clavulanic acid) are also effective, but do not have significant advantages over the recommended regimens.[70]

Many other compounds have also been studied. The most interesting of the newer agents is azithromycin, because of its activity against *C. trachomatis* in a single dose of 1g.[119-125] However, its activity against *N. gonorrhoeae* is still uncertain: a 1g dose of azithromycin has usually, but not reliably, eradicated *N. gonorrhoeae*.[125-127] A 2g dose is more effective, but is associated with a level of adverse effects such that it is not currently a viable alternative, even if it were less expensive.[126] More experience is needed with the 1g dose, particularly in the light of its activity against chancroid[128] in addition to *C. trachomatis*. This combined activity could have tremendous benefit for treatment of STDs in Africa, with an impact on decreasing the spread of HIV.

#### 3.1.3 Concurrent Therapy for Chlamydia trachomatis Infection

When a single-dose regimen is used for *N. gonorrhoeae*, concurrent therapy to eradicate *C. trachomatis* is also recommended.[75] In those infected with *N. gonorrhoeae*, *C. trachomatis* can be detected in the urethra of 20 to 30% of men and in the genital tract of 40 to 50% of women. None of the recommended single-dose regimens for gonorrhoea (see section 3.1.2) will reliably or even frequently eradicate *C. trachomatis*;[70,81,82] this includes ofloxacin, which appears to eradicate it with multiple-dose therapy.[129]

The choice of regimens to eradicate *C. trachomatis* is discussed in more detail in section 3.2. However, except in pregnancy, the recommended regimen is doxycycline 100mg orally twice daily for 7 days. Azithromycin, either used alone to treat both, or used in conjunction with a regimen active against *N. gonorrhoeae*, is also an option. However, a concern with the use of azithromycin in conjunction with single-dose oral regimens for gonorrhoea is the possibility of enhanced adverse reactions.

#### 3.1.4 Treatment of Gonococcal Infection in Pregnancy

In pregnancy, the regimen of choice is one of the cefalosporins, with adjunctive erythromycin for *C. trachomatis*. Since the fluoroquinolones are contraindicated, if a cefalosporin cannot be given, spectinomycin 2g intramuscularly as a single dose remains the best alternative, with erythromycin being used for the portion of the regimen active against *C. trachomatis*.

#### 3.1.5 Treatment of Conjunctivitis Due to Neisseria gonorrhoeae in Adults

There is minimal experience in treating this condition but ceftriaxone 1g in a single intramuscular dose in conjunction with lavage of the infected eye with saline once, appears effective.[75]

#### 3.1.6 Treatment of Disseminated Gonococcal Infection

There is little current experience with disseminated gonococcal infection in the era of penicillin- and tetracycline-resistant *N. gonorrhoeae*. Based on past experience, treatment of disseminated *N. gonorrhoeae* infection is more difficult and requires multiple-dose treatment, preferably initiated in hospital. The CDC recommendations are for initial therapy in hospital, particularly if there are concerns about compliance with therapy, where the diagnosis is uncertain, or where there are purulent synovial effusions or other complications. The recommended regimen is ceftriaxone 1g intramuscularly or intravenously every 24 hours, with alternative initial regimens being cefotaxime 1g intravenously every 8 hours or ceftizoxime 1g intravenously every 8 hours.[75] For patients allergic to cefalosporins, spectinomycin 2g intramuscularly every 12 hours is recommended.

The initial regimen should be continued for 24 to 48 hours after improvement begins, with therapy then switched to either cefixime 400mg orally twice daily or ciprofloxacin 500mg orally twice daily to complete a total combined course of at least 7 days. In all cases, a 7-day regimen effective against *C. trachomatis* (see section 3.1.3) should also be used.

#### 3.1.7 Treatment of Complicated Gonococcal Infection

Treatment of complicated *N. gonorrhoeae* infections such as pelvic inflammatory disease and epididymitis are discussed in sections 4.3 and 4.4, respectively. In the current era of penicillin- and tetracycline-resistant *N. gonorrhoeae*, there is minimal experience in treating gonococcal endocarditis or meningitis. Recommended therapy is ceftriaxone 1 to 2g intravenously every 12 hours given for 10 to 14 days for meningitis and at least 28 days for endocarditis.[75]

#### 3.1.8 Treatment of Gonococcal Infection in Children

Children who weigh 45kg or more should receive the same doses as adolescents and adults, with the exception that those under 17 years should not receive fluoroquinolones and those under 9 years should not receive tetracyclines (for the component of therapy active against *C. trachomatis*).

For children under 45kg, the recommended regimen for children with uncomplicated gonococcal vulvovaginitis, cervicitis, urethritis, pharyngitis or proctitis is ceftriaxone 125mg intramuscularly in a single dose.[75] Cefixime can also be used, but supporting data are meagre. The alternative is spectinomycin 40 mg/kg intramuscularly in a single dose, which should not exceed 2g.

For those under 45kg with bacteraemia, arthritis or meningitis, the recommended regimen is ceftriaxone 50 mg/kg intramuscularly or intravenously in a single daily dose (not to exceed 1g for bacteraemia or arthritis, or 2g for meningitis).[75] The duration of treatment is 7 days for bacteraemia or arthritis and 10 to 14 days for meningitis.

#### *3.1.9 Treatment of Neonatal Gonococcal Infection*

Because of the neonatal morbidity and risk of septicaemia, in areas where the incidence of gonorrhoea is high, all pregnant women should have endocervical cultures examined as part of routine antenatal care. Babies born to mothers with gonorrhoea should routinely have orogastric and rectal cultures taken,[41] and blood cultures should be taken if septicaemia is suspected, especially if the membranes have ruptured prematurely. If cultures or Gram-stained smears from the mother show gonococci at birth, or cultures or Gram-stained smears from the conjunctiva show gonococci, ceftriaxone 25 to 50 mg/kg should be given intravenously or intramuscularly in a single dose that should not exceed 125mg.[75] Topical antibacterial eye drops are not needed in conjunction with parenteral therapy. However, some continue to treat conjunctivitis until cultures are negative.

Treated infants should be followed in hospital for evidence of disseminated infection. If sepsis, arthritis or meningitis are diagnosed or strongly considered, treatment is recommended with ceftriaxone 25 to 50 mg/kg/day intravenously or intramuscularly in a single daily dose, or cefotaxime 25 mg/kg intravenously or intramuscularly every 12 hours.[75] These are given for 7 days unless meningitis is documented, in which case the duration of therapy should be at least 10 to 14 days.

Recommended regimens to prevent gonococcal ophthalmia neonatorum continue to be a single application of 1% silver nitrate aqueous solution, 0.5% erythromycin ophthalmic ointment, or 1% tetracycline ophthalmic ointment.[75] However, none of these prevents nasopharyngeal colonisation with *C. trachomatis* and they are of uncertain benefit in preventing chlamydial ocular infection. The best way to prevent transmission of *N. gonorrhoeae* and *C. trachomatis* to the infant is to detect and treat the infection in the mother prior to delivery.

#### *3.1.10 Follow-up and Management of Sexual Partners*

In patients who take the recommended treatments and improve, test-of-cure evaluations are not recommended.[75] Those who do not respond or whose symptoms recur should be re-evaluated.

Ideally, all sexual partners, whether symptomatic or not, should be evaluated and treated with a regimen active against *N. gonorrhoeae* and *C. trachomatis* as soon as possible, whether or not diagnostic tests are positive. In some circumstances it is more realistic to try to have partners treated even without testing. As guidelines for which sexual partners to treat, the CDC recommends that where the index case is symptomatic, all sexual partners within the last 30 days should be sought.[75] When the index case is asymptomatic, it should be those within the last 60 days, and where there has not been any contact in the last 60 days, it should be the last sexual partner.

### 3.2 *Chlamydia trachomatis* Infection

#### *3.2.1 Goals of Treatment*

The first goal of treatment is to use a regimen which has an efficacy against *C. trachomatis* as close to 100% as possible. A second goal is to prevent the development of complications. In women, this is often impossible because spread of infection to the upper genital tract may have already occurred. Between 20 to 40% of women with apparently uncomplicated cervical infection already have endometrial infection.[130,131] With regard to *C. trachomatis* and pelvic inflammatory disease, there is little or no evidence that treatment reverses sequelae that have already arisen, and the mouse model suggests that the window of opportunity for an effect of antimicrobials in preserving fertility is very narrow.[132,133] This is substantiated by clinical data showing that delay in initiation of therapy for pelvic inflammatory disease is associated with a worsened outcome.[35] A large proportion of women develop complications of ectopic pregnancy or infertility without ever knowing that they were infected.[34,39] Despite these concerns, there is evidence that attempts to detect and treat infection with *C. trachomatis* do decrease the overall rate of recognised pelvic inflammatory disease, so that this goal may sometimes be met.[105]

A third goal is to decrease spread of the infection in the community.

### 3.2.2 Effective Antimicrobial Agents

The tetracyclines have traditionally been the drugs of choice for treatment of uncomplicated *C. trachomatis* genital infections.[80,134,135] Among the tetracyclines, doxycycline 100mg orally twice daily for 7 days has become the preferred agent.[75,100] This is not because of increased efficacy *versus* other tetracyclines in those who take their medications, but rather because of improved patient acceptance. The benefits of less frequent administration due to the longer half-life of doxycycline, better penetration of body sites, the ease of administration due to twice daily therapy, the ability to take the drug with food, and possibly lower rates of adverse effects are felt to outweigh the minimally increased cost compared with tetracycline hydrochloride. There is little convincing evidence that more than 7 days of treatment with tetracyclines is required to eradicate *C. trachomatis* in uncomplicated genital infection.[80,136] However, a disquieting observation has been that some isolates of *C. trachomatis* demonstrate *in vitro* and in some cases *in vivo* resistance to the tetracyclines[137,138] and also to erythromycin.[139] Furthermore, the DNA of *C. trachomatis*, but not usually positive cultures, can be detected in the upper genital tract long after treatment.[140-142] The overall significance of such findings is uncertain, and has not altered recommendations for treatment.

The macrolide drug erythromycin is an effective alternative to the tetracyclines. The advent of the newer macrolide *azithromycin* has been a major advance in the treatment of uncomplicated infection with *C. trachomatis*; in studies with reasonable (though still possibly too short) follow-up, azithromycin has provided efficacy equivalent to that of doxycycline with a single 1g oral dose.[119-125] Although it has not yet been fully evaluated, its effectiveness is likely to be better than that of doxycycline because treatment need only be taken once rather than over a period of 1 week. The major problem with azithromycin is its cost, which is much greater than that of the tetracyclines or the older macrolide erythromycin. Azithromycin appears safe in children, but data on its efficacy against *C. trachomatis* in this age group are meagre. Although it should theoretically be safe in pregnancy, supporting data are lacking.

Several studies that have attempted to evaluate the potential cost effectiveness of azithromycin compared with other regimens suggest that in selected populations, its use is cost effective when all relevant costs are considered.[62,63] These studies, however, assume 100% compliance with the drug, which might be correct in settings where it is directly administered, but may not apply where individuals are given prescriptions and asked to fill them.

Another newer regimen for uncomplicated *C. trachomatis* disease is ofloxacin 300mg orally twice daily for 7 days.[129] Ofloxacin has the advantage of high activity against *N. gonorrhoeae*, but is expensive. It should not be used in pregnancy or in those under 17 years of age.

Alternative regimens include a sulfonamide such as sulfafurazole (sulfisoxazole) in a dose of 500mg orally 4 times daily, or sulfamethoxazole in a dose of 1g orally twice daily for 10 days.[143] Cotrimoxazole (trimethoprim/sulfamethoxazole) 960mg (2 tablets) twice daily for 7 days can also be used but has no advantage over sulfonamides alone. Clindamycin, typically given as part of regimens for pelvic inflammatory disease[144,145] or during pregnancy,[146,147] is effective in women but may not be in men.[80] In pregnancy, clindamycin may also have an advantage in decreasing the risk of premature rupture of membranes and premature labour due to *C. trachomatis* and other pathogens.[49]

Multiple-dose penicillin regimens have some activity against *C. trachomatis* but are not reliable and therefore are not indicated for routine use, although they do have a role in pregnancy.[148,149] While not a standard regimen, rifampicin 600mg orally once daily for 7 days is also active.[80]

### 3.2.3 Treatment of Uncomplicated Genital Chlamydial Infection in Adolescents and Adults

The currently recommended regimens for uncomplicated genital *C. trachomatis* infection in adolescents and adults are either doxycycline 100mg orally twice daily for 7 days, or azithromycin 1g orally as a single dose.[75]

The alternatives are ofloxacin 300mg orally twice daily for 7 days, erythromycin base 500mg orally 4 times daily for 7 days, or erythromycin ethyl succinate 800mg orally 4 times daily for 7 days. A further (albeit inferior) alternative is sulfafurazole 500mg orally 4 times daily for 10 days.

#### 3.2.4 Treatment of Genital Chlamydial Infection in Pregnancy

In pregnancy, options are much more restricted, and treatment of *C. trachomatis* infection remains problematic, as does the question of the effect of such treatment on pregnancy outcome.[45] At present, erythromycin base 500mg orally 4 times daily for 7 days is still the preferred regimen, with other erythromycin formulations as alternatives.[75] Erythromycin is recommended primarily because of inadequate experience with azithromycin in this group. Frequently, however, erythromycin cannot be tolerated, and a high proportion of treated individuals are unable to complete the prescribed course.[80,146-150] In such cases, amoxicillin 500mg orally 3 times daily for 7 to 10 days is recommended.

Erythromycin estolate is contraindicated during pregnancy because of possible drug-related hepatotoxicity.

#### 3.2.5 Treatment of Infection With *Chlamydia trachomatis* in Infants and Children

For children under 45kg, the recommended therapy is erythromycin 50 mg/kg/day in 4 divided doses for 10 to 14 days;[75] for those over 45kg but under 8 years of age, adult doses of erythromycin are recommended.

For children over 45kg and 8 years of age or older, adult regimens of doxycycline are recommended. It is likely that azithromycin would also be an acceptable alternative, but supporting data are lacking.

In infancy, the recommended regimen is erythromycin 50 mg/kg/day in 4 divided doses for 10 to 14 days.[75] Previous recommendations also included a sulfonamide such as sulfafurazole 150 mg/kg/day in divided doses for at least 14 days.[114] As with *N. gonorrhoeae* infections, treatment of the mother and her sex partner(s) is very important.

#### 3.2.6 Treatment of Reiter's Syndrome Associated with *Chlamydia trachomatis* Infection

There is increasing evidence that a portion of cases of Reiter's syndrome or sexually-acquired arthritis are due directly or indirectly to infection with *C. trachomatis*.[42,43] Long term treatment with a tetracycline appears to improve outcome.[44,151]

#### 3.2.7 Follow-up and Management of Sexual Partners

For those who take the recommended treatments and improve, routine test-of-cure evaluations are not recommended[75] and are not cost effective.[93] Those who do not respond or whose symptoms recur should be re-evaluated.

A high proportion of infected sexual partners will be asymptomatic.[92] Ideally, all sexual partners should be evaluated and treated with a regimen active against *C. trachomatis* as soon as possible; in some circumstances it is more realistic to try to have them treated even without testing. As guidelines for which sexual partners to treat, the CDC recommends that where the index case is symptomatic, all sexual partners within the last 30 days should be sought.[75] Where the index case is asymptomatic, it should be those within the last 60 days, and where there has not been any contact in the last 60 days, it should be the last sexual partner.

### 3.3 Syphilis

Although studies that meet current criteria for scientifically acceptable study design have not been performed, based on extensive experience, penicillin remains the drug of choice for treatment of syphilis.[73,75,152,153] A serum penicillin concentration of only 0.03 U/ml is treponemicidal, but it must be continuous, and must extend over a period of 8 to 14 days in infectious syphilis and 21 days in all late and latent cases. In contrast to the gonococcus, no increased resistance of the treponeme has been shown, but there is increasing evidence that standard doses may be less effective in the treatment of some patients with concurrent infection with HIV.[18,75]

An unusual feature of the treatment of syphilis is the Jarisch-Herxheimer reaction which can occur within the first 24 hours of any therapy for syphilis. It is an acute febrile reaction often associated with headache, myalgias and flare-up of rashes. Although not a contraindication to treatment in pregnancy, it can precipitate labour or cause fetal distress. Its development is unpredictable, but can be ameliorated with antipyretics.

#### 3.3.1 Treatment of Early Syphilis

Early syphilis (e.g. primary, secondary or latent syphilis of less than 1 year's duration) can be treated with a single intramuscular injection of benzathine benzylpenicillin (benzathine penicillin G) 2.4MU.[75] Doxycycline 100mg orally twice daily or tetracycline hydrochloride 500mg orally 4 times daily for 14 days are alternatives in penicillin-allergic individuals, but the tetracyclines (and erythromycin) are much less efficient antitreponemal drugs and should only be used where penicillin is contraindicated, and where compliance is assured. If compliance with therapy or follow-up cannot be assured, desensitisation and treatment with penicillin is recommended.[75]

Ceftriaxone in multiple-dose, but not single-dose regimens, has been successful, but the optimal dose and duration have not been established.[113]

#### 3.3.2 Treatment of Syphilis of More than 1 Year's Duration (Excluding Neurosyphilis)

With the exception of neurosyphilis, patients with syphilis of over 1 year's duration (e.g. latent syphilis of unknown or more than 1 year's duration, cardiovascular syphilis, or late benign syphilis) should receive 3 doses of intramuscular benzathine benzylpenicillin 2.4MU at weekly intervals.[75] As with early syphilis, the alternatives are doxycycline 100mg orally twice daily or tetracycline hydrochloride 500mg orally 4 times daily, but for a duration of 4 weeks. However, there are few published data on these alternative choices.

#### 3.3.3 Treatment of Neurosyphilis

Diagnosis and treatment of symptomatic or asymptomatic neurosyphilis is more controversial. The diagnostic yield from cerebrospinal fluid examination is low even in syphilis of more than 1 year's duration. Accepted criteria for cerebrospinal fluid examination include neurological or ophthalmic signs or symptoms, other evidence of active syphilis (e.g. aortitis, gumma), previous treatment failure, infection with HIV, serum nontreponemal titre ≥1 : 32 unless the duration of syphilis is known to be under 1 year, and situations where penicillin will not be used (unless the duration of syphilis is under 1 year).[75]

In terms of treatment, even in those without HIV, failures have occurred on both benzathine and procaine penicillin regimens. The CDC recommends benzylpenicillin (aqueous crystalline penicillin G) 2 to 4MU intravenously every 4 hours for 10 to 14 days.[75] An alternative approach, when compliance can be assured, is to give procaine penicillin G 2.4MU intramuscularly once daily, in conjunction with probenecid 500mg orally 4 times daily, both for 10 to 14 days. Some authorities would follow either of these regimens with at least one dose of benzathine benzylpenicillin 2.4MU intramuscularly.

These penicillin regimens are still recommended even for those with penicillin allergy, after appropriate testing and desensitisation if needed.

#### 3.3.4 Treatment of Syphilis in Pregnancy

During pregnancy, penicillin is the drug of choice. The recommended penicillin regimens are the same as for nonpregnant individuals, except that some authorities would add an additional dose of benzathine benzylpenicillin 2.4MU for treatment of primary or secondary syphilis.[75]

If the woman has a penicillin allergy, desensitisation and treatment with penicillin is preferred over use of other regimens such as erythromycin. The tetracyclines are contraindicated in pregnancy because of the risk of hepatotoxicity and their adverse effects on the fetal skeleton and tooth development. If penicillin use is not an option, and compliance and follow-up can be assured, erythromycin base 500mg orally 4 times daily for 14 days can be considered, but there are minimal data on its efficacy. Since erythromycin cannot be relied upon to cure syphilis in the fetus, the infant should be treated with penicillin at birth.[75]

#### 3.3.5 Treatment of Congenital Syphilis

The selection of infants to evaluate for congenital syphilis, the evaluation itself, and the criteria on which to make the diagnosis of congenital syphilis can be quite difficult. Infants should not leave hospital without the serological status of the mother being known, and the indications for treatment should be liberal if test results cannot exclude syphilis in the infant. Infants born to mothers who were treated for syphilis in pregnancy with erythromycin should be treated.[75]

For infants, the recommended treatment regimens are 10 to 14 days of either benzylpenicillin (aqueous crystalline penicillin G) 100,000 to 150,000 U/kg/day intravenously (as 50,000 U/kg every 12 hours for the first 7 days of life and every 8 hours subsequently), or procaine penicillin G 50,000 U/kg intramuscularly once daily.[75]

For older infants and children, the recommended dose is benzylpenicillin (aqueous crystalline penicillin G) 200,000 to 300,000 U/kg/day intravenously or intramuscularly (as

50,000 U/kg every 4 to 6 hours) for 10 to 14 days.

#### 3.3.6 Treatment of Syphilis in Infants and Children Where Congenital Syphilis Has Been Excluded

Children with syphilis need to be thoroughly evaluated clinically and need to be assessed to distinguish between congenital syphilis and acquired syphilis. For treatment, the recommended regimen is benzathine benzylpenicillin 50,000 U/kg intramuscularly, up to a maximum of 2.4MU, given in a single dose for early latent syphilis, and as 3 doses at weekly intervals for late latent syphilis or latent syphilis of unknown duration.

#### 3.3.7 Treatment of Syphilis in Patients with HIV Infection

In general, the formal recommendations for treatment in the presence of HIV infection are identical to those stated above, but follow-up is more frequent and longer, and some recommend inclusion of initial and follow-up cerebrospinal fluid examinations.[75] Where experts differ, some would treat primary and secondary syphilis with additional doses of benzathine benzylpenicillin 2.4MU. As in pregnancy and neurosyphilis, only penicillin therapy is recommended.

#### 3.3.8 Follow-up

Treatment failures can occur with any regimen, and those treated can acquire new infection. Hence all individuals treated must be followed carefully clinically and serologically. In those without HIV infection, serological studies should be performed at least at 3, 6 and 12 months after treatment for early syphilis, and in addition at 24 months for syphilis of over 1 year's duration or for neurosyphilis.

Nontreponemal test titres should decrease over time, and in most cases of the first episode of primary, secondary or early latent syphilis should revert to negative or low stable levels. In these individuals there should be at least a 4-fold fall in 3 months. Seroreversal of the nontreponemal tests takes 6 to 12 months if the patient is treated in the infectious stage. Those who fail should be evaluated for infection with HIV. Failures without evidence of neurosyphilis should be treated with three weekly intramuscular injections of benzathine benzylpenicillin 2.4MU.

In late syphilis, nontreponemal tests may remain positive despite successful treatment, although if initially high, they should fall. The indications for repetition of cerebrospinal fluid serology are controversial, but if initially abnormal they should be repeated at 6-month intervals to demonstrate at least an improvement.

If surveillance is not intended to be performed, initial treatment should be with an augmented dose of penicillin. In those with HIV infection, surveillance should be carried on longer than in those without.

#### 3.3.9 Treatment of Sexual Partner(s)

Sexual transmission of syphilis is unusual after the first year of infection, since it occurs through mucocutaneous lesions. However, all sexual partners should be evaluated clinically and by serology, and in some cases treated presumptively. If the sexual contact occurred within the preceding 90 days, presumptive treatment with a single intramuscular injection of benzathine benzylpenicillin 2.4MU should be given to those who have had sexual contact with someone with primary, secondary or latent infection of less than 1 year's duration, or with someone whose nontreponemal test titre is ≥1 : 32 and the syphilis is of unknown duration.[75] Because infection could be present without detectable antibodies, treatment is warranted even if the individual is seronegative.

Treatment should also be given if the sexual contact occurred over 90 days ago and serological results are not immediately available and follow-up may not be certain.

Long term sexual partners of those with syphilis of longer duration should be assessed and treated according to their own clinical and serological findings.

## 4. Optimum Treatment of Clinical Syndromes

### 4.1 Urethritis

#### 4.1.1 Types of Urethritis and their Causes

Sexually acquired urethritis in men is separated into gonococcal and non-gonococcal urethritis.[68,154,155] Non-gonococcal urethritis is diagnosed when urethritis (increased numbers of polymorphonuclear leucocytes in urethral material) is detected, but *N. gonorrhoeae* is absent. A special case of non-gonococcal urethritis is postgonococcal urethritis, which is diagnosed when urethritis develops after treatment for gonorrhoea which successfully eradicates *N. gonorrhoeae*.[155]

In men who present with acute non-gonococcal urethritis and have not received treatment for non-gonococcal urethritis within the last several months, the major causes of the condition are *C. trachomatis* (15 to 50% of cases) and *Ureaplasma urealyticum* (30 to 40%). In 30 to 50% of cases, no cause is detected. Over the period from the late 1970s to the present, the portion of cases attributable to *C. trachomatis* has been falling in many countries, with rates of detection now closer to 15 to 25%.[6,123]

#### 4.1.2 Symptoms and Signs

Non-gonococcal urethritis is probably the most common form of STD encountered in males in clinical practice in developed countries.[80,134] However, in many less developed countries, and even in inner city populations in some developed countries, gonococcal urethritis may still be more frequent than non-gonococcal urethritis. The clinical symptoms of non-gonococcal urethritis, which occur at varying times after sexual intercourse (usually from 1 to 5 weeks), differ quantitatively but not qualitatively from those of gonococcal disease. The dysuria tends to be less severe and the urethral discharge is less profuse and tends to be watery or mucoid rather than purulent. If the discharge is purulent, it is indistinguishable clinically from gonorrhoea.

Although it is often possible to suspect clinically whether an individual has non-gonococcal or gonococcal urethritis, physical examination alone is not a satisfactory means of differentiating the two conditions. There are no clinical clues to differentiate men with non-gonococcal or gonococcal urethritis who do or do not have *C. trachomatis* or *U. urealyticum*.

#### 4.1.3 Initial Treatment of Urethritis

In the past, the distinction between gonococcal and non-gonococcal urethritis was very important because of the tendency to use penicillins for gonorrhoea and tetracyclines for non-gonococcal urethritis. Now that tetracyclines (or erythromycin) are advocated as part of the treatment for gonorrhoea, the distinction between causes of urethritis has less influence on initial treatment, except that a single-dose antigonococcal regimen is not used for non-gonococcal urethritis.

Treatment for gonorrhoea (see section 3.1.2) should be given when gonococcal urethritis has been diagnosed or not excluded. For non-gonococcal urethritis, the tetracyclines are considered the drugs of choice, with erythromycin regimens as the alternatives. Although the optimum dose and duration of treatment have not been determined, initial management should be with a 7-day course of a tetracycline, usually doxycycline. There is no difference in ultimate outcome when men are given a longer initial course of treatment.[156]

Partners should be treated with a tetracycline or with erythromycin, as for *C. trachomatis* infections (see section 3.2.3). The CDC recommends that when the index case is symptomatic, partners from the last 30 days should be evaluated and treated. If the index case is asymptomatic, partners during the last 60 days should be evaluated and treated, or if there were no partners in that time, the most recent partner should be evaluated and treated.

Currently, the balance of published and unpublished experience with azithromycin 1g orally as a single dose for treatment of non-gonococcal urethritis suggests that it is equivalent to doxycycline for patients with and without *C. trachomatis*.[121,122] This is important since most men with chlamydial urethritis are managed on a syndromic basis and the results of tests for *C. trachomatis* are not known at the time of treatment.

#### 4.1.4 Management of Urethritis when Initial Treatment Fails

As discussed in section 3.2, *C. trachomatis* infection is relatively easily eradicated by tetracyclines or erythromycin, but if followed carefully, 30 to 40% of men with non-gonococcal urethritis will have persistence or recurrence of urethritis after such treatment.[156] In these men, the cause is usually not detected but *C. trachomatis* is rarely isolated unless medication is taken incorrectly or the individual is exposed to a new or inadequately treated partner.

Diagnosis of persistent or recurrent urethritis after initial treatment requires objective evidence of urethritis clinically or by laboratory evidence of urethral inflammation. The presence of symptoms alone does not establish a diagnosis of a recurrent or persistent urethritis and should not by itself lead to further treatment.

If no cause is found or only *U. urealyticum* is isolated in a compliant patient who has not been re-exposed, the usual next treatment is erythromycin 500mg orally 4 times daily for 2 weeks to the individual only and not to the partner.[68] In the 5 to 10% of men who still have urethritis after both these courses, even extensive investigations do not usually reveal the cause. The optimum management at this stage is not certain; although these men usually suffer considerable psychological distress, there is little evidence for long term sequelae in them or their partners, even if sexual intercourse is resumed and no further treatment is given. In most of these men, the urethritis resolves without further antimicrobial treatment, but the possibility of alternative diagnoses, including infection with organisms such as *T. vaginalis* must always be considered. *T. vaginalis* is identified infrequently in men with urethritis in North America, but is reported more frequently in Africa, South America, and Eastern Europe. Herpes simplex virus also causes urethritis, but not persistent urethritis.

In some cases, studies for prostatitis or urethroscopy need to be undertaken, although these are usually not helpful.[157] In exceptional circumstances, patients should be given a 4- to 6-week course of a tetracycline or erythromycin. However, it is not known if this truly improves the ultimate outcome.

## 4.2 Cervicitis

### 4.2.1 Causes and Clinical Presentation

Cervical infection is the female counterpart of urethritis in the male.[158-160] The three main causes of cervicitis are *N. gonorrhoeae, C. trachomatis* and primary infection with herpes simplex virus. Symptomatic primary herpes simplex virus infection is usually readily differentiated. The diagnosis of cervicitis is more difficult than that of urethritis because the criteria are less well established and accepted, and the presence of polymorphonuclear leucocytes in endocervical secretions is less useful diagnostically than in urethritis.[161] However, a relatively easily recognised sign is the presence of pus or mucopus in the cervical os, seen as a yellow or off-white exudate in the cervical os or on a white swab used to obtain an endocervical specimen.[148] Mucopus is associated with an increased number of polymorphonuclear leucocytes on Gram stain, but the presence of polymorphonuclear leucocytes in the absence of other findings is not very useful for the diagnosis of infection. Friability (induced mucosal bleeding from the cervical os when the first swab is obtained) and oedema and/or erythema in an area of ectopy on the exocervix are often present.

Unfortunately, just as with urethritis, many infections with *N. gonorrhoeae* and *C. trachomatis* are not associated with any symptoms, signs or evidence of an inflammatory response.

### 4.2.2 Consequences of Cervical Infection

Infection with *C. trachomatis* or *N. gonorrhoeae* in the cervix is much more important than infection in the male urethra. Whereas most men can be infected with urethral pathogens for a long time without any significant physical sequelae, at least 10% of women with *C. trachomatis* or *N. gonorrhoeae* in the cervix will develop ascending infection of the fallopian tubes.[37,38] In women with *C. trachomatis* infection in the cervix but without any evidence of pelvic inflammatory disease, spread of infection to the endometrium can be documented in 20 to 40%.[130,131]

Pelvic inflammatory disease can arise within days. This is associated with a 10 to 20% risk of involuntary infertility secondary to tubal inflammation, a 10-fold increased risk of tubal pregnancies, and perhaps a 15 to 20% risk of chronic pelvic pain.[37-39] Pelvic inflammatory disease associated with *C. trachomatis* tends to be less acute and harder to recognise than that associated with *N. gonorrhoeae*,[162] and delay in initiation of therapy correlates with an increased risk of long term sequelae.[35]

Women with *N. gonorrhoeae, C. trachomatis* or herpes simplex virus in the cervix also expose their infants to significant sequelae after vaginal delivery, and are a major reservoir of infection in the community. Cervicitis can also be associated with cervical atypia and may play a role in the development of cervical cancer.[56]

### 4.2.3 Initial Treatment of Cervicitis

The initial treatment of cervicitis not considered to be complicated by endometritis or pelvic inflammatory disease is determined by the clinical findings, laboratory evidence, clinical suspicion that gonococcal infection may be present, or a concern that individuals will not return for treatment if a decision is made to defer treatment until the results of laboratory tests are available.

Treatment should be with a single-dose antigonococcal regimen (see section 3.1.2) *plus* a regimen active against *C. trachomatis* (see section 3.2.3) if cervicitis is diagnosed and gonococcal infection is detected or there is a strong possibility of gonococcal infection (e.g. detection of cervicitis in a woman attending a clinic with high prevalence of gonococcal infection), or there is a suspicion of gonococcal cervical infection and a concern that the person will not return for follow-up.[75,163] If cervicitis is detected in a woman with a low likelihood of having gonococcal infection, or tests to detect *N. gonorrhoeae* are negative, then treatment as for chlamydial infection alone, i.e. with doxycycline, azithromycin[123,124] or ofloxacin,[129] is appropriate (see further section 3.2.3). Where the prevalence of both *N. gonorrhoeae* and *C. trachomatis* is low, a diagnostic test with high sensitivity and specificity could be used, and if the person is likely to be available for follow-up, treatment may be deferred until the results of tests are available.

#### 4.2.4 Expected Response to Treatment

If the treatment regimens are taken as prescribed and there is no sexual re-exposure to a new or untreated partner, failure to eradicate *N. gonorrhoeae* or *C. trachomatis* is unusual. The clinical response has been less well evaluated, but many women continue to have cervical inflammation even when proven *N. gonorrhoeae* or *C. trachomatis* infections have been eradicated. However, over time, findings of cervicitis usually improve.

As in non-gonococcal urethritis not due to *C. trachomatis*, cervicitis not due to *C. trachomatis* or *N. gonorrhoeae* will often improve on similar regimens.

#### 4.2.5 Treatment of Sexual Partner(s)

Partners of women with cervicitis should be evaluated for STDs and then treated as appropriate for uncomplicated gonococcal and/or chlamydial infection. Since it is often not clear how long the woman has been infected, sexual partners for at least the last 60 days should be evaluated and treated.

### 4.3 Pelvic Inflammatory Disease

#### 4.3.1 Causes

Microbiological studies tend not to be very helpful in the initial management of acute pelvic inflammatory disease, in part because of the numerous potential causes. The major causes of acute pelvic inflammatory disease are *N. gonorrhoeae*, *C. trachomatis*, vaginal organisms such as coliforms, group B streptococci, *Gardnerella vaginalis* and anaerobes, *Haemophilis influenzae*, and *Mycoplasma hominis*.[39,162,164-167] Documentation that one or more of these are the causative agents in pelvic inflammatory disease is difficult. The presence of organisms in the vagina or cervix does not necessarily indicate that they will be found in the upper genital tract. Ideally, specimens for diagnosis should be obtained from the fallopian tubes and the endometrium,[39,166-168] but this is usually not feasible. Even if it is, for some of these bacteria, rapid diagnosis is not possible.

Because of this combination of circumstances, and the hope that early initiation of therapy might decrease the risk of long term sequelae,[35] treatment should be started as soon as the diagnosis of pelvic inflammatory disease is considered, and should be with antimicrobials providing a broad spectrum of activity against all potential causes.

#### 4.3.2 Diagnostic/Treatment Criteria

Infection that ascends to the uterus, fallopian tubes or adnexa should be treated more aggressively than uncomplicated genital infection because the patient may be more toxic, and because of concerns about the long term sequelae. However, a considerable proportion of tubal infections are never suspected by the patient or the clinician.[34,39,167] Because treatment at the time pelvic inflammatory disease is recognised may do little to reverse damage that has already occurred, in general it is safer to be liberal with the diagnosis in an attempt to decrease the proportion of cases that are missed. It is important for the woman and her partner(s) to be aware that when using very liberal criteria for diagnosis, initiation of treatment does not prove that the woman has pelvic inflammatory disease.

Treatment should be initiated for pelvic inflammatory disease if the woman is sexually active and has the minimal symptoms of recent onset of low abdominal pain or abnormal vaginal bleeding in conjunction with tenderness of the uterus or adnexa.[163] The minimal criteria advocated by the CDC are slightly different and include all of lower abdominal tenderness, adnexal tenderness and cervical motion tenderness.[75] Atypical presentations of pelvic inflammatory disease are frequent.[39]

A series of additional criteria increase the specificity of the diagnosis. They include fever (oral temperature over 38.3°C), abnormal cervical or vaginal discharge, an adnexal mass or abscess, an elevated erythrocyte sedimentation rate or C-reactive protein, and laboratory evidence of cervical infection with *C. trachomatis* or *N. gonorrhoeae*.[39,75,167] However, none of these are required to make a clinical diagnosis.

Definitive criteria, which are often not attainable and are not required for initiation of therapy, include histopathological evidence of endometritis on endometrial biopsy,[166] tubo-ovarian abscess documented by ultrasound or another imaging technique, or laparoscopic abnormalities consistent with pelvic inflammatory disease.[38,162]

It should be emphasised that no microbiological evidence is required to establish the diagnosis.

#### 4.3.3 Indications for Hospitalisation

Although in many circumstances, hospitalisation for the initiation of treatment will not be feasible, it is desirable.[24] It is mandatory when:

1) The diagnosis is uncertain and surgical emergencies such as ectopic pregnancy or appendicitis cannot be excluded.

2) A pelvic abscess is suspected.

3) When the patient is an adolescent or is pregnant.

4) The woman has infection with HIV.

5) Severe illness or nausea and vomiting preclude outpatient management.

6) The woman is thought to be unable to follow or is unable to tolerate an outpatient regimen.

7) The woman does not improve or cannot be followed within 48 to 72 hours of initiating outpatient treatment.[75,163]

Infection with HIV is included since it appears that pelvic inflammatory disease is more frequent and possibly more aggressive in those with HIV infection.[169]

In some places, early laparoscopy may be performed, but the logistics of arranging a laparoscopy should not be allowed to delay treatment. It is important for the clinician and the woman to recognise that a clinical diagnosis of pelvic inflammatory disease not confirmed by direct visualisation or documentation of a tubal or adnexal mass or endometritis must be considered only a tentative diagnosis, and other diagnostic possibilities must be remembered.[39,167]

#### 4.3.4 Inpatient Treatment of Pelvic Inflammatory Disease

Inpatient regimens recommended by the CDC in 1993[75] have not changed substantially over the last decade and there is increasing support for their effectiveness, at least in the short term.[145,170] The recommended regimens are:

1) Doxycycline 100mg intravenously or orally every 12 hours *plus* cefoxitin 2g intravenously every 6 hours or cefotetan 2g intravenously every 12 hours. [Other cefalosporins with equivalent antianaerobic activity could be used instead of cefoxitin or cefotetan].

2) Clindamycin 900mg intravenously every 8 hours *plus* standard gentamicin doses intravenously or intramuscularly (2 mg/kg loading dose followed by 1.5 mg/kg every 8 hours).

These regimens should be given for at least 48 hours after the woman shows substantial clinical improvement. The first regimen is then followed by oral doxycycline 100mg twice daily to complete 14 days of therapy, and the second regimen is followed by the same oral doxycycline course or clindamycin 450mg orally 4 times daily to complete a total of at least 14 days. Continuation with clindamycin is preferred if the woman has a tubo-ovarian abscess.

Numerous alternative regimens have been partially evaluated, and theoretically should provide broad-spectrum coverage. Examples include ampicillin/sulbactam *plus* doxycycline, or ofloxacin *plus* clindamycin or metronidazole.[75,145,170]

#### 4.3.5 Outpatient Treatment of Pelvic Inflammatory Disease

When the woman is not hospitalised, there is considerable debate about what constitutes an acceptable outpatient regimen. As a minimum, there must be coverage against *N. gonorrhoeae* and *C. trachomatis*, but in an era where many strains of *N. gonorrhoeae* are tetracycline-resistant, there are theoretical concerns that a single dose of therapy directed against *N. gonorrhoeae* may not cure upper genital tract infection.[163] Similar concerns arise with respect to eradication of Gram-negative aerobes, and anaerobes.

The CDC has proposed two regimens:[75]

1) A single dose of an antigonococcal agent (cefoxitin 2g intramuscularly plus probenecid 1g orally in a single dose, or ceftriaxone 250mg intramuscularly, or another parenteral single-dose third-generation cefalosporin) followed by doxycycline 100mg orally twice daily for 14 days. Others would consider use of ciprofloxacin, ofloxacin or cefixime for the single-dose component in this approach.[163]

2) Multiple-dose regimens active against *N. gonorrhoeae*, Gram-negative aerobes and anaerobes, i.e. ofloxacin 400mg orally twice daily for 14 days, *plus* either clindamycin 450mg orally 4 times daily or metronidazole 500mg orally twice daily for 14 days.

As with the inpatient regimens, there are other possible regimens, but for all there is little objective information available, particularly in the current era of increasing resistance to tetracyclines.[163]

There is no role in the treatment of sexually transmitted pelvic inflammatory disease for a penicillin or a cefalosporin as single drug therapy. Tetracycline hydrochloride may be substituted for doxycycline, but is less desirable as it is less active against certain anaerobes, is less well tolerated, and requires more frequent administration.

Women receiving oral therapy must be reassessed 48 to 72 hours after the initiation of treatment and hospitalised if the response is suboptimal. This situation would usually require more definitive attempts to specifically establish the diagnosis. An additional advantage of follow-up is to verify that the woman has filled her prescription and is taking the medication.[85]

#### *4.3.6 Expected Response to Therapy*

Because the ultimate means of assessing the efficacy of treatment is proof of normal tubal patency and function (i.e. uterine pregnancy), studies demonstrating the long term efficacy of the suggested treatment regimens are not available. There is considerable evidence of short term clinical improvement and eradication of key pathogens with numerous regimens.[145,170,171] However, a considerable proportion of women still develop irreversible tubal damage. This is increased in women with non-gonococcal pelvic inflammatory disease, and when there is a delay in initiation of treatment.[35,38] The situation is further complicated because short term clinical improvement does not mean that the key pathogens have been eradicated.[172]

#### *4.3.7 Treatment of Sexual Partner(s) and Follow-up*

As with all proven or potential *N. gonorrhoeae* or *C. trachomatis* infections, partners should be evaluated and treated as for uncomplicated gonococcal and chlamydial infection. Women with pelvic inflammatory disease should be carefully followed clinically and microbiologically at 7 to 10 days and again at 4 to 6 weeks after treatment.

### 4.4 Acute Epididymitis

Complications of gonococcal or chlamydial infections in men are quite infrequent even without treatment, but in less than 1% of men, acute epididymitis will develop. In older men, or men with structural abnormalities, the usual causes of epididymitis are classical urinary tract pathogens.[173,174] However, in younger men the main causes are *N. gonorrhoeae* and *C. trachomatis*. When epididymitis is suspected, as well as evaluating for classical urinary tract pathogens, men should be carefully evaluated for urethritis clinically and by smear, and have diagnostic tests for *N. gonorrhoeae* and *C. trachomatis*. Particularly in younger men, torsion of the testicle should be considered.

Sexually acquired acute epididymitis should be treated with a single-dose antigonococcal regimen (see section 3.1.2) followed by 10 days of doxycycline 100mg orally twice daily. However, the CDC still recommends the higher dose of ceftriaxone (250mg intramuscularly) in this setting.[75] An alternative regimen recommended by the CDC is ofloxacin 300mg orally twice daily for 10 days. This latter regimen would be expected to be more effective than the first regimen if the epididymitis was due to coliform bacteria. Adjunctive measures of therapy include bed rest and scrotal elevation. Partners should be evaluated and managed as for contacts of individuals with *N. gonorrhoeae*, with treatment directed against both *N. gonorrhoeae* and *C. trachomatis*.

### 4.5 Sexual Assault

For the antimicrobial component of management of sexual assault victims, the CDC recommends prophylaxis with a combination of ceftriaxone 250mg intramuscularly as a single dose, metronidazole 2g orally as a single dose, and doxycycline 100mg orally twice daily for 7 days.[75,175] However, some reject the use of an injectable agent in this setting and substitute an oral agent for the component active against *N. gonorrhoeae*.[163]

## 5. Optimum Treatment of Other Sexually Transmissible Diseases

### 5.1 Vulvovaginitis

Vulvovaginitis is an exceedingly frequent condition. Although in some circumstances it may be very difficult to distinguish between a normal discharge and one that is abnormal, diagnosis and initial management is usually quite straightforward.[48,159,176,177]

#### Symptoms and Evaluation

Symptoms suggestive of vaginitis include an increased vaginal discharge, genital itch, external dysuria, an unpleasant or fishy vaginal odour, and introital dyspareunia.[48,159,177] Though not diagnostic alone, the presence of specific genital pathogens is often suggested by the symptoms. Accepted causes of vaginitis include *Trichomonas vaginalis* and genital yeasts. A less accepted entity is bacterial vaginosis in which *Gardnerella vaginalis* (formerly called *Corynebacterium vaginale* or *Haemophilus vaginalis*) is present in conjunction with a marked increase in the number of vaginal anaerobes.[176]

A specific diagnosis of the cause of vaginitis is usually made by a combination of symptoms, physical findings, the vaginal pH, vaginal Gram stains, and direct methods like saline preparations to detect motile trichomonads and 'clue cells' and potassium hydroxide preparations to detect yeasts. Cultures are useful for detection of *T. vaginalis* but are too sensitive for the detection of yeasts and *G. vaginalis*. Thus, positive cultures for these latter two organisms in the absence of other features of the disease are not indications for treatment.[163]

Treatment should not be given blindly when the clinical and laboratory features do not indicate a specific infection. Many women with 'excessive' discharge undoubtedly have physiological reasons for the discharge and do not benefit from treatment. The presence of a low vaginal pH (less than 4.5) and predominantly epithelial cells and lactobacilli on a Gram stain of vaginal material are strong indicators of normality in such women. Since cervical discharge can also contribute to what is considered by patients to be vaginal discharge, the possibility of cervicitis (see section 4.2) must also be considered.

##### *5.1.1 Trichomoniasis*

Trichomoniasis is due to infection with the flagellate protozoan *Trichomonas vaginalis*.[23] Although there are probably other means of transmission, trichomoniasis should be considered to be sexually transmitted. Its detection in the asymptomatic male sex partner, in whom it is thought to persist only transiently, is difficult.

Trichomoniasis frequently coexists with gonorrhoea and other sexually transmissible pathogens. Typical symptoms include vaginal or introital itch plus discharge. The classical clinical features (a bright red vaginal mucosa and a yellow or green, frothy, malodorous discharge) are often evident, but some cases merely present as a mildly inflamed vagina of nonspecific appearance, or even without any abnormalities. Though most women with trichomoniasis do not develop significant sequelae, there is now increasing evidence that it can be associated with adverse pregnancy outcomes, particularly premature rupture of membranes and preterm delivery.[46,159]

###### Treatment Regimens

Symptomatic and asymptomatically infected individuals and their sexual partners should be treated.[23,48] The standard treatment, especially in clinical settings, is metronidazole 2g orally as a single dose.[75] This achieves a comparable cure rate to longer courses of metronidazole and the taking of tablets is assured, at least if the dose is given under supervision. Moreover, the convenience of the single-dose regimen is more likely to be accepted by the male sex partner who is often asymptomatic and may see no need to take treatment, let alone a multiple-dose course. Alternative single-dose oral regimens that have comparable efficacy are tinidazole 2g or ornidazole 1.5g. Where patient compliance is likely, some prefer multidose regimens such as metronidazole 500mg orally twice daily for 7 days, or 3 doses of 1g of nimorazole or tinidazole 12 hours apart.

Follow-up is unnecessary for those who become and remain asymptomatic after treatment. However, an increasing proportion of strains are becoming relatively resistant to these regimens. In cases of true treatment failure, many will still respond to metronidazole 500mg orally twice daily for 7 days or metronidazole 2g once daily for 3 to 5 days.[23] Very occasionally, the maximum tolerated dose of metronidazole orally (750mg orally 3 times daily) *plus* either metronidazole or ornidazole 500mg intravaginally daily for 10 days is required to retreat patients who repeatedly fail on lower doses. There have been some failures on even this regimen.

Most authorities consider the nitroimidazole drugs to be contraindicated in the first trimester of pregnancy, but are now less concerned about using them later in pregnancy (see also chapter 2; sect. 1.3.6). After the first trimester, the recommended treatment is metronidazole 2g in a single dose.[75] Although clotrimazole 100mg intravaginally at bedtime for 7 days was previously recommended, the data supporting this regimen are meagre. Lactating women can be treated with a single 2g dose of metronidazole if breast feeding is stopped for at least 24 hours after treatment.

Patients taking nitroimidazole drugs such as metronidazole, tinidazole, ornidazole and nimorazole should not drink any alcoholic beverages because of a possible disulfiram-like intolerance reaction. Fear of possible carcinogenicity following the use of metronidazole in trichomoniasis has not been substantiated.[178]

#### *5.1.2 Vulvovaginal Candidiasis*

*Candida albicans* and other yeasts are often present in the female genital tract without causing infection.[159] They can be found in the vagina in about a fifth of sexually active women, being most common in the younger age groups. Clinical infection usually occurs when a suitable environment is produced hormonally (e.g. in pregnancy, with oral contraceptive use, or premenstrually), in diabetic patients, or following alteration of the normal bacterial flora by antibiotic treatment. Women with HIV infection, even without significant decreases in the number of CD4 cells, also commonly have vulvovaginal candidiasis.[179] Approximately 20% of sexually active women harbour *C. albicans* in the anorectum and there is a strong association between rectal and vaginal candidiasis. Though considered in the differential diagnosis of sexually-acquired vulvovaginitis, yeasts are not generally sexually transmitted and the woman does not need to be sexually active to develop clinical infection.

Typical symptoms include itch and often oedema and erythema of the introital region. Discharge is often not a symptom, although on examination, a white or cheesy discharge is usually noted. Many women are asymptomatic despite clinically evident disease. In women with clinically significant candidal vaginitis or vulvovaginitis, yeasts or pseudohyphae can be seen on Gram stain, saline preparations or potassium hydroxide preparations. If not detected or if detected and the woman is asymptomatic, treatment should, in general, not be offered.

##### Treatment Regimens

Treatment of this common and recurring infection is far from satisfactory, as shown by the large number of drugs available for treatment and the differing lengths of treatment courses recommended.[177] Previously, the standard treatment was with nystatin, but the imidazole derivatives such as miconazole, clotrimazole, econazole, tioconazole, isoconazole, butoconazole and terconazole in the doses recommended by the CDC (see below) are significantly more effective and usually result in relief of symptoms and negative cultures in 80 to 90% of women. Various different regimens of the same medication have been used, ranging in duration from single-dose therapy to 7 to 14 days. Single-dose regimens should usually be reserved for minimally to moderately symptomatic women with a first or infrequent episode of yeast vulvovaginitis. Longer courses are indicated in those with more severe symptoms or a history of frequent recurrences.

Regimens suggested by the CDC[75] are:

- *Butoconazole* 2% cream 5g intravaginally for 3 days.
- *Clotrimazole* 1% cream 5g intravaginally for 7 to 14 days, or one 100mg vaginal tablet daily for 7 days, or two 100mg vaginal tablets daily for 3 days, or one 500mg vaginal tablet as a single dose.
- *Miconazole* 2% cream 5g intravaginally for 7 days, or one 200mg vaginal tablet daily for 3 days, or one 100mg vaginal tablet daily for 7 days.
- *Tioconazole* 6.5% ointment 5g intravaginally in a single application.
- *Terconazole* 0.4% cream 5g intravaginally for 7 days, or 0.8% cream 5g intravaginally for 3 days, or one 80mg vaginal tablet daily for 3 days.

Some of these creams and vaginal tablets are oil-based and hence may weaken latex condoms and diaphragms. Some are available as over-the-counter preparations which has the potential advantage of decreased cost, but the potential disadvantage of inappropriate use by women whose symptoms are not due to candidiasis. As a reasonable compromise, such regimens are probably best used by women who have previously had a documented episode, and then experience an episode with the same symptoms.

***Oral regimens*** of ketoconazole, fluconazole and itraconazole are also effective for vulvovaginal candidiasis and numerous regimens have been used.[75,177] There is a lack of consensus as to which is the most appropriate; regimens typically range from single-dose to 5-day courses. The symptomatic response to these agents tends to be slightly slower than with intravaginal treatments. The principal concerns associated with their use are adverse reactions, particularly hepatotoxicity with ketoconazole, and also clinically significant interactions with numerous other drugs (see appendix B).

***Recurrent candidal infections*** are common and in most cases are true treatment failures.

Sometimes they are the result of too short a course of treatment, associated with the predisposing factors listed above, or are due to reinfection from a male sex partner. For the treatment of recurrences, it is imperative that the woman be instructed to take the full course of treatment if this was not the case initially. Treatment may be with an alternative regimen, but often doubling the duration of use of the initial medication will be effective. Treatment of women with very frequent recurrences is suboptimal and no regimen has been shown to be ideal.[177]

Although the yeast is found on the penis of up to 20% of even circumcised males, only in uncircumcised males is candidal balanitis common. Routine treatment of male partners does not improve the outcome in women;[75] treatment of males with a topical antifungal cream is reserved for those with symptoms or signs suggestive of balanitis.

#### *5.1.3 Bacterial Vaginosis*

Bacterial vaginosis has a relatively characteristic clinical and laboratory pattern, and symptomatic patients benefit from treatment.[48,176,177,180] Although initially *Gardnerella vaginalis* was thought to be the cause, it is clear that numerous bacteria must interact to produce this syndrome, and cultures for *G. vaginalis* are not useful for its detection or management. Classical symptoms include an offensive fishy odour, particularly after unprotected intercourse, and an often profuse, thin discharge. Vaginal inflammation is usually absent, but typically there is a thin, homogeneous discharge that uniformly coats the vaginal wall and introitus. The vaginal pH is greater than 4.5, a fishy odour is released with 10% potassium hydroxide, vaginal epithelial cells are coated with large numbers of small Gram variable coccobacillary bacteria ('clue cells'), and vaginal lactobacilli are absent or greatly reduced in number.

There is increasing evidence that bacterial vaginosis is associated with premature rupture of membranes and premature labour, and ascending uterine or pelvic infection after surgical or obstetric procedures.[47,48,159] Nevertheless, the accepted indication for treatment is relief of symptoms, even in pregnancy.[75] Hence women with clinical and laboratory signs of bacterial vaginosis, but without symptoms should not usually be treated. Subsequent studies may expand these indications.

##### Treatment Regimens

The recommended treatment for bacterial vaginosis has traditionally been metronidazole 500mg orally twice daily for 7 days.[114] Many still consider this to be the treatment of choice, but the 1993 CDC guidelines propose as an alternative, metronidazole 2g as a single oral dose.[75] Other alternatives which have been effective in clinical trials include clindamycin 2% cream 5g intravaginally for 7 days, metronidazole 0.75% gel 5g intravaginally twice daily for 5 days, or clindamycin 300mg orally twice daily for 7 days.[75] The clindamycin cream regimen is preferred in the first trimester of pregnancy.

These regimens are usually associated with significant improvement, but the recurrence rate may be up to 15%, which is not altered by treating sex partners.[48] The optimum management of women with repeated treatment failures is not certain, but they should not receive numerous courses of metronidazole. One of the other regimens will often be successful.

### 5.2. Viral Infections

#### *5.2.1 Genital Herpes*

##### Clinical Presentation and Course

Infection due to genital herpes simplex virus has become increasingly common, unlike the decrease in prevalence noted for sexually transmitted infections for which curative treatments are available.[26,27] Lesions are typically single or grouped, painful, and associated with tender inguinal lymphadenopathy.[50,51] Although typical lesions go through a pattern of vesicles followed by ulceration and then scabbing, in women often only ulcers are noted. Genital herpes has a marked tendency to recur, recurrences being more likely and more frequent with herpes simplex virus type 2 infection in the genital tract, and less frequent with herpes virus type 1.[27,50,181] New lesions tend to form for up to 2 weeks in the initial episode, but for only days in recurrent episodes. These recurrences may be infrequent or frequent and can produce marked physical and psychological distress.[52] The major risk of spread is from clinically apparent lesions, but the virus can be isolated intermittently from some individuals without lesions.

Diagnosis of symptomatic disease is by exclusion of *T. pallidum* and *Haemophilus ducreyi*, and, where available, the demonstration of herpes simplex virus from the lesion by culture or a direct nonculture test. Serology is usually not helpful, especially in recurrent disease.[27,181] In those with a first episode, serology may be more helpful.

There is no effective cure for genital herpes. None of the available treatments eradicates the virus; at best, they merely shorten the duration of each episode. The psychological distress associated with the onset of attacks and variation in the course of lesions makes assessment of treatment difficult. Hence rigidly controlled studies are required to evaluate regimens.[182] It is critical that treatments of unproven benefit be avoided, despite the zeal to help these often desperate individuals.

#### Treatment of Initial Episodes

Numerous antiviral regimens have been evaluated, and many have shown promise in decreasing the severity and duration of symptoms.[183] The antiviral agent most often used for genital herpes is *aciclovir* which should be given either orally or intravenously as early as possible after the start of an infection;[55,75,184] topical aciclovir is of little benefit. For the first clinical episode of genital herpes, the recommended regimen is oral aciclovir 200mg 5 times daily for 7 to 10 days or until clinical resolution is attained. For a first episode of herpes proctitis, a dose of 400mg orally 5 times daily for 10 days or until clinical resolution is recommended. For very severe disease with associated aseptic meningitis, urinary retention, or severe local discomfort and extensive lesions, intravenous aciclovir 5 to 10 mg/kg 8-hourly is given for 5 to 7 days or until clinical resolution.

If initiated early enough, all of these regimens decrease the duration of lesions and the magnitude of symptoms; however, none alters the risk of recurrent disease.

#### Treatment of Recurrent Episodes

There are two general approaches to treatment of those who have frequent recurrences of genital herpes. Episodes treated within 2 days of the onset of lesions with 5 days of oral aciclovir 200mg 5 times daily, 400mg 3 times daily, or 800mg twice daily have about a 1-day shorter clinical course.[55,75,172,183] Because of this marginal benefit, such an approach is not usually recommended in immunocompetent individuals. The alternative approach is long term suppression with oral aciclovir 400mg twice daily or 200mg 3 to 5 times daily,[55,75] which will usually decrease the frequency of lesions by at least 75%, but is expensive, and does not alter the propensity for the condition to recur once aciclovir has been stopped.[185] Safety and efficacy have been documented in those who have received such regimens for durations as long as 5 years.[55] To determine that the individual's pattern of recurrences has not changed, long term suppressive therapy should be stopped at approximately yearly intervals to determine the frequency of recurrences.

Although it would seem likely, there is no definitive evidence that suppressive therapy decreases the risk of transmission to partners.

#### Ancillary Measures

Although aciclovir treatment has some benefit, in many circumstances management should be conservative, and even those on aciclovir can be helped symptomatically by additional measures. The lesions should be kept dry, and opioid analgesics should be avoided. Severe dysuria can be helped by urinating in the shower or a bath.

All individuals, no matter how they are managed, should be informed about the natural history of herpes simplex virus and its implications. Its tendency to recur and the fact that it is most readily spread when lesions are present must be clearly stated. Condoms provide incomplete protection against spread of genital (and oral) herpes, but their use is recommended by many to decrease the spread of herpes. Women should also be told about the implications for pregnancy and the need for an increased frequency of Papanicolaou (Pap) smears because of the statistical association with an increased risk of cervical cancer.[56]

#### Management of Sexual Partner(s)

Though herpes is sexually transmitted, there is no benefit in treating sexual partners unless they have their own indications for treatment. Nevertheless, partners should usually be evaluated and counselled. If they become more widely available, one of the serologic tests that detects type-specific antibodies should be useful in informing partners of their risk of acquiring infection from symptomatic or asymptomatic infected partners.[27]

#### Treatment of Genital Herpes in Pregnancy

This has been a very confusing and controversial area, but several advances have been made. The first is that although aciclovir use is not recommended in pregnancy, an ongoing registry has so far not shown an increase in birth defects.[55,75] On balance therefore, it appears reasonable to use aciclovir during pregnancy for life-threatening maternal herpes infection.

The management of maternal herpes to prevent perinatal transmission has also become more clear. Numerous studies have now shown that the greatest risk of transmission is with primary genital herpes occurring near or at term.[53] Among women with recurrent herpes who have lesions at the time of vaginal delivery, the risk of transmission is under 3%.[27] Routine herpes cultures taken during pregnancy do not help in assessing risk at the time of delivery. Instead, all women at term should be carefully questioned and examined for evidence of possible genital herpes. Those with a history of genital herpes, or those whose partners have genital herpes should have an intrapartum culture obtained to aid subsequent management of the infant.

Infants delivered through an infected birth canal of a woman with recurrent herpes should be followed prospectively without aciclovir treatment, unless cultures obtained from the infant 24 to 48 hours after birth become positive, or the infant develops evidence of clinical disease.[54] If treated, aciclovir 30 mg/kg/day is recommended for 10 to 14 days.

#### Management of Genital Herpes in Individuals with HIV Infection

There is a statistical association between the prevalence of antibody to herpes simplex virus type 2 and antibody to HIV.[186] The two major issues that relate to treatment are the need for more aggressive treatment in immunocompromised individuals, and the increased prevalence of aciclovir-resistant strains of herpes simplex in those with HIV infection. Recommended oral doses of *aciclovir* are 400mg 3 to 5 times daily.[75] If the disease is particularly severe, intravenous aciclovir therapy is recommended.

If the disease does not respond to aciclovir, resistance to the drug should be suspected, and hospitalisation considered to administer *foscarnet* 40 mg/kg intravenously every 8 hours until there is clinical resolution.

### *5.2.2 Genital and Anorectal Warts (Condylomata Acuminata)*

#### Causes and Clinical Presentation

This troublesome and increasingly common condition caused by human papilloma viruses is usually sexually transmitted. There are numerous types of human papilloma viruses, with some having a greater predilection for external sites (e.g. types 6 and 11), and others for more subclinical cervical involvement (e.g. types 16, 18, 31, 33, and 35).[57,58] However, individual types can affect any site. The incubation period is long, about 1 to 3 months in some, but much longer in many. A high proportion, probably the majority, of those infected do not develop visible lesions.

Detection of genital warts requires a careful search. In women, they are typically pale and moist, with a cauliflower-like surface, and occur most commonly in the vestibule near the fourchette, but also around the hymen, on the inside of the labia, and in the vagina. They also occur, with a horny surface, on the dry perivulval and perianal skin. Though the cervix is often infected, clinically evident disease is unusual. In males, warts occur on the scrotum, perianal skin and penis, and in the meatus and urethra. In individuals who practise anal intercourse, they can also occur within the anal canal and even the lower rectum. Under certain conditions, especially during pregnancy, there can be rapid growth and extension of the lesions, which can form masses several centimetres across on the vulva, in the vagina, on the cervix or around the anus. The oral contraceptive pill seems to have a milder but similar effect on their progression.

There is rapidly mounting evidence that human papilloma viruses are a major factor in the development of many cases of cervical carcinoma and probably also vulvar, perianal and penile squamous cell carcinomas.[56] The frequency and severity of cervical dysplasia and neoplasia is increased in women with HIV infection, particularly with advancing immunosuppression.[187,188]

#### Outcomes of Therapy

Although there are associations between certain types of human papilloma virus and increased risk of cervical cancer, this information cannot be readily applied to an individual woman. There are no treatments that will eradicate the virus.[189,190] Recommended regimens will result in disappearance of most, but not all visible lesions, but usually at least 25% will recur within 3 months. At present, most authorities suggest that the goal of treatment is removal of visible genital warts for aesthetic reasons,[75] but this treatment is not likely to reduce the risk of cervical malignancy. For prevention of cervical dysplasia and cancer, reliance should be placed on regular Papanicolaou smears and colposcopic biopsy.

It is not known if removal of visible warts decreases the risk of transmission of human papilloma virus.

#### Treatment Measures

Treatment is by destruction of the lesions, but because of the association with malignancy, atypical or persistent warts should be biopsied, and Papanicolaou smears should be obtained from women prior to treatment. All treatments have disadvantages that include some combination of toxicity, expense or propensity for scarring.[75,189,190]

Until recently, the most frequently used treatment was *podophyllin.* Its use is contraindicated in pregnancy, but otherwise podophyllin is relatively inexpensive, relatively simple to use, and generally safe. However, if misused, it can result in significant inflammation to normal skin. There are numerous methods for application of podophyllin. The CDC recommends 10 to 25% podophyllin in compound tincture of benzoin applied only to the wart and not to the normal skin, and not in excess of 0.5ml or coverage of 10 $cm^2$, to be washed off in 1 to 4 hours.[75] If used in the vagina, <2 $cm^2$ should be treated and the area should be dry before removal of the speculum. In the urethral meatus, it should also be allowed to dry before there is contact with the normal mucosa and it should be washed off in 1 to 2 hours. Treatments are repeated once weekly, with the duration of exposure to podophyllin sometimes increased depending upon patient compliance and tolerance. If warts persist after 6 applications, other treatments are indicated. Podophyllin is most often used for external genital or perianal lesions, but can also be used with great care for vaginal, meatal and anal warts if the treated area is allowed to dry before there is contact with normal mucosa. It is not recommended for cervical or intraurethral warts.

For self-treatment of genital warts, *podophyllotoxin* (podofilox) 0.5% solution is simpler to use, safe, and can be self-applied, but should only be used for lesions visible to the person, and should not be used in pregnancy.[75] It is a pure compound with a stable shelf-life, and does not require washing off after application. Although heavily keratinised lesions may not respond quite as well, initial efficacy and recurrence rates are similar to those seen with podophyllin. It is applied to the wart with a cotton swab twice daily for 3 days, followed by no treatment for 4 days. This cycle can be repeated for up to 4 cycles. Treatments should not exceed 0.5ml per day or coverage of >10 $cm^2$.

*Cryotherapy* with liquid nitrogen or dry ice is recommended for external genital, perianal, vaginal, urethral meatus, anal and oral warts.[75] It is relatively inexpensive, does not require anaesthesia, and does not result in scarring if done correctly, but it requires special equipment and most treated individuals experience mild to moderate local pain during and after treatment.

*Trichloroacetic acid* 80 to 90% can also be used for external genital, perianal, vaginal and anal warts.[75] It is applied weekly for up to 6 weeks, with application of talc or baking soda to remove unreacted acid. If 6 weeks of application fails, alternative treatments should be used. However, less data are available on its effectiveness than with the above treatment.

*Electrodesiccation* or *electrocautery* may sometimes be used but are contraindicated in those with cardiac pacemakers or lesions proximal to the anal verge.[75] Experience with these methods is limited, they require local anaesthesia, and discomfort is moderate. They can be used for external genital, perianal or oral warts.

*Carbon dioxide laser* and *conventional surgery* are useful for management of extensive warts or when other methods have failed.[75] They should not be used for limited lesions, are expensive, and like other regimens do not eradicate human papilloma viruses.

*Interferon-α*, given systemically, has provided varying results and is not currently recommended as first-line therapy because of its expense, toxicity and limited efficacy.[75,190] Results are slightly better with intralesional injection but this approach is also not recommended. Similarly, therapy with topical fluorouracil is no longer recommended.

#### Follow-up and Management of Sexual Partner(s)

Once warts have responded to treatment, routine additional follow-up in excess of usual recommendations for individuals without warts is not necessary. Sexual partners with exophytic warts may wish to be treated, but otherwise special examination for detection of warts is not indicated. Though condoms can be recommended, it is unlikely that they will have significant, if any, benefit because of the high frequency of subclinical infection that may already have occurred, and persistence of the human papilloma virus despite treatment at sites that may not be protected by the condom.

#### Treatment of Genital Warts in Pregnancy and in Patients with HIV Infection

Lesions may progress in pregnancy. Podophyllin and podophyllotoxin use is contraindicated. Caesarean section to reduce the minimal risk of laryngeal papillomatosis in infants is not recommended.[75]

In patients with HIV infection, the regimens discussed above are used, but the response is often poorer.

## 5.3 Ectoparasitic Infestations

### *5.3.1 Pubic Lice*

Pediculosis pubis due to the pubic or crab louse *Phthirus pubis* is usually self-evident, but on occasions tends to be missed by both the clinician and patient, unless a thorough search is made in good light for nits and adult lice. These are semitransparent and very variable in size.[191] They lie tightly applied to the skin of the pubic area by their specially hooked claws, but can spread to the leg, abdominal and axillary hairy areas. Sometimes the nits or eggs attached to the hairs like tiny 'grains of wheat' are the only visible signs.

#### Treatment Regimens

Recommended treatment regimens are 1% lindane (gamma benzene hexachloride) shampoo applied for 4 minutes to the infested and adjacent hairy areas, and then thoroughly washed off; *or* permethrin 1% cream rinse applied to the affected area and washed off after 10 minutes; *or* pyrethrins with piperonyl butoxide shampoo applied to the infested and adjacent hairy areas and washed off after 10 minutes.[75,191] Lindane is not recommended for pregnant or lactating women or children <2 years of age. Lindane is the least expensive agent and toxicity is not reported with the 4-minute application.

Treatment should be repeated in 7 days if lice are found or eggs are observed at the hair-skin junction. Clothing or bed linen which has been contaminated within 3 days of initiation of treatment should be washed and/or dried by machine (hot cycle for each) or else drycleaned.

### *5.3.2 Scabies*

Scabies is an increasingly common condition caused by the mite *Sarcoptes scabiei* var. *hominis*.[191] It should be suspected in any person without a history of allergy or eczema who complains of a persistent severe generalised itching, especially at night. The rash is nonspecific, consisting mainly of scratch marks and a few small papules. Typical scaly plaques can occur on the periareolar area of the breast and on the glans penis, with papules on the shaft. Scabies is commonly acquired through the close bodily contact associated with sexual activity, and in this context is usually seen in adolescents and young adults. As the incubation period is about a month, and the mite can be transferred by normal social contact among a group of people living together, all members of the household or residence, whether symptomatic or not, should be treated, as well as the sexual partner(s).

#### Treatment Regimens

All treatments are applied to the entire body from the neck down. The recommended regimens are permethrin cream 5% applied and washed off after 8 to 14 hours, or lindane 1% as 30ml of lotion or 30g of cream and washed off after 8 hours.[75,191] An alternative treatment is crotamiton 10% cream or lotion applied nightly for 2 consecutive nights, and washed off 24 hours after the second application. Lindane should not be used after a bath, in those with extensive dermatitis, in pregnant or lactating women, or in children <2 years of age. Lindane is relatively inexpensive but there is some resistance to its effect and some toxicity. Permethrin is effective and safe, but is more expensive.

Disinfection of clothing and bedding should be carried out as for pubic lice. Itching does not stop for a week or more despite cure. Corticosteroid creams should be avoided, as they may mask the condition. Treatment may be applied again after a week if there is no clinical improvement. Thereafter, it should not be repeated unless live mites are identified.

## 5.4 Genital Ulcer/Lymphadenopathy Syndrome

In developed countries, genital ulcers are much less frequent than urethritis or vaginitis.[71,72] In contrast, particularly in Southeast Asia and Africa, genital lesions with or without lymphadenopathy are one of the most frequent manifestations of STD.[9] The major genital lesions without lymphadenopathy are warts, molluscum contagiosum, scabies and granuloma inguinale (see below, section 5.4.3). Traumatic lesions, if secondarily infected, might present with lymphadenopathy. Classical STD presentations with lymphadenopathy include syphilis, herpes simplex virus, chancroid and lymphogranuloma venereum.[71] In industrialised countries, the most frequent cause is herpes simplex virus, followed by syphilis, with an increasing prevalence of chancroid in selected areas. In developing countries, the most frequent cause is chancroid followed by syphilis. Chancroid, syphilis and herpes all facilitate the transmission of HIV,[15,192-194] and control of chancroid and syphilis are one means of slowing the spread of HIV.[9,10]

Although initiation of treatment should ideally be based on a specific diagnosis, in many circumstances where the prevalence of chancroid and syphilis is high, and diagnostic tests are not available or are suboptimal, management may need to be directed towards both. Furthermore, mixed infection is frequent.

#### *5.4.1 Chancroid (Haemophilus ducreyi Infection)*

Chancroid is caused by the Gram-negative bacillus *H. ducreyi*.[9,195] Clinically, it is associated with 1 to 3 large, painful, undermined, irregular ulcers with a grey base.[71,72,195] There is usually a single, tender and ultimately fluctuant inguinal mass. Constitutional symptoms are unusual. Without a specific diagnosis, a suitable indication for treatment is the presence of one or more painful genital ulcers and no evidence of syphilis by a dark field examination or serology, and the lesion is not typical of herpes or tests for herpes are negative.

The susceptibility of *H. ducreyi* to antimicrobial drugs varies in different locales and has been changing over time.[128] Successful treatment cures the infection, resolves symptoms and signs of ulcers and lymphadenopathy, and prevents transmission to others. There may be residual scarring, especially if buboes drain spontaneously.

##### Treatment Regimens

The recommended regimens for chancroid are azithromycin 1g orally as a single dose, ceftriaxone 250mg intramuscularly as a single dose, or erythromycin 500mg orally 4 times daily for 7 days.[75] Alternative regimens include amoxicillin 500mg plus clavulanic acid 125mg orally 3 times daily for 7 days, or ciprofloxacin 500mg orally twice daily for 3 days. Cotrimoxazole (trimethoprim-sulfamethoxazole) is no longer recommended. If there is not marked improvement within 7 days, the diagnosis should be reassessed, and if further treatment is required, a different regimen should be used.

In patients with HIV infection, treatment may be more difficult and individuals should be followed closely; multiple-dose rather than single-dose therapy is preferred.[75] Erythromycin is currently the drug of choice in this setting, but a recent study has shown azithromycin 1g to have equal efficacy.[128] With both regimens, failure has been associated with seropositivity for HIV, and with lack of circumcision.

##### Adjunctive Measures

If buboes are fluctuant, they should be aspirated for diagnosis and as an adjunct to treatment. Individuals should also be tested for HIV infection at initial diagnosis, and for HIV and syphilis at 3 months if the initial tests were negative.

Sexual partners from within the last 10 days before onset of symptoms should be evaluated and treated, even if disease is not found.

#### *5.4.2 Lymphogranuloma Venereum*

Lymphogranuloma venereum is caused by 3 serovars of *C. trachomatis* that are unusual in that they result in more invasive disease and constitutional symptoms. In most cases, the most obvious manifestation of disease is matted, tender, ultimately fluctuant, and often bilateral inguinal lymphadenopathy in conjunction with constitutional symptoms. Although a genital lesion may be present, it is usually transient. As with chancroid, buboes should be aspirated for diagnosis and symptomatic management.

##### Treatment Regimens

Antimicrobial treatment is with multidose agents active against *C. trachomatis* (see section 3.2.2), but treatment should be given for 21 days. Doxycycline 100mg twice daily is the regimen of choice, with the alternatives being erythromycin 500mg 4 times daily or sulfafurazole 500mg 4 times daily (or equivalent).[75] Sexual partners should be treated with a similar regimen.

Systemic symptoms should respond relatively quickly, although the inguinal mass may take longer to respond. Late complications may respond only minimally.

#### *5.4.3 Granuloma Inguinale (Calymmatobacterium granulomatis Infection)*

Granuloma inguinale or donovanosis is caused by *C. granulomatis*, a bacterium that has not been grown *in vitro* and hence has been difficult to study. The ulcer is chronic, non-painful, raised, beefy, irregular and indurated, and may ultimately cause considerable destruction. Pain, inguinal lymphadenopathy, and constitutional symptoms are rare.

#### Treatment Regimens

The preferred treatment is cotrimoxazole 960mg (2 tablets) twice daily for 14 days, or tetracycline 500mg orally 4 times daily for at least 14 days.[114] If treatment is going to be successful, there should be a significant response within 7 days.

## 5.5 Acquired Immune Deficiency Syndrome (AIDS)

HIV infection and AIDS are discussed further in chapter 32 (sect. 3.1). However, AIDS and classical STDs are inextricably linked.[10,12,15,192-194,196] Sexual transmission is the dominant means of spread of HIV, and in the absence of a cure for infection with this virus, preventive measures are very similar.[194,197-202] Furthermore, several STDs facilitate the transmission of HIV and infection with HIV makes treatment of several sexually transmissible diseases more difficult.[18,75,128] Even in North America, where sexual transmission was predominantly associated with male homosexual activity, for several years the fastest rates of increase have been linked to heterosexual activity and spread to infants.[28]

### 5.5.1 Altered Manifestations of STDs in Patients with HIV Infection

In association with the immunosuppression of HIV infection, but possibly for additional reasons, the presentation of several STDs is more dramatic or more frequent. Even in those without AIDS, there are associations with excessive antibody to herpes simplex virus type 2 in heterosexual individuals who are HIV positive.[186] In a group of women with pelvic inflammatory disease in an HIV endemic area, there was much more antibody to HIV than expected, and a trend towards greater need for surgical intervention in those who were HIV positive.[169] Even before there is significant diminution in numbers of CD4 cells, women with HIV infection may develop recurrent vaginal yeast infections.[179] Several studies have shown a significant relationship with cervical dysplasia or neoplasia in women who are HIV positive, with more aggressive disease occurring with advancing immunosuppression.[187,188] Some authorities believe that manifestations of syphilis are also altered in those who are HIV positive.[18]

There is also evidence for decreased effectiveness of standard therapies, not only for diseases like genital herpes and candidiasis (which are known to respond less well to treatment in anyone who is profoundly immunosuppressed), but also for primary syphilis[18] and chancroid.[128]

### 5.5.2 Facilitation of Spread of HIV by STDs

There is overwhelming evidence that transmission and acquisition of HIV is facilitated by genital ulcer disease, particularly chancroid and syphilis.[10,15,192-194] However, there is also evidence linking infection with *C. trachomatis*, *N. gonorrhoeae* and herpes simplex virus with an increased risk of HIV transmission.[13-15,186,194]

### 5.5.3 Treatment for STDs as a Means of Decreasing the Spread of HIV

Because of the significant association between several STDs and transmission of HIV, and the lack of any curative treatment for HIV infection, aggressive detection and treatment of STDs is one way to try to decrease the spread of HIV.[197] This can be predicted from theoretical models,[12-14] but also from clinical studies.[10,192,193] In a study in Africa, a population of over 1000 predominantly HIV positive female prostitutes was enrolled in an STD/HIV control programme to assess the benefits of a programme in which the major components were diagnosis and treatment of STD and promotion of condom use.[10] It was estimated that between 6000 and 10,000 cases of HIV were prevented yearly, at a cost of US$8 to 12 per case prevented.

New drugs like azithromycin either alone, or combined with a single dose of another oral agent like ciprofloxacin, have tremendous appeal for single visit treatment of common STDs like *N. gonorrhoeae*, *C. trachomatis*, *H. ducreyi* and possibly syphilis. Should this approach be successful, it lends itself to trials of mass treatment of selected populations. Previously, this has been done on a limited scale to combat gonorrhoea and syphilis.[203,204] Such an approach is contrary to usual wishes to restrict the administration of antimicrobials to those who do not need them, but if done successfully might actually lead to less overall administration of antimicrobials and also impede the spread of HIV.[77]

### 5.5.4 Common Preventive Measures for STDs and HIV Infection

Many of the preventive measures for STDs and HIV infection are similar. Educational programmes that promote delay in onset of coital activity, reduction in numbers of sexual partners, and use of condoms or other barrier methods are important for both.[75,194,198,199,201,202] Use of agents with virucidal and spermicidal activity may have some additional benefit, but there are concerns that overuse of such agents intravaginally may increase the risk of transmission of HIV.[198,200,201]

## 6. Future Treatments for STDs

As with most infectious diseases, the quality of data on which to base treatment recommendations for STDs varies widely. It is imperative that future studies be rigorous, including addressing issues of compliance, multiple concurrent infections, and special populations. Recommendations for the design and performance of studies for the evaluation of treatments for STDs have been proposed.[126,152,171,182,205-209] Although not fully practical for many places where most disease is seen, they should help to standardise key elements of studies.

Two big issues that influence overall effectiveness are compliance-related concerns and the development of resistance to standard regimens which necessitates development of new agents or new regimens. Cost is a relevant concern, particularly the cost of drugs to individuals, and to programmes where budgets are assigned to specific envelopes. However, in the wider perspective, the cost of drugs tends to be only a small component of overall costs in cost-effectiveness or cost-benefit studies.[62,63,83,84] At an individual level, the cost of diagnostic tests often exceeds the cost of medication, and drugs are administered to only a fraction of those who are tested.

Despite problems with compliance and drug resistance, available treatments have contributed significantly to the decrease in numbers of treatable STDs. Effective treatments have had a dramatic effect on the reproductive rates of infections.[77,210,211] However, with the important exception of zidovudine use during pregnancy to decrease transmission of HIV to infants,[212] available drugs used for treatment of viral STDs do not dramatically affect the numbers of viral STDs and do not cure them. Pending development of curative regimens, the current focus for these infections must be on preventive measures which include educational efforts, use of barrier methods, treatment of susceptible STDs to decrease transmission of HIV, and, where available, use of vaccines such as hepatitis B vaccines.

## References

1. Cates Jr W. The epidemiology and control of sexually transmitted diseases in adolescents. Adolescent Medicine, State of the Art Reviews 1990; 1: 409-27
2. Centers for Disease Control and Prevention. Summary of notifiable diseases, United States, 1993. Morbidity and Mortality Weekly Report 1993; 42: 1-73
3. Gully PR, Rwetsiba DK. Trends in gonorrhea in Canada: 1980-1989. Canada Diseases Weekly Report 1991; 17: 105-9
4. Gully PR, Rwetsiba DK. Chlamydial infection in Canada. Canada Diseases Weekly Report 1991; 17: 282-91
5. Bell TA, Hein K. Adolescents and sexually transmitted diseases. In: Holmes KK, Mardh PA, Sparling PF, et al., editors. Sexually transmitted diseases. New York: McGraw-Hill Book Co, 1984: 73-84
6. Patrick DM, Bowie WR. The epidemiology of *Chlamydia trachomatis* infection in British Columbia. In: Orfila J, Bryne GI, Chernesky MA, et al., editors. Eighth International Symposium on Human Chlamydial Infections. Bologna: Societa Editrice Esculapio, 1994: 32-5
7. Handsfield HH, Rice RJ, Roberts MC, et al. Localized outbreak of penicillinase-producing *Neisseria gonorrhoeae:* paradigm for introduction and spread of gonorrhea in a community. Journal of the American Medical Association 1989; 261: 2357-61
8. Rothenberg RR. The geography of gonorrhea: empirical demonstration of core group transmission. American Journal of Epidemiology 1983; 117: 688-94
9. Jessamine PG, Ronald AR. Chancroid and the role of genital ulcer disease in the spread of human retroviruses. Medical Clinics of North America 1990; 74: 1417-31
10. Moses S, Plummer FA, Ngugi EN, et al. Controlling HIV in Africa: effectiveness and cost of an intervention in a high-frequency STD transmitter core group. AIDS 1991; 5: 407-11
11. de Muylder X, Laga M, Tennstedt C, et al. The role of *Neisseria gonorrhoeae* and *Chlamydia trachomatis* in pelvic inflammatory disease and its sequelae in Zimbabwe. Journal of Infectious Diseases 1990; 162: 501-5
12. Boily M-C, Brunham RC. The impact of HIV and other STDs on human populations: are predictions possible? Infectious Disease Clinics of North America 1993; 7: 771-92
13. Brunham RC, Cheang M, McMaster J, et al. *Chlamydia trachomatis*, infertility, and population growth in sub-Saharan Africa. Sexually Transmitted Diseases 1993; 20: 168-73
14. Brunham RC, Garnett GP, Swinton J, et al. Gonococcal infection and human fertility in sub-Saharan Africa. Proceedings of the Royal Society of London, Series B 1992; 246: 173-7
15. Clottey C, Dallabetta G. Sexually transmitted diseases and human immunodeficiency virus: epidemiologic synergy? Infectious Disease Clinics of North America 1993; 7: 753-70
16. Walckiers D, Piot P, Stroobant A, et al. Declining trends in some sexually transmitted diseases in Belgium between 1983 and 1989. Genitourinary Medicine 1991; 67: 374-7
17. Finelli L, Budd J, Spitalny KC. Early syphilis: relationship to sex, drugs, and changes in high-risk behavior from 1987-1990. Sexually Transmitted Diseases 1993; 20: 89-95
18. Hook III EW, Marra CM. Acquired syphilis in adults. New England Journal of Medicine 1992; 326: 1060-9
19. Hillis S, Nakashima A, Amsterdam L, et al. *Chlamydia trachomatis* infections: trends in prevalence, incidence,

incidence of recurrent infection, pelvic inflammatory disease and ectopic pregnancy following a comprehensive program. In: Orfila J, Bryne GI, Chernesky MA, et al., editors. Eighth International Symposium on Human Chlamydial Infections. Bologna: Societa Editrice Esculapio, 1994: 67-70

20. Piot P, Van den Hoek JAR, Van Damme L, et al. Epidemiology and control of genital chlamydial infection. In: Orfila J, Bryne GI, Chernesky MA, et al., editors. Eighth International Symposium on Human Chlamydial Infections. Bologna: Societa Editrice Esculapio, 1994: 7-16
21. Ripa T. Epidemiologic control of genital *Chlamydia trachomatis* infections. Scandinavian Journal of Infectious Diseases 1990 Suppl. 69: 157-67
22. Harry TC, Rashid S, Saravanamuttu KM, et al. Trichomoniasis: perspectives in declining prevalence in a GUM clinic. Sexually Transmitted Diseases 1994; 21: 357-9
23. Lossick JG, Kent HL. Trichomoniasis: trends in diagnosis and management. American Journal of Obstetrics and Gynecology 1991; 165: 1217-22
24. Westrom L. Decrease in incidence of women treated in hospital for acute salpingitis in Sweden. Genitourinary Medicine 1988; 64: 59-63
25. Centers for Disease Control. Ectopic pregnancy - United States 1988-1989. Morbidity and Mortality Weekly Report 1992; 41: 591-4
26. Johnson RE, Nahmias A, Madger LS, et al. A seroepidemiologic survey of the prevalence of herpes simplex virus type 2 infection in the United States. New England Journal of Medicine 1989; 321: 7-12
27. Mertz GJ. Epidemiology of genital herpes infection. Infectious Disease Clinics of North America 1993; 7: 825-39
28. Centers for Disease Control. Mortality attributable to HIV infection/AIDs - United States, 1981-1990. Morbidity and Mortality Weekly Report 1991; 40: 41-4
29. Kipke MD, Hein K. Acquired immunodeficiency syndrome (AIDS) in adolescents. Adolescent Medicine, State of the Art Reviews 1990; 1: 429-49
30. Persson K, Mansson AS, Nordenfelt E. Similar change of antibody pattern for herpes simplex virus type 2 and *Chlamydia trachomatis* from 1970 to 1993. In: Orfila J, Bryne GI, Chernesky MA, et al., editors. Eighth International Symposium on Human Chlamydial Infections. Bologna: Societa Editrice Esculapio, 1994: 36-9
31. World Health Organization. Control of sexually transmitted diseases. Geneva: World Health Organization, 1985
32. Donders GGG, Desmyter J, de Wet DH, et al. The association of gonorrhoea and syphilis with premature birth and low birth weight. Genitourinary Medicine 1993; 69: 998-1001
33. Stoll BJ, Glover S, Freed G, et al. Cost of congenital syphilis. Pediatric Infectious Disease Journal 1993; 12: 621
34. Gump DW, Gibson M, Ashikaga T. Evidence of prior pelvic inflammatory disease and its relationship to *Chlamydia trachomatis* antibody and intrauterine contraceptive device use in infertile women. American Journal of Obstetrics and Gynecology 1983; 146: 153-9
35. Hillis SD, Joesoef R, Marchbanks PA, et al. Delayed care of pelvic inflammatory disease as a risk factor for impaired fertility. American Journal of Obstetrics and Gynecology 1993; 168: 1503-9
36. Mueller BA, Luz-Jimemez M, Daling JR, et al. Risk factors for tubal infertility: influence of history of prior pelvic inflammatory disease. Sexually Transmitted Diseases 1992; 19: 28-34
37. Westrom L. Incidence, prevalence, and trends of acute pelvic inflammatory disease and its consequences in industrialized countries. American Journal of Obstetrics and Gynecology 1980; 138: 880-92
38. Westrom L, Joesoef R, Reynolds G, et al. Pelvic inflammatory disease and fertility: a cohort study of 1,844 women with laparoscopically verified disease and 657 control women with normal laparoscopic results. Sexually Transmitted Diseases 1992; 19: 185-92
39. Westrom L, Mardh PA. Acute pelvic inflammatory disease (PID). In: Holmes KK, Mardh PA, Sparling PF, et al., editors. Sexually Transmitted Diseases. 2nd ed. New York: McGraw-Hill Book Co, 1989: 593-613
40. Chow JM, Yonekura ML, Richwald GA, et al. The association between *Chlamydia trachomatis* and ectopic pregnancy: a matched-pair, case-control study. Journal of the American Medical Association 1990; 263: 3164-7
41. Handsfield HH, Hodson WA, Holmes KK. Neonatal gonococcal infection. 1. Orogastric contamination with *Neisseria gonorrhoeae*. Journal of the American Medical Association 1973; 225: 697-701
42. Keat A. Sexually transmitted arthritis syndromes. Medical Clinics of North America 1990; 74: 1617-31
43. Keat A, Thomas BJ, Taylor-Robinson D. Chlamydial infection in the aetiology of arthritis. British Medical Bulletin 1983; 39: 168-74
44. Lauhio A, Leirisalo-Repo M, Lahdevirta J, et al. Double-blind, placebo-controlled study of three-month treatment with lymecycline in reactive arthritis, with special reference to *Chlamydia* arthritis. Arthritis and Rheumatism 1991; 34: 6-14
45. Cohen I, Veille J-C, Calkins BM. Improved pregnancy outcome following successful treatment of chlamydial infection. Journal of the American Medical Association 1990; 263: 3160-3
46. Nugent RP, Hillier SL, for the Investigators of the Johns Hopkins Study of Cervicitis and Adverse Pregnancy outcome. Mucopurulent cervicitis as a predictor of chlamydial infection and adverse pregnancy outcome. Sexually Transmitted Diseases 1992; 19: 198-202
47. Gravett MG, Nelson HP, DeRouen T, et al. Independent association of bacterial vaginosis and *Chlamydia trachomatis* infection with adverse pregnancy outcome. Journal of the American Medical Association 1986; 256: 1899-903
48. Hillier S, Holmes KK. Bacterial vaginosis. In: Holmes KK, Mardh PA, Sparling PF, et al., editors. Sexually transmitted diseases. 2nd ed. New York: McGraw-Hill Book Co, 1989: 547-59
49. McGregor JA, French JI, Seo K. Adjunctive clindamycin therapy for preterm labor: results of a double-blind, placebo-controlled trial. American Journal of Obstetrics and Gynecology 1991; 165: 867-75
50. Corey L, Adams HG, Brown ZA, et al. Genital herpes simplex virus infections: clinical manifestations, course and complications. Annals of Internal Medicine 1983; 98: 958-72
51. Corey L, Holmes KK. Genital herpes simplex virus infection: current concepts in diagnosis, therapy, and prevention. Annals of Internal Medicine 1983; 98: 973-83
52. Catotti DN, Clarke P, Catoe KE. Herpes revisited: still a cause for concern. Sexually Transmitted Diseases 1993; 20: 77-80
53. Brown ZA, Benedetti J, Ashley R, et al. Neonatal herpes simplex virus infection in relation to asymptomatic maternal infection at the time of labor. New England Journal of Medicine 1991; 324: 1247-52
54. Stagno S, Whitley RJ. Herpesvirus infection in the neonate and children. In: Holmes KK, Mardh PA, Sparling PF, et al., editors. Sexually transmitted diseases. 2nd ed. New York: McGraw-Hill Book Co, 1989: 863-87
55. Whitley RJ, Gnann Jr JW. Acyclovir: a decade later. New England Journal of Medicine 1992; 327: 782-9
56. Paavonen J, Koutsky LA, Kiviat N. Cervical neoplasia and other STD-related genital and anal neoplasias. In: Holmes KK, Mardh PA, Sparling PF, et al., editors. Sexually transmitted diseases. 2nd ed. New York: McGraw-Hill Book Co, 1989: 561-92

57. Oriel D. Genital human papillomavirus infection. In: Holmes KK, Mardh PA, Sparling PF, et al., editors. Sexually transmitted diseases. 2nd ed. New York: McGraw-Hill Book Co, 1989: 433-41
58. Shah KV. Biology of human genital tract papillomaviruses. In: Holmes KK, Mardh PA, Sparling PF, et al., editors. Sexually transmitted diseases. 2nd ed. New York: McGraw-Hill Book Co, 1989: 425-31
59. Alter MJ, Margolis HS. The emergence of hepatitis B as a sexually transmitted disease. Medical Clinics of North America 1990; 74: 1529-41
60. Bratos MA, Eiros JM, Orduna A, et al. Influence of syphilis in hepatitis B transmission in a cohort of female prostitutes. Sexually Transmitted Diseases 1993; 20: 257-61
61. Estany A, Todd M, Vasquez M, et al. Early detection of early chlamydial infection in women - an economic evaluation. Sexually Transmitted Diseases 1989; 16: 21-7
62. Genc M, Ruusuvaara L, Mardh P-A. An economic evaluation of screening for *Chlamydia trachomatis* in adolescent males. Journal of the American Medical Association 1993; 270: 2057-64
63. Haddix AC, Hillis SD, Kassler WJ. The cost-effectiveness of single-dose therapy for *Chlamydia trachomatis* infections in women. In: Orfila J, Bryne GI, Chernesky MA, et al., editors. Eighth International Symposium on Human Chlamydial Infections. Bologna: Societa Editrice Esculapio, 1994: 55-8
64. Nettleman MD, Jones RB. Cost-effectiveness of screening women at moderate risk for genital infections caused by *Chlamydia trachomatis*. Journal of the American Medical Association 1988; 260: 207-13
65. Todd MJ, Estany A, McLaren R. Cost of pelvic inflammatory disease and associated sequelae in Canada. Canada Diseases Weekly Report 1988; 14: 206-8
66. Washington AE, Arno PS, Brooks MA. Economic cost of pelvic inflammatory disease. Journal of the American Medical Association 1986; 255: 1735-8
67. Washington AE, Johnson RE, Sanders Jr LL. *Chlamydia trachomatis* infections in the United States: what are they costing us? Journal of the American Medical Association 1987; 257: 2070-2
68. Bowie WR. Urethritis in males. In: Holmes KK, Mardh PA, Sparling PF, et al., editors. Sexually transmitted diseases. 2nd ed. New York: McGraw-Hill Book Co, 1989: 627-39
69. Schachter J. Diagnosis of *Chlamydia trachomatis* infection. In: Orfila J, Bryne GI, Chernesky MA, et al., editors. Eighth International Symposium on Human Chlamydial Infections. Bologna: Societa Edsitrice Esculapio, 1994: 293-302
70. Moran JS, Zenilman JM. Therapy for gonococcal infections: options in 1989. Reviews of Infectious Diseases 1990; 12 Suppl. 6: S633-44
71. Kraus SJ. Evaluation and management of acute genital ulcers in sexually active patients. Urologic Clinics of North America 1984; 11: 155-62
72. Schmid GP. Approach to the patient with genital ulcer disease. Medical Clinics of North America 1990; 74: 1559-72
73. Hutchinson CM, Hook III EW. Syphilis in adults. Medical Clinics of North America 1990; 74: 1389-416
74. Bowie WR, MacDonald NE, editors. Canadian guidelines for the diagnosis and management of sexually transmitted diseases, by syndrome, in children, adolescents and adults. Canada Diseases Weekly Report 1989; March, 15S1
75. Centers for Disease Control and Prevention. Sexually transmitted diseases treatment guidelines. Morbidity and Mortality Weekly Report 1993; 42 (RR-14): 1-102
76. Hook III EW, Spitters C, Reichart CA, et al. Chlamydia screening in STD clinic patients: positive tests do not ensure treatment of infection. In: Orfila J, Bryne GI, Chernesky MA, et al., editors. Eighth International Symposium on Human Chlamydial Infections. Bologna: Societa Editrice Esculapio, 1994: 44-7
77. Bowie WR. Antibiotics and sexually transmitted diseases. Infectious Disease Clinics of North America 1994; 8: 841-57
78. Evans AJ, Morrison GD, Price DJ. Prolonged use of the Greenland method of treatment of gonorrhea. British Journal of Venereal Diseases 1980; 56: 88-91
79. Willcox RR. How suitable are available pharmaceuticals for the treatment of sexually transmitted diseases? 1: conditions presenting as genital discharges. British Journal of Venereal Diseases 1977; 53: 314-23
80. Bowie WR. Epidemiology and therapy of *Chlamydia trachomatis* infections. Drugs 1984; 27: 459-68
81. Bowie WR, Ast J, Sibau L, et al. Need for treatment of gonorrhea to be effective against *Chlamydia trachomatis*. Canadian Journal of Infectious Diseases 1993; 4: 347-51
82. Stamm WE, Guinan ME, Johnson C, et al. Effect of treatment regimens for *Neisseria gonorrhoeae* on simultaneous infection with *Chlamydia trachomatis*. New England Journal of Medicine 1984; 310: 545-9
83. Begley CE, McGill L, Smith PB. The incremental cost of screening, diagnosis, and treatment of gonorrhea and chlamydia in a family planning clinic. Sexually Transmitted Diseases 1989; 16: 63-7
84. Nettleman MD, Jones RB, Roberts SD, et al. Cost-effectiveness of culturing for *Chlamydia trachomatis*: a study in a clinic for sexually transmitted diseases. Annals of Internal Medicine 1986; 105: 189-96
85. Brookoff D. Compliance with outpatient antibiotics among women treated in the emergency department for pelvic inflammatory disease [Abstract No. 106]. 22nd Annual Meeting of the Society for Academic Emergency Medicine, Toronto, Ontario, May 26-29, 1992
86. Katz BP, Zwickl BW, Caine VA, et al. Compliance with antibiotic therapy for *Chlamydia trachomatis* and *Neisseria gonorrhoeae*. Sexually Transmitted Diseases 1992; 19: 351-4
87. Jordan WC. Doxycycline vs. tetracycline in the treatment of men with gonorrhea. Sexually Transmitted Diseases 1981; 8 Suppl: 105-9
88. Washington AE, Browner WS, Korenbrot CC. Cost-effectiveness of combined treatment for endocervical gonorrhea. Considering co-infection with *Chlamydia trachomatis*. Journal of the American Medical Association 1987; 257: 2056-60
89. Bowie WR, Willetts V, Jewesson PJ. Adverse reactions in a dose-ranging study with a new long-acting fluoroquinolone, fleroxacin. Antimicrobial Agents and Chemotherapy 1989; 33: 1778-82
90. Katz BP, Danos CS, Quinn TS, et al. Efficiency and cost-effectiveness of field follow-up for patients with *Chlamydia trachomatis* infection in a sexually transmitted disease clinic. Sexually Transmitted Diseases 1988; 15: 11-6
91. Handsfield HH, Lipman TO, Harnisch JP, et al. Asymptomatic gonorrhea in men. Diagnosis, natural course, prevalence and significance. New England Journal of Medicine 1974; 290: 117-23
92. Thelin I, Wennstrom A-M, Mardh P-A. Contact-tracing in patients with genital chlamydial infection. British Journal of Venereal Diseases 1980; 56: 259-62
93. Schiotz HA, Csango PA. Test-of-cure for asymptomatic genital chlamydial infections in women: a cost-benefit analysis. Sexually Transmitted Diseases 1992; 19: 133-6
94. Katz BP, Batteiger BE, Jones RB. Effect of prior sexually transmitted disease on the isolation of *Chlamydia trachomatis*. Sexually Transmitted Diseases 1987; 14: 160-4
95. Alexander ER. Is it cost-beneficial to screen adolescent males for *Chlamydia*? American Journal of Public Health 1990; 80: 531-2

96. Aronson MD, Phillips RS. Screening young men for chlamydial infection. Journal of the American Medical Association 1993; 270: 2097-8
97. Randolph AG, Washington AE. Screening for *Chlamydia trachomatis* in adolescent males: a cost-based decision analysis. American Journal of Public Health 1990; 80: 545-50
98. Shafer M-A, Schachter J, Moncada J, et al. Evaluation of urine-based screening strategies to detect *Chlamydia trachomatis* among sexually active asymptomatic young males. Journal of the American Medical Association 1993; 270: 2065-70
99. Buhang H, Skjeldestad FE, Halvorsen LE, et al. Should asymptomatic patients be tested for *Chlamydia trachomatis* in general practice? British Journal of General Practice 1990; 40: 142-5
100. Centers for Disease Control and Prevention. Recommendations for the prevention and management of *Chlamydia trachomatis* infections, 1993. Morbidity and Mortality Weekly Report 1993; 42 (RR-12): 1-39
101. Hart G. Risk profiles and epidemiologic interrelationships of sexually transmitted diseases. Sexually Transmitted Diseases 1993; 20: 126-36
102. Humphreys JT, Henneberry JF, Rickard RS, et al. Cost-benefit analysis of selective screening criteria for *Chlamydia trachomatis* infection in women attending Colorado family planning clinics. Sexually Transmitted Diseases 1992; 19: 47-53
103. Nettleman MD, Bell TA. Cost-effectiveness of prenatal testing for *Chlamydia trachomatis*. American Journal of Obstetrics and Gynecology 1991; 164: 1289-94
104. Phillips RS, Aronson MD, Taylor WC, et al. Should tests for *Chlamydia trachomatis* cervical infection be done during routine gynecologic visits? An analysis of the costs of alternative strategies. Annals of Internal Medicine 1987; 107: 188-94
105. Scholes D, Stergachis A, Heidrich FE, et al. Selective screening for Chlamydia reduces the incidence of pelvic inflammatory disease: results from a randomized intervention trial. In: Orfila J, Bryne GI, Chernesky MA, et al., editors. Eighth International Symposium on Human Chlamydial Infections. Bologna: Societa Editrice Esculapio, 1994: 28-31
106. Sellors JW, Pickard L, Gafni A, et al. Effectiveness and efficiency of selective vs universal screening for chlamydial infection in sexually active young women. Archives of Internal Medicine 1992; 152: 1837-44
107. Trachtenberg AI, Washington AE, Halldorson S. A cost-based decision analysis for Chlamydia screening in California family planning clinics. Obstetrics and Gynecology 1988; 71: 101-8
108. Hook III EW, Holmes KK. Gonococcal infections. Annals of Internal Medicine 1985; 102: 229-43
109. Judson FN. Gonorrhea. Medical Clinics of North America 1990; 74: 1353-66
110. Centers for Disease Control and Prevention. Decreased susceptibility of *Neisseria gonorrhoeae* to fluoroquinolones - Ohio and Hawaii, 1992-1994. Morbidity and Mortality Weekly Report 1994; 43: 325-7
111. Jaffe HW, Schroeter AL, Reynolds GH, et al. Pharmacokinetic determinants of penicillin cure of gonococcal urethritis. Antimicrobial Agents and Chemotherapy 1979; 15: 587-91
112. Nettleman MD, Smith V, Moyer NP. Penicillin resistant *Neisseria gonorrhoeae* in low prevalence areas: implications for cost-effective management. Sexually Transmitted Diseases 1990; 17: 175-80
113. Peterman TA, Zaidi AA, Lieb S, et al. Incubating syphilis in patients treated for gonorrhea: a comparison of treatment regimens. Journal of Infectious Diseases 1994; 170: 689-92
114. Centers for Disease Control. 1989 Sexually transmitted diseases treatment guidelines. Morbidity and Mortality Weekly Report 1989; 38 (S-8): v-43
115. Handsfield HH, Hook III EW. Ceftriaxone for treatment of uncomplicated gonorrhea: routine use of a single 125-mg dose in a sexually transmitted disease clinic. Sexually Transmitted Diseases 1987; 14: 227-30
116. Handsfield HH, McCormack WM, Hook III EW, et al. A comparison of single-dose cefixime with ceftriaxone as treatment for uncomplicated gonorrhea. New England Journal of Medicine 1991; 325: 1337-41
117. Verdon MS, Douglas JM, Wiggins SD, et al. Treatment of uncomplicated gonorrhea with single doses of 200 mg cefixime. Sexually Transmitted Diseases 1993; 20: 290-3
118. Echols RM, Heyd A, O'Keeffe BJ, et al. Single-dose ciprofloxacin in the treatment of uncomplicated gonorrhea: a worldwide summary. Sexually Transmitted Diseases 1994; 21: 345-52
119. Hammerschlag MR, Golden NH, Oh MK, et al. Single dose of azithromycin for the treatment of genital chlamydial infections in adolescents. Journal of Pediatrics 1993; 122: 961-5
120. Johnson RB. The role of azalide antibiotics in the treatment of Chlamydia. American Journal of Obstetrics and Gynecology 1991; 164: 1794-6
121. Lauharanta J, Saarinen K, Mustonen M-J, et al. Single-dose oral azithromycin versus seven-day doxycycline in the treatment of non-gonococcal urethritis in men. Journal of Antimicrobial Chemotherapy 1993; 31 Suppl. E: 177-83
122. Lister PJ, Balechandran T, Ridgway GL, et al. Comparison of azithromycin and doxycycline in the treatment of non-gonococcal urethritis in men. Journal of Antimicrobial Chemotherapy 1993; 31 Suppl. E: 185-92
123. Martin DH, Mroczkowski TF, Dalu ZA, et al. A controlled trial of a single dose of azithromycin for treatment of chlamydial urethritis and cervicitis. New England Journal of Medicine 1992; 327: 921-5
124. Ossewaarde JM, Plantema FHF, Rieffe M, et al. Efficacy of single-dose azithromycin versus doxycycline in the treatment of cervical infections caused by *Chlamydia trachomatis*. European Journal of Clinical Microbiology and Infectious Diseases 1992; 11: 693-7
125. Steingrimsson O, Olafsson JH, Thorarinsson H, et al. Single dose azithromycin treatment of gonorrhea and infections caused by *C. trachomatis* and *U. urealyticum* in men. Sexually Transmitted Diseases 1994; 21: 43-6
126. Handsfield HH, McCutchan JA, Corey L, et al. Evaluation of new anti-infective drugs for the treatment of uncomplicated gonorrhea in adults and adolescents. Clinical Infectious Diseases 1992; 15 Suppl. 1: S123-30
127. Waugh MA. Open study of the safety and efficacy of a single oral dose of azithromycin for the treatment of uncomplicated gonorrhea in men and women. Journal of Antimicrobial Chemotherapy 1993; 31 Suppl. E: 193-8
128. Tyndall MW, Agoki E, Plummer FA, et al. Single dose azithromycin for the treatment of chancroid: a randomized comparison with erythromycin. Sexually Transmitted Diseases 1994; 21: 231-4
129. Hooton TM, Batteiger BE, Judson FN, et al. Ofloxacin versus doxycycline for treatment of cervical infection with *Chlamydia trachomatis*. Antimicrobial Agents and Chemotherapy 1992; 36: 1144-6
130. Jones RB, Mammel JB, Shepard MK, et al. Recovery of *Chlamydia trachomatis* from the endometrium of women at risk for chlamydial infection. American Journal of Obstetrics and Gynecology 1986; 155: 35-9
131. Paavonen J, Kiviat N, Brunham RC, et al. Prevalence and manifestations of endometritis among women with cervicitis. American Journal of Obstetrics and Gynecology 1985; 152: 280-6

132. Landers DV, Sung ML, Bottles K, et al. Does addition of anti-inflammatory agents to antimicrobial therapy reduce infertility after murine chlamydial salpingitis? Sexually Transmitted Diseases 1993; 20: 121-5
133. Tuffrey M. The use of animal models to study human chlamydial diseases. In: Orfila J, Bryne GI, Chernesky MA, et al., editors. Eighth International Symposium on Human Chlamydial Infections. Bologna: Societa Editrice Esculapio, 1994: 513-24
134. Martin DH. Chlamydial infections. Medical Clinics of North America 1990; 74: 1367-87
135. Toomey KE, Barnes RC. Treatment of *Chlamydia trachomatis* genital infection. Reviews of Infectious Diseases 1991; 12 Suppl. 6: S645-55
136. Workowski KA, Lampe MF, Wong KG, et al. Long-term eradication of *Chlamydia trachomatis* genital infection after antimicrobial therapy: evidence against persistent infection. Journal of the American Medical Association 1993; 270: 2071-5
137. Shepard MK, Jones RB. Recovery of *Chlamydia trachomatis* from endometrial and fallopian tube biopsies in women with infertility of tubal origin. Fertility and Sterility 1989; 52: 232-8
138. Jones RB, Van der Pol B, Martin DH, et al. Partial characterization of *Chlamydia trachomatis* isolates resistant to multiple antibiotics. Journal of Infectious Diseases 1990; 162: 1309-15
139. Mourad A, Sweet RL, Sugg N, et al. Relative resistance to erythromycin in *Chlamydia trachomatis*. Antimicrobial Agents and Chemotherapy 1980; 18: 696-8
140. Bevan CD, Siddle NC, Mumtaz G, et al. *Chlamydia trachomatis* in the genital tract of women with acute salpingitis identified by a qualitative and quantitative polymerase chain reaction before and after treatment. In: Orfila J, Bryne GI, Chernesky MA, et al., editors. Eighth International Symposium on Human Chlamydial Infections. Bologna: Societa Editrice Esculapio, 1994: 350-3
141. Lehtinen M, Paavonen J. Heat-shock proteins in the immunopathogenesis of chlamydial pelvic inflammatory disease. In: Orfila J, Bryne GI, Chernesky MA, et al., editors. Eighth International Symposium on Human Chlamydial Infections. Bologna: Societa Editrice Esculapio, 1994: 599-610
142. Patton DL, Cosgrove Sweeney YT, Plier PK, et al. Detection of *Chlamydia trachomatis* by cell culture, polymerase chain reaction (PCR) and ligase chain reaction (LCR) in upper and lower tract reproductive tissues in an experimental monkey model of PID. In: Orfila J, Bryne GI, Chernesky MA, et al., editors. Eighth International Symposium on Human Chlamydial Infections. Bologna: Societa Editrice Esculapio, 1994: 314-7
143. Bowie WR, Alexander ER, Floyd J, et al. Differential response of chlamydial and ureaplasma-associated urethritis to sulfafurazole (sulfisoxazole) and aminocyclitols. Lancet 1976; 2: 1276-8
144. Landers DV, Wolner-Hanssen P, Paavonen J, et al. Combination antimicrobial therapy in the treatment of acute pelvic inflammatory disease. American Journal of Obstetrics and Gynecology 1991; 164: 849-58
145. Walker CK, Kahn JG, Washington AE, et al. Pelvic inflammatory disease: metaanalysis of antimicrobial regimen efficacy. Journal of Infectious Diseases 1993; 168: 969-78
146. Alger LS, Lovchik JC. Comparative efficacy of clindamycin versus erythromycin in eradication of antenatal *Chlamydia trachomatis*. American Journal of Obstetrics and Gynecology 1991; 165: 375-81
147. Campbell WF, Dodson MG. Clindamycin therapy for *Chlamydia trachomatis* in women. American Journal of Obstetrics and Gynecology 1990; 162: 343-7
148. Crombleholme WR, Schachter J, Grossman M, et al. Amoxicillin therapy for *Chlamydia trachomatis* in pregnancy. Obstetrics and Gynecology 1990; 75: 752-6
149. Magat AH, Alger LS, Nagey DA, et al. Double-blind randomized study comparing amoxicillin and erythromycin for the treatment of *Chlamydia trachomatis* in pregnancy. Obstetrics and Gynecology 1993; 81: 745-9
150. Schachter J, Sweet RL, Grossman M, et al. Experience with the routine use of erythromycin for chlamydial infections in pregnancy. New England Journal of Medicine 1986; 314: 276-9
151. Rahman MU, Hudson AP, Schumacher Jr HR. Chlamydia and Reiter's syndrome (reactive arthritis). Rheumatic Disease Clinics of North America 1992; 18: 67-79
152. Ronald AR, Silverman M, McCutchan JA, et al. Evaluation of new anti-infective drugs for the treatment of syphilis. Clinical Infectious Diseases 1992; 15 Suppl. 1: S140-7
153. Zenker PN, Rolfs RT. Treatment of syphilis, 1989. Reviews of Infectious Diseases 1990; 12 Suppl. 6: S590-609
154. Bowie WR. Effective treatment of urethritis: a practical guide. Drugs 1992; 44: 207-15
155. Holmes KK, Handsfield HH, Wang S-P, et al. Etiology of nongonococcal urethritis. New England Journal of Medicine 1975; 292: 1199-205
156. Bowie WR, Alexander ER, Stimson JB, et al. Therapy for nongonococcal urethritis: double-blind randomised comparison of two doses and two durations of minocycline. Annals of Internal Medicine 1981; 95: 306-11
157. Krieger JN, Hooton TM, Brust P, et al. Evaluation of chronic urethritis: defining the role for endoscopic procedures. Archives of Internal Medicine 1988; 148: 703-7
158. Brunham RC, Paavonen J, Stevens CE, et al. Mucopurulent cervicitis: the ignored counterpart in women of urethritis in men. New England Journal of Medicine 1984; 311: 1-6
159. Holmes KK. Lower genital tract infections in women: cystitis, urethritis, vulvovaginitis, and cervicitis. In: Holmes KK, Mardh PA, Sparling PF, et al., editors. Sexually transmitted diseases. 2nd ed. New York: McGraw-Hill Book Co, 1989: 527-45
160. Paavonen J, Critchlow CW, DeRouen T, et al. Etiology of cervical inflammation. American Journal of Obstetrics and Gynecology 1986; 154: 556-64
161. Moscicki B, Shafer M-A, Millstein SG, et al. The use and limitations of endocervical Gram stains and mucopurulent cervicitis as predictors for *Chlamydia trachomatis* in female adolescents. American Journal of Obstetrics and Gynecology 1987; 157: 65-71
162. Svennson L, Westrom L, Ripa KT, et al. Differences in some clinical and laboratory parameters in acute salpingitis related to culture and serologic findings. American Journal of Obstetrics and Gynecology 1980; 138: 1017-21
163. Gully PR, Bowie WR, MacDonald NE, et al., editors. 1992 Canadian guidelines for the prevention, diagnosis, management and treatment of sexually transmitted diseases in neonates, children, adolescents and adults. Canada Communicable Diseases Report, 1992: 18S1
164. Peterson HB, Galaid EI, Cates Jr W. Pelvic inflammatory disease. Medical Clinics of North America 1990; 74: 1603-15
165. Soper DE, Brockwell NJ, Dalton HP. Microbial etiology of urban emergency department acute salpingitis: treatment with ofloxacin. American Journal of Obstetrics and Gynecology 1992; 167: 653-60
166. Wasserheit JN, Bell TA, Kiviat NB, et al. Microbial causes of proven pelvic inflammatory disease and efficacy of clindamycin and tobramycin. Annals of Internal Medicine 1986; 104: 187-93
167. Wolner-Hanssen P, Kiviat NB, Holmes KK. Atypical pelvic inflammatory disease: subacute, chronic, or subclinical upper genital tract infection in women. In: Holmes KK, Mardh PA, Sparling PF, et al., editors. Sexually Transmit-

ted Diseases. 2nd ed. New York: McGraw-Hill Book Co, 1989: 615-20
168. Paavonen J, Teisela K, Heinonen PK, et al. Microbiological and histopathological findings in acute pelvic inflammatory disease. British Journal of Obstetrics and Gynaecology 1987; 94: 454-60
169. Hoegsberg B, Abulafia O, Sedlis A, et al. Sexually transmitted diseases and human immunodeficiency virus infection among women with pelvic inflammatory disease. American Journal of Obstetrics and Gynecology 1990; 163: 1135-9
170. Peterson HB, Galaid EI, Zenilman JM. Pelvic inflammatory disease: review of treatment options. Reviews of Infectious Diseases 1990; 12 Suppl. 6: S656-64
171. Sweet RL, Bartlett JG, Hemsell DL, et al. Evaluation of new anti-infective drugs for the treatment of acute pelvic inflammatory disease. Clinical Infectious Diseases 1992; 15 Suppl. 1: S53-61
172. Sweet RL, Schachter J, Robbie MO. Failure of β-lactam antibiotics to eradicate *Chlamydia trachomatis* in the endometrium despite apparent clinical cure of acute salpingitis. Journal of the American Medical Association 1983; 250: 2641-5
173. Berger RE. Acute epididymitis. In: Holmes KK, Mardh PA, Sparling PF, et al., editors. Sexually transmitted diseases. 2nd ed. New York: McGraw-Hill Book Co, 1989: 641-51
174. Berger RE, Alexander ER, Harnisch JP, et al. Etiology, manifestations, and therapy of acute epididymitis: prospective study of 50 cases. Journal of Urology 1979; 121: 750-4
175. Schwarcz SK, Whittington WL. Sexual assault and sexually transmitted diseases: detection and management in adults and children. Reviews of Infectious Diseases 1990; 12 Suppl. 6: S682-90
176. Amsel R, Totten PA, Spiegel CA, et al. Nonspecific vaginitis: diagnostic criteria and microbial and epidemiologic associations. American Journal of Medicine 1983; 74: 14-22
177. Sobel JD. Vaginal infections in adult women. Medical Clinics of North America 1990; 74: 1573-602
178. Beard CM, Noller KL, O'Fallon WM, et al. Lack of evidence for cancer due to use of metronidazole. New England Journal of Medicine 1979; 301: 519-22
179. Imam N, Carpenter CCJ, Mayer KH, et al. Hierarchical pattern of mucosal candida infections in HIV-seropositive women. American Journal of Medicine 1990; 89: 142-6
180. Lossick JG. Treatment of sexually transmitted vaginosis/vaginitis. Reviews of Infectious Diseases 1990; 12 Suppl. 6: S665-81
181. Mertz GJ. Genital herpes simplex virus infections. Medical Clinics of North America 1990; 74: 1433-54
182. Corey L, McCutchan JA, Ronald AR, et al. Evaluation of new anti-infective drugs for the treatment of genital infection due to herpes simplex virus. Clinical Infectious Diseases 1992; 15 Suppl. 1: S99-107
183. Stone KM, Whittington WL. Treatment of genital herpes. Reviews of Infectious Diseases 1990; 12 Suppl. 6: S610-9
184. Bryson YJ, Dillon M, Lovett M, et al. Treatment of first episodes of genital herpes simplex virus infection with oral acyclovir: a randomized double-blind controlled study in normal subjects. New England Journal of Medicine 1983; 308: 916-21
185. Douglas JM, Critchlow C, Benedetti J, et al. A double-blind study of oral acyclovir for suppression of recurrence of genital herpes simplex infection. New England Journal of Medicine 1984; 310: 1551-6
186. Hook III EW, Cannon RO, Nahmias AJ, et al. Herpes simplex virus infection as a risk factor for human immunodeficiency virus infection in heterosexuals. Journal of Infectious Diseases 1992; 165: 251-5
187. Schafer A, Friedmann W, Mielke M, et al. The increased frequency of cervical dysplasia-neoplasia in women infected with the human immunodeficiency virus is related to the degree of immunosuppression. American Journal of Obstetrics and Gynecology 1991; 164: 593-9
188. Vermund SH, Kelley KF, Klein RS, et al. High risk of human papillomavirus infection and cervical squamous intraepithelial lesions among women with symptomatic human immunodeficiency virus infection. American Journal of Obstetrics and Gynecology 1991; 165: 392-400
189. Brown DR, Fife KH. Human papillomavirus infections of the genital tract. Medical Clinics of North America 1990; 74: 1455-85
190. Kraus SJ, Stone KM. Management of genital infection caused by human papillomavirus. Reviews of Infectious Diseases 1990; 12 Suppl. 6: S620-32
191. Billstein SA, Mattaliano Jr VJ. The 'nuisance' sexually transmitted diseases: molluscum contagiosum, scabies, and crab lice. Medical Clinics of North America 1990; 74: 1487-505
192. Pepin J, Plummer FA, Brunham RC, et al. The interaction of HIV infection and other sexually transmitted diseases: an opportunity for intervention. AIDS 1989; 3: 3-9
193. Plourde PJ, Pepin J, Agoki E, et al. Human immunodeficiency virus type 1 seroconversion in women with genital ulcers. Journal of Infectious Diseases 1994; 170: 313-7
194. Wasserheit JM. Epidemiological synergy: interrelationships between human immunodeficiency virus infection and other sexually transmitted diseases. Sexually Transmitted Diseases 1992; 19: 61-71
195. Schmid GP. Treatment of chancroid, 1989. Reviews of Infectious Diseases 1990; 12 Suppl. 6: S580-9
196. Toomey KE, Moran JS, Rafferty MP, et al. Epidemiological considerations of sexually transmitted diseases in underserved populations. Infectious Disease Clinics of North America 1993; 7: 739-52
197. Cates Jr W. The 'other STDs': do they really matter? Journal of the American Medical Association 1988; 259: 3606-8
198. Cates Jr W, Stone KM. Family planning, sexually transmitted diseases and contraceptive choice: a literature update - part 1. Family Planning Perspectives 1992; 24: 75-84
199. Centers for Disease Control and Prevention. Update: barrier protection against HIV infection and other sexually transmitted diseases. Morbidity and Mortality Weekly Report 1993; 42: 589-97
200. Rosenberg MJ, Holmes KK, and the WHO Working Group on Virucides. Virucides in prevention of HIV infection: research priorities. Sexually Transmitted Diseases 1993; 20: 41-4
201. Stratton P, Alexander NJ. Prevention of sexually transmitted infections: physical and chemical barrier methods. Infectious Disease Clinics of North America 1993; 7: 841-59
202. Weller SC. A meta-analysis of condom effectiveness in reducing sexually transmitted HIV. Social Science and Medicine 1993; 36: 1635-44
203. Jaffe HW, Rice DT, Voigt R, et al. Selective mass treatment in a venereal disease control program. American Journal of Public Health 1979; 69: 1181-2
204. Potterat JJ, Rothenberg R, Bross DC. Gonorrhea in street prostitutes: epidemiology and legal implications. Sexually Transmitted Diseases 1979; 6(2): 58-63
205. Beam Jr TR, Gilbert DN, Kunin CM. General guidelines for the clinical evaluation of anti-infective drug products. Clinical Infectious Diseases 1992; 15 Suppl. 1: S5-32
206. Handsfield HH, McCutchan JA, Corey L, et al. Special issues in clinical trial of new anti-infective drugs for the treatment of sexually transmitted diseases. Clinical Infectious Diseases 1992; 15 Suppl. 1: S96-8

207. Handsfield HH, Ronald AR, Corey L, et al. Evaluation of new anti-infective drugs for the treatment of sexually transmitted chlamydial infections and related clinical syndromes. Clinical Infectious Diseases 1992; 15 Suppl. 1: S131-9
208. McCutchan JA, Ronald AR, Corey L, et al. Evaluation of new anti-infectives for the treatment of vaginal infections. Clinical Infectious Diseases 1992; 15 Suppl. 1: S115-22
209. Ronald AR, Corey L, McCutchan JA, et al. Evaluation of new anti-infective drugs for the treatment of chancroid. Clinical Infectious Diseases 1992; 15 Suppl. 1: S108-14
210. Brunham RC. The concept of core and its relevance to the epidemiology and control of sexually transmitted diseases. Sexually Transmitted Diseases 1991; 18: 67-8
211. Brunham RC, Plummer FA. A general model of sexually transmitted disease epidemiology and its implications for control. Medical Clinics of North America 1990; 74: 1339-51
212. Connor EM, Sperling RS, Gelber R, et al. Reduction of maternal-infant transmission of human immunodeficiency virus type 1 with zidovudine treatment. New England Journal of Medicine 1994; 331: 1173-80

Chapter 34

# Diseases of a Tropical Environment

*K. Krishnaswamy*

## Synopsis of Important Principles

1) Although modern drugs have contributed to improved health standards in tropical countries, because of other closely linked detrimental environmental factors, tropical diseases and the problems associated with them continue to pose an increasing threat to human welfare.

2) Dosages of drugs based on Western populations may not be appropriate for use in tropical countries because of differences in genetic profiles, bodyweight, nutritional status and environments in which peoples of a tropical country are placed. Of all factors that influence drug response in a tropical environment, nutrition is probably the most important.

3) Diet accounts for a considerable proportion of inter- and intraindividual variability. Drug dosages may have to be altered depending on the nutritional status of an individual, the type of nutrient deficiency (proteins, calories, vitamins, minerals or trace metals), and the extent of change in pharmacokinetics of a drug.

4) The interplay between malnutrition and infection is of considerable importance in developing countries, one leading to the other through a vicious cycle. Malnourished children are particularly susceptible to infectious diseases; tuberculosis and pertussis, for example, are common and occur at an earlier age, and measles is much more severe in children in tropical countries than in well-nourished children living in a Western environment.

5) Better drugs are needed to treat tropical diseases, but control or eradication of these diseases will only result from measures such as vector control, immunisation and improvement in public health and sanitation practices.

6) The choice of an appropriate drug regimen in a tropical country to control diseases such as tuberculosis, leprosy and malaria is not only determined by each country's financial and personnel resources, but also by studying the factors in a given population that influence drug response and the infrastructure available for healthcare.

7) Nutritional deficiency disorders encountered in developing countries require appropriate therapy. Food fortification such as iodine- and iron-fortified salt to prevent goitre and anaemia, and supplementation of nutrients such as intermittent large doses of retinol (vitamin A) to prevent blindness in children, and iron and folate to prevent nutritional anaemias in pregnant women, are some of the major programmes currently being undertaken by governments in these countries.

8) Glucose-6-phosphate dehydrogenase (G6PD) deficiency is common and severe in a number of ethnic groups in tropical countries and should be excluded before certain drugs are given [e.g. primaquine, dapsone, sulfonamides, cotrimoxazole (trimethoprim/sulfamethoxazole), nitrofurantoin]. Folate deficiency is common in tropical countries and drugs that impair folate metabolism (e.g. pyrimethamine, cotrimoxazole) should be given with caution in patients with folate deficiency or folate-deficient diets.

9) It is important to consider the effects of drugs on nutrients since large segments of populations are deficient in a number of nutrients. Nutritional status must be evaluated, particularly in relation to specific nutrients depleted by long term usage of antituberculosis, antiepileptic and antifolate agents, and hormonal contraceptives.

The importance of geographical and environmental factors in determining the prevalence, incidence, progress, recovery and relapse of tropical diseases are well recognised. However, to tackle the health problems and lessen the burden of diseases in overpopulated, overcrowded, poorly developed and economically poor countries, a multidisciplinary approach is needed. Measurement of health needs in the tropics is beset with problems. Although enough is known about the nature of the problem, quantitative data about its extent are not always available. Health problems and diseases in the tropics are closely linked with social and economic structures, culture and religion, food production and distribution, and factors such as unhygienic surroundings, illiteracy, overpopulation, and the lack of transportation and communication facilities. Health resources in underprivileged countries are difficult to compare with those in well developed countries and are certainly inadequate with respect to the health needs of the population.

The World Health Organization recommends that a minimum of 7% of the GDP be allocated towards public health expenditure. However, several developing countries are unable to achieve this level of expenditure. For example, India spends only 0.8 to 1% of GDP on public health, whereas Brazil spends 0.5%, Mexico 0.4% and Turkey 0.3% of GDP on public health.

Medical practice in developing areas has involved some crude extracts, powders and juices from animal, plant and other sources. Even today, the practice of traditional medicine continues in many parts. For example, in Sri Lanka, India, China and Japan, professional education and practice have been adapted to indigenous medical traditions. The WHO recommends that traditional medicines continue to form a part of healthcare in these countries. However, there are very few guidelines to assist in assessment of the quality, safety or effectiveness of traditional therapies, and there is little regulatory control of the use of these therapies.

Advances in physiology, chemistry, biochemistry and other related disciplines, an increase in world travel, and infiltration of Western medicine have brought modern pharmacology to the tropics. Although the flow of drugs has been large and has greatly contributed towards improved health standards, due to other closely linked detrimental factors, tropical diseases and the problems associated with them continue to pose a threat to human welfare. For example, due to multidrug-resistant microbes and parasites, several tropical diseases such as malaria, trypanosomiasis, schistosomiasis, leishmaniasis, leprosy and tuberculosis are still prevalent today despite the use of modern medicines. The advent of acquired immune deficiency syndrome (AIDS) has clearly compounded the problem.

Nevertheless, morbidity and mortality arising from tropical diseases is on the decline in most countries. The marked improvement in health standards is due to some extent to disease-controlling drugs made available by local governmental organisations and by the support of international organisations.

## 1. Drugs and Developing Countries

Prescription of drugs in tropical and underdeveloped countries is determined to a large extent by factors such as the existence and development of a local pharmaceutical industry, the availability and cost of drugs, the production and distribution of medicines in rural and urban health centres, the purchasing power of the community, the health structure itself, and the availability of healthcare and related programmes.

### 1.1 Development of Pharmaceuticals

With the advent of modern medicine, drug manufacturing facilities are being established in many countries and, with the help of foreign collaborations, bulk drugs are produced from raw materials available in the country. India, for example, is a major drug-producing nation in the third world and has around 6000 licensed drug manufacturing units. These include multinational, private sector and public sector organisations involved in the production of drugs and dosage forms. Research, development and available technological facilities in the drug industry affect the cost of drugs in developing countries.

Research and development are crucial for growth and development of drugs to combat diseases. The world average outlay on research and development is 12% of drug sales, but it is only 2% in India and much less in other countries such as Bangladesh, Pakistan and Thailand. In the long term, this is detrimental to local interests and expenditures on drugs will increase further because of the high costs of production and importation.

Despite controls on prices, many drugs are beyond the financial means of the common person, especially in rural areas. In some cases, domestic production of bulk drugs and raw materials may not be sufficient to meet requirements, so that they must be imported. 25 years ago, 90% of requirements were met by imports, whereas current imports account for barely 10% of local production in a country like India. Even so, a number of essential drugs such as antibiotics, antituberculosis and antileprotic drugs, vitamin preparations, etc. must still be imported to meet requirements.

### 1.2 Production and Distribution of Drugs

Drugs manufactured by local industry in the tropics cover a wide therapeutic spectrum. For example, India produces antibiotics, sulfonamides, vitamins, hormones, antihistamines, tranquillisers, anaesthetics, antituberculosis, antileprotic, antimalarial, antidiarrhoeal and antidysentery drugs, analgesics, antipyretics, antidiabetic drugs and vaccines. These drugs are manufactured using mostly indigenous raw materials and chemicals. However, the cost of production of basic and intermediate products are sometimes higher than would be seen in more developed nations, because of inadequate technology. The technology is not modern and, because of a lack of trained personnel or financial resources, and difficulty in transfer of technology, it is not on a par with that seen in developed nations.

The industry in India has built a system of distribution that ensures availability of medicines throughout the country. However, due to the low profits and variable demand, manufacturers often do not produce large enough quantities of essential drugs to meet the requirements. In the 1980s, 25% of total pharmaceutical production in India was of vitamins, tonics, health restoratives and enzyme digestants consumed mostly by the wealthy urban population who generally do not need these drugs.[1] Distribution of medicines is mediated through pharmacists and general merchants holding drugs licences (public and private sector). Despite these developments, the vast rural population (about 70 to 80%) does not receive the full benefits of modern medicine. The organisation of medical stores (equipment, temperature used to safeguard shelf life, accessibility) naturally has a great influence on drug consumption patterns. Pharmacies in rural areas are scarce because of geographical remoteness, the isolated population for which a pharmacy would cater, the low purchasing power of the people, and the absence of trained personnel.

In many tropical countries, a problem exists in that there are too many different drugs and too many brands, but inadequate bulk supplies of essential drugs.[2,3,4] Often, large urban hospitals or patients of doctors with private practices in urban areas receive most of the available drugs.

### 1.3 Consumption of Drugs

Despite the rapid and major advances made in local drug industries in countries such as India, the per capita consumption of medicines is only about Rs14 to 18/year (US$0.4 to 0.7/year), mostly consumed by 20 to 30% of the population. In rural India, per capita drug consumption is only Rs 0.40/year. This contrasts with Rs 100-300/year (US$10 to 30) in developed countries. This pattern is similar to that in other developing countries such as Indonesia, Pakistan, Egypt, Korea, Thailand, Brazil and Mexico. Even doubling the production of drugs will result in a per capita consumption of no more than Rs 12 to 14/year (less than US$2/year) and a population coverage of no more than 40%. However, the projected figure for per capita drug consumption is Rs 76/year, which is based on the estimated total production of drugs.

It is evident that there must be sustained and progressive growth in production and distribution to reach the rural populations. Simultaneously, other health facilities (doctors, hospitals, dispensaries, clinics, rural health centres) and allied services must be developed. However, most tropical diseases are preventable either by chemoprophylaxis, immunisation and/or improvement in environmental sanitation. In rural India, no villages have sanitation facilities and only 10 to 15% have safe drinking water. Hence, although drug production, particularly of essential drugs, may have to be increased in the immediate future, if prevention programmes are successful, drug requirements, consumption and production may be lessened.

### 1.4 Problems Associated With Drug Usage

The pattern of drug consumption in a developing country varies widely within the same country,[5] use of antibacterial and antiparasitic drugs being maximal in district hospitals, while national teaching hospitals spend most drug funds on tranquillisers, sedatives and antidepressants. The majority of drug prescriptions in teaching hospitals are for expensive proprietary preparations. This may not be true if teaching hospitals supply drugs. In some countries, pat-

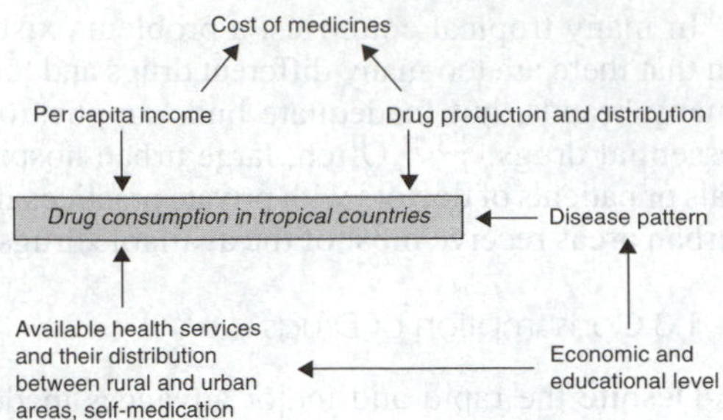


**Fig. 1.** Inter-related factors in drug consumption patterns in tropical countries.

terns of drug consumption may be widely different between high and low income groups and depend on prescribing habits of general practitioners and the purchasing power of individuals.[6] Many surveys have indicated that clinicians prescribing habits in urban environments are often inappropriate and that there is a high self-medication rate, with liberal dispensing of scheduled drugs by pharmacists.[7,8] Also, there is a wide gap between precepts and practices prevailing among clinicians.[9]

Inadequate communication, low standards of medical care, low clinician to population ratios, levels of availability of low-cost drugs, marketing practices, economic status and educational levels all affect drug consumption in developing countries.[6,10] Indiscriminate use of intravenous fluids and inappropriate prescribing of drugs, including excessive demands on drug supplies by medical personnel and their families, also influence drug use in developing countries.[11] Inappropriate use of medicines (e.g. prescription of broad-spectrum antibiotics in inadequate doses),[12] uninhibited sales of potentially toxic analgesics, and use of non-essential vitamin/mineral preparations should be viewed with great caution.[7,8] Such practices may surface as iatrogenic problems in the future. Use of local herbal medicines also contributes to the pattern of drug use, as well as to adverse drug reactions.[13,14]

Figure 1 illustrates factors that affect drug consumption in tropical countries.

## 2. Clinical Pharmacological Considerations

### 2.1 Determinants of Drug Dosages in a Tropical Environment

Drug therapy in tropical countries has a profound influence on health statistics. However, rational use of drugs based on pharmacokinetic and pharmacodynamic studies in these populations is lacking, so drug dosages recommended by textbooks and pharmaceutical manufacturers are followed. Most of these regimens are standardised for Western populations that are genetically different and located in a different environment. Populations differ widely in physiological and/or biochemical constitution. The genetic profile, bodyweight, nutritional status and environment are 4 major factors that have a direct bearing on drug dosages (table I). The inter-relation of these factors as they affect drug action is shown in figure 2.

#### *2.1.1 Genetic Profile*

The literature is replete with evidence that genetic factors profoundly influence drug metabolism, efficacy and toxicity.[15] It has been estimated that about a third of known enzymes in the human system exist in a polymorphic form and 2 or more variants of each enzyme are recognised. Polymorphic acetylation of drugs like isoniazid and dapsone may determine not only the clinical response, but also the likelihood of toxicity (see further chapter 1; sect. 5.2.1). Isoniazid is the most effective and widely used antituberculosis drug in Asia, Africa and South America. There are large interindividual differences in the rates of isoniazid metabolism. Meticulously controlled clinical trials have indicated that the clinical response is identical between individuals with different capacities to acetylate isoniazid, provided the drug is given on a daily basis. However, once-weekly treatment in rapid acetylators is inadequate as compared with slow acetylators.[16] On the other hand, the development of some toxic effects such as peripheral neuropathy with isoniazid appears to be more common in slow acetylators of the drug.

Polymorphism in the rate of oxidation of a number of drugs, including debrisoquine, has been demonstrated in some populations. While the incidence of the poor metaboliser phenotype appears to be low (less than 2%) in Egyptians and Saudi Arabians, in Nigerians and Ghanaians the incidence is similar to that in Europeans (between 5 and 10%) [see further chapter 1; sect. 5.2.2]. As yet, information on the incidence of this polymorphism in different ethnic groups and also on its significance in clinical practice is far from complete, but it may account for the significant interindividual variation in steady-state plasma concentrations observed

**Table I.** Determinants of drug dosages in tropical countries

| |
|---|
| Genetic profile |
| Bodyweight |
| Nutritional status and dietary habits |
| Tropical environment: |
| • Climatic factors |
| • Infections and infestations |
| • Environmental pollutants (e.g. mycotoxins and other food poisons) |

with some of these drugs. In the case of perhexiline, the incidence of peripheral neuropathy may be increased in individuals who are poor metabolisers of the drug.

Toxic reactions to drugs due to genetic variation may be encountered in certain populations. One of the best known and most common examples is enzyme deficiency of glucose-6-phosphate dehydrogenase (G6PD). Different types of G6PD deficiency predominate in different ethnic groups.[17] The use of the antimalarial drug primaquine, even in therapeutic doses, can precipitate haematological abnormalities. In Africans, usually a mild deficiency (enzyme activity 8 to 20% of normal) is encountered, whereas in Mediterranean regions, the deficiency is severe (zero to 4% enzyme activity). A number of variants have been described in East and Southeast Asia and it is likely that at least some of these may be as severe as the Mediterranean types.

The incidence of haemolytic episodes varies in different ethnic groups. Several drugs, such as the sulfonamides and sulfones, dapsone, phenacetin, furazolidone, nitrofurantoin, etc., can precipitate significant haemolysis if used for a long duration. Indigenous drugs may also cause haemolysis. For example, in Singapore, the herb 'Chuan Lian' (*Coptis teeta*) is a potent haemolytic agent in G6PD-deficient infants, with resultant brain damage due to kernicterus. Similarly, naphthalene from moth balls may cause haemolysis in enzyme-deficient neonates clothed with apparel stored in drawers containing moth balls.[14] Fava beans, which are widely consumed in Southeast Asia, are also a well known trigger of acute haemolysis, the oxidant alkaloid varying in concentration depending on the time the bean is harvested and its mode of preparation.

The effect of drugs in populations at risk will be determined by factors like sex of the patient, severity of G6PD deficiency, the need for the drug and duration of therapy, and the presence of other factors such as infections that can also precipitate haemolysis in enzyme-deficient individuals. Drug-induced cyanosis and hereditary methaemoglobinaemia (for methaemoglobin-forming drugs such as dapsone, primaquine and chloroquine) are also important genetically-determined drug reactions.[18]

Other genetic abnormalities with varying modes of inheritance are prevalent in some developing countries. Most studies are of hospitalised patients who have experienced adverse reactions, so it is not possible to identify groups that are more prone to such disorders. There have been reports of prolonged suxamethonium (succinylcholine) apnoea in individuals with low plasma cholinesterase concentrations. For

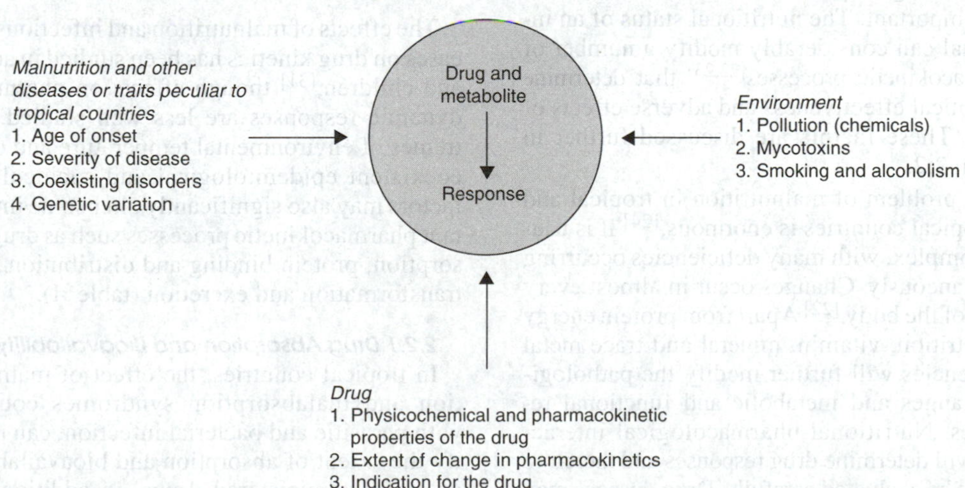


**Fig. 2.** Factors determining drug response (therapeutic and toxic) in a tropical environment.

example, in a specific community of India (Vaishyas) the plasma cholinesterase concentrations are low, hence doses of suxamethonium must be decreased. It has also been reported that extensive metabolisers of drugs (e.g. debrisoquine) that are metabolised by oxidation may be more prone to certain cancers in African countries.[19]

#### 2.1.2 Bodyweight

Many studies of drugs have established doses on the basis of an average bodyweight of 70kg. These doses are often extrapolated to other populations, usually following absolute doses without considering changes in average bodyweight. Since the mean weight of an adult in developing countries is about 55kg, most Asians, for example, receive about 30% more drug per dose when dosages are based on recommendations for populations in developed countries.[20] This problem may be more acute in children, since the dosage of many drugs is based on age. For the same age, bodyweight and growth patterns are entirely different in developed countries and developing nations.[21] Thus, drug dosages should be recommended on a bodyweight basis, rather than on the basis of age or an absolute fixed quantity. In India, for example, rifampicin dosages are reduced from 600 to 450mg because mean bodyweights are between 45 and 55kg, or the dose can be calculated as 10 mg/kg.

#### 2.1.3 Nutritional Status

Of all the environmental factors that may influence drug response, nutrition is one of the most important. The nutritional status of an individual can considerably modify a number of pharmacokinetic processes[22,23] that determine the clinical effectiveness and adverse effects of drugs. These factors are discussed further in section 2.2.

The problem of malnutrition in tropical and subtropical countries is enormous.[24] It is usually complex, with many deficiencies occurring simultaneously. Changes occur in almost every organ of the body.[22] Apart from protein energy malnutrition, vitamin, mineral and trace metal deficiencies will further modify the pathological changes and metabolic and functional responses. Nutritional-pharmacological interactions will determine drug responses and therefore have to be evaluated carefully. Drug dosages may have to be altered depending on the nutritional status, the type of nutrient deficiency, and the extent of change in the pharmacokinetics of a drug.[25]

#### 2.1.4 Environment

Some factors that determine the metabolism of and response to drugs are related to the physical and chemical environment.[26] Higher altitudes have been shown to alter drug responses. For example, impairment in performance due to the antihistamine chlorpheniramine (chlorphenamine) increases as a function of increasing altitude.[27] Light has also been shown to modify metabolism and the response to drugs,[28] and relative humidity in an environment can alter phototoxic responses to topically applied drugs.[29]

Changes in ambient temperature have a pronounced effect on the toxicity of drugs. For example, griseofulvin concentrations in the skin are higher in summer than in winter months.[30] Therefore, it seems likely that in extreme weather conditions, such as those experienced in tropical and subtropical areas, drug distribution, phototoxicity and metabolic disposition may be altered by climatic factors. Further, epidemiological differences in disease pattern, intestinal microflora, atmospheric contamination and mycotoxins may be associated with changes in drug response. However, while the need for systematic studies of drug response in relation to the physical and chemical environment, particularly in tropical countries, has been recognised for years, these studies have yet to be undertaken.

### 2.2 Pharmacokinetic Processes Influenced by a Tropical Environment

The effects of malnutrition and infectious diseases on drug kinetics has been studied in adults and children,[31] though effects on pharmacodynamic responses are less well studied. Extremes of environmental temperature and other coexistent epidemiological and sociocultural factors may also significantly alter some important pharmacokinetic processes such as drug absorption, protein binding and distribution, biotransformation and excretion (table II).

#### 2.2.1 Drug Absorption and Bioavailability

In tropical countries, the effect of malnutrition and malabsorption syndromes coupled with parasitic and bacterial infection, can modify the extent of absorption and bioavailability of orally administered drugs. In addition, the gastrointestinal tract, both histologically and functionally, is said to be different in a tropical

**Table II.** Processes likely to be altered by malnutrition, infection and the environment

| |
|---|
| Absorption of drugs |
| Binding and distribution of drugs |
| Excretion of drugs (biliary, renal) |
| Tissue uptake, localisation and response to drugs (drug-receptor interaction) |

environment (see Rosenberg & Scrimshaw).[32] Atrophic changes in the villus membrane occur due to malnutrition, infection and infestation, which are frequent in tropical countries. Studies with antibiotics such as tetracycline and rifampicin have indicated that there is a defect in the absorption of such drugs in malnutrition.[23] Therefore, the absorption of nutrients and drugs is altered. The extent of tetracycline and rifampicin absorption is reduced. Tetracycline absorption was quantified using intravenous and oral preparations,[33] while urinary excretion was used as an index of absorption for rifampicin.[34] Further absorption studies should be undertaken, particularly in the presence of parasitic and bacterial infections.

### 2.2.2 Drug Protein Binding and Distribution

Protein-energy malnutrition alters plasma and tissue proteins quantitatively and probably also qualitatively. The rate of albumin synthesis is directly related to the level of protein intake and amino acid supply, and the profile of plasma proteins (albumin, globulins and other carrier proteins) is altered in protein-energy malnutrition. Similarly, glycoproteins, particularly $\alpha_1$-acid glycoprotein which transports basic drugs (see chapter 1; sect. 3.2), are also altered in malnutrition.[35] Studies have shown that the protein binding of a number of drugs such as salicylate, warfarin, digoxin and thiopental is altered in malnourished children.[36] However, the clinical implications, particularly in actual clinical use situations, have yet to be evaluated in most cases.

In other studies, the tissue uptake of tetracycline has been shown to be poor in under-nutrition.[37] In febrile conditions, cardiovascular changes associated with fever result in lower gentamicin plasma concentrations, owing to a shift of the drug from plasma to other body fluid compartments.[38] This may result in therapeutic failure.

### 2.2.3 Drug Biotransformation

Most drugs are metabolised in the liver by metabolising enzymes present in the microsomal, mitochondrial and soluble fractions. The therapeutic effectiveness and toxicity of many drugs are closely related to the rate of metabolism by the liver.

The implications of liver disease for drug therapy are discussed in chapter 22 (sect. 12.4) and appendix F, so only those conditions common to tropical countries are elaborated here. These may be broadly divided into 4 groups:

1. Malnutrition
2. Parasitic infestation
3. Liver injury due to mycotoxins
4. Cirrhosis and/or malignancy.

Malnutrition is a major public health problem in tropical countries. Fatty infiltration with impaired synthesis of lipoproteins is a characteristic feature of severe protein-calorie malnutrition.[22] Most commonly, however, only liver vacuolation is encountered. Involvement of the endoplasmic reticulum is a feature in protein-energy malnutrition. Thus, it is important to evaluate whether such changes impair the mixed-function oxidases involved in drug metabolism.

Table III summarises studies in children and adults in developing countries such as India and Africa where varying grades of malnutrition are encountered. Studies in adults using drugs such as antipyretic/analgesics, antibacterial, antimalarial and antituberculosis drugs, and oral contraceptives[25] indicate that in mild and moderate forms of malnutrition, drug biotransformation is enhanced and excretion by the kidney is more rapid, thus decreasing steady-state drug concentrations to levels that may lead to therapeutic failure. However, in most studies, only total drug clearance values are documented. The clearance of phenazone, a substance which is not protein bound, is elevated in mild and moderate forms of malnutrition and decreased in severe malnutrition in adults.[43] However, studies in severe protein-energy malnutrition in children[40,42] show that clearances are decreased and accumulation of some drugs may occur, requiring alterations in dosage schedules to avoid toxicity. For example, in kwashiorkor, the clearance of chloramphenicol, sulfadiazine, phenazone and several other antibiotics is decreased. Deficiencies of micronutrients such as zinc and ascorbic acid (vitamin C) may also decrease drug metabolism, whereas iron and thiamine (vitamin $B_1$) deficiency may accelerate metabolism.[44,45]

The field of nutritional-pharmacological interactions is a relatively young area of science and only recently have nutritionists in many

**Table III.** Influence of nutritional disorders and dietary changes on drug clearance in people from developing countries (after Anderson;[39] Buchanan;[40] Krishnaswamy;[31,41] Mehta[42])

| Drugs | Nutritional status/condition | Effect on drug clearance | % Change |
|---|---|---|---|
| **1. Children** | | | |
| *Analgesics/antipyretics:* | | | |
| Phenazone (antipyrine) | Kwashiorkor | Decreased | 46[a] |
| | Less than 75% of normal weight for age | Decreased | 30[a] |
| *Antibacterial drugs:* | | | |
| Cefoxitin | Kwashiorkor | Decreased | 28[a] |
| Chloramphenicol | Less than 60% of normal weight for age | Decreased | 27[b] |
| Benzylpenicillin (penicillin G) | Kwashiorkor | Decreased | 36[a] |
| Gentamicin | Kwashiorkor | Decreased | 55[a] |
| Sulfadiazine | Less than 60% of normal weight for age | Decreased | 47[c] |
| *Antituberculosis drugs:* | | | |
| Isoniazid | Kwashiorkor | Decreased | 62[a] |
| *Other drugs:* | | | |
| Chloroquine | Kwashiorkor | Decreased | 19[b,c] |
| **2. Adults** | | | |
| *Analgesic/antipyretics:* | | | |
| Phenazone (antipyrine)[b] | Undernutrition | Increased | 6[b] |
| | Nutritional oedema | Decreased | 21[b] |
| | Low protein diet | Decreased | 32[b,e] |
| | High protein diet | Increased | 46[b,e] |
| | Charcoal broiled beef | Increased | 38 |
| *β-Adrenoceptor blocking drugs:* | | | |
| Propranolol | High protein diet | Increased | 60[e] |
| | High carbohydrate diet | Decreased | 37[e] |
| *Antibacterial drugs:* | | | |
| Tetracyclines | Undernutrition | Increased | 45[b] |
| | Nutritional oedema | Decreased | 43[b] |
| Sulfadiazine | Undernutrition | Increased | 41[b] |
| *Antituberculosis drugs:* | | | |
| Rifampicin (rifampin) | Undernutrition | Increased | 63[b] |
| *Antimalarial drugs:* | | | |
| Chloroquine | Undernutrition | Increased | 60[b] |
| *Nonsteroidal anti-inflammatory drugs:* | | | |
| Phenylbutazone | Undernutrition | Increased | 62[b] |
| *Bronchodilator drugs:* | | | |
| Theophylline | High protein diet | Increased | 28[e] |
| | Low protein diet | Decreased | 22[e] |
| | Charcoal broiled beef | Increased | 32 |

a Comparisons between before and after rehabilitation.
b Comparisons between normal and malnutrition.
c Based on urinary excretion of acetylated drug.
d Based on renal clearance.
e Compared with high carbohydrate/low protein diet and *vice versa*.

countries become aware of such interactions.[46] Metabolic studies involving alterations in dietary macronutrients indicate that a protein diet increases the clearance of drugs, whether caloric intake is low or high.[47,48] However, protein intake must contribute 20 to 50% of energy; a high carbohydrate intake associated with low protein intake decreases drug clearance. Very low calorie intake, even if the protein intake is around 10% of total energy, leads to decreased drug clearance, which is similar to the finding in severely malnourished individuals. On a carbohydrate intake of 59 to 63% and protein intake of 5% of total energy, clearance decreased by 33% from that seen with 15% protein intake and by 24% from that seen with 10% protein intake. In other studies, induction of drug metabolism has been observed with substances such as brussels sprouts, cabbage and charcoal broiled beef in the diet.[49] These findings indicate that drug therapy in malnourished patients must be based on the severity of the nutritional state, the presence of coexisting nutritional disorders and infection, and on common dietary practices that may induce or inhibit drug metabolism.

The relationship between malnutrition and liver diseases has been overemphasised;[50] several studies have shown that there is no cause and effect relationship.[51,52] However, cirrhosis of the liver is commonly encountered in adults in the tropics, and childhood cirrhosis and idiopathic portal hypertension predominate in certain areas. Naturally occurring hepatotoxins (especially aflatoxin), as well as viral hepatitis and probably a host of other unknown factors, may be causally related to liver dysfunction, particularly in relation to drug biotransformation. Hepatic blood flow and hepatic extraction of drugs may also be different in such conditions.

Haemochromatosis, parasitic diseases with liver involvement (amoebiasis, leishmaniasis, schistosomiasis and yellow fever may also considerably modify drug metabolism, depending on the duration and degree of infection and concomitant pathological changes. In *Schistosoma mansoni* infection, portal systemic vascular shunts can develop through which drugs can initially bypass the liver. In such cases, oral bioavailability of highly extracted drugs such as niridazole will be markedly increased.[53]

The prevalence of primary hepatic carcinoma is highest in Africa. Mycotoxins, particularly aflatoxin, and its association with malignancy has been repeatedly stressed. Aflatoxin itself is metabolised by liver enzymes and has an inhibitory effect on carcinogen metabolism.[54] The effects on drug and xenobiotic metabolism will obviously be determined by factors such as the amount and duration of exposure and the individual's inherent capacity to eliminate the toxin.

#### *2.2.4 Excretion*

Tropical disease can result in kidney involvement (renal lithiasis) and has the potential to interfere with glomerular filtration, tubular secretion and reabsorption of drugs eliminated by renal mechanisms – depending on the protein binding of the drug, renal plasma flow, urinary pH and the extent of tubular involvement (reabsorption). *Schistosoma haematobium* infection for example, is often complicated by abnormal kidney function. Some drugs used to treat schistosomiasis, such as antimonials, are eliminated mostly unchanged in the urine, necessitating assessment of renal function and great care with dosage. Further, on high protein diets, renal clearance of drugs is faster than on low protein diets.[55]

### 2.3 Altered Tissue Responsiveness to Drugs in Tropical Environments

A difficult area of study in clinical pharmacology is the quantification of drug effects in relation to plasma concentrations so as to indicate tissue uptake and response to a drug. The clinical response is determined by a number of factors and hence objective methods of evaluation must be developed for each drug before the tissue response can be discussed. However, studies have indicated that the disposition of drugs can be altered by factors such as infection and pyrexia.

Influenza A and adenovirus infection have been shown to increase the risk of toxicity with theophylline during the acute stages.[56]

The antihypertensive response to propranolol seems to be lower in Kenyan patients, particularly in the present of severe undernutrition.[57] Similarly, some Black patients require higher doses of prazosin to control blood pressure than do Caucasian patients,[58,59] probably indicating a higher tissue requirement. Such isolated studies indicate an altered tissue response that may not necessarily be accompanied by changes in pharmacokinetics. More recent studies of theophylline and lung function in malnutrition indicate that pharmacodynamic responses to this drug are decreased in malnourished individuals.

Nutritional status is also an important determinant of drug toxicity. Anthracycline chemotherapy is more frequently associated with cardiomyopathy in malnourished than in normal children.[60] In very severe protein deficiencies in experimental animals,[61] a decrease in toxic reactions was noted with xenobiotics with metabolites that are more toxic than the parent compound. However, in mild and moderate forms of malnutrition, where the enzyme systems are intact and metabolism is normal or increased, toxicity reactions were found to be greater. There are little human data about toxicity of drugs in nutritional disorders. However, in general, it can be stated that tissue sensitivity and toxic responses are likely to vary depending on the severity of the nutritional deficiency and the chemical nature of the metabolite toxicity. Hepatic injury due to paracetamol (acetaminophen) has been shown to be less severe in anorexia nervosa patients.[62] In children receiving theophylline, better therapeutic responses were observed when they received a very low protein diet (3% protein energy).[63]

The incidence of pre-eclampsia and eclampsia is higher in undernourished pregnant women. When drugs such as diuretics and diazepam are given, the outcome of pregnancy, in terms of prematurity and prenatal deaths, is higher in this group than in their healthy counterparts.[64]

## 3. Vitamin Deficiencies

### 3.1 Vitamin A (Retinol) Deficiency

Human vitamin A (retinol) deficiency has a global distribution and is one of the most important aetiological factors contributing to preventable blindness, particularly in young children in all developing countries. Inadequate intake of retinol is the primary cause of the widespread prevalence of retinol deficiency. Dietary intake of retinol in general is inadequate in all segments of the population among the poor communities and therefore infants born to mothers with low intakes have relatively low hepatic reserves. These infants further develop a deficiency due to low concentrations of retinol in breastmilk. In addition, infection impairs retinol absorption. Retinol deficiency is more commonly associated with protein-calorie malnutrition, which is much more widely prevalent. Conjunctival xerosis, bitot spots, and night blindness are the commonly encountered signs. Corneal involvement (keratomalacia) is the final stage of xerophthalmia and is often associated with protein-energy malnutrition and infection.[65]

#### Optimum Treatment

Retinol, being a fat-soluble vitamin, is stored in the liver. It is administered both orally and parenterally for therapeutic effect. However, intramuscular administration of oily retinol 1000IU (30,000μg) failed to increase serum retinol concentrations in children with protein-energy malnutrition.[66] In contrast, a single intramuscular injection of water-miscible retinol resulted in a rapid and striking increase in serum retinol concentrations, and rapid clinical improvement.[67] Corneal xerosis improves and vision is normalised within a few days after administration. Conjunctival lesions and night blindness respond to a dosage of 1000μg daily for a week. However, in severe cases involving the cornea, water miscible parenteral preparations are indicated, since many children have associated gastroenteritis. Corneal involvement also requires local treatment with antibiotics to prevent and control secondary infection.

#### Prevention and Prophylaxis

Since inadequate dietary intake of retinol (both preformed and provitamin) is the major aetiological factor, the most rational approach for control and prevention is to improve the diet. Consumption of inexpensive and rich sources of β-carotene (a retinol precursor) such as green leafy vegetables should be encouraged in the population. This, however, involves nutrition education and at present may be considered as a long term approach.

Since retinol can be stored in the body, massive doses (i.e. 2000IU or 60,000μg) can be administered at infrequent intervals for a prolonged effect. With such doses, more than 50% is retained in the body[68] and significant concentrations of serum retinol are maintained for nearly 6 months.[67] Results of a massive dose programme in India (60,000μg retinol orally twice a year) indicate a significant reduction in the incidence of xerophthalmia.[69,70] Such programmes are also being implemented on a large scale in other countries like Indonesia, Thailand and Bangladesh.

### 3.2 Vitamin D Deficiency

The role of vitamin D in calcium transport from the intestine and in bone metabolism has long been known. Clinical manifestations and pathology of vitamin D deficiency in humans are confined to the skeletal and muscular systems. Rickets and osteomalacia are disorders of phosphorus and calcium metabolism, characterised by defective mineralisation and resulting in bending and distortion of bones, skeletal deformities and tetanic spasms of muscles. Dietary deficiency, defective absorption, liver abnormalities and renal defects can lead to vitamin D deficiency. Vitamin D resistant rickets due to a genetically determined metabolic abnormality has also been described. Vitamin D deficiency occurs in overcrowded localities with limited exposure to sunlight and in women who practice the habit of covering the entire body with cloth.

Cholecalciferol (vitamin $D_3$) synthesised in the skin is converted to 25-hydroxycholecalciferol (calcifediol) in the liver, which is then further hydroxylated in the kidney to the active hormone 1α,25-dihydroxycholecalciferol (calcitriol). Calciferol (vitamin $D_2$) from the diet is metabolised in an identical manner. 1α,25-Dihydroxycholecalciferol is necessary for the synthesis of a (binding) protein in the intestine which is responsible for calcium absorption.[71]

**Optimum Treatment**

Vitamin D may be administered orally or parenterally. Oral administration is effective as a cure of rickets. Daily administration of calciferol (vitamin $D_2$) 1500 to 5000IU will produce healing, demonstrable on x-ray, within 2 to 4 weeks. Parenteral administration is indicated in cases of malabsorption. Massive doses of calciferol (600,000IU) in 2 or 3 divided doses at fortnightly intervals have also been tried in the cure of rickets.

Although calciferol is a good therapeutic agent for dietary deficiency, in cases of chronic liver disease and renal failure, the biologically active metabolites of vitamin D are more beneficial. Direct administration of the vitamin D metabolites 25-hydroxycholecalciferol (calcifediol) or 1α,25-dihydroxycholecalciferol (calcitriol) will also help treat rickets and osteomalacia resistant to calciferol. The more readily synthesised 1α-hydroxycholecalciferol (alfacalcidol) [1 to 2 μg/day], an analogue of calcitriol, and calcitriol itself (1 to 1.5 μg/day) are commonly used to promote calcium absorption, particularly in the osteodystrophy of chronic renal failure (see also chapter 24; sect. 7.1.2).[72,73]

## 3.3 Vitamin B Complex Deficiencies

Vitamin B complex deficiency diseases such as beri beri, pellagra, orolingual lesions, peripheral neuropathy and central nervous system manifestations contribute significantly towards morbidity among the poorer segments of populations of developing countries. The prevalence of clinical and subclinical deficiency of these vitamins is high, particularly in vulnerable groups such as pregnant and lactating women, children of growing age and adolescents. Clinical symptoms such as neurological manifestations, with or without oral lesions, are often encountered in adults. The main causes of vitamin B complex deficiency disorders are inadequate intake, malabsorption, excessive requirement during physiological stress (pregnancy, fever), increased excretion due to tissue depletion as a result of diseases and drugs, and, rarely, due to defective utilisation of the vitamin.

### *3.3.1 Thiamine (Vitamin $B_1$) Deficiency*

The severe forms of thiamine (aneurine or vitamin $B_1$) deficiency leads to beri beri, which has diverse manifestations. It may present as cardiac beri beri (acute and chronic forms), atrophic beri beri or polyneuritis, infantile beri beri, Wernicke's encephalopathy, and/or Korsakoff's psychosis. The disease is encountered commonly in rice-eating populations of Southeast Asian countries and in patients with chronic alcoholism.

Thiamine is absorbed from the upper small intestine by a specialised saturable transport process. Oral doses above 2.5mg appear to be largely unabsorbed.[74]

The capacity to retain thiamine is also low. Alcoholism and concomitant folate deficiency decrease thiamine absorption. Although both thiamine and riboflavin are absorbed by saturable intestinal transport mechanisms, the 2 vitamins do not share a common specialised absorption pathway.[75] Certain thiamine derivatives (thiamine allyl disulfide, thiamine propyl disulfide, *S*-diacetyl thiamine, dibenzoyl thiamine), are absorbed more easily than thiamine hydrochloride[76] and are useful in the treatment of thiamine deficiency when a rapid and sustained response is needed.

Thiamine in doses of 5 to 10mg daily is curative for most manifestations. Doses larger than this administered by oral or parenteral routes may be wasted. Treatment for 4 to 6 weeks may be necessary, depending on the deficiency and the type of clinical manifestation. Neurological manifestations of dietary deficiency and chronic alcohol use are treated for 4 to 6 weeks while loss of appetite and calf-muscle tenderness are treated for 1 to 2 weeks.

### *3.3.2 Riboflavin (Vitamin $B_2$) Deficiency*

Clinical manifestations of ariboflavinosis are orolingual lesions, seborrhoeic dermatitis and scrotal dermatitis. Riboflavin (vitamin $B_2$) is absorbed from the proximal intestine in a capacity-limited process. Its absorption is increased in the presence of food.[77] If a large dose is administered, nearly all of it is recovered in the urine. Renal clearance of riboflavin exceeds the glomerular filtration rate, suggesting that renal tubular secretion of riboflavin occurs.

Clinical recovery of ariboflavinosis is complete with doses of 5 to 10 mg/day of riboflavin given for 14 to 21 days.

#### *3.3.3 Pyridoxine (Vitamin $B_6$) Deficiency*

The prevalence of pyridoxine (vitamin $B_6$) deficiency in humans is not well documented. Oral lesions, convulsions in infants, peripheral neuropathy, sideroblastic anaemia, dermatitis and behavioural changes have been reported to occur in pyridoxine deficiency (natural or induced).

Pyridoxine, pyridoxal phosphate and pyridoxamine are equally useful and are rapidly absorbed by passive diffusion from the jejunum. More than 30% of pyridoxine in plasma is in the form of pyridoxal phosphate bound to albumin. The tissue content of pyridoxal phosphate is regulated by the binding of this coenzyme with the protein moiety. Riboflavin and pyridoxine are closely inter-related. Clinical signs and response are identical, irrespective of whether pyridoxine or riboflavin is administered in patients with oral lesions. The biochemical basis for these deficiencies has been reviewed by Bamji and Faizy.[78]

Although clinical signs of pyridoxine deficiency are not clearly delineated, pyridoxine has been used to treat a number of clinical disorders like hyperemesis in pregnancy, myoclonic epilepsy, muscular dystrophy, depression induced by oral contraceptives, homocystinuria and cystathioninuria. Oral or parenteral pyridoxine 20 to 50 mg/day has been used to treat various clinical conditions. Conditions that are pyridoxine-dependent, however, require larger amounts (100 to 200 mg/day).

#### *3.3.4 Nicotinic Acid Deficiency*

Nicotinic acid (niacin) deficiency results in pellagra, which is characterised by bilateral symmetrical dermatitis on the exposed extensor surfaces, orolingual manifestations, gastrointestinal disturbances and dementia. Nicotinic acid is absorbed readily from the intestinal tract. Little is stored in the body. It is metabolised and the metabolites are excreted in urine. Nicotinic acid is present in tissues, largely as the coenzymes nicotinamide-adenine dinucleotide (NAD) and nicotinamide-adenine dinucleotide phosphate (NADP).

Nicotinic acid is administered in daily doses of 50 to 300mg to treat pellagra. All manifestations respond to therapy, with 4 to 6 weeks' therapy required for completed clinical cure.[79]

### 3.4 Ascorbic Acid (Vitamin C) Deficiency

Severe ascorbic acid (vitamin C) deficiency leads to scurvy and is characterised by weakness, anaemia, spongy gums, mucocutaneous and subperiosteal haemorrhages, pseudoparalysis and marked irritability. Repeated infections are common in ascorbic acid deficiency.

Absorption of ascorbic acid occurs mainly from the proximal small intestine by a nonpassive saturable process.[80] In the blood, ascorbic acid is almost exclusively present in its reduced form. It is excreted as oxalic acid, unchanged ascorbic acid and very little as dehydroascorbic acid.

#### Optimum Treatment

Oral administration of ascorbic acid in scurvy gives satisfactory results and the condition responds to as little as 10mg daily. However, in infants, 100 to 200mg daily in divided doses will produce a clinical response much faster. Large doses of ascorbic acid have also been used for the common cold, atherosclerosis, infections and fluorosis, though it is of doubtful clinical effectiveness in these conditions.

### 3.5 Toxicity of High-Dose Vitamins

Although vitamin deficiency states are of prime concern, it is important to consider possible effects of excessive vitamin intake. Toxic manifestations are more often encountered with fat-soluble vitamins (e.g. vitamins A, D, E), since water-soluble vitamins (e.g. B complex, C) have a renal threshold that allows excess amounts to be excreted by the kidneys. The following toxic manifestations have been described (see DiPalma & Ritchie[81]):

- *Retinol* (vitamin A): increased intracranial pressure associated with headache, vomiting, drowsiness, bulging of fontanelles, diplopia and papilloedema occur in acute hypervitaminosis A (doses greater than 300,000IU). Chronic hypervitaminosis A manifests as anorexia, pruritus, increased irritability, swelling of bones, seborrhoeic cutaneous lesions and hepatomegaly. x-Rays reveal hyperosteosis after ingestion of excessive doses for several weeks or months.
- *Vitamin D*: symptoms develop after 1 to 3 months of large intakes of vitamin D (e.g. >4000 IU/day calciferol), and include hypotonia, anorexia, irritability, constipation, polydipsia and polyuria. Hypercalcaemia and hypercalciuria are characteristic features.

Aortic valvular stenosis may occur. x-Rays reveal metastatic calcification and generalised osteoporosis.

- *Thiamine*: anaphylactic reactions have been described due to sensitisation to the vitamin. Toxic doses of thiamine affect the cardiovascular system, producing symptoms of peripheral circulatory failure.[82]
- *Nicotinic acid:* in doses of 50 to 100mg, this agent produces flushing and pruritus, whereas nicotinamide is free from such reactions. The most common serious toxicity reported for nicotinic acid is abnormal liver function and jaundice with doses of 3 g/day given for at least a year.
- *Ascorbic acid*: excess ascorbic acid (1 to 3g daily) may result in acidosis, gastrointestinal complaints, glycosuria, oxaluria, renal stones (particularly in individuals prone to develop oxalosis, hyperuricaemia and cystinuria), and a state of conditioned need.

## 4. Anaemias

Nutritional anaemias are highly prevalent almost all over the world. Iron deficiency anaemia is one of the important public health problems facing many developing countries. Anaemias due to deficiency of folic acid and cyanocobalamin (vitamin $B_{12}$) are also common in developing countries, as well as in some developed countries.

### 4.1 Iron Deficiency Anaemias

Dietary inadequacy, poor absorption of iron from diets primarily based on plant foods, hookworm infestation and repeated pregnancy are common causes of iron deficiency in the tropics and subtropics.

#### Optimum Treatment

As in developed countries, patients can be treated with oral iron. Most will respond readily to the least expensive preparation, ferrous sulfate. If adverse effects are troublesome, ferrous gluconate may be tried. Ferrous fumarate and ferrous succinate are alternatives. The properties and dosages of the various oral iron preparations and the limited indications for parenteral iron therapy are discussed in chapter 26 (sect. 5.1).

In view of the widespread nature of iron deficiency in tropical countries, it is important that major public health measures are undertaken to prevent anaemia. Routine iron supplementation for pregnant women and preschool children, in whom anaemia is a serious problem, has been advocated. Another practical measure is fortification of foods with iron. A number of vehicles have been proposed and used for iron fortification in several countries. In India, table salt is a suitable vehicle since it is universally consumed, centrally processed and produced in bulk. Iron salts selected for this purpose must be stable, colourless and their availability should be satisfactory when ingested with food. Studies indicate that ferric orthophosphate, together with a promotor of absorption such as sodium sulfate, is ideal for salt fortification.[83] Long term community studies indicate that iron-fortified salt is a simple and effective public health measure to control iron deficiency anaemia in any population.[84]

### 4.2 Folate Deficiency Anaemia

Deficiency of folic acid leads to megaloblastic anaemia, which is quite often seen in pregnant women and in infants and children in tropical countries (due to dietary deficiency or increased requirements of folate as a consequence of malarial haemolysis or haemoglobinopathies), in malabsorption syndromes and in patients on antiepileptic drugs. Megaloblastic anaemia may also occur in association with poverty, malnutrition and infection/infestation.

Folic acid is rapidly absorbed from the upper part of the small intestine (jejunum) by active transport. About 65% of folic acid in plasma is protein bound and the free folate is cleared by the kidney by glomerular filtration. There is tubular reabsorption of folate at plasma concentrations less than 10 μg/L. When given in large doses, folic acid is cleared at a fast rate and excreted.

#### Optimum Treatment

In patients with folate deficiency anaemia, a dose of 5mg folic acid given orally once daily is more than adequate, even in patients with malabsorption. The duration of folate therapy depends on the nature of the underlying disorder. Long term folic acid administration is indicated only in sickle cell anaemias and thalassaemias. In tropical countries, prophylactic doses of folic acid (300μg) are required for prevention of pregnancy anaemias.[85]

Although folic acid is relatively non-toxic, a few examples of sensitivity reactions to it have been recorded. Long term folate therapy may increase fit frequency in some epileptics and precipitate vitamin $B_{12}$ neuropathy (see further chapter 26; sect. 5).

### 4.3 Vitamin $B_{12}$ Deficiency Anaemia

Vitamin $B_{12}$ (cyanocobalamin) deficiency in humans occurs due to dietary inadequacy or malabsorption. Dietary inadequacy occurs only among vegetarian populations, since there are no plant sources of vitamin $B_{12}$. However, this deficiency is not as common as other vitamin B complex deficiencies in people living in tropical environments. Possibly due to poor hygiene, vitamin $B_{12}$ synthesised by bacteria may be available to this population. Pernicious anaemia, on the other hand, is genetically determined and is characterised by failure to absorb vitamin $B_{12}$. Other causes include gastrectomy and ile-ectomy anaemias, intestinal disorders like tropical sprue, blind loop syndromes, fish tapeworm infestation, and drugs that interfere with absorption. In addition to anaemias, neurological manifestations are encountered in vitamin $B_{12}$ deficiency.

#### Optimum Treatment

Treatment of vitamin $B_{12}$ deficiency anaemia is discussed in chapter 26 (sect. 5.2.1).

## 5. Tropical Parasitic Infections

Parasitic infestation usually implies infection caused by protozoa and helminths prevalent under conditions of overcrowding, poverty and poor sanitation. Although parasitic infestations are not usually responsible for producing fulminant, life-threatening situations, the potential hazards of such infections lie in their marked and chronic effects on nutrition, growth and mental acuity. Chronic disability may have far reaching effects on society in hyperendemic areas where there is also substantial undernutrition.

Treatment of tropical parasitic diseases is complicated by several factors. The size of the population infected with parasites is enormous. The possibility of frequent reinfection is always present as long as the environmental conditions permit repeated exposure. Mass treatment and control measures must, as far as possible, run in parallel. However, treatment is not always successful because patients are often not sufficiently well educated to understand the need for prolonged therapy. Noncompliance with treatment is the rule rather than the exception.

Since there are still no effective immunisation procedures for protection against protozoal and helminthic diseases, clinicians must rely on drugs for treatment. Unfortunately, many of the drugs used are toxic both to the parasite and the host and their mechanisms of action are little known in most cases. With some drugs, such as antimonials and arsenicals, the toxic dose for humans is near the therapeutic dose. Since many patients with parasitic infestations are also malnourished, toxic antiparasitic drugs become more hazardous, with patients more likely to experience severe adverse reactions as a result of an altered drug response (see section 2). It is clear that many existing toxic antiparasitic drugs should be replaced by better and safer remedies.

Drugs for parasitic diseases in general have not been developed systematically. Pharmacokinetic data are lacking for several agents in current use. Limitations of effectiveness and problems of severe toxicity further compound the problem. The use of these drugs is based on clinical trial and error. The WHO has helped by setting up a programme for research and training in tropical diseases. This has helped development and testing of a number of important new disease control tools, chemotherapy, vaccine development and vector control.[86] Malarial control programmes, chemotherapy for diseases, praziquantel for schistosomiasis, free supply of pentamidine for trypanosomiasis, ivermectin for onchocerciasis, diethylcarbamazine for lymphatic filariasis, and multidrug regimens for leprosy and tuberculosis have received attention. However, while the importance of effective and safe chemotherapeutic agents for management of tropical parasitic diseases is obvious, eradication of these diseases will only result from measures such as vector control, immunisation and improvement in public health and sanitation practices. The issues involved are complex.

### 5.1 Malaria

Malaria is the most important tropical disease, affecting over 2200 million people with more than 2 million deaths per year.[87] It is transmitted by the bite of female anopheles mosquitoes and needs systematic treatment. Drug resistance in the treatment of malaria is well documented.[88] Four species of the genus plasmodium infect humans: *Plasmodium vivax*, *Plasmodium ovale*, *Plasmodium malariae* and *Plasmodium falciparum*. Deaths are usually due to *P. falciparum*. The protozoan has several stages of development and cycles. The merozoites deposited in the blood after the mosquito bite are rapidly carried via the bloodstream to the liver where they multiply asexually. This is known as pre-erythrocytic schizogony. A single sporozoite produces several merozoites. The merozoites are released into blood in the symptomatic stage. Some intrahepatic forms are dormant for months (hypnozoites) before they multiply. Such sleeping forms in *P. vivax* and *P. ovale* infection are responsible for relapses.

Merozoites in the blood stream enter the red cell and the erythrocyte cycle begins. Erythrocytic schizogony releases the merozoites to continue the cycle. After the asexual cycle, some of these develop into gametocytes which are long-lived and relatively inert. Gametocytes are sucked by the female mosquito, where they mature and form merozoites which are inoculated back into the human host.

#### 5.1.1 Clinical Pharmacology of Drugs Used in Treatment

The classification of antimalarial drugs is as follows:[89]

1) *Tissues schizonticides* which inhibit the growth of pre-erythrocytic stages of the parasite in the liver. Proguanil, primaquine and pyrimethamine with or without sulfonamides act as causal prophylactics to prevent infection.

2) *Antirelapse drugs* such as primaquine and 8-aminoquinolones which kill the dormant hypnozoites and are mainly indicated for *P. vivax* and *P. ovale* malaria.

3) *Blood schizonticides* (e.g. chloroquine, quinine, mefloquine) which kill the erythrocytic forms and can also be used as suppressive prophylactics. Pyrimethamine, proguanil, sulfonamides, antibiotics and, to a small degree, primaquine have schizonticidal effects.

4) *Gametocytocides* which destroy the asexual stage of the parasite in the blood, including that of *P. falciparum*. Primaquine is considered the first-line agent.

5) *Sporozonticides* (e.g. pyrimethamine, proguanil) which inhibit formation of oocyst and sporozoites in mosquitoes.

Sporozonticides and gametocytocidal drugs are not of any direct use to the infected person, but limit spread of infection in endemic areas.

The clinical pharmacological properties of the more commonly used antimalarial drugs are shown in table IV.

#### Chloroquine

Chloroquine, a 4-aminoquinoline derivative, has no effect against the exoerythrocytic tissue stage of malaria. It is highly effective against asexual erythrocytic stages of all forms except drug-resistant *P. falciparum*, and it can also kill the gametocytes of *P. vivax*, *P. ovale* and *P. malariae*. Chloroquine inhibits parasite growth by forming a complex with haeme (ferriprotoporphyrin IX) released during degradation of haemoglobin in parasitised erythrocytes. It may also intercalate with plasmodium DNA.

***Pharmacokinetic characteristics:*** chloroquine is well absorbed from the gastrointestinal tract and from muscle and subcutaneous tissue. Following oral administration, its bioavailability is increased by food. With daily doses of 300mg, steady-state concentrations of 125 μg/L are produced. Therapeutic concentrations are 30 μg/L for *P. falciparum* and 15 μg/L for *P. vivax*. Chloroquine has a large apparent volume of distribution[90,91] and a long half-life of 41 to 50 days. It has extensive tissue distribution and concentrates in the liver, spleen, kidney, lung and melanin-containing tissues. Parasitised erythrocytes also concentrate chloroquine,[92] and its distribution in red blood cells parallels that in plasma.

Chloroquine is metabolised to monodeacetyl chloroquine, which has antimalarial activity. Unchanged chloroquine accounts for about 50% of the drug excreted in the urine while 20% is accounted for by its metabolite. The renal clearance of chloroquine is about half of its total systemic clearance.

***Clinical use:*** chloroquine phosphate or sulfate is given along with food by the oral route, while the hydrochloride is given by the parenteral route. It appears to be well tolerated in pregnancy and childhood. Chloroquine is also used as an anti-inflammatory agent (e.g. in rheumatoid arthritis). It should be used with caution in liver disease and its dosage should be reduced in renal impairment.

***Tolerability:*** when chloroquine is administered by the oral route for acute malarial attacks, gastrointestinal disturbances, pruritus and visual disturbances may occur; however, prolonged administration once weekly for suppressive purposes does not usually result in untoward reactions. Chloroquine may cause discolouration of nail beds and mucous membranes, and may produce a lichenoid skin eruption. High doses of the drug can produce retinopathy, myopathy, cardiomyopathy and peripheral neuropathy.

**Table IV.** Comparative clinical pharmacological properties of drugs commonly used in the treatment and prevention of malaria

| Feature | Chloroquine | Pyrimethamine | Sulfadoxine | Mefloquine | Primaquine | Halofantrine |
|---|---|---|---|---|---|---|
| Mechanism of action | Forms a toxic complex with ferriprotoporphyrin IX (haeme) | Inhibits dihydrofolate reductase | Inhibits dihydropteroate synthetase | Forms a toxic complex with ferritoprotoporphyrin IX (haeme) | Interferes with plasmodial mitochondrial function, and binds to DNA | Forms a toxic complex with ferritoprotoporphyrin IX (haeme) |
| Sensitive species | *P. vivax*<br>*P. falciparum*<br>*P. ovale*<br>*P. malariae* | P. vivax<br>P. falciparum (resistant) | *P. vivax*<br>*P. falciparum*<br>*P. ovale*<br>*P. malariae* | *P. falciparum*<br>*P. vivax* (suppressive) | Exoerythrocytic forms<br>*P. virax*<br>*P. ovale*<br>Gametocides (all forms) | *P. falciparum* |
| Class of drug | Blood schizonticide and gametocide | Tissue schizonticide, sporonticide | Blood schizonticide | Blood schizonticide | Tissue schizonticide/ blood gametocide | Blood schizonticide |
| Onset of drug effects (h) | 3 | 2-6 | 3-6 | 6 | 1-2 | 5-8 |
| **Pharmacokinetic characteristics:** | | | | | | |
| F (%) | 90 | 85 | | 85 | 90-100 | ?(poor) |
| Linear kinetics | Yes | Yes | Yes | Yes | Yes | Yes (nonlinear at high doses) |
| $t_{½β}$ (h) | 1220 (41-50d) | 80-95 | 125 | 530 | 4-5 | 91-113 |
| Vd (L)[a] | 57,400 | 203 | | 1330 | 322 | 5124 |
| CL (L/h)[a] | 65 | 1.7 | 2.4 | 2.0 | 56 | 42 |
| Protein binding (%) | 55 | 87 | 90 | 98 | | |
| Principal route of elimination | Renal | Renal | Renal | Biliary/faecal and renal | Renal and faecal | Faecal |
| Form eliminated | Unchanged | Metabolites | Unchanged | Unchanged and as carboxylic acid metabolite | Metabolites | Unchanged and as *N*-desbutyl metabolite |
| Metabolite activity relative to parent drug | Less active | Metabolites not characterised, but found in urine | | Carboxylic acid metabolite is inactive | Less active | Less active |
| Route of administration | PO or parenteral | PO | PO | PO | PO | PO |
| Treatment dosage (adults) | 600mg (base) initially, then 300mg 6-8h later and 300mg on 2 consequent days (1.5g total) | 75mg (with sulfadoxine) as a single dose | 1500mg (with pyrimethamine) as a single dose | 750mg initially, then 500mg 6-8h later and 250mg after a further 6-8h | 15mg (base) daily | 3 × doses of 500mg 6-hourly |
| Duration of treatment (days) | 3 | 1 | 1 | 1 | 14 | 1 |
| Prophylactic/ suppressive dosage (adults) | 300mg (base)/week | 25 mg/week (in combination with sulfadoxine) | 500 mg/week (in combination with pyrimethamine) | 250 mg/week for 4 weeks, then 125 mg/week | 45mg (base) per week for 8 weeks | |
| Adverse effects | GI upset, pruritus, headache, fatigue, visual disturbances, dyskinesias, neurovascular disease | Skin rashes, megaloblastic anaemia | Stevens-Johnson syndrome, epidermal necrolysis, hepatitis, haemolysis | GI upset, dizziness, headache, pruritus, skin rashes, CNS toxicity | Mild anaemia, methaemoglobinaemia, depression, confusion, cardiac arrhythmia; granulocytopenia, agranulocytosis | Abdominal pain, nausea, vomiting, headache, pruritus, skin rashes |

**Table IV.** *[Continued]*

| Feature | Chloroquine | Pyrimethamine | Sulfadoxine | Mefloquine | Primaquine | Halofantrine |
|---|---|---|---|---|---|---|
| Patient benefits | PO administration is effective and less costly than other routes | Effective against resistant strains of *P. falciparum* | Effective in multiresistant forms | Effective in multiresistant falciparum malaria | Provides radical cure of *P. vivax* infection | Effective in multiresistant falciparum malaria |
| Limitations | Resistance | Toxicity | Toxicity | Resistance now established in some areas. Expensive | | Cross-resistance with mefloquine has been noted in some areas. Expensive |

a Per 70kg (with normal renal function).

*Abbreviations:* PO = oral; GI = gastrointestinal; F = oral bioavailability; $t_{½β}$ = elimination half-life; CL = total body clearance; Vd = apparent volume of distribution.

#### Proguanil

Proguanil is a biguanide derivative that is well tolerated when given by the oral route. It is mainly used as a prophylactic agent, particularly for chloroquine-resistant *P. falciparum* malaria. Proguanil selectively inhibits plasmodial dihydroreductase. It is slowly but adequately absorbed from the gastrointestinal tract. Peak plasma concentrations occur within 5 hours and the elimination half-life is 16 to 20 hours. The drug is metabolised to active and inactive metabolites; 40 to 60% of a dose is excreted in the urine as either the unchanged drug or as the active metabolite. Proguanil is associated with few adverse reactions. Occasionally, it produces nausea and diarrhoea, and large doses may produce vomiting and haematuria.

#### Amodiaquine

This 4-aminoquinoline drug has been used as a prophylactic and therapeutic agent for chloroquine-resistant *P. falciparum* malaria. Amodiaquine is well absorbed orally and is eliminated in 2 phases with an initial half-life of 10 hours followed by a prolonged elimination phase.[93] The drug and its active metabolite are detected in urine for many months after a single dose. For non-immune patients with acute infection, a 600mg dose followed by 300mg doses at 6, 24 and 48 hours later is recommended. For suppression, the usual dose is 300 to 400mg every 7 days. Due to toxicity, its use as prophylactic agent is no longer advocated. Hepatotoxicity and agranulocytosis limit its therapeutic usefulness.

#### Pyrimethamine/Sulfadoxine

***Pyrimethamine*** is a diaminopyrimidine derivative used in the prophylaxis, suppression and combined chemotherapy of chloroquine-resistant strains (table IV). Suppression of *P. vivax* is possible if medication is continued 6 to 10 weeks after leaving a malarial area. It inhibits dihydrofolate reductase activity, and when given in combination with a sulfonamide (e.g. sulfadoxine), is very useful for multiresistant strains.

Pyrimethamine is slowly but nearly completely absorbed after oral administration. Peak plasma concentrations occur 2 to 6 hours after an oral dose, and the plasma half-life is 80 to 95 hours.[92] The drug accumulates mainly in the kidneys, lungs, liver and spleen, and suppressive concentrations are maintained in plasma for 2 weeks.[94] It is metabolised and excreted in the urine; it is also excreted in breastmilk.

***Sulfadoxine*** is well absorbed following oral administration, has a mean half-life of 123 hours, and is excreted unchanged in the urine.[91] It inhibits dihydropteroate synthetase. Thus, a combination of pyrimethamine and sulfadoxine has a synergistic inhibitory effect on development of resistance.

Large doses of sulfadoxine produce megaloblastic anaemia. The combination of sulfadoxine with pyrimethamine can produce skin reactions (erythema multiforme), Stevens-Johnson syndrome, toxic epidermal necrolysis and hepatitis. It can also produce haemolysis.

Pyrimethamine is also available in combination with *dapsone* (12.5mg + 100mg, respectively) which can be given weekly for prophylaxis and suppressive therapy.

#### Mefloquine

Mefloquine is a 4-quinoline methanol derivative used both for prophylaxis and treatment of malaria. Mefloquine probably acts by forming a complex with haeme (ferriprotoporphyrin IX) which results from digestion of host cell haemoglobin by the parasite. This complex is toxic to membranes and parasitic enzymes. The antimalarial activity of mefloquine depends on the ability of the drug to form hydrogen bonds with parasite proteins.

***Pharmacokinetic characteristics:*** there is considerable variation in the pharmacokinetics of mefloquine. Oral mefloquine is 85% bioavailable. Peak concentrations occur 6 to 24 hours after administration and are 2 to 3 times higher in Asians than in Western populations.[95] The elimination half-life is 2 to 3 weeks.[96] Mefloquine has extensive tissue distribution and a large volume of distribution. Concentrations in the liver and lung are high. The drug has a high affinity for erythrocyte membranes and concentrates in red cells. It is mainly excreted in the faeces with small amounts appearing in the urine. Several metabolites are formed.

***Tolerability:*** most adverse effects of mefloquine are mild, e.g. nausea, vomiting, diarrhoea, and require no specific treatment. The drug may worsen orthostatic hypotension and has produced cardiac abnormalities such as sinus arrhythmia and bradycardia. Dysphonia and neuropsychiatric disturbances have also been documented.

#### Primaquine

Primaquine is the only commonly used 8-aminoquinoline derivative. Its mechanism of action is not clear but may involve interfering with plasmodial mitochondrial function and binding to DNA.

Absorption of primaquine is complete after oral administration. Peak plasma concentrations occur within 3 hours and the elimination half-life is 4 to 5 hours. It has a large volume of distribution. Primaquine is rapidly metabolised and only a small fraction (<1%) is excreted unchanged in the urine. Metabolites have less antimalarial activity than the parent drug.[97] Primaquine is the least toxic of the antimalarial drugs. Adverse effects are generally mild, but methaemoglobinaemia and haemolytic anaemia may occur in G6PD-deficient individuals. Granulocytopenia and agranulocytosis are rare adverse reactions.

#### Halofantrine

Halofantrine, an arylamino alcohol, is a relatively new schizonticide active against both chloroquine-sensitive and chloroquine-resistant malaria. Its mode of action is through formation of a halofantrine-ferriprotoporphyrin IX complex and inhibition of the proton pump at the host-parasite interface.

Halofantrine is poorly and variably absorbed after oral administration. Peak plasma concentrations after the third dose are achieved after 16 hours. It is metabolised to *N*-debutyl-halofantrine, and its plasma half-life is between 91 to 113 hours. Halofantrine is distributed widely in tissues and excreted mainly in faeces.[98]

Common adverse effects of halofantrine include abdominal pain, pruritus, vomiting, diarrhoea, headache and rash.

#### Artesunate

Artesunate is a derivative of the Chinese medicinal herb Quinghaosu, which has long been used for in traditional Chinese medicine for treating fever. The drug has a sesquiterpene lactone ring with an endoperoxide bridge.[99] It acts by increasing the oxidant stress on intra-erythrocytic forms and is active against both *P. falciparum* and *P. vivax*. Artesunate is rapidly hydrolysed to its principal active metabolite dihydroartemisinin, which is rapidly eliminated. The pharmacokinetics of artesunate are not fully characterised because methods of detection are still being developed. Limited information indicates that the elimination of half-life of artesunate is 23 minutes, while that of dihydroartemisinin is 45 minutes.[88] Peak plasma concentrations of artesunate are 2.64 mg/L and dihydroartemisinin 2.02 mg/L after intravenous administration. After oral administration, peak concentrations are seen within 3 hours. Fever and parasitaemia respond to artesunate administration within 8 to 18 hours and 20 to 38 hours, respectively.

Quinghaosu drugs are less toxic than quinolones. Commonly reported adverse reactions are nausea, vomiting and diarrhoea. No serious toxicity has been noted in humans.[100,101]

### *5.1.2 Optimum Treatment*

The drugs used in malarial treatment act in several ways:

- As tissue schistozontocides, inhibiting the growth of the pre-erythrocytic stage of the parasite in the liver
- As hypnozoitocides, killing the dormant liver stages
- As blood schistozontocides, acting on the erythrocytic state while gametocytocides destroy the sexual stages of the parasite in the blood
- As sporontocides, which act on the oocysts and sporontocides injected into the blood.

A combination of drugs is required for prevention of acute illness and relapses. Chloroquine-resistant malaria found in several areas is treated either with quinine or pyrimethamine/sulfadoxine combinations or with mefloquine; proguanil is used for prophylaxis. For severe malaria, particularly of the cerebral type, intravenous drugs should be considered. In patients with renal insufficiency, dosage adjustments of antimalarial drugs are required. The new agent artesunate (see section 5.1.1 above) is currently being used for resistant cases of *P. falciparum* malaria.

*Chloroquine:* for treatment of acute malarial attacks, an initial loading dose of 600mg chloroquine (base) is followed 6 hours later by 300mg and then 300mg on each of the 2 following days. For infants and children, the initial dose should not exceed 10 mg/kg bodyweight, followed by 5 mg/kg. For chemoprophylactic or suppressive therapy, 300mg chloroquine base (equivalent to 500mg chloroquine phosphate) is given once each week starting 2 weeks before and continued for 8 weeks after the last exposure in endemic areas.

Gastrointestinal disturbances can be avoided if chloroquine is taken with food. Acute toxicity with cardiac dysfunction is treated with mechanical ventilation, adrenaline, diazepam, etc. Generally, the toxic symptoms disappear when therapy is stopped. Retinal examination is recommended during therapy with chloroquine.

*Pyrimethamine/sulfadoxine:* for acute malarial attacks, pyrimethamine 75mg with sulfadoxine 1500mg (i.e. 3 tablets) are given orally as a single dose. Paediatric doses range from one-quarter tablet (<1 year) to 1 tablet (4 to 8 years); two tablets are given for children 9 to 14 years of age.

Because of potential toxicity, long term prophylaxis with pyrimethamine/sulfadoxine is not recommended except in areas of marked resistance. If skin or mucous membrane lesions occur, prophylactic usage should be discontinued. Calcium folinate (leucovorin calcium) 10 mg/day is recommended to reduce or avert haematological toxicity.

*Mefloquine:* for curative treatment, 1 to 3 doses of oral mefloquine 1200 to 1500mg are given. In children, a dose of 25 mg/kg is given. For prophylaxis, a schedule of 250mg weekly for 4 weeks, followed by 125mg weekly has been used successfully in adults.

*Primaquine* 15 mg/day in combination with chloroquine is given for 14 days for radical cure of malaria due to sensitive strains of *P. vivax*. *Proguanil* is used as long term prophylaxis for chloroquine-resistant *P. falciparum* malaria as an alternative to pyrimethamine/sulfadoxine. Dosages of proguanil are 200 to 300 mg/day.

*Halofantrine* is given as 3 doses of 500mg every 6 hours for treatment of acute malarial attacks; parasitaemia is cleared between 34 and 78 hours. Paediatric doses are 8 mg/kg administered 3 times 6-hourly. A second course is given after 7 days for non-immune patients (those who lack antiplasmodial antibodies). There is some cross resistance between mefloquine and halofantrine.

*Quinine*, though not in common use, is used to treat resistant strains.[89] Quinine sulfate 650mg 3 times daily for 3 to 5 days followed by a single dose of pyrimethamine 50 to 75mg combined with sulfadoxine 1 to 1.5g or mefloquine 1 to 1.5g will eradicate infection completely. If quinine resistance is encountered, a 7-day course of tetracycline 1 to 2 g/day may be given.

*Artesunate* is available in preparations for oral and rectal administration and for injection.[100] There is still no consensus regarding its dosage regimen. If the treatment schedule is short, recrudescences are common.

The WHO recommends that artesunate be given for a minimum of 3 days, followed by a single dose of mefloquine. If mefloquine cannot be given, artesunate monotherapy is given for at least 5 or preferably 7 days. A dose of 100 to 200mg initially is followed by 100 mg/day for 4 to 6 days. For the treatment of severe infections, artesunate can be administered by the intravenous or intramuscular routes. The initial dose is 2 mg/kg, followed by 1 mg/kg every 12 hours until oral treatment can be given. Artesunate therapy should be followed by mefloquine.[88,99]

#### Treatment of Cerebral Malaria

For cerebral malaria, chloroquine 200 to 300mg may be given as a slow intravenous infusion. No more than 900mg should be given in 24 hours by the intravenous route. In resistant infections, quinine dihydrochloride 20 mg/kg can be infused over 4 hours, followed by maintenance doses of 10 mg/kg given as 2-hour infusions every 8 hours for 7 days. Quinidine has also been recommended for cerebral malaria. Supportive therapy such as dialysis for renal failure, mechanical respiratory assistance, and corticosteroids for cerebral oedema are also indicated.

#### 5.1.3 Prevention of Malaria

The resurgence of malaria in many parts of the world due to development of resistance, particularly in malignant species of *P. falciparum*, has caused great concern. Chemoprophylaxis is therefore advisable for all travellers to countries where malaria exists. In areas where there is multidrug resistance, measures of personal protection are considered to be much better and safer than drugs, although chemoprophylaxis provides some degree of protection.

Malarial chemoprophylaxis with the drugs shown in table IV should begin 1 week before travel and continued for 4 weeks after departure from the risk area. This will kill the parasites in circulation and those that are released from the liver. However, it may not kill dormant hypnozoites in the liver. It is believed that bodyweight-adjusted dosages of antimalarials may give better protection. In *P. falciparum* areas, pyrimethamine/sulfadoxine (or pyrimethamine/dapsone) and mefloquine are recommended. Alternatively, doxycycline (100mg daily starting 1 to 2 days before travel and continued for 4 weeks after departure from the risk area) may be given.

For chloroquine-sensitive species, chloroquine, proguanil or mefloquine are first-line agents. For chloroquine-resistant species, mefloquine, doxycycline, proguanil or pyrimethamine with sulfadoxine or dapsone are recommended.[102] Prophylaxis with pyrimethamine/sulfadoxine should be restricted to chloroquine-resistant areas.[103,104]

### 5.2 Filariasis

Filariasis is a general term for a large group of parasitic infections. They are produced by nematodes of the family filarioidea. The 4 species most prevalent in humans are *Wuchereria bancrofti, Brugia malayi, Onchocerca volvulus* and *Loa loa*. Depending on the species, the slender filarial worms are found in the circulatory and lymphatic systems, muscles and connective tissues of the host. They are transmitted by blood sucking insects by ingestion of microfilariae from human donors. The insects act as intermediate hosts to larval development. The infected larvae are transmitted to a new host, where they migrate to specific sites and produce different clinical entities. *W. bancrofti* is the most widespread of all filarial diseases and is found in most tropical and subtropical countries. It is also seen in Central and South America. The second most prominent species is *B. malayi* and is found in Asia, particularly in Southern India and Sri Lanka. *O. volvulus* occurs throughout the tropical zone and is the major cause of blindness.

Filariasis is essentially an endemic disease. *W. bancrofti* is transmitted by the mosquito *Culex fatigens* and other species. *O. volvulus* is transmitted by black flies of the genus Simulium. Since the flies are usually found near rivers and streams, the blindness is called river blindness. *L. loa* is transmitted by the bites of flies of the genus Chysops. The adult worms of *W. bancrofti* and *B. malayi* reside in the lymphatic system and microfilariae are found in the circulatory system. Adult worms of *O. volvulus* and *L. loa* are seen in muscle and connective tissue; the microfilariae are found in the dermis and subcutaneous tissue. Lymphatic filariasis (elephentiasis) is caused by *W. bancrofti* and *B. malayi*. *L. loa* causes loiasis characterised by transient subcutaneous swellings (calabaz) while *O. volvulus* produces blindness and skin rashes.

#### 5.2.1 Clinical Pharmacology of Drugs Used in Treatment

##### Diethylcarbamazine

Diethylcarbamazine, a piperazine derivative, causes rapid disappearance of microfilariae of *W. bancrofti*, *B. malayi*, *L. loa* and *O. volvulus*. However, it does not kill microfilariae of *O. volvulus* in nodules. The mechanism of action of diethycarbamazine is via a reduction in muscular activity, immobilising the organisms and dislocating the parasites from their normal habitats. It also alters surface membranes, rendering the worms susceptible to host defences. Adult worms of *L. loa*, *W. bancrofti* and *B. malayi* are also killed by diethylcarbamazine. Intracellular processing and transport of certain macromolecules is affected by the drug.

***Pharmacokinetic characteristics:*** diethylcarbamazine is rapidly absorbed from the gastrointestinal tract, reaching peak plasma concentrations in 1 to 2 hours. The half-life of the drug is 10 to 12 hours with an alkaline urine and 2 hours with an acidic urine.[105] The apparent volume of distribution is 200 to 240L. It is metabolised rapidly and extensively excreted in the urine as both the parent drug and a diethylcarbamazine-*N*-oxide metabolite which accounts for 50% of the oral dose.

***Tolerability:*** dose-related adverse effects with diethylcarbamazine *per se* are not severe and disappear quickly. They include anorexia, nausea, vomiting, weakness, dizziness, lethargy and headache. Most adverse effects are due to death of the parasite caused by the drug. In patients with onchocerciasis, a Mazzotti reaction consisting of itching, skin rashes, enlargement of lymph nodes and papular rash, with fever, tachycardia and arthralgia may occur. Ocular complications such as punctate keratitis, uveitis and atrophy of retinal pigment epithelium can also occur,[106] as can leucocytosis, proteinuria and eosinophilia. Adverse reactions are less common in bancroftian filariasis than in brugian filariasis. Local reactions such as lymphadenitis, lymphangitis and lymphoedema may also be seen

Diethylcarbamazine is a first-line agent for treating lymphatic filariasis. It is relatively well tolerated in large scale use in lymphatic filariasis.

#### 5.2.2 Optimum Treatment

The prevalence and incidence of adenolymphangitis decrease significantly after treatment with diethylcarbamazine. Attacks of funiculitis, epididymitis and orchitis are reduced and the drug reduces the occurrence of chronic obstructive lesions. Transient lymphoedema, hydrocele and chyluria usually respond to treatment with diethylcarbamazine, which is first-line therapy for tropical pulmonary eosinophilia.

The dose of diethylcarbamazine in bancroftian filariasis is 6 mg/kg/day given orally in divided doses for 12 to 21 days. For brugian filariasis, the dose ranges from 3 to 6 mg/kg/day for 21 days. Doses as high as 18 to 72 mg/kg/day have also been given. Repeated courses at intervals of 4 to 6 weeks are usually necessary to ensure complete parasitological cure.

### 5.3 Onchocerciasis

Onchocerciasis is a systemic filarial infection caused by *O. volvulus*. The prevalence and severity of the disease vary widely. The major endemic areas are Africa and Latin America and 20 to 40 million people appear to be at risk and 18 million are affected.[107] It is a leading cause of blindness and also results in dermatitis and lymph node involvement. The infection is transmitted by the bite of female black flies of the Simulium species.

#### 5.3.1 Clinical Pharmacology of Drugs Used in Treatment

Despite much research, a limited number of drugs are available for the treatment onchocerciasis. Diethylcarbamazine (see section 5.2.1) is the most widely used agent. Ivermectin is a new compound that can be considered superior to other drugs used to treat the disease.

##### Ivermectin

Ivermectin, a mixture of monocyclic lactones, is an orally effective antifilarial agent used for the treatment of onchocerciasis. It is also active against *W. bancrofti*, *L. loa* and gastrointestinal helminths such as hookworms and *Strongyloides stercoralis*. Its mechanism of action appears to be through a direct toxic effect, causing immobility of the microfilaria and facilitating clearance by lymphatic drainage. Ivermectin is an agonist of the neurotransmitter $\gamma$-aminobutyric acid (GABA). It potentiates GABA release and results in postsynaptic blockade of neurotransmission, with consequent inhibition of mobility and paralysis. It produces intrauterine degeneration within developing microfilariae.

***Pharmacokinetic characteristics:*** following oral administration, ivermectin has a bioavailability of about 60% and reaches peak plasma concentrations within 3 to 4 hours. It has an apparent volume of distribution of 47L, and is 9% bound to plasma protein. The elimination half-life is 28 hours and oral clearance is 1.2 L/h.[108] Metabolites of the drug have been detected in the urine and faeces.

***Clinical use and tolerability:*** the aim of treatment with ivermectin is to reduce the microfilariae load in the skin and eyes to prevent blindness and prevent morbidity, particularly chronic itching. It is generally well tolerated. Most of the unwanted effects of the drug are due to immunological reactions to dead microfilariae. The severity of adverse effects is therefore related to the degree of parasitic infestation. Adverse effects reported include myalgia, rash, lymph node tenderness, sweating, itching, fever and chills, joint and facial swelling. Severe symptomatic postural hypotension has been reported associated with sweating, tachycardia and confusion. Adverse effects can be treated with analgesics, antihistamines and hydrocortisone as soon as the symptoms are noted. The dosages of drugs will depend on the severity of toxicity.

**Benzimidazoles**

The benzimidazoles *mebendazole* and *flubendazole* have shown promising results in onchocerciasis.[109] Their mechanism of action appears to involve disruption of microtubular formation, resulting in cessation of maturation of oocytes to the early morula stage. These compounds are extremely useful against helminthic infections such as ascariasis, trichuriasis and hookworm infection. In onchocerciasis, they sterilise the female worm.

Mebendazole is poorly absorbed, with rapid first-pass metabolism resulting in low plasma concentrations. It is 95% bound to plasma protein and is extensively metabolised. Very little unchanged drug appears in the urine while the metabolites are excreted in bile and urine. It does not cause significant systemic toxicity, though transient abdominal pain and diarrhoea occur often. Rare adverse effects of mebendazole include allergic reactions, alopecia, neutropenia and agranulocytosis.

Flubendazole is also poorly absorbed and must be given by intramuscular injection.

#### 5.3.2 Optimum Treatment

*Diethylcarbamazine* is used as a suppressive agent but has no effect on adult worms. New microfilaria therefore repopulate the skin and the eye a few months after diethylcarbamazine treatment, and repeated administration may be necessary. Reactions are invariable and can be life-threatening in heavily infected patients. Symptoms of existing ocular lesions may be aggravated.[110] The recommended dosage regimen of diethylcarbamazine for a 50kg adult is an initial dose of 50mg on day 1, 50mg twice daily on day 2, and then a maintenance dose of 100mg twice daily for 3 to 8 days, the total dose being 1350mg over a period of 8 days. This dosage may have to be repeated after 4 months.

As onchocerciasis affects the skin and eyes, transdermal applications of diethylcarbamazine as a 1 to 2% lotion have been tried. This local application kills skin microfilaria without serious adverse effects. Diethylcarbamazine eye drops have also been tried, but while killing ocular microfilaria, this form of treatment has been associated with severe reactions. The administration of corticosteroids to overcome adverse reactions is beneficial, but requires medical supervision. The use of moderate urinary alkalinisation to reduce the elimination of diethylcarbamazine and hence reduce dosages and adverse reactions has resulted in higher microfilarial deaths, but in long term treatment, manipulation of urinary pH is of little practical value.

*Ivermectin* is an effective agent and is suitable for mass treatment. Single doses of 150 µg/kg result in a decrease in the microfilariae count by 85 to 95% within 2 months. Doses of 100 to 200 µg/kg can suppress the disease for several months.[111] For heavy ocular involvement, it is better to give ivermectin every 6 months rather than once yearly.[112] Ocular parasites decrease in parallel with the reduction in skin microfilaria. By reducing the prevalence of microfilariae, ivermectin also influences the rate of disease transmission.

*Mebendazole* 30 to 50 mg/kg/day given orally for 2 to 4 weeks has also proved effective, but is not commonly used nowadays.

### 5.4 Schistosomiasis

Schistosomiasis is a chronic debilitating disease, geographically distributed widely in several parts of the world. It is caused by 3 major schistosome species: *S. mansoni*, *S. haematobium* and *S. japonicum*, and there are other less prevalent species implicated as well. Worldwide, as many as 200 million persons are estimated to be infected.[113] However, while infection is common, only a small minority develop significant disease. Adult forms of *S. mansoni* and *S. japonicum* reside in the venules of the intestines and the disease mainly manifests as hepatic disease. *S. haematobium* adults are found in venules of the urinary tract and present primarily as a disease of the ureters and bladder. The eggs are responsible for tissue injury, a granulomatous response and fibrosis.

The intermediate host is a snail in which the eggs develop into cercariae, which are infective to both humans and animals. These penetrate the skin with specific proteolytic enzymes and enter the lymph vessels or veins. Schistosomes then migrate to the heart and lungs and are carried by the bloodstream to the liver. In the portal circulation, depending on the species, mature male and female schistosomes begin to migrate to various tissues and lay eggs. In the case of *S. mansoni* and *S. japonicum*, the adult worms lay eggs around 45 weeks after infection, while for *S. haematobium*, it takes 8 to 12 weeks. Adult worms do not multiply in humans. The eggs laid are either retained in the tissue or swept back into the portal system or to the bladder. Mature schistosome ova excreted from intestines and bladder release the miracidium that enters the intermediate host, the snail, and the life cycle continues. Cercariae are most infectious immediately after shedding and are not viable 48 hours after release into water.

The duration and intensity of infection, the location of the eggs and some host factors govern the disease manifestations.

#### *5.4.1 Clinical Pharmacology of Drugs Used in Treatment*

The clinical pharmacological properties of drugs used in the treatment of schistosomiasis are shown in table V.

##### Metrifonate

Metrifonate, an organophosphorus compound, is a relatively safe and effective schistosomicide that can be administered orally. Its major mechanism of action appears to be via inhibition of cholinesterase. Metrifonate is mainly active against *S. haematobium* and the reasons for its specificity for this species are not yet clear. In the body, metrifonate rearranges itself nonenzymatically to dichlorvos[114] and this metabolite is a more potent inhibitor of cholinesterase. After single oral doses, the plasma concentration of metrifonate is 31 μmol/L while that of dichlorvos is 0.3 μmol/L. At this concentration, the enzyme is inhibited within 15 minutes.[115] Enzyme inhibition results in the worms being transported to the lungs where development is not possible.[116] The plasma half-life of both metrifonate and dichlorvos is 1.5 hours. Metrifonate also undergoes extensive metabolism.

***Tolerability:*** adverse effects with metrifonate are generally mild or transient and include colic, diarrhoea, nausea or vomiting. Others such as headache, fatigue, muscular weakness, sweating, fainting, muscular tremors, bronchospasm and vertigo have also been noted. Patients treated with metrifonate should avoid insecticide exposure, since it can reduce cholinesterase activity.

##### Oxamniquine

Oxamniquine, a tetrahydroquinoline derivative, is a potent schistosomicide that kills *S. mansoni*, particularly the male worms. It is first-line therapy for *S. mansoni* infection but is not effective against the other 2 species. Oxamniquine is well absorbed when given orally and is metabolised to inactive acidic metabolites that are primarily excreted in urine. About 70% is excreted in the urine as metabolites. Oxamniquine is enzymatically converted to an ester which produces an ion responsible for alkylating DNA. It causes marked reductions in worm recovery and egg counts.

***Tolerability:*** the most common adverse effects of oxamniquine are drowsiness, dizziness and headache, while convulsions, fever, vomiting and diarrhoea also occur occasionally. Dizziness does not last long and hence the drug is often prescribed at bedtime.

##### Hycanthone

Hycanthone is an active metabolite of lucanthone and is a methylthioxanthine derivative. It is effective against *S. haematobium* and *S. mansoni* when given by intramuscular injection. Hycanthone is metabolised in the liver and excreted in the bile and faeces as conjugated metabolites. It binds to acetylcholine receptors and paralyses the worms, preventing them from feeding, which ultimately results in their death.

The disadvantage of hycanthone is that it has a very high incidence of adverse effects such as nausea, vomiting, abdominal pain, weakness, dizziness, headache and anorexia. Hepatic damage has resulted in restricted use of the drug.

##### Niridazole

Niridazole, a nitrothiazole derivative, is effective against almost all schistosome species. It is an active schistosomicide and binds covalently to macromolecules in the schistosomes. When, administered by the oral route, it is absorbed rapidly and metabolised in the liver. Peak plasma concentrations are seen after 6 hours. Niridazole is uniformly distributed and eliminated largely in urine and bile. Its availability is increased in patients with schistosomiasis of *S. mansoni* origin, due to portosystemic shunts. Since it has several toxic effects, niridazole has been superseded by other drugs.[117]

Niridazole is carcinogenic to hamsters and mice, but associations between niridazole and cancer have not been established in humans. It produces a high incidence of adverse effects such as neuropsychiatric disturbances, convulsions, hyperexcitability, mania and depression. Other adverse effects include nausea, skin rashes and nonspecific electrocardiographic changes. Testicular damage has also been reported, as has haemolysis in patients with G6PD deficiency.

##### Praziquantel

Praziquantel is a newly developed and relatively expensive drug with a broad spectrum of activity against the 3 major species of schistosomes.[118] Its mechanism of action is via alter-

**Table V.** Comparative clinical pharmacological properties of drugs used in the treatment of schistosomiasis

| Feature | Amoscanate | Hycanthone | Metrifonate | Niridazole | Oltipraz | Oxamniquine | Praziquantel |
|---|---|---|---|---|---|---|---|
| Mechanism of action | Accumulation of cyclic-AMP | Inhibits cholinesterase | Inhibits cholinesterase | Binds to macromolecules | Reduces glucose utilisation, and glutathione levels | Alkylates DNA | Alters ion concentrations |
| Sensitive species | *S. haematobium* *S. japonicum* *S. mansoni* | S. haematobium S. mansoni | *S. haematobium* | *S. mansoni* *S. haematobium* *S. japonicum* | *S. mansoni* *S. haematobium* | *S. mansoni* | *S. mansoni* *S. japonicum* *S. haematobium* |
| Principal route of elimination | Renal | Biliary and faecal | Renal | Renal | Renal and faecal | Renal | Renal |
| Form eliminated | ? | Inactive metabolites | Inactive metabolites | Active and inactive metabolites | Metabolites and unchanged | Inactive metabolites | Inactive metabolites |
| Dosage | 300 mg/kg once | 2.5 mg/kg once | 7.5-10 mg/kg every other week for 2-3 wks | 25 mg/kg/d in 2-3 divided doses for 7d | 1-1.5g tid for 2-3d | 15-20 mg/kg/d in 2 divided doses for 1-3d *or* 40-60 mg/kg/d[a] in 2 divided doses for 2-3d | 20-25 mg/kg q4h (see text) |
| Route of administration | PO | IM | PO | PO | PO | PO | PO |
| Adverse effects | CNS disturbances, jaundice | Headache, nausea, vomiting, dizziness, abdominal pain, hepatic damage | Colic, diarrhoea, nausea, vomiting, headache, muscular weakness, sweating, bronchospasm, tremors, vertigo | Neuropsychiatric disturbances, convulsions, testicular damage, GI disturbances, headache, skin rash | Nausea and vomiting, abdominal pain, dizziness, headache, phototoxicity | Drowsiness, dizziness, headache, seizure, eosinophilia, convulsions | Abdominal discomfort, anorexia, nausea, headache, dizziness, urticaria, diarrhoea |
| Relative clinical effectiveness | ++ | +++ | ++++ | ++++ | ++++ | ++++ | ++++ |
| Reduction in egg counts[b] (%) | | 50-90 | 95 | 85-90 | 90 | 95 | 96 |
| Parasitological cure (%) | | | 44-93 | | | Does not eradicate the parasite | 80 |

a African dosage.

b Treatment is given until the absence of live eggs in the rectal tissue and stool, after 3 to 5 months of treatment.

*Abbreviations:* bid = twice daily; tid = 3 times daily; GI = gastrointestinal; PO = oral; IM = intramuscular.

ations of inorganic ion transport (calcium and potassium) as well as glucose metabolism in the parasite. Praziquantel also increases the binding of IgG and IgM to the surface of the parasite.

***Pharmacokinetic characteristics:*** praziquantel is readily absorbed after oral administration and reaches peak plasma concentrations after 1 to 2 hours. However, its systemic availability is reduced by first-pass metabolism. Conjugated metabolites are formed and 80% of an administered dose is recovered in the urine as metabolites within 4 days. The elimination half-life is 1.5 hours. The drug is detected in bile, faeces, cerebrospinal fluid and breastmilk.[91]

***Tolerability:*** adverse effects of praziquantel are generally mild or transient and include abdominal discomfort, nausea, headache, dizziness, drowsiness, anorexia and skin eruptions. Fever and diarrhoea are relatively rare. The bioavailability and adverse effects of the drug are increased in the presence of liver disease.

#### Oltipraz

Oltipraz is a broad-spectrum orally effective antischistosomal drug. It reduces schistosomal glutathione concentrations and glucose utilisation, and produces degenerative changes in the structure of both male and female worms. It also causes an hepatic shift of the worms and decreases egg counts. The worms lose their attachment to host tissues and from the mesenteric vein shift to the liver.

***Tolerability:*** the most frequent adverse effect of this drug is nausea followed by vomiting and pain in the abdomen. Insomnia, headache, weakness and dizziness also may occur. Paraesthesias of the extremities and phototoxicity have been reported.

#### Amoscanate

Amoscanate, an amine, has a broad spectrum of activity. Its particle size and formulation considerably influence its effectiveness. Little is known about the pharmacokinetics and mode of action of amoscanate. It may cause an accumulation of cyclic-AMP and disturb metabolism in schistosomes. Its adverse effects such as central nervous system disturbances, jaundice and hepatotoxicity limit its use.

### *5.4.2 Optimum Treatment*

Although many drugs are available to treat schistosomiasis, praziquantel and oxamniquine are first-line therapy. They are relatively safe and effective and praziquantel appears to be better in individuals resistant to oxamniquine. Even patients with portal fibrosis are able to use one of these agents. These drugs have completely replaced antimonials which were used earlier. Hycanthone and niridazole are also used. However, both the latter drugs are contraindicated in patients with portosystemic shunts.

*Praziquantel:* dosage schedules for praziquantel differ depending on the species involved. Cure rates range from 75 to 100%.[119] It is effective against double infections of *S. mansoni* and *S. haematobium* and more recently has been shown to be useful in *S. mekongi* infection. For *S. japonicum* and *S. mekongi* infections, praziquantel is given orally as 3 doses of 20 mg/kg at 4-hour intervals. For *S. haematobium*, single oral doses of 40 mg/kg result in a cure rate of 72 to 100%. For *S. mansoni*, 2 doses of 25 mg/kg given 4 hours apart produce a cure rate of 63 to 97%. Praziquantel can be used in advanced cases where portal hypertension and ascites are seen. However, its cost is an important limiting factor in treatment.

*Oltipraz:* for *S. mansoni* infection, oltipraz is given in doses of 3 to 4.5 g/day in 3 divided doses which achieves cure rates of around 90%. For *S. haematobium* infection, a total dose of 25 mg/kg is given over 1 to 2 days with cure rates of 90%.

*Amoscanate* is effective against *S. mansoni*, *S. japonicum* and *S. haematobium*. The single doses necessary for complete elimination of both worms and eggs are 300 mg/kg if the drug particle size is 30 to 50μm, or 5 to 10 mg/kg with a particle size of 0.5μm. More clinical trials are needed to determine the optimum particle size for formulation.

*Metrifonate* is given as a single dose of 7.5 to 10 mg/kg every other week for 2 to 3 weeks. It is first-line therapy for *S. haematobium* infection and reduces egg counts by approximately 90 to 95%, with a parasitological cure in 44 to 93% of patients.[120] Monthly doses of metrifonate are reported to have a prophylactic effect against *S. haematobium*.

*Oxamniquine* is the best drug available for treatment of acute, subacute, chronic and complicated infections caused by *S. mansoni*. The dose is 20 mg/kg/day for 1 to 3 consecutive days which cures 60 to 90% of patients. In children, 20 mg/kg is given in 2 divided doses 4 to 6 hours apart, preferably after meals. It reduces eggs counts, but does not eradicate the parasites. In double infections with *S. mansoni* and *S. haematobium*, patients can be treated concomitantly with oxamniquine and metrifonate.

*Hycanthone* is administered as single intramuscular injections of 3 to 3.5 mg/kg, resulting in cure rates for *S. mansoni* and *S. haematobium* infection of 50 to 90%. Hycanthone treatment causes regression of the hepatosplenomegaly that occurs due to *S. mansoni* infection. It reduces egg output and kills worms. Hycanthone is contraindicated in patients with hepatosplenic involvement or other forms of liver disease. Because of its high rate of adverse reactions, it must be used with great caution.

*Niridazole* treatment is effective against all major schistosome species. The dosage is 25 mg/kg/day for 7 days or 35 mg/kg/day for 5 days in 2 or 3 divided doses each day. Cure rates vary from 85 to 100% for *S. haematobium* infection and 30 to 70% for *S. mansoni* infection. With doses of 20 mg/kg/day for 5 days, the cure rate is only 55% for *S. japonicum* infection. Niridazole is contraindicated in portosystemic shunting and in individuals with psychotic disturbances.

Older drugs such as metrifonate and hycanthone are being replaced by oltipraz and praziquantel.[121] Clinical trials are still being conducted to determine the most cost-effective dosages. Resistance to drugs is emerging. Currently, praziquantel appears to be the best tolerated broad-spectrum schistosomicide, and can be administered for as few as 5 days.

#### 5.4.3 Prevention and Control of Schistosomiasis

For control of schistosomiasis, the emphasis is shifting away from control of the snail host to a direct attack on the parasite by chemotherapy.[122,123] Careful follow-up for egg outputs and parasitological cure can be used to judge the outcome of therapy. Retreatment with alternative drugs is practised in heavily infected areas.

*Metrifonate* is useful for prophylaxis (see above). Though expensive, treating all individual in a community with a single-dose regimen of *praziquantel* appears to be an attractive alternative.

### 5.5 Leishmaniasis

Leishmaniasis affects 13 million people and is a protozoal disease caused by the genus leishmania and has 4 major clinical syndromes: visceral leishmaniasis (kala azar), cutaneous leishmaniasis, mucocutaneous leishmaniasis (espundia), and diffuse cutaneous leishmaniasis. The parasites are transmitted from animal reservoirs to human hosts by the bite of sandflies. Leishmania is a zoonotic infection that involves rodents, canines and various forest mammals. The sandflies, while sucking blood, ingest amastigotes that transform into promastigotes in the gut of the insect. These migrate into the proboscis and are deposited on the skin of the new host.

Person-to-person transmission is infrequent. The course of the subsequent disease is determined by the host's cellular immunity and the species of the parasite. Pathogenesis is related to lymphocytic infiltration in the skin, hypersensitivity to the parasite antigens, and the ability of the organism to suppress T cells. Cure of leishmaniasis requires activation of infected macrophages by lymphokines released from sensitised T cells. The organism can be demonstrated by smear or by culture of aspirates. Antibodies are detectable for all forms of leishmaniasis.

Leishmania species cause a diverse group of diseases. *Leishmania tropica* and *Leishmania major* cause cutaneous disease, *Leishmania mexicana* and *Leishmania braziliensis* cause cutaneous and mucosal disease, and infection with *Leishmania donovani* results in visceral leishmaniasis. The cutaneous disease is characterised by a slow progression through papular, nodular, ulcerative and healing stages, which results in scar tissue. *L. major* and *L. braziliensis* spread through the lymphatic system to regional lymph nodes. *L. braziliensis* also causes mucocutaneous disease. It can destroy the oral nasal mucosa and septum.

*L. donovani* complex causes kala azar, characterised by parasitisation of the macrophages of the spleen, lymph nodes, liver and bone marrow. Splenomegaly, hepatomegaly, lymphadenopathy, scaly and grayish skin, and anaemia characterise the disease. Kala azar is found in Africa, Asia, the Mediterranean, the Middle East and Latin America.

*L. braziliensis* is often treated to prevent mucosal spread of disease. The cutaneous leishmaniasis caused by *L. tropica* and *L. major* heal spontaneously and, hence, chemotherapy is not always considered except when infection occurs on the face and may lead to scars, when lesions fail to heal within 4 to 6 months, or if infections metastasise.

#### 5.5.1 Clinical Pharmacology of Drugs Used in Treatment

First-line therapies for leishmaniasis are pentavalent antimonials, pentamidine, amphotericin B, allopurinol and ketoconazole.[124] Their clinical pharmacological properties are summarised in table VI.

##### Pentavalent Antimonials

The pentavalent antimonial drugs *sodium stibogluconate* (sodium antimony gluconate) and *meglumine antimonate* inhibit amastigote bioenergetics, glycolytic and fatty acid oxidation, and interfere with energy production (ATP) and the antioxidant defence system.

***Pharmacokinetic characteristics:*** the pharmacokinetics of these drugs are remarkably similar.[125] They are rapidly absorbed from intramuscular injection sites and peak plasma concentrations occur 2 hours after the initial

**Table VI.** Comparative clinical pharmacological properties of drug used to treat leishmaniasis

| Feature | Allopurinol | Amphotericin B | Ketoconazole | Pentamidine | Pentavalent antimonials[a] |
|---|---|---|---|---|---|
| Mechanism of action | Analogue of ATP, ADP: competes with ATP | Inhibits folate synthesis. Increases membrane permeability | Inhibition of membrane function | DNA binding, polyamine biosynthesis | Inhibition of bioenergetics, glycolytic and fatty acid oxidation |
| Sensitive species | *L. donovani* | *L. braziliensis*<br>*L. donovani* | *L. braziliensis* | *L. donovani* | *L. donovani*<br>*L. braziliensis*<br>*L. mexicana* |
| Principal route of elimination | Renal | Renal | Faecal and renal | Renal | Renal |
| Form eliminated | Unchanged and as active metabolite (oxypurinol) | Unchanged | Inactive metabolites | Unchanged | Unchanged |
| Dosage | 21 mg/kg/d in 3 divided doses for 14-70d | Test dose, then 0.5-1 mg/kg/d for 15-20d (max. total dose 1g) | 400-600 mg/d for 10-14d | 4 mg/kg on alternate days for 30d (second course) | 20-30 mg/kg/d IV (or 850 mg/d IM) for 20-30d[b] |
| Route of administration | PO | IV infusion (in 5% dextrose) | PO | IV | IV or IM |
| Common adverse effects | Rash, hypersensitivity | Nephrotoxicity, fever, chills, hypokalaemia, hypomagnesaemia, phlebitis, anaemia | Liver enzyme abnormalities, gynaecomastia, decreased libido, nausea, vomiting | Rash, fever, phlebitis, hypotension, hypoglycaemia, leucopenia, neutropenia, thrombocytopenia, anaemia | Sterile abscesses, venous thrombosis, organotoxicity (kidney, liver), myalgias, arthralgia, headache, GI disturbances |
| Occasional adverse effects | Stevens-Johnson syndrome, neutropenia, thrombocytopenia, anaemia | Hypotension and shock | Hepatotoxicity | Hypocalcaemia, pancreatitis and diabetes, ECG changes, arrhythmias | Hypersensitivity reactions, fever, tachycardia weakness, insomnia, sudden death |

a Sodium stibogluconate and meglumine antimonate.

b As sodium stibogluconate.

*Abbreviations:* IM = intramuscular; IV = intravenous; PO = oral; tid = 3 times daily; bid = twice daily; ECG = electrocardiographic; GI = gastrointestinal.

dose. Plasma concentration data are best described by a 2-compartment model with an initial absorption phase with a half-life of 0.85 hours, followed by a rapid elimination phase with a mean half-life of 2 hours and a slow elimination phase with a half-life of 76 hours. Sodium stibogluconate is highly protein bound and more than 98% of the dose is excreted in the urine within 24 hours. It has a volume of distribution of 15.4L. Trough concentrations of sodium stibogluconate of 0.04 to 0.08 mg/L occur after the first dose of 10 mg/kg and increase to 0.19 to 0.33 mg/L 24 hours after the 30th dose. The slow terminal elimination phase may be related to its *in vivo* toxicity. It is not clear whether a favourable response to treatment depends on peak concentrations or maintenance of inhibitory concentrations.

***Tolerability:*** adverse effects of these drugs include sterile abscesses, venous thrombosis, and organ toxicity such as renal and hepatic damage, and cardiotoxicity. Myalgias, arthralgias, anorexia, headache and vomiting occur commonly. Occasionally, hypersensitivity reactions, palpitations, weakness, dizziness and insomnia occur. Sudden deaths are usually due to arrhythmias. In general, untoward reactions are less frequent and severe than with trivalent antimonial compounds, such as antimony potassium tartrate.

**Pentamidine**

Pentamidine, an aromatic diamidine, interacts with DNA or inhibits polyamine biosynthesis required for replication. It is generally useful as a salvage therapy when kala azar fails to respond to antimonials. Pentamidine is well absorbed from parenteral sites of administration and has a plasma half-life of 6 hours, a volume of distribution of 210L, and clearance of 4.3 L/h/kg (72 ml/min/kg). Oral bioavailability is low, as are CNS concentrations of the drug.[126] Pentamidine is largely excreted unchanged in urine; however, renal clearance accounts for only 2% of total plasma clearance.

***Tolerability:*** the adverse effects of pentamidine, in particular arrhythmias, diabetes, frequently-occurring myelosuppression and anaemia preclude its regular use.

#### Amphotericin B

This is a polyene antibiotic used as a systemic antifungal agent (see further chapter 31; sect. 6.1.1). It is not a water-soluble compound and hence is solubilised with sodium deoxycholate to form a micelle. Amphotericin B has a half-life of 15 days, clearance of around 1.8 L/h, volume of distribution of about 280L and is more than 90% is protein bound. Peak concentrations reached are 1 mg/L after a 50mg dose, with less than 5% entering the CNS.[127] The drug binds to tissue proteins and membranes and is concentrated in the liver, spleen, kidney and lung. Its slow elimination compounds its adverse effects.

Amphotericin B is a useful treatment of mucocutaneous leishmaniasis, with a 93% response rate and less than 10% relapse rate after 1 to 10 years of follow-up.

***Tolerability:*** a major adverse reaction that frequently occurs with amphotericin B therapy is nephrotoxicity. Hypokalaemia, hypomagnesaemia, fever and chills, with phlebitis and anaemia also occur frequently. Hypotension and stroke occur occasionally.

#### Allopurinol

Allopurinol, a structural analogue of hypoxanthine, is toxic to amastigotes and forms analogues of AMP, ADP and ATP. These analogues inhibit parasite metabolism by competing with ATP.

***Pharmacokinetic characteristics:*** allopurinol is rapidly absorbed after oral administration. It has a half-life of about 0.83 hours, clearance of 46 L/h and forms oxypurinol as the major metabolite. Oxypurinol is eliminated extensively by the kidney and the dose of allopurinol should be reduced in proportion to renal function. Peak plasma concentrations are reached within 30 to 60 minutes. Less than 30% is excreted as unchanged drug.

***Tolerability:*** the major adverse effect of allopurinol, which occurs frequently, is a hypersensitivity reaction, including skin rash and occasional Stevens-Johnson syndrome. Neutropenia, thrombocytopenia and anaemia have also been documented.

#### Ketoconazole and Itraconazole

These drugs are azoles that demethylate sterols in the parasite and interfere with membrane function. They are most useful in cutaneous leishmaniasis.

Oral absorption of ketoconazole is variable; an acidic environment is required for absorption. Ketoconazole has an elimination half-life of 7 to 8 hours, which rises with increases in dosage. Adverse effects include abnormalities in liver enzymes, gynaecomastia, decreased libido, nausea and vomiting, while occasionally severe progressive fatal hepatotoxicity is observed.

### *5.5.2 Optimum Treatment*

Cutaneous leishmaniasis spontaneously remits in months to years. However, because of local morbidity and the possibility of the mucosal spread, it should be treated. Visceral disease progresses rapidly and needs prompt treatment. Disease of the nasal mucosa progresses slowly but results in destruction of nasal septum; laryngeal and pharyngeal disease may progress to suffocation. Thus, all forms of leishmaniasis other than very mild cutaneous forms must be treated.

*Pentavalent antimonial compounds* are effective and are given in doses of 20 mg/kg/day (as sodium stibogluconate) by the intravenous route or 850 mg/day by the intramuscular route once a day for 20 days, or until 2 weeks after parasitological cure. A cure rate of 92% is achieved for mucocutaneous lesions with 20 mg/kg/day given for 30 days and identical treatment is adopted for systemic leishmaniasis.[128] Children are generally given the same dose. The main disadvantages of this treatment are the long courses of therapy required, the necessity for parenteral administration and its high cost. With lower dosages, the cure rate is much lower. For cutaneous lesions, antimony therapy is given until lesions heal. It has been suggested that multiple injections maintain high tissue concentrations and might be superior to once-daily regimens. However, they are not in common clinical use. Parasitological cure is generally confirmed by biopsy or splenic aspiration.

*Pentamidine* is effective for kala azar in 90% of cases. It is given in doses of 4 mg/kg on alternate days for 6 to 8 doses and is usually considered in patients who do not respond to pentavalent antimonial therapy. A second course is given after an interval of 1 to 2 weeks in areas where the infection is known to be less responsive.

*Amphotericin B* is given intravenously after a test dose and is increased from 0.5 to 1 mg/kg/day administered over 1 to 2 hours in 5% dextrose. The total dose is dependent on the clinical response, but is usually less than 1g. It is given for kala azar and mucocutaneous leishmaniasis (cure rate 93%).[129]

*Allopurinol* is given in doses of 21 mg/kg/day orally in 3 divided doses for 2 to 10 weeks. *Ketoconazole* is also administrated orally, the usual adult dose being 400 to 600mg once daily. The duration of therapy varies depending on the severity of the illness and may last from 10 to 14 days.

Monitoring of toxicity, electrocardiograms, and hepatic and renal function may aid in decreasing the severity of adverse reactions. In patients with hypersensitivity reactions and Stevens-Johnson syndrome, administration of prednisolone may be considered. Blood counts must be repeated often.

## 5.6 Trypanosomiasis

African trypanosomiasis or sleeping sickness is due to infection by *Trypanosoma brucei rhodesiense* and *Trypanosoma gambiense* which are transmitted by tsetse flies (Glossina species). The parasites are detectable in blood, lymph and spinal fluid of the infected human host. Both forms of the disease are fatal if untreated. The Gambian form (West African chronic) is characterised by low parasitaemia, gradual onset of neurological symptoms, lymphadenopathy and death around 2 years after initial infection. The Rhodesian form (East African acute) is characterised by high parasitaemia, rapid onset of neurological symptoms and death within weeks or months of infection. Somnolence and Parkinsonism characterises both forms. More than 35 million people appear to be at risk of infection.[130]

The trypanosomes are extracellular and develop antigenic variations of the thick outer glycoprotein layer, leading to cyclical variation of the surface protein and waves of parasitaemia, with new surface antigen, after immunity to the last surface antigen has already developed. Thus, the infection has a prolonged course. Therapy is aimed at killing the parasites in the blood stream. Once a spinal tap and neurological examinations are negative, patients are given less toxic drug therapy. However, if there is an indication that the brain is infected, more toxic drugs that can penetrate the blood-brain barrier need to be considered.

In addition to African trypanosomiasis, American trypanosomiasis or Chagas' disease is a zoonosis caused by *T. cruzi* that produces cardiomyopathy, mega-oesophagus, megacolon and death. It is commonly encountered in Southern California, Argentina and Chile and is transmitted by blood sucking insects. *T. cruzi* is vulnerable to drugs that form intracellular free radicals.

### 5.6.1 Clinical Pharmacology of Drugs Used in Treatment

Chemotherapy of African trypanosomiasis currently centres on drugs such as pentamidine for chemoprophylaxis and early stages of the disease, suramin to treat early stage of the disease, and melarsoprol to treat late stages (table VII).[131] Alternative drugs include eflornithine (difluoromethylornithine, DFMO). Diminazene is currently not recommended for humans. Several trypanocidal agents lack effectiveness against all stages of the disease and activity against all strains of pathogen, and are not orally bioavailable.

#### Pentamidine

The mechanism of action of pentamidine, though not well characterised, includes inhibition of dihydrofolate reductase, binding to DNA, inhibition of replication and RNA polymerase, and consequent reduced nucleic acid biosynthesis.[132] Drug concentrations in trypanosomes are many times that of blood. Pentamidine is not well absorbed from the gastrointestinal tract and hence is usually given parenterally. It is rapidly taken up by tissues and its slow excretion by the kidney (unchanged) seems to be the important factor in its use as a prophylactic agent in trypanosomiasis. Its plasma half-life is 6 hours, volume of distribution 210L, clearance 4.3 L/h/kg, and the CNS to plasma concentration ratio is low. Pentamidine is effective for as long as 6 months after a single intramuscular dose.

***Tolerability:*** the use of pentamidine is limited by adverse effects such as hypotension, diabetes and renal damage. Adverse reactions to pentamidine occur in a high proportion (43 to 83%) of patients.[133] Apart from serious hypotension and renal insufficiency, drug fever, hypersensitivity reactions, leucopenia, anaemia, and electrocardiographic abnormalities may occur. Fatal pancreatitis and ventricular arrhythmias have been noted. Most adverse effects occur between 7 and 14 days after starting therapy.

**Table VII.** Comparative clinical pharmacological properties of drugs used in trypanosomiasis

| Feature | Benznidazole | Eflornithine | Melarsoprol | Nifurtimox | Pentamidine | Suramin |
|---|---|---|---|---|---|---|
| Mechanism of action | Inhibits nucleic acid synthesis | Inhibition of ornithine decarboxylase and polyamine biosynthesis | Inhibition of pyruvate kinase; disruption of energy generation | DNA damage and inhibition of parasite specific antioxidant defence | Inhibition of dihydrofolate reductase, RNA polymerase binding to DNA | Inhibition of NADH oxidation |
| Sensitive species | *T. cruzi* | *T. gambiense* | *T. gambiense* *T. rhodesiense* (CNS forms) | *T. cruzi* | *T. gambiense* | T. gambiense T. rhodesiense |
| Dosage | 5 mg/kg od for 30-120d | 100 mg/kg qid initially then 75 mg/kg qid for 42d | 3.6 mg/kg od for 3d, repeated after 10d | 2-2.5 mg/kg qid for 90-120d | 3-4 mg/kg od for 7-10d (every 90d for prophylaxis) | 100-200mg test dose, then 1g/wk for 7 wks |
| Route of administration | PO | IV for 2 wks then PO for 4 wks | IV | PO | IV or IM | IV |
| Route of elimination | Renal | Renal | Renal | Renal | Renal | Renal |
| Form eliminated | Metabolite | Unchanged | Unchanged | Unchanged | Unchanged | Unchanged |
| Relative clinical effectiveness | +++ | ++++ | +++ | +++ | ++++ | +++ |
| Common adverse effects | Peripheral neuropathy, purpuric dermatitis, GI disturbance, haemolytic anaemia | GI disturbance, anaemia | Highly toxic (encephalopathy, fever, vasodilatation) | GI disturbance, peripheral neuropathy, haemolytic anaemia | Hypotension, hypoglycaemia, sterile abscess, phlebitis, renal damage, GI disturbance | Idiosyncratic reactions, nephrotoxicity, proteinuria, GI disturbance, chest and abdominal pain |
| Occasional adverse effects | Myelosuppression, disorientation, seizures, malaise, rash | Neutropenia, thrombocytopenia, decreased auditory acuity, seizures, haematuria, rash | Herxheimer reactions, jaundice, conjunctival irritation | Disorientation, seizures, rash, malaise, insomnia | Abortions, anaemia, ECG changes, ventricular arrhythmia, pancreatitis and diabetes | Optic atrophy, neuropathy, rash, adrenal insufficiency, myelosuppression, haemolytic anaemia |

*Abbreviations:* IM = intramuscular; IV = intravenous; PO = oral; od = once daily; qid = 4 daily; ECG = electrocardiograph; GI = gastrointestinal.

**Suramin**

Suramin is a divalent cationic agent administered by the intravenous route. It does not cross the blood-brain barrier and is ineffective against disease in the nervous system. Suramin has a slow onset of action (24 hours delay)[134] as the parasite takes the drug up by pinocytosis. It is trypanocidal at high concentrations (4 mol/L). Suramin is excreted slowly in unchanged form by the kidney. Total plasma clearance is less than 0.03 L/h, volume of distribution is 40L and the elimination half-life is 50 days.[135] It can be detected in blood 3 months after administration.

***Tolerability:*** suramin is highly toxic and produces adverse effects on the fetus. Idiosyncratic reactions with vomiting, shock, convulsions, collapse and death can occur.[131] Delayed reactions such as blindness, peripheral neuropathy, adrenal insufficiency, nephrotoxicity, haemolytic anaemia and agranulocytosis can also occur. Heavy proteinuria and kidney damage are common adverse reactions. Malnutrition and renal insufficiency further increase the toxicity of the drug.[136]

**Melarsoprol**

Melarsoprol is a trivalent arsenical that acts primarily by inhibiting parasite pyruvate kinase, thus disrupting parasite glycolysis. This drug can cure all stages of both Gambian and Rhodesian forms. It is administered intravenously and is rapidly excreted in the urine. Reasonable concentrations are seen by day 3 of treatment (day 4 in the CSF) and patients feel better within 3 to 4 days of starting therapy.

***Tolerability:*** melarsoprol causes severe toxicity and leads to death in 1% of patients. Immediate reactions include fever, chest pain, vasodilatation and skin reactions. Encephalopathy occurs in 1 to 10% of patients.[137] Other adverse effects include jaundice, diarrhoea and conjunctival irritation.

#### Eflornithine

Eflornithine inhibits the synthesis of ornithine, which is needed for polyamine synthesis and protozoan replication. Rapidly dividing trypanosomes are sensitive to eflornithine. It has an oral bioavailability of approximately 50%, plasma half-life of 3 hours and is predominantly excreted by the kidney. CSF concentrations are 25 to 45% of serum concentrations.

Eflornithine is useful as a treatment of African sleeping sickness.[138] Oral administration is complicated by diarrhoea and thrombocytopenia. Currently, the drug is given by the intravenous route.

#### Nifurtimox

Nifurtimox is the only drug active against American trypanosomiasis. Nifurtimox is a 5-nitrofuran that is believed to act by causing breaks in parasite DNA by inhibiting parasite-specific antioxidant defence enzyme systems. Concentrations of 1 μmol/L damage intracellular amastigotes *in vitro* and stop development. Nifurtimox is absorbed after oral administration, but results in low concentrations (10 to 20 μmol/L) in plasma.[134] It is rapidly metabolised and several unidentified metabolites are present in urine.

***Tolerability:*** it is rare for a patient to undergo a full course of treatment with nifurtimox because adverse effects such as gastrointestinal discomfort, peripheral neuritis, disorientation, restlessness, insomnia, seizures and rashes occur. Haemolytic anaemia can be precipitated in patients with G6PD deficiency.

#### Benznidazole

Like nifurtimox, benznidazole inhibits nucleic acid and protein synthesis. Free radical generation, however, is less than with nifurtimox. At higher doses (5 mg/kg), it frequently produces peripheral neuropathy and purpuric dermatitis. Lower doses result in gastrointestinal disturbances and myelosuppression.

#### Other Drugs

*Tryparsamide* is a pentavalent arsenical compound effective against both forms of trypanosomiasis. However, optic nerve toxicity may lead to irreversible blindness. *Melarsonyl* can be given by subcutaneous or intramuscular injection, but is toxic.

### 5.6.2 Optimum Treatment

First-line drugs for trypanosomiasis without CNS involvement are pentamidine and suramin. The dosage of *pentamidine* is 3 to 4 mg/kg daily intravenously or intramuscularly for 7 to 10 days. Pentamidine has also been given for prophylaxis every 3 to 6 months in doses of 4 mg/kg intramuscularly. (*NB.* intramuscular injections can result in local abscess). Pentamidine is highly efficacious against the Gambian form.

After a test dose of 100 to 200mg, *suramin* is administered intravenously in 1g doses weekly for 5 weeks.[139] The paediatric dosage is 20 mg/kg weekly. *Melarsoprol* is given for infections with abnormal CSF in doses of 2 to 3.6 mg/kg/day intravenously for 3 days (maximum dose 180mg); in children, the dose is 1.8 mg/kg/day. The 3-day regimen is repeated after 10 days. In some countries, 3 doses/week are repeated for 4 weeks and a total dose of 37.5 mg/kg is considered. Suggested dosages of *tryparsamide* are 30 mg/kg given 10 to 12 times by the intravenous route at 5- to 7-day intervals.

*Eflornithine* is given in doses of 400 mg/kg/day intravenously in 4 divided doses initially, followed by 75 mg/kg orally every 6 hours for a total of 6 weeks. In most studies, the drug has been given by the intravenous route for the first 2 weeks and then changed to the oral form. *Nifurtimox* is given in doses of 8 to 10 mg/kg/day in adults and 15 mg/kg/day in children in 4 divided doses; therapy is recommended for 90 to 120 days. *Benznidazole* is given orally at 5 mg/kg/day for 30 to 120 days for *T. cruzi* infection.

In general, the above dosage regimens have been based more on trial and error than on sound pharmacokinetic considerations. Adverse reactions are serious with this group of drugs. Prednisolone 1 mg/kg/day (up to 40 mg/day) given along with melarsoprol (continued through the second course and tapered thereafter) has reduced the incidence of encephalopathy from 11 to 4%. The dosages of most of these drugs must be adjusted in patients with renal failure. To avoid serious toxic reactions, kidney and liver function and blood tests (including platelets and blood sugar) should be monitored regularly.

### 5.6.3 Prevention of Trypanosomiasis

Pentamidine has been considered for prophylaxis, but most other drugs are too toxic for prophylactic use. No effective prophylaxis exists for Chagas' disease.

## 5.7 Toxoplasmosis

Toxoplasmosis caused by the intracellular protozoan *Toxoplasma gondii* is a common cause of latent infection worldwide. Humans are affected by ingesting oocysts excreted by cats or by consuming undercooked meat with tissue cysts. Transplacental transmission occurs and infection during pregnancy is responsible for congenital toxoplasmosis. Infection can be reactivated from a dormant stage in immunocompromised hosts, AIDS patients and recipients of transplant organs from infected patients. Acute and reactivated infections require treatment.

Though infection is common worldwide, only some individuals suffer from the disease toxoplasmosis. IgG antibodies are sensitive and specific for the detection of toxoplasma infection. Detection of acute acquired infections are more difficult, but specific IgM antibody or high titres of IgG may be useful in diagnosis.

### 5.7.1 Clinical Pharmacology of Drugs Used in Treatment

#### Pyrimethamine

Pyrimethamine (see also section 5.1.1) given with a sulfonamide (e.g. sulfadiazine or trisulfapyrimidines) is the first-line treatment for toxoplasmosis. This combination has synergistic activity against toxoplasma trophozoites both *in vivo* and *in vitro*. However, no drug or combination is known to be effective against tissue cysts that characterise chronic latent infection. Serum concentrations of 1 to 4.5 mg/L are usually observed after pyrimethamine dosages of 25 to 75 mg/day. Serum concentrations >0.75 mg/L in the presence of sulfonamides and >3.0 mg/L in their absence are required.[140]

In view of its erratic absorption and variable serum concentrations, daily administration of pyrimethamine is advisable. A predictable adverse effect is bone marrow suppression. Pyrimethamine is teratogenic and should be avoided in pregnancy.

#### Sulfonamides

Sulfonamide drugs inhibit dihydrofolic acid synthetase. In the treatment of toxoplasmosis, trisulfapyrimidines (i.e. equal parts of sulfadiazine, sulfamerazine and sulfadimidine) and sulfadiazine alone are given in combination with pyrimethamine.

Adverse reactions to sulfonamides may limit their use. Nausea and diarrhoea are common. Skin rashes, including Stevens-Johnson syndrome are also a concern, as are nephrolithiasis and reversible renal failure. Renal damage is usually reversed when the patient is hydrated and the urine is alkalinised. Urological complications with trisulfapyrimidines appear to occur less frequently than with sulfadiazine.

#### Spiramycin and Clindamycin

The macrolide antibiotic *spiramycin* is effective in toxoplasmosis and may be used to treat pregnant women. It is concentrated in tissues and therefore may have greater activity in this infection than other macrolides. Spiramycin is slowly eliminated and biliary excretion is significant. It is better tolerated than the combination of pyrimethamine and sulfadiazine.

*Clindamycin* is concentrated in the eye (choroid) and is effective in ocular toxoplasmosis.

#### Other Drugs

*Roxithromycin* has proved effective in a murine model of toxoplasmosis. *Erythromycin* has also proved effective in preventing death in an encephalitis murine model. *Immunomodulators* used in human trials to treat neoplastic diseases and AIDS-related illnesses have proved moderately effective in acute systemic toxoplasmosis. The lack of adequate clinical pharmacological and therapeutic information for the treatment of toxoplasmosis is due to the slow methods of evaluating the activity of drugs, the absence of controlled clinical trials, and the currently imprecise diagnosis and therapy of the condition.

### 5.7.2 Optimum Treatment

Immunocompetent children or adults with lymphadenitis require therapy. In those with signs of vital organ involvement and prolonged symptoms, treatment is continued until signs and symptoms of acute disease are controlled. Generally this takes 4 to 6 weeks but in immunodeficient patients therapy may need to be continued for 6 months or more. A loading dose of *pyrimethamine* of 200 mg/day in 2 divided doses is given, followed by 50 to 100 mg/day once daily for suppressive and maintenance therapy. The loading dose of *sulfadiazine* is 75 mg/kg up to a maximum of 4g, followed by 150 mg/kg/day for 8 days in 2 divided daily doses. For *spiramycin,* the dose is 2 to 4 g/day in 4 divided doses. No controlled trials have been conducted to demonstrate the effectiveness of one regimen over another.

In patients who cannot tolerate sulfonamides or spiramycin, *clindamycin* is used at doses of 2.4 to 4.8 g/day intravenously in 3 to 4 divided doses, followed by 300mg orally every 6 hours for 3 weeks. In immunocompromised patients, clindamycin has gained some attention for toxoplasmosis encephalitis. A dose of 2.4 to 4.8 g/day intravenously followed by 1.2 to 2.4 g/day orally is administered for toxoplasmosis encephalitis. Clindamycin 300mg orally every 6 hours for 3 weeks is given for toxoplasmic chorioretinitis. Relapses are noted in around 80% of patients and occur within 7 weeks of discontinuing therapy. The combination of pyrimethamine and a sulfonamide usually controls relapses.

In immunodeficient patients, long term suppressive therapy with pyrimethamine (25 to 50 mg/day) and sulfadiazine (2 to 4 g/day) is recommended. Corticosteroids are not recommended for routine treatment but may be considered for toxoplasmosis encephalitis. Calcium folinate (leucovorin calcium) 5 to 10 mg/day can be given to reduce the adverse effects of pyrimethamine (without inhibiting its action on toxoplasma). Sulfonamides are not used in patients with encephalitis.

For prevention of toxoplasma infection during kidney transplantation, pyrimethamine 25 mg/day for 6 weeks is administered after transplantation is completed. To cure toxoplasmosis infection during pregnancy, pyrimethamine (50 mg/day), sulfadiazine (3 g/day) and calcium folinate are administered for 3 weeks alternating with 3 weeks of spiramycin (3 g/day).

#### Congenital Toxoplasmosis

Congenital toxoplasmosis is treated with a combination of pyrimethamine and a sulfonamide. The dose of pyrimethamine is 1 mg/kg every 2 days while that of sulfadiazine is 100 mg/kg/day in 2 divided doses with calcium folinate 5 mg every second day. Three-week courses of this combination may be alternated with 4- to 6-week courses of spiramycin 100 mg/kg/day in 2 to 3 divided doses daily.

#### Chorioretinitis

For chorioretinitis, corticosteroids are given for 6 months. Pyrimethamine and sulfadiazine are also used in active chorioretinitis, with treatment usually administered for 1 month. Clindamycin 300mg orally 4 times a day is very effective for human toxoplasmosis chorioretinitis.

## 5.8 *Pneumocystis carinii* Pneumonia

*Pneumocystis carinii* is an opportunistic pathogen found in the lungs. It produces pneumonia, particularly in immunosuppressed patients. In over 75% of patients with AIDS, *Pneumocystis carinii* pneumonia (PCP) develops on more than 1 occasion and is the cause of death in 25% of patients.[141] *P. carinii* is more closely related to fungi than to protozoa. It has a worldwide distribution among humans and animals, and is often found in premature malnourished infants and in immunosuppressed patients. Antibodies are produced locally and systemically, but have little protective role.

### *5.8.1 Clinical Pharmacology of Drugs Used in Treatment*

Several drugs are available to treat and prevent PCP. Trimethoprim and sulfamethoxazole (cotrimoxazole) or pentamidine are regularly used. Other drugs under investigation include dapsone and trimethoprim, trimetrexate, eflornithine, atovaquone and the combination of primaquine and clindamycin.

#### Cotrimoxazole

Cotrimoxazole (trimethoprim/sulfamethoxazole) is a broad-spectrum antibacterial agent that inhibits synthesis of tetrahydrofolic acid. The trimethoprim component inhibits dihydrofolate reductase while sulfamethoxazole inhibits its incorporation of aminobenzoic acid into dihydrofolate. The optimal plasma concentrations ratio of trimethoprim to sulfamethoxazole is 1 : 20 for maximal synergistic effects.

### *5.8.2 Optimum Treatment*

The treatment schedule for PCP is indicated in table VIII. Adult and paediatric dosages are the same. Three weeks of therapy is usual for AIDS patients. The drugs are generally administrated orally and if necessary by the intravenous route. If creatinine clearance is below 1.8 L/h (30 ml/min), dosages must be adjusted. If evidence of toxicity such as decreasing neutrophil or platelet counts and progressive hepatic or renal dysfunction develops, treatment with cotrimoxazole should be discontinued and pentamidine administrated.

Immunosuppressed patients can be protected by prophylactic administration of cotrimoxazole (150 mg/m$^2$ trimethoprim and 750 mg/m$^2$ sulfamethoxazole per day).[142] Intermittent prophylaxis with the same dosage given in 2 divided doses on 3 consecutive days per week is effective in preventing PCP in patients with cancer. Prophylaxis should be considered in AIDS patients, patients who have been treated for PCP, those in whom immune competence is poor, or patients with candidiasis. The optimum duration of prophylaxis is not clear.

*Pentamidine* is given in doses of 4 mg/kg intravenously as a single dose over 1 to 2 hours.

**Table VIII.** Treatment of *Pneumocystis carinii* pneumonia (PCP) [see also chapter 23; sect. 10.1]

| Drug of choice | Dosage |
|---|---|
| Cotrimoxazole [trimethoprim (TMP)/ sulfamethoxazole (SMX)] | TMP 20 mg/kg/d + SMX 100 mg/kg/d PO or IV in 4 divided doses for 14-21d<br>Paediatric dose same |
| Pentamidine | 4 mg/kg/d IV for 14-21d; nebuliser delivery under investigation |
| Dapsone/trimethoprim (TMP) | Dapsone 100mg PO od + TMP 20 mg/kg/d in 4 divided doses for 14-21d |
| Trimetrexate/calcium folinate ± sulfadiazine | Trimetrexate 30-60 mg/m$^2$ od for 21d; calcium folinate 80 mg/m$^2$/d in 4 divided doses for 23d; ± sulfadiazine 1 g/d PO in 4 divided doses for 21d |
| Eflornithine | 400 mg/kg/d IV in 4 divided doses for 14d, then 300 mg/kg/d in 4 divided doses for up to 42d or more |

*Abbreviations:* IV = intravenous; PO = oral; od = once daily.

The duration of treatment with this agent is 10 days to 3 weeks. Nebulised pentamidine for both treatment and prophylaxis of PCP may also be used. Nebulised drug is not absorbed systemically and its bioavailability is only 5%. However, severe pulmonary haemorrhage, rash, acute renal failure and spontaneous pneumothorax have been seen with nebulised pentamidine.[134] Prophylactically, pentamidine 30 to 60mg is nebulised over 30 minutes every 2 weeks.

The next choice of drug is *dapsone* and combinations of *dapsone* and *trimethoprim*. Dapsone in doses of 100mg orally once daily together with trimethoprim (20 mg/kg/day in 4 divided doses) given for 14 to 21 days is effective in 100% of patients. The dosage of dapsone must be adjusted if there is renal impairment. Adverse reactions with this drug include anaemia, methaemoglobinaemia, anorexia, nausea and vomiting.

*Trimetrexate,* an inhibitor of dihydrofolate reductase, has been used in combination with calcium folinate with or without sulfadiazine. Trimetrexate has a half-life of 10 to 32 hours, is biotransformed in the liver and excreted in urine. Occasionally, peripheral neuropathy and elevations of transaminases and serum creatinine have been reported.[134]

*Eflornithine* is given either orally or intravenously and has been used in patients unresponsive to conventional therapy. Adverse effects of this drug include haematological and gastrointestinal reactions. It may be used as a salvage therapy.

*Pyrimethamine and sulfadoxine have synergistic activity on folate metabolism. This combination has a prolonged action due to the long plasma half-lives of the two drugs (pyrimethamine 80 to 95 hours and sulfadoxine 125 hours). It is most useful for prophylaxis of PCP.[143] However, hypersensitivity reactions have occurred.[144] Studies of primaquine* in combination with *clindamycin* are in progress, and preliminary results are encouraging.

## 6. Leprosy

Leprosy is a chronic infection caused by *Mycobacterium leprae*, and affects colder parts of the body such as the skin, upper respiratory tract, anterior surfaces of the eyes, testes and superficial segments of peripheral nerves. According to the WHO,[145] there are 5.5 million people with leprosy in the world. The highest prevalences are seen in tropical Africa, South America, South Asia (India), Southeast Asia (the Philippines), and coastal Pacific Islands. There are 2 main varieties, lepromatous and tuberculoid, and the predominant type varies in different populations. It develops in all age groups. Unfavourable, unhygienic surroundings and overcrowding undoubtedly play an important role in determining susceptibility.

### 6.1 Clinical Pharmacology of Drugs Used in Treatment

Although chemotherapy of leprosy began in the 1940s with the sulfones, treatment has not advanced much and dapsone remains the drug of choice. However, due to emerging resistance patterns and the advent of other drugs, the WHO[122] recommends 4 drugs for combined chemotherapy. Progress in the chemotherapy of leprosy has been slow due to inefficient animal models, methods of diagnosis, the chronic nature of the disease, and inadequate treatment and control measures. Financial and administrative difficulties in implementing multidrug regimens compound the problem. Although there is adequate knowledge of the bacilli and host responses, social aspects in terms of patient and societal attitude need more emphasis.

First-line drugs in treatment are dapsone[146] rifampicin, clofazimine, ethionamide and prothionamide.[147] Thioacetazone, isoniazid and pyrazinamide have also been used (table IX).

### *6.1.1 Dapsone*

Dapsone is a bacteriostatic drug that inhibits folic acid synthesis. It has only weak bactericidal activity; however, *M. leprae* are extremely sensitive to dapsone. Steady-state concentrations are twice as high as concentrations resulting from a single dose[148] and are 150 times the minimum inhibitory concentration (MIC).

**Pharmacokinetic Characteristics**

Dapsone is slowly but completely absorbed after oral administration and is 70 to 80% bound to plasma proteins. It is well distributed in total body water and present in all tissues of the body, especially in liver, muscle, kidney and skin. Following intramuscular injection of 375mg in an oily vehicle, dapsone concentrations of 1 mg/L were found. Salivary glands are highly permeable to dapsone and the concentrations there are 18 to 27% of blood concentrations. Dapsone crosses the placental barrier and is secreted in breastmilk, but does not have major adverse effects on the fetus or infant.[149]

Dapsone is metabolised by acetylation (to acetyldapsone) and by *N*-hydroxylation. However, deacetylation also occurs and metabolites are not detected to a significant extent in plasma. Acetylation polymorphism is known to occur in dapsone metabolism (see chapter 1; sect. 5.2.1), but does not affect its pharmacokinetics or clinical effectiveness as acetylation is not the only route of metabolism. Therapeutic responses are seen in both acetylator phenotypes. *N*-Hydroxydapsone is excreted as both

**Table IX.** Comparative clinical pharmacological properties of drugs used in the treatment of leprosy

| Feature | Dapsone | Rifampicin (rifampin) | Clofazimine | Ethionamide/ prothionamide |
|---|---|---|---|---|
| Mechanism of action | Primarily bacteriostatic; inhibition of folate synthesis | Bactericidal; inhibits DNA-dependent RNA polymerase | Bacteriostatic; binds to DNA | Bactericidal |
| Onset of action (h) | 2-6 | 2-3 | 4-8 | 0.5-1.5 |
| **Pharmacokinetic characteristics:** | | | | |
| F (%) | 95 | 90 | 70-85 | 90 |
| Linear kinetics | Yes | Yes | Yes | Yes |
| $t_{½β}$ (h) | 30 | 4 | 70 days | 2 |
| Vd (L)[a] | 69 | 68 | | |
| CL (L/h)[a] | 3 | 10 | | |
| Protein binding (%) | 73 | 80 | | 30 |
| Principal route of elimination | Hepatic/renal | Renal | Renal (conjugated metabolite) and faecal (free drug) | Renal |
| Active metabolites | Yes | Yes | No | Yes |
| Metabolite activity relative to parent drug | Less active | Equal | ? | Less active or equal |
| Route of administration | PO | PO | PO | PO |
| Dosage | 50-100mg od | 600mg once/month | 50 mg/d[b] | 250-375 mg/d[c] |
| Relative clinical effectiveness | ++++ | ++++ | ++++ | +++ |
| Potential drug interactions | Probenecid | Anticoagulants, oral antidiabetics, oral contraceptives, corticosteroids, halothane (see also appendix B) | | Alcohol (ethanol), antihypertensives, cycloserine |
| Patient benefits | Inexpensive and freely available; less toxic | Single dose | Single dose | Single dose |
| Limitations | Resistance | Expensive | Expensive<br>Skin discolouration | Expensive<br>Skin discolouration |

a Per 70kg (with normal renal function).

b In multibacillary disease, 300 mg once/month is also given.

c Ethionamide dosage.

*Abbreviations:* od = once daily; bid = twice daily; F = oral bioavailability; $t_{½β}$ = elimination half-life; CL = total body clearance; Vd = apparent volume of distribution; PO = oral.

the free form (2 to 7%) and a conjugated form (30 to 50%). A high renal clearance has been suggested.[150] The *N*-hydroxylated forms are less active in leprosy.

#### Tolerability

The most frequent adverse effects of dapsone are haematological in nature and dose-related. Methaemoglobinaemia caused by the hydroxylated metabolites is more severe in G6PD deficient patients. Haemolysis occurs when dosages of 50 mg/day are exceeded in G6PD deficient patients.

Dapsone allergy occurs rarely (1 in 400 patients) but results in exfoliative dermatitis, generalised lymphadenopathy, jaundice and fever in patients with a known history of sulfone allergy. Mild gastrointestinal reactions such as nausea, vomiting and abdominal pain also may occur when doses exceed 100 mg/day. Dapsone has very few drug interactions, but probenecid increases its toxicity/effectiveness by blocking renal tubular excretion.[151,152]

### 6.1.2 Clofazimine

Clofazimine is a bacteriostatic agent with some anti-inflammatory effects that is useful in lepromatous leprosy in the reaction phase. It is most active when administered daily or 3 times a week.

#### Pharmacokinetic Characteristics

Absorption of clofazimine is 85% when a micronised form in oil suspension is used for oral administration and appears to be dose-related, with increased absorption after food.[153] Clofazimine is extensively distributed in tissues. It is highly lipophilic and is therefore distributed into fatty tissue and macrophages. Although, it does not cross the blood-brain barrier, it crosses the placenta and is excreted in breastmilk. The elimination half-life of clofazimine has been estimated at 70 days (based on urinary recovery). Steady-state plasma concentrations are not reached until after 30 days and therefore loading doses are useful.[154] Urinary metabolites have been identified but their biological activity is unknown. Much of a dose is excreted unchanged in the faeces. Clofazimine is used only in combination therapy, although resistance is rare.

#### Tolerability

The most common adverse effects of clofazimine are red-brown hyperpigmentation of the skin and conjunctiva, and abdominal pain. Cutaneous pigmentation can fade within 6 to 12 months of treatment. Milder gastrointestinal symptoms and generalised xeroderma and ichthyosis have been noted.

Clofazimine has also been recommended for HIV patients with disseminated *Mycobacterium avium* complex infection.[154]

### 6.1.3 Rifampicin

Of the available drugs, rifampicin possesses the highest bactericidal activity against *M. leprae*. Its absorption is rapid and nearly complete and peak plasma concentrations occur 2 to 4 hours after oral administration. Both the peak concentration and area under the plasma concentration-time curve (AUC) are greater if the drug is given before food. During continuous administration, plasma concentrations of rifampicin and its elimination half-life are usually higher after the first dose than after subsequent doses, due to induction of its own metabolism. It crosses both the blood-brain and placental barriers, but does not adversely affect the fetus. The drug is metabolised in the liver and its metabolites are excreted in both the bile and urine. Deacetyl-rifampicin, the major metabolite, is as active as the parent compound.

Rifampicin, due to its potent effect in inducing drug metabolising enzymes, decreases the effectiveness of several other drugs that may be given concomitantly (table IX) [see also chapter 23; sect. 9.1.1 and appendix B].

### 6.1.4 Thionamides (Ethionamide and Prothionamide)

The thionamide drugs ethionamide and prothionamide are virtually interchangeable. They are bactericidal in nature, but less potent than rifampicin. Peak concentrations are reached within 30 minutes after oral administration, elimination half-lives are about 2 hours, and both drugs are converted to *S*-oxides in the body. Resistance develops rapidly and the thionamides are currently used as alternatives to clofazimine. The most serious adverse effect of these drugs is hepatitis, particularly when they are used in combination with rifampicin. They potentiate the CNS effects of alcohol, cycloserine and antihypertensives (resulting in hypotension).

### 6.1.5 Other Drugs

The skin discolouration provoked by clofazimine, the hepatotoxicity of thionamides, and the emergence of resistant strains have stimulated further research on antileprotic drugs. A phenazine derivative of clofazimine that is as active as clofazimine in mice but with low toxicity is awaiting clinical trials in leprosy patients. Two fluoroquinolones, pefloxacin (800mg daily) and ofloxacin (400mg daily) inhibit bacterial DNA transcription with few adverse effects.[155] The macrolide antibiotics clarithromycin and roxithromycin are also potentially useful, as is minocycline which is currently undergoing short term clinical trials.[155]

#### *6.1.6 Vaccines*

Trials are in progress comparing the effectiveness of autoclaved *M. leprae* alone and in combination with bacille Calmette-Guérin (BCG). The Indian Cancer Research Center (ICRC) has developed a vaccine employing the cultivable ICRC mycobacteria. This vaccine has been tested in several clinical trials, with no reports of serious adverse effects.[156] A highly immunogenic cell protein peptidoglycan complex of *M. leprae* offers promise as a purified vaccine for leprosy and is also being evaluated.[157]

### 6.2 Optimum Treatment

From a clinical point of view, combination drug therapy appears to be safe and effective in the treatment of leprosy. Since adverse drug reactions may occur, some of which may be serious, it is necessary to monitor liver and kidney function during therapy. For effective treatment there must be good patient compliance, and supervised administration of drugs such as rifampicin and clofazimine given as a single monthly dose is essential. Clofazimine appears to be useful for controlling lepromatous reactions as well, while rifampicin or the thionamides are extremely useful for killing *M. leprae*.

Dapsone is well tolerated but clofazimine, due to its effect in causing skin discolouration, is not as well accepted. Most gastrointestinal reactions with dapsone are not serious and may disappear on prolonged therapy. Although concomitant administration of rifampicin may decrease the elimination half-life and steady-state plasma and tissue concentrations of dapsone, in terms of effectiveness, this pharmacokinetic interaction does not appear to be important. Similarly, concomitant administration of antituberculosis drugs has not resulted in important drug interactions with clofazimine or prothionamide. However, one important drug interaction appears to be that between rifampicin and corticosteroids; when rifampicin is administered, corticosteroid plasma concentrations are reduced markedly.

No drug is used as monotherapy in leprosy as this would promote emergence of resistant strains. The WHO recommends multidrug therapy with the following goals: to treat disease, prevent bacterial resistance, and interrupt transmission by rapidly eliminating viable *M. leprae*.

Treatment depends on the type of leprosy. The borderline lepromatous leprosy and polar lepromatous leprosy are referred to as *multibacillary* leprosy. Borderline tuberculoid and polar tuberculoid and indeterminant classes are grouped together as *paucibacillary* disease. Treatment of multibacillary leprosy is continued for nearly 2 years or until smears are negative, whichever is longer. In paucibacillary disease, treatment is for 6 months or until clinical inactivity is achieved. Relapse in multibacillary cases is easy to recognise. It can be confirmed bacteriologically by slit skin smear examination. Relapse in paucibacillary cases is difficult to diagnose and needs confirmation by slit skin smear examination or biopsy. For surveillance, it is recommended that paucibacillary cases be examined clinically once a year for a minimum of 2 years and multibacillary cases be examined both clinically and bacteriologically once a year for a minimum of 5 years.[122]

In paucibacillary patients, rifampicin 600mg once a month is administered under supervision along with dapsone 100 mg/day for 6 months. Multibacillary patients should receive dapsone 100 mg/day and clofazimine 50 mg/day unsupervised with rifampicin 600mg and clofazimine 300mg once a month under supervision. If clofazimine cannot be used, ethionamide 250 to 375 mg/day is given.

There are variations of multidrug therapy.[156] Multidrug therapy in the US for both paucibacillary and multibacillary leprosy patients consists of rifampicin 600 mg/day with dapsone 100 mg/day, with paucibacillary patients receiving treatment for 6 months and multibacillary patients receiving it for 3 years. Clofazimine 50 mg/day may be added to the regimen for patients with resistant multibacillary and paucibacillary leprosy. In an Indian government programme, rifampicin 600 mg/day for 14 days is followed by 600mg pulses every month.[158]

Mild *lepromatous reactions* are often encountered and can be treated with aspirin to control pain and reduce inflammation. Chloroquine 150mg 3 times a day as an anti-inflammatory drug has been tried. Corticosteroids, clofazimine and thalidomide are the standard drugs used to manage severe reactions. *Clofazimine* is generally effective in erythema nodosum leprosum (ENL), and a dosage of 100 to 200 mg/day for up to 3 months may eliminate or reduce corticosteroid requirements. *Thalidomide* helps to control the neuritis and iritis of ENL and is the drug of choice for ENL in men and nonfertile women. The dose of thalidomide is 400mg 4 times daily reduced gradually to an effective daily dose of 100 mg/day, given for 6 months. Cyclosporin and immunomodulators have also been used in ENL.

Corticosteroids are the first-line treatment for reversal reactions and prednisolone is given in doses of 40 to 80 mg/day for 3 to 4 days initially, then reduced by 50%. The dose is then further reduced by 10mg each week. Corticosteroids are used as long as there is active neuritis. Weaning patients with chronic ELN off corticosteroids can be difficult and they may require clofazimine.

In certain individuals, despite adequate bacterial concentrations of antileprotic drugs, some *M. leprae* persist. These are termed 'persisters'. Pyrazinamide has been used as a companion antileprosy drug to overcome these 'persister' bacilli.[159]

## 7. Tuberculosis

Tuberculosis is a chronic bacterial infection caused by *Mycobacterium tuberculosis*, and is characterised by granuloma in infected tissues and cell-mediated hypersensitivity. It is transmitted from person to person via the respiratory route and spreads by haematogenous dissemination. The site of the disease is the lungs. Extrapulmonary tuberculosis in the nervous system, bone, gastrointestinal system, lymph nodes, etc. is well known. Tuberculosis produces acute disease that kills young and old alike. Current estimates indicate that one-third of the world's population is infected with *Mycobacterium tuberculosis*, making it the most prevalent infection in the world.[160] It is a slow progressive worldwide epidemic. Tuberculosis bacilli grow slowly, dividing approximately every 18 to 24 hours. Once cell-mediated immunity develops, infection with *M. tuberculosis* is arrested. In individuals in whom cell-mediated immunity cannot contain the infection, it progresses to disease. Thus, the clinical manifestations of the disease are a result of a balance between the host response and bacterial virulence. Tuberculosis is prominent among patients with AIDS.

Current treatment of tuberculosis is based on administration of effective drug treatment. The drugs most commonly used to treat tuberculosis are isoniazid, rifampicin, ethambutol, pyrazinamide, ethionamide/prothionamide, cycloserine, thioacetazone, *p*-aminosalicylic acid and streptomycin. Others such as amikacin, ciprofloxacin, ofloxacin, clofazimine, kanamycin, capreomycin and rifabutin have also been tried. Although efficacious drugs are available, treatment is often not successful because of poor compliance, drug resistance and toxicity, and the high cost of medication.[161]

The clinical pharmacology of antituberculosis drugs and the optimum treatment/prevention of the disease are discussed in chapter 23 (sect. 9). The cost of treatment and its implications for controlling tuberculosis in a community are also discussed in chapter 23 (sect. 9.4).

## 8. Whooping Cough in a Tropical Environment

Whooping cough (pertussis) is a highly infectious disease spread by droplet infection. It may be very debilitating to the child because of the long duration of illness. The incidence of whooping cough in most tropical countries is high and infection occurs at an earlier age than in developed countries due to earlier exposure. Since morbidity and mortality in whooping cough is closely related to the age at which the child is infected, the lower age incidence in developing countries is significant.

Although malnourished children will not withstand severe attacks of whooping cough as well, the disease is not much more severe in undernourished than in well-nourished children. However, whooping cough may cause malnutrition because of the long duration of debility. While antibiotics are useful in the first week of the disease, and when bronchopneumonia develops, management of the disease and its successful outcome depend largely on the standard of nursing and maternal care, which may be lacking in tropical countries.

#### Optimum Treatment/Prevention

There are few effective measures to prevent pertussis. Vaccination and antimicrobial prophylaxis (e.g. with erythromycin) along with corticosteroids and $\beta_2$-adrenoceptor agonists such as salbutamol in the paroxysmal stage will decrease the severity of the disease.[162] Pertussis vaccine has a high protection rate (85 to 94%), but does not confer permanent immunity. Protection lasts for 3 years, declining slowly thereafter. However, immunised persons who develop pertussis usually have milder disease and fewer complications than non-immunised persons. Occasionally, untoward reactions are observed with the presently available whole cell pertussis vaccine. A cell-free pertussis vaccine that is stated to produce fewer adverse effects is currently being developed.[163] Acellular pertussis vaccine appears to cause fewer adverse reactions than whole cell vaccine.[164]

Cough suppressants, antispasmodics, expectorants, mucolytic agents and sedatives have not been shown to be effective in the management of pertussis. Humidified oxygen is indicated for patients with sustained hypoxaemia. There is evidence that erythromycin, tetracycline and chloramphenicol may be effective in aborting or attenuating the illness if administered in the preparoxysmal stage of the disease. These antibiotics may also render patients non-infectious. The dose of erythromycin for treatment is 50 mg/kg/day in divided doses for 14 days.[165]

## 9. Measles in a Tropical Environment

Measles is a severe disease in many tropical countries and has a high mortality rate. It is a good example of the interaction between nutrition and infection in children. Measles is more severe in infants and young children. Earlier studies indicated that measles is much more severe and the mortality rate higher in undernourished children.[166] However, community-based studies in India indicate that the incidence, disease course, degree of immune suppression, and occurrence of complications such as bronchopneumonia and diarrhoea are similar in well-nourished and undernourished children.[167] Cellular and humoral responses to measles infection in malnourished children are also adequate and similar to those in well-nourished children. While nutritional status does not influence antibody titres to measles vaccine,[168] measles infection does have a deleterious effect on the nutritional status of the child.[169,170]

#### Optimum Treatment/Prevention

Morbidity and mortality from measles can be considerably reduced by adequate healthcare.[171] Where there are complications and secondary bacterial infection, antibiotic therapy is essential.

With properly designed protocols for local situations, vaccination programmes can eradicate measles. It is, however, necessary to have a proper administrative structure to ensure that the vaccine is preserved in cold at all levels of delivery (cold chain) until it is administered to the patient.[172] A seroepidemiological study indicated 9 months as the minimum and 5 years as the maximum age for vaccination for effective control of the disease.[173]

## 10. Use of Drugs in a Tropical Environment

Problems in the use and availability of drugs in tropical environments are many and complex. In terms of prescribing, these problems relate in particular to the dosage and administration of drugs, and the use of drugs in the presence of diseases and coexisting conditions encountered in a tropical environment.

### 10.1 Dosage and Administration of Drugs

The first problem is the danger of toxicity from overdosage if Western dosage schedules are followed. On the basis of bodyweight alone, people in Asia would receive about 30% more drug per dose than their heavier Western counterparts. This is more significant if a drug with a low therapeutic index is used or when drugs are given on a long term basis. Signs of overdosage will soon develop. The problem is more acute in children, as the dosage of many drugs is recommended on the basis of age, but bodyweight in developing countries may be as much as 40% lower than in same-aged Western children. Malnutrition contributes further to low bodyweight. Thus, overdosage may result from failure to consider bodyweight in prescribing and is particularly likely in children.

Although malnutrition and other tropical diseases would not be expected to have a major effect on the response to drugs, knowledge in this field is limited. Nevertheless, prescribers should be aware that protein deficiency may lead to decreased metabolism of drugs eliminated by the liver. Similarly, many parasitic infections are associated with liver or kidney complications that may affect drug clearance. Changes in response may become a major problem of treatment with some drugs, for example, in *Schistosoma mansoni* infection treated with niridazole and hycanthone. Protein-energy malnutrition may profoundly affect the protein binding and distribution of drugs.

Malnutrition can also lead to problems of drug administration and absorption.[40] Children with kwashiorkor often have oedema of the lower limbs, which makes intramuscular injections into the quadriceps difficult and may affect the absorption of some drugs. They also have diminished muscle mass, making recurrent intramuscular injections difficult. Oral administration of drugs can also be affected by vomiting and diarrhoea that occur in protein-calorie malnutrition. Drugs are poorly retained and absorption may be impaired due to the short intestinal transit time. Mucosal atrophy of the bowel, which occurs in severe cases, may also impair drug absorption.

Many diseases in a tropical environment other than malnutrition can give rise to difficulty of absorption of drugs after oral administration. This can occur in patients with a primary malabsorption syndrome of unknown aetiology such as tropical sprue or in patients with infections caused by *Giardia lamblia, Capillaria phillipinensis* or *Strongyloides stercoralis*. These parasitic infections can give rise to similar events as in tropical sprue. Such difficulties must be borne in mind when oral administration of drugs is considered in these conditions.

### 10.2 Use of Drugs in the Presence of Folic Acid Deficiency

Folate deficiency is a common problem in tropical environments. The small body store of folate can easily be depleted during growth, in pregnancy, or in the presence of infections or increased production of red blood cells, as in haemolytic anaemia. In addition, many drugs can adversely affect folate metabolism and in combination with these factors, may eventually precipitate folate deficiency into frank megaloblastic anaemia.

Drugs that may affect folate metabolism include pyrimethamine and cotrimoxazole. Pyrimethamine inhibits the enzyme dihydrofolate reductase, which converts dihydrofolate to tetrahydrofolate. In the case of cotrimoxazole, the sulfamethoxazole component inhibits formation of *p*-aminobenzoic acid, while trimethoprim, like pyrimethamine, blocks dihydrofolate reductase, leading to impaired folate formation in bacterial cells. Pyrimethamine and cotrimoxazole are often used in tropical areas where malnutrition is common, but usual doses are unlikely to lead to impaired folate metabolism, except in patients actually or potentially folate deficient.[174] Clearly, simultaneous use of cotrimoxazole to treat bacterial infection in a patient receiving pyrimethamine for malaria prophylaxis would further impair a folate deficiency state and possibly lead to megaloblastic anaemia.[175] Where diet is inadequate, folate supplements may be given with these drugs.

### 10.3 Use of Drugs in Populations with G6PD Deficiency

Several ethnic groups in tropical countries have a deficiency of glucose-6-phosphate dehydrogenase (G6PD) that makes their red blood cells susceptible to haemolysis by oxidant drugs such as primaquine, dapsone, many sulfonamides and nitrofurantoin. The deficiency is severe in Northwest India, East and Southeast Asia. Any patient with haemolytic episodes (haemoglobinuria is the usual presentation), particularly following use of an oxidant drug, should be suspected of G6PD deficiency. Affected individuals should be given advice about medications to avoid. In some situations, the greater likelihood of acute haemolysis may influence the choice of drug or the need to exclude G6PD deficiency before a drug is given. For example, cotrimoxazole is more likely than chloramphenicol to induce haemolysis when used in typhoid fever in Hong Kong Chinese patients with G6PD deficiency[176,177] and phenacetin is best avoided in Southeast Asian patients because of the severe haemolysis it commonly causes in enzyme-deficient individuals.[14]

### 10.4 Use of Corticosteroids

Corticosteroids have many therapeutic applications and indications for their use are increasing. However, indiscriminate administration of corticosteroids to patients in a tropical environment can be hazardous, especially in patients with occult *Strongyloides* or amoebic infection. In the case of *Strongyloides*, a massive autoinfection with widespread dissemination of larvae to intestinal organs may occur.[178] This hyperinfection is often associated with severe enterocolitis and Gram-negative septicaemia. Unrecognised, it may lead to death.

*Amoebiasis* is often unrecognised. Corticosteroids prescribed for other disorders may exacerbate amoebiasis, acute amoebic dysentery and fulminate progression of hepatic amoebiasis. Since amoebiasis can mimic almost any abdominal or hepatic disorder (especially ulcerative colitis), use of corticosteroids to treat mis-

**Table X.** Drug-induced nutritional deficiencies

| Drug | Affected nutrients | Possible mechanism | Effect |
|---|---|---|---|
| Anorectic drugs | All nutrients | Anorexia | Decreased food intake |
| Antacids | Phosphates | Decreased absorption | Osteomalacia |
| Antiepileptic drugs (phenytoin, phenobarbital, primidone, valproic acid) | Folate | Decreased absorption | Megaloblastic anaemia |
| | Vitamin D | Enzyme induction | Osteomalacia |
| | Vitamin E | Excess utilisation? | Haemolysis |
| | Zinc | Chelation | Anorexia, cerebellar dysfunction |
| | Selenium | Peroxide damage | Hepatotoxicity |
| | Vitamin K | ? | Haemorrhage |
| Antifolate drugs (e.g. methotrexate, pyrimethamine, trimethoprim) | Folic acid | Dihydrofolate reductase inhibition | Megaloblastic anaemia, cytopenia |
| Biguanides (e.g. metformin) | Cyanocobalamin (vitamin $B_{12}$) | Decreased absorption | Megaloblastic anaemia |
| Cefalosporins[a] (cefamandole, cefoperazone, latamoxef) | Vitamin K | Decreased prothrombin synthesis | Bleeding episodes |
| Cholestyramine | Fat, fat-soluble vitamins, iron | Complex formation | Anaemia, osteomalacia, bleeding, steatorrhoea |
| Colchicine | Fat, β-carotene, $Na^+$, $K^+$, cyanocobalamin (vitamin $B_{12}$) | Mucosal damage | Anaemia, lethargy |
| Corticosteroids | Calcium | Decreased $Ca^{++}$ transport, vitamin D metabolism | Bone disorders |
| Coumarin anticoagulants | Vitamin K | ? | Haemorrhage |
| Diuretics | $Zn^{++}$, $Ca^{++}$, $K^+$, $Mg^{++}$ | Urinary loss | Weakness, electrolyte depression |
| Furosemide (frusemide) | Thiamine | Urinary loss | Cardiac muscle weakness |
| Glutethimide | Calcium | Enzyme induction, altered calcium metabolism | Osteopenia |
| Hormonal steroid contraceptives[b] | Riboflavin, folic acid, pyridoxine, ascorbic acid, thiamine | Enzyme induction, decreased absorption, competition for binding of the enzymes | Metabolic errors, depression |
| Hydralazine | Pyridoxine | Complex formation | Peripheral neuropathy |
| Isoniazid | Pyridoxine | Complex formation | Peripheral neuropathy, convulsions, psychiatric manifestations |
| | Vitamin D | Enzyme induction | Osteopenia |
| | Nicotinic acid | Competitive inhibition of coenzymes and pyridoxine deficiency | Pellagra |
| Laxatives (mineral oils) | Fat-soluble vitamins; $Ca^{++}$ | Malabsorption | Osteomalacia |
| Levodopa | Pyridoxine | Complex formation | Peripheral neuropathy |
| Neomycin | Vitamins A, D, $B_{12}$ | Malabsorption | Osteomalacia |
| *p*-Aminosalicylic acid | Cyanocobalamin (vitamin $B_{12}$) | Decreased absorption | Megaloblastic anaemia |
| Penicillamine | Pyridoxine, $Zn^{++}$, $Cu^{++}$ | Complex formation | Peripheral neuropathy, anaemia |
| Potassium chloride | Cyanocobalamin (vitamin $B_{12}$) | Decreased ileal pH | Decreased absorption |
| Rifampicin | Vitamin D | Enzyme induction | Osteomalacia |
| Salicylates | Ascorbic acid, folic acid | Increased excretion, decreased uptake | ?Anaemia, infection |
| Sulfasalazine | Folic acid | Mucosal block | Decreased absorption |
| Tetracycline | Iron, ascorbic acid | Chelation | Decreased absorption |

a Agents with an *N*-methylthiotetrazole side chain.
b Combined estrogen-progestagen preparations.

diagnosed ulcerative colitis may have a disastrous effect. Patients with 'colitis', are often treated, rightly or wrongly, with corticosteroids at some stage. Apparently, amoebae become more invasive after corticosteroid administration. A possible explanation is that suppression of the inflammatory and immunological response interferes with the host-parasite equilibrium.[179] It is wise to investigate a patient who has lived in the tropics for amoebiasis whenever corticosteroid therapy is considered. The best laboratory procedure is serological investigation together with repeated stool examination.

## 11. Drug-Induced Nutritional Deficiencies

The risk of drug-induced nutritional deficiencies varies, depending on the chemistry and pharmacological actions of the drugs concerned. Drugs can affect protein, carbohydrate, fat, vitamin and mineral requirements.[180] The variables that determine the incidence of drug-induced deficiencies are nutrient intake and storage, genetic variability in drug handling, dose and duration of treatment, combinations of drugs used, disease states, certain physiological situations (pregnancy, growth) and other environmental factors. Many changes are not often clinically significant under circumstances of normal nutrition, but clearly become important where malnutrition or undernutrition exist in a tropical environment.

The common symptoms of drug-induced malnutrition are weight loss, growth retardation, diarrhoea, dermatitis, paraesthesias, bone pain, bleeding gums, anorexia and anaemia. These effects are induced when drugs interfere with the intake, absorption, binding, metabolism and excretion of nutrients (table X).[181]

Anorectic drugs suppress appetite and food intake. Many antibiotics decrease appetite by causing gastrointestinal disturbances. A variety of compounds decrease absorption of nutrients such as amino acids, vitamins, and minerals through effects on intestinal motility, intestinal mucosal changes, specific inhibition of active transport mechanisms, suppression of bacterial growth, and intraluminal interactions. Malabsorption (primary or secondary) can lead to deficiencies of vitamins A, D, E, K, folate and cyanocobalamin. A number of drugs (e.g. phenytoin, phenobarbital, primidone, prednisone, isoniazid) may result in vitamin D-mediated hypocalcaemia. Metabolic antagonists such as purine or folic acid antagonists, antimalarials, isoniazid and hydralazine are known antivitamins, resulting in folic acid or pyridoxine deficiency. Oral contraceptives produce metabolic alterations, particularly involving B complex vitamins and vitamins A and C.[182,183] Hepatic enzyme-inducing drugs such as antiepileptics can lead to faster metabolism of vitamins A and D. A number of drugs interfere with vitamin K and its action. Broad-spectrum antibiotics, analgesics, antiepileptics and corticosteroids, for example, may interfere either with absorption, binding or synthesis of vitamin K-dependent clotting factors.[184]

Hyperexcretion and tissue depletion of nutrients can lead to mineral and trace nutrient deficiencies.[185] It is usually seen with long term usage of antacids, diuretics, chelating agents, etc. In addition, a number of agents (corticosteroids, antibiotics, contraceptives, phenothiazines, thiazides) interfere with amino acid absorption, nitrogen balance, or carbohydrate and fat metabolism.

## Acknowledgements

I thank my colleague Dr B. Dinesh Kumar at the National Institute of Nutrition for help rendered during the preparation of the manuscript, and Mrs Lakshmi Rani and Mrs Sailaja for typing the manuscript.

## References

1. Melrose D. Bitter pills. Oxford: Oxfam Publications, 1983: 31
2. World Health Organization. The selection of essential drugs. Technical Report Series No. 615. Geneva: World Health Organization, 1977
3. World Health Organization. Selection of essential drugs. Technical Report Series No. 641. Geneva: World Health Organization, 1979
4. Habiyamber V, Wertheimer AI. Programme on essential drugs. World Health Forum 1993; 14: 140
5. Yudkin JS. Provision of medicines in a developing country. Lancet 1978; 1: 810
6. Dineshkumar B, Raghuram TC, Radhaiah G, et al. Profile of drug use in urban and rural India. PharmacoEconomics 1995; 7: 332
7. Tomson Y, Wessling A, Tomson G. General practitioners for rational use of drugs. European Journal of Clinical Pharmacology 1994; 47: 213
8. Greenhalgh T. Drug prescription and self medication in India: an exploratory survey. Social Science in Medicine 1987; 25: 307
9. Krishnaswamy K, Kumar BD, Radhaiah G. Drug survey precepts and practices. European Journal of Clinical Pharmacology 1985; 29: 363
10. Kaldor A. Patterns and problems of drug consumption in a developing country. Clinical Pharmacology and Therapeutics 1976; 19: 657
11. Bygbjerg IC. Use of drugs in developing countries. Tropical Doctor 1978; 8: 174
12. Schwartz RK, Soumarai SB, Avorn SJ. Physicians' motivations for non-scientific drug prescription. Social Science in Medicine 1989; 28: 577
13. Teoh PC. Hospital admissions due to adverse reactions to drug therapy. Australian Family Physician 1975; 4: 191
14. Wong HB. Acute haemolysis in Southeast Asia. Medical Progress 1977; 4(3): 12
15. Vesell E. Relationship between drug distribution and therapeutic effects in man. Annual Review of Pharmacology and Toxicology 1974; 14: 249
16. Ellard GA. The potential clinical significance of the isoniazid acetylator phenotype in the treatment of pul-

monary tuberculosis. Tubercle and Lung Disease 1984; 65: 211

17. World Health Organization. Pharmacogenetics - the influence of heredity on the response to drugs. World Health Chronicle 1974; 28: 25
18. Kaeda JS, Chnotray GP, Ranjit MR, et al. A new glucose-6-phosphate dehydrogenase variant G6PD Orissa is the major polymorphic variant in tribal populations in India. American Journal of Human Genetics 1995; 57: 1335
19. Idle JR, Mahgoub A, Sloan TP, et al. Some observations on the oxidation phenotype status of Nigerian patients presenting with cancer. Cancer Letters 1981; 11: 331
20. Salafsky B. Dangers of drug toxicity due to overdosage in Southeast Asia. Journal of Tropical Medicine and Hygiene 1976; 79: 49
21. Teoh PC. Drug dosage for Southeast Asian patients. Medical Progress 1977; 4: 11
22. Krishnaswamy K. Drug metabolism and pharmacokinetics in malnutrition. Clinical Pharmacokinetics 1978; 3: 216
23. Krishnaswamy K. Drug metabolism and pharmacokinetics in malnourished children. Clinical Pharmacokinetics 1989; 17: 68
24. World Health Organization. Food and nutrition strategies in national development. Technical Report Series No. 584. Geneva: World Health Organization, 1976
25. Krishnaswamy K. Drug metabolism and pharmacokinetics in malnutrition. Trends in Pharmacological Sciences 1983; 4: 295
26. Sanvordekar DR, Lambert HJ. Environmental modification of mammalian drug metabolism and biological response. Drug Metabolism Reviews 1972; 3: 201
27. Higgins EA, Davis Jr AW, Fiorica V, et al. Effects of two antihistamine containing compounds upon performance at three altitudes. Aerospace Medicine 1968; 19: 1167
28. Nair V, Casper R. The influence of light on daily rhythm in hepatic drug metabolizing enzymes in rat. Life Sciences 1969; 8: 1291
29. Levine GM, Harber LC. The effect of humidity on the phototoxic response to 8-methoxy psoralen in guinea pigs. Acta Dermato-Venerologica 1969; 49: 82
30. Epstein WL, Shah VP, Riegelman S. Griseofulvin levels in stratum corneum. Study after oral administration in man. Archives of Dermatology 1972; 106: 344
31. Krishnaswamy K. The effect of nutritional status on drug action. Pharmacy International 1985; 6: 41
32. Rosenberg IH, Scrimshaw NS. Workshop on malabsorption and malnutrition. American Journal of Clinical Nutrition 1972; 25: 2046-25
33. Raghuram TC, Krishnaswamy K. Influence of nutritional status on plasma levels and relative bioavailability of tetracycline. European Journal of Clinical Pharmacology 1977; 12:281
34. Polasa K, Murthy KJR, Krishnaswamy K. Rifampicin kinetics in undernutrition. British Journal of Pharmacology 1984; 17: 481
35. Jagadeesan V, Krishnaswamy K. Drug binding in undernourished: a study on the binding of propranolol to $\alpha_1$-acid glycoprotein. European Journal of Clinical Pharmacology 1985; 27: 657
36. Buchanan N. Drug protein binding and protein-energy malnutrition. South African Medical Journal 1977; 52: 733
37. Shastri RA, Krishnaswamy K. Undernutrition and tetracycline half life. Clinica Chimica Acta 1976; 66: 157
38. Pennington JE, Dale DC, Reynolds HY, et al. Gentamycin sulfate pharmacokinetics lower levels of gentamycin in blood during fever. Journal of Infectious Diseases 1975; 77: 1253
39. Anderson KE. Influence of diet and nutrition on clinical pharmacokinetics. Clinical Pharmacokinetics 1988; 14: 325
40. Buchanan N. Drug kinetics in protein energy malnutrition. South African Medical Journal 1978; 53: 327
41. Krishnaswamy K. Effects of malnutrition on drug metabolism and toxicity in humans. In: Hathcock JN, editor. Nutritional toxicology. New York: Academic Press, 1985: 105
42. Mehta S. Drug disposition in children with protein energy malnutrition. Journal of Paediatric Gastroenterology and Nutrition 1983; 2: 407
43. Krishnaswamy K. Nutrition and drug metabolism. Indian Journal of Medical Research 1978; 68: 109
44. Langman MJS, Smithard DJ. Antipyrine metabolism in iron deficiency. British Journal of Clinical Pharmacology 1977; 4: 631P
45. Smithard DJ, Langman MJS. The effect of vitamin supplementation upon antipyrine metabolism in the elderly. British Journal of Clinical Pharmacology 1978; 5: 181
46. Hathcock JN, Coon J. Nutrition and drug interrelations. New York: Academic Press, 1978
47. Anderson KE, Conney AH, Kappas A. Nutrition and oxidative drug metabolism in man: relative influence of dietary lipids, carbohydrates and proteins. Clinical Pharmacology and Therapeutics 1979; 26: 493
48. Krishnaswamy K, Kalamegham R, Nadamuni Naidu A. Dietary influences on the kinetics of antipyrine and aminopyrine in human subjects. British Journal of Clinical Pharmacology 1984; 17: 139
49. Conney AH. Induction of microsomal enzymes for foreign chemicals and carcinogenesis by polycyclic aromatic hydrocarbons. Cancer Research 1982; 42: 4875
50. Rubin E, Lieber CS. Malnutrition and liver diseases - an over emphasised relationship. American Journal of Medicine 1968; 45: 1
51. Keet MP, Hansen JDL, Moddie AD, et al. Kwashiorkor, a ten year follow up study. Proceedings of the Twelfth International Congress of Pediatrics, Vienna 1971; 2: 387
52. Ramalingaswami V, Nayak NC. Liver disease in India. In: Popper and Schaffner, editors. Progress in liver disease, Vol. III. New York: Grune and Stratton, 1970: 222
53. Faigle JW. Blood levels of a schistosomicide in relation to liver function and side effects. Acta Pharmacologica Toxicologica Copenhagen 1971; 29 Suppl. 3: 233
54. Gurtoo GM, Campbell TC, Webb RE, et al. Effect of aflatoxin and benzpyrene pretreatment upon the kinetics of benzpyrene hydroxylase. Biochemical and Biophysical Research Communications 1968; 31: 588
55. Berlinger WG, Park GF, Spector R. The effect of dietary protein on the clearance of allopurinol and oxypurinol. New England Journal of Medicine 1985; 313: 771
56. Chang KC, Bell TD, Lauer BA, et al. Altered theophylline pharmacokinetics during acute respiratory viral illness. Lancet 1978; 1: 1132
57. Obel AOK, Vere DW. Antipyrine and propranolol disposition in malnutrition. East African Medical Journal 1978; 55: 20
58. Falase AO, Salako LA, Aminee JM. Lack of effect of low doses of prazosin in hypertensive Nigerians. Current Therapeutic Research 1976; 19: 603

59. Mroczek WJ, Fotiu S, Davidov ME, et al. Prazosin in hypertension: a double-blind evaluation with methyldopa and placebo. Current Therapeutic Research 1974; 16: 769
60. Obama M, Cangir A, Van Eys J. Nutritional status and anthracycline cardiotoxicity in children. Southern Medical Journal 1983; 76: 577
61. Varma DR. Protein deficiency and drug interactions: a review. Drug Development Research 1981; 1: 183
62. Newman TJ, Bergman GJ. Acetaminophen hepatotoxicity and malnutrition. American Journal of Gastroenterology 1979; 72: 647
63. Feldman CH, Hutchinson VE, Pippenger CE, et al. Effect of dietary protein and carbohydrate on theophylline metabolism in children. Pediatrics 1980; 66: 956
64. Raman L, Kumar S, Venkatesh PR, et al. Influence of different various drug regimes in pre-eclampsia on foetal outcome. Proceedings of the 2nd International Congress of ISSHIP. Cairo: Ainshams University Press, 1982
65. Reddy V. Vitamin A deficiency and blindness in Indian children. Indian Journal of Medical Research 1978; 68: 48
66. Reddy V, Srikantia SG. Serum vitamin A in kwashiorkor. American Journal of Clinical Nutrition 1966; 18: 105
67. Srikantia SG, Reddy V. Effect of a single massive dose of vitamin A on serum and liver levels of the vitamin. American Journal of Clinical Nutrition 1970; 23: 114
68. Reddy V, Sivakumar B. Studies on vitamin A absorption in children. Indian Pediatrics 1972; 9: 307
69. Vijayraghvan K, Sarma KVR, Rao PN, et al. Impact of massive doses of vitamin 'A' on incidence of nutritional blindness. Lancet 1984; 2: 149
70. Vijayraghvan K, Brahamam GNV, Gal Reddy V. Linking periodic dosing of vitamin 'A' with universal immunization programme. An evaluation report submitted to UNICEF, 1966
71. Deluca HF. The kidney as an endocrine organ involved in the function of vitamin D. American Journal of Medicine 1975; 58: 39
72. Chalmer TM, Darie MW, Hunter JO, et al. 1-Alphahydroxycholecalciferol as a substitute for the kidney hormone, 1,25-dihydroxycholecalciferol in chronic renal failure. Lancet 1973; 2: 696
73. Madsen S, Olgaard K, Ladefoged J. Bone mineral content in chronic renal failure during long-term treatment of 1α-hydroxycholecalciferol. Acta Medica Scandinavica 1978; 203: 385
74. Campbell JA, Morrison AB. Some factors affecting the absorption of vitamins. American Journal of Clinical Nutrition 1963; 12: 162
75. Levy G, Hewitt RR. Evidence in man for different specialized intestinal transport mechanism for riboflavin and thiamine. American Journal of Clinical Nutrition 1971; 24: 401
76. Thompson AD, Frank O, Baker H, et al. Thiamine propyl disulfide: absorption and utilisation. Annals of Internal Medicine 1971; 74: 529
77. Jusko WJ, Levy G. Plasma protein binding of riboflavin and riboflavin-5'-phosphate in man. Journal of Pharmaceutical Sciences 1968; 56: 58
78. Bamji MS, Faizy A. Vitamin deficiency in man - recent studies on fat soluble vitamins, thiamin, riboflavin, pyridoxine and vitamin C. Journal of Scientific and Industrial Research 1978; 37: 42
79. Narasinga Rao BS, Gopalan C. Niacin. In: Olson RE, editor. Present knowledge in nutrition, 5th ed. Washington DC: Nutrition Foundation, 1984: 318
80. Hornig D. Metabolism of ascorbic acid. World Review of Nutrition and Dietetics 1975; 23: 225
81. DiPalma JR, Ritchie DM. Vitamin toxicity. Annual Review of Pharmacology and Toxicology 1977; 17: 133
82. Haley JJ, Flesha AM. A toxicity study of thiamine hydrochloride. Science 1946; 104: 567
83. Narasinga Rao BS. Studies on iron deficiency anaemia. Indian Journal of Medical Research 1978; 68: 58
84. Srikantia SG. Use of iron fortified common salt and its effects on the prevalence of anaemia. Proceedings of the Nutrition Society of India 1983; 28: 7
85. Iyengar L, Rajalakshmi K. Effect of folic acid supplement on birth weights of infants. American Journal of Obstetrics and Gynecology 1975; 122: 332
86. World Health Organization. Tropical disease research: a global partnership. In: Maurice J, Pearcl AM, editors. Eighth Programme Report. Geneva: World Health Organization, 1987
87. World Health Organization. Vector control for malaria and other mosquito-borne diseases. WHO Technical Report Series No. 857, 1995
88. World Health Organization. International travel and health: vaccination requirements and health advice. Geneva: World Health Organization, 1995
89. Bruce-Chwatt LJ, Black RH, Canfield CJ, et al. In Bruce-Chwatt, editor. Chemotherapy of malaria. 2nd ed. Geneva: World Health Organization, 1981
90. Gustafsson LL, Walker O, Alvan G, et al. Disposition of chloroquine in man after single intravenous and oral doses. British Journal of Clinical Pharmacology 1983; 15: 471
91. Webster Jr LT. Drugs used in the chemotherapy of protozoal infections. In: Gillman AG, et al., editors. The pharmacological basis of therapeutics. London: Pergamon Press, 1990: 892
92. White NJ. Clinical pharmacokinetics of antimalarial drugs. Clinical Pharmacokinetics 1985; 10: 187
93. White NJ. Drug treatment and prevention of malaria. European Journal of Clinical Pharmacology 1988; 34: 1
94. Stickery DR, Simmons WS, De Angeles RL, et al. Pharmacokinetics of pyrimethamine and 24-diamino-6-pyrimidine relevant to meningeal leukaemia. Proceedings of the American Association of Cancer Research 1973; 14: 52
95. Palmer KJ, Holliday SM, Brogden RN. Mefloquine: a review of its antimalarial activity, pharmacokinetic properties and therapeutic efficacy. Drugs 1993; 45: 430-75
96. Karbwang J, Bunnag D, Breckenridge AM, et al. The pharmacokinetics of mefloquine and pyrimethamine in Thai male and female subjects. European Journal of Clinical Pharmacology 1987; 32: 173
97. Mihaly GW, Ward SA, Edwards G, et al. Pharmacokinetics of primaquine in man: identification of the carboxylic acid derivative as a major plasma metabolite. British Journal of Clinical Pharmacology 1984; 17: 441
98. Bryson H, Goa KL. Halofantrine: a review of its antimalarial activity, pharmacokinetic properties and therapeutic potential. Drugs 1992; 43: 236-58
99. Barradell LB, Fitton A. Artesunate: a review of its pharmacology and therapeutic efficacy in the treatment of malaria. Drugs 1995; 50: 714
100. Nosten F, Price RN. New antimalarials: a risk benefit analysis. Drug Safety 1995; 12: 264
101. Looareesuwan S, Kyle DE, Viravan C, et al. Treatment of patients with recrudescent malaria with a sequential combination of artesunate and mefloquine. Amer-

ican Journal of Tropical Medicine and Hygiene 1992; 47: 794
102. Keystone JS. Prevention of malaria. Drugs 1990; 39: 337
103. Miller KD, Lobel HO, Satriale RF, et al. Severe cutaneous reactions among anaemia travellers using pyrimethamine/sulfadoxine for malaria prophylaxis. American Journal of Tropical Medicine and Hygiene 1986; 35: 451
104. Struchler C, Mittelholzer Kerr L. How frequent are notified severe cutaneous adverse reactions to Fansidar? Drug Safety 1993; 8: 163
105. Edwards G. Recent advances in the chemotherapy of onchocerciasis. Trends in Pharmacological Sciences 1984; 192: 195
106. Greene BM. Ocular and systemic complications of diethylcarbamazine for onchocerciasis: association with circulating immune complexes. Journal of Infectious Diseases 1983; 147: 890
107. Hopkins DR. Honing in on helminths. American Journal of Tropical Medicine and Hygiene 1992; 46: 626
108. Goa KL, McTavish D, Clissold SP. Ivermectin: a review of its antifilarial activity, pharmacokinetic properties and clinical efficacy in onchocerciasis. Drugs 1991; 42: 640
109. Taylor HR. Recent developments in the treatment of onchocerciasis. Bulletin of the World Health Organization 1984; 62: 509
110. Awadzi K, Gilles HM. Diethylcarbamazine in the treatment of patients with onchocerciasis. British Journal of Clinical Pharmacology 1992; 34: 281
111. Newland HS, White AT, Green BM, et al. Effect of single dose ivermectin therapy on human *Onchocerca volvulus* infection with onchocercal ocular involvement. British Journal of Ophthalmology 1988; 72: 561
112. Rothova A, Vandertelilzi A, Stitma JS, et al. Ocular involvement in patients with onchocerciasis after repeated treatment with ivermectin. American Journal of Ophthalmology 1990; 110: 6-16
113. World Health Organization. Bridging the gaps. WHO Report. Geneva: World Health Organization, 1995
114. Holmstedt B, Nordgren I, Sandoz M, et al. Summary of toxicological and pharmacological information available. Archives of Toxicology 1978; 41: 3
115. Reiner E. Estrases in schistosomes. Reaction with substrate and inhibitors. Acta Pharmacologica et Toxicologia 1981; 5 Suppl. 49: 72
116. James C, Webber G, Preston JM. A comparison of the susceptibility to metrifonate of *Schistosoma haematobium, S. matthei* and *S. mansoni* in hamsters. Annals of Tropical Medicine and Parasitology 1972; 66: 467
117. De Cock KM. Hepatosplenic schistosomiasis: a clinical review. Gut 1986; 27: 734
118. Katz M. Anthelmintics: current concepts in the treatment of helminthic infection. Drugs 1986; 32: 358
119. King CH, Mahmoud AAF. Drugs five years later: praziquantel. Annals of Internal Medicine 1989; 110: 290
120. King CH, Lombardi G, Lombardi C, et al. Chemotherapy based control of schistosomiasis haematobia I: metrifonate versus praziquantel in control of intesity and prevalence of infection. American Journal of Medicine and Hygiene 1988; 39: 295
121. Chandrashekhar K. Schistosomiasis drug therapy and treatment considerations. Drugs 1991; 42: 379
122. World Health Organization. WHO Expert Committee on Leprosy. Technical Report Series No. 768. Geneva: World Health Organization, 1988
123. World Health Organization. Control of schistosomiasis. WHO Technical Report Series No. 830. Geneva: World Health Organization, 1993
124. Berman JD. Chemotherapy for leishmaniasis: biochemical mechanisms, clinical efficacy and future strategies. Reviews of Infectious Diseases 1988; 10: 560
125. Chulay JD, Fleckenstein L, Smith DH. Pharmacokinetics of antimony during treatment of visceral leishmaniasis with sodium stibogluconate or meglumine antimonate. Transactions of the Royal Society of Tropical Medicine and Hygiene 1988; 82: 69
126. Berman JD, Fleckenstein L. Pharmacokinetic justification of antiprotozoal therapy: a US perspective. Clinical Pharmacokinetics 1991; 21: 479
127. Gallis HA, Drew RH, Pickard WW. Amphotericin B: 30 years of clinical experience. Reviews of Infectious Diseases 1990; 12: 308
128. Marsden PD. Mucosal leishmaniasis (Espundia ascomel, 1911). Transaction of the Royal Society of Tropical Medicine and Hygiene 1986; 80: 859
129. Sampaio SAP, Castro RM, Dillon NL, et al. Treatment of mucocutaneous (American) leishmaniasis with amphotericin B: report of 70 cases. International Journal of Dermatology 1971; 10: 179
130. World Health Organization. African trypanosomiasis. In: Tropical Disease Research, 7th Programme Report. Geneva: World Health Organization, 1985: 5/1-5/19
131. Gutteridge WE. Existing chemotherapy and its limitations. British Medical Bulletin 1985; 41: 162
132. Goa KL, Campoli-Richards DM. Pentamidine isethionate: a review of its antiprotozoal activity, pharmacokinetic properties and therapeutic use in *Pneumocystis carinii* pneumonia. Drugs 1987; 33: 242
133. Andersen R, Boedicker M, Ma M, et al. Adverse reactions associated with pentamidine isethionate in AIDS patients: recommendations for monitoring therapy. Drug Intelligence and Clinical Pharmacy 1986; 20: 862
134. Van Voorhis WC. Therapy and prophylaxis of systemic protozoan infections. Drugs 1990; 40: 176
135. Collins JM, Klecker JRW, Yarchoan R, et al. Clinical pharmacokinetics of suramin in patient with HTLV-III/LAV infection. Journal of Clinical Pharmacology 1986; 26: 22
136. World Health Organization. The African trypanosomiasis. Technical Report Series No. 635. Geneva: World Health Organization, 1979
137. Molyneux DH. Selective primary health care: strategies for control of disease in the developing world. VIII. African trypanosomiasis. Reviews of Infectious Diseases 1983; 5: 945
138. Taleman H, Schechter PJ, Marcelis L, et al. Difluoromethylornithine, and effective new treatment of Gambian trypanosomiasis: results in five patients. American Journal of Medicine 1987; 82: 607
139. Rew RS. African trypanosomiasis. In: Campbell WC, Rew RS, editors. Chemotherapy of parasitic diseases. New York: Plenum Press, 1986: 129-37
140. Weiss LM, Harris C, Beerger M, et al. Pyrimethamine concentrations in serum and cerebrospinal fluid during treatment of acute toxoplasmosis encephalitis in patients with AIDS. Journal of Infectious Diseases 1988; 157: 580
141. Hughes WT. *Pneumocystis carinii* pneumonitis. New England Journal of Medicine 1987; 317: 1021
142. Editorial. Treatment of *Pneumocystis carinii* pneumonia. Medical Letter 1987: 29: 103

143. Levine SJ, White DA. *Pneumocystis carinii*. Clinics in Chest Medicine 1988; 9: 395
144. Kovacs JA, Hiemenz JW, Macher AM, et al. *Pneumocystis carinii* pneumonia: a comparison between patients with the acquired immunodeficiency syndrome and patients with other immunodeficiencies. Annals of Internal Medicine 1984; 100: 663
145. World Health Organization. The world health report. Geneva: World Health Organization, 1995
146. World Health Organization. Chemotherapy of leprosy for control programmes. Technical Report Series No. 675. Geneva: World Health Organization, 1982
147. Waters MFR. New approaches to chemotherapy for leprosy. Drugs 1983; 26: 465
148. Modderman ESM, Mercus FWHM, Zuidema J, et al. Dapsone levels after oral therapy and weekly oily injections in Ethiopian leprosy patients. International Journal of Leprosy 1983; 51: 191
149. Sanders SW, Zone JJ, Foltz RL, et al. Hemolytic anaemia induced by dapsone transmitted through breast milk. Annals of Internal Medicine 1972; 96: 465
150. Zuidema J, Modderman ESM, Mercus FWHM. Clinical pharmacokinetics of dapsone. Clinical Pharmacokinetics 1986; 11: 299-315
151. Zuidema J, Modderman H, Merkus FWHM. Clinical pharmacokinetics of dapsone. Clinical Pharmacokinetics 1986; 11: 299
152. Goodwin CS, Sparell G. Inhibition of dapsone excretion by probenecid. Lancet 1969; 2: 884
153. Mathur A, Venkatesan K, Bharadwaj VP, et al. Evaluation of effectiveness of clofazimine therapy - monitoring of absorption from gastrointestinal tract. Indian Journal of Leprosy 1985; 57: 146
154. Holdiness MR. Clinical pharmacokinetics of clofazimine: a review. Clinical Pharmacokinetics 1989; 16: 74
155. World Health Organization. Tropical diseases - progress in international research 1987-88 (3). The disease leprosy. UNDP/World Bank/WHO/ Special Program for Research and Training in Tropical Diseases, 9th Program Report. Geneva: World Health Organization, 1989
156. Meyers WM, Marty AM. Current concepts in the pathogenesis of leprosy. Drugs 1991; 41: 832
157. Editorial. Vaccine against leprosy. National Medical Journal of India 1994; 7: 153
158. Venkatesan K. Clinical pharmacokinetic consideration in the treatment of patient with leprosy. Clinical Pharmacokinetics 1989; 16: 365
159. Katoch K, Ramu G, Ramanatham U. Pyrazinamide as a part of combination. Therapy for BL-LL patients - a preliminary report. International Journal of Leprosy 1988; 56: 1
160. Bloom BR, Murray GL. Tuberculosis commentary on re-emergent killer. Science 1992; 257: 1055
161. World Health Organization. Tuberculosis control. Technical Report Series No. 671. Geneva: World Health Organization, 1982
162. Basu JW. Pertussis: current status of prevention and treatment. Pediatric Infectious Disease Journal 1985; 4: 614
163. Sato Y, Fukumi H, Kimura M. Development of a pertussis component vaccine in Japan. Lancet 1984; 1: 122
164. Wintermeyer SM, Nahata MC, Kyllomen KS. Whole cell and acellular pertussis vaccines. Annals of Pharmacotherapy 1994; 28: 925
165. Henry RL, Dorman DC, Skinner JA, et al. Antimicrobial therapy in whooping cough. Medical Journal of Australia 1981; 2: 27
166. Morley DC. Severe measles. In: Paediatric priorities in the developing world. London: Butterworths, 1973: 207
167. Bhaskaram P, Madhusudan J, Radhakrishnan KV, et al. Immune response in malnourished children with measles. Journal of Tropical Paediatrics 1986; 32: 123
168. Bhaskaram P, Madhusudan J, Radhakrishnan KV, et al. Immunological response to measles vaccination in poor communities. Human Nutrition and Clinical Nutrition 1986; 40: 295
169. Axton JHM. Measles and the state of nutrition. South African Medical Journal 1979; 55: 125
170. Bhaskaram P, Reddy V, Shyam R, et al. Effect of measles on the nutritional status of pre-school children. Journal of Tropical Medicine and Hygiene 1984; 87: 21
171. John TJ, Joseph A, Goerge T, et al. Epidemiology and prevention of measles in rural South India. Indian Journal of Medicine Research 1986; 72: 153
172. Dudgeon JA. Prospect for worldwide control of measles. Reviews of Infectious Diseases 1983; 5: 621
173. Bhaskaram P, Radhakrishnan KV, Madhusudan J. Sero-epidemiological study to determine age for measles vaccination. Indian Journal of Medical Research 1986; 83: 480
174. Chanarin I, England JM. Toxicity of trimethoprim-sulphamethoxazole in patients with megaloblastic haemopoiesis. British Medical Journal 1972; 1: 651
175. Ansdell VE, Wright SG, Hutchinson DBA. Megaloblastic anaemia after pyrimethamine and co-trimoxazole. Lancet 1976; 2: 1257
176. Chan TK, McFadzean AJS. Haemolytic effect of trimethoprim sulphamethoxazole in G-6-PD deficiency. Transactions of the Royal Society of Tropical Medicine and Hygiene 1974; 68: 61
177. Chan TK, Todd D, Tso SC. Drug induced haemolysis in glucose-6-phosphate dehydrogenase deficiency. British Medical Journal 1976; 2: 1227
178. Plorde JJ, Ivan LB, Petersdorf RG. Other intestinal nematodes: strongyloidiasis. In: Harrison's principles of internal medicine, 6th ed. New York: McGraw-Hill, 1971: 1050
179. Stuiver PC, Goud ThJLM. Corticosteroids and liver amoebiasis. British Medical Journal 1978; 2: 394
180. Roe DA, Campbell TC, editors. Drugs and nutrients. New York: Marcel Dekker Inc., 1984: 299-505
181. Hathcock JN, Coon J, editors. Nutrition and drug interrelations. New York: Academic Press, 1976
182. Faizy A, Bamji MS, Iyengar L. Effect of oral contraceptive agents on vitamin nutrition status. American Journal of Clinical Nutrition 1975; 28: 606
183. Briggs M. Biochemical effects of oral contraceptives. Advances in Steroid Biochemistry and Pharmacology 1976; 5: 65
184. Koch-Weser J, Sellers EM. Drug interactions with coumarin anticoagulants. New England Journal of Medicine 1971; 285: 487
185. Thomas JA. Drug nutrient interactions. Nutrition Reviews 1995; 53: 271

# Pharmacokinetic Drug Data

*W. Taeschner* and *S. Vožeh*

This appendix compiles physicochemical properties of drugs and representative values for selected pharmacokinetic parameters. Five parameters are included in the tables which follow: total clearance (CL), apparent volume of distribution (Vd), half-life ($t^1\!/_2$), protein binding, and normal nonrenal drug clearance fraction [$f_{NR(n)}$ or $P_o$]. Drugs have been classified according to their predominant pharmacological action or therapeutic use so that differences and similarities between individual agents within a class can be readily seen.

***Clearance*** (CL) reflects the relationship between drug elimination rate and its serum or plasma concentration (i.e. rate of elimination = concentration • clearance), and is calculated either by the dose divided by the area under the serum or plasma concentration *versus* time curve from time zero to infinity (AUC), or by the dose rate divided by the average serum or plasma concentration at steady-state. Although, strictly speaking, clearance can only be calculated from serum concentration measurements obtained after intravenous administration, *apparent* clearances after oral or intramuscular administration are reported if intravenous data are not available. The most important practical application of the total clearance derives from the fact that this pharmacokinetic parameter determines the average concentration at steady-state for a given dose rate (i.e. average concentration at steady-state = dose rate divided by clearance).

***Half-life*** ($t^1\!/_2$) and ***apparent volume of distribution*** (Vd) values refer to the terminal elimination phase half-life and the volume of distribution obtained by dividing the clearance by the elimination rate constant associated with the terminal elimination phase ($Vd_{area}$ or $V_z$). This choice is based on practical considerations. Firstly, the terminal elimination phase half-life and $Vd_{area}$ represent the relevant parameters for deriving a dose regimen (i.e. dose interval and loading dose) for drugs whose pharmacokinetics can, for clinical purposes, be approximated by a 1-compartment model (see chapter 1, sect. 2.2.4). In addition, even for drugs with multicompartmental characteristics, the terminal elimination phase half-life can be used for a conservative estimate of the time required to reach steady-state at a constant dosage (4 to 5 half-lives of the drug). The second practical reason for this choice is the simple fact that these two parameters are the most frequently reported ones in pharmacokinetic studies. This applies in particular to the parameter $Vd_{area}$. For theoretical reasons, $Vd_{ss}$ (the volume of distribution at steady-state) is the preferred parameter as it better reflects the relationship between the amount of drug in the body and the serum or plasma concentration at steady-state and is, for most realistic pharmacokinetic models, independent of the elimination rate, whereas $Vd_{area}$ changes when the elimination rate constant decreases or increases. Where these parameters (terminal elimination phase half-life and $Vd_{area}$) are not reported or not appropriate, this is indicated in the 'notes' column.

The normal ***nonrenal drug clearance fraction*** [$f_{NR(n)}$ or $P_o$] is defined as the nonrenal drug clearance divided by the total clearance (normalised for creatinine clearance of 100 ml/min). The parameter has been derived either from the intercept of the linear relationship between creatinine clearance and the drug plasma clearance (see also nomogram method of dose estimation in renal failure in appendix E) or from the fraction of drug excreted unchanged in the urine. *Thus, 1 – $f_{NR(n)}$ is an estimate of the fraction of drug excreted unchanged in the urine* in individuals with normal renal and hepatic function.

## 1. Selection of 'Representative' Values

Ideally, pharmacokinetic parameters should be determined in the patient who is treated with the drug. This is unfortunately often not the case. The typical pharmacokinetic study is usually performed in a group of healthy volunteers or in a selected subpopulation of patients with a specific characteristic (e.g. old age or cirrhosis) with or without a control group which, again, often consists of healthy individuals. It is, therefore, difficult to determine a representative value on the basis of such studies. In compiling the parameter values for this appendix, the following approach was taken:

1) Where studies in patients representative of the general population treated with the drug are available, these results have been included.

2) Values obtained in healthy individuals are cited only if pharmacokinetic studies yielding the necessary information in patients are not available.

3) If several studies on the same drug are available, a 'typical' value has been chosen, usually a weighted average or a median.

Results for different subpopulations with a specific characteristic have not been included for two reasons: (a) space limitations do not allow the listing of results of individual studies investigating the influence of a specific factor on drug kinetics; and (b) more importantly, many of the factors reported to affect the pharmacokinetics of individual therapeutic agents are difficult to quantify. (An important exception is the impairment of renal function which is dealt with in chapter 24 and in appendices D and E.) Quantitative changes in nonrenal elimination rate and distribution characteristics are, therefore, difficult to predict on the basis of a readily available parameter.

Readers requiring information on pharmacokinetics in renal or hepatic diseases or in breastmilk should refer to appendices D and E, F, and C, respectively, or to the original literature for other pathophysiological conditions. It is also important to remember that various factors can be expected to influence the kinetics of most drugs, not only those for which the appropriate pharmacokinetic investigations have been performed.

For a discussion of the various factors that may be expected to influence the pharmacokinetic characteristics of a drug, see chapter 1, section 3.

## 2. Limitations Imposed by Interindividual Variability

Although it is well known that pharmacokinetic parameters vary between patients for most drugs, very little quantitative information is available concerning the extent of the unpredictable interindividual variability. The main reason for this is the large number of patients that must be studied if reliable and representative estimates are to be obtained. The problem of estimation and control of interindividual variability in drug therapy represents an important research area in applied pharmacokinetics (for a review, see Rowland et al. 1985). Several methods have been proposed for estimation of the variability in pharmacokinetic parameters, but results have been reported for only a few drugs. However, the available information does allow two important conclusions to be drawn concerning interindividual pharmacokinetic variability:

1) In patients, the interindividual variability of pharmacokinetic parameters is usually very large. For example, a standard deviation of the total clearance as large as 50% of the population mean is not unusual. Since this may not be true for a homogeneous group of healthy individuals, the interindividual pharmacokinetic variability has often been underestimated.

2) A large part of the interindividual variability cannot be explained by disease states, drug interactions or other patient characteristics that are readily accessible to measurement. In other words, even after correcting for all measurable factors known to influence drug disposition, interindividual variability remains large.

Because the number of drugs for which a quantitative estimate of the interindividual patient variability is available is very small, this information could not be included in the table. We also excluded ranges of values found in different studies, because they cannot be interpreted as representative estimates of the interindividual variability. On the basis of present knowledge concerning the extent of interindividual pharmacokinetic variability, it seems prudent to assume for the total clearance and elimination half-life of a drug an interindividual coefficient of variation of about 50% of the population average (this implies a 5-fold range). The interindividual variability of the volume of distribution is usually somewhat smaller. With this in mind, the values presented here can be interpreted *only as guidelines* indicating the range in which pharmacokinetic parameters for an individual patient may lie.

The data cited were obtained from many different sources, including reviews, original articles and compilations of physicochemical properties. The major journals that were systematically searched for data are listed below. Although great care has been taken in compiling the values, some 'incorrect' data may have been included. We would be very grateful to readers who advise us of any missing or incorrect values.

## Further Reading

Herzfeldt CD. Dissoziationskonstanten von Arzneistoffen: eine Uebersichtstabelle. Pharmazeutische Zeitung 1980; 125: 608

Ritschel WA. Biological half-lives and their clinical application: pKa values and some clinical applications. In: Francke & Whitney, editors. Perspectives in clinical pharmacy. Hamilton, IL: Drug Intelligence, 1972: 286 and 325

Rowland M, Sheiner LB, Steimer J-L, editors. Variability in drug therapy: description, estimation and control. New York: Raven Press, 1985

Various authors. British Journal of Clinical Pharmacology

Various authors. Clinical Pharmacokinetics

Various authors. Clinical Pharmacology and Therapeutics

Various authors. Current Therapeutic Research

Various authors. Drugs

Various authors. European Journal of Clinical Pharmacology

Various authors. European Journal of Drug Metabolism and Pharmacokinetics

Various authors. Journal of Clinical Pharmacology

Various authors. Journal of Pharmacokinetics and Biopharmaceutics

**Appendix A.** Index to drugs listed (see under group heading in the following tables)

| Drug | Group |
|---|---|
| Acebutolol | β-Adrenoceptor antagonists |
| Acecainide | Antiarrhythmic drugs |
| Acenocoumarol (nicoumalone) | Anticoagulants |
| Acetaminophen | *see* paracetamol |
| Acetazolamide | Diuretics |
| Acetylsalicylic acid | *see* aspirin |
| Acetohexamide | Antidiabetic drugs |
| Acitretin | Miscellaneous drugs |
| Acetylcysteine | Miscellaneous drugs |
| β-Acetyldigoxin | Cardiac glycosides |
| *N*-Acetylprocainamide | *see* acecainide |
| Aciclovir | Antiviral drugs |
| Acrivastine | Antihistamines |
| Actinomycin D | *see* dactinomycin |
| Ademetionine (*S*-adenosyl-L-methionine) | Antidepressants |
| Adenine arabinoside | *see* vidarabine |
| Adenosine | Antiarrhythmic drugs |
| *N*-Ajmaline hydrogen tartrate | *see* prajmaline |
| Albuterol | *see* salbutamol |
| Alclofenac | Analgesics, NSAIDs |
| Alcohol | *see* ethanol |
| Alcuronium chloride | Muscle relaxants, skeletal |
| Alfaxalone | Anaesthetics, intravenous |
| Alfentanil | Analgesics |
| Alfuzosin | Miscellaneous drugs |
| Alglucerase | Miscellaneous drugs |
| Allopurinol | Gout drugs |
| Alprazolam | Antianxiety drugs/ hypnosedatives, benzodiazepines |
| Alprenolol | β-Adrenoceptor antagonists |
| Amantadine | Anti-Parkinsonian drugs |
| Amdinocillin | *see* mecillinam |
| Amidopyrine | *see* aminophenazone |
| Amikacin | Antibacterial drugs, aminoglycosides |
| Amiloride | Diuretics |
| Aminocaproic acid | Miscellaneous drugs |
| Aminoglutethimide | Antineoplastic and immunosuppressive drugs |
| Aminophenazone | Analgesics |
| 5-Aminosalicylic acid | *see* mesalazine |
| *p*-Aminosalicylic acid (PAS) | Antituberculosis drugs |
| Amiodarone | Antiarrhythmic drugs |
| Amitriptyline | Antidepressants |
| Amlodipine | Calcium antagonists |
| Amoxicillin | Antibacterial drugs, penicillins |
| Amphetamine | Miscellaneous drugs |
| Amphotericin B | Antifungal agents |
| Ampicillin | Antibacterial drugs, penicillins |
| Amrinone | Inotropic agents |
| Anistreplase (APSAC) | Miscellaneous drugs |
| Aprindine | Antiarrhythmic drugs |
| APSAC | *see* anistreplase |
| Aspirin (acetylsalicylic acid) | Analgesics |
| Astemizole | Antihistamines |
| Atenolol | β-Adrenoceptor antagonists |
| Atracurium besilate | Muscle relaxants, skeletal |
| Atropine | Anticholinergics |
| Auranofin | Miscellaneous drugs |
| Aurothioglucose (gold thioglucose) | Miscellaneous drugs |
| Aurothiomalate sodium (gold sodium thiomalate) | Miscellaneous drugs |
| Azapropazone | Analgesics, NSAIDs |
| Azathioprine | Antineoplastic and immunosuppressive drugs |
| Azelastine | Antihistamines |
| Azithromycin | Antibacterial drugs, macrolides |
| Azlocillin | Antibacterial drugs, penicillins |
| Aztreonam | Antibacterial drugs, others |
| Bacampicillin | Antibacterial drugs, penicillins |
| Baclofen | Miscellaneous drugs |
| BCNU | *see* carmustine |

| Drug | Group |
|---|---|
| Beclomethasone dipropionate | Corticosteroids |
| Benazepril | ACE inhibitors |
| Bendroflumethiazide (bendrofluazide) | Diuretics |
| Benzylpenicillin (penicillin G) | Antibacterial drugs, penicillins |
| Betamethasone | Corticosteroids |
| Betaxolol | β-Adrenoceptor antagonists |
| Bevantolol | β-Adrenoceptor antagonists |
| Bezafibrate | Lipid-lowering drugs |
| Bishydroxycoumarin | *see* dicoumarol |
| Bisoprolol | β-Adrenoceptor antagonists |
| Bleomycin | Antineoplastic and immunosuppressive drugs |
| Bopindolol | β-Adrenoceptor antagonists |
| Bretylium | Antiarrhythmic drugs |
| Brodimoprim | Antibacterial drugs, others |
| Bromazepam | Antianxiety drugs/ hypnosedatives, benzodiazepines |
| Bromocriptine | Anti-Parkinsonian drugs |
| Bromperidol | Antipsychotic drugs |
| Brotizolam | Antianxiety drugs/ hypnosedatives, benzodiazepines |
| Budesonide | Corticosteroids |
| Buflomedil | Miscellaneous drugs |
| Bumetanide | Diuretics |
| Bupivacaine | Anaesthetics, local |
| Buprenorphine | Analgesics |
| Buserelin | Miscellaneous drugs |
| Buspirone | Antianxiety drugs/ hypnosedatives, others |
| Busulfan | Antineoplastic and immunosuppressive drugs |
| Butabarbital | *see* secobutabarbital |
| Butorphanol | Analgesics |
| Cadralazine | Antihypertensive drugs |
| Caffeine | Miscellaneous drugs |
| Captopril | ACE inhibitors |
| Carbamazepine | Antiepileptic drugs |
| Carbenicillin | Antibacterial drugs, penicillins |
| Carbimazole (*see* thiamazole) | Antithyroid and thyroid drugs |
| Carboplatin | Antineoplastic and immunosuppressive drugs |
| Carmustine | Antineoplastic and immunosuppressive drugs |
| L-Carnitine | *see* levocarnitine |
| Carteolol | β-Adrenoceptor antagonists |
| Carumonam | Antibacterial drugs, others |
| Carvedilol | β-Adrenoceptor antagonists |
| Cefacetrile | Antibacterial drugs, cefalosporins |
| Cefaclor | cefalosporins |
| Cefadroxil | cefalosporins |
| Cefalexin | cefalosporins |
| Cefaloridine | cefalosporins |

| Drug | Group |
|---|---|
| Cefalothin | Antibacterial drugs, cefalosporins |
| Cefamandole | cefalosporins |
| Cefanone | cefalosporins |
| Cefapirin | cefalosporins |
| Cefatrizine | cefalosporins |
| Cefazolin | cefalosporins |
| Cefepime | cefalosporins |
| Cefetamet pivoxil | cefalosporins |
| Cefixime | cefalosporins |
| Cefmenoxime | cefalosporins |
| Cefodizime | cefalosporins |
| Cefonicid | cefalosporins |
| Cefoperazone | cefalosporins |
| Ceforanide | cefalosporins |
| Cefotaxime | cefalosporins |
| Cefotiam | cefalosporins |
| Cefoxitin | cefalosporins |
| Cefpirome | cefalosporins |
| Cefpodoxime proxetil | cefalosporins |
| Cefprozil | cefalosporins |
| Cefradine | cefalosporins |
| Cefsulodin | cefalosporins |
| Ceftazidime | cefalosporins |
| Ceftibuten | cefalosporins |
| Ceftizoxime | cefalosporins |
| Ceftriaxone | cefalosporins |
| Cefuroxime | cefalosporins |
| Celiprolol | β-Adrenoceptor antagonists |
| Cetirizine | Antihistamines |
| Ciclacillin | Antibacterial drugs, penicillins |
| Chloral hydrate | Antianxiety drugs/ hypnosedatives, others |
| Chlorambucil | Antineoplastic and immunosuppressive drugs |
| Chloramphenicol | Antibacterial drugs, others |
| Chlordiazepoxide | Antianxiety drugs/ hypnosedatives, benzodiazepines |
| Chlormethiazole | *see* clomethiazole |
| Chlorodeoxyadenosine | *see* cladribine |
| Chloroquine | Antimalarial drugs |
| Chlorothiazide | Diuretics |
| Chlorpheniramine (chlorphenamine) | Antihistamines |
| Chlorphentermine | Anorexiants |
| Chlorpromazine | Antipsychotic drugs |
| Chlorpropamide | Antidiabetic drugs |
| Chlortetracycline | Antibacterial drugs, tetracyclines |
| Chlorthalidone | Diuretics |
| Cibenzoline | Antiarrhythmic drugs |
| Cicloprolol | β-Adrenoceptor antagonists |
| Cilastatin | Antibacterial drugs, others |
| Cilazapril | ACE inhibitors |
| Cimetidine | Antiulcer drugs |
| Cinoxacin | Antibacterial drugs, others |
| Ciprofloxacin | Antibacterial drugs, fluoroquinolones |

| Drug | Group |
|---|---|
| Cisapride | Miscellaneous drugs |
| Cisplatin | Antineoplastic and immunosuppressive drugs |
| Citalopram | Antidepressants |
| Cladribine (chlorodeoxyadenosine) | Antineoplastic and immunosuppressive drugs |
| Clarithromycin | Antibacterial drugs, macrolides |
| Clavulanic acid | Antibacterial drugs, others |
| Clindamycin | Antibacterial drugs, others |
| Clobazam | Antianxiety drugs/ hypnosedatives, benzodiazepines |
| Clodronate disodium (clodronic acid) | Miscellaneous drugs |
| Clofibrate | Lipid-lowering drugs |
| Clomethiazole (chlormethiazole) | Antianxiety drugs/ hypnosedatives, others |
| Clomipramine | Antidepressants |
| Clonazepam | Antiepileptic drugs |
| Clonidine | Antihypertensive drugs |
| cis(Z)-Clopenthixol | *see* zuclopenthixol |
| Clorazepate (dipotassium clorazepate) | Antianxiety drugs/ hypnosedatives, benzodiazepines |
| Cloxacillin | Antibacterial drugs, penicillins |
| Clozapine | Antipsychotic drugs |
| Codeine | Analgesics |
| Codergocrine mesylate | *see* ergoloid mesylates |
| Colchicine | Gout drugs |
| Cortisone | Corticosteroids |
| Cromoglycate sodium (cromolyn sodium) | *see* sodium cromoglycate |
| Cyclophosphamide | Antineoplastic and immunosuppressive drugs |
| Cyclosporin (cyclosporin A) | Antineoplastic and immunosuppressive drugs |
| Cytarabine (cytosine arabinoside) | Antineoplastic and immunosuppressive drugs |
| Dacarbazine | Antineoplastic and immunosuppressive drugs |
| Dactinomycin (actinomycin D) | Antineoplastic and immunosuppressive drugs |
| Dantrolene | Miscellaneous drugs |
| Dapsone | Antimalarial drugs |
| Daunorubicin | Antineoplastic and immunosuppressive drugs |
| Debrisoquine | Antihypertensive drugs |
| Deferoxamine (desferrioxamine) | Miscellaneous drugs |
| Defibrotide | Miscellaneous drugs |
| Demeclocycline (demethylchlor-tetracycline) | Antibacterial drugs, tetracyclines |
| *N*-Desalkylflurazepam | Antianxiety drugs/ hypnosedatives, benzodiazepines |
| Desipramine | Antidepressants |
| Deslanoside | Cardiac glycosides |
| *N*-Desmethyldiazepam | *see* nordazepam |
| Dexamethasone | Corticosteroids |

| Drug | Group |
|---|---|
| Dexfenfluramine | Anorexiants |
| Dextropropoxyphene (propoxyphene) | Analgesics |
| Dezocine | Analgesics |
| Diazepam | Antianxiety drugs/ hypnosedatives, benzodiazepines |
| Diaziquone | Antineoplastic and immunosuppressive drugs |
| Diazoxide | Antihypertensive drugs |
| Diclofenac | Analgesics, NSAIDs |
| Dicloxacillin | Antibacterial drugs, penicillins |
| Dicoumarol (bishydroxycoumarin) | Anticoagulants |
| Didanosine | Antiviral drugs |
| Diethylcarbamazine | Miscellaneous drugs |
| Diflunisal | Analgesics, NSAIDs |
| Digitoxin | Cardiac glycosides |
| Digoxin | Cardiac glycosides |
| Diltiazem | Calcium antagonists |
| Diphenhydramine | Antihistamines |
| Diphenoxylate | Antidiarrhoeals |
| Diphenylhydantoin | *see* phenytoin |
| Diphenylpyraline | Antihistamines |
| Disopyramide | Antiarrhythmic drugs |
| Dipotassium clorazepate | *see* clorazepate |
| Disulfiram | Miscellaneous drugs |
| Dobutamine | Inotropic agents |
| Dopamine | Inotropic agents |
| Dopexamine | Inotropic agents |
| Dothiepin | Antidepressants |
| Doxacurium | Muscle relaxants, skeletal |
| Doxapram | Miscellaneous drugs |
| Doxazosin | Antihypertensive drugs |
| Doxepin | Antidepressants |
| Doxorubicin | Antineoplastic and immunosuppressive drugs |
| Doxycycline | Antibacterial drugs, tetracyclines |
| Ecogramostim | *see* granulocyte macrophage colony-stimulating factor |
| Edatrexate | Antineoplastic and immunosuppressive drugs |
| Enalapril | ACE inhibitors |
| Encainide | Antiarrhythmic drugs |
| Enoxacin | Antibacterial drugs, fluoroquinolones |
| Enoxaparin sodium | Anticoagulants |
| Enoximone | Inotropic agents |
| Enprofylline | Bronchodilators |
| Enprostil | Antiulcer drugs |
| Epalrestat | Antidiabetic drugs |
| Epirubicin | Antineoplastic and immunosuppressive drugs |
| Epoetin (erythropoietin) | Miscellaneous drugs |
| Ergoloid mesylates (codergocrine mesylate) | Miscellaneous drugs |
| Ergotamine | Miscellaneous drugs |
| Erythromycin | Antibacterial drugs, macrolides |
| Erythropoietin | *see* epoetin |

| Drug | Group |
|---|---|
| Esmolol | β-Adrenoceptor antagonists |
| Ethacrynic acid | Diuretics |
| Ethambutol | Antituberculosis drugs |
| Ethanol | Miscellaneous drugs |
| Ethchlorvynol | Antianxiety drugs/ hypnosedatives, others |
| Ethinylestradiol | Estrogens and progestagens |
| Ethionamide | Antituberculosis drugs |
| Ethosuximide | Antiepileptic drugs |
| Ethylbiscoumacetate | Anticoagulants |
| Ethynodiol diacetate | Estrogens and progestagens |
| Etidocaine | Anaesthetics, local |
| Etodolac | Analgesics, NSAIDs |
| Etomidate | Anaesthetics, intravenous |
| Etoposide | Antineoplastic and immunosuppressive drugs |
| Etretinate | Miscellaneous drugs |
| Famotidine | Antiulcer drugs |
| Felodipine | Calcium antagonists |
| Fenbufen | Analgesics, NSAIDs |
| Fenfluramine | Anorexiants |
| Fenofibrate | Lipid-lowering drugs |
| Fenoprofen | Analgesics, NSAIDs |
| Fentanyl | Analgesics |
| Filgrastim | *see* granulocyte colony-stimulating factor |
| Finasteride | Miscellaneous drugs |
| Flecainide | Antiarrhythmic drugs |
| Fleroxacin | Antibacterial drugs, fluoroquinolones |
| Flucloxacillin | Antibacterial drugs, penicillins |
| Fluconazole | Antifungal agents |
| Flucytosine | Antifungal agents |
| Fludarabine | Antineoplastic and immunosuppressive drugs |
| Fludrocortisone | Corticosteroids |
| Flufenamic acid | Analgesics, NSAIDs |
| Flumazenil | Miscellaneous drugs |
| Flunarizine | Miscellaneous drugs |
| Flunisolide | Corticosteroids |
| Flunitrazepam | Antianxiety drugs/ hypnosedatives, benzodiazepines |
| Fluorouracil (5-fluorouracil) | Antineoplastic and immunosuppressive drugs |
| Fluoxetine | Antidepressants |
| Flupirtine | Analgesics |
| Flurazepam | Antianxiety drugs/ hypnosedatives, benzodiazepines |
| Flurbiprofen | Analgesics, NSAIDs |
| Flutamide | Antineoplastic and immunosuppressive drugs |
| Fluvoxamine | Antidepressants |
| Formestane | Antineoplastic and immunosuppressive drugs |
| Foscarnet | Antiviral drugs |
| Fosinopril | ACE inhibitors |

| Drug | Group |
|---|---|
| Furosemide (frusemide) | Diuretics |
| Gabapentin | Antiepileptic drugs |
| Gallium nitrate | Miscellaneous drugs |
| Ganciclovir | Antiviral drugs |
| Gemfibrozil | Lipid-lowering drugs |
| Gentamicin | Antibacterial drugs, aminoglycosides |
| Glibenclamide (glyburide) | Antidiabetic drugs |
| Glibornuride | Antidiabetic drugs |
| Gliclazide | Antidiabetic drugs |
| Glipizide | Antidiabetic drugs |
| Glutethimide | Antianxiety drugs/ hypnosedatives, others |
| Glyburide | *see* glibenclamide |
| Glyceryl trinitrate | *see* nitroglycerin |
| Gold sodium thiomalate | *see* aurothiomalate sodium |
| Gold thioglucose | *see* aurothoglucose |
| Goserelin | Miscellaneous drugs |
| Granisetron | Antiemetics |
| Granulocyte colony-stimulating factor (rG-CSF) | Miscellaneous drugs |
| Granulocyte macrophage colony-stimulating factor (rGM-CSF) | Miscellaneous drugs |
| Griseofulvin | Antifungal agents |
| Guanabenz | Antihypertensive drugs |
| Guanethidine | Antihypertensive drugs |
| Guanfacine | Antihypertensive drugs |
| Halofantrine | Antimalarial drugs |
| Haloperidol | Antipsychotic drugs |
| Haloperidol decanoate | Antipsychotic drugs |
| Heparin | Anticoagulants |
| Hexobarbital | Antianxiety drugs/ hypnosedatives, barbiturates |
| Hydralazine | Antihypertensive drugs |
| Hydrochlorothiazide | Diuretics |
| Hydrocortisone | Corticosteroids |
| Hydroflumethiazide | Diuretics |
| Hyoscine | *see* scopolamine |
| Ibopamine | Inotropic agents |
| Ibuprofen | Analgesics, NSAIDs |
| Idarubicin | Antineoplastic and immunosuppressive drugs |
| Ifosfamide | Antineoplastic and immunosuppressive drugs |
| Iloprost | Miscellaneous drugs |
| Imipenem | Antibacterial drugs, others |
| Imipramine | Antidepressants |
| Indapamide | Diuretics |
| Indobufen | Antiplatelet agents |
| Indomethacin | Analgesics, NSAIDs |
| Indoramin | Antihypertensive drugs |
| Inosine pranobex | Miscellaneous drugs |
| Insulin | Antidiabetic drugs |
| Interferon-α | Miscellaneous drugs |
| Interferon-γ1b | Miscellaneous drugs |
| Interleukin-2 | Miscellaneous drugs |

| Drug | Group |
|---|---|
| Ipratropium bromide | Bronchodilators |
| Isepamicin | Antibacterial drugs, aminoglycosides |
| Isoniazid | Antituberculosis drugs |
| Isoprenaline (isoproterenol) | Bronchodilators |
| Isosorbide dinitrate | Antianginal agents |
| Isosorbide 2-mononitrate | Antianginal agents |
| Isosorbide 5-mononitrate | Antianginal agents |
| Isotretinoin (13-*cis*-retinoic acid) | Miscellaneous drugs |
| Isradipine | Calcium antagonists |
| Itraconazole | Antifungal agents |
| Ivermectin | Miscellaneous drugs |
| Kanamycin | Antibacterial drugs, aminoglycosides |
| Ketamine | Anaesthetics, intravenous |
| Ketanserin | Antihypertensive drugs |
| Ketobemidone | Analgesics |
| Ketoconazole | Antifungal agents |
| Ketoprofen | Analgesics, NSAIDs |
| Ketorolac | Analgesics, NSAIDs |
| Ketotifen | Antihistamines |
| Labetalol | β-Adrenoceptor antagonists |
| Lamotrigine | Antiepileptic drugs |
| Lanatoside C | Cardiac glycosides |
| Lansoprazole | Antiulcer drugs |
| Latamoxef (moxalactam) | Antibacterial drugs, cefalosporins |
| Lenograstim | *see* granulocyte colony-stimulating factor |
| Leuprorelin | Miscellaneous drugs |
| Levamisole | Miscellaneous drugs |
| Levocarnitine (L-carnitine) | Miscellaneous drugs |
| Levodopa | Anti-Parkinsonian drugs |
| Levonorgestrel | Estrogens and progestagens |
| Lidocaine (lignocaine) | Antiarrhythmic drugs |
| Lincomycin | Antibacterial drugs, others |
| Liothyronine | Antithyroid and thyroid drugs |
| Lisinopril | ACE inhibitors |
| Lisuride | Anti-Parkinsonian drugs |
| Lithium | Antipsychotic drugs |
| Lofepramine | Antidepressants |
| Lomefloxacin | Antibacterial drugs, fluoroquinolones |
| Loperamide | Antidiarrhoeals |
| Loprazolam | Antianxiety drugs/ hypnosedatives, benzodiazepine |
| Loracarbef | Antibacterial drugs, others |
| Loratadine | Antihistamines |
| Lorazepam | Antianxiety drugs/ hypnosedatives, benzodiazepine |
| Lorcainide | Antiarrhythmic drugs |
| Lovastatin | Lipid-lowering drugs |
| Lynestrenol | Estrogens and progestagens |
| Lysuride | *see* lisuride |

| Drug | Group |
|---|---|
| Maprotiline | Antidepressants |
| Marograstim | *see* granulocyte colony-stimulating factor |
| Mazindol | Anorexiants |
| Mebendazole | Miscellaneous drugs |
| Mebhydrolin | Antihistamines |
| Mecillinam (amdinocillin) | Antibacterial drugs, penicillins |
| Medroxyprogesterone | Estrogens and progestagens |
| Mefenamic acid | Analgesics, NSAIDs |
| Mefloquine | Antimalarial drugs |
| Melphalan | Antineoplastic and immunosuppressive drugs |
| Mepacrine | Antimalarial drugs |
| Meperidine | *see* pethidine |
| Mepivacaine | Anaesthetics, local |
| Meprobamate | Antianxiety drugs/ hypnosedatives, others |
| Meproscillarin | Cardiac glycosides |
| Mesalazine | Miscellaneous drugs |
| Mesna | Miscellaneous drugs |
| Metformin | Antidiabetic drugs |
| Methadone | Analgesics |
| Methaqualone | Antianxiety drugs/ hypnosedatives, others |
| Methicillin | Antibacterial drugs, penicillins |
| Methimazole | *see* thiamazole |
| Methohexital | Anaesthetics, intravenous |
| Methotrexate | Antineoplastic and immunosuppressive drugs |
| β-Methyldigoxin | *see* metildigoxin |
| Methyldopa | Antihypertensive drugs |
| Methylphenidate | Miscellaneous drugs |
| Methylprednisolone | Corticosteroids |
| Metildigoxin | Cardiac glycosides |
| Metoclopramide | Antiemetics |
| Metolazone | Diuretics |
| Metoprolol | β-Adrenoceptor antagonists |
| Metronidazole | Antitrichomonal drugs |
| Mexiletine | Antiarrhythmic drugs |
| Mezlocillin | Antibacterial drugs, penicillins |
| Mianserin | Antidepressants |
| Miconazole | Antifungal agents |
| Midazolam | Antianxiety drugs/ hypnosedatives, benzodiazepines |
| Midecamycin (miocamycin) | Antibacterial drugs, macrolides |
| Midodrine | Miscellaneous drugs |
| Mifepristone | Miscellaneous drugs |
| Milrinone | Inotropic agents |
| Minocycline | Antibacterial drugs, tetracyclines |
| Minoxidil | Antihypertensive drugs |
| Miocamycin | *see* midecamycin |
| Misoprostol | Antiulcer drugs |
| Mitoxantrone | Antineoplastic and immunosuppressive drugs |

| Drug | Group |
|---|---|
| Mivacurium chloride | Muscle relaxants, skeletal |
| Moclobemide | Antidepressants |
| Molgramostim | *see* granulocyte macrophage colony-stimulating factor |
| Moracizine (moricizine) | Antiarrhythmic drugs |
| Morphine | Analgesics |
| Moxalactam | *see* latamoxef |
| Moxonidine | Antihypertensive drugs |
| Nabumetone | Analgesics, NSAIDs |
| Nadolol | β-Adrenoceptor antagonists |
| Nadroparin calcium | Anticoagulants |
| Nafarelin | Miscellaneous drugs |
| Nafcillin | Antibacterial drugs, penicillins |
| Nalbuphine | Analgesics |
| Nalidixic acid | Antibacterial drugs, others |
| Naloxone | Analgesics, antagonists |
| Naltrexone | Analgesics, antagonists |
| Naproxen | Analgesics, NSAIDs |
| Nedocromil | Miscellaneous drugs |
| Nefopam | Analgesics |
| Neostigmine | Miscellaneous drugs |
| Netilmicin | Antibacterial drugs, aminoglycosides |
| Nicardipine | Calcium antagonists |
| Nicorandil | Antianginal agents |
| Nicotinic acid (niacin) | Lipid-lowering drugs |
| Nicoumalone | *see* acenocoumarol |
| Nifedipine | Calcium antagonists |
| Nilutamide | Antineoplastic and immunosuppressive drugs |
| Nimesulide | Analgesics, NSAIDs |
| Nimodipine | Calcium antagonists |
| Nisoldipine | Calcium antagonists |
| Nitrazepam | Antianxiety drugs/hypnosedatives, benzodiazepines |
| Nitrendipine | Calcium antagonists |
| Nitrofurantoin | Antibacterial drugs, others |
| Nitroglycerin (glyceryl trinitrate) | Antianginal agents |
| Nitroprusside sodium | *see* sodium nitroprusside |
| Nizatidine | Antiulcer drugs |
| Nordazepam | Antianxiety drugs/ hypnosedatives, benzodiazepines |
| Norethisterone (norethindrone) | Estrogens and progestagens |
| Norethynodrel | Estrogens and progestagens |
| Norfloxacin | Antibacterial drugs, fluoroquinolones |
| Nortriptyline | Antidepressants |
| Octreotide | Miscellaneous drugs |
| Ofloxacin | Antibacterial drugs, fluoroquinolones |
| Olsalazine | Miscellaneous drugs |
| Omeprazole | Antiulcer drugs |
| Ondansetron | Antiemetics |
| Ornidazole | Antitrichomonal drugs |
| Orphenadrine | Anti-Parkinsonian drugs |
| Ouabain | Cardiac glycosides |
| Oxacillin | Antibacterial drugs, penicillins |
| Oxaprozin | Analgesics, NSAIDs |
| Oxatomide | Antihistamines |
| Oxazepam | Antianxiety drugs/ hypnosedatives, benzodiazepines |
| Oxcarbazepine | Antiepileptic drugs |
| Oxpentifylline | *see* pentoxifylline |
| Oxprenolol | β-Adrenoceptor antagonists |
| Oxyphenbutazone | Analgesics, NSAIDs |
| Oxytetracycline | Antibacterial drugs, tetracyclines |
| Paclitaxel (taxol) | Antineoplastic and immunosuppressive drugs |
| Pamidronate disodium (pamidronic acid) | Miscellaneous drugs |
| Pancuronium | Muscle relaxants, skeletal |
| Papaverine | Miscellaneous drugs |
| Paracetamol (acetaminophen) | Analgesics |
| Paraldehyde | Antianxiety drugs/ hypnosedatives, others |
| Paroxetine | Antidepressants |
| Pefloxacin | Antibacterial drugs, fluoroquinolones |
| Penbutolol | β-Adrenoceptor antagonists |
| Penicillamine (D-penicillamine) | Miscellaneous drugs |
| Penicillin G | *see* benzylpenicillin |
| Penicillin V | *see* phenoxymethylpenicillin |
| Pentamidine | Miscellaneous drugs |
| Pentazocine | Analgesics |
| Pentobarbital | Antianxiety drugs/ hypnosedatives, barbiturates |
| Pentostatin | Antineoplastic and immunosuppressive drugs |
| Pentoxifylline (oxpentifylline) | Miscellaneous drugs |
| Pergolide | Anti-Parkinsonian drugs |
| Perhexiline | Antianginal agents |
| Perindopril | ACE inhibitors |
| Perphenazine | Antipsychotic drugs |
| Pethidine (meperidine) | Analgesics |
| Phenacetin | Analgesics |
| Phenformin | Antidiabetic drugs |
| Phenobarbital | Antiepileptic drugs |
| Phenoxymethylpenicillin (penicillin V) | Antibacterial drugs, penicillins |
| Phenprocoumon | Anticoagulants |
| Phenylbutazone | Analgesics, NSAIDs |
| Phenylephrine | Miscellaneous drugs |
| Phenylethylmalonamide (PEMA) | Antiepileptic drugs |
| Phenytoin (diphenylhydantoin) | Antiepileptic drugs |
| Pimozide | Antipsychotic drugs |
| Pinacidil | Antihypertensive drugs |
| Pindolol | β-Adrenoceptor antagonists |

| Drug | Group |
|---|---|
| Piperacillin | Antibacterial drugs, penicillins |
| Piracetam | Miscellaneous drugs |
| Pirenzepine | Antiulcer drugs |
| Piretanide | Diuretics |
| Pirmenol | Antiarrhythmic drugs |
| Piroxicam | Analgesics, NSAIDs |
| Pirprofen | Analgesics, NSAIDs |
| Pivampicillin | *see* ampicillin |
| Pivmecillinam (*see* mecillinam) | Antibacterial drugs, penicillins |
| Polythiazide | Diuretics |
| Prajmaline | Antiarrhythmic drugs |
| Pravastatin | Lipid-lowering drugs |
| Prazepam | Antianxiety drugs/ hypnosedatives, benzodiazepines |
| Praziquantel | Miscellaneous drugs |
| Prazosin | Antihypertensive drugs |
| Prednisolone | Corticosteroids |
| Prednisone | Corticosteroids |
| Prenalterol | Inotropic agents |
| Primidone | Antiepileptic drugs |
| Primaquine | Antimalarial drugs |
| Probenecid | Gout drugs |
| Probucol | Lipid-lowering drugs |
| Procainamide | Antiarrhythmic drugs |
| Prochlorperazine | Antipsychotic drugs |
| Promethazine | Antihistamines |
| Propafenone | Antiarrhythmic drugs |
| Propantheline | Anticholinergics |
| Propiram | Analgesics |
| Propofol | Anaesthetics, intravenous |
| Propoxyphene | *see* dextropropoxyphene |
| Propranolol | β-Adrenoceptor antagonists |
| Propylthiouracil | Antithyroid and thyroid drugs |
| Proquazone | Analgesics, NSAIDs |
| Proscillaridin | Cardiac glycosides |
| Pyrazinamide | Antituberculosis drugs |
| Pyridostigmine | Miscellaneous drugs |
| Pyrimethamine | Antimalarial drugs |
| Quazepam | Antianxiety drugs/ hypnosedatives, benzodiazepines |
| Quinalbarbitone | *see* secobarbital |
| Quinapril | ACE inhibitors |
| Quinidine | Antiarrhythmic drugs |
| Quinine | Antimalarial drugs |
| Ramipril | ACE inhibitors |
| Ranitidine | Antiulcer drugs |
| Reserpine | Antihypertensive drugs |
| Rifampicin (rifampin) | Antituberculosis drugs |
| Risperidone | Antipsychotic drugs |
| Rolitetracycline | Antibacterial drugs, tetracyclines |
| Roxatidine | Antiulcer drugs |
| Roxithromycin | Antibacterial drugs, macrolides |
| *S*-Adenosyl-L-methionine | *see* ademetionine |
| Salbutamol | Bronchodilators |

| Drug | Group |
|---|---|
| Salicylate | Analgesics, NSAIDs |
| Sargramostim | *see* granulocyte macrophage colony-stimulating factors |
| Scopolamine (hyoscine) | Anticholinergics |
| Scopolamine *N*-butylbromide | Anticholinergics |
| Secobarbital | Antianxiety drugs/ hypnosedatives, benzodiazepines |
| Secobutabarbital (butabarbital) | Antianxiety drugs/ hypnosedatives, barbiturates |
| Selegiline | Anti-Parkinsonian drugs |
| Sertraline | Antidepressants |
| Simvastatin | Lipid-lowering drugs |
| Sisomicin | Antibacterial drugs, aminoglycosides |
| Sodium aurothiomalate | *see* aurothiomalate sodium |
| Sodium cromoglycate | Miscellaneous drugs |
| Sodium nitroprusside | Antihypertensive drugs |
| Sodium valproate | *see* valproic acid |
| Sotalol | β-Adrenoceptor antagonists |
| Spectinomycin | Antibacterial drugs, others |
| Spironolactone | Diuretics |
| Streptomycin | Antituberculosis drugs |
| Sufentanil | Analgesics |
| Sulbactam | Antibacterial drugs, others |
| Sulindac | Analgesics, NSAIDs |
| Sulfadoxine | Antimalarial drugs |
| Sulfadiazine | Antibacterial drugs, sulfonamides |
| Sulfadimidine (sulfamethazine) | sulfonamides |
| Sulfafurazole (sulfisoxazole) | sulfonamides |
| Sulfamethizole | sulfonamides |
| Sulfamethoxazole | sulfonamides |
| Sulfamethoxydiazine | sulfonamides |
| Sulfamethoxypyridazine | sulfonamides |
| Sulfapyridine | sulfonamides |
| Sulfasalazine | sulfonamides |
| Sulfathiazole | sulfonamides |
| Sulfinpyrazone | Gout drugs |
| Sumatriptan | Miscellaneous drugs |
| Tacrolimus (FK 506) | Antineoplastic and immunosuppressive drugs |
| Tamoxifen | Antineoplastic and immunosuppressive drugs |
| Teicoplanin | Antibacterial drugs, others |
| Temazepam | Antianxiety drugs/ hypnosedatives, benzodiazepines |
| Temocillin | Antibacterial drugs, penicillin |
| Teniposide | Antineoplastic and immunosuppressive drugs |
| Tenoxicam | Analgesics, NSAIDs |
| Terazosin | Antihypertensive drugs |
| Terbutaline | Bronchodilators |
| Terfenadine | Antihistamines |
| Tetracycline | Antibacterial drugs, tetracyclines |

| Drug | Group |
|---|---|
| Tetroxoprim | Antibacterial drugs, others |
| Theophylline | Bronchodilators |
| Thiamazole (methimazole) | Antithyroid and thyroid drugs |
| Thiamphenicol | Antibacterial drugs, others |
| Thiopental (thiopentone) | Anaesthetics, intravenous |
| Thioridazine | Antipsychotic drugs |
| Thyroxine | Antithyroid and thyroid drugs |
| Tiapride | Antipsychotic drugs |
| Tiaprofenic acid | Analgesics, NSAIDs |
| Ticarcillin | Antibacterial drugs, penicillins |
| Ticlopidine | Antiplatelet agents |
| Timolol | β-Adrenoceptor antagonists |
| Tinidazole | Antitrichomonal drugs |
| Tobramycin | Antibacterial drugs, aminoglycosides |
| Tocainide | Antiarrhythmic drugs |
| Tolamolol | β-Adrenoceptor antagonists |
| Tolazamide | Antidiabetic drugs |
| Tolbutamide | Antidiabetic drugs |
| Tolfenamic acid | Analgesics, NSAIDs |
| Tolmetin | Analgesics, NSAIDs |
| Torasemide | Diuretics |
| Tramadol | Analgesics |
| Trandolapril | ACE inhibitors |
| Tranexamic acid | Miscellaneous drugs |
| Trazodone | Antidepressants |
| Tri-iodothyronine | *see* liothyronine |
| Triamcinolone | Corticosteroids |
| Triamterene | Diuretics |

| Drug | Group |
|---|---|
| Triazolam | Antianxiety drugs/ hypnosedatives, benzodiazepines |
| Trimethoprim | Antibacterial drugs, others |
| Trimipramine | Antidepressants |
| Tropisetron | Antiemetics |
| Tubocurarine | Muscle relaxants, skeletal |
| Urapidil | Antihypertensive drugs |
| Ursodeoxycholic acid | Miscellaneous drugs |
| Valproic acid (sodium valproate) | Antiepileptic drugs |
| Vancomycin | Antibacterial drugs, others |
| Vecuronium bromide | Muscle relaxants, skeletal |
| Verapamil | Calcium antagonists |
| Vidarabine (adenine arabinoside) | Antiviral drugs |
| Vigabatrin | Antiepileptic drugs |
| Vinblastine | Antineoplastic and immunosuppressive drugs |
| Vincristine | Antineoplastic and immunosuppressive drugs |
| Vindesine | Antineoplastic and immunosuppressive drugs |
| Warfarin | Anticoagulants |
| Zalcitabine | Antiviral drugs |
| Zidovudine | Antiviral drugs |
| Zolpidem | Antianxiety drugs/ hypnosedatives, others |
| Zonisamide | Antiepileptic drugs |
| Zopiclone | Antianxiety drugs/ hypnosedatives, others |
| Zuclopenthixol | Antipsychotic drugs |

**Appendix A.** Pharmacokinetic drug data

| Drug | Nature[a] | pKa[b] | F[c] (%) | CL[c] (L/h) | $t_{1/2}$[c] (h) | Vd[c] (L) [per 70kg] | Protein binding[c] (%) | $f_{NR(n)}$[c,d] [$P_o$] | Notes |
|---|---|---|---|---|---|---|---|---|---|
| **ACE (angiotensin-converting enzyme) inhibitors** | | | | | | | | | |
| Benazepril[e*] | | | | 1.5 | 3(22**) | 8.4 | >95 | | * Prodrug; data shown are for active metabolite benazeprilat<br>** Terminal elimination half-life |
| Captopril[f] | | 3.7/9.8 | 65 | ≈56 | ≈1.9 | ≈49[g] | 30 | 0.55[f] | |
| Cilazapril[e*] | | | 57-77 | 7 | 1.8(40-50**) | 35 | | 0.1 | * Prodrug; data shown are for active metabolite cilazaprilat<br>** Terminal elimination half-life |
| Enalapril[e*] | | 3.0/5.4 | 40 | 6.1 | 5(35**) | | 50 | 0.1 | * Prodrug; data shown are for active metabolite enalaprilat<br>** Terminal elimination half-life |
| Fosinopril[e*] | | | | 1.5 | 2(12**) | 10.5 | 95 | 0.5 | * Prodrug; data shown are for active metabolite fosinoprilat<br>** Terminal elimination half-life |
| Lisinopril | | 2.5/4/6.7/10 | 25-50 | ≈6 | 30* | | <1 | 0.2 | * Terminal elimination half-life |
| Perindopril[e*] | | | 66-95 | ≈40 | ≈5(25**) | ≈15.4 | 60 | | * Prodrug; data shown are for active metabolite perindoprilat<br>** Terminal elimination half-life |
| Quinapril[e*] | | | | ≈13 | ≈2 | | 97 | | * Prodrug; data shown are for active metabolite quinaprilat |
| Ramipril[e*] | | | | | ≈3(110**) | | 56 | | * Prodrug; data shown are for active metabolite ramiprilat<br>** Terminal elimination half-life |
| Trandolapril[e*] | | | | | 24 | | 94 | | * Prodrug; data shown are for active metabolite trandolaprilat |
| β-**Adrenoceptor antagonists** (β-blockers) | | | | | | | | | |
| Acebutolol[e] | B | 9.67 | 40 | 20 | 7 | 84 | ≈20 | 0.8[e] | |
| Alprenolol[e] | B | 9.7 | 10 | 27 | 2.5 | 77 | 76 | 1.0[e] | |
| Atenolol | B | 9.55 | 55 | 11 | 6.7 | 77 | 3 | 0.06 | |
| Betaxolol | | 9.38 | 80-89 | 19.6 | 18 | 577.5 | 50 | 0.85 | |
| Bevantolol | B | 8.1 | 60 | | 2* | 105 | 95 | 0.95 | * Terminal phase with $t_{1/2}$ up to 11h in some individuals |
| Bisoprolol | | | >90 | 15[h] | 10 | 210[h] | 30 | 0.5 | |
| Bopindolol | | | 70 | 31 | 8* | 203 | | 1.0 | * Two hydroxylation phenotypes |
| Carteolol[e] | | | | | 5.4 | | | 0.3[e] | |

[Continued over]

*For footnotes, see final page of table (p.1664)*

**Appendix A.** *[Continued]*

| Drug | Nature[a] | pKa[b] | F[c] (%) | CL[c] (L/h) | $t_{½}$[c] (h) | Vd[c] (L) [per 70kg] | Protein binding[c] (%) | $f_{NR(n)}$[c,d] [$P_o$] | Notes |
|---|---|---|---|---|---|---|---|---|---|
| **β-Adrenoceptor antagonists** *[continued]* | | | | | | | | | |
| Carvedilol | | | 25 | | 5.8 | 105-140 | | 0.98 | |
| Celiprolol | | 9.68 | | | 4.5 | | 25 | | |
| Cicloprolol | | | 90 | | 10 | | | | |
| Esmolol | B | 9.5 | | 1200 | 0.15 | 238 | 56 | 1.0 | |
| Labetalol | B | 7.38 | 33 | 90 | 3.9 | 392 | 50 | 0.95 | |
| Metoprolol[e] | B | 9.7 | 50 | 68 | 3.5 | 385 | 8 | 0.95[e] | |
| Nadolol | B | 9.67 | 25 | 12 | 19 | 133 | 28 | 0.25 | |
| Oxprenolol | B | 9.5 | 30 | 12 | 2.2 | 91 | 92 | 0.95 | |
| Penbutolol[e] | B | 9.3 | 100 | | 26 | | >95 | 0.95[e] | |
| Pindolol | B | 8.8 | 100 | 32 | 2.5 | 84 | 50 | 0.5 | |
| Propranolol[e] | B | 9.45 | ≈30 | 63 | 4 | 196 | 93 | 1.0[e] | |
| Sotalol | B | 8.3/9.8 | >60 | 10 | 7.5* | 91 | <1 | 0.2 | * Terminal elimination phase $t_{½}$ ≈15h |
| Timolol[f] | B | 8.8 | 61 | 32 | 2.7 | 119 | 60 | 0.8[f] | |
| Tolamolol | B | 7.94 | | 45 | 2.5 | 147 | 91 | 0.9 | |
| **Anaesthetics, intravenous** | | | | | | | | | |
| Alfaxalone | S | | | 85 | 0.5 | 56 | 46 | | |
| Etomidate | A | 4.24 | | 44 | 4.6 | 315 | 75 | 1.0 | |
| Ketamine[f] | | 7.5 | 20* | 60 | 3 | 140 | 12 | 1.0[f] | *IM |
| Methohexital | A | 8.3 | | 50 | 1.5 | 70 | | 1.0 | |
| Propofol | | | | 104 | 0.05; 0.5; 4* | 280[g] | | 1.0 | * Triexponential |
| Thiopental | A | 7.45 | | 8 | 10 | 210[g] | 80 | 1.0 | |
| **Anaesthetics, local** | | | | | | | | | |
| Bupivacaine | B | 8.1 | | 35 | 2.7 | 70[g] | 96 | 0.95 | |
| Etidocaine | B | 7.7 | | 67 | 2.7 | 133[g] | 94 | 1.0 | |
| Mepivacaine | B | 7.7 | | 47 | 1.9 | 84[g] | 77 | 0.95 | |
| **Analgesics** | | | | | | | | | |
| Alfentanil | | 6.5 | | 20 | 1.5 | 49 | 90 | | |
| Aminophenazone (amidopyrine) | B | 5.0 | 75 | 29 | 1.5-2.3* | 60.2 | 30 | 1.0 | * Dose-dependent |

| | | | | | | | | | |
|---|---|---|---|---|---|---|---|---|---|
| Aspirin[e] | A | 3.5 | 68 | 39 | 0.25* | 10.5 | ≈70 | 1.0* | * Active metabolite (salicylate) has a longer $t_{½}$ (2-30h) |
| Buprenorphine | B | 8.49/10.03 | 30* | 70 | 2.5 | 140 | ≈96 | 1.0 | * Sublingual |
| Butorphanol | | | | | 3 | | 80 | 1.0 | |
| Codeine[e] | B | 7.95 | 55 | 98* | 2.8 | 378* | ≈7 | 1.0[e] | * After oral administration, corrected for bioavailability |
| Dezocine | | | 100 | 200 | 2.6 | 742 | | | |
| Dextropropoxyphene | B | 6.3 | | 66 | 2.7 | 189 | 78 | ≈1.0 | |
| Fentanyl[f] | B | 8.43 | | 47 | 3 | ≈210 | 83 | 0.95[f] | |
| Flupirtine[e] | | | 90 | 6.8 | 8.5 | 80.5 | 80 | | |
| Ketobemidone | B | | 34 | 7 | 2.1 | 259 | | 0.95 | |
| Methadone | B | 8.25 | 92 | 7.5 | 29 | 280 | 80 | 0.6 | |
| Morphine[f] | Amp | 9.85/7.87 | 20-33 | 72 | 2.5 | 245 | 35 | 0.9[f] | |
| Nalbuphine[e] | | | | | 3.5 | | | 0.9[e] | |
| Nefopam[f] | | 8.35 | | | 4 | | 75 | 0.95[f] | |
| Paracetamol[e] (acetaminophen) | A | 9.5 | 70-90 | 19.3 | 2.5 | 65.8 | low* | 1.0[e] | * At therapeutic doses |
| Pentazocine | B | 8.8 | | 79 | 3 | 392 | 65 | 0.8 | |
| Pethidine (meperidine)[e] | B | 6.3 | 54 | 38 | 6.9 | 280 | 70 | 0.9[e] | |
| Phenacetin[e] | Sa | | | 87 | 1.2 | 105 | 33 | 1.0[e] | |
| Propiram | | | >97 | 26.6 | 7 | 161 | | | |
| Sufentanil | | 8.01 | | 44 | 2.6 | 140 | 93 | | |
| Tramadol[e] | | | | 26 | 6 | 231 | 4 | 0.7[e] | |
| • *Nonsteroidal anti-inflammatory drugs (NSAIDs)* | | | | | | | | | |
| Alclofenac | A | 4.6 | | | 3 | 7 | >99 | 0.7 | |
| Azapropazone | A | | | 0.6 | 13 | 11.2 | 99 | 0.4 | |
| Diclofenac[f] | A | | 60 | 15.6 | 1.5 | 10.5 | >99 | 1.0[f] | |
| Diflunisal | A | | 100 | 0.35-0.49* | 5-20* | 7.7 | 99 | 0.95 | * Dose-dependent |
| Etodolac | | | | 2.8 | 6 | 28.7 | >99 | 1.0 | |
| Fenbufen[e] | A | | >85 | | 10 | 210[h] | >99 | 0.95[e] | |
| Fenoprofen[f] | A | 4.5 | >85 | 3.9[h] | 2.8 | 6.3[h] | >99 | 0.95[f] | |
| Flufenamic acid | A | | | | 9 | | >90 | 1.0 | |
| Flurbiprofen | A | | >85 | 1.3[h] | 3.5 | 7[h] | >99 | 0.9 | |
| Ibuprofen | A | 4.4/5.2 | >80* | 3.5[h] | 2.5 | 9.8[h] | 99 | 1.0 | * Dose-dependent |
| Indomethacin | A | 4.5 | >85 | 6.3 | 6 | 14 | >90 | 0.85 | |
| Ketoprofen | A | | >85 | 5.2 | 1.4 | 7.7 | <94 | 0.75 | |

[Continued over]

*For footnotes, see final page of table (p.1664)*

**Appendix A.** *[Continued]*

| Drug | Nature[a] | pKa[b] | F[c] (%) | CL[c] (L/h) | $t_{½}$[c] (h) | Vd[c] (L) [per 70kg] | Protein binding[c] (%) | $f_{NR(n)}$[c,d] [$P_o$] | Notes |
|---|---|---|---|---|---|---|---|---|---|
| **Analgesics** *[continued]* | | | | | | | | | |
| Ketorolac | | 3.49 | 80 | 2 | 5.6 | 17.5 | 99 | | |
| Mefenamic acid | A | 4.2 | | | 3.5 | | high | 0.9 | |
| Nabumetone[e] | | | 35 | 0.24* | 24* | 7* | >99* | | * Data shown are for pharmacologically active metabolite (6-MNA) |
| Naproxen | A | 4.15 | 99 | 0.3 | 14 | 7 | 99 | 0.9 | |
| Nimesulide | | | | | 4.8 | | 99 | | |
| Oxaprozin | | | 100 | 0.18 | 56 | 14 | >99.5 | | |
| Oxyphenbutazone | A | 4.7 | | | 45 | | 99 | 1.0 | |
| Phenylbutazone[e] | A | 4.5 | >85 | | 70 | 11.9 | 99 | 1.0[e] | |
| Piroxicam | A | 6.3 | | 0.14[h] | 45 | 9.8[h] | 99 | 0.9 | |
| Pirprofen[f] | | | | 1.4 | 6.5 | 12.6 | > 99 | 0.95[f] | |
| Proquazone[e] | | | | 40 | 0.6-1.3 (6.7-13*) | 39.2[g] | >98 | 1.0 | * Data for pharmacologically active metabolite |
| Salicylate | A | 2.97/12.5 | | 0.6-3.6* | 2-30* | 11.9* | 85* | 0.9 | * Dose-dependent |
| Sulindac[e] | A | 4.5 | >88 | | 7* | | 96 | 1.0* | * Active sulfide metabolite has a longer $t_{½}$ (18h) |
| Tenoxicam | | | | 0.13 | 72 | 14 | 99 | 1.0 | |
| Tiaprofenic acid | A | | | 4.5 | 2 | * | 98 | 0.55 | * ≈ Plasma volume |
| Tolfenamic acid | A | | 56-63 | 9.3 | 2.5 | 11.2 | >99 | 0.9 | |
| Tolmetin | A | 3.5 | | 6[h] | ≈1 | ≈7[h] | ≥99 | 0.95 | |
| • *Analgesic antagonists* | | | | | | | | | |
| Naloxone[f] | B | 7.94 | 2 | 104 | 1.5 | 210 | | ≈1.0[f] | |
| Naltrexone | | | 5-60* | 94 | 2.7 | 994 | 20 | 1.0 | * Dose-dependent |
| **Anorexiants** | | | | | | | | | |
| Chlorphentermine[f] | B | 9.6 | | | ≈41 | 168 | | 0.8[f] | |
| Dexfenfluramine[e] | | | | | 18.2 | 910 | | 0.9[e] | |
| Fenfluramine | B | 9.9 | | | 18 | | 34 | | |
| Mazindol | | 8.6 | | | ≈36 | | | | |
| **Antianginal agents** (see also β-adrenoceptor antagonists and calcium antagonists) | | | | | | | | | |
| Isosorbide dinitrate[e] | | | 30 | 147 | 0.3 | 105 | | 1.0[e] | |
| Isosorbide 2-mononitrate | | | 100 | 21 | 2.5 | ≈49 | | 1.0 | |

| | | | | | | | | | |
|---|---|---|---|---|---|---|---|---|---|
| Isosorbide 5-mononitrate | | | 93 | 7.6 | 4.4 | 49 | 0 | 0.8 | |
| Nicorandil | | | >75 | 52-69 | 0.75 | 84 | 24 | 1.0 | |
| Nitroglycerin (glyceryl trinitrate) | | | | ≈1260 | 0.05 | ≈210 | | | |
| Perhexiline | B | | | | ≈66/157* ≈280/395** | | | 1.0 | * Rapid metabolisers: (–) enantiomer/(+) enantiomer ** Poor metabolisers: (–)enantiomer/(+) enantiomer |
| **Antianxiety drugs/hypnosedatives** | | | | | | | | | |
| • *Barbiturates* | | | | | | | | | |
| Hexobarbital | A | 8.34 | >90 | 14[h] | 5 | 105[h] | | 1.0 | |
| Pentobarbital[f] | A | 8.11 | 100 | 1.5 | 25 | 70 | 55 | 1.0[f] | |
| Secobarbital (quinalbarbitone) | A | 7.92/12.5 | | | ≈25 | ≈105 | 50 | 1.0 | |
| Secobutabarbital (butabarbital) | A | 7.9 | | ≈1[h] | ≈40 | ≈56[h] | 26 | 1.0 | |
| • *Benzodiazepines* | | | | | | | | | |
| Alprazolam[f] | B | 2.4 | | 4.0[h] | 16 | 70[h] | 70 | 0.9[f] | |
| Bromazepam | Amp | 2.8. 11 | | 2.5 | 12 | 70 | | 1.0 | |
| Brotizolam[e] | | | | 7 | 5 | 49 | 90 | 1.0[e] | |
| Chlordiazepoxide[e] | B | 4.8 | >86 | 1 | 20 | 28 | 96 | 1.0[e] | |
| Clobazam[e] | | | | 2[h] | 35 | 98[h] | 90 | 1.0[e] | |
| Clorazepate[e] (dipotassium clorazepate) | | 3.5/12.5 | | | 2 | | | 1.0[e] | Active metabolite: nordazepam (*N*-desmethyldiazepam, see below) |
| *N*-Desalkylflurazepam | | | | 0.5* | 80 | 49* | 98 | | * After oral flurazepam |
| Diazepam[e] | B | 3.3 | 100 | 1.8 | 40* | 140 | 98 | 1.0 | * Active metabolite nordazepam (*N*-desmethyldiazepam) has a longer $t_{½}$ |
| Flunitrazepam[f] | B | 1.84 | 85 | 8[h] | 29 | 259[h] | | 1.0[f] | |
| Flurazepam[e] | Amp | 1.9/8.16 | | | 2/80* | 238 | 97 | 1.0 | * Parent drug/active metabolite (*N*-desalkylflurazepam) |
| Loprazolam | | 6 | | | 9.7 | | 80 | 1.0 | |
| Lorazepam | Amp | 1.3/11.5 | 93 | 3[h] | 20 | 105[h] | 90 | 1.0 | |
| Midazolam | B | 6.1 | 35 | 20 | 3.0 | 84 | 95 | 1.0 | |
| Nitrazepam | Amp | 3.4/10.8 | 78 | 4 | 30 | 175 | 85 | 1.0 | |
| Nordazepam[e] (*N*-desmethyldiazepam) | Amp | 11.65/3.35 | 50 | 1.5 | 80 | 175 | 97 | 1.0[e] | |
| Oxazepam | Amp | 11.51/1.56 | >90 | 8[h] | 7 | 70[h] | >95 | 1.0 | |

*[Continued over]*

*For footnotes, see final page of table (p.1664)*

**Appendix A.** *[Continued]*

| Drug | Nature[a] | pKa[b] | F[c] (%) | CL[c] (L/h) | $t_{1/2}$[c] (h) | Vd[c] (L) [per 70kg] | Protein binding[c] (%) | $f_{NR(n)}$[c,d] [$P_o$] | Notes |
|---|---|---|---|---|---|---|---|---|---|
| **Antianxiety drugs/hypnosedatives** *[continued]* | | | | | | | | | |
| Prazepam[e] | B | 2.74 | 86 | 10[h] | 1.3* | 980[h] | | 1.0* | * Active metabolite nordazepam (*N*-desmethyldiazepam) has a longer $t_{1/2}$ |
| Quazepam[e] | | | | | 37 | 476 | >95 | 1.0[e] | |
| Temazepam | B | 1.31 | >80 | 4[h] | 13 | 70[h] | 97 | 1.0 | |
| Triazolam[e] | | | 55 | 20[h] | 3 | 70[h] | 80 | 1.0[e] | |
| • *Others* | | | | | | | | | |
| Buspirone[e] | | | 4 | 92.5 | 2.4 | 371 | 95 | 1.0[e] | |
| Chloral hydrate[e] | A | 10.04 | | | 8* | | ≈35* | 1.0 | * Trichloroethanol (active metabolite) |
| Clomethiazole | B | 3.2 | 10 | 100 | 6 | 840(210[g]) | 64 | 0.95 | |
| Ethchlorvynol | | | | | ≈25 | ≈175 | | | |
| Glutethimide[e] | A | 4.52 | | | ≈10 | | 54 | 1.0[e] | |
| Meprobamate[f] | | | | 3[h] | 10 | | | 0.9[f] | |
| Methaqualone[f] | Sa | 2.5 | | ≈8[h] | 35 | 420[h] | 80 | 0.9[f] | |
| Paraldehyde | | | | | ≈6 | | | | |
| Zolpidem | | | 70 | 18.2 | 2 | 37.8 | 90 | 1.0 | |
| Zopiclone | | | 80 | 14.8 | 4.9 | 98 | 45 | 1.0 | |
| **Antiarrhythmic drugs** (see also β-adrenoceptor antagonists) | | | | | | | | | |
| Acecainide* (*N*-acetylprocainamide) | | | 83 | 8.3 | 8 | 91 | 10 | 0.2 | * Recommended therapeutic serum concentration 15-25 mg/L |
| Adenosine | | 3.8/6.2 | | | 0.003 | | | | |
| *N*-Ajmaline hydrogen tartrate[f] | B | 8.2 | | 20 | 5.5 | 140 | 61 | 0.85[f] | |
| Amiodarone[e] | B | 6.56 | 50 | 8.6 | 14*/1300** | 4970 | 96 | 1.0[e] | * Single dose IV<br>** Multiple doses |
| Aprindine | | | | 13-68* | 8-10.1* | 280-1120* | 96 | 1.0 | * Dose-dependent, after oral administration |
| Bretylium[f] | $B_4$ | | 23 | 47 | 7.8 | 574 | | 0.2[f] | |
| Cibenzoline | | | 85 | 40 | 7.2 | 392 | 50-60 | 0.4 | |
| Disopyramide[e]* | B | 10.4 | 83 | 40** | 5.5** | 182** | 54-81† | 0.4[e] | * Recommended therapeutic serum concentration 2-8 mg/L<br>** Calculated from unbound plasma concentrations<br>† Concentration-dependent |

| | | | | | | | | | |
|---|---|---|---|---|---|---|---|---|---|
| Encainide | | | 42 | 55.4 | 3.0/8.7* | 189 | ≈75 | | * Slow demethylators |
| Flecainide[e]* | | | 95 | 42.8** | 12**/19.5† | 588** | 52 | 0.7[e] | * Recommended therapeutic serum concentration < 800 µg/L<br>** Healthy volunteers<br>† Arrhythmia patients |
| Lidocaine* (lignocaine) | B | 7.86 | 35 | 40 | 3.9 | 210 | 60 | 0.95 | * Recommended therapeutic serum concentration 2-5 mg/L |
| Lorcainide[e] | B | | 5-65* | 60 | 9 | 700 | 85 | 1.0[e] | * Dose-dependent, nonlinear |
| Mexiletine[f]* | | 8.75 | 85 | 27 | 10 | 350 | 70 | 0.8[f] | * Recommended therapeutic serum concentration 0.8-2 mg/L |
| Moracizine | | | 36 | 66 | 2.15 | 206.5 | 95 | 1.0 | |
| Pirmenol[f] | | | 87 | 12.6 | 7 | 91 | 87 | 0.7[f] | |
| Procainamide[e]* | B | 9.2 | 83 | ≈37** | 3** | 154 | 15 | 0.3[e] | * Recommended therapeutic serum concentration 4-10 mg/L<br>** Acetylator phenotype-dependent |
| Propafenone[e] | | | 5-12† | 47* | 5* | 210 | >95 | 1.0[e] | * Hydroxylator phenotype-dependent.<br>† Dose-dependent |
| Quinidine[e]* | B | 4.0/8.6 | 78 | 18 | 6 | 175 | 90 | 0.8[e] | * Recommended therapeutic serum concentration 2-5 mg/L |
| Tocainide | B | 7.7 | 100 | 10.9 | 14 | 224 | ≈12 | 0.5 | |
| **Antibacterial drugs** | | | | | | | | | |
| • *Aminoglycosides* | | | | | | | | | |
| Amikacin | B | | | 4* | 3** | 17.5 | <10 | 0.02 | * ≈60% of creatinine clearance<br>** Terminal elimination phase $t_{1/2}$ ≈100h |
| Gentamicin | B | 8.2 | | 4* | 3.0** | 17.5 | <10 | 0.02 | * ≈60% of creatinine clearance<br>** Terminal elimination phase $t_{1/2}$ ≈100h |
| Isepamicin | | | | 4.2 | 1 | 6.65[g] | 3-8 | | |
| Kanamycin | B | 7.2 | 100* | 6 | 2.5 | ≈21 | 0 | 0.03 | * IM |
| Netilmicin | B | | | 4* | 3.0** | 17.5 | low | 0.01 | * ≈70% of creatinine clearance<br>** Terminal elimination phase $t_{1/2}$ ≈100h |
| Sisomicin | B | | | 4* | 3** | 17.5 | low | 0.01 | * ≈60% of creatinine clearance<br>** Terminal elimination phase with long $t_{1/2}$ must be assumed |
| Tobramycin | B | 6.7/8.3/9.9 | 0 | 4* | 3** | 17.5 | <10 | 0.02 | * ≈60% of creatinine clearance<br>** Terminal elimination phase $t_{1/2}$ ≈100h |
| • *Cefalosporins* | | | | | | | | | |
| Cefacetrile[f] | A | 1.97 | | 12 | 2 | 42 | 20 | 0.04[f] | |
| Cefaclor[f] | | | 90 | 30[h] | 0.6 | 35[h] | | 0.25[f] | |

[Continued over]

*For footnotes, see final page of table (p.1664)*

**Appendix A.** *[Continued]*

| Drug | Nature[a] | pKa[b] | F[c] (%) | CL[c] (L/h) | $t_{1/2}$[c] (h) | Vd[c] (L) [per 70kg] | Protein binding[c] (%) | $f_{NR(n)}$[c,d] [$P_o$] | Notes |
|---|---|---|---|---|---|---|---|---|---|
| **Antibacterial drugs** *[continued]* | | | | | | | | | |
| Cefadroxil | | | | 12[h] | 1.5 | 28[h] | | 0.1 | |
| Cefalexin | A | 2.5/7.3 | 90 | 15 | 1 | 21 | 15 | 0.04 | |
| Cefaloridine | A | 3.4 | | 10 | 1 | 14 | 20 | | |
| Cefalothin[e] | A | 2.5 | | 20 | 0.5 | 14 | 70 | 0.04[e] | |
| Cefamandole | A | 3.0 | | 10 | 1 | 14 | 75 | 0.04 | |
| Cefanone | A | | | 3.5 | 2.5 | 14 | 88 | 0.05 | |
| Cefapirin[f] | A | 2.15 | | 25 | 0.7 | 49 | 45 | 0.4[f] | |
| Cefatrizine | A | | | | 1.4 | | 58 | 0.2 | |
| Cefazolin | A | 2.1 | | 3 | 2 | 9.1 | 85 | 0.06 | |
| Cefepime | | | | 8 | 2 | 14 | 16-19 | 0.2 | |
| Cefetamet pivoxil | | | 50 | 8.2 | 2.5 | 21 | 22 | | |
| Cefixime | | | 40 | 4.4 | 3.5 | 16.8 | 70 | 0.85 | |
| Cefmenoxime | | | | 14.4 | 1 | 28[g] | 77 | 0.15 | |
| Cefodizimee | | | 90-100* | 2.7 | 4.9 | 11.2 | 81 | 0.47 | * IM |
| Cefonicid | | | | 1.3 | 3.6 | 7.7[g] | 98 | 0.03 | |
| Cefoperazone | A | 2.55 | | 4.5 | 2 | 14 | 90 | 0.75 | |
| Ceforanide | | | 100* | 3 | 2.8 | 10.5 | 80 | 0.1 | * IM |
| Cefotaxime | A | 3.5 | 90-95* | 15 | 1.2 | 25.2 | 25-40 | 0.5 | * IM |
| Cefotiam | A | | | 20 | 1 | 21 | 40 | 0.35 | |
| Cefoxitin[e] | A | 2.2 | | 15 | 1 | 14 | 75 | 0.3[e] | |
| Cefpirome | | | | | 2 | | | 0.1 | |
| Cefpodoxime proxetil | | | 50 | 17.8 | 2.6 | 49 | 18-23 | 0.2 | |
| Cefprozil | | | 90 | | 1.3 | | 45 | | |
| Cefradine | Amp | 2.6/7.3 | >90 | 17 | 0.8 | 17.5 | 10 | 0.15 | |
| Cefsulodin | | | | 8.7 | 1.5 | 24.5 | 30 | 0.2 | |
| Ceftazidime | | | | 6.7 | 2.0 | 17.5 | ≈15 | 0.05 | |
| Ceftibuten | | | | | 2.5 | | | | |
| Ceftizoxime | | | | 8 | 1.7 | 21 | 30 | 0.05 | |

| | | | | | | | | |
|---|---|---|---|---|---|---|---|---|
| Ceftriaxone | A | 2.6/3.2 | | 0.5-1.2* | 7 | 7-14* | 83-96* | 0.5 | * Concentration-dependent due to saturable protein binding |
| Cefuroxime | A | ≈2.5 | | 8 | 1.3 | 17.5 | ≈40 | 0.07 | |
| Latamoxef (moxalactam)[e] | | | 70-100* | 6 | 2 | 21 | 50 | 0.05[e] | * IM |
| • *Fluoroquinolones* | | | | | | | | | |
| Ciprofloxacin | | | 69-85 | 30 | 5 | 210 | ≈30 | 0.3 | |
| Enoxacin | | | 80 | 20 | 6 | 175 | ≈35 | 0.4 | |
| Fleroxacin | | | 99 | 7.8 | 11 | 91[g] | 23-32 | 0.2 | |
| Lomefloxacin | | | | 20 | 7.5 | 147 | 10 | 0.25 | |
| Norfloxacin | | | 31-45 | | 4.8 | | 15 | 0.7 | |
| Ofloxacin | | | 100 | 16[h] | 7 | 210[h] | | 0.25 | |
| Pefloxacin | Amp | 6.3/7.6 | 90-100 | 8 | 12 | 133 | ≈25 | 0.9 | |
| • *Macrolides* | | | | | | | | | |
| Azithromycin | | | 37 | 5[h] | 10-57* | 1890 | 7-50* | | * Dose-dependent |
| Clarithromycin[e] | | | 55 | 52 | 3 | 245 | 40-70 | | |
| Erythromycin | B | 8.8 | 35 | 26 | 1.3-2.4* | 35-70* | 73 | 0.8 | * Dose-dependent |
| Midecamycin | | | | | 0.98 | 280 | 47 | 1.0 | |
| Roxithromycin | | | | | 11 | | | 0.7 | |
| • *Penicillins* | | | | | | | | | |
| Amoxicillin | A | 2.4/7.4/9.6 | 75 | 15 | 1 | 28 | 18 | 0.06 | |
| Ampicillin | A | 2.5/7.2 | | 13 | 1 | 21 | 18 | 0.1 | |
| Azlocillin | A | 2.8 | | 9* | 1* | 14 | ≈30 | 0.4 | * Dose-dependent |
| Bacampicillin, see ampicillin | | | | | | | | | |
| Benzylpenicillin (penicillin G) | A | 2.8 | | 30 | 0.7 | 28 | 65 | 0.08 | |
| Carbenicillin | A | 3.3 | | 8 | 1.2 | 14 | 50 | 0.02 | |
| Ciclacillin | | 2.68/7.5 | | | | | | | |
| Cloxacillin[e] | A | 2.7 | 43 | 12 | 0.5 | 7 | 95 | 0.25[e] | |
| Dicloxacillin | A | 2.7 | | 8 | 0.8 | 14 | 98 | 0.5 | |
| Flucloxacillin[e] | A | 2.7 | | 5 | 1.5 | 10.5 | 93 | 0.3[e] | |
| Mecillinam (amdinocillin)[f] | A | 3.4/8.9 | | 51* | 1.0* | ≈70* | ≈20 | 0.4[f] | * After oral dose of pivmecillinam |
| Methicillin | A | 3 | | 30 | 0.6 | 28 | 40 | | |
| Mezlocillin | A | 2.7 | | 12 | 1 | 17.5 | 35 | 0.4 | |

[Continued over]

*For footnotes, see final page of table (p.1664)*

**Appendix A.** *[Continued]*

| Drug | Nature[a] | pKa[b] | F[c] (%) | CL[c] (L/h) | $t_{1/2}$[c] (h) | Vd[c] (L) [per 70kg] | Protein binding[c] (%) | $f_{NR(n)}$[c,d] [$P_o$] | Notes |
|---|---|---|---|---|---|---|---|---|---|
| **Antibacterial drugs** *[continued]* | | | | | | | | | |
| Nafcillin | A | 2.7 | 36 | 30 | 1 | 70 | 90 | | |
| Oxacillin | A | 2.84 | 33 | 27 | 0.6 | 28 | 94 | 0.6 | |
| Phenoxymethylpenicillin (penicillin V) | A | 2.73 | | | 0.5 | ≈35 | 80 | 0.6 | |
| Piperacillin | A | 4.0 | | 10 | 1 | 14 | 22 | >0.25 | |
| Pivmecillinam, see mecillinam | | | | | | | | | |
| Temocillin | | | | | 5 | | | 0.3 | |
| Ticarcillin | A | 2.5/3.42 | | 8.5 | 1.2 | 14 | 60 | 0.1 | |
| • *Sulfonamides* | | | | | | | | | |
| Sulfadiazine | Amp | 6.48/2.0 | 100 | 1.5 | 10 | 24.5 | 60 | 0.45 | |
| Sulfadimidine (sulfamethazine) | Amp | 7.38/2.36 | | 2[h]* | 6* | 14[h] | 80* | 0.2 | * Dose-dependent |
| Sulfafurazole (sulfisoxazole) | A | 5.0 | | 1.8 | 7.7 | 24.5[h] | 88 | 0.5 | |
| Sulfamethizole | Amp | 5.45/2.0 | | ≈7 | 1.5 | 24.5[h] | 90 | 0.5 | |
| Sulfamethoxazole | A | 5.6 | 100 | 1.57[h] | 10 | 14[h] | 68 | 0.8 | |
| Sulfamethoxydiazine | A | 7 | | | 36 | 17.5 | 87 | | |
| Sulfamethoxypyridazine | A | 6.7 | | | 40 | 14 | 65 | 0.5 | |
| Sulfapyridine | Amp | 8.43/2.58 | | | 5/15* | | | 0.95 | * Rapid/slow acetylators |
| Sulfasalazine | A | | | | 10* | <70 | >95 | 0.9 | * Probably represents the absorption half-life |
| Sulfathiazole | Amp | 7.12/2.36 | | | ≈3 | | | | |
| • *Tetracyclines* | | | | | | | | | |
| Chlortetracycline[f] | Amp | 3.3/7.4/9.3 | | | 6 | 84 | 55 | 0.8[f] | |
| Demeclocycline (demethylchlortetra-cycline) | Amp | 3.3/7.2/9.4 | | | 12 | 126 | ≈70 | | |
| Doxycycline | Amp | 3.4/7.7/9.7 | 93 | 1.7 | 16 | 49 | 90 | 0.7 | |
| Minocycline | Amp | 2.8/5.0/9.5/7.8 | 100 | 5 | 15 | 105 | 70 | 0.85 | |
| Oxytetracycline | Amp | 7.3/3.3/9.1 | | | 10 | ≈105 | ≈30 | 0.2 | |
| Rolitetracycline | A | 7.4 | | | 10 | 70 | ≈50 | 0.3 | |

| | | | | | | | | | |
|---|---|---|---|---|---|---|---|---|---|
| Tetracycline | Amp | 7.7/3.3/9.5 | 77 | 15[h] | 6 | 140[h] | | 0.12 | |
| • *Others* | | | | | | | | | |
| Aztreonam | | | | ≈6 | 1.5 | 14 | 56 | 0.3 | |
| Brodimoprim | | 7.15 | | | | | | | |
| Carumonam | | | | 6.6 | 1.4 | 12.6 | 20 | 0.2 | |
| Chloramphenicol | Alc | 5.5 | 76-93 | 12 | 4 | 56 | ≈60 | 0.95 | |
| Cilastatin* | | 2/4.4/9.2 | 0† | 14 | 0.9 | 17.5 | 35** | 0.2 | * See also imipenem<br>** *In vitro*<br>† IM: 100% |
| Cinoxacin | A | 4.7 | | 13 | 1.5 | 17.5 | 63 | 0.3 | |
| Clavulanic acid | | | | 13 | 1 | 14 | 27 | 0.55 | |
| Clindamycin[f] | B | 7.45 | 87 | 12 | 3 | 56 | 93 | 0.9[f] | |
| Imipenem* | | 3.2/9.9 | | 14 | 0.9 | 17.5 | 10-20** | 0.3 | * See also cilastatin (pharmacokinetics determined in combination with cilastatin)<br>** *In vitro* |
| Lincomycin[f] | B | 7.5 | | | 5 | 35 | 72 | 0.6[f] | |
| Loracarbef | | | | 15 | 1.1 | 23.8 | | 0.1 | |
| Nalidixic acid[e] | A | 6.7 | | ≈10[h] | ≈6 | ≈70[h] | 95 | 0.8[e] | |
| Nitrofurantoin[e] | A | 7.2 | 87 | 41 | 1 | 56 | ≈40 | 0.7[e] | |
| Spectinomycin | B | 7.0/8.7 | | 6 | 2 | 14 | low | 0.08 | |
| Sulbactam | | | | 17 | 1 | 17.5 | | 0.9 | |
| Teicoplanin | | | | 1.1 | 50 | 77 | 90 | 0.35 | |
| Tetroxoprim | B | 8.25 | | 5 | 7 | 56 | ≈15 | 0.45 | |
| Thiamphenicol | | 7.2 | | | ≈2 | | <10 | 0.1 | |
| Trimethoprim | B | 7.2 | 100 | 4.5[h] | 11 | 91[h] | 45 | 0.45 | |
| Vancomycin | B | | | 4.0 | 10 | 42[g] | <10-55* | 0.03 | * Largely deviating values reported by different investigators |
| **Anticholinergics** | | | | | | | | | |
| Atropine | B | 9.25 | | 70 | 2.2 | 231 | 50 | 0.45 | |
| Propantheline[f] | $B_4$ | | | 79 | 1.8 | | | 0.85[f] | |
| Scopolamine (hyoscine) | B | 7.55 | 23 | 45 | 2.5 | 140 | | 0.45 | |
| Scopolamine *N*-butylbromide | $B_4$ | | | | 14 | | 11* | | * Albumin |

[Continued over]

For footnotes, see final page of table (p.1664)

**Appendix A.** *[Continued]*

| Drug | Nature[a] | pKa[b] | F[c] (%) | CL[c] (L/h) | $t_{½}$[c] (h) | Vd[c] (L) [per 70kg] | Protein binding[c] (%) | $f_{NR(n)}$[c,d] [$P_o$] | Notes |
|---|---|---|---|---|---|---|---|---|---|
| **Anticoagulants** (see also antiplatelet agents) | | | | | | | | | |
| Acenocoumarol (nicoumalone) | A | 5.05 | | 1.4/15*<br>2.5** | 10/3*<br>10** | 14/21*[g]<br>35** | 98.5 | 1.0 | *R(+)/S(−) enantiomers<br>** Racemate (after oral administration) |
| Dicoumarol (bishydroxycoumarin) | A | 4.4/8.0 | | | ≈70 | ≈10.5 | >99 | 1.0 | |
| Enoxaparin sodium | | | 91 | 1.24 | 4.2* | 7 | | | * Anti-factor Xa activity (antithrombin activity, 2.1h) |
| Ethylbiscoumacetate | A | 3.1/7.5 | | | 2 | 7 | 90 | | |
| Heparin | A | | 0 | 2.5* | 1.5* | 4.9 | 95** | 0.8 | * Dose- and assay-dependent<br>** Lipoproteins |
| Nadroparin calcium | | | 98† | 1.2 | 3.5(2.6)* | 350(3.5)* | | | * Subcutaneous (intravenous) administration<br>† After subcutaneous administration |
| Phenprocoumon | A | 4.2 | | 0.07[h] | 110 | 11.2[h] | 99 | | |
| Warfarin[e] | A | 5.0 | 100 | 0.2/0.15*[h] | 35/50* | 10.5[h] | 99 | 1.0[e] | *S(−)/R(+) enantiomers |
| **Antidepressants** | | | | | | | | | |
| Ademetionine (S-adenosyl-L-methionine) | | | 93* | | 1.5 | 28 | <5 | | * IM (very low after oral administration) |
| Amitriptyline[e] | B | 9.4 | 48 | 51 | 19 | 1085[g] | 95 | 1.0[e] | |
| Citalopram | | | | 21 | 33 | 980 | 50 | 0.9 | |
| Clomipramine[e] | B | | | 45 | 20 | 1162 | 98 | 1.0[e] | |
| Desipramine[e] | B | 10.2 | 51 | 130[h] | 22 | 1568[h] | 80 | 1.0[e] | |
| Dothiepin | | | 30 | 146 | 25 | 4900 | | | |
| Doxepin[e] | B | 8 | 27 | 65* | 17 | 1400* | | 1.0[e] | * After oral administration (assuming calculated bioavailability of 27%) |
| Fluoxetine | | | | 40(10) | 48(96) | 1400(2940) | 94 | 0.97 | Single (multiple) doses |
| Fluvoxamine | | | 77 | | 20 | 1400 | | 0.95 | |
| Imipramine[e] | B | 9.5 | 27 | 58 | 18 | 1470 | 89 | 1.0[e] | |
| Lofepramine[e] | | | <10 | 686[h] | 2.2 | | >99 | 1.0 | Active metabolite is desipramine |
| Maprotiline[e] | B | 10.5 | 68 | 63.5 | 40 | 3640 | 88 | 1.0[e] | |
| Mianserin[e] | | 7.1 | 63 | 19 | 33 | 441 | 95 | 0.95[e] | |
| Moclobemide | | | 55 | 58 | 1.7 | 84 | 50 | 1.0 | |
| Nortriptyline[e] | B | 9.73 | 51 | 40 | 28 | 1470 | 93 | 1.0[e] | |

| | | | | | | | | | |
|---|---|---|---|---|---|---|---|---|---|
| Paroxetine | | | 50 | | 24 | | 95 | 0.98 | |
| Sertraline | | | | | 26 | >1400 | 99 | 1.0 | |
| Trazodone | | | | | 8 | - | 93 | 1.0 | |
| Trimipramine[f] | B | | 41 | 67 | 23 | 2170 | 95 | 1.0[f] | |
| **Antidiabetic drugs** | | | | | | | | | |
| Acetohexamide[e] | | | | | 1.5/6* | 14[h] | ≈75 | 0.6[e] | * Parent drug/active metabolite |
| Chlorpropamide[e] | A | 4.8 | >90 | 0.13[h] | 40 | ≈10.5[h] | 90 | 0.2[e] | |
| Epalrestat | | | | | 1 | | | | |
| Glibenclamide (glyburide)[e] | | 5.3 | | 5.5 | 1.5-10* | 10.5 | >99 | 1.0[e] | * Largely deviating values reported by different investigators |
| Glibornuride[f] | A | | | | 8 | 17.5[h] | 95 | 1.0[f] | |
| Gliclazide | A | 5.8 | | 0.8 | 12 | 21 | 90 | 1.0 | |
| Glipizide[f] | A | | | ≈2.5[h] | 5 | 14[h] | >98 | 1.0[f] | |
| Insulin | Pep | | | 10-40* | 0.25-2* | | ≈5 | 0.4 | * Largely deviating values reported by different investigators |
| Metformin | | | 50 | 26-42* | 1.5-4.5*† | 70-280* | <5 | 0.01 | * Largely deviating values reported by different investigators<br>† Terminal elimination phase $t_{1/2}$ ≈10h |
| Phenformin | B | 3.1/11.8 | | 45[h] | 5 | 350[h] | ≈20 | 0.3 | |
| Tolazamide | A | 3.5/5.7 | | | 7 | | 94 | | |
| Tolbutamide | A | 5.43 | | ≈1[h] | 7 | 10.5[h] | 95* | | * Concentration-dependent |
| **Antidiarrhoeals** | | | | | | | | | |
| Diphenoxylate | B | 7.07 | | | 2.5 | 322 | | | |
| Loperamide[f] | B | 8.7 | | | 10 | | 97 | 1.0[f] | |
| **Antiemetics** | | | | | | | | | |
| Granisetron | | | | 14.7 | 11 | 231 | | 0.9 | Wide interindividual differences |
| Metoclopramide | | | 85 | 38/23* | 4/7* | 210 | 30 | 0.7 | * Possibly dose-dependent |
| Ondansetron | | | 60 | 29 | 3 | 161 | 70-76 | | |
| Tropisetron | | | 52-66** | 60/12* | 8/35 | 546 | 59-71** | 0.9 | * Two hydroxylation phenotypes.<br>** Dose-dependent |
| **Antiepileptic drugs** | | | | | | | | | |
| Carbamazepine[e] | Sa | | >70 | 1.1/4.5[h] | 36/16* | 84[h] | 75 | 1.0[e] | * Single dose/long term treatment |
| Clonazepam | Amp | 1.5/10.5 | 98 | ≈6[h] | 25 | 210[h] | 85 | 1.0 | |
| Ethosuximide[f] | A | 9.3 | | 0.7 | 54 | 49 | <10 | 0.8[f] | |

[Continued over]

*For footnotes, see final page of table (p.1664)*

**Appendix A.** *[Continued]*

| Drug | Nature[a] | pKa[b] | F[c] (%) | CL[c] (L/h) | $t_{½}$[c] (h) | Vd[c] (L) [per 70kg] | Protein binding[c] (%) | $f_{NR(n)}$[c,d] [$P_o$] | Notes |
|---|---|---|---|---|---|---|---|---|---|
| **Antiepileptic drugs** *[continued]* | | | | | | | | | |
| Gabapentin | | | 60 | 7.5 | 5-7 | 49 | 0 | | |
| Lamotrigine | | | 98 | 1.9 | 30 | 80.5 | 55 | 0.9 | |
| Oxcarbazepine[e] | | | | | 8* | 52.5* | 40* | 1.0 | * Data shown are for active metabolite (10, 11-dihydro-10-OH-carbamazepine) |
| Phenobarbital* | A | 7.2 | 100 | 0.3 | 100 | 49 | 50 | 0.7 | * Recommended therapeutic serum concentration 10-35 mg/L |
| Phenylethylmalonamide (PEMA) | | | 90 | 2 | 16 | 49 | low | | |
| Phenytoin* (diphenylhydantoin) | A | 8.33 | 98 | ** | ** | 56 | 90 | 1.0 | * Recommended therapeutic serum concentration 10-20 mg/L<br>** Dose-dependent: $V_{max}$ = 415 mg/day; Km = 5.7 mg/L |
| Primidone[e] | A | | 86-96 | 2[h] | 10* | 42[h] | 20 | 0.6 | * $t_{½}$ of metabolites (phenylethylmalonamide and phenobarbital) is longer (see above) |
| Valproic acid (sodium valproate)[e*] | A | 4.95 | 100 | 0.5 | 13 | 10.5 | 90 | | * Recommended therapeutic serum concentration 50-100 mg/L |
| Vigabatrin | | | | 5.6 | 7 | 56 | <1 | 0 | |
| Zonisamide | | | | 1.24 | 75 | 105 | 49 | | |
| **Antifungal agents** | | | | | | | | | |
| Amphotericin B[f] | Amp | 5.5/10.0 | | ≈1.8 | ≈360 | 280 | >90 | 0.95[f] | |
| Fluconazole | | | 90 | | 30 | 56 | 11 | 0.3 | |
| Flucytosine | | | 84 | 0.8 | 4.2 | 55.3 | low | 0.03 | |
| Griseofulvin | | | | | ≈22 | ≈105 | | 1.0 | |
| Itraconazole | | | 40 | | 30* | | >99 | | * At steady-state |
| Ketoconazole | | 2.9/6.5 | | | 8 | | 99 | 1.0 | |
| Miconazole[f] | | 6.65 | 27 | 46 | 23 | 1400 | 99 | 1.0[f] | |
| **Antihistamines** ($H_1$-receptor antagonists) | | | | | | | | | |
| Acrivastine | | | 18 | 18.2 | 2.1 | 52.5 | 50 | | |
| Astemizole[e] | | | | | ≈20 | ≈17,500 | 97 | 1.0[e] | Pharmacologically active metabolite has a longer $t_{½}$ (240h) |
| Azelastine | | | >80 | | 25/35* | | 83 | | * At steady-state |
| Cetirizine | | | | 3 | 7-10 | 35 | 93 | 0.4 | |

| | | | | | | | | | |
|---|---|---|---|---|---|---|---|---|---|
| Chlorpheniramine[e] (chlorphenamine) | B | 9.2 | | 7.2 | 20 | 238 | 72 | 0.8[e] | |
| Diphenhydramine[f] | B | 8.3 | 42 | 47 | 5 | 280 | 98.5 | 0.9[f] | |
| Diphenylpyraline[f] | B | 9.1 | | | 32 | | | 0.9[f] | |
| Ketotifen[e] | | | 50 | | 22 | | 75 | 1.0[e] | |
| Loratadine[e] | | | | 720 | 14.4* | | 98 | | * After multiple doses |
| Mebhydrolin | | 6.7 | | | 4 | | 4 | | |
| Oxatomide | | | | | 14 | | 91 | 1.0 | |
| Promethazine | B | 9.1 | 25 | 68 | 12 | 910[g] | | | |
| Terfenadine[e] | | | | | 20 | | 97 | 1.0[e] | |
| **Antihypertensive drugs** (see also ACE inhibitors, β-adrenoceptor antagonists, calcium antagonists and diuretics) | | | | | | | | | |
| Cadralazine[e] | | 6 | | 10.9[h] | 1 | 46.9 | 70-80 | 0.2[e] | |
| Clonidine[f] | B | 8.25 | 90 | 0.16-0.6* | 6.2-12.8* | 241.5 | 20 | 0.4[f] | * Dose-dependent |
| Debrisoquine* | | | | | 3.2 | | | | * Two hydroxylation phenotypes |
| Diazoxide[f] | A | 8.74 | 86-96 | | 36 | 15.4 | 91 | 0.8[f] | |
| Doxazosin | | | 65 | 7.3 | 15.6* | 98 | >98 | 1.0 | * At steady-state |
| Guanabenz | | | | | 13 | 7350-13,370* | 90 | 0.95 | * Dose-dependent |
| Guanethidine[e] | B | 9.0/12.0 | 20 | | ≈150 | | | 0.5[e] | |
| Guanfacine | | | | 11-22 | 12-23 | 455 | 64 | 0.75 | |
| Hydralazine[e] | B | 7.1 | 16/35[†] | 200* | 2.5 | 350 | 89 | 0.85[e] | * Two acetylation phenotypes<br>† Rapid/slow acetylators |
| Indoramin | B | 7.8 | | 66 | 5-15* | 518 | 90 | 0.95 | * Interindividual variability |
| Ketanserin[f] | | | 50 | 25 | 13 | 434 | 94 | 0.95[f] | |
| Methyldopa[e] (α-methyldopa) | Aac | 2.2/9.2/ 10.6/12 | 25 | ≈24 | ≈1.3 | ≈42 | <15 | 0.4[e] | |
| Minoxidil[e] | B | 4.6 | 95 | 35 | 3.5 | 210[h] | 0 | 0.9[e] | |
| Moxonidine | | | 88 | 43-69 | 3 | 210 | 7 | 0.4 | |
| Pinacidil[e] | | | | 37[h] | 2.6 | 98 | 40-60 | 0.95[e] | |
| Prazosin | B | 6.5 | 57 | 10 | 3 | 35 | 94 | 1.0 | |
| Reserpine[f] | B | 6.6 | 50 | 15 | 60-270* | | 96 | 1.0[f] | * Largely deviating values reported by different investigators |
| Sodium nitroprusside | | | 0 | | very short* | | | | * At therapeutic doses not detectable in plasma. Toxic metabolites |
| Terazosin | | | 82 | 3.3 | 12 | 21 | 90 | 0.9 | |

[Continued over]

For footnotes, see final page of table (p.1664)

**Appendix A.** *[Continued]*

| Drug | Nature[a] | pKa[b] | F[c] (%) | CL[c] (L/h) | $t_{1/2}$[c] (h) | Vd[c] (L) [per 70kg] | Protein binding[c] (%) | $f_{NR(n)}$[c,d] [$P_o$] | Notes |
|---|---|---|---|---|---|---|---|---|---|
| **Antihypertensive drugs** *[continued]* | | | | | | | | | |
| Urapidil | | 7.1 | 78 | 12 | 2.7 | 42 | 80 | 0.8 | |
| **Antimalarial drugs** | | | | | | | | | |
| Chloroquine[e] | B | 8.4/10.8 | 100 | 65[h] | 1220 | 57,400[h] | 55 | 0.3[e] | |
| Dapsone[f] | A | 1.2 | | 3* | 30 | 105* | 73 | 0.9[f] | * Two acetylation phenotypes |
| Halofantrine[e] | | | | 40 | 102 | 5110 | | | |
| Mefloquine[f] | | | | 1.8[h] | 530 | 1330[h] | 98.3 | 0.9[f] | |
| Mepacrine (quinacrine) | B | 7.7/10.3 | | | 120 | | 90 | | |
| Primaquine[e] | | | 74-100 | 27[h] | 5.5 | 231 | | >0.95[e] | |
| Pyrimethamine[f] | B | 7.2 | | 1.7[h] | 82 | 203 | 87 | 1.0[f] | |
| Quinine | B | 4.3/8.4 | | 5.5 | 14 | 112 | 90 | 0.8 | |
| Sulfadoxine | | | | | 200 | | | | |
| **Antineoplastic and immunosuppressive drugs** | | | | | | | | | |
| Aminoglutethimide | | | | 3.5/4.5[h]* | 15/11* | 70 | 24 | | * Single dose/long term treatment |
| Azathioprine[e] | | | 60 | | 0.2* | | | 1.0[e] | * Active metabolite (mercaptopurine) has a $t_{1/2}$ ≈0.7h |
| Bleomycin[f] | Pep | | | 5.2 | 3 | 24.5 | | 0.45[f] | |
| Busulfan[f] | | | | | 2.5 | | | 1.0[f] | |
| Carboplatin | | | | 4.5 | 3 | 18.2 | >15(85)* | | * Dose/time-dependent |
| Carmustine (BCNU) | | | | 235 | 0.3* | 231 | | | * Highly reactive intermediates |
| Chlorambucil[f] | Amp | 5.8/8.0 | | | 1.5 | | | 1.0[f] | |
| Cisplatin (*cis*-platinum) | | | | 0.3 | 40-240* | | ≈90 | | * Total platinum: largely deviating values reported by different investigators |
| Cladribine | | | 55 | 60 | 6.7 | 644 | | | |
| Cyclophosphamide[e] | B | | 74-97* | 4.4 | 7 | 49 | 13 | 0.5[e] | * Dose-dependent |
| Cyclosporin (cyclosporin A) | | | 34 | 17* | 10* | 245* | 98 | 1.0 | * Determined from concentration in blood |
| Cytarabine (cytosine arabinoside)[f] | B | 4.3 | <20 | 55 | 2.3 | 175 | 13 | 0.9[f] | |
| Dacarbazine | | 4.42 | | 12 | 0.7 | 44.1 | | 0.3 | |
| Dactinomycin (actinomycin D) | Pep | | | | 36 | | | | |

| | | | | | | | | | |
|---|---|---|---|---|---|---|---|---|---|
| Daunorubicin[e] | Gly | 9.45 | | | 27 | 1610 | | 0.9[e] | |
| Diaziquone | | | | 22[h] | 0.5 | 8.4[g] | 79 | | |
| Doxorubicin (Adriamycin)[e] | B | 8.34 | | | ≈30 | ≈3010 | 71 | 0.6[e] | |
| Edatrexate | | | | 25 | 0.8 | | | | |
| Epirubicin | | | | 89 | 39 | 3500 | | ≈1.0 | |
| Etoposide (VP 16-213) | | | 50 | 2.3 | 5.6 | 16.1 | 94 | 0.9 | |
| Fludarabine | | | 70 | 7-15.5 | 6.9-12.4 | 77-161 | | | |
| Fluorouracil[e] (5-fluorouracil) | B | 8.1 | 28* | 63 | 0.25 | 17.5 | | 1.0[e] | * Wide range (0-78%) |
| Flutamide[e] | | | | | 6.6-22* | | | | * Dose-dependent |
| Formestane | | | 20-25* | | 120-240 | | 84 | | * IM |
| Idarubicin | | | 30 | 51-207 | 6-35 | 3220 | 96 | | |
| Ifosfamide | | | 100 | 3.6 | 6.5 | 33.6 | | | |
| Melphalan[e] | B | | 78 | 31 | 1.5 | 35 | 55 | 0.9[e] | |
| Methotrexate[e] | A | 4.3/5.5 | 65 | 12 | 10 | | 95 | 0.06[e] | |
| Mitoxantrone | | | | 45 | 57 | 1960 | 78 | 0.95 | |
| Nilutamide[e] | | | | | 58 | | | | |
| Paclitaxel | | | | ≈20 | ≈8 | ≈140 | 90 | | |
| Pentostatin | | 5.2 | | 3.5 | 3-9 | 39.9 | <5 | | |
| Tacrolimus (FK 506) | | | 5-67* | 143 | 8.7 | 1295 | 88 | 1.0 | * Dose-dependent |
| Tamoxifen[e] | | | | | ≈91 | | >99 | | |
| Teniposide (VM 26) | | | | | 19 | | >90 | | |
| Vinblastine[f] | B | 5.4/7.4 | | 52 | 25 | 1890 | 75 | 0.95[f] | |
| Vincristine[f] | | 5/7.4 | | 7.7 | 85 | 588 | 75 | 0.95[f] | |
| Vindesine | | | | 17.5 | 24 | 616 | | | |
| **Anti-Parkinsonian drugs** | | | | | | | | | |
| Amantadine[f] | B | 10.1 | | 16.5[h] | 15 | 560[h]* | | 0.1[f] | * Possibly dose-dependent |
| Bromocriptine[f] | Pep | 4.9 | 6 | 56 | 3 | ≈238 | 90 | 1.0[f] | |
| Levodopa[e] | Aac | 2.3/8.7 | | | 1.4 | | | 1.0[e] | |
| Lisuride[f] | | | 10-15 | 48 | 2.2 | 140 | 70 | 1.0[f] | |
| Orphenadrine | B | 8.4 | | | 18 | | 20 | | |
| Pergolide | | | | | 27 | | 90 | | |
| Selegiline | | | | | | 301 | 94 | | |

[Continued over]

For footnotes, see final page of table (p.1664)

**Appendix A.** *[Continued]*

| Drug | Nature[a] | pKa[b] | F[c] (%) | CL[c] (L/h) | $t_{½}$[c] (h) | Vd[c] (L) [per 70kg] | Protein binding[c] (%) | $f_{NR(n)}$[c,d] [$P_o$] | Notes |
|---|---|---|---|---|---|---|---|---|---|
| **Antiplatelet agents** | | | | | | | | | |
| Indobufen | | | | 1.3 | 7* | 14 | >99 | 0.9 | * 13h in elderly |
| Ticlopidine | | | | | 96* | | 98 | | * At steady-state |
| **Antipsychotic drugs** | | | | | | | | | |
| Bromperidol | | 8.6 | 50 | | 24 | | 90* | | * *In vitro* |
| Chlorpromazine[e] | B | 9.3 | 32* | 38** | 30 | 1470** | 98 | 1.0[e] | * After oral administration<br>** After IM administration |
| Clozapine | | | 50 | 45.6[h] | 16 | | 95 | | |
| Haloperidol | B | 8.3 | 65 | 46 | 20 | 1400 | 90 | 1.0 | |
| Haloperidol decanoate | | | | | 500* | | | | * After IM injection (depot preparation of haloperidol) |
| Lithium* | | | >85 | 1.6 | 27 | 56 | | 1.02 | * Therapeutic serum concentration 0.4-1.2 mmol/L |
| Perphenazine | B | 3.7/7.8 | | 107 | ≈21 | | | | |
| Pimozide | B | 7.32 | | | 50 | | 99 | | |
| Prochlorperazine | B | 3.73/8.1 | | | ≈23 | | | | |
| Risperidone[e] | | | | | 3* | 105 | 90 | | * $t_{½}$ of pharmacologically active metabolite (9-OH-risperidone) is 24h |
| Tiapride | | | 75 | | 3-5 | 100.1 | <4 | 0.25 | |
| Thioridazine[e] | | | | | ≈20 | | 99* | 1.0[e] | * Concentration-dependent |
| Zuclopenthixol [cis(Z)-clopenthixol] | | | 50* | | 20 | | | | * IM |
| **Antithyroid and thyroid drugs** | | | | | | | | | |
| Carbimazole, see thiamazole | | | | | | | | | |
| Liothyronine (tri-iodothyronine) | | | | 1 | ≈48 | ≈35 | >99 | | |
| Propylthiouracil | A | 7.8 | | 7 | 1.5 | ≈28 | 80 | 0.9 | |
| Thiamazole (methimazole) | | | | 10[h] | 4 | ≈42 | Low | 0.9 | |
| Thyroxine | | | | 0.1 | 150 | ≈14 | >99 | | |

| | | | | | | | | | |
|---|---|---|---|---|---|---|---|---|---|
| **Antitrichomonal drugs** | | | | | | | | | |
| Metronidazole[e] | B? | 2.62 | 100* | 3 | 8 | 49 | <20 | 0.85[e] | * Rectal: 70% |
| Ornidazole[e] | | 2.6 | | | 14 | 63[h] | <15 | 0.95[e] | |
| Tinidazole | | | >90 | 3 | 13 | 45.5 | 12 | 0.75 | |
| **Antituberculosis drugs** | | | | | | | | | |
| *p*-Aminosalicylic acid (para-aminosalicylic acid; PAS) | A | 3.25 | | | ≈1 | ≈14 | ≈15 | 0.9 | |
| Ethambutol[f] | B | 6.9/9.5 | 73 | 30 | 4* | 175 | 6.30 | 0.2[f] | * Terminal elimination phase $t_{½}$ ≈15h |
| Ethionamide[f] | B | | | | 2 | | ≈30 | 1.0[f] | |
| Isoniazid | B | 2.0/3.85 | | ≈20/10* | 1.2/3* | 42 | low | 0.6 | * Rapid/slow acetylators |
| Pyrazinamide | | | | | 10 | | 50 | | |
| Rifampicin (rifampin)[e] | Amp | 1.7/7.9 | | 10[h] | 4* | 70[h] | 80 | 0.85[e] | * Dose- and time-dependent |
| Streptomycin | | | | | 3 | ≈21 | ≈50 | 0.04 | |
| **Antiulcer drugs** | | | | | | | | | |
| Cimetidine | B | 6.8 | 70* | 36 | 2 | 91 | 20 | 0.3 | * IM: >90% |
| Enprostil | | | | | 34 | | | | |
| Famotidine | | | 37-43 | 25 | 3 | 84[g] | 16 | 0.2 | |
| Lansoprazole | | | | | 2 | | | 1.0 | |
| Misoprostol[e] | | | | | 1.5* | | 85 | | * Active metabolite. Parent drug undetectable in plasma after oral dose |
| Nizatidine | | | 98 | 47 | 1.4 | 91 | 30 | 0.4 | |
| Omeprazole | Amp | 3.97/8.8 | 67 | 35 | 0.5 | 24.5 | 95 | 1.0 | |
| Pirenzepine | | | 26 | 15 | 11 | | 12 | 0.50 | |
| Ranitidine[e] | B | 2.7 | 50 | 35 | 2 | 105 | 15 | 0.3[e] | |
| Roxatidine[e] | | | | 25* | 6* | 1190* | 6 | 0.4 | * Data shown are for active metabolite (parent drug not detected) |
| **Antiviral drugs** | | | | | | | | | |
| Aciclovir | B | 2.27 | 15-30 | 12 | 3 | 49 | 15 | 0.1 | |
| Didanosine[e] | | | 40 | 48 | 0.6-1.4* | 70 | <5 | 0.5 | * Pharmacologically active metabolite has longer $t_{½}$ (12h) |
| Foscarnet | | 7.27/3.41/ 0.4 | | 12.8 | 88 | 357[g] | | 0.1 | |
| Ganciclovir | | | 6 | 12 | 2-4 | 39.2 | 2 | 0 | |

[Continued over]

For footnotes, see final page of table (p.1664)

**Appendix A.** *[Continued]*

| Drug | Nature[a] | pKa[b] | F[c] (%) | CL[c] (L/h) | $t_{1/2}$[c] (h) | Vd[c] (L) [per 70kg] | Protein binding[c] (%) | $f_{NR(n)}$[c,d] [$P_o$] | Notes |
|---|---|---|---|---|---|---|---|---|---|
| **Antiviral drugs** *[continued]* | | | | | | | | | |
| Vidarabine (adenine arabinoside)[e] | | | | | ≈3.5 | | | 0.98[e] | |
| Zalcitabine | | | 88 | 13.6 | 1.2 | 37.8 | <4 | 0.25 | |
| Zidovudine | | | 64 | 100* | 1-2 | 98-147 | 7-38 | 0.85 | * High interpatient variability |
| **Bronchodilators** | | | | | | | | | |
| Enprofylline | | | | 15 | 1.8 | 35 | | 0.1 | |
| Ipratropium bromide | B | | | | ≈3.5 | | | 0.3 | |
| Isoprenaline (isoproterenol) | B | 8.6 | | | ≈2 | | 65 | | |
| Salbutamol (albuterol) | B | 9.3. 10.3 | | | ≈5 | | | | |
| Terbutaline | Amp | 10.1/11.2/ 8.8 | | 13 | 15 | 112[g] | 25 | 0.45 | |
| Theophylline[e]* | Amp | 8.6/3.5 | 96 | 3 | 8 | 35 | 50 | 0.9[e] | * Recommended therapeutic serum concentration 10-20 mg/L |
| **Calcium antagonists** | | | | | | | | | |
| Amlodipine | | 8.6 | 60 | 21.5 | 38 | 1470 | 95 | 0.9 | |
| Diltiazem | | 7.7 | 41 | 60 | 5.1 | 315 | 98 | 1.0 | |
| Felodipine | | | 16 | 69 | 11.4 | 679 | 99 | 1.0 | |
| Isradipine | | | 16 | 40 | 8.8 | 203[g] | 97 | 1.0 | |
| Nicardipine | | | 15-45* | 42 | 1 | 52.5 | >98 | 1.0 | * Dose-dependent |
| Nifedipine | | | 50 | 42 | 1.8 | 98 | 97 | 1.0 | |
| Nimodipine | | | | 60 | 1.7 | 63 | 98 | 1.0 | |
| Nisoldipine | | | 8 | 50 | 11.3 | 245 | 99 | 1.0 | |
| Nitrendipine | | | 30 | 80 | 6.3 | 378 | >99 | 1.0 | |
| Verapamil[e] | B | 8.75 | 25 | 52* | 4.8* | 308 | 90 | 1.0[e] | * Nonlinear kinetics after multiple oral doses; racemate (enantiomers have different pharmacokinetic properties) |
| **Cardiac glycosides** | | | | | | | | | |
| β-Acetyldigoxin | Gly | | | | 46 | | 15 | 0.3 | |
| Deslanoside | Gly | | | | ≈36 | | 25 | | |

| | | | | | | | | | |
|---|---|---|---|---|---|---|---|---|---|
| Digitoxin[e] * | Gly | | >90 | 0.2 | 134 | 31.5 | >90 | 0.7[e] | * Recommended therapeutic serum concentration 15-25 µg/L |
| Digoxin* | Gly | | 70 | 4.5 | 40 | 420 | 27 | 0.3 | * Recommended therapeutic serum concentration 0.8-2 µg/L |
| Lanatoside C[e] | Gly | | | | 40* | 280 | 20 | 0.3[e] | * Active metabolite (digoxin) |
| Meproscillarin[f] | Gly | | | | 46 | | 96 | 0.8[f] | |
| Metildigoxin (β-methyldigoxin) | Gly | | | | 62 | | 10 | 0.35 | |
| Ouabain (strophanthin G)[e] | Gly | | | | 21 | | 42 | 0.25[e] | |
| Proscillaridin | Gly | | | | 40 | | | 1.0 | |
| **Corticosteroids** | | | | | | | | | |
| Beclomethasone dipropionate | S | | 60-90 | | 15 | | | | |
| Betamethasone | S | | 72 | 11 | 6.5 | 126 | 6.4 | 0.95 | |
| Budesonide | S | | 10† | 84* | 2.7* | 308* | 88* | | * Racemate<br>† High first-pass metabolism |
| Cortisone | S | | | | 1.5 | | | | |
| Dexamethasone | S | | 80 | 14.7 | 3 | 52.5 | 77 | 1.0 | |
| Fludrocortisone | | | | | 0.5 | | 75 | | |
| Flunisolide | S | | | | 1.8 | 126 | | 0.95 | |
| Hydrocortisone | S | | | 21-30* | 1.3-1.9* | 21-35* | 75-95* | | * Dose-dependent |
| Methylprednisolone | S | 4.6 | 82 | 15 | 3 | 49 | | 1.0 | |
| Prednisolone | | | 80 | 6.3-15* | 3.6 | 28-91* | 65-91* | 1.0 | * Concentration-dependent |
| Prednisone (see prednisolone) | | | 78 | | | | | | |
| Triamcinolone | S | | | 45-70* | 1.4 | 98-147* | | 1.0 | * Dose-dependent |
| **Diuretics** | | | | | | | | | |
| Acetazolamide | A | 7.2 | | ≈2,7 | ≈1.7 | | 95 | 0.2 | * Dose-dependent |
| Amiloride[f] | B | 8.7 | 50 | ≈31[h] | ≈9.6 | ≈350[h] | | 0.25[f] | |
| Bendroflumethiazide[f] (bendrofluazide) | A | 8.5 | | 15 | 3.9 | 84 | 94 | 0.7[f] | |
| Bumetanide[f] | A | | 90 | 12 | 1.75 | 16.8 | 96 | 0.35[f] | |
| Chlorothiazide | A | 6.7/9.5 | 100* | | ≈13 | | | | * Dose-dependent |
| Chlorthalidone[f] | | 9.4 | 65 | 6 | 47 | 294 | 76 | 0.5[f] | |
| Ethacrynic acid | A | 3.5 | | | ≈0.8 | | | | |
| Furosemide (frusemide) | A | 3.9 | 65 | 8 | 1 | 21 | 97 | 0.35 | |

[Continued over]

For footnotes, see final page of table (p.1664)

**Appendix A.** *[Continued]*

| Drug | Nature[a] | pKa[b] | F[c] (%) | CL[c] (L/h) | $t_{1/2}$[c] (h) | Vd[c] (L) [per 70kg] | Protein binding[c] (%) | $f_{NR(n)}$[c,d] [$P_o$] | Notes |
|---|---|---|---|---|---|---|---|---|---|
| **Diuretics** *[continued]* | | | | | | | | | |
| Hydrochlorothiazide | A | 7.0/9.2 | 66-75 | 22 | 10 | 210 | 40 | 0.05 | |
| Hydroflumethiazide | A | 8.9/10.7 | 50 | | ≈10* | | 95 | | * Calculated from urine data |
| Indapamide[e] | A | 8.3 | | 1.3[h] | 17 | | 77 | 0.95[e] | |
| Metolazone | A | 9.7 | | 6.6 | 20 | 112 | 95 | 0.2 | |
| Piretanide | A | | 57-80 | 12 | 1.4 | 21 | >90 | 0.55 | |
| Polythiazide | A | | | | 26 | | 84 | 0.75 | |
| Spironolactone[e] | S | | 70 | | 19* | | 98* | 1.0[e] | * Active metabolite (canrenone) |
| Torasemide | | 6.44 | 76-92 | 2.5 | 3.3 | 11.2 | 98 | 0.7 | |
| Triamterene | B | 6.1 | 52 | 97[h] | ≈3 | | 56 | 0.95 | |
| **Estrogens and progestagens** | | | | | | | | | |
| Ethinylestradiol | S | | 40 | 23 | 13 | 203 | 97 | | |
| Ethynodiol, see norethisterone | | | | | | | | | |
| Levonorgestrel | S | | 100 | 7.7 | 28 | 203 | 94 | | |
| Lynestrenol, see norethisterone | | | | | | | | | |
| Medroxyprogesterone[f] | S | | | ≈76* | ≈36 | ≈42* | 94 | 0.55[f] | * After oral and IM administration |
| Norethisterone (norethindrone) | S | | 64 | 27 | 10 | 280 | 80 | | |
| Norethynodrel, see norethisterone | | | | | | | | | |
| **Gout drugs** | | | | | | | | | |
| Allopurinol[e] | B | 9.4 | 90 | 46 | 0.83* | ≈42 | 0.45 | 0.85[e] | * Active metabolite (oxypurinol) $t_{1/2}$ ≈40h |
| Colchicine[f] | B | 1.65 | | 36 | ≈1 | 49 | 31 | 1.0[f] | |
| Probenecid[e] | A | 3.4 | 100 | 1.4 | 6-12* | 11.2 | 89 | 0.9[e] | * Dose-dependent |
| Sulfinpyrazone[e] | A | 2.8 | | 1.4 | 3 | 4.2 | 98 | 0.55[e] | |
| **Hypoglycaemic drugs** (see antidiabetic drugs) | | | | | | | | | |
| **Inotropic agents** (see also cardiac glycosides) | | | | | | | | | |
| Amrinone | | | 93 | 1.4[h] | 5 | 7[h] | | | |

| | | | | | | | | | |
|---|---|---|---|---|---|---|---|---|---|
| Dobutamine | B | 9.45 | | 244 | 0.04 | 14 | | | |
| Dopamine | | | | 234-330* | 0.12 | | | | * Dose-dependent |
| Dopexamine | | | | 151 | 0.12 | | | | |
| Enoximone | | | 53-60 | 50 | 7 | 413 | 80 | 1.0 | |
| Ibopamine[e] | | | | | 0.016 (1.5-3.1*) | | | | * Pharmacologically active metabolite (epinine) |
| Milrinone | | | 85-92 | 10 | 2.2 | 28 | | 0.15 | |
| Prenalterol | | | 50 | 48 | 2.4 | 168 | low | 0.4 | |
| **Lipid-lowering drugs** | | | | | | | | | |
| Bezafibrate | A | | | 8[h] | 1.7 | 19.6[h] | 95 | 0.15 | |
| Clofibrate | A | 2.95 | | 0.4 | 15/54* | 8.4 | 97** | 0.8 | * After single/multiple doses<br>** Concentration-dependent |
| Fenofibrate[e] | | | | 1.9* | 22* | 62.3* | >99* | | * Values are for the active metabolite fenfibric acid |
| Gemfibrozil[e] | | | | | 7.6 | | 97 | 1.0[e] | |
| Lovastatin[e] | | | <5 | | | | >95 | | |
| Nicotinic acid (niacin) | A | 4.8 | | | 0.75 | | | 0.1 | |
| Pravastatin | | | 17 | 57 | 1.95 | 32.2[g] | 55 | 0.5 | |
| Probucol | | | | | 1100 | | | | |
| Simvastatin[e] | | | <5 | | 2 | | >95 | 1.0[e] | |
| **Muscle relaxants, skeletal** | | | | | | | | | |
| Alcuronium chloride | | | | 5 | 3 | 24.5 | | 0.2 | |
| Atracurium besilate[e] | | | | 28 | 0.3* | 11.9 | 82 | 1.0* | * Pharmacologically active metabolites |
| Doxacurium chloride | | | | 9.4 | 1.5 | 14.7 | 32 | | |
| Mivacurium chloride | | | | 300* | 0.03* | 14* | | | * Data are for 2 most active isomers |
| Pancuronium bromide[e] | | | | 7 | 1.5 | 16.1 | | <0.4[e] | |
| Tubocurarine (*d*-tubocurarine) | $B_4$ | 8.1/9.1 | | 6.2 | 3.8 | 24.5 | 56 | 0.4 | |
| Vecuronium bromide[e] | | | | 12 | 1.5 | 14[g] | | ≈0.8[e] | |
| **Miscellaneous drugs** | | | | | | | | | |
| Acetylcysteine (*N*-acetylcysteine) | | | 9 | 58*/8** | 2*/5.5** | 42*/35**[g] | | 0.7* | * Reduced acetylcysteine<br>** Total acetylcysteine |
| Acitretin | | | 60 | 6.8-16 | 51* | 245 | >99 | 1.0 | * After multiple doses, small amounts of etretinate ($t_{½}$ 120 days) detected in blood of some patients treated with acitretin |
| Alfuzosin | | 8.13 | 64 | 25 | 4.8* | 175 | 90 | 0.9 | * Large interindividual variation ($t_{½}$ 1-27h) |

[Continued over]

*For footnotes, see final page of table (p.1664)*

**Appendix A.** *[Continued]*

| Drug | Nature[a] | pKa[b] | F[c] (%) | CL[c] (L/h) | $t_{1/2}$[c] (h) | Vd[c] (L) [per 70kg] | Protein binding[c] (%) | $f_{NR(n)}$[c,d] [$P_o$] | Notes |
|---|---|---|---|---|---|---|---|---|---|
| **Miscellaneous drugs** *[continued]* | | | | | | | | | |
| Alglucerase | | | | 27-106 | 0.05-0.18 | 3.5-19.6 | | | Great interindividual variability |
| Aminocaproic acid | Amp | 4.43/10.75 | | 11.4 | 4.9 | 28 | | 0.3 | |
| Amphetamine[e] | B | 9.9 | | | 5-21* | | | 0.5[e] | * Urinary pH dependent |
| Anistreplase (APSAC) | | | | | 1.5* | | | | * Determined from fibrinolytic activity |
| Auranofin | | | 24 | | 400/600* | | 60 | | * Single/multiple doses |
| Aurothioglucose | | | | | 600* | | 90 | | * After multiple doses |
| Aurothiomalate sodium (gold sodium thiomalate) | | | | | ≈550 | | ≈95 | | |
| Baclofen[f] | A | 3.9/9.6 | | | 3.5 | | 30 | 0.15[f] | |
| Buflomedil | | | 50-80 | 27 | 3 | 91 | 70 | 0.8 | |
| Buserelin | | | 3 | | 1.6 | | 15 | | |
| Caffeine | | | | 9[h] | 4 | 49 | 35 | >0.95 | |
| Cisapride | | | 40-50 | | 10 | 168 | 98 | 1.0 | |
| Clodronate disodium | | | | 6 | 2* | | | ≈0.1 | * Slow elimination phase with $t_{1/2}$ 13h |
| Dantrolene[e] | A | 7.5 | | | ≈9 | | | 0.95[e] | |
| Deferoxamine | | | | | 6 | | | | |
| Defibrotide | | | 3-13 | | 0.3 | 3.5 | | | |
| Diethylcarbamazine | | | | 12[h] | 12 | 175[h] | | 0.15 | |
| Disulfiram | | | | 55[h] | 7.3 | 574[h] | | | |
| Doxapram | | | | 25 | 7 | 245 | | | |
| Epoetin (erythropoietin) | Pep | | 21.5 | 0.18*† | 8*† | 2.1*† | | 0.9 | * In dialysis patients<br>† After IV dose |
| Ergoloid mesylates (codergocrine mesylate) | | | | | 1.5-4.1 | | | | |
| Ergotamine | B | 6.4 | 2/46* | 45 | 1.9 | 126 | | 0.5 | * Oral/IM |
| Ethanol | Alc | | | * | * | 35 | | >0.95 | * Dose-dependent ($V_{max}$ = 120 mg/kg/h; Km ≈50 mg/L) |
| Etretinate | | | 40 | | ≈5* | 140 | 98 | 1.0 | * Terminal elimination half-life 2880h (120 days) |
| Finasteride | | | 80 | | 8.4 | 77 | 90 | 1.0 | |
| Flumazenil | | | 16 | 60 | 0.9 | 73.5[g] | 45 | 1.0 | |

| | | | | | | | | | |
|---|---|---|---|---|---|---|---|---|---|
| Flunarizine | | | | | 430 | 3010 | 90 | | |
| Gallium nitrate | | | | 2.8 | 25(-196) | 88.9 | | | |
| Goserelin | | | | 8.2* | 4-5* | 14 | | | * After subcutaneous administration |
| Granulocyte colony-stimulating factor (rG-CSF) | | | | | 5* | | | | * Dose-dependent |
| Granulocyte macrophage colony-stimulating factor (rGM-CSF) | | | | 6 | 1.5 | | | | |
| Iloprost | | | <20 | 67 | 0.6 | 49 | | 1.0 | |
| Inosine pranobex | | | | | 0.8 | | | | |
| Interferon-α | | | >80* | ≈10 | ≈5 | ≈70 | | | * IM, SC |
| Interferon-γ1b | | | | | 0.6 | | | | |
| Interleukin-2 | | | | 3-11 | 1.5-12 | 441-553 | | | Great interassay (30)% and inter/intrapatient variability |
| Isotretinoin[e] (13-*cis*-retinoic acid) | | | 21 | 21[h] | 20 | | 99.9 | 1.0[e] | |
| Ivermectin | | | 60 | 1.2 | 28 | 46.9 | 93 | | |
| Levamisole | B | 8.0 | | 18.6 | 4.3 | 98 | | | |
| Levocarnitine (L-carnitine) | | | | | 2-15 | 18.2 | | | |
| Leuprorelin | Pep | | | 8.3 | 2.9 | 35 | | | |
| Mebendazole[f] | | | 17 | | ≈1 | ≈140 | ≈90 | 0.95[f] | |
| Mesalazine | | | | 17 | 1.5 | 42 | 43 | 0.8 | |
| Mesna | | | 63 | 74 | 1.2 | 49 | | 0.7 | |
| Methylphenidate | | | 25/5* | 28/51.1* | 5.6/3.7* | 185.5/126*[g] | | | **D*/*R* enantiomer |
| Midodrine[e] | | | 90 | 102* | 3 (0.5)* | 294* | | 0.95 | * Active metabolite (parent drug) [metabolite is deglymidodrine] |
| Mifepristone | | | 69 | 3[h] | 16 | 25.9[g] | 98 | | |
| Nafarelin | | | | | 2-3 | | 80 | | |
| Nedocromil | | | 3 | 4.2 | 0.9 | | 80 | | |
| Neostigmine[f] | | | | 28 | 1.3 | 49 | | 0.45[f] | |
| Octreotide | Pep | | <5 | 11.4 | 1.5 | 23.8 | - | 0.9 | |
| Olsalazine | | | | | 1 | | | | |
| Pamidronate disodium | | | | | 27 | | | | |
| Papaverine | B | 5.93 | | ≈50 | ≈1.6 | ≈105 | | | |
| Penicillamine (D-penicillamine) | B | 1.8/10.5 | | 60[h] | 2.5 | | | 0.85 | |

[Continued over]

*For footnotes, see final page of table (p.1664)*

**Appendix A.** *[Continued]*

| Drug | Nature[a] | pKa[b] | F[c] (%) | CL[c] (L/h) | $t_{½}$[c] (h) | Vd[c] (L) [per 70kg] | Protein binding[c] (%) | $f_{NR(n)}$[c,d] [$P_o$] | Notes |
|---|---|---|---|---|---|---|---|---|---|
| **Miscellaneous drugs** *[continued]* | | | | | | | | | |
| Pentamidine | | | | | >7 | 210 | | 0.95 | |
| Pentoxifylline (oxpentifylline)[e] | | 9.2 | 30 | | 1* | 168 | | 1.0 | * Active metabolite |
| Phenylephrine | Amp | 9.8/18.77 | 38 | 126 | 2.5 | 343[g] | | 0.85 | |
| Piracetam | | | 100 | | 5.5 | | | 0.02 | |
| Praziquantel[f] | | | 80 | | ≈1.5 | | | 1.0[f] | |
| Pyridostigmine[f] | | | 14 | 30 | 2 | 70[g] | | 0.25[f] | |
| Sodium cromoglycate | A | 2.0 | | | 0.1 | | 7.0 | 0.6 | |
| Sumatriptan | | | 14/96* | 72 | 2 | 168 | 14-21 | 0.8 | * Oral/SC |
| Tranexamic acid | A | 4.3/10.6 | 34 | 6.7 | 10 | | | 0.03 | |
| Ursodeoxycholic acid | A | ≈6.0 | | | ≈100 | | | | |

a A = acid; Aac = amino acid; Alc = alcohol; Amp = ampholyte; B = base; $B_4$ = base with quaternary ammonium group; Gly = glycoside; Pep = peptide; S = steroid; Sa = substituted amide.

b The pH at which the drug is 50% ionised. For clinical application of this value see chapter 1 (sect. 1.1).

c 'Representative' values found in human pharmacokinetic studies. Note that the interindividual variability of pharmacokinetic parameters in patients is usually very large; for example, the typical range for the total clearance of various drugs is 4- to 5-fold (see introduction for further information and references).

F = bioavailability (oral, unless stated otherwise). ***NB.*** Oral bioavailability values are largely dependent on the galenic formulation. Values after intramuscular (IM) administration are indicated separately.

CL = total clearance, calculated either by the dose divided by the total area under the serum or plasma concentration *versus* time curve *or* by the dose rate divided by the average steady-state concentration.

$t_{½}$ = half-life of the terminal elimination phase (unless stated otherwise).

Vd = apparent volume of distribution obtained by dividing the total clearance by the elimination rate constant associated with the terminal elimination phase.

d $f_{NR(n)}$ (also referred to as $P_o$ value) = *normal* nonrenal drug clearance fraction [ = nonrenal drug clearance divided by total (plasma) clearance in individuals with normal renal function (creatinine clearance = 100 ml/min), i.e. the fraction of the dose eliminated by nonrenal pathways in normal individuals]. See nomogram method of dose estimation in renal failure in appendix E for clinical application of this value.

***NB.*** $1 - f_{NR(n)}$ is an estimate of the fraction of the drug excreted unchanged in the urine in normal individuals.

e Pharmacologically active metabolite(s).

f Metabolite(s) with possible pharmacological activity.

g Apparent volume of distribution at steady-state.

h After oral administration.

Appendix B

# Guide to Clinically More Important Drug Interactions

*D.I. Quinn* and *R.O. Day*

The potential number of drug interactions increases with each release of a new drug onto the market. Each new agent has the theoretical potential to interact with all those that preceded it. The pharmacokinetic and pharmacodynamic mechanisms underlying adverse drug interactions are discussed in chapters 1 and 7 and from these discussions it will be apparent that many predicted reactions are not manifest as such in clinical practice. The reasons for this are more complex than the putative mechanisms of the interactions themselves, but involve such difficult to define variables as the patients' ability to absorb, metabolise and excrete drugs, and their ability to compensate for the adverse effects of drugs or drug interactions through homeostatic mechanisms.

When the pharmacokinetic or pharmacodynamic behaviour of one drug is altered by another, it will only become clinically apparent when such an alteration reaches a threshold where the changed efficacy or toxicity of the drug is significant. The extent to which a drug's pharmacokinetic and/or pharmacodynamic behaviour can vary before the threshold is reached and an adverse effect is seen varies with the therapeutic and toxic indices of the drug and with the competency of the individual's homeostatic mechanisms to compensate for the resultant changes. Thus, clinicians will only see the tip of the iceberg with drug interactions: although many drug combinations will produce alterations in measurable parameters (including plasma concentrations), they are not always of sufficient magnitude to be of clinical significance.

While clinicians generally view drug interactions for their potential to produce harm, not all interactions are harmful. The inhibition of cyclosporin metabolism by diltiazem and other calcium antagonists has been utilised in transplant recipients to reduce the amount of ingested cyclosporin required to produce immunosuppressive plasma concentrations and thereby significantly reduce the cost of therapy.[1] In addition, calcium antagonists provide a further advantage of diminishing the nephrotoxic effects of cyclosporin which can lead to hypertension and renal impairment in a proportion of transplant recipients.

Adverse drug interactions of most importance occur as the end result of either decreased drug activity with diminished efficacy, or increased drug activity with exaggerated or unusual effects. Nonsteroidal anti-inflammatory drugs (NSAIDs) diminish the efficacy of virtually all antihypertensive agents with resultant reduced control of blood pressure and increased antihypertensive dose requirements.[2,3] Erythromycin increases the plasma concentration of terfenadine to levels where terfenadine produces prolongation of the QT interval on the electrocardiogram and, in some patients, life-threatening ventricular arrhythmias, including torsades de pointes.[4] However, with the plasma concentrations of terfenadine usually seen in the absence of cytochrome P450 enzyme inhibition, abnormalities of cardiac rhythm and prolongation of the QT interval are rarely seen.

The table in this appendix must be used with discrimination and with a knowledge of the principles of clinical pharmacology (see chapter 1) and drug interactions (see chapter 7). Significant interactions do not occur in every patient given a combination listed, and in this regard the table is intended only as a guide to the more significant interactions likely to occur in clinical practice. Predicting significant drug interactions in individuals is difficult and this task is made more difficult by the plethora of new agents released onto the market each year.

Generally, where a serious drug interaction between two agents has been reported in the literature or has occurred in a particular patient, then one should be cautious about using agents from similar classes in combination. Knowledge of the mechanisms involved in interactions with earlier agents of a class of drugs can help predict whether such a reaction is likely to occur with newer members of that class. For example, cimetidine is a potent inhibitor of the cytochrome P450 hepatic microsomal enzyme system which is important in the metabolism of many drugs. This results in multiple drug interactions with altered pharmacokinetics and increased plasma concentrations of the metabolised drug when cimetidine is included in the regimen. The newer $H_2$-receptor antagonist ranitidine also inhibits the cytochrome P450 enzyme system but its potency in this respect is less than 10% of that of cimetidine. The difference is that while cimetidine produces many clinically important interactions, ranitidine produces virtually none related to its effects on hepatic metabolism.

Omeprazole, an acid pump inhibitor, also has the potential to inhibit some cytochrome P450 enzymes, but its effects on plasma concentrations of most drugs and, in the case of warfarin, on blood coagulability as measured by the international normalised ratio (INR) have been of marginal clinical significance. The result is that concurrent therapy with omeprazole may potentiate the effect of warfarin in some patients to a small degree but this is rarely significant in clinical practice, particularly with close monitoring of warfarin therapy by INR estimations.[5] All of these potential interactions must be taken into account when choosing between drugs for acid-peptic disease.

One approach to predicting whether new agents will produce altered function of hepatic microsomal enzymes is to evaluate the nature and intensity of the binding of these agents to the enzymes *in vitro*.[6] Where a previous agent in the class has produced a clinically significant alteration in the function of a cytochrome P450 subtype, the newer agent should be evaluated against this enzyme subtype for relative binding affinity and for reversibility of binding. The mere presence of an *in vitro* binding pattern similar to that of drugs known to have been involved in important interactions does not prove that an interaction will occur or is even likely to, but rather provides a preclinical indication that such interactions should be watched for and documented *in vivo*.

Some pharmacodynamic drug interactions may be predicted. Fluoxetine, a selective serotonin reuptake inhibitor, may induce a 'serotonergic syndrome' (consisting of cerebellar signs, myoclonus, hyperreflexia, confusion, hypomania, shivering, sweating, tachycardia and mild to moderate hypertension with nausea, diarrhoea and abdominal cramps) when given to patients receiving or who have previously received a nonselective monoamine oxidase (MAO) inhibitor.[7] This syndrome has also been described in patients in whom L-tryptophan or clomipramine were added to a nonselective MAO inhibitor. The theoretical cause of this syndrome is an excess serotonin effect, presumably because of potentiation of the actions of the respective drugs on serotonergic transmission. Increasing the postsynaptic serotonergic effect is thought to be important in the efficacy of these antidepressant drugs. However, the syndrome has also been described in some patients in whom fluoxetine has been combined with carbamazepine or lithium.[8,9] The implications of this in terms of the action of carbamazepine and lithium on serotonin and its receptors, and for the pharmacodynamic mechanism underlying the induction of the serotonergic syndrome are unclear, although at least part of the antidepressant effect of lithium may be mediated through serotonergic effects.

Thus, in clinical practice, one should be cautious when combining any of the selective serotonin reuptake inhibitors with tricyclic antidepressants, MAO inhibitors, lithium or carbamazepine until further information about this syndrome becomes available. This has particular relevance in situations where combinations of antidepressant drugs may be considered to augment antidepressant efficacy, e.g. in nonresponsive or only partially responsive cases.[10] Recent reports have described the serotonergic syndrome subsequent to combination of the selective MAO inhibitors selegiline and moclobemide with other proserotonergic drugs.[11] Death has been a not uncommon outcome of these interactions and this serves to emphasise the need for caution and vigilance when such combinations are considered and used.[12,13]

## 1. Which Drug Interactions Are of Most Importance?

Drug interactions are likely to be of major clinical importance where:

1) Commonly used drugs are involved. For example, digoxin, warfarin and antiepileptic drugs are commonly involved in interactions.

2) Common combinations of drugs, perhaps used to treat the same or often coexisting conditions, are involved. An example is the interaction between quinidine and digoxin where the plasma concentration of digoxin may be increased to toxic levels following the addition of quinidine.[14]

3) The interaction has serious or potentially fatal consequences. For example, when pethidine (meperidine) is administered to patients receiving nonselective MAO inhibitors, a rare but

dramatic reaction involving excitation, sweating, rigidity of muscles, marked fluctuations in blood pressure, coma and, on occasions, death, may occur.[15] Other interactions may have particular social and legal implications such as when patients on long term verapamil therapy assume they can consume a certain amount of alcohol and be within the legal limit to drive a motor vehicle but are in fact over that limit because of inhibition of the metabolism of alcohol by verapamil.[16]

The table is not intended as a comprehensive guide to potential drug interactions but rather lists those likely to be of major clinical importance. As such, it provides information on interactions that all clinicians should be aware of. Serious or life-threatening interactions should be committed to memory, particularly if they fall into areas commonly confronted in a particular clinician's practice.

It should also be noted that many major interactions can be avoided by close monitoring of therapy, reduction of drug dosage to a minimum effective level, planning the timing of administration of particular agents, or substituting an alternative agent.

## 2. What Factors Make Drug Interactions More Likely to Occur?

Factors that make drug interactions more likely include:

- The number of drugs taken by a patient
- The dosage administered
- The duration of therapy
- The patient's ability to metabolise and excrete drugs and their metabolites (i.e. hepatic and renal function plus genetic factors)
- The patient's ability to compensate for increased, decreased or altered drug activity (homeostasis)
- The patient's understanding and ability to act appropriately in the face of loss of therapeutic control or an adverse event.

Interactions that compromise therapeutic control are far more likely to be confronted by the clinician than interactions producing discrete adverse events. In this regard, oral anticoagulants, antiepileptic drugs, theophylline, digoxin, antihypertensives, methotrexate and cyclosporin are particularly susceptible to meaningful changes in therapeutic effect or toxicity due to the effect of other drugs on their activity. Certain drugs have a tendency to produce significant interactions by altering the absorption, metabolism, distribution and excretion of other concurrently administered drugs (see chapter 7).

## 3. Minimising the Occurrence of Drug Interactions

As discussed in chapter 7, an awareness of the more important interactions and knowledge of the mechanisms involved can help avoid, or at least minimise, adverse drug effects or ineffective therapy.

The following guidelines provide a framework for the avoidance or reduction of drug interactions:

1) Take a careful history from the patient, but when asking patients about drugs they may be taking remember to ask not only about prescription drugs but also over-the-counter medication, illicit drugs, and herbal, home or traditional remedies. It is also important to use terms that patients can readily understand, and in this regard it is often useful to identify the condition being treated with the medication, e.g. blood pressure tablets for antihypertensives, heart tablets for digoxin, and so on. Many valuable clues can be gleaned from a well taken history from patients or their carers, with special attention to the introduction or withdrawal of drug therapy in relation to important symptoms.

2) Avoid multiple drug therapy whenever possible, or at least limit the number of drugs prescribed for concurrent use by a patient, since the incidence of adverse drug reactions increases with the number of drugs prescribed. One way of doing this is set a limit on the period of use of prescribed drugs, particularly antibiotics.

3) If multiple drug therapy is required, avoid drugs that predictably cause clinically important interactions or make control of therapy difficult. Some drug combinations are best avoided, while with others, alternative therapy that can be more safely given may be substituted, e.g. with oral anticoagulants, substitute paracetamol (acetaminophen) for aspirin or NSAIDs, ranitidine for cimetidine, and a short-acting benzodiazepine for barbiturates used as hypnosedatives – or consider a course of cognitive or relaxation therapy as an alternative to drug therapy altogether. Drug combinations that can cause serious reactions should be avoided wherever possible (e.g. those with non-selective MAO inhibitors).

Other interactions where there may be potential for altered rates and degrees of absorption such as those with cholestyramine, iron and zinc supplements, antacids, tetracyclines or didanosine can be avoided by spacing doses of the drugs a number of hours apart. If fixed combinations of drugs are used, the composition of the product must be known and the possibility of an interaction with one of the components considered.

Always keep in mind genetic factors, associated diseases and organ dysfunction, particularly of the liver and kidneys, which may make an interaction more likely – for example, the interaction of phenytoin and isoniazid in patients who are slow acetylators of isoniazid (see chapter 1, sect. 5.2.1).

4) Changes of drug therapy should be kept to a minimum. If changes are necessary and involve known interacting drugs, some dosage alteration can be anticipated, but the time course and extent of the interaction varies with the drugs and the individual patient. Any dosage adjustment should be made only on the basis of results derived from close observation of therapy over a period of time after the change. This is particularly important with oral anticoagulants (see chapter 26) and antiepileptic drugs (see chapter 29).

5) Use special care with 'problem' drugs. The treatment of patients receiving agents such as oral anticoagulants, oral antidiabetic drugs, digoxin, cytotoxic drugs, cyclosporin, antiepileptic drugs, antihypertensives or drugs with CNS depressant or excitatory effects should be closely supervised because of the known risks of interactions leading to unwanted toxicity or interference with therapeutic control.

6) Educate and instruct the patient. Warn patients of the possible dangers that may arise if they change (stop taking or alter the dosage) or add to their intake of medication, whether prescribed, over-the-counter, herbal or illicit, without making their doctor aware. This applies particularly to patients being discharged from hospitals, as well as to outpatients receiving the 'problem' drugs listed above.

Specific patient instructions may be desirable in some cases, e.g. regarding the risks of combining nonselective MAO inhibitors with certain foodstuffs, common cold remedies, and pethidine (meperidine). Provision of written guidelines or consumer product information (which is becoming increasingly available around the world) may also help. Warnings against giving pethidine to patients receiving nonselective MAO inhibitors could also be inscribed onto a permanently worn bracelet, along with information on any allergies the patient may have. Another example of an interaction of a particular group of drugs with a foodstuff is the increased effect of dihydropyridine calcium antagonists seen when patients ingest grapefruit or its juice.[17]

Alcohol is often forgotten as a significant drug until it produces clinical dysfunction. Similarly, one should not forget the additive CNS depressant effects that often occur within the first few days of adding antianxiety or antidepressant drugs (see chapter 30) or the unpleasant disulfiram-like reaction that may result from the ingestion of alcohol with a number of drugs including metronidazole and certain cefalosporins (see table).

## 4. Steps in Researching a Possible Drug Interaction

Important steps in researching a possible drug interaction in a patient include:

1) Be suspicious when a change in clinical status or an unusual clinical syndrome follows a change in the therapeutic regimen.

2) Use the table as a starting point to define common clinically relevant drug interactions. In using the table, it is important to note that it does not attempt to represent all potential drug interactions. It is also important to note that interactions involving drugs or drug combinations that are not in common usage or interactions involving newer drugs may not be included.

3) If there is still significant suspicion of a drug interaction, more detailed references such as those cited below should be consulted (see 'Further Reading'). The next or concurrent step is to do a literature search through one of the on-line or volume subscribed databases such as 'Medline' or 'Reactions' CD-ROM which often yield up-to-date information.

## 5. Documenting and Reporting a Possible New Drug Interaction

There are a number of criteria for documenting a drug interaction. These include:

1) A temporal relationship between the *commencement* of a drug combination and alteration in therapeutic control or onset of a new symptom complex.

2) A temporal relationship between the *cessation* of a drug combination and the compensa-

tory change in therapeutic control or offset of a symptom complex.

3) Renewed alteration of therapeutic control or recurrence of a symptom complex on re-challenge with the drug combination. (NB. This is advisable or necessary only in rare situations where non-interacting alternatives are not available and the drug to be added is essential to the patient's well being).

4) A formal clinical study to establish the pharmacokinetic basis of the interaction in healthy controls and define the 'population at risk'.

Most countries have regulatory agencies to receive reports of possible adverse drug reactions and interactions (e.g. the Food and Drug Administration in the US, the Committee on Safety of Medicines in the UK, the Adverse Drug Reactions Advisory Committee in Australia, the Centre for Adverse Reactions Monitoring in New Zealand, and the Adverse Drug Reaction Monitoring Division of the Drugs Directorate of Health in Canada). Each of these agencies contributes to a World Health Organization (WHO) database which provides feedback to member countries. These systems are ideally accessible by clinicians. Most reports are of single patients with peculiar reactions but a collation of reports by the body concerned allows for early identification of new problems with particular drugs.

Clinicians, however, tend to be reluctant to report interactions or reactions that are well described, and this results in an underestimate of the incidence of reactions by the regulatory agencies. Similarly, many clinicians view a single case seen by them as inconsequential when in fact, the reporting of their experience into a system that allows correlation with others and feedback to the wider medical and paramedical community contributes greatly to our knowledge of and ability to prevent such reactions.

## 6. Use of the Table

The table has been arranged by pharmacological action or therapeutic use classification. The listings have been organised so that the effects of the interaction are described *under the drug for which a change in activity can lead to an increased risk of adverse effects or reduced efficacy.* For example, the effect of antacids in markedly decreasing the plasma concentrations of simultaneously administered tetracyclines is described under antibacterial agents (tetracyclines) and not under antacids. In this way, the clinician can become aware of the consequences of adding (or withdrawing) other drugs to the important primary agent. Cross references to all drugs involved are, however, provided in the main index of the book.

In many cases, potential interacting drugs can be given concurrently, provided the possibility of an interaction is kept in mind and appropriate modification of dosage or therapy is anticipated and instituted promptly. In some select cases, however, concurrent use of the interacting drugs should be avoided altogether.

### Acknowledgements

The authors would like to acknowledge the contributions of Drs Jane Adcock (Neurology), Gregory Dore (Infectious Diseases), Edgar Freed (Psychiatry), David Rees (Cardiology), and Ken Williams (Pharmacology) of St Vincent's Hospital for advice on the manuscript.

### Further Reading

Hansten PD, Horn JR. Drug interactions and updates, 8th ed. Vancouver: Applied Therapeutics, 1993

Jankel CA, Fitterman LK. Epidemiology of drug-drug interactions as a cause of hospital admissions. Drug Safety 1993; 9: 51-9

McInnes GT, Brodie MJ. Drug interactions that matter: a critical appraisal. Drugs 1988; 36: 83-110

Medline® CD ROM Database. National Library of Medicine. Peabody, MA: EBSCO Publishing, 1994

Reactions® Weekly and CD-ROM Database. Auckland: Adis International

### References

1. Wagner K, Phillip T, Heinemeyer HH, et al. Interaction of cyclosporin and calcium antagonists. Transplantation Proceedings 1989; 21: 1453-6
2. Sahloul MZ, al-Kiek R, Ivanovich P, et al. Nonsteroidal antiinflammatory drugs and antihypertensives. Nephron 1990; 56: 345-52
3. Johnson AG, Nguyen TV, Day RO. Do nonsteroidal anti-inflammatory drugs affect blood pressure? A meta-analysis. Annals of Internal Medicine 1994; 112: 289-300
4. Honig PK, Woolsley RL, Zamani K, et al. Changes in the pharmacokinetics and electrocardiographic pharmacodynamics of terfenadine with concomitant administration of erythromycin. Clinical Pharmacology and Therapeutics 1992; 52: 231-8
5. Creutzfeldt W. Risk-benefit assessment of omeprazole in the treatment of gastrointestinal disorders. Drug Safety 1994; 10: 66-82
6. Houston JB. Utility of in vitro drug metabolism data in predicting in vivo metabolic clearance. Biochemical Pharmacology 1994; 47: 1469-79
7. Sternbach H. The serotonin syndrome. American Journal of Psychiatry 1991; 148: 705-13
8. Dursun SM, Mathew VM, Reveley MA. Toxic serotonin syndrome after fluoxetine and carbamazepine [letter]. Lancet 1993; 342: 442

9. Muly EC, McDonald W, Steffens D, et al. Serotonin syndrome produced by a combination of fluoxetine and lithium. American Journal of Psychiatry 1993; 150: 1565
10. Price LH, Heninger MD. Lithium in the treatment of mood disorders. New England Journal of Medicine 1994; 331: 591-8
11. Livingston MG. Interactions with selective MAOIs. Lancet 1995; 345: 533-4
12. Neuvonen PJ, Pohjola-Sintonen S, Tacke U, et al. Five fatal cases of serotonin syndrome after moclobemide - citalopram and moclobemide - clomipramine overdoses. Lancet 1993; 342: 1419
13. Lefebvre H, Noblet C, Moore N, et al. Pseudophaeochromocytoma after multiple drug interactions involving the selective monoamine oxidase inhibitors selegiline. Clinical Endocrinology 1995; 42: 92-9
14. Angelin B, Arvidssen A, Dahlqvist R, et al. Quinidine reduced biliary clearance of digoxin in man. European Journal of Clinical Investigation 1987; 17: 262-5
15. Stack CG, Rogers P, Linter SPK. Monoamine oxidase inhibitors and anaesthesia: a review. British Journal of Anaesthesia 1988; 60: 222-7
16. Bauer LA, Schumock G, Horn J, et al. Verapamil inhibits ethanol elimination and prolongs the perception of intoxication. Clinical Pharmacology and Therapeutics 1992; 52: 6
17. Bailey DG, Spence JD, Munoz C, et al. Interaction of citrus juices with felodipine and nifedipine. Lancet 1991; 337: 357-62

**Appendix B.** Guide to clinically more important drug interactions (by drug class).

*NB.* Bold type in column two denotes interactions that: (1) involve commonly used drugs; (2) involve common drug combinations used to treat the same condition or conditions that often coexist; or (3) may have serious or potentially fatal consequences

| Primary drug | May interact with | **Potential result** (see introductory notes) | Implications for management and how to avoid |
|---|---|---|---|
| **Alcohol** (ethanol) | **Analgesics**<br>**Antianxiety drugs**<br>**Antidepressants**<br>**Antihistamines** (some compounds)<br>**Antipsychotics**<br>**Hypnosedatives**<br>Marijuana | Enhanced CNS depressant effects with acute alcohol ingestion | Instruct the patient. Warn about possible adverse effect on performance skills particularly related to driving motor vehicles or operating heavy machinery, especially within the first few days of new therapy. Among the antidepressants, some selective serotonin reuptake inhibitors do not significantly enhance the sedative effects of alcohol and may be the preferred drugs for patients who wish to take alcohol periodically.<br>**Note:** Caffeine or other stimulants do not reverse the adverse effects of alcohol or other CNS depressants on psychomotor function |
| | Cisapride<br>Metoclopramide | More rapid absorption of alcohol with a resultant early elevated peak in blood alcohol concentrations | Instruct the patient. Warn about possible adverse effects on performance skills and that general warnings regarding safe levels of alcohol ingestion prior to driving or coordination of crucial activities may not apply to them |
| | Biguanide oral antidiabetic drugs (e.g. metformin) | Risk of hyperlacticacidaemia | Instruct the patient to avoid excessive quantities (moderate to large) of alcohol and to be aware of and to report early symptoms of lactic acidosis (vomiting and malaise, abdominal pain, diarrhoea) |
| | Sulphonlyurea oral antidiabetic drugs (e.g. chlorpropamide, tolbutamide, etc.) | Disulfiram-like intolerance (facial flushing and headache) of alcohol in some cases (particularly with chlorpropamide). Hypoglycaemic activity may be increased with acute alcohol ingestion if food intake is restricted (e.g. malnutrition, prolonged fasting) | Instruct the patient about possibility of intolerance of alcohol and to avoid moderate to large quantities of alcohol. Intolerance of small quantities of alcohol is more likely with chlorpropamide. Educate patient to maintain adequate nutrition |
| | **Nonselective monoamine oxidase inhibitors** (e.g. phenelzine, isocarboxazid, tranylcypromine) | Enhanced CNS depressant effects with acute alcohol ingestion. Hypertensive crises with high tyramine content wines (e.g. Chianti, Alicante type) and some beers and cheeses | Advisable to avoid all alcoholic beverages since tyramine content not likely to be known to patient, but generally, spirits and white wines are safer than red wines, liqueurs and beers for patients who cannot or do not wish to abstain from alcohol |
| | Some cefalosporins (e.g. latamoxef, cefamandole, cefoperazone, cefotetan)*<br>Ketoconazole<br>Metronidazole<br>Nifuratel<br>Procarbazine | Disulfiram-like intolerance of alcohol in some cases | Instruct the patient about possibility of reaction and to avoid excessive alcohol consumption.<br>* The 3-methythiotetrazole side chain in the cefem nucleus is thought to confer disulfiram-like activity |
| | Verapamil | Modest increase in blood alcohol concentrations for a given quantity of acute alcohol ingestion in patients on long term verapamil therapy | Instruct the patient. Warn about possible adverse effects on performance skills and that general warnings regarding safe levels of alcohol ingestion prior to driving or coordination of crucial activities may not apply to them |
| **Anaesthetics, general** (see also chapter 12) | | | |
| Cyclopropane<br>Enflurane<br>Halothane<br>Isoflurane | Alfentanil<br>Fentanyl<br>Morphine<br>Sufentanil | Decreased mean alveolar concentrations of volatile anaesthetics with reduced effect | Titrate volatile anaesthetic dosage to desired level of anaesthesia |

[Continued over]

**Appendix B.** *[Continued]*

| Primary drug | May interact with | **Potential result** (see introductory notes) | Implications for management and how to avoid |
|---|---|---|---|
| **Anaesthetics, general** *[continued]* | | | |
| | β-Adrenoceptor antagonists (β-blockers)<br>Diltiazem<br>Verapamil | Negative inotropic effect and varying degrees of atrioventricular block reported | Avoid these combinations or monitor the patient closely if the combination is unavoidable |
| | Antihypertensive agents | Hypotension on induction of anaesthesia, especially in patients receiving ACE inhibitors, adrenergic neuron blocking drugs, and α-adrenoceptor blockers | Titrate concentrations of volatile anaesthetics to blood pressure in patients receiving antihypertensive drugs |
| | **Catecholamines** (e.g. adrenaline) | Anaesthetic sensitises myocardium to catecholamines with risk of severe ventricular arrhythmias | Avoid intravenous use of adrenaline. Dilute adrenaline solutions may be given intramuscularly or subcutaneously with appropriate precautions |
| Halothane<br>Sevoflurane<br>Trichloroethylene | Soda lime | Anaesthetic agent may be adsorbed or absorbed and neurotoxic products may be formed, particularly if soda lime is dry | Ensure adequate water content of soda lime, or avoid its use altogether |
| Ketamine | Diazepam<br>Hydroxyzine<br>Secobarbital (quinalbarbitone) | Prolonged recovery time (by around 30-40%) with use of these drugs as premedication | Be aware of extended recovery when used for short surgical procedures |
| | **Thyroid hormones** | Severe hypertension and tachycardia | Try to control with a β-blocker. Avoid this combination |
| Methoxyflurane | Tetracycline | Risk of renal failure increased | Avoid this combination. Substitute another antibacterial agent |
| Thiopental (thiopentone) | Atracurium<br>Ketamine<br>Pancuronium<br>Pethidine (meperidine)<br>Suxamethonium (succinylcholine) | Chemically incompatible (precipitate) | Mix in separate syringes |
| | Opioid analgesics | Increased respiratory depression and hypnotic effects | Use combination carefully, titrating dose to clinical effect |
| Trichloroethylene | Catecholamines | See above (as for cyclopropane, etc.) | See above |
| **Analgesics** (see also chapter 12) | | | |
| Aspirin and salicylates | **Alcohol** | Potentiation of aspirin-induced gastric mucosal damage and prolongation of bleeding time | Warn patients of the possible consequences of this combination (avoid long term use) |
| | Antacids | Therapeutic plasma salicylate concentrations not maintained in rheumatoid arthritis and rheumatic fever with concurrent use of aluminium and magnesium hydroxides, calcium carbonate, and sodium bicarbonate | Avoid this combination in treatment of rheumatoid arthritis and rheumatic fever. Alternatively, substitute another anti-inflammatory analgesic in rheumatoid arthritis patients if plasma salicylate concentration cannot be maintained in therapeutic range (150-300 mg/L) by adjusting aspirin dosage |
| | Corticosteroids | Reduced plasma salicylate concentrations (therapeutic concentrations may not be attained). Accumulation of salicylate with risk of toxicity when corticosteroid dosage reduced and dose of salicylate not altered | Monitor salicylate concentrations and adjust dose if necessary when adding or withdrawing corticosteroid |

| | | | |
|---|---|---|---|
| Alfentanil (see also opioids, below) | Erythromycin | Increased plasma concentrations and protracted clinical effects of alfentanil | Avoid this combination, if possible. Consider alternative antibiotics. Use naloxone to reverse the effects of alfentanil; review regularly to assess dose interval of naloxone |
| Fentanyl (see also opioids, below) | Carbamazepine | Decreased effect of fentanyl given during anaesthesia for craniotomy | Titrate dose of fentanyl to required anaesthetic effect |
| Methadone (see also opioids, below) | Carbamazepine<br>Phenytoin<br>**Rifampicin** (plus other enzyme-inducing agents) | Decreased plasma concentrations of methadone and symptoms of opioid withdrawal in those receiving the drug in maintenance programmes | Dosage of methadone in maintenance programmes will need to be increased if enzyme-inducing agents are given concurrently. On some occasions, a manifold increase in dosage will not produce significant plasma methadone concentrations. Consider use of an alternative antiepileptic drug such as valproic acid (no interaction reported) |
| | **Diazepam**<br>Erythromycin<br>Fluvoxamine | Increased plasma methadone concentrations with possible potentiation of opioid effects | Avoid these combinations if possible. Monitor for enhanced effects of methadone when adding erythromycin, diazepam or fluvoxamine, and opioid withdrawal symptoms when ceasing them |
| Opioids (strong analgesics) | **Alcohol**<br>**Butyrophenones**<br>**Hypnosedatives**<br>**Phenothiazines**<br>Thiopental | Enhanced CNS depressant effects | Instruct patient. Modify dosage of antipsychotic if necessary. Warn about possible effect on performance skills |
| | Cimetidine | Potential for increased plasma concentrations and duration of action of opioids | Avoid these combinations, if possible. Substitute ranitidine, famotidine or nizatidine for cimetidine.<br>Antagonise opioid effect with naloxone if necessary |
| | Hydroxyzine | Enhanced analgesia and sedation without additional respiratory depression | May be advantageous in the perioperative period |
| | Tricyclic antidepressants (e.g. desipramine, amoxapine, amitriptyline) | Prolongation and potentiation of analgesic and respiratory depressant effect. Desipramine plasma concentrations may be increased | Use this combination with caution. Generally tricyclic antidepressants should be started at a low dosage and increased while monitoring for adverse effects (including sedation) |
| Paracetamol (acetaminophen) | **Alcohol** (chronic use)<br>Barbiturates<br>Isoniazid | Increase susceptibility to acute hepatic necrosis with large doses of paracetamol | Limit paracetamol ingestion to 4 g/day. If prolonged therapy with the combination is needed, check plasma paracetamol concentrations and liver enzymes regularly |
| Pethidine (meperidine) [see also opioids, above] | Barbiturates<br>Chlorpromazine<br>Phenytoin | Decreased plasma pethidine concentrations and relatively increased plasma norpethidine concentrations, with diminished analgesic effect and CNS hyperactivity and possible seizures | Avoid this combination, especially in patients with renal or liver disease. Consider alternative analgesic, e.g. morphine<br>**Note:** Enhanced CNS depressant effects may occur with phenobarbital doses over 120 mg/day |
| | **Nonselective monoamine oxidase inhibitors** (e.g. phenelzine, isocarboxazid, tranylcypromine)<br>**Selegiline** | Severe reactions with pethidine in some patients (see also under antidepressants and anti-Parkinsonian drugs) | Avoid pethidine. Substitute (with caution) another strong analgesic such as morphine |
| **Anthelmintic drugs** (see also chapter 22) | | | |
| Mebendazole | Carbamazepine<br>Phenytoin | Decreased plasma mebendazole concentrations | Little relevance when mebendazole is used to treat intestinal nematodes but may be important where there is tissue involvement; substitute another antiepileptic drug such as valproic acid |
| Praziquantel | Carbamazepine<br>Corticosteroids<br>Phenytoin | Decreased bioavailability of praziquantel by 75% with phenytoin, and more than 90% with carbamazepine | Either consider alternative antiepileptic therapy or increase dose of praziquantel with titration to response |

[Continued over]

**Appendix B.** *[Continued]*

| Primary drug | May interact with | **Potential result** (see introductory notes) | Implications for management and how to avoid |
| --- | --- | --- | --- |
| **Antianxiety drugs/hypnosedatives** (see also chapter 30) | | | |
| Alprazolam (see also benzodiazepines, below) | Dextropropoxyphene | Increased plasma concentrations of alprazolam with increased sedation | Avoid this combination |
| Barbiturates<br>Benzodiazepines<br>Chloral hydrate<br>Glutethimide | β-Adrenoceptor antagonists<br>**Alcohol** (acute ingestion)<br>**Analgesics, strong (opioids)**<br>**Antihistamines** (some)<br>**Antidepressants**<br>**Antipsychotics**<br>Erythromycin | Increased CNS depressant effects, either by central effect or inhibition of metabolism resulting in increased plasma concentrations of drug concerned | Instruct the patient. Warn about possible adverse effects on performance skills, especially with first few days of therapy, and to avoid excessive quantities of alcohol. Avoid use of chloral hydrate or glutethimide because of toxicity profiles.<br>Avoid use of barbiturates as occasional hypnotics. If a hypnotic is required, use short-acting agents (e.g. temazepam, oxazepam, or lorazepam) for short periods. Consider cognitive or relaxation therapies as alternatives to hypnosedatives and anxiolytics |
| Benzodiazepines | Fluoxetine | Increased plasma concentrations of diazepam, alprazolam and possibly midazolam (but not clonazepam) with increased CNS depressant effects | Benzodiazepines are often required to counteract the agitation seen with the commencement of fluoxetine therapy. Instruct the patient. Warn about possible adverse effects on performance skills, and monitor clinically for excess sedation and adjust benzodiazepine dose accordingly. Alternatively, use clonazepam |
| Diazepam (see also benzodiazepines, above) | β-Adrenoceptor antagonists<br>Omeprazole | Increased plasma concentrations of diazepam in some patients | Instruct the patient. Warn about possible adverse effects on performance skills, and monitor clinically for excess sedation and adjust diazepam dose accordingly |
| Midazolam (see also benzodiazepines, above) | **Cimetidine**<br>**Ranitidine**<br>**Diltiazem**<br>**Dipyridamole**<br>**Erythromycin**<br>**Fluoxetine** (possible)<br>**Verapamil**<br>**Ketoconazole**<br>**Itraconazole** | Increased plasma concentrations of midazolam with increased level and protracted length of sedation | Either avoid use of midazolam in patients on these drugs or use sparingly in small increments |
| **Antiarrhythmic drugs** (see also chapter 20) | | | |
| Adenosine | **β-Adrenoceptor antagonists**<br>**Digoxin**<br>**Diltiazem**<br>Dipyridamole<br>Disopyramide<br>Tacrine<br>**Verapamil** | Increased sensitivity of cardiovascular system to adenosine | Use incremental dose of adenosine until supraventricular tachycardia responds; smaller doses than usual may be needed |
| | Caffeine<br>Theophylline | Reduced sensitivity of cardiovascular system to adenosine | Use incremental dose of adenosine until supraventricular tachycardia responds; larger doses than usual may be needed |
| Amiodarone | **β-Adrenoceptor antagonists** | Addition of a β-blocker to amiodarone therapy may induce bradycardia, cardiac arrest or ventricular fibrillation after initial doses | Avoid this combination or commence β-blocker in hospital with cardiac monitoring |

| | | | |
|---|---|---|---|
| | Cimetidine | Increased plasma amiodarone concentrations with increased risk of toxicity | Avoid this combination; substitute ranitidine, famotidine or nizatidine for cimetidine |
| | **Diltiazem**<br>**Verapamil** | Bradycardia and decreased cardiac output | Monitor closely for signs of cardiotoxicity when these drugs are combined |
| | Halofantrine | Possible increased incidence of ventricular arrhythmias | Avoid this combination if possible |
| Disopyramide<br>Mexiletine | Barbiturates<br>Phenytoin<br>Rifampicin (and other enzyme-inducing agents) | Plasma concentrations of antiarrhythmic drugs decreased | Monitor plasma concentrations and patient's clinical status and adjust dosage accordingly |
| Flecainide | Amiodarone<br>Cimetidine<br>Fluoxetine | Increased plasma flecainide concentrations | Reduce the dose of flecainide by 50% when adding amiodarone and monitor plasma concentrations of both drugs.<br>Monitor plasma flecainide concentrations when fluoxetine is added.<br>Use ranitidine, famotidine or nizatidine instead of cimetidine |
| Lidocaine (lignocaine) | Cimetidine | Plasma concentrations of lidocaine increased | Reduce maintenance dose of lidocaine and monitor patient's clinical status or, alternatively, substitute ranitidine, famotidine or nizatidine |
| | Phenytoin | Decreased plasma lidocaine concentrations, while adding to myocardial depressant effects | Do not infuse phenytoin and lidocaine simultaneously. Watch for lidocaine toxicity in patients on long term phenytoin |
| | Propranolol<br>Other β-blockers | Plasma concentrations of lidocaine increased | Reduce lidocaine dosage and monitor patient's clinical status |
| Mexiletine<br>(see also above) | Quinidine<br>Theophylline | Increased plasma mexiletine concentrations in some patients | Avoid these combinations or monitor plasma mexiletine concentrations and ECG effects and adjust mexiletine dose accordingly |
| Procainamide | Amiodarone<br>Cimetidine<br>Ranitidine<br>Trimethoprim | Plasma concentrations of procainamide and N-acetylprocainamide increased | Monitor for signs of toxicity, especially in the elderly who have a decreased ability to excrete these drugs. Dosage modification may be necessary |
| Propafenone | **Cimetidine**<br>**Quinidine** | Increased plasma concentrations of propafenone with potential for ventricular arrhythmia | Avoid combination if possible, or monitor plasma propafenone concentrations and adjust dosage accordingly |
| | Rifampicin | Decreased plasma concentrations of propafenone with potential lack of efficacy | Avoid this combination if possible, or monitor plasma propafenone concentrations and adjust dosage accordingly |
| Quinidine | Acetazolamide<br>Antacids<br>Urinary alkalinisers | Increased plasma concentrations of quinidine with potential toxicity | Administer antacids and urinary alkalinisers cautiously. Monitor plasma quinidine concentrations if any evidence of toxicity is suspected |
| | Amiodarone | Marked increase in plasma quinidine concentrations (with case reports of torsades de pointes) | Avoid combination if possible; otherwise, measure quinidine plasma concentrations frequently after commencement of amiodarone and adjust doses of quinidine and amiodarone accordingly |
| | Cimetidine<br>Verapamil | Plasma concentrations of quinidine increased in some patients | Monitor for signs of quinidine toxicity if these drugs used concurrently. Consider substituting ranitidine, famotidine or nizatidine for cimetidine, or another antihypertensive for verapamil |
| | Kaolin-pectin | Decreased quinidine plasma concentrations | Separate administration of the two drugs and monitor plasma quinidine concentrations, with dosage adjustment accordingly |
| | Phenobarbital<br>Phenytoin<br>Rifampicin | Plasma concentrations of quinidine significantly decreased | Avoid use of barbiturates as occasional hypnotics; substitute a benzodiazepine. Monitor plasma concentrations of quinidine with use of phenytoin and phenobarbital as antiepileptics and rifampicin in antituberculosis regimens, and adjust dose accordingly |

*[Continued over]*

**Appendix B.** *[Continued]*

| Primary drug | May interact with | **Potential result** (see introductory notes) | Implications for management and how to avoid |
|---|---|---|---|
| **Antibacterial drugs** (see also chapter 31) | | | |
| Ampicillin/amoxicillin | **Allopurinol** | Incidence of ampicillin/amoxicillin-induced rash may be increased in patients receiving allopurinol | Avoid this combination |
| Aminoglycosides (amikacin, gentamicin, kanamycin, netilmicin, streptomycin, tobramycin) | **Amphotericin B**<br>**Cefalothin**<br>Cisplatin<br>Clindamycin<br>Methoxyflurane<br>**Vancomycin** | Increased risk of nephrotoxocity and, in the case of cisplatin and vancomycin, ototoxicity | Avoid combination if possible or monitor renal function closely in patients receiving these drugs concurrently or subsequent to one another |
| | Loop diuretics (bumetamide, ethacrynic acid, furosemide, piretanide) | Increased risk of ototoxicity when combined with loop diuretics in renal failure | If possible, avoid this combination; or reduce the aminoglycoside dosage to the minimum effective level (monitor by plasma assay), and regularly check renal function |
| | **Nonsteroidal anti-inflammatory drugs (NSAIDs)** | Increased plasma aminoglycoside concentrations with potential for toxicity, especially in the elderly | Avoid combination or monitor plasma aminoglycoside concentrations closely and adjust dose accordingly |
| | Penicillins | Most penicillins can inactivate aminoglycosides if mixed together | Do not mix together and hang in a slow intravenous infusion bottle. Administration of the drugs by slow intravenous push separated by a fluid flush does not result in inactivation |
| Cefalothin | **Amikacin**<br>**Gentamicin**<br>**Kanamycin**<br>**Streptomycin**<br>**Tobramycin**<br>**Ethacrynic acid** (large doses)<br>**Furosemide** (large doses) | Increased risk of nephrotoxicity, particularly in the elderly | If possible, avoid this combination, or reduce dosage of one or both agents and check renal function regularly |
| Clarithromycin | Rifabutin | Decreased plasma concentrations of clarithromycin | Keep rifabutin dosage below 300 mg/day (see also under rifabutin below) |
| Chloramphenicol<br>Doxycycline | Barbiturates<br>Carbamazepine<br>Phenytoin<br>Rifampicin | Plasma concentrations of chloramphenicol and doxycycline decreased to subtherapeutic levels with potential for compromised efficacy | Avoid this combination, if possible. Use an alternative antiepileptic drug such as valproic acid or monitor plasma concentrations of chloramphenicol or doxycycline, if possible, and adjust dose accordingly |
| Dapsone (see also entry below) | Rifampicin | Decreased plasma concentrations of dapsone with possible loss of efficacy | Either avoid combination or increase dose of dapsone and observe response of infection to therapy |
| Dapsone<br>Pyrimethamine<br>Trimethoprim | Didanosine (ddl) | Decreased dapsone, pyrimethamine and trimethoprim absorption | Avoid combination, if possible; otherwise give dapsone, pyrimethamine or trimethoprim at least 2 hours before didanosine |
| Fluoroquinolones | **Antacids**<br>Antineoplastics<br>Calcium salts<br>**Didanosine (ddl)**<br>**Ferrous sulfate**<br>Sucralfate<br>Zinc sulfate | Decreased plasma concentrations of fluoroquinolones due to decreased absorption | Avoid combination, if possible; otherwise give drugs as far apart as possible |

| | | | |
|---|---|---|---|
| Methenamine (hexamine) | Acetazolamide<br>Urinary alkalinisers | Loss of methenamine effect as urinary antiseptic | Avoid combination or use alternative urinary antiseptic or antibiotic |
| Rifabutin | Clarithromycin | Increased plasma concentrations of rifabutin with risk of uveitis | Avoid this combination if possible or keep rifabutin dosage below 300 mg/day and monitor patients for uveitis |
| Sulfonamides | *p*-Aminobenzoic acid | Decreased sulfonamide antibacterial efficacy | Avoid this combination |
| Tetracyclines | Antacids<br>Didanosine (ddl) | Plasma concentrations of tetracyclines markedly decreased by simultaneous administration of aluminium, sodium, calcium and magnesium-containing liquid antacids and by didanosine | Give drugs 1 to 2 hours apart, if possible |
| | Colloidal bismuth subcitrate (tripotassium dicitrato bismuthate) | Plasma concentrations of tetracyclines decreased | Uncertain whether dose or time-related absorption mechanism involved. Avoid this combination if possible |
| | Iron haematinics | Plasma concentrations of tetracyclines and absorption of iron markedly decreased | Give conventional iron tablets 3 hours after tetracyclines.<br>? May not be a problem with slow release iron preparations |
| | Zinc sulfate | Plasma concentrations of tetracyclines markedly decreased | Not a problem with doxycycline |
| **Anticholinergic drugs** | **Antidepressants**<br>Antihistamines<br>**Anti-Parkinsonian drugs** (anticholinergics)<br>**Antipsychotics**<br>Disopyramide<br>Marijuana | Anticholinergic side effects increased by nonselective monamine oxidase inhibitors, tricyclic antidepressants, some antihistamines (e.g. diphenhydramine, phenindamine, promethazine), anti-Parkinsonian drugs (e.g. orphenadrine, trihexphenidyl, procyclidine) and antipsychotics, particularly in the elderly | Modify dosage if necessary, particularly in the elderly. Watch for urinary retention, constipation, blurred vision, delirium and pyrexia |
| **Anticholinesterases** (e.g. pyridostigmine, neostigmine, ambenonium) | Anticholinergic drugs<br>Aminoglycosides<br>Quinidine | The therapeutic effects of anticholinesterases may be antagonised in patients being treated for myasthenia gravis | Use anticholinergic drugs, aminoglycosides and quinidine with caution in patients with myasthenia gravis being treated with anticholinesterase drugs.<br>**Note:** Anticholinergic drugs are used to diminish certain autonomic and peripheral cholinergic side effects from anticholinesterases in some patients with myasthenia gravis. When these agents are combined, careful clinical assessment and titration of the dosage of both drugs is required |
| **Anticoagulants** (see also chapter 26) | | | |
| ***1. Drugs which increase anticoagulant action***<br>(**Note:** increased anticoagulant action may be manifest by a relative increase in the international normalised ratio [INR] or by potentiation of bleeding by effects of other drugs on parts of the clotting mechanism not affected by warfarin) | | | |
| Coumarins (e.g. warfarin, dicoumarol, acenocoumarol, phenprocoumon, ethylbiscoumacetate) | Alcohol, acute | May markedly increase warfarin effect | Advise patients on warfarin not to binge drink.<br>See comments on chronic alcohol ingestion below |
| | Severe alcoholic liver disease | May be extremely sensitive to warfarin due to impaired clotting factor synthesis | Generally recognised as a contraindication to any form of anticoagulation due to the risk of variceal haemorrhage |
| | Allopurinol | Very variable increase in warfarin effect, ranging from nonsignificant to life-threatening increases in effect | Monitor INR closely after addition of allopurinol to a stable warfarin regimen |
| | **Amiodarone** | Marked potentiation of effect of warfarin | Reduce dose of warfarin. Monitor INR closely for several weeks after amiodarone started until control is re-established |
| | Anabolic steroids<br>**Danazol** | Marked potentiation of coumarin anticoagulants (warfarin, dicoumarol) | Modify dose of coumarin when adding danazol to a stable warfarin regimen.<br>? Avoid by use of non C-17 alkylated anabolic steroid such as nandrolone |

*[Continued over]*

**Appendix B.** *[Continued]*

| Primary drug | May interact with | **Potential result** (see introductory notes) | Implications for management and how to avoid |
|---|---|---|---|
| **Anticoagulants** *[continued]* | | | |
| Coumarins *[continued]* | Ancrod<br>Heparin | Marked potentiation of anticoagulant effect | Avoid use of full-dose anticoagulants affecting different parts of the clotting system together. When switching from one anticoagulant to another, monitor the effects of each closely and scale doses accordingly |
| | **Aspirin**<br>**Nonsteroidal anti-inflammatory drugs (NSAIDs)** | Increased risk of bleeding due to effect on platelet function and damaging action on gastric mucosa. No effect on degree of hypoprothrombinaemia with NSAIDs or at low doses of aspirin, although high doses of aspirin can produce hypoprothrombinaemia in their own right | Where possible, avoid this combination; substitute paracetamol. If aspirin or NSAIDs are essential, consider adding a cytoprotective agent such as misoprostol |
| | Azapropazone<br>Oxyphenbutazone<br>Phenylbutazone | Predictably and markedly potentiate effect of warfarin (by 50 to 75%) as well as other coumarins (phenprocoumon, dicoumarol) | Avoid this combination. Substitute another NSAID, e.g. indomethacin, ibuprofen or naproxen (do not affect warfarin kinetics or anticoagulant control but may still increase risk of bleeding due to antiplatelet aggregating activity or risk of gastrointestinal bleeding) |
| | Cefalosporins | Some cefalosporins (cefamandole, cefoperazone, cefotetan, latamoxef) markedly potentiate warfarin effect | Monitor INR closely where a cefalosporin is added to a stable warfarin regimen |
| | Chloramphenicol<br>Erythromycin<br>Nalidixic Acid | Potentiation of effect of warfarin | Monitor INR closely and adjust dosage of warfarin accordingly |
| | **Cimetidine** | Variable degrees of potentiation of warfarin effect, ranging from minimal to marked | Avoid this combination. Use ranitidine, famotidine or nizatidine instead |
| | Ciprofloxacin<br>Enoxacin<br>Norfloxacin | Potentiation of effect of warfarin | Monitor INR closely and adjust dosage of warfarin accordingly |
| | **Clofibrate**<br>**Gemfibrozil**<br>**Lovastatin** | Markedly potentiate effect of anticoagulant (warfarin, ethylbiscoumacetate) in many patients | Reduce dose of coumarin (e.g. by 25 or 30% with warfarin) when clofibrate or lovastatin added. Monitor INR daily for a few days. Consider simvastatin as an alternative lipid-lowering agent (no reported interaction) |
| | Cotrimoxazole (trimethoprim/ sulfamethoxazole)<br>Sulfinpyrazone<br>Other sulfonamides | Potentiation of effect of warfarin | Monitor INR closely and adjust dosage of warfarin accordingly |
| | **Dextropropoxyphene** + **paracetamol** | Potentiation of effect of warfarin | Avoid this combination. Substitute paracetamol alone |
| | Disulfiram | Potentiation of effect of warfarin | Monitor INR closely and adjust dosage of warfarin accordingly |
| | Fluoxetine<br>Fluvoxamine | Potentiation of effect of warfarin | Avoid this combination or monitor INR closely when adding these drugs to a stable warfarin regimen. Paroxetine appears to have less potential for interaction, although clinical experience is lacking |
| | Flutamide | Potentiation of effect of warfarin | Monitor INR closely and adjust dosage of warfarin accordingly |
| | Azole antifungals (ketoconazole, fluconazole, miconazole, itraconazole) | Potentiation of effect of warfarin in some patients | Anticipate need to adjust dosage of warfarin if azole antifungal therapy is commenced, ceased or dosage is altered. Monitor INR closely |

| | | | |
|---|---|---|---|
| | **Metronidazole** | Markedly potentiates effect of warfarin | Reduce dose of warfarin. Monitor INR for a few days or more, or substitute alternative antimicrobial agent |
| | Omeprazole | Potentiation of effect of warfarin in some patients | Monitor INR closely after commencing, ceasing or changing doses of omeprazole |
| | Proguanil | Potentiation of effect of warfarin | Monitor INR when proguanil is commenced or ceased |
| | Propafenone | Potentiation of effect of warfarin | Monitor INR when propafenone is commenced or ceased |
| | **Quinidine** | Markedly potentiates effect of warfarin in some patients | Avoid this combination. Substitute procainamide or sotalol |
| | **Tamoxifen** | Marked potentiation of warfarin effect in some patients | Monitor INR closely when tamoxifen is added to a stable warfarin regimen |
| | **Thyroid hormones** | Markedly potentiate effect of warfarin and dicoumarol in virtually all patients | Reduce dose of coumarin (e.g. by one-third with warfarin) when D-thyroxine added. Monitor INR daily for a few days or more |
| | Vitamin A and retinoids<br>Vitamin E (tocopherol) | Potentiation of effect of warfarin | Avoid these combinations |
| Indanediones (phenindione) | **Aspirin** | Increased risk of bleeding due to effect on platelet function and damaging action on gastric mucosa. No effect on degree of hypoprothrombinaemia at low doses of aspirin, although high doses can produce hypoprothrombinaemia in their own right | Where possible, avoid this combination. Substitute paracetamol. If aspirin is essential, consider adding a cytoprotective agent such as misoprostol |

***2. Drugs which decrease anticoagulant action***
(**Note:** manifest by a relative decrease in the international normalised ratio [INR])

| | | | |
|---|---|---|---|
| Coumarins<br>(e.g. warfarin, dicoumarol, acenocoumarol, phenprocoumon, ethylbiscoumacetate) | Alcohol, chronic | May result in decreased warfarin effect due to hepatic enzyme induction | Advise patients with significant alcohol intake to drink moderate amounts regularly rather than binging, and check INR regularly |
| | Aminoglutethimide<br>Mitotane | Marked decrease in effect of warfarin | Monitor INR closely and adjust dose of warfarin accordingly |
| | **Barbiturates**<br>**Phenobarbital**<br>**Primidone** | Marked decrease in effect of coumarins (warfarin, dicoumarol, acenocoumarol, ethylbiscoumacetate, phenprocoumon) in many patients. Dose requirement may be increased many-fold (even up to 10×) | Avoid use of barbiturates as occasional hypnotics; substitute a benzodiazepine or consider use of behavioural or relaxation therapies. Barbiturates taken regularly as antiepileptics (i.e. in steady-state) do not affect anticoagulant control, unless the barbiturate is withdrawn or its dosage altered without modifying the dose of anticoagulant |
| | **Carbamazepine**<br>Dicloxacillin<br>Nafcillin<br>Sucralfate | Decrease in effect of warfarin | Monitor INR closely when these drugs are commenced, ceased or there is a change in dosage |
| | Cholestyramine | Markedly reduces absorption or warfarin when given up to 3 hours after its administration | Give warfarin 2 or more hours before cholestyramine if possible, but monitor INR as an increase in dosage may still be required |
| | Etretinate | Case reports of warfarin resistance | Monitor INR closely when etretinate is commenced or ceased |
| | Griseofulvin | Decrease in effect of warfarin in some patients | Monitor INR closely and adjust dose of anticoagulant carefully |
| | Phenytoin | Changes in warfarin effect may be variable with an initial increase in effect followed by a decrease in effect from 7 to 10 days onwards | Monitor INR closely in the 4 weeks following addition of phenytoin to a stable warfarin regimen |

*[Continued over]*

**Appendix B.** *[Continued]*

| Primary drug | May interact with | **Potential result** (see introductory notes) | Implications for management and how to avoid |
|---|---|---|---|
| **Anticoagulants** *[continued]* | | | |
| Coumarins *[continued]* | **Rifampicin** | Marked decrease in effect of warfarin, acenocoumarol and phenprocoumon | Monitor INR and adjust dose of warfarin carefully, or avoid rifampicin in antituberculosis regimens (e.g. if compliance can not be guaranteed). **Note:** Any adjustment of coumarin dosage should only be made on the basis of results derived from close observation of therapy and INR estimations over a period of time after the change |
| **Antidepressants** (see also chapter 30) | | | |
| Nonselective monoamine oxidase (MAO) inhibitors (e.g. phenelzine, isocarboxazid, tranylcypromine) | **Alcohol**<br>**Analgesics, strong (opioids)**<br>**Hypnosedatives** | CNS depressant effects increased | Instruct patient. Warn about possible adverse effect on performance skills, especially with first few days of therapy. Advisable to avoid alcoholic beverages since tyramine content not likely to be known by patient |
| | Amphetamines (including MDMA [Ecstacy])<br>Cocaine<br>Dextromethorphan<br>**Ephedrine**<br>Fenfluramine<br>**Levodopa**<br>**Phenylephrine**<br>**Pseudoephedrine**<br>**Foodstuffs containing tyramine** (Chianti and Alicante type wines, some beers, matured cheese, yoghurt, pickled herrings, chicken liver, vegetables, yeast, and meat extracts) or **dopamine** (broad bean pods) | Acute adrenergic crisis (marked headache, severe hypertension, subarachnoid haemorrhage) if monoamine oxidase inhibitors (MAOIs) given with these agents | Avoid these combinations. Treat crises with intravenous phentolamine 5mg |
| | Tricyclic antidepressants (imipramine, clomipramine, etc.) | Agitation, tremor, hyperpyrexia and coma if given inadvertently with tricyclic antidepressants | Allow space of 2 to 3 weeks after withdrawal of MAOI. These agents can be given together if commenced simultaneously after a washout period and the dosage of each is carefully tailored. This reaction is not seen with all tricyclic antidepressants and amitriptyline may actually protect against its occurrence |
| | **Fluoxetine** (and probably other selective serotonin reuptake inhibitors) Tryptophan | 'Serotonergic syndrome' (abdominal cramping, cerebellar signs, myoclonus, confusion, sweating, tachycardia and hypertension) | Wait 5 weeks after fluoxetine discontinuation before commencing nonselective monoamine oxidase inhibitors, and wait 2 weeks after ceasing the MAOI before commencing fluoxetine. Alternatively, consider use of the reversible selective MAO-A inhibitor moclobemide (no reported interaction) |
| | **Pethidine (meperidine)**<br>Tryptophan | Severe reaction (excitation, sweating, rigidity, hyper- or hypotension, coma) in some patients | Avoid this combination. Cautious use of other strong analgesics (e.g. morphine) in reduced dosage |
| Reversible inhibitors of MAO-A (moclobemide) | **Selective serotonin reuptake inhibitors (SSRIs)**<br>**Tricyclic antidepressants** | 'Serotonergic syndrome' (abdominal cramping, cerebellar signs, myoclonus, confusion, sweating, tachycardia and hypertension) | Wait 2 weeks after ceasing tricyclic antidepressants or SSRIs before commencing moclobemide, or monitor closely if combination is essential |

| | | | |
|---|---|---|---|
| Selective serotonin reuptake inhibitors (SSRIs) [fluoxetine, paroxetine, fluvoxamine, sertraline] | Tryptophan | Agitation, restlessness, poor concentration and nausea | Avoid this combination |
| | Carbamazepine<br>**Lithium**<br>**Moclobemide**<br>**Selegiline** | 'Serotonergic syndrome' (abdominal cramping, cerebellar signs, myoclonus, confusion, sweating, tachycardia and hypertension) in some patients | Consider alternative antiepileptic drugs such as valproic acid. If therapy with these combinations is necessary, monitor the patient clinically and cease both drugs at the first sign of the 'serotonergic syndrome'.<br>Lithium or moclobemide may be added to SSRI therapy to achieve an augmented antidepressant effect |
| Tricyclic antidepressants (amitriptyline, imipramine, etc.) | Adrenaline (epinephrine)-containing local anaesthetics<br>Noradrenaline (norepinephrine) | Prolonged pressor response; possible arrhythmias | Use plain local anaesthetics |
| | Anticholinergics<br>Antihistamines (some)<br>Anti-Parkinsonian drugs (anticholinergics)<br>Amantadine | Increased risk of troublesome anticholinergic side effects in the elderly if given with anticholinergics, anti-Parkinsonian drugs or some antihistamines (e.g. diphenhydramine, phenindamine, promethazine) | Use conservative doses of tricyclic antidepressants in the elderly. Monitoring of plasma concentrations may be helpful |
| | Alcohol | Increased risk of paralytic ileus and CNS depressant effects when given with alcohol | Instruct patient to limit consumption of alcohol. Warn about possible adverse effects on performance skills, especially with first few days of therapy on amitriptyline |
| | Barbiturates<br>Carbamazepine<br>Phenytoin | Decreased tricyclic plasma concentrations | Titrate tricyclic antidepressant dose to response and adverse effects being aware that patients on hepatic enzyme-inducing agents may require a higher tricyclic dose for response |
| | Quinidine<br>Cimetidine | Marked increase in plasma concentrations of tricyclic drugs with associated clinical toxicity | Monitor patients clinically for increased adverse effects and adjust dose of antidepressant if needed. Use ranitidine, famotidine or nizatidine instead of cimetidine |
| | **Fluoxetine**<br>**Fluvoxamine**<br>**Paroxetine**<br>**Sertraline** | Marked increase in plasma concentrations of tricyclic drugs with associated clinical toxicity | Decrease dose of tricyclic antidepressant by 25 mg per day until the dose is 25% of the original or less than 75 mg before commencing fluoxetine, or decrease planned tricyclic dose by 75% if concurrent therapy is planned and monitor for toxicity. Monitoring plasma tricyclic drug concentrations may be helpful |
| | **Nonselective monoamine oxidase inhibitors** (e.g. phenelzine, isocarboxazid, tranylcypromine) | Agitation, tremor, hyperpyrexia and coma if given inadvertently with monoamine oxidase inhibitors | Allow interval of 2 to 3 weeks after withdrawal of MAOI. These agents can be given together if commenced simultaneously after a washout period and the dosage of each is carefully tailored |
| **Antidiabetic drugs** (see also chapter 19) | | | |
| Biguanides (metformin) | Alcohol | Risk of hyperlacticacidaemia | Instruct the patient to avoid excessive quantities (moderate to large) of alcohol, and to be aware of and to report early symptoms of lactic acidosis (vomiting and malaise, abdominal pain, diarrhoea) |
| Sulphonylureas (tolbutamide, chlorpropamide, tolazamide, acetohexamide, glibenclamide [glyburide], glipizide, gliclazide) | **ACE inhibitors**<br>**Perhexiline** | Increased insulin sensitivity with potential for hypoglycaemia (case reports) | Monitor for hypoglycaemia when ACE inhibitors or perhexiline are added to stable antidiabetic therapy |

[Continued over]

**Appendix B.** *[Continued]*

| Primary drug | May interact with | **Potential result** (see introductory notes) | Implications for management and how to avoid |
|---|---|---|---|
| **Antidiabetic drugs** *[continued]* | | | |
| Sulphonylureas *[continued]* | **β-Adrenoceptor antagonists** (β-blockers) | Hypoglycaemic activity may be increased in some patients and early symptoms of hypoglycaemia may be masked (less likely with $\beta_1$-selective agents). Hyperglycaemia may occur in some patients due to decreased insulin sensitivity and release | Altered doses of sulphonylureas may be needed in some patients. β-Blockers prevent the release of lactate from muscle which is normally subsequently converted in the liver to glucose. In the absence of lactate, hypoglycaemia may result, particularly when the liver contains little or no glycogen (e.g. after prolonged fasting, in ketosis, in any patient with liver disease, or in alcoholics) |
| | Alcohol | Disulfiram-like intolerance (facial flushing, headache) of alcohol in some cases, particularly with chlorpropamide. Hypoglycaemic activity may be increased with acute alcohol ingestion if food intake is restricted (e.g. malnutrition, prolonged fasting) | Instruct the patient about the possibility of alcohol intolerance and to avoid moderate to large quantities of alcohol; intolerance of small quantities of alcohol more likely with chlorpropamide. Educate patient to maintain adequate nutrition |
| | Anabolic steroids | Increased hypoglycaemic activity of some sulphonylureas induced by some anabolic steroids | Advise diabetic patient on sulphonylureas against usage of anabolic steroids |
| | **Antacids**<br>**$H_2$-Receptor antagonists**<br>**Omeprazole** | Increased absorption of tolbutamide, glibenclamide (glyburide) and glipizide with potential for hypoglycaemia | Avoid these combinations or monitor for hypoglycaemia closely |
| | Barbiturates<br>Phenytoin<br>Rifampicin<br>(and other enzyme-inducing drugs) | May make diabetic control more difficult by decreasing the hypoglycaemic effect of the sulphonylurea | Likely to be a problem with compounds extensively metabolised in the liver (e.g. tolazamide, tolbutamide, glibenclamide, acetohexamide). Avoid occasional use of barbiturates as hypnosedatives. Substitute a benzodiazepine or consider cognitive or relaxation therapies as alternatives |
| | Chloramphenicol | Hypoglycaemic activity of tolbutamide and chlorpropamide markedly increased | Avoid this combination. Substitute another antibacterial drug (but not sulfonamides or ciprofloxacin; see below) |
| | Ciprofloxacin | Reports of hypoglycaemia after commencement of ciprofloxacin in patients on glibenclamide | Avoid combination if possible. Warn patient of possible increased risk of hypoglycaemia and increase frequency of blood glucose monitoring |
| | **Clofibrate** | Severe hypoglycaemia has been reported with tolbutamide and clofibrate | A reduced dose of tolbutamide may be needed in some patients. Increase frequency of blood glucose monitoring |
| | Corticosteroids<br>Diuretics (e.g. thiazides) | May make diabetic control more difficult | Modify dose of sulphonylurea if necessary |
| | Dicoumarol | Hypoglycaemic activity of tolbutamide and chlorpropamide markedly increased | Avoid this combination; use of warfarin may decrease risk of interaction |
| | Fluconazole<br>Ketoconazole | Hypoglycaemia reported with fluconazole at a dose of 100 mg/day and various sulphonylureas, and with ketoconazole and tolbutamide | Use alternative antifungal such as itraconazole if possible, or instruct patient to anticipate hypoglycaemia with dose adjustment to sulphonylurea based on blood glucose monitoring |
| | **Fluoxetine**<br>**Nonselective monoamine oxidase inhibitors** (e.g. phenelzine, isocarboxazid, tranylcypromine) | Enhanced or prolonged hypoglycaemic response to sulphonylureas | Monitor blood glucose closely when MAOIs or fluoxetine are added to a stable oral antidiabetic drug regimen |

| | | | |
|---|---|---|---|
| | Oxyphenbutazone<br>Phenylbutazone | Hypoglycaemic coma has been reported on many occasions with phenylbutazone and chlorpropamide, acetohexamide, glibenclamide or tolbutamide | Avoid this combination. Substitute another NSAID such as ibuprofen, indomethacin or naproxen |
| | Salicylates (large doses) | Hypoglycaemic activity of chlorpropamide enhanced | Avoid this combination. Substitute another NSAID such as ibuprofen, indomethacin or naproxen |
| | **Sulfonamides**<br>Sulfinpyrazone | Hypoglycaemia secondary to decreased clearance of tolbutamide, chlorpropamide, glipizide and glibenclamide (glyburide) | Avoid these combinations. Substitute another antibacterial agent (except chloramphenicol or ciprofloxacin which, under certain circumstances, can increase the activity of the sulphonylureas)<br>**Note:** The risk of drug-induced hypoglycaemic reactions is increased in the presence of associated renal impairment or liver dysfunction, with restricted food intake, and in the elderly |
| **Antiemetic/prokinetic agents** (see also chapter 22, sect. 5.1) | | | |
| Cisapride | **Ketoconazole**<br>**Itraconazole** | Increased plasma concentrations of cisapride (prolongation of QT interval and ventricular arrhythmias reported) | Avoid these combinations |
| Metoclopramide | Ranitidine | Increased incidence of akathisia | Monitor for occurrence and avoid combination subsequently |
| **Antiepileptic drugs** (see also chapter 29) | | | |
| Barbiturates (e.g. phenobarbital, primidone) | Phenytoin | Decrease in plasma concentrations of phenobarbital by 30% over 1 to 4 weeks | Monitor plasma concentrations of phenobarbital and phenytoin when phenytoin added to stable phenobarbital or primidone regimen, and adjust doses of both drugs accordingly |
| | Sulthiame | Marked increase in plasma concentrations of phenobarbital in many patients | Monitor plasma concentrations of phenobarbital when sulthiame is added to stable regimens, and reduce dose of phenobarbital or primidone if necessary |
| | Urinary alkalinisers | Decreased plasma concentrations through inhibition of renal tubular resorption | Useful therapeutic manoeuvre in severe toxicity or overdose |
| | Valproic acid | Increased plasma concentrations of phenobarbital with marked sedation | Reduce dose of phenobarbital or primidone when valproic acid is added to a stable regimen |
| Carbamazepine | Cimetidine | Variable increase in plasma carbamazepine concentrations by up to 30% | Avoid this combination; substitute ranitidine, famotidine or nizatidine |
| | Danazol<br>Fluoxetine<br>Fluvoxamine<br>Isoniazid<br>Nicotinamide | Marked increase in plasma carbamazepine concentrations with toxicity and, in the case of fluoxetine, extrapyramidal symptoms and 'serotonin syndrome' (shivering, agitation, incoordination, hyperreflexia, myoclonus) | Monitor carbamazepine plasma concentrations when these drugs are added to stable carbamazepine regimen and reduce dose if necessary. Either avoid the combination of fluoxetine and carbamazepine or watch for features of extrapyramidal symptoms or serotonin syndrome and cease one or both drugs at onset |
| | **Dextropropoxyphene (propoxyphene)** | Marked increase in plasma concentrations of carbamazepine with toxicity | Avoid use of dextropropoxyphene for pain relief for more than 1 day. Substitute aspirin or paracetamol and codeine |
| | Diltiazem<br>Verapamil | Marked increases in plasma carbamazepine concentrations | Monitor carbamazepine plasma concentrations when diltiazem or verapamil are added to stable carbamazepine regimen and reduce dose if necessary.<br>**Note:** not reported with nifedipine or felodipine |
| | Erythromycin<br>Clarithromycin<br>Troleandomycin | Marked increase in plasma concentrations of carbamazepine with toxicity | Avoid use of these combinations if possible. Substitute another antibacterial drug or monitor plasma carbamazepine concentrations closely when commencing or ceasing erythromycin, clarithromycin or troleandomycin |

*[Continued over]*

**Appendix B.** *[Continued]*

| Primary drug | May interact with | **Potential result** (see introductory notes) | Implications for management and how to avoid |
|---|---|---|---|
| **Antiepileptic drugs** *[continued]* | | | |
| Carbamazepine *[continued]* | **Phenytoin** | Decrease in plasma carbamazepine concentrations with concurrent increase in plasma carbamazepine 10, 11-epoxide levels and possible clinical toxicity | Monitor both carbamazepine and phenytoin plasma concentrations closely when commencing, ceasing or altering dosage of either. Perform a plasma carbamazepine 10, 11-epoxide determination (if available) if toxicity suspected in the presence of a normal range of carbamazepine concentrations |
| | **Lamotrigine**<br>Loxapine<br>**Valproic acid** | Marked increases in plasma carbamazepine 10, 11-epoxide concentrations with clinical toxicity in the presence of normal plasma carbamazepine concentrations | Monitor the patient clinically for carbamazepine toxicity when used concurrently with either valproic acid or lamotrigine. Perform a plasma carbamazepine 10, 11-epoxide determination (if available) if toxicity suspected and adjust carbamazepine dose accordingly |
| Lamotrigine | **Barbiturates**<br>**Carbamazepine**<br>? Paracetamol<br>**Phenytoin** | Decreased plasma lamotrigine concentrations | Monitor plasma lamotrigine concentrations closely when these drugs are commenced, ceased or their dosages are altered |
| | **Valproic acid** | Increased plasma lamotrigine concentrations | Monitor plasma lamotrigine concentrations closely when valproic acid is commenced, ceased or its dosage altered |
| Phenytoin | Alcohol, acute | Increased plasma phenytoin concentrations with heavy binges; little effect from mild to moderate intermittent alcohol ingestion | Instruct patient to avoid large binges |
| | Alcohol, chronic | Decreased plasma phenytoin concentrations with heavy long term use of alcohol; little effect from mild to moderate chronic ingestion | Advise patient to keep alcohol intake moderate or, if this is not possible, to ingest at a constant level and have frequent plasma level monitoring |
| | Amiodarone | Increased plasma phenytoin concentration | Monitor plasma phenytoin concentrations when amiodarone added to stable phenytoin regimen.<br>**Note:** Amiodarone CNS toxicity can clinically mimic that produced by phenytoin so that obtaining plasma levels of both drugs may be advisable when clinical toxicity is present |
| | Antacids<br>Sucralfate | Significant reduction in plasma phenytoin concentrations in some patients | Space administration of phenytoin and either antacids or sucralfate as much as possible, and by at least 2 hours |
| | Chloramphenicol | Marked increase in plasma concentrations of phenytoin | Avoid use of chloramphenicol, or if essential, monitor plasma concentrations of phenytoin and adjust dose accordingly |
| | **Cimetidine**<br>**Fluconazole**<br>Omeprazole | Marked increase in plasma phenytoin concentrations | Monitor plasma phenytoin concentrations and adjust dose accordingly; or substitute ranitidine, famotidine or nizatidine (no significant interaction reported) for cimetidine or omeprazole, and consider alternative antifungal or antiepileptic drugs.<br>**Note:** The combination of cimetidine and phenytoin has been implicated in the development of life-threatening thrombocytopenia in patients undergoing neurosurgical procedures. This mitigates strongly against this combination in this setting |
| | Diazoxide (oral) | Mutual antagonism. Marked decrease in plasma concentration of phenytoin. Hyperglycaemic effect of diazoxide antagonised | Avoid this combination |

| | | | |
|---|---|---|---|
| | Dicoumarol | Marked increase in plasma concentration of phenytoin when dicoumarol added | Avoid this combination; substitute warfarin |
| | Disulfiram | Marked increase in plasma concentration of phenytoin in many patients | If possible, avoid this combination; or monitor plasma concentrations of phenytoin and reduce dose if necessary |
| | Fluoxetine<br>Fluvoxamine | Increased plasma phenytoin concentrations | Avoid combination, or monitor plasma phenytoin concentrations closely and adjust dose accordingly |
| | Isoniazid | Marked increase in plasma concentrations of phenytoin in some patients who are slow acetylators of isoniazid | Monitor plasma concentration of phenytoin when isoniazid added to stable phenytoin regimen, and reduce dose if necessary |
| | **Nutrient formulae** (for nasogastric feeding) | Decreased plasma phenytoin concentrations by up to 75% | Monitor plasma phenytoin concentrations closely when commencing, ceasing or changing nutrient formulae. Plasma phenytoin levels may be better maintained by giving a single daily dose during a period when enteral feeding is not taking place such as at night |
| | Phenobarbital | Variable effect on plasma phenytoin concentrations and also dependent on dosage; occasionally a marked increase may occur on adding phenobarbital or after its withdrawal (substrate competition for metabolism occurs immediately phenobarbital is started but a more slowly developing enzyme induction reverses this effect) | Monitor plasma concentrations of phenytoin whenever phenobarbital is added to a stable phenytoin regimen or if phenobarbital is withdrawn |
| | Phenylbutazone | Marked increase in plasma concentrations of phenytoin in some patients | Avoid this combination. Substitute another NSAID such as ibuprofen, indomethacin or naproxen |
| | Paroxetine<br>Rifampicin | Decreased plasma phenytoin concentrations | Monitor plasma phenytoin concentrations closely when paroxetine or rifampicin are commenced or ceased in patients on a stable phenytoin regimen |
| | Sulfonamides (sulfaphenazole, sulfamethizole) | Marked increases in plasma concentrations of phenytoin in a few patients | Avoid this combination. Substitute another antibacterial drug (except chloramphenicol) |
| | Sulthiame | Marked increases in plasma concentrations of phenytoin in many patients | Monitor plasma concentrations of phenytoin when sulthiame added to stable phenytoin regimen and reduce dose if necessary |
| | Valproic acid | Marked but temporary increase in the free (unbound) plasma phenytoin concentration and in drug effects | Monitor plasma concentrations of phenytoin when valproic acid added to a stable regimen. Free phenytoin concentration will initially be higher than expected for a given total plasma phenytoin concentration. Monitor for signs of phenytoin toxicity. An initial temporary reduction in phenytoin dosage may be necessary |
| | **Vigabatrin** | Decreased plasma phenytoin concentrations by 30% over 4 weeks | Monitor plasma phenytoin concentrations when commencing, ceasing or altering dosage of vigabatrin.<br>**Note:** Most clinically significant interactions with phenytoin become manifest within 1 to 6 weeks after addition of the other drug. Interactions with phenytoin may not always be detrimental. Modest elevation of a low plasma concentration of phenytoin may actually improve seizure control. However, a marked increase in the plasma concentration increases the risk of toxicity |
| Valproic acid | **Barbiturates**<br>**Carbamazepine**<br>Chlorpromazine<br>**Phenytoin** | Decreased plasma valproic acid concentrations by up to 50% | Monitor plasma valproic acid concentrations when these drugs are added to a stable valproic acid regimen.<br>**Note:** The incidence of hepatotoxicity and hyperammonaemia may be increased when hepatic enzyme-inducing drugs are used concurrently with valproic acid |

*[Continued over]*

**Appendix B.** *[Continued]*

| Primary drug | May interact with | **Potential result** (see introductory notes) | Implications for management and how to avoid |
|---|---|---|---|
| **Antiepileptic drugs** *[continued]* | | | |
| Valproic acid *[continued]* | Doxorubicin<br>Cisplatin | Decreased plasma valproic acid concentrations due to decreased absorption | Monitor plasma valproic acid concentrations when these drugs are used concurrently |
| | Cimetidine<br>Erythromycin<br>Isoniazid | Increased plasma valproic acid concentrations | Monitor plasma valproic acid concentrations when cimetidine, erythromycin or isoniazid are added to a stable valproic acid regimen, or consider ranitidine or famotidine or alternative antimicrobials |
| | Salicylates | Increased plasma valproic acid concentrations with reports of acute psychosis on coadministration | Avoid this combination; substitute paracetamol or another NSAID |
| Zonisamide | Carbamazepine<br>Phenytoin | Decreased plasma zonisamide concentrations | Monitor zonisamide plasma concentrations if concurrent therapy with phenytoin or carbamazepine is necessary |
| **Antifungal agents** (see also chapter 31) | | | |
| Amphotericin B | **Aminoglycosides**<br>**Cefalothin**<br>**Cyclosporin** | Increased incidence and severity of renal impairment | Avoid these combinations if possible, or monitor renal function closely |
| Griseofulvin | Phenobarbital | Absorption of griseofulvin impaired | Give griseofulvin in 3 divided doses or avoid phenobarbital if possible |
| Ketoconazole<br>Itraconazole | Antacids<br>Cimetidine<br>**Didanosine (ddI)**<br>Omeprazole<br>Ranitidine<br>Sucralfate | Absorption of ketoconazole and itraconazole significantly decreased | Anticipate need to increase dose of ketoconazole or itraconazole (plasma itraconazole concentrations may be useful, if available) or, if possible, use fluconazole (no reported interaction) |
| | **Carbamazepine**<br>**Phenytoin**<br>Phenobarbital<br>Primidone<br>**Rifabutin**<br>**Rifampicin** | Decreased plasma concentrations of ketoconazole and itraconazole with potential for antifungal treatment failure | Avoid these combinations, if possible, or use fluconazole (no reported interaction). If itraconazole is essential then plasma concentrations (if available) may assist in dose modification |
| **Antihistamines** | | | |
| Terfenadine<br>Astemizole | **Erythromycin**<br>**Clarithromycin**<br>**Troleandomycin**<br>**Fluoxetine**<br>**Itraconazole**<br>**Ketoconazole**<br>Halofantrine<br>Grapefruit juice | Markedly increased plasma concentrations of terfenadine and astemizole with resultant QT interval prolongation and risk of potentially fatal ventricular arrhythmias, including torsades de pointes | Avoid these combinations. Substitute cetirizine or loratadine (or sedating antihistamines) for terfenadine or astemizole, or consider alternative therapy (e.g. other antibacterial agents or fluconazole or amphotericin B as antifungal therapy) |
| Sedating agents (e.g. promethazine, diphenhydramine, chlorphenamine, cyclizine) | **Alcohol**<br>**Hypnosedatives** | CNS depressant effects increased | Instruct patient. Warn about possible adverse effects on performance skills, especially with first few days of therapy |

| | | | |
|---|---|---|---|
| **Antihypertensive drugs** (see also chapter 21) | | | |
| ACE inhibitors | **Azathioprine** | Increased risk of neutropenia | Monitor white blood cell count. Neutropenia generally occurs in first three months of combination therapy |
| | **Epoetin (erythropoietin)**<br>**Potassium supplements**<br>**Potassium-sparing diuretics** | Increased risk of hyperkalaemia, especially in patients with renal impairment | Avoid these combinations or monitor plasma potassium concentration carefully |
| | Nonsteroidal anti-inflammatory drugs (NSAIDs) | Attenuation of antihypertensive effects of ACE inhibitors with possible loss of blood pressure control | Monitor blood pressure regularly and modify ACE inhibitor dose if necessary |
| | **Plasma protein solutions** | Increased incidence of reactions to the plasma protein solution (often manifest as severe hypotension, possibly due to bradykinin effect) | Avoid combination if possible. If not, monitor patient closely and be aware of the potential need for cessation of the plasma protein infusion and inotropic support |
| Adrenergic neuron blockers (bethanidine, debrisoquine, guanethidine) | Amphetamines<br>Chlorpromazine<br>Ephedrine<br>Phenylephrine<br>Phenylpropanolamine<br>Pizotifen<br>Pseudoephedrine<br>(NB. anorexiants, except fenfluramine; common cold remedies)<br>Tricyclic antidepressants | Antihypertensive effect antagonised and control of blood pressure may be lost | Avoid these combinations, especially oral common cold remedies. Substitute a β-blocker or use an antidepressant with little or no effect on the noradrenaline (norepinephrine) uptake pump such as mianserin or trazodone.<br>**Note:** Sympathomimetic drugs, including cold remedies, should be used with caution in all hypertensive patients |
| β-Adrenoceptor antagonists (β-blockers) | **Adrenaline** | Enhanced pressor response to adrenaline due to unopposed peripheral α-receptor effects | Avoid this combination or use adrenaline cautiously in patients on β-blockers |
| | Barbiturates<br>Carbamazepine<br>Rifampicin | Decreased plasma concentrations of propranolol, metoprolol and alprenolol with diminished clinical response | Watch for loss of β-blocker effect; consider use of atenolol, nadolol or sotalol which are not likely to be affected |
| | **Calcium antagonists (diltiazem, verapamil)**<br>**Disopyramide** | Enhanced depression of myocardial function and atrioventricular conduction | A combination of a β-blocker and calcium antagonist can be beneficial (e.g. in patients with angina pectoris), but use low doses initially and monitor carefully for left ventricular failure and bradyarrhythmia. Avoid this combination in patients with a sinus node syndrome, sinus bradycardia or atrioventricular block. If unavoidable, use nifedipine (less likely to affect atrioventricular conduction), and monitor patient closely.<br>Use quinidine instead of disopyramide |
| | Cimetidine<br>Dextropropoxyphene | Increased plasma concentrations and clinical effect of alprenolol, metoprolol, propranolol and oxprenolol | Substitute ranitidine, famotidine or nizatidine for cimetidine, and another analgesic for dextropropoxyphene; use atenolol as an alternative β-blocker |
| | **Digitalis glycosides**<br>Tacrine | Increased risk of atrioventricular block and bradycardia | Monitor patient for bradycardia and atrioventricular conduction delay on ECG |
| | Fluoxetine | Increased plasma concentrations of metoprolol and propranolol (case reports) with resultant bradycardia and atrioventricular block | Monitor for bradycardia and hypotension when adding fluoxetine to a stable β-blocker regimen |
| | Nonsteroidal anti-inflammatory drugs (NSAIDs) | Attenuation of the antihypertensive effect of β-blockers with possible loss of blood pressure control | Monitor blood pressure regularly and modify β-blocker dose if necessary. The effects of indomethacin and phenylbutazone on blood pressure are well documented but the effect of other NSAIDs is less clear; sulindac appears to have little adverse effect on blood pressure control |

*[Continued over]*

**Appendix B.** *[Continued]*

| Primary drug | May interact with | **Potential result** (see introductory notes) | Implications for management and how to avoid |
|---|---|---|---|
| **Antihypertensive drugs** *[continued]* | | | |
| Calcium antagonists | Carbamazepine<br>Phenobarbital<br>Primidone<br>Phenytoin | Decreased plasma concentrations of felodipine and nimodipine | Consider alternative antihypertensive or antiepileptic therapy |
| | Cimetidine | Increased plasma concentrations of verapamil, diltiazem and nifedipine (and possibly other dihydropyridines) | Substitute ranitidine (except in the case of nifedipine and other dihydropyridines where ranitidine may increase bioavailability) |
| | Fluoxetine | Reports of increased effect of nifedipine and verapamil | Monitor for hypotension when adding fluoxetine to a stable calcium antagonist regimen |
| | Grapefruit juice | Increased plasma levels of felodipine, nifedipine, nitrendipine and nisoldipine in most patients | Advise patients to avoid grapefruit juice while on these medications |
| | Rifampicin | Marked decrease in diltiazem, verapamil and nifedipine plasma concentrations and effect | Avoid this combination; consider alternative antihypertensives or antianginals |
| | Valproic acid | Increased plasma concentrations of nimodipine | Titrate nimodipine to blood pressure and adjust dosage accordingly |
| Clonidine | Tricyclic antidepressants | Decreased antihypertensive effect | In hypertensive patients use an alternative antihypertensive agent. Clonidine (decreased autonomic symptoms) and tricyclic antidepressants (sedative and antidiarrhoeal) may be used together in the therapy of opioid withdrawal |
| Methyldopa | Amphetamines<br>Other CNS stimulants<br>Tricyclic antidepressants | Antihypertensive effect may be antagonised and control of blood pressure may be lost | Interaction not as predictable or as well documented as with adrenergic neuron blocking drugs (see above) |
| | Iron haematinics | Decreased plasma concentrations and antihypertensive efficacy of methyldopa | Avoid this combination |
| Prazosin | **β-Adrenoceptor antagonists**<br>**Diuretics** | Increased first-dose hypotensive effect | Begin prazosin at the lowest possible dose and at night |
| All antihypertensive agents | **Anaesthetics, general** | Hypotension, particularly on induction of anaesthesia and especially in patients receiving ACE inhibitors, adrenergic neuron blocking drugs, and α-adrenoceptor blockers | Titrate concentrations of volatile anaesthetics to blood pressure in patients receiving these drugs |
| | Sympathomimetic bronchodilators<br>Liquorice<br>**Nonsteroidal anti-inflammatory drugs (NSAIDs)** | Can sometimes make antihypertensive therapy more difficult | Monitor blood pressure regularly. Modify therapy if necessary. The effects of indomethacin and phenylbutazone on blood pressure are well documented. The effect of other NSAIDs is less clear, although sulindac may have less influence and may be the NSAID of choice in patients on antihypertensive therapy |
| | Contraceptives, oral | Increased risk of vascular damage and difficulty in controlling blood pressure | It may be preferable to avoid oral contraceptives in patients needing antihypertensive therapy, but difficulties with blood pressure control are less pronounced with formulations containing low doses of constituent hormones |
| | Fenfluramine<br>Nitrates<br>Phenothiazines | Can lower blood pressure considerably (especially fenfluramine with Rauwolffia and methyldopa) | Avoid these combinations if possible. Monitor blood pressure regularly. Modify therapy if necessary |

| | | | |
|---|---|---|---|
| **Antimalarial drugs** (see also chapter 34) | | | |
| Chloroquine<br>Halofantrine<br>Mefloquine<br>Quinine | Amiodarone<br>Flecainide<br>Quinidine<br>Sotalol<br>Astemizole<br>Terfenadine<br>Quinine | Risk of QT prolongation and ventricular arrhythmia | Avoid these combinations if possible. If quinine is required to treat a patient with a malarial crisis who has recently received chloroquine, halofantrine or mefloquine, monitor closely for DT prolongation and arrhythmia |
| **Antineoplastic drugs** (see also chapter 27) | | | |
| Bleomycin | **Oxygen** | Acute respiratory failure in patients previously exposed to bleomycin | Use oxygen concentrations of less than 35% when giving anaesthetics to patients previously treated with bleomycin |
| Carmustine | **Cimetidine** | Increased length and severity of myelosuppression | Avoid this combination; substitute ranitidine, famotidine or nizatidine |
| Cisplatin | Ifosfamide | Increased renal dysfunction, particularly in children, manifest as hypokalaemia and hypomagnesaemia | Monitor plasma potassium and magnesium concentrations and supplement as required |
| Doxorubicin | **Cyclosporin**<br>**Streptozocin** | Increased plasma concentrations of doxorubicin with increased toxicity | Either avoid these combinations or decrease the dose of doxorubicin when combination therapy is required |
| Etoposide (VP 16) | **Cyclosporin** | Increased plasma concentrations of etoposide with increased bone marrow toxicity | Avoid this combination or decrease dose of etoposide if concurrent therapy is contemplated |
| Etoposide (VP 16)<br>Tenoposide (VM 26) | Phenobarbital<br>Phenytoin<br>Possibly other enzyme-inducing agents | Decreased plasma concentration of etoposide and tenoposide with possible loss of antitumour efficacy | Avoid these combinations, if possible. Consider an alternative antiepileptic drug such a valproic acid, or adjust dose of etoposide or tenoposide based on response and toxicity |
| Fluorouracil | Metronidazole | Increased fluorouracil toxicity without increased antitumour effect | Avoid this combination |
| Mercaptopurine | **Allopurinol** | Increased plasma concentrations of mercaptopurine with enhanced toxicity | Decrease dose of mercaptopurine to 25% of usual |
| | Cotrimoxazole (trimethoprim/ sulfamethoxazole) | Decreased plasma concentrations of mercaptopurine with loss of efficacy | Avoid this combination |
| Methotrexate | **Cisplatin**<br>**Nonsteroidal anti-inflammatory drugs (NSAIDs)**<br>Penicillins, high-dose<br>Probenecid<br>Retinoids<br>**Salicylates**<br>**Sulfonamides** | Markedly increased plasma concentrations of methotrexate with severe toxicity in some patients (particularly those receiving high-dose methotrexate therapy) | Avoid these combinations, if possible, and consider substitution of paracetamol for pain relief. The combination of low-dose methotrexate with NSAIDs for rheumatoid arthritis is acceptable but care needs to be taken to monitor for clinical and haematological toxicity. Monitor plasma methotrexate concentrations and clinical toxicity, and use folinic acid as an antidote where necessary. Exercise particular care in patients with renal impairment |
| | Broad-spectrum antibiotics | Decreased plasma methotrexate concentrations after oral administration with resultant loss of efficacy | Either avoid these combinations or monitor plasma methotrexate concentrations and adjust dose accordingly, or give methotrexate parenterally for duration of antibiotic therapy |
| Tamoxifen<br>Medroxyprogesterone | Aminoglutethimide | Decreased plasma tamoxifen and medroxyprogesterone concentrations with possible decreased efficacy | Avoid these combinations; there is no proven benefit of combination over single endocrine drug therapy in breast cancer |

*[Continued over]*

**Appendix B.** *[Continued]*

| Primary drug | May interact with | **Potential result** (see introductory notes) | Implications for management and how to avoid |
|---|---|---|---|
| **Anti-Parkinsonian drugs** (see also chapter 29) | | | |
| Levodopa | **Nonselective monoamine oxidase inhibitors** (e.g. phenelzine, isocarboxazid, tranylcypromine) | Acute adrenergic crisis | Avoid this combination |
| | Papaverine | Therapeutic efficacy of levodopa gradually reduced over some weeks | Avoid this combination |
| | Pyridoxine | Therapeutic efficacy of levodopa reduced (except when given with a decarboxylase inhibitor) | Avoid this combination or use levodopa plus a decarboxylase inhibitor |
| | Spiramycin<br>Iron haematinics | Marked decrease in plasma concentrations of both carbidopa and levodopa with loss of efficacy | Avoid these combinations. Consider an alternative antibacterial or separate dose of iron supplement and levodopa/carbidopa by as much time as possible |
| | Tiapride | Mutual antagonism of effect | Avoid this combination |
| Selegiline | **Fluoxetine**<br>**Pethidine (meperidine)** | 'Serotonergic syndrome' (abdominal cramping, cerebellar signs, myoclonus, confusion, sweating, tachycardia and hypertension) in some patients | Avoid these combinations |
| **Antipsychotic and antimanic drugs** (see also chapter 30) | | | |
| Butyrophenones (haloperidol) | **Alcohol**<br>**Analgesics, strong (opioids)**<br>**Hypnosedatives** | Increased CNS depressant effects | Instruct patient. Warn about possible adverse effect on performance skills, especially with the first few days of therapy |
| | Carbamazepine<br>Rifampicin (rifampin) | Decreased plasma haloperidol concentrations and probable decreased efficacy | Monitor patients clinically and consider dosage increase of haloperidol where carbamazepine is added to the regimen |
| | Fluoxetine<br>Tiapride | Increased incidence of extrapyramidal adverse effects | Avoid these combinations if possible. Modify therapy early if extrapyramidal effects are evident. Paroxetine may be an alternative to fluoxetine |
| | Lithium<br>Methyldopa | Toxic extrapyramidal syndrome in some patients (with normal range of lithium concentrations) | When haloperidol or methyldopa and lithium are given in combination, keep doses to a minimum and watch for extrapyramidal signs |
| Clozapine | Fluoxetine | Increased plasma clozapine and norclozapine concentrations | Monitor for clinical clozapine toxicity and adjust dose accordingly |
| Lithium | **ACE inhibitors** | Case reports of lithium toxicity, presumably due to decreased renal clearance of lithium, and of renal impairment | Monitor plasma lithium concentrations and adjust dosage accordingly. Monitor renal function in patients on this combination |
| | Carbamazepine<br>Phenytoin | Cerebellar syndrome with hyperreflexia in some patients | This may result from toxic plasma concentrations of any of these drugs but most often is **not** associated with elevated plasma levels. Lithium does, however, inhibit the potential of carbamazepine to induce syndrome of inappropriate antidiuretic hormone (ADH) secretion and agranulocytosis |
| | **Diuretics** (especially thiazides and thiazide-like agents, including metolazone) | With loss of sodium, lithium retention and toxicity may occur | Use reduced doses of lithium and monitor plasma lithium concentrations regularly (probably more frequently than usual). Thiazides may be useful in reversing nephrogenic diabetes insipidus produced by lithium |

| | | | |
|---|---|---|---|
| | **Fluoxetine** | 'Serotonergic syndrome' (abdominal cramping, cerebellar signs, myoclonus, confusion, sweating, tachycardia and hypertension) in some patients, which may or may not be associated with toxic plasma lithium concentrations | Monitor clinically for 'serotonergic syndrome' features and cease fluoxetine and/or lithium at first sign of onset; monitor plasma lithium concentrations frequently after the addition of fluoxetine to a stable lithium regimen |
| | Fluvoxamine | Possible induction of seizures as well as other CNS symptoms | Avoid this combination |
| | Diltiazem<br>Methyldopa<br>Verapamil | Toxicity at normal plasma lithium concentrations (perhaps due to pharmacodynamic potentiation) | Avoid these combinations |
| | **Nonsteroidal anti-inflammatory drugs (NSAIDs)** | Increased plasma concentrations of lithium with risk of lithium toxicity | Monitor plasma lithium concentrations regularly and adjust lithium dose accordingly |
| | Sodium chloride<br>Sodium bicarbonate | The lower the sodium intake, the greater the lithium retention; the higher the sodium intake the greater the lithium excretion | Instruct the patient. Warn about conditions leading to sodium loss and hence lithium retention (e.g. excessive sweating in hot weather, vomiting, intercurrent infection, low sodium diet, long term diuretics) |
| Phenothiazines | **Alcohol**<br>**Analgesics, strong (opioids)**<br>**Hynosedatives** | Increased CNS depressant effects | Instruct patient. Modify dosage of antipsychotic if necessary. Warn about possible effect on performance skills |
| | Antacids | Absorption of chlorpromazine may be impaired by concurrent aluminium hydroxide gel or aluminium hydroxide plus magnesium trisilicate antacids | Give drugs a few hours apart if possible |
| | Fluoxetine<br>Tiapride | Increased incidence of extrapyramidal adverse effects | Avoid combination if possible. Modify therapy early if extrapyramidal adverse effects evident |
| | Lithium | Decreased bioavailability of chlorpromazine | Anticipate increased dosage requirement of chlorpromazine when lithium is added, or reduced dosage requirement when lithium is withdrawn |
| **Antispasticity/muscle protective drugs** (see also chapter 29) | | | |
| Dantrolene | Verapamil | Diminution of muscle protective effect of dantrolene in patient with previous malignant hyperthermia | Avoid this combination in patients with a history of malignant hyperthermia. Use an alternative antihypertensive |
| **Antituberculosis drugs** (see also chapter 23) | | | |
| Isoniazid | Aluminium hydroxide gel | Decreased absorption of isoniazid | Only likely to be significant with intermittent isoniazid regimens. Give isoniazid 1 hour before antacid if possible |
| | Corticosteroids | Decreased plasma concentrations of isoniazid | Increase in isoniazid dose may be appropriate |
| Rifampicin (rifampin) | **Antacids**<br>**Didanosine (ddI)**<br>**Ketoconazole**<br>**Itraconazole** | Decreased absorption of rifampicin | Give didanosine or antacids at least 2 hours after rifampicin and space ketoconazole and itraconazole administration as far away from rifampicin as possible; consider increasing the dose of rifampicin if long term antituberculosis/antifungal therapy is necessary |
| | *p*-Aminosalicylic acid (bentonite as excipient) | Plasma concentrations of rifampicin markedly decreased | Give *p*-aminosalicylic acid preparations containing bentonite 8 to 12 hours after rifampicin |
| | Phenobarbital | Plasma concentrations of rifampicin markedly decreased | Avoid occasional use of barbiturates. Substitute a benzodiazepine for occasional hypnotic use. Increase dosage of rifampicin if long term antituberculosis/antiepileptic therapy is necessary |
| **Antiulcer drugs** (see also chapter 22) | | | |
| Cimetidine<br>Ranitidine | Antacids | Reduced absorption of $H_2$-receptor antagonists | Give antacids 1 hour after $H_2$-receptor antagonist |

*[Continued over]*

**Appendix B.** *[Continued]*

| Primary drug | May interact with | **Potential result** (see introductory notes) | Implications for management and how to avoid |
|---|---|---|---|
| **Antiviral drugs** (see also chapter 32) | | | |
| Didanosine (ddI) | **Alcohol**<br>**Corticosteroids**<br>**Cotrimoxazole, high-dose**<br>**Pentamidine** | Increased incidence of pancreatitis and hyperamylasaemia | Avoid these combinations if possible, or monitor plasma amylase levels and symptoms closely |
| Foscarnet | Aminoglycosides<br>Radiographic contrast media | Increased incidence and severity of renal impairment | Avoid these combinations or monitor serum creatinine closely and cease if renal function deteriorates |
| | Pentamidine | Increased risk of hypocalcaemia and possibly hypomagnesaemia | Avoid combination if possible. Monitor plasma calcium and magnesium levels |
| Ganciclovir | Imipenem/cilastatin | Increased risk of seizures (? by decreasing clearance of imipenem) | Avoid this combination |
| | **Antineoplastics**<br>**Cotrimoxazole (trimethoprim/ sulfamethoxazole)**<br>**Zidovudine** | Increased incidence and severity of neutropenia | Cease zidovudine and possibly cotrimoxazole for the duration of ganciclovir therapy.<br>Avoid antineoplastic therapy while on ganciclovir or consider use of colony stimulating factors |
| Vidarabine | Allopurinol<br>Interferon-α | Increased neurotoxicity (cerebellar, behavioural and psychiatric syndromes) | Either avoid combination or watch closely for clinical toxicity and cease one or both agents at onset |
| Zalcitabine | Dapsone<br>Isoniazid<br>Vincristine<br>and other agents known to induce neuropathy | Increased incidence of neuropathy which may be painful and only partially reversible | Avoid these combinations if possible and cease one or both agents at the first sign of peripheral neuropathy (diminished vibration sensation in the toes); neuropathy may worsen after cessation and take weeks to settle |
| Zidovudine | Interferon-α | Synergistic effect in response of Kaposi's sarcoma but increased incidence and severity of neutropenia | Monitor neutrophil count closely and cease one or both agents if neutrophil count is less than $1000 \times 10^6$ cells/L, or otherwise consider use of colony stimulating factors |
| | Amphotericin B<br>**Antineoplastic drugs**<br>**Cotrimoxazole, high-dose**<br>Flucytosine<br>Foscarnet<br>**Ganciclovir**<br>Pyrimethamine | Additive haematological toxicity | Monitor blood count indices closely in patients on combinations of these drugs |
| | Clarithromycin | Decreased absorption of zidovudine | Administer drugs 4 hours apart |
| | **Methadone**<br>Probenecid<br>Trimethoprim<br>**Valproic acid** | Increased plasma concentrations of zidovudine and possibly the toxic metabolite 3'-amino 3'-deoxythymidine (AMT) | Monitor clinically for increased zidovudine toxicity, particularly anaemia |
| | Ribavirin | Antagonism of antiviral effect as well as increased haematological toxicity | Avoid this combination |
| | **Rifabutin**<br>**Rifampicin** | Decrease in plasma zidovudine concentrations | Monitor plasma zidovudine levels when either rifabutin or rifampicin are commenced or discontinued |

| | | | |
|---|---|---|---|
| **Bronchodilators** (see also chapter 23) | | | |
| Theophylline | **Cimetidine**<br>? Famotidine<br>Fluvoxamine | Significantly increased theophylline plasma concentrations with possible toxicity | Avoid these combinations; use ranitidine instead of cimetidine (effect of ranitidine on plasma theophylline concentrations not clinically significant) or an alternative antidepressant for fluvoxamine such as fluoxetine (no interaction reported) |
| | Amiodarone<br>Clarithromycin<br>Contraceptives, oral<br>Erythromycin<br>Fluoroquinolones (ciprofloxacin, enoxacin, pefloxacin)<br>Interferon-α<br>Pentoxifylline<br>Tacrine<br>Thiabendazole<br>Ticlopidine<br>Troleandomycin<br>Verapamil | Increased theophylline plasma concentrations. Toxicity may result if concentrations already in upper therapeutic range | Avoid these combinations, if possible. Otherwise, monitor plasma theophylline concentrations and reduce dose accordingly (approx. 25% reduction may be needed with erythromycin and 50% reduction with troleandomycin) |
| | Phenobarbital<br>Phenytoin<br>Rifampicin<br>(and other enzyme-inducing drugs including tobacco) | Decreased theophylline plasma concentrations | Larger than normal doses of theophylline may be needed in epileptics or tuberculosis patients. Monitor plasma theophylline concentrations and adjust dose accordingly |
| **Cardiac glycosides** (see also chapter 20) | | | |
| Digitoxin<br>Digoxin<br>(see also below) | Aminoglutethimide<br>Phenobarbital<br>**Phenytoin**<br>Rifampicin | Decreased plasma digoxin or digitoxin concentrations | Monitor plasma digoxin or digitoxin concentrations closely on commencing, ceasing or altering dosage or aminoglutethimide, phenytoin or rifampicin. Avoid use of barbiturates for occasional sedation; substitute a benzodiazepine or consider behavioural or relaxation therapy |
| | Amphotericin B<br>Carbenoxolone<br>**Diuretics** | Risk of digitalis toxicity increased in presence of hypokalaemia | Ensure adequate intake of potassium or use a potassium-sparing diuretic. Monitor plasma potassium levels |
| | **Cholestyramine**<br>**Colestipol**<br>Sucralfate | Decreased bioavailability of digoxin and digitoxin possible | Give drugs 8 hours after digoxin or digitoxin |
| | **Quinidine** | Marked increase in digoxin plasma concentrations with real risk of toxicity, with lesser but still potentially significant effects on plasma digitoxin concentrations | Anticipate need to reduce dosage if quinidine added. Monitor plasma digoxin or digitoxin concentrations and the patient's clinical status closely |
| | Suxamethonium (succinylcholine) | Risk of dangerous arrhythmias due to sudden release of potassium | More likely to be a problem in presence of trauma, burns, wounds, muscular disorders. Avoid suxamethonium in such cases |
| Digoxin<br>(see also above) | Alprazolam | Increased plasma digoxin concentrations with risk of toxicity, particularly in the elderly | If possible avoid combination by using alternative benzodiazepines or behavioural or relaxation therapies; if not, monitor plasma digoxin concentrations and the patient's clinical status |
| | **Amiodarone**<br>Propafenone | Marked increase in digoxin plasma concentrations with risk of toxicity | Anticipate need to reduce digoxin dosage if propafenone or amiodarone added. Monitor plasma digoxin concentrations and patient's clinical status closely |

[Continued over]

**Appendix B.** *[Continued]*

| Primary drug | May interact with | **Potential result** (see introductory notes) | Implications for management and how to avoid |
|---|---|---|---|
| **Cardiac glycosides** *[continued]* | | | |
| Digoxin *[continued]* | Antacid liquids (aluminium hydroxide or magnesium-containing) | Decreased bioavailability of digoxin with concomitant administration of aluminium hydroxide or magnesium salts | Give drugs about 6 hours apart if possible. More likely to be a problem with slowly dissolving digoxin tablets |
| | Antidiarrhoeals (adsorbent type) | Decreased bioavailability of digoxin with concurrent administration of kaolin-pectin suspension | Give drugs about 6 hours apart if possible. More likely to be a problem with slowly dissolving digoxin tablets |
| | **Calcium antagonists** (verapamil, nifedipine, diltiazem) | Marked increase in digoxin plasma concentrations as well as potential for prolonged atrioventricular conduction, particularly with verapamil and diltiazem | Anticipate need to reduce digoxin dosage if calcium antagonists added. Nifedipine may not interact to same extent as verapamil and diltiazem but close observation is advisable. Amlodipine or felodipine may be useful alternatives (no interaction reported) |
| | Cyclosporin<br>Itraconazole<br>Omeprazole | Increased plasma concentrations of digoxin | Monitor plasma digoxin concentrations and adjust dose accordingly |
| | Erythromycin<br>Fluoroquinolones<br>Tetracyclines | Increased plasma digoxin concentrations in 10% of patients (by eradicating degradative gut bacteria) | Monitor plasma digoxin concentrations closely when commencing or ceasing erythromycin, fluoroquinolones or tetracyclines, and adjust dose accordingly |
| | **Nonsteroidal anti-inflammatory drugs (NSAIDs)**<br>**Salicylates** | Increased plasma concentrations of digoxin with potential for toxicity in some patients | Monitor plasma digoxin concentrations and adjust dose accordingly |
| **Contraceptives, oral** (see also chapter 18) | | | |
| | Ascorbic acid (vitamin C)<br>Didanosine (ddI)<br>**Ferrous sulfate**<br>Sucralfate | ? Interference with absorption or enterohepatic circulation of estrogen. Case reports of pregnancy and menstrual irregularities | Consider advising additional or alternative contraception when these drugs are used in patients on oral contraceptives. In the case of ascorbic acid, the bioavailability of ethinylestradiol may be increased, producing symptoms or signs of estrogen excess |
| | Broad-spectrum antibiotics | ? Interference in enterohepatic circulation of estrogen. Case reports of pregnancy and menstrual irregularities, although controlled studies have often failed to show a significant interaction | This interaction appears to affect only a small proportion of women. Whether additional contraception should be recommended is a matter for individual clinical judgement |
| | Barbiturates<br>**Carbamazepine**<br>Griseofulvin<br>Oxcarbazepine<br>**Phenytoin**<br>Rifampicin (rifampin) | Increased metabolism of estrogen. Pregnancy and a high incidence of menstrual irregularities have resulted | Consider alternative forms of contraception. Avoid occasional use of barbiturates. Substitute a benzodiazepine if necessary.<br>**Note:** Bleeding disturbances in a previously regular contraceptive cycle indicate that the method is no longer reliable. Increasing the dose or a change of contraceptive does not eliminate the risk of bleeding disturbances or pregnancy. The offending drug should be withdrawn, the disturbed contraceptive cycle stopped and a new one started, along with an additional method of contraception for the new course. When the offending drug cannot be withdrawn, an alternative method of contraception is advised. Any enzyme-inducing drug is a potential source of risk to contraceptive efficacy in users of oral contraceptives |
| | Troleandomycin | Cholestatic jaundice | Avoid this combination |

| | | | |
|---|---|---|---|
| **Corticosteroids, systemic** (see also chapter 19) | | | |
| Dexamethasone<br>Hydrocortisone<br>Methylprednisolone<br>Prednisone<br>Prednisolone | Barbiturates (e.g. phenobarbital, primidone)<br>Phenytoin<br>Carbamazepine<br>Aminoglutethimide<br>Rifampicin (rifampin) | Dexamethasone, hydrocortisone, methylprednisolone, prednisolone and prednisone metabolism enhanced. Efficacy of steroid reduced with increased dose requirement | Increased corticosteroid dosage needed, particularly with the longer acting steroids (e.g. dexamethasone). A doubling of the usual steroid dosage may be necessary; careful follow-up with further adjustments according to clinical response is essential.<br>Avoid occasional use of barbiturates. Substitute a benzodiazepine or consider cognitive or relaxation therapy.<br>Interpret dexamethasone suppression tests cautiously.<br>Adjust dosage when rifampicin is withdrawn (e.g. in patients with tuberculosis as a consequence of long term immunosuppressive therapy with corticosteroids).<br>In Addison's disease, consider alternative agent to rifampicin |
| Dexamethasone | Ephedrine | Dexamethasone metabolism enhanced | Avoid this combination. Substitute a $\beta_2$-adrenoceptor agonist bronchodilator |
| Methylprednisolone | Contraceptives, oral<br>Ketoconazole<br>Troleandomycin | Methylprednisolone metabolism reduced with possible increased incidence of adverse effects | Avoid this combination; otherwise anticipate dosage reduction of methylprednisolone |
| **Diuretics** (see also chapter 24) | | | |
| Acetazolamide | Salicylates | Increased plasma acetazolamide concentrations with risk of CNS toxicity (lethargy, confusion, tinnitus, somnolence, anorexia), particularly if renal impairment is present | Avoid this combination if possible, or monitor for CNS effects and reduce dose of acetazolamide at first sign of toxicity |
| Amiloride<br>Spironolactone<br>Triamterene | **ACE inhibitors** | Increased risk of hyperkalaemia, especially in patients with impaired renal function | In general, avoid these combinations and certainly in presence of impaired renal function. Monitor plasma potassium levels closely |
| Loop diuretics (bumetamide, ethacrynic acid, furosemide) | **Aminoglycosides** (amikacin, gentamicin, kanamycin, netilmicin streptomycin, tobramycin) | Increased risk of ototoxicity when combined with loop diuretics in renal failure | If possible, avoid this combination; or reduce the aminoglycoside dosage to the minimum effective level (monitor by plasma assay) and regularly check renal function |
| | **Cefalothin** | Increased risk of nephrotoxicity with large doses of ethacrynic acid or furosemide | If possible, avoid this combination; or reduce dosage of one or both agents and check renal function regularly |
| Thiazide diuretics<br>Furosemide | **Nonsteroidal anti-inflammatory drugs (NSAIDs)** | Attenuation of diuretic and antihypertensive response | Anticipate increased dose requirements of diuretics. Particular caution required in elderly patients with heart failure and those with renal impairment |
| Triamterene (see also above) | Indomethacin | Acute renal failure possible (case report) | Monitor renal function in patients receiving this combination |
| **Endocrine drugs** (see also chapter 19) | | | |
| Bisphosphonates (e.g. etidronate) | Calcium supplements | Decreased absorption of bisphosphonates with possible compromise of antiosteoporotic effect | Avoid concurrent use. Administer bisphosphonates in the morning and calcium supplements at night, or otherwise alternate each type of agent at 2-weekly intervals |
| Bromocriptine | Erythromycin | Increased plasma concentrations of bromocriptine with potential for increased incidence of adverse effects | Avoid this combination if possible. Use roxithromycin as an alternative to erythromycin |
| | Antipsychotic drugs | Mutually inhibitory | Avoid this combination |
| Thyroid hormones | **Carbamazepine** | Increased requirement for thyroid hormone replacement in hypothyroid patients | Check thyroid function tests monthly in patients on commencing, ceasing or altering dose of carbamazepine |
| | Cholestyramine | Absorption of thyroid hormone impaired | Give drugs 4 to 5 hours apart if possible |

*[Continued over]*

**Appendix B.** *[Continued]*

| Primary drug | May interact with | **Potential result** (see introductory notes) | Implications for management and how to avoid |
|---|---|---|---|
| **Endocrine drugs** *[continued]* | | | |
| Thyroid hormones *[continued]* | **Ketamine** | Severe hypertension and tachycardia | Avoid this combination. Try control with propranolol |
| **Gout drugs** (see also chapter 25) | | | |
| Probenecid<br>Sulfinpyrazone | Salicylates (low doses) | Therapeutic efficacy of probenecid and sulfinpyrazone markedly inhibited | Avoid low doses of salicylates. Occasional small analgesic doses seem to be without significant effect on uricosuric action |
| | Thiazide diuretics | Therapeutic efficacy of urate-altering drugs may be inhibited | An increase in dosage of the uricosuric agent may be needed |
| **Immunosuppressive agents** (see also chapter 28) | | | |
| Azathioprine<br>Mercaptopurine | **Allopurinol** | Biotransformation of active metabolite (mercaptopurine) impaired, leading to increased plasma concentrations | Decrease azathioprine dose to 33% of usual and decrease dose of mercaptopurine to 25% of usual, and monitor for haematological toxicity when used in combination with allopurinol |
| Cyclosporin (cyclosporin A) | Allopurinol<br>ACE inhibitors (possible)<br>**Aminoglycosides**<br>**Amphotericin B**<br>**Azole antifungals**<br>**Chloroquine**<br>**Ciprofloxacin**<br>Clarithromycin<br>Contraceptives, oral<br>**Corticosteroids**<br>**Cotrimoxazole (trimethoprim/ sulfamethoxazole)**<br>Danazol<br>Erythromycin<br>Fluoxetine<br>Grapefruit juice<br>Hydroxychloroquine<br>Imipenem/cilastatin<br>Melphalan<br>Methyltestosterone<br>Norethisterone<br>**Nonsteroidal anti-inflammatory drugs (NSAIDs)**<br>**Tacrolimus (FK 506)**<br>Trimethoprim | Potentiation of cyclosporin nephrotoxicity (due either to increased cyclosporin plasma concentrations or pharmacological potentiation of nephrotoxicity) | Close monitoring of renal function and plasma cyclosporin concentrations essential in patients receiving these combinations.<br>**Note:** Azole antifungals, particularly ketoconazole, and calcium antagonists such as diltiazem are used to decrease the cyclosporin dose required to produce immunosuppressive plasma concentrations of cyclosporin |
| | Diltiazem<br>Verapamil<br>Nicardipine | Increased cyclosporin plasma concentrations but with relative sparing of nephrotoxicity | Monitor cyclosporin plasma concentrations on commencing, ceasing or altering dose of calcium antagonist.<br>**Note:** This interaction is often used to produce an immunosuppressive plasma concentration of cyclosporin at a lower ingested dose to reduce therapy cost. If a calcium antagonist that does not increase plasma cyclosporin concentrations is required, then nifedipine or nitrendipine may be used (no interaction reported) |

| | | | |
|---|---|---|---|
| | Nifedipine | Increased incidence of gingival hyperplasia | Observe for this adverse effect and cease nifedipine on onset |
| | Barbiturates<br>**Carbamazepine**<br>Griseofulvin<br>Nafcillin<br>?Octreotide<br>**Omeprazole**<br>**Phenytoin**<br>Pyrazinamide<br>Rifampicin | Decreased cyclosporin plasma concentrations with associated rejection of transplanted organs | Monitor cyclosporin concentrations. Increase cyclosporin dose as necessary to maintain plasma concentrations and transplant organ function. Valproic acid may be a useful alternative where anticonvulsant therapy is required (no interaction reported) |
| Penicillamine | Iron haematinics | Decreased plasma penicillamine concentrations | Avoid this combination |
| **Iron haematinics** | Antacid liquids<br>Colloidal bismuth subcitrate | Absorption of iron may be impaired by magnesium or carbonate-containing antacids and by colloidal bismuth subcitrate | Give drugs as far apart as possible |
| | Tetracyclines | Plasma concentrations of tetracyclines and absorption of iron markedly decreased | Give conventional iron tablets 3 hours apart if possible.<br>? May not be a problem with slow release iron preparations |
| **Lipid-lowering drugs** | | | |
| Cholestyramine<br>Colestipol | Acidic drugs (e.g. digoxin, warfarin)<br>Gemfibrozil<br>Pravastatin<br>Many others | Because it is an anion exchange resin, cholestyramine may bind acidic drugs in the gut, delaying or impairing their absorption | Give other drugs an hour or more before cholestyramine or colestipol, if possible. Administration of the ion exchange resin with meals and other lipid-lowering agents at bedtime or before breakfast is advised. |
| Lovastatin<br>? Simvastatin | **Cyclosporin**<br>Erythromycin<br>**Gemfibrozil**<br>**Nicotinic acid (niacin)** | Increased plasma concentration of lovastatin with increased risk of adverse effects, in particular myositis | Avoid these combinations. Case reports suggest similar interactions involving simvastatin. Pravastatin may be a safer alternative to lovastatin or simvastatin when combination with gemfibrozil is required |
| **Migraine drugs** (see also chapter 29) | | | |
| Ergotamine | **Adrenaline (epinephrine)**<br>**β-Adrenoceptor antagonists**<br>**Dopamine**<br>Erythromycin<br>**Sumatriptan**<br>Troleandomycin | Increased risk of peripheral ischaemia | Avoid these combinations in patients with peripheral vascular disease; observe others for signs of vascular insufficiency.<br>Consider sumatriptan as an alternative to ergotamine in patients on β-blockers.<br>Use an alternative antibiotic for erythromycin and troleandomycin |
| Flunarizine | Carbamazepine<br>Phenytoin | Marked decrease in plasma flunarizine concentrations | Monitor therapeutic effect and adjust dose accordingly |
| **Muscle relaxants, skeletal** (see also chapter 12) | | | |
| Depolarising<br>(e.g. suxamethonium [succinylcholine]) | **Aminoglycosides**<br>**Furosemide**<br>**Magnesium infusions**<br>Polymixins | Neuromuscular blocking activity may be increased. Also danger of respiratory arrest | Give these antibiotics with extreme caution during surgery or postoperative period. Anticipate prolongation of block. Interaction has most often followed streptomycin and neomycin and appears most predictable if antibiotics are given intraperitoneally or if usual doses are used in a patient with impaired renal function or muscle weakness. The block can often be antagonised by neostigmine and calcium |

*[Continued over]*

**Appendix B.** *[Continued]*

| Primary drug | May interact with | **Potential result** (see introductory notes) | Implications for management and how to avoid |
|---|---|---|---|
| **Muscle relaxants, skeletal** *[continued]* | | | |
| Depolarising *[continued]* | Anticholinesterases (e.g. ecothiopate eye drops, pesticides)<br>Cyclophosphamide<br>Phenelzine<br>Tacrine<br>Thiotepa | Serum cholinesterase levels decreased and neuromuscular blocking activity may be prolonged | Desirable to assess serum cholinesterase activity prior to use of suxamethonium. Avoid suxamethonium if serum cholinesterase levels significantly decreased (as likely with ecothiopate eye drops). If suxamethonium is necessary, use with extreme caution |
| | Digoxin | Increased risk of various bradyarrhythmias with suxamethonium | Avoid this combination |
| | Procainamide<br>Procaine (large doses)<br>Propanidid<br>Quinidine | Neuromuscular blocking activity may be increased | Give these combinations with caution and anticipate prolongation of block. Large doses of procaine seem necessary to enhance block |
| | Lithium | Neuromuscular blocking activity may be prolonged | Anticipate prolongation of block. Generally, lithium should be ceased prior to elective surgery and electroconvulsive therapy (it may diminish response to electroconvulsant therapy) |
| Non-depolarising (e.g. tubocurarine, pancuronium, vecuronium, atracurium) | Anticholinesterases<br>Immunosuppressive drugs<br>Long term antiepileptics | Neuromuscular blocking activity may be decreased in some patients | Anticipate need to modify dose of relaxant; monitor patient clinically for level of neuromuscular blockade |
| | **Aminoglycosides**<br>Amphotericin B<br>Azlocillin<br>Clindamycin<br>**Cyclosporin**<br>**Furosemide**<br>**Magnesium infusions**<br>Polymixins<br>Quinidine<br>Tetracyclines | Neuromuscular blocking activity may be increased. Also danger of respiratory arrest | Give these combinations with caution and anticipate prolongation of block |
| | Inhalational anaesthetics (e.g. enflurane, isoflurane) | Neuromuscular blocking activity may be increased | Decreased doses of muscle relaxant required in patients receiving these agents. Halothane appears to have less potentiating effect than isoflurane and enflurane |
| | **Hypokalaemia** | Neuromuscular blocking activity may be increased | Correct potassium deficit |
| Pancuronium (see also above) | Lithium<br>Verapamil<br>?Other calcium antagonists | Neuromuscular blocking activity may be increased | Anticipate prolongation of block. Edrophonium may be more effective in reversing blockade than neostigmine in the presence of calcium antagonists |
| | Corticosteroids | Rapid termination of action by large doses of corticosteroids | Careful monitoring of neuromuscular transmission is required if this combination is used |
| **Potassium supplements** | **ACE inhibitors**<br>**Amiloride**<br>**Spironolactone**<br>**Triamterene** | Increased risk of hyperkalaemia, especially in patients with impaired renal function | In general, avoid these combinations and certainly in the presence of impaired renal function; monitor plasma potassium levels |

| | | | |
|---|---|---|---|
| **Vasopressor agents** | | | |
| Noradrenaline (levarterenol) | Amitriptyline<br>Imipramine<br>Guanethidine<br>Methyldopa<br>Selegiline | Marked increase in pressor response (NB. does not occur with MAOIs) | Give noradrenaline only with caution, beginning with very small doses |
| | Antipsychotics | Reduced pressor effect | Avoid this combination |
| Metaraminol<br>Methoxamine<br>Mephentermine | Nonselective monoamine oxidase inhibitors (e.g. phenelzine, isocarboxazid, tranylcypromine) | Marked increase in pressor response | Avoid this combination. Noradrenaline may be preferable |
| | Tricyclic antidepressants | Circulatory effect enhanced | Give indirect-acting vasopressors only with caution |
| Phenylephrine | Guanethidine | Marked increase in pressor response, even from eye drops of either agent | Avoid this combination |
| | Nonselective monoamine oxidase inhibitors (e.g. phenelzine, isocarboxazid, tranylcypromine) | Slight to moderate increase in pressor response (only a real problem with oral phenylephrine) | Avoid oral and probably also nasal phenylephrine. Give parenteral phenylephrine with caution |
| | Tricyclic antidepressants | Circulatory effect enhanced | Give phenylephrine only with caution |

# Guide to Safety of Drugs in Breast Feeding

*E.J. Begg, H.C. Atkinson* and *B.A. Darlow*

Clinicians are frequently called upon to advise mothers about the safety to the infant of drug ingestion during breast feeding. This appendix provides guidelines which may enable rational decisions to be made.

A number of factors affect the passage of drugs into breast milk.[1-3] Drugs pass from maternal plasma into milk by passive diffusion and are distributed within the aqueous, protein and lipid phases of milk. The total amount of drug that enters the milk is therefore affected by the composition of milk and by the physicochemical characteristics of the drug itself, such as its acid-base characteristics, protein binding and lipid solubility. It is probable that all drugs in maternal plasma will be present in milk to some extent, but it is clearly the actual amount ingested along with the oral availability and clearance of a drug in the infant that are of most importance in determining the likely plasma concentrations attained.

The most commonly quoted index of drug distribution into milk is the milk : plasma concentration ratio (M/P). It is, however, more appropriate to calculate the daily dose of drug ingested by the infant in milk, which can then be compared with doses used therapeutically or with maternal doses corrected for weight. Best of all, of course, are actual concentrations observed in suckling infants, but unfortunately these are rarely available.

## 1. Use of the Tables

### 1.1 Table I

Table I summarises reports quantifying the distribution of drugs into human breast milk.

*M/P ratio:* the M/P ratios quoted are based on comparisons of areas under the milk and plasma concentrations-time curves ($M/P_{AUC}$), except where indicated. M/P ratios based on single time points have not been included, because they rely on the often erroneous assumption that milk and plasma drug concentrations parallel each other throughout the dosage interval.[4]

*Time of peak concentration in milk*, i.e. the $t_{max}$ $^{milk}$: this is the time after drug ingestion at which concentrations in milk are at their highest. In general, it is safest for an infant to feed at the time of the trough maternal plasma concentration (i.e. just prior to the next dose of the drug) to minimise the dose ingested.

*Infant dose:* the infant dose (per kg per day) [$D_{inf}$] is calculated from the maximum maternal plasma concentration, unless stated otherwise, and represents the maximum likely exposure. The calculation is made as follows. Firstly, the maternal steady-state plasma concentration ($C^{ss}$) is calculated from:

$$C^{ss} = \frac{\text{Dose/hour} \cdot F}{CL} \qquad \text{(Eq. 1)}$$

where F is the oral availability and CL the total drug clearance. The infant dose (mg/kg/day) is then calculated from[4]:

$$D_{inf} = C^{ss} \cdot M/P_{AUC} \cdot V_{milk} \qquad \text{(Eq. 2)}$$

where $V_{milk}$ is the volume of milk ingested (usually 150 ml/kg/day).

*Percentage maternal dose:* the infant dose can be compared with the maternal dose ($D_{mat}$) on a mg/kg basis as an index of comparative exposure to the drug:

$$\text{Percentage } D_{mat} = \frac{D_{inf}}{D_{mat}} \cdot 100 \qquad \text{(Eq. 3)}$$

*Comments:* in this column, doses used therapeutically in infants are included, so that comparisons can be made with doses ingested via milk. Other notes are self-explanatory.

*Infant concentrations:* the final $C^{ss}$ achieved in infants is determined by the dose rate, oral availability (F) and clearance (CL) in the infant, as in Equation 1. Any differences in F or CL between mother and infant will be reflected in different $C^{ss}$ values relative to dose. Although the literature on the subject is sparse, there is little to indicate that F values in infants differ enough to be an important consideration. In order to err on the side of safety, we have assumed total oral availability (i.e. F = 1) in our calculations. CL, however, is subject to considerable change during the early period of infant maturation. In infants aged 28 to 34 weeks postconceptual age, CL can be as little as one-tenth of adult values; at 34 to 40 weeks, one-third; at 40 to 44 weeks, one-half; and at 44 to 68 weeks, two-thirds of adult values (per kg). Adult values of CL are approximated at postconceptual ages of >68 weeks. This means that concentrations in infants might be 10, 3, 2 or 1.5 times higher than maternal concentrations, relative to the same dose, in these age groups (for a detailed review, see Atkinson et al.[1]).

### 1.2 Table II

Table II is a quick reference table in which all the above considerations have been incorporated.

- Drugs rated **'1'** are probably safe for the infant during breast feeding, on the basis that maximum plasma concentrations in the infant are likely to be <10% of maternal plasma concentrations.
- Drugs rated **'2'** might, under some circumstances, achieve infant plasma concentrations up to 50% of maternal values. While this may be too high for the drug to be recommended as safe during breast feeding, there should be some flexibility in this group. The risk : benefit ratio must be considered in each individual case.
- Drugs rated **'3'** are probably not safe for the infant during breast feeding, because infant plasma concentrations may approach and (rarely) exceed those of the mother.
- Drugs rated **'4'** should be avoided because they are particularly toxic and the risk : benefit ratio is too unfavourable for the infant.
- Drugs rated **'5'** are contraindicated in infants with known or likely deficiency of glucose-6-phosphate dehydrogenase (G6PD).

## 2. Limitations

The decision that infant concentrations of <10% of maternal concentrations are tolerable is somewhat arbitrary, and has no scientific basis. The mother is (usually) receiving her drugs because of a therapeutic need, while the infant does not require the drug at all (an 'innocent bystander'). We have selected 10% as a practical cut-off limit, but more studies are needed to clarify this issue.

The non-inclusion of drugs in the tables is due to the absence of reliable data. Those that do not have a reliable M/P estimate (e.g. those with single time-point estimates only) have not been included. Studies involving such drugs could, however, be useful in making decisions about individual cases, using the equations above to estimate likely infant exposure. If there is absolutely no information about the distribution into breast milk of a particular drug, it is recommended that an alternative drug from the same class is used, chosen on the basis of information provided in the tables.

Table II is based on the regular use of standard doses. Where doses are unusually high, or uncontrolled (e.g. social drug abuse), erring on the side of caution is recommended. Isolated doses, as opposed to regular doses, pose less of a problem for the infant.

## 3. General Guidelines for Increasing Safety During Breast Feeding

It is always prudent to follow some general guidelines to increase the safety of drug use during breast feeding:

1) Feeding of the infant should take place just prior to the next dose of a drug, or as late as possible after drug ingestion.

2) For drugs labelled '2' in table II, alternating breast feeding with cow's milk or formula may enable the risk : benefit ratio to swing towards allowing breast feeding to continue.

3) During short courses of drugs that are considered unsafe during breast feeding, milk can be expressed and discarded and breast feeding resumed after the drug is discontinued (making allowance for clearance of the drug from the mother, e.g. a period of 4 half-lives after the last dose will bring maternal concentrations to <10% of steady-state concentrations).

**Table I.** Summary of reports quantifying the distribution of drugs into human breast milk

| Drug | No. of study participants | M/P$_{AUC}$ | $t_{max}$ milk (h) | Infant dose (per kg/day) | % Maternal dose | Comments | Reference |
|---|---|---|---|---|---|---|---|
| **ACE (angiotensin-converting enzyme) inhibitors** | | | | | | | |
| Captopril | 12 | 0.031 | 3.8 | 0.705μg | 0.014* | *$C_{milk}$ reported as unbound drug, which would be an underestimation of dose | 5 |
| Enalapril | 3 | ID | | 0.03μg* | <0.02 | *Measured as enalaprilat. Postdose $C_{milk}$ value <0.2 μg/L (detection limit) | 6 |
| | 5 | 0.02* | | 0.34μg | 0.1 | *Using estimated maternal plasma AUC | 7 |
| **β-Adrenoceptor antagonists** (β-blockers) | | | | | | | |
| Acebutolol | 3 | ID | | 0.618mg | 3.5 | | 8 |
| Atenolol | 7 | 4.5 | 6 | 0.26mg | 16 | | 9 |
| | 4 | 2.32 | 2-8 | 0.32mg | 19.2* | *Infant : maternal C ratios 0.04 to 0.67 | 10 |
| | 5 | ID | 1 | 95μg | 5.7* | *$C_{milk}$ measured at 2h. $t_{max}$ is probably greater (see above) | 11 |
| Dilevalol | 6 | 0.46 | 1 | 22μg | 0.3 | | 12 |
| Labetalol | 21 | ID | | 4.1-5.9μg (mean) | 0.07 | | 13 |
| | 3 | 1.5 | 2.5 | 99μg | 0.5* | *Infant C <20 μg/L (detection limit) and 21 μg/L (n = 1) | 14 |
| Mepindolol | 5 | ID | | 3.7μg | 1.1* | *Infant C undetectable (n = 4). Infant : maternal C ratio = 0.05 (n = 1) | 15 |
| Metoprolol | 8 | ID | | 58μg | 1.7* | *Mean infant : maternal C ratio = 0.044 | 16 |
| | 3 | 2.81 | 2-6 | 30μg | 1.8* | *Infant C <2.7 μg/L (n = 3) | 10 |
| | 3 | 3.6 | | 54.6μg | 3.3 | | 9 |
| | 9 | ID | | 63μg | 1.9 | | 17 |
| Nadolol | 12 | 4.6 | 6 | 66μg | 5.1 | | 18 |
| Oxprenolol | 12 | 0.29* | | 71μg | 0.45-0.70 | *Mean M/P ratio (n = 3) | 19 |
| | 9 | 0.45* | | 61μg | 1.5 | *Mean M/P ratio (n = 9) | 20 |
| Propranolol | 5 | ID | | 4μg | 0.3 | | 11 |
| | 1 | 0.76 | 2-3 | 6.3μg | 0.24 | | 21 |
| | 1 | 0.32 | 2-3 | 1.4μg | 0.2 | | 22 |
| | 3 | ID | 2.8-5 | 11.2μg | 0.9 | | 23 |
| Sotalol | 5 | ID | | 1.6mg | 22* | *No bradycardia noted in suckling infants | 24 |
| Timolol | 11 | ID | | 13.2μg | 3.3 | | 19 |
| Timolol eye drops | 1 | ID | | 0.75μg | | | 25 |
| **Anaesthetics, local** | | | | | | | |
| Bupivacaine | 1 | ID | | 0.17mg | 1.7 | | 26 |
| **Analgesics** | | | | | | | |
| Butorphanol | 6* | ID | 1 | 0.23μg | 0.7 | *IM dose | 27 |
| | 6 | ID | 1 | 0.54μg | 0.4 | | 27 |
| Codeine | 1 | 2.16 | 1.5 | 68μg* | 6.8 | *Infant therapeutic dose 1-3 mg/kg/day | 28 |
| Dextropropoxyphene | 6 | 0.4* | 2 | 42μg | 0.6 | *Norpropoxyphene also 0.4 | 29 |
| Methadone | 2 | 0.47* | | 10.5μg | 2.2 | *M/P ratio, but milk concentrations approximately parallel plasma concentrations | 30 |
| Morphine | 1 | 2.46 | | 2.9μg* (mean) | 0.4** | *Infant therapeutic dose 100-200 μg/kg/dose SC or IV<br>**Drug given as codeine, with the morphine metabolite measured, and assuming 100% conversion of codeine to morphine | 28 |
| | 5 | 2.45 | 0.75 | 37.5μg | 2.5 | | 31 |
| Nalbuphine | 7 | 0.46 | | 0.8μg (mean) | 0.2 | | 32 |
| Nefopam | 5 | ID | | 22μg (mean) | 0.4 | | 33 |
| Paracetamol (acetaminophen) | 1 | 0.81* | | 0.133mg (mean)** | 2.9 | *Drug given as phenacetin, with paracetamol metabolite measured assuming 100% conversion<br>**Infant therapeutic dose 30-40 mg/kg/day | 28 |
| | 3 | 0.76 | 2 | 0.66mg | 7.9 | | 34 |
| • *Nonsteroidal anti-inflammatory drugs (NSAIDs)* | | | | | | | |
| Azapropazone | 4 | 0.003 | 4 | 0.4mg | 1.5 | | 35 |
| Fenbufen | 15 | 0* | | <0.075mg | <0.75 | *$C_{milk}$ 0.5 mg/L (limit of assay sensitivity) | 36 |
| Flufenamic acid | 10 | ID | | 18μg | 0.1 | | 37 |

*[Continued over]*

*For abbreviations and symbols, see final page of table (p. 1713)*

**Table I.** *[Continued]*

| Drug | No. of study participants | $M/P_{AUC}$ | $t_{max}$ milk (h) | Infant dose (per kg/day) | % Maternal dose | Comments | Reference |
|---|---|---|---|---|---|---|---|
| **Analgesics** *[continued]* | | | | | | | |
| Flurbiprofen | 10 | 0.02 | 3 | 13.8μg (mean) | 0.8 | | 38 |
| | 12 | ID | | 12μg | 0.5 | | 39 |
| Ibuprofen | 12 | 0* | | <1.15mg | <0.6 | *$C_{milk}$ <1 mg/L (limit of assay sensitivity) | 40 |
| Indomethacin | 16 | 0.37* | | <17μg | <1 | *Mean of multiple single point estimations | 41 |
| Indoprofen | 4 | ID | | 102μg | 0.6 | | 42 |
| Ketorolac | 10 | <0.037* | | <2mg | <0.4 | | 43 |
| Mefenamic acid | 10 | ID | | 4.5μg | 0.3 | | 44 |
| Naproxen | 1 | ID | 4 | 0.134mg | 1.1 | | 45 |
| Piroxicam | 2 | ID* | | 33μg | 5-10** | *Mean M/P ratio + 0.012 ± 0.002 (n = 3)<br>**None detected in plasma of 1 infant | 46 |
| Salicylate | 1 | 0.05 | 3 | 0.168mg | 2.2 | | 28 |
| | 1 | ID | 3 | 1.5mg | 1.5-4.6 | | 47 |
| | 6 | ID | 2.6 | 7mg | 4 | | 48 |
| Suprofen | 6 | 0.014 | 1-2 | 24μg | 0.7 | | 49 |
| Tolmetin | 1 | 0.0055 | 1 | 21μg | 0.3 | | 50 |
| **Antianxiety drugs/hypnosedatives** | | | | | | | |
| • *Benzodiazepines* | | | | | | | |
| Clorazepate (dipotassium clorazepate) | 7 | ID | | 2.3μg* | ID** | *$C_{milk}$ values measured as clorazepate and nordazepam 'equivalents'. Sampling times not specified and $C_{milk}$ values may be greater<br>**Infant : maternal C ratio (mean) = 0.14 in infants where $C_{inf}$ > detectable limit | 51 |
| Diazepam | 4 | 0.16* | | 3.3μg | 2.0 | *Mean M/P = 0.16, some variation | 52 |
| | 3 | ID | | 11.7μg | 2.3 | | 53 |
| Flunitrazepam | 5 | 0.39 | <2 | 0.12μg | 0.6 | | 54 |
| Lorazepam | 4 | ID | | 1.3μg* | 2.2 | *$C_{milk}$ values reported as unbound concentrations | 55 |
| Lormetazepam | 4 | ≈0 | | <30mg | <0.1 | | 56 |
| Metaclazepam | 10 | 0.3 | | <30μg | 6 | | 57 |
| Midazolam | 2 | 0.16 | 2 | <0.5μg | 0.7 | | 58 |
| Nitrazepam | 1 | ID | | 15μg* | ID | *$C_{milk}$ values measured as nitrazepam and metabolites | 59 |
| | 12 | 0.27* | | 3μg | 3 | *Based on multiple paired samples, not AUC | 58 |
| Oxazepam | 1 | ID | 1.5 | 4.5μg | 0.9 | | 60 |
| Pinazepam | 9 | ID | | 1μg* | 1.4** | *$C_{milk}$ (pinazepam) exceeds detectable limit. Nordazepam (*N*-desmethyldiazepam) metabolite measured<br>**Assuming 100% conversion to metabolite. $C_{milk}$ measured 2 days after stopping drug. Infant exposure may be greater | 61 |
| Prazepam | 5 | 0.11* | 22** | 13.4μg** | 3.2† | *Mean M/P ratio, relatively constant<br>**Metabolite nordazepam (*N*-desmethyldiazepam) measured<br>†Assuming 100% conversion to metabolite | 62 |
| Quazepam | 4 | 4.13 | 3 | 14.4μg | 5.8 | | 63 |
| • *Others* | | | | | | | |
| Chloral hydrate | 50 | ID | | 0.47mg* | 2.0 | *Infant therapeutic dose 15-50 mg/kg/day. Maternal dose administered as 1.3g suppository | 64 |
| Clomethiazole (chlormethiazole) | 4 | 0.73 | | 0.5mg* | 1.2**† | *$C_{milk}$ values reported as μg/g milk. Converted to volume terms using density of milk.<br>**Maternal dose adjusted to allow for dosage form, chlormethiazole edisylate<br>†Infant : maternal C ratios <0.02 | 65 |
| Glutethimide | 13 | ID | 8-12 | 41μg* | 0.5 | *No $C_{milk}$ values measured before 8h | 66 |
| Trichloroethanol | 50 | ID | 0.75-6 (variable) | 0.47mg | 2.4* | *Given as rectal chloral hydrate, assuming 100% conversion, to trichloroethanol | 64 |
| Zopiclone | 12 | 0.51 | 2.4 | 1.7μg | 4.1 | | 67,68 |

*For abbreviations and symbols, see final page of table (p. 1713)*

**Table I.** *[Continued]*

| Drug | No. of study participants | M/P$_{AUC}$ | $t_{max}^{milk}$ (h) | Infant dose (per kg/day) | % Maternal dose | Comments | Reference |
|---|---|---|---|---|---|---|---|
| **Antiarrhythmic drugs** | | | | | | | |
| Acecainide (*N*-acetylprocainamide) | 1 | 2.86 | | 0.8mg | 2* | *Metabolite of procainamide. Assuming 100% conversion to metabolite | 69 |
| Amiodarone | 1 | ID | | 2.5mg | 37*† | *Infant : maternal C ratio = 0.4 †Desethyl metabolite excreted in milk. Infant : maternal C ratio = 0.15 | 70 |
| Disopyramide | 1 | ID | | 0.66mg | 6.6* | *Disopyramide and metabolite undetectable in infant plasma | 71 |
| | 1 | ID | | 0.26mg | 3.1* | *Infant C <650 μg/L (detection limit) | 72 |
| Flecainide | 1 | ID | | 0.16mg | 5 | | 73 |
| Lidocaine (lignocaine) | 1 | ID | | 0.12mg | 0.34 | | 74 |
| Mexiletine | 1 | ID | | 0.12mg | 0.6* | *Infant C <0.05 mg/L (n = 2) | 75 |
| | 1 | 1.48 | | 0.158mg | 1.6 | | 76 |
| Procainamide | 1 | 3.2 | | 1.5mg* | 4.5 | *Infant therapeutic dose 50 mg/kg/day | 69 |
| Quinidine | 1 | ID | | 1.23mg* | 4.1 | *Infant therapeutic dose 30 mg/kg/day | 77 |
| **Antibacterial drugs** | | | | | | | |
| • *Aminoglycosides* | | | | | | | |
| Amikacin | 2-3 | ≈0 | 4-6 | * | | *Trace C$_{milk}$ values only | 78 |
| Gentamicin | 10 | 0.166* | 3-5 | 67.5** | 2.2 | *Calculated from data given. **Newborn serum concentration 0.41 μg/L | 79 |
| • *Cefalosporins* | | | | | | | |
| Cefaclor | 7 | ID | | 53μg* | 0.7 | *Infant therapeutic dose 20 mg/kg/day | 80 |
| Cefadroxil | 6 | ID | 5 | 0.19mg | 1.1 | | 81 |
| Cefalexin | 2-3 | 0.09 | 4 | 0.105mg* | 1.2 | *Infant therapeutic dose 100 mg/kg/day | 78 |
| | 6 | ID | 4 | 75μg | 0.5 | | 81 |
| Cefalothin | 6 | ID | 2 | 71mg | 0.4 | | 81 |
| Cefapirin | 6 | ID | 2 | 65μg* | 0.4 | | 81 |
| Cefazolin | 20 | ID | 3 | 0.23mg | 0.7 | | 82 |
| | | ID | | 24μg | 0.14* | *Milk concentration only measured at 1h, $t_{max}^{milk}$ may be <1h; % maternal dose may be greater | 83 |
| Cefmenoxime | 5 | ID | <12 | 0.26mg* | 1.6* | *C$_{milk}$ values measured 12-72h. $C_{milk}^{max}$ would be expected to occur before 12h postdose | 84 |
| Cefonicid | 10 | ID | | 24μg | 0.14* | *C$_{milk}$ values measured at 1h only. $C_{milk}^{max}$ would be expected to occur after 1h postdose | 83 |
| Cefotaxime | 12 | ID | 2 | 48μg | 0.3 | | 85 |
| Cefoxitin | 6 | ID | 1-4 | 53μg | 0.16 | | 86 |
| | 18 | ID | | 0.14mg* ** | 0.2 | *C$_{milk}$ <0.5 mg/L (limit assay sensitivity) for all samples except 1 **Infant therapeutic dose (>3 months) 80-160 mg/kg/day | 87 |
| Cefprozil | 9 | 0.6 | 6 | <1mg | 0.3 | | 88 |
| Cefradine | 6 | 0.2 | 1 | 93μg* | 0.005 | *Infant therapeutic dose 25-30 mg/kg/day | 89 |
| Ceftazidime | 11 | ID | 1 | 0.7mg | 0.7 | | 90 |
| Ceftriaxone | 20 | 0.04 | 4-7 | 0.11mg | 0.7 | | 91 |
| | 1 | 0.04 | 10 | 1.2mg | 4.7 | | 92 |
| Latamoxef (moxalactam) | 8 | ID | | 0.55mg | 0.6 | | 93 |
| • *Fluoroquinolones* | | | | | | | |
| Ciprofloxacin | 10 | 2.17 | <2 | 0.6mg | 4.8 | | 94 |
| Fleroxacin | 7 | 0.61 | 2.6 | 0.7mg | 10 | | 95 |
| Ofloxacin | 10 | 1.30 | <2 | 0.36mg | 5.4 | | 94 |
| Pefloxacin | 10 | 0.98 | <2 | 0.53mg | 8 | | 94 |
| • *Macrolides* | | | | | | | |
| Clarithromycin | 12 | 0.25 | 2.2 | 0.5mg | 1.8 | M/P hydroxy metabolite (active) 0.66 | 96 |
| Erythromycin | 2-3 | 0.41 | 4 | 0.180mg* | 2.1 | *Infant therapeutic dose 30-40 mg/kg/day | 78 |
| • *Penicillins* | | | | | | | |
| Amoxicillin | 6 | ID | 5 | 0.121mg* | 0.7 | *Infant therapeutic dose 20 mg/kg/day | 81 |

*[Continued over]*

*For abbreviations and symbols, see final page of table (p. 1713)*

**Table I.** *[Continued]*

| Drug | No. of study participants | M/P$_{AUC}$ | $t_{max}$ milk (h) | Infant dose (per kg/day) | % Maternal dose | Comments | Reference |
|---|---|---|---|---|---|---|---|
| **Antibacterial drugs** *[continued]* | | | | | | | |
| Ampicillin | 2-3 | 0.04 | 4-6 | 21µg* | 0.25 | *Infant therapeutic dose 50-100 mg/kg/day | 78 |
| | 10 | 0.23 | | 0.21mg | 2.5 | | 97 |
| Benzylpenicillin (penicillin G) | 2-3 | 0.37 | 2 | 45µg | 0.8 | *Infant therapeutic dose 10-50 mg/kg/day | 78 |
| Carbenicillin | 2-3 | 0.02 | 4 | 36µg | 0.001 | | 78 |
| Epicillin | 6 | 0.18 | 6 | 26µg | 0.08 | | 89 |
| Phenoxymethyl-penicillin (penicillin V) | 12 | ID | | 0.11mg* ** | 0.25 | *No significant differences observed in the *extent* of drug transfer into milk in mastitis patients compared with healthy controls<br>**Infant therapeutic dose 20-60 mg/kg/day | 98 |
| Pivampicillin | 6 | ID | | 0.14mg* ** | 0.37 | *Measured as ampicillin<br>**Infant therapeutic dose (ampicillin) 50-100 mg/kg/day | 99 |
| Ticarcillin | 2-3 | ≈0 | | <15µg | <0.09 | | 78 |
| • *Sulfonamides* | | | | | | | |
| Sulfasalazine | 3 | ID | | 0.41mg*;<br>11.5mg** | 1.2;<br>4.5** | *Infant therapeutic dose 50-100 mg/kg/day<br>**Assuming 100% conversion of sulfasalazine to sulfapyridine (SP) and 5-aminosalicylic acid | 100 |
| | 12 | ID | | | 7* | *As sulfapyridine; sulfasalazine detected in only 5/31 milk samples | 101 |
| • *Tetracyclines* | | | | | | | |
| Chlortetracycline | 8 | ID | | 0.15-0.3mg | 0.5-0.9 | | 102 |
| Minocycline | 1 | ID | | 0.12mg* | 3.6 | *Infant therapeutic dose (>8 years) 4 mg/kg/day | 103 |
| Tetracycline | 2-3 | 0.58 | 4 | 0.12mg | 4.8 | | 78 |
| • *Others* | | | | | | | |
| Aztreonam | 6 | 0.009;<br>0.005 | 6 IM;<br>4 IV | 45µg<br>33µg | 2.7<br>2.0 | | 104 |
| Chloramphenicol | 2-3 | 0.73 | 4-6 | 0.62mg* | 7.4 | *Infant therapeutic dose: 25 mg/kg/day (neonate), 50-70 mg/kg/day (infant) | 78 |
| | 4 | 0.58 | 2 | 0.49mg | 6 | | 105 |
| Clindamycin | 5 | 0.21 | | 0.21mg* | 2.8 | *Infant therapeutic dose 8-12 mg/kg/day | 106 |
| | 2-3 | 0.3 | 4 | 0.14mg | 5.4 | | 78 |
| Imipenem/cilastatin | 12 | | | | | | 107 |
| a) Imipenem | | ID | 2-4 | 0.28mg | 3.4 | | |
| b) Cilastatin | | ID | | <75µg | <0.9 | | |
| Lincomycin | 9 | ID | | 0.2mg | 0.6 | | 108 |
| Methenamine | 4 | ID | | 1.4mg* | 8.3 | *Infant therapeutic dose 20-50 mg/kg/day | 109 |
| Nalidixic acid | 13 | ID | | 0.10mg* (mean) | 0.3 | *Infant therapeutic dose 50-60 mg/kg/day | 110 |
| Nitrofurantoin | 9 | ID | | 0.08mg | 0.6 | | 111 |
| | * | ID | | <0.3mg** | <4.5 | *Number of patients not specified<br>**Infant therapeutic dose 6 mg/kg/day | 112 |
| | 6 | ID | | <0.3mg | <6 | | 113 |
| Rosaramicin | 10 | 0.12 | 2-4 | 6.7µg | 0.2 | | 114 |
| Thiamphenicol | 7 | 0.92 | 4 | 0.3mg | 3.6 | | 105 |
| **Anticoagulants** | | | | | | | |
| Phenprocoumon | 1 | ID | | 11.4µg* | | *Infant therapeutic dose 50µg/kg/day | 115 |
| Warfarin | 6 | ≈0 | | <3.75µg* | <4.4 | *$C_{milk}$ <25 µg/L (assay detection limit). Infant C <25 µg/L | 116 |
| **Antidepressants** | | | | | | | |
| Amfebutamone (bupropion) | 1 | 4.5 | 2 | 28µg | 0.6* | *None detected in infant | 117 |
| Amitriptyline | 1 | ID | | 16µg | 0.9 | | 118 |
| | 1 | ID | | 10.3µg | 0.6* | *Infant C <10 µg/L (limit of assay sensitivity) | 119 |
| | 1 | 0.83 | 1.5 | 15.5µg | 0.9 | | 120 |
| Amoxapine | 1 | ID | | <3mg | <0.07 | | 121 |
| Desipramine | 1 | ID | | 40.2µg | 1.0* | *Infant C <1 µg/L | 122 |

*For abbreviations and symbols, see final page of table (p. 1713)*

**Table I.** *[Continued]*

| Drug | No. of study participants | M/P$_{AUC}$ | $t_{max}$ milk (h) | Infant dose (per kg/day) | % Maternal dose | Comments | Reference |
|---|---|---|---|---|---|---|---|
| **Antidepressants** *[continued]* | | | | | | | |
| | 1 | ID | | 18μg | 0.5** | *Dose: Imipramine 200 mg/day. Desipramine is an active metabolite<br>**Assuming 100% conversion to desipramine | 123 |
| Dothiepin | 2 | ID | | 1.7μg | 0.2 | | 124 |
| | 8 | 0.8-1.6* | | 50μg | <1.5*† | *Fore- (0.8) and hind- (1.6) milk. Single point estimation.<br>†Infant C <10μg/L | 125 |
| Doxepin | 1 | ID | | 0.25μg | 0.01 | | 126 |
| Fluoxetine | 1 | ID | | 10.5μg* | 3* | *Fluoxetine + norfluoxetine | 127 |
| | 1 | ID | | 17.8μg* | 5.3* | *Fluoxetine + norfluoxetine | 128 |
| Imipramine | 1 | ID | 1 | 4.4μg | 0.13 | | 123 |
| Maprotiline | 1 | ID | | 39μg | 1.6 | | 129 |
| Mianserin | 2 | ID | | 12μg | 1.4 | | 130 |
| Moclobemide | 6 | 0.72 | <3 | 80μg | 1.6 | | 131 |
| Nortriptyline | 1 | ID | | 8.3μg* | 0.53**† | *Resulting from 100mg maternal dose of amitriptyline.<br>**Calculated assuming 100% conversion of amitriptyline to nortriptyline<br>†Infant C <10 μg/L | 119 |
| | 1 | ID | | 27μg* (mean) | 1.3 | *Infant therapeutic dose (>6 years) 1-2 mg/kg/day | 132 |
| Sertraline | 1 | ≈0.6 | 5 | 4.3μg | 0.26 | Undetectable in infant's serum | 133 |
| Trazodone | 6 | 0.14 | 2 | 9μg | 1.1 | | 134 |
| **Antidiabetic drugs** | | | | | | | |
| Tolbutamide | 2 | ID | | 3mg* | 18 | *Wide variations in milk concentrations after 500mg twice daily | 135 |
| **Antiemetics** | | | | | | | |
| Domperidone | 10 | ID | | 0.165μg | 0.05 | | 136 |
| Metoclopramide | 23 | ID | 1-2 | 24μg* | 4.7** | *Infant therapeutic dose 0.3-0.5 mg/kg/day<br>**1 in 5 infants had detectable C of 20 μg/L | 137 |
| | 10 | ID | | 19μg | 11.3 | | 138 |
| **Antiepileptic drugs** | | | | | | | |
| Carbamazepine | 1 | ID | | 0.39mg* (mean) | 4.9** | *Infant therapeutic dose 10-20 mg/kg/day<br>**Infant : maternal C = 0.52 | 139 |
| | 4 | 0.39* | | 0.75mg | 3.5-7.3** | *Based on multiple samples<br>**Infant : maternal steady-state C = 0.1-0.47 | 140 |
| | 16 | 0.36* | | 0.38mg (mean) | 2.8 | *Mean M/P ratio = 0.36 (n = 16) | 141 |
| Clonazepam | 1 | ID | | 2μg | 1.5-3** | *Infant therapeutic dose 20-200 μg/kg/day<br>**Maternal dose not specified. Assumed 4-8mg daily maintenance dose | 142 |
| Ethosuximide | 5 | 0.86* | | 7.4mg | 29.6** † | *Mean M/P ratio, relatively constant<br>**Maternal dose not specified, assumed 25 mg/kg/day<br>†Infant therapeutic dose 15-50 mg/kg/day | 143 |
| | | 0.79* | | 3.2mg | 13 | *Mean M/P ratio | 144 |
| Phenobarbital | 8 | ID* | | 1.56mg** | 23-156† | *Wide variation in M/P ratio<br>**Infant therapeutic dose 4-5 mg/kg/day<br>†Maternal dose not specified, assumed 1-6 mg/kg/day | 144 |
| | 6 | ID | | 2.2mg | 27-133* | Infant : maternal steady-state C = 0.48<br>*Maternal dose not specified, assumed 1.6mg/kg/day | 145 |
| Phenytoin | 6 | 0.13 | | 0.24mg* | 3.6-7.2** | *Therapeutic dose: 6-8 mg/kg/day (neonates), infants 8-10 mg/kg/day<br>**Detectable C in 2/6 infants: 0.12 and 0.18 mg/L (assay sensitivity 0.12 mg/L) | 146 |
| | | 0.18* | | 0.12mg | 3.0** | *Mean M/P ratio, relatively constant<br>**Maternal dose not specified, assumed 4-7 mg/kg/day | 144 |
| Primidone | 8 | 0.18* | | 0.35mg | 1.4-2.8** | *Mean M/P ratio, n = 12<br>**Maternal dose not specified, assumed 1-2 mg/kg/day | 144 |

*[Continued over]*

*For abbreviations and symbols, see final page of table (p. 1713)*

**Table I.** *[Continued]*

| Drug | No. of study participants | M/P$_{AUC}$ | $t_{max}$ milk (h) | Infant dose (per kg/day) | % Maternal dose | Comments | Reference |
|---|---|---|---|---|---|---|---|
| **Antiepileptic drugs** *[continued]* | | | | | | | |
| Primidone *[continued]* | 2 | ID | | | | Infant : maternal steady-state C = 0.1-0.25 | 145 |
| Valproic acid (sodium valproate) | 16 | 0.05* | | 0.27mg** | 1.8† | *Mean M/P ratio, relatively constant<br>**Therapeutic dose for neonates 20-40 mg/kg/day<br>†Infant : maternal C ratios <0.04-0.40 | 147 |
| **Antifungal drugs** | | | | | | | |
| Fluconazole | 1 | 0.75 | ≈ | 0.27mg | 11 | | 148 |
| **Antihistamines** (H$_1$-receptor antagonists) | | | | | | | |
| Clemastine | 1 | ID | | 1.5μg | 9* | *Likely to be greater as based on single milk sample 20 hours after the dose. Infant C <2mg/L. Child reported to be drowsy | 149 |
| Loratadine | 6 | 1.2 | 2 | 4.4μg | 0.7 | | 150 |
| Terfenadine | 4 | 0.21 | 4.25 | 0.01mg | 0.45 | Active metabolite only. No parent drug detected | 151 |
| Triprolidine | 3 | 0.53 | 1-2 | 0.36μg* (mean) | 0.9 | *Infant therapeutic dose 1.25 mg/kg/day | 152 |
| **Antihypertensive drugs** (see also ACE inhibitors, β-adrenoceptor antagonists, calcium antagonists and diuretics) | | | | | | | |
| Clonidine | 9 | ID | | 0.41μg | 7.8 | | 153 |
| Dihydralazine | 1 | ID | | 4.6μg | 0.3 | | 154 |
| Hydralazine | 1 | ID | | 20μg* | 0.8 | *Infant therapeutic dose 0.75-7.5 mg/kg/day | 155 |
| Methyldopa | 3 | ID | | 30μg | 0.09 | | 156 |
| | 3 | 0.22 | 4.5 | 0.17mg | 1.2 | | 157 |
| Minoxidil | 1 | 0.76 | 1 | 6.3μg | 2.5 | | 158 |
| **Antimalarial drugs** | | | | | | | |
| Chloroquine | 3 | 2.86 | | ID | 3.1* | *Authors concluded that it is very unlikely that low concentrations of chloroquine in milk would protect a breast-fed infant against malaria | 159 |
| | 6 | ID | 7 | 0.66mg | 11 | | 160 |
| | 5 | ID | 3 | 0.6mg | 12 | | 161 |
| | 6 | 0.36* | | 48μg** | 1 | *M/P ratios relatively constant<br>**Infant prophylactic dose 5 mg/kg once weekly | 162 |
| Dapsone | 3* | 0.35 | | ID | 9.6 | *Dapsone and pyrimethamine were coadministered as 'Maloprim' (see entry for pyrimethamine) | 159 |
| Hydroxychloroquine | 1 | ID | | 170μg (mean) | 3.3 | | 163 |
| | 1 | ID | | 1.6μg | 0.05* | *Milk sampled 15-48h after dose | 164 |
| Mefloquine | 2 | 0.15 | | 8μg | 0.2 | | 165 |
| Pyrimethamine | 3 | 5.46 | | ID | 30.2* | *Authors concluded that although significant amounts of pyrimethamine were excreted, protection against malaria would not be expected for a breast-fed infant | 159 |
| **Antineoplastic and immunosuppressive drugs** | | | | | | | |
| Azathioprine | 2 | ID | 2-8 | 2.7μg* | 1.2 | *C$_{milk}$ values measured as metabolite mercaptopurine | 166 |
| Cisplatin | 1 | ≈0 | | | <0.7* | *C$_{milk}$ below detectable limit, measured as platinum | 167 |
| | 1 | 0.06 | <1 | 22μg | 0.3 | | 168 |
| Cyclosporin | 1 | 1.9* | | 62μg** | | *Estimated at steady-state<br>**<5% of an immunosuppresive dose | 169 |
| Doxorubicin | 1 | | 24 | 19μg | 1.3 | | 167 |
| Hydroxycarbamide (hydroxyurea) | 1 | 10 | | 1.26mg* | 5 | *Milk sampled at 2h after dose. C$_{milk}$ may not represent a peak value | 170 |
| Methotrexate | 1 | 0.04 | 10 | 3.5μg | 0.93 | | 171 |
| **Antipsychotic drugs** | | | | | | | |
| Chlorpromazine | 1 | ID | 2 | 44μg* | 0.2 | *Single dose 1200mg. Infant therapeutic dose 2 mg/kg/day | 172 |

*For abbreviations and symbols, see final page of table (p. 1713)*

**Table I.** *[Continued]*

| Drug | No. of study participants | $M/P_{AUC}$ | $t_{max}^{milk}$ (h) | Infant dose (per kg/day) | % Maternal dose | Comments | Reference |
|---|---|---|---|---|---|---|---|
| **Antipsychotic drugs** *[continued]* | | | | | | | |
| Chlorprothixene | 1 | 1.6 | 4 | 31μg | 0.3 | | 173 |
| Flupenthixol | 2 | ID | | 0.22μg* | 0.46 | *After IM depot preparation | 174 |
| | 1 | ID | | 0.27μg | 0.8 | | 174 |
| | 1 | ID | | 0.42μg (mean) | 0.63* | *Infant C <0.2 μg/L and 0.3 μg/L | 132 |
| Haloperidol | 1 | ID | | 3.2μg | 2* | *Infant urine concentration 1.5 μg/L | 175 |
| | 1 | ID | | 0.75μg | 0.15 | | 176 |
| Lithium | 1 | 0.42* | | 0.41mg | 1.8** | *Based on a review of the literature M/P ratios (n = 6)<br>**Calculated assuming maternal dose of 20-25 mg/kg/day | 177 |
| Perphenazine | 1 | 0.8 | | 0.5μg | 0.1 | | 178 |
| Sulpiride | 20 | ID | | 0.15mg* | 9 | *$C_{milk}$ values measured 2h postdose | 179 |
| | 45 | ID | | 0.22mg* | 13.2 | *$C_{milk}$ values measured 4h postdose. $t_{max}^{milk}$ may be greater | 180 |
| Zuclopenthixol | 5 | ID | | 0.3μg* | 0.5 | *Predose $C_{milk}$ value. Likely to represent the minimum dose | 181 |
| | 1 | ID | | 1.4μg* | 1.6 | *Dose: 72mg IM/2 weeks | 181 |
| | 1 | ID | | 3μg (mean) | 1.3 | | 132 |
| **Antithyroid and thyroid drugs** | | | | | | | |
| Carbimazole | 1 | 0.9 | 1 | 45μg | 27 | | 182 |
| | 1 | ID | | 6.5μg | ID* | *Infant Cs (n = 2), 45 and 52 μg/L compared with C associated with adult thyroid suppression of 50-100 μg/L | 183 |
| Liothyronine (triiodothyronine) | 12 | ID | | 0.116μg | 11.6 | | 184 |
| Propylthiouracil | 9 | ID | 1.5 | 0.12μg (mean) | 1.8 | | 187 |
| | 1 | 0.23 | 1-6 | 45μg | 2.6 | | 182 |
| Thiamazole (methimazole) | 1 | ID | | 10μg* | 12 | *Infant therapeutic dose 200 μg/kg/day. Maternal dose 2.5mg twice daily | 185 |
| | 4 | 1.03* | 1 | 0.11μg (mean) | 16.6 | *Mean M/P ratio | 186 |
| Thiouracil | 2 | ID | | 18mg | 113 | | 188 |
| Thyroxine | 16 | ID | | 0.17μg* ** (mean) | 5.9-11.8† | *Measured as $T_3$. Thyroxine ($T_4$) converted to $T_3$ (active). $C_{milk}$ ($T_4$) <7 μg/L (limit assay sensitivity)<br>**Infant therapeutic dose (0-6 months) 8-10 μg/kg/day<br>†Infant thyroxine dose > adult dose $D_{inf}$ represents only 2.5% of infant therapeutic dose | 189 |
| | 12 | ID | | <0.04μg | <1.6 | | 184 |
| **Antitrichomonal drugs** | | | | | | | |
| Metronidazole | 3 | ID | 2-4 | 8.7mg | 0.4 | | 190 |
| | 15 | 0.98* | | 2.2mg** | 11† | *M/P ratios relatively constant<br>**Infant therapeutic dose 15-35 mg/kg/day<br>†Infant : maternal C ratio 0.13 and 0.1 (n = 2) | 191 |
| | 8 | ID | 0.5 | 3.75mg | 0.13 | | 192 |
| | 10 | 1.08 | 4 | 1.2mg | 36* | *Detectable C in 5 infants; simultaneous infant : maternal Cs = 0.14 (range 0.02-0.21); remaining infant C <0.05 mg/L | 193 |
| | 12 | 0.91* | 2 | 2.3mg | 11.5** | *Mean M/P ratio, relatively constant<br>**Infant : maternal C ratio (mean) = 0.125 | 194 |
| Tinidazole | 5 | ID | | 0.27mg (mean) | 1 | | 195 |
| | 24 | ID | | 0.9mg* ** | 11 | *Milk sampled at 12 and 24h postdose $C_{milk}^{max}$ would be expected to occur before 12h postdose<br>**Infant therapeutic dose 50 mg/kg (single) | 196 |

*[Continued over]*

*For abbreviations and symbols, see final page of table (p. 1713)*

**Table I.** *[Continued]*

| Drug | No. of study participants | M/P$_{AUC}$ | $t_{max}$ milk (h) | Infant dose (per kg/day) | % Maternal dose | Comments | Reference |
|---|---|---|---|---|---|---|---|
| **Antituberculosis drugs** | | | | | | | |
| Aminosalicylic acid (*p*-aminosalicylic acid) | 1 | ID | 3 | 0.17mg* | 0.25 | *Infant therapeutic dose 200 mg/kg/day | 197 |
| Isoniazid | 1 | ID* | 3 | 2.5mg | 50 | *Drug appears to concentrate in milk | 198 |
| Pyrazinamide | 1 | ID | 3 | 0.23mg* | 1.4 | *Infant therapeutic dose 30 mg/kg/day | 197 |
| **Antiulcer drugs** | | | | | | | |
| Cimetidine | 1 | 1.7* | | 0.9mg | 5.4 | *Variable M/P ratios reported | 199 |
| | 12 | 5.77 | 3.3 | 1-1.5mg | 6.7 | Active transport into milk | 200 |
| Famotidine | 8 | 1.5* | 6 | 11μg | 1.6 | *Estimated from data given | 201 |
| Nizatidine | 3 | 1.2 | 1-2 | 0.1mg | 4 | | 202 |
| Ranitidine | 6 | 2.8* | Variable | 0.5mg | 5** | *Medium (range 1-13) **Median | 203 |
| | 1 | ID | 5.5 | 0.4mg | 7.8 | | 204 |
| Roxatidine | 1 | | | 0.15mg | 4 | | 205 |
| **Antiviral drugs** | | | | | | | |
| Aciclovir | 1 | ID | >3 | 0.196mg | 1.2 | | 206 |
| | 1 | ID | 4 | 0.2mg* | 1.1 | *Infant therapeutic dose 15-30 mg/kg/day | 207 |
| **Bronchodilators** | | | | | | | |
| Diprophylline (dyphylline) | 20 | 2.08 | <2-4 | 2.12mg** | 42 | *Estimate only. Assumed $t_{max}$ = 2h and $C_{milk}$ calculated from C and M/P$_{AUC}$ **$C_{milk}$ and C parallel. Infant therapeutic dose (>6 years) 6-11 mg/kg/day | 208 |
| Enprofylline | 6 | 0.81* | | 1.32mg (mean) | 2.2 | *Mean M/P ratio, relatively constant | 209 |
| Pseudoephedrine | 3 | 2.5 | 1-1.5 | 40μg* | 4 | *Infant therapeutic dose 2.5-4 mg/kg/day | 151 |
| Terbutaline | 2 | ID | Variable | 0.6μg | 0.5 | | 210 |
| | 2 | 1.04 | | 0.6μg | 0.24* | *Infant C <0.1 μg/L (n = 1) | 211 |
| | 4 | ID | Variable | 0.70μg | 0.6* | *Infant C <0.1 μg/L (n = 1) | 212 |
| Theophylline | 3 | 0.67 | | 1-2mg* | 19-63** | *Infant therapeutic dose 5-20 mg/kg/day; neonatal dose 3-6 mg/kg/day **$C_{milk}$ not specified, assumed maternal C of 10-20 mg/L | 213 |
| | 4 | 0.76 | 1-3 | 1.1-2.3mg | 8-54* | *$C_{milk}$ not specified, assumed maternal C of 10-20 mg/L | 214 |
| **Calcium antagonists** | | | | | | | |
| Diltiazem | 1 | 0.98 | 2-3 | 34μg | 0.9 | | 215 |
| Nifedipine | 1 | 0.74 | 1 | 7μg | 0.8 | | 216 |
| | 1 | ID | 1 | 7.5μg | 1.2 | | 217 |
| Nitrendipine | 3 | 0.8 | 1-2 | 0.4μg | 0.1 | | 218 |
| Nimodipine | | 0.25* | | 0.25μg | <0.1 | *Mean of 7 single points | 219 |
| Tiapamil | 6 | 0.44 | <1 | 18μg | 0.2 | | 220 |
| Verapamil | 1 | ID | | 25μg | 0.42 | | 221 |
| | 1 | ID | | 5.7μg | 0.14 | | 222 |
| | 1 | ID | 1.5 | 45μg | 0.84 | | 223 |
| | 1 | 0.60 | 1 | 11.9μg* | 0.3** | *Infant therapeutic dose 0.5-1 mg/kg IV (single dose) **Infant C <1 μg/L for verapamil and norverapamil | 224 |
| **Cardiac glycosides** | | | | | | | |
| Digoxin | 2 | ID | 4-6 | 0.12μg | 2.9* | *Infant C <0.1 μg/L (n = 2) | 225 |
| | 5 | 0.86* | | 0.1μg (mean) | 2.3 | *Mean M/P ratio | 226 |
| | 11 | 0.55 | | 97ng (mean) | 2.3 | | 227 |
| | 1 | ID | | 0.29μg | 2.3* | *Infant : maternal C ratio = 0.095 | 228 |
| | 11 | 0.62 | | 0.45μg* | 5.6 | *Maximum, after 0.5mg IV to mother | 229 |

*For abbreviations and symbols, see final page of table (p. 1713)*

**Table I.** *[Continued]*

| Drug | No. of study participants | M/P$_{AUC}$ | $t_{max}$ milk (h) | Infant dose (per kg/day) | % Maternal dose | Comments | Reference |
|---|---|---|---|---|---|---|---|
| **Corticosteroids** | | | | | | | |
| Methylprednisolone | 1 | ID | 8 | 1.13μg* | 1.1 | *Infant dose (physiological effect 0.12 mg/kg/day; pharmacological effect 2.42-1.67 mg/kg/day) | 166 |
| Prednisolone | 6 | 0.13 | 1 | 0.148μg*† | 3.6 | *For high dose, i.e. 80 mg/kg/day. M/P$_{AUC}$ increased with dose, possibly due to increased plasma unbound fraction of prednisolone with increasing dose †Infant therapeutic dose 0.35-2 mg/kg/day | 230 |
| | 7 | ID | | 2.6ng | 3.1 | | 231 |
| | 3 | 0.25 | | 12μg* | 1.4 | *After 50mg IV | 232 |
| Prednisone | 1 | ID | | 4.3ng* | 0.26 | *Combined prednisone and active metabolite of prednisolone | 233 |
| **Diagnostic agents** | | | | | | | |
| Diatrizoic acid | 1 | ID | | <0.3mg* | <0.05 | *C$_{milk}$ <2 mg/L (detection limit) | 234 |
| Iodamide | 1 | ID | | <0.3mg* | <0.06 | *C$_{milk}$ <2 mg/L (detection limit) | 234 |
| Iohexol | 3 | ID | 3-6 | 6.8mg | 0.9 | | 235 |
| Iopanoic acid | 11 | ID | 15 | 7.5mg | 11.2 | | 236 |
| Metrizamide | 1 | ID | | * | | *Maternal dose 5.06g to subarachnoid space; 0.65mg excreted in milk over 24h | 237 |
| Sodium metrizoate | 2 | ID | 1.5-6 | 2.7mg | 0.5 | | 235 |
| **Diuretics** | | | | | | | |
| Acetazolamide | 1 | 0.3* | | 315μg** | 1.9 | *Mean M/P ratio **Infant therapeutic dose 5 mg/kg/day | 238 |
| Chlorothiazide | 11 | ID | | <0.15mg* | <1.8 | *C$_{milk}$ <1 mg/L (detection limit) | 239 |
| Chlorthalidone | 7 | ID | | 56μg* | 6.7 | *Infant therapeutic dose 2mg 3 times/week | 240 |
| Hydrochlorothiazide | 1 | 1.03 | 3-4 | 18μg* | 2.2 | *Infant therapeutic dose (<6 months) 3 mg/kg/day | 241 |
| Spironolactone | 1 | ID | | 15.6μg | 1.2* | *Measured as canrenone (active metabolite) assuming 100% conversion from spironolactone | 242 |
| **Estrogens and progestagens** | | | | | | | |
| Estradiol | 6 | ID | Variable 3-11 | 0.15μg* | 0.004 | *Dose as 50 or 100mg suppository | 243 |
| Ethinylestradiol | 4 | ID | | 2.3ng | 0.3 | | 243 |
| Levonorgestrel | 10 | ID | | 8.6ng | | | 244 |
| | 100 | ID | | 18ng* | 1.1 | *Dose 100 μg/day implant | 245 |
| Lynestrenol | 6 | ID | | 0.5μg | 0.6 | | 246 |
| Medroxyprogesterone | 10 | 0.72 | | 1μg | 3.4* | *IM depot injection with assumption of constant release of drug from depot | 247 |
| | 6 | ID | | 1.5μg | 5* | *IM depot injection with assumption of constant release of drug from depot | 247 |
| | 7 | ID | | 261ng | 0.87 | | 248 |
| Mestranol | 4 | ID | | 36ng | 1.4 | | 249 |
| Norethisterone (norethindrone) | 5 | ID | | 36ng* | | *Maternal dose = 40mg silastic implant | 250 |
| | 20 | 0.26* | | 0.75μg | 0.02** | *Mean M/P ratio (n = 77) **Dose deep IM injection | 251 |
| | 5 | 0.19 | | 0.112μg | 1.9 | | 248 |
| | 5 | 0.35 | | 1.2μg | 2 | | 247 |
| | 12 | 0.18 | 4-8 | 2.2μg | 0.26 | Infant : maternal C ratio 0.12 | 252 |
| Norgestrel | 15 | ID | | 0.117μg | 2.8* | *Infant : maternal C ratio 0.023 (n = 2) | 253 |
| **Hypoglycaemic drugs** (see antidiabetic drugs) | | | | | | | |
| **Lipid-lowering drugs** | | | | | | | |
| Pravastatin | 11 | 0.16 (0.26)* | 3.3 (3.4)* | 1μg | <0.4 | *Values for the isomeric metabolite. Negligible secretion in breast milk | 254 |

*[Continued over]*

*For abbreviations and symbols, see final page of table (p. 1713)*

**Table I.** *[Continued]*

| Drug | No. of study participants | M/P$_{AUC}$ | $t_{max}$ $^{milk}$ (h) | Infant dose (per kg/day) | % Maternal dose | Comments | Reference |
|---|---|---|---|---|---|---|---|
| **Radiopharmaceuticals** | | | | | | *See Mountford & Coakley [255] for guidelines for breast feeding following radiopharmaceutical administration. The following comments are the recommendations of these authors | |
| Chromic $^{32}$P-phosphate | | | | | | Discontinue breast feeding | |
| $^{67}$Ga-Gallium citrate | | | | | | Discontinue breast feeding | |
| $^{125}$I-Fibrinogen | | | | | | Discontinue breast feeding | |
| $^{125}$I-MAA | | | | | | Discontinue breast feeding | |
| Na$^{131}$I | | | | | | Discontinue breast feeding | |
| $^{75}$Se-Methionine | | | | | | Discontinue breast feeding | |
| Sodium $^{32}$P-phosphate | | | | | | Discontinue breast feeding | |
| $^{125}$I-Hippuran | | | | | | Discontinue breast feeding for 24h | |
| $^{131}$I-Hippuran | | | | | | Discontinue breast feeding for 24h | |
| Sodium $^{89m}$Tc-pertechnatate | | | | | | Discontinue breast feeding for 12h | |
| $^{99m}$Tc-MAA | | | | | | Discontinue breast feeding for 6h | |
| $^{51}$Cr-Edetic acid | | | | | | Discontinue breast feeding for 4h | |
| $^{111}$In-Leucocytes | | | | | | Discontinue breast feeding for 4h | |
| $^{99m}$Tc-DTPA | | | | | | Discontinue breast feeding for 4h | |
| $^{99m}$Tc-Edetic acid | | | | | | Discontinue breast feeding for 4h | |
| $^{99m}$Tc-MDP | | | | | | Discontinue breast feeding for 4h | |
| $^{99m}$Tc-Erythrocytes | | | | | | Discontinue breast feeding for 4h | |
| **Miscellaneous drugs** | | | | | | | |
| Baclofen | 1 | 0.66 | 4 | 18μg | 5.4 | | 256 |
| Carbetocin | 5 | 0.02 | 2 | ≈1ng* | 0.08* | *Single dose | 257 |
| Cyproterone | 6 | 0.39 | | 39μg | 0.9 | | 258 |
| Fluoride (sodium fluoride) | 1 | ID | 2 | 0.86mg* ** | | *Dose includes base fluoride concentration contained in milk after high dose fluoride, NaF 25 mg/day. Low dose NaF 1.5 mg/day in 5 women did not result in a demonstrable increase in breast milk fluoride concentrations over background concentrations. **Recommended dose of fluoride in infants <6 months is 0.55 mg/day in areas without fluoridation | 259 |
| Gold salts (e.g. sodium aurothiomalate) | 1 | ID | | 3.3μg* | 5.5** | *Based on milk concentration 66h after final dose of a course of a single 20mg dose, followed by 7 weekly 50mg doses of IM sodium aurothiomalate **Infant urine gold concentration 0.4 μg/L at 66h and <0.4 μg/L after 5 weeks. | 260 |
| | 2 | ID | 17-69 | 28μg* | 8.4 | *After 50mg total dose of IV aurothiomalate | 261 |
| Iodine | 1 | ID | | 82.5μg | 9.9** | *Concentrated in milk. Single M/P ratio = 6.3 **After 50mg free iodine applied topically to vagina, assuming complete absorption | 262 |
| Ivermectin | 4 | 0.57* | 4-6 | 2.75μg | 1.8 | *Calculated from data given | 263 |
| Magnesium sulfate | 1 | ID | | 2.4mg* | 0.5 | *$MgSO_4$ given as 4g loading dose and 1 g/h for 24h IV. Infant dose calculated above background $MgSO_4$ content in milk | 264 |
| Methylergometrine | 8 | ID | | 0.2μg | 4.6 | | 265 |
| Noscapine | 8 | 0.37 | 1-2 | 8.3μg | 0.5 | | 266 |
| Pentoxifylline (oxpentifylline) | 5 | 0.87* | | 11μg | 0.2 | *Based on 4-hour sample pairings | 267 |
| Praziquantel | 5 | 0.32 | 2-3 | 0.06mg | 0.1 | Milk concentrations parallel plasma | 268 |
| Pyridostigmine | 2 | 0.66* | 3.5-4 | 3.8μg** | 0.05-0.12 | *Measured M/P ratios **Infant C <2 μg/L after maternal dose of 60mg 5 times/day (n = 2) | 269 |
| Sennosides A & B ('Senokot') | 25 | * | | * | | *$C_{milk}$ <0.34 mg/L as sennosides A and B (minimum detection level) | 270 |
| Tranexamic acid | 1 | ID | | 12μg | 0.012-0.024 | *Maternal dose not stated. Assumed to be 1-1.5g 3-4 times daily | 271 |
| **Miscellaneous 'social' drugs** | | | | | | | |
| Amphetamine | 1 | ID* | | 20.7μg | 6.2 | *Mean M/P ratio = 5 | 272 |

*For abbreviations and symbols, see final page of table (p. 1713)*

**Table I.** *[Continued]*

| Drug | No. of study participants | $M/P_{AUC}$ | $t_{max}^{milk}$ (h) | Infant dose (per kg/day) | % Maternal dose | Comments | Reference |
|---|---|---|---|---|---|---|---|
| **Miscellaneous 'social' drugs** *[continued]* | | | | | | | |
| Caffeine | 5 | 0.51 | 0.5 | 0.24mg | 9.6 | | 273 |
| | 1 | ID | | 0.17mg | 0.63* | *Maternal dose 20 cups of coffee/day. Estimated caffeine intake 1600 mg/day | 47 |
| | 6 | 0.83 | 1.5 | 0.35mg | 21 | | 274 |
| | 1 | 0.76 | 2.2 | 0.33mg | 13.2 | | 275 |
| Cocaine | 1 | 10 | | 3.8μg* ** | ID† | *Maternal dose: a 'dab' of cocaine applied to the gum *$C_{milk}$ values measured 12-60h postdose $t_{max}^{milk}$ would be expected to be 12h †Infant had clinical signs of cocaine toxicity | 276 |
| Ethanol | 12 | 0.89 | 1 | 117mg | 4 | 0.6g/kg to mother | 277 |
| | 11 | 0.93* | | 60mg | 3 | *Milk and plasma concentrations parallel | 278 |
| Nicotine | 23 | 2.92* | | 9.3μg** | ID | *Mean M/P ratio **Highest milk concentration | 279 |
| | 54 | ID | | 5.9μg** | ID | | 280 |
| | 9 | ID | | 77μg | ID | | 281 |
| Phencyclidine (PCP) | 1 | ID | | 0.6μg* | ID | *41 days after PCP dose | 282 |
| Tetrahydrocannabinol (THC) | 2 | ID* | | 9μg** | ID | *THC concentrated in milk. Single M/P ratio = 8 **From milk of a long term smoker, 7 pipes of cannabis/day | 283 |
| Theobromine | 6 | 0.82 | 2-7 | 0.8mg* | 20 | *240mg dose given as 113g of chocolate | 284 |

*Abbreviations:* $M/P_{AUC}$ = milk : plasma concentration ratio based on comparison of areas under milk and plasma concentration-time curves; $t_{max}^{milk}$ = time to peak concentration in milk; C = plasma drug concentration; $C_{milk}$ = concentration of drug in milk; $C_{milk}^{max}$ = peak concentration of drug in milk; $t_{max}$ = time to peak plasma concentration; $D_{inf}$ = infant dose; ID = insufficient data; IM = intramuscular; IV = intravenous; SC = subcutaneous.

*For table II (summary of safety of drugs during breast feeding), see pages 1714 - 1716*

**Table II.** Summary of safety of drugs during breast feeding. Classification and advice: **1** = Probably safe. Maximum infant plasma concentrations <10% of maternal plasma concentrations; **2** = Weigh up risk : benefit ratio. Maximum infant plasma concentrations between 10 and 50% of maternal plasma concentrations; **3** = Breast feeding not generally advisable. Maximum infant plasma concentrations possibly >50% of maternal plasma concentrations; **4** = Breast feeding contraindicated because of potential toxicity; **5** = Breast feeding contraindicated in infants with known or possible glucose-6-phosphate dehydrogenase deficiency

| Drug | Age of infant (weeks)[a] | | | |
|---|---|---|---|---|
| | <34 | 34-44 | >44-68 | >68 |
| **ACE (angiotensin-converting enzyme) inhibitors** | | | | |
| Captopril | 1 | 1 | 1 | 1 |
| Enalapril | 2 | 1 | 1 | 1 |
| **β-*Adrenoceptor antagonists* (β-blockers)** | | | | |
| Acebutolol | 2 | 2 | 1 | 1 |
| Atenolol | 3 | 3 | 2 | 2 |
| Dilevalol | 1 | 1 | 1 | 1 |
| Labetalol | 1 | 1 | 1 | 1 |
| Mepindolol | 2 | 1 | 1 | 1 |
| Metoprolol | 2 | 1 | 1 | 1 |
| Nadolol | 3 | 2 | 1 | 1 |
| Oxprenolol | 2 | 1 | 1 | 1 |
| Propranolol | 1 | 1 | 1 | 1 |
| Sotalol | 3 | 3 | 2 | 2 |
| Timolol | 2 | 2 | 1 | 1 |
| Timolol eye drops | 1 | 1 | 1 | 1 |
| **Anaesthetics, local** | | | | |
| Bupivacaine | 2 | 1 | 1 | 1 |
| **Analgesics** | | | | |
| Butorphanol | 1 | 1 | 1 | 1 |
| Codeine | 3 | 2 | 2 | 1 |
| Dextropropoxyphene | 1 | 1 | 1 | 1 |
| Methadone | 2 | 1 | 1 | 1 |
| Morphine | 1 | 1 | 1 | 1 |
| Nalbuphine | 1 | 1 | 1 | 1 |
| Nefopam | 1 | 1 | 1 | 1 |
| Paracetamol (acetaminophen) | 2 | 2 | 2 | 1 |
| • *Nonsteroidal anti-inflammatory drugs (NSAIDs)* | | | | |
| Azapropazone | 2 | 1 | 1 | 1 |
| Fenbufen | 1 | 1 | 1 | 1 |
| Flufenamic acid | 1 | 1 | 1 | 1 |
| Flurbiprofen | 1 | 1 | 1 | 1 |
| Ibuprofen | 1 | 1 | 1 | 1 |
| Indomethacin | 1 | 1 | 1 | 1 |
| Indoprofen | 1 | 1 | 1 | 1 |
| Ketorolac | 1 | 1 | 1 | 1 |
| Mefenamic acid | 1 | 1 | 1 | 1 |
| Naproxen | 2 | 1 | 1 | 1 |
| Piroxicam | 3 | 2 | 2 | 2 |
| Salicylate | 2,5 | 2,5 | 1,5 | 1,5 |
| Suprofen | 1 | 1 | 1 | 1 |
| Tolmetin | 1 | 1 | 1 | 1 |
| **Antianxiety drugs/hypnosedatives** | | | | |
| • *Benzodiazepines* | | | | |
| Diazepam | 2 | 1 | 1 | 1 |
| Flunitrazepam | 1 | 1 | 1 | 1 |
| Lorazepam | 2 | 1 | 1 | 1 |
| Lormetazepam | 1 | 1 | 1 | 1 |
| Metaclazepam | 3 | 2 | 1 | 1 |
| Midazolam | 1 | 1 | 1 | 1 |
| Oxazepam | 1 | 1 | 1 | 1 |
| Pinazepam | 2 | 1 | 1 | 1 |
| Prazepam | 2 | 1 | 1 | 1 |
| Quazepam | 3 | 2 | 1 | 1 |
| • *Others* | | | | |
| Chloral hydrate | 2 | 1 | 1 | 1 |
| Clomethiazole (chlormethiazole) | 2 | 1 | 1 | 1 |
| Glutethimide | 1 | 1 | 1 | 1 |
| Trichloroethanol | 2 | 1 | 1 | 1 |
| Zopiclone | 2 | 2 | 1 | 1 |
| **Antiarrhythmic drugs** | | | | |
| Acecainide (*N*-acetylprocainamide) | 2 | 1 | 1 | 1 |
| Amiodarone | 3 | 3 | 3 | 1 |
| Disopyramide | 3 | 2 | 2 | 1 |
| Flecainide | 3 | 2 | 1 | 1 |
| Lidocaine (lignocaine) | 1 | 1 | 1 | 1 |
| Mexiletine | 2 | 1 | 1 | 1 |
| Procainamide | 2 | 2 | 1 | 1 |
| Quinidine | 2 | 2 | 1 | 1 |
| **Antibacterial drugs** | | | | |
| • *Aminoglycosides* | | | | |
| Amikacin | 1 | 1 | 1 | 1 |
| Gentamicin | 2 | 1 | 1 | 1 |
| • *Cefalosporins* | | | | |
| Cefaclor | 1 | 1 | 1 | 1 |
| Cefadroxil | 2 | 1 | 1 | 1 |
| Cefalexin | 2 | 1 | 1 | 1 |
| Cefalothin | 1 | 1 | 1 | 1 |
| Cefapirin | 1 | 1 | 1 | 1 |
| Cefazolin | 1 | 1 | 1 | 1 |
| Cefmenoxime | 2 | 1 | 1 | 1 |
| Cefonicid | 1 | 1 | 1 | 1 |
| Cefotaxime | 1 | 1 | 1 | 1 |
| Cefoxitin | 1 | 1 | 1 | 1 |
| Cefprozil | 1 | 1 | 1 | 1 |
| Cefradine | 1 | 1 | 1 | 1 |
| Ceftazidime | 1 | 1 | 1 | 1 |
| Ceftriaxone | 2 | 1 | 1 | 1 |
| Latamoxef (moxalactam) | 1 | 1 | 1 | 1 |
| • *Fluoroquinolones* | | | | |
| Ciprofloxacin | 2 | 2 | 1 | 1 |
| Fleroxacin | 3 | 2 | 2 | 1 |
| Ofloxacin | 3 | 2 | 1 | 1 |
| Pefloxacin | 3 | 2 | 1 | 1 |
| • *Macrolides* | | | | |
| Clarithromycin | 2 | 1 | 1 | 1 |
| Erythromycin | 2 | 1 | 1 | 1 |
| • *Penicillins* | | | | |
| Amoxicillin | 1 | 1 | 1 | 1 |
| Ampicillin | 1 | 1 | 1 | 1 |
| Benzylpenicillin (penicillin G) | 1 | 1 | 1 | 1 |
| Carbenicillin | 1 | 1 | 1 | 1 |

*For footnotes, see final page of table (p. 1716)*

**Table II.** *[Continued]*

| Drug | Age of infant (weeks)[a] | | | |
|---|---|---|---|---|
| | <34 | 34-44 | >44-68 | >68 |
| **Antibacterial drugs** *[continued]* | | | | |
| Epicillin | 3 | 2 | 1 | 1 |
| Phenoxymethyl-penicillin (penicillin V) | 1 | 1 | 1 | 1 |
| Pivampicillin | 1 | 1 | 1 | 1 |
| Ticarcillin | 1 | 1 | 1 | 1 |
| • *Sulfonamides* | | | | |
| Sulfasalazine | 3,5 | 2,5 | 2,5 | 1,5 |
| • *Tetracyclines* | | | | |
| Chlortetracycline | 1 | 1 | 1 | 1 |
| Minocycline | 2 | 2 | 1 | 1 |
| Tetracycline | 2 | 2 | 1 | 1 |
| • *Others* | | | | |
| Aztreonam | 2 | 1 | 1 | 1 |
| Chloramphenicol | 3,4,5 | 2,4,5 | 2,5 | 1,5 |
| Clindamycin | 3 | 2 | 1 | 1 |
| Imipenem/cilastatin | 2 | 2 | 1 | 1 |
| Lincomycin | 1 | 1 | 1 | 1 |
| Methenamine | 3 | 2 | 2 | 1 |
| Nalidixic acid | 1,5 | 1,5 | 1,5 | 1,5 |
| Nitrofurantoin | 1,5 | 1,5 | 1,5 | 1,5 |
| Rosaramicin | 1 | 1 | 1 | 1 |
| Thiamphenicol | 2 | 2 | 1 | 1 |
| **Anticoagulants** | | | | |
| Warfarin | 2 | 2 | 1 | 1 |
| **Antidepressants** | | | | |
| Amfebutamone (bupropion) | 1 | 1 | 1 | 1 |
| Amitriptyline | 1 | 1 | 1 | 1 |
| Amoxapine | 1 | 1 | 1 | 1 |
| Desipramine | 2 | 1 | 1 | 1 |
| Dothiepin | 1 | 1 | 1 | 1 |
| Doxepin | 1 | 1 | 1 | 1 |
| Fluoxetine | 3 | 2 | 1 | 1 |
| Imipramine | 1 | 1 | 1 | 1 |
| Maprotiline | 2 | 1 | 1 | 1 |
| Mianserin | 2 | 1 | 1 | 1 |
| Moclobemide | 2 | 1 | 1 | 1 |
| Nortriptyline | 2 | 1 | 1 | 1 |
| Sertraline | 1 | 1 | 1 | 1 |
| Trazodone | 2 | 1 | 1 | 1 |
| **Antidiabetic drugs** | | | | |
| Tolbutamide | 3 | 3 | 2 | 2 |
| **Antiemetics** | | | | |
| Domperidone | 1 | 1 | 1 | 1 |
| Metoclopramide[b] | 2 | 2 | 1 | 1 |
| **Antiepileptic drugs** | | | | |
| Carbamazepine | 2 | 2 | 1 | 1 |
| Clonazepam | 2 | 1 | 1 | 1 |
| Ethosuximide | 3 | 3 | 2 | 2 |
| Phenobarbital | 3 | 3 | 3 | 3 |
| Phenytoin | 3 | 2 | 2 | 1 |
| Primidone | 2 | 1 | 1 | 1 |
| Valproic acid (sodium valproate) | 2 | 1 | 1 | 1 |
| **Antifungal drugs** | | | | |
| Fluconazole | 3 | 3 | 2 | 2 |

| Drug | Age of infant (weeks)[a] | | | |
|---|---|---|---|---|
| | <34 | 34-44 | >44-68 | >68 |
| **Antihistamines** ($H_1$-receptor antagonists) | | | | |
| Clemastine | 3 | 2 | 2 | 1 |
| Loratadine | 1 | 1 | 1 | 1 |
| Terfenadine | 1 | 1 | 1 | 1 |
| Triprolidine | 1 | 1 | 1 | 1 |
| **Antihypertensive drugs** (see also ACE inhibitors, β-adrenoceptor antagonists, calcium antagonists and diuretics) | | | | |
| Clonidine | 3 | 2 | 2 | 1 |
| Dihydralazine | 1 | 1 | 1 | 1 |
| Hydralazine | 1 | 1 | 1 | 1 |
| Methyldopa | 1 | 1 | 1 | 1 |
| Minoxidil | 2 | 1 | 1 | 1 |
| **Antimalarial drugs** | | | | |
| Chloroquine | 3 | 2 | 2 | 2 |
| Dapsone | 3,5 | 2,5 | 2,5 | 1,5 |
| Hydroxychloroquine | 2 | 2 | 1 | 1 |
| Mefloquine | 1 | 1 | 1 | 1 |
| Pyrimethamine | 3,5 | 3,5 | 2,5 | 2,5 |
| **Antineoplastic and immunosuppressive drugs** | | | | |
| Azathioprine | 2 | 1 | 1 | 1 |
| Cisplatin | 1,4 | 1,4 | 1,4 | 1,4 |
| Doxorubicin | 2,4,5 | 1,4,5 | 1,4,5 | 1,4,5 |
| Hydroxycarbamide (hydroxyurea) | 3,4 | 2,4 | 1,4 | 1,4 |
| Methotrexate | 1,4 | 1,4 | 1,4 | 1,4 |
| **Antipsychotic drugs** | | | | |
| Chlorpromazine | 1,5 | 1,5 | 1,5 | 1,5 |
| Chlorprothixene | 1 | 1 | 1 | 1 |
| Flupenthixol | 1 | 1 | 1 | 1 |
| Haloperidol | 2 | 1 | 1 | 1 |
| Lithium | 2 | 1 | 1 | 1 |
| Perphenazine | 1 | 1 | 1 | 1 |
| Sulpiride[b] | 3 | 2 | 2 | 2 |
| Zuclopenthixol | 2 | 1 | 1 | 1 |
| **Antithyroid and thyroid drugs** | | | | |
| Carbimazole | 3,4 | 3,4 | 2,4 | 2,4 |
| Liothyronine (tri-iodothyronine) | 3 | 2 | 2 | 2 |
| Propylthiouracil | 2 | 1 | 1 | 1 |
| Thiamazole (methimazole) | 3 | 2 | 2 | 2 |
| Thiouracil | 3 | 2 | 2 | 2 |
| Thyroxine | 3 | 2 | 2 | 2 |
| **Antitrichomonal drugs** | | | | |
| Metronidazole | 3 | 3 | 2 | 2 |
| Tinidazole | 3 | 2 | 2 | 2 |
| **Antituberculosis drugs** | | | | |
| Aminosalicylic acid (*p*-aminosalicylic acid) | 1 | 1 | 1 | 1 |
| Isoniazid | 3 | 3 | 3 | 3 |
| Pyrazinamide | 2 | 1 | 1 | 1 |
| **Antiulcer drugs** | | | | |
| Cimetidine | 3 | 3 | 2 | 1 |
| Famotidine | 2 | 1 | 1 | 1 |
| Nizatidine | 2 | 2 | 1 | 1 |
| Ranitidine | 3 | 2 | 2 | 1 |
| Roxatidine | 2 | 2 | 1 | 1 |

*[Continued over]*

*For footnotes, see final page of table (p. 1716)*

**Table II.** *[Continued]*

| Drug | Age of infant (weeks)[a] | | | |
|---|---|---|---|---|
| | <34 | 34-44 | >44-68 | >68 |
| **Antiviral drugs** | | | | |
| Aciclovir | 2 | 1 | 1 | 1 |
| **Bronchodilators** | | | | |
| Diprophylline (dyphylline) | 3 | 3 | 3 | 2 |
| Enprofylline | 2 | 1 | 1 | 1 |
| Pseudoephedrine | 2 | 2 | 1 | 1 |
| Terbutaline | 1 | 1 | 1 | 1 |
| Theophylline | 3 | 3 | 3 | 3 |
| **Calcium antagonists** | | | | |
| Diltiazem | 1 | 1 | 1 | 1 |
| Nifedipine | 1 | 1 | 1 | 1 |
| Nimodipine | 1 | 1 | 1 | 1 |
| Nitrendipine | 1 | 1 | 1 | 1 |
| Tiapamil | 1 | 1 | 1 | 1 |
| Verapamil | 1 | 1 | 1 | 1 |
| **Cardiac glycosides** | | | | |
| Digoxin | 2 | 1 | 1 | 1 |
| **Corticosteroids** | | | | |
| Methylprednisolone | 2 | 1 | 1 | 1 |
| Prednisolone | 2 | 2 | 1 | 1 |
| Prednisone | 1 | 1 | 1 | 1 |
| **Diagnostic agents** | | | | |
| Diatrizoic acid | 1 | 1 | 1 | 1 |
| Iodamide | 1 | 1 | 1 | 1 |
| Iohexol | 1 | 1 | 1 | 1 |
| Iopanoic acid | 3 | 2 | 2 | 2 |
| Metrizamide | 1 | 1 | 1 | 1 |
| Sodium metrizoate | 1 | 1 | 1 | 1 |
| **Diuretics** | | | | |
| Acetazolamide | 2 | 1 | 1 | 1 |
| Chlorothiazide[b] | 2 | 1 | 1 | 1 |
| Chlorthalidone | 3 | 2 | 2 | 2 |
| Hydrochlorothiazide[b] | 2 | 1 | 1 | 1 |
| Spironolactone | 2 | 1 | 1 | 1 |
| **Estrogens and progestagens** | | | | |
| Estradiol | 1 | 1 | 1 | 1 |
| Ethinylestradiol | 1 | 1 | 1 | 1 |
| Levonorgestrel | 2 | 1 | 1 | 1 |
| Lynestrenol | 1 | 1 | 1 | 1 |
| Medroxyprogesterone | 2 | 2 | 1 | 1 |
| Mestranol | 2 | 1 | 1 | 1 |
| Norethisterone (norethindrone) | 2 | 1 | 1 | 1 |
| Norgestrel | 2 | 1 | 1 | 1 |
| **Lipid-lowering drugs** | | | | |
| Pravastatin | 1 | 1 | 1 | 1 |
| **Radiopharmaceuticals[b]** | | | | |
| **Miscellaneous drugs** | | | | |
| Baclofen | 3 | 2 | 1 | 1 |
| Carbetocin | 1 | 1 | 1 | 1 |
| Cyproterone | 2 | 1 | 1 | 1 |
| Gold (aurothiomalate sodium) | 3,4 | 2,4 | 2,4 | 1,4 |
| Iodine | 3,4 | 2,4 | 2,4 | 1,4 |
| Ivermectin | 2 | 1 | 1 | 1 |
| Magnesium sulfate | 1 | 1 | 1 | 1 |
| Methylergometrine | 2 | 2 | 1 | 1 |
| Noscapine | 1 | 1 | 1 | 1 |
| Pentoxifylline (oxpentifylline) | 1 | 1 | 1 | 1 |
| Praziquantel | 1 | 1 | 1 | 1 |
| Pyridostigmine | 1 | 1 | 1 | 1 |
| Tranexamic acid | 1 | 1 | 1 | 1 |
| **Miscellaneous 'social' drugs** | | | | |
| Amphetamine | 3 | 2 | 1 | 1 |
| Caffeine | 3 | 3 | 2 | 2 |
| Cocaine | 4 | 4 | 4 | 4 |
| Ethanol | 3 | 3 | 2 | 2 |
| Theobromine | 3 | 3 | 2 | 2 |

a Refers to postconceptual age.

b May suppress lactation.

**Classification and advice:**

**1** = Probably safe. Maximum infant plasma concentrations <10% of maternal plasma concentrations.

**2** = Weigh up risk : benefit ratio. Maximum infant plasma concentrations between 10 and 50% of maternal plasma concentrations.

**3** = Breast feeding not generally advisable. Maximum infant plasma concentrations possibly >50% of maternal plasma concentrations.

**4** = Breast feeding contraindicated because of potential toxicity.

**5** = Breast feeding contraindicated in infants with known or possible glucose-6-phosphate dehydrogenase deficiency.

## References


1. Atkinson HC, Begg EJ, Darlow BA. Drugs in human milk: clinical pharmacokinetic considerations. Clinical Pharmacokinetics 1988; 14: 217-40
2. Begg EJ, Atkinson HC. Modelling of the passage of drugs into milk. Pharmacology and Therapeutics 1993; 59: 301-10
3. Bennett PN, editor. Drugs and human lactation. Amsterdam: Elsevier, 1988
4. Wilson JT, Brown RD, Hinson JL, et al. Pharmacokinetic pitfalls in the estimation of the breast milk plasma ratio for drugs. Annual Review of Pharmacology and Toxicology 1985; 25: 667-89
5. Devlin RG, Fleiss PM. Captopril in human blood and breast milk. Journal of Clinical Pharmacology 1981; 21: 110-3
6. Huttunen K, Gronhagen-Riska C, Fyhrquist F. Enalapril treatment of a nursing mother with slightly impaired renal function. Clinical Nephrology 1989; 31: 278
7. Redman CWG, Kelly JG, Cooper WD. The excretion of enalapril and enalaprilat in human breast milk. European Journal of Clinical Pharmacology 1990; 38: 39
8. Boutroy MJ, Bianchette G, Dubruc C, et al. To nurse when receiving acebutolol: is it dangerous for the neonate? European Journal of Clinical Pharmacology 1986; 30: 737-9
9. Liedholm H, Melander A, Bitzen PO, et al. Accumulation of atenolol and metoprolol in human breast milk. European Journal of Clinical Pharmacology 1981; 20: 229-31
10. Kulas J, Lunell NO, Rosing U, et al. Atenolol and metoprolol: a comparison of their excretion into human breast milk. Acta Obstetricia et Gynecologica Scandinavica 1984; 118: 65-9
11. Thorley KJ, McAinsh J. Levels of the beta-blockers atenolol and propranolol in the breast milk of women treated for hypertension in pregnancy. Biopharmaceutics and Drug Disposition 1983; 4: 299-301
12. Radwanski E, Nagabhushan N, Affrime MB, et al. Secretion of dilevalol in breast milk. Journal of Clinical Pharmacology 1988; 28: 448-53
13. Michael CA. Use of labetalol in the treatment of severe hypertension during pregnancy. British Journal of Clinical Pharmacology 1979; 8: 211S-5S
14. Lunell NO, Kulas J, Rane A. Transfer of labetalol into amniotic fluid and breast milk in lactating women. European Journal of Clinical Pharmacology 1985; 28: 597-9
15. Krause W, Stoppelli I, Milia S, et al. Transfer of mepindolol to newborn by breast-feeding mothers after single and repeated daily doses. European Journal of Clinical Pharmacology 1982; 22: 53
16. Sandstrom B, Lindeberg S, Lundborg P, et al. Disposition of the adrenergic blocker metoprolol in late pregnant women, the amniotic fluid, the cord blood and the neonate. Clinical and Experimental Hypertension 1983; B2: 75-82
17. Sandstrom B. Metoprolol excretion into breast milk. British Journal of Clinical Pharmacology 1980; 9: 518-9
18. Devlin RG, Duchin KL, Fleiss PM. Nadolol in human serum and breast milk. British Journal of Clinical Pharmacology 1981; 12: 393-6
19. Fidler J, Smith V, De Swiet M. Excretion of oxprenolol and timolol in breast milk. British Journal of Obstetrics and Gynaecology 1983; 90: 961-5
20. Sioufi A, Hillion D, Lumbroso P, et al. Oxprenolol placental transfer, plasma concentrations in newborns and passage into breast milk. British Journal of Clinical Pharmacology 1984; 18: 453-6
21. Levitan A, Manion J. Propranolol therapy during pregnancy and lactation. American Journal of Cardiology 1973; 32: 247
22. Bauer J, Pape B, Zajicek J, et al. Propranolol in human plasma and breast milk. American Journal of Cardiology 1979; 43: 860-2
23. Smith M, Livingstone I, Hooper W, et al. Propranolol, propranolol glucuronide, and naphthoxylactic acid in breast milk and plasma. Therapeutic Drug Monitoring 1983; 5: 87-93
24. O'Hare MF, Murnaghan GA, Russel CJ, et al. Sotalol as a hypotensive agent in pregnancy. British Journal of Obstetrics and Gynaecology 1980; 87: 814-20
25. Lustgarten JS, Podos SM. Topical timolol and the nursing mother. Archives of Ophthalmology 1983; 101: 1381-2
26. Baker PA, Schroeder D. Interpleural bupivacaine for postoperative pain during lactation. Anesthesia and Analgesia 1989; 69: 400-2
27. Pittman KA, Smyth RD, Losada M, et al. Human perinatal distribution of butorphanol. American Journal of Obstetrics and Gynecology 1980; 138: 797-800
28. Findlay JWA, Deangelis RL, Kearney MF, et al. Analgesic drugs in breast milk and plasma. Clinical Pharmacology and Therapeutics 1981; 29: 625-33
29. Kunka RL, Venkataramanan R, Stern RM, et al. Excretion of propoxyphene and norpropoxyphene in breast milk. Clinical Pharmacology and Therapeutics 1984; 35: 675-80
30. Pond SM, Kreek MJ, Tong TG, et al. Altered methadone pharmacokinetics in methadone-maintained pregnant women. Journal of Pharmacology and Experimental Therapeutics 1985; 233: 1-6
31. Feilberg VL, Rosenborg D, Christensen CB, et al. Excretion of morphine in human breast milk. Acta Anaesthesiologica Scandinavica 1989; 33: 426-8
32. Wischnik A, Wetzelsberger N, Lucker PW. Elimination von Nalbuphin in die Muttermilch. Arzneimittel-Forschung 1988; 38: 1496-8
33. Liu DTY, Savage JM, Donnell D. Nefopam excretion in human milk. British Journal of Clinical Pharmacology 1987; 23: 99-101
34. Bitzen PO, Gustafsson KG, Melander A, et al. Excretion of paracetamol in human breast milk. European Journal of Clinical Pharmacology 1981; 20: 123-5
35. Bald R, Bernbeck-Betthauser EM, Spahn H, et al. Excretion of azapropazone in human breast milk. European Journal of Clinical Pharmacology 1990; 39: 271-3
36. Chicarreli FS, Eisner HJ. Metabolic and pharmacokinetic studies with fenbufen in man. Arzneimittel-Forschung 1980; 30 (4A): 728-35
37. Buchanan RA, Eaton CJ, Koeff ST, et al. The breast milk excretion of flufenamic acid. Current Therapeutic Research 1969; 11: 533-8
38. Cox SR, Forbes KK. Excretion of flurbiprofen into breast milk. Pharmacotherapy 1987; 7: 211-5
39. Smith IJ, Hinson JL, Johnson VA, et al. Flurbiprofen in post-partum women: plasma and breast milk disposition. Journal of Clinical Pharmacology 1989; 29: 174-84
40. Townsend RJ, Benedetti TJ, Erickson SH, et al. Excretion of ibuprofen into breast milk. American Journal of Obstetrics and Gynecology 1984; 149: 184-6

41. Lebedevs TH, Wojnar-Horton RE, Yapp P, et al. Excretion of indomethacin in breast milk. British Journal of Clinical Pharmacology 1991; 32: 751-4
42. Lakings DB, Lizarraga C, Haggerty WJ, et al. High-performance liquid chromatographic determination of indoprofen in human milk. Journal of Pharmaceutical Sciences 1979; 68: 1113-6
43. Wischnik A, Manth SM, Lloyd J, et al. The excretion of ketorolac tromethamine into breast milk after multiple oral dosing. European Journal of Clinical Pharmacology 1989; 36: 521-4
44. Buchanan R, Eaton C, Keoff S, et al. The breast milk excretion of mefenamic acid. Therapeutic Research 1968; 10: 592-6
45. Jamali F, Stevens D. Naproxen excretion in milk and its uptake by the infant. Drug Intelligence and Clinical Pharmacy 1983; 17: 910-11
46. Ostensen M. Piroxicam in human breast milk. European Journal of Clinical Pharmacology 1983; 25: 829-30
47. Bailey DN, Weibert RT, Naylor AJ, et al. A study of salicylate and caffeine excretion in the breast milk of two nursing mothers. Journal of Analytical Toxicology 1982; 6: 64-8
48. Jamali F, Keshavarz G. Salicylate in breast milk. International Journal of Pharmaceutics 1981; 8: 285-90
49. Chaikin P, Chasin M, Kennedy B, et al. Suprofen concentrations in human breast milk. Journal of Clinical Pharmacology 1983; 23: 385-90
50. Sagraves R, Waller ES, Goehrs HR. Tolmetin in breast milk. Drug Intelligence and Clinical Pharmacy 1985; 19: 55-6
51. Rey E, Giraux P, d'Athis P, et al. Pharmacokinetics in placental transfer and distribution of clorazepate and its metabolite nordiazepam in the feto-placental unit and in the neonate. European Journal of Clinical Pharmacology 1979; 15: 181-5
52. Brandt R. Passage of diazepam and desmethyldiazepam into breast milk. Arzneimittel-Forschung 1976; 26: 454-7
53. Erkkola R, Kanto J. Diazepam and breast feeding. Lancet 1972; 1: 1235-6
54. Jensen OH, Bredesen JE, Lindbaek G. Transfer of flunitrazepam to mother's milk. Tidsskrift For Den Norske Laegeforening 1981; 101: 504
55. Summerfield RJ, Nielsen MS. Excretion of lorazepam into breast milk. British Journal of Anaesthesia 1985; 57: 1042-3
56. Humpel M, Stopelli I, Milia S, et al. Pharmacokinetics and biotransformation of the new benzodiazepine, lormetazepam, in man. European Journal of Clinical Pharmacology 1982; 21: 421-5
57. Schotter A, Mueller R, Gunther C, et al. Transfer of metaclazepam and its metabolites into breast milk. Arzneimittel-Forschung 1989; 39: 1468-70
58. Matheson I, Lunde PKM, Bredesen JE. Midazolam and nitrazepam in the maternity ward: milk concentration and clinical effects. British Journal of Clinical Pharmacology 1990; 30: 787-93
59. Reider J, Wendt G. Pharmacokinetics and the metabolism of the hypnotic nitrazepam. In: Garattini S, et al. editors. The benzodiazepines. New York: Raven Press 1973: 99-127
60. Wretlind M. Excretion of oxazepam in breast milk. European Journal of Clinical Pharmacology 1987; 33: 209-10
61. Pacifici GM, Cuoci L, Guarneri M, et al. Placental transfer of pinazepam and its metabolite N-desmethyldiazepam in women at term. European Journal of Clinical Pharmacology 1984; 27: 307-10
62. Brodie RR, Chasseaud LF, Taylor T. Concentrations of N-descyclopropyl-methylprazepam in whole blood, plasma and milk after administration of prazepam to humans. Biopharmaceutics and Drug Disposition 1982; 2: 59-68
63. Hilbert J, Gural R, Symchowicz S, et al. Excretion of quazepam into human breast milk. Journal of Clinical Pharmacology 1984; 24: 457-62
64. Bernstine JB, Meyer AE, Bernstine RL. Maternal blood and breast milk estimation following the administration of chloral hydrate during the puerperium. Journal of Obstetrics and Gynaecology of the British Empire 1956; 63: 228-31
65. Tunstall ME, Campbell DM, Dawson BM, et al. Chlormethiazole treatment and breast feeding. British Journal of Obstetrics and Gynaecology 1979; 86: 793-8
66. Curry SH, Ridall D, Gordon SJ, et al. Disposition of glutethimide in man. Clinical Pharmacology and Therapeutics 1971; 12: 849-57
67. Matheson I, Sande HA, Gaillot J, et al. Zopiclone excretion in breast milk. British Journal of Clinical Pharmacology 1985; 20: 290P-1P
68. Matheson I, Sande HA, Gaillot J. The excretion of zopiclone into breast milk. British Journal of Clinical Pharmacology 1990; 30: 267-71
69. Pittard WB, Glazier H. Procainamide excretion in human milk. Journal of Pediatrics 1983; 102: 631-3
70. McKenna WJ, Harris L, Rowland E, et al. Amiodarone therapy during pregnancy. American Journal of Cardiology 1983; 51: 1231-3
71. Barnett DB, Hudson SA, McBurney A. Disopyramide and its N-monodesalky metabolite. British Journal of Clinical Pharmacology 1982; 14: 310-2
72. MacIntosh D, Buchanan N. Excretion of disopyramide in human breast milk (letter). British Journal of Clinical Pharmacology 1985; 19: 856-7
73. Wagner X, Jouglard J, Moulin M, et al. Coadministration of flecainide and sotalol during pregnancy: lack of teratogenic effects, passage across the placenta and excretion in human breast milk. American Heart Journal 1990; 119: 700-2
74. Zeisler JA, Gaarder TD, Mesquita SA. Lidocaine excretion in breast milk. Drug Intelligence and Clinical Pharmacy 1986; 20: 691-3
75. Timmis AD, Jackson G, Holt DW. Mexiletine for control of ventricular dysrhythmias in pregnancy. Lancet 1980; 2: 647-8
76. Lewis A, Johnston A, Patel L, et al. Mexiletine in human blood and breast milk. Postgraduate Medical Journal 1981; 57: 546-7
77. Hill LM, Malkasian GD. The use of quinidine sulfate throughout pregnancy. Obstetrics and Gynecology 1979; 54: 366-8
78. Matsuda S. Transfer of antibiotics into maternal milk. Biological Research in Pregnancy 1984; 5: 57-60
79. Celiloglu M, Celiker S, Guven H, et al. Gentamicin excretion and uptake from breast milk by nursing infants. Obstetrics and Gynecology 1994; 84: 263-5
80. Takase Z, Shirafuji H, Uchida M. Clinical and laboratory studies of cefaclor in the field of obstetrics and gynecology. Chemotherapy (Tokyo) 1979; Suppl. 27: 666-71
81. Kafetzis DA, Siafas CA, Georgakopoulos PA, et al. Passage of cephalosporins and amoxicillin into breast milk. Acta Paediatrica Scandinavica 1981; 70: 285-8

82. Yoshioka H, Kazuhiko C, Takimoto M, et al. Transfer of cefazolin into human milk. Journal of Pediatrics 1979; 94: 151-2
83. Lou MA, Wu YH, Jacob LS, et al. Penetration of cefonicid into human breast milk and various body fluids and tissues. Reviews of Infectious Diseases 1984; 6: S816
84. Weissenbacher ER, Adams D, Gutschow K, et al. Clinical results and concentrations of cefmenoxime in serum, amniotic fluid, mother's milk and umbilical cord. American Journal of Medicine 1984; 77 Suppl. 6A: 11-2
85. Kafetzis DA, Lazarides CV, Siafas CA, et al. Transfer to cefotaxime in human milk and from mother to foetus. Journal of Antimicrobial Chemotherapy 1980; 6 Suppl. A: 135-41
86. Dresse A, Lambotte R, Dubois M, et al. Transmammary passage of cefoxitin: additional results. Journal of Clinical Pharmacology 1983; 23: 438
87. Roex AJM, van Loerner AC, Puyenbroek JI, et al. Secretion of cefoxitin in breast milk following short-term prophylactic administration in caesarian section. European Journal of Obstetrics Gynecology and Reproductive Biology 1987; 25: 299-302
88. Shyu WC, Shah VR, Campbell DA, et al. Excretion of cefprozil into human breast milk. Antimicrobial Agents and Chemotherapy 1992; 36: 938-41
89. Mischler TW, Corson SL, Larranga A, et al. Cephradine and epicillin in body fluids of lactating and pregnant women. Journal of Reproductive Medicine 1978; 21: 130-6
90. Blanco JD, Jorgensen JH, Castaneda YS, et al. Ceftazidime levels in human breast milk. Antimicrobial Agents and Chemotherapy 1983; 23: 479-80
91. Kafetzis DA, Brater DC, Fanourgakis JE, et al. Ceftriaxone distribution between maternal blood and foetal blood and milk postpartum. Antimicrobial Agents and Chemotherapy 1983; 23: 870-3
92. Bourget P, Quinquais-Desmaris V, Fernandez H. Ceftriaxone distribution and protein binding between maternal blood and milk postpartum. Annals of Pharmacotherapy 1993; 27: 294-7
93. Miller R, Keegan K, Thrupp L, et al. Human breast milk concentration of moxalactam. American Journal of Obstetrics and Gynecology 1984; 148 (3): 348-9
94. Giamarellou H, Kolokythas E. Pharmacokinetics of three newer quinolones in pregnant and lactating women. American Journal of Medicine 1989; 87 Suppl. 5A: 49S-51S
95. Dan M, Weidekamm E, Sagiv R, et al. Penetration of fleroxacin into breast milk and pharmacokinetics in lactating women. Antimicrobial Agents and Chemotherapy 1993; 37: 293-6
96. Sedlmeyr T, Peters F, Raasch W, et al. Clarithromycin, a new macrolide antibiotic. Effectiveness in pueperal infections and pharmacokinetics in breast milk. Geburtshilfe und Frauenheilkunde 1993; 53: 488-91
97. Campbell AC, McElnay JC, Passmore CM. The excretion of ampicillin in breast milk and its effect on the suckling infant. British Journal of Clinical Pharmacology 1991; 31: 230
98. Matheson I, Samseth M, Loberg R, et al. Milk transfer of phenoxymethylpenicillin during puerperal mastitis. British Journal of Clinical Pharmacology 1988; 25: 33-40
99. Matheson I, Samseth M, Sande HA. Ampicillin in breast milk during puerperal infections. European Journal of Clinical Pharmacology 1988; 34: 657-9
100. Khan AZA, Truelove SC. Placental and mammary transfer of sulphasalazine. British Medical Journal 1979; 2: 1553
101. Jarnerot G, Into-Malmberg MB. Sulphasalazine treatment during breast feeding. Scandinavian Journal of Gastroenterology 1979; 14: 869-71
102. Guilbeau JA, Schoenbach EB, Schaub IG, et al. Aureomycin in obstetrics: therapy and prophylaxis. Journal of the American Medical Association 1950; 143: 520-6
103. Mizuno S, Takata M, Sano S, et al. Studies on minocycline [in Japanese]. Japanese Journal of Antibiotics 1969; 22: 473-9 [Cited in: Bennett PN, editor. Drugs and human lactation. Amsterdam: Elsevier, 1988]
104. Fleiss PM, Richwald J, Gordon J, et al. Aztreonam in human serum and breast milk. British Journal of Clinical Pharmacology 1985; 19: 509-11
105. Plomp TA, Thiery M, Maess RAA. The passage of thiamphenicol and chloramphenicol into human milk after single and repeated oral administration. Veterinary and Human Toxicology 1983; 25: 167-72
106. Steen B, Rane A. Clindamycin passage into human milk. British Journal of Clinical Pharmacology 1982; 13: 661-4
107. Ito K, Izumi K, Takagi H, et al. Fundamental and clinical evaluation of imipenem/cilastatin sodium in the perinatal period. Japanese Journal of Antibiotics 1988; 41: 1778-85
108. Medina A, Fiske N, Hjelt-Harvey I, et al. Absorption diffusion, and excretion of a new antibiotic, lincomycin. Antimicrobial Agents and Chemotherapy 1963; 3: 189-96
109. Allgen LG, Holmberg G, Persson B, et al. Biological fate of methenamine in man. Acta Obstetricia et Gynecologica Scandinavica 1979; 58: 287-93
110. Traeger A, Peiker G. Excretion of nalidixic acid via mother's milk. Archives of Toxicology 1980; Suppl. 4: 388-90
111. Varsano I, Fischl J, Shochet SB. The excretion of orally ingested nitrofurantoin in human milk. Journal of Pediatrics 1973; 82: 886-7
112. Hosbach RE, Foster RB, Norwich NY. Absence of nitrofurantoin from human milk. Journal of the American Medical Association 1967; 202: 1057
113. Pons G, Rey E, Richard M-O, et al. Nitrofurantoin excretion in human milk. Developmental Pharmacology and Therapeutics 1990; 14: 148-52
114. Stoehr G, Juhl R, Veals J, et al. The excretion of rosaramicin in breast milk. Journal of Clinical Pharmacology 1985; 25: 89-94
115. Von Kries R, Nocker D, Schmitz-Kummer E, et al. Transfer of phenprocoumon in breast milk. Is oral anticoagulation with phenprocoumon a contraindication for breastfeeding? Monatsschr Kinderheilkunde 1993; 141: 505-7
116. Baty JD, Breckenridge A, Lewis PJ, et al. May mothers taking warfarin breast feed their infants? British Journal of Clinical Pharmacology 1976; 3: 969
117. Briggs GG, Samson JH, Ambrose PJ, et al. Excretion of bupropion in breast milk. Annals of Pharmacotherapy 1993; 27: 431-3
118. Brixen-Rasmussen L, Halgrener J, Jorgenson A. Amitriptyline and nortriptyline excretion in breast milk. Psychopharmacology 1982; 76: 94-5
119. Bader T, Newman K. Amitriptyline in human breast milk and the nursing infant's serum. American Journal of Psychiatry 1980; 137: 855-6

120. Pittard WB, O'Neal W. Amitriptyline excretion in human milk. Journal of Clinical Psychopharmacology 1986; 6: 383-4
121. Gelenberg AJ. Amoxapine, a new antidepressant, appears in human milk. Journal of Nervous and Mental Disease 1979; 167: 635
122. Stancer HC, Reed KL. Desipramine and 2-hydroxydesipramine in human breast milk and the nursing infants serum. American Journal of Psychiatry 1986; 143: 1597-600
123. Sovner R, Orsulak PJ. Excretion of imipramine and desipramine in human breast milk. American Journal of Psychiatry 1979; 136: 451-2
124. Rees JA, Glass RC, Sporne GA. Serum and breast milk concentrations of dothiepin. Practitioner 1976; 217: 686
125. Ilett KF, Lebedevs TH, Wojnar-Horton RE, et al. The excretion of dothiepin and its primary metabolites in breast milk. British Journal of Clinical Pharmacology 1993; 33: 635-9
126. Kemp J, Illet KF, Booth J, et al. Excretion of doxepin and N-desmethyldoxepin in human milk. British Journal of Clinical Pharmacology 1985; 20: 497-9
127. Isenberg KE. Excretion of fluoxetine in human breast milk. Journal of Clinical Psychiatry 1990; 51: 169
128. Burch KJ, Wells BG. Fluoxetine/norfluoxetine concentrations in human milk. Pediatrics 1992; 89: 676-7
129. Lloyd AH. Practical considerations in the use of maprotiline (Ludiomil) in general practice. Journal of International Medical Research 1977 Suppl. 4: 122-9
130. Buist A, Norman TR, Dennerstein L. Mianserin in breast milk. British Journal of Clinical Pharmacology 1993; 36: 133-4
131. Pons G, Schoerlin MP, Tam YK, et al. Moclobemide excretion in human breast milk. British Journal of Clinical Pharmacology 1990; 29: 27-31
132. Matheson I, Skjaeraasen J. Milk concentrations of flupenthixol, nortriptyline and zuclopenthixol and between-breast differences in two patients. European Journal of Clinical Pharmacology 1988; 35: 217
133. Altshuler LL, Burt VK, McMullen M, et al. Breastfeeding and sertraline: a 24-hour analysis. Journal of Clinical Psychiatry 1995; 56: 243-5
134. Verbeeck RK, Ross SG, McKenna EA. Excretion of trazodone in breast milk. British Journal of Clinical Pharmacology 1986; 22: 367-70
135. Moiel RH, Ryan JR. Tolbutamide Orinase in human breast milk. Clinical Pediatrics 1967; 6: 480
136. Hofmeyr GJ, Iddekinge B, Blott JA. Domperidone: secretion in breast milk and effect on puerperal prolactin levels. British Journal of Obstetrics and Gynaecology 1985; 92: 141-4
137. Kauppila A, Arvela P, Koivisto M, et al. Metoclopramide and breast feeding: transfer into milk and the newborn. European Journal of Clinical Pharmacology 1983; 25: 819-23
138. Lewis P, Devenish C, Kahn C. Controlled trial of metoclopramide in the initiation of breast feeding. British Journal of Clinical Pharmacology 1980; 9: 217-9
139. Pynnonen S, Sillanpaa M. Carbamazepine and mothers milk. Lancet 1975; 1: 63
140. Kuhnz W, Jäger-Roman E, Rating D, et al. Carbamazepine and carbamazepine-10, 11-epoxide during pregnancy and postnatal period in epileptic mothers and their nursed infants: pharmacokinetics and clinical effects. Pediatric Pharmacology 1983; 3: 199-208
141. Froescher W, Eichelbaum M, Niesen M, et al. Carbamazepine levels in breast milk. Therapeutic Drug Monitoring 1984; 6: 226-71
142. Fisher JB, Edgren BE, Mammel MC, et al. Neonatal apnea associated with maternal clonazepam therapy: a case report. Obstetrics and Gynecology 1985; 66: 34S-5S
143. Kuhnz W, Koch S, Jakob S, et al. Ethosuximide in epileptic women during pregnancy and lactation period: placental transfer, serum concentrations in nursed infants and clinical status. British Journal of Clinical Pharmacology 1984; 18: 671-7
144. Kaneko S, Sato T, Suzu K. The levels of anticonvulsants in breast milk. British Journal of Clinical Pharmacology 1979; 7: 624-7
145. Kuhnz W, Koch S, Helge H, et al. Primidone and phenobarbital during lactation period in epileptic women: total and free drug serum levels in the nursed infants and their effects on neonatal behaviour. Developmental Pharmacology and Therapeutics 1988; 11: 147-54
146. Steen B, Rane A, Lonnerholm G, et al. Phenytoin excretion in human breast milk and plasma levels in nursed infants. Therapeutic Drug Monitoring 1982; 4: 331-4
147. Von Unruh G, Froescher W, Hoffman F, et al. Valproic acid in breast milk: how much is really there? Therapeutic Drug Monitoring 1984; 6: 272-76
148. Force RW. Fluconazole concentrations in breast milk. Pediatric Infectious Diseases 1995; 14: 235-6
149. Kok TH, Taitz HG, Bennet MJ, et al. Drowsiness due to clemastine transmitted in breast milk. Lancet 1982; 1: 914
150. Hilbert J, Radwanski E, Affrime MB, et al. Excretion of loratadine in human breast milk. Journal of Clinical Pharmacology 1988; 28: 234-9
151. Lucas BD, Scarim SK, Benjamin S, et al. Terfenadine pharmacokinetics in breast milk in lactating women. Clinical Pharmacology and Therapeutics 1995; 57: 398-402
152. Findlay JWA, Butz RF, Sailstead JM, et al. Pseudoephedrine and triprolidine in plasma and breast milk of nursing mothers. British Journal of Clinical Pharmacology 1984; 18: 901-6
153. Hartikainen-Sorri AL, Heikkinen JE, Koivisti M. Pharmacokinetics of clonidine during pregnancy and nursing. Obstetrics and Gynecology 1987; 69: 598-600
154. Franke G, Pietsch P, Schneider T, et al. Studies on the kinetics and distribution of dihydralazine in pregnancy. Biological Research in Pregnancy 1986; 7: 30
155. Liedholm H, Wahlin-Boll E, Hanson A, et al. Transplacental passage and breast milk concentrations of hydralazine. European Journal of Clinical Pharmacology 1982; 21: 417-9
156. Jones HMR, Cummings AJ. A study of the transfer of $\alpha$-methyldopa to the human foetus and newborn infant. British Journal of Clinical Pharmacology 1978; 6: 432
157. White WB, Andreoli JW, Cohn RD. Alpha-methyldopa disposition in mothers with hypertension and in their breast-fed infants. Clinical Pharmacology and Therapeutics 1985; 37: 387-90
158. Valdivieso A, Valdes G, Spiro TE, et al. Minoxidil in breast milk. Annals of Internal Medicine 1985; 102: 135
159. Edstein MD, Veenendaal RJ, Newman K, et al. Excretion of chloroquine, dapsone, and pyrimethamine in human milk. British Journal of Clinical Pharmacology 1986; 22: 733-5
160. Ogunbona FA, Onye CO, Bolaji OO, et al. Excretion of chloroquine and desethylchloroquine in human milk. British Journal of Clinical Pharmacology 1987; 23: 473-6

161. Ette EI, Essien EE, Ogonor JI, et al. Chloroquine in human milk. Journal of Clinical Pharmacology 1987; 27: 499-502
162. Akintonwa A, Gbajumo SA, Mabadeje AFB. Placental and milk transfer of chloroquine in humans. Therapeutic Drug Monitoring 1988; 10: 147-9
163. Nation RL, Hackett LP, Dusci LJ, et al. Excretion of hydroxychloroquine in human milk. British Journal of Clinical Pharmacology 1984; 17: 368-9
164. Ostensen M, Brown ND, Chiang PK, et al. Hydroxychloroquine in human breast milk. European Journal of Clinical Pharmacology 1985; 28: 357
165. Edstein MD, Veenendaal JR, Hyslop R. Excretion of mefloquine in human breast milk. Chemotherapy 1988; 34: 165-9
166. Coulam CB, Moyer TP, Jiang NS, et al. Breast feeding after renal transplantation. Transplantation Proceedings 1982; 14: 605-9
167. Egan PC, Costanza ME, Dodion P, et al. Doxorubicin and cisplatin excretion into human milk. Cancer Treatment Reports 1985; 69: 1387-9
168. Ben-Baruch G, Menczer J, Goshen R, et al. Cisplatin excretion in human milk. Journal of the National Cancer Institute 1992; 84: 451-2
169. Behrens O, Kohlhaw K, Gunter H, et al. Cyclosporin A in blood and breast milk. Geburtshilfe und Frauenheilkunde 1989; 49: 207-9
170. Sylvester RK, Lovell Teresi ME, Brundage D, et al. Excretion of hydroxyurea into milk. Cancer 1987; 60: 2177-8
171. Johns D, Rutherford L, Leighton P, et al. Secretion of methotrexate into human milk. American Journal of Obstetrics and Gynecology 1972; 112: 978-80
172. Blacker KH, Weinstein BJ, Ellman GL. Mother's milk and chlorpromazine. American Journal of Psychiatry 1962; 19: 178-9
173. Matheson I, Evang A, Overo KF, et al. Presence of chlorprothixene and its metabolites in breast milk. European Journal of Clinical Pharmacology 1984; 27: 611-3
174. Kirk L, Jorgenson A. Concentrations of CIS (Z)-flupentixol in maternal serum, amniotic fluid, umbilical cord serum and milk. Psychopharmacology 1980; 72: 107-8
175. Whalley LJ, Blain PG, Prime JK. Haloperidol secreted in breast milk. British Medical Journal 1981; 282: 1746-7
176. Stewart RB, Karas B, Springer PK. Haloperidol excretion in human milk. American Journal of Psychiatry 1980; 137: 849-50
177. Schou M, Amdisen A. Lithium and pregnancy: III. British Medical Journal 1973; 2: 138
178. Olesen OV, Bartels U, Poulsen JH. Perphenazine in breast milk and serum. American Journal of Psychiatry 1990; 147: 1378-9
179. Aono T, Shioji T, Aki T, et al. Augmentation of puerperal lactation by oral administration of sulpiride. Journal of Clinical Endocrinology and Metabolism 1979; 48: 478-82
180. Polatti F. Sulpiride isomers and milk secretion in puerperium. Clinical and Experimental Obstetrics and Gynaecology 1982; 9: 144-7
181. Aaes-Jorgensen T, Bjorndal F, Bartels U. Zuclopenthixol levels in breast milk. Psychopharmacology 1986; 90: 417-8
182. Low LCK, Lang J, Alexander WD. Excretion of carbimazole and propylthiouracil in breast milk. Lancet 1979; 2: 1011
183. Rylance GW, Woods CG, Donnelly MC, et al. Carbimazole and breast feeding. Lancet 1987; 1: 928
184. Jansson L, Ivarsson S, Larsson I, et al. Tri-iodothyronine and thyroxine in human milk. Acta Paediatrica Scandinavica 1983; 72: 703-5
185. Tegler L, Lindstrom B. Antithyroid drugs in milk. Lancet 1980; 2: 591
186. Cooper D, Bode H, Nath B, et al. Methimazole pharmacology in man: studies using a newly developed radioimmunoassay for methimazole. Journal of Clinical Endocrinology and Metabolism 1984; 58: 473-9
187. Kampmann J, Johansen K, Hansen J, et al. Propylthiouracil in human milk. Lancet 1980; 1: 736-8
188. Williams RH, Kay GA, Jandorf BJ. Thiouracil: its absorption, distribution and excretion. Journal of Clinical Investigation 1944; 23: 613-27
189. Mizuta H, Amino N, Ichihara K, et al. Thyroid hormones in human milk and their influences on thyroid function of breast fed babies. Pediatric Research 1983; 17: 468-71
190. Eriksson G, Oppenheim G, Smith G. Metronidazole in breast milk. Obstetrics and Gynecology 1981; 57: 48-50
191. Heisterberg L, Branebjerg P. Blood and milk concentrations of metronidazole in mothers and infants. Journal of Perinatal Medicine 1983; 11: 114-20
192. Moore B, Collier J. Drugs and breast feeding. British Medical Journal 1979; 2: 211
193. Gray MS, Kane P, Squires S. Further observations on metronidazole (Flagyl). British Journal of Venereal Diseases 1961; 37: 278-9
194. Passmore CM, McElnay JC, Rainey EA, et al. Metronidazole excretion in human milk and its effect on the suckling neonate. British Journal of Clinical Pharmacology 1988; 26: 45-51
195. Evaldson GR, Lindgren S, Nord CE, et al. Tinidazole milk excretion and pharmacokinetics in lactating women. British Journal of Clinical Pharmacology 1985; 19: 503-7
196. Mannisto PT, Karhunnen M, Koskela O, et al. Concentrations of tinidazole in breast milk (letter). Acta Pharmacologica et Toxicologica 1983; 53: 254-6
197. Holdiness MR. Antituberculosis drugs and breast feeding. Archives of Internal Medicine 1984; 144: 1888
198. Berlin CM, Lee C. Isoniazid and acetylisoniazid disposition in human milk and plasma. Federation Proceedings 1979; 38: 426
199. Somogyi A, Gugler R. Cimetidine excretion into breast milk. British Journal of Clinical Pharmacology 1979; 7: 627-8
200. Oo CY, Kuhn RJ, Desai N, et al. Active transport of cimetidine into human milk. Clinical Pharmacology and Therapeutics 1995; 58: 548-555
201. Courtney TP, Shaw RW, Cedar E, et al. Excretion of famotidine in breast milk. British Journal of Clinical Pharmacology 1988; 26: 639P
202. Obermeyer BD, Bergstrom RF, Callaghan JT, et al. Secretion of nizatidine into human breast milk after single and multiple doses. Clinical Pharmacology and Therapeutics 1990; 47: 724-30
203. Riley AJ, Crowley P, Harrison C. Transfer of ranitidine to biological fluids, milk and semen. In: Misiewicz JJ, Wormsley KG, eds. The clinical use of ranitidine. Oxford: Medicine Publishing Foundation 1981; 5: 77-86
204. Kearns GL, McConnell RF, Trang JM, et al. Appearance of ranitidine in breast milk following multiple dosing. Clinical Pharmacy 1985; 4: 322-4
205. Burrows JL, Jolley KW, Sullivan DJ. Determination of roxatidine in human plasma, urine and milk by capil-

lary gas chromatography using nitrogen-selective detection. Journal of Chromatography 1988; 432: 199-208
206. Lau RJ, Emery MG, Galinsky E. Unexpected accumulation of acyclovir in breast milk with estimation of infant exposure. Obstetrics and Gynecology 1987; 69: 468-71
207. Meyer LJ, Miranda P, Sheth N, et al. Acyclovir in human breast milk. American Journal of Obstetrics and Gynecology 1988; 158: 586-8
208. Jarboe CH, Cook LN, Malesic I, et al. Dyphylline elimination kinetics in lactating women: blood to milk transfer. Journal of Clinical Pharmacology 1981; 21: 405-10
209. Laursen LC, Borga O, Ljungholm K, et al. Transfer of enprofylline into breast milk. Therapeutic Drug Monitoring 1988; 10: 150-2
210. Boreus LO, De Chateau P, Lindberg C, et al. Terbutaline in breast milk. British Journal of Clinical Pharmacology 1982; 13: 731-2
211. Lonnerholm G, Lindstrom B. Terbutaline excretion into breast milk. British Journal of Clinical Pharmacology 1982; 13: 729-30
212. Lindberg C, Boreus LO, De Chateau P, et al. Transfer of terbutaline into breast milk. European Journal of Respiratory Diseases 1984; 65 Suppl. 134: 87-91
213. Stec GP, Greenberger P, Ruo T, et al. Kinetics of theophylline transfer to breast milk. Clinical Pharmacology and Therapeutics 1980; 28: 404-8
214. Yurchak AM, Jusko WJ. Theophylline secretion into breast milk. Pediatrics 1976; 57: 518-20
215. Okada M, Inoue H, Nakamura Y, et al. Excretion of diltiazem in human milk. New England Journal of Medicine 1985; 312: 992-3
216. Penny WJ, Lewis MJ. Nifedipine is excreted in human milk. European Journal of Clinical Pharmacology 1989; 36: 427-8
217. Ehrenkranz RA, Ackerman BA, Hulse JD. Nifedipine transfer into human milk. Journal of Pediatrics 1989; 114: 478-80
218. White WB, Yeh SC, Krol GJ. Nitrendipine in human plasma and breast milk. European Journal of Clinical Pharmacology 1989; 36: 531-4
219. Tonks AM. Nimodipine levels in breast milk. Australia and New Zealand Journal of Surgery 1995; 65: 693-4
220. Hartmann D, Lunell NO, Friedrich G, et al. Excretion of tiapamil in breast milk. British Journal of Clinical Pharmacology 1988; 26: 183-6
221. Miller MR, Withers R, Bhamra R, et al. Verapamil and breast-feeding. European Journal of Clinical Pharmacology 1986; 30: 125-6
222. Anderson HJ. Excretion of verapamil in human milk. European Journal of Clinical Pharmacology 1983; 25: 279-80
223. Inoue H, Unno N, Ou MC, et al. Level of verapamil in human milk. European Journal of Clinical Pharmacology 1984; 26: 657
224. Anderson P, Bondesson U, Mattiasson I, et al. Verapamil and norverapamil in plasma and breast milk during breast feeding. European Journal of Clinical Pharmacology 1987; 31: 625-7
225. Loughnan PM. Digoxin excretion in human breast milk. Journal of Pediatrics 1978; 92: 1019-20
226. Levy M, Granit L, Laufer N. Excretion of drugs in human milk. New England Journal of Medicine 1975; 297: 789
227. Chan V, Tse TF, Wong V. Transfer of digoxin across the placenta and into breast milk. British Journal of Obstetrics and Gynaecology 1978; 85: 605-9
228. Finley JP, Waxman MB, Wong PY, et al. Digoxin excretion in human milk. Journal of Pediatrics 1979; 94: 339-40
229. Reinhardt D, Richter O, Genz T, et al. Kinetics of the translactal passage of digoxin from breast feeding mothers to their infants. European Journal of Pediatrics 1982; 138: 49-52
230. Ost L, Wettrell G, Bjorkhem I, et al. Prednisolone excretion in human milk. Journal of Pediatrics 1985; 106: 1008
231. McKenzie S, Selley J, Agnew J. Secretion of prednisolone into breast milk. Archives of Disease in Childhood 1975; 50: 894-6
232. Greenberger PA, Odeh YK, Frederiksen MC, et al. Pharmacokinetics of prednisone transfer to breast milk. Clinical Pharmacology and Therapeutics 1993; 53: 324-8
233. Katz F, Duncan B. Entry of prednisone into human milk. New England Journal of Medicine 1975; 293: 1154
234. Fitzjohn TP, Williams DG, Laker MF, et al. Intravenous urography during lactation. British Journal of Radiology 1982; 55: 603-5
235. Nielsen ST, Matheson I, Rasmussen JN, et al. Excretion of iohexol and metrizoate in human breast milk. Acta Radiologica 1987; 28: 523-6
236. Holmdahl KH. Cholecystography during lactation. Acta Radiologica 1956; 45: 305-7
237. Ilett K, Hackett L, Paterson J. Excretion of metrizamide in milk. British Journal of Radiology 1981; 54: 537-8
238. Soderman P, Hartvig P, Fagerlund C. Acetazolamide excretion into human breast milk. British Journal of Clinical Pharmacology 1984; 17: 599
239. Werthmann MW, Krees SV. Excretion of chlorothiazide in human breast milk. Journal of Pediatrics 1972; 81: 781-3
240. Mulley BA, Parr GD, Pau WK, et al. Placental transfer of chlorthalidone and its elimination in maternal milk. European Journal of Clinical Pharmacology 1978; 13: 129-31
241. Miller MR, Cohn RD, Burghart PH. Hydrochlorothiazide disposition in a mother and her breast-fed infant. Journal of Pediatrics 1982; 101: 789-91
242. Phelps D, Karim A. Spironolactone: relationship between concentrations of dethioacetylated metabolite in human serum and milk. Journal of Pharmaceutical Sciences 1977; 66: 1203
243. Nilsson S, Nygren K, Johansson EDB. Transfer to estradiol to human milk. American Journal of Obstetrics and Gynecology 1978; 132: 653-7
244. Heikkila M, Haukkamaa M, Luukkainen T. Levonorgestrel in milk and plasma of breast-feeding women with a levonorgestrel-releasing IUD. Contraception 1982; 25: 41-9
245. Diaz S, Herreros C, Juez G, et al. Fertility regulation in nursing women. Contraception 1985; 32: 53-74
246. Van Der Molen HJ, Hart PG, Wijmenga HG. Studies with 4-$^{14}$C-lynestrenol in normal and lactating women. Acta Endocrinologica 1969; 61: 255-74
247. Koetsawang S, Nukulkarn P, Fortherby K, et al. Transfer of contraceptive steroids in milk of women using long-acting gestagens. Contraception 1982; 25: 321
248. Saxena B, Schrimanker K, Grudzinskas J. Levels of contraceptive steroids in breast milk and plasma of lactating women. Contraception 1977; 16: 605-13
249. Wijmenga H, Van Der Molen H. Studies with 4-$^{14}$C-mestranol in lactating women. Acta Endocrinologica 1969; 61: 655-77

250. Bhaskar A, Schulze P, Acksteiner B, et al. Quantitative analysis of norethindrone in milk using deuterated carrier and gas chromatography-mass spectrometry. Journal of Steroid Biochemistry and Molecular Biology 1979; 11: 1323-8
251. Fotherby K, Towobola D, Muggeridge J, et al. Norethisterone levels in maternal serum and milk after intramuscular injection of norethisterone oenanthate as a contraceptive. Contraception 1983; 28 (5): 405
252. Cooke ID, Back DJ, Shroff NE. Norethisterone concentration in breast milk and infant and maternal plasma during ethynodiol diacetate administration. Contraception 1985; 31: 611-20
253. Nilsson S, Nygren K-G, Johansson E. d-Norgestrel concentrations in maternal plasma, milk and child plasma during administration or oral contraceptives to nursing women. American Journal of Obstetrics and Gynecology 1977; 129: 178
254. Pan H, Fleiss P, Moore L, et al. Excretion of pravastatin, an HMG CoA reductase inhibitor in breast milk of lactating women. Journal of Clinical Pharmacology 1988; 28: 908-59
255. Mountford PJ, Coakley AJ. Guidelines for breast feeding following maternal radiopharmaceutical administration. Nuclear Medicine Communications 1986; 7: 399-401
256. Eriksson G, Swahn CG. Concentrations of baclofen in serum and breast milk from a lactating woman. Scandinavian Journal of Clinical and Laboratory Investigation 1981; 41: 185-7
257. Silcox J, Schulz P, Horbay GLA, et al. Transfer of carbetocin into human breast milk. Obstetrics and Gynecology 1993; 82: 456-9
258. Stopelli I, Rainer E, Humpell M. Transfer of cyproterone acetate to the milk of lactating women. Contraception 1980; 22: 485-93
259. Ekstrand J, Spak CJ, Falch J, et al. Distribution of fluoride to human breast milk. Caries Research 1984; 18: 93-5
260. Bell RAF, Dale IM. Gold secretion in maternal milk. Arthritis and Rheumatism 1976; 19: 1374
261. Ostensen M, Skavdal K, Myklebust G, et al. Excretion of gold into human breast milk. European Journal of Clinical Pharmacology 1986; 31: 251
262. Postellon DC, Aronow R. Iodine in mothers milk. Journal of the American Medical Association 1982; 247: 463
263. Ogbuokiri JE, Ozumba BC, Okonkwo PO. Ivermectin levels in human breast milk. European Journal of Clinical Pharmacology 1994; 46: 98-0
264. Cruikshank DP, Varner MW, Pitkin RM. Breast milk magnesium and calcium concentrations following magnesium sulfate treatment. American Journal of Obstetrics and Gynecology 1982; 143: 685-8
265. Erkkola R, Kanto J, Allonem H, et al. Excretion of methylergometrine (methylergonovine) into the human breast milk. International Journal of Clinical Pharmacology 1978; 16: 579-80
266. Olsson B, Bolme P, Dahlstrom B, et al. Excretion of noscapine in human breast milk. European Journal of Clinical Pharmacology 1986; 30: 213-5
267. Witter FR, Smith RV. The excretion of pentoxifylline and its metabolites into human breast milk. American Journal of Obstetrics and Gynecology 1985; 151: 1094-7
268. Putter J, Held F. Quantitative studies on the occurrence of praziquantel in milk and plasma of lactating women. European Journal of Drug Metabolism and Pharmacokinetics 1979; 4: 193-8
269. Hardell LI, Lindstrom B, Lonnerholm G, et al. Pyridostigmine in human breast milk. British Journal of Clinical Pharmacology 1982; 14: 565-7
270. Werthmann M, Kress S. Quantitative excretion of Senokot in human breast milk. Medical Annals of the District of Columbia 1973; 42: 4-5
271. Verstraete M. Clinical application of inhibitors of fibrinolysis. Drugs 1985; 29: 236-61
272. Steiner E, Villen T, Hallberg M, et al. Amphetamine excretion in breast milk. European Journal of Clinical Pharmacology 1984; 27: 123-4
273. Tyrala EE, Dodson WE. Caffeine secretion into breast milk. Archives of Disease in Childhood 1979; 54: 787-800
274. Stavchansky S, Combs A, Sagraves R, et al. Pharmacokinetics of caffeine in breast milk and plasma after single oral administration of caffeine to lactating mothers. Biopharmaceutics and Drug Disposition 1988; 9: 285-99
275. Hildebrandt R, Gundert-Remy U. Lack of pharmacologically active saliva levels of caffeine in breast-fed infants. Pediatric Pharmacology 1983; 3: 237-44
276. Chasnoff IJ, Lewis DE, Squires L. Cocaine intoxication in a breast-fed infant. Pediatrics 1987; 80: 836
277. Kesaneimi YA. Ethanol and acetaldehyde in the milk and peripheral blood of lactating women after ethanol administration. Journal of Obstetrics and Gynaecology of the British Commonwealth 1974; 81: 84-6
278. Flores-Huerta S, Hernandez-Montes H, Argote RM, et al. Effects of ethanol consumption during pregnancy and lactation on the outcome and postnatal growth of the offspring. Annals of Nutrition and Metabolism 1992; 36: 121-8
279. Luck W, Nau H. Nicotine and cotinine concentrations in serum and milk of nursing smokers. British Journal of Clinical Pharmacology 1984; 18: 9-15
280. Trundle JI, Skellern GG. Gas chromatographic determination of nicotine in human breast milk. Journal of Clinical Hospital Pharmacy 1983; 8: 289-93
281. Fergusson BB, Wilson DJ, Schaffner W. Determinations of nicotine concentrations in human milk. American Journal of Diseases of Children 1976; 130: 837-9
282. Kaufman KR, Petrucha RA, Pitts FN, et al. PCP in amniotic fluid and breast milk: case report. Journal of Clinical Psychiatry 1983; 44: 269-70
283. Perez-Reyes M, Wall ME. Presence of delta-9 tetrahydrocannabinol in human milk. New England Journal of Medicine 1982; 307: 819-20
284. Resman BH, Blumenthal P, Jusko WJ. Breast milk distribution in theobromine chocolate. Journal of Pediatrics 1977; 91: 477-80

Appendix D

# Guide to Drug Dosage in Renal Failure

*W.M. Bennett*

The dosage of many drugs must be adjusted in patients with renal dysfunction to avoid adverse reactions and to ensure efficacy. In addition, the biochemical abnormalities present in renal failure may alter the pharmacodynamics of agents not normally excreted by the kidneys, resulting in heightened pharmacodynamic effects.

The theoretical basis for adjusting drug dosage in renal failure is discussed in other chapters in this book (see chapter 1, sect. 5.4.4; and chapter 24, sect. 1.4). Because data on individual drug kinetics are collected in relatively few patients, extrapolation to other patient groups is difficult. Although drug level monitoring may provide a more precise tool to ensure therapeutic efficacy and safety, these services are not always available. Furthermore, for some drugs, such as the aminoglycoside antibiotics, control of blood concentrations has not always reduced the incidence of toxicity because of the poor correlation between blood concentrations and uptake into target tissues such as the inner ear and kidneys.

The table (table I) that follows provides *rough guidelines* on which to base drug therapy in patients with varying degrees of renal insufficiency. The recommendations are derived from a large literature base which is often conflicting and seldom based on prospective validation of data derived under controlled conditions. Thus, the clinician needs to carefully weigh factors present in the individual patient using the information in the table as a starting point.

An alternative approach to estimation of maintenance doses by use of a nomogram is presented in appendix E.

## 1. Use of the Table

Drugs are listed in alphabetical order according to their predominant pharmacological action or therapeutic use. An 'anti' classification has been used in most cases. The maintenance dosage recommendations are based on the excretion or metabolism of the drug or a pharmacologically active metabolite, as well as the normal elimination (plasma) half-life of the parent drug and/or active metabolite. Where data were available, an indication is given of the plasma half-life of the drug in the anuric patient and of the percentage of drug excreted unchanged in the urine under normal circumstances.

- *Loading dose:* in general, all patients are given a loading dose which is the same as the 'usual' dose for a patient with normal renal function.
- *Maintenance dose:* the table is prepared on the basis of two methods of dose modification: (a) the 'usual' maintenance dose given at variable increased intervals according to the estimated prolongation in plasma half-life with renal insufficiency; and (b) reduction of the size of the maintenance dose leaving the normal dose interval unchanged. The dose reduction method is used in particular for drugs for which a relatively constant plasma concentration is desired.

In the table, following identification of the method used (**D** for dose reduction or **I** for interval extension), recommendations are given for various levels of renal function as estimated by the glomerular filtration rate (GFR). For the dose reduction method, the percentage of the usual dose that should be given at the normal dose interval is shown, whereas for the interval extension method, the number of hours between doses of normal size is given. No controlled clinical trials have been performed to establish the relative efficacy of these two methods for drug dosage alterations in patients with renal insufficiency. The interval extension method provides the benefits of convenience and decreased cost, while the dose reduction method produces more constant blood concentrations.

The qualitative effect of standard clinical dialysis on drug removal is shown for haemodialysis (**H**) and peritoneal dialysis (**P**). The designation 'yes' refers to the removal of enough drug to require a dosage supplement to ensure adequate therapeutic blood concentrations, whereas 'no' refers to the lack of need for dosage adjustment with dialysis. Drug removal by more permeable membranes such as those used in continuous arteriovenous haemofiltration is not included, and dosage adjustments for patients on continuous ambulatory peritoneal dialysis (CAPD) are not given.

It should be emphasised that some drugs that have high dialysis clearances could be designated 'no' if the amount of drug removed does not necessitate supplemental postdialysis doses. This usually occurs when the apparent volume of distribution is large, e.g. digoxin. 'No' does not apply to high flux dialysis membranes and continuous therapies used in acute renal failure where drug loss is by convective transport and thus highly dependent on protein binding. To ensure efficacy when information about dialysis loss is not available, maintenance doses should be given after dialysis. The designation 'no' in the table does not preclude the use of dialysis or haemoperfusion for drug overdoses.

Toxic effects in patients with renal failure as well as comments pertinent to therapy in these patients and representative reference material are also included in the table.

## 2. Limitations of the Table

When using the dosage guidelines, the following points must be considered:

1) *The status of renal function must be determined not only before but also during the entire period of treatment* - the appropriate maintenance dose for a patient is not a stable characteristic if the kidney function is not stable. It can change as dramatically as kidney function; a dose which was carefully calculated yesterday may have become excessive overnight, because in the meantime, the patient has stopped making urine.

2) *The dosage guidelines do not necessarily apply to elderly patients* - even when creatinine concentrations and blood urea nitrogen are normal, since elderly patients with low muscle mass can have 'normal' serum urea or creatinine in the presence of reduced renal function. A drug that is largely eliminated by the kidney may therefore accumulate in an elderly patient. Other changes in drug disposition in the elderly patient may also be important, e.g. in the apparent volume of distribution (see further chapter 4; sect. 1.4).

3) *Many aspects of individual patients influence drug response in uraemia* - the complexity of the clinical status in individual uraemic patients, as well as variables such as possible altered absorption, protein binding or metabolism, liver function, other drug therapy, etc, makes any fixed approach to drug dosage subject to error (see further chapter 1, sect. 5.4.4; and chapter 24, sect. 2). Individual patients must always be followed for clinical evidence of drug toxicity or lack of efficacy. The dosage guidelines given may therefore require frequent reappraisal to ensure effective and safe therapy.

4) *Monitoring of drug plasma concentrations is useful* - particularly for drugs with a low therapeutic ratio such as the antiarrhythmics (see further chapter 1, sect. 6.2.1; and chapter 5, sect. 3).

5) *Uraemic patients should always be observed carefully for unexpected drug toxicity* (see further chapter 6, sect. 6; and chapter 24, sect. 1.5).

### Further Reading

Anderson RJ, Schrier RW, Gambertoglio JG. Clinical use of drugs in patients with kidney and liver disease. Philadelphia: WB Saunders, 1981

Bennett WM, Aronoff GR, Morrison G, et al. Drug prescribing in renal failure: dosing guidelines for adults. American Journal of Kidney Diseases 1983; 3: 155

Chennavasin P, Brater DC. Nomograms for drug use in renal disease. Clinical Pharmacokinetics 1981; 6: 193

Golper TA, Wedel SK, Kaplan AA, et al. Drug removal during continuous arteriovenous hemofiltration: theory and clinical observations. International Journal of Artificial Organs 1985; 8: 307-12

Golper TA, Bennett WM. Drug removal by continuous arteriovenous hemofiltration: a review of the evidence in poisoned patients. Medical Toxicology 1988; 3: 341-9

Knepshield JH, Winchester JF. Hemodialysis and hemoperfusion for drugs and poisons. Transactions of the American Society of Artificial Internal Organs 1982; 28: 666

Maher JF. Pharmacokinetics in patients with renal failure. Clinical Nephrology 1984; 21: 39

Reidenberg MM, Drayer DE. Drug therapy in renal failure. Annual Review of Pharmacology and Toxicology 1980; 20: 45

Van Scoy RE, Wilson WR. Antimicrobial agents in patients with renal insufficiency. Mayo Clinic Proceedings 1983; 58: 246

Wenk M, Vožeh S, Follath F. Serum level monitoring of antibacterial drugs. Clinical Pharmacokinetics 1984; 9: 475

**Appendix D.** Guide to drug dosage in renal failure

| Drug | Elimination half-life ($t_{1/2}$) [adults] | | Excreted unchanged (%) | Extra-renal excretion[a] (normal) | Normal dose interval (h) | Dose adjustment for renal failure[b] | | | | Dialysis[d] | Toxic effects in renal failure/ Notes[e] | References |
|---|---|---|---|---|---|---|---|---|---|---|---|---|
| | normal (h) | ESRD (h) | | | | method[c] | creatinine clearance (ml/min) | | | | | |
| | | | | | | | > 50 | 10-50 | < 10 | | | |
| **ACE (angiotensin-converting enzyme) inhibitors** | | | | | | | | | | | | |
| Benazepril | 21-22 | Prolonged | 15 | | 12 | D | Unch | 25-75 | 25-50 | No (H) | | 1 |
| Captopril | 1.9 | 21-32 | 50-70 | | 12 | D | Unch | Unch | 50 | Yes (H) | Proteinuria, nephrotic syndrome, granulocytopenia, hyperkalaemia | 2 |
| Enalapril | 24-36 | 40-60 | 50 | | 12 | D | Unch | 75-100 | 50 | Yes (H) | | 3 |
| Fosinopril | 15 | 19-28 | 50 | | 12 | D | Unch | Unch | 75 | No (H,P) | Avoid in patients with combined liver and kidney failure | 4 |
| Lisinopril | 12-36 | 36-48 | 70 | | 24 | D | Unch | 75 | 50 | Yes (H) | | 5 |
| Perindopril | 11 | 26-36 | 80-90 | | 12-24 | D, I | 50-100 q12-24h | 25-75 q18-24h | 25 q48h | Yes (H) | | 6 |
| Quinapril | 2.3 | 12 | 50 | | 12 | D | Unch | 50-75 | 50 | No (H,P) | | 7 |
| Ramipril | 5-8 | 15 | 30 | | 12-24 | D | Unch | 50-75 | 50 | Yes (H) | | 8, 9 |
| β-**Adrenoceptor antagonists** (see chapters 20, sect. 6.1.2 and 21, sect. 3.2) | | | | | | | | | | | | |
| Acebutolol | 7-9 | 7 | 55 | He | 12 or 24 | D | Unch | 50 | 25* | No (H) | *Active metabolite with long $t_{1/2}$ (diacetolol) accumulates | 10 |
| Atenolol | 6-9 | 15-35 | < 90 | | 24 | D<br>I | Unch<br>24 | 50<br>48 | 25<br>96 | Yes (H)<br>No (P) | Accumulates in ESRD | 11, 12 |
| Betaxolol | 14-22 | 31 | 15 | He | 24 | D | Unch | Unch | 50 | No (H,P) | | 13 |
| Bevantolol | 1.4 | 1.4 | Low | He | 12 | D | Unch | Unch | Unch | ? | Has α-adrenoceptor blocking action | 14 |
| Bisoprolol | 10-12 | 18-24 | 50 | | 24 | D | Unch | Unch | 50 | No (H,P) | | 15-17 |
| Bopindolol | 6-8 | 10.4 | Low | He | 24 | D | Unch | 25-50 | 25 | Yes (H,P) | | 18 |
| Carteolol | 7 | 33 | 60-70 | | 12 | D | Unch | 50 | 25 | No (H,P) | | 19 |
| Carvedilol | 3-6 | ? | Low | He | 12 | D | Unch | Unch | 75 | No (H) | Half-life prolonged in the elderly to 15h | 20 |
| Celiprolol | 3-5 | 5-8 | 20 | NR | 24 | D | Unch | Unch | 50 | No (H,P) | | 21 |
| Esmolol | 9 min | 9 min | < 5 | NR | IV infusion | D | Unch | Unch | Unch | No (H,P) | Rapidly hydrolysed by red cell esterases | 22 |
| Labetalol | 3-8 | 3-8 | 0-5 | He | 12 | D | Unch | Unch | Unch | No (H) | | 23 |
| Metoprolol | 2.5-4.5 | 2.5-4.5 | 5 | He | 12 | D | Unch | Unch | Unch | Yes (H) | Bioavailability may increase and caution advised; metabolites spuriously increase bilirubin by assay interface | 24 |
| Nadolol | 14-24 | 45 | 90 | | 24 | D | Unch | 50 | 25 | Yes (H) | Accumulates in ESRD | 25 |
| Pindolol | 2.5-4 | 3-4 | 40 | He | 12 | D | Unch | Unch | Unch | ? | | 26 |

[Continued over]

For footnotes, see final page of table (p. 1747)

**Appendix D.** *[Continued]*

| Drug | Elimination half-life ($t_{1/2}$) [adults] | | Excreted unchanged (%) | Extra-renal excretion[a] (normal) | Normal dose interval (h) | Dose adjustment for renal failure[b] | | | | Dialysis[d] | Toxic effects in renal failure/ Notes[e] | References |
|---|---|---|---|---|---|---|---|---|---|---|---|---|
| | normal (h) | ESRD (h) | | | | method[c] | creatinine clearance (ml/min) | | | | | |
| | | | | | | | > 50 | 10-50 | < 10 | | | |
| **β-*Adrenoceptor antagonists*** *[continued]* | | | | | | | | | | | | |
| Propranolol | 2-6 | 1-6 | < 5 | He | 6-12 | D | Unch | Unch* | Unch* | No (H) | *Bioavailability may increase and caution advised; metabolites spuriously increase bilirubin by assay interface | 27, 28 |
| Sotalol | 5-15 | 56 | 60 | He | 12 | D | Unch | 30 | 15-30 | Yes (H) | | 29 |
| Timolol | 2.5-4 | 4 | 15 | He | 8-12 | D | Unch | Unch | Unch | No (H) | | 12 |
| **Anaesthetics, intravenous (**see chapter 12; sect. 2.1) | | | | | | | | | | | | |
| Thiopental (thiopentone) | 10 | 6-18 | 10-15 | He | Infusion | D | Unch | Unch | 75 | ? | | 30, 31 |
| **Analgesics** (see chapter 12, sect. 7.1) | | | | | | | | | | | | |
| • *Nonsteroidal anti-inflammatory drugs* | | | | | | | | | | | These agents may reduce renal function as well as causing interstitial nephritis, nephrotic syndrome and hyperkalaemia, and may decrease the effect of diuretics | |
| Diclofenac | 1-2 | 1-2 | < 5 | He | 12 | D | Unch | Unch | Unch | No (H,P) | May cause sodium retention, aggravation of hypertension, reduced GFR | 32 |
| Diflunisal | 5-20* | 115 | < 5 | He | 12 | D | Unch | Unch | 50 | No (H) | *Dose-dependent | 33, 34 |
| Fenoprofen | 2-3 | ? | 2-5 | He | 6-8 | D | Unch | Unch | Unch | No (H) | May cause sodium retention, aggravation of hypertension, reduced GFR | 33, 34 |
| Ibuprofen | 2.5 | Unch | 10 | He | 6 | D | Unch | Unch | Unch | No (H) | May cause sodium retention, reduced GFR | 33-36 |
| Indomethacin | 4-12 | 4-12 | 15 | He | 8-12 | D | Unch | Unch | Unch | No (H) | May cause sodium retention, aggravation of hypertension, reduced GFR | 33, 34, 37 |
| Ketoprofen | 1-3 | 3-6 | 10 | He | 12 | D | Unch | 50 | 25 | No (H,P) | May cause sodium retention, aggravation of hypertension, reduced GFR | 38 |
| Naproxen | 14-17 | 15 | < 1 | He | 12 | D | Unch | Unch | Unch | No (H) | May cause sodium retention, reduced GFR | 33, 34, 39 |
| Piroxicam | 45 | 44 | 2-5 | He | 24 | D | Unch | Unch | Unch | No (H,P) | May cause sodium retention, aggravation of hypertension, reduced GFR | 40 |
| Pirprofen | 5-10 | 10-15 | < 5 | He | 12 | D | Unch | Unch | 50 | No (H,P) | May cause sodium retention, aggravation of hypertension, reduced GFR | 41 |
| Proquazone | 5-14 | 10-16 | 50 | He | 24 | D | Unch | Unch | 50 | No (H,P) | May cause sodium retention, aggravation of hypertension, reduced GFR | |

| | | | | | | | | | | | | |
|---|---|---|---|---|---|---|---|---|---|---|---|---|
| Sulindac | 7* | ? | 7 | He | 12 | D | Unch | Unch | Unch | No (H) | *Active metabolite (sulfide) t½ = 16 hours. Appears less likely to reduce GFR than congeners; metabolic activation of prodrug to active metabolite | 33, 34, 42 |
| Tenoxicam | 70 | 70 | < 1 | He | 24 | D | Unch | Unch | Unch | No (H,P) | May cause sodium retention, aggravation of hypertension, reduced GFR | 43 |
| Tolmetin | 1-2 | 2-4 | 2-3 | He | 12 | D | Unch | Unch | 50-75 | No (H,P) | May cause false-positive urinary test for protein | 43 |
| • *Simple analgesics* | | | | | | | | | | | | |
| Aspirin | 2-30* | 2-30* | 10* | He | 4-6 | I | 4 | 4-6 | Avoid** | Yes (H,P) | *Salicylate (dose-dependent elimination). Nephrotoxic in overdoses; may decrease GFR; excretion enhanced in alkaline urine. **Adds to uraemic platelet dysfunction and gastrointestinal symptoms | 44 |
| Codeine | 2.5-3.5 | 19 | 16 | He | 4-6 | D | Unch | Unch | Unch | No (H) | Excessive sedation, respiratory depression | 45 |
| Dextropro-poxyphene | 12 | 12-20 | < 20 | He | 4-6 | D | Unch | Unch | 25* | No (H,P) | *Active metabolite (norpropoxyphene) accumulates; excessive sedation | 46 |
| Paracetamol (acetamino-phen) | 2 | 2 | < 10 | He | 4-6 | I | 4 | 6 | 8 | Yes (H) No (P) | Nephrotoxic as well as hepatotoxic in overdosage due to formation of a reactive alkylating metabolite | 47 |
| • *Strong analgesics (opioids)* | | | | | | | | | | | | |
| Butorphanol | 2.2-3.5 | ? | < 5 | He | 4 | D | Unch | Unch | Unch | ? | Excessive sedation, respiratory depression | 48 |
| Fentanyl | 3-14 | Unch | 10 | He | Single dose | D | Unch | Unch | Unch | ? | Excessive sedation, respiratory depression | 49, 50 |
| Methadone | 18-97 | 13-55 | 25 | G | 6-8 | D | Unch | Unch | 50-75 | No (H,P) | Excessive sedation, respiratory depression. Excretion enhanced in acid urine | 51 |
| Morphine | 2.3-2.5 | 3-4 | 10-15 | He, G | 4 | D | Unch | Unch | 50-75* | No (H,P) | Excessive sedation, respiratory depression. *Renal metabolism decreases in ESRD resulting in enhanced pharmacological effect | 52-54 |
| Pentazocine | 2-3 | ? | 12 | He | 4-6 | D | Unch | Unch | Unch | Yes (H) | Respiratory depression, excessive sedation | 55 |
| Pethidine (meperidine) | 2.4-7 | Unch* | ≈ 5 | He | 4 | D | Unch | Unch | 50-75 | No (H) | *Active metabolite accumulates which may produce seizures, excessive sedation, respiratory depression. Excretion increased 20-30% in acid urine | 56, 57 |
| Sufentanil | 2-4 | 2-4 | < 10 | He | Single dose | D | Unch | Unch | Unch | ? | | 58 |
| Tramadol | 6 | 6-10 | 50 | | 6 | D | Unch | Unch | 50 | ? | | 59 |
| • *Analgesic antagonists* | | | | | | | | | | | | |
| Naloxone | 1-1.5 | ? | Low | He | 2-4 | D | Unch | Unch | Unch | ? | | 60 |
| Naltrexone | 1.1-2.7 | ? | Low | He | 2-4 | D | Unch | Unch | Unch | ? | | 61 |

*[Continued over]*

*For footnotes, see final page of table (p. 1747)*

**Appendix D.** *[Continued]*

| Drug | Elimination half-life ($t_{1/2}$) [adults] normal (h) | ESRD (h) | Excreted unchanged (%) | Extra-renal excretion[a] (normal) | Normal dose interval (h) | Dose adjustment for renal failure[b] method[c] | creatinine clearance (ml/min) > 50 | 10-50 | < 10 | Dialysis[d] | Toxic effects in renal failure/ Notes[e] | References |
|---|---|---|---|---|---|---|---|---|---|---|---|---|
| **Antianxiety drugs/hypnosedatives** (see chapter 30, sect. 6.1) | | | | | | | | | | | | |
| • *Barbiturates** | | | | | | | | | | | *Drugs in this group may increase osteomalacia in haemodialysis patients; $t_{1/2}$ decreases with long term therapy; excessive sedation | |
| Hexobarbital | 3.5-5 | ? | 20-30 | He | 12-24 | D | Unch | Unch | Unch | No (H) | | 30 |
| Pentobarbital | 18-48 | Unch | 20 | He | 8-24 | D | Unch | Unch | Unch | No (H) | | 30 |
| Phenobarbital | 60-150 | 117-160 | 30* | He | 8 | I | Unch | Unch | 12-16 | Yes (H,P) | *Up to 50% excreted unchanged in alkaline urine | 30 |
| Secobarbital (quinalbarbitone) | 20-35 | ? | 10-20 | He | 24 | D | Unch | Unch | Unch | No (H,P) | | 30 |
| • *Benzodiazepines** | | | | | | | | | | | *Agents in this group may cause excessive sedation or encephalopathy in dialysis patients | |
| Alprazolam | 10-19 | 10-19 | 20 | He | 12-24 | D | Unch | Unch | Unch | ? | | 62 |
| Brotizolam | 4-8 | 7-9 | 1 | He | 24 | D | Unch | Unch | Unch | ? | | 63 |
| Chlordiazepoxide | 5-30 | Unch | < 1 | He | 8-24 | D | Unch | Unch | 50 | No (H) | Active metabolites accumulate; excessive sedation | 64-66 |
| Clorazepate | 36-200 | 150-300* | < 1 | He | 24 | D | Unch | Unch | Unch | ? | *Long-acting active metabolite | 67 |
| Diazepam | 24-48 | Unch | < 1 | He | 8-24 | D | Unch | Unch | Unch | No (H) | Excessive sedation; active metabolite (*N*-desmethyldiazepam) accumulates | 64, 65, 68 |
| Flurazepam | 47-100* | Unch | < 1 | He | 24 | D | Unch | Unch | Unch | No (H) | Excessive sedation. * Principal active metabolite | 64, 65 |
| Lorazepam | 8-25 | 32-70 | <1 | He | 8-24 | D | Unch | Unch | 50 | No (H) | Excessive sedation | 64, 65, 69, 70 |
| Midazolam | 9-16 | 32-70 | < 1 | He | 24 | D | Unch | Unch | Unch | No (H) | Protein binding decreased in uraemia | 71 |
| Nitrazepam | 21-40 | | < 1 | He | 24 | D | Unch | Unch | Unch | ? | | 72 |
| Oxazepam | 6-25 | 25-90 | < 1 | He | 8-24 | D | Unch | Unch | 75 | No (H) | Excessive sedation; glucuronide metabolite accumulates | 69, 73 |
| Prazepam | 36-200 | 150-300* | < 1 | He | 24 | D | Unch | Unch | Unch | ? | *Long-acting metabolite | |
| Triazolam | 2-5 | ? | < 1 | He | 24 | D | Unch | Unch | Unch | ? | | 74, 75 |

| | | | | | | | | | | | | |
|---|---|---|---|---|---|---|---|---|---|---|---|---|
| • *Others* | | | | | | | | | | | | |
| Buspirone | 2-5 | 5-6 | 1 | He | 12 | D | Unch | Unch | Unch* | ? | *Active metabolite accumulates | 76 |
| Meprobamate | 6-17 | Unch | 8-19 | He | 6 | I | 6 | 9-12 | 12-18 | Yes (H,P) | Excessive sedation | 77 |
| **Antiarrhythmic drugs** (see chapter 20, sect. 8.2 and also β-adrenoceptor antagonists) | | | | | | | | | | | | |
| Acecainide (*N*-acetyl-procainamide) | 6-8 | 42-70 | 75 | | 4-6 | I | Unch | 6 | 12 | Yes (H) | | 78 |
| Amiodarone | 3-100 days | Unch | < 1 | He | 24 | D | Unch | Unch | Unch | No (H) | Thyroid dysfunction peripheral neuropathy; increases plasma digoxin concentration | 79, 80 |
| Bretylium | 6-13.6 | 16-32 | 75 | | 6-8 | D | Unch | 25-50 | Avoid* | No (H) | *Little specific data on ESRD | 81 |
| Cibenzoline | 5-8 | 22-24 | 75 | | | D, I | Unch q6-12h | 70 q12-24h | 50 q24h | No (H) | | 82 |
| Disopyramide | 5-8 | 10-18 | 50-60 | He | 6-8 | I | Unch | 12-24 | 24-40 | Yes (H) | Urinary retention | 83 |
| Encainide | 1-3 | 1-3 | < 10 | He | 4 | D | Unch | Unch | Unch | ? | Metabolites accumulate | 79 |
| Flecainide | 12-20 | 19-26 | 7-45* | He | 12 | D | Unch | Unch | 75 | No (H) | *Excretion enhanced in acid urine; metabolites accumulate | 79, 84, 85 |
| Lidocaine (lignocaine) | 1.2-4 | 1.3-3.0 | 20* | He | Infusion | D | Unch | Unch | Unch | No (H) | $t_{1/2}$ dependent on hepatic blood flow; active metabolite accumulates during prolonged infusion.<br>*Excretion enhanced in acid urine | 86 |
| Lorcainide | 7-13* | ? | < 3 | He | 12-24 | D | Unch | Unch | Unch | ? | *Active metabolite (norlorcainide) has a longer $t_{1/2}$ and may accumulate | 79, 87 |
| Mexiletine | 8-13 | 16 | 10-20 | He | 12 | D | Unch | Unch | 75 | ? | Excretion enhanced in acid urine | 79, 88 |
| Procainamide | 2.5-4.9 | 5.3-5.9 | 45-65* | He | 4-6 | I | 4-6 | 6-12 | 8-24 | Yes (H) | May cause lupus syndrome.<br>*Active metabolite (*N*-acetylprocainamide) has a longer $t_{1/2}$ and accumulates more than parent drug | 89 |
| Propafenone | 2.2-9.5 | 7-20 | < 1 | He | 8 | I | Unch | 8-24* | 8-24* | No (H,P) | *Enzymatic genetic polymorphism results in variable metabolism | 90 |
| Quinidine | 3-16 | 3-16 | 10-50* | He | 6-12 | I | Unch | Unch | Unch | Yes (H,P) | Active metabolite; may cause lupus syndrome; increases plasma digoxin.<br>*Excretion enhanced in acid urine | 91 |
| Tocainide | 11-19 | 22 | 40 | He | 8 | D | Unch | Unch | 50 | Yes (H) | | 92, 93 |
| **Antibacterial drugs** (see chapter 31, sect. 1) | | | | | | | | | | | | |
| • *Aminoglycosides** | | | | | | | | | | | *All agents in this group are ototoxic and nephrotoxic, and rarely may cause respiration paralysis. Monitor serum levels to ensure efficacy | 94, 95 |
| Amikacin | 2.5-3 | 30 | 95 | | 8-12 | D<br>I | 60-90<br>12 | 30-70<br>12-18 | 20-30<br>24 | Yes (H,P) | | 96, 97 |

[Continued over]

*For footnotes, see final page of table (p. 1747)*

**Appendix D.** *[Continued]*

| Drug | Elimination half-life ($t_{1/2}$) [adults] normal (h) | Elimination half-life ($t_{1/2}$) [adults] ESRD (h) | Excreted unchanged (%) | Extra-renal excretion[a] (normal) | Normal dose interval (h) | Dose adjustment for renal failure[b] method[c] | creatinine clearance (ml/min) > 50 | creatinine clearance (ml/min) 10-50 | creatinine clearance (ml/min) < 10 | Dialysis[d] | Toxic effects in renal failure/ Notes[e] | References |
|---|---|---|---|---|---|---|---|---|---|---|---|---|
| **Antibacterial drugs** *[continued]* | | | | | | | | | | | | |
| Gentamicin | 2.5-3 | 30-50 | 90-98 | | 8 | D<br>I | 60-90<br>8-12 | 30-70<br>12 | 20-30<br>24 | Yes (H,P) | | 94, 98 |
| Kanamycin | 2-5 | 72-96 | 50-90 | | 8 | I | 8-12 | 12-24 | 48-72 | Yes (H,P) | | 94, 98 |
| Netilmicin | 2.2-3 | 40 | 90-95 | | 8-12 | D<br>I | 60-90<br>8-12 | 30-70<br>12 | 20-30<br>24 | Yes (H,P) | | 99, 100 |
| Sisomicin | 2-3 | 35-80 | 90-95 | | 8 | I | 8-12 | 12 | 24 | Yes (H) | | 95 |
| Streptomycin | 2.5 | 100 | 30-90 | | 12 | I | 24 | 24-72 | 72-96 | Yes (H) | Minimal nephrotoxicity | 94 |
| Tobramycin | 2.5-3 | 56 | 90-98 | | 8 | D<br>I | 60-90<br>8-12 | 30-70<br>12 | 20-30<br>24 | | | 101 |
| • *Cefalosporins** | | | | | | | | | | | *Rare allergic interstitial nephritis; absorbed well when administered intraperitoneally. Some agents with 3- methylthiotetrazole side chains (e.g. latamoxef, cefamandole, cefoperazone) may cause bleeding in patients with renal failure | 102-104 |
| Cefacetrile | 0.5-2 | 16 | 75 | He | 6-8 | I | 6 | 6-8 | 8-12* | Yes (H) | *Usual doses required to treat urinary tract infections | 103, 105 |
| Cefaclor | 0.6-1 | 3 | 90-95 | | 8 | D | 100 | 50-100 | 50 | Yes (H,P) | | 106 |
| Cefadroxil | 1.5 | 20-25 | 70-90 | | 8 | I | 8 | 12-24 | 24-48 | Yes (H) | | 107 |
| Cefalexin | 1 | 20-40 | 90-46 | | 6 | I | 6 | 6 | 8-12* | Yes (H,P) | *Usual doses required to treat urinary tract infections | 105 |
| Cefalothin | 0.5-1 | 3-18 | 60-90 | He | 6 | I | 6 | 6-8 | 12* | Yes (H) | *Convulsions in large doses; may falsely raise creatinine by interference with assay | 105 |
| Cefamandole | 1 | 11 | 100 | | 4-6 | I | 6 | 6-8 | 12 | Yes (H) | Bleeding due to hypoprothrombinaemia | 108 |
| Cefapirin | 0.6-0.8 | 2.4-2.7 | 50 | He | 6 | I | 6 | 6-8 | 12 | Yes (H) | | 105, 109 |
| Cefazolin | 1.8-2 | 40-70 | 80 | | 6 | I | 8 | 12 | 24-48* | Yes (H)<br>No (P) | *Ineffective for urinary infection when GFR <10 ml/min | 110 |
| Cefepime | 2.2 | 18 | 80 | | 8 | I | 12 | 18-24 | 24-48 | Yes (H) | | 111 |
| Cefixime | 3.1 | 12 | 20-50 | He | 12 | D | 100 | 75 | 50 | Yes (H,P) | | 112 |
| Cefmenoxime | 1.1-1.6 | 6-26 | 80 | | 6 | I | 6-8 | 8-12 | 12-24 | Yes (H) | | 113 |
| Cefmetazole | 1.2 | 2.1 | 85 | | 6-12 | I | 16 | 24 | 48 | Yes (H) | Concomitant probenecid doubles half-life | 114 |

| | | | | | | | | | | | | |
|---|---|---|---|---|---|---|---|---|---|---|---|---|
| Cefonicid | 3.5-4.5 | 17-56 | 90-99 | | 24 | D | 50 | 20-50 | 10-20 | Yes (H) | | 102, 115 |
| Cefoperazone | 1.6-2.4 | 2.1 | 20 | He | 12 | I | Unch | Unch | Unch | Yes (H) | Bleeding due to hypoprothrombinaemia; reduce dose 50% for jaundice | 116 |
| Ceforanide | 2.2-3.0 | 25 | 85-90 | | 12 | I | 12 | 12-24 | 24-48 | Yes (H) | | 117 |
| Cefotaxime | 1 | 2.6* | 50-60 | He | 6-8 | I | 6-8 | 8-12 | 12-24 | Yes (H) | *$t_{1/2}$ of active metabolite in ESRD | 118 |
| Cefotetan | 3.5 | 13-25 | 75 | | 12 | D | 100 | 50 | 25 | Yes (H,P) | | 119 |
| Cefotiam | 0.9-1.1 | 2.7-13 | 65-93 | | 6-8 | D | Unch | Unch | 50-75 | Yes (H) | | 120 |
| Cefoxitin | 1 | 13.20 | 77-90 | | 6-8 | I | 8 | 8-12 | 24-48 | Yes (H) No (P) | May falsely raise creatinine by interference with assay | 121 |
| Cefpodoxime proxetil | 2.5 | 26 | 30 | | 12 | I | 12 | 16 | 24-48 | Yes (H) | | 122 |
| Cefprozil | 1.7 | 6 | 65 | He | 12 | | 12 | 12-18 | 24 | Yes (H) | | 123 |
| Cefradine | 1.3 | 6-15 | 100 | | 6 | D | 100 | 50 | 25 | Yes (H,P) | | 124 |
| Cefroxadine | 0.8-1 | 40 | 90-98 | | 6 | D | 65-100 | 15-65 | 10-15 | Yes (H) | | 125 |
| Cefsulodin | 1.7 | 13 | 64 | He | 6 | | 6 | 12-24 | 24 | Yes (H) | | 126 |
| Ceftazidime | 1.2-2 | 13 | 60 | He | 8-12 | I | 8-12 | 24-48 | 48-72 | Yes (H.P) | | 127 |
| Ceftizoxime | 1.4-1.7 | 30 | 70-100 | | 8-12 | D | 50-100 | 15-50 | 10-15 | Yes (H) | | 128 |
| Ceftriaxone | 7-9 | 12-24 | 30-65 | He | 12-24 | D | Unch | Unch | Unch | Yes (H) | | 129 |
| Cefuroxime | 1.1-1.4 | 17 | > 90 | | 6-8 | D | 100 | 50-75 | 50 | Yes (H) | | 130 |
| Latamoxef (moxalactam) | 2-2.3 | 18-23 | 61-79 | He | 8 | I | 8 | 12 | 12-24 | Yes (H) | Bleeding due to hypoprothrombinaemia; contains 3.8 mmol $Na^+$ per g | 131 |
| • *Fluoroquinolones** | | | | | | | | | | | *Most agents in this group malabsorbed in presence of Mg, Ca, Al and Fe ions; theophylline metabolism impaired | |
| Ciprofloxacin | 3-6 | 6-9 | 50-70 | He | 12 | D | 100 | 50-75 | 50 | No (H,P) | | 132-135 |
| Enoxacin | 6-9 | <30h | | He | | D* | Unch | Unch | 25 | ? | May be reduced clearance of metabolites. Dosages should commence at lower end of therapeutic range | 136, 137 |
| Fleroxacin | 13 | 21-28 | 70 | He | 12 | D | 100 | 50-75 | 50 | Yes (H) | | 138 |
| Lomefloxacin | 8 | 44 | 76 | He | 24 | D | 100 | 50-75 | 50 | No (H,P) | | 139 |
| Norfloxacin | 3.5-6.5 | 8 | 30 | He | 12 | D | 12 | 12-24 | Avoid | Not applic-able | | 140 |

[Continued over]

*For footnotes, see final page of table (p. 1747)*

**Appendix D.** *[Continued]*

| Drug | Elimination half-life ($t_{1/2}$) [adults] normal (h) | Elimination half-life ($t_{1/2}$) [adults] ESRD (h) | Excreted unchanged (%) | Extra-renal excretion[a] (normal) | Normal dose interval (h) | Dose adjustment for renal failure[b] method[c] | creatinine clearance (ml/min) > 50 | creatinine clearance (ml/min) 10-50 | creatinine clearance (ml/min) < 10 | Dialysis[d] | Toxic effects in renal failure/ Notes[e] | References |
|---|---|---|---|---|---|---|---|---|---|---|---|---|
| **Antibacterial drugs** *[continued]* | | | | | | | | | | | | |
| Ofloxacin | 5-8 | 28-37 | 68-80 | | 24 | D | Unch | 50 | 25-50 | No (H,P) | | 141, 142 |
| Pefloxacin | 10 | 15 | 11 | He | 24 | D | Unch | Unch | Unch | No (H,P) | | 143, 144 |
| • *Macrolides* | | | | | | | | | | | | |
| Azithromycin | 10-60 | ? | 6-12 | He | 24 | D | Unch | Unch | Unch | No (H,P) | | 145 |
| Clarithromycin | 2.5-6 | ? | 15 | He | 12 | D | Unch | 75 | 50-75 | Yes (H) | | 146 |
| Erythromycin | 1.4 | 5-6 | 15 | He | 6 | D | Unch | Unch | 50-75* | No (H,P) | *Ototoxicity with large doses | 147 |
| • *Penicillins** | | | | | | | | | | | *Agents in this group may cause allergic interstitial nephritis; seizures and coagulopathy at high blood levels | 148-150 |
| Amoxicillin | 0.9-2.3 | 5-20 | 50-70 | He | 8 | I | 8 | 8-12 | 12-18* | Yes (H) No (P) | Skin rash. *High doses needed for urinary infection in ESRD | 151 |
| Ampicillin | 0.8-1.5 | 7.20 | 30-90 | He | 6-8 | I | 8 | 8-12 | 12-18* | Yes (H) No (P) | Skin rash. *High doses needed for urinary infection in ESRD Injection contains 3 mmol $Na^+$ per g | 148, 149 |
| Azlocillin | 0.8-1.5 | 5-6 | 50-60 | He | 4-6 | I | 4-6 | 6-8 | 8 | Yes (H) | Contains 2.7 mmol $Na^+$ per g. May cause hypokalaemic metabolic alkalosis | 150, 152, 153 |
| Benzyl-penicillin (penicillin G) | 0.5 | 6-20 | 60-85 | He | 6-8 | D | Unch | 75 | 25-50* 12-16 | Yes (H) | Convulsions, false-positive urine protein reactions. | 148, 149 |
| | | | | | | I | 6-8 | 8-12 | | No (P) | *Upper dose limit of 4-6 MU per day in severe renal failure; potassium salt contains 1.7 mmol $K^+$/MU | |
| Carbenicillin | 1.2-1.5 | 10-20 | 80-85 | He | 4-6 | I | 8-12 | 12-24 | 24-48* | Yes (H) | *Inactivates aminoglycosides; contains 4 to 7 mmol $Na^+$ per g. May cause hypokalaemic alkalosis | 148, 149, 154, 155 |
| Cloxacillin | 0.5 | 1 | 30-65 | He | 6 | D | Unch | Unch | Unch | No (H) | | 148, 149, 156 |
| Dicloxacillin | 0.8 | 1-2 | 35-70 | He | 6 | I | Unch | Unch | Unch | No (H) | | 148, 149, 156 |

| | | | | | | | | | | | | |
|---|---|---|---|---|---|---|---|---|---|---|---|---|
| Mecillinam (amdinocillin) | 1 | 4-6 | 70 | He | 4-6 | D | Unch | 50 | 25 | Yes (H) | | 157 |
| Methicillin | 0.5-1.0 | 4 | 25-80 | He | 4-6 | I | 4-6 | 6-8 | 8-12 | No (H,P) | | 148, 149 |
| Mezlocillin | 0.6-1.2 | 2.6-5.4 | 60-70 | He | 4-6 | I | 4-6 | 6.8 | 8 | Yes (H) | Contains 1.9 mmol $Na^+$ per g | 150, 152, 158 |
| Nafcillin | 0.5-1 | 1.2 | 35 | He | 6 | D | Unch | Unch | Unch* | No (H) | Coagulopathy. *Dose must be reduced in combined renal and liver failure | 159 |
| Piperacillin | 0.8-1.5 | 3.3-5.1 | 75.90 | He | 6 | I | 4-6 | 6-8 | 8 | Yes (H) | Contains 1.9 mmol $Na^+$ per g | 160 |
| Ticarcillin | 1.2 | 16 | 80-90 | He | 4-6 | I | 8-12 | 12-24 | 24-48 | Yes (H) No (P) | As for carbenicillin (see above) | 161 |
| • *Tetracyclines** | | | | | | | | | | | *Agents in this group potentiate acidosis, raise BUN and phosphorus, and increase catabolism | |
| Doxycycline | 15-24 | 18-25 | 33-45 | He | 24 | I | Unch | Unch | Unch | No (H,P) | Group drug of choice for extrarenal infection | 162 |
| Minocycline | 12-16 | 12-18 | 6-10 | G | 12 | D | Unch | Unch | Unch | No (H,P) | Can be used for extrarenal infections | 162, 163 |
| Tetracycline | 6-10 | 57-108 | 48-60 | He | 6 | I | 8-12 | 12-24 | 24* | No (H,P) | *Avoid (aggravates renal insufficiency) | 164 |
| • *Others* | | | | | | | | | | | | |
| Aztreonam | 1.5-2.9 | 6-8 | 75 | He | 8-12 | D | Unch | 50-75 | 25 | Yes (H,P) | | 165, 166 |
| Chloramphenicol | 1.6-4 | 3-7 | 5-15 | He* | 6 | D | Unch | Unch | Unch | No (H,P) | *$t_{1/2}$ markedly prolonged with combined liver and kidney dysfunction | 167, 168 |
| Cilastatin | 1 | 12 | 60 | | Given with imipenem | D | Unch | Unch | Avoid | No (H) | Unnecessary in renal failure | 169, 170 |
| Cinoxacin | 1.2 | 12 | 55 | He | 12 | D | 100 | 50 | Avoid | Avoid | | 171 |
| Clavulanic acid | 1 | 3-4 | 30-40 | | 6-8 | D | Unch | Unch | 50-75 | Yes (H) | Combined with amoxicillin or ticarcillin for clinical use | 172, 173 |
| Clindamycin | 2-4 | 3-5 | 5-15 | He | 6 | D | Unch | Unch | Unch | No (H,P) | | 174 |
| Imipenem | 1 | 4 | 20-70 | He | 6 | D | Unch | 50 | 25 | Yes (H) | | 169, 170 |
| Lincomycin | 4-5 | 10-20 | 10-15 | He | 6 | I | 6 | 6-12 | 12-24 | No (H,P) | | 175 |
| Meropenem | 1.1 | 6-8 | 65 | He | 6 | D, I | 100 q6h | 50-75 q12h | 50-75 q24h | Yes (H) | | 176 |
| Metronidazole | 6-14 | 8-15 | < 10 | He* | 8 | I | 8 | 8-12 | 12-24* | Yes (H) No (P) | Neurotoxic and gastrointestinal symptoms may mimic uraemia *Some active metabolites | 177, 178 |
| Nalidixic acid | 6-7 | 21 | 20 | He | 6 | D | Unch | Avoid | Avoid* | ? | *Metabolites accumulate; rare drug-induced lupus syndrome | 179 |

[Continued over]

For footnotes, see final page of table (p. 1747)

**Appendix D.** *[Continued]*

| Drug | Elimination half-life ($t_{1/2}$) [adults] normal (h) | Elimination half-life ($t_{1/2}$) [adults] ESRD (h) | Excreted unchanged (%) | Extra-renal excretion[a] (normal) | Normal dose interval (h) | Dose adjustment for renal failure[b] method[c] | creatinine clearance (ml/min) > 50 | creatinine clearance (ml/min) 10-50 | creatinine clearance (ml/min) < 10 | Dialysis[d] | Toxic effects in renal failure/ Notes[e] | References |
|---|---|---|---|---|---|---|---|---|---|---|---|---|
| **Antibacterial drugs** *[continued]* | | | | | | | | | | | | |
| Nitrofurantoin | 0.3-1 | 1 | 30-40 | NR | 8 | D | Unch | Avoid* | Avoid** | Yes (H) | *Peripheral sensory neuropathy due to metabolites. **Ineffective | 180 |
| Spectinomycin | 1.6-2 | 16.29 | 35-90 | | Single dose | D | Unch | Unch | Unch | Yes (H) | | 181 |
| Sulbactam | 1 | 10-21 | 50-80 | | 6-8 | I | 6-8 | 12-24 | 24-48 | Yes (H) | β-Lactamase inhibitor (combined with ampicillin) | 182 |
| Sulfafurazole (sulfisoxazole) | 3-8 | 6-12 | 60-80 | He | 6 | I | 6 | 8-12 | 12-24* | Yes (H,P) | *If high urinary levels desired use normal intervals | 183 |
| Sulfamethoxazole | 9-11 | 20-50 | 60-80 | He | 12 | I | 12 | 18 | 24* | Yes (H) No (P) | *If high urinary levels desired use normal intervals | 183 |
| Tazobactam | 1 | 7 | 65 | | 24 | D | Unch | 75 | 50 | Yes (H) | Combined with piperacillin | 184 |
| Teicoplanin | 9-13 | 20-49 | 40-60 | | 24 | I | 24 | 48 | 72 | No (H,P) | | 185 |
| Trimethoprim | 9-13 | 20-49 | 40-70 | He | 12 | I | 12 | 18 | 24* | Yes (H) | *Haematological effects (antifolate action); may increase serum creatinine due to competition for secretion | 186 |
| Vancomycin | 6-10 | 200-250 | 90-100 | | 6 | I | 24-72 | 72-240 | 240 | No (H,P) | Ototoxic at serum concentrations >50 mg/L | 187, 188 |
| **Anticholinesterases** | | | | | | | | | | | | |
| Neostigmine | 0.5-2.1 | Prolonged* | 75 | NR | 1-2 | I | 2 | 2 | 6-8 | ? | Bladder atony. *ESRD patients may have prolonged action due to low cholinesterase levels. Active metabolites | 189, 190 |
| Pyridostigmine | 1.5-2 | 6* | High | NR | 3-8 | D | Unch | Unch | Unch | ? | Bladder atony. *ESRD patients may have prolonged action due to low cholinesterase levels | 191 |
| **Anticoagulants** (see chapter 26, sect. 3.1.4, 3.1.5) | | | | | | | | | | | | |
| Heparin | 1-2 | 0.5-3 | Negligible | NR | 4-6 | D | Unch | Unch | Unch | No (H,P) | May potentiate uraemic bleeding | 192, 193 |
| Nadroparin | 2.2-3 | 3-5 | 50 | | 12 | D | Unch | 50-100 | 25-50 | Yes (H) | Monitor factor Xa inhibition in ESRD | 194 |
| Warfarin | 42 | 30* | Negligible | He | 24 | D | Unch | Unch | Unch | No (P) | Metabolites with anticoagulant properties excreted by the kidney; may potentiate uraemic bleeding | 195 |

| | | | | | | | | | | | | |
|---|---|---|---|---|---|---|---|---|---|---|---|---|
| **Antidepressants, tricyclic*** (see chapter 30, sect. 5.1) | | | | | | | | | | | *Agents in this group are anticholinergic and may cause urinary retention; also excessive sedation | 77, 196, 197 |
| Amitriptyline | 21 | ? | < 5 | He* | 12 | D | Unch | Unch | Unch | No (H,P) | *Metabolised to nortriptyline | 197, 198 |
| Desipramine | 12-54 | ? | < 5 | He | 8-12 | D | Unch | Unch | Unch | No (H,P) | | 197 |
| Doxepin | 8-25 | 10-18 | < 5 | He | 12 | D | Unch | Unch | Unch | No (H,P) | | 197, 199 |
| Imipramine | 6-20 | ? | < 5 | He* | 12 | D | Unch | Unch | Unch | No (H,P) | *Metabolised to desipramine | 197 |
| Nortriptyline | 15-90 | 15-66 | < 5 | He | 12 | D | Unch | Unch | Unch | No (H,P) | | 197, 200 |
| Protriptyline | 54-98 | ? | < 5 | He | 24 | D | Unch | Unch | Unch | No (H,P) | | 197 |
| **Antidiabetic drugs** (see chapter 19, sect. 3.2) | | | | | | | | | | | | |
| Acetohexamide | 6-8 | 31 | Low | He | 12 | I | 12-24 | Avoid | Avoid | No (P) | Accumulation of metabolite with hypoglycaemic action may falsely increase serum creatinine | 201, 202 |
| Chlorpropramide | 24-42 | 50-200 | 10-60 | NR | 24 | I | 24-36 | Avoid | Avoid* | No (P) | *Prolonged hypoglycaemia in azotaemic patients; impairs renal water excretion | 201, 202 |
| Glibenclamide (glyburide) | 10-16 | ? | 50 | He | 24 | D | Unch | Unch | Unch | ? | | 203 |
| Glipizide | 3-7 | ? | 3-10 | He | 24 | D | Unch | Unch | Unch | ? | | 201, 204 |
| Insulin (regular) | 2-3 | Pro-longed | < 5 | He | 8* | D | Unch | 75 | 50 | ? | *Dosage dependent on blood sugar level | 205 |
| Tolazamide | 6-8 | ? | 15 | He | 24 | D | Unch | Unch | Unch | ? | | 201, 202 |
| Tolbutamide | 4-7 | Unch | < 1 | He, NR | 8 | D | Unch | Unch | Unch | No (H) | May impair renal water excretion | 201, 202, 206 |
| **Antiemetics** (see chapter 22, sect. 5.1) | | | | | | | | | | | | |
| Metoclopramide | 4 | 14-18 | 7-20 | He | 8 | D | Unch | 75 | 25-50 | No (H) | Extrapyramidal movements, dyskinesia | 207, 208 |
| Ondansetron | 3.5 | 5-9 | < 10 | He | 8-12 | D | Unch | Unch | Unch | ? | | 209 |
| **Antiepileptic drugs** (see chapter 29, sect. 4.1) | | | | | | | | | | | | |
| Carbamazepine | 20-36* | ? | 2-3 | He | 24 | D | Unch | Unch | 75 | No (H) | May cause inappropriate ADH secretion; active metabolites are renally excreted. *Single doses. $t_{1/2}$ shorter during long term therapy (10-20h) due to induction of own metabolism | 210-212 |
| Clonazepam | 20-60 | Unch | < 1 | He | 8-12 | D | Unch | Unch | Unch | ? | Excessive sedation | 64, 65 |

[Continued over]

*For footnotes, see final page of table (p. 1747)*

**Appendix D.** *[Continued]*

| Drug | Elimination half-life ($t_{1/2}$) [adults] normal (h) | ESRD (h) | Excreted unchanged (%) | Extra-renal excretion[a] (normal) | Normal dose interval (h) | Dose adjustment for renal failure[b] method[c] | creatinine clearance (ml/min) > 50 | 10-50 | < 10 | Dialysis[d] | Toxic effects in renal failure/ Notes[e] | References |
|---|---|---|---|---|---|---|---|---|---|---|---|---|
| **Antiepileptic drugs** *[continued]* | | | | | | | | | | | | |
| Phenytoin (diphenyl-hydantoin) | 20-30* | 8 | < 5 | He | 8 | D | Unch | Unch | Unch | No (H) | *Dose-dependent. Decreased protein binding and increased volume of distribution in ESRD; may cause folate deficiency | 210, 211, 213 |
| Primidone | 6-12* | 12 | 15-60 | He** | 8-12 | I | 8 | 8-12 | 12-24 | Yes (H) | Excessive sedation, folic acid deficiency, nystagmus. *Parent drug. **Partially converted to phenobarbital and PEMA which have longer half-lives | 210, 211, 214 |
| Trimethadione (troxidone) | 12-24 | ? | 1 | He* | 12 | I | 8 | 8-12 | 12-24 | ? | Nephrotic syndrome. *Active metabolites have long $t_{1/2}$ | 210, 211 |
| Valproic acid/ sodium valproate | 8-15 | 10 | 2-3 | He | 8 | D | Unch | Unch | Unch | No (H,P) | Hepatotoxicity; other antiepileptic drugs induce metabolism and decrease $t_{1/2}$ | 210, 211, 215, 216 |
| Vigabatrin | 7 | 15 | 70 | | 8 | D | Unch | 50-75 | 25-50 | ? | May lower serum phenytoin concentrations | 217 |
| ***A*ntifungal agents** (see chapter 31, sect. 6.1) | | | | | | | | | | | | |
| Amphotericin B | 24* | 24* | 5 | He, NR | 24 | I | 24 | 24 | 24-36** | No (H,P) | Nephrotoxicity; renal tubular acidosis, hypokalaemia, nephrogenic diabetes insipidus. *Terminal phase $t_{1/2}$ 15 days. **Ineffective for renal parenchymal infections | 218, 219 |
| Fluconazole | 22 | ? | 70 | He | 24 | I | 24 | 24-48 | 48-72 | Yes (H) | Interferes with cyclosporin metabolism | 220 |
| Flucytosine (5-fluorocytosine) | 3-6 | 75-200 | > 90 | | 6 | I<br>D | 6<br>50 | 12-24<br>30-50 | 24-48<br>20-30 | Yes (H,P) | Hepatic dysfunction; marrow suppression more common in azotaemic patients | 218, 219 |
| Griseofulvin | 14 | 20 | 1 | He | 6 | D | Unch | Unch | Unch | No (H,P) | | |
| Itraconazole | 21 | 25 | 35 | He | 12 | D | Unch | Unch | 50-100 | No (H,P) | | 221 |
| Ketoconazole | 1.5-8 | 1.8 | 1 | He | 24 | D | Unch | Unch | Unch | No (H) | Interferes with cyclosporin metabolism and enhances its nephrotoxicity | 222 |
| Miconazole | 20-24* | 20-24 | 1 | He | 8 | D | Unch | Unch | Unch | No (H,P) | Hyponatraemia *Initial rapid elimination rate | 218, 219 |
| **Antihistamines** | | | | | | | | | | | | |
| Astemizole | 9-10 days | Unch | < 5 | He | 24 | D | Unch | Unch | Unch | ? | | 223 |

| | | | | | | | | | | | | |
|---|---|---|---|---|---|---|---|---|---|---|---|---|
| Cetirizine | 9-10 | 16-25 | 50 | | 24 | D | Unch | 75 | 50 | No (H) | | 224 |
| Chlorpheniramine (chlorphenamine) | 13-31 | Prolonged | < 7 | He | 6-8 | D | Unch | Unch | Unch | Yes (H) No (P) | Excessive sedation | 225, 226 |
| Diphenhydramine | 4-7 | ? | < 4 | He | 6-8 | I | 6 | 6-12 | 10-18 | ? | Excessive sedation; may cause urinary retention (anticholinergic activity) | 227 |
| Terfenadine | 16-22 | ? | < 10 | He | 12-24 | D | Unch | Unch | Unch | No (H,P) | | 228 |
| **Antihypertensive drugs*** (see chapter 21, sect. 3; see also ACE inhibitors, β-adrenoceptor antagonists, calcium antagonists and diuretics) | | | | | | | | | | | *Blood pressure best guide to dosage | |
| Clonidine | 6-23* | 39-42 | 45 | NR | 6-8 | D | Unch | Unch | Unch | No (H) | Excessive sedation. *Dose-dependent | 229 |
| Diazoxide | 21-36 | 20-53 | 50 | NR | Bolus* | D | Unch | Unch | Unch | Yes (H,P) | *Rapid IV bolus injection (10-30 seconds) | 230 |
| Doxazosin | 9.5-12.5 | 13 | < 5 | | 12 | D | Unch | Unch | Unch | No (H) | | 231 |
| Guanabenz | 12-14 | ? | < 5 | He | 12 | D | Unch | Unch | Uncg | ? | | 232 |
| Guanadrel | 10 | ? | 50 | | 24 | D | Unch | Unch | Unch | ? | | 233 |
| Guanethidine | 120-240 | ? | 25-50 | NR | 24 | I | 24 | 24 | 24-36 | ? | Orthostatic hypotension | 234 |
| Guanfacine | 12-23 | 15-25 | 33 | He | 24 | D | Unch | Unch | Unch | No (H) | | 235 |
| Hydralazine | 2.0-2.5* | 7-16 | 25 | He,G | 8-12 | I | 8-12 | 8-12 | 8-16 12-24* | No (H,P) | *Slow acetylators | 236, 237 |
| Methyldopa | 1-1.7 | 7-16 | 20-60 | He** | 6 | I | 6 | 9-18 | 12-24* | Yes (H,P) | *Retention of active metabolites; excessive sedation. **Renal excretion more important with intravenous use | 238 |
| Minoxidil | 2.8-4.2 | 2.8-4.2 | 15-20 | He | 8-12 | D | Unch | Unch | Unch | Yes (H) | Fluid retention; pericardial effusion | 239 |
| Moxonidine | 2-3 | 6-9 | 50 | | 24 | D | Unch | 50-75 | Avoid | No (H) | | 240 |
| Prazosin | 1.8-4.6 | ? | < 5 | He | 8-12 | D | Unch | Unch | Unch* | No (H,P) | May produce profound hypotension with first dose. *Patients with ESRD may respond to a lower dose | 241, 242 |
| Reserpine | 46-168 | 87-323 | < 1 | He | 24 | D | Unch | Unch | Avoid | No (H,P) | Excessive sedation; gastrointestinal bleeding | 243 |
| Sodium nitroprusside | < 10 min | < 10 min | < 10 | NR | Constant IV infusion | D | Unch | Unch | Unch* | Yes (H)* | *Toxic metabolite thiocyanate is dialysable; level should be kept <100 mg/L to avoid seizures, coma | 244, 245 |
| Terazosin | 9-12 | 8-12 | 30 | | 12 | D | Unch | Unch | Unch | ? | | 246 |
| Urapidil | 2.7-4.8 | 6.2 | 10-15 | He | 12 | D | Unch | Unch | 75 | No (H,P) | | 247 |
| **Antimalarial drugs** | | | | | | | | | | | | |
| Chloroquine | 2-4 | 5h-50 days | 50 | He, NR | 12 | D | Unch | Unch | 50* | No (H) | *If prolonged treatment necessary, 50-100 mg/day | 248 |

[Continued over]

*For footnotes, see final page of table (p. 1747)*

**Appendix D.** *[Continued]*

| Drug | Elimination half-life ($t_{1/2}$) [adults] normal (h) | Elimination half-life ($t_{1/2}$) [adults] ESRD (h) | Excreted unchanged (%) | Extra-renal excretion[a] (normal) | Normal dose interval (h) | Dose adjustment for renal failure[b] method[c] | creatinine clearance (ml/min) > 50 | creatinine clearance (ml/min) 10-50 | creatinine clearance (ml/min) < 10 | Dialysis[d] | Toxic effects in renal failure/ Notes[e] | References |
|---|---|---|---|---|---|---|---|---|---|---|---|---|
| **Antimalarial drugs** *[continued]* | | | | | | | | | | | | |
| Pyrimethamine | 1.5-7.3 days | 1.5-7.3 days | 16-30 | NR, He | Weekly | D | Unch | Unch | Unch | No (H,P) | Metabolites excreted for weeks because of tissue storage | 248 |
| Quinine | 4-16 | Unch* | 20 | NR, He | 8 | D<br>I | 8<br>100 | 8-12<br>75 | 24<br>30-50 | Yes (H) | *Marked tissue accumulation | 248 |
| **Antineoplastic and immunosuppressive drugs*** (see chapters 27 and 28) | | | | | | | | | | | *Most agents in this group cause marrow depression which adds to uraemic bleeding and infection | |
| Azathioprine | 0.2-1 | Slightly pro-longed | 50 | He* | 24 | I | 24 | 24 | 24-36 | Yes (H) | *Converted to mercaptopurine. Allopurinol increases drug activity | 249, 250 |
| Bleomycin | 1.3-9 | 2-30 | 60 | He | Twice a week | D | Unch | Unch | 50 | No (H) | Pulmonary toxicity enhanced; hyperuricaemia | 251, 252 |
| Busulfan | 2.5 | ? | 1 | He | 24 | D | Unch | Unch | Unch | ? | May cause haemorrhagic cystitis | 253, 254 |
| Carboplatin | Biphasic 1 & 2-3 | Pro-longed | 85 | | 24 | D | Unch | 75 | 50 | Yes (H) | Nephrotoxic | 255 |
| Cisplatin | 2-72 | 1-240 | 25-75 | ?NR | 24 | D | Unch | 75 | 50 | Yes (H)* | Nephrotoxic; toxicity decreased by hydration; renal Mg wasting.<br>*Dialysis only effective up to 3h after dose | 256-258 |
| Cyclophos-phamide | 5-7 | 4-12 | <25 | NR* | 12 | I | 12 | 12 | 18-24 | Yes (H) | Haemorrhagic cystitis, bladder fibrosis, bladder carcinoma, sterility, alopecia, inappropriate ADH secretion.<br>*Active metabolite | 254, 259 |
| Cyclosporin (cyclosporin A) | 10-24 | 12-24 | < 2 | He | 24 | D | Unch | Unch | Unch | No (H,P) | Nephrotoxic; hypertension, hyperkalaemia, seizures, hirsutism | 260 |
| Cytarabine (cytosine arabinoside) | Biphasic 0.1 & 2.5 | ? | 10 | | 24 | D | Unch | Unch | Unch | ? | Renal excretion of metabolites | 261 |
| Doxorubicin | 16-30 | 16-24 | 25 | He* | 24 | D | Unch | Unch | 75 | ? | *$t_{1/2}$ of active metabolite 36h; rare acute renal failure, nephrotic syndrome; cardiotoxicity | 254, 262 |
| Etoposide | 3-6 | 3-6 | 30 | He | 24 | D | Unch | 75 | 50 | ? | | 263 |
| Fluorouracil | 20* | 20* | 15 | NR | 24 | D | Unch | Unch | Unch | Yes (H) | *Active metabolites | 261 |
| Idarubicin | 11-35 | ? | 15 | NR | 24 | D | Unch | Unch | Unch | ? | | 264 |
| Ifosfamide | 7-16 | ? | 20 | He | 24 | D | Unch | 50 | 50 | ? | Nephrotoxic; haemorrhagic cystitis reduced by concomitant sulfhydryl (mesna) | 265 |

| | | | | | | | | | | | | |
|---|---|---|---|---|---|---|---|---|---|---|---|---|
| Melphalan | 1.5-2 | 4-6 | 13 | NR | 24 | D | Unch | Unch | 50-75 | ? | | 254, 266 |
| Methotrexate | 3.5-60 | Pro-longed | 90 | He | 24 | D | Unch | 50 | Avoid | Yes (H) No (P) | Folate deficiency; high doses nephrotoxic due to tubular precipitation of metabolite | 267, 268 |
| Mitomycin C | Short | ? | 15-30 | He | 24 | D | Unch | Unch | 75 | ? | Nephrotoxic | 270, 271 |
| Nilutamide | 40 | ? | < 10 | He | 24 | D | Unch | Unch | Unch | ? | | 272 |
| Plicamycin (mithramycin) | 2 | ? | 50 | | 24 | D | Unch | 75 | 50 | ? | Cumulative nephrotoxicity | 269 |
| Semustine | Biphasic 5 & 27 | ? | 50 | | 24 | D | Unch | Unch | Avoid* | ? | Dose-related cumulative nephrotoxicity | 269 |
| Tamoxifen | 18-120 | ? | < 10 | NR | 24 | D | Unch | Unch | Unch | ? | | 273 |
| Vinblastine | Tri-phasic | ? | 35 | He | 24 | D | Unch | Unch | Unch | ? | May cause inappropriate ADH secretion | 269 |
| Vincristine | 0.8-2.6/ 85* | Unch | High | He | 7 days | D | Unch | Unch | Unch | ? | Neurotoxicity; inappropriate ADH secretion. *Terminal elimination phase $t_{1/2}$ | 274 |
| **Anti-Parkinsonian drugs** (see chapter 29, sect. 7.1.1) | | | | | | | | | | | | |
| Bromocriptine | 3 | ? | 6-7 | He | 6-8 | D | Unch | Unch | Unch | ? | Orthostatic hypotension; digital vasospasm at high doses | 275 |
| Carbidopa | 15* | ? | 40 | He | 12 | D | Unch | Unch | Unch | ? | *Half-life is for levodopa in combination preparation | 276 |
| Levodopa | 0.8-1.6 | ? | < 5 | NR | 8-12 | D | Unch | Unch | Unch | ? | Active metabolites have long $t_{1/2}$; may darken urine | 277, 278 |
| Selegiline | 12-24 | ? | < 10 | He | 12 | D | Unch | Unch | Unch | ? | | 279 |
| Trihexphenidyl (benzhexol) | 13 | Pro-longed | Prob. Low | NR | 12 | D | Unch | Unch | Unch | ? | May cause urinary retention (anticholinergic activity) | 276 |
| **Antipsychotic drugs*** (see chapter 30, sect. 3.1) | | | | | | | | | | | *Prototype chlorpromazine. Agents in this group have anticholinergic activity and may cause urinary retention, orthostatic hypotension | |
| Chlorpromazine | 16-30 | Unch | 5 | He | 8-12 | D | Unch | Unch | Unch* | No (H,P) | *Excessive sedation may require dosage decrease; toxic psychosis reported | 77, 280-282 |
| Clozapine | 6-30 | ? | 15 | He | 24 | D | Unch | Unch | Unch | No (H,P) | | 283 |
| Haloperidol | 10-36 | ? | < 5 | He, G | 24 | D | Unch | Unch | Unch | No (H,P) | Excessive sedation, hypotension | 284 |
| Lithium carbonate | 14-28 | Pro-longed | 100 | | 8 | D | Unch | 50-75 | 25-50 | Yes (H,P) | Nephrogenic diabetes insipidus, renal tubular acidosis, chronic interstitial fibrosis. Toxicity when serum levels > 1.2 mmol/L; toxicity enhanced by volume depletion, diuretics and nonsteroidal anti-inflammatory drugs | 285-287 |

[Continued over]

*For footnotes, see final page of table (p. 1747)*

**Appendix D.** *[Continued]*

| Drug | Elimination half-life ($t_{½}$) [adults] | | Excreted unchanged (%) | Extrarenal excretion[a] (normal) | Normal dose interval (h) | Dose adjustment for renal failure[b] | | | | Dialysis[d] | Toxic effects in renal failure/ Notes[e] | References |
|---|---|---|---|---|---|---|---|---|---|---|---|---|
| | normal (h) | ESRD (h) | | | | method[c] | creatinine clearance (ml/min) | | | | | |
| | | | | | | | > 50 | 10-50 | < 10 | | | |
| **Antipsychotic drugs** *[continued]* | | | | | | | | | | | | |
| Tiapride | 3-5 | 22 | 90-95 | | 8 | D | Unch | 75 | 50 | ? | | 288 |
| **Antithyroid drugs** | | | | | | | | | | | | |
| Propylthiouracil | 1-2 | 8.5 | 30 | He | 8 | D | 100 | 75 | 50 | ? | Cardiotoxicity, leucopenia | 289, 290 |
| Thiamazole (methimazole) | 2-4 | 9 | 7-12 | G, He | 12 | D | 100 | 75 | 50 | ? | Leucopenia | 289, 290 |
| **Antituberculosis drugs** (see chapter 23, sect. 9.1) | | | | | | | | | | | | |
| *p*-Aminosalicylic acid (para-aminosalicylic acid; PAS) | 1.5 | 23 | 40 | He* | 8 | I | 8 | 12 | Avoid* | Yes (H) | Adds to acidosis, gastrointestinal symptoms. *Active metabolites | 291 |
| Capreomycin | 2 | ? | 50 | | 24 | I | 24 | 24 | 48 | No (H,P) | | 292 |
| Cycloserine | 12-20 | Prolonged | 60 | He | 12 | I | 24 | Avoid | Avoid | Yes (H) | Mood disturbances | 291 |
| Ethambutol | 4 | 7-15 | 75-90 | | 24 | I | 24 | 24-36 | 48 | Yes (H,P) | Decreased visual acuity, peripheral neuritis | 291 |
| Ethionamide | 2 | Unch | 1 | He* | 12 | I | Unch | Unch | Unch | No (H,P) | *Active metabolite | 291 |
| Isoniazid | 0.7-4 | 17 | 5-30* | He | 8 | I | 8 | 8 | 8(12)* | Yes (H,P) | *Slow acetylators | 291, 293 |
| Pyrazinamide | 9 | 26 | 1-3 | | 24 | D | 100 | Avoid | Avoid | Avoid | | 294 |
| Rifampicin (rifampin) | 1.5-5 | 1.8-3.1 | 15-30 | He* | 24 | D | Unch | 50-100 | 50 | No (H) | May cause acute renal failure, potassium wasting and renal tubular defects. *Active metabolite (desacetylrifampicin) | 291, 295 |
| **Antiulcer drugs** (see chapter 22, sect. 4.1) | | | | | | | | | | | | |
| Cimetidine | 2 | 5 | 40-70 | He | 12 | D | 100 | 75 | 50 | No (H,P) | Confusion; rare acute interstitial nephritis; may increase serum creatinine due to competition for renal excretion | 296, 297 |
| Famotidine | 2.5-4 | 12 | 80 | | 24 | D | Unch | 75 | 50 | No (H) | | 298, 299 |
| Lansoprazole | 1.3-1.7 | 1.6-2 | < 5 | He | 24 | D | Unch | Unch | Unch | No (H) | | 300 |
| Nizatidine | 1.1-1.6 | 6-9 | 60 | | 24 | D | Unch | 50 | 25 | No (H) | | 301, 302 |

| | | | | | | | | | | | | |
|---|---|---|---|---|---|---|---|---|---|---|---|---|
| Omeprazole | 1.5-3 | 2-4 | < 5 | He | 24 | D | Unch | Unch | Unch | No (H) | | 303, 304 |
| Ranitidine | 1.5-3 | 6-9 | 25-70 | He | 12 | D | 100 | 75 | 50 | Yes (H) | | 305-307 |
| **Antiviral drugs** (see chapter 32, sect. 2) | | | | | | | | | | | | |
| Aciclovir | 2.1-3.8 | 20 | 40-70 | | 8 | I | 8 | 12-24 | 48 | Yes (H) | Neurotoxic in patients with renal failure; may cause acute renal failure if injected rapidly intravenously | 308, 309 |
| Amantadine | 12-15 | 500 | 90 | | 12-24 | I | 12-24 | 48-72 | 168 | No (H,P) | | 308, 310 |
| Didanosine | 1.6 | ? | 40 | | 12 | I | 12 | 24 | 48 | Yes (H) | | 311 |
| Foscarnet | 3 | Pro-longed | 85 | | 8 | D | 75 | 50 | 25 | Yes (H) | Nephrotoxic, seizures, hypomagnesaemia | 312 |
| Ganciclovir | 3-6 | 30 | 95-100 | | 12 | I | 12 | 24-48 | 48-96 | Yes (H) | Marrow toxicity | 313 |
| Ribavirin | 30-60 | Un-known | 50 | He | 24 | D | 100 | 100 | 75 | Yes (H) | Active metabolite (renally excreted) | 314 |
| Vidarabine (adenine arabinoside) | 3-3.5* | 5* | 50 | He* | Daily 12h infusion | D | 100 | 100 | 75 | Yes (H)* | *Active hypoxanthine metabolite excreted by the kidney | 315 |
| Zidovudine | 1-1.4 | 1.4-3 | 8-25 | He | 8 | D, I | 100 q8h | 100 q8h | 50 q12h | Yes (H) | | 316 |
| **Bronchodilators** | | | | | | | | | | | | |
| Terbutaline | 3-4 | 3-4 | 60 | He | 8 | D | Unch | 50 | Avoid | ? | IV or subcutaneous doses cleared by kidney | 317 |
| Theophylline | 3-12 | ? | 7-13 | He | 6-8 | D | Unch | Unch | Unch | Yes (H,P) | | 318-320 |
| **Calcium antagonists** (see chapters 20, sect. 6.1.3 and 21, sect. 3.4) | | | | | | | | | | | | |
| Amlodipine | 35-50 | 50 | < 10 | He | 24 | D | Unch | Unch | Unch | No (H,P) | | 321, 322 |
| Bepridil | 24-48 | 24-48 | < 10 | He | 24 | D | Unch | Unch | Unch | No (H,P) | | 323 |
| Diltiazem | 2-8 | 3.5 | < 10 | He* | 6-8 | D | Unch | Unch | Unch | No (H,P) | *Active metabolites | 324, 325 |
| Felodipine | 7-21 | 15-29 | < 10 | He | 12 | D | Unch | Unch | Unch | No (H,P) | | 326 |
| Isradipine | 2.5-12 | 9-14 | < 10 | He | 12 | D | Unch | Unch | Unch | No (H,P) | | 327, 328 |
| Nicardipine | 1 | 1 | < 10 | He | 12 | D | Unch | Unch | Unch | No (H,P) | | 329 |
| Nifedipine | 4-5.5 | 5-7 | < 10 | He* | 8 | D | Unch | Unch | Unch | No (H,P) | *Active metabolites. Can cause oedema, acute renal dysfunction | 324, 330 |
| Nimodipine | 1-3 | 22 | < 10 | He | 12 | D | Unch | Unch | Unch | No (H,P) | | 331, 332 |
| Nitrendipine | 12 | 12 | < 10 | He | 12 | D | Unch | Unch | Unch | No (H,P) | | 333 |

*[Continued over]*

*For footnotes, see final page of table (p. 1747)*

**Appendix D.** *[Continued]*

| Drug | Elimination half-life ($t_{1/2}$) [adults] normal (h) | ESRD (h) | Excreted unchanged (%) | Extra-renal excretion[a] (normal) | Normal dose interval (h) | Dose adjustment for renal failure[b] method[c] | creatinine clearance (ml/min) > 50 | 10-50 | < 10 | Dialysis[d] | Toxic effects in renal failure/ Notes[e] | References |
|---|---|---|---|---|---|---|---|---|---|---|---|---|
| **Calcium antagonists** *[continued]* | | | | | | | | | | | | |
| Verapamil | 3-7 | 2.4-4 | < 10 | He* | 8 | D | Unch | Unch | Unch | No (H,P) | *Active metabolites. Acute renal dysfunction reported | 324, 330 |
| **Cardiac glycosides*** (see also chapter 20, sect. 5.4.3) | | | | | | | | | | | *Can add to uraemic gastrointestinal symptoms. Serum concentrations best guide to dosage; loading dose 50-75% of normal in ESRD because of decreased volume distribution. Toxicity enhanced by dialysis removal of potassium and magnesium | |
| Digitoxin | 134-192 | 240 | < 30 | He* | 24 | D | Unch | Unch | 50-75 | No (H,P) | *8-10% converted to digoxin. Serum concentration rises with quinidine coadministration | 334, 335 |
| Digoxin | 30-40 | 87-100 | 76-85 | G* | 24 | D | Unch | 25-75 | 10-25* | No (H,P) | Radioimmunoassay may overestimate serum concentrations in ESRD. Renal clearance reduced by quinidine, spironolactone, amiodarone.<br>*Serum concentration 12h after dose best guide in ESRD | 336-338 |
| Ouabain (strophanthin G) | 21 | 60-70 | 37-50 | G | 12-24 | I | 24 | 24-36 | 36-48 | No (H,P) | | |
| **Diuretics*** (see chapters 21, sect. 3.1; and chapter 24, sect. 5.1) | | | | | | | | | | | *Agents in this group may produce extracellular fluid volume depletion | |
| Acetazolamide | 1.7-5.8 | ? | 100 | | 6 | I | 6 | 12 | Avoid* | ? | *Ineffective. May potentiate acidosis, produce urolithiasis | 339, 340 |
| Amiloride | 6-9.6 | 8-140 | 50 | He | 12-24 | D | Unch | 50 | Avoid* | ? | *Hyperkalaemia common with GFR < 30 ml/min; may produce hyperchloraemic metabolic acidosis | 341, 342 |
| Bumetanide | 1.2-1.5 | 1.5 | 33 | N | 6 | D | Unch | Unch | Unch | ? | Cramps, muscle weakness, gynaecomastia | 343-345 |
| Chlorthalidone | 47-80 | ? | 50 | N | 24 | I | 24 | 24 | 48 | ? | | 339, 346 |
| Ethacrynic acid | 0.8-4 | ? | 20 | He | 6 | I | 6 | 6 | Avoid* | No (H) | *Ototoxic, particularly in combination with aminoglycosides and with large doses | 339 |
| Furosemide (frusemide) | 0.3-1.6 | 1.3-14 | 67 | He | 6 | D | Unch | Unch | Unch* | No (H) | Allergic interstitial nephritis; ototoxic, particularly in combination with aminoglycosides<br>*High doses useful in ESRD | 339, 347 |

| | | | | | | | | | | | | |
|---|---|---|---|---|---|---|---|---|---|---|---|---|
| Hydrochloro-thiazide | 6-15 | Pro-longed | > 95 | | 12 | D | Unch | Unch* | Avoid* | ? | Hyperuricaemia. *Ineffective with GFR < 30 ml/min | 348, 349 |
| Indapamide | 14-18 | 14-18 | 7 | He | 24 | D | Unch | Unch | Unch | No (H) | | 350 |
| Metolazone | 20 | ? | 70 | | 24 | D | Unch | Unch | Unch* | No (H) | *High doses may be useful in ESRD | 351 |
| Piretanide | 1.4 | 1.6-3 | 75 | | 12 | D | Unch | Unch | Unch | No (H) | | 352 |
| Spironolactone | 10-35* | 10-35* | 20-30 | He | 6 | I | 6 | 6 | Avoid** | ? | *Active metabolite (canrenone). **Hyperkalaemia with GFR < 30 ml/min; may produce hyperkalaemic metabolic alkalosis | 339, 353 |
| Torasemide | 2-4 | 3-60 | 75 | | 12 | D | Unch | Unch | Unch | No (H) | | 354 |
| Triamterene | 1.5-3 | 10 | 5-10 | He | 12 | I | 12 | 12 | Avoid* | ? | *Hyperkalaemia with GFR < 30 ml/min; renal calculi, folic acid antagonist | 355, 356 |
| **Gout drugs*** (see chapter 25, sect. 13.1] | | | | | | | | | | | *Most agents in this group add to uraemic bleeding and gastrointestinal symptoms | |
| Allopurinol | 0.7-1.6 | Pro-longed | Low | NR* | 24 | D<br>I | Unch<br>24 | 50<br>24-48 | 30<br>48-72 | Yes (H) | *Principal active metabolite (oxypurinol) has a long $t_{1/2}$ (13-29h) and accumulates in renal failure, causing fever, eosinophilia, skin desquamation and decreased renal function. Rare xanthine stones | 357, 358 |
| Colchicine | 0.3-1 | 0.7 | 5-17 | He | 12 | D | Unch | Unch | 50* | No (H) | Aggravates gastrointestinal symptoms. *Unchanged dose for acute use | 359 |
| Probenecid | 4-12 | ? | 1-5 | NR | 12 | D | Unch | Unch | Avoid* | ? | *May precipitate urolithiasis; ineffective at low GFR | 360, 361 |
| Sulfinpyra-zone | 3-5 | Unch | 50 | NR | 6-8 | I | Unch | Unch | Avoid* | ? | *May precipitate urolithiasis; rare acute renal failure; ineffective at low GFR | 362 |
| **Hypoglycaemic drugs** (see antidiabetic drugs) | | | | | | | | | | | | |
| **Lipid-lowering drugs** (see chapter 20, sect. 4.2) | | | | | | | | | | | | |
| Bezafibrate | 2 | 5-9 | 20 | He | 12 | D | Unch | 50-70 | 10-30 | No (P) | Myositis, rhabdomyolysis reported | 363 |
| Clofibrate | 6-54 | 110 | 18-32 | He, G | 6 | I | 6-12 | 12-18 | 24-48 | No (H) | Myopathy; reduce dose in nephrotic syndrome; impairs renal water excretion | 364, 365 |
| Gemfibrozil | 1.5 | Unch | < 10 | He | 12 | D | Unch | Unch | Unch | No (H,P) | | 366 |
| Lovastatin | 6-8 | ? | < 5 | He | 24 | S | Unch | Unch | Unch | ? | Rhabdomyolysis reported in transplant patients receiving cyclosporin | 367 |
| Pravastatin | 1.3-2.6 | ? | < 5 | He | 24 | D | Unch | Unch | Unch | ? | Rhabdomyolysis reported in transplant patients receiving cyclosporin | 368 |
| **Muscle relaxants, skeletal*** (see chapter 12, sect. 2.1) | | | | | | | | | | | *Aminoglycosides, hypokalaemia, acidosis and hypermagnesaemia enhance neuromuscular blocking effects | |
| Atracurium besilate | 20 min | Unch | Low | NR | IV infusion | D | Unch | Unch | Unch | ? | Can be used safely in renal failure | 369, 370 |
| Doxacurium chloride | 1-2.5 | 3-6 | 30 | | Single dose | D | Unch | 50-75 | 25-50 | ? | Prolonged neuromuscular blockade in ESRD | 371 |

[Continued over]

*For footnotes, see final page of table (p. 1747)*

**Appendix D.** *[Continued]*

| Drug | Elimination half-life ($t_{1/2}$) [adults] normal (h) | ESRD (h) | Excreted unchanged (%) | Extra-renal excretion[a] (normal) | Normal dose interval (h) | Dose adjustment for renal failure[b] method[c] | creatinine clearance (ml/min) > 50 | 10-50 | < 10 | Dialysis[d] | Toxic effects in renal failure/ Notes[e] | References |
|---|---|---|---|---|---|---|---|---|---|---|---|---|
| **Muscle relaxants, skeletal** *[continued]* | | | | | | | | | | | | |
| Gallamine triethiodide | 2-3 | 9 | 53-95 | | Single dose | D | Unch | Avoid* | Avoid* | Yes (H,P) | *Prolonged apnoea | 372 |
| Mivacurium chloride | 0.2-0.4 | 0.3-0.8 | < 10 | NR | Single dose | D | Unch | Unch | Unch | No (H,P) | | 373 |
| Pancuronium bromide | 1.5-2.2 | 4.3 | 40 | He | Single dose | D | Unch | Unch | Avoid* | ? | *Active metabolites accumulate in ESRD; duration of action prolonged | 190, 374 |
| Suxamethonium chloride (succinylcholine) | 3 | ? | Low | NR* | Single dose | D | Unch | Unch | Unch** | ? | *Renal excretion of active metabolites. **Acute hyperkalaemia with large doses in ESRD; prolonged apnoea | 375 |
| Tubocurarine | 0.1-3.8 | 5 | 75 | He | Single dose | D | Unch | Unch | Unch* | ? | *Prolonged effects with large or repeated doses | 376, 377 |
| Vecuronium bromide | 1 | 1.5 | 10-25 | He | Single dose | D | Unch | Unch | Unch | ? | Can be used safely in renal failure | 369, 378 |
| **Miscellaneous drugs** | | | | | | | | | | | | |
| Auranofin | 17-25 | ? | 12 | NR | 12-24 | D | Unch | Unch | Unch | ? | Nephrotoxic; proteinuria and rare nephrotic syndrome | 379 |
| Aurothiomalate sodium (gold sodium thiomalate) | 10-35 days* | ? | 60-90 | NR | 24 | D | Unch | Unch | Avoid | No (H) | *Prolonged $t_{1/2}$ in tissues. Nephrotoxic; proteinuria, membranous glomerulonephritis | 380 |
| Epoetin (recombinant human erythropoietin) | 6-9 | 6-9 | < 10 | He | after each diaylsis IV in ESRD | D | Unch | Unch | Unch | No (H) | Doses lower with subcutaneous administration | 381 |
| Ergoloid mesylates (codergocrine mesylate) | 1.5-4.1 | ? | < 10 | He | 8 | D | Unch | Unch | Unch | ? | | 382 |
| Etidronate disodium | 6 (plasma) 3-6 mos (bone) | Prolonged | < 5 | NR | 24 | D | Unch | Unch | Avoid | ? | Can elevate creatinine. $t_{1/2}$ dependent on bone turnover rate | 383 |
| Goserelin | 4-5 | 12 | < 10 | NR | 24 | D | Unch | Unch | Unch | ? | | 384 |

| | | | | | | | | | | | | |
|---|---|---|---|---|---|---|---|---|---|---|---|---|
| Leuprorelin | 3-4 | ? | NR | | Sustained release depot injection | D | Unch | Unch | Unch | ? | | 385 |
| Levamisole | 4-6 | Unch | < 5 | | 8 | D | Unch | Unch | Unch | ? | | 386 |
| Pamidronate disodium | 2-5 (plasma) 3-6 mos (bone) | Pro-longed | < 5 | NR | 24 | D | Unch | 50-100 | Avoid | ? | Lymphopenia, leucopenia, pyrexia common with initial dose. $t_{1/2}$ dependent on bone turnover rate | 387 |
| Penicillamine (D-penicill-amine) | 1.5-3 | Unch | 3-25 | He | 8-24* | D | Unch | Avoid | Avoid | ? | Nephrotic syndrome proteinuria *Depends on indication | 388, 389 |
| Pentamidine | 29* | 118 | 20 | | 24 | I | 24 | 24-36 | 48 | No (H,P) | Nephrotoxic. *Extensive tissue uptake | 390 |
| Pentoxifylline (oxpentifylline) | 0.8 | Pro-longed | < 10 | He | 8 | D | Unch | Unch | 50-75 | ? | | 391 |
| Piracetam | 5-6 | Pro-longed | 90 | | 6 | D | Unch | 75 | 50 | ? | | 392 |
| Sodium cromogly-cate (cromolyn sodium) | 1.2 | 1.2 | < 10 | NR | Inhaled | D | Unch | Unch | Unch | No (H,P) | | 393 |

a He = hepatic; G = gastrointestinal; NR = non-renal (precise route unknown or not clear). Although some antibacterial agents may not require any dosage modification because of extrarenal excretion, adequate urinary concentrations may not be obtained when treating urinary infections (e.g. erythromycin, doxycycline).

b *See also introduction. Plasma concentrations should always be used to monitor therapy whenever feasible, especially when the agent is potentially toxic and/or when lengthy intervals are required between doses.* These intervals, which reflect the 'usual' maintenance dose, are based on typical dosage regimens and should only be considered as a representative *rough* guide. Other dosage regimens for an individual drug can be modified in proportion to the dose adjustments shown. Associated liver disease for most drugs with an hepatic route of elimination would generally have to be severe to alter dosage schedules further (see also appendix F).

c I = interval extention method of dosage adjustment (values given are hours between 'usual' maintenance doses); D = dose reduction method of dosage adjustment (values given indicate percentage of usual maintenance dose); Unch = unchanged.

d 'Yes' indicates removal of enough drug to require dosage supplement to ensure adequate therapeutic blood concentrations; 'No' indicates lack of need for dosage adjustment with dialysis (see also introduction). *NB.* A lack of requirement for supplemental dosage in therapeutic situations does not necessarily preclude the use of dialysis or haemoperfusion for drug overdoses. H = haemodialysis; P = peritoneal dialysis.

e See also discussion in chapter 1 (sect. 5.4.4), chapter 6 (sect. 5.2), chapter 24 (sect. 1, 11), and specifically for the drugs listed in the chapters given by the cross reference alongside the drug class heading.

*Abbreviations:* $t_{1/2}$ = elimination half-life; ESRD = end stage renal disease; I = interval extension method of dosage adjustment (values given are hours between 'usual' maintenance doses); D = dose reduction method of dosage adjustment (values given indicate percentage of usual maintenance dose); He = hepatic; G = gastrointestinal; NR = non-renal; H = haemodialysis; P = peritoneal dialysis; Unch = unchanged.

## References


1. Balfour JA, Goa KL. Benazepril: a review of its pharmacodynamic and pharmacokinetic properties, and therapeutic efficacy in hypertension and congestive heart failure. Drugs 1991; 42: 511-39
2. Duchin KL, Pierides AM, Heald A, et al. Elimination kinetics of captopril in patients with renal failure. Kidney International 1984; 25: 942
3. Todd PA, Goa KL. Enalapril: a reappraisal of its pharmacology and therapeutic use in hypertension. Drugs 1992; 43: 346-81
4. Murdoch D, McTavish D. Fosinopril: a review of its pharmacodynamic and pharmacokinetic properties, and therapeutic potential in essential hypertension. Drugs 1992; 43: 123-40
5. Lancaster SG, Todd PA. Lisinopril: a preliminary review of its pharmacodynamic and pharmacokinetic properties and therapeutic use in hypertension and congestive heart failure. Drugs 1988; 35: 646
6. Todd PA, Fitton A. Perindopril: a review of its pharmacological properties and therapeutic use in cardiovascular disorders. Drugs 1991; 42: 90-114
7. Wadworth AN, Brogden RN. Quinapril: a review of its pharmacological properties and therapeutic efficacy in cardiovascular disorders. Drugs 1991; 41: 378-99
8. Shionori H, Ikeda Y, Kimura K, et al. Pharmacodynamics and pharmacokinetics of single dose ramipril in hypertensive patients with various degrees of renal function. Current Therapeutic Research 1986; 40: 74-85
9. Todd PA, Benfield P. Ramipril: a review of its pharmacological properties and therapeutic efficacy in cardiovascular disorders. Drugs 1990; 39: 110-35
10. Singh BN, Thoden WR, Ward A. Acebutolol: a review of its pharmacological properties and therapeutic efficacy in hypertension, angina pectoris and arrhythmia. Drugs 1985; 29: 531
11. Kirch W, Gorg ER. Clinical pharmacokinetics of atenolol - a review. European Journal of Drug Metabolism and Pharmacokinetics 1982; 7: 81
12. Frishman WH. Atenolol and timolol, two new systemic β-adrenoreceptor antagonists. New England Journal of Medicine 1982; 306: 1456
13. Beresford R, Heel RC. Betaxolol: a review of its pharmacodynamic and pharmacokinetic properties, and therapeutic efficacy in hypertension. Drugs 1986; 31: 6-28
14. Frishman WH, Goldberg RJ, Benfield P. Bevantolol: a preliminary review of its pharmacodynamic and pharmacokinetic properties, and therapeutic efficacy in hypertension and angina pectoris. Drugs 1988; 35: 1-21
15. Payton CD, Fox FG, Pauleau NF, et al. The single dose pharmacokinetics of bisoprolol (10mg) in renal insufficiency: the clinical significance of balanced clearance. European Heart Journal 1987; 8 Suppl. M: 15-22
16. Kirch W, Rose I, Demers HG, et al. Pharmacokinetics of bisoprolol during repeated oral administration to healthy volunteers and patients with kidney or liver disease. Clinical Pharmacokinetics 1987; 13: 110-7
17. Lancaster SG, Sorkin EM. Bisoprolol: a preliminary review of its pharmacodynamic and pharmacokinetic properties and therapeutic efficacy in hypertension and angina pectoris. Drugs 1988; 36: 256-85
18. Harron DWG, Goa KL, Langtry HD. Bopindolol: a review of its pharmacodynamic and pharmacokinetic properties and therapeutic efficacy. Drugs 1991; 41: 130-49
19. Hasenfuss G, Schafer-Korting M, Knauf H, et al. Pharmacokinetics of carteolol in relation to renal function. European Journal of Clinical Pharmacology 1985; 29: 461-5
20. McTavish D, Campoli-Richards D, Sorkin EM. Carvedilol: a review of its pharmacodynamic and pharmacokinetic properties, and therapeutic efficacy. Drugs 1993; 45: 232-58
21. Milne RJ, Buckley MMT. Celiprolol: an updated review of its pharmacodynamic and pharmacokinetic properties, and therapeutic efficacy in cardiovascular disease. Drugs 1991; 41: 941-69
22. Benfield P, Sorkin EM. Esmolol: a preliminary review of its pharmacodynamic and pharmacokinetic properties, and therapeutic efficacy. Drugs 1987; 33: 392-412
23. Carter BL. Labetalol. Drug Intelligence and Clinical Pharmacy 1983; 17: 704
24. Regardh CG, Johnsson G. Clinical pharmacokinetics of metoprolol. Clinical Pharmacokinetics 1980; 5: 557
25. Frishman WH. Nadolol: a new beta adrenoreceptor antagonist. New England Journal of Medicine 1981; 305: 678
26. Galeazzi RL, Gugger M, Weidmann P. Beta blockade with pindolol: differential cardiac and renal effects despite similar plasma kinetics in normal and uremic man. Kidney International 1979; 15: 661
27. Stone WJ, Walle T. Massive propranolol metabolic retention during maintenance hemodialysis. Clinical Pharmacology and Therapeutics 1980; 28: 448
28. Wood AJ, Vestal RE, Spannuth CL. Propranolol disposition in renal failure. British Journal of Clinical Pharmacology 1980; 10: 561
29. Blair AD, Burgess ED, Maxwell BM, et al. Sotalol kinetics in renal insufficiency. Clinical Pharmacology and Therapeutics 1981; 29: 457
30. Affrime MB, Lowenthal DT. Analgesics, sedatives and sedative-hypnotics. In: Anderson et al., editors. Clinical use of drugs in patients with liver and kidney disease. Philadelphia: WB Saunders, 1981: 199-210
31. Christensen JH, Andreasen F, Jansen J. Pharmacokinetics and pharmacodynamics of thiopental in patients undergoing renal transplantation. Acta Anaesthesiologica Scandinavica 1983; 27: 513
32. Todd PA, Sorkin EM. Diclofenac sodium: a reappraisal of its pharmacodynamic and pharmacokinetic properties, and therapeutic efficacy. Drugs 1988; 35: 244-85
33. Verbeeck RK, Blackburn JL, Loewen GR. Clinical pharmacokinetics of nonsteroidal anti-inflammatory drugs. Clinical Pharmacokinetics 1983; 8: 297
34. Nickander R, McMahon FG, Ridolfo AS. Nonsteroidal antiinflammatory drugs. Annual Review of Pharmacology and Toxicology 1979; 19: 469
35. Albert KS, Gernaat CM. Pharmacokinetics of ibuprofen. American Journal of Medicine 1984; 76: 40
36. Kantor TG. Ibuprofen. Annals of Internal Medicine 1979; 91: 877
37. Stein G, Kunze M, Zaumseil J, et al. Pharmacokinetics of indomethacin and indomethacin metabolites administered continually to patients with healthy and damaged kidneys. International Journal of Clinical Pharmacology and Biopharmaceutics 1977; 15: 470
38. Williams RL, Upton RA. The clinical pharmacology of ketoprofen. Journal of Clinical Pharmacology 1988; 28: S13-22
39. Antila M, Haatja M, Kasanen A. Pharmacokinetics of naproxen in subjects with normal and impaired renal function. European Journal of Clinical Pharmacology 1980; 18: 263
40. Verbeeck RK, Richardson CJ, Blocka KLN. Clinical pharmacokinetics of piroxicam. Journal of Rheumatology 1986; 13: 789-96
41. Todd PA, Beresford B. Pirprofen: a review of its pharmacodynamic and pharmacokinetic properties, and therapeutic efficacy. Drugs 1986; 32: 509-37

42. Rhymer AR. Sulindac. Clinics in Rheumatic Diseases 1979; 5: 553
43. Todd PA, Clissold SP. Tenoxicam: an update of its pharmacology, and therapeutic efficacy in rheumatic diseases. Drugs 1991; 41: 625-46
44. Levy G. Pharmacokinetics of salicylate in man. Drug Metabolism Reviews 1979; 9: 13
45. Barnes JN, Williams AJ, Tomson MJ, et al. Dihydrocodeine in renal failure: further evidence for an important role of the kidney in the handling of opioid drugs. British Medical Journal 1985; 290: 740
46. Gibson TP, Giacomini KM, Briggs WA. Pharmacokinetics of d-propoxyphene in anephric patients. Clinical Pharmacology and Therapeutics 1977; 21: 103
47. Forrest JA, Clements JA, Prescott LF. Clinical pharmacokinetics of paracetamol. Clinical Pharmacokinetics 1982; 7: 93
48. Heel RC, Brogden RN, Speight TM, et al. Butorphanol: a review of its pharmacologic properties and therapeutic efficacy. Drugs 1978; 16: 473
49. Mather LE. Clinical pharmacokinetics of fentanyl and its newer derivatives. Clinical Pharmacokinetics 1983; 8: 422
50. Fung DL, Eisele JH. Fentanyl pharmacokinetics in awake volunteers. Journal of Clinical Pharmacology 1980; 20: 652
51. Berkowitz BA. The relationship of pharmacokinetics to pharmacological activity: morphine, methadone, naloxone. Clinical Pharmacokinetics 1976; 1: 219
52. Don HG, Dieppa RA, Taylor P. Narcotic analgesics in anuric patients. Anesthesiology 1976; 42: 745
53. Inturrisi CE. Disposition of narcotics in patients with renal disease. American Journal of Medicine 1977; 62: 528
54. Boerner U, Abbott S, Roe RL. The metabolism of morphine and heroin in man. Drug Metabolism Reviews 1975; 4: 39
55. Payne IP. The clinical pharmacology of pentazocine. Drugs 1973; 5: 1
56. Szeto HH, Inturrisi CE, Houde R, et al. Accumulation of normeperidine, an active metabolite of meperidine, in patients with renal failure or cancer. Annals of Internal Medicine 1977; 86: 738
57. Edwards DJ, Svensson CK, Visco JP, et al. Clinical pharmacokinetics of pethidine: 1982. Clinical Pharmacokinetics 1982; 7: 421
58. Monk JP, Beresford R, Ward A. Sufentanil: a review of its pharmacological properties and therapeutic use. Drugs 1988; 36: 286-313
59. Lee CR, McTavish D, Sorkin EM. Tramadol: a preliminary review of its pharmacodynamic and pharmacokinetic properties, and therapeutic potential in acute and chronic pain states. Drugs 1993; 46: 313-40
60. Bullingham RE, McQuay HJ, Moore RA. Clinical pharmacokinetics of narcotic agonist-antagonist drugs. Clinical Pharmacokinetics 1983; 8: 332
61. Gonzalez JP, Brogden RN. Naltrexone: a review of its pharmacodynamic and pharmacokinetic properties, and therapeutic efficacy in the management of opioid dependence. Drugs 1988; 35: 192-213
62. Garzone PD, Kroboth PD. Pharmacokinetics of the newer benzodiazepines. Clinical Pharmacokinetics 1989; 16: 337-64
63. Langley MS, Clissold SP. Brotizolam: a review of its pharmacodynamic and pharmacokinetic properties, and therapeutic efficacy as an hypnotic. Drugs 1988; 35: 104-22
64. Breimer DD, Jochemsen R. Clinical pharmacokinetics of hypnotic benzodiazepines. British Journal of Clinical Pharmacology 1983; 16: 2775
65. Greenblatt DJ, Shader RI. Clinical use of the benzodiazepines. Rational Drug Therapy 1981; 15: 1
66. Greenblatt DJ, Shader RI, MacLeod SM. Clinical pharmacokinetics of chlordiazepoxide. Clinical Pharmacokinetics 1978; 3: 381
67. Ochs HR, Rauh HW, Greenblatt DJ, et al. Clorazepate dipotassium and diazepam in renal insufficiency: serum concentrations and protein binding of diazepam and desmethyldiazepam. Nephron 1984; 37: 100-4
68. Mandelli M, Tognoni G, Garattini S. Clinical pharmacokinetics of diazepam. Clinical Pharmacokinetics 1978; 3: 72
69. Greenblatt DJ. Clinical pharmacokinetics of oxazepam and lorazepam. Clinical Pharmacokinetics 1981; 6: 89
70. Morrison G, Chiang ST, Koepke HH, et al. Effect of renal impairment and hemodialysis on lorazepam kinetics. Clinical Pharmacology and Therapeutics 1984; 35: 646
71. Calvo R, Suarez E, Rodriguez Sasiain JM, et al. The influence of renal failure on the kinetics of intravenous midazolam - an in vitro and in vivo study. Research Communications in Chemical Pathology and Pharmacology 1992; 78: 311-20
72. Ochs HR, Oberem U, Greenblatt DJ. Nitrazepam clearance unimpaired in patients with renal insufficiency. Journal of Clinical Psychopharmacology 1992; 12: 183-5
73. Murray TG, Chiang ST, Koepke HH. Renal disease, age and oxazepam kinetics. Clinical Pharmacology and Therapeutics 1981; 30: 805
74. Greenblatt DJ, Divoll M, Abernethy DR, et al. Clinical pharmacokinetics of the newer benzodiazepines. Clinical Pharmacokinetics 1983; 8: 233
75. Roth T, Roehrs TA, Zonck FJ. Pharmacology and hypnotic efficacy of triazolam. Pharmacotherapy 1983; 3: 137
76. Goa KL, Ward A. Buspirone: a preliminary review of its pharmacological properties and therapeutic efficacy as an anxiolytic. Drugs 1986; 32: 114-29
77. Gambertoglio JG, Laver RM. Use of neuropsychiatric drugs. In: Anderson & Schrier, editors. Clinical use of drugs in patients with kidney and liver disease. Philadelphia: WB Saunders, 1981: 276-95
78. Harron DWG, Brogden RN. Acecainide: a review of its pharmacodynamic and pharmacokinetic properties, and therapeutic potential in cardiac arrhythmias. Drugs 1990; 39: 720-40
79. Gillis AM, Kates RE. Clinical pharmacokinetics of the newer antiarrhythmic agents. Clinical Pharmacokinetics 1984; 9: 375
80. Latini R, Tognoni G, Kates RE. Clinical pharmacokinetics of amiodarone. Clinical Pharmacokinetics 1984; 9: 136
81. Rapeport WG. Clinical pharmacokinetics of bretylium. Clinical Pharmacokinetics 1985; 10: 248
82. Harron DWG, Brogden RN, Faulds D. Cibenzoline: a review of its pharmacological properties, and therapeutic potential in arrhythmias. Drugs 1992; 43: 734-59
83. Shen DD, Cunningham JL, Shudo I. Disposition kinetics of disopyramide in patients with renal insufficiency. Biopharmaceutics and Drug Disposition 1980; 1: 133
84. Conard GJ, Ober RE. Metabolism of flecainide. American Journal of Cardiology 1984; 53: 41B
85. Holmes B, Heel RC. Flecainide: a preliminary review of its pharmacodynamic properties and therapeutic efficacy. Drugs 1985; 29: 1
86. Waller ES. Pharmacokinetic principles of lidocaine dosing in relation to disease state. Journal of Clinical Pharmacology 1981; 21: 181
87. Eiriksson CE, Brogden RN. Lorcainide: a preliminary review of its pharmacodynamic properties and therapeutic efficacy. Drugs 1983; 27: 279

88. Baudinet C, Henrard L, Quinaux N, et al. Pharmacokinetics of mexiletine in renal insufficiency. Acta Cardiologica 1980; Suppl. 25: 55
89. Gibson TP, Atkinson AJ, Matusik E. Kinetics of procainamide and N-acetyl-procainamide in renal failure. Kidney International 1977; 12: 422
90. Bryson HM, Palmer KJ, Langtry HD. Propafenone: a reappraisal of its pharmacology, pharmacokinetics and therapeutic use in cardiac arrhythmias. Drugs 1993; 45: 85-130
91. Ochs HR, Greenblatt DJ, Woo E. Clinical pharmacokinetics of quinidine. Clinical Pharmacokinetics 1980; 5: 150
92. Hasegawa GR. Tocainide: a new oral antiarrhythmic. Drug Intelligence and Clinical Pharmacy 1985; 19: 514
93. Oltmanns D, Pottage A, Endell W. Pharmacokinetics of tocainide in patients with combined hepatic and renal dysfunction. European Journal of Clinical Pharmacology 1983; 25: 787
94. Pechere J, Dugal R. Clinical pharmacokinetics of aminoglycoside antibiotics. Clinical Pharmacokinetics 1979; 4: 170
95. Noone P. Sisomicin, netilmicin and dibekacin: a review of their antibacterial activity and therapeutic use. Drugs 1984; 27: 548
96. Ristuccia AM, Cunha BA. An overview of amikacin. Therapeutic Drug Monitoring 1985; 7: 12
97. Meyer RD. Amikacin. Annals of Internal Medicine 1981; 95: 328
98. Hallynek T, Soep HH, Dehli L. Influence of age and renal disease on aminoglycoside dosage. Journal of Antimicrobial Chemotherapy 1981; 8 Suppl. A: 1
99. Craig WA, Gudmauadsson S, Reich RM. Netilmicin sulfate a comparative evaluation of antimicrobial activity, pharmacokinetics, adverse reactions and clinical efficacy. Pharmacotherapy 1983; 3: 305
100. Guay DR. Netilmicin. Drug Intelligence and Clinical Pharmacy 1983; 17: 83
101. Brogden RN, Pinder RM, Sawyer PR, et al. Tobramycin: a review of its antibacterial and pharmacokinetic properties and therapeutic use. Drugs 1976; 12: 166
102. Tartaglione TA, Polk RE. Review of the new second generation cephalosporins: cefonicid, ceforanide and cefuroxime. Drug Intelligence and Clinical Pharmacy 1985; 19: 188
103. Balant L, Dayer P, Auckenthalaer R. Clinical pharmacokinetics of the third generation cephalosporins. Clinical Pharmacokinetics 1985; 10: 101
104. Clark J, Hochman R, Rolla AR, et al. Coagulopathy associated with the use of cephalosporin or moxalactam antibiotics in acute and chronic renal failure. Clinical and Experimental Dialysis and Apheresis 1983; 7: 177
105. Thompson RL, Wright AJ. Cephalosporin antibiotics. Mayo Clinic Proceedings 1983; 58: 79
106. Derry JE. Evaluation of cefaclor. American Journal of Hospital Pharmacy 1981; 38: 54
107. Leroy A, Humben G, Godin M, et al. Pharmacokinetics of cefadroxil in patients with impaired renal function. Journal of Antimicrobial Chemotherapy 1982; 10 Suppl. B: 39
108. Czerwinski A, Federson J. Pharmacokinetics of cefamandole in patients with renal impairment. Antimicrobial Agents and Chemotherapy 1979; 15: 161
109. Bergan T, Orjavik O, Brodwall EK. Pharmacokinetics of cefapirin in patients with normal and impaired renal function. Arzneimittel-Forschung 1981; 10: 1773
110. Quintiliani R, Nightingale CH. Cefazolin. Annals of Internal Medicine 1978; 89: 650
111. Barradell LB, Bryson HM. Cefepime: a review of its antibacterial activity, pharmacokinetic properties and therapeutic use. Drugs 1994; 47: 471-505
112. Brogden RN, Campoli-Richards DM. Cefixime: a review of its antibacterial activity, pharmacokinetic properties and therapeutic potential. Drugs 1989; 38: 524
113. Gambertoglio JG, Alexander DP, Barriere SL. Cefmenoxime pharmacokinetics in healthy volunteers and subjects with renal insufficiency and on hemodialysis. Antimicrobial Agents and Chemotherapy 1984; 26: 845
114. Schentag JJ. Cefmetazole sodium: pharmacology, pharmacokinetics, and clinical trials. Pharmacotherapy 1991; 11: 2-19
115. Pontzer RE, Kaye D. Cefonicid: a long acting, second generation cephalosporin. Pharmacotherapy 1985; 4: 325
116. Lyon JA. Cefoperazone. Drug Intelligence and Clinical Pharmacy 1983; 17: 7
117. Barriere SL, Mills J. Ceforanide: antibacterial activity, pharmacology, and clinical efficacy. Pharmacotherapy 1982; 2: 322
118. Doluiso JT. Clinical pharmacokinetics of cefotaxime in patients with normal and reduced renal function. Reviews of Infectious Diseases 1982; 4: S333
119. Martin C, Thomachot L, Albanese J. Clinical pharmacokinetics of cefotetan. Clinical Pharmacokinetics 1994; 26: 248-58
120. Konishi K, Ozawa Y. Pharmacokinetics of cefotiam in patients with impaired renal function and in those undergoing hemodialysis. Antimicrobial Agents and Chemotherapy 1984; 26: 647
121. Kampf D, Shurig R, Korsukewitz I, et al. Cefoxitin pharmacokinetics: relation to three different renal clearance studies in patients with various degrees of renal insufficiency. Antimicrobial Agents and Chemotherapy 1981; 20: 741
122. Frampton JE, Brogden RN, Langtry HD, et al. Cefpodoxime proxetil: a review of its antibacterial activity, pharmacokinetic properties and therapeutic potential. Drugs 1992; 44: 889-917
123. Wiseman LR, Benfield P. Cefprozil: a review of its antibacterial activity, pharmacokinetic properties, and therapeutic potential. Drugs 1993; 45: 295-317
124. Solomon AE, Buggs JD, McGleachey R. The administration of cephradine to patients with normal and impaired renal function. British Journal of Clinical Pharmacology 1975; 2: 443
125. Ohkawa M, Takamae K, Shimamura M, et al. Pharmacokinetics of cefroxadine in healthy volunteers and patients with impaired renal function. Chemotherapy 1981; 27: 149
126. Matzke GR, Keane WF. Cefsulodin pharmacokinetics in patients with various degrees of renal function. Antimicrobial Agents and Chemotherapy 1983; 23: 369
127. Richards DM, Brogden RN. Ceftazidime: a review of its antibacterial activity, pharmacokinetic properties and therapeutic use. Drugs 1985; 29: 105
128. Richards DM, Heel RC. Ceftizoxime: a review of its antibacterial activity, pharmacokinetic properties and therapeutic use. Drugs 1985; 29: 281
129. Richards DM, Heel RC, Brogden RN, et al. Ceftriaxone: a review of its antibacterial activity, pharmacodynamic properties and therapeutic use. Drugs 1984; 27: 469
130. Walstad RA, Nilsen OG, Berg ICJ. Pharmacokinetics and clinical effects of cefuroxime in patients with severe renal insufficiency. European Journal of Clinical Pharmacy 1983; 24: 391
131. Carmine AA, Brogden RN, Heel RC, et al. Moxalactam (latamoxef): a review of its antibacterial activity, pharmacokinetic properties and therapeutic use. Drugs 1983; 26: 279

132. Gasser TC, Ebert SC, Graversen PH, et al. Ciprofloxacin pharmacokinetics in patients with normal and impaired renal function. Antimicrobial Agents and Chemotherapy 1987; 31: 709-12
133. Gasser TC, Ebert SC, Graversen PH, et al. Pharmacokinetics of ciprofloxacin in patients with impaired renal function. Reviews of Infectious Diseases 1988; 10 Suppl. 1: 110
134. Drusano GL, Weir M, Forrest A, et al. Pharmacokinetics of intravenously administered ciprofloxacin in patients with various degrees of renal function. Antimicrobial Agents and Chemotherapy 1987; 31: 860-4
135. Campoli-Richards DM, Monk JP, Price A. Ciprofloxacin: a review of its antibacterial activity, pharmacokinetic properties and therapeutic use. Drugs 1988; 35: 373-447
136. Bury RW, Becker GJ, Kincaid-Smith PS, et al. Elimination of enoxacin in renal disease. Clinical Pharmacology and Therapeutics 1987; 41: 434-8
137. Henwood JM, Monk JP. Enoxacin: a review of its antibacterial activity, pharmacokinetic properties and therapeutic use. Drugs 1988; 36: 32-66
138. Weidekamm E. Pharmacokinetics of fleroxacin in renal impairment. American Journal of Medicine 1993; 94 Suppl. 3A: 70S
139. Wadworth AN, Goa KL. Lomefloxacin: a review of its antibacterial activity, pharmacokinetic properties and therapeutic use. Drugs 1991; 42: 1018-60
140. Holmes B, Brogden RN, Richards DM. Norfloxacin: a review of its antibacterial activity, pharmacokinetic properties and therapeutic use. Drugs 1985; 30: 482-513
141. Mignot A, Couet W, Lefebvre MA, et al. Pharmacokinetics of ofloxacin in patients with renal failure. Reviews of Infectious Diseases 1988; 10: S109
142. Todd PA, Faulds D. Ofloxacin: a reappraisal of its antimicrobial activity, pharmacology and therapeutic use. Drugs 1991; 42: 825-76
143. Höffler D, Schäfer L, Koeppe P, et al. Pharmacokinetics of pefloxacin in normal and impaired renal function. Arzneimittel-Forschung 1988; 38: 739-43
144. Gonzalez JP, Henwood JM. Pefloxacin: a review of its antibacterial activity, pharmacokinetic properties and therapeutic use. Drugs 1989; 37: 628
145. Peters DH, Friedel HA, McTavish D. Azithromycin: a review of its antimicrobial activity, pharmacokinetic properties and clinical efficacy. Drugs 1992; 44: 750-99
146. Barradell LB, Plosker L, McTavish D. Clarithromycin: a review of its pharmacological properties and therapeutic use in *Mycobacterium avium-intercellulare* complex infection in patients with acquired immune deficiency syndrome. Drugs 1993; 46: 289-312
147. Welling PG, Craig W. Pharmacokinetics of intravenous erythromycin. Journal of Pharmaceutical Sciences 1978; 67: 1057
148. Wise R. Penicillins and cephalosporins: antimicrobial and pharmacological properties. Lancet 1982; 2: 140
149. Wright AJ, Wilkowske CJ. The penicillins. Mayo Clinic Proceedings 1983; 58: 21
150. Eliopoulos GM, Moellering RC. Azlocillin, mezlocillin and piperacillin: new broad spectrum penicillins. Annals of Internal Medicine 1982; 97: 755
151. Neu HC. Amoxicillin. Annals of Internal Medicine 1979; 90: 356
152. Bergan T. Overview of acylureidopenicillin pharmacokinetics. Scandinavian Journal of Infectious Diseases 1981; Suppl. 29: 33
153. Whelton A, Stout RL, Delgado FA. An azlocillin dosing nomogram for renal insufficiency. Journal of Antimicrobial Chemotherapy 1983; 11 Suppl. B: 97
154. Latos DS, Bryan CS, Stone WJ. Carbenicillin therapy in patients with normal and impaired renal function. Clinical Pharmacology and Therapeutics 1975; 17: 692
155. Lipner HL, Ruzany F, Dasgupta M. The behaviour of carbenicillin as a nonreabsorbable anion. Journal of Laboratory and Clinical Medicine 1975; 86: 183
156. Nauta EH, Mattie H. Dicloxacillin and cloxacillin: pharmacokinetics in healthy and hemodialysis subjects. Clinical Pharmacology and Therapeutics 1976; 20: 98
157. Neu HC. Amdinocillin: a novel penicillin. Antibacterial activity, pharmacology and clinical use. Pharmacotherapy 1985; 5: 1
158. Bergan T. Review of the pharmacokinetics of mezlocillin. Journal of Antimicrobial Chemotherapy 1983; 11 Suppl. C: 1
159. Rudnick M, Morrison G, Walker G. Renal failure, hemodialysis and nafcillin kinetics. Clinical Pharmacology and Therapeutics 1976; 20: 413
160. Holmes B, Richards DM, Brogden RN, et al. Piperacillin: a review of its antibacterial activity, pharmacokinetic properties and therapeutic use. Drugs 1984; 28: 375
161. Parry MF, Neu HC. Pharmacokinetics of ticarcillin in patients with abnormal renal function. Journal of Infectious Diseases 1976; 133: 46
162. Heany D, Eknoyan G. Minocycline and doxycycline kinetics in chronic renal failure. Clinical Pharmacology and Therapeutics 1978; 24: 233
163. Brogden RN, Speight TM, Avery GS. Minocycline: a review of its antibacterial and pharmacokinetic properties and therapeutic use. Drugs 1975; 9: 251
164. Siegal D. Tetracyclines: a new look at old antibiotics. New York State Journal of Medicine 1978; 78: 950, 1115
165. Hopefl AW. Aztreonam - an overview. Drug Intelligence and Clinical Pharmacy 1985; 19: 171
166. Fillastre JP, Leroy A, Baudoin C, et al. Pharmacokinetics of aztreonam in patients with chronic renal failure. Clinical Pharmacokinetics 1985; 10: 91
167. Slaughter RL, Cerra FB, Koup JR. Effect of hemodialysis on total body clearance of chloramphenicol. American Journal of Hospital Pharmacy 1980; 37: 1083
168. Ambrose PJ. Clinical pharmacokinetics of chloramphenicol and chloramphenicol succinate. Clinical Pharmacokinetics 1984; 9: 222
169. Gibson TP, Demetriades JL, Bland JA. Imipenem/cilastatin: pharmacokinetic profile in renal insufficiency [abstract]. American Journal of Medicine 1985; 78: 54
170. Buckley MM, Brogden RN, Barradell LB, et al. Imipenem/cilastin: a reappraisal of its antibacterial activity, pharmacokinetic properties and therapeutic efficacy. Drugs 1992; 44: 408
171. Sisca TS, Heel RC, Romankiewicz JA. Cinoxacin: a review of its pharmacological properties and therapeutic efficacy in the treatment of urinary tract infections. Drugs 1983; 25: 544-69
172. Smith BR, LeFrock J. Amoxicillin-potassium clavulanate: a novel β-lactamase inhibitor. Drug Intelligence and Clinical Pharmacy 1985; 19: 415
173. Munch R, Luthy R, Blaser J, et al. Human pharmacokinetics and CSF penetration of clavulanic acid. Journal of Antimicrobial Chemotherapy 1981; 8: 29
174. Roberts AP, Eastwood JB, Gower PE, et al. Serum and plasma concentration of clindamycin following a single intramuscular injection of clindamycin phosphate in maintenance hemodialysis patients and normal subjects. European Journal of Clinical Pharmacology 1978; 14: 435
175. Malacoff RF, Finkelstein FO, Andriole VI. Effect of peritoneal dialysis on serum levels of tobramycin and

lincomycin. Antimicrobial Agents and Chemotherapy 1975; 8: 574

176. Leroy A, Fillastre JP, Etienne I, et al. Pharmacokinetics of meropenem in subjects with renal insufficiency. European Journal of Clinical Pharmacology 1992; 42: 535-8
177. Houghton GW, Dennis MJ, Gabriel R. Pharmacokinetics of metronidazole in patients with varying degrees of renal failure. British Journal of Clinical Pharmacology 1985; 19: 203
178. Ralph ED. Clinical pharmacokinetics of metronidazole. Clinical Pharmacokinetics 1983; 8: 43
179. Barbeau G, Belanger PM. Pharmacokinetics of nalidixic acid in old and young volunteers. Journal of Clinical Pharmacology 1982; 22: 491
180. Conklin JD. The pharmacokinetics of nitrofurantoin and its related bioavailability. Antibiotics and Chemotherapy 1978; 25: 233
181. Kusumi R, Metzler C, Fass R. Pharmacokinetics of spectinomycin in volunteers with renal insufficiency. Chemotherapy 1981; 27: 95
182. Campoli-Richards DM, Brogden RN. Sulbactam/ampicillin: a review of its antibacterial activity, pharmacokinetic properties, and therapeutic use. Drugs 1987; 33: 577-609
183. Reeves D. Sulphonamides and trimethoprim. Lancet 1982; 2: 370
184. Bryson HM, Brogden RN. Tazobactam: a review of its antibacterial activity, pharmacokinetic properties and therapeutic potential. Drugs 1994; 47: 506-35
185. Campoli-Richards DM, Brogden RN, Faulds D. Teicoplanin: a review of its antibacterial activity, pharmacokinetic properties and therapeutic potential. Drugs 1990; 40: 449-86
186. Patel R, Welling PG. Clinical pharmacokinetics of co-trimoxazole (trimethoprim-sulphamethoxazole). Clinical Pharmacokinetics 1980; 5: 403
187. Kucers A. Chloramphenicol, erythromycin, vancomycin, tetracyclines. Lancet 1982; 2: 425
188. Moellering RC, Krogstad DJ, Greenblatt W. Vancomycin therapy in patients with impaired renal function: a nomogram for dosage. Annals of Internal Medicine 1981; 94: 343
189. Cronnelly R, Stanski DR, Miller RD. Renal function and the pharmacokinetics of neostigmine in anesthetized man. Anesthesiology 1979; 51: 22
190. Ramzam MI, Somogyi AA, Walker JS, et al. Clinical pharmacokinetics of the nondepolarizing muscle relaxants. Clinical Pharmacokinetics 1981; 6: 25
191. Cronnelly R, Stanski DR, Miller RD, et al. Pyridostigmine kinetics with and without renal function. Clinical Pharmacology and Therapeutics 1980; 28: 78
192. Tien AN, Bjornson J. Heparin elimination in uremic patients on hemodialysis. Scandinavian Journal of Haematology 1977; 17: 29
193. Estes JW. Clinical pharmacokinetics of heparin. Clinical Pharmacokinetics 1980; 5: 204
194. Barradell LB, Buckley MM. Nadroparin calcium: a review of its pharmacology and clinical applications in the prevention or treatment of thromboembolic disorders. Drugs 1992; 44: 858
195. Kelly JG, O'Malley K. Clinical pharmacokinetics of oral anticoagulants. Clinical Pharmacokinetics 1979; 4: 1
196. Amsterdam J, Brunswick D, Mendels J. The clinical application of tricyclic antidepressant pharmacokinetics and plasma levels. American Journal of Psychiatry 1980; 137: 653
197. Lieberman JA, Cooper TB, Suckow RF, et al. Tricyclic antidepressant and metabolite levels in chronic renal failure. Clinical Pharmacology and Therapeutics 1985; 37: 301
198. Sandoz M, Vandel S, Vandel B, et al. Metabolism of amitriptyline in patients with chronic renal failure. European Journal of Clinical Pharmacology 1984; 26: 227
199. Faulkner RD, Senekjian HO, Lee CS. Hemodialysis of doxepin and desmethyl doxepin in uremic patients. Artificial Organs 1984; 8: 151
200. Dawling S, Lynn K, Rosser R. Nortriptyline metabolism in chronic renal failure: metabolite elimination. Clinical Pharmacology and Therapeutics 1982; 32: 322
201. Balant L. Clinical pharmacokinetics of sulphonylurea hypoglycaemic drugs. Clinical Pharmacokinetics 1981; 6: 215
202. Skillman TG, Feldman JM. The pharmacology of sulfonylureas. American Journal of Medicine 1981; 70: 361
203. Feldman JM. Glyburide: a second generation sulfonylurea hypoglycemic agent. Pharmacotherapy 1985; 5: 43
204. Lebovitz HE. Glipizide: a second generation sulfonylurea hypoglycemic agent. Pharmacotherapy 1985; 5: 63
205. Rabkin R, Simon NM, Steiner S. Effect of renal disease on renal uptake and excretion of insulin in man. New England Journal of Medicine 1970; 282: 182
206. Nelson E. Rate of metabolism of tolbutamide in test subjects with liver disease or impaired renal function. American Journal of the Medical Sciences 1964; 248: 657
207. Harrington RA, Hamilton CW, Brogden RN, et al. Metoclopramide: an updated review of its pharmacologic properties and clinical use. Drugs 1983; 25: 451
208. Lehmann CR, Heironimus JD, Collins CB, et al. Metoclopramide kinetics in patients with impaired renal function and clearance by hemodialysis. Clinical Pharmacology and Therapeutics 1985; 37: 284
209. Markham A, Sorkin EM. Ondansetron: an update of its therapeutic use in chemotherapy-induced and postoperative nausea and vomiting. Drugs 1993; 45: 931-52
210. Eadie MJ. Anticonvulsant drugs: an update. Drugs 1984; 27: 328
211. Penry JK, Newmark ME. The use of antiepileptic drugs. Annals of Internal Medicine 1979; 90: 207
212. Bertilsson L. Clinical pharmacokinetics of carbamazepine. Clinical Pharmacokinetics 1978; 3: 128
213. Richens A. Clinical pharmacokinetics of phenytoin. Clinical Pharmacokinetics 1979; 4: 153
214. Lee CS, Marbury TC, Perchalski RT, et al. Pharmacokinetics of primidone elimination by uremic patients. Journal of Clinical Pharmacology 1982; 22: 301
215. Marbury TC, Lee CS, Bruni J, et al. Hemodialysis of valproic acid in uremic patients. Dialysis and Transplantation 1980; 9: 961
216. Rimmer EM, Richens A. An update on sodium valproate. Pharmacotherapy 1985; 5: 171
217. Grant SM, Heel RC. Vigabatrin: a review of its pharmacodynamic and pharmacokinetic properties and therapeutic potential in epilepsy and disorders of motor control. Drugs 1991; 41: 889-926
218. Graybill JR, Craven PC. Antifungal drugs used in systemic mycoses. Drugs 1983; 25: 41
219. Daneshmend TK, Warnock DW. Clinical pharmacokinetics of systemic antifungal drugs. Clinical Pharmacokinetics 1983; 8: 17
220. Grant SM, Clissold SP. Fluconazole: a review of its pharmacodynamic and pharmacokinetic properties and therapeutic potential in superficial and systemic mycoses. Drugs 1990; 39: 877-916
221. Grant SM, Clissold SP. Itraconazole: a review of its pharmacodynamic and pharmacokinetic properties, and therapeutic use in superficial and systemic mycoses. Drugs 1989; 37: 310-44
222. Van Tyle JF. Ketoconazole mechanism of action, spectrum of activity, pharmacokinetics, drug interactions, adverse reactions and therapeutic use. Pharmacotherapy 1984; 4: 343

223. Richards DM, Brogden RN, Heel RC. Astemizole: a review of its pharmacodynamic properties and therapeutic efficacy. Drugs 1984; 28: 38-61
224. Campoli-Richards DM, Buckley MM, Fitton A. Cetirizine: a review of its pharmacological properties and clinical potential in allergic rhinitis, pollen-induced asthma, and chronic urticaria. Drugs 1990; 40: 762-81
225. Peets EA, Jackson M, Symchowics S. Metabolism of chlorpheniramine maleate in man. Journal of Pharmacology and Experimental Therapeutics 1972; 180: 464
226. Rumore MM. Clinical pharmacokinetics of chlorpheniramine. Drug Intelligence and Clinical Pharmacy 1984; 18: 701
227. Glazko AJ, Dill WA, Young RM. Metabolic disposition of diphenhydramine. Clinical Pharmacology and Therapeutics 1974; 16: 1066
228. McTavish D, Goa KL, Ferrill M. Terfenadine: an updated review of its pharmacological properties and therapeutic efficacy. Drugs 1990; 39: 522-74
229. Houston MC. Clonidine hydrochloride: review of pharmacological and clinical aspects. Progress in Cardiovascular Diseases 1981; 23: 337
230. Pearson RM. Pharmacokinetics and response to diazoxide in renal failure. Clinical Pharmacokinetics 1977; 2: 198
231. Young RA, Brogden RN. Doxazosin: a review of its pharmacodynamic and pharmacokinetic properties, and therapeutic efficacy in mild or moderate hypertension. Drugs 1988; 35: 525-41
232. Holmes B, Brogden RN, Heel RC, et al. Guanabenz: a review of its pharmacodynamic properties and therapeutic efficacy in hypertension. Drugs 1983; 26: 212
233. Halstenson CE, Opsahl JA, Abraham PA, et al. Disposition of guanadrel in subjects with normal and impaired renal function. Journal of Clinical Pharmacology 1989; 29: 128-32
234. Rahn KH. The influence of renal function on plasma levels, urinary excretion, metabolism and antihypertensive effects of guanethidine in man. Clinical Nephrology 1973; 1: 14
235. Sorkin EM, Heel RC. Guanfacine: a review of its pharmacodynamic and pharmacokinetic properties, and therapeutic efficacy in the treatment of hypertension. Drugs 1986; 31: 301
236. Ludden TM, McNay JL, Shephard A, et al. Clinical pharmacokinetics of hydralazine. Clinical Pharmacokinetics 1982; 7: 185
237. Reece PA, Cozamanis I, Zacest R. Kinetics of hydralazine and its main metabolites in slow and fast acetylators. Clinical Pharmacology and Therapeutics 1980; 28: 769
238. Myhre F, Rugstad HE, Hansen T. Clinical pharmacokinetics of methyldopa. Clinical Pharmacology and Therapeutics 1982; 7: 221
239. Campese VM. Minoxidil: a review of its pharmacological properties and therapeutic uses. Drugs 1981; 22: 257
240. Chrisp P, Faulds D. Moxonidine: a review of its pharmacology, and therapeutic use in essential hypertension. Drugs 1992; 44: 993-1012
241. Stanaszek WF, Kellerman D, Brogden RN, et al. Prazosin update: a review of its pharmacological properties and therapeutic use in hypertension and congestive heart failure. Drugs 1983; 25: 339
242. Lowenthal DT, Hobbs D, Affrime MB. Prazosin kinetics and effectiveness in renal failure. Clinical Pharmacology and Therapeutics 1980; 27: 779
243. Zsotér TT, Johnson GE, DeVeber GA. Excretion and metabolism of reserpine in renal failure. Clinical Pharmacology and Therapeutics 1973; 14: 325
244. Cohn JN, Buke LP. Nitroprusside. Annals of Internal Medicine 1979; 91: 752
245. Schulz V. Clinical pharmacokinetics of nitroprusside, cyanide, thiosulphate. Clinical Pharmacokinetics 1984; 6: 239
246. Titmarsh S, Monk JP. Terazosin: a review of its pharmacodynamic and pharmacokinetic properties, and therapeutic efficacy in essential hypertension. Drugs 1987; 33: 461-77
247. Langtry HD, Mammen GJ, Sorkin EM. Urapidil: a review of its pharmacodynamic and pharmacokinetic properties, and therapeutic potential in the treatment of hypertension. Drugs 1989; 38: 900-40
248. White NJ. Clinical pharmacokinetics of antimalarial drugs. Clinical Pharmacokinetics 1985; 10: 187
249. Bach JF, Dardenne M. The metabolism of azathioprine in renal failure. Transplantation 1971; 12: 253
250. Nanlin S, Jessup K, Floyd M, et al. Quantitation of plasma azathioprine and 6-mercaptopurine levels in renal transplant patients. Transplantation 1980; 29: 290
251. Crooke ST, Prestakayo AW. Bleomycin pharmacokinetics in patients with varying renal function. Cancer Research 1977; 18: 286
252. Crooke ST, Comis RL, Einhorn LH, et al. Effects of variations in renal function on the clinical pharmacology of bleomycin administered as an IV bolus. Cancer Treatment Reports 1977; 61: 1631
253. Ehrsson H, Hassan M, Ehrnebo M, et al. Busulfan kinetics. Clinical Pharmacology and Therapeutics 1983; 34: 86
254. Balis FM, Holcenberg JS, Bleyer WA. Clinical pharmacokinetics of commonly used anticancer drugs. Clinical Pharmacokinetics 1983; 8: 202
255. Wagstaff AJ, Ward A, Benfield P. Carboplatin: a preliminary review of its pharmacodynamic and pharmacokinetic properties, and therapeutic efficacy in the treatment of cancer. Drugs 1989; 37: 162-90
256. Blachey JD, Hill JB. Renal and electrolyte disturbances associated with cisplatin. Annals of Internal Medicine 1981; 95: 628
257. Gormley PE, Bull JM, LeRoy AF. Kinetics of cis-dichlorodiammineplatinum. Clinical Pharmacology and Therapeutics 1979; 25: 351
258. Himmelstein KJ, Patton TF, Belt RJ, et al. Clinical kinetics of intact cisplatin and some related species. Clinical Pharmacology and Therapeutics 1981; 29: 658
259. Grochow LB, Colvin M. Clinical pharmacokinetics of cyclophosphamide. Clinical Pharmacokinetics 1979; 4: 380
260. Follath F, Wenk M, Vozeh S, et al. Intravenous cyclosporine kinetics in renal failure. Clinical Pharmacology and Therapeutics 1983; 34: 638
261. Peters GJ, Schornagel JH, Milano GA. Clinical pharmacokinetics of anti-metabolites. Cancer Surveys 1993; 17: 123-56
262. Benjamin RS, Riggs CE, Bachur NR. Plasma pharmacokinetics of adriamycin and its metabolites in humans with normal hepatic and renal function. Cancer Research 1977; 37: 1416
263. Henwood JM, Brogden RN. Etoposide: a review of its pharmacodynamic and pharmacokinetic properties, and therapeutic potential in combination chemotherapy of cancer. Drugs 1990; 39: 438-90
264. Hollingshead LM, Faulds D. Idarubicin: a review of its pharmacodynamic and pharmacokinetic properties, and therapeutic potential in the chemotherapy of cancer. Drugs 1991; 42: 690-719
265. Dechant KL, Brogden RN, Pilkington T. Ifosfamide/mesna: a review of its antineoplastic activity, pharmacokinetic properties and therapeutic efficacy in cancer. Drugs 1991; 42: 428-67

266. Alberts DS, Chang SY, Chen HS, et al. Oral melphalan kinetics. Clinical Pharmacology and Therapeutics 1979; 26: 73
267. Shen DD, Azarnoff DL. Clinical pharmacokinetics of methotrexate. Clinical Pharmacokinetics 1978; 3: 1
268. Jolivet J, Cowan KH, Curt GA, et al. The pharmacology and clinical use of methotrexate. New England Journal of Medicine 1983; 309: 1094
269. Black DJ, Livingston RB. Antineoplastic drugs in 1990: a review. Drugs 1990; 39: 489-501, 652-73
270. Hartigh JD, McVie JG, Van Oon WJ, et al. Pharmacokinetics of mitomycin C in humans. Cancer Research 1983; 43: 5017
271. Hanna WT, Knauss S, Regester RF. Renal disease after mitomycin C therapy. Cancer 1981; 48: 2583
272. Harris MG, Coleman SG, Faulds D. Nilutamide: a review of its pharmacodynamic and pharmacokinetic properties, and therapeutic efficacy in prostate cancer. Drugs & Aging 1993; 3: 9-25
273. Buckley MM, Goa KL. Tamoxifen: a reappraisal of its pharmacodynamic and pharmacokinetic properties, and therapeutic use. Drugs 1989; 37: 451-90
274. Owellen RJ, Road MA, Hains FO. Pharmacokinetics of vinblastine and vincristine in humans. Cancer Research 1977; 37: 2603
275. Spark RF, Dickstein G. Bromocriptine and endocrine disorders. Annals of Internal Medicine 1979; 90: 949
276. Berg MJ, Ebert B, Willis DK, et al. Parkinsonism - drug treatment: Part 1. Drug Intelligence and Clinical Pharmacy 1987; 21: 10-21
277. Nutt JG, Fellman JH. Pharmacokinetics of levodopa. Clinical Neuropharmacology 1984; 7: 35
278. Doller HJ. Levodopa pharmacokinetics. Drug Metabolism and Disposition 1978; 6: 164
279. Chrisp P, Mammen GJ, Sorkin EM. Selegiline: a review of its pharmacology, symptomatic benefits and protective potential in Parkinson's disease. Drugs & Aging 1991; 1: 228-48
280. Sheehan J, White A, Wilson R. Hazards of phenothiazines in chronic renal failure. Irish Medical Journal 1982; 75: 335
281. Loo JC, Midha KK, McGilveray IJ. Pharmacokinetics of chlorpromazine in normal volunteers. Communications in Psychopharmacology 1980; 4: 121
282. McAllister CJ, Scowden EB, Stone WJ. Toxic psychosis induced by phenothiazine administration in patients with chronic renal failure. Clinical Nephrology 1978; 10: 191
283. Fitton A, Heel RC. Clozapine: a review of its pharmacological properties, and therapeutic use in schizophrenia. Drugs 1990; 40: 722-47
284. Forsman A, Ohman R. Pharmacokinetic studies on haloperidol in man. Current Therapeutic Research 1976; 20: 319
285. Lydiard RB, Gelenberg AJ. Hazards and adverse effects of lithium. Annual Review of Medicine 1982; 33: 327
286. Procci WR. Mania during maintenance hemodialysis successfully treated with oral lithium carbonate. Journal of Nervous and Mental Diseases 1977; 164: 355
287. Amdisen A. Serum level monitoring and clinical pharmacokinetics of lithium. Clinical Pharmacokinetics 1977; 2: 73
288. Steele JW, Faulds D, Sorkin EM. Triapride: a review of its pharmacodynamic and pharmacokinetic properties, and therapeutic potential in geriatric agitation. Drugs & Aging 1993; 3: 460-78
289. Kampmann JP, Hansen JM. Clinical pharmacokinetics of antithyroid drugs. Clinical Pharmacokinetics 1981; 6: 401
290. Cooper DS. Antithyroid drugs. New England Journal of Medicine 1984; 311: 1353
291. Holdiness MR. Clinical pharmacokinetics of the antituberculosis drugs. Clinical Pharmacokinetics 1984; 9: 511
292. Lehmann CR, Garrett LE, Winn RE, et al. Capreomycin kinetics in renal impairment and clearance by hemodialysis. American Review of Respiratory Disease 1988; 138: 1312-3
293. Weber WW, Hein DW. Clinical pharmacokinetics of isoniazid. Clinical Pharmacokinetics 1976; 4: 287
294. Lacroix C, Hermelin A, Guiberteau R, et al. Haemodialysis of pyrazinamide in uraemic patients. European Journal of Clinical Pharmacology 1989; 37: 309-11
295. Acocella G. Pharmacokinetics and metabolism of rifampin in humans. Reviews of Infectious Diseases 1983; 5 Suppl. 3: S428
296. Larsson R, Erlanson P, Bodemar G, et al. Pharmacokinetics of cimetidine and its sulfoxide metabolite during hemodialysis. European Journal of Clinical Pharmacology 1982; 21: 325
297. Somogyi AA, Gugler R. Clinical pharmacokinetics of cimetidine. Clinical Pharmacokinetics 1983; 8: 463
298. Campoli-Richards DM, Clissold SP. Famotidine: pharmacodynamic and pharmacokinetic properties and a preliminary review of its therapeutic use in peptic ulcer disease and Zollinger-Ellison syndrome. Drugs 1986; 32: 197-221
299. Langtry DH, Grant SM, Goa KL. Famotidine: an updated review of its pharmacodynamic and pharmacokinetic properties, and therapeutic use in peptic ulcer disease and other allied diseases. Drugs 1989; 38: 551-90
300. Barradell LB, Faulds D, McTavish D. Lansoprazole: a review of its pharmacodynamic and pharmacokinetic properties and its therapeutic efficacy in acid-related disorders. Drugs 1992; 44: 225-50
301. Aronoff GR, Bergstrom RJ, Bopp RJ, et al. Nizatidine disposition in subjects with normal and impaired renal function. Clinical Pharmacology and Therapeutics 1988; 43: 688-95
302. Price AH, Brogden RN. Nizatidine: a preliminary review of its pharmacodynamic and pharmacokinetic properties, and its therapeutic use in peptic ulcer disease. Drugs 1988; 36: 521-39
303. Naesdal J, Andersson T, Bodemar G, et al. Pharmacokinetics of [$^{14}$C] omeprazole in patients with impaired renal function. Clinical Pharmacology and Therapeutics 1986; 40: 344-51
304. Clissold SP, Campoli-Richards DM. Omeprazole: a review of its pharmacodynamic and pharmacokinetic properties, and therapeutic potential in peptic ulcer disease and Zollinger-Ellison syndrome. Drugs 1986; 32: 15-47
305. Brogden RN, Carmine AA, Heel RC, et al. Ranitidine: a review of its pharmacology and therapeutic use in peptic ulcer disease and other allied disease. Drugs 1982; 24: 267
306. Gaginella TS, Bauman JH. Ranitidine hydrochloride. Drug Intelligence and Clinical Pharmacy 1983; 17: 873
307. Roberts C. Clinical pharmacokinetics of ranitidine. Clinical Pharmacokinetics 1984; 9: 211
308. Hirsch MD, Swartz MN. Antiviral agents. New England Journal of Medicine 1980; 302: 903-49
309. Gnann JW, Barton NH, Whitley RJ. Acyclovir: mechanism of action, pharmacokinetics, safety and clinical applications. Pharmacotherapy 1983; 3: 275
310. Wu MJ, Ing TS, Soung S, et al. Amantadine hydrochloride pharmacokinetics in patients with impaired renal function. Clinical Nephrology 1982; 17: 19
311. Faulds D, Brogden RN. Didanosine: a review of its antiviral activity, pharmacokinetic properties and thera-

peutic potential in human immunodeficiency virus infection. Drugs 1992; 44: 94-116
312. Chrisp P, Clissold SP. Foscarnet: a review of its antiviral activity, pharmacokinetic properties and therapeutic use in immunocompromised patients with cytomegalovirus retinitis. Drugs 1991; 41: 104-29
313. Faulds D, Heel RC. Ganciclovir: a review of its antiviral activity, pharmacokinetic properties and therapeutic use in immunocompromised patients with cytomegalovirus infections. Drugs 1990; 39: 597-638
314. Kramer TH, Gaar GG, Ray CG, et al. Hemodialysis clearance of intravenously administered ribavirin. Antimicrobial Agents and Chemotherapy 1990; 34: 489-90
315. Aronoff GR, Szwed JJ, Nelson RL, et al. Hypoxanthine-arabinoside pharmacokinetics after adenine arabinoside administration to a patient with renal failure. Antimicrobial Agents and Chemotherapy 1980; 18: 212
316. Wilde MI, Langtry HD. Zidovudine: an update of its pharmacodynamic and pharmacokinetic properties, and therapeutic efficacy. Drugs 1993; 46: 515-78
317. Morgan DJ. Clinical pharmacokinetics of β-agonists. Clinical Pharmacokinetics 1990; 18: 270-94
318. Ogilvie RI. Clinical pharmacokinetics of theophylline. Clinical Pharmacokinetics 1978; 3: 267
319. Kradjan WA, Martin TR, Delaney CJ, et al. Effect of hemodialysis on the pharmacokinetic of theophylline in chronic renal failure. Nephron 1982; 32: 40
320. Bauer LA, Bauer SP, Blouin RA. The effect of acute and chronic renal failure on theophylline clearance. Journal of Clinical Pharmacology 1982; 22: 65
321. Laher MS, Kelly JG, Doyle.GD, et al. Pharmacokinetics of amlodipine in renal impairment. Journal of Cardiovascular Pharmacology 1988; 12 Suppl. 7: 60-3
322. Murdoch D, Heel RC. Amlodipine: a review of its pharmacodynamic and pharmacokinetic properties, and therapeutic use in cardiovascular disease. Drugs 1991; 41: 478-505
323. Hollingshead LM, Faulds D, Fitton A. Bepridil: a review of its pharmacological properties and therapeutic use in stable angina pectoris. Drugs 1992; 44: 835-57
324. McAllister RG, Hamann SR, Blouin RA. Pharmacokinetics of calcium-entry blockers. American Journal of Cardiology 1985; 55: 30B
325. Chaffman M, Brogden RN. Diltiazem: a review of its pharmacological properties and therapeutic efficacy. Drugs 1985; 29: 387
326. Todd PA, Faulds D. Felodipine: a review of the pharmacology and therapeutic use of the extended release formulation in cardiovascular disorders. Drugs 1992; 44: 251-77
327. Chandler MHH, Schran HF, Cutler RE, et al. The effects of renal function on the disposition of isradipine. Journal of Clinical Pharmacology 1988; 28: 1076-80
328. Fitton A, Benfield P. Isradipine: a review of its pharmacodynamic and pharmacokinetic properties, and therapeutic use in cardiovascular disease. Drugs 1990; 40: 31-74
329. Sorkin EM, Clissold SP. Nicardipine: a review of its pharmacodynamic and pharmacokinetic properties, and therapeutic efficacy, in the treatment of angina pectoris, hypertension and related cardiovascular disorders. Drugs 1987; 33: 296-345
330. Kates RE. Calcium antagonists: pharmacokinetic properties. Drugs 1983; 25: 113
331. Kirch W, Ramsch KD, Duhrsen U, et al. Clinical pharmacokinetics of nimodipine in normal and impaired renal function. International Journal of Clinical Pharmacology Research 1984; 4: 381-4
332. Langley MS, Sorkin EM. Nimodipine: a review of its pharmacodynamic and pharmacokinetic properties, and therapeutic potential in cerebrovascular disease. Drugs 1989; 37: 669-99
333. Goa KL, Sorkin EM. Nitrendipine: a review of its pharmacodynamic and pharmacokinetic properties, and therapeutic efficacy in the treatment of hypertension. Drugs 1987; 33: 123-55
334. Vohringer HF, Rietbrock N. Digitalis therapy in renal failure with special regard to digitoxin. International Journal of Clinical Pharmacology Therapy and Toxicology 1981; 19: 175
335. Graves PE, Fenster PE, MacFarland RT, et al. Kinetics of digitoxin and the bis-monodigitoxosides of digitoxigenin in renal insufficiency. Clinical Pharmacology and Therapeutics 1984; 36: 607
336. Aronson JK. Clinical pharmacokinetics of digoxin. Clinical Pharmacokinetics 1980; 5: 137
337. Kramer HJ, Pennig J, Klingmuller D, et al. Digoxin-like immunoreacting substances in the serum of patients with chronic uremia. Nephron 1985; 40: 297
338. Gault MH, Vasdev SC, Longerich LL. Endogenous digoxin-like substances and combined hepatic and renal failure. Annals of Internal Medicine 1984; 101: 567
339. Lant A. Diuretics: clinical pharmacology and therapeutic use. Drugs 1985; 29: 57, 162
340. Morsil DN, Brown RD. Acetazolamide and symptomatic metabolic acidosis in mild renal failure. British Medical Journal 1981; 283: 1527
341. George CF. Amiloride handling in renal failure. British Journal of Clinical Pharmacology 1980; 9: 94
342. Hansten PD. Potassium supplement interactions. Drug Interactions Newsletter 1982; 2: 1
343. Marcantonio LA, Auld WHR, Murdoch WR, et al. The pharmacokinetics and pharmacodynamics of the diuretic bumetanide in hepatic and renal disease. British Journal of Clinical Pharmacology 1983; 15: 245
344. Halstenson CE, Matzke GR. Bumetanide: a new loop diuretic. Drug Intelligence and Clinical Pharmacy 1983; 17: 786
345. Ward A, Heel RC. Bumetanide: a review of its pharmacodynamic and pharmacokinetic properties and therapeutic uses. Drugs 1984; 28: 426
346. Mulley BA, Parr GD, Rye RM. Pharmacokinetics of chlorthalidone. European Journal of Pharmacology 1980; 17: 203
347. Benet LZ. Pharmacokinetic/pharmacodynamics of furosemide in man: a review. Journal of Pharmacokinetics and Biopharmaceutics 1979; 7: 1
348. Beermann B, Groschinsky-Grind M. Clinical pharmacokinetics of diuretics. Clinical Pharmacokinetics 1980; 5: 221
349. Niemeyer C, Hasenfuss G, Wais U, et al. Pharmacokinetics of hydrochlorothiazide in relation to renal function. European Journal of Clinical Pharmacology 1983; 24: 661
350. Chaffman M, Heel RC, Brogden RN, et al. Indapamide: a review of pharmacodynamic properties and therapeutic efficacy in hypertension. Drugs 1984; 28: 189
351. Tilstone WJ, Dargie H, Dargie EN. Pharmacokinetics of metolazone in normal subjects and in patients with cardiac or renal dysfunction. Clinical Pharmacology and Therapeutics 1974; 16: 322
352. Clissold SP, Brogden RN. Piretanide: a preliminary review of its pharmacodynamic and pharmacokinetic properties, and therapeutic efficacy. Drugs 1985; 29: 489-530
353. Gabow PA, Moore S, Schrier RW. Spironolactone-induced hyperchloremic acidosis in cirrhosis. Annals of Internal Medicine 1979; 90: 338
354. Friedel HA, Buckley MM. Torasemide: a review of its pharmacological properties, and therapeutic potential. Drugs 1991; 41: 81-103

355. Ettinger B, Oldroyd NO, Sorgel F. Triamterene nephrolithiasis. Journal of the American Medical Association 1980; 244: 2443
356. Hasegawa J, Lin ET, Williams RL, et al. Pharmacokinetics of triamterene and its metabolite in man. Journal of Pharmacokinetics and Biopharmaceutics 1982; 10: 507
357. Hande KR, Noone RM, Stone WJ. Severe allopurinol toxicity. Description and guidelines for prevention in patients with renal insufficiency. American Journal of Medicine 1984; 76: 47
358. Hande KR, Reed E, Chabner B. Allopurinol kinetics. Clinical Pharmacology and Therapeutics 1978; 23: 598
359. Levy M, Spino M, Read SE. Colchicine: a state-of-the-art review. Pharmacotherapy 1991; 11: 196-211
360. Cunningham RF, Israili ZH, Dayton PG. Clinical pharmacokinetics of probenecid. Clinical Pharmacokinetics 1981; 6: 135
361. Dayton PG, Perel JM. The metabolism of probenecid in man. Annals of the New York Academy of Sciences 1971; 179: 399
362. Lecaillon JB, Souppart C, Schroeller IP, et al. Sulfinpyrazone kinetics after intravenous and oral administration. Clinical Pharmacology and Therapeutics 1979; 26: 611
363. Monk JP, Todd PA. Bezafibrate: a review of its pharmacodynamic and pharmacokinetic properties, and therapeutic use in hyperlipidaemia. Drugs 1987; 33: 539-76
364. Gugler R. Clinical pharmacokinetics of hypolipidaemic drugs. Clinical Pharmacokinetics 1978; 3: 425
365. Sherrard DJ, Goldberg AB, Hass LB, et al. Chronic clofibrate therapy in maintenance hemodialysis patients. Nephron 1960; 25: 219
366. Todd PA, Ward A. Gemfibrozil: a review of its pharmacodynamic and pharmacokinetic properties, and therapeutic use in dyslipidaemia. Drugs 1988; 36: 314-9
367. Henwood JM, Heel RC. Lovastatin: a preliminary review of its pharmacodynamic properties and therapeutic use in hyperlipidaemia. Drugs 1988; 36: 429-54
368. McTavish D, Sorkin EM. Pravastatin: a review of its pharmacological properties and therapeutic potential in hypercholesterolaemia. Drugs 1991; 42: 65-89
369. Conner CS. Atracurium and vercuronium: two unique neuromuscular blocking agents. Drug Intelligence and Clinical Pharmacy 1984; 18: 714
370. Fahey MR, Rupp SM, Fisher DM, et al. The pharmacokinetics and pharmacodynamics of atracurium in patients with and without renal failure. Anesthesiology 1984; 61: 699
371. Faulds D, Clissold SP. Doxacurium: a review of its pharmacology and clinical potential in anaesthesia. Drugs 1991; 42: 673-89
372. Ramzam MI, Shanks CA, Triggs EJ. Gallamine disposition in surgical patients with chronic renal failure. British Journal of Clinical Pharmacology 1981; 12: 141
373. Frampton JE, McTavish D. Mivacurium: a review of its pharmacology and therapeutic potential in general anaesthesia. Drugs 1993; 46: 1066-89
374. Somogyi AA, Shanks CA, Triggs EA. The effects of renal failure on the disposition and neuromuscular blocking effects of pancuronium bromide. European Journal of Clinical Pharmacology 1977; 12: 23
375. Bishop MJ, Hornbein TF. Prolonged effect of succinylcholine after neostigmine and pyridostigmine administration in patients with renal failure. Anesthesiology 1983; 58: 384
376. Miller RD, Maheo RS, Benet LZ. The pharmacokinetics of d-tubocurarine with and without renal failure. Journal of Pharmacology and Experimental Therapeutics 1977; 202: 1
377. Matteo RS, Nichitateno K, Pua EK, et al. Pharmacokinetics of d-tubocurarine in man. Anesthesiology 1980; 52: 335
378. Miller RD. Vecuronium: a new nondepolarizing neuromuscular blocking agent. Pharmacotherapy 1984; 4: 238
379. Chaffman M, Brogden RN, Heel RC, et al. Auranofin: a preliminary review of its pharmacological properties and therapeutic use in rheumatoid arthritis. Drugs 1984; 27: 378
380. Lorber A. Monitoring gold plasma levels in rheumatoid arthritis. Clinical Pharmacokinetics 1977; 2: 127
381. Faulds D, Sorkin EM. Epoetin (recombinant human erythropoietin): a review of its pharmacodynamic and pharmacokinetic properties, and therapeutic potential in anaemia and the stimulation of erythropoiesis. Drugs 1989; 38: 863-99
382. Wadworth AN, Chrisp P. Co-dergocrine mesylate: a review of its pharmacodynamic and pharmacokinetic properties, and therapeutic use in age-related cognitive decline. Drugs & Aging 1992; 2: 153-73
383. Etidronate for postmenopausal osteoporosis. Medical Letter on Drugs and Therapeutics 1990; 32: 111
384. Chrisp P, Goa KL. Goserelin: a review of its pharmacodynamic and pharmacokinetic properties, and clinical use in sex-hormone-related conditions. Drugs 1991; 41: 254-88
385. Chrisp P, Sorkin EM. Leuprorelin: a review of its pharmacology and therapeutic use in prostatic disorders. Drugs & Aging 1991; 1: 487-509
386. Plante GE, Erian R, Petitclerc C. Renal excretion of levamisole. Journal of Pharmacology and Experimental Therapeutics 1981; 216: 617-23
387. Fitton A, McTavish D. Pamidronate: a review of its pharmacological properties and therapeutic efficacy in resorptive bone disease. Drugs 1991; 41: 289-318
388. Lange K. Nephropathy induced by D-penicillamine. Contributions to Nephrology 1978; 10: 63
389. Bergstrom RF, Kay DR, Harkcom TM, et al. Penicillamine kinetics in normal subjects. Clinical Pharmacology and Therapeutics 1981; 30: 404
390. Pentamidine for *Pneumocystis carinii* pneumonia. Medical Letter on Drugs and Therapeutics 1985; 27: 6
391. Ward A, Clissold SP. Pentoxifylline: a review of its pharmacodynamic and pharmacokinetic properties and therapeutic efficacy. Drugs 1987; 34: 50-97
392. Vernon MW, Sorkin EM. Piracetam: an overview of its pharmacological properties and a review of its therapeutic use in senile cognitive disorders. Drugs & Aging 1991; 1: 17-35
393. Shapiro GG, König P. Cromolyn sodium: a review. Pharmacotherapy 1985; 5: 156-70

Appendix E

# Nomogram Method of Dose Estimation in Renal Failure

*L. Dettli*

For drugs excreted entirely or partly unchanged by the kidneys, the nomogram method for calculating dosage in renal failure is based on the linear relationship which exists between the total (plasma) drug clearance (or elimination rate constant) and glomerular filtration rate (GFR) as determined by the endogenous creatinine clearance ($CL_{CR}$). Normal renal function is defined by $CL_{CR}$ = 100 ml/min = 6 L/hour.

## 1. Graphic Estimation of Individual Drug Elimination Parameters

The *individual drug clearance fraction* (P), which describes the total clearance of the drug in the patient with renal failure as a fraction of its normal clearance, is determined in the following way by means of the nomogram depicted in figure 1:

The value of the *normal non-renal drug clearance fraction, $f_{NR}(n)$* ($P_o$), obtained from appendix A, is plotted on the left ordinate of the nomogram and connected with its upper right corner by a straight estimating line. The point of intersection between the patient's endogenous creatinine clearance ($CL_{CR}$) [lower abscissa], and the estimating line indicates at the left ordinate the individual drug clearance fraction (P) in the patient.

The *half-life* of the drug in the individual patient ($\hat{t}_{1/2}$) is calculated from the normal half-life ($t_{1/2}$) [see appendix A] according to the following relationship:

$$\hat{t}_{1/2} = t_{1/2}/P \qquad \text{(Eq. 1)}$$

## 2. Dosage Rules

The *individually adapted* dosage regimen, i.e. loading dose ($\hat{D}*$), maintenance dose ($\hat{D}$) and dosage interval ($\hat{T}$), is calculated from the *normal* dosage regimen, i.e. loading dose (D*), maintenance dose (D) and dosage interval (T), by means of one of the following simple dosage rules:

| **Rule 1:** | **Rule 2:** |
|---|---|
| $\hat{D}* = D*$ | $\hat{D}* = D*$ |
| $\hat{D} = D \cdot P$ | $\hat{D} = D$ |
| $\hat{T} = T$ | $\hat{T} = T/P$ |

Expressed verbally, these rules are interpreted as follows:

In both rules the normal loading dose (D*) remains unchanged.

According to rule 1, the dosage regimen is adapted by *reducing the maintenance dose:* the normal maintenance dose (D) is multiplied by the individual drug clearance fraction (P). The normal dosage interval (T) remains unchanged.

According to rule 2, the dosage regimen is modified by *prolonging the dosage interval:* the normal dosage interval (T) is divided by the individual drug clearance fraction (P). The normal maintenance dose (D) remains unchanged.

In the case of continuous intravenous drug infusion, the maintenance dose (D) is the amount of drug administered per dosage interval. Irrespective of the functional capacity of the kidneys, the correct loading dose is calculated as follows:

$$\hat{D}* = D* = 1.44 \cdot D \cdot t_{1/2}/T \qquad \text{(Eq. 2)}$$

## 3. Estimating Renal Function

In daily practice, creatinine clearance ($CL_{CR}$) is usually estimated from the plasma creatinine concentration ($C_{CR}$) rather than measured. For this purpose, the following estimating equation of Cockcroft and Gault[1] which considers sex, age, and bodyweight of the patient is recommended:

$$\underset{\text{(ml/min)}}{CL_{CR}} = \frac{(140 - \text{age}) \cdot \text{bodyweight (kg)}}{72 \cdot C_{CR}\ \text{(mg/dl)}} \qquad \text{(Eq. 3)}$$

Equation 3 is valid for males; in females the result is multiplied by 0.85.

*Note:* Conventional units (mg/dl) may be calculated from SI units (μmol/L), and *vice versa,* based on the following relationship: 1 mg/dl = 88.4 μmol/L.

Alternatively, if SI units are to be used, the following equation is recommended:

$$\underset{\text{(ml/min)}}{CL_{CR}} = \frac{(150 - \text{age}) \cdot \text{bodyweight (kg)}}{C_{CR}\ (\mu\text{mol/L})} \qquad \text{(Eq. 4)}$$

In males 10% is added to, and in females 10% subtracted from the value estimated according

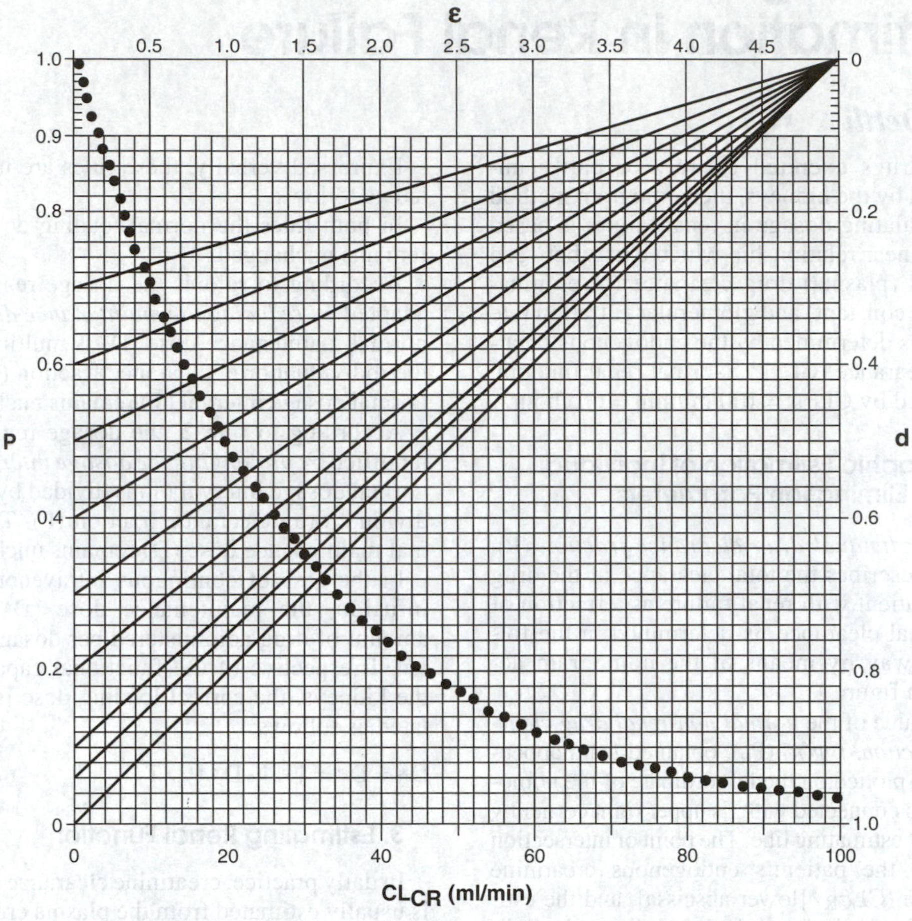


**Fig. 1.** Nomogram for the graphic determination of the individual drug clearance fraction of a drug in a patient with renal failure, P (left ordinate) from the endogenous creatinine clearance, $CL_{CR}$ (lower abscissa), and of the decay fraction, d (right ordinate) from the relative dosage interval, $\varepsilon = T/t_{1/2}$ (upper abscissa). Use of the nomogram is explained in the text (after Spring;[2] by permission of the author and editor). For drug $P_o$ [$f_{NR}(n)$] values, see appendix A.

to equation 4. This equation results in very similar estimates of creatinine clearance to equation 3.

Example

Administration of cimetidine in a 60-year-old female patient with a bleeding gastric ulcer. Bodyweight = 70kg, plasma creatinine concentration ($C_{CR}$) = 2 mg/dl. According to equation 3, the estimated endogenous creatinine clearance is:

$$CL_{CR} = \frac{(140 - 60) \cdot 70}{72 \cdot 2} \cdot 0.85$$

$$= 33 \text{ ml/min}$$

In appendix A one finds $P_o$ [$f_{NR(n)}$] = 0.25 for the non-renal clearance fraction of cimetidine. The value $P_o$ = 0.25 is plotted on the left ordinate and connected with the upper right corner of the nomogram by a straight line. The point of intersection between $CL_{CR}$ = 33 (lower abscissa) with this estimating line results in the individual drug clearance fraction P = 0.5 at the left ordinate.

If it is assumed that in these circumstances D* = 200mg, D = 200mg and T = 4 hours represents the normal dosage regimen of cimetidine, rules 1 and 2 result in the following individually adjusted dosage regimens:

**Rule 1:**

$\hat{D}* = D* = 200mg$

$\hat{D} = D \cdot P = 200 \cdot 0.5 = 100mg$

$\hat{T} = T = 4$ hours

**Rule 2:**

$\hat{D}* = D* = 200mg$

$\hat{D} = D = 200mg$

$\hat{T} = T/P = 4/0.5 = 8$ hours

## 4. A More Complex Dosage Rule

The dosage regimen of most drugs can be adjusted satisfactorily to the functional capacity of the kidneys by means of the simple rules 1 and 2. Exceptions are drugs such as the aminoglycosides and several penicillins and cefalosporins, and various other drugs (see table I) which have in common the following characteristics:

a) The therapeutic effect is irreversible (e.g. bactericidal, cytotoxic)

b) The value of $P_o$ [$f_{NR(n)}$] is extremely small (< 0.1; see appendix A)

c) The normal dosage interval is much longer than the normal half-life.

According to the following rule 3, the same normal loading dose ($\hat{D}* = D*$) is administered to all patients; the dosage interval ($\hat{T}$) is freely chosen by the clinician, the maintenance dose ($\hat{D}$) is equal to the so-called *decay fraction* (d), i.e. to the fraction of the loading dose eliminated during the dosage interval:

**Rule 3:**

$\hat{D}* = D*$

$\hat{D} = D \cdot d$

In order to find the decay fraction (d), the clinician determines first the so-called *relative dosage interval* ($\hat{\varepsilon} = \hat{T}/\hat{t}_{1/2}$), i.e. the dosage interval expressed in half-lives. The point of intersection between ε (upper abscissa of the nomogram) and the curved interrupted line read off from the right ordinate is the decay fraction (d).

### Example

Adjustment of the normal dosage regimen D* = 80mg, D = 80mg, T = 8 hours of gentamicin to a patient with a creatinine clearance ($CL_{CR}$) = 35 ml/min. From the non-renal clearance fraction [$f_{NR(n)}$] $P_o = 0.02$ of gentamicin (see appendix A), the individual drug clearance fraction (P) is determined by means of the nomogram as described above. The result is P = 0.38. From the normal half-life ($t_{1/2} = 3.0$ hours) of gentamicin (see appendix A), equation 1 predicts the individual half-life $\hat{t}_{1/2} = t_{1/2}/P = 3.0/0.38 = 8$ hours. The clinician decides to use the dosage interval $\hat{T} = 24$ hours. This results in a relative dosage interval $\hat{\varepsilon} = \hat{T}/\hat{t}_{1/2} = 24/8 = 3$. In the nomogram, the point of intersection between ε = 3 (upper abscissa) and the curved interrupted line results in d = 0.88 at the right ordinate. The adjusted dosage regimen reads now as follows:

$\hat{T} = 24$ hours

$\hat{D}* = D* = 80mg$

$\hat{D} = D \cdot d = 80 \cdot 0.88 = 70mg$

**Table I.** Some drugs for which rule 3 should be used (see text)

| | | |
|---|---|---|
| Amoxicillin | Cefalexin | Dibekacin |
| Ampicillin | Cefaloridine | Epicillin |
| Astromicin (fortimicin A) | Cefalothin | Fosfomycin |
| | Cefamandole | Gentamicin |
| Bacampicillin | Cefazolin | Hetacillin |
| Bacmecillinam | Cefonicid | Latamoxef (moxalactam) |
| Benzylpenicillin (penicillin G) | Cefoperazone | |
| | Cefroxadine | Lividomycin |
| Carbenicillin | Ceftazidime | Netilmicin |
| Carfecillin | Ceftezole | Sisomicin |
| Carindacillin | Ceftizoxime | Spectinomycin |
| Cefacetrile | Cefuroxime | Streptomycin |
| Cefadroxil | Ciclacillin | Tobramycin |

## 5. Limitations of the Nomogram

1) Serum creatinine ($C_{CR}$) should never be used as an estimating parameter in patients with acute renal failure or changing kidney function, or in patients undergoing haemodialysis, *until* the steady-state serum concentration of creatinine is reached again. In patients with severe acute renal failure, it may take some weeks before the steady-state concentration of creatinine corresponding to the functional state of the kidneys is eventually reached. Serum creatinine is also inaccurate as an estimating parameter in the presence of severe uraemia ($C_{CR}$ > 8 mg/dl) or systemic muscular disease.

2) For reasons discussed in chapter 1 (sect. 5.4.4) and chapter 24 (sect. 2.1), a dosage schedule calculated by the nomogram method does not obviate the need to monitor therapy by plasma concentration estimations.

3) Uraemic patients should always be carefully observed for signs of unexpected drug tox-

icity (see chapter 6, sect. 5.2; and chapter 24, sect. 1.5).

4) *Note:* Since creatinine is partly eliminated by tubular secretion, $CL_{CR}$ markedly overestimates GFR in patients with severe renal impairment ($CL_{CR}$ < 30 ml/min). As a result, drugs such as the aminoglycosides that are eliminated almost entirely by the renal pathway (i.e. $P_o$ [$f_{NR(n)}$] ≤ 0.1, see table I and appendix A) will be underdosed when $CL_{CR}$ is used as an estimate of GFR.[3]

## Further Reading

### Basis of Nomogram

Spring P. Calculation of drug dosage regimens in patients with renal disease: a new nomographic method. International Journal of Clinical Pharmacology and Biopharmacy 1975; 11: 76

### Background Theory

Cockcroft DW, Gault MH. Prediction of creatinine clearance from serum creatinine. Nephron 1976; 16: 31

Dettli L. Drug dosage in renal disease. Clinical Pharmacology and Therapeutics 1974; 16: 274

Dettli L. Drug dosage in renal disease. Clinical Pharmacokinetics 1976; 1: 126

Dettli L. Elimination kinetics and dosage adjustment of drugs in patients with kidney disease. Progress in Pharmacology. Vol. 1, No. 4. Stuttgart: Fischer, 1977

Dettli L. The kidney in pre-clinical and clinical pharmacokinetics. Japanese Journal of Clinical Pharmacology and Therapy 1984; 15: 241

Lesar TS. Gentamicin dosing errors with four commonly used nomograms. Journal of the American Medical Association 1982; 248: 1190

## References

1. Cockroft DW, Gault MH. Prediction of creatinine clearance from serum creatinine. Nephron 1976; 16: 31
2. Spring P. Calculation of drug dosage regimens in patients with renal disease: a new nomographic method. International Journal of Clinical Pharmacology and Biopharmacy 1975; 11: 76
3. Lesar TS. Gentamicin dosing errors with four commonly used nomograms. Journal of the American Medical Association 1982; 248: 1190

# Guide to Drug Dosage in Hepatic Disease

*M.F. Hebert*

The use of drugs in patients with liver disease may pose a number of problems for the clinician, the nature and extent of which depend on the pharmacological and pharmacokinetic characteristics of the drug administered and the type and severity of the liver disease. As liver disease progresses, the ability to hepatically eliminate drugs can become impaired. The ability to eliminate a specific drug may or may not correlate with the organ's synthetic capacity for substances such as albumin or clotting factors which tend to decrease as hepatic function declines. Unlike renal disease, where estimates of renal function based on endogenous (creatinine) or exogenous (inulin) substances correlate with pharmacokinetic parameters of drug elimination such as clearance and half-life (see appendices D and E), so-called 'liver function tests' such as AST, ALT and alkaline phosphatase do not reflect actual liver function, but rather are markers of liver cellular damage. Consequently, these markers are not useful for predicting changes in drug metabolism, and our ability at present to make dosage changes based on such markers is limited.

Despite this, information about the ways in which hepatic impairment can alter drug disposition is clinically useful and can serve as a guide for developing dosage regimens in the presence of hepatic dysfunction.

## 1. Use of the Tables

The tabular data in appendix F provide information about changes in estimated pharmacokinetic parameters that have been reported in the presence of hepatic disease. The tables indicate 5 major pharmacokinetic variables (clearance, volume of distribution, elimination half-life, percentage of drug unbound, and bioavailability) and provide, when available, the observed mean values (± SD) for each variable in a group of patients with hepatic disease relative to healthy controls. Use of the tables requires some knowledge of all the pharmacokinetic variables shown. A detailed consideration of these variables is beyond the scope of this discussion, and the reader is referred to the references listed below for a comprehensive discussion of their derivation and significance.

In practice, the most important of these variables is *clearance*, which may be defined as the rate of drug elimination relative to a concentration, where the concentration selected (plasma, blood or unbound) determines the clearance. The relevance of clearance lies in the way it can be used to determine a dosage regimen (see further appendix G). At steady-state, when the rate of drug administration (i.e. the dosage regimen) equals the rate of drug elimination, the clinician can select a dosage regimen for a drug if its total systemic clearance (CL) and a desired steady-state plasma or blood concentration ($C^{ss}$) are known:

Rate of drug administration = $CL \cdot C^{ss}$

For example, if a desired steady-state concentration of theophylline is 10 mg/L and the clearance of the drug is 3 L/h, the dosage rate required to achieve this average steady-state concentration will be 180mg every 6 hours (3 L/h · 10 mg/L = 30 mg/h or 180 mg/6h). An important point regarding clearance is that it is additive. Clearance from each eliminating organ (liver, kidney, other) can be summed to provide an estimate of total systemic clearance. For a drug eliminated entirely by the liver, hepatic clearance is thus equal to total systemic clearance. Many of the drugs listed in the tables are eliminated entirely via hepatic processes, so the total systemic clearance value shown also reflects hepatic clearance.

*The volume of distribution* of a drug at steady-state ($Vd_{ss}$) may be used to estimate the amount of drug in the body at steady-state ($A^{ss}$) when a specific plasma concentration is known or desired ($Vd_{ss} \cdot C^{ss} = A^{ss}$). End-stage liver disease can significantly alter the volume of distribution of drugs. For example, water soluble drugs with relatively small volumes of distribution will have a significant increase in their volumes of distribution in patients with ascites. The volume of distribution of an aminoglycoside, for example, could be 20L in an individual patient which would be increased to 30L if that same patient developed 10L of ascites. On the other hand, a drug like digoxin would not be expected to have a significant change in volume of distribution due to ascites since it has a very large volume of distribution (420L).

*Half-life* ($t_{1/2}$) data presented in the table are useful in estimating the time to attain and decay from steady-state. Four half-lives are required to reach steady-state once a stable dosage regimen is instituted, and a similar period is required to approach negligible amounts of drug in the body once a stable dosage regimen is discontinued.

The *percentage of drug unbound* ($f_u$) in blood or plasma represents the ratio of the free drug concentration to total drug concentration. This ratio is determined in plasma or serum unless otherwise indicated.

*Bioavailability* (F) refers to the percentage of drug reaching the systemic circulation after oral administration.

Altered pharmacokinetics of drugs in liver disease can include all or some of the following changes:

1) Impaired intrinsic hepatic eliminating capacity due to lack of or impaired function of hepatocytes.

2) Impaired biliary elimination due to biliary obstruction or transport abnormalities.

3) Impaired hepatic blood flow due to surgical shunting, collateral circulation or poor hepatic perfusion with cirrhosis and portal hypertension.

4) Altered volume of distribution due to differences in body composition with increased extracellular fluid (ascites, oedema) and decreased muscle mass.

5) Decreased protein binding due to impaired albumin production or drug displacement from accumulated substances normally cleared by the liver.

6) Increased bioavailability through decreased first-pass metabolism; and/or

7) Decreased bioavailability due to malabsorption of fats in cholestatic liver disease.

As far as changes in plasma protein binding are concerned, one of the most crucial considerations will be the interpretation of measured concentrations of drugs, since most clinical laboratories report total concentrations rather than unbound concentrations. When evaluating concentrations of drugs that have significantly altered protein binding in liver disease (e.g. phenytoin), it is important to either correct the measured concentration or the target therapeutic concentration for protein binding (see further chapter 5).

There is considerable variation in the efficiency with which different drugs are normally removed from the blood by the liver. Table I provides several examples of drugs which are highly extracted by the liver (efficiently removed from the blood) and those which are not, and indicates the influence of liver disease on their clearance. The hepatic clearance of highly extracted drugs is influenced more by changes in hepatic blood flow than by other determinants of hepatic drug elimination (intrinsic hepatic clearance and protein binding). The converse is true for poorly extracted drugs. Because hepatic disease usually results in reduced hepatic blood flow, often with extensive portosystemic shunting of blood, the hepatic clearance of highly extracted drugs is most consistently reduced by hepatic illness.

Because of the many factors that can affect intrinsic hepatic eliminating capacity (clearance), the influence of hepatic disease on the clearance of poorly extracted drugs is less predictable (table I).

**Table I.** Effect of liver disease on the clearance of highly and poorly extracted drugs

| Drug | Change in total systemic clearance in liver disease (%) |
|---|---|
| **Highly extracted** | |
| Lidocaine (lignocaine) | –40 |
| Metoprolol | –25 |
| Morphine | –7 |
| Pentazocine | –46 |
| Pethidine (meperidine) | –50 |
| Propranolol | –62 |
| Verapamil | –50 |
| **Poorly extracted** | |
| Ampicillin | –16 |
| Atenolol | +23 |
| Chloramphenicol | –65 |
| Chlordiazepoxide | –54 |
| Cimetidine | –9 |
| Diazepam | –53 |
| Furosemide (frusemide) | –15 |
| Lorazepam | +8 |
| Naproxen | +2 |
| Oxazepam | +14 |
| Prednisone | +9 |
| Tolbutamide | +44 |
| Warfarin | 0 |

*Symbols:* – = reduction in clearance; + = an increase in clearance.

## 2. Limitations of the Tables

The data in appendix F are generated in small numbers of patients, mostly those with alcoholic cirrhosis. The influence on drug disposition of other forms of hepatic disease and of the variability in hepatic function that almost certainly occurs over time with a single type of hepatic disease has not been well studied. The data presented in the tables should thus be used as a first approximation in developing a dosage regimen for patients with evidence of hepatic impairment. For some agents, there is a great deal of variability in the estimated pharmacokinetic parameters in liver disease with some patients demonstrating severely impaired ability to clear the drug and others having clearance comparable to healthy controls. This problem makes it particularly difficult to make dosage recommendations for a specific patient with liver disease. Another complicating factor in developing dosage regimens for a specific patient is that in any given patient, the ability to metabolise one drug may not be predictive of their ability to metabolise another agent since multiple enzyme systems are involved in drug metabolism. One enzyme system may be significantly impaired while another may remain intact.[1]

When selecting a dosage regimen for an hepatically eliminated agent in a patient with liver disease, it is essential to weigh the severity of illness and the risk of inadequate dosage against the therapeutic index and potential for drug toxicity for the specific patient.

The volume of distribution data in appendix F is not sufficient to permit general guidelines regarding the selection of loading doses of drugs in the presence of hepatic impairment. When the clinical situation requires the use of hepatically eliminated agents for patients with liver disease, close observation for desired effects and toxicity, and reliance wherever possible on the services of a competent therapeutic drug monitoring laboratory, will remain important in defining and adjusting a dosage regimen in a particular patient.

Finally, it is important to recognise that, quite independently of abnormalities in drug disposition, liver disease may cause substantial alterations in pharmacodynamic effects. The best recognised example of this is the apparent increase in cerebral sensitivity to a variety of strong analgesics, antianxiety and hypnosedative drugs in patients with liver disease, particularly those with hepatic encephalopathy. An attempt has been made to indicate such drugs in appendix F, and avoidance of these agents is strongly advised, within reason, in patients with severe liver disease.

### Further Reading

Blaschke TF. Protein binding and kinetics of drugs in liver disease. Clinical Pharmacokinetics 1977; 20: 32

Bond WS. Clinical relevance of the effect of hepatic disease on drug disposition. American Journal of Hospital Pharmacy 1978; 35: 406

Brockmoller J, Roots I. Assessment of liver metabolic function: clinical implications. Clinical Pharmacokinetics 1994; 27: 216-48

McLean AJ, Morgan DJ. Clinical pharmacokinetics in patients with liver disease. Clinical Pharmacokinetics 1991; 21: 42-69

Pang KS, Rowland MR. Hepatic clearance of drugs. Journal of Pharmacokinetics and Biopharmaceutics 1977; 5: 625

Roberts RK, Desmond PV, Schenker S. Drug prescribing in hepatobiliary disease. Drugs 1979; 17: 198

Secor JW, Schenker S. Drug metabolism in patients with liver disease. Advances in Internal Medicine 1987; 32: 379

Wilkinson GR, Shand DG. A physiological approach to hepatic drug clearance. Annual Review of Pharmacology and Toxicology 1980; 20: 389

Williams RL. Drug administration in hepatic disease. New England Journal of Medicine 1983; 309: 1616

*Appendix F continued overleaf*

**Table II.** Guide to drug dosage in hepatic disease (values in normal/control individuals are given in parentheses; * indicates values differ significantly from normal individuals)

| Drug | Disease | No. of patients | Pharmacokinetic parameters in hepatic disease[a]<br>CL[b] (L/h) | Vd[c] (L) | $t_{1/2}$ (h) | $f_u$ (%) | F (%) | Dose adjustment/ comments | References |
|---|---|---|---|---|---|---|---|---|---|
| **ACE (angiotensin-converting enzyme) inhibitors** | | | | | | | | | |
| Cilazapril | C | 9<br>(10) | CL/F:<br>9.6<br>(16.8) | | | | | Start with a reduced dose and titrate to response.<br>Patients' renal function not stated | 2 |
| Enalapril | C | 7<br>(10) | | | 0.84 ± 0.45<br>(0.78 ±0.41) | | | Highly variable pharmacokinetics of enalapril and enalaprilat in liver disease; some studies have noted increased enalaprilat concentrations in liver disease possibly related to impaired renal function. If used, start with a reduced dose and titrate to response | 3 |
| | C | 7<br>(7) | CL/F:<br>39.2 ± 12.2*<br>(91.6 ± 32.3) | | 0.63 ± 0.21<br>0.63 ± 0.32 | | | | 4 |
| **β-Adrenoceptor antagonists** (β-blockers) | | | | | | | | | |
| Acebutolol | LD | 13<br>(8) | | | Range:<br>1.44-4.8*<br>(1.02-2.55) | | | Reduced dose in patients with impaired hepatic function | 5 |
| Atenolol | C | 9<br>(12) | 12.7 ± 7.9<br>(10.3 ± 4.2) | 98 ± 25†<br>(76 ± 32) | 6.0 ± 1.4<br>5.0 ± 1.4 | | | Unchanged | 6 |
| Bisoprolol | LD<br>moderate | 5 | CL/F:<br>8.3* | Vd/F:<br>164.5 | 14.2* | | | Reduced dose necessary in some patients. Start with a low dose and titrate to response | 7 |
| | severe | 7<br>(11) | 13.4<br>(14.6) | 348<br>(197) | 16.7*<br>(8.7) | | | | |
| | AH<br>C | 5<br>11<br>(8) | CL/F:<br>10.5 ± 2.2<br>9.5 ± 3.5<br>(12.5 ± 3.5) | Vd/F:<br>237.2 ± 67.5<br>178.6 ± 59.2<br>(180.5 ± 36.6) | 12.5 ± 2.2<br>13.5 ± 3.6<br>(10.0 ± 2.5) | | | | 8 |
| Bopindolol | C | 14<br>(15) | | | 9.7 ± 3.6*<br>(6.0 ± 1.4) | | | Reduced dose necessary in some patients. Start low and titrate to response | 9 |
| Cicloprolol | LD | 12<br>(134) | | | 14.5 ± 0.7*<br>(10.9 ± 0.2) | | | Reduced dose necessary in some patients. Start low and titrate to response | 10 |
| Esmolol | C | 9<br>(3) | 634.2 ± 184.8<br>(516.6 ± 38.6) | 228.2 ± 58.8<br>(170.1 ± 18.9) | 0.27 ± 0.04<br>(0.21 ± 0.06) | | | No dose adjustment necessary | 11 |
| Labetalol | LD | 10<br>(7) | | 526 ± 98*<br>(805 ± 241) | 2.8 ± 1.3<br>(3.1 ± 1.1) | | 63 ± 8*<br>(33 ± 22) | Reduced dose probably necessary | 12 |
| Metoprolol | C | 10<br>(6) | 36.6 ± 24.7<br>(48.0 ± 16.1) | 280 ± 66‡<br>(224 ± 34) | 7.2 ± 3.8<br>(4.2 ± 2.7) | | 84 ± 32<br>(50 ± 27) | Reduced dose probably necessary | 13 |

| | | | | | | | | | |
|---|---|---|---|---|---|---|---|---|---|
| Propranolol | C | 6 (15) | $CL_T$: 33.5 ± 21.0* (53.9 ± 15.6) $CL_H$: 80.8 ± 57.0* (162.7 ± 64.4) | 375 ± 100.7* (293 ± 59.3) | 11.8 ± 8.5* (3.9 ± 0.9) | 9.7 ± 2.9* (6.7 ± 1.2) | 60 ± 7* (36 ± 9) | Reduced dose in cirrhosis. Marked slowing of heart rate may occur in cirrhosis with conventional doses. Low initial dose and regular heart rate monitoring recommended. | 14 |
| | C | 7 (9) | 34.8 ± 22.2* (51.6 ± 16.2) | 380 ± 108* (290 ± 51) | 11.2 ± 8.5* (4.0 ± 0.9) | 10.2 ± 4.2* (6.6 ± 1.2) | 54 ± 16 (38 ± 9) | May rarely precipitate HE | 15 |
| | C | 5 (6) | 37.6* (54.2) | 355‡ (194) | 7.15* (2.92) | 79 (54) | | | 16 |
| **Anaesthetics, intravenous** | | | | | | | | Due to increased cerebral sensitivity, these agents should be used cautiously in liver disease | |
| Etomidate | C | 13 (10) | | | | 44.2 ± 7.6*§ (24.9 ± 4.4) | | Insufficient information to make dosage recommendation. § Unbound fraction highly correlated with serum albumin | 17 |
| Methohexital | AVH | 10 (5) | 71.0 ± 42.5 (50.0 ± 8.5) | 289‡ (69) | 3.6 (1.4) | | | No dose adjustment necessary | 18 |
| | C | 8 (8) | 54 ± 22 (60 ± 14) | 163 ± 97‡ (146 ± 48) | 3.4 ± 2.4 (2.3 ± 0.7) | | | | 19 |
| Propofol | C | 10 (10) | 119 ± 41* (138 ± 37) | 476 ± 287‡ (384 ± 222) | 0.6 ± 0.4 (0.5 ± 0.3) | 1.9 ± 0.6 (2.2 ± 0.6) | | No dose adjustment necessary in cirrhosis | 20 |
| Thiopental (thiopentone) | C | 8 (9) | 18.5 ± 9.2 (16.4 ± 5.0) | 245 ± 133 (161 ± 35) | 11.9 ± 4.2 (8.8 ± 1.6) | 25.2 ± 3.9* (14.5 ± 3.4) | | Although data are unclear, it appears that no dose reduction is necessary. Increased $f_u$ may lead to increased pharmacological effect and some individuals with liver disease may experience toxicity with induction | 21 |
| **Analgesics** | | | | | | | | | |
| • *Simple analgesics* | | | | | | | | | |
| Aspirin | ALD | 8 (13) | CL/F: 2.0 (2.0) | Vd/F: 14.8 ± 8.4 (12.5 ± 2.6) | 7.3 ± 2.5 (7.9 ± 2.0) | 18.6 ± 10.5* (8.5 ± 2.6) | | Unchanged, but avoid in severe liver disease. Values shown are for salicylate | 22 |
| Paracetamol (acetaminophen) | LD | 23 | | | 2.9 ± 0.3 | | | Unchanged, but total daily dose should be reduced in cirrhosis to avoid toxicity | 23 |
| | C | | | | | | | | 24 |
| | + ascites | 14 | | | 5.2 ± 2.7 | | | | |
| | − ascites | 7 | | | 3.9 ± 1.4 | | | | |
| | + shunt | 4 | | | 5.3 ± 0.8 | | | | |
| | − shunt | 17 (14) | | | 4.6 ± 2.7 (2.9 ± 1.5) | | | | |
| | C | 11 (12) | CL/F: 9.72 ± 3.06* (21.30 ± 4.08) | | 3.7 ± 0.8 (2.1 ± 0.6) | | | | 25 |

[Continued over]

For footnotes, see final page of table (p. 1785)

**Table II.** *[Continued]*

| Drug | Disease | No. of patients | Pharmacokinetic parameters in hepatic disease[a] | | | | | Dose adjustment/ comments | References |
|---|---|---|---|---|---|---|---|---|---|
| | | | CL[b] (L/h) | Vd[c] (L) | $t_{1/2}$ (h) | $f_u$ (%) | F (%) | | |
| **Analgesics** *[continued]* | | | | | | | | | |
| Paracetamol *[continued]* | C | 6 | | | 3.42 ± 2.5 | | | | 26 |
| | C | 11<br>(6) | CL/F:<br>13.9 ± 2.2*<br>(28.2 ± 6.8) | | 3.1 ± 0.6*<br>(2.0 ± 0.5) | | | | 27 |
| | AVH | 10<br>(20) | CL/F:<br>13.4 ± 7.0<br>(17.0 ± 7.0) | Vd/F:<br>51.9 ± 11.1<br>(48.1 ± 13.3) | 3.2 ± 1.4*<br>(2.1 ± 0.5) | | | | 28 |
| • *Nonsteroidal anti-inflammatory drugs (NSAIDs)* | | | | | | | | This group of drugs should be used with caution in end-stage liver disease due to antiplatelet activity, gastrointestinal irritation and renal effects | |
| Etodolac | C | 10<br>(10) | | | 6.0 ± 1.9<br>(5.7 ± 1.3) | 1.07<br>1.01 | | No dose adjustment necessary | 29 |
| Ibuprofen | ALD<br>mild<br>severe | 9<br>6<br>(29) | | | 1.9 ± 0.3<br>2.6 ± 0.6<br>(2.2 ± 0.4) | | | Avoid in severe liver disease | 30 |
| | C moderate-severe | 8 R(–)<br>S(+)<br>(8) R(–)<br>S(+) | | | 3.1 ± 1.7*<br>3.4 ± 1.0*<br>(1.7 ± 0.3)<br>(1.8 ± 0.5) | | | | 31 |
| Mefenamic acid | C | 12<br>(10) | | | 2.46 ± 0.7*<br>(1.73 ± 0.31) | | 41% > control | Reduced dose may be necessary in cirrhosis | 32 |
| Naproxen | CLD | 11<br>(7) | | Vd/F:<br>5.73‡<br>(5.74) | 20.36<br>(14.14) | | | Reduce dose (by ≈ 50%) in cirrhosis | 33 |
| | C | 10<br>(10) | CL/F:<br>Single dose:<br>0.339 ± 0.108<br>(0.416 ± 0.06)<br>Steady-state:<br>0.556 ± 0.102<br>(0.547 ± 0.083) | Vd/F:<br>Single dose:<br>10.8 ± 2.1†<br>(9.25 ± 1.03)<br>Steady-state:<br>16.8 ± 4.8<br>(12.1 ± 1.7) | | ≈ 60% > control<br>(0.2) | | | 34 |
| Phenylbutazone | C | 6<br>(5) | | | 94.5<br>(81.8) | | | Avoid in severe liver disease | 35 |

| | | | | | | | | | |
|---|---|---|---|---|---|---|---|---|---|
| | CAH<br>C | 4<br>5<br>(5) | CL/F:<br>0.52 ± 0.15*<br>0.36 ± 0.13<br>(0.16 ± 0.03) | Vd/F:<br>36.4 ± 15.4<br>38.5 ± 12.5*<br>(19.6 ± 7.8) | 52.4 ± 12.0*<br>96.8 ± 47.0<br>(88.1 ± 21.9) | | | | 36 |
| Tenoxicam | C | 6<br>(14) | CL/F:<br>0.14 ± 0.05<br>(0.09 ± 0.03) | | 53 ± 19<br>(69 ± 19) | 0.8 ± 0.3<br>(0.8 ± 0.1) | | No dose adjustment necessary | 37 |
| • *Strong analgesics* | | | | | | | | Excessive sedation may occur with this group of drugs in cirrhosis. Extreme caution should be used when administering them in patients with a history of hepatic encephalopathy | |
| Dextropro-poxyphene (propoxy-phene) | C | 8<br>(7) | | | | 27.0 ± 6.0<br>(25.0 ± 3.0) | | Avoid.<br>Markedly increased sedation in cirrhosis | 38 |
| Fentanyl | C | 8<br>(13) | 47.5 ± 19.0<br>(45.4 ± 18.2) | 299‡<br>(241) | 5.1 ± 3.4<br>(4.4 ± 2.9) | | | Unchanged | 39 |
| Methadone[d] | CLD<br>mild<br>moderate<br>severe | <br>4<br>5<br>5<br>(5) | <br>18.8 ± 4.7<br>23.6 ± 12.3<br>14.2 ± 4.1<br>(18.5 ± 5.9) | | <br>11.3 ± 3.8<br>13.0 ± 3.6<br>35.5 ± 17.0*<br>(18.9 ± 6.7) | | | Avoid in severe liver disease | 40 |
| Morphine[d] | C | 8<br>6 | 88.2 ± 31.5*<br>140.7 ± 33.6 | 313.6 ± 61.6*<br>294.7 ± 65.1 | 3.35 ± 0.65*<br>1.85 ± 0.53 | | | Reduce dose in cirrhosis.<br>Unchanged in mild liver disease.<br>Substantial extrahepatic metabolism may occur. | 41 |
| | C | 7<br>(6) | 47.9 ± 14.4*<br>(117.6 ± 23.7) | 287 ± 93<br>(280 ± 171) | 4.2 ± 0.5*<br>(1.7 ± 0.7) | | 101 ± 43.4*<br>(47 ± 14.2) | Excessive sedation may occur in cirrhosis, particularly in patients with a history of HE | 42 |
| | C | 6<br>(6) | 69.2 ± 20.7<br>(74.0 ± 25.6) | 161 ± 91‡<br>(203 ± 168) | 2.2 ± 1.3<br>(2.5 ± 1.5) | 84.0<br>(80.2) | | | 43 |
| Pentazocine[d] | C | 4<br>(4) | 23.9 ± 7.3*§<br>(46.1 ± 7.8) | 370 ± 81†<br>(387 ± 74) | 12.0 ± 3.0*<br>(5.7 ± 1.4) | | 70 ± 19*<br>(21 ± 7) | Reduce dose or avoid.<br>§ CL is based on whole blood | 44 |
| | C | 8<br>(4) | 40.5 ± 17.8*<br>(74.8 ± 14.2) | 306 ± 77‡<br>(342 ± 188) | 6.6 ± 1.9*<br>(3.8 ± 0.5) | | 68 ± 21*<br>(18 ± 5) | | 45 |
| Pethidine (meperidine)[d] | AVH | 14<br>(15) | 38.9 ± 13.7*<br>(75.7 ± 31.6) | 389 ± 126‡<br>(416 ± 186) | 6.99 ± 2.74*<br>(3.37 ± 0.82) | 44.0<br>(41.7) | | Reduce dose or avoid.<br>Increased narcotic effect in cirrhosis.<br>May precipitate HE due to increased cerebral sensitivity. | 46 |
| | C | 10<br>(8) | 39.8 ± 17.6*<br>(79.0 ± 23.0) | 403 ± 179‡<br>(292 ± 93) | 7.04 ± 0.92*<br>(3.21 ± 0.80) | 35.0 ± 6.0<br>(36.0 ± 14.0) | | | 47 |
| | C | 8<br>(4) | 34.4 ± 9.5*§<br>(54.0 ± 19.0) | 263 ± 28‡<br>(232 ± 53) | 6.0 ± 1.3*<br>(3.6 ± 0.4) | | 87 ± 27*<br>(48 ± 13) | § CL is based on whole blood | 45 |
| | C | 6<br>(8) | 22.4 ± 7.0*§<br>(45.3 ± 12.6) | 331 ± 73†<br>(381 ± 125) | 10.9 ± 4.6*<br>(6.4 ± 1.2) | | 80 ± 15*<br>(57 ± 13) | | 44 |
| | C | 5<br>(6) | 23.5 ± 6.3*<br>(50.4 ± 11.8) | 364 ± 21‡<br>(329 ± 49) | 11.4 ± 4.4*<br>(5.2 ± 0.9) | | 85 ± 12*<br>(53 ± 7) | | 48 |

[Continued over]

*For footnotes, see final page of table (p. 1785)*

**Table II.** *[Continued]*

| Drug | Disease | No. of patients | Pharmacokinetic parameters in hepatic disease[a] | | | | | Dose adjustment/ comments | References |
|---|---|---|---|---|---|---|---|---|---|
| | | | $CL^b$ (L/h) | $Vd^c$ (L) | $t_{1/2}$ (h) | $f_u$ (%) | F (%) | | |
| **Analgesics** *[continued]* | | | | | | | | | |
| Sufentanil | C, ALD | 12<br>(9) | 46.2 ± 19.3<br>(47.5 ± 10.5) | 280 ± 112†<br>231 ± 49† | 4.1 ± 0.6<br>(3.5 ± 0.9) | 9.6 ± 1.8<br>(8.3 ± 1.5) | | Unchanged | 49 |
| Tramadol | LD | 12<br>(10) | 16.3*<br>(42.6) | | 13.3<br>(55.1) | | | Reduce dose in patients with liver disease | 50 |
| **Antianginal agents** (see also β-adrenoceptor antagonists and calcium antagonists) | | | | | | | | | |
| Isosorbide 5-mononitrate | C | 3<br>(2) | 5.16<br>(7.39) | 34.9<br>(47.8) | 4.66<br>(4.77) | | 77.6<br>(98.8) | Unchanged. | 51 |
| Nicorandil | C | 8<br>(8) | 40.7 ± 10.1<br>(30.7 ± 7.6) | 84 ± 98‡<br>(35 ± 7) | 1.7<br>(1.1) | | 69 ± 29<br>(80 ± 8) | No dose adjustment necessary. Some patients with cirrhosis have a substantially reduced bioavailability | 52 |
| **Antianxiety drugs/hypnosedatives** | | | | | | | | | |
| • *Barbiturates* | | | | | | | | Due to increased sensitivity, these drugs are probably best avoided in severe liver disease | |
| Amobarbital | C<br>Alb <3.5<br>Alb >3.5 | <br>4<br>5<br>(10) | <br>2.46 ± 0.68<br>7.13 ± 1.68<br>(5.52 ± 1.33) | <br>79.5 ± 35.8<br>114.0 ± 43.4<br>(91.3 ± 32.3) | | <br>69.0*<br>39.5<br>(39.3) | | Reduce dose in cirrhosis | 53 |
| Cyclobarbital | AVH<br>C | 10<br>8<br>(8) | 1.4 ± 0.5*<br>1.0 ± 0.2*<br>(2.3 ± 0.5) | | 22.4 ± 8.3*<br>35.2 ± 7.3*<br>(13.4 ± 2.8) | | | Reduce dose in cirrhosis | 54 |
| Hexobarbital | AVH | 13<br>(14) | 8.1 ± 3.6*<br>(15.0 ± 3.5) | 77 ± 28‡<br>(77 ± 8) | 8.2 ± 3.1*<br>(4.4 ± 1.2) | | | Reduce dose in cirrhosis.<br>Avoid in severe liver disease | 55 |
| | C<br>mild<br>severe | <br>8<br>22<br>(22) | <br>7.9 ± 2.9*<br>5.3 ± 2.1*<br>(13.9 ± 4.2) | <br>79.8 ± 18.2‡<br>109.9 ± 44.8<br>(87.5 ± 16.8) | <br>8.5 ± 2.9*<br>17.0 ± 7.5*<br>(5.7 ± 1.8) | | | | 56 |
| • *Benzodiazepines* | | | | | | | | These drugs may exacerbate or precipitate HE in patients with cirrhosis or severe acute liver disease. They are best avoided or used with care and in reduced doses | |
| | | | CL/F: | Vd/F: | | | | | |
| Alprazolam | C | 17<br>(17) | 2.35 ± 1.34*<br>(5.12 ± 2.23) | 71.4 ± 17.5<br>(81.2 ± 10.5) | 19.7 ± 14.3*<br>(11.4 ± 4.9) | 23.2 ± 4.2*<br>(29.0 ± 2.5) | | Reduce dose by 50-60% or avoid in cirrhotic patients | 57 |
| Brotizolam | C | 8<br>(8) | 2.7<br>(3.8) | 43.4*<br>(27.3) | 12.8*<br>(6.9) | 12.4*<br>(9.2) | | Reduce dose | 58 |

| | | | | | | | | | |
|---|---|---|---|---|---|---|---|---|---|
| Chlordiaze-<br>poxide | AVH<br>C | 5<br>8<br>(8) | 0.4 ± 0.3*<br>0.5 ± 0.1*<br>(0.9 ± 0.3) | 30.8 ± 12.6*<br>33.6 ± 9.8‡*<br>(23.1 ± 4.2) | 91.0 ± 99.5*<br>62.7 ± 27.3*<br>(23.8 ± 11.6) | 8.1*<br>5.4*<br>(3.5) | | Use with caution.<br>Reduce dose or avoid in ALD | 59 |
| | | | | | | | | § Drug administered IM | |
| | C | 11<br>(14) | 0.8 ± 0.5*<br>(2.3 ± 2.0) | 24.0 ± 5.6<br>(26.8 ± 9.7) | 34.9 ± 28.9*<br>(9.99 ± 3.40) | | | | 60 |
| | ALD§ | 11<br>(5) | CL/F:<br>0.53 ± 0.25*<br>(0.97 ± 0.19) | Vd/F:<br>30.0 ± 25.1<br>(22.5 ± 12.1) | 40.1 ± 16.9*<br>(16.5 ± 8.0) | | | | 61 |
| Clotiazepam | C | 10<br>(12) | CL/F:<br>9.0 ± 2.5*<br>(13.2 ± 6.1) | Vd/F:<br>128 ± 31*<br>(180 ± 73) | 10.0 ± 1.6<br>(10.2 ± 4.8) | | | Reduce dose or avoid in cirrhotic patients | 62 |
| Diazepam | C | 9<br>(5) | 0.828 ± 0.144*<br>(1.596 ± 0.246) | 121.8 ± 14.7*‡<br>(79.1 ± 19.6) | 105.6 ± 15.2*<br>(46.6 ± 14.2) | 4.7*<br>(2.2) | | Reduce dose (by ≈ 50%) in cirrhosis and avoid in severe or acute liver disease | 63 |
| | CAH,C<br>+ ascites<br>– ascites | <br>7<br>10<br>(5) | <br>0.38 ± 0.24*<br>0.75 ± 0.44<br>(1.02 ± 0.47) | <br>41.4 ± 20.0<br>48.1 ± 31.2<br>(68.6 ± 28.8) | <br>77.4 ± 11.4*<br>48.7 ± 38.3<br>(43 ± 7.2) | | | | 64 |
| | AVH, C<br>IC, OJ<br>Ca | 12<br>6<br>12<br>(18) | 0.59 ± 0.11*<br>1.01 ± 0.19<br>0.65 ± 0.06<br>(0.9 ± 0.11) | | 116.0 ± 9.8*<br>59.0 ± 14.5<br>77.1 ± 9.8*<br>(53.1 ± 5.6) | | | | 65 |
| | C, LD | 4<br>(4) | 0.5<br>(1.9 ± 0.7) | 49.7<br>(72.8 ± 7.7) | 60.0<br>(32.6 ± 11.3) | | | | 66 |
| | C | 9<br>(4) | 1.13*<br>(2.26) | 214.2<br>(91.7) | 164.0*<br>(32.1) | | | | 67 |
| Lorazepam | C<br>AVH | 13<br>9<br>(11) | 3.4 ± 2.0<br>3.1 ± 1.4<br>(3.2 ± 1.0) | 140.7 ± 57.4*†<br>106.4 ± 42.2*<br>(89.6 ± 23.8) | 41.2 ± 24.5*<br>28.3 ± 8.9<br>(21.7 ± 7.6) | 11.4 ± 2.5*<br>9.0 ± 1.9*<br>(6.8 ± 1.8) | | As with other benzodiazepines, HE may be exacerbated or precipitated; avoid or use with care and in reduced doses | 68 |
| Midazolam | C | 7<br>(8) | 22.7 ± 9.4*<br>(43.7 ± 15.4) | 106.2 ± 26.6<br>(80.7 ± 29.1) | 3.9 ± 1.8*<br>(1.6 ± 0.8) | | | Reduce dose by 50% in cirrhosis | 69 |
| | C | 7<br>(7) | 14.0 ± 6.7*<br>(23.6 ± 4.8) | 83.3 ± 35.2‡<br>(98.7 ± 16.7) | 7.4 ± 3.2*<br>(3.8 ± 1.6) | 3.16 ± 2.17<br>(1.68 ± 0.98) | 76 ± 37*<br>(38 ± 16) | | 70 |
| | C | 10<br>(9) | 24.1 ± 10.2*<br>(38.2 ± 13.4) | 82 ± 27‡<br>(99 ± 27) | 2.8 ± 0.5*<br>(2.3 ± 0.7) | | | | 71 |
| Nitrazepam | C | 12<br>(9) | 3.5 ± 1.0<br>(3.8 ± 0.8) | 152 ± 41<br>(132 ± 18) | 30.5 ± 9.3<br>(25.5 ± 3.3) | 18.9 ± 4.3<br>(13.0 ± 1.8) | | Reduce dose | 72 |
| Oxazepam | AVH<br>C | 7<br>6<br>(8)y<br>(8)o | CL/F:<br>8.2 ± 3.3<br>9.3 ± 4.6<br>(6.8 ± 2.0)<br>(8.2 ± 3.0) | Vd/F:<br>51.7 ± 18.5<br>60.9 ± 23.3<br>(47.7 ± 32.8)<br>(61.2 ± 13.0) | 6.1 ± 1.3<br>7.8 ± 2.0<br>(7.1 ± 3.4)<br>(6.4 ± 1.1) | 14.0<br>12.4<br>(13.3)<br>(10.7) | | Unchanged.<br>(y = young control; o = older control) | 73 |

[Continued over]

For footnotes, see final page of table (p. 1785)

**Table II.** *[Continued]*

| Drug | Disease | No. of patients | Pharmacokinetic parameters in hepatic disease[a] | | | | | Dose adjustment/ comments | References |
|---|---|---|---|---|---|---|---|---|---|
| | | | CL[b] (L/h) | Vd[c] (L) | $t_{1/2}$ (h) | $f_u$ (%) | F (%) | | |
| **Antianxiety drugs/hypnosedatives** *[continued]* | | | | | | | | | |
| Oxazepam *[continued]* | C | 5 (7) | | | 7.1 ± 2.2 (5.6 ± 1.9) | | | | 60 |
| Temazepam | C | 16 (15) | CL/F: 5.63 ± 4.28 (5.80 ± 24.65) | Vd/F: 76 ± 27‡ (114 ± 88) | 12.8 ± 5.7 (16 ± 5.8) | 5.54 ± 1.66* (3.85 ± 0.36) | | As with other benzodiazepines, HE may be exacerbated or precipitated; avoid or use with care and in reduced doses | 74 |
| Triazolam | C | 8 (18) | CL/F: 62.2*§ (100.4) | | 9.7*§ (3.9) | 16.9 ± 2.4* (13.8 ± 1.6) | | Reduce dose or avoid in cirrhosis. § Apparent oral clearance and $t_{1/2}$ reported for free drug | 75 |
| | C | 8 (8) | CL/F (range): 21.0 (8.4-41.5)* 28.1 (14.0-41.9) | | 4.10 (2.69-7.7)* 3.63 (2.58-5.87) | | | | 76 |
| | C | 6 (6) | CL/F: 15.9 ± 5.5 (17.1 ± 5.3) | | 4.07 ± 3.50 (2.27 ± 1.69) | | | | 77 |
| • *Others* | | | | | | | | | |
| Clomethiazole (chlormethiazole) | C | 8 (6) | 45.4 ± 17.8* (63.4 ± 9.3) | 519 ± 240 (585 ± 187) | 8.7 ± 4.0 (6.6 ± 2.4) | 44.2* (35.6) | 116 ± 25* (10 ± 7) | Reduce oral dose by 50% in cirrhosis | 78 |
| Zolpidem | C | 8 (8) | | | 9.9 ± 8.2 (2.2 ± 0.3) | | | Reduce dose in cirrhosis | 79 |
| | C | 12 (6) | | | | 11.3 ± 2.4* (8.1 ± 0.5) | | | 80 |
| Zopiclone | C | 7 (8) | | | 8.53 ± 2.20* (3.50 ± 0.93) | | | Avoid in cirrhosis. May exacerbate HE | 81 |
| **Antiarrhythmic drugs** (see also β-adrenoceptor antagonists) | | | | | | | | | |
| Encainide | C | 6 (8) | 60 ± 15* (108 ± 34) | 303 ± 103 (254 ± 68) | 3.6 ± 1.2 (2.7 ± 0.8) | 24 (30) | 76 ± 42* (26 ± 20) | Although metabolism of encainide is impaired in cirrhosis, dose adjustment may not be necessary since production of more active metabolites is not affected | 82 |
| | C-EM (EM) C-PM (PM) | 8 (8) 1 (2) | 51 ± 30* (55.8 ± 30.0) 5.4 (13.8 ± 6.0) | 139 ± 59‡ (137 ± 66) 165 (201 ± 5.6) | 3.3 ± 2.7 (3.3 ± 2.5) 21.4 (11 ± 4.9) | | 48 ± 18* (29 ± 14.7) 105 (95 ± 30) | | 83 |
| Lidocaine (lignocaine) | AVH | 6§§ | 54.6 ± 16.4§ (84.0 ± 16.4) | 217 ± 126‡§ (140 ± 35) | 2.7§ (1.5) | | | Reduce dose in acute hepatitis and in cirrhosis. | 84 |

| | | | | | | | | | |
|---|---|---|---|---|---|---|---|---|---|
| | C | 8<br>(10) | 25.1*<br>(42.2) | 162‡<br>(93) | 4.9*<br>(1.8) | | | Monitor lidocaine concentrations. | 85 |
| | C | 6<br>(9) | 87.0 ± 24.9*<br>(60.0 ± 11.6) | 206 ± 69*†<br>(129 ± 25) | 1.6 ± 0.3<br>(1.5 ± 0.4) | | 26 ± 20<br>(33 ± 33) | § Pharmacokinetic parameters are in whole blood. | 86 |
| | CPH<br>CAH<br>C-mild<br>C-severe | 13<br>11<br>10<br>11<br>(17) | 74.5 ± 54.1<br>83.2 ± 35.5<br>58.0 ± 27.8<br>29.5 ± 7.0*<br>(62.6 ± 15.7) | 131 ± 83<br>151 ± 83<br>131 ± 60<br>133 ± 40<br>(135 ± 41) | 1.3 ± 0.7<br>1.3 ± 0.7<br>1.6 ± 0.6<br>3.2 ± 0.7*<br>(1.6 ± 0.8) | | 14 ± 40<br>26 ± 27<br>14 ± 19<br>50 ±20*<br>(25 ± 206) | §§ Patients served as their own controls following recovery | 87 |
| | CAH<br>C | 22<br>22<br>(6) | 55.8 ± 23.9<br>39.1 ± 18.1<br>(53.5 ± 24.8) | | 1.9 ± 1.3<br>3.4 ± 2.4*<br>(1.5 ± 0.7) | | | | 88 |
| Lorcainide | C, ALD | 8<br>(12) | 48.8 ± 8.6<br>(60.1 ± 18.2) | 665 ± 196‡<br>(546 ± 203) | 12.5 ± 4.5*<br>7.7 ± 2.2 | 20.0<br>(17.0) | | Reduce dose (by ≈ 25%).<br>Due to reduced clearance, use cautiously in patients with cirrhosis | 89 |
| Mexiletine | C | 6<br>(6) | 9.7 ± 3.3*<br>(34.7 ± 12.7) | 363 ± 127‡<br>(414 ± 70) | 28.7 ± 9.8*<br>(9.9 ± 3.9) | | 49.0<br>(55.0) | Reduce maintenance dose to 0.25-0.3 of usual dose | 90 |
| Moracizine | C | 8<br>(12) | | | 7.7 ± 3.5*<br>(3.2 ± 1.7) | 5.9 ± 0.9<br>(4.9 ± 0.8) | | Reduce dose in cirrhosis | 91 |
| Propafenone | ALD,C | 8<br>(4) | Range:<br>21.0-64.7<br>(47.9-59.6) | | Range:<br>3.9-11.5<br>(2.0-3.7) | Range:<br>4.6-12.3<br>(3.2-4.5) | Range:<br>36-143<br>(5-60) | Some patients require reduced dose in alcoholic liver disease | 92 |
| Quinidine | CAH | 1<br>(11) | 7.7<br>(19.6 ± 7.0) | 455<br>(168 ± 70) | 41.5<br>(6.3 ± 1.7) | | | Reduce dose in severe liver disease | 93 |
| | C | 8<br>(8) | CL/F:<br>21.8 ± 7.1<br>(21.0 ± 4.8) | Vd/F:<br>266 ± 79*<br>(175 ± 20) | 9 ± 3*<br>(6 ± 1) | 14.7-54.5<br>(10.5-65.0) | | | 94 |
| | ALD<br>C | 11<br>6<br>(6) | CL/F:<br>24.9 ± 16.3<br>15.6 ± 8.6<br>(13.5 ± 4.7) | | 6.6 ± 2.3<br>12.8 ± 4.4*<br>(6.5 ± 1.0) | | | | 95 |
| Tocainide | C | 6 | 7.73 ± 3.23§ | 267 ± 77† | 27.4 ± 15.4 | | | Monitor plasma concentrations.<br>§ Non-renal CL unchanged | 96 |
| **Antibacterial drugs** | | | | | | | | For antibacterial agents that may require dose reduction in liver disease, careful consideration of the severity of infection and the adverse effects of the agent (i.e. its therapeutic index) is necessary when selecting the dose | |

[Continued over]

*For footnotes, see final page of table (p. 1785)*

**Table II.** *[Continued]*

| Drug | Disease | No. of patients | Pharmacokinetic parameters in hepatic disease[a] CL[b] (L/h) | Vd[c] (L) | $t_{½}$ (h) | $f_u$ (%) | F (%) | Dose adjustment/ comments | Refer-ences |
|---|---|---|---|---|---|---|---|---|---|
| **Antibacterial drugs** *[continued]* | | | | | | | | | |
| • *Aminoglycosides* | | | | | | | | Due to the nephrotoxicity of the aminoglycosides, careful use or avoidance is recommended. Increased volume of distribution in ascites may necessitate larger loading doses. Impaired clearance in hepatorenal syndrome and increased volume of distribution may necessitate longer dosage intervals. Monitor plasma concentrations | |
| Amikacin | LD | 8 | | 9.8<br>(3.13) | 2.55<br>(2.37) | | | See above | 97 |
| Gentamicin | C | 6 | 3.5 | 21 | 2.4 | | | See above | 98 |
| • *Cefalosporins* | | | | | | | | | |
| Cefetamet | C | 12<br>(12) | 7.38 ± 1.73<br>(7.68 ± 0.61) | 22.7 ± 4.6‡<br>(23.2 ± 2.2) | 2.35 ± 0.41<br>(2.42 ± 0.21) | | 50.1 ± 12.9<br>(44.6 ± 9.1) | No dose adjustment necessary | 99 |
| Cefodizime | C | 6<br>(6) | 5.1 ± 1.8*<br>(3.0 ± 0.4) | 38.5 ± 14.0<br>(12.0 ± 21.0) | 6.4 ± 0.8*<br>(2.7 ± 0.2) | | | Limited information prevents dosage recommendation.<br>Pharmacokinetic changes suggest there may be some protein binding alterations | 100 |
| Cefoperazone | LD | 6<br>(8) | 2.0*<br>(4.7) | 11.7<br>(10.4) | 4.30*<br>(1.60) | | | Reduce dose (by ≈ 50%) in advanced cirrhosis. | 101 |
| | C | 6<br>(6) | 3.8 ± 1.9[§]<br>(3.7 ± 0.8) | 15.9 ± 4.2*‡[§]<br>(6.3 ± 1.2) | 4.5 ± 2.7*<br>(1.5 ± 0.2) | | | Moderate dose reduction in severe liver disease.<br>[§] CL and Vd normalised to body surface area of $1.73m^2$ | 102 |
| | C | 11<br>(10) | 2.10 ± 0.61*<br>(3.63 ± 0.67) | 12.36 ± 2.58*<br>(9.22 ± 1.87) | 4.29 ± 1.16*<br>(1.77 ± 0.25) | 74.27 ± 13.91*<br>(31.78 ± 7.55) | | | 103 |
| Cefotaxime | C | 9 | 9.86[§]<br>3.50-17.80 | 18.1‡[§]<br>11.6-32.4 | 2.30[§]<br>1.15-4.10 | | | Modest dose adjustment may be necessary in cirrhosis. | 104 |
| | C | | | | | | | Moderate dose reduction in severe liver disease | 105 |
| | + ascites[§§] | 6 | 11.6 ± 5.5 | 124 ± 191 | 7.5 ± 3.9 | | | | |
| | – ascites | 6 | 28.5 ± 9.2 | 57 ± 22 | 1.3 ± 0.4 | | | | |
| | LD | 6 | 13.0 ± 4.0 | 28.0 ± 12.6 | 1.49 ± 0.41* | | | [§] Mean and range given; no controls. CL reduced 30-40%.<br>[§§]Therapeutic concentrations in ascites fluid for ≈ 20 hours | 106 |
| | LD + ascites | 6 | 11.2 ± 2.7 | 27.3 ± 9.1 | 1.69 ± 0.42* | | | | |
| | LD + jaundice | 8 | 8.7 ± 3.5* | 22.4 ± 7.7 | 1.84 ± 0.37* | | | | |
| | LD + jaundice + ascites | 7 | 10.0 ± 3.2* | 28.7 ± 9.1 | 2.42 ± 1.87* | | | | |
| | | (4) | (18.9 ± 5.7) | (20.3 ± 3.5) | (0.78 ± 0.19) | | | | |

| | | | | | | | | | |
|---|---|---|---|---|---|---|---|---|---|
| | C-ALD | 8<br>(8) | | 11.1 ± 5.3*<br>(17.5 ± 5.4) | 60.9 ± 28.0*<br>(34.3 ± 14.0) | 4.79 ± 3.00<br>(1.59 ± 0.57) | | | 107 |
| Cefprozil | C | 12<br><br>(12) | cis<br>trans<br>cis<br>trans | CL/F:<br>14.8 ± 5.7<br>16.8 ± 8.0<br>(15.5 ± 4.1)<br>(18.8 ± 7.7) | | 2.2 ± 0.7<br>1.5 ± 0.5<br>(1.6 ± 0.5)<br>(1.2 ± 0.1) | | No dose adjustment necessary | 108 |
| Ceftazidime | IC[§] | | | 7.98 ± 1.02 | 20.0 ± 2.91 | 1.74 ± 0.41 | | Modest dose adjustment may be necessary in cirrhosis.<br>[§] T-tube study | 109 |
| | CLD | 12 | | 5.5 ± 2.6 | 10.5 ± 2.8‡ | 2.8 ± 0.8 | | | 110 |
| | C | 11<br>(6) | | 5.7 ± 2.2<br>(5.9 ± 1.7) | 42.5 ± 14.9*<br>(16.4 ± 4.5) | 5.40 ± 1.03*<br>(1.98 ± 0.24) | | | 111 |
| Ceftriaxone | C<br>– ascites<br>+ ascites | <br>4<br>6 | | <br>1.0 ± 0.2<br>1.4 ± 0.4 | <br>10.6 ± 0.8<br>19.1 ± 4.8* | <br>8.0 ± 2.0<br>9.7 ± 1.8 | | No dose adjustment necessary | 112 |
| | C-ALD | 8<br>(8) | | 1.2 ± 0.6<br>(0.8 ± 0.3) | 16.1 ± 4.2*<br>(9.1 ± 2.1) | 10.69 ± 4.27<br>(9.05 ± 1.73) | | | 107 |
| Cefuroxime | C | 6<br>(5) | | 13.6 ± 4.0<br>(10.5 ± 0.9) | 15.3 ± 2.7<br>(18.1 ± 3.6) | 1.0 ± 0.3*<br>(1.8 ± 0.4) | | Unchanged | 113 |
| • *Fluoroquinolones* | | | | | | | | | |
| Ciprofloxacin | C: single dose<br><br>C: steady-state | 7<br>(7)<br>7<br>(7) | | CL/F:<br>45.88 ± 14.01<br>(50.42 ± 14.43)<br>39.75 ± 13.39<br>(39.78 ± 5.42) | Vd/F:<br>198.1 ± 41.3<br>(243.6 ± 70.0)<br>197.4 ± 40.6<br>(196.7 ± 40.6) | 3.47 ± 1.23<br>(3.71 ± 0.41) | | No dose adjustment necessary | 114 |
| | C | 5<br>(5) | | CL/F:<br>26.9 ± 6.7<br>(31.9 ± 10.1) | Vd/F:<br>140 ± 49<br>(168 ± 35) | 3.6 ± 0.3<br>(3.8 ± 0.7) | | | 115 |
| Fleroxacin | C<br>– ascites<br>+ ascites | <br>6<br>6<br>(12) | | <br>5.5 ± 1.0<br>3.0 ± 1.4*<br>(6.8 ± 1.3) | <br>94 ± 14‡<br>98 ± 18<br>(100 ± 22) | <br>16.6 ± 2.7<br>29.6 ± 8.5*<br>(14.1 ± 1.8) | <br>100 ± 7<br>99 ± 8<br>(103 ± 11) | Reduced dose may be necessary in patients with cirrhosis and ascites | 116 |
| Norfloxacin | C | 3<br>(6) | | | | 5.47 ± 0.84<br>(4.28 ± 1.33) | | Unchanged | 117 |
| Ofloxacin | C | 8<br>(8) | | CL/F:<br>9.7 ± 1.3<br>(12.2 ± 4.6) | Vd/F:<br>105 ± 21*<br>(77 ± 21) | 7.6 ± 1.0*<br>(4.9 ± 0.9) | | Reduced dose may be necessary in cirrhosis | 115 |
| | C,ALD | 12<br>(12) | | CL/F:<br>5.8 ± 2.9*<br>(13.3 ± 2.6) | Vd/F:<br>84 ± 28*<br>(126 ± 14) | 11.6 ± 3.4*<br>(7.0 ± 1.4) | | | 118 |
| Pefloxacin | C | 10<br>(8) | | CL/F:<br>2.71 ± 1.71*<br>(6.85 ± 1.4) | Vd/F:<br>78.4 ± 20.3*<br>(116.9 ± 14.0) | 29.0 ± 18.1*<br>(12.3 ± 2.4) | | Reduced dose may be necessary in cirrhosis | 119 |

[Continued over]

*For footnotes, see final page of table (p. 1785)*

**Table II.** *[Continued]*

| Drug | Disease | No. of patients | Pharmacokinetic parameters in hepatic disease[a] CL[b] (L/h) | Vd[c] (L) | $t_{½}$ (h) | $f_u$ (%) | F (%) | Dose adjustment/ comments | References |
|---|---|---|---|---|---|---|---|---|---|
| **Antibacterial drugs** *[continued]* | | | | | | | | | |
| Pefloxacin *[continued]* | C | 25<br>(11) | 1.76 ± 1.31*<br>(6.03 ± 2.99) | 79.8 ± 32.5<br>(90.2 ± 30.2) | 46.3 ± 42.5*<br>(11.3 ± 3.5) | | | | 120 |
| | C | 16<br>(12) | 2.66 ± 1.85*<br>(8.19 ± 2.80) | 107.8 ± 18.2<br>(131.6 ± 25.9) | 35.1 ± 19.0*<br>(11.0 ± 2.6) | | | | 121 |
| Rufloxacin | C | 13<br>(5) | CL/F:<br>1.68 ± 0.43*<br>(2.46 ± 0.54) | Vd/F:<br>96 ± 7<br>(103 ± 29) | 40.0 ± 9.0<br>(30.1 ± 8.7) | 49.8 ± 6.9<br>(42.9 ± 4.2) | | No dose adjustment necessary | 122 |
| • *Macrolides* | | | | | | | | | |
| Azithromycin | C-Pugh A<br>C-Pugh B | 10<br>6<br>(6) | CL/F:<br>13.5 ± 4.2<br>14.3 ± 3.5<br>(17.2 ± 4.5) | Vd/F:<br>661.3 ± 100.2<br>640.7 ± 134.0<br>(659.7 ± 121.8) | 60.6 ± 19.2<br>68.1 ± 13.2<br>(53.5 ± 7.1) | | | No dose adjustment necessary | 123 |
| Erythromycin | C | 6<br>(6) | | | 3.2 ± 0.5*<br>(2.0 ± 0.7) | | | Dose reduction necessary in some patients, but weigh the risk of inadequate treatment (relatively large therapeutic range) | 124 |
| | C | 5<br>(6) | 24.2 ± 8.3<br>(34.2 ± 12.1) | 85.5 ± 23.8*‡<br>(57.6 ± 14.8) | 2.24 ± 0.89<br>(1.36 ± 0.43) | 58.3 ± 17.7*<br>(30.5 ± 2.8) | | | 125 |
| Midecamycin (miocamycin) | C | 6<br>(6) | | | 1.78 ± 0.36*<br>(1.18 ± 0.29) | | | Reduced dose may be necessary in cirrhosis | 126 |
| Rokitamycin | C (mild) | 12 single dose<br>(12) single dose | CL/F:<br>307.0 ± 789.8<br>(348.2 ± 721.6) | | 1.33 ± 3.05<br>(1.02 ± 0.90) | | | No dose adjustment necessary in mild cirrhosis | 127 |
| | C (mild) | 12 steady-state<br>(12) steady-state | 353.9 ± 405.0<br>(282.0 ± 389.4) | | 1.45 ± 3.33<br>(1.02 ± 0.69) | | | | |
| Roxithromycin | C-ALD | 10<br>(12) | | | 25.2 ± 6.0*<br>(10.5 ± 4.8) | | | Insufficient information to make dosage recommendation | 128 |
| • *Penicillins* | | | | | | | | | |
| Ampicillin | C | 9<br>(8) | 16.8 ± 8.2<br>(20.5 ± 4.8) | 59.1 ± 43.1*‡<br>(19.5 ± 4.6) | 1.9 ± 0.6*<br>(1.3 ± 0.2) | | | Unchanged | 129 |
| | C | 9<br>(8) | | 13.8 ± 1.1*<br>(9.4 ± 1.1) | 1.8 ± 0.2*<br>(1.4 ± 0.1) | | | | 130 |
| Carbenicillin | LD | 9<br>(5) | | | 1.9 ± 0.6*<br>(1.0 ± 0.3) | | | Unchanged | 131 |

| | | | | | | | | |
|---|---|---|---|---|---|---|---|---|
| Mezlocillin | C | 4<br>(8) | 7.5 ± 1.8*<br>(14.9 ± 3.6) | | 2.62 ± 0.48*<br>(0.96 ± 0.08) | | Reduce dose by 50% in cirrhosis | 132 |
| Nafcillin | C<br>OJ | 12<br>5<br>(12) | 17.5 ± 8.9*<br>9.8 ± 3.4*<br>(35.0 ± 8.7) | 19.9 ± 5.8*‡<br>15.9 ± 2.4*<br>(27.1 ± 7.3) | 1.23 ± 0.31<br>1.73 ± 0.44*<br>(1.02 ± 0.20) | | Reduce dose | 133 |
| • *Others* | | | | | | | | |
| Aztreonam | C-ALD<br>PBC | 6<br>6<br>(6) | 3.4 ± 0.0<br>4.2 ± 0.4<br>(4.2 ± 0.4) | 14 ± 0‡<br>14 ± 0<br>(11 ± 0) | 3.2 ± 0.6*<br>2.2 ± 0.1*<br>(1.9 ± 0.2) | | Unchanged in PBC. Reduce dose in C-ALD by 20-25% (must weigh risk *vs* benefit) | 134 |
| Brodimoprim | C (children - Pugh A & B) | 10<br>(12) | CL/F:<br>2.4 ± 0.5<br>(2.3 ± 0.4) | Vd/F:<br>189 ± 70<br>(105 ± 14) | 56 ± 14<br>(34 ± 7) | 10.2 ± 3.6*<br>(5.7 ± 0.9) | No dose adjustment necessary | 135 |
| Chloramphen-icol | AH<br>C | 6<br>6<br>(8) | 3.14 ± 0.50*<br>3.55 ± 1.23*<br>(10.12 ± 1.54) | 51.9 ± 4.1*<br>50.0 ± 10.0*<br>(65.9 ± 11.3) | 11.60 ± 1.62*<br>10.45 ± 2.79*<br>(4.61 ± 0.93) | | Avoid.<br>Increased toxicity may occur in cirrhosis | 136 |
| Clindamycin | AH<br>CAH<br>C | 7<br>6<br>9<br>(8) | | | 2.6<br>2.1<br>2.5<br>(1.8) | | Insufficient information to make dosage recommendation | 137 |
| Metronidazole | C | 6<br>(5) | 4.83 ± 2.67<br>(4.45 ± 0.38) | 51.8 ± 6.9<br>(42.0 ± 1.6) | 10.8 ± 5.9<br>(7.4 ± 0.7) | | Unchanged in mild liver disease but reduce dose in severe liver disease | 138 |
| | C<br>severe | 10<br>(9) | 1.05 ± 0.46*<br>(3.11 ± 1.57) | 26.60 ± 6.64*<br>(33.60 ± 6.30) | 19.9 ± 7.9*<br>(7.9 ± 2.1) | | | 139 |
| | C | 8<br>(8) | 1.7 ± 0.6*<br>(5.0 ± 0.8) | 44 ± 9<br>(48 ± 7) | 20 ± 9*<br>(7.3 ± 0.9) | | | 140 |
| | ALD | 8 | 2.1 ± 0.5 | 53.9 ± 11.2 | 18.31 ± 6.06 | | | 141 |
| Ornidazole | AH<br>C<br>OJ | 10<br>10<br>10 | 33.5 ± 7.3*<br>37.3 ± 15.8*<br>26.1 ± 5.1 | 53.7 ± 12.0‡<br>52.3 ± 20.2<br>36.8 ± 2.3* | 19.3 ± 2.2*<br>19.3 ± 5.7*<br>17.4 ± 2.5* | | Reduce dose in liver disease | 142 |
| Vancomycin | LD | 9<br>(6) | 2.9 ± 2.9*<br>(9.7 ± 3.7) | 22 ± 12†<br>(32 ± 16) | 37.0 ± 74.3*<br>(2.6 ± 1.3) | | Reduce dose in liver disease.<br>Monitor plasma concentrations | 143 |
| **Anticoagulants** | | | | | | | | |
| • *Parenteral* | | | | | | | | |
| Heparin | C | | | | 1.96 ± 0.51*<br>(1.23 ± 0.06) | | Monitor effect.<br>May require lower doses due to impaired clotting factor production | 144 |

[Continued over]

For footnotes, see final page of table (p. 1785)

**Table II.** *[Continued]*

| Drug | Disease | No. of patients | Pharmacokinetic parameters in hepatic disease[a] | | | | | Dose adjustment/ comments | References |
|---|---|---|---|---|---|---|---|---|---|
| | | | CL[b] (L/h) | Vd[c] (L) | $t_{1/2}$ (h) | $f_u$ (%) | F (%) | | |
| **Anticoagulants** *[continued]* | | | | | | | | | |
| • *Oral* | | | | | | | | The response to oral anticoagulants may be markedly enhanced in obstructive jaundice (due to reduced vitamin K absorption) and also in hepatitis and cirrhosis (due to decreased production of vitamin K- dependent clotting factors). Prothrombin index should be closely monitored | 145 |
| Phenprocoumon | C | 9 (7) | CL/F: 0.115 ± 0.034* (0.063 ± 0.013) | Vd/F: 11.4 ± 2.5 (9.3 ± 0.9) | 74.2 ± 25.8* (105.5 ± 17.2) | 1.14 ± 0.12* (0.80 ± 0.03) | | See above | 146 |
| Warfarin | AVH | 5 (5) | CL/F: 0.43 ± 0.06 (0.43 ± 0.05) | Vd/F: 13.3 ± 2.8 (14.7 ± 1.4) | 23 ± 5 (25 ± 3) | 1.2 ± 0.1 1.2 ± 0.1 | | Start with low doses and titrate to response | 147 |
| **Antidepressants** | | | | | | | | | |
| Amitriptyline | C + shunt | 1 | | | 37.7 | | | Reduce dose in patients with cirrhosis and portocaval shunt | 148 |
| Fluoxetine | C | 13 (12) | 5.0 ± 9.7* (40.3 ± 29.0) | 3570 ± 3430 (2450 ± 1470) | 158.4 ± 117.6* (52.8 ± 40.8) | 8.8 ± 1.3 (9.1 ± 1.6) | | Reduce dose in cirrhosis | 149 |
| Fluvoxamine | C, ALD | 13 | CL/F: 54.8 | | 24.7 ± 10.6 | | | Reduce dose in cirrhosis | 150 |
| Moclobemide | LD | 9 | 14.6 ± 11.2* | 75.7 ± 40.3 | 3.87 ± 2.62 | | 84 ± 25 | Reduce dose in liver disease | 151 |
| Paroxetine | C-ALD | 12 (6) | | | 83 ± 82 (36 ± 20) | | | Reduce dose in cirrhosis | 152 |
| Tranylcypromine | C | 5 (7) | | | | | | Avoid. Marked cerebral depressant effect may occur in cirrhosis | 153 |
| **Antidiabetic drugs** | | | | | | | | | |
| Tolbutamide | C | 5 (7) | | | 9.3 (4.4 ± 0.7) | | | Use with care in cirrhosis. Increased risk of hypoglycaemia. | 154 |
| | AVH | 5 (5)[§] | $CL_T$: 1.8 ± 0.4* (1.3 ± 0.2) $CL_U$: 21 ± 3 (18 ± 3) | 10.5 ± 2.1 (10.5 ± 2.1) | 4.0 ± 0.9* (5.9 ± 1.4) | 8.7 ± 0.8* (6.8 ± 0.6) | | [§] Controls were same patients after recovery | 155 |

| | | | | | | | | |
|---|---|---|---|---|---|---|---|---|
| **Antiemetics** | | | | | | | | |
| Ondansetron | LD-mild<br>LD-moderate<br>LD-severe | 6<br>6<br>7<br>(6) | 12.7*<br>17.9*<br>5.8*<br>(28.7) | 224*‡<br>230*<br>179*<br>(153) | 9.1*<br>9.2*<br>20.6*<br>(3.6) | | Reduce dose in patients with hepatic impairment | 156 |
| **Antiepileptic drugs** | | | | | | | | |
| Phenobarbital | AVH<br>C | 8<br>6<br>(6) | | | 104<br>130 ± 37*<br>(86 ± 7) | | Increased adverse effects (e.g. ataxia) may occur in severe liver disease. Monitor plasma concentrations and adjust dose accordingly. May worsen HE | 157 |
| Phenytoin | AVH | 5<br>(5) | 2.55<br>(2.16) | 47.9<br>(44.5) | 13.2<br>(12.6) | 12.6<br>(9.9) | Safe in usual doses in mild liver disease. Clearance may be substantially reduced in cirrhosis, and plasma level monitoring with dose adjustment advisable. | 158 |
| | AVH,C | 15 | Reduced in 4/15 | | | | Phenytoin concentrations must be corrected for low albumin levels | 159 |
| Primidone | AVH | 7<br>(7) | CL/F:<br>2.9 ± 1.0<br>(2.5 ± 0.6) | Vd/F:<br>76.3 ± 27.3<br>(60.2 ± 15.4) | 18.0 ± 3.1<br>(17.0 ± 2.4) | | Unchanged.<br>Monitor effect | 160 |
| Valproic acid/ sodium valproate | C | 7<br>(6) | CL/F:<br>0.5 ± 0.1<br>(0.5 ± 0.1) | Vd/F:<br>15.4 ± 6.3*†<br>(9.8 ± 3.5) | 18.9 ± 5.1*<br>(12.2 ± 3.7) | 29.3*<br>(11.3) | Reduce dose (50% reduction in mean $CL_u/F$) | 161 |
| **Antihistamines** ($H_1$-receptor antagonists) | | | | | | | | |
| Cetirizine | C-ALD<br>PBC, OJ | 5<br>5<br>(16) | CL/F:<br>2.0 ± 1.0<br>1.7 ± 0.4<br>(3.1 ± 0.8) | Vd/F:<br>46.9 ± 32.2<br>32.9 ± 4.2<br>(40.6 ± 11.2) | 14.32 ± 2.30*<br>13.86 ± 3.14*<br>(9.42 ± 2.40) | | Reduce dose in liver disease | 162 |
| | PBC | 6<br>(13) | CL/F:<br>1.8 ± 0.4<br>(2.5 ± 0.2) | Vd/F:<br>30.8 ± 2.8<br>(35.0 ± 4.9) | 13.8 ± 1.8*<br>(7.4 ± 1.6) | | | 163 |
| Diphenhydramine | C | 9<br>(8) | $CL_T$: 33.5 ± 13.7<br>(41.7 ± 12.8)<br>$CL_U$: 1.6 ± 0.9*<br>(2.8 ± 1.0) | 595 ± 435‡<br>(455 ± 214) | 15.2 ± 4.4*<br>(9.3 ± 2.0) | 33.3*<br>(21.9) | Unchanged.<br>Generally safe in liver disease | 164 |
| Hydroxyzine | PBC | 8 | CL/F:<br>36.33 ± 31.33 | Vd/F:<br>1589 ± 931 | 36.6 ± 13.1 | | Reduce dose in PBC | 165 |
| **Antihypertensive drugs** (see also ACE inhibitors, β-adrenoceptor antagonists, calcium antagonists and diuretics) | | | | | | | | |
| Ketanserin | C | 26 | 17.5 ± 1.9 | 175 ± 35‡ | 10.1 ± 2.9 | | Reduce dose in cirrhosis | 166 |
| **Antineoplastic and immunosuppressive drugs** | | | | | | | | |
| Cyclophosphamide | LF | 7<br>(10) | Reduced ≈ 30% | | 12.5 ± 1.0*<br>(7.6 ± 1.4) | 87.5<br>(87.5) | Reduce dose in severe liver disease | 167 |

[Continued over]

*For footnotes, see final page of table (p. 1785)*

**Table II.** *[Continued]*

| Drug | Disease | No. of patients | Pharmacokinetic parameters in hepatic disease[a] | | | | | Dose adjustment/ comments | References |
|---|---|---|---|---|---|---|---|---|---|
| | | | CL[b] (L/h) | Vd[c] (L) | $t_{½}$ (h) | $f_u$ (%) | F (%) | | |
| **Antineoplastic and immunosuppressive drugs** *[continued]* | | | | | | | | | |
| Cyclosporin (cyclosporin A) | LD<br>mild<br>moderate | <br>9<br>7<br>(25) | CL/F:<br>211 ± 140<br>124 ± 79*<br>(220 ± 139) | Vd/F:<br>2072 ± 1638<br>1484 ± 1130<br>(1596 ± 1085) | <br>5.8<br>8.7*<br>(3.5) | | | Monitor blood concentrations.<br>Oral dose may need to be increased in cholestasis due to poor absorption.<br>Intravenous doses may need to be decreased in some patients with liver disease and impaired clearance | 168 |
| Etoposide | OJ | 6<br>(15) | 2.7 ± 1.1<br>(1.9 ± 0.6) | | | 27 ± 15*<br>(9 ± 3) | | Reduce dose in cholestatic liver disease.<br>Increased unbound AUC | 169 |
| | OJ | 11<br>(23) | 2.5 ± 0.7<br>(2.8 ± 1.0) | 21.5 ± 6.3<br>(23.7 ± 13.4) | 5.7 ± 1.7<br>(6.4 ± 2.4) | | | | 170 |
| **Antipsychotic drugs** | | | | | | | | | |
| Chlorpromazine | C | 21<br>(13) | | | 24<br>(31) | | | Avoid.<br>May precipitate HE in cirrhosis due to increased cerebral sensitivity | 171 |
| **Antituberculosis drugs** | | | | | | | | Risk of inadequate treatment must be weighed against risk of toxicity when choosing a dose | |
| *p*-Aminosalicylic acid (para-aminosalicylic acid; PAS) | C, AVH | 7<br>(7) | 10.8 ± 1.8<br>(11.0 ± 1.9) | 6.79 ± 0.98<br>(6.86 ± 1.40) | 0.45 ± 0.09<br>(0.44 ± 0.09) | | | Unchanged | 172 |
| Isoniazid | C | 13<br>(12) | | | 6.74 ± 1.19*<br>(3.24 ± 0.48) | | | Reduce dose in severe liver disease.<br>Increased risk of hepatotoxicity if usual doses used in those with impaired liver function | 173 |
| Rifabutin | LD-mild<br>LD-moderate<br>LD-severe | 6<br>6<br>4<br>(12) | | | 16 ± 11<br>11 ± 10<br>42 ± 18<br>(67 ± 45) | | | Insufficient information to make dosage recommendation | 174 |
| Rifampicin (rifampin) | C | 13<br>(12) | | | 5.42 ± 1.98*<br>(2.80 ± 0.76) | | | Reduce dose in severe liver disease | 173 |
| **Antiulcer drugs** | | | | | | | | | |
| Cimetidine | LD | 12<br>(6) | 27.8 ± 8.7<br>(30.7 ± 5.6) | 98 ± 42‡<br>(77 ± 28) | 2.9 ± 1.1<br>(2.3 ± 0.7) | | | Usual dose safe in mild liver disease but use with caution and in reduced dosage in severe liver disease. | 175 |
| | C | 9<br>(11) | 36.4 ± 11.5<br>(33.4 ± 8.8) | | 2.0 ± 0.4<br>(2.3 ± 0.4) | | 97 ± 21<br>(84 ± 13) | | 176 |

| | | | | | | | | | |
|---|---|---|---|---|---|---|---|---|---|
| | C | 14<br>(12) | CLT: 29.2 ± 14.9<br>(26.7 ± 11.4)<br>CLH: 4.4 ± 6.1*<br>(11.4 ± 2.8) | 71.5 ± 12.0*‡<br>(55.7 ± 16.7) | 2.23<br>(1.99) | | 76.8 ± 18.3*<br>(59.9 ± 22.6) | | 177 |
| | C | 11<br>(11) | 29.8 ± 9.7*<br>(45.4 ± 11.4) | 105 ± 31*<br>(150 ± 39) | 2.53 ± 0.63<br>(2.33 ± 0.40) | | 82.5 ± 37.6<br>(59.6 ± 21.5) | § Inverse correlation between $CL_H$ and prothrombin time. | 178 |
| | C | 11 | $CL_T$: 34.5 ± 13.3<br>$CL_H$: 16.3 ± 7.3§ | 95.2 ± 139.3‡ | | | 91 ± 20 | §§ Reduced $CL_T$ in patients with HE; lowered dosage recommended | 179 |
| | C<br>+ HE<br>– HE | <br>8<br>8<br>(4) | <br>21.2 ± 4.1§§<br>41.4 ± 14.3<br>(36.8 ± 19.7) | <br>54.0 ± 16.0<br>78.4 ± 13.9<br>(67.8 ± 39.3) | <br>2.3 ± 0.3<br>2.3 ± 0.6<br>(1.7 ± 0.1) | | | | 180 |
| | C (severe) | 8 | $CL_T$: 21.4 ± 10.9*<br>$CL_H$: 5.8 ± 6.7* | 56 ± 18‡ | 2.5 ± 1.0 | | 70 ± 39 | | 181 |
| | C | 8<br>(7) | $CL_T$: 17.9 ± 13.9*<br>(40.3 ± 14.9)<br>$CL_H$: 12.3 ± 4.8*<br>(16.9 ± 8.4) | 53.9 ± 9.9*‡<br>(88.2 ± 31.5) | 2.25 ± 0.38*<br>(1.55 ± 0.44) | | 79.5 ± 17.5 | | 182 |
| | LD | 10<br>(19) | 25.3 ± 6.0*<br>(50.2 ± 13.0) | 95.9 ± 26.6<br>(124.6 ± 47.6) | 2.08 ± 0.45*<br>(1.50 ± 0.41) | | | | 183 |
| Famotidine | CAH<br>Compensated-C<br>Decompensated-C | 6<br>11<br>3<br>(7) | 17.3 ± 7.6<br>14.8 ± 5.8<br>7.6 ± 0.4*<br>(14.8 ± 2.5) | 74.2 ± 18.9<br>67.2 ± 16.1<br>92.4 ± 44.8<br>(86.8 ± 20.3) | 3.47 ± 1.96<br>3.50 ± 1.23<br>7.70 ± 3.33*<br>(3.83 ± 1.06) | | | Reduce dose in decompensated cirrhosis (some individuals with decompensated cirrhosis have substantially prolonged $t_{1/2}$; caution with use of high doses) | 184 |
| | Decompensated-C | 10<br>(6) | 24.9 ± 8.6<br>(25.3 ± 8.2) | 109 ± 24.8‡<br>(88.6 ± 19.4) | 4.24 ± 1.72<br>(2.96 ± 0.48) | | 47.8 ± 13.2<br>(39.8 ± 19.1) | | 185 |
| Lansoprazole | H<br>Compensated-C<br>Decompensated-C | 8<br>8<br>8<br>(18) | CL/F:<br>13.3 ± 9.8<br>2.8 ± 1.4*<br>4.9 ± 4.2*<br>(18.2 ± 9.8) | Vd/F:<br>39.9 ± 17.5<br>24.5 ± 4.2<br>38.5 ± 16.1<br>(31.5 ± 12.6) | 3.2 ± 2.1*<br>6.1 ± 1.5*<br>7.2 ± 2.5*<br>(1.4 ± 0.8) | | | Reduce dose in cirrhosis | 186 |
| Omeprazole | C | 8<br>(8) | CL/F:<br>5.85 ± 2.58*<br>(48.3 ± 17.8) | | 2.85 ± 1.68*<br>(0.73 ± 0.04) | | | Although there is a significant decrease in CL/F in cirrhosis, the q24h dosage interval will minimise accumulation. Smaller doses may be used to achieve the same effect | 187 |
| | C | 8 | 4.0 ± 0.8 | 14.7 ± 2.0 | 2.8 ± 0.6 | | 98 ± 14 | | 188 |
| Pirenzepine | C | 8<br>(12) | 10.0 ± 1.8<br>(10.8 ± 2.8) | 121 ± 35‡<br>(111 ± 22) | 14.3 ± 3.9<br>(11.1 ± 3.8) | | | No dose adjustment necessary | 189 |

[Continued over]

For footnotes, see final page of table (p. 1785)

**Table II.** *[Continued]*

| Drug | Disease | No. of patients | Pharmacokinetic parameters in hepatic disease[a] CL[b] (L/h) | Vd[c] (L) | $t_{1/2}$ (h) | $f_u$ (%) | F (%) | Dose adjustment/ comments | References |
|---|---|---|---|---|---|---|---|---|---|
| **Antiulcer drugs** *[continued]* | | | | | | | | | |
| Ranitidine | C | 9<br>(10) | 28.6 ± 7.9*<br>(32.6 ± 7.6) | 115 ± 30<br>(106 ± 35) | 2.8 ± 0.7*<br>(2.1 ± 0.3) | | 70 ± 21*<br>(51 ± 13) | Dose adjustment not usually required but some patients with alcoholic cirrhosis may require a reduced dose | 190 |
| | C | | | | | | | | 191 |
| | + ascites | 5 | $CL_T$: 28.8 ± 9.6<br>$CL_H$: 19.3 ± 5.1 | 130 ± 67 | 3.0 ± 0.7* | | | | |
| | – ascites | 5 | $CL_T$: 43.5 ± 5.9<br>$CL_H$: 22.9 ± 6.9 | 124 ± 9 | 2.0 ± 0.3 | | | | |
| | C | 9 | 28.2 ± 10.2 | 84 ± 14‡ | 2.9 ± 0.4 | 95.4 | 58 ± 11 | | 192 |
| | C-ALD | 11<br>(5) | 15.4 ± 7.2*<br>(31.9 ± 5.5) | 44.8 ± 24.5‡<br>(57.4 ± 12.6) | 2.53 ± 0.46*<br>(1.40 ± 0.20) | | | | 193 |
| **Antiviral drugs** | | | | | | | | | |
| Zidovudine | C | 14<br>(6) | CL/F:<br>41.2 ± 14.6*<br>(153.7 ± 48.8) | Vd/F:<br>136 ± 58*<br>(216 ± 73) | 2.4 ± 1.2*<br>(1.0 ± 0.4) | | | Reduced dose may be necessary in some patients with cirrhosis | 194 |
| **Bronchodilators** | | | | | | | | | |
| Theophylline | C | 9<br>(19) | 2.94*<br>(4.34) | 55.0‡<br>(35.6) | 25.6*<br>(6.7) | 63.2<br>(47.4) | | Reduce dose.<br>Higher incidence of toxic effects (including seizures) in cirrhosis. Plasma concentrations should be monitored closely during long term administration in cirrhosis and during acute hepatitis, with dose adjustment as necessary | 195 |
| | C | 8<br>(57) | CL/F:<br>1.32 ± 0.79*<br>(4.41 ± 2.00) | Vd/F:<br>39.4 ± 5.6*<br>(33.7 ± 5.6) | 28.8 ± 14.3*<br>(6.0 ± 2.1) | 71.0 ± 16.0*<br>(35 ± 6.0) | | | 196 |
| | AVH<br>IC<br>C | 4<br>7 | 1.5 ± 0.2*<br>2.7 ± 1.7 | 40.6 ± 7.0*<br>40.6 ± 7.7* | 19.2 ± 1.3*<br>14.4 ± 8.7* | | | | 197 |
| | mild<br>severe | 5<br>7<br>(6) | 2.7 ± 1.8<br>2.5 ± 0.2*<br>(2.7 ± 1.0) | 31.5 ± 3.5<br>41.3 ± 9.8<br>(28.7 ± 8.4) | 11.9 ± 7.4<br>65.4 ± 29*<br>(7.7 ± 1.3) | | | | |
| | LD | 24<br>(26) | CL/F:<br>2.4 ± 1.6*<br>(2.7 ± 0.8) | Vd/F:<br>36.8 ± 11.5<br>(37.0 ± 5.5) | 17.6 ± 14.1*<br>(7.6 ± 2.3) | | | | 198 |
| | CAH<br>C | 6<br>20<br>(10) | 2.52 ± 0.91*<br>1.89 ± 0.77*<br>(5.25 ± 0.77) | | | | | | 199 |

| | | | | | | | | | |
|---|---|---|---|---|---|---|---|---|---|
| **Calcium antagonists** | | | | | | | | | |
| Amlodipine | LD | 10<br>(8) | CL/F:<br>30.1<br>(43.4) | | 55.9<br>(34.1) | | | Reduce dose in liver disease | 200 |
| Diltiazem | C | 7<br>(7) | | Vd/F:<br>548 ± 148<br>(554 ± 235) | 7.2 ± 1.6<br>(5.3 ± 2.4) | | | Reduced dose necessary in some patients with cirrhosis. Start low and titrate to response | 201 |
| Felodipine | C | 9 | 29.0 ± 13.9 | 392 ± 231‡ | 16.3 ± 8.3 | | | Reduce dose in cirrhosis | 202 |
| Gallopamil | C | 6<br>(6) | CL/F (range):<br>109 (42-234)<br>(492) | | 11.6 (5.1-20.2)<br>([3-6]) | | | Reduce dose by 50% in cirrhosis and titrate to response | 203 |
| Isradipine | LD<br>C | 7<br>8<br>(8) | 54 ± 16<br>38 ± 19*<br>(66 ± 12) | 210 ± 147<br>322 ± 203<br>(490 ± 217) | 5.8 ± 3.7<br>11.9 ± 6.1*<br>(5.1 ± 2.4) | | 15.6 ± 7.6<br>36.9 ± 16.2*<br>(16.5 ± 9.9) | Reduce dose in cirrhosis | 204 |
| Nicardipine | C | 10<br>(6) | CL/F:<br>75.6<br>(344.4) | Vd/F:<br>1610<br>(840) | 19.4<br>(3) | | | Reduce dose in cirrhosis | 205 |
| | C-ALD | 9<br>(9) | 24.3 ± 7.5*<br>(53) | 769 ± 296*‡<br>(297) | 30 ± 10<br>(7.5) | | | | 206 |
| | C | 9<br>(8) | | | 13.7 ± 19.2<br>(1.6 ± 1.1) | | | | 207 |
| Nifedipine | C | 7<br>(7) | 14.0 ± 6.5*<br>(35.3 ± 8.4) | 90.3 ± 42.0*‡<br>(58.2 ± 25.2) | 7.0 ± 4.2*<br>(1.9 ± 0.4) | 8.5 ± 2.5*<br>(4.4 ± 0.8) | 90.5 ± 26.2*<br>(51.1 ± 17.1) | Reduce oral dose by 50-60% in cirrhosis. Reduce dose in other patients with impaired liver function | 208 |
| | C | 7<br>(10) | | | 7.2 ± 3.3*<br>(1.7 ± 0.6) | | | | 209 |
| | LD | 13<br>(8) | | | Range:<br>0.93-8.2<br>(0.65-1.85) | | | | 5 |
| Nimodipine | C<br><br>C | 6 PO<br>(5 PO)<br>6 SL<br>(5 SL) | CL/F:<br>217 ± 222*<br>(519 ± 176)<br>158 ± 85*<br>(420 ± 226) | | | | | Reduce dose in cirrhosis | 210 |
| Nisoldipine | C | 8<br>(8) | 29.6 ± 7.0*<br>(50.8 ± 18.4) | 448 ± 161<br>(287 ± 147) | 16.6 ± 4.6*<br>(9.7 ± 5.4) | | 14.7 ± 10.1*<br>(3.7 ± 2.1) | Reduce dose in cirrhosis | 211 |

[Continued over]

*For footnotes, see final page of table (p. 1785)*

**Table II.** *[Continued]*

| Drug | Disease | No. of patients | Pharmacokinetic parameters in hepatic disease[a] CL[b] (L/h) | Vd[c] (L) | $t_{½}$ (h) | $f_u$ (%) | F (%) | Dose adjustment/ comments | References |
|---|---|---|---|---|---|---|---|---|---|
| **Calcium antagonists** *[continued]* | | | | | | | | | |
| Nitrendipine | CLD | 12 | CL/F:<br>Single dose:<br>2.1<br>Steady-state:<br>0.65 | Vd/F:<br>Single dose:<br>36.5<br>Steady-state:<br>10.5 | Single dose:<br>23.4<br>Steady-state:<br>11.8 | | | Reduced dose may be necessary in cirrhosis. Dosage adjustment during long term therapy may be necessary in patients with combined cardiac and hepatic disease.<br>Adjust dosage according to haemodynamic response | 212 |
| | ALD | 6<br>(6) | | | 19.57 ± 4.28<br>(15.29 ± 7.25) | | Increased<br>≈ 300% | | 213 |
| | AH<br>CAH<br>C | 5<br>5<br>11<br>(6) | 63.4 ± 21.7*<br>50.4 ± 16.9*<br>51.2 ± 23.3*<br>(77.4 ± 27.2)* | 78.1 ± 17.0*<br>30.4 ± 20.8*<br>65.3 ± 41.5*<br>(13.4 ± 8.3) | 4.28 ± 2.2<br>3.79 ± 3.2<br>7.67 ± 13.5*<br>(2.19 ± 1.1) | | 0.26 ± 0.16<br>0.48 ± 0.36<br>0.54 ± 0.33<br>(0.40 ± 0.27) | | 214 |
| Tiapamil | C | 8<br>(8) | 43.9<br>(56.7) | 171 ± 53‡*<br>(101 ± 28) | 3.5 ± 0.9*<br>(1.7 ± 0.3) | 47.6 ± 7.9 | 52 (n=2) | Reduced dose necessary in some patients with cirrhosis. Recommend starting low and titrating to response | 215 |
| Verapamil | C | 7<br>(6) | 37.0*<br>(75.5) | 642‡<br>(431) | 14.2*<br>(3.7) | | 52.3*<br>(22.0) | Reduce dose in cirrhosis (IV x 0.5; PO x 0.2) | 216 |
| | C | 5<br>(7) | | | | | 16 ± 5*<br>(9.9 ± 1.5) | | 217 |
| **Cardiac glycosides** | | | | | | | | | |
| Digitoxin | CAH | 6 | | | 105.6*<br>(194.4) | | | Unchanged in mild liver disease. In severe liver disease, elimination may be substantially reduced requiring dose reduction. | 218 |
| | C | 8[§]<br>(8) | 0.22 ± 0.05<br>(0.23 ± 0.05) | 51.8 ± 11.9<br>(57.4 ± 4.0) | 168 ± 52<br>(187 ± 54) | 4.9<br>(4.4) | No difference | In cirrhosis, no change in digitoxin pharmacokinetics but the potential for accumulation of metabolites warrants cautious use. | 219 |
| | C | 9<br>(8) | 0.315 ± 0.113<br>(0.302 ± 0.083) | 71.4 ± 21.0<br>(59.5 ± 5.9) | 175.2 ± 93.6<br>(151.2 ± 26.4) | | | [§] Patients had hepatorenal insufficiency | 220 |
| Digoxin | C | 3<br>(4) | | | 43.2<br>(43.2) | | | Insufficient information to make dosage recommendation.<br>Monitor digoxin concentrations | 221 |
| **Corticosteroids** | | | | | | | | | |
| Prednisolone | CAH | 6<br>(10) | | | 3.42 ± 0.56<br>(3.58 ± 0.35) | | | Unchanged | 222 |

| | | | | | | | | | |
|---|---|---|---|---|---|---|---|---|---|
| | CAH<br>+ remission<br>– remission | <br>5<br>5<br>(7) | | | <br>5.2 ± 2.2<br>4.5 ± 1.3*<br>(4.1 ± 0.8) | | | | 223 |
| | C | 7<br>(8) | | | 2.66 ± 0.48<br>(3.06 ± 0.38) | 28.6 ± 3.6*<br>(17.7 ± 3.5) | | | 224 |
| Prednisone | CAH | 6<br>(10) | 16.7 ± 4.7<br>(15.4 ± 3.4) | 69 ± 13<br>(70 ± 8) | 3.0 ± 1.0<br>(3.3 ± 1.0) | | | Same as prednisolone in CAH | 222 |
| | CAH<br>+ remission<br>– remission | <br>5<br>5<br>(7) | | | <br>3.8 ± 2.5<br>4.7 ± 2.5<br>(4.3 ± 2.1) | | | | 223 |
| **Diuretics** | | | | | | | | Overvigorous therapy with loop diuretics may precipitate HE in patients with cirrhosis. Use with care and monitor serum potassium | |
| Bumetanide | C | 8<br>(8) | $CL_T$: 2.33 ± 0.98*<br>(7.74 ± 1.75)<br>$CL_M$: 0.72 ± 0.83<br>(2.76 ± 1.04) | 6.36 ± 2.83*‡<br>(9.45 ± 2.77) | 2.0 ± 1.0*<br>(1.1 ± 0.2) | | 92<br>(89) | Monitor effects. Increased concentrations and prolonged $t_{½}$ in cirrhosis. Patients with cirrhosis may require higher levels to achieve the same response | 225 |
| Furosemide<br>(frusemide) | C | 8<br>(7) | $CL_T$: 13.0 ± 4.6<br>(10.4 ± 1.9)<br>$CL_H$: 5.6 ± 3.1<br>(3.4 ± 1.7) | 15.9 ± 5.2<br>(12.7 ± 2.4) | 0.87 ± 0.13<br>(0.85 ± 0.13) | | | Diminished natriuretic effect with increased sensitivity to hypokalaemia and volume depletion in cirrhosis.<br>Increased risk of HE.<br>Monitor effects, particularly with high doses | 226 |
| | C | 7<br>(4) | 7.2 ± 2.1<br>(8.5 ± 2.5) | 12.0 ± 3.5‡<br>(9.3 ± 3.7) | 2.2 ± 1.3*<br>(1.2 ± 0.3) | 6.5 ± 2.7<br>(4.4 ±1.9) | 59 ± 22<br>(51 ± 14) | | 227 |
| | C | 7<br>(7) | 6.6 ± 1.74*<br>(10.0 ± 3.24) | 10.7 ± 2.2*‡<br>(8.0 ± 1.5) | 1.32 ± 0.31*<br>(0.75 ± 0.02) | | | | 228 |
| | C | 8<br>(10) | 8.52 ± 2.7<br>(9.36 ± 1.32) | 12.1 ± 3.7*‡<br>(8.5 ± 1.3) | 1.35 ± 0.38*<br>(1.00 ± 0.31) | | | | 229 |
| Spironolactone | C | 9<br>(15) | | | 10.0<br>(6) | | | Safe at usual doses. | 230 |
| | LD | 6<br>(5) | | | 3.88 ± 3.33[§]<br>(2.75 ± 0.60) | | | [§]No change in canrenone $t_{½}$ compared with controls | 231 |
| Torasemide<br>(torsemide) | C | 12 | 2.3 ± 0.8 | 24.0 ± 6.2 | 8.1 ± 3.4 | | 96.3 | No dose adjustment necessary. Increased drug concentrations seen in cirrhosis are compensated by decreased pharmacodynamic response | 232 |
| Triamterene | C | | | | Increased<br>(x 4) | | | Start with a low dose and titrate to response in severe liver disease. | 233 |
| | C | 7<br>(8) | CL/F:<br>8.04 ± 6.7*<br>(97.0 ± 37.2) | | | 38 ± 8<br>(44 ± 6) | | | 234 |

[Continued over]

For footnotes, see final page of table (p. 1785)

**Table II.** *[Continued]*

| Drug | Disease | No. of patients | Pharmacokinetic parameters in hepatic disease[a] CL[b] (L/h) | Vd[c] (L) | $t_{½}$ (h) | $f_u$ (%) | F (%) | Dose adjustment/ comments | References |
|---|---|---|---|---|---|---|---|---|---|
| **Diuretics** *[continued]* | | | | | | | | | |
| Triamterene<br>*[continued]* | C | 6<br>(7) | CL/F:<br>20.5 ± 17.5[§]<br>(220.2 ± 105.4) | | | | | [§] Low CL/F in cirrhosis as well as decrease in response to drug in some patients | 235 |
| **Lipid-lowering drugs** | | | | | | | | | |
| Clofibrate | AVH<br>C | 6<br>6<br>(6) | CL/F:<br>0.40 ± 0.13<br>0.47 ± 0.16<br>(0.43 ± 0.12) | Vd/F:<br>11.9 ± 3.5†<br>14.0 ± 2.1*<br>(9.8 ± 1.4) | 20.9 ± 5.9<br>19.3 ± 6.6<br>(17.5 ± 4.3) | 2.8<br>7.2*<br>(2.8) | | Unchanged | 236 |
| Gemfibrozil | C | 8<br>(6) | | | 2.1<br>(1.5) | | | Insufficient information to make dosage recommendation | 237 |
| **Muscle relaxants, skeletal** | | | | | | | | | |
| Atracurium besilate | LF | 6[§]<br>(6) | 27.3 ± 6.3<br>(22.3 ± 3.4) | 14.5 ± 3.4*[§§]<br>(11.1 ± 1.5) | 0.4 ± 0.1<br>(0.4 ± 0.03) | | | Unchanged.<br>[§] Patients also had renal failure.<br>[§§] Volume of distribution = $Vd_{area}$ | 238 |
| | CAH, PBC<br>ALD, C | 7<br>(7) | 33.6 ± 7.1*<br>(27.7 ± 5.0) | 19.7 ± 5.0*†<br>(14.1 ± 5.0) | | | | | 239 |
| Pancuronium bromide | C | 14<br>(12) | 6.1 ± 1.7*<br>(7.8 ± 1.7) | 29.1 ± 15.2*<br>(19.5 ± 3.6) | 3.5 ± 1.5*<br>(1.9 ± 0.6) | | | Use with caution in cirrhosis. Larger loading doses may be necessary.<br>Prolonged effects can be expected | 240, 241 |
| Mivacurium chloride | LD | 9<br>(9) | 2.0 ± 0.8*<br>(4.2 ± 1.7) | 8.7 ± 3.6‡<br>(7.8 ± 5.0) | | | | Reduce dose in end-stage liver disease | 242 |
| Vecuronium bromide | ALD | | 18.5 ± 3.8<br>(18.9 ± 8.4) | 15.4 ± 3.5‡<br>(12.6 ± 4.2) | 0.86 ± 0.21<br>(0.96 ± 0.30) | | | No dose adjustment necessary | 243 |
| **Miscellaneous drugs** | | | | | | | | | |
| Fazadinium | C<br>IC | 8<br>8<br>(11) | 7.8 ± 1.7<br>8.5 ± 2.7<br>(10.0 ± 4.3) | 31.4 ± 10.7*<br>24.5 ± 5.9<br>(20.1 ± 7.7) | 2.6 ± 0.9*<br>1.7 ± 0.4*<br>(1.4 ± 0.3) | | | Unchanged | 244 |
| Flumazenil | C | 8<br>(8) | 42.3 ± 21.2*<br>(72.1 ± 11.2) | 63.7 ± 18.9‡<br>(67.9 ± 13.3) | 1.4 ± 0.5*<br>(0.8 ± 0.2) | | 65.2 ± 25.7*<br>(27.8 ± 6.0) | No dose adjustment necessary for loading dose.<br>Reduce dose if repeated doses are necessary.<br>May induce seizures in alcoholic cirrhosis | 245 |
| | C-moderate<br>C-severe | 8<br>8<br>(8) | 29.6 ± 6.6*<br>19.0 ± 5.3*<br>(73.6 ± 11.2) | 49.39 ± 13.10*<br>62.30 ± 10.80*<br>(47.86 ± 12.37) | 1.26 ± 0.39*<br>2.36 ± 0.46*<br>(0.76 ± 0.14) | | | | 246 |
| Iloprost | C | 8 | 41.2 ± 20.2 | | 0.47 ± 0.40 | | | Reduce dose in cirrhosis | 247 |

**Miscellaneous drugs** *[continued]*

| | | | | | | | | | |
|---|---|---|---|---|---|---|---|---|---|
| Testosterone | C | 13<br>(9) | | | | | | Insufficient information to make dosage recommendation.<br>Increased oral AUC in cirrhosis | 248 |
| Xamoterol | LD | 6<br>(6) | 10.3 ± 4.4<br>(14.6 ± 4.1) | 65 ± 22<br>(60 ± 13) | 15.3 ± 6.4<br>(8.4 ± 2.8) | | 6.1 ± 4.1<br>(6.9 ± 3.4) | Some patients with liver disease may require a reduced dose.<br>Start with a low dose and titrate to response | 249 |

a Whenever possible, values are given as mean (± SD), or single mean or median values. In a few instances, ranges are given. Values in normal/control individuals are given in parentheses; * indicates values significantly different from normal individuals.

b Clearance (CL) values are all corrected for 70kg bodyweight. Values for clearance are total systemic plasma clearance ($CL_T$) unless otherwise indicated. **NB:** CL/F values have been given for studies which administered the drug only via a route other than intravenously. CL can only be estimated when the intravenous route has been used. Otherwise, an apparent CL value can be calculated which contains an inverse bioavailability factor (CL/F).

c Values for apparent volume of distribution (Vd) are corrected for 70kg bodyweight, and unless otherwise indicated, are derived assuming monoexponential plasma decay kinetics. † indicates values derived from the β-phase, and ‡ indicates values derived from the steady-state volume of distribution. **NB:** Vd/F values have been given for studies which administered the drug only via a route other than intravenously. Vd can only be estimated when the intravenous route has been used. Otherwise, an apparent Vd value can be calculated which contains an inverse bioavailability factor (Vd/F).

d Due to increased sensitivity, this agent should be used cautiously in patients with cirrhosis.

*Abbreviations:* Alb = serum albumin (g/dl); AH = acute hepatitis; ALD = alcoholic liver disease; AVH = acute viral hepatitis; C = cirrhosis; Ca = liver cancer; CAH = chronic active hepatitis; CL = clearance [total systemic plasma clearance ($CL_T$) unless otherwise indicated]; $CL_u$ = clearance based on the concentration of the unbound drug; $CL_R$ = renal clearance; $CL_H$ = hepatic (metabolic) clearance where $CL_R + CL_H = CL_T$; CL/F = oral clearance; CLD = chronic liver disease; CNS = central nervous system; CPH = chronic persistent hepatitis; DIH = drug-induced hepatitis; EM = extensive metaboliser; $f_u$ = free (unbound) fraction of drug in plasma; F = bioavailability (oral); FL = fatty liver; H = hepatitis; HE = hepatic encephalopathy; IC = intrahepatic cholestasis; LD = undefined liver disease; LF = liver failure; OJ = obstructive jaundice; PBC = primary biliary cirrhosis; PM = poor metaboliser; PO = oral; RF = renal failure; shunt = surgical portosystemic anastomosis; + = with; – = without; SL = sublingual; Vd = apparent volume of distribution; Vd/F = volume of distribution after oral administration; $Vd_{ss}$ = volume of distribution at steady-state; $Vd_{area}$ = volume of distribution (calculated from the area under the curve); $t_{1/2}$ = elimination half-life; IM = intramuscular; IV = intravenous.

## References


1. Kroemer HK, Klotz U. Glucuronidation of drugs: a re-evaluation of the pharmacological significance of the conjugates and modulating factors. Clinical Pharmacokinetics 1992; 23: 292-310
2. Gross V, Schölmerich J, Treher E, et al. Altered kinetics of cilazapril (Ro 31-2848) and cilazaprilat (Ro 31-3113) in patients with liver cirrhosis. Hepatology 1988; 8: 1382
3. Baba T, Murabayashi S, Tomiyama T, et al. The pharmacokinetics of enalapril in patients with compensated liver cirrhosis. British Journal of Clinical Pharmacology 1990; 29: 766-9
4. Ohnishi A, Tsuboi Y, Ishizaki T, et al. Kinetics and dynamics of enalapril in patients with liver cirrhosis. Clinical Pharmacology and Therapeutics 1989; 45: 657
5. Lejeune P, Desager JP, Meunier H, et al. Kinetics of a single dose combination of nifedipine/acebutolol in patients with chronic liver disease. International Journal of Clinical Pharmacology Therapy and Toxicology 1988; 26: 513-6
6. Kirch W, Schafer-Korting M, Mutschler E, et al. Clinical experience with atenolol in patients with chronic liver disease. Journal of Clinical Pharmacology 1983; 23: 171
7. Hayes PC, Jenkins D, Vavianos P, et al. Single oral dose pharmacokinetics of bisoprolol 10mg in liver disease. European Heart Journal 1987; 8 Suppl. M: 23-9
8. Kirch W, Rose I, Demers HG, et al. Pharmacokinetics of bisoprolol during repeated oral administration to healthy volunteers and patients with kidney or liver disease. Clinical Pharmacokinetics 1987; 13: 110-7
9. Wensing G, Branch RA, Humbert H, et al. Pharmacokinetics after a single oral dose of bopindolol in patients with cirrhosis. European Journal of Clinical Pharmacology 1990; 39: 569-72
10. Dubruc C, Bianchetti G, Mondini L, et al. Influence of hepatic and renal insufficiency on the pharmacokinetic profile of cicloprolol. European Journal of Drug Metabolism and Pharmacokinetics 1990; 15: 44
11. Buchi KN, Rollins DE, Tolman KG, et al. Pharmacokinetics of esmolol in hepatic disease. Journal of Clinical Pharmacology 1987; 27: 880-4
12. Homeida M, Jackson L, Roberts CJC. Decreased first-pass metabolism of labetalol in chronic liver disease. British Medical Journal 1978; 2: 1048
13. Regårdh CG, Jordo L, Ervik M, et al. Pharmacokinetics of metoprolol in patients with hepatic cirrhosis. Clinical Pharmacokinetics 1981; 6: 375
14. Branch RA, Kornhauser DM, Shand DG, et al. Biological determinants of propranolol disposition in normal subjects and patients with cirrhosis. British Journal of Clinical Pharmacology 1977; 4: 630P
15. Wood AJJ, Kornhauser DM, Wilkinson GR, et al. The influence of cirrhosis on steady-state blood concentrations of unbound propranolol after oral administration. Clinical Pharmacokinetics 1978; 3: 478-87
16. Watson RGP, Bastain W, Larkin KA, et al. A comparative pharmacokinetic study of conventional propranolol and a long acting preparation of propranolol in patients with cirrhosis and normal controls. British Journal of Clinical Pharmacology 1987; 24: 527
17. Carlos R, Calvo R, Erill S. Plasma protein binding of etomidate in patients with renal failure or hepatic cirrhosis. Clinical Pharmacokinetics 1979; 4: 144-8
18. Richter E, Gallenkamp H, Heusler H, et al. Plasma clearance von methohexital bei akuter hepatitis. Medizinische Klinik 1980; 74: 1584
19. Duvaldestin P, Chauvin M, Lebrault C, et al. Effect of upper abdominal surgery and cirrhosis upon the pharmacokinetics of methohexital. Acta Anaesthesiologica Scandinavica 1991; 35: 159-63
20. Servin F, Desmonts JM, Haberer JP, et al. Pharmacokinetics and protein binding of propofol in patients with cirrhosis. Anesthesiology 1988; 67: 887-91
21. Pandele G, Chaux F, Salvadori C, et al. Thiopental pharmacokinetics in patients with cirrhois. Anesthesiology 1983; 59: 123
22. Roberts MS, Rumble RH, Wanwimolruk S, et al. Pharmacokinetics of aspirin and salicylate in elderly subjects and in patients with alcoholic liver disease. European Journal of Clinical Pharmacology 1983; 25: 253
23. Forrest JAH, Finlayson NDC, Adjepon-Yamoah KK, et al. Antipyrine, paracetamol, and lignocaine elimination in chronic liver disease. British Medical Journal 1977; 1: 1384
24. Arnman R, Olsson R. Elimination of paracetamol in chronic liver disease. Acta Hepato-Gastroenterologica 1978; 25: 283
25. Andreasen PB, Hutters L. Paracetamol (acetaminophen) clearance in patients with cirrhosis of the liver. Acta Medica Scandinavica 1979; Suppl. 624: 99
26. Benson GD. Acetaminophen in chronic liver disease. Clinical Pharmacology and Therapeutics 1983; 33: 95
27. Villeneuve JP, Raymond G, Bruneau J, et al. Pharmacocinetique et metabolisme de l'acetaminophene chez des sujets normaux, alcoholiques et cirrhotiques. Gastroenterologie Clinique et Biologique 1983; 7: 898
28. Jorup-Ronstrom C, Beermann B, Wahlin-Boll E, et al. Reduction of paracetamol and aspirin metabolism during viral hepatitis. Clinical Pharmacokinetics 1986; 11: 250-6
29. Lasseter K, Shamblen E, Murdoch A, et al. Pharmacokinetics of etodolac in patients with hepatic cirrhosis. Journal of Clinical Pharmacology 1988; 28: 933
30. Juhl RP, Van Theil DH, Dittert LW, et al. Ibuprofen and sulindac kinetics in alcoholic liver disease. Clinical Pharmacology and Therapeutics 1983; 34: 104
31. Li G, Treiber G, Maier K, et al. Disposition of ibuprofen in patients with liver cirrhosis: stereochemical considerations. Clinical Pharmacokinetics 1993; 25: 154-63
32. Tkaczewski W, Adamska-Dyniewska H, Bozenna G, et al. Farmakokinetyka kwazu mefenaminowego u chorych z marskocia watroby. Polski Tygodnik Lekarski 1978; 33: 1997
33. Calvo MV, Dominquez-Gil A, Macias JG, et al. Naproxen disposition in hepatic and biliary disorders. International Journal of Clinical Pharmacology Therapy and Toxicology 1980; 18: 242-6
34. Williams RL, Upton RA, Cello JP, et al. Naproxen disposition in patients with alcoholic cirrhosis. European Journal of Clinical Pharmacology 1984; 27: 291
35. Hvidberg EF, Andreasen PB, Ranek L. Plasma half-life of phenylbutazone in patients with impaired liver function. Clinical Pharmacology and Therapeutics 1973; 15: 171
36. Adithan C, Shashindran CH, Gandhi IS, et al. Pharmacokinetics of phenylbutazone in chronic liver disease. Indian Journal of Medical Research 1980; 71: 316
37. Crevoisier CH, Zaugg PY, Heizmann P, et al. Influence of liver cirrhosis upon the pharmacokinetics of tenoxicam. International Journal of Clinical Pharmacology Research 1989; 9: 327-4
38. Giacomini KM, Giacomini JC, Gibson TP, et al. Propoxyphene in cirrhotic patients with and without sur-

gically constructed portacaval shunt. Clinical Pharmacology and Therapeutics 1980; 28: 417

39. Haberer JP, Schoeffler P, Couderc E, et al. Fentanyl pharmacokinetics in anaesthetized patients with cirrhosis. British Journal of Anaesthesia 1982; 54: 1267
40. Novick DM, Kreek MJ, Fanizza AM, et al. Methadone disposition in patients with chronic liver disease. Clinical Pharmacology and Therapeutics 1981; 30: 353
41. Mazoit J-X, Sandouk P, Zetlaoui P, et al. Pharmacokinetics of unchanged morphine in normal and cirrhotic subjects. Anesthesia and Analgesia 1987; 66: 293-8
42. Hasselström J, Eriksson S, Persson A, et al. The metabolism and bioavailability of morphine in patients with severe liver cirrhosis. British Journal of Clinical Pharmacology 1990; 29: 289-97
43. Patwardhan RV, Johnson RF, Hoyumpa A, et al. Normal metabolism of morphine in cirrhosis. Gastroenterology 1981; 81: 1006
44. Pond SM, Tong T, Benowitz NL, et al. Enhanced bioavailability of pethidine and pentazocine in patients with cirrhosis of the liver. Australian and New Zealand Journal of Medicine 1980; 10: 515
45. Neal EA, Meffin PJ, Gregory PB, et al. Enhanced bioavailability and decreased clearance of analgesics in patients with cirrhosis. Gastroenterology 1979; 77: 96
46. McHorse TS, Wilkinson GR, Johnson RF, et al. Effect of acute viral hepatitis in man on the disposition and elimination of meperidine. Gastroenterology 1975; 68: 775
47. Klotz U, McHorse TS, Wilkinson GR, et al. The effect of cirrhosis on the disposition and elimination of meperidine in man. Clinical Pharmacology and Therapeutics 1974; 16: 667
48. Pond SM, Tong T, Benowitz NL, et al. Presystemic metabolism of meperidine to normeperidine in normal and cirrhotic subjects. Clinical Pharmacology and Therapeutics 1981; 30: 193
49. Chauvin M, Ferrier C, Haberer JP, et al. Sufentanil pharmacokinetics in patients with cirrhosis. Anesthesia and Analgesia 1989; 68: 1-4
50. Lee CR, McTavish D, Sorkin EM. Tramadol: a preliminary review of its pharmacodynamic and pharmacokinetic properties and therapeutic potential in acute and chronic pain states. Drugs 1993; 46: 313-40
51. Steudel HC, Volkenandt M, Steudel AT. Pharmacokinetics of isosorbide-5-mononitrate after oral and intravenous administration in patients with liver cirrhosis: first results. Zeitschrift fur Kardiologie 1983; Suppl. 3: 24
52. Jungbluth GL, Della-Coletta AA, Blum RA, et al. Comparative pharmacokinetics (PK) and bioavailability of nicorandil (NIC) in subjects with stabilized cirrhosis and matched healthy volunteers. Clinical Pharmacology and Therapeutics 1991; 49: 181
53. Mawer GE, Miller NE, Turnberg LA. Metabolism of amylobarbitone in patients with chronic liver disease. British Journal of Pharmacology 1972; 44: 549-60
54. Breyer-Pfaff U, Seyfert H, Weber M, et al. Assessment of drug metabolism in hepatic disease: comparison of plasma kinetics of oral cyclobarbital and the intravenous aminopyrine breath test. European Journal of Clinical Pharmacology 1984; 26: 95
55. Breimer DD, Zilly W, Richter E. Pharmacokinetics of hexobarbital in acute hepatitis and after apparent recovery. Clinical Pharmacology and Therapeutics 1975; 18: 433
56. Zilly W, Breimer DD, Richter E. Hexobarbital disposition in compensated and decompensated cirrhosis of the liver. Clinical Pharmacology and Therapeutics 1978; 23: 525
57. Juhl RP, Van Theil DH, Dittert LW, et al. Alprazolam pharmacokinetics in alcoholic liver disease. Journal of Clinical Pharmacology 1984; 24: 113-9
58. Jochemsen R, Joeres RP, Wesselman JGJ, et al. Pharmacokinetics of oral brotizolam in patients with liver cirrhosis. British Journal of Clinical Pharmacology 1983; 16: 315S
59. Roberts RK, Wilkinson GR, Branch RA, et al. Effect of age and parenchymal liver disease on the disposition and elimination of chlordiazepoxide. Gastroenterology 1978; 75: 479
60. Sellers EM, Greenblatt DJ, Giles HG, et al. Chlordiazepoxide and oxazepam disposition in cirrhosis. Clinical Pharmacology and Therapeutics 1979; 26: 240
61. Morgan DD, Robinson JD, Mendenhall CL. Clinical pharmacokinetics of chlordiazepoxide in patients with alcoholic hepatitis. European Journal of Clinical Pharmacology 1981; 19: 279
62. Ochs HR, Greenblatt JD, Knuchel M. Effect of cirrhosis and renal failure on the kinetics of clotiazepam. European Journal of Clinical Pharmacology 1986; 30: 89-92
63. Klotz U, Avant GR, Hoyumpa A, et al. The effects of age and liver disease on the disposition and elimination of diazepam in adult man. Journal of Clinical Investigation 1975; 55: 347
64. Branch RA, Morgan MH, James J, et al. Intravenous administration of diazepam in patients with chronic liver disease. Gut 1976; 17: 975-83
65. Hepner GW, Vesell ES, Lipton A, et al. Disposition of aminopyrine, antipyrine, diazepam, and indocyanine green in patients with liver disease or on anticonvulsant drug therapy: diazepam breath test and correlations in drug elimination. Journal of Laboratory and Clinical Medicine 1977; 90: 440
66. Klotz U, Antonin KH, Brugel H, et al. Disposition of diazepam and its major metabolite desmethyldiazepam in patients with liver disease. Clinical Pharmacology and Therapeutics 1977; 21: 430
67. Greenblatt DJ, Harmatz JS, Shader RI, et al. Factors influencing diazepam pharmacokinetics: age, sex and liver disease. International Journal of Clinical Pharmacology Research 1978; 16: 177
68. Kraus JW, Desmond PV, Marshall JP, et al. Effects of aging and liver disease on disposition of lorazepam. Clinical Pharmacology and Therapeutics 1978; 24: 411
69. MacGilchrist AJ, Birnie GG, Cook A, et al. Pharmacokinetics and pharmacodynamics of intravenous midazolam in patients with severe alcoholic cirrhosis. Gut 1986; 27: 190-5
70. Pentikäinen PJ, Välisalmi L, Himberg J-J, et al. Pharmacokinetics of midazolam following intravenous and oral administration in patients with chronic liver disease and in healthy subjects. Journal of Clinical Pharmacology 1989; 29: 272-7
71. Trouvin J-H, Farinotti R, Haberer J-P, et al. Pharmacokinetics of midazolam in anaesthetized cirrhotic patients. British Journal of Anaesthesia 1988; 60: 762-
72. Jochemsen R, Van Beusekon BR, Spoelstra P, et al. Effect of age and liver cirrhosis on the pharmacokinetics of nitrazepam. British Journal of Clinical Pharmacology 1983; 15: 295
73. Shull HJ, Wilkinson GR, Johnson R, et al. Normal disposition of oxazepam in acute viral hepatitis and cirrhosis. Annals of Internal Medicine 1976; 84: 420

74. Ghabrial H, Desmond PV, Watson KJR, et al. The effects of age and chronic liver disease on the elimination of temazepam. European Journal of Clinical Pharmacology 1986; 30: 93-7
75. Bakti G, Fisch HU, Karlaganis G, et al. Mechanism of the excessive sedative response of cirrhotics to benzodiazepines: model experiments with triazolam. Hepatology 1987; 7: 629-38
76. Kroboth PD, Smith RB, Van Thiel DH, et al. Nighttime dosing of triazolam in patients with liver disease and normal subjects: kinetics and daytime effects. Journal of Clinical Pharmacology 1987; 27: 555-60
77. Robin DW, Lee M, Hasan SS, et al. Triazolam in cirrhosis: pharmacokinetics and pharmacodynamics. Clinical Pharmacology and Therapeutics 1993; 54: 630-7
78. Pentikäinen PJ, Neuvonen PJ, Jotell KG. Pharmacokinetics of chlormethiazole in healthy volunteers and patients with cirrhosis of the liver. European Journal of Pharmacology 1980; 17: 275
79. Bianchetti G, Dubruc C, Thiercelin JF, et al., editors. Clinical pharmacokinetics of zolpidem in various physiological and pathological conditions, imidazopyridines in sleep disorders. New York: Raven Press, 1988
80. Pacifici GM, Viani A, Rizzo G, et al. Plasma protein binding of zolpidem in liver and renal insufficiency. International Journal of Clinical Pharmacology Therapy and Toxicology 1988; 26: 439-
81. Parker G, Roberts CJC. Plasma concentrations and central nervous system effects of the new hypnotic agent zopiclone in patients with chronic liver disease. British Journal of Clinical Pharmacology 1983; 16: 259
82. Bergstrand RH, Wang T, Roden DM, et al. Encainide disposition in patients with chronic cirrhosis. Clinical Pharmacology and Therapeutics 1986; 40: 148-54
83. Wensing G, Mönig H, Ohnhaus EE, et al. Pharmacokinetics of encainide in patients with cirrhosis. Cardiovascular Drugs and Therapy 1991; 5: 733-40
84. Williams RL, Blaschke TF, Meffin PJ, et al. Influence of viral hepatitis on the disposition of two compounds with high hepatic clearance: lidocaine and indocyanine green. Clinical Pharmacology and Therapeutics 1976; 20: 290
85. Thomson PD, Melmon KL, Richardson JA, et al. Lidocaine pharmacokinetics in advanced heart failure, liver disease, and renal failure in humans. Annals of Internal Medicine 1973; 78: 499
86. Huet PM, Lelorier J. Effects of smoking and chronic hepatitis B on lidocaine and indocyanine green kinetics. Clinical Pharmacology and Therapeutics 1980; 28: 208
87. Villeneuve JP, Thibeault MJ, Ampelas M, et al. Drug disposition in patients with HBsAg-positive chronic liver disease. Digestive Diseases and Sciences 1987; 32: 710-4
88. Testa R, Borzone S, Risso D, et al. Formation kinetics of the lidocaine metabolite (MEGX) in patients with chronic active hepatitis and cirrhosis. European Journal of Gastroenterology and Hepatology 1993; 5: 845-51
89. Klotz U, Fischer C, Muller-Seydlitz P, et al. Alterations in the disposition of differently cleared drugs in patients with cirrhosis. Clinical Pharmacology and Therapeutics 1979; 26: 221
90. Pentikäinen PJ, Hietakorpi S, Halinen MO, et al. Cirrhosis of the liver markedly impairs the elimination of mexiletine. European Journal of Clinical Pharmacology 1986; 30: 83
91. Pieniaszek HJ, McEntegart CM, Davidson AF, et al. Moricizine pharmacokinetics in patients with hepatic cirrhosis. Journal of Clinical Pharmacology 1991; 31: 864
92. Lee JT, Yee Y-G, Dorian P, et al. Influence of hepatic dysfunction on the pharmacokinetics of propafenone. Journal of Clinical Pharmacology 1987; 27: 384-9
93. Powell JR, Okada R, Conrad KA, et al. Altered quinidine disposition in a patient with chronic active hepatitis. Postgraduate Medical Journal 1982; 58: 82
94. Kessler KM, Humphries WC, Black M, et al. Quinidine pharmacokinetics in patients with cirrhosis or receiving propranolol. American Heart Journal 1978; 96: 627
95. Debruyne D, Gram LF, Grollier G, et al. Quinidine disposition in relation to antipyrine elimination and debrisoquine phenotype in alcoholic patients with and without cirrhosis. International Journal of Clinical Pharmacology Research 1989; 9: 319-25
96. Oltmanns D, Pottage A, Endell W. Pharmacokinetics of tocainide in patients with combined hepatic and renal dysfunction. European Journal of Clinical Pharmacology 1983; 25: 787-90
97. Lanao JM, Dominguez-Gil A, Macias JG, et al. The influence of ascites on the pharmacokinetics of amikacin. International Journal of Clinical Pharmacology Therapy and Toxicology 1980; 18: 57
98. Petitjean A, Astier A, Louchahi M, et al. Pharmacocinetique de la gentamicine chez le cirrhotique decompense consequences therapeutiques. Pathologie Biologie 1983; 31: 399
99. Hayton WL, Kneer S, Blouin RA, et al. Pharmacokinetics of intravenous cefetamet and oral cefetamet pivoxil in patients with hepatic cirrhosis. Antimicrobial Agents and Chemotherapy 1990; 34: 1318-22
100. El Touny M, El Guinaidy MA, Abdel Barry M, et al. Pharmacokinetics of cefodizime in patients with liver cirrhosis and ascites. Chemotherapy 1992; 38: 201-5
101. Cochet B, Belaieff J, Allaz AF, et al. Decreased extrarenal clearance of cefoperazone in hepatocellular diseases. British Journal of Clinical Pharmacology 1981; 11: 389
102. Boscia JA, Korzeniowdki OM, Snepar R, et al. Cefoperazone pharmacokinetics in normal subjects and patients with cirrhosis. Antimicrobial Agents and Chemotherapy 1983; 23: 385
103. Saudek F, Moravek J, Modr Z. Cefoperazone pharmacokinetics in patients with liver cirrhosis: a predictive value of the ujoviridin test. International Journal of Clinical Pharmacology Therapy and Toxicology 1989; 27: 82-7
104. Höffken G, Lode H, Koeppe P, et al. Pharmacokinetics of cefotaxime and desacetyl-cefotaxime in cirrhosis of the liver. Chemotherapy 1984; 30: 7
105. Vincent P, Colombel JF, Husson MO, et al. Pharmacokinetics of cefotaxime in cirrhotic patients with or without ascites. Presse Medicale 1988; 17: 2331-4
106. Ko RJ, Sattler FR, Nichols S, et al. Pharmacokinetics of cefotaxime and desacetylcefotaxime in patients with liver disease. Antimicrobial Agents and Chemotherapy 1991; 35: 1376-80
107. Hary L, Andrejak M, Leleu S, et al. The pharmacokinetics of ceftriaxone and cefotaxime in cirrhotic patients with ascites. European Journal of Clinical Pharmacology 1989; 36: 613-
108. Shyu WC, Wilber RB, Pittman KA, et al. Pharmacokinetics of cefprozil in healthy subjects and patients with hepatic impairment. Journal of Clinical Pharmacology 1991; 31: 372-6

109. Walstad RA, Wiig JN, Thurmann-Nielsen E, et al. Pharmacokinetics of ceftazidime in patients with biliary tract disease. European Journal of Clinical Pharmacology 1986; 31: 327
110. Pasko MT, Beam TR, Spooner JA, et al. Safety and pharmacokinetics of ceftazidime in patients with chronic hepatic dysfunction. Journal of Antimicrobial Chemotherapy 1985; 15: 365-74
111. El Touny M, El Guinaidy MA, Abdel Barry M, et al. Pharmacokinetics of ceftazidime in patients with liver cirrhosis and ascites. Journal of Antimicrobial Chemotherapy 1991; 28: 95-100
112. Stoeckel K, Koup JR. Pharmacokinetics of ceftriaxone in patients with renal and liver insufficiency and correlations with a physiologic nonlinear protein binding model. American Journal of Medicine 1984; 77 (4c): 26
113. Okolicsanyi L, Venuti M, Orlando R, et al. Pharmacokinetic studies of cefuroxime in patients with liver cirrhosis. Arzneimittel Forschung 1982; 32: 777
114. Frost RW, Lettieri JT, Krol G, et al. The effect of cirrhosis on the steady-state pharmacokinetics of oral ciprofloxacin. Clinical Pharmacology and Therapeutics 1989; 45: 608-16
115. Miglioli PA, Palatini P, Orlando R, et al. Evaluation of ciprofloxacin and ofloxacin pharmacokinetics in liver cirrhosis. Drugs 1993; 45 Suppl. 3: 270
116. Blouin RA, Hamelin BA, Smith DA, et al. Fleroxacin pharmacokinetics in patients with liver cirrhosis. Antimicrobial Agents and Chemotherapy 1992; 36: 632-8
117. Eandi M, Viano I, De Nola F, et al. Pharmacokinetics of norfloxacin in healthy volunteers and patients with renal and hepatic damage. European Journal of Clinical Microbiology and Infectious Diseases 1983; 2: 253-9
118. Silvain C, Bouquet S, Breux JP, et al. Oral pharmacokinetics and ascitic fluid penetration of ofloxacin in cirrhosis. European Journal of Clinical Pharmacology 1989; 37: 261-5
119. Cardey J, Silvain C, Bouquet S, et al. Oral pharmacokinetics and ascitic fluid penetration of pefloxacin in cirrhosis. European Journal of Clinical Pharmacology 1987; 33: 469-72
120. Galtier M, Bressolle F, de la Coussaye J-E, et al. Multiple-dose pharmacokinetics of pefloxacin in patients with hepatocellular deficiency. Clinical Pharmacokinetics 1993; 25: 415-23
121. Danan G, Montay G, Cunci R, et al. Pefloxacin kinetics in cirrhosis. Clinical Pharmacology and Therapeutics 1985; 38: 439-2
122. Triger DR, Granai F, Woodcock J, et al. Multiple-dose pharmacokinetics of rufloxacin in patients with cirrhosis. Hepatology 1993; 18: 847-52
123. Mazzei T, Surrenti C, Novelli A, et al. Pharmacokinetics of azithromycin in patients with impaired hepatic function. Journal of Antimicrobial Chemotherapy 1993; 31: 57-63
124. Hall KW, Nightingale CH, Gibaldi M, et al. Pharmacokinetics of erythromycin in normal and alcoholic liver disease subjects. Journal of Clinical Pharmacology 1982; 22: 321
125. Barre J, Mallat A, Rosenbaum J, et al. Pharmacokinetics of erythromycin in patients with severe cirrhosis. Respective influence of decreased serum binding and impaired liver metabolic capacity. British Journal of Clinical Pharmacology 1987; 23: 753
126. Miglioli PA, Pivetta P, Orlando R, et al. Pharmacokinetics of miocamycin in patients with liver cirrhosis. Chemotherapy 1989; 35: 330-2
127. Orlando R, Fragasso A, Benvenuti C, et al. Pharmacokinetics of rokitamycin after single and repeated dose oral administration to patients with liver cirrhosis. Drug Investigation 1991; 3: 162-6
128. Lebrec D, Benhamou JP, Fourtillan JB, et al. Roxithromycin: pharmacokinetics in patients suffering from alcoholic cirrhosis. British Journal of Clinical Practice 1987; 41: 63
129. Lewis GP, Jusko WJ. Pharmacokinetics of ampicillin in cirrhosis. Clinical Pharmacology and Therapeutics 1975; 18: 475
130. Chalas J, Labayle D, Macarrio J, et al. Metabolisme et cinetique de l'elimination de l'ampicilline dans la cirrhose. Semaine des Hôpitaux de Paris 1980; 56: 464
131. Hoffman TA, Cestero R, Bullock WE. Pharmacodynamics of carbenicillin in hepatic and renal failure. Annals of Internal Medicine 1970; 73: 173
132. Bunke CM, Aronoff GR, Brier ME, et al. Mezlocillin kinetics in hepatic insufficiency. Clinical Pharmacology and Therapeutics 1983; 33: 73
133. Marshall JP, Salt WB, Elam RO, et al. Disposition of nafcillin in patients with cirrhosis and extrahepatic biliary obstruction. Gastroenterology 1977; 73: 1388
134. MacLeod CM, Bartley EA, Payne JA, et al. Effects of cirrhosis on kinetics of aztreonam. Antimicrobial Agents and Chemotherapy 1984; 26: 493
135. Stockis H, Borzio F, Deroubaix X, et al. Pharmacokinetics of brodimoprim in special populations. Journal of Chemotherapy 1993; 5: 480-7
136. Narang APS, Datta DV, Nath N, et al. Pharmacokinetic study of chloramphenicol in patients with liver disease. European Journal of Clinical Pharmacology 1981; 20: 479
137. Hinthorn DR, Baker LH, Romig DA, et al. Use of clindamycin in patients with liver disease. Antimicrobial Agents and Chemotherapy 1976; 9: 498
138. Daneshmend T, Homeida M, Kaye CM, et al. Disposition of oral metronidazole in hepatic cirrhosis and in hepatosplenic schistosomiasis. Gut 1982; 23: 807
139. Farrell G, Baird-Lambert J, Cvejic M, et al. Disposition and metabolism of metronidazole in patients with liver failure. Hepatology 1984; 4: 722-6
140. Loft S, Sonne J, Dossing M, et al. Metronidazole pharmacokinetics in patients with hepatic encephalopathy. Scandinavian Journal of Gastroenterology 1987; 22: 117-23
141. Lau AH, Evans R, Chang C-W, et al. Pharmacokinetics of metronidazole in patients with alcoholic liver disease. Antimicrobial Agents and Chemotherapy 1987; 31: 1662-4
142. Taburet AM, Attali P, Bourget P, et al. Pharmacokinetics of ornidazole in patients with acute viral hepatitis, alcoholic cirrhosis, and extrahepatic cholestasis. Clinical Pharmacology and Therapeutics 1989; 45: 373-9
143. Brown N, Ho DHW, Fong KLL, et al. Effect of hepatic function on vancomycin clinical pharmacology. Antimicrobial Agents and Chemotherapy 1983; 23: 603
144. Teien AN. Heparin elimination in patients with liver cirrhosis. Thrombosis and Hemostasis 1977; 38: 701
145. Kliesch WF, Young PC, Davis WD. Dangers of prolonged anticoagulant therapy in hepatic disease. Journal of the American Medical Association 1960; 172: 103
146. Kitteringham NR, Bustgens L, Brundert E, et al. The effect of liver cirrhosis on the pharmacokinetics of phenprocoumon. European Journal of Clinical Pharmacology 1984; 26: 65

147. Williams RL, Schary WL, Blaschke TF, et al. Influence of acute viral hepatitis on disposition and pharmacologic effect of warfarin. Clinical Pharmacology and Therapeutics 1976; 20: 90
148. Hdrina PD, Lapierre YD, Koranyi EK. Altered amitriptyline kinetics in a depressed patient with porto-caval anastamosis. Canadian Journal of Psychiatry 1985; 30: 111
149. Schenker S, Bergstrom RF, Wolen RL, et al. Fluoxetine disposition and elimination in cirrhosis. Clinical Pharmacology and Therapeutics 1988; 44: 353-9
150. van Harten J, Duchier J, Devissaguet J-P, et al. Pharmacokinetics of fluvoxamine maleate in patients with liver cirrhosis after single-dose oral administration. Clinical Pharmacokinetics 1993; 24: 177-82
151. Stoeckel K, Pfefen JP, Mayersohn M, et al. Absorption and disposition of moclobemide in patients with advanced age or reduced liver or kidney function. Acta Psychiatrica Scandinavica 1990; 82: 94-7
152. Dalhoff K, Almdal TP, Bjerrum K, et al. Pharmacokinetics of paroxetine in patients with cirrhosis. European Journal of Clinical Pharmacology 1991; 41: 351-4
153. Morgan MH, Read AE. Antidepressants and liver disease. Gut 1972; 13: 697
154. Ueda H, Sakurai T, Ota M, et al. Disappearance rate of tolbutamide in normal subjects and in diabetes mellitus, liver cirrhosis, and renal disease. Diabetes 1963; 12: 414
155. Williams RL, Blaschke TF, Meffin PJ, et al. Influence of acute viral hepatitis on disposition and plasma binding of tolbutamide. Clinical Pharmacology and Therapeutics 1977; 21: 301
156. Blake JC, Palmer JL, Minton NA, et al. Pharmacokinetics of intravenous ondansetron in patients with hepatic impairment. British Journal of Clinical Pharmacology 1993; 35: 441-3
157. Alvin J, McHorse T, Hoyumpa A, et al. The effect of liver disease in man on the disposition of phenobarbital. Journal of Pharmacology and Experimental Therapeutics 1975; 192: 224
158. Blaschke TF, Meffin PJ, Melman KL, et al. Influence of acute viral hepatitis on phenytoin kinetics and protein binding. Clinical Pharmacology and Therapeutics 1975; 17: 685
159. Kutt H, Winters W, Scherman R, et al. Diphenylhydantoin and phenobarbital toxicity. The role of liver disease. Archives of Neurology 1964; 11: 649
160. Pisani F, Perucca E, Primerano G, et al. Single-dose kinetics of primidone in acute viral hepatitis. European Journal of Clinical Pharmacology 1984; 27: 465
161. Klotz U, Rapp T, Muller WA, et al. Disposition of valproic acid in patients with liver disease. European Journal of Clinical Pharmacology 1978; 13: 55
162. Horsmans Y, Desager JP, Hulhoven R, et al. Single-dose pharmacokinetics of cetirizine in patients with chronic liver disease. Journal of Clinical Pharmacology 1993; 33: 929-32
163. Simons FER, Watson WTA, Minuk GY, et al. Cetirizine pharmacokinetics and pharmacodynamics in primary biliary cirrhosis. Journal of Clinical Pharmacology 1993; 33: 949-54
164. Meredith CG, Christian DC, Johnson RF, et al. Diphenhydramine disposition in chronic liver disease. Clinical Pharmacology and Therapeutics 1984; 35: 474
165. Simons FER, Watson WTA, Chen XY, et al. The pharmacokinetics and pharmacodynamics of hydroxyzine in patients with primary biliary-cirrhosis. Journal of Clinical Pharmacology 1989; 29: 809-15
166. Lebrec D, Hadengue A, Gaudin C, et al. Pharmacokinetics of ketanserin in patients with cirrhosis. Clinical Pharmacokinetics 1990; 19: 160-6
167. Juma FD. Effect of liver disease on the pharmacokinetics of cyclophosphamide. European Journal of Clinical Pharmacology 1984; 26: 591
168. Yee GC, Kennedy MS, Storb R, et al. Effect of hepatic dysfunction on oral cyclosporine pharmacokinetics in marrow transplant patients. Blood 1984; 64: 1277
169. Stewart CF, Arbuck SG, Fleming RA, et al. Changes in the clearance of total and unbound etoposide in patients with liver dysfunction. Journal of Clinical Oncology 1990; 8: 1874-9
170. Hande KR, Wolff SN, Greco FA, et al. Etoposide kinetics in patients with obstructive jaundice. Journal of Clinical Oncology 1990; 8: 1101-7
171. Maxwell JD, Carrella M, Parkes JD, et al. Plasma disappearance and cerebral effects of chlorpromazine in cirrhosis. Clinical Science 1972; 43: 143
172. Held H, Fried F. Elimination of para-aminosalicylic acid in patients with liver disease and renal insufficiency. Chemotherapy 1977; 23: 405
173. Acocella F, Bonnollo L, Garimoldi M, et al. Kinetics of rifampicin and isoniazid administered alone and in combination to normal subjects and patients with liver disease. Gut 1972; 13: 47
174. Benedetti MS, Edwards DMF, Poggesi I, et al. Pharmacokinetics of rifabutin in hepatic insufficiency. 9th International Conference on AIDS 1993: 501
175. Schentag JJ, Cerra FB, Calleri BM, et al. Age, disease, and cimetidine disposition in healthy subjects and chronically ill patients. Clinical Pharmacology and Therapeutics 1981; 29: 737
176. Sonne J, Poulsen HE, Dossing M, et al. Cimetidine clearance in hepatic cirrhosis. Clinical Pharmacology and Therapeutics 1981; 29: 191
177. Gugler R, Muller-Liebenau B, Somogyi A. Altered disposition and availability of cimetidine in liver cirrhotic patients. British Journal of Clinical Pharmacology 1982; 14: 421
178. Albin H, Couzigou P, Vincon G, et al. Pharmacocinetique de la cimetidine chez le cirrhotique ascitique. Gastroenterologie Clinique et Biologique 1983; 7: 251
179. Cello JP, Oie S. Cimetidine disposition in patients with Laennec's cirrhosis during multiple dosing therapy. European Journal of Clinical Pharmacology 1983; 25: 223
180. Ziemniak JA, Bernhard J, Schentag JJ. Hepatic encephalopathy and altered cimetidine kinetics. Clinical Pharmacology and Therapeutics 1983; 34: 375
181. Grahnen A, Jameson S, Loof L, et al. Pharmacokinetics of cimetidine in advance cirrhosis. European Journal of Clinical Pharmacology 1984; 26: 347
182. Villeneuve JP, Fortunet-Fouin H, Arsene D. Cimetidine kinetics and dynamics in patients with severe liver disease. Hepatology 1983; 3: 923
183. Yamasaki H, Arima T, Nagashima H. Pharmacokinetic studies of cimetidine in patients with liver disease. Gastroenterologia Japonica 1987; 22: 440-7
184. Ohnishi K. Effects of hepatic disease on the pharmacokinetics of famotidine and effects of famotidine on hepatic hemodynamics and peptic ulcer. Hepato-Gastroenterology 1990; 37: 6-10
185. Vincon G, Baldit C, Couzigou P, et al. Pharmacokinetics of famotidine in patients with cirrhosis and ascites.

European Journal of Clinical Pharmacology 1992; 43: 559-62

186. Delhotal-Landes B, Flouvat B, Duchier J, et al. Pharmacokinetics of lansoprazole in patients with renal or liver disease of varying severity. European Journal of Clinical Pharmacology 1993; 45: 367-71

187. Rinetti M, Regazzi MB, Villani P, et al. Pharmacokinetics of omeprazole in cirrhotic patients. Arzneimittel Forschung 1991; 41: 420-2

188. Andersson T, Olsson R, Regårdh C-G, et al. Pharmacokinetics of [$^{14}$C] omeprazole in patients with liver cirrhosis. Clinical Pharmacokinetics 1993; 24: 71-8

189. Krakamp B, Tanswell P, Leidig P, et al. Steady-state intravenous pharmacokinetics of pirenzepine in patients with hepatic insufficiency and combined renal and hepatic insufficiency. European Journal of Clinical Pharmacology 1989; 36: 71-3

190. Young CJ, Daneshmend TK, Roberts CJC. Effects of cirrhosis and ageing on the elimination and bioavailability of ranitidine. Gut 1982; 23: 819

191. Bretagne JF, Reymann JM, Tassou JJ, et al. Pharmacocinetique de la ranitidine par voie intravenineuse et son effet sur la secretion gastrique acide stimulee par la pentagastrine chez le cirrhotique. Gastroenterologie Clinique et Biologique 1983; 7: 355

192. Smith IL, Ziemniak JA, Bernhard H, et al. Ranitidine disposition and systemic availability in hepatic cirrhosis. Clinical Pharmacology and Therapeutics 1984; 35: 487

193. Gonzalez-Martin G, Paulos C, Veloso B, et al. Ranitidine disposition in severe hepatic cirrhosis. International Journal of Clinical Pharmacology Therapy and Toxicology 1987; 25: 139-42

194. Taburet A-M, Naveau S, Zorza G, et al. Pharmacokinetics of zidovudine in patients with liver cirrhosis. Clinical Pharmacology and Therapeutics 1990; 47: 731-9

195. Piafsky DM, Sitar DS, Rangno RE, et al. Theophylline disposition in patients with hepatic cirrhosis. New England Journal of Medicine 1977; 296: 1495

196. Mangione A, Imhoff TE, Lee RV, et al. Pharmacokinetics of theophylline in hepatic disease. Chest 1978; 73: 616

197. Staib AH, Schuppan D, Lissner R, et al. Pharmacokinetics and metabolism of theophylline in patients with liver disease. International Journal of Clinical Pharmacology Therapy and Toxicology 1980; 18: 500

198. Schellens JHM, Janssens AR, Van Der Wart JHF, et al. Relationship between the metabolism of antipyrine, hexobarbital and theophylline in patients with liver disease as assessed by a 'cocktail' approach. European Journal of Clinical Investigation 1989; 19: 472-9

199. Amodio P, Lauro S, Rondana M, et al. Theophylline pharmacokinetics and liver function indexes in chronic liver disease. Respiration 1991; 58: 106-1

200. Darnis F, Poupon R. Pharmacokinetics and safety of single oral doses of amlodipine in patients with and without hepatic impairment: an open study. International Journal of Clinical Pharmacology Research 1993; 13: 29-33

201. Kurosawa S, Kurosawa N, Owada E, et al. Pharmacokinetics of diltiazem in patients with liver cirrhosis. International Journal of Clinical Pharmacology Research 1990; 6: 311-8

202. Regårdh CG, Edgar B, Olsson R, et al. Pharmacokinetics of felodipine in patients with liver disease. European Journal of Clinical Pharmacology 1989; 36: 473-9

203. Kaim AAH, Farker K. Pharmacokinetics and pharmacodynamics of gallopamil in patients with liver cirrhosis. Naunyn-Schmiedebergs Archives of Pharmacology 1992; 345: R9

204. Cotting J, Reichen J, Kutz K, et al. Pharmacokinetics of isradipine in patients with chronic liver disease. European Journal of Clinical Pharmacology 1990; 38: 599-603

205. D'Heygere F, Ling T, Waddell G, et al. Evaluation of steady state plasma levels of nicardipine hydrochloride in patients with impaired liver function. British Journal of Clinical Pharmacology 1988; 25: 96P

206. Salazar TA, Chang MM, McEntegart C, et al. Pharmacokinetics of intravenous nicardipine in patients with hepatic cirrhosis or renal failure. Clinical Pharmacology and Therapeutics 1992; 51: 132

207. Razak TA, McNeil JJ, Sewell RB, et al. The effect of hepatic cirrhosis on the pharmacokinetics and blood pressure response to nicardipine. Clinical Pharmacology and Therapeutics 1990; 47: 463-9

208. Kleinbloesem CH, van Harten J, Wilson JPH, et al. Nifedipine: kinetics and hemodynamic effects in patients with liver cirrhosis after intravenous and oral administration. Clinical Pharmacology and Therapeutics 1986; 40: 21-8

209. Ene MD, Roberts CJC. Pharmacokinetics of nifedipine after oral administration in chronic liver disease. Journal of Clinical Pharmacology 1987; 27: 1001-4

210. Gengo FM, Fagan SC, Krol G. Nimodipine disposition and haemodynamic effects in patients with cirrhosis and age-matched controls. British Journal of Clinical Pharmacology 1987; 23: 47-53

211. van Harten J, van Brummelen P, Wilson JHP, et al. Nisoldipine: kinetics and effects on blood pressure and heart rate in patients with liver cirrhosis after intravenous and oral administration. European Journal of Clinical Pharmacology 1988; 34: 387-94

212. Saris SD, Porter RS, Lowenthal DT, et al. Effect of chronic vs acute dosing of nitrendipine in chronic liver disease [abstract]. Clinical Pharmacology and Therapeutics 1986; 39: 226

213. Lasseter KC, Shamblen EC, Murdoch AA, et al. Steady-state pharmacokinetics of nitrendipine in hepatic insufficiency. Journal of Cardiovascular Pharmacology 1984; 6: S977-81

214. Dylewicz P, Kirch W, Santos SR, et al. Bioavailability and elimination of nitrendipine in liver disease. European Journal of Clinical Pharmacology 1987; 32: 563

215. Hinderling PH, Eckert M, Gasic S, et al. Comparative pharmacokinetics and cardiovascular effects of tiapamil in healthy volunteers and patients with hepatic cirrhosis. European Journal of Clinical Pharmacology 1986; 31: 397-404

216. Somogyi A, Albrecht M, Kliems G, et al. Pharmacokinetics, bioavailability and ECG response of verapamil in patients with liver cirrhosis. British Journal of Clinical Pharmacology 1981; 12: 51

217. Giacomini KM, Massoud N, Wong FM, et al. Decreased binding of verapamil to plasma proteins in patients with liver disease. Journal of Cardiovascular Pharmacology 1984; 6: 924-8

218. Storstein L, Amlie JP. Digitoxin pharmacokinetics in chronic active hepatitis. Digestion 1975; 12: 353

219. Kirch W, Ohnhaus EE, Dylewicz P, et al. Bioavailiability and elimination of digitoxin in patients with hepatorenal insufficiency. American Heart Journal 1986; 111: 325-9

220. Nokhodian A, Santos SRCJ, Kirch W. Digitoxin and its metabolites in patients with liver cirrhosis. European Journal of Drug Metabolism and Pharmacokinetics 1993; 18: 207-13
221. Marcus FI, Kapadia GG. The metabolism of tritiated digoxin in cirrhotic patients. Gastroenterology 1964; 47: 517
222. Schalm SW, Summerskill WHJ, Go VLW. Prednisone for chronic active liver disease: pharmacokinetics, including conversion to prednisolone. Gastroenterology 1977; 72: 910
223. Uribe M, Summerskill WHJ, Go VLW. Comparative serum prednisone and prednisolone concentrations following administration to patients with chronic active liver disease. Clinical Pharmacokinetics 1982; 7: 452
224. Bergrem H, Ritland S, Opedal I, et al. Prednisolone pharmacokinetics and protein-binding in patients with portosystemic shunt. Scandinavian Journal of Gastroenterology 1983; 18: 273
225. Marcantonio LA, Auld WHR, Murdoch WR, et al. The pharmacokinetics and pharmacodynamics of the diuretic bumetanide in hepatic and renal disease. British Journal of Clinical Pharmacology 1983; 15: 245
226. Keller E, Hoppe-Seyler G, Mumm R, et al. Influence of hepatic cirrhosis and end-stage renal disease on pharmacokinetics and pharmacodynamics of furosemide. European Journal of Clinical Pharmacology 1981; 20: 27
227. Sawhney VK, Gregory PB, Swezey SE, et al. Furosemide disposition in cirrhotic patients. Gastroenterology 1981; 81: 1012
228. Gonzalez G, Arancibia A, Rivas MI, et al. Pharmacokinetics of furosemide in patients with hepatic cirrhosis. European Journal of Clinical Pharmacology 1982; 22: 315
229. Verbeeck RK, Patwardhan RV, Villeneuve JP, et al. Furosemide disposition in cirrhosis. Clinical Pharmacology and Therapeutics 1982; 31: 719
230. Varadi A, Feher T, Bodrogi L, et al. Spironolactone metabolism in normal subjects and in patients with liver cirrhosis. Arzneimittel Forschung 1977; 27: 1618
231. Abshagen U, Rennekamp H, Luszpinski G. Disposition kinetics of spironolactone in hepatic failure after single doses and prolonged treatment. European Journal of Clinical Pharmacology 1977; 11: 169-76
232. Schwartz S, Brater C, Pound D, et al. Bioavailability, pharmacokinetics and pharmacodynamics of torsemide in patients with cirrhosis. Clinical Pharmacology and Therapeutics 1993; 54: 90-7
233. Mutschler E, Gilfrich HJ, Knauf H, et al. Pharmacokinetics of triamterene. Clinical and Experimental Hypertension 1983; A5 (2): 249
234. Villeneuve JP, Rocheleau F, Raymond RT. Triamterene kinetics and dynamics in cirrhosis. Clinical Pharmacology and Therapeutics 1984; 35: 831
235. Dao MT, Villeneuve J-P. Kinetics and dynamics of triamterene at steady-state in patients with cirrhosis. Clinical and Investigative Medicine 1988; 11: 6-9
236. Gugler R, Kurten JW, Jensen CJ, et al. Clofibrate disposition in renal failure and acute and chronic liver disease. European Journal of Clinical Pharmacology 1979; 15: 341
237. Knauf H, Kolle EU, Mutschler E. Gemfibrozil absorption and elimination in kidney and liver disease. Klinische Wochenschrift 1990; 68: 692-8
238. Ward S, Neill EAM. Pharmacokinetics of atracurium in acute hepatic failure (with acute renal failure). British Journal of Anaesthesia 1983; 55: 1169-72
239. Parker CJR, Hunter JM. Pharmacokinetics of atracurium and laudanosine in patients with hepatic cirrhosis. British Journal of Anaesthesia 1989; 62: 177-83
240. Duvaldestin P, Agoston S, Henzel D, et al. Pancuronium pharmacokinetics in patients with liver cirrhosis. British Journal of Anaesthesia 1978; 50: 1131
241. Ward ME, Adu-Gyamfi Y, Strunin L. Althesin and pancuronium in chronic liver disease. British Journal of Anaesthesia 1975; 47: 1199
242. Cook DR, Freeman JA, Lai AA, et al. Pharmacokinetics of mivacurium in normal patients and in those with hepatic or renal failure. British Journal of Anaesthesia 1992; 69: 580
243. Arden JR, Lynham DP, Castagnoli KP, et al. Vecuronium in alcoholic liver disease: a pharmacokinetic and pharmacodynamic analysis. Anesthesiology 1988; 68: 771-6
244. Duvaldestin P, Saada J, Henzel D, et al. Fazadinium pharmacokinetics in patients with liver disease. British Journal of Anaesthesia 1980; 52: 789
245. Janssen U, Walker S, Maier K, et al. Flumazenil disposition and elimination in cirrhosis. Clinical Pharmacology and Therapeutics 1989; 46: 317-23
246. Pomier-Layrargues G, Giguere JF, Lavoie J, et al. Pharmacokinetics of benzodiazepine antagonist Ro 15-1788 in cirrhotic patients with moderate or severe liver dysfunction. Hepatology 1989; 10: 969-72
247. Hildebrand M, Krause W, Angeli P, et al. Pharmacokinetics of iloprost in patients with hepatic dysfunction. International Journal of Clinical Pharmacology Therapy and Toxicology 1990; 28: 430-4
248. Nieschlag E, Cuppers HJ, Wickings EJ. Influence of sex, testicular development and liver function on the bioavailability of oral testosterone. European Journal of Clinical Investigation 1977; 7: 145
249. Nicholls DP, Taggart AJ, McCann JP, et al. The pharmacokinetics of xamoterol in liver disease. British Journal of Clinical Pharmacology 1989; 28: 718-21

# Clearance and Volume Method of Dose Prediction

*N.H.G. Holford*

A major goal of therapeutics is to individualise treatment so that optimum benefit is obtained. One of the more obvious means of individualisation is to vary the dose of a drug, and several methods have evolved that are more or less based on a mixture of practical empiricism and academic theory. This appendix describes a method for dose prediction which uses the concepts of drug clearance and volume of distribution to relate concentration to drug elimination and distribution. Clearance and its pharmacokinetic companion, volume of distribution, are the cornerstones of a method of dosage selection which incorporates demographic information and feedback from responses to the drug.

## 1. Target Concentration Concept

Pharmacokinetically guided dose individualisation is based on the target concentration concept (see also chapter 5). This concept assumes that the desired clinical response will be more readily achieved at the same *concentration* in different individuals than if the same *dose* is given. This is because the variability in the dose-concentration relationship will be removed from the overall dose-concentration-effect relationship, e.g. patients with different degrees of renal impairment will need different doses of gentamicin to achieve similar average steady-state concentrations.

There is also a pharmacodynamic component to the target concentration concept. Differences between individuals in the concentration-effect relationship may be predictable and thus a different target concentration may be appropriate, e.g. a patient who is hypokalaemic will be more sensitive to the action of digoxin and should be treated with a lower target concentration.

## 2. Clearance and the Target Concentration

In most cases, important differences in clinical effects arising from differences in drug concentration between patients given the same dose will be proportional to the average steady-state concentration ($C^{ss}$). While important differences in effect may arise from concentrations achieved after the first (loading) dose (see chapter 5; sect. 1.2), these instances are less common. The principles of the target concentration concept apply equally well to the selection of both maintenance doses (by use of clearance) and loading doses (by use of volume of distribution), and the theoretical basis for both methods is discussed in turn. This section and sections 3 to 7 below deal with the prediction of maintenance doses by the clearance method, the procedure for which is summarised in figure 1. Prediction of loading doses by the volume of distribution method is discussed in sections 8 to 12.

The $C^{ss}$ is determined by the rate of drug input and clearance. The target $C^{ss}$ can therefore be achieved by knowing clearance and using the product of these parameters to predict the required drug input rate. However, differences between individuals in factors affecting clearance are responsible for major differences in drug dosage rate. If these factors can be identified and used to predict differences in clearance, then a change in drug dosage rate can be readily calculated (table I).

## 3. Clearance, Drug Elimination and Concentration

Clearance reflects the relationship between drug elimination rate and drug concentration, i.e.:

$$\text{Elimination rate} = \text{Concentration} \cdot \text{Clearance}$$

Most commonly, the drug elimination rate is linearly proportional to the serum concentration (first-order elimination kinetics). In some cases, however, clearance changes with concentration, in which case the drug elimination rate does not increase in proportion to concentration and may eventually reach a maximum when the elimination capacity is reached (mixed-order elimination kinetics).

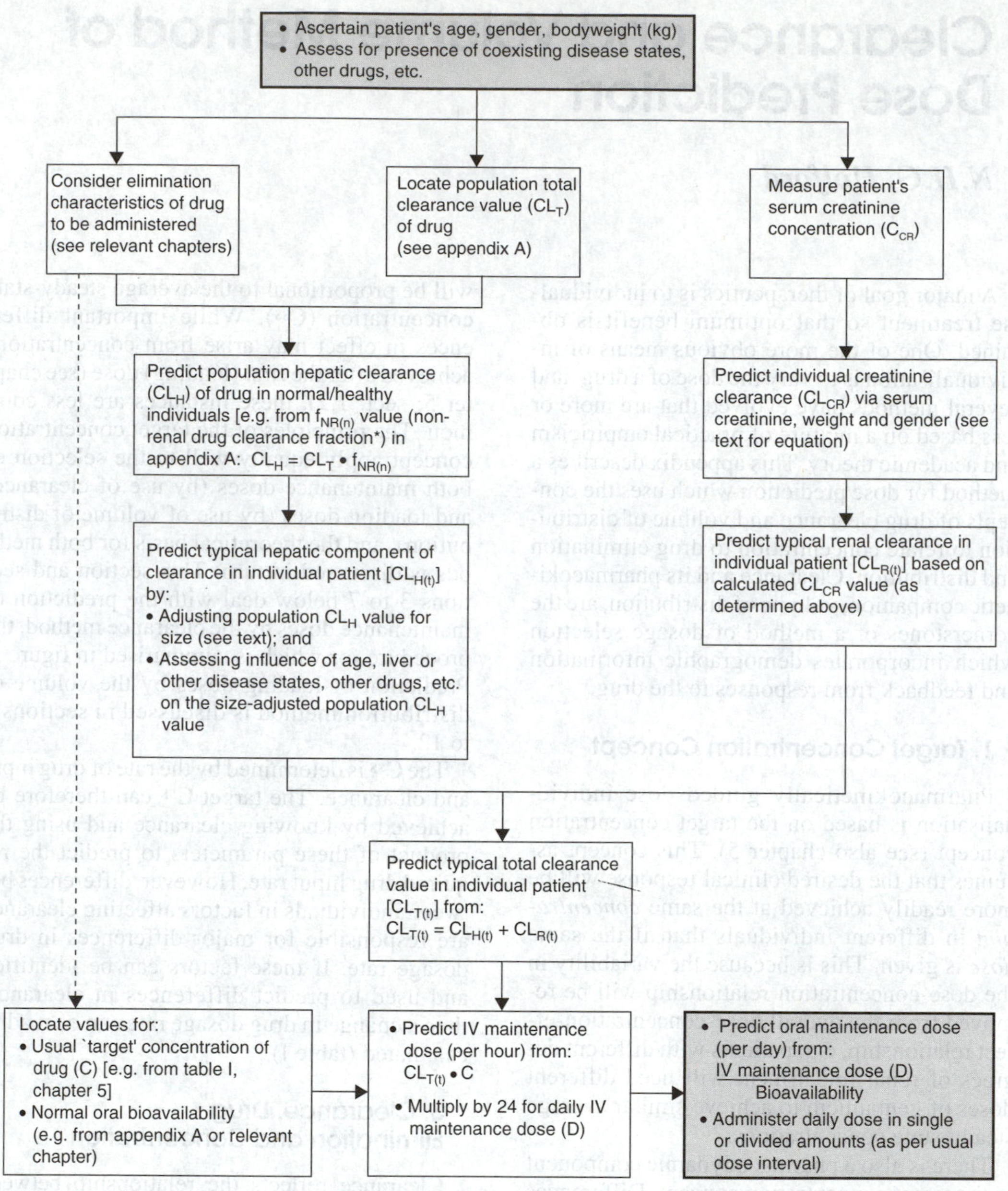

• Ascertain patient's age, gender, bodyweight (kg)
• Assess for presence of coexisting disease states, other drugs, etc.
Consider elimination characteristics of drug to be administered (see relevant chapters)
Locate population total clearance value ($CL_T$) of drug (see appendix A)
Measure patient's serum creatinine concentration ($C_{CR}$)
Predict population hepatic clearance ($CL_H$) of drug in normal/healthy individuals [e.g. from $f_{NR(n)}$ value (non-renal drug clearance fraction*) in appendix A: $CL_H = CL_T \bullet f_{NR(n)}$
Predict individual creatinine clearance ($CL_{CR}$) via serum creatinine, weight and gender (see text for equation)
Predict typical hepatic component of clearance in individual patient [$CL_{H(t)}$] by:
• Adjusting population $CL_H$ value for size (see text); and
• Assessing influence of age, liver or other disease states, other drugs, etc. on the size-adjusted population $CL_H$ value
Predict typical renal clearance in individual patient [$CL_{R(t)}$] based on calculated $CL_{CR}$ value (as determined above)
Predict typical total clearance value in individual patient [$CL_{T(t)}$] from:
$CL_{T(t)} = CL_{H(t)} + CL_{R(t)}$
Locate values for:
• Usual 'target' concentration of drug (C) [e.g. from table I, chapter 5]
• Normal oral bioavailability (e.g. from appendix A or relevant chapter)
• Predict IV maintenance dose (per hour) from: $CL_{T(t)} \bullet C$
• Multiply by 24 for daily IV maintenance dose (D)
• Predict oral maintenance dose (per day) from: IV maintenance dose (D) / Bioavailability
• Administer daily dose in single or divided amounts (as per usual dose interval)
* May be assumed to equal hepatic clearance fraction for most drugs


**Fig. 1.** Procedure for predicting maintenance drug dosage by the clearance method (see also chapter 5). *Abbreviation*: IV = intravenous.

Because first-order elimination is most common, it is usual to regard clearance in an individual as a fixed quantity. However, even if a drug has mixed-order elimination, the target concentration concept can still be applied by calculating clearance at the target concentration. This concentration-specific clearance is then used in exactly the same way to calculate the maintenance dose rate as it would be for a drug with a constant clearance. For example, the clearance of phenytoin at its target concentration of 10 mg/L is calculated as follows:

$$\text{Clearance} = \frac{V_{max}}{K_m + \text{Concentration}}$$

$$= \frac{415\ \text{mg/day}}{5\ \text{mg/L} + 10\ \text{mg/L}}$$

$$= 27.6\ \text{L/day}$$

$$= 1.15\ \text{L/h}$$

where $V_{max}$ is the maximum rate of metabolism of the drug and Km is the concentration at which its rate of metabolism is one-half maximum (typical values for phenytoin shown in the above equation).

## 4. Total Clearance Reflects the Sum of All Elimination Processes

The maintenance dose rate can be predicted from the total drug clearance. The total clearance is determined by the sum of clearances from all elimination processes. The major elimination pathways are:

1) Liver – by metabolism or excretion in the bile

2) Kidneys – by glomerular filtration or tubular secretion

3) Lungs – a major route of elimination for gaseous anaesthetics

4) Gut – elimination can take place via the gut but unless drug is trapped in the gut lumen, e.g. by activated charcoal, the faecal route is not an effective elimination pathway once drug has been absorbed

5) Dialysis – some drugs are readily dialysable so that substantial quantities of drug can be eliminated during haemodialysis. Clearance by dialysis is known as dialysance.

By considering each component of clearance separately, it is straightforward to predict the total clearance, even in complex situations with multiple organ disease:

Total clearance = Liver clearance + renal clearance + lung clearance + gut clearance + dialysance.

## 5. Prediction of Hepatic Clearance

Hepatic clearance is influenced directly by liver blood flow, intrinsic liver disease, drugs and other factors affecting liver function. Hepatic function is difficult to predict precisely because there are no readily available clinical markers of function that quantitatively predict drug elimination. Hypoalbuminaemia is a late marker of decreased hepatic function. Markers of liver damage such as serum alanine aminotransferase (ALT) do not reflect hepatic function and are not predictors of drug elimination by the liver.

Congestive heart failure appears to decrease the hepatic clearance of many drugs through a combination of hypoxaemia and congestion. Acute uncompensated heart failure can decrease hepatic clearance by 50%, even for low extraction ratio drugs (see also chapter 1). Even more dramatic decreases (to 20% of normal) may be seen with high extraction ratio drugs whose elimination is also dependent on liver blood flow.

**Table I.** Important principles in individualising drug dosage by the clearance method

1. Pharmacokinetically guided dose individualisation is based on the target concentration concept (see chapter 5)
2. The same target concentration can be achieved in individuals by predicting the clearance
3. Clearance reflects the relationship between drug elimination rate and drug concentration
4. The major determinants of clearance are hepatic and renal function. Total clearance can be calculated from the sum of hepatic (or nonrenal) and renal components
5. Hepatic clearance is influenced directly by liver blood flow, intrinsic liver disease, drugs and other factors affecting liver function, and indirectly by heart failure. Hepatic function is difficult to predict because there are no readily available clinical markers of function that quantitatively predict drug elimination
6. Renal clearance has glomerular and tubular components. Renal disease tends to change these components to a similar degree, although some drug interactions may selectively modify the tubular secretion component. Renal function can be readily predicted by creatinine clearance, which in turn, can be adequately predicted from the serum creatinine concentration and simple patient data
7. The rate of drug elimination is predicted by the product of clearance and drug concentration. At steady-state, the rate of elimination is equal to the intravenous maintenance dose rate (for oral maintenance dose rate, the intravenous dose rate must be divided by the drug's oral bioavailability). The maintenance dose rate can therefore be predicted from the product of clearance and the target drug concentration

## 6. Prediction of Renal Clearance

Renal clearance has glomerular and tubular components. Renal disease tends to change these components to a similar degree, although some drug interactions may selectively modify the tubular secretion component, e.g. probenecid blocks penicillin's renal tubular secretion. Renal function can be readily predicted from creatinine clearance ($CL_{CR}$) which, in turn, can be adequately predicted from the serum creatinine concentration ($C_{CR}$) and simple patient data such as weight, age and gender (see below). Comparison of these prediction methods with those based on attempts to collect urine over 24 hours have shown that the serum creatinine prediction is more reliable.[1]

It should be borne in mind that formulae such as those described by Cockcroft and Gault[2] or Bjornsson[3] predict creatinine production rate in a quite empirical fashion. Further empirical adjustment is necessary for patients with diminished muscle mass. Muscle is the primary source of creatinine. Patients with wasting diseases may produce 50% or less creatinine than would be predicted from their weight, age and gender.

## 7. Prediction of Maintenance Dose Rate

The rate of drug elimination is predicted by the product of clearance and drug concentration:

Elimination rate = Clearance • Concentration

Elimination rate is sometimes confused with clearance. The above equation should make the difference clear, i.e. clearance predicts the rate of elimination at any given concentration.

At steady-state, the rate of elimination is equal to the intravenous (IV) maintenance dose rate. The IV maintenance dose rate can therefore be predicted from the product of clearance and the target drug concentration:

IV maintenance dose rate = Clearance • Target concentration

If another route of drug administration is used, e.g. oral, then the IV maintenance dose rate must be divided by the drug's oral bioavailability:

Oral maintenance dose rate = IV maintenance dose rate/Oral bioavailability

## 8. Volume of Distribution and the Target Concentration

The target concentration approach may also be used to predict the size of a *loading dose*. Most commonly the loading dose will be the first dose but in general, the term is applied to an additional dose, or series of doses, which are larger than the maintenance dose and are intended to achieve the target concentration more rapidly.

## 9. Volume of Distribution, Amount of Drug in the Body and Concentration

The volume of distribution reflects the relationship between the amount of drug in the body and drug concentration, i.e.:

Amount in body = Concentration • Volume of distribution

The volume is an *apparent* volume because it does not necessarily reflect a physical space in the body. It is determined by body composition and is almost always independent of drug concentration.

## 10. Prediction of Volume of Distribution

The apparent volume of distribution is usually directly proportional to bodyweight. The proportionality to bodyweight will vary, however, with differences in body composition. Polar drugs, e.g. gentamicin, typically have small volumes of distribution that approximate extracellular fluid volume (15 to 20 L/70kg) because these compounds have difficulty crossing cell membranes. If extracellular fluid volume is increased, e.g. due to ascites or pleural effusion, then the apparent volume of distribution will be increased in direct proportion to the additional fluid. On the other hand, in obesity, fat soluble drugs may have a volume of distribution which is proportionately greater than total bodyweight because of partitioning into adipose tissue.

## 11. Prediction of Loading Dose

### 11.1 Prior to a Constant Rate Maintenance Dose

The dose of a drug needed to increase its concentration in the body is readily predicted from the apparent volume of distribution. The simplest form of loading dose is one designed to reach the target concentration immediately and will be followed by a maintenance dose infusion.

Loading dose = Volume of distribution • Target concentration

### 11.2 Prior to an Intermittent Maintenance Dose

When the maintenance dose is given intermittently on a regular basis, there will be predictable peak and trough concentrations achieved at steady-state. The ratio of the concentration of

**Table II.** The accumulation factor for typical values of half-life and dosage interval

| Dosage interval | Half-life | | | |
|---|---|---|---|---|
| | 6h | 12h | 24h | 72h |
| 6h | 2.00 | 3.41 | 6.29 | 17.82 |
| 8h | 1.66 | 2.70 | 4.85 | 13.49 |
| 12h | 1.33 | 2.00 | 3.41 | 9.17 |
| 24h | 1.07 | 1.33 | 2.00 | 4.85 |

drug at steady-state to the first such maintenance dose (at the same time after the dose) is known as the accumulation factor. The accumulation factor (AF) is determined solely by the dosage interval and the elimination half-life:

$$AF = \frac{1}{1 - e^{-0.7/t_{1/2} \cdot \text{Dosage interval}}}$$

The expression in the denominator of this equation reflects the fraction of drug lost after each dose at steady-state because $e^{-0.7/t_{1/2} \cdot \text{Dosage interval}}$ is the fraction of drug remaining (assuming bolus drug input) at the end of the dosage interval. Typical values of the accumulation factor are shown in table II.

The maintenance dose size for intermittent dosage is determined by the desired maintenance dose rate and the dosage interval:

Maintenance dose = Maintenance dose rate • Dosage interval

The loading dose which will exactly match the peak and trough steady-state concentration can be predicted from:

Loading dose = Accumulation factor • Maintenance dose

In general, a loading dose is not considered unless the accumulation factor is 2 or greater, i.e. the dosage interval is less than one elimination half-life.

## 12. Influence of Body Size

The influence of body size on volume of distribution and clearance can be approximated in adults in simple proportion to bodyweight (over 50kg). However, this approach may seriously overpredict clearance if applied naively to small adults or children.[4] Clearance is quite well predicted over a wide range of sizes by using weight and the general allometric equation:

$$CL = CL_{std} \cdot (Weight/Weight_{std})^{0.75}$$

where $CL_{std}$ is the clearance in an individual who weighs $Weight_{std}$ (i.e. 70kg). An alternative is to use predicted body surface area (SA) using the formula of Du Bois and Du Bois:[5]

$$CL = CL_{std} \cdot (SA/SA_{std})$$

The surface area standard ($SA_{std}$) is $1.9m^2$.[4]

## 13. Clinical Application

### Example 1

*A 60kg, 80-year-old man has acute congestive heart failure. His serum creatinine concentration ($C_{CR}$) is 0.1 mmol/L. What oral maintenance dose of digoxin would be expected to reach a target concentration of 1 μg/L?*

#### Relevant Pharmacokinetic Parameters and Assumptions

Total digoxin clearance is 9 L/h in a healthy 70 kg person. About 6 L/h of total clearance is due to renal clearance if kidney function is normal [i.e. creatinine clearance of 6 L/h (100 ml/min)]. The normal liver clearance is therefore 3 L/h/70kg.

#### Prediction of Individual Creatinine Clearance

The predicted creatinine clearance ($CL_{CR}$) in this patient can be obtained from a formula based on the concepts developed by Cockcroft and Gault[2] and extended by Bjornsson:[3]

$$CL_{CR}\,(L/h) = \frac{160 - \text{age (y)}}{C_{CR}\,(\text{mmol/L}) \cdot 250} \cdot \frac{\text{Bodyweight (kg)}}{70}$$

(the value should be multiplied by 0.9 for female patients)

From the above equation, the predicted $CL_{CR}$ for this elderly male patient is 2.7 L/h.

#### Prediction of Individual Drug Clearance

Normal digoxin liver clearance in a 60kg person would be expected to be about 3 • 60/70 = 2.57 L/h. However, in this man with congestive heart failure, the liver clearance is probably reduced to about half this value, i.e. 1.3 L/h. Since digoxin renal clearance is very similar to creatinine clearance (see above), the renal clearance of the drug will be 2.7 L/h. Thus, the total digoxin clearance in this patient will be equal to the sum of the predicted liver and renal clearances, i.e.:

Total clearance = 1.3 L/h (Liver clearance) + 2.7 L/h (Renal clearance) = 4 L/h

### Prediction of Expected Maintenance Dose

For a target concentration of 1 μg/L, the expected intravenous (IV) maintenance dose rate is:

IV maintenance dose rate = 4 L/h • 1 μg/L
= 4 μg/h = 96 μg/day

Because the oral bioavailability of digoxin is about 70%, the oral maintenance dose is about 50% larger:

Oral maintenance dose rate = 96 μg/day/0.7
≈ 140 μg/day

A practical dose would be to give two 62.5μg tablets daily. With appropriate treatment, this patient's heart failure should improve over a few days and along with this, the hepatic component of digoxin elimination should also improve. The total clearance when the heart failure is compensated might then be 5.3 L/h even if no improvement in renal function takes place. This would suggest that an additional 32% (5.3/4) increase in the oral dose would be warranted to 185 μg/day. A practical dose would be to give three 62.5μg tablets daily.

### Example 2

*What oral loading dose would be appropriate for the patient described above?*

### Relevant Pharmacokinetic Parameters

Digoxin volume of distribution is 500L in a 70kg person. The volume of distribution is diminished in renal failure but in heart failure it is proportional to the total bodyweight. Extra water due to oedema contributes negligibly to the apparent volume of distribution of digoxin.

### Prediction of Individual Drug Volume of Distribution

The volume of distribution in a 60kg person would be expected to be about 500 · 60/70 = 420L.

### Prediction of Expected Loading Dose

If an intravenous infusion of digoxin was being given to achieve a target concentration of 1 μg/L, the loading dose would be:

IV loading dose = 420L • 1 μg/L = 420μg

If an oral maintenance dose of 125 μg/day had been chosen (see above), then the expected elimination half-life should be considered to predict the loading dose (see above for calculation of maintenance dose and clearance):

$$\text{Half–life} = \frac{0.7 \cdot \text{Volume of distribution}}{\text{Clearance}}$$

$$= \frac{0.7 \cdot 420\text{L}}{4\ \text{L/h}}$$

$$= 74\text{h}$$

Table II shows that with a dosage interval of 24 hours and a half-life of 72 hours, the accumulation factor is 4.85. The predicted loading dose is therefore:

Loading dose = 4.85 • 125μg = 606μg

A practical dose would be to give two 250μg tablets initially followed by a further 250μg 24 hours later, i.e. a total of 750μg. This is quite close to the desired total of a 606μg loading dose plus 125μg for the first maintenance dose.

It should be noted that as the accumulation factor gets bigger, the fluctuation from peak to trough at steady-state becomes smaller and a loading dose calculated using the accumulation factor and maintenance dose becomes closer to the dose predicted by simply multiplying the volume of distribution and the target concentration.

## 14. Follow-up Measurement of Concentration

It should be recognised that dose prediction based on patient features such as size and renal function can only be partly successful. For drugs with a narrow therapeutic index, such as digoxin, it is sensible to measure drug concentration when steady-state is thought to have been achieved. This measured concentration can then be used to estimate the patient's clearance more precisely and a reasoned decision made to modify the dose if necessary (see further chapter 5; sect. 3).

### References


1. Wheeler LA, Sheiner LB. Clinical estimation of creatinine clearance. American Journal of Clinical Pathology 1979; 72: 27-31
2. Cockcroft DW, Gault MH. Prediction of creatinine clearance from serum creatinine. Nephron 1976; 16: 31-41
3. Bjornsson TD. Use of serum creatinine concentrations to determine renal function. Clinical Pharmacokinetics 1979; 4: 200-2
4. Holford NHG. A size standard for pharmacokinetics. Clinical Pharmacokinetics 1996; 30: 329-32
5. Du Bois D, Du Bois EF. Clinical calorimetry. Tenth paper. A formula to estimate the approximate surface area if height and weight be known. Archives of Internal Medicine 1916; 17: 863

# Subject Index

## A

## B

## D

## E

## F

## G

## N

## O

## P

## T

# U

## V

Dep. Legal: B-1.639-97